Textbook of
Anesthesia
for Postgraduates

Complimentary Slides

Available complimentary PPTs for easy understanding of the following topics:

- Anesthetic Machine
- Anesthetic Delivery System
- Anesthetic Instruments
- Vaporizers
- Capnography
- Oxygen
- ECG
- Local Anesthetic Agents
- Intravenous Anesthetics
- Inhalational Anesthetics
- Muscle Relaxants
- Mechanical Ventilation

To access the PPTs, simply scan this QR code.

Textbook of Anesthesia for Postgraduates

Second Edition

VOLUME 2

TK Agasti

MBBS (Kol) DGO (Kol) DA (Kol) MD (Guj)

Consultant Anesthetist
Zenith Super Specialist Hospital
Midland Multidisciplinary Hospital
Disha Eye Hospital
Kolkata, West Bengal, India

Foreword
Atul Prabhakar Kulkarni

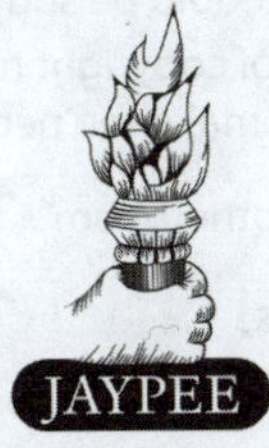

JAYPEE BROTHERS MEDICAL PUBLISHERS
The Health Sciences Publisher
New Delhi | London

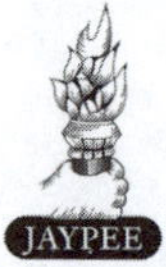 **Jaypee Brothers Medical Publishers (P) Ltd**

Headquarters
Jaypee Brothers Medical Publishers (P) Ltd
EMCA House, 23/23-B
Ansari Road, Daryaganj
New Delhi 110 002, India
Landline: +91-11-23272143, +91-11-23272703
+91-11-23282021, +91-11-23245672
Email: jaypee@jaypeebrothers.com

Corporate Office
Jaypee Brothers Medical Publishers (P) Ltd
4838/24, Ansari Road, Daryaganj
New Delhi 110 002, India
Phone: +91-11-43574357
Fax: +91-11-43574314
Email: jaypee@jaypeebrothers.com

Overseas Office
JP Medical Ltd.
83, Victoria Street, London
SW1H 0HW (UK)
Phone: +44 20 3170 8910
Fax: +44 (0)20 3008 6180
Email: info@jpmedpub.com

Website: www.jaypeebrothers.com
Website: www.jaypeedigital.com

© 2024, Jaypee Brothers Medical Publishers

The views and opinions expressed in this book are solely those of the original contributor(s)/author(s) and do not necessarily represent those of editor(s) or publisher of the book.

All rights reserved. No part of this publication may be reproduced, stored or transmitted in any form or by any means, electronic, mechanical, photocopying, recording or otherwise, without the prior permission in writing of the publishers.

All brand names and product names used in this book are trade names, service marks, trademarks or registered trademarks of their respective owners. The publisher is not associated with any product or vendor mentioned in this book.

Medical knowledge and practice change constantly. This book is designed to provide accurate, authoritative information about the subject matter in question. However, readers are advised to check the most current information available on procedures included and check information from the manufacturer of each product to be administered, to verify the recommended dose, formula, method and duration of administration, adverse effects and contraindications. It is the responsibility of the practitioner to take all appropriate safety precautions. Neither the publisher nor the author(s)/editor(s) assume any liability for any injury and/or damage to persons or property arising from or related to use of material in this book.

This book is sold on the understanding that the publisher is not engaged in providing professional medical services. If such advice or services are required, the services of a competent medical professional should be sought.

Every effort has been made where necessary to contact holders of copyright to obtain permission to reproduce copyright material. If any have been inadvertently overlooked, the publisher will be pleased to make the necessary arrangements at the first opportunity.

Inquiries for bulk sales may be solicited at: jaypee@jaypeebrothers.com

Textbook of Anesthesia for Postgraduates (2 Volumes)

First Edition: 2011
Second Edition: **2024**

ISBN: 978-93-5696-265-1

Printed in India at Rajkamal Electric Press, Kundli, Haryana.

Contents

Mechanical Ventilation

■ INTRODUCTION AND HISTORY

For centuries, it has been felt that failure to breathe should not be allowed to cause any death to any person. So, expired air ventilation (mouth-to-mouth resuscitation) has been used throughout the ancient history, in an effort to revive the apparently dead person, especially from drowning. So, in the Second Book of Kings, there is a vivid description of such a successful mouth-to-mouth breathing by prophet Elisha. He performed this on a child who appeared to be dead from drowning. But, the actual date of this event is not known. Then, during the period of 12th and 13th century, tracheostomy was usually used to perform for ventilation for the treatment of drowned persons, instead of by mouth-to-mouth breathing. After that, in between 1493 and 1541, Paracelsus and Vesalius were credited for the introduction of bellows and a pipe to ventilate the lungs through this tracheostomy wound. But, only for ventilation, tracheostomy was not accepted by the people during this era. Then, Elisha's mouth-to-mouth breathing was rediscovered by Tossach, in 1743. But, that method of ventilation was later condemned, as an unhygienic maneuver, by the newly founded Royal Humane Society. After that, in 1763, the "Society for the Recovery of Drowned Persons" was formed in Amsterdam. They declared to offer medals and prizes, for new ideas and apparatuses for ventilation, other than mouth-to-mouth unhygienic breathing. Hence, many designs of pumps, bellows, and tubes were introduced to ventilate the lungs through larynx or tracheostomy wound. In 1811, Brodie and Waterton employed the "*curare (muscular paralysis) plus bellows*" principle for positive pressure ventilation on experimental animals and also suggested that artificial breathing by bellows could be used to treat severe respiratory depression in opium poisoning.

Then, in 1827, Leroy demonstrated the dangers of this positive pressure ventilation such as rupture of alveoli, pneumothorax, etc. which was later confirmed by Magendie's report, in 1829. So, after that, positive pressure ventilation for resuscitation, using bellows, fell into disrepute. In 1837, Royal Humane Society also criticized positive pressure ventilation by bellows and recommended the manual compression of chest (negative pressure ventilation), if artificial ventilation was necessary. So, for the next century, positive pressure ventilation by bellows went into oblivion, but mouth-to-mouth resuscitation and chest compression for ventilation continued. Then, again 100 years later, bellows for resuscitation or ventilation reappeared, when Kreiselman introduced his own apparatus during the Second World War. Within this period of 100 year (1840–1940), most of the mechanical aids for artificial ventilation were depended on the application of subatmospheric pressure from outside the thorax (negative pressure ventilation).

During that period, using the principle of subatmospheric (negative) pressure from outside the thorax for ventilation, the *tank ventilator*, and *cuirass ventilator* were invented which were later claimed as a very successful apparatus for the treatment of respiratory paralysis and respiratory failure due to poliomyelitis. The schematic diagram of tank and cuirass ventilator is shown in **Figures 1 and 2**. First tank ventilator was patented in America, in 1864. After that, different modifications to this basic design of tank ventilator were introduced over the next few years. In 1929, Drinker and his colleagues first introduced their tank ventilator for prolonged artificial respiration (ventilation). This apparatus subsequently was known as the "*iron lung*". The first patient to be treated with the iron lung was a victim of paralytic bulbar poliomyelitis. The tank ventilator, introduced by Dinker and his colleagues, was also the first ventilator driven by power. In this tank ventilation, the patient was placed on a mattress inside an air tight cabinet, from which only his or her head is protruded. A padded collar, around the neck, formed an effective air tight seal. The pressure inside the cabinet was lowered rhythmically by a system of pumps or

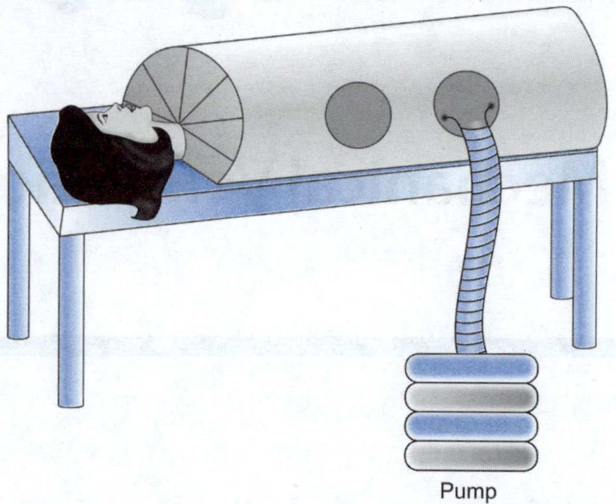

Fig. 1: The tank ventilator. Inside the ventilator the patient is placed in a body shaped shell. Head is outside the tank.

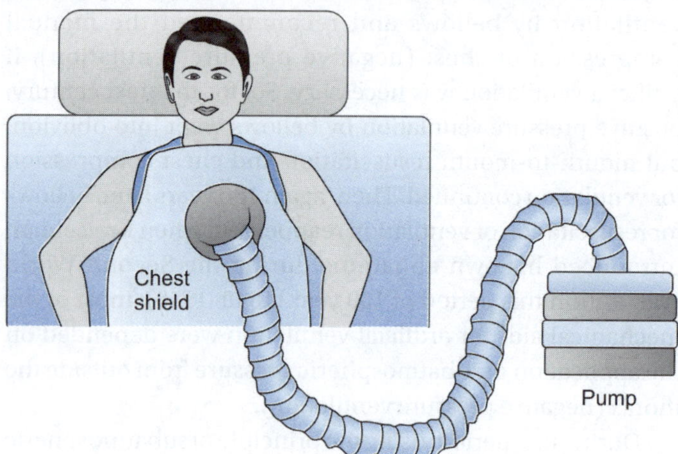

Fig. 2: Cuirass ventilator with chest shield (red) which is connected with pump.

a set of bellows during inspiration and was next allowed to return to atmospheric level slowly during expiration. There were *"portholes"* at the sides of the tank, through which the patient could be observed and *"sealed ports"* to allow the use of manometers, blood pressure cuffs, and stethoscopes. *The two main disadvantages of these tank ventilators were:* (i) Access to the patient for nursing care and physiotherapy was restricted and (ii) the airway was not usually protected. So, the vomiting and regurgitation are particularly hazardous in respect to the chance of aspiration, during this intermittent negative pressure ventilation (INPV) by tank ventilators, even for patients who have normal laryngeal and pharyngeal reflexes. If vomiting occurs, then an emergency port should be opened immediately to equalize the pressure between the inside and the outside of the tank and thus reduce the risk of aspiration.

Cuirass ventilator was named after the piece of a 15th century body armor which was used during war.

It is consisted of a breast and back plate, which were joined together at their sides by hinges, forming a rigid shell around the thorax. This rigid shell was fitted over the thorax and upper abdomen and a padded rim at the periphery, around the neck and upper abdomen, made contact with the skin to form an air-tight seal. A bellow was connected by a flexible tubing to the airspace, situated between the skin of thorax and rigid shell. The expansion of bellow was able to create a subatmospheric (negative) pressure in the airspace between the chest wall and the armor plates, during inspiration and allowed the chest wall to inflate and the air to rush into lungs through airways. During expiration, the pressure in the air space again became atmospheric and the chest wall deflated with the lungs and the air came out. Cuirass ventilators though work on the same principle as tank ventilator (negative pressure ventilation which physiologically occurs during our normal respiration), but left patient's arms and legs free and causes less circulatory embarrassment than tank ventilators. But, they were less efficient than tank ventilators and the tidal volume, obtained by a given subatmospheric pressure, was smaller. So, this cuirass ventilator was used as an assistant for patients who were suffering from chronic respiratory impairment, with some respiratory efforts, but not had complete respiratory paralysis or who were recovering from some acute episode of paralysis.

After 1940, due to multiple disadvantages of tank and cuirass ventilators, positive pressure ventilation again resurfaced by the work of Krliselman, during the Second World War, in 1939. During that period, Krliselman's work was also supported by the development of nondepolarizing neuromuscular blocking agents by Griffith, in 1942. He was the first to use curare in anesthesia. This development initiated the need for new positive pressure ventilators in anesthesia which could be combined with newly developed endotracheal intubation techniques by Magill and Macintosh. These were more convenient for operating theater environment and also solving the problem of oropharyngeal and gastric secretions, entering the trachea in negative pressure ventilation. Another cause for losing the popularity of negative pressure ventilations, by tank and cuirass ventilators, was that these were large and awkward devices. The poliomyelitis epidemic which occurred in Copenhagen in 1952 also had enormous influence on the development of newer positive pressure ventilation techniques and ventilators. By this time, controlled positive pressure ventilation was well established in anesthesia.

During that epidemic of poliomyelitis, an eminent anesthetist, named Ibsen, was called in by Professor Lassen to help him for the ventilator management of polio patients in Blegdam Hospital. Then, Ibsen developed the procedure of positive pressure ventilation by manual method (hand) through tracheostomy tube and almost all the students of his medical school were appointed to help him with this manual positive pressure ventilation. So, medical teaching (academic) activities were temporarily suspended, until polio epidemic was over. After that, Lassen and Ibsen established some basic principles for long-term positive pressure ventilation. These were (i) the careful control of airway pressure, (ii) the protection of airway during intubation, (iii) the humidification of inspired air, (iv) the avoidance of high inspired O_2 concentration for ventilation, and (v) meticulous physiotherapy.

Once the acute phase of poliomyelitis disease was over, then weaning was accomplished by a forerunner intermittent mandatory ventilation (IMV). Then, the adequacy of ventilation was assessed by the oximetry and end-tidal CO_2 concentration measurement. So, after the Second World War, in 1945, there were two stimuli for the further development of positive pressure mechanical ventilation. The first was the introduction of curare into anesthesia. The second was the fear of health authorities that if another epidemic of poliomyelitis occurred, then large number of patients might require artificial ventilations which in turn need huge manpower. So, in 1940, the first commercial automatic mechanical ventilator for anesthesia was manufactured in Sweden for intermittent positive pressure ventilation (IPPV).

A dramatic fall in the mortality from polio epidemic was occurred, after this new technique of automatic IPPV had been introduced for its management and this ensured that IPPV would become the standard method of artificial ventilation than negative pressure ventilation, made by the tank and cuirass ventilator. Later, the superiority of automatic IPPV was also confirmed by Stockholm polio epidemic, in the following year and New England polio epidemic, in 1955. After the introduction of poliomyelitis vaccine (Salk and Sabin), the incidence of poliomyelitis fell sharply. So, the ventilation skill which had been developed to fight polio epidemic, was diverted to other good uses, such as anesthesia, and for the management of polyneuritis, drug over doses, trauma, asthma, and complicated surgeries where the prolonged artificial positive pressure ventilation was needed. After that, in 1960, the indications for IPPV were broadened further and its cardiovascular effects were also investigated. The value of mechanical positive pressure ventilation in anesthesia was also soon recognized simultaneously in Sweden, Britain, and many other European countries. But, during that period, it (rampant use of IPPV) was still disputed in USA, where the reliance on manual IPPV was just germinating. However, later, the more stringent (essential) ventilator requirements for cardiac surgery change this view in USA.

After the successful establishment of automatic IPPV, as the ideal mode of treatment for respiratory failure, a group of patients went on to develop a lung condition, which were characterized by certain specific radiological changes and severe impairment of gas exchange, due to prolonged ventilation. At that time, such changes in lung condition were called by many names, such as shock lung, acute respiratory distress syndrome (ARDS), and respirator lung. But, in 1970, the pathophysiology of such lung condition was studied intensively and positive end-expiratory pressure (PEEP) was introduced. The PEEP was added to IPPV to aid better gas exchange in patients with shock lung or ARDS. But, gradual recognition of the adverse effects of PEEP on circulation (CVS) started the quest for an ideal level of it (PEEP) which would balance between the respiratory advantages against the circulatory disadvantages of it. The year of 1970 also saw the development of extracorporeal circulation techniques which could ensure adequate gas exchange for several weeks.

At that period, high-frequency ventilation (HFV) was also developed, but its true role in long-term mechanical ventilation was not established. In 1960, pulmonary oxygen toxicity was also blamed for the pathology of ARDS or shock lung, because toxic effects of pure oxygen on lung, at standard atmospheric pressure, was known for over 50 years. Hence, an inspired O_2 concentration of 50% or less was considered safe. So, after 1960, most ventilators which are in use in North America employed a Venturi device to entrain air and to mix it (air) with the principal gas flow of O_2. This evidence, together with the experience which was already gained from polio patients, established that IPPV with *modest level of O_2* in inspired gas and a *modest level of inspiratory and expiratory pressure* may be continued indefinitely, without any adverse effects on lungs. Then, the subsequent evolution of ventilators had taken two paths. One was to fulfil the need for cheap, simple, and reliable method which could be used for anesthesia and for the majority of patients needing short-term ventilation. The other was to provide increasingly sophisticated and versatile ventilators with the facilities, necessary for treating patients with severe respiratory failure or suffering from other life-threatening condition.

ARTIFICIAL INTERMITTENT POSITIVE PRESSURE VENTILATION

After the Second World War, in 1939, positive pressure ventilation was established which certainly was artificial and intermittent. So, this artificial intermittent positive pressure ventilation (AIPPV) can be employed and classified by three ways:

1. AIPPV requiring no apparatus, e.g., expired air ventilation (e.g., mouth-to-mouth resuscitation)

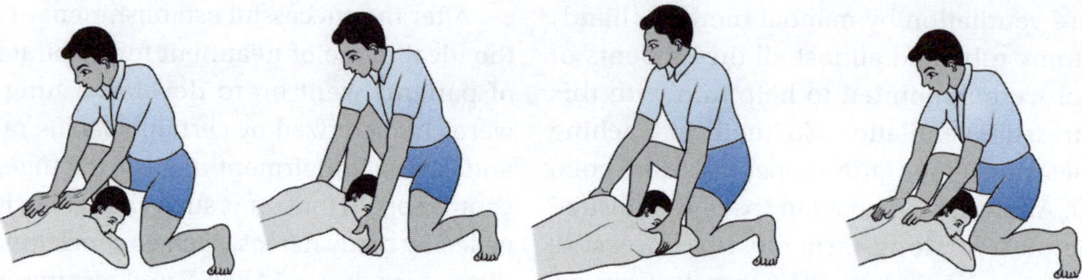

Fig. 3: Holger–Nielsen's manual method for artificial respiration.

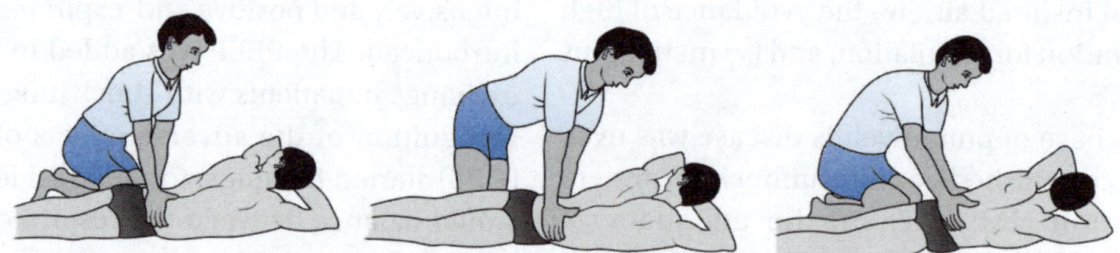

Fig. 4: Schaffer's manual method for artificial respiration.

2. AIPPV using simple devices or apparatuses, e.g., artificial manual breathing unit (AMBU) bag
3. AIPPV using sophisticated instruments such as manual ventilation by Boyle's machine or automatic ventilation by ventilators.

Artificial Intermittent Positive Pressure Ventilation by using no Apparatus (Mouth-to-mouth Resuscitation)

It was previously described that Elisha's mouth-to-mouth positive pressure ventilation, which was gone out of vogue today, due to the development of tracheostomy and bellows, was rediscovered by Tossach, in 1743. But, again as the mouth-to-mouth method of breathing was unhygienic, so Royal Humane Society had condemned it and recommended some other methods of ventilation, described below. But, in 1954, Elam and in 1958, Safar showed that the other methods of non-mouth resuscitation, (recommended at that time by Royal Humane Society), such as Holger–Nielsen method, Schaffer's method, or Sylvester's method failed to provide adequate ventilation. So, since that time mouth-to-mouth breathing or expired air resuscitation had again become the method of choice when any equipment were not available. But, that mouth-to-mouth resuscitation was not applicable for those who have inhaled toxic gases or who are the victims of cyanide poisoning **(Figs. 3 and 4)**.

Artificial Intermittent Positive Pressure Ventilation by using Simple Devices

Many simple devices had made the positive pressure ventilation through mouth easier, more acceptable, more hygienic, and more effective than mouth-to-mouth

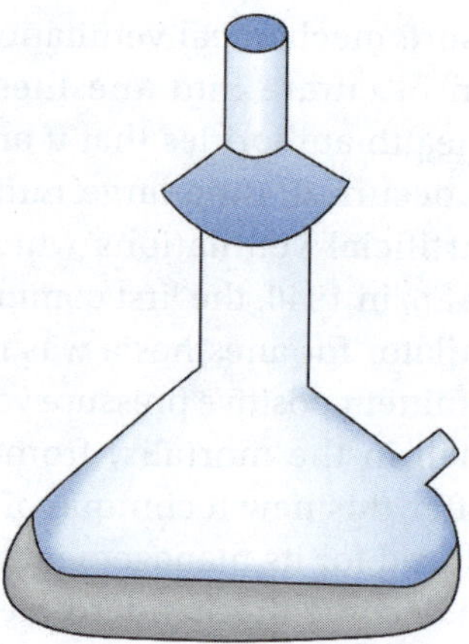

Fig. 5: Laerdal pocket mask.

ventilation. This devices are so simple that it can be carried in pocket. AIPPV, using these simple devices are of the following types. This may be expired air ventilation or fresh air ventilation, enriched with O_2.

Mouth Ventilation by Mask

Here, the device is nothing but a simple transparent *Laerdal pocket face mask* which is shown in **Figure 5**. In this device, the angle piece is replaced by a short, straight tube to which the resuscitator's lips can be applied for forceful blow. A nipple can be added on the body of the mask, so that through it O_2 can be added to the inspired gas. This device makes the IPPV procedure more hygienic and O_2 enriched expired air (when O_2 is added) can be used to ventilate the patient.

Mouth Ventilation by Airway Devices

Here, different types of airways are used for expired air ventilation by mouth. These different types of airways are

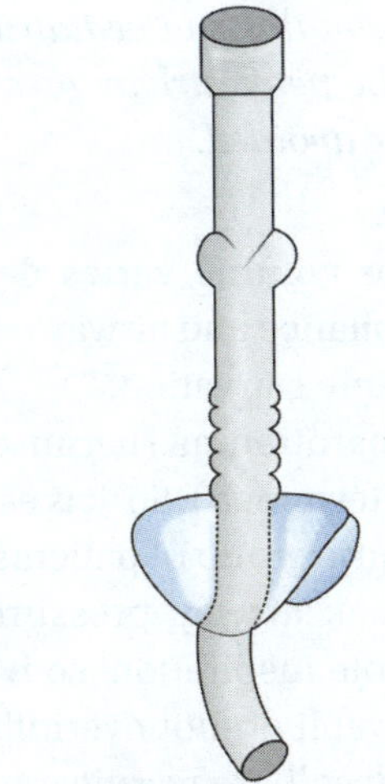

Fig. 6: Safar-S-tube.

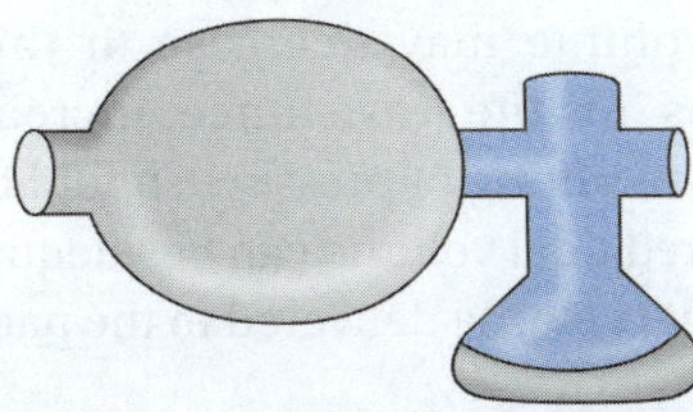

Fig. 7: Artificial manual breathing unit (AMBU) bag with mask.

Safar S-tube, Brook airway, esophageal obturator airway, etc. The Safar S-tube is a double Guedel airway and is used both as a pharyngeal airway and for ventilation. The Brook airway is slightly sophisticated where a nonreturn value in used and which allow the expired air from patient to pass out into environment. In esophageal obturator airway, a large cuffed tube is designed to obstruct the esophagus which prevents the reflux of gastric contents during ventilation. **Figure 6** shows Safar S-tube.

Bag-valve-mask Ventilation

Here, resuscitator's mouth is not used for expired air ventilation. Instead, a *self-refilling bag* is used to ventilate the patient by mask. Between the bag and the mask, a nonrebreathing valve is incorporated which helps the expired air from patient to pass out. O_2 can be administered, if available, through a side tube, but a reservoir tube is necessary to deliver 100% O_2. Example of one such ventilation is by AMBU bag, which is shown in **Figure 7**.

Artificial Intermittent Positive Pressure Ventilation using Sophisticated Instrument

Artificial intermittent positive pressure ventilation, using sophisticated instrument, can be conducted manually or automatically. When it is conducted manually, then the best example is bag-mask ventilation by Boyle's apparatus. Automatic, artificial, intermittent, positive pressure ventilation also can be performed by ventilators.

The power mechanism (electric or pneumatic) forms an important part of driving system of an automatic ventilator. The only electrically driven ventilator uses only electrical source for its complete working. Here, both the electronic and mechanical components of ventilator uses only the electrical source for its complete working. These only electric driven ventilators find a good application, typically, during transport of a patient. On the other hand, both pneumatically and electrically operated ventilators need a source of highly compressed, pressurized air to operate the mechanical components of ventilator, in addition to electrical source which operate its electronic components and ultimate for the complete control of it. The source of compressed air can be provided from external or internal sources. The *external source* of compressed air is available either (i) from a cylinder or (ii) from an *air compressor* which is permanently built in the ventilator or (iii) through an *air compressor*, available for the use of hospital. Some ventilators incorporate piston assembly or turbine technology in their system, as the *internal source* of compressed air. This turbine compresses the room air, after it is sucked inside the ventilator. In such ventilator systems, there is no need for an external source of compressed air for their function. Except the anesthetic ventilator which uses the anesthetic gas mixture from Boyle's machine, the air is sucked inside the other type of ventilators (which are used in critical care unit) from the atmosphere, and this is blended then with the external source of O_2 to meet the desired FiO_2.

An automatic, intermittent, positive, pressure ventilation has four stages:

- *Inspiration:* Inflation of lungs.
- *Changing over from inspiration to expiration:* Cycle.
- *Expiration:* Deflation of lungs.
- *Changing over from expiration to inspiration:* Trigger.

The term "cycling" is referred to the changing over from inspiration to expiration and the term "triggering" is referred to the changing over from expiration to inspiration. The classification of different types of ventilators is given in **Box 1**.

Inspiration

In positive pressure ventilation, inspiration can be instituted by presenting a preset pressure or a preset volume of air to the patient's upper airways. So, as a result of the difference between the upper airway pressure and the alveolar pressure, gas flows into the lungs of a patient. Now, this flow of gas results in delivery of a fixed volume of air [in

BOX 1: Classification of ventilators.

- *According to power and control mechanism:*
  - Pneumatically driven and operated
  - Electrically driven and operated
  - Both
- *According to cycling mechanism:*
  - Time cycling
  - Volume cycling
  - Flow cycling
  - Pressure cycling
  - Combinational cycling
- *According to trigger mechanism:*
  - Time or ventilator triggered
  - Patient triggered

volume-controlled ventilation (VCV)] or variable volume of air [in pressure-controlled ventilation (PCV)] in patient's lung. So, according to the preset pressure presentation or preset volume presentation the *ventilators can be first classified into:*

- *Pressure-controlled (or generated) ventilator:* Here, ventilator applies a fixed pressure, set by the operator, in the upper airway of a patient during inspiration. So, due to this *fixed pressure* pattern, the *volume of air* delivered to the patient during inspiration may vary according to the condition of lungs.
- *Volume- or flow-controlled (generated) ventilator:* Here, ventilator delivers a fixed volume of air, set by the operator in the lungs of a patient during inspiration. Like PCV, as *fixed volume* of air is delivered to the patient, so the *pressure in the airway* may vary according to the conditions of the lungs.

Pressure-controlled ventilation: In pressure-controlled or generated or limited ventilation, the peak inspiratory pressure (PIP or P_{max}) is preset by the operator and is maintained for the whole set (fixed) inspiratory time. So, the flow or volume of air, entering the patient's lungs, will depend on the set pressure, lung compliance, airway resistance, and the time allowed (set) for inspiration. The flow of air in alveoli decreases as the alveolar pressure gradually increases with the increasing alveolar volume and ceases when the alveolar pressure equals to the applied set airway pressure. So, the delivered tidal volume will depend on all the factors which affect the flow of air.

In PCV, the normal airway pressure is typically set in the range of 15–30 cmH$_2$O, while pressure above 50 cmH$_2$O can be associated with an increased risk of barotrauma. However, high pressure (even above 50 cmH$_2$O) is sometimes set in cases of ARDS, to inflate the stiff lungs and *here the PCV is preferred mode of ventilation. The PCV is also used for obstructive lung diseases, where resistance for airflow into the*

lungs is very high. In neonatal and pediatric patients, PCV is also indicated, since the peak airway pressure is controlled and barotrauma can be avoided.

Advantages of PCV are:

- As the flow rate or volume varies depending on the patient's lung compliance and airway resistance, so there may be flow or volume starvation.
- It protects against barotrauma (because the higher limit of pressure is predetermined). So, it is essentially used for neonatal and pediatric group of patients.
- Since the fixed peak airway pressure is maintained throughout the whole inspiration, so it ensures that not only the healthy alveoli do not overinflate, but also, the *nonparticipating alveoli are recruited* resulting in better gas exchange.

Disadvantages of PCV are:

- The tidal volume may decrease, if the compliance deteriorates or the resistance increases. In such situations, the setting of pressure should be changed, as if the delivered tidal volume can be adequate.
- Required tidal volume delivered to the patient cannot be assured.
- Minute ventilation (flow or volume) should be closely observed to ensure adequate alveolar ventilation.

In PCV, adequate alveolar ventilation and oxygenation can be achieved by the manipulation of various ventilator settings. Patient's alveolar ventilation depends on minute volume. Minute volume depends on tidal volume and respiratory rate. *In PCV, tidal volume cannot be controlled directly by knob as it will vary.* Tidal volume depends on pressure (PIP-PEEP) and time constant. Time constant depends on resistance and compliance. Time constant cannot be controlled by knob, while only preset pressure is controlled by knob, thus controlling the tidal volume indirectly. Respiratory rate depends on inspiratory time and expiratory time and I:E ratio, all of which can be controlled by knob. So, in *PCV, ventilation is controlled by controlling the knob of* (i) pressure (PIP-PEEP), (ii) respiratory rate, (iii) inspiratory time, (iv) expiratory time, and (v) I:E ratio, according to the resistance and compliance of airways and lung tissues. The last four respiratory parameters are integrated and when *any two* of these four is changed, then other two will change automatically. Therefore, in PCV, only three knobs are regulated and these are: *one* pressure controlling knob and *any two* respiration controlling knob.

Oxygenation can be improved by increasing FiO$_2$. *In PCV, pressure is the independent variable and volume is the dependable variable.* In lung pathology, when compliance decreases and resistance increases, then the pressure is set such that an adequate volume of air is delivered according to that set pressure. In PCV, the amount of delivered air (minute or tidal volume) will be shown on the screen of ventilator, but there will be no knob to control it. *The ultimate arterial oxygenation and ETCO$_2$ is maintained by setting the knob of (i) pressure, (ii) inspiratory time, (iii) expiratory time, (iv) I:E ratio, (v) FiO$_2$, (vi) PEEP, and (vii) flow pattern.*

Pressure-controlled ventilation differs from *pressure-cycled ventilation* and *pressure support ventilation (PSV)*. In pressure-cycled ventilation, the inspiration is terminated when the peak set pressure level is reached, whereas in PCV, the peak pressure is held constant in the form of plateau, until the inspiratory time has elapsed. Difference of PCV from PSV will be discussed later in the next paragraph. The most salient feature of PCV is that the maximal airway and alveolar pressures are controlled. Whereas the tidal volume and subsequently the minute volume and alveolar ventilation cannot be controlled which depend on the compliance of lungs, resistance of airways, and ventilatory pattern. The effective tidal volume is the result of the product of compliance and P$_{max}$. The level of P$_{max}$ which is the necessary inspiratory pressure level, is chosen or set, depending on the tidal volume required, but the pressure exceeding 35 cmH$_2$O should generally be avoided.

In both, pressure-controlled and pressure support ventilation, a set or fixed pressure is controlled by the machine. But, the difference between the two involves the inspiratory time which is machine controlled in the former (PCV) and patient controlled in the latter (PSV).

The special advantages of PCV for its decelerating flow are:

- Since the flow of air (volume) during PCV is decelerating, so the peak airway pressure *due to airway frictional resistance* occurs early in inspiration, and the peak airway pressure *due to elastic recoil resistance* (compliance of lungs) does occur at the end of inspiration. This produces less variability of peak airway pressure than during VCV.
- Effective ventilation in cases of air flow distribution disorders in lungs. The decelerating inspiratory flow characteristic of PCV reduces overinflation of well ventilated "faster alveoli".
- Improved gas exchange due to characteristic of decelerating flow.
- PCV, like PSV, is also especially suited for ventilation during losses due to leakage (e.g., fistula and uncuffed tracheal tube) as an increased flow to maintain the preselected pressure can automatically compensate these losses to a certain degree.

In reality, PCV or PSV refers to how the different type or mode of breaths are modified by pressure, rather than specifying it as a particular mode or type of breath. PCV can be delivered in conjunction with controlled mechanical ventilation (CMV), assist control mechanical ventilation (ACMV), synchronized intermittent mandatory ventilation (SIMV), etc. It was actually been available for many years in conjugation with IMV in neonatal ventilators. A number of variants of PCV have recently been introduced into the clinical practice which includes pressure-controlled-inverse ratio ventilation (PC-IRV), airway pressure release ventilation (APRV), intermittent mandatory pressure release ventilation, and bilevel positive airway pressure (BIPAP) ventilation.

The initial settings for PCV include FiO$_2$, airway pressure level (P$_{max}$) and the end-expiratory pressure, as well as backup mode and rate. P$_{max}$ is adjusted to ensure adequate tidal volume. Backup mode and rate is chosen to provide adequate minute ventilation in the event of decreased intrinsic respiratory drive and may be supplied either in pressure control or SIMV mode.

Volume-controlled ventilation: In a volume-controlled or limited ventilation, a preset amount of minute volume is delivered to the patient in a fixed inspiratory time, set by the respiratory rate and tidal volume in machine. The breath (inspiration) is triggered on by the timing interval determined by the set respiratory rate. Then, it cycles off into the expiratory phase when the inspiratory time has elapsed. By controlling the respiratory rate and tidal volume knob (inspiratory time and I:E ratio will automatically be set), the minute volume should be fixed or preset. That prefixed minute volume should be delivered during fixed inspiratory time. The alveolar and upper airway pressure that is developed due to this inspired volume will depend on the volume and flow pattern of gas delivered by the ventilator, lung compliance, airway resistance, and the time allowed for inspiration.

Volume (or flow) controlled (or generated) ventilators are thought as *strong ventilators than PCV*, because the minute volume (set by the tidal volume and respiratory rate) delivery will not change with the patient's lung characteristic, i.e., lung compliance and airway resistance. Here, the minute volume is independent or fixed factor and the airway or alveolar pressure is dependent or variable factors which are affected by the changes in lung compliance and airway resistance. If lung compliance decreases and resistance increases, then airway or alveolar pressure will also increase, as ventilators will try to ventilate the preset volume of gas within the preset time. So, barotrauma can happen. Thus, to avoid barotrauma, minute volume (by tidal volume and respiratory rate) should be set carefully according to the compliance and the resistance of lungs and should not be used in pediatric patients (mainly neonates and infants) and pathological lung conditions. Here, as the pressure is variable so it cannot be controlled directly according to wish. Indirectly it can be controlled by adjusting the preset tidal volume level and inspiratory time (independent variable). In normal lungs with normal compliance and resistance, if volume is set wrongly, then barotrauma can also occur.

In contrast, *pressure-controlled ventilators are thought as weak ventilators* because the minute volume will change as the patient's lung characteristic changes. So, to maintain the adequate ventilation independent variable such as pressure should be controlled accordingly. In these ventilators, airway pressure is the independent variable, volume is dependent variable (cannot be controlled directly, can be controlled through pressure), and are affected by the changes in lung compliance and airway resistance.

The main indications of VCV are intraoperative IPPV, restrictive lung diseases, and patients weighing >10 kg (where lung's compliance and resistance are thought to be normal). Adequate ventilation and oxygenation can be achieved in VCV by manipulation of minute volume (tidal volume and respiratory rate) and FiO_2. Tidal volume can be set according to patient's body weight (10–12 mL/kg) and minute volume can be set by controlling tidal volume and respiratory rate knob. After setting a minute volume, if airway pressure goes to the allowable maximum limit (not causing barotrauma) and *still oxygenation is not adequate, then oxygenation can be improved by increasing the FiO_2. In VCV, oxygenation cannot be improved by further increasing the minute volume in fear of barotrauma. In such situation for better oxygenation, PEEP can be used with increasing FiO_2.*

Advantages of VCV are:

- *Pressure time waveform* of a VCV *should be ramped one.* Because the ramped pressure time waveform helps to maintain minimum mean airway pressure (MAP).
- Guaranteed preset volume (minute volume) is delivered during each breath which ensures proper ventilation.

Disadvantages of VCV are:

- The resulting high distending peak airway pressure can cause barotrauma.
- Distending or peak airway pressure will increase, if compliance of lung decreases and resistance of airway increase. So, it is mandatory to correctly set the high pressure alarm limit.
- Unequal ventilation of different alveoli, with their different resistances and different time constant, can occur. The flow of air takes the path of least resistance. Hence, the alveoli with lower resistance (compliance) and short time constant will be overinflated. Whereas the alveoli with higher resistance and longtime constant will be under inflated (will not be recruited). However, *in case*

of PCV, since the fixed peak airway pressure is maintained throughout the whole inspiration, so it ensures that not only the healthy alveoli do not overinflate (healthy alveoli will overinflate), but also, the *nonparticipating alveoli are recruited,* resulting in better gas exchange.

- Since, the flow and subsequently the volume is fixed in VCV, so an improper flow setting can cause flow hunger for the patient. This may cause discomfort and hypoxemia to the patient. In VCV, if lung's characteristics change frequently, then you will have to keep eye continuously on pressure gauge and according to that you have to control or preset the minute volume by controlling the tidal volume knob and respiratory rate knob for avoidance of barotrauma.

Whereas in PCV, if lung's characteristics change frequently, then *you will have to keep your eye continuously* on computer screen, giving tidal volume/minute volume data or the breathing bag of ventilator or SPO_2 level for adequate tidal volume and according to that you have to adjust the pressure setting knob for proper ventilation and oxygenation. On the contrary, in VCV, if the characteristics of lungs change frequently, then *you will have to keep your eye continuously on pressure gauge* to prevent barotrauma. In some VCV, there is no pressure gauge. In such circumstances, an idea of airway pressure, produced by preset volume on the background of certain compliance and resistance of lungs, should work in mind.

In a ventilator, the distinction between the pressure generated and volume or flow generated is important. A cheap and simple ventilator use a weighted concertina bag to generate a constant volume during inspiration. Even today these ventilators remain adequate for the majority of patients who require artificial ventilation during anesthesia. The more sophisticated modern ventilators are fitted with devices which instantaneous measure the flow of gas during inspiration. This information can be incorporated into the feedback loop of ventilator to ensure the delivery of some predetermined volume and flow pattern. As a result, there is now greater emphasis on the flow pattern, produced by a ventilator during inspiration. In theory, ventilator can produce any inspiratory flow pattern or waveform. But, the four main waveforms which are shown in **Figure 8** are sine wave, ramp or accelerating flow, top hat or constant flow, and reverse ramp or decelerating flow. No matter, what flow pattern is chosen, but the inspiratory flow in any pattern can be modified further by adding an end-inspiratory pause (EIP). Toward the end of inspiration, the flow of gas ceases, but the lungs are held inflated for a variable period which is called the "pause time". This pause time and expiratory flow pattern is shown in **Figure 9**.

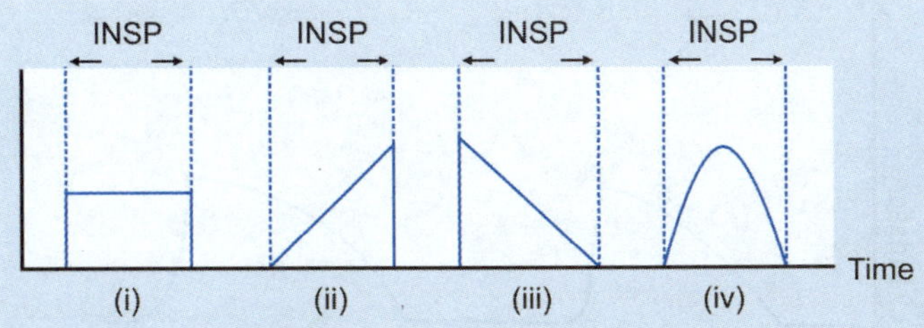

Fig. 8: (i) Constant flow, (ii) Accelerating flow (ramp), (iii) Decelerating flow, and (iv) Sine flow.

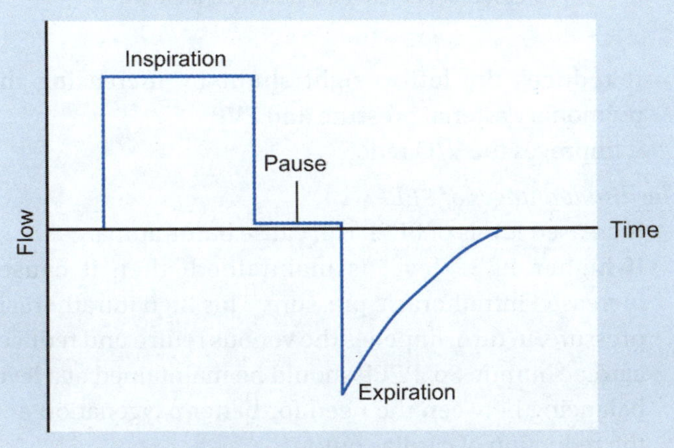

Fig. 9: Flow-time waveform (square pattern) with end-inspiratory pause.

Changing Over from Inspiration to Expiration

Changing over form inspiration to expiration may be *time cycled, volume cycled, pressure cycled, flow cycled, or combination of them.* But, among these, time cycled changing over from inspiration to expiration is commonly used. In time-cycled ventilation, expiration occurs after a predetermined duration of inspiration. It is most popular. The time cycle may be of electronic, mechanical or pneumatic controlled. If a ventilator is time cycled, then the change from inspiration to expiration will occur after a fixed time interval, no matter what airway pressure has been reached or tidal volume has been delivered. But, in volume-controlled and time-cycled ventilator, minute volume is preset by tidal volume and respiratory rate (PCV is usually time cycled, but may or may not be. However, VCV is always time cycled). So, inspiratory time (time cycled) is fixed by I:E ratio, leaving the airway pressure is only variable. Sometimes confusion arises by seeing the excursion of inflating bellows, which create the optical illusion of being volume cycled, though in fact they are time cycled and volume controlled. To ensure delivery of a preset volume in a preset time, the ventilator

must have sufficient power to overcome the circumstances where there is increase in airway resistance or decrease in lung compliance.

In volume-cycled ventilators, there is some confusions as to what volume cycling really means. Ideally, a volume-cycled ventilator would changeover to expiration, when the desired tidal volume had been delivered to the patient's lung, whatever may be the time needed. Unfortunately, lung expansion is not easy to measure and volume-cycled ventilators rely on measuring the volume of gas leaving the ventilator. So, if there are leaks in the apparatus or if the connecting tubes are distensible, then the volume leaving the ventilator may be very different from the volume which reaches the lungs. It has been suggested that the meaning of true volume cycling should apply to those ventilators which measure the gas volume leaving the ventilator and compare it with the volume which the patient exhales. This comparison would be regarded as a better form of volume cycle during ventilation than the volume of gas leaving the ventilator. But, unfortunately very few ventilators have these facilities.

Others forms of cycling, such as flow cycling, pressure cycling, and combination cycling are also possible. But, neither of these are commonly used. In flow cycling, the end of inspiration will depend on the inspiratory flow. The moment when the inspiratory flow reaches the level of a predetermined flow, then the inspiration is terminated and the expiratory phase begins. *Flow cycling is generally used for PSV.* In pressure cycling, when the airway pressure reaches a preset PIP, set beforehand by the operator, then the ventilator will end the inspiratory phase. Other parameters such as inspiration time, tidal volume and flow are variable. The time taken to reach the peak pressure level will depend on the airway resistance and lung compliance. In such circumstances (pressure-cycled ventilation), before adequate inspiratory volume, expiration will start. *This is the difference between a pressure-cycled and pressure-controlled ventilation. Therefore, it is important that a pressure cycling ventilation must be differentiated form a PCV.* If an adjustable pressure safety value is set to low value, then the changeover from the inspiration to expiration may become pressure cycled in some ventilators that would otherwise be time cycled or volume cycled.

The present day ventilators offer the facility to use a combination of the above four cycling mechanisms. One cycling mechanisms is used as the basic mechanism and the second one is used as a secondary backup. *PSV is an example of combination cycle. In PSV, flow cycling is the primary, whereas time and pressure cycling forms the secondary backup.*

Expiration

The majority of ventilators allow passive expiration to atmosphere and the pressure created in the upper airway at the end of expiration is atmospheric. But, this atmospheric pressure at the end of expiration can be modified by applying: (i) negative end-expiratory pressure (NEEP), (ii) expiratory retard (ER), or (iii) PEEP.

During the early development of old ventilators, the use of negative pressure (subatmospheric) at the end of expiration was advocated to expedite the expiration. But, this NEEP is not used now, though many ventilators still provide this facility. The main disadvantage of NEEP is that it causes the early closing of bronchiole of smaller diameter and subsequently air trapping in alveoli. So, in the second phase of evolution of ventilator, to prevent this peripheral airway collapse during expiration, in chronic lung disease with obstructive airway, a variable resistance is placed during expiration in the expiratory limb of ventilator which reduce the expiratory flow rate. This is called the *expiratory retard*. It tries to maintain a pressure above atmospheric level in alveoli and peripheral airways of smaller diameter and so prevents their early closure. Thus, the idea of positive pressure during expiration had developed.

Positive end-expiratory pressure is the positive pressure above atmospheric level (atmospheric level is regarded as baseline or "0" cmH$_2$O) which is presented artificially in the expiratory phase of respiratory cycle. This above atmospheric pressure level (positive pressure) is preset by operator and is generated by the ventilator. *This set positive pressure, during expiration, prevents the early closure of alveoli and peripheral airways. Thus, they try to maintain a patent airway with inflated alveoli and gaseous exchange. However, the ideal level of this PEEP does (should) offer no resistance to expiratory flow.* The PEEP can be used as a stand-alone mode or in combination with other modes. *The physiological level of PEEP is 0–5 cmH$_2$O. The PEEP ≥10 cmH$_2$O can be used in the treatment of ARDS. Though, the PEEP improves ventilation and thus oxygenation, but the disadvantage is it reduces cardiac output. The graphical representation of PEEP is shown in* **Figure 10**.

The mechanism of action and advantages of PEEP:
- It helps to prevent the collapse of smaller airways and alveoli and also try to inflate the already collapsed alveoli
- Thus, it helps in the better participation of gas exchange. It reduces the dead space to tidal volume ratio.
- It prevents atelectasis as positive pressure is maintained at the end of expiration and increases the expiratory time.
- It gradually lowers the alveolar distending pressure due to more and more alveolar recruitment
- It helps to improve the functional residual capacity (FRC)

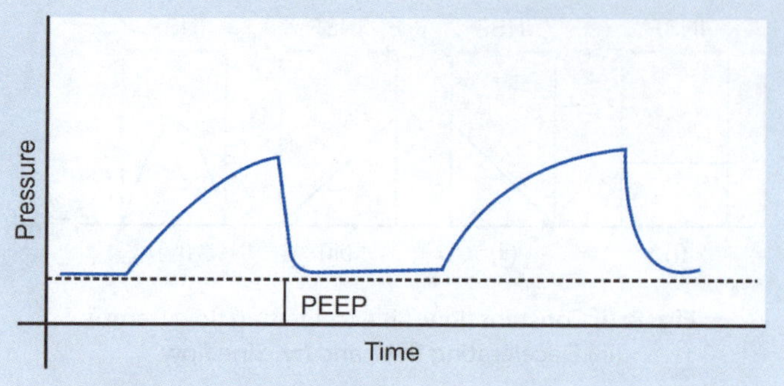

Fig. 10: Pressure time curve shows positive end-expiratory pressure (PEEP) in mechanical ventilation.

- It reduces the left-to-right shunt by increasing the pulmonary arterial pressure and PVR
- It improves the V/Q ratio.

The disadvantages of PEEP:
- Increased levels of PEEP can cause barotrauma.
- If higher PEEP level is maintained, then it causes increased intrathoracic pressure. This high intrathoracic pressure, in turn, impedes the venous return and reduces cardiac output. So, PEEP should be maintained at a level balancing between the need for better oxygenation and the reduction of cardiac output.
- It decreases renal perfusion (from increased renal venous pressure)
- Since higher level of PEEP reduces the venous return, so it causes increased intracranial pressure
- It increases hepatic congestion (from increased hepatic venous pressure)
- It worsens the right-to-left intracardiac shunts.

Sometimes, in few circumstances positive airway pressure is developed automatically at the end of expiration. This is called *auto-PEEP*. Auto-PEEP is also known as the *intrinsic PEEP*. It occurs due to air trapping in alveoli, caused by inadequate expiratory time, due to high respiratory rate or severe airway obstruction with high expiratory airway resistance. *The auto-PEEP means the presence of PEEP that is automatically created at the end of expiration due to any obstruction (spasm) in conducting part of airway or due to inadequate expiration for high respiratory rate. The difference between auto-PEEP and extrinsic PEEP is that in auto-PEEP there is peripheral airway closure first (due to airway spasm) resulting air trapping in alveoli and PEEP in alveoli. These trapped air does not help in gas exchange. But in extrinsic PEEP, which is created by machine artificially, airway pressure is maintained above the atmospheric level at the end of expiration and thus prevents the closure of peripheral airway and alveoli (with positive pressure in alveoli) which helps in gas exchange.

Auto-PEEP is not reflected or detected in ventilator manometer which will continue to show either zero (if extrinsic PEEP is not applied) or set PEEP level (if extrinsic PEEP is applied and in such case if auto-PEEP is again developed). To monitor the level of auto-PEEP, the expiratory port of ventilator should be occluded before the start of inspiration in next breath. *Auto-PEEP can increase the work of breathing, since the patient has to overcome the auto-PEEP level to trigger the ventilator. It also more increases the intrathoracic pressures, leading to more reduction of venous return and cardiac output. Auto-PEEP can be eliminated or kept under control by increasing the expiratory time or by reducing the inspiratory time or by reducing the airway obstruction by bronchodilator.*

In extrinsic PEEP, when used correctly, the peak airway pressure may significantly be less than the predicted sum of peak end-inspiratory pressure measured prior to application of PEEP and positive airway pressure applied. If positive end-expiratory airway pressure (PEEP) is applied in a situation where additional alveolar recruitment cannot or does not occur, then it can have detrimental effects on both hemodynamics and lung mechanics. A decrease in lung compliance still with the addition of PEEP indicates that additional gas exchanging units or alveoli are not being recruited and that the PEEP is unlikely to be of clinical benefit. *The useful effect of PEEP is exhausted at about 15 cmH$_2$O. At pressure exceeding 15 cmH$_2$O, the alveolar diameter does not increase more with increasing PEEP level.* The alveolar tissue cannot be stressed further by applying more high pressure, so that there is a danger of overdistention and alveolar rupture (barotrauma). This effect begins at the level of PEEP which is about 15 cmH$_2$O. *When addition of PEEP results in improvement in lung compliance and oxygenation, but a decrease in cardiac output, then it may be that the intravascular volume depletion is present. The PEEP level should be selected such that sufficient oxygenation is provided with FiO$_2$ not exceeding 0·6 (or 60%)* and is most commonly employed when FiO$_2$ ≥0.5 (50%) is needed for more than few hours to avoid hypoxia. During its application as PEEP is increased in small steps, titrated against the effect, similarly it should also be decreased slowly. Abrupt termination of PEEP therapy can result in pleural effusion, in addition to hypoxia. The extubation of patient is usually done at the PEEP level of 3–5 cmH$_2$O, because "*physiological PEEP*" is held at this level by the closure of glottis.

Changing Over from Expiration to Inspiration

Changing over of ventilation from expiration to inspiration needs some trigger factors which determine the start of inspiration after a period of expiration. This changing over is called trigger and is either determined by ventilator (ventilator triggered and can be preset) or by patient (patient triggered). On the contrary, during changing of from inspiration to expiration, there is no patient initiated cycling, like patient trigger. In a ventilator triggered breath, inspiration starts depending on the timing (time triggered), set on the ventilator by clinician. Ventilator triggers inspiration after a preset duration of expiration or after a preset duration of entire respiration (inspiration + expiration). This should not be confused with the time-cycled changeover from inspiration to expiration (I → E = cycling, E → I = triggering). If the entire respiratory cycle is used for triggering, then any increase in inspiratory time will lead to corresponding decrease in expiratory time. This change may have a profound effect on inspiratory/expiratory ratio and results in auto-PEEP. In a *ventilator triggered*, the time is preset (time triggered) and the patient is completely paralyzed. There is no patient's effort to inspiration and this type of time trigger is used in CMV mode of ventilation. On the other hand, in patient triggered, the breath is initiated by patient's own effort and then immediately ventilator changes over from expiration to inspiration. Assisted ventilation, provided by ventilator, is not possible without patient triggering.

Patient-triggered ventilation has the following advantages:
- It reduces the duration of ventilatory support
- It reduces the weaning time
- It improves the level of blood gases
- It lowers the oxygen dependency.

Patient trigger mechanisms are of various types such as: (1) pressure triggering, (2) flow triggering, (3) chest wall impedance triggering, and (4) abdominal wall motion triggering. The last two patient triggering mechanisms are not commonly used. The two most common types of patient triggering mechanisms are: (i) pressure triggering and (ii) flow triggering. Whereas, *in ventilator trigger, time triggering* is the most commonly used mechanism.

Patient pressure triggering: The pressure triggering is used when the patient tries to take breath spontaneously. When the patient tries to take breath, then there is drop in the airway pressure. This drop in airway pressure is sensed by the ventilator and results in start of inspiration which is delivered by the ventilator. The trigger level on the ventilator is set as unit of cmH$_2$O. The ventilator continuously monitors and senses the airway pressure. For the ventilator to be triggered and deliver a breath, it is essential that the drop in airway pressure by the patient's own respiratory effort must exceed the set pressure trigger or sensitivity level. If the pressure drop in the patient's airway (initiated by the patient's own inspiratory effort) which is transmitted to the ventilator's circuit is not sufficient enough, then the ventilator cannot sense it and will not be triggered to deliver a breath.

In the commercially available ventilators, the sites for pressure sensing are: (i) inside the ventilator, (ii) at the patient's airway (proximal triggering), or (iii) at the carina (distal triggering). The proximal and distal triggering are more sensitive as compared to the drop of pressure being sensed inside the ventilator. The commonly used values for pressure triggering are in the range of -0.5 cmH_2O to -3 cmH_2O. It must be noted that the negative value indicates the drop in pressure below the zero or atmospheric level, when PEEP is not set. But, when PEEP is applied then this negative triggering pressure should be calculated from the set level of PEEP pressure. For example, if PEEP is set at $+10$ cmH_2O and pressure trigger sensitivity is set at -3 cmH_2O, then patient must generate a drop of pressure up to $+7$ cmH_2O $(10 - 3 = 7)$ from $+10$ cmH_2O to trigger the ventilation by ventilator.

The triggering sensitivity is referred to the negative pressure which is generated by the patient to stimulate the ventilator to deliver a breath. Trigger sensitivity is reduced means at more negative pressure, ventilator will be stimulated and this will increase the work of breathing of patient. On the other hand, trigger sensitivity is increased means at slight negative pressure ventilator will be stimulated. When the trigger sensitivity is increased, then the ventilator delivers the breath at slight initiation of patient's effort to take breath, so the patient's capability of taking its own full breath will be diminished and wearing from ventilator will be delayed. *If the trigger is set at maximum (highest) sensitivity level, then the ventilator will often perform an autocycle. So, the trigger should be set at such maximum sensitivity level that does not cause autocycling and usually this pressure is -0.5 to -3 cmH$_2$O.*

Patient flow triggering: In this patient initiated flow triggering, a continuous flow is present in ventilator circuit during the expiratory phase. Due to continuous flow in ventilator circuit during expiration, there is also a continuous flow at the exhalation valve. But, when the patient tries to make a spontaneous effort for inspiration, then the flow is suddenly interrupted at the exhalation valve of ventilator. Hence, the machine senses this interruption of flow and initiates a delivery of breath. *For flow triggering to be functional, the anesthetist needs to set a flow sensitivity setting in liters per minute. When the patient breaths spontaneously, the generated flow gradient must be higher than the flow trigger level, set by the clinician for the ventilator to sense and to initiate a breath delivery. The commonly used values of flow triggering are in the range of 0.6–4 L/min.* In some ventilators, the trigger flow

may need to be set, whereas in some ventilators there is a fixed preset flow to trigger the machine.

However, it is very important to note that triggering is not just a method, but rather the application of a method that affects the patient's work of breathing and ventilator synchrony. The trigger sensitivity setting must be optimized after proper assessing the patient's own ability to trigger. In the initial stages of the ventilatory support, the trigger must be set at more sensitive level. *It means at less negative value, as for example, -1 cmH$_2$O for pressure triggering or 0.5 L/min for flow triggering. As the patient's condition improves, the trigger sensitivity should be decreased, because the patient will gradually try to take breath by himself.*

Inspiratory/Expiratory Time Ratio (I:E)

The I:E ratio have an important effect on the removal of expired gases and on the mean intrathoracic pressure which again have an implication on oxygenation and cardiac output. Usually, an adequate time is required for the removal of expired gases without any air trapping. So, the expiratory time is greater than inspiratory time. Normally, the I:E ratio is about 1:2, i.e., the duration of expiration is twice than that of inspiration. It limits gas trapping and optimizes the mean intrathoracic pressure. In obstructive lung disease, this I:E ratio is <1:2, i.e., the expiration becomes more prolonged than normal. In such circumstance, there also occurs gas trapping due to spasm of peripheral airways and reduction of cardiac output. For volume-cycled ventilators, I:E ratio can be achieved by adjusting V_T, respiratory rate, and inspiratory flow rate. Whereas, in time cycled ventilators, the I:E ratio is adjusted by controlling the respiratory rate and inspiratory time. Most of the ventilators are time cycled.

While setting respiratory rate on ventilator for a spontaneously breathing patient the following points should be kept in mind; these are: (i) The patient's actual rate demand, (ii) The patient's anticipated ventilatory requirement, and (iii) The impact of rate setting on breathing time. The ventilators are not capable of varying inspiratory time and flow which is set by the operator. For example, with machine backup at a rate setting of 12 breaths/minute, the total cycle time (T_{Tot}) for each breath is 5 seconds. If the I:E ratio is set at 1:2 or if V_T and flow have been set at 0.5 L and 0.34 L/sec, respectively, then T_I (inspiratory time) is fixed at 1.5 seconds and expiratory time (T_E) will be 3.5 seconds. If the patient actually triggers at 24 breaths/min, then T_{Tot} declines to 2.5 seconds. T_I remains fixed at 1.5 seconds, because it is determined by the preset machine (backup) rate, the I:E ratio or the inspiratory flow settings. The T_E must now decrease from 3.5 seconds to 1 second and the actual I:E ratio will increase from 1:2 to near about 2:1. At a rate of

40 breaths/min ($T_{Tot} = 1.5$ seconds), T_E becomes "0" and then "fighting with the ventilator" must result. For these reasons, the machine backup rate should always be set close to the patient's actual respiratory rate. If the actual respiratory rate initiated by patient is very high that effective ventilation cannot be achieved, then the patient needs additional sedation and possibly neuromuscular blockade.

Tidal Volume (V_T)

It is generally accepted that V_T should be in the range of 10–15 mL/kg of body weight for most of the patients. Because, the small tidal volume (6–8 mL/kg) promotes the development of microatelectasis, while very large tidal volume can cause barotrauma and cardiovascular decompensation.

However, in some conditions such as obstructive lung disease and ARDS, it is probably safer to choose a relatively low tidal volume (5–7 mL/kg) to avoid complications. While setting V_T, it is important to consider the role of compliance of the connecting tube of ventilator circuit. This is approximately 3–4 mL/cmH$_2$O during peak pressure. So, during inflation certain amount of tidal volume will not be delivered to the patient. But, as the airway pressure falls and the tubes return to its original size, then this volume will be measured as exhaled volume, if a spirometer is attached on the expiratory limb of ventilator circuit.

Inspiratory Flow

The *inspiratory flow rate* is the measurement of *velocity* at which the breathing gas is supplied to patient. It is an important determinant of patient's work of breathing. If the ventilator's inspiratory flow rate is chosen less than the patient's flow demand, then the patient will increase his inspiratory efforts in an attempt to improve his gas delivery. Thus, it will increase the patient's work of breathing. *So, to minimize this work of breathing, the ventilator's inspiratory flow rate should be fixed above the patient's peak flow demand. On the other hand, if the inspiratory flow rate is very high during VCV, then it can lead to increased inspiratory peak pressure.* Thus, overinflation of healthy lung leads to an impaired V/Q ratio and increased intrapulmonary shunt. So, a balance has to be reached. Constant flows of 60–70 L/min are well tolerated in ventilator-dependent patients and it does not manifest significant levels of auto-PEEP. Flow rates may require modification in certain circumstances such as chronic obstructive pulmonary disease (COPD) or asthma. Here, higher flow rates (70–100 L/min) are often used to shorten the inspiratory time and to lengthen the expiratory time. Thus, potentially it reduces the degree of auto-PEEP and hyperinflation.

Pressure-controlled and pressure support ventilation can deliver the high initial flow rates. This may be advantageous for patients with high initial flow demands or those with severe lung disease, demanding high minute ventilations.

FiO$_2$

The principle for setting FiO$_2$ is like that it (FiO$_2$) should be selected, as high as necessary, to save the patient's life when emergency condition arise and as low as possible to prevent O$_2$ toxicity when patient's condition is stable. The increased inspired O$_2$ concentration to maintain PaO$_2$ should always be understood as symptomatic treatment. In case of respiratory failure, it is common practice to initiate ventilatory support with FiO$_2$ of 1 (i.e., 100% O$_2$). In such circumstance, it is advised to ignore the potential for oxygen toxicity, during the first few hours of ventilatory management by 100% O$_2$. Then, it should be decreased gradually. *One instance, where clinician must minimize FiO$_2$ at all costs, is a patient who has received bleomycin or amiodarone. Because, these drugs make the lungs extremely susceptible to injury (oxygen toxicity), mediated by O$_2$ radicals.*

DIFFERENT MODES OF MECHANICAL VENTILATION

The mode of mechanical ventilation is defined as the configuration of flow, pressure, and volume of gas which is delivered to the patient in a specific characteristic manner, coupled with cycling and triggering mechanisms. Thus, the ventilation mode also specifies the manner in which the ventilator breaths are controlled, cycled, and triggered. The controlled factors are operator specified values such as airway pressure, volume, and flow that cannot be exceeded during inspiration and expiration. If the specific values of any of the parameter are exceeded, then inspiratory flow is immediately stopped and the ventilator circuit is vented to atmospheric pressure or to the specified PEEP value. Cycle refers to the factors that determine the end of inspiration and trigger defines what the ventilator senses to initiate an inspiration.

The modes of ventilation are:
- Controlled mechanical ventilation: It may be of two types (1) VCV and (2) PCV.
- Assisted mechanical ventilation (AMV)
- Assist control mechanical ventilation
- IMV
- Synchronized intermittent mandatory ventilation (SIMV)
- Positive end-expiratory pressure
- Continuous positive airway pressure (CPAP)
- Bilevel positive airway pressure
- Pressure support ventilation

- Inverse ratio ventilation
- Airway pressure release ventilation
- Spontaneous ventilation
- Apnea backup ventilation
- Dual mode ventilation.

Controlled Mechanical Ventilation: VCV and PCV

Here, all the breaths, delivered to patient, are totally controlled by ventilator and ventilatory pattern is totally independent of patient's breathing effort. In CMV mode, the ventilator is totally nonresponsive to patient's spontaneous respiratory efforts and requirements, still if the patient starts to take breath by himself. So, CMV is usually used in totally paralyzed patient. If this mode is used in a partially paralyzed patient or the patient starts to take breath spontaneously, then there will be a fight between the ventilator and patient (i.e., breath stacking or starvation—anyone can occur). So, this mode is not useful for spontaneously (even slightly) breathing patients. In this controlled mode of ventilation, the breath is delivered to the patient by ventilator at a preset fixed respiratory rate and pattern (volume or pressure), determined by the ventilator controls. *Here, in VCV every breath is time cycled and time triggered.* For volume-controlled breaths or ventilation (VCV), the set volume is delivered to the patient in the set inspiratory time, irrespective of developed airway pressure which are determined by lung mechanics (lung compliance and airway resistance). The fixed minute volume is totally controlled by the ventilator. Since, very high pressure (if it develops due to altered lung mechanics as pressure is dependent variable) can cause barotrauma. *So, to ensure patient's safety the VCVs should be equipped with a pressure release valve and high pressure alarm to alert the clinician.*

Whereas, in pressure-controlled breaths or ventilation (PCV), the set pressure plateau is maintained for the set inspiratory time for each breath. *Like VCV, PCV is also time cycled and time triggered.* In PCV, during inspiratory phase, a given pressure is immediately imposed at airway opening and this set pressure remains at this user specified level throughout the inspiration. Since, the inspiratory airway pressure in PCV is specified by the operator, so the tidal volume and inspiratory flow rate are dependent variables and are not user specified. PCV is the preferred mode of ventilation for neonates and infants and for patients with increased risk of barotrauma and for postoperative thoracic surgical patients in whom the shear forces across a fresh suture line should be limited. When using PCV, minute ventilation and tidal volume must be monitored by seeing the amount of gas delivered on control panel of ventilator,

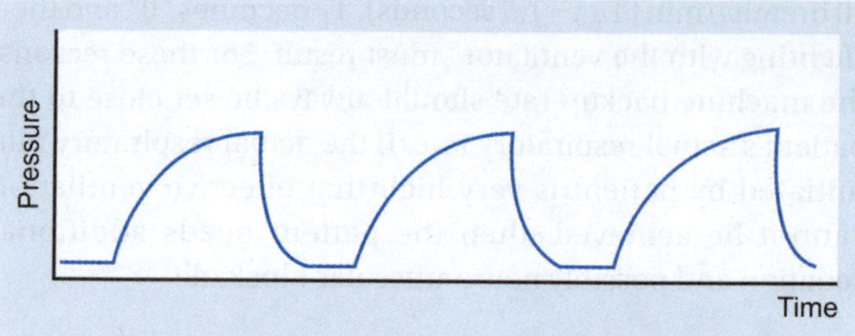

Fig. 11: Controlled mechanical ventilation and time cycled.

to ensure adequate ventilation (whereas in VCV airway pressure should be monitored by seeing the pressure gauge of monitor). Inadequate or over adequate minute ventilation can be altered through changes in respiratory rate or through changes of set pressure by pressure control knob in PCV **(Fig. 11)**.

The PCV mode is used as a control mode with a normal I:E ratio or with increase I:E ratio. It could also be used in combination with PSV mode of ventilation. *At present, the primary indication for PCV is ARDS patient* to whom the conventional IPPV with PEEP is not effective, i.e., specifically those patients, who are on an FiO_2 of 1 (100%), have a peak inspiratory pressure (PIP) of >50 cmH_2O, higher PEEP levels of >15 cmH_2O, higher assist control rates >16 respiratory rate, have low PaO_2 and low lung compliance. Now a special form of CMV, i.e., the pressure regulated volume control (PRVC) mode of ventilation is available on many sophisticated ventilators. This mode has advantageous features of both the VCV and PCV mode of ventilation. It incorporates tidal volume as a servo parameter to ensure adequate volume delivery in PCV mode. *Usually in our anesthesia practice, we administer a constant flow, pressure-limited or regulated, volume-controlled, time-cycled ventilation that is often regulated up to 35 cmH_2O to prevent barotrauma.*

Some common indications for the use of CMV mode of ventilations are:

- *Neuromuscular paralysis:* This may be drug induced as in general anesthesia (commonly the VCV), or neuromuscular pathology such as myasthenia gravis and paralytic poliomyelitis.
- Prolonged apnea
- Severe central nervous system depression due to such as high-dose narcotic, brain trauma, and spinal cord injury
- Postoperative patients with complete paralysis
- Patients who have fatigue of respiratory muscles and need for maximal rest of it.

Some complications or disadvantages associated with CMV mode are:

- During incomplete paralysis as the patient's triggering efforts are not sensed and supported by the ventilator, so it can cause patient's discomfort and agitation during recovery.

- This CMV mode is unresponsive to the changing minute ventilation and airway pressure requirements of patient.
- Total CMV for a longer period can inhibit the contraction of respiratory muscles which are then prone to atrophy. Because this mode is generally used in patients, who are fully paralyzed with muscle relaxants or in patients with poor or no spontaneous attempts to respiration. It is also used when the patient's respiratory drive is suppressed with heavy doses of narcotics and sedatives due to any reasons for therapeutic purposes.

Assisted Mechanical Ventilation

Here, every breath of patient is assisted by mechanical ventilator, but breath rate is completely controlled by the patient. Ventilator only supplements the patient initiated or triggered breath, during changing over from expiration to inspiration (E → I). But, the initiation of expiration (I → E) is time cycled. The initiation of breath by ventilator (E → I) occurs as a consequence of a sensing device which detects patient's initiated breath as a fall in airway pressure below the end-expiratory pressure (pressure triggered). This amount of fall in patient's airway pressure required to trigger a breath by ventilator is referred to as trigger sensitivity, which can be adjusted. So, for the proper functioning of this mode, it is essential to set the optimum trigger level sensitivity, so that all the patient's efforts to inspiration (from expiration) are recognized by the ventilator. Thus, every recognized patient's effort is assisted by ventilator, either by a volume-controlled breath (VCV) or by a pressure-controlled breath (PCV). As this ventilatory mode is time cycled, so the spontaneous respiratory rate of patient must exceeds the control backup respiratory rate of ventilator or the ventilator's set respiratory rate should be kept below the patient's spontaneous effort rate. *In this mode, ventilator does not respond to patient's apnea, as there is no system for control or mandatory breath* (**Figs. 12A and B**).

Assist Control Mechanical Ventilation

Assist control mechanical ventilation is a combination mode where "assist" refers to the ventilator's supplementation of patient initiated breaths and "control" refers to the mandatory preset (backup) ventilation when there is no patient's initiation of breath (patient is completely apneic). An inspiratory cycle is initiated either by patient's inspiratory effort or by ventilator itself, if patient's effort is not detected within a specified time window by a timer signal (patient is completely apneic or the respiratory rate of patient is very low). If the breath which is delivered by ventilator is

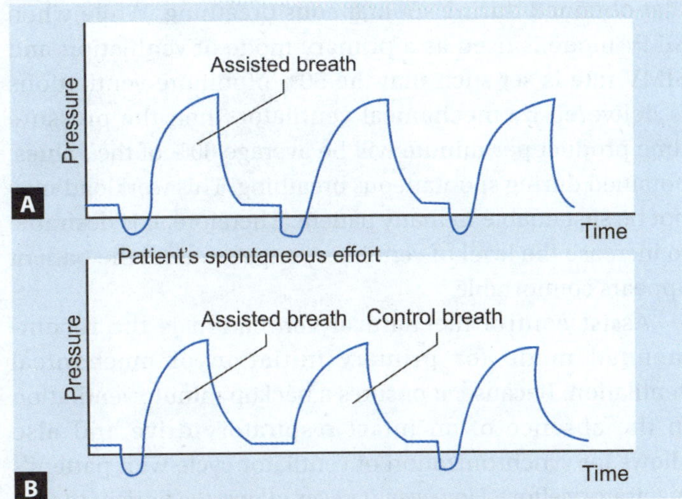

Figs. 12A and B: (A) Assisted mechanical ventilation; (B) Assist control mechanical ventilation.

due to patient's spontaneous efforts, then it is called the assisted ventilation and if the breath delivery is due to set respiratory rate in ventilator in the presence of apnea, then it is called the controlled ventilation. As every breath (assisted or controlled) is a mechanical breath, hence volume or pressure-controlled delivery will be as per the ventilator's settings. It is important to set the proper trigger sensitivity and backup respiratory rate, matching with the patient for proper working of this mode. An insensitive trigger setting will inadvertently change the ACMV mode to CMV mode. If the spontaneous respiratory effort rate of patient exceeds the control backup rate, then no control breaths are delivered and the ventilator will function completely in assisted mode. However, if the patient's spontaneous effort is less than the control backup rate, then the volume or pressure control breaths by ventilator will be provided at appropriate intervals. As compared to CMV mode, in patient with slight spontaneous efforts, this ACMV mode allows for better synchrony between the patient and the machine. So, it can be applied to awake, sedated or fully paralyzed unconscious patients. Since, it has been shown that CMV mode used for >48 hours results in the reduction of diaphragmatic muscle mass and diaphragmatic twitch tension, so it has been suggested that a minimal amount of diaphragmatic work is required to prevent the reduction in diaphragmatic strength and endurance. During ACMV mode, with optimum ventilator settings, the load faced by the inspiratory muscles, should not be enough to cause fatigue of inspiratory muscles or respiratory distress, but should be sufficient enough to prevent muscle atrophy.

With assisted ventilation on optimal ventilator settings, the pressure-time product of inspiratory muscles which is the measure of work of breathing, will be average 50% of that obtained during spontaneous breathing. While when SIMV mode is used as a primary mode of ventilation and SIMV rate is set such that the 50% of minute ventilations is delivered by mechanical ventilator, then the pressure time product per minute will be average 80% of the values, obtained during spontaneous breathing. This workload may not be sustainable in many patient. Therefore, it is desirable to increase the level of ventilatory support, until the patient appears comfortable.

Assist control mechanical ventilation is the recommended mode for primary initiation of mechanical ventilation. Because, it ensures a backup minute ventilation in the absence of an intact respiratory drive and also allows for synchronization of ventilator cycle with patient's inspiratory effort. *However, it never allows the patient to take a full breath by himself (difference from SIMV)*. Problems can arise when ACMV is used in patients with tachypnea due to nonrespiratory or nonmetabolic factors such as anxiety, pain, or airway irritation. In such situation, respiratory alkalemia due to high respiratory rate (which is due to full ventilatory assistance for each patient initiated breath) and excessive washout of CO_2 may produce trigger myoclonus or seizures. Also COPD patients who are tachypneic may develop auto-PEEP on ACMV mode of ventilation, with potential for barotrauma. Auto-PEEP also limits venous return, decreases cardiac output, and increases airway pressure. ACMV mode is not effective for weaning the patients from mechanical ventilation, because it provides full ventilator assistance for each patient initiated breath. Hence, now for weaning ACMV is replaced by SIMV mode of ventilation.

Indications for use of ACMV mode are:
- Patients who are earlier put on CMV mode for complete muscular paralysis or apnea, but now are gradually initiating spontaneous respiratory efforts.
- Patients who have own stable respiratory drive with any capability of triggering the ventilator.
- The ventilator should be set to achieve minimum 80% of minute ventilation. This is prove to be a good setting of ACMV mode.
- Postoperative patients coming out of the effects of complete muscular paralysis and anesthesia.

Advantages of ACMV mode are:
- Atrophy of respiratory muscles seen in CMV and AMV mode can be prevented in ACMV mode. This is due to spontaneous efforts (initiated by patient), being assisted and supported by ventilator.
- It avoids patient agitation (fighting between patient and ventilator). This is because the patient can now get assisted ventilation for his or her spontaneous efforts from the ventilator.

- As the patient is allowed to control his or her respiratory rate, so the minute volume, and the $PaCO_2$ of patient can be normalized.

Complications of ACMV mode are:
- If the patient's respiratory rate increases in ACMV mode, then an auto-PEEP will develop. This will cause the mean intrathoracic pressure to increase, affecting the venous return and cardiac output.
- Increased respiratory rate will increase the minute volume and subsequently the mean alveolar pressure causing barotrauma.
- If the patient respiratory rate is high and is being assisted at higher rates, then it can result into hyperventilation causing hypocapnea and respiratory alkalosis.

Intermittent Mandatory Ventilation

In IMV, the ventilator delivers intermittent mandatory breaths in a predetermined pattern (volume- or pressure-controlled ventilation, time cycled with set respiratory rate) and allows the patient to breath spontaneously in between the mandatory breath. This mode is a combination of CMV mode with a facility to support the patient's spontaneous efforts fully (not assisted). The point where IMV differs from CMV is that in between the ventilator's breath, the breathing circuit is open and patient can breathe fresh gas at his own rate and tidal volume. There is no option of synchronization between the ventilator's breath and the patient's breath. All spontaneous breaths are fully patient's controlled or all controlled breaths are fully ventilator's control. So, ACMV = CMV + AMV (not a single full spontaneous breathing is allowed). But IMV = CMV + full patient's spontaneous breathing (not a single spontaneous breathing is assisted). In ACMV, all the ventilation is machine controlled, but some are triggered and some are not triggered. But, in IMV, there is no trigger and all or none principle is followed (i.e., if patient breaths he will take his full breath, otherwise machine will force him to take breath).

"Breath stacking" is the major limitation of this IMV mode. This is because as the ventilator is allowed to deliver some mandatory breath, the rate of which is set by operator and the patient is also permitted to breathe spontaneously, so at times, it is seen that the patient is fighting with the ventilator. This is due to sometimes patient's exhalation is superimposed by ventilator's inspiration. Hence, the patient faces a high expiratory resistance which is called the "breath stacking". So, due to the problems of breath stacking, the IMV mode is now replaced with a mode which delivers the mandatory breath when necessary and synchronizes the ventilator's breaths with patient's efforts, i.e., SIMV. The IMV can be used as a full ventilatory support mode or as a weaning mode.

Advantages of IMV mode are:

- Decreased requirement of sedation and muscle relaxation
- Better ventilation to perfusion (V/Q) matching
- Lower MAP
- Avoidance of respiratory alkalosis
- Expedited weaning
- Prevention of respiratory muscle atrophy or discoordination
- Reduced likelihood of cardiac decompensation

Disadvantages of IMV mode are:

- Increased risk of CO_2 retention
- Increased work of breathing and respiratory muscle fatigue
- Stacking of breath

  Setting of this IMV mode include mandatory rate, mandatory tidal volume/minute volume, I:E ratio, trigger sensitivity, high and low pressure alarm, respiratory rate, and tidal volume display.

Synchronized Intermittent Mandatory Ventilation (SIMV)

SIMV = CMV + AMV + patient's full spontaneous breathing or ACMV + patient's full spontaneous respiration. In SIMV mode, the patient spontaneously breaths and intermittent ventilator's breaths are synchronized and if there is no spontaneous breath by patient, then ventilator takes over the whole responsibility, producing mandatory ventilation (CMV). Synchronization means ventilator waits for patient's spontaneous inspiration. If the inspiration is not sufficient enough (measured by triggered sensitivity), then machine assist the ventilation (AMV). In between CMV and AMV, patient takes full spontaneous respiration if he can. In SIMV, it is important to set an optimal trigger sensitivity level, so that the patient can have optimum amount of spontaneous respiration and this optimum amount of ventilation is assisted and the next optimum amount is fully controlled. So, to achieve this the ventilator must create a *timing window* which divides the expiratory time into nonsynchronization interval and synchronization interval. Synchronization interval is responsible for mandatory breath by ventilator and nonsynchronization interval is for ventilator-assisted spontaneous breath. If the patient's spontaneous efforts occur in the synchronization interval, then the next schedule mandatory breath will be shifted accordingly and will be delivered as assisted ventilation to the patient in response to patient trigger. In the absence of patient's effort during synchronization interval, the mandatory breath is delivered as per the set breath rate interval. On the other hand, any

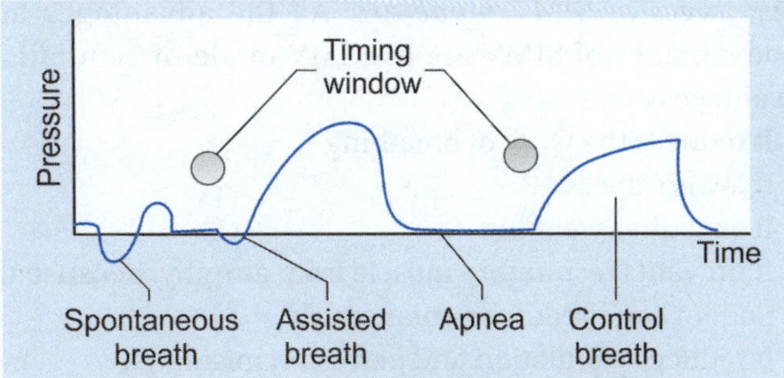

Fig. 13: Synchronized intermittent mandatory ventilation (SIMV), volume controlled.

patient's effort in nonsynchronization interval will result in a ventilator-assisted breath which is completely patient controlled (**Fig. 13**). The mandatory breaths, which are delivered to patient, will not exceed the set SIMV rate. Usually, the mandatory rate in SIMV is set such that even if the patient has no spontaneous attempts, still adequate minute ventilation is delivered to the patient. Usually, a minimum rate of 8–10 breaths/min with a tidal volume of 8–10 mL/kg is set for mandatory breaths. When the spontaneous attempts are rigorous and adequate, the patient is weaned off this mode.

The major difference between SIMV and ACMV is that in SIMV the patient is allowed fully to breathe spontaneously, i.e., without ventilator assistance, in between the delivered breaths by ventilator (assisted or control). However, mandatory breaths are delivered in synchrony with the patient's inspiratory efforts at a frequency, determined by the operator. If the patient fails to initiate a breath, the ventilator delivers a fixed tidal volume breath and resets the internal timer for the next cycle of respiration. SIMV also differs from ACMV in that only the preset number of breaths is ventilator assisted.

SIMV allows patients with an intact respiratory drive to exercise inspiratory muscles in between the assisted breaths. This characteristic makes the SIMV a very useful mode of ventilation for both supporting and weaning of an intubated patient. SIMV may be difficult to use in patients with tachypnea, because they may attempt to exhale during the ventilator programmed inspiratory cycle. When this occurs, then the airway pressure may exceed the inspiratory pressure limit or the ventilator's assisted breath will be aborted or minute volume may drop below that programmed by operator (anesthetist). In such setting, if tachypnea occurs in response to respiratory or metabolic acidosis, then a change to ACMV will increase minute ventilation and will help to normalize pH, while the underlying pathology is further evaluated.

Advantages of SIMV mode are: All the advantages and disadvantages of SIMV are like IMV mode of ventilation. Advantages are:

- It reduces the work of breathing
- It lowers the MAP
- It expedites weaning
- It prevents respiratory muscle from atrophy, because the patient can breathe spontaneously.
- It reduces ventilation and perfusion mismatch
- It avoids breath stacking.

Limitations of SIMV mode are: Sometimes, the mandatory respiratory rates, which are set in ventilator, do not provide adequate minute ventilation, if the patient develops apnea. In such circumstances, respiratory rates delivering lower than adequate minute ventilation, should be closely monitored. Otherwise, the ventilator is set with an appropriate apnea backup mode, if available, on ventilator.

Mandatory Minute Ventilation (MMV)

This is also a servo controlled (i.e., feedback controlled) ventilation mode, similar to that of SIMV. But, it differs from SIMV in that instead of predetermined respiratory rate (as in SIMV respiratory rate is preset), a predetermined fixed minimum amount of minute volume, that the ventilator is bound to deliver to patient, is the criteria for the mode of this mechanical breath. So, this mode of ventilation also can be called SIMMV (synchronised intermittent mandatory minute ventilation). Like SIMV, the MMV (or SIMMV) mode is also useful for partially spontaneously breathing patients. During MMV, the ventilator continuously measures the actual patient's spontaneous minute volume that he or she inhales and compares it with the clinician set minimum minute volume. If the patient's spontaneous minute ventilation goes below the set mandatory minute ventilation, then the ventilator automatically takes over the responsibility and the difference between these two minute volumes is then delivered as mandatory breaths by ventilator. If the patient's spontaneous minute ventilation is higher than the set mandatory minute ventilation, then no ventilator breaths will be delivered.

MMV (SIMMV) may be a useful method of ventilation for patients with fluctuations in ventilatory drive or who are being weaned from mechanical ventilation. During weaning, as the patient can contribute gradually more control over the spontaneous portion of his tidal volume, so the mandatory minute ventilation, can be decreased automatically gradually. A good strategy of MMV mode is to set the MMV value, as little as below the desired minute ventilation of patient. If the patient experiences apnea episode, then the ventilator automatically takes over the responsibility and delivers additional mandatory breaths. In some ventilators,

the function of MMV is replaced by "apnea backup" mode which works on the criteria of low minute volume alarm limit.

The advantages of MMV is that it is useful in preventing hypoventilation and simultaneously permits complete spontaneous breathing. The disadvantages of MMV is that under distress the patient may have a breathing pattern of rapid respiratory rates and shallow tidal volume. This rapid breathing pattern of the patient may be identified by the ventilator as the predetermined minimum minute ventilation is met. Thus, this rapid shallow respiration cause inadequate alveolar ventilation and muscle fatigue.

Pressure Support Ventilation

The PSV combines the advantages of PCV with spontaneous breathing. As the breathing is spontaneously maintained in PSV, so the patient himself determines the respiratory rate, inspiratory time, tidal volume. Each inspiratory effort of the patient is assisted by the ventilator at a preset level of inspiratory pressure. So, PSV is a patient or pressure triggered and pressure or flow-cycled ventilation. Because as the chosen pressure is constant, so the flow decreases as more and more the lungs are filled (decelerating flow). Thus, when flow comes to zero against a certain elevated pressure, inspiration ends and expiration starts. *Flow cycling forms the primary criteria for termination of breath in PSV.* The other safety backup criteria are time and pressure. During PSV, the inspiratory phase is terminated when inspiratory air flow falls below a certain level. In most ventilators, this flow rate cannot be adjusted by the operator. If PSV is used, patient receives ventilatory help, only when the ventilator detects an inspiratory effort (patient or pressure triggered) **(Figs. 14A and B)**.

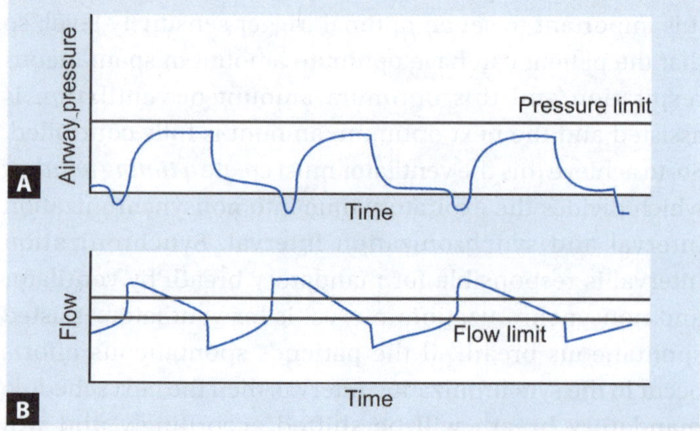

Figs. 14A and B: Airway pressure and airway flow versus time during pressure support ventilation. All the breaths are patient triggered and flow cycled. Inspiration is cycled off when the inspiratory flow drops below a predetermined threshold level which is internally set in ventilation circuit.

Thus patient initiates a pressure support when:

- There is fall in pressure of airway.
- The spontaneous inspiratory flow touches the value of certain limit (e.g., between 1 and 15 L/min)
- The inhaled volume is <25 mL during spontaneous breathing.

Pressure support ventilation can be used as an independent mode or in combination with SIMV and CPAP modes. In combination with SIMV, it ensures volume-cycled backup for patients whose respiratory drive is depressed, either spontaneously or as a result of various therapeutic maneuvers.

The pressure support stops when:

- The inspiratory flow goes back to zero or the patients actively exhales
- The inspiratory flow goes below 25% of the maximum flow
- The above criteria become inoperative or when the time of exhalation takes >4 seconds—a safety mechanism.

The advantages of PSV are:

- Maximally reducing the work of breathing this mode enhances the patient's comfort on ventilator
- Maximize patient's control on respiration
- No hemodynamic consequences
- With the change in work of breathing, pressure support can be adjusted (decreasing the level of pressure support during weaning and increasing the levels of pressure support when patient gradually deteriorates). Normally, to overcome the airway resistance [including the tubing system of ventilator, endotracheal (ET) tube, etc.] a pressure support of 5–10 cmH$_2$O is required.
- A preferred mode of weaning from mechanical ventilator. PSV is well tolerated by most of the patients who are being weaned. PSV parameters can be set in such a way that it can provide a full or a nearly full ventilatory support and can be withdrawn slowly over a period of days in a systemic fashion, where gradually load is applied on respiratory muscles.
- Provide an insight of patient's respiratory status, i.e., if patient is in the state of normal work of breathing (weaning) or not. For example, a patient with COPD, exhibiting good clinical status and normal gas exchange with normal pressure support (3–7 cmH$_2$O), is a good candidate for tracheal extubation.

It is observed that addition of PSV mode to the spontaneous breathing pattern causes an increase in tidal volume and decrease in respiratory rate. Increased tidal volume and decreased respiratory rate cause increased alveolar ventilation. Increased tidal volume (V_T) produces a decrease in the ratio between dead space and tidal volume (V_D/V_T)

and thus better gas exchange. Studies have demonstrated that addition of PEEP can increase the efficacy of PSV and much reduces the work of breathing in patients with COPD, presenting with intrinsic PEEP. So, combination of PSV with PEEP may be the optimum way to support the ventilation.

The limitations of PSV mode are:

- It is applied only to the patients who breathe spontaneously.
- When high pressure support is needed then PSV mode is not good. Then, PCV is far better mode.
- As PSV is a flow-cycled ventilation, so if there is any circuit leak, then it causes continuous flow and continuous delivery of airway pressure, even during patient's spontaneous expiration. This can lead to severe hemodynamic compromise. Thus, autocycling caused by circuit leak allows inspiration to be triggered.
- With this mode, patient with unreliable inspiratory effort may receive inadequate ventilation.
- High airway pressure, if there is high level of pressure support.

Continuous Positive Airway Pressure

Like PEEP, it is not a true mode of ventilation, because patient is already breathing spontaneously with full effort. The ventilator provides fresh gas flow to breathing circuit during the whole cycle of respiration and produces in the circuit a constant operator specified pressure that can range from 0 to 25 cmH$_2$O. Basically, *CPAP is like PEEP (which is maintained only at the end of expiration), but it differs from later in that CPAP is applied continuously both during inspiration and expiration and only during spontaneous breathing. Unlike PEEP, the CPAP cannot be applied during controlled ventilation, whereas PEEP can be applied both during controlled and spontaneous ventilation.* CPAP can also be administered to the patient noninvasively by using a mask attached to the patient's face with harness. It is also a popular weaning mode **(Figs. 15A and B)**.

Bilevel (or Biphasic) Positive Airway Pressure

Bilevel positive airway pressure is a unique ventilatory mode which covers the entire spectrum from complete mechanical ventilation to full spontaneous breathing. It is a variation of PCV, but differs from it that in BIPAP spontaneous breaths is possible. BIPAP ventilation indicates two levels of positive pressure and thus it is named so. Among the two levels of positive pressure, one level is maintained during inspiration (inspiratory positive airway pressure or IPAP) and the other level is maintained during expiration (expiratory positive airway pressure or EPAP). IPAP is always greater than EPAP

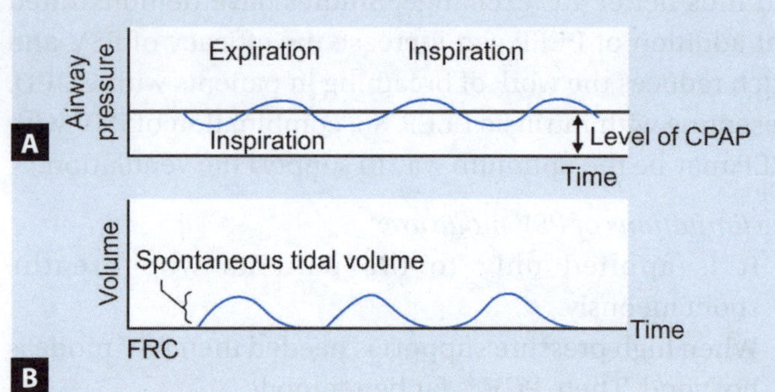

Figs. 15A and B: Airway pressure and lung volume versus time profiles during CPAP. Breathing is spontaneous and no ventilator assist is provided. The spontaneous profile is superimposed on an elevated mean airway pressure that the user specifies. (CPAP: continuous positive airway pressure; FRC: functional residual capacity)

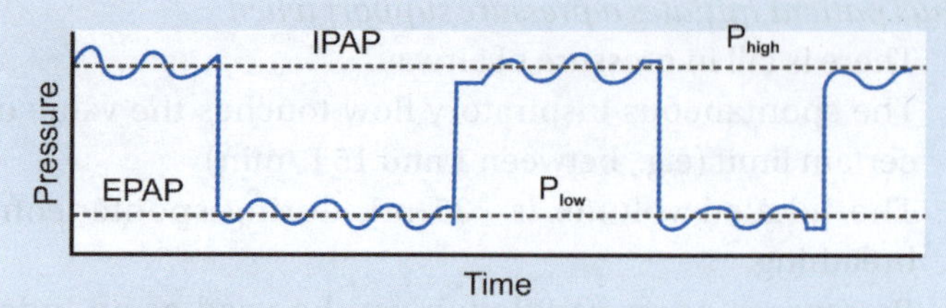

Fig. 16: Biphasic positive airway pressure. (EPAP: expiratory positive airway pressure; IPAP: inspiratory positive airway pressure)

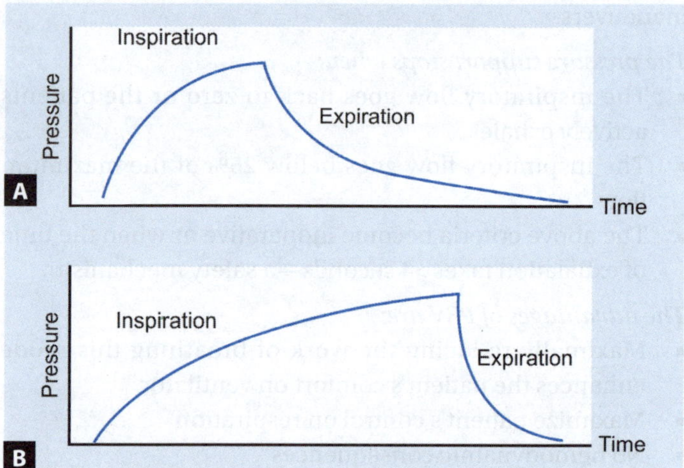

Figs. 17A and B: Inverse ratio ventilation (IRV). (A) Normal inspiration: expiration ratio; (B) Inverse inspiration: expiration ratio.

in BIPAP. *But, when IPAP is equal to EPAP, it results in CPAP otherwise EPAP is similar to PEEP.* Patient can breathe spontaneously at both IPAP and EPAP. BIPAP is available on ventilators or as separate BIPAP machine. The various forms of BIPAP are classified according to the respective proportions of mechanical ventilation and spontaneous breathing present in it. These classification include:

- There is no spontaneous breathing → CMV + BIPAP.
- There is spontaneous breathing at the upper pressure level → APRV + BIPAP.
- There is spontaneous breathing at the lower pressure level → IMV + BIPAP.
- Continuous spontaneous breathing, both equal pressure levels = CPAP
- There is spontaneous breathing at both the pressure level = Genuine BIPAP

On a ventilator, BIPAP is possible by administering PCV (a type of CMV) in conjugation with PEEP or PSV in conjugation with CPAP. For the BIPAP mode, two levels of pressure and inspiratory plus expiratory time have to be set. BIPAP mode also can be used by noninvasive ventilation via a facemask.

This BIPAP mode is said to have a number of advantages over conventional modes of ventilation. Because as EPAP is applied during expiration, so it enhances alveolar recruitment, improves FRC, and oxygenation. On the other hand, IPAP improves hypoxemia and/or hypercapnia by improving tidal volume delivery by pressure support or PCV. Other advantages of BIPAP include: it allows spontaneous breathing, require less sedation, need higher inspiratory drive, and reduce atelectasis **(Fig. 16)**.

Inverse Ratio Ventilation

During normal spontaneous respiration or in conventional mechanical ventilation (pressure or volume controlled), the inspiratory time is lesser than the expiratory time, i.e., I:E ratio is ≤1 (normally it varies between 1:1 and 1:4). But, IRV refers to a special type of mechanical ventilation in which the I:E ratio is set to greater than one (i.e., I:E is ≥1 which varies between 1:1 and 4:1). By increasing this ratio to more than one, inspiratory time is made to prolong and expiratory time is made to reduce. When this IRV is used in conjunction with PCV or VCV, then it is called PC-IRV or VC-IRV **(Figs. 17A and B)**.

There are certain advantages after increasing the inspiratory time than expiratory. These advantages are:

- Increase in inspiratory time causes increase in MAP, but without increasing the peak airway pressure, despite a constant tidal volume and PEEP level. This helps to open the collapsed alveoli. Within a certain range of increased MAP, there is a direct linear relationship between MAP and oxygenation.
- In poorly compliant lungs such as ARDS, acute lung infections, etc., the alveoli are become of long "time constant" (i.e., slow alveoli). It means they require longer inspiratory time for full inflation which is not possible by standard duration of inspiration, during

conventional ventilation. So, prolonged inspiratory time in such circumstances sustains the alveolar inflation and improves alveolar ventilation. This also decreases the dead space in diseased lung (V_D/V_T is reduced) and improves the oxygenation with better matching of ventilation-perfusion ratio.

The decrease in expiratory time also has certain effects. Due to the reduction of expiratory time, tidal volume cannot be expired completely, so intrinsic PEEP or auto-PEEP develops automatically. This intrinsic PEEP also avoids the end-expiratory alveolar collapse of slower lung compartments which give rise to an increase in FRC, increase in gas exchange area, and reduction of intrapulmonary R to L shunt. The intrinsic or auto-PEEP has its own disadvantages, but here only the advantageous part of it is taken into account. It is important to say that IRV (or auto-PEEP) is not a substitute for extrinsic PEEP. The extrinsic PEEP is very important. It helps for the stability of those faster alveoli that empty completely under IRV. Also the effect of external PEEP is additive to the effect of internal PEEP and helps for a damaged lung compartment.

In PCV and VCV in conjunction with IRV (PC-IRV and VC-IRV), inspiratory time can be extended or modified by:
- Applying an end-inspiratory pause
- Decreasing the inspiratory flow rate
- Changing from a constant to a decelerating flow pattern. The inspiratory flow during PCV is initially high. Then it decreases gradually as the alveolar pressure rises with lung inflation. This decelerating inspiratory flow pattern results in a better distribution of ventilation. It is also associated with increased MAP for any given tidal volume, inspiratory time, and improved gas exchange.

Methods of setting IRV are:
- The IRV is likely to be most effective, only during early period, in the course of the development of ARDS, when the recruitable lung units are still there.
- The decision of IRV is to be taken, only when the patient is unable to be properly oxygenated at acceptable levels of PEEP, FiO_2, and peak alveolar pressure on conventional PCV or VCV with CMV or ACMV mode of ventilation.
- With IRV the arrangement for extensive monitoring should be started including blood gas analysis, central venous pressure (CVP), arterial line, etc.
- With IRV deep sedation and neuromuscular paralysis should be added to prevent (i) asynchronous breathing, (ii) to enhance comfort, and (iii) to allow the measurement of MAP which reflect the lung distension.
- If patient is already in VCV, then as a first step to changeover to VC-IRV from VCV constant flow should be changed to decelerating flow. This will approximate

the inspiratory flow pattern of PCV with its possible gas exchange advantages. In many ventilators, this will decrease the mean inspiratory flow rate, extend the inspiratory time and increase the MAP.

Airway Pressure Release Ventilation

Airway pressure release ventilation is a new ventilatory mode and is not well understood till now. Presently, only one ventilator (Drager Evita) can provide this APRV mode of ventilation. In this mode of ventilation, the patient is allowed to breathe spontaneously, during which high CPAP is applied. It is used on patients with decreased lung compliance, such as ARDS, acute lung injury (ALI), etc. and on those patients who had decreased FRC. This is because in APRV mode airway pressure is much lower than conventional ventilatory mode, if the conventional modes are applied in such pathological conditions of lungs. This mode should not be used on patients with high airway resistance (such as in bronchospasm), because success of this mode depends on rapid increase and decrease in airway pressure and rapid emptying of the lungs **(Fig. 18)**.

Airway pressure release ventilation is nothing but a CPAP mode at high pressure level in which release valve is opened for a short time (1–2 seconds). When the release valve is opened for short time (automatically at a set pressure level), the high ventilatory CPAP pressure comes to a lower level (or zero) allowing lungs to exhale. Thus, the APRV breaths dance between the high and low CPAP levels. The gas delivery to the patient depends on pressure gradient, patient's lung compliance, and airway resistance.

The, APRV combines the features of CPAP and PCV mode. In this mode, the inspiratory flow valve is opened throughout the ventilatory cycle such that the patient is allowed to breathe spontaneously at any point during the high CPAP breathe. Through short pressure release, expiration and CO_2 elimination is ensured and again it returns to the original CPAP levels which provide mechanical inspiration. If the patient is not breathing spontaneously, PC-IRV and APRV are indistinguishable.

CPAP breathe. Through short pressure release, expiration and CO_2 elimination is ensured and again it return to the

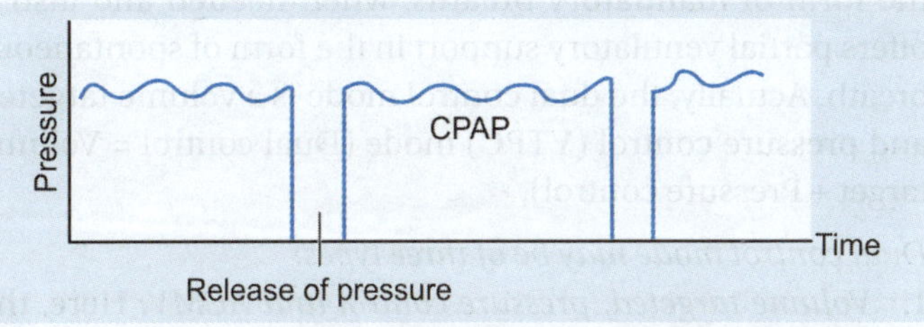

Fig. 18: Airway pressure release ventilation. (CPAP: continuous positive airway pressure)

original CPAP levels which provides mechanical inspiration. If the patient is not breathing spontaneously, PC-IRV and APRV are indistinguishable.

Apnea Backup Ventilation

This mode of ventilation provides mandatory breaths when the patient suddenly goes in apnea due to any cause. So this mode of ventilation is also known as the *safety mode of ventilation*, because it provides a mandatory ventilatory support during unpredicted apnea. *It is used in combination with all the modes and especially with SIMV and CPAP for spontaneously breathing patients.* In completely controlled mode such as CMV, patient is automatically apneic and thus this mode is not needed. So, apnea backup ventilation mode must be set for spontaneously breathing patients. The ventilators monitor the time period continuously, during which the patient is taking spontaneous breathing and/or there is sufficient inspiratory mandatory minute ventilation (MMV). When either of the criteria is violated, then the ventilator immediately starts delivering mandatory breaths to the patient. This will continue still the patient resumes spontaneous breathing and/or there is an increase in inspiratory minute volume. *In some ventilators this mode needs to be set, while in others it is automatically set.*

Dual Control Mode (Dual Mode Ventilation)

It is one of the newer mode of ventilation and provides the advantages of both volume control and pressure-controlled or pressure support ventilation. *As it is a volume controlled, so ventilation guarantees the calculated volume delivery and also as it is PCV, so also, it provides fine control over distending pressure of alveoli.* It also provides more patient and ventilator flow synchrony for spontaneously breathing patient. Hence, combination of both the volume and pressure control can offer better ventilation solution to the patient. Even though it is called the dual control, still the ventilator actually controls either pressure or volume, but not both at the same time. In this mode, the target volume is set and the maximum pressure limit is also set. *The ventilator automatically make changes in pressure level breath by breath, but within a limit (set by the clinician) ventilator achieve the target volume at least possible pressure.* It offers a full ventilatory support in the form of mandatory breaths, when needed and also it offers partial ventilatory support in the form of spontaneous breath. Actually, the dual control mode is a volume targeted and pressure control (VTPC) mode (Dual control = Volume target + Pressure control).

Dual control mode may be of three types:

1. *Volume targeted, pressure control and ACMV:* Here, the breaths are patient or time triggered, time cycled, and VTPC.

2. *Volume targeted and pressure support:* Here, all the spontaneous breaths are supported by ventilator. The breaths are patient triggered, volume targeted, pressure supported, and flow or pressure or time cycled.
3. *Volume targeted, pressure control and SIMV:* Here, the user sets a number of time or patient-triggered mandatory breaths which are VTPC. In between these mandatory breath, there are also spontaneous breaths which are also volume targeted and pressure supported.

The advantages of dual control mode are:
- Better ventilator and patient synchrony
- Reduces the need for sedation
- Keeping distending pressure under control, this mode assures delivery of adequate tidal volume
- Reduces work of breathing
- Helps quicker weaning.

■ WAVEFORM IN MECHANICAL VENTILATION

To optimize the mechanical ventilation, proper monitoring of four parameters of it (ventilation) is essential. These four parameters of ventilation are *pressure, flow, volume, and time*. The real-time graphic displays of these parameters as *waveform and loop* on the ventilator front panel offers the clinician to evaluate the adequacy of ventilator settings and to monitor the patient's response to ventilator therapy. So, the all newer mechanical ventilators are now equipped with a graphic package that displays many selected (by clinician) ventilator waveforms and loops, facilitating the assessment of patient's condition **(Figs. 19A to C)**.

Any single variable parameter displayed against time is known as waveform graphic. When viewing the waveform graphics which is also called "scalar", the time is conventionally shown on horizontal (X) axis, whereas the flow, volume and pressure are plotted on vertical (Y) axis. Therefore, there are three main waveforms: (1) flow versus time, (2) pressure versus time, and (3) volume versus time and each waveform has its own characteristic which is shown in **Figures 19A to C**. Flow itself is again of four patterns: (i) square (constant), (ii) accelerating, (iii) decelerating, and (iv) sine. Therefore, the pressure and volume waveforms also differ for each flow pattern which is also shown in **Figures 20A to C**.

There are two graphic displays in loops: (1) Pressure-volume loop and (2) flow-volume loop. Loops are the two-dimensional graphic display of two parameters. When the pressure-volume loop is viewed, the horizontal (X) axis is used to indicate pressure (in cmH_2O) and volume (in mL) is displayed on vertical (Y) axis. On the other hand, when viewing the flow-volume loop, then the horizontal (X) axis is used to indicate volume, whereas the flow is displayed on

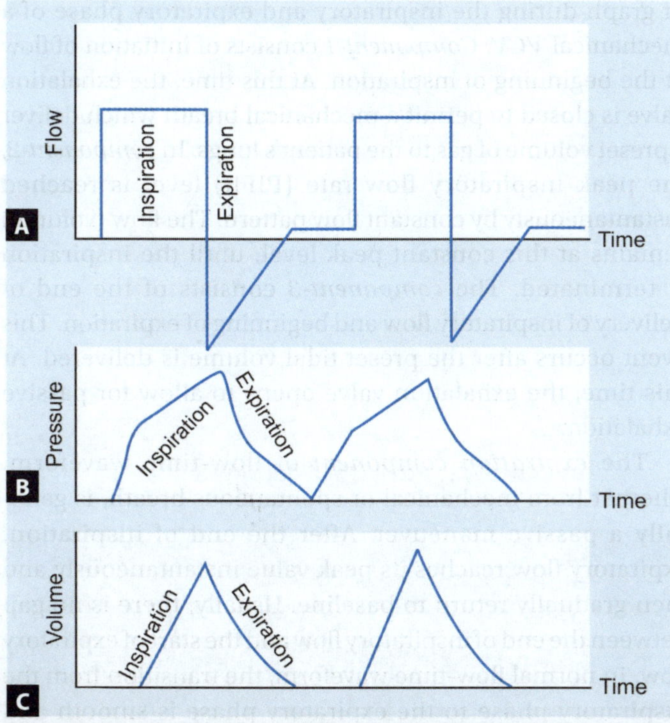

Figs. 19A to C: The typical flow-time, pressure-time, and volume-time waveform. Among these only the flow-time waveform has negative deflection below the baseline and helps in proper interpretation of expiration. These waveforms also differ during mechanical and spontaneous ventilation, during volume-controlled and pressure-controlled ventilation, and during different flow patterns.

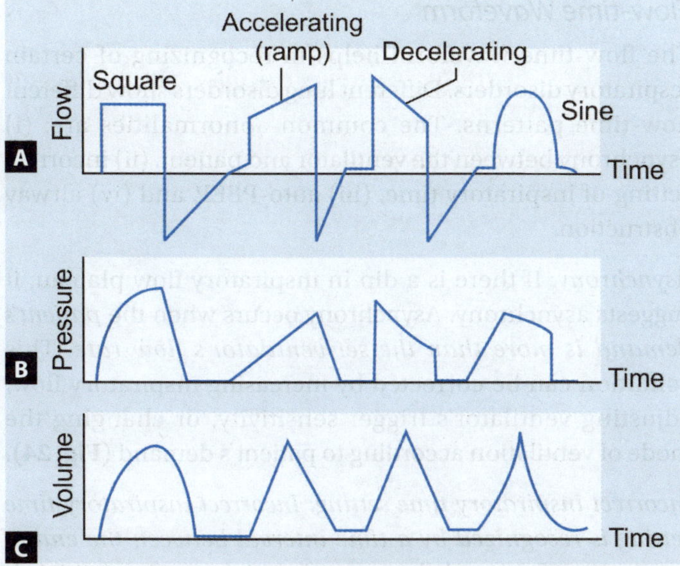

Figs. 20A to C: Flow-time, pressure-time, and volume-time waveform which corresponds with different flow patterns during mechanical (not spontaneous) volume-controlled and time-cycled ventilation.

vertical (Y) axis. In vertical flow axis, the inspiratory curve is plotted above the baseline and the expiratory curve is traced below the baseline. However, it is not unusual to

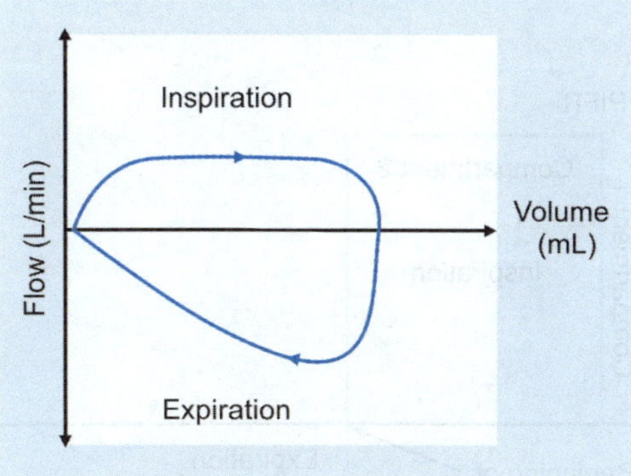

Fig. 21: Flow-volume loop.

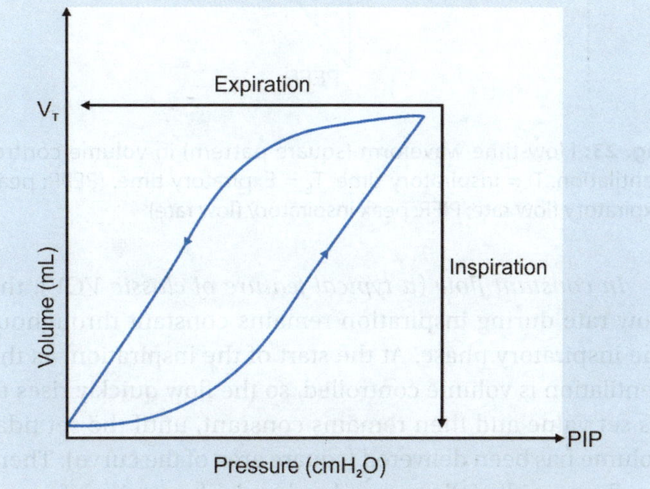

Fig. 22: Pressure-volume loop. (PIP: peak inspiratory pressure).

see a completely reverse pattern, where the inspiratory component is presented below the baseline **(Figs. 21 and 22)**.

Flow-time Waveform

This waveform shows the gradual changes in flow during inspiration and expiration with time. In the graph, time is represented by the horizontal X-axis (in second) and the flow is represented by the vertical Y-axis (in liters per minute). The flow above the X-axis represents inspiratory flow and the flow below the X-axis represents the expiratory flow. Commonly, the two types of flows are used in clinical practice: (1) Constant or square flow and (2) decelerating flow. *The constant or square waveform of flow is the characteristic of VCV, whereas the decelerating waveform of flow is the characteristic of PCV.* However, most of the ventilator allow a clinician to select a specific flow pattern that is most suitable to that patient. *Flow-time waveform is similar for both mechanical and spontaneous breath.* The flow-time curve for a spontaneous breath resembles a sine wave flow pattern.

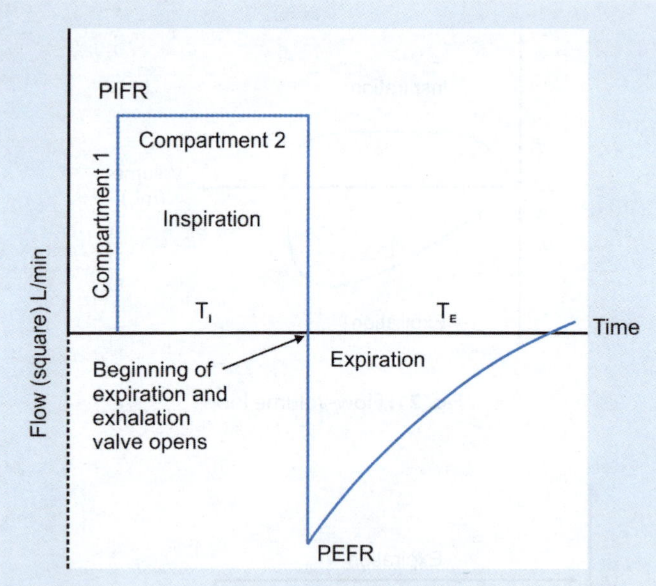

Fig. 23: Flow-time waveform (square pattern) in volume control ventilation. T$_I$ = Inspiratory time, T$_E$ = Expiratory time. (PEFR: peak expiratory flow rate; PIFR: peak inspiratory flow rate)

In constant flow (a typical feature of classic VCV), the flow rate during inspiration remains constant throughout the inspiratory phase. At the start of the inspiration, as the ventilation is volume controlled, so the flow quickly rises to its set value and then remains constant, until the set tidal volume has been delivered (square area of the curve). Then, the flow rapidly falls to zero level at the beginning of pause time. At the end of this pause time, the expiratory flow begins, the course of which depends on the resistances in ventilator system and on the parameters of lungs and airways **(Fig. 23)**.

In decelerating flow (a typical feature of PCV mode), the flow falls constantly after having reached an initial high value. This is because in initial phase at set fixed pressure the filling volume in lungs increases. Then at this set constant pressure the flow of gas in alveoli starts to fall. Then at the end of inspiration the pressure in the lung is equal to the set pressure in breathing system, so there is no further flow.

In flow-time wave graphic, the tracing below the baseline, representing the expiratory flow is significant, because it shows the lung's characteristic and airway resistance. Moreover, only the flow-time waveform demonstrates a significant tracing below the baseline. The other waveforms stay above the baseline except pressure-time waveform where a very small deflection occurs below the baseline when the patient initiates inspiration spontaneously.

Components of Flow-time Waveform

The *square form of a flow-time wave pattern* will be used here, throughout this discussion, to identify the each component of graph during the inspiratory and expiratory phase of a mechanical *VCV*. *Component-1* consists of initiation of flow at the beginning of inspiration. At this time, the exhalation valve is closed to permit a mechanical breath which deliver a preset volume of gas to the patient's lungs. In *component-2*, the peak inspiratory flow rate (PIFR) level is reached instantaneously by constant flow pattern. The flow (volume) remains at this constant peak level, until the inspiration is terminated. The *component-3* consists of the end of delivery of inspiratory flow and beginning of expiration. This event occurs after the preset tidal volume is delivered. At this time, the exhalation valve opens to allow for passive exhalation.

The *expiration component* of flow-time waveform, whether from mechanical or spontaneous breath, is generally a passive maneuver. After the end of inspiration, expiratory flow reaches its peak value instantaneously and then gradually return to baseline. Usually, there is no gap between the end of inspiratory flow and the start of expiratory flow. In normal flow-time waveform, the transition from the inspiratory phase to the expiratory phase is smooth and there is no time interval. The components of expiratory flow are: *initiation of expiration, peak expiratory flow rate (PEFR), and duration of declining expiratory flow (or expiratory time T$_E$)*.

Recognition of Common Abnormalities of Flow-time Waveform

The flow-time waveform helps in recognizing of certain respiratory disorders. Different lung disorders show different flow-time patterns. The common abnormalities are: (i) asynchrony between the ventilator and patient, (ii) incorrect setting of inspiratory time, (iii) auto-PEEP, and (iv) airway obstruction.

Asynchrony: If there is a dip in inspiratory flow plateau, it suggests asynchrony. Asynchrony occurs when the *patient's demand is more than the set ventilator's flow rate*. This condition can be corrected by increasing inspiratory flow, adjusting ventilator's trigger sensitivity, or changing the mode of ventilation according to patient's demand **(Fig. 24)**.

Incorrect inspiratory time setting: Incorrect inspiratory time setting is recognized by a time interval between the end of inspiratory flow and the start of expiratory flow which is not present in the normal flow-time waveform, where the transition from inspiration to expiration is smooth. This can be corrected by increasing the set inspiratory time and increasing the flow rate. If inspiratory time is set very short, then the inspiratory flow is suddenly stopped due to the start of expiratory flow. Compare this with a smooth transition

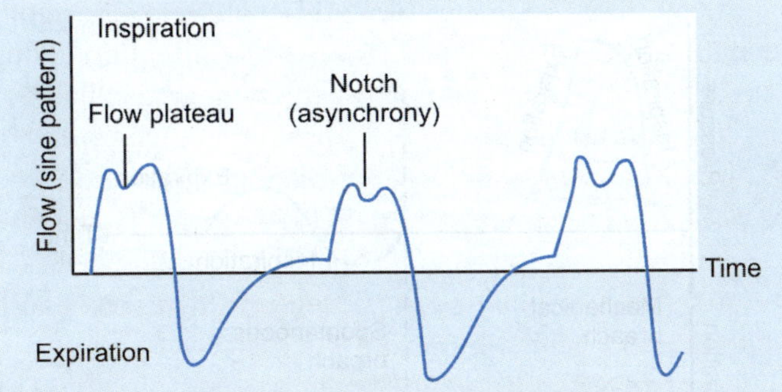

Fig. 24: Flow-time waveform (sine pattern) shows asynchrony between the ventilator and patient. In normal flow-time waveform, the flow plateau is smooth and no notch indicates adequate flow.

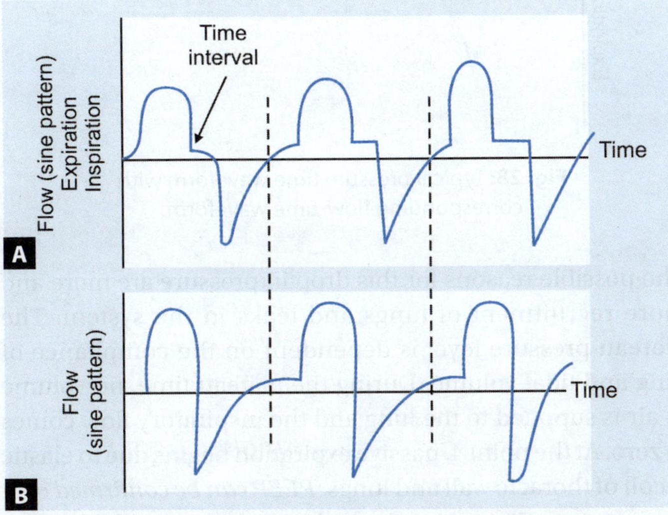

Figs. 25A and B: (A) Incorrect inspiratory time setting in flow-time waveform (sine pattern); (B) Rectification has been done.

from inspiratory phase to expiratory phase in normal condition. This short inspiratory phase can be corrected by increasing the inspiratory time **(Figs. 25A and B)**.

Airway obstruction and active exhalation: Exhalation is normally passive. The expiratory flow pattern and PEFR depend upon the changes in patient's lung compliance, airway resistance, as well as patient's active efforts to exhale. Increased airway resistance due to *bronchospasm or accumulation of secretions in the airway* may result in *decreased PEFR and a prolonged expiratory flow* (T_E). If the patient begins to exhale actively using accessory expiratory muscles, this may result in an increase in PEFR and a shorter duration of expiratory flow. Flow waveform can also verify the clinically *suspected bronchoconstriction*. In such cases, the PEFR is reduced and the expiratory flow returns to baseline very slowly. The *administration of bronchodilator* improves PEFR and allows for an expiratory flow to return to the baseline within normal time period **(Figs. 26A and B)**.

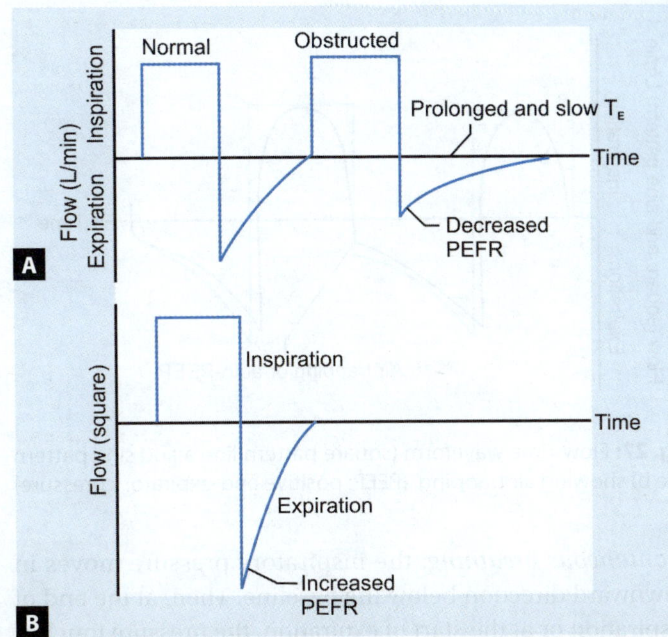

Figs. 26A and B: (A) Flow-time waveform (square pattern) normal and obstructed; (B) Response to bronchodilator, it has the same effect like active exhalation. (PEFR: peak expiratory flow rate)

Air trapping or auto-PEEP: Normally, the expiratory flow returns to baseline prior to next breath. In the event, when the patient is unable to exhale completely leading to air trapping in alveoli, then the expiratory flow does not return to zero level or baseline and the subsequent inspiration begins below the baseline. It indicates insufficient expiration and the presence of auto-PEEP. *The presence of auto-PEEP or air trapping may result from* (i) inadequate expiratory time, (ii) too high respiratory rate, (iii) long inspiratory time, and (iv) prolonged exhalation due to bronchoconstriction. Even though the auto-PEEP is best detected from flow-time waveform, but its magnitude is not directly measured from this graphic. *A higher inspiratory flow rate (in volume-cycled ventilators) or short T_I (in time-cycled ventilators) allows for a longer T_E and may eliminate auto-PEEP. Auto-PEEP can also be eliminated by increasing the PEEP level and bronchodilator therapy* **(Fig. 27)**.

Pressure-time Waveform

This waveform shows the gradual changes in airway pressure with time. In typical pressure-time waveform, the horizontal X-axis represents time in seconds and the vertical Y-axis represents the changes in pressure of airway in cmH₂O. During *mechanical ventilation*, the inspiratory pressure rises in an upward direction from the baseline. Then, with the start of expiration pressure starts to fall, while at the end of expiratory pressure returns to baseline level. But, during

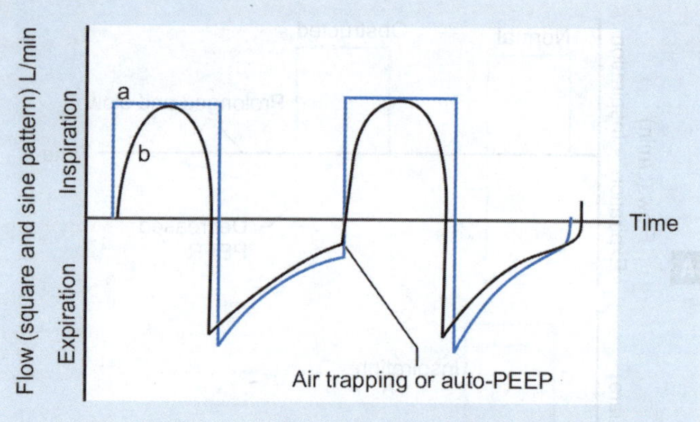

Fig. 27: Flow-time waveform (square pattern line a and sine pattern line b) showing air trapping. (PEEP: positive end-expiratory pressure)

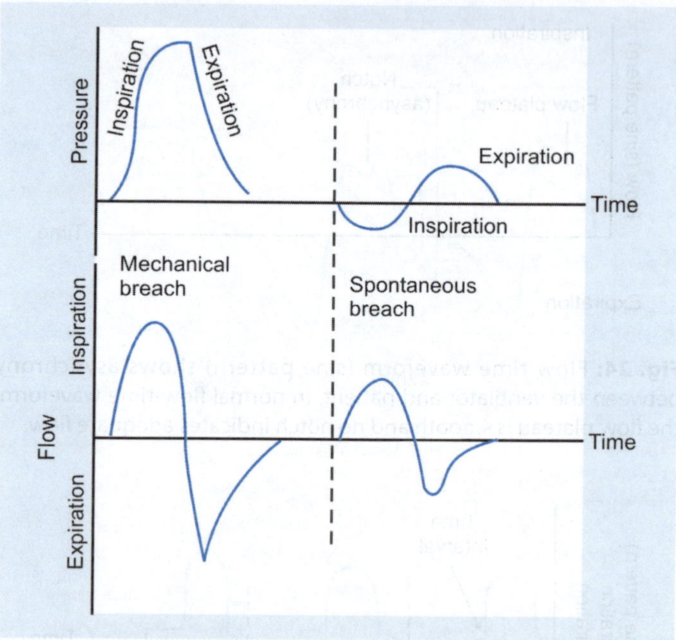

Fig. 28: Typical pressure time waveform with corresponding flow-time waveform.

spontaneous breathing, the inspiratory pressure moves in downward direction below the baseline. Then, at the end of inspiration or at the start of expiration, the pressure touches the base line. While with the continuation of expiration, pressure rises above the baseline and then again returns to baseline at the end of expiration or beginning of inspiration. Thus, this pressure-time waveform during spontaneous ventilation is not same, as that of controlled ventilation. Again in controlled ventilation, pressure-time waveform differs in *volume-controlled and pressure controlled ventilation. In VCV, the pressure-time waveform again changes according to the types of flow pattern, such as constant (square), decelerating, accelerating, and sine.*

A typical pressure versus time waveform in a *volume-controlled mechanical ventilation,* (not in spontaneous breathing) *with constant or square flow,* is shown in **Figure 28**. Here, the inspiration starts at *point 1*. At the beginning of inspiration, the pressure between the points 1 and 2 increases instantly due to the resistances in system. The level of the pressure at *point 2* is equivalent to the product of resistance and flow. After point 2, the pressure increases further gradually in straight line till the *point 3* **(Fig. 28)** is reached (the peak pressure point). At point 3, the peak or maximum pressure is called the PIP. The gradient of this curve is dependent on the inspiratory flow, airway resistance, and the overall compliance of lungs. Increased airway resistance (Raw) and/or decreased lung compliance result in an increased PIP. Up to point 3, the ventilator applies the set tidal volume and thereafter no further flow is delivered. So, as there is no flow at this point (point 3), the pressure level quickly falls to the plateau pressure (*point 4*). This drop in pressure is equivalent to the rise in pressure, caused by the resistance at the beginning of inspiration and finally shows the compliance of lungs. After that, there may be slight decrease in pressure *between the points 4 and 5.*

The possible reasons for this drop in pressure are more and more recruitment of lungs and leaks in the system. The plateau pressure level is dependent on the compliance of lung and tidal volume. During the plateau time, no volume of air is supplied to the lung and the inspiratory flow comes to zero. At the point 4, passive expiration begins due to elastic recoil of thoracic wall and lungs. *PEEP can be confirmed only by a pressure-time waveform and pressure-volume loop. PEEP is present only when the baseline pressure remains above zero. The pressure-time waveform also varies with the triggering mechanism of mechanical breath. If the breaths are initiated at the baseline at fixed intervals, the mode is definitely time triggered and a control mode. In an assisted mode, the patient initiates the breath by generating a negative pressure. This event can be observed on the pressure-time waveform where a small negative deflection below the baseline precedes a mechanical breath. The ventilator sensor recognizes the patient's effort and delivers a mechanical breath* **(Fig. 29)**.

Although the dynamic mechanics of lungs can be observed from this pressure-time waveform, still the addition of an inspiratory pause provides some more information to calculate the static mechanics. For example, the plateau pressure (P_{Plat}) or alveolar pressure is obtained by the activation of an inspiratory pause control knob which can produce a pause. During this maneuver, the exhalation valve is kept in closed position and the volume is held constant in lungs for a moment. For clinical purposes, plateau pressure is same as alveolar pressure at the end of inspiration. This measurement provides a means of measuring the static

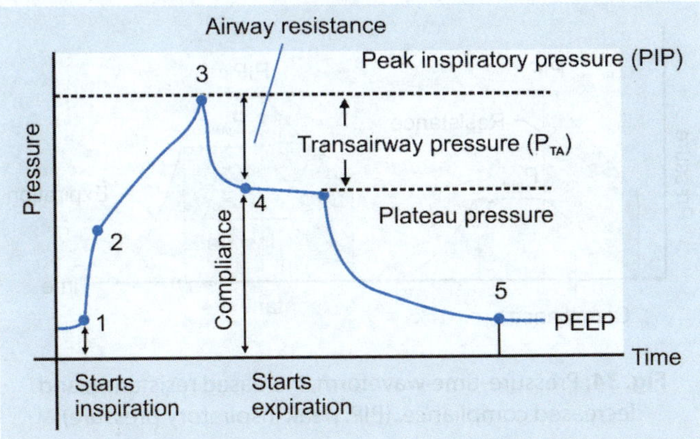

Fig. 29: A typical pressure time waveform, in a volume-controlled, constant flow, mechanical ventilation. (PEEP: positive end-expiratory pressure)

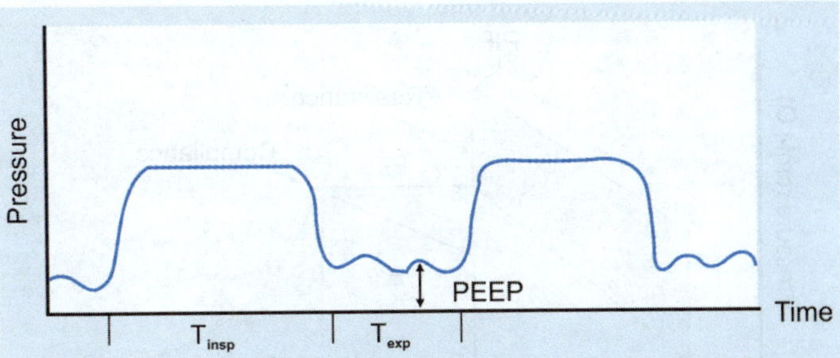

Fig. 30: Pressure-time waveform in pressure-controlled ventilation. (PEEP: positive end-expiratory pressure)

lung compliance. The transairway pressure which can be calculated by deducting the plateau pressure from PIP (P_{TA} = PIP − P_{Plat}) reflects the pressure required to overcome the airway resistance. In bronchospasm, the pressure required to overcome the recoiling force (lung compliance) can be determined. The static lung compliance can be obtained by dividing the volume of lung by plateau pressure minus (*see* **Fig. 7**) PEEP, if present **(Fig. 30)**.

In PCV, the pressure-time waveform has a different shape. Pressure increases rapidly from the lower pressure until it reaches the upper pressure level and then remain constant for the set inspiratory time. The drop in pressure during the expiratory phase follows the same curve as in VCV.

The pressure-time waveform is useful in:
- Evaluating the PIP
- Determining the PEEP or CPAP level
- Setting the ventilator trigger sensitivity levels
- Indicating the changes in airway resistance and lung compliance.

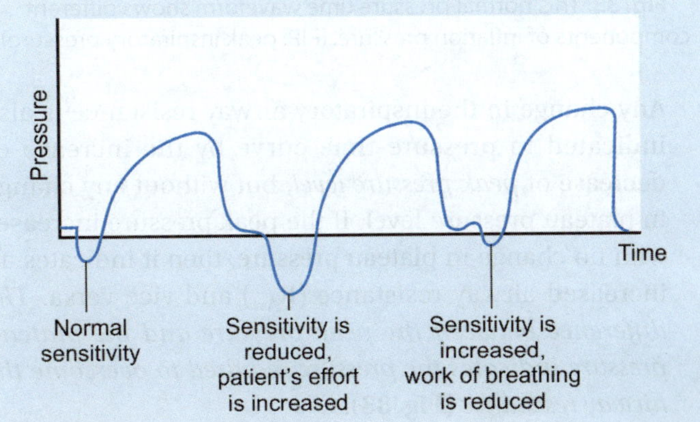

Fig. 31: Pressure-time waveform (when flow-time is sine pattern) shows different trigger sensitivity.

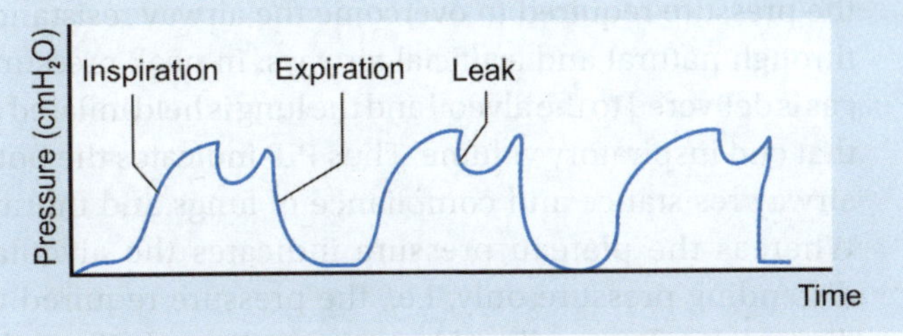

Fig. 32: Pressure-time waveform (with flow-time sine pattern) shows leak as peak inspiratory pressure level is not maintained.

Recognition of Common Abnormalities

From the diagnostic point of view, some changes in pressure-time curve have profound clinical significance. The common abnormalities which are found in clinical practice in pressure time waveform during VCV are described here:

- The large negative movement below the baseline of a pressure-time waveform in mechanical VCV indicates excessive trigger work. It increases patient's work of breathing, because patient needs to do excessive work to trigger the ventilator to deliver a breath. This condition can be corrected by adjusting the trigger sensitivity setting in such a manner that the ventilator is made more sensitive to patient's effort and thus reduces the work of patient. But, during recovery the trigger sensitivity is reduced gradually to increase the work of breathing of patient which helps in weaning **(Fig. 31)**.

- In normal pressure-time waveform during VCV, the peak pressure is achieved quickly and then a plateau pressure is maintained steadily. Failure to maintain a steady plateau pressure with a notch indicates a leak or an inability to deliver the required flow. This condition can be corrected by identifying and rectifying the leak in ET tube or in ventilator circuit or by increasing the inspiratory flow **(Fig. 32)**.

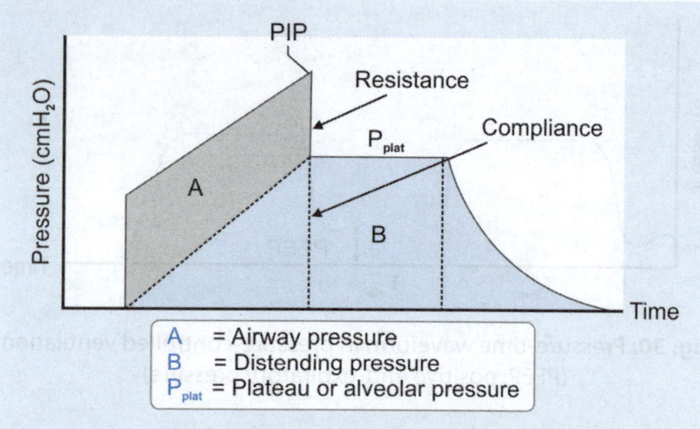

Fig. 33: This normal pressure time waveform shows different components of inflation pressure. (PIP: peak inspiratory pressure)

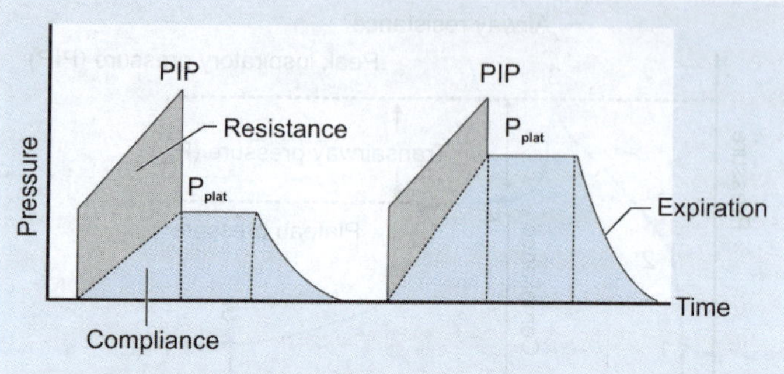

Fig. 34: Pressure-time waveform, increased resistance, and decreased compliance. (PIP: peak inspiratory pressure)

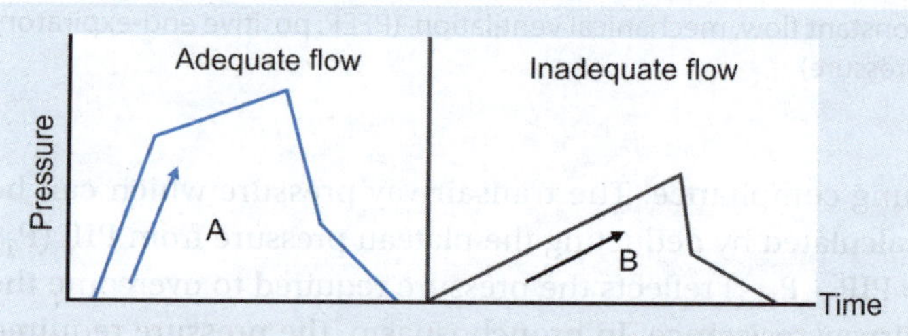

Fig. 35: Pressure-time waveform (in volume-controlled ventilation) with adequate (A) and inadequate inspiratory flow (B).

■ Any change in the inspiratory airway resistance is also indicated in pressure-time curve by the increase or decrease of *peak pressure level,* but without any change in plateau pressure level. If the peak pressure increases with no change in plateau pressure, then it indicates an increased airway resistance (R_{Aw}) and vice versa. *The difference between the peak pressure and the plateau pressure indicates the pressure required to overcome the airway resistance* (**Fig. 33**).

■ The total pressure generated at the airway during mechanical ventilation is comprised of two components: (1) pressure required to distend the respiratory system (lung) which is determined by the compliance and (2) the pressure required to overcome the airway resistance through natural and artificial airways. In peak pressure, gas is delivered to the alveoli and the lung is held inflated at that end inspiratory volume. Thus PIP indicates the both airway resistance and compliance of lungs and thorax. Whereas the plateau pressure indicates the alveolar distending pressure only, i.e., the pressure required to distend the chest wall and lungs (compliance) (**Fig. 34**).

So, (i) Peak inspiratory pressure (PIP) = Resistance + Compliance and (ii) Plateau Pressure = Compliance. Thus, if both peak pressure and plateau pressure increase or decrease in same direction, then it reflects the changes in lung compliance. On the other hand, if both the pressure increase in a similar proportions simultaneously, then it indicates decrease in lung compliance and vice versa (in increased airway resistance only peak pressure will increase).

■ When the pressure does not return to baseline, before the next inspiration, then it indicates that expiratory time is inadequate (inspiration starts before completion of expiration) or PEEP is applied. If expiratory time is not adequate, then it can be corrected by increasing the expiratory time.

■ During VCV, in inspiration the rate of rise of pressure (slope) is related to PIFR settings and can be used to adjust the peak flow rates. Inadequate flow rate is indicated when the pressure rises (slope) very slowly, or sometimes is indicated when there is a depression in the inspiratory limb of pressure contour (**Fig. 35**).

■ High-flow rate also can be determined by pressure-time waveform. It is indicated by shorter inspiratory time than normal.

Volume-time Waveform

This waveform shows the gradual changes in volume of lungs during its inspiratory and expiratory phase of respiration. In a mechanical ventilator, the total inspiratory volume is derived from the integration of flow over time. In this waveform, the horizontal X-axis represents time in seconds and the vertical Y-axis represents volume of lungs in cubic centimeters (cm). During the phase of inspiratory flow, the volume of lungs increases continuously. Then, during the pause it remains constant and next during expiration the transferred volume decreases as a result of passive (**Fig. 36**) exhalation. *The volume-time waveform for mechanical and spontaneous breath is similar in pattern. Again the volume-time waveform in mechanical volume-controlled and pressure-controlled ventilation is more or less is same.* Information obtained from this volume-time

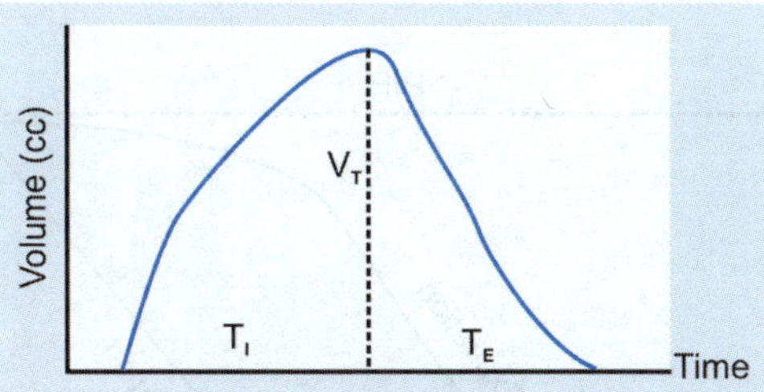

Fig. 36: Volume-time waveform without any inspiratory pause.

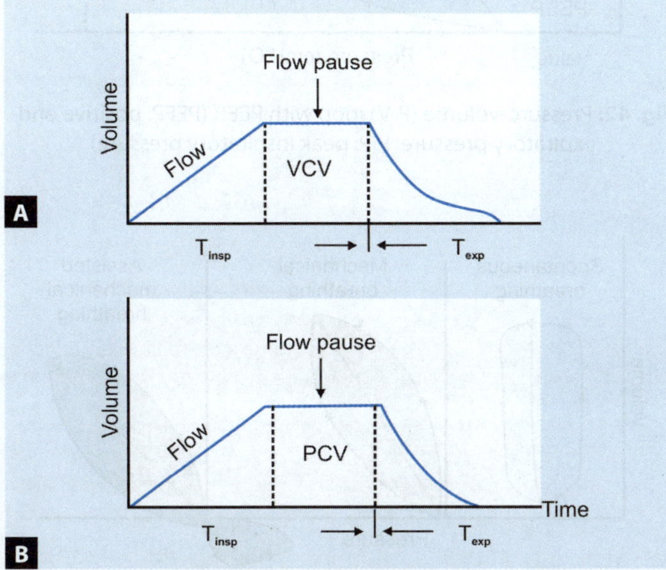

Figs. 37A and B: The volume-time waveform where there is gradual change in volume during inspiration and expiration in volume-controlled and pressure-controlled ventilation. Here an inspiratory pause is used. (PCV: pressure-controlled ventilation; VCV: volume-controlled ventilation)

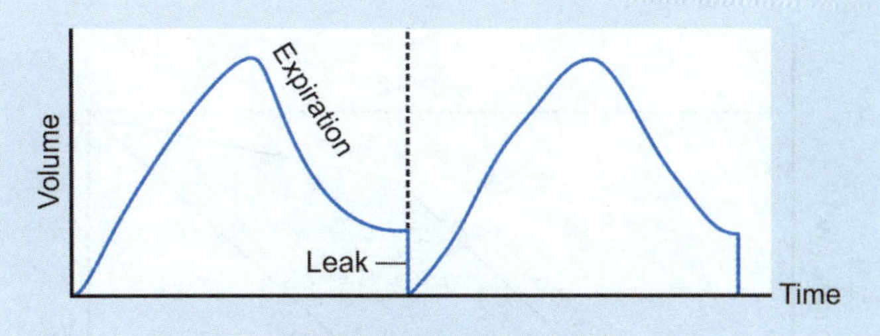

Fig. 38: Volume-time waveform, showing leak.

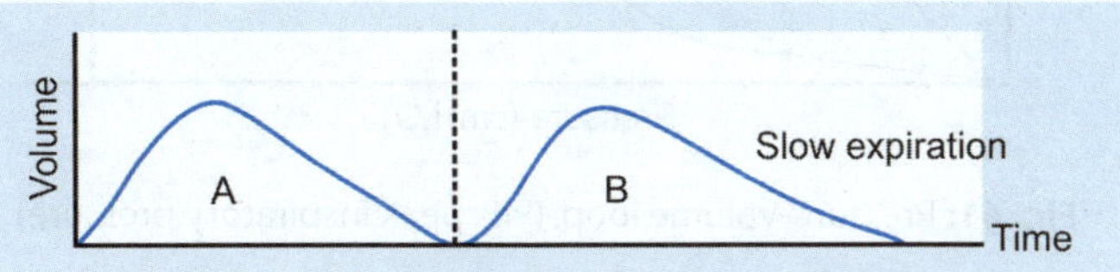

Fig. 39: Volume-time waveform. (A) Normal expiration and (B) Slow expiration.

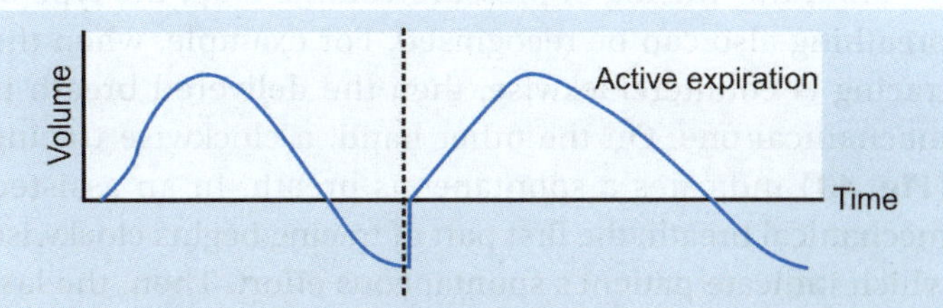

Fig. 40: Volume-time waveform, showing active expiration due to cough, agitation or severe obstruction.

waveform includes: a visual representation of inspiratory time, tidal volume, inspiratory pause, expiratory phase, and expiratory time (**Figs. 37A and B**).

Interpretation

- If the expiratory volume tracing does not return to baseline at the end of expiration, then it indicates leaks anywhere in endotracheal tube or in ventilator breathing circuit. By graphic pattern, the site of this leak can also be located. The amount of leak also can be easily estimated by measuring the distance from plateau to the end of expiratory tracing (**Fig. 38**).
- If the expiratory volume tracing moves very slowly toward baseline, then it indicates the slow movement of expiratory gases due to any obstruction. Hence, it can lead to an auto-PEEP, since the exhalation is not completed. It can be corrected by administering the bronchodilators or increasing the expiratory time or decreasing the inspiratory time (**Fig. 39**).
- If the expiratory volume tracing goes downward, touches the baseline, and then further goes below the baseline, then it indicates that the expired volume is more than the inspired volume and it is due to coughing, patient's agitation, or auto-PEEP. It can also occur, if the flow transducer is not properly calibrated (**Fig. 40**).

Pressure-Volume Loop (Fig. 41)

The pressure-volume loop indicates the changes in pressure and the corresponding changes in volume of lungs. Initially, inspiration begins from the level of FRC which corresponds to the crossing of X- and Y-axis. Then, inspiration terminates when the preset volume or pressure (in VCV and PCV respectively) is achieved. After that, expiration begins and the tracing returns again to FRC level at the end of exhalation (expiration). From this pressure volume loop, we can get the PIP and tidal volume (V_T). Usually, the FRC level is situated at the junction of X- and Y-axis. But, when PEEP is applied,

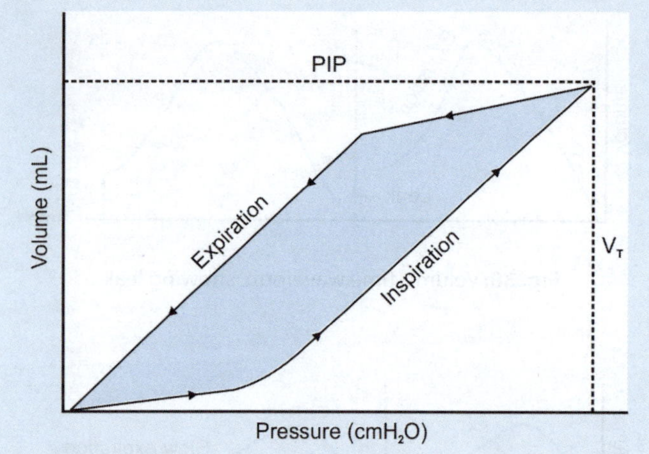

Fig. 41: Pressure-volume loop. (PIP: peak inspiratory pressure)

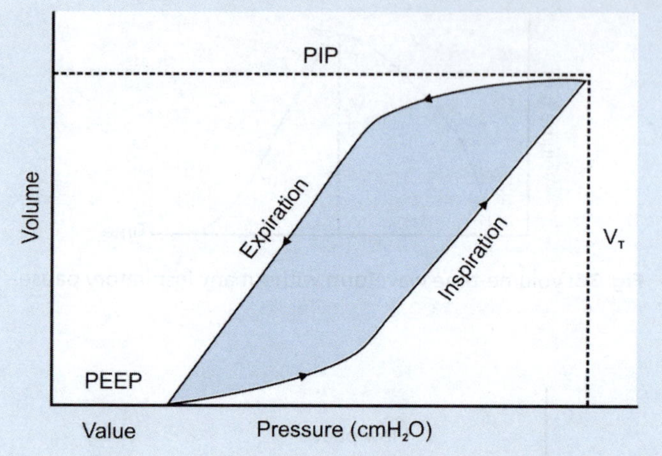

Fig. 42: Pressure-volume (P-V) loop with PEEP. (PEEP: positive end-expiratory pressure; PIP: peak inspiratory pressure)

then the level of FRC increases and shifts rightward along the X-axis, from where the inspiration begins **(Fig. 42)**.

From this tracing of pressure-volume loop, the type of breathing also can be recognized. For example, when the tracing is counterclockwise, then the delivered breath is mechanical one. On the other hand, a clockwise tracing **(Fig. 43)** indicates a spontaneous breath. In an assisted mechanical breath, the first part of tracing begins clockwise which indicate patient's spontaneous effort. Then, the last part of this tracing shows the counterclockwise direction which indicates mechanical breath **(Fig. 44)**.

The major advantage of this loop is that it can provide a quick assessment of work of breathing. Because, the work of breathing is calculated from the product of pressure and volume (work of breathing = pressure × volume). Within this work of breathing, elastic and resistive part also can be classified. Both on the inspiratory and expiratory limb of pressure-volume tracing, there is a point where the slope is suddenly changed. This point is called the *inflection point*. It represents sudden changes in pressure responsible for the opening and closing of alveoli. *The lower inflection point means the opening pressure of alveoli and the upper inflection point means the closing pressure of alveoli. The higher opening pressure indicates the decreased compliance of lungs (stiffer lungs) and causes the loop moving laterally toward right along the pressure axis. During setting of PEEP, the lower inflection point is recommended to optimize the recruitment of alveoli and it will prevent the repeated opening and closing of alveoli* **(Figs. 45 and 46)**.

A shift of loop toward right indicates decreased lung compliance and toward left indicates increased lung compliance. This can be judged by observing the pressure, required to deliver the same tidal volume in three loops. This is applicable only in volume-targeted ventilation.

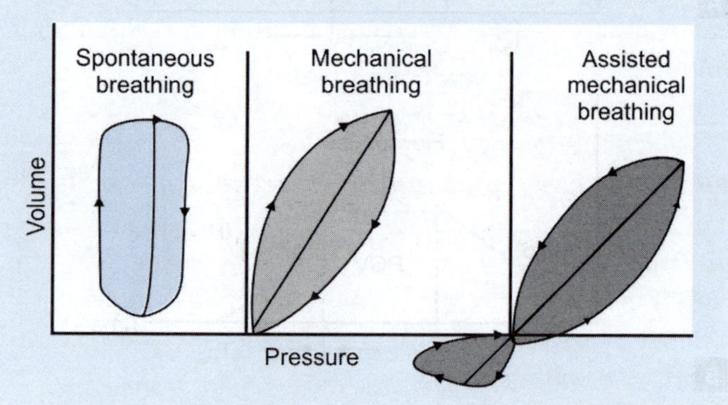

Fig. 43: Different types of breathing in P-V loop.

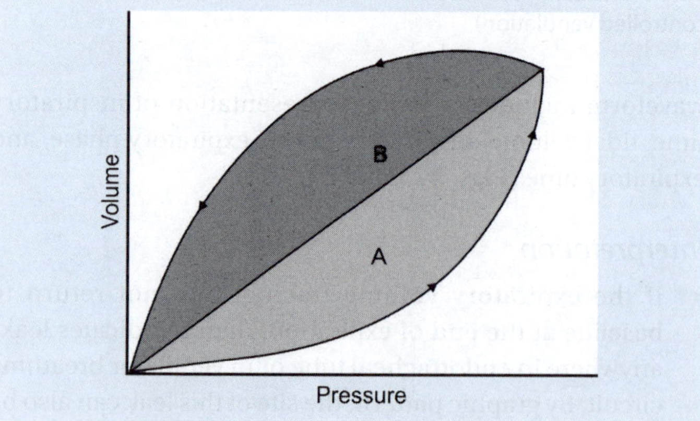

Fig. 44: Assessment of work of breathing by P-V (pressure-volume) loop. (A) Normal resistive work and (B) Normal elastic work.

But, in pressure-targeted ventilation the tidal volume (V_T) is the changing variable, where PIP is constant.

An increased resistance of airway due to obstructive lung disease is responsible for abnormal widening of only

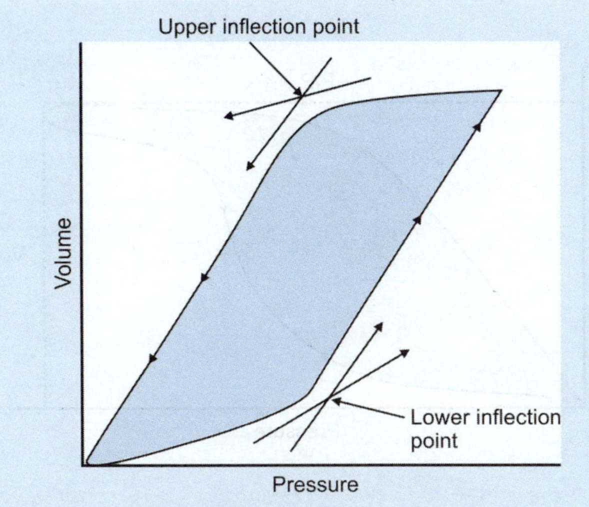

Fig. 45: Inflection points in P-V loop.

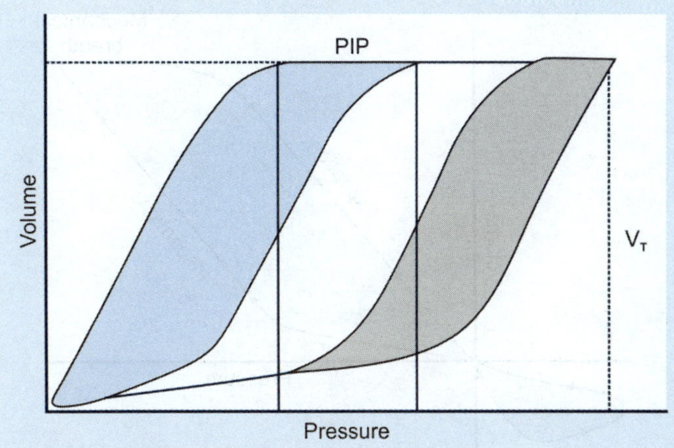

Fig. 46: Changes of lung compliance in P-V loop (volume-controlled ventilation). PIP is different, but VT is same. (PIP: peak inspiratory pressure)

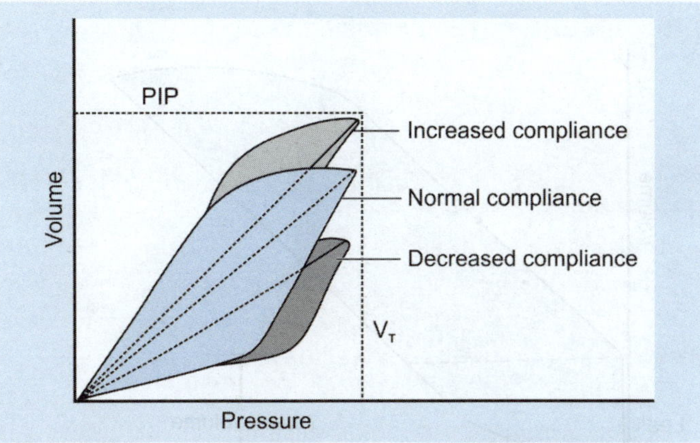

Fig. 47: Changes of lung compliance in P-V loop (controlled ventilation). PIP is same but V_T is different. (PIP: peak inspiratory pressure)

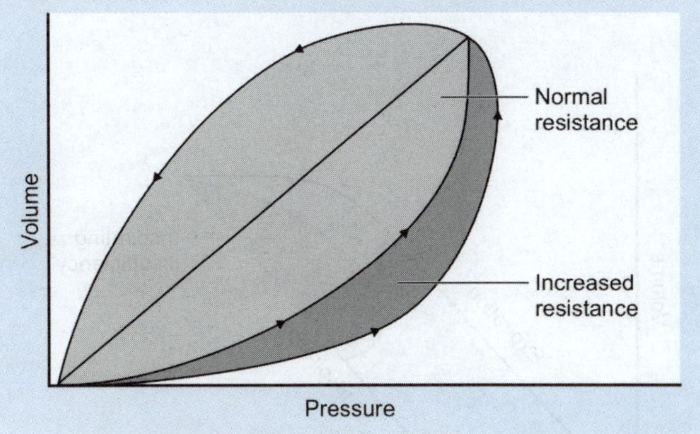

Fig. 48: Increased resistance shown in P-V loop.

the inspiratory part of tracing and exhibits a wide pressure-volume loop. This abnormal widening of pressure-volume loop is known as the increased *"hysteresis"*.

Normally, the direction of a pressure-volume loop is counterclockwise and indicates mechanical breath. But a clockwise direction before mechanical breath indicates patient's effort for breathing. Adjusting the sensitivity of ventilator one can decrease (minimize) or increase the effort of breathing and thus decrease or increase the work of breathing. In pressure-volume loop it is recognized by a significant clockwise deflection of tracing, below the baseline **(Figs. 47 and 48)**.

When the expiratory tracing (limb) of a pressure-volume loop does not return to zero level on the axis of volume, then it suspects an air leak. On the other hand, an insufficient inspiratory flow is recognized by a scooped-out pattern in the middle of inspiratory limb, exhibiting a notch, during mechanical breath **(Figs. 49 and 50)**.

Alveolar overdistention is a common manifestation, during ventilation of patient with ARDS, by VCV mode and is detrimental to patients. This is classically seen in pressure-volume loop which is known as "beak effect" or "duckbill" effect. It is characterized by an increase in airway pressure without an appreciable increase in volume. In such circumstances, switchover to pressure-targeted ventilation (PCV) with appropriate safe pressure level or reduction of tidal volume are indicated **(Figs. 51 and 52)**.

Flow-Volume Loop

In this loop, there is no set convention in assigning the inspiratory and expiratory component around the volume or X-axis.

Some ventilators produce flow-volume loop with inspiration on the upper half and expiration on the lower

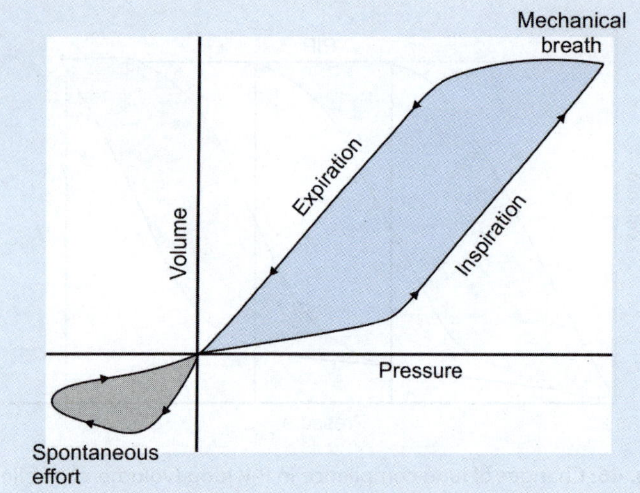

Fig. 49: P-V loop showing spontaneous breathing effort and mechanical breath.

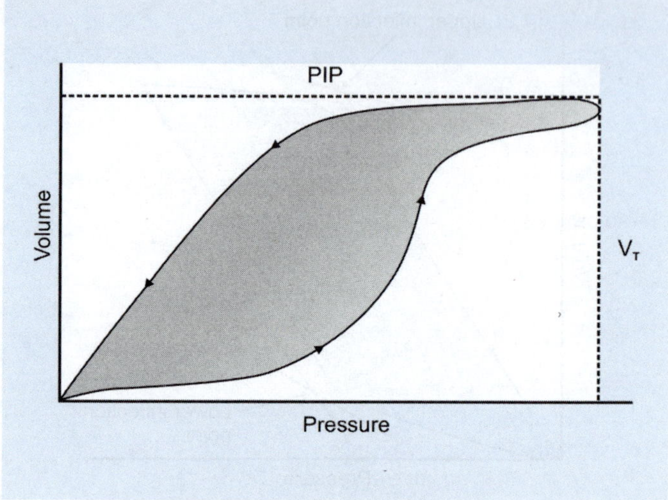

Fig. 52: Duckbill effect of P-V loop.

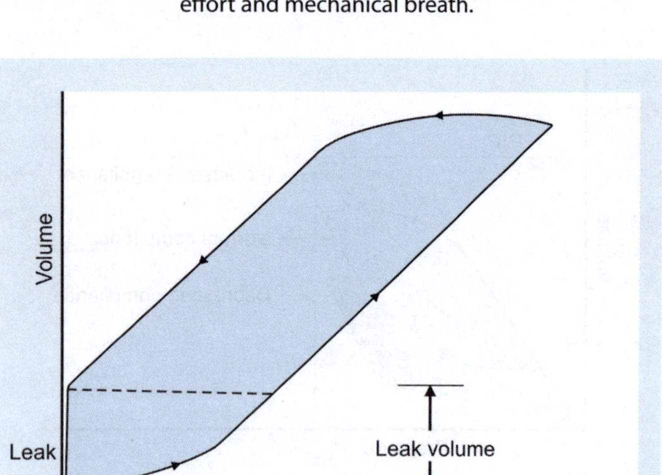

Fig. 50: Air leak in P-V loop.

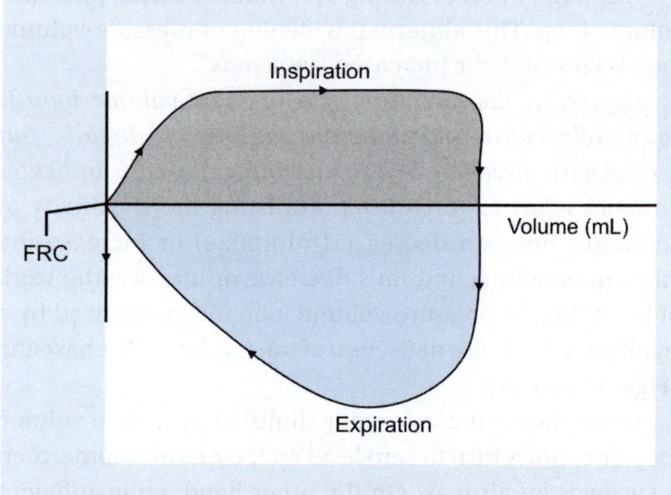

Fig. 53: A normal flow-volume (F-V) loop. (FRC: functional residual capacity)

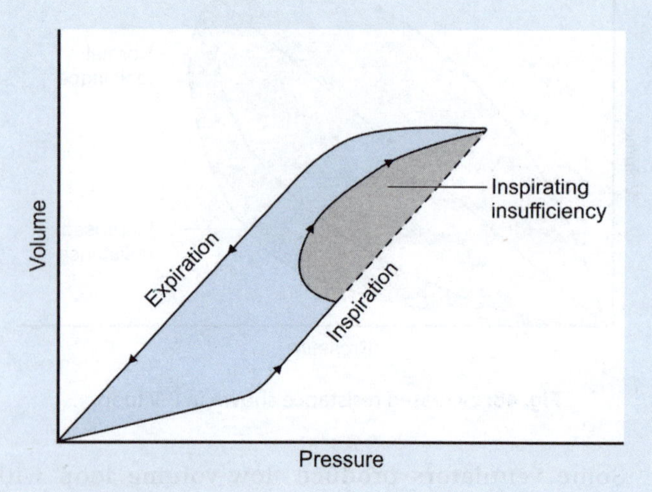

Fig. 51: P-V loop with inadequate inspiratory flow.

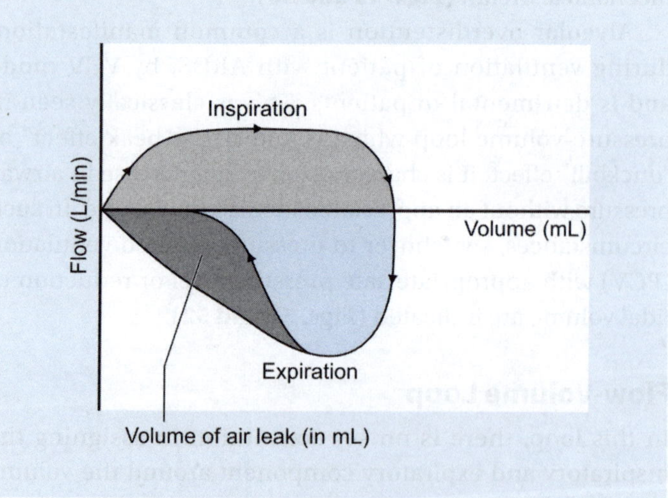

Fig. 54: Air leak in a flow-volume (F-V) loop.

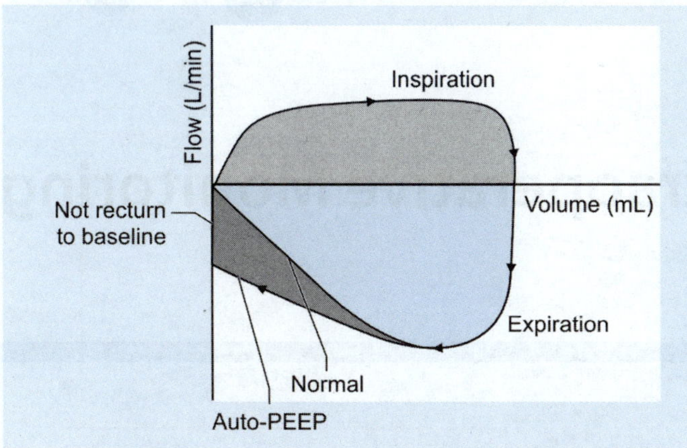

Fig. 55: Auto-PEEP in flow-volume (F-V) loop. (PEEP: positive end-expiratory pressure)

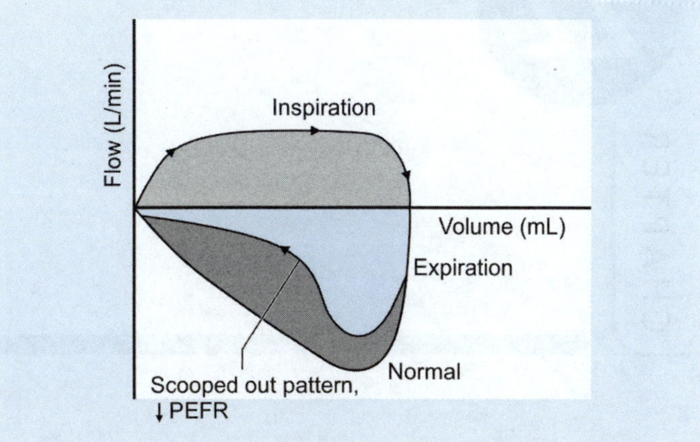

Fig. 56: Increased airway resistance in flow-volume (F-V) loop. (PEFR: peak expiratory flow rate)

half. While in others it is reverse. A flow-volume loop provides information such as tidal volume, beginning of inspiration and end of expiration, PIFR, and PEFR (**Fig. 53**).

Ideally, the inspired and expired volume should be equal. But, with an air leak the expired volume will be less than an inspired volume. This can be identified from a flow-volume loop, when the volume indicates the magnitude of air leak (**Fig. 54**).

In an air trapping or auto-PEEP condition, the expiratory flow does not return to zero level. But, the inspiration must begin from the zero flow level. So, the expiratory tracing will jump abruptly from the trapped level to zero level for next inspiration (**Fig. 55**).

An increased airway resistance due to bronchospasm also can be diagnosed by a flow-volume loop. It is characterized by a scooped-out pattern of expiratory limb and decreased PEFR. The administration of bronchodilator may show an improvement in both the configuration of expiratory tracing and PEFR. A continued scooped-out configuration of expiratory tracing and low PEFR suggest the ineffectiveness of bronchodilator therapy (**Fig. 56**).

Intraoperative Monitoring

■ INTRODUCTION

Monitoring of a patient is the key aspect of anesthesiology. But, with more and more development in the subject of anesthesia, the range and complexity of the available monitors used in this discipline have also been increased rapidly. For example, the stethoscope, sphygmomanometer, and electrocardiogram (ECG) are now supplemented by pulse oximeter, capnometer, expired gas analyzer, processed electroencephalogram (processed EEG) and evoked potential monitor, transesophageal echocardiography, and a host of many others. While these have brought undoubted benefits, but their sophistication and complexity have also brought additional problems. The main problem is that they are very costly to use in every case and is not available in small hospitals and rural areas. So, till now, there has been little progress toward an international consensus, regarding their use.

During the use of different monitors, high index of suspicion should always be kept in mind regarding their accuracy. So, this requires a constant comparison with clinical observation. Monitors may be tired by the end of the day. Calibration may slip and zeros may drift. So, they cannot always provide a sleepless vigilance that we would like. Also, many problems in instrumental monitoring arise due to the patient machine interference at the site of contact. For this reason, repeated clinical examination and its corroboration with the instrument monitoring is still of primary importance.

But, the most primary equipment for clinical monitoring is the various special senses of the attending anesthetist. The anesthesiologist also develops a special sixth sense. This is a subconscious mental computation, resulting from the observation, and previous experience which warns him of the impending wrong events and allows him to take a prompt action before hand to meet the need of a patient.

The basic clinical monitoring of patients during anesthesia is:
- Noninvasive blood pressure by sphygmomanometer
- Pulse by clinical palpation
- Peripheral circulation
- Degree of the filling of the jugular vein
- Color of the skin, mucous membrane, and blood coming out of the surgical exposure
- Temperature
- Urine output (>0.5 mL/kg/h)
- Respiratory movement of chest and movement of anesthetic bag
- Depth of anesthesia by heart rate (HR), BP, perspiration, lacrimation, movement of the body, etc.
- Muscle tone
- Pupils.

As per definition, a "monitor" is an instrument which is used continuously or at intervals to measure the condition or the parameters of a patient that should be kept within prescribed limits and it reminds or gives us warnings when this condition or parameter goes beyond that limit. In a monitor, the mechanical energy within a physiological variable is converted into an electrical signal by a transducer. Then, it is processed and transmitted on the screen for display and to an automatic recording system for recording. In a monitor the physiological electrical signal, such as in ECG, is also amplified, processed, and displayed on the screen. Accurate detailed recording of parameter is also a fundamental of monitoring.

Pen and paper are still the most reliable tools for anesthetic records. Although automated recording is available nowadays, but the automated records are not regarded as infallible. The anesthetist should initialize all the monitoring errors on any automated record sheet.

The manufacturers of early monitors generally paid little attention to the type of presentation. So, during that period the OT clinicians or anesthesiologists were presented with a collection of boxes for monitoring of each parameter or physiological events of the body. In addition, an increase in the number of sensors attached to the patients for each parameter also led to a progressive increase in the number of boxes which cause predictably confusing results.

Recently, the tendency has changed with the development of a single central display unit, which allows a single monitor screen to provide a wide range of items for measurements. Also, the addition and omission of information can easily be done by just changing the modules of a single multimonitor. In such central display, unit faulty modules too can be changed easily. While there are many benefits of this multimonitor approach in terms of clarity and consistency, but the threat of information overload is still present. The current multimonitor may display up to six waveforms and digital values of different physiological parameters with different colors and sizes which are alterable by the operator. In a stressful situation, there is limited ability for an operator to absorb all the information. So, a complex and crowded multimonitor is almost useless in acute crisis. Therefore, it is vital that the most important information is easily seen during crisis and not obscured by a mass of interesting, but nonessential lifesaving data.

Before taking any steps for the treatment of a patient with the help of the results of a monitor, some points should always be kept in mind. These are:

- Different companies use different methods to measure the same parameter in their instruments. So, the results may not be the same in different instruments. Unfortunately, companies are usually reluctant to disclose the details of how their machine operates. They only do this to protect their market.

- During the measurement of some physiological variables such as the depth of anesthesia, the electrical activity of brain is measured and is then transformed into mathematical data. This is then compared to a reference value, which is different for different companies. So, the accuracy of result may vary.

- A monitor which functions well in the OT may give faulty results in an aircraft or ambulance due to the noise or vibrations.

- Monitors may also provide additional hazards for a patient. Because, they are usually made of potentially magnetic material. When such a monitor is taken into the vicinity of a MRI machine, then its magnetism is likely to be accelerated by the huge magnetic field of MRI machine and may cause severe injuries to the patient or may even give inaccurate results. The strong magnetic field may also induce electrical current in the wires placed near the monitor with the possibility of burning of patient due to heat. So, all the anesthetic equipment used in radiology unit should, therefore, be made of nonmagnetic material or moved outside the magnetic field with long cable to monitor the patient from the outside of radiology room. Several manufacturers now make specific MRI compatible equipment.

- Monitors should be checked, serviced, and calibrated at regular intervals, set by the manufacturer. Because, many components used in the monitors may degrade with time and lead to suboptimal performance.

- Many types of equipment have been designed to be used for adults only. Their use in children, especially in neonates, may produce unreliable results.

NEUROMUSCULAR MONITORING

■ INTRODUCTION

Muscle power in an awake and nonanesthetized patient can easily be evaluated through some voluntary tests. But, in an anesthetized patient, this is impossible. So, in an anesthetized patient, the muscle power is tested directly by nerve stimulation and indirectly by muscle tone, movement of anesthetic bag, tidal volume, head lifting (for 5 seconds), just after recovery by anticholinesterase, etc. The other indicators of adequate recovery of muscle strength include the ability to generate an inspiratory pressure of at least -25 cmH$_2$O and a forceful hand grip. But, all these indirect methods are influenced by multiple factors other than the neuromuscular blockade by muscle relaxants. For example, twitch tension is reduced due to hypothermia of monitored

muscle group by about 6°C. So, for accurate information about the status of neuromuscular function, a direct method by using a nerve stimulator is employed. This assesses the muscle power by the response of muscle to electrical nerve stimulation.

But, till now only a few anesthesiologists use nerve stimulator to assess the neuromuscular function or muscle power during anesthesia. Instead, they use only clinical criteria for the evaluation of neuromuscular block, during and after anesthesia. But, the interest in monitoring neuromuscular block by nerve stimulator during anesthesia has been growing over the past few years due to:

- Increase in awareness regarding the problems of postoperative residual neuromuscular blockade

- Variations in patient's sensitivity (response) to different neuromuscular blocking agents and also variations in sensitivity (response) among different group of muscles to neuromuscular blocking agents in a same patient.
- Use of long-acting muscle relaxants
- Use of continuous infusion of short-acting muscle relaxants
- Patients suffering from neuromuscular diseases and muscular dystrophies

There is no contraindication for the use of nerve stimulator for neuromuscular monitoring. But, certain sites may be excluded for surgical procedures.

GENERAL PRINCIPLES

The reaction of a single muscle fiber, causing contraction to an electrical stimulus, is an all-or-none phenomenon. But, the response of whole muscle does not follow this all-or-none rule. Here, the response depends on the number of muscle fibers that are activated by electrical stimulus or blocked by drugs and the amount or intensity of stimulus. If a nerve is stimulated with sufficient or maximum electrical intensity, then all the muscle fibers supplied by that nerve will react. So, during neuromuscular monitoring, all the stimuli should be of maximum strength or above it. In practice, the electrical stimulus which is applied to a nerve is usually 20–25% above its maximum intensity to achieve maximum response. This electric stimulus is called as the *supramaximal stimulus*. To deliver a supramaximal stimulus, the peripheral nerve stimulator must be capable of generating at least 50 mA current with 100-Ω load.

But, one of the *disadvantages of supramaximal stimulus* is pain and discomfort. Though this drawback of supramaximal stimulus does not cause much problem during intraoperative period, as the patient is under anesthesia. But, it causes definite problem during recovery, as the patient is awake enough to feel the pain. So, some researchers advocate electrical stimulus little below the maximum level. This is called as the *submaximal stimulus*. However, the *disadvantage of this submaximal stimulus* is its poor accuracy which is not acceptable in clinical practice. So, the usual recommendation is to use a supramaximal stimulus, whenever possible.

The *character of an electrical stimulus* to a nerve fiber should not only be of supramaximal, but will also be of square wave, i.e., monophasic and rectangular. The biphasic electric stimulus will cause repetitive firing or burst of action potential and will increase the response to subsequent stimulation, leading to inaccurate results.

The *standard optimal duration of stimulus* (or pulse) should be of 0.2–0.3 millisecond. The duration of stimulus exceeding 0.5 millisecond will cause direct stimulation of muscle and will give inaccurate results.

So, the electrical stimulus for monitoring of neuromuscular functional status should be a monophasic, rectangular pulse of 0.2–0.3 millisecond duration and of supramaximal intensity (100–200 mV).

SITES OF NERVE STIMULATION AND MUSCLE RESPONSIVENESS

For the stimulation of a nerve in neuromuscular monitoring, either silver chloride pads (used in ECG) or subcutaneous needles are used over the superficial peripheral motor nerve. Any superficially located peripheral motor nerve may be used for neuromuscular monitoring. But, it must be remembered that different muscle groups, supplied by a motor nerve, have different sensitivities to neuromuscular blocking drugs. For neuromuscular monitoring, the evoked mechanical response (i.e., contraction) or electrical response (EMG) of the innervated muscle is observed. However, the direct stimulation of muscles should be avoided. So, the electrodes should be placed over the course of the nerve, but not directly on the muscle itself. Ulnar nerve stimulation to see the response of adductor pollicis and facial nerve stimulation to see the response of orbicularis oculi and corrugator superficialis are the two most commonly monitored motor nerves and their supplying muscles respectively. The effect of corrugator superficialis and orbicularis oculi supplied by ulnar nerve parallel with laryngeal muscles. So, they are considered as the ideal muscles (corrugator superficialis is considered more ideal than orbicularis oculi) for the monitoring of laryngeal muscles paralysis, during intubation. However, due to technical infeasibility of applying electrodes over face, they are not used routinely. So, the most commonly used muscle for neuromuscular monitoring is adductor pollicis, supplied by the ulnar nerve.

Ulnar nerve is the most popular nerve for neuromuscular monitoring and the elbow and wrist are the most convenient sites. But, the median, posterior tibial, and common peroneal are also sometimes used. When the ulnar nerve at the site of the wrist is selected for neuromuscular monitoring, then the electrodes are placed over the volar side of the wrist. One electrode is placed 1 cm proximal to a point, where the proximal flexion creases of wrist cross the tendon of flexor carpi ulnaris muscle. The second electrode is placed 2–3 cm proximal to previous one. The stimulation of ulnar nerve at the wrist causes only the flexion of fingers and adduction of thumb. When the ulnar nerve is selected at elbow, then the second electrode is placed over the ulnar groove at elbow.

While placing the electrodes, two things have to be kept in mind. These are: (i) Avoid placing the stimulating electrode too close to the recording electrode, and (ii) Avoid the direct stimulation of long flexors of forearm. When the ulnar nerve stimulation is selected at elbow (this site is mainly chosen for pediatric patients), the active negative electrode should be placed at wrist to ensure maximal response. When the electrodes are placed close to each other at wrist, then the polarity of electrodes is not important. When the temporal branch of facial nerve is selected for neuromuscular monitoring, then the negative electrode is placed over the nerve directly and the positive electrode is placed anywhere over the forehead.

Regarding muscle responsiveness, the different groups of muscle have different sensitivity to neuromuscular blocking drugs, and the results obtained from one group of muscles cannot be extrapolated to other groups of muscles. For example, the diaphragm is most resistant to neuromuscular blocking drugs than any other group of muscles of our body. In the second order, the muscles which will come in reference to resistance are the abdominal and respiratory muscles. This is followed by the laryngeal muscles and lastly the muscles of face. The most sensitive muscles to neuromuscular block are facial muscles, laryngeal or upper airway muscles, adductor pollicis muscle, abdominal muscles, the muscles of limbs and masseter. So, keeping in mind about different sensitivities of different group of muscles to muscle relaxant, we can say that the neuromuscular functional status or intensity of block in adductor pollicis will not be the same as in diaphragm. Thus, during anesthesia and surgery the total elimination of response of adductor pollicis to single twitch or train-of-four (TOF) stimulation does not exclude the possibility of movement of diaphragm, causing cough, hiccup, etc. On the other hand, if the most sensitive muscle, such as adductor policies, is chosen for neuromuscular monitoring guide for the administration of muscle relaxants during surgery, then there will be less chance of an overdose of muscle relaxants. Again, the advantage of taking the most sensitive adductor pollicis muscle, as a monitoring sample, is that sufficient recovery of adductor pollicis (i.e., when TOF ratio exceeds 0.7) signifies there is no residual block in the diaphragm.

■ PATTERNS OF ELECTRICAL STIMULUS

Five patterns of electrical stimulation for neuromuscular monitoring, which are shown in **Figure 1**, are used in clinical anesthesia. These are:

  i.   Single-twitch stimulation
  ii. Train-of-four stimulation
  iii. Tetanic stimulation
  iv. Posttetanic count (PTC) stimulation
  v.   Double-burst stimulation

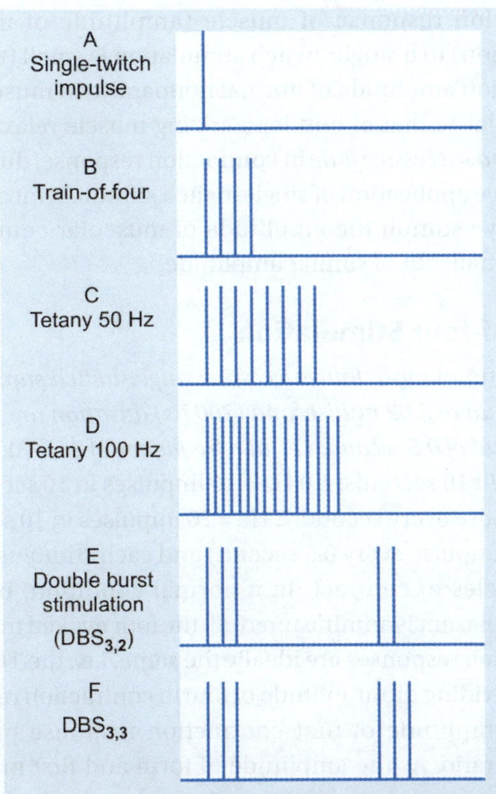

Fig. 1: Various patterns of electrical stimulus for monitoring of neuromuscular function.

Single-twitch Stimulation

In a single-twitch stimulation, a single supramaximal electrical stimulus of duration 0.2 milliseconds and of frequency 1–0.1 Hz (one stimulation after every 1 second interval = 1 Hz and 1 impulse in every 10 seconds interval = 0.1 Hz) is generally used. After very intense or complete neuromuscular block (i.e., after 100% block) by both the depolarizing or nondepolarizing muscle relaxants, there will be no contraction response of muscle to any electrical stimulus (whatever may be the intensity of stimulus) and this phase is called as the *"period of no response"*.

Then, when the neuromuscular block gradually dissipates (i.e., intensity of block is going down) from its 100% intensity of block or after incomplete paralysis by *nondepolarizing agents* after its administration, the evoked contraction response of muscle (amplitude of muscle's contraction) to a single-twitch stimulation is small (than the contraction amplitude of normal nonparalyzed muscle) and there is *successive fade* in contraction response during the successive application of single-twitch stimuli. In contrast, when the neuromuscular block gradually dissipates (i.e., the intensity of block is going down) from its 100% intensity of block or after incomplete paralysis by *depolarizing agents* after its administration, the evoked contraction response of muscle (amplitude of muscle's contraction) to a single-twitch stimulation is small (than the contraction amplitude of normal nonparalyzed muscle) and it is similar to that of nondepolarizing muscle relaxant, but there is *no successive fade* in contraction response, during the successive application of single-twitch stimuli. It means after successive stimuli the amplitude of muscular contraction will be small, but of similar amplitude.

Train-of-four Stimulation

In TOF stimulation, *four successive single-twitch supramaximal stimuli of 0.02 millisecond (200 μs) duration are given at an interval of 0.5 second, i.e., at a frequency of 2 Hz* (0.1 Hz = 1 impulse in 10 seconds, 1.0 Hz = 10 impulses in 10 seconds or one impulse every second, 2 Hz = 20 impulses in 10 seconds, i.e., one impulse every 0.5 second) and each stimulus causes the muscles to contract. In a normal condition, before a muscle relaxant is administered, all the four evoked muscular contraction responses are ideally the same, i.e., the TOF ratio is one (dividing the amplitude of fourth contraction response by the amplitude of first contraction response provides the TOF ratio. As the amplitude of forth and first muscular contraction is same, so the ratio is one). During intense or 100% complete neuromuscular block (both by depolarizing and nondepolarizing agents), there is no evoked muscular contraction response to TOF, like single-twitch stimulus. Hence, as before, this phase is also called as the "period of no response" and indicates intense or near about 100% neuromuscular block.

After administration of *nondepolarizing muscle relaxant*, when the intensity of block is gradually increasing before reaching 100% block or "period of no response", then the *TOF response shows the characteristic fade* (i.e., the amplitude of muscular contraction response gradually decreases and then the 4th, 3rd, 2nd, and 1st response gradually one after one disappears) and this amplitude of muscular contraction response is inversely proportional to the degree of block. *The disappearance of fourth response indicates >75% block, the disappearance of third response indicates >80% block and the disappearance of second response indicates >90% block. When, there is no response, even against first stimulus of TOF, then the block is 100%.* Surgical relaxation (muscular relaxation needed for surgical operation) usually requires 70–90% neuromuscular block. Sometimes, it is difficult to estimate the TOF ratio. So, it is more convenient to visually observe the sequential disappearance of muscle responses or twitches, as this also correlates well with the degree of block. Disappearance of four responses one after another with increase in intensity of block is called as *TOF-4 score*. If out of four responses of TOF, only one response is seen,

then the TOF score is 1. If two responses are seen, then the TOF score is 2 and so on.

The reason for fading, seen with nondepolarizers are: (i) Slow and progressive blockage of acetylcholine receptors at neuromuscular junction. (ii) Slow and progressive blockage of acetylcholine secretion from prejunctional level.

After the administration of *nondepolarizing muscle relaxant* in an intubating dose, intense neuromuscular blockade (>90% block or ±100% block) occurs initially. In this phase, the patient is intubated. In this intense phase of blockade (±100% of block), there is no muscular contraction (response) to any stimulus of TOF or single-twitch stimulation or any other type of electrical stimulation. Duration of this "no response period" depends on the type of muscle relaxant, the dose and the sensitivity of patient to that drug. After this "phase of no response" which lasts only for a few minutes, a single contraction response (4th response of TOF) appears first, after TOF stimulation. Surgical relaxation phase begins now and surgery is started. Gradually 3rd, 2nd, and 1st responses appear to TOF stimulation and a good correlation exists between the degree of neuromuscular blockade and the number of responses reappearing to TOF stimulation. When only one response appears against the four stimuli of TOF, then, the block is 90–95% and when all the four responses appear, then the block is 60–85%. The presence of one or two responses by TOF stimulus indicates sufficient relaxation for most surgical procedures. The reversal of *nondepolarizing neuromuscular block* should not be attempted, when it (neuromuscular block) is in intense or in no-response phase. Reversal should be tried, when at least two or preferably three responses (muscular contraction) appear by TOF stimulation. Reversal in the intense phase will often be inadequate, regardless of the dose of reversal.

The appearance of 4th (last) response in TOF stimulation heralds the recovery phase. When the TOF ratio is more or less 0.4 (40% recovery), then the tidal volume is normal. But, the vital capacity and inspiratory force are below the normal and the patient cannot raise his head or arm. When, the TOF ratio is around 0.6 (60% recovery), the patient can lift the head for 3 seconds, but vital capacity and inspiratory force are still below the normal. At a TOF ratio around 0.7 (70% recovery), the patient can lift the head for 5 seconds, cough, protrude the tongue and open his eyes. Vital capacity and inspiratory force become normal at TOF ratio of 0.8. Adequate recovery from neuromuscular block in clinical anesthesia is considered, when the TOF ratio varies in between 0.5 and 0.7. The TOF ratio of 0.8 indicates absence of residual neuromuscular block.

After the administration of *depolarizing muscle relaxant,* when the intensity of block is gradually increasing before reaching 100% block or "period of no response", then the

TOF response *does not show the characteristic fade* (i.e., the amplitude of muscular contraction response does not gradually decrease, but the amplitude of 1st to 4th response *decreases* and remains *same* (no fade) and then the 4th, 3rd, 2nd, and 1st response will gradually *disappear* one after one) and this amplitude of response is inversely proportional to the degree of block. *Like the nondepolarizing block, the disappearance of fourth response in depolarizing block, indicates >75% block, the disappearance of third response indicates >80% block and the disappearance of second response indicates >90% block. When, there is no response, even against first stimulus of TOF, then the block is 100%.* Surgical relaxation (muscular relaxation needed for surgical operation) usually requires 70–90% neuromuscular block.

During *depolarizing neuromuscular block (phase I block)*, in its intense phase (100% block), there is also no response to TOF stimulus, like the nondepolarizing muscle relaxant. Then, when the intense phase (100% block) gradually dissipates, the 4th, 3rd, 2nd, and 1st response to TOF stimulus starts to appear. But, these responses do not show characteristic fade, instead shows a sustained response (amplitude of incoming all the responses are same), though of *low amplitude* than the nonparalyzed muscle. In contrast, when some patients who have genetically determined abnormal plasma cholinesterase activity, are given the same dose of succinylcholine, then they show a *nondepolarizing* like block, characterized by fade in response to TOF stimulus. Such a block is called as the *phase II block*. Also, when succinylcholine is given at repeated intervals, or by prolonged infusion, then phase II block also sometimes precipitates **(Fig. 2)**.

Phase II block, due to the prolonged infusion or excessive dose of succinylcholine in normal genotype (with normal cholinesterase activity), should be differentiated from phase II block by the normal dose of succinylcholine due to abnormal genotype (with abnormal cholinesterase activity). Phase II block with normal genotype with normal cholinesterase activity, but by high doses of succinylcholine can be reversed by cholinesterase inhibitors. But, the effect of cholinesterase inhibitors in phase II block with abnormal genotype, with abnormal cholinesterase activity is unpredictable and should not be used or used with extreme caution. This unpredictability can vary from repotentiation of block to temporary improvement to full reversal. So, even if the neuromuscular function improves promptly, still patient's surveillance should continue for at least an hour.

The advantages of TOF stimulation in monitoring neuromuscular block are that the degree of block can be read directly from TOF ratio, even though a preoperative value is lacking. It is less painful and does not affect the degree of block, like tetanic stimulation. It has a great advantage mainly during nondepolarizing block.

TOF is best utilized: (i) To assess reversal after neuromuscular block at the end of surgery. The ratio of 0.7 (i.e., fourth response has 70% height of first response) indicates adequate recovery, but recovery is guaranteed only at a ratio of >0.9. (ii) To diagnose phase II block (succinyl overdosage or abnormal plasma (pseudo) cholinesterase). If the patient on succinylcholine shows fading, it is pathognomonic of phase II block.

Tetanic Stimulation

The tetanic stimulation consists of multiple and very rapid single-twitch electrical stimulation, given successively. It is commonly used at a frequency of 50–100 Hz for 5 seconds (1 Hz = 10 stimuli in 10 seconds. So, the 50 Hz = 500 stimuli in 10 seconds. So, the duration of every stimulus is 20 milliseconds). The effect or evoked response of tetanic stimulus on normal muscle is a sustained contraction, without posttetanic facilitation or fade. The effect of tetanic stimulation on a *depolarizing block* is same as that of normal muscle, i.e., sustained contraction, but of low amplitude (according to the intensity of block, no response when block is 100%) and no posttetanic facilitation or fade (when small muscular response is found with <100% block). During *nondepolarizing and phase II block,* when the block is intense, then obviously there is no response to tetanic stimulation, like the single twitch and TOF stimulation (period of no response). But, when intensity of block progresses after the administration of muscle relaxant, then the response to tetanic stimulation also shows the gradual fade and posttetanic facilitation which ultimately shows no response with 100% block. Similarly, after 100% block with full doses of nondepolarizing agent, with the passage of time when the intense block gradually disappears after the no response phase, then the response to tetanic stimulation with fade and posttetanic facilitation reappears. Thus, in nondepolarizing and phase II block, the response to tetanic stimulation is not sustained contraction, but fade occurs and posttetanic facilitation is seen. This is seen in **Figure 3**.

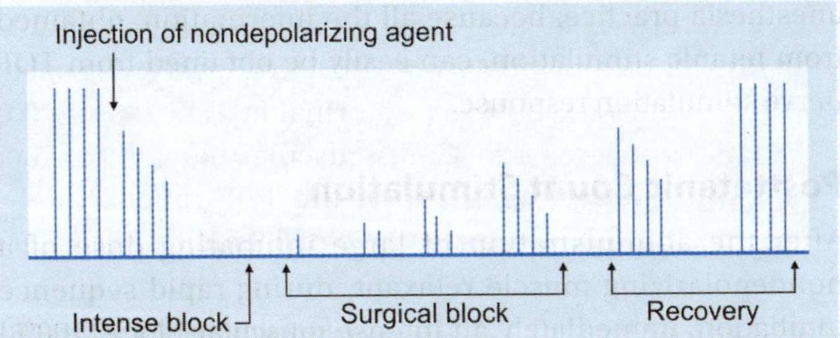

Fig. 2: Changes in response to train-of-four (TOF) stimulation during block, and recovery from nondepolarizing muscle relaxants.

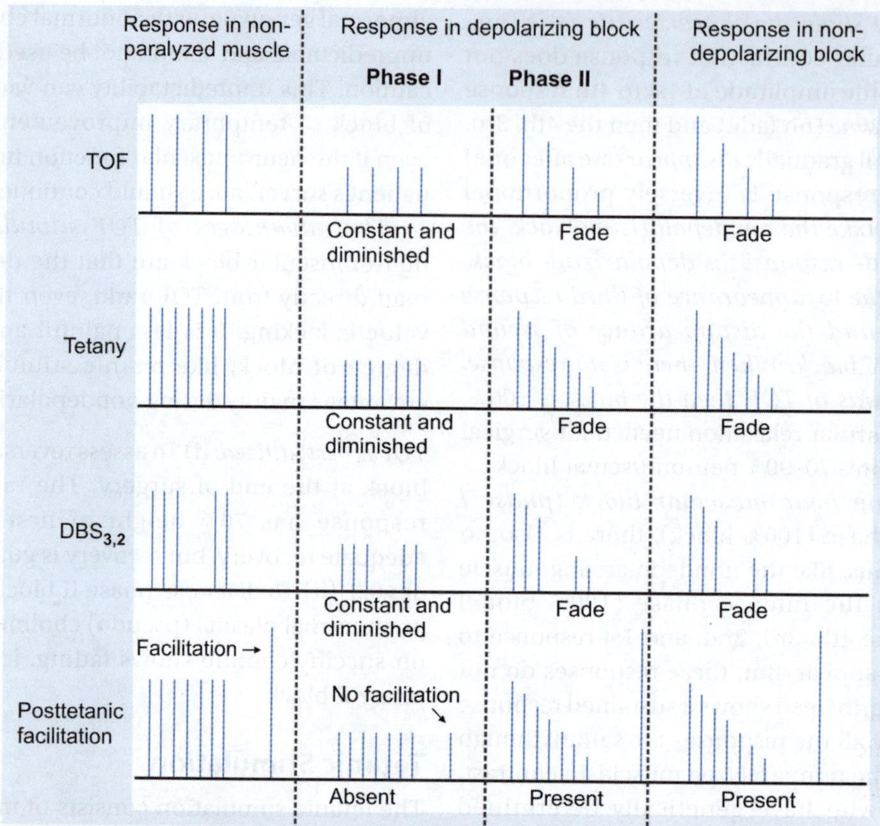

Fig. 3: Different responses of muscle to different stimuli in nonparalyzed state and both depolarizing and nondepolarizing blocks.

Probable Mechanism of "Fade" After Tetanic Stimulus

In normal circumstances when tetanic stimulation is given, then a large amount of ACh is released from the stored site. This causes the depletion of store of ACh and so its release gradually decreases. Thus, at the end of the process of tetanic stimulation an equilibrium is settled, when the release and synthesis of ACh becomes equal. At this stage of equilibrium, muscle response to tetanic stimulation is still sustained and does not show any fade. This is simply because the amount of ACh and the number of postsynaptic receptors where ACh acts is much greater than what is necessary to evoke a response. It means that there is a great margin of safety at the postsynaptic membrane. When this margin of safety is reduced by nondepolarizing neuromuscular blocking agents, or phase II block, then the decrease in release of ACh during tetanic stimulation produces "fade".

Another explanation of fade is that it may be due to the prejunctional effect of nondepolarizing agents. It reduces the amount of Ach, available for release, at nerve terminals during stimulation. This is called as the *blockade of ACh mobilization*. The absence of fade in case of nondepolarizing neuromuscular block correlates well with clinical recovery. Fade is more obvious during double-burst or sustained tetanic stimulation than following repeated single twitch stimulation or TOF stimulus. So, the first two methods are more preferred to determine the adequacy of recovery.

The posttetanic increase in twitch (contraction) response is called as the posttetanic facilitation. This is due to the increase in the synthesis and mobilization of ACh, caused by a tetanic stimulation which continues for some time, even after the discontinuation of stimulus. The degree and duration of posttetanic facilitation depends on the degree of neuromuscular block by nondepolarizing agents. It is evident in partial depolarizing block and disappears within 60 seconds of tetanic stimulation.

The disadvantage of tetanic stimulation is that it is very painful and cannot be used in an unanesthetized patient. Tetanic stimulation has very little place in everyday clinical anesthesia practice, because all the information, obtained from tetanic stimulation, can easily be obtained from TOF nerve stimulation response.

Posttetanic Count Stimulation

After the administration of large intubating dose of a nondepolarizing muscle relaxant, during rapid sequence intubation, immediately an intense muscular block (100%) occurs within 30–60 seconds in which single-twitch, TOF, tetanic stimulation, or any type of electrical stimulation to nerve does not create any response (twitch or contraction) in its supplying muscle (no-response phase). So, to know the degree of block in this "intense or no response phase" of block, the PTC stimulation method is used. However, during very intense block, there is no response to posttetanic stimulation also. As the intensity of block gradually dissipates and before the first response to TOF stimulation reappears, the response to a single-twitch stimulation after a tetanic stimulation (so, it is called as the posttetanic stimulation) appears. Then, with more passing of time the number of responses to single-twitch stimulus, after a tetanic stimulus, gradually increases and is counted. The increase in the number of count indicates the gradually waning of block, and then the first-single response to TOF stimulus will appear. As the block further wanes, the consecutive four responses to four TOF stimulation appear. So, the PTC stimulation is used to quantify the intensity of no response phase of neuromuscular block of peripheral muscles, when the other types of stimuli (single twitch, TOF, and tetanic) fail to respond in "no-response phase". The PTC is used by applying tetanic stimulation (50 Hz for 5 seconds), and then observing the posttetanic response by giving a single-twitch stimulation at 1 Hz frequency for 3 seconds after the end of tetanic stimulation.

Explanation of PTC: Tetanic stimulation will increase ACh level at neuromuscular junction. This increased ACh will replace some molecules of nondepolarizers from its binding site on receptors, producing a response. While, on the other hand, the depolarizer will produce more muscular relaxation by continuous availability of ACh due to continuous tetanic stimulation and PTC will be absent. *Absence of PTC with nondepolarizers indicates a very intense block. However, this is not applicable for depolarizing agent.*

Double-burst Stimulation

Without a recording instrument, muscular response (contraction) to a stimulus (single-twitch, TOF or PTC) always cannot be visualized or felt by touch or any tactile means, which may help to evaluate or exclude the small degree of residual neuromuscular block. So, DBS was developed with the specific aim of allowing manual detection of small amounts of residual neuromuscular block, after recovery. With DBS, it is easier to feel "fade" in the muscular response (contraction) against electrical stimulus.

DBS consists of *two groups of short bursts* of *high-frequency tetanic stimulation* at an interval of 750–780 milliseconds. It represents two variations. The DBS-3 pattern consists of first group of three short (0.2 milliseconds or 200 µs duration) high frequency tetanic bursts, separated by an interval of 20 milliseconds (50 Hz), followed by another group of three bursts of 50 Hz, applied 750–780 milliseconds later after first group of three stimulus. DBS-3, 2 consists of three 50 Hz impulses of 0.2 milliseconds duration, followed by two such impulses, 750 milliseconds later. The DBS-3, 3 pattern is more in clinical use than DBS-3, 2 pattern. It is more sensitive than TOF stimulation for clinical (i.e., visual) evaluation of fade. In control study on nonparalyzed muscle, the feel of two muscle contractions in response to DBS is equal. In a paralyzed condition, the second response is weaker than the first (i.e., "fade"), which can be felt easily. Thus, the absence of fade in response to DBS usually means absence of clinically significant residual neuromuscular blockade. Measured mechanically by tactile mean (feeling muscular contraction), the TOF ratio correlates closely well with DBS. The feeling and tactile evaluation of response to DBS is superior to tactile evaluation of response to TOF stimulation.

Further, tetanic, PTC and DBS are very high intensity stimuli, therefore are used to assess the deep blocks or where neuromuscular monitoring is done by visual observation of movement (like adduction of thumb after stimulating ulnar nerve) or by tactile means.

To conclude: Adductor pollicis (supplied by ulnar nerve) is the most commonly chosen muscle and TOF is the most commonly used stimulus for neuromuscular monitoring. Fading, posttetanic facilitation, and PTC are only exhibited by nondepolarizing muscle relaxants.

RECORDING OF EVOKED MUSCULAR RESPONSE

By three methods we can record and measure the evoked muscular response to an electrical stimulus.

i. Recording of evoked mechanical response of muscle (i.e., contraction) to electrical stimulus [mechanomyography (MG)].
ii. Recording of evoked electrical response of muscle to electrical stimulus [electromyography (EMG)]
iii. Recording of evoked acceleration response of muscle to electrical stimulus [acceleromyography (AMG)]

Mechanomyography

Here, the evoked *contraction response*, developed by a muscle, due to an electrical stimulus is recorded and measured. This is most easily achieved in clinical anesthesia by measuring the thumb movement, due to an electrical stimulation. When the ulnar nerve is stimulated by a nerve stimulator, the adductor pollicis muscle of thumb contracts and acts on a *force displacement transducer* which converts this mechanical force into an electrical signal. Then this signal is amplified, displayed, and recorded.

Electromyography

Here, the compound *action potential* of muscular contraction, produced by the stimulation of a peripheral nerve, is recorded. In clinical anesthesia, the evoked electrical response from the contraction of a muscle is most often obtained from the muscles of thenar and hypothenar eminences of hand, innervated by the ulnar or median nerve. Both the surface and needle electrodes can be used, but the needle electrodes have no extra advantage over the surface electrodes. In commercially available machines for evoked EMG, the results are displayed either as a percentage of control or as a TOF ratio and the results may also be given as "twitch height" in the print-out.

Advantages of EMG over MG are:

- Easier to set up
- Response reflects only those factors which influence the neuromuscular transmission.
- Response can also be obtained from muscles which are not accessible to mechanical recording.

The disadvantages of EMG are:

- EMG response is very sensitive to electrical interference, i.e., diathermy.
- Placement of electrodes is very critical and may cause false negative results with the slightest variations.
- If the stimulating electrodes lie closer to the muscle than the nerve, then the muscle is stimulated directly and the recording electrode picks up the signal directly from the muscle even when neuromuscular transmission is completely blocked.

Acceleromyography

It is a newer and simpler method of measuring and recording the neuromuscular function. It measures the *acceleration of contraction* of thumb muscles instead of force produced by contraction of muscle, after stimulation of a motor nerve. When the muscle mass of thumb is fixed, then the acceleration of contraction of thumb muscle is directly proportional to the force of contraction (Newton's Second Law) and this evoked acceleration of contraction is measured. In clinical practice, an accelerometer is fixed to thumb and the ulnar nerve is stimulated. Then the exposure of electrode of an accelerometer to the force of contraction of muscle generates an electrical voltage which is proportional to the acceleration of contraction of thumb muscles in response to nerve stimulation. This voltage signal is then analyzed and displayed on a recording system.

It is a small handy instrument which fulfills most of the requirements of a neuromuscular monitoring unit and so, it is used routinely during and after operation.

■ STIMULATING ELECTRODES

The electrodes which transmit electrical impulses from a stimulator to a nerve are classified into *surface electrodes and needle electrodes.* Surface electrodes are most commonly used and are made up of rubber or disposable pregelled silver chloride, like the ECG electrodes. The minimum conducting area of an electrode for monitoring of neuromuscular block should be 7–8 mm in diameter which is needed to transmit adequate current for the underlying nerve. Skin should be properly cleaned before using the electrodes and the old rubber electrodes should not be reused as it increases impedance.

Needle electrodes are used when the supramaximal responses cannot be obtained by surface electrodes. The needles should be placed subcutaneously and not within the nerve. If specially-coated commercially made needle electrodes are not available, then the ordinary steel needles made for injection can also be used as electrodes.

MONITORING OF THE RESPIRATORY SYSTEM

■ INTRODUCTION

During anesthesia, in addition to its normal function, i.e., O_2 uptake and CO_2 excretion, the respiratory system also transfers the inhalational anesthetic agents into the circulation. So, the function of respiratory system can be monitored clinically by the (i) examination of patient and also instrumentally by measuring the different volumes and capacity of lungs during ventilation, (ii) the concentration of gases in inspiratory and expiratory gas mixture, and (iii) the tension of different gases in blood-by-blood gas analysis.

The measurement of total minute ventilation is simple. But, the most relevant portion of minute volume, i.e., alveolar ventilation is much more difficult to measure. The alveolar ventilation can be considered as a relatively fixed portion of minute volume. Because, the physiological dead space, which is invariably increased during anesthesia, remains a reasonably constant fraction of the tidal volume.

Over a wide range of tidal volume, the alveolar ventilation can be calculated from the equation which is written as: $V_A = V_E - V_D$ (V_A = Alveolar ventilation, V_E = Respiratory minute volume or minute ventilation, V_D = Dead space ventilation).

The alveolar ventilation can also be calculated from PCO_2 of the exhaled gases, or alveolar PCO_2 (P_ACO_2) and arterial PCO_2 (P_aCO_2) from the following equations: $P_ACO_2 = K (P_aCO_2/VA)$. So, if the PCO_2 of the exhaled gas (P_ACO_2) is known in relation to the arterial PCO_2 (P_aCO_2), then the alveolar ventilation can be calculated from the above equation.

The alveolar ventilation can also be calculated from another equation. $P_ACO_2 = K(VCO_2/VA)$, where $VCO_2 = CO_2$ production. In this equation, P_ACO_2 is a function of only two variables. Since in clinical practice, the VCO_2 is relatively constant, therefore P_ACO_2 is only the determinant factor of alveolar ventilation (VA), to which it is inversely proportional, i.e., $P_ACO_2 \propto 1/VA$. So, the measurement of end-tidal CO_2 tension (P_tCO_2), which indicates P_ACO_2 is another way of monitoring the function of respiratory system.

Till now, the relationship between P_ACO_2 and ventilation has been discussed. Now, the relationship between the P_ACO_2 and P_aCO_2 shall be discussed. If the CO_2 production remains constant, then the difference between P_ACO_2 and P_aCO_2 is dependent on the following factors, such as: (i) diffusion nonequilibrium, (ii) ventilation/perfusion (V_A/Q) mismatching, and (iii) right to left shunting.

Diffusion Nonequilibrium

It is the difference between the pulmonary capillary blood CO_2 tension and the P_ACO_2. This can occur under two conditions: (i) increased pulmonary blood flow to such a level that the blood lacks sufficient time in the alveoli, disabling gas tension to reach its equilibrium, and (ii) thickening of the alveolar capillary membrane, such that the rate of diffusion of gas from capillary to alveolus is slowed. In practice, there has never been any evidence of diffusion nonequilibrium for CO_2. Similarly, diffusion nonequilibrium of O_2 very rarely exists. It exists in patients with interstitial fibrosis or in patients with normal lung function, but undergoes severe exercise.

V_A/Q Mismatch

The CO_2 dissociation curve in blood is a monotonically increasing one. Therefore, it is possible for a lung unit with low P_ACO_2 to compensate for lung units with high P_ACO_2, producing a normal P_aCO_2 in the face of substantial V_A/Q mismatch. On the other hand, unlike the CO_2 dissociation curve, the O_2 dissociation curve in blood has a plateau at the point at which Hb is fully saturated. Therefore, V_A/Q mismatch always results in arterial hypoxemia, but not hypercarbia.

Right to Left Shunt

Discussed elsewhere.

CLINICAL MONITORING OF RESPIRATORY SYSTEM

The continuous direct clinical observation of the color of a patient (such as the mucous membrane, skin, lips, color of blood, etc.), the respiratory rate of it, the movement of chest and breathing bag, etc. help us to judge the adequacy of ventilation. The color of mucous membrane of a patient can be used to assess the oxygenation. But anemia, polycythemia, changes in the shape of O_2 dissociation curve, or poor lighting may lead to mistakes. Different anesthetic agents, sedatives and opioid analgesics are potent depressants of respiration. Thus, hypoxic brain damage can occur within few minutes, if the respiratory system of a patient is not monitored properly and treated efficiently. So, in cases where the anesthetized patient is breathing spontaneously, then a constant observation of patient by the anesthetist is needed to detect any tracheal tug, paradoxical chest movement, or the failure of reservoir bag to move adequately, etc. Because, it indicates partial or complete airway obstruction.

Free passage of air through airways can also be confirmed clinically by hearing the sound of clear airflow through the nose or mouth. It also can be confirmed by feeling the warmth of expired air at the back of the hand, if it is placed by the anesthetist himself. Snoring and rattles or complete silence indicate impending or complete airway obstruction. Maintaining a clear airway in an anesthetized patient is a great skill. It requires much practice with constant vigilance to every detail and a pair of strong forearm muscles to push the mandible *upward and forward toward the roof* in a nonintubated patient. Clinically, periodic auscultation of chest by a stethoscope also confirms the position of endotracheal tube (ET) and detects any accumulation of secretions, pneumothorax or bronchospasm, if present. Thus, we can ensure the monitoring of respiratory system clinically.

MONITORING OF THE RESPIRATORY FUNCTION BY PRECORDIAL AND ESOPHAGEAL STETHOSCOPE

Many anesthetists still believe that during anesthesia a patient's respiratory system should be monitored by a precordial or esophageal stethoscope even in the presence of many electronic gadgets. But, though they (precordial stethoscope and esophageal stethoscope) have many advantages, still they are being gradually replaced by modern pulse-oximetry and capnography for better bedside monitoring of the respiratory function. Esophageal stethoscope is a very simple, cheap, and much informative instrument for clinical monitoring of respiratory system. It has the advantage of ensuring that the anesthetist stays in close contact with the patient. It is a small balloon-tipped probe that is inserted into the esophagus through mouth and connected to either a standard stethoscope head-piece or a molded ear-piece. When the length of an esophageal stethoscope has been adjusted, so that the balloon is opposite to the heart, then it also provides a constant monitoring of heart rate and breath sounds together. It is especially very useful in children, because it may detect any air embolism by hearing the characteristic mill-wheel murmur. By a precordial or esophageal stethoscope, we can also detect the bronchospasm, moist sounds, or any other adventitious sound of the lungs early, before it is reflected through pulse-oximetry and capnography. ECG leads, pacemaker electrodes, temperature probe and/or ultrasound probe for continuous intraoperative esophageal echocardiography can also be incorporated with the esophageal stethoscope. The information provided by the precordial or esophageal stethoscope is: confirmation of ventilation, quality of breath sound, confirmation of heartbeat (even when there are multiple artifacts in cardiac monitors) and quality heart sound [a soft tone is associated with hypotension and low cardiac output (CO)]. The main disadvantages of esophageal stethoscope are that it cannot confirm the bilateral equal breath sound after endotracheal intubation or cannot exclude the bronchial intubation. It should be avoided in patients with esophageal varices or strictures.

MONITORING OF RESPIRATORY SYSTEM BY MEASURING THE RESPIRATORY RATE, AIRWAY PRESSURE, TIDAL VOLUME, AND DISCONNECTION ALARM

Measurement of Respiratory Rate

It is usually measured clinically. It can also be obtained from the capnography or continuous ECG monitoring. When the ECG leads are used to monitor the respiratory rate, then a very high-frequency electrical current is passed across the thorax of patient from the chest electrodes and then the electrical impedance which changes cyclically with the respiratory movement of chest is measured. From this cyclical changes of electrical impedance, the respiratory rate is calculated and displayed.

Measurement of Airway Pressure

High airway pressure may cause damage to the alveoli, reduce the cardiac output, and predispose to pneumothorax in all the patients, receiving positive pressure ventilation. So, the airway pressure should be measured continuously or intermittently. The airway pressure is usually measured by simple mechanical pressure gauges or electronic gadgets which are attached to the ventilators or even to the Boyle's

---

BOX 1: Causes of changes in airway pressure.

- *Causes of increase in airway pressure:*
  - Bronchospasm
  - Pneumothorax
  - Pulmonary edema
  - ARDS
  - Less surfactant
  - Consolidation and collapse
  - Reversal of neuromuscular paralysis
  - Laparoscopy
  - Head down tilt
  - Kinking of breathing tube
  - Plug of sputum
- *Causes of decrease in airway pressure:*
  - Sudden disconnection
  - Low gas flow

(ARDS: acute respiratory distress syndrome)

---

machine. However, the narrow tracheal tube, long breathing system, or high respiratory rate may not accurately reflect the correct airway pressure, measured by the mechanical gauges.

Airway pressure is increased due to bronchospasm, pulmonary edema, pneumothorax ($\downarrow$ lung compliance), head down position, reversal of neuromuscular block, laparoscopy ($\downarrow$ thoracic compliance), plug of airway by sputum, or kinked tracheal tube (equipment problem), etc. On the other hand, airway pressure is suddenly decreased due to disconnection of breathing system, any leak in the circuit or empty cylinder **(Box 1)**.

Measurement of Tidal Volume

The measurement of tidal volume is an important way of monitoring the function of respiratory system. It confirms the ventilation of patient and optimizes the ventilator settings. For the measurement of tidal volume by bedside method, such as a spirometer has been used for many years. But, although this device is small and provides accurate result, still it has some disadvantages. The disadvantages are: (i) water vapor in expired air causes inaccuracies, (ii) weight of spirometer dictates its use at the machine end of breathing circuit, resulting in accurate result, (iii) its use is restricted mainly to the circle system when the volume of expired gas is measured as tidal volume, and (iv) its tendency to under-read at low tidal volume and over-read at high tidal volume.

In modern tidal volume monitors, there is a small connector which is attached to the ET tube. Two tubes lead from this connector to the pressure sensors which is situated in the body of main TV monitor. Measurement of small and differential pressure changes between the two tubes allows the calculation of airway pressure and inspired-expired tidal volume. The modern anesthetic machines which have an integrated circuit and ventilator have a *hot-wire anemometer* for the measurement of tidal volume. It uses an electrically heated hot wire, placed across the flow of air. Airflow cools the wire and thus decreases its electrical resistance, from where the amount of airflow during each breath (tidal volume) can be calculated. These devices are simple and reliable. But, they are delicate enough and need great protection.

Most multimonitors now have the facility to integrate the measurement of flow, pressure, and time in order to produce the *real-time measurement of compliance, flow-volume loops, and pressure-volume loops* along with the tidal volumes and other parameters of lung volume. These displays are especially useful in patients whose lungs are difficult to ventilate. It is also helpful where there are rapid changes in compliance of lungs, such as during one-lung anesthesia.

Disconnection Alarm

Most breathing systems have a disconnection alarm, as they have multiple connections which are dislodged easily, causing failure of ventilation and harm to the patient. Disconnection alarm detects the cyclical changes in airway pressure and gives an alarm, if there is any unexpected change (high or low) in pressure during ventilation. They are usually battery-powered and some need to have the alarm limits, set manually. But, most of the machines automatically detect the normal range of every parameter and then set off an alarm, if any significant change in respiratory rate, tidal volume, or airway pressure occurs. They may also set off an alarm, if high airway pressure is sensed somewhere.

MONITORING OF RESPIRATORY SYSTEM BY THE MEASUREMENT OF THE QUANTITY OF O_2 IN BLOOD

One of the most important functions of respiratory system is the delivery of O_2 from air to blood. So, the measurement of O_2 level in blood by measuring the (a) oxygenation saturation, (b) oxygen tension, (c) total oxygen content, (d) mixed venous O_2 tension, etc. are among the some methods of monitoring the respiratory function.

Measurement of Oxygen Saturation in Blood

The O_2 saturation of blood is usually measured noninvasively by pulse oximeter which works on the principles of oximetry and plethysmography.

Oximetry

When light passes through a solute which is dissolved in solvent, then it (light) is partly transmitted, partly absorbed, and partly reflected back which depends on the concentration of solute. This principle of transmission, absorption, and reflection of light is used in several monitoring devices to estimate the concentration of this dissolved solutes. In an oximeter, the absorption of infrared light is used to estimate the concentration of oxy-Hb (as solute) which remains in plasma (solvent) by using the *Beer Lambert's law.*

The Beer's law dictates that the solvent (e.g., plasma) is transparent to a particular frequency of light which is used for oximetry. Whereas, the solute (hemoglobin—reduced or oxygenated) absorbs this light and that absorption is directly proportional to the concentration of this solute (Hb).

On the other hand, the Lambert's law states that when a beam of light falls on a semitransparent, homogeneous substance, then due to absorption the intensity of transmitted light decreases exponentially, as the distance (depth) traveled through the solute increases and is proportional to the distance. So, the two laws (i.e., Beer and Lambert laws) can be combined and reproduced as:

$$A = d\,C\,E \qquad (1)$$

Where, A = absorbance of light, d = distance, C = concentration of solute, E = absorption coefficient of solute, which is constant for a given molecular weight and specified wavelength of a light.

The absorption coefficients of most of the common four types of Hb [oxyhemoglobin (O_2Hb), carboxyhemoglobin (CO-Hb), met-hemoglobin (met-Hb) and reduced hemoglobin carrying CO_2 (HHb)] at the working range of wavelength of red and infrared light which are used for oximetry are obtained from a graph which is given next. So, for the four types of Hb, the equation will be:

$$A = d\,(C_1E_1 + C_2E_2 + C_3E_3 + C_4E_4) \qquad (2)$$

The normal blood contains nil or negligible amount of Met-Hb and CO-Hb, and they do not take part in O_2 carrying. In a normal individual the blood contains mainly the reduced Hb and Oxy-Hb which takes part in transport O_2. So, to measure the O_2 saturation, we can shorten the equation (2) to equation (3) by measuring the absorption of light by the only two relevant hemoglobin such as oxyhemoglobin, and reduced hemoglobin. Now, the equation is:

$$A = d\,(C_1E_1 + C_2E_2) \qquad (3)$$

So, if the Met-Hb and CO-Hb were not present in the blood sample, then the concentration of O_2Hb and HHb, i.e., C_1 and C_2 could be determined by using the light of two wavelengths only, instead of four wavelengths which is required to measure the concentration of four types of Hb. From the **Figures 4 and 5**, it is observed that in case of a light of wavelength of 800 nm, the coefficient for O_2Hb and reduced Hb (HHb) are same. So, if an oximeter uses this wavelength of light and no Met-Hb or CO-Hb were present in blood, then the equation would be reduced to: A = d E800 $(C_1 + C_2)$.

Thus, the total sum of Oxy-Hb and reduced Hb could be determined by using the light of a single wavelength only. Using the lights of two wavelengths, the concentration of the two types of Hb can be determined separately and from there the percentage of individual Hb may be calculated easily. So, the percentage of saturation of total Hb by the O_2 is: O_2Hb/Total Hb $(O_2Hb + HHb) \times 100$. This is the value of SpO_2 in percentage, where the S stands for saturation and the P stands for pulsatile. Certain other abbreviations related to it are: SaO_2 = arterial O_2 saturation and SvO_2 = venous O_2 saturation. The abbreviation SpO_2 is used, because the oximeter cannot differentiate an artery from a vein, but can only recognize the O_2 saturation of pulsatile tissues which is usually of the arterial system, i.e., capillary. So, practically the SpO_2 and SaO_2 are equivalent. This Beer-Lambert's law can also be applied to measure the concentration (in percentage) of other mixture of gases and vapor in blood. If in any pathological condition, the concentration of Met-Hb and CO-Hb increases, then this equation will be: SpO_2 = $O_2Hb/(O_2Hb + HHb + Met-Hb + CO-Hb) \times 100\%$.

Now, we are considering the equation (2). If absorbance is measured by a single light of a specific wavelength (h), and the coefficient for the four types of Hb at that wavelength is known from the graph **(Fig. 4)**, then the preceding equation would contain four unknowns: C_1, C_2, C_3, C_4 (as E_1, E_2, E_3, and E_4 are known from graph). So, to solve this problem of four unknowns the light of four different wavelengths is needed. Similarly, to know the two unknown such as C_1 and C_2 in equation (3) we need two lights of different wavelength, considering that CO-Hb and met-Hb are absent in blood. *In vitro*, the concentration of four or more types of Hb is measured by a special type of *laboratory oximeter* which uses light of four or more wavelengths passing through a cuvette, filled with a solution of lysed red blood cells. Therefore, theoretically, an oximeter will require light of four different wavelengths to measure the fractional saturation of each type of hemoglobin, otherwise it may lead to erroneous results. But, this is not available clinically.

In clinical noninvasive oximetry, the red and infrared lights of two separate wavelengths are transmitted through a tissue bed. There are many light absorbers, i.e., different types of tissues are present in the pathway of transmitted light. These are skin, soft tissues, muscles, bones, venous blood, etc. (nonpulsatile part), and the arterial or capillary blood (pulsatile part). But, the pulse oximetry does not take into account the effect of absorption of light by these nonpulsatile tissue, because by some intelligent calculation it is deducted from the pulsatile tissue, which is described later **(Figure 5)**.

On one side of the probe which is used in pulse oximeter, there are two light emitting diodes (LED) which release red

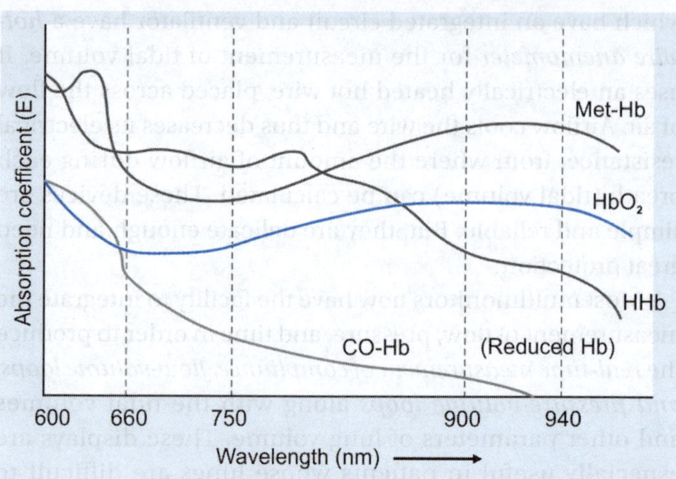

Fig. 4: Absorption coefficients of four types of Hb are plotted on vertical axis against the transmitted light of wavelength of different ranges.

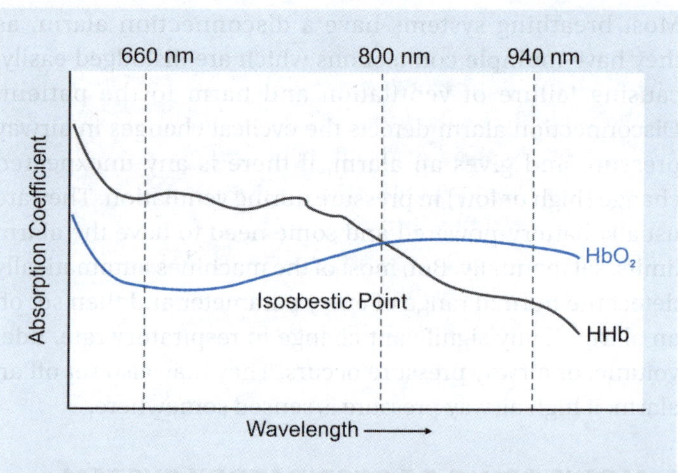

Fig. 5: Absorption spectra of oxy-Hb and reduced hemoglobin. For two types of Hb, two lights of different wavelengths (660 nm and 940 nm) are needed to get their absorption coefficient, respectively. By the light with a wavelength of 800 nm, we get a single coefficient, where the respective coefficients of HbO_2 and HHb are same and measures the total H.

(of wavelength 660 nm) and infrared (of wavelength 940 nm) light respectively. On the other side of the probe there is a photo cell which detects the transmitted light after passing through the tissues and its absorption. The electrical output from the photodetector or cell consists of a steady signal (X), which results from the absorption of light by the nonpulsatile tissues, such as bones, muscles, fat, venous blood, etc. On this steady nonpulsatile signal, a pulsatile signal (Y) is superimposed, resulting from the absorption of light by the pulsatile arterial or capillary blood, coming in the light-path. These two raw signals of which one is nonpulsatile and another is pulsatile are then processed complexly by the microprocessor. The Y component is measured relative to the X component which is independent of the intensity of incident light. Then, the ratio (R) of amplitude of the red and infrared pulsatile signal is determined (using an algorithm), which is related to arterial O_2 saturation.

The pulsatile expansion of the capillary arterial bed increases the length (depth) of absorption path and thereby increases the absorption. As the pulse oximetry uses only the light of two wavelengths – red light (of 660 nm wavelength) and infrared light (of 940 nm wavelength), so the pulse oximeter first determines the Y component of absorption for each wavelength of light, and then divides this value by the corresponding X component of absorption for each wavelength of light to obtain a "pulse-added" absorption. The oximeter, then, calculates the ratio (R) of this "pulse added" absorption which is empirically related to the percentage of arterial O_2 saturation (SaO_2). $R = (Y_{660}/X_{660})/(Y_{940}/X_{940}) = (Y_{660}/Y_{940}) \times (X_{940}/X_{660})$. Here, $Y_{660}/Y_{940} =$ the ratio of pulsatile components of absorption for the light of 660 and 940 nm of wavelength, and $X_{940}/X_{660} =$ the ratio of nonpulsatile components of absorption for the light of 940 and 660 nm of wavelength **(Figure 6)**.

The curves, used in different commercial devices, are prepared by different companies. These are based on their experimental studies, and conducted by the companies on different group of human volunteers. Although each curve is the property of this manufacturer, but the system being used is similar. So, the curves are very similar. For example, when the ratio of red to infrared absorbance is 1, the saturation of O_2 is 85% for all the machines.

For the best sensitivity, the difference between the ratio of absorption of red and infrared light by HbO_2 (oxyhemoglobin) and HHb (reduced hemoglobin) at the two wavelengths should be maximized. At a wavelength of 660 nm, the HbO_2 absorbs light 10 times less than that of reduced Hb and at a wavelength of 940 nm, the absorption coefficient of HbO_2 is much greater than that of reduced hemoglobin (HHb).

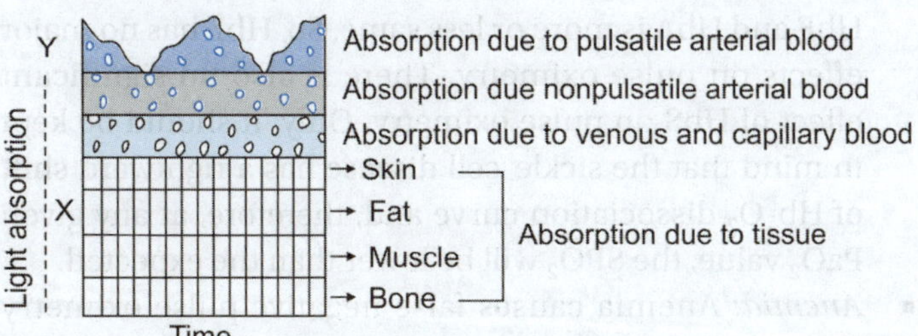

Fig. 6: This is a diagrammatic representation of all the components of a living tissue which absorbs the light. The Y component represents both the pulsatile and the nonpulsatile components of a living tissue which absorbs light. The X component represents only the nonpulsatile absorbing component of a living tissue.

Ear oximeter (which acts on the principle of simple oximetry, but not on pulse oximeter) has no ways of differentiating between the pulsatile arterial SO_2 of hemoglobin and nonpulsatile venous SO_2 of hemoglobin. So, it is applied on the ear with the idea that the earlobe contains predominantly arterial blood, and the reading shows the arterial SO_2. But, one cannot be sure that the earlobe contains only arterial blood. So, the other pulse oximeters, except the ear oximeter, are able to make this differentiation by assuming that the pulsatile portion of signal is entirely that of arterial blood. This is almost always true, except under unusual clinical conditions such as high venous pulsation in tricuspid regurgitation.

Pulse Oximeter in Practice

In practice, on one side of the probe of the pulse oximeter there is the LED which transmits two lights such as a red light at 660 nm of wavelength and an infrared light at 940 nm of wavelength from one side of the finger. It also has one photo diode, i.e., a sensing transducer on the opposite side of the finger. When the two LEDs are activated, it transmits two lights through the finger alternatively. Then, passing through the different tissues of finger the absorbed light on the opposite side is transduced into an electrical signal by the photo diode and is passed on to the computer. There, the ratio of absorption of these two lights by oxy- and reduced Hb is calculated electronically by a microprocessor, from where the SPO_2 is derived by an internally stored algorithm.

The measurement of SO_2 by light absorption technique was in existence for many years like ear oximeters, but it could not determine the pulsatile portion of the O_2 saturation. So, the development of pulse principle or plethysmography has increased substantially the reliability of such monitors and resulted in their extremely widespread use. However, the main drawback of this pulse oximetry is its insensitivity to the large changes in arterial PO_2 at the higher end of Hb-O_2 dissociation curve, i.e., after reaching 100% saturation it cannot be increased further with the increase in O_2 tension in blood.

In neonates, when the repeated arterial puncture is not technically feasible to measure the arterial PO_2, then capillary PO_2 which is very close to arterial O_2 is measured by this pulse oximeter. But, capillary PO_2 is definitely lower than arterial PO_2. This difference can be reduced by taking capillary blood sample from prewarmed heel site, where there is abundance of local blood flow relative to the local tissue O_2 consumption. In contrast, in capillaries where PO_2 is significantly lower than arterial PO_2, but there the capillary SO_2 approximates arterial SO_2. This is because of the shallow slope of the lower part of the Hb-O_2 dissociation curve.

The other technical problems of pulse oximeter and their solutions are:

- The LED in the probe does not emit light of a very fixed wavelength (monochromatic light), but usually emits light which wavelength runs in a spectrum and it should be narrow. But, certain companies use light which wavelength varies in the range of wide spectrum. The central wavelength of this emission spectrum varies among the diodes of different manufacturers. But, this variation should not be >5 nm (e.g., 660 ± 5 nm). A shift in the center of the wavelength of light spectrum, emitted by LED, causes changes in the measured absorption coefficient and results in an error in the estimation of oxygen saturation. A light of narrow spectrum, within its acceptable range of wavelength, increases the accuracy. If a light of wide range of wavelength is used for emission, then the pulse oximeter should be programmed accordingly to accept the center wavelength of both the red and infrared light and also allow the device to correct internally and automatically the values for the different wavelengths. But, this will be a very costly affair.
- Another problem of pulse oximeter is that the photodiodes, which are used opposite to the LED in the sensor probe, cannot differentiate the light of different wavelengths, i.e., whether the light is coming from red, infrared, or room light source. This problem is eliminated by alternating the red and infrared LED light sources on and off, at a frequency of 100 times per second. After absorption through tissues, when the red light is on the photo diode detector, it produces a current in which room light also takes part. Then, similarly after absorption through tissues, when the infrared light is on the photo-diode or detector, it also produces a current with the room light. Finally, when both the LEDs are turned off, then the photodiode detector produces the signal from room light only. Computer in the pulse oximeter eliminates all these common factors of light interference by calculating the ratio. This is a very clever design, but sometimes different sources of light produce different artifacts which can be minimized by covering the sensor with an opaque shield.
- Another problem arises when the amplitude of signal ratio is very low. Usually, all the oximeters have devices to amplify their signals. But, with the amplification of signal, the noise is also amplified. So, to prevent this type of artifact, a minimum value for signal to noise ratio is incorporated, below which level the device displays no value for SPO_2. Some oximeters display low-signal strength error message and some others display a plethysmographic wavelength for the visual identification of noise.

- Patient's motion, which is equivalent to high AC to DC signal ratio, also produces artifacts. These artifacts are eliminated by increasing the signal averaging time (i.e., the device averages its measurements over a longer period of time). But, the longer averaging time also slows the response time to an acute change in SO_2. So, many pulse oximeters have a system to select one from several time-average modes. Some oximeters use sophisticated algorithms to identify and reject the spurious signals.

Causes of Errors in Pulse Oximetry

As clinically the pulse oximeter takes the help of two lights of two different wavelengths, so the presence of Hb species other than the reduced Hb and oxy-Hb may cause erroneous readings. In a research laboratory, the sophisticated pulse oximeter uses multiple lights of separate wavelengths and by this device this error can be reduced.

- *Carboxyhemoglobin (CO-Hb):* The carboxyhemoglobin is formed during carbon monoxide (CO) poisoning. In the presence of CO-Hb, there is *falsely high* pulse oximeter reading. When the concentration of CO-Hb is 50%, then the pulse oximeter reading is about 95%. The probable explanation is that the light of 940 nm wavelength has no absorption in CO-Hb and therefore does not contribute to the total absorbance of light. At 660 nm of wavelength, CO-Hb has an absorbance close to that of O_2Hb. So, the O_2 saturation becomes falsely high.
- *Met-hemoglobin (Met-Hb):* At 940 nm of wavelength the absorption of light by Met-Hb is highest among other species of Hb, and at 660 nm of wavelength the absorption of light by Met-Hb is very close to reduced Hb. Thus, the absorption ratio of 1:1 of Met-Hb corresponds to the O_2 saturation of 85%. Therefore, SpO_2 is *falsely low* when it is truly high (>85%) and SpO_2 is falsely high when it is truly low (<85%). Independent of actual arterial O_2 saturation, SpO_2 shows to be 85% in the presence of high Met-Hb concentration.
- *Structural hemoglobinopathies:* Absorption spectrum of HbF and HbA is more or less same. So, HbF has no major effects on pulse oximetry. There is also no significant effect of HbS on pulse oximetry. Only, it should be kept in mind that the sickle-cell disease has a rightward shift of Hb-O_2 dissociation curve and, therefore, at any given PaO_2 value, the SPO_2 will be lower than the expected.
- *Anemia:* Anemia causes false negative pulse oximetry result. Polycythemia has no apparent effect on pulse oximetry.
- *Nail-polish:* Blue nail-polish with an absorption spectrum near about 660 nm causes a *false negative* result. Nail polishes of other colors have minimum effects.

- *Jaundice:* Bilirubin has no significant effect on pulse oximetry. But, nonpulsatile oximetry may measure a falsely low value.
- *Skin:* Very thick skin and deep pigmentation can result in reduced signals and cause slightly *low false* results. Otherwise, no significant effect is reported.
- *Movement:* Movement, especially shivering, can falsely depress the SpO_2 reading.
- *Blood flow:* Reduced amplitude of pulsation, due to low-tissue perfusion, can cause difficulty in obtaining signals and thus gives a *false low* SpO_2 reading. The causes of low-tissue perfusion are low cardiac output, severe anemia, hypothermia, increased systemic vascular resistance, etc. So, in addition to SpO_2 the pulse oximeter also provides an indication of tissue perfusion from pulse amplitude. Again, as SpO_2 is normally close to 100%, so only gross abnormalities are detected. Depending on a particular O_2-Hb dissociation curve in a patient, the 90% saturation reading in a pulse oximeter indicates the PaO_2 of <65 mm of Hg. This compares with clinically detectable cyanosis, which requires 5 g of reduced Hb and usually corresponds to the SpO_2 of <80%. In the absence of gross pulmonary diseases and low FiO_2, the bronchial intubation will usually go undetected by pulse oximeter.
- *Other causes:* The other causes of artifacts in pulse oximetry are: excessive ambient light, methylene blue dye, venous pulsation in a dependent limb, malpositioned sensor with leakage of light from LED to photodiode, bypassing arterial bed (optical shunting), etc.

Special Uses of Pulse Oximeter

Other than the measurement of O_2 saturation in capillary blood the two special uses of pulse oximeter are: (i) measurement of mixed venous oxygen saturation (SVO_2), and (ii) noninvasive brain oximetry. SVO_2 continuously varies with the changes of Hb concentration, cardiac output, arterial O_2 saturation, and the whole body O_2 consumption. So, interpretation of SVO_2 is much informative but is very complex. It requires the placement of a PAC containing fiber-optic sensor in pulmonary artery that continuously measures the SVO_2 in a manner similar to a pulse oximeter.

A special type of noninvasive pulse oximetry can also measure the regional O_2 saturation (rSO_2) of hemoglobin in brain. Unlike ordinary pulse oximetry, it measures the venous, capillary, and arterial blood O_2 saturation of brain tissue and represents an average reading. So, it is helpful to know the O_2 status or circulation of the brain during hypothermia, cerebral embolism, hypotension, hypoxia, etc. where there is a dramatic decrease of rSO_2. In this type of special noninvasive pulse oximetry, a sensor is placed on the forehead which emits light of a specific wavelength and then measures the amount of reflected light after absorption by brain tissue. It works on the principle of infrared optical spectroscopy.

Measurement of O_2 Tension (PO_2) in Blood

Other than the measurement of saturation of O_2 in blood by noninvasive method, the most straightforward method of assessing the respiratory function is to measure directly the arterial O_2 tension (PaO_2) from blood sample. This is done by the following methods.

By Oxygen Electrode: The Polarographic Method

This is usually done by Clark polarographic O_2 electrode. The Clark's polarographic O_2 electrode consists of a platinum cathode and a silver anode. They are connected to a battery through a meter which measures the flow of current and this flow of current is proportional to the amount of O_2 present in solution.

As in any resistive circuit and according to the Ohm's law an increase in voltage increases the flow of current. However, this polarographic electrochemical cell which measures the O_2 concentration or tension does not obey this Ohm's law ($E = I \times R$), but rather exhibits a plateau. That means with in certain range the increase in voltage does not increase the flow of current, but the increase in O_2 tension increases the flow of current. This is called polarogram. The platinum and silver electrodes are immersed in an electrolyte cell. A membrane, permeable to O_2 only but not to the electrolyte, covers one surface of the cell. A polarizing voltage, ranging between 600 and 800 mV is applied in the circuit. O_2 diffuses through this membrane and reacts at the platinum cathode producing hydroxyl ions. For this reaction, electron is needed and it is supplied by the silver chloride anode. Thus, the reduction of O_2 which occurs at the platinum cathode corresponds with the oxidation which occurs at the silver chloride anode by the following reactions.

$$O_2 + 4e \rightarrow 2O_2^-$$
$$2O_2^- + 2H_2O \rightarrow 4OH^-$$
$$4Ag \rightarrow 4Ag^+ + 4e^-$$
$$4Ag^+ + 4Cl^-$$

Thus, multiple small cells are setup and tiny electrical circuits are generated which is dependent on the O_2 tension at the platinum cathode. The current meter measures the current produced by the consumed electrons in the reaction at the cathode and this consumption of electron is proportional to the local PO_2 **(Fig. 7)**.

This polarographic method needs withdrawal of blood sample to measure PO_2. To obviate this need of drawing

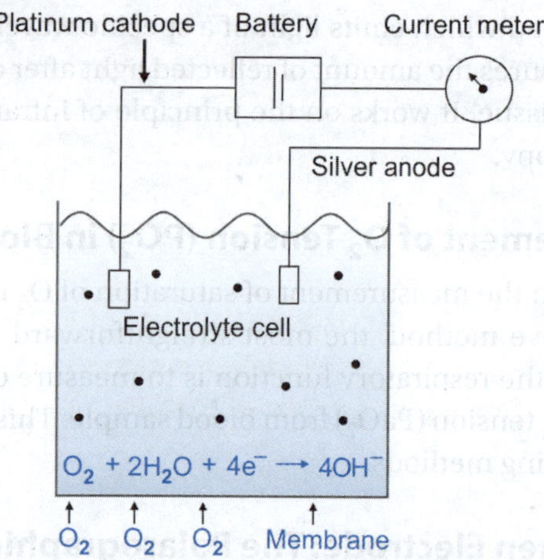

Fig. 7: Clark polarographic O_2 electrometer. The circuit consists of a current meter which is connected to a platinum cathode, a silver anode, and a battery (voltage source). These electrodes are immersed in an electrolyte cell, which have a membrane, permeable only to O_2 but not to the electrolytes. O_2 diffuses through the membrane and reacts with the platinum cathode. Here, it receives electrons (e^-) and reacts with water and produces OH^- ion. This OH^- ion reacts with the silver anode and gives up electrons. Thus, small electrical circuit is generated. The current meter measures the current produced by these two electrodes and the concentration of O_2 which is responsible for this production of current.

blood samples, intra-arterial PO_2 monitors have also been developed recently by using fiber-optic technique. This technique uses a particular property of O_2. This particular property of O_2 is to absorb energy from excited electrons of a fluorescent dye. To elevate the electrons in the dye to a higher energy state an incident light is used. These excited or highly energized electrons may then return to a lower energy level by emitting photons. Molecular O_2 by absorbing the energy inhibits this photon emission. This process of inhibition which is called fluorescent quenching is related to the concentration of O_2 and is used to measure the PO_2.

By Galvanic or Fuel Cell

A galvanic cell converts chemical energy (oxidation – reduction by O_2) into electrical energy and thus the generated potential is dependent on the O_2 concentration needed for the chemical reaction. At the cathode end (made by gold mesh) O_2 is reduced to hydroxyl ions by its reaction with electron and water and at the anode the lead is oxidized by removing electron. This chemical reaction produces a potential gradient and hence a flow of electrical current. This is measured and read out digitally on the screen of monitor with audible alarms. Unlike O_2 electrode in polarographic method, this fuel cell does not need any battery and is also cheap, portable, and reliable. This also needs little maintenance. But, inaccurate response to calibration with O_2

and air suggests that the fuel cell is exhausted and should be replaced. The chemical reaction which takes place in fuel cell uses up the components of the cell. So, its life depends on the concentration of O_2 to which it is exposed and on the duration of exposure. Usually, a fuel cell lasts for 6–12 months.

By Transcutaneous Electrodes

This is a noninvasive method of measuring PO_2 of blood. This device also consists of a small or miniaturized Clark O_2 electrode. The probe of this device is attached to the skin with an adhesive tape through a contact liquid to form an airtight seal and the area is also heated to 43°C by this probe. At this temperature, the blood flow to the skin is increased and the capillary O_2 diffuses out of the skin. This allows the accurate measurement of PO_2 by the attached electrode. Actually, the measurement of PO_2 by this transcutaneous method ($PtCO_2$) reflects the capillary PO_2 which is lower than the PaO_2. So, the skin is warmed to 43°C to increase the capillary blood flow and then $PtCO_2$ correlates well with PaO_2. The main disadvantage of heating the probe electrically to improve the cutaneous circulation is burning of skin on prolonged use. Also, unlike the original electrode in blood-gas machine, this miniaturized probe contains only one drop of electrolyte. So, when the sensor is heated continuously to 43°C, then this elevated temperature causes the electrolyte to evaporate very quickly and reduces the life span of this device.

Peripheral vasoconstriction, thick adult skin, and reduction of cardiac output cause a decrease in $PtCO_2$ level. This is because of cutaneous hypoxia due to hypoperfusion and may produce erroneous results. However, this technique is particularly useful in infants, in whom the local skin blood flow tends to be high and capillary PO_2 is as close as to the arterial PO_2 and in whom repeated drawing of arterial blood is technically difficult and may cause anemia. Another disadvantage of transcutaneous O_2 electrodes is that the time constant of PO_2 measurement is nearly a minute. So, sudden decrease in PaO_2 cannot be detected quickly enough to take any appropriate measure. Prolonged application may also cause skin burn. Problems also occur with surgical diathermy. Because, the heated circuit provides a return path for the cutting current which may overheat the transcutaneous electrode and cause burn.

Measurement of O_2 Content

The measurement of total O_2 content in blood is also a type of monitoring of the respiratory function. It can be measured from the value of O_2 saturation of the Hb, Hb concentration and the tension of O_2 in blood, using the formula below:

Oxygen content of blood (mL/dL) = [SO_2(%) × Hb(g/dL) × 1.34] + [0.0225 + PO_2(KPa)]

The oxygen content in blood can also be measured by Van Slyke technique, using chemical and volumetric analysis.

Measurement of Mixed Venous O_2 Saturation

Mixed venous O_2 saturation is obtained from the equation:

$SvO_2 = SaO_2 - VO_2/13.9 \times Q \times (Hb)$

Q = Cardiac output, (Hb) = Hemoglobin concentration

VO_2 = Oxygen consumption

Mixed venous O_2 saturation is decreased in circumstances where there is low SaO_2, low cardiac output, low (Hb), elevated VO_2, etc., low SVO_2 is also found in all those conditions which produce impairment of O_2 delivery to the tissues. So, measurement of SVO_2 is very helpful in detecting any condition that may impair tissues oxygenation. The SVO_2 can be measured intermittently by taking blood sample from pulmonary artery catheter or continuously by a pulmonary artery catheter which is equipped with a fiber-optic bundle and oximeter. Low level of SVO_2, usually <60%, may sensitively indicate an abnormality of any of the factors which are mentioned above.

Measurement of Tissue Oxygenation

Till now, the measurement of arterial oxygen level (saturation, tension, or content) has been discussed which is an indicator of the status of respiratory function. But, adequate arterial oxygenation does not always indicate adequate tissue oxygenation, because there are many other factors which determine the tissue O_2 level, such as local tissue blood flow, rate of O_2 consumption by tissues, acid base status, temperature, etc. So, for appropriate monitoring of the respiratory function of a patient, measurement of the level of O_2 in tissues or tissue-oxygenation is important.

Tissue oxygenation or O_2 level in tissues is measured by the tissue PO_2 measuring electrodes which have certain problems. These problems are:

- Tissue destruction by electrodes
- Since different tissues have different blood flow and different O_2 consumption levels. So different tissues have different PO_2 level, rather than a single-standard value as in blood.
- Area within the same tissue, changes in oxygenation have been demonstrated under varying local conditions.

Recently, tissue oxygenation is being measured by using light which wavelength falls within the near infrared band (wavelength 650–1,100 nm) and which can penetrate the tissue reasonably well. Commercially, such an instrument is available which using this technique can measure the O_2 saturation of brain tissue. To measure the brain tissue O_2 level, the incident light is applied on the scalp from where it enters the brain. Then, a small proportion of light is scattered and returns back after its absorption by brain tissues to the analyzer by a fiber-optic bundle. The absorption and the intensity of this reflected light depends on the O_2 level of tissues and thus the machine measures the O_2 level of it. The measured O_2 saturation of brain includes arterial, capillary, and venous blood. But, it is heavily weighted toward the values of venous blood. Whereas, pulse oximetry measures only the arterial O_2 saturation, as it only measures the pulsatile portion of the tissue. So, it indicates the amount of O_2 delivered to the tissues, but does not indicate the amount of O_2 diffused in it or the consumption and need of O_2 by it.

Recently, it has also become possible to measure the tension of oxygen at the intracellular level by mixing the light of different wavelengths. This is more likely to provide a better estimation of O_2 availability at the cellular level than the currently available clinical monitoring parameters. This technique has been used to monitor the intracellular changes of muscle and brain tissue during respiratory acidosis, hypoxia, and cardiopulmonary bypass.

▌ MEASUREMENT OF INSPIRED O_2 CONCENTRATION

An anesthetic apparatus usually supplies O_2 and anesthetic gases to the patient. Thus, it regulates the arterial PO_2, and the uptake and elimination of inhalational anesthetic agents by lungs. So, the knowledge of the composition of inspired gases, at least the concentration of O_2 in it, is important for the routine monitoring of a patient.

Therefore, it is mandatory to analyze the inspired gases for its O_2 concentration constantly during the all forms of anesthesia. This will ensure that hypoxic mixtures are not used and will also confirm that the desired concentration of anesthetic agents are being delivered. Thus, the delivery of an adequate amount of O_2 is so crucial for safe anesthesia that multiple safety monitoring systems including using of an oxygen analyzer in the circuit are considered mandatory.

During low-flow closed circuit anesthesia, the inspired concentration of O_2 cannot be calculated from the rotameter, if nitrous oxide is being used. So, the measurement of inspired O_2 concentration becomes mandatory, as part of the intraoperative patient monitoring. The O_2 concentration in inspired gases can be measured by the following ways:

Paramagnetic O_2 Analyzer

Most of the monitors have a paramagnetic sensor. It uses the property of O_2 which is based on its weak attraction by a magnetic field. As most of the anesthetic gases are diamagnetic, so they are weakly repelled by a magnetic field. Two unpaired electrons, spinning at the same direction in the outer electron shell of an O_2 atom, make this molecule strongly paramagnetic, i.e., attracted toward a magnetic field.

In the chamber of a paramagnetic monitor, there is a small sphere, filled with nitrogen. The sphere is suspended from a bar that is free to rotate by a strong magnetic field. In a normal condition, i.e., when exposed to air, the bar finds a position where the force exerted on the sphere by the magnetic field is balanced by the torsion of the suspending wire. If the O_2 concentration in the chamber increases, then the O_2 is attracted toward the magnetic field. This inward movement of O_2 displaces the sphere and causes the bar to rotate. This small twisting movement of the bar is measured and then amplified. Thus, when calibrated, the O_2 concentration in the chamber may be calculated easily from the position of the bar. This instrument identifies and accurately measures the O_2 concentration in a mixture of gases over a wide range. It is a very reliable and a fast method. But, unfortunately, it cannot measure continuously the breath-by-breath changes of O_2 concentration in inspired gas mixture and its sample volume is large.

Polarographic O_2 Electrode and O_2 Fuel Cell

Some monitors use polarographic O_2 electrodes and some use O_2 fuel cell for the measurement of the concentration of O_2 in inspired gases. Although the response time for both of these instruments is long, but they are cheap, compact, portable, and are of sufficient accuracy for clinical use, as a continuous way of monitoring for inspired O_2 concentration. The fuel cell measures the partial pressure of O_2, instead of its concentration and its accuracy is usually around ±2% with a response time < 10 seconds. The long life (2,000 hours, when exposed to 100% O_2) and the robustness of fuel cell lends it a valuable device for this role and it should be available with all the anesthetic machines. Before each use, the analyzer should be calibrated by exposure to air and 100% O_2.

MONITORING OF RESPIRATORY SYSTEM BY MEASUREMENT OF CO$_2$ IN BLOOD

Measurement of CO$_2$ Tension in Blood

Like O_2 tension, measurement of CO_2 tension in the blood also reflects the status of respiratory function. So, the monitoring of PCO_2 in blood is another way of monitoring the respiratory function of a patient. But except monitoring of respiratory function, measurement of PCO_2 of blood also monitors the acid-base status, cardiac function, function of anesthetic machine, etc. Blood PCO_2 can be measured directly or indirectly in different ways, some of which are described below.

Directly by CO$_2$ Electrode

It is also called the Severinghaus CO_2 electrode and is used in the blood gas analyzer to measure the PCO_2 of blood.

This CO_2 electrode acts by measuring the changes of pH in blood. As a pH electrode, it is kept in contact with a thin layer of bicarbonate buffer solution which is separated from blood or plasma by a thin teflon or silicone membrane. This membrane is only permeable to CO_2 but not to blood cells, plasma or charged ions. The whole unit is maintained at 37°C. The CO_2 diffuses from blood into the buffer solution through this membrane, and causes a change in H^+ concentration of solution which is reflected as CO_2 tension on the screen of monitor. The electrode is calibrated by equilibrating the buffer solution with two known CO_2 concentrations which establish the relationship between pH and PCO_2.

Indirectly by Transcutaneous Measurement of PCO$_2$

Transcutaneous CO_2 electrode is nothing but a miniature modification of Severinghaus electrode which is used in the blood gas machine to measure the CO_2 tension of blood. Here, the CO_2 diffuses through a membrane into the cell, where it reacts with water and produces carbonic acid. The pH sensitive glass electrode, then, reacts to this change in concentration of hydrogen ions by producing a small electromotive force which can then be measured as the partial pressure of CO_2. After the introduction of Severinghaus CO_2 electrode in 1958, it was first used in a blood-gas analyzing machine. Then, in 1970, this electrode was miniaturized and incorporated into a transcutaneous probe to measure the blood CO_2 tension through skin noninvasively **(Figure 8)**.

The advantages and disadvantages of this transcutaneous CO_2 probe is similar to that of transcutaneous Clark O_2 probe or an electrode which is used to measure the blood O_2

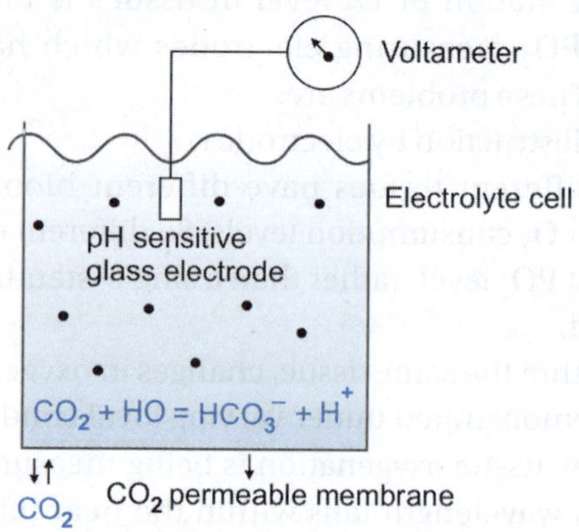

Fig. 8: Diagrammatic representation of a Severinghaus CO_2 electrode. This device consists of a pH sensitive glass electrode and an electrolyte cell, having a CO_2 permeable membrane covering on the surface. The gas electrode is immersed in the electrolyte cell. Through the permeable membrane, CO_2 diffuses into the cell. Then, it reacts with water producing carbonic acid and changes the pH. The pH electrode then detects the change in pH, which is directly proportional to the CO_2 concentration.

tension. Actually, transcutaneous CO_2 electrode measures the capillary PCO_2. So, to get the actual arterial PCO_2, the blood flow should be increased in the capillaries by warming the skin to 44°C through the probe. Again, heating of Severinghaus CO_2 electrode and applying it to the surface of skin increases the metabolic production of CO_2 in the tissue, resulting in a higher PCO_2 than the actual arterial PCO_2. Another disadvantage is that unlike the CO_2 electrode used in blood-gas machine in transcutaneous electrodes, the used electrolyte is only a few millimeter in amount. So, the continuous heating of probe to 44°C causes quick evaporation of water from the electrolyte, and hence results in a short lifespan of the transcutaneous probe. However, in the newer transcutaneous probes all these disadvantages are removed by incorporating some newer technologies and electronic calibration. The main advantage of this transcutaneous CO_2 probe is that repeated withdrawal of blood to measure the blood PCO_2 is not required which is very helpful for children.

Measurement of End-tidal CO_2 Tension by Capnography

The measurement of end-tidal CO_2 tension by capnography (ETPCO$_2$) is another way of monitoring the respiratory function. The ETPCO$_2$ is used as an estimation of P_ACO_2 and hence P_aCO_2, because the level of P_ACO_2 and P_aCO_2 runs parallel and is very close to each other, except in some rare circumstances, where the arterial and alveolar CO_2 tension difference is high. The normal gradient between the P_ACO_2 and P_aCO_2 is 2–5 mm Hg. It reflects the volume of alveolar dead space, i.e., the number of alveoli which is ventilated, but not perfused. Thus, any increase in the alveolar dead space by reduction in lung perfusion, such as, air embolism, ↓BP, ↓cardiac output, etc. decrease the expired CO_2 concentration and lessens the ETCO$_2$ tension and increases the P_ACO_2 – P_aCO_2 gradient. This gradient is also increased when there are other causes of impairment of lung perfusion and the end-tidal CO_2 level does not reach the arterial level. So, sometimes the ETCO$_2$ value should be checked with arterial blood samples, especially in more complex situations. These include: severe pulmonary diseases and situations where the accurate control of arterial CO_2 level is critical to save the life. So, the end-tidal CO_2 (ETCO$_2$) analysis has achieved a high degree of popularity. The **Box 2** shows different conditions where the ETCO$_2$ increased and decreased. The indications for the use of capnometer are listed in **Box 3**.

A variety of techniques can be used for the measurement of ETCO$_2$ concentration and its tension, such as, *mass spectrometry, Raman's analysis, infrared absorption technique*, etc. But, the last is used in majority of capnometers.

BOX 2: Conditions for high, low, and nil end-tidal CO_2 tension.

- Conditions of raised end-tidal CO_2 tension
  - Hypoventilation, due to neuromuscular diseases, central respiratory depression by opioid, thoracic surgeries, etc. leading to retention of CO_2
  - *Rebreathing:* Exhausted sodalime or defective valves of closed circuit, faulty equipment, etc. which impair the absorption of CO_2 or cause inhalation of expired CO_2
  - Malignant hyperthermia, pyrexia, thyrotoxicosis, malignant neuroleptic syndrome, sepsis, etc. due to increased production of CO_2 in hypermetabolic state
  - CO_2 inhalation
  - Laparoscopy by CO_2
  - After release of tourniquet
  - Bicarbonate IV administration, producing CO_2 in plasma
  - Bronchial intubation, due to increase in ventilation and perfusion mismatch (V/Q)
- Conditions of low end-tidal CO_2 tension
  - Hyperventilation
  - Bronchial intubation
  - Hypothermia
  - Hypometabolism
  - Hypoperfusion of lungs (decrease delivery of CO_2 to lungs) due to hypotension
  - Pulmonary embolism by air, fat, or thrombus (It may become zero if the embolus is large enough to occlude the total pulmonary circulation)
  - Leak in breathing circuit
- *No tracing of graph of end-tidal CO_2 tension (ETCO$_2$)*
  - Esophageal intubation
  - Accidental extubation
  - Complete obstruction of ET tube or circuit
  - Disconnection of breathing circuit
  - Complete stoppage of ventilation
  - Cardiac arrest, causing failure to carry CO_2 from tissue to lungs

No change in ETCO$_2$: In bronchospasm or COPD, there is increase in upsloping (phase II) of wave form. But, due to high diffusibility of CO_2 the net value of ETCO$_2$ (endpoint of phase III) remains normal even in severe bronchospasm

---

BOX 3: Indications of the use of capnometer.

- Confirmation of tracheal intubation
- Confirmation of adequate ventilation
- Detection of hyperthermia (malignant or not)
- Detection of rebreathing
- Detection of V_A/Q mismatch
- Detection of pulmonary embolism
- Detection of malfunctions of inspiratory and expiratory valve
- Confirmation of continued ventilation or detachment at any part of circuit
- Detection of cardiac activity during CPR or to assess the performance of CPR: The CPR is considered as gross failure, if it is not able to generate ETCO$_2$ of at least 10 mm Hg.
- Control the level of hypocapnia, during hyperventilation in neurosurgery.

Infrared radiation of 1–15 μm (1,000–15,000 nm) wavelength is absorbed by all the gases which have two or more dissimilar electrons at the outer orbit of their atoms. In the infrared absorption method, an infrared light beam is projected through the gas sample and then the intensity of this transmitted light is measured, after its absorption, while passing through it. However, this absorption of infrared light is different in intensity, depending on the concentration and the absorption spectrum of the gas to be analyzed. CO_2 absorbs infrared light with a characteristic peak at the wavelength close to 4.3 μm (4,300 nm). Several other molecules, such as, N_2O, CO, water vapor, and O_2 can also absorb the light in this area of wavelength spectrum (absorption spectrum of N_2O and CO is 4.5 and 4.7 μm respectively). Thus, they may interfere with CO_2 measurement, especially if the composition of incident light includes wavelengths, other than those in a very narrow spectrum around the CO_2 absorption peak. But in practical use, the fixed geometry of this gas (CO_2) sampling cell, a narrow band infrared light source and a compensating electronic circuit of a computer can often automatically correct the interference by other gases. After absorption, a special photocell detects and transduces the absorbed infrared radiation to a continuous electrical output. The modern CO_2 analyzers for clinical use are very stable, but it requires calibration to its zero point routinely at a regular time interval.

To ensure the accuracy, most monitors modify the principles of infrared absorption technique by different methods (described below) to measure the CO_2 content accurately in several ways. Sometimes the beam is usually turned on and off up to 4,000 times per minute to provide a zero-light reference. Sometimes the infrared light from a single light source is usually split and passed through two identical chambers: one contains the gas mixture to be analyzed and the other is empty. The absorption of CO_2 is then calculated by comparing the two beams. Lastly, each beam may be reflected through the chamber for several times by a series of mirrors to increase the amount of absorption and make it easier to measure.

The modern multimonitors for the measurement of $ETPCO_2$ use infrared light of several wavelengths and are, therefore, able to automatically detect the concentration of various other gases which are present in the mixture. This method is also used to monitor different anesthetic agents during inspiration and expiration. Estimation of the end-tidal O_2 tensions ($ETPO_2$) can also be used as a monitoring parameter for respiratory function, because $ETPO_2$ is equivalent to P_AO_2 and hence PaO_2. But, this is not always true, because of the variable alveolar and arterial oxygen tension gradient (A-a). In a normal individual, the gradient is <10 mm Hg. But, in a V_A/Q mismatch, this A-a oxygen tension gradient will be very high, resulting in an arterial hypoxemia which is not reflected by $ETPO_2$. But, usually the V_A/Q mismatch has no effect on the relation between the $ETPCO_2$ and P_aCO_2. Furthermore, if a patient receives high inspired O_2 concentration, then the $ETPO_2$ will be falsely high and shall overestimate the PaO_2. Even a dead patient may show high $ETPO_2$, if he is ventilated with 100% O_2.

A capnometer is usually of two types:

(i) Side-stream capnometer and (ii) Mainstream capnometer.

i. *Side-stream capnometer:* In a side-stream capnometer, the main infrared analyzer module is situated out of the anesthetic circuit at a distance from the patient within the multimonitor unit. So, it constantly drains the gas sample of around 150 mL/min by a small pump via a fine-gauge tubing. But, the main analyzer which is placed in a multimonitor unit should be placed as close to the patient as possible. This will reduce the amount of gas drained out from the circuit. This infrared analyzer module or sensor may be a separate unit or may be housed in the main multimonitor which measures the other parameters of the patient. The side-stream capnometer is less reliable, but is less liable to accidental damage. The infrared measuring cell, i.e., the core of the instrument should be protected from water vapor and other particulate matters, as they may cause erroneous readings, due to their higher infrared absorption. Usually, water vapor present in the expired air condenses at room temperature in the sampling tube and accumulates in a water trap which is then filtered out from the sampling gas before entering in the main analyzing module. In critical care settings or in very long cases, where inspired gases are warmed and humidified properly, then the workload increases on the water-separating system of the capnometer as the inspired air has high water content. The disadvantages of side-stream capnometer are:

• There is some delay in detection and measurement of PCO_2. This is further increased if the tubing, leading from the anesthetic circuit is too long or too wide. This delay is called as the *"CO_2 flight time"*. It can be minimized and the sensitivity can be increased by using high gas flow rates (up to 250 mL/min) for sampling and narrow short tubing (low dead space) assemble, compatible with the position of equipment with respect to the patient breathing circuit. On the other hand, if the tidal volume is small such as in a pediatric patient, then this high rate of aspiration (gas sampling) may draw much fresh gas from the circuit and dilute the $ETCO_2$ reading. Low aspiration rates (<50 mL/min) can also delay $ETCO_2$ measurement and underestimate it during rapid ventilation by drawing fresh gas from the circuit.

- Multiple connection sites in the assembly of sidestream capnometer such as sampling gas pump, flow regulation, water-trap, etc. may cause increased incidence of gas leakage or breakage and erroneous result.
- If the sampling flow exceeds the expired gas flow, then contamination from the fresh gas source may occur which may give inaccurate reading. The rate of gas sampling can be adjusted from 50 to 500 mL/min, but the usual volume of the gas sample is maintained between 50 and 150 mL/min.
- In certain circumstances such as during pediatric anesthesia, the removal of 150 mL of gas from the circuit may affect ventilation. So, most monitors incorporate the facility to return the measured gas to the circuit through a second tube. Thus, this second tube also helps to prevent the OT pollution by anesthetic gases coming out from capnometer.

ii. *Mainstream capnometer:* In a mainstream capnometer, there is no system of continuously drawing of sample gas by a pump. The sensor or the main infrared analyzing module of the mainstream capnometer is placed along the breathing circuit itself, resulting in a quick and accurate measurement of PCO_2 from expired gases. The analysis of end-tidal PCO_2 correlates well with the concentration of CO_2 in the alveoli and hence in the arterial blood. So, to get a correct result, the mixing of expired gas with the fresh gas should be prevented. So, the instrument should be placed as close to the alveoli as possible. Hence, the measuring head is placed in close proximity to an ET tube.

The *advantages* of mainstream capnometer are:

- No gas is subtracted from the breathing circuit, so it does not affect the ventilation.
- No suction pump or other device is required for sampling which adds complexities to the mechanical system.
- No uncertainty in gas sampling
- Response time is faster.

The *disadvantages* of mainstream capnometer are:

- The measuring chamber is usually heated to about 40°C to prevent water condensation in the chamber window. So, the heated sensing head should be kept away from direct contact with the patient's skin.
- It is relatively heavy and must be supported to prevent ET tube kinking.
- Sensor's window must be kept clean of mucus and other particles to prevent false reading.
- Calibration is problematic.

Periodically, the capnometer should be calibrated by using the gases of known concentration, guided by the respective companies. Mainstream capnometers are often equipped with calibration sample cells, sealed with a mixture of CO_2 and N_2 of known concentration. In some instruments, the room air is sampled in the mainstream cuvette for calibration and bring the CO_2 level automatically to zero.

Capnographic Waveform

Different capnographic waveforms are shown in **Figures 9A to H**. In capnographic waveform or tracing there are four phases. Among these, the phases I, II, and III corroborate with expiration and phase IV corroborates with inspiration. In phase I (dead-space phase) the expired gas, which comes out from anatomical dead space, such as ET-tube and large airways, is devoid of CO_2. This is because they contain only the previous fresh gas which does not take part in gaseous exchange. So, in this phase I there is no rise in PCO_2 in tracing which follows the base line. This phase I is followed by phase II. In this short phase II, as the expiration continues, so a rapid upstroke of PCO_2 level is recognized. This is because the anatomical dead space gases, coming from the lower part of the conducting part of airways, containing no CO_2 mixed with the alveolar gases containing CO_2 now, starts to excrete and the concentration of CO_2 increases rapidly. This phase II is also called as the "transition or the rising front of CO_2" and is followed by phase III which is called as the alveolar or plateau phase.

This phase III represents the constant, but a slowly rising part of the graph and reaches a peak at the final phase of expiration. This represents final $ETCO_2$ tension value. The cause of this constant slowly rising of PCO_2 in phase III is that gradually expired gases, containing more and more CO_2 coming purely from alveoli (not mixed with anatomical dead space gases, the gas of phase II is a mixture of dead space and alveolar gas) reaches the analyzer. This is because CO_2 excretion from pulmonary capillaries into alveoli continues at a nearly constant rate during expiration and this CO_2 molecule is not diluted by the lung volume which becomes progressively smaller by the exhalation process. This gradual and relative increase in the concentration of CO_2 in smaller lung volume is responsible for this constant and slowly rising part of the graph or phase III. Slow exhalation, as in the acute asthma patient, induces a steeper alveolar plateau. Thus, the end of the phase III or alveolar plateau represents the final $ETCO_2$ tension. In a normal individual the $ETCO_2$ tension is 2–3 mm Hg less than P_aCO_2. But, the chronic pulmonary diseases and acute V_A/Q mismatch wide this difference. At the end of phase III, when the expiration still continues and lung volume [functional residual capacity (FRC)] goes below the closing capacity, then the expired CO_2 concentration

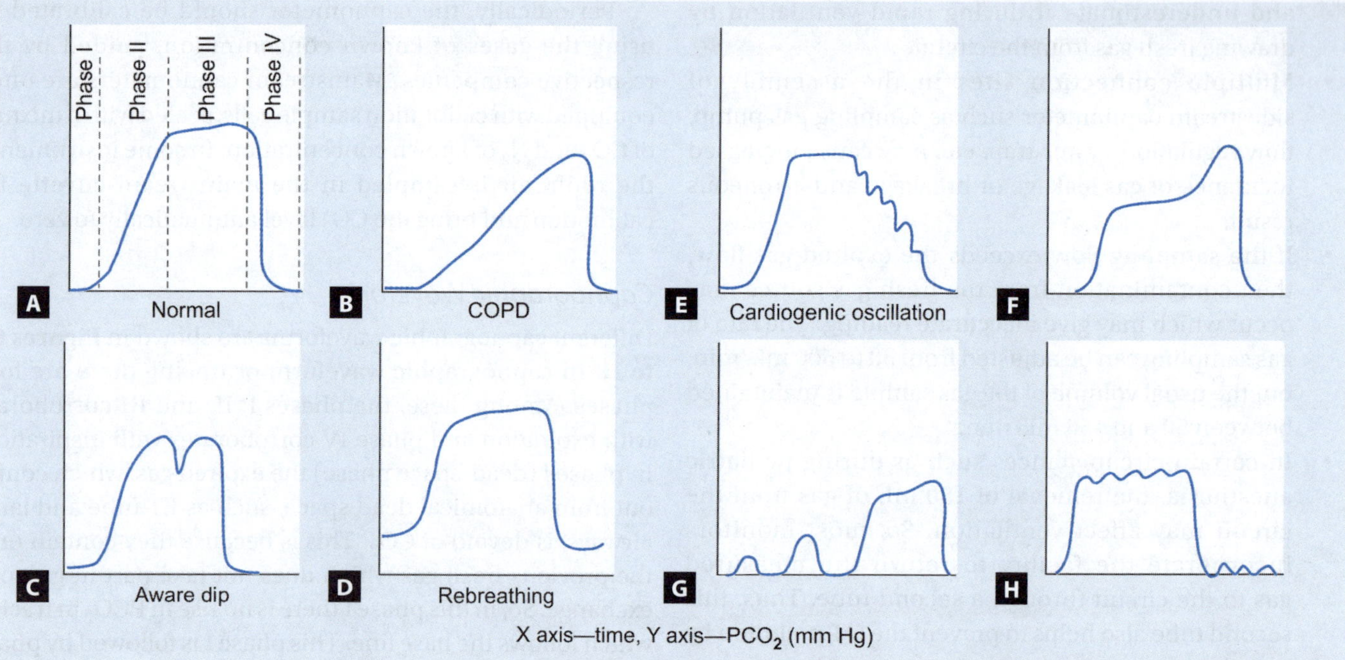

Figs. 9A to H: Analysis of ETCO$_2$ tension waveform. Phase I represents the gas of anatomical dead space. So, it does not contain any CO$_2$ and is seen as flat phase running along the base line. A raised phase I **(Fig. D)** suggests rebreathing or malfunctioning of inspiratory and expiratory valve or an exhausted soda lime. Phase II represents the rapid rise of tracing, after phase I. This is due to the exhaled gases coming first from anatomical dead space and then alveoli and so containing gradually more and more CO$_2$. This corresponds to beginning of expiration. A slanted upstroke **(Fig. B)** represents the obstruction of airway during expiration. This obstruction may be due to asthma, COPD, kinking of airway, secretions, etc. No plateau is reached before next inspiration and the gradient between ETPCO$_2$ and P$_a$CO$_2$ will increase. Phase III consists of a nearly horizontal plateau which corresponds with exhalation of gas coming entirely from alveoli. During expiration, the gas leaving the alveoli comes from the different parts of alveoli. Hence, this phase represents the average concentration of CO$_2$. The end of plateau represents the end-tidal CO$_2$ concentration or tension when it attains fairly a constant level. In a normal individual, it is usually 3–5 mm Hg lower than P$_a$CO$_2$. The measurement of the slope of Phase III is a noninvasive method for estimating cardiac output, since the mixed venous blood flow contributes to the generation of this slope. The appearance of dips **(Fig. C)** in this phase indicates spontaneous respiratory efforts in a paralyzed patient or artifacts from the surgical manipulation in abdomen. Phase IV represents the beginning of inspiration which shows the rapid fall of CO$_2$ tension toward the base line. One may see **(Fig. E)** some oscillations, called the "cardiogenic oscillation" in this down stroke. They are believed to be due to the contraction and relaxation effect of heart and intrathoracic great vessels on the lungs, causing air to flow in and out in an oscillating manner. **Figure F** indicates some leak in sampling line during IPPV. It results in a plateau of long duration and a brief upswing at the end of phase III. The plateau height is inversely proportional to the size of leak. The brief upswing is due to the next inspiration when positive pressure transiently pushes undiluted end-tidal gas through the sampling line. **Figure G** shows return to spontaneous ventilation. The first breath is small. The subsequent breath increases in height with gradual resumption of normal waveform. **Figure H** shows irregular plateau and/or base line. It may be due to the displacement of ET-tube in the upper larynx or lower pharynx. It may also be due to the pressure on chest which causes the small volume of gas to move in and out of the lungs.

rises sharply at the end of phase III or alveolar plateau. This is also responsible for the peak of phase III. The phase III is followed by phase IV which is characterized by the rapidly decreasing value of CO$_2$ tension toward the inspired value. This is caused by the inspired gas being sucked into the analyzing site.

The capnograph value, during inspiration, represents the CO$_2$ tension or its concentration in the inspired air which depends on the type of the breathing circuit, fresh gas flow, respiratory rate, and the amount of rebreathing. Rebreathing of the expired gas containing CO$_2$ due to any reason causes an inspired level of CO$_2$ tension above the baseline. The probable causes of rebreathing are: improper circuit with increased dead space, low fresh gas flow, exhaustion of CO$_2$ absorber, high respiratory rate, etc.

In a side-stream capnometer, the sampling flow rate has a greater impact on the capnograph value. So, it should be taken into account during interpretation. Sampling flow rate by suction pump in a capnometer can vary between 50 mL and 400 mL/min, but usually in an adult it is adjusted to 150 mL/min. When the respiratory fresh gas flow decreases below the sampling value, such as in pediatric anesthesia or low-flow anesthesia, then the capnometer contributes significantly to the bulk flow, in and out of the respiratory circuit. In this situation, for sampling the monitor should aspirate the gas alternatively from the trachea or the inspiratory limb, causing an oscillatory graph in phase III and phase IV which is known as "cardiogenic oscillation". It appears as a small, tooth like, regular wave at the end of expiratory phase.

The other probable explanations of cardiogenic oscillations are:

i. It is due to the contraction and relaxation of heart and the movement of intrathoracic great vessels of lungs which forces the air out of the lungs in oscillating fashion. So, this rate of oscillation matches with the heart rate.

ii. Negative intrathoracic pressure, low respiratory rate, reduction of vital capacity, increased heart size ratio, low tidal volume, low inspiratory and expiratory ratio, muscular relaxation, etc. may cause cardiogenic oscillations. But, in most of the cases it can be corrected by increasing the flow rate, respiratory rate, tidal volume or by applying positive end-expiratory pressure (PEEP). It is very common in the pediatric group of patients, because the size of infant's heart is relatively greater than the thorax. If the capnometer is less sophisticated or the wave of oscillations are large, then the instrument may count each wave as a breath and display an erroneously high respiratory rate.

The inaccurate reading by a capnometer is also produced, if the sampling gas is diluted with the fresh gas from the circuit. This occurs:

- If the fresh gas flow is too high.
- If the gas sampling site is far away from the patient.
- If there is high respiratory rate.
- If the tidal volume is small (particularly in neonates and infants) in comparison to the size of breathing system.

Normally, the end-tidal CO_2 tension (ETPCO$_2$) varies between 35 and 45 mm of Hg. The PCO_2 above 45 mm Hg is called hypercapnia and below 35 mm Hg is called hypocapnia.

Causes of hypercapnia:
- Fever and malignant hyperpyrexia
- Depression of the respiratory center due to any cause with concomitant reduction of total ventilation and elevation of PCO_2
- Reduction of ventilation, caused by partial paralysis of the respiratory muscles, neuromuscular transmission disorders, high spinal anesthesia, etc.
- Acute respiratory distress including acute asthma, pulmonary edema, acute exacerbation of COPD, respiratory failure, etc.
- Inadequate ventilation in a controlled ventilated patient
- Insufflation of CO_2 in the peritoneal cavity, during laparoscopy

- Defects in mechanical ventilation setting
- IV administration of bicarbonate
- Inadequate fresh gas flow

Causes of hypocapnia:
- Hyperventilation
- Increased dead space in presence of normal P_aCO_2. In some alveoli where there is no blood flow, there is no transfer of CO_2 from blood to alveoli. Thus, the gas emanating from such alveoli containing no CO_2, dilutes the exhaled gas with CO_2 coming from other region of the lungs and ETCO$_2$ tension decreases.
- High sampling rate in presence of an elevated fresh gas flow rate for side-stream capnometer.
- In atelectasis, where alveoli are perfused but are ventilated, then there is a shunting of mixed venous blood and no diffusion of CO_2 from blood to alveoli.

In atelectasis, there is high P_aCO_2, but a normal or low ETCO$_2$ tension. This causes high arterial and alveolar end-tidal CO_2 tension difference (P_aCO_2 - PETCO$_2$), which ensures one of the indications for the delivery of PEEP ventilation. This low ETCO$_2$ tension in atelectasis is due to the impairment of the diffusion of CO_2 from the blood into alveoli. However, excessive PEEP again causes the over distention of alveoli which will hamper perfusion and CO_2 exchange, causing high P_aCO_2 and PETCO$_2$ difference. So, an optimum PEEP should be maintained.

Sometimes, a sudden dip in alveolar plateau phase or phase III, during controlled ventilation, indicates initiation of spontaneous respiration. This is due to the passing of a small bolus of fresh inspired gas (not containing any CO_2) into sampling site by the sudden onset of spontaneous inspiration. This dip can be interpreted as (i) the partial recovery from anesthesia, (ii) the activation of respiration, induced by sudden stimulation from surgical site, (iii) the inadequate inspiratory power, during switching over from mechanical to spontaneous ventilation, and (iv) the first sign for the need of reversal of neuromuscular blockade.

MONITORING OF APNEA FOR NONINTUBATED PATIENT

Apnea is defined as the cessation of respiration for >10 seconds. It should be detected as soon as possible to save a patient's life. For the intubated patients, this apnea can be easily detected within a second by capnography or airway pressure monitor. But, in nonintubated patient this detection of apnea is challenging. In nonintubated patient, this detection of apnea is performed either by monitoring airflow through nostril or by monitoring chest movement.

- *Monitoring airflow at nostril:* Airflow at nostril is detected (i) by placing an acoustic probe in nasal cavity, or (ii) by encasing the patient's head and neck in tight canopy (very claustrophobic for conscious patient), or (iii) by noninvasive capnography by placing a special $ETCO_2$ probe in nasal cavity.

- *Monitoring of chest movement:* The methods, employed to detect chest movements, are:
  - *Impedance plethysmography:* This is also called as *respiratory inductance plethysmography*. Here, the thorax is encircled by elastic bands, containing conductor coil and movements are detected by the changes in impedance (resistance). A modified version of impedance plethysmography, called as the *photoplethysmography* is more sensitive for this purpose.
  - *Transthoracic impedance pulmonometry*: It is also known as *electrical impedance pulmonometry*. Here, a small amount of current is delivered continuously through ECG leads. It detects continuously the change in transthoracic electrical impedance, accompanied by chest movement due to respiration and is converted to respiratory rate by software present in monitor. All advanced ECG monitor have this parameter, incorporated in them. Electrical impedance pulmonometry is the simplest and most commonly used method to detect apnea in a nonintubated patient. However, the measurement of respiratory rate by using nasal $ETCO_2$ cannulas have yielded more accurate results than thoracic impedance technology.

The major limitation of these monitors is that they cannot detect obstructive apnea. The patients with upper airway obstruction produce paradoxical chest movements and monitor cannot differentiate these paradoxical movements from normal chest movements. Pulse oximeter does not directly detect apnea. But, by indirect way (decrease in O_2 saturation of pulsatile blood) to detect apnea, it is very important, not only in intubated patient, but also in nonintubated patient.

By these impedance plethysmography or impedance pulmonometry, not only respiratory rate is measured, but also tidal volume is measured and from these two parameters minute volume and other respiratory volumes are also measured (which is discussed below).

■ MONITORING OF ANESTHETIC GASES

For three reasons each component of a mixture of anesthetic gases or vapors is analyzed and measured in practice, both during inspiration and expiration. These reasons are:
  i. To establish the identity and the concentration of individual anesthetic agent which is required for the

better control and delivery of anesthesia to patient, including the judgment of depth of anesthesia and also the stability of hemodynamic system.
  ii. To detect and reduce the atmospheric pollution
  iii. To assess the metabolic or cardiorespiratory function by measuring the cardiac output, either by analyzing the respired gases (O_2, CO_2, and N_2) or by using inert tracer gases, such as helium, argon, etc.

The concentration of different anesthetic gases or agents such as nitrous oxide, halothane, isoflurane, sevoflurane, etc., used during anesthesia (including O_2 and CO_2 also), are measured by the following various methods.

Mass Spectrometry

The mass spectrometer, which once upon a time was a special laboratory tool for research purposes only, has now become a common operating room instrument for measuring the concentration of anesthetic gases. It measures the concentration of individual gases in a mixture, largely depending on the basis of their molecular weight. The basic principle on which the mass spectrometer works is based on the ratio in between the quantity of charge of a molecule after its ionization (q) to its mass (m), i.e., (q/m).

The mechanism of action of a mass spectrometry is shown in **Figure 10**. Here, the gas samples are passed through an electron beam (ionizer) which strips one or more electrons from the individual gas molecule and gives them a positive charge.

Then, after ionization the ions of individual gas molecules are passed through a magnetic field, oriented perpendicular to their direction of motion. Now, the magnetic force situated at right angle to the ions deflects each ion by an angle "α", and falls on the photodetectors. The deflecting angle (i.e., the path of the ion becomes curved) is proportional to the charge "q", and the sideways acceleration from this force

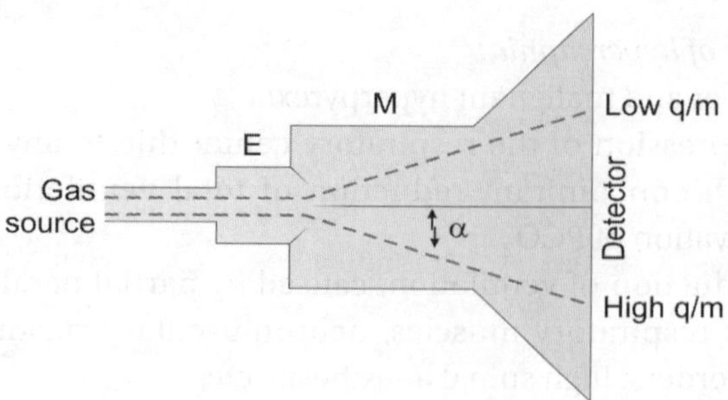

Fig. 10: Schematic diagram of a mass spectrometer. Gas molecules at low pressure are ionized and accelerated by an electrical field (E). The ions are then passed through a perpendicular magnetic field (M) that deflects their path through an angle α. This deflection angle is determined by the ratio of charge to mass (q/m) of the ions and is used to identify the species of the gas.

is inversely proportional to the mass "m" of the molecule. Therefore, the angle of deflection "α" is the function of q/m. Thus, photodetectors which are placed at specific locations measure the individual gas concentration, which is proportional to the count of molecules deflected per minute.

During the measurement of the concentration of gases in a gas mixture, the gas samples are drawn from the anesthetic circuit into an evacuated ionizing chamber, where they are bombard by electron beams. Then, the positively charged ions are passed through a slit from the ionizing chamber to the next chamber. In the next chamber, these ions are accelerated by a plate to which negative voltage is applied. The magnetic field from the plate deflects the ions according to their charge and mass ratio (q/m). Then, the number of ions that strike on the detector is proportional to the partial pressure (which again depends on the concentration of the gas in the mixture) of the gas in the sample. Thus, the streams of ions of different gases are detected by varying the accelerating and focusing voltage. Hence, a mass spectrum is produced by relating the detector output on the Y-axis (calibrated to the concentration of gas) and by accelerating the voltage on the X-axis (calibrated to the molecular weight).

The ability of a mass spectrometer to measure the concentration of different individual gases depends upon the charge/mass ratio of that gases. Since, most of the ions created by the ionization are singly charged due to the missing of a single electron, so the most important variable is, therefore, the molecular weight. Hence, the two different gases of same molecular weight such as N_2O and CO_2 are not distinguishable ordinarily by a mass spectrometer, using the principles outlined above.

During ionization, some molecules also lose two electrons, instead of one and become doubly charged. So, they behave like ions, with half of their mass. Also, during ionization some molecules become fragmented causing a secondary peak, rather than a single peak for each gas molecule, such as during the identification and quantification of CO_2 and N_2O. Both the CO_2 and N_2O produce a parent peak at 44 Da, but also produce a secondary peak at 12 Da and 30 Da, respectively.

Mass spectrometer is a bulky and expensive instrument, but has a very short response time which is approximately 100–200 milliseconds. So, the original implementation of its use in anesthesia has placed (located) it in a remote-central location. Hence, the samples are conveyed by tubes from multiple operation theaters to the remote-centrally located spectrometer for the analysis of gases, used in anesthesia on a time-sharing basis. This time-sharing basis increases the delay time and because of the greater length of the tubing

necessary to convey the sample gases from the patient to the machine. Recently, a number of small spectrometer instruments are available for use in individual operating rooms. These instruments typically can measure the gases, like O_2, CO_2, N_2O, N_2, halothane, enflurane, isoflurane, etc., simultaneously.

Raman Scattering Analyzer

When a photon particle, from the source of a light, collides with a molecule of any gas, then there is some absorption of kinetic energy from the photon. After that, this photon is scattered sideways, having a lower energy level and longer wavelength. This phenomenon is called as the "Raman scattering". In this phenomenon, the degree of the absorption of energy by this gas molecule from the falling photon particle and the wavelength of the scattered photon or light depends upon the molecular weight and the structure of the gas molecule. Spectral analysis of that scattered light may, therefore, be used to measure the concentrations of individual gas in the mixture. As a photon source the light which is usually used is argon laser with the wavelength of 488 nm. This type of gas analyzer is fast, accurate, and relatively compact for the measurement of CO_2, N_2, O_2 and other anesthetic gases.

Infrared Absorption Technique

This technique is used in most of the modern anesthetic monitors, with the same principle, as for the measurement of CO_2 in a capnometer and with the same problems. The advantages of this technique are rapid and accurate analysis with the identification of each gas, present in the mixture. In this method, the infrared light beam is first projected through the gas sample and then the intensity of the transmitted light, after its absorption, is measured by a detector. Gases, which molecules contain two dissimilar atoms or more than two electrons in their outer orbit, absorb infrared radiation in the same region of spectrum.

The CO_2 absorbs the infrared light with a characteristic peak at the wavelength of this light close to 4.3 μm (4,300 nm). Several other molecules of anesthetic gases such as N_2O, O_2, CO, and water vapor also absorb the infrared light in this area of the spectrum of wavelength of infrared light. Thus, CO_2 measurement is disturbed, especially if the composition of incident light includes wavelength, other than those of a very narrow spectrum around the CO_2 absorption peak. See **Figure 11**.

As discussed above, the infrared absorption technique is used to analyze the molecules having only a dipole atom, therefore, it cannot be used to identify O_2 and nitrogen.

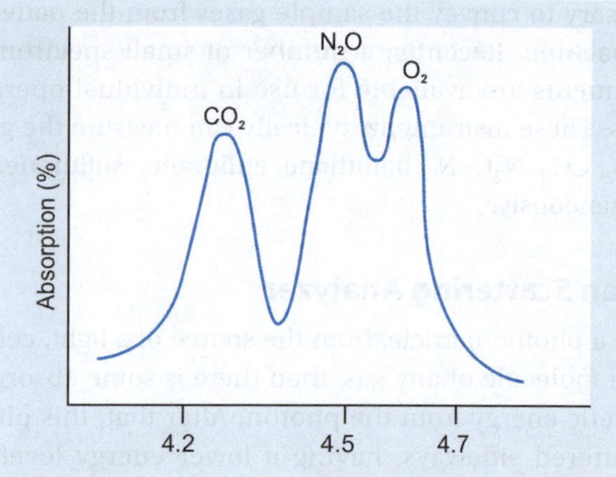

Fig. 11: Infrared analyzer is an instrument which gives a continuous recording of the concentration or tension of CO_2 in a mixture of gases. It is also used to measure the other volatile anesthetic agents by careful selection of the infrared wavelength which depends on the potential components of the gas mixture. The use of a specific infrared wavelength of 4.2 µm for the analysis of CO_2 should avoid the interference from the presence of N_2O and O_2. The infrared radiation is emitted from a hot wire and a particular wavelength is obtained by passing it through an interference filter. There may be a rotating disk which permits the passing of infrared light of different specific wavelengths and simultaneous analysis of various types of gases. Basically, the amount of absorption of radiation is proportional to the concentration of CO_2 and other gases present in the analyzing chamber. After passing through the sample analyzing chamber and absorption of it (infrared light) by the gases, the radiation is focused on the photodetector situated on the opposite site. Greater the absorption of infrared radiation by the gas sample, lesser will be the radiation detected by the detector. Consequently, it is possible to process the detector output electronically to indicate the concentration of the gas present. Most of the newer instruments use a second beam, which passes through the reference chamber. Any changes in the output which are not due to the changes in CO_2 concentration in the sample cell, also appear at a reference detector, and are subtracted from the output of the sample detector. Such an analyzer is called a double beam instrument.

Gas-liquid Chromatography

Chromatography was originally introduced, in 1906, by a Polish botanist, named Tswett, for the separation of different color pigments, present in a plant extract. It is of four different types such as: (i) Paper chromatography, (ii) Thin layer chromatography, (iii) Column chromatography, and (iv) Gas-liquid chromatography. The gas-liquid chromatography is a very helpful instrument to separate and analyze the components of gases in a mixture. Not only that, in addition, it may be used to analyze blood samples, containing different solute, such as the volatile, intravenous, local anesthetic, and anticonvulsant agents, etc. In combination with the mass spectrometer, it is also an important analytic tool, because the mass spectrometer identifies the molecular fragments, present in any concentration, which are eluded from chromatography.

MEASUREMENT OF CENTRAL RESPIRATORY DRIVE FOR MONITORING OF RESPIRATORY FUNCTION

The main causes of respiratory failure are: depressed central ventilatory drive, abnormalities of pulmonary mechanics, and impairment of respiratory gas exchange. Among these, the depressed central ventilatory drive is the most common cause of respiratory failure. So, the measurement of ventilatory drive is very important for the assessment of the function of respiratory system, particularly in anesthesia where most of the anesthetic agents are respiratory depressants and also in the process of weaning of patients from mechanical ventilators. Ventilatory drive is measured directly by minute ventilation (Ve) and indirectly by P_aCO_2 level. But, clinically, the measurement of Ve and P_aCO_2 is very difficult. So, various measures for the assessment of neural respiratory central drive have been sought. These are:

- By dividing and examining the respiratory waveform into inspiratory and expiratory components.
- *By measuring the inspiratory flow rate:* This is obtained by dividing the tidal volume by inspiratory time (tidal volume/inspiratory time). The drawback in this method is that many patients have high ventilatory drive, but is not able to translate this drive into a respiratory output, because of their impaired ventilatory mechanics.
- *By measuring the rate of respiration:* It is also a method of monitoring the respiratory drive. But, the main disadvantage is that respiratory depression does not always indicate the reduction of respiratory rate. In narcotic-induced respiratory depression, tidal volume is mainly depressed with a little change in the respiratory rate.
- *By measuring the value of P_{100}:* It is another sophisticated method for assessing the respiratory drive. The P_{100} is defined as the maximum negative inspiratory airway pressure, which is obtained 100 milliseconds after the temporary occlusion of airway in a spontaneously breathing patient. It is a very useful index of respiratory drive without being affected by any voluntary effort and changes in respiratory mechanics. The normal value of P_{100} is 1–2 cmH_2O and is not appreciably noticed by a patient during its measurement. Possibly, one could also use P_{100} as a guide to the discontinuation of mechanical ventilation, after general anesthesia.

MONITORING OF PULMONARY MECHANICS

Till now, we were monitoring the function of respiratory system by measuring the concentration of O_2, CO_2, and other anesthetic gases or agents in blood, inspiratory air, and expiratory air. Also, we have tried to monitor the function of respiratory system by measuring the ventilatory drive which are described just before. But, now we will discuss the monitoring of the functions of respiratory system by measuring the respiratory mechanics.

There are four principal determinants for the measurement of pulmonary mechanics. These are: *flow, pressure, volume,* and *time.* From these, we can monitor the respiratory mechanics by measuring the *lung compliance* and *airway resistance* and by drawing the different loops such as *flow-volume loop, pressure-volume loop,* etc. But, it should be kept in mind that all these parameters are interrelated.

Flow

The measurement of the rate of flow of air or gases (both during inspiratory and expiratory phase of respiration) is useful for two reasons: (i) the measurement of airway resistance and lung compliance requires the measurement of both the rate of flow of air or gases and the pressure in airway or lungs, and (ii) from the measurement of flow the most ventilators calculate the different lung volumes, such as: tidal volume, minute volume, etc. by multiplying it with time. Again, from these volumes, the computers of modern ventilators can also calculate the volume-pressure curve, the flow-volume curve, lung compliance, airway resistance, etc. So, before the measurement of any parameter, the measurement of flow and pressure is most important. The flow is measured by the following methods.

Rotameter

It is a variable orifice (but constant pressure) type of flowmeter. Another type of variable orifice type of flowmeter is a peak flowmeter. Rotameter consists of a vertical glass tube, inside of which a metal alloy-made bobbin rotates. At the bottom of the rotameter there is fine flow control valve which controls the flow of gas. When this bottom valve is opened, then the pressure of the gas forces the bobbin up in the tube and gas starts to flow. The inner wall of the rotameter tube is cone-shaped. This causes the pressure to remain constant throughout the range of flow into tube. The tube is calibrated according to the amount of gas flow, keeping the pressure constant and so the bobbin rotates freely. Each rotameter and its calibration is specific for a specific gas. The laminar flow in a rotameter is found at low-flow rates and depends on the viscosity of that gas. But, turbulent flow predominates at a higher flow rate and it depends on the density of that gas. It is the most common type of flowmeter which is used in all the anesthesia machines to measure the flow of gas.

Peak Flowmeter

This instrument can measure the peak flow rate maximum up to 1,000 L/min and is very useful clinically. In this instrument there is a vane, which rotates during the flow of air through it or a piston which moves against a constant force, produced by a light spring. The maximum position, adopted by the vane or piston, depends on the peak expiratory flow rate and this position is held by a ratchet. Then, the reading is obtained from a mechanical pointer which is attached to the vane or the piston. The serial measurement of peak expiratory flow rate is useful to assess the prognosis in asthmatic patients. This measurement may be performed by using a handheld Wright's peak flowmeter.

Bourdon Gauge Flowmeter

It is already said that the two above-mentioned flowmeters are of variable-orifice, but of constant pressure type. But, this Bourdon gauge flowmeter and pneumotachograph (discussed next) are of variable pressure, but a fixed-orifice flowmeter. This gauge is calibrated to the gas flow rate according to the pressure changes across a fixed orifice. However, these rugged flowmeters are useful for measuring the flow of gas from cylinders at high pressure.

Pneumotachograph

When patients are being ventilated mechanically, then the respiratory parameters are easily measured. It is also relatively easy to make such measurements continuous by a pneumotachograph. The pneumotachograph measures the rate of flow by sensing the pressure changes across a small, but fixed orifice. Usually, the tidal volume is measured by observing the displacement of inflating bellows, or by passing the respired (inspired + expired) gas through a respirometer. But, in some machines, the gas flow is also measured by pneumotachograph.

In pneumotachograph, a pressure transducer records the changes in pressure due to obstruction to the flow of gas. Then, the pressure-transducer transduces it into a continuous electrical output to give the amount of flow and volume digitally. The obstruction produced in pneumotachograph may be in the form of a gauge screen (screen type pneumotachograph), or a bundle of small tubes aligned along the airway (Fleisch pneumotachograph or vitalograph). The pressure change against the obstruction in pneumotachograph is related to the flow rate and from this pressure change the flow is measured in a pneumotachograph. The pneumotachographs are not accurate over a very wide range of gas flow and are also affected by the humidity of flowing gas, its temperature, gas composition, etc. So, it requires frequent calibration, correction, and compensation. In some ventilators, the measured minute volume is compared with the selected or set volume and an alarm starts to buzz, whenever there is a discrepancy. A vortex type pneumotachograph, which is also frequently used in modern mechanical ventilators, works by measuring the interruptions of an ultrasonic beam, which is placed across a tube and is continuously disrupted by the laminar flow, resulting in vortices.

Ultrasonic Flowmeter

This instrument works (measures the rate of flow of air or gases) by measuring the speed of ultrasonic waves, propagated parallel to the direction of flow of air or gases.

Hot-wire Anemometers

It consists of an electrically heated wire, placed across the flow of a gas stream. The flow of gas tends to cool the wire and changes the electrical conductivity, thus sending changes in electrical signal. The changing electrical signal reads the amount of gas flow.

Flow is also measured by the amount of additional electrical current, necessary to maintain the wire at a constant temperature during flow of gases, because when gases flow over a wire, it cools down. This method is highly sensitive for the measurement of gas flow, but is highly dependent on the original temperature of flowing gas and the contamination of gas with water droplets.

Volume

Different lung volumes or air/gases entering or coming out of the lungs are measured by the following ways.

Drager Volumeter

This is a very simple and accurate device to measure the volume of dry gases entering or coming out of the lungs. But, it is affected by moisture. Here, the volume of gas that flows through this volumeter is measured by measuring the rotation of two light, interlocking, dumbbell-shaped rotor which is directly proportional to the flow of gas.

Wright Spirometer

This device contains a light vane which is made of mica and rotates within a small cylinder. Then, the inflowing volume of air, which is to be measured, is directed to it by a tangential slit. Thus, during the flow of air through this wright spirometer, the rotation of this mica vane drives a gear chain which is attached with a pointer on a dial, from where the flow rate can be measured. From this flow rate, the machine calculates the volume of air or gases that flow through it. Thus, the minute volume can be read directly and then the tidal volume can be calculated from this reading and respiratory rate.

It has dead space of only 25 mL and is of low resistance which is self-rectifying. Although the response in this type of spirometer is nonlinear, but still it is reasonably accurate in the relevant range of minute volume (4–15 L/min). But, the Wright spirometer seriously over-reads at high-minute volume (>15 L/min) and under reads at low-minute volume (<4 L/min). This is due to the inertia of the moving parts of machine. As with many other devices, its accuracy also deteriorates, when it becomes wet. Clinically, it is also a very useful and convenient instrument for cooperative and unanesthetized patients. But, for the most accurate measurement of lung volumes in a cooperative patient, dry gas meters and other sophisticated electronic pulmonary function analyzers may be employed. However, these instruments are not in common use in ITU. Alternatively, a bellows type of dry gas spirometer (e.g., the vitalograph) can be brought to bedside to measure the peak expiratory flow rate, vital capacity, and timed expiratory volume (e.g., FEV_1).

Integration from Flow Signal

The volume of air or gases, flowing in and out of the lungs, is also measured indirectly from the flow rate. The flow signal (electrical signals originating from flow rate) from different flowmeters is integrated electronically over the time to measure the volume of air or gases entering the lungs.

Indirect Method to Measure Volume

In an unintubated but anesthetized patient, the volume of ventilation can also be measured by monitoring the changes in external dimensions of thorax and abdomen, either clinically by direct observation or by using one of the techniques mentioned below.

In an unintubated but anesthetized patient, the volume of thorax is measured from the movement of thorax and abdomen by a magnetometer. This works by measuring the anteroposterior thoracic, lateral thoracic, and abdominal dimensions are called as the pneumography. Here, some nonelastic tapes are placed around the chest and abdomen. Then, the ends of these tapes are connected to a displacement sensor and the volume is measured. Another method of measurement of volume is from the movement of the thorax and abdomen by using coils of wire, sewn into an elasticated strap that encircles the thorax and abdomen. The expansion of the chest and the abdomen increases the space between the coils. So, it alters the inductance, generated by a high frequency AC current and converts it into electrical signal. This method is called the "Respiratory Inductance Plethysmography". The self-inductance of the coils which changes in proportion to the changes of the encircled areas can be calibrated to provide continuous monitoring of the volume of ventilation. As the result of this method is sensitive to the changes in posture and position of the body, so it cannot be used during surgery on thorax and abdomen.

In an intubated patient, the measurement of tidal volume, respiratory rate, and from these the measurement of minute ventilation is easy. Now, these parameters are routinely measured by modern mechanical ventilators. The measurement of ventilatory volume in a conscious patient has been discussed before and during the discussion of flow and volume measurement (by spirometer, vitalograph, etc.)

Pressure

Methods of measurement of pressure have been discussed before (See the measurement of airway pressure).

Pulmonary Compliance

During the process of expiration, when the lung volume reaches at the level of functional residual capacity (FRC), then the pressure at the level of mouth and alveoli is same and atmospheric. So, in such position, there is no tendency of gas to flow in and out of the lungs. In such position, the tendency of the lungs to collapse (due to the *elastic tissue* of *lungs* and *chest wall* and the *surface tension* of *alveoli*, all of which constitute the elastic resistance) is exactly counterbalanced by the outward pull of chest wall.

After that, during the process of inspiration gas may, now, start to flow into the lungs by (i) reducing the pressure in alveoli by primary expansion of chest wall, due to the *spontaneous breathing,* caused by the contraction of inspiratory muscles which constitutes the work of breathing, or (ii) increasing the air pressure at the mouth by *IPPV.*

So, each method of inspiration causes a development of pressure gradient between the mouth and alveoli, resulting in the flow of gas into lungs and thus causing volume changes of it (lung). Hence, the relationship between the change in the volume (Δv) of lungs and thorax, and the pressure gradient (Δp) between the mouth and alveoli is known as compliance (c). At the end of inspiration, gas flow stops and the pressure in all the alveoli again becomes same as that of the mouth and atmosphere. The force acting to impede this flow of gas during inspiration into the lungs are: (i) the elastic resistance of lung parenchyma and soft tissue of chest wall, (ii) the nonelastic resistance of chest wall, comprising the movements of bones at joints, and (iii) the nonelastic frictional resistance due to the flow of gas through air passage. So, for air to flow into the lungs, a pressure gradient has to be developed to overcome all these elastic and nonelastic resistances of the lungs and the chest wall.

Thus, from the point of view of inspiration and to produce tidal airflow, the lungs are passive organs and rely solely on the work, done actively by the diaphragm and the intercostal muscles. Under normal *resting* conditions all the work is done *actively* during inspiration, while expiration is *passive* (during exertion or dyspnea the expiration becomes *active*). During IPPV, the work is done by the breathing machine and again this is also usually done during inspiration, while the expiration is generally passive.

Hence, during inspiration, the expansion of both the lungs and chest wall requires a *distending force* which is *expressed as volume change (in mL) per unit change of distending pressure (in cmH$_2$O),* and this is called as the *compliance* (C). Therefore, compliance (C) = Increase of volume (Δv) in mL/Pressure gradient (Δp) in cmH$_2$O. $C = \Delta v / \Delta p$.

For air to flow into the lungs and to make a volume change, a pressure gradient (a negative or positive, i.e., negative in normal spontaneous breathing, and positive in IPPV) should be developed to overcome the elastic, nonelastic resistance, and frictional resistance. So, the relationship between compliance (C) and resistance (E) is reciprocal, i.e., $C = 1/E$. (E is the change of pressure per unit change of volume or $\Delta p / \Delta v$).

The *total resistance* includes both (i) the elastic and nonelastic resistance of the lungs and the chest wall, and also (ii) the frictional resistance. The total compliance (C_T) is the sum of the compliance of the lungs (C_L) and the compliance of the chest wall (C_{CW}). The relationship between the total compliance (C_T) and the individual compliance of lungs (C_L) and chest wall (C_{CW}) is $1/C_T = 1/C_L + 1/C_{CW}$ or $C_T = (C_L C_{CW}) (C_L + C_W)$.

The individual compliance of the lungs and the chest wall in a normal healthy person is approximately same and it is about 0.2 L/cmH$_2$O (200 mL/cmH$_2$O). Thus, the final and the total change in the volume of *chest wall with lungs* (i.e., thorax) is 0.2 L and this is obtained by pressure gradient of 1 cmH$_2$O, exerted both by the *chest wall and lungs* each. So, the total pressure gradient exerted together by the chest wall and the lungs is 2 cmH$_2$O. Thus, the total thoracic compliance is 0.1 L/cmH$_2$O or 100 mL/cmH$_2$O. However, the normal average value of this is 50–100 mL/cmH$_2$O.

To detect *only the lung compliance* (C_L), the volume change (Δv) and transpulmonary pressure gradient (which is $P_A - P_{PLU} = \Delta p$) should be measured. To detect only the *chest wall compliance* (C_{cw}), the volume change Δv and transmural pressure gradient ($P_{PLU} - P_{ENVIORNMENT} = \Delta p$) should be measured. Thus, to determine the total compliance (C_T), the volume changes (Δv) and the transthoracic pressure gradient Δp ($\Delta p = P_A - P_{ENVIORNMENT}$) should be measured. In clinical practice, the individual CL and CW are not measured, but only the CT is measured.

The compliance is approximately linear over most of its normal ranges. But, it is lower when the volume of lung is very small, i.e., almost fully deflated or when the volume of lung is very high, i.e., almost fully inflated. The former is due to the added force needed to expand the collapsed areas of lung, and also to overcome the surface tension effects. The latter is due to the elastic fibers of the lung reaching their maximum limit.

The lung exhibits *hysteresis*, i.e., the compliance differs both during inflation and deflation. If the compliance is measured when the flow of air has ceased, as during breathholding or apnea in anesthesia, then it is known as the *static compliance* (CSTAT). But, when the volume changes of the lung and the thorax in relation to pressure changes is measured during the process of respiration, then it is known as the *dynamic compliance* (CDYN). For example, during inspiration the work is done to expand the lungs and the thorax from their resting position at FRC. In a healthy supine, paralyzed patient, a sustained inflation pressure of 1 kpa (10 cmH$_2$O) will increase the lung volume to about 0.85 L. So, the static compliance is 0.85 L/kpa or 85 mL/cmH$_2$O, or 0.085 L/cmH$_2$O. However, during an inflation if it is necessary to consider the dynamic compliance, then it is nearly about 70% of the static compliance.

Measurement of Compliance

We can measure both the static (C$_{STAT}$) and dynamic compliances (C$_{DYN}$). It is measured by the pressure-volume relationship, through curves or loops. In these curves and loops, the *changes in lung volume* are displayed on the *vertical axis* against the inspiratory or expiratory *pressure changes* which are displayed on the *horizontal axis*. It is important to know that the pressure, which is used to calculate the *total compliance*, may be of the end of the inspiration or plateau pressure (P$_{PLAT}$). This is for the determination of *static compliance*. However, during the period of inspiratory gas flow, the peak airway inspiratory pressure (P$_{PK}$) is necessary for determination of *dynamic compliance*. For calculation of compliance always the positive end-expiratory pressure (PEEP) must be subtracted from the peak pressure or plateau pressure. The PEEP value is usually obtained from the airway pressure monitor at the end of expiration. So, the C$_{DYN}$ = V$_T$/(P$_{PK}$ - PEEP) and C$_{STAT}$ = V$_T$/(P$_{PLAT}$ - PEEP).

V$_T$ is the tidal volume, which is fixed in volume-cycled ventilators. When there is a development of auto-PEEP, then it should be considered in the place of external PEEP in the above-mentioned equation. Otherwise, the measurement of compliance shall be affected. Auto-PEEP is developed when there is insufficient expiratory time. This is because, it prevents complete emptying of the lungs and elevates the end-expiratory alveolar pressure. This is not detected directly by the airway pressure monitor. Auto-PEEP causes ↓cardiac output, ↓BP, and even EMD (electromechanical dissociation), when the patient is on a ventilator.

The auto-PEEP is most likely to be present, when there is an increase in airway resistance or decrease in compliance causing the prolongation of **(Fig. 12)** the expiratory time. It also occurs when high ventilation rates are required. The measurement of auto-PEEP is accomplished by obstructing the exhalation port of ventilator, while waiting for the onset of next ventilator breath. Alveolar pressure will then become equal to that of the ventilator circuit and auto-PEEP can be measured on the airway pressure monitor (gauze). During the measurement of auto-PEEP, it is important to prevent the fresh gas flow from entering the circuit, which shall falsely elevate the auto-PEEP.

The *total static compliance of thorax (lungs and chest wall)* can also be measured in an intubated patient by occluding the tube and measuring the pressure in the system. After that, the tube is unclamped and the volume of air or gas expired is collected and measured in a spirometer. From this, a pressure-volume curve can be plotted and the total static compliance can be measured. For the measurement of *only static compliance of lung*, the pressure gradient between the airway and the pleural space has to be measured. The direct measurement of intrapleural pressure by placing the tip of a sampling catheter within the pleural space is not possible practically. So, the esophageal pressure, which closely parallels the intrapleural pressure is measured. Since this measurement is a static one, so it is made with the patient holding his breath, after having inspired a known volume of air from the spirometer. The procedure is then repeated a number of times with different volumes, so that a pressure

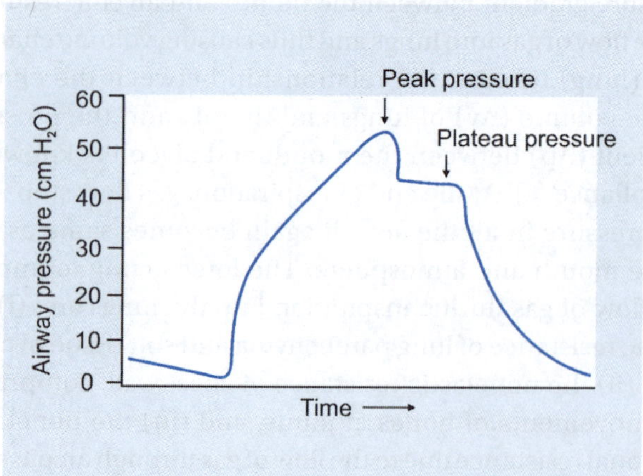

Fig. 12: Airway pressure waveform against time. Decrease in the static compliance causes increase in the plateau pressure. Whereas the decrease in the dynamic compliance results in an increase of peak airway pressure. Peak airway pressure is related to both the airway resistance and the thoracic compliance, whereas plateau pressure is only related to the compliance.

volume curve can be constructed. This is usually linear and gives an average value of static lung compliance. The *compliance of chest wall* is obtained *by the subtraction of lung compliance from the total thoracic compliance.* During the measurement of compliance, the compliance of anesthetic circuit, including the humidifier and gas warming system (which may be as high as 10 mL/cmH$_2$O) must be accounted too, for an accurate result.

The values of measured compliance should always be read in relation to the predicted normal value of a person of same sex, age, height, weight, lung volume, and FRC. Any change in FRC, such as, a simple change in posture can produce a change in compliance. The *total static compliance is decreased* during atelectasis, pulmonary edema, pneumothorax, emphysema, mitral stenosis, external compression on chest, ↑intra-abdominal pressure due to any cause, ↑pressure on rib cage, ↑intrathoracic pressure (pleural effusion), etc. The total *dynamic compliance is decreased* by an elevated airway resistance, such as, due to bronchospasm, mucous plug, kinking of airway or tubes, induction of anesthesia, etc. It has been known for many years that the induction of anesthesia itself causes a decrease in compliance, which is due to the increased elastic recoil property of lungs after induction. A typical value of static compliance of lungs and chest wall in an anesthetized and paralyzed patient is 85 mL/cmH$_2$O. Whereas in a supine position, for the conscious patient it is about 120 mL/cmH$_2$O.

Decreased thoracic compliance to <25 mL/cmH$_2$O is unlikely to result in successful weaning off from mechanical ventilation. During anesthesia, many factors operate at the same time, affecting the compliance, and the situation changes so often that it is frequently impossible to relate any change in compliance to a specific single agent or procedure. For example, drugs may affect the muscles of thorax and change the compliance. The secretions in respiratory tract, alterations in cardiac output, constriction of bronchioles or dilatation of pulmonary vessels, etc.—also alter the compliance.

Resistance

For air to flow in and out of the lungs, a pressure gradient, between the alveoli and the environment, has to be developed at the cost of energy. The work of breathing supplies this energy and is responsible for this propulsion of air. But, the flow of air in and out of the lungs is opposed by some factors or force which is called as the resistance (R). So, the function of the work of breathing is to supply energy which will overcome this resistance to create the pressure gradient, and thus helps the air to flow in and out of the lungs. Hence, the relationship between the pressure gradient (Δp) and the flow of air into the lungs or the rate of change of volume

(Δv) is influenced by the resistance. So, the resistance (R) is defined as the change in pressure for (per) unit change in volume, or R = Δp/Δv.

This equation of resistance is equal to the equation of elasticity, but is reciprocal to compliance. The normal value of total resistance in respiratory system is 1.5 cmH$_2$O/L. But, under anesthesia, it may rise as high as 9 cmH$_2$O/L.

There are three essential components of resistance and these are:

i. Elastic resistance, due to lung parenchyma and soft tissues of thoracic wall.
ii. Nonelastic resistance, due to the friction as well as due to the movement of the bony structure of chest wall.
iii. Frictional resistance in airway due to the movement of air.

Elastic Resistance of the Lungs

During inflation, the changes (increase) in the lung volume occur, as a result of the expansion *forces* applied to the lungs, which is expressed as *pressure.* This is the concept of compliance. Whereas, the concept of elastance or elastic resistance is opposite to the compliance which prevents this change in volume of lung (expansion of lung). Thus, to summarize, the compliance *which is the change in volume per unit change of pressure* works against the resistance, *which is change in pressure per unit change in volume.*

The elastic resistance of lungs is also the force which tends to return the lungs to its original size after stretching or inflation and is responsible for the air to exit. It should not be thought of as the force required to expand the lungs. One of the principal factors, causing the elastic recoil of the lung, is the presence of elastic fibers within the pulmonary tissue. Another important factor, contributing to the elastic resistance, is the surface tension of the fluid, lining the alveolar walls. *At larger lung volumes,* connective or elastic tissue elements predominate in the elastic resistance. Whereas, *at lower lung volumes* the effects of the surface tension in alveoli predominate in elastic resistance. The important role of surface tension of the fluid, lining the alveolar walls, is to draw the opposing walls closer together, so that the alveoli collapse. If this fluid, lining the alveoli, is only water, then it would exert a considerable elastic pull of about 70 dynes/cm. But, fortunately, the presence of surfactant (detergent-like agent which reduces surface tension) within this water, lining the alveolar wall, reduces this collapsing pull to as little as 2–8 dynes/cm.

The alveolar wall is always lined with a thin layer of fluid and the curved surface of the lining fluid on the alveolar wall creates a tension. This tends to make the surface area of the alveoli which is exposed to the air as little as possible, and hence the alveoli collapse. Thus, this collapsing force or tension in alveoli (on alveolar wall) is called as the surface tension. It follows the Laplace rule, i.e., $P = 2T/R$ or $T = \frac{1}{2}PR$. Where, P is the alveolar pressure, T is the surface tension, and R is the alveolar radius.

From the above equation it is clear that radius is directly proportional to the surface tension. If the radius of the alveoli decreases, i.e., when the alveolar size reduces during expiration, then the surface tension tending to collapse the alveoli will increase and a vicious cycle will be established. It can be explained simply by the fact that liquid molecules are crowded much closer together on the curved lining surface, when the alveoli decrease in size and thus gradually increase the collapsing or pulling surface tension force (elastic resistance).

But, in fact, this does not happen. Because, the alveoli are coated with a detergent like chemical, called surfactant, which reduces the surface tension or the elastic recoiling property of alveoli. As the alveoli deflate and the size decreases (during expiration), the amount of surfactant per unit area of alveolar membrane increases, and so the surface tension is more and more reduced, which is proportional to the increase in surfactant concentration per unit area of alveolar surface, due to the reduction of alveolar radius. In this way, the action of surfactant becomes more efficient, when the alveoli decrease in size. Therefore, contrary to what would be predicted on the basis of Laplace's law, the elastic recoiling (collapsing) resistance of the smaller alveoli is lesser than the larger alveoli, and hence the smaller alveoli can be inflated more easily than the larger ones.

Nonelastic Structural Resistance

The nonelastic structural resistance of thorax is composed of the thoracic wall, the diaphragm, and the abdominal contents and is due to the movement (friction) of these structures among them.

Airway Frictional Resistance (Nonelastic)

Airway resistance is important, because it is dependent on the length and the size of the lumen of bronchial tree. This airway nonelastic frictional resistance also depends on the type of flow. The flow of air through the bronchial tree may be *turbulent* or *laminar*. Laminar flow occurs at low flow rates and in the smaller bronchi. Laminar flow rate (V) is related to the driving pressure (δp) by Poiseuille's law or equation, i.e., $V = \delta p \, \pi \, r^{4}/8 \, nL$. Where, r is the radius of the tube, L is the length of the tube, and n is the viscosity of gas.

Radius of the tube is critical. Halving of the tube diameter reduces the flow by a factor of 16, for the same driving pressure (δp). This has a very important implication in pediatric practice. Because, to maintain the same flow in a tube which is reduced half in diameter, the driving force should be increased by 16 times.

Laminar flow occurs when the gas passes down the tube, less than a certain critical velocity. When flow exceeds the critical velocity, it becomes turbulent. Airway resistance in turbulent flow can be lowered by density. This explains why low-density gas such as helium diminishes the resistance to flow in severe upper airway obstruction.

The total crosssectional area of the airway increases as branching occurs. Therefore, velocity of airflow decreases. Laminar flow is therefore chiefly confined to the airways, below the main bronchi. The flow in the trachea is turbulent during most of the respiratory cycle. Airway resistance is estimated indirectly by monitoring the flow-time or volume-time relationship, in a passive exhalation after manual inflation of the lungs.

MONITORING OF CENTRAL NERVOUS SYSTEM

■ INTRODUCTION

The central nervous system (CNS) is monitored during intraoperative period by three methods: (1) EEG monitoring, (2) evoked responses monitoring, and (3) cerebral blood-flow monitoring.

Electroencephalogram Monitoring

- *Uses of EEG:* During the monitoring of CNS by EEG, it is used (i) to monitor the depth of anesthesia and (ii) to assess the cerebral ischemia during neurovascular surgeries, especially during carotid endarterectomy.

- *Effect of anesthetic agents on the modalities of EEG:*
  - All the inhalational and intravenous anesthetic agents produce biphasic pattern on EEG. It means at lower doses, they cause excitation (high frequency and low amplitude waves), followed by depression (low frequency and high-amplitude waves) at higher doses. But, the exceptions are: (i) opioids produce only depression, (ii) ketamine and N_2O produce only excitation, (iii) benzodiazepines, opioids, and dexmedetomidine cannot produce complete suppression of EEG (isoelectric line or electrocortical silence) even at higher doses.

- Similar biphasic pattern of EEG is also seen with hypoxia and hypercarbia. It means early (mild) hypoxia or hypercarbia causes the excitation of CNS (high frequency and low amplitude waves in EEG), while severe hypoxia or hypercarbia causes the depression of CNS (low frequency and high amplitude waves in EEG).
- Hypothermia and cerebral ischemia produce progressive depression of EEG, without any initial excitation.

Evoked Responses Monitoring

Types of Evoked Responses

- *Somatosensory evoked responses:* The tests, detecting the somatosensory evoked responses, are useful for surgeries which put the sensory tracts at risk, e.g., spine surgery, exploration of brachial plexus, brain surgery (involving sensory tract and thalamus), and repair of aneurysm on thoracic or abdominal aorta.
- *Brainstem auditory evoked response (BAER):* Monitoring and detecting the responses, arising from brainstem auditory pathway, are useful for the surgical procedures, involving the auditory pathway in brainstem, e.g., posterior fossa surgeries and resection of acoustic neuroma.
- *Visual-evoked response (VER):* Monitoring of these evoked responses is useful for the surgical procedures which put the visual tract at risk, e.g., optic glioma surgery and pituitary tumor surgery.

- *Motor-evoked response (MER):* These types of monitoring are useful for that surgeries which put the motor tracts (both at the brain and spinal cord level) at risk.

Effects of Anesthetic Agents on Evoked Responses

- All the inhalational agents, propofol, barbiturates, benzodiazepine, neurological injury, ischemia, hypoxia, and hyperthermia inhibit the evoked responses, i.e., decrease the amplitude, and increase the latency (response time) of them (evoked responses).
- Ketamine, opioids, and dexmedetomidine do not have any clinical significant effect on evoked responses.

Cerebral Blood Flow Monitoring

- *Xenon wash-out technique:* It is very cumbersome technique and is not used generally.
- *Transcranial Doppler technique:* To monitor cerebral blood flow, it is very simple, useful, and noninvasive method.
- *Jugular venous oxygen saturation technique:* It is simple but invasive technique.
- Cerebral oximetry by special probe, applied on forehead.
- *Thermodilution technique:* For this invasive method, two thermistors of different temperature are placed in brain and from the difference in temperature of the two areas of brain blood flow is calculated.

MONITORING OF DEPTH OF ANESTHESIA

■ INTRODUCTION

The conceptualization of the depth of anesthesia is very complex. It ranges from in-depth scientific discussion of MAC (minimum alveolar concentration of the anesthetic) to the clinical assessment of light, moderate, and deep anesthesia.

Horace Wells failed to demonstrate the anesthetic properties of N_2O in 1845, when his patient screamed out of pain during dental extraction, even though he later could not recall the sensation of pain (*loss of memory, but no loss of pain sensation*). One year later, WTG Morton succeeded in anesthetizing a patient named Gilbert with ether. Gilbert later reported that he had been aware of the surgery, but had experienced no pain (*loss of pain sensation, but no loss of memory*). Thus, it seems that Well's patient was aware of pain, but had no postoperative recall. While Morton's patient had some postoperative recall, but there was no awareness of pain. After that, 158 years have passed. But, still the assessment and the monitoring of the depth of anesthesia, which includes both the depth of analgesia and the depth of loss of memory, remains evasive. Even now, despite the fact that *awareness under anesthesia* is terrifying both to the patients and also to the anesthesiologists, still the general notion, regarding the *awareness under anesthesia* remains cloudy.

■ HISTORY

A Greek philosopher, in 100 BC, had first described the analgesic and amnesic properties of Mandogra. The word *"Anesthesia"* was also first used by him. Then, after a long gap, in 1721, the word *"Anesthesia"* first appeared in Bailey's English Dictionary. There, it was described as *"the loss of sensation, but not the loss of consciousness."* After that, in 1771, in Encyclopedia Britannica the word "anesthesia" was defined as *"the privation of senses"*. Now, *anesthesia is defined as the triad of analgesia, hypnosis, and skeletal muscle relaxation, with recent addition of the depression of autonomic nervous system.*

For long time, the immobility in response to a noxious stimulus has been used as the measure of the depth of anesthesia. But, it was before the appearance of muscle relaxants. So, after the routine use of muscle relaxants in practice of anesthesia, there appears many problems regarding the assessment of the depth of anesthesia, as the movement part is removed by the paralysis of muscles. So, to circumvent these vexing problems, the anesthetists have turned toward the most easily quantifiable EEG changes, as the measurement of depth of anesthesia.

In 1847, after the introduction of ether in 1846, Plomley had first defined the depth of anesthesia by describing it in different stages, starting from the onset of anesthesia to the surgical endpoint. These stages, described by Plomley were: intoxication, excitement, and the deeper levels. In the same year, a Paris physiologist, named Marie Flourens, concluded that ether with the deepening of anesthesia causes the gradual depression of CNS in order of (from earlier to later) the higher cerebral centers, the cerebellum, the spinal cord, and finally the medulla oblongata, where the respiratory and cardiovascular centers are located. Then, in 1847, John Snow who became very interested on ether soon after its (ether) introduction, described five stages of etherization (ether anesthesia) as a concept of depth of anesthesia in his publication. Among these five stages, the first three were of *light anesthesia*. The fourth stage is comprised of what we would regard as *surgical anesthesia* and in the fifth stage respiration became progressively impaired and is stopped. In the same year, two deaths were reported from ether anesthesia. So, the early 19th century saw the introduction of premedication, different sedatives and opioids and more other rapid acting anesthetics such as N_2O, ethylene, etc., as the anesthetic excitement phase could be traversed more rapidly by them. So, the attempt to measure the depth of anesthesia by only the degrees of etherization, described by John Snow, soon became blunted.

Then, in 1911, the concept of a balanced anesthesia had come, when George Washington taught that psychic stimuli could be obliterated by light general anesthesia, while noxious impulses (stimuli) due to surgery could be blocked by local analgesia. After that, in 1926, John S. Lundy of Mayo clinic first introduced the term "*Balanced Anesthesia*" by combining different methods such as premedication, regional analgesia and general anesthesia, so that pain relief was obtained by judicious mixing of agents and techniques.

Then, in 1937, Guedel's book, named "Inhalational Anesthesia", was published. In this publication, he described the depth of anesthesia in four stages in case of an unpremedicated ether anesthesia, with additional four

planes of stage III. Then, in 1954, Artusio expanded this Guedel's stage I, describing it more into three planes:

1. In plane 1 of stage 1, the patient had no amnesia or analgesia.
2. In plane 2 of stage 1, the patient had total amnesia, but partial analgesia.
3. In plane 3 of stage 1, the patient had complete analgesia and amnesia.

After that, for a long time, the clinical signs to measure the depth of anesthesia, defined by Guedel and Artusio, for intraoperative monitoring, had significant practical utility, during the administration of ether and chloroform anesthesia.

■ MEMORY AND AWARENESS

Before the introduction of ether, in 1846, any surgical operation was like a dream to the physician and a nightmare to the patient. So, there are many stories of torture and suffering by the victims of surgical operation, performed before the introduction of ether. But, even with the passage of time and dramatic improvement of medical science, with the introduction of many potent drugs, equipment and methods till now the vivid descriptions of *pain and recall* during surgery *have not been eliminated completely*.

The *two degrees* of inadequate depth of anesthesia have been described by Vickers. The *first degree* involves the retention of memory of an event that occurred while under anesthesia. This retention of memory or awareness is termed as the "*recall*" and represents a conscious or explicit memory. This conscious memory involves spontaneous recall without the aid of any clue. This positive information may help in enhanced patient recovery. The *second degree* of inadequate depth of anesthesia involves patients with no memory of events, i.e., no recall, but have the responsiveness to the auditory input or verbal command, which is termed as the "*wakefulness*". This "wakefulness" has been described as the response of a patient to a verbal command during and after surgery without recall. This detection of meaningful auditory input under anesthesia has also been termed as the *memory in unconsciousness* or *implicit memory*. This implicit memory or memory in an unconscious state may alter the behavior or performance of a patient. This negative information could have deleterious psychological effects postoperatively. Although, a lot of literature exist regarding the intraoperative recall and wakefulness, but much of it is anecdotal. As a result, our understanding of the factors relevant to the patient's recall or wakefulness is limited.

The incidence of memory (explicit or implicit) during anesthesia is probably underestimated. This is because, very often only the conscious recall is taken as an evidence, but the implicit memory or memory in unconscious state are not taken into account. The incidence of intraoperative awareness or wakefulness has been reported to be about 0.2–2%, but it may be as high as 40% in high-risk situations such as trauma, cesarean section, etc., where narcotics and sedatives are used less judiciously. The incidence of intraoperative memory or recall is similar to both the volatile agents and TIVA technique. *The incidence of recall is high in patients who are given anesthesia with only N_2O, O_2, and muscle relaxants than with potent inhaled anesthetics. However, the use of potent inhaled anesthetics does not guarantee the lack of recall. The intraoperative awareness or recall can also occur with high dose of opioid anesthesia, though it was not thought so previously.*

There are many ways of rendering the adequate depth of anesthesia. But, what is the *"adequate"* is difficult to define. We do not have definite endpoints to measure the adequacy, unlike analgesia. The only reliable endpoint for consciousness is the *absence of response to a voice command, but this does not distinguish light sleep from a deeper one.* However, most patients end up with more hypnotic effect than necessary during intraoperative period and probably is the cause of postoperative drowsiness and delay in discharge from the hospital. At the same time, when large doses of opioids and muscle relaxants are used to suppress the somatic and autonomic responses, then this hypnosis is usually inadequate. It has been shown that even maximum doses of opioids fail to suppress the conscious awareness or memory formation. In a recent study, even at bispectral index (BIS) values of 60–70 which correspond to adequate hypnosis, two-thirds of the patients respond to voice commands, though fortunately only one-fourth of patients recall the episodes of awareness.

Unfortunately, there is no "gold standard" to compare the different states of anesthesia. So, some argue that the "depth" is a wrong term. It is better to know whether the patient is adequately anesthetized or not. So, to divide these states into various levels seems practically inappropriate.

Grades of awareness:

- Explicit memory with recall.
- Explicit memory without recall.
- Implicit memory.
- Not aware.

The last stage is only obtained in deep anesthesia with no sign of awareness or recall at all.

The memory may be *explicit* (needs effort to recall) or *implicit* (effortless). An explicit memory system is *more sensitive* to the effects of GA. With increasing anesthetic concentration, there is little effect on conscious awareness, but explicit memory is lost. Further increase of anesthetic concentration abolishes *conscious awareness*, but implicit memory may be present, leading to postoperative psychosomatic dysfunctions.

Pharmacodynamics and Depth of Anesthesia

Actually, the process of anesthesia and its depth are nothing but the pharmacological responses (pharmacodynamics) of an anesthetic agent. The pharmacodynamics of anesthetic agents again depend on the pharmacokinetic properties of them. So, before discussing the clinical and electrophysiological methods of measuring the depth of anesthesia, we must try to understand the pharmacological concepts of it, i.e., pharmacokinetics and pharmacodynamics of the anesthetic agent which is related to the depth of anesthesia. *Actually, anesthesia is the pharmacological response of an anesthetic drug (pharmacodynamics) and its depth, i.e., the intensity of action depends on the administered dose, the concentration of it in blood, and the elimination of that drug (pharmacokinetics) from the body.* So, measurement of the depth of anesthesia is governed by the pharmacokinetics of that agent and is nothing but the pharmacodynamic measurement of it.

Though, the continuous measurement of depth of anesthesia is actually the continuous measurement of the pharmacodynamics of an anesthetic agent being used, but we indirectly measure it by measuring the blood concentration of that drug (pharmacokinetic factor) and plotting the concentration versus effect relationship on a graph of that drug. Actually, the concentration and effect (kinetic-dynamic) relationship of a drug is a sigmoid-shaped curve **(Figs. 13A and B)**.

The lower minimal or baseline effect and the upper maximal effect of an anesthetic agent are the extremes of drug response. However, the mid-point between the baseline and the maximal effect is commonly referred to as the CP_{50}. This indicates the plasma concentration of a drug that results in 50% of its maximal effect. This parameter indicates the potency of the drug and the sensitivity of the individual to that drug. Although, CP_{50} can be measured and the concentration-versus-effect curve of a drug can be generated, but there are some limitations of this methodology. Because, the concentrations-effect curves of two drugs have two different curves, and if the maximal effects differ, then the CP_{50} values cannot be used to compare the drug potency or the individual sensitivity to it. There are also some other limitations, such as the type of stimulus given to measure the response of a drug **(Table 1)**.

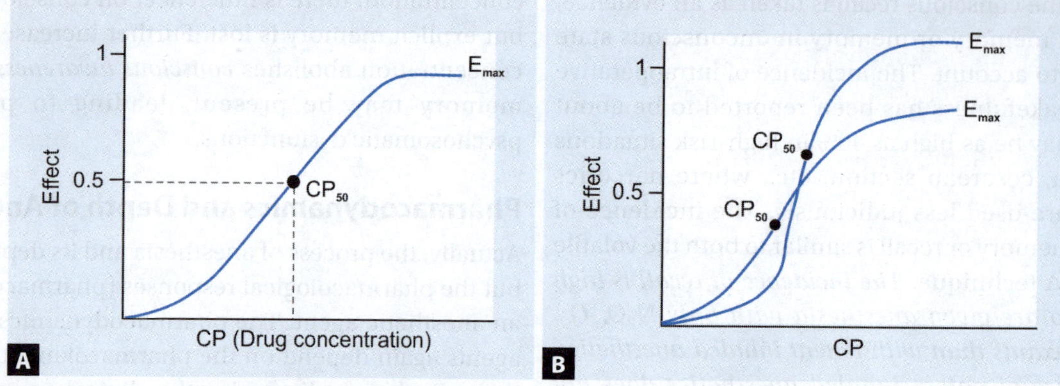

Figs. 13A and B: (A) The relationship between the plasma concentration of a drug (CP) and its effect is like a sigmoidal curve, where: E_{max} = maximal drug effect, CP_{50} = the plasma concentration of drug that produces 50% of its maximal effect. The slope of curve = the rate of change; (B) Two anesthetic agents have different concentration-response curves, with different maximal effects. Their CP_{50} values are also different.

TABLE 1: Pharmacokinetic and pharmacodynamic components of the dose-response relationship.	
Dose of a drug → Concentration in blood → Response in tissue	
↑	↑
pharmacokinetics	*pharmacodynamics*
• Initial volume of distribution	• Concentration or response relationship
• Distributional clearance	• Threshold effect
• Steady state level	• Maximal effect
• Metabolic clearance	• Slope factor
• Terminal elimination	• Equilibrium delay or hysteresis

THE MAC CONCEPT FOR THE MEASUREMENT OF DEPTH OF ANESTHESIA FOR VOLATILE ANESTHETIC AGENTS

At the equilibrium of distribution, the partial pressure of inhaled anesthetic agents should be similar in all the body tissues, e.g., alveolus, blood, and brain. Thus, the measurement of end-tidal concentration of a volatile anesthetic agent which is the representative of the alveolar concentration of it, is nothing but an indirect measurement of the concentration of this agent in brain which is again parallel to the depth of anesthesia. This is because the cerebral perfusion of volatile anesthetic agents is very large and most of the volatile anesthetic agents are highly lipid soluble. So, it is possible to achieve easily an equilibrium between the end-tidal alveolar, arterial and brain concentration (or partial pressure) within 15 minutes of their exposure to a constant alveolar anesthetic concentration.

So, the *MAC is defined* as the minimum alveolar concentration of inhaled anesthetic agent, which is required to prevent in 50% of the subjects from responding to a painful stimulus with gross powerful movement. In this definition, there are two things which are not properly explained: (i) *the nature of the stimulus,* and (ii) the *extent of the response.* Therefore, for the determination of MAC in human beings initially surgical *skin incision* is taken as the standard noxious stimulus, because skin incision represents a reproducible form of supramaximal surgical stimulation. Again, the response to stimulation must entail a positive, gross, purposeful muscular movement, usually of the head or extremities, and this is taken as the *standard response.*

Regarding the type of stimulus and the type of response to the stimulus, there is some controversy in MAC concept, for measuring the depth of anesthesia. For responses, twisting and jerking of head is also considered as positive, but twitching or grimacing is not. Coughing, swallowing, and chewing response are not considered as positive movement for responses. Similarly, there are also other stimuli which are stronger than the initial skin incision. These are: (i) intraoperative profound surgical manipulation, (ii) peritoneal traction, (iii) endotracheal intubation, etc.

Thus, MAC concept has been expanded by using different noxious stimuli and observing their different clinical response. These are MAC-awake, MAC-intubation, MAC-skin incision, MAC-BAR, etc.

MAC-awake

"MAC-awake" is the minimum alveolar concentration of an inhaled anesthetic agent that would allow the opening of eyes on verbal command. This type of stimulus (verbal command) and response (opening of eyes) is used during emergence from anesthesia. Thus, this stimulation (verbal command) is less intense than surgical skin incision, and response (opening of eyes) occurs at lower concentrations of anesthetics than movement to skin incision.

MAC-intubation

"MAC-intubation" is the minimum alveolar concentration of an inhaled anesthetic agent that would inhibit the movement and coughing during endotracheal intubation. Here, the stimulation is more intense and the response is inhibited by minimum alveolar concentration of the anesthetic agent which is necessary for that strong stimulus.

MAC-BAR

"MAC-BAR" is the minimum alveolar concentration of an anesthetic agent which is necessary to prevent the adrenergic response (catecholamine secretion) to skin incision and is measured by the concentration of catecholamines in venous blood.

All the MAC values are nothing but the representation of concentration or dose-effect relationship curves (i.e., pharmacokinetic-pharmacodynamic relationship) of that inhaled agent. But the difference of it depends on the type of the noxious stimuli, used to elicit the different types of responses. However, for measuring the depth of anesthesia, the MAC concepts have other limitations also (which cannot be discussed fully here).

METHODS OF MEASURING AND/OR MONITORING THE DEPTH OF ANESTHESIA

The depth of anesthesia is measured and/or monitored by the following methods:

- Clinical or conventional methods of monitoring
- Brain electrical activity (EEG) monitoring.

Clinical or Conventional Methods of Monitoring of Depth of Anesthesia

This is performed by (i) some clinical techniques (signs), (ii) isolated forearm technique, (iii) lower esophageal contractility (LOC) technique, (iv) heart rate variability (HRV) technique, etc.

Clinical Signs

Among the clinical signs that are used to assess the depth of anesthesia are: change in heart rate, change in blood pressure, body movement, eyelash reflex, pupillary reflex, perspiration, tearing, change in respiratory rate, etc. against different types of stimuli. The clinical signs of *light anesthesia* are: (i) tachycardia, hypertension, (ii) lacrimation, perspiration, (iii) body movement, (iv) tachypnea, breathholding, coughing, laryngospasm, and bronchospasm, (v) eye movement, and (vi) presence of reflexes. For the measurement of depth of anesthesia by clinical signs the most commonly used scoring system is the Evan's score (or PRST system).

This scoring system assesses: (i) the autonomic activity, related to the changes in systolic pressure (P), (ii) the changes in heart rate (R), (iii) sweating (S), and (iv) tear (T). It is a very simple system and does not require any sophisticated instrument. But, these parameters are not specific for the type of anesthesia or the anesthetic agent and the results can vary widely among the individuals. The score ranges from 0 to 8. But, the midpoint seldom exceeds which reflects the inadequacy of this scoring system. This can be explained by the fact that tachycardia secondary to anticholinergic drugs such as atropine makes the heart rate uninterpretable. This is also applicable to β-blockers, opiates, etc. which obtund the sympathetic system activity producing bradycardia and stops response to pain.

Isolated Forearm Technique

This technique of detecting awareness (depth of anesthesia) was used previously in clinical practice and in some experiments during research. Here, a tourniquet is applied on upper arm and is inflated above systolic blood pressure, before the administration of muscle relaxant. Movement of hand either to command or spontaneously or after skin incision indicates awareness. But, the absence of movement does not indicate the absence of wakefulness. Because, some argue that a response to command intraoperatively is a late sign of attempting to prevent awareness. However, not all responding patients have a recall. One limitation of this technique is the available fixed time due to tourniquet-induced ischemia, before patients are unable to move their hands.

Lower Esophageal Contractility

After full skeletal muscle relaxation by a neuromuscular blocking agent, the smooth muscles of the lower half of the esophagus still retain their potential contractile activity. This activity is related to the CNS depression and so is used to measure the depth of anesthesia. Two types of smooth muscle activity in the lower esophagus are detected: one is the spontaneous lower esophageal contractions (SLOC) and another is the provoked lower esophageal contraction (PLOC). SLOC is under the control of higher centers and can be induced spontaneously by emotion and stress in an awake individual. It arises spontaneously and is not affected by muscle relaxants. It can be detected only by a pressure transducer. On the other hand, PLOC is induced by a provoked stimulation by inflating the balloon in the lower esophagus and the interpretation is similar to SLOC.

Both SLOC and PLOC are reduced in latency and amplitude during general anesthesia. But, the published data about its use in the monitoring of depth of anesthesia is limited. One way of improving the available information is by combining the measurement of SLOC frequency with PLOC amplitude which leads to the derivation of the esophageal contractility index (OCI). The OCI is easy to interpret and can be used in the presence of muscle relaxants. However, the general opinion is against this method and it is now considered unreliable in measuring the depth of anesthesia.

Heart Rate Variability

It is postulated that the anesthetic agents first act directly or indirectly on the brainstem. Then, it inhibits the cerebral cortex through the ascending efferent projections from the midbrain. Therefore, the measurement of one of the important brainstem mediated autonomic activity, such as, heart rate, which is not affected by any factor other than the anesthetic agent is a good method to monitor the depth of anesthesia. The special analysis of HRV reveals three components: (i) Circadian low frequency fluctuation, (ii) Baroreceptor attributed medium frequency fluctuation, and (iii) the respiration induced high-frequency fluctuation. The last component is also called as the respiratory sinus arrhythmia (RSA), which is manifested by an increased heart rate during inspiration and a decreased heart rate during expiration. This is mediated by a parasympathetic reflex, connecting the stretch receptors in lungs to the vagal motor neurons, innervating the heart. The RSA is easily recognized by an ECG monitor, which is time locked to R-wave peak. Using an online analysis of RSA, it is found that RSA is reduced during anesthesia and is increased during recovery, while it is also related to the depth of anesthesia.

Though RSA is useful for monitoring the depth of anesthesia, but needs a healthy myocardial conducting system and an intact autonomic nervous system. Any factor which affects these two systems, such as, β-blocker, conduction block, autonomic neuropathy, etc., may interfere with the result.

Electrophysiological Approaches to Monitor the Depth of Anesthesia

The realization that the anesthetic drugs affect the EEG dates back to the discovery of electrical activity in brain. The electrical activity of brain in animals was first noted by Richard Caton of Liverpool, in 1875. But, he was unable to record it. Then, in 1920, the development of electronic amplifiers allowed the recording of low-voltage electrical activity of brain. Berger, in 1929, recorded the changes in electrical potential by placing the electrodes on the scalp of human beings. In 1930, Berger also measured the influence of chloroform on EEG. Then, in 1931, he described the alpha rhythm in EEG. In 1934, Adrian and Matthews developed the clinical use of EEG. Then, Gibbs postulated that EEG might be used to measure the depth of anesthesia and also reported, in 1937, that the anesthetic agents change EEG activity from a high frequency-low voltage to a low frequency-high voltage character. In 1952, Faulconer demonstrated the relationship between the concentration of ether in blood and the pattern of EEG with the increased depth of anesthesia.

The electrical activity of the cerebral cortex or EEG is mainly of two types: *spontaneous* and *evoked*. The spontaneous EEG which is used to measure the depth of anesthesia is again classified into *raw* and *processed*.

Spontaneous EEG to Measure the Depth of Anesthesia

Raw EEG: The record of spontaneous electrical activity of brain is known as the *electroencephalogram* (EEG). Whereas the process of the recording of changes in electrical potential between the different areas of brain by means of electrodes, placed on the scalp, is known as the *electroencephalography*, and the instrument used in this recording of electrical potential is known as the *electroencephalograph*. An EEG record may be *bipolar* or *unipolar* and consists of different types of rhythmic waves. The bipolar EEG is the record of the fluctuations of potential between the two cortical electrodes. Whereas the unipolar EEG is the record of potential difference between a cortical electrode and an indifferent electrode, placed on any part of the body. EEG is a more complex signal with very low amplitude of 50–200 μv and with frequency that is classified conventionally into four categories: δ waves (0–4 Hz), θ waves (4–8 Hz), α waves (8–13 Hz), and β waves (>13 Hz).

The EEG is more or less a noninvasive indicator of cerebral function. When the patient is unresponsive or unconscious, then this EEG helps to assess the cerebral physiology. But, the recording of this electrical activity of brain, with acceptable low level of artifacts and interferences, is very difficult. This is because EEG signals are very small and easily masked by some extraneous activities, such as, muscular contraction. So, it requires very careful, secure, and correct placement of electrodes for correct recording and interpretation. Then, they have to be amplified and filtered from frequencies which are outside of the optimal range. Again, multiple channels are required and the interpretation can be tedious and time consuming.

All the anesthetic agents can cause changes in cortical neural activity, reflected by EEG. However, these changes of frequency are never accurate diagnostic tools and they have to be interpreted with a particular relevant context. For example:

- Induction of anesthesia—increases the β-activity with decrease in α-rhythm.

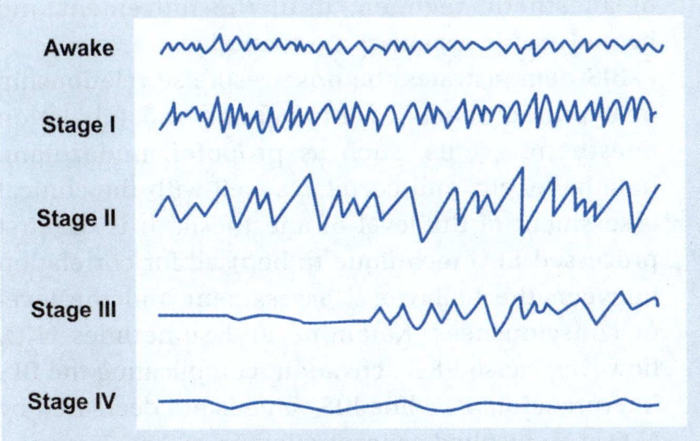

Fig. 14: Increase in plasma concentration of thiopentone, produces a characteristic change in EEG. Stage I: Frequency and amplitude of waveforms are increased. Stage II: Decrease in frequency but increase in amplitude is observed. Stage III: Burst suppression pattern is seen. Stage IV: It shows an isoelectric EEG.

- Deepening of anesthesia—"θ" or "δ" activity predominates.
- Further deepening of anesthesia—results in a burst suppression **(Fig. 14)**.

Processed EEG: Actually, the unprocessed raw EEG is not a practical tool for monitoring the depth of anesthesia. Hence, many techniques are developed to process and analyze this raw EEG. So, gradually the sophisticated and automated analysis of various processed EEG have generated several potentials for measuring the depth of anesthesia. But, still there are two generic problems with these processed EEGs.

These are: (i) dissimilar anesthetic agents generate different EEG patterns, and (ii) various pathophysiological events, other than anesthesia, also affect the EEG such as hypotension, hypoxia, hypercarbia, etc. Such events may also modify both the patient's level of consciousness and the expected EEG pattern, which can be generated by any given anesthetic agent and thus confuse the interpretation.

The recording of raw EEG involves the accumulation of large amount of information on the EEG paper. But, newer computer analysis techniques can distill and summarize the raw EEG into a condensed (data reduction), descriptive format which is called the *"processed EEG".* In a processed EEG, after distillation or filtration and amplification, the analog signal is converted to a digital signal. Then, various signal processing algorithms are applied to the frequency, amplitude and latency of the signal to derive a phase-relationship data which generates a single number. This single number system is often referred to as "index" which is typically scaled between 0 and 100. This index represents the progression of the clinical states of consciousness such as *awake, sedated, light anesthesia, deep anesthesia,* etc. Artifact

recognition algorithm which is used to avoid contamination and spurious index is an important component of the software in most monitors. Although EMG activity from the scalp muscles (as electrodes are placed on it) is considered as an artifact from the viewpoint of pure EEG analysis, but it may be a very important source of clinically relevant information. Because, sudden appearance of the frontal EMG activity suggests somatic responses to noxious stimuli, resulting from inadequate analgesia and may give a warning of impending arousal. For these reasons, some monitors separately provide information on the level of EMG activity.

For the processed EEG, two methods of data reduction such as: (i) Fast fourier analysis and (ii) Aperiodic analysis are used. The "Fast Fourier Analysis" method measures the *power* of EEG and is used to derive the *spectral* edge. So, by this *power spectral analysis* of EEG by Fast Fourier method, the measurement of the depth of anesthesia is performed on the blocks of EEG and the result is displayed either as a spectral array or as a power, in a series of frequency bands. The median power frequency (MPF) with 50% of power above or below its value; or the spectral edge frequency (SEF) with 95% of power below its value, both have been used routinely to measure the anesthetic depth. For example, MPF of <4.8 Hz predicts the loss of consciousness and is the basis of its use in closed-loop delivery of drugs in TIVA. Most of the newer anesthetic monitors, used to measure the depth of anesthesia, include a module for monitoring EEG and its processed forms like SEF, MPF, etc. Then, periodic analysis is performed by serially examining each wave, recording its wavelength and its peak-to-peak amplitude. Another method of data reduction, such as *bispectral* analysis has been used to predict the movement as response to surgical stimulation, i.e., depth of anesthesia.

Other processed EEG's: Other than median power frequency (MPF) and spectral edge frequency (SEF), which have been already discussed, the other processed EEGs which are used for the monitoring of depth of anesthesia are: Bispectral EEG, narcotrend, patient state analyzer, evoked potential monitor, entropy, etc.

As ketamine, N₂O, and dexmedetomidine do not cause the depression of EEG, therefore these EEG based monitoring cannot be applied to measure the depth of anesthesia with these agents.

i. *Bispectral (BIS) EEG monitors:* Bispectral index (BIS) monitor is the first scientifically validated commercially available monitor to measure the depth of anesthesia. It analyzes the multiple facets of real-time EEG and generate a score by set algorithm. It exhibits a score of 100 for fully awake state and 0 for completely silent brain. BIS score of 45–60 indicates adequate depth of anesthesia.

The characteristics of this bispectral (BIS) EEG monitoring system include:

- It is a more advanced EEG signal processing approach than the traditional fast fourier EEG signal processing methodology.
- It has greater correlation among the huge collection of clinical data (patient's movement, hemodynamics, and drug concentrations), EEG data, and advanced multivariate statistical data to create a BIS parameter.
- BIS analysis specially measures or is more sensitive to the hypnotic component of anesthetic agent. But, it does not measure or is less sensitive to the analgesic components of anesthetic agent.
- BIS monitoring definitely improves the quality of anesthetic regimen.

BIS has been validated for many commonly used anesthetic drugs. It shows a good correlation with the end-tidal sevoflurane concentration, as well as the blood propofol concentration. Studies have shown that the use of BIS can decrease the consumption of anesthetic agents. So, it also helps in speed of awakening and in a faster discharge. The utility of BIS is maximal when the anesthetic regimen is a combination of low doses of opiate analgesia with high doses of hypnotic drugs which is titrated to the bispectral response. For the BIS to reflect maximally, higher doses of hypnotic drugs with lower doses of opiates should be used. The higher doses of opiates result in a significant synergistic interaction with the hypnotic drugs. Also, the reduced amount of hypnotic drugs result in less profound hypnotic EEG effects on CNS and therefore a less sensitive BIS response. It appears that the synergistic interaction of opiates and hypnotics, to reach the clinical endpoint, does not correlate well with the EEG effects of hypnotics. The pharmacodynamic relationship of BIS to hypnotic drug concentration is unchanged (i.e., lowering of BIS with increasing hypnotic drugs) if opiate concentration increases.

The clinical use of BIS monitoring involves separating the hypnotic and analgesic components of an anesthetic regimen. During routine anesthesia with small to moderate doses of analgesic drugs, an adequate dose of hypnotic agents is used and it keeps the BIS level at the range of 50–60. During intense surgical manipulation if the BIS increases and patient exhibits movement or hemodynamic responses, then it should be corrected by increasing the dose of hypnotic agent and thus lowering the BIS value to 50–60 range. On the contrary, if the BIS remains lower, but the movement and hemodynamic responses continue, then incremental doses of opiates should be added to increase the analgesic component

of anesthetic regimen, until the movement and hemodynamic responses are controlled.

BIS demonstrates the dose-response relationship of hypnotic effects of intravenous and inhalation anesthetic agents, such as propofol, midazolam, halothane, etc. and correlates well with the clinical assessment of the level of anesthesia. It is the first processed EEG technique to be used for correlation between the behavioral assessment and the level of consciousness. Ketamine and sometimes N_2O, however, cause EEG activation, complicating the BIS interpretation. Baseline BIS value is not decreased by N_2O at an inspired concentration up to 50%. However, during surgery, the antinociceptive effect of N_2O may be responsible for the observed decrease in value of BIS. As the pediatric EEG only approaches the adult pattern by about 5 years of age, so it cannot automatically be extrapolated to young children. But still, healthy adult EEG data are used to authenticate the BIS algorithm of children, because early investigation suggests that BIS may be valid in children, older than 1 year of age. Comparison of BIS values at various clinical endpoints between the adults and children suggests that BIS performs similarly in adults and children in respect to dose-response relationship of anesthetic agents. Its use is also rapidly expanding, especially during care of a critically ill patient admitted in the ICU.

BIS has also been used in cardiopulmonary bypass, vegetative states, CPR, hypoglycemic coma, etc. But, here an increase or decrease in BIS may not always reflect adequate awareness or lack of it. Recently, it has been seen that when BIS is used along with ECT, then values fall to 26–28. This is due to the postictal EEG depression after ECT. Hence, in such circumstances correlation of BIS with the awakening is affected. It may be unreliable in conditions like dementia. Also, electromagnetic operating systems used in surgeries might affect the BIS monitoring.

Like an EEG signal, BIS is also subject to interference and artifacts, particularly from EMG activity which can artificially elevate the BIS value. So, some monitors also show a display of signal quality index and an indicator of EMG interference. As there is no "gold standard" monitor against which BIS can be compared, so studies have used predictive probability that is likely to occur in various clinically relevant endpoints such as the loss of consciousness, recovery, recall, etc., at different BIS values. The probability of postoperative recall is very low when BIS is kept <60 intraoperatively.

ii. *Narcotrend monitor:* This EEG derived monitor, used for the assessment of depth of anesthesia, performs automatic computer analysis of raw EEG during anesthesia. In this system two electrodes are placed on the forehead of patient and a third electrode serves as a reference. It uses a 6-letter classification with 14 sub-classifications. The letters are A to F, where A represents an awake patient and F denotes burst suppression. In-between all these, the B and C represent the sedated and light anesthesia of patient, respectively. With this system the stages D and E are aimed (D = general anesthesia and E = general anesthesia with deep hypnosis) at steady-state anesthesia. During practice, B and C should be avoided and F is considered unnecessarily deep. The relationship (comparison) between BIS and Narcotrend is shown in **Box 4.**

iii. *Patient-state analyzer:* The patient-state analyzer is also an EEG-derived color-coded patient safety index (PSI) which is recorded on a scale in between 0 and 100. Green color indicates the hypnotic state and comes in the 25–50 PSI range. Yellow indicates deep hypnosis and involves an index below 25. Blue indicates burst suppression **(Table 2)**. Whereas the white indicates artifacts which the analyzer machine identifies and discards. The main advantage claimed with this system is that there is little interference with cautery, electromagnetic operating system, or noise pollution.

iv. *Cerebral state monitor:* It is a handheld device that analyzes a single-channel EEG and presents a cerebral state index (CSI) which is also scaled in between 0 and 100. In addition, it also provides EEG suppression percentage and measurement of EMG activity. The monitor is also on-line and evaluates the amount of instantaneous burst suppression (BS) during each 30-seconds period. The CSI is a unit-less scale from 0 to 100, where 0 indicates a flat EEG and 100 indicates EEG activity corresponding to awake state. The range

of adequate anesthesia is defined to be between 40 and 60.

Evoked Potential (EEG) to Monitor the Depth of Anesthesia

The evoked response or activity in the cerebral cortex is elicited directly by stimulating the cortical surface (Direct Cortical Evoked Response) or indirectly by stimulating the peripheral sense organs like: the retina—by photostimulation (Visual Evoked Potential—VEP), the ear—by auditory click (Auditory Evoked Potential—AEP) or the peripheral sensory nerve endings (Somato Sensory Evoked Potential—SSEP). Here, we will discuss only the AEP. Because, others are not used to monitor the depth of anesthesia.

The type of stimulation may be sensory, electrical, magnetic, or even cognitive in nature. The two major types of evoked potentials are sensory (SEP) and motor (MEP), which assess the functional integrity of sensory and motor pathways respectively and is greatly influenced by the effect of narcotics, drugs, and physiological conditions, like sleep, etc. The most commonly used evoked potential for assessing the depth of anesthesia is SEP. Here, the stimulus is applied at the peripheral nerves and the resulting response is recorded centrally at the cerebral or cortical level.

The evoked waves consist of some positive, followed by a few small negative and then by many larger and more prolonged positive deflection. The *first* positive-negative wave sequence is called as the *primary* evoked response, while the *second* one is called as the diffuse *secondary* response. This evoked response can be separated by means of a special computer from the underlying spontaneous EEG.

The computer techniques (which process the EEG signals) first extract the evoked potential from the underlying spontaneous cortical electrical activity after the respective stimulus. The evoked responses are used primarily (i) to monitor the functional integrity of neural structures, (ii) to identify the anatomical integrity of neural structures, and (iii) to diagnose the neurophysiological conditions. As evoked response is sensitive to anesthetic drugs, so they have been used to measure the effect of anesthetic drugs on brain and also the depth of anesthesia.

There are several advantages and disadvantages of using evoked potentials for monitoring the effects of anesthetic drugs and the depth of anesthesia.

Advantages:
- Body's response to some form of stimulation forms the pivot (central point) for assessing the depth of anesthesia.
- Measuring the evoked potential is a noninvasive and continuous method of measuring the body's response to appropriate stimuli.

BOX 4: Comparison between BIS and Narcotrend.

1. BIS ≈ 100 to 85 = A and B levels of Narcotrend system
   (A = Awake, B = Sedated)
2. BIS ≈ 85 to 65 = C levels of Narcotrend system
   (C = Light anesthesia)
3. BIS ≈ 65 to 40 = D and E levels of Narcotrend system
4. BIS ≈ <40 = F (burst suppression)

TABLE 2: Color-coding of PSI.

Green (25–50)	Hypnotic state
Yellow (<25)	Deep hypnosis
Blue	Burst suppression
White (artifacts)	Discarded
(PSI: patient safety index)	

Disadvantages:

- Though all the anesthetic agents cause changes in evoked response, but there is no standard to measure the drug effect that enables one to identify or characterize this drug effect or the depth of anesthesia.
- There is no known parameter to measure the evoked response.
- There are also technical, clinical, and practical complexities of recording the evoked responses, like stimulus characteristics (intensity, duration, etc.), electrode placement, recording equipment, recording technique, etc.

Auditory-evoked response or potential (AEP): Among all the evoked response, AEP is the most important. So, it is only discussed here. Sense of hearing is the last to be lost and first to be recovered during induction of anesthesia and return of consciousness respectively. This is the basis of using the auditory evoked response for measuring the consciousness and depth of anesthesia. The applied auditory impulses hit the cochlea of the ear, then it travels via the eighth nerve and reaches the brainstem. The auditory stimuli are given as clicks from earphones. Normally, 1,024 clicks at the rate of 6 per second are given, depending on the background noise. Any disturbance in hearing could affect the ability of AEP to reflect the depth of anesthesia.

The auditory-evoked response is again divided into (i) the brainstem response, (ii) the early cortical response, and (iii) the late cortical response.

i. *Brainstem responses:* This is also termed as "Brainstem Auditory Evoked Potential (BAEP)". These occur within first 10 milliseconds and consist mainly of six waves, labeled as I to VI. The BAEP is presented as a smooth curve, therefore, typically only the wave V can be detected. They are preserved with all the volatile anesthetic agents and change very little with anesthesia. So, they are not so useful to us.

ii. *Early cortical responses:* This is also termed as "Middle Latency Auditory Evoked Potential (MLAEP)". These occur within 10–80 milliseconds and are designed as PoNo, PaNa, PbNb, etc. These responses, especially Nb, show graded changes with the effect of anesthetic agents and are so useful to grade the depth of anesthesia. Nb with a frequency of 47 seconds is 100% sensitive and specific for explicit memory during isoflurane anesthesia. All the volatile anesthetic agents suppress the early cortical response component of AEP to a similar extent at equipotent MAC. All the volatile anesthetics increase the latency and decrease the amplitude in a reversible dose-concentration related manner. N_2O decreases it in a progressive dose-related manner due to an increase in the auditory threshold. Intravenous anesthetic agents also change the evoked potential similar to the inhaled anesthetics, except benzodiazepines. Ketamine does not affect the early cortical response. Opioids produce only the partial suppression, even in high doses. High doses of opioids do not suppress the consciousness or sensory function. Thus, benzodiazepines, ketamine, opioids, and MAC 0.5 volatile agents preserve the early cortical response and so cannot be used to prevent the intraoperative awareness.

Reversible headphones or earphones *deliver the active auditory stimulus.* Cost-effective disposable surface electrodes are *used to measure the AEP* and the subsequent result enables to measure the patient's level of consciousness. From the mathematical analysis of AEP waveform, the device generates an AEP index that provides a correlation between the depth of anesthesia with the anesthetic drug concentration. The AEP index is scaled from 0 to 100. In contrast to other EEG indices, the AEP corresponds with low probability of consciousness at <25, rather than the higher numeric threshold associated with the other monitors. More recently AEP index is scaled from 0 to 60. When using this 0–60 range, fewer oscillations are observed, while the patient is awake. When asleep, the graphical resolution of the lower index value is higher. It is recommended to use the AEP index in 0–60 range. AEP index is very specific and sensitive. When compared to SEF, MPF, and BIS, then AEP index is most sensitive in distinguishing transition from consciousness to unconsciousness.

iii. *Late cortical responses:* This is also termed as "Long Latency Auditory Evoked Potential (LLAEP)". These occur after 80 milliseconds and are designated as P_1N_1, P_2N_2, etc. These evoked responses are very less sensitive to anesthetic drugs and volatile agents. Hence, they are of no practical use. The disappearance of P_1N_1 indicates transition from consciousness to unconsciousness. Other single derivative derived from the late cortical response like second differential, first differential, coherent frequency, ARX index, etc. are all being evaluated, but are not so promising.

Other Monitors to Measure the Depth of Anesthesia

The other equipment which is used to monitor the depth of anesthesia has been listed below:

i. Positron emission tomography (PET)
ii. Super conductive quantum interference device (SQUID)
iii. Ocular microtremor monitoring (OMT)

PET

PET scanning is an invasive method and cannot be used in routine cases.

SQUID

It is noninvasive, measuring the functional activity of the brain, but is very expensive.

Oculomicrotremor Monitoring

Oculomicrotremor is a high frequency physiological tremor of eye. It is present in all the subjects and is related to the toxic activity of oculomotor neurons, and is also present in brainstem. It has been shown that OMT correlates well with the level of consciousness. OMT is suppressed by thiopentone, propofol, and sevoflurane. It is measured by a piezoelectric strain gauge technique where the probe is placed on conjunctiva or closed eye. Earlier, the probe was placed on anesthetized sclera. But, nowadays, it can be placed on closed eyelid. End-tidal sevoflurane concentration of 1–2% does neither decrease OMT nor decrease BIS, though it shows a falling trend. When compared to BIS, the OMT may exclude an aware patient more accurately than BIS, though the graded measure of emergence is better, seen with BIS. The OMT remains depressed, until just before the first response to verbal command appear. *Hence, it is more useful as an awareness monitor than the depth of hypnosis monitor.*

MONITORING OF CARDIOVASCULAR SYSTEM

■ INTRODUCTION

The cardiovascular system is responsible for the transport of different substrates and their metabolites to different tissues and it also supplies the adequate oxygen from lungs to tissues and CO_2 from tissues to lungs in order to support their (organs) continued normal function. Thus, an adequate organ function reflects the adequacy of the performance of a cardiovascular system. So, clinically sometimes, we measure the urine output, skin color, body temperature, mental status, sensory or motor functions (cerebral indices), etc. for the monitoring of the adequacy of the function of a cardiovascular system. But, these clinical monitoring is not always true or possible due to the presence of some intrinsic end-organ dysfunction. Because, this kind of *clinical indirect monitoring of CVS* requires the absence of intrinsic end-organ dysfunction. So, the direct monitoring of the different facets of CVS by instruments is more practical and reliable than the only clinical monitoring of the function of different end organs. But, both the complexity and the diversity of the multiple nonclinical indirect or direct monitoring (both noninvasive and invasive) of CVS by instruments, depends on many variables, such as the nature of surgical procedure, the fragility of patient's cardiovascular system, the considerations of the risks and costs of various monitoring techniques, etc. So, the ultimate and final decision, regarding the extent of the nonclinical monitoring of CVS by different sophisticated electronic instruments, depends on the judgment of anesthetist who will choose the particular technique or instrument for the monitoring of CVS and which will provide the maximum information with minimum risks and cost to the patient and will optimize the management of this particular patient.

■ HISTORY

It was 28th January of 1848, when the first death, due to anesthesia during a surgery, was reported and this surgery was a simple excision of ingrowing toenail under the administration of chloroform. This was just 2 years, after the first public demonstration of anesthesia by ether and the patient was only 15 years old lady, named Hannah Greener. However, before that, another two deaths were also reported unofficially in the March of 1847. Among these two deaths, the first one was a young woman of 30 years old, named Lincs of Yrantham and the second was a 52-year-old man of Essex whose name is not known.

So, nearly a full and a half century later, these incidents still remind us that even a rudimentary awareness and a minimum monitoring of patient's cardiovascular system can avert many of these mishaps. Also, the development of newer and far less toxic anesthetic drugs than chloroform, like sevoflurane, enflurane, etc., emphasizes that the necessity of adequate and careful monitoring of CVS is still not less important today or in future, than it was thought previously, at the time of invention of anesthesia. At that time, the assessment of patient's cardiac performance was entirely subjective, i.e., without any equipment. Then, the next part of 19th century saw little or no advancement in the development of objective monitoring by equipment, during anesthesia.

In 1860, Joseph Clover had first started the monitoring of patient by keeping his fingers on patient's pulse while administering chloroform. Then, at the end of that century, a feather was added to the vulcanite face-piece to monitor the respiration of a patient by observing its movement. Then, in 1894, Earnest A Codman, a surgeon of Harvard, had developed a system of intraoperative monitoring and a record-keeping system at the Massachusetts General Hospital. After that, in 1903, a routine and a new form of cardiac monitoring protocol was first introduced in anesthesia practice in the USA. This had included (i) the measurement of systolic blood pressure by Riva-Rocci's sphygmomanometer, (ii) the measurement of heart rate, (iii) the measurement of respiratory rate, etc. The mercury manometer was first used to measure the blood pressure by Poiseuille, in 1828. Then, in 1834, Herrison developed a crude instrument which was placed directly over an artery to measure the blood pressure. Vierordt was the first to estimate the amount of counter pressure which is just necessary to obliterate the arterial pulse. After that, Jules Marey and Von Basch had become the pioneer in clinical sphygmomanometry ("sphygmo" means pulse, and "manometer" means measurement of pressure of liquid or gas in a container). Riva Rocci first introduced the blood pressure cuff in 1896, although the breadth of the cuff, he used, was only 5 cm. Then, Von Recklinghausen had drew attention to the importance of the width of cuff to get better results.

Then, in 1905, Korotkoff, a Russian physician, had described the sphygmomanometric sounds using stethoscope, from large a peripheral artery, during the deflation of cuff. This was called as the Korotkoff sounds and it (hearing of Korotkoff sound by stethoscope, for the measurement of BP, during the deflation of cuff) still remains, even today, the standard technique for blood pressure measurement, manually, in all the spheres of medical care. After that, in 1911, Mckesson added the measurement of respiratory rate and the measurement of inspired O_2 concentration in the monitoring armamentarium of anesthesia. The oximetry was first performed, as early as, in 1913. Then, there was a steady development in the sphere of monitoring, during anesthesia, with the Einthoven's discovery of ECG. This was the early 1960 and this ECG monitoring was done, during this period, by using a cathode ray oscilloscope. Gradually, this monitoring of CVS by ECG, using cathode ray oscilloscope, was introduced into the anesthetic practice.

The oscillotonometer principle which was first developed in 1931 by Von Recklinghausen, by using an inflated cuff to sense the arterial pulsations, as the oscillatory changes of cuff pressure, has now become the cornerstone of methodology for most of the today's automated noninvasive blood pressure measuring devices. Originally, Von Recklinghausen had used a needle to sense the changes (or oscillations) in cuff pressure, indicating the systolic and diastolic blood pressure. Later, in 1970, different automatic oscillotonometer were developed by various equipment companies, where the changes in the pressure of cuff is detected by electronic transducer and this electrical signal, produced by transducer, is analyzed and presented digitally as systolic, diastolic, and mean arterial pressure (MAP).

Though, the intra-arterial BP was first measured invasively by Stephen Hales, in 1733, by direct cannulation of an artery of an animal, but it was not in practice till 1949, when Peterson and Dripps developed a safe and percutaneous arterial cannulation method. However, in the next few decades, the development of transducer technology and better arterial catheters made the invasive BP monitoring a standard and widely accepted method in all the areas of critical care.

Venous pressure was also first measured by Stephen Hales, in 1733, on a mare. But, then, after a long interval, it was first measured on a man by Fray in 1902 and was first used clinically in 1910. Then, in 1929, Forssman's pioneering work on human cardiac catheterization, which was first done on himself, stimulated the progress of this chapter. This landmark achievement and also the development of many better materials for manufacturing of catheter allowed the subsequent completion of many important cardiac investigations which have formed the basis of understanding of our current use of central venous pressure (CVP) monitoring. The first plastic (polythene) intravenous catheter was used in 1945, and after this, the plastic central venous catheter was developed rapidly.

Lagerlof and Werko had first reported the value of pulmonary capillary wedge pressure (PCWP) as a reflection of the left ventricular filling pressure (actual preload). Finally, in 1970, the development of flexible, balloon tipped and flow directed Swan-Ganz catheter by Swan had made the pulmonary artery catheterization possible routinely. After that, Seldinger had developed a guidewire directed deep vascular cannulation technique which added a great safety and ease to this type of cardiac monitoring. Now, the modern pulmonary artery catheters provide a variety of additional diagnostic and therapeutic tools, such as the determination of cardiac output by thermodilutional technique, determination of mixed venous oxygen saturation by oximetry, atrial or ventricular pacing, and many others. Thus, gradually it (vascular cannulation) became the hallmark of a "full" invasive cardiac monitoring system in anesthesia and critical care unit.

Blood gas analysis was first started by Pflunger, as early as, in 1872. Then, Leland Clark developed polarographic oxygen electrode, in 1956, which forms the basis of modern oxygen electrode. At the same time, the polio epidemic in Copenhagen had stimulated the search for different methods of measuring arterial PCO_2. At first, Astrup had measured the pH of blood with different CO_2 concentration to determine its PCO_2. But, later, the development of CO_2 electrode greatly facilitated this measurement and a full acid-base picture could be derived from the Siggaard-Andersen nomogram. However, today, these calculations are performed by a microprocessor. Capnography was first used clinically in 1960, although the infrared analyzer was first employed as early as in 1865.

However, the most unique addition, in the armamentarium of intraoperative cardiac monitoring system, took place in 1954 with the first use of ultrasound in cardiology by Edler and Hertz. But, their one-dimensional motion (M-mode) analysis has rapidly given way to the two-dimensional (2D) echocardiography. It displays different cardiac anatomy in various planes, even in real time. The development and the use of transesophageal transducer was first established, in 1980, by Hisanaga. Then, gradually TEE has gained significant popularity in anesthesiology and has built a stable platform for continuous, noninvasive, and high-quality intraoperative monitoring of cardiac functions. Moreover, the addition of Doppler technology and color-flow imaging has further established TEE as an important tool in modern anesthesia practice.

Clinical Monitoring of Cardiovascular System

The principal aim of function of cardiovascular system (CVS) is to ensure adequate supply of O_2 to tissues. The supply of adequate amount of O_2 to tissues (or O_2 content) is the product of cardiac output (CO), hemoglobin concentration, and hemoglobin saturation by O_2. Clinically, the hemoglobin concentration and the hemoglobin saturation by O_2 may be estimated by looking at the mucous membrane and skin. The CO may be estimated clinically by the volume of pulse, output of urine, and the warmth of extremities. Therefore, the observation of a good pulse, pink skin, and warm extremities, plus or especially when these are combined with urine output of >0.5 mL/kg/h, then these findings imply that there is unlikely to be any cardiovascular problem, provided there is no peripheral vascular disease.

In children, the observation of capillary circulation by capillary refill time provides a valuable indication of a stable cardiac status, as peripheral vascular diseases are rare in children. The capillary refill time is the time, taken by the capillaries to be refilled, after the digit has been exsanguinated by firm pressure. When a finger has been kept under pressure for 3 seconds, then a capillary refill time of <1.5 seconds is considered normal. But, a time >5 seconds is indicative of impaired circulation or shock. While the patients, presented with complex cardiovascular problems may require more sophisticated monitors, but still the value

of direct observation of patient and the examiner's fingers on the patient's pulse can never be underestimated. But, in practice, sometimes dimmed theater light and surgical drapes may cause difficulties for the direct observation of patient and clinical monitoring. So, in such situation electronic monitors become essential. But, still, the direct observation of patient should always be maintained as far as possible and should be taken as the supplementary to instrumental monitoring. Therefore, for many healthy patients who are undergoing minor procedures, the above-mentioned physical signs and clinical monitoring may provide a considerable important portion of total cardiovascular monitoring. But, when the operation becomes more complex or the patient presents with more advanced unstable CVS, then the extent of this supplementary electronic monitoring grows accordingly. However, still, the careful clinical assessment of patient helps the clinician to confirm or refute the information, derived from the important monitoring systems.

Monitoring by Stethoscope

In 1818, Rene Theophile Laennec had first introduced the stethoscope in general medical practice. After that, 100 years had passed. Then, in 1908, Harvey Cushing had first proposed that this stethoscope could be used for continuous routine monitoring of CVS during surgery.

Two types of stethoscopes are used for continuous cardiovascular monitoring during surgery. These are the *precordial stethoscope* and the *esophageal stethoscope*. They provide simple breath sounds and heart sounds continuously throughout the operation. In a precordial stethoscope, the metal bell is strapped on the precordium. Then, both the heart sounds and breath sounds are heard through a long tube and a custom-molded mono-aural plastic earpiece. Electronically amplified stethoscopes also have been designed in an attempt to improve the quantity and the clarity of heart rounds and breath sounds. Stethoscope with wireless system, using radio-transmitted signals, has also been developed. These wireless stethoscopes also allow the continuous monitoring of CVS, while the anesthetist pays attention to the other monitors, instead of sitting by the side of patient.

An esophageal stethoscope is minimally invasive, but provides clear breath sounds and distinct heart sounds, when its tip is positioned into esophagus at 28–30 cm from the incisors. By this, the core body temperature can also be measured via a thermistor which is incorporated into the tip of this esophageal stethoscope. Specially configured esophageal stethoscopes also permit the recording of transesophageal ECG which sometimes may become useful in diagnosing atrial arrhythmias, right ventricular ischemia, or posterior left ventricular ischemia. Transesophageal atrial pacing also can be accomplished by these transesophageal stethoscopes, which is equipped with bipolar pacing electrodes on its outer surface.

But, the routine use of pulse oximeter, capnometer, and other electronic monitors, driven by their ubiquitous usefulness and imposed law, has diminished recently the widespread application of precordial and esophageal stethoscopes in clinical practice, despite their immense utility in basic patient monitoring. Currently, the precordial and esophageal stethoscopes are used intraoperatively in institutions, where there are no electronic monitors. Then, their role in diagnosing important respiratory problems, such as bronchospasm, crepitation, etc., probably exceed their value as continuous monitors for the circulatory system.

Failure of these stethoscopes to detect untoward events is more frequent than the electronic monitors and it is due to the difficulty to concentrate continuously or to listen to both the heart and breath sounds simultaneously.

Heart Rate Monitoring

It is the most simple and noninvasive (or rather least invasive) form of monitoring of CVS. It acts as an important guide in determining the influence of anesthetic agents on CVS, reaction of CVS to surgical stimuli, and any underlying cardiovascular pathology. The monitoring of the heart rate (pulse rate) by keeping "fingers on pulse" is ubiquitous and is fundamental of all the monitoring. But practically, it is not always possible due to other engagements of an anesthesiologist. However, fortunately most of the monitors (invasive or noninvasive) used during anesthesia practice provide a continuous audio and numerical display of the heart rate.

In ECG monitors, the heart rate is displayed by measuring the QRS interval by recognizing the peak of R-wave on a beat-to-beat basis. The electrocardiographic measurement of heart rate begins with the accurate detection of R-wave and the measurement of R-R interval, which is displayed and updated by every 5–15 seconds. The automatic *noninvasive* blood pressure measuring devices also usually display the heart rate by counting the cuff oscillation. The *invasive* blood pressure monitoring system derives the heart rate from the arterial and as well as from the pulmonary artery waveform. The pulse oximeter computes and displays the heart rate from capillary pulsation.

All the heart rate monitors, like other monitors, are also subjected to errors from artifacts, pathological states, or other therapies. Some common errors in heart rate monitoring are listed in **Box 5**.

BOX 5: Some common errors in heart rate monitors.

1. The ECG monitors often count the pacemaker artifacts (especially atrial) resulting, the faulty heart rate
2. When the T-waves are exceptionally tall, then the ECG monitor counts these T-waves in addition to QRS complexes, causing an apparent doubling of the actual heart rate. Intra-aortic balloon pump, the counter pulsation also can cause the same doubling error in blood pressure (from arterial form) derived heart rate
3. The presence of pulsus paradoxus apparently reduces the actual heart rate to half
4. The electrocautery invariably interferes the counting of heart rate by ECG monitor

Pulse Rate Monitoring

The electrical depolarization and the systolic contraction of heart per minute is called as the *heart rate*. It generates a palpable peripheral arterial pulsation and its rate per minute is called as the *pulse rate*. Pulse deficit is the difference between this heart rate and the pulse rate. So, the monitoring of pulse rate is more important than the heart rate and is very helpful to make an idea of the peripheral organ perfusion. This is because all the cardiac systoles (which produce the heart rate) do not produce sufficient cardiac output which is responsible to produce a palpable pulse and peripheral circulation. The typical example of pulse deficit is AF in which the short R-R intervals compromise cardiac filling during diastole and results in a reduced stroke volume with an imperceptible peripheral arterial pulse. Thus, all the cardiac systoles do not end in palpable peripheral pulses and there is a deficit between the heart rate and the pulse rate in AF.

Another extreme example of difference between the heart rate and the pulse rate is EMD (electromechanical dissociation). This is actually a condition where the electrical activity and contraction of heart is present, but there is no or minimal stroke volume and cannot produce any palpable pulse. Therefore, there is presence of heart rate, but absence of pulse rate. This is usually seen in patients with cardiac tamponade, extreme hypovolemia, extreme peripheral vasodilatation, anaphylactic shock, etc.

On the monitor's screen, we get the heart rate from ECG tracing and the pulse rate from different pulse sources. For example, pulse oximeter uses the capillary pulsation (pulse source) where an optical transducer measures the capillary volume changes (plethysmograph) and provides the pulse rate for most patients, except in patients with severe arterial occlusive diseases or marked peripheral vasoconstriction. Pulse rate is also obtained by electromechanical transducers in NIBP devices, which determine the pulse rate, by counting the oscillations in the pressure cuff. When, during the direct and invasive arterial pressure measurement, a catheter is placed inside the arterial lumen, then the arterial pressure waveform also provides a reliable pulse rate. The piezo-electric devices of Doppler probes are also used for accurate pulse rate monitoring. The output of these monitors is displayed upon an oscilloscope. A qualitative index of pulse volume and its flow may be obtained from this oscilloscope.

Pulse rate counting, using the intra-arterial pressure tracings, may sometimes be misleading, when the nonsystolic arterial pulsations are detected by the monitor and are counted separately. For example, when a patient is treated with an intra-aortic balloon pump, then the pressure pulse resulting from the balloon inflation during diastole may be detected, producing a fictitiously high pulse rate. When the morphology of pulse becomes double peaked, (which is called "bisferiens pulse"), such as those arising in patients with aortic valve regurgitation, then it may also produce a similarly increased (doubled) pulse rate. In contrast, patients with pulsus alternans may have an inappropriately low pulse rate (half), due to the diminished magnitude of every alternate arterial pulsation. In such cases, the counting of pulse rate from the pulmonary artery pressure waveform can provide a reliable pulse rate.

Monitoring of Cardiovascular System by ECG

Electrocardiography, during the monitoring of CVS, warns us about the changes in heart rate, its rhythm, and the development of any ischemia which may precede to the bad hemodynamic changes. The disturbances in the potassium and calcium levels of blood may also be recognizable from ECG during the monitoring of CVS. However, a major limitation of ECG in cardiovascular monitoring is that there is no indication of cardiac output, which may fall to be zero in spite of a normal ECG tracing. The quality and the ease with which the electrical signals of heart are be obtained, is due to the improvement in electronics and electrode design. Thus, the "mat" electrode has greatly reduced the time, required to establish a good interface. With many systems, however, the signal is interfered following the use of electrosurgical diathermy. But, recently many commercially available ECG monitors are capable of rejecting the diathermy interference **(Fig. 15)**.

The standard lead II is the commonly used lead for the monitoring of CVS, because it allows the excellent detection of any intraoperative arrhythmias. But, it does not always show the myocardial ischemic changes, which may only be visible in lead V_5. So, the unusual bipolar lead, named as the CM_5 lead (central manubrium to the fifth intercostal space in the left anterior axillary line) allows an excellent

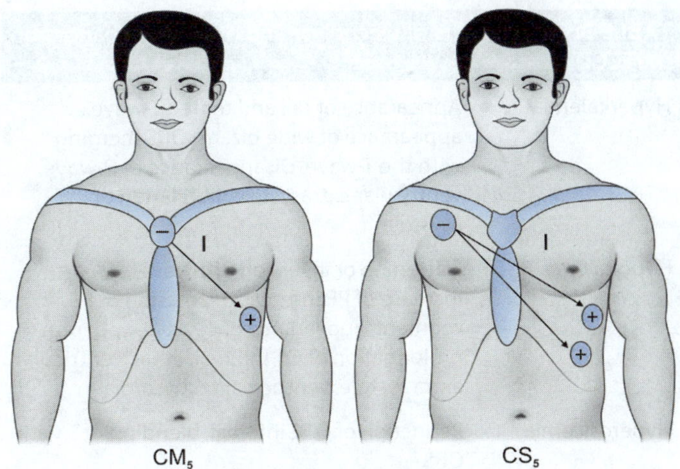

Fig. 15: Monitoring of the CVS by ECG.

detection of both the ischemia and arrhythmias. Therefore, it is always recommended for continuous intraoperative ECG monitoring. The CM_5 and the CS_5 leads are shown in **Figure 15**.

Another lead, named CS_5 (central subclavicle) is also very important for the intraoperative ECG of CV monitoring. Here, the right arm (RA) electrode is placed under the right clavicle, the left arm (LA) electrode is placed in the V_5 position and the left leg (LL) electrode is placed in its usual position. In this CS_5 lead arrangement, the lead I is selected for the detection of anterior myocardial wall ischemia and the lead II is selected for the detection of inferior wall ischemia or arrhythmia. If a unipolar precordial V_5 lead is not available, then this CS_5 bipolar lead is the best and easiest alternative for monitoring of myocardial ischemia and arrhythmia. The **Table 3** shows the effects of the disturbances of electrolytes and others on ECG.

Arterial Blood Pressure Monitoring

The measurement of blood pressure is one of the most fundamental parameters for the monitoring of cardiovascular function.

It represents the force of contraction of heart that drives the blood to flow from center to periphery (systolic pressure) and also represents the load against which heart has to work (diastolic pressure). The peak pressure, generated within the vessels during the systolic contraction of ventricle, is called as the *systolic blood pressure* and the continuous pressure within the blood vessels during the diastolic relaxation of ventricle is called the *diastolic blood pressure*. The *pulse pressure* is the difference between these two pressures. The average arterial pressure over a period of full cardiac cycle is termed as the *mean arterial pressure*. It is a time-weighted average pressure, which prevails throughout the whole

TABLE 3: Some effects of electrolyte and other disturbances on the ECG.

Hyperkalemia	Appearance of tall and tented T-wave, appearance of wide bizarre QRS merging with the T-wave. Disappearance of P-wave, ventricular extrasystole, fibrillation or asystole
Hypokalemia	Flattening or inversion of T-wave, increase of PR interval, depression of ST segment, appearance of U-wave, apparent prolongation of QT interval, atrial, ventricular extra systole, ventricular tachycardia
Hypercalcemia	Reduction of QTC interval, blending of T with QRS
Hypocalcemia	Prolongation of QTC interval
Hypomagnesemia	Prolongation of QTC interval
Venous air embolism	Right heart strain pattern, atrial and ventricular extrasystole

The QT interval varies with the heart rate. So, when it is corrected to a heart rate of 60 beats per minute, then it is signified as "QTC" (QT corrected).

cardiac cycle. So, the mean blood pressure is approximately equal to the diastolic pressure plus one-third of the pulse pressure, i.e., Mean BP = DP + 1/3 (SP – DP).

The monitoring of the function of CVS is aimed at to assess the amount of cardiac output, which is required to maintain the oxygen-flux. So, the most important parameter for the monitoring of CVS is the cardiac output or flow. But, it is very difficult to measure the cardiac output clinically and it has been discussed in the last part of this chapter. So, to monitor the perfusion of organs which is the most important function of CVS, we measure HR and BP. But, fortunately the most easily monitored parameter such as HR and BP bear some constant relationship with CO, by the following equations, such as: Pulse rate = CO ÷ Stroke Volume, and Blood pressure = Cardiac Output × SVR.

The arterial blood pressure is generally affected by the site, where it is measured. This is because the *pulse wave* moves peripherally along the wall of the arterial tree. So, this pulse wave may distort the *pressure waveform* which moves along the column of blood, leading to an exaggeration of the systolic and pulse pressure. The *level of the measuring site* of BP relative to the level of the heart also affects the value of BP. This is because of gravity. In patients with severe peripheral vascular disease, there may be a significant difference in the value of measured blood pressure between the right and left arm and between the arms and legs. However, in such circumstances, the higher value should be taken for these patients **(Figure 16)**.

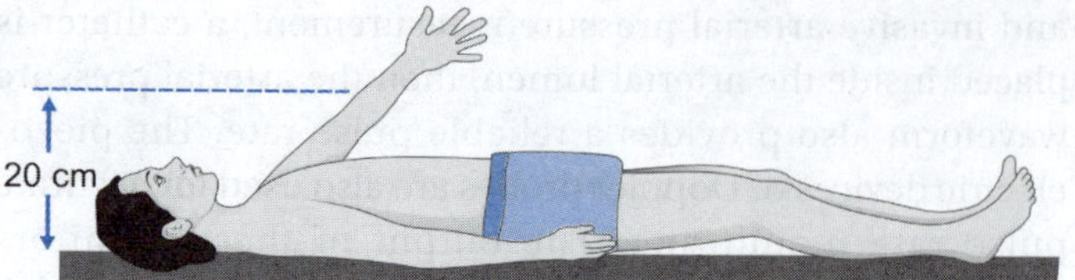

Fig. 16: Difference of arterial BP (in mm Hg) at the different sites of measurement in relation to BP, measured at the level of heart. This difference is equal to the height of the interposed column of water (in cmH_2O). This difference is obtained by multiplying the numerical value of the height of water column (in cmH_2O) by the conversion factor, i.e., 0.74. (1 cmH_2O = 0.74 mm Hg).

The easily measured parameters of cardiovascular function such as the BP and pulse rate are less reliable than the CO and SVR, which are more reliable, but difficult to measure. For example, if the SVR is high, then the BP will also be high, but the cardiac output will be low, which cannot be understood by the level of the blood pressure only. Thus, the arterial pressure should be viewed as an indicator, but not always as the measurement of organ perfusion. All types of anesthesia, no matter how "trivial", is an indication for the measurement of BP. But, its frequency and the technique of measurement depend on the gravity of surgery, the condition of patient, and the experience of anesthetist. Generally, the measurement of BP, which is based on noninvasive oscillometric principle and is measured after every 3–5 minutes interval, is adequate in most cases.

Blood pressure is measured mainly by two techniques: indirect (noninvasive) and direct (invasive). The noninvasive method for the measurement of BP is based on the technique of palpation, Doppler, auscultation, oscillometry, and plethysmography.

Indirect or Noninvasive Methods

The most common indirect methods for the measurement of BP are based on the principle of *Riva-Rocci sphygmomanometer*. The use of this method consists of the inflation of a pneumatic cuff, leading to the occlusion of blood flow of a large artery and then sensing the sequence of physical changes that occur in and around this just opened large artery, as the pressure occluding the artery is released and the blood begins to flow through it. Originally, Riva-Rocci described the measurement of systolic blood pressure by the disappearance of radial pulse, when the cuff was inflated (cuff inflation technique). But, nowadays a *variation of this Riva-Rocci method* is employed where both the systolic and/or diastolic pressures are measured during the deflation of cuff and when the pulse reappears (cuff-deflation or return-to-flow technique). This reappearance of pulse, which helps in the detection of systolic and diastolic blood pressure, is detected by the method of palpation, Doppler, auscultation, or oscillometry method. This indirect (noninvasive) methods of BP measurement may be *intermittent or continuous.* This intermittent noninvasive method of BP measurement again may be of *manual or automated.*

Noninvasive intermittent techniques: BP can be measured intermittently and noninvasively either by *manually* or by an *automatic machine.*

Manual method: This is the simplest way of measurement of BP and is based on the auscultation of Korotkoff sounds. Using a Riva-Rocci sphygmomanometer cuff, Korotkoff, an another scientist, applied a stethoscope on the artery, directly below the cuff to auscultate the sound which is generated as the cuff was slowly deflated and the blood starts to flow through the just opened arteries. This sound is created by a complex series of audible frequencies, produced by the (i) turbulent flow of blood, (ii) vibration of unstable arterial wall, and (iii) shock wave formation, as the external occluding pressure on a major artery is reduced. When the cuff pressure is deflated gradually, after its initial inflation, then the pressure level where the completely occluded artery just opened and blood starts to flow through a narrow opening of arterial lumen, the first producing sound (Phase I) by the above-mentioned mechanism is considered as the *systolic pressure.* Then, gradually the character of this sound changes (phases II and III). Finally, the sound becomes muffled (phase IV) and becomes absent (phase V). The pressure where the sound becomes muffled or absent (phases IV and V) is taken as the *diastolic pressure.* In certain pathological conditions, such as in aortic incompetence, the phase V may not occur and phase IV is continuous.

The accuracy of BP, measured by this noninvasive intermittent manual method, depends on the width of cuff and the rate of the release of pressure. The width of cuff should be at least 20–30% of the circumference of the limb and the pneumatic bladder should cover at least half of the circumference of arm. A cuff of 14 cm wide and 30 cm long is considered satisfactory for the accurate measurement of BP in adult. An excessively narrow cuff produces a *falsely high value* and an excessively wide cuff shows a *falsely low value.* Similarly, the optimal rate of the release of pressure for accurate result is 3 mm of Hg/sec. The rapid release of pressure also causes the falsely low value. If we calculate the rate of deflation of cuff with the HR, then the deflation of pressure of 2 mm Hg per beat will further increase the accuracy. As the generation of Korotkoff sounds depends on the blood flow, so the pathological or iatrogenic causes which decrease the blood flow, such as cardiogenic shock or the use of vasopressor agents, etc. can result in a falsely low blood pressure reading. The aneroid manometer needs

frequent calibration for correct results. During shivering, the pneumatic cuff may need a high occluding pressure due to the low compliance of underlying tissues. So, it may result in pseudohypertension.

Sometimes, only the systolic pressure is estimated by inflating the cuff around the upper arm to a high pressure above the systolic level and then detecting the return of radial pulse when the cuff is deflated (*palpation method*). When the cuff pressure is gradually decreased, then the pressure level at which the pulse is first palpated is taken as the systolic pressure. Despite its crudeness, this method is very helpful in situations where other monitoring devices are not available and where a patient has suddenly deteriorated, necessitating only systolic pressure measurement as life-saving.

Automatic method: The standard auscultatory method which is used manually to measure the blood pressure often fails, when the arterial blood pressure is <60 mm Hg. This is because the Korotkoff sounds are of too low-pitch to be audible at that pressure. In that situation, BP can be measured intermittently by automatic noninvasive methods based on the oscillotonometric (oscillometric) principle or ultrasound technology (Doppler principle and arteriosonade). This automatic noninvasive blood pressure (ANIBP) measurement devices provide consistent and reliable data. Again, many of these machines can compute an accurate mean arterial pressure (MAP) from the systolic and diastolic pressure which is a very valuable hemodynamic parameter. Though, the BP measured by this oscillometric principle is reliable, still there are some disadvantages which are given in **Box 6**.

In the oscillotonometric principle, the variations or oscillation of pressure within the cuff, which is transmitted into the air within the cuff, from the arterial pulsation during the deflation of cuff, are sensed by the electronic monitor and are used to determine the values of arterial blood pressure. Originally, in Von Recklinghausen's BP measuring device (sphygmomanometer) this principle of oscillotonometer

---

BOX 6: Disadvantages of oscillometry.

- Inaccurate, if systolic BP is <60 mm Hg
- Inaccurate, if arrhythmia is present
- Inaccurate in the presence of a wrong-sized cuff
- Inaccurate during movement of limbs
- Discomfort in an awake patient
- Does not provide continuous or beat-to-beat result
- If the interval between the two measurements is too short, there is chance of skin and nerve damage
- Back flow of blood into the IV cannula, if it is in the same arm
- Delay in drug reaching the circulation
- Malfunctioning of the pulse oximeter, if it is used on the same limb

was used which senses the arterial wall motion and displays this (arterial wall motion) as an oscillation of a pointer on a scale. The systolic blood pressure is that at which small oscillations of needle suddenly increase in amplitude when the cuff pressure is gradually reduced and blood starts to flow.

Unfortunately, at that time the interpretation of diastolic point was controversial and subjective. Later, the second cuff which was originally used in Von Recklinghausen's device, is replaced by stethoscope with hearing the sound first by Korotkoff (Korotkoff's sound). But, now this technique has become even more accurate than the conventional sphygmomanometry, and has been improved by electronic devices. Arterial pulsations make small oscillations in the completely sealed air of the cuff, when the cuff starts to be inflated and the arterial diastolic pressure becomes equal to the cuff pressure (in the empty cuff there will be no oscillation). These oscillations are absent or very small, if the cuff is inflated above the systolic pressure and the artery is completely occluded with no flow of blood through it. Mercury or aneroid manometer provides an unreliable and gross measurement of these small oscillations.

But, when the intracuff pressure is decreased to the systolic blood pressure, after its initial inflation to a higher than systolic pressure, then the oscillations are markedly increased. Maximum oscillation occurs at MAP after which it again decreases **(Fig. 17)**. The electronic devices measure the pressure at which the amplitude of oscillation changes. Then from these changes, a microprocessor calculates the systolic, mean, and diastolic blood pressure, using an algorithm. Thus, oscillometric principle needs identical consecutive pulse waves for its measurement. So, it is unreliable during arrhythmias.

The ultrasound technology for the measurement of ANIBP uses the Doppler principle to determine the

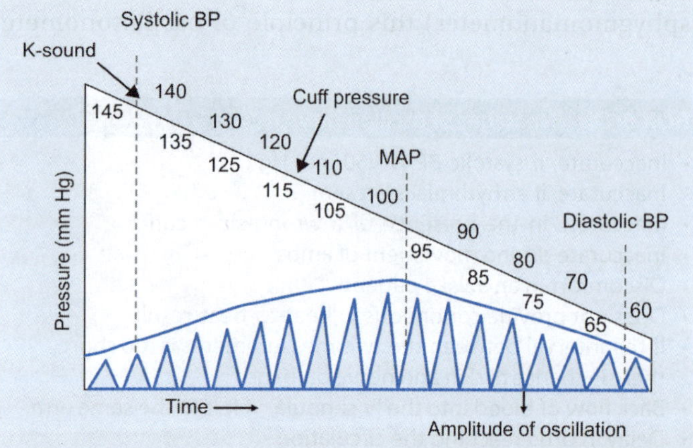

Fig. 17: The principle of oscillometric method for determination of arterial BP.

blood flow or the arterial wall motion distal to the cuff. In Doppler principle, the motion of the arterial wall is sensed by ultrasound when blood starts to flow through the large arteries, during the deflation of cuff, after its initial occlusion by the inflation of cuff above the systolic blood pressure. The main drawback of this ultrasound technology is that it requires an extreme attention to the placement and securing of ultrasound transducer directly over the artery. Because, the dislodgment of transducer probe from just over the arterial site leads to the sudden loss of information and disturbs the attention of anesthetist who has to quickly decide whether the cause of this failure is within the machine or with the patient. The ultrasound technique is not suitable for the measurement of diastolic BP, but the systolic pressure can reliably be determined by the Doppler technique. It has the added advantage of using the probe as a pulse monitor. However, it is useful for the obese patients, pediatric patients and the patients in shock.

Recently, a modification of Doppler technology is done by using piezoelectric crystal. By this technique, the lateral arterial wall movement, during the intermittent opening and closing of artery between the systolic and diastolic pressure is detected. Therefore, this Doppler instrument detects both the systolic and diastolic pressure accurately.

What is Doppler effect?
It is the shifting (changing) of the frequency of reflected ultrasound wave, when the reflecting source (blood) moves relative to the point from where the ultrasound is originating (i.e., comes nearer to the source of ultrasound or goes distant to it). It can be explained in this way that the pitch of a moving vehicle (train) increases or decreases as it approaches to the station or departs from the station. Similarly, the frequency of the reflected ultrasound wave will increase or decrease from a moving object (blood), causing a shift (change) in the frequency. A Doppler probe transmits an ultrasonic signal, which is reflected from the underlying moving tissue which may be the blood flow. Then, the shift of reflected frequency is detected by the detector incorporated within the same probe. Thus, the difference between the transmitted and received (reflected) frequency causes the characteristic changes of sound, which indicates the nature of blood flow.

Noninvasive continuous technique: In this technique, the BP is measured *continuously* and *noninvasively* by an *automated* technique from the finger by using a microprocessor and servo-technology (arterial-volume-clamp method). This is better known as the *servo-plethysmo-manometer.* In this device, there is a cuff within which there is an infrared photoelectric probe. This probe produces a photoplethysmograph and continuously measures the size (diameter) of the digital arteries by transillumination

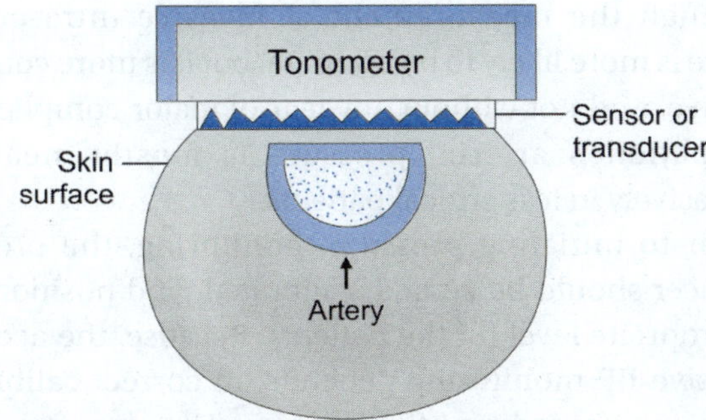

Fig. 18: Tonometer for continuous beat-to-beat measurement of the arterial BP noninvasively.

method. The cuff pressure and the photoplethysmograph interact through a sophisticated servo-controlled mechanism and tracks the arterial pressure throughout the cardiac cycle which is displayed on the monitor screen as a numerical value and a continuous waveform.

Recently, the BP is also measured noninvasively and continuously by devices which use the changes in arterial wall elasticity by arterial tonometry **(Fig. 18)**. Arterial tonometry actually is a version of "applanation tonometry". Here, a superficial artery (usually radial) is compressed and partially flattened against the underlying bone. Then, this flattened arterial surface serves as a transducer for intravascular pressures, acting perpendicularly against the vessel wall. An array of piezoelectric crystals, positioned on the skin overlying this flattened portion of artery senses these changes of perpendicular arterial pressure and translates them into a continuous arterial pressure waveform. Previously, it was thought that this arterial tonometry is better than other forms of continuous noninvasive pressure monitoring. But, unfortunately the most recent clinical studies have identified the limitations of this device, particularly in pediatric patients and in patients receiving the vasodilating drugs.

So, now, in the terms of absolute accuracy of blood pressure measurement, the intermittent oscillometry technique appears to be superior than the radial artery tonometry.

The role of these newer, continuous, and noninvasive BP monitors is still unclear. This is because there is still some doubt about the accuracy of their result (compared with the invasive method). Again, though, it is still controversial whether these devices can actually supplement the continuous invasive monitoring or not, but certainly there are a population of patients in whom these techniques shall find a niche and become an important part in their monitoring armamentarium.

Direct or invasive method: This requires an intra-arterial cannula of 20 G to 22 G in diameter (a Teflon catheter causes less thrombosis than a catheter made of polypropylene) to be inserted directly into an artery for the direct measurement of

BOX 7: Technique of radial artery cannulation.

For radial artery cannulation, the supination and extension of wrist joint makes the radial artery at its optimum position for cannulation. The tube and transducer system should be ready, flushed with saline, for quick connection after cannulation. By ultrasound or palpation (by lightly pressing the artery with the tips of the index and middle fingers of nondominant hand over the area of maximum impulse) the course of the radial artery is determined. Now, after cleaning the skin by antiseptic solution, 1% lignocaine is infiltrated into the skin of an awake patient, directly over the artery with a small-gauge needle

Now, an 18-G needle with a catheter, surrounding the needle, is used directly to puncture the skin and the artery at 45° angle, directing toward the point of palpation. Then, the needle is lowered to 30° angle and is advanced to another 1–2 mm, making sure that the tip of the catheter is well within the lumen of the vessel. After that, the needle is withdrawn, keeping the catheter in place and blood will start to flash back through the catheter. In such situation, firm pressure can be applied over the artery, proximal to the catheter tip, to prevent the blood from spurting from the catheter. Now, a guidewire is advanced through the catheter into the artery and this catheter is withdrawn. Next, the intra-arterial cannula (tube) is advanced over the guidewire and the guidewire is withdrawn. Now, the tube with transducer system is attached with the intra-arterial cannula

blood pressure. The radial artery is usually first chosen in an adult for direct invasive intra-arterial BP monitoring and the femoral artery is used more often in children. The radial artery is commonly chosen for intra-arterial cannulation, because of its superficial location and collateral flow. The collateral circulation is very important to prevent distal ischemia and necrosis due to arterial injury by any unsuccessful attempt. Only 5% of total population have incomplete palmar arches and inadequate collateral flow to radial artery and these individuals are more prone to ischemia and necrosis of hand, distal to the radial artery. The technique for radial artery cannulation is described in **Box 7**.

Ulnar artery cannulation is more difficult, because of its deeper position and more tortuous in nature. If a patient's radial artery is punctured, but cannulation is unsuccessful, then the ipsilateral ulnar artery should never be tried for the fear of compromised blood flow to the portion of hand, distal to it.

The anesthetists are also very fond of brachial artery cannulation, for invasive measurement of blood pressure. Because: (i) it is easily identified in antecubital fossa, and (ii) its proximity to the aorta provides less waveform distortion (more peripheral is the position of artery, the most is the waveform distortion). But, as it is nearer to the elbow, so it is more predisposed to kinking during the flexion of forehand. On the other hand, the femoral artery provides an excellent access to intra-arterial cannulation for continuous invasive

BP monitoring. But, it is more prone to pseudoaneurysms, sepsis, thrombosis, and atheroma. As the dorsalis pedis and posterior tibial artery are far away from the aorta, so they have the most distorted waveforms and are not chosen for invasive intra-arterial BP monitoring. The another chosen site for intra-arterial BP monitoring is the axillary artery. But, the axillary artery is surrounded by the nerves of brachial plexus. So, any unsuccessful cannulation can produce hematoma and nerve damage.

After insertion into the artery, the cannula is attached to a transducer (fluid-filled electromechanical strain gauge) by a narrow-bore, low-compliance pressure tubing. Then, the entire system is attached to a flushing system through a stopcock for flushing the catheter and to prevent thrombus formation within the catheter. Many systems incorporate an automatic flushing device with a continuous slow (1–3 mL/h) infusion of heparinized saline (1 unit/mL), or a spring-controlled valve that allows a periodic high-pressure flushing, for clearing the arterial line, after a blood sample is taken. The practice of using heparinized saline may unnecessarily expose the patient to extra heparin and hence increase the risk of immune-mediated thrombocytopenia. The stopcock in the system provides a site for blood sampling and allows the transducer to be exposed to atmospheric pressure which establishes a zero-reference value. But, the newer systems include a needleless sampling port and an in-line aspiration system. These permit blood sampling without the use of sharp needles and allow the aspirated waste blood to be returned to the patient within a closed system.

The accuracy of transducer depends on the correct calibration and zeroing procedure. This calibration of two types: internal calibration and external calibration. The internal calibration and the zeroing procedure is done by the following way which is described below. The external calibration of a transducer compares the transducer's reading with a manometer or any other measuring instrument. But, the modern transducers now rarely require any external calibration.

The pressure transducer is set at the level of patient's left ventricle and is opened to air to obtain a reference pressure which is taken as zero. When the pressure is zeroed, then the transducer converts the pressure changes directly into the changes of electrical resistance which are measured by the monitor. Thus, the transducer is internally calibrated and on this zero level, the arterial pressure is superimposed and measured. A real-time arterial pressure waveform is usually displayed, in addition to the digital values of pulse rate and the systolic, diastolic, and mean arterial pressure on the screen of monitor. In a few patients, there is marked discrepancy between the arterial pressure, measured invasively and noninvasively.

Though the measurement of invasive intra-arterial pressure is more likely to be accurate, but it is more complex, expensive, and not without any fear of major complication. So, a patient's arterial pressure is mostly measured noninvasively in less critical patients.

Prior to initiating pressure monitoring, the pressure transducer should be zeroed, calibrated, and positioned to an appropriate level (of the patient). Because, the accuracy of invasive BP monitoring depends on correct calibration and zeroing procedure of transducer. The stopcock at the level of desired point of measurement is opened, which is usually at the midaxillary line. This activates the zero trigger in the monitor. Then, if the patient's height is altered by lowering or raising the OT table, then the transducer should also be moved accordingly, or should be zeroed to the new level of midaxillary line. The zero-reference point of the transducer should be checked regularly to eliminate the drift. In the sitting position of patient, the arterial pressure in brain differs significantly from that of the left ventricle. In such a position, the arterial pressure of brain is determined by setting the transducer to zero at the level of ear.

The damping effect, during the monitoring of invasive BP, is caused by some parts of the measuring system. It may be caused by (i) the bubbles of air in tubing, (ii) too long or too elastic tubes, (iii) a kinked cannula or arterial spasm, etc. The damping produces a graph, which reduces the amplitude of measurement of systolic and diastolic pressure, tending toward the mean pressure.

The direct or invasive arterial pressure measurement has become a standard monitoring procedure for any high-risk patient, during anesthesia or in patients with severe circulatory instability, caused by an underlying medical condition, or when the planned operative procedure causes large and sudden cardiovascular changes. The other indications for intra-arterial cannulation for invasive BP measurement include: induced hypotension, end-organ diseases necessitating precise beat-to-beat pressure measurement, and the need for repeated blood gas analysis. It is also commonly used for the patients in intensive care unit (ICU) and in high dependency areas (HDU). Extensive experience with this technique over the years has demonstrated its value and safety, so that current indications for its use have become numerous. Also, the threshold, for applying it, has been lowered to encompass its use in nearly all seriously ill patients, or complicated surgical procedures. Few indications for arterial cannulation are listed later.

Limiting the blood flow in vessels and thus, causing ischemia distally, is the chief complication of intra-arterial cannulation and the measurement of BP invasively. This usually does not happen due to the presence of a collateral blood supply. So, before a radial intra-arterial cannulation,

BOX 8: Indications of arterial catheterization for continuous beat-to-beat measurement of BP.

- Anticipated CVS instability such as severe cardiovascular disease, major trauma, massive transfusion, major surgery, etc
- Direct manipulation of CVS, such as during cardiac surgery, major vascular surgery, induced hypotension, etc
- Surgery with severe cardiovascular diseases, such as valvular diseases, history of MI, severe angina, etc
- Massive obesity where indirect measurement of BP is not possible or inaccurate
- When frequent blood sampling is required such as for blood gas analysis, severe acid-base disturbance, severe electrolyte imbalance, severe sepsis, coagulopathies, etc

it is advisable to check the efficiency of collateral circulation (for radial and ulnar artery it is done) by Allen's test or Weber's test. Allen's test is simple, but not so reliable. In this test, the patient first makes a tight fist and exsanguinates his hand. Then, the operator occludes both the radial and the ulnar arteries by his finger. After that the operator releases only the ulnar artery and the collateral flow through the radial artery and the palmar arterial arch is confirmed by flushing of thumb within 5 seconds.

The delayed return of the color of thumb in-between 5 and 10 seconds indicates an equivocal test. If the delay is >10 seconds then insufficient collateral circulation is confirmed. Alternatively, collateral circulation distal to the radial artery occlusion can be diagnosed by a Doppler probe, plethysmography, or pulse oximetry.

The advantages of direct arterial pressure measurement (Box 8):

- Accuracy.
- Beat-to-beat observation or continuous real time monitoring of the changes in blood pressure.
- Very essential when there is a very rapid swinging of blood pressure.
- Also accurate even at very low-pressure level, where cuff-based measurement techniques may prove impossible.
- Helpful in some morbidly obese patients or those with burned extremities.
- Arterial cannulation also helps to obtain blood samples frequently. New devices also allow the continuous monitoring of arterial blood gas values, using the fiber-optic sensors, placed directly into the artery through vascular catheter. The analysis of intra-arterial pressure waveform also allows for the estimation of CO (cardiac output) and other hemodynamic parameters, derived from this CO value, such as the CI (cardiac index), SV (stroke volume), and SI (stroke index), etc.
- Intentional pharmacological or mechanical cardio-vascular manipulation, such as intra-aortic balloon counterpulsation, deliberate-induced hypotension, and administration of vasoactive drug infusions are possible.
- The shape of the arterial wave also provides several clues of hemodynamic variables. For example, (i) the rate of upstroke indicates the contractility of myocardium, (ii) the rate of downstroke indicates the peripheral vascular resistance, (iii) the exaggerated variation of the size of waveform during respiratory cycle indicates hypovolemia, and (iv) the MAP is calculated by integrating the area, under the pressure curve.

Various physiological and pathological states can produce a generalized arterial pressure gradient, i.e., different levels of blood pressure at different sites of body. Thus, the difference in BP in mm Hg at the different heights of measurement can be equalized by the addition or subtraction of the height of an interposed column of water (cmH_2O) multiplied by a conversion factor (1 cmH_2O = 0.74 mm Hg). Larger differences are seen between the peripheral and the central arterial pressures, in patients with shock. For example, the femoral artery systolic pressure may exceed the radial artery systolic pressure by >40 mm Hg in septic shock, patients receiving norepinephrine infusions, etc. This difference in pressure at different sites has significant therapeutic implications during the management of critically-ill patients. Other vasoactive drugs, neuraxial block, different patient's position and changes in the patient's temperature also produce gradients that alter the relation between the central and the peripheral arterial pressure measurements. Hypothermia and thermoregulatory vasoconstriction also cause the radial arterial systolic pressure to exceed the femoral artery systolic pressure.

The complications of direct arterial cannulation are:

- Bleeding
- Thrombosis and arterial damage
- Ischemia of tissues distal to artery
- Embolization
- Sepsis
- Needs high skill to insert
- Expensive

The intra-arterial blood pressure monitoring is the gold standard for the management of critically ill patients. Because, it provides a continuous beat-to-beat accurate pressure measurement. So, the quality of waveform, which depends on the dynamic characteristics of intra-arterial catheter, tubing, and transducer system, is very important. Because, a false reading leads to inappropriate therapeutic intervention and disaster **(Table 4)**.

An arterial pressure waveform is the expression of the summation of simple sine and cosine of waves (Fourier analysis). So, for accurate results the catheter-tube-transducer

TABLE 4: Pressure at different sites of cardiovascular system.

	Site	Range (mm Hg)	
SVC		0–5	4
RA	Systolic	4–8	6
	Diastolic	0–5	4
RV	Systolic	15–30	20
	Diastolic	0–10	5
PA	Systolic	15–30	25
	Diastolic	5–15	10
PCWP	Mean	5–15	10
LA	Systolic	10–15	10
	Diastolic	5–0	5
LV	Systolic	80–120	110
	Diastolic	5–10	8

(LA: left atrium; LV: left ventricle; PA: pulmonary artery; RA: right atrium; RV: right ventricle; SVC: superior vena cava)

system must respond adequately to the highest frequency of arterial waveform, or the frequency of measuring system must exceed that of the arterial waveform (average 16–24 Hz). The frequency of a modern measuring catheter-tube-transducer system is >200 Hz (this frequency is much higher than the frequency of radial arterial waveform which is 16–24 Hz) and so it gives very accurate results.

The damping coefficient of transducer and the other parts of the arterial pressure measuring system should be optimum which ranges in between 0.6 and 0.7 Hz. Because, underdamping is a serious problem and may lead to overshooting with a falsely high BP. The over dampening, caused by the addition of more tubes, stopcock, tube of low compliance or air in tube, etc. will reduce the frequency of system and will cause falsely low systolic pressure. On the other hand, the under damping will lead to the overshooting of the frequency of system and falsely high systolic BP.

The dynamism of the catheter-tube-transducer system can be improved and damping can be reduced by: eliminating the unnecessary stopcocks, minimizing the tube length, using the low compliance tubes and removing any air bubble from the system.

What is a pressure transducer?

The transducer is a device where the any form of mechanical energy is converted into an electrical energy or signal. The pressure transducer is a device where the mechanical energy of pressure wave is converted into an electrical signal. It contains a diaphragm which is distorted by an arterial or venous pressure wave. Most of the transducers are of resistance type and work on the strain gauge principle.

Here, the diaphragm is made of multiple silicone crystals which are arranged as a Wheatstone bridge circuit. The stretching or pressure on these silicone crystals causes a change in their resistance and subsequently causes a change in voltage output, which is proportional to the pressure applied on the diaphragm. Now, the pressure transducers have been changed from bulky and reusable one to a small and disposable one.

Central Venous Pressure Monitoring

The overall cardiac performance depends on the filling of heart at the end of its diastole, i.e., (i) the end-diastolic filling volume and pressure of right atrium for the right ventricular function, and (ii) the end-diastolic filling volume and pressure of left atrium for the left ventricular function, provided there is no abnormality of tricuspid and mitral valve. So, the monitoring of CVP at the junction of SVC and right atrium reflects the filling and the function of the right side of the heart directly and also the filling and the performance of the left side of the heart, indirectly. Whereas, the measurement of PCWP from the pulmonary capillary which is connected to the left atrium without any valve reflects more or less indirectly the pressure of the left atrium and the function of the left side of the heart. This is because the Sterling's law relates the stroke volume or cardiac function (right or left ventricle) with their end-diastolic filling volume and pressure. Again, the relationship of these two parameters, i.e., the end-diastolic filling pressure and volume (which are directly proportional) and stroke volume depend on the state of the intrinsic myocardial performance, i.e., the contractility of heart and the status of pulmonary vasculature.

Although the CVP or right heart filling pressure is the indicative of circulatory volume or right heart function, but it is often possible with appropriate assumption to use CVP for the monitoring and the management of left heart function. For example, the low left ventricular output or low systemic BP due to blood or fluid loss or due to any condition causing reduction of preload can be diagnosed by measuring the CVP. However, the measurement of pulmonary capillary wedge pressure has drawn attention to the inadequacy of CVP as a measurement of left heart function, because there are major differences between these two right and left pressure systems of heart. Such discrepancies are particularly common during pump failure due to endotoxemia, myocardial infarction, etc. Here, CVP is highly elevated, but cardiac output is very low due to the intrinsic failure of myocardial contractility or performance. Rapid infusion of small amount of fluid may also be a useful clinical test for the determination of cause of failure, i.e., whether due to reduction of preload or intrinsic pump failure. The measurement of CVP by catheterization of SVC, not only helps to measure directly the pressure of the right side of the heart or indirectly the pressure of the left side of the heart but, also has some other functions such as:

- *Fluid management in shock:* Rapid infusions of fluid to correct severe hypovolemia and shock.
- *As a venous access:* To administer some vasoactive and caustic drugs that might irritate and injure the smaller peripheral veins.
- For hyperalimentation and total parenteral nutrition
- For aspiration of air from air emboli during craniotomy in sitting position.
- For comprehensive cardiac monitoring during major vascular surgery, and during all cardiac surgery for placement of pulmonary artery catheter (PAC).
- For insertion of transcutaneous pacing leads.
- Gaining venous access in patients with poor peripheral veins, such as in severe burn.
- With specialized catheter, the central venous catheterization can be used for the continuous monitoring of $ScVO_2$ (central venous O_2 saturation).
- Through central venous line, pulmonary artery catheter (PAC) can be introduced to measure CO, pulmonary artery occlusion pressure (LVEDP).

In a normal individual, the average value of CVP varies in-between 3 and 10 cmH_2O (2–8 mm Hg). In children, the CVP is 3–6 cmH_2O. The CVP > 20 cmH_2O indicates right heart failure. It depends on the intravascular volume status, the intrinsic tone of the musculature of the vessels and the functional integrity of the right side of the heart. It reflects the filling pressure or volume and subsequently the stroke volume of right ventricle. As the tip of the CVP catheter is located at the junction of SVC and RA, so it is exposed to the changes in intrathoracic pressure. Hence, inspiration will increase or decrease the CVP, depending on whether the ventilation is controlled or spontaneous. But, whatever may be the pressure, it should be measured at the end of expiration.

It is *reduced* in (i) hypovolemia due to any cause, (ii) venodilatation, (iii) spinal/epidural anesthesia, and (iv) general anesthesia causing venodilatation. But, it is *increased* during (i) congestive heart failure, (ii) pulmonary embolism, (iii) IPPV and PEEP, (iv) cardiac tamponade (v) constrictive pericarditis, (vi) pleural effusion and hemothorax, (vii) coughing and straining, and (viii) fluid overload, etc. *A low CVP with low BP indicates hypovolemia, while a high CVP with low BP indicates pump (heart) failure.*

Ideally for the measurement of CVP, the tip of the central venous catheter should be placed, just above the right atrium or at the junction of the right atrium and SVC. Advancing the catheter too far may cause arrhythmias and even damage to the myocardium. If the monitoring of the pulmonary arterial pressure and the left atrial pressure is planned, only then the pulmonary artery catheter (PAC) should be advanced, beyond the right atrium and the right ventricle, into the pulmonary artery. Because of the large swings in the intrapleural pressure, which may accompany the mechanical ventilation, it is preferable that all the measurements of CVP should be made with the ventilator disconnected or IPPV is stopped.

There are usually *three techniques* which are adapted by anesthetists for central venous cannulation to monitor CVP. These are:

- A catheter over a needle technique. This is similar to simple peripheral venous catheterization.
- A catheter through a needle technique, which requires a large-bore needle stick.
- A catheter over guidewire technique, which is commonly known as Seldinger technique or method.

The central venous cannulation for the measurement of CVP is also usually done by any of the *three routes*.

i. *Long catheter through the brachial or femoral vein:* The most peripheral veins, such as the brachial veins in antecubital fossa or the femoral vein in femoral triangle is also chosen for the central venous cannulation, using a long catheter. Sometimes, the cephalic or basilic vein, on the outer upper arm, may also be used. But, here success is less likely due to the long tortuous route of these veins. Otherwise, this method is relatively easy and has a very low incidence of acute and serious complications. But, unfortunately, the tip of the cannula commonly fails to reach the central vein, if these peripheral superficial veins are used. Infection and thrombophlebitis are common, if the catheters left in-situ for >48 hours in any route.

ii. *Subclavian vein:* As the subclavian is a large vein and quite close to SVC, so a short central venous catheter can be inserted easily through the skin into this vein. For subclavian cannulation, either the supra- or infraclavicular approach is adopted. But, the infraclavicular approach to this vein for central venous cannulation is most commonly accepted. During cannulation, the angle of the needle should be low and tangential to the ribs in order to avoid the perforation of pleura. The subclavian artery is situated posterior to the vein in this line of approach. So, its puncture may result in significant hemomediastinum and hemothorax. In this approach, the overlying clavicle affords the easy fixation of catheter to the skin and this is comfortable for the patients too. But, unfortunately as the needle, wire and the catheter are not inserted under direct vision, so accidental perforation of the adjacent subclavian artery or pleura is common. Importantly, if arterial bleeding occurs, it may not be evident and cannot be controlled by external pressure because of the position of clavicle. Damage may also be caused to the brachial plexus, which runs along the main vessels. Because of the higher incidence of these major complications, subclavian cannulation is generally used only where specific clinical advantages are evident.

iii. *Internal jugular veins (IJV):* This route is the safest and most reliable for central venous cannulation. The ideal vein for the monitoring of CVP is right jugular vein (RJV) among the right and left jugular vein, because:

- It is valveless and is in direct communication with right atrium.
- The vein is close to the skin.
- The consistent predictable anatomic location of IJV within a palpable landmark.
- The short, straight (right IJV), and valveless course of IJV to the SVC and right atrium.
- Bleeding, if occurs, can be controlled by direct external pressure.
- Success rate is >90% in both adults and children.

Technique of CVP catheterization through right internal jugular vein: It is most commonly done by Seldinger technique. The patient is placed in Trendelenburg position, because this position reduces the chance of air embolism. First the cannula with the stylet is introduced through the skin at the tip of the triangle, formed by the two heads of sternomastoid muscle and clavicle. The direction of the needle should be slightly lateral and toward the ipsilateral nipple. However, the majority of clinician now use the ultrasound to locate the internal jugular vein and in some institutions the use of ultrasound for this purpose is mandatory. Next, when the internal jugular vein is once punctured, then the stylet is withdrawn and a J-wire is passed through the cannula into the IJV and cannula is withdrawn. Next, the CVP catheter is railroad over the J-wire. The tip of the catheter should be at the junction of the SVC and right atrium which is usually 15 cm from the point of entry. At the end of the procedure, an X-ray of chest must be performed to check the position of the catheter and to exclude the pneumothorax.

However, due to the proximity of internal jugular vein to the common carotid artery, cervical spine, major nerves and pleura, the life-threatening complications are still relatively common during central venous cannulation through this route.

Whatever is the route, the central venous catheter should be inserted only when a clear indication for the measurement of CVP is present. For central venous cannulation, always the safest route should be chosen and catheter should be removed at the earliest opportunity. Careful technique and adequate observation of the patient is mandatory, including a mandatory chest X-ray, after insertion of catheter. During the central venous cannulation, ECG should be continuously monitored in order to observe any dysrhythmias which can occur if the tip of catheter crosses the SVC and right atrial junction, or when the catheter is more advanced into the right ventricle and PA to monitor the other filling pressures. If the direct pulmonary arterial pressure monitoring is planned, then it should be established prior to the central venous cannulation.

The *complications* of central venous catheterization are: (i) *Immediate* → carotid artery puncture (most common acute complication), arrhythmias, bleeding, pneumothorax, hemothorax, damage to the thoracic duct (chylothorax), damage to esophagus and damage to other vital structures, such as brachial plexus, phrenic nerve, cardiac puncture, cardiac tamponade, air embolization, etc. (ii) *Delayed* → sepsis, thrombosis, kinking of catheter, displacement of catheter, etc. **(Box 9)**.

The CVP measurement can be made either by a simple water-filled manometer, connected to a running fluid line via a stopcock or by an electronic transducer and digital display. The measurement of CVP by water manometer is simplest, least expensive, and sufficient in many cases for general assessment of intravascular volume status. When CVP is measured by water manometer, then the right atrium of patient's heart and the zero point of manometer scale should be kept at the same level. As the normal value of CVP varies in between 3 and 10 cmH$_2$O (due to low pressure system), so a small change in the relative height of reference, e.g., when an operating table is moved up and down, may lead to an appreciable error. In practice, a single measurement of CVP is unreliable, as this value may be altered in an unpredictable manner by several factors, such as positive pressure ventilation, patient's position, etc. The response of CVP to a fluid challenge is more valuable. In hypovolemic patients the initial change in CVP is small with a rapid infusion of fluid. But, with continued infusion the CVP increases more quickly as normovolemia is achieved. Contrary, in patients who are overloaded with fluid or have a heart failure, even a small amount of intravenous fluid causes a marked increase in CVP at initial phase. Sudden increase in CVP may also be caused by events, such as pulmonary embolism, myocardial infarction, pneumothorax, etc.

The CVP monitoring during anesthesia and surgery are very useful in determining the overall fluid volume status of patient, the effect of fluid or blood loss and in guiding the fluid replacement therapy. The responses of CVP to fluid replacement therapy can also provide information, regarding the venous compliance and the functional efficiency of the right side of the heart.

When a pressure transducer is used for monitoring of CVP, then the device displays the pressure unit in millimeter of Hg, but not in centimeters of H_2O as in a water manometer (1.36 cmH$_2$O = 1 mm Hg). It is also important to understand that during monitoring of this low-pressure system, the transducer should be placed and zeroed at correct level, i.e., the right atrial level. The zero reference at the level of right atrium or the manubriosternal joint and the manometer scale or the transducer must bear a constant relationship. The waveform of CVP which is displayed on the screen of an electronic device is actually a wealth of information. The venous pressure waves reflect the normal sequences of the mechanical events of cardiac cycle. The first large positive deflection "A" wave is caused by atrial contraction, which is quickly followed by a small positive "C" wave due to the bulging of tricuspid valve in right atrium, with the onset of ventricular systole. Then, this "C" wave is followed by "X" descent due to the atrial relaxation which is again followed by a late positive deflection "V" wave, due to the gradual accumulation of blood in the superior vena cava and the right atrium. Finally, the "Y" descent is caused by the opening of tricuspid valve and rapid right ventricular filling. In atrial fibrillation the "A" wave is absent, as there is no effective atrial contraction. However, sometimes large "A" waves (cannon waves) also occur in some arrhythmias, such as complete heart block, nodal rhythm, etc. when atrium contracts against a closed tricuspid valve. The tricuspid regurgitation, ventricular overfilling or heart failure, etc. cause distortion and an increased size of "V" wave **(Fig. 19)**.

Pulmonary Arterial Pressure Monitoring

Starling first demonstrated that the left ventricular flow or cardiac output is directly proportional to LVED fiber length, which is again proportional to LVEDV. This LVEDV is again directly proportional to LVEDP which we try to measure indirectly by pulmonary artery pressure (PAP). Thus, one of the main determinants of CO and hence O_2 delivery to tissues is the left ventricular end-diastolic volume (LVEDV),

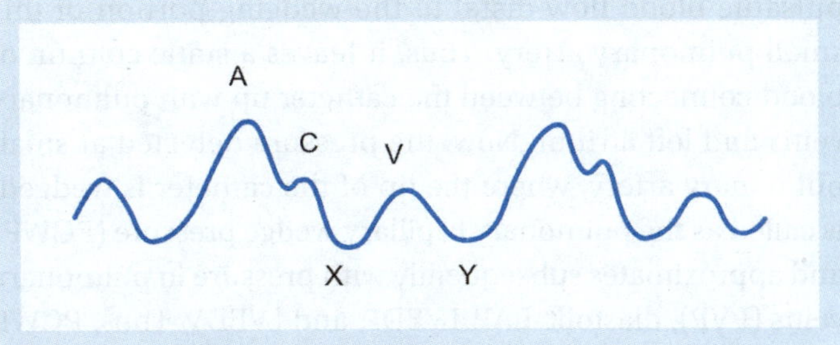

Fig. 19: Central venous pressure wave.

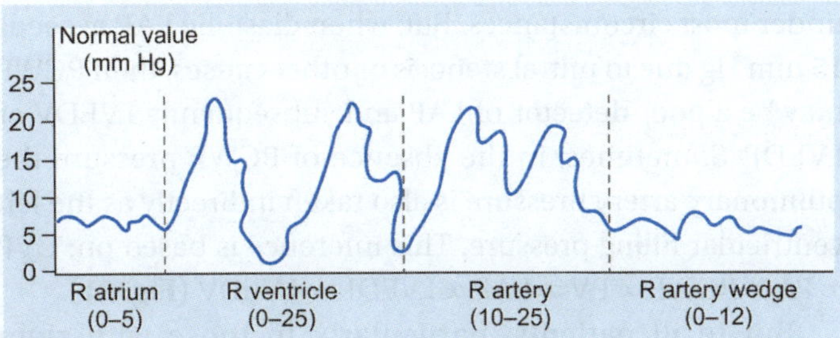

Fig. 20: This is a diagrammatic representation of the pressure waveform which is seen on the monitor, while the tip of the pulmonary artery catheter is advanced through the right atrium and right ventricle and ultimately to lie in the pulmonary artery. The right atrial pressure wave is characterized by low systolic and low diastolic value. The right ventricular pressure wave is characterized by high systolic and low diastolic value. The main pulmonary artery pressure wave is characterized by high systolic and high diastolic value. Pulmonary artery wedge wave is characterized by low systolic but high diastolic value. When the balloon is inflated with the tip of the catheter wedged in a branch of a pulmonary artery, immediately the pulmonary artery wedge pressure waveform is seen on the monitor. The pressure values, shown here, represent in a normal spontaneously breathing patient.

which assumes the amount of blood ready to be pumped out, during left ventricular systole. But it cannot be measured directly. So, if left ventricular compliance is normal, then the left ventricular end-diastolic pressure (LVEDP) can be used as an indicator of LVEDV. Thus, the measurement of LVEDP is very vital for determination or assessment of left ventricular performance and CO.

Again, unless an abnormal pressure gradient exists across the mitral valve, then the left atrial pressure (LAP) and pulmonary venous pressure (PVP) reflect LVEDP. On the other hand, the measurement of pressure in the small pulmonary artery reflects the PVP which ultimately reflects **(Fig. 20)** the LAP, LVEDP, and CO. So, the measurement of pressure in a small pulmonary artery by wedging the tip of a pulmonary artery catheter which is known as PCWP gives us a vital clue of CO. The entry and wedging (by inflation of a balloon) of the tip of a pulmonary artery catheter into small pulmonary artery (capillary) ceases the phasic and pulsatile blood flow distal to the wedging portion of this small pulmonary artery. Thus, it leaves a static column of blood connecting between the catheter tip with pulmonary veins and left atrium. Now, the pressure detected at small pulmonary artery, where the tip of the catheter is wedged, is called as the pulmonary capillary wedge pressure (PCWP) and approximates subsequently with pressure in pulmonary veins (PVP), diastolic LAP, LVEDP, and LVEDV. Thus, PCWP which is also termed as PAOP (pulmonary artery occlusion pressure), provides an indirect nearly accurate estimation of preload or diastolic filling of the left side of the heart under most circumstances. But, when diastolic LAP exceeds 15 mm Hg due to mitral stenosis or other causes, then PCWP may be a poor detector of LAP and subsequently LVEDV or LVEDP. Sometimes, in the absence of PCWP pressure the pulmonary artery pressure is also taken indirectly as the left ventricular filling pressure. This inference is based on: CVP $\propto$ PA $\propto$ PCWP $\propto$ PV $\propto$ LAP $\propto$ LVEDP $\propto$ LVEDV **(Fig. 21)**.

But in ill patients, particularly in those with right ventricular failure, pulmonary edema, mitral valve diseases, and those receiving positive pressure ventilation, etc.; the relation between the pulmonary artery pressure (or pressure of the right side of the heart) and LAP or PVP (pressure of the left side of the heart) is uncertain. Unfortunately, as it is not possible to cannulate the left atrium easily, so we try to estimate or measure indirectly the LVEDP (proportional to LVEDV—which is again the main determinant of CO) by measuring the pressure of the right side of the heart by measuring the PCWP, PAP, RVP, CVP, etc.

On the basis of relationship between the PA pressure, PV pressure, and alveolar pressure (PALV), the lung is divided into three zones (I, II, and III). For the measurement of PAP and PCWP, the tip of the pulmonary artery catheter (PAC) should be in zone III, where PVP exceeds alveolar pressure and the capillary conduit is completely opened being capable of directly transmitting the pressure of blood from left side of heart to the right side. In the supine position, as a large portion of lung remains in zone III, so it is assumed that the tip of PAC always remains in zone III. When the patient is ventilated with high positive pressure or PEEP, then most of the zone III will be converted to zone II or I. In this situation, the relationship between PCWP and LAP is lost. The maximum limit of PEEP is 10 cmH$_2$O, below which the relationship is maintained.

In an average the pulmonary artery diastolic pressure (PADP) which is about 10 mm Hg is often used as a good indicator of PCWP which is about 9 mm Hg. But in some situations, where the pulmonary artery diastolic pressure increases such as in pulmonary hypertension (or $\uparrow$ PVR) due to hypoxia, hypercarbia, chronic obstructive lung diseases or vasoactive drugs, etc., then PADP does not correlate well with PCWP or pressure of the left side of heart. Therefore, to summarize, it can be stated that in conditions where the left heart function correlates well with the right heart function and there is no condition suggesting grossly abnormal PVR, then CVP can be trusted as sole indicator of the overall left-sided cardiac filling pressure and cardiac output.

The *old pulmonary artery catheter* (PAC) (or *Swan-Ganz* catheter) usually has three lumens and a thermistor

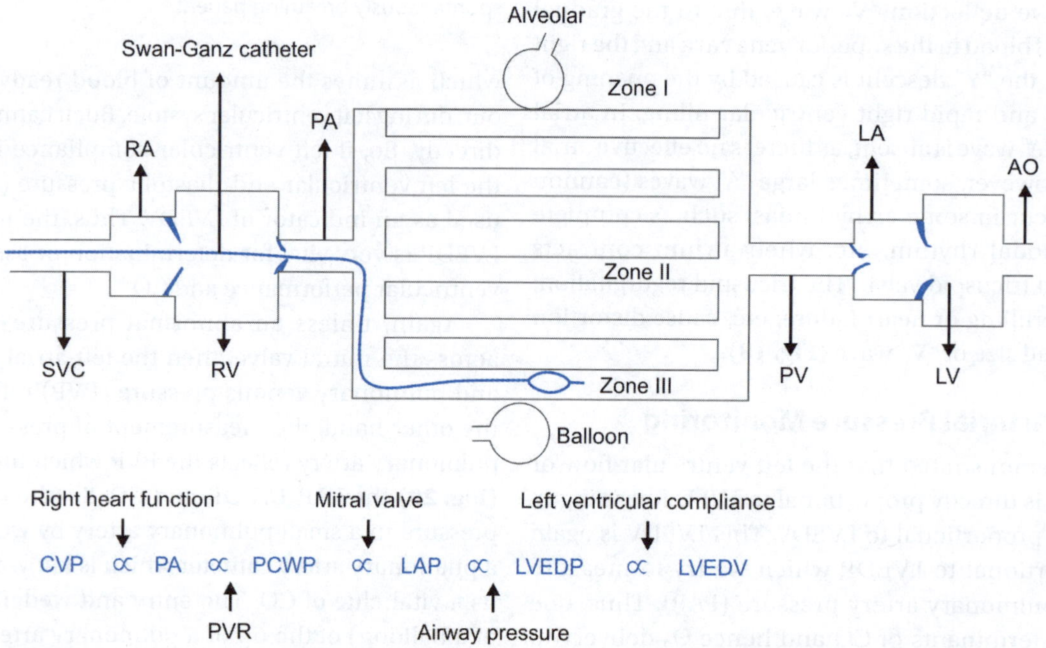

Fig. 21: Relationship between various determinants of cardiac output.

near at the tip. This thermistor is connected by a wire to CO measuring computer by thermodilution technique. The most distal lumen opens at the tip and is connected proximally to a pressure transducer which displays the pressure waveform on monitor screen. Proximal to the tip, there is another lumen which is used to inflate the balloon. There is another proximal lumen, which is used for the measurement of CO. In addition to the measurement of CO, the PAC is also used for sampling of mixed venous blood. However, *the modern PAC has five lumens* with provisions for CVP monitoring port, extravenous infusion ports, a fiber-optic bundle for blood O_2 saturation measurement, and a lumen for the passage of wire for ECG recording and atrial or ventricular pacing. The balloon-tipped Swan–Ganz catheter is flow directed, i.e., its movement through different chambers of heart is directed by the flow of blood. The presence of this catheter in the different parts of the heart is confirmed by pressure recording, pressure tracing (waveform) and distance from catheter tip. Entry of the catheter tip into right ventricle is confirmed by the sudden increase in systolic BP (systolic pressure in right atrium is 0–8 mm Hg, while in right ventricle it is 15–30 mm Hg. The entry of catheter tip into pulmonary artery is best indicated by sudden increase in diastolic pressure (diastolic pressure in right ventricle is 0–8 mm Hg, while in pulmonary artery it is 5–15 mm Hg.

Because of cost, technical feasibility, complications ranging from minor arrhythmias (most common complications, incidences are around 30%) to life-threatening situations such as pulmonary artery rupture, severe arrhythmias and death and availability of noninvasive (or less invasive) monitors, pulmonary artery catheterization is hardly done nowadays.

Procedure of pulmonary artery catheterization: Insertion of PAC first requires the insertion of a central venous cannula at any site. Then, PAC can be placed successfully through any of the central venous cannulation sites. But, the right IJV is preferred by most of the clinicians. External jugular vein may also be used. But, the success rate is less than IJV. If neck veins are not available, then left subclavian vein is next preferred to right subclavian vein. Because, the left subclavian vein courses to SVC in a smooth gradual turn than its right counterpart. Prior to insertion of every PAC, it should be checked by inflating and deflating the balloon and irrigating all the three or five intracatheter lumen with heparinized saline. The distal lumen is connected to an electronic pressure transducer which is zeroed at the mid-axillary line. After the introduction of PAC through its valved port of introducer, used for central venous cannulation, the distal port of PAC is connected to pressure transducer. When the catheter is first placed into SVC and a central venous waveform is seen on monitor, then the balloon is inflated. If the central

venous waveform varies with respiration, then it confirms that the tip of the catheter is in intrathoracic position, but either in superior vena cava or in RA. At approximately 15 cm distance from the insertion point, the distal tip should enter the RA. The balloon is inflated with air, the volume of which is according to the manufacturer's recommendation (usually 1.5 mL). It protects the myocardium and endocardium from injury by the tip of the catheter. It also allows the flow of blood or the right ventricular output to direct the catheter forward from chamber to chamber and from chamber to main artery. On the other hand, the balloon is always deflated during withdrawal or for any manipulation.

After its introduction, the pulmonary artery catheter is first advanced toward the RA and then toward the tricuspid valve from SVC. From this point onward ECG monitoring for detection of any dysrhythmias is very important. This is because premature ventricular contractions (PVC) are often seen during PAC insertion and its passage through the different chambers of heart which may require intervention. As the PAC advances, then the ballooned tip of the catheter tends to move toward the pulmonary artery from the right ventricle by the direction of the flow of blood. Although some manipulation may be required, but it usually advances easily through the right atrium and the right ventricle into the pulmonary artery. However, the corresponding changes in the measured pressure can be observed over the screen as the catheter advances. The location of the tip of the PAC is also determined by identifying the characteristics of the pressure waves of that cardiac chambers and vessels which are encountered during its passage. The advancement of catheter tip from chamber to chamber is facilitated by the different phases of cardiac cycle and also by the flow of blood as PAC is a flow-directed catheter. For example, the catheter tip with balloon passes from the SVC into the right atrium and then to the right ventricle during diastole. But, the catheter passes from the right ventricle to the pulmonary artery during systole.

The location of catheter tip into right ventricle is characterized by a sudden increase in systolic pressure and a wide pulse pressure. Then, from right ventricle to pulmonary artery (PA), the catheter passes on during systole, and the location of the tip of PAC at PA is characterized by a sudden increase in diastolic pressure and a narrow pulse pressure. The entry of the tip of the catheter into the PA normally occurs by 35–45 cm distance from the entry site. The catheter further advances through the pulmonary artery, until it eventually fills the lumen of a small pulmonary artery to become wedged and to lose much of its pulsatile character as seen in the small PA. In this position, the tip of the catheter is isolated from the proximal part of this small PA by the balloon. The transducer then measures the pressure of the pulmonary capillaries which are in continuity with the pulmonary veins and hence the left atrium in front. This is then taken as the measurement of the left atrial pressure at diastole. If the balloon is deflated at this wedged position, then the pulmonary artery waveform is restored again and at the end of each measurement of left atrial pressure the balloon must be deflated to avoid pulmonary infarction. During passage of catheter through the right atrium, right ventricle, and pulmonary artery, there is chance of knotting. So, to prevent knotting the balloon should be deflated and the catheter is withdrawn, till the pressure changes do not occur at the expected distance. In very difficult cases, such as, in low cardiac output, pulmonary hypertension, congenital heart diseases, etc., the catheter advancement by flotation of the balloon can be enhanced: (i) by the deep breaths of patient, (ii) by positioning of patient in a right lateral or head-up position, (iii) by increasing the cardiac output, (iv) by administering a small dose of inotropic agent, etc.

If the wedging of catheter occurs before the maximum inflation of balloon, then it signals its over-wedged position. In such condition, the catheter should be withdrawn slightly because there is a chance of pulmonary artery rupture which may carry 50–70% mortality rate. So, the PAP should continuously be monitored to detect any over-wedged position which is an indication of catheter migration. The correct position of catheter is also confirmed by the lateral chest X-ray. Usually, most catheter migrate caudally (basal portion of lungs) and to the right side (right lung). But, sometimes it wedges anterior to the vena cava, where the true pulmonary capillary pressure is less than the alveolar pressure. This results in a spuriously elevated pressure measurement during IPPV.

The relative contraindications of pulmonary artery catheterization are: complete LBBB which may lead to complete heart block, WPW syndrome and Ebstein malformation which may lead to severe arrhythmias. The risk of complications increases with the duration of catheterization. So, it should not be kept for >72 hours.

Though, the PAC can provide invaluable information for the care of critically ill patients, but still there are several pitfalls in the procedure of measurement and interpretation of these data. So, it sometimes makes the PAC a counterproductive and even hazardous tool. For example, the balloon of the catheter is inflated blindly only by the observing the PA pressure tracing, which guides the balloon's position. But, unfortunately the PA pressure waveform can be distorted by artifacts and can misguide the actual position of the catheter balloon, whether it is properly wedged or not. This confusion may result in an erroneous and dangerous overinflation of balloon, causing severe complications.

TABLE 5: Complications of pulmonary artery catheterization with reported incidence (in %).

Bleeding	5–10%
Mural thrombus	25–60%
Thrombophlebitis	6–10%
Arterial puncture	1–3%
Pneumothorax	0.3–4%
Air embolism	0.5–1%
Minor arrhythmia	4–68%
Severe arrhythmia (VT and VF)	0.5–60%
RBBB	0.1–4%
LBBB	0.1–8%
Pulmonary artery rupture	0–1%
Pulmonary infarction	0.1–5%
Positive culture at catheter tip	1–34%
Endocarditis	2–9%
Catheter knotting	1–2%

(LBBB: left bundle branch block; RBBB: right bundle branch block; VF: ventricular fibrillation; VT: ventricular tachycardia)

So, the routine use of PAC should not be performed, till the benefits over balance the risks. Thus, the decision of monitoring with a PAC depends on the clinical judgment of the anesthetist who must weigh all the pros and cons of this process in the background of the status of the particular patient, the proposed surgical procedure and the particular process setting.

The complications of pulmonary artery catheterization are: tachydysrhythmias (such as PVC, VT, VF, etc.), heart block (RBBB, LBBB, or complete AV block in patients with prior LBBB), endocarditis, pulmonary embolism, pulmonary infarction, pulmonary artery rupture, sepsis (positive catheter tip culture), tricuspid and/or pulmonary regurgitation, etc. **(Table 5)**.

Uses of Pulmonary Artery Catheterization:
- Measuring the pressure in different chambers of heart, except left ventricle.
- *Calculating CO (cardiac output) and stroke volume:* The most commonly used method to calculate CO is thermodilution method. Here, ice-cold saline is injected in PA and then the change in temperature of blood in PA is noted by thermistor. The processor, then, calculates the CO by computerized algorithm. The alternative to this thermodilution method is dye-dilution method and Fick principle. The Fick principle is discussed below in details. In dye-dilution method, in place of ice-cold saline the idocyanine green or lithium is injected and like the change of temperature, the change of color is noted.

Next, from this change of color, processor calculates the CO by computerized algorithm.

To decrease the invasiveness of pulmonary artery catheterization, a modified approach such as transpulmonary thermodilution method may be used where the ice-cold saline is injected in SVC through CVP catheter and thermistor is placed in femoral artery, instead of PA, to record the change in temperature.

- *Measuring pulmonary artery occlusion pressure (PAOP):* It is also called as pulmonary capillary occlusion pressure or pulmonary capillary wedge pressure (PCWP). It represents left atrial pressure. Normally, the PAOP is 4–12 mm Hg. This PAOP is best utilized to differentiate between cardiogenic and noncardiogenic pulmonary edema [acute respiratory distress syndrome (ARDS)]. The PAOP < 18 mm Hg indicates noncardiogenic pulmonary edema. While the PAOP < 25 mm Hg indicates cardiogenic pulmonary edema.
- *Taking mixed venous blood sample:* PA is considered as the best site for mixed venous blood sample. Oxygen saturation in mixed venous blood indicates the amount of O_2 extracted by tissue. Therefore, O_2 saturation of mixed venous blood determines the tissue perfusion or CO. The normal mixed venous O_2 saturation is 75%. Because, 25% is consumed by tissues (let the arterial O_2 saturation is 100%). The mixed venous O_2 saturation < 60% indicates significant deficiency in tissue perfusion. Special pulmonary artery probe is also available which can continuously measure the O_2 saturation of mixed venous blood.
- *Monitoring fluid therapy:* CVP measures the preload of the right side of heart, whereas the PAOP measures the preload of the left side of heart. For the monitoring of fluid therapy, measurement of preload of left heart is definitely better than that of right heart. Therefore, PAOP is better guide than CVP for the management of fluid therapy. Low PAOP and low stroke volume indicates hypovolemia (less preload to left heart, so less stroke volume). High PAOP and low stroke volume represent pump failure, i.e., cardiogenic shock (adequate preload to left heart, still due to inadequate myocardial contraction less stroke volume).

Monitoring of Left Atrial Pressure

Directly the LAP is measured only during open cardiac surgeries. This parameter affords a more definite data of the left ventricular filling pressure. Thus, it provides a definite direct assessment of the left ventricular filling volume and performance of the left side of the heart. The LAP monitoring also directly helps in the diagnosis of malfunctions of the mitral valve prosthesis. Direct LAP monitoring is usually performed by putting a thin catheter into the left atrium through a purse-string suture in the right superior pulmonary vein. The catheter is then brought out of a wound through the infra-xiphoid portion of the chest wall and is connected to a pressure transducer.

Monitoring of Cardiac Performance

The principal function of CVS is to supply the oxygenated blood to the tissues. So, the principal aim of monitoring of cardiovascular system should be the monitoring of the efficiency of performance of the heart as a pump. Efficiency of the performance of the heart as a pump is only assessed by measuring the following parameters such as cardiac output, mixed venous O_2 saturation (SVO_2) and SVR.

Cardiac Output Measurement

The measurement of CO is a straightforward method for the assessment of efficiency of cardiac function, because CO is the revealing indicator of the entire functional efficiency of CVS. The importance of knowing the CO can also be explained from the fact that a patient with normal BP and PCWP may have poor vital organ perfusion if there is high SVR, causing low CO and SVR cannot be measured easily. So, the knowing of cardiac output is very vital, and is measured by the following methods: invasive and noninvasive.

Invasive Methods

i. *Fick's principle:* It was shown by Fick that the total amount of O_2 consumed per minute (VO_2) by an individual is equal to the difference between the arterial and venous O_2 content ($C_aO_2 - CVO_2$) multiplied by the cardiac output (CO) per minute.

Therefore, $VO_2 = (C_aO_2 - CVO_2) \times CO$, or $CO = (VO_2)/(C_aO_2 - CVO_2)$

The total O_2 consumption can be calculated from the difference between the O_2 content in the inspired air and the expired air. Again, from the arterial line, we can measure the arterial O_2 content and from PAC the venous O_2 content. Alternatively, instead of O_2 this cardiac output can also be measured by the Fick's principle using CO_2. The steps are as follows:

- CO_2 output per minute is determined with Douglas bag.
- Alveolar air is collected and its CO_2 tension is determined which is identical to that of arterial blood.
- Alveolar air is again collected after holding of the breath for 5 seconds, which is identical to that of venous blood.

Therefore, $CO = CO_2$ output in minute/$(P_aCO_2 - PVCO_2)$

Cardiac output can also be measured invasively by the indicator-dilution technique and the thermodilution technique. But, the variations of Fick's principle are the basis of these indicator dilution and thermodilution method for the measurement of CO.

ii. Indicator dilution method: This method is not used in clinical practice, so is not discussed here.

iii. Thermodilution method: This is a gold standard invasive method for the measurement of CO. In this method a bolus of cold water is injected through the proximal lumen of PAC in the right atrium. Then, when the cold water passes from the right atrium through the right ventricle to the pulmonary artery, then a thermistor, present at the tip of the PAC measures the difference in temperature of blood in the pulmonary artery, before and after the injection of cold water. Now, we know that the degree of the changes in temperature is inversely proportional to the output of the right ventricle which is equal to the cardiac output of the left ventricle, and it is determined from this change in temperature. The temperature change is high, if the flow or cardiac output is high and the temperature change is low, when the flow or cardiac output is low. Thus, a plotting of the changes of temperature against time produces a thermodilution curve. Computer in the device computes (determines) the CO from this temperature difference data.

Though, it is the gold standard method for the measurement of CO, but it has some drawbacks and these are:

- The injection of bolus cold water may be too slow or too fast.
- There are possibilities of poor mixing of cold water within the blood.
- There are chances of ectopic heart beats, causing the variation of CO.
- Variability of CO with each breath
- Time consuming.
- All the drawbacks of pulmonary artery catheterization.

Practically, several measurements are taken. But, the most extreme results are discarded and the average of three closely paced results are taken.

Recently, through PAC a small filament or a coil is used at its tip which is electronically heated periodically and provides some small pulses of heat into the blood, proximal to the pulmonary valve, instead of bolus cold water. It also contains a thermistor that measures the change in temperature of the blood of pulmonary artery. Then, the computer in monitoring device determines the CO by cross-correlating the heat production and the change in temperature. Thus, these monitors provide a continuous measurement of CO and also gives us the record of the changes of CO with time, graphically.

Though, this method has multiple benefits, still PAC is an invasive technique and has all the complications similar to pulmonary artery catheterization (listed above) which leads to a search for a more safe and easier method.

Noninvasive methods

- *Doppler–ultrasound technology:* The measurement of CO by Fick's principle is invasive and an expensive one. The popular and gold standard thermodilution technique for the measurement of CO also uses the Fick principle and needs PA catheterization with all its risks. So, these limitations led to the exploration and the development of newer noninvasive method for the determination of CO by ultrasound. The Doppler ultrasound technology measures the blood velocity by using the principal that the frequency of a transmitted wave changes if it is reflected off from a moving object. Thus, the Doppler ultrasound technology measures the velocity of blood in the ascending or descending aorta (according to the route and the position of probe) over a period of ejection time (TEJ), and determines an average velocity value (V_{AVG}) for each heartbeat. It also measures the cross-sectional area of ascending or descending aorta ($Area_{AO}$). Then, the device calculates the CO by multiplying the V_{AVG}, with the $Area_{AO}$, TE_J and HR. Thus, $CO = V_{AVG} \times Area_{AO} \times TE_J \times HR$.

The ultrasound probes are placed on the suprasternal notch or in the esophagus, or in the trachea with ET-tube. The probe emits an ultrasonic sound wave that is then reflected off the red cells in aorta. The machine, then, measures the velocity of blood, the cross-sectional area of the aorta and various patterns of flow to calculate the CO. The estimation of stroke volume and cardiac contractility are also possible by this method. If the descending aorta is used, then the proportion of CO directed to the upper arms, head and neck must be assumed and the calculated flow through the descending aorta should be adjusted accordingly to determine the CO. When the probe is placed on the suprasternal notch, it measures the velocity of blood at the aortic valve. It can also emit continuous waves (CW) and pulse waves (PW) for continuous and intermittent measurement of the CO. Through transesophageal route the probe is attached to the tip of the standard esophageal stethoscope and determines the velocity of the blood flow in the descending or thoracic aorta. The transtracheal device uses a special type of ET tube with a PW Doppler ultrasound transducer incorporated in its tip and measures the velocity of blood flow in ascending aorta.

The great advantage of this ultrasound device is that it is noninvasive, easy to use, and provides an almost instantaneous measurement of CO with a very low incidence of complications. But, the disadvantage is that, unfortunately, the probe usually has a very narrow angle of detection, and the calculated velocity is much dependent on the angle between the direction of sound waves and the direction of red cells in which they travel. (Since, the cosine of this angle Q is a part of Doppler formula for velocity measurement). So, a constant alignment between the probe and the blood flow through aorta is necessary. Small movements of probe, therefore, change the calculated CO markedly.

The recent clinical trials have shown that these Doppler ultrasound monitors are unable to determine an absolute value of CO reliably. So, this technique has been dismissed as inaccurate and impractical for routine use. They are used more now to provide a trend with time. They are, therefore, very useful in guiding perioperative fluid management, but have a limited scope in the intensive care unit.

- *Transthoracic impedance plethysmography technology:* This technique was first reported by Kubicek and his colleagues. This technique uses the principle that, as the amount of blood in the thoracic wall varies with each heartbeat, so it causes a corresponding change in the electrical conductance or impedance of the thorax. From these changes in the impedance of the thorax, an impedance plethysmograph is developed, from which CO is determined (using an algorithm and the computer). Due to its *high noninvasiveness* and *more or less accurate results*, it has an increased acceptability in the intraoperative and critical care cases. In practice, the *main disadvantage* of this method is interference from other electrical equipment and changes in electrode conductance, which may produce unreliable results.

Measurement of Mixed Venous O_2 Saturation

The SVO_2 is possibly a more comprehensive measurement of cardiac performance, than the CO itself. This is because, it also reflects whether the CO is adequate enough to meet the tissue metabolic needs or not. The SVO_2 is the function of: (i) the level of arterial O_2 saturation (SaO_2), (ii) the rate of O_2 consumption (VO_2), and (iii) the concentration of hemoglobin (Hb).

So, the $SVO_2 = (SaO_2 - VO_2)/(CO \times 1.34\ Hb)$. An *advantage* of this method is its ability to provide a continuous assessment of cardiac performance. The *disadvantage* is that SVO_2 depends on multiple variable parameters (as the above equation says). So, when any of these variables changes significantly, then one cannot assume that a change in venous O_2 saturation results solely from a change in CO or cardiac performance.

Measurement of Systemic Vascular Resistance

Cardiac performance also can be assessed indirectly by the measurement of systemic vascular resistance (SVR). It is measured from the formula:

SVR = (MAP – CVP)/CO × 80
MAP = Mean arterial pressure (mm Hg)
CVP = Central venous pressure (mm Hg)
CO = Cardiac output (L/min)
[× 80] = Factor to convert Wood units (mm Hg/L/min) to (dynes/s/cm^5)

The normal value of SVR is 15 Wood units (range 10–20 Wood units) or 1,200 dynes/s/cm^5 (range 800–1,600 dynes/s/cm^5).

Peripheral Nerve Block

INTRODUCTION AND HISTORY

In 1880, two American surgeons, named Halsted and Hall, had first injected cocaine by the side of peripheral nerves such as the ulnar, musculocutaneous, supratrochlear, and infratrochlear nerves, and produced peripheral nerve block for minor surgical procedures. Then, in 1885, James Leonard Corning used Esmarch elastic bandage, with a peripheral nerve block and had tried to prolong the duration of action of a local anesthetic (LA) agent by arresting the circulation and reducing the absorption of it (LA agent) from tissues. This idea was further advanced by Barun, by using epinephrine, mixed with an LA agent, as a chemical tourniquet in 1903.

At the beginning of civilization, though the surgeons were pioneers, regarding the early discoveries of regional anesthesia (RA), but the developing specialty of anesthesiology had gradually dominated over it. So, after that, the role of RA or peripheral nerve block has expanded from the room of operating theater to the arena of the postoperative recovery room and then pain management clinic, by holding the hand of the anesthetist. Previously, the peripheral nerve block was applied only on adults and selected group of patients, but later it was proved that with appropriate selection of patients and with the help of sedation, the regional techniques of peripheral nerve block can also be used for all the age groups of patients. There are different techniques of RA for extremities. But the duration of surgery mainly influences both the type of regional technique, selected and the choice of the LA agent, used. The plans for postoperative pain relief (analgesia) also influence the approach to peripheral nerve block or technique of RA.

Any anesthesiologist does not underestimate the role of sedation, during the surgery, under RA or peripheral nerve block, for example, many perfect brachial plexus (BP) blocks have been undone (failed) due to inadequate management of sedation. The regional blockade on extremities or peripheral nerve block has wide application, by not only providing surgical anesthesia and analgesia but as well as treating chronic pain syndromes, involving the extremities. Regional anesthesia on the extremity (upper or lower) or other RA on a trunk, including sympathetic ganglion blockade have also several other advantages during the postoperative period, compared with general anesthesia (GA). These include (1) decreased requirement of sedation, (2) decreased nausea and vomiting, (3) minimum stay in the hospital, and (4) early discharge and a smooth transition from parenteral to oral analgesics or other drugs as the block or anesthetic effects dissipate gradually. During the peripheral nerve block, continuous infusion of the LA agents near a peripheral plexus of nerve via a percutaneous catheter has also become an increasingly common form of RA, if surgery is prolonged or postoperative analgesia is needed.

The success of the RA technique was first dependent on only paresthesia seeking technique, which was first described by Winnie, but later the stimulation of nerve by any nerve stimulator technique was popularized. However, now RA under ultrasound guidance is the choice. The purpose of RA has also now expanded from intraoperative purpose and reduction of requirement of general anesthesia to (1) perioperative pain management, (2) acceleration of convalescence, (3) reduction of stress response, (4) reduction of systemic analgesic requirements, and (5) reduction of opioid-related side effects.

The *selection of patients* for the RA technique is very crucial. It starts from thorough history taking and physical examination to a thorough analysis of risk-benefit ratio, if this surgery is done under RA, for example, patient's intolerance to opioids, e.g., those with obstructive sleep apnea (OSA) or high risk of nausea and vomiting may be benefitted from opioid-sparing effects of RA. Patients with chronic pain and opioid tolerance also receive optimal doses with RA. For the success of RA, the compulsory requirements are (1) comprehensive knowledge regarding regional anatomy,

(2) a complete plan regarding surgical procedure, (3) according to surgical procedure selection of appropriate RA technique, and (4) a review of various other considerations (e.g., tourniquet placement, bone grafting, and probable extension of surgical procedure and its duration).

■ RISKS AND CONTRAINDICATIONS

The risks and contraindications of RA are more or less similar to that of neuraxial (spinal and epidural) block and are discussed in details in chapter 24. Here, we will go through a short discussion, regarding the risks and contraindications of RA.

- Patient's cooperation is the key to the success of RA. Without the patient's full cooperation, RA cannot be administered, plus though it can be administered, surgery cannot be performed. Patient's cooperation is also a key to the safety of RA when it is administered. Patients who cannot remain still during the procedure of RA may be at an increased risk. Examples of such patients are younger patients and some developmentally delayed patients, as well as patients with dementia or movement disorders.
- Hemorrhage and local hematoma formation increase the risk of RA in patients who have bleeding disorders and are taking anticoagulant medications. In such circumstances, the risks of RA must be balanced against the possible benefits of RA.
- Risks during lumbar plexus and paravertebral block due to their proximity to retroperitoneal space and neuraxis should be weighed against the benefits of these blocks.
- Placement of a block by a needle through a site of infection can track infection deep into the body near the target nerve tissue and its surrounding structures. Therefore, the presence of local infection is a relative contraindication for performing RA.
- Nerve injury is always a possibility in RA. But some patients with preexisting medical conditions such as peripheral neuropathy and diabetic neuropathy are at an increased risk and may have higher incidences of complications, including prolonged and/or permanent loss of sensory and motor function. The exact cause for this damage of nerve tissue is not known, but the probable explanations are (1) local ischemia from high injection pressure, (2) vasoconstrictors, (3) neurotoxic effects of the LA agent, and (4) direct trauma.
- Other risks associated with RA include systemic toxicity of the LA agent, resulting from intravascular injection or perivascular absorption. In the event of systemic LA toxic reaction, seizure activity, and cardiovascular collapse may occur. In case of cardiovascular collapse (1) treatment should be started immediately, (2) may call for the assistance of "Code Blue", (3) initiate cardiopulmonary resuscitation, (4) administer incremental doses of epinephrine, (4) infuse intravenous (IV) lipid emulsion, and if all fails, (5) prepare for cardiopulmonary bypass.
- Site-specific risks should also be considered for each individual patient. In a patient with severe pulmonary compromise or hemidiaphragmatic paralysis, for example, a contralateral interscalene or deep cervical plexus block with resultant phrenic nerve block can be catastrophic.

■ TECHNIQUES FOR NERVE LOCALIZATION

Placement of the needle tip close to a target nerve or a plexus of nerves is the key to the success of RA. So, this placement of the needle tip as close as possible to the target nerve of the plexus is facilitated by several techniques and these techniques are the paresthesia technique, nerve stimulator technique, and ultrasound technique.

- *Paresthesia technique:* Formerly, before the development of nerve stimulator and ultrasonography (USG), elicitation of paresthesia by touching the nerve by needle tip was the mainstay of RA, but this technique is now rarely used for nerve localization. Applying surface landmark and anatomical relationship as a guide, a needle used for RA is advanced through the skin and its underlying tissues toward the target nerve. When the needle makes a direct contact with the nerve, paresthesia is elicited in its area of sensory distribution, supplied by this sensory nerve. However, this principle of nerve localization will not be applicable for motor nerve.
- *Nerve stimulation technique:* In this technique, an insulated needle is used whose hub is connected to a nerve stimulator. Nerve stimulator is a battery-operated machine that emits a small amount (0–5 mA) of electric current at a set frequency (usually 1–2 Hz). The tip of this insulated needle concentrates the electric current, generated by a nerve stimulator, as it is insulated. A grounding electrode is attached to the patient to complete the circuit. When the insulated needle tip is placed in proximity to a motor nerve, then a specific muscle contraction is induced and an LA agent is injected. Here, the principle is that more close is the needle tip to a nerve, less amount of current will induce muscular contraction. Generally, when 0.5 mA current induces muscle contraction, then it is thought that needle tip is very close to nerve and an LA agent is injected. On the other hand, when 0.2 mA current induces muscle contraction, then it is thought that the placement of the needle tip is intraneural, though there is little evidence to support this specific cutoff. Most practitioners inject an

LA agent when current between 0.2 and 0.5 mA results in muscular response. For most of the blocks, using this technique in adults, 30–40 mL of the LA agent is injected with gentle aspiration between divided doses.

- *Ultrasound technique:* Ultrasound uses piezoelectric crystal which emits high-frequency (1–20 MHz) sound waves. These sound waves travel through different tissues of different densities with different rates. Therefore, different amounts of waves reflect (echo) from different tissues of different densities and these amount of waves, which are echoed, is directly proportional to the densities of tissues, i.e., tissues of more density transmit less sound and echo more waves. Now, these echoed sound waves are received by the transducer and are converted by transducer into electrical signal. The degree of efficiency, with which sound waves passes through a substance, determines its echogenicity. The structures through which sound waves passes easily and echoes less waves, are described as *hypoechoic* and appear as dark or black on screen. On the other hand, structures through which sound waves do not pass easily and echo more sound waves, are described as *hyperechoic* and appear as bright or white on screen.

Peripheral nerve localization by ultrasound is now becoming increasingly popular. It may be used either alone or combined with other modalities such as nerve stimulation. The frequency (type) of the transducer, used for nerve location, depends on the depth of the target nerve and the approach angle of needle relative to transducer. The high-frequency transducer provides poor tissue penetration and is therefore used for more superficial nerves, but it offers a high-resolution picture with a relatively clear image. On the other hand, the low frequency transducer provides good tissue penetration and is therefore used for far deeper nerves, but it offers a low-resolution picture with poor quality.

According to the array, the ultrasound transducer is again of two types (1) linear array transducer and (2) curved array transducer. The curved array (curvilinear) transducer is used for deeper target nerves that require a more acute angle between the needle and the long axis of the transducer because this acute angle maximizes the returning ultrasound waves. In contrast, the linear array transducer is used for superficial target nerves that do not require a more acute angle between the needle and the long axis of the transducer. Moreover, this linear array transducer offers an undistorted image and is therefore often the first choice among practitioners.

Needle insertion can pass either parallel (in-plane) or not parallel (out of plane) to the plane of ultrasound waves. Nerves are best imaged when it falls at the right angle to the plane of ultrasound waves, i.e., in the cross-sectional view of the nerve where they have a characteristic honeycomb appearance.

■ CONTINUOUS PERIPHERAL NERVE BLOCK

In this procedure, a thin catheter is placed through the percutaneous route by the side of the target nerve and the LA agent is administered by this catheter to prolong nerve block. So, this procedure is also called the perineural LA infusion. The advantages of this continuous nerve block are (1) improved continuous analgesia, (2) reduction in resting and dynamic pain, (3) reduction in supplemental analgesic requirements, (4) reduction in opioid-related side effects, (5) reduction in sleep disturbance, (6) improved ambulation and functioning of limb, (7) accelerated resumption of passive joint movement for physiotherapy, etc. Recent evidence suggests that continuous sciatic, femoral, and paravertebral perineural LA infusion in the immediate postoperative period decreases the risk of persistent postsurgical pain.

There are many types of catheters for continuous peripheral nerve block. These are (1) very flexible and relatively rigid, (2) through the needle and over the needle, and (3) nonstimulating (without nerve stimulator) and stimulating (with nerve stimulator). However, there is little evidence that any single design results in better effects. Long-acting LA agent, for example, ropivacaine is more commonly used, because it provides a more favorable (high) sensory-to-motor block ratio, i.e., more analgesia than muscular paralysis. In an attempt to further minimize muscular paralysis (motor block); diluted LA solution is used (differential block). However, unlike a single-shot (injection) peripheral nerve block, in continuous peripheral nerve block by catheter no adjuvant, added to LA solution, has been demonstrated to be of benefit. Local anesthetic solution is administered as repeated bolus doses or continuous infusion (by a portable infusion pump) or as a combination of these two methods.

Complications due to continuous peripheral nerve block by a catheter are similar to that of other peripheral nerve block. These complications are systemic LA toxicity, infection, nerve injury, catheter retention, hematoma formation, etc. In addition, femoral or sciatic nerve block increases the risk of falling, due to motor block; whatever maybe its degree. Hence, this continuous peripheral nerve block by a catheter is usually reserved for patients having procedures expected to result in postoperative pain that is difficult to control with oral analgesics and will not resolve in less time than the duration of a single injection peripheral nerve block.

UPPER EXTREMITY BLOCK OR BRACHIAL PLEXUS BLOCK

Applied Anatomy

The brachial plexus provides a complete motor and nearly a total sensory innervation to the upper limb. It is formed by the anterior primary (ventral) rami of C_5, C_6, C_7, C_8, and T_1 spinal nerves with variable contribution from the anterior primary (ventral) rami of C_4 and/or T_2 spinal nerves. These anterior primary (ventral) rami are called the roots **(Fig. 1)** of the brachial plexus. After the exit from the respective intervertebral foramen, these spinal nerves first cross the transverse process of their corresponding cervical vertebra at the same level and lie between the anterior and middle scalene muscle. The *anterior scalene muscle* arises from the anterior tubercle of the transverse process of the upper seven cervical vertebrae (C_1 to C_7) and takes insertion on the scalene tubercle of the first rib in front of the subclavian artery. The *middle scalene muscle* arises from the posterior tubercle of the transverse process of seven cervical vertebrae (C_1 to C_7) and takes insertion on the first rib, behind the subclavian artery.

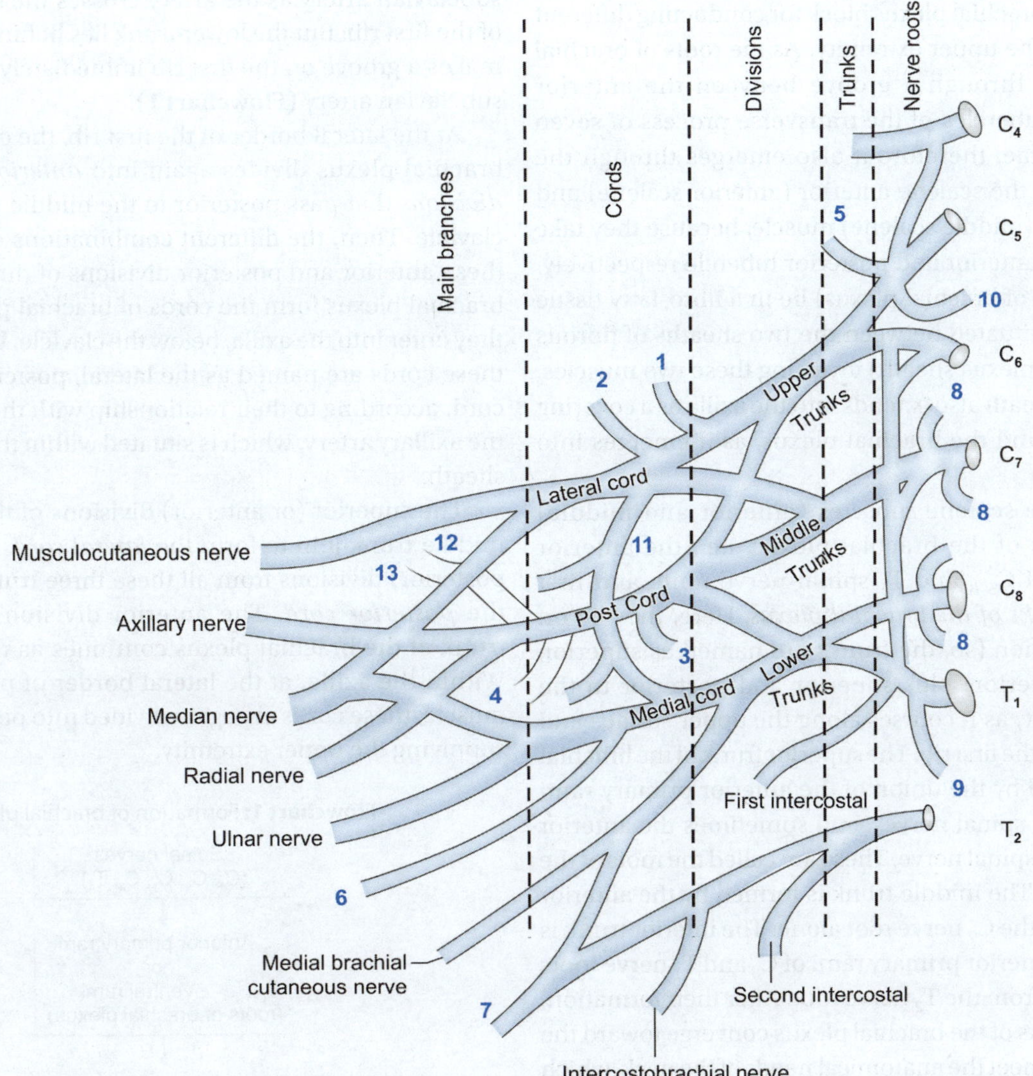

Fig. 1: The brachial plexus.

Notes:

1. Nerve to subclavian muscle
2. Suprascapular nerve
3. Subscapular nerve
4. Thoracodorsal nerve (or nerve to latissimus dosri)
5. To phrenic nerve
6. Medial antebrachial cutaneous nerve
7. Medial brachial cutaneous nerve
8. To longus cervicis and scalene muscles
9. Long thoracic nerve (or nerve to serratus anterior)
10. Dorsal scapular nerve
11. Anterior thoracic nerve
12. and 13. Upper and lower subscapular nerve

The prevertebral fascia which arises from the anterior and the posterior tubercle of the transverse processes of seven cervical vertebrae, after first investing both the muscles of scalene, fuses laterally and encloses the brachial plexus in a fascial sheath. This is called the *sheath of the brachial plexus* (or brachial plexus sheath). Thus, the *brachial plexus sheath* is continuous from its origin at the level of the seven transverse processes of cervical vertebrae in the neck to its (brachial plexus sheath) distal insertion at the level of the origin of the coracobrachialis muscle. Hydrostatically this brachial plexus sheath is intact throughout its course. So, the filling of this sheath with an LA agent at its various levels is the basis of the brachial plexus block for conducting different types of RA on the upper extremity. As the roots of brachial plexus emerge through a groove between the anterior and posterior tubercles of the transverse process of seven cervical vertebrae, therefore it also emerges through the groove between the scalene anterior (anterior scalene) and scalene medius (middle scalene) muscle, because they take origin from the anterior and posterior tubercle respectively. So, they (nerves of brachial plexus) lie in a fibro-fatty tissue space which is situated between the two sheaths of fibrous tissue (brachial plexus sheath) investing these two muscles. Laterally, this sheath also extends into the axilla as a covering membrane around the brachial plexus, as it emerges into the axilla.

Between the scalene muscles (anterior and middle) the nerve roots of the brachial plexus, i.e., the anterior primary rami of C_{5-8} and T_1 spinal nerve unite and first form three *trunks of the brachial plexus*. Here, they lie on vertical orientation (so, the trunks are named as superior, middle, and inferior) plus superior and posterior to the subclavian artery, as it courses along the upper surface and lateral border of the first rib. The superior trunk of the brachial plexus is formed by the union of the anterior primary rami of the C_5 and C_6 spinal nerves, and sometimes the anterior primary rami C_4 spinal nerve. These are called the roots of the brachial plexus. The middle trunk is formed by the anterior primary rami of the C_7 nerve root alone. The inferior trunk is formed by the anterior primary rami of C_8 and T_1 nerve roots and sometimes from the T_2 nerve root. After their formation, these three trunks of the brachial plexus converge toward the apex of axilla to meet the anatomical needs of the neck, which requires hypermobility in all directions. This convergence of nerve trunks is maximally tightest, just medial to the first rib, which is about 4 cm lateral to the transverse processes of C_6 vertebra. At this point, the brachial plexus assumes its most compact arrangements, and block of it (brachial plexus) at this level cause rapid and complete surgical anesthesia and analgesia of the upper limb.

The *trunks of the brachial plexus* lie in the posterior triangle of the neck and are also invested by the sheath of the prevertebral fascia. In this posterior triangle, the trunks of the brachial plexus are superficially placed and covered only by skin, platysma muscle, and the investing layer of deep cervical fascia. In such a position, they are also crossed by a number of structures such as the inferior belly of the omohyoid muscle, external jugular vein, transverse cervical artery, and supraclavicular nerves. Within the posterior triangle of neck, in a thin subject, the trunks of the brachial plexus can also easily be palpated by the fingers. The upper and middle trunks of the brachial plexus lie above the subclavian artery as the artery crosses the superior surface of the first rib. But the lower trunk lies behind the artery and makes a groove on the first rib immediately posterior to the subclavian artery **(Flowchart 1)**.

At the lateral border of the first rib, the each trunk of the brachial plexus divides again into *anterior and posterior divisions* that pass posterior to the middle one-third of the clavicle. Then, the different combinations of the joining of these anterior and posterior divisions of three trunks of the brachial plexus form the cords of brachial plexus just when they enter into the axilla, below the clavicle. Within the axilla, these cords are named as the lateral, posterior, and medial cord, according to their relationship with the second part of the axillary artery, which is situated within the same brachial sheath.

The superior (or anterior) divisions of the superior and middle trunk join to form the *lateral cord*. The inferior (or posterior) divisions from all these three trunks join to form the *posterior cord*. The anterior division of the inferior trunk of the brachial plexus continues as the *medial cord*. Within the axilla, at the lateral border of pectoralis minor muscle, these cords are again divided into peripheral nerves, supplying the upper extremity.

Flowchart 1: Formation of brachial plexus.

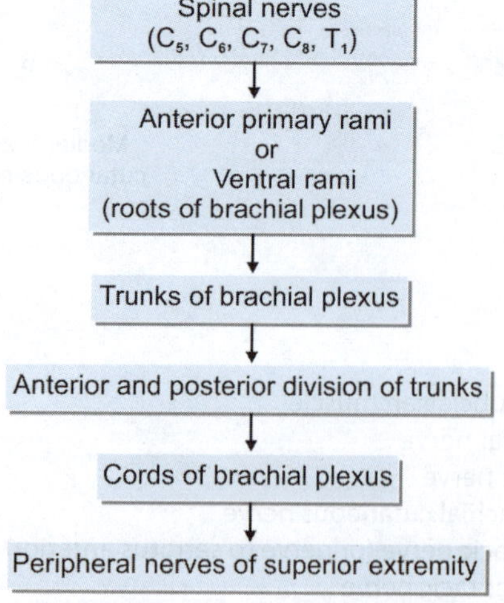

Among the peripheral nerves of upper extremity, the *musculocutaneous nerve* which arises from the lateral cord of brachial plexus is the most proximal branch of it (brachial plexus). So, this maximum proximity of this nerve explains why it is most commonly spared, during the axillary approach of the brachial plexus block. The next proximal branch of brachial plexus, after the musculocutaneous nerve, is the *axillary nerve*, and it arises from the posterior cord. Its position also explains why it is also commonly spared during the axillary approach of the brachial plexus block. Therefore, the surgical procedures, requiring the widespread total upper extremity motor and sensory paralysis by the brachial plexus block are conducted most often by the approach (technique) which is more proximal than the axillary approach of the brachial plexus block. After axillary nerve, the *median nerve* arises from the lateral and medial cord of the brachial plexus. The *radial nerve* arises from the posterior cord and the *ulnar nerve* arises from the medial cord of the brachial plexus, respectively.

Beside the terminal branches or peripheral nerves (ulnar, radial, median, etc.) that arise from the cords of brachial plexus, several terminal branches also arise from the roots of brachial plexus, providing motor innervations to the rhomboid muscle (C_5), subclavian muscle (C_5 and C_6), serratus anterior muscle (C_5, C_6, and C_7), etc. The suprascapular nerve arises from the C_5 and C_6 nerve roots and supplies the muscles of the dorsal aspect of scapula and sensory to the shoulder joint. So, to block these nerves, the higher approaches for brachial plexus block, such as the *intescalene approach* is necessary. No branches arise from the trunks and the divisions of the brachial plexus **(Fig. 2)**.

For the brachial plexus block, four sites or approaches for the injection of the LA agents are chosen such as (1) *interscalene*, (2) *supraclavicular*, (3) *infraclavicular*, and (4) *axillary*. The indications, results, technique, and complications of brachial plexus block are specific for each of these sites or approaches. Hence, the site or the approach for the brachial plexus block should be selected according to (1) surgical requirement, (2) potential complications, and (3) anesthesiologist's ability or skill. The proximal branches of the brachial plexus, arising from its roots at cervical region, are usually blocked only by interscalene approach of the brachial plexus block. The axillary approach of the brachial plexus block takes place at the site of the origin of the terminal branches of plexus. At this level the, terminal branches have a constant relationship with the axillary artery, for example, *the median nerve is lateral to the artery, the ulnar nerve is medial to the artery, and the radial nerve is posterior to the artery. This constant relationship of these terminal nerves helps in easy identification and complete block of these nerves through the axillary route.* By using this

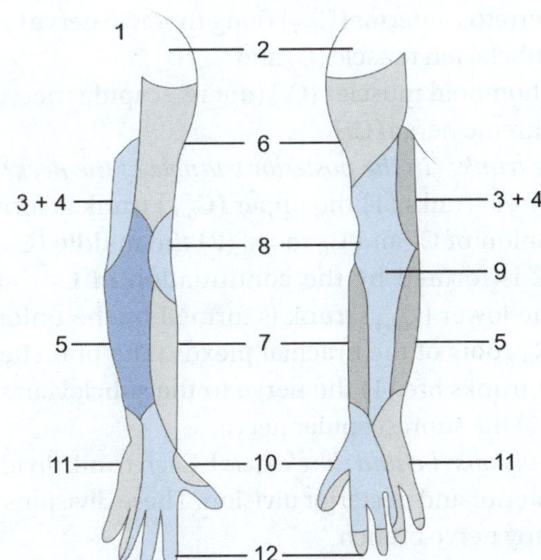

Fig. 2: The cutaneous distribution of peripheral nerves over the upper extremity.

Notes:
1. Supraclavicular nerve
2. Upper lateral cutaneous nerve of the arm
3. Medial cutaneous nerve of the arm
4. Intercostobrachial nerve
5. Medial cutaneous nerve of the forearm
6. Lower lateral cutaneous nerve of the arm
7. Lateral cutaneous nerve of the forearm
8. Posterior cutaneous nerve of the arm
9. Posterior cutaneous nerve of the forearm
10. Radial nerve
11. Ulnar nerve
12. Median nerve

axillary approach, the proximal branches of the brachial plexus, which are blocked only by the interscalene approach, cannot be blocked.

Now, the composition of the brachial plexus can be summarized as follows:
- *Five roots:* These roots are made by the anterior primary (ventral) rami of C_5 to T_1 spinal nerves and are situated between the anterior and medial scalene muscles. These roots receive only gray rami communication, carrying postganglionic sympathetic fibers, from the cervical sympathetic chain, for example, the C_5 and C_6 roots receive postganglionic sympathetic fibers from the middle cervical sympathetic ganglion, the C_7 and C_8 roots receive postganglionic sympathetic fibers from the inferior cervical sympathetic ganglion, and the T_1 root receives postganglionic sympathetic fibers from the T_1 sympathetic ganglion.

The roots of the brachial plexus give branches to:
- Longus cervicis muscle (C_{5-8})
- Scalene muscles (C_{5-8})

- Serratus anterior (C_{5-7}) (long thoracic nerve)
- Subclavian muscle (C_5 and C_6)
- Rhomboid muscles (C_5) (dorsal scapular nerve)
- Phrenic nerve (C_5)

■ *Three trunks (in the posterior triangle of the neck):* There are three trunks (1) the upper (C_{5-6}) trunk is formed by the union of C_5 and C_6 roots, (2) the middle (C_7 alone) trunk is formed by the continuation of C_7 root, and (3) the lower (C_{8-1}) trunk is formed by the union of C_8 and T_1 roots of the brachial plexus. The branches from these trunks are (1) the nerve to the subclavian muscle and (2) the suprascapular nerve.

■ *Six divisions (behind the clavicle):* Each trunk divides into an anterior and posterior division. These divisions do not give any nerve branch.

■ *Three cords (within the axilla):*
1. *Lateral cord:* It is formed by the union of anterior divisions of upper and middle trunks. It gives the following branches: Lateral pectoral nerve, the musculocutaneous nerve, and the lateral head of the medium nerve.
2. *Medial cord:* It is the continuation of anterior division of lower trunk. It gives the following branches: Medial pectoral nerve, medial cutaneous nerve of arm, medial cutaneous nerve of forearm, medial head of medium nerve, and ulnar nerve.
3. *Posterior cord:* It is formed by the union of postdivisions of all the three trunks. It gives the following branches: Upper subscapular nerve, nerve to the latissimus dorsi muscle (thoracodorsal nerve), lower subscapular nerve, axillary nerve, and radial nerve.

The branches of the brachial plexus, arising from the roots and trunks of the brachial plexus are situated in neck above the clavicle, and so these are called the *supraclavicular branches*. But the major distribution of the brachial plexus is derived from its cords and is situated below the clavicle. Therefore, they are called the *infraclavicular branches*.

Interscalene Approach of the Brachial Plexus Block

Among all the approaches of brachial plexus block, it is the most proximal and cephalic approach. So, all the complications related to this approach of the brachial plexus block, are due to its proximity to the vital structures in neck. It is performed at the level of the roots and the trunks of the brachial plexus, and most often at the level of superior trunk over the transverse process of C_6 vertebra.

Indications: The principal indication for the interscalene approach of the brachial plexus block is the surgeries over the proximal part of upper extremity, e.g., shoulder and upper

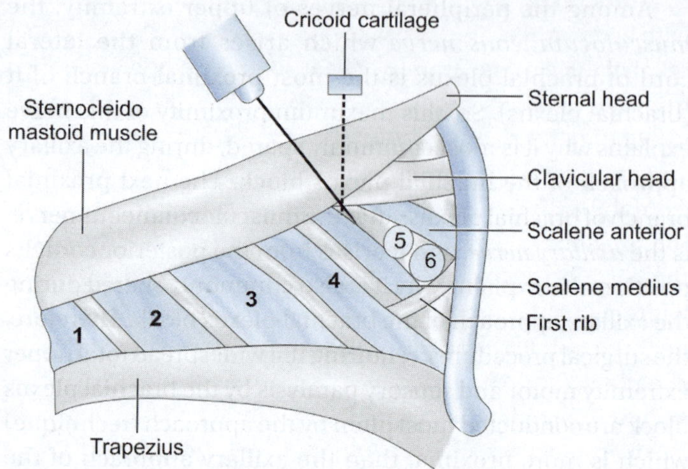

Fig. 3: The site of interscalene approach of the brachial plexus block.
Notes:
1. Semispinalis capitis 2. Splenius capitis
3. Levator scapulae 4. Scalene posterior
5. Brachial plexus 6. Subclavian artery

arm (upper one-third of the humerus). Supraclavicular, infraclavicular, and axillary approach for brachial plexus block is reserved for surgeries distal to midhumerus. This is because surgery over the shoulder requires block of C_3 and C_4 cutaneous branches, which need partial cervical plexus block with full brachial plexus block and this is only achieved by the interscalene approach of the brachial plexus block. On the other hand, for the forearm and hand surgery this approach can also be used, but block will be incomplete and is not necessary **(Fig. 3)**, because by the interscalene approach, the block of inferior trunk of the brachial plexus which supply mainly the forearm and hand (C_8, T_1) is often incomplete and frequently require supplementation by *isolated ulnar nerve bock* for adequate surgical anesthesia, along its (ulnar) distribution. The nerves responsible for thoracic innervation from the brachial plexus enter into the thorax through the axilla, but they remain outside the brachial plexus sheath. So, if the surgical incision, for surgeries on the upper extremity, involves the medial side of the upper part of thorax and axilla, as in the transdeltoid approach for the surgeries on the upper extremity, then these areas might remain unblocked by this interscalene approach of the brachial plexus block. Similarly, if the skin surfaces, which are innervated by the nerves arising from C_2 to C_4 segment of spinal cord, is involved in surgery, it may not be blocked by this approach of the brachial plexus block and may require supplementation block by paravertebral LA injection. An inferior axillary surgical approach for the operation on shoulder joint may also require too large skin area to be blocked. So this approach of the brachial plexus block is of no help in such cases.

Sometimes, the brachial plexus block may still be used with light general anesthesia for extended postoperative pain relief of the upper extremity, because the scarring developed from the previous surgery could be another obstacle to the use of pure RA (brachial plexus block) for repeated shoulder surgery. This is due to the isolation of some nerve structure from the action of the LA agent by developed fibrosis from the previous surgeries. So, the use of nerve stimulator and the elicitation of paresthesia are sometimes recommended with this technique, in order to place the needle accurately near the nerve. In the posterior triangle, the brachial plexus sheath is very thin and so the feeling of piercing this thin sheath of brachial plexus at that site by the blocking needle is very difficult to perceive, during interscalene approach of the brachial plexus block.

Technique of interscalene approach: The anatomical background for this correct interscalene approach for brachial plexus block is the exact identification (of the location) of brachial plexus in the groove which is formed by the overlapping of anterior and middle scalene muscles at the level of cricoid cartilage. This overlap of anterior and middle scalene muscles occurs over the transverse process of C6 vertebra. The entire brachial plexus is accessible at this point from outside, because the complete sheath of brachial plexus is formed here. Any injection within the plexus sheath, at this level of nerve trunk of brachial plexus, will have access to the entire brachial plexus, including its roots and cords. By the use of nerve locator and elicitation of motor-evoked response or paresthesia, felt in arm, the origin of specific nerve is also identified. This will help in specific nerve block. But any injection of an LA drug outside the sheath of brachial plexus will not result in its block. So, the knowledge, regarding the branches of the brachial plexus, which lie outside the plexus sheath, will prevent these potential failures of blocks. The examples of such instances are the suprascapular nerve, axillary nerve, long thoracic nerve, etc., which leave the sheath at this level. So, the paresthesia to the anterior chest (pectoral area) or the area of scapula or acromion region which are due to the stimulation of these nerves, lying outside the plexus sheath, should not be mistaken as a confirmatory sign of brachial plexus entry of needle at this level.

For the interscalene approach of the brachial plexus block, patient should lie in the supine position and the head will be turned away 30° or less from the side of block (on contralateral side). After that, the posterior border of *sternocleidomastoid* muscle is palpated first, by asking the patient to lift his head. Then, the interscalene groove (where middle and anterior scalene muscle cross each other) can be palpated by rolling the finger of anesthetist laterally from the posterior border of *sternocleidomastoid* muscle, over the belly of anterior scalene muscle. Then, a line is drawn laterally from cricoid cartilage to intersect the interscalene groove. This indicates the level of transverse process of C_6 vertebra. The external jugular vein often crosses the interscalene groove at the level of cricoid cartilage. The interscalene groove should not be confused with the groove between the sternocleidomastoid and anterior scalene muscle which lies further anterior.

After proper sterile skin preparation, a 4 cm and 24 G short-beveled needle is inserted slowly perpendicular to the skin, with 45° caudal and slightly posterior angulation. Needle is then advanced in that direction, until the paresthesia is felt. This usually occurs at very superficial level. A click may be felt, if the blunt (short-beveled) needle is used, when it goes through the prevertebral fascia. If bone is encountered within 2 cm of skin, then it is likely to be the transverse process of C6 vertebra. *Nerve stimulator* may be helpful to identify individual nerve of brachial plexus or the whole plexus itself. Motor response of deltoid and biceps muscle indicates stimulation of superior trunk. A motor response of the diaphragm indicates that the needle is placed in too anterior direction while a motor response of trapezius or serratus anterior muscle indicate that the needle is placed in too posterior direction.

In *paresthesia technique*, the perceived feeling anywhere in the arm is a reliable indicator of the superior trunk of the brachial plexus. However, the appreciation of paresthesia over the region of scapula, acromion, or pectoral area indicates the suprascapular, axillary, or long thoracic nerve, respectively which is not located within the sheath of the brachial plexus and there is a chance of failure. After getting paresthesia over arm (which indicates that the tip of the needle within the sheath) the needle should be fixed at that position. It also can be helped by using a flexible extension tubing. After negative aspiration, 10–40 mL of LA drug is injected incrementally, depending on the desired extent of block. There is a definite relationship between the volume of the LA agent and the extent, depth, and duration of RA (block), for example, 40 mL of an LA solution is associated with complete cervical and brachial plexus block for prolonged period.

In *ultrasound technique*, a needle "out of plane" or "in plane" can be used and an insulated needle, attached to a nerve stimulator, can be used to confirm the accuracy of the target structure. For both techniques, after the identification of sternocleidomastoid and interscalene groove, approximately at C_6 level, a high-frequency linear transducer is placed perpendicular to the course of interscalene muscles. Hence, the anterior and middle scalene muscles with brachial plexus in between them will be visualized in cross section. The internal jugular vein and internal carotid artery will be seen lying anterior to the anterior scalene muscle. For an "out of plane" technique, the block needle is inserted in a direction at a right angle to the ultrasound beam and just cephalad to transducer and is advanced caudally toward the visualized plexus. However, for an "in plane" technique, the needle is inserted in a direction parallel to the ultrasound beam and just posterior to the transducer. The advancement of needle should be visualized during the entire procedure. Depending on the visualization of the spread of LA drug, a lower volume (10 mL) is employed for postoperative analgesia, whereas a large volume (20–30 mL) of an LA agent is commonly used for surgical anesthesia.

Complications: Ipsilateral phrenic nerve block, with diaphragmatic paralysis, occurs in almost all the patients during the interscalene approach of the brachial plexus block. It causes a 25% reduction in pulmonary function. This is due to the anterior spread of LA solution over the anterior scalene muscle, and blocking the phrenic nerve. This may cause dyspnea, hypercapnia, and hypoxemia in respiratory compromised patient. Therefore, the sedation required for these patients to tolerate these symptoms, also has a negative impact. On the other hand, the ipsilateral involvement (block) of the vagus nerve, recurrent laryngeal nerve, and stellate ganglion with the concomitant block of brachial plexus through the interscalene approach has little or no significance, but the related symptoms may require assurance or sedation. Ipsilateral recurrent laryngeal nerve involvement often induces hoarseness of voice. In patients with contralateral vocal cord paralysis, respiratory distress may ensue. Stellate ganglion block results in Horner syndrome, manifesting myosis, ptosis, and anhidrosis.

For postoperative pain relief, after a total shoulder replacement surgery under GA, this interscalene approach for brachial plexus block can be adopted, but only after confirming that there is no nerve damage during surgery. Otherwise, later this block should be blamed for any nerve injury, what was actually done during surgery under general anesthesia. Other site specific risks include vertebral artery injection, and it is suspected if immediate seizure activity is observed. As little as 1 mL of an LA agent delivered into the vertebral artery, may induce a seizure. If the needle is long enough and the direction of the needle is caudal, then any of the epidural or subarachnoid block can be precipitated during this interscalene approach of the brachial plexus block. This is due to the close proximity of dural sleeve over spinal nerves and the site of interscalene approach for brachial plexus block. As several important vascular structures are also in close proximity to the site of LA injection, so during the interscalene approach of the brachial plexus block, repeated aspiration and incremental dose of

an LA agent should be given which will guard against the inadvertent intravascular injection of drug. In this approach of the brachial plexus block, the nerve damage or neuritis can also occur like any other peripheral nerve block.

Supraclavicular Approach for Brachial Plexus Block

The advantage of this approach, over interscalene approach, for brachial plexus block is that a small volume of LA drug can be delivered, directly near the three trunks, where they are compactly arranged, resulting in rapid onset and reliable dense brachial plexus block. So, once it was described as the "spinal anesthesia of arm". But the higher rate of complication may restrict this approach for brachial plexus block. However, recently, it has seen the resurgence with the use of ultrasound guidance. During the application of this technique, the incidences of complications (risks) should be balanced with the benefits (rapid and dense block), achieved by it. Distal to the transverse processes of cervical vertebrae, the prevertebral fascia invests the nerve of brachial plexus, forming the brachial plexus sheath. When the nerves of brachial plexus pass over the lateral border of the first rib, then this brachial plexus sheath of them becomes complete and formed a neurovascular bundle, which lies posterior and inferior to the clavicle, at about its midpoint. For this approach of the brachial plexus block, the striking of first rib with needle is the most important landmark. Then, the walking of needle in the correct plane on the superior surface of first rib will lead to the identification of brachial plexus. Another landmark for this approach of the brachial plexus block is the apex of palpable subclavian artery, which can be traced in cephalic direction to identify the interscalene muscular interval. Lateral to this subclavian pulse, at the level of midclavicle, the supraclavicular part of brachial plexus can be found. During interscalene block, if the crossing of anterior and middle interscalene muscle is traced distally toward the clavicle, then the brachial plexus also can be approached at the supraclavicular level **(Fig. 4)**.

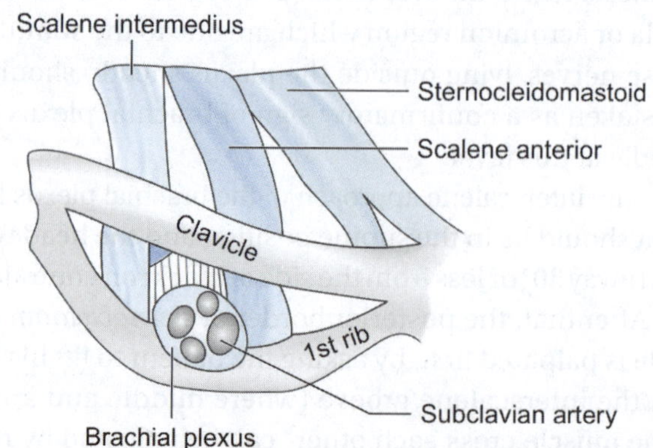

Fig. 4: The brachial plexus with subclavian artery on the first rib.

Indications of supraclavicular approach: This approach for brachial plexus block is applicable for any surgical procedures of upper extremity, where the brachial plexus block can be used theoretically. But due to the sparing of most proximal part of brachial plexus by this approach, and thus not blocking the nerves, which arise from its roots and supply over the shoulder, somebody would recommend the interscalene approach, when the surgical procedure is performed on shoulder. The supraclavicular brachial plexus block also does not reliably anesthetize the axillary and suprascapular nerves. However, practically the supraclavicular approach for brachial plexus block with adequate amount of LA drug usually provide adequate anesthesia for any surgical procedure on shoulder, with reasonably high success rate. This is because large amount of LA drugs, placed at this site, can easily spread in cranial direction and block the roots and its branches of the brachial plexus.

Technique: Three anatomical points are most important for the performance of supraclavicular approach of the brachial plexus block. These are:

1. The three trunks of the brachial plexus are clustered vertically over first rib and they lie above and posterior to the subclavian artery which often can be palpated in a thin patient.
2. The neurovascular bundle lies posterior to the clavicle at about its midpoint.
3. The first rib acts as a barrier for the needle, piercing the pleural dome.

The patient is first placed in the supine position with the head turned toward the opposite site. Then, at the midpoint of clavicle, the pulse of subclavian artery is felt, and the point just lateral to this pulse is the site of injection of the LA agent. If the pulse of subclavian artery is not palpable, then the midpoint of clavicle is also the landmark for the site of injection of the LA agent for this approach of the brachial plexus block. Proper aseptic measure is taken. Then, for this block, a 22–25 G and 1″ long blunt beveled needle is selected. It is advanced through the skin wheal in a caudal, but slightly medial and posterior direction, toward the subclavian pulse, until a paresthesia is encountered. If no paresthesia is elicited, then the needle is advanced more, until the superior surface of the first rib is encountered by the tip of the needle. If the artery is encountered, then the needle is withdrawn, till the blood is no longer aspirated.

After encountering with first rib, the needle is walked on this rib, first lateral, and then at medial direction, until the paresthesia is elicited. When paresthesia is encountered, then 20–30 mL of LA drug is injected. The caudal direction of needle must be avoided which increases the **(Fig. 5)**

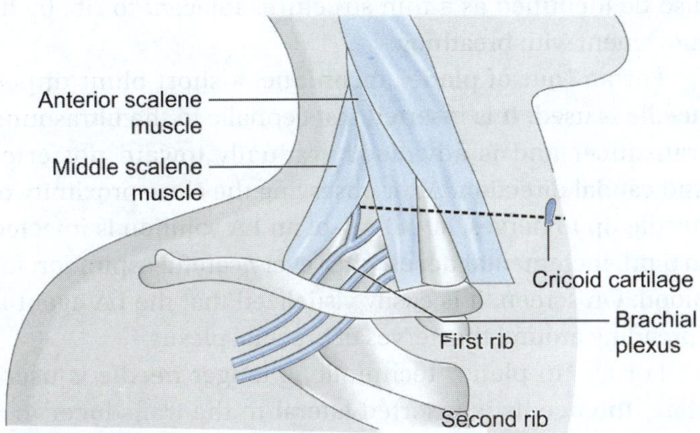

Fig. 5: The site of interscalene block, supraclavicular block, and infraclavicular block.

incidence of entry of the tip of the needle into the pleural cavity and lung parenchyma at their apex and development of pneumothorax. Advancing the needle deeper than the reasonable length to encounter the first rib must be avoided for the fear of also pneumothorax. If any air is aspirated, then the chest X-ray is mandatory. Air aspiration does not preclude complicating the block, because fine needle usually prevents significant air leak from the lung, producing pneumothorax. So, it is unwise to discharge an outpatient without overnight observation, after brachial plexus block through the supraclavicular approach, particularly if there is an increased chance of pneumothorax.

The modified *plumb-bob* technique, for this approach of the brachial plexus block, needs the same patient position. The needle entry site is at the point where the lateral border of the sternocleidomastoid muscle inserts on (takes origin from) the clavicle. After aseptic preparation, a 22 G and 4 cm long, but short bevel needle is inserted through the skin while mimicking a plumb-bob suspended over needle entry site. Often paresthesia is encountered prior to contacting the first rib or subclavian artery. If no paresthesia is elicited, needle is directed in cephalic direction. If still no paresthesia is elicited then the needle tip is directed caudal until the first rib is contacted.

Ultrasound technique: For supraclavicular block by ultrasound technique, the patient should lie in the supine position with his head turned 30° toward the contralateral side. In the supraclavicular fossa, superior to clavicle, a high-frequency linear transducer is placed with an angle slightly toward thorax. On screen, the subclavian artery is easily identified. Just superficial and lateral to this subclavian artery, the nerves of brachial plexus are seen as multiple hypoechoic disks-like structures. Deep to the artery, the first rib is also seen as hyperechoic structure. Visceral pleura can also be identified as a thin structure, adjacent to rib, by its movement with breathing.

For an "out of plane" technique, a short blunt tipped needle is used. It is inserted just cephalic to the ultrasound transducer and is advanced gradually toward posterior and caudal direction. After observing the close proximity of needle tip to nerves, 30–40 mL of an LA solution is injected in 5 mL incremental doses, after every careful aspiration for blood. On screen, it is easily visualized that the LA agent is spreading around the nerves of brachial plexus.

For an "in plane" technique, a longer needle is used. Here, the needle is inserted lateral to the transducer in a direction parallel to the ultrasound beam. Gradually, the needle is advanced medially toward the subclavian artery, until the tip is visualized near brachial plexus, just lateral and superficial to the artery. Then, after negative aspiration for blood, 20–30 mL of LA drug is injected in incremental doses. The spread of drug around the plexus will be seen on screen.

Complications: The incidence of pneumothorax, after supraclavicular approach of the brachial plexus block, is very high (0.5–0.6 %) and is most common in this approach. The incidence of pneumothorax, even in experienced hands, is more if the routine diagnosis is sought by X-ray than clinical findings for the diagnosis of pneumothorax. Subclinical pneumothorax is more common than symptomatic pneumothorax. The onset of symptoms is sometimes delayed and may take 24 hours. Therefore, routine X-ray just after the block, for the diagnosis of pneumothorax, is not justified. The injury of subclavian artery and subclavian vein are also possible in this approach, like the injury to the thoracic duct (on the left side). Injury to the nerves of brachial plexus may also happen from the direct traumatic needle insertion within the nerve or intraneural injection of the LA agent. Other complications of this approach of the brachial plexus block include phrenic nerve block (40–60%), Horner's syndrome, and neuropathy due to nerve injury, and cervical sympathetic block which only requires reassurance.

Infraclavicular Approach for Brachial Plexus Block

This approach of the brachial plexus block is only described for historical reasons. The infraclavicular approach for brachial plexus block offers the same advantages as that of supraclavicular approach, but the high complication rate due to (1) the long distance crossed by the needle, (2) the very closeness of the needle to the parenchyma of lungs and great vessel, and (3) the scarcity of experienced anesthetist to teach this technique has made its application limited **(Fig. 6).** So, the excessive high rate of complication for potential pneumothorax, trend to limited hospitalization time, quick discharge of patient and increasing the number

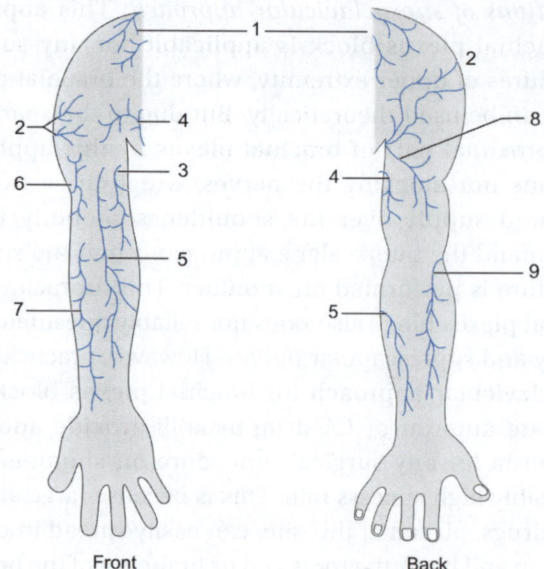

Fig. 6: Infraclavicular approach for brachial plexus block.

Notes:
1. *Lateral supraclavicular nerve ($C_{3,4}$):* It arises from the cervical plexus and divides into three parts, i.e., medial, intermediate, and lateral pierces the deep fascia of neck and descends over clavicle that supplies skin over deltoid, pectoralis major as far down as the level of a horizontal line drawn from the second costal cartilage.
2. *Upper lateral cutaneous nerve of the arm ($C_{5,6}$):* It is a branch of axillary nerve that supplies skin over the lower half of the deltoid muscle.
3. *Medial cutaneous nerve of the arm ($T_{1,2}$):* It arises from the medial cord of brachial plexus that supplies skin on the medial side of the arm.
4. *Intercostobrachial nerve (T_2):* It arises from the second intercostal nerve, crosses the axilla, thereafter pierces deep fascia of the upper arm; and supplies the floor of axilla and medial side of the upper arm.
5. *Medial cutaneous nerve of forearm (C_8, T_1):* It arises from the medial cord of brachial plexus, pierces deep fascia at the middle of the arm, supplies skin over the front of upper arm between basilic and cephalic vein, and also supplies the medial half of the forearm.
6. *Lower lateral cutaneous nerve of the arm ($C_{5,6}$):* It is a branch of radial nerve that arises from the radial nerve before, it leaves the radial groove of humerus, and pierces the deep fascia 2–3 cm below the deltoid tuberosity. It supplies skin of the front, lateral, and posterior side of the upper arm.
7. *Lateral cutaneous nerve of the forearm ($C_{5,6}$):* It is the continuation of musculocutaneous nerve. It pierces the deep fascia lateral to biceps muscle, 2 cm above the elbow. It supplies the skin of both the front and back of lateral side of the forearm. It also supplies the skin over the ball of thumb.
8. *Posterior cutaneous nerve of the arm (C_5):* It arises from the radial nerve in axilla. It pierces the deep fascia a little below the posterior fold of axilla. It supplies a wide area of skin on the back of the arm from the level of deltoid tuberosity to the elbow.
9. *Posterior cutaneous nerve of the forearm ($C_{6–8}$):* It arises from radial nerve. It pierces deep fascia 2–3 cm above the elbow. It passes downward behind the lateral epicondyle. It descends on the back of the forearm up to the wrist. It supplies the skin of the back of the forearm from elbow to wrist.

of outpatient extremity procedures under RA have made this approach now obsolete.

As the anterior and posterior divisions of brachial plexus pass over the first rib and move toward the posterior surface of clavicle, their tight and vertical disposition is still maintained. Then, the plexus (cords) passes under the clavicle and move toward to axilla, passing just inferior to the coracoid process. At this point, the brachial plexus is still directly over the first rib in horizontal plane and this rib theoretically prevents any needle, approaching the plexus at this site, from entering into the thorax. The infraclavicular part of brachial plexus is also tightly arranged within its sheath and any access of this brachial plexus at this level will result in the rapid exposure of entire plexus to an LA agent. The disadvantage of this approach for brachial plexus block at this site is that it lies 2–3" deep to the skin surface, making it more difficult to approach.

Indications: Like supraclavicular, in this approach of the brachial plexus block, there is also high failure rate in blocking the branches, arising from the proximal part of brachial plexus which is only possible by interscalene method. So, the block of brachial plexus through this route is not the choice for shoulder and upper arm surgery which need the block of brachial plexus more proximally, because only the most proximal approach for brachial plexus, such as the interscalene approach, can block the nerves or branches of the brachial plexus, arising from its root, which supply the shoulder. But in contrast to interscalene approach, high success rate is anticipated of ulnar nerve block in this approach. So, like supraclavicular approach, this infraclavicular approach of the brachial plexus block is indicated for surgeries on superior extremity at elbow and distal to the elbow. The shoulder and upper arm are not anesthetized by this approach. As with other brachial plexus block, the intercostobrachialis nerve (T_2 dermatome) is spared.

This approach is also relatively contraindicated for outpatients, because of its potential risk for subclinical pneumothorax like supraclavicular approach, which may be manifested after the patient has left the hospital. Like supraclavicular brachial plexus block, the distinct advantage of this approach is that rapid higher density block can be achieved without requiring movement of hand prior to the onset of anesthesia. This is unlike the axillary approach where hand is moved before the block which causes pain, (1) due to the injury for which this surgery is advised, or (2) due to the presence of any contracture which prevents the abduction and circumduction of axilla.

Technique of infraclavicular block: The patient is positioned supine and the head is turned toward the opposite side. After proper aseptic measure, a skin wheal is raised on the inferior border at the midpoint of clavicle. The insertion point of needle should be just lateral to the subclavian pulse, if it can be identified. Then, a 22 G and 3" long needle is advanced at 45° angle toward the humeral head, through this skin wheal. Always the needle should be advanced away from the chest wall to reduce the chances of entry of needle into the apex of lung, producing pneumothorax. The right position of the needle can be identified by elicitation of paresthesia. If bone (coracoid) is encountered by the needle, then it should be withdrawn and advanced again with slightly different direction. During aspiration test, by a fluid-filled syringe if air is aspirated, then the chest X-ray is must. If a long insulated needle is available, then the nerve stimulator can also be used to elicit motor-evoked response for the better identification of brachial plexus **(Fig. 7)**.

- *Nerve stimulation technique:* The patient is positioned supine and the head is turned toward contralateral side. Coracoid process is identified by palpation as bony prominence between the acromioclavicular joint and the deltopectoral groove. The nerves of brachial plexus and subclavian artery run deep to the coracoid process and their location can be found 2 cm medial, 2 cm caudal to it and 4–5 cm deep to the skin. A relatively long (8 cm) insulated needle is inserted perpendicular to the skin and is advanced directly posterior, until a motor response is elicited. An acceptable motor response is finger flexion or extension but not elbow flexion and extension.

- *Ultrasound technique for infraclavicular brachial plexus block:* The patient is kept in supine position with 90 degree arm abduction. A small curvilinear transducer

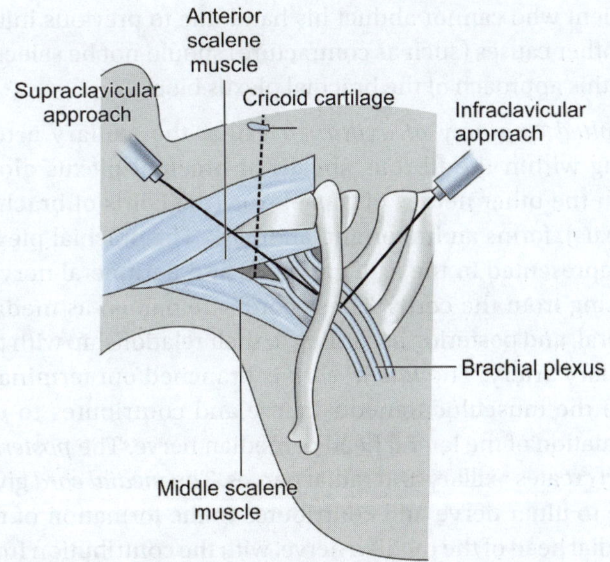

Fig. 7: Using nerve stimulator to elicit motor-evoked response for identifying brachial plexus.

is placed on parasagittal plane over the point which is 2 cm caudal and 2 cm medial to coracoid process. The lateral, medial, and posterior cords of brachial plexus are seen as hyperechoic area above, below, and posterior to the artery respectively. Now, a long 10 cm needle is introduced through the point which is 2 cm cephalad to the transducer. The optimum position of the tip of the needle is in-between the axillary artery and the posterior cord of brachial plexus. 20–30 mL of local anesthetic agent is now injected in this position. For continuous infusion of local anesthetic agent, catheter can be placed in this location, i.e. behind the axillary artery.

Complication: The most common complication of this approach of the brachial plexus block is pneumothorax and hemothorax which may not be detected at the time of block, but can be serious later on. Thoracic duct injury, on the left side, would be an insidious occurrence. The injury of other great vessels and nerves of chest are also common.

Axillary Approach for Brachial Plexus Block

It is the most common approach of the brachial plexus block for surgery on upper extremity (at and below the elbow). This is because (1) easy performance, (2) reliability for hand and forearm anesthesia, (3) widespread familiarity of this approach, and (4) low complication rate. This block is ideally suited for outpatients and can also easily be adopted for pediatric group. The axillary approach for brachial plexus block is *unsuitable for upper arm and shoulder surgery,* because the axillary, musculocutaneous, and medial brachial cutaneous nerves, arising from the proximal part of brachial plexus, are often spared by this approach and should be supplemented separately at the axilla or elbow. Patient who cannot abduct his hand due to previous injury or other causes (such as contracture) should not be selected for this approach of the brachial plexus block.

Applied anatomy of axilla: In axilla, the axillary artery lying within the fibrous sheath of brachial plexus along with the other nerves of this plexus (the cords of brachial plexus), forms an important landmark. The brachial plexus is represented in the axilla as cords and peripheral nerves, arising from the cords. These cords are named as medial, lateral, and posterior, according to their relationship with the axillary artery. The *lateral cord* is branched out terminally into the musculocutaneous nerve and contributes to the formation of the lateral head of median nerve. The *posterior cord* creates axillary and radial nerves. The *medial cord* gives rise to ulnar nerve and contributes to the formation of the medial head of the median nerve, with the contribution from the lateral cord. These terminal branches of the brachial plexus cord also maintain the same relationship with the

axillary artery, like their primary contributors (cords). Thus, the radial nerve remains posterior to the artery, ulnar nerve remains medial to the artery, and median nerve remains lateral to the artery.

When the brachial plexus block is performed most proximally (interscalene approach), then the most distal nerve, such as the ulnar nerve is spared frequently. On the other hand, when the brachial plexus block is performed distally (axillary approach), then the most proximal branches such as the axillary and musculocutaneous nerves are spared frequently. The medial part of the upper arm gets sensory innervation from the branches of T_1 and T_2 spinal nerves which lies outside the brachial plexus and comes from the thoracic wall. These nerves are called the *medial brachial cutaneous* and *intercostobrachialis nerve* and are found in the subcutaneous tissues of axilla. These nerves cannot be blocked by the axillary approach of the brachial plexus block. These are only can be blocked by a *separate subcutaneous field block* at the medial site of the upper arm. For this a vertical line, created by the skin wheal is infiltrated upward to the deltoid prominence and downward to the edge of the triceps. Then about 5 mL of an LA agent is deposited at this straight line in the subcutaneous tissue. A 25 G spinal needle can be a convenient tool for this injection **(Fig. 8)**.

The neurovascular bundle in axilla, formed by (1) the nerves of brachial plexus, (2) axillary artery, and (3) axillary vein, is a multicompartmental structure. It makes no complete, but a partial barrier, for the diffusion of LA drug among the compartments. So, due to this multicompartmental structure, some recommend multiple injections through different sites within the axilla, for this axillary approach of the brachial plexus block, to produce better results, But some practitioners are reluctant to reenter the sheath of brachial plexus within the axilla for

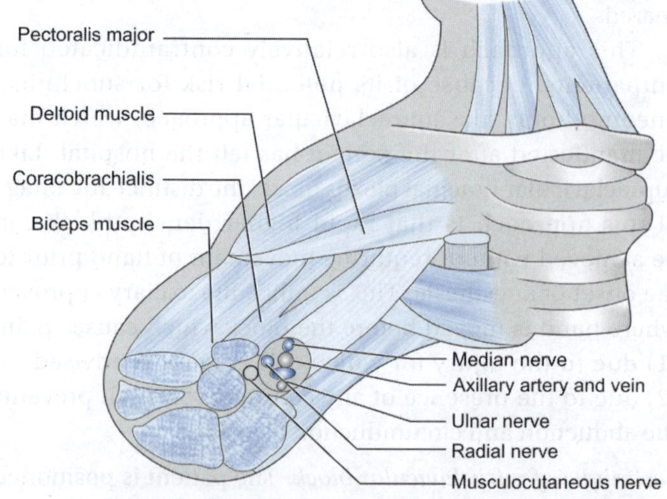

Fig. 8: The brachial plexus in axilla.

the second time, after a bolus of the LA agent has already been injected, because they fear that if the nerve is pierced during the entry of sheath by needle in second time, it will leave the patient unaware (due to the first time block) of pain and will cause potential severe nerve damage. So, a great controversy surrounds between the single versus multiple-injection technique for this axillary approach of the brachial plexus block and still it remains unresolved. The elicitation of paresthesia for successful axillary block is also controversial, because of reportedly higher risk of nerve damage. Although actual data are limited, but motor-evoked response by the nerve locator is very helpful for the success of axillary block.

There are few contraindications to the axillary brachial plexus block. Local infection, neuropathy, and bleeding risk are common, like the other peripheral nerve blocks, as the axilla is highly vascularized, so there is more risk of an LA uptake through the small veins, traumatized by the needle placement.

Technique of axillary block: There are four different techniques for the axillary approach of the brachial plexus block, depending on the different methods of confirmation of the placement of needle tip within the sheath of brachial plexus. These are (1) *transarterial technique,* (2) *"sheath-pop" technique,* (3) *elicitation of paresthesia technique,* and (4) *nerve stimulator technique.*

The patient should be first placed in the supine position. Then, the arm is positioned at right angle to his body and elbow is flexed to 90°. The dorsum of the hand should rest on the bed or pillow. This is called the neutral position of arm. Any further dorsal or ventral displacement of arm, from this neutral position, will cause the palpation of axillary artery's pulsation difficult. The more dorsal displacement of arm may accentuate the prominence of the underlying head of humerus and flattens the contents of the overlying sheath of brachial plexus which may make the palpation of pulsation of axillary artery difficult.

Now, the axillary artery is first palpated in axilla and then it is fixed against the head of the humerus. After that a skin wheal is raised directly over the artery by the LA agent. Whenever possible, the most proximal area for the appreciation of pulse is selected. This is because the sheath, surrounding the brachial plexus, begins to loss distally from this point. The best proximal site for the injection of the LA agent for the brachial plexus block in axilla is the site of skin fold, formed by the crossing of pectoralis complex (major), arising from the thorax with the arm.

After the injection of the LA agent, the arm should be returned to the patient's side. This will allow the head of the humerus to move further from the sheath and will ensure the maximum proximal spread of the LA agent. This is because the filling of sheath, as far proximally as possible, with the anesthetic agent from the site of injection, results in better regional block. After a time span of 2–3 minutes, arm can be repositioned and any supplemental blocks, (for medial brachial cutaneous nerve, intercostobrachialis nerve, and musculocutaneous nerve) if indicated can be performed.

Methods of Identifying the Brachial Plexus Sheath

As previously described, there are four different techniques or methods for identifying the brachial plexus sheath, but all these techniques that have in common in them is the positioning of arm which allows the best palpation of axillary artery and maximizes the gathering of information from the palpation of this surface anatomy of axillary artery.

Transarterial Technique

In this technique, a skin wheal is raised first by the LA agent, at the most proximal site, where the pulsation of axillary artery is appreciated as best. The anesthetist's nondominant hand is positioned at this site in such a way that it can identify the pulse as best, but will not occlude the arterial flow. For easy operation of this technique, the needle is usually connected first to an extension tubing and then to the syringe. It will help for the maximum needle control and fixation of it, if needed. In this transarterial technique, the needle will pierce the artery and blood is to be aspirated during the passage of its tip through the arterial lumen. The needle will advance gently through the palpable pulse, perpendicular to the plane of artery while a constant gentle aspiration by syringe is applied by the assistant. When aspiration of blood ceases, then it implies a sign that the tip of the needle is just beyond the arterial wall at its posterior surface.

Now, the 40 mL solution of the LA agent is injected posterior to the artery. Alternatively, the half of the LA solution is injected posterior and the half of the LA solution is injected anterior to the artery, but a great care must be taken to avoid intravascular injection of the LA agent, by using a test dose or using epinephrine as a marker in it. Some investigators report nearly 100% success of axillary brachial plexus block with this transarterial technique, but some practitioners avoid this transarterial technique in the belief that it is unnecessarily traumatic. Whatever is the controversy, now this technique has fallen out of favor due to the trauma of twice purposefully penetrating the axillary artery, along with a theoretically increased risk of inadvertent intravascular LA injection **(Fig. 9)**.

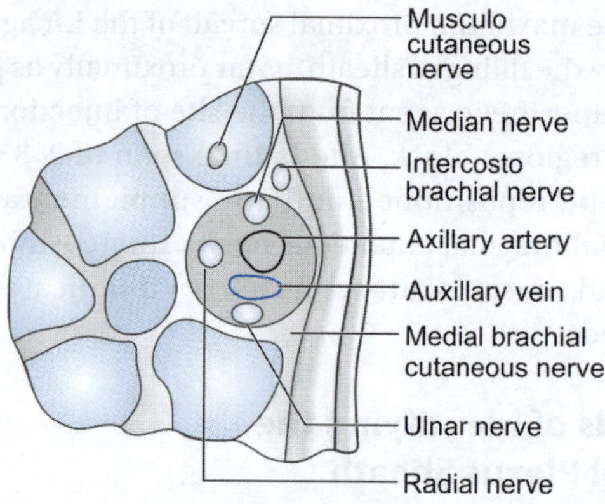

Fig. 9: Axillary block.

"Sheath Pop" Technique

This axillary approach for brachial plexus block is developed by identifying the brachial plexus sheath, during the entry within it, without piercing the axillary artery or eliciting paresthesia, i.e., not injuring the vessels and nerves. However, this technique is facilitated, due to the development of new, small, blunt, and short beveled regional needles. This new, blunt, and short beveled regional needle maximizes the tactile information, during its insertion through the brachial plexus sheath. Due to the superficial nature of axillary artery, the short length of the needle is selected. After appropriate positioning of hand and creation of a sterile field, the needle is directed toward a position which is next to the medial or lateral side of the underlying pulse. Usually, the sheath surrounding the brachial plexus is approached lateral to the axillary pulse. Then, the blunt-bevel needle is advanced through the skin until the axillary sheath is entered by the side of axillary artery, as evidenced by a "fascial click" (sheath pop). Then, the needle is advanced 1 mm further into the sheath, where up to 40 mL drug is injected, after negative aspiration. By this technique the success rate is very high, but it is most difficult to teach. Benefit of this technique is elimination of persistent paresthesia or compressive hematoma of axillary artery which is occurred due to the direct prick of nerve and artery.

Elicitation of Paresthesia

It is one of the oldest methods for the identification of nerve or its plexus for conduction block. The elicitation of paresthesia also can be applied easily for brachial plexus block, like other nerve blocks and the result can also be improved by anatomical approach, based on the dermatomes, involved in the proposed surgical procedure. So, the knowledge for the proper location of the nerves of brachial plexus in axilla is essential. The success of block for a given terminal (peripheral) nerve of plexus is further improved by the injection only at that site, from where the paresthesia is elicited. The axillary artery is the correct constant landmark, creating a fixed relationship with these nerves. Again, the correct identification of paresthesia requires extensive knowledge of terminal (peripheral) sensory components of these nerves, for example, the elicited paresthesia in hand must easily be identified by its origin. If it is located in the dorsal aspect of thumb, then the radial nerve is implicated. If the paresthesia is located in the midpalm, especially on the palmar surface, then the median nerve is implicated.

However, the selection of needle, used to elicit paresthesia, is controversial. Some thought that the blunt needle pushes the nerve away from its tip, causing less chance of piercing it, whereas the fine needle may more likely enter the substance of nerve and can cause more injury to the nerve. But some thought that fine needle will cause less nerve injury, if the nerve substance is inadvertently entered at all, than the blunt needle.

During the initial injection of the LA agent, paresthesia perhaps is slightly increased due to the pressure, caused by the LA agent on nerve. This pressure initially induces activation of nerve fibers (i.e., action potential of nerve fibers) and increases conduction through it, before Na^+ channels are blocked. Thus, it increases paresthesia initially. The advantage of this technique is that it relatively increases the success rate of block in selected dermatomes, but the potential complication rate may increase due to the intentional elicitation of paresthesia by piercing the nerve, whether this technique of elicitation of paresthesia would influence the rate of persistent paresthesia postoperatively is unknown.

Nerve Stimulator Technique

With minimum required frequency and voltage, it is possible to stimulate and elicit the motor activity of a nerve with little or no painful sensation. Thus, it helps to verify the placement of the tip of a needle very close to a nerve. In axilla, the nerves are identified by their specific motor activities which are like that (1) *median nerve:* Wrist flexion, thumb opposition, and forearm pronation; (2) *ulnar nerve:* Wrist flexion, thumb adduction, and fourth/fifth digit flexion; and (3) *radial nerve:* Digit/wrist/elbow extension and forearm supination. Again, the use of variable voltage nerve stimulator, combined with insulated needle, also increases the success rate, because this combination guarantees that current can be delivered only to the tissues, near to the desired nerve, adjacent to the injecting port of needle, but the disadvantage of this variable voltage nerve stimulator, combined with the insulated needle it is difficult to prick the blunt insulated needle through dermis.

So, after raising a skin wheal, the passage of an insulated needle through the dermis is facilitated by the passage of a similar gauge sharp needle before and thereby avoiding the bending of regional insulated needle or the folding of its insulating layer over the needle. The nerve stimulator unit is turned on, after the skin is penetrated by the needle and during the search for nerve. The current is kept at 1 mA or less and at 2 Hz frequency to avoid the recruitment of nociceptive fibers, when the nerves are searched for. If pain occurs, simultaneously with the motor-evoked response, then the patient may move his or her limbs involuntarily and may displace the needle. Gentle muscle movement, elicited from an appropriate nerve muscle unit, confirms the correct needle placement. Then, the decrease of voltage to 0.5 mA or less and still the elicitation of muscle movement indicate the very closeness of the needle tip to the nerve and high probability of successful block. The further confirmation of the correct placement of needle is also possible, if the equipment allows the injection of the LA agent during the delivery of current. If injection is given during the stimulation of nerve, initially there is an increase in the magnitude of motor-evoked response, analogous to pressure paresthesia. This increase of motor-evoked response should be followed quickly by the decrease and the gradual abolition of the movements of muscles as injection proceeds.

If the nerve stimulator technique is employed, without the use of an insulated needle, then the current density, flowing along the entire shaft of the needle, must be considered and a large area will be stimulated. There is also another technique to increase the probability or success rate that the injecting port of needle will be close to the part of the nerve, eliciting motor-evoked response. For that, the needle is advanced gradually till the response occurs, then the needle is withdrawn until it (response) just disappears and again moves forward in the same track, until the response barely occurs again.

The complications of nerve stimulator technique are same as others. Insulated or noninsulated needle may encounter the artery, vein, or nerve and may be the potential for injury.

Ultrasound Technique

Using a high-frequency linear array ultrasound transducer, the axillary artery and the axillary vein are visualized in cross section. On screen, the brachial plexus can be identified, surrounding the axillary artery. The needle is inserted superior (lateral) to the transducer and is advanced inferiorly (medially) toward the plexus, under direct visualization. Then, 10 mL of LA solution is injected around the each nerve, including the musculocutaneous nerve, if is indicated.

Continuous Brachial Plexus Block with Catheter

Since 1940s, the continuous brachial plexus block has been described. It is usually obtained by placing and securing a catheter in the vicinity of the nerves of brachial plexus. This can be performed by technique, using both the catheter "over" the needle and "through" the needle methods. Catheter "through" and "over" the needle method means, it can be passed through the needle, after it pierces the skin, or the needle can be threaded through the catheter, before piercing the skin. The longer catheters are helpful for better fixation and provide superior blockade, if the tip of the catheter lies more proximal to the nerve plexus. However, stimulating electrode with catheter is not available still now for continuous brachial plexus block.

Comments: The axilla is a suboptimal site for perineural catheter placement, because of greatly inferior analgesia versus an infraclavicular infusion, as well as theoretically increased risks of infection and catheter dislodgment.

The advantages of this technique are:
- Potential prolongation of surgical anesthesia, if needed
- Decreased risk of toxicity of the LA agent, as small incremental doses are used
- Postoperative pain relief
- Sympathectomy

The disadvantages of this technique are:
- Increased incidences of inadequate surgical anesthesia, as repeated small does are given
- Infection
- Difficulty in securing catheter, causing kinking, migration, etc.

Indications for continuous brachial plexus block with catheter are:
- Upper extremity or digit replantation
- Total elbow arthroplasty
- Reflex sympathetic dystrophies for which prolonged pain relief by sympathectomy are advantageous.

Supplemental Brachial Plexus Blocks—Medial Brachial Cutaneous and Intercostobrachialis Nerve Block (Fig. 10)

The brachial plexus block, by any route, alone cannot anesthetize some area, over the medial upper part of the arm, which is supplied by the T_1 and T_2 segments of spinal cord through the medial brachial cutaneous and intercostobrachialis nerve. They remain outside the brachial plexus sheath. So, sometimes to make the brachial plexus block complete, the supplemental peripheral block of these nerves is necessary. The *medial brachial cutaneous*

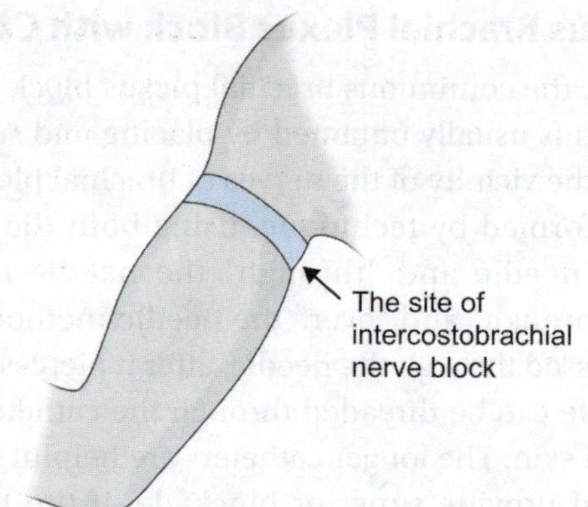

Fig. 10: Medial brachial cutaneous and intercostobrachialis nerve block.

nerve and the *intercostobrachialis nerve* are found in subcutaneous tissue over the medial part of upper arm. So, they can only be blocked by subcutaneous tissue field block over the medial part of the upper arm. For this field block, a skin wheal is created along a transverse line, which extends anteriorly up to the deltoid prominence and posteriorly up to the edge of the triceps. Then, about 5–10 mL of an LA agent is deposited along this straight line in subcutaneous tissue to block the medial brachial cutaneous and intercostobrachialis nerve.

DISTAL UPPER EXTREMITY CONDUCTION BLOCK OF INDIVIDUAL NERVE

This (block of individual nerve of upper extremity) can be performed as a sole anesthetic technique for the small surgical procedures on the upper extremity with limited dermatomes or as a supplemental for partial (inadequate) brachial plexus block. Each of the peripheral nerve (musculocutaneous nerve, radial nerve, median nerve, and ulnar nerve) is identified and can be blocked at the level of elbow or wrist according to the need. Intravenous upper extremity RA is also a type of peripheral upper extremity block **(Fig. 11)**.

Musculocutaneous Nerve Block

The conduction block of this nerve, performed separately, is frequently used to supplement the inadequate primary brachial plexus block, because there is high incidence of sparing this nerve, when the axillary route is approached for brachial plexus block. It is especially useful in surgical procedure where the complete motor block of the upper arm is required by brachial plexus block through the axillary route. It is also equally effective in blocking this nerve on the radial and dorsal surface of the forearm and hand where the terminal sensory supply of this nerve is located **(Fig. 12)**.

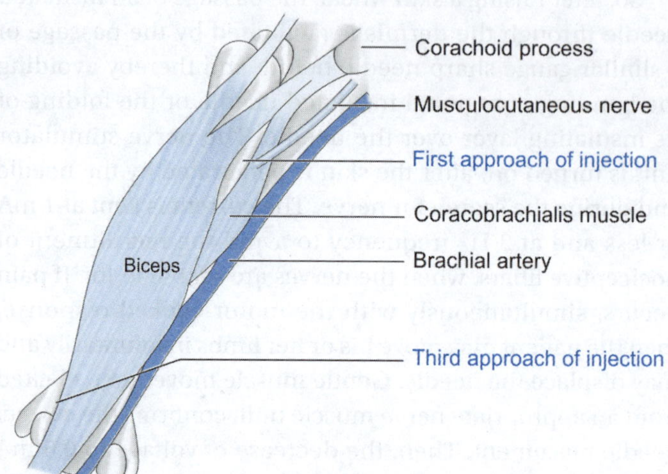

Fig. 11: Musculocutaneous nerve block (right arm).

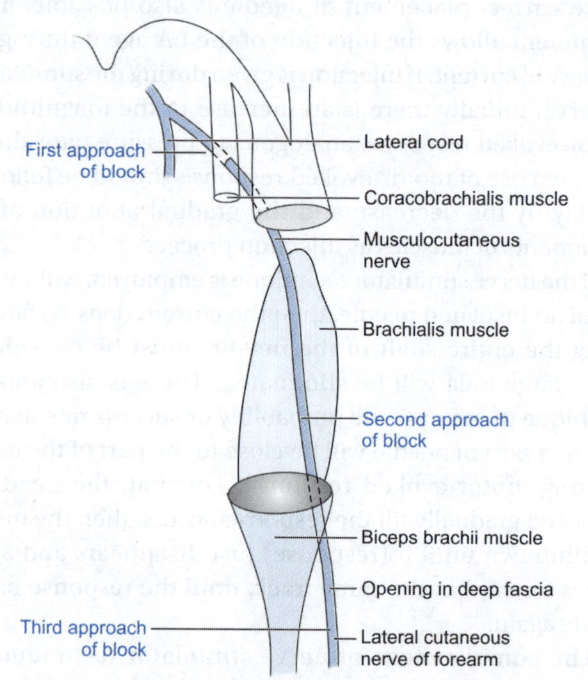

Fig. 12: The course of left musculocutaneous nerve.

Anatomy of Musculocutaneous Nerve

This nerve is the terminal (peripheral) continuation of the lateral cord of brachial plexus. It lies external to the brachial plexus sheath and passes through the substance of coracobrachialis muscle, lying posterior to the axillary artery. It leaves the axilla by piercing the coracobrachialis muscle. This site (where it leaves the axilla by piercing the coracobrachialis muscle) is the *first site of block* of this musculocutaneous nerve, but when it lies within the coracobrachialis muscle. Then, the nerve follows the axillary artery toward the arm where it gives of numerous motor branches, supplying (1) the coracobrachialis muscle, (2) the both heads of biceps, and (3) the medial part of brachialis muscle. The nerve then exits the coracobrachialis muscle and runs downward and laterally between the biceps and brachialis muscles to reach the lateral side of the arm. This (when it runs downward between the biceps and brachialis muscle) is the *second site of block* of this musculocutaneous nerve. It then extends up to the elbow. At the elbow, it pierces the deep fascia on the lateral side of the tendon of biceps and continued as the lateral cutaneous nerve of forearm and supplies the skin on the radial side of the anterior surface of forearm. At the level of the elbow, where this nerve pierces the deep fascia is the *third site of block* of this musculocutaneous nerve block of this nerve at the first approach causes complete motor loss of biceps and coracobrachialis muscle, weakness (partial motor loss) of brachialis muscle and sensory loss over the lateral half of the forearm **(Fig. 13)**.

For the first approach of block, the substance of coracobrachialis muscle is palpated and pulled upward first. Then, a 22 G blunt, short-beveled needle is inserted into the substance of muscle (coracobrachialis) and 5 mL of an LA agent is injected locally. For the second approach of block, the biceps muscle is found between the skin and the nerve. So, the biceps muscle is pulled upward by the fingers of operator hand and the nerve is left behind over the brachialis muscle and humerus **(Fig. 14)**.

Then, the needle is inserted perpendicular to the surface of the skin down up to the humerus. After contact with the bone by needle, 5 mL of drug is injected. For the third approach of block, the lateral cutaneous nerve of forearm, which is the continuation of musculocutaneous nerve of arm, can be blocked at 1 cm proximal to the intercondylar line, immediately lateral to the tendon of biceps muscle. The infiltration of 5 mL of LA solution subcutaneously at this site provides an excellent block of this nerve **(Fact file I)**.

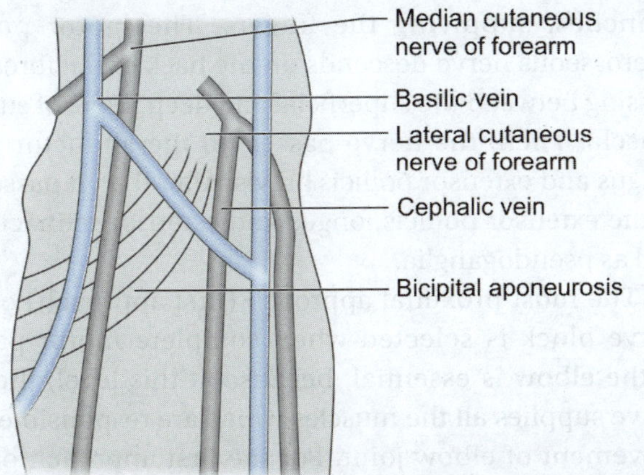

Fig. 13: Structure over the roof of cubital fossa.

FACT FILE I: Musculocutaneous nerve.

- *Branches:*
  - *Muscular:*
    - To the coracobrachialis muscle
    - To the both heads of biceps muscle
    - To the medial part of brachialis (lateral part of brachialis muscle is supplied by radial nerve)
  - *Articular:*
    - To the elbow joint
  - *Sensory:*
    - Lateral cutaneous nerve of forearm
- *Effect of block:*
  - *Motor loss:* Biceps and coracobrachialis are paralyzed. The brachialis is weakened, because a part of it is also supplied by the radial nerve. So, due to the paralysis of these muscles, the flexion of the elbow joint becomes weak. But still it is possible by the unaffected part of brachialis and the superficial flexors of elbow joint in the supine position of hand
  - *Sensory loss:* It is present only over the lateral half of the forearm, but clinically this area of sensory loss is less due to the overlapping of adjacent cutaneous nerve which are not affected

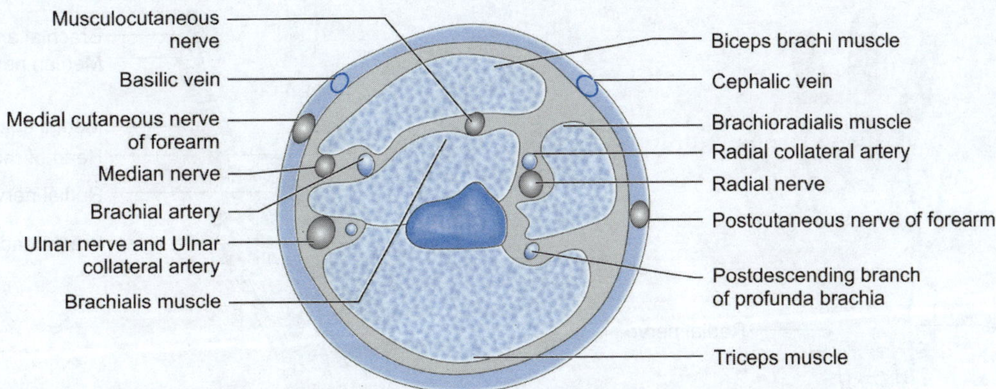

Fig. 14: Transverse section passing through the lower one third of arm.

Radial Nerve Block

The radial nerve can be blocked proximally at the level of the arm and also distally at the level of the elbow and **(Fig. 15)** wrist. It depends on the purpose (1) either for the supplementation of brachial plexus block, or (2) for individual block of this nerve. Above the elbow, the nerve is a mixed one and contains both the motor and sensory component. But at the level of wrist, the block of radial nerve is purely sensory.

Anatomy of Radial Nerve (Fig. 16)

The radial nerve is the continuation of the posterior cord of brachial plexus. After its exit from the axilla, the nerve enters into a spiral groove on the post surface of the humerus, in between the long and the medial head of triceps. This is the *first approach of block* of this nerve. In the spiral groove, it gives off branches as the *lower lateral cutaneous nerve of arm* and the *posterior cutaneous nerve of forearm*. Then, after running through the spiral groove with arteria profunda brachialis artery, the radial nerve pierces the later intermuscular septum and enters the anterior compartment of arm, 4–6 cm above the elbow. In the anterior compartment of the arm, the radial nerve reaches in front of the lateral epicondyle where it passes between the epicondyle and the head of the radius bone. This is the *second approach of block* of radial nerve at the level of elbow. Here, the nerve divides into the deep motor branch (*posterior interosseous nerve*) and *superficial sensory branch*. Then, the superficial sensory branch descends with the radial artery along the lateral side of the forearm **(Fig. 17)**.

Then, 7 cm above the wrist joint or the styloid process of radius, this nerve winds round the lateral border of the forearm, deep to the tendon of brachioradialis muscle and passes to the back on the dorsal surface of the forearm. Then, going to the base of the forearm, it pierces the deep fascia and passes superficial to the extensor reticulum, medial to the cephalic vein. This is the *third approaches of block* of radial nerve at the level of wrist. Finally, it reaches on the back of the hand, where it divides into five digital sensory branches, supplying the fingers. The motor posterior interosseous nerve descends on the back of the forearm, by passing between the superficial and deep fibers of supinator muscle. Then, the nerve passes on the abductor pollicis longus and extensor pollicis brevis. After that, it passes deep to the extensor pollicis longus and extensor retinaculum to end as pseudoganglia.

The most proximal approach (first approach) of radial nerve block is selected when complete motor paralysis of the elbow is essential, because at this level, the radial nerve supplies all the muscles which are responsible for the movement of elbow joint. For the first approach of radial

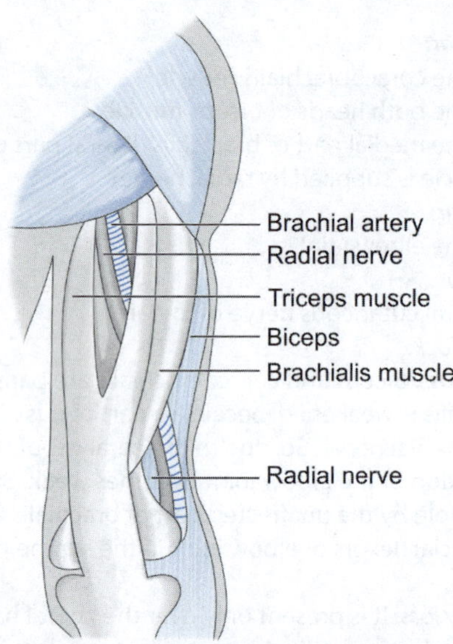

Fig. 15: The radial nerve block under the triceps muscle and at the proximal site of elbow in the right arm (posterior surface of nerve).

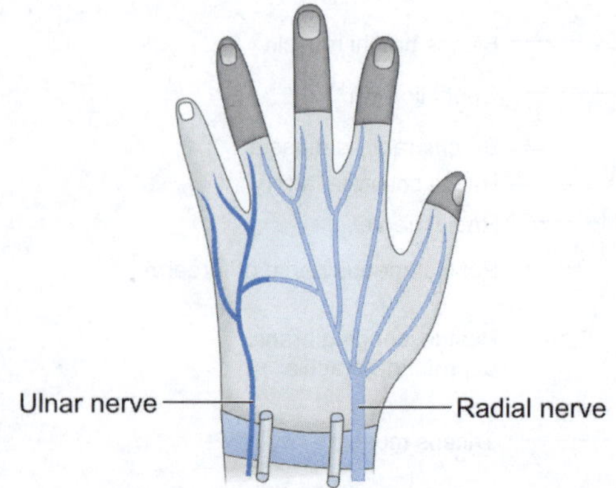

Fig. 16: Ulnar and radial nerve.

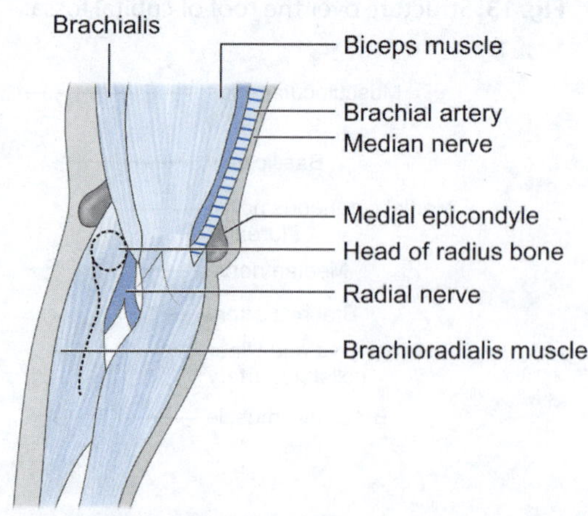

Fig. 17: Radial nerve block at antecubital fossa.

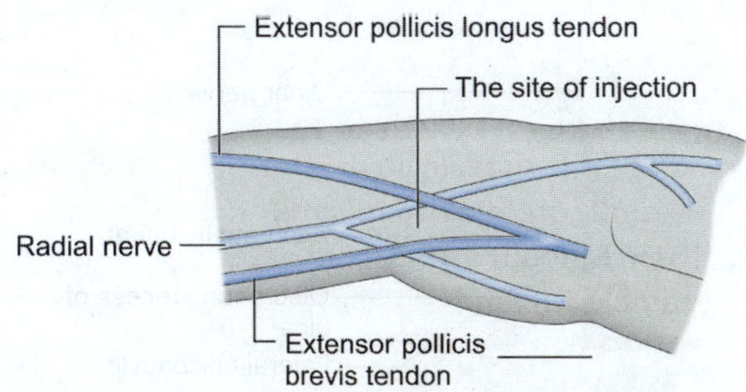

Fig. 18: Radial nerve block at the left wrist.

nerve block, the lateral edge of triceps muscle and the musculospiral groove of humerus are palpated first. Then, a blunt needle is introduced between the two heads of this triceps muscle toward the humerus and 5–8 mL of LA drug is injected, after the contact of needle tip with bone on spiral groove is felt. Like other field blocks, the needle is withdrawn and again advanced forward with different directions for one or more injections, close to the spiral groove of humerus at different locations **(Fig. 18)**.

For the second approach, the radial nerve can be blocked at elbow, as it passes over the anterior aspect of lateral epicondyle in antecubital fossa. In such position, the tendon of biceps is identified first. Then, a 22 G and 4 cm long insulated needle is inserted at the intercondylar line, 2 cm lateral to the tendon of biceps and is advanced directing toward the lateral epicondyle till the bone in encountered or the extension of wrist or fingers is elicited. Then, the area between the lateral epicondyle of humerus and the head of radius is infiltrated by the LA agent as a field block. To avoid nerve injury, elicitation of paresthesia should be avoided. If paresthesia is elicited, the needle should be relocated prior to any injection.

The terminal part of radial nerve is purely sensory and is subcutaneous in the distal part of the forearm. At the distal part of the forearm, it first runs overs the radius, then sweeps from the ventral to the dorsal surface of wrist and supply the area shown in **Figure 16**. At the level of wrist, the radial nerve can be blocked at the site where it is subcutaneous and palpable. In such position, the radial nerve is situated just lateral to the radial artery which can be easily palpated lateral to the flexor carpi radialis tendon.

For the third approach of radial nerve block (i.e., at the wrist), the extensor pollicis longus tendon is identified first, when the patient extends his thumb or the pulsation of radial artery is identified. Then, the needle is inserted subcutaneously over the tendon (but does not pierce the tendon) at the base of the first metacarpal bone or just lateral to the artery. The injection of LA agent should be subcutaneous and superficial to the tendon. About 2 mL of the LA agent is injected proximally subcutaneously along

the tendon and 1 mL is injected, as the needle passes at right angle across the "anatomical snuff box." Alternately, the LA solution can be injected as a field block in the dorsal subcutaneous tissue proximal to the base of the thumb and index finger. Ultrasound may be used at the level of wrist or midforearm to identify the radial nerve just lateral to the radial artery. The motor branches, sensory branches and the effects of block of radial nerve at different levels are shown in **Fact file II**.

Ulnar Nerve Block

Among all the peripheral nerve blocks of upper extremity, the block of ulnar nerve at the level of the elbow is most easily performed, but it is most likely to cause nerve injury from the incorrect technique. It (ulnar nerve block) can also easily be accomplished in Guyton's canal at wrist, in the same way as the block of median nerve in the carpal tunnel. The block of ulnar nerve is usually performed for the anesthesia of hypothenar region, the fifth finger and the ulnar half of fourth finger, which is depicted in **Figure 19**.

FACT FILE II: Radial nerve.

- *Branches:*
  - *Motor:*
    - To long and medial head of triceps muscle
    - To lateral part of brachialis muscle
    - To brachioradialis muscle
    - To extensor carpi radialis longus and brevis muscle
    - To supinator muscle
    - All the extensor group of muscle of forearm
  - *Sensory:*
    - Posterior cutaneous nerve of the arm
    - Lower lateral cutaneous nerve of the arm (upper lateral cutaneous nerve of arm is the branch of axillary nerve)
    - Posterior cutaneous nerve of forearm
    - Dorsal digital branches, supplying the lateral and medial side of thumb, lateral side of the index finger up to the middle phalanx, adjacent sides of index and middle finger up to the middle phalanx and adjacent sides of middle and ring finger up to the middle phalanx
- *Effect of block:*
  - *At the wrist:*
    - Only sensory loss of digits is supplied by this nerve
  - *At the elbow:*
    - Sensory loss at the wrist
    - *Motor loss:* All the extensor of wrist, causing wrist drop. When an attempt is made to extend the fingers, the proximal phalanx remains flexed, but the middle and distal phalanges will be extended by the unaffected interossei and lumbricals
  - *At the spiral groove:*
    - Sensory loss as wrist
    - Motor loss as elbow
    - Plus the muscles of the back of the arm

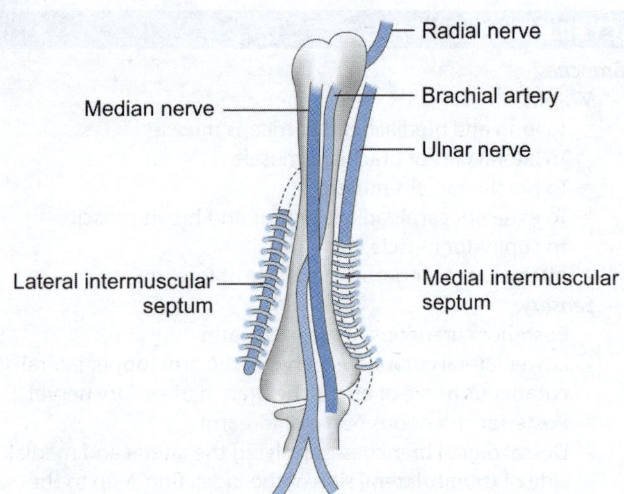

Fig. 19: The course of different nerves in the right arm (anterior aspect).

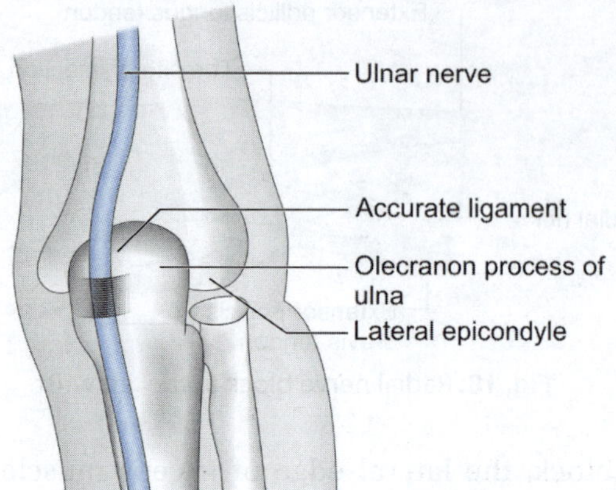

Fig. 20: Ulnar nerve block at the elbow.

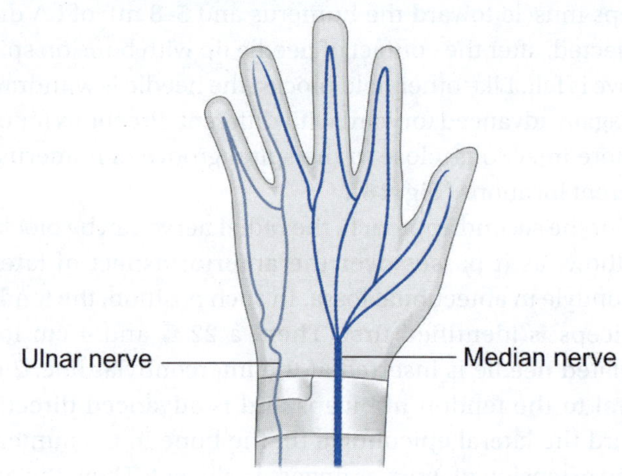

Fig. 21: Location of ulnar and median nerve.

Anatomy of Ulnar Nerve

After exit from the axilla, the ulnar nerve first runs along the medial side of the brachial artery which is a continuation of the axillary artery. Then, at the middle of the arm, the ulnar nerve pierces the medial intermuscular septum from anterior to posterior and runs down on the back of the medial epicondyle of humerus where it is covered by the arcuate ligament. It is the *site of block of ulnar nerve* at the elbow. The ulnar nerve, then, enters the **(Fig. 20)** anterior aspect of forearm by running between the two heads of origin of the *flexor carpi ulnaris* muscle and descends downward lying on *flexor digitorum profundus* muscle. Here (at the anterior aspect of forearm), it (ulnar) is overlapped by flexor carpi ulnaris muscle in the upper part, and by the skin and deep fascia in the lower part of forearm. The nerve, then, enters the hand along with the ulnar artery, running in front of the flexor retinaculum, but lateral to the pisiform bone. It is the site of the block of ulnar nerve at the wrist. Here, the ulnar nerve is located in the interval between ulnar artery and flexor carpi ulnaris tendon **(Fig. 21)**.

On entering the hand, it (ulnar nerve) divides into terminal muscular and sensory branches. The terminal muscular branches of ulnar nerve supply the following muscles, such as the palmaris brevis muscle, all the hypothenar muscles, adductor pollicis muscle, all the dorsal interossei muscles, and the third and fourth lumbrical muscles. The terminal sensory branches of the ulnar nerve supply the palmar medial side of the little finger and the adjacent palmar sides of the ring and little finger. At the middle of the forearm, the ulnar nerve gives a cutaneous branch which pierces the deep fascia and descends in front of the flexor retinaculum and supply the skin of the medial half of the palm. Another dorsal cutaneous branch arises from the ulnar nerve, 5 cm above the wrist and

it supplies the medial side of the dorsum of hand, the medial dorsal side of the little finger and the adjacent dorsal sides of the little and ring finger. The block of ulnar nerve at this side provides only the sensory loss along the ulnar side of the hand, little finger, and ulnar half of the ring finger.

The ulnar nerve can most easily be blocked at its subcutaneous position which is situated posterior to the medial epicondyle of elbow (ulnar nerve block at the elbow). But the block of ulnar nerve at this site is associated with high incidence of neuritis. So, the use of very fine needle, the avoidance of intraneural injection, and the small amount of drug reduces these incidences of neuritis. At the elbow, the LA agent should be injected in a fanwise fashion, without eliciting the sign of paresthesia. The technique to block the ulnar nerve at the level of elbow is like that. An insulated 22 G needle is inserted approximately one finger breath proximal to the arcuate ligament and is advanced, until the flexion of fifth/forth finger or the adduction of thumb is elicited. Then, 35 mL of an LA solution is injected at that site **(Fig. 20)**.

At the wrist, the nerve is located in between the ulnar artery (laterally) and the flexor carpi ulnaris tendon

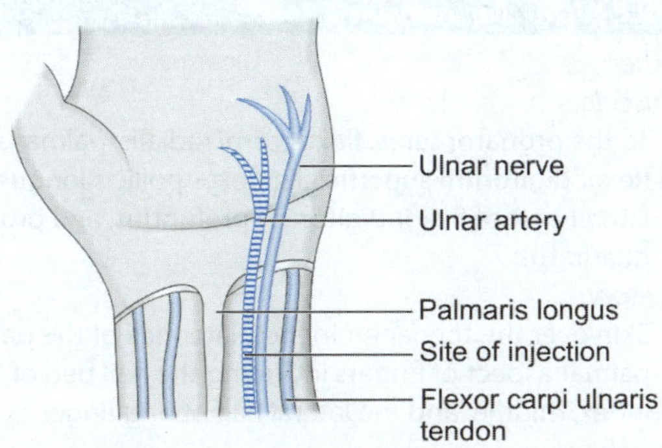

Fig. 22: Ulnar nerve block at wrist.

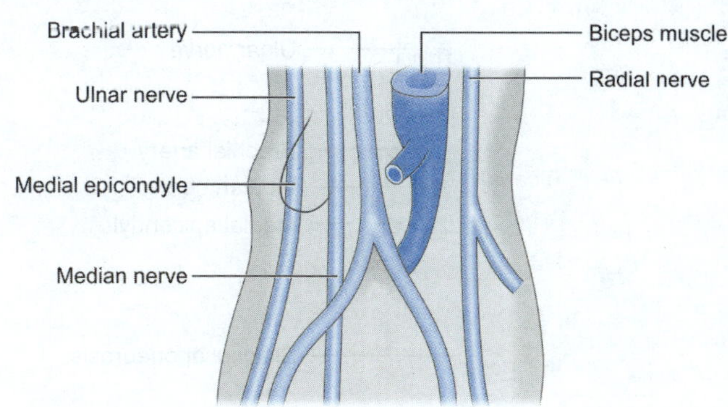

Fig. 23: Antecubital fossa and its contents (left arm).

FACT FILE III: Ulnar nerve.

- *Branches:*
  - *Muscular:* To flexor carpi ulnaris, medial part of flexor digitorum profundus, hypothenar muscles, all dorsal interossei, third and fourth lumbricals, and adductor pollicis
  - *Sensory:* Palmar and dorsal surface of hand, little finger, and medial side of ring finger
- *Effect of block:*
  - *At the wrist:*
    - *Motor loss:* All the intrinsic muscles of hand except those supplied by the median nerve, i.e., all interossei, third and fourth lumbricals, hypothenar muscle. Thus, it produces *claw hand*, loss of power of abduction of second to fifth digits, loss of power of adduction of thumb.
    - *Sensory loss:* Loss of sensation of little finger and medial side of ring finger.
  - *At the elbow:*
    - *Motor loss:* Same as block at wrist plus paralysis of the medial part of flexor digitorum profundus going to the little and ring finger. So, the distal phalanges of these fingers are not acutely flexed as in claw hand.
    - *Sensory loss:* Same as loss at wrist plus medial side of dorsal and palmar aspect of forehand.

(medially), which can easily be defined by the forced flexion of wrist. Then, the needle is inserted perpendicular to the skin; just medial to the artery and 35 mL of drug is injected in a fan wise fashion (*see* **Fig. 22**). The motor and sensory branches of ulnar nerve and the effects of block of this nerve at different levels are given in **Fact file III**.

Median Nerve

The median nerve can easily be blocked in antecubital space (fossa) at the level of the elbow or in carpal tunnel at the level of the wrist. The anatomical landmarks for median nerve are almost constant and are readily accessible for conduction block. The median nerve block is performed for anesthesia for surgeries on median dermatomes of hand which is depicted in **Figure 23**.

Anatomy of Median Nerve

The median nerve is formed by the union of (1) medial head, coming from the medial cord and (2) lateral head, coming from the lateral cord of the brachial plexus. In the axilla, this nerve first runs along the lateral side of axillary artery. Then, it exits the axilla and descends by resting on brachialis muscle, still lying at the lateral side of the axillary artery. At the insertion of coracobrachialis muscle on humerus, the median nerve crosses in front of the artery and then further descends down resting on brachialis muscle to reach the cubital fossa, where it is covered only by the bicipital aponeurosis (**Fig. 24**).

After that, from cubital fossa, the median nerve enters the forearm, between the two heads of pronator teres muscle. Then, it runs downward in the forearm, resting on flexor digitorum profundus muscle, but deep to the flexor digitorum superficialis muscle. About 5 cm above the flexor retinaculum, it becomes more superficial, by running only deep to the deep fascia of the forearm. Now, the nerve enters the palm, deep to the flexor retinaculum and through the carpal tunnel, i.e., through the space, bounded between the flexor retinaculum in front and carpal bones behind. On entering the palm, the median nerve now supplies the muscles of thenar eminence, the first and second lumbricals and the sensory to the palmar aspect of thumbs, index finger, middle finger, and lateral side of the ring finger. In the lower part of the forearm, a cutaneous branch arises from the median nerve. It pierces the deep fascia and enters the palm superficial to flexor retinaculum to supply the skin of the lateral aspect of palm.

The median nerve can be blocked at elbow in antecubital fossa or at the wrist. At cubital fossa, where the nerve is only covered by bicipital aponeurosis, the relation of median nerve with the vessels, from lateral to medial, is biceps tendon, brachial artery, and median nerve. This is the major landmark for median nerve block in antecubital fossa, at the intercondylar line of elbow. For the median nerve block, in antecubital fossa, the brachial artery is palpated first and then a short 22 G insulated needle is inserted just medial

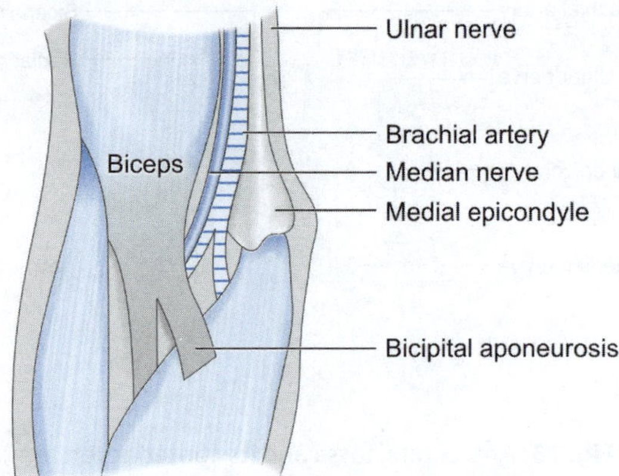

Fig. 24: Median nerve block at elbow.

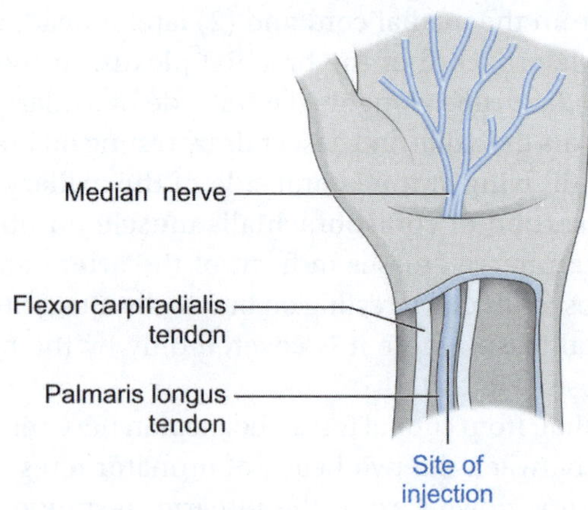

Fig. 25: Median nerve block at wrist.

to the artery and is directed toward the medial epicondyle, until the wrist flexion and thumb opposition is elicited. Then, 35 mL of an LA drug is injected medial to the artery. If *ultrasound* is used, the median nerve is identified in cross section, just medial to the brachial artery and an LA solution is injected to surround it.

At wrist, the median nerve is located in between the palmaris longus and flexor carpi radialis tendon **(Fig. 25)**. To block the median nerve at wrist, the tendon of palmaris longus is first identified by asking the patient to flex the wrist against resistance. Then, a short 22 G needle is inserted adjacent and lateral to the tendon of palmaris longus and is advanced about 0.5 cm. A "pop" is usually felt when the needle traverses the flexor retinaculum and the median nerve can be blocked by injecting 23 mL of an LA agent in between these two tendons, proximal to the wrist crease. A superficial palmar branch of the median nerve, supplying the skin over thenar eminence, does not pass below the flexor retinaculum. This branch should also be blocked separately by injecting 0.51 mL of LA solutions, subcutaneously above

FACT FILE IV: Median nerve.

- *Branches:*
  - *Muscular:*
    - To the pronator teres, flexor carpi radialis, palmaris longus, flexor digitorum superficialis, flexor pollicis longus, lateral part of flexor digitorum profundus, and pronator quadratus
  - *Sensory:*
    - Skin over the thenar eminence, later half of the palm and palmar aspect of fingers including the nail bed of thumb, index, middle; and the lateral half of ring finger
- *Effect of block:*
  - *At the wrist:*
    - *Motor loss:* Thenar muscles and first and second lumbricals are paralyzed. Thus, it causes wasting of thenar prominence and in ability to oppose the thumb
    - *Sensory loss:* Loss of sensation of digits supplied by this nerve. *Carpal tunnel syndrome* affects this nerve producing wasting of thenar muscles and pain in digits supplied by this nerve
  - *At the elbow:*
- *Motor loss:* All the muscles of palm supplied by this nerve, all the flexors of wrist, pronator teres, and pronator quadratus. Thus, it causes the loss of flexion of wrist, and loss of pronation
- *Sensory loss:* Same as loss at wrist

the retinaculum. The motor and sensory branches of median nerve and the effects of block of this nerve at different levels are given in **Fact file IV**.

INTRAVENOUS REGIONAL ANESTHESIA OF EXTREMITY

This technique was first described by a German surgeon, named August Bier, in 1908. So, this type of RA of extremity is also called the *Bier's block*. During that period, after its introduction, it was very much popular in clinical practice, but it had gradually lost its popularity, due to the evaluation (appearance) of other less risky procedures of conduction block, such as the brachial plexus block and the other individual nerve blocks with the help of nerve stimulator and ultrasound guidance.

General Consideration

The Bier's block is an excellent technique (type) of RA for short surgical procedures (<90 minutes, usually 45–60 minutes) over the extremities, mainly the superior extremity. When the peripheral venous system of extremity is filled with the LA agents, then the backward diffusion of these LA agents into the tissue spaces provides dense motor and sensory block. The duration of this type of anesthesia is mainly limited by the length of time that the pneumatic tourniquet can be inflated (applied) without any ischemic injury to limbs, which is usually about 60–90 minutes.

In Bier's block, the patient's safety completely depends on the integrity of this pneumatic tourniquet, because it must be inflated to a pressure which will be high enough to prevent the reaching of the LA agent in systemic circulation and this pressure is maintained, until a safe time interval between the inflation and deflation is reached, regardless of the duration of surgery, during which period the drug is completely diffused into the tissue. It is because though a very low concentration of the LA agent is used, still a bolus high volume is injected into the venous part of circulatory system directly, after the tourniquet is inflated. This technique or this type of RA can be applied to any surgical procedure distal to the elbow or knee, provided its expected duration is 1 hour or less and provided it allows a site for placing a small intravenous catheter in the distal part of the hand (dorsum) or leg (foot).

Due to any surgical reasons, when an anesthetist becomes reluctant to deflate the tourniquet, even after exceeding an hour from the time of inflation, then pain elicited by the tourniquet which is usually a normal phenomenon after a specific time interval, can result in failure of this type of RA, even though the sensory anesthesia at the surgical site is still in effect. On the other hand, very short surgical procedures (under 10–15 minutes) should be taken into account and the pneumatic tourniquet should not be deflated within 45 minutes, after the injection of LA agent, even though the surgery has been completed long before. In orthopedic procedures where vigorous manipulations are required, then attention must also be given to the potentiality of disrupting the integrity of tourniquet (looseness of tourniquet) and the distribution of drug in systemic circulation, after its absorption from the affected limb, causing cardiovascular system (CVS) and central nervous system (CNS) toxicity. However, the bupivacaine is not recommended for this Bier's procedure, due to the high incidences of its systemic toxicity and death. Other rare complications of Bier's block are compartmental syndrome and loss of limb.

Advantages of Bier's Block

- Easy administration
- Rapid onset
- Rapid recovery
- Complete muscular relaxation
- No special skill
- Controllable extent of anesthesia.

Disadvantages of Bier's Block

- Tourniquet discomfort
- Rapidity of recovery leading to the postoperative pain

- Difficulty in providing blood less field
- Difficulty in exsanguination for painful hand
- Sudden, accidental, or early deflation of tourniquet may lead to toxic reaction.

Technique of Bier's Block

As a first step in this technique, an intravenous cannula is placed, as distally as possible, for giving an LA agent on upper or lower extremity which is to be blocked. Another intravenous cannula is also placed on the opposite limb for giving intravenous fluids, drugs, etc., in emergency. A double pneumatic tourniquet is applied on the operated limb, proximal to the surgical field, on thigh or arm. After exsanguination of limb by elastic Esmarch bandage, the proximal pneumatic cuff is inflated first to approximately 50–100 mm Hg higher than the systolic pressure of this patient. Then, calculated total dose of LA agent (4–6 mg/kg of 0.5% lignocaine without epinephrine and preservative, e.g., 25 mL for forearm or ankle and 50 mL for below knee) is injected intravenously slowly through the cannula, placed on the operated limb. Then, the onset of the effect of RA starts within 5 minutes.

If the patient complains of tourniquet pain (usually after 20–30 minutes), then the distal tourniquet, which overlies the anesthetized skin, is inflated and the previous proximal tourniquet, which is situated on the nonanesthetized skin, is released or deflated. Patients usually tolerate the distal tourniquet for an additional 15–20 minutes, because it is inflated over an anesthetized area. The use of a single wide cuff pneumatic tourniquet, during intravenous RA, allows the lower inflation pressure which causes the less incidences of neurological complications in contrast to a high inflation pressure with narrow double pneumatic tourniquet cuffs. Somebody inflates and deflates the proximal and distal cuffs alternately to increase the patient's tolerance.

At the end of the surgical procedure, care must also be taken in deflating the tourniquet, so that the patient is not suddenly exposed to the bolus dose of an LA agent which is absorbed from the affected limb, causing CVS and CNS toxicity. Even for the surgical procedures of a very short duration, the tourniquet must be left inflated for a total of at least 15–20 minutes to avoid a rapid intravenous bolus of local anesthetic, resulting in systemic toxicity. The tourniquet can safely be released, minimum after 25 minutes, from its application. It may also be deflated for 1 or 2 seconds and reinflated again. Thus, these maneuvers are repeated several times, with certain pause between each step, to reduce the systemic LA toxicity. If minor CNS or CVS sign appear at any time, between the two consecutive deflations, then the interval between the deflations of cuff is increased.

■ DIGITAL BLOCK

The digital branches of radial, ulnar, and median nerves first run through the intermetacarpal intervals or spaces. Then, they divide and enter the base of each digit from its four corners, close to the palmar and dorsal surfaces of each digit. The duplication of dorsal and palmar digital nerves demands that the injection technique for digital block must take into account this duplication of digital nerves. In addition, these digital nerves are small and only sensory and would be very intolerant to the intraneural injection of an LA agent or hydrostatic pressure, produced from outside on the nerve, due to the increased volume of LA drug. A 25 G (or more fine) blunt bevel needle is selected for the digital block with a length of about 1 " or less.

The injection usually starts with the entry of needle on the dorsal surface, proximal to the web space. Then, the needle is directed to the palmar side, close to the peritoneum of the metacarpal head. The elicitation of paresthesia is avoided and if it occurs, the needle is redirected. Then, 2–3 mL of an LA agent is injected, as the needle is gradually withdrawn. A good digital block is assured by a gentle massage of the web space after injecting the drug and withdraws of the needle **(Figs. 26A and B)**. The *LA agents with vasoconstrictors should not be used for the digital block, due to the fear of ischemia and necrosis of the fingers.* The maximum volume of drug which is usually 2–3 mL, on each side, should not exceed. The excessive volume of drug can cause vascular insufficiency and gangrene, as a result of digital artery occlusion by its mechanical pressure effect. The digital nerve blocks are commonly used and are very effective method for the wide varieties of minor outpatient surgical procedures on digits.

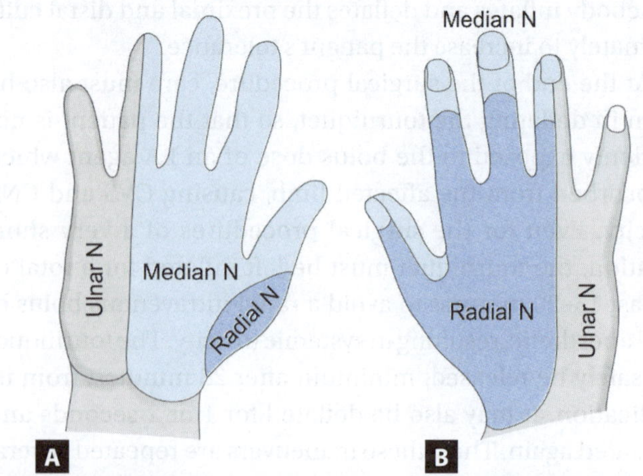

Figs. 26A and B: Sensory innervation of radial, ulnar, and median nerve of the hand. (A) Palmar surface and (B) Dorsal surface.

■ WRIST BLOCK

Wrist block is a very superficial and an easy-to-perform technique. It is devoid of any systemic complications. So, it should be in the armamentarium of every anesthesiologist. Actually, the wrist block is nothing but the ulnar, medial, and radial nerve block, on same sitting, at the level of the wrist. The wrist block is commonly performed for any hand surgery where tourniquet is not required or as a supplementation for incomplete brachial plexus block.

At the wrist, the median nerve is located between the tendons of palmaris longus (medially) and flexor carpi radialis (laterally).The palmaris longus tendon is often made most prominent, among all the tendons at wrist and the median nerve passes immediately lateral to it. At the wrist, this median nerve can be blocked by inserting a needle at that position (by the lateral side of the tendon of palmaris) and going deep, until it pierces the deep fascia or the retinaculum, when the fascial "click" is appreciated. If the "click" is not felt, then the needle is further inserted deep, until it contacts the bone. After contact with bone, the needle is slightly withdrawn for 2–3 mm and the local anesthetic agent is injected.

At wrist, the ulnar nerve is situated between the ulnar artery (pulsation may be felt) and the tendon of flexor carpi ulnaris at the level of ulnar styloid process. At this level, the ulnar nerve is blocked by inserting a needle under the tendon of flexor carpi ulnaris muscle, close to its styloid attachment. The needle is then advanced further for 5–10 mm and 3–5 mL of local anesthetic agent is injected at that site.

At the level of wrist, the radial nerve (superficial branch) runs along the medial aspect of brachioradialis muscle and lateral to the radial artery. It quits the artery about 7 cm above the styloid process of radius. At that level, the nerve winds round the lateral border of forearm between the tendon of brachioradialis and radius, and then pass to the back of the forearm. Going to the back of the forearm, it pierces the deep fascia and descends superficial to the extensor retinaculum, medial to the cephalic vein. Above the styloid process, it gives off the digital branches for the skin of the *dorsal aspect of thumb, index finger, middle finger, and lateral half of the ring finger.* Several of its branches pass superficially over the anatomical *"snuff box."* The radial nerve block requires a more extensive infiltration, because it has less predictable anatomical location and divides into multiple smaller cutaneous branches. A subcutaneous infiltration of 5 mL of local anesthetic agent, just above the radial styloid process is done aiming medially. This infiltration of an LA agent is then extended further laterally, using another 5 mL of an LA agent.

LOWER EXTREMITY BLOCKS

Unlike the blocks of upper extremity which is more popular, the lower extremity blocks are less popular. This is because:

- There is a widespread acceptance and safety of spinal and epidural anesthesia for lower extremity.
- Like brachial plexus, nerves supplying the lower limbs are not anatomically clustered at one place, where they can easily be blocked
- With anatomical consideration these blocks are technically more difficult and require more training
- Persistent block of any major nerve of lower extremity makes the patient unambulatory and causes an unacceptable side effect for outpatients.

But still there are some advantages of lower extremity block and these are:

- Postoperative pain relief
- Lack of complete sympathectomy (as is occurred in central neuraxial block) which make it ideal for very ill patients.

The nerves supplying the lower extremity are *sciatic, femoral, lateral femoral cutaneous,* and *obturator nerve.* These nerves can be blocked, as proximal as at lumbosacral plexus or as distal as at toes, depending on the surgical procedure and the postoperative plan for analgesia.

Anatomy of Lumbar Plexus

The nerves, supplying lower extremity, are derived either from lumber plexus **(Fig. 27)** and/or sacral plexus. The lumbar plexus is formed by the anterior (ventral) rami of the upper four lumbar spinal nerves (L_1, L_2, L_3, and L_4). The ventral rami of first lumbar spinal nerve receive a contribution from the anterior (ventral) rami of T_{12} spinal (subcostal) nerve. And the anterior (ventral) rami of fourth lumbar spinal nerve gives a contribution to the anterior (ventral) rami of L5 spinal nerve, forming *lumbosacral trunk* which take part in the formation of *sacral plexus.* The lumbar plexus lies in the space which is situated between the psoas major (in front) and quadratus lumborum (behind) muscle. This space, between the psoas major muscle in front and the quadratus muscle behind, is called the *psoas compartment.* So, the lumbar plexus block at this level is also called the *"psoas compartment block."* The ventral ramus of first lumbar spinal nerve (L_1), after receiving a twig from the ventral ramus of the T_{12} spinal nerve, divides into two branches that are (1) a large upper branch and (2) a small lower branch. The large upper branch again divides and forms the *iliohypogastric and ilioinguinal nerves.* The small lower branch joins with a twig from the second lumbar nerve (L_2) and forms the *genitofemoral nerve.* The rest of the ventral

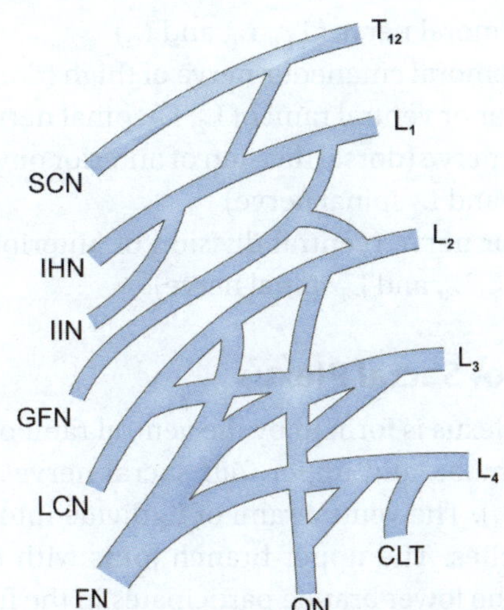

Fig. 27: Formation of lumbar plexus. (CLT: contribution to lumbosacral trunk; FN: femoral nerve; GFN: genitofemoral nerve; IHN: iliohypogastric nerve; IIN: ilioinguinal nerve; LCN: lateral cutaneous nerve of thigh; ON: obturator nerve; SCN: subcostal nerve)

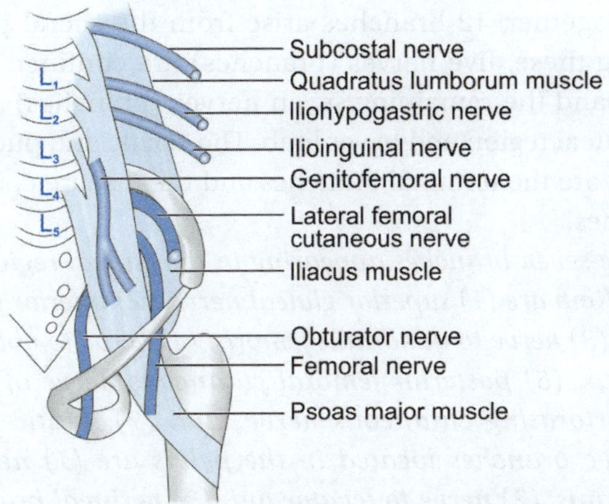

Fig. 28: Nerves arising from the lumbar plexus.

rami of second, third, and fourth lumbar nerves divide each into the dorsal and ventral branches. The dorsal branches of the second and third lumbar nerves unite to form the *lateral femoral cutaneous nerve of thigh.* The dorsal branches of the second, third, and fourth lumbar nerves unite to form the *femoral nerve.* The ventral branches of the second, third, and fourth lumbar nerves unite to form the *obturator nerve* **(Fig. 27)**. The branches of the lumbar plexus come out along the lateral margin of psoas muscle, under the covering of psoas fascia **(Fig. 28)**.

The branches of lumbar plexus emerge from the lateral border of psoas muscle. These branches are:

- Iliohypogastric nerve (T_{12}, L_1)
- Ilioinguinal nerve (T_{12}, L_1)

- Genitofemoral nerve (T_{12}, L_1, and L_2)
- Lateral femoral cutaneous nerve of thigh (dorsal division of anterior or ventral rami of L_2, L_3 spinal nerve)
- Femoral nerve (dorsal division of anterior or ventral rami of L_2, L_3, and L_4 spinal nerve)
- Obturator nerve (ventral division of anterior or ventral rami of L_2, L_3, and L_4 spinal nerve).

Anatomy of Sacral Plexus

The sacral plexus is formed by the ventral rami of the fourth and fifth lumbar, and upper four sacral nerves (L_4, L_5, S_1, S_2, S_3, and S_4). The ventral rami of L_4 divide into upper and lower branches. The upper branch joins with the lumbar plexus and the lower branch participates in the formation of sacral plexus by joining with the ventral rami of L_5 and thus forming lumbosacral trunk. So, the L_4 nerve is called the nervi furcalis. The ventral ramus of S_4 divides into upper and lower branches. The lower branches join with the ventral ramus of S_5 and form the coccygeal plexus.

Altogether, 12 branches arise from the sacral plexus. Among these, five nerves (branches) are confined to the pelvis and the remaining seven nerves (branches) supply the gluteal region and lower limb. The sciatic and pudendal nerves are the terminal branches and the rest are collateral branches.

The seven branches appearing in the gluteal region and lower limb are (1) superior gluteal nerve, (2) inferior gluteal nerve, (3) nerve to quadratus femoris, (4) nerve to obturator internus, (5) posterior femoral cutaneous nerve of thigh, (6) perforating cutaneous nerve, and (7) sciatic nerve. The five branches located in the pelvis are (1) nerve to pyriformis, (2) nerve to levator ani, (3) perineal branch of S4 nerve, (4) pelvic splanchnic nerve, and (5) pudendal nerve.

The sciatic nerve is one of the terminal branch of sacral plexus. It is the thickest nerve of our body. It is formed by the combination of two major nerve trunks (1) *tibial nerve* (ventral branches of L_4, L_5, S_1, S_2, and S_3) and (2) *common peroneal nerve* (dorsal branches of L_4, L_5, S_1, S_2, and S_3). Both the components assemble and emerge through the greater sciatic foramen below the pyriformis.

■ LUMBAR PLEXUS BLOCK

The lumbar plexus block is usually indicated for (1) knee surgery, (2) any surgery on the thigh (only anterolateral aspect), (3) saphenous vein stripping, (4) chronic pain management of lower extremity, etc. It eliminates the need for individual nerve block, such as the femoral nerve, lateral femoral cutaneous nerve of thigh and obturator nerves. By lumbar plexus block, the sciatic nerve cannot be blocked. When combined with sciatic nerve block, then this lumbar plexus block can be used for any surgery on lower extremity.

The lumbar plexus can be blocked by two approaches (1) psoas compartmental approach or block and (2) "3-in-1" approach or perivascular block.

Psoas Compartment (Block) Approach

This is also called *posterior lumbar plexus block*. In this technique, needle is placed into the space between psoas major and quadratus lumborum muscle and a large volume of LA drug is injected into this space to block the iliohypogastric, ilioinguinal, genitofemoral, femoral, obturator, and lateral femoral cutaneous nerve of thigh, causing surgical anesthesia of groin, hip, and anterolateral portion of thigh. Therefore, this block is useful for surgical procedures involving hip joint, knee joint, and anterior thigh. Complete anesthesia of knee can be attained with proximal sciatic nerve block. This technique must be combined with sciatic nerve block for the complete RA of entire lower limb. The lumbar plexus is relatively close to the multiple sensitive structures and reaching it requires a very long needle. Hence, this posterior lumbar plexus block has one of the highest complication rates, among all the peripheral nerve blocks.

Technique of Psoas Compartment Block

The patient is first placed in lateral position with the hips are flexed and the operated side is up. Then, the intercristal line (horizontal line drawn across the highest points of both the iliac crests) is identified which corresponds to the fourth lumbar spine or L_3–L_4 intervertebral space. From the fourth lumbar spine, a point which is situated 3 cm caudal and 5 cm lateral, is marked. This is the site of injection for psoas compartmental block. Then, after proper antiseptic skin preparation, a 22 G and 15 cm long needle is advanced, perpendicular to the skin, from the site of entry, till it contacts with the transverse process of the fifth lumbar vertebra.

After that, the needle is slightly withdrawn and is redirected in cephalad direction, till it slips off the transverse process of fifth lumbar vertebra. Now, it is sure that the needle is within the substance of psoas muscle. At this position, high resistance should be felt, if a glass syringe, filled with air or saline, is connected with this introducing needle and piston is pushed. Now, the needle which is already attached with the 20 mL air or saline filled syringe, is slowly advanced till the loss of resistance is detected, as like the epidural anesthesia technique. Nerve stimulator offers further confirmation of this point by motor-evoked response from the femoral (quadriceps contraction) or obturator (thigh adduction) nerve.

The needle is manipulated until the twitches of quadriceps muscle are seen or felt at 0.5 mA or less voltage. Thus, following successful identification of lumbar plexus in psoas compartment, 30–40 mL of local anesthetic agent of choice is injected with intermittent aspiration, to rule out any intravascular injection. Another technique for this posterior lumbar plexus block is like that in the midline lumbar spinous processes are palpated and first a line is drawn through these spinous processes. Next, both the iliac crests are identified and are connected by a line which approximates the level of L_4. Posterior superior iliac spine is then palpated and a line is drawn which is parallel to the first-line. Now, the point of intersection between the transverse (intercristal) line and the intersection of the lateral and middle thirds of the two sagittal lines is the point of needle entry. If available, the ultrasound imaging of transverse process may be helpful to estimate the lumbar plexus depth.

The *complications* of psoas compartment block are (1) increased risk of possible epidural block, (2) subarachnoid block (the dural sleeve over the nerve root containing subarachnoid space is no >2–4 cm from the site of injection), (3) intravascular injection; (4) peripheral nerve damage, (5) block secondary to extravasation of local anesthetic agent, (6) retroperitoneal hematoma, (7) renal capsular puncture with subsequent hematoma, etc. Though unilateral sympathetic block has a little significance, still one of the advantage of psoas compartment block, over the spinal or epidermal anesthesia, is that the incidence of hypotension is less, if this occurs. The proximity of pelvis and pelvic viscera to this psoas compartment makes the infection a potential issue of this type of block especially, if the needle makes undetected contact with the lumen of these viscera.

This psoas compartment block requires adequate sedation and analgesia, as these are very deep invasive procedure and the needle traverses the multiple muscular planes. The success rate of this block is dependent on the volume of an LA agent. A volume of <30 mL, in an adult patient of 70 kg weight, are less reliable in achieving anesthesia of the entire lumbar plexus. When surgery requires the use of tourniquet or anesthesia is required on the posterior aspect of leg, then the sciatic nerve block must accompany the psoas compartment block. This can easily be achieved in the same patient with the same position as psoas compartment block.

Perivascular Approach (3-in-1 Femoral Block)

The femoral nerve innervates the main hip flexors and knee extensors and provides much of the sensory innervation of hip and thigh. Its most medial branch is the saphenous nerve. It innervates much of the skin of the medial side of leg and ankle joint. The term "3-in-1 block" refers to anesthetizing the femoral, lateral femoral cutaneous, and obturator nerve by a single injection, below the inguinal ligament. Now, this term has largely been abandoned, because evidence accumulated demonstrating the failure of most single injections to consistently affect all three nerves. A femoral nerve block alone will seldom provide adequate surgical anesthesia, but it is often used to provide postoperative analgesia for hip, thigh, knee, and ankle (via saphenous nerve) procedures.

Technique of 3-in-1 Femoral Block

This technique is the modification of the classic approach of a single femoral nerve block in femoral triangle. The idea of this modified technique of femoral nerve block is that femoral sheath, surrounding the nerve roots while arising from the lumbar plexus, extends downward as femoral sheath in the femoral triangle **(Fig. 29)**. So, it acts as an enclosed conduit around the femoral nerve, artery, and vein for the spread of local anesthetic agent proximally, if it (LA agent) is injected within this femoral sheath, below the inguinal ligament at the femoral triangle, maintaining a distal pressure. Thus, it results in proximal spread of an LA solution into the psoas compartment from femoral triangle.

The femoral sheath is confluent, all the way proximally up to the origin of their nerves, from the lumbar plexus in the prevertebral area of lumbosacral region. At the same proximal location, the lateral femoral cutaneous nerve and the obturator nerves are also formed and are situated within this sheath. So, if local anesthetic drugs track proximally, it will also bathe these three nerves at their origin; resulting in "3-in-1" blocks (femoral nerve, lateral femoral cutaneous nerve, and obturator nerves).

The modification of this technique which converts the only femoral nerve block into the "3-in-1" block, mainly

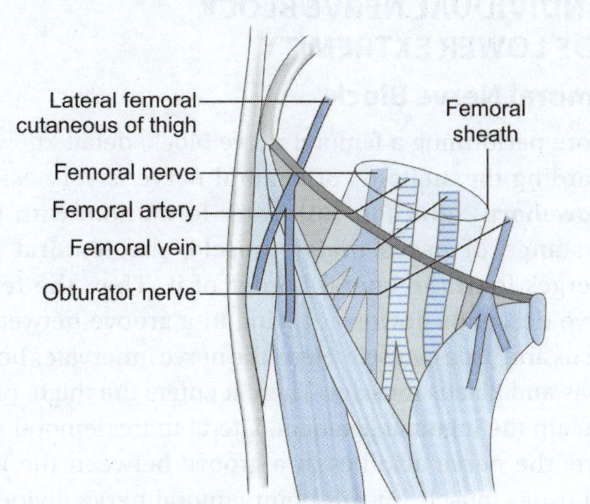

Fig. 29: The site of femoral nerve block.

involves the pressure, applied distal to the injection site in the femoral triangle and the increased volume of local anesthetic agent (20 vs. 40 mL). This method also requires selecting the site of injection, as close to the inguinal ligament as possible. The sheath covering the femoral nerve, artery, and vein becomes incomplete distally at a variable distance, just below the inguinal ligament. So, beyond this point, any attempt to fill the sheath and try to induce proximal spread of an LA agent will be unsuccessful. The placement of pressure, distal to the injection site in femoral triangle, must be as complete as possible, but without disrupting the placement of needle within femoral sheath. The confirmation of needle placement within the femoral sheath is not different from that of the classical approach of individual femoral nerve block.

A continuous "3-in-1" femoral block can also be accomplished with insertion of a catheter within the femoral sheath at femoral triangle. If the femoral sheath is catheterized correctly and the catheter is advanced for up to 5–8 cm proximally, then the injected LA solution will be very close to the lumbosacral plexus and the complete block of all the nerves of the plexus becomes a high probability.

The inguinal ligament is marked as a line, connecting the pubic tubercle and the anterior superior iliac spine. Then, the femoral artery is marked by its pulsation just below the inguinal ligament. After that, a short beveled, 22 G and 5 cm long needle is advanced, lateral to the artery in cephalad direction, after piercing the skin, subcutaneous tissue, and femoral sheath. Then, 20–40 mL of an LA drug is injected incrementally, after the negative aspiration test while applying pressure by fingers distally on the femoral sheath. By 20 mL drug, femoral and lateral femoral cutaneous nerve blocks can be predicted. But the obturator nerve block may require a minimum 30 mL of drug.

INDIVIDUAL NERVE BLOCK OF LOWER EXTREMITY

Femoral Nerve Block

Before performing a femoral nerve block, detail knowledge regarding the anatomy of femoral nerve is very essential **(Flowchart 2 and Fig. 30)**. After formation, with in the substance of psoas major muscle, the femoral nerve emerges from the lateral border of it. Then the femoral nerve descends downward lying in a groove between the iliacus and psoas muscle. Here, the nerve innervates both the psoas and iliacus muscles. Then, it enters the thigh, passing beneath the inguinal ligament, lateral to the femoral artery. Here, the nerve also lies in a groove between the iliacus and psoas muscle. At this point femoral nerve divides into anterior and posterior divisions which then subsequently

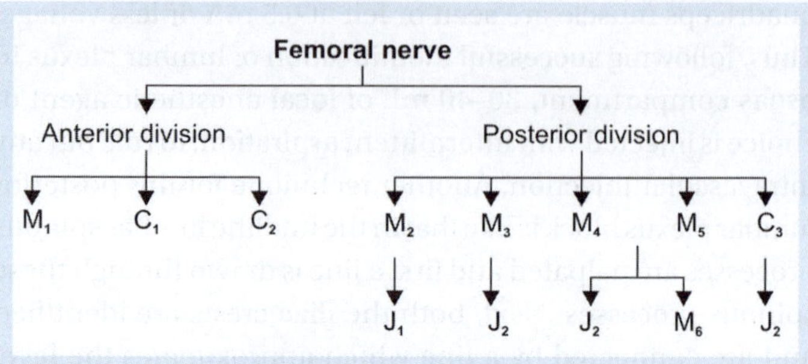

Flowchart 2: The cutaneous nerves of lower extremity.

(C_1: intermediate cutaneous nerve of thigh; C_2: medial cutaneous nerve of thigh; C_3: saphenous nerve; J_1: hip joint; J_2: knee joint; M_1: sartorius; M_2: rectus femoris; M_3: vastus lateralis; M_4: vastus intermedius; M_5: vastus medialis; M_6: articularis genu)

break into multiple branches and supply (1) the motors to the quadriceps group of muscles and sartorius muscles, (2) the sensory over the skin of anterior thigh from inguinal ligament to knee, (3) as saphenous nerve (sensory) on the medial side of the leg from knee to big toe, and (4) supplies the articular branches to the hip and knee joint. Beyond the inguinal ligament, the femoral nerve does not represent as a discreet structure, but has split into a bundle of spaghetti strands.

Practical Application of Femoral Nerve Block

The only femoral nerve is blocked for virtually some minor specific surgical procedures on the upper part of thigh and for any lower extremity procedure, where the immobility of knee joint is necessary or the use of pneumatic tourniquet is essential. Practically, the isolated femoral nerve block is primarily used in combination with other peripheral nerve block. It can be used alone for (1) small surgical procedures, limited only on the anterior thigh, for example, small muscle biopsy, skin grafting, etc.; (2) knee arthroscopy and any operation on patella; (3) surgical repair of midfemoral shaft fracture, e.g., acute pain relief, reduction, and traction placement in the setting of an acute fracture of the shaft of femur; (4) surgical procedure on the knee; and (5) postoperative pain relief for surgical procedures on the medial side of the leg.

Technique of Femoral Nerve Block

For the classical individual femoral nerve block, the important anatomical landmark is the point which is situated below the inguinal ligament and immediately lateral to the pulsation of femoral artery **(Fig. 31)**. After a proper antiseptic skin preparation, a skin wheal is created by the LA agent, just 1–2 cm lateral to the femoral pulse, at the level of femoral crease. It

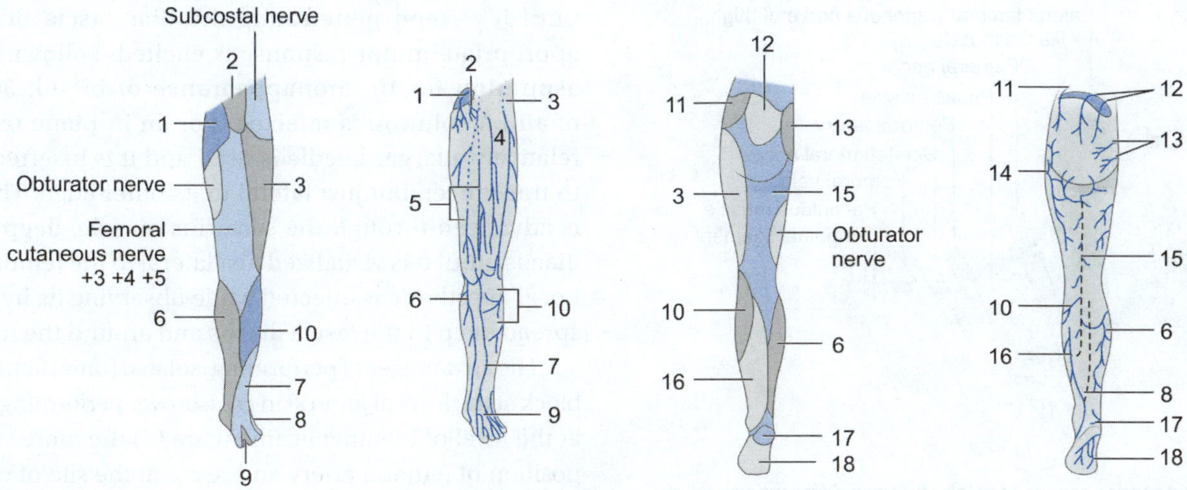

Fig. 30: Division of femoral nerve.

Notes:

1. *Ilioinguinal nerve (L_1):* It escapes through the lateral part of superficial inguinal ring. Most of its branches go to the scrotum or labia majora. Some of its branches supply the skin over the medial adjacent part of the thigh.
2. *Femoral branch of genitofemoral nerve (L_1, L_2):* It pierces the deep fascia, 2 cm below the inguinal ligament, and is slightly lateral to the saphenous opening. It supplies an area of skin, about the size of a palm of a hand, immediately below the inguinal ligament.
3. *Lateral (femoral) cutaneous nerve of thigh (L_2, L_3):* Discussed in the text.
4. *Intermediate femoral cutaneous nerve (L_2, L_3):* It is a branch of femoral nerve. It pierces the deep fascia in the midline of thigh. It extends up to the knee.
5. *Medial femoral cutaneous nerve (L_2, L_3):* It is also a branch of femoral nerve. It pierces the deep fascia on the medial side of the thigh. Then, it divides into two branches (1) anterior and (2) posterior branch. Both extend up to the knee.
6. *Saphenous nerve (L_3, L_4):* Discussed in the text.
7. *Superficial peroneal nerve (L_4, L_5, and S_1):* Discussed in the text.
8. *Sural nerve:* It supplies the lateral part of the dorsum of the foot.
9. *Deep peroneal nerve:* It supplies the adjacent sides of first and second toes.
10. *Lateral cutaneous nerve of calf:* It arises from the common peroneal nerve on the lateral head of gastrocnemius. It pierces the deep fascia almost at once and descends to supply the skin over the lateral and anterior surface of upper part of leg.
11. *Lateral cutaneous branch of subcostal and iliohypogastric nerve:* They supply the upper and lateral gluteal region of thigh.
12. *Lumbar nerves:* They are the branches of dorsal rami (not ventral rami which take part in the formation of lumbar plexus) of L_1, L_2, and L_3 lumbar spinal nerves and supply the upper medial region of thigh.
13. *Sacral nerves:* They are the branches of dorsal (posterior) rami of S1, S2, S3 sacral spinal nerves and supply the upper medial region of thigh.
14. *Lateral (femoral) cutaneous nerve of thigh (it is the same nerve numbered in figure as 3):* It supplies the lower lateral region of the thigh.
15. *Posterior cutaneous nerve of thigh (S1, S2, and S3):* It arises from sacral plexus. It comes out of pelvis through the greater sciatic foramen, under coverage of gluteus maximus muscle. Then, it lies on the medial border of sciatic nerve and leaves the gluteal region and enters the back of thigh. After that, it runs downward under the deep fascia. It pierces the deep fascia at the back of knee. The terminal branches descend downward up to halfway of the back of leg. It supplies gluteal region, peroneal region, back of the thigh, and upper part of the back of the leg.
16. *Peroneal (sural) communicating branch:* It arises from the common peroneal nerve in the popliteal fossa together with lateral cutaneous nerve of calf and pierces the deep fascia. Then, it passes downward to join with sural nerve. It supplies skin over proximal two-thirds of the back of the leg with sural nerve.
17. *Medial calcaneal branch:* It arises from the tibial nerve at the ankle. It pierces the flexor retinaculum. It supplies the skin of the posterior and lateral surfaces of the heel.
18. *Medial and lateral plantar nerves:* They are the terminal branches of posterior tibial nerve. They supply the whole sole and planter surface of digits.

is also to be noted that the femoral crease is located 2–4 cm below the inguinal ligament. For a "single shot femoral block," a short (<1 inch) blunt bevel needle is usually used and it will allow good appreciation of needle's entry into the femoral sheath. The needle is first inserted lateral to the femoral artery and is then further moved parallel to the artery in a cephalad and posterior direction, within the sheath at an angle of 45° to skin. The proximity of the needle to the femoral nerve can be confirmed by the feeling of the entry of needle into the femoral sheath. An alternative to this technique is the field block by injection of an LA agent at multiple sites.

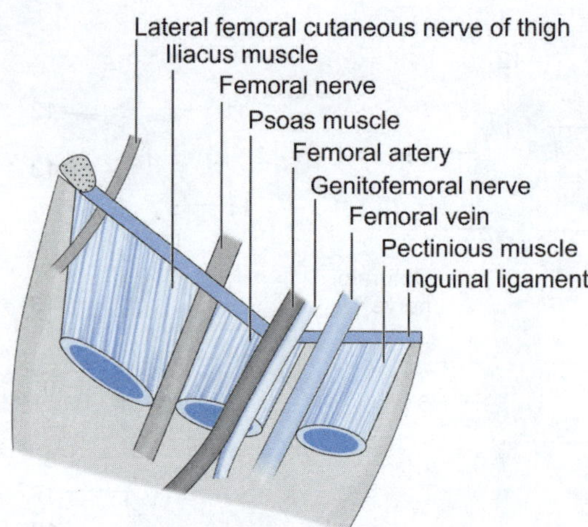

Fig. 31: Anterior aspect of thigh showing different site for the injection of different nerve blocks.

The confirmation of the proximity of nerve to the needle is also done by the elicitation of paresthesia or by the use of nerve stimulator, by eliciting the motor-evoked response (twitch) in the quadriceps group of muscles (look for the motion of patella). The ultimate goal of this nerve stimulation is to obtain twitches in quadriceps muscle or patella at the minimal voltage of 0.5 mA or less. The success with nerve stimulator technique requires differentiation between the evoked-motor response and the direct stimulation of the muscles by current, due to the immediate vicinity of the tip of the needle to muscle, from where the current is discharged directly to the muscle.

When the sartorius twitches are obtained first, as the motor-evoked response, then the needle should be redirected which subsequently and promptly results in the stimulation of quadriceps muscle. The injection of local anesthetic agent, only after the stimulation of sartorius muscle, may result in failure to achieve femoral block. For isolated (or only) femoral nerve block, 10–20 mL of local anesthetic drug within the femoral sheath at the femoral triangle will accomplish the complete block, whereas a larger volume of an LA agent with some modification of technique will result in "3-in-1" block **(Fig. 31)**.

For femoral nerve block by *ultrasound technique*, a high-frequency linear ultrasound transducer is placed over the area of inguinal crease and parallel to crease itself. On screen the femoral artery and the femoral vein will be visualized in cross section, with overlying iliac fossa. Just lateral to artery and deep to iliac fascia, on screen the femoral nerve appears as a spindle-shaped structure with a "honey comb" texture. For an out-of-plane technique, the block needle is inserted just lateral to the femoral nerve and is directed in cephalic direction at an angle approximately 45° to the skin. The needle is advanced

until it is seen penetrating the iliac fascia or until an appropriate motor response is elicited. Following careful aspiration for the nonappearance of blood, 30–40 mL of an LA solution is injected. For an in-plane technique, relatively a larger needle is used and it is inserted parallel to transducer, but just lateral to its outer edge. The needle is advanced through the sartorius muscle, deep to fascia iliacus, until it is visualized just lateral to the femoral nerve. Local anesthetic is injected while observing its hypoechoic spread deep to the fascia iliacus and around the nerve.

The advantages of performing isolated (only) femoral nerve block at the level of groin skin crease, over performing the block at the level of inguinal ligament are (1) the more superficial position of femoral artery and nerve at the site of crease, (2) the greater width of femoral nerve at the site of crease, (3) the more consistent femoral nerve–artery relationship at the site of crease, and (4) the more consistent results of block at this site. The isolated femoral nerve block is a superficial one and does not result in significant patient discomfort. Thus, light premedication is usually sufficient.

Because of the proximity of femoral artery and vein, the most likely complication of attempted femoral nerve block would be hematoma due to the puncture of vessels. In this procedure, the intravascular injection of an LA agent is also very likely. Intraneural injection is also possible, but unlikely because of the extensive branching of femoral nerve at the site of attempted block. Poor site preparation or poor care of continuous catheter (if it is used) would make the infection of the injection site common and it is also due to its proximity of injection site to groin.

The femoral nerve is fully enclosed in a sheath which is extended downward up to or just below inguinal ligament. This is an ideal site for the placement of catheter within the sheath for continuous femoral blockade. The most common technical approach to this catheter procedure is the Seldinger technique. In this method, a smaller pliable, nontraumatic catheter is inserted through a larger, nonpermanent catheter. The proper intrasheath placement of catheter is most commonly confirmed by motor-evoked response using a nerve stimulator. However, the ideal confirmation of the placement of catheter is accomplished with the injection of an LA agent through catheter, while the stimulation is still performed and augmentation, followed by the extinction of muscular contraction, is observed.

The continuous femoral nerve block by catheter has a unique place for long-term postoperative pain relief after surgery over the anterior aspect of thigh. Low concentration local anesthetics can provide pain relief without motor block. Bupivacaine of 0.125% concentration is ideally suited for only pain relief with minimal resultant toxicity or motor block. Due to the close proximity to the groin, the site of the insertion of needle and catheter for femoral nerve block mandates sterile procedure and proper dressing to avoid infection. Like other catheter technique, nerve trauma and catheter breakage are also potential complications here.

Lateral (Femoral) Cutaneous Nerve Block

The lateral (femoral) cutaneous nerve of thigh (L_2 and L_3) is a pure sensory nerve and originates from the dorsal branches of the ventral rami of second and third lumbar spinal nerves. It provides only sensory innervation to the lateral side of thigh, above the knee. After its origin, it moves ventrally and laterally through the psoas compartment, between the psoas and iliacus muscles, immediately caudal to the ilioinguinal nerve. Then, after emerging from the lateral border of psoas muscle, it descends over the iliacus muscle, but under its (iliac) fascia. Then, it enters the thigh deep to the inguinal ligament, 1–2 cm medial to the anterior superior iliac spine. Distal to the inguinal ligament, the nerve divides into anterior and posterior branches in thigh. The anterior branch becomes superficial after piercing the deep fascia, about 10 cm distal to the anterior superior iliac spine and supplies the skin over the anterior and lateral side of thigh, as far as up to the knee. The posterior branch pierces the fascia lata at a higher position than the anterior branch and directly supply the skin over the lateral surface of the thigh, extending from greater trochanter to about half of the thigh. This nerve has no motor supply. So, the stimulation of this nerve by a stimulator does not produce any motor-evoked response and is not helpful **(Fig. 32)**.

The site of injection, for the block of this nerve, is 2 cm medial and 2 cm caudal to the anterior superior iliac spine. After proper antiseptic skin preparation, for the block of this nerve, a 22 G and 4 cm long needle is inserted perpendicularly through the skin, until a sudden loss of resistance is felt, which indicates the passage of needle through the fascia lata. Then, the needle is gently advanced, just slightly beyond this resistance, and a volume of 10–15 mL of an LA solution is injected fanwise below and above the fascia. This procedure is again repeated for the second time, with a slightly different direction of the needle. Multiple injection sites make this field block technique successful. This lateral femoral cutaneous nerve block is indicated only for some superficial minor surgical procedures which require only sensory, but no motor block of the lateral side of the thigh, for example, a small simple muscle biopsy from vastus lateralis, skin graft harvesting from the upper part of the lateral thigh, meralgia paresthetica (it means sensation of pricking, tingling, numbness, and burning pain, etc. on the outer part of thigh that has no objective cause), etc.

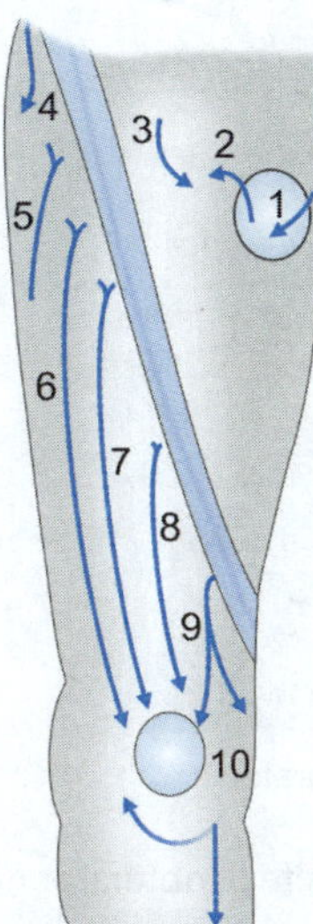

Fig. 32: Lateral (femoral) cutaneous nerve of thigh.

Notes:
1. Femoral branch of genitofemoral nerve
2. Branch of ilioinguinal nerve
3. Branch of medial femoral cutaneous nerve
4. Branch of subcostal nerve
5. Posterior division of lateral cutaneous nerve of thigh (not the branch of femoral nerve)
6. Anterior division of lateral cutaneous nerve of thigh (not the branch of femoral nerve)
7. Lateral division of intermediate femoral cutaneous nerve (branch of femoral nerve)
8. Medial division of intermediate femoral cutaneous nerve (branch of femoral nerve)
9. Anterior and posterior divisions of the medial femoral cutaneous nerve (branch of femoral nerve)
10. Saphenous nerve (branch of femoral nerve).

Obturator Nerve Block

The obturator and genitofemoral nerves are rather the large branches of lumbar plexus. They provide (1) *sensory* innervation over the inguinal area, the area over the femoral triangle, the medial part of the thigh, knee joint, hip joint and (2) *motor fibers* to the adductors of thigh such as the adductor longus, adductor brevis, adductor magnus, obturator internus, and obturator externus. This relatively large area of sensory and motor coverage, by this nerve, has proved the potentiality or the wide applications of block of only this nerve in surgical anesthesia, postoperative analgesia, and chronic pain management over these areas.

Anatomy of Obturator Nerve

The obturator nerve arises from the ventral division of the anterior (ventral) rami of L_2, L_3, and L_4 lumbar spinal nerves. It descends first through the substances of psoas

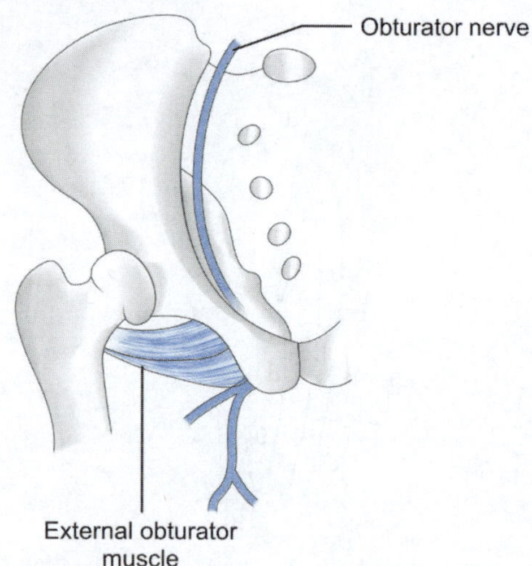

Fig. 33: The site of obturator nerve block.

major muscle up to the sacroiliac joint, where it pierces out the medial border of this muscle (psoas major) and passes down behind the bifurcation of the common iliac vessel. It then descends over the fascia, covering obturator internus muscle and subsequently runs directly on the periosteum of the ischium bone. Then, it descents through the pelvis along with its lateral wall and in close proximity to the inferolateral wall of the bladder, bladder neck, and the lateral wall of the prostatic (membranous) part of the urethra. Here, it accompanies with obturator artery and vein. Finally, it reaches the obturator canal through the obturator foramen and exits into the thigh from the pelvis, after dividing into anterior and posterior divisions **(Fig. 33)**.

The *anterior branch* of obturator nerve provides (1) sensory supply to the skin over the inner part of thigh, hip joint, (2) a branch to the subsartorial plexus, and (3) several motor branches to the adductors of thigh (pectineus, adductor longus, and adductor brevis). The *posterior branch* of the obturator nerve supplies motor to the posterior group of adductors of thigh (adductor brevis, adductor magnus, and obturator externus) and an articular branch (sensory) to the knee.

Clinical Application of Obturator Nerve Block

The obturator nerve can most easily be blocked, along with other nerves, by using the same approach, for the block of lumbosacral plexus, but it can also separately (individually) be blocked for the following simple procedures such as:

- For some superficial surgical procedures over the medial part of the thigh
- To relief the spasm of the adductors of hip which causes the relaxation of midthigh
- To relieve the intractable pain of hip joint due to osteoarthritis

- As a diagnostic aid for the pain syndromes in hip joint, inguinal area, or lumbar spine
- For muscle biopsy and tendon transfer or release from midthigh
- Any lower extremity procedure requiring the prolonged use of a pneumatic tourniquet
- A block of adductor nerve is usually required for complete anesthesia of knee and is most often performed in combination with femoral and sciatic nerve blocks for this purpose.

The individual or the only block of obturator nerve is very difficult for any anesthesiologist and is also very uncomfortable for patients, even under ideal conditions. Usually, the obturator nerve block is combined with other nerve block in following conditions such as (1) the superficial surgery of thigh (combined with femoral and lateral femoral cutaneous block) and (2) knee surgery (combined with femoral, lateral femoral cutaneous and/or sciatic nerve block).

Technique of Obturator Nerve Block

The patient is placed in the supine position and the anesthesiologist should stand at that patient's side which is to be blocked. The patient's leg should be flexed at the knee joint and should be slightly abducted, to make the tendon of adductor longus prominent, close to its attachment to the pubic bone, i.e., pubic tubercle. The site of injection or the needle's entry point through the skin for this obturator nerve block is demarcated as the point which is situated 2 cm lateral and 2 cm caudal to the pubic tubercle. At this point, the needle will enter medial to the femoral artery and above the tendon of adductor longus, but midway between the pubic tubercle and femoral artery and 2–3 cm below the inguinal ligament.

To avoid patient discomfort, a skin wheal should be created which is followed by injection of an LA agent at deeper level. Once the tissues have been prepared, one long (10 cm) needle, used for this block, is first directed from the skin surface toward the inferior pubic ramus, until a contact is made by the needle with the bone. When the contact with bone is made, then the needle should be "walked off" the inferior ramus of pubis in a dorsal and distal direction, until it begins to slip into the obturator canal. Then, the proximity of needle tip to the obturator nerve can be confirmed by three ways (1) creating field block with relatively more volume of drug and repositioning the needle, (2) eliciting paresthesia on the medial part of the thigh, and (3) using a nerve stimulator to elicit the movement of the adductor group of muscles (adduction of thigh). Any of these strategies requires 10–20 mL of drug.

The complications of obturator nerve block are same as that of other nerve block such as nerve damage, intravascular injection, hematoma, and sepsis. The most common complication of attempting this obturator nerve block is the excessive patient discomfort. The failure rate for successful block of this obturator nerve is also high and this is because of the location of it. Higher infection rate may also be a concern with this nerve block than with others.

Sciatic Nerve Block

Combined with other nerves, the sciatic nerve block is also required (1) for most of the surgeries over lower extremity and (2) for all the surgical procedures, requiring the application of pneumatic tourniquet on lower extremity. The nerve can be *blocked at the level of hip* both from the anterior and posterior approach and this is known as the *sciatic block*. The terminal branches of sciatic nerve also can be *blocked individually at the level of knee* and below of it (knee). At the level of knee, the block of both the component of sciatic nerve is called the *popliteal block*. The individual peripheral branches of sciatic nerve also can be approached, such as the *common peroneal nerve* near fibular head and the other branches at the level of the ankle as a component of ankle block.

Anatomy of Sciatic Nerve

The sciatic nerve is the thickest and the largest nerve in our body, with root value of L_4, L_5, S_1, S_2, and S_3. Its width is 2 cm. It leaves the pelvis with posterior femoral cutaneous nerve of thigh (a branch of sacral plexus), through greater sciatic foramen, below the muscle named pyriformis, but within the sciatic notch. Then, it descends between the greater trochanter of femur on the lateral side and ischial tuberosity on the medial side and passes gradually distally under the covering of gluteal muscles in sciatic groove, running just over the lesser trochanter of femur. Then, it becomes superficial at the lower border of gluteus maximus muscle and descends further downward along the posterior aspect of the thigh, lying on adductor magnus muscle up to the popliteal fossa. At the popliteal fossa, the common trunk of sciatic nerve splits into two distinct entities such as the *tibial nerve* and *common peroneal nerve*, although they run together within a fibrous sheath, until just above the knee. The branches of sciatic nerve are depicted in **Flowchart 3**.

The sciatic nerve block provides (1) motor paralysis to the hamstring group of muscles, (2) sensory anesthesia (loss) over the posterior aspect of the thigh, and (3) the sensory loss over the entire leg below the knee, except a medial strip of skin which is innervated by saphenous nerve, a branch of femoral nerve. Since the branches of sciatic nerve to the hamstring group of muscles depart the sciatic

Flowchart 3: Branches of sciatic nerve.

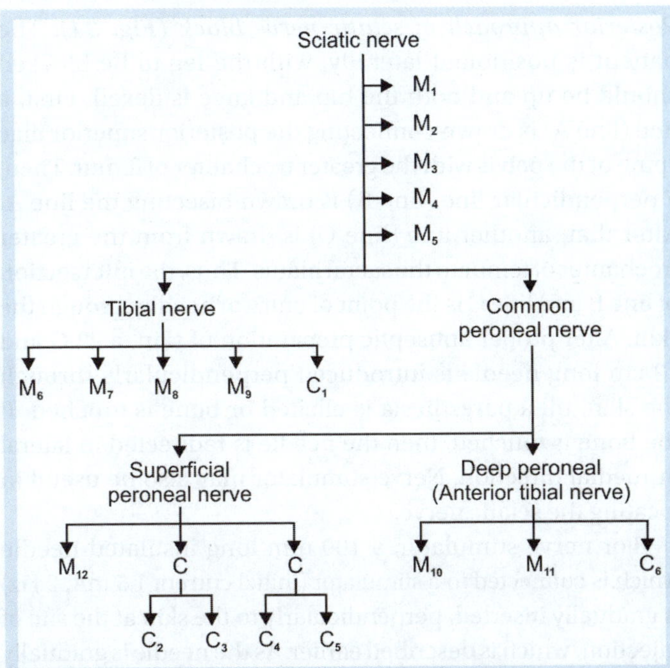

(C_1: sural nerve; C_2: adjacent sides of third and fourth toes; C_3: adjacent sides of fourth and fifth toes; C_4: medial side of great toe; C_5: adjacent sides of second and third toes; C_6: adjacent sides of great toe and second toe; M_1: semimembranosus; M_2: ischial fibers of adductor magnus; M_3: semitendinosus; M_4: long head of biceps femoris; M_5: short head of biceps femoris; M_6: both heads of gastrocnemius; M_7: plantaris; M_8: soleus; M_9: popliteus; M_{10}: tibialis anterior; M_{11}: extensor digitorum longus and brevis, extensor hallucis longus, first and second interossei; M_{12}: peroneus longus and brevis)

nerve significantly below the level of blockade, therefore the twitches of these hamstring groups of muscles can be accepted as a sign of reliable localization of sciatic nerve by nerve stimulator.

Clinical Application of Sciatic Nerve Block

The sciatic nerve block, together with the femoral or saphenous nerve block, can be used for any surgical procedure below the knee that does not require tourniquet. Tourniquet cannot be applied in this type of combination of block, because the sensory supply of thigh remains intact. However, this type of combination of the peripheral nerve block avoids sympathectomy and its complications, which are commonly found as the consequences of central neuraxial block. So, this type of combination of sciatic, femoral, and saphenous nerve block can be taken as an alternative to the central neuraxial block for the surgical procedures below the knee. Therefore, its use may be advantageous in cases in which any shift in hemodynamics may be deleterious, such as a patient with significant aortic stenosis. The sciatic nerve can be blocked by two approaches; *posterior approach, anterior approach, and subgluteal approach.*

Technique of Sciatic Nerve Block

*Posterior approach of sciatic nerve block **(Fig. 34)**:* The patient is positioned laterally, with the leg to be blocked should be up and both the hip and knee is flexed. First, a line (line A) is drawn connecting the posterior superior iliac spine of the pelvis with the greater trochanter of femur. Then, a perpendicular line (line B) is drawn bisecting the line A. After that, another line (line C) is drawn from the greater trochanter of femur to the sacral hiatus. Thus, the intersection of line B and line C is the point of entry of needle through the skin. After proper antiseptic preparation of skin, a 22 G and 12 cm long needle is introduced perpendicularly through the skin, till a paresthesia is elicited or bone is touched. If the bone is touched, then the needle is redirected in lateral or medial direction. Nerve stimulator may also be useful in locating the sciatic nerve.

For nerve stimulator, a 100 mm long insulated needle which is connected to a stimulator (initial current 1.5 mA, 2 Hz) is gradually inserted, perpendicularly to the skin at the site of injection, which is described earlier. As the needle is gradually advanced to the deeper plane, then a twitch of gluteus muscles is observed first. This is due to the direct stimulation of muscle by current. Once the twitching of gluteus muscle disappears with the further needle advancement, then the stimulation of sciatic nerve is obtained. The stimulation of sciatic nerve is recognized by the contraction of the hamstring group of muscles, supplied by the tibial component of sciatic nerve. Typically, the twitching of the hamstring group of muscles is observed first. Then, with the minimal further advancement of needle, the twitches of foot are also readily observed. When this maneuver fails to localize the sciatic nerve, the needle is withdrawn up to the skin and is again redirected. The sciatic nerve is typically located at the depth of 5–8 cm from skin in an average size adult patient. Once, the stimulation of foot is obtained by 0.2–0.4 mA or less amount of current, then it is thought that the needle is in correct position and 20–30 mL of an LA agent is injected. The sciatic nerve block is of very deep in nature. So, adequate analgesia and sedation is necessary during this procedure to ensure the patient's satisfaction and comfort.

*Anterior approach of sciatic nerve block **(Fig. 35)**:* This approach is applicable when the patient cannot be positioned laterally, due to the pain or lack of cooperation. The another advantage of this anterior approach for sciatic nerve block is that this approach is very convenient and also allows the performance of femoral nerve block in same position which subsequently shortens the time required to complete the block of both these nerves. With patient in supine position, a line (line A) is drawn over the inguinal ligament from the anterior superior iliac spine to the public tubercle of pelvis.

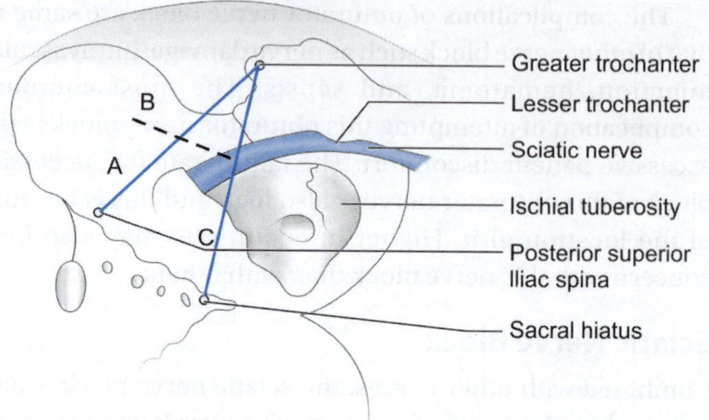

Fig. 34: Sciatic nerve block. Posterior approach.

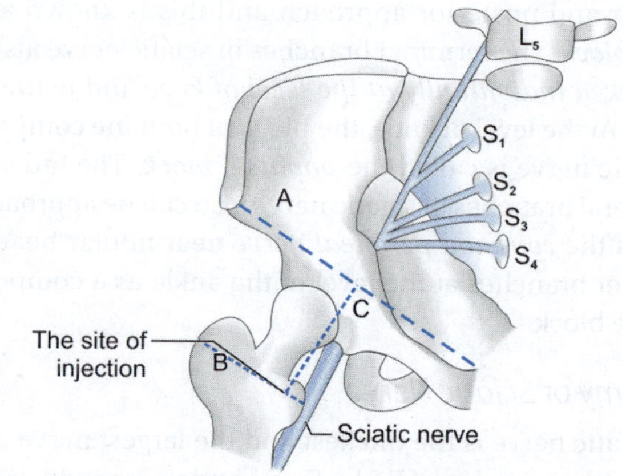

Fig. 35: Sciatic nerve block, anterior approach.

Then, a second-line (line B) is drawn parallel to the previous line, beginning at the tuberosity of greater trochanter. After that, a third-line (line C) is drawn which is perpendicular to line A, and at the juncture of its lateral two-thirds and medial one-third. Then, the intersection of line B and line C is the point of the entry of needle through the skin for the block of sciatic nerve by anterior approach. After proper antiseptic skin preparation, a 22 G and 12 cm long needle is advanced gradually, perpendicular to the skin, till it contacts with the bone which is lesser trochanter. Needle is then redirected medially passing the femur and paresthesia is sought. At that position, 20 mL of an LA drug is injected incrementally, after a negative aspiration test.

If the nerve stimulator is used, then the proper position of the needle is recognized by the stimulation of sciatic nerve which results in rhythmic movements of the foot (simultaneous plantar or dorsiflexion).

- *Ultrasound technique:* The patient is positioned supine and the leg is rotated externally. A low frequency curvilinear transducer is placed transversely over the midthigh at the level of lesser trochanter. On screen, the structures such as femur, femoral vessels, adductor muscles, and gluteus maximus are identified. Posterior to femur and between these adductor and gluteus muscles, sciatic nerve as an elliptical hyperechoic structure is also identified. Using a long needle, now the sciatic nerve is approached from anterior to posterior (in the plane) or cephalad to caudal (out of the plane), taking care not to touch the femoral vessels. When the needle tip reaches very nearer to the sciatic nerve, then the solution of an LA agent is injected.

Subgluteal approach of sciatic nerve block: At subgluteal region the landmarks are often more easily identified and less tissues are traversed. Hence, the sciatic nerve block through the subgluteal approach is another useful alternative to the conventional posterior approach for sciatic nerve block. At subgluteal region, the sciatic nerve is more superficially located. So, the exclusive use of ultrasound in this approach of sciatic nerve block is more practical as well.

- *Nerve stimulation technique:* The patient is kept in Sim's position and the greater trochanter and ischial tuberosity are identified first. Now, a line is drawn between them. Next, from the midpoint of this first-line a second-line is drawn, perpendicular to it (first-line) and it is extended caudally for 4–5 cm. Now, the end of this second-line is the needle entry point and a long insulated needle is introduced and is progressed slightly cephalad, until the plantar flexion or the inversion of foot is elicited. Now, 25 mL of an LA solution is injected at that position of the needle tip.
- *Ultrasound technique:* Like above, patient is kept in Sim's position and the greater trochanter and ischial tuberosity are identified first. Now, a linear high frequency or curvilinear low frequency ultrasound transducer is placed over the midpoint, between these ischial tuberosity and greater trochanter in a transverse orientation. Now, on screen, both these bony structures along with the gluteal muscles, with their fascial layer, defining their deep border, will be seen. The sciatic nerve, as an elliptical hyperechoic structure will be visible in cross section, just deep to this layer, in a location approximately midway between the ischial tuberosity and greater trochanter, but superficial to the quadratus femoris muscle.

For an *"out of plane"* technique, the insulated needle is introduced just caudal to the transducer and is advanced in an anterior with slight cephalad direction. Once the needle passes through the gluteus muscles and its tip reaches next to the sciatic nerve, LA solution is injected, after the careful aspiration for the nonappearance of blood. The spread of LA solution around the sciatic nerve will also be visualized on screen. For an *"in plane"* technique, the insulated needle is introduced lateral to the ultrasound transducer. It is advanced through the field of ultrasound beam, until the tip is visible deep to the gluteus maximus and next to the sciatic nerve. Now, in such position of needle tip, LA solution is injected and its spread around the sciatic nerve will also be visible on the screen.

■ NERVE BLOCK AROUND KNEE

Just as the terminal branches of the brachial plexus can be blocked distally around the elbow and wrist joint, similarly the individual terminal branches of the nerves of lower extremity, arising from the lumbosacral plexus, can be blocked around the knee, ankle, and foot depending on the objectivity.

Popliteal Block

By this technique, the components of sciatic nerve such as the tibial and common peroneal nerve can be blocked together in the popliteal fossa behind the knee. In this block, as the hamstring muscles are spared, so it (popliteal block) allows the lifting of foot with the flexion of knee and thus it facilitates the ambulation. As the sciatic nerve block fails to provide complete sensory anesthesia for the cutaneous innervation of the medial side of the leg and the ankle joint capsule (which is supplied by saphenous nerve), so with the saphenous nerve block, this popliteal block of sciatic nerve (tibial and common peroneal nerve) can also be used for any surgery at any site on the leg, ankle and foot (complete anesthesia, both motor and sensory, below the knee). The popliteal fossa is formed *above* by the tendon of semitendinosus and semimembranosus muscles *medially* and by the tendon of biceps muscle *laterally* and *below* by the two heads of the gastrocnemius muscle *medially* and *laterally* (**Fig. 36**).

Within the popliteal fossa, from medial to lateral; the popliteal vein, popliteal artery, and sciatic nerve are situated. Proximal to the flexion crease of knee, the terminal branches of sciatic nerve, i.e., the tibial and common personal nerves are bundled together by some fibrous sheath and this is the site for the injection of an LA agent for popliteal block. This posterior approach of popliteal block is performed with the patient in prone position and the leg is fully extended. About 2 cm, proximal to the flexion crease of knee, the pulsation of popliteal artery is identified first. Then, the site, 1 cm lateral to this pulsation, is the needle entry point for popliteal block. After proper antiseptic skin preparation, a 22 G but 4 cm long blunt beveled needle is inserted, perpendicular to the skin first. Then, it is advanced till the paresthesia or motor-evoked response (if nerve stimulator is used) is elicited which

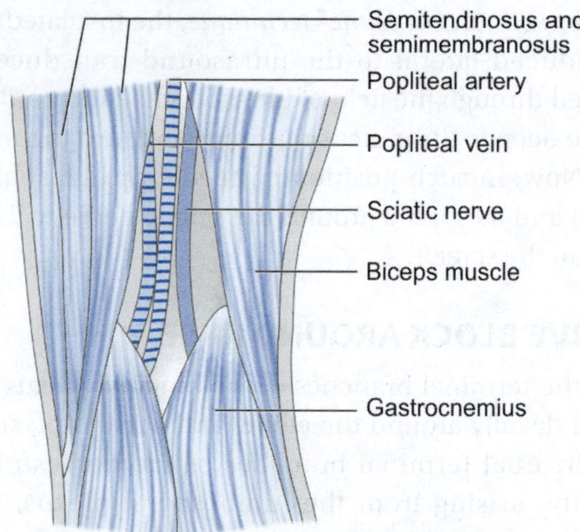

Fig. 36: The popliteal block (right leg).

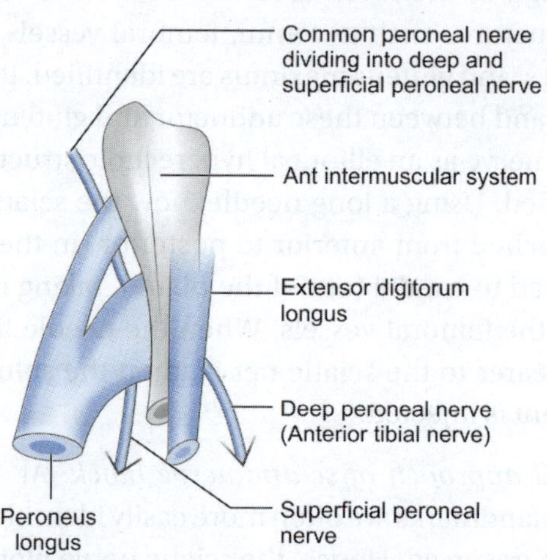

Fig. 37: Block at the level of fibular head.

is plantar flexion or dorsiflexion of foot. Then, 10–20 mL of LA drug is deposited.

Ultrasound Technique

For popliteal block (block of sciatic nerve in popliteal fossa) the patient is positioned prone and the apex of popliteal fossa is identified first. Then, a high-frequency linear ultrasound transducer is placed in transverse orientation over the apex of popliteal fossa and on the screen the femur, biceps femoris tendon, sciatic nerve, and popliteal vessels are identified in cross section. In this position, the nerve is usually situated posterior and lateral (or immediately posterior) to the vessels and is often located in close relationship to the tendon of biceps femoris, just at its medial edge. For an "out of plane" technique, the needle is introduced just caudal to the transducer and is directed anteriorly and slightly cephalad. When the needle is in close contact with the sciatic nerve, then after negative aspiration for blood, LA solution is injected and its spread is observed on screen. For an "in plane" technique, the needle is introduced lateral to the ultrasound transducer and is advanced traversing or just anterior to the biceps femoris muscle. This whole process is observed on screen and when the needle tip comes in close contact with the nerve, then LA solution is injected.

Tibial Nerve Block

It is one of the two terminal divisions of sciatic nerve (another division of sciatic nerve is common peroneal nerve) and comes out of it (sciatic nerve) at the level of the junction of upper two-thirds and lower one-third on the back of the thigh. But they (these two terminal divisions of sciatic nerve) lie side by side in a common fibrous sheath. After that, it descends through the upper part of popliteal fossa, along the lateral side of the popliteal vein. Then, at the middle of the popliteal fossa, it crosses superficial to the popliteal vein and artery at the back of the knee and descends on the fascia, covering the popliteus muscle. Now, at the lower part of the popliteal fossa, this tibial nerve lies medial to the popliteal vein and artery. It, then, now continues downward finally as the posterior tibial nerve (PTN) from the lower border of the popliteus muscle on the back of the leg, with posterior tibial artery within the posterior compartment of the leg.

At ankle, it reaches the midpoint between the medial malleolus and calcaneus, under the flexor retinaculum and divides into the lateral and medial plantar nerves. The posterior tibial nerve (the continuation of tibial nerve into leg) innervates all the muscles of the posterior compartment of leg and supplies the sensory to ankle and skin over the heel. The medial and the lateral plantar nerves which are the terminal branches of posterior tibial nerve innervate all the intrinsic muscles of sole and supply the sensory to the entire sole and many of the tarsal and metatarsal joints.

Common Peroneal Nerve Block

It is one of the two terminal divisions of sciatic nerve. It runs downward and laterally through the upper part of popliteal fossa, along the medial margin of biceps femoris muscle. It then comes in direct contact with the lateral surface of the neck of the fibula, between the two heads of the origin of peroneus longus muscle. Here, it divides into *superficial peroneal* (or *musculocutaneous*) and *deep peroneal* (or *anterior tibial*) nerves **(Fig. 37)**.

The superficial peroneal nerve is the nerve of the lateral (peroneal) compartment of leg. It supplies the peroneus group of muscles and the skin over the lower part of the leg. After supplying the peroneal group of muscles, it pierces the deep fascia at the junction of the medial and lateral third of the lateral surface of the leg and becomes a superficial

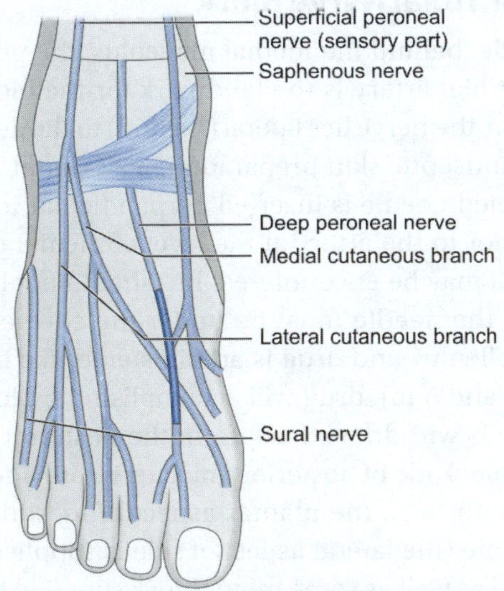

Fig. 38: Ankle block.

sensory nerve. Then, it passes to the front of the leg and divides into the *medial and lateral cutaneous branches of leg*. Both of these divisions, then, reach the dorsum of the foot in front of the superior and inferior extensor retinaculum and then are distributed as follows. The *medial division sends two digital nerves:* (1) One goes to the medial side of the great toe, up to its tip and (2) the other divides to supply the adjacent sides of the second and third toes. The nail bed of any toe is not supplied by the digital branches of the nerves of the dorsum of foot. The nail beds are supplied by the plantar digital nerves. The *lateral divisions again divide into two dorsal digital nerves*. One divides to supply the adjacent sides of the third and fourth toes. Other divides to supply the adjacent sides of the fourth and fifth toes **(Fig. 38)**.

The deep peroneal or anterior tibial nerve is one of the branches of the common peroneal nerve and originates at the lateral surface of the neck of the fibula. It first enters the anterior compartment of the leg and then descends on the interosseous membrane. It innervates all the muscles of the anterior compartment of the leg. On reaching the front of the ankle, it divides into lateral and medial branches. The lateral branch supplies the tarsal joints, metatarsophalangeal joints, and interossei muscles. The medial branch runs along the lateral side of the arteria dorsalis pedis and supply motor to the first dorsal interosseous muscle and sensory to the adjacent sides of the great toe and the second toe.

The block of this common peroneal nerve is appropriate only for surgery on the lateral side of the foot, when popliteal block is difficult. The site of injection or block is just distal to the head of the fibula below knee, where this nerve crosses the head of the fibula from posterior compartment to lateral compartment of leg. The nerve can be blocked by field block technique or with the help of nerve stimulator.

Relatively a small volume of 5–10 mL of drug is required for this block.

Saphenous Nerve Block

It is one of the branches of the posterior division of femoral nerve and is purely a sensory nerve. It descends through the femoral triangle, lateral to femoral artery and then, enters the adductor canal through the apex of femoral triangle. Here, it superficially crosses the femoral artery from lateral to medial side and pierces the aponeurotic roof of the adductor canal. It then descends along the medial side of the knee. On the medial side of the knee, it pierces the deep fascia between the tendon of sartorius and the tendon of gracilis muscles and becomes superficial. It now descends superficially over the deep fascia, along the medial surface of the tibia (bone) with great saphenous vein, but in front of it (great saphenous vein). At lower one-third of the leg, it divides into two branches which include (1) one descends along the medial border of the tibia to end over the skin of the medial side of the ankle and (2) the other enters the foot, in front of the medial malleolus and then runs along the medial border of the foot up to the ball of the great toes. Thus, the saphenous nerve is the terminal sensory continuation of the femoral nerve on the medial side of the leg and foot, up to the ball of the great toe.

Individual saphenous nerve is blocked for minor surgeries over the skin on the medial side of the leg. For complete anesthesia of foot, it is blocked with other nerves around the ankle, but this block is used mainly in conjunction with a sciatic nerve block to provide a complete anesthesia/analgesia below the knee.

It can be blocked by the infiltration of subcutaneous tissue with an LA agent in a straight line, perpendicular to the course of this nerve, at any one of the several easily identified sites such as (1) *at the medial side of the knee joint* (above the joint), over the femoral condyle by a transverse skin infiltration with 5–10 mL of an LA agent, which can be confirmed by testing by pinprick between the first and second toes on the dorsal surface of the foot, (2) *over the medial prominence of tibia* (below the knee joint), just distal to the knee joint, and (3) as a routine *part of full block around the ankle*, medial malleolus is identified and 5 mL of LA solution is infiltrated in a line, running anteriorly around the ankle.

Above the knee joint, this saphenous nerve can be blocked deep to the sartorius muscle in sartorial canal (*trans-sartorial technique for saphenous nerve block*). For this procedure, a *high-frequency linear ultrasound probe* is used to identify the junction between the sartorius, vastus medialis, and adductor muscles in cross section, just distal to the adductor canal. A long needle is inserted from medial to lateral (in the plane of ultrasound) or angled cephalad (out of the plane of ultrasound) and 5–10 mL of LA solution is deposited within this fascial plane.

■ NERVES BLOCK AROUND THE ANKLE

For the surgical procedures on foot, an ankle block is a fast, low risk, and low technology procedure. For ankle block, the excessive volume of LA solution and the use of vasoconstrictor, such as epinephrine should be avoided to minimize the risk of ischemic complications. Since this block includes five separate injections, it is often uncomfortable for patients and adequate sedation and analgesia as premedication is advised.

In ankle block, the complete anesthesia of foot (both motor and sensory) requires the blockade of five separate nerves, supplying it, around the ankle. These include the *posterior tibial and sural nerve* (branch of the tibial nerve), the *superficial and deep peroneal nerve* (branch of the common peroneal nerve), and the *saphenous nerve* (branch of the femoral nerve). Depending on the site of surgical procedure, it may also be possible to block less than five nerves with accurate knowledge of their sensory and motor supply **(Fig. 38)**.

Saphenous nerve is the only innervation of foot that is not a part of the sciatic nerve. It supplies the superficial skin sensation on the anteromedial aspect of foot up to the ball of the great toe of foot. Deep peroneal nerve, arising at the lateral surface of the neck of fibula from common peroneal nerve, enters the anterior compartment of the leg and runs downward. Then, it entering the ankle between the extensor hallucis longus and extensor digitorum longus tendon, supplies the extensor muscles of toes and skin sensation to the first dorsal web space. The superficial peroneal nerve, arising at the lateral surface of the neck of fibula from common peroneal nerve, descends toward the ankle through the lateral compartment of leg. It gives motor branches to the muscles of eversion. It enters the ankle just lateral to extensor digitorum longus tendon and provides cutaneous sensation to the dorsum of foot and toes. The posterior tibial nerve is a direct continuation of tibial nerve. It enters the foot by running posterior to the medial malleolus. Here, it is located behind the posterior tibial artery and gives the branches calcaneal, medial plantar, and lateral plantar nerves. It provides sensory innervation to the heel, the medial of the sole (medial plantar nerve), the lateral part of sole (lateral plantar nerve), as well as the tips of all the toes. The *sural nerve* is a branch of tibial nerve and enters the foot between the Achilles tendon and the lateral malleolus to provide the sensation of the lateral part of the foot.

The ankle block is selected, especially in patients who are too sick for central neuraxial block, or unable to handle higher volume of an LA agent required for other regional anesthetic techniques for the block of lower extremity, but need surgery on foot, distal to the malleoli.

Posterior Tibial Nerve Block

At the ankle, behind the medial malleolus, the pulsation of posterior tibial artery is the landmark for the block of this nerve. Here, the nerve lies lateral (behind) to the artery. After a proper antiseptic skin preparation, a 22 G and 3 cm long blunt beveled needle is inserted perpendicular to the skin, but posterior to the artery at the level of medial malleolus. Paresthesia may be encountered, but should not be sought. The tip of the needle must be under the covered edge of medial malleolus and drug is administered like field block technique and 5 mL drug will accomplish the block. Then, the needle is withdrawn back from the posterior aspect of tibia. The blockade of posterior tibial nerve provides the loss of sensory on heel, the plantar aspect of toes, the medial aspect of sole (the lateral aspect of sole is supplied by sural nerve), and as well as some motor block supplied by it.

Sural Nerve Block

It is the cutaneous branch of the tibial nerve and arises from it (tibial nerve) in popliteal fossa. It is also joined by a sural communicating branch, coming from the common peroneal nerve. The sural nerve pierces the deep fascia and becomes superficial at the level of the lower one-third on the back of the leg. Then, it passes behind the lateral malleolus, along with the small saphenous vein and goes along the lateral border of foot up to the tip of little toe. At the level of ankle, it is located superficially between the lateral malleolus (anteriorly) and Achilles tendon (posteriorly).

After proper antiseptic skin preparation, a 25 G and 3 cm long needle is inserted through the skin, lateral to the Achilles tendon, directing toward the lateral malleolus and then 5 mL of LA solution is injected subcutaneously. This block provides anesthesia of the lateral aspect of foot and the lateral aspect of the proximal part of sole.

Deep Peroneal, Superficial Peroneal, and Saphenous Nerve Block

These three nerves can be blocked through a single needle entry point at intermalleolar line (between medial and lateral malleolus) in front of ankle. At intermalleolar line, the tendon of extensor hallucis longus is identified first by asking the patient to dorsiflex his big toe. At this intermalleolar line, the tendon of extensor digitorum longus can also be palpated easily on the lateral side of extensor hallucis longus tendon. Between these two tendons the anterior tibial artery is situated and is palpable at this level. The needle is inserted perpendicular to the skin on intermalleolar line by the side of anterior tibial artery between these two tendons and 5 mL of LA drug is deposited under the extensor retinaculum.

This will block the deep peroneal nerve and anesthetize the skin between the first and second toes.

During the withdrawal of needle, it is again directed laterally along the intermalleolar line through the same entry site of skin and 5 mL of LA drug is deposited subcutaneously blocking the superficial peroneal nerve, resulting in anesthesia of the dorsum of foot, excluding the first interdigital cleft which is already anesthetized by the block of deep peroneal nerve. The same maneuver can now be performed in the medial direction along the intermalleolar line, anesthetizing the saphenous nerve, supplying a strip of skin along the medial aspect of foot.

ILIOHYPOGASTRIC, ILIOINGUINAL, AND GENITOFEMORAL NERVE BLOCK

Indications

Iliohypogastric (L_1), ilioinguinal (L_1), and genitofemoral (L_1, L_2) nerves are the branches of lumbar plexus and lies in the muscular layers of abdominal wall. They mainly supply the skin of groin and genital areas. So, blockade of these nerves is used for surgical procedures on inguinal and genital areas, such as herniorrhaphy, orchidopexy, chronic pain, postoperative pain relief over this area, etc. The block of these three nerves is also done along with femoral nerve block for long saphenous vein stripping. The block of these nerves has also been used to diagnose and treat pain due to nerve entrapment, neuralgias, neuromas, etc., on their site of sensory supply **(Fig. 39)**.

Anatomy

The ventral ramus of first lumbar spinal nerve (L_1), after receiving a twig from the ventral ramus of twelfth thoracic spinal nerve (T_{12}), divides into two branches, the upper and lower. The upper branch again divides into two branches. These include (1) *iliohypogastric* and (2) *ilioinguinal nerve*. The lower branch unites with a branch from the ventral ramus of second lumbar spinal nerve (L_2) and form the *genitofemoral nerve*.

After formation, the *iliohypogastric nerve* first emerges from the lateral border of psoas major muscle by piercing it. Then, it runs downward and laterally in front of quadratus lumborum and transversus abdominis muscle, but behind the kidney. Here, this nerve is embedded in the fascia covering the quadratus lumborum. Now the nerve pierces the transversus abdominis muscle and runs obliquely forward between it and internal oblique muscle of anterior abdominal wall. Here, it supplies both the muscles. Then, the nerve divides into lateral and anterior cutaneous branches. The lateral cutaneous branch pierces the internal and external oblique muscles above the iliac crest and supplies the posterolateral area of gluteal skin. On the other hand, the anterior cutaneous branch runs further forward between the transversus abdominis and internal oblique muscles, and pierces the internal oblique muscle 2 cm medial to the anterior superior iliac spine and runs between it and the external oblique aponeurosis toward the inguinal region. Then, it pierces the external oblique aponeurosis 3 cm above the superficial inguinal ring and supplies the skin over the suprapubic region.

The *ilioinguinal nerve* after its formation also runs like iliohypogastric nerve but below it. It is smaller in size **(Fig. 40)** than the previous one and pierces the internal oblique muscle close to anterior superior iliac spine. Then, the nerve runs medially on internal oblique muscle and enters the inguinal canal from above. This nerve is the only content of canal which does not pass through the deep inguinal ring. It then traverses along the medial part of canal to come out through the superficial inguinal ring and supplies (1) the skin over symphysis pubis, (2) the skin over the root of scrotum and penis in male or labia majora in female, and (3) the skin over the superomedial angle of femoral region.

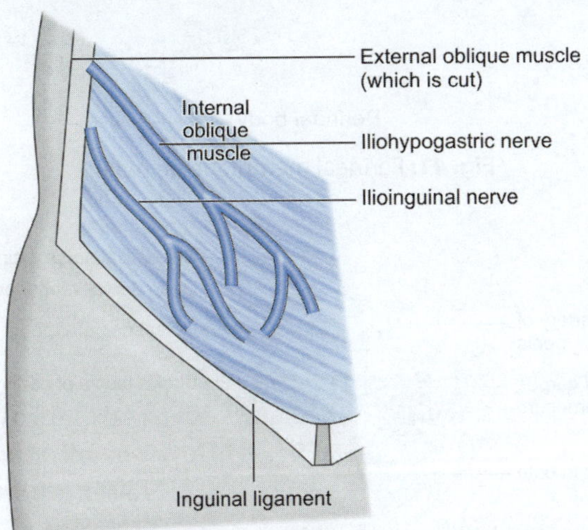

Fig. 39: Iliohypogastric and ilioinguinal nerve block.

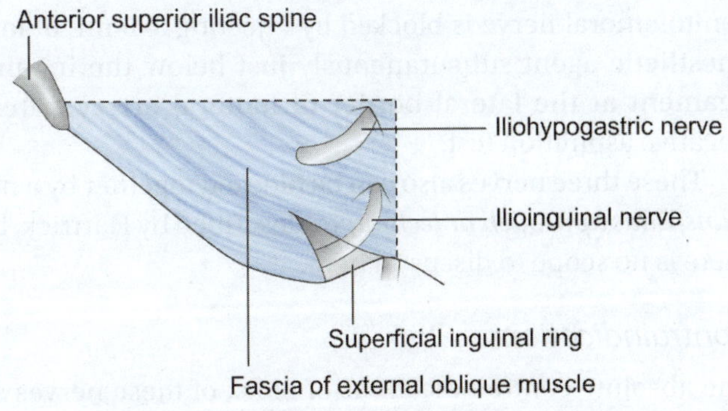

Fig. 40: Iliohypogastric and ilioinguinal nerve.

After its formation the genitofemoral nerve pierces the psoas major muscle and emerges from its abdominal surface at its medial border, opposite to the body of L_3 or L_4 vertebra. It then descends subperitoneally on psoas major muscle behind the ureter. Here, it divides into genital and femoral branches above the inguinal ligament at variable distance. Then, this genital branch enters the inguinal canal through its deep inguinal ring and becomes the content of spermatic cord. In the spermatic cord, it is also known as the nerve to the cremaster, supplying the cremaster muscle and scrotal skin (in male). In female, this genital branch in inguinal canal accompanies the round ligament and supplies the skin of labia majora and mons pubis. Now, the femoral branch of genitofemoral nerve descends lateral to the external iliac artery. It then passes behind the inguinal ligament and enters the femoral triangle lateral to the femoral artery, but within its sheath. It supplies the skin of the upper part of femoral triangle, but below the inguinal ligament.

Technique

Iliohypogastric and Ilioinguinal Nerve Block

For the block of these two nerves the patient is first positioned in supine and then the anterior superior iliac spine is identified. After that an imaginary line is drawn from it to the umbilicus. From this line a point is marked which is 2 cm medial and 2 cm cephalad to the anterior superior iliac spine. This is the entry point of needle to block the aforementioned nerves. After proper skin preparations, a 22–25 G needle which is 3.5″ long is inserted perpendicular to the skin until it just pierces and cross the external oblique aponeurosis below which these nerves lie. Then, 8–10 mL of local anesthetic agent is injected fanwise at that site to the block both the iliohypogastric and ilioinguinal nerves.

Genitofemoral Nerve Block

For the block of this nerve, the patient is first positioned supine and then hips are extended. The genital branch of genitofemoral nerve is first blocked by infiltrating 3–5 mL of local anesthetic agent, just lateral to the pubic tubercle, below the inguinal ligament. Similarly, the femoral branch of genitofemoral nerve is blocked by injecting 3–5 mL of local anesthetic agent subcutaneously just below the inguinal ligament at the lateral border of femoral artery, after a negative aspiration test.

These three nerves also can be blocked together by a new *transpsoas approach or technique*, described by Hartrick, but there is no scope to discuss it here.

Contraindications

The absolute contraindications of block of these nerves are sepsis, local infection, coagulopathy, lack of consent, etc.

If there is coagulopathy but presence of strong indication, then the procedure can be executed very cautiously using a 27 G fine spinal needle.

■ PENILE BLOCK (FIG. 41)

The penile block is performed (1) for any surgical procedure over the penis or (2) for postoperative pain relief, after any surgery over penis, under general anesthesia. Penis is actually innervated by the dorsal nerve of penis or clitoris. It is the branch of pudendal nerve and gives this branch while it runs in pudendal canal. Then, the dorsal nerve of penis enters into the penis deep to its Buck's fascia under the symphysis pubis and divides into dorsal and ventral branches. The genital branch of genitofemoral nerve and the terminal branches of ilioinguinal nerve also supply the skin over the root of the penis, near symphysis pubis **(Fig. 42)**.

Bilaterally, the dorsal nerve of penis is blocked by injecting 2–3 mL of an LA agent, under the Buck's fascia at 10 and 2 o'clock position, using a 25 G needle which is 1″ long. The whole penis also can be anesthetized by giving a fan-shaped (triangular or rounded) field block around the root of the penis with 10 mL local anesthetic agent. For penile block epinephrine or any other vasoconstricting agents, mixed with local anesthetic solution always should have to be avoided to prevent the end artery spasm, leading to ischemic injury of penis **(Fig. 43)**.

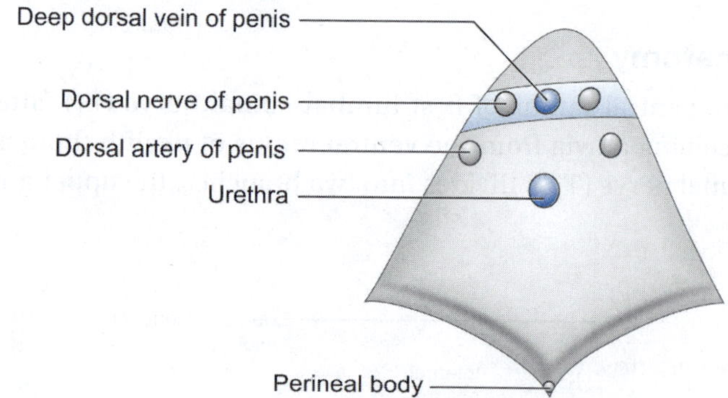

Fig. 41: Perineal membrane (in male).

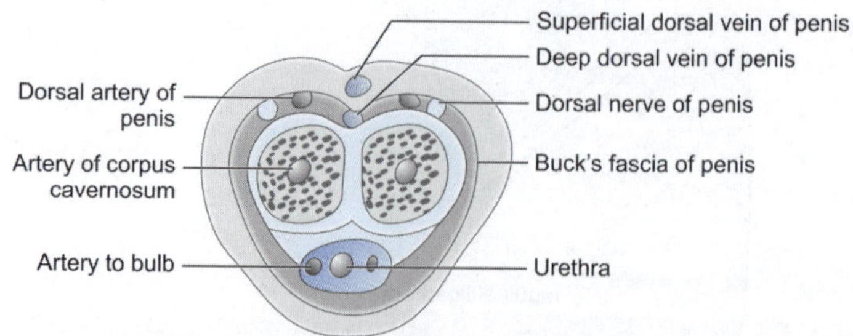

Fig. 42: Transverse section through the body of penis.

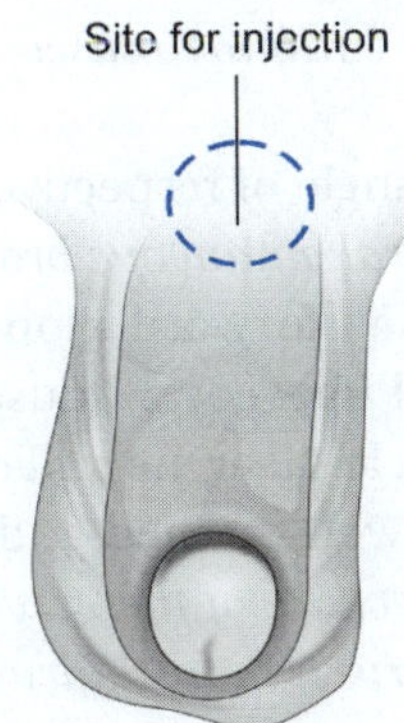

Fig. 43: Penile field block.

As the penis is a very vascular structure, therefore careful aspiration before every injection is mandatory to avoid any inadvertent intravascular administration of the LA agent.

■ INTERCOSTAL NERVE BLOCK

Indication

The intercostal nerve block is very useful in many circumstances, though it has some inherent disadvantages. The bilateral blockade of sixth to twelfth intercostal nerves provides both the motor block and sensory loss of the anterior abdominal wall, extending from the xiphoid process to the symphysis pubis. The bilateral blockade of intercostal nerve is always necessary, because there is some overlap of innervation, over the midline, from each side. The muscles of anterior abdominal are relaxed, but there is no anesthesia of visceral peritoneum. So, light general anesthesia or supplemental bilateral celiac plexus block is necessary, if any intra-abdominal procedure is attempted by only intercostal nerve block. This combined technique (bilateral intercostal block plus celiac plexus block) is ideally suited for upper abdominal surgery such as cholecystectomy, gastrectomy, and splenectomy. But for the midabdominal surgery this intercostal block and celiac plexus block is further supplemented by the paravertebral block of the first and second spinal nerve roots.

In a similar fashion, intrathoracic surgery also can be performed by the combination of upper intercostal nerve block and stellate ganglion block, with or without light general anesthesia. However, though these are not generally used, but they are very useful for severe debilitated patients. Thus, the intercostal nerve block with the plexus or ganglionic block provides an alternative approach to the spinal and epidural anesthesia for intra-abdominal or intrathoracic surgical procedures, if the central neuraxial blocks are contraindicated. On the other hand, only intercostal nerve block without plexus or ganglion block also can replace the spinal or epidural anesthesia for surgical procedures

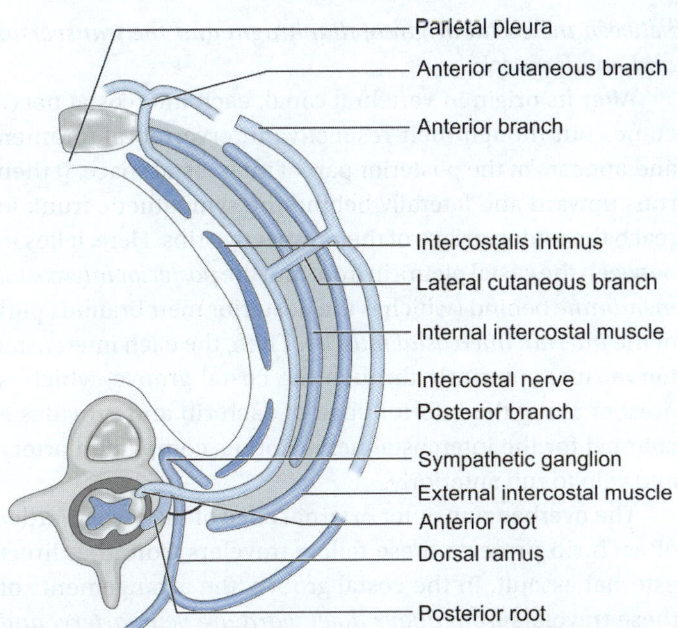

Fig. 44: The intercostal nerve with its origin and branches.

performed only on the abdominal or chest wall without the price of sympathectomy, which is associated with central neuraxial block.

The unilateral intercostal nerve block of three or more ribs at a time provides an excellent pain relief for fractured ribs, herpes zoster, pleurisy, chest tube insertion or replacement, percutaneous biliary drainage, etc. This technique is also useful to relieve the acute post-thoracotomy pain, midline abdominal surgical incisional pain, subcostal incisional pain, etc. It improves the ventilatory function and reduces the narcotic requirements, but this intercostal nerve block does not provide analgesia, as effective as continuous epidural infusions. On the other hand, it needs frequent and repeated injection to relief the pain.

Anatomy of Intercostal Nerve (Fig. 44)

Each intercostal nerve is the direct *continuation of the ventral ramus* of a thoracic spinal nerve. They are twelve in number on each side. Among these, the third to sixth intercostal nerves are accounted (termed) as the *typical intercostal nerves*, because they are only confined to the thoracic wall. The major portion of the first thoracic spinal nerve (first intercostal nerve) joins with the ventral ramus of C_8 spinal nerve and forms the lower trunk of brachial plexus. The lateral cutaneous branch of the second intercostal nerve remains undivided. Rather, it becomes the *intercostobrachial* nerve and supply the *medial side of the upper arm and arm pit*. The seventh to elevnth intercostal nerves enter the anterior abdominal wall by passing through the *digitation between the costal origin of diaphragm and the transversus abdominis muscle.*

After its origin in vertebral canal, each intercostal nerve comes out though their respective intervertebral foramen and appears in the posterior part of intercostal space. It then runs upward and laterally behind the sympathetic trunk to reach the undersurface of their respective ribs. Here, it lies in between the costal pleura in front and the *posterior intercostal membrane* behind (which is the posterior membranous part of the *internal intercostal muscle*). Then, the each intercostal nerve runs anteriorly through the costal groove, which is present along the inferior edge of each rib and provides a channel for the intercostal nerve and its companion artery and vein to run anteriorly.

The overhanging outer external edge of the lower border of each rib protects these fellow travelers from the direct external assault. In the costal groove, the arrangements of these travelers *from above downward are vein, artery, and nerve (VAN)* (**Figs. 45 and 46**). When these neurovascular structures run under the lower edge of respective rib in their costal groove, then it runs between the *external intercostal and internal intercostal muscle lying externally and the*

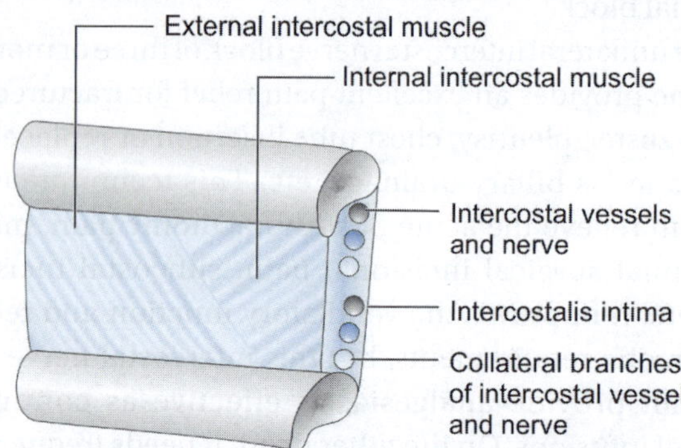

Fig. 45: The contents of intercostal space.

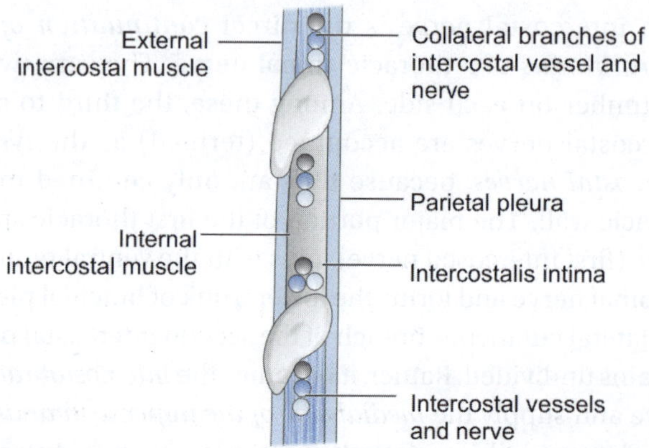

Fig. 46: Vertical section through an intercostal space.

intercostalis intimus (intima) muscle and parietal pleura lying internally.

On reaching the angle of respective rib, each intercostal nerve gives off a *lateral cutaneous branch.* Then, the main trunk of nerve passes forward along the costal groove between the internal intercostal muscle and intercostalis intimus (intima) muscle. Near the midaxillary line, the costal grove becomes less well-defined and the nerve migrates away from the rib. *Because of these two factors, the reliable block of intercostal nerve is more difficult beyond the anterior axillary line.*

In the anterior part of intercostal space, the nerve passes in front of sternocostalis muscle and crosses the internal thoracic artery anteriorly. Then, it pierces the intercostalis internus, anterior intercostal membrane (the anterior membranous part of intercostalis externus or *external intercostal muscle*), pectoralis major, and comes out as the *anterior cutaneous nerve* to supply the skin of the anterior chest wall (T_2–T_6) and the anterior abdominal (T_7–T_{12}) wall.

The ventral ramus of the *first thoracic spinal nerve* is not entirely the intercostal nerve. It divides into upper and lower branches. The large upper branch crosses the neck of the first rib and joins with the ventral ramus C8 nerve to form the *lower trunk of brachial plexus.* The smaller lower branch is continued as the *first intercostal nerve.*

The 12th intercostal or subcostal nerve is unique in that it is not closely associated with its corresponding rib. *The branches of it depart early and join with L1 spinal nerve to form the iliohypogastric and ilioinguinal nerve.* So, the standard subcostal injection technique is less likely to produce anesthesia of this nerve.

The *lateral cutaneous branch* of each intercostal nerve arises near the angle of each rib and pierces the muscle in midaxillary line. After being cutaneous, this branch again divides into two branches (1) anterior and (2) posterior branch. The *anterior branch* runs anteriorly and unites by the side of the sternum with the anterior cutaneous nerve which is the terminal part of the main intercostal nerve. The *posterior branch* runs posteriorly and unites with the cutaneous branch of the dorsal ramus of same thoracic spinal nerve which also supplies the paravertebral group of muscles and the skin over it. Both these branches supply the skin over their corresponding area.

A *collateral branch* also arises from each intercostal nerve, near the angle of each corresponding rib. It also passes forward through the same intermuscular plane like the main nerve, but along the upper border of the next lower rib. Anteriorly, it terminates as the *additional anterior cutaneous nerve* by piercing the muscle, like the terminal part of the main intercostal nerve.

Each intercostal nerve is connected with the corresponding sympathetic ganglion of sympathetic chain by white and gray rami communicantes. The white ramus carries the preganglionic sympathetic fibers, while the gray ramus carries the postganglionic sympathetic fibers from the ganglion.

Technique of Intercostal Block

The anatomy of every rib may themselves vary. Posteriorly, by the side of the midline, all the ribs are well protected by the paravertebral group of muscles. The lower six ribs are broad, flat, and more superficial than the upper six ribs. So, they are easily palpated lateral to these paravertebral groups of muscles. The upper ribs are narrower, deeper, and are more protected by scapula and paravertebral muscles. So, they are not easily palpated and technically more difficult to reach by the needle. As the upper ribs are protected laterally by the scapula, so paravertebral approach is more practical in this region.

The intercostal nerves can readily be blocked at the angle of rib, just lateral to the sacrospinalis group of muscles. The patient may be placed in lateral, sitting, supine, or prone position, but prone position is more practical and technically easy to block the intercostal nerve. In prone position, a pillow is placed under the abdomen to provide slight flexion of thoracic spine. The arms will hang over the edge of the operating table, so that the scapula falls away laterally from the angle of the ribs.

First a line is drawn along the thoracic vertebral spines. Then, the ribs are identified along the line of their most extreme posterior angulation. For the 12th rib, this is usually 7 cm away from the midline, whereas for the sixth rib, this is usually 5 cm away from the midline. Thus, a line is drawn connecting the posterior angles of these two ribs which

will run upward lying 3–5 cm away from the midline and is angled medially at the upper level. The posterior angles of the remaining ribs will come on this line and inferior border of each rib is marked on this line.

Then, after an appropriate skin preparation, sedation, and analgesia, a 22 G and 4 cm long needle is inserted perpendicular to the skin, until it rests on the rib. Then, the needle is directed in caudal direction, until it passes below the inferior border of the rib, where 3–5 mL of local anesthetic agent is injected. This process is repeated for each rib, starting with lower most and moving gradually upward.

The six or seven designated ribs on each side are blocked in this process. The ribs of the opposite side also can be blocked in similar manner. Alternatively, the intercostal block can also be performed on a supine patient at midaxially line. In practical situation, the lateral cutaneous branch of the intercostal nerve is not targeted for block, because in reality, CT studies show that the injected solution spreads several centimeters along the costal groove and block this lateral cutaneous branch automatically.

If this intercostal nerve block is to be supplemented by somatic paravertebral nerve blockade and sympathetic celiac plexus blockade, then these should be performed at the completion of intercostal anesthesia, but care should be taken to adjust the total dose of LA drug, so that the maximum recommended doses does not exceed.

Complications of Intercostal Block

The probable complications of intercostal block are pneumothorax (most common), hemothorax, perforation of lung, and collapse of lobe of a lung, sepsis, respiratory inadequacy, systemic toxicity of an LA agent, hypotension, etc.

Spinal, Epidural, and Caudal Anesthesia or Central Neuraxial Block

■ HISTORY

It was 1855, when Friedrich Gaedcke (FG) of Germany had first isolated cocaine (alkaloid) from coca plant (*Erythroxylon coca*). This plant usually grew as bush in Bolivia and Peru. Before that discovery, the leaves of this plant were well-known to the local Indians (Red Indians) as euphoriant and central nervous system (CNS) stimulant. But, they did not know the local anesthetic (LA) property of the leaves of this plant. The modern local or regional anesthesia (RA) began with the introduction of cocaine into medical practice, in September 1884, by Karl Koller **(Fig. 1)**, after its isolation from plant by FG. Karl Koller was then only a 27-year-old trainee ophthalmologist in Vienna. He was also the first medical man who used and published the analgesic and local anesthetic properties of cocaine in different journals, by applying it as topical drop, during ophthalmic surgery.

Before the discovery of analgesic and local anesthetic property of cocaine by him, Karl Koller was working under an ophthalmic professor, named, Carl Ferdinand. He (Carl Ferdinand) was then considerably dissatisfied with the standard and the condition of general anesthesia (GA), for ophthalmic surgery, during that period. Karl Koller also soon began to share the same dissatisfaction with his professor, regarding the restlessness, coughing, vomiting, etc. during the operative and postoperative period after ophthalmic surgeries under GA. So, he began to realize that this problem would only be solved, if any local anesthetic agent could be invented, which when will be instilled as a drop into the conjunctional sac, would abolish pain and would allow painless surgery. With this aim, Koller also tried with morphine and other sedatives, by instillating them as topical drop into conjunctival sac. But, he was unsuccessful for this purpose. So, turbulent ophthalmic operating conditions, under GA, continued.

Sigmund Freud, a friend and contemporary of Karl Koller, was also working as junior colleague in the neurology

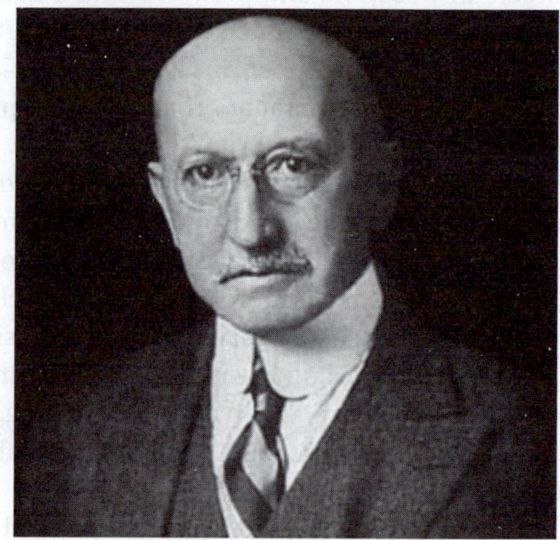

Fig. 1: Karl Koller.

department of same hospital. He later achieved world fame as the originator of psychoanalysis. In a fine summer of 1884, Freud was working with cocaine, what was at that time a fairly new drug, and had reached Europe from South America. It was then in and around 1860. As cocaine produced euphoria and CNS stimulation, so it led Freud to believe that cocaine might be a remedy for morphine addiction and as well as can be used as tonic for his psychoneurotic patients. He also knew that cocaine deadened mucous membrane. But, Sigmund Freud never thought that it was due to the local anesthetic property of cocaine. He was also not clear about the effects of cocaine on muscular contraction. Then, once Freud went on holiday, asking Koller to do some experiments on cocaine and to elucidate the problem.

Thus, when Freud was on holiday, Karl Koller had started same experiments by applying cocaine on his own tongue. But, he was astonished by cocaine's strange power to deaden all the sensation of his tongue. In a flash, he realized that this might be that agent, he had been looking for long period, to act as local anesthetic agent for his eye operations. Then, he started serial experiments to investigate the analgesic and local anesthetic properties of cocaine, in his experimental laboratory, on animals. Later, Koller used cocaine on his friends and lastly on his patients. He was extremely satisfied with his own work and had lost no time in making his discovery public. Then, he wrote a short preliminary report and asked his friend, Dr Josef Brettaver, to read it for him at the forthcoming meeting of German Ophthalmological Society which is to be held in Heidelberg where Koller himself was not be able to attend it.

In 15th September of 1884, Brettaver's paper made a sensation. After that, Koller had given many lectures on the local anesthetic property of cocaine. He also gave many clinical demonstrations on the local anesthetic property of 2% cocaine solution in the outpatient clinic. In the following months, Koller read two full papers on the local anesthetic property of cocaine before the Imperial Medical Society. But, Freud, whose interest in surgical anesthesia was minimal, made no claim to this discovery by Koller.

However, before the work of Koller, in 1849, Simpson had also recorded some history on local anesthesia and himself had done some experiments on local anesthesia. But, in-between 1849 and 1884 and before Koller's discovery, *ether spray* was also used for local anesthesia and it acts by freezing the skin. Later, *ethylchloride spray* was also used for same purpose, in 1880, by Rothenstein.

After Koller's work on topical anesthesia, in 1884 and in the early part of 1890, Reclus of Paris and Karl Ludwig of Berlin, had first popularized *infiltration anesthesia* using cocaine. But, the first direct nerve block with cocaine had been employed by WS Halsted and RJ Hall and the mandibular nerve was their first target nerve. Then, Halsted extended his work on this concept, by blocking other nerves. Subsequently, he was the first surgeon who had tried to block the nerves of face, brachial plexus, internal pudendal nerve, and posterior tibial nerve, using the cocaine. He also first showed that the reduction of circulation in any part of our body, by an Esmarch bandage, would prolong the effects of local anesthetic agent. After that, when the use of cocaine was popularized, then gradually its toxicity became evident, due to the use of it (cocaine) in higher doses. These toxicities of cocaine were CNS stimulation, addiction among general surgical patients, and clouding of cornea, when it is used as topical anesthesia in ophthalmic surgery.

So, subsequently, the relatively less toxic substitutes, for the highly toxic cocaine, as local anesthetic agent, was searched for. Hence, in 1890, in dentistry, the oil of cloves (eugenol) was first used as local analgesic and anesthetic agent, instead of cocaine. Then, gradually *Giesel's tropacocaine* was appeared, in 1891, and subsequently

Fourneau's stovocaine was marketed, in 1904. *Einhorn's novocaine (procaine)* was described in 1899, but was first used clinically, in 1904. Then, it was popularized by H Braun, in 1905. Subsequently, Miescher and Uhlmann introduced *nupercaine (cinchocaine)* in 1929. *Amethocaine* was first described in 1931. Then, first important milestone, about local anesthetic agent, came when Lofgren and Lundqvist first synthesized *lignocaine*, in 1943. But, Gordh was the first to use it clinically in Stockholm, in 1948. Then, the local anesthetic agents which were appeared chronologically are *chloroprocaine* in 1952, *mepivacaine* in 1956, *prilocaine* in 1959, *bupivacaine* in 1963, *etidocaine* in 1972, and *ropivacaine* in 1993.

H Braun had first introduced *adrenaline* in clinical practice, in 1902 (which was first isolated in pure form, in 1897) with cocaine to retard its absorption and to prolong its effect. The term "block" was first used, in 1897, by Crile and the term "regional anesthesia" was first used by Cushing, in 1901.

The existence of cerebrospinal fluid (CSF) was first discovered by Domenico Cotugno, in 1764. But, its circulation was first described by F Magendie, in 1825. He gave its name of this fluid as CSF. In 1885, when JL Corning was experimenting with the effect of cocaine on the spinal nerve on his dog, he accidentally pierced the dura and gave first spinal anesthesia by injecting cocaine in subarachnoid space. Later, deliberately he had repeated the subdural injection of cocaine and called it as spinal anesthesia. Then, he suggested that this type of anesthesia might be used in surgery. After that, this lumbar dural puncture was standardized as clinical procedure by HI Quincke in Germany, in 1891 **(Fig. 2)**.

The first planned spinal anesthesia on human being for surgery was performed by August Bier, on 16th August, in 1898. In this surgery, the patient was a 34-year-old parturient and Bier courageously injected 3 mL of 5% cocaine solution in CSF through the lumbar spinal route. However, this experiment became a great success. Then, subsequently Mr Bier had used spinal anesthesia on six patients. After that, to prove his faith on his method, Bier and his assistant each injected 2 mL of 1% cocaine solution into each other's subarachnoid space. The name of Bier's assistant was Hildebrandt. This procedure was actually first attempted on Bier by his assistant. However, after successfully locating the subarachnoid space, Hildebrandt was unable to attach the syringe with its needle and a considerable amount of CSF was lost on floor. So, in order to salvage the experiment, Hildebrandt volunteered himself as the research subject to Bier. This time the intrathecal injection of cocaine was successfully completed by Bier. Then, Bier and Hildebrandt celebrated their achievement

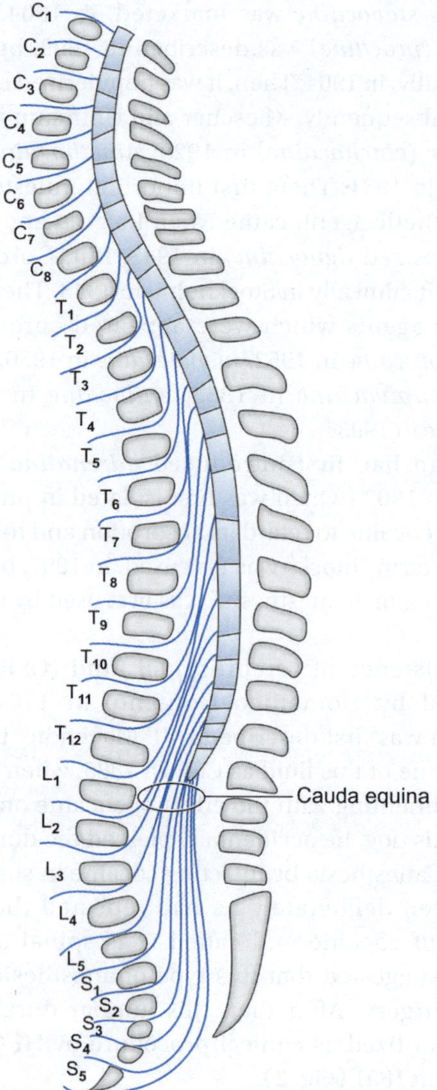

Fig. 2: Longitudinal section of vertebral column.

with wine and cigars. Unfortunately, on the next day, Bier complained of severe headache which was resolved after 9 days. However, Hildebrandt had also suffered from headache significantly more. While anesthetized, their degree of analgesia and anesthesia had been tested and monitored by being kicked on their shin bone by other and pinched with instruments. As a result, they not only developed a postdural puncture headache (PDPH), but also suffered from severe bruises over their legs, due to repeated assessment of their sensory block by kick and pinched with instruments. Then, this work was published, in April 1899, under the title "Research on the cocainization of spinal cord". Then, the popularity of spinal anesthesia had quickly spread. August Bier had also described in this book that his own postspinal headache is due to the excessive leakage of CSF. Bier also advised spinal anesthesia for operation on legs. But, later he gave it up, owing to the high toxicity of cocaine.

Soon after that, Tuffier and Sicard of Paris had extended the scope of spinal anesthesia in the other field of surgeries including the operation on external genitalia and lower abdomen. In 1903, adrenaline was introduced with local anesthetic agents to increase the duration and to reduce the toxicity of cocaine, used in spinal anesthesia. Due to the toxicity of cocaine, stovocaine was first used in spinal anesthesia, in 1904, and novocaine (procaine) in 1905, soon after their discovery. In 1907, A. E. Barker, a surgeon of London, was the first to realize the importance of the curvature of vertebral column and the use of gravity in controlling the level of spinal anesthesia. He first introduced "heavy" or hyperbaric solution of stovocaine in 5% glucose. Contrary, the Babcock of Philadelphia was the first to use hypobaric solution of stovocaine. His hypobaric formula was stovaine containing alcohol, lactic acid, etc.

G Labat, in 1921, had first used novocaine crystals, which was dissolved in CSF for barbotage technique. In the meantime, during 1923, ephedrine was introduced in the practice of medicine. Then, its use in spinal anesthesia had also gained popularity. So, ephedrine was first used to control hypotension and to maintain blood pressure (BP) in spinal anesthesia, in 1927.

For the surgeries on head, neck, and thorax, the spinal anesthesia was also first used, in 1909. After discovery of nupercaine, in 1929, it was first used as hyperbaric solution by McLelland of New York, in 1930, with great success. It was partly due to the longer duration of action of it. At that time, nupercaine was also used as hypobaric solution. Then, gradually amethocaine (tetracaine), lignocaine, and bupivacaine were used in spinal anesthesia, shortly after their discovery.

In UK, spinal anesthesia was under cloud for many years, though it was used rampantly worldwide, during that period. It was partly because of high tendency for court litigation, if complication occurred. A burning example of this was the Woolley and Roe case, in early 1950, in which paraplegia had occurred, followed by spinal anesthesia in two patients, operated on same day. At that time, it was thought that this complication was due to the contamination of anesthetic solution by phenol which entered the ampoules through a minute crack in the glass. But, after prolonged investigation, a much more likely explanation was that the used needle and its accessories was sterilized by boiling in a sterilizer which had been contaminated with acid substances, used to prevent scale formation.

In 1901, F Cathelin and A Sicard of Paris were the first to attempt sacral approach for the epidural space independently. This was some years before the lumbar route for epidural space came into use. Sacral block was, next, employed in Germany, in 1909, and was popularized by

G Labat, in 1923, by his book. The use of sacral analgesia in infants was first described by Campbell, in 1933. The method of continuous caudal analgesia by catheter was developed by Hingson, in 1943.

The history of lumbar epidural block is somewhat cloudy. It was not certain, whether Corning had deposited cocaine into intradural or extradural space, in 1885. Although the interspinous approach for epidural space has also been demonstrated at the beginning of this century, but Pages of Madrid, in 1921, was the first to describe the practical application of lumbar epidural anesthesia. Later, in 1931, Dogliotti of Italy had popularized this lumbar epidural technique. This is followed by other clinical exponents, such as Hess (1934), Odom (1936), and Harger and his associates (1941). The Curbelo of Cuba was the first to insert a ureteric catheter into the epidural space to perform the continuous epidural block, using the Tuohy needle. This needle was first designed for intrathecal use, but later it was adapted to allow the passage of smaller bore catheter through it (needle) into epidural space. The first report of the injection of opiates into epidural space came from Jerusalem, in 1979.

◼ INTRODUCTION

The central neuraxial block (CNB) (spinal or epidural anesthesia) results in chemical sympathectomy, sensory block, and motor paralysis. The procedure of spinal anesthesia is devoid of any systemic pharmacological effect of local anesthetic drug, due to its small volume. On the other hand, the epidural block is not always devoid of any systemic pharmacological effect of used local anesthetic agent, as it needs large volume (dose). Both the individual spinal and epidural or continuous epidural block have their own advantages and disadvantages. But, the combined spinal and epidural (CSE) anesthesia had blurred the differences between these two types of CNB (spinal and epidural), covering the disadvantages of each other and added flexibility of wide range for their clinical use.

Cocaine was the first drug used in spinal anesthesia. Gorton had first promoted very high spinal anesthesia for head and neck surgery. However, Koster had first used total spinal block for intrathoracic and intracranial procedures.

In previous days, spinal block was also used for medical therapy, e.g., pulmonary edema, due to its hypotensive effect. During that period and till now, the anesthesiologists continue to face the confusion, regarding the balance between the risks and the benefits of spinal anesthesia, especially those involving continuous spinal anesthesia (CSA) or the use of 5% xylocaine. In USA, the Food and Drug Administration (FDA) had withdrawn the very fine spinal catheter and 5% xylocaine, due to the perceived association between them (5% xylocaine and fine spinal catheter) and cauda equina syndrome. It seems likely that the more spinal and epidural blocks have failed, due to the inadequate IV sedation, and anxiolysis, rather than due to technical failure.

The continuous epidural block, used for postoperative analgesia, decreases the length of hospital stay and allows the more efficient use of continuously increasing stretched (over burden) healthcare service. There is a common believe that in epidural block there is less reduction of BP and is slower in onset. But, this is not always correct. The ephedrine which is used to check the hypotension, due to RA, is a mixed adrenergic agonist and is preferred than a pure adrenergic agonist. Gradually, the days are coming, when the infusion of large amount of crystalloid solution, as the preload, to minimize the spinal or epidural hypotension, should be rethought. Sometimes, during epidural anesthesia, due to large amount of drug, the level of anesthetic agent in blood may reach a concentration (toxic level) which is sufficient enough to produce systemic effects.

◼ ANATOMY

To form the vertebral column, multiple vertebrae are arranged in a column. Hence, it is so named. The whole vertebral column consists of 23 fibrocartilaginous disks and 33 vertebrae of which seven are cervical, 12 are thoracic, five are lumbar, five are sacral, and four are coccygeal. The cervical, thoracic, and lumbar vertebrae are called the free vertebrae and each of them presents their regional characteristics. On the other hand, the sacral and coccygeal vertebrae are called the fixed vertebrae. This is because the five sacral vertebrae are fused to form the sacrum and the four rudimentary coccygeal vertebrae are united to form the coccyx.

The functions of vertebral column are:
- Support of trunk
- Transmission of body weight
- Protection of spinal cord, spinal nerves, and its meninges
- Attachment of muscles and ligaments for various movements of trunk.

There is very slight movement between two adjacent vertebrae. But, a very wide range of movements of vertebral column are possible, when the multiple small movements between the two vertebrae are considered as a whole.

◼ PARTS OF VERTEBRA

Body

The body of a vertebra transmits body weight and is connected to the bodies of adjacent upper and lower vertebrae by intervertebral disks, forming secondary cartilaginous joints. The body of a vertebra is enclosed by a shell of compact bone, except at its upper and lower surfaces, where it is composed of spongy bone and is covered by a plate of a hyaline cartilage. The front and sides of the body of a vertebra are somewhat concave in shape and pierced by blood vessels. The posterior surface of the body of a vertebra presents one or more centrally placed basivertebral foramina, through which the basivertebral vein and some nutrient arteries pass. Along the entire mobile part of vertebral column, the anterior and the posterior surfaces of the body of each vertebra are connected respectively by a continuous flow of anterior and posterior longitudinal ligaments of which the anterior ligament is stronger than the posterior **(Fig. 3)**.

Vertebral Arch

It is situated behind the body of each vertebra and is composed of one pedicle and one lamina on each side. This pedicle and lamina present on each side of a vertebra, joins together posteriorly at the midline and forms a vertebral arch. This vertebral arch forms the lateral and posterior boundary of vertebral foramen. This vertebral foramen is also bounded anteriorly by the posterior surface of the body of respective vertebra. Thus, both the body and the vertebral arch of a piece of vertebra complete a vertebral foramen. The vertebral foramen of adjacent upper and lower vertebra joins continuously to form a canal, known as vertebral canal. This vertebral canal lodges and protects spinal cord, spinal nerve, its meninges, and CSF. In cervical region, the vertebral canal is triangular in shape and is more larger for the accommodation of cervical enlargement of spinal cord. However, in thoracic region,

the vertebral canal is comparatively smaller and circular. In lumbar region, this vertebral canal is again somehow more larger and triangular in shape to accommodate the lumbar enlargement of spinal cord. *In adults, the spinal cord ends usually at the level of the lower border of L_1 vertebra and the subdural and subarachnoid spaces (containing CSF) end at the level of S_2 vertebra.* After the end of spinal cord, the vertebral canal contains a bunch of spinal nerves, called the *cauda equina* and a non-nervous pial thread known as the *filum terminale (FT) interna*. This pial thread (FT interna) is nothing but the continuation of pial membrane as thread, after the end of nervous tissue of spinal cord **(Fig. 4)**.

An area called the *epidural space (or extradural space)* intervenes between the periosteum of vertebral canal and the dura mater, covering the spinal cord. This epidural space extends from the foramen magnum above to the sacral hiatus below and contains (1) *loose fibrofatty tissues* with valveless (2) *internal vertebral venous plexus*. This epidural space is also traversed by the (3) *roots of spinal nerves with their covering meningeal sheaths* after coming out from spinal cord and crossing over the subarachnoid space. Two deficiencies are present at the lateral and posterior walls of vertebral column. The former is called the *intervertebral foramen* and the later is called the *interlaminar foramen (space)*.

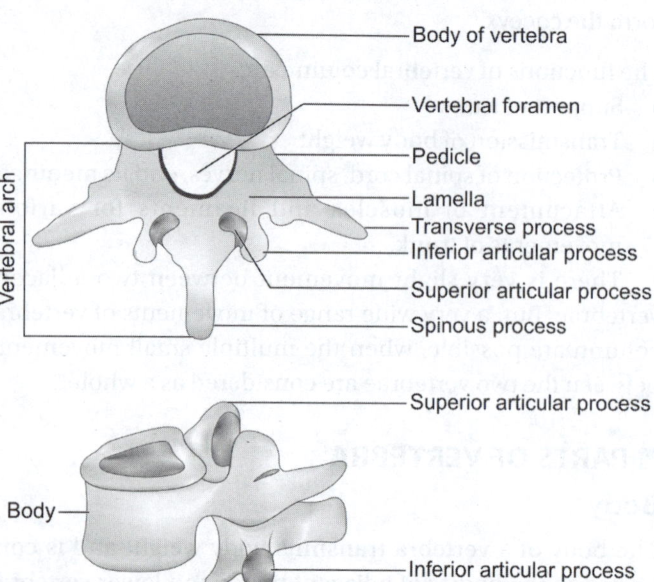

Fig. 3: Typical lumbar vertebra.

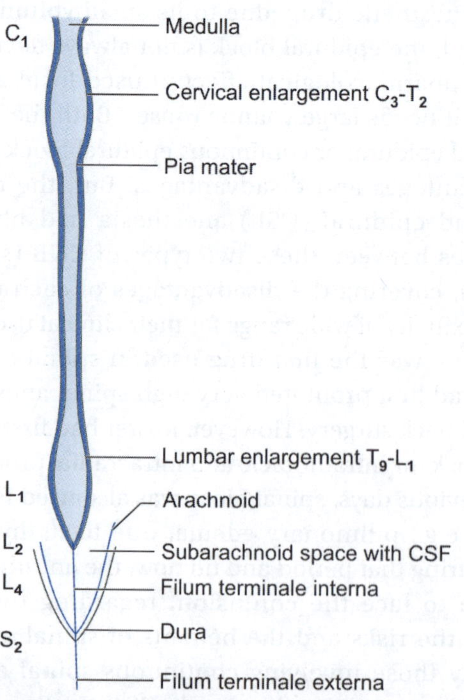

Fig. 4: Important vertebral levels of (i) the end of spinal cord, (ii) the end of pia mater, (iii) the end of arachnoid mater, and (iv) the end of dura mater. (CSF: cerebrospinal fluid).

Pedicle

Each pedicle springs from the posterolateral surface of vertebral body, and is situated at somewhat midway between its upper and lower surfaces. It projects backward with slight lateral inclination. Each pedicle is grooved above and below and these grooves are called the *superior and inferior vertebral grooves* or notch, respectively. Inferior groove is more deeper than the superior. Each groove together with the groove of the pedicle of upper and lower vertebra forms the *intervertebral foramen.* Thus, each intervertebral foramen is bounded above and below by the pedicles of adjacent vertebrae, behind by the interarticular joint, and in front by the lower part of the body of upper vertebra and the intervertebral disk. *The intervertebral foramens are narrowest in cervical and upper thoracic regions. It gradually increases in size and becomes widest in relation to fifth lumbar vertebra. Along with the gradual increase in the size of intervertebral foramens, the thickness of spinal nerves (which are coming out through the intervertebral foramina) is also increased in craniocaudal direction. So, the lower lumbar nerves are more vulnerable to compression within the lumber intervertebral foramens.*

Each intervertebral foramen contains (1) both the ends of the anterior and posterior nerve root with dorsal root ganglia, (2) the beginning of mixed spinal nerve, (3) the beginning of two rami of spinal nerve—anterior and posterior, (4) a spinal artery, and (5) an intervertebral vein. In cervical region, the superior vertebral notches transmit the numerically corresponding cervical nerves and the inferior notches transmit the immediately succeeding cervical nerves. But, in rest of the vertebral column, however, the superior notches transmit the immediately preceding spinal nerves and the inferior notches are occupied by the numerically corresponding spinal nerves. This is because cervical vertebrae are seven in number, whereas the cervical spinal nerves are eight in number on each side.

Lamina

Each lamina arises from the dorsal or posterior end of each pedicle. Then, it passes medially and backward and fuses with its fellow of opposite site at the midline. Now, from this fused laminae, an elongated spinous process projects backward, with a slight downward inclination. The laminae of adjacent upper and lower vertebrae, which are situated above and below of the present vertebra, are connected with each other by a series of fibroelastic membrane called the *ligamentum flavum.* In the midthoracic region, the adjacent laminae of upper and lower vertebrae partially overlap with one another. The space between the laminae of two upper and lower adjacent vertebrae and the interarticular joint is called

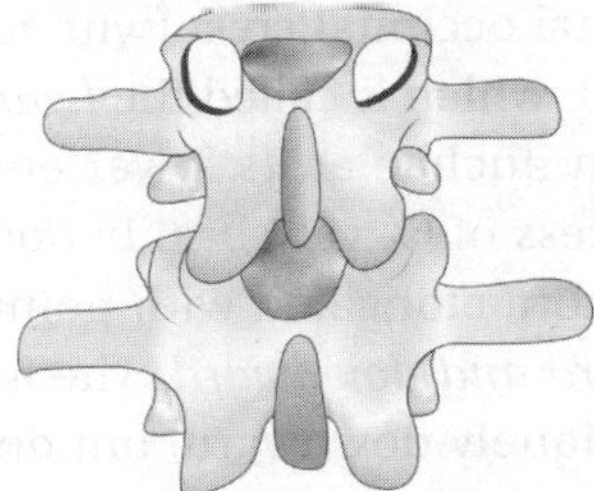

Fig. 5: Lumbar vertebrae and its posterior view.

the *interlaminar foramen.* So, the interlaminar foramen is bounded above and below by the adjacent laminae and at the sides by the inner aspect of the articular process of upper and lower vertebra (or the posterior aspect of interarticular joint). *During the extension of vertebral column, it becomes narrow, but during flexion, it enlarges and provides an easy access to spinal or epidural needle* **(Fig. 5)**.

Processes

They are seven in number, such as two transverse, one spinous, and four articular processes, arising from each vertebra. The transverse and spinous processes give attachment to different ligaments and muscles, acting on vertebral column.

Transverse process: The transverse process of each vertebra projects laterally on each side of it, arising from the junction of pedicle and lamina. *In cervical vertebrae,* the transverse processes present a foramen, which is called the *foramen transversarium. It transmits: the second part of vertebral artery (except in seventh cervical vertebra), a plexus of vertebral veins and a plexus of sympathetic nerves. In thoracic vertebrae,* the transverse processes present a costal facet (except the last two thoracic vertebrae) on its anterior surface, close to their tip, for the articulation with the tubercle of numerically corresponding rib and forms a *costotransverse joint. In lumbar vertebrae,* the transverse processes are relatively slender. The transverse processes of all the free vertebrae are connected with each other by intertransversus muscles. In some regions, these transverse processes give attachment to erector spinae and paravertebral group of muscles which help in the flexion, extension, and rotation of trunk.

Spinous process: The unpaired spinous process of each vertebra projects backward in the midline, from the fused laminae of both sides. *In the cervical region,* the spines are *horizontal, short and present a bifid tip,* except the second and seventh cervical spine, *which are not bifid, elongated, and prominent.* The seventh cervical spine is called the cervical prominence. The tip of the spinous process of cervical vertebrae is connected to one another and to the external occipital crest (with its protuberance) by a fibrous band, which is called the *ligamentum nuchae*. This ligamentum nuchae at its lower end is attached to the spinous process of C_7 vertebra. *In the thoracic region, the spines are more elongated with pointed tips and are inclined backward and downward.* The first four thoracic spines slope obliquely downward, but do not overlap on one another. While the fifth to eighth thoracic spines overlap on one another. The lower four thoracic spines from eighth to twelfth are almost horizontal. *In the lumbar region, the spine are broad, quadrilateral, and horizontal* in direction **(Figs. 6A to C)**. All the thoracic and lumbar spines are connected with each other by the *interspinous ligament*, along their shaft and *supraspinous ligament* along their tip. The lumbar spines also provide attachments to the posterior layer of thoracolumbar fascia and the extensor muscles of trunk. *Since, considerable spaces are available in the interval between the horizontally directed lumbar spines, so the spinal (subarachnoid) or epidural anesthesia*

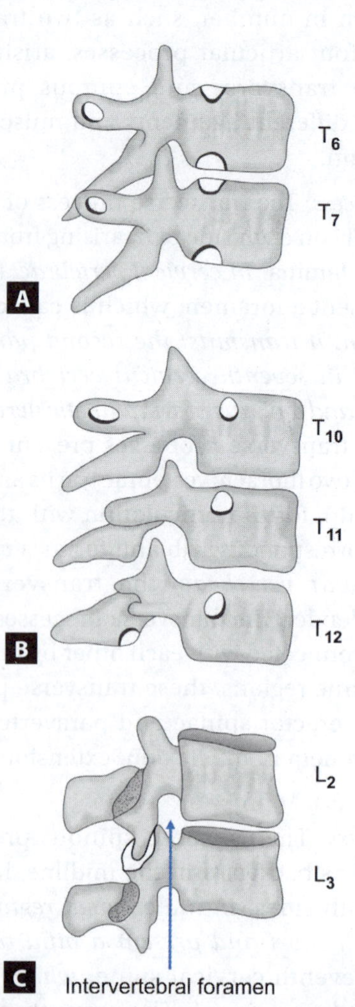

is often made through these intervals of lumbar spines. This lumbar subarachnoid puncture is usually performed distal to the caudal end of spinal cord (below L_1) to avoid its injury.

Articular process: There are four articular processes, arising from each vertebra, from the point of junction between their pedicle and lamina. Among these, each pair of superior and inferior (two superior and two inferior) articular processes project respectively above and below, from the junctions of pedicles and laminae. These articular processes are meant for the articulation with the articular processes of the immediately upper and lower vertebra. When viewed from behind, it is shown that the vertebral spines occupy the median line and there are two vertebral grooves, each lying lateral to this vertebral spine. These vertebral grooves, lying on each side of vertebral spines, are occupied by the deep extensor muscles of back. In the cervical and lumbar regions, these grooves are shallow and formed by the laminae of vertebra. In the thoracic region, these grooves are deep, wide, and formed by the laminae and the transverse processes of vertebra also.

Some landmarks of vertebral column are **(Fig. 7):**

- T_3 spine corresponds with the level of scapular spine
- T_7 spine corresponds with the inferior angle of scapula
- L_4 spine corresponds with the summits of iliac crest (useful for lumbar puncture)
- S_2 spine corresponds with the posterior superior iliac spine (end of the spinal subarachnoid space)
- The upper end of natal cleft, between the two buttocks, corresponds with the sacral hiatus, and it is useful for sacral epidural anesthesia.

Figs. 6A to C: (A) Lateral view of sixth and seventh thoracic vertebrae; (B) Lateral view of 10th, 11th, and 12th thoracic vertebrae; and (C) Lateral view of second and third lumbar vertebrae.

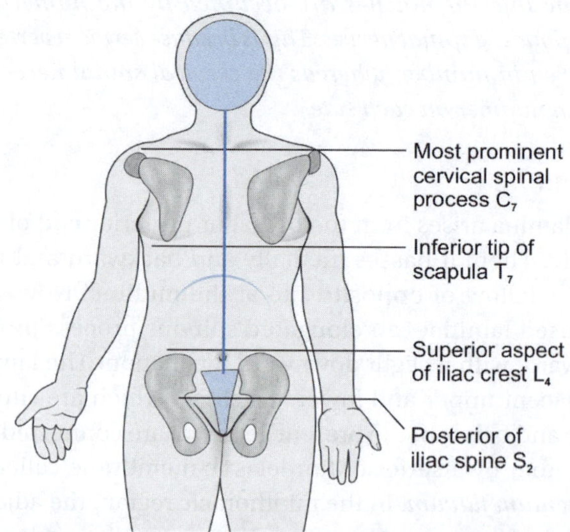

Fig. 7: The surface landmarks for identifying the spinal vertebral levels.

Ligaments of the Vertebral column

All the parts (body, articular process, lamina, and transverse process) of a bony vertebra are held together by a series of overlapping ligaments. These ligaments not only bind the vertebrae together, but also assist in protecting the spinal cord. These ligaments are:

Anterior and Posterior Longitudinal Ligaments

It runs in front and behind of the bodies of vertebra, extending from the axis (second cervical vertebra) to the sacrum.

Ligamentum Flavum

As this name says, it is made up of yellow elastic fibers. Above, it is attached to the anterior and inferior aspect of the lamina of upper vertebra and below it is attached to the superior and posterior aspect of the lamina of lower vertebrae. It blends posteriorly and medially with interspinous ligaments and with the ligamentum flavum of opposite side. Laterally and anteriorly, it blends with the capsule of interarticular joint of that side. It is thinnest at the cervical region and thickest at the lumbar region. These ligaments are muscle sparers and assist in the straightening of vertebral column, after bending forward. It also helps in maintaining the erect posture of body. It comprises half of the total length of the posterior wall of vertebral column **(Table 1)**.

Interspinous Ligaments

It extends forward from the tip of the spinous process of each vertebra, where it fuses with the supraspinous ligament, to the point where the two laminae from the opposite sides of a vertebra fuse in the midline. Here, it (interspinous ligament, not supraspinous ligament) blends with the ligamentum flavum. Above, it is attached to the inferior border of the spine of upper vertebra and below it is attached to the superior border of the spine of lower vertebra. In lumbar region, it is most wide and dense.

Supraspinous Ligament

It extends from the tip of seventh cervical spine to the sacrum (first sacral vertebra), joining the tip of all thoracic and lumbar spinous processes. From seventh cervical spine and above, it is continuous with the ligamentum nuchae. It is thickest and widest in lumbar region.

Curvature of Vertebral Column

There are four curvatures in vertebral column (1) two concave ventrally: one at thoracic and another at sacrococcygeal regions and (2) two concave dorsally: one at cervical and another at lumbar regions. The thoracic and sacral curvatures are the remnants of the flexion attitude of fetus in uterus. So, they are called the *primary curvatures*. Whereas, the cervical curvature appears after birth when the child lifts his head and lumbar curvature appears at the end of 1st year when the child learns to stand. So, they are called the *secondary curvatures*. The cervical and lumbar curvatures (secondary curvature) are caused by the unequal thickness of intervertebral disks (thicker anteriorly and thinner posteriorly) and the thoracic and sacral curvatures (primary curvatures) are caused by the bony configuration. The accentuated pathological ventral curvature of vertebral column at thoracic region is called the *kyphosis* and the accentuated dorsal curvature of vertebral column at lumbar region is called the *lordosis*. Scoliosis is the exaggerated form of lateral curvature of vertebral column. The dorsally concave *cervical curvature* extends from the atlas (C_1) to the second thoracic vertebra. The ventrally concave *thoracic curvature* extends from the second thoracic vertebrae to the 12th thoracic vertebrae. The dorsally concave *lumbar curvature* extends from the first lumbar vertebra to the fifth lumbar vertebra. And, the ventrally concave *pelvic curvature* or sacrococcygeal curvature extends from the lumbosacral joint to the tip of the coccyx and faces downward and forward.

Intervertebral Disk

The intervertebral disks connect the upper and lower surfaces of the bodies of adjacent upper and lower vertebrae and are present from the second cervical vertebra (axis) up to the first sacral vertebra. They actually intervene between the plates of hyaline cartilages which cover the upper and lower surfaces of the adjacent vertebral bodies. Each intervertebral disk is made up of a central gelatinous part, called the *nucleus pulposus* and a peripheral fibrocartilaginous part, called the *annulus fibrosus*. It accounts for one-fourth to one-fifth of the total length of vertebral column.

It is thicker at cervical and lumbar region where the vertebral column needs more mobility and is thinner at thoracic region where the vertebral column needs less mobility. In cervical and lumbar regions, it is more thickened anteriorly than posteriorly. So, it also gives rise to

TABLE 1: Characteristics of ligamentum flavum at different level of vertebral column.

Site of vertebral column	Distance from skin to ligament (in cm)	Thickness of ligament (mm)
Cervical	2–3	2–3
Thoracic	3–5	3–5
Lumbar	3–8	5–6

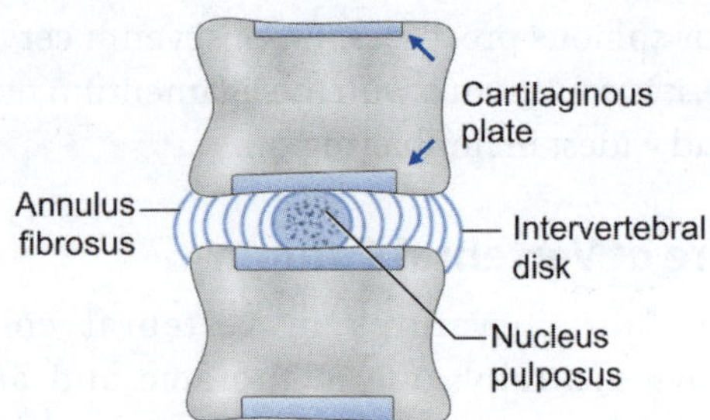

Fig. 8: Intervertebral disk.

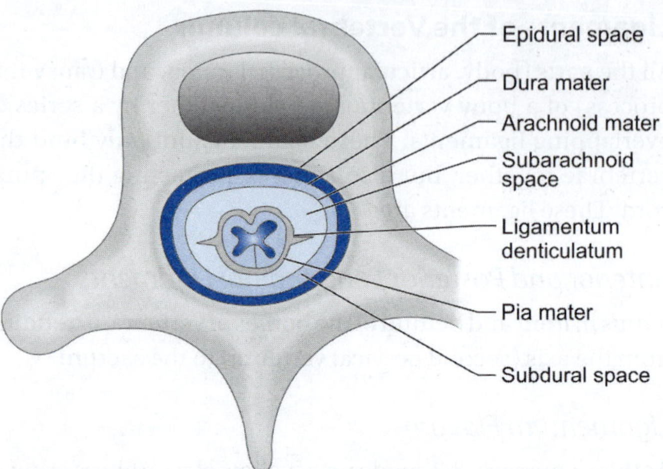

Fig. 9: Relationship of spinal cord to the meninges and vertebra.

the ventral convexity of vertebral column at these regions. It also functions as shock absorber when is placed between two vertebral bodies and connects them strongly. The intervertebral disk also provides resiliency to the vertebral column and ensure equal distribution of compressive forces on the upper and lower surfaces of the body of a vertebra. If during spinal block, the needle hits the peripheral annular fibrosus, then the nucleus pulposus may prolapse through it and may cause sciatica **(Fig. 8)**.

The peripheral annulus fibrosus is composed of series of fibers, arranged in concentric laminae. These concentric fibers in each lamina of annulus fibrosus are arranged in parallel to each other, but run obliquely between the bodies of two adjacent vertebrae. The posterior fibers of this lamina are predominantly vertical which predisposes to herniation of nucleus pulposus. The peripheral fibers of annulus fibrosus consists of collagenous tissue and the inner fibers are made of fibrocartilages tissue which blend with nucleus pulposus without any demarcation. At the front and the behind of the vertebral bodies, the annulus fibrosus blends with the anterior and posterior longitudinal ligaments, respectively. Some fibers of annulus fibrosus sink deeply into the bone and the others are attached to the epiphyseal ring of vertebral bodies.

The nucleus pulposus is a gelatinous mucoidal mass, containing abundant water, cartilage cells, and a few multinucleated notochordal cells in children. In young persons, the water content of nucleus pulposus is about 90%. This produces great turgor or fullness of the disk. In healthy young adults, these intervertebral disks are so strong that the vertebrae may break before the disks are ruptured, during a fall. By the end of the first decade, the notochordal cells disappear and the mucoidal materials are replaced by fibrocartilage. The water content of disks also diminishes with the advancement of age.

Contents of Vertebral Canal from Outward to Inward

- Epidural space (or extradural space)
- Spinal dura mater
- Subdural potential capillary space
- Spinal arachnoid mater
- Spinal subarachnoid space with CSF
- Spinal pia mater (arachnoid mater and pia mater together from leptomeninges)
- Spinal cord, spinal nerves, and cauda equina.

Epidural Space (Extradural Space)

Anatomy of epidural space: It is the space which is bounded between the spinal dura mater and the periosteum of vertebrae **(Fig. 9)**. The periosteum of bony vertebrae is also called the *periosteal dura* and the true dura mater of spinal cord is known as the *spinal dura*. Therefore, it (spinal epidural space) is bounded on one side by spinal dura mater and on another side by (1) the posterior surface of the bodies of vertebrae with posterior longitudinal ligament *(anteriorly)*, (2) the pedicles and intervertebral foramina *(laterally)*, and (3) the lamina and ligamentum flavum *(posteriorly)*. Superiorly, it is closed by the fusion of spinal dura mater with the periosteum of skull bone and vertebral bone (periosteal dura) at the margin of foramen magnum. So, the epidural space does not extend upward into the cranium beyond the foramen magnum. So, the epidural space, present in the vertebral canal, is called the *spinal epidural space*. Below, the spinal dura mater extends only up to the level of S_1 vertebra, so the *subarachnoid space* also extends up to that level inferiorly, but the epidural space extends beyond that level up to the level of sacral hiatus, where it is closed by the sacrococcygeal ligament **(Fig. 10)**.

Through intervertebral foramen, the spinal epidural space communicates with paravertebral space, outside the vertebral canal. The fibrous strands, anchoring the spinal dura mater posteriorly with periosteum (periosteal dura), partly divide the spinal epidural space into two half at

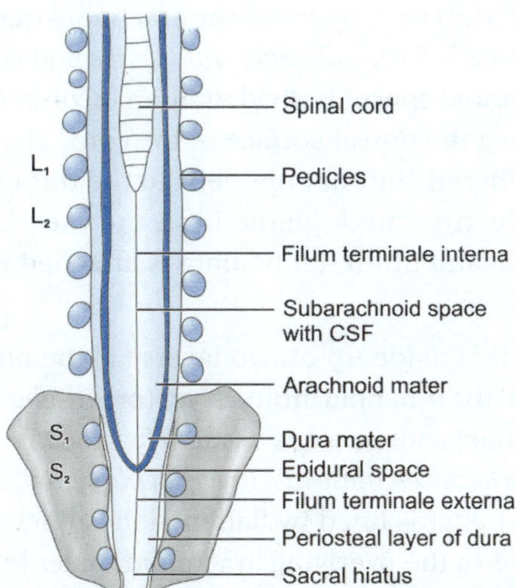

Fig. 10: Diagrammatic longitudinal section through the lower end of vertebral column. (CSF: cerebrospinal fluid)

midline. Actually, in undisturbed state, the spinal epidural space is a potential one, with some loose areolar tissue in the midline and some epidural venous plexus by the side of midline. The spinal dura or the investing layer of dura is in contact with the ligamentum flavum (where periosteum is absent) or with periosteum (where bone is present), but is not adhere to it. After any inflammatory disease, the spinal dura is adhered to the periosteum (periosteal dura) of vertebral bone and the epidural space is obliterated. When an epidural needle passes through ligamentum flavum, then the blunt edge of the needle can contact with spinal dura and push it away. Thus, pushing away the spinal dura from periosteum (or periosteal dura) creates a negative pressure which can be used to verify the proper placement of needle into epidural space. It (pushing away the spinal dura from periosteum) also creates a space which can accept the local anesthetic agent or a catheter pushed into spinal epidural space. The epidural space at each vertebral level must be filled with local anesthetic agent to ensure a complete anesthesia, while the general rule is that 1 mL of anesthetic agent is required for each vertebral segment. But, the range for a normal human being is wide which may vary from 0.8 to 2 mL for each segment, while a catheter with a titrated dose is most commonly used.

The contents of spinal epidural space are:

- Loose areolar tissue
- Loose areolar fat
- 31 pairs of spinal nerves, with dural cuff, on their way to intervertebral foramen
- Sacral and coccygeal nerves
- Spinal arteries, arising from different sources at different levels, enter the epidural space through intervertebral

foramen and supply the spinal cord, spinal nerves, meninges, periosteum, and ligaments.

- *Vertebral venous plexus:* It forms a network of veins, running vertically in epidural space. It can be divided into *anterior epidural venous plexus* and *posterior epidural venous plexus*. The anterior venous plexuses lie anteriorly on the either sides of midline and basivertebral veins empty into it. The posterior venous plexuses lie posteriorly on the either side of midline. These epidural venous plexuses communicate above with intracranial venous sinuses and below with pelvic, portal, and caval system of veins. They also connect with intervertebral veins which pass out through intervertebral foramina and so communicate with (1) vertebral, (2) ascending cervical, (3) deep cervical, (4) intercostals, (5) iliolumbar, and (6) lateral sacral veins. These epidural venous plexuses have no valves. So, these epidural veins become distended during coughing, straining, pregnancy, etc. when the venous pressure rises. Through these valveless veins, blood also can flow in opposite direction during increased intrathoracic and intra-abdominal pressure.

Meninges

The brain and the spinal cord are enveloped by three connective tissue membranes. These are called the meninges and are named from outside inward as the *dura mater, arachnoid mater,* and *pia mater.* The space outside the dura mater is called the *epidural space.* It is bounded between periosteal where bone (lamina) is present and ligamentum flavum where bone is not present on one side and the dura mater on another side. A potential space, which is called the subdural space and is filled with a capillary layer of fluid, intervenes between the dura mater and arachnoid mater. A subarachnoid space appears between the arachnoid mater and the pia mater and is filled with CSF. In some parts of the brain and spinal cord, the subarachnoid space is significantly enlarges forming the *cisterns.* These three meninges primarily support and protect the soft tissues of the brain and spinal cord. Hence, they are surnamed by the word "mater" which means *"the mother for protection".*

Dura mater: It is a thick, fibrous, and nonelastic membrane. In the cranial cavity, this dura mater is arranged in two layers which are called *the periosteal and the investing layer of dura mater.* Here, the periosteal layer of dura mater represent the inner periosteum layer of skull bones and is adhered firmly with the investing layer of dura mater, except where they split to enclose the venous sinuses of cranium. So, *in cranial cavity, there is no epidural space* (as the periosteal and the investing layer of dura mater adhere firmly). In the vertebral column, this cranial periosteal layer of dura mater represents (continuous with) the inner periosteum layer of the bony part of vertebral canal and the cranial investing layer of dura mater represents (continuous with) the dura mater proper of spinal cord (or spinal dura mater) and the space between them is called the *epidural space.*

The investing layer of dura is continued from the cranium into the vertebral canal as spinal dura, but is firmly adhered at the margins of foramen magnum with the periosteal layer. Hence, the epidural space of the vertebral column is closed above at the level of foramen magnum and local anesthetic solution deposited into spinal epidural space of vertebral canal can never enter into the cranial cavity.

Below, this investing layer of dura mater or spinal dura mater ends with arachnoid mater as a tube at the level of first or second sacral vertebra, so that CSF is not found below this level. At the level of S_2 vertebra, the investing layer of dura mater or spinal dura mater ends with arachnoid mater, by giving a covering layer to the *FT interna.* This FT interna is now known as the *filum terminale externa* with the coverings of dura and arachnoid mater and goes down to blend with the periosteum on the back of coccyx. The anterior and the posterior nerve roots issuing from the spinal cord pierce the dura and carry a tubular prolongation of dural sheath (dural cuffs) which blends ultimately with the perineurium of mixed spinal nerve. In the vertebral canal, the spinal dura is loosely attached anteriorly by fibrous stands to the posterior longitudinal ligaments and thus anchors its place anteriorly. Similarly, it is loosely attached posteriorly by fibrous strands to the vertebral arch and thus anchors its place posteriorly.

Arachnoid mater: The word "arachnoid mater" owes its name from a Greek word named "arachnes" which means "spider". In the cranial cavity and vertebral canal, this meningeal layer is so named, because the *numerous spiders like trabecular structures extend between the arachnoid and the pia mater through CSF in subarachnoid space.* It does not follow the pia mater so intimately to line the every indentation of brain and spinal cord which the pia mater does. The arachnoid mater is a thin, delicate, and transparent structure. It constitutes the middle of the three investing membranes (dura, arachnoid, and pia), covering the brain, and spinal cord. *The spinal arachnoid mater is the continuation of cerebral arachnoid mater* and is closely applied (but, not yet attached) to dura mater. The *subdural space* (between the dura and arachnoid mater) is a potential capillary space, containing little serous fluid (but not CSF) and possibly such a thin film of fluid exerts a negative force of traction which keeps the arachnoid mater in contact with dura mater and prevents the arachnoid mater from projecting inward from

dura mater. The space between the arachnoid mater and the pia mater is called the *subarachnoid space* and contain CSF. It (subarachnoid space) is divided by an incomplete midline septum along the dorsal surface of the cord. The arachnoid mater is adhered (but not applied) to the dura mater only where some structures pierce both the membranes and where the ligamentum denticulata is attached to the dura mater.

Pia mater: It is made up of two layers (1) the outer *epi-pia layer* and (2) the inner pia intima layer (or *pia-glia layer*) lying in close contact with nervous tissue. *The blood vessels of CNS actually run between these two layers of pia mater.* The epi-pia layer of pia mater is lined by flattened mesothelial cells and is connected to the overlying arachnoid mater by a number of trabecular structures through CSF in subarachnoid space. These trabeculae are called the *arachnoid trabeculae. The blood vessels enter the tissue of CNS by piercing the dura and arachnoid mater and then extend through these trabecular structures (arachnoid trabeculae) from arachnoid mater to pia mater through CSF in subarachnoid space and finally ramify between the epi-pia and pia-glia layer of pia mater.* The intercommunicating space around the arachnoid trabeculae in subarachnoid space, contains CSF.

The pia intima or pia-glia layer of pia mater covers intimately the surfaces of nervous tissue of brain and spinal cord. It (pia-glia layer) consists of mesothelial cells, held on a mesh work of reticular, elastic, and collagen fibers and ultimately rests on a basement membrane which is lined internally by the foot plates of astrocytes. Posteriorly, the pia mater is adherent to the posterior medial septum of spinal cord and is also connected to arachnoid mater through the CSF of subarachnoid space by a fenestrated subarachnoid septum. Anteriorly, the pia mater is folded into the anterior median fissure of spinal cord. On each side, between the ventral and dorsal root of spinal nerve, the pia mater forms a narrow vertical ridge, with tooth-like processes, projecting from its lateral free border. This is called the *ligamentum denticulatum* (**Fig. 9**) and is attached to the dura mater through arachnoid mater, between the two roots of spinal nerves. These processes help to suspend the spinal cord in the middle of subarachnoid space. The blood vessels, going to brain and spinal cord, lie in the subarachnoid space along the trabecular structure, before piercing the pia. They (blood vessels) carry with them a sleeve of pia mater in the tissue of brain and spinal cord.

Filum terminale: It starts as a thread-like structure, at the level of L_1 or L_2 vertebra, from the terminal end of spinal cord (conus medullaris). It has two parts. The first part of FT is named as *FT interna* and the second part of FT is named as the *FT externa.* The FT interna is composed of only pia mater and its length is about 15 cm. It extends from the apex of conus medullaris to S_2 vertebra. It then continues below S_2 vertebra as FT externa, by piercing the arachnoid and dura mater at the level of S_2 vertebra and then ends eventually by blending with periosteum at the back of coccyx. The FT externa is about 5 cm in length and is composed of dura, arachnoid, and pia mater.

Subarachnoid Space

It is a CSF-filled wide space lying between the pia and arachnoid mater and surrounds the entire CNS like water a bath. The spinal subarachnoid space is wider than its cerebral counterpart. In spinal or vertebral canal, it is widest below L1 vertebra where spinal cord ends to continue as cauda equina. Below L_1 vertebra, the subarachnoid space contains CSF and cauda equina **(Fig. 11)**.

Cerebrospinal Fluid: Cerebrospinal fluid is a clear, colorless liquid with pH of 7.4. The average volume of CSF in adult is near about 135 mL, of which 35 mL is in the ventricle, 25 mL is in the cerebral subarachnoid space, and 75 mL is in the spinal subarachnoid space. Choroid plexus in the ventricles secrets CSF at a rate of 0.3–0.4 mL/min. The normal glucose content of CSF is 2.5–4.4 mmol/L (45–80 mg/dL) and protein content is 20 mg/dL. The normal albumin and globulin ratio in CSF is 1:1. After spinal anesthesia, the albumin level in CSF rises and becomes double of its normal value on 18th day. The normal CSF pressure varies from 70 to 180 mm H_2O in lateral position to 375–550 mm H_2O in vertical posture. During epidural anesthesia, the increased pressure in the epidural space is transmitted to the subarachnoid space and hence the sensation of dizziness is felt by the patient. The specific gravity of CSF at body temperature, compared to

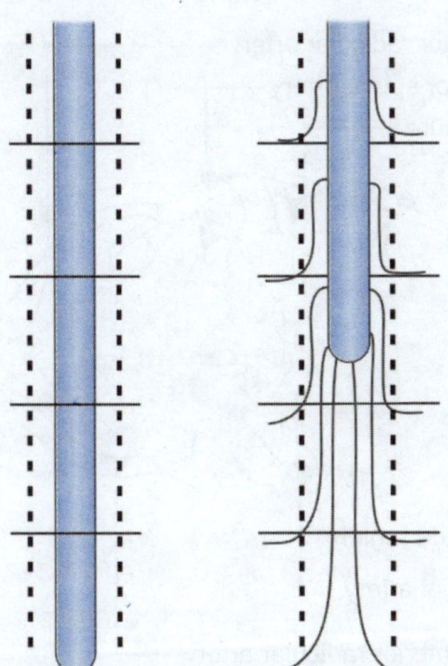

Fig. 11: The effect of recession of spinal cord, during its development, on the course of spinal nerves.

water is 1.007, whereas the specific gravity of 10% dextrose which is commonly used to make the anesthetic solution hyperbaric is 1.034.

Spinal Cord

The spinal cord, as a part of CNS, is the continuation of brain. It is an elongated and cylindrical neural structure and is contained within the upper two-thirds of vertebral canal. Although cylindrical, it is somewhat flattened ventrodorsally (anteroposteriorly). It retains actually the primitive form of CNS which is present in all the animals. The spinal cord is mainly concerned with the reception of different sensory impulses (information), their integration and association of these sensory impulses, and then production (output) of reflex (motor) responses of basic characters. It is the direct continuation of medulla oblongata of brain. *Spinal cord begins at the upper border of atlas at the level of foramen magnum and ends, in adult, as a conical structure named conus medullaris, at the level of lower border of L_1 vertebra or upper border of L_2 vertebra.* The apex of conus meduladris is continued down as FT interna at first part and then as FT externa in second part.

The length of a spinal cord is about 42–45 cm in an adult individual. Sometimes, it extends up to the second or even, more rarely, up to the third lumbar vertebra. In newborn the spinal cord extends up to the third lumbar vertebra and in fetal life the cord extends the entire length of vertebral canal up to the last sacral vertebra. At the 3rd month of fetal life, the length of the spinal cord is as long as the vertebral canal and each spinal nerve arises from the cord at the level of their corresponding intervertebral foramen. During the subsequent development, the spinal cord does not grow as fast as the vertebral column. Therefore, the lower end of spinal cord gradually ascends to reach the level of third lumbar vertebra at the time of birth, and the lower border of first lumbar vertebra in adult.

As a result of this relative upward migration of spinal cord, the roots of spinal nerves have to follow an oblique and downward course to reach their appropriate (corresponding) intervertebral foramen **(Fig. 11)**. This obliquity is most marked in the lumbar spinal nerves and many of these roots occupy the vertebral canal below the level of the terminal end of spinal cord. So, below the first lumbar vertebra the vertebral canal is occupied by the leash of lumbar, sacral, and coccygeal spinal nerve roots, termed as the *cauda equina.* Another result of this upward recession of spinal cord is that the *spinal segments do not lie opposite to their corresponding number of vertebrae.* In estimating the position of spinal segment and spinal nerves in relation to the surface of the body and spine of vertebra, it is found that the later (the spine of vertebrae) is always lower than their corresponding spinal segment. *As a rough guide, it may be stated that in the cervical region there is a difference of one segment (e.g., the fifth cervical spine overlies the sixth cervical spinal segment), in the upper thoracic region there is a difference of two segments (e.g., the fourth thoracic spine overlies the sixth thoracic spinal segment), in the lower thoracic region there is a difference of three segments (e.g., the ninth thoracic spine lies opposite the 12th thoracic spinal segment).* The spinal cord has two enlargements, such as cervical and lumbar, corresponding to their increased nerve supply to the upper and lower limbs. The cervical enlargement extends from C_3 to T_2 spinal segment and the lumbar enlargement extends from T_9 to L_1 spinal segment.

Blood Supply of Spinal Cord

The spinal cord is mainly supplied by *two posterior and one anterior spinal artery*. The posterior spinal arteries, one on each side of the midline, arise from the *posterior inferior cerebellar arteries* at the level of the base of the skull. It supplies the posterior horn of gray matter and the posterior columns of white matter and is reinforced by the numerous posterior radicular arteries, arising from the ascending cervical artery, deep cervical artery, intercostal artery, and the lumbar artery. The single anterior spinal artery is formed by the union of two small branches, each of which arises from the vertebral artery of that side at the level of foramen magnum **(Figs. 12 and 13)**.

The reinforcement of anterior spinal artery, at the level of every vertebra, is few and irregular. But, one radicular artery, reinforcing the anterior spinal artery at the level of T_{11} segment, supplies the lumbar enlargement of spinal cord and is constant. This is called the *radicular magna or artery of Adamkiewicz*. The anterior spinal artery supplies the anterior and the lateral columns of white matter and most of the gray matter. The branches of anterior and posterior spinal arteries do not anastomose with each other and thus creates three distinct vascular areas in spinal cord, with no anastomoses between them. Hence, this arrangement makes the cord more prone to damage by hypotension, thrombosis, vasoconstriction, aortic clamping, etc. **(Fig. 14)**.

Anterior Spinal Artery Syndrome

It is due to the damage of the anterior and lateral columns of cord, due to the thrombosis of anterior spinal artery and is manifested as paraplegia. But, there is retention of the sensation of posterior column which includes touch, pain, pressure, temperature, joint position, vibration, etc.

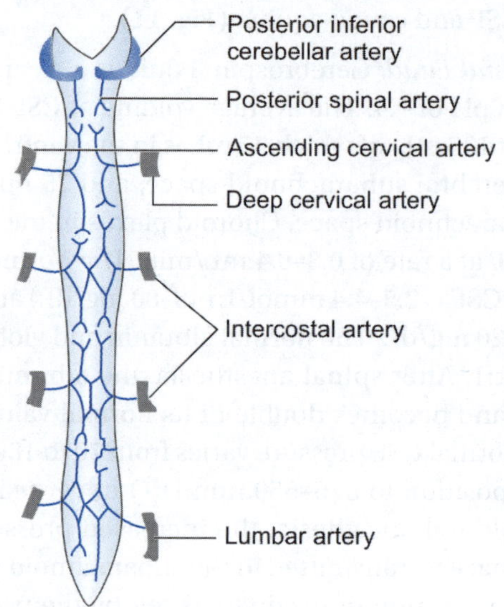

Fig. 13: Posterior arterial trunk of spinal cord.

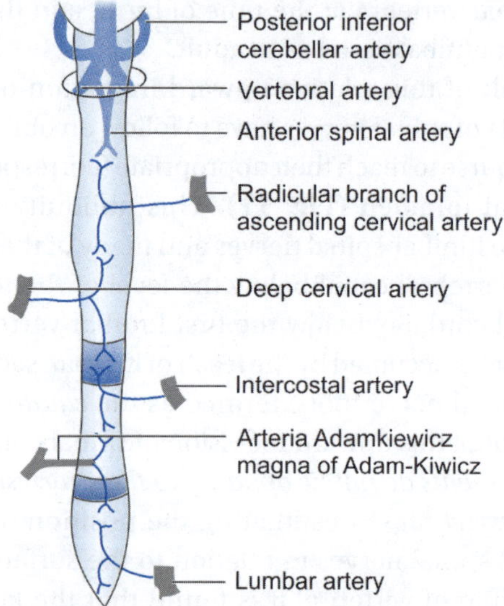

Fig. 12: Anterior arterial trunk of spinal cord.

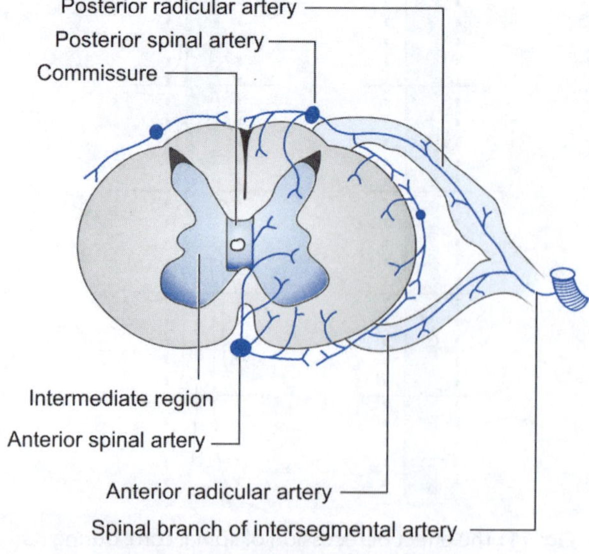

Fig. 14: Arterial supply of spinal cord.

Venous Drainage of Spinal Cord

It is done by the anterior and posterior venous plexuses of spinal cord. These venous plexuses of spinal cord ultimately drain into the vertebral, azygos, and lumbar veins by some small veins which are passed through the intervertebral foramina. The normal intraspinal capillary pressure is 30 mm Hg. The deprivation of blood supply of spinal cord for 2 minutes may result in the infarction of cord.

■ SPINAL NERVES

The spinal cord gives attachment on its either side to a series of *31 pairs of spinal nerves.* These spinal nerves are eight cervicals, 12 thoracics, five lumbars, five sacrals, and one coccygeal. Each spinal nerve arises from spinal cord by two roots—anterior (or ventral) and posterior (or dorsal). Again each nerve root is formed by the aggregation of several numbers of rootlets that arise from the cord over a certain length **(Fig. 15)**. The length of the spinal cord, giving origin to the rootlets for one spinal nerve, constitutes one spinal segment. So, the spinal cord is made up of (divided into) 31 spinal segments, such as eight cervical, 12 thoracic, five lumbar, five sacral, and one coccygeal. The anterior or ventral root of a spinal nerve contains motor fibers (both intrafusal and extrafusal) to the skeletal muscles of trunk and limbs and in some places preganglionic autonomic sympathetic (motor) fibers to the glands, smooth muscles of internal organs, and blood vessels. The dorsal or posterior or sensory roots convey the sensory fibers from the peripheral general exteroceptive receptors from the skin and subcutaneous tissues carrying sensation of pain, temperature, touch, pressure, etc. and general proprioceptive sensations from the muscles, bones, and joints. Some fibers convey, in addition, general visceral sensations including visceral pain from internal organs and blood vessels.

Both the anterior (ventral) and posterior (dorsal) roots of spinal nerve receive a small tubular prolongation from the spinal meninges (arachnoid and dura mater, not pia mater) and enter their corresponding intervertebral foramen. Then, there (in intervertebral foramen) they unite to form a mixed spinal nerve and comes out of foramen. Just before joining with the ventral root, the dorsal root presents a spinal ganglion (dorsal root ganglion) and it usually lodges in the corresponding intervertebral foramen. After coming out of the spinal cord and piercing the pia mater within the vertebral (spinal) canal, the spinal nerve roots first run in the subarachnoid space and carry a sleeve of CSF within the tubular prolongation of meninges (arachnoid mater and dura mater) up to the intervertebral foramen where they (spinal nerves) pierce the arachnoid and dura mater. After piercing the arachnoid mater and dura mater in the intervertebral foramen, when the spinal nerves come out, then the arachnoid covering blends with the perineurium and the dura covering blends with the epineurium of the spinal nerves.

Each spinal ganglion which is present on the dorsal root of spinal nerves contains 50,000–100,000 unipolar neurons. The axon of each neuron of these spinal roots (dorsal) ganglion sends a single *peripheral process* into the mixed spinal nerve to carry the sensory impulses from the target organs of periphery and sends *a central process* to the dorsal horn of spinal cord, through their dorsal root. It is roughly estimated that the number of sensory fibers in a dorsal nerve root is about 50,000–100,000, whereas the number of motor fibers in a ventral nerve root is about 5,000. In more than half of the population, the first cervical and the coccygeal spinal nerve present no dorsal root.

The upper seven cervical spinal nerves leave their respective intervertebral foramina above the pedicles of their respective vertebrae. The eighth cervical nerve emerges below the pedicles of seventh cervical vertebra. Then, eventually all the thoracic, lumbar, and sacral spinal nerves emerge below the pedicles of their corresponding vertebrae. Due to the cranial shift of spinal cord, during its development with increased age, the spinal nerve roots become progressively oblique from above downward. In the lumbosacral regions, the roots of spinal nerve descend almost vertically and form a bunch of nerves, known as the cauda equina. It is so named because it resembles to the tail of a horse. *This cauda equina is formed (around the non-nervous pial filament which is called the filum terminale interna), by the roots of five pairs (below L_1 or L_2) of lumbar, five pairs of sacral and one pair of coccygeal spinal nerves.*

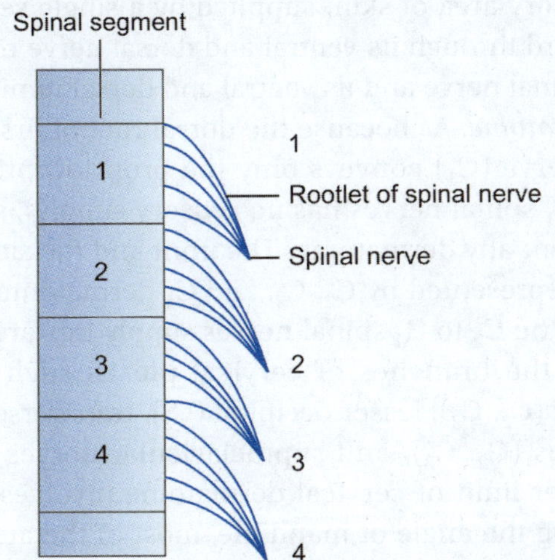

Fig. 15: Scheme to illustrate the concept of spinal segment and spinal nerve.

After emerging through the intervertebral foramen, each mixed spinal nerve (formed by the joining of ventral motor and dorsal sensory root—so called mixed nerve) divides immediately into its dorsal and ventral primary rami. Thus, each ramus receives fibers from both the motor (ventral) and sensory (dorsal) roots, i.e., each ramus has both the sensory and motor fibers. Immediately after division, the *dorsal primary ramus* passes backward and supplies the muscles (motor) and the skin (sensory) of back. It is to be noted that the C_1 spinal nerve has no cutaneous branch (dorsal root) and the dorsal rami of C_7, C_8, L_4, and L_5 spinal nerves do not supply the skin. In the neck, the dorsal ramus of cervical spinal nerves supplies the splenius and other neck muscles deep to it. After piercing and supplying the muscles, the dorsal ramus again divides into medial and lateral branches to supply the skin segmentally. In general, the extensor muscles of vertebral column (motor), the scalp, and the varying extent of skin over these muscles (sensory) are supplied by the dorsal ramus.

The *ventral ramus* (not root) supplies (1) the prevertebral flexor group of muscles of neck and trunk, (2) the muscles of thorax and abdominal wall, (3) the muscles of upper and lower extremities (motor), and (4) the skin of the sides and the front of the neck and trunk and extremities (sensory). The prevertebral flexor group of muscles include the longus capitis, longus colli, scalene, psoas, quadratus lumborum, etc. and piriformis. *In neck*, the ventral rami of eight cervical spinal nerves supply to the prevertebral group of muscles in neck. *In the trunk*, the ventral ramus of 12 thoracic and first lumbar spinal nerves supplies the intercostal muscles and their overlaying skin, segmentally. The ventral rami of upper 11 thoracic spinal nerves form the intercostal nerves and that of 12 thoracic spinal nerves form the subcostal nerve. The ventral ramus of first lumbar spinal nerve is distributed via the iliohypogastric and ilioinguinal nerve. Each intercostal nerve supplies the muscles of intercostal space. But, the lower six intercostal nerves pass beyond the costal margin to supply the flat muscles of anterior abdomen and rectus abdominis. Moreover, the ventral rami of spinal nerves (which are also called the roots of plexus) form the cervical, brachial, lumbar, and sacral plexuses at their respective places. The skin and the muscles of upper limbs are supplied from *brachial plexuses* and those of lower limbs are supplied from *lumbosacral plexuses*.

Out of these 31 pairs of spinal nerves, only 14 pairs (12 thoracic and 2 lumbar) of spinal nerves are connected with the sympathetic chain by white rami communicantes, containing preganglionic sympathetic fibers. While all the spinal nerves (including these above 14 pairs) are connected with the sympathetic chain by their gray rami communicantes, containing postganglionic sympathetic fibers. The white rami communicantes contain the preganglionic sympathetic fibers, arising from the lateral horn cells of spinal cord, extending between T_1 and L_2 segment of it. After arising from the lateral horn cells of spinal cord, the preganglionic sympathetic fibers reach the sympathetic chain by the white rami communicantes and make connection with the postganglionic sympathetic fibers at the corresponding ganglion in the sympathetic chain or pass uninterruptedly to the upper or lower ganglion of this sympathetic chain, where they make synapses with the postganglionic fibers. Thus, the postganglionic fibers arise from all the sympathetic ganglia, situated on the sympathetic chain, and are then carried by the gray rami communicantes to all the mixed spinal nerves. Thus, the sympathetic chains get its inflow from only the 14 pairs of white rami communicantes from 14 pairs of spinal nerves (T_1-L_2), but have 31 pairs of gray rami communicantes for outflow to all the spinal nerves. Hence, each of the 31 pairs of spinal nerves receive the gray rami communicantes from sympathetic trunk and conveys the postganglionic sympathetic fibers (nonmyelinated) to supply throughout the whole body, except the abdominal and thoracic visceras and the structures of head and neck. The structures of head and neck get their sympathetic supply by cranial nerves. The thoracic visceras get their sympathetic supply through pulmonary and cardiac plexus and abdominal visceras get their sympathetic supply through splanchnic nerves. These sympathetic fibers supplying the thoracic and abdominal visceras arise directly from the ganglion of sympathetic chain. They do not pass through spinal nerves. Thus, the sympathetic system innervates the entire body wall and all the four limbs through 31 pairs of spinal nerves.

■ DERMATOMES

The sensory area of skin, supplied by a single segment of spinal cord through its ventral and dorsal nerve root, i.e., a single spinal nerve and its ventral and dorsal rami, is called the *dermatome*. As because the dorsal root of first cervical spinal nerve (C_1) conveys only the proprioceptive fibers (or the C_1 spinal nerves has no sensory supply), so it does not present any dermatome. The front and the sides of the neck is represented by C_2, C_3, and C_4 dermatomes. This is because the C_2 to C_4 spinal nerves supply this area of skin through the branches of cervical plexus such as great auricular (C_2, C_3), lesser occipital (C_2), transverse cervical cutaneous (C_2, C_3), and supraclavicular nerves (C_3, C_4). The upper limit of cervical dermatome involves the skin overlaying the angle of mandible, most of the auricle and the occipital region of scalp. Above that limit, the cervical dermatome meets with the sensory area supplied by the Vth cranial nerve (trigeminal N). Below, the cervical dermatome

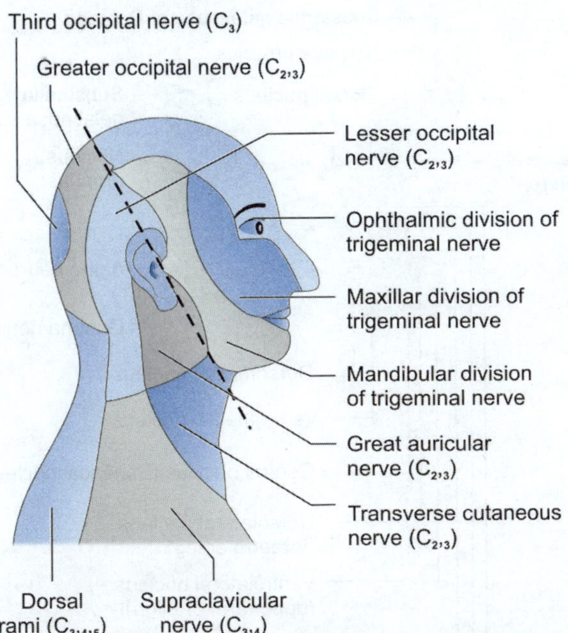

Fig. 16: The segmental innervation of scalp, neck, and face. One side of the dashed line is supplied by cranial trigeminal nerve and another side is by spinal nerves.

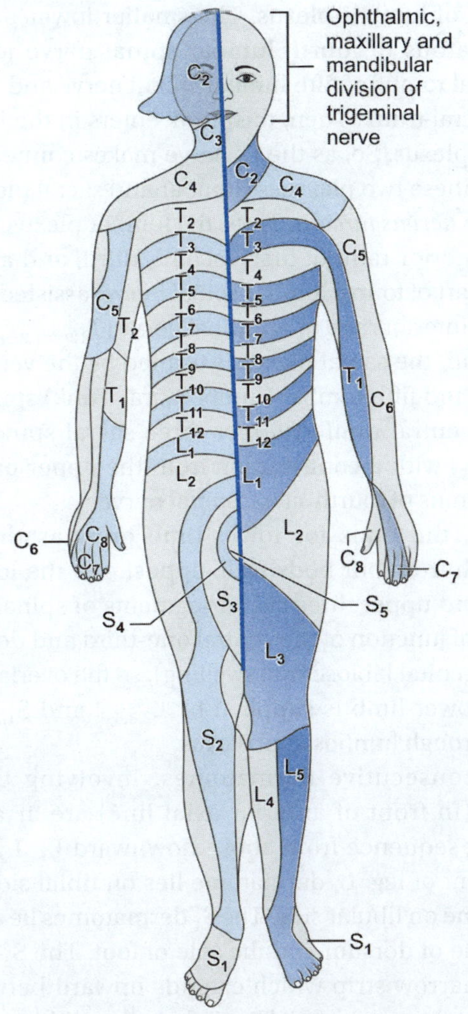

Fig. 17: The illustration of dermatomes.

extends up to the sternal angle in front and over the rounded shoulder laterally **(Fig. 16)**.

The dermatomes of trunk are represented by T_2 to L_1 spinal nerves and are arranged in regular series, like strips. On the body, the adjacent dermatomes overlap on each other considerably. So, the interruption of a single dermatome does not produce any effect on RA. At the level of sternal angle, the C_4 and T_2 dermatomes meet. This is because, the missing C_5, C_6, C_7, C_8, and T_1 dermatomes are carried over by the branches of brachial plexus and supply the upper limb which develops as the lateral outgrowth from body wall.

The upper limb is supplied by the nerves of brachial plexus which is formed by the spinal nerves, arising from the cervical enlargement of spinal cord. The brachial plexus is formed by the ventral rami (which form the root or starting point of plexus) of C_5, C_6, C_7, C_8, and T_1 spinal nerves. The brachial plexus consists of roots (the ventral ramus of spinal nerve), trunks, and cords. The five roots (the ventral rami of spinal nerves) of brachial plexus which extend from C_5 to T_1 emerge through the interval between scalenus anterior and scalenus medius muscles.

The anterior division of brachial plexus supplies the flexor compartment and the posterior division supplies the extensor compartment of the muscles of upper limb. The flexor group of muscles possesses richer innervation than that of the extensor group of muscles, because their actions are more powerful and precise. This explains why the most caudal roots of the brachial plexus which is derived from T_1, is distributed entirely to the muscles of flexor compartment. This same principle is also applicable to the lumbosacral plexus, where the S_3 root supplies all the muscles of the flexor compartment of lower limb **(Fig. 17)**.

The extreme peripheral end of upper limb is supplied by the central dermatomes. Thus, (1) the radial side of the arm of upper limb is supplied by C_5, (1) the radial side of the forearm is supplied by C_6, (3) the middle three fingers with their adjacent palmar and their dorsal surfaces is supplied by C_7, (4) the little finger with the ulnar side of forearm is supplied by C_8, and (4) the ulnar side of arm is supplied by the T_1 segments. The dermatomes overlaying the deltoid and the bottom of axilla are borrowed from neck and trunk and are supplied respectively by the C_4 and T_2 spinal segments.

Each lower limb is supplied by lumbar and sacral plexus of that side which is formed by the spinal nerves, arising from the lumbar enlargement of spinal cord. The lumbar plexus is formed by the ventral rami of upper three lumbar spinal nerves and the larger upper part of the ventral ramus of fourth lumbar spinal nerve (L_1 to L_4). These are called the roots of lumbar plexus. The smaller lower part of the ventral ramus of fourth lumbar spinal nerve joins with the ventral ramus of fifth lumbar spinal nerve and forms the lumbosacral trunk. Then, this trunk enters in the formation of sacral plexus. So, as the L_4 nerve makes connecting link between these two plexuses (lumbar and sacral plexus), it is called the *nervus furcalis*. Thus, the lumbar plexus is formed by the anterior rami of first, second, third, and ascending (larger) part of fourth lumbar spinal nerve, assisted by a twig from the anterior rami of T_{12} spinal nerve (T_{12}, $L_{1,2,3,4}$). On the other hand, the sacral plexus is formed by the ventral rami of fourth and fifth lumbar (lumbosacral trunk) spinal nerve and the ventral rami of upper three sacral spinal nerves ($L_{4,5}$, $S_{1,2,3}$) with a contribution from the upper part of the ventral ramus of fourth sacral spinal nerve.

Since, the buds for lower limb grow as the lateral outgrowth from our body wall, opposite to the lower four lumbar and upper three sacral segments of spinal cord (at the level of junction of the ventral one-third and dorsal two-thirds of genital labioscrotal swelling), so the overlaying skin of each lower limb is supplied by $L_{2,3,4,5}$, and $S_{1,2,3}$ spinal nerves through lumbosacral plexus.

The consecutive dermatomes, involving the front of thigh (in front of anterior axial line) are arranged in following sequence from above downward L_1, L_2, and L_3. In the front of leg, L_4 dermatome lies on tibial side and L_5 dermatome on fibular side. The S_1 dermatomes lie along the lateral side of dorsum and the sole of foot. The S_2 segment forms a narrow strip which extends upward between the anterior and posterior axial lines along the middle of the calf and the back of the thigh. The S_3 segment involves a wide semicircular area around the anus and between the axial lines of two sides. The S_4 segment supplies the adjacent perianal skin.

MICROSCOPIC STRUCTURE OF THE SPINAL CORD

On cross section the spinal cord presents a white matter at its periphery and a butterfly like gray matter at its center.

Gray Matter

The gray matter consists of nerve cells, neuroglial cells, and blood vessels. In the center of the spinal cord, this gray matter is arranged as H-shaped manner. So, it is butterfly in shape. All the nerve cells in this area are nonmyelinated, and so it is gray in color. The gray matter presents (1) a pair of ventral horns, (2) a pair of dorsal horns, (3) an intermediate region which intervenes between the ventral and dorsal horns, and (4) a commissure which connects the symmetrical halves of gray matter of each side, across the midline. The *ventral horns* are broader than the dorsal horns and are further broader in

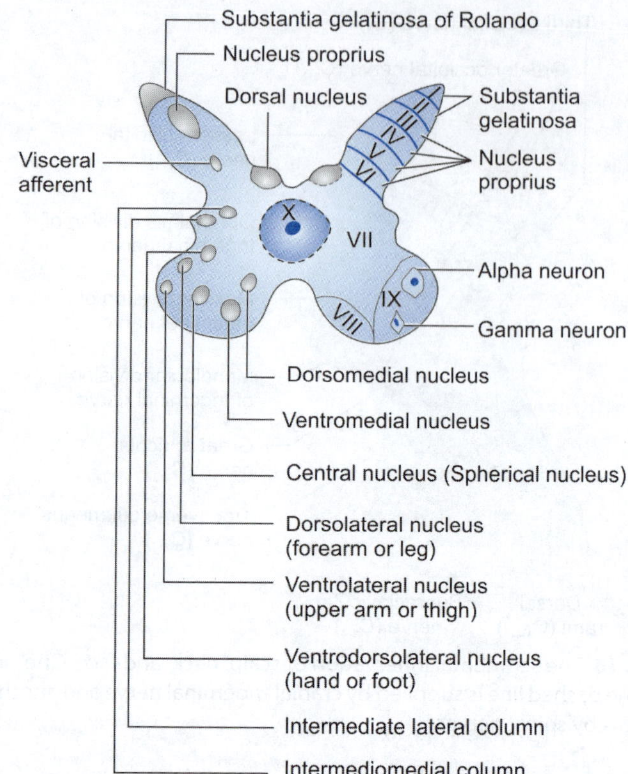

Fig. 18: Schematic representation of gray matter.

the cervical and lumbar region than the thoracic region to accommodate the numerous motor neurons, suppling the muscles of upper and lower limbs. The *dorsal horn* consists of an apex, head, neck, and a base. The base is continuous with the intermediate region of gray matter. The apex of dorsal horn is caped with a translucent mass of nerve tissue, called the *substantia gelatinosa of Rolando* which allows the entry of sensory impulses through dorsal nerve roots. The intermediate region of gray matter intervenes between the bases of the ventral and dorsal horns and lies lateral to the commissure. In thoracic and upper two lumbar regions, this intermediate region forms some lateral projections, which are called the *lateral horns*. These lateral horns are the center of peripheral sympathetic output (**Fig. 18**).

The gray commissure is longitudinally traversed by a *central canal,* containing CSF. It is lined by ependymal cells and is continuous above with the cavity of fourth ventricle, through the central canal of medulla oblongata. Within the conus medullaris of spinal cord, at lumbar region, the central canal is dilated to form the terminal ventricle. It may also extend for a distance of about 4–5 mm into the proximal part of the FT interna. The central canal is surrounded by neuroglial tissue, called the *substantia gelatinosa centralis.*

The anterior or ventral horn of gray matter contains *motor neurons* and *interneurons* (internuncial or connector neurons. *Renshaw cell* is a type of interneuron). The motor neurons send axon fibers to the muscles. The interneurons or internuncial neurons possess small cell bodies and their processes are confined within the gray matter. They connect between the axons of sensory neurons situated in the dorsal horns and the cell body of motor neurons situated in the ventral horn, and is responsible for reflex activities. Their reflex activities may be intrasegmental or intersegmental, and ipsilateral or contralateral. Sometimes, the axons of sensory neurons, present in dorsal horn, make direct connection with the motor neurons of ventral horn, without the intervention of internuncial neurons. This is called the *monosynaptic relays*. The interneuron or internuncial neurons may be *excitatory or inhibitory*. But a particular interneuron cannot act in both ways. *The Renshaw cell is the classical example of inhibitory interneuron*. The neurochemical transmitter substance of inhibitory synapses within the spinal cord is usually glycine while the inhibitory neurotransmitter substance in the brain is γ-aminobutyric acid (GABA).

The motor neurons in the anterior horn of gray matter is of three types, i.e., *(1) alpha (α), (2) beta (β), and (3) gamma (γ)*. The axons of these motor neurons leave the spinal cord through the ventral *root* of their corresponding spinal nerve and then reach the effector striated muscles through the ventral and dorsal *ramus* which are the branches of this (mixed) spinal nerve (mixed spinal nerve, commonly called the spinal nerve, is formed by the union of the ventral root and the dorsal root which are coming out of the spinal cord). The cell bodies of α-neuron are large and their axons are thickly myelinated, conducting at a velocity of about 15–120 m/second. These axons end on striated muscles by forming *motor end plate* over the individual muscle fiber *(extrafusal fiber)*. The number of muscle fibers or muscle cells supplied by a single α (alpha) neuron is known as the *motor unit*, which may be large or small. The larger motor unit includes 100–200 muscle fibers or more (supplied by one motor neuron) and is concerned with the gross voluntary body muscle movements. The smaller motor unit is comprised of 5–10 muscle fibers and appears in skillful muscle movements, such as the movements of the fingers of hand and eyeballs.

On the other hand, a *single α-neuron* may receive 1,000 or more synaptic connections from (1) interneurons or (2) from the sensory fibers of dorsal roots with their cell bodies lying at dorsal root ganglia or (3) from the descending fibers of upper motor neurons. These synapses may be excitatory or inhibitory. The α-motor neurons also receive connections from (4) muscle spindles, corticospinal tract and vestibulospinal tract. Sometimes, the axons of α-neurons provide collateral branches which make synapses with the cell body of *Renshaw cell type of interneurons*, situated in the anterior gray column (ventral horn). In turn, the axons

of Renshaw cells send impulse to inhibit the corresponding α-neurons and prevent excessive α firing. On occasions, the Renshaw cells also inhibit the adjacent α-neurons and suppress the action of antagonistic muscles at the same time.

The *γ-neurons* are small in size and their axons are thinly myelinated, conducting at velocity of 10–45 m/second. The simple act of picking up a pencil from the table not only employs the α-motor pathways, but also engage (send impulses through) some afferent pathways which reach the spinal cord from the sensory endings of skin, joints, and the muscles spindle of hand and fingers muscle to control the total skeletal muscle movement of hand and to pick up the pencil. In fact, the *muscles spindles* are the *sensory end-organ* of skeletal muscles and are responsible for signaling the degree of shortening or lengthening of whole skeletal muscle. In this way, they can provide information, so that only the exact amount of skeletal muscle activity which is required for the task is used.

Histologically, the muscle spindle is an elongated and encapsulated structure which lies in parallel with the skeletal muscle fibers and shares its attachment **(Fig. 19)**. This latter point is of particular importance, as its principle function is to signal the exact length of skeletal muscle fiber. Within the capsule of muscle spindle, small specialized *intrafusal fibers* can be recognized as *(1) the nuclear bag fiber and (2) the nuclear chain fiber*. The γ-neuron (motor), present at the anterior horn of gray matter, supplies to the contractile polar regions of both the nuclear bag and nuclear chain type of intrafusal fibers of muscle spindle. The noncontractile equatorial region of intrafusal fibers are supplied by the general sensory nerve endings which act as stretch receptors and convey the sensory impulses when the polar regions contract, subsequent to the (1) excitation of γ-neuron, and control the amount of contraction, or (2) when the entire muscle is passively stretched to control the amount of the length of muscle.

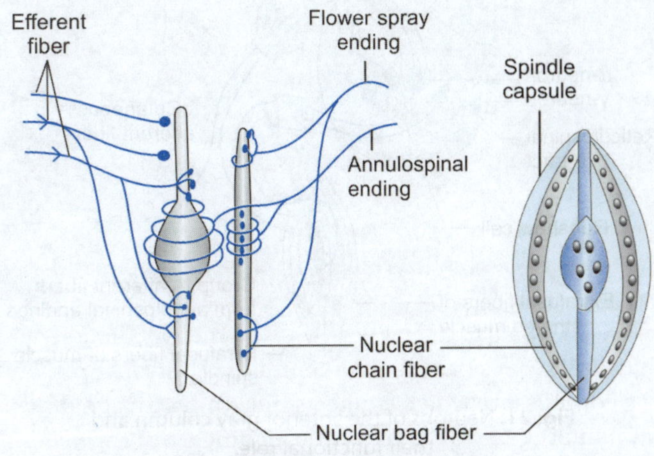

Fig. 19: Neuromuscular spindle.

The cell bodies of both the sets of sensory afferent fibers are located in the dorsal root ganglia of posterior nerve root and their central process reach the spinal cord through the dorsal nerve root and make the monosynaptic connection directly or through internuncial neurons with the α-neurons which supply the extrafusal fibers of corresponding skeletal muscle **(Figs. 20 and 21)**. Therefore, the α-neurons are excited and the whole muscle is thrown into contraction, until it shortens to equal with the degree of the contraction of muscle spindle, controlled by γ-neuron. This method of control of contraction of a voluntary muscle fiber, by the γ-reflex loop, maintains its residual length, even in resting condition and without any influence from higher center.

The γ-loop acts as a servomechanism and forms the basis of the reflex control of residual muscle tone. The function of intrafusal fibers is to inform the CNS, through the γ-loop, about the length and the rate of change in the length of extrafusal fibers, whereas the α-neurons on stimulation produce the final shortening of muscles without limit, but the γ-neurons cause the muscle to contract to a predetermined length. The activities of γ-neurons are controlled by both the pyramidal and extrapyramidal fibers which may be excitatory or inhibitory. Considerable control of these motor neurons is exerted directly by reticular system and indirectly by cerebellum and basal ganglia.

The cell body and the axon of β-neurons are intermediate in size and diameter. Their axons supply both the extrafusal muscle fibers and the intrafusal fibers of muscle spindle.

There are four sets of neuronal column in the dorsal horn of gray matter. From the apex to the base of it, they (the sets of neuronal column) are named as follows: (1) *Substantia gelatinosa of Rolando*, (2) *nucleus proprius (NP)*, (3) *Clarke's column (nucleus dorsalis)*, and (4) *visceral afferent nucleus (VAN)* **(Fig. 22)**. The *substantia gelatinosa (SG)* is composed of cell body of sensory neurons and the small- and medium-sized cell body of interneurons. It extends along the entire length of spinal cord. Traced above, it is continuous with the nucleus of the spinal tract of trigeminal nerve. The SG

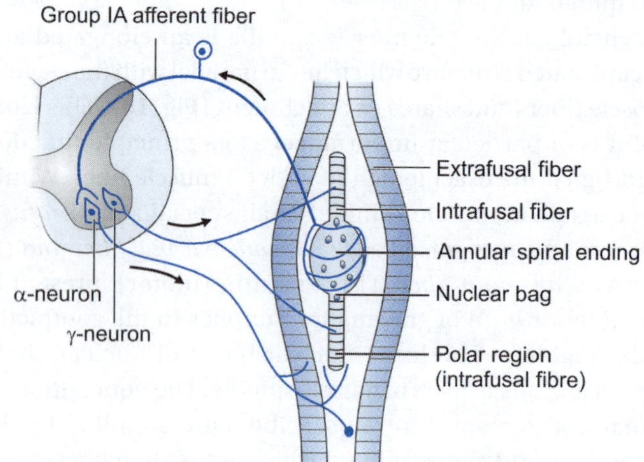

Fig. 20: Pathways of active stretch reflex.

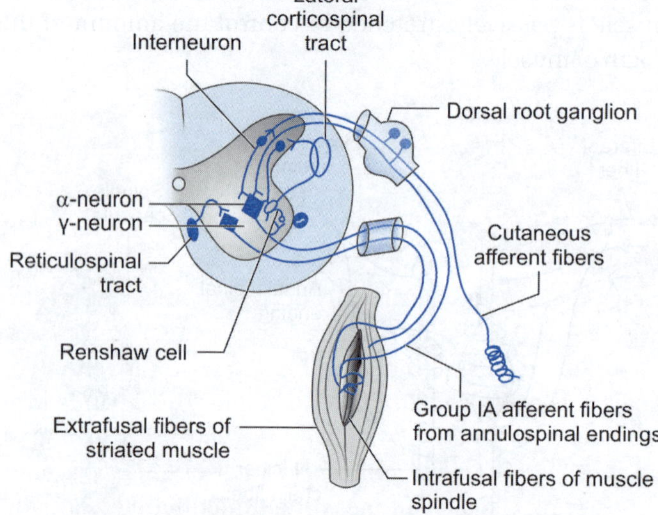

Fig. 21: Neurons of the anterior gray column and their functional role.

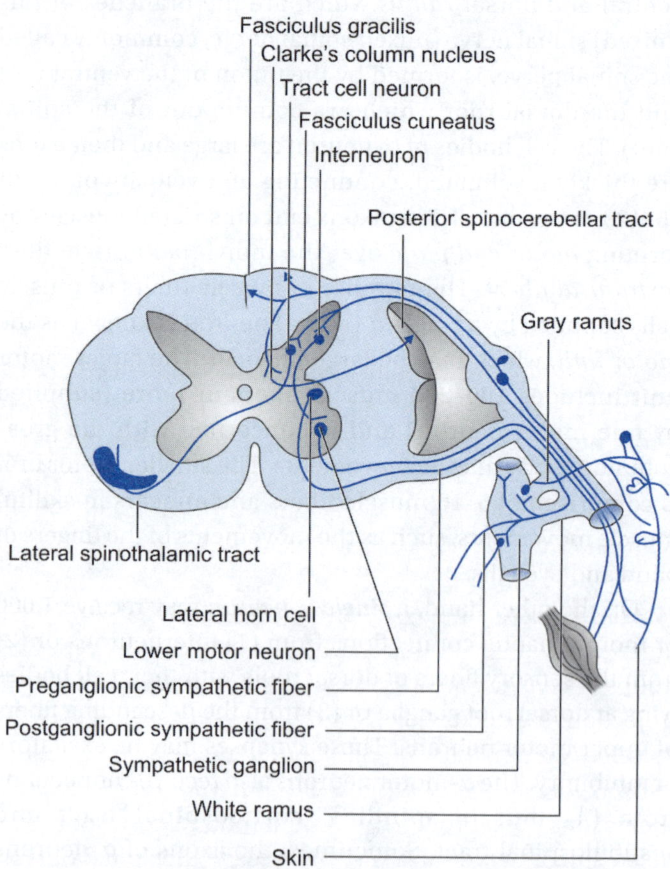

Fig. 22: The neurons of posterior gray column and lateral horn cells with their functional role.

is traversed by the fibers of dorsal nerve roots which are the axons of neurons situated in dorsal root ganglia and carry the peripheral sensation. Some of these fibers make synapses with the cells of SG, while others pass more deeply to the cells of NP. The *NP* lies deep to SG and constitutes the head and neck of the dorsal horn of gray matter. It extends along the entire length of spinal cord and is composed of the cell body of interneurons and tract cells. The axons of these tract cells contribute to form the ascending tracts of anterolateral white funiculi. The sensory afferent fibers of dorsal root which pass through SG and do not make synapses there, make synapses with the cells of NP or make tract. The *nucleus dorsalis (Clarke's column)* occupies the base of dorsal horn and extends from C_8 to L_2 segments of spinal cord. The nucleus dorsalis is also consists of interneuron and tract cells. The cells of SG and NP areas are responsible for pain and temperature sensation, whereas the Clarke's column or nucleus dorsalis receives the proprioceptive afferent (i.e., muscle and joint sensation), touch, and pressure sensation. The axons of cell body of dorsal nucleus or Clarke's column pass ipsilaterally and form the posterior spinocerebellar tracts. The *VAN* is situated at the base of the dorsal horn and extends from T_1 to L_2 and S_2 to S_4 segments of spinal cord. The cell bodies situated within this VAN receive visceral afferent fibers through the dorsal nerve roots and project fibers to the preganglionic visceral efferent nuclei of autonomic system which are located in the lateral horn of the corresponding segments of spinal cord.

The lateral horn of the intermediate region of gray matter extends from T_1 to L_2 segments of spinal cord. It is composed of intermediolateral and intermediomedial columns of cells and these cells *act as the preganglionic motor neurons of sympathetic* system (thoracolumbar outflow, **Fig. 22**). The preganglionic sympathetic fibers, arising from these cell bodies of sympathetic motor neurons, are thinly myelinated and pass successively through ventral roots and mixed spinal nerve trunk and reach the corresponding ganglia of sympathetic chain via *white rami communicates.* So, T_1 to L_2 spinal nerves have white rami communicantes in addition to gray rami communicantes which are present in all the spinal nerves, carrying the nonmyelinated postganglionic sympathetic fibers which arises from the ganglion of sympathetic chain. These intermediomedial groups of cells reappear in sacral region without any lateral projection. It extends from S_2 to S_4 segments of spinal cord. *These cells also act as the cell body of preganglionic motor neurons for the sacral outflow of parasympathetic system.* Their axons pass through the ventral roots of corresponding mixed spinal nerves and then they leave the spinal nerves to form the pelvic splanchnic nerves or nervi erigentes (parasympathetic).

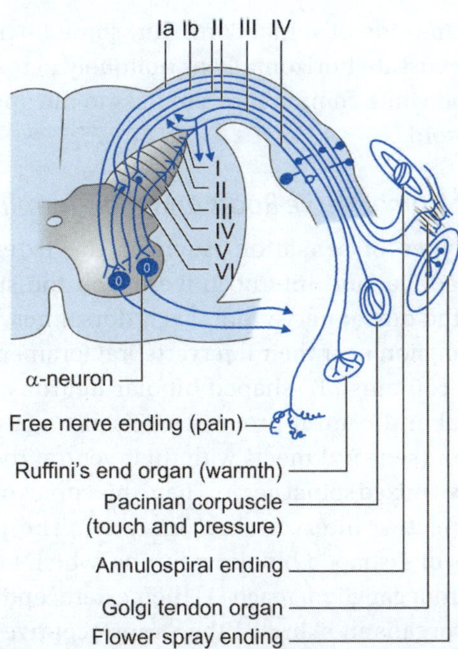

Fig. 23: Arrangements of sensory fibers at the root entry zone and their immediate termination.

Recently, the entire spinal gray matter is mapped out by *Rexed into ten laminae,* according to cytoarchitecture and packing density of neurons **(Fig. 23)**. The *laminae I to VI* are confined in dorsal horns. Among these, the lamina I and II corresponds with SG and the lamina III to VI corresponds with NP. The *lamina VII* occupies the intermediate region of gray matter. It includes nucleus dorsalis, intermediomedial and intermediolateral nucleus of autonomic system. The *lamina VIII* is located in the medial part of ventral gray column in the cervical and lumbosacral enlargements of spinal cord. In the other segments of spinal cord, lamina VIII is located at the base of ventral horn. The *lamina IX* is located in the lateral part of ventral horn, in the enlarged segment of spinal cord, for limbs. Whereas in the rest of the segments of spinal cord (except the enlarge segment of spinal cord for limbs, such as cervical and lumbar segment), it occupies the head of the ventral horn. The *lamina X* occupies the area around the central canal which consists mostly of neuroglial cells.

White Matter

The white matter of spinal cord consists of nerve fibers (but, not the nerve cell bodies), neuroglial cells, and blood vessels. It is white because the nerve fibers here are myelinated. In spinal cord, the white matter occupies the periphery of the butterfly-shaped central gray matter and is arranged into *three pairs of white funiculi* (1) anterior, (2) lateral, and (3) posterior. Usually, all the white funiculi are essentially composed of longitudinal nerve fibers which are grouped into different *functional tracts* and runs upward or downward on the same side of spinal cord. But, some fibers of white matter decussate horizontally or obliquely across the gray matter and white commissure and pass to the opposite side of spinal cord.

Fibers of Dorsal Nerve Roots and their Termination

All the types of sensation, such as the exteroceptive, proprioceptive, and interoceptive, reach the spinal cord through the dorsal nerve root. Each dorsal nerve root has its one ganglion near their intervertebral foramen and each ganglion contains "T"-shaped bipolar neurons with their peripheral and central processes. Distal to ganglion, the dorsal root (sensory) meets with their ventral root (motor) and forms a mixed spinal nerve. Then, this comes out through their respective intervertebral foramen. The peripheral processes of T-shaped bipolar neurons, which are situated in dorsal root ganglion, reach (1) their exteroceptive sensory receptor organs in skin, (2) the proprioceptive receptors in muscles, bones, and joints, and (3) the interoceptive or visceroceptive receptors in blood vessels and viscera. The central process of these T-shaped bipolar neurons forms the dorsal nerve root and fans out centrally into six or eight rootlets and enters the spinal cord. At the entry zone of dorsal root, each rootlet presents medial and lateral divisions or bundles.

The medial divisions consist of thickly myelinated group I and group II fibers. The fibers of group I are again subdivided into group Ia and group Ib fibers. The fibers of group Ia convey the primary afferents from muscle spindle. The fibers of group Ib carry the afferents from Golgi tendon organs, touch, and pressure. The fibers of group II convey the secondary afferents from muscle spindle, touch receptors, pressure receptors, and vibratory receptors (Pacinian corpuscles). All the fibers of medial division enter into the posterior fasiculi and joint with the ascending tracts.

The lateral divisions consist of thinly myelinated group III and unmyelinated goup IV fibers. The group III fibers conduct fast and discriminative pain and temperature sensation. The group IV fibers are concerned with slow (aching) pain and visceral sensation. On reaching the spinal cord, the fibers of lateral division divide into short ascending and descending branches in the dorsolateral tract of Lissauer. Then, it extends one or two segments cranially and/or caudally and provides collateral and terminal branches which enter into the dorsal horn of gray matter.

BLOOD–CEREBROSPINAL FLUID AND BLOOD–BRAIN BARRIER

The projection of vascular pial fringes into the ventricles of brain, such as the lateral, third and fourth ventricle, is called the *choroidal plexus*. The *ependyma* is a single layer of ciliated columnar cells. This lines the ventricles of brain including the choroidal plexus and the central canal of spinal cord. The ependyma, lining the choroidal plexuses of ventricles, helps actively in the formation of CSF. Actually, it presents the *blood–CSF barrier*. The choroidal plexus presents numerous villi-like projections in the ventricle as. These are called the choroidal villi. Each villus-like projection contains capillary plexus. Each capillary plexus is formed by afferent and efferent vessels, a small amount of connective tissue stroma derived from pia mater, and few nerve fibers. These aforesaid structures of choroidal villi are enveloped by ependymal cells, which are simple ciliated columnar resting on a basement membrane and are connected to one another by a tight junction **(Fig. 24)**.

Thus, the blood–CSF barrier consists of the following:
- Fenestrated endothelial cell layer of choroid capillaries, resting on a basement membrane
- A tissue space intervening between the vascular endothelial cell layer and the ependymal cell membrane
- A continuous layer of ependymal cells connected by tight junctions.

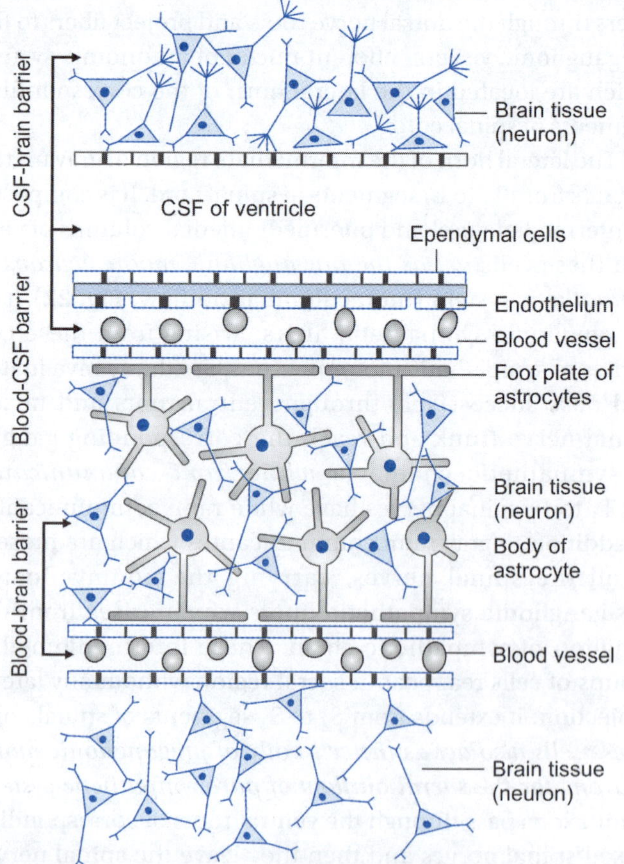

Fig. 24: The blood–CSF, CSF–brain, and blood–brain barrier. (CSF: cerebrospinal fluid)

The ependymal cells are actually the cells which are derived from the germinal layer of primitive neural tube and give rise to the development of neuroblasts and spongioblast. The spongioblast differentiates into astrocyte and oligodendrocytes.

The arterial blood of choroidal plexus is derived from anterior and posterior choroidal arteries. The former (anterior choroidal artery) is the branch of internal carotid artery. The latter (posterior choroidal artery) is usually three or four in number and is derived from the posterior cerebral artery. The venous blood from the choroid plexus is assembled on each side to form a single choroid vein. The choroid veins join with the thalamostriate veins and ultimately drain into straight sinus through internal cerebral and great cerebral veins. The mechanism for the control of circulation of blood through choroidal plexuses is not yet established.

The ependymal cells on ventricular surface exhibits numerous microvilli. The structures of ependymal cells suggest that they are concerned with transcellular and bidirectional transport of solvents and solutes between choroidal capillaries and ventricular CSF. The total surface area of choroidal plexuses ranges from 150 to 300 cm^2. The active transport, through ependymal cells, provides higher concentrations of Na^+ and Cl^- and lower concentrations of other substances in the CSF than that of plasma.

It is important to mention at this stage about the existence of two more brain barrier. These are *CSF–brain barrier and blood–brain barrier*. The *CSF–brain barrier* intervenes between the CSF and extracellular (neuron or glial cells) space. It includes extrachoroidal ependymal cells of ventricles which have gap junctions between them, basement membrane, and subependymal glial cell membrane. The *blood–brain barrier* includes the tissues that intervene between the blood in capillaries and neurons.

The blood–brain barrier consists of the following:
- The nonfenestrated endothelium of the capillaries connected by tight junctions
- The basement membrane for vascular endothelium on which it rests
- The perivascular feet and the cell bodies of astrocytes
- The network of intercellular spaces between the astrocytes and the neurons, having an interval of about 200A wide.

The blood–brain barrier permits the entry of water, O_2, CO_2, some drugs like sulfadiazine, erythromycin, etc. readily into the brain. But proteins, bile salt, catecholamines, and drugs like penicillin, etc. cross the barrier to a limited extend.

The CSF–brain barrier is weaker than the blood–brain barrier. This is because vital dyes and isotopes injected into the CSF gain quick access into neurons and neuroglia. In general, substances possessing high lipid solubility, such as CO_2, volatile anesthetics, and barbiturates pass from the blood to the brain and ultimately to the CSF. On the other hand, substances with limited lipid solubility, such as electrolytes, sugar, and amino acids pass from the blood to the CSF and ultimately to the brain.

SELECTION OF THE PATIENT FOR REGIONAL ANESTHESIA

Psychological Factors

During training period, many anesthetists have the experience of successfully placing the LA agent in the subarachnoid or epidural space. But, the effect of this RA fails. In such circumstances, one of the most common reasons for this unfortunate event is that the regional anesthetic technique, that is selected, was not suitable for that patient. These patients, which are not suitable for RA, are easy to identify. So, in such circumstance, it is a great mistake, from the side of an anesthetist, to try to coerce with such patients to accept RA, without providing heavy sedation or GA because it is likely to be very difficult to manage these groups of patients in operation theater (OT) room, only with RA. So, RA without heavy sedation or GA is impossible or rarely provided to children. The patients of adolescent age group can be difficult to evaluate how they will behave in OT under only RA, without heavy sedation or GA. Patients with psychiatric diseases, e.g., schizophrenia, manic depression, claustrophobia, Alzheimer's, dementia, etc. are not suitable for RA.

Some orthopedic surgeries require special position during operation. This does not cause problems for short surgeries. But, this can become extremely uncomfortable over long period of time, especially for patients who are suffering from body arthritic changes. Then, the gradual movement of patient that results from restlessness, during lengthy procedures, can require excessive sedation and spoil the advantage of RA. Some procedures, for example, shoulder surgery, surgery over head and neck area, retinal ophthalmic surgery, etc. require the patient to be drapped over his head for a considerable period of time. But, some patients may not be able to tolerate this situation and RA is not suitable for these groups of patients. Another problem of RA is if the patient does not understand the principal language, which is used in the OT by staffs to communicate with patient, and the anesthetists are not fluent with the language of the patient to communicate with him or her. Sometimes, RA without supplement of sedation or GA is also probably not wise. Some surgeons prefer to work with RA and modify their surgical techniques to accommodate it.

So, to make RA successful, they also explain to the patient about the benefits of RA over GA, before the patient meets with anesthetists. Contrary, some surgeons are uncomfortable to work with RA. So, they become reluctant to convey their patient regarding the benefit of RA. Then, the preparation for RA may become more complicated or even impossible by anesthetist.

Physical Factors

- Regional anesthesia should not be attempted when patient has any signs of systemic infection. So, general sepsis should be considered as absolute contraindication for RA.
- Psoriasis and hidradenitis are the two conditions, in which although the skin is not infected, but this area must be avoided for needle prick. So, another site for regional technique should be selected, otherwise GA is preferred.
- Herpes, found at preoperative examination, may pose problems. Secondary and subsequent recurrence of this disease is not contraindication for RA. But, primary herpes is often associated with viremia and so is a contraindication for RA.
- Chronic osteomyelitis does not show any evidence of bacteremia and so RA is not contraindicated. However, the presence of bacteremia in an acute case of osteomyelitis is contraindication for RA and should be avoided.
- Pelvic infection presents controversy when RA is considered. The confluence of lymphatic drainage from pelvis and epidural space makes the placing of a needle (a potential nidus for infection) into vertebral canal, during such infective condition controversial.
- For RA to be considered—no systemic signs of sepsis or clinical signs of pyelonephritis should be present.
- Many human immunodeficiency virus (HIV)-positive patients are severely ill and might be considered ideally suited for RA due to severe illness. However, the invasion of CNS by HIV virus is of particular concern for RA. This is because the virus has property to cause demyelination. So, it is now generally agreed that any disease state which cause demyelination is an absolute contraindication for RA, since local anesthetic agent too accelerates this demyelination. Here, the risk benefit ratio must be calculated.

Neurological Diseases

- For diseases with central demyelination, such as amyotrophic lateral sclerosis and Guillain–Barrè syndrome, the RA is an unwise choice.
- The diabetic peripheral neuropathy is an area, where there is less consensus between RA and GA. Patients with this type of peripheral neuropathy often have other end-organ diseases which make them ideal for RA. But, however, due to medicolegal issues, for postoperative changes in the extent of neuropathy, due to diabetes (but, not due to anesthesia), some anesthetists are reluctant to use RA in such cases. So, though mechanism of diabetic neuropathy is unknown and unaffected by the action of local anesthetic agents, still proper preoperative evaluation for any neurological deficit of such patient by thorough physical examination and risk/benefit analysis of this situation should be clarified before taking any decision for RA.
- Any history of old stroke, especially any old embolic event, is not a contraindication for RA. The patient requiring urgent surgery in the period, immediately after a hemorrhagic stroke, RA is strongly contraindicated. It (RA) is also contraindicated for any patient with a potential risk for increased intracranial pressure. The gray zone is the time interval between an acute condition and a chronic one. So, a risk/benefit analysis and complete documentation of patient status is mandatory.

Coagulopathy

The actual incidences of neurological dysfunction, associated with CNB, resulting from cord compression due to hemorrhagic complications, such as hematoma, paraplegia, and abscess are unknown. But, the incidences which are cited in different literatures vary from 1 in 150,000 in epidural to less than 1 in 220,000 in spinal anesthesia. Among these complications, the epidural hematoma is the most common and 68% of patients have the history of coagulation abnormality, due to intravenous heparin, antiplatelet medication, oral anticoagulants intake, dextran 70 administration, etc. Like the introduction of needle and/or catheter, the epidural hematoma also can occur immediately after the removal of epidural catheter. These suggest that the removal of catheter is not entirely atraumatic. So, the determination of patient's coagulation status at the time of catheter removal is perhaps as critical as that at the time of catheter placement.

Neurological outcome is good only in 38% of patients who underwent laminectomy within 8 hours of the diagnosis of epidural hematoma. But, routine screening for coagulation profile in healthy patients, who are not taking any medicine that influences coagulation cascade, is no longer advised before RA. But, practitioner of RA must take proper history of symptoms and signs of any coagulation defect. History of taking any anticoagulants, antiplatelets [aspirin and nonsteroidal anti-inflammatory drugs (NSAIDs)], a prior history of surgical bleeding diathesis, etc. should not be excluded from the indication of RA, but should be evaluated carefully.

The most valuable tools to detect potential bleeding problems during RA are bleeding time (BT), prothrombin time (PT), partial thromboplastin time (PTT), and now international normalized ratio (INR) which are the gold standard indicators for the integrity of an intrinsic and extrinsic pathways of coagulation. Salicylation of platelet, by antiplatelet aggregating factors such as aspirin, is irreversible and the effect of aspirin is not resolved till new generation of platelets is synthesized. Thus, 1 week withholding of aspirin and NSAID makes preoperative choice easier. However, not every patient could be prepared in this manner. Coagulopathy from this medication should be considered unusual. Prophylaxis of deep vein thrombosis (DVT) may involve low-dose heparin/warfarin/coumarin, etc. and should be titrated against a defined prolongation of PT/PTT ratio. In such cases of prophylaxis, coagulation cascade is usually not altered, keeping in mind that a small percentage of patients will always have abnormal coagulation test.

So, laboratory testing should be minimal for preoperative preparation of anesthesia. Withholding the medication for a period and documenting their normal coagulation tests after withdrawal is best choice. Preparing a risk/benefit ratio for these patients is mandatory. For a patient with clinically documented embolism and in need of urgent surgery of stopping the anticoagulant must be a joint decision by surgeon and anesthesia team. Rarely, an indication for RA is so strong that active reversal of anticoagulation is executed with blood component therapy (fresh frozen plasma, cryoprecipitate, and vitamin K) to allow anesthetists to use RA technique. Resumption of heparin is decided by surgeon when surgical bleeding is stable in postoperative period.

Regional Anesthetic Management of Patients who are on Oral Anticoagulants (Warfarin)

The anesthetic management of patients, who are orally anticoagulated preoperatively with warfarin, is dependent on the dosage and the timing of initiation of therapy. The PT and INR value (normal value of PT—9.6–11.1 seconds which corresponds to an INR value of 1.4) of patients, who are on chronic oral anticoagulation, will require at least 3–5 days to become normal, after the discontinuation of anticoagulant therapy. Therefore, except in extraordinary circumstances, the spinal or epidural needle or catheter placement and removal of it should not be performed in dully anticoagulated patients. It is, therefore, recommended that the documentation of patient's normal coagulation status should be achieved, prior to the implementation of neuraxial block.

The patients, who are getting warfarin as thromboprophylaxis preoperatively, have significantly higher PTs and complication rate. On the other hand, many orthopedic surgeons administer the first dose of warfarin on the night before surgery. For these patients, the PT and INR should be checked prior to any neuraxial block, if the first dose was given >24 hours earlier or a second dose of oral anticoagulant has been administered.

The patients, receiving low dose of warfarin therapy for long period, should have their PT and INR monitoring, during their CNB, on daily basis and also should be checked before the removal of catheter, especially if the initial dose of warfarin is >36 hours before hand. There is large variability in patient's response to warfarin. For example, usually the mean PT, by low dose (5 mg) of warfarin given postoperatively, does not increase beyond the normal range, until 48 hours is passed.

Again, the average therapeutic value is not achieved, until the 7th postoperative days have passed. But, few patients have PT value >12.8 seconds after a single dose of warfarin. Higher dose of warfarin may require more intensive monitoring of coagulation status. Reduced doses of warfarin should be given to patients who are likely to have an enhanced response to this drug. An INR >3 should prompt the physician to withhold or reduce the dose of warfarin in patients with indwelling neuraxial catheters. There is no definitive recommendation for removal of neuraxial catheters in patients with therapeutic levels of anticoagulation status during a neuraxial catheter infusion. But caution must be exercised in taking decision about the removing and maintaining these catheters.

Regional Anesthetic Management of Patients who are Receiving Heparin

The safety of CNB with intraoperative heparinization is well documented, provided no other coagulopathies are present. But, the concurrent use of other medications that affect the coagulation status may increase the risk of bleeding complications for patients receiving standard heparin.

Intravenous heparin administration should be delayed for at least 1 hour after needle placement. Indwelling catheter should be removed 1 hour before a subsequent heparin administration or 2-4 hours after the last heparin dose. The evaluation of coagulation status may be appropriate or mandatory prior to the placement of catheter or removal of it in patients who have demonstrated enhanced response to anticoagulants or are on higher doses of heparin. Although, the occurrence of a bloody or difficult needle placement may increase the risk, but there are no data to support the mandatory cancellation of a schedule dose. If the decision is made to proceed for CNB in a patient, who is receiving heparin, then a full discussion with the surgeon and careful postoperative monitoring is warranted.

There is no contraindication to use of spinal or epidural block after administration of subcutaneous standard dose of heparin, provided the coagulation parameters remain within the recommended level and close monitoring is performed.

Regional Anesthetic Management of Patients who are Receiving Low Molecular Weight Heparin

The patients, on preoperative low molecular weight heparin (LMWH), should be thoroughly assessed to have altered coagulation profile at the time of spinal or epidural needle or catheter placement. A single short spinal anesthesia may be the safest neuraxial block in patients, receiving preoperative LMWH. In these patients, needle placement should occur at least 10–12 hours after the last LMWH dose. The patients, receiving higher doses of LMWH, will require longer delays (24 hours). Neuraxial block should be avoided in patients, where a dose of LMWH is administered 2 hours preoperatively. This is because needle placement coincides with the peak anticoagulant activity of LMWH. Antiplatelet, oral anticoagulant, standard heparin, or dextran, administered in combination with LMWH, may increase the risk of spinal hematoma.

Patients, who are not receiving any anticoagulant, heparin, or LMWH at present, but with proposed postoperative initiation of LMWH for thromboprophylaxis, may safely undergo single dose and continuous catheter techniques. But, the first dose of LMWH should not be administered earlier than 24 hours postoperatively. In addition, it is recommended that the indwelling catheter should be removed at least 24 hours, after the last dose of LMWH.

The decision to implement LMWH therapy, in the presence of an indwelling catheter, must be made with care. The extreme vigilance of patient's neurological status is warranted. A minimum dose of opioid or very dilute local anesthetic solution which does not block the motor is recommended in these patients, in order to allow the frequent monitoring of neurological function. If epidural analgesia is anticipated to continue for >24 hours, LMWH administration may be delayed or an alternative method of thromboprophylaxis may be selected, based on the risk profile for this individual patient. These decisions should be made preoperatively to allow optional management of both postoperative analgesia and thromboprophylaxis.

Regional Anesthetic Management of Patients who are Receiving Antiplatelet Medication

The antiplatelet medications are now frequently used as primary agents for thromboprophylaxis. The only antiplatelet drugs, by themselves, appear to represent no added significant risk, for the development of spinal hematoma, in patients having epidural or spinal anesthesia. Several large studies have demonstrated the relative safety of neuraxial blockade in both the obstetric and surgical patients, receiving these medications. However, the concurrent use of medications that affect the other components of clotting mechanisms, such as oral anticoagulants, standard heparin, and LMWH, may increase the risk of bleeding complications for the patients, receiving antiplatelet agents. Assessment of platelet function prior to the performance of neuraxial block is not recommended.

Ticlopidine and clopidogrel are also used as platelet aggregation inhibitors. These agents interfere with the platelet fibrinogen binding and subsequent platelet-platelet interactions. The effect of these drugs is irreversible for the whole lifespan of platelet. Ticlopidine and clopidogrel have no effect on platelet cyclooxygenase and act independently of aspirin. The risk of spinal hematoma in patients receiving ticlopidine and clopidogrel is unknown.

◼ EQUIPMENT REQUIRED FOR REGIONAL ANESTHESIA

A failure of an anesthetist to provide basic resuscitation, immediately after the development of any complication, due to the toxicity of LA agent from any regional block, may accentuates the toxicity of LA agent. This is because the toxicity of LA agent is magnified by hypoxia, hypotension, and acidosis. Thus, a vicious cycle may set up. The LA agent-induced grand mal seizure should also be promptly identified and treated by securing the patients airway and giving a dose of thiopental intravenously. It is followed by an intubating dose of succinylcholine and subsequent intubation and ventilation. This prevents hypoxia and meets the excessive demand of O_2 for skeletal muscles due to seizure. By the time, the action of drugs, used for the induction of anesthesia wear off, and the seizure precipitated by the local anesthetic agent, used for RA, will also be resolved.

So, the minimum equipment requirement for a safe performance of regional anesthesia (both peripheral nerve block and central neuraxial block) are:

- Emergency resuscitation drugs
- Appropriate needles, syringes, intravenous cannulas, etc.
- Access to circulation and IV fluids
- Thiopental, succinylcholine, atropine, adrenaline, and other emergency drugs
- Oxygen and device for assisted positive pressure ventilation
- Suction, laryngoscope, and tracheal tubes
- Monitoring devices

- All facilities for GA
- Trained assistance.

Many anesthetists do not routinely wear sterile gown or face mask for regional techniques. But, *it is mandatory* to wear sterile gown and mask for the central neuraxial blockade and introduction of catheter. However, this *may not be mandatory for other regional blockade,* such as plexus block or field block. There is some controversy regarding the routine extensive monitoring during the injection of any regional block. But, this is mandatory during central neural blockade.

INDICATIONS AND CONTRAINDICATIONS OF CENTRAL NEURAXIAL BLOCK

As a general rule, the CNB is only indicated for the surgical procedures, which can be accomplished on awake or slightly sedated patient, with sensory and motor block that is appropriate for this surgical procedure and the level of block does not produce any adverse patient's outcome. Therefore, low spinal or epidural anesthesia (block up to T_{10} spinal level or below it) carries different implication than the high (block up to T_4 spinal level) spinal or epidural anesthesia. The neuraxial blocks are used without conjunction of GA, usually for the surgical procedures on the lower half of the body or in conjunction with GA usually for the procedures on the upper half of the body (upper abdomen, thorax, and neck). Indeed in some European centers, cardiac surgery has also been routinely performed under thoracic epidural anesthesia, typically with light GA.

Indications

Spinal anesthesia may be an especially good choice than any other regional anesthetic procedure. This is because the total dose of local anesthetic drug, to achieve this block up to the level of T_{10} is quite small and will not push its total dose, as occurs during epidural anesthesia or different plexus blocks, close to toxic level. The CNB, as a primary anesthetic procedure, is most commonly used to provide surgical anesthesia for all procedures, carried out on the lower half of our body. Hence, *the usual indications for CNB include* the surgeries on lower limbs, pelvis, genitals, rectum, perineum, obstetric, and most of the urological procedures.

The RA in the form of CNB is also used for the upper abdominal surgery, but in combination with GA or sedation. It is *less commonly used as a primary anesthetic procedure* for the upper abdominal surgeries. Because, it can be difficult to achieve safely an upper level of sensory block which is adequate for patient's comfort. Recently, the RA technique has found in favor of analgesia in obstetric practice (obstetric analgesia) and also provides anesthesia for both the elective and emergency obstetric procedures. The patients, with respiratory diseases, may definitely get benefit from RA by avoiding GA. But, only if the block does not extent beyond the level of T_{10} spinal segment. So, the *caution should be exercised in patients with severe respiratory and cardiac diseases,* if the level of block extends high up above the level of T_{10}. Because, in acute respiratory disease, the motor block of accessory respiratory muscles by RA may impaired the pulmonary mechanics and aggravate the impairment of ventilation.

If a neuraxial anesthetic procedure is being considered, then its risks and benefits must be discussed with the patient. With it an informed consent should also be obtained. The patient must be mentally prepared for neuraxial blocked and the type of neuraxial blockade must be appropriate for the type of surgery. Patients should keep in their mind that they have no or little motor function on their lower extremities until the block resolves. Surgical procedures that require maneuvers, compromising respiratory function (for example, pneumoperitoneum or pneumothorax) or surgical procedures that are unusually of long duration are typically performed under GA, with or without neuraxial blockade.

Except the lumbar approach, the other approaches for spinal or subarachnoid block (SAB), such as thoracic and cervical approach, are not used for the fear of damage to spinal cord. So, the dural puncture, for spinal block, is usually performed below the level of first lumbar vertebra to prevent the damage of spinal cord which terminates at this level. But, this is not true for epidural anesthesia which can be approached through any route such as cervical, thoracic, lumbar, and sacral.

A relatively uncommon, but useful indication for spinal anesthesia is elective surgical procedures over spine, especially lumbar, such as laminectomy, spinal stenosis revision, and lumbar fusion. Usually, majority of these cases are performed under GA. But, there have been a number of reports of successful application of spinal anesthesia for the abovementioned surgical procedures on spine. The reluctance to use spinal anesthesia for lumbar spine surgery is based on several factors which are discussed later. Many surgeons are unaccustomed to perform spine surgery on an awake patient. Occasionally, the movement of patients and any change in the pattern of ventilation of an awake patient can be very disturbing. Many anesthetists are also reluctant to employ any regional technique on a prone patient. This is because, if GA is needed intraoperatively, then the intubation of such patient in prone position is difficult and potentially very dangerous. So, some anesthesiologists prefer to have control over patient's airway under GA, before the patient is placed in prone position.

On the other hand, surgery on lumbar spine requires sensory block up to T_{12} segment. Further, an awake patient with block up to T_{12} level is capable of safely positioning his upper part of body, including his head and neck and can maintain his or her own airway, unless oversedated or the sensory level of spinal block is too high. If the duration of operation is too prolonged and the effect of original spinal anesthesia recedes, then the dura will be in view and an enthusiastic surgeon can perform another second subarachnoid injection of LA agent. But, except periosteum, the rest of the spinal tissue where the surgery is going on, is insensitive. So, the need for supplementation of anesthesia, when the effect of original spinal anesthesia recedes, is only confined to infiltration of skin by LA agent only for wound closure.

Contraindications

The contraindication for spinal and epidural anesthesia are grouped under two headings *(1) absolute and (2) relative*. But, at some points the demarcation between these two groups of contraindication is blurred.

Absolute Contraindications

- Patient's refusal, lack of consent, and proved allergy to local anesthetic agent
- Patient's inability to maintain stillness due to any medical causes
- Lack of cooperation and understanding from patient's side
- Intracranial lesion, due to any cause, resulting ↑ICP. It is a very important contraindication for spinal anesthesia, because it may result in brain stem herniation, due to excessive leakage of CSF. Epidural is also contraindicated (relative) in such patients, because the inadvertent intrathecal puncture, during the procedure of epidural anesthesia, may result in a sudden fall in CSF pressure with herniation of brain stem through foramen magnum.
- Coagulopathy and untreated clotting defect
- Skin infection at prick point of needle
- Severe spinal and neurological abnormality causing it technically impossible
- Fixed cardiac output (CO) states, e.g., severe mitral stenosis (MS), MI, AS, etc. with very low left ventricular ejection fraction
- Absence of resuscitation equipment and no intravenous access to meet emergency
- Severe hypovolemia, due to massive hemorrhage, for example, central placenta previa, road traffic accident, etc.

Relative Contraindications

- *Coagulopathy (intrinsic or idiopathic):* In a patient taking anticoagulant, the risk must be weighed against the benefit of RA. Well-controlled anticoagulant treatment is not always a contraindication for spinal or epidural anesthesia.
- *Fever:* General sepsis is an absolute contraindication for spinal or epidural anesthesia, because infection may settle at the point of injection, if there is any hematoma. But, all the types of fever, for example, simple fever without any general sepsis, are not an absolute contraindication.
- Uncooperative patient
- Lack of anesthetist's experience
- The potential for major blood loss during surgery, e.g., grade IV placenta previa
- Previous laminectomy is not an absolute contraindication for spinal or epidural anesthesia. It may be relative contraindication.
- *Heparin for DVT:* Activated partial thromboplastin time (APTT) ratio up to 2 and in case of coumarin, INR up to 2 is safe ground for epidural or spinal anesthesia.
- Preexisting neurological deficits and demyelinating lesions
- Hypertrophic obstructive cardiomyopathy (left ventricular outflow obstruction).

Controversial

- Prior back surgery at the site of introduction of spinal or epidural needle
- Complicated surgery
- Prolonged surgery
- Major blood loss
- Maneuvers that compromise respiration.

Spinal or Epidural

The choice, between the spinal and epidural anesthesia for a patient, depends on the following multiple factors:

- Predictability of the length of surgery—epidural with catheter is preferred for prolonged surgery and where the duration of surgery is unpredictable.

  Spinal anesthesia is preferred where the duration of surgery is short and highly predictable.
- Where there is need for prolonged postoperative analgesia, then the epidural (with or without catheter) is preferred.
- Where both the spinal or epidural is applicable, then the chances of postspinal headache should be considered.
- If patient is discharged immediately, then the single-shot epidural without catheter is preferred.

- For the short surgical procedures, waiting for epidural to take effect makes spinal more practical.
- For the more sick patients, epidural block with catheter is preferred than spinal. Because, it avoids the sudden physiological changes which occurred during spinal anesthesia.
- For obstetric analgesia (not anesthesia), SAB has no role.

PHYSIOLOGICAL EFFECTS OF CENTRAL NEURAXIAL BLOCK (SPINAL AND EPIDURAL)

The CNB is associated with certain physiological changes in our body and these are described below. When these physiological changes in our body cross their limits, then complications occur. For example, the physiological effects of neuraxial block such as hypotension is not a complication. It becomes a complication when the hypotension is severe and produces damage, because complications imply damage to the patient.

Cardiovascular Effects

The CNB, i.e., spinal or epidural anesthesia produces pharmacological sympathectomy. The effect of this pharmacological sympathectomy, due to the spinal or epidural anesthesia, is similar to that of α- and β-adrenergic blocking agent. However, the level of this sympathectomy and its effects depends on the height of block. *In spinal anesthesia, the level of sympathectomy is 2–4 dermatomes above the level of sensory block and in epidural anesthesia it is at the same level of sensory block. Sympathetic block, i.e., sympathectomy causes both venous and arterial dilatation. But the effect of venodilatation predominates as the 75% of total blood volume is on the venous side. In general, the dilatation of arteries and resistance vessels (arterioles) cause the reduction of afterload and increase in CO (provided, preload is maintained). Whereas, the dilation of venous capacitance vessel cause reduction of preload and decrease in CO. But, the resultant effect of this arteriolar (resistance vessels) dilatation against venous dilatation in spinal or epidural block is decrease in CO and hypotension. This is due to the preponderance of venodilatation.*

The decrease in myocardial contractility and heart rate also lead to the decrease in CO and hypotension, but this occurs in a very high spinal or epidural block. This happens when the block extends above the level of T_1 spinal segment and there is blockade of all the cardioaccelerator sympathetic fibers which arise from the T_1 to T_4 segment of spinal cord (sympathetic outflow is from T_1 to L_2). This causes the decrease in compensatory sympathetic outflow from the cardiac spinal sympathetic center, in response to afferent impulses from intrinsic chronotropic stretch receptor of

the right atrium and great veins which in turn decreases the chronotropic and inotropic drive of heart, leading to the further reduction of CO and hypotension. Thus, a vicious cycle starts.

There is also decrease in coronary blood flow. This is because, the coronary blood flow parallels with the mean arterial pressure and due to the fall of this mean arterial pressure (MAP), there is also the fall of coronary flow. Here, the decrease in coronary blood flow is not due to the coronary vasoconstriction. The myocardial O_2 consumption rate also varies. When there is fall of systemic vascular resistance and MAP without tachycardia, then there is also the reduction of afterload and subsequent reduction of O_2 consumption by heart. But, when there is compensatory tachycardia, then O_2 consumption by myocardium tremendously increases.

Usually, there is no change in the rate of blood flow in organs, when the sensory block extends only up to the level of T_{10}. This is because the reduction of preload, due to venodilatation, causing decrease in CO and simultaneously reduction of afterload, due to arterial dilatation, causing increase in CO, balance each other. But, when the block extends above T_{10} level, then the balance tilts toward hypotension and the blood flow in different organs are impaired. Till up to 20% fall of MAP cerebral blood flow does not fall. But, until now it is still controversial and unanswered that up to which level the decrease of mean arterial BP is acceptable. However, the reduction of BP below 30% of MAP is not advisable.

In summary, the sympathetic outflow to the capacitance vessels of our whole body originates from T_1 to L_2 segments of spinal cord. Among these, the sympathetic cardioaccelerator fibers arise from the T_1 to T_4 segment of spinal cord. The degree of compensatory sympathetic response to the CNB is proportional to the number of segments blocked. In spinal and epidural block, due to pharmacological sympathectomy, the decrease in venous return decreases cardiac preload and hence CO. In response to this changes, there is a compensatory increase in heart rate (provided the cardioaccelerator fibers are not blocked) which tries to maintain CO and BP. This is mediated by the sinoaortic baroreceptors. On the other hand, the decreased afterload, due to the dilatation of arteriolar resistance vessels, due to pharmacological sympathectomy in spinal or epidural block, may improve the performance of left ventricle (LV) (provided preload is maintained by fluid), CO, BP, and visceral perfusion. But, the ultimate result regarding the CO, BP, and organ perfusion depends on the severity of the reduction of preload and afterload which again depends on the extent of the block of sympathetic outflow. Coronary flow increases as long as the CO and the pressure head in aorta are maintained. If the CO and pressure head is not increased, then the vasopressor agents are required to maintain BP, tissue perfusion, and patient's well-being by constricting the capacitance vessels and the arteriolar resistance vessels. Compensatory increase in heart rate to maintain CO and BP requires the intactness of sympathetic efferent fibers to heart, which originate from the T_1 to T_4 segment of spinal cord. If sympathetic block extends above this height, then the compensatory increase in heart rate and myocardial contractility will not occur and this will result in severe hypotension. It is also possible in such situation that the increased and the unopposed dominance of vagal tone to heart may drive the heart rate slow, causing bradycardia and hypotension. So, to counteract this increased and unopposed vagal tone, anticholinergic agents (atropine) are also helpful.

Respiratory Effect

The spinal or epidural anesthesia, with sensory block up to the lower thoracic dermatomes, i.e., more or less around the T_{10} level, has little clinical significance (effect) on the mechanics of respiratory system. Up to this T_{10} level of block, the tidal volume remains unchanged, as most of the intercostal muscles and diaphragm (supplied by phrenic nerve; root value $C_{3,4,5}$) remains unaffected. But, the vital capacity may decrease, due to the reduction in inspiratory and expiratory reserve volume. This is again due to the paralysis of some accessory respiratory muscles of abdomen.

Rarely, the respiratory arrest occurs in spinal and epidural anesthesia and if it (respiratory arrest) occurs, then it is due to the hypoperfusion and hypoxia of respiratory center in brain stem, due to severe hypotension or due to the paralysis of all respiratory muscles including the diaphragm. This occurs when the block extends up to a very higher level or due to total spinal block. *Hence, the CNB should be used cautiously in the respiratory compromised patients, because the unintentional extension of block to higher level will cause the paralysis of accessory respiratory muscles* and the further deterioration of pulmonary function, and even respiratory arrest, due to the hypoperfusion and hypoxia of central respiratory center, due to severe hypotension plus paralysis of all respiratory muscles.

As the level of the block rises, an increasing proportion of muscles, involved in respiration, is affected. The principal muscle of respiration, i.e., the diaphragm, usually remains unaffected, except in extreme cases of very high spinal anesthesia, extending to cervical region or total spinal block. As the block ascends, gradually more and more intercostal muscles become paralyze after the paralysis of abdominal muscles. But, most healthy patients remain able to maintain normal ventilation by the remaining unaffected muscles. Although the subjective feeling of immobility of chest wall

and suffocation may be alarming, if they are not informed in advance. In such situation, mild sedation may be needed to increase the tolerance of patient. But, this subjective distress may be early and greatly magnified in patients, suffering from respiratory disease and if heavy sedation is used. So, the panicky sense of suffocation may sometimes make the central neuraxial blockade a poor choice for some patients. *The degree of sedation, necessary for the patient to tolerate anxiety, could cause further respiratory depression in a patient who has limited respiratory reserve.* In order to achieve the goal of avoiding instrumentation of airway (i.e., intubation) by using spinal or epidural anesthesia, the general rule is to keep the motor level of blockade below T_7. If higher spinal or epidural block is necessary for surgical procedure, then the selection of GA with controlled airway should be considered, with or without combination of CNB.

Patients with severe chronic lung disease rely upon the accessory muscles of respiration (intercostal and abdominal muscles) to actively inspire or exhale. In such patients, the high level of neural blockade will impair their pulmonary functions by hindering the activity of these accessory muscles. Similarly, effective coughing and clearing of airway secretions require these muscles. Therefore, the CNB should be used with caution in patients with limited respiratory reserve in chronic lung diseases. Hence, the chronic pulmonary diseases are the relative contraindications for CNB. These deleterious effects of neuraxial block on chronic lung diseases need to be weighted against the advantage of avoiding airway instrumentation and positive pressure ventilation by neuraxial block. For the surgical procedures, above the umbilicus, a pure regional technique may not be the best choice in patients with severe lung disease. On the other hand, these patients become benefited from the effects of thoracic epidural analgesia by low concentration LA agent and opioids or intrathecal opioids in postoperative period, particularly following upper abdominal or thoracic surgery.

Some evidences suggest that the postoperative thoracic epidural analgesia, in high-risk patients, can improve pulmonary outcome by (1) decreasing the incidence of pneumonia and respiratory failure, (2) improving the oxygenation, and (3) decreasing the duration of mechanical ventilatory support.

Gastrointestinal Effect

The sympathetic supply to gastrointestinal (GI) tract originates from the T_5 to L_1 segment of spinal cord. So, when the spinal anesthesia, extending up to T_5 segment, results in chemical sympathectomy supplying GI tract, then the vagal tone over the GI tract dominates and sympathetic tone disappears. This results in hyperperistalsis and early emptying of GI tract. So, the gastric emptying is facilitated with the reduction of gastric emptying time. The nausea and vomiting also result due to the hyperperistalsis of gut and vagal stimulation. Hence, atropine is effective in the treatment of this type of nausea and vomiting, by blocking the vagus. The spinal or epidural anesthesia provides excellent surgical condition of GI tract, due to the contracted gut. Hepatic blood flow decreases in proportion to decrease in MAP. But, its function remains unaffected and there is no hepatic ischemia, provided there is no severe hypotension for prolonged period. Hepatic function is less impaired in CNB than GA. In postoperative stage of epidural analgesia and anesthesia, the intramucosal pH of stomach remains high (alkaline) and provides a protective effects from gastric ulceration.

Renal Effects

Renal blood flow is maintained through autoregulation plus due to wide physiological reserve. So, the decrease of renal blood flow, due to the reduction of BP, following CNB, has little physiological importance with less effect on kidney function. But, the loss of autonomic control of bladder (because block both at lumbar or sacral level cut both the sympathetic and parasympathetic control of bladder) results in urinary retention, till this block wears off. Hence, the neuraxial block is a frequent cause of urinary retention, causing delayed patient discharge from hospital and frequent catheterization. However, urine production is unaffected by the spinal or epidural block, as long as the MAP is not significantly reduced. During the regression from spinal or epidural block, it starts from higher level and the thick nerve fibers are freed first. Hence, as the center of bladder innervation is situated at S_{2-4}, spinal segment and some of the nerve fiber, involved in urination, are thin and easily blocked, so they may be the last to regress. Therefore, the passing of urine may be one of the last effects of regression from the spinal or epidural anesthesia.

Neurological Effects

The preoperative anxiety before surgery leads to sympathetic stimulation and increased release of catecholamine. These result in gluconeogenesis and myocardial stress. This sympathetic stimulation also causes increased heart rate and increased myocardial oxygen demand. But, the sympathectomy, resulting from spinal anesthesia, interrupts this catecholamine release and causes the reduction of its level. The plasma level of adrenocorticotropic hormone (ACTH) varies from unknown to decrease in the presence of sympathetic block.

Metabolic and Endocrine Effects

Any surgical trauma *induces* systemic neuroendocrine *stress responses*, due to the activation of sympathetic system via the somatic and visceral afferent (sensory) impulses, in addition to the local *inflammatory responses*. This systemic neuroendocrine stress responses include elevated concentration of ACTHs, such as the cortisol, epinephrine, norepinephrine, vasopressin as well as the activation of renin–angiotensin–aldosterone system. The clinical manifestations of this systemic neuroendocrine stress responses include the tachycardia, intraoperative and postoperative hypertension, hyperglycemia, etc. The neuraxial blockade totally or partially suppresses these neuroendocrine stress responses and improves the cardiovascular, pulmonary, and renal functions.

PREOPERATIVE PREPARATION, PREMEDICATION, AND INTRAOPERATIVE MANAGEMENT OF PATIENT FOR REGIONAL ANESTHESIA

The patients, scheduled for RA, should also be prepared like GA, because all the regional techniques have certain failure rate (though small) and patients may require GA at any moment. Therefore, all the protocols regarding history, fasting, premedication, preoperative investigation, etc. are the same for regional and general anesthesia. Reassurance is the cornerstone of the successful outcome of a regional anesthetic technique. Many patients prefer to go to sleep during operation. These patients should be reassured that sedation will be available, if required. Some patients have the fears of development of backache or neurological complications, particularly paralysis in future, following spinal and epidural anesthesia. These patients should also be reassured, regarding the safety of this technique.

The risks and benefits of a proposed regional anesthetic technique should also be discussed in advance with the patient. This discussion and written consent should be recorded in patient's chart. Already, there is considerable anxiety in patients regarding the outcome of proposed surgery. With it, anxiety for the procedure of spinal or epidural anesthesia is added. Hence, mild anxiolytic premedication is very essential. If the patients have previous back pain, then it will increase, when the patient is positioned for spinal or epidural anesthesia. Hence, the patient cannot be positioned properly, leading to the difficulty in positioning needle in proper place and the failure of procedure. So, this pain can be relieved by any narcotics given in small doses. This will help in better positioning of patient and will facilitate anesthetist to give spinal or epidural block easily. But, whatever may be given, it has to keep in mind that overpremedication does not allow the patient to maintain the needed position for extradural or dural puncture, particularly if sitting position is selected. The level of anxiolysis to the point of disinhibition should also be avoided, because it can lead to sudden untoward movements and agitation of patient, resulting difficulty for RA.

The site of injection or block must be cleaned with an appropriate antiseptic agent according to local hospital or institution policy. The anesthetists must wear sterile gown and face mask, especially during any CNB. If the patient is awake, then the procedure can be made more tolerable by subcutaneous infiltration of small amount of local anesthetic agent by a very fine 30 G needle or by applying eutectic local anesthetic mixture on skin, before pricking by needle. However, during the delivery of local anesthetist drug in spinal canal (spinal or epidural) care must be taken to avoid any inadvertent intravenous injection of local anesthetic agent. So, prior to injection, aspiration must be performed to detect any blood into syringe. The aspiration should also be repeated, when large volume of drug is used in epidural technique. At the end, it is most important to say that the whole procedure should be appropriately documented.

Aspects, other than the technical part of regional block, should also be carefully considered and the overall experience of patient, regarding RA, should be as much pleasant as possible. Most patients, except those undergoing minor surgical procedure, expect to be sleepy or unconscious. So, attention must be paid to patient's desire with overall comfort and warmth feeling while lying on a hard table and the provision of a relaxed environment. The patient should be protected from viewing the operation by the use of screens and towels, if needed. In some operations the position of patient may itself give rise to some discomfort and embarrassment due to exposure. So, adequate sedation may make such procedures more tolerable.

Supplementation of Regional Anesthetic Technique

It may be done by the following methods:

- *By distraction of mind:* The diversion of patient's attention from surgery is the major adjunct of RA. This can be performed by the use of personal stereos. Alternatively, a member of operating room staff may engage patient's mind by continuous chatting.
- *By use of sedation:* Properly titrated sedation can be used to supplement the RA. The provision of amnesia and hypnosis, for the events in operating room, can be an advantage for many patients. But, the extensive use of sedation, in conjunction with RA, is illogical at best and dangerous at worst. In such situation, anesthesiologist

must justify yourself for the use of excessive sedative drugs. Theoretically, the choice of sedative drugs during RA appears to be wide. But, in practice, only a few drugs are used. Among all the sedatives, benzodiazepine is the first choice. Midazolam, the water-soluble benzodiazepine, offers considerable advantages over its predecessor diazepam. It may be administered by intravenous bolus (0.15–0.17 mg/kg) or by continuous infusion (0.25 mg/kg/hour) technique. There is wide variation of dose-response relationship of midazolam. The abovementioned dose is for the primary guidance only. So, great care and caution are required during the use of midazolam.

The newer anesthetic agent, propofol, can also be used in place of midazolam. The continuous infusion of propofol is probably the best method for the administration of sedation with RA throughout the whole surgical procedure. An infusion of propofol at the rate of 2–4 mg/kg/hour will provide sedation with rapid recovery. Now, some newer methods of administration of propofol are also of interest. For this, a software algorithm is attached within the infusion pump with the aim to maintain the blood levels of propofol at the selected level (*target-controlled infusion*). By this technique, precise degree of sedation may be maintained. Another method of administration of propofol is to allow the patient to self-administer it (propofol) in anxiolytic doses. This is called the *patient-controlled sedation* and is analogous to the patient-controlled analgesia (PCA). The advantages of propofol over midazolam are that the drug is easier to titrate. Oversedation is probably less common and recovery is more rapid, though the amnestic effect of propofol is not as powerful, as that provided by midazolam. However, great care and caution with regard to cardiorespiratory system should also be maintained in case of propofol, like that of midazolam.

The small doses of short-acting opioids, such as fentanyl (1–2 µg/kg) or sufentanil (0.2–0.6 µg/kg), also can be used for analgesia in addition to or instead of sedative drugs. The supplementary analgesia has synergistic action with sedatives and may help to relief the discomfort during RA. During the use of sedatives and analgesics, it is mandatory to monitor the saturation of oxyhemoglobin and to administer oxygen, whenever necessary.

- *By use of general anesthesia:* It may seem unlogistic to render deliberately a patient insensible by applying GA or heavy sedation, when the CNB is providing perfect operating condition. But, sometimes the anxiety or doubt, concerning the efficacy of block provided or inadequate block, may force the anesthetist to apply GA in addition to CNB. In such circumstances, very light plane of GA is needed. The combination of GA with CNB will give excellent operating condition, as well as a prolonged postoperative analgesia. But, while combining GA with CNB, an anesthetist must keep in his mind that this combination may sometimes produce a potential problem, in which the sudden onset of sympathetic block from CNB and cardiac depression effect from GA, together can cause considerable hemodynamic compromise.

Awake Versus Asleep in RA

There has been recent controversy, regarding the performance of central neuraxial blockade (CNB) in the awake, sedated, or anesthetized state of a patient. The reason for controversy evolves from the fact that awake patient will tell and warn the anesthetist when the neural tissue is deemed to be damaged by a needle or catheter or injecting solution. But, there is no clear-cut evidence that always CNB or any other plexus and peripheral nerve block should be performed with the patient awake. Because, there are multiple reports when neural damage has occurred in an awake patient and the patient did not complain at the time of institution of regional block. On the other hand, there is no doubt that warning signs such as paresthesia and pain, associated with nerve damage, will be masked by sedation or anesthesia. Again, it is easier to perform RA on a patient who is asleep or anesthetized, particularly in children.

The thoracic epidural blockade, with or without catheter, is the most difficult situation to resolve. The technique of thoracic epidural anesthesia is very challenging and the success is more likely, when the patient is asleep. So, the careful use of nerve stimulators (when a nerve with motor function is to be blocked) is imperative during RA in an anesthetized patient. But, this cannot be performed when the nerve to be blocked is purely sensory. So, at the conclusion, it can be said that the question, regarding the use of spinal, epidural, or any regional block in awake and sedated patient, is still remain unresolved. But, always we will have to keep in mind that if any nerve damage occurs in sedated or anesthetized patient, then it may be very difficult to defend in the court, though it is widely used all over the world.

Position of Patient

Usually, three positions of patient are used for spinal or epidural anesthesia. These are lateral, sitting, and prone. Before positioning patient, to lateral or prone, it is mandatory to secure an intravenous line with a large bore indwelling cannula and monitoring devices are connected. The preintervention administration of 0.5–1 L of intravenous crystalloid or colloid solution, as bolus to limit the hypotension, induced by CNB, is considered as standard practice. But, care may be required for those patients with severe pulmonary disease, heart disease, renal disease, etc. Treatment of CNB induced hypotension with vasoactive drugs is an alternative approach to IV fluid loading. But, controversy surrounds in this topic.

Lateral Position

This position is also known as the "fetal position". It is the most common position which is practiced now for CNB and does not need any well-trained assistant. It is useful for more sedated patient also. Patient should be positioned with head slightly tilted down or up, so that the spread of hypo-, iso- or hyperbaric local anesthetic solution to operative site (dermatomes) is optimized. The spinal column has two ventral concavity, i.e., (1) thoracic and (2) sacral. So, when the patient is placed in supine after lateral position, then the movement of hyperbaric local anesthetic solution within the spinal subarachnoid space is not always toward the dependent part (caudal direction), if the injection is given at the mid lumbar region (L_2 or L_3 space). This is because the LA agent (in thoracolumbar kyphosis) will move cephalad from the maximum lumbar prominence, situated at the level of L_2-L_3 vertebra, toward the most dependent part of thoracic curvature in supine position, situated at about the level of T_4 or T_5 vertebra **(Fig. 25)**.

If the dural puncture is performed in lateral position and this position is maintained for few minutes, then there is a slight tendency for the dependent limb to be influenced or paralyzed more by unilateral manner, although due to CSF mechanics both sides are ultimately affected equally. Leaving the patient on lateral position for 5–10 minutes, after the injection of hyperbaric solution, there is more likely to produce a unilateral denser block on dependent side, but not the complete unilateral block. Only at higher spinal segmental level, there is preferential unilateral blockade. With regard to the cephalad and caudal spread, the lateral position functions in same way as the supine position. In any position (lateral, sitting, or prone), few moments should

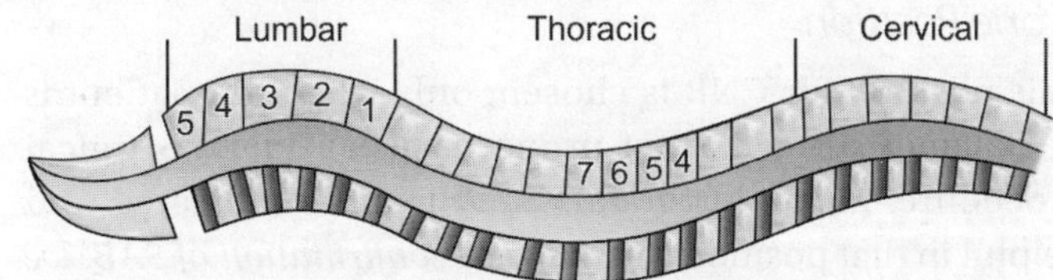

Fig. 25: The most prominent part of lumbar lordosis and the most dependent part of thoracic curvature (concavity) in supine position is shown in this figure.

always be spent for careful identification of most appropriate interspinous space for dural puncture or epidural anesthesia (EA) which may save much time, increases the chances of successful block and will ensure that the procedure is as speedy and comfortable as possible for the patient.

Sitting Position

It is chosen only when the lower lumbar and sacral levels of anesthesia are required or is adequate for the proposed surgical procedures on perineal, lower urinary tract, vaginal tract, etc. Sometimes, the obesity and scoliosis may make the identification of spinous process and interspinous spaces at the midline more difficult in lateral position. So, if only for the obesity and scoliosis, the sitting posture is chosen, but the higher sensory anesthesia is needed, then the patient should be made supine immediately, after the procedure in sitting position.

Some anesthetists also prefer the sitting position than lateral position for routine spinal or epidural anesthesia. This is because the sitting position has the following advantages (1) the identification of anatomic midline is often easier, when the patient is sitting; (2) generally the vertebra column remain in a straight line in such position; (3) the flexion of spine in sitting position maximizes the target area between the two adjacent spinous process; and (4) the identification of interspinous spaces is easier and so the technique of block is easier to perform in sitting position. On the other hand, some patients may find difficult to sit for lumbar puncture (e.g., fractured neck of femur) and in such situation the lateral position will be more appropriate. However, the care may be required during the performance of RA in sitting position, if premedication has been administered and there should be an assistant for positioning of such patient. After giving block at L$_{2-3}$ interspinous space, if sitting position is maintained for 5–10 minutes, then it blocks the lower lumbar (below the puncture site), all sacral (S$_{1-4}$) and coccygeal spinal nerves, i.e., cauda equina only, which is called the saddle block. It also depends on the lumbar level where dura is punctured. If dura is punctured at higher thoracic level and sitting position is maintained for 5 minutes then more higher spinal segments will be blocked.

Prone Position

This position for CNB is chosen, only when the patient is to be maintained in that prone position during surgical procedure. *Paramedian approach* is more indicated and helpful in that position (prone). *For confirmation of SAB, we have to aspirate CSF, because CSF pressure is minimum in that position.* In some circumstances, the spinal or epidural anesthesia is given in lateral position and then patient is made prone. In such situation, if the patient is placed in prone position, before fixation of drug, then the movement of drug through CSF is determined by the same factors, such as (1) the change in the compliance of subarachnoid space, (2) the degree of the tilting of vertebral column, (3) as well as the gravity of drug. As the thoracolumbar kyphosis is reversed, when the patient is in prone position and the degree of flexion- extension, achieved by prone position, influences the location of most dependent site of vertebral column, as well as the movement of drugs, so the placement of patient into prone position, with downward direction of head, before the onset of a gravity dependent spinal anesthesia, could result in dangerously high cephalad spread.

■ SPINAL ANESTHESIA

Technique of Intrathecal (Spinal) Anesthesia through Lumbar Puncture Route

Worldwide, the intrathecal (spinal or subarachnoid) anesthesia is the most commonly performed regional anesthetic technique, whereas the extradural (or epidural) blockade is used to provide labor analgesia and post-operative analgesia, in addition to any surgical anesthesia. For intrathecal anesthesia, the thoracic or cervical route is not used for fear of spinal cord injury, except when the dura is inadvertently punctured, during the thoracic or cervical extradural analgesia/anesthesia. So, for intrathecal or spinal anesthesia, only the lumbar puncture is conducted, under strict aseptic technique, with all the required equipment for resuscitation.

Most anesthetists perform *intrathecal lumbar puncture in the midline* and the space is selected between the spine of L$_3$ and L$_4$ or L$_2$ and L$_3$ vertebrae. Once, the anesthetist is happy with the position of the patient, then the skin of the back should be cleaned with an antiseptic solution or spray, guided by the protocol of that institution, and allowed to dry. Then, the patient should be drapped properly. After that, the skin and its deeper structures, over the targeted interspinous space, can be infiltrated with local anesthetic agent, prior to the insertion of spinal needle, but this will depend on the anesthetist's choice. Some anesthetists do not infiltrate the skin by LA agent, prior to the main technique. Now, the anesthetists have several choice for several types of needle for lumbar puncture, i.e., from the traditional cutting needle (Quincke) to the more recently introduced pencil tip (Whitacre and Sprotte) needle. However, the pencil tip needle is now the first choice of many anesthetists for intrathecal anesthesia, as it is associated with reduced incidences of PDPH.

Most anesthetists perform the intrathecal lumbar puncture in the midline *(median approach)* and the space is selected between the spine of L_3 and L_4 or L_2 and L_3 vertebrae. Now, the vertebral spinous processes and interspinous space are identified and selected. Then, the spinal needle is inserted through the area of the anesthetized skin, by making an angle cranially to compensate for the angle of spinous process and keeping the needle parallel to the floor. Now, *the needle will pass gradually through the skin, subcutaneous tissue, supraspinous ligament, interspinous ligament, ligamentum flavum, and finally through the epidural space, dura mater, and arachnoid mater before entering the subarachnoid space (Fig. 26)*. During the passage of needle, the skin and subcutaneous tissue will offer little resistance initially. As the needle courses deeper, it will enter the supraspinous ligament, interspinous ligament, and ligamentum flavum subsequently. During this passage of needle, increased resistance will be felt.

If bone is contacted superficially by needle, then it is probably that the needle is hitting the lower spinous process. On the contrary, if any bone is contacted by

needle at deeper plane, then it is probably that the needle is hitting the upper spinous process. In both the condition, needle should be redirected. When the needle will cross the ligamentum flavum, then there is often a characteristic "give" sensation, due to the loss of resistance. After getting this loss of resistance, the needle is advanced slightly more and the tip of the needle will gradually passes through the epidural space and pierce the dura and arachnoid mater. The *successful intrathecal puncture of needle is confirmed*, when the removal of the stylet is followed by the appearance of CSF at the hub of the needle. However, the appearance of CSF may be delayed, if a very fine needle, such as 27 G needle, is used. Again, if there is any doubt regarding the authenticity of fluid, then the *use of a bedside glucose testing strip* may be helpful. If a cutting tip spinal needle is used, then it is recommended that the needle should be inserted with the bevel parallel to the fibers of ligamentum flavum and dura mater, so that the fibers are parted away rather than are cut by the needle tip, as it is advanced. Inserting the needle in this fashion also reduces the chances of PDPH.

The *lateral or paramedian approach* to the subarachnoid space is also useful when the midline approach is difficult due to some scar tissue or arthritic changes. That means when the patient cannot be positioned easily due to severe arthritis, kyphosis, or prior spine surgery, then paramedian approach for spinal block is useful. The abnormal curvatures of spine, such as scoliosis and kyphoscoliosis have multiple effects on neuraxial anesthesia. Placing the block becomes more difficult because of the rotation and the angulation of vertebral bodies and spinous process. Finding the midline and interlaminar space may be difficult. So, the paramedian approach to neuraxial anesthesia may be preferable in patients with severe scoliosis and kyphoscoliosis.

Many anesthetists use routinely the paramedian approach for neuraxial anesthesia. After proper skin preparation and sterile draping, skin is infiltrated with LA solution, for paramedian approach, 2 cm lateral to the inferior aspect of the superior spinous process of the desired level. As the needle does not pass through the supraspinous and interspinous ligaments and penetrates the paravertebral muscles, so initially the needle will encounter little resistance. The needle is directed and advanced at a 10–25° angle toward the midline. If any bone is encountered by the needle at a shallow depth in this paramedian approach, then we will have to think that the needle has touched the medial part of lower lamina. In such situation, the needle should be redirected mostly upward and slightly laterally. On the other hand, if any bone is encountered by the needle at deeper plane, then we will have to think that the needle has touched the lateral part of lower lamina. In such situation, the needle

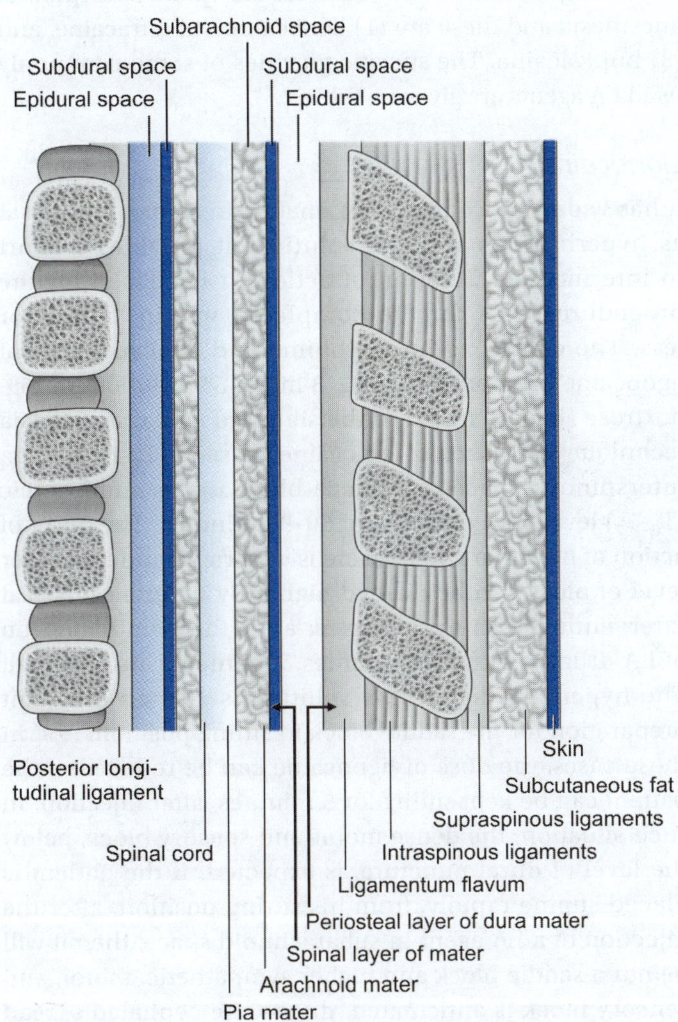

Fig. 26: The sagittal section through lumbar vertebrae.

should be redirected slightly cranially and more toward the midline. Once, the tip of the needle is confirmed to be lying in subarachnoid space, then the local anesthetic solution is injected. It is a good practice to confirm that the tip of the needle will not move during the aspiration of CSF or at some point during the injection of LA agent. Once the block has been established, then the upper level of anesthesia should be identified with the loss of sensation by pin prick (a common measurement), although some would suggest that the touch is a more reliable method for the assessment of the level of block.

Choice of Local Anesthetic Agent for Spinal Anesthesia

For the spinal or subarachnoid anesthesia, various drugs with different volumes, concentration, doses, baricity, along with the various sites of lumbar puncture, and the position of patient, are used to meet the aim. Therefore, there are multiple and multiple studies regarding all these variables. Hence, the comparison of these multiple studies is also very difficult, as the different parameters for the measurements of the efficacy of neural block (both sensory and motor) have been used. The most important factor for the choice of local anesthetic drug in spinal block is its duration of action which also varies according to the concentration, volume, and the total dose (in milligram) of drug with the site of injection and the position of patient.

Among these, the most important factor for the duration of action of a LA agent is the drug itself. From the beginning of spinal anesthesia and till now, many different drugs have been used for spinal block. But, recently only a few drugs remain in current practice. However, in the more recent years, the choice of drug, available to anesthesiologist for spinal anesthesia in India, has been reduced only to the most commonly used 0.5% bupivacaine in 8% dextrose. Other drugs that are available for SAB in other countries (not in India) include procaine, lignocaine, mepivacaine, and tetracaine. The duration of action of these drugs varies (the reason of which is described above), but in general, procaine has a short duration of action, lignocaine and mepivacaine have a moderate duration of action, and the tetracaine and bupivacaine have a longer duration of action. The action of hypobaric solution persists for longer period than that of its isobaric solutions which in turn have a more prolonged action than that of its hyperbaric solutions. Sometimes, the epinephrine is added with local anesthetic agents to extend their duration of action. It undoubtedly doubles the duration of action of LA agents. The epinephrine may also has some direct antinociceptive effect on the spinal cord and this is due to the direct activation of descending

TABLE 2: Specific gravities of some spinal anesthetic agents.

Agent	Specific gravity
• *Bupivacaine:*	
– 0.5% plain	0.99–1
– 0.5% in 8.25% dextrose	1.02–1.03
• *Lignocaine:*	
– 2% plain	1
– 5% in 7.5% dextrose	1.02–1.03
• *Tetracaine:*	
– 0.5% in water	0.99
– 0.5% in dextrose	1.01–1.02
• *Procaine:*	
– 10% plain	1.01
– 2.5% in water	0.99

adrenergic inhibitory systems that ultimately modulate the neural activity of dorsal horn. If patient plans to go home after outpatient surgical procedure, then the short-acting LA drug is preferred. In most of the countries of the world, three drugs are commonly used for the spinal and epidural anesthesia and these are (1) lignocaine, (2) tetracaine, and (3) bupivacaine. The specific gravities of some commonly used LA agents are given in **Table 2**.

Lignocaine

It has wide application in RA, mainly in spinal anesthesia as hyperbaric or isobaric solution. It provides a short to intermediate duration of action. It is chosen for the procedures that can be completed within 1 hour or less. The commonly used volume and concentration of lignocaine in spinal block is 2–3 mL of 5% solution in 7.5% dextrose (hyperbaric). For the standard spinal anesthesia technique 50–100 mg of lignocaine is used at L_2-L_3 or L_3-L_4 interspinous space to achieve block up to midthoracic (T_6-T_7) level for a duration of 60–90 minutes. The onset of action of hyperbaric lignocaine is vary rapid and the upper level of block can be pushed higher by different physical intervention within 5 minutes, after the administration of LA drug or within 10 minutes, if epinephrine is added. The hyperbaric lignocaine solution is also an excellent preparation for the saddle block in sitting position. And in these cases, the dose of lignocaine can be reduced, if the patient can be kept sitting for 5 minutes, after injection. In such situation, the dense motor and sensory block, below the level of dural puncture, is expected. If the patient is placed supine rapidly, from his sitting position, after the injection of a LA agent in subarachnoid space, then it will be not a saddle block and higher sympathetic, motor, and sensory block is anticipated, due to the cephalad spread of LA agent. It was found in different studies that there is higher incidence of transient radicular irritation with the use of 5% lignocaine in subarachnoid space. But, the relation between 5% lignocaine and transient radicular irritation is controversial. So, the reduction of concentration of lignocaine in hyperbaric spinal preparation is under trial.

Till now, there is also some controversy, regarding the use of vasoconstrictor with different local anesthetic drugs, such as lignocaine, tetracaine, and bupivacaine, during spinal anesthesia. The addition of 0.1–0.2 mg epinephrine (adrenaline) or 5 mg phenylephedrine prolongs the duration of action of lignocaine and increases its efficacy during the CNB. Here, with the passing of time, the two spinal segments regression from the cephalic end is taken as the parameter for the measurement of the duration of neuraxial block. But, the addition of adrenaline in spinal LA drugs, to increase their duration of action, may increase the risk of anterior spinal artery syndrome and cord ischemia, particularly if associated with hypotension.

The SAB by isobaric solution is also possible by using 2% plain solution of lignocaine (isobaric lignocaine), without added preservative. But, the standard dose of isobaric lignocaine solution in SAB is 3–4 cc with or without 0.2 mg epinephrine. It provides anesthesia (motor and sensory block) up to the level of T_{10} for 60–90 minutes, if the drug is administered at L_3-L_4 space in supine horizontal position. However, *the level of anesthesia by isobaric lignocaine solution does not depend on the physical position of the patient after injection. But, the level of anesthesia in isobaric solution depends only on the volume, total dose, the direction of the needle bevel and the speed of injection of local anesthetic drug. Mixed with sterile water, the preservative free 2% lignocaine also can be used as hypobaric solution for the subarachnoid block.*

The allergy, caused by LA agent, is commonly due to para-aminobenzoic acid (PABA) which is the breakdown product of ester-linked LA agents, such as *procaine,* by plasma enzymatic cleavage. It (PABA) is thought to trigger an allergic reaction in certain individual who may have previous immunological sensitization to PABA, as it is a common ingredient in many fragrances and cosmetics. Thus, the immunoglobulin G (IgG) or immunoglobulin M (IgM)-mediated anaphylaxis is a possibility of some ester-linked LA agent. True allergy to amide local anesthetic agent is uncommon, except the multidose preparations that have methylparaben as preservative. Methylparaben is a common allergen and is related to PABA. Even skin testing conducted under optimum circumstances to identify allergy of LA agent does not totally eliminate this concern. So, reasonable caution is mandatory. The dose, concentration, and the volume of lignocaine, used in epidural anesthesia, are discussed in separate section.

Bupivacaine

Like lignocaine, it is also a very commonly used LA agent for spinal anesthesia and in some country, it is the only available drug for SAB. Commonly used hyperbaric concentration of bupivacaine for SAB is 0.75% and 0.5% in 8.25% dextrose. The 2 cc of these hyperbaric bupivacaine solution, injected at L_3-L_4 interspinous space in supine horizontal position, can block sensory level up to the T4 or T6 spinal segment (dermatomes). However, lower dose is used in some extreme age group of patients, due to the reduced compliance of subarachnoid space. The expected duration of action of 2 cc hyperbaric bupivacaine in subarachnoid space is average 2 hours. This duration of action of bupivacaine can be reduced, if the drug is made to spread over a wide area and diluted with CSF by the change of physical position of patient. However, as the spread of LA agent reduces the duration of action, but it increases the level of block of spinal segment. The isobaric form, i.e., 0.5% and 0.75% bupivacaine in plain aqueous solution (without preservative) are also used in spinal anesthesia. Different studies indicate that there is no difference in the duration of action over a wide range of concentration from 0.25 to 0.75% as long as the total dose (in milligram) of isobaric bupivacaine is kept constant. Below the 0.25%, the intensity and the duration of motor block by bupivacaine is decreased. With isobaric solutions, the onset of action of bupivacaine is also slow, taking 10 minutes or more for the full sensory and motor block. As with other isobaric techniques, the level of block for the isobaric bupivacaine is typically up to the T_{12} spinal segment and the hemodynamic alterations are minimal due to lower level and the slow onset of anesthesia which allows the adequate time for endogenous hemodynamic compensation. When the isobaric form of bupivacaine is used, then the injected total dose of drug (i.e., total dose in milligram) is more important in determining the height of block than the volume of drug and position of the patient. The action of bupivacaine lasts for 2–2.5 hours. The typical subarachnoid dose of bupivacaine is 15–20 mg. Addition of epinephrine with bupivacaine for spinal anesthesia has minimal clinical significance (epidural dose of bupivacaine is further discussed in separate chapter).

Tetracaine (Amethocaine)

It is available in package as both crystal (20 mg) and 1% solution (20 mg) which can be mixed with sterile water (hypobaric), dextrose solution (hyperbaric), or CSF (isobaric). Thus, an anesthetist will prepare their own solution (baricity) of tetracaine, according to their need. The onset of action of tetracaine is 5–10 minutes and the duration of action of it is 2–3 hours with epinephrine. Its duration of action may persist for 5 hours in lower extremity. It is the most commonly used agent for spinal anesthesia in USA. In some countries, the readymade preparation of tetracaine, with different baricity, is also available. Previously prepared tetracaine spinal kits contain 1% tetracaine solution in 2 cc ampoule which is mixed with 10% dextrose for hyperbaric solution. Some anesthesiologists do not prefer premade preparation. Instead, they constitute the solution themselves immediately before their use. Because, as tetracaine is an ester local anesthetic, so it loses its potency in premixed solution, after exposure to heat, which explains occasional failure of block after the use of premade tetracaine. The usual dose of hyperbaric tetracaine for spinal anesthesia is 6–20 mg, depending on the patient's height, weight, age, and other factors that decrease the compliance of subarachnoid space. The level of sensory and motor block usually extends up to the level of T_4-T_6 spinal segment, after the lumbar spinal of 20 mg tetracaine at L_2-L_3 interspinous space in supine position. The onset of action of tetracaine is relatively rapid than that of bupivacaine, but somewhat slower than that of lignocaine. The addition of 0.2 mg epinephrine with tetracaine increases the duration of action by 20–50%. The classic isobaric tetracaine solution can be prepared by mixing its crystal with CSF, drawn from patient after dural puncture. Like other isobaric solutions, the speed of injection, total dose, the orientation of the bevel of spinal needle, etc. influence the level of block, produced by tetracaine, but not the patient's position or posture (physical condition). The dose of isobaric tetracaine solution is same as that of its hyperbaric solution.

Choice of Needle for Spinal Anesthesia

- The first question, regarding the choice of spinal needle is if it should be disposable or reusable. But, most anesthetists accept disposable tray, though there is no indication that the disposable set shifts the risk-benefit equation in patient's favor.
- The second question, regarding the choice of spinal needle, is cutting or noncutting pencil tipped. The cutting tipped needle, such as Quincke or Babcock, cut the dural fiber during their introduction through the dural membrane, causing more leakage of CSF and the most incidences of postspinal headache. Whereas, the noncutting conical pencil tipped spinal needle, such as the Greene/Whitacre/Sprotte, does not cut the dural fibers (only separate the fibers of dura mater) and is associated with the decreased incidences of PDPH, when the needle sizes are same.
- The third question, regarding the choice of needle, is if it should be fine (thin) or thick. Fine needles, such as 25 G or above, are preferred by most of the anesthetists for spinal anesthesia, due to the less incidences of

postspinal headache. But, the introduction of these fine needles into the subarachnoid space, passing through multiple tough fibrous tissues, is technically difficult and so the incidence of failure rate is high. Very fine needles may be inserted through an introducer or a 20 G needle. These spinal needle introducer aids the passage of a very fine spinal needle through tough ligamentous structures of vertebral column. In older patients, in whom the ligamentous structure of vertebral column become calcified, it may be impossible to insert a very fine pencil tipped needle into subarachnoid space through the tough structure without the use of an introducer. The introducer also has an additional advantage that spinal needle does not touch the skin and so also reduces the chances of infection.

- The fourth question, regarding the choice of spinal needle, is if it should be long or short beveled and sharp or blunt pointed. The standard sharp pointed but long beveled needles are suitable for repeated spinal blocks and may permit the smooth passage of needle through the tissues. This enables the fine control of needle tip, but the less recognition of tissue plane. Whereas, the short-beveled blunt needle (e.g., Sprotte needle) may enable tissue planes to be identified more easily, but the passage of needle through the tissues is not so smooth.

The nerve damage caused by this type of needle is controversial. It is assumed that the standard *sharp* long beveled needles *cause less nerve damage*, if it (nerve) is pierced by the needle accidentally. But, there is more chance to pierce the nerve by this type of needle. On the other hand, the *blunt* short-beveled needle has less chance to pierce the nerve. But, if it happens (pierces the nerve), will cause more damage to the nerve. The less nerve damage by a sharp long-beveled needle is due to the nerve fibers being separated, rather than torn.

Spinal Needles

The standard hypodermic needle has a sharp pointed tip with a bevel <20°. This is called the needle with "A" type of bevel. But, the needle which is used for the nerve block in RA, is designed to be less traumatic to nerve tissues. So, it is made slightly blunt with the bevel >45° and is called the needle with "B" type of bevel. Depending on the purpose of the needle, for which it will be used, the bevel of the needle can be either *sharp,* polished, or *dull* **(Fig. 27)**. The usual site for the exit of drug from needle is the tip of it (needle). But, for some special applications, the exit site is sometimes kept not exactly at the tip of the needle, but slightly distal to the tip of the needle. Some other modifications of the needle may also improve the dexterity of the operator. These are wings

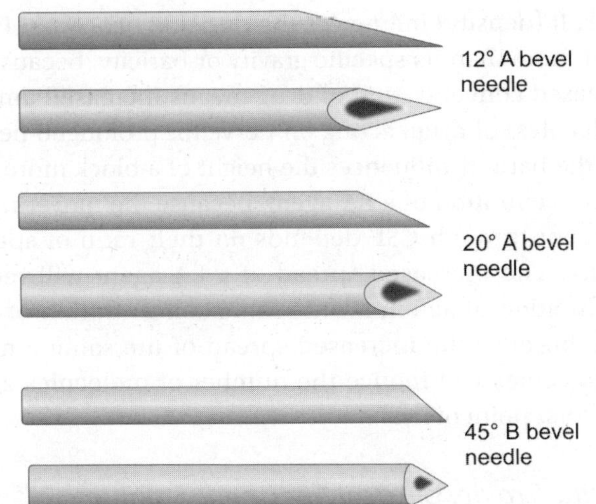

Fig. 27: The different types of A and B needle used for regional block.

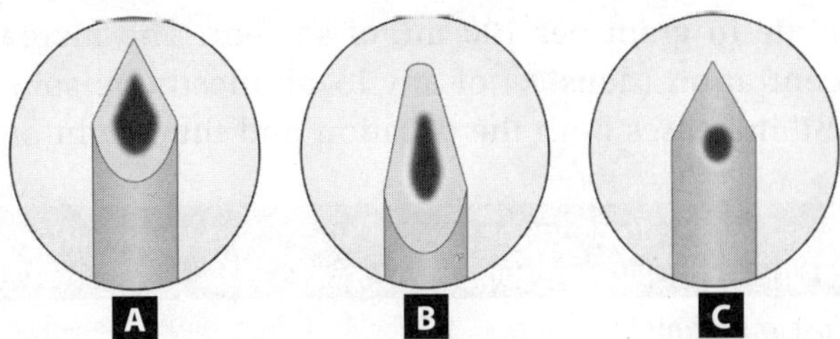

Figs. 28A to C: Spinal needle. (A) Quincke; (B) Sprotte; and (C) Whitacre.

that can be attached to the hub of the needle. This allows the two-handed better grip of the needle and enables the operator to feel the tissues better during its (needle) passage through the tissues. Some needles have alternating polished and dull surface along the shaft of it for better tissue feeling. The shape, sharpness, bevel, and the hole at the tip of the needle are all variable that can be manipulated to suit its special needs. The Tuohy and Hustead modification are such examples of altering the tip of needle for special task such as for the epidural anesthesia. The 2–4 mm area at the tip of Tuohy needle is gently curved, which is designed to pass the needle through the soft tissue smoothly and make contact with dura, without penetrating it.

The spinal needles are also classified (1) according to the size of the needle and (2) according to the shape of the needle tip. According to the size, the type of spinal needle extends from 20 to 30 G. Thicker wide-bore needle helps to feel the tissue structures better, during its passage through it and after piercing the dura, the flow of CSF through wide-bore needle is faster. So, it helps in easy recognition of proper placement of needle in subarachnoid space. Another advantage of thicker wide-bore needle is less failure rate in compare to finer needle. But, the incidence of PDPH is high in case of thicker wide-bore needles, due to the large dural hole and significant CSF leak. On the other hand, these advantages of thick needle become the disadvantages of fine needle. So, in fine thin narrow-bore needle, there is less feeling (recognition) of tissue structure, during its passage through it (tissues). Further, the flow of CSF through a fine needle is not easy. So, the recognition of the placement of it (needle) in subarachnoid space is difficult, and failure rate is high. But, one distinct advantage of fine needle is the less incidences of PDPH. Sometimes, very fine spinal needles (25 to 30 G) need introducer (18 to 20 G) to facilitate their insertion through

skin, ligaments, and other structures of vertebral column. The introducer also prevents the deflection, bending or the breaking of needle, while passing through the tissues. The introducer also helps to keep the spinal needle sterile, as it does not come in contact with skin and other structures.

According to the shape of the tip of spinal needle, it is again subclassified into (1) cutting tip spinal needle and (2) noncutting pencil tip spinal needle (**Figs. 28A to C**).

- *Cutting tipped spinal needle:*
  - *Pitkin needle:* It has short, cutting bevel, and eccentric sharp pointed tip.
  - *Howard Jones:* It is a metallic spinal needle with cutting tip, available in size ranging between 20 and 24 G.
  - *Quincke–Babcock:* It is the most widely used spinal needle, with cutting tip and long sharp bevel. It has an exit point at its tip and is available from 16 to 30 G.
  - *Atraucan:* It is a cutting tip needle with double bevel.
- *Noncutting pencil tipped spinal needles:*
  - *Green needle:* Long sharp bevel and rounded tip with orifice at end.
  - *Whitacre needle:* Solid pencil tip with small lateral orifice, 2 mm proximal to the tip—proximal injecting needle.
  - *Sprotte needle:* Solid pencil tip with large lateral orifice whose diameter is equal to the internal diameter of the needle with proximal injecting point.

Factors Affecting the Height and Duration of Block in Spinal Anesthesia

The factors affecting the height and the duration of the action of block in spinal anesthesia are listed in **Box 1** and the factors that probably do not affect the height of spinal block are listed in **Box 2**. The duration of action of different LA agents are given in **Table 3**.

Density of Local Anesthetic Solution

The density of any solution is the weight of solute in gram per 1 mL of solvent. Concentration is nothing but density, but concentration in weight/volume (w/v) means weight of solute in gram per 100 mL of solvent. The increased concentration (density) of any local anesthetic solution in CSF increases both the duration and the height of the

> **BOX 1:** Factors affecting the level of spinal anesthesia (arranged according to their importance from more to less).
>
> - *Most important factors:*
>   - Site of injection
>   - Baricity of anesthetic solution
>   - Position of patient:
>   - During injection
>   - Immediately after injection
>   - Drug dose
> - *Less important factors:*
>   - Drug volume
>   - Patient height
>   - Curvature of spine
>   - Pregnancy
>   - Needle direction
>   - Age
>   - Intra-abdominal pressure
>   - Volume of cerebrospinal fluid (CSF)

> **BOX 2:** Factors that probably do not affect the height of spinal block.
>
> - Rate of injection
> - Addition of vasoconstrictor
> - Barbotage technique
> - Cough or any strain, like bearing down during labor
> - Bevel of needle
> - Weight of patient
> - Gender

block. It (density) influences the duration of action of a LA agent more than its specific gravity or baricity, because the increased concentration of drug means increased amount (molecules) of drug, acting on nerve for prolonged period. But, the baricity influences the height of a block more than the concentration of a LA agent, because the movement of LA agent through CSF depends on their ratio of specific gravity. The increased spread of a LA agent will reduce the duration of action for the same concentration of a LA drug, because the increased spread of the same amount of molecules will reduce the number of molecules at the particular point of nerve.

Specific Gravity of Local Anesthetic Solution

It is the ratio of density of a solution compared to the density of water. It also influences both the duration and the height of block, like the baricity of the solution of a LA drug by influencing the spread.

Baricity of Local Anesthetic Solution

Baricity is the ratio of comparing the specific gravity of one solution to another. Baricity of LA solution is classified as hyperbaric, isobaric and hypobaric in reference to the specific gravity of CSF which varies between 1.003 and 1.005. The plain LA solutions, such as 2% lignocaine and 0.5% bupivacaine, which are available commercially for the local infiltration of subcutaneous tissue are prepared at a specific gravity nearly identical to CSF (isobaric) at room temperature and hence they are isobaric. When they are warmed to body

TABLE 3: The dosages and the duration of action of commonly used spinal local anesthetic (LA) drugs.

		(Doses in mg)			(Duration in minute)	
Drug	**Preparation**	**Perineum and lower limbs**	**Lower abdomen (up to T_{10})**	**Upper abdomen (up to T_4)**	**Plain**	**With adrenaline (0.1 to 0.2 mg)**
Lignocaine	5% in 7.5% dextrose	20–50	50–70	70–100	60–90	90–120
Bupivacaine	0.5% in 8.25% dextrose	5–10	10–15	15–20	90–120	120–150
Ropivacaine	0.5% and 0.75% solution	6–12	12–16	16–18	90–120	90–120
Tetracaine	1% in 10% dextrose (0.5% hyperbaric)	5–10	10–15	15–20	90–120	120–150

Dosages and duration of adjuvants in subarachnoid space			
Drugs	**Dose (µg)**	**Duration (hour)**	**Side effects and comments**
Fentanyl	10–25	1–2	Nausea, vomiting, urinary retention, itching, sedation, respiratory depression, and ileus
Sufentanil	1.5–5	1	Do
Morphine	150–250	4–24	Do
Epinephrine	100–200		Ischemia of cord
Clonidine	15–150		Sedation, hypotension, and prolongation of action of LA agents

temperature before injection, then they become slightly hypobaric. The classical isobaric LA injection can also be prepared from crystal of local anesthetic agent such as the tetracaine after mixing it in patient's CSF. The hypobaric solutions of tetracaine also can be made by mixing the crystal of local anesthetic agent in preservative-free sterile water. Hyperbaric solutions are created by mixing the LA agent with 7.5–10% dextrose (in order to achieve the specific gravity of 1.02 or above).

Hyperbaric solution: The hyperbaric solutions of LA agents are made by adding 7.5–10% dextrose with it. They move downward in CSF and block the roots of nerve below the level of dural puncture. Spinal anesthesia in sitting position and if it is maintained for 5–10 minutes, after the administration of LA agent, then the LA agent will move caudally and block the coccygeal, sacral, and lumbar spinal nerves (below the puncture site) only. This is called the *saddle block*. The hyperbaric solution of LA agent also moves toward the dependent side in lateral position and cephalad up to the midpoint of thoracic anteriorly concave curvature in supine position, if the site of dural puncture is at the height of lumbar lordosis and the patient is in slightly Trendelenburg position. Otherwise (if the patient is in anti-Trendelenburg position and the site of dural puncture is at the height of lumbar lordosis), the drug will accumulate caudally in the sacral hollow and will produce inadequate height of block. In supine position, the hyperbaric solution causes more higher block than the isobaric or hypobaric solution. In lithotomy position, the baricity of LA solution have little effect on the height of block. The hyperbaric solution acts in a more predictable manner than the hypobaric or isobaric plain solution of LA agent. The peripheral nerve toxicity of local anesthetic agents is increased in the presence of dextrose. But, it is uncertain, whether this is a direct effect of dextrose on nerve or whether the presence of dextrose enhances the toxic effect of local anesthetic agent.

Isobaric solution: They are the simplest solutions of LA agent. They are commonly marketed for infiltration anesthesia, such as 2% xylocaine and 0.5% bupivacaine in vial with preservative and are also used in epidural block. An isobaric LA solution tends to remain at the level of injection. The spread and consequently the height of the block by isobaric local anesthetic solution in spinal anesthesia does not depend on the position or the posture of patient. So, the height of blocking effect of a LA agent is more unpredictable, when it (LA agent) is made isobaric from hyperbaric. Tetracaine (amethocaine) isobaric formulation is made by diluting the tetracaine crystal (20 mg) in CSF at 1:1 ratio. The distribution of isobaric local anesthetic solution and consequently the height of block produced by it mainly depends on the volume of drug, the temperature, and the direction of injection.

Hypobaric solution: They are usually used and most useful in prone positions for anorectal procedures or in lateral positions for hip surgery. Theoretically, the 2% lignocaine has been investigated as a "clinically" hypobaric spinal drug. But, practically, the physiochemical properties of 2% lignocaine are more isobaric than hypobaric. Still, some anesthesiologists find it (2% lignocaine) more useful in situations, reserved for hypobaric techniques.

Lipid and Water Solubility of Drug

The most lipid soluble anesthetic agent, such as the fentanyl spreads less than the less lipid soluble anesthetic agent, such as the morphine in spinal anesthesia. This is because when a LA agent becomes more and more lipid soluble, then it is absorbed more and more quickly by the local lipid rich nervous system at the site of injection, impairing the spread of it.

Volume of Local Anesthetic Solutions

Like baricity, position of patient and site of injection, the volume and the total dose of drug (in milligram) have same effect on the height of spinal anesthesia. But increased dose in milligram certainly prolongs the duration of block. On the other hand, the greater spread of a large volume of local anesthetic agent (same in milligram) may brief its duration of effect due to the quick absorption of it by the blood vessels of large area. So, the spread of LA agent, increased by the baricity, posture or other means, curtailed the duration of effect of LA agent, provided the amount of drug (concentration) remain same.

Barbotage

This term is derived from a French word, named "barboter", which means to paddle or mix. The repeated aspiration of CSF by syringe and injection of local anesthesia in the subarachnoid space cause mixing and dispersing of the original dose of local anesthetic agent with CSF. This is called the barbotage technique. Thus, the spread of a given dose of local anesthetic drug and subsequently the height of anesthesia can be increased by barbotage, which is now hardly used.

Site of Injection

Any site (or interspinous space) for injection can be chosen for the administration of local anesthetic agent for spinal or epidural anesthesia. But, obviously the higher will be the site of injection, the higher will be the height of block. This is applicable to both the spinal and epidural anesthesia. But, in spinal anesthesia, the higher will be the site of injection, the higher will be the chance of cord injury and severe hypotension. Hence, the L_{3-4}/L_{4-5} is the safer intervertebral space to restrict the dural puncture for spinal block in order to avoid the possible damage of spinal cord. But, the epidural block can be given at any site, such as the cervical, thoracic, lumbar, and sacral region.

Position of Patient during and Immediately after Subarachnoid Injection

Like the abovementioned factors, the position of patient during and immediately after injection in subarachnoid or epidural space is also very important in determining the height of block. But, (1) the baricity of LA solution, (2) the concentration and volume of drug, along with (3) the position of patient, and (4) the site of injection are all interrelated and can be modulated, according to the necessity of the height of block. After placement in subarachnoid space, the local anesthetic agent is very rapidly taken up by the nerve tissues of spinal cord and disappears from the CSF. So, the first 5 minutes after administration of drug are very crucial for the local anesthetic agent for tissue fixation. In lateral position, the vertebral column is more or less horizontal. However, in lateral position in some women, the vertebral column is inclined toward the head and it is due to the increased width of pelvis, relative to the shoulder. In some men, the vertebral column is inclined toward the coccyx, because of the increased width of shoulder relative to the pelvis. So, the operating table should be inclined, during CNB in the lateral position of patient, according to the necessity, keeping all the factors in mind **(Fig. 29)**.

For anorectal, perineal, genital, and bladder neck surgeries, 1 mL hyperbaric solution in sitting position (maintained for 5 minutes) at L_{4-5} space is useful which blocks

only the sacral, coccygeal, and L_{4-5} spinal nerves with little or no fall of BP. This is known as the saddle block. Increasing the volume and concentration of LA agent the duration of this type of block can be increased according to the duration of surgery. But for lower abdominal surgery 1.5–2 mL drug (hyperbaric) at L_{3-4} space is injected in lateral position and the patient is turned immediately in supine position. This is sufficient for 45 minutes to 1 hour surgery in lower abdomen. L_{3-4} interspace forms the apex of the lumbar curvature. So, the administration of heavy drug in that space in supine position causes the spread of LA agent up to the midthoracic segment, as T_5 is the most dependent part of thoracic curvature in supine position. Sometimes, after injection of LA drugs may fall in the hollow of sacrum, leading to the block of only sacral and coccygeal spinal nerve roots.

For the upper abdominal operations, block up to the T_4 or T_5 spinal segment, is required. This is obtained when the 2–3 mL of hyperbaric LA drug is injected at L_{2-3} interspace, with slight head-down position. For upper abdominal surgeries, the level of anesthesia is needed up to T4 segment along with the greater splanchnic nerve ($T_{4,5,6,7,8}$) block supplying the omentum and mesentery. So, intraoperative paraesophageal vagus block is also given by surgeon for upper abdominal surgery along with the spinal or epidural anesthesia. *Some landmarks of segmental supply which is very useful for spinal anesthesia are perineum: S_{2-4}, groin: L_{1-2}, umbilicus: T_{10}, xiphoid: T_7, nipple: T_{4-5}, second intercostals space: T_2, clavicle: C_3-C_4, and subcostal arch: T_{6-8}.*

Factors which decrease the size of subarachnoid space also cause the compression and the decrease of the compliance of subarachnoid space. For example, increased intra-abdominal pressure and transmitted via intervertebral foramen to epidural space cause compression and the reduction of subarachnoid space. Thus pregnancy, obesity, ascites, huge ovarian tumor, or any other factors that increase the intra-abdominal pressure cause the reduction of the volume of subarachnoid space. The reduction of CSF volume or the volume of subarachnoid space inversely correlates well with the dermatomal spread of spinal anesthesia. Therefore, the pregnancy, obesity, ascites, etc. cause the increase in the height of block with the same volume of drug. Age decreases the compliance of subarachnoid space and increases the height of block also. The decrease of compliance of subarachnoid space with increase of age is due to the increase of stiffness and decrease of the size of subarachnoid space.

Pregnancy

Pressure over inferior vena cava by gravid uterus causes the dilatation of the epidural veins which in turn decreases

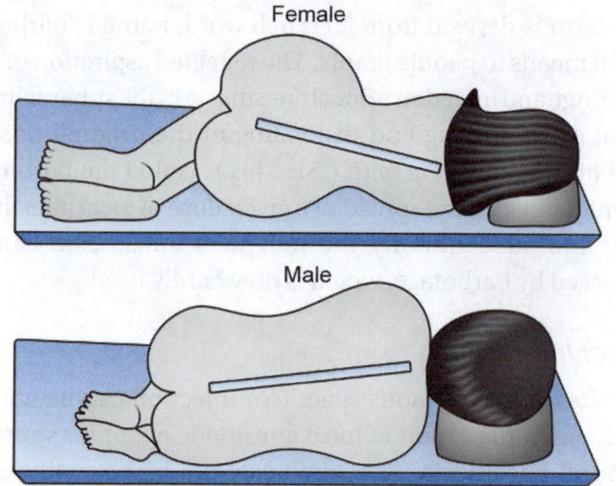

Fig. 29: The natural tendency of inclination of vertebral column in lateral position of male and female patient.

the volume of epidural space and increases the epidural pressure. Thus, the compression of subarachnoid space from increased epidural pressure causes the lower volume of it (subarachnoid space) and the higher spread of LA solution. Progesterone also potentiate LA action, which is also responsible for the increase in spread (height) of action of local anesthetic agent in pregnancy.

Ascites

It has also the same effect as gravid uterus on inferior vena cava and in turn on epidural vessels and epidural space. Also increased intra-abdominal pressure from ascites is transmitted directly into the epidural space through the intervertebral foramen and thus increases the epidural pressure. Hence, the increase in pressure in epidural space in turn decreases the size of subarachnoid space and increases the spread and the action of local anesthetic agent in spinal anesthesia.

Obesity

Obese patients also have decreased subarachnoid compliance, particularly when the patient is in supine position, where the weight of anterior abdominal wall acts, much in the same way, as a gravid uterus or ascites.

Spinal Stenosis

For the same reasons, decreased compliance of subarachnoid space in spinal stenosis causes wider spread and increased height of action of LA agent in spinal anesthesia.

Age

The age influences the conduct and outcome of subarachnoid anesthesia to some extent. Geriatric patients have the decreased compliance of subarachnoid space and reduced CSF volume which causes greater spread and increased extent of the level of spinal anesthesia with same volume of drug. This is applicable to hyperbaric as well as to isobaric and hypobaric anesthetic solutions.

Geriatric patients rarely develop PDPH. So, the use of fine, noncutting spinal needle to minimize this complication is not necessary. On the other hand, the thick and cutting sharp spinal needle have definite advantage for the geriatric patients, since these patients have difficult dural puncture, due to the calcification of ligaments, such as the supraspinous, interspinous ligaments which will offer greater resistance for the passage of needle through these calcified ligaments. The low incidence of spinal headache in geriatric patient is probably related to the advanced degenerative arthritis which is common in

the geriatric spine and makes the continued leak of CSF unlikely, due to inflammation that induces the sealing of dural puncture.

Temperature

It also acts for the movement of drug. Hyperthermia increases the height of block and hypothermia decreases the height of block.

Height of Block Necessary for Few Common Operations

(1) Prostate, bladder, and upper thigh: block up to the T_{10} dermatomes; (2) Inguinal hernia: block up to the T_{10} dermatomes; (3) Umbilical operation: block up to the T_{6-7} dermatome; (4) Lower abdominal operation: block up to the T_7 dermatome; and (5) Upper abdominal surgeries (cholecystectomy, gastrectomy, transverse colectomy, etc.): block up to the T4 dermatome.

For gut surgery, some afferent stimuli pass through the vagus nerve. So, such type of surgeries require paraesophageal block of vagus nerve or GA along with spinal or epidural block. Here, the CNB helps by producing an ischemic field, gut retraction, good relaxation, reduction of stress, and postoperative analgesia.

Fate of Local Anesthetic Agent in CSF

Anatomically, it is likely that the exposure of spinal cord and its nerve roots to local anesthetic agent which is injected in the CSF, results in the blockade of conduction of impulses through them, before they exit through the intervertebral foramen. However, though there is also exposure of spinal cord to local anesthetic agent, but the conventionally used concentration and doses of LA drug make the penetration of it (LA drug) into the deeper parts of intact spinal cord unlikely. The termination of the action of LA agent after spinal anesthesia is likely to occur by the dissociation of drug into the spinal fluid from the cord and its roots first and later by the absorption of it (LA agent) into the vascular space. The principal site of action of epidural block is also the spinal nerve roots while they are passing through the epidural space. The direct injection of local anesthetic agent into CSF for spinal anesthesia allows a relatively small dose and volume of local anesthetic agent to spread over a wide area spinal cord and to achieve dense sensory and motor blockade. In contrast, the same concentration, but the much higher volume of local anesthetic agent is injected into epidural space, as there is no influence of spread of drug by CSF. Moreover, the injection site (level) for epidural anesthesia must be close to the nerve roots that must be anesthetized. The termination of action of LA agent after epidural block is likely to occur by the absorption of drug by epidural venous plexuses and partly by passing of the drug into the subarachnoid space.

First very quick, then gradual fall of concentration of local anesthetic drug in CSF is seen in spinal block. The first steep fall in concentration of local anesthetic agent in CSF is due to the mixing of drug with CSF and then the rapid intake of this drug by the nerve root and spinal cord. The second gradual decrease of drug concentration in CSF is due to the vascular absorption of drug from CSF and nervous tissue. The CSF flows into venous sinuses via arachnoid villi may also contribute, to some extent, in the clearance of local anesthetic agent. The lymphatic drainage has also contribution in the clearance of drug. Local anesthetic acts both on the spinal cord and nerve roots, but opioids act only in the substance of cord.

ORDER OF BLOCKING OR SENSITIVITY OF DIFFERENT NERVE FIBERS TO LOCAL ANESTHETIC AGENTS

All the types of fibers within a mixed nerve (motor + sensory + proprioceptive + autonomic) are affected by local anesthetic agents during the spinal or epidural anesthesia. But, within one mixed nerve, there is a tendency for the smaller (thin) and slow conducting fibers (sensory) to be *more readily blocked* than the larger (thick) and fast conducting fibers (motor), though always this rule does not hold good, because it is well established that the myelinated autonomic preganglionic sympathetic B fibers, which are larger and have a faster conduction time, are *about three times more sensitive* to local anesthetic agent than the thinner and slower conducting nonmyelinated postganglionic C fibers. **Figure 30** shows the longitudinal section of a myelinated nerve fiber and **Figure 31** shows the cross section of individual nerve fiber and a nerve trunk. The LA agents have to penetrate the barrier of epineurium, perineurium, endoneurium, and myelin sheath (if present), before they work on nerve fibers.

The preganglionic autonomic B fibers are the most sensitive of all the nerve fibers, causing early vasodilation and consequent hypotension which is a well-recognized early sequel to epidural, spinal, or paravertebral block. Large (or thick), rapid conducting, and motor A-α fibers are the *most resistant* to local anesthetic agents. It is probable that the A-δ fibers, responsible for the pain and temperature sensation are more sensitive than the C pain fibers, although it (A-δ fibers) is larger and more rapid conducting than the C fibers. This explains why sometimes the pathological pains, such as the impending uterine rupture or placental separation, conducted by C fibers, may

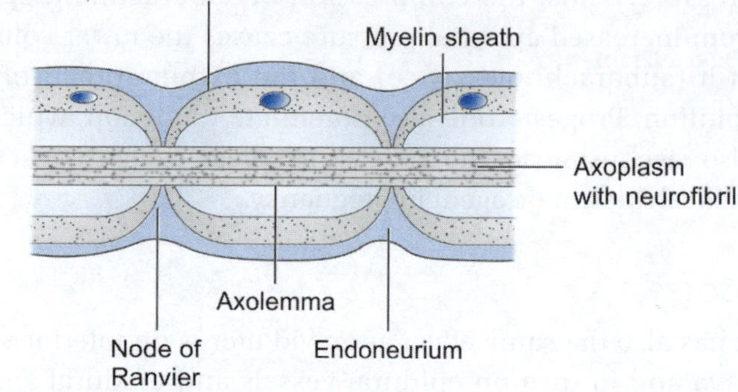

Fig. 30: Longitudinal section of myelinated peripheral nerve.

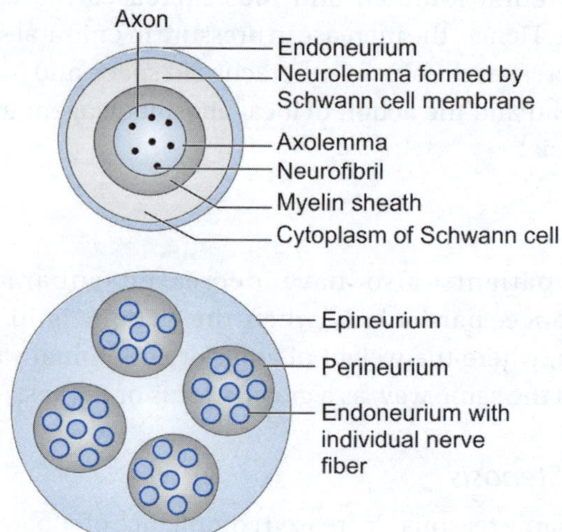

Fig. 31: Organization of a trunk of peripheral nerve.

break through an epidural block which is relieving the physiological labor pain conducting through A-δ fibers. This is called the *"epidural sieve"*. The sensory (proprioceptive) A-α fibers appear to be more sensitive to blockade than the motor A-α fibers, although both have the same conduction velocity. This is because the sensory fibers conduct at a higher frequency **(Table 4)**.

All the local anesthetic agent block the small and slow conducting sensory fibers more rapidly than motor fibers. The varying ability of different LA agents, to produce the sensory and motor block, would appear to be related largely to their epidural use. Thus, bupivacaine, the most selective for sensory fibers on epidural use, produces profound motor block on peripheral and intrathecal use. In summary, the order of sensitivity of nerve fibers to be blockade (starting from the most sensitive) is like that sympathetic preganglionic B fibers, pain and temperature (A-δ) fibers, touch (A-β) fibers, and proprioception and motor (A-α) fibers **(Table 4)**.

TABLE 4: Characteristic features of various nerve fibers.

Fiber type	Diameter (mm)	Conduction velocity (m/s)	Function	
			Sensory	**Motor**
A-α	13–20	70–120	Proprioception	Somatic
A-β	5–12	30–70	Touch, pressure	–
A-γ	4–11	15–30	–	Muscle spindle
A-δ	1–4	12–30	Pain, temperature	–
B	1–4	3–15	–	Preganglionic sympathetic
C	0.5–1	0.5–2.5	Pain, reflex	Postganglionic sympathetic

Explanation of feeling of some pain or failure of RA after technically correct procedure:

The probable explanations of failure after a technically good spinal or epidural block are:

- A given concentration of local anesthetic solution may block the fine fibers carrying the ordinary or sharp pain sensation, but may not be adequate to block some large fibers, responsible for carrying pressure and dull pain sensation. Increasing the concentration of local anesthetic agent will solve this problem.
- Some pain fibers pass via sympathetic nerve and then via sympathetic chain to reach the spinal cord at higher level than the site of injection and may be the cause of failure.
- Dura can be punctured in the midline as well as laterally and even possibly at the dural investment of nerve root, resulting in the false feeling of the placement of needle tip in the subarachnoid space.
- The tip of the needle may be moved further during the pushing of injection after the proper placement of it (needle) in the subarachnoid space and the local anesthetic agent has not been deposited into the CSF of proper subarachnoid space.
- Rarely, the fluid-filled cyst in the subarachnoid space, where the needle tip is entered, may be responsible for failure. The membrane of the cyst limits the spread of local anesthetic agent.
- A problem with the potency of local anesthetic solution may be responsible and possible.

Sometimes, the local anesthetic agent accumulates in the sacral hollow from the highest injecting point at the summit of lumbar lordosis, during the dural puncture in lateral position, followed by supine position, through lumbar route, due to the anti-Trendelenburg position of patient. In such situation, inadequate level of anesthesia up to the groin results.

The partial failure is a more common problem than the complete failure and is mainly due to insufficient dose and improper position of patient, rather than the individual variation. In partial or complete failure, the block can be repeated. But, often GA is more appropriate.

During spinal anesthesia before injecting drug, it is wise to verify that the spinal needle is surely located in the subarachnoid space and is freely communicating with CSF. To confirm this, the needle should be rotated 360° with observation of free flow of CSF in all quadrants. If dural puncture is oblique or at the dural sleeve, there may be one or more quadrant where free flow of CSF does not occur. This may signal inadequate or partial dural puncture and in such cases the needle should be removed and is placed again correctly. Failure to replace the needle correctly results in two adverse outcomes. In an oblique puncture, an inadequate level of spinal anesthesia may result. If injection is into the dural sleeve, hydrostatic injury to the nerve root may occur. Intense searing paresthesia at the time of CSF withdrawal, during test, may signal the nerve root damage and is early enough to avoid the morbidity.

CONTINUOUS SPINAL ANESTHESIA

Continuous spinal anesthesia is a comparatively newer concept of RA and is performed by the introduction of microcatheter into the spinal subarachnoid space. But, it is always remained in controversy due to many neurological complications. The history of CSA can be dated back to 1907 when Dean, a British surgeon, first used this technique to prolong the duration of spinal anesthesia. He first performed the CSA by the repeated injection of local anesthetic agents into the subarachnoid space, through a lumbar puncture needle, which was left in situ after its successful entry. But, the needle breakage and spinal cord trauma were some of the ominous complications of this procedure. Then, in 1940, Lemmon introduced malleable needle and split mattress technology for this procedure. After that in 1944, Edward Tuohy used a malleable spinal catheter, i.e., a number 4 ureteral catheter for CSA and had popularized this technique. But during that period, PDPH due to large needle and thick catheter was very rampant in CSA, which led to the introduction of microcatheters in 1990. Then, different sizes of microcatheters, varying from 27 to 32 G were made available and could be introduced into the subarachnoid space via 22–27 G spinal needle for CSA. But surprisingly, this did not reduce the incidence of PDPH. On the contrary, it causes increased neurological complication, termed the cauda equina syndrome. Hence, in 1992, FDA in USA had banned CSA with spinal catheters, thinner than 24 G.

Before discussing more about CSA, let us first to innumerate its various advantages and disadvantages.

Advantages and Disadvantages of CSA

Advantages of CSA

- Reduced failure rate as CSF flowed into the catheter can be visualized.
- Prolonged anesthesia which further can be extended, even in the postoperative period, for adequate analgesia.
- Requires low doses of local anesthetic agent, especially when compared to continuous epidural anesthesia (CEA).
- Extreme hemodynamic and cardiovascular stability, due to the use of low and gradual incremental dosage of local anesthetic agent.
- May be used for prolonged pain relief, as in cancer patients, by allowing the subarachnoid administration of narcotics for its long duration of action.

Disadvantages of CSA

- Increased incidence of PDPH
- Increased incidences of nerve injury, causing sensory loss, or motor loss or both
- Increased chances of infection and hemorrhage
- Increased incidence of cauda equina syndrome
- Very fine spinal needles (27 G and 29 G) and very fine catheters (30 G and 32 G) have made the technique possible without the risk of severe PDPH. But, these sizes of needles and catheters make the successful lumbar puncture more difficult.

Hemodynamic Stability in CSA

Perhaps the most undisputable indication for CSA is very elderly or critically ill patients who are scheduled for surgeries on lower abdomen or inferior extremities. The elderly patients generally have some cardiovascular compromise due to hypertension, ischemic heart disease, heart failure, etc. or have some respiratory compromise due to low respiratory reserves or both. The critically ill patients are also similarly compromised. Hence, they require very good hemodynamic stability during anesthesia, which is offered best only by CSA. The CSA offers a very good hemodynamic stability, because very low dose of local anesthetic agent is given at a time which prevents very rapid and widespread of drug and thus causes slower onset of action. This helps in gradual slow sympathetic block and easy gradual cardiovascular adaptability (compensation). It also gives enough time to an anesthetist for adequate fluid infusion and vasopressor therapy, if required. The low incidences of hypotension, the low requirement of vasopressors, and the low failure rate of this procedure are some of the indications of hemodynamic stability in CSA.

Postdural Punctural Headache in CSA

Though it was first thought that the incidences of PDPH were low with microcatheters in CSA, yet this topic is still now very controversial. The various studies, at various times, have proved that the microcatheters not always lower the incidences of PDPH. In fact, one study also showed that severity of PDPH was more in microcatheters and maximum patients required epidural blood patch for the treatment of it. Also PDPH was observed to be more in younger age group of patients who had gone through surgeries under CSA. Hence, it was inferred that PDPH was more frequently seen in lower age group patients (especially parturients) with microcatheters and with longer duration (especially for postoperative analgesia by microcatheter).

Cauda Equina Syndrome

Microcatheters for CSA were initially introduced with the aim for decreasing the incidences of PDPH. But, in reality, it hardly did so. On the contrary, it more commonly causes neurological deficit, termed as the *"cauda equina syndrome"*. A local anesthetic agent, when introduced into the CSF through a conventionally used spinal needle, then it causes *a turbulence* which helps in mixing of the drug in CSF. But, when the microcatheters are used, then the lack of this turbulence causes an improper mixing of drug into CSF. Hence, if there is no turbulence and proper mixing, then the hyperbaric local anesthetic agents, thus, will settle at the bottom of the spinal theca depending on the position of the patient. Therefore, a higher concentration of local anesthetic agent is found, near the caudal portion of spinal cord, exposing the nerves of cauda equina long enough to the high concentration of these drugs which sometimes become toxic to these nerve fibers. This causes some serious neurological defects, which is known as the *cauda equina syndrome*.

Failure of CSA

One of the causes of the failure of CSA is its technical difficulty, during the introduction of catheter in the subarachnoid space, through the needle successfully. (1) The inability to inject local anesthetic agent, (2) the knotting of catheters inside the spinal canal, (3) broken catheters, etc. are the other major causes of frequent inability of producing adequate anesthesia by CSA. Therefore, very thin microcatheters such as 32 G are also supplied by a steel wire stylet to help in threading it (the microcatheter) through a 25–27 G spinal needle. These catheters would bend very easily during their introduction in the spinal canal. Then, the straightening or even the removing of them, would often pose a problem. Sometimes, the threading of catheter becomes difficult, even though the spinal needle is in place. This is due to the dura which may cover the opening of the spinal needle or needle touches the lateral or the anterior wall of the spinal cord.

In such cases, a little withdrawal of the needle may help in threading of microcatheter through it into the CSF. The spinal microcatheters should not be introduced >2–3 cm inside the dural sac. More than 4 cm insertion of microcatheter often changes the direction of the catheter caudally, causing frequent cauda equina syndrome. The 22 G Sprotte spinal needle prevents the caudal migration of a 28 G spinal microcatheter. Often, the spinal catheter may also get entangled in the nerve roots or may even enter the intervertebral foramen along with the nerve roots, causing low backpain, radicular pain, or even transient paresthesia during the procedure. This may result in the transient or permanent neurological damage.

During any failure or difficulty in threading the catheter through a fine spinal needle, the procedure should be reassessed or abandoned. In such situation, GA is better option than facing the grave neurological defects in postoperative periods.

Present Status of CSA

For the very elderly or compromised patients with severe systemic complication, the CSA may still be the best and safest opted technique. It gives a stable hemodynamic platform, and thus decreases both the morbidity and mortality of patient. As small, slow, and gradual incremental doses of LA agents are given in CSF, so hemodynamic status remains almost unaltered. Hence, high-risk patients with chronic bronchitis, emphysema, hypertension, coronary artery diseases, myocardial ischemia, myocardial infarction, congestive cardiac disease, etc. tolerate this method of CSA much better. PDPH is the main disadvantage of CSA with the incidence of 6–9% with 20 G catheters. But, it is more common in younger age group of patients and incidence becomes almost nil after 60 years of age. Neurological injuries are more common with microcatheters. But, by abandoning the technique, whenever there is some technical difficulty during insertion (as discussed before), the possibility of neurological trauma can be avoided.

Thus, it can be concluded that CSA is the choice of anesthesia in elderly and very high-risk patients with many systemic complications or a severely compromised state. It is best avoided in young and obstetric age group of patients where CEA is still the choice. The ultrathin

microcatheters need not be used as they have no added advantages. The anesthetist should be well prepared to abandon the technique and goes for a GA, whenever there is some problem in insertion and threading of a microcatheter through the fine spinal needle, especially if patient complains of radial pain or paresthesia. This shall avoid neurological damage and postoperative neurological deficits.

■ EPIDURAL ANESTHESIA

Though, the *epidural anesthesia and analgesia* had lead its journey from a small arena like labor ward and/or the obstetric operating room, but now it has spread a strong foot hold over a wide area and become a common practice in surgical patients including neck, thoracic, abdominal, and cardiothoracic surgeries. Recently, it has also made its strong presence in the pain clinic. However, at present, epidural anesthesia and analgesia for obstetric surgeries have been superseded by spinal anesthetic technique in some underdeveloped countries. But, the painless labor by walking epidural analgesia and subsequent obstetric surgery (if needed) by epidural anesthesia is still the routine practice in many developed countries. On the other hand, the postoperative epidural analgesia following major surgery is now the best means of analgesia in the modern postoperative care. The indications for the epidural anesthesia and analgesia are listed in **Box 3**.

Epidural anesthesia is provided by the effect of local anesthetic agent on the spinal nerve roots, as they pass from the spinal cord to the intervertebral foramen, through the extradural or epidural space. Some part of the local anesthetic agent which is deposited in the epidural space also penetrates the dura and arachnoid mater and passes into the CSF to act directly on the spinal cord and the spinal nerve roots, bathed by CSF. The epidural analgesia, provided by the low concentration of LA agent, also acts by the same mechanism as epidural anesthesia. But, the addition of other drugs such as opioids, clonidine, benzodiazepine, etc. acts only through the receptors on spinal cord. This proves that the drug placed in the epidural space diffuses through CSF.

The indications and the contraindications for epidural anesthesia and analgesia are similar to those of intrathecal anesthesia. But, the most common indication for epidural technique is where the duration of surgery is prolonged, the patient is very ill and high-quality postoperative analgesia is needed. Because, all these requirements can be provided only by the intermittent bolus injections or by the continuous infusion of LA agent or narcotics into the epidural space, using an epidural catheter.

BOX 3: Indications of epidural block.

- *Surgical, obstetric, diagnostic, and prognostic:*
  - Surgical anesthesia and analgesia
  - Obstetric anesthesia and analgesia
  - Differential neural blockade to evaluate pain
  - Prognostic indicator before destruction of nerve
- *Acute pain:*
  - Palliation of acute pain in any emergency
  - Patients with multiple fractured ribs by thoracic epidural
  - Management of pain due to acute pancreatitis
  - *In cervical epidural:* To evaluate head, neck, face, shoulder, and upper extremity pain
  - *In lumbar epidural:* To evaluate lower abdominal, back, groin, pelvic, bladder, perineal, genital, rectal, anal lower extremity pain
  - Postoperative pain
  - Pain due to acute herpes zoster
  - Pain due to vascular insufficiency of the extremities
- *Prophylactic and preemptive pain:*
  - Before amputation of ischemic limbs
- *Chronic benign pain:*
  - Radiculopathy
  - Spinal stenosis
  - Spondylosis
  - Vertebral compression fracture
  - Diabetic polyneuropathy
  - Postherpetic neuralgia
  - Reflex sympathetic dystrophy
  - Phantom limb syndrome
  - Peripheral neuropathy
- *Cancer-related pain:*
  - Pain secondary to malignancies
  - Pain due to bony metastases
  - Chemotherapy-related peripheral neuropathy

Some Important Characteristics of Epidural Anesthesia and Analgesia

- It needs more skill
- Sitting position is only preferred, when it is absolutely necessary. Otherwise, increased pressure of CSF in sitting position increases the risk of dural puncture, leading to spinal anesthesia.
- Absolute stillness of patient's posture, during this procedure is very necessary.
- During this procedure, any movement, cough, cry, etc., can cause increased CSF pressure and enhance the chances of dural puncture.
- The intervertebral space, such as L_{2-3}, L_{3-4}, L_{4-5} is preferred for epidural anesthesia and analgesia, though any interspinous space can be chosen. The choice of site for the introduction of Tuohy needle or any epidural needle is determined by the surgical incision site. The insertion of needle should be at the level of the middle of dermatomes (spinal segments) that innervate the area of the skin in which the incision will lie.

During any difficulty, the best interspinous space may be one vertebra above or below the ideal level. The anesthetist should balance the practical problems of a potentially difficult space, against the benefit of a successful first time identification of an epidural space, which is one or two vertebra below or above. In difficulty of flexing spine or lumbar lordosis, upper spaces can be chosen. Thoracic approach for epidural block is generally used by skilled person for upper abdomen and thoracic surgery and/or postoperative analgesia.

- At the site of the entry of an epidural needle, the prior application of an eutectic LA mixture over the skin or the infiltration of skin by local anesthetic agent is very important for the use of a thick 16–18 G Tuohy needle or any epidural needle in awake patient.
- In the lumbar approach of epidural anesthesia, the depth of ligamentum flavum from the skin for most of the patient is 3.5–6 cm (average 4 cm). On the other hand, the ligamentum flavum is itself 5–6 mm thick in midline.
- Patients with the history of previous spinal surgery at the site of planned epidural anesthesia have more chance of failure or partial block. It is either due to technical difficulty in identifying the space or an anatomical distortion of the space by scaring, hematoma, adhesion, etc. which prevents the spread of local anesthetic agent in the epidural space. Even in patient without previous spine surgery or disease, repeated epidural anesthesia at the same site becomes less effective with each application. Explanation of this failure is that repeated entry of needle and injection of local anesthetic agent into the same small epidural space cause anatomical changes (due to bleeding, hematoma, inflammation, and scar formation) and obliterate some parts of epidural space.
- One of the probable causes of one-sided epidural anesthesia is the migration of catheter into the dural sleeve or the moving out of epidural space with outgoing nerve root, through the intervertebral foramen.
- Another important characteristic of the epidural anesthesia and analgesia is that there is relatively large absorption of LA agent from this space due to large absorption area, dense epidural venous plexus, and large volume of drug.

Needle of Epidural Anesthesia

The standard epidural needle is typically 17–18 G in thickness and 3–3.5 inches in long. The two types of needle used for epidural anesthesia and analgesia are Tuohy and Crawford **(Fig. 32)**. Most commonly the Tuohy needle is used for epidural anesthesia and analgesia. The important feature of this needle is its rounded Huber point tip which

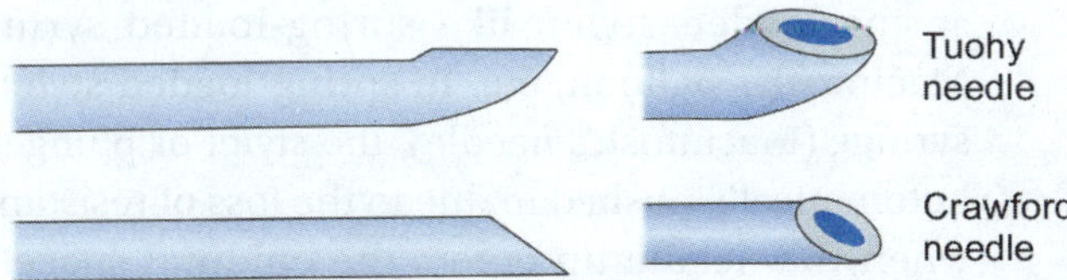

Fig. 32: Epidural needle.

is curved and blunt. The curvature of this bevel tip is 15–30°. The curvature of this tip directs the passage of the catheter and the bluntness of its tip reduces the risk of dural puncture by pushing away the dura from ligamentum flavum, when the needle just enter the epidural space, passing through the ligamentum flavum. The large caliber of this Tuohy needle helps in the easy detection of epidural space, particularly by the loss of resistance. The Tuohy needle is graduated in centimeter and so it can also help to assess the depth of epidural space. For single-shot epidural technique, where the catheter is not used, the Crawford epidural needle is also very much appropriate. It is a modification of Tuohy needle with a small sharp area at its tip.

Approach for Epidural Space

Our approach for epidural space may be in the midline (median approach) or from the lateral side (paramedian approach). In midline approach, once the tip of the needle enters into the supraspinous ligament, after crossing the skin and subcutaneous tissue, then a considerable resistance during the advancement of needle and injection of fluid is felt. This resistance is due to the advancement of needle through the interspinous ligament and ligamentum flavum. After that as soon as the tip of the needle enters the epidural space, then there is a feeling of sudden loss of resistance **(Fig. 33)**. The advancement of the needle, just under and parallel to the spinous process of the vertebra above, will yield the easiest entry of it (needle) into the epidural space in the midline. The contact of the tip of the needle with bone close to the skin usually suggests obstruction due to spinous process, whereas the contact of the tip of the needle with bone at deeper level suggests obstruction due to lamina or pedicle and signals the possibility that needle has perhaps strayed away from the midline or is angled too cephalad or caudal.

During lateral or paramedian approach of epidural space the sacrospinal and other paravertebral group of muscles are encountered first after the skin and subcutaneous tissue. It offers a doughy feeling, as supraspinous and interspinous ligaments are bypassed. Strong resistance only felt when the paravertebral groups of muscles are crossed and the tip of the needle hits the ligamentum flavum. After crossing the ligamentum flavum, there is a sudden loss of resistance.

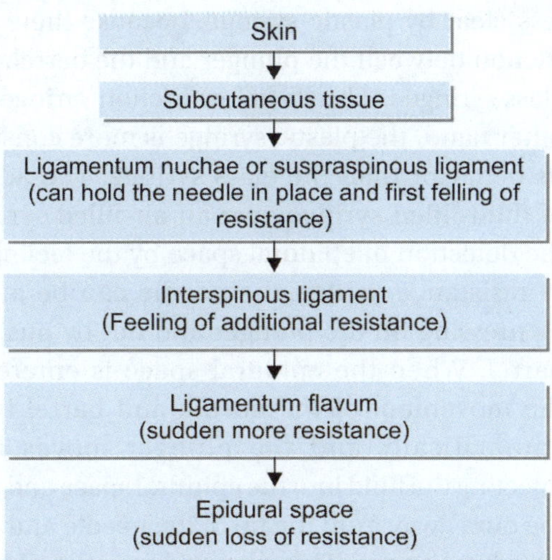

Fig. 33: Resistance offered to the needle during passage to epidural space.

It indicates that the tip of the epidural needle has entered the epidural space. The key to successful insertion of needle in epidural space in this approach is the change from doughy soft feeling to tough gritty feeling (resistance), due to the change from the muscle to ligamentum flavum, followed by the loss of resistance. The too abrupt advancement of the needle in any approach may result in accidental dural puncture and subdural block. The chances of the traumatic damage to nerve roots and epidural vein is more during epidural anesthesia in lateral approach because the two posterior epidural venous plexuses lie by the side of the midline. Like spinal anesthesia, the lateral approach for epidural block is also applicable (1) only when the interspinous space is narrow and (2) there is difficulty to approach the epidural space through midline due to any cause.

Methods of Identifying Epidural Space

The epidural space can be identified by different methods. These are as follows:

- *By feeling the loss of resistance:* This is the most commonly used clinical practice for the detection of epidural space. The feeling for the loss of resistance, for the detection of epidural space (when the tip of the epidural needle enters the epidural space), can be tested by two ways, either by *fluid-filled syringe* or by *air-filled syringe* with epidural needle.
  - *Advantage/disadvantage of fluid-filled syringe (glass or plastic) for the detection of epidural space:* The question between the glass or plastic syringe for detection of epidural space by the feeling of loss of resistance depends on the individual anesthetist's choice and experience. The loss of resistance is

less clear by plastic syringe, because there is more friction between the plunger and the barrel. But, the glass syringe is always of low friction syringe. On the other hand, the plastic syringe is more consistent in its behavior than the glass syringe. The advantage of fluid-filled syringe over an air-filled syringe, for the detection of epidural space by the feeling of loss of resistance, is that the needle can be advanced by pressing on the plunger and not by pushing the barrel. When the epidural space is entered, then the movement of the needle and barrel is halted automatically and the plunger moves forward injecting the fluid into the epidural space and pushing the dura away from the tip of the needle and creating an actual space. This also reduces the chances of dural puncture.

The advancement of the needle must be at the right angle to the hip and shoulder. However, being parallel to the floor has no importance. The hole at the needle tip pointing cephalad will minimize the angle at which the needle tip encroaches the epidural space and thus will reduce the chances of dural puncture. The advancement of the needle should be smooth and continuous. The disadvantage of a fluid-filled syringe is that sometimes a few drops of fluid drip back from the needle hub, after its proper entry into the epidural space and can create a confusion for CSF as dural puncture occurs.

- *Advantage/disadvantage of air-filled syringe for detection of epidural space:* Here, the epidural needle cannot be advanced by giving pressure on the plunger of the syringe alone. But, the needle must be advanced step by step by holding the needle shaft or the barrel of the syringe, rather than in a continuous fashion, like a fluid-filled syringe, described before. Thus, the use of an air-filled syringe needs the elicitation of the bounce of plunger with every millimeter of the advancement of needle to feel the loss of resistance for the detection of epidural space. It is a more slower process and there is more chance of dural puncture, because like fluid the air does not automatically remove the dura from the tip of the needle when it enters the epidural space. But, as no fluid drips back from the needle hub, after the entry of the tip of the needle into epidural space, so no confusion is created for dural puncture. However, here are the more chances of emphysema and air embolism (if the needle enters into a vein).

There are other many mechanical helps (methods) to feel the sign of loss of resistance by an air-filled syringe. These are Macintosh's needle with spring-loaded stylet, like spring-loaded syringe, Macintosh's balloon, etc. In spring-loaded stylet or syringe (Macintosh's needle), the stylet or plunger is automatically pushed in due to the loss of resistance, when the needle tip enters the epidural space. In Macintosh's balloon, it is automatically deflated, when the tip of the epidural needle enters the epidural space. But, they are usually not used now, because they are more complicated, produce more false-negative and false-positive result, and cause more distractions.

After entering the epidural space, the air or fluid-filled syringe is disconnected. If a small amount of fluid (in case of air-filled syringe) leaks back, it may raise concern about the partial dural puncture. But, it can be resolved by two ways. If the fluid is of room temperature and flow is self-limiting, it is surely fluid of epidural space, whereas CSF would feel warm, if it is allowed to drop on the forearm of anesthesiologist. Because, it (CSF) is coming from the core of patient's body and its flow is not self-limiting. The use of test sticks for glucose would also make the distinction between the CSF and other fluids, since CSF would contain some glucose, whereas other fluid such as fluid of the epidural space, saline, or local anesthetic agents would not.

- *By negative pressure sign:* A negative pressure is detected in 50–80% of cases in the epidural space. There are three explanations which have been put forward to account for this negative pressure in the epidural space.
  - The first theory is that the negative pressure which is normally present in the pleural cavity is transmitted from this cavity via the thoracic paravertebral spaces and through the intervertebral foramen to the epidural spaces.
  - The second theory is that negative pressure is created by expanding the volume of vertebral canal and consequently that of the epidural space by the flexion of the spine.
  - The third theory is that the negative pressure is simply created by indenting the dura with the tip of the needle. This is the most probable explanation of negative pressure in epidural space. The negative pressure is obliterated once the fluid is injected and then the epidural pressure may rise to as high as 30 cm of water during an epidural injection. Clinically, the negative pressure in the epidural space has been demonstrated in a number of ways.
    - *Hanging drop method:* While the needle is progressing toward the epidural space, a drop of fluid (saline or LA agent) is deposited at the hub of

the needle, until the drop is hanging. Then, as soon as the tip of the needle reaches the epidural space, then due to the negative pressure, created by pushing the dura away, the fluid will be sucked into the hub. However, this technique should be limited to the experienced hands, because heavy skill is required to interpret the feel of tissue during very slow approach to the epidural space and to see the drop movement simultaneously. This technique is further limited by the possibility of tiny bit of tissue or blood clot at the needle tip which may prevent the passive transmission of negative pressure from the epidural space to the hub of the needle. Very slow approach and the increased feel of tissue is mandatory, when the epidural anesthesia is applied in thoracic or cervical spine.

- *Odom's indicator:* A drop of fluid being contained in a small glass capillary tube is attached with the epidural needle. As the epidural space is entered by the tip of the needle, then the fluid moves inward to the negative pressure of the space. This is Odom's indicator. This negative pressure sign has also the distinct advantage in lateral approach.

Technique of Epidural Anesthesia

Usually, the epidural anesthesia is applied by two methods (1) single-shot epidural without catheter or (2) continuous epidural by catheter.

Single-shot Epidural Anesthesia

The single-shot epidural anesthesia, without any catheter, is rarely used nowadays, except for few outdoor or day-case surgeries. It is unjustified, if the epidural anesthesia is used for any surgery, but the patient is not allowed to enjoy a good postoperative analgesia by repeated doses or by continuous infusion of local anesthetic or narcotic agents in the epidural space through the epidural catheter later on.

Continuous Epidural Anesthesia by Catheter

The ability to insert a catheter, safely into the epidural space, allows the slow injection of local anesthetic agents and/or narcotics, intermittently by bolus or continuously through infusion (1) to control the rate of neural blockade, (2) to decrease the hemodynamic side effects, and (3) to reinject the drug when necessary and thus maintaining anesthesia and/or analgesia indefinitely. There are multiple positive points about the CEA using catheter.

The safe access to the epidural space in thoracic and cervical regions will also create the possibility of *selective block in limited dermatomes* and thus will accomplish

the only analgesic objective (pain control), minimizing the side effects of widespread motor block and widespread pharmacological sympathectomy. For orthopedic anesthesia, the control (relief) of postoperative pain is valuable, especially where the orthopedic surgical indication requires the excellent postoperative pain control for continuous passive or active motion of limbs (physiotherapy) after fracture repair, joint replacement, release of frozen joint, etc.

The obstetric analgesia and postoperative pain control are the ideal conditions for continuous epidural analgesia. Here, the surgical anesthesia is not sought for, as it will hamper the objective of obstetric analgesia by hindering the vaginal delivery. The ideal situation would be only analgesia in the restricted dermatomes of surgical site with no or minimal motor block. When used alone or in conjunction with a low concentration of local anesthetic agent (e.g., 0.25% bupivacaine) and a lipophilic narcotic (e.g., morphine, fentanyl, sufentanil, etc.), this catheter technique should make possible near total relief of postoperative and labor pain. It does not interfere with pulmonary mechanics [in chronic obstructive pulmonary disease (COPD)] and allows a patient of enough motor strength to take self-care. In instances, where the complete motor function is essential, the use of only narcotic drug without local anesthetic agent can achieve analgesia without even slight degree of motor block.

Epidural Catheter

The size of epidural catheter varies from 19 G wide-bore to 30 G microbore. Typically, a 19 G or 20 G epidural catheter is introduced through a 17 G or 18 G epidural needle. The wide-bore large catheters are used for adult patients and fine microcatheters are used for the pediatric patients. When using a curved tipped needle, the bevel opening of needle should be directed either cephalad or caudal. And the catheter is advanced 2–6 cm into epidural space. The shorter the distance the catheter is advanced, the more likely it is to become dislodged. Conversely, the further the catheter is advanced, the greater the chance of penetrating epidural vein and unilateral block. Because, the catheter may either exit the epidural space through intervertebral foramen or may course into the anterolateral recesses of epidural space. Catheters that will remain in place for prolonged period (>1 week) may be tunneled under the skin.

The objective regarding the use of epidural catheter is to pass largest possible catheter through a given needle, since the tensile strength of a catheter decreases with its higher number (or fine/bore). Impregnating the walls of catheter with a special chemical substance, which increases the tensile strength of it, is another approach to use the fine catheters, without decreasing its (catheter) tensile strength. The goal is to minimize the risk of catheter loss under the skin (in vertebral canal or at anywhere between the skin to ligamentum flavum) or long-term follow-up for evaluation, if a part of a catheter is lost and cannot be removed. The material selected for the construction of catheter is determined by many factors. When a catheter is made up of Teflon, then the advantages are (1) increased-firmness causes easy insertion, (2) greatest possible resistance to prevent kinking, (3) during continuous use, the linear shear strength is maximal and does not soften when it reaches the body temperature. The disadvantage of Teflon catheter is (1) the increased rigidity and (2) the absence of increased flexibility at body temperature which increases the risk of trauma to nerves and blood vessels by this catheter. Some catheters have stylet for easy insertion or to help to steer the passage of catheter in epidural space with fluoroscopic guidance. Spiral wire reinforced catheters are very resistant to kinking.

Spinal nerve roots are usually located in tight epidural compartment with minimal mobility. Thus, a rigid less flexible catheter which is made of Teflon and is inserted in this tight epidural space, can lacerate or penetrate the surface of these rigid nerve roots. In that situation, if a catheter is left in place when the patient is mobile or in anticoagulant, the gradual softening of a catheter, when is made of polyvinyl chloride (PVC) would be a distinct advantage. Teflon lacks this softening property. So, PVC catheters are thought better for softness and flexibility during insertion and use. But, this material causes (1) the decreased resistance to breakage and (2) the increased chances of kinking. The chance of breakage is even more for a catheter which has multiple exit ports at their tip and this is because of their inherent weakness at the site of these ports.

The catheters with a single orifice at the most distal end are selected for accurate delivery of anesthetic solutions at the exact site of placement of it. But, there is more chance of occlusion of this type of catheter with single distal orifice by blood clot or tissues. Whereas, the multiorificed catheter cannot deliver the injecting anesthetic solution accurately at the site of its placement, but minimize the potential for occlusion of it by blood clot or tissues that can occur with single port catheter. The size of port around the diameter of the catheter also theoretically increases the area of spread of the solution at the site of injection, but at the cost of decreased shear strength of catheter. Some epidural catheters are designed with fine metal stylet inside it which makes them quite rigid, and helps to guide the catheter easily. In such situation besides potential nerve injury, there is higher risk of dural puncture with stylet catheter,

even after the successful placement of needle. This risk can be decreased by withdrawing the stylet so that the 1–2 cm tip of the catheter is free of stylet and is not rigid any more. But, still the stylet gives the necessary rigidity to the catheter within the hub of epidural needle during the initial entry into the epidural space and helps its insertion. Epidural catheter increases the versatility and the duration of CNB.

Catheter tip emerges from the tip of the needle, if the 10 cm mark on the catheter disappears at the hub. A resistance, during the passage of catheter through the epidural needle, may be felt at this point. If any resistance during the passage of catheter is felt beyond this point, then it should never be withdrawn without needle, neither should it be forced onward. The withdrawal of catheter alone without the needle, once it has emerged from the tip of the needle, may cause the end of the catheter to be sheared off by the tip of the needle and remain in the epidural space. If a piece of an epidural catheter is accidentally left behind in the epidural space, then there has been some debate over whether the patient should be informed or not. It is probably best to be honest. So, it should be explained what has happened. But, the patient will be very anxious after this explanation. Hence, the patients should be reassured that the chances of long-term adverse sequelae are remote.

The obstruction during passage of catheter through the epidural needle may be due to:
- Catheter tip hits against nerve root
- Catheter tip hits against blood vessel
- It hits against the dura
- The needle or the catheter tip is not in the epidural space at all.

Catheter tip should not be passed >15 cm from the needle hub. Once catheter enters into the epidural space in the midline, it will generally pass freely. If resistance is encountered well before this, the needle may be carefully rotated through 90°. If this still does not enable the catheter to pass then increasing the spinal flexion of patient may be helpful. Sometimes, the catheter may run a short distance into the epidural space and then is curled back or pass out through the intervertebral foramen. The tendency for a catheter to pass in one side of the epidural space increases the likelihood of an asymmetrical or unilateral block which, if resistant to treatment, may necessitate removal and reinsertion of the catheter. If blood is aspirated, the catheter is slightly withdrawn. If flow of blood still persists, then another space is tried. As the aspiration of blood or CSF does not give 100% guarantee that if the catheter is in the blood vessels or in the subarachnoid space or not, so a test dose is mandatory before giving the full clinical dose. Epidural catheter should be inserted only 2–3 cm in the epidural space from the tip of the needle. There are no advantages in passing the catheter for more than 4 or 5 cm from the tip of the needle into the epidural space. The migration of catheter into the anterior epidural space is the most common misposition of it. The use of multi- or uniport catheter depends on the anesthetist's choice. The multiport catheter has the less chances of unilateral and unblocked spinal segments than the single port catheter.

Epidural Test Dose

The quantity (volume and concentration) of LA agent in solution needed for epidural anesthesia is highly larger than that needed for spinal anesthesia. Therefore, toxic side effects are almost guaranteed if a full epidural dose is injected intrathecally or intravascularly. Hence, the safeguards against these adverse events are *test dosing and incremental dosing.* These safeguards are applied whether the drugs (injections) are administered through the needle or catheter.

An epidural test dose is designed to detect both the subarachnoid and intravascular injection. Therefore, after the proper placement of an epidural catheter, the administration of test dose before delivering the full anesthetic dose of LA agent has in common the objective of decreasing the incidence of inadvertently injecting a large volume of anesthetic agent, scheduled for epidural anesthesia into the intravascular or subarachnoid spaces. A variety of agents and strategies have been described for this test dose procedure, but the ultimate choice depends on the experience of an anesthetist.

Any evidence of epidural anesthesia, even partial, signals an extremely low probability that the needle or catheter is fully within the subarachnoid space or within the lumen of a blood vessel. On the contrary, extended anesthesia than expected by the test dose, signals the probability that the needle or catheter is in the subarachnoid space. The 2–3 mL of local anesthetic drug (a dose insufficient for epidural blockade, but sufficient for spinal effect and expected to occur within 2 minutes) is used as the test dose, before giving the total dose, scheduled for this epidural anesthesia.

However, the correct period of timing, between the test dose and the next principal injection, is very important and is determined by the type of LA agent used. There is no reliability in this procedure, if correct time interval (2–3 minutes for lignocaine's onset of action) is not maintained prior to the next main injection. If bupivacaine is selected as the epidural agent, then the time interval between the test dose and the principal anesthetic doses would need to be longer or initial test dose would have to be performed

with another agent, e.g., lignocaine. During continuous epidural anesthesia and analgesia, each subsequent epidural injection should also be preceded by aspiration and epidural test dose, because catheter migration into vessel or subarachnoid space does occur at any time.

The intravascular injection of LA agent, during the administration of test dose or principal dose, is identified by the systemic signs, based on the occurrence of cranial nerve paresthesia and this is due to the disinhibition of limbic system of brain, curved by LA agent. Thus, the intravascular injection of LA agent can be identified by the (1) general ill feeling, (2) unexplained fear, (3) perioral paresthesia, (4) lingual paresthesia (metal taste), (5) ocular paresthesia (scotoma), (6) aural events (roaring in the ear), etc. These symptoms are very obvious with 2-chloroprocaine, but less obvious with lignocaine and absent with bupivacaine, because of its very high protein-binding property.

The CNS toxicity as signs of intravascular injection is reported being unreliable, following small doses of LA agent alone. So, the vasoactive substances are often injected with LA agent as the indicators or markers and their systemic effects are used as the signs of intravascular injection of LA agent. The classical choice of vasoactive substance as marker is epinephrine. The most common test dose is 3 mL of LA agent with 15 µg of epinephrine (adrenaline) preferably 1.5% lignocaine (45 mg lignocaine) with 1: 200,000 epinephrine (0.005 mg/mL). This dose of epinephrine will produce 20–30% increase in patient's heart rate within 20–30 seconds of injection. It will last for a brief period (1–2 minutes) and is unlikely to harm patient. To detect the increase in heart rate, caused by epinephrine which is used as test dose, electrocardiography monitoring is mandatory and mere symptom like palpitation is unreliable. The use of epinephrine as test dose is contraindicated in cardiac patients and parturients (potential risk of uterine artery vasoconstriction).

Some clinicians have suggested that even the use of this low dose LA agent (45 mg lignocaine), as test dose for epidural anesthesia and analgesia, is also problematic, because the inadvertent injection of this 45 mg lignocaine in subarachnoid space, during epidural *labor analgesia* can be difficult to manage in labor room. Unfortunately, the epinephrine, as a marker of intravenous injection, is not ideal. *False positive* (for example, a uterine contraction causing pain or an increase in heart rate coincident to test dosing) and *false negative* (bradycardia and exaggerated hypertension in response to epinephrine in patients taking β-blockers) can occur. Simply aspirating, prior to injection, is insufficient to avoid inadvertent intravenous injection. Most experienced practitioners have encountered false-negative aspirations through both the needle and catheter.

Incremental dosing (if aspiration is negative, a fraction of total intended dose, typically 5 mL, is injected) is a very effective method of avoiding serious complications, because here every dose is test dose. Here, every incremental dose is large enough for symptoms (tinnitus or metallic taste) or signs (slurred speech, altered mentation) for intravascular injection, if occur, but small enough to avoid seizure or cardiovascular compromise.

At last, in conclusion, it can further be told that a false sense of security does not develop, if a test dose has no adverse effects. Although it is rare, still it is not uncommon for epidural catheters to migrate into the blood vessels or into the subarachnoid space, after satisfactory test doses. Therefore, the anesthetist must be vigilant at all times. If a clinician (1) uses an initial test dose, (2) is very serious about aspirating, prior to each injection, and (3) always uses incremental dosing, then the major systemic toxic side effects and the total spinal anesthesia from accidental intrathecal injection will be rare. Rescue lipid emulsion (20% intralipid 1.5 mL/kg) must be available, whenever epidural blocks are performed, in the event of local anesthetic systemic toxicity.

Drugs and their Doses for Epidural Block

The common drugs and their doses are described below and also listed in the **Table 5**.

Lignocaine

For epidural anesthesia, initially 15–18 mL of 1.2–2% (commonly 1.5%) lignocaine hydrochloride is used with or without adrenaline in the dose of 5 μg/mL. The action of this dose lasts for 1–1.5 hours. If adrenaline is used with LA agent, then some prolongation of this local anesthetic action occurs. The subsequent repeated doses of lignocaine cause tachyphylaxis and so it is impossible to maintain a continuous analgesia and/or anesthesia by lignocaine by infusion or repeated bolus doses, without ultimately producing any serious systemic toxicity of it. The 0.5% solution of lignocaine gives sensory block without affecting the motor and 1.5% solution of it gives good both the sensory

and motor block, while 2% solution causes the intense motor and sensory block. So, for the epidural anesthesia and analgesia, the dose of lignocaine varies according to the *volume, concentration, site of injection, and the desired effect.*

Bupivacaine

The 0.5–0.75% solution of bupivacaine HCl is usually used in a dose of 2 mg/kg or 0.4 mL/kg for epidural anesthesia. The action of surgical anesthesia of this dose and concentration of bupivacaine lasts for about 4 hours. However, the only analgesic or sensory action may last for 8 hours. A concentration of 0.125–0.25% bupivacaine is also used only for the postoperative analgesia, avoiding the motor block and the analgesic action of this concentration lasts only for about 4 hours. A concentration of 0.25% solution of bupivacaine is usually satisfactory only for sensory block, but the duration and reliability of 0.125% solution are not usually acceptable. On the other hand, in 0.25% solution of bupivacaine there may, however, be minor degrees of motor block and some risk of hemodynamic instability. So, such a concentration of bupivacaine would be unsuitable for upper abdominal or thoracic analgesia which may produce a high incidence of hypotension. Again in general, the lower concentration (0.125%) of bupivacaine does not cause motor block by any degree, but necessitate larger volume of drugs and consequently increases the spread which may result in higher incidence of hypotension. Unlike lignocaine, the epidural dose of bupivacaine can be repeated for an indefinite period, without producing tachyphylaxis and any risk of systemic toxicity. The 0.75% of bupivacaine is not recommended in USA.

The dose of continuous epidural infusion by bupivacaine is 0.125–0.375% solution at the rate of 10–20 mL/hour. Levobupivacaine may be used in place of bupivacaine.

Chloroprocaine

The preservative-free 2–3% chloroprocaine is also used both for the spinal and epidural block. But, the duration of the action of chloroprocaine is very short and only 45 minutes. So, combining of chloroprocaine with continuous catheter technique allows a good matching of surgical procedure with minimal recovery time. It is mainly used in USA. However, it antagonizes the action of fentanyl.

Ropivacaine HCl

Ropivacaine has less CNS and CVS toxicity than bupivacaine, but more or less has the same onset and duration of action, like it (bupivacaine). It causes better differential block, i.e., at lower concentration the ropivacaine profoundly blocks only sensory, but completely preserve the motor. So, the 0.05–0.1%

TABLE 5: Onset and duration of action of local anesthetic agents administered epidurally in 20–30 mL of volumes.

Drug	Concentration (%)	Onset (min)	Duration of action	
			Plain (min)	Adrenaline 1:2,00,000 (min)
Lignocaine	2	10–20	60–90	90–180
Bupivacaine	0.5	15–25	160–240	160–240
Chloroprocaine	3	10–15	45–60	60–90

solution of ropivacaine is used for only sensory block, but 0.3% for profound sensory and slightly motor block and 1% for both profound sensory and motor block. Therefore, it is best suited for obstetric anesthesia and analgesia and postoperative pain relief by infusion technique.

Method of Injection of Anesthetic Agent through Epidural Catheter

There are many methods or sequences for the injection of anesthetic agent, during the CEA, using catheter. Among these, the *first choice* is after an appropriate test dose, the calculated first schedule dose of local anesthetic agent is injected through the epidural needle prior to the placement of catheter through the needle. The advantage of this method is allowing the time for the onset of anesthesia while the catheter is being placed and when the catheter placement is complete, then there is already enough anesthesia to begin the surgical procedure without wasting any time. Also the bolus first dose of local anesthetic agent, injected through the needle, will expand the epidural space and make the catheter placement much easier and successful.

But, the disadvantages of this method are found in those cases, where even the correct placement of needle and injection of anesthetic agent through this needle, will not allow the subsequent successful insertion of catheter. In such cases, the replacement of needle in another space is much riskier as local anesthetic has already filled the epidural space, which may confuse the detection of epidural and subarachnoid space and once epidural anesthesia has been set up, the absence of paresthesia does not indicate needle contact with neural tissue and cannot prevent the trauma of nerves.

The *second choice* is after the test dose of drug through needle (which expands the epidural space), the catheter is inserted first. Then, after positioning the patient, the first bolus dose of local anesthetic agent is injected through the catheter, followed by the subsequent doses or continuous infusion. *Another choice* is that some anesthesiologists prefer to give the first dose of local anesthetic agent through the epidural needle, before the catheter placement with patient in sitting position. This approach offers maximum bathing of large nerve roots (L_5-S_1) by gravitating down the anesthetic agent for those cases where the dermatomes supplied by these nerve roots are a major part of surgery. Due to the downward movement of LA agent, subsequent insertion of catheter does not produce confusion like first technique. Although uncommon, it is also possible to thread a catheter caudally by directing the tip of the needle caudally. This is because the needle may be rotated caudally, after its entry into the epidural space. But, this entails more risk, because the needle is directed against the dura and the rotation of needle would cause a corkscrew-like effect in which case the needle would advance either partially or completely from epidural space into the subdural or subarachnoid space.

Mechanism of Action and Fate of Local Anesthetic Agent in Epidural Space

Till now this discussion is full of a controversy and unclear, but some postulated hypothesis exists. The *principal site* of action of LA agent in epidural anesthesia is the portion of nerve roots which are present in the epidural space. The local anesthetic agents, injected in the epidural space, also can pass out of the intervertebral foramina and act on the mixed spinal nerve in the intervertebral foramina. As these foramina are generally occluded by the spinal nerves and accompanying vessels, so with the increased age these foramina become narrower and thus confine the anesthetic solution more in the epidural space and cause much higher block by increased spread with same volume of drug. Also the substantial amount of drug diffuses in the subarachnoid area from the epidural space for its action. But, the two modes of block, i.e., in the epidural space and in the subarachnoid space are different.

This is explained by the fact that the epidural block works segmentally, nearest to the injection site which would be impossible, if the intrathecal route of distribution was the only factor for the mechanism of action of epidural anesthesia. The local anesthetic agent in epidural anesthesia also penetrates the dural cuff to block the nerve roots and transmit centrally along the nerve to block their conduction in the spinal cord. Now, whatever may be the destination of the epidurally administered local anesthetic agent, they must ultimately be absorbed into the bloodstream. The absorption of local anesthetic agents into the circulation takes place more rapidly from the epidural than from the subarachnoid space. The speed with which they are absorbed depends upon the local vascularity, which may again be influenced by the injected adrenaline and by the characteristics of drug itself.

Epidural Anesthesia using Catheter and CVS/RS

Epidural anesthesia (EA) has unique effect on CVS. If the patient is properly prepared with volume expander and the level of anesthesia is properly titrated by catheter, then the influence of epidural anesthesia on LV performance is favorable, even in patients with cardiac disease, with decreased CO and decreased LVEF. The multiple experimental work demonstrates the reversal of myocardial ischemia with segmental thoracic epidural analgesia. This is because the epidural anesthesia allows the suitable placement of catheter and then the proper titration of anesthetic drug with the level of block, which results in controlled rate and degree of sympathetic block, allowing the adequate time for compensation for the decreased venous return, and reduced CO, by activating the cardiac acceleration fibers.

The CEA by catheter controls the respiratory mechanics more easily than the SAB. The decrease of pulmonary function is proportionate to the height of motor block achieved. Even the lowest level of lumbar epidural anesthesia causes abdominal muscular paralysis which is only involved in active expiration. The impairment of active expiration has no clinical significance on respiration in the absence of COPD. As the level of motor block ascends, it affects the increasing amount of muscles involved in quiet respiration. The intercostal muscles act by stabilizing and expanding the bony thorax and thus help in respiration by creating a negative intrathoracic pressure. As more and more intercostal muscles are blocked, then the respiration becomes more dependent on diaphragm alone. Block of high sensory level in epidural anesthesia, blunts the normal endocrine response to surgical stress and also the respiratory response to increased level of arterial PCO_2.

Factors Controlling the Spread of Epidural Block

The factors controlling the spread (extend) of epidural block are:

- *Volume and concentration of local anesthetic agent:* The volume and concentration of LA agent influence the epidural anesthesia as spinal anesthesia which has been discussed earlier. However, in epidural anesthesia the spread of LA agent and the involvement of more and more dermatomes depends more on the volume of drugs. But, the intensity of sensory and motor block depends on the concentration of drug.

- *Posture of patient:* Though 0.5% bupivacaine and 2% lignocaine is isobaric, still it tends to spread in epidural space according to the gravity (like a falling feather through air toward the earth), but not so reliably, as the hyperbaric solutions given intrathecally (like a stone dropping in water). As the fat has a lower specific gravity than the aqueous local anesthetic solutions, but the very thin film of it in the epidural space is unlikely to be sufficient to account for such positive geotropism. Gravity is more effective for epidural spread in obese than in normal subject. This is because there is more presence of fat in epidural space in an obese patient than in a normal individual. The height of block is not so clinically predictable by the position and posture changes in epidural anesthesia, because the gravity and the baricity are not so intimately related to the spread of block in

epidural anesthesia. Here, the volume of drug is more determining factor to determine the height of block. Still, it is apparent that tilting can determine the caudal and cephalad spread in epidural anesthesia. Thus, the lateral position produces a block which is significantly higher on the dependent side. In most subjects, it is possible to induce only sacral spread of local anesthetic solution in epidural anesthesia with the aid of sitting position. But, it may be necessary to use a low space and/or a large volume.

- *Site of injection:* Epidural anesthesia mainly works segmentally at the roots, which is nearest to the injection site. So, the site of injection is very important for the level of anesthesia in epidural procedure. As for example, during the upper abdominal surgery, where the dermatomes are supplied by thoracic spinal nerves, very large volume of drug (which may reach toxic level) is necessary to reach the thoracic segments, if the epidural is given by lumbar route. So, in such cases higher interspinal space is preferable and ideally thoracic epidural approach greatly reduces the dose requirement and unnecessary lumbar anesthesia. For the lower extremities and perineal block, the lower lumbar interspaces are preferred. For obstetric analgesia, a very lower lumbar approach than L_2-L_3 interspinal space causes the standard volume of solution to be ineffective and has too much effect on the legs.

- *Age of patient:* The total dose requirement of local anesthetic agent, during epidural anesthesia, is inversely related to the age of a patient. The age-related arteriosclerosis and osteoarthritis changes cause the gradual closure of intervertebral foramen and thus prevents the leak of anesthetic solutions in the paravertebral space, from epidural area, through the intervertebral foramen, causing the increased spread of it along the vertebral column and the higher level of block with the same volume of LA agent.

- *Pregnancy or intra-abdominal tumors:* Increased pressure on inferior vena cava by gravid uterus or any other intra-abdominal tumors or ascites leads to the diversion of venous return from the lower part of the body through the vertebral and epidural venous plexuses. Therefore, the distension of these venous plexuses, within the vertebral canal, causes the reduction of epidural space and so the higher spread by the same volume of LA drug results in the higher level of block and more hypotension. But, some schools do not believe in it. They believe that the pregnant patients are more sensitive to hypotensive effect of LA agents. This is because there is already vasodilation, due to the high level of progesterone. Thus, for the pain relief in labor, a small volume of drug is adequate (where very few segments have to be blocked) than obstetric anesthesia.

- *Height and weight of patient:* The obesity reduces and the height of patient increases the dose requirement of local anesthetic agent for the same level of epidural block.
- *Nerve root size:* The general principle regarding the relationship between the effect of epidural anesthesia and the diameter of nerve root is that their relationship is inversely proportional. Hence, the S_1 nerve root is thickest of all the spinal nerves and is notoriously resistant to epidural block. So, the S_1 dermatome has a very long latency and shorter duration of block.

INDIVIDUAL EPIDURAL BLOCK

Thoracic Epidural

The thoracic epidural space extends from the lower margin of C_7 vertebra to the upper margin of L_1 vertebra. The vertebral column in the thoracic area normally has a kyphotic curvature (concave ventrally) with its apex at the level of approximately T_6 vertebra in supine position. The inclination of the spinous processes of thoracic vertebrae is different at different levels. The spines from T_1 to T_4 vertebrae have very little downward inclination, whereas those of T_5-T_8 vertebrae tilt significantly downward, making a midline approach to the epidural space practically impossible in that area. The T_9-T_{12} spines direct dorsally without any significant inclination **(Fig. 34)**. So, the midline approach for epidural space is possible in that T_9-T_{12} spaces.

The ligamentum flavum in the thoracic region is not as thick as in the lumbar region. So, in the thoracic region, the epidural space can be entered without encountering much resistance. In thoracic area, the epidural space is only 3–4 mm wide and like other space contains loose areolar tissue, fat, and vertebral venous plexuses. The lumbar enlargement of the spinal cord is situated within the thoracic vertebra between T_9 and T_{12} segment. The pressure in

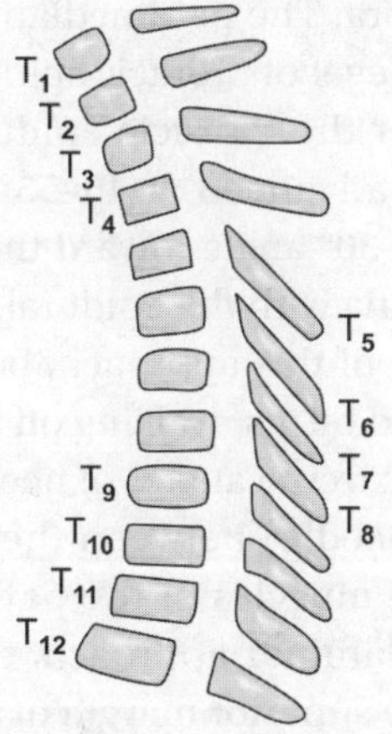

Fig. 34: The inclination of spine of different thoracic vertebrae.

the thoracic epidural space is approximately –15 cmH$_2$O (negative) and is very close to that of the negative intrapleural pressure. It is more pronounced in the sitting position. However, the negative pressure in the epidural space is also considered to be secondary to the tenting of the dura by the blunt epidural needle, during the procedure. However, in 12% of cases, the pressure in the epidural space is not negative.

The cardiovascular effect of thoracic epidural anesthesia depends on the upper level of block. The preganglionic sympathetic fibers, as white rami communicantes, are present in all the thoracic spinal nerve. Sympathetic block up to T_{10} level, extending from L_2 produce minimal cardiovascular changes. The degree of hypotension, due to sympathetic block up to that level, will depend on the existing blood volume. The hypotension, if occur, usually will be partly compensated by the vasoconstriction of upper extremities and will be partly compensated by cardiac stimulation, producing tachycardia and increased myocardial contraction, as the T_1-T_4 cardiac sympathetic fibers are not blocked. If the block extends up to the segment T_6 from L_2 then the hypotension will not be compensated by the abovementioned mechanisms and it (hypotension) will be revealed.

This hypotension is primarily due to venodilatation, causing the pooling of blood in venous side, and subsequently decreased right heart filling and decreased CO. Blocking of the sympathetic fibers to the abdominal viscera, including those to the adrenal medulla, also can reduce the response to stress during the lower abdominal and pelvic surgical procedures. If the block extends up to the T_1 segment, then the sympathetic fibers innervating the heart will also be affected. Therefore, the cardioaccelerator fibers, coming out of the T_1-T_4 segment will be blocked, producing severe bradycardia and hypotension due to the nonavailability of cardiac compensatory mechanism and also due to the unopposed action of parasympathetic fibers derived from the vagus nerve.

Sometimes, it results in cardiac standstill. So, the response is manifested primarily by the combined effects of the degree of sympathetic denervation and the degree of unopposed vagal nerve dominance. Sympathetic denervation produces arterial and, more important, arteriolar dilatation. But, this arterial or arteriolar dilatation is not complete. Because, the vascular smooth muscle on the arterial side maintains a significant degree of residual autonomous tone which is not dependent on sympathetic system. The venous system has very little smooth muscle, present within its walls, and maintains no significant residual autonomic tone, due to the complete sympathectomy. Thus, venodilatation and severely reduced preload result in a reduction in CO with severe hypotension, but without any compensation as the cardioacceleratory fibers are blocked. Bradycardia or cardiac standstill also can occur after blockade of the cardioacceleratory fibers arising from T_1 to T_4 segment or the failure of the activation of great veins and right arterial cardiac receptors, which usually occurs due to the decreased venous return and reflexly increase the heart rate (Bainbridge reflex). During sympathetic block below the level of T_4, the baroreceptors on the wall of carotid sinus and aortic arch normally respond to the fall in BP by producing a compensatory tachycardia (Marey's law) through vagal afferent (withdrawal) and efferent pathways.

Bainbridge Reflex

The venous engorgement of the right atrium and great veins reflexly increase the heart rate. The afferent fibers arising from the roots of the great veins and right atria pass along the trunk of the vagus to the cardiac center. The engorgement of these parts stimulates the nerve endings and *reflexly inhibits the vagal tone* and also stimulates the sympathetic to some extent. Thus, the heart rate rises and CO increases. This reflex is called the Bainbridge reflex or more appropriately the *venous reflex*.

Cardioinhibitory Reflex (Sinoaortic or Marey's Reflex)

There are multiple stretch receptors on the wall of carotid sinus and aortic arch. When the BP rises, then these nerve endings become stimulated due to stretching and cause the sensory impulses to pass through the sinoaortic nerves and *increase the vagal tone.* So, the heart rate falls. On the other hand, when the BP falls, then no inhibiting impulse passes up and heart rate rises. Thus, the heart rate and BP have an inverse relation. This is known as the *Marey's law.*

The paralysis of intercostal muscles by thoracic epidural block can affect the respiratory volumes. When this block affects all the intercostal muscles, then the normal ventilation and $PaCO_2$ can still be maintained by the activity of diaphragm only, since the phrenic nerve is not affected. But, the patient suffers from a severe feeling of suffocation. So, sedation is very much needed which again reduces the central ventilatory drive. On the other hand, secondary to intercostal muscle paralysis, the increased diaphragmatic activity improves the tidal volume. But, the inspiratory reserve volume and functional reserve capacity are significantly decreased with the decrease of vital capacity.

Thoracic epidural with Tuohy needle and catheter can be performed by the patient sitting, lateral, or prone position. The sitting position provides the better alignment of spine and facilitates the better identification of landmarks. But,

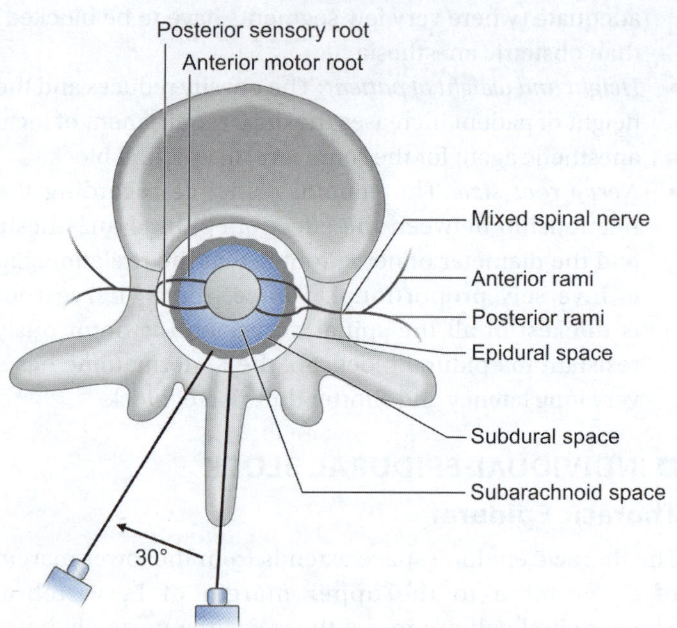

Fig. 35: Cross section of median and paramedian approach to the thoracic epidural space. The black color circle indicates the dura mater and the blue color circle indicates the arachnoid mater.

a patient who is anxious may have a strong vasovagal and hypotensive reaction. So, for them, lateral decubitus is preferred. The flexion of patient contributes very little by expanding the interlaminar space in the thoracic region **(Fig. 35)**.

Thoracic epidural space also can be approached from three directions, such as midline, paramedian, and laminar. The midline approach is applicable in the upper part of thoracic spine between the C_7 and T_5 vertebrae and in the lower part of thoracic spine between the T_9 and T_1 2 vertebrae, because in these areas, the spinous processes are more or less horizontal and project directly to the posterior with minimal downward inclination. In these segments, the level of the spinous process corresponds to the same level of vertebra. The paramedian or lateral approach can be used at any level of thoracic spine. In paramedian or lateral approach for the thoracic epidural anesthesia, the epidural needle is advanced at 45–55° angle in cephalad direction and at 15–30° angle toward the midline **(Fig. 35)**. Contacting the lamina with the epidural needle significantly increases the safety of this approach, because the epidural space can be entered by just walking off the superior margin of the lamina. The extreme angles of needle can result in the passing of it (the needle) between the spinous processes into the paraspinal muscles of the paravertebral space of opposite side. For laminar approach, the starting point is 1–2 cm lateral to the superior margin of the spinous process (like paramedian approach), but the needle is not angled

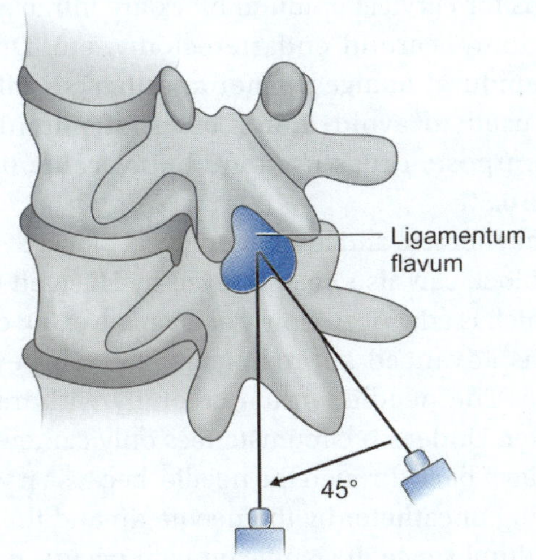

Fig. 36: Median and paramedian approach to the lumbar epidural space.

toward the midline. It runs parallel to the spinous process and enters the interlaminar foramen medial to the interarticular process. Here, only the lateral portion of the epidural space is entered **(Fig. 36)**.

The complications of thoracic epidural technique or approach are similar to those of lumbar epidural. There are many indications for thoracic epidural block. Among them, a few are stated below. Thoracic epidural catheters are increasingly utilized for providing the intraoperative and especially postoperative analgesia for thoracic and upper abdominal surgical procedures, such as the mastectomy, cholecystectomy, gastrectomy, repair of diaphragmatic hernia, etc. It has also been utilized for thoracotomy and cardiac surgery in conjunction with light GA. Patients with multiple fractured ribs get excellent analgesia by thoracic epidural with catheter at selected segments.

Local anesthetic agent, such as 0.125% bupivacaine and/or an opioid can be used without any motor block and hypotension. Catheters placed in the thoracic epidural space can also be used to provide only long-term analgesia using opioids, local anesthetic agents, phenol, or alcohol in alone or with combination of them for chronic pain, due to many causes or acute pain in nonoperable malignancy. The catheter should be placed in the area of the involved nerve roots. If alcohol is used, it should be injected through the catheter in 0.5 mL incremental doses to a maximum of 5 mL. The injection has to be repeated daily for at least 3 days. The phenol is used in concentration of 5% with dextrose or with normal saline.

Cervical Epidural

The cervical epidural space is bounded above by the fusion of the investing layer of dura mater (vertebral periosteum) and the spinal layers of dura mater at the level of foramen magnum and below it is continuous with the thoracic epidural space at the level of T_1 vertebra. The cervical epidural space is bounded anteriorly by the posterior surface of the body of cervical vertebra with posterior longitudinal ligament and posteriorly by the cervical vertebral laminae and ligamentum flavum. The ligamentum flavum is thin in the cervical region and gradually becomes thicker caudally. It is thickest at the lumbar region. This fact has direct clinical implication, because the loss of resistance felt during cervical epidural block is more subtle than it is in the lumbar and lower thoracic region. The vertebral pedicles and intervertebral foramina form the lateral boundary of cervical epidural space.

The degenerative changes and the narrowing of these intervertebral foramina, associated with aging, may be marked in the cervical region. Such changes reduce the leakage of local anesthetic solution out of the intervertebral foramina and account for the reduced anesthetic dose requirement in elderly patients, undergoing cervical epidural block. At the level of C_7 vertebra, the distance between the ligamentum flavum and the dura mater is only about 1.5–2 mm. It is due to the presence of the cervical enlargement of spinal cord, serving the upper extremities, whereas the distance between the ligamentum flavum and the dura mater is greatest at the level of L_2 interspace, measuring about 5–6 mm in adults. It should also be noted that the flexion of the neck moves this cervical enlargement more toward the cephalad direction, resulting in the widening of epidural space up to 3–4 mm at the level of C_7-T_1 interspace. This fact has important clinical implications for the cervical epidural block.

Like other epidural space, cervical epidural space also contains loose areolar tissue, fat, epidural veins, arteries, and lymphatics. Fat in the epidural space serves as a shock absorber for other contents of the space and as a depot for injected drugs. The amount of epidural fat varies in direct proportion to the amount of fat, stored elsewhere in the body. The epidural fat is relatively vascular and appears to change to a denser consistency with aging. This change in consistency may account for the significant variations in required dose of a drug in adults, especially with the cervical approach to the epidural space. The valveless epidural veins are concentrated principally at the anterolateral portion of the epidural space and transmit both the intrathoracic and intra-abdominal pressures.

When pressure in either of these body cavities increases, such as during the Valsalva's maneuver or the compression of inferior vena cava in the abdomen by a gravid uterus, ascites, or a tumor mass, etc. then the cervical epidural veins distend and reduce the volume of this epidural space. This decrease in the volume of cervical epidural space can directly affect (decrease) the amount of LA drug, needed to obtain a given level of neural blockade. Most of the epidural arteries with their significant anastomoses lie in the lateral portions of cervical epidural space. The arteries enter the epidural space via two routes (1) through the intervertebral foramina and (2) via the direct anastomoses from the intracranial portion of vertebral arteries. Trauma to these epidural arteries can result in the formation of epidural hematoma and compromise the blood supply to the spinal cord itself.

Cervical epidural block can be carried out with the patient in the sitting, lateral or prone position and each position has its advantages and disadvantages. The *sitting position* for cervical epidural block is most preferred, because (1) it enhances the operator's ability to identify the midline, (2) it also ensures that the cervical spine is flexed which widens the lower cervical epidural space, (3) the sitting position avoids the rotation of the spine which is inherent in the lateral position and makes the identification of cervical epidural space difficult. But, sitting position is not always an option for patients with acute vertebral compression fracture or with the history of vasovagal syncope or sedated, where lateral position is preferred.

For the patient's comfort, *lateral decubitus or position* is more suitable and also for those who cannot assume the sitting position. If lateral position for the cervical epidural block is selected, then care must be taken to ensure that there is no rotation of the patient's spine, because it will make the cervical epidural block extremely difficult or impossible or produce complications. During cervical epidural, it will have to be kept in mind that the flexion of cervical spine is mandatory to maximize the width of the cervical epidural space.

Another important point for cervical epidural anesthesia is that the needle entry site should be exactly in the midline. Failure to accurately identify the midline is the most common cause of difficulty in performing the cervical epidural block. The *prone position* for cervical epidural block is selected in special cases such as during the placement of epidural catheters with spinal stimulation electrodes. However, this prone position should be avoided if sedation is required, because the access to the airway is limited.

For the purposes of diagnostic and/or prognostic cervical epidural block, 1% preservative-free lignocaine is most suitable as local anesthetic agent. For therapeutic purpose, 0.25% preservative-free bupivacaine in combination with 80 mg of depot methylprednisolone is injected. Subsequent dose of methylprednisolone is 40 mg daily, with or without local anesthetic agent, to treat the acute painful conditions. The chronic painful conditions, such as the cervical radiculopathy and diabetic neuropathy are treated by daily or every alternate day or once in a week injection through the catheter, as the clinical situation dictates. The other indications for cervical epidural block are intractable pain, thyroidectomy, carotid endarterectomy, etc. During the cervical epidural analgesia (not anesthesia), differential block is used to avoid motor block of phrenic nerve. For this purpose, drugs used are bupivacaine 0.125% or lignocaine 0.5%.

Like the thoracic and lumbar epidural block, the cervical epidural block can also be employed by Hustead or Tuohy needle which is advanced slowly at an angle of 30° cephalad. Catheter is advanced approximately 2–3 cm beyond the needle tip. The needle is then carefully withdrawn over the catheter. Under no circumstances only catheter should be withdrawn back through the needle, because it will cause the shearing of catheter by the needle tip and the lost of it in the epidural space. If significant pain occurs, during the placement of epidural needle or catheter or during the injection of drug, then the physician should immediately stop the procedure and will ascertain the cause of pain to avoid the possibility of neural trauma. So, intravenous sedation or GA before the initiation of cervical or other epidural nerve block renders the patient unable to provide accurate verbal feedback, if the needle is misplaced. Like other CNB, during cervical epidural block, if an epidural needle or catheter is accidentally placed in the subarachnoid space and the problem goes unrecognized, then injection of a fraction of epidural doses of local anesthetics solution will cause immediate total spinal anesthesia and its consequences. So, implication of test dose in cervical epidural anesthesia is not as helpful as thoracic and lumbar epidural anesthesia.

The administration of opioids and local anesthetic agents into the cervical epidural space may be associated with a greater incidence of urinary retention. This side effect is more common in elderly male and multiporous females whose bladders are prolapsed. Overflow incontinence may occur when such patients are unable to void or bladder catheterization is not done. So, all patients must empty their bladder before their discharge from the pain clinic, if they get cervical epidural anesthesia or analgesia.

■ CAUDAL (SACRAL) EPIDURAL ANESTHESIA

Anatomy of Sacrum, Sacral Canal, and Hiatus

The sacrum represents the fusion of five sacral vertebrae. However, many variations of this fusion are common and have an important bearing on the incidences of failure rate of caudal epidural anesthesia. The sacrum is triangular in shape. The apex of this triangle is directed below and is formed by the fifth sacral vertebra which articulates with the coccyx. The base of the triangle is formed by the first sacral vertebra and articulates with the body of fifth lumbar vertebra. The anterior surface of the sacrum is concave and is characterized by four anterior sacral foramina on both sides of midline (total four pairs) through which the anterior primary rami of four sacral spinal nerves pass out. The posterior surface of the sacrum which has a greater interest for anesthetist is convex. A bony ridge with three or four rudimentary spinous processes runs in the midline and is called the median sacral crest. On both sides of this median sacral crest, there are four posterior sacral foramina (total four pairs), corresponding with the anterior one, through which the posterior primary rami of four spinal sacral nerves pass out **(Fig. 37)**. The local anesthetic solutions, injected into the sacral epidural space or sacral canal, can pass freely through these foramina and this is an important factor for the unpredictability of the height to which caudal anesthesia may extend. The canal in the sacrum is called the sacral canal. It is also triangular in shape and continuous above with the lumbar portion of vertebral canal and terminates below at the sacral hiatus.

The sacral canal contains:

- The epidural space with its venous plexuses and fibrofatty tissue. This sacral epidural space extends below throughout the whole sacral canal up to the sacral hiatus and it is continuous above with the lumbar epidural space.
- The dural sac which is made of spinal dura mater.
- *The arachnoid mater and under it the subarachnoid space:* It contains CSF and ends between the S_1 and S_3 vertebrae (usually at the lower border of S_2)
- The five sacral nerve roots
- Coccygeal nerve
- Filum terminale externa.

The epidural venous plexus in sacral canal generally ends at S_4 level, but may also continue caudally. Most of these vessels are concentrated in the anterior portion of the sacral canal. Both, the dural sac and the epidural vessels are susceptible to trauma, during the excessive cephalad advancement of epidural needles and catheters, used for caudal block through the sacral canal. The remainder of the

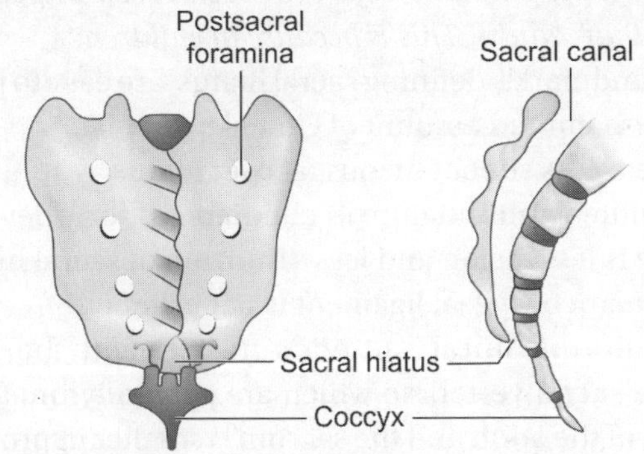

Fig. 37: Posterior and sagittal view of sacrum and coccyx.

sacral canal is filled with fibrofatty tissue which is subjected to age-related increase in density.

The *sacral hiatus* is actually a deficiency on the posterior wall at the lower end of the sacrum. It results from the failure of the fusion of laminae of fifth sacral vertebrae. It is triangular in shape. The apex of the hiatus is formed by the spine of fourth sacral vertebrae. The lateral margin of hiatus bears a prominence on each side and is called the sacral cornu. This sacral cornu represents the articular process of fifth sacral vertebrae. The base of the sacral hiatus is formed by the superior surface of coccyx and is covered by posterior sacrococcygeal membrane. In surface marking, the sacral hiatus forms an equilateral triangle with the two posterior superior iliac spines.

There may be multiple anatomical variations of sacral hiatus. Some of which are described below. (1) The apex of the hiatus may be formed by the spine of second or third sacral vertebrae, due to the absence of the laminae of third and fourth sacral vertebrae, respectively. (2) Occasionally, the whole bony post wall of the sacrum remains deficient. (3) On the other hand, when the lamina of fifth sacral vertebra is present, then this sacral hiatus becomes very small with the diameter as narrow as 2 mm and makes the introduction of needle for caudal epidural anesthesia almost impossible. There are many fibrous bands in the sacral canal which divide the sacral epidural space into multiple loculi, causing the incomplete spread of local anesthetic agents in the sacral canal and incomplete epidural anesthesia. Nowadays, the caudal epidural anesthesia is often combined with GA for pediatric patients to decrease the amount of intraoperative anesthetic agents and/or to provide the postoperative analgesia for the surgeries on inguinal region, perineal region, lower extremities, and sometimes lower abdomen.

Technique of Sacral Epidural Anesthesia

It is better to see and practice than to read the technique of caudal epidural anesthesia. Usually, the needle selected for caudal anesthesia should be malleable enough to adapt itself with the curvature of the sacral canal and will not break. A wide-bore needle gives a better feel of the structures, as it passes through the sacral hiatus and its canal, while a short bevel at the tip of the needle minimizes the risk of puncturing the dura. However, nowadays many operators use an ordinary disposable hypodermic needle for caudal epidural block.

The ideal position of patient for caudal block is prone or lateral. The sacral hiatus is identified first by sacral cornu. The needle then pierces the skin and sacrococcygeal ligament at right angle. After that, the needle should be depressed in the intergluteal fold and is advanced cranially in the sacral canal, maximally up to the line joining the two posterior superior iliac spine, where the dural sac (with the subarachnoid space) ends. Then, the aspiration for blood or CSF is done. During aspiration, the flow of blood through needle indicates the puncture of epidural vein and in that case needle should be withdrawn for a few millimeters. If CSF comes through needle, then this epidural procedure should be abandoned or converted it to spinal block. For test dose (test for the confirmation whether the tip of the needle has entered the dural sac or remains outside the dural sac in the epidural space), 2 mL of local anesthetic drug is used first. If patient can move his toes, then it is sure that the tip of the needle is in epidural space and not in the subarachnoid area. Then, the rest of the drug is injected.

Problems of Sacral Epidural Anesthesia

The needle may miss the sacrococcygeal ligament and may pass dorsal to the sacrum under the skin or may pass under the periosteum of the posterior surface of sacrum. This can be tested by injecting a few milliliters of air and palpating the crepitus under the skin. The needle may slip under the base of the coccyx and can pierce the rectum or fetal head (in pregnancy). The needle may run beneath the periosteum of the sacral canal, causing more marked resistance to injection and the complaint of severe backache. Any feeling of resistance, during the injection of LA agent, indicates that needles are not placed in proper position.

Doses of Drugs used for Sacral Epidural Anesthesia

The level of the block by caudal epidural anesthesia depends on the volume of local anesthetic solution and the position of the patient. With the patient in horizontal position, 20–30 mL of local anesthetic drug is required to block up to L_{4-5} level. It is used for the operations on anus, perineum, and vagina. The 40 mL drug is needed for analgesia and anesthesia up to the umbilical level. But, with the patient in horizontal position such a large dose may risk the systemic toxic reaction. However, the Trendelenburg position helps in upward extension of the drug and reduces the dose of LA drugs.

Indications for Sacral Epidural

The main indication of epidural anesthesia through this caudal route is the production of conduction block of only the lower lumbar and sacral spinal nerve roots for the procedures, such as the urinary bladder operation, anal-vulval-vaginal operation, operation on inguinal region, and circumcision without affecting BP and much systemic conditions. In some conditions where the caudal-epidural

anesthesia is highly indicated due to the severe illness of patient, but sacral approach is technically very difficult, then it may be easier to perform lumbar epidural block in sitting position. Postoperative analgesia by caudal epidural procedure in conjunction with GA is a good choice, particularly in children and obstetric analgesia.

Continuous Caudal Epidural Anesthesia using Catheters

An epidural catheter may be placed into the sacral canal in a manner, analogous to that of continuous lumbar, thoracic or cervical epidural anesthesia, through an epidural needle placed in the sacral canal though sacral hiatus. The epidural catheter is advanced through the needle approximately 2–3 cm beyond its tip and then the needle is carefully withdrawn over the catheter. But, under no circumstances, the catheter is withdrawn back through the needle to avoid the shearing of catheter tip.

A test dose of 3–4 mL of local anesthetic agent is, then, given via the catheter and the patient is observed for any sign of local anesthetic toxicity, due to the inadvertent intravascular or subarachnoid injection. If no sign of side effects or toxicity of LA agent is noted, then the intermittent boluses or continuous infusion of local anesthetic agent, with or without opioids, are administered through the catheter. Because of the proximity to the anus, the risk of infection limits the long-term use of caudal epidural catheters.

Pediatric Caudal Block

Though, the placement of an epidural catheter allows for continuous infusion of local anesthetic agent, with or without opioid or opioid alone, for continuous caudal block for various reasons, till the single-injection caudal or sacral block is one of the most popular pediatric regional anesthetic techniques for the intra- and postoperative analgesia. A combination of caudal block, supplemented with light GA, allows for a quicker recovery due to lesser need of volatile and other general anesthetic agent.

Technically, the caudal blocks are much easier to perform in children than adults. This is because in children:

- The landmarks, defining sacral hiatus, are easy to palpate.
- There is limited amount of gluteal pad of fat.
- There is less subcutaneous fat over hiatus.
- The gluteal musculature in children is poorly developed.
- There is less fusion and less distortion of sacral hiatus.
- The sacrococcygeal ligament is not calcified.

In children, dural sac ends in-between the second and third sacral vertebrae which are generally much lower than that of the adult and the sacrum is smaller in proportion to the overall size of the body of children. So, there is much higher possibility to pierce the dura during caudal block in children.

It is previously stated that when the caudal block is combined with GA, then it provides excellent perioperative analgesia. So, the common indications for pediatric caudal epidural block are (1) sacral segment surgeries—circumcision, rectal operation, club foot repair, etc.; (2) groin surgeries—herniorrhaphy, orchidopexy, hydrocele, etc.; (3) urologic procedures; and (4) lower extremity orthopedic procedures. By increasing the volume of drug, the level of caudal block can be increased high by which the different lower abdominal surgeries can also be performed.

For caudal epidural, 0.25% bupivacaine is the commonly used drug which provides minimal motor blockade with adequate sensory blockade. But, the total dose of bupivacaine should not exceed 3 mg/kg. An easy calculation for the volume of 0.25% bupivacaine is 0.5 mL/kg for only sacral blockade, 0.75 mL/kg for the blockade of lumbar segments, and 1.25 mL/kg for the blockade of thoracic segments. Test dose is unreliable for sacral epidural block in children, so close observation, frequent aspiration, and fractionated injection of drug is the best safeguard against the undetected subarachnoid and intravascular injection.

CAUSES OF FAILED EPIDURAL BLOCKS

In spinal anesthesia, the procedural end point is very clear (i.e., free flowing of CSF), the onset of anesthesia is very fast and the technical success rate is very high. Whereas, in epidural anesthesia, the procedural end point is not so clear (dependent on detection of loss of resistance and negative pressure), the onset of anesthesia is slower, and the less predictable spread of LA agent makes the epidural anesthesia inherently less predictable than the spinal anesthesia.

In epidural anesthesia, the misplaced injection of LA agent can occur in a number of situations. (1) In some patients, the spinal ligaments (supraspinous and interspinous) are soft and so either good resistance is never appreciated or a false loss of resistance is encountered. (2) Sometimes, the epidural needle may enter into the paraspinous muscles, when the needle goes away from midline in median approach and may cause a false loss of resistance. (3) A unilateral block can occur, if the LA agent is delivered through a catheter that has either passed through an intervertebral foramen or is coursed laterally. The chances of this occurring (passing of catheter through intervertebral foramen) increase when a longer length of catheter is introduced into the epidural space. (4) The large size of L_5, S_1, and S_2 spinal nerves may delay the adequate penetration of LA agent and is thought to be responsible for sacral sparing. This type of problem is particularly found during surgery on knee, ankle, and foot.

(5) Despite a seemingly good epidural block, patients may complain of visceral pain where afferent fibers are carried through autonomic system (vagus and sympathetic). For example, pain due to traction on spermatic cord or peritoneum can be alleviated by high thoracic sensory block or intravenous supplementation with opioids or other agents

The problem of unilateral block (point 3) can be solved by withdrawing the catheter 1–2 cm and reinjecting LA agent through catheter with the patient turned with unblocked side down. The segmental sparing of block, which may be due to the septations within the epidural space, may also be corrected by injecting an additional dose of local anesthetic agent with the unblocked segment positioned down. The problem of point 4 is solved by elevating the head end of the OT table and reinjecting additional dose of LA agent through the catheter to achieve a more intense block of these nerve roots.

COMPLICATIONS OF SPINAL AND EPIDURAL BLOCK

As some complications are common for both the spinal and epidural anesthesia, so they are discussed together first. Specific complications for spinal or epidural will be discussed later or at specific places **(Box 4)**.

Hypotension

Vasodilation and hypotension is the most predictable and desirable feature of central neuraxial blockade when the nerve roots above the levels of L_2 segment are affected, from where the preganglionic sympathetic fibers originate. Severe hypotension is expected more likely in the older patients and in the patients with higher level of block (T_5 and above). The definition of hypotension during CNB varies, but a systolic BP of <90 mm Hg is challengeable. It is more appropriate to consider a fall in BP of 25–30% from its preoperative MAP level as a practical guide to dictate the treatment. The incidence of hypotension, following CNB, has been reported to be 92% in an untreated control group, undergoing cesarean section with spinal anesthesia. It is a very serious problem in spinal anesthesia and is due to its very rapid onset and giving no time for adequate cardiovascular compensation. More quick acting anesthetic drugs cause more quick and severe fall of BP. In continuous epidural, this incidence of hypotension can be reduced by giving the full dose of LA agent in multiple small incremental doses, when an extensive epidural block is needed and thus giving the CVS adequate time for compensation. This complication can be managed by intravenous preloading with crystalloid (1–2 L) or colloid solution.

> **BOX 4:** Complications of central neuraxial block (CNB).
>
> - *Related to needle and/or catheter introduction:*
>   - *Trauma:*
>   - Nerve root damage
>   - Spinal cord damage
>   - Cauda equina syndrome
>   - Dural puncture leak causing postdural puncture headache (PDPH), tinnitus, diplopia, etc.
>   - Cranial nerve injury
>   - Backache
>   - *Bleeding:*
>   - Intraspinal hemorrhage
>   - Epidural hematoma
>   - *Infection:*
>   - Meningitis
>   - Epidural abscess
>   - *Displacement of needle or catheter:*
>   - Inadvertent intravascular injection
>   - Inadvertent subarachnoid block or total spinal (epidural block)
>   - Inadequate block
>   - No effect
>   - *Shearing and retention of catheter*
> - *Exaggerated physiological responses:*
>   - Total spinal anesthesia (in case of epidural block)
>   - Higher block than expected
>   - Respiratory arrest and cardiac arrest
>   - Urinary retention
>   - Anterior spinal artery syndrome
>   - Horner's syndrome
> - *Toxicity of drugs:*
>   - Systemic toxicity
>   - Transient neurological symptoms
>   - Cauda equina syndrome

Colloid solutions are more effective in reducing the incidences of hypotension at their lower volumes than the crystalloid solution. But, the colloids are more expensive and carry a slightly increased risk of allergic reaction. So, the crystalloids are generally preferred for IV preloading as routine prophylaxis against hypotension. However, caution is required for the patients with cardiac diseases, where the smaller volumes of IV fluids plus earlier use vasopressors are advisable. The administration of only large volumes of IV fluid, as the only treatment of persistent hypotension, produced by central neuraxial blockade, is potentially dangerous and is not recommended. Pressure-rising drugs such as ephedrine, mephentermine, or methoxamine are used where preloading (moderate amount, e.g., 1–1.5 L) fails to maintain MAP. Combination of preloading and vasoconstrictor had maximum effect and is the best in preventing spinal hypotension. This is followed by the sole use of vasoconstrictor which is the second choice. Preloading alone offers least protection against spinal hypotension,

do not believe only on the preloading to control the severe spinal or epidural hypotension.

The optimal treatment of hypotension, induced by central neural blockade, remains still unresolved. A correction of the fall of systemic vascular resistance generally includes the treatment with α-adrenergic agonist such as the methoxamine, mephentermine, or ephedrine, whereas the impaired venous pooling is corrected by IV fluids and β-adrenergic agonists. A slight head-down tilt and elevation of legs encourage venous return. Methoxamine, as an α-adrenergic agonist, increases the peripheral vascular resistance and restores the BP, but perhaps at the expense of reduced organ blood flow. This drug may produce or extend bradycardia and is preferable to ephedrine when tachycardia is present. So, some cautions should be exercised when there is a normal or lower than normal heart rate, as more reflex bradycardia due to the increase of vascular resistance may follow the administration of methoxamine or other vasoconstrictive agents. The initial intravenous bolus dose of methoxamine should be 2 mg. Ephedrine is a predominantly β-adrenergic agonist. It acts both directly and indirectly on both α- and β-receptors. But, its indirect action is more than its direct action and its β action is more than its α action. It has little direct effect on peripheral resistance. It mainly acts on heart. Thus, it maintains the BP by increasing the heart rate with some effect on the venous pooling. Ephedrine is also advantageous over methoxamine in pregnancy, because here the preservation of uterine blood flow in the presence of hypotension is more important. It is administered in repeated bolus dose of 3–6 mg intravenously according to the situation.

Sometimes, the simple treatment of bradycardia by atropine may restore the BP to an acceptable level. The raising of legs i) to increase the venous drainage and ii) thus to reduce the chance of hypotension, may also encourage the further cranial spread of local anesthetic block, if this is under taken at the very early stages of anesthesia, and will cause more hypotension.

Postdural Puncture Headache

It is the complication of spinal block only and in epidural anesthesia it occurs only when the needle inadvertently punctures the dura. The principal cause of PDPH in spinal anesthesia is low CSF pressure and it is due to its continuous seepage through the punctured hole on dura or aseptic meningeal irritation. It also may herald the onset of infective meningitis. The rate of the leakage of CSF from subarachnoid space to epidural space, causing PDPH should be above 10 mL/hour. The loss of CSF up to 10 mL/hour has no symptom or headache. The healing of dural puncture usually takes 3 weeks. So, PDPH usually lasts for 1–2 weeks. But, it may last for days, weeks, or even months. In traumatic leakage, the choroid plexus can form CSF maximum at the rate of 500 mL/day.

The mechanism of PDPH is, when the rate of the leakage of CSF through the dural hole exceeds its rate of formation, then it leads to some change in hydrodynamics of CSF. This causes the loss of the cushioning effect of brain and produce traction on vessels, basal dura, tentorium, and other sensitive brain structure. Attachment of these structures to the cranium on one hand and the meninges on the other hand leads to the stretching of meninges and blood vessels, causing pain. The PDPH is mainly posturally mediated and is being worse in upright position. This is due to the increase in downward traction of brain tissue by the gravity. The typical PDPH starts 6–12 hours after the puncture of dura and lasts for weeks. It is worse in sitting up position and disappears after lying down. The pain is typical and different from any other previously experienced headache by the patient. Usually, the pain is experienced at the frontal region or behind the eyeball. Nausea and vomiting may accompany this pain. Tinnitus and deafness may also accompany the PDPH and is due to the low CSF pressure, resulting in fall of intralabyrinthine pressure. The normal CSF pressure is 150 mm H_2O. When PDPH precipitates, it drops to 50 mm H_2O. It is most common in obstetric patient, because during contraction of uterus and bearing down there is more leakage of CSF. The PDPH is also more commonly associated with young female patient, large-bore spinal needle, cutting-tip needle, passing of the bevel of needle tip at right angle to dural fibers, etc. Other factors that increase the rate of PDPH are those that increase CSF pressure and subsequently it is leaked, e.g., obesity, ascites, and pregnancy **(Figs. 38A and B)**.

Classification of Postdural Puncture Headache

Postdural puncture headache is classified into mild, moderate, and severe form:

- *Mild PDPH:* Here PDPH is slight and does not restrict daily activities. The patient is not bedridden at any time during the day. There are no other associated symptoms like nausea, vomiting, etc. with PDPH.
- *Moderate PDPH:* Here PDPH is significant and restricts daily activities. The patient is bedridden for some part of the day. Associated symptoms may or may not be present.
- *Severe PDPH:* Here PDPH is very intense and forced the patient to stay in bed throughout the whole day. Associated symptoms are always present.

   In one study, it is found that 86% of patients who developed PDPH have associated symptoms, such as the

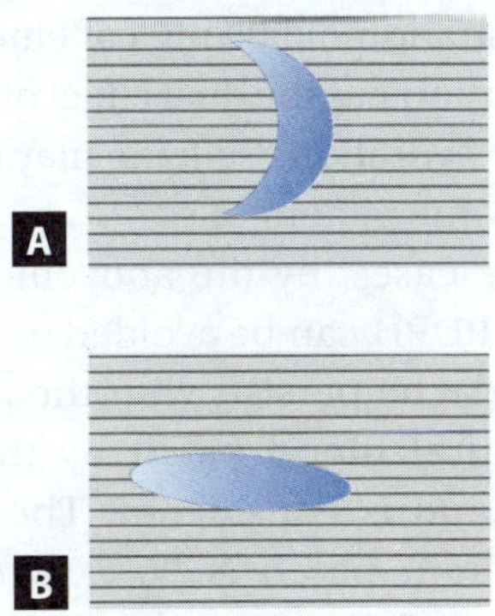

Figs. 38A and B: (A) The aperture of hole in dura made by the bevel of spinal needle which is perpendicular to the direction of dural fiber. (B) The aperture of hole in dura made by bevel of spinal needle which is parallel to the direction of dural fiber.

nausea (60%), vomiting (24%), stiffness of neck (43%), ocular symptoms (13%), and auditory symptoms (12%). Other symptoms associated with PDPH are:

- Vestibular symptoms: Nausea, vomiting, vertigo, dizziness, etc.
- Cochlear symptoms: Hearing loss, hyperacusis, tinnitus, etc.
- Ocular symptoms: Photophobia, diplopia, difficulty in accommodation, etc.
- Musculoskeletal symptoms: Stiffness of neck, scapular pain, etc.

Prophylaxis and the Management of PDPH

Prophylaxis and management of PDPH are:

- The use of more and more fine and pencil tipped needle
- The bevel of the needle tip should be parallel to the dural fiber during its puncture.
- The lateral position of the patient during the spinal procedure is associated with the less incidences of PDPH.
- The postoperative monitoring should be done in lying down position, at least for 24 hours in bed. In case of the use of wide-bore needle, the postoperative rest in bed should be at least for 72 hours. This rest will help in the repair of hole of dural puncture and will reduce the incidence of PDPH.
- Avoiding all types of straining activities and trying to lie down in prone position
- Analgesics, adequate oral intake of water which ensures maximum production of CSF, the use of DDAVP in the dose of 4 mg/day, etc. are other methods by which the incidence of PDPH can be reduced. Another conservative method for the management of PDPH is use of IV caffeine and sodium benzoate. Caffeine is a potent vasoconstrictor and may relieve the symptoms of PDPH by preventing the traction on blood vessel of brain stem.

Rapid administration of 500 mg caffeine mixed in 1 L of crystalloid solution has the dual effect of caffeine in bolus and aggressive hydration. Caffeine may be an adrenergic stimulant for some patients also.

- In most of the cases, by the abovementioned simple measures, the PDPH can be avoided or treated. But, still when the headache persists with the above measures, then an epidural blood patch by the 10–20 mL of autologous blood is considered. The success rate of autologous blood patch is 90%. With the possible accumulation of CSF under the ligamentum flavum, the successful epidural placement of needle during the placement of blood patch may yield small amount of clear or straw colored liquid and confuse. However, it may frequently produce mild headache, neckache, and paresthesia. Also the introduction of infection by such a means would be disastrous. So, this procedure should be reserved only for the severe refractory cases of PDPH.

Sometimes, the excessive leakage of CSF can cause death, due to the herniation of uncus against the tentorium cerebelli. This is due to the high intracranial pressure (ICP) for any cerebral lesion which was present before dural puncture.

Differential Diagnosis of PDPH

Other causes of postoperative headache, not related to the dural puncture, should be differentiated from PDPH. These are migraine, meningitis, dehydration, hyponatremia, neck muscle spasm due to stiffness of operating room table, withdrawal from caffeine, etc.

Cranial Nerve Paralysis

Any cranial nerve can be affected by CNB. This is possibly due to the result of excessive spread of local anesthetic agent in the brain, causing direct neural toxicity or as a result of the downward traction of brain, along with the cranial nerves, due to the low CSF pressure from leakage. Among all the cranial nerves, VIth cranial nerve is more prone to injury and it is due to its long and tortuous course. Due to the low CSF pressure from leakage, there is descent of medulla and pons which causes the stretching of this nerve and the injury of it between its origin at pons and anchoring site at cavernous sinus, over the apex of the petrous temporal bone. VIth cranial nerve injury causes photophobia and diplopia due to lateral rectus muscle paralysis.

Accidental Total Spinal Block

The total spinal block results when the full epidural dose of local anesthetic solution is inadvertently placed in the subarachnoid space, during an attempted epidural anesthesia. In total spinal, the large doses of local anesthetic solution, scheduled for epidural anesthesia, spread all over the spinal and cranial CSF and blocks (1) all the nerve roots including the cranial nerves, (2) vital centers on the fourth ventricle, and (3) all the sympathetic outflows, causing complete cardiopulmonary shut down. The effects of these are severe hypotension, severe bradycardia, apnea, aphonia, unconsciousness, dilatation of pupil, and even cardiac arrest. The appearance of the patient resembles like death, even if the cardiac arrest does not occur. Usually, it comes soon after the injection of drug in the wrongly diagnosed epidural space, but it may be delayed for 30–45 minutes.

The cornerstone of the management of this total spinal block is quick diagnosis, intubation, ventilation with 100% O_2, aggressive management of hypotension by pressure rising drugs, correction of bradycardia, IV fluids, etc. Patients usually recover completely after the LA drug is withdrawn from the cranial CSF which usually occurs within 1–2 hours. Then, surgery can also be carried out, when the patient's condition becomes stable. Hypotension should not be allowed to persist for long time. Due to the hypotension and ischemia of neural tissue or due to the irritant effect caused by the large volume of anesthetic drug in intrathecal space (which is in direct contact with nerve tissue) prolonged (delayed) neurological disturbances may occur.

Epidural analgesia for labor pain (obstetrics analgesia) can be made safely via adjacent interspinous space after an inadvertent dural puncture during the first epidural attempt. But, this cannot be applied for lower uterine cesarean section (LUCS) (obstetrics anesthesia). Because large dose of LA agent is needed for cesarean section and this may cause total spinal block after passing through the previous dural hole which is made inadvertently by the epidural needle in previous attempt. If the level of block ascends high up, then consciousness is gradually lost as afferent impulses reaching cortex, becomes fewer and fewer.

Respiratory Failure

It is due to the higher spread of spinal or epidural block and may be due to the deliberate or inadvertent attempt. When the height of the block reaches up to the level of T_1 spinal segment, then the gradual progressive paralysis of all the intercostal muscles, the reduction of voice to whisper, the increased diaphragmatic activity, the increased activity of the accessory respiratory muscles of neck and tracheal tug, etc. are some of the common features of peripheral respiratory failure. But, as the central respiratory drive persists and the cervical spinal segment, from where the phrenic nerve originates, is not blocked, so the patient continues the respiration, which is only accomplished by diaphragm. If local anesthetic drug spreads in the cervical segment, then the apnea may also supervene, due to the phrenic nerve paralysis. There may be warning of this development and this warning is that the patient will complain of tingling or numbness in their hands. This is due to the involvement of brachial plexus as it is formed by the cervical spinal nerve roots.

This higher spinal anesthesia, causing peripheral respiratory failure, is also associated with severe hypotension which causes reduced cerebral circulation. The apnea may also be due to this hypotension and reduced blood supply to the cerebral respiratory center, but may or may not be due to the direct spread of drug to the brain stem. So, the immediate restoration of BP is the primary physiological consideration during the higher CNB. The management of complete respiratory failure is like that of total spinal block. But, the speed is very vital in this treatment, as the cardiac arrest may rapidly follows the respiratory arrest, in cases of ischemic medullary paralysis.

If the respiratory difficulties are reported, then the anesthetist should be prepared to intubate and ventilate the patient. It is important to remember that although the patient may be unable to breathe, due to phrenic paralysis, he or she still may be conscious and a small dose of an intravenous anesthetic agent is indicated to render the patient unconscious. Sometimes, the upper airway reflexes may also still be active and muscle relaxants may be needed to facilitate the intubation. The patient may require some form of GA to maintain unconsciousness, until the block wanes and spontaneous respiration returns. If the block is high enough into the cerebral cortex, then unconsciousness will occur spontaneously, but the consciousness may return before the patient can breathe spontaneously.

Back Pain

The back pain resulting from the spinal or epidural anesthesia is mainly related to the needle puncture, causing tissue trauma and mild bleeding into the tissues. The tissues include supraspinous ligament, interspinous ligament, ligamentum flavum, and intervertebral disk. With fine needle, the backache is uncommon. Further, the potential changes due to the injury in tissues are altered by the previous presence of any degenerative processes. The probability of back pain increases, when the large bore needles are used and/or repeated attempts in same space or tissues are made. Patients with existing back pain should be made aware that a brief moderate increase in the back pain may occur.

However, any back pain after CNB should be thought of as possible sign of more serious complication. For example, severe back pain within the first several hours, after the resolution of anesthesia, should be considered as the early sign of accumulating hematoma. When a progressively worsening back pain is accompanied by further conduction blockade, after returning from primary anesthesia, then the possibility of neural compression by rapidly expanding epidural hematoma must be investigated. But, severe back pain which begins after 24–48 hours of CNB and gradually progresses, then it must be evaluated as the possible cause of epidural abscess, especially if there are signs of systemic sepsis.

Previously, a local anesthetic agent such as 2-chloroprocaine preparation had contained sodium bisulfite as preservative which has neurotoxic property. So, in the past, many permanent neurological defects have been reported, following the inadvertent massive subarachnoid injection of this preparation during attempted epidural anesthesia. Therefore, in newer preparations of 2-chloroprocaine, sodium bisulfate is replaced by ethylenediaminetetraacetic acid (EDTA) as preservative. Hence, the use of this newer preparation of 2-chloroprocaine sometimes causes severe persistent back pain and it is due to its low pH and the influence of EDTA on skeletal muscle which begin shortly after the resolution of epidural anesthesia. This back pain is described as the severe muscle spasm of the paravertebral group of muscle mass and is thought to be caused by the backtracking of EDTA solution along the path around the needle or catheter or through the intervertebral foramen to the paravertebral space.

During the flexion of spine, the intervertebral disk is protruded into the spinal canal due to the increased pressure on it by vertebral body. Thus, it becomes more prone to damage by the needle, causing back pain, due to cord compression by the prolapsed disk. The backache also may be simply due to the musculoskeletal and sacroiliac strain which is common during obstetric delivery and if this patient has received CNB, then it is sometimes blamed. However, sometimes back pain is as common in patients who have not received spinal or epidural anesthesia, as in those who have received it.

Hematoma

It results from the injury of epidural venous plexuses or subarachnoid vessels by needle or catheter. Damage to the epidural vessels is more likely to occur with an epidural catheter than with a needle. In patients with untreated clotting defects and "unmonitored anticoagulant therapy", hematoma may be so large, as to produce cord compression and neurological damage. So, a clotting defect should be considered as a contraindication to epidural or spinal block. This hematoma may be a nidus for infection in preexisting bacteremia and may lead to abscess formation, causing epidural abscess. The metastatic blood-borne infection may also occur, particularly in a small epidural hematoma, originating from some other focal source of sepsis. Large hematoma, producing symptoms, needs early surgical intervention. The hematoma and abscess almost produce the same symptoms, but the differentiating point is that the symptoms of hematoma develop much more quickly than abscess. Laminectomy is urgently required to evacuate the hematoma or abscess and to avoid permanent neurological defect from cord compression.

Cord or Nerve Root Damage

Nerve roots or spinal cord can be damaged at any space during epidural or spinal anesthesia by the needle or catheter. It may be temporary or permanent. In the distribution area, due to this damage of nerves, there may be pain, paresthesia, numbness, etc. which may gradually recover, if the injury is minor in nature and reversible.

Meningitis

Meningitis, which means an infection of meninges, is a very prognostically bad sequelae of spinal or epidural anesthesia. It can be prevented by rigid aseptic technique during the procedure. On the other hand, meningism which means aseptic meningitic reaction can also occur due to the blood or injection of irritant agents in CSF. The irritant agents, responsible for this aseptic meningitis (meningism), may be chemical antiseptics, starch powder from gloves, detergent, high concentration of drug, alcohol, phenol, preservatives, radiopaque agents, etc. which enter in the epidural space or CSF during the CNB procedure. Blood responsible for meningism comes from punctured vessels present in the subarachnoid space or epidural space.

Ischemic Cord Damage

As the spinal cord is supplied by some end arteries, so it is more prone to ischemic damage due to different causes. One of such cause is the addition of adrenaline in local anesthetic solution, which produces vasoconstriction and ischemia of cord. This ischemic cord damage by adrenaline is also aggravated, if it is associated with severe hypotension in arteriosclerotic subjects. Some space occupying lesion in spinal canal, such as hematoma, abscess, and neoplasm also can cause the compression of functional end arteries and ischemia of cord. When the anterior spinal artery which supplies the large part of the cord is obliterated or jeopardized, then it produces anterior spinal artery syndrome. This syndrome is characterized predominantly by the motor disturbance with sometimes loss of sphincter control and sensation. Hypotension from any cause may

predispose to cord ischemia. Preexisting arterial diseases (aorta/radicular arteries) may also aggravate this functional ischemia of cord.

Paraplegia

After central neuraxial blockade, sometimes paraplegia has also been reported. This paraplegia can be caused by hematoma, abscess formation, chemical irritant, direct needle trauma, etc. Except CNB, various anatomical abnormalities of spinal cord and vertebral column, such as the developmental laminar stenosis, narrow spinal canal, and extradural spinal tumor may be the principal cause of paraplegia by compromising the circulation of cord. But, when these are aggravated by spinal or epidural anesthesia, then the regional block had to take the blame, though it is merely a coincidence.

Adhesive Arachnoiditis

It may be due to:

- The injection of contaminated local anesthetic
- The mistaken injection of irritant solution in epidural and subarachnoid space instead of local anesthetic agent
- The injection of full epidural dose of LA agent intrathecally.

Cauda Equina Syndrome

It is due to the injury of cauda equina by the needle, catheter, or toxic effect of high concentration of local anesthetic agent leading to:

- Paraplegia, loss of leg reflexes
- Incontinence of faces or retention of urine
- Loss of sexual function
- Paralysis of perineal nerve.

The causes of injury of cauda equina are the same as cord or root damage or paraplegia.

Nerve Damage due to Chemical Irritant

A number of chemical substances such as antiseptic, alcohol, phenol, preservatives, drugs, etc. can cause definite nerve damage (spinal cord and nerve roots) or their irritation, when these are injected in the epidural or intrathecal space. Pain is felt immediately and one is forced to abandon the procedure, as soon as possible, if analgesia or anesthesia does not follow the spinal or epidural block which suggests that local anesthetics or appropriate drugs has not been injected. Also highly concentrated local anesthetic agent in contact with nerve for a long time can also cause irreversible nerve damage, with histological change in nerve fiber. So, the hypobaric or isobaric technique is largely abandoned, because it causes the deposition of large volume of drug around the nerves, displacing CSF, which is the normal environment of nerve roots. In total spinal, not only hypotension, but also disturbances of pH, electrolyte, and osmotic factors around the nerve fibers for longer time help to damage the nerve as large volume of drug has suddenly come in direct contact with the nerve.

Persistent Paresthesia

Any neurological defect should be evaluated, after the complete resolution of the effect of local anesthetic drug, keeping in mind that in case of bupivacaine, the complete resolution may take 24 hours or longer. If the resolution of neural blockade is followed by the return of neural deficit, then a more aggressive approach is necessary. This complication first suggests the development of compressive damage to central axis. The evaluation for neurological defect should include some predisposing factors (coagulopathy, antiplatelet medication, etc.), the details of the procedure, (blood via needle/catheter, paresthesia during needle placement, or catheter insertion, etc.) and the history of the aggressive positioning of patient with catheter in place. Investigations should also look (search) for the other possible etiologies, such as the surgical procedure, the positioning of patients, the devices, and traction used during surgery or to position the patient. Electromyography (EMG) before anesthesia can detect the preexisting neurological defects, but the exact location of defect from an acute injury of nerve is not possible with EMG, until axonal degeneration has occurred. Therefore, this is not valid until 3 weeks have elapsed.

An isolated, unilateral lesion, distributed over some definite dermatomes is more easily attributed to epidural anesthesia than patchy multidermatomal lesion. The direct compression of cord often crosses several dermatomes and causes multidermatomal lesion. Therefore, it can be differentiated from the isolated nerve root injury. The absence of accompanying motor defect absolves epidural/spinal anesthesia. Cauda equina syndrome is occurred due to either transverse chemical meningitis or vascular embarrassment of antispinal artery.

Epidural Abscess

The actual incidence of intraspinal abscess, after the epidural or spinal anesthesia, is very low. It is unusual for an epidural abscess to form and accumulate enough to present symptoms within 12 hours, except for unusually very virulent organisms. When the excessive back pain, after 24–48 hours of central neuraxial blockade, is accompanied by neurological irritation, focal deficit, systemic signs of toxicity, etc., then investigation is mandatory. The definitive

diagnosis for intraspinal abscess is made by computed tomography (CT) scan or magnetic resonance imaging (MRI). Definitive treatment of it requires decompressive laminectomy and aggressive IV antibiotic therapy to prevent the permanent neurological defect.

Wet Tap

During an attempted epidural anesthesia, the inadvertent passage of a large epidural needle in subarachnoid space through the dura mater is called the wet tap. The response of an anesthetist to a possible wet tap should start immediately with its confirmation and followed by next anesthetic plan and strategies, with keeping in mind of severe PDPH. After a wet tap, there are several options. In *first option*, the local anesthetic agent with spinal dose can be injected into subarachnoid space to create a spinal anesthesia (converting epidural into spinal anesthesia), if it fits with the proposed surgical procedure. The *second option* is needle and can be replaced at a different interspinous space and the epidural anesthesia may be tried again in this different interspinous space. The second attempt of epidural anesthesia at the same level might not be a wise choice, even if a clean reentry of an epidural needle into the epidural space through the same interspinous space is possible. This is because of the potential for massive subarachnoid deposition of local anesthetic agent through the previous dural hole. After a wet tap, epidural anesthesia can be followed by some maneuvers to decrease the incidence of headache. These maneuvers are the injection of saline and blood patch through the catheter, prior to its removal, which will resist the further leakage of CSF through the previous puncture site. Early epidural patch of blood is probably not indicated, because the success of this treatment is considerably higher even when applied after 24 hours.

Local Anesthetic Toxicity

Despite proper safeguard, it is also possible to have a toxic blood level of local anesthetic agent from a properly calculated dose in epidural anesthesia, mainly in continuous form. For local anesthetic agents with low protein binding, the signs of toxicity should be quite obvious and early. For example, the symptoms of cranial nerve paresthesia such as the lingual paresthesia or perioral tingling would likely to be reported rapidly by almost every patient who are given procaine (low protein binding). If the LA agent is of intermediate protein binding, for example, lignocaine and mepivacaine, then the gradual report of aura due to CNS toxicity could be missed, especially if the patient is not in constant communication with anesthesiologist during dosing. Generally, the signs of gradual accumulation of local anesthetic agent in CNS include perioral numbness, gustatory paresthesia, ringing in the ear, visual scotoma, etc. In LA agents with high protein binding, for example, bupivacaine and etidocaine, the aura may be very short or even absent.

Other Neurological Complication

Other than paraplegia, spinal cord and nerve root damage and ischemic cord injury, the other possible neurological complications are pruritus, trigeminal nerve palsy, radiculitis, ascending myelitis, transverse myelitis, meningoencephalitis, intraocular hemorrhage, Horner's sign, unmasking of spinal cord neoplasm, etc.

Failed Epidural Anesthesia

Sometimes, after the successful location of epidural space and the injection of the full dose of local anesthetic agent in this space, it may produce no result or anesthesia. This is called the *failed epidural anesthesia*. The speculation of such failure is that needle may pass off the midline into the paravertebral muscle mass and simulate the false loss of resistance during the testing and injection of drug. Another speculation for failed epidural anesthesia is that though the needle is placed correctly at midline, but any cystic degeneration in the epidural space (congenital or degenerative process) can create a false space, where this phenomenon may occur. One way for the identification of such false space is that the loss of resistance during the administration of the initial dose of injection gives way to a rapid increase in resistance, as the false space becomes filled, or the injection through the needle is easy, but the catheter placement is not possible.

Urinary Retention

Although, the action of central neural blockade, provided by a single-shot subarachnoid or epidural anesthesia (not continuous postoperative epidural analgesia), usually lasts only for few hours, but urinary retention can sometimes be a problem, even after the block has been regressed. This retention of urine is a particular problem in the older male patients who may have preexisting pathology related to prostate enlargement. This problem is again exaggerated, if large amounts of intravenous fluids have been administered, as the part of the management of hypotension associated with the central neural blockade. So, many anesthetists routinely catheterize the bladder in patients, having central neural blockade, either before or after the block has been instituted. But, bladder catheterization is often associated with a transient bacteremia. This itself does not usually cause problems, but there are certain groups of patients in whom the

administration of prophylactic IV antibiotics is advisable. These groups of patients include those having valvular heart disease, prosthetic joint replacements, etc.

■ DIFFERENTIAL BLOCKADE

The concentrations of local anesthetic agents, required to achieve conduction blockade, are different for each nerve fiber. These differences are influenced by (1) the size of nerve fiber, (2) myelination, and (3) various other tissue factors, such as (i) the rate of diffusion of LA agents through the tissues, (ii) the location of fiber within the nerve trunk (those on the surface are easier to block than those in the center), (iii) fibrous diffusion barriers around the nerve trunk, (iv) the ability of LA agent to move through the extracellular fluid, etc. There is a general principle that the nerve fibers with smaller diameter will be blocked first than the nerve fiber with larger diameter and the nonmyelinated nerve fibers are blocked earlier than the myelinated nerve fibers. So, the sensory fibers are blocked with the lesser concentration of LA agents than that of the motors. Hence, there is only one type of nonmyelinated group C fiber which is theoretically most easy to block than the myelinated groups of nerve fibers with comparable size. But, practically these C fibers are bundled in groups with significant amount of neural connective tissue (Schwann cells) around this bundle, requiring the higher concentration of LA agent to block these fibers than the comparable myelinated A-δ fibers.

The fibers *earliest to be blocked* are preganglionic B-fibers (though myelinated) that create pharmacological sympathectomy and hypotension, associated with spinal or epidural anesthesia. After these B group of fibers, the nerve fibers which are *next sensitive* to be blocked are the A group of fibers. Within the fibers of group A, the concentration of local anesthetic agent that is required to block the motor A-α fibers is double than that required to block the sensory A-δ fibers. If LA agent is injected at lower concentration or at a considerable distance from the site of action (i.e., nerve fiber), then it is found that the sensory fibers are blocked earlier, leaving the motor fibers. This explains the separation of motor block (A-α fiber) from the sensory block (A-δ fiber) which thus can be elicited. So, at the margin of any area, where the RA is given, due to the gradual fall of the concentration of LA drug at the margin, the A-α fiber will not be blocked there, causing the separation of motor block from the sensory and autonomic block. This is called the differential blockade.

Similarly, in spinal or epidural block, the injection of LA agent at the lumbar region delivers a relatively high concentration of it to the cauda equina which has very limited diffusion barrier. Hence, the blockade at this level is uniformly dense for all the types of nerve fibers. Then, as the agent spreads by the influence of gravity within the CSF and as it moves in cephalad direction against the gravity, then the relative concentration of LA agent drops with increasing cephalad movement, and finally at a higher distance, the agent reaches a concentration at which the myelinated largest and thickest A-α fibers are no longer blocked and there is no interruption of the conduction of motor nerve. But, the nerve fibers carrying the pain, touch, temperature, and preganglionic sympathetic fibers are blocked. This is called the differential block. As the block precedes more cephalad, then the nerve fibers carrying the touch and pressure sensation (A-β, γ fibers) are remain unblocked, but the pain, temperature, and preganglionic (A-δ, C, B fiber) fibers are blocked. This explains the common experience with spinal anesthesia, when the patient retains a sense of pressure at the site of surgery, while having no feeling of sharp pain at the margin of the upper limit of the achieved block. So, the classic teaching is that there are different of two spinal segments between the motor, sensory, and sympathetic block depending on the local anesthetic agent for spinal anesthesia and the method of measurement of block. The simplest method for the evaluation of block of different fibers (which is generally used), usually brings no dissimilarity between the level of anesthesia produced by the blockade of A-δ and C-fiber. But, to reflect the blockade of B fiber, the clinical tool for its evaluation is the cold sensation of the patient. If actually sympathectomy is measured by thermography or galvanometry, the levels of it can be as much as five segments higher than the light touch.

- A fibers:
  - A-α fibers: 13–20 µm in diameter, myelinated, and carry motor impulse.
  - A-β fibers: 5–12 µm in diameter, myelinated, carry touch, and pressure sensation.
  - A-γ fibers: 4–11 µm in diameter, myelinated, carry impulse to muscle spindle.
  - A-δ: 1–4 µm in diameter, myelinated, carry pain, and temperature sensation.
- B fibers: 1–4 µm in diameter, myelinated, and preganglionic sympathetic.
- C fibers: 0.5–2 µm in diameter, nonmyelinated, postganglionic sympathetic, carry pain, and temperature sensation.

■ COMBINED SPINAL-EPIDURAL ANESTHESIA

This technique combines the advantages of both the spinal and epidural anesthesia and thus makes it more versatile and flexible by (1) removing the disadvantages of each other and (2) adding the advantages of both. This method

of combined spinal-epidural anesthesia (CSEA) describes the placement of epidural needle in epidural space first, followed by an epidural catheter or a spinal needle through the previous needle. The history of CSEA dates back to 1937, when Soresi, a New York surgeon, first performed an epidural block with a fine-gauze needle and then he pushed the needle through the dura and arachnoid to make it a spinal block. There is no control of clinical trials at that time and Soresi had claimed that his technique had produced 24–48 hours postoperative pain relief from the single injection of procaine, both into the epidural and spinal spaces. But, his claim was clearly over optimistic and failed to impress others.

Then CSEA was attempted by Curelaru, a Romanian anesthetist, who performed both the spinal and epidural blocks in a same patient, but through separate interspinous spaces. Almost simultaneously with Curelaru's work and unaware of it, Brownridge in Adelaide also performed combined spinal and epidural block for cesarean section, using separate interspinous spaces by the spinal and epidural needles like Curelaru. But, the Brownridge's reasons, for combining both the techniques, were very much same as in keeping with the modern aims of combining the rapid onset, reliability, and low toxicity of the spinal block, with the ability of an epidural catheter to extend or prolong the block, if necessary and use it for the postoperative pain relief. In the following years, Coates was the first to describe the spinal needle through the epidural needle, using a single interspinous space. He used an available long spinal needle which could protrude past the tip of the epidural needle, the prototype for customized CSE sets, which is now provided by the manufacturers.

This variety of CSEA has now become the most popular. However, this *needle through needle* technique does not allow the placement and testing of the epidural catheter, prior to the spinal injection. But, when this (test dose) is regarded as essential, then either a separate interspinous space may be used or another variety requiring specialized equipment can be employed. This is the *needle beside needle or "double-barrel" needle*. This equipment consists essentially of an epidural needle with a spinal needle channel which is soldered or incorporated in the wall of epidural needle. After the epidural needle has been placed and the catheter is inserted through its channel, the spinal needle is introduced through its channel into the subarachnoid space.

At present, there are *different technical combinations* for CSEA. These are:

- *Use of separate intervertebral space for each epidural and spinal needles:* Here, catheter is negotiated through the epidural needle first and test dose is given. Then, through another intervertebral space, dura is punctured by spinal needle and in subarachnoid space of this intervertebral space LA drug is deposited. The patient is then turned supine and according to the necessity of the height of block, drug is injected through the epidural catheter. The same epidural catheter can be used for postoperative analgesia too.

- *Use of the same intervertebral space for epidural and spinal needle:* Here, the epidural needle is placed first. Then, through the epidural needle a spinal needle is introduced (needle through needle) and the dura and arachnoid is punctured. After the spinal drug is given in this subarachnoid space through the spinal needle, it is withdrawn and the catheter is introduced through the epidural needle in epidural space. Then, the epidural needle is withdrawn and patient is turned supine **(Fig. 39)**. The disadvantages of this second technique are:
  - It does not allow the placement and testing of epidural catheter prior to the spinal injection. So, anxiety may arise about the movement of the heavy (hyperbaric) spinal LA solution which is already injected and may spread toward the cephalad or caudal direction, especially if there is delay in the positioning of patient due to the difficulties, arising from the later insertion of catheter. This problem can be readily avoided by performing the CSEA in the Oxford position which had been introduced since 1984. Other ways of avoiding this problem are to perform the epidural first, using a separate intervertebral space or needle beside needle method. Where spinal injection is given after catheter is introduced.
  - There is controversy about the maximum possible protrusion of the spinal needle beyond the tip of the epidural needle when the hubs are opposed. If spinal needle is too short it is less likely to puncture the dura, if too long it may transfix the dura and injure the cord.
  - The grazing of the tip of the spinal needle against the bend of Tuohy needle
  - Catheter may pass through the hole in dura, made by the spinal needle, in the subarachnoid space, though this possibility is very remote.

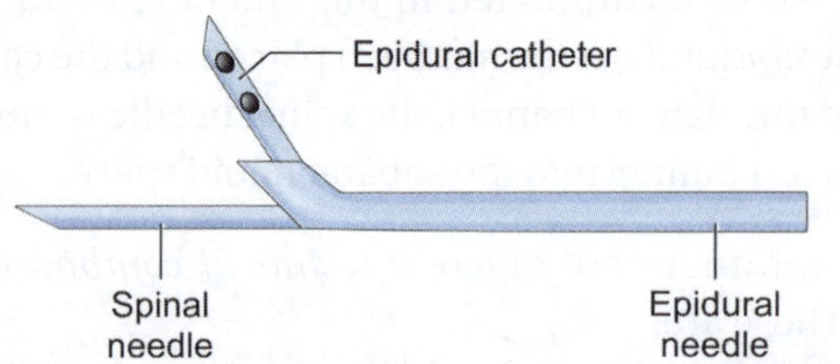

Fig. 39: Combined spinal-epidural needle which allows the placement of 20 G epidural catheter through the modified Tuohy needle and placement of a 27 G spinal needle via an addition lumen.

- To remove the above disadvantages, "needle beside needle" technique is introduced. This equipment consists essentially of an epidural needle with a spinal needle guide channel, incorporated in its wall. After the epidural needle has been placed and catheter is inserted (also tested by test dose), spinal needle is inserted through its side channel.

Uses of CSEA

The *advantages* of CSEA include rapid onset, profound neuraxial block, the ability to titrate the block with the reduction of BP, long duration of blockade according to the necessary, postoperative analgesia, and lower the total drug dose. The possible *disadvantages* of CSEA include increased failure rate of SAB (approximately 5%), intrathecal migration of epidural drug and/or catheter, and decreased ability and reliability of epidural test dosing. The CSEA has been most widely accepted in obstetric population. So, the concept of *"walking epidural"* has become popular among the patients, when the intrathecal opioid allows the rapid onset of analgesia without motor blockade and the extrathecal (epidural) low concentration of bupivacaine (0.125–0.25%) allows prolonged analgesia.

The lipid soluble opioids such as fentanyl or sufentanil are most commonly used for this purpose. The use of CSEA may (1) reduce the incidences of instrumental vaginal delivery, (2) lower the anxiety, and (3) decrease the incidences of PDPH. It is demonstrated that compared with epidural block, constituted by lignocaine and fentanyl for cesarean section, the CSEA constituted by hyperbaric bupivacaine in subarachnoid space and fentanyl in epidural space provides more rapid onset, better motor blockade, decreased anxiety levels, decreased shivering, and greater patient satisfaction.

The potential advantages of CSEA are now well known. The main uses of it are for orthopedic and obstetric purposes. The great flexibility of CSEA has also provided its use in many other different situations.

Obstetrics

Today obstetrics is the most common indication for CSEA, both (1) as a method of pain relief during labor and (2) for operative obstetrics. The introduction of CSEA, as pain relief during labor, had lagged behind its use for cesareans section. The intrathecal use of local anesthetics for the relief of labor pain went back as early as 1900 and the intrathecal use of morphine for the relief of labor pain went back, as late as 1980. However, a single short intrathecal local anesthetics are only effective for limited period and a single short intrathecal morphine is only effective during the first stage of labor and has a high incidence of side effects. However, the CSA has always been associated with an unacccptably high incidence of severe PDPH. Consequently, the ability of CSEA to provide quick and reliable control of labor pain with the injection of local anesthetic or more lipid soluble opioids than morphine or their combination in subarachnoid space and then continue the pain relief by epidural catheter provides the distinct advantage of CSEA over a single-shot spinal anesthesia or continuous lumbar epidural analgesia and anesthesia. There are two situations in which CSEA is particularly advantageous. The first of these is the delayed call for analgesia, where the pain relief by epidural block is slower on onset and requires high motor blocking concentrations of local anesthetic. Secondly, CSEA has proved to be one of the most effective ways of providing analgesia with minimal motor block which is called "walking epidural".

The indication of CSEA for operative obstetrics essentially means cesarean section. Use of CSEA for cesarean section has two distinct advantages. The first is to use an adequate dose of spinal drug to achieve an adequate height and depth of anesthesia for the operation and then to use the epidural catheter to modify or prolong the block, if the spinal is inadequate and/or to provide postoperative analgesia. The second is called the "sequential technique" in which in an attempt to reduce the hypotension a minimum amount of spinal dose which is intentionally made to be inadequate for surgery is used. The block is then deliberately extended cephalad with the epidural dose through catheter. In this two stage technique (sequential technique), the epidural catheter is not just act as a reserve for rescue anesthesia or postoperative analgesia, but it served as a conduit for routine local anesthetic to gradually raise the level of an intentional low SAB.

The epidural block has achieved wider acceptance as an alternative to SAB in obstetrical patients who are chronically hypovolemic such as in preeclampsia. This is because incrementally giving the drugs through the epidural catheter increases the epidural sensory and motor blockade in stages and thus minimizes the risk of hypotension. However, one large prospective study which compared the epidural and CSEA for severely preeclamptic patient undergoing LUCS had concluded that the changes in BP are similar after epidural block or CSEA. Similarly, another study concluded that SAB produced reductions in BP similar to epidural block in severely preeclamptic patients requiring LUCS. But, spinal anesthesia is widely used for obstetrical surgery for technical simplicity, high success rate, minimal maternal and fetal drug exposure, minimal risk of maternal aspiration, and an awake cooperative postoperative patient. However, recently many anesthesiologist can place an epidural needle and catheter faster than they locate CSF with a small gauge spinal needle.

So, subsequently administration of an epidural anesthesia need not significantly expand operative room time.

Orthopedics

Orthopedic cases are the second most popular indication for the use of CSEA after obstetric cases. When CSEA is compared with individual epidural or spinal block for major orthopedic surgeries, then it is found that CSEA has a quicker onset, better quality control, and lower failure rate than the individual spinal or epidural anesthesia alone. CSEA is also very useful for outpatient orthopedic surgeries. It allows a minimal amount of spinal local anesthetic agent to be used and thus hastens recovery, but with the ability of the epidural catheter to prolong the block if necessary.

Now, there are increasing number of indications for the use of CSEA other than obstetric and orthopedic cases.

■ ADJUVANTS TO REGIONAL ANESTHESIA

There was a time, in few days before, when our concept about pain was guided only by the simple *"doorbell theory"*. This theory expresses that press the switch, the bell rings and cut the wire, the ringing stops. But later, we have come to understand that such an old perception is a wrong guide to pain treatment and invariably leads to unsatisfactory results or frank failure of pain management. After the doorbell theory, the *"gate control theory"* of Melzack and Wall and the concept of *"central sensitization"* have revolutionized the current management of pain. The preemptive analgesia, although proven and disproven by voluminous data, has stood the time, because the clinicians have repeatedly shown satisfactory results in the preemptive analgesia from the points of view of patients and caregivers.

Based on the current data, it is proved that the acute painful stimuli create many changes, not only in the periphery at the site of origin, but also in the neurochemical and molecular milieu of dorsal root ganglion and the dorsal horn cells of spinal cord. Additionally, an increased neuronal metabolic activity in the other parts of central neurons system has been noted during acute pain, suggesting multiple dimension of pain. In 1993, Dickinson summarized the role of endogenous neurotransmitter systems in modulating and processing the pain, coming from peripheral nervous system to the CNS and includes more than 25 such neurotransmitter systems in his summary. Then, if we multiply this formidable, but incomplete list of neurotransmitters, by the potential sites of action within the spinal cord, then a visionary can conjure up a wealth of potential ways to enhance the spinal analgesia. So, inspired by many rapidly changing knowledge, regarding the peripheral, spinal, and supraspinal responses to pain, investigators have reacted similarly by searching for the correct agonists or antagonists, and stimulants and inhibitors of pain. Thus, the drugs and all the pain control modalities are mixed and matched to achieve an optimal relief of pain with least complications.

Acting directly on the proverbial doorbell wire theory, the RA is a mainstay in the armamentarium of an anesthesiologist for the management of pain. In the last few years, several pain relieving drugs have been studied and combined with other drugs, with the objective of producing optimum analgesia and the least possible side effects. The combination of analgesic therapy in search of synergistic effect has been a common practice. Therefore, different neurotransmitter system was targeted with a combination of drugs to achieve the optimum therapeutic outcome with lower doses of drugs, thereby resulting in reduced side effects.

Hence, as adjuvants, many things can be added with local anesthetic agents in RA. These are narcotics, benzodiazepines, α_2-adrenergic agonists (i.e., clonidine), cholinesterase inhibitors (neostigmine), and phencyclidine (ketamine).

The aim of using adjuvants with or without local anesthetic agent in spinal and epidural spaces is to:
- Improve the analgesic intensity
- Increase the duration of action
- Achieve the faster onset of action
- Achieve the acceptable analgesia with the lower doses of LA drug and thus to reduce the risks and side effects.

Intraspinal or Epidural Opioids or Narcotics

Following the initial reports, in 1979, of clinical efficacy of intrathecal and epidural opioids, they have subsequently been used to control the pain following a wide variety of surgical procedures, as sole analgesic agents or in combination with low dose of local anesthetic agent. Bypassing the blood and blood–brain barrier, the small doses of opioids, administered either in the subarachnoid or epidural spaces, act directly on the spinal cord to provide profound and prolonged segmental analgesia. This undoubtedly represents a major breakthrough in pain management. Numerous studies have shown that spinal or epidural opioids can provide profound postoperative analgesia with less central and systemic adverse effects than the opioids administered systemically. Then, a large number of nonopioid analgesics have also been administered in epidural or subarachnoid space to achieve the pain relief, without the risk of respiratory depression. This technique has been employed successfully to treat intraoperative, postoperative, traumatic, obstetric, chronic, and acute cancer pain. Among these, the management

of postoperative and obstetric pain is the most common indication for the spinal or epidural opioid analgesia.

The unique feature of spinal or epidural opioid analgesia is the lack of other sensory (except pain), sympathetic and motor block that allows the patients to ambulate without the risk of orthostatic hypotension or motor incoordination (walking epidural) which is usually associated with local anesthetic agents, administered spinally or epidurally or opioids administered parenterally. These advantages of spinal or epidural opioids are particularly beneficial in high-risk patients, undergoing major surgery, such as the patients with severely compromised pulmonary or cardiovascular function, grossly obese patients, and very elderly patients.

For intrathecal or epidural administration, the analgesic doses of morphine are only 2–5% of the parenteral dose. Thus, patients can be expected to be less drowsy, more cooperative, and more ambulatory. Intrathecal opioids are very easy for administration, either at the time of injection of local anesthetic drug during spinal anesthesia or as a separate technique when GA is administered. With catheter, the epidural route for opioids with local anesthetic has been used much more extensively for intraoperative surgical analgesia and anesthesia, and for postoperative pain control with or without local anesthetic agents. The reasons for popularity of epidural opioids include epidural opioids provide excellent analgesia alone or in combination with local anesthetic agent with or without GA, willingness to leave an epidural catheter in place for extended periods to maintain analgesia and freedom from the risk of PDPH (only in epidural route).

The synergistic effects of both opioid and local anesthetic agent are best seen at their low doses. At higher doses, the clinical synergistic effect becomes blurred and the toxic effects of both of them supervene. When the effects of IM or IV narcotics and epidural or spinal narcotics are compared in respect to analgesia, ambulation, GI motility, early and late pulmonary function, duration of hospitalization, occurrence of DVT in the postoperative period, etc., then it is found that the average doses of IV or IM narcotics is seven times greater than that required by the epidural or spinal route. Patients, receiving epidural or spinal narcotics report superior analgesia, ambulate sooner, have fewer pulmonary complications, have earlier return of bowl function, and are discharged from the hospital earlier than the patients receiving IM or IV narcotics. Mortality, overall complication, infection, time of extubation, and hospital costs are all significantly lower when the narcotics are given intrathecally or epidurally than the parenteral group. Although, the intraspinal or epidural opioid is not as effective as regional analgesia, provided by the local anesthetic agents for controlling the pain during vaginal delivery, but intraspinal or epidural only opioids for control of pain following cesarean section is widely used. These may be offered when spinal or epidural anesthesia is chosen for surgery.

The rational for the combination of local anesthetic agent with the small doses of opioids, for the relief of labor pain is that these two types of drugs eliminate pain by acting at two different distinct sites: The local anesthetic agents act at the nerve roots and the opioids act at the receptor site of the dorsal horn of spinal cord. The spinal opioids alone provide good relief of pain at rest, but may not be adequate during physiotherapy and mobilization. Although the combinations of local anesthetic agents and opioids are used for postoperative and labor pain, but the results are more impressive in the relief of labor pain. Because, it is well recognized that the labor pain is different from the postoperative pain, as it is not relieved by the epidural opioids alone. Patients receiving epidural injections of local anesthetics, combined with opioids, report more rapid onset, more profound and long-lasting relief of labor pain and less motor blockade (due to the lower concentration of LA agent, for example, 0.125% bupivacaine, instead of 0.5% bupivacaine, as the opioid is combined with LA agent for the synergistic analgesic action) than the patients receiving either drug alone. As a part of combined spinal-epidural technique intrathecal opioids (e.g., fentanyl 25 µg, sufentanil 5–7 µg) combined with very small doses of local anesthetic (e.g., bupivacaine 1 mg) provide almost instantaneous pain relief during labor and the epidural catheter is used if labor is prolonged. These low doses of narcotics and local anesthetic agents through both the thecal and the extrathecal route allow the parturients to ambulate which is called the "walking epidurals".

The only preservative-free morphine preparations have been used epidurally or intrathecally in a wide range of concentrations with no apparent differences in efficacy. The addition of epinephrine to morphine is not recommended. The dose of intrathecal morphine varies between 0.1 and 0.2 mg. Epidural morphine can be used as intermittent injection or as continuous infusion both through the catheter. The effective doses of continuous infusion of epidural morphine may range from 0.1 to 0.5 mg/hour. Elderly patients may require remarkably small doses of epidural morphine. The relationship between the age and the total dose of epidural morphine to achieve analgesia is effective 24-hour morphine dose (mg) = 18 – Age (0.15).

A more lipophilic opioid drug, such as fentanyl is also useful when rapid onset of epidural or intrathecal analgesia is important. The dose of intrathecal fentanyl is 20–25 µg. The intermittent boluses of 50–75 µg fentanyl through epidural route can also be used to achieve analgesia, promptly in the immediate postoperative period, if the initial epidural dose of morphine is not adequate. When the fentanyl is used as the sole opioid analgesia, then 25–100 µg bolus of fentanyl in epidural space is given first, followed by continuous infusion of 25–100 µg/hour fentanyl with a pump **(Table 6)**.

The adverse effects of central neuraxial narcotics are respiratory depression, pruritus (particularly face and upper trunk), urinary retention, nausea, vomiting, and sedation (uncommon). The incidence of respiratory depression is about 0.3% at low doses of opioid which is usually used. At higher doses, the incidence of respiratory depression may be higher. It results from the migration of these narcotic agents to the brain stem. So, it is more frequent with the more hydrophilic opioids than the more lipophilic opioids. This is

TABLE 6: Dose and duration of action of adjuvants to regional anesthesia.

Single dose (mg)		Rate of infusion (mg/h)	Onset of action (min)	Duration of action of single dose (in hour)
Epidural:				
Morphine	1–5	0.1–1	30	10–24
Meperidine	20–50	10–50	10	5–10
Diamorphine	5	–	5	12
Methadone	1–8	0.2–0.5	10	5–10
Fentanyl	0.025–0.1	0.025–0.1	5	2–6
Sufentanil	0.01–0.06	0.01–0.06	5	2–6
Alfentanil	0.5–1	0.2–0.5	10	1–2
Intraspinal:				
Morphine	0.1–0.3	–	10	10–24
Meperidine	10–30	–	5	10–24
Fentanyl	0.01–0.025	–	5	3–5

because the more hydrophilic opioids are less absorbed by the nervous tissue which is rich in fat and remains in more water soluble form in CSF which helps it to flow more to cephalad direction.

Therefore, a very high level of vigilance is mandatory during the use of intrathecal or epidural opioids. Intensive care facilities should be used for high-risk patients, e.g., advanced age, serious underlying diseases, extensive surgery, etc. Early respiratory depression occurs within the first 2 hours, following epidural narcotic injection. It is due to the result of vascular uptake from epidural and subarachnoid space and redistribution of opioid (i.e., the same mechanism that follows the IV or IM injection). Delayed respiratory depression, occurring within 6–12 hours, following the spinal or epidural injection, is likely the consequence of cranial spread of opioid in CSF. Pruritus is common and sometimes becomes bothersome in few patients receiving central neuraxial opioids. This incidence is particularly high in obstetric patients. The itching may be generalized or localized, with the face being a common site. Although, the pruritus caused by intrathecal or epidural opioid is probably not due to the release of histamine, still antihistamines often provide symptomatic relief.

Nausea and vomiting caused by the intrathecal or epidural opioid is believed to be due to the cranial spread of opioid, through the CSF to the vomiting and CTZ center, located superficially in the floor of fourth ventricle. This can be frequently treated by antiemetics.

The sedation produced by epidural or intraspinal opioid rarely becomes a significant problem. It is due to the result of the spread of the drug through CSF to the receptors in the thalamus, limbic system, or cortex.

Mechanism of Action of Epidural or Spinal Opioids

The perception of pain and the reaction to it are both altered by the opioids, so that the pain is no longer taken as unpleasant or distressing sensation and patient tolerates it better. The analgesic actions of systemic opioids have both the spinal and supraspinal components. But, the central neuraxial opioids have only spinal components. The intrathecal or extrathecal injection of opioids has been shown to cause segmental analgesia without affecting other modalities. This is because it acts only on the opioid receptors in the SG (lamina I and II) of dorsal horn and inhibits the release of excitatory neurotransmitters from the primary afferent fibers, carrying the pain impulses. The action of opioid also appears to be exerted through the interneurons at the dorsal horns which are involved in the gating of pain impulses. The release of substance P from the primary afferent pain fibers in the spinal cord and its postsynaptic

action on the dorsal horn neurons is also inhibited by the opioids. Normally, the action of systemic opioid (not the spinal and epidural opioids) at supraspinal sites, such as in the medulla, midbrain, limbic system, and cortical areas is to alter the processing and the interpretation of pain impulses as well as to send the inhibitory impulses from these centers through the descending pathways along the spinal cord. Several other aminergic and neuronal systems appear to be involved in the action of systemic opioids and simultaneous action at spinal and supraspinal sites greatly amplifies the analgesic action of it.

When given through the epidural or spinal route, the uptake of opioids by the spinal cord is proportional to their lipid solubility. The highly lipid-soluble opioids are quickly absorbed by the cord, resulting in lesser cephalad spread of it. So, the highly lipophilic opioid drugs have the faster onset of action and quicker elimination than the hydrophilic opioid agents. Reversely, the hydrophilic opioids are taken up by the spinal cord to a lesser extent and, therefore, they show their greater cephalad spread than the lipophilic opioids. It also shows delayed onset of action and elimination. Opioids from the subarachnoid or epidural space are eliminated by the vascular uptake.

Intrathecal or Intraepidural Midazolam

Gamma-aminobutyric acid is a simple amino acid molecule which is found as an inhibitory neurotransmitter in about 40% of the synapses, both in the central and peripheral nervous system. Tissue trauma causes release of variety of chemical substances into the vicinity of injury, such as the P-substances, bradykinin, leukotrienes, 5-hydroxytryptamine (5HT), prostaglandins, etc. These substances sensitize the peripheral nociceptor, so that the transduction threshold of sensitivity is decreased. Therefore, the peripheral C fibers tend to fire spontaneously and even fire in response to non-noxious stimulation such as touching the skin. This causes a condition of primary hyperalgesia around the wound and subsequently the total spinal cord sensitization. As a result, the pain perception gradually increases in strength even though the stimulus remains the same or absent. This phenomenon is called the "wind up" phenomenon.

Pain due to spinal cord sensitization and wind-up phenomenon is resistant to opioid. But, we know that GABA reduces this sensitization and dampen this wind up phenomenon. The GABA receptors are of two types (1) GABA-A and (2) GABA-B. Among these, the GABA-A receptors are present in presynaptic or primary afferent fibers and postsynaptic fibers. It is specially found in lamina II of dorsal horn of spinal cord, whereas GABA-B receptors are found in the interneurons. So, inhibitions of selective

GABA-A receptors would be ideal for analgesic action, causing powerful analgesia with no sedation. Benzodiazepines act on these GABA-A receptors and inhibit them.

Midazolam, a water-soluble benzodiazepine, when injected intrathecally, causes spinally mediated antinociceptive effects without any CNS effect, by combining with the spinal cord GABA-A receptors. It also suppresses the visceral pain. The intrathecal midazolam probably also releases an endogenous opioid which acts on delta receptors of spinal cord and thus produces analgesia. The intrathecal midazolam causes segmental cord level analgesia and has almost no neurotoxicity or major side effects, up to the doses of 2 mg by bolus in spinal or epidural space or up to the doses of 6 mg/day by continuous infusion in epidural space. There is no significant nausea, vomiting, sedation, amnesia, itching, urinary retention, hypotension, bradycardia, etc. with intrathecal BZD.

Intrathecal or Intraepidural Clonidine

The clonidine's analgesic property is known for last few years and is used extensively by veterinarians without proper knowledge of its mechanism of action. Initially, it was used in humans for the control of BP. Then, it was tested through epidural route on animals for analgesia, with much promising results and no neurotoxicity. After that, ice was broken when Tamsen and Gordh first used clonidine epidurally on two chronic pain patients, in 1984, and the result was very promising. The adrenergic α2-receptors are present on both the pre- and postsynaptic area. Clonidine is α2-adrenergic agonist and the stimulation of presynaptic α2-adrenergic receptors causes the inhibition of the release of norepinephrine from the sympathetic terminals at periphery and noradrenergic neurons in CNS. These α2-receptors are also located on the superficial laminae of spinal cord and brain stem nuclei, responsible for pain. So, the analgesia, caused by systemic clonidine, may be produced at spinal and brain stem level. The intrathecal or intraepidural clonidine acts only at the spinal level.

Clonidine like local anesthetic agents also causes the blockade of conduction of nerve fibers. At spinal cord level, it also decreases the noxious afferent inputs through its interaction with the α2-adrenoreceptors. It also reduces the release of substance P and excitatory amino acid in spinal cord in response to the peripheral nerve stimulation by noxious stimuli, suggesting presynaptic inhibitory mechanism. It also hyperpolarizes the neurons in the dorsal horn and render them less responsible to afferent stimuli. In addition to brain stem and peripheral site of action, the neuraxial administration of clonidine inhibits the sympathetic preganglionic neurons in spinal cord, resulting in hypotension. The sedative property of clonidine also reduces the requirement of hypnotics and is often a desirable feature.

Analgesic, hypnotic, and hemodynamic effects of clonidine after central neuraxial or systemic administration begins within 30 minutes and reaches maximum within 1–2 hours, but these actions last for 6–8 hours.

Doses of Clonidine

For RA and analgesia, through epidural route, the dose of clonidine with 0.5% bupivacaine is 0.5–1 µg/kg. It does not produce respiratory depression and does not suppress the neurohumoral secretion during stress, but produce analgesia. Postoperatively, 3–10 µg/kg extradural clonidine, as the sole agent, results in 4–6 hours analgesia, but at the expense of bradycardia, hypotension, and sedation.

Uses of Clonidine

Clonidine may be used through intrathecal or extrathecal (epidural) route for analgesia with or without local anesthetic agents. It may also be used with bupivacaine, lignocaine, ropivacaine for peripheral nerve blocks, such as for the molar extractions, intercostal block, and brachial plexus block. It gives early onset, prolonged duration of action and satisfactory analgesia and anesthesia, when it is used with local anesthetic agent. In case of sympathetically maintained pain, the prolonged relief of pain (9–10 times longer duration) is achieved by bupivacaine and clonidine combination than the bupivacaine alone after stellate ganglion block.

Intrathecal Ketamine

Ketamine, which is available in market, is a racemic mixture of its two enantiomers, such as (R-) and (S-) form of it. Its α-elimination phase is few minutes, but the β-elimination phase of it is 2–3 hours. One of its metabolites, such as norketamine, is one-third to one-fifth as potent as the original drug and is responsible for the prolonged analgesic effect of ketamine. It produces a dissociation state (catalepsy) in patient by the electrophysiological inhibition of the thalamocortical pathways, and the stimulation of limbic system. It has good bronchodilating and minimal respiratory depression effect. The protective airway reflexes are preserved by ketamine, but in noncoordinated way. It also increases oral secretion.

The analgesic and anesthetic properties of ketamine are mainly attributed by interaction of it with N-methyl-D-aspartate (NMDA) receptors and other non-NMDA glutamate receptors. By blocking the action of other non-NMDA receptors, such as the opioid receptors, cholinergic receptors, muscarinic and nicotinic receptors, adrenergic receptors, and GABA receptors, ketamine plays a minimal role in analgesia. The NMDA is the most abundant excitatory neurotransmitter causing pain sensation in CNS, where the ketamine acts. "Wind up" phenomenon in dorsal horn is responsible for chronic pain and it acts through NMDA receptors where ketamine also acts.

The reduction of polysynaptic stimulation in the CNS by ketamine which is also responsible for analgesic effect of it acts through NMDA receptor at postsynaptic sites. Ketamine binds to the phencyclidine part of the NMDA receptor channel and thus inhibits the activation of glutamate and blocks NMDA receptor. Nitric oxide (NO) plays important role in pain perception. NMDA and non-NMDA receptor activation stimulate NO synthesis. So, inhibition of NO synthesis by the blocking of NMDA and non-NMDA receptors by ketamine may be involved in its analgesic effect.

For the ubiquitous character of ketamine, it is suggested that the combination of systemic ketamine with regional or peripheral nerve block or combining ketamine with local anesthetic agent for regional or peripheral nerve block may cause more optimal pain relief.

Intrathecal and Intraepidural Neostigmine

The laboratory studies have suggested that the spinal cholinergic activation produces analgesia, because the cholinergic receptors have been found in spinal cord and have been shown to have a potent antinociceptive action. So, considerable evidences exist to implicate the role of cholinergic agonists acetylcholine (Ach) and anticholinesterase agents (neostigmine), which increases the level of Ach by inhibiting the breakdown of it in the spinal cord, in the inhibition of nociceptive transmission, by stimulating these cholinergic receptors and cause analgesia. They do not act on opioid receptor, NMDA receptor or non-NMDA receptor. It does not cause any axonal conduction blockade such as the local anesthetic agents. It is also found that the intrathecal analgesia produced by neostigmine is mediated through the M_1 and M_2 muscarinic cholinergic receptor which can be blocked by atropine. The autoradiographic studies reveal the existence of muscarinic receptors, such as both M_1 and M_2 in the lamina II and III of spinal cord. Neostigmine, as an anticholinesterase inhibitor, causes an accumulation of ACh at the muscarinic receptors in the dorsal horn, when it enters into the CSF and thus causes analgesia.

Neostigmine is used both through intrathecal and epidural route with local anesthetic agents where the duration of analgesia becomes prolonged. The intrathecal dose of neostigmine is 50 µg. The 50 µg neostigmine in epidural route is less effective in prolonging the duration of analgesia. Neostigmine in a dose of 100 µg as an additive to epidural lignocaine is proved to be best in prolonging the duration of analgesia, through this epidural route. The increased dose of neostigmine (150 µg epidurally) prolongs the duration of postoperative analgesia, but at the cost of increased incidences of side effects. The common side effects of neuraxial neostigmine are nausea, vomiting, hypotension, sweating, etc.

Epinephrine

When the epinephrine is administered centrally, it may also potentiate the action of local anesthetic agents. The mechanisms of action are:

- Like clonidine, the low doses of extradural epinephrine have direct α2-activity on the dorsal horn cells.
- The vasoconstrictor properties of epinephrine reduce the vascular uptake of local anesthetic agents and thus it helps to prolong their action.

CENTRAL NEURAXIAL BLOCKADE VERSUS GENERAL ANESTHESIA

The CNB is less forgiving than GA for anything less than perfection. The choice of any anesthetic technique, such as CNB or GA is a complex medical decision which depends on many factors, such as patient's characteristics, type of surgery, type of anesthetic technique and its risks, anesthetist's choice, surgeon's choice, etc. The assessment of anesthetic risk both in CNB and GA include the consideration of anesthetic technical factors, toxicities of anesthetic agent, intraoperative or postoperative events, management of postoperative pain, etc. However, with proper planning and sufficient experience, it is possible to do CNB and GA with same risk and CNB as rapidly as GA. But, there is one distinct advantage of CNB over GA is that the patient can be immediately transferred to recovery room on completion of surgery after CNB. However, GA cause prolonged emergence which can delay the next postoperative procedure.

Cardiorespiratory Effect

Many anesthesiologists think that CNB is preferable to GA for patients with pulmonary diseases. But, many published studies, comparing the pulmonary complications, observed after CNB and GA, have not established any consistent benefit of CNB over GA. Some studies suggested the beneficial effects of CNB over GA in patients with lung disease with respect to decreased morbidity from respiratory complication. However, other studies have not established the superiority of either anesthetic technique in the elderly and in patients with chronic lung disease. There is also definite evidence that the excellent postoperative analgesia with continuous extradural analgesia leads to a reduction in respiratory complications. It is also possible that high quality analgesia from other than epidural (e.g., PCA) may also lead to the reduction in pulmonary complication. So, the provision of adequate analgesia may be more important than the method of analgesia employed.

CNB acts directly on the nerve pathway and avoids the surgical stress with its hemodynamic demands. Thus, it directly avoids the myocardial depressant effect of inhalational agents of GA, whereas the GA acts indirectly through CNS to avoid the surgical stress with its hemodynamic demands. Hypotension, following CNB, is not always preventable and is not always without any adverse effects. So, the CNB is not always a safer alternative to careful GA for heart patient, particularly in inexperienced hands. CNB is particularly hazardous for patients who require well-maintained preload (e.g., aortic stenosis). It is also very crucial in many cardiac patients (coronary disease) causing sudden fall in diastolic pressure with resultant fall in coronary perfusion.

Conversely, the reduction of afterload by CNB may be beneficial for patients with regurgitant valves. But, an epidural block with catheter and the simultaneous intelligent use of IV fluids with vasoconstrictor can carefully titrate this fall of BP. So, always the CNB may not be more hazardous in a patient then GA. Appropriate invasive monitoring of filling pressure, CO, and systemic vascular resistance sometimes may make CNB more safer than GA. Several studies have shown that the CNB in comparison to GA is associated with less cardiac morbidity. This might be related to the reduction in thromboembolic manifestation and the reduction in catecholamine levels in plasma and the avoidance of cardiac depression. But, later studies concluded that the CNB does not reduce the rate of cardiac complications than GA. Contrary, still, many practitioners argue that the individual subgroups of patients should benefit from CNB and so they continue to offer spinal or epidural anesthesia, with or without catheter to their high-risk patients.

Metabolic and Endocrine Alterations

Surgical procedures performed under GA result in increased plasma concentration of glucose, lactate, cortisol, aldosterone, renin, vasopressin, growth hormone, epinephrine, norepinephrine, etc. But, these changes do not occur under CNB, because it completely abolishes the stress response to surgery by blocking the nerve pathway. It is observed that in CNB the markers for surgical stress, i.e., increase in protein degradation and decrease in protein synthesis were typically arrested as compared to GA. The mechanism by which CNB inhibits the metabolic and endocrine alterations during surgery is probably related to the blockade of afferent and efferent pathways for nociceptive impulses. The CNB also prevents central sensitization of pain and provides preemptive analgesia.

Blood Loss

In CNB, decreased bleeding is observed during surgery, especially during the procedure on the lower abdomen and lower part of the body. But, there seems to be little reduction in bleeding associated with upper abdominal and thoracic surgery. The reduction of bleeding during surgery is probably due to (1) the hypotension caused by sympathetic block, (2) the reduction of venous pressure, leading to reduced venous oozing, and (3) the relaxation of capillary sphincters, causing the reduction of arteriolar bleeding. This results in decreased requirement of transfusion and its related complications in CNB as compared to GA.

Nausea and Vomiting

Nausea and vomiting can occur with both the techniques. But, the incidence is more with GA than CNB. In CNB, as laryngeal reflexes are intact (if the patient is not deeply sedated), there is less chance of aspiration, if vomiting occurs. But, in GA, if larynx is not properly guarded, then there is every chance of aspiration if vomiting occurs. Another point is that during CNB if vomiting occurs, then it is very much distressing, because the abdominal and a part of thoracic muscles are paralyzed.

Postoperative Pain Relief

Central neuraxial anesthesia can easily be converted to postoperative analgesia. Hence, many of the prescribed benefits of CNB are actually due to this analgesia, which can be extended into the postoperative period.

Thromboembolism

The CNB is associated with decrease in blood viscosity and less alterations in coagulation factors, such as the inhibition of coagulation and the stimulation of fibrinolysis which commonly occurs in GA. One can see the inhibition of platelet aggregation from local anesthetic drugs during CNB. In the postoperative period, CNB also limits the increase in factor VIII or von Willebrand factor. Thus, CNB increases the total limb blood flow, which is responsible for the reduction in the incidence of thromboembolic events (mainly DVT and pulmonary embolism). This effect of CNB may be as great as 50% in the reduction of thromboembolic incidences during hip surgery. In multiple studies, it is found that the arterial blood flow, the venous emptying rate, and the venous capacitance are all higher in patients, receiving CNB. Intraoperatively, the breathing pattern may also have a profound influence on the blood flow in legs. The spontaneous breathing during CNB promotes the better venous return and this results in higher CO and better blood flow in legs. While intermittent positive pressure ventilation (IPPV) during GA impedes the venous return and this results in low CO and reduced blood flow in legs. Thus, the CNB is associated with the less incidences of thromboembolic phenomenon than GA.

Coagulation Profile

In GA, the aggregation of platelets and the hypercoagulable state of blood is triggered by some neurohumoral changes which is due to the stress responses during surgery. But, this is completely attenuated in CNB. On the other hand, the RA and analgesia also effectively attenuates the increase in plasminogen activity as compared to GA.

Hypothermia

Both the GA and CNB impair the homeostasis of temperature. Hypothermia, during CNB, can nearly be as severe as that which is observed during GA. The thermoregulatory activity is impaired with advancing age during CNB, but no age-related differences regarding thermoregulation were found during GA. On the other hand, the CNB decreases vasoconstriction and shivering thresholds, possibly by producing a substantial increase in apparent leg temperature. This explains why the CNB is associated with severe hypothermia.

Mortality

A number of large studies have been performed to evaluate the postoperative mortality rate following CNB or GA after major surgical procedures. The short-term mortality rate (up to 3 months postoperatively) is better after CNB as compared to GA. But, there is no difference in long-term survival rate (up to 1 year postoperatively) with both the techniques. Many of the deaths, occurring in GA group during the 1st postoperative month were related to the thromboembolic complications. However, large retrospective cohort study of elderly patients with hip fracture is unable to demonstrate that CNB is associated with better outcome than GA.

There is no general consensus that certain types of patients undergoing certain types of surgery benefit more from regional or general anesthesia. The ultimate outcome of surgery depends on how a technique is performed rather than which technique is selected. The outcome also depends on the skill of the practitioner, patient's factor and the occurrence of side effects or complications. For many anesthetists, the benefits of RA appear to be self-evident and worth attaining, while other practitioner virtually perform no regional technique throughout their whole life.

Discharge Criteria

The use of CNB for ambulatory surgery (or day case or outpatient surgery) has gradually become more popular. The introduction of higher gauzes (more fine) pencil point spinal needles has reduced the incidence of PDPH to approximately 1% and has increased the discharge criteria. The ideal CNB for day-case surgery would combine the rapid and adequate surgical anesthesia with rapid achievement of discharge criteria, such as ambulation and urination.

Combined spinal-epidural anesthesia can also be used for day-case surgery with early discharge criteria. Availability of the epidural catheter for a rescue anesthesia in CSEA allows the use of minimal doses of spinal local anesthetic agent with resultant rapid recovery and discharge. However, no current data is available to assess the relative cost benefit ratio versus decreased recovery time with CSEA. CSA may also have applicability in an ambulatory setting, because it has the ability to use lower amount of local anesthetic agent which can lead to faster recovery time, especially in the elderly who are less prone to PDPH. However, with the introduction of laryngeal mask airway (LMA) and newer anesthetic agents with faster and more pleasant recovery profiles, such as propofol, remifentanil, sevoflurane, and desflurane have reduced the stress of GA and shortened the length of stay in postanesthetic care unit than that seen for CNB.

SUBARACHNOID BLOCK VERSUS EPIDURAL BLOCK

Technical Aspect

From the technical point of view, SAB is easier to perform and has a definite objective endpoint, i.e., the flow of CSF through the spinal needle. Conversely, the epidural block (EB) is not easy to perform and there is no definite objective end point, i.e., location of epidural space is confusing. The end point of identification of epidural space is loss of resistance and the presence of negative pressure. The loss of resistance is proved by the sudden easy movement of piston within the barrel. And the presence of negative pressure in the epidural space is proved by the inward movements of a drop of fluid in the hub of the needle. This is called the hanging drop technique. But, neither of these methods of locating the epidural space guarantees the proper location of the needle tip in all the patients.

Another difference between the SAB and EB from the technical point of view is that SAB is administered through the lumbar site only, whereas EB can be administered through the multiple sites such as lumbar, thoracic, cervical, or caudal.

Onset and Spread

The onset of anesthesia is much more rapid in SAB than EB. The spread of level of anesthesia is more predictable and controlled in SAB than EB. The level of anesthesia in SAB can be controlled initially by using the baricity of anesthetic solutions and then by adjusting the patient's position. However, neither of these factors is much helpful in controlling the level in EB. The level of anesthesia in EB is controlled only by the use of epidural catheter and the volume of drug though the position of patient helps little.

Duration of Anesthesia and Analgesia

The failure to produce anesthesia and analgesia to a desired degree (level) and duration are the inherent deficiency of a single sort technique of SAB or EB, whereas the epidural catheter technique provides a prolonged anesthesia and analgesia, removing the previous deficiencies. The catheter technique for CSA is also available. It requires 10–15 times less amount of local anesthetic agent than is needed for epidural blockade and thus virtually eliminates the possibility of systemic toxic reactions of local anesthetic agents. The other advantages of CSA over the conventional SAB are the ability of it to prolong the anesthesia, if it is needed, for long surgical procedures or even for postoperative analgesia with fewer episodes of hypotension and less need for vasopressors. With the advent of 32 G catheter that can be threaded through 26 G needle, the incidence of PDPH has decreased. But, though it (PDPH) is reduced, still there is potential for infection, hemorrhage, and nerve trauma in CSA.

Depth of Surgical Anesthesia

The SAB provides a more profound depth of surgical analgesia and anesthesia than EB. On the other hand, the requirement for supplemental parenteral analgesia or sedation is more for EB than compared to SAB. One of the advantages of SAB over EB is that it (SAB) does not suffer from the patchiness of anesthesia which is sometimes exhibited by EB.

Unilateral Block

The SAB can be manipulated to achieve predominantly a unilateral block, by keeping the patient in lateral position for 5–10 minutes after the administration of anesthetic agent and by controlling the baricity of anesthetic solutions. The unilaterality in SAB also can be maximized by using a side port spinal needle and a small dose of local anesthetic agent. However, this facility is not available in EB.

Hemodynamic Stability

Hemodynamic parameters are better preserved during EB, particularly when catheter is used, than SAB. The degree of change in MAP, stroke volume, CO, and heart rate is quick and more following SAB than EB.

Postdural Puncture Headache

The PDPH is a troublesome complication of SAB, whereas the EB is completely devoid of this problem. However, the potential for accidental dural puncture by a thick epidural needle ever present in EB and it results in severe headache, particularly in young patients. A higher incidence of PDPH is observed in parturients after SAB.

Systemic Toxicity

One of the main advantages of SAB over EB is that small amount of local anesthetic agent produces the desired level and effective depth of anesthesia. Thus, the potential for CNS toxicity and systemic cardiovascular toxicity due to LA agents is almost nonexistent in SAB. On the other hand, in EB as large amount of local anesthetic solution is used, so there is more chance of systemic and cardiovascular toxicity, caused by LA agents. Also, the accidental intravascular or intrathecal injection of large amount of local anesthetic agent in EB can lead to severe systemic toxicity or total spinal block, respectively.

Blood Loss

The SAB and EB both reduce the loss of blood during surgery. But, the EB reduces more blood loss than SAB and results in more reduced number of transfused blood units. With hypotensive epidural anesthesia, there is approximately 50% decrease in intraoperative blood loss as compared to SAB. The coagulation function is partly better preserved during epidural block than SAB. This is indicated by the higher PT in SAB. This is mainly because the blood loss, the dilution of circulating coagulation factors, and the fibrinogen activation are greater during SAB than EB.

Spinal Cord Injury

Both the SAB and EB are associated with spinal cord and nerve root injury from mechanical trauma. But, in SAB, the spinal cord and nerve root damage may also result from chemical injury by local anesthetic solution which is not found in EB. The transient neurological symptoms (TNSs) have been described after SAB with any local anesthetic agent, but it is found most commonly with lignocaine. However, the recent retrospective, prospective, and closed claim studies report that the incidences of postoperative neurological injury in patients undergoing SAB is in-between 0.7 and 1%. It has been rarely seen after epidural block and GA.

Pediatric Anesthesia

■ INTRODUCTION

Strictly speaking, though all the patients, who are below the age of 14 years, fall into the pediatric group, but only the patients who are below the age 5 years or with weight of <20 kg, need specialized anesthetic management. This is because the newborn and infant have a number of especial physiological features which differ from the adult and these differences are of much relevance to an anesthetist and *the anesthetic management to this later group of patients (below 5 years) is known as the pediatric anesthesia.*

The difference in anatomy and physiology between the pediatric and the adult group of patients have many important consequences on anesthesia, mainly with the babies of 27 weeks gestation (birth weight as low as 600 g) with some peculiarities which may persist for more longer than the defined period, after birth. Some of these peculiarities result from the fact that the newborns and infants at birth has to possess some machineries which are required to adapt the environment in mother's womb which is totally different from the outside of it. Another important peculiarity is that such a small creature requires some very special protective mechanisms to meet the hostile world outside after birth. Other peculiarities are merely the result of adult functions, being as yet underdeveloped. Thus, the neonate should not be regarded merely as an incomplete small adult, but rather, as a totally different organism. So, the provisions of a safe pediatric anesthesia depend on the clear understanding of these anatomical, physiological, pharmacological, and psychological differences between the pediatric and the adult group of patients.

A full-term neonate is one whose gestational age at birth is 37 weeks or more, whereas a preterm neonate is one whose gestational age at birth is lesser than 37 weeks. But, with the passing of days, the medical and technological advances have pushed the gestational age closer and closer to 20 weeks, at which the preterm neonates can be made

TABLE 1: Classification and nomenclature of pediatric patients according to their ages.

Premature	<37 weeks
Neonate	First 4 weeks after birth
Infant	From fifth week after birth up to first year
Toddler	1–3 years
Preschool	3–6 years
School age	6–10 or 12 years
Prepubescent	10–12 years (girl), 12–14 years (boy)
Pubescent	12–14 years (girl), 14–16 years (boy)

viable and their care should be taken by an anesthetist. The classification and the nomenclature according to the age of the pediatric patients are given in **Table 1**.

■ NORMAL WEIGHT GAIN

During the first few days after birth, the newborn infant loses up to 10% of its original birth weight. This is because of the loss of their extracellular fluid. However, then, the most full-term infants regain this lost birth weight by the age of 10 days, after birth. Subsequently, they gain weight at the rate of 25–30 g/day for their first 3 months of life. Thereafter, they gain weight at the rate of about 400 g by every month, for the remaining part of their first year. An infant usually doubles its birth weight by the age of 6 months and triples its birth weight at the end of 1 year. Subsequently, the birth weight becomes four times at the end of 2 years and 5 times at the end of 3 years of their age. At 5 years, the expected weight of a child is calculated by multiplying the birth weight with 6 and at 10 years with 10, respectively.

Here is another easy formula for calculating the weight of a baby. (1) Weight of a baby = [Age (in years) + 4] × 2 in kg, for 1–6 years and (2) weight of a baby = [Age (in years)] × 3 in kg, for 7–12 years. There are also many other formulae described in different books.

TABLE 2: The normal important milestones of pediatric patients.	
4–6 weeks	Social smile
3 months	Head holding
6 months	Sits and supports, transfers object from one hand to other
8–10 months	Crawls
9 months	Stands holding furniture
12 months	Walks holding furniture, says one word
13 months	Walks without much support, says three words with meaning, feed itself
15–18 months	Joins 2–3 words into a sentence

The most important difference between the pediatric and the adult age group of patients is the size of their body which varies with age. But, weight is the most important determinant factor for the difference between the pediatric and the adult age group of patients, because for any therapy drugs are always prescribed per kilogram of body weight. Although it is rational to express the body size and to administer the therapeutic agents in terms of body weight, but many physiological processes are measured in relation to their body surface area. But, the total body surface area to body weight ratio of an infant is approximately twice than that of an adult. So, the metabolic rate, water, and electrolyte requirement and the requirements of ventilation are proportionately greater in pediatric age group of patients than that of an adult, when expressed on the basis of body weight. But, gradually these differences decrease, as the neonate and infant passes through their childhood to an adult. Some important milestones are listed in **Table 2** by which an anesthetist can assess the age of the pediatric patients.

■ CARDIOVASCULAR SYSTEM

Fetal Circulation and its Changes after Birth

In fetal life, blood is oxygenated in placenta and is then returned back to fetal heart by umbilical vein. The umbilical vein enters the fetus at umbilicus through umbilical cord and then courses through liver to join with the left portal vein. There is another vein called *ductus venosus*, which connects the left portal vein with inferior vena cava (IVC) and provides a low resistance pathway (bypass) between the left portal vein and IVC **(Fig. 1)**. Thus, the oxygenated blood coming from placenta through umbilical vein has two pathways before entering the right atrium. Most of the oxygenated blood coming from the placenta shunts through ductus venosus to IVC and only a small portion of oxygenated blood passes through portal vein, liver parenchyma, and hepatic vein and ultimately reaches to IVC.

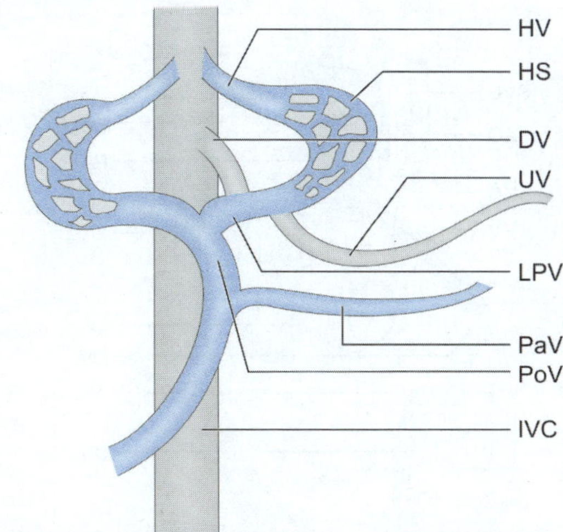

Fig. 1: Fetal circulation and its changes after birth. (DV: ductus venosus; HS: hepatic sinusoid; HV: hepatic vein; IVC: inferior vena cava; LPV: left portal vein; PaV: pancreatic vein; PoV: portal vein; UV: umbilical vein)

Thus, the blood of IVC comprises (1) blood coming from the liver parenchyma through hepatic vein, (2) blood coming directly from placenta through ductus venosus, and (3) blood coming directly from lower extremities. On reaching the right atrium, the oxygenated blood of IVC is divided into two portions (streams) by the inferior margins of septum secundum, which is called the crista dividens. About one-third of this total oxygenated blood of IVC enters left atrium through the foramen ovale, and the remaining two-thirds of the blood of IVC mixes with the deoxygenated venous blood coming from the superior vena cava (SVC) and enters the right ventricle **(Fig. 2)**.

The oxygenated blood, then reaching the left atrium from right atrium through foramen ovale, again mixes with the small amount of deoxygenated blood, coming from the lungs through pulmonary vein without any oxygenation and passes to the left ventricle. The left ventricle then pumps out this oxygenated plus small amount of deoxygenated blood into the ascending aorta for distribution to coronary arteries, head, neck, and upper extremities.

The deoxygenated blood, coming to the right atrium from head, neck, and superior extremities through SVC, after mixing with the two-thirds of IVC blood (that does not run through foramen ovale to left atrium), passes almost directly into the right ventricle. Then, right ventricle pumps out this deoxygenated blood into pulmonary trunk. A small amount of this blood (10%) of pulmonary trunk enters the pulmonary circulation and returns to the left atrium through pulmonary veins without taking any oxygen from the lungs. The rest of the blood (90%) of pulmonary trunk passes through the ductus arteriosus into descending aorta and mixes with the small amount of blood reaching the descending aorta from

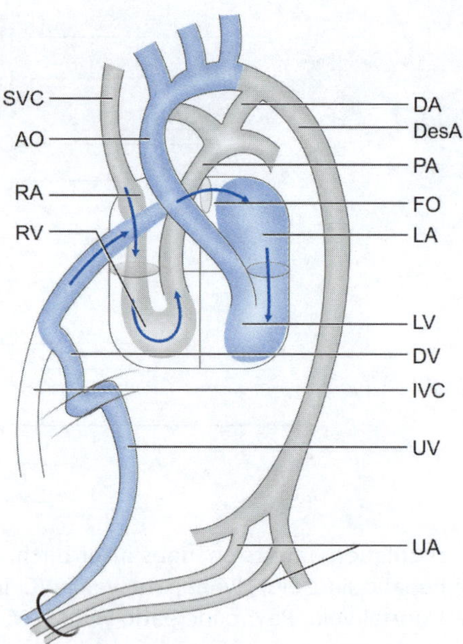

Fig. 2: Fetal circulation. (AO: aorta; DA: ductus arteriosus; DesA: descending aorta; DV: ductus venosus; FO: foramen ovale; IVC: inferior vena cava; LA: left atrium; LV: left ventricle; PA: pulmonary artery; RA: right atrium, RV: right ventricle; SVC: superior vena cava; UV: umbilical vein; UA: umbilical artery)

aortic arch. In fetal life, the largest branch of descending aorta is the umbilical artery. So, the 80% of blood of descending aorta flows through the umbilical artery to placenta, through the umbilical cord for oxygenation. This is favored by the low resistance of circulation of placenta. The remaining portion of the blood of descending aorta flows to lower extremities.

Therefore, in fetal circulation there are two right-to-left shunts. One is at the level of *ductus arteriosus* and the other is at the level of *foramen ovale.* And this right-to-left shunt (flow of blood from right to left side of heart) is due to higher pulmonary vascular resistance (PVR) than the systemic vascular resistance (SVR). It is also because the pressure, developed in the right atrium and right ventricle, exceeds than that of the left atrium and left ventricle which is again due to the handling of large amount of blood by the right side of the heart than its left counterpart.

As a result of this pressure difference between the two ventricles, the wall thickness of them may be the same, or the right ventricle may be thicker than that of the left ventricle. This is in contrast to the adult situation, where the wall-thickness of right ventricle is about one-quarter of the left. As a consequence, the electrocardiographic (ECG) pattern of the neonate and infant is comparable to that of an adult who has right ventricular hypertrophy.

The summary of major differences between the fetal (predelivery) and neonatal or adult (postdelivery) circulation. In these differences, the fetal circulation is characterized by:

- The presence of placental circulation which acts like adult pulmonary circulation provides the gas exchange for fetus
- The presence of gas exchange in a collapsed fetal lung
- There is very little flow of blood through fetal lungs and consequently there is very little pulmonary venous return to the fetal left atrium. So, the left side of heart in fetus is a low pressure system.
- The presence of ductus venosus, which joins the portal vein with IVC, provides a low resistance bypass passage for the umbilical oxygenated blood to reach IVC
- The presence of crista dividens and widely open foramen ovale provides a route for the oxygenated blood to reach the left atrium and left ventricle from the umbilical vein and IVC for distribution to coronary arteries and brain
- The presence of a widely open ductus arteriosus which allows the right ventricular blood to reach the descending aorta and the umbilical arteries for further oxygenation, bypassing the nonfunctioning lungs.

After the clamping of umbilical cord and after the first breath, the high PVR, which was present during fetal life, falls and at the same time the SVR rises. This causes the pressure at the right side of the heart to become less than that of the left side of the heart. These changes stop the flow of blood through foramen ovale and ductus arteriosus which was still maintained up to the period of birth, due to the higher pressure at the right side of the heart than the left. The rise in SVR after birth is due to the elimination of low resistance placental vascular bed from systemic circulation, because of the clamping of umbilical cord.

The factors responsible for the fall in PVR after birth are:
- The unfolding of pulmonary vasculature due to the expansions of lungs
- The development of negative interstitial pressure, arising from the surface tension forces
- An increase in arterial oxygen tension, associated with decreased CO_2 tension, following the onset of pulmonary breathing which causes the diminished hypoxic pulmonary vasoconstriction and reduced PVR. The maximum decrease in PVR occurs rapidly during the first day of life and then continues to decrease gradually during the next several years, as the architecture of pulmonary vessels change slowly.

After the first breath, lungs become inflated with air and PVR falls. This causes the sudden increased pulmonary blood flow and subsequently increased left atrial pressure. This change in right and left atrial pressure causes the stoppage of blood flow through the foramen ovale and ductus arteriosus and subsequently closes these right-to-left shunts in most cases.

As the functional or the physiological closure of ductus arteriosus results from the fall in PVR and the increase in SVR, but it is also caused by the contraction of the smooth muscles of ductus arteriosus. This is due to the increase in PaO_2 after first breath. The sensitivity of the contraction of the smooth muscle cells of ductus arteriosus to PaO_2 depends on the gestational age of neonate and is parallel. This means as the gestational age of fetus and neonate will increase, the sensitivity of the contraction of the smooth muscle cells of ductus arteriosus to PaO_2 will also increase. This closure of ductus arteriosus is completed within 10–15 hours after birth. But, during this period, this closure of ductus arteriosus is *reversible as it is physiological, not anatomical.* Its anatomical closure is delayed by another 2–3 weeks.

This closure of ductus arteriosus is also influenced (inhibited) by prostaglandin E (PGE) which relaxes the ductal smooth muscles and contraction occurs with the inhibition of prostaglandin synthesis. The prevention of ductal closure by the administration of PGE is used therapeutically in certain congenital heart diseases, where there is reduced pulmonary blood flow such as pulmonary atresia. In these circumstances, deliberately delaying the ductal closure clinicians serve to maintain an increased pulmonary blood flow, until a surgical aortopulmonary anastomosis is established. Contrary, prostaglandin inhibitors are sometimes used to induce early ductal closure where continued ductal shunting is undesirable.

This neonatal circulation (ductus arteriosus is physiologically closed, but anatomically is not closed) is usually labile and sometimes may revert from neonatal to fetal type of circulation, with blood flowing from right to left side of heart, through the functionally closed (not anatomically) ductus arteriosus or foramen ovale. *So, this circulatory state of neonate is called the transitional circulation and the reverse from postdelivery to predelivery state is initiated by hypoxia, hypercarbia, acidosis, anesthesia-induced changes in pulmonary, or peripheral vascular tone, etc.* This reversal state is caused by either an increase in PVR, or decrease in SVR in response to hypoxia, hypercarbia, acidosis, and anesthetic drugs. It is especially important in patients with hyaline membrane disease or congenital diaphragmatic hernia which are especially responsible for the abovementioned conditions. Thus, a vicious cycle is set up between hypoxia, hypercarbia, acidosis, and right-to-left shunt, leading to central cyanosis, more hypoxia, gradual fall of cardiac output (CO) and subsequently death. This explains why the hypoxemic events in infants during anesthesia are dangerous and often prolonged, despite when the treatment appears to be adequate.

The risk factors that prolong this transitional circulatory state include prematurity, infection, acidosis, hypothermia, hypoxia, congenital heart diseases, etc. So, care must be taken to keep the neonates and infants warm to maintain normal arterial O_2 and CO_2 tension and to avoid anesthetic-induced myocardial depression. The myocardial structure of heart, particularly the volume of ventricular cellular mass which is responsible for myocardial contractility and CO is significantly underdeveloped in neonates and infants than adults. So, the ventricles are less compliant in neonates and infants. This developmental ventricular myocardial immaturity of the pediatric group of patients accounts for the early tendency to cause biventricular failure. This also accounts for the high sensitivity of neonatal myocardium to volume overload, poor tolerance to an increase in afterload, and heart-rate dependent CO.

Summary of Fetal Circulation and Changes at Birth

The circulation in a fetus is essentially same as that in an adult, except for certain special differences. Here, this fetal circulation is summarized with some differences from an adult.

- The source of oxygenated blood in fetus is not the lungs, but instead the placenta.
- The oxygenated blood from placenta comes to the fetus through umbilical vein and joins the left branch of the portal vein. Then, ductus venosus joins the left branch of the portal vein with the IVC. So, a large portion of oxygenated blood from placenta passes through the left branch of portal vein, ductus venosus, and IVC and reaches the right atrium. The deoxygenated blood coming from the gut and spleen passes through the substance of the liver. Then, it passes to the IVC through hepatic vein. Here, at the level of the hepatic vein, the IVC also receives deoxygenated blood from the lower extremities.
- The oxygen-rich blood reaches the right atrium through IVC from placenta through the left branch of portal vein and ductus venosus. It also carries deoxygenated blood from the gut, spleen, and lower limbs. Then, the oxygenated blood of IVC is directed by the valve of the IVC toward the foramen ovale. After that, the oxygen-rich blood reaching at foramen ovale is directed into the left atrium by the lower edge of septum secundum (crista dividens). The deoxygenated blood returning to the right atrium (1) from the upper limbs, head, and neck through the SVC and (2) from the lower limbs, gut, spleen, and the parenchyma of the liver through the IVC passes into the right ventricle.
- From the right ventricle, this deoxygenated blood enters into the pulmonary trunk. Then, from the pulmonary trunk, only a small portion of this blood reaches the lungs

and passes through it to the left atrium by pulmonary vein without oxygenation. The greater part of this deoxygenated blood from pulmonary trunk is short-circuited by ductus arteriosus into descending aorta.

- Now, we have seen that the left atrium receives mainly the oxygenated blood from the placenta through the right atrium and foramen ovale and a small amount of deoxygenated blood from the lungs through the pulmonary veins. The blood in left atrium is, therefore, fairly rich in oxygen. This blood passes into the left ventricle and then into the ascending aorta. Now, this oxygen-rich blood passes into the carotid artery, coronary arteries, and the subclavian arteries from ascending aorta and supply the brain, heart, the structures of head and neck, and the upper extremities. The rest of the blood gets mixed up with the deoxygenated blood coming from the right ventricle through the ductus arteriosus and supplies the placenta and lower extremities. Therefore, the parts of our body that are supplied by the branches of descending aorta, distal to its junction with the ductus arteriosus, receive blood with less oxygen content from right ventricle.

- Much of the blood of aorta, after its junction with the ductus arteriosus, is carried by the umbilical arteries to the placenta where it is again oxygenated and returned to the heart through umbilical vein, ductus venosus, and IVC. Soon after birth, several changes take place in fetal blood vessels, which lead to the establishment of adult type of circulation. The changes in fetal blood vessels, leading to the establishment of adult type of circulation after birth are: (1) The muscles in the wall of the umbilical arteries contract immediately after birth and occludes their lumen. This prevents the loss of fetal blood into placenta. (2) The lumens of umbilical veins and ductus venosus are also occluded. But, this takes place a few minutes after birth, so that all the fetal blood in placenta gets time to be drained back into the fetus. Though, the umbilical artery, umbilical vein and ductus venosus occlude immediately or within few minutes after birth, but this closure is physiological (functional) and not anatomical. Anatomical closure takes about 2 months. A patent ductus venosus decreases the delivery of drugs to liver, and may prolong their elimination half-life. (3) The ductus arteriosus is now occluded, so that all the blood from right ventricle, now, flows to the lungs, where it can be oxygenated. (4) The pulmonary blood vessels increase in size after birth due to their (pulmonary vasculature) unfolding and consequently a much larger volume of blood reaches the left atrium through lungs.

- As a result, the pressure inside of left atrium is greatly increased. Simultaneously, the pressure inside of right atrium is gradually diminished, because the extra amount blood from placenta no longer reaches it. The net result of these pressure changes causes (1) the pressure in left atrium to exceed than that of right atrium and (2) the closure of foramen ovale. The vessels that are occluded soon after birth are in due course replaced by fibrous tissue and form ligaments. The ligaments formed by the occlusion of fetal vessels are:
  - Umbilical arteries → Medial umbilical ligaments
  - Left umbilical veins → Ligamentum teres of liver
  - Ductus venosus → Ligamentum venosum
  - Ductus arteriosus → Ligamentum arteriosum.

Differences in Cardiovascular System Between the Pediatric and Adult Group of Patients

The cardiovascular system (CVS) of pediatric and adult group of patients differs enormously. At birth, the size and the thickness of the wall of right and left ventricle are similar. But, within first few days of life, after birth, the thickness of the wall of left ventricle starts to increase gradually in response to the increased SVR and workload of left ventricle. On the other hand, the thickness of the wall of right ventricle remains unchanged. So, by 3 months after birth, the mass of the left ventricle exceeds than that of the right ventricle and approaches the relative proportions of an adult (in adult, the ratio of the thickness of the wall of right and left ventricle is 1:3). The weight of a heart of an infant becomes double in their first year of life, while the body weight becomes triple. Again, the weight of this heart becomes double between the age of 4 and 5 years and between the age of 12 and 13 years of their life. Thus, it gradually reaches the adult weight.

The myocardium of a newborn contains less contractile tissue and more connective tissue than that of an adult. This is reflected by the less active contraction of ventricular myocardium and the decreased compliance of pediatric heart. It is also suggested that the limitation of the myocardial contractility of a pediatric heart is due to the decreased intracellular calcium influx and the decreased calcium sensitivity of the myocardial contractile proteins. All these limitations of myocardial contractility of a pediatric heart tend to decrease or fix the size of stroke volume and maintain a fixed CO, depending on the heart rate (HR) (CO = stroke volume × HR). In neonates and infants, the resting stroke volume remains fairly constant at about 1 mL/kg. Shortly after birth, the resting CO is about 200 mL/kg/min depending mainly on heart rate which declines gradually to 100 mL/kg/min by pubescent.

Although, the basal heart rate is high in neonates and infants than in adults, but in these groups of patients, the sudden activation of parasympathetic system, anesthetic over dose, hypoxia, etc. can suddenly trigger the bradycardia and profound reduction in CO. Very sick neonates and infants, undergoing emergency or prolonged surgical procedures, are particularly prone to the sudden episode of severe bradycardia that can lead to hypotension, asystole and intraoperative death. The other reasons behind these serious events are that the sympathetic system and the baroreceptor reflexes are not fully mature in these patients. Their CVS displays a blunted response to the exogenous catecholamines. So, the myocardium of neonates and infants are less able to respond to hypovolemia with compensatory vasoconstriction. Therefore, the intravascular volume depletion in neonates and infants may be signaled by hypotension without tachycardia. The immature heart is more sensitive to depression by volatile anesthetics and opioid-induced bradycardia.

The cardiac output (CO) and cardiac index (CI = CO divided by body surface area) in pediatric patients are higher than that of adults and this is due to their high metabolic rate. So, the O_2 and other nutrients can be delivered easily to their actively growing tissues by increased circulation, according to their increased metabolic need. In pediatric patients, this high CO and subsequent high CI are dependent mainly on heart rate than ventricular filling and the force of myocardial contraction, because ventricles of neonates and infants are poorly compliant. So, even though, the ventricles of a pediatric heart follow the Frank–Starling law, but the main determinant factor of CO is heart rate. Thus, the neonates and infants can tolerate higher heart rate (even 200 beats/min) with ease. Therefore, during pediatric anesthesia, bradycardia should be avoided at any cost, because it represents a fall in CO (as CO is heart rate dependent). So, sudden decrease of heart rate from 200 beats/min to 50 beats/min in an infant should be considered as cardiac arrest or as a severely compromised CO. Therefore, it should be treated immediately with cardiac massage, O_2, atropine, and adrenaline. In pediatric patients, cardiac arrhythmias are rare in absence of any persisting cardiac diseases and the most common form of cardiac arrest in such age group of patients is asystole or electromechanical dissociation (EMD) [not ventricular tachycardia (VT) or ventricular fibrillation (VF)].

The afterload of CVS is determined by the resistance of large arterial blood vessels and the tone of systemic peripheral vascular bed. As the sympathetic tone is poorly developed in neonates and infants, so the afterload or SVR of them is usually low. But, it increases in parallel with the increase in systemic blood pressure with age. So, the systemic arterial pressure of neonates and infants tends to be low than that of the adults and it is due to ↓SVR. The standard arterial pressure in neonate, during their first day of life, is about 70/50 mm Hg, although immediately after delivery, it is slightly greater than this. Then, it rises gradually over their first week of life to approximately 90/50 mm Hg and to normal adult value of 120/70 mm Hg by the age of 14–16 years **(Table 3)**. In asphyxiated neonates, the arterial pressure at birth may be higher. The rate of increase in blood pressure, during the first week of life after birth, will be lower. In preterm neonate, between 27 and 30 weeks of gestational age, the systolic pressure ranges between 45 and 55 mm Hg. The ability of an infant to maintain his blood pressure in response to various circulatory stress is more difficult to assess than in adults. It is, therefore, not surprising that the CVP is raised even by the head-up tilt of neonates and this is reflected by the rise in aortic pressure in some infants and never by a fall (difference from adults).

The response of neonates and infants to blood loss is perhaps that aspect of circulatory physiology which is of greatest interest to an anesthesiologist. All the evidences suggest that human neonates and infants have a less active baroreceptor system, which normally helps in compensatory mechanism to blood loss. Also, it has been suggested that the liver serves as a great buffer in the face of increase in blood volume load in neonate. It is also evidenced by the fact that gross liver enlargement may occur with little or no rise in CVP after overblood transfusion which would indicate the ability of liver to take up the large volume of blood from venous system, without increasing blood pressure and manifesting heart failure.

The sympathetic system is also less developed in neonates and infants and venodilatation occurs at rest. Thus, the sympathetic system cannot be blocked further, causing more venodilatation which is maximum at rest. So, the pediatric patients who are normovolemic at the start of anesthesia, do not exhibit fall in arterial pressure when spinal anesthesia is administered. Moreover, they do not require preloading like an adult to avoid hypotension, as the further venous pooling does not occur and the venous capacitance does not further increase from sympathectomy by spinal or epidural anesthesia.

At birth, the autonomic innervation of heart is primarily parasympathetic, with sparse contribution from sympathetic nervous system. But, this balance of autonomic innervation gradually matures as the child grows with the parallel increase in innervation from sympathetic nervous system. Thus, the infant's CVS maintains a lower catecholamine store and displays a blunted response to exogenous catecholamines. Hence, due to this reason the pediatric vascular tree is less able to respond to hypovolemia and vasoconstriction than adult.

TABLE 3: Heart rate and blood pressure of pediatric patients at different ages.

Age	Heart rate	Systolic pressure	Diastolic pressure
<1 months	110–160 beats/min	70–90 mm Hg	45–50 mm Hg
2–5 months	90–140 beats/min	80–100 mm Hg	50–60 mm Hg
5–12 months	80–120 beats/min	90–110 mm Hg	60–65 mm Hg
>12 months	90–100 beats/min	100–120 mm Hg	65–70 mm Hg

The decreased sympathetic neural output also explains the normally reduced blood pressure in neonates, infants, and children, and their increased susceptibility to reflex bradycardia and hypotension. Again, the diminished baroreceptor activity in infants may reduce their ability to adapt hypotension by an increase in heart rate. So, the hallmark of intravascular fluid depletion in neonates and infants is profound hypotension without tachycardia.

The potent causes of reflex bradycardia and hypotension, in pediatric age group of patients during anesthesia, include easy vagal stimulation by laryngoscopy, tracheal intubation, tracheal suctioning, traction on eye muscles, viscera, etc. This is due to high parasympathetic tone in the pediatric group of patients. Bradycardia may also easily be caused by a variety of anesthetic drugs, such as suxamethonium, halothane, and neostigmine. These effects can be successfully treated by IV atropine (20 μg/kg).

The immature neonatal and infantile heart is also more sensitive to the calcium channel blocking properties of volatile anesthetic agents and opioid-induced bradycardia.

◼ HEMOGLOBIN AND BLOOD VOLUME

The postdelivery hemoglobin (Hb) concentration of a neonate ranges from 13 to 20 g/dL (average 18 g/dL). Then, this concentration of Hb decreases gradually during infancy, reaching a level of 10 g/dL by 10–15 weeks of age after birth in full-term neonates and 8 g/dL by 4–8 weeks of age after birth in preterm neonates. This decrease in Hb concentration in early infancy is due to their decreased erythropoiesis and shorter lifespan of red cells. This is called the *"physiological anemia of infancy"*. Then, after reaching its plateau, the Hb concentration again increases steadily throughout their infancy, touching the adult value by the end of first year. A preoperative Hb concentration of less than 10 g/dL is abnormal and should always be investigated. Normally, the concentration of fetal hemoglobin (HbF) at 30 weeks of gestation is 95% of its total Hb. But, at birth this HbF constitutes about 80% of total hemoglobin. By 4 months, this falls to 10–15% and by 6 months this HbF disappears completely from the circulation which is replaced by HbA. The synthesis of adult hemoglobin (HbA) is fully established by the age of 6 months.

The differences between the HbF and HbA are:
- A higher affinity of HbF for O_2 than HbA
- A reduced affinity of 2,3-diphosphoglycerate (2,3-DPG) to HbF than HbA
- The leftward shifting of oxygen dissociation curve of HbF.

The higher affinity of HbF for O_2 in pediatric group of patients is due to the poor affinity for binding of 2,3-DPG with the γ-chain of HbF, allowing the O_2 to bind strongly with it. This is reflected by low P50 value of fetal Hb-O_2 (oxyhemoglobin) dissociation curve, which is only 20 mm Hg (at 20 mm Hg PaO_2 the HbF is 50% saturated with O_2). This is due to high-binding affinity of HbF to O_2) in a full-term neonate. This low P_{50} value helps the fetus to optimize (increase) the uptake of O_2 from placenta.

It also prevents the release of O_2 from HbF at tissue level, due to the leftward shifting of O_2 dissociation curve. The other factors that shift the O_2 dissociation curve toward the left (i.e., low P50) include alkalosis, hypothermia, and hyperventilation which also limit the availability of O_2 at tissue level. However, these demerits of HbF are removed by the increase in Hb concentration, increase in CO, expanded blood volume, etc., in the neonates and infants. On the other hand, the low PO_2 and increased metabolic acidosis at tissue level due to the hypermetabolic state of pediatric patients help in the downloading of O_2 into the tissues and shift the oxygen dissociation curve toward the right at tissue level. Hence, as the leftward shifting of O_2 dissociation curve prevents in O_2 downloading, while the rightward shifting of O_2 dissociation curve helps in the same, thus compensating each other. Hyperventilation produces alkalosis and discourages the downloading of O_2 at the tissue level. So, hyperventilation should be avoided and normocapnia should be maintained during pediatric anesthesia.

The normal blood volume of a neonate at birth is about 90 mL/kg. It gradually decreases to 80 mL/kg in infants and young children. By the age of 6–8 years, an adult level of 75 mL/kg blood volume is attained. The decision to transfuse blood in pediatric group of patients should be balanced against all other risks. In case of blood loss, usually the children can tolerate hematocrit value up to 25%. Blood loss of >10% of total red cell mass should be replaced by transfusion of blood, especially if the initial Hb is less than normal and further losses are expected. However, otherwise the most children who have a normal Hb concentration at the beginning of surgery, can tolerate losses of up to 20% of their total red cell mass.

■ RESPIRATORY SYSTEM

During intrauterine life, the lungs begin to develop from 4th to 5th week of gestation. By the 6th week of intrauterine life, the lobar or secondary bronchi are developed. By the 7th week, the segmental or tertiary bronchi start to develop and by the 8th week, the subsegmental airways start to grow. By the 16th week of gestation, the tracheobronchial tree undergoes division up to the 16th order, terminating into terminal bronchioles and acini. At the 16th week of intrauterine life, the number of airways and the number of pulmonary blood vessels in a fetus is similar to that of an adult, but the number of alveoli is less in number and this number gradually increases toward the term. From the 16 weeks of gestation, the lungs begin to mature as a potential gas exchange organ, because after that and onward the pulmonary capillaries start to interdigitate among the alveoli.

Gradually, the type II pneumocytes begin to appear after 20 weeks of gestation. It is nothing, but the differentiated epithelial cells of alveoli. The type I pneumocytes are derived from these type II cells. In mature adult lungs, these type I cells cover 25 times more surface area of alveoli than the type II cells. At birth, the total number of alveoli is 20–50 million and each terminal bronchiole opens into a single alveolus, instead of a fully developed cluster of alveoli. In neonates, the alveoli are thick-walled and its numbers constitute only 10% of that of an adult. Then, these alveoli increase in number by multiplication and also increase in size, until the child reaches the age of 8 years. Thus, at the end of 8 years, the total number of alveoli in children is 300 million which is equal to that of an adult. Subsequently, the growth of lung occurs by an increase in only of alveolar and airway size, but without any increase in their number by multiplication. The granules of surfactants are produced and appear in the alveolar lining cells (type II pneumocytes) as early as at 24 weeks of intrauterine life. So, after 24 weeks, an independent life, outside the uterine cavity, becomes theoretically possible. The surfactants are lipoproteins in nature and reduce the surface tension of the lining fluid of alveoli below the 10–15 dynes/cm.

The fluid-air interface at the surface of alveoli which develops after the first breath of a newborn cannot be maintained without this surfactant. So, the lungs are unable to retain air within the alveoli without the surfactant and collapses. If the pressure is measured within the alveoli of different sizes without surfactant, then it is found that the smaller alveoli have higher intra-alveolar pressure than the larger ones which is explained by the *Laplace law*.

The Laplace law says that the pressure in each sphere (alveoli) varies inversely with the radius of it (if the tension at the wall of alveoli is constant). If a lung is considered as a large cluster of bubbles or alveoli in communication with each other, then it is expected that the smaller alveoli without surfactant would expand less readily on inspiration and empty more completely on expiration, than the larger ones. This is due to the high inward collapsing surface tension force of the smaller alveoli than the larger ones. Thus, the larger ones would become over distended and the smaller ones would collapse, because the smaller alveoli gradually drain into the larger ones. But, fortunately, this does not happen due to the presence of surfactant at their alveolar fluid-air interface, which reduces the surface tension to a degree that is inversely proportional to the surface area of the alveoli. Thus, the reduction of surface tension in smaller alveoli is greater than the larger ones and they remain distended or open, giving rise to a stable condition.

This *Laplace phenomenon* is not restricted to the consideration of just the surface tension of alveoli. But, it is applicable to any other hollow viscera of our body also. For example, a smaller heart does not have to develop the same tension in its wall, as a larger one, in order to produce the same given pressure within its cavities. A small diaphragm with a small radius can produce a larger negative intrathoracic tension, despite its paper-thin musculature which is found during the first breath, and this negative intrathoracic pressure is as high as in adults (–70 mmH$_2$O).

The active constituents of this intra-alveolar surfactant are phospholipids, 85% of which is lecithin. Lecithin appears in amniotic fluid toward the term. This terminal increase of lecithin in amniotic fluid is greater than that of sphingomyelin, which is another phospholipid surfactant and is present in amniotic fluid from the 24th week of gestation. When the ratio of lecithin to sphingomyelin is above 2, then the risk of collapse of the alveoli is less. If the child is born prematurely and these surfactant phospholipids are insufficient, then respiratory failure may follow. Glucocorticoids accelerate the production of these pulmonary surfactants. This is proved by the fact that neonates who develop hyaline membrane disease have a low blood cortisol level, than the neonates who have a pulmonary disease.

The lungs in utero are filled with fluid. However, the composition of this fluid differs from both the amniotic fluid and serum, since the pH of intra-alveolar fluid is lower and the chloride content is higher than the both amniotic fluid and serum. This alveolar fluid is formed by active secretory and absorption process of alveolar epithelial cells. In the course of delivery, this alveolar fluid is expressed out of the lungs by the force, exerted on the chest wall of fetus by birth canal and presumably it is replaced by air, when the chest wall expands during the first breath or first cry. The volume of fluid expressed in this way from lungs may be as much as 42 mL. With the first forceful respiratory effort after birth, most of the alveoli are recruited. Then, gradually more and more alveoli are recruited in the subsequent respirations and they are expanded. Then, the residual fluid in the lung is readily absorbed, as it has an extremely low colloidal osmotic pressure. This absorption of alveolar fluid takes nearly about 24–72 hours after birth and occurs through the transcapillary and translymphatic routes.

Within 1 minute of the clamping of umbilical cord, the first breath of neonate is established. For establishment of this first breath, many sensory factors, such as sound, touch, and temperature are needed. But, the major factor for the establishment of this first breath in newborn is sudden resetting of respiratory center to a new level of PaO_2 and $PaCO_2$, and the hypercapnia and hypoxia had pronounced effect in this resetting. During this establishment of first respiration, the sensory impulses first strike on the reticular system of brain and cause a resetting of respiratory center to a new level of arterial O_2 and CO_2 concentration, so that the levels of O_2 and CO_2 tension, which had no effect on respiration before, now start effecting. The ventilatory response to CO_2 tension increases with increasing age. The ventilatory response to hypoxemia in the neonate is more complex than its response to CO_2. The tension of O_2 in carotid blood rises after the first few breaths from 35 mm Hg to >60 mm Hg and the CO_2 tension falls from 65 mm Hg to 35 mm Hg.

The tidal volume of first breath in a newborn is about 20–80 mL and generates an extremely negative intrapleural pressure which as about –70 cmH_2O during inspiration. The first expiration is also active and assists in the expulsion of lung fluid. Then, progressively, each respiratory cycle shows a *smaller pressure-volume loop,* with steadily decreasing the effort of breathing and retention of air in alveoli with every inspiration. The normal functional residual volume which is about 70–80 mL in a neonate is established within 60 minutes of birth **(Fig. 3)**.

The respiratory system of neonates and infants is less efficient and has low reserve volumes than that of adults. But, its O_2 consumption is 2–3 times as high as an adult. The two respiratory reflexes are seen in a neonate: (1) paradoxical reflex of head and (2) Hering–Breuer reflex. The first one is the inspiratory response which occurs after a partial inflation of the lungs. The second one is the passive expiratory response that occurs after inflation. The respiratory pattern of some premature neonates is described as "periodic", characterized by the occasional episodes of apnea, extending for 5–15 seconds. When apnea is prolonged for >15 seconds, then there is bradycardia and Hb desaturation (<90%). The frequency of apnea is directly related to the degree of prematurity and 70% of preterm neonates show such periodic respiration. Among this, 50% have prolonged apneic

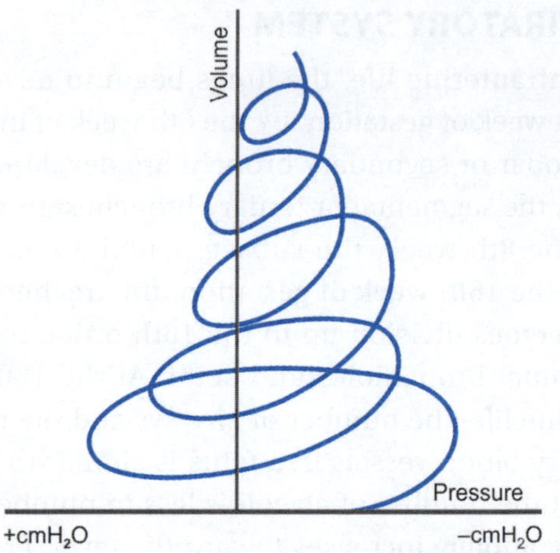

Fig. 3: The first few breaths of a neonate, where there is a high negative intrapulmonary pressure and low tidal volume. This is followed by a gradual reduction of this negative intrapulmonary pressure and an increase in the tidal volume.

episodes (>15 seconds). Between two apneic episodes, there is normal respiratory rate or tachypnea. The management of this apnea of prematurity is theophylline. Periodic breathing and apnea may be associated with full-term neonates, but they are rarely associated with perioperative complications.

Causes of Less Efficiency and Low Reserve of Respiratory System in Neonates and Infants

Compared to older children and adults, the neonates and infants have less efficient system for ventilation. This is because of their week intercostal and diaphragmatic musculature which is again due to: (1) the paucity of mature adult type I muscle fibers in pediatric intercostal and diaphragmatic muscles, (2) horizontal and more pliable ribs, and (3) a protuberant abdomen. The protuberant abdomen of neonates and infants pushes the diaphragm upward, beyond its optimal curvature for maximum contraction. This increases the total load against which the diaphragm has to work, and reduces its efficiency. So, the respiratory system of pediatric group of patients is less efficient, with a low reserve than adults **(Box 1)**.

The other causes for the less efficiency of respiratory system in pediatric group of patients are:

- The diameter of airways in neonates and infants is smaller. This increases the resistance to air flow, which is inversely proportional to the radius of the lumen of airways and raised to its power of five (r^5). The airway resistance in neonates is 30 cmH_2O/L/second, whereas in adults, it is only 2 cmH_2O/L/second. Thus, the narrow airway in pediatric group of patients results in an increased resistance to the flow of air up to the age of

BOX 1: Causes of low respiratory reserve in neonates and infants.

- High respiratory rate
- Narrow airways and high resistance to airflow
- High compliance of airways and chest wall
- Low compliance of lung
- Sole reliance on diaphragmatic function due to weak and underdeveloped intercostal muscles
- High O_2 consumption and metabolic rate
- High dead space to tidal volume ratio
- Infantile configuration of respiratory muscles (type I fibers)
- Alveolar ventilation twice than adult
- Large physiological shunt
- Small lung volume
- Low vital capacity (half of an adult)
- Weak intercostal and diaphragmatic

TABLE 4: Comparison of respiratory parameters between neonates and adults.

Parameters	Adult	Neonate
Tidal volume (mL/kg, during spontaneous respiration)	7–10	7
Dead space (mL/kg)	2	2
Respiratory rate/min	15	30
V_D:V_T	0.3	0.3
Compliance (mL/cmH$_2$O)	100	6
Airway resistance (cmH$_2$O/L/S)	2	30
Time constant (S)	1.1	0.5
O_2 consumption (mL/kg/min)	4	7

8 years. In children, the nasal resistance represents almost 50% of the total airway resistance. So, it accentuates the problem in children with nasal congestion, as they are obligatory nasal breathers **(Table 4)**.

- In children, the compliance of airways and the chest wall is high and this is due to the poor development of the structures of airway and chest wall. Thus, the high compliance of chest wall provides a little support to the lungs and so the negative intrathoracic (intrapleural) pressure is poorly maintained during inspiration. Hence, it reduces the efficacy of respiratory system in pediatric group of patients. The high compliance of airways also causes the early closure of it and the closing volume occurs within the tidal breathing, i.e., functional airway closure occurs during each breath [functional residual capacity (FRC) $\leq$ CC]. Therefore, it causes an increase in the alveolar and arterial O_2 tension difference (P_A-PaO$_2$). This explains why the PaO$_2$ in neonates and infants is lower than that of the adults and the children are more at the risk of respiratory failure. On the other hand, the lung compliance in neonates and infants is also very low. This is only about 6 mL/cmH$_2$O (adult value is 100 mL/cmH$_2$O) and is due to the poor development of elastic tissue in alveoli. This also accounts for the greater closing capacity (CC) of lungs and thus, predisposes the neonate to the increased intrapulmonary shunting of blood and higher PaCO$_2$. Thus, the combination of the higher compliance of airways and chest wall and the lower compliance of alveoli (lung) promotes the collapse of chest wall, during inspiration and relatively low residual lung volume at expiration. These result in the decrease in FRC and limit the reserve of O_2 content in blood, during the period of apnea (e.g., intubation attempts) and predispose the neonates and infants to atelectasis and hypoxemia.

- In neonates and infants, there is also high metabolic rate and high O_2 consumption which need increased ventilation. So, to fulfill this high metabolic rate and O_2 consumption rate and subsequently to achieve adequate alveolar ventilation, the neonates and infants have to maintain high respiratory rate and subsequently increased work of breathing. This high respiratory rate increases alveolar minute ventilation. Alveolar minute volume (MV) is therefore rate-dependent, but not tidal volume dependent in neonates and infants. Thus, the normal resulting increased respiratory rate in neonates and infants becomes approximately double than that of the adults. In neonates and infants, the average respiratory rate is 30–40 breaths/min which is already at higher limit of respiratory reserve. While in adult, it is just 15 per minutes with much reserve. This explains the cause of low efficiency and low reserve of respiratory system in neonates and infants. The high alveolar minute ventilation in neonates and children also explains why the induction and emergence from inhalational anesthesia are relatively rapid in small children. Also, a high metabolic rate explains why desaturation occurs very rapidly in children.

- Until the infant reaches the second year of age, the fibers of main respiratory muscles, (diaphragm, and intercostal) do not achieve the configuration of adult type 1 muscle fiber. The adult type 1 muscle fibers have an ability to perform repeated exercise without fatigue. As the newborns and infants are somewhat deficient in this adult type 1 muscle fiber, so any factor that increases the work of breathing, results in an early fatigue of these pediatric types of respiratory muscles and causes respiratory failure.

- In neonates and infants, there is already higher dead space to tidal volume ratio (V_D/V_T). So, any modest increase in dead space (V_D) by equipment, such as by the facemasks, breathing tubes, humidifiers, or due to any other causes may have a disproportionately greater effect and reduces the efficiency of respiratory system in this group of patients.

- In children, the ventilation is solely dependent on diaphragmatic function. This is because the ribs are soft, horizontal (i.e., perpendicular to vertebral column), and noncalcified and the intercostal muscles are poorly developed. Due to this horizontal disposition, there is no bucket handle type of movement of ribs in children, as in the adults. So, there is less expansion of chest wall and less ventilation. The diaphragm is also more horizontally attached to the ribs, reducing its mechanical advantages, during contraction. Furthermore, the slight abdominal distension may also easily cause the splinting of diaphragm, resulting in the less efficient contraction of it, leading to the easy respiratory failure in pediatric patients.
- In neonates and infants, the alveolar ventilation per kilogram of body weight is twice than that of the adults. Thus, it already depletes the reserve and reduces the efficiency of respiratory system during emergency in neonates and infants. The normal alveolar ventilation in neonates is 150 mL/kg/min, whereas the alveolar ventilation in adults is about 60 mL/kg/min.
- The another important cause for the less efficiency of respiratory system in pediatric group of patients is their large physiological shunt, the value of which is nearly about 20% on day-one after birth.
- The volumes of lungs in infants and neonates are disproportionately smaller, in relation to their body size, in comparison to the adults. But, the metabolic rate in infants and neonates is nearly twice than that of the adults. Therefore, the ventilatory requirement for per unit volume of lung is enormously high in neonates and infants. Thus, they have far less reserve for gas exchange than adults.
- The normal O_2 consumption, normal CO_2 production and normal tidal volume (mL/kg) in neonates and infants are almost double than that of the adults. The average neonatal O_2 consumption is about 7 mL/kg/min, as compared to 4 mL/kg/min in the adults, whereas the average normal neonatal CO_2 production is 6 mL/kg/min as compared to 3 mL/kg/min in the adults. Tidal volume of a neonate is 6 mL/kg, whereas in an adult it is 3 mL/kg. All these data explain how the respiratory system of neonate and infant is using its reserve and depletes it (this reserve) and is less efficient than adult.
- The vital capacity of a neonate and infant is half than that of an adult, i.e., only 35 mL/kg for a neonate, whereas 70 mL/kg for an adult.

TABLE 5: Respiratory rate and age in children.

Preterm neonate	40–70/min
Neonate	40 per minute
2–5 years	25–30/min
5–12 years	20–25/min
>12 years	15–20/min

- The FRC of a neonate is 30 mL/kg, whereas the adult has an FRC of 35 mL/kg.
- Moreover, hypoxic and hypercapnic ventilatory drives are not well developed in neonates and infants. In fact, unlike adults, hypoxia and hypercapnia depress the respiration in these groups of patients.
- *Respiratory rate:* It varies with the age **(Table 5)**.

The different lung volumes of neonates and infants differ from adults. It is definitely smaller in neonates and infants than that of adults, but when compared with respect to their body weight and metabolic rate, it is higher than that of adults. The gas exchange area of neonatal and infantile lungs is 50 times less than that of adults. The gas exchange area of neonatal lung is only 3 m^2 in comparison to that of an adult, which is about 150 m^2, though the metabolic rate of neonates is twice than that of adult. The FRC per kilogram of body weight reaches the adult value during the first 48 hours after birth, but still the closing volume exceeds the FRC during normal breathing and explains the cause of low PaO_2 in neonates. When normalized for body weight, the tidal volume for both the groups is same. Dead space volume per kilogram of body weight is also same for both the groups and it is about 30% of tidal volume.

Spontaneous respiratory rate decreases, as the age increases. This reflects the age-related decrease in ventilatory requirement which is parallel to the decrease in metabolic rate with age. This is explained by O_2 consumption rate in neonates which is about 7 mL/kg/min and is twice than that of adult. The normal adult value of O_2 consumption rate is about 3.5 mL/kg/min. Although, the respiratory rate of neonates and infants is high, alveolar ventilation is still inefficient than adults. Consequently, when the trachea is intubated and ventilation is constituted by mechanical ventilator, then the normocapnia is only maintained by high tidal volume of 10–15 mL/kg and the low respiratory rate of 20–25 breaths/min in healthy neonates and infants. This explains why in neonates and infants, the energy is mainly utilized to maintain the spontaneous respiration and is the major source of CO_2 production. To maintain normocapnia and a normal PaO_2 in neonates with poor respiratory gas exchange, higher respiratory rate (>15–25 breaths/min) is required. The neonatal and infantile lungs continue to grow and mature throughout their childhood and adolescence, and reach the adult value by 16 years of age.

The airway of pediatric patients differs from adults in following ways:

- The tongue of the pediatric group of patients is relatively larger than adults in relation to the oropharynx. So, there is every possibility of an upper airway obstruction by this large tongue in this age group of patients. It (large tongue) also causes technical difficulties during laryngoscopy and intubation.
- The larynx of the pediatric age group of patients is located high up in the neck. In neonates and infants, it is situated at the level of C_{3-4} vertebrae, whereas, in adults, it is situated at the level of C_{5-6} vertebra. This is because, the neck is short, and the hyoid cartilage lies in close proximity to thyroid cartilage in pediatric patients. So, a straight blade of a laryngoscope, behind the epiglottis, becomes frequently successful to expose the vocal cords.
- The epiglottis of neonates and infants is long, floppy, and acutely angled over laryngeal inlet. It projects posteriorly at an angle of 45° to the base of the tongue. Whereas, the epiglottis of an adult is short, broad, flat, and projects posteriorly at an angle of only 15–25° to the base of the tongue. So, the control of epiglottis and the exposure of larynx by the blade of laryngoscope is more difficult in pediatric group of patients than adults.
- The pediatric larynx is funnel shaped and the position of cricoid cartilage in this larynx marks its *narrowest portion up to the 5 years of age*. In contrast, the adult larynx is tubular in shape and is narrowest at the level of vocal cords which is much above the cricoid cartilage **(Fig. 4)**. In adults, an endotracheal (ET) tube which passes the vocal cord (glottic opening) will readily pass into trachea without any hindrance at the level of cricoid cartilage.

But, in neonates and infants an ET tube that easily passes the vocal cords, may be tight in subglottic region at the level of cricoid cartilage and may not pass into trachea. This is due to the maximum narrowing of pediatric larynx at this level, due to the presence of cricoid cartilage, from where the trachea begins. Hence, the uncuffed ET tubes are preferred in patients <10 years of age.

The cricoid cartilage is covered with loose pseudostratified *columnar epithelium*. So, it is easily susceptible to inflammation and edema, when traumatized by cuffed or tight tubes. When the epithelium of cricoid cartilage swells due to inflammation and trauma, then it occludes the lumen of cricoid ring and severely obstructs the airflow through it. The *resistance of airflow* through a pipe is inversely proportional to the fifth power of the radius of the lumen of a tube. So, a small amount of swelling of the mucous membrane of cricoid cartilage will cause a little decrease in the radius of its lumen, but will cause a tremendous increase in the *resistance to airflow* and a tremendous decrease in the flow of gas through it in the pediatric group of patients. For example, when the radius of cricoid lumen decreases twofold, the resistance to airflow increases by 32 folds (i.e., $2^5 = 32$).

- The head of the neonates and infants is relatively large in comparison to their body size than that of an adult. The occiput of it is most prominent and the chin is retrognathic. So, the prominence of occiput and the largeness of the head of the pediatric group of patient keeps it already in a "sniffing" position without pillow which facilitates tracheal intubation. Therefore, any pillow under the head during intubation may disturb this sniffing position and may make intubation difficult in neonates and infants **(Box 2)**.
- The nasal passage of the neonates and infants is relatively narrow and accounts for >50% of the total airway resistance. On the other hand, the neonates and infants are obligatory nasal breathers. So, they are highly predisposed to obstruction in the presence of even a very small amount of secretion in the airway.

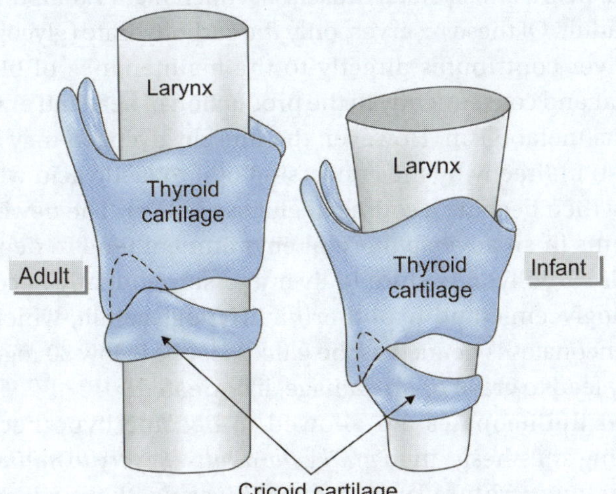

Fig. 4: Adult and infant larynx.

BOX 2: Characteristics of the pediatric airway.

- Relatively large tongue
- High up larynx
- Long, soft, and acutely angled epiglottis
- Funnel-shaped larynx
- The narrowest part of larynx is the cricoid cartilage
- Obligatory nasal breathers
- High compliance and easy to collapse chest wall and airway
- Retrognathic chin
- Short trachea and neck
- Prominent adenoids and tonsils

- The neck of neonates and infants is short. So, the trachea of neonates and infants is also short and is made up of soft (compliant), and less number (4–5 cm) of noncalcified cartilaginous rings. Whereas, the trachea of an adult is long (10–11 cm) and made up of relatively less soft (noncompliant) cartilaginous ring, most of which may be calcified. So, it does not easily collapse during any airway obstruction such as pediatric patients.

Thus, the combination of these two characteristics, i.e., a high compliance of chest wall and airway and a low compliance of lung tissue in neonates and infants (opposite to that of an adult) promotes the chest wall to collapse easily during the inspiration and maintains a relatively low residual lung volume at expiration, which results in a decreased FRC and low oxygen reserves.

TEMPERATURE REGULATION AND ITS MAINTENANCE IN PEDIATRIC PATIENTS

Pediatric patients have a larger body surface area per kilogram of their body weight than adults (smaller body mass index). Therefore, the (1) metabolism, (2) O_2 consumption, (3) CO_2 production, (4) thermogenesis, (5) CO, (6) alveolar ventilation, etc. are better correlated with their body surface area than the body weight of a neonate and infant.

The neonates and infants are particularly vulnerable to hypothermia. This is due to (1) their large body surface area to weight ratio, (2) poor insulation of their body due to their thin skin and limited fat stores, (3) their immature sweat function, (4) their initial low basal metabolic rate (BMR), and (5) their inability to move away from any adverse hypothermal environment. This vulnerability to hypothermia in pediatric group of patients causes the early arterial desaturation by increasing their cellular metabolism and O_2 consumption. Previously, it was thought that this vulnerability to hypothermia is due to the ill-developed temperature regulating mechanism in pediatric patients. But, this is incorrect because, actually, they do not have any well-developed mechanism for increasing heat production in response to cold.

The infants are able to raise their heat production in response to cold only up to 70 cal/kg/min, as compared to an adult, who can achieve the heat production up to 90 cal/kg/min. Again, this vulnerability to hypothermia in neonates and infants is due to their greater heat losing surface area than the mass of heat producing tissues, i.e., larger body surface area (heat-losing) to body weight (heat-producing) ratio than adult. The premature infant is even more susceptible to hypothermia. This is because of their very thin skin and limited fat stores than a mature neonates and infants and so losing more heat.

The three processes of thermogenesis producing heat in infants are:
1. Voluntary muscle activity
2. Involuntary muscle activity
3. Nonshivering (by cellular metabolism) thermogenesis

The minimal ability of the neonates and infants to shiver (voluntary muscle activity) during their first 3 months of life makes the metabolism of brown fat (cellular thermogenesis) the *principal method* of heat production for this age group of patients. Brown fat is a specialized adipose tissue, capable of metabolizing fat in situ, and is present in the newborn of most species. It develops between 25 and 30 weeks of gestation and constitutes about 25–30% of the total body weight. The distribution of this brown fat varies from species to species, but in humans it is mainly found largely around the axilla, kidneys, adrenal glands, between the scapulae, and around the blood vessels of the neck, mediastinum, and the loin. *The differences between these brown and white fat are:*
- The blood supply is copious in brown fat.
- In brown fat, the nerve supply is abundant.
- The cells of brown fat are multinucleated and judiciously equipped with mitochondria.

The activities of tissues in brown fat to produce heat are mediated by catecholamines and can be abolished by sympathetic blockers. The substrate used for heat production in brown fat is mainly the fatty acids and the temperature of this tissue rises markedly when the subject is exposed to cold. The metabolism of brown fat is severely limited in premature infants and sick neonates who are deficient in stores of this brown fat. Furthermore, volatile anesthetic agents inhibit thermogenesis in brown adipocyte cells.

The newborn infants, however, cannot maintain their temperature only at the expense of their brown fat consumption, but also burn their carbohydrate reserve for thermogenesis. At birth, the glycogen content in the cells of liver, heart, and skeletal muscles is much higher than that of an adult. Of these reserves, only the carbohydrate (glycogen) of liver contributes directly to the maintenance of blood sugar and consequently to the production of heat and energy by its metabolism. However, the muscle glycogen may also do so indirectly by the conversion of it to lactic acid which may then become a source of glucose in liver. The newborn infants in an adverse thermal environment tend to deplete their carbohydrate store in liver and subsequently become hypoglycemic and hypothermic. Hypoglycemia, which in the neonates is defined as the glucose levels below 30 mg/dL, may lead to grave brain damage, if untreated.

If the neonates are allowed to become hypothermic during anesthesia, then *unlike the adults they try to maintain their temperature only by nonshivering thermogenesis, i.e., by cellular metabolism.* Therefore, as the metabolic rate increases, O_2 consumption also increases. Then, this increased O_2 consumption puts an additional burden on their cardiopulmonary system and this may become critical in neonates with a limited reserve. On the other hand, the release of norepinephrine in response to cold stress causes vasoconstriction, which in turn causes further tissue hypoxia and lactic acidosis in the face of increased O_2 consumption and demand. This acidosis in turn favors an increase in right-to-left shunt which further causes hypoxemia. As a result, a vicious positive feedback loop of hypoxemia and acidosis is set up. This problem of hypothermia is further compounded by cold operating room environment, wound exposure, IV fluid administration, dry cool anesthetic gases, and the direct effect of anesthetic agents on their temperature regulatory mechanism. Thus, hypothermia (even mild) is a serious problem in pediatric group of patients, during perioperative period and can cause (1) delayed awakening from anesthesia, (2) cardiac irritability (arrhythmias), (3) respiratory depression, (4) increased PVR, (5) increased susceptibility to anesthetic agents and neuromuscular blockers, etc.

The *homeothermic* animals have the ability to generate and lose heat and thus maintain their core temperature in a fixed range. Heat loss from body occurs by one or more of the following four processes: (1) *radiation,* (2) *convection,* (3) *evaporation, and* (4) *conduction.* Environment around a patient controls the loss of heat by these four processes. The *neutral thermal environment* is defined as the range of ambient temperature at which the loss of temperature by evaporation does not occur. In this neutral thermal environment, the metabolic rate is minimal. The temperature of such an environment is 34°C for premature neonates, 32°C for term neonates and 28°C for an adult. These are also the temperature settings of an incubator.

Among the four processes of heat loss, radiation, convection, and evaporation are the most important processes, responsible for heat loss in an operation theater (OT). Radiation accounts for about 60% of heat loss from a neonate or an infant placed in a 21°C room temperature. If the room temperature is raised to a thermoneutral environment of 34°C, then the loss of heat by radiation will decrease to about 40% of their total heat loss. The reason for this is that the heat loss by radiation is a function of the difference between their skin and room temperature. So, if room temperature is raised, then the heat loss by radiation is minimum. The second major source of heat loss in neonate is convection and this also can be reduced by increasing the room temperature to skin temperature. Evaporative loss also can be reduced by keeping the environmental temperature at a neutral level. The neonate possesses minimum subcutaneous fat that cannot act as thermal insulation.

Many procedures and precautions can be undertaken in OT to maintain the body temperature of a neonate and an infant, mainly by reducing the heat loss. *Thus, the procedures taken to maintain the body temperature of a neonate and an infant by heat loss are:*

- The neonate should be transported to the theater wrapped up by an insulator or in an incubator, set at thermoneutral temperature. Ideally, few hours before surgery, the theater should be warmed to the thermoneutral temperature. This causes the walls and the equipment of the theater to warm up and reduces the net heat loss by radiation. Heat loss by radiation is a two-way process. The child loses heat by radiation to the walls and equipment and it also gains heat from the walls and equipment provided they are properly heated previously.

- All the body parts of a child that are not needed for surgical and monitoring purposes should be covered. Overhead radiant heaters should be used, if the child has to be exposed.

- During surgery, the child should lie on a thermostatically controlled heated blanket.

- Forced air-warming system by blowing filtered warm air into quilted blankets with perforations are effective in maintaining the child's temperature during surgery. This allows warm air to come into direct contact with the child.

- Other measures such as using bonnets to reduce heat loss from the exposed head are very effective. IV fluids and fluids used for lavage of the body cavities should be warmed to the body temperature. Anesthetic gases should be humidified and warmed, in order to reduce the heat loss from lungs. The newborn in the cold OT or labor room is very vulnerable to cold stress, because some heat loss is inevitable. This also can be reduced by warm wrappings, heated mattresses, overhead heaters, aluminum covers, etc.

■ RENAL FUNCTION AND FLUID BALANCE

The kidneys and subsequently all its functions are immature at birth. The maturation of renal tissues occurs by hyperplasia during the first 6 weeks of life and then by hypertrophy during the next first year of life after birth.

However, the complete maturation of renal tissues occurs by about 2 years of age. Due to low perfusion pressure and immaturity of glomerular and tubular functions, both the glomerular filtration rate (GFR) and subsequently the renal tubular reabsorption rate are low in neonates and infants. At birth, the GFR is only about 45 mL/min/1.7 m^2, which increases rapidly to about 65 mL/min/1.7 m^2 by 6 months. Then, gradually it approaches to an adult value of

125 mL/min/1.7 m^2 by the age of 2 years. Thus, the kidneys of neonates and mainly of premature are unable to handle excessive water and solute load, especially the Na$^+$ and K$^+$. The half-life of medicines that are excreted by glomerular filtration, are also prolonged. Hence, there is more chance of overtransfusion which may lead to pulmonary edema and cardiac failure in this age group of patients. Because of low GFR, poor capacity to concentrate urine, and no diuretic response to water load, the infant's kidney is also less well equipped to deal with the effects of dehydration.

At birth, in neonate the urine volume is about 25 mL/kg/day. This gradually rises to about 100–120 mL/kg/day by the end of first week. The insensible loss in normal babies is about 25–30 mL/kg/day. To maintain normal serum electrolyte concentration, the neonates and infants require Na$^+$ about 3–5 mmol/kg/day and an equivalent amount of K$^+$ per day. The ability of an immature kidney in neonate and infant to eliminate excess Na$^+$ is limited. So, an extra load of Na$^+$ in the absence of loss, easily results in hypernatremia and its sequel. The premature neonates often possess multiple renal defects including decreased creatinine-clearance, increased glucose-excretion, decreased bicarbonate reabsorption, and poor diluting-concentrating ability.

A great difference exists in the distribution of water in their body as a percentage of body weight among the neonates, infants, and adults **(Table 6)**. In premature infants, the water constitutes about 85% of their total body weight. In neonates, infants, and adults, this percentage is about 80%, 75%, and 65% respectively. In neonates, most of their total body water remains in extracellular compartment in contrast to adults, where most of their total body water remains in intracellular compartment. The plasma volume in percentage of body weight remains constant throughout the life and this is at about 5% of total body weight.

The approach to IV fluid therapy in pediatric group of patients should be considered in the light of their high metabolic rate, high O$_2$ demand, and a high body surface area to their body weight ratio. In first week of life, the requirement of fluid for maintenance increases every day **(Table 7)**. When we relate the daily water requirement with the metabolic or caloric demand, then the general rule is that 100 mL of water is required for each 100 calories of spent energy.

On the other hand, when we relate the fluid requirement to body weight, then in infants with body weight up to 10 kg, the fluid requirement is 100 mL/kg/day or 4 mL/kg/hour. For neonates and infants with body weight between 10 kg and 20 kg, this calculation requires an addition of water of 2 mL/kg/hour for each kilogram increase in body weight **(Table 8)**.

As for example, for a neonate with body weight of 15 kg, the fluid requirement is $(10 \times 4) + (5 \times 2) = 50$ mL/hour or 1,200 mL/day. Between 20 and 30 kg, the daily fluid requirement needs an addition of 1 mL/kg/hour, for each kilogram increase in body weight above 20 kg to the previous requirement. As for example, for a neonate or infant of 25 kg, the fluid requirement is $(10 \times 4) + (10 \times 2) + (5 \times 1) = 65$ mL/hour or 1,600 mL/day. Of the total fluid deficit, 50% is replaced in the first hour and 25% in each of the next 2 hours. However, this calculation does not include the previous deficit, third space loss due to surgical procedures, hyperthermia, hyperventilation, etc. The third space loss depends on surgical procedures and may vary from 1 mL/kg/hour for a minor surgical procedure to as much as 15 mL/kg/hour for major surgical procedures.

We also have to think about the composition of IV fluid. There is still some controversy regarding the requirement of glucose in IV fluid. Some reports of hypoxic brain damage have been published, due to high blood glucose

TABLE 7: Fluid requirements in the first week of life.

Rate (mL/kg/day)	Day after birth
0	1
50	2, 3
70	4, 5
100	6
125	7

TABLE 8: Calculation of the fluid requirement (only for maintenance) in pediatric patients.

Weight (kg)	Hourly requirement (mL/kg/hour)	Daily requirement (mL/day)
Up to 10 kg	4 mL/kg/hour	100 mL/kg/day
10–20 kg	$10 \times 4 + 2$ (weight in kg − 10) mL/hour	$1,000 + 48$ (weight in kg − 10) mL/day
Above 20 kg	$(10 \times 4) + (10 \times 2) + 1$ (weight in kg − 20) mL/hour = $60 + 1$ (weight in kg − 20) mL/hour	$1,000 + 48 \times 10 + 24$ (weight in kg − 20) mL/day = $1,480 + 24$ (weight in kg − 20) mL/day

TABLE 6: Distribution of water as percent of body weight.

	ICF (%)	ECF (%)	Plasma (%)	Total (%)
Premature	30	50	5	85
Neonate	40	35	5	80
Infant	40	30	5	75
Adult	40	20	5	65

(ECF: extracellular fluid; ICF: intracellular fluid)

levels. So, some anesthesiologists do not recommend the routine use of glucose-containing solutions as IV fluid. This is also true that unrecognized hyperglycemia, ketosis, and high metabolic rate of neonates and infants are the motivating factors for discarding the routine use of glucose containing solutions in pediatric patients. But, this is not always true for those who have not food or fluid for a long time and also those who have a diminished glycogen store. The neonates who are at greater risk of hypoglycemia are: (1) premature babies or babies of small for gestational age, (2) babies receiving hyperalimentation, and (3) babies born to diabetic mothers. So, the current practice is to avoid the risk of hypoglycemia. But, routine use of only 5% dextrose or lactated Ringer's solution is discouraged. Instead, 5% dextrose in 0.45% normal saline is used in a piggyback infusion at maintenance rates with lactated Ringer's solution (or any balanced salt solution) for all deficits and third space losses. The IV fluids should also be administered by using a system that allows small volume to be given accurately. Anesthesiologists usually perform this by injecting fluid using a syringe or by a microprocessor-controlled syringe-driven infusion pump. The later method is preferable, as fluid is given at a slow but steady and accurate rate.

The anesthesiologists must assess the blood loss during surgery. In minor surgical procedures, this blood loss is minimal and the assessment is performed by the visual inspection of surgical field, swabs, mops, suction bottle, etc. But, for major surgeries where the blood loss is more, then the weighing of swabs and colorimeter is helpful. The estimated circulating blood volume in neonates, infants, and children is near about 70–80 mL/kg. In general, the blood loss <10% of total blood volume, either requires no replacement or can be replaced by crystalloid solutions. Blood loss in-between 10% and 20% should always be replaced by colloids or blood. But, over 20% of loss must always be replaced by blood. The adequacy of blood replacement should always be assessed on the background of normal blood pressure, pulse rate, and central venous pressure **(Table 9)**.

TABLE 9: Some important parameters of a new born weighing 4 kg.

Heart rate	120–140 minutes
Mean blood pressure	70 mm Hg
Respiratory rate	35–40 breaths/min
Tidal volume	16 mL
Alveolar ventilation	400 mL/min
Hb concentration	18–20 g/100 mL
Urinary output	20–30 ml/kg/24 hours
Fluid requirement	100 mL/kg/24 hours

■ HEPATIC FUNCTION

The maturity of liver function is somewhat incomplete during birth at term. The ability to detoxify drugs and the carbohydrate metabolism system in liver are both poorly developed during birth. But, the capability to synthesize albumin and coagulation factors is normal at birth. By 6 weeks of age, the enzyme systems of liver function develop as per the adult levels, though they (enzyme system) are not induced (stimulated) by agents which they metabolize. The conjugation reactions are often impaired in neonates, resulting in jaundice. Because of low glycogen stores and hepatic immaturity, hypoglycemia (defined as blood glucose level of 30 mg/dL or less) in a term baby is common. In low birth weight or premature babies, hypoglycemia (defined as blood glucose level 20 mg/dL or less) is more common. In neonates and infants, this hypoglycemia is usually without symptoms, unless the level is very low when the apneic attacks or convulsions may occur. Hypothermia also causes hypoglycemia and vice versa. The plasma levels of albumin and other plasma proteins (necessary for binding of drugs) are low in term newborns and even lower in premature infants. This is responsible for the greater level of free drug in the plasma and neonatal coagulopathy (e.g., hence the need for vitamin K at birth). As the infant gradually grows, the function of liver matures in two ways: (1) the enzyme system slowly develops and (2) the hepatic blood flow gradually increases delivering more blood to the liver.

■ HYPOCALCEMIA

This condition commonly occurs during the first 2 days of life and this is mainly due to the immaturity of parathyroid glands and high phosphate content of some milk formulae which are usually available in market. The nonspecific neurological signs, such as the irritability causing tetany or convulsions, due to the low level of blood calcium are usually treated by intravenous infusion of 2% solution of calcium gluconate at the dose of 5 mg/kg/hour.

■ GASTROINTESTINAL SYSTEM

Gastric secretion in a fetus begins from the second trimester of pregnancy or 16 weeks of intrauterine life. The gastric pH is alkaline at birth. Then, it decreases approximately to a pH of 4 by the 8 hours after birth. On the second day of life, the gastric pH reaches within the range of an adult. Till 4–5 months of age after birth, coordination between the respiration and swallowing does not develop. So, it frequently causes gastroesophageal reflux, laryngeal aspiration, and coughing. The developmental abnormalities of upper intestine often manifest as vomiting and regurgitation, but the developmental abnormalities lower intestine often manifest as the distension of abdomen and failure to pass meconium. Any developmental anomaly of gastrointestinal tract manifests as early as within 24–36 hours after birth.

CENTRAL NERVOUS SYSTEM

The anatomical developments of nervous system in a newborn are complete at term. But, the functional development of nervous system including myelination, synaptic connections, synthesis of neurotransmitters, etc. continues for 2 years after the commencement of extrauterine life. The cranium of a newborn is soft and pliable. It has many nonfused cranial sutures, two open fontanels (the posterior fontanel closes by 6–9 months and the anterior fontanel closes by 18 months of postnatal life), poorly developed cerebral cortex, fragile subependymal blood vessels, a spinal cord that ends at L4 level, etc. All these peculiarities that differ from the central nervous system (CNS) of an adult have many important implications in the management of pediatric anesthesia.

Water is the predominant constituent of neonatal and infantile brain tissue. Then, due to more and more myelination and dendritic proliferation, the water content of the brain tissue of the pediatric group of patient gradually decreases and the fat content increases throughout the infancy and childhood. The modern inhalational anesthetic agents are less soluble in water than fat. So, their (volatile anesthetic agents) partition coefficient is lowest in premature and newborn babies. This gradually increases with the passage of time after birth and this is due to the decrease in the concentration of water as body constituent. This explains the more rapid wash-in (induction) and wash-out (recovery) of inhalational anesthetic agents from the brain tissue of neonates and infants, when compared to the adults and hence the altered requirements of it for this age group of patients. The blood–brain barrier is immature and more permeable in the neonates and infants. So, the barbiturates, opioids, antibiotics, bilirubin, etc. cross this more permeable blood–brain barrier more rapidly.

In asphyxiated neonates and also in preterm babies, the autoregulation of cerebral blood flow is compromised, i.e., the cerebral blood flow varies directly with the systemic mean arterial pressure. But, still it is autoregulated over a wide range of change in arterial blood pressure in healthy neonates and infants. The neuroendocrine axis of stress for pain and surgery, and the mechanism responsible for perception of noxious stimuli are well developed in neonates and infants like the adults. So, an inadequate level of analgesia and anesthesia in the perioperative period can result in marked stress response and its consequences in this pediatric group of patients.

PHARMACOLOGICAL (PHARMACOKINETIC AND PHARMACODYNAMIC) STATUS OF DRUGS IN PEDIATRIC PATIENTS

The dosing of drugs in any age group of patient, also in pediatric group of patient, is typically (conventionally) adjusted on per kilogram of body weight basis for convenience. But, actually the dosing of drugs in neonates, infants, and younger children should be on allometric design *(allometric dosing)* where patient's allometric body weight is approximated according to their age. This allometric body weight of a neonate or infant is 50th percentile body weight (in kg) = (Age × 2) + 9. In contrast to the conventional body weight adjusted drug dosing, the allometric drug dose calculation (calculation of dose of a drug according to allometric body weight) takes into account the age-related physiological differences, such as (1) the disproportionately larger pediatric intravascular and extravascular fluid compartments, (2) the immaturity of hepatic biotransformation pathways, (3) the increased organ blood flow, (4) the decreased protein for drug binding, and (5) the higher metabolic rate.

The pharmacological status of different drugs in pediatric patients differ from that of the adults due to the following reasons. These reasons are:

- Due to the difference in composition of body fluids and tissues between the pediatric and adult patients
- Due to the difference in cardiac index and distribution of CO to different tissues between the pediatric and adult patients
- Due to the difference in protein-binding capacity of drugs between the pediatric and adult patients
- Due to the difference in maturation of blood–brain barrier between the pediatric and adult patients
- Due to the difference in functional maturity of liver and kidneys between the pediatric and adult patients. The neonates and infants have a relatively (1) decreased GFR, (2) decreased hepatic blood flow, (3) impaired renal tubular function, and (4) immature hepatic enzyme systems.

In neonates and infants, the total body water content (due to the large extracellular fluid and large blood volume) is disproportionately higher than adults. For example, the total body water content in neonates and infants is 70–75% of their body weight, whereas the total water content of in adult is 50–55% of their body weight. Then, it (water content in neonates and infants) gradually decreases with increasing their age and this is due to the gradual increase in fat and muscle content in the body of pediatric group of patients **(Fig. 5)**. So, the water-soluble highly ionized drugs have a larger volume of distribution and require a larger initial

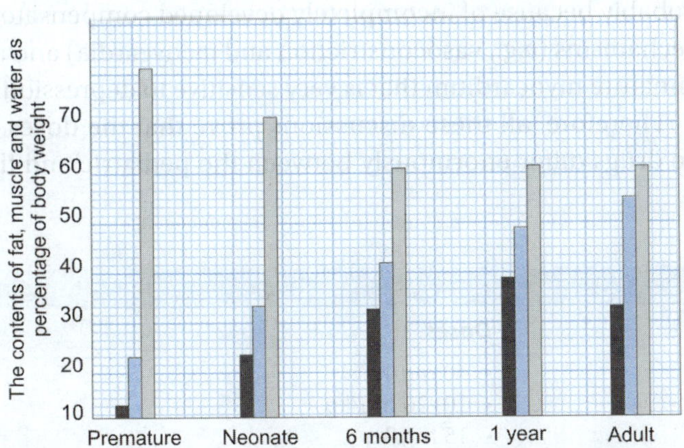

Fig. 5: Changes in body composition from a premature neonate to an adult. The high water content in the body of a premature neonate causes a large volume of distribution of water soluble drugs and thus an increase in their dose requirement. Whereas a low fat and muscle content provides less redistribution of fat soluble drugs and hence prolongs their duration of action (as their effects are terminated by the redistribution of water) Grey: total body water, Black: muscle mass, Blue: fat.

dose on weight basis in neonates and infants to achieve the desired blood level, e.g., succinylcholine. On the other hand, in neonates and infants there is much less fat and muscle tissue than in older children and adults. So, the drugs which depend on redistribution into fat and muscle for the termination of their actions (e.g., thiopentone, propofol, and fentanyl) have a longer duration of action.

In general, when compared to an adult, the potency of many drugs is greater in neonates and infants, requiring a lower does, but this potency is lesser in older children and adults, requiring higher dose. Similarly, many drugs which have prolonged elimination half-life require lower dose in neonates and infants than adults, but contrary the drugs which have shorter elimination half-life require a higher dose in neonates and infants than an adult. These differences gradually equalize as the pediatric patients march toward their adulthood.

In premature babies and neonates, there is lower plasma concentration of albumin. Therefore, the ability of albumin to bind with drugs is also lower than in an adult. So, most of the IV drugs in these groups of patients remain in a free-active form, requiring a lower dose. The concentration of $\alpha 1$ acid glycoprotein which is the major binding protein in plasma for opioids and local anesthetics is also lower in pediatric patients, resulting in exaggerated and prolonged actions of these two groups of drugs in this age group of patients.

At birth the blood–brain barrier is immature and it gradually matures with increasing age. Again, the brain of neonates and infants receives a large proportion of CO than the brain of adults. So, the brain is exposed to more drugs and the concentration of drugs in brain is higher in neonates and infants than in adults. Thus, it explains why narcotics should be used with caution and in reduced amounts in this age group of patients.

In pediatric group of patient, the renal functions reach an adult level by the age of 3 months and by that time the clearance of most of the drugs by kidney reaches its adult values. The activity of liver function reaches its adult value by 6 weeks after birth. But, the volume and the weight of liver and kidney are disproportionately more than an adult, and hence receive more percentage of CO. This explains why most medications have a shorter half-life in children older than 2 years than in neonates and adults. In general, most medications will have prolonged elimination half-life in premature and term infants, shorter half-life in children and again prolonged of half-life in those approaching adulthood.

Some special characteristics of pharmacology (pharmacokinetics and pharmacodynamics) of inhalational anesthetic agents in neonates and infants are:

- Higher alveolar and minute ventilation (due to high respiratory rate) in relation to reduced FRC ($\uparrow$minute ventilation to FRC ratio) in neonates, infants, and younger children → $\uparrow$alveolar concentration of inhalational agents.
- High CI, i.e., high CO in relation to body weight increases the rate of equilibrium of inhalational anesthetic agents in tissues → $\uparrow$brain concentration of any inhalational anesthetic agent.
- Preponderance of vessel-rich tissues (e.g., brain) and greater proportional distribution of CO to these vessel-rich organs (brain) → $\uparrow$brain concentration of any inhalational anesthetic agent.
- Reduced water solubility of inhaled anesthetic agents in blood, i.e., blood/gas coefficients of volatile anesthetics are lower in neonates and infants than in adults → $\uparrow$brain concentration of inhalation anesthetic agent.

All these factors cause alveolar and brain concentration of inhalational anesthetic agents to increase rapidly and fall rapidly. This increased rate of equilibration of inhalational agents in neonates and infants correlates well with the earlier development of cardiovascular side effects and explains why the induction and recovery, during inhalation anesthesia by volatile anesthetic agents, are more rapid in children.

The minimum alveolar concentration (MAC) values of inhalational anesthetic agents change with age. It is lower for premature infants and increases to its peak value at their age of 3 months. Then, it gradually declines again, until the adult value is reached. So, the infants are known to have greater anesthetic requirement than the older children and adults. Hence, the infants are in a precarious condition between the higher requirement of inhaled anesthetic agents (say, for ET intubation) and anesthetic overdose (from cardiovascular standpoint). Use of narcotics and muscle relaxants usually widen this gap.

The blood pressure of neonates and infants tends to be more sensitive to volatile anesthetics agents. This is probably because of incompletely developed compensatory mechanisms (e.g., vasoconstriction and tachycardia) and an immature myocardium that is very sensitive to depression.

Therefore, all these discussions prove that the doses of the drugs differ enormously between the pediatric and the

TABLE 10: Pediatric drug dosages.

Drugs	Comment	Doses
Acetaminophen (paracetamol)	• Rectal • Oral • Intravenous (>2 years) • Maximum per day	• 40 mg/kg • 10–20 mg/kg • 15 mg/kg • 60 mg/kg
Atracurium	IV (intubation)	0.5 mg/kg
Alfentanil	• Anesthetic supplementation • Maintenance infusion	• 20–25 µg/kg • 1–3 µg/kg
Atropine	• IV • IM	• 0.01–0.02 mg/kg • 0.02 mg/kg
Cisatracurium	IV for intubation	0.15 mg/kg
Calcium gluconate	IV slowly	15–100 mg/kg
Dexamethasone	IV	0.1–0.5 mg/kg
Dopamine	Infusion	2–20 µg/kg/ min
Dobutamine	Infusion	2–20 µg/kg/ min
Ephedrine	IV	0.1–0.3 mg/kg
Epinephrine	• IV bolus • Endotracheal • Infusion	• 10 µg/kg • 100 µg/kg • 0.05–1.0 µg/kg/min
Esmolol	• IV bolus • Infusion	• 100–500 µg/kg • 25–200 µ
Fentanyl	• Pain relief (IV) • Pain relief (intranasal) • Main anesthetic (IV) • Maintenance (infusion) • Anesthetic adjunct	• 1–2 µg/kg • 2 µg/kg • 50–100 µg/kg • 2–4 µg/kg • 1–5 µg/kg
Glycopyrrolate	IV	0.01
Hydrocortisone	IV	1.0 mg/kg
Ibuprofen	Oral	4–10 mg/kg
Ketamine	• IV induction • IM induction • Oral induction • Per rectum induction	• 1–2 mg/kg • 5–10 mg/kg • 5–10 mg/kg • 10 mg/kg
Magnesium sulfate	• IV (slowly) • Maximum	• 25–50 mg/kg • 2.0 g
Mannitol	IV	0.25–1.0 g/kg
Metoclopramide	IV	0.15 mg/kg
Midazolam	• Sedation (IV) • Sedation (IV) • Premedication (oral) • Maximum (oral)	• 0.05 mg/kg • 0.1–0.15 mg/kg • 0.5 mg/kg • 20 mg

Contd…

Contd...

Drugs	Comment	Doses
Methylprednisolone	IV	2–4 mg/kg
Meperidine	IV	0.2–0.5 mg/kg
Methohexital	• Induction (IV) • Induction (IM)	• 1–2 mg/kg • 10 mg/kg
Neostigmine	IV (according to degree of paralysis)	0.04–0.07 mg/kg
Norepinephrine	Infusion	0.05–2 µg/kg/ min
Nitroprusside	Infusion	0.5–4.0 µg/kg/ min
Ondansetron	IV	0.1 mg/kg
Pancuronium	IV	0.1 mg/kg
Phenylephrine	IV	1–10 µg/kg
Propofol	• Induction • Maintenance (infusion)	• 2–3 mg/kg • 0.06–0.250 mg/kg/min
Remifentanil	• IV bolus • IV infusion	• 0.25–1.0 µg/kg • 0.05–2 µg/kg/min
Rocuronium	IV for intubation	0.6–1.2 mg/kg
Succinylcholine	• Intubation (IV) • Intubation (IM)	• 1–2 mg/kg • 4 mg/kg
Sugammadex	IV (according to degree of paralysis)	2–4 mg/kg
Sodium bicarbonate	IV	1 mEq/kg
Sufentanil	• Main anesthetic induction (IV) • Maintenance infusion (IV) • Anesthetic adjunct (IV) • Premedication (intranasal)	• 10–15 µg/kg • 0.5–2.0 µg/kg • 0.5–1.0 µg/kg • 2.0 µg/kg
Thiopentone	IV induction	5–6 mg/kg

adult group of patients and the doses of commonly used drugs used in pediatric patients are given in **Table 10**.

VARIOUS ANESTHETIC AGENTS USED IN PEDIATRIC ANESTHESIA

Volatile Anesthetic Agents

Halothane

Although the use of halothane in western countries has declined gradually, but still it is the gold standard volatile anesthetic agent for the induction of anesthesia in pediatric patients in most of the underdeveloped countries, due to its least pungent odor (it is less pungent than sevoflurane) and less costly. It allows a very smooth induction, maintenance, and emergence from anesthesia. The low blood–gas solubility coefficient of halothane (2.3) and its high potency also permits rapid onset, as well as rapid recovery from anesthesia. But, many anesthetists now consider sevoflurane as the gold standard for this purpose. However, it is very costly (relatively) for the underdeveloped and developing countries. The airway-related problems like coughing, laryngospasm, secretions, etc. occur less frequently with halothane and sevoflurane than with the other volatile anesthetic agents, such as enflurane, isoflurane, and desflurane. Thus, halothane like sevoflurane is the anesthetic agent of choice for the induction of anesthesia by mask, with airway problems, in pediatric group of patients.

As most of the vaporizers allow high concentration (like $5 \times$ MAC) of any volatile anesthetic agent to be administered, if needed, so it can be given with almost 100% O_2 without any nitrous oxide (N_2O). This is also very helpful in children with an airway problem. The potency of halothane varies with age. In neonates, the MAC value of halothane is about 0.9%. But, it increases rapidly to a maximum of 1.2% at 6 months of age and, thereafter, it declines gradually to its adult value of 0.8%. The lower MAC value of halothane in neonates in comparison to infants is due to the immaturity of CNS in neonates. The higher value of MAC in infants, compared to older children and adults, is due to the increase in brain water content in the previous group of patients. The prolonged duration of action of halothane than other newer volatile agents (sevoflurane and desflurane) make it sometimes also especially useful in pediatric anesthesia, as the plane of anesthesia does not quickly reduce, during intubation or instrumentation of airway, after induction by it.

Halothane depresses the myocardium, reduces the heart rate, and decreases the CO. The hypotension produced by halothane is primarily due to its direct myocardial depression effects and bradycardia. It is, therefore, prudent to give an anticholinergic agent to prevent the reduction of heart rate, prior to halothane administration. Another concern with halothane is that it sensitizes the myocardium to exogenous and endogenous catecholamines, causing arrhythmia. But, most arrhythmias associated with halothane in pediatric anesthesia are due to either hypoxia, hypercarbia or inadequate level of anesthesia. Thereafter, a prudent pediatric anesthetist will must control hypercarbia, prevents hypoxia, and maintain an adequate level (depth) of anesthesia to prevent the halothane-induced arrhythmia. The maximum recommended dose of epinephrine with local anesthetic solutions during halothane anesthesia is 5–10 μg/kg. The effect of LA agent is also aggravated in pediatric anesthesia by hypercarbia, and an inadequate level of anesthesia. The potent myocardial depressant effect of halothane can have profound effect on neonates and children with congenital heart diseases. It is also responsible for the occasional inability to give sufficient concentration of halothane to critically ill patients to provide anesthesia, without inducing severe hypotension. In these circumstances, the lower concentrations of halothane and the liberal doses of short-acting newer narcotics generally provide better response.

Approximately, the 20% of absorbed halothane is metabolized in liver, mainly by the oxidation and produce its higher degree of metabolites. This higher degree of metabolism of halothane in liver appears to be an important factor for the etiology of halothane hepatitis. So, the repeated administration of halothane within a period of <3–6 months may be associated with hepatic dysfunction and occasionally with fulminant hepatic failure. Though, the exact mechanism of this hepatitis, induced by halothane, is not known, but it is speculated that the oxidative metabolites of halothane acts as an antigen and are responsible for this hepatitis, inducing Ag-Ab reaction. These oxidative hepatic metabolites of halothane are poorly developed in children and this explains extreme rarity of halothane-induced hepatitis in pediatric patients, though the incidence of halothane hepatitis in adults when exposed to this drug (halothane) is 1:10,000–1:30,000. However, if a child needs a second anesthesia within 3–6 months of first halothane anesthesia, then a risk-benefit assessment has to be undertaken. The physical characteristics and the physiological effects of inhalational anesthetic agents are shown in **Table 11**.

Isoflurane

Isoflurane is one of the important agents in the series of halogenated volatile ether compound such as halothane and chemically it is a halogenated methyl ether. It was originally developed in the place of ether, in order to improve its molecular stability and also to reduce its metabolism in liver, when compared to halothane. The metabolism of isoflurane in liver is about 1/100th of that of halothane (0.2%), and therefore, there is no report of hepatotoxicity of isoflurane in children, after its prolonged use.

Like ether, isoflurane has an irritant and pungent odor. Thus, it is associated with an increased incidence of airway problems, such as coughing, secretions, and laryngospasm. during induction, maintenance (with or without muscle. relaxant), and recovery from anesthesia. So, despite the low blood gas solubility coefficient (1.4) of isoflurane, when compared to halothane which dictates a rapid induction and recovery from anesthesia, the speed of induction of anesthesia by this agent (isoflurane) is significantly lower in clinical practice. The recovery characteristics of isoflurane

TABLE 11: Physical characteristics and physiological effects of volatile anesthetic agents.					
	Agents				
	Ether	*Halothane*	*Sevoflurane*	*Isoflurane*	*Desflurane*	*N$_2$O*
Odor	Most pungent	Sweet	Minimum pungent	Markedly pungent	Markedly pungent	Nil
Minimum alveolar concentration (MAC)	2	1.2	2.5	1.9	9.9	105
Blood gas partition coefficient	12	2.1	0.7	1.2	0.4	0.47
Myocardial depression	↑↑	↓↓	↑↓	↓	↓	↓
Vessel dilatation	↑↑	↓	↓↓	↓↓	↓↓	↑
Respiratory depression	↑	↓	↓↓	↓↓	↓↓	Nil
Rate of metabolism (%)	4	20	2	0.2	0.02	Nil

are poorer than halothane. But, the advantage of isoflurane over halothane is that an equipotent concentration of isoflurane produces similar reduction of blood pressure, without reducing the heart rate and myocardial contractility (myocardial depression), like halothane. The reduction of arterial blood pressure during isoflurane anesthesia is due to decrease in peripheral vascular resistance, rather than myocardial depression (like halothane) by isoflurane. This suggests that despite similar reduction in blood pressure, isoflurane is associated with greater cardiovascular reserve than halothane, especially in neonates, infants, and children where heart rate and myocardial contractility is more important to maintain CO and blood pressure.

Like halothane, the MAC value of isoflurane also varies with age. It is about 1.6% in neonates, 1.9% in infants (1–6 months) and then declines gradually to approximately 1.2% in adults.

Sevoflurane

Like isoflurane, the sevoflurane also belongs to the series of halogenated volatile ether anesthetics agent, but it is halogenated solely by fluorine. The presence of only fluorine reduces the solubility of sevoflurane in both fat and blood. Thus, this reduces the anesthetic potency of sevoflurane, while increases the rate of uptake and elimination of it. So, as a volatile anesthetic agent, it has the property of causing very rapid induction and recovery, due to its very low blood-gas partition coefficient (0.68), though it is a less potent volatile anesthetic agent. The eye lash reflex is lost within 60–90 seconds, after the beginning of the administration of sevoflurane at 5–6%. The blood gas partition coefficient of desflurane is 0.42, which also suggests that induction of anesthesia by desflurane should be more rapid than sevoflurane. But, this not so true, because the desflurane is also very irritant to the upper airway, causing breath holding, coughing, laryngeal spasm, etc. just like isoflurane which results in delayed induction by desflurane.

The smell of sevoflurane is least pungent (but according to some agents, halothane is least pungent) than all other currently available volatile anesthetic agents. So, higher concentrations of sevoflurane up to a maximum of about 8% can be given to pediatric patients without cough, increase in secretion, breath holding, laryngeal spasm, and other airway problems. There is little to be gained by adding N_2O with sevoflurane during induction, as the MAC sparing effect of sevoflurane is not so great as like other agents. The MAC value of sevoflurane also changes with age. In neonates, it is 3.3%, in infants, it is 2.5%, and in adults, it is 2%. The incidences of cardiac depression, bradycardia, and arrhythmias are minimal during the induction and

maintenance of anesthesia by sevoflurane than halothane. So, all these favorable points of sevoflurane make it the anesthetic agent of choice for induction and maintenance in pediatric patients. But, only the higher cost of sevoflurane restrains its use and this economic consideration dictates that sevoflurane should mainly be used for induction, followed by other cheaper halogenated agents, such as halothane and isoflurane. for maintenance.

The other areas of concern with sevoflurane during anesthesia, regarding its lesser safety are higher rate of metabolism of sevoflurane in liver which is about 2% (isoflurane 0.2%) and its instability with soda lime. It is found that after 60–90 minutes of anesthesia with sevoflurane, the peak concentration of fluoride ion in plasma rises from 1/3rd to 2/3rd of its proposed nephrotoxic level (50 mmol/L). With soda lime, the sevoflurane also produces a chemical, named *Compound A*, which is nephrotoxic and is mainly found during the use of circle absorber system with low gas flow anesthesia (0.5 to 1 L/min, in experimental animals). But, fortunately the formation of compound A in humans is much lower than in experimental animals, with the abovementioned flow and there is no reported cases of nephrotoxicity in human till now. So, the use of sevoflurane with soda lime in low-flow circle system is still debatable, but not totally condemned [above 2 L/min of fresh gas flow (FGF)].

Desflurane

Desflurane is another halogenated volatile ether anesthetic agent, where a single chlorine atom of isoflurane is replaced by fluorine. So, like isoflurane, it has also a markedly pungent odor and is unsuitable for induction of anesthesia, like isoflurane, due to the high incidence of airway complications, such as breath holding, laryngospasm, cough, and increased secretion. The blood–gas partition coefficient of desflurane is lowest (0.4) among all the inhalational anesthetic agents (for N2O it is 0.47). Thus, the induction of anesthesia and recovery from it is fastest with desflurane, when compared to that of other inhalational anesthetic agents. The drug is stable in soda lime and the hemodynamic responses are similar to that of halothane. But, unlike halothane, the metabolism of desflurane in liver is very minimum, which is approximately 0.02% (halothane 20%) and so has not the incidences of hepatotoxicity. This advantage of desflurane clearly sets it apart from the other currently available potent volatile anesthetic agents. The MAC value of desflurane also changes with age, such as in neonates, it is 9.2%, in infants, it is 9.9%, and in adults, it is 6%. As the desflurane is stable in soda lime and provides a rapid recovery, so it is also a suitable agent for the maintenance of anesthesia in pediatric patients, using close circuit with soda lime. But, its high cost bars its use which can be mitigated by the use of low-flow rates in circle system.

The rate of emergence from anesthesia is fastest, following desflurane and sevoflurane. But, both these agents are associated with the increased incidences of agitation or delirium, after rapid emergence, particularly in young children. So, many anesthesiologists switch over to either isoflurane or halothane for the maintenance of anesthesia, following an induction by desflurane or sevoflurane.

Nitrous Oxide

Nitrous oxide is a very less potent (MAC 105%), nonirritant, noninflammable, sweet smelling inhalational anesthetic agent. Due to its low potency as an anesthetic agent, it is used as an adjunct with other potent anesthetic agents and is not used as a sole anesthetic agent. It is very stable with little biotransformation and produces rapid induction as well as recovery, due to its low blood–gas partition coefficient (0.47).

At the equipotent anesthetic concentrations, it is half as potent as halothane in depressing the myocardium. So, in premature babies and neonates the N_2O should not be used. In such cases, air may be substituted as a carrier gas for O_2 and other inhalational agents. N_2O also should not be used in some pediatric surgeries, such as bowel obstruction, diaphragmatic hernia, lobar emphysema, and Eustachian tube obstruction and the cause of which is given in relevant chapter.

Intravenous Inducing agents

All the commonly used intravenous inducing agents, like thiopentone, propofol, benzodiazepine, ketamine, etc. can safely be used in pediatric group of patients.

Thiopentone

It produces smooth induction of anesthesia in one arm-brain circulation time and the termination of this anesthetic effect of thiopentone occurs through distribution and redistribution of it in the muscle, fat, and different tissue compartments. Termination of anesthetic effect of thiopentone does not occur through quick metabolism of it, like that of propofol. But, gradually it accumulates in different body compartments with increasing doses. So, it cannot be used as continuous infusion for maintenance of anesthesia and should be used very cautiously in premature neonates and malnourished infants who have less muscle mass and low fat stores.

The dose of thiopentone varies with age. In neonates, the dose of thiopentone is only 3.5 mg/kg. But, it increases rapidly to 6–7 mg/kg in infants and then it again declines gradually throughout the childhood to an adult value of 4–5 mg/kg. The increased requirement of thiopentone in infants and early childhood is due to the increased CO which reduces the first pass concentration of thiopentone, arriving at brain. The reduced requirement of thiopentone in neonates is explained by its decrease in plasma protein binding capacity in them. The induction doses of thiopentone also can be reduced by 50% with the use of different other sedative premedications. The most important drawback of thiopentone in pediatric use is its cardiovascular and respiratory depression effect. The cardiovascular depression effect of thiopentone includes the reduction of myocardial contractility and arterial blood pressure by about 15–20%. So, it should be avoided in pediatric group of patients who are dehydrated, have significant amount of blood loss, or have heart failure. The other side effects of thiopentone are hiccup, cough, laryngospasm, etc.

Propofol

Like propofol, it also produces a rapid and smooth induction of anesthesia in pediatric age group of patients with low incidence of serious side effects. Chemically, it is an alkyl phenol compound and marketed as 1% emulsion, in a white soybean oil base, with egg phosphatide and glycerol. Like thiopentone, it is also a highly lipophilic and protein-bound compound, but without any analgesic properties. *The dose requirement of propofol for pediatric patients is higher than adults.* This is because (1) the volume of central compartment of pediatric patients, which is responsible for the distribution and redistribution of propofol, is 50% larger in pediatric patients than that of adults, plus (2) 25% shorter elimination half-life and 25% higher plasma clearance rate of propofol than that of adults in pediatric group of patients.

The beauty of propofol in pediatric anesthesia lies in its use, as both for induction by bolus doses and for maintenance by continuous infusion. The propofol is now licensed for use as an induction agent in children over 1 month. But, it is not recommended for prolonged sedation by continuous infusion in critically ill pediatric patients in neonatal intensive care unit (NICU). Till now, the target-controlled infusion (TCI) pump for propofol is not configured for pediatric use, like that of use in adults. The children up to the 8 years of age may require almost double the adult dosage (3–5 mg/kg) of propofol. The dose of propofol for continuous infusion is 100–300 µg/kg/min. Pain may occur during bolus injection of propofol for induction. But, this can be minimized by using a larger vein, injecting the solution slowly, and administering IV lignocaine in the dose of 0.2 mg/kg, before the administration of propofol. There is reduction in heart rate with propofol, particularly below the 2 years of age and this is due to the attenuation of baroreceptor reflex. There is also a larger fall in blood pressure, compared to the equipotent doses of thiopentone. Respiratory depression and the incidence of apnea are greater with propofol than thiopentone, although laryngeal mask insertion is easier due to more depression of laryngeal reflexes by propofol.

Propofol is not contraindicated in epilepsy, though involuntary movements may be seen during the induction with propofol. These involuntary movements, induced by propofol, are usually due to the inadequate induction dose and early stimulation. Because of its prompt wake-up characteristic, antiemetic effect, usability as continuous infusion and low incidence of serious side effects, propofol is gradually displacing the short-acting barbiturates, as the induction agent of choice for pediatric outpatients. It is particularly useful for maintenance of sedation during radiotherapy, or in children undergoing a radiological diagnostic procedure. Although not common in pediatric anesthetic practice, still the technique of total intravenous anesthesia (TIVA) using propofol is very useful in children who are prone to malignant hyperthermia or children with history of porphyria (in porphyria the thiopentone is absolutely contraindicated). Strict aseptic technique is recommended during the handling of propofol as any contamination of its intralipid and preservative free preparation and its subsequent use may produce sepsis.

Propofol is not recommended for the prolonged maintenance of the sedation of critically ill pediatric patients in NICU. Because, this drug has been associated with higher rate of mortality in NICU, compared to other intravenous anesthetic agents and a controversial *"propofol infusion syndrome"* which is caused by propofol and is responsible for these NICU deaths, has been described. The essential features of this propofol infusion syndrome are metabolic acidosis, hemodynamic instability, hepatomegaly, rhabdomyolysis, multiorgan failure, etc. Although this syndrome has been seen primarily in critically ill children, but this rare syndrome has also been reported in adults and in patients undergoing long-term propofol infusion (>48 hours) for sedation at high doses (>5 mg/kg/hour).

Ketamine

Like the thiopentone and propofol, it is also helpful as a very good inducing agent for pediatric anesthesia. But, unlike the thiopentone and propofol, it has a strong analgesic property. The intravenous administration of ketamine in the doses, as low as 1–2 mg/kg, produces adequate analgesia and sedation (induction). The lack of cardiovascular depression effect of ketamine allows it to be used as an ideal agent for the induction of anesthesia in very sick children. So, it is widely used as a sole anesthetic agent in many developing countries. The dose of ketamine should be reduced in neonates and infants, because of the reduced clearance and prolonged metabolism of it in them. The emergence phenomenon from ketamine anesthesia is less common in children, especially when it is used in combination with midazolam. But, the incidence of postoperative nausea and vomiting (PONV) and salivation is higher with ketamine than any other inducing agents. The increased production of both the bronchial and salivary secretion by ketamine is the major side effect of it and usually requires prior administration of an antisecretory agent before the use of it (ketamine).

During ketamine anesthesia, even though the upper airway reflexes are relatively well preserved, but still the aspiration of gastric contents may occur during anesthesia induced by it. So, it should not be used as a sole anesthetic agent for infants with full stomach or with hiatus hernia. The emergence phenomenon from ketamine anesthesia is accompanied by strong hallucination and unpleasant dreams. But, this is well marked in adult patients and not so prominent in pediatric patients, as the children are almost always dreaming. The current available formulation of ketamine in market is a racemic mixture of S (+) and R (−) enantiomers. Though, it is possible to separate the two enantiomers, but there is no such commercially viable technology which can separate them for their individual clinical use. The aim to separate these two isomers of ketamine and to make it commercially available is the S (+) enantiomer of ketamine is twice potent, recovery is quicker, and the incidence of emergence reaction is also low in comparison to R (−) enantiomer of it.

The contraindications for the use of ketamine in pediatric patients include presence of active upper respiratory tract infection (URTI), increased intracranial pressure (ICP), open globe injury, seizure disorders, severe hypertension, severe ischemic heart disease, etc.

Narcotics

Due to the immaturity of blood–brain barrier in neonates and infants, the higher lipophilicity and the lower clearance rate of the newer fentanyl group of narcotics and its congeners have made the neonates and infants, below the 6 months of age, very sensitive to this group of drugs. Hence, the opioids appear to be more potent in neonates and early infants than in the older children and adults. So, the narcotics should be used with caution in premature neonates, term infants, and infants below the age of 6 months who are not in intensive care unit and whose ventilation need not be controlled postoperatively. Infants older than 6 months and the children probably have a response to narcotics similar to that of adults.

Morphine

It is least lipophilic than meperidine and all the other members of this group of drugs. So, the entry of morphine in CNS is mainly controlled by the degree of the maturity of CNS's blood–brain barrier. Hence, in an immature blood–brain barrier, morphine enters the CNS most readily than all the other narcotics. In contrast, meperidine is more lipophilic than morphine. Therefore, it is able to cross the blood–brain barrier more readily, but only after its maturation, because its penetration into CNS does not depend on the maturity of blood–brain barrier, but depends on the lipophilicity of this drug. Thus, the effects of an immature blood–brain barrier would be much less significant for meperidine than for morphine, but the lipophilicity would be much more significant for meperidine than that of morphine. On the other hand, in case of morphine this is reverse. Meperidine may not be appropriate for long-term administration in pediatric group of patients. This is due to the accumulation of its active and toxic metabolites such as normeperidine.

Morphine and other narcotics (except remifentanil) are metabolized mainly in liver and their actions (the actions of these metabolites) are terminated by conjugation with glucuronide in liver and subsequently by its renal clearance. But, other than metabolism in liver and subsequent renal excretion (which is responsible for the termination and shorter duration of action of morphine), the very high lipid solubility of some other newer narcotics of fentanyl group has a shorter duration of action and it is due to their rapid distribution and redistribution in tissues, like muscles and fat, like thiopentone and propofol. So, in neonates and infants, the deficiency of microsomal enzymes in liver, responsible for glucuronide conjugation may be responsible for the prolongation of the clinical effects of morphine and other older narcotics whose termination of actions depend only on conjugation with glucuronide in liver.

The newborns and the infants have a lower rate of metabolism and clearance of morphine. Therefore, a standard dose of morphine will result in higher plasma values of it, due to longer elimination half-life of it. In spite of all these disadvantages, still morphine remains the most commonly used opioid for the management of severe pain in children and is the gold standard with which the other potent analgesics are compared.

In neonates and infants who are below 6 months old and undergoing relatively brief procedures (near about 1 hour), a single dose of 25 µg/kg of morphine usually provides adequate intraoperative and postoperative analgesia. After a more prolonged and complex surgery, the postoperative analgesia is supplemented with a continuous infusion of morphine of 5–10 µg/kg/hour. For children and infants above 6 months of their age, the adult doses of morphine are recommended. For continuous infusion or patient-controlled analgesia (PCA), due to its long half-life, morphine in a loading dose of 100 µg/kg/hour is used first (if not used intraoperatively, which is usually done), followed by a maintenance dose of 25 µg/kg/hour.

Fentanyl

It is a synthetic, highly lipid-soluble, pure opioid agonist and is 100 times more potent than morphine. Because of its high lipid solubility and large volume of distribution, a single dose of fentanyl has more rapid onset and shorter duration of action than morphine. The termination of effects of an initial single standard low bolus dose of fentanyl is due to the redistribution of it in peripheral tissues, like muscles and fat. Whereas, the termination of effects of a high or continuous infusion dose of fentanyl depends on its elimination through liver by metabolism and kidney by filtration, when the redistribution sites of fentanyl are saturated and come in an equilibrium. So, if fentanyl is used as an infusion or in multiple repeated doses, then the progressive saturation of peripheral tissues by it, lead to the prolonged duration of action of it, as the clearance of it by metabolic process in liver is slow like morphine.

Due to the rapid onset and brief duration of action, fentanyl now is the most commonly used narcotic in pediatric anesthesia in short bolus doses, but not by infusion. As fentanyl is more lipophilic than morphine and meperidine, so its CNS action does not depend on the maturity of blood–brain barrier. The maturity of blood–brain barrier dictates the entry of water soluble (hydrophilic) narcotics only such as morphine. The immature blood–brain barrier of neonates and infants permits only the entry of hydrophilic morphine, but not lipophilic fentanyl. Thus, this explains fentanyl's lesser sensitivity in premature infants and neonates than the older ones.

The volume of distribution of fentanyl in infants is similar to that of adults, but the plasma clearance and elimination half-life of fentanyl are greater in neonates and infants. This is due to high hepatic blood flow in infants than adults. The dose of fentanyl producing an anesthetic state also produces a stable cardiovascular response. Fentanyl can be used in the dose of 2–10 µg/kg with other anesthetic agent mainly volatile agent in a surgery where postoperative ventilation is not needed. Usually, it is administered in the dose of 1–2 µg/kg at the start of anesthesia which is followed by further bolus doses as clinically indicated, or by a continuous infusion in the dose of 1 µg/kg/hour.

Higher doses of fentanyl such as 30 µg/kg can be used only in cardiac and other surgeries, where postoperative

BOX 3: Advantages of remifentanil.

- It is metabolized by nonspecific esterase enzyme in plasma and tissues
- The metabolites of remifentanil are inactive
- Half-life of this drug is short and is independent of the duration of infusion
- Lack of cumulative effect

TABLE 12: Guidelines of doses of muscle relaxants and their antagonists in pediatric patients.

Agents	Dose for tracheal intubation (2 × ED95) (mg/kg)	Maintenance dose (mg/kg)	
		With N_2O/O_2	With halothane
Succinylcholine	2.00	—	—
Atracurium	0.5–0.6	0.3	0.2
Rocuronium	0.6–0.7	0.4	0.3
Pancuronium	0.6–0.7	0.08	0.06
Vecuronium	0.1–0.15	0.08	0.06
Cisatracurium	0.1–0.15	0.06	0.03
Mivacurium	0.2–0.25	0.1	0.1
Pipecuronium	0.08–0.12	0.08	0.08
Reversal agents			
Neostigmine	20–60 µg/kg + Atropine (10–20 µg/kg)		
Edrophonium	0.3 mg/kg + Atropine (10–20 µg/kg)		

ventilation is mandatory or to produce a full state of anesthesia with stable hemodynamic conditions without other anesthetic agents, mainly volatile agents. Since, the CO of neonates is determined by their heart rate, so the fentanyl-induced bradycardia may require concomitant administration of vagolytic drugs, such as atropine or pancuronium. Fentanyl is sometimes associated with chest wall rigidity impairing adequate ventilation.

Remifentanil

It is the newest of all the synthetic narcotics. It is an ultra-short-acting drug and its methyl ester linkage makes this drug susceptible to metabolism by the nonspecific plasma and tissue esterase enzymes. The clearance of remifentanil is high (increased) in neonates and infants, but its elimination half-life is same (unaltered) compared to adults. The pharmacokinetic profile of remifentanil in children, between 2 and 12 years of age, is similar to that of an adult. It has rapid distribution phases, small volume of distribution, and an elimination half-life of only 2–10 minutes. The dose of remifentanil is 1 µg/kg, followed by infusion of 0.25 µg/kg/min. Still now, there is very few data regarding the use of remifentanil in neonates and infants. At present, it is not licensed for use in children under the age of 2 years **(Box 3)**.

Muscle Relaxants

The use of neuromuscular blocking drugs has a definite place in pediatric anesthesia. But, the responses of these groups of drugs on pediatric patients differ markedly from those in adults. All the muscle relaxants generally have a *faster onset of action* (up to 50%) in pediatric patients. This is because of their shorter circulation time than adults and it (shorter circulation time) is due to the increased CO in proportion to their body surface area in neonates and infants. In general, due to this increased CO in proportion to the body surface area, the neonates and infants are also *resistant to the depolarizing drugs (require higher doses), but sensitive to nondepolarizing agents (require lower doses).* The explanation for this sensitivity of nondepolarizing agents is immaturity of neuromuscular junction in neonates, infants, and younger group of patients. However, this sensitivity is slightly counterbalanced by the larger extracellular

compartment of these groups of patients which reduce the concentration of drug at their neuromuscular junction **(Table 12)**, where the doses of different muscle relaxants are given.

Succinylcholine

Because of its high water solubility, succinylcholine is widely and rapidly distributed into the extracellular fluid volume of neonates and infants, containing more water which is greater than adults. This accounts for decreased sensitivity of succinylcholine in neonates and infants than the older ones and needs higher doses of succinylcholine in neonates and infants. So, the dose of succinylcholine, required for muscle relaxation and intubation in neonates and infants, is approximately twice than that of children and adults. Thus, the dose of succinylcholine for neonates and infants is 2 mg/kg through IV and for adults it is 1 mg/kg through IV. This dose of succinylcholine will produce 95% neuromuscular block within 30 seconds which is followed by 90% recovery within 5–10 minutes. Children are more susceptible than adults to cardiac arrhythmias, hyperkalemia, rhabdomyolysis, myoglobinemia, masseter spasm, malignant hyperthermia, etc., after the administration of succinylcholine.

Succinylcholine frequently causes cardiac arrhythmia in pediatric patients, mainly when it is used with halothane. Sometimes, severe bradycardia and sinus arrest may follow the first dose of succinylcholine. But, it is more common after repeated bolus doses. So, atropine (20 µg/kg) should be given through IV prior to the first dose of succinylcholine in children. If a child unexpectedly experiences cardiac arrest, following the administration of succinylcholine, then immediate treatment for hyperkalemia should be instituted. However, prolonged and heroic cardiopulmonary resuscitative efforts must also be instituted immediately.

There is always a tendency to develop phase II block in neonates and infants with succinylcholine. It is also one of the most potent triggering agents for the development of malignant hyperthermia. The incidence of malignant hyperthermia increases, if succinylcholine is preceded by halothane induction. Fatal cardiac arrest may also occur in a small number of patients, following administration of succinylcholine. It is presumed that, these patients may have unsuspected muscular dystrophies and the drug causes massive breakdown of muscle cells, causing hyperkalemia and cardiac arrest. It is also not possible to predict this group of patients who are prone to exhibit this response. So, all these complications make the routine use of succinylcholine on pediatric patients a controversy. On the other hand, succinylcholine is the only commercially available shortest acting muscle relaxant that provides a dependable and a very rapid onset of action.

So, the present status of succinylcholine in pediatric anesthesia is that it should only be reserved for patients with full stomach, necessitating rapid sequence intubation in emergency cases or in cases of difficult intubation or for the treatment of intractable laryngospasm which does not respond to positive pressure ventilation, causing severe hypoxia, and impending cardiac arrest. For the later, intramuscular succinylcholine in the dose of 4–6 mg/kg is also used if IV line is not already secured. In such situation, atropine in the dose of 20/kg IM should be administered at the same time to prevent bradycardia. Some anesthesiologists also advocate intralingual administration of succinylcholine (2 mg/kg in the midline) as an alternate emergency route, if IV line is not available.

In contrast to depolarizing muscle relaxants (e.g., succinylcholine), the nondepolarizing muscle relaxants show higher sensitivity in neonates and infants than children and adults. So, full neuromuscular blockade occurs at a lower blood concentration and this is true for all the nondepolarizing muscle relaxants. The probable explanations of this fact are: (1) the immaturity of neuromuscular junction in neonates and infants, or (2) the difference in the bioavailability of drug, or (3) the lesser binding of nondepolarizing muscle relaxant with plasma proteins whose concentration is less in neonates and infants than adults.

On the other hand, the clinical significance of this higher sensitivity may not be great enough, owing to the larger volume of distribution of these nondepolarizing neuromuscular blocking drugs, due to the large extracellular fluid volume in the neonates and infants than adults. The immaturity of renal and hepatic function in neonates and infants also cause slower excretion of nondepolarizing drugs and hence the prolongation of blocking effect of these agents. Only the action of nondepolarizing drugs, those are metabolized in plasma (e.g., atracurium and mivacurium), does not vary greatly with age. So, the specific choice of a nondepolarizing muscle relaxants in neonates and infants depends on the onset of action, duration of action required, and the desired or undesired side effects of this relaxant. If a prolonged action and tachycardia is desired, then pancuronium is the best choice, otherwise atracurium is still the chosen one for the shorter procedures. Hoffmann elimination and ester hydrolysis of atracurium make it (atracurium) particularly useful in newborns and infants.

Atracurium

After a standard dose of 0.5 mg/kg through IV, the atracurium produces 95% depression of twitch response in voluntary muscles and then full intubating condition occurs within 0.9 minutes after its administration in neonates and infants. But, the recovery to the 10% of controlled twitch height, after the administration of atracurium, occurs within 20 minutes. The volume of distribution of atracurium in neonates and infants is 0.18 L/kg in contrast to adults which is 0.14 L/kg. The plasma clearance of atracurium has also been found to be greater in neonates and infants (9 mL/kg/min) than that of adults (5 mL/kg/min). The adverse effects associated with atracurium are related mainly to the release of histamine. These are probably hypotension, tachycardia, and/or bronchospasm. The cardiovascular changes, caused by the atracurium, are dose related, and usually occur at the doses >2 ED95 value of atracurium.

Vecuronium

Vecuronium is also chosen in pediatric patients for surgical procedures which are of longer duration and also where the tachycardia is not desired. This is because the vecuronium-induced neuromuscular block is characterized by the lack of histamine release and marked cardiovascular stability in all these age group of patients. It is a very long-acting nondepolarizing muscle relaxant in neonates and infants than adults. Vecuronium, in its standard intubating dose of 100 µg/kg, maintains over 90% neuromuscular blockade for almost an hour in neonates and infants, compared to just 30–40 minutes in adults.

Mivacurium

Mivacurium is another very short-acting nondepolarizing muscle relaxant. It offers the advantage of producing satisfactory surgical conditions (muscle relaxation) for the brief surgical procedures, like succinylcholine. But, vary rapid intubating conditions, as produced by succinylcholine, is not provided by it. Mivacurium has the shortest duration of action among all the currently available nondepolarizing drugs and its action is terminated like succinylcholine by plasma pseudocholinesterase. So, like succinylcholine, very occasionally a patient may be cholinesterase deficient, when its (mivacurium) duration of action may be prolonged. In a dose of 0.2 mg/kg through IV, mivacurium provides an excellent muscular relaxation within 2 minutes. Then, 20% recovery of twitch response occurs after 8–9 minutes and spontaneous 95% recovery of twitch response occurs within 20 minutes. Mivacurium is also an ideal nondepolarizing muscle relaxant which can be administered by constant infusion, since there does not appear to be any accumulation of this drug. As mivacurium is structurally similar to that of atracurium, so it has significant histamine releasing properties, which may be evident even at therapeutic doses. So, the standard dose of mivacurium which is 0.2 mg/kg should not be exceeded.

Rocuronium

Many clinicians consider rocuronium is the drug of choice for routine intubation in pediatric patients because it has the most rapid onset of action among all the currently available nondepolarizing muscle relaxants. An IV dose of rocuronium in 0.6 mg/kg produces the 90% depression of twitch response and an ideal intubating condition within 30 seconds, after its administration, like succinylcholine, but without any significant changes in blood pressure and heart rate. So, it may therefore be used as an alternative to succinylcholine, when rapid tracheal intubation is desired and succinylcholine is considered as contraindicated, whereas the duration of the clinical effects of rocuronium, following a standard intubating dose (0.6 mg/kg), is longer and is near about 40 minutes. Therefore, the atracurium, rocuronium, and vecuronium, have a short, intermediate, and long duration of action, making them the most commonly used muscle relaxants in pediatric anesthesia. The larger doses of rocuronium (0.9–1.2 mg/kg) may be used for rapid sequence induction, if a prolonged duration of muscle relaxation is not a concern.

Rapacuronium

Rapacuronium is a currently used new aminosteroid nondepolarizing muscle relaxant. It is gradually being evaluated in pediatric practice. Multiple data suggest that its onset action is similar to that of succinylcholine and its duration of action is comparable that of mivacurium.

Reversal of Neuromuscular Blockade

The general rule for the use of nondepolarizing muscle relaxants in neonates and infants is the careful titration of dose due to extreme variability of their response. So, the initial dose of nondepolarizing muscle relaxants should be one-third to one-half of calculated total dose for the pediatric patient. The antagonism of neuromuscular blockade by anticholinesterase in all the neonates and small infants is mandatory, even if the spontaneous recovery is complete clinically. This is because any compensatory increase in the work of breathing due to residual neuromuscular block may cause fatigue and respiratory failure. Nondepolarizing blockade in pediatric patients are usually reversed by neostigmine (0.03–0.07 mg/kg) or edrophonium (0.5–1 mg/kg) along with an anticholinergic agent, like glycopyrrolate (0.01 mg/kg) or atropine (0.01–0.02 mg/kg). The *sugammadex,* a specific antagonist for rocuronium and vecuronium, is recently released to reverse the action of all nondepolarizing muscle relaxant, even in the face of neuromuscular blockade that could not be reversed with conventional cholinesterase inhibitors. The useful signs for the reversal of neuromuscular blockade in neonates and infants are the ability to lift their legs and arms and the recovery of train-of-four response to peripheral nerve stimulation.

■ PEDIATRIC ANESTHETIC RISK FACTORS

The pediatric anesthetic risk is best assessed from the database of a register, which is made by an investigating group. This register was made on reports, based on approximately one million pediatric anesthetic cases, administered since 1994. From this register, all the cardiac arrests and deaths were investigated and analyzed to find out the possible causes during anesthesia with these incidents. It was found that approximately 300 cardiac arrests had occurred and among them 150 arrests were directly related to anesthesia. Thus, the incidences of risk for cardiac arrest in pediatric anesthesia are 1.5 in 10,000 cases and among these the mortality rate is 30%. Another 6% patients had suffered from permanent injury. But, the majority 64% patients either did not suffer from any injury or only temporary injury. It is also important to note that the age is responsible for 50% of all the anesthesia-related cardiac arrests. Among them, the <1 month age babies, i.e., neonates have the highest risk. About 40% babies, with a physical status of American Society of Anesthesiologists (ASA) 3–5, had suffered anesthesia-related cardiac arrest. So, like the adults, the major predictors for mortality in the cases of pediatric anesthesia are age, ASA physical status, and emergency surgery.

Among all the cardiac arrests, 80% had occurred during the induction of anesthesia and is most frequently preceded by bradycardia, hypotension, and low SPO_2 levels. The most common cause of cardiac arrest during the induction of anesthesia is cardiovascular depression due to medications. Among the medicines, halothane alone or in combination with other drugs is believed to be responsible in 60% of cases. In another 10% cases, the inadvertent intravascular injection of local anesthetic agent during caudal injection (still following a negative aspiration test) is blamed. In about 50% cases of cardiac arrest in pediatric anesthesia, patients have congenital heart disease. The respiratory causes for cardiac arrest are most often due to laryngospasm, airway obstruction, and difficult intubation (in a decreasing order). In most cases, laryngospasm occurs during induction.

SOME IMPORTANT CONSIDERATIONS IN PEDIATRIC ANESTHESIA

Preoperative Assessment

A preoperative visit to an anesthetic clinic, followed by the preoperative preparation for surgery of pediatric patients of all the ages by an anesthetist, is very crucial. Prior to surgery, the baby's condition should be properly evaluated to determine (1) any abnormality in CVS, (2) the degree of respiratory distress, if any, (3) airway problems in respect to intubation, (4) metabolic disturbances, (5) temperature variations, (6) the extent of planned surgical procedure matching with patient's condition, etc. Among these, a detailed history and physical examination of patient, with special emphasis on the assessment of cardiovascular and respiratory function, is most important. The neonatal history should also include the problems during delivery, the severity of prematurity, the history of admission in NICU after birth, etc. The infants born prematurely, especially those with history of apneic periods, are more likely to develop apnea following anesthesia. So, they should not be accepted for day-case procedures, until they are at least 60 weeks of gestational age (20 weeks after birth). The respiratory history includes asthma, frequent colds, obstructive sleep apnea, etc.

The cardiovascular assessment for the pediatric group of patients mainly includes *cyanosis, heart murmur, and whether dyspnea is present during exercise or not*. The majority of pathological murmurs are diagnosed in their neonatal age and these children are already under the care of a cardiologist. The previously unreported murmurs were commonly heard between the ages of 2–4 years and the majority of them were functional. Mild murmurs in a child with normal heart sounds and normal oxygen saturation and without any limitation in exercise tolerance can be assumed to be innocent, if they are not pansystolic.

Most asymptomatic patients with murmurs do not have significant cardiac pathology.

The *innocent murmurs* may occur in >30% of normal children. They are usually soft, short systolic, and ejection murmurs and are best heard along the left lower or left upper sternal borders without any significant radiation. The innocent murmurs situated at the *left upper sternal border* are due to the flow of blood across the pulmonary valve, whereas those at the *left lower sternal border* are due to the flow of blood from the left ventricle into the aorta (Still's vibratory murmur). In case of any doubt, surgery should be deferred until a formal assessment has been made by a pediatric cardiologist. The pediatrician and possibly a cardiologist should carefully evaluate the patients with a newly diagnosed murmur, particularly in infancy. An echocardiogram or a color Doppler should be obtained if (1) the patient is symptomatic (e.g., poor feeding, failure to thrive, or easy fatigability); (2) the murmur is a harsh, loud, holosystolic or holodiastolic, and radiates widely; or (3) if the pulses are either bounding or markedly diminished.

The *previous family history,* regarding the anesthesia of pediatric patients, is also important which includes *malignant hyperpyrexia* and *prolonged apnea,* caused by suxamethonium. The problems during previous anesthesia, such as PONV, poor pain relief, and difficult venous access are also important. The laboratory tests required for surgery depend on the severity of existing illnesses and also the preexisting diseases (outlined from history and full clinical examination). For example, if a *healthy neonate or infant* is scheduled for a minor elective surgery such as repair of an inguinal hernia, then only routine blood count with Hb and serum glucose estimation is needed. Some pediatric centers require no preoperative laboratory tests in healthy children undergoing minor procedures. *However, obviously, this puts more responsibility on anesthetist, surgeon, and pediatrician to correctly identify the patients who require preoperative testing or not for anesthesia and surgical procedures.* On the other hand, if the patient presents with *some chronic illness or any congenital defect*, then extensive investigations including complete blood count, blood biochemistry, electrolytes, coagulation profiles, etc. are required, according to the defect and surgery planned.

Mere failure to urinate within 24 hours of birth, which is a very common event for a neonate, usually should not direct any renal function testing. However, in the presence of other concurrent congenital anomalies such as presence of some congenital renal anomalies, then this absence of urine output should be considered as serious. In such circumstances, extensive investigations should be undertaken including serum potassium, blood urea nitrogen, creatinine, ultrasound, etc.

If children suffer from upper and lower respiratory tract infection (RTI), surgery should be delayed. The standard recommendation for this delay is 4–6 weeks, after an episode of acute RTI, however bearing in mind that some children have frequent RTI (5–10 times/year). In such circumstances, each case should be dealt on the basis of its own merits, for example, whether the child has nasal discharge, inflamed tonsil, infected eardrums, fever, etc. In rare cases, the viremic phase of illness may be associated with myocarditis. So, children who have active viral illness or children who have recently been immunized using live vaccines should not have elective anesthesia and surgery, as these children may develop a viral myocarditis. In such circumstances, surgery should be avoided for a week, especially following DTP and *Haemophilus influenzae* vaccination and for 2 weeks after measles, mumps, and rubella MMR. A diagnosis of bronchiolitis and measles warrants a delay of at least 6 weeks.

However, a child suffering from mild cold possesses maximum difficulty in taking decisions by an anesthetist. The history in such cases is crucial, because it is important to decide whether the child is at the beginning or at the end of the process of URTI. A child who is (1) apyrexial, (2) has no chest signs, and (3) constitutionally well, is probably at the end of an attack of URTI and fit for surgery too, even with a running nose. Actually, the decision to anesthetize children with RTI remains controversial and depends on (1) the presence of other coexisting diseases, (2) the severity of symptoms of RTI, and (3) the urgency for surgery. If the surgery cannot be deferred, then much consideration should be given to (1) an anticholinergic agent and bronchodilator during premedication, (2) mask ventilation or use of laryngeal mask airway (LMA), avoiding tracheal intubation, if possible, (3) humidification of inspired gases, and (4) a longer than usual stay in recovery room. Anesthesia in the presence of RTI is associated with higher incidence of laryngospasm, bronchospasm, postoperative croup, pneumonia, and hypoxemia. All these are due to the increased incidence of secretions and airway obstructions in the presence of RTI. These risks are increased fivefold using an LMA, and by a factor of 10 if the child is intubated. But, still some anesthetists prefer to use ET tube, considering that it is wise and easy to control the airway, using an ET tube which will minimize the risk of cough or laryngospasm during anesthesia. However, generally, for minor procedures where muscle relaxants are not needed, then LMA is the best choice according to my view.

During preoperative assessment of pediatric group of patients, the anesthetist should also keep in mind the *possible intubation difficulties*, due to recent trauma, inflammation, tumor, congenital syndrome **(Table 13)**, etc., like the

TABLE 13: Some common congenital syndromes associated with difficult intubation.

Syndrome	Clinical features
Down	Small mouth, large tongue, small subglottic area, and congenital heart diseases
Pierre Robinson	Small mouth, retrognathia, large tongue, cleft palate, and subglottic stenosis
Turner	Short and webbed neck, narrow- and high-arched palate, small mandible, and epicanthic fold
Klippel–Feil	Cervical vertebral fusion, less number of cervical vertebra, and rigid and short neck
Goldenhar	Cervical spine abnormality and mandibular hypoplasia
Treacher Collins	Hypoplasia of malar bone, micrognathia, coloboma, preauricular ear tags, cleft palate, malocclusion of the teeth, and deformity of the middle auricles causing deafness

adult patients which are discussed in details in respective chapter. The other possible conditions and syndromes which are common to pediatric group of patients and are responsible for difficult intubation, should also be looked for. Some patients also may present with respiratory distress which can only be alleviated by surgery and for which this surgery is proposed. These include (1) choanal atresia, (2) laryngeal cysts or webs, (3) congenital diaphragmatic hernia, (4) esophageal atresia with or without tracheoesophageal (TE) fistula, (5) pulmonary cysts producing lobar emphysema or compression of lung tissues. On the other hand, patients may present with respiratory distress due to concomitant causes which are not related to proposed surgery. But, whatever may be, the degree of this respiratory distress should always be evaluated clinically by (1) observing the color of mucous membrane, (2) observing the degree of intercostal and sternal recession, and (3) auscultation of lung fields before starting anesthesia. Radiological examination of chest should always be undertaken in such conditions and the blood–gas status is estimated (if needed) by using blood from an arterial puncture preoperatively. Pneumothorax, which is often present in severe cases of diaphragmatic hernia on contralateral side (or in the cases of severe respiratory distress) should always be drained before anesthesia, by inserting a cannula into pleural space through second intercostal space and connecting it to an underwater drain. Metabolic disturbances due to hypovolemia, hypoglycemia, acidosis, etc. should also be corrected preoperatively by the intravenous infusion of appropriate IV solutions.

All the children should be accurately weighed after admission, because body weight is the simplest and most reliable guide to drug doses. Hemoglobin estimation should be performed routinely. A perioperative Hb of <10 g/dL does not necessarily entail cancelation of surgery, if the child is otherwise fit and the surgery is not much blood-losing. All children above the 3 months of age, coming from Africa or Mediterranean countries, are likely to be the carriers of sickle cell disease. So, they should be screened by sickle cell test and then Hb electrophoresis should be undertaken, if the screening test is positive.

A nasogastric tube should always be passed in all the sick pediatric patients, because during the intraoperative or postoperative period, gastric distension occurs readily in them and may jeopardize their normal respiratory function and may cause regurgitation with subsequent pulmonary aspiration, leading to acidosis and pneumonia.

Fasting

The purpose of fasting of any patient, before anesthesia and surgery, is to decrease the risk of aspiration pneumonitis from regurgitation of gastric acidic juice and asphyxia from the presence of solid food in vomitus. The aspiration pneumonitis occurs, if the pH of gastric fluid is <2.4 and the volume aspirated is >0.8 mL/kg. The neonates, scheduled for surgery within 24 hours after birth, are usually not fed by mouth and so they do not need any fasting protocol. But, the neonates or infants, who are presented for surgery after feeding, need a fasting protocol which is extensively reviewed and different from the previous protocol. Recently, a number of studies have shown that there is no difference between the residual gastric volume and pH in children who are allowed to fast for 2–3 hours prior to the induction of anesthesia, and those who are allowed to fast overnight or a standard fasting for 6 hours. *It is also demonstrated that fasting for >2 hours after oral, clear fluid ingestion does not decrease the risk of aspiration and pneumonitis, if aspiration occurs.* Again, the half-life of water in the stomach is only about 12 minutes which implies that 95% of ingested water leaves the stomach within 1 hour. The half-life for breast milk is about 25 minutes and that for formulated milk is 51 minutes. So, the breast milk leaves the stomach more rapidly than the formulated milk. Hence, a moderate approach of allowing the children to drink clear fluid (water, apple juice, etc.), 3 hours before the induction of anesthesia, has several advantages. *These recommendations are, however, for the healthy neonates, infants and children who are without any risk factors for decreased gastric emptying or aspiration.* For preoperative fasting protocol see the **Table 14**.

The advantages of allowing the children to drink clear fluid, three hours before the induction of anesthesia, are:
- From psychological point of view, this approach is more human and is also more satisfactory for both the parents

TABLE 14: Preoperative fasting guidelines for pediatric patients (fasting time in hours).

Age (months)	Clear fluid	Breast milk	Cow/formulated milk	Solid
<3	2	4	4	6
3–6	2	4	4	6
6–36	2–3	4–6	6	6
>36	2–3	4–6	6	6

Note: A clear fluid is defined as a fluid through which a newspaper can be read.

and the children, without increasing the risk of pulmonary aspiration of gastric contents and pneumonitis.
- As pediatric patients have higher metabolic rate and larger body surface area/weight ratio than adults, therefore, there are more chances of dehydration and metabolic acidosis in prolonged fasting than adults. But, 2–3 hours fasting decreases the chances of dehydration, hypoglycemia, and acidosis.
- There is less chance of hypovolemia during the induction of anesthesia.
- The incidences of aspiration are very low and are reported to be approximately 1:1,000 in pediatric patients. So, the prolonged fasting does not necessarily decrease this risk.

However, these recommendations are only for the healthy neonates, infants, and children, without the risk factors of decreased gastric emptying or aspiration.

The formulated milk should be considered as solid food. So, for any form of milk, other than breast milk, the standard fasting of 6 hours or more is advised. But, there is also some evidence that infants <3 months may safely be given infant formula feed or cow's milk up to 4 hours, preoperatively. Infants who are breastfed may have their last feed 4 hours prior to the anesthetic induction. In emergency settings, e.g., in a child, who has sustained trauma shortly after having food, it is probably best (if possible) to wait for 6 hours, before the induction of anesthesia. Clearly in this situation, risk-benefit judgment has to be made, especially, if the surgery is a dire emergency.

Premedication

The *aim of premedication* in pediatric anesthesia is (1) to produce a calm and cooperative child, before the induction of anesthesia. Premedication is also used (2) to reduce the stress of anesthesia and surgery and also (3) to reduce the risk of postoperative nausea/vomiting and behavioral disturbances. The *psychological preparation* of pediatric patients is an important aspect of preoperative care, especially for the younger children. So, preoperative counseling is the best form of premedication for younger children. The anesthesiologist should avoid wearing a white coat and will explain in great details to the family and this child, how the anesthesia will be administered to the children and what will be done to ensure the utmost safety. The more the information the parents and this child have, the more easily they can be dealt with the stress of surgery and hospitalization. Presurgical programs, such as videotapes, literature, and booklets are also very helpful and make easy the preoperative counseling and physiological preparation. After the admission in hospital, but before anesthesia and surgery, every effort should be made to help the child to adjust the new hospital environment by friendly interior design, availability of toys, collection of photographs, etc. But, unfortunately, outpatients and morning-of-admission surgery, together with a busy operating room schedule often make it difficult for an anesthesiologist to have enough time for this preoperative counseling and psychological preparation. For this reason, premedication in the form of medicine can be extremely helpful.

Sometimes, sedative premedication is required, especially for children who in spite of good preoperative counseling remains apprehensive. They include the (1) excessively upset child, (2) children with previous unpleasant experiences of anesthesia and surgery, and (3) certain children with developmental delays, such as with cerebral palsy and Down syndrome. The preschool children are mostly at risk. They are more vulnerable to separation anxiety in a strange hospital environment, but without the ability to reason himself. Older children or adolescents may request premedication. Sometimes, even when the anesthesia and surgery are uneventful, still there may be a disturbingly high incidence of postoperative psychological problems which include nightmares, sleeping disturbances, bed-wetting, eating disorders, behavioral changes, etc.

The prior use of local anesthetic cream, such as the eutectic mixture of local anesthetic (EMLA), Ametop, or tetracaine gel has some advantages and reduces the necessity of sedative premedications for the establishment of an IV cannula. The availability of these abovementioned topical local anesthetic creams reduces the pain of venipuncture and greatly facilitates the intravenous induction. EMLA cream is a eutectic mixture of 5% lignocaine and 5% prilocaine in 1:1 ratio. It should be applied at least 40–50 minutes before any needle prick and can produce vasoconstriction. The EMLA cream should be avoided in children, below the 1 year of age and this is because of the risk of methemoglobinemia from absorbed prilocaine, due to the reduced levels of methemoglobin reductase enzyme in infants. *Ametop* is a 4% gel formulation of amethocaine. It is licensed to be used above the age of 4 weeks and has vasodilating property.

It has a shorter onset of action which is about 30 minutes and a prolonged duration of action which is about 4 hours. But, it has a higher incidence of allergic reactions.

Sedative premedication should not be used at the expense of respiratory depression. Sedative premedication is contraindicated (not absolute) in patients with respiratory insufficiency or airways obstruction. In some surgeries, like cleft palate, neurosurgery, tonsillectomy, etc. sedative premedication are usually not used, because it delays the recovery of laryngeal or other reflexes which is not at all desirable for these types of surgeries for the pediatric group of patients. But, this rule is not mandatory. However, much less sedation is required if the child has been carefully prepared by preanesthetic counseling.

Sedative premedication is not used in neonates and infants usually below 6 months of age, as separation anxiety is not a concern in this age group and this group of patients is more sensitive to respiratory and cardiovascular depressant effects of the sedative agents. But, this protocol is not followed by some group of anesthesiologists, because the time interval between the last feed and the scheduled timing for surgery cannot be controlled properly in a busy hospital. So, the children usually cry and disturb their parents. Hence, to reduce the anxiety of parents some anesthetists break the protocol and premedication is given to make the baby sleep.

Atropine or glycopyrrolate is sometimes used as an antisialagogue during premedication, because increased secretion in narrow pediatric airways may cause airway obstruction and respiratory distress in the pediatric group of patients. Though the vagal tone is low in neonates, but in some centers atropine is given IV routinely during induction of anesthesia, particularly if suxamethonium and halothane is used. But, atropine is also omitted in some centers because of low vagal tone, especially in the newborns and also because of the danger of increasing the viscosity of bronchial secretions, particularly in babies with dehydration or mucoviscidosis which may lead to the plugging of bronchioles or even the main bronchi with inspissated mucus. They also do not use atropine routinely, because modern anesthetic agents do not require antisialagogue (anticholinergic) agent due to their minimal irritating and secreting effects. The absorption of orally administered atropine (40 µg/kg) is variable. So, to ensure efficacy atropine (20 µg/kg) or glycopyrrolate (10 µg/kg) is administered intramuscularly 30 minutes before OT. Many anesthesiologists prefer atropine IV at or shortly after induction. If the baby is pyrexial and toxic, then atropine should be used in small doses or may even be omitted, balancing between the risk of febrile convulsions and necessity.

Almost all the sedatives are effective as premedication. But, the choice depends on individual anesthetist and the protocol of institution. The need for sedative premedication must be individualized, according to the underlying medical conditions of patients, the length of surgery, and the desired induction procedures of anesthesia. Sedative premedications may be administered through oral, IM, rectal, sublingual, nasal, or IV route and doses are based on the body weight of child. Among them the oral route is mostly preferred in pediatric patients. The disadvantage of rectal route is that the effect of such administration is likely to be unpredictable. IM route provides accuracy of doses and certainty of actions, but very few children welcome this route.

For sedation as premedication midazolam, given orally (0.3–0.5 mg/kg, 15 mg maximum), is gaining widespread popularity. The effect of this oral preparation of midazolam occurs within 10 minutes and its peak effect reaches 20–30 minutes after its oral administration. However, it does not influence the discharge time in day-case surgeries as one of the disadvantages of sedative premedication is that it prolongs the discharge time. Though, there is oral preparation of midazolam, but it is not available in all countries. Hence, the parenteral preparation of midazolam can also be given orally, but it has a very bitter taste. This can be eliminated by diluting it in concentrated sweet fruit juice. The paracetamol elixir is also suitable for mixing with injectable form of midazolam for oral administration and has the merit of incorporating an analgesic component to the premedicant. Smaller doses of midazolam have been used in combination with oral ketamine (4–6 mg/kg) for inpatients. As an alternative to midazolam, in some centers the parenteral preparation of ketamine is also used orally in a dose of 3–10 mg/kg as premedication. But, ketamine causes excessive salivation and increases PONV. So, an antisialagogue and an antiemetic should always be used with ketamine premedication. If a profound degree of sedation is required during the preoperative preparation of patient, then it is also possible to combine midazolam with ketamine. A relatively new route for administration of midazolam and ketamine as premedication is the intranasal route. But, at this stage it is still unknown, how much of the drug applied through intranasal route, is absorbed directly into CNS through the cribriform plate and how much is absorbed through nasal mucosa. But, it will have to keep in mind that preservatives present in injectable preparations of these two drugs (as preservative free special preparation for use through nasal rouse is not available) are neurotoxic when passes directly to neural tissues through cribriform plate. So, it is better not to use this preservative added preparation of these two agents, through this nasal route, at present.

The nasal and rectal doses of midazolam are respectively 0.2–0.3 mg/kg and 0.4–0.5 mg/kg. The nasal and rectal doses of ketamine are respectively 3 mg/kg and 6 mg/kg. Because of the decrease in bioavailability of these drugs through oral and rectal route, the doses of these agents must be significantly higher when using these routes than with other routes.

The use of fentanyl as premedicant through oral transmucosal route is very popular, though it can also be used through any other routes. For absorption through buccal mucosa, it is prepared by incorporating fentanyl in a lozenge, like lollipop and the children are allowed to suck it. It is available in doses of different ranges. The swallowing of saliva decreases its efficacy, because the first pass metabolism of fentanyl, i.e., when it passes through liver, is high. The onset of action of fentanyl through transmucosal route is 20–30 seconds and the duration of action of fentanyl through this route is 30 minutes for a dose of 10–15 µg/kg of fentanyl. The disadvantages of fentanyl as premedication are pruritus, nausea, vomiting, respiratory depression, and frequent oxygen desaturation. Respiratory rate decreases within 10 minutes. So, constant observation and monitoring of patient is required and it should be administered only in a monitored clinical setting. The principal advantage of fentanyl as premedication is decrease in intra- and postoperative analgesic requirement, but it does not delay the discharge of patient from hospital.

Sufentanil also can be used as a premedicant, like fentanyl. But, it is most successful when it is used through intranasal route. However, the intranasal dose of sufentanil is 1.5–3 µg/kg and it sedates the child within 10 minutes. However, the disadvantages of sufentanil are same as fentanyl. Traditionally, the children undergoing cardiac surgery need heavy premedication. Here, naturally, the choice is morphine, because it can prevent the spasm of right ventricular infundibulum in uncorrected Fallot's tetralogy.

There are many other drugs which also can be used for sedative premedication. These are diazepam (0.4 mg/kg orally), lorazepam, trimeprazine (vallergan, 3–4 mg/kg orally), chloral hydrate, promethazine (1 mL/kg), etc. The injection of vitamin K1 in the dose of 1 mg should always be given through IM to all the newborns, in view of the immaturity of hepatic production of prothrombin. The longer duration of action makes lorazepam unsuitable as premedicant for daycare surgery. The chloral hydrate and triclofos are used as more for sedation than premedication. The oral doses of chloral hydrate and triclofos are 25–50 mg/kg and 50 mg/kg, respectively.

Induction of Anesthesia

The method of induction of anesthesia, in pediatric group of patients, is most colorful and is determined by a number of factors, such as (1) the age of the patient, (2) the behavior or the psychological setup of the child, (3) the ability of the child to cooperate with anesthetist, (4) the medical conditions of the patient, (5) the proposed surgical procedure, and (6) the presence or the absence of full stomach. But, among these, the last and the *most important factor is the anesthetic procedure with which the anesthesiologist is most convenient or competent.*

When the infants are younger (less) than 10–12 months of age, then the induction of anesthesia by volatile anesthetic agents, through face masks, is the procedure of choice. Fortunately, the modern, potent, volatile anesthetic agents can render the small children unconscious within minutes. This is also usually easier in children who have been sedated prior to entering the operating room and who are sleepy enough without ever knowing what his happening *(steal induction)*. There are also some other healthy alternatives to the abovementioned inhalational technique, for induction of anesthesia, without frightening the children and these are described in the **Box 4**.

Typically, during inhalational induction, the child coax for breathing an odorless mixture of N_2O (70%) and O_2 (30%). Sevoflurane or halothane is added to this anesthetic gas mixture, gradually in increasing concentration of 0.5%, after every 3–5 breaths. Many, if not most, pediatric anesthetists consider sevoflurane as the agent of choice for inhalational induction rather than halothane, because sevoflurane has a wider therapeutic safety window in terms of cardiovascular depression and has no unpleasant smell. The desflurane and

isoflurane are not used for induction, because they have more pungent smell and are associated with increased coughing, breath holding, laryngospasm etc. during the induction of anesthesia. Some clinicians use a *single-breath induction technique* with the sevoflurane of initial 7–8% concentration to speed up the induction. It produces unconsciousness very rapidly, after 4–6 breaths, without any excitement. But, this single-breath technique should not be used with halothane, as it has severe cardiodepressant effects. When the single-breath technique, using the high concentration of halothane and sevoflurane, is not used, then the patients typically pass through an excitement stage, during which period, any stimulation by premature attempt of laryngoscopy or even IV cannulation can induce laryngospasm.

There are many differences between an adult and pediatric anatomy of airway that influence the mask ventilation and intubation. Equipment, appropriate for age and size **(Table 15)**, should be selected. The neonates and most young infants are obligate nasal breathers and obstruct easily. Nasal airways, which are useful for adults, traumatize the small nares and prominent adenoids in small children. Oral airway will help to displace the oversized tongue. Compression of submandibular soft tissues should be avoided during mask ventilation to prevent upper airway obstruction. Positive pressure ventilation during mask induction and prior to intubation sometimes causes gastric distension with impairment of lung expansion. Sucking with an orogastric or nasogastric tube will decompress the stomach.

In older children, who allow an IV line before induction of anesthesia, then, in such circumstances intravenous induction is preferred. Intravenous induction is also preferred, if the patient comes to the operating room with a previously inserted intravenous catheter, due to some other reasons. Intravenous cannulation on premature, neonates, and infants can be a vexing ordeal. This is more true for them who have spent few days in a NICU and have no intact

---

BOX 4: More healthy options of induction without frightening the child.

- Insufflation of anesthetic gases over the child's face
- Substituting a clear, scented face mask in the place of a traditional black one
- Placing a drop of food flavoring oil inside the mask (e.g., oil of orange)
- Allowing the child to sit during the early stages of induction

---

TABLE 15: Equipment appropriate for age.

	Premature	Neonate	Infant	Toddler	Young child	Old child
Age	0–1 months	0–1 months	1–12 months	1–3 years	3–8 years	8–12 years
Weight (kg)	0.5–2.5	2.5–5	5–10	10–15	15–30	30–50
Mask size	00	0	0	1	2	3
Oral airway size	000–00	00	0 (40 mm)	1 (50 mm)	2 (70 mm)	3 (80 mm)
Laryngoscope blade size	00	0	1	1.5	2.0	3.0
Endotracheal tube (ET) tube (ID in mm)	2.5–3.0	3.0–3.5	3.5–4.0	4.0–4.5	4.5–5.0	5.0–6.0
Laryngeal mask airway (LMA) size	1.0	1.0	1.0	2.0	2.5	3.0

veins. Even healthy children can prove a challenge because of extensive subcutaneous fat. The saphenous vein has a consistent location at ankle and it can easily be cannulated, even if it is not visible or palpable. The transillumination technique or ultrasonography often helps in such difficult situation. In emergency situations, where repeated attempts for intravenous cannulation have failed, then the parenteral fluids can effectively be infused through an 18-G needle inserted into the medullary sinusoids of tibial bone. This intraosseous infusion can be used for all medications which are given normally intravenously. The drugs act in this route, as rapidly as IV route, and is considered as a part of standard trauma resuscitation, advanced cardiac life support (ACLS), and pediatric advanced life support (PALS) protocols when intravenous access cannot be obtained.

Patients, with full stomach, always need intravenous rapid induction and intubation, with or without succinylcholine. In such situation, induction by inhalational agents, even by single-breath technique, is never tried to prevent aspiration of gastric contents. For IV induction of anesthesia, the thiopentone, propofol, ketamine, midazolam, diazepam, etc., can be used. The induction of anesthesia by *intramuscular ketamine* injection (5–10 mg/kg) is only reserved for some specific situations, such as (1) the handling of a very violent child who will not take any oral premedicant, (2) the patient refuses to cooperate during the induction of anesthesia by volatile inhalational agents, (3) the patient is younger and healthy enough who requires many assistant to apply force for the inhalation of volatile anesthetic agents, (4) there is no IV line before hand for intravenous induction, and (5) those involving combative, particularly mentally challenged or autistic patients.

The child should be accompanied by parents (or someone with whom he or she is comfortable) to the anesthesia room. The person, accompanying the child, should be informed beforehand what to expect in anesthesia room. He should be made aware of the excitation state of child, when the inhalational induction by mask is initiated or he should be made aware of how to assist the anesthetist when IV induction is planned by distracting the child. During mask induction by volatile anesthetic agents, breath holding by the patient is very common and if so, then one should not attempt to assist respiration by squeezing the bag because this often elicits cough and laryngospasm. Breath holding should be differentiated from airway obstruction or laryngospasm by an anesthetist by observing the movements of bag, chest wall and abdomen. Airway obstruction, most commonly due to the falling of tongue, can be managed by the extension of neck and by an upward thrust of mandible, applied at its angle. But, if laryngospasm occurs, then the closing of pop-off valve of anesthetic circuit and simple creation of positive

airway pressure of about 10 cmH$_2$O (while allowing the child to breathe spontaneously and not squeezing the bag) will often help to overcome the laryngospasm and will allow the entry gas into lungs. Still, if this procedure is ineffective, then administration of positive pressure ventilation by squeezing the bag, but avoiding the inflation of stomach, often will disrupt the laryngospasm. However, in very emergency conditions, the intravenous muscle relaxant is the only answer. But, if IV line is not yet instituted, then only the puncture of cricothyroid membrane for ventilation can save the life of child.

In children, where difficult airway is anticipated, the induction by mask should be done very slowly, gradually increasing the concentration of inhalational anesthetic agent and maintaining spontaneous respiration. As the level of anesthesia deepens, then gentle manual assistance of ventilation by anesthetist, corroborating with spontaneous respiration, may be done. This allows an anesthesiologist to assess whether he will be able or not to ventilate successfully by mask, when muscle relaxant is used and intubation fails. Muscle relaxant should be used, only if an anesthetist feels that he can ventilate the patient successfully by mask, if intubation fails too. A child with an airway obstruction should have a slow and prolonged induction of anesthesia before allowing laryngoscopy and ET intubation. In some emergency conditions, when the patient presents with full stomach and airway problem, then the issue of full stomach is secondary to the airway problem. Rapid sequence induction of anesthesia and intubation is indicated in these patients. A surgical team should be prepared to perform an emergency tracheostomy, if the total airway obstruction occurs and mask ventilation or ET intubation fails.

Induction of anesthesia through rectal route is also a unique technique in pediatric group of patients and has many advantages over oral route. Many different medications are used rectally for induction of anesthesia. The main advantage of this approach is that the child falls asleep in parent's arms and hence the separation of patient from his or her parent is atraumatic. This technique (administration of inducing agent through oral route) is no more intimidating than taking a rectal temperature. Oxygen desaturation is usually not a problem, unless the child's head flexes forward causing airway problem.

Other than inhalational, intravenous, and rectal route, many medications are also used intramuscularly for induction of anesthesia, like premedication. But, here the only difference between the induction of anesthesia and premedication is the doses of drugs used. The main advantage of this route for induction of anesthesia over rectal and oral route is its reliability but its main disadvantage is being a painful procedure.

A child with a full stomach should be treated like an adult with full stomach. As metabolic rate is much greater in pediatric patients, so O_2 desaturation occurs more rapidly in neonates and infants than children and more rapidly in children than adults. However, the added problem in this group of patient is that the children are usually uncooperative and refuse to breathe 100% O_2 prior to induction (preoxygenation) for denitrogenation. Like an adult, all the steps of rapid induction and intubation should be followed in pediatric patients with full stomach. During induction of pediatric group of patients with full stomach, injection of atropine is mandatory. This is because atropine will prevent anesthesia induced reflexes, succinylcholine-induced bradycardia and delay the bradycardia due to hypoxemia. During induction and intubation of a patient with full stomach, cricoid pressure is also mandatory and is applied gently after the child loses consciousness. Awake or sedated awake intubation with topical anesthesia should be considered for emergency procedures in neonates and small infants when they are critically ill or a potential difficult airway is present.

Unlike adult practice, it is not possible to have all the necessary monitoring devices placed on the child before induction. So, the appropriate monitoring should be placed as soon as possible, after the induction of anesthesia.

For mask induction, different types of face masks are also used. Face masks with different sizes and different flavors or scents are now also available to reduce the unpleasant smell of anesthetic vapors. Scented transparent silicon or plastic masks are much more acceptable to little children than the traditional Rendell-Baker or Soucek masks which are made up of black rubber or polyvinyl chloride (PVC). But, the advantage of these later masks is that they have very small dead space of only 4 mL. On the other hand, the transparent clear plastic masks allow an anesthetist to observe the presence of vomitus, though they have high dead space volume. In fact, the Rendell-Baker mask was originally developed to fit around the facial anatomy of a child in an attempt to minimize equipment dead space. But, the flow of fresh gas in a clear mask is such that the advantage of using a Rendell-Baker mask has now become minimal. On the other hand, these Rendell-Baker masks are much more difficult to use than the transparent ones with pneumatic cushion. An alternative way for induction of anesthesia, in the absence of face mask, is cupping of anesthesiologists hand over the face of a child, while holding and directing the T-piece carrying anesthetic gases toward the nose of the patient.

Airway Management

The ratio of the dead space and tidal volume ($V_D/V_T = 0.4$) remains constant throughout the life of a healthy patient. But, any increase in the dead space by anesthetic apparatus, circuits, connectors, humidifiers, etc., also significantly increases the V_D and V_T ratio and this has significant effect on ventilation. Therefore, always this (increment of dead space by anesthetic apparatus, circuits, connectors, etc.) should be kept at a minimum level. Further, this is very important for a child who breaths spontaneously and has a compromised cardiovascular and respiratory systems. The anesthetic circuit which is most commonly used in children under 5 years of age or below 20 kg of body weight throughout the world, is the Jackson Rees modification of Ayres T-piece. This is also called the Mapleson F system.

The original Ayer's T-piece was made up of a light metal T-tube with a main lumen of 1 cm in diameter. A smaller side tube was attached at right angles to the main lumen through which the anesthetic gas mixture was introduced. Then, a length of a rubber tube was attached to the open end of the main lumen of this T-piece and it acts as a reservoir of anesthetic gases. This rubber tubing is called the expiratory limb. This is the modification of the Ayer's T-piece to the Mapleson E circuit. To prevent the dilution of FGF by air and to avoid rebreathing, the capacity of this expiratory limb must be greater than the tidal volume and the FGF must be twice than the MV of the patient.

In 1950, Jackson Rees again modified this system by attaching an open-tailed breathing bag to the reservoir tube in order to facilitate the controlled ventilation and to observe the spontaneous ventilation. This is called the Mapleson F circuit **(Fig. 6)**. The reservoir bag in the Mapleson F circuit helps (1) to observe the respiration, (2) to assess the tidal volume of a patient and the compliance of lung, (3) to reduce the dead space during spontaneous ventilation (as the FGF washes out the expired gas during the pause after each expiration), and (4) allows the application of continuous

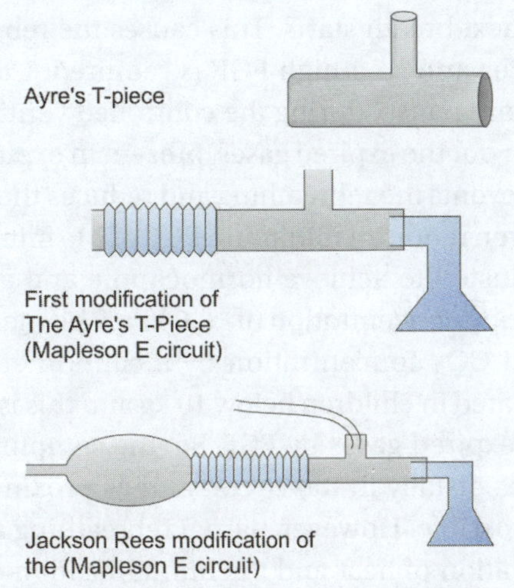

Fig. 6: Ayre's T-piece and modification over it.

positive airway pressure (CPAP) in a spontaneous ventilation or positive end-expiratory pressure (PEEP) in controlled ventilation which helps in improving oxygenation.

The main *advantages* of this valve less circuit are: simplicity, light weight, low resistance, and minimal apparatus dead space and helping in manual ventilation (if needed) by the open-ended reservoir bag. This circuit may be used both for the spontaneous and controlled ventilation. Controlled ventilation (manually or by a ventilator) is the most satisfactory mode of ventilation for neonates and infants, because any changes in compliance, air leak, tube displacement, etc. can easily be detected. For mechanical ventilation, the bag is removed and an appropriate ventilator is attached to the expiratory limb. Scavenging system may be connected indirectly to the circuit which prevents the possibility of blockage of the expiratory flow.

The *disadvantage* of this circuit is the absence of a pressure relief valve in it. It is very popular both for the induction and the maintenance of anesthesia for short duration. The recommended FGF to maintain normocarbia in a Mapleson F circuit, during spontaneous respiration, is 200–300 mL/kg. But, FGF of only 70 mL/kg produces normocarbia (normocapnia) during controlled ventilation. The FGF, approximately equal to normal MV, is also sufficient to maintain normocapnia in controlled ventilation. This is because CO_2 rebreathing has no consequence during controlled ventilation in this circuit and an anesthetist can control $PaCO_2$ by increasing ventilation.

Another recommendation for FGF rate, necessary to prevent rebreathing: 2.5 times the minute ventilation, for spontaneous breathing or 1,000 mL + 200 mL/kg in controlled ventilation.

This discrepancy for this recommendation of FGF rate is dependent on respiratory pattern. A high respiratory rate, with minimal expiratory pause, allows no time for the FGF to flush out the expired gases through expiratory limb before the next breath starts. This causes the rebreathing of expired gases and so a high FGF is required. Contrary, an end expiratory pause, during the controlled ventilation, will help to flush out the expired gases, present in expiratory limb and thus prevents the rebreathing and reduces the FGF. Most of the children require a minimum FGF of 3 L/min which can then be adjusted to achieve normocapnia and an inspired carbon dioxide concentration of <0.6 kPa. The measurement of end tidal CO_2 concentration by a capnometer may be underestimated in children below 10 kg and this is due to the dilution of expired gases by FGF. So, the sampling of gases should be as distally in the circuit and as proximally to the patient as possible. However, partial rebreathing also allows the conservation of heat and the humidification of inspired gases in ventilators.

The MV should be calculated by: MV = tidal volume (10 mL/kg) × RR. After tracheal intubation, controlled ventilation (if it is decided) can be conducted either manually or mechanically by ventilators. Traditionally, many institutions still prefer manual controlled ventilation, because it allows a breath-by-breath estimation of the changes in chest compliance. But, gradually the need for manual assessment of chest compliance is pushed back and to assure adequacy of ventilation the modern noninvasive monitoring techniques, such as oximetry, capnography, and pressure-volume loops are now in widespread.

Moreover, the manual ventilation limits the activities of an anesthetist and may provide a false sense of security in detecting the changes in compliance by hand. But, still the ability to hand-ventilate using the Ayre's T-piece (Mapleson F circuit) is essential in pediatric practice and such circuit should always be available at hand in cases of the failure of mechanical ventilation by ventilator (when patient is mechanically ventilated) or unexpected desaturation. In a baby with gastroschisis or exomphalos, manual ventilation can be used to assess the changes in lung compliance and can determine the volume of abdominal contents that can be reduced back into abdominal cavity. Manual ventilation, during the repair of TE fistula, can be timed properly which allows the surgeon to get maximum exposure and time for the repair.

Standard adult ventilators are also suitable for pediatric patients with weight >20 kg. But, below 20 kg, a pediatric version is needed with the ability to deliver small tidal volumes, rapid respiratory rate, variable inspiratory flow rate, and different I:E ratio. However, the always measurement of this small inspired tidal volume is meaningless, because the compression of gases in the ventilator tubing and variable leaks around the ET tube gives a false security. But, the more sophisticated ventilators may, however, be capable of measuring the expired tidal volume which is of more practical value.

Two modes of controlled ventilation are commonly used for the neonates and infants. These are (1) Volume controlled/time cycled and (2) Pressure controlled/time cycled. The volume controlled/time cycled ventilation deliver a fixed tidal volume which is based on inspiratory time and inspiratory flow, but is independent of peak inspiratory pressure. It makes an allowance for changes in lung compliance, but at the potential cost of high peak airway pressure. With decrease in compliance of lungs, the tidal volume does not change, but the peak airway pressure changes. However, in contrast to the volume controlled/time cycled ventilation, the pressure controlled/time cycled ventilation delivers a variable tidal volume, under a fixed inspiratory peak pressure. Here, the tidal volume or MV varies directly with the compliance of chest wall and lung and is indicated by the movement of bellow or is seen directly on the panel screen. As the compliance decreases, the tidal volume also decreases and vice versa. However, both these ventilatory modes should be used with caution, when there are chances of marked variation in lung's compliance, due to surgery or pathological conditions, such as bronchoconstriction and pulmonary edema. To account for the changes in lung compliance, when using a pressure-controlled ventilation, the adequacy of alveolar ventilation can only be assessed by using a breath-by-breath capnography.

The ultimate setting of a ventilator's parameters depends on the clinical observation and the results from monitors. The inspiratory flow, by changing the pressure or volume, can be gradually increased or decreased, until the optimum chest movement is observed. The measurement of capnography and pulse oximetry confirms normocapnia and adequate oxygenation. The peak airway pressure should always be kept at minimum level and an alarm at both the upper and lower limits of expected peak pressure is mandatory in all ventilators. Most of the children are ventilated adequately with a respiratory rate in-between 20 and 30 breaths/min and inspiratory peak pressure in-between 15 and 20 cmH$_2$O. The respiratory rate should be adjusted accordingly to achieve the normocapnia.

In a ventilator, the respiratory rate is set electronically between 20 and 30 breaths/min and inspiratory: expiratory ratio varies from 1:1 to 1:3. The gas flow rate required to produce a given MV is obtained by using a nomogram. This takes into account the volume of gas which is lost during the expiratory phase. PEEP may be applied to the expiratory limb of the ventilator. This can also be used as a constant pressure device (CPAP) by incorporating a pressure-limiting relief valve **(Fact file I)**.

Nonrebreathing valves are also used in pediatric anesthesia. But, they tend to stick and produce more resistance and dead space. Circle absorber is used in pediatric anesthetic circuit in some countries (e.g., USA). They have light tubing, silicone rubber valves, low gas flow with efficient humidification, warming, and scavenging systems.

FACT FILE I

The tidal volume of neonates is only 20 mL and the physiological dead space is just its one-third. So, the amount of alveolar ventilation in neonates is only 14 mL. Hence, the addition of even a very small dead space from the anesthetic apparatus (even a few milliliter) represents a very large proportional increase in dead space and tidal volume ratio. Masks are not suitable for neonates and infants for prolonged periods, because they usually require intubation. However, good fitting of the face mask is more important than its low dead space, because the latter can be reduced by increasing the FGF within the mask. The Rendell-Baker and Soucek masks do not make a good air seal on the face, though their dead space is very low.

For the older children, over 20 kg, it is satisfactory to use the Bains, Humphrey ADE, or the circle absorber system. The Humphrey ADE circuit is a hybrid system, incorporating Mapleson A, D, and E types of circuits in one breathing system (circuit). Here, the E mode behaves similar to T-piece. The A mode is efficient in children over 10 kg of weight. Both the D and E modes are suitable for controlled ventilation. The circle absorber system offers economic advantages, because a low FGF required for it. It also conserves warmth and moisture, as the reaction of CO$_2$ with soda lime is exothermic, producing heat and water. While using the circle absorber system, in a completely close circuit, then the ability to monitor the inspiratory and expiratory levels of O$_2$, N$_2$O, CO$_2$, and volatile anesthetic agents is mandatory. The unidirectional valves may increase the resistance to breathing and should not be allowed to become damp. Pediatric circle system, using a 15-mm light-weight hose, is suitable for children over 5 kg. Till now, there is no evidence of nephrotoxicity in children due to compound A formed by the action of sevoflurane with soda lime.

In the past, much interest had been given to the resistance of breathing system and the dead space volume of apparatus, during the use of circle CO$_2$ absorber system which led pediatric anesthesiologists to use nonabsorber (Mapleson F circuit) systems mainly. However, recently the attitude has changed and there is renewed interest in the use of circle system with CO$_2$ absorber in pediatric anesthesia practice.

The recent research works do not support the opinion that the circle system with CO$_2$ absorber imposes more resistance to breathing in infants and children during controlled ventilation. In contrast, it appears that the mechanical dead space, imposed by some T-piece connectors, can be excessive during spontaneous respiration. Some problems, such as muscle fatigue, inefficient ventilation, and tendency for lung collapse which were observed previously with circle absorber system, were due to spontaneous breathing with this system. So, it can be advised that if ventilation is either controlled or assisted in neonates or infants, then a standard adult circle system which is fitted with low dead space connectors, small bore tubing, and a reduced capacity reservoir bag, is appropriate for the maintenance of anesthesia in pediatric patients of all ages **(Box 5)**. Again, it is easy to scavenge the waste gases from all these systems, with the resultant benefit of reducing the pollution of theater environment.

An appropriately sized Guedel's airway is an important and useful adjunct in maintaining the airway when a child is being anesthetized, but not intubated. A too small airway is ineffective and a too large airway may obstruct the larynx itself. So, an airway of correct length is used and this length is

<table>
<tr><td colspan="2">BOX 5: Reasons for a renewed interest in the use of circle system with CO₂ absorber in pediatric practice.</td></tr>
</table>

BOX 5: Reasons for a renewed interest in the use of circle system with CO_2 absorber in pediatric practice.

- Increased concern about economy
- Environmental pollution
- Improvement in the design of anesthetic machines and ventilators
- Use of the small bore anesthetic circuits, reducing the anatomical dead space
- Increase in availability and use of multigas analyzers
- The desire to use standard anesthetic breathing circuits for patients of all ages

BOX 6: Estimation of laryngeal mask airway (LMA) size in pediatric patients.

Size of LMA	Weight (kg)	Cuff volume (mL)
1	0–5	2–5
1.5	5–10	5–7
2	10–20	7–10
2.5	20–30	12–14
3	Large child >30	15–20

measured which is equivalent to the distance from the angle of mouth to the angle of mandible.

Depending on the surgical and patient requirements, general anesthesia (GA) in pediatric group of patients can be maintained with face mask, ET tube, or LMA. But, the introduction of LMA offers a healthy alternative to face mask anesthesia with Guedel's airway in patients, scheduled for minor surgery. Both the indication and the insertion technique of LMA for pediatric patients are similar to that of an adult. For the preterm neonates who require GA, the spontaneous ventilation with face mask or LMA is avoided, because they are more prone to periodic breathing and apnea during GA. Nevertheless, the role of LMA in neonatal surgery is limited. This is because in most instances, the neonatal airway should be secured to prevent aspiration and to facilitate positive pressure ventilation, but neither of which can be properly assured with LMA. Infants are also poor candidates for anesthesia with spontaneous ventilation by LMA and higher doses of volatile anesthetics. It is because of poor pulmonary mechanics, causing early respiratory failure and increased susceptibility to cardiovascular depressant effects of volatile anesthetic agents. These groups of patients are likely to be benefited best from balanced anesthesia, offered by the full dose of muscle relaxant, intubation, controlled ventilation, minimum concentration of volatile anesthetic agents, and the optimum doses of opioids. Balanced anesthesia should also be applied to older children undergoing surgeries for >45 minutes duration. The surgeries, lasting for <30–40 minutes of duration, may be allowed to continue in children under spontaneous ventilation by LMA, with the mixture of N_2O, O_2, and volatile anesthetic agents, and is supplemented by the appropriate doses of opioids and local or regional block, where necessary.

For the maintenance of anesthesia and the maintenance of proper airway (from falling of tongue on larynx), the LMA is one step ahead of facemasks with Guedel's oropharyngeal airway, but one step behind the ET tube. So, it is in an intermediate position between the face mask with oropharyngeal airway (Guedel) and ET tube. During the maintenance of an anesthetized airway, the LMA has certain advantages over the face mask with Guedel's airway, but also has some disadvantages, when compared to ET tube. The LMA is generally used only when spontaneous breathing is planned in a child during surgery, though controlled ventilation can be performed with LMA when necessary. It does not protect the airway against aspiration of gastric contents, like ET tube. So, it is unwise to use the LMA in a patient with full stomach. The LMA is also displaced easily, causing airway obstruction. So, the present status of LMA is that it can be used in a variety of operations with spontaneous respiration or controlled ventilation, where the airway pressure is kept below 15–20 cmH_2O.

Laryngeal mask airways are available in different sizes (**Box 6**) to fit all the children, including neonates. But the neonatal (size 1) LMA is not popular for different reasons, such as difficulty to insert, easy displacement, and increased apparatus dead space resulting in rebreathing and hypercapnia. On the other hand, due to the large cross-sectional area of the LMA tube, airway resistance increases very little. The success rate for insertion of LMA in the neonates and infants is less. In 70% unsuccessful cases, it is seen that the epiglottis is not in the normal anatomical position. In most instances, the epiglottis is down folded over the laryngeal inlet or within the bowl of the LMA. This is because the LMA, used for the neonates and infants, is not designed according to their airway. Actually, the LMA designed for the adult airway is simply scaled down in size to fit the neonates, infants, and young children.

Endotracheal Tube

Though, previously it was mandatory to intubate the trachea, during the artificial ventilation in neonates and infants, but now with the advent of LMA, it is no more mandatory. Tracheal intubation with controlled respiration has several advantages. These *advantages* are (1) by tracheal intubation bronchial toileting becomes easy, (2) it protects the lungs against aspiration of gastric contents, and (3) if high pressure controlled ventilation is needed, then it will be possible by tracheal intubation. But, although when the patient is properly prepared and premedicated, then the incidences of aspiration is very low. Hence, the LMA is no longer contraindicated medicolegally from the points of view of aspiration, when the patient is prepared properly. However, the operations in oral cavity are not possible without tracheal intubation and with or without controlled ventilation. Even for the operations outside the oral cavity, it becomes very difficult to maintain an airway of a neonate by only using airway devices and a face mask, even for the shortest surgical procedures, requiring GA. So, it is usually wise to intubate trachea electively in most situations. But, intubation results in the reduction of cross-sectional area of airway. For example, a 3.5-mm ET tube causes an increase in resistance by a factor of 16. So, the tracheal intubation should not be followed by spontaneous ventilation. It always should be followed by controlled ventilation in order to reduce the work of breathing in pediatric patient.

There are different types of ET tubes which are used for pediatric patients. These are cuffed/uncuffed/Magill/Oxford/preformed [Ring-Adair-Elwyn (RAE)]/Armored/Cole, etc., and may be made of different materials, such as PVC, silicone, rubber, and plastic. The RAE tubes are not recommended routinely for the infants, because of the frequent inadvertent bronchial intubation caused by it. They are frequently used to facilitate the surgery around the head and neck. In RAE tube, there is a preformed bend that may be temporarily straightened during intubation. Both the cuffed and uncuffed versions of nasal and oral RAE tubes are also available in various sizes. As the diameter of RAE tube increases, the total length and the distance from the distal tip to the curve of the tube also increases. Frequently, there is a mark at the bend. In majority of cases, when this mark is at the level of teeth (in oral version) or naris (in nasal version), then the tip of the tube will be satisfactorily positioned in the midtrachea, provided the proper size of the tube for this patient is selected. However, this is just a guideline and should not be used as the sole criteria for judging the correct positioning of the tube **(Fact file II)**.

The curvature of the nasal RAE tube is opposite to the curvature of the oral RAE tube, so that when in place the outer portion of the tube is directed over the patient's forehead. This helps to reduce the pressure on the nares. This tube may also be useful for oral intubation of patients who are to be operated in prone position. The oral RAE tubes are shorter than the nasal ones. The external portion of the oral RAE tube is bent at an acute angle, so that when in place it rests on the patient's chin. These tubes are easy to secure and their use may reduce the risk of unintended extubation. The curvature of the RAE tube allows the breathing system

FACT FILE II

After ET intubation, controlled ventilation is the choice in neonates, infants, and in all babies up to 5–10 kg of body weight, even for minor surgical procedures. This is because:

- Small babies are very sensitive to respiratory depressant effects of anesthetic agents.
- Controlled ventilation provides adequate alveolar ventilation
- Controlled ventilation maintains the normal residual lung volume
- Unintentional delivery of large tidal volume to a small child can generate excessive peak airway pressure and cause barotrauma. So, pressure control ventilation, which is found on nearly all newer anesthetic ventilators, should be used for neonates, infants, and toddlers.
- Nonetheless, because breathing circuit resistance is easily overcome by positive pressure ventilation, the circle system can be safely used in patients of all ages, if ventilation is controlled.
- During spontaneous ventilation, even the low resistance of a circle system can become a significant resistance, because of unidirectional valves, breathing tubes and CO_2 absorber.
- Pediatric breathing circuits are usually short, lighter, and stiffer in contrast to adult circuit which are long, heavy, and complaint.
- Additional dead space contributed by the tube and circle system consists only of the volume of distal limb of Y-connector and the portion of ET tube that extends proximal to airway
- Condenser humidifiers or heat and moisture exchanger (HME) can add considerable dead space, depending on the size of patient. They either should not be used or an appropriately sized, pediatric HME should be employed.

The ventilation rate is maintained at 30–40 breaths/min, adequate tidal volume with peak inspiratory pressure of 15–20 cmH_2O, PEEP of 5 cmH_2O, and FGF of 4 L/min to preserve the FRC. For babies above 10 kg of body weight, spontaneous respiration with or without intubation may be allowed if the surgical procedure permits.

and its connections to be placed away from the surgical field during operations, especially around the head and neck without using special connectors. The disadvantages of RAE (preformed) tubes include difficulty in passing a suction catheter down them and these tubes offer more resistance than the comparable sized conventional ET tubes.

The spiral embedded armored tube has a spirally winded reinforcing wire which is made up of metal or nylon and is covered internally and externally by rubber, PVC, or silicone. Spirally embedded or armored tubes are especially useful in situations where bending or compression of the ET tube is likely to occur.

The ET tubes may be either disposable or reusable. The reusable red rubber ET tubes, though possibly more irritant to mucosa, are less liable to kinking and are easier to insert. Generally, uncuffed tubes are used in children below the age of 5 years. This is because cuff pressure may cause ischemic injury to the underlying tracheal mucosa which subsequently may lead to postintubation croup or severe postintubation laryngeal edema leading to obstruction. This postintubation laryngeal edema may also require further intubation or even tracheostomy. However, currently, most of the anesthesiologists do not use uncuffed tubes whose sizes are >4.0.

Another crucial point of pediatric anesthesia by intubation is the determination of the size or internal diameter (ID) of an ET tube, appropriate for the given patient. The general formula to calculate the ID or the appropriate size of tube is ID (in mm) = Age (years) ÷ 4 + 4. Now, for example, a 4-year-old child would be predicted to require a 5-mm ET tube. When using the above formula, any fractional sizes should be rounded up. This formula is only used as a rough guide to determine the size of a tracheal tube in children aged 4 years or above. But, the determination of the size of tube for neonates is guided by their body weight. It is better to recall that a neonate weighing ±3 kg will require a 3–3.5-mm (ID) tube. Low birth weight or premature babies need a 2.5–3.0-mm (ID) tube. Now, it will not be very difficult to determine the size of ET tube for the age group between the newborns and 4 years old child and it should be determined by the interpolation of sizes between 3 and 5 mm (ID) tube.

It is advisable to keep in hand the tubes of one size both larger and smaller (0.5 mm larger or smaller) than the selected tube during intubation. For neonates, the best guide in choosing the ET tube is weight. In pediatric patients, the ideal size of a tube will be like that when it is in place there should have a small air leak around it to prevent the damage of mucous membrane of the rigid subglottic region, i.e., the cricoid ring, which is the narrowest part of the child's airway. A correctly sized tube is one in which ventilation is adequate, but a small audible leak of air is present when the positive pressure is applied at 20 cmH$_2$O.

However, this view has recently been challenged. But whatever may be the debate, it is clear that an appropriate sized tracheal tube should pass easily through the cricoid ring and there should not be excessive air leak in the working range. An alternative rough guide for the determination of the size of an ET tube is to use a tube with an external diameter similar to that of the child's little finger. As the children have a relatively short trachea, so the tube may easily enter either the right or the left main bronchus, or may even come out of the trachea easily when the neck is extended. Certain care to be taken during intubation:

- After intubation and intermittently during operation auscultation of both the lungs is mandatory.
- Tube should be well secured by adhesive tapes with the immobile maxilla, rather than the movable mandible.
- The length of the tip of an ET tube from the alveolar margin (i.e., the length of the tube in the air passage) should be calculated from the formula: Age/2 + 12 cm.

This above formula is applicable only for the patients who are >2 years of age. However, the length of an orotracheal tube from the alveolar ridge (in centimeter) to the tip of the tube for patients aged <2 years is produced in the **Table 16** and should be memorized. But, whatever may be the length, it should allow the tip of the tube to reach the midtracheal point, while 2–3 cm of the tube should protrude out from the mouth for fixation. Some disposable tubes have a special marking 2 cm away from the patient's end to indicate the adequate insertion of tube into the trachea, passing below the vocal cord. Correct positioning of the tracheal tube should also always be checked by capnography and auscultation of the lung fields. The ET tube is connected with the anesthetic machine by a connector. However, a pediatric 8.5-mm connectors are usually used, instead of the standard 15 mm connector. The catheter mount should be avoided in pediatric anesthesia because a large dead space is involved. An alternative calculation for the measurement of the length of the ET tube from the alveolar margin to the midtrachea point is three times of the internal diameter of the ET tube and for nasal intubation this measurement of length is [Age (years) ÷ 2 + 15] cm **(Table 16)**.

If intubation is preceded by a period of difficult mask ventilation, then it is very common for the stomach to become inflated by ventilating gas. The inflated stomach decreases the tidal volume of the lungs, causing arterial desaturation. So, in this situation the stomach should be deflated by passing a nasogastric tube and removing it after operation.

In first year of life, Magill's laryngoscope with a straight blade of infant size, placed behind or posterior to epiglottis, is more helpful for the visualization of larynx and vocal cord. Because, in pediatric patients the larynx is situated more anteriorly and high up in the neck, opposite to C$_{3-4}$ vertebral body (in older children and adults it lies opposite to C$_{5-6}$ vertebral body) and is covered by a large, soft, and floppy (as the cartilaginous support is not yet fully developed) epiglottis, inclined at an angle of 45° with glottis. So, the

TABLE 16: Estimation of endotracheal tube size in neonates and infants.

Weight or age	Length from alveolar ridge	Internal diameter
1–2 kg	7 cm	2.5 mm
2–4 kg	8 cm	3 mm
Term neonate	9–10 cm	3.5 mm
3 months to 1 year	10–12 cm	4 mm
2 years	11–12 cm	4.5 mm
4 years	12–13 cm	Age ÷ 4 + 4 = 5 mm

visualization of vocal cord with a curved blade (Mackintosh) laryngoscope is difficult. The straight blade of Magill's laryngoscope flattens out the curvature of epiglottis and lifts it by pushing forward directly and thus exposes the larynx. Pediatric version of Polio and McCoy blades are also available for pediatric laryngoscopy and intubation in difficult cases. For visualization of larynx, an anesthesiologist has to align the three imaginary axes: one through trachea, one through pharynx, and one through mouth. In adults and older children, this is usually achieved by placing a pillow under the head (familiar "sniffing the morning air position") and putting the tip of laryngoscope blade into vallecula in front of epiglottis. But, in neonates and infants, due to a larger head and shorter neck relative to their body, instead of placing the pillow under the head, it is usually necessary to place it under the shoulder. Laryngoscopy should be done very gently in pediatric group of patients and proper care should also be taken to avoid the trapping of lips between the teeth and laryngoscope blade which will cause injury and bleeding and distract the concentration of anesthetist. The blade of laryngoscope also should not be levered against the upper incisor teeth which may cause dislodging or even breaking them. Certain considerations prior to ET intubation are:

- Whether an awake, a traumatic intubation is possible and can be achieved easily.
- The possible presence of conditions making intubation difficult or impossible (e.g., TE fistula)
- The difficulty in maintaining an unobstructed airway with a face mask after induction and difficulty of maintaining ventilation by face mask after muscle relaxants
- The presence of intestinal obstruction
- A very poor general condition of the patient **(Table 17)**.

It should also be noted that the concept of conscious intubation depends entirely on the clinical state of patient and bears no relationship with age. However, in a vigorous infant and provided there is no possibility of aspiration of pharyngeal content, anesthesia always should be induced prior to intubation. After intubation by an uncuffed ET tube, the laryngopharynx is lightly packed with ribbon gauze, moistened with water or liquid paraffin, to stabilize the ET tube and to prevent its kinking as well as leaking of gas.

Monitoring

The best monitoring device during pediatric anesthesia is that which increases a contact between an anesthetist and his patient. So, there is no substitute for an experienced and vigilant anesthetist observing a child, and it is complimented with some instrumental monitoring by modern electronic devices. Hence, for this instrumental monitoring, conventional adult electronic gadgets are

TABLE 17: Suggested size (ID) and length of the oral ET tube.

Age	Length from alveolar ridge	Internal diameter
2 years	11–12 cm	4.5 mm
4 years	12–13 cm	5 mm
5 years	13–14 cm	5.5 mm
6–7 years	14–15 cm	6 mm
8–9 years	15–16 cm	6.5 mm
10 years	16–17 cm	7 mm
11–12 years	17–18 cm	7.5 mm
13–14 years	18–19 cm	8 mm

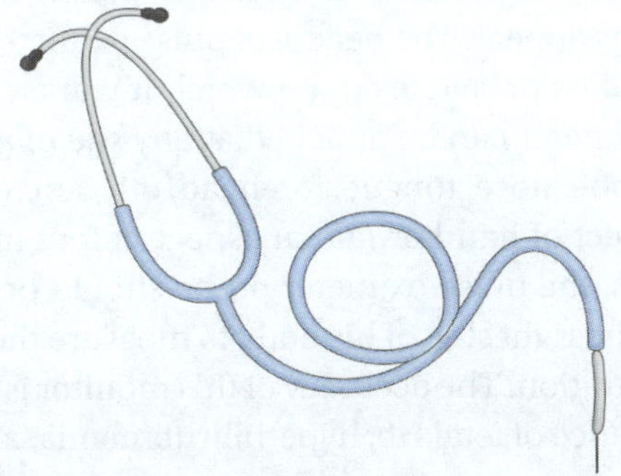

Fig. 7: Esophageal stethoscope.

applicable, but with some special modifications for smaller infants and neonates. With these electronic monitoring, color changes of skin and mucous membrane, movement of chest and breathing bag, changes of respiratory pattern, peripheral arterial pulses, etc. should also closely be observed clinically. It provides information about the present status of patient's oxygenation, ventilation, and circulation.

The routine instrumental monitoring of pediatric patient always include a precordial or esophageal stethoscope **(Fig. 7)**, a blood pressure cuff of suitable width, pulse oximetry, ECG, temperature, end tidal CO_2 tension, and a peripheral nerve stimulator, if muscle relaxants are administered. A precordial stethoscope and pulse oximetry should always be attached after induction, if not possible before. The precordial stethoscope should be changed to an esophageal one, after the trachea has been intubated. The precordial or esophageal stethoscopes assist in monitoring heart rate, quality of heart sounds, and pulmonary ventilation. The esophageal stethoscope is also used for a qualitative measurement of CO, because a volume-depleted infant has soft heart sounds and an increase in intensity of heart sounds, after volume repletion, may be recognized easily.

The sphygmomanometry method of measuring blood pressure in small baby is difficult and this is because of the inaudibility of Korotkoff sounds. But, the blood pressure can be measured by automatic devices accurately, provided the width of measuring cuff covers at least two-thirds of upper arm and surrounds at least the three-fourths of limb. Many of the mechanical automatic sphygmomanometer devices are calibrated to the size of patient, so it is important to select the proper "neonate" mode for accurate measurement of noninvasive blood pressure.

The greatest advancement of this century, in the sphere of monitoring in pediatric anesthesia, is the development of pulse oximetry by which O_2 saturation of Hb can be measured continuously and noninvasively by a transcutaneous method. It is an extremely sensitive apparatus giving very early warning signs of impending hypoxia, long before clinical signs appear. The beauty of pulse oximetry lies in the simplicity of its principles upon which it works. The sensor of pulse oximeter can be attached at any site of patient, like finger, earlobe, nose, tongue, forehead, etc., and even on the medial aspect of hand or lateral aspect of foot in neonates. In neonates, the pulse oximeter probe should preferably be placed on the right side of his body to measure the preductal oxygen saturation. The accuracy of this monitor is unaffected by the presence of fetal Hb, hyperbilirubinemia, anemia, etc. However, accuracy is affected by several other factors, such as the presence of met- and carboxyhemoglobin, nail polish, extraneous infrared lights (from radiant overhead heaters), hypothermia, and hypotension. Sometimes, the pulse oximetry results may not be accurate in cold neonates with poorly perfused extremities, due to vasoconstrictions. In such situations, the application of oximeter probe to earlobe or nose may yield an accurate result. In addition, the use of an overhead radiant light for warming the baby may result in inaccurate oximeter results. So, the oximeter sensor should be shielded from radiant light. The artifacts, due to the movement of patient, always give inaccurate measurement of O_2 saturation in neonates and infants during anesthesia. But, now, newer algorithms have virtually eliminated motion artifacts and enable the accurate measurement of O_2 saturation of Hb in pediatric patients in spite of spontaneous movement.

The ECG monitoring is used for almost all pediatric patients during their surgical procedures. The direct monitoring of arterial and central venous pressure is also easily achieved after cannulation of radial artery and internal jugular vein. However, such invasive direct arterial and central venous pressure monitoring are only be used in pediatric patients when such monitoring are absolutely necessary for the management of safe anesthesia during complicated surgery or in high-risk patients. During central venous and/or arterial cannulation, all air bubbles should be removed from pressure tubing and only small volume of flushes should

be used to prevent air embolism and circulating overload, respectively in pediatric group of patient. The right radial artery is often chosen for cannulation in neonates, because its preductal location mirrors the actual oxygen content of carotid and retinal arteries. A femoral artery catheter may be a suitable alternative in very small neonates when radial artery is not easily assessed. The critically ill neonates may still have an umbilical artery catheter in situ. The anesthetists should not use these monitors simply because the patient is small or he is inexperienced. If these monitors are needed, then it can be inserted by an anesthetist or a surgeon or even a cardiologist or a neonatologist. Pulmonary artery catheter is rarely indicated in pediatric patients, as the pressures of right and left side of heart are almost identical.

The end tidal CO_2 tension correlates well with alveolar and subsequently arterial CO_2 tension. So, the measurement of end tidal CO_2 tension, using a capnometer with a pediatric cuvette, is mandatory in pediatric anesthesia. Thus, the analysis of end tidal CO_2 allows the assessment of adequacy of ventilation, confirmation of ET tube placement, and early warnings of malignant hyperthermia. The CO_2 partial pressure in blood can also be estimated noninvasively by transcutaneous methods. But, this technique of measurement of CO_2 tension by transcutaneous route is not commonly used in the OT, because it requires a long calibration period, responds slowly to the changes of CO_2 partial pressure in blood and does not provide breath-by-breath analysis, like the end tidal CO_2 tension. For the measurement of alveolar CO_2 tension which correlates well with arterial CO_2 tension, two types of capnometers are available. These are (1) sidestream and (2) mainstream capnometers. The accuracy of capnometer reading depends on several factors, such as type of capnometer, the location of end-tidal gas sampling port in anesthetic circuit, the type of anesthetic circuit being used, and the cardiopulmonary dysfunction of patient. The sidestream capnometer aspirates gas continuously from the breathing circuit through a fine bore tubing and the main analyzer lies at a distance. So, for an accurate result this sidestream analyzer must aspirate gas at a sufficient rate, compared to respiratory rate and the gas should be sampled from within tracheal tube. For this purpose, an 18-G or a 20-G IV catheter may be inserted into a 3- or 3.5-mm ID ET tube.

On the other hand, the mainstream capnometer is placed directly at the junction between an ET tube and the patient end of anesthetic circuit and it directly analyzes the expired gas as it passes through the sensor of it. Hence, it does not need to aspirate the gas continuously. Thus, these capnometers provide more accurate results about end tidal CO_2 tension than sidestream capnometers. But, these are heavier than the light-weight pediatric circuits and add more dead space. Nevertheless, the small tidal volume and rapid respiratory rate of small infants can present difficulties with both the capnometer models. The end tidal CO_2 tension which is similar to alveolar CO_2 tension does not correlate well with arterial CO_2 tension in the presence of right-to-left cardiac shunt. But, in contrast the end tidal CO_2 tension accurately reflects arterial CO_2 tension in the presence of left-to-right shunt. Also, the end tidal CO_2 tension does not accurately reflect the arterial CO_2 tension in lung diseases. In such situations, the end tidal CO_2 tension should not be relied upon for accurate assessment of the adequacy of alveolar ventilation. Here, the arterial blood gases should always be analyzed to document the actual gas tension.

The body temperature should always be monitored, during the surgery of small babies by nasopharyngeal, esophageal, or rectal probes due to their increased susceptibility to iatrogenic hypothermia and hyperthermia and also for early detection of malignant hyperthermia. Hypothermia can be prevented by maintaining a warm operating room environment (26°C or higher), warming and humidifying the inspired gases, using a warm blanket, and also by warming all the IV fluids. The room temperature required for a neutral thermal environment varies with age. It is highest with premature newborns. However, it should also be kept in mind that during the maintenance of temperature of pediatric patients, utmost care also must be taken to prevent unintentional skin burns and iatrogenic hyperthermia from overzealous warming efforts.

Among all these routes, the nasopharyngeal thermal probe provides an accurate reflection of body core temperature. The esophageal temperature may not accurately reflect the core temperature, because it is usually affected directly by the temperature of inspired gases. The rectal temperature also can reflect accurately the core temperature, but it changes very slowly. The body core temperature also can be measured accurately from external auditory meatus. But, it is not commonly used, because of the risk of trauma to tympanic membrane. Axillary temperature does not provide the actual core temperature of patient's body and it is very difficult to maintain the position of probe over axillary artery.

Extubation and Postoperative Care

At the end of surgery, when extubation is planned, then the administration of volatile anesthetic agents should be stopped and the neuromuscular block should be antagonized, if they are used at all. The neuromuscular block should be antagonized in all the pediatric group of patients, especially in neonates (preterm or full term) and infants. Because, even with the use of modern short-acting neuromuscular blocking agents, the recovery from muscular

paralysis in neonates and infants remain unpredictable and any residual neuromuscular blockade may quickly lead to respiratory failure. Following anesthesia with spontaneous ventilation, under volatile anesthetic agents for short surgical procedures, extubation should be performed under deep anesthesia. It is not advisable to extubate this group of patients under light anesthesia, as severe laryngospasm is very frequent. Therefore, to maintain the level of deep anesthesia volatile anesthetic agents are continued till the child has been extubated successfully. The ET tube is extubated after thorough oropharyngeal suctioning and then the child is given 100% O_2 to breathe.

During the reversal of neuromuscular block by neostigmine (40–50 µg/kg), atropine (20 µg/kg), and glycopyrrolate (10 µg/kg), the patients tend to follow three phases. In the beginning, the patient begins to breathe irregularly and tries to strain on ET tube. Next, the patients hold their breath for a variable period. At that time, they are at the greatest risk of hypoxia. Then, finally the regular respiration is resumed. After that, the patient begins to gag on ET tube, move his limbs, and contract the rectus abdominis muscle. Extubation is done after thorough oropharyngeal suctioning at this phase and 100% O_2 is administered with utmost attention for further occurrence of laryngospasm.

After extubation, the postoperative management of pediatric patient depends on the grade and the complications of surgery and anesthesia and the associated medical conditions of patient. After any surgery, the patients should be monitored with pulse oximeter, apnea monitor, and ECG in recovery room, because the neonates are very prone to postanesthetic apnea. The 20% of preterm neonates may develop postoperative apnea after GA and the risk of which increases in the presence of anemia and decreases with increasing postconceptual age. The risk of postanesthetic apnea is also high in the presence of congenital heart disease, severe respiratory distress, intracranial hemorrhage, and any other major organ dysfunction. This postoperative apnea usually occurs within 6 hours after discontinuation of anesthesia. Though, the process of maturation of respiratory center is a dynamic process, still due to individual variations it is not surprising to face postoperative apnea, even in full-term neonates. Caffeine is recommended for the management of postanesthetic apnea. A single dose of caffeine of 10 mg/kg is sufficient for 18–24 hours to prevent postoperative apnea. However, all patients who are prone to postanesthetic apnea are observed with an apnea monitor for 24 hours or at least 12 hours, after the last apneic episode.

■ NEONATAL ANESTHESIA

Children, younger than 1 year, have the higher incidences of complications in anesthesia than the older children. The reasons for these higher incidences of complications in anesthesia for children younger than 1 year are:

- Usually, the neonates who are presented for surgery are of ASA grade 3 and 4.
- The cardiovascular and respiratory system of the neonates, particularly the premature ones, function between the adult or extrauterine and the fetal or intrauterine type. So, any type of surgical stress or hypoxia can convert this adult type of circulation to its fetal type and as a consequence worsen the hypoxemia and acidosis and cause death, unless the cycle is broken immediately.
- Immaturity of organ systems (especially the cardiovascular, pulmonary, renal, hepatic, and nervous system), high metabolic rate, high ratio of body surface area to weight, miscalculation of drug doses, etc. make the taking care of neonates and premature babies technically very difficult.
- The care of neonates is also always confronted with sudden physiological changes, unexpected responses, and some unknown congenital problems.

Most of the complications that arise during neonatal anesthesia are due to the lack of understanding of their special considerations, prior to the induction of anesthesia. So, the neonatal anesthesiologist has to be prepared for these unexpected situations and has to be ready with the varieties of equipment and of proper sizes to provide the highest level of care.

The controlled ventilation, after ET intubation, is the technique of choice for neonates and for most of the babies, up to the 5 kg of body weight, even for minor procedures. The small babies are very sensitive to respiratory depressant effects of inhalational anesthetic agents. So, the controlled ventilation ensures adequate alveolar ventilation and maintains a normal residual lung volume. But, recently many operations are done under spontaneous respiration with LMA. During spontaneous ventilation, even the low resistance of circle system can become a significant obstacle for the sick neonate. Unidirectional valves, long breathing tube, and absorbers account for most of this resistance. For patients weighing <10 kg, some anesthesiologists prefer the Mapleson D circuit, because of their low resistance and lightweight. Nevertheless, as the resistance of breathing circuit can easily be overcome by positive pressure ventilation, so the circle system can safely be used in patients of all ages, if ventilation is controlled. Monitoring of airway pressure may provide an early evidence of obstruction caused by a kinked ET tube or advancement of the tube into the main stem bronchus.

For controlled ventilation in neonates, a respiratory rate of 30–40 breaths/min with inspiratory and expiratory ratio

of 1:2 (it is occasionally necessary to reverse the inspiratory: expiratory ratio from 1:2 to 2:1 to improve gas exchange) is used with a peak inflation pressure of 25–30 cmH_2O (but not >30 cmH_2O). PEEP of 5 cmH_2O (not >10 cmH_2O) is also used to preserve FRC with a FGF of 4 L/min. Using PEEP and peak inflation pressure up to 30 cmH_2O, we should keep the inspired O_2 concentration as low as possible to maintain a PaO_2 just between 60 and 80 mm Hg. Early application of PEEP to the patients with hyaline membrane disease improves the gas exchange and may also decrease the severity of the disease by reducing the surfactant consumption. The net effect of PEEP on tissue oxygenation depends on the degree to which the CO is reduced (PEEP than 10 cmH_2O reduces CO). For the babies over 5 kg of body weight, anesthesia by spontaneous breathing without intubation is possible, but only if the surgery permits and is of very short procedure.

Every effort should be made to maintain the neonate's temperature by minimizing thermal loss. OT should be warmed. Electric warmer, warming blankets, and heated humidification of inspired gases, particularly when nonbreathing circuit is used, minimizes the heat loss.

Pulse oximeter is extremely important, not only to prevent hypoxia, but also to prevent hyperoxia and retinopathy of prematurity (ROP). Oxygen saturation should be maintained between 93 and 95% (PaO_2 between 60 and 80 mm Hg), which keeps the patient on the steep side of oxy-hemoglobin dissociation curve. Keeping the O_2 saturation at this level, an anesthetist will maintain a delicate balance between the potential rapid O_2 desaturation due to absence of any reserve, and the potential development of ROP due to higher inspired O_2 concentration. So, an anesthesiologist should be extremely vigilant and should respond quickly to any changes in O_2 saturation.

Premature neonates are deficient in surfactant production, which results in alveolar instability and atelectasis. This results in an increased intrapulmonary shunting and decreased compliance of lungs. Mild cases can be treated conservatively with humidified O_2. But, severe cases require tracheal intubation and mechanical ventilation. The decision to provide mechanical respiratory support is always made on clinical grounds, such as apneic attacks, respiratory rate above 60 breaths/min, signs of increasing work of breathing (nasal flaring and subcostal recession), increasing O_2 dependence (needs increased inspiratory O_2 concentration to maintain normal arterial O_2 saturation), and failure to clear secretion. Such babies are unable to maintain an arterial O_2 tension between 50 and 80 mm Hg with increasing inspired O_2 concentration and the CO_2 tension rises above 50 mm Hg. On the other hand, high pressure and high inspired O_2 concentration which is sometimes required for mechanical ventilation may result in retrolental fibroplasia and damage to lung parenchyma. Factors that cause this progressive destruction of lung architecture and function (with fibrosis and cyst formation) due to high pressure and high O_2 concentration are pulmonary hypoplasia, surfactant deficiency, the presence of left-to-right shunt, high ventilatory pressures (>30 cmH_2O), high inspired O_2 concentration (>60%), chronic infection, and poor mucociliary function. This condition is progressive and vicious in cycle, as increased V/Q mismatching demands higher inspired O_2 concentration and falling lung compliance needs even higher inflation pressure. This high peak inspiratory pressure causes more shear injury of the lung parenchyma, creating a vicious cycle. This can be reduced only by the judicious use of PEEP and other ventilatory modes. A significant number of children who have had this type of treatment develop chronic lung disease of prematurity (previously termed "bronchopulmonary dysplasia"). So, the measurement of cutaneous O_2 and CO_2 tension is increasingly important and satisfactory, and is particularly helpful even when it may be difficult to obtain arterial blood for blood gas analysis. A reasonable correlation exists between the transcutaneous and arterial gas levels, when the peripheral circulation is good. But significant discrepancy may occur in patients with poor tissue perfusion and with arterial O_2 tension at extremes of hypoxia and hyperoxia.

Weaning from the ventilator takes place after achievement of the cardiovascular and biochemical stability with inflation pressure of <25 cmH_2O, $PaCO_2$ of <50 mm Hg, and PaO_2 of >80 mm Hg at FiO_2 of 0.5 (i.e., the inspired oxygen concentration being 50%). Neonates must never breathe through an ET tube without PEEP, because the zero end-expiratory pressure allows the small lungs to collapse progressively, so that the closing volume comes closer to the FRC in subsequent respirations with increased right-to-left intrapulmonary shunting and hypoxia. As the lung volume falls, the airway resistance to gas flow rises, so that the work of breathing and oxygen consumption also rises. With the ET tube in place, the normal mechanism is lost, whereby the glottis generates 2–3 cmH_2O pressure in terms of respiratory distress.

■ SOME SPECIAL PEDIATRIC SURGICAL CASES

Congenital Diaphragmatic Hernia

In this condition, which occurs in 1 out of 4,000 live births, the abdominal viscera herniate through a defect in the diaphragm, most commonly through the *foramen of Bochdalek*. Another name for this foramen of Bochdalek is the persistent pleuroperitoneal canal. It is a free communication between the peritoneal and pleural cavities, causing a posterolateral hernia of the abdominal viscera

into thorax. It is due to the failure of diaphragm to develop from the lateral arcuate ligament on one or both sides, forming a triangular gap. So, a congenital diaphragmatic hernia takes place through that opening and abdominal viscera herniate into the thorax due to the positive intra-abdominal pressure. In severe degree of congenital diaphragmatic hernia almost all the abdominal viscera, including the stomach, intestine, liver, and spleen, may be above the diaphragm and impair the development of lungs, causing hypoplasia of it. The intrauterine gestational age at which herniation begins to occur determine the severity of hernia which in turn determines the degree of lung hypoplasia.

So, along with this congenital diaphragmatic hernia, there is also concomitant pulmonary hypoplasia associated with ↑PVR, ↑PAP, and pulmonary hypertension. If the defect starts at an early gestational age, then the mediastinum is also shifted to the right and the growth of the contralateral lung is also stunted. The degree of respiratory distress at birth is related mainly to the degree of associated pulmonary hypoplasia which is indirectly related to the degree of the herniation of abdominal viscera into the thoracic cavity. The neonates and infants who present with respiratory distress soon after birth, indicates severe degree of herniation and severe degree of lung hypoplasia. Usually, they do not survive as they have inadequate amount of lung tissue to sustain life. After birth, the midgut starts to fill with air, causing the further distension of gut and the compression of lungs which further increases the respiratory and cardiovascular distress. The diagnosis of congenital diaphragmatic hernia is suspected by respiratory distress after delivery and a scaphoid empty abdomen. This is confirmed by a chest X-ray.

The repair of diaphragmatic hernia is not an emergency one and the child should be managed medically first. The surgery is considered only when the child's condition is optimized medically. The pulmonary hypertension should be treated with tolazoline and PGE inhibitor, before the administration of anesthesia for better result **(Box 7)**. The intraoperative $PaCO_2$, reflected as $ETCO_2$ tension, reflects the severity of lung pathology and the chances of survival. It is the anesthesiologist's duty to control the $PaCO_2$ to improve the hypoxemia and to check the hypotension.

The defect of diaphragmatic hernia is usually repaired through an abdominal incision. The use of muscle relaxant

BOX 7: Problems faced by an anesthetist during perioperative management of congenital diaphragmatic hernia.

- Hypoxemia, due to pulmonary hypoplasia, gut distension and pulmonary hypertension
- Acidosis due to hypercapnia
- Hypotension caused by kinking of major blood vessels, particularly those of the liver

and ventilation of patient by mask and bag before intubation may cause the inflation of stomach and more herniation of gut into thorax. So, an awake intubation without bag and mask ventilation is ideal (only if possible) and prevents the over distension of gut which cause the further herniation of abdominal viscera into the thoracic cavity. N_2O also should not be used for the same reason, as it overdistends the gut and increases the herniation of abdominal viscera into thoracic cavity. An intra-arterial line is helpful in this type of surgery for blood gas analysis and continuous beat-to-beat monitoring of blood pressure. The anesthetic agents that depress the myocardium should always be avoided and stress response should be blunted by narcotics, such as fentanyl or remifentanil, which helps to establish a stable hemodynamic system. It is not always possible to introduce back all the viscera totally from thorax into the peritoneal cavity. In such cases, a silastic silo may be used to introduce the contents gradually into the abdomen. Postoperative ventilation is essential for the management of such patients.

Esophageal Atresia and Tracheoesophageal Fistula

The esophageal atresia, with or without tracheal fistula (communication) with esophagus which is called the TE fistula, occurs in about 1 out of 3,000 live births. It should be suspected especially when the hydramnios complicates the pregnancy. Different types of TE fistula are shown in **Figures 8A to E**.

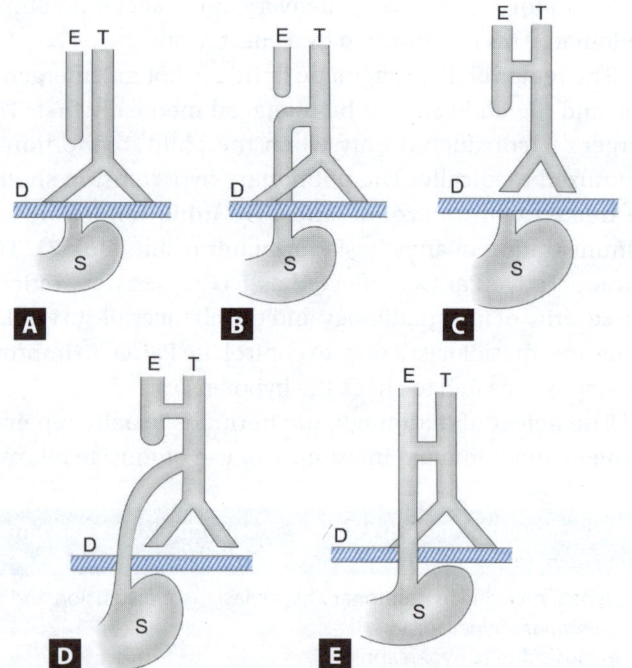

Figs. 8A to E: Varieties of tracheoesophageal fistula. (E: esophagus; T: trachea; S: stomach; D: diaphragm)

The infants, suffering from this disease, are of low birth weight and this anomaly may be the part of a larger constellation of many other congenital anomalies of the structures, such as vertebrae (V), anus (A), trachea (T), esophagus (E), and renal (R) which are abbreviated shortly as VATER. Among these, the cardiovascular anomalies, such as the septal defects and the coarctation of aorta, most often coexist with this condition. So, echocardiography should always be performed before surgery of such patients. Other anomalies, described above, should also be excluded by thorough clinical examination and full investigations. Usually, after birth, a baby who is suffering from esophageal atresia and associated TE fistula, presents with respiratory distress or symptoms of choking during feeding and distended abdomen. Usually, the six types of TE fistulae with esophageal atresia (from A to E) are described, and most of them present with an inability to swallow, because of the esophageal atresia, except type E. The diagnosis of this congenital anomaly is confirmed only by passing a nasogastric tube, which cannot be passed into stomach. The main risk of life in TE fistula comes from the soiling of lungs with saliva or gastric contents, causing pneumonitis and lack of nutrition **(Box 8)**.

After birth, the corrective surgery for TE fistula should be performed as one stage repair and as soon as possible. The delay will usually result in more soiling of lungs, causing more pneumonitis which makes the patient gradually inoperable.

Preoperatively, the child should not receive any feeding and a large bore catheter is placed in the blind esophageal diverticulum in the A, B, C, and D types of TE fistula. It will help to drain saliva continuously, so that the child does not swallow it. The child should be nursed in prone position, with head-up tilt to prevent the soiling of lungs by gastric fluid in B, D, and E types of TE fistula. If the lungs are soiled and the child has pneumonia or pneumonitis, then the operation should be postponed, until the pneumonitis improves by antibiotic and physiotherapy. The operation should be performed as soon as the child's condition is optimized medically. Sometimes, if operation is delayed for a long time, due to severe illness of baby, then initially a palliative gastrostomy should be performed to provide the means of nutrition during recovery from pneumonitis and to prevent further pneumonitis.

BOX 8: The major issues for the management of safe anesthesia in tracheoesophageal (TE) fistula repair.

- Aspiration pneumonitis
- Overdistension of stomach by air coming through fistula
- Ventilatory problems, as gases pass through trachea and fistula to further distend the stomach
- Problems due to other concomitant congenital anomalies

Awake intubation or inhalational induction by volatile anesthetic agents, followed by intubation, is the choice of anesthesia. Intubation after an adequate dose of a muscle relaxant and followed by intermittent positive pressure ventilation (IPPV) is contraindicated. Because, the positive pressure ventilation causes the huge distension of stomach, due to the passage of gas through trachea and fistula, and subsequent the compression of diaphragm and lungs. Initially, the ET tube should be inserted intentionally to the deeper level beyond the fistula, than predicted, in any main bronchus, right or left. ET tube is then withdrawn slowly, until the breath sounds are heard equally on both sides. This technique of ET intubation usually ensures that the tip of ET tube is placed beyond the level of fistula, but proximal to carina. The leak of gas into the stomach, caused by the placement of ET tube proximal to the fistula, is easily diagnosed by auscultation of abdomen with a precordial stethoscope. The ET tube should be inserted with the bevel facing up, so that the posterior wall of ET tube occludes the fistula. This is because the fistula is usually situated on the posterior wall of trachea. After the inhalational induction by volatile anesthetic agents and intubation by muscle relaxant, controlled ventilation is always recommended for the surgical repair of TE fistula.

After the intubation, the determination of O_2 saturation by pulse oximeter is the most useful monitoring. Because, any intraoperative change in the position of ET tube, as little as 1–2 mm from its previous position, may determine, whether the anesthesiologist is ventilating both the lungs, or one lung or the fistula. The ventilation also must be monitored very carefully during the surgical dissection of fistula, as the trachea may kink during traction or manipulation and the ET tube may be dislodged during this traction and kinking of trachea. Postoperatively, the neonates especially the premature ones, may have repeated apneic spells and this is may be due to the residual effect of anesthesia, hypoxia, hypoglycemia, anemia, hypocalcemia, hypothermia, etc. Therefore, the patient should not be reversed to spontaneous respiration postoperatively for at least 12 hours. The postoperative care of a neonate, after the surgical repair of TE fistula, should be given in a NICU with full monitoring facilities.

Pyloric Stenosis

The incidence of pyloric stenosis is about 1 in 400 live births and males are affected in about 80% cases. It presents usually, during the first 4–6 weeks of life after birth and is not a surgical emergency. The pathology of pyloric stenosis is the gross thickening of the pyloric circular smooth muscle, like a hard tumor, causing obstruction to food with increased vomiting. If untreated, the infant loses weight and becomes severely dehydrated with hypokalemia, hypochloremia, and metabolic alkalosis. This is due to repeated vomiting of gastric secretions, containing H^+ and Cl^- ions. As the obstruction is at the level of pylorus, so there is no loss of alkaline intestinal secretions. The body is thus loaded with bicarbonate and the kidney has to take this load. Therefore, this bicarbonate load on the kidney at its glomerular level exceeds its absorption power at tubular level. Thus, the urine becomes alkaline and indicates a compensatory phase. If the dehydration remains uncorrected, then hypovolemia activates renin-angiotensin-aldosterone axis to preserve the circulating volume by absorbing Na^+ and water from the renal tubules. This results in an exchange of Na^+ for H^+ and K^+ (Na^+ enters, H^+ and K^+ released), which leads to the paradoxical acidic urine with worsening of hypokalemia and metabolic alkalosis. This indicates decompensatory phase. In compensatory phase, Na^+ will be absorbed only in exchange of K^+ and H^+ will be retained to compensate loss of H^+ from stomach.

The surgery for pyloric stenosis (pyloromyotomy) is not an emergency one. So, it should be preceded by the complete correction of fluid and electrolyte imbalance. The initial management of pyloric stenosis is (1) gastric suction through a nasogastric tube and (2) IV cannulation for parenteral therapy. The nasogastric suction is very important, because the stomach is always filled up with old food, debris, barium sulfate (if it is used for radiological diagnosis), etc. The initial intravenous infusion of fluid should be 5% dextrose in 0.45% saline to which the 40 mmol/L of KCl is added (2 mL/kg of 0.9% NaCl raises the serum chloride by 1 mmol/L). Usually, the rate of infusion of fluid is 6 mL/kg/hour. During the preoperative preparation of patient, the gastric residue is drained off continuously by nasogastric suction and stomach is washed with 0.9% saline every 4 hourly, until the aspirate becomes clear and odorless. Surgery should not take place, until the plasma chloride level is at least 90 mmol/L and the potassium bicarbonate concentration is 25 mmol/L.

Usually, the child becomes ready for surgery within 24–48 hours, after the commencement of treatment. Before induction of anesthesia, stomach should always be aspirated and as the children are sick but lusty, so awake intubation is not possible. However, the induction should be smooth by either inhalation or intravenous route according to the experience of anesthesiologist. Cricoid pressure must be used, which should be as effective in infants as in adults to prevent the aspiration of gastric contents in lungs if there is any, even after aspiration by nasogastric tube. The postoperative oral feeding is usually re-established immediately after the patient returns to the ward. The postoperative analgesia is provided by wound infiltration with local anesthetic agents and rectal or oral paracetamol, depending on when the surgeon decides to feed the child.

Omphalocele and Gastroschisis

Omphalocele and *gastroschisis* are the protrusion of the part of small intestine, through a defect in the anterior abdominal wall, at the level of umbilicus (not through umbilical cord), resulting in the exposure of viscera that are either covered (omphalocele) or uncovered (gastroschisis) by peritoneum, whereas the *exomphalos* is the herniation of abdominal viscera into the umbilical cord of varying degree, without any defect in the anterior abdominal wall. However, though the omphalocele or gastroschisis and the exomphalos are embryologically two separate conditions, but still, they present the similar challenges to anesthesiologists **(Box 9)**.

These conditions are always surgical emergencies. It is imperative that the abdominal contents should be placed in a clear sterile polythene bag, as soon as possible, after birth to prevent the infection, heat loss, and fluid loss. Adequate intravenous access and extensive intraoperative invasive monitoring are usually necessary during surgical correction of these congenital anomalies. This is because (1) hypotension secondary to the tension on major organs or (2) inferior caval compression during the surgical manipulation is common. The N_2O should be avoided during the maintenance of anesthesia. Muscle relaxants should be used liberally to provide optimal surgical conditions and relaxation for closure of the defect on anterior abdominal wall, through which herniation has occurred. Nasogastric tube should always be in place to decompress the stomach which will help in the reduction of viscera and easy closure of anterior abdominal wall. In such cases, postoperative controlled ventilation is mandatory, because of the reduction in compliance of lungs, due to increased intra-abdominal pressure postoperatively, caused by the return of viscera into peritoneal cavity and to provide adequate time to abdominal wall to stretch and to accommodate the viscera slowly. The intravenous alimentation plays a vital role for the rapid recovery of these patients. Sometimes, it

is not possible to close the defect in one sitting, then staged surgical procedures may be planned.

Meningomyelocele

It is the herniation of a part of meninges and spinal cord through a defect in vertebral column. It is a common neonatal congenital abnormality and requires an emergency surgery. **Box 10** listed the points which should be kept in the mind of an anesthetist, during the surgery of a meningomyelocele.

Cleft lip and Cleft palate

Though in some centers, the total repair of both cleft lip and cleft palate is carried out in neonatal period, but usually the primary repair of a cleft lip is performed, during the first few weeks of life and that of a cleft palate is performed between 1 and 3 years of age. The cleft lip and cleft palate are also often accompanied by other congenital anomalies. Among them, the defects of cardiac and CNS are of particular relevance to an anesthesiologist. These conditions are also often associated with Pierre–Robin syndrome (micrognathia, cleft palate, and glossoptosis), Treacher–Collins syndrome (cleft palate and hypoplasia of first bronchial arch) and Klippel–Feil syndrome (fused cervical vertebrae). These congenital anomalies may cause incipient or actual respiratory obstruction and make the intubation very difficult. In Pierre–Robin syndrome, the periodic episodes of respiratory obstruction occur, due to a relatively oversized tongue, blocking the airway. So, they have to be nursed in prone position, in order to overcome this obstruction. Failure to thrive as a consequence of difficulties in feeding and repeated respiratory infections is common in this group of patients.

The ideal collaboration of surgeon, pediatrician, and anesthesiologist is very much desirable in treating the preoperative anemia, malnutrition, respiratory infection, etc., which are commonly associated with these congenital anomalies and also in judging the optimal time for operation for this group of patients.

Sedative premedication should be avoided during the surgery of cleft palate. The induction of anesthesia by inhalation of N_2O, O_2 together with the halothane or sevoflurane is simple and effective, although some anesthesiologists prefer an intravenous induction. Once the child is asleep by

BOX 9: The challenges in management of omphalocele and gastroschisis.

- Massive fluid loss and dehydration. It results from exposed visceral surfaces and from third space loss, caused by partial bowel obstruction
- Heat loss
- Infection
- Difficulty in surgical closure without causing severe increase in intra-abdominal pressure and severe compression on lungs
- Frequent association of these conditions with prematurity
- Other associated congenital defects with these conditions

BOX 10: Points to be kept in mind during anesthesia of meningomyelocele.

- Possible association of meningomyelocele with hydrocephalus
- Possibility of cranial nerve injury during surgery
- Possibility of brain herniation during and after surgery
- Possibility of underestimation of fluid and blood loss

inhalational anesthetic agents, then an intravenous infusion line can conveniently be set up. The intubation of trachea can be performed under deep inhalational anesthesia, but the use of muscle relaxants intravenously provides an optimum condition. But, before giving relaxants of any sort, it is wise to ensure that the facial configuration of patient will allow effective artificial ventilation with a bag and mask. It is particularly important to avoid trauma to the lips or gums in children, waiting for repair of cleft lip during intubation. So, a "tooth guard" made of several layers of sticking plaster or a custom made soft plastic mold is used. It will not only protect the gums, but also prevents the laryngoscope blade from falling into the maxillary defect. Sometimes, the use of a wad of gauze, placed in the roof of the mouth, will prevent the blade of the laryngoscope from slipping into the cleft.

There should be a wide range of ET tubes, available to anesthesiologist, for intubation, during the surgery of cleft lip and cleft palate. The surgeon requires the tube to be as unobtrusive as possible, while the anesthesiologist requires a non-kinkable secure airway. During operation, the use of one of the various modifications of Dott Mouth Gag will allow a good access to the surgeon, and the ET tube is retained in position by the lower (tongue) blade. But, care must be taken to check the patency of the ET tube, after the insertion of gag, as the latter may occlude the tube by pressing it on the mandible. A preformed ET tube such as Oxford tube is preferred in these cases, because it is strengthened proximal segment and built in pharyngeal curve offers greater resistance to kinking than the standard Magill's tube. The Oxford tube is, however, more difficult to introduce than the gently curved Magill's tube. But, using a fine gum elastic bougie, threaded inside the tube as an introducer, greatly facilitates the intubation. The Oxford tube is tapered at the patient's end. It is, therefore, possible unintentionally to force an overlarge tube through the glottis and through the narrowest part of the trachea at the level of cricoid cartilage which may give rise to laryngeal edema and postoperative croup. So, particular care must be taken to select a well-fitting tube with minimal gas leak. A small gas leak is of no significance, because particularly as a pharyngeal pack is invariably used in such cases to protect against the inhalation of blood.

Many anesthesiologists allow spontaneous ventilation during surgery and maintain anesthesia by N_2O, O_2 with any potent inhalational anesthetic agent. Provided, the concentration of halothane is kept low and hypercarbia is not allowed to occur, then an infiltration of local anesthetic with 1:200,000 adrenaline is not a concern. Controlled ventilation using N_2O, O_2, and nondepolarizing relaxants and/or opioids is a useful alternative, particularly when an anesthesiologist is reluctant to use the halothane.

With the completion of surgery after pharyngeal suction, extubation should be done carefully in an awake and semiprone position which will protect against the aspiration of slightly oozed blood from the operation site. Prior to extubation, auscultation of chest is mandatory which may reveal any retained secretion and occasionally a poorly expanding or a blocked segment of the lung. In such conditions, the careful suction of ET tube, followed by the gentle hyperinflation of lungs is usually all that is needed. The children who are accustomed to breathe through the large defects in palate have little time to accommodate the diminished airway, following operative repair. So, a bag, mask, and an airway should be ready to treat any temporary obstruction of the airway, following extubation. An anesthetic technique which will ensure the rapid recovery of pharyngeal reflexes should be selected. Blood should be crossmatched as the surgical loss may exceed 10% of the total blood volume.

The postoperative airway problems, after the surgical correction of cleft palate, are not infrequent, particularly in the cases of small mandible, where the effectiveness of genioglossus muscle is lost and the tongue falls back, partially or completely blocking the airway. In such circumstances, the nursing of child in prone position is usually sufficient, although the forward traction of tongue, by means of a tongue stitch, may be required in refractory cases.

Inguinal Hernia

This is one of the most common operations like circumcision in the pediatric age group of patients. At present, the regional anesthesia (RA) (spinal, epidural, or caudal) combined with light GA is the chosen mode of anesthesia for repair of inguinal hernia in pediatric patients. Only GA is indicated where the RA is absolutely contraindicated. RA combined with GA has several advantages over only GA.

The advantages of regional anesthesia combined with GA are:
- Decreased dose of general anesthetic agent required for surgery
- Rapid pain free recovery
- Early ambulation
- Early discharge.

For RA, the type of blocks and techniques chosen should have minimal side effects and should not interfere with the motor function. All the techniques of RA, such as spinal, caudal, or lumbar epidural with or without catheter and with or without adjunct may be applied. The child should have an IV cannula in place before the RA is applied. But, unlike the adult practice, the volume preloading is not needed. The administration of vasoactive drugs such as ephedrine is also not required. *Spinal anesthesia* has a very quick onset of action with profound muscle relaxation, but its duration of action is short. *Caudal anesthesia* and analgesia have a slower onset, but lasts for a longer time. Therefore, *under GA combined with caudal block,* the bilateral inguinal hernia can also be repaired and can provide postoperative analgesia too. The combined spinal-epidural (CSE) anesthesia has both the advantages of spinal and caudal anesthesia. Hence, in conclusion, it can be said that all types of regional anesthetic techniques adopted in adults can be administered safely in pediatric patients, combined with GA. But, only strict attention has to be paid to the route of administration, the dose of local anesthetic agent, and the size of proper equipment (e.g., miniature needle, fine catheter, etc.).

Caudal block with 0.25% bupivacaine, in a dose of 0.75–1 mL/kg with or without catheter, is effective for inguinal hernia repair or orchidopexy. For *circumcision or hypospadias* repair, the caudal dose of bupivacaine is 0.5 mL/kg as 0.25% solution. For the volumes over 20 mL, the bupivacaine is diluted to 0.15%. For all the abovementioned percentage and doses of bupivacaine, analgesia lasts for 4–6 hours. Bupivacaine concentration, higher than 0.25%, offers no added advantage about sensory blockade, except adverse motor blockade. Also 0.125% bupivacaine solution is reported to produce the same quality and the duration of intraoperative and postoperative analgesia, as its 0.25% solution and the lower concentration resulted in lesser motor blockade. *For inguinal hernia repair and orchidopexy* the ilioinguinal and iliohypogastric nerve block, which is achieved by infiltrating 0.25% bupivacaine, medial to the anterior superior iliac spine, also has been used successfully in pediatric patients. The penile nerve block for circumcision or hypospadias operation or any other surgical procedure on the penis, which is achieved by the infiltration of 1–3 mL of adrenaline-free 0.25% bupivacaine or adrenaline-free 1% lignocaine, provides excellent intraoperative and postoperative analgesia.

The direct local infiltration of the surgical wound by long-acting local anesthetic agents is another effective method of providing pain relief (postoperative analgesia) in all children. In most institutions, it is now rare for a pediatric patient to awaken from anesthesia without some form of regional block. Parents are advised to start analgesia (oral or parenteral) when the child begins to become irritable, but prior to the complete dissipation of the block. This procedure usually provides a smooth transition and a pain-free postoperative period.

■ POSTOPERATIVE PAIN RELIEF IN CHILDREN

Many adverse pathophysiological changes occur in children due to the acute postoperative pain. These are the increase

BOX 11: Misconception governing the postoperative pain relief in children.

- Due to immaturity of the nervous system, children experience no or little pain than adults. But the nerves responsible for pain are fully developed by 27 weeks of gestation
- Pediatric patients, especially neonates and infants, have no memory of pain
- Pain is not a character building for children, which is incorrect

in anxiety, avoidance, and the certain adverse somatic signs and symptoms, such as ↑HR, ↑BP, metabolic acidosis, RR causing respiratory alkalosis, and catecholamines and the increase in parent's distress. But, unfortunately the acute pain experienced by children is often inadequately assessed and treated, in spite of our sincere efforts.

This is because pain in children had been often underestimated and undertreated. This is due to an exaggerated fear of respiratory depression caused by narcotics which are used as postoperative analgesics and other misconceptions. Regarding this misconception see the **Box 11**.

But, modern pediatric anesthesia asserts on the controlling and decreasing the postoperative pain, as far as possible, without causing any harm to the child. The severity of the pain dictates the choice of the analgesic. Mild pain is treated with nonopioids, whereas the moderate and severe pain is treated with opioids and/or RA.

The adequate pain management in pediatric patients requires the following methodical approach:
- Pain evaluation
- Routes of administration
- Selection of drugs.

Pain Evaluation

The pain in pediatric patients can be assessed by using self-report, behavioral observation, and psychological changes, depending on the age of the child and his or her communication skills. In the school going age, the children can give the verbal description of severity of their pain, but it is more difficult to evaluate it (pain) in a preverbal child. So, the different ages demand the different methods of evaluation of pain. However, the behavioral and physiological scales are important for newborns, infants, and preschool children. Their score is based on the changes in physiological parameters, such as the heart rate, blood pressure, respiratory rate, sweating, crying, patient's position, and facial expressions.

The most popular scales for the assessment of pain in preverbal children are the Children's Hospital of Eastern Ontario Pain Scale (CHEOPS), the Objective Pain Scale (OPS) of Hannallah and Broadman, and the Children and Infants Post-operative Pain Scale (CHIPPS). In older children, the self-evaluation scores are much more suitable. Therefore, the visual analog scales (VAS) can be used for this group of patient. The "Smiling Faces" scale (from smiling to sad and then to crying faces, corresponding to increasing pain) and "the Color's Scale" (from red to green—highest pain to no pain) are also routinely applied according to the age, verbal communication skill, and intelligence of patient.

Routes of Administration

Oral analgesia is always desirable for children, whenever is possible. The standard doses of analgesics and adequate intervals through oral route provide excellent analgesia in the majority of patients. The *intravenous route* of administration of drugs provides rapid onset of analgesia with the advantage of incremental intravenous titration, but with no discomfort to the child. The *intramuscular injections should be avoided*, as children often deny repeated intramuscular injections and also because of unpredictable pharmacokinetics.

Patient-controlled analgesia also provides excellent analgesia for pediatric group of patients. However, preoperative education is valuable for children using PCA. This is because the patient needs the control of button to self-administer the bolus of analgesics and before using PCA adequate intravenous loading dose of the opioid is required to achieve the adequate blood levels. The two modes of PCA are used. These are (1) bolus only and (2) bolus with continuous infusion. Various nerve blocks and epidural block are also often can be used for postoperative analgesia. **Table 18** shows the different routes of administration of analgesic drugs.

Selection of Drugs

The *nonsteroidal anti-inflammatory drugs (NSAIDs) are taken as the first line of therapy for analgesia* in pediatric group of patients. This is followed by the opioids and then local anesthetics. Recently, the local anesthetic agents have become the drug of choice for the postoperative analgesia.

However, most recently a multimodal approach, using a combination of drugs, provides effective analgesia with lower doses of every drugs than any single drug.

Among the *NSAIDs,* the paracetamol is the agent of first-line management for pediatric pain control. Their action is linked to their anti-inflammatory, antipyretic, and analgesic effects by inhibiting cyclo-oxygenase and thus reducing the production of pain mediators, such as thromboxanes and prostaglandins. Their main efficacy is in *mild to moderate pain*. But, they also have an opioid-sparing effect. They are metabolized in the liver and excreted by the kidneys. They should be used with caution in newborns, because their organs are still immature. Other side effects of NSAIDs are gastric irritation and inhibition of platelet function. They also have a *ceiling effect* which means that above a certain higher dose there is only an increase in their side effects, without increasing the analgesic effect.

The NSAIDs must be avoided in infants <1 year. Most NSAIDs can be administered by the oral or rectal route, while ketorolac and paracetamol can be used through IV. Paracetamol is the most commonly used pediatric analgesic in daily practice. A recent paper recommends the following doses of paracetamol in children 40 mg/kg as rectal suppositories (PR) initially, followed by 20 mg/kg orally, followed by 30 mg/kg orally at every 8 hours interval. The 90 mg/kg/day dosage is not always sufficient for pain relief and 100–200 mg/kg/per rectum may be necessary, keeping in mind that the toxicity is connected with the cumulative action of repeated doses.

In the newborn, the dosage of paracetamol is reduced to 40 mg/kg/PR, followed by 30 mg/kg/12 hours orally. *Propacetamol,* the injectable water soluble prodrug of paracetamol is useful for faster onset of analgesia. The recommended IV dose of ketorolac, another NSAID whose effectiveness has been demonstrated successfully in acute pain management, is 0.75 mg/kg and provides analgesia similar to 0.1 mg/kg of morphine. Diclofenac is used as 0.5–1 mg/kg/rectal and ibuprofen as 10 mg/kg orally, every 8 hours.

The *opioids* are the basis of postoperative treatment for *moderate to severe pain*. Their action is at the specific receptors along the CNS, inhibiting the release of neurotransmitters. The major concern for the use of narcotics in the pediatric age group of patients is the proportional increase in side effects with increased doses. These are respiratory depression, nausea, vomiting, pruritus, urinary retention, delay in gastrointestinal function, etc. The respiratory depression can occur even several hours after the administration of opioids. So, the accurate monitoring of all the vital parameters such as the respiratory rate and oxygen saturation is mandatory.

TABLE 18: Common routes of administration.	
Oral	Transmucosal preparation of fentanyl lollipop (8–10 µg/kg)
Rectal	• Paracetamol (80–170 mg) • Diclofenac (12.5 mg)
Parenteral	• Intramuscular • Intravenous • Bolus, continuous infusion, patient-controlled analgesia (PCA), epidural, and subcutaneous

The evaluation of sedation score is also important for pediatric group of patients because a slight overdose of narcotics may easily cause deep sedation which is not desirable. Morphine is the gold standard opioid with which all other opioids are compared and is frequently used for postoperative pain relief in children. The doses of morphine depend on the route of administration, for example: (1) SC → 0.01–0.02 mg/kg, (2) IV → 0.02–0.1 mg/kg, (3) continuous infusion: loading dose of 0.1–0.2 mg/kg, followed by 0.01 mg/kg/hour; (4) Epidural → 0.03 mg/kg/8 hours. However, the abovementioned doses of morphine must be reduced in newborns and infants.

Fentanyl is 100 times more potent than morphine. It has a rapid onset of action and shorter half-life. So, it is useful for short-term therapy in acute pain, in the dose of 1–4 µg/kg through intravenous. Fentanyl also can be administered epidurally at the dose of 1–2 µg/kg. Remifentanil is the most recent synthetic opioid which is mainly metabolized by a specific plasma esterase. It has a very short elimination half-life of 3–5 minutes. Alfentanil and sufentanil are two other important synthetic opioids. The commonly prescribed adjuvant drug for opioid's complication is naloxone (5–10 µg/kg through IV) and ondansetron (0.1–0.2 mg/kg/8 hourly by IV or PO).

The RA has wide application for the management of postoperative pain in pediatric group of patients. The regional analgesia can involve epidural block, subarachnoid block, different plexus block, different peripheral nerve block wound infiltration, and topical application. Blocks are safe and effective in children with the use of different local anesthetic agent with or without adjuvants, like clonidine,

TABLE 19: Common regional block.

Caudal	0.5–1.2 mL/kg of 0.25% bupivacaine for sacral or lumbar nerves
Penile block	0.1 mL/kg of 0.25% bupivacaine on each side
Ilioinguinal block	
Lumbar epidural	0.5 mL/kg of 0.5% bupivacaine
Brachial plexus block	0.3 mL/kg of 0.25% bupivacaine

opioids, etc. in both as single shot or as continuous infusion technique, according to the type of surgery and the quality and intensity of the postoperative pain. It is the best technique for reducing the surgical stress. All the local anesthetics, used for adults, may be applied in pediatric practice too, provided the appropriate dosing regimens are followed. The lignocaine and mepivacaine are suitable for short time surgeries and mild postoperative pain, while bupivacaine is used for long-term analgesia. Ropivacaine is the new amino-amide local anesthetic agent with lesser cardiac and CNS toxicity than bupivacaine. **Table 19** shows the doses of bupivacaine in different regional analgesic technique.

To conclude for the postoperative pain management in pediatric patients, we can always say that the presence of a tender and loving care of mother, by the side of the child, reduces the pain to a great extent. The anticipation of pain and its pre-emptive intervention is very helpful. Using the multimodal (pharmacological, cognitive, behavioral, and physical) and the multidisciplinary approach for the relief of pain, whenever possible, offers the best postoperative pain relief in children.

Perioperative Arrhythmia and its Management

■ INTRODUCTION

The incidences of perioperative cardiac arrhythmia varies from center to center and it depends on many factors. These factors are:

- The types of arrhythmias (because all the types of arrhythmias are not taken into account or their incidences, as all are not potentially so harmful)
- The types of surveillance (extensive surveillance increases the incidences of arrhythmias and less sensitive surveillance decreases the incidences of arrhythmias)
- The characteristics of patients and underlying diseases
- The nature of surgery
- The nature of anesthesia itself with its different variabilities.

The perioperative arrhythmias are nothing different or special in type. These are the same arrhythmias that we see in everyday cardiological practice. But, these are just named such (perioperative arrhythmia), because they are associated with the operative and anesthetic procedures. Even the management of these arrhythmias remains more or less the same, except the stoppage or the alterations of some anesthetic drugs and the stoppage of some surgical procedures, such as the traction on viscera, muscles (especially ocular), and peritoneum. The incidence of perioperative arrhythmias in *cardiothoracic surgery* with extensive monitoring exceeds 90% and in most of these cases requires no treatment whereas this incidence of perioperative arrhythmia in *elective cesarean section* is very low. The factors that determine how a patient tolerates these perioperative arrhythmias include: (1) the heart rate, (2) the type of arrhythmia, (3) the duration of this arrhythmia, (4) the presence and the severity of any underlying cardiac disease with this arrhythmia, (5) the effects of that specific arrhythmia (cardiac rhythm) on the cardiac output (CO), and (6) the possible interaction of antiarrhythmic drugs with the drugs which are administered to produce and maintain the anesthesia.

■ HEART RATE

The measurement of heart rate and the identification of cardiac arrhythmia go hand in hand. This is because many abnormalities of heart rate measurement (incorrect measurement of heart rate) results from arrhythmias and also any wrong measurement of heart rate may seem arrhythmia. Hence, to begin with, I shall describe ways (methods) how to measure the heart rate from electrocardiogram (ECG) tracing and how to diagnose the abnormalities that can affect it. It will have to remember that, when there is talk of measuring the heart rate, it will mean the ventricular rate which corresponds to the patient's pulse and not the atrial rate.

Measurement of Heart Rate

The measurement of heart rate from an ECG tracing is simple and can be done in several ways:

- When the paper speed is 25 mm/second, then 1 second ECG tracing covers 25 mm length of paper or 25 small squares, or 5 large squares (every small square is 1 mm and every large square containing 5 small squares is 5 mm) **(Fig. 1)**. Therefore, 1 minute ECG tracing covers 1,500 small squares or 300 large squares (60 second × 5 large squares). If patient's cardiac rhythm is regular, then that have to do is to count the number of large squares between two QRS complexes and divide 300 (1 minutes or 60 seconds cover 300 large squares) by this number which will give the heart rate.

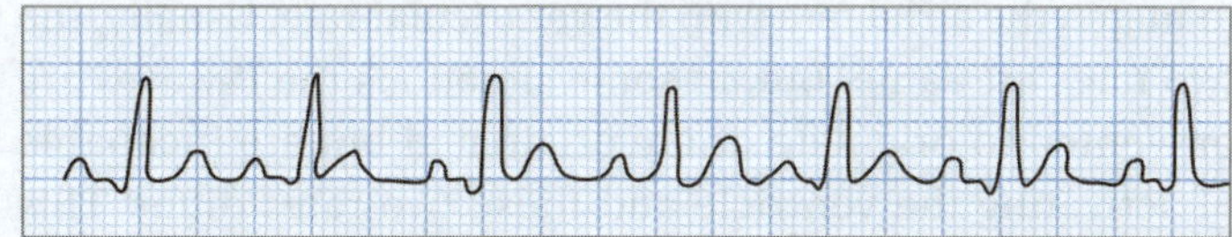

Fig. 1: Electrocardiogram (ECG) with sinus rhythm at heart rate of 100 beats/min, because there are three large squares between two QRS complexes.

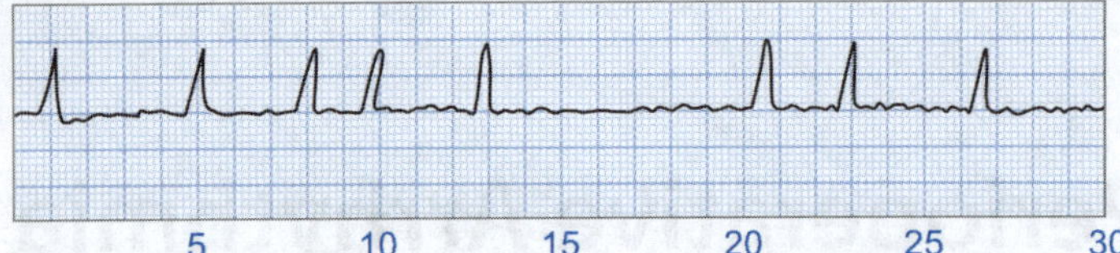

Fig. 2: This graph shows irregular cardiac rhythm. Here, the heart rate is calculated like that: we know that the 5 large square is 1 second, or 1 second = 5 large squares. So, the 60 seconds or 1 minute = 60 × 5 = 300 large squares. The 30 large squares contain 8 QRS complexes. So, the 300 large squares contain 8 × 10 = 80 QRS complexes. Thus, the heart rate is 80 beats/min.

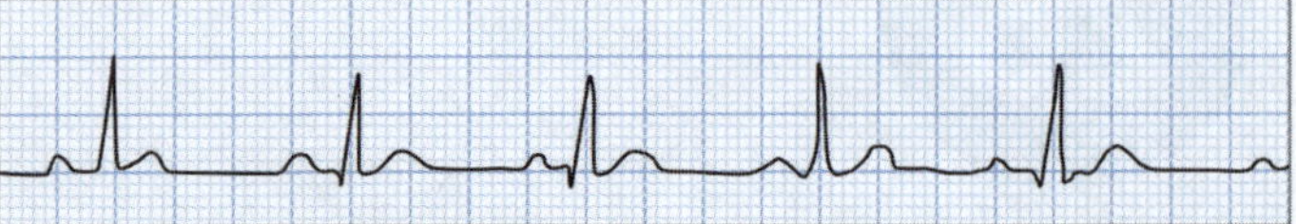

Fig. 3: This electrocardiogram (ECG) graph indicates 20 small squares between two R-waves. So, 20 small squares indicate one heartbeat. Therefore, 1,500 small squares (or 1 minute) indicate 1,500 ÷ 20 = 75 heartbeats.

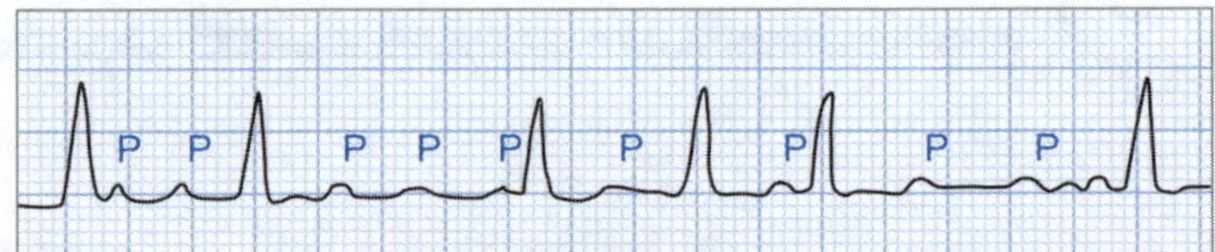

Fig. 4: This electrocardiogram graph shows different P-wave rate and QRS complex rate. To calculate the P-wave rate and QRS complex rate separately, we have to take the help of 30 large squares.

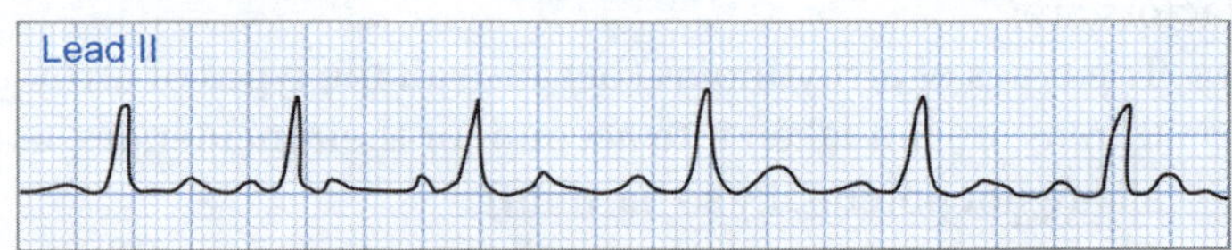

Fig. 5: This is an electrocardiogram graph of sinus rhythm which is characterized by: (1) regular heart beat by any rate, (2) P-waves are upright in lead II, and (3) QRS complex after every P-wave.

For example, if there are four large squares between two QRS complexes, then the heart rate is 300 ÷ 4 = 75 per minute. The explanation is like that the 300 large squares mean 1 minute timing and the number of large squares between two QRS complexes mean the interval between two heart beats. So, the division of 300 (i.e., 1 minute) by the interval (time in second) between two heart beats will give the heart rate.

- When the rhythm is irregular, this method does not work well, because the number of large squares, between two QRS complexes, varies from beat to beat. Here, that have to do is to count the number of QRS complexes within the total duration of 30 large squares which indicates the number of QRS complexes in 6 seconds (1 second means 5 large squares) **(Fig. 2)**.

  Now, the heart rate can simply be workout by multiplying the number of QRS complexes in 6 seconds (which is equivalent to 30 large squares) with 10. As for example, if the number of QRS complexes within 30 large squares is 6, then the heart rate is 6 × 10 = 60 per minute.

- When the ECG paper speed is 25 mm/second (i.e., 25 small squares per second because every small square is 1 mm or 0.04 second), then within 1 minute the tracing covers 1,500 small squares (1 second covers 25 small squares, therefore, 60 seconds cover 60 × 25 = 1,500 small squares). Then the heart rate can easily be calculated by dividing 1,500 with the number of small squares between two R-waves. As for example, let the number of small squares between two R-waves is 20. Then the heart rate is 1,500 ÷ 20 = 75 per minute **(Fig. 3)**.

These above methods of the measurement of ventricular rate also can be used to measure the atrial or P-wave rate and to match the atrial rate with the ventricular rate. Usually, the two rates are same. But, in some situations the P-waves are prevented to originate or are originated but are incapable of activating the ventricle and these two rates differ. This situation will be discussed later on **(Fig. 4)**.

After the measurement of heart rate, one has to decide is whether: (1) it is regular or irregular, (2) there is bradycardia or tachycardia, (3) QRS complex is narrow or broad, and (4) it is supraventricular or ventricular in origin. As a general rule, a regular cardiac rhythm with heart rate between 60 and 100 beats/min is considered normal. If the heart rate is regular, but below 60 beats/min, then it is called the bradycardia and if the heart rate is regular, but above 100 beats/min, then it is called the tachycardia.

Sinus Rhythm

Sinus rhythm is the normal cardiac rhythm in which the sinoatrial (SA) node acts as the natural pacemaker and discharging the impulses at the rate of 60–100 times per minute **(Fig. 5)**.

Sinus Arrhythmia

It is the normal physiological variation of heart rate with respiration, i.e., increase in heart rate during inspiration and decrease in heart rate during expiration. Heart rate increases during inspiration as a reflex response to the increased blood volume returning to the heart during inspiration. But, during expiration, reverse occurs and heart rate decreases. It is harmless and no treatment is necessary. It is uncommon after the age of 40 years. The characteristics of sinus arrhythmia in ECG tracing are that every P-wave is

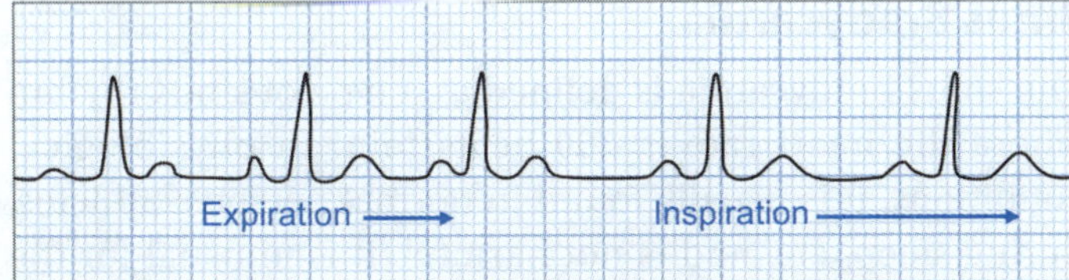

Fig. 6: This is an electrocardiogram (ECG) graph of sinus arrhythmia, characterized by the heart rate of 100 beats/min during inspiration and 75 beats/min during expiration.

followed by QRS complex and the heart rate varies with the respiration **(Fig. 6)**.

CLASSIFICATION OF PERIOPERATIVE DIFFERENT TYPES OF CARDIAC RHYTHM

The following types of cardiac rhythms (normal or abnormal) are usually encountered during the perioperative period **(Box 1)**:

- *Rhythms arising from sinoatrial node:* Sinus rhythm, sinus arrhythmia, sinus bradycardia, sinus tachycardia, sick sinus syndrome (SSS), and sinus arrest.
- *Rhythms arising from atrial musculature:* Atrial tachycardia [supraventricular tachycardia (SVT) and paroxysmal supraventricular tachycardia (PSVT)], atrial flutter, atrial fibrillation (AF), and atrial ectopic.
- *Rhythms arising from atrioventricular node:* Atrioventricular (AV) nodal re-entry tachycardia, AV re-entry tachycardia [Wolff–Parkinson–White (WPW) syndrome], AV nodal or junctional rhythm, and AV junctional tachycardia.
- *Ventricular rhythms arising from ventricular musculature:* Ventricular extrasystoles, ventricular tachycardia (VT), accelerated idioventricular rhythm, torsades de pointes, ventricular flutter, and ventricular fibrillation (VF).
- *Rhythm due to conduction disturbances:* Escape rhythm, ectopic beats [right bundle branch block (RBBB) or left bundle branch block (LBBB) are not varieties of rhythm. These are only due to conduction defects].

The following questions should be asked for the diagnosis or identification of various types of cardiac rhythms:
The diagnosis of various types of cardiac rhythm, from the tracing of ECG, is not usually difficult. But, sometimes it may become difficult. Then, the following questions should be asked which will facilitate to diagnose the different arrhythmias. These are:
- *From where the impulses are arising?*
  SA node, atria, AV node, or ventricles.
- *How the impulses are conducted?*
  Normal conduction, accelerated conduction (WPW syndrome), or blocked conduction.

<table>
<tr><td>BOX 1: Different types of cardiac rhythms.</td></tr>
</table>

- *Sinoatrial (SA) nodal rhythms:*
  - Sinus rhythm
  - Sinus arrhythmia
  - Sinus tachycardia
  - Sinus bradycardia
  - Sick sinus syndrome
  - Sinus arrest
  - Sinus block
- *Atrial rhythms:*
  - Atrial tachycardia
  - Paroxysmal atrial tachycardia
  - Atrial flutter
  - Atrial fibrillation
- *Atrioventricular (AV) rhythms:*
  - AV nodal or junctional rhythms
  - AV junctional tachycardia
  - AV re-entry tachycardia
  - AV nodal re-entry tachycardia
- *Ventricular rhythms:*
  - Ventricular tachycardia
  - Accelerated idioventricular rhythms
  - Torsades de pointes
  - Ventricular fibrillation
- *Conduction disturbances:*
  - RBBB
  - LBBB, LAHB, and LPHB
  - Bifascicular block
  - Complete block
- Escape rhythms
- Ectopic beats

(LBBB: left bundle branch block; LAHB: left anterior hemiblock; LPHB: left posterior hemiblock; RBBB: right bundle branch block)

- *If the rhythm is regular or irregular?*
  To determine whether the cardiac rhythm is regular or not, the distance between the two consecutive R-waves is measured. If the RR intervals vary, then the rhythm is irregular. The causes of irregular rhythm is sinus arrhythmia, atrial flutter with varying degree of blocks, AF, any supraventricular rhythm with intermittent block, escape rhythm, ectopic beats, and VF.
- *If the rhythm is supraventricular (including the AV junction) or ventricular?*
  The supraventricular rhythm means when it originates from the site above the ventricle. All the supraventricular rhythms produce narrow QRS complexes, provided there is no conduction defects. If supraventricular rhythm is associated with bundle branch block or an accessary pathway, then the QRS complexes will be broad. The ventricular rhythm by itself originating from ventricular musculature are associated with broad QRS complex (>3 small squares). This is due to the conduction of

impulses through ventricular musculature, instead of through the specified high conducting Purkinje fibers which takes less times.

- *If the P-waves are present or not?*

The presence of P-waves indicates atrial activity. So, the careful examination of P-waves and QRS complexes gives an idea of the relationship between the atrial and ventricular activity. The shape of P-wave also provides an idea of the origin of atrial depolarization. For example, if it is upright in lead II, then it is sure that the atrial depolarization origins in or near the SA node. On the contrary, an inverted P-waves in lead II suggest its origin closer to or within the AV node. This is because, here, the impulses pass from AV node to SA node whose direction is upward and opposite to the direction of lead II. If all the P-waves are followed by QRS complexes, then it indicates that the conduction from atrium to ventricle is normal and there is no AV block. If there are more P-waves than QRS complexes, then the conduction between atria and ventricles is being either partly blocked or completely blocked or atrial activity is such increased that it is beyond the normal conduction capability of the AV node. More QRS complexes than P-waves indicate AV dissociation with higher ventricular rate than atrium. During the identification of P-wave, always, we have to bear in our mind that sometimes the P-waves may be difficult or even impossible to identify clearly. Therefore, it can be difficult to say firmly that the atrial activity is present or absent.

- *If there is bradycardia or tachycardia?*

CAUSES OF PERIOPERATIVE BRADYCARDIA AND ITS MANAGEMENT

In the previous page, all the arrhythmias are classified according to the site of their origin. But, here from the aspect of management, all the arrhythmias are classified under the two broad headings: (1) arrhythmias, causing bradycardia and (2) arrhythmias, causing tachycardia.

The common causes of perioperative arrhythmias, causing bradycardia are:

- Sinus bradycardia
- Sinus arrest
- Sinoatrial block
- Sick sinus syndrome
- Conduction defects—second- and third-degree AV block
- Escape rhythm—AV junctional escape rhythms, ventricular escape rhythm
- Ectopic
- Asystole

Sinus Bradycardia

The sinus bradycardia is defined as a type of sinus rhythm where the heart rate is <60 beats/min. In physiological conditions, it is usually found in normal persons, athletes, during sleep, etc. and is not harmful. It is unusual for the sinus bradycardia to be slower than 40 beats/min, otherwise the alternative causes like heart block, drug effect, etc. should be considered. The probable pathological causes of sinus bradycardia are drugs (digoxin, β-blockers, antiarrhythmic agents, adenosine, verapamil, diltiazem, anesthetic drugs, etc.), ischemic heart disease (IHD), M1-leading to conduction defects, SSS, hypothyroidism, hypothermia, electrolyte imbalance, obstructive jaundice, uremia, raised intracranial pressure (ICP), etc.

The characteristic features of sinus bradycardia in ECG **(Fig. 7)** are:

- Heart rate is <60 beats/min.
- Every P-wave is followed by a QRS complex.
- The P-wave is upright in lead II and inverted in lead aVR.

If the bradycardia is severe, i.e., <40 beats/min, then one has to consider sinus arrest, SA block, SSS, and complete heart block, etc. If this sinus bradycardia is severe, then escape beats or escape rhythms, from the AV node or ventricles, may also occur (start to originate) as a safeguard (compensatory) mechanism.

For sinus bradycardia, due to physiological conditions, no treatment is needed. But, for the management of symptomatic severe sinus bradycardia, the first step is to assess the urgency of situation, such as the syncope, falls, dizziness or breathlessness. This is usually done by proper history taking, careful examination, and further investigations (e.g., thyroid function, plasma electrolytes, etc.). It (investigations) will also help to identify the underlying pathological causes for this severe bradycardia and to correct it (1) by where possible by the discontinuation or the reduction of the dose of responsible drugs, (2) by the identification of abnormal cardiac rhythm and its management, (3) by the identification and the treatment of hypothyroidism, etc. When the bradycardia is severe and symptomatic with the evidence of severe hemodynamic disturbances, then more urgent treatment is instituted immediately, such as (1) injection atropine—300–600 µg given slowly intravenously, and/or

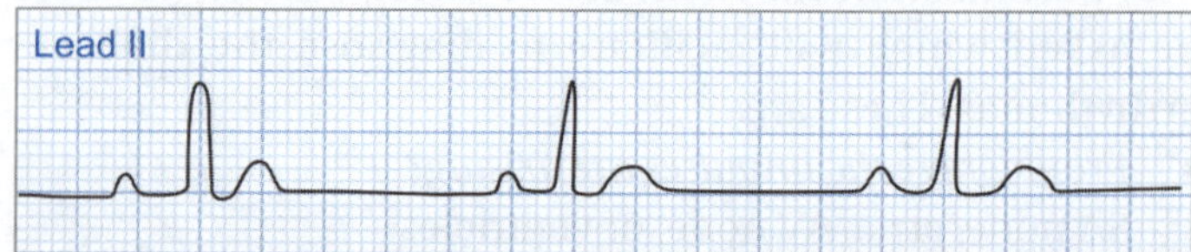

Fig. 7: This is an electrocardiogram (ECG) graph of sinus bradycardia, characterized by: (1) heart rate 50 beats/min, (2) upright P-wave in lead II, and (3) QRS complex after every P-wave.

(2) injection isoprenaline—0.5–10 µg/min by intravenous infusion very slowly.

However, the insertion of temporary pacemaker, later on permanent if indicated, is preferred than the prolonged infusion of isoprenaline. So, isoprenaline infusion should only be used as a short-term measure, while arranging for temporary or permanent pacing. Chronic severe bradycardia, due to any cause, may also be an indication for a permanent pacemaker, particularly, when it is causing symptoms or hemodynamic disturbance, even after the removal of the etiologies.

Sick Sinus Syndrome

The SSS refers to some conditions which are characterized by the combination of (1) abnormal impulse generation and (2) its conduction problems related to the dysfunction of sinus node. As the name (syndrome) suggests, it is a collection of symptoms, such as dizziness, fatigue, confusion, syncope, and congestive heart failure. Any of the following ECG findings can be seen in patient with SSS with different combination. These are *sinus bradycardia, SA block, sinus arrest,* and *brady-tachy syndrome.*

Sinoatrial Block (SA Exit Block)

Here, the SA node depolarizes as normal rate, but some impulses fail to reach the atria from the SA node. Here, the pathology lies in the junction between the SA node and atrial muscle. The SA block may be of three degrees:

1. *First-degree SA exit block:* It denotes a *prolonged exit time* of all the impulses from SA node to the surrounding atrial tissue. It cannot be diagnosed by standard surface ECG, but requires invasive intracardiac recording.
2. *Second-degree SA exit block:* It denotes the intermittent failure of exit of impulses from the SA node to the atrium. It is manifested in ECG as the *intermittent absence of P-wave.* This is because, the P-wave fails to appear in the expected place. But, the *next usually appears, exactly where it is expected.*
3. *Third-degree SA exit block or complete SA block:* Here, all the impulses originating from SA node are blocked and fails to pass to atrium. So, it is characterized by complete lack of SA node activity in ECG and the presence of a subsidiary ectopic atrial or AV junctional pacemaker **(Fig. 8).**

Sinus Arrest

Here, the SA node fails to depolarize itself, but there is no abnormality of passing the impulses from the SA node to the atrium, once it originates. So, all the manifestations of sinus arrest are like that of third-degree SA exit block. By looking

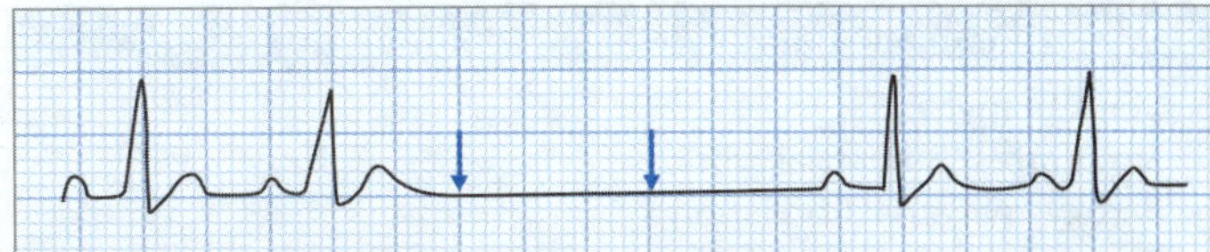

Fig. 8: This is an electrocardiogram (ECG) graph of sinoatrial block, characterized by two P-waves fail to appear, but the next P-wave appears where it is expected.

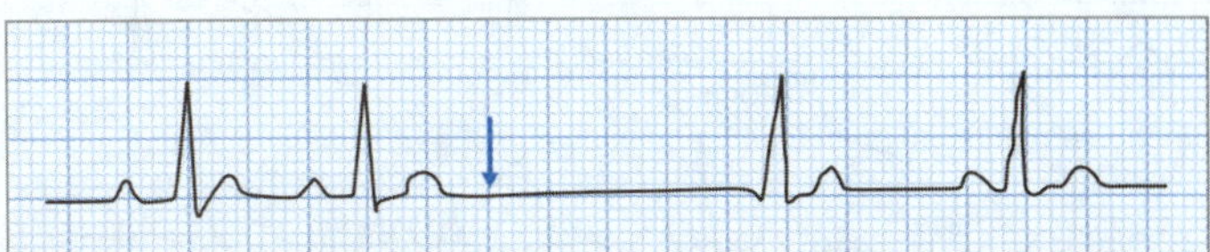

Fig. 9: This is an electrocardiogram (ECG) graph of sinus arrest, characterized by P-wave fails to appear, but the next P-wave does not appear where expected.

at the ECG strip, we can find that a P-wave will suddenly fail to appear in the expected place and there is a gap of variable length, until the sinus node fires again, which is irregular and a P-wave appears **(Fig. 9).**

Brady-tachy Syndrome

It refers to a combination of sinus bradycardia, SA block, sinus arrest (all the components of SSS) with PSVT **(Box 2).** In this syndrome the tachycardia often emerges as an escape rhythm in response to the episode of bradycardia and then it usually terminates with prolonged sinus pause. So, there is alternate periods of tachycardia and bradycardia. Moreover, any atrial tachycardia, during which the atrial ectopic site is activated, may cause an overdrive suppression of the sinus node, resulting in the clinical appearance of this syndrome **(Fig. 10).**

The SSS usually coexists with AF, atrial flutter, atrial tachycardia, AV conduction disorder, etc.

The degeneration and the fibrosis of SA node and its conducting system, due to aging, is the most common cause of this SSS. The probable other causes of SSS are IHD, drugs (antiarrhythmic), cardiomyopathy, myocarditis, etc. The diagnosis of this syndrome usually requires 24 hours Holter monitoring. While looking at the ECG strip, a P-wave will suddenly fail to appear in the expected place and there is a gap of variable length, until the sinus node fires again and a P-wave appears. The conduction problems become apparent, when a patient with brady-tachy syndrome develops AF. During tachycardia, the AV node fails to conduct all the atrial impulses at this unusual high atrial rate. Thus, AV block precipitates and the ventricular rate remains slow.

An asymptomatic patient with SSS does not require any treatment. But, the symptomatic patients need the

BOX 2: Common features of sick sinus syndrome.

- Sinus bradycardia
- Sinus arrest, sinoatrial block
- Paroxysmal atrial fibrillation
- Paroxysmal supraventricular tachycardia
- Atrioventricular block

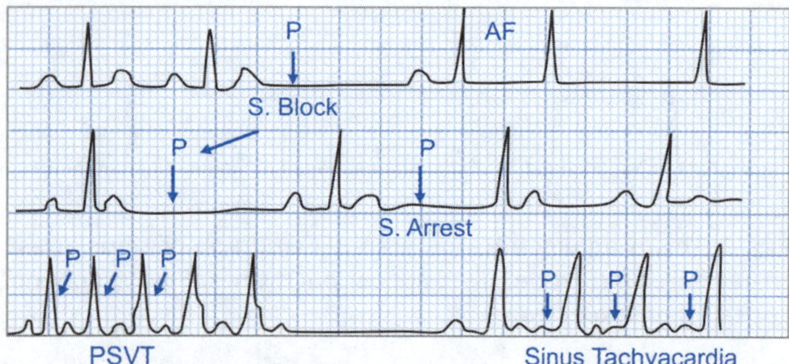

Fig. 10: This is an electrocardiogram (ECG) graph of sick sinus syndrome, characterized by: (1) sinus block, (2) sinus arrest, (3) atrial fibrillation (AF), (4) paroxysmal supraventricular tachycardia (PSVT), and (5) sinus tachycardia.

consideration for permanent pacemaker. This is particularly important, if they also have paroxysmal tachycardia that require antiarrhythmic drugs (which can worsens the episodes of bradycardia). On the other hand, the paroxysmal tachycardia, which arise as an escape rhythm in response to the episodes of bradycardia, may improve, as the consequence of pacing and thus the vicious cycle is cut.

ATRIOVENTRICULAR CONDUCTION DEFECTS

Introduction

The specialized conducting system (AV bundle, bundle of His, and Purkinje fibers), running between the atrium and the ventricle, ensures the smooth conduction of sinus impulses from the atrium to the ventricle, resulting in the synchronous contraction of these two chambers. Hence, any abnormalities of this conducting system may lead to the incomplete or complete block of the passage of impulses from the atrium to the ventricle, causing cardiac stand still or escape ventricular beat. The discussion on these conduction abnormalities has three significant clinical points and these are

1. The detection of the site of conduction disturbance
2. The chance of the risk of the progression of incomplete block to complete block
3. The probability of the electrophysiological and hemodynamic stability of the subsidiary escape rhythm, arising distal to the block.

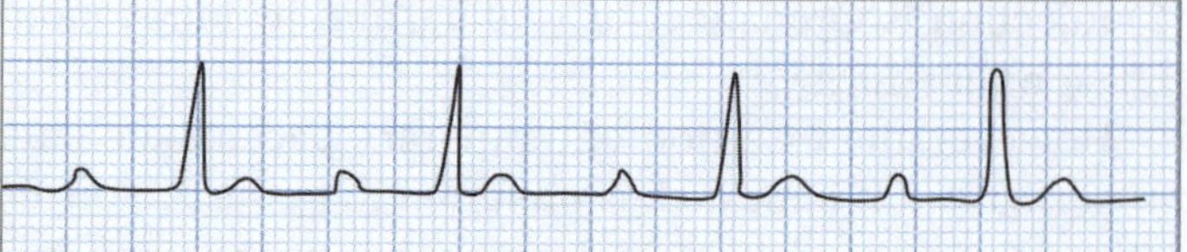

Fig. 11: This is an electrocardiogram (ECG) graph of first-degree atrioventricular (AV) block. It is characterized by the long PR interval (0.32 second).

This last point is very important, because the symptoms which will develop, depend on the stability of this escape rhythm. After the AV block, the subsidiary escape beat can arise from the bundle of His or distal to the bundle in the Purkinje system. The difference between these two types of escape rhythm is that the impulses, arising from the bundle of His, are of 50–60 beats/min, whereas the impulses, arising from the distal Purkinje system, are 30–40 beats/min and unstable with broad QRS complex.

Classification

Atrioventricular conduction defects or block can be classified into three degrees:

1. *First-degree AV block:* It is also called the *prolonged AV conduction defect,* which is characterized by the PR interval of >0.2 second **(Fig. 11)**. The PR interval is the period that extends from the beginning of P-wave to the beginning of R-wave and includes (1) the time for atrial depolarization, (2) the time for impulse passing through the AV node with physiological delay, and (3) the time for the impulse passing through the His-Purkinje conducting system. The delay in passing of impulses through any of these structures can contribute to the prolonged PR interval.

   The delay in atrial depolarization has no clinical significance, whereas the delay within the AV node results in the prolonged PR interval (>0.24 second) with normal QRS complex. And the delay in His-Purkinje system results in the prolonged QRS duration or broad QRS complex, in addition to the prolonged PR interval. *However, the first-degree heart block does not usually need any management.*

2. *Second-degree AV block:* This is also called the intermittent AV block, as the some but not all the atrial impulses fail to conduct to the ventricles through AV node. The second-degree AV block is again of two types, such as *Mobitz type I and Mobitz type II.*

   In Mobitz type I (Wenckebach block) variety of second-degree AV block, there is gradual prolongation of PR interval, followed by a complete block of conduction of an atrial impulse to the ventricle. This type of second-degree AV block is almost always localized in the AV node and is associated with normal QRS duration. This type of AV block is usually found with inferior wall infarction, β-blockers, calcium channel antagonists, drug intoxication particularly digitalis, normal individual with high vagal tone, etc. So, this phenomenon may be physiological and is sometimes observed at rest or during sleep in athletic young adults. Sometimes, this Mobitz type I category of second-degree AV block can progress to third-degree complete heart block, but it is uncommon, except in acute inferior wall myocardial infarction (MI). But, still, if the Mobitz type I category of AV block progresses to complete block, it is well tolerated, This is because, the escape pacemaker usually arises in the proximal bundle of His and provides a stable rhythm. So, the Mobitz type I block rarely necessitates any aggressive therapy. If the ventricular rate as a consequence of Mobitz type I block is adequate and the patient is asymptomatic, then only observation is sufficient **(Fig. 12)**.

In Mobitz type II variety of second-degree AV block, there is sudden complete block of the conduction of impulses from the atrium to the ventricle through AV node, without any previous warning of prolonged PR interval. In some varieties of this type of conduction defect, the block is localized in the His-Purkinje system, but not in the AV node and is associated with the prolonged duration of QRS complexes. Clinically, it is very important, because it has the high incidences of progression to the complete AV block, with the unstable escape pacemaker rhythm below the block. So, cardiac pacing is necessary in this type of block **(Fig. 13)**.

3. *Third-degree AV block:* In third-degree AV block, no atrial impulse propagates to ventricles from atrium. So, the escape beat may arise from the AV node or His-Purkinje system. When the escape beat arise from the AV node, then the block is proximal to the origin of this escape beat in AV node and this block is called the AV nodal block. In such situation, the escape ventricular beat is of normal QRS complex (as it passes through the normal Purkinje fibers) with the rate of 40–50 beats/min and is responsive to exercise or atropine. This is usually of congenital type. If the block is situated in the His-Purkinje system, then the escape rhythm arises from the ventricular musculature and is unreliable. It is characterized by broad QRS complexes, with the rate of <40 beats/min and is usually unresponsive to atropine and exercise. This type of complete AV block mandates pacemaker implantation **(Fig. 14)**.

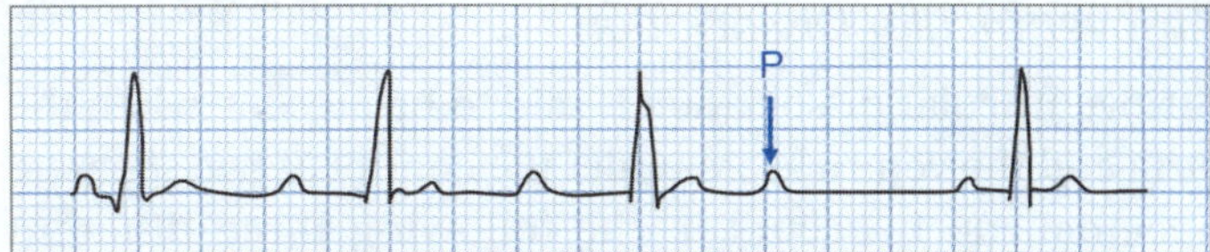

Fig. 12: This is an electrocardiogram (ECG) graph of Mobitz type I AV block. It is characterized by: (1) the progressive lengthening of PR interval (0.16 second, then 0.28 second, then 0.32 second), (2) followed by a P-wave fails to be conducted with no QRS complex, and (3) then PR interval resets with repeated cycle.

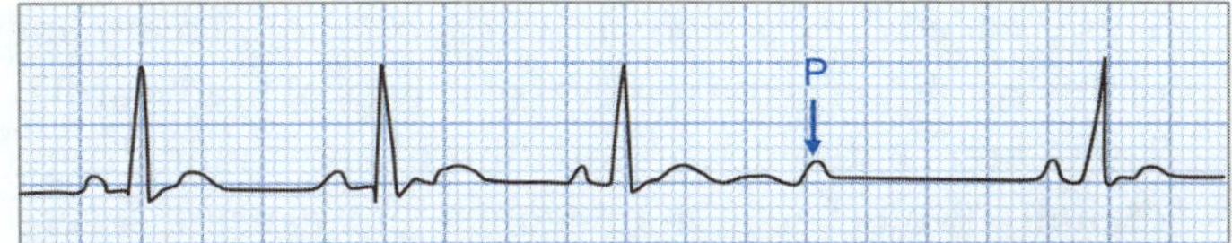

Fig. 13: This is an electrocardiogram (ECG) graph of Mobitz type II block. It is characterized by: (1) all the normal and constant PR intervals and (2) occasional P-wave fails to be conducted.

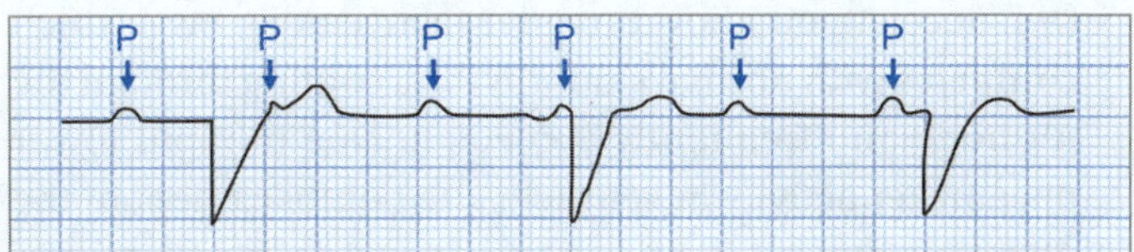

Fig. 14: This is a graph of third-degree atrioventricular (AV) block. It is characterized by: (1) P-wave (atrial) rate is 100 beats/min, (2) QRS complex (ventricular) rate is 42 beats/min, (3) broad QRS complexes, and (4) no relationship between the P-waves and QRS complexes. There is no relationship between the P-waves and QRS complexes, because no P-wave is conducted to the ventricle through AV node, due to the complete AV block. The QRS complexes are broad, because they arise from the ventricular musculature.

Adams–Stokes Attack (Stokes-Adams Syndrome)

The episodes of ventricular asystole, in the absence of escape beat, may complicate the complete heart block or Mobitz type II second-degree AV block or the SSS. This may be recurrent and cause syncope which is called the *"Adams–Stokes" attack*. A typical episode of Adams–Stokes syndrome is characterized by the sudden loss of consciousness (which frequently occurs) without warning and may result in the sudden fall of patient on ground. Convulsions (due to cerebral ischemia) can occur, if there is prolonged asystole. There is also death-like appearance during the attack. But, when the heart starts to beat again, then there is characteristic regain of consciousness and flush. In contrast to epilepsy, the recovery in Adams–Stokes attack is rapid. Other diseases, like the *hypersensitive carotid sinus syndrome* and the *malignant vasovagal syndrome*, may also cause similar symptoms and should be differentiated from Adams–Stokes attack.

Atrioventricular Dissociation

Atrioventricular dissociation is said to be present, when the atria and the ventricle are under the control of two separate pacemakers. It occurs in the following three different conditions:

1. When there is complete AV block—discussed before.
2. There is no AV block, but due to severe sinus bradycardia, the escape AV junctional rhythm starts. In such case, when the sinus rate and the escape rate are same, then the P-wave occurs just before the following QRS complex. This is called the *isorhythmic AV dissociation*. Treatment of this condition is the removal of causes of bradycardia. These are: (1) the discontinuation of anesthetic drugs, digitalis, β-blockers, Ca-antagonist, etc. causing severe bradycardia, (2) the use of vagolytic agents, and (3) pace making, only if the patient becomes symptomatic due to severe bradycardia.
3. There is no AV block, but enhanced lower pacemaker rate (VT, accelerated idioventricular tachycardia, etc.) which competes with normal sinus rhythm, coming through the AV node and frequently exceeds it. Due to rapid lower pacemaker activity in ventricle, the bombardment of the AV node by impulses arising from ventricle in a retrograde fashion, renders it refractory to the normal sinus impulse. Thus, the atrium and the ventricle beat independently. This is called interference AV dissociation, and is usually happened during myocardial ischemia, infarction, after cardiac surgery, etc. The treatments of such condition are: (1) the administration of antiarrhythmic agent, (2) the removal of offending drugs, and (3) the correction of metabolic abnormalities or ischemia.

Role of Intracardiac ECG in Diagnosis of AV Conduction Defects

The main indication for performing an intracardiac ECG or His bundle ECG is to determine the proper indication for pacing or to select the proper patient who will be benefited from pacing:

- *A symptomatic third-degree AV block:* In such patient, the His bundle ECG will be helpful to assess the stability of the junctional *pacemaker*, if it is present. If His bundle escape rhythm is unstable, then pacing is indicated, though the patient is asymptomatic.
- *Patient with syncope and bundle branch or fascicular block:* If such patient shows infra-His bundle conduction disturbance then they are indicated for pacing. But nodal conduction disturbance are not indication for pacing. Bifascicular block with asymptomatic patient are not indicated for intracardiac ECG as these group of patients are very unusually associated with AV conduction disturbances.
- *Symptomatic second- and third-degree AV block:* These are always the indications for pacing without intracardiac ECG.
- *Asymptomatic second-degree AV block:* It is always indicated for intracardiac or His bundle ECG. If the block is established at the intra- or infra-His bundle level, then pacing is indicated though the patient is asymptomatic.

Management of AV Conduction Defects

Pharmacological Therapy

It is only indicated in acute situations of AV conduction defect. Atropine in the dose of 0.6–2 mg IV and isoprenaline in the dose of 1–4 µg/min by infusion increases the heart rate, by removing the AV block. But, they have insignificant effect, only if the block is below the AV node. Moreover, the result of pharmacological therapy is not always consistent and long term. So, pacing is the only answer for long-term management of conduction defect.

CAUSES OF PERIOPERATIVE TACHYCARDIA AND ITS MANAGEMENT

The tachycardia is defined as the heart rate above 100 beats/min. The *sinus tachycardia* is sinus rhythm (i.e., regular impulses arising from SA node) with heart rate above 100 beats/min. The *nonsinus tachycardia* means tachycardia where the impulses do not arise from the sinus node, but from anywhere else. The physiological causes of sinus tachycardia are anxiety, pain, fever, exercise, etc. It is rare for sinus tachycardia to exceed 180 beats/min, except in fit athlete. *At this heart rate, it may be difficult to differentiate the P-waves from the previous T-waves, as they march on each other and then this the rhythm can be mistaken for an AV nodal re-entry tachycardia or PSVT.*

Some pathological causes for sinus or nonsinus tachycardia are: (1) drugs, such as atropine and adrenaline, (2) heart failure, (3) fluid loss, (4) anemia, (5) hyperthyroidism, (6) MI, (7) pulmonary embolism, etc.

The characteristic features of sinus tachycardia **(Fig. 15)** in ECG are:

- Heart rate is >100 beats/min.
- The P-wave is upright in lead II and inverted in lead aVR.
- Every P-wave is followed by a QRS complex, though sometimes it is very difficult to identify the P-wave **(Fig. 16)**.

The management of sinus tachycardia is the management of its cause. When a patient has a compensatory tachycardia, such as in blood loss, fluid loss, anemia, and low BP in such

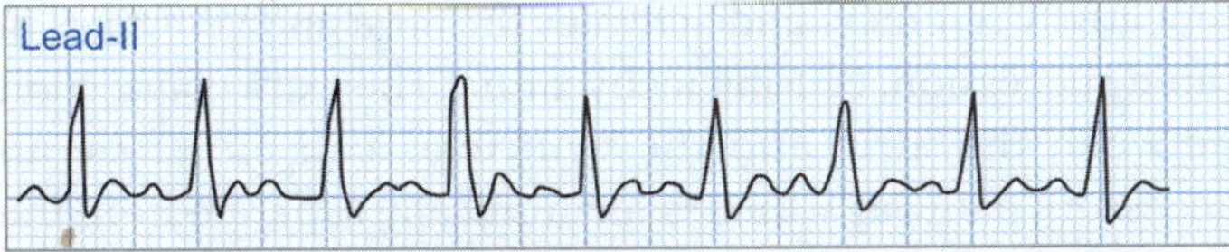

Fig. 15: This is an electrocardiogram (ECG) graph of sinus tachycardia. It is characterized by: (1) heart rate 150 beats/min, (2) QRS complexes after every P-wave, and (3) upright P-waves in lead II.

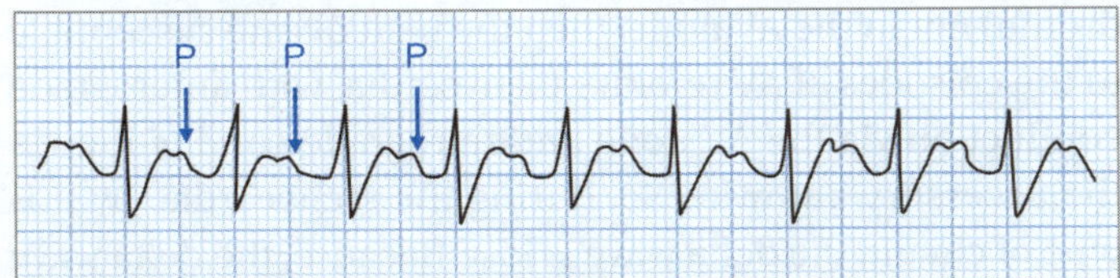

Fig. 16: This is an electrocardiogram (ECG) graph of sinus tachycardia with P-waves hidden within the previous T-waves.

situations the slowing of heart rate with β-blockers can lead to disastrous decompensation. However, if the sinus tachycardia is inappropriate or noncompensatory in nature, as in anxiety, heart failure, or hyperthyroidism, etc. then the treatment of this tachycardia with β-blockers may be helpful or lifesaving.

Tachycardia also can be classified into:
- *Narrow QRS complex tachycardia* (<3 small squares)
- *Broad QRS complex tachycardia* (>3 small squares)

In *narrow complex tachycardia,* the impulses always arise from above the ventricular level, i.e., they are supraventricular in origin. The QRS complexes formed by impulses arising from the supraventricular level are narrow, because these impulses pass, after their origin, through the normal fast conducting tissues, such as the AV node, bundle of His, and lastly through the Purkinje fibers. But, when any impulse arises from the ventricular level and does not pass through these normal conducting path, instead goes through the myocardium, then these QRS complexes become broad. This is because this conduction through myocardium is not as fast as the normal conducting tissues. The *causes of narrow complex tachycardia are* sinus tachycardia, atrial tachycardia, AV nodal re-entrant tachycardia, AV re-entry tachycardia, AV junctional tachycardia, atrial flutter with high AV conduction, AF with high AV conduction, WPW syndrome, etc.

In *broad complex tachycardia,* the impulses always arise below the level AV node, except supraventricular origin with bundle branch block. The *causes of broad QRS complex tachycardia are* VT, accelerated idioventricular tachycardia, torsades de pointes, ventricular flutter, VF, SVT with bundle branch block, etc.

Narrow Complex Tachycardia and its Management

Paroxysmal Supraventricular Tachycardia or (Atrial Tachycardia)

It is not a sinus tachycardia, as the impulse originates from an ectopic focus, somewhere within the atrial myocardium, except the SA node. The characteristic features of PSVT in ECG are:
- Heart rate >100 beats/min
- Abnormally shaped P-waves **(Fig. 17)**.

The atrial rate (P-wave) in PSVT is usually 150–250 beats/min. But, when the atrial rate is above 200 beats/min, then the AV node struggles to keep up with the conduction of impulses through it and AV block may precipitate.

The management of PSVT depends on the urgency of the situation, i.e., the evidence of any hemodynamic disturbance, such as hypotension, cardiac failure, and poor peripheral perfusion. However, the general rule is that the SVT, causing hemodynamic disturbance, requires urgent diagnosis and treatment. Initially, carotid sinus massage (vagal stimulation) reduces the heart rate by increasing the degree of AV block and in 80% of cases, it is effective. When the hypotension is present with PSVT, then IV phenylephrine in the dose of 0.1 mg in incremental rate may correct the hypotension and subsequently tachycardia (alone) or in combination with carotid sinus massage which correct tachycardia **(Fact file I)**.

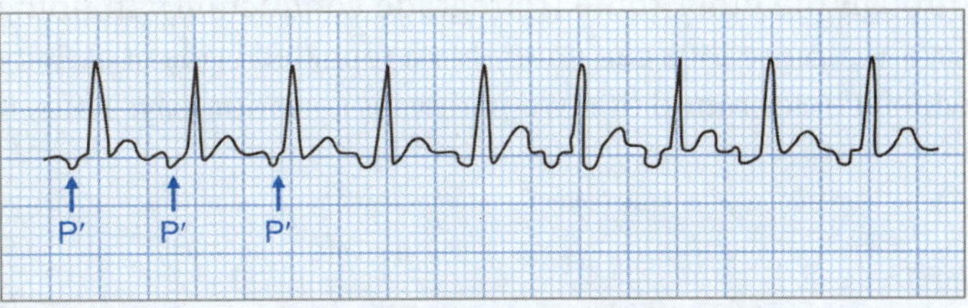

Fig. 17: This is an electrocardiogram (ECG) graph of atrial tachycardia. It is characterized by: (1) heart rate 150 beats/min and (2) abnormally shaped P-waves.

FACT FILE I

Supraventricular tachycardia

The term SVT is often misused. So, it frequently leads misunderstanding. Literally, it refers to any tachycardia which originates above the ventricle (supraventricle). Thus, it encompasses: sinus tachycardia, atrial tachycardia, AF, AV re-entry, nodal re-entry tachycardia, etc. But, some people use this term specifically to mean only AV nodal re-entry tachycardia. So, now it is recommended that all the arrhythmias should be diagnosed as specifically as possible and the term SVT should be reserved only for those whose are not diagnosed specifically, but its origin is above the ventricle.

If this fails, then verapamil in the dose of 2.5–10 mg IV or adenosine in the dose of 6–12 mg IV stat is used as second step of management. Adenosine is preferred than verapamil, because of its extremely short half-life and without any side effects. The adenosine should not be used, if the patient has asthma or obstructive airway diseases. Verapamil should not be used, if patient has recently taken β-blocker, otherwise severe bradycardia can result.

The β-blockers can also be used to slow or terminate the tachycardia of PSVT, but these are the agents of third choice. Digitalis also reduces the rate of atrial tachycardia, but produces slower onset of action and has no role in acute therapy of tachycardia of PSVT.

If pharmacological treatment of PSVT fails or when this tachycardia is recurrent, in spite of good pharmacological treatment, then temporary pacing may be used to terminate the arrhythmia. As the last resort, if severe ischemia and/or hypotension are caused by tachycardia, then direct current (DC) cardioversion should be considered.

AV Re-entry and AV Nodal Tachycardia

Atrioventricular re-entry tachycardia may arise, when there is a second alternate pathway for the passing of impulses from the atria to the ventricles. This is in addition to the normal route through the AV node for the conduction of impulses. The presence of two different routes for the conduction of impulses from the atrium to the ventricle creates the possibility that impulses can travel down through one route (anterograde conduction) and then return back through the other route (retrograde conduction). In doing so, an impulse thus can enter into a repeated cycle of activity which circles round the two pathways continuously. Thus, it

repeatedly re-enters and activates the atria and ventricles in rapid succession, causing tachycardia. The extra connection between the atria and the ventricles can either be an accessory pathway which is anatomically separate from the AV node (*AV re-entry tachycardia, e.g., WPW syndrome*) or through the AV node itself in which both the pathways lie in the AV node but are different from their electrical activity (*AV nodal re-entry tachycardia*) (**Figs. 18A and B**).

When the accessory pathways are found (like in WPW syndrome) not in the AV node, then the patients are susceptible to the episodes of AV re-entry tachycardia, with anterograde conduction via the AV node and retrograde conduction via the accessory pathway. So, during the tachycardia, by this type of circuit, the delta wave is lost. Because, the delta wave is only formed, when the anterograde conduction occurs through the accessory pathway and retrograde conduction occurs through the AV node. An AV re-entry tachycardia taking this route, i.e., down the accessory pathway and up the AV node is very rare. Hence, when it does occur, then only the delta waves are seen.

Patients with AV nodal dual pathway, i.e., when both the pathways (accessory and normal) exist within the AV node, are also at the increased risk of AV re-entry tachycardia. This is called the *AV nodal re-entry tachycardia* in which the anterograde conduction usually occurs down the normal AV nodal pathway and the retrograde conduction occurs via the abnormal additional pathway within the AV node.

Both the AV re-entry and AV nodal re-entry tachycardia have the following characteristics:
- Heart rate is 150–250 beats/min.
- There is one abnormal P-wave (P^1) per QRS complex (although P-waves are not always clearly seen).
  - There are regular QRS complexes.

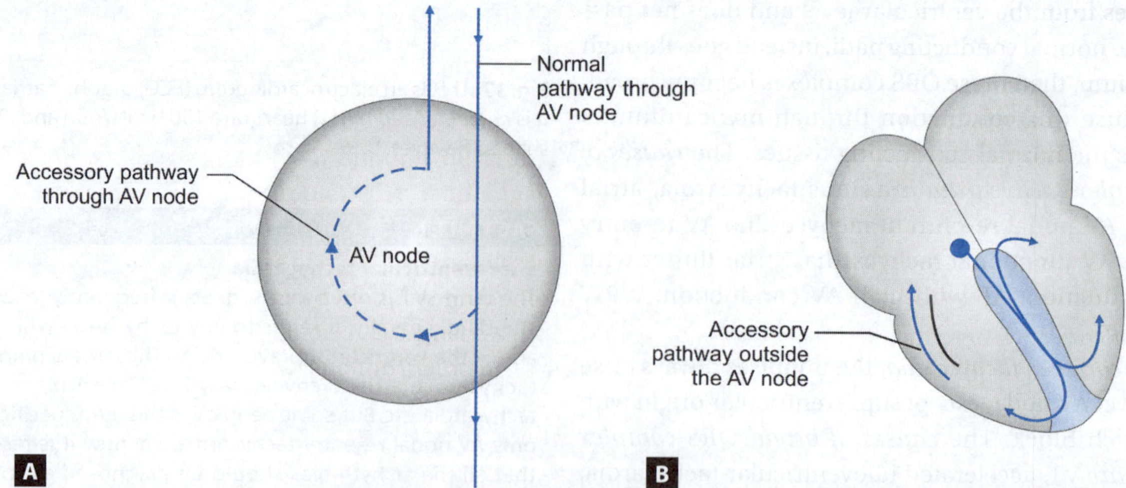

Figs. 18A and B: (A) Accessory pathway through the atrioventricular (AV) node (AV nodal re-entry tachycardia); (B) Accessory pathway outside the AV node (AV re-entry tachycardia).

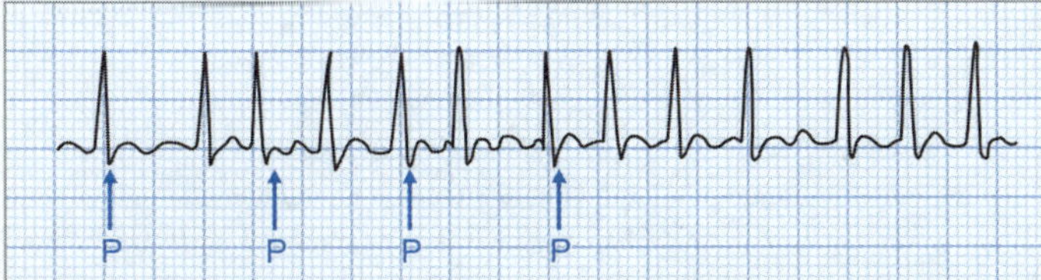

Fig. 19: This is an electrocardiogram (ECG) graph of atrioventricular (AV) re-entry tachycardia in Wolff–Parkinson–White (WPW) syndrome. It is characterized by: (1) ventricular rate is 225 beats/min, (2) narrow QRS complexes, and (3) inverted P-waves after QRS complexes.

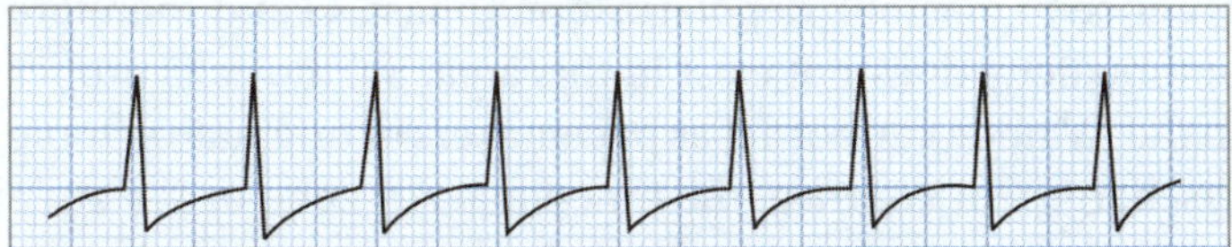

Fig. 20: This is an electrocardiogram (ECG) graph of atrioventricular (AV) nodal re-entry tachycardia. It is characterized by: (1) ventricular rate 150 beats/min, (2) narrow RS complexes, and (3) invisible P-wave.

- QRS complexes are narrow (in the absence of aberrant conduction).
- There may have delta waves or not. The *delta wave is present* in the AV re-entry tachycardia, where the accessory pathway is present outside the AV node and the anterograde conduction occurs through this accessory pathway and retrograde conduction occurs through the AV node. *Delta wave is absent* in AV re-entry tachycardia, if the anterograde conduction occurs through AV node and retrograde conduction occurs through the accessory pathway which is situated outside the AV node. The *delta wave is also absent* in the AV nodal re-entry tachycardia, where the accessory pathway is present within the AV node **(Figs. 19 and 20)**.

In AV re-entry tachycardia, the inverted P¹-waves are often seen in the middle between two QRS complexes. But, in AV nodal re-entry tachycardia the inverted P¹-waves are often difficult or impossible to find out, as they follow the QRS complexes closely or are buried within them. Although, the actual position of P¹-waves may be helpful to distinguish between the AV re-entry tachycardia and AV nodal re-entry tachycardia, but an ECG in sinus rhythm (i.e., when tachycardia is not present) is more diagnostic, as it may reveal a short PR interval or delta wave, suggesting WPW syndrome. Truly speaking, the definite diagnosis of AV re-entry and AV nodal re-entry tachycardia is very difficult and need electrophysiological studies.

Management of AV nodal re-entry and AV re-entry tachycardia: The AV nodal re-entry tachycardia can be prevented by increasing the block within the AV node and thereby breaking the repetitive cycle of electrical activity by β-blocker or by Valsalva maneuver. Valsalva maneuver works by increasing the vagal inhibition on AV nodal conduction. Alternative of this maneuver is carotid sinus massage.

AV nodal re-entry can also be prevented by the use of drugs. The drugs with degree of preference are adenosine, digitalis, β-blocker, and Ca-channel antagonist such as verapamil. Adenosine should not be used, if the patient suffers from asthma or any other obstructive airway disease. In emergency situation when the patient is hemodynamically compromised, then urgent DC cardioversion or overdrive atrial pacing is done.

The management of AV re-entry tachycardia is also same like that of AV nodal re-entry tachycardia. The patient with AV re-entry tachycardia, who requires pharmacological agents for chronic therapy, should also be considered as the candidates for the radiofrequency catheter ablation of the bypass tract.

Wolff–Parkinson–White Syndrome

Normally, in most people the impulses pass from the atrium to the ventricle through a distinct normal path, such as AV node, bundle of His, and Purkinje fibers. But, some people have additional or accessory conducting path between the atria and the ventricles. This accessory path is called the *bundle of Kent* and the conduction of impulses through this accessory pathway is faster than the AV node. So, the wave of depolarization reaches the ventricle from atrium more quickly (when it only passes anterogradely through this accessory pathway) than usual and thus the PR interval becomes short. A part of the ventricle is activated first by the accessory path, giving rise to Delta wave—the first part of the QRS complex. Shortly after that, the rest of the ventricle is depolarized rapidly with the arrival of the normally conducted wave of depolarization via the AV node from the atrium and complete the rest of the QRS complex **(Fig. 21)**.

The key diagnostic point of WPW syndrome in ECG is the short PR interval and the delta waves.

The WPW syndrome without tachycardia is found incidentally and may be asymptomatic. In these cases, no action is needed. Some patients with WPW syndrome have symptoms of palpitation due to tachycardia or arrhythmia. If a symptomatic patient with WPW syndrome due to tachycardia requires surgery of any kind, then the anesthetist must be informed of the ECG finding.

The protocol for the management of tachycardia in WPW syndrome is similar to that of PSVT. The pharmacological aim of therapy for WPW syndrome is the increase of refractoriness and the reduction of conduction velocity through the components of re-entrant circuit. If there is life-threatening

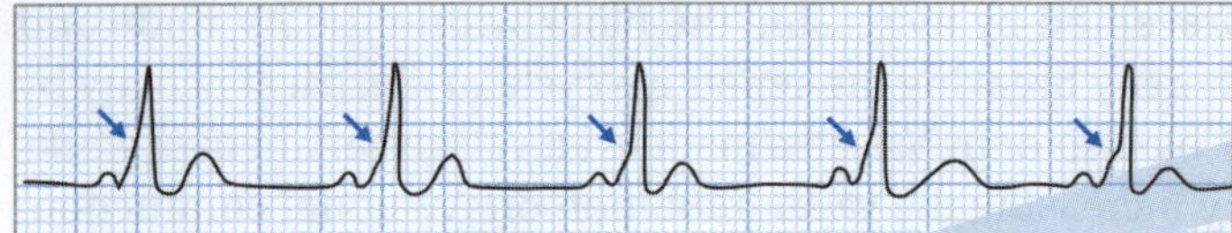

Fig. 21: This is an electrocardiogram (ECG) of Wolff–Parkinson–White (WPW) syndrome, characterized by ventricular rate 75 beats/min, short PR interval (0.08 second), and delta waves shown by arrow.

FACT FILE II

Atrial fibrillation and WPW syndrome

Not only the AV re-entry tachycardia complicates the WPW syndrome, but also the AF may be precipitated. In AF, due to the AV re-entry tachycardia, the conduction of impulses to the ventricle can occur via either the accessory pathway (most common) or the AV node or both. When the conduction of impulses through accessory pathway takes place, it causes rapid and potentially lethal ventricular rate. Therefore, the drugs, such as verapamil and adenosine, which block the AV node are detrimental in such patient and increase the conduction through accessory pathway. In such circumstances, the DC cardioversion is the treatment of choice. These conditions also can be treated by drugs which slow the conduction through accessory pathway, such as sotalol, disopyramide, and amiodarone. The ablation of accessory path also can be thought.

rapid ventricular rate in response to WPW syndrome, then DC cardioversion is carried out. Alternatively, lignocaine (3–5 mg/kg) or procainamide (15 mg/kg) can be used, slowly intravenously over 15–20 minutes to reduce the ventricular rate. Sometimes, the WPW syndrome is associated with AF. Then, the IV verapamil or digitalis should not be used and if used, then, it should be given very cautiously, because these drugs decrease the refractoriness of accessory path and increase the ventricular rate, causing VT. In chronic therapy, verapamil is not associated with increased risk.

In patient with WPW syndrome and AF, the use of β-blockers are of no utility in controlling the ventricular response, when the conduction proceeds through the bypass tract. In patient with WPW syndrome and PSVT, atrial and ventricular pacing almost always terminate the PSVT immediately and regularize the ventricular rate.

The radiofrequency catheter ablation of the bypass tract offers a permanent cure of WPW syndrome and is effective in 90% patients. It is the treatment of choice of WPW syndrome in patient with symptomatic arrhythmias **(Fact file II)**.

AV Junctional Tachycardia

The AV node is divided in three regions: (1) The central N region, (2) the peripheral AN region, where the atrial fibers enter the AV node, and (3) the peripheral NV region, where the AV node extends into the bundle of His

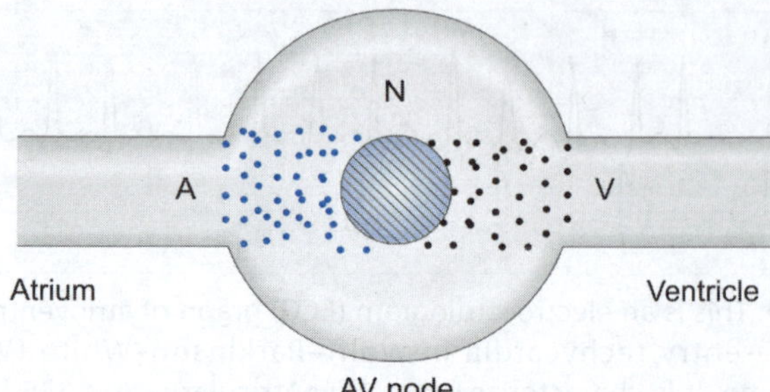

Fig. 22: Atrioventricular (AV) node.

(Fig. 22). It had been said that the central N region show the absence of diastolic depolarization (phase 4) and therefore automaticity does not exist in this area. So, the cells proper in the AV node cannot act as pacemakers or originate ectopic discharges. In contrast, the junctional AN zone or NV zone are the zones of automaticity and can act as pacemakers or may be the site of ectopic discharge of impulses. Hence, the older terminology of AV nodal rhythms had been replaced by AV junctional rhythms. However, the more recent studies also have demonstrated the diastolic depolarization in the N regions of AV node. Therefore, the older designation of AV nodal rhythms can be justified **(Fig. 22)**.

In junctional beat **(Fig. 23)**, the ectopic impulse arises from any junctional sites (AN or NV zones) of AV node. The impulse then spreads upward into the atrium and downward into the ventricle. This usually produces an upright P^1 wave in aVR and high esophageal leads, and an inverted P^1 wave in aVF and low esophageal leads. This P^1 wave can be buried in the QRS complex during tachycardia and may not be visible. The atrium is activated in a retrograde fashion prior to the activation of ventricle. This produces a normal or short P^1R interval. Such a beat is not distinguishable from an atrial ectopic beat, arising from a low atrial focus near the AV node and therefore is best referred to as the supraventricular beat. The finding of a short P^1R interval (<0.12 second) with an inverted P^1 wave **(Box 3)** in lead aVF may favor in the diagnosis of the junctional origin of impulses. The P^1R interval longer than 0.12 second with an inverted P^1 in aVF may favor ventricular excitation.

In AV junctional rhythm and tachycardia, the QRS-T complexes are of normal configuration. The junctional beats may be either premature, i.e., occurring earlier than the next anticipated sinus beat or escape beats. The previous one occurs, when the increased automaticity of junctional sites develops (e.g., digitalis toxicity) and the later occurs when the sinus rate slows. When the junctional beats act as escape rhythm, then it is regular and the rate may vary from 40 to 80 beats/min.

The junctional escape rhythms are the form of safety net for heart. Without escape rhythms, the complete failure

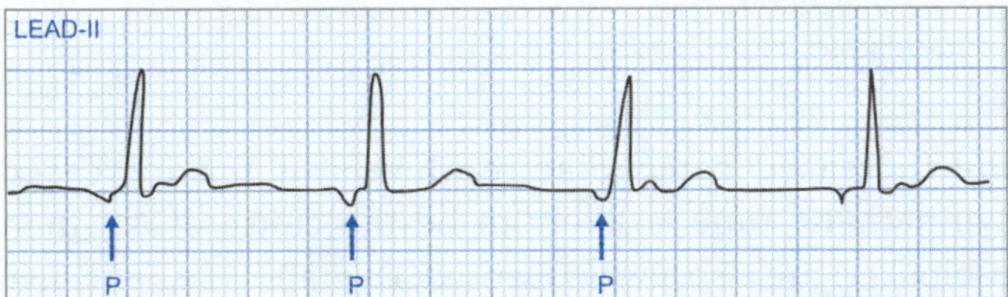

BOX 3: Causes of inverted P-waves.

- Incorrectly positioned electrodes
- Change of axis of heart
- Dextrocardia
- *Abnormal atrial depolarization:*
  - Atrial ectopic
  - AV junctional rhythm
  - Retrogradely conducted ventricular ectopic
  - Retrogradely conducted ventricular tachycardia

Fig. 23: This is an electrocardiogram (ECG) of atrioventricular (AV) junctional rhythm, characterized by: (1) inverted P-waves in lead II, (2) abnormally short PR interval, and (3) narrow QRS complexes.

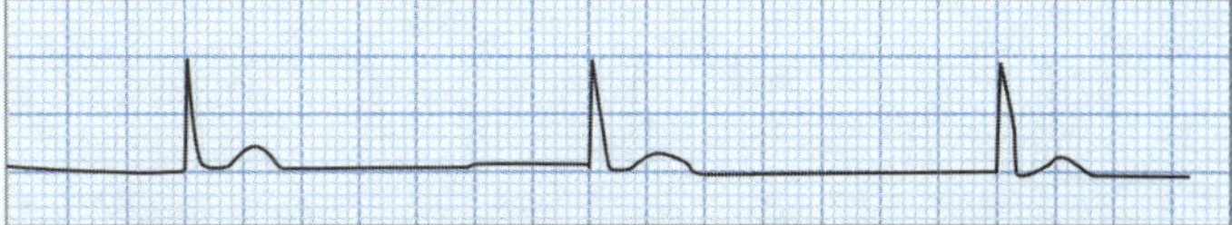

Fig. 24: This is an electrocardiogram (ECG) of atrioventricular (AV) junctional escape rhythm, characterized by: (1) heart rate 43 beats/min, (2) absent P-waves, and (3) narrow QRS complexes.

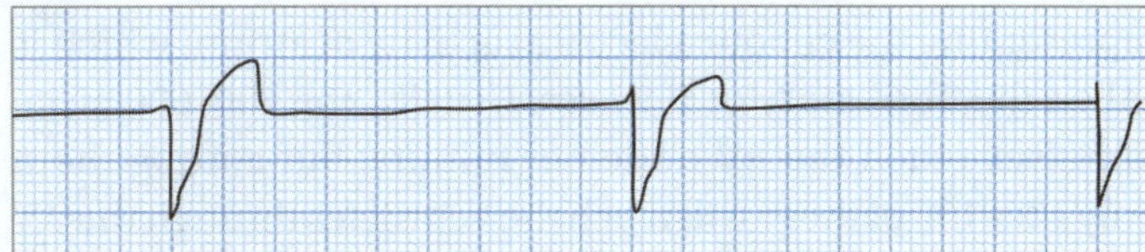

Fig. 25: This is an electrocardiogram (ECG) of ventricular escape rhythm, characterized by: (1) heart rate 33 beats/min, (2) absent P-waves, and (3) broad QRS complexes.

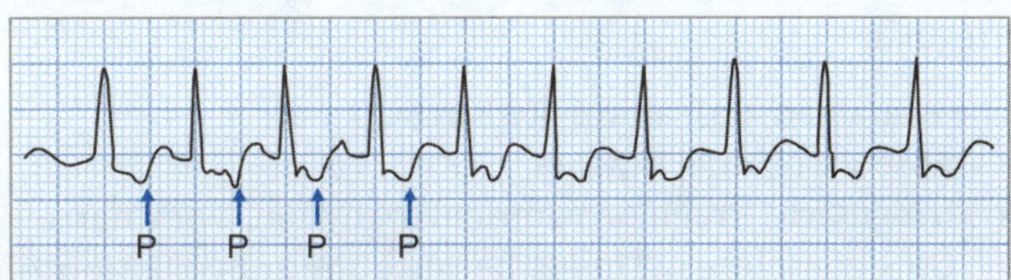

Fig. 26: This is an electrocardiogram (ECG) of atrioventricular (AV) junctional tachycardia. It is characterized by: (1) heart rate 150 beats/min, (2) narrow QRS complexes, and (3) P-waves hidden within the ST segments.

of the generation of impulses from the SA node and its conduction through AV node at any moment would lead to the ventricular asystole and death. So, the heart has a number of *subsidiary pacemaker site* that can take over the responsibility, if normal impulse generation from SA node or its conduction fails. The subsidiary pacemaker site are located in the AV junction or in the ventricular myocardium. If the AV junction fails to receive impulse, as a result of SA arrest or block or even during severe sinus bradycardia, then it will take over as the cardiac pacemaker. The QRS complexes generated from ventricular depolarization by AV junctional rhythm will have the same morphology as normal, but at a slower rate of around 40–60 beats/min. The AV junctional pacemaker will continue, until it is inhibited by the impulses from the SA node. If the AV junctional pacemaker fails or its impulses are blocked to pass to ventricle, then a ventricular pacemaker (from ventricular myocardium or Purkinje fiber) will take over the responsibility and this QRS complexes will be broad **(Figs. 24 and 25)**.

The AV junctional rhythm may be transient or permanent. The transient AV junctional rhythm may sometimes be seen in normal people. It may be produced by carotid sinus pressure (protective escape phenomenon) or may result from digitalis (increased automaticity of junctional site) or quinidine administration. This transient or permanent junctional rhythm also results from varieties of organic heart diseases, e.g., rheumatic fever, coronary artery disease, other acute infectious myocarditis, etc.

In AV junction tachycardia (which is due to the increased automaticity of AV junctional rhythm), the rate can vary from 120 to 200 beats/min. The ventricular rhythm is regular. The P^1 waves may precede or be buried in or follow QRS complexes. The ECG pattern of QRS complex is identical with that of a junctional premature beat. With a rapid rate it is impossible to tell whether any given P^1 wave is related to the preceding QRS complex or to the following complex **(Fig. 26)**. Actually one cannot differentiate the ECG pattern produced by junctional tachycardia from that produced by an atrial tachycardia arising from a low atrial ectopic focus near AV node. Therefore, the general term such as SVT is more applicable than the specific term AV junctional tachycardia. Thus, management of AV junctional tachycardia is like that of atrial tachycardia.

Atrial Fibrillation

Atrial fibrillation is much more common than atrial flutter. It affects 5–10% of elderly people and may be permanent or paroxysmal. The electrophysiological characteristic of AF is the local, multiple, rapid, and chaotic depolarization of atrial musculature which divides the atria into multiple small islands. Hence, no P-waves are seen in ECG. Instead, the baseline of ECG consists of low amplitude oscillations,

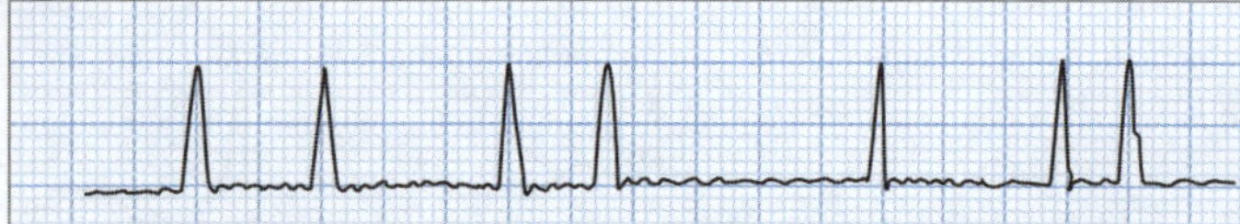

Fig. 27: This is an electrocardiogram (ECG) of atrial fibrillation. It is characterized by: (1) absent of P-waves and (2) irregularly irregular QRS rhythm as AV node fails to pass all the impulses, coming from high atrial activity (>300 beats/min).

representing the chaotic electrical activity of atrium which is called the fibrillatory or F-waves. Usually, the 400–600 atrial impulses reach the AV node per minute, but among them only 120–150 of these will reach the ventricles through the AV node to produce the tachycardia of narrow QRS complexes. This is due to the block of AV node, with the traffic jam of impulses. However, due to this traffic jam and as the block of AV node conduction of atrial impulses through AV node is erratic, so it makes the ventricular rhythm irregularly irregular.

The characteristic features of AF in ECG are:

- Absence of atrial P-waves
- Irregularly irregular ventricular rhythm, with narrow QRS complexes. This is because the transmission of atrial impulses through AV node is erratic which makes the ventricular complexes irregularly irregular **(Fig. 27)**.

Once the AF has been diagnosed perioperatively, then the cause of it should always be sought with careful patient's history and examination. This is because, the AF may be the first manifestation of many forms of organic heart diseases, particularly those that are associated with the enlargement or the dilatation of atria. The common causes of AF are hypertension, IHD, hyperthyroidism, SSS, consumption of alcohol, rheumatic mitral valvular disease, cardiomyopathy, atrial septal defect (ASD), pericarditis, myocarditis, pulmonary embolism, pneumonia, cardiac surgery, etc. **(Box 4)**. When such factors are present, then the therapy of AF should be directed toward the primary abnormality.

The aims of treating AF are:

- To control the ventricular rate
- To reduce the risk of thromboembolism
- If possible, restoration of sinus rhythm.

If patient's clinical status is severely compromised perioperatively by AF, due to high ventricular rate, then the electrical cardioversion is the treatment of choice. In the absence of severe cardiovascular compromised state, the slowing of ventricular rate in AF can be achieved by β-blockers, verapamil or digitalis. Both the β-blockers and verapamil prolongs the refractory period of AV node and thus slows the conduction through it. Where

BOX 4: Common causes of atrial fibrillation.
- Valvular heart disease (rheumatic mitral valve)
- Coronary artery disease
- Hypertension
- Sick sinus syndrome
- Hyperthyroidism
- Alcohol
- Cardiomyopathy
- Pericardial disease
- Congenital heart disease
- Pulmonary embolism
- Chest infection
- Idiopathic

the increased catecholamine levels or the increased sympathetic tone is likely to be the cause of AF, then β-blockers are also always favored. Digitalis is less effective in controlling ventricular rate in AF, because it takes longer time for the onset of action and associated with more toxicity. Pharmacological cardioversion to sinus rhythm in AF also can be attempted by quinidine, flecainide, sotalol, propafenone, or amiodarone. Among them, the amiodarone is probably more effective than other agents, but can lead to troublesome side effects.

If medical cardioversion fails, the electrical cardioversion is useful. The DC cardioversion for AF is successful, when it is not long-standing, and atrium is not enlarged. In patients, where cardioversion is unsuccessful or in whom AF is likely to recur, then it is better to allow the patient to remain in AF and to control the ventricular response only with β-blockers or verapamil. Anticoagulation therapy appears to decrease the incidences of systemic embolization, associated with AF and cardioversion. Some advocate transesophageal echocardiography to locate the clot in atrium, before the cardioversion who is suffering from AF. In the absence of clot, cardioversion can be undertaken and anticoagulation started immediately.

The risk of stroke, due to thrombi in AF, can be reduced up to 60% by anticoagulant therapy using warfarin. The use of anticoagulant in nonrheumatic AF is controversial. Patients without risk factors for thromboembolic events (previous thromboembolic episode, age >75 years, hypertensive, diabetes mellitus, heart failure, large left atrium, impaired left ventricular function) may require only aspirin. In patients, below the age of 65 years, no anticoagulation therapy is required. The use of warfarin is most controversial in the elderly who have both the highest risk of stroke and the highest risk of bleeding when taking warfarin. The benefits and the risks of anticoagulant therapy for AF must always be weighted up, before initiating treatment.

Resistant AF can also be treated by electrical AV nodal ablation (to prevent conduction from atria to ventricle) with insertion of permanent ventricular pacemaker.

Atrial Flutter

The characteristic features of atrial flutter in ECG are:

- Atrial rate is around 300 beats/min. This is in-between atrial tachycardia and AF (atrial tachycardia < atrial flutter < atrial flutter).
- *Sawtooth baseline:* This is because of the undulating P-wave, due to the rapid atrial rate which gives a characteristic undulating appearance to the baseline of the ECG. This is also called the *flutter waves* **(Fig. 28)**.
- AV block, usually of 2:1, 3:1, and 4:1.

The atrial flutter differs from atrial tachycardia. The difference is that atrial rate or P-wave is higher (usually 250–350 beats/min) in flutter than tachycardia and is often, almost, exactly 300 beats/min. The AV node cannot keep up with such high atrial rate. So, the AV block occurs. This is most commonly 2:1, although 3:1, 4:1 or other variable degrees of block may also occur. Thus, the ventricular rate is less than atrial rate and may be 150, 100, or 75 beats/min.

The causes of atrial flutter are the same as those of AF. The most effective treatment of atrial flutter in emergency condition is DC cardioversion. In patients, who develop atrial flutter following an open heart surgery or recurrent flutter in the setting of acute MI, then atrial pacing can usually convert the atrial flutter to sinus rhythm. Atrial pacing may also be tried. It may also convert the atrial flutter to AF which allows for the easier control of ventricular response. If the immediate control of atrial flutter is not mandated by the patient's clinical status, then the ventricular response should first be slowed by blocking the AV node with the β-blockers, or Ca-antagonist (verapamil). Once, the AV nodal conduction is slowed with any of these drugs, then an attempt to convert the flutter to sinus rhythm using sotalol, flecainide, propafenone, or amiodarone should be tried. The doses of these drugs which are selected are gradually increased, until the rhythm converts or side effects occur.

Broad QRS Complex Tachycardia and its Management

The causes of broad complex tachycardia are VT, accelerated idioventricular rhythm, idioventricular tachycardia, VF, ventricular flutter, torsades de pointes, and SVT with bundle branch block.

Ventricular Tachycardia

It is defined as broad, abnormal QRS complexes, with rate >100 beats/min (usually in-between 140 and 220 beats/min) **(Box 5)**. Usually, the episodes of VT can be self-limiting. But, sometimes it may be sustained or can degenerate into VF. *From the managemental point of view VT can be classified into sustained and nonsustained type. Sustained VT is* defined as VT that persists >30 seconds with severe hemodynamic compromise. It generally accompanies with some form of serious underlying cardiac pathology, such as acute MI, IHD, cardiomyopathies, myocarditis, congenital heart diseases, metabolic disorders, drug toxicity, and prolonged QT syndrome.

The *nonsustained VT* is defined as three or more successive ectopic ventricular beats and is sustaining <30 seconds. It is usually not associated with any serious underlying cardiac diseases and does not produce any symptoms, i.e., without any hemodynamic compromise.

The ECG diagnosis of VT is suggested by tachycardia with broad QRS complexes (rate exceeding 100 beats/min) **(Fig. 29)**. The QRS configuration may be uniform (monomorphic) or it may vary from beat to beat (polymorphic) as

BOX 5: Causes of ventricular tachycardia.
• Ischemic heart disease
• Acute myocardial infarction (MI)
• Cardiomyopathy
• Myocarditis
• Congenital heart disease
• Mitral valve prolapse
• Drugs
• Electrolyte disturbance
• Hypoxia
• Idiopathic

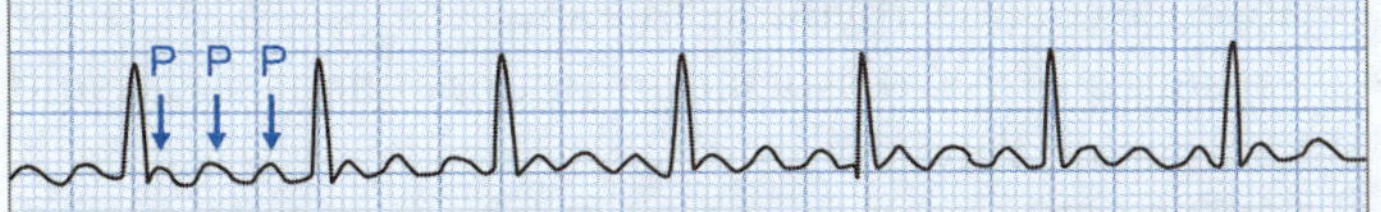

Fig. 28: This is an electrocardiogram (ECG) of atrial flutter with 3:1 atrioventricular (AV) block. It is characterized by: (1) flutter P-waves at the rate of 300 beats/min, (2) QRS complexes at the rate of 100 beats/min, and (3) 3:1 AV block (when atrial rate is above 200 beats/min, AV node struggles to keep up with the impulse conduction and AV block may occur).

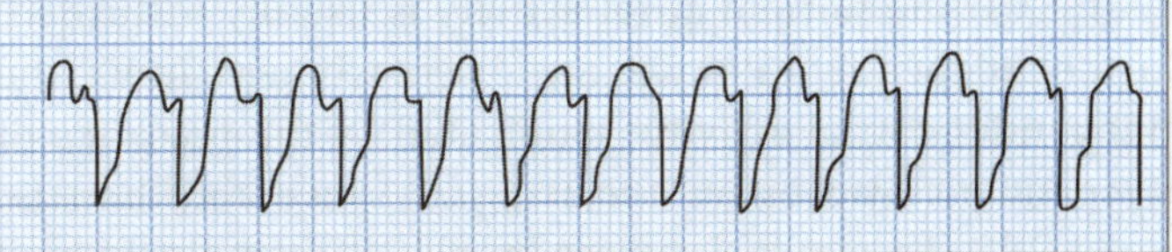

Fig. 29: This is an electrocardiogram (ECG) of ventricular tachycardia (VT). It is characterized by: (1) broad complex tachycardia at a rate of 200 beats/min, (2) QRS duration >0.14 second (3.5 small squares), and (3) concordance (same QRS direction) in all the leads from V_1 to V_6.

in "torsades de pointes". The bidirectional VT refers to VT that shows an alternation in QRS amplitude and axis, e.g., VT with RBBB with alternating superior (leftward) and inferior axis (rightward).

Sometimes, the onset of VT is generally abrupt and this paroxysmal VT is usually initiated by sudden multiple ventricular premature contraction (VPC). In nonparoxysmal tachycardia, the onset is gradual.

The SVT with RBBB or LBBB may also resemble VT, due to the broad QRS complex and increased heart rate. But, it should be distinguished from original VT. Because, the clinical implications and management of these two arrhythmias are totally different.

These two conditions (true VT and SVT with bundle branch block) can be differentiated apparently by:

- The observation of intermittent canon waves in the tracing of central venous pressure monitoring and the varying intensity of first heart sounds which suggest AV dissociation and the presence of VT.
- The close observation of 12-lead ECG which may also be helpful.
- The pharmacological maneuvers, such as the IV administration of verapamil or adenosine (these agents terminate only the SVT, but not the VT). But, this procedure to differentiate them can be hazardous and should be avoided.
- It is always useful to have a 12-lead ECG, during sinus rhythm or nontachycardia condition (i.e., before the development of VT) for comparison with that during tachycardia. If the QRS morphology during tachycardia is same with the previous QRS complex in ECG, i.e., when there is no tachycardia, then the diagnosis of PSVT with conduction defect is favored.
- An infarction pattern on the sinus rhythm tracing suggests the potential presence of VT.

A characteristic feature of VT due to ventricular cause is the presence of independent atrial activity with it. This is suggested by:

- Independent P-wave
- Fusion beats **(Fact file III)**
- Capture beats **(Fact file IV)**

In SVT, the normal atrial activity is usually disturbed. So, the independent P-waves are absent whereas, in VT, the independent atrial activity is indicated by the presence of independent P-waves, but occurring at a slower rate than the broad QRS complexes. So, these broad QRS complexes bear no relationship to P-wave. Thus, through theoretically there is definite P-wave, but it can be difficult or even impossible to find out these P-waves in the jungle of multiple broad QRS complexes, originating from ventricle during VT.

FACT FILE III

Fusion beat

Sometimes, the captured sinus impulse invades the ventricle through AV node, when the ectopic ventricular impulse also tries to invade the whole ventricle, originating from ventricle. Then, each impulse will activate part of the ventricles and the resulting QRS complex will have a configuration which is in-between that of the pure sinus conducted ventricular beat and the pure ectopic ventricular beat. Thus, the combination or summation of these two types of beats is *known as the ventricular fusion beats*. The ventricular capture and fusion beats are the most reliable diagnostic pointer to the ventricular origins of the basic VT.

FACT FILE IV

Capture beat

When there are both independent sinus and ventricular rhythm, then their impulses meet at the AV node and here interfere each other's mutual progress. So, the AV node always remains in a state of refractoriness and this is due to the prior passing of either the sinus impulses from SA node or the ectopic impulses from ventricles. But, sometimes, with critical timing and due to slow ventricular ectopic rate, a sinus impulse may reach the AV node during a nonrefractory phase of it and is conducted to the ventricle. Thus, it immediately *activates or captures* the ventricle for that beat only. This conducted sinus impulse, resulting in ventricular contraction and normal QRS complex, during continuous ectopic broad QRS ventricular rhythm, is known as the capture beat. The QRS complex of capture beat is easily recognized, because it resembles a normal narrow sinus conducted ventricular beats, in-between the broad QRS complexes originating from ventricular ectopic site. Furthermore, the capture beat is always related to a preceding sinus P-wave.

The fusion beats occur when the ventricles are activated and contracted by an atrial impulse and by an ectopic ventricular impulse at a time arriving simultaneously **(Fig. 30)**. The capture beats occur when an atrial impulse manages to "capture" the ventricles for a normal contraction, causing a normal QRS complex in the jungle of broad, rapid, and QRS complexes. This may be preceded by a normal P-wave **(Fig. 31)**.

The characteristics of ECG that suggest tachycardia of ventricular origin (VT) are:

- Broad complex QRS > 0.14 S or 3 small squares, in the absence of antiarrhythmic therapy
- Presence of AV dissociation (independent atrial and ventricular activity)
- Similar QRS pattern or axis in all the precordial leads
- Left axis deviation with RBBB morphology or northwest axis deviation (extreme left axis deviation) with LBBB morphology
- Capture/fusion beat
- No response to carotid sinus massage or IV adenosine

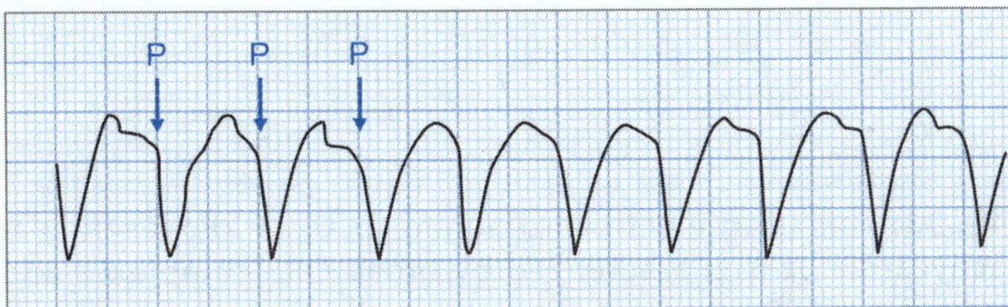

Fig. 30: This is a graph of fusion beat ventricular tachycardia (VT). It occurs when the atrial and ventricular impulses arrive in the ventricle simultaneously.

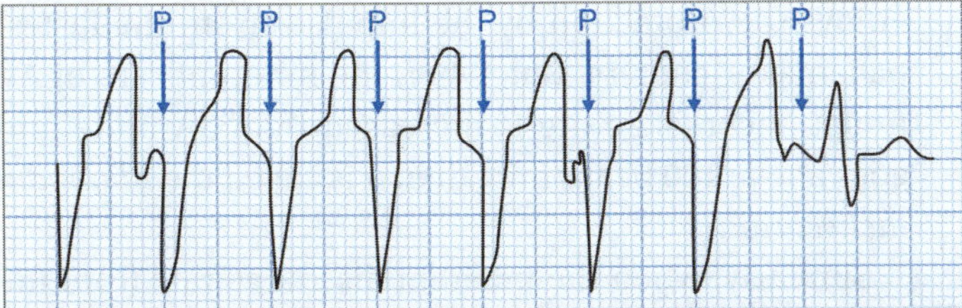

Fig. 31: This is an electrocardiogram (ECG) of captured beats in ventricular tachycardia (VT). It is characterized by: (1) broad complex VT, (2) arrows show independent P-waves deforming the QRS complexes, and (3) the last beat is the capture beat.

The symptoms, resulting from VT, depend on the CO which again depends on the ventricular rate, the duration of tachycardia, and the presence and the extent of the underlying cardiac pathology. When the tachycardia (ventricular) is very rapid and is associated with severe myocardial dysfunction, then CO tremendously decreases producing hypotension, syncope, and unconsciousness. Contrary, it will have to keep in mind that the presence of hemodynamic stability does not preclude the diagnosis of VT. Decrease in CO, during VT, may also be attributed by the loss of atrial contribution to ventricular filling (especially if AF is present) and by the abnormal sequence of ventricular activation.

Ventricular tachycardia without heart disease has a good prognosis with extremely low risk of sudden death. On the other hand, VT within first 6 weeks of MI has poor prognosis.

The episodes of VT can be terminated by using: (1) DC cardioversion, (2) drugs, and (3) pacing. But, the management of VT depends mainly on the risk-benefit ratio, because the antiarrhythmic agents can also produce or exacerbate the ventricular arrhythmias, when they are given to prevent it. A patient with nonsustained VT without any organic heart disease and without any symptoms should not be treated, because the prognosis will not be affected. However, the patient with sustained VT, but without any heart disease, may become symptomatic and require treatment (due to very low CO producing hypotension and symptoms).

The tachycardia responds well to β-blockers, vera-pamil, procainamide, sotalol, amiodarone, etc. For the pharmacological termination of VT, the procainamide is the most effective agent. If it cannot terminate the tachycardia, it will always at least slow the rate. For the selection of appropriate antiarrhythmic pharmacological agent to prevent recurrence, programmed stimulation is the most effective way. In stable patients, when the pharmacological therapy fails, a pacing catheter can be inserted percutaneously into the right ventricular apex and the VT can be terminated by overdrive pacing. Ventricular pacing to terminate VT is effective, but may sometimes also precipitate VF. The VT caused by severe sinus bradycardia should also be treated by pacing at first hand. A patient with sustained VT with organic heart disease and severe hemodynamic compromise, the rhythm should be promptly terminated by DC cardioversion. Automatic implantable cardioverter defibrillator (AICD) devices can be implanted to deliver low energy shocks for recurrent episodes of VT or VF. The development of endocardial catheter, intraoperative mapping, and the localization of the site of the origin of arrhythmia by electrophysiological testing and then subsequent surgical ablation can better cure the VT.

Some specific types of VT:

- *Torsades de pointes (twisting points):* It is an unusual form of VT which is associated with long QT interval and undulating pattern (polymorphic) in the direction of QRS axis (the axis of QRS is always changing). The ECG shows rapid, irregular, and broad QRS complexes that oscillate from an upright to an inverted position and seem to twist around the baseline. So, it is named as the twisting point, because the mean QRS axis changes. The arrhythmia is usually nonsustained and repetitive, but may degenerate into VF.

  It can occur during the treatment with certain antiarrhythmic drugs (quinidine, phenothiazines, tricyclic antidepressant, etc.), electrolyte abnormalities (particularly hypokalemia and hypomagnesemia), hereditary syndromes (Jervell and Lange–Nielsen Syndrome, Romano–Ward syndrome), intracranial events, and bradyarrhythmias particularly third-degree AV block **(Box 6)**.

The hallmarks of torsades de pointes in ECG **(Fig. 32)** are:
- Broad complex tachycardia with polymorphic QRS complexes
- Marked QT prolongation
- Variation in QRS axis.

These patients, with torsades de pointes, often have the multiple episodes of sustained or nonsustained VT, with recurrent syncope and the risk of the development of VF with sudden cardiac arrest. So, urgent assessment

BOX 6: Causes of long QT interval and torsades de pointes.

- *Electrolyte disturbances:*
  - Hypokalemia
  - Hypocalcemia
  - Hypomagnesemia
- *Bradycardia:*
  - Complete heart block
  - Sinus node disease
- *Drugs:*
  - Class Ia antiarrhythmic drugs (e.g., disopyramide)
  - Class III antiarrhythmic drugs (e.g., sotalol and amiodarone)
  - Tricyclic antidepressants (e.g., amitriptyline), phenothiazines (e.g., chlorpromazine), erythromycin, and other macrolides
- *Congenital syndrome:*
  - Jervell and Lange–Nielsen syndrome
  - Romano–Ward syndrome (autosomal dominant) (autosomal recessive associated with congenital deafness)

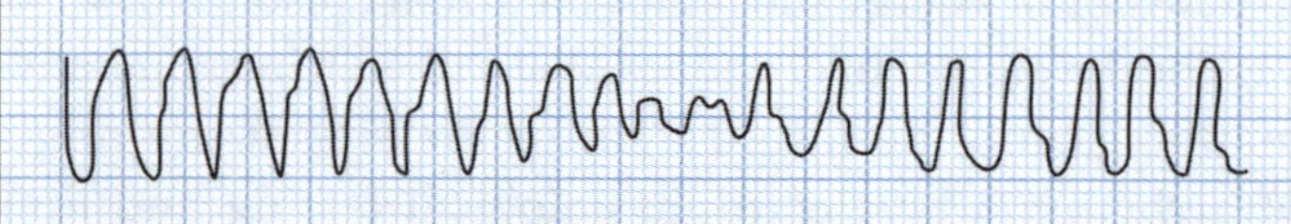

Fig. 32: This is an electrocardiogram (ECG) of torsades de pointes. It is characterized by: (1) broad complex tachycardia (300 beats/min) and (2) variations in QRS axis.

is warranted with the identification and the withdrawn of causative drugs, prolonging QT interval, and the correction of electrolyte abnormalities. The management is like that:

- The drug-induced torsades de pointes is treated by atrial or ventricular pacing which increases the heart rate and thereby shortens the QT interval.
- For patients with congenital prolonged QT syndrome, β-adrenergic blocking agent is the mainstay of therapy.
- Cervicothoracic sympathectomy is also indicated as a form of therapy in torsades de pointes by interrupting the sympathetic supply to heart.

- *Idioventricular tachycardia:* The idioventricular tachycardia results from the accelerated ventricular depolarization, originating from the ectopic foci, situated in ventricle. The heart has many potential pacemaker cells. These are situated in the SA node, AV node, atria, His bundle, and the ventricles. But, only one of these sites with highest automaticity controls the heart rate. It is because the impulses arising from the pacemaker cells of higher automaticity reaches the lower potential subsidiary pacemaker's site and abolishes their immature impulses, before they have the time to fire. Thus, the subsidiary pacemaker center with lower automaticity

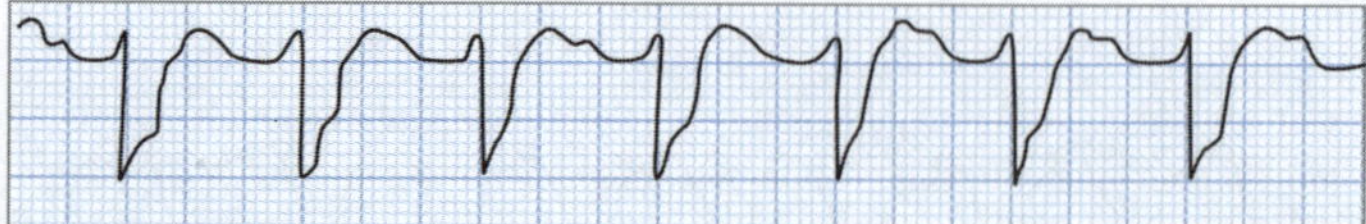

Fig. 33: This is an electrocardiogram (ECG) of idioventricular tachycardia. It is characterized by broad QRS complexes and heart rate is 100 beats/min. When the broad QRS complex rate is <100 beats/min, but >40 beats/min, it is called the accelerated idioventricular rhythm. When the broad QRS complex rate is <40 beats/min, then it is called the escape ventricular rhythm.

enjoys the protection by the impulses from the fastest pacemaker centers. But, when the inherent rate of AV nodal pacemaker site is increased than SA node and goes above 100 beats/min, then it is called the *idionodal tachycardia*.

Similarly, when the inherent discharge rate from the ectopic ventricular pacemaker site is increased more than SA node, and goes above 100 beats/min, then it is also called the *idioventricular tachycardia*. But, when the discharge rate from the idioventricular pacemaker site is below the rate of SA node, then it is called the *accelerated ventricular rhythm*. So, it is commonly found in incomplete AV dissociation or found in the presence of causes, which decrease the sinus rate or increase the expression of nonspecific ventricular pacemaker site, such as fever and carditis. It is not a sudden, precipitous, dramatic event like VT, and does not precipitate in VF. The idioventricular tachycardia whose rate varies around 100 beats/min is not so pathognomonic and rarely causes much decrease in CO and hemodynamic embarrassment. The only difference between the idioventricular tachycardia and VT is the ventricular rate (in VT the heart rate is 150–220 beats/min) **(Fig. 33)**.

The diagnosis of idioventricular tachycardia is based on the following criteria:

- Evidence of ventricular origin—broad, bizarre QRS complexes
- Presence of captured beats—the captured beats are due to the relatively slow rate of idioventricular tachycardia than VT and the relatively long cycle of ventricular ectopic action potential which permits adequate recovery time and therefore a greater opportunity to capture a sinus beat. With very fast ventricular rates, as occur in VT, the refractory period frequently occupies the whole ventricular cycle and therefore, the opportunity to capture a sinus beat becomes minimal or absent.
- As the rate of idioventricular tachycardia is not so high, so the ectopic ventricular rhythm also begins

with several consecutive fusion beats. This is also called the *incomplete capture beat*. Since, the rate of two rhythms (atrial and ventricular) are close to each other, so the idioventricular tachycardia tends to terminate, after the few successive fusion complexes.

- AV dissociation may be present or not. If it is present, fusion or captured beats will not be found.
- The ectopic pacemaker site for idioventricular tachycardia has great protection. This is evident from the fact that it is abolished when the sinus rhythm regains its dominance. This is in contrast to VT, where the ectopic rhythm is not abolished by the faster sinus rhythm.

Ventricular Flutter

The ventricular flutter is the expression of:
- A very rapid and regular ectopic ventricular discharge like VT but the rate is higher than VT.
- Grossly abnormal intraventricular conduction **(Fig. 34)**.

In ECG, the QRS and T deflection of ventricular depolarization are very wide and bizarre, one merging with the other. So that it is difficult to define or separate the QRS complex, ST segment, and T-wave. This is the difference between the ventricular flutter and VT. In VT, this separation is possible. This results in the appearance of a continuous *sine-like wave form* in ventricular flutter.

The bizarre sine-like wave of ventricular flutter also may result from the abnormal intraventricular conduction alone. In ventricular flutter, the coordinated activation of ventricular myocardium and the sufficient contraction of it to produce a stable hemodynamic condition, by giving

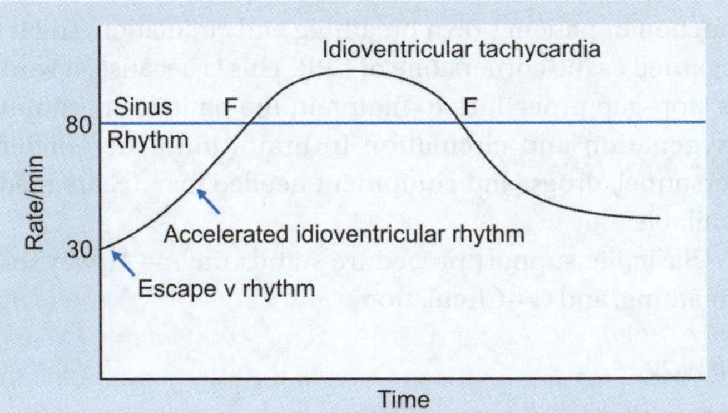

Fig. 34: Mechanism of ventricular tachycardia. A potential ventricular escape rhythm (the beginning of black curved line) is enhanced to accelerated idioventricular rhythm. When it exceeds the the rate of sinus rhythm, then it becomes manifested as a ventricular tachycardia. At the point F, both the sinus and idioventricular rhythm will be at the same rate. Thereby, after that ventricular beat results in ventricular fusion beats. Before the point F, the ventricular beats are captured.

some CO, is still present. However, the change from VT to ventricular flutter is associated with a fall in blood pressure (BP) and CO.

Ventricular flutter is uncommon in clinical practice. It acts as a phase of transition lying between VT and VF **(Fig. 34)**. So, only few examples are recorded, since the condition usually progresses or changes rapidly from VT to VF. Ventricular flutter differs from VF in the uniformity, constancy, regularity, and relatively large amplitude of QRS deflection, whereas the deflections of VF are small and completely chaotic and irregular.

It is well known that ventricular flutter and VT are the expressions of same mechanism. So, their separation may nevertheless serve a useful purpose, since a diagnosis of ventricular flutter immediately connotes a very rapid ventricular rate and/or grossly abnormal intraventricular conduction and reflects an ominous clinical state with a drop in BP and a low CO.

Ventricular Fibrillation

Ventricular fibrillation is a very fatal condition and so it requires an immediate diagnosis and treatment. The onset of this type of arrhythmias is rapidly followed by the loss of consciousness, as the CO falls tremendously or becomes nil and if untreated, then death ensues. The three-fourths of all cardiac arrest are in the form of VF.

Ventricular fibrillation is most commonly seen: (1) after acute MI, (2) in severe IHD, (3) following the administration of antiarrhythmic drugs, (4) after electrical accidents, (5) in severe electrolytes and acid-base imbalance, etc.

Genesis of VF:
- The nonischemic VF begins after a short run of very rapid VT, which is again initiated by subsequent multiple VPC. The VT ultimately breaks down into multiple wavelets of re-entry circuit within the ventricular myocardium leading to VF.
- In infarction or in ischemia, the VF is usually precipitated by a premature, single, early ventricular depolarization or a QRS complex falling on T-wave (vulnerable period), which produces a rapid VT that degenerate into VF. The onset of VF, within the 48 hours of infarction, is called the primary VF and has a good long-term prognosis. Because, once corrected by DC shock, this primary VT does not require prophylactic treatment (i.e., low rate of recurrence). On the other hand, the onset of VF after 48 hours of infarction is called the secondary VF and it merits bad prognosis due to its high recurrence rate.

Electrocardiographically, the VF is recognized by grossly irregular undulation of waves (ventricular complexes) in ECG which is of varying amplitudes, contours, and rates **(Fig. 35)**.

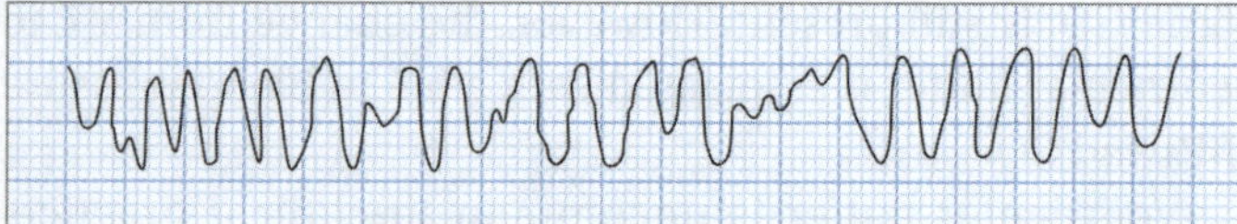

Fig. 35: This is an electrocardiogram (ECG) of ventricular fibrillation. It is characterized by chaotic ventricular activity.

The management of VF is as cardiac arrest, i.e., institution of cardiopulmonary resuscitation (CPR) immediately.

CARDIAC ARREST AND CARDIOPULMONARY RESUSCITATION

Cardiac arrest is defined as the sudden and complete loss of cardiac function. In this condition, the patient immediately loses consciousness, pulse is not palpable and respiration ceases quickly. So, death is virtually inevitable, unless an effective treatment is provided promptly. Therefore, any effective treatment which is tried immediately to start the cardiac function is called the CPR.

Most frequently many cardiac arrests are managed very poorly. This is because (1) there is lack of immediate organization of an efficient team, (2) lack of proper knowledge about the recommended procedures, (3) immediate lack of proper equipment and drugs, and (4) very frequently, different types of arrhythmias that occur during cardiac arrest are incorrectly diagnosed and treated. So, the management of cardiac arrest which is called the CPR is described in a stepwise manner to prevent the haphazard way of working.

Step I

If it is seen that a patient has been suddenly collapsed and becomes unresponsive or unconscious due to cardiac arrest, then immediate help is sought. This is because, the chances of successful outcome from CPR decline rapidly with the passing of time (every second). The cardiac arrest which is manifested as unresponsiveness or unconsciousness should be confirmed first by shaking the patient and asking the questions loudly, while keeping the fingers on pulse (first on radial, then if not palpable on brachial or carotid artery) and examining the eyelash or corneal reflexes. Simultaneously, the respiration should also be checked, when unresponsiveness is confirmed and pulse is not palpable. If the respiration is not felt then cardiac arrest is *confirmed clinically* and immediate help is sought and precordial thump is delivered. If precordial thump is started within 30 seconds of confirmation of cardiac arrest, then the energy delivered by this precordial thump is sufficient enough to restore an effective rhythm in 2% cases of VF and up to 40% cases of VT (provided the cardiac arrest is

Flowchart 1: Algorithm of adult basic life support (BLS).

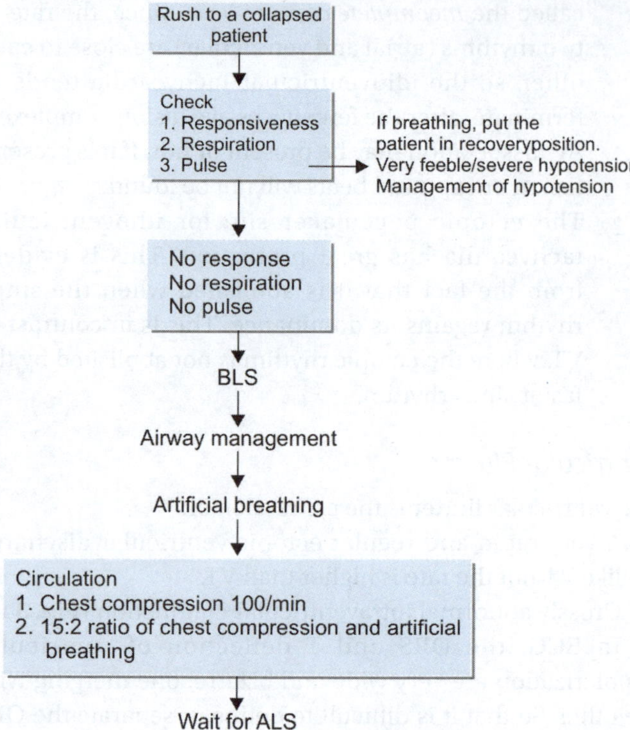

presented in the form of VF or VT and we know >90% of cardiac arrest is in these forms) **(Flowchart 1)**.

If precordial thump fails to work, (usually fails) then the next steps of CPR are:
- Basic life support (BLS).
- Advanced life support (ALS).

Step II

Though the BLS itself very rarely restores the cardiac function or patient's own breathing and circulation, still it is regarded as the cornerstone of CPR. This is because, it works as stop-gap procedure to maintain the patient's minimum oxygenation and circulation in brain, until the efficient personnel, drugs, and equipment needed for ALS are made available.

Basic life support procedure stands on: A—Airway, B—Breathing, and C—Circulation.

Airway

Airway should be maintained by:
- Opening the mouth
- Removing or loosing any clothing around the patient's neck
- Removing foods, blood, froth, etc. from the mouth and cleaning the airway
- Lifting the chin in order to lift the tongue from the back of the throat (oropharynx and laryngopharynx).

Breathing

Breathing of the patient should be assessed by looking at the chest and/or by listening the mouth of the patient for breath sound and/or by feeling the patient's exhaled air on the dorsal surface of the examiner's hand. This is actually the part of the diagnosis of cardiac arrest. If the patient does not breathe, then immediate *mouth-to-mouth* artificial breathing should be started or *artificial ventilation should be started by any device which is available at hand (pocket mask and mouth or Ambu bag).* The different types of devices which are in use for artificial ventilation have been discussed in separate chapter.

Circulation

When breathing of the patient is assessed, then peripheral pulse (brachial and carotid) also should be palpated simultaneously without wasting any time. This is the part of the diagnosis of cardiac arrest, not its management. If there is no palpable peripheral pulse, then the diagnosis of cardiac arrest is confirmed and immediately full BLS is started, i.e., with mouth-to-mouth or bag and mask breathing, and cardiac compression. Classical cardiac compression is performed by placing the heal of one hand on the middle of the lower half of the patient's sternum and placing the heel of other hand over the first and then interlocking the fingers. After that, pressure should be given vertically downward, so that sternum is depressed for 4–5 cm. The rate of the chest compression should be maintained at 100–120 beats/min. The time taken for each chest compression should be equal to the time taken to release the pressure. Every 15 chest compression should be followed by two ventilations at a ratio of 15:2. The idea behind this chest compression is that the cerebral blood flow of at least 20% of normal is needed to be maintained for a full neurological recovery and this is possible by this type of properly performed cardiac compression and artificial ventilation. The recovery of spontaneous respiration and peripheral pulse should be checked after every 10 breaths.

Step III

Advanced life support is the main part of this step. ALS is commenced as soon as there is availability of proper equipment, such as the intubating aids, monitors, defibrillator, ventilating equipment, drugs, and trained cardiac arrest management team. BLS should be continued till ALS is available and applied. Now, as the part of ALS, the defibrillator or cardiac monitor should be attached and the cardiac rhythm disorder should be studied by the other members of the team, when BLS is going on.

There are four types of arrhythmias that are usually encountered during or shortly after cardiac arrest. These are:

- Ventricular fibrillation
- Pulseless VT or sustained VT with no CO
- Asystole
- Electromechanical dissociation (EMD).

Ventricular Fibrillation

It is the most common form of arrhythmia in cardiac arrest and appears as a chaotic rhythm on ECG. If the monitor is faulty or the gain is turned too low, then it can also be mistaken as asystole.

Pulseless VT

It appears as broad, rapid, ventricular complexes (QRS complex) with severe hemodynamic compromise, characterized by nil or very low CO (pulseless). In such type of arrhythmia, causing cardiac arrest, DC shock is very helpful to convert VF or VT to normal cardiac electrical activity or to such a cardiac electrical activity which is capable of maintaining a workable CO.

Asystole

It implies that there is no electrical cardiac activity and thus the ECG is simply shown as a flat or straight line. DC shock is not helpful in asystole, rather it potentiates the asystole **(Fig. 36)**.

Electromechanical Dissociation

In such condition, the cardiac electrical activity is normal and the heart contracts normally. But, it fails to produce any CO or any effective circulation. This is mainly due to the severe reduction of preload. The DC shock is also not helpful in EMD **(Fig. 37)**.

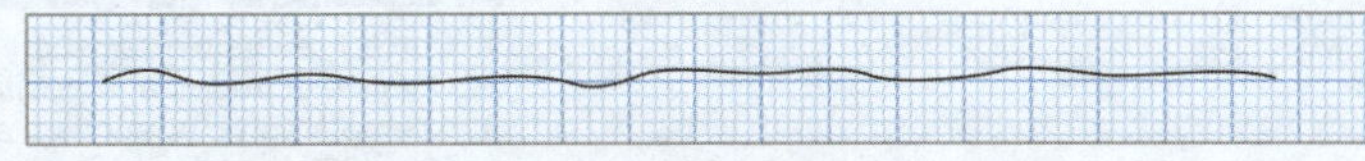

Fig. 36: This is an electrocardiogram (ECG) of asystole. It is characterized by flat line in ECG (no spontaneous electrical activity).

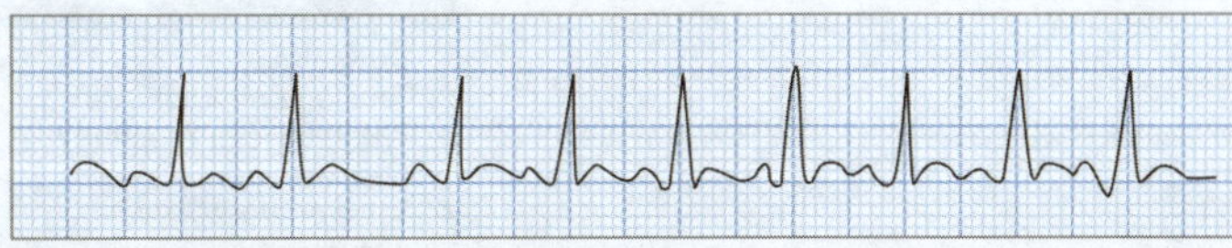

Fig. 37: This is an electrocardiogram (ECG) of electromechanical dissociation. It is characterized by normal QRS complexes, even in the absence of cardiac output.

Management of VF and VT in Cardiac Arrest

Defibrillation converts the abnormal cardiac rhythm, i.e., VF and VT (which is the most common, i.e., >95%) to sinus rhythm or at least to a rhythm that restores some CO. So, the first step of ALS is defibrillation, even before the diagnosis of specific electrical activity in cardiac arrest **(Flowchart 2)**. Defibrillation is also the choice of management for VF and VT in intensive care unit (ICU). In addition, defibrillation can also be used, if there is asystole because it cannot be entirely confirmed that it is not due to the small complex (fine) VF. So, in *doubt of benefit*, defibrillation should be used even in asystole as VF and VT is the most common (in >95% of cases) and treatable form of cardiac arrest. *However, there is no reason in defibrillating a patient, if it is confirmed that there is asystole.* Because, defibrillation just changes one type of cardiac rhythm to another, but it will not restart the heart, where there is no initial electrical activity as in asystole.

In case of EMD, the defibrillation also has no role, because by the definition of EMD the heart is working normally electrically, but without any CO due to some mechanical reasons such as the absolute reduction of preload.

During defibrillation the following steps should be under taken and these are:

- All nitrate patches should be removed from the patient's body.
- The paddles always should be placed at least 15 cm away from the permanent pacemaker.
- Electrode gel always should be used on the skin below the paddles.
- Electrode gel should not spread between the paddles as this can cause a short circuit.
- Everybody attaining this patient should stand clear of the patient and his bed, just during discharging of electrical energy.

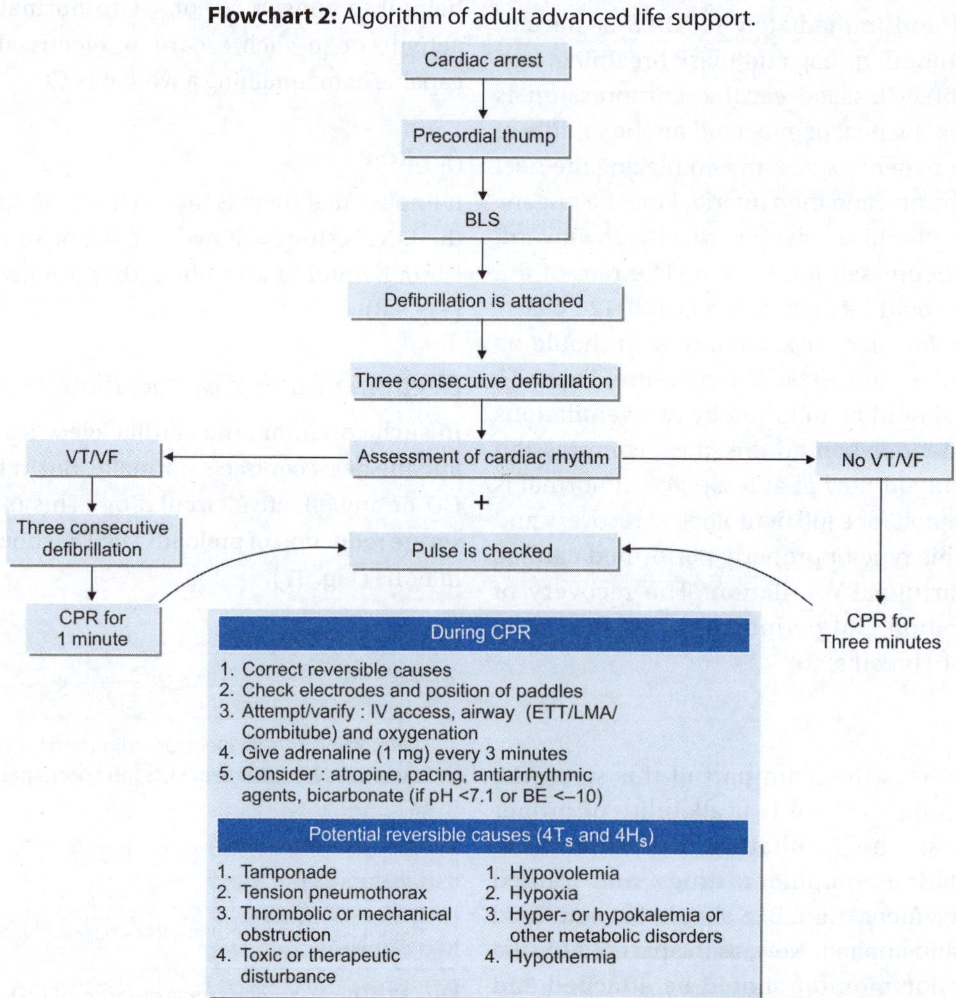

Flowchart 2: Algorithm of adult advanced life support.

(BE: base excess; CPR: cardiopulmonary resuscitation; ETT: endotracheal tube; IV: intravenous; LMA: laryngeal mask airway; VF: ventricular fibrillation; VT: ventricular tachycardia)

Then, in rapid succession (i.e., one after another, not measuring the time interval between the two), three DC shocks are given with the energy of 200 J, 200 J, and 300 J respectively. After that, a brief pause (few seconds) is given to assess the patient's cardiac rhythm on monitor's screen and/or pulse and to recharge the defibrillator. These three successive DC shocks should be delivered within 45 seconds and it is not necessary to resume the BLS as a part of ALS (i.e., ventilation and chest compression) between each of these three successive DC shocks.

After the first round of three DC shock, BLS is again started for a minute and the cardiac rhythm and pulse are assessed at the end of this minute. At this point, the intravenous line is instituted and patient is intubated by others. BLS should not be interrupted for >15 seconds, due to any reason, when attempting intravenous line and/or intubation. If access to the IV line and intubation fails in first attempt, then it should not be tried again, till the end of the next set (second round) of three DC shocks. In-between the failed attempt for line and intubation and DC shock, BLS should be continued for another 1 minute.

The second set of three DC shocks should be with energy of 300 J each. Before the second set of DC shock, 1 mg adrenaline is given intravenously (if line is procured) or through endotracheal tube. It is not necessary to give time to adrenaline to circulate, before giving the second set of DC shocks, because adrenaline does not aid in defibrillation. But it only improves the cerebral and coronary circulation by constricting the peripheral vasculature and reducing the blood flow to the skin and skeletal muscle. If adrenaline is used by endotracheal route, then the total dose should be diluted to 10 mL in isotonic saline and should be used by five ventilations.

After the administration of adrenaline and the second set of DC shocks, the BLS should be continued again for a minute and at the end of this minute the patient's cardiac rhythm and pulse should be assessed again. If still satisfactory cardiac rhythm has not been restored, then the third set of three DC shocks should be delivered with energy of 360 J each.

Thus, each loop [DC shock → BLS (it means chest compression and ventilation) → assessment → drug] should take no >2 or 3 minutes and should be repeated, until either an effective cardiac rhythm maintaining some CO is restored or it is decided that CPR would be abandoned.

After the third set of DC shocks, if VF is still continuing, then the following things can be done:

- Antiarrhythmic agents, such as lignocaine, bretylium, or amiodarone can be started.
- K^+, Ca^{2+}, magnesium should be checked and corrected.
- Paddle position should be changed.

Actually the benefit of the use of antiarrhythmic drugs are lacking in the management of CPR. Again the routine use of sodium bicarbonate to correct the acidosis, following cardiac arrest, is not recommended, because paradoxically it worsens the intracellular acidosis and does not improve the final outcome. If bicarbonate is to be used, then dose should be calculated from arterial pH and blood gas analysis that is discussed in acid-base balance chapter.

Management of Asystole in Cardiac Arrest

Following the cardiac arrest, BLS is started immediately, while looking for ALS and if possible the causes should be treated simultaneously with BLS and ALS. The management of asystole in cardiac arrest is not the DC shock, because the DC shock does not regenerate (work), when there is no electrical cardiac activity. But, sometimes very fine electrical activity in the form of VF may be *misdiagnosed as asystole,* due to the faulty equipment or too low gain setting on the monitor. So, this wrong diagnosis is very dangerous and if there is any doubt, then for *benefit of doubt* three DC shocks at energy level of 200 J, 200 J, and 360 J each should be given successively to avoid missing of a potentially reversible VF. On the other hand, application of DC shock in a confirmed asystole has no adverse effect.

Following DC shocks, the BLS and ALS should be continued again like the management of VT or VF in CPR. Intubation and access to the intravenous lines should be tried. Cardiac rhythm should be diagnosed as confirmed asystole. Adrenaline 1 mg should be administered intravenously and BLS should be maintained for 3 minutes with chest compression to ventilation ratio of 15:2. Then second dose of adrenaline is given and the patient's cardiac rhythm and pulse is again assessed. If still the asystole persists, then 3 mg atropine in a single bolus dose is given through IV. The cycle should be repeated, maintaining BLS, and giving further doses of adrenaline every 3 minutes. After three repeated cycle, if the patient is still in asystole, pacing should be done using transvenous pacing wire or transthoracic pacing. In the meantime, all the causes for cardiac asystole are searched for and removed.

Management of EMD in Cardiac Arrest

In cardiac arrest, if rhythm is diagnosed as EMD, then always the underlying remediable causes should be immediately looked for and treatment is started. The few causes of EMD are cardiac tamponade, drug overdose, electrolyte disturbance, hypothermia, hypovolemia, pulmonary embolism, tension pneumothorax, etc.

Immediately the BLS is started, while looking for ALS and if possible treating the causes. After intubating the patient and gaining the intravenous access, the adrenaline in the dose of 1 mg is administered through IV in bolus and then BLS is continued for 3 minutes with chest compression to ventilation ratio of 15:2. After that, the cardiac rhythm and pulse is assessed. If still EMD persists, then one bolus dose of 3 mg atropine is given through IV. These cycles should be repeated, maintaining BLS and ALS and giving the further doses of adrenaline after every 3 minutes interval.

Although the high doses of adrenaline (5 mg through IV), alkalizing agents, calcium, and pressor rising agents can be given, still there is no confirmed evidence for their routine use in cardiac arrest and better prognosis.

Nondrug Therapy of Cardiac Arrhythmia

External Defibrillation or Cardioversion

The cardioversion is the process of the restoration of normal electrical rhythm of heart by electrical shock (current) and the device by which this process of cardioversion by electric shock is accomplished is known as the defibrillator. This process of cardioversion can be accomplished by passing the sufficiently large amount of direct electrical current through the heart from an external or internal sources. The mechanism of action of this DC shock is that it will completely depolarize the heart from outside for a fraction of a second and will temporarily interrupt any internal arrhythmia (electrical activity). Thus, it will produce a brief period of asystole which is usually followed by the resumption of normal sinus rhythm.

The defibrillator usually delivers a high energy DC of short duration via two metal paddles or gel pad, positioned over the upper right sternal edge and the apex of the heart. When this technique is used to treat *organized rhythms* such as AF or VT, then the shock should be synchronized with the ECG and is normally given *at 0.02 seconds after the peak of R-wave*. Otherwise, if energy is applied during a critical period around the peak of T-wave, then it may provoke VF. But, this precise timing of discharge of shock is not important in VF, as it is not an organized electrical cardiac rhythm.

In ventricular and other emergencies, the energy of the first shock should be minimum of 200 J. There is no need for anesthesia, if the patient is unconscious such as VF in cardiac arrest. But, usually an *elective cardioversion* requires a general anesthesia or sedation for conscious subject such as for the correction of atrial arrhythmia. High energy shocks may cause the myocardial damage also. So, if there is no urgency, it is appropriate to begin with a low amplitude shock, i.e., 50–100 J and gradually going to larger shocks, if necessary.

Digoxin toxicity increases the risk of untoward arrhythmias after cardioversion. So, it is conventional practice to withhold the drug for 24 hours before any elective cardioversion. Patients with long-standing atrial arrhythmias such as AF are at the increased risk of systemic embolism before and after the cardioversion. So, it is wise to ensure that the patient is adequately anticoagulated for at least 4 weeks on either side of the procedure.

Implantable Cardioverter Defibrillators

These are expensive and sophisticated devices which can automatically sense and terminate the life-threatening different types of ventricular arrhythmias by pacing or synchronized cardioversion with low energy shock or defibrillation with high energy shock. But, this automatic high energy shock can be painful, if the patient is still conscious. These devices also can pace the ventricles in the event of severe bradycardia and asystole. Implantable cardioverter defibrillators (ICDs) are implanted transvenously like a permanent pacemaker and are subject to similar complications. Clinical trials among the high risk patients have shown that the devices are more effective than antiarrhythmic drugs in preventing sudden death from severe cardiac arrhythmia. An ICD is used to treat the patient who present with cardiac arrest due to VT or VF or sustained VT causing syncope or severe hemodynamically compromised VT associated with poor left ventricular function [left ventricular ejection fraction (LVEF) <35%]. These devices may also be used prophylactically in selected patients who are thought to be at the high risk of sudden cardiac death, such as long QT syndrome, hypertrophic cardiomyopathy, and arrhythmogenic right ventricular dysplasia.

Radiofrequency Catheter Ablation

The aim of this technique is to interrupt the re-entry circuit by selectively damaging the accessory path for conduction of cardiac impulses with endocardial tissue by radiofrequency energy, delivered through a catheter that is passed into the heart through a peripheral artery or vein. This procedure is often time consuming and the patient may experience some discomfort during the time of ablation. But, it does not require any anesthesia. Serious complications are rare and subject to similar of pacing. The radiofrequency ablation eliminates the need for long-term drug therapy and is an attractive form of treatment for many arrhythmias offering the prospect of a lifetime cure. The technique has revolutionized the management of many cardiac arrhythmias and is now the treatment of choice for atrial tachycardia, AV nodal re-entry tachycardia, WPW syndrome, and AF. The applications of this technique are now expanding. So, it has also been used to treat some forms of VT.

■ PACEMAKER

The process of artificial electrical depolarization of heart, which is known as *cardiac pacing*, is a valuable clinical means of therapies of different types of arrhythmias. The device by which this cardiac pacing is done is known as the *cardiac pacemaker.* So, its major uses include (1) to control the rate and rhythm of heart and thus correcting some arrhythmias and (2) to deliver counter shock by DC current (cardioversion) for the correction of some arrhythmias which is already discussed.

The anesthesiologists must learn about pacemakers due to two reasons: (1) in the perioperative period, pacing is the mode of treatment for a large number of cardiac arrhythmias facing emergencies and (2) pacing affects the appearance of ECG which may sometimes confuse an anesthetist to diagnose a cardiac arrhythmia from ECG reading. Due to the advancement of technology more and more sophisticated kinds of pacemakers are coming out, so that a wide range of pacemaker with different mode of functions are now available. But, the two most basic functions of pacemakers for the control of cardiac rate and rhythm are:

- It provides a safety in patients who are at risk of bradycardia or asystole.
- It terminates tachycardia.

Classification of Pacing

There are three methods of pacing:

1. *External pacing:* It is effective only in very emergency situation, where the internal temporary pacing is not available or if available but has no time to implant it. However, it becomes ineffective after several hours and it is painful to the conscious patient. So, the patients must be sedated. Transthoracic pacing is the example of such an external pacing, and is also called the *transcutaneous pacing.* It functions by delivering an electrical stimulus that is sufficient to induce cardiac contraction from outside through two large adhesive gel pad or electrodes, placed over the apex and the upper right sternal edge, like defibrillation. These two electrodes also can be placed over the precordium and the back of the patient. It has the advantage of being easy and quick to set up, but may cause discomfort and skeletal muscle contraction. Some sophisticated ECG monitor or defibrillator machines incorporate this type of transcutaneous pacing system which can be used as a temporary measure, until the temporary transvenous pacing is established.

2. *Internal pacing with power source outside the body:* This is also called the *temporary pacing.* It can be accomplished by inserting an electrode into the heart through a large vein in neck, or arm, or leg, or by the direct puncture of myocardium through the chest wall. These techniques are effective for emergency situations and short-term therapy. Its status lies between the external pacing and the permanent pacing. Here, the electrode which is placed within the cardiac cavity, is connected to an external pulse generator (power source) which can be adjusted time to time to alter the energy output and pacing rate. The threshold of pacing should be the lowest output that will reliably pace the heart and it should be <1 mV, during the initial period of implantation. It may require daily adjustment, because the threshold of myocardium tends to rise, due to the inflammation and edema of cardiac tissue, around the tip of the electrode.

3. *Internal pacing with power source implanted in the body:* This is also called the permanent pacing. Again it can be of two types:

   i. *Left ventricular epicardial pacemaker:* Here, the electrodes are sutured directly into the left myocardium under the epicardium. This is done via thoracotomy or subxiphoid approach. The power source is embedded in the abdominal wall.

   ii. *Right ventricular endocardial pacemaker:* Here, the electrodes are introduced into the apex of the right ventricle via an axillary or subclavian vein and the power source is implanted at the pectoral or axillary area. Because of the relative simplicity and better efficacy of this procedure, the insertion of this type of permanent pacemaker is preferred.

The temporary pacemaker provides pacing in an emergency situation, until a permanent pacemaker is implanted. In temporary pacing, the electrodes are introduced usually through the transvenous route. But, the transesophageal and transcutaneous temporary pacing also can be used. Here, the battery and the electronics part of pacemaker remain outside the body, whereas in permanent pacemaker, the battery, electronics, and the electrodes are all implanted within the patient's body. Both the temporary and the permanent pacemakers are such set that they monitor the patient's cardiac activity (senses the electric activity of patient's heart) continuously and provide impulses when necessary, because patients seldom need pacing impulse from pacemaker continuously. This helps to prolong the life of battery of pacemakers. This is called the *demand pacing.*

All the pacemaker units mentioned above can function in an unipolar or bipolar manner. The unipolar circuit consists of a cathode end which is inserted into the myocardium and an anode end which is situated at a remote site, usually on the surface of the implanted power unit. But, the bipolar pacemaker has both the cathode and anode end within the heart which are usually at 1–2 cm apart.

Indications for Temporary Pacing

The indications for temporary pacing are:

- Patients waiting for permanent pacing
- *Acute MI:* In acute inferior wall MI complete heart block is usually developed due to the damage of artery which supplies the AV node. So, extensive infarction causes severe bradycardia or second and third-degree AV block due to the damage of the bundle branches in the interventricular septum. In such situation mortality is high. So, immediate temporary pacing and inotropic support are very essential.
- Some tachycardia such as AV re-entry tachycardia and VT can be terminated by overdrive temporary pacing in emergency situations.
- Perioperative pacing.

Indications for Permanent Pacing

The indications for permanent pacing are:

- Second-degree AV block with an episode of symptomatic bradycardia (syncope) regardless of whether it is Mobitz type I or II.
- Third-degree AV block
- Bifascicular block with a history of syncope or documented intermittent failure of the remaining fascicle. Asymptomatic patients with bifascicular block are not indicated for pacing.
- Sick sinus syndrome with symptoms only. Asymptomatic patients with SSS are not indicated for pacemaker.
- Malignant vasovagal syndrome
- Carotid sinus syndrome.

DESCRIPTION OF PERMANENT PACEMAKER

The permanent pacemakers are usually described by internationally accepted code of five letters. Each letter describes an individual aspect of the pacemaker's different function that is shown in the **Table 1**. There are different types of pacemaker available in the market. Among them, some commonly available pacemakers are described here.

VVI

This pacemaker senses ventricle (V) by single lead placed within the ventricle (V). It also paces ventricle via the same lead when no cardiac electrical activity is detected. So, this is also called the ventricular demand pacemakers. Otherwise, the pacemaker always senses and is inhibited (I) by normal ventricular activity and does not send impulses for ventricular contraction.

TABLE 1: Letter codes for different functions of pacemaker.

Letter refers to	Code	Meaning
1. Chamber paced	V	Ventricle
	A	Atrium
	D	Dual or both the chambers
2. Chamber sensed	V	Ventricle
	A	Atrium
	D	Dual or both the chambers
	O	None
3. Mode of response or sensing	T	Triggering of pacemaker (ventricular synchronous)
	I	Inhibition of pacemaker (ventricular demand)
	D	Inhibition or triggering
	O	None
	R	Rate responsiveness and reverse function (this pacemaker is silent at slow rates and activated by fast rates)
4. Programmable functions	P	Programmable for rate or output or both
	M	Multiprogrammable
	O	None
	E	External control
5. Special antitachycardia functions	P	Pacing of tachycardia
	S	Shock delivered
	D	Dual (pacing and shock)
	O	None
	B	Bursts of impulses

VVT

This is a triggered (T) type of ventricular pacemaker. During sinus conducted rhythm (or other spontaneous rhythm), the pacemaker also continuously discharges impulses approximately 0.04–0.08 second after the onset of normal QRS complex. Thus, it can be seen as an artifact in the ECG and indicates pacemaker function. But, it plays no role in ventricular depolarization, because the artifact constantly falls in the absolute refractory period of the normal action potential of the ventricle. Whenever, the spontaneous sinus rhythm falls below the preset rate, fixed by the pacemaker, then the pacemaker assumes its function. This is not a demand pacemaker.

AAI

The single lead of this pacemaker is situated in atrium (A) and senses atrial (A) activity. If the normal atrial activity is detected, then the pacemaker is inhibited (I). But, whenever atrial activity is not detected, then it takes over the function by pacing the atria. It is also a type of *demand atrial pacemaker*.

AAO

This is not a demand pacemaker and the electrode is placed in the atrium. It is not a demand pacemaker, because it does not sense (O) the atrial electrical activity and is not inhibited. It continuously sends impulses according to a prefixed rate for atrial depolarization and subsequently ventricle contracts. If the patient's problem, requiring pacing, is due to the SA node or atrial disease, but AV nodal and His-Purkinje system conduction is normal, then this transvenously inserted atrial pacemaker is effective.

DVI

This unit paces both the atrium and the ventricle, but senses only the ventricle (V). As this pacemaker paces both the chambers of heart, so it is designated as double (D) chamber pacemaker. The pacemaker is inhibited (I) by an earlier spontaneous ventricular depolarization. But, since there is no atrial sensing, so atrial pace impulse will not be inhibited and atrial pace artifacts will appear regularly in the ECG at the programmed rate, even though the P-waves precede them. *It cannot be used in the presence of AF.*

DDD

This pacemaker has two leads, one in the atrium and other one in the ventricle. So, it is called the dual chamber (D) pacemaker. It senses both the atrial and ventricular activity (D). It is inhibited, if it senses the activity in ventricle. In complete AV block, if it senses atrial activity without ventricular activity, it can pace ventricle in sequence with atria. It can also pace the atria alone or atria and ventricle both in sequence (D).

AAIR, VVIR, DDDR

"R" indicates the rate of responsiveness. The rate of responsiveness means pacemakers adjust the heart rate or pacing rate according to the need of the patient during activity which mimic the physiological response. Here, the patient's level of activity is continuously monitored by pacemaker through several parameters, such as vibration, respiration, or temperature of blood. Thus, heart rate is adjusted by pacemaker according to the activity.

Programmable Pacemaker

The advancement of technology in the manufacture of pacemaker permits future modifications or change of many of its functions (programme) by external means, thereby sparing the need for an invasive procedure. Thus, the changes of different parameters can be made in the pacemaker from outside. These are the pacing rate, sensing interval (rate hysteresis), pulse width, amplitude, etc. This facility allows the cardiologist to prolong the life of a pacemaker by choosing the optimum settings and providing the means to overcome a wide range of pacing problems. For example, programming can be used to increase the output in the face of an unexpected increase in threshold or to altered sensitivity, if the pacemaker is inappropriately inhibited by electrical potentials, generated in the pectoral muscles.

The *atrial pacing is appropriate* for the patients with SSS (SA disease) without AV block. *Ventricular pacing is the only suitable mode* for the patients with continuous AF. In DDD (dual chamber pacing), the atrial electrode can be used to detect the spontaneous atrial activity and trigger the ventricular pacing. Thereby, it preserves the AV synchrony and allows the ventricular rate to increase together with the atrial rate during exercise and other forms of stress. Thus, though DDD is more expensive, but has many *advantages* when compared to only ventricular pacing. These include: (1) superior hemodynamics with better effort tolerance, (2) a lower prevalence of atrial arrhythmias in patients with SSS, and (3) the ability to prevent and cure the "pacemaker syndrome". The *pacemaker syndrome* consists of fall in BP and dizziness, precipitated by the start of ventricular pacing.

VVIMB

This is similar to VVI pacemaker, but is multiprogrammable with pacing bursts for tachyarrhythmias.

DVIM

This is an atrioventricular pacemaker which paces both the atrium and the ventricle. It is ventricular inhibited and is multiprogrammable.

■ ECG FINDINGS IN PACEMAKER

The pacemaker depolarizes atrium and/or ventricle by electrical impulses which are generated within it (pacemaker) and appear in the ECG tracing as *"pacing spikes"*. In atrial pacing, the pacing spikes will be followed by P-wave and in ventricular pacing, the pacing spikes will be followed by broad QRS complexes (broad complex is due to the conduction of electrical impulse through the ventricular muscles like ectopic foci, but not through the normal conducting Purkinje tissue). Therefore, the recognition of any specific disease state of the myocardium and its conducting system by ECG analysis, during the pacing, is usually impossible. In only atrial pacing, the spikes are

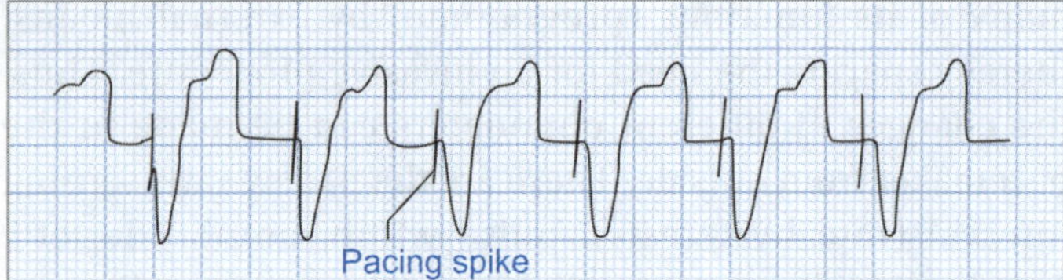

Fig. 38: Graph of the ventricular pacing, it is characterized by ventricular pacing spikes and followed by broad QRS complex.

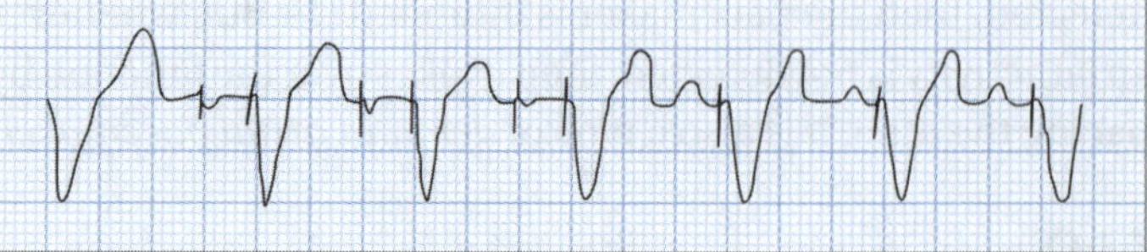

Fig. 39: Dual chamber pacing. The first three cardiac cycles show the atrial and ventricular pacing with narrow pacing spikes in front of each P-wave and QRS complex. The last three beats show spontaneous P-waves with a different morphology and no pacing spikes. The pacemaker senses or tracks these P-waves and maintains an AV synchrony by pacing the ventricle after an appropriate interval.

followed by P-waves and normal QRS complexes (without ventricular spike) as the impulses conduct via the normal conducting pathway (AV node, bundle of His, and Purkinje fibers). In dual chamber pacing, both the spikes will be seen. The failure of a pacing spike to be followed by depolarization of heart indicates a problem with "capture" **(Fig. 38)**.

The ECG tracing also can help: (1) in localizing the site of electrode placement and (2) in detecting the change of position of electrode by the dislodgement of it, if occurs. In right ventricular apical endocardial pacing, the depolarization wave of heart will flow from right to left (R → L) and from apex to base. The resulting QRS vector, therefore, will be oriented to the left and superiorly. Thus, the QRS complexes in lead I will be positive and in lead II, III, and aVF will be negative. On the other hand, if the electrode is displaced from the apex to the outflow of right ventricle, then the direction of depolarization wave will be R → L, but from base to apex. So, the QRS complex remains upright in lead I, but now becomes upright in lead II, III, and aVF.

Interpreting of an ECG of a patient with functioning pacemaker, the pacemaker rate should be accurately measured. Any change in rate indicates the early battery failure.

In unipolar pacemaker as the distance between the anode and the cathode is long, so the pacing spike will be large. But in bipolar unit due to the close position of anode and cathode, the spike (pacemaker artifact) will be small in ECG tracing.

For the detection of any changes in the pacemaker position by dislodgement, the determination of the spatial orientation of the pacing spike is also helpful. This is especially applicable to a bipolar right ventricular endocardial pacemaker. The cathode is usually distal to the anode. So, as a result of its position in the right ventricular apex, the vector of electrical artifact or spike will be oriented to the right and superiorly. Thus, it will produce negative artifact in lead I, II, and aVF. If due to any cause, the electrode becomes detached and floats into the right ventricular outflow tract, then the vector of this artifact will be directed inferiorly. Then, it will produce an upright artifact in II, III, and aVF lead. The explanation is like that the anode-cathode

relation in the right ventricular pacemaker will be reversed, i.e., the distal pole will be the anode. In this instance, the artifact for pacing will be oriented to the left and inferiorly, producing an upright signal in lead I, II, and aVF **(Fig. 39)**.

During the management of VT, when the antiarrhythmic drugs fail, then the ventricular pacing has been successfully used to prevent the recurrent VT and VF. The mechanism is like that when the repolarization of ventricular muscle becomes asymmetrical, due to some reasons (ischemia, infarction), leading to the local potentiation of ectopic discharge, then the pacing of heart at the rate of 130–150 beats/min, causes the ventricular repolarization to become synchronous throughout the entire myocardium and eliminate the local potentials with arrhythmias. This type of pacing is called the *"overdrive pacing"*. In the treatment of refractory VT, ventricular pacing at rates slower than the tachycardia (which is called the *underdrive pacing*) may also abolish arrhythmia by interrupting the re-entry circuit that causes the tachycardia.

If the entire heart is depolarized for a moment by sufficient current, introducing in the myocardium, then the normal cardiac rhythm is re-established after depressing or breaking the cycle of arrhythmia. This countershock is delivered externally by defibrillation. This is called DC shock. But, it can be applied internally during cardiothoracic surgery or through pacemaker. It is a major lifesaving process by eliminating VF and VT during resuscitation process of cardiac arrest. In emergency, the countershock or DC shock is also preferable to drug therapy to terminate the atrial flutter and fibrillation. This DC defibrillator introduces an electrical charge for 0.0025 second (AC defibrillation introduces an electrical charge for 0.25 second and due to this long duration, the charge could fall on supernormal phase of any rhythm and can produce any type of arrhythmia) and is now coupled with synchronizing device that prevents the discharge at the critical phase of cardiac cycle and thus avoids any serious arrhythmia.

Surgically implanted defibrillator are also now available which are programmed to recognize VT and VF spontaneously and discharge an internal DC shock automatically.

■ PACEMAKER AND SURGERY

The importance of pacemaker from the anesthetic point of view during surgery are:

- The original indication for the insertion of pacemaker should be known to an anesthetist, which may modify the mode and outcome of anesthesia.
- The type of pacemaker also should be known, which will help to diagnose the intraoperative arrhythmia.
- Checking of pacemaker before and after surgery for any "capture beat"
- To avoid any interference or damage to the pacemaker from diathermy

- Inappropriate pacemaker inhibition, due to any intraoperative measures, can cause bradycardia or even asystole.
- To minimize the pacemaker damage or its inhibition, the active diathermy electrode should be placed at least 15 cm away from the pacemaker generator box and the indifferent electrode as far from the box as possible.

Patients with certain cardiac conduction disorders who do not have a permanent pacemaker should be considered for a temporary pacemaker, if they are about to undergo general anesthesia. These indications for temporary pacing are: (1) third-degree AV block and (2) second-degree AV block. Pacing is not usually necessary for bifascicular block unless the patient has a history of syncope.

Ischemic Heart Diseases and Anesthesia

INTRODUCTION, ETIOLOGY, AND PATHOPHYSIOLOGY

Ischemia refers to the lack of O_2 due to inadequate perfusion (blood flow). It may be absolute or relative and results from an imbalance between the decrease in supply of O_2 and/or increase in its (O_2) demand. Therefore, myocardial ischemia occurs either from a decrease in coronary blood flow (e.g., variant angina) and/or from a disproportionate increase in myocardial O_2 demand (e.g., exertional angina).

The myocardial *O_2 supply* is primarily determined by the volume of coronary blood flow. The volume of coronary blood flow (supply) is dependent both on the perfusion pressure (pressure in aorta) and the coronary vascular resistance which ultimately depends on the diameter of the lumen of coronary artery. On the other hand, the four major factors which govern myocardial *O_2 demand* or consumption are: ventricular wall tension, afterload, heart rate (HR), and ventricular contractility. Another term such as the *"double product"* is a clinically useful index of myocardial O_2 demand. This is obtained from multiplying the systolic blood pressure (BP) (afterload) with HR.

With increasing age, the people mainly suffer from cardiovascular diseases. The cardiovascular diseases account for the majority of perioperative morbidity and mortality (deaths) with increasing age. Now, in a population, the persons with advanced age is increasing gradually and so more and more patients are coming for surgery with coexisting cardiovascular diseases, among which the *ischemic heart disease (IHD) is most common.* The first and the foremost common presentation of IHD is acute myocardial infarction (MI) in 50% of patients.

The *main cause* of *decrease in coronary blood flow (supply),* causing myocardial ischemia and infarction with increased age, is the reduction of the diameter of the lumen of coronary arteries by atherosclerosis. The atherosclerosis of coronary arteries causes an absolute decrease in coronary blood flow in basal state or may also limit the appropriate increase in coronary blood flow, when the demand for this flow is increased, e.g., during exercise. The important *risk factors* for the development of atherosclerosis are male gender, increasing age, hypercholesterolemia, high plasma low-density lipoprotein (LDL) and low plasma high-density lipoprotein (HDL), systemic hypertension, cigarette smoking, diabetes, obesity, sedentary lifestyle, and a positive family history, etc.

The *coronary blood flow can also be limited by arterial thrombi, spasm, or the narrowing of coronary ostium due to aortitis.* The reduction of O_2-carrying capacity of blood (e.g., severe anemia, presence of carboxyhemoglobin, etc.) is a rare cause of myocardial ischemia and infarction. Myocardial ischemia can also occur, if *myocardial O_2 demands are abnormally increased,* e.g., exercise, tachycardia, severe myocardial (ventricular) hypertrophy due to hypertension, or aortic stenosis, etc. Not infrequently, two or more causes of ischemia coexist, such as an increase in O_2 demand due to left ventricular hypertrophy and a reduction in O_2 supply, secondary to coronary atherosclerosis. Often such a combination leads to early clinical manifestation of myocardial ischemia. The *manifestation of myocardial ischemia* (coronary arterial disease) are symptoms (usually angina), characteristic changes in electrocardiogram (ECG), characteristic changes in echocardiography, biochemical evidences of myocardial necrosis (infarction), ventricular dysfunction, arrhythmias, or sudden death.

The *most common cause* of myocardial ischemia is atherosclerotic disease, affecting the epicardial coronary arteries. In healthy persons, these epicardial coronary arteries serve largely as conduits. They undergo little constriction and relaxation. So, these vessels are referred to as the *conductance vessels.* On the contrary, the intramyocardial vessels normally exhibit striking changes in their tone and radius. The normal flow of blood through coronary arteries is controlled according to the myocardial own O_2 demand, and this O_2 demand is meet by the dilatation and the constriction properties of coronary vessels. Normally, the intramyocardial resistance vessels demonstrate an immense capacity of dilatation during needs, e.g., exercise, emotion, stress, etc. This manner of regulation of myocardial O_2 supply, by myocardium itself, is called the *myocardial metabolic regulation (chemical regulation)*. The intramyocardial coronary resistance vessels also adapt physiological alterations with BP within its certain range, in order to maintain the coronary blood flow constant, according to myocardial needs. This is also called the *coronary autoregulation (physical regulation)*.

The atherosclerosis is caused by (i) the dysfunction of vascular endothelium in dyslipidemia and (ii) the abnormal interaction of endothelium with blood monocytes and platelets. This leads to the subintimal collection of abnormal fat, debris, and cells (i.e., *atherosclerotic plaque*) at the different segments of coronary artery (*mainly epicardial*), resulting in the segmental reductions of cross-sectional area of coronary artery. *The anginal symptoms are generally absent, until the atherosclerotic lesions cause 50–70% block of coronary circulation.* When this occlusion of a lumen reaches 70%, then maximum compensatory dilatation of the resistance vessels occur distally. Now, the blood flow through coronary artery may be adequate at rest, but becomes inadequate with increased metabolic demand. In such circumstances, an extensive collateral blood supply allows some patients to remain relatively asymptomatic, despite severe coronary disease.

Coronary vasospasm is also an important cause of transient transmural ischemia in some patients. However, the most vasospastic episodes of the coronary arteries occur at their preexisting stenotic lesions in epicardial vessels. When the luminal area is reduced by more than approximately 80%, then the blood flow at rest may also be reduced and after that any further minor decrease in stenotic orifice can reduce the coronary flow dramatically, causing ischemia at rest. Severe coronary narrowing and myocardial ischemia are frequently accompanied by the development of collateral vessel. Usually this occurs, when the narrowing develops gradually. But, when this collateral is well developed, then such collaterals can provide sufficient blood flow to sustain the viability of myocardium at rest. But, this is not possible during the conditions of increased demand.

The IHDs are often manifested as angina pectoris, acute MI, cardiac arrhythmias, heart failure, or sudden death. Among these, the angina pectoris is the most common symptom of myocardial ischemia and is classified into the following clinical syndromes such as *(i) classical or stable angina, (ii) variant angina (Prinzmetal angina), (iii) mixed angina, (iv) unstable angina, (v) nocturnal, postprandial, and walkthrough angina, and (vi) silent angina.*

Classical angina: It is also called stable angina. It is the most common form of angina. The underlying pathology of this angina is obstruction of large coronary arteries, which are running epicardially and send perforating branches to supply the deeper myocardium, by atherosclerotic plug. Here, the coronary obstruction is fixed and the blood flow fails to increase during increased demand, despite the local factors mediated dilatation of resistance vessels. This type angina is predictably provoked by increased demand (exercise, emotion, etc.), so is named as *stable angina*. The drugs which reduce cardiac work load (*directly* by acting on heart or *indirectly* by reducing *preload*, hence ventricular end-diastolic pressure and *afterload*) are useful for this type of angina. They also arrange favorable redistribution of blood flow to ischemic areas.

Variant angina: It is also called *vasospastic or Prinzmetal angina*. It is an uncommon form of angina. The underlying pathology of this angina is recurrent localized coronary vasospasm which may be superimposed on atherosclerotic coronary artery. The time of occurrence of this type of angina is unpredictable and may occur at rest, during sleep, etc. The drugs which relief coronary artery spasm (glyceryl trinitrate) are useful for this type of angina.

Unstable angina: It is defined as an abrupt increase in severity, frequency, or the duration of anginal attacks, which may occur even at rest. It is mostly due to the intraluminal partial rupture of an atheromatous plaque, causing the gradual aggregation of platelets and progressive occlusion of coronary artery. Occasionally, it is also associated with coronary spasm. Critical stenosis (>70% occlusion of lumen) in one or more major coronary arteries is present in more than 80% of patients with this angina symptom. It reflects severe underlying coronary disease and may be followed by MI.

Silent angina: Here, the myocardium is suffering from ischemia, but there is no anginal pain (asymptomatic). This type of ischemia is fairly common following general surgery. Patients with diabetes have an increased incidence of this type of silent ischemia (angina).

■ DIAGNOSIS OF MYOCARDIAL ISCHEMIA

History

The most important aspect of history, regarding myocardial ischemia which is a part and parcel of diagnosis, is the description by patient of his own chest discomfort, i.e., character, location, radiation, duration, precipitating, and palliative factors of this chest discomfort, etc. Typically, the patients describe the angina pectoris as an unusual *sensation of tightness or heaviness* over his own left precordium. The others commonly used adjectives of chest discomfort, by the patient himself due to this myocardial ischemia, include *squeezing, constricting, suffocating, and crushing sensation, etc.* Some patients make a tight fist over their chest to show what the pain or discomfort is. The myocardial ischemic pain may radiate to the inner aspects of left arm, or to the inner aspect of both arms or shoulders, or to the neck and jaw. The radiation of pain toward lower abdomen is unusual and one should be caution about making this as diagnosis of angina.

The chest pain which is sharp, stabbing, and comes and goes in seconds, but not dull and continuous are unlikely to represent angina. The anginal syndrome usually begins from low intensity and then gradually goes to a peak, before subsiding over several minutes. The resolution of ischemic pain is usually due to the cessation of precipitating factors, such as the exercise, tension, cold exposure, etc., or due to the use of nitroglycerine. Patients with (i) the classical history of angina pectoris, (ii) male gender, and (iii) old age, increase the likelihood for the affection of left main coronary artery or multivessel disease.

The noncardiac (nonanginal) chest pain is usually transient. *It is exacerbated by the movement of chest wall.* It is also associated with the tenderness over involved area which is often a costochondral joint. The retrosternal sharp pain which is exacerbated by deep breathing, coughing, or changing in body position, *suggests pericarditis.* The esophageal spasm can produce severe substernal pain. It may be confused with the angina pectoris. In such condition, administration of nitroglycerine is also likely to relieve pain, because esophagus also contents smooth muscles.

From the severity of history, the patient's myocardial functional capacity can be determined and this has been shown to correlate well with the result of treadmill test. This patient's myocardial functional capacity is prognostically very important and can be quantified as MET (metabolic equivalents). One MET is defined as *the rate of O_2 consumption* by a normal person which is 3–5 mL/kg/min. However, any mobility problems, due to skeletal dysfunction, limit this test or assessment. Patients who can exercise at 4 MET or greater present a low risk for perioperative morbidity due to ischemia:

1. One MET = eating and dressing
2. Three MET = light work or walk (3–4 km/hour)
3. Four MET = climb a flight of stairs
4. Six MET = short run.

A patient who had a coronary artery bypass graft (CABG) operation within 5 years and has no symptoms may be considered of normal perioperative risk.

Physical Examination

The physical examination is often normal in the patient with stable angina. Although, these physical examinations are frequently normal, but a careful examination may reveal some important contributory information, regarding the prognostically significant comorbidities, such as, the hypertension, peripheral vascular diseases, diabetes mellitus, renal diseases, pulmonary diseases, xanthelasma, arcus senilis, etc. There may also be some signs of associated anemia, thyroid disease, etc. The physical examination by palpation can also reveal thickened peripheral arteries, signs of cardiac enlargement, etc. The examination of the fundus of retina may also reveal the increased light reflexes and arteriovenous nicking, as the evidence of hypertension. Examination during an episode of chest pain may reveal a transient S_4 or S_3 heart sound and it is due to the altered left ventricular compliance or a murmur of mitral regurgitation, resulting from papillary muscle dysfunction. The aortic stenosis, aortic regurgitation, pulmonary hypertension, and hypertrophic cardiomyopathy must be excluded, since these disorders may cause angina, even in the absence of coronary artery disease.

During physical examination, the signs of left ventricular failure (LVF) also should be searched for. The peripheral edema is usually a late finding in patients with LVF. It is often due to the venous insufficiency. The examination of jugular venous pulse for abnormalities reflects the right ventricular failure.

Laboratory Studies

Although the diagnosis of IHD is made with confidence from typical history, but a number of simple laboratory tests can be helpful to correlate between the history and the diagnosis. The urine should be examined for the evidence of diabetes mellitus and renal diseases, since both these conditions may accelerate the atherosclerosis and myocardial ischemia. During laboratory investigations, the examination of blood should include the measurement of lipids (total cholesterol, LDL, HDL), glucose, creatinine, hematocrit, thyroid function, and any special test, indicated (directed) by the physical examination. A chest X-ray is important, since it may show the consequences of IHD, i.e., the cardiac enlargement, signs of heart failure, etc. The calcification of coronary artery can sometimes be identified by X-ray.

ECG

An ECG should be performed on all the patients over 50 years of age who are scheduled for surgery and in younger patients who are with risk factors of IHD. Always the changes from previous ECG tracing should be investigated. The bundle branch block may predispose to bradyarrhythmias or atrial fibrillation. But, 24 hours ECG monitoring is only necessary, if there is any history of palpitations or blackouts.

If patients with a known prior history of MI are excluded, then nearly 60% of patients, presenting with the history of angina pectoris, have a normal ECG. But, the absence of abnormalities in resting ECG does not eliminate the possibility of IHD. The repolarization abnormalities, i.e., the T-wave and ST-segment changes and intraventricular conduction disturbances at rest are suggestive of IHD. But, they are nonspecific, because they can occur in any pericardial, myocardial, and valvular heart diseases also. These are also found in anxiety, changes in posture, drugs, and esophageal diseases. The more specific ECG changes, associated with myocardial ischemia, are the ST-segment and T-wave changes, which usually accompany the episode of angina and disappear thereafter **(Table 1)**.

The characteristic of ST-segment changes in myocardial ischemia is the displacement of its normal axis from neutral electrical base line. The ST-segment is usually depressed during angina, but may be elevated in its Prinzmetal form. Along with ST-segment, the T-wave changes in ECG, during ischemia, include the symmetrical T-wave inversion which may be transient. In a patient with consistent inverted T-waves, in association with prior pathological Q-wave from previous MI, may manifest a return of T-wave to its normal upright position during ischemic attack. This is called the *pseudonormalization.*

Summary of ECG changes related to IHD: Without prior MI, the base line ECG is normal in 50–60% of patients with IHD. The evidence of ischemia by ECG is often become apparent only during angina. The most common baseline abnormality in ECG, affected by ischemia, is nonspecific changes in ST-segment and T-wave. The prior MI may be manifested by Q-waves or loss of R-waves in leads closest to infarction area. The first-degree heart block, bundle branch block, or hemiblock may be manifested as ischemia of myocardium. The persistent ST-segment elevation, following MI, may be indicative of a left ventricular aneurysm. A long rate corrected QT interval (QTc >0.44 S) usually reflects underlying ischemia, drug toxicity, electrolyte imbalances, autonomic dysfunction, etc. These patients with long QT interval are at increased risk for developing ventricular arrhythmias. Because, long QT interval reflects long duration of ventricular repolarization which predisposes patients to re-entry phenomenon. Chest X-ray can be used to exclude cardiomegaly for correlation of ischemic finding in ECG.

Exercise ECG (stress testing): 12 leads ECG before, during, and after exercise on a treadmill is the most widely used test for the diagnosis of IHD **(Box 1)**. It is useful for establishing patient's left ventricular functional reserve and thus the prognosis. The program is usually *symptoms limited.* So, the test is discontinued with the evidence of chest pain,

TABLE 1: Relation between areas of myocardial ischemia and electrocardiogram (ECG) leads.

ECG leads	Coronary artery	Area of ischemia
• I, aVL • II, III, aVF • V_3–V_5	• Circumflex artery • Right coronary artery • Anterior descending artery	• Lateral aspect of left ventricle • Right atrium, right ventricle • Anterolateral aspect of left ventricle

BOX 1: Indications of exercise electrocardiogram testing.

- Diagnosis of chest pain
- Assessing of exercise tolerance
- Assessing the response to treatment
- Risk stratification of stable angina
- Risk stratification after myocardial infarction
- Assessing the exercise-induced arrhythmias

discomfort, shortness of breath, dizziness, fatigue, and ST-segment depression >0.2 mV. The test is also discontinued when there is fall in HR (fall exceeding >10 beats/min), fall in systolic BP (exceeding >20 mm Hg) and development of ventricular tachycardia or arrhythmia.

The *significant diagnostic* ischemic ST-segment response is defined as the flat depression of it (ST-segment) for >0.1 mV below the baseline and lasting longer than 0.08 second. The junctional or up sloping of ST-segment changes are not considered as diagnostic of myocardial ischemia. It does not constitute a positive test. *The abnormalities of T-wave alone are also not considered as diagnostic of ischemia.* This stress ECG test has a high negative, but a low positive predictive value. This test is useful for assessing ischemic patients, possessing high- or intermediate-risk than low-risk group. The overall, false +ve or false –ve results is 15%. A positive treadmill test indicates that the likelihood of IHD is 98% in males over 50 years of age with a history of typical angina pectoris.

The likelihood of IHD decreases progressively, if the patient has atypical or no chest pain. The incidence of false +ve test is significantly increased in asymptomatic male, under the age of 40 years, with no risk factor for premature atherosclerosis. The false +ve result also increases, when there is (i) previous changes or abnormality of ST-segment and T-wave at rest, (ii) patient taking drugs like digitalis, quinidine, etc., (iii) with intraventricular conduction disturbances, (iv) myocardial hypertrophy, and (v) abnormal serum potassium level. Since the overall sensitivity of exercise stressed ECG is only about 75%, a negative result does not exclude IHD. In negative result, the likelihood of three vessels disease or left main coronary artery disease is extremely unlikely.

The normal response to exercise or stress-induced ECG includes a progressive increase in HR and BP. But an important adverse prognostic part of this test is failure of BP to increase with sign of ischemia, because it reflects ischemia-induced global left ventricular dysfunction.

The presence of chest pain or severe ST-segment depression (>0.2 mV) at low workload, which persists for >5 minutes, after the premature termination of exercise, *increases the specificity* of this test. It suggests severe IHD and high risk with further adverse events. Exercise ECG testing is not always possible or cannot be performed, because of the presence of many noncardiac causes, such as peripheral vascular diseases and associated claudication, lung disease, arthritis, other orthopedic causes, etc. In the presence of following conditions such as artificially paced ventricular rhythm, preexisting ST-segment depression, left ventricular hypertrophy, digitalis therapy, preexcitation syndrome, etc. which interfere the interpretation of exercise ECG test, it should not be performed. Other contraindications of this exercise ECG testing are given in the **Boxes 2 and 3**.

More about exercise ECG: The usefulness of this test is limited in patients with baseline ST-segment abnormalities and those who are unable to increase their HR (>85% of maximal predicted), because of fatigue, dyspnea, or drug therapy. The overall sensitivity and specificity of this test is 65% and 90% respectively. This test is most sensitive, near about 80%, in patients with three vessels disease or left main coronary artery disease. Diseases that are limited to left circumflex artery may also be missed, because ischemia in its distribution may not be evident on the standard surface ECG. A normal test does not necessarily exclude coronary artery disease, but suggests absence of severe disease. To assess risk, the degree of ST-segment depression, the time of onset of this depression, and the time required for reversal of this depression after stoppage of exercise are very important. Development of ischemia in ECG at low level of exercise is associated with significantly increased risk and cardiac complications. Exercise-induced ventricular ectopic frequently indicates severe myocardial ischemia with ventricular dysfunction.

Echocardiography

The exercise-induced ECG test and associated ST-segment changes indicate the presence of IHD. But, it cannot locate the site of obstruction in coronary vessels and its associated ventricular wall motion abnormalities. So, an initial, *without any stress, cardiac wall motion analysis by echocardiography* and then *cardiac wall motion analysis by echocardiography, performed after stressing the heart by dobutamine infusion (stress echocardiography),* correspond to the site of myocardial ischemia. Thus, it tremendously helps to localize the obstructive coronary lesion. The stress echocardiography

BOX 2: Absolute contraindications to stress electrocardiogram.

- Unstable angina (pain within 48 hours of test)
- Myocardial infarction (within 7 days)
- Acute pericarditis
- Acute fever
- Severe aortic stenosis
- Hypertrophic obstructive cardiomyopathy
- Uncontrolled hypertension
- (Systolic > 200 mm Hg, diastolic > 120 mm Hg)
- Heart failure

BOX 3: Relative contraindications to stress electrocardiogram.

- Myocardial infarction (after 7 days to 1 month)
- Mild-to-moderate aortic stenosis
- Known severe coronary artery disease
- Significant left ventricular dysfunction
- Known serious risk of arrhythmia

also can be done by artificial cardiac pacing which enhances the accuracy of stress echocardiography and helps to localize the obstructive coronary lesion.

Nuclear Stress Imaging

The nuclear stress imaging is very useful for assessing the coronary perfusion. After administration, the tracers like thallium, technetium, etc. can be detected and their concentration into myocardium can be measured by positron emission computed tomography (PECT) that correspond to coronary blood flow. When there is lesser tracer activity, it suggests a significant coronary obstructive lesion. Exercise or stress increases the difference in tracer concentration between the normal and the underperfused regions. This is because the coronary blood flow increases markedly with exercise, except in regions which are distal to the obstruction in coronary artery. The magnitude of perfusion abnormality is most important prognostic indicator of ischemia.

Both of these, i.e., echocardiography and nuclear stress imaging are indicated for the diagnosis of IHD when the exercise-induced ECG is not possible or when it is difficult to interpret the ST-segment changes on ECG. The intravenous infusion of dobutamine or artificial cardiac pacing provides progressively adequate cardiac stress for patients who cannot exercise. Alternatively, the effects of cardiac stress on the extent of coronary dilatation can be assumed by artificially producing coronary dilatation by administration of coronary vasodilator such as adenosine or dipyridamole which dilates the normal coronary arteries, but evokes minimal to no change in the diameters of atherosclerotic coronary arteries.

Coronary Angiography (or Arteriography)

Coronary arteriography is the most definitive investigation for diagnosis, localization, and quantitation of IHD. It provides the most important information about the condition of coronary arteries. The *common indications for cardiac catheterization and arteriography are* chronic stable or unstable angina, markedly positive exercise or stress-induced ECG test, postinfarction angina, inconclusive noninvasive studies, frequent hospitalization due to cardiac causes, unexplained cardiomyopathy, high risk of IHD, angina following thrombolytic therapy, valve replacement in patient with high risk of IHD, etc. It is also helpful for establishing the diagnosis of nonatherosclerotic coronary artery disease such as coronary artery spasm.

Although coronary angiography is an invasive procedure, still the risk of this test is very low in relation to the potential information which is yielded from the study. The overall mortality of angiography is 0.2%. Patients >55 years of age and with an ejection fraction <30% or with left main coronary artery disease have the greatest risk for complications.

■ TREATMENT OF ISCHEMIC HEART DISEASE

The general guidelines for treating the patients with IHD are: (1) The correction of risk factors with the hope of slowing the progression of IHD; (2) The modification of patient's lifestyle to reduce the stress and to improve the exercise tolerance; (3) The treatment of medical conditions that aggravate ischemia, e.g., hypertension, hyperthyroidism, anemia, etc.; (4) The pharmacological manipulation to increase coronary supply and to reduce myocardial O_2 demand; (5) The prevention of the formation of platelet plug or thrombus formation; (6) The removal of coronary occlusion by percutaneous coronary intervention (e.g., angioplasty with or without stenting).

Medically, IHD is treated mainly by the following drugs such as *antiplatelets, antithrombin, β-blockers, Ca^{2+} channel blockers, and nitrates.* So, the preoperative awareness of an anesthetist about these drugs is important, because these drugs may exert potentially adverse effects during anesthesia. *The aim of medical treatment of IHD is to decrease myocardial O_2 requirement or demand and to improve coronary blood flow or supply.* When the optimal medical therapy fails to control the symptoms of IHD, then revascularization of myocardium by CABG, percutaneous transluminal coronary angioplasty (PTCA) or placement of coronary stent is indicated. Among these, the CABG is the most promising and is performed when the occluded coronary artery is of reasonable size, free of distal plaque and has a high-grade proximal stenosis. It is likely to improve the survival of patient with EF <40% and multivessel disease.

But, the presence of hypokinetic or akinetic area declares poor prognosis.

If not contraindicated, then low-dose aspirin, as antiplatelet agent, is recommended for all the IHD patients. It is used in the dose of 75–325 mg/day and decreases the risk of cardiac events. Clopidogrel inhibiting platelet aggregation acts more effectively than aspirin. For patients, in whom the placement of intracoronary stent is anticipated, platelet glycoprotein IIb/IIIa receptor antagonists are more useful. It acts by inhibiting the adhesion, activation, and aggregation of platelet.

As antithrombin, the *unfractionated heparin* is recommended for the treatment of unstable angina. But, it has many disadvantages, such as the variability in their dose response relationship, due to its variable binding with plasma protein. So, instead of unfractionated heparin, the *low molecular weight-fractionated heparin* (LMWH) provides a more predictable and long half-life pharmacological profile as antithrombin. It has also advantages that it does not need monitoring by activated partial thromboplastin time (APTT) measurement and can be administered easily by through subcutaneous route. During the weeks, following the initial presentation of unstable angina, the combination of warfarin and aspirin can be used. It is superior to monotherapy with aspirin or warfarin alone.

The β-*adrenergic blocking agents* (mainly the cardio-selective $β_1$-blocker) are the first-line agents for the patients with stable IHD **(Table 2)**. Because, they decrease myocardial O_2 demand or consumption by reducing HR and myocardial contractility. The chronic administration of $β_1$-blocker also decreases the risk of MI and sudden death. They also increase the survival after MI and reduce the likelihood of a subsequent infarction. Now, it has been used in low doses in patients in whom the β-blockers have traditionally been considered to be contraindicated such as congestive heart failure, pulmonary disease, advanced age, etc. The $β_1$-blocker induced decrease in HR and contractility is maximum during activity than at rest. The decrease in HR also increases the diastolic cardiac perfusion time which may also contribute to improved myocardial perfusion.

The $β_2$-blockers can increase the risk of bronchospasm in patients with reactive airway disease and can increase the manifestations of peripheral vascular resistance. So, it ($β_2$-blocker) is not used in IHD patients. The most common side effects of β-blocker therapy are fatigue and insomnia. It is *contraindicated* in heart block, but not in diabetes mellitus, though (i) it may mask the signs of sympathetic nervous system activity during hypoglycemia, (ii) delay metabolic recovery from hypoglycemia, and (iii) impair the handling of large K^+ load.

TABLE 2: Pharmacodynamic properties of different beta blockers.

Drugs	β_1-selective blocker	β_2-selective blocker	a-blocking action	Sympathomimetic	Membrane stabilizing	Half-life (hour)
Atenolol	+ +					10
Metoprolol	+ +				+	6
Bisoprolol	+					12
Nebivolol	+					
Esmolol	+ +					10 minutes
Labetalol	+	Agonism	+		+	10
Carvedilol	+	+	+		+	10
Propranolol	+	+ +			+ +	6
Oxprenolol	+	+		+	+	2
Alprenolol	+	+		+	+	4
Timolol	+	+				6
Sotalol	+	+				10

TABLE 3: Effects of beta blockers, Ca channel blockers, and nitrates on cardiac action.

Drugs	Preload	Afterload	Contractility	SA node	AV conduction	Coronary dilatation	Systemic vasodilatation
β-blockers	$-/\uparrow$	$-/\downarrow$	$\downarrow\downarrow\downarrow$	$\downarrow\downarrow\downarrow$	$\downarrow\downarrow$	No effect	No effect
Nitrates	$\downarrow\downarrow$	$\downarrow$	No effect	No effect	No effect	$\uparrow$	$\uparrow\uparrow$
Verapamil	No effect	$\downarrow$	$\downarrow\downarrow$	$\downarrow\downarrow$	$\downarrow\downarrow\downarrow$	$\uparrow$	$\uparrow$
Diltiazem	No effect	$\downarrow$	$\downarrow$	$\downarrow\downarrow$	$\downarrow\downarrow$	$\uparrow$	$\uparrow$
Amlodipine	No effect	$\downarrow\downarrow$	No effect	No effect	No effect	$\uparrow$	$\uparrow$

(AV: atrioventricular; SA: sinoatrial)

The β_1-blockers with membrane stabilizing property result in antiarrhythmic activity. Agents with intrinsic sympathomimetic property are better tolerated by patients with mild to moderate ventricular dysfunction. Certain β-blockers (bisoprolol, carvedilol, and extended duration metoprolol) improve survival in patients with chronic heart failure. Patients on long-standing β-blocker therapy should continue it preoperatively. Because, acute withdrawal of it will place the patient at increased risk of cardiac morbidity and mortality. It should also be continued in postoperative period who take these agents chronically.

The use of long-acting *calcium channel blockers (CCBs)* for IHD are not as effective as β_1-blockers for decreasing the incidence of M1, but are comparable to β-blockers in terms of relieving the frequency and the severity of angina pectoris which is due to coronary artery spasm. These agents are especially chosen, when a patient cannot take a β-blocker due to contraindication or insufficient. They *reduce myocardial O_2 demand by decreasing the cardiac afterload and augment myocardial O_2 supply by coronary vasodilatation.* Verapamil and diltiazem also reduce myocardial O_2 demand by slowing HR. The short-acting Ca^{2+} channel blocker, such as nifedipine, is not recommended for management of IHD, as they increase sympathetic activity with associated adverse cardiac events. So, only the long-acting Ca^{2+} channel blockers are used **(Table 3)**.

There are adverse interactions between the CCBs and anesthetic drugs. For example, the myocardial depression and peripheral vasodilatation effect, produced by volatile anesthetic drugs, could be exaggerated by the similar effects of CCBs. The CCBs may also potentiate the effects of depolarizing and nondepolarizing muscle relaxants and exaggerate the diseased states, associated with skeletal muscle weakness. The pharmacological antagonism of neuromuscular transmission may be impaired in the presence of Ca^{2+} channel blocker. This is because of diminished presynaptic release of acetylcholine. Verapamil and diltiazem can potentiate depression of cardiac contractility and conduction in atrioventricular (AV) node by volatile anesthetics.

The *nitrates* can be used for both the treatment of acute ischemia and prophylaxis against frequent anginal episodes. They dilate the coronary and its collateral arteries and thus improve coronary blood flow, preferentially subendocardial blood flow in ischemic area. It also decreases the peripheral vascular resistance, resulting in the decrease in left ventricular outflow impedance and myocardial O_2 consumption. The prominent venodilating property of nitrates decreases the venous return and thus preload also. Thereby, it decreases the left ventricular filling pressure, filling volume, force of contraction (Frank–Starling law), and myocardial O_2 consumption.

All the above mentioned properties of organic nitrates, thus, help to decrease the frequency, duration, and severity of angina pectoris. It also helps to increase the amount of exercise needed, before the onset of ST-segment depression. Nitrates are relatively contraindicated in hypertrophic obstructive cardiomyopathy and severe aortic stenosis. The sublingual tablet or oral spray of nitroglycerine is recommended for prompt relief of angina pectoris, but not for long-term therapy. For later, long-acting nitrate preparation is effective and recommended. The therapeutic value of organic nitrate is compromised or dampened by the rapid development of tolerance during sustained therapy of it. So, for long-term use, nitrates should be administered with one daily nitrate-free interval of at least 8 hours to prevent this development of nitrate tolerance.

ANESTHETIC MANAGEMENT OF PATIENTS WITH KNOWN OR SUSPECTED IHD UNDERGOING NONCARDIAC SURGERY

Assessment

The goal of the preoperative anesthetic assessment of a patient, with IHD, is to identify the individuals with increased risk of adverse perioperative cardiological outcome. The risk of perioperative death, due to cardiac complications, is <2% for the patients who do not have IHD. On the other hand, *this risk is doubled or tripled* in patients with known or suspected coronary or other sclerotic vascular diseases. The most reliable indicator for adverse perioperative cardiac events in patients, who is suffering from IHD and undergoing noncardiac surgery, is *myocardial ischemia* during operation and within first 48 hours following surgery.

The *perioperative risk for patients with IHD is usually estimated* on the basis of patient's exercise tolerance. The patients who can perform strenuous activities like walking, running, climbing, etc., but without any cardiac symptoms, have lower risk of cardiac complications than patients who are unable to perform such strenuous exercise. The

limited exercise tolerance, in the absence of significant lung disease, is the most striking evidence of decreased cardiac reserve. The patients should always be evaluated against the background of exercise, because the symptoms of IHD may be absent at rest. In stable patients with angina pectoris and undergoing elective major noncardiac surgery, there are few independent predictors of cardiac complications. *These predictors are* current complaints of angina pectoris, use of nitrate therapy, history of positive exercise test, history of M1, Q-wave in ECG, history of congestive heart failure, history of pulmonary edema, history of paroxysmal nocturnal dyspnea, etc. The previous CABG surgery, preoperative ST-T-wave changes on ECG, presence of critical aortic stenosis, presence of abnormal cardiac rhythm, advanced age, etc. are also the valuable predictors. It is also important to recognize the presence of incipient congestive heart failure preoperatively, as the added stress of anesthesia, surgery, and postoperative pain may convert this incipient preoperative congestive heart failure to overt congestive heart failure.

Physical examination and investigations for preoperative assessment of patient with IHD are like physical examination and investigation of an IHD patient who is not going for any surgical procedure which is described before.

Preoperative Preparation and Medication

The high risked myocardial ischemic patients, undergoing noncardiac surgery, are probably best benefited from optimal preoperative anti-ischemic treatment which is described before. This preoperative anti-ischemic treatment or the preparation of patients can be achieved by pharmacological and psychological method. The patient suffering from severe myocardial ischemia can also be treated preoperatively by CABG operation or angioplasty with or without stent before any elective noncardiac surgery.

Anxiety which is a part and parcel of a surgery is another important precipitating factor of ischemia. It acts by evoking the activity of sympathetic nervous system with accompanying increase in systemic BP and HR. Both of these increase myocardial O_2 demand which may manifest as myocardial ischemia in ECG and may be first recognized when these patients arrive in operation theater (OT). These ECG changes are usually taken as the silent sign of ischemia, because they are not accompanied by angina pectoris or hemodynamic abnormalities. This silent ischemia is not different from those that occur in same patients during their normal daily activities.

Anxiety is managed by both psychological and pharmacological approaches. The psychological approach for the reduction of anxiety is attempted by preoperative visit of a patient to an anesthetic clinic, during which the fearless anesthetic sequences are explained in details. The pharmacological approach for reduction of anxiety can be achieved by many drugs. But, the choice of drug depends on the personal preference and the experience of anesthetist. The aim of premedication for a myocardial ischemic patient is to produce maximum sedation and amnesia without any undesirable degree of circulatory and ventilatory depression. For this purpose benzodiazepine (BZD) is a very useful drug. It can be combined with morphine (10–15 mg IM in an adult) plus scopolamine (0.4–0.6 mg IM adult dose). Because, scopolamine produces profound sedative and amnestic effect without any undesirable changes in HR. So, it is very valuable as a premedicant for IHD patients. Overmedication is equally detrimental and should be avoided, because it may result in hypoxemia, respiratory acidosis, and hypotension.

Drugs used for medical management of patients with IHD should not be withdrawn abruptly and are continued throughout the perioperative period. For example, the sudden withdrawal of antihypertensive agents, mainly β-blocker, may result in rebound increase in sympathetic nervous system activity. Nitrates should be given preoperatively, intraoperatively, and postoperatively. In high-risk patients, they can be continued as IV also. Otherwise, oral and transdermal route for nitrate is sufficient for low-risk groups. Prophylactic administration of nitrates intravenously or transdermally to patients with coronary arterial disease in perioperative period provides no benefit to patients those are not previously on long-term nitrate therapy and without any ongoing ischemia.

The calcium antagonists should be given postoperatively. The dihydropyridine group of calcium antagonist (nifedipine), especially short-acting, adds to the risk of acute MI. Therefore, these should be substituted to another class such as phenylalkylamine (verapamil) or benzothiazepine (diltiazem) group of Ca^{2+} antagonist. The angiotensin-converting enzyme (ACE) inhibitors improve survival in patients with left ventricle dysfunction due to IHD. So, they should be given preoperatively and also should be resumed postoperatively as soon as gastrointestinal (GI) absorption resumes. If they have been stopped for several days, then restarting at reduced doses may be prudent, as most of these drugs are associated with first dose hypotension. There is theoretical possibility of H_2 receptor antagonist to produce coronary artery vasoconstriction. Because, this is mediated by unopposed H1 receptors activity. But practically, it does not seem to produce any adverse side effects in IHD patients.

Induction of Anesthesia

The anesthetic technique for induction in IHD patients is aimed at to minimize the incidences and severity of myocardial ischemia by preventing the factors which predispose it, such as tachycardia, hypotension, hypertension, hypoxia, etc. Induction of anesthesia for patients with IHD can be achieved by intravenous administration of several common inducing agents such as propofol, thiopentone, BZD, etc. Among these, ketamine is not the choice, as it increases myocardial O_2 consumption or demand by increasing HR and systemic BP. Direct laryngoscopy and tracheal intubation may initiate sympathetic nervous system stimulation and subsequent myocardial ischemia. It is aggravated more when there is previous existence of systemic hypertension. So, the sympathetic pressure response, produced by direct laryngoscopy and tracheal intubation, can be minimized by the addition of following drugs. Lignocaine in the dose of 1–2 mg/kg, administered intravenously about 90 seconds before direct laryngoscopy, decreases the magnitude and the duration of the elevation of systemic BP. An alternative to lignocaine is nitroprusside. It is administered 15 seconds before laryngoscopy and intubation in the dose of 1–2 µg/kg/min by infusion. Like lignocaine, nitroprusside also effectively attenuates the pressure response related to intubation, but not the HR. Another alternative to attenuate the sympathetic pressure response in patients with IHD is infusion of esmolol in the dose of 100–300 µg/kg/min before and during the laryngoscopy and intubation. It is especially useful for blunting the increase in HR, evoked by intubation. A small dose of fentanyl (1–2 mg/kg by IV) or equivalent doses of other short-acting opioids, administered before direct laryngoscopy and intubation, may also be useful for blunting the circulatory responses, evoked by laryngoscopy and tracheal intubation. The continuous infusion of nitroglycerine in the dose of 0.25–1 µg/kg/min by IV may also be used as prophylaxis against the development of coronary vasospasm and subsequent development of myocardial ischemia in vulnerable patients. But, many controlled studies do not consistently confirm that this approach decreases the incidence of intraoperative myocardial ischemia.

Maintenance of Anesthesia

The choice of drugs, used for maintenance of anesthesia, depends upon the preoperative evaluation of patient and the presumed left ventricular function. Sympathetic activation due to surgical stimulation is not detrimental for normal left ventricular function. But, in patients with IHD, sympathetic activation by surgical stimulation is harmful due to increased O_2 demand (due to ↑HR, ↑afterload, and ↑preload) in an already compromised heart. From this point of view, volatile anesthetics (sevoflurane, isoflurane, and desflurane) are useful by minimizing this sympathetic stimulation and subsequent decreasing the myocardial O_2 requirement. The volatile anesthetic may be administered alone or in combination with N_2O and opioids. If the use of volatile anesthetics is associated with much reduction of systemic BP, then it will decrease the coronary perfusion pressure (due to reduction of aortic pressure) and its flow which will be detrimental for IHD patients. So, excessive reduction of BP by volatile anesthetic agents is never desirable in IHD patients.

In patients with severely impaired LV function, if slight myocardial depression by volatile anesthetic agents is associated with much reduction of cardiac output, then in such circumstances short-acting opioids in liberal doses are selected, instead of volatile anesthetics. For severely myocardium compromised patients due to ischemia, high doses of opioid such as fentanyl 50–100 µg/kg/IV or equivalent doses of other short-acting opioids are used as sole anesthetic agent. In such circumstances, BZD or N_2O or low-dose volatile anesthetics can be used, if adequate amnesia cannot be ensured with this high dose of opioid alone. In such situation, you will have to keep in mind that addition of N_2O and volatile anesthetic agent to opioid are associated with myocardial depression which is not found when any of these drugs is administered alone.

Regional anesthesia is a well-accepted technique for patients with IHD. But, the reduction of systemic BP should be maintained strictly within 20% of preanesthetic mean arterial pressure (MAP) value. In one sense, regional anesthesia is beneficial for IHD patients, because it reduces myocardial O_2 requirement by producing sympathetic nervous system blockade. In another sense, regional anesthesia is not beneficial for IHD patients, because flow through coronary arteries, narrowed by atherosclerosis, is pressure dependent. So, much decrease of MAP (<20% of preanesthetic value) is associated with severe reduction of blood flow through coronary arteries which is greater than the reduction of O_2 requirement. So, prompt treatment of hypotension (that exceeds 20% of preanesthetic value) by IV administration of ephedrine, phenylephrine, or any other vasoconstrictive agent which is very well known to a working anesthetist is often recommended. A disadvantage of using IV fluid load to treat hypotension, induced by regional anesthesia, is the interval which is necessary to become effective and the preloading by IV fluid to maintain BP is not such effective as vasoconstrictive agent.

Regarding muscle relaxants, vecuronium, rocuronium, atracurium, and cisatracurium are the drug of choice for patients with IHD. Because, they are associated with minimal to no effects on HR and systemic BP. Atracurium and mivacurium release histamine and there is transient alteration of BP. Pancuronium increases HR with BP and may precipitate myocardial ischemia. However, it has been used, without any apparent adverse effects in many patients, with IHD for many decades. Pancuronium is especially used to offset the negative inotropic and negative chronotropic effect of other anesthetic drugs such as volatile anesthetic agents. The idea that simultaneous use of β-blocker therapy prevents pancuronium induced increase in HR, but it is not always correct, as this drug most likely increase the HR by its vagolytic property, but not by sympathomimetic mechanism.

Glycopyrrolate is preferred as anticholinergic drug, during the reversal of nondepolarizing neuromuscular blockade, if excessive increase in HR is a great concern. The combination of anticholinesterase and anticholinergic agent can be used safely for reversal of muscular paralysis in IHD patients. Myocardial ischemia should also be anticipated during emergence and extubation due to hypertension and tachycardia. So, extubation at deep plane of anesthesia or the use of short-acting β-blocker during extubation should be considered. To prevent intraoperative myocardial ischemia, intraoperative blood loss needs accurate replacement and hemoglobin should be maintained by regular measurement.

Monitoring During Anesthesia

The aim of intraoperative monitoring, for patients with IHD, is the early detection of myocardial ischemia which is influenced both by the complexity of operative and anesthetic procedure and the severity of disease. During the routine use of expensive and complex monitors, to detect intraoperative ischemia, one should keep in mind that most of the myocardial ischemia is not associated with minor intraoperative hemodynamic abnormalities in a healthy patient and so such complex monitoring should not be used routinely. Intraoperative intra-arterial pressure monitoring is reasonable in patients with severe coronary arterial disease and with multiple major cardiac risk factors who are undergoing major surgeries. Central venous pressure can be monitored during prolonged or complicated procedures involving large fluid shifts and blood loss.

Electrocardiogram is the most acceptable and the most cost-effective methods for detecting the intraoperative myocardial ischemia. But, the sensitivity and the specificity of it vary greatly. Early ischemic changes are subtle and involve the changes in morphology of T-waves including inversion, tenting, or both. More obvious ischemic changes in ECG are seen in the form of progressive ST-segment depression. The down sloping and the horizontal ST-segment depression are of greater specificity for ischemia than its upsloping depression. New ST-segment elevation is rare during noncardiac surgery and is indicative of severe ischemia, vasospasm, or infarction.

There is good correlation between the lead of ECG used to monitor the myocardial ischemia and the anatomical distribution of ischemia. The sensitivity of ECG in detecting ischemia is related to the number of leads monitored. Studies suggest that the V_5, V_4, II, V_2, and V_3 leads in decreasing order are sensitive and most useful. Usually, the lead II likely reflects the area of ischemia supplied by right coronary artery. It is also useful in identifying the P-waves and subsequent cardiac rhythm disturbances due to ischemia. Whereas, the lead V_5 reflects the area of ischemia supplied by the anterior descending coronary artery. The lead I and lead aVL reflect the area supplied by the circumflex coronary artery.

The diagnosis of ischemia by ECG mainly depends on the changes in ST-segment. These changes are characterized by the depression or elevation of it (ST-segment) by at least 1 mm. The depth of the changes of ST-segment is parallel to the severity of myocardial ischemia. This is also associated with T-wave changes. But, there are numerous factors which can produce these changes without ischemia. *Except ischemia, the other factors which can produce ST-segment changes are* conduction defect, arrhythmia, electrolyte imbalance, digitalis therapy, etc. The visual detection of ST-segment changes is sometimes unreliable. So, the computerized analysis of ST-segment changes is incorporated in some machine and offers a high modality for the detection of ischemia by a very simple and noninvasive method in high-risk patient **(Figs. 1A and B)**.

Transesophageal echocardiography (TEE) and the measurement of pulmonary capillary wedge pressure (PCWP) are also sometimes used during complex operative procedures for the detection of ischemia. TEE is gradually becoming accepted standard procedure for the intraoperative diagnosis of myocardial ischemia. It is based on the principle that ventricular wall motion abnormalities occur before the changes in ST-segment takes place in ECG. Whereas, the other conditions, responsible for ventricular wall motion changes, should be excluded preoperatively. The limitation of TEE for monitoring of ischemia is its cost and the need for extensive training for its interpretation. Another limitation of it is that the TEE probe cannot be introduced before induction of anesthesia. So, there is a critical period of induction during which myocardial ischemia may develop in the absence of this monitoring. The present status of TEE for the monitoring of ischemia is that it provides minimal additive value over analysis of ST-segment on ECG.

The value of the measurement of PCWP for random or routine monitoring of ischemia is questionable. Only in selected patients, the value and the safety of this PCWP monitoring is accepted. The monitoring of PCWP and the diagnosis of ischemia correlates well, when the left ventricular ejection fraction is >0.5 (or 50%) and there is no previous evidence of left ventricular dysfunction. Contrary, when the ejection fraction is <0.5, then there is no longer

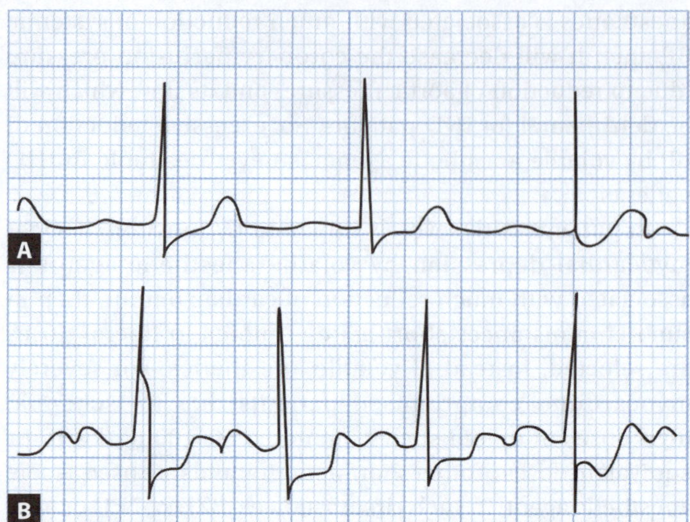

Figs. 1A and B: Electrocardiogram (ECG) of lead V5 at rest. (A) ECG of lead V5 after 5 minutes of exercise. (B) Here, the ST-segment is depressed horizontally 3 mm (0.3 mV), indicating a positive test for ischemia.

a predictable correlation between the findings of PCWP monitoring and the diagnosis.

The increasing number of individuals, treated with coronary stenting, can be problematic perioperatively, especially when the antiplatelet therapy is must discontinued for major surgeries. Such patients are at very increased risk of thrombosis and perioperative MI. In such situation, anesthesia providers should never discontinue antiplatelet or antithrombotic agents perioperatively *without discussing the risks and benefits of discontinuation of these drugs* with patient and his or her cardiologist.

Postoperative Care

During postoperative period, the myocardial ischemic patients should be cared on the following aspects:

- The relief of postoperative pain in ischemic patient is very vital. Because, otherwise, it will activate the sympathetic nervous system, leading to increased myocardial oxygen demand and ischemia. Adequate relief of pain also facilitates deep breathing and coughing which may decrease the likelihood of atelectasis and the development of pneumonia.

- In intraoperative period, patient's body temperature decreases which may predispose to shivering on awakening. This shivering leads to the abrupt increase in myocardial O_2 demand and ischemia. So, in postoperative period, all the attempts should be made to check the shivering and O_2 administration is mandatory. It is of interest that postoperative MI most often occurs within 48–72 hours after operation and this is a period that usually corresponds to the discontinuation of supplemental O_2 and less aggressive treatment of pain. So, following major surgery, all the patients at risk should have supplemental O_2 for 3–4 days postoperatively, particularly at night. Continuous ECG monitoring is also useful for detecting postoperative myocardial ischemia which is often though asymptomatic.

Perioperative Acute Myocardial Infarction

Perioperative MI most frequently occurs around 3–4 days after surgery. Symptoms may be typical or atypical. In 20% cases, the symptoms may be silent. In perioperative MI, the mortality rate is very high and may rise up to 50%. The diagnostic criteria for MI may vary, but the sole reliance on CK-MB assay for the diagnosis of MI will overestimate the incidence of it, especially in patients with ischemic limbs or after aortic surgery. During the management of perioperative MI, the therapeutic options are reduced or limited. This is because thrombolysis is generally contraindicated during perioperative period. Other noncontraindicated possible treatment of MI is aspirin and β-blockers. Emergency angioplasty for MI is probably at least as effective as thrombolysis.

Valvular Heart Diseases and Anesthesia

■ INTRODUCTION

The perioperative management of patients with valvular heart diseases is a very important aspect for anesthetists during his clinical practice. So, for the proper management of this group of patients, he must know the hemodynamic changes associated with every particular type of valvular lesion. The valvular lesion produces hemodynamic burden (overload) on left or right ventricle (RV) or on both the ventricles or on atrium with or without ventricles. Initially, the cardiovascular system (CVS) tolerates this burden and tries to compensate this overload. Always, the aim of this compensation, performed by myocardium, is to maintain adequate cardiac output. So, during the examination of such patient, an anesthetist will get many findings which are due to this compensatory changes, but are not due to the actual pathology of heart. Then, this hemodynamic burden gradually leads to cardiac muscle (myocardial) dysfunction and failure, when this compensatory mechanism is crossed. So, at this decompensatory stage, during the examination of a patient, an anesthetist will get only the signs of heart failure.

More or less, all the valvular lesions produce two types of hemodynamic overload such as the pressure overload [mitral stenosis (MS) and aortic stenosis (AS)] and the volume overload [mitral regurgitation (MR) and aortic regurgitation (AR)] on the left or right ventricle and the left or right atrium (RA). Pressure overload produces more damage on heart and morbidity than that of the volume overload. Other than the knowledge, regarding the compensatory hemodynamic changes, perioperative management of these group patients with valvular heart disease, depends also on the knowledge, regarding the effects of different anesthetic drugs (used for perioperative anesthesia purpose), on the different hemodynamic parameters of the heart such as the heart rate (HR), rhythm, blood pressure (BP), systemic vascular resistance (SVR), peripheral vascular resistance (PVR), etc.

■ MITRAL STENOSIS

Etiology and Pathophysiology (Fig. 1)

An acquired MS is almost always *rheumatic in origin* (as its delayed complication) and particularly affects the female (two-thirds of rheumatic MS patients are female). However, in some elderly patients, the heavy *calcification* of mitral valve apparatus can also produce an acquired form of MS. There is also a rare form of congenital MS. However, MS can also occur in dialysis-dependent patients. The stenotic process of mitral valve is estimated to begin after a minimum of 2 years, following rheumatic heart disease and results from progressive fusion and calcification of valve leaflets. Symptoms usually develop after 20–30 years.

In MS, the normal left ventricular filling is restricted by the decreased area of flow from left atrium (LA) to left ventricle (LV) across the stenosed mitral valve. The normal cross-sectional area of mitral valve is 4–6 cm^2. Cardiac symptoms appear, when this area is reduced to about 2.5 cm^2 (<50% of

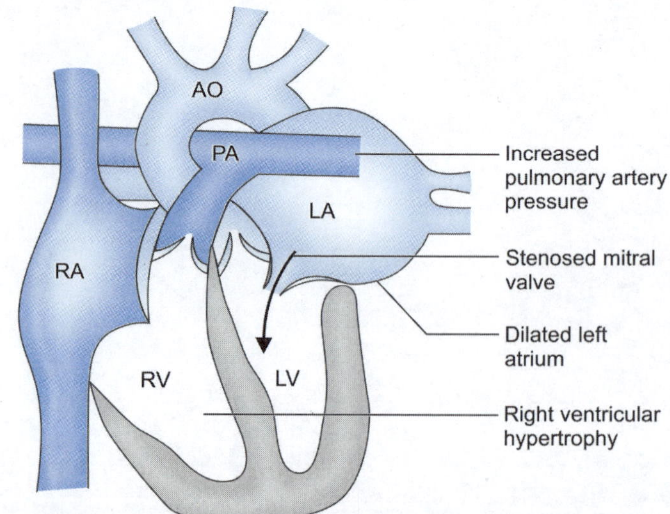

Fig. 1: Mitral stenosis. (AO: aorta; LA: left atrium; LV: left ventricle; PA: pulmonary artery; RA: right atrium; RV: right ventricle)

normal). When the mitral valve area is measured in between 2.5 cm and 1 cm, then this MS is recognized as *moderate*. But, when the valve area is measured below 1 cm^2, then this MS is recognized as *severe* and the symptoms are also severe. At this level, the left intra-atrial pressure is >25 mm Hg and pulmonary hypertension sets up.

Normally, the mitral transvalvular (between LA and LV) pressure gradient is 5 mm Hg. When, it exceeds than 10 mm Hg, then this MS is considered as severe. Less than 50% of patients have isolated MS. The remaining patients also have MR. Up to the 25% of patients also have rheumatic involvement of aortic valve (AS or AR). The rheumatic process causes the valve leaflets to be thickened, funnel shaped, and calcified. Annular calcification of mitral valve is also found. The mitral commissures are fused. The chordae are also fused and shortened. The valve cusps become rigid. As a result, the valve leaflets typically display the bowing or doming, during ventricular filling (diastole) on echocardiography.

In the early phase of MS, the *compensation* that is aimed at for proper LV filling and subsequently good cardiac output is normally achieved by (i) increasing the pressure gradient,

between the LA and LV, across the stenosed mitral valve, (ii) maintaining the normal HR or preventing tachycardia which reduces the ventricular filling time, and (iii) maintaining the sinus cardiac rhythm. This *increased pressure gradient* across the stenosed mitral value increases the flow of blood from the LA to LV and compensates this stenosis. In this stage of MS, this good LV filling and good cardiac output also dependent (other than increased pressure gradient) upon the increased *atrial contraction* or kick (atrial contraction is responsible for 20–30% of ventricular feeling) and the *duration of ventricular diastole*. So, this valvular obstruction produces increased left atrial volume and left arterial pressure (mechanism of compensation). Thus, with this increased volume and pressure, the dilatation and the hypertrophy of LA occur. The LA is often markedly dilated, promoting supraventricular tachycardia (SVT), particularly atrial fibrillation (AF). Blood flow stasis in LA also promotes the formation of thrombi in its (atrium) appendage or auricle **(Flowchart 1)**.

The stroke volume or cardiac output may decrease (*decompensation*) during stress-induced tachycardia by reducing the duration of ventricular diastole and thus by reducing the time of LV diastolic filling or when an

Flowchart 1: Compensatory changes in MS.

Mitral stenosis

↓

Decreased flow through mitral valve

↓ Decreased cardiac output → cold calm periphery

Increased volume and pressure of LA

↓

Increased force of contraction of LA

↓ Compensatory increase in cardiac output

Increased flow through mitral valve

↓

Hypertrophy and dilatation of LA

↓

But is limited due to the thin wall of LA chamber

↓

No valve in pulmonary vein

↓

So pressure is directly transmitted to the pulmonary vasculature

↓

Development of pulmonary congestion

↓

So dyspnea by slight exertion (most common symptom of MS)

↓

Pulmonary hypertension

↓

Concentric RV hypertrophy without the increase of its size

(LA: left atrium; MS: mitral stenosis; RV: right ventricle)

effective atrial contraction is lost by huge atrial dilatation or by the development of AF.

The symptomatic patients, with MS, typically exhibit dyspnea on exertion or orthopnea (dyspnea in lying position) or paroxysmal nocturnal dyspnea, although the left ventricular contractility is usually normal. In *acute cases,* actually, this dyspnea in MS is due to the acute increase in pulmonary venous pressure, in response to the increased left atrial pressure. This results in the transudation of fluid into the pulmonary interstitial space, leading to the pulmonary edema, decreased pulmonary compliance, and increased work of breathing, which ultimately lead to progressive dyspnea on exertion, orthopnea, or paroxysmal nocturnal dyspnea. With the gradual progress of disease in *chronic cases,* when the pulmonary venous pressure exceeds the oncotic pressure of plasma proteins (25–30 mm Hg), then incipient pulmonary edema develops. During compensation, with the increase of pulmonary venous pressure, there is also concomitant increase in the lymphatic drainage from lungs. This will also cause the thickening of capillary basement membrane (as compensatory mechanism) which enables the patients to tolerate the increased pulmonary vascular pressure without the development of frank (overt) pulmonary edema. Eventually, all these will lead to the pulmonary vascular changes, resulting in the irreversible increase in PVR, pulmonary hypertension, reduce lung compliance, increased work of breathing, and chronic dyspnea.

The embolic events are common in patients with MS and AF. The dislodgment of clots from LA results in systemic emboli, commonly to cerebral circulation. Patients also have an increased incidence of pulmonary emboli, pulmonary infarction, hemoptysis, etc. The chest pain occurs in 10–15% of patients with MS, even in the absence of CAD. The patients may also develop the hoarseness of voice as a result of the compression of left recurrent laryngeal nerve by the enlarged LA. The function of LV is usually preserved in the majority of patients with pure MS. The LV is chronically underloaded in patients with MS and the stroke volume may be reduced. At the same time, the LA, RV, and RA are frequently dilated and dysfunctional. Vasodilation that occurs following general anesthesia (GA) can lead to venous pooling and reduction of preload. This may precipitate hemodynamic collapse.

The surgical correction of MS is indicated, when the symptoms increase, and/or there is evidence of the development of pulmonary hypertension. Otherwise, the mild symptoms of MS are treated by diuretics which act by decreasing the preload and subsequently the left atrial pressure. In the presence of AF, due to LA hypertrophy and enlargement, which is commonly found as a compensatory mechanism to MS, the HR is controlled by digoxin, β-blockers, or Ca^{2+} channel blockers. Patients with history

of emboli and those at high risk (age older than 40 years, a large atrium with chronic AF) are usually anticoagulated. If pulmonary hypertension and right ventricular failure develop as a consequence to severe MS, then inotropic support by dopamine or dobutamine in the dose of 1 µg/kg/min through IV and reduction of pulmonary pressure by nitroprusside in the dose of 0.1–0.5 µg/kg/min through IV may be useful. The percutaneous trans-septal catheter balloon mitral valvotomy often provides mechanical relief in selected young or pregnant patients, as well as older patients who are not fit for cardiac surgery. In the presence of heavy valvular calcification or when the surgery is indicated, then the treatments are open commissurotomy or valve reconstruction or mitral valve replacement.

Preoperative Abnormalities

On examination of patient with MS, the pulse may be found irregular, if AF develops and this is due to the left atrial hypertrophy and dilatation. The palpation of precordium of a patient, suffering from MS, may also reveal a palpable first heart sound. On auscultation, there may be an *opening snap* that occurs during the early period of diastole. When this "snap" is more close to the second heart sound, then it is assumed that the MS is more severe. The calcification of mitral valve also may result in the disappearance of opening snap. In MS, this opening snap is followed by a rumbling *mid-diastolic murmur* with *presystolic accentuation* **(Fig. 2)**. The loudness of this murmur is not a guide to the severity of MS and may be inaudible, if still the stenosis is severe and cardiac output is low. The AF may cause the decompensation of the hemodynamic changes of MS by decreasing the left ventricular filling volume, due to the ineffectual contraction of LA and by decreasing the left ventricular filling time. Thus,

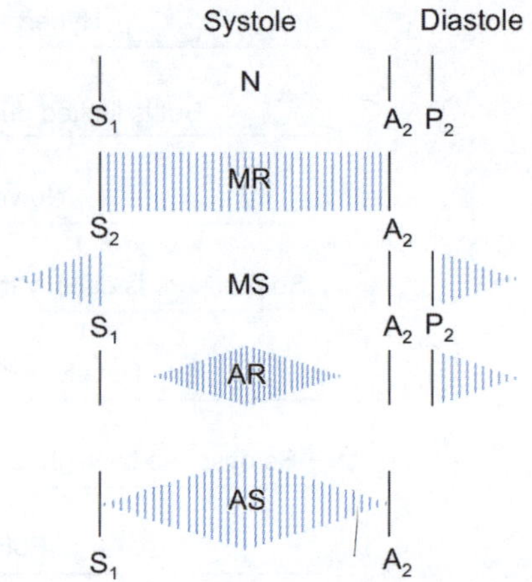

Fig. 2: Comparison of systolic and diastolic heart sounds in various abnormalities. (AR: aortic regurgitation; AS: aortic stenosis; MR: mitral regurgitation; MS: mitral stenosis)

it reduces the cardiac output. This is manifested clinically by the cool, cyanosed peripheries, and low volume pulse.

The chest X-ray in MS shows left atrial enlargement with prominent left atrial appendage and a *double contour* on the right border of the heart. The left atrial enlargement is also often visible on chest radiograph as (i) the straightening of the left border of the heart, (ii) the widening of cardinal angle, and (iii) the displacement of barium-filled esophagus on a lateral view. The *Kerley B lines* may be present. The electrocardiogram (ECG) may show *P mitrale* (large biphasic p-wave) and it is due to the left atrial enlargement. The definitive diagnosis of MS is made by *echocardiography*, which allows (i) the precise measurement of mitral valve ring, (ii) left atrial dimensions, and (iii) the demonstration of any abnormal movement of thickened and calcified mitral valve cusps. It also permits the assessment of transvalvular pressure gradients.

In the presence of AF which is common for MS, the systemic thromboembolism may occur. This is because of the stasis of blood in the distended LA which predisposes to the formation of thrombi, especially with the onset of AF. The venous thrombosis is also encouraged by low cardiac output and decreased physical activity, which are the characteristics of these patients.

The patient with symptomatic MS, when comes for anesthesia for any noncardiac surgery, usually takes digoxin, diuretics, β-blockers, and anticoagulants. The digitalis is most often administered to increase the myocardial contractility and to slow the ventricular rate in responses to AF, as it reduces the rate of conduction through atrioventricular (AV) node. The slowing of ventricular rate, caused by digitalis, also prolongs the duration of diastole and thus improves the left ventricular filling with increased cardiac output. An adequate digitalis effect on heart is indicated by the ventricular rate, which is slower than 80 beats/min at rest. During the chronic digitalis therapy, the toxicity caused by digitalis is suggested by the prolongation of PR interval in ECG. The concomitant use of diuretics with digitalis increases the vulnerability of the development of digitalis toxicity and it is due to the total body depletion of potassium.

Symptomatic history is a good guide to assess severity of disease like MS. Dyspnea on mild exertion with episodes of paroxysmal nocturnal dyspnea indicates the left atrial pressure is of 15–20 mm Hg or greater.

Anesthetic Problem in Mitral Stenosis

The anesthetic management of a patient with MS, scheduled for noncardiac surgery, includes the avoidance of events which may further decrease the cardiac output. The tachycardia and AF reduces the LV diastolic filling time, LV filling volume, and subsequently the cardiac output and thus

precipitate the pulmonary edema. So, they (tachycardia and AF) should be avoided at any cost during the perioperative period. Simultaneously, the large decrease in SVR, due to any cause, may result in severe hypotension. Because, there is limited capacity to increase the cardiac output by compensation. So, sudden decrease in SVR, due to any cause during anesthesia, may not be tolerated well, as the systemic BP is maintained only by the compensatory increase in HR (which is also not tolerated in MS). Hence, if necessary, the systemic BP and SVR should be maintained by sympathomimetic vasoconstricting drugs, like the ephedrine or phenylephrine. The advantage of ephedrine is its β-adrenergic effect, which increases myocardial contractility without increasing the HR. Because, any drug-induced tachycardia would be undesirable. Phenylephrine also eliminates this increase in HR. But, the increase in left ventricular afterload, which follows the administration of this predominantly α-agonist drug, could decrease the left ventricular stroke volume.

In MS, the volume overload may easily produce pulmonary edema. Contrary, the hypovolemia accentuated by diuretics or due to any other causes, may easily reduce the cardiac output. So, a fine balance should be maintained between the hyper- and hypovolemia. The myocardial depressant drugs can cause severe hypotension and should be avoided in MS. The Trendelenburg position may easily result in pulmonary edema, hypoxia, and acidosis in patients, suffering from MS. Then, this hypoxia and acidosis may further cause pulmonary vasoconstriction with pulmonary hypertension and thus they set a vicious cycle. N_2O may be unsafe, if pulmonary vascular resistance is increased, because it causes pulmonary vasoconstriction. Otherwise, it is not contraindicated. Bacteremia during surgery or any instrumentation carries the increased risk of bacterial endocarditis in MS, like other valvular heart diseases.

Anesthetic Management

The objective of (anesthetic) management when giving anesthesia on a patient, suffering from MS, for a noncardiac surgery are: (i) to maintain a sinus rhythm, (ii) to avoid tachycardia, (iii) to avoid hypovolemia, and (iv) to avoid fluid overload. The extend of *intraoperative monitoring*, during anesthesia of a patient suffering from MS, depends on the extent of noncardiac surgery and the severity of MS. The invasive hemodynamic monitoring, transesophageal echocardiography (TEE), and noninvasive cardiac output monitoring are used only for the major surgical procedures and where there are chances of large fluid shift. The measurement of PCWP, in the presence of MS, reflects the transvalvular (LA to LV) pressure gradient and not necessarily the left ventricular end-diastolic pressure (LVEDP) or cardiac output. A prominent "a" waves and a decreased "y" descent are typically present on the pulmonary capillary wedge pressure (PCWP) wave form in patients who are in sinus rhythm. A prominent "cv" wave on central venous pressure (CVP) waveform is usually indicative of secondary tricuspid regurgitation. The ECG, noninvasive blood pressure (NIBP), SPO_2, $ETCO_2$, etc. should be used routinely in all the cases. The ECG typically shows a "notched P-wave" in patients who are in sinus rhythm and have enlarged LA, due to MS.

Prophylaxis against infective endocarditis is the only preoperative medical therapy for MS in asymptomatic patients. So, prophylactic antibiotics are required for any surgery, performed on mitral stenotic patient which carries the increased risk of producing bacteremia. This usually includes the dental, genitourinary, intestinal, and perineal surgeries, etc. If high ventricular rate, due to AF, accompanies with MS preoperatively, then it (HR) should be controlled before surgery. It is acceptable to continue the anticoagulant therapy for minor surgeries, if it is started preoperatively. Whereas for the major surgeries, which are likely to be associated with significant blood loss, then the common practice is to discontinue warfarin 3–5 days before surgery and it is substituted with heparin. Atropine should be avoided in MS, as the tachycardia further reduces the LV filling, by reducing the ventricular filling time, through the already compromised stenosed mitral valve. A sedative premedication reduces the anxiety and any associated bad circulatory responses produced by tachycardia, due to anxiety.

The *induction of anesthesia* on patient, in the presence of MS, can be achieved by any commonly available intravenous inducing agent. There is no "ideal" general anesthetic agent for MS. The vasopressors are often needed to maintain vascular tone, following anesthetic induction. But, the ketamine should be avoided, because it has a great tendency to increase the afterload and HR. The tracheal intubation is usually performed by the administration of muscle relaxants that are unlikely to induce undesirable cardiovascular changes due to the release of histamine or affecting the conduction of cardiac impulses. The use of succinylcholine on patient with MS and taking digoxin is sometimes associated with ventricular arrhythmias, but it is not a consistent observation. So, the use of succinylcholine is not an absolute contraindication in MS. In this regard, pancuronium is also not the choice, as it causes tachycardia **(Box 1)**.

During the maintenance of anesthesia, an adequate depth of analgesia, amnesia, and muscle relaxation is essential. This goal is most closely reached by using the combination of N_2O, opioids, and low concentration of volatile anesthetics agents. However, the N_2O can produce

increased pulmonary vascular resistance by pulmonary vascular constriction. But, it seems unlikely that the magnitude of this change, caused by N_2O, would justify the avoidance of this drug in asymptomatic patients with MS. On the other hand, when the coexisting pulmonary hypertension is severe, then N_2O may more likely to increase the pulmonary vascular resistance and should be avoided. For adequate intraoperative analgesia, the high doses of short-acting opioids such as fentanyl, alfentanil, remifentanil, etc. are used for severe mitral stenotic patients. If the high doses of short-acting opioids are used for cesarean section with severe MS, then the baby may suffer from severe respiratory depression, but responds well to a single dose of naloxone.

Like the other valvular diseases of heart, in MS, the light general anesthesia (which is due to not properly titrated with the level of surgical stimulation) may also produce tachycardia, systemic hypertension, and decrease cardiac output due to the increased systemic and pulmonary vascular resistance. In such circumstances, the infusion of nitroprusside in the dose of 0.5–1 µg/kg/min may effectively decrease this SVR and increase the cardiac output, particularly when the severe pulmonary hypertension or MR coexist with MS.

The intraoperative tachycardia is usually controlled by deepening anesthesia with an opioid (except pethidine) or β-blocker (esmolol or metoprolol). In the presence of AF, the ventricular rate should be controlled by the appropriate drugs. Marked intraoperative hemodynamic deterioration, in MS, from sudden SVT necessitates cardioversion. Phenylephrine is preferred over ephedrine as a vasopressor, because the former lacks the β-adrenergic activity. Vasopressin may also be employed to restore vascular tone, if hypotension develops secondary to anesthetic induction. There is no contraindication for the use of anticholinesterase and anticholinergic agent for the reversal of nondepolarizing muscle relaxants, though the adverse effects of tachycardia deserve consideration. In this respect, glycopyrrolate is better than atropine.

The use of regional anesthesia in patient, suffering from MS, bears the same advantages, disadvantages, and precaution as the patient suffering from ischemic heart disease. Patients remain very sensitive to vasodilating effects of spinal and epidural anesthesia. In theory, epidural anesthesia may be easier to manage than spinal anesthesia. Because, in epidural there is slow and gradual onset of sympathetic blockade and its advantages.

The *degree of intraoperative monitoring* of patient with MS depends upon the severity of lesion and the magnitude of surgery. The monitoring of asymptomatic patients does not need any special comment. On the other hand, the symptomatic patients, undergoing major surgery, may need extensive monitoring including the intra-arterial BP, TEE, pulmonary artery catheterization, etc. These monitorings are helpful in confirming the adequacy of cardiac functions including the cardiac output, intravascular fluid volume, ventilation, oxygenation, etc. In the absence of pulmonary hypertension, the changes in CVP will mirror the left atrial pressure changes. However, if it is present, then PAWP does not correlate very well with the left atrial pressure. In the absence of pulmonary hypertension, though CVP shows correctly the left atrial pressure, still it poorly reflects the left ventricular filling. This is due to the presence of stenosis in mitral valve. Intraoperative tachycardia should be treated rapidly. In such situation esmolol is very effective and easily titrable. During operation any negative inotropic effects are easily outweighed by the benefits of controlling the rate. If the tachycardia is due to new AF, then direct current (DC) cardioversion should be considered.

■ MITRAL REGURGITATION

Etiology and Pathophysiology

The MR can develop insidiously (chronically) or acutely as the result of a large number of disorders. The *chronic MR* is usually the result of rheumatic disease, and congenital anomaly. In rheumatic disease, the mechanisms of development of MR are destruction, dilatation, or calcification of mitral annulus and it is developed often concomitant with MS. The *acute MR* is usually due to myocardial infarction (rupture of chorda tendinae or dysfunction of papillary muscles), infective endocarditis, or chest trauma. Again the MR may be primary or secondary. The *primary MR* is present when only the components of mitral valve are responsible for the development of MR and the correction of the structure of mitral valve corrects MR. On the other hand, the *secondary MR* is present, when other than the components of mitral valve, other factors are responsible for the development of MR, e.g., ventricular dilatation where the apposition of the leaflets of mitral valve is prevented. In such circumstances, the correction (repair) of mitral valve is not effective.

The causes of MR are again classified as *acquired* and *congenital*. All the acute and chronic causes of MR are

acquired, except the congenital or developmental causes. The rheumatic disease is the principal cause of MR in *underdeveloped countries* like MS. So, the MR is almost always associated with MS. But, in *developed countries,* the principal causes of this MR are mitral valve prolapse (MVP), myocardial infarction causing damage to papillary muscles, and chordae tendinae, and the dilatation of mitral ring due to the dilatation of heart. The MR may also follow, after the successful surgery of MS by valvotomy or valvoplasty.

The MVP is the most common cause of MR in *developed countries.* In developed countries, the MR is also caused by the congenital anomalies, myxomatous degenerative changes, bacterial endocarditis, etc. The MR is sometimes a feature of connective tissue disorders such as Marfan's syndrome. The efficacy of mitral valve depends on the proper function of chordae tendinae and their papillary muscles, attached to the valve cusps. So, the dilatation of LV, due to any cause, distorts the geometry of the supporting structures of valve (i.e., chordae tendinae and papillary muscles) and may cause MR. The progressive elongation of chordae tendinae, due to any cause, may also lead to the gradual development of MR. But, if the MI occurs, then due to the rupture of chordae tendinae, MR suddenly develops in acute form. However, this complication is rare before the fifth and sixth decade of life. In developed countries, MR is also due to dilated cardiomyopathy, and impaired ventricular function that results from coronary artery disease. Endocarditis may also lead to the distortion of the leaflets of valve and is an important cause of acute or chronic MR.

The *basic hemodynamic derangement of MR* is the decrease of left ventricular stroke volume in forward direction through aortic valve. This is because a part of left ventricular stroke volume is regurgitated back through the incompetent mitral valve into the LA. Patients with regurgitation fraction of >0.6 (>60%) toward the LA are considered to have severe MR. The patients with regurgitation fraction of 30–60% generally cause moderate symptoms. Whereas, the patients with regurgitation fraction of <30% of total stroke volume toward LA generally have mild symptoms **(Fig. 3)**.

The *fraction of left ventricular stroke volume that regurgitates into LA depends* on the (i) size of mitral valve orifice, (ii) pressure gradient across the mitral valve, and (iii) duration of ventricular ejection, i.e., HR. On the other hand, *the ventricular ejection through aorta depends on* (a) the impedance of aorta, i.e., SVR and (b) the previous factors which control the amount of regurgitation. So, the pharmacological interventions that increase or decrease the SVR have an important impact on the forward ejection fraction and the backward regurgitation fraction of the left ventricular stroke volume. The pharmacological reduction of SVR increases the LV ejection fraction in the aorta and decreases the LV regurgitation fraction in the LA and vice versa.

The *chronic MR* causes the gradual dilatation of LA with little increase in intra-atrial pressure and hypertrophy. Therefore, chronic MR is associated with relatively few symptoms. Atrial compliance determines the clinical symptoms. Patients with normal atrial compliance (does not get time to dilate, such as in *acute MR*) have primarily pulmonary vascular congestion and pulmonary edema. On the other hand, patients with increased atrial compliance (long-standing MR, resulting in a large dilated LA, i.e., chronic MR) primarily show the signs of reduced cardiac output. Most patients are in between these two extremes and exhibit symptoms of both pulmonary congestion and low cardiac output.

However, the rheumatic fever-induced MR is associated with marked left atrial enlargement and AF. Nevertheless, the LV dilates slowly in MR as the left ventricular and the left atrial pressures increase gradually as the result of chronic volume overload. Then, the breathlessness, pulmonary hypertension, and pulmonary edema gradually supervene. These symptoms depend on how suddenly the regurgitation develops. The chronic MR produces a symptom complex that is similar to that of MS. But, the sudden onset of isolated MR due to MI or rupture chordae tendinae usually presents with acute pulmonary edema **(Flowchart 2)**.

In MR, left ventricular filling is less dependent on atrial contraction than MS. So, the conversion of AF to normal sinus rhythm is of little help and produces the minimal changes in cardiac output in MR. Left ventricular hypertrophy (LVH) and myocardial ischemia is unlikely in the presence of isolated MR (i.e., when not associated with MS or AS),

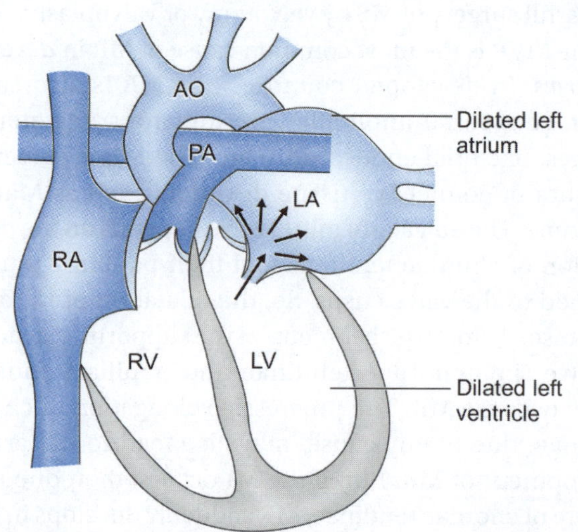

Fig. 3: Mitral regurgitation. (AO: aorta; LA: left atrium; LV: left ventricle; PA: pulmonary artery; RA: right atrium; RV: right ventricle)

Flowchart 2: Compensatory changes in MR.

Mitral regurgitation

↓

Systolic leak from LV to LA

↓

No obstruction of flow through mitral valve

↓

So, the blood flow freely from LA to LV during diastole

↓

Therefore, the mean LA pressure remain normal or slight increased

↓

No increase in pulmonary venous pressure

↓

No pulmonary venous congestion

↓

Dilatation of LA and LV due to the handling of large blood volume

↓

Forward flow from LV to aorta is less than regurgitation from LV to LA due to high systemic BP

↓

So, the patient complain more of fatigue (due to low CO) than dyspnea (due to pulmonary congestion)

↓

Dyspnea occurs, if MR is severe and is associated with pulmonary hypertension or LV myocardial failure

↓

So, the presence of pulmonary hypertension in MR indicates: (i) severe MR, (ii) LVF, and (iii) acute MR

(BP: blood pressure; CO: cardiac output; LA: left atrium; LV: left ventricle; LVF: left ventricular failure; MR: mitral regurgitation)

because the left ventricular wall tension is rapidly dissipated through the incompetent mitral valve. But, when the MR is a severe one, then due to the handling of large amount of blood by the left side of the heart, along with the dilation and hypertrophy of LA, there is also eccentric hypertrophy of LV and the progressive impairment of contractility of it. In time, the stress on left ventricular wall increases, resulting in an increased demand for myocardial oxygen supply.

When MR is combined with MS, then the impairment of the flow of large amount of blood from the LA to LV (the normal amount of blood drained through pulmonary veins into the LA plus the regurgitate blood from the LV to LA) across the stenotic valve tremendously increases the left atrial pressure and its hypertrophy. In such patient AF, pulmonary hypertension, and pulmonary edema develop more early than those with isolated MR.

Diagnosis of Mitral Regurgitation

On clinical examination, MR is recognized by the presence of *apical pansystolic murmur which often radiates toward the axilla and is often accompanied by thrill. The first heart sound is faint or silent, because mitral valve closure is abnormal.* During ventricular filling, increased forward flow of blood (due to normal amount of blood coming from the lungs plus the regurgitate blood) through mitral valve from LA to LV may give rise to prominent third heart sound. The chronic MR is compensated by the development of eccentric atrial and ventricular hypertrophy and enlargement. This is detected by the apex beat which is usually displaced toward the left (as a result of dilatation of LV) and feels active and rocking (due to LV hypertrophy for overload).

The radiograph and ECG in MR may show the features of left atrial and/or LVH **(Figs. 4A and B)**. Like the MS, the AF

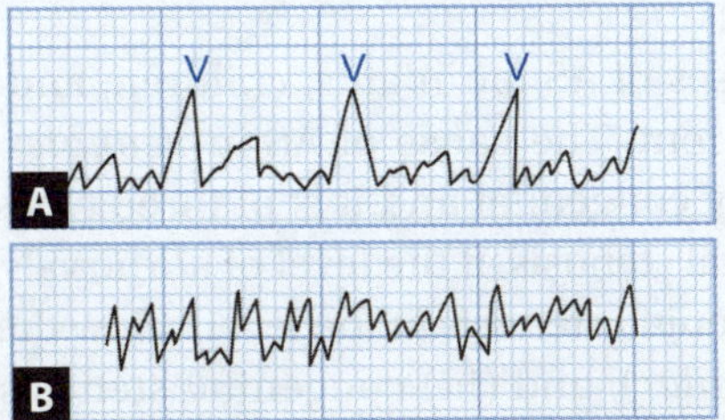

Figs. 4A and B: The picture shows the tracing of pulmonary artery occlusion pressure from a patient with mitral regurgitation. (A) When blood regurgitate back into the left atrium through incompetent mitral valve produce large "V" waves on tracing; (B) It shows that the magnitude of the V-waves are decreased or abolished. It is due to administration of vasodilator-like hydralazine. Vasodilators decrease resistance to forward ejection of the left ventricular stroke volume. As a result, the stroke volume into the aorta increases and the volume of regurgitate flow into the left atrium decreases with the magnitude of the "V" wave.

is also common in MR as a consequence of atrial dilatation. Echocardiography provides information about the state of mitral valve, left ventricular function, and left atrial size. The severity of MR is best assessed by echocardiography. But, it should be realized that the left ventricular ejection fraction, as a reflection of LV performance, will be overestimated in the presence of MR. So, Doppler echocardiography is required to estimate the extent of regurgitation. In echocardiography, the motion of the leaflet of mitral valve is often described as normal, prolapsing, or restrictive. The excessive motion or the prolapse of valve is defined by the systolic movement of leaflets beyond the plane of mitral valve and into LA.

During cardiac catheterization, for the tracing of PCWP, the severity of MR may be indicated by the size of "V" waves, produced by LA. The size of "V" wave parallels with the severity of MR. It also can be assessed by left ventricular angiography.

Anesthetic Management for Mitral Regurgitation

Unlike the stenotic mitral valvular lesions in MS, the chronic MR causes few symptoms. So, it progresses insidiously causing LV and left atrial damage, before the symptoms have developed. Thus, the surgical treatment of MR is recommended, when the regurgitation fraction is <0.6 (60%), i.e., before the patient becomes symptomatic. The progressive radiological cardiac enlargement or the echocardiographic evidence of the deterioration of left ventricular function is also the indications of surgical intervention of mitral valve. In mild-to-moderate cases of MR (diagnosed by echo), the reduction of SVR increases the forward stroke volume and decreases the regurgitation volume. Surgical treatment is usually reserved for the patients with moderate-to-severe symptoms. In this regard (surgical management of MR), mitral valve repair or valvuloplasty is preferred than the mitral valve replacement to avoid its related problems (e.g., thromboembolism, hemorrhage, and prosthetic failure). This is because, in mitral valve repair the mortality is less and the outcome is better than MS. Catheter-mediated valve repairs are continually being refined, potentially reducing the need for "open" surgery.

The principles of anesthetic management of a patient with MR for noncardiac surgery are the avoidance of events that cause increase of regurgitation and reduction of cardiac output. This is achieved by (i) avoiding decrease in HR (bradycardia), (ii) avoiding increase in SVR (afterload), and (iii) avoiding myocardial depression (myocardial contractility). Unlike MS, in MR the left ventricular forward stroke volume through aorta is increased when the HR is increased. Contrary in MS, tachycardia is not desirable as it

> **BOX 2:** Goals of anesthetic management of patients with mitral regurgitation (MR).
>
> - Prophylactic antibiotic to avoid infective endocarditis.
> - Prevent decrease in heart rate (bradycardia)
> - Avoid increase in blood pressure (BP) (afterload)
> - Avoid depression of myocardial contractility
> - Avoid fluid overload and pulmonary congestion
> - Monitoring of amount of regurgitation by echo or other invasive method

reduces the LV filling by reducing the diastolic ventricular filling time and subsequent reduces the cardiac output. But, in MR bradycardia is not desirable as it reduces the forward LV stroke volume and increases the regurgitation volume by increasing the left ventricular end-diastolic volume (LVEDV) and acutely dilating the mitral annulus. So, sudden bradycardia may result in abrupt LV volume overload and the HR should ideally be kept in between 80 and 100 per minute **(Box 2)**.

Likewise, sudden increase in SVR (afterload), such as during endotracheal (ET) intubation and surgical stimulation under light anesthesia, causes reduction of LV stroke volume and causes increase in regurgitation from LV to LA. This produces acute decompensation of LV. So, overall anesthetic management of a MR patient is drug-induced afterload reduction with nitroprusside, combined with a cardiac inotrope such as dopamine or dobutamine, and maintenance of (avoiding of bradycardia) HR.

Like MS, in the patient, suffering from MR, the prophylactic antibiotic is also started in the preoperative period to prevent the development of infective endocarditis. GA is the usual choice for MR. The induction of anesthesia for patient in the presence of MR can be achieved with any available intravenous inducing agent with possible exception of ketamine which should be avoided. This is because, the ketamine has great propensity to increase the SVR and systemic BP. Thus, it will reduce the forward flow from LV to aorta. The succinylcholine for intubation is not contraindicated. The anesthetic points of view, regarding the choice of nondepolarizing muscle relaxants, are same as that of MS, but *pancuronium which generally produces a modest increase in HR is beneficial for MR.*

The low doses of volatile anesthetic agents can also be administered to attenuate the undesirable increase in SVR and systemic BP, associated with the intubation and surgical stimulation, but without depressing the myocardium. Although, any specific volatile anesthetic agent is not considered as superior than other, but the isoflurane, sevoflurane, or desflurane (not halothane) are the choice. Because, they decrease the SVR with minimum depressant effect on myocardial contractility. In the presence of acute or severe MR,

when the myocardial function is severely compromised, then the sole use of opioid as anesthetic agent, which minimizes the likelihood of drug-induced myocardial depression, is the choice. In such situation, inodilator such as milrinone may be employed to improve the ventricular function (by increased myocardial contraction) and to reduce the systemic resistance (by vasodilatation) and ultimately to promote the forward, as opposed to regurgitant, blood flow.

The intraoperative anesthetic management and the maintenance of intravascular fluid volume in MR are same as that of intraoperative management of MS. The GA and the alterations of SVR (afterload) are well tolerated, unless the regurgitation through mitral valve is very severe. Other anesthetic approaches are also well tolerated by MR. Fluid overload is a major risk factor in MR, but less than with MS. The intraoperative monitoring of MR is also same as that of MS. The minor operations, performed on patients with asymptomatic MR, probably do not require any invasive monitoring. The *complex invasive monitoring* (such as the transesophageal echocardiography, use of pulmonary artery catheter, measurement of cardiac output by thermodilution technique, etc.) is necessary for the patients with severe MR, undergoing a complex surgical procedure. In the tracing of pulmonary artery pressure, the presence of *prominent V-waves* indicates appreciable regurgitation through the mitral valve. The changes in V-wave amplitude can also assist in estimating the magnitude of MR. *Spinal and epidural anesthesia are well tolerated by MR patients than MS patients, provided bradycardia is avoided.*

■ AORTIC STENOSIS

Etiology and Pathophysiology

Aortic stenosis is usually idiopathic in origin and results from the degeneration and the calcification of the cusps of aortic valve. The likely etiologies of AS vary with the age of the patients:

- The causes of AS for infants, children, and adolescents are different. The cause of AS in *neonates and infants* is usually congenital and it is of three types, such as (i) congenital stenosis at the level of aortic valve (*valvular*), (ii) congenital stenosis at the level below the aortic valve (*subvalvular*), and (iii) congenital stenosis at the level above the aortic valve (*supravalvular*);
- The causes of AS for *young adults* and middle-aged patients are early calcification and fibrosis of congenitally present bicuspid aortic value and rheumatic disease. Rheumatic AS is rarely isolated. It is more commonly associated with AR or mitral valve disease. Abnormalities in the number of cusps (bicuspid valve) or their architecture produce turbulence that traumatizes the valve and eventually leads to stenosis;

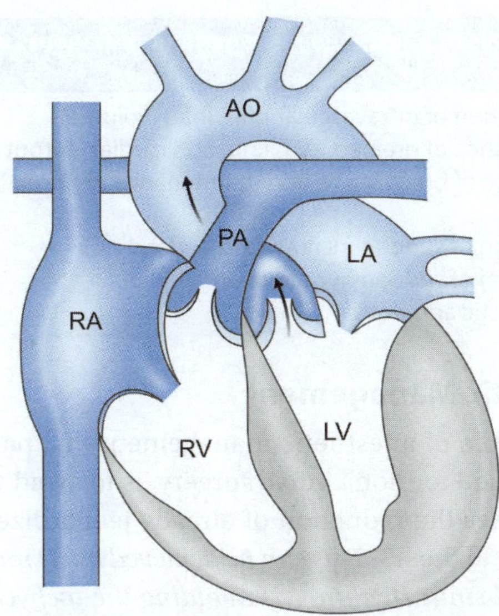

Fig. 5: Aortic stenosis. (AO: aorta; LA: left atrium; LV: left ventricle; PA: pulmonary artery; RA: right atrium; RV: right ventricle)

- The causes of AS for *elderly patients* are senile degeneration of aortic valve, calcification of bicuspid valve, and rheumatic disease **(Fig. 5)**.

The AS is more likely to occur at earlier age (below 30–40 years) in persons, who are born with bicuspid aortic valve than in those with normal tricuspid aortic valve. Otherwise, except the congenital forms, the AS develops slowly in older age. As compensatory mechanism, initially the cardiac output in AS is maintained at the cost of steadily increasing pressure gradient across the aortic valve due to the outflow obstruction. Then, the LV gradually becomes hypertrophied and maintains the cardiac output. So, the prominent features of AS are (i) decrease in left ventricular compliance as a result of hypertrophy, (ii) diastolic dysfunction as a result of an increase in ventricular muscle mass with fibrosis, and (iii) myocardial ischemia as a result of LV hypertrophy and increased workload.

In contrast to LVEDV, which remains normal until very late in AS (it increases early in MR), LVEDP is elevated early in the disease. This leads to the decreased diastolic pressure gradient between the LA and LV, resulting in impaired LV filling. Now, the LV filling is quite dependent on normal left atrial contraction and any loss of LA systole (e.g., AF) can precipitate congestive heart failure.

After that when the AS becomes more severe and cardiac output gradually falls, then the coronary blood flow gradually becomes inadequate and patient develops angina, even in the absence of any coronary artery disease. It indicates increased myocardial O_2 requirement, due to increased concentric myocardial hypertrophy which is again due to increased outflow obstruction. Furthermore, the myocardial O_2 delivery is decreased due to the compression of subendocardial coronary blood vessels by increased intracavity left ventricular systolic pressure which increase up to 300 mm Hg. So, AS is associated with same risk factors, as those of IHD.

The fixed outflow obstruction, at aortic level, limits the increase in cardiac output, which is required for increased activity. So, the effort or activity related hypotension and syncope may occur. Gradually, the LV can no longer be able to overcome the outflow tract obstruction and the left ventricular outflow failure supervenes. Classically, the patients with advanced (end-stage) AS have the *triad of heart failure, angina, and syncope.* This syncope may be exertional or at rest. The exertional syncope is thought to be due to (i) decreased cardiac output not matching according to need due to AS, plus (ii) an inability to tolerate the vasodilatation in muscle tissue during exertion. In contrast to MS which tends to progress very slowly, the AS typically remains asymptomatic for many years. But, then it deteriorates rapidly when the symptoms develop. *Thus, death usually ensures within 3–5 years of the onset of symptoms.*

The severity of AS is best assessed by measuring the pressure gradient across aortic valve by echocardiography. But, poor exercise tolerance and especially the syncope suggest severe stenosis. The critical or severe AS, capable of causing symptoms and sudden death, is characterized by transvalvular pressure gradient higher than 50 mm Hg and an aortic orifice area is lesser than 0.8 cm^2 (the normal aortic valve area is 2.5–3.5 cm^2). The long-term prognosis of AS depends upon the degree of stenosis (i) the area of aortic valve is <0.7 cm^2—*severe AS*, (ii) the area of aortic valve is 0.7–1.5 cm^2—*moderate AS*, and (iii) the area of aortic valve is >1.5 cm^2—*mild AS*. The transvalvular pressure gradient of 50 mm Hg is critical because, further increase in transvalvular pressure gradient does not significantly increase the stroke volume (pressure gradient up to 50 mm Hg as a compensatory mechanism, increase in stenosis increases transvalvular pressure gradient, and increases stroke volume).

A pressure gradient across the aortic valve of >50 mm Hg is considered to be *severe AS* and pressure gradient across the aortic valve of <20 mm Hg is considered as *mild AS.* The pressure gradient between 50 and 20 mm Hg, across the aortic valve is considered as *moderate AS.* These pressure gradients are increased by tachycardia and exercise.

This pressure gradient across the aortic valve should be interpreted with the measurement of LV function because with time the function of LV will start to fail and the measured transvalvular pressure gradient will then *start to fall again. But it does not mean that AS is not severe.* Aortic stenosis is almost always associated with AR. It is also associated with LV systolic dysfunction, due to the increase in afterload. This leads to ventricular hypertrophy and gradually progress to diastolic dysfunction, due to increased LV wall thickness.

In contrast to MS which tends to progress very slowly, AS typically remains asymptomatic for many years. But, then, it deteriorates rapidly when symptoms develop. Thus, death usually ensures within 3–5 years, after the onset of symptoms, without valve replacement. Percutaneous balloon valvuloplasty is generally used in younger patients with congenital AS. It can also be used in elderly patients with calcific AS who are poor candidates for valve replacement surgery. Surgical replacement of stenotic aortic valve till remains the mainstay of therapy.

Diagnosis of Aortic Stenosis

The mild and moderate degree of AS is usually asymptomatic. The classical clinical symptoms of AS (which indicate severe form) are angina pectoris, exertional dyspnea, exertional syncope, episodes of acute pulmonary edema, etc. On clinical examination, the carotid pulse is felt as low volume and slow rising. A radial pulse is also of slow rising and of decreased amplitude. *A pulse pressure of <30 mm Hg reflects severe AS. Contrary, if the systolic BP is >180 mm Hg, then the AS is not significant.* The auscultation of patient with AS reveals a characteristic systolic ejection murmur over the precordium, radiating toward the neck. It is best heard on aortic area, i.e., on second right parasternal intercostal space and is "diamond" in shape. The aortic component of second heart sound is inaudible. An ejection click may be present in young patients, but not in older patients, due to the calcified valves. The chest X-ray may show a prominent ascending aorta due to poststenotic dilatation of aortic arch. The ECG demonstrates the evidence of LVH with the changes of ST-segment. Left bundle branch block (LBBB) is also common in AS. In advanced cases of AS, the features of LV hypertrophy are often gross and the depression of ST-segment with T-wave inversion (strain pattern) may be seen in leads, reflecting LV.

The echocardiography examination provides a more accurate assessment of the severity of AS. It also provides information regarding the thickening and the calcification of aortic valve combined with decreased mobility of the valve cusps. It is also useful in determining the left ventricular ejection fraction and its extent of hypertrophy.

The Doppler study of heart permits the calculation of systolic pressure gradient across the aortic value and detects the presence or absence of AR. Cardiac catheterization and coronary angiography is indicated if echocardiography studies are unsatisfactory or if it is necessary to assess the state of coronary arteries.

- Optimization of intravascular fluid load (volume)
- Maintenance of preload, LV filling, and cardiac output
- Avoidance of bradycardia and maintenance of normal sinus rhythm
- Prevention of sudden increase in afterload
- Prevention of sudden hypotension
- Prophylactic antibiotic

Anesthetic Management

The principle of anesthetic management of a patient with AS, scheduled for noncardiac surgery, is to avoid the events which causes the reduction of already jeopardized cardiac output due to the AS. *This can be achieved by (i) maintaining the normal sinus rhythm, (ii) avoiding the tachycardia and bradycardia, (iii) avoiding the sudden increase in SVR, (iv) avoiding the sudden severe hypotension, and (v) optimizing the intravascular fluid volume (to maintain optimum venous return and left ventricular filling).* Like anesthetic management of other valvular disease, GA is also the choice in AS **(Box 3)**.

Regional anesthesia is not preferred because the blockade of peripheral sympathetic nervous system (SNS) can lead to the both undesirable sudden and severe hypotension (i) due to the decrease in venous return (preload) and subsequently cardiac output and (ii) due to the decrease in afterload (BP) due to arterial dilatation in an already compromised patient who has limited outflow from LV, due to AS. However, a vasoconstrictor medication must be immediately available, if regional anesthetic techniques are applied. *But, RA is not absolutely contraindicated and epidural catheter technique is often used.* It (epidural anesthesia by catheter) is preferred to single shot spinal anesthesia because of its slower onset of hypotension which allows more timely correction. Continuous spinal catheter can similarly be used to gradually increase the level of block and slow the onset of hypotension.

During the anesthetic management of a patient, suffering from severe AS, the choice of anesthetic agents and techniques is less important than the effective management of their hemodynamic effects (on HR and BP). Intraoperative optimum maintenance of HR is important because it determines the time available for diastolic filling of LV and then subsequently the amount of ejection of blood into the aorta. Sustained tachycardia can decrease the time for left ventricular diastolic filling and forward ejection, leading to the reduction in CO. On the other hand, sudden severe bradycardia can also lead to acute overdistention of LV. This is because the ventricle gets more time for diastolic filling. It is important to recognize that the increase in SVR and BP (i.e., afterload) can lead to the further reduction of stroke volume and cardiac output through obstructed orifice. Contrary, the sudden large decrease in SVR may be associated with large decrease in systemic BP, because cardiac output is relatively fixed. This fall in BP reduces the coronary perfusion of LV which is hypertrophied and may result in ischemia and reduced contractility. Thus, a vicious cycle sets in causing further left ventricular myocardial dysfunction, fall in BP, and fall in coronary circulation.

The indications for preoperative prophylactic antibiotic and premedication for the patients with AS is like the other cardiac valvular diseases. During the induction of patients with AS, ketamine should not be used. All the anesthetic drugs must be given with caution. The exact method of anesthesia is probably less important than the care with which it is administered and the extensive monitoring of patient. The intraoperative monitoring also depends on the severity of this disease and the complexity of surgery.

If the patient is symptomatic, then cardiological advice should be obtained. In symptomatic patients, the aortic valve replacement or balloon valvoplasty may be more important than the proposed elective nonsurgical operation. This is because mortality approaches to near about 75% within 3 years, after the AS becomes symptomatic, unless the valve is surgically replaced. Aortic valve replacement usually relieves the symptoms of AS dramatically and the ejection fraction increases. The dangerous feature of AS is that the signs and symptoms appear late in this disease. But, once they occur, the prognosis is poor. So, an anesthetist must be cautious during dealing of such a patient.

■ AORTIC REGURGITATION

Etiology and Pathophysiology

Aortic regurgitation may be due to the disease of aortic valve cusps or the dilatation of aortic root. *The diseases of aortic valve cusps that cause AR are* congenital bicuspid valve, rheumatic fever, infective endocarditis, etc. *The causes of aortic root dilatation, leading to AR are* rheumatic fever, endocarditis, idiopathic root dilatation associated with systemic hypertension, aging, dissection of aorta, aneurysm of aorta, syphilis, collagen vascular disease, Marfan's syndrome, trauma, etc. *Acute AR* is usually due to infective endocarditis, aortic dissection, and trauma. Except endocarditis, trauma and dissection, the other above-mentioned causes are responsible for *chronic AR* **(Fig. 6)**.

In AR, there is ultimate decrease in the forward propulsion of LV stroke volume, due to the regurgitation of a part of the ejected blood from aorta, back into the LV, after its ejection. Then, this regurgitated blood volume in LV is added to that volume of blood which enters into LV from LA

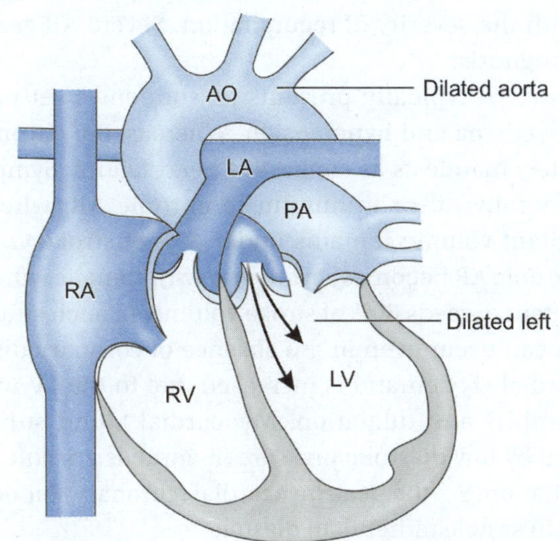

Fig. 6: Aortic regurgitation. (AO: aorta; LA: left atrium; LV: left ventricle; PA: pulmonary artery; RA: right atrium; RV: right ventricle)

and this combined volume of blood is next further ejected out into aorta. Thus, by this compensatory mechanism, the cardiac output is maintained by the increase in LVEDV during subsequent contraction. So, gradually both the LVH and dilatation occur.

Patients with severe AR have the largest end-diastolic volume of any heart disease. LVEDP usually remains normal or is slightly elevated. The magnitude of the regurgitation of blood from the aorta into LV depends on (i) the time available for the regurgitation to occur, i.e., HR, and (ii) the pressure gradient across the aortic valve which again depends on the SVR and the diastolic ventricular pressure. Thus, the magnitude of AR can be decreased (i) by increasing the HR, but up to a certain limit and (ii) by the reduction of SVR by peripheral vasodilatation.

With *chronic AR*, the LV gradually dilates and hypertrophies to compensate the regurgitation. Thus, it results in large stroke volume that is entirely ejected into aorta and a part of it is regurgitated back. So, the stroke volume of LV may eventually be *doubled or tripled* and the major arteries are then conspicuously become pulsatile. In some cases, the stroke volume may be increased to >200 mL. As the disease progresses, then the left ventricular diastolic pressure gradually rises, at first only with exercise and then breathlessness develops. Later, the myocardium becomes stiff, the LVEDP increases, premature mitral valve closure occurs and finally the cardiac failure supervenes. A helpful indicator for left ventricular function in AR is the echocardiographic determination of end-systolic LV volume and the ejection fraction. However, both of which remain normal, until the LV function does not deteriorate. The symptoms appear late in this disease and do not correlate well with the severity of regurgitation. Severe AR carries a poor prognosis.

Acute AR typically presents as sudden onset of pulmonary edema and hypotension. Whereas, the chronic AR ultimately manifests as congestive heart failure. Symptoms are generally nil or minimum in chronic AR, when the regurgitant volume remains under 40% of stroke volume. But, chronic AR becomes severe and symptomatic, when the regurgitant exceeds 60% of stroke volume. In such situation, angina can occur even in the absence of coronary disease. Myocardial O_2 demand is increased due to the LV muscle hypertrophy and dilatation. Myocardial blood supply is reduced by low diastolic pressure in aorta as a result of the regurgitation. So, the peak myocardial (coronary) blood flow occurs in systole rather than diastole.

Diagnosis of Aortic Regurgitation

Clinically, the AR is diagnosed by its characteristic *pan diastolic blowing murmur*. It is best heard along the left sternal border on chest and is accompanied by an ejection systolic murmur due to increased stroke volume. The peripheral signs of *hyperdynamic circulation* such as (i) a widened pulse pressure, (ii) decreased diastolic BP, (iii) bounding and collapsing peripheral pulses, (iv) heaving apical impulse (volume overload), etc. are found during the clinical examination of patient. Until the onset of breathlessness, the only symptom of AR may be the awareness of own heartbeat, particularly when the patient is lying on his left side. This is only due to the hyperdynamic circulation and increased stroke volume. Clinically, the dyspnea and pulmonary edema suggest advancement of disease. In such circumstances, the diastolic BP falls in proportion to the severity of valvular lesion. In *acute severe AR* (e.g., perforation of aortic cusps due to acute endocarditis), there may be no time for the compensatory LVH and dilatation to develop and the features of acute heart failure predominates. Like MR, the symptoms of AR may not appear until the LV dysfunction is advanced. In contrast to AS, sudden death due to AR is rare.

The chest radiograph in AR characteristically shows the cardiac and aortic dilatation together with the signs of left heart failure. When the AR is marked, then the ECG may show the LVH and the changes in ST-segment. Echocardiography in AR typically shows a dilated LV with its vigorous contraction until the heart failure ensues. The amount of regurgitation through the aortic valve is readily detected by Doppler echocardiography. Cardiac catheterization and aortography can also be helpful in assessing the severity of regurgitation and the dilatation of aorta.

Treatment: Most patients with chronic AR remain asymptomatic for 10–20 years. Then, once symptoms appear, the expected life expectancy is reduced and the patients usually die within 5 years, if valve replacement is not done. Diuretics and angiotensin-converting enzyme (ACE) inhibitors or angiotensin receptor blockers (ARBs) for the reduction of afterload generally benefit patients with advanced chronic AR. The decrease in diastolic pressure reduces diastolic gradient for regurgitation. Patients with chronic AR should receive valve replacement, before any irreversible ventricular dysfunction is established. Percutaneous aortic valve replacement is now increasingly used for high-risk patients with AR.

Anesthetic Management

The preanesthetic management of AR includes (i) the treatment of underlying conditions such as endocarditis or syphilis and (ii) prophylactic antibiotic. Aortic valve replacement is indicated, if the patient is symptomatic. However, surgery is also advised for asymptomatic patients, if there is progressive radiological evidence of cardiomegaly and echocardiographic evidence of deteriorating LV function. ACE-inhibitors (as vasodilator) have been shown to prevent progressive LV dilatation and are recommended for asymptomatic patients **(Box 4)**.

The anesthesia-induced fall in SVR is better tolerated by AR than with AS. The fall in SVR decreases the flow of regurgitation. Contrary, an increase in SVR increases the flow of regurgitation and precipitate heart failure. Up to a certain degree, tachycardia shortens the diastole and therefore, reduces the regurgitation. As the ventricle is less hypertrophied in AR, it is less at risk from tachycardia-induced ischemia. So, the goal of anesthetic management for noncardiac surgery in patients with AR is to maintain adequate forward LV stroke volume: (i) by avoiding sudden decrease in HR, (ii) by avoiding sudden increase in SVR, and (iii) minimizing the drug-induced myocardial depression. During the whole intraoperative period, HR should be maintained above 80 beats/min. Because, bradycardia can lead to acute left ventricular increasing the volume overload by increasing the duration of ventricular diastole and thus increasing the volume of regurgitation.

The sudden increase in SVR may also precipitate the left ventricular failure (LVF), requiring treatment with peripheral vasodilators, such as nitroprusside. Like other

> **BOX 4:** Goals of anesthetic management of patients with aortic regurgitation (AR).
>
> - Prophylactic antibiotic
> - Avoidance of sudden increase in afterload
> - Prevent decrease in HR and maintain at higher side
> - Use vasopressor carefully

valvular diseases, GA is the choice for patients with AR. Although, reduction of SVR due to regional anesthesia is theoretically beneficial, but the uncontrolled nature of this response detracts an anesthetist from the use of it in such patient. Then still if RA is decided, then epidural is safer than spinal as it can be slowly induced allowing appropriate measures to take if the BP falls. Vasopressors should be used carefully to avoid excessive increases in SVR. Induction, intubation, maintenance, and perioperative monitoring of anesthesia in AR is like other cardiac valvular diseased patient.

■ MITRAL VALVE PROLAPSE

Etiology and Pathophysiology

Mitral valve prolapse is defined as the billowing of mitral leaflets into the LA during ventricular systole. It is currently the most commonly diagnosed cardiac valve abnormality and the progressive degeneration of this valve now represents the primary cause for mitral valve dysfunction that requires replacement or repair. It is also known as *Barlow syndrome*. Pathologically, it is due to the myxomatous degeneration of one or both the leaflets of mitral valve. So, they become enlarged, redundant, thick, rubbery, and floppy and prolapse back into the LA during ventricular systole. The tendinous cords also tend to be elongated, thinned, and occasionally ruptured. The posterior mitral leaflet is more commonly affected than its anterior leaflet. The mitral annulus may also be dilated. It is relatively a common abnormality, affecting 1–3% of general population and the women are seven times more frequently affected than men. In MVP, the concomitant tricuspid valve involvement is common (20–40% cases) and the aortic and pulmonary valves can also be affected.

The basis for this *primary myxomatous* degeneration of mitral valve is unknown. Probably, there is some underlying intrinsic defect of synthesis or remodeling of connective tissue. So, this myxomatous degeneration of mitral valve is a common feature of Marfan's syndrome and occasionally occurs in other connective tissue disorders. The most cases of MVP are sporadic or familial, affecting otherwise normal persons. *Secondary myxomatous* degeneration of mitral valve is due to regurgitation of it by another etiology (ischemic dysfunction).

Most patients, with MVP, are asymptomatic and in small percentage of cases, this myxomatous degeneration is progressive. The valvular abnormality, associated in MVP, is usually discovered only incidentally on physical examination. A minority of patients complain of palpitation, dyspnea, or atypical chest pain. In extreme cases arrhythmias, embolic events, florid MR, infective endocarditis, and sudden death may occur. Among the arrhythmias, both atrial and ventricular arrhythmias are common. Paroxysmal supraventricular tachycardia (PSVT) is the most commonly encountered sustained arrhythmia. An increased incidence of abnormal AV bypass tracts is reported in patients with MVP. Auscultation discloses midsystolic click caused by abrupt tension on the redundant valve leaflets and chordae tendineae as the valve attempts to close. There may or may not be an associated regurgitant murmur.

The *diagnosis of MVP* is usually made preoperatively by the auscultation of characteristic "click" with or without associated regurgitant murmur. This diagnosis is confirmed by echocardiography which shows systolic prolapse of mitral valve leaflets into LA. This prolapse of mitral valve leaflets is accentuated by maneuvers that decrease ventricular volume (preload).

Most patients with MVP have a normal life span. About 10–15% of patients develop progressive MR. A smaller percentage of patients develop embolic phenomenon or infective endocarditis. Patients with both a click and a systolic murmur seem to be at the greater risk of developing complications. The anticoagulation or antiplatelet agents may be used for the patients with the history of emboli. Whereas, the β-adrenergic blocking drugs are commonly used for arrhythmias.

Anesthetic Management of Mitral Valve Prolapse

The management of patients, suffering from MVP, depends on the clinical course of this disease and the present condition of the patients. Most patients are asymptomatic and do not require any special care. The key to anesthesia in MVP is to minimize the excessive contraction of LV (e.g., SNS stimulation, decreased SVR, hypovolemia, or unusual surgical positioning]. Multiple case reports suggest an association between the MVP and intraoperative arrhythmias. Premedication should produce anxiolysis without causing excessive tachycardia which may reduce ventricular volume and possibly may worsen the valve prolapse and regurgitation. The ventricular arrhythmias, if occur intraoperatively, particularly following sympathetic stimulation, are usually treated by lignocaine and β-adrenergic blocking drugs. The MR caused by MVP is generally exacerbated by the decrease in left ventricular size. So, hypovolemia and factors that increase ventricular emptying or decrease afterload should be avoided. Vasopressor with pure α-adrenergic activity, such as phenylephrine, is preferred to those that are primarily β-adrenergic agonists.

Congenital Heart Diseases and Anesthesia

■ INTRODUCTION

Congenital heart diseases (CHDs), the incidences of which are listed in **Table 1**, are usually manifested in neonate, infant, or childhood. But, sometimes, they may pass unrecognized and are not diagnosed until the adult life. Some congenital defects of heart [e.g., atrial septal defect (ASD)] may cause no symptoms throughout the whole life and may first be detected incidentally during the routine preoperative examination by an anesthetist. However, the most patients with CHD present with cyanosis or congestive heart failure. *Cyanosis* is typically the result of an abnormal intracardiac communication that allows the deoxygenated blood to reach the systemic arterial circulation (*right-to-left shunt*). *Congestive heart failure* is most prominent with defects that either obstruct the left ventricular outflow or markedly increase the pulmonary blood flow. The latter (increased pulmonary blood flow) is usually due to an abnormal intracardiac communication that returns the oxygenated blood to the right side of the heart [*left-to-right shunt*, e.g., patent ductus arteriosus (PDA)]. Whereas, the right-to-left shunt generally decreases pulmonary blood flow. In many cases, more than one lesion is present.

A very few years back, some CHDs, which were refused to be operated, are now undergoing cardiac surgery. This is due to: (i) the better development of surgical technology, (ii) better intraoperative myocardial protection, and (iii) major advances in the field of pediatric cardiac anesthesia. Such many patients who have undergone corrective cardiac surgery may remain well for many years, with full correction or under correction, and subsequently are presented for anesthesia during noncardiac surgery. Therefore, their number is now gradually steadily increasing. But, many patients will still have residual problems.

A study, in 1992, had reported an incidence of 47% of adverse perioperative events in CHD patients, undergoing noncardiac surgical procedures who were operated before. The pediatric cardiac surgical procedures for CHDs can be divided into three groups: (i) *curative procedures,* (ii) *corrective procedures,* and (iii) *palliative procedures.* In *curative procedures,* the patients are completely cured from congenital abnormalities of their heart without any residual problem and have a normal life expectancy, e.g., PDA, ASD, ventricular septal defect (VSD), etc. In *corrective procedures,* the patient's hemodynamic status is markedly improved, but there is some residual problems in their heart and the life expectancy of the patients may not have returned to normal, e.g., tetralogy of Fallot (TOF). In *palliative procedures,* after cardiac surgery, the patients may still have distinct abnormal circulations and cardiac physiology, but avoid the consequences, if CHD remains untreated (unoperated). Their life expectancy is not normal, but many are expected to reach the mid adulthood, e.g., Fontan procedures. The number of such surviving adults with palliated CHDs is also steadily increasing with advances in surgical and medical treatment.

The total incidence of CHD is about 7–10 per 1,000 live births. About 85% of these children reach their adult life. Among all the other congenital anomalies (cardiac and noncardiac) in our body, the CHD is the most common. It constitutes about 30% of all the congenital diseases. Previously, the acquired rheumatic heart disease was the

TABLE 1: Incidences of congenital heart disease.	
Disease	**Incidence (%)**
VSD	40
ASD	10
Pulmonary stenosis	7
PDA	6
Coarctation of aorta	5
Tetralogy of Fallot	5
Transposition of the great vessels	3

(ASD: atrial septal defect; PDA: patent ductus arteriosus; VSD: ventricular septal defect)

principal cause of all the heart diseases. But, with the decline of rheumatic disease, the CHD has become the principal cause of total heart diseases. Among the CHDs, 10–15% of patients have other associated congenital anomalies such as in the skeletal, genitourinary, or gastrointestinal system, etc.

Congenital heart diseases can be classified into:
- *Acyanotic defects:* Ventricular septal defect, ASD, PDA, pulmonary stenosis (PS), coarctation of aorta (CA), and atrioventricular septal defect (AVSD), etc.
- *Cyanotic defects:* Tetralogy of Fallot, transposition of the great vessels (TOGV), Eisenmenger's complex, etc.
  For complete classification of CHD, Refer **Table 2**.

These above-mentioned nine congenital forms of heart diseases constitute about 80% of all the total CHDs. Other wide range of more unusual and complex congenital lesions of heart comprises the remainder 20% of CHDs.

The proper understanding of the *development of heart* and fetal circulation helps us to understand how the CHDs occur. The heart develops from a single tube. First, from mesoderm a single tube is formed and it folds back on itself and then divides into two tubes for separate circulation. Failure of this separation can lead to some forms of atrial and VSDs. The failure of the alignment of great vessel with the ventricles contributes to the TOGV, TOF, and truncus arteriosus, etc. Due to high pulmonary vascular resistance and as the fetus cannot breath in uterus, so it has little blood flow through lungs during intrauterine life.

The fetal circulation, therefore, allows the oxygenated blood from placenta to pass directly to the left side of heart through foramen ovale without flowing through lungs.

This oxygenated blood, then, from left ventricle (LV) passes to the ascending aorta. On the other hand, the deoxygenated blood from right ventricle (RV) passes through the ductus arteriosus to descending aorta and reaches the placenta through umbilical arteries for oxygenation. The CHDs may also arise, if the changes from intrauterine fetal circulation to extrauterine circulation are not properly completed. The ASD occurs at the site of foramen ovale, if it does not close. The ductus arteriosus may remain open as PDA, if it fails to close after birth. The failure of the aorta to develop at the point of aortic isthmus can lead to the narrowing or CA.

Among the causes of CHDs, (i) the antenatal maternal infection, (ii) the antenatal exposure of mother and fetus to drugs or toxins, and (iii) the genetic or chromosomal abnormalities are the most important factors. Maternal rubella is associated with PDA, pulmonary and/or aortic stenosis, and ASD. Maternal alcohol abuse is associated with septal defects. Maternal systemic lupus erythematosus (SLE) is responsible for the different forms of congenital heart block of fetus and newborn, causing CHD. However, the major advancement in molecular biology have also much helped us to understand the genetic basis of CHDs. Genetic abnormalities are responsible for 10% of all the congenital cardiovascular lesions. Among these, two-thirds is due to trisomy-21 (Down syndrome) and one-third is due to trisomy-13, trisomy-18, and Turner's syndrome.

Maternal diabetes and use of lithium are also associated with the high incidences of CHDs. A widely used abbreviation such as CATCH-22 depicts a syndrome of CHD which is due to the defects in chromosome 22. CATCH-22 syndrome consists of (i) cardiac defects, (ii) abnormal faces, (iii) thymus hypoplasia, (iv) cleft palate, and (v) hypocalcemia. Another common genetic disorder is Marfan's syndrome which results from the mutations of gene, responsible for the formation of fibrin and a component of extracellular matrix. Marfan's syndrome is characterized by skeletal disproportion (arm span greater than height), arachnodactyly (long, thin, spider like fingers), sternal depression, generalized hypermobility of joints, lens dislocation, and a high-arched palate. The mitral valve prolapse, aortic incompetence, and aortic dissection are the most serious complication associated with Marfan's syndrome (*See* **Table 2**).

The symptoms of CHD may be absent or the child may be symptomatic and dyspneic. He may fail to attain normal growth and development. *Chronic hypoxemia* in patients with cyanotic heart disease typically results in *erythrocytosis*. This increase in red cell mass (hematocrit value) which is due to excess renal erythropoietin secretion, serve to restore normal tissue O_2 delivery. Unfortunately, due to erythrocytosis, *blood viscosity* is also increased. When the tissue oxygenation is restored to normal, then

TABLE 2: Classification of congenital heart disease.

Lesions causing outflow obstruction	*Left ventricle:* • Coarctation of aorta • Aortic stenosis • *Right ventricle:* Pulmonic valve stenosis
Lesions causing left-to-right shunt	• Ventricular septal defect • Patent ductus arteriosus • Atrial septal defect • Endocardial cushion defect
Lesions causing right-to-left shunt	*With decreased pulmonary blood flow:* • Pulmonary atresia • Tetralogy of Fallot • Eisenmenger's syndrome • Ebstein's anomaly • Tricuspid atresia *With increased pulmonary blood flow:* • Truncus arteriosus • Transposition of the great vessels • Single ventricle • Double-outlet right ventricle • Hypoplastic left heart

hematocrit or blood viscosity becomes stable and the symptoms of hyperviscosity syndrome are absent and the patient is said to have compensated. Patients with uncompensated erythrocytosis and hyperviscosity will not establish this equilibrium and they have *hyperviscosity syndrome (thromboembolic complications).* This risk of stroke (thromboembolic complications) is aggravated by dehydration. Children younger than 4 years of age are at greater risk of stroke.

Coagulation abnormalities are also common in patients with cyanotic heart disease. In these patients, platelet counts tend to be low normal and many patients have defects in coagulation cascade. In these patients, *hyperuricemia* is also common. Because, there is increased urate reabsorption, secondary to renal hypoperfusion and results in progressive *impaired kidney function* **(Box 1).**

The diagnosis of CHD is apparent during the first week of life in about 50% of affected neonates and before the 5 years of age is apparent in virtually all the remaining patients. Some congenital defects of heart are not compatible with extrauterine life or if compatible, it is only for a short period. The clinical signs and the severity of symptoms of CHD may vary with the type, complexity, and the degree of complexity of anatomical lesion. Early diagnosis is important because many types of CHD are amenable to surgical treatment. But, this opportunity may be lost, if the secondary changes such as the pulmonary vascular damage and pulmonary hypertension develops. The persistently raised pulmonary flow (e.g., with left-to-right shunt) leads to increased pulmonary resistance, followed by *pulmonary hypertension.* Then, progressive changes (including the obliteration of distal vessels) take place in pulmonary vasculature and once these changes are established, this increased pulmonary resistance becomes irreversible. Hence, if the severe pulmonary hypertension develops, then a left-to-right shunt, which is present from early may reverse, resulting in right-to-left shunt and marked cyanosis (Eisenmenger's syndrome). This is more common with large VSD or persistent ductus arteriosus than with ASD.

> **BOX 1:** Common problems in patients with congenital heart disease.
>
> - Growth impairment
> - Hypoxemia
> - Cyanosis
> - Erythrocytosis
> - Blood hyperviscosity
> - Pulmonary hypertension
> - Thromboembolic phenomenon
> - Infective endocarditis
> - Hyperuricemia
> - Impairment of renal function

The patients with Eisenmenger's syndrome are at particular risk from abrupt changes in afterload that exacerbates right-to-left shunt during anesthesia. The younger the patient will be at the time of corrective cardiac surgery, the greater is the likelihood that pulmonary vascular resistance will normalize. In older patients, if pulmonary vascular resistance is greater than one-third of SVR during corrective cardiac surgery, then progressive pulmonary vascular changes cannot be stopped. Cardiac arrhythmias are not usually a prominent feature of CHD. *Infective endocarditis* is the most common risk factor associated with CHD. Sudden death sometimes occurs in patient with CHD who have undergone some surgical correction. It reflects the myocardial scarring or damage to cardiac conducting system.

Echocardiography is the initial diagnostic step, if CHD is suspected. Both, the transthoracic and transesophageal route for echocardiography facilitate the early and accurate diagnosis of CHD. Recently, three-dimensional echocardiography, Doppler, and magnetic resonance imaging (MRI) have increased the understanding of complex cardiac malformation accurately. They also allow the visualization of abnormal blood flow and transposition of vascular structures. Cardiac catheterization and angiocardiography are also definitive diagnostic procedure for patients with CHD.

PREOPERATIVE ASSESSMENT OF PATIENTS WITH CHD FOR NONCARDIAC SURGERY

It helps to gain a clear understanding regarding the anatomy and pathophysiology of patient's congenital cardiac defect.

History

At first, the patient should be asked about the limitations of his daily activities. It will try to define clinically the nature and the severity of his or her cardiac lesion. This history may also provide some clue regarding the presence of other anomalies in his or her body and syndromes associated with CHD.

Examination

To diagnose and to assess the severity of CHD, the patient should be properly inspected, palpated, and auscultated. The cyanosis, peripheral edema, and hepatosplenomegaly should be searched for. The peripheral pulses, heart, and lungs are assessed for murmur, signs of heart failure, and any infection. Cyanosed patients should have a brief neurological examination also **(Box 2).**

Investigations

The laboratory tests obviously depend on the type of proposed noncardiac surgery and the severity of cardiac

BOX 2: Signs and symptoms of congenital heart disease.

- Asymptomatic
- Dyspnea, tachypnea
- Cyanosis
- Failure to gain weight
- Decreased exercise tolerance
- Murmur and thrill
- Thromboembolism
- Erythrocytosis
- Heart failure
- Sudden death

BOX 3: Factors indicating high risks of patients.

- Unexplained dizziness or syncope
- Fever and recent CVA
- Recent worsening of symptoms of myocardial ischemia
- Signs and symptoms of cardiac failure
- SpO_2 <75% while breathing air
- Hematocrit value >60%, indicating severe polycythemia
- Recent onset of arrhythmia
- Severe aortic or pulmonary stenosis
- Uncorrected tetralogy of Fallot or Eisenmenger's syndrome

(CVA: cerebrovascular accident)

disease. But, the most patients will require complete blood count (CBC), coagulation profile, liver function test (LFT), and electrolytes estimation. Recent chest radiograph, electrocardiogram (ECG), echocardiography, and Doppler are done routinely. Transesophageal echocardiography (TEE), MRI, and other investigations are done according to the need (extend of congenital cardiac abnormalities and the extend of noncardiac surgery). For example, some patients may need pulmonary function tests. In some patients, baseline SpO_2 level, while breathing air, is also recorded. Data from cardiac catheterization and angiocardiography should also be kept in mind.

Factors Indicating High Risk

When a patient with CHD is undergoing a noncardiac surgery, they should be balanced between the potential risks and the benefits of proposed surgery. The admission of patient in intensive care unit (ICU) or high-dependency care unit (HDU) or he should be removed to any specialized cardiac center will depend on the risk factors, playing in individual **(Box 3)**.

SPECIFIC PROBLEMS FOUND IN PATIENTS WITH CONGENITAL HEART DISEASE

The specific problems which are usually encountered during anesthesia in patients with CHD are described here.

Myocardial Dysfunction

Primarily some forms of myocardial dysfunction, mainly of ventricle, are usually present in all forms of CHD which may lead to perioperative cardiac failure. Superimposed on it is secondary cardiac dysfunction which is due to the poor intraoperative myocardial protection.

Arrhythmias

In perioperative period, all types of arrhythmias may be precipitated during noncardiac surgery on patients, suffering from CHD. This may be due to original disease or due to some iatrogenic (surgery and medications) factors. Some patients, suffering from CHD, develop complete heart block following cardiac surgery and have pacemakers in situ.

Air Embolism

All CHD patients are at potential risk from systemic air embolism, particularly in ASD, PDA, and VSD with right-to-left shunt. So, all intravascular lines should be free of air.

Cyanosis

Perioperative cyanosis is common in patients suffering from CHD. It is generally due to the intracardiac mixing of oxygenated and deoxygenated blood (e.g., complete AVSD) or the shunting of blood from right side to the left side of heart (e.g., TOF and Eisenmenger's syndrome) or heart failure.

Anticoagulation

Most CHD patients are under anticoagulants such as aspirin, warfarin, etc. So, the perioperative management of these patients undergoing noncardiac surgery is very difficult.

Endocarditis

Most patients with CHD are at increased risk from the development of endocarditis during perioperative period. So, preoperative antibiotic prophylaxis is very important.

Myocardial Ischemia

Development of perioperative myocardial ischemia with or without myocardial infarction (MI) in patients with CHD is very common. So, it should be protected and treated immediately.

■ ATRIAL SEPTAL DEFECT

Atrial septal defect is the second most common (one-third) form among all CHDs and occurs twice as frequently in females than in males. The ASD is of two types *ostium secundum* (most common, 70%) and *ostium primum (30%)*.

The ostium secundum type of ASD results in single or multiple (fenestrated) openings between the two atria and involves the fossa ovalis, which in intrauterine life remains as foramen ovale. Whereas, the ostium primum type of ASD is located at the lower part of interatrial septum and overlie the mitral and tricuspid valve. It results from the defect of endocardial cushion or from the defect of atrioventricular valves, which are associated with "left mitral valve" and mitral regurgitation (MR). The more severe form of ASD is the AVSD, which is associated with Down's syndrome and results in severe pulmonary hypertension, if not treated in infancy. On the other hand, ostium secundum is associated with mitral value prolapse. The surgical repair of these forms of ASD occasionally results in complete heart block. Most of the ASDs occur as the result of spontaneous genetic mutation.

Most children with ASDs are asymptomatic or minimally symptomatic. Some have recurrent pulmonary infections. Congestive heart failure and pulmonary hypertension are more commonly encountered in adults with ASD. Patients with ostium primum defects often have large shunts and may also develop significant MR **(Fig. 1)**.

The right side of the heart (right atrium and RV) is much more compliant than the left side of the heart (left atrium and LV). So, a large volume of blood shunts through this defect from the left atrium to the right atrium (left-to-right shunt) and then through the RV to pulmonary artery and lungs. As a result, there is gradual increased pressure and the enlargement of the right side of the heart and pulmonary artery. Thus, gradually pulmonary hypertension and sometimes shunt reversal (right to left) occur in long-standing cases of ASD. But, it is less common and tends to occur later in life than with other types of left-to-right shunt such as VSD and PDA. The magnitude and the direction of blood flow through this defect are determined by the size of the defect and the relative compliance of the two atrium and two ventricles.

A small defect in the interatrial septum which is <0.5 cm in diameter is associated with no hemodynamic sequelae. But, when the defect approaches ±2 cm in diameter, then clinical features appear. The ASD in which the pulmonary flow is 50% or above the systemic flow, is often considered as large enough to be clinically recognizable and should be closed surgically or through transarterial catheter technique. Severe pulmonary hypertension and shunt reversal are both taken as contraindication to corrective surgery of ASD.

The chest radiograph of ASD typically shows an enlargement of heart and the pulmonary artery. The ECG usually shows right axis deviation and incomplete right bundle branch block (RBBB). This is because right ventricular depolarization is delayed as a result of its hypertrophy and dilatation. Echocardiography can directly demonstrate the defect of ASD. Sometimes atrial fibrillation and supraventricular tachycardia may accompany an ASD.

The anesthetic management of a patient who is suffering from ASD and left-to-right shunt and is scheduled for noncardiac surgery has minimal implication. The prophylactic antibiotics are needed to protect against infective endocarditis, if ASD is associated with other valvular abnormalities. During intraoperative management, the change in SVR has an important implication on ASD. Any increase in SVR favors an increase in the magnitude of left-to-right shunt and right heart failure. So, it should be avoided during perioperative period. On the other hand, any decrease in SVR tends to decrease the magnitude of left-to-right shunt or sometimes becomes reverse, if SVR falls to a great extent. Meticulous avoidance of air entry into intravenous line is imperative in ASD patient.

■ VENTRICULAR SEPTAL DEFECT

Ventricular septal defect is one of the common causes (25–30%) of all the CHD, occurring one in every 500 live births. It occurs as a result of incomplete septation (division) of primitive ventricle. Embryologically, the intraventricular septum has a membranous and a muscular portion. The muscular portion is further divided into inflow, trabecular, and outflow part. Most VSDs are of "perimembranous" type, i.e., at the junction of membranous and muscular portions (70%). Another 20% of VSD is situated in the muscular portion of interventricular septum at its middle or apical area. Next 5% of VSD is situated just below the aortic valve,

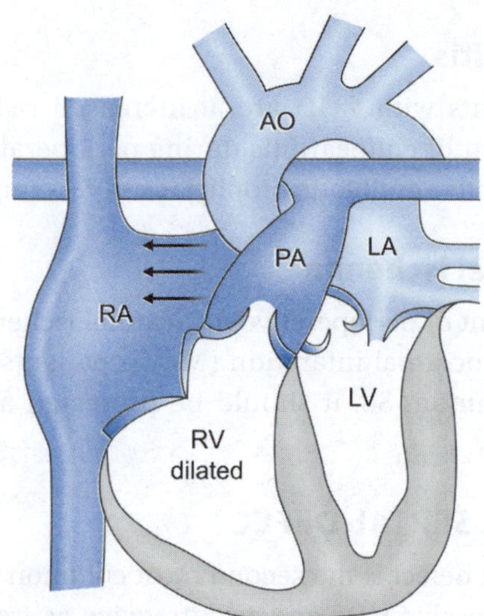

Fig. 1: Atrial septal defect. (AO: aorta; LA: left atrium; LV: left ventricle; PA: pulmonary artery; RA: right atrium; RV: right ventricle)

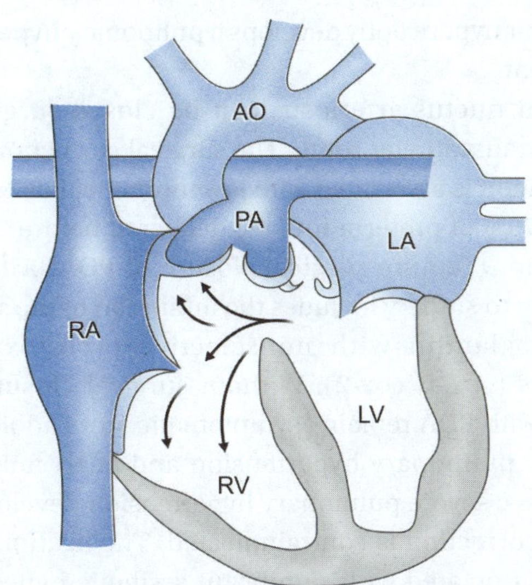

Fig. 2: Ventricular septal defect. (AO: aorta; LA: left atrium; LV: left ventricle; PA: pulmonary artery; RA: right atrium; RV: right ventricle)

causing aortic regurgitation and near the junction of mitral and tricuspid valve **(Fig. 2)**.

The VSD may be an isolated case or becomes a part of a complex CHD. It may be congenital or acquired. Acquired VSD may result from the rupture of interventricular septum, as a complication of acute MI or rarely from trauma. The resulting functional abnormality of a VSD is dependent on the size of the defect, and the presence or absence of pulmonary vascular resistance (PVR) and other cardiac abnormalities. The maximum number of small VSDs, which are present at birth, close spontaneously, when a child reaches 2 years of age. The restrictive defects of VSD are associated with small left-to-right shunt. The patients with small VSD are treated medically and followed with ECG (for signs of right ventricular hypertrophy) and echocardiography. The surgical closures are usually undertaken in patients with large VSD before pulmonary vascular disease and Eisenmenger physiology develop.

In VSD, the blood flows from high pressure of LV to the low pressure of RV, during the whole period of ventricular systole, producing a pansystolic murmur. This is usually heard best at left sternal edge and also radiates all over the precordium. A small defect often produces a loud murmur but contrary a large defect often produces a softer murmur, particularly if pressure in RV is elevated. This may be found immediately after birth, when the pulmonary vascular resistance remains high or when the shunt is reversed, e.g., in Eisenmenger's syndrome.

The symptoms, signs, and pathology produced by VSD depend on: (i) the size of the defect, (ii) the difference between the systemic and pulmonary vascular resistance (the difference between the pressure of LV and RV), and (iii) the rate of flow through the defect of VSD. (a) If the defect is small, (b) the pulmonary and systemic flow ratio is <1.5:1, and (c) there is no pulmonary hypertension, then there is minimal increase in pulmonary blood flow and patient is asymptomatic. On the other hand, if the defect is large enough and the pressure in the two ventricles is equal, then the flow through the pulmonary and systemic circulation depends on their relative resistance.

Initially, SVR is higher than pulmonary vascular resistance and the blood flows from the LV toward the RV (L-to-R shunt). These moderate-sized VSDs often present with congestive cardiac failure (CCF) due to markedly increased pulmonary blood flow with pulmonary and systemic flow ratio 3:1 or more. These patients require early operation for closure of VSD. However, if they require anesthesia for another noncardiac surgical procedure, prior to their definitive cardiac operation, then they may present severe problems. They should be intubated in all cases, except the very minor procedures. One should always try to avoid increasing the left-to-right shunt (e.g. avoid hyperventilation and unnecessary high inspired oxygen levels). Care should be taken regarding the fluid administration. Inotropic support is often required. Over the time, the pulmonary vascular resistance gradually increases and the pulmonary hypertension develops, causing a decline in the magnitude of left-to-right (L to R) intracardiac shunt. Gradually, the shunt become reverse flowing right to left (R to L) with the development of cyanosis and arterial hypoxemia. Before the development of pulmonary hypertension, these large VSD patients often require pulmonary artery banding to protect their pulmonary circulation. This band may tighten as the child grows, resulting in cyanosis. The VSDs often close spontaneously and the band may then be removed. Like ASD, the intraoperative anesthetic management of VSD for noncardiac surgeries includes the control of systemic and pulmonary vascular resistance on which will depend the magnitude of left-to-right or reverse shunt. When left to right shunting is present, then abrupt increase in PVR and decrease in SVR are poorly tolerated and should be avoided.

PATENT DUCTUS ARTERIOSUS

The ductus arteriosus is a connection which arises from the arch of the aorta, just distal to left subclavian artery, and connects the arch of the aorta with the left pulmonary artery. In fetal life, the pulmonary vascular resistance is high than the systemic vascular resistance. So, the blood from pulmonary artery, which is ejected out from the RV, bypassing the deflated lungs, runs through this ductus arteriosus and enters the descending aorta for oxygenation in placenta.

Normally, the ductus arteriosus closes within 24–48 hours after birth in a full-term neonate. But, in preterm neonates, it frequently fails to close and also sometimes it fails to close in full-term infants. Occasionally, the persistence of this ductus arteriosus may be associated with other congenital abnormalities in body and is much more common in females. When this ductus arteriosus fails to close spontaneously after birth, then it results in continuous flow of blood from aorta to pulmonary artery (opposite to fetal circulation) due to the reduction of pulmonary vascular resistance than systemic resistance after birth.

Then, the flow of blood through this PDA after birth will depend on: (i) the pressure gradient between the aorta and pulmonary artery, (ii) the ratio of systemic and pulmonary vascular resistance, and (iii) the diameter and the length of the duct. As much as, 50% of left ventricular output may be recirculated through the lungs with a consequent increase in pulmonary artery pressure which leads to progressive pulmonary vascular damage and pulmonary hypertension. If the pulmonary vascular resistance increases and the pulmonary artery pressure rises exceeding the aortic pressure, then the shunt will be reversed, flowing from pulmonary artery to aorta, causing central cyanosis (Eisenmenger's syndrome) **(Fig. 3)**.

With small shunt, there may be no symptoms for many years. This small defect of PDA is often detected accidentally, during the routine preoperative physical examination of patient, scheduled for any noncardiac surgery in their later part of life. During this time, a characteristic continuous systolic and diastolic murmur is heard with late systolic accentuation, which is heard maximally in the second left intercostal space below the clavicle. Gradually, the right ventricular hypertrophy develops if pulmonary hypertension is apparent.

Patent ductus arteriosus can be closed surgically or through transcatheter route. The surgical correction of PDA by its ligation is associated with low mortality. It is estimated that the 75% of preterm infants, delivered before 28 weeks of gestation, require surgical closure of PDA. Alternative procedure to surgery includes the inhibition of the synthesis of prostaglandin with nonselective cyclo-oxygenase inhibitors (cox-1, cox-2). Without surgical closure, most patients with PDA remain asymptomatic, until adolescence, when the pulmonary hypertension and heart failure may occur. Once severe pulmonary hypertension develops, then surgical correction is contraindicated. The ligation of PDA is often associated with significant systemic hypertension during the immediate postoperative period, which is managed by continuous infusion of vasodilator drugs, such as nitroprusside. If this systemic hypertensive persists, then long-acting antihypertensive drugs will gradually substitute the nitroprusside.

The first step of anesthetic management of an uncorrected PDA patient, scheduled for noncardiac surgery, is preoperative prophylaxis by antibiotic for the protection against infective endocarditis. The principal of intraoperative anesthetic management of PDA patient, scheduled for noncardiac surgery, is also same like that of ASD and VSD, i.e., maintaining a balance between the systemic vascular resistance and the pulmonary vascular resistance. The decrease of systemic vascular resistance improves the systemic blood flow by decreasing the magnitude of left-to-right shunt. But, this decrease of SVR will not go below the pulmonary part, when the reverse shunt will flow and cyanosis will develop. Contrary, the increase in SVR and decrease in pulmonary vascular resistance would increase the magnitude of the left-to-right shunt and should be avoided. Invasive positive pressure ventilation (IPPV) of the patient's lung is well tolerated, as increased airway pressure increases the pulmonary vascular resistance and subsequently decreases the pressure gradient between the left and the right side of the heart and the flow across the PDA.

■ TETRALOGY OF FALLOT

These patients have (i) pulmonary or infundibular stenosis (right ventricular outflow obstruction), (ii) VSD, (iii) overriding of aorta on the right and left ventricle, and (iv) right ventricular hypertrophy **(Fig. 4)**. Right ventricular obstruction, present in most of the TOF patients (80%) is due to *infundibular stenosis,* which is due to the hypertrophy

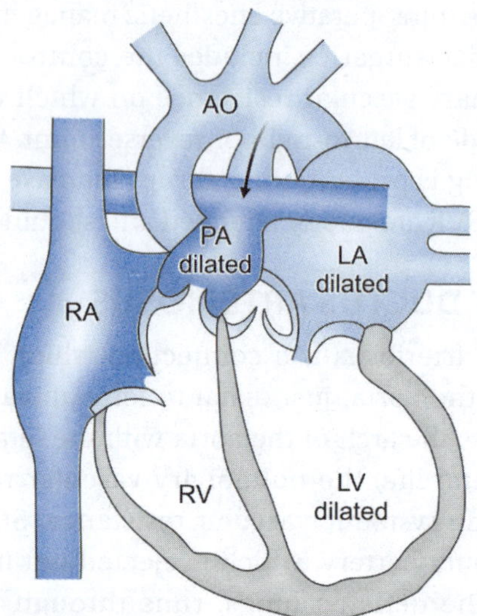

Fig. 3: Patent ductus arteriosus. (AO: aorta; LA: left atrium; LV: left ventricle; PA: pulmonary artery; RA: right atrium; RV: right ventricle)

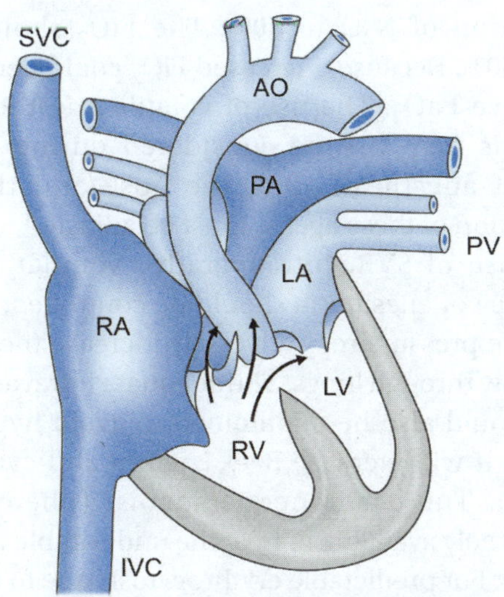

Fig. 4: Tetralogy of Fallot (TOF). (AO: aorta; IVC: inferior vena cava; LA: left atrium; LV: left ventricle; PA: pulmonary artery; PV: pulmonary vein; RA: right atrium; RV: right ventricle; SVC: superior vena cava)

of subpulmonic muscles. In next 20% of patients, suffering from TOF, there is *PS.* The pulmonary valve is often *bicuspid* or less commonly *atretic.* The infundibular obstruction is not a static (permanent) one. It is aggravated by sympathetic tone and is therefore dynamic. This obstruction is likely responsible for the *hypercyanotic spells*, observed in very young patients.

Tetralogy of Fallot is the most common *cyanotic* CHD. Right ventricular hypertrophy occurs, because (a) the VSD permits the RV to a continuous exposure to the high pressure of LV and (b) the pulmonary or infundibular stenosis causing right ventricular outflow obstruction. Several other anomalies may be associated with TOF. These are right aortic arch, ASD (TOF plus ASD is known as pentalogy of Fallot), anomalies of coronary arteries, etc.

The *cyanosis in TOF is due to* intracardiac right-to-left shunt which is again due to the right ventricular hypertrophy. The magnitude of RV hypertrophy determines the severity of shunt and the severity of cyanosis. Due to pulmonary or infundibular stenosis, the flow across the right ventricular outflow tract is relatively fixed. So, the changes in SVR (drug induced) may severely affect the magnitude of this shunt. The decrease in SVR increases the right-to-left intracardiac shunt and increases the cyanosis with arterial hypoxemia. Reversely, increase in SVR decreases the right-to-left shunt and decreases the cyanosis with increased pulmonary blood flow.

The diagnosis of TOF is usually established by echocardiography and Doppler. It assesses (i) the presence of other associated abnormalities, (ii) the level and the severity of right ventricular outflow obstruction, (iii) the magnitude of right ventricular hypertrophy, (iv) the size of main pulmonary artery and its branches, and (v) the number, location, and size of VSD. Cardiac catheterization further confirms the diagnosis of TOF by providing the different anatomical and hemodynamic data. The MRI of heart can also provide much of the information.

Most patients with TOF present with cyanosis from birth. On examination, murmur is heard along the left sternal border due to the turbulent flow of blood across the stenotic pulmonic valve and VSD. Chest radiograph shows the evidence of decreased lung vascularity and the heart is "boot shaped". The right axis deviation and the RV hypertrophy is the common finding in ECG. Squatting position is the common picture of children with TOF. Because, it is speculated that this squatting position increases the SVR by kinking the large arteries in inguinal area and subsequently this increased SVR decreases the intracardiac right-to-left shunt and increases the pulmonary blood flow. The arterial O_2 tension is usually <50 mm Hg. Arterial O_2 desaturation is present, even when the patient is breathing with 100% O_2.

Sometimes, paroxysmal cyanotic spells occur with severe arterial hypoxemia, tachypnea, seizures, and loss of consciousness or even death. These attacks can occur without obvious provocation. But, it is often associated with crying and exercise. The mechanism of this paroxysmal cyanotic spells is not properly known. The probable explanation is like that sometimes there is sudden decrease in pulmonary blood flow due to the spasm of infundibular cardiac muscle or sudden decrease in SVR. The management of this paroxysmal cyanotic spell is administration of β-blocker such as esmolol or propranolol. It removes the dynamic infundibular obstruction by relieving its smooth muscle spasm. Cyanotic spell is also managed by intravenous administration of fluids and/or phenylephrine. It helps by (i) increasing SVR, (ii) decreasing intracardiac right-to-left shunt, and (iii) increasing pulmonary blood flow. The sympathomimetic agents with β-agonistic properties are not used. Because, they may accentuate the spasm of infundibular cardiac muscle and cyanosis.

The definitive treatment of TOF is complete surgical correction. Without surgery, mortality exceeds 50% by the age of 3 years. In the past, three palliative procedures were done to improve the pulmonary arterial blood flow. These palliative procedures are (i) the side-to-side anastomosis of ascending aorta and right pulmonary artery, (ii) the side-to-side anastomosis of descending aorta and left pulmonary artery, and (iii) the end to side anastomosis of subclavian and pulmonary artery (Blalock–Taussig operation). Now, the correction of TOF is done by (i) the closure of VSD with Dacron patch and (ii) the relief of right ventricular outflow obstruction by placing a synthetic graft.

The aim of anesthetic management during noncardiac surgery of a patient with TOF is to reduce R → L intracardiac shunt and, thus, in turn to increase pulmonary blood flow and PaO_2. The magnitude of R → L shunt also alters the pharmacokinetics of both injected and inhaled drugs that bypass the lungs. The severity of R → L intracardiac shunt can be increased by (i) decreased SVR, (ii) increased PVR, and (iii) increased myocardial contractility which accentuates the infundibular obstruction to blood flow. Contrary, the R → L intracardiac shunt can be reduced by the reversal of abovementioned actions. So, the pharmacological agents that decrease SVR such as volatile anesthetics, nitroprusside, histamine-releasing muscle relaxants, α-adrenergic blocking agents, etc, should be avoided. Pulmonary blood flow can be decreased by increasing PVR that accompany many intraoperative ventilatory maneuvers such as IPPV, positive end-expiratory pressure (PEEP), etc. So, all these should be regulated and controlled. Furthermore, the loss of negative intrapleural pressure on opening the chest increases PVR and severity of shunt. But, indeed, PaO_2 does not predictably deteriorate, either with the institution of IPPV or after the opening of chest, in patients with TOF and many advantages of intraoperative controlled ventilation usually offset its potential hazard.

During preoperative anesthetic preparation of patients, suffering from TOF, crying should be avoided which may precipitate the hypercyanotic attack. The β-adrenergic blocker should be continued, till the induction of anesthesia to prevent cyanotic spell. The induction of anesthesia is usually accomplished with ketamine which improve arterial oxygenation by increasing SVR and thus decreasing R → L intracardiac shunt. Ketamine also increases PVR which is undesirable in Fallot patients. But, this concern is not clinically significant. Tracheal intubation is facilitated by administration of muscle relaxants. During the use of IV drugs, it should be kept in mind that the onset and magnitude of action of drugs is more rapid in Fallot due to the R → L shunt which decreases pulmonary dilutional effects of drugs and the metabolism of drug like fentanyl in lungs. For this reason, it is prudent to decrease the dose of intravenous cardiac and respiratory depressant drugs in these patients.

For intraoperative muscular paralysis, pancuronium is the agent of choice, as it maintains high SVR and blood pressure (BP). Pancuronium also increases heart rate (HR) which is helpful for maintaining left ventricular output. The use of N_2O for the maintenance of anesthesia in TOF has many disadvantages. These disadvantages are: it (N_2O) increases PVR and decreases inspired O_2 concentration. But, the advantages of N_2O are: it does not decrease SVR like volatile agents. So, balancing the advantages and disadvantages, it seems prudent to limit the inspired concentration of N_2O to 50%. The FiO_2 should not be reduced <50%. Because, increased FiO_2 could decrease PVR and improve PaO_2. The use of volatile anesthetic agents and opioids may also be considered during the maintenance of anesthesia. But, the dose and the rate of administration of these agents must be adjusted to minimize the decrease of SVR. Intraoperative ventilation for the maintenance of anesthesia should be controlled, but excessive positive pressure may adversely increase the resistance to blood flow through lungs. The adequate intravascular fluid volume should also be maintained to avoid hypovolemia. Otherwise, it will increase R → L shunt and cyanosis and hypoxemia. The α-adrenergic agonist (phenylephrine) should be freely available to treat the undesirable decrease in SVR and BP. For predictable erythrocytosis due to cyanosis, it is probably not necessary to consider blood transfusion until about 30% of patient's blood volume has been lost. Meticulous care should be taken to avoid infusion of air through tubing which is used to deliver intravenous solutions as it could lead to systemic air embolization.

The patients, who have undergone successful surgical correction of TOF, are usually asymptomatic. But, still their life expectancy is not so hopeful. The survival rate of them is shortened, due to the sudden unexplained death. Cardiac arrhythmias, particularly ventricular, are common in patients following the surgical correction of the TOF. Pulmonary regurgitation may develop, as a result of surgical repair, leading to right ventricular hypertrophy and dysfunction.

■ EISENMENGER'S SYNDROME

The persistently raised pulmonary blood flow, due to left-to-right (L → R) intracardiac shunt in large VSD, ASD, etc., leads to increased pulmonary resistance followed by pulmonary hypertension. Then, progressively the changes like obliteration of distal vessels take place in pulmonary vasculature due to the presence of persistent pulmonary hypertension. Thus, once established, this increased pulmonary resistance is irreversible and pulmonary hypertension becomes unavoidable and permanent. Hence, when severe pulmonary hypertension develops to a level that equals or exceeds the SVR, then L → R intracardiac shunt is reversed, resulting in right-to-left (R → L) intracardiac shunt and marked cyanosis which is called as the Eisenmenger's syndrome. Shunt reversal occurs in about 60% of patients with an untreated VSD, 30% of patients with an untreated PDA, and about 20% of patients with an untreated ASD. The murmur which was previously present associated with these cardiac defects gradually disappears when the Eisenmenger's syndrome develops. Patients with Eisenmenger's syndrome are particularly at increased risk from abrupt changes in afterload that exacerbate right to left (R → L) shunting such as vasodilatation, anesthesia, pregnancy, etc. Central cyanosis appears and digital clubbing develops. The chest radiograph shows the enlarged central pulmonary arteries and peripheral pruning of pulmonary vessels. The ECG shows hypertrophy of RV. Palpitation is common and is most often due to the onset of atrial fibrillation or atrial flutter. Sudden death is also not uncommon in patients with Eisenmenger's syndrome.

There are many palliative surgeries, but no treatment has proved effective in producing sustained decrease in PVR. The presence of irreversible increased PVR contraindicates the surgical correction of the original CHD that was responsible for Eisenmenger's syndrome.

The Eisenmenger's patients should be managed in a specialist center whenever possible. The aim of anesthetic management for patients with Eisenmenger's syndrome undergoing noncardiac surgery is to strictly maintain the preoperative levels of SVR and to avoid the vasodilatation by any cost. This is because the degree of shunting depends on PVR:SVR ratio. So, the reduction of SVR (epidural/spinal anesthesia) and rise of PVR (hypoxia, hypercarbia, acidosis, and cold) should be avoided. Decreasing the SVR or increasing the PVR leads to deterioration of blood oxygen saturation rather like in patients with TOF. Desaturation episode can be treated as like TOF. To maintain SVR, continuous intravenous infusions of norepinephrine can be administered during the perioperative period. The inotropic support may be required even for the shortest procedures. All the possible cares for the minimization of blood loss with the development of hypovolemia should be taken. So, preoperative administration of antiplatelet drugs is not encouraged. Opioids can be used safely for perioperative analgesia.

Laparoscopic procedures are not recommended for Eisenmenger's syndrome patients. Because, the insufflation of peritoneal cavity with CO_2 may cause increase in $PaCO_2$ resulting in acidosis and hypotension. Acidosis and hypotension increase the PVR:SVR ratio, causing more R → L shunt, cyanosis, and hypoxia. Thus, a vicious cycle sets-up. Efforts to maintain normocapnia may be accompanied by hyperventilation, increase in airway pressure, and PVR which further increases R → L shunt. The whole thing is further aggravated when intra-abdominal pressure (IAP) increases and the patients are placed in head-down position. Early extubation in these patients is better to avoid the deleterious effects of IPPV.

TRICUSPID ATRESIA

Due to congenital tricuspid atresia, blood cannot flow from right atrium to RV. During intrauterine life, in a fetus blood flows from RA to LA through foramen ovale and then through LV to aorta. Next, blood flows from aorta through PDA into pulmonary circulation. After birth, this route is necessary for survival of a neonate. Hence, early survival is dependent on prostaglandin E-1 as infusion to maintain the patency of PDA with percutaneous balloon atrial septostomy, if foramen ovale closes. If foramen ovale remains patent, then septostomy is not necessary. Cyanosis is evident at birth and its severity depends on the amount of pulmonary blood flow that is achieved through PDA. Severe cyanosis requires a modified Blalock–Thomas–Taussig shunt operation early in life. The preferred surgical management is a modified Fontan procedure, in which the venous drainage is directed to pulmonary circulation. In some centers, a shunt is made between SVC and PA instead of Fontan procedure. In these both procedures, blood flows from systemic veins to pulmonary circulation and then to LA without the assistance of RV. The success of these procedures depends on a high systemic venous pressure and maintaining the both low PVR and a low LA pressure. Heart transplantation is necessary for a failed Fontan procedure.

TRANSPOSITION OF THE GREAT VESSELS

Here, systemic veins drain into RA and aorta arises from RV and pulmonary veins drain into LA and pulmonary artery arises from LV. Thus, deoxygenated blood runs through systemic circulation and oxygenated blood runs through pulmonary circulation. Therefore, survival is possible only through mixing of oxygenated and deoxygenated blood across the foramen ovale and a PDA. Hence, for the patency of PDA, the infusion of prostaglandin E1 is essential. The presence of a VSD increases this mixing of oxygenated and deoxygenated blood and reduces the level of hypoxemia and the chances of survival.

In TOGV, the corrective surgical treatment involves the procedures in which the aorta is divided and reanastomosed with LV and the pulmonary artery is divided and reanastomosed with RV. The coronary arteries must also be reimplanted into the old pulmonary artery root. If a VSD is present, it should be closed. Less commonly and alternately, an atrial switch (retransposition) procedure (Senning) may be carried out, if an arterial switch (retransposition) is not possible.

The TOGV may occur with VSD and pulmonic stenosis. This combination of defects mimics the TOF. However, the obstruction affects the LV but not the RV. Here, the corrective surgery involves the patch closure of VSD, directing the left ventricular outflow into the aorta, the ligation of proximal pulmonary artery, and connecting the right ventricular outflow with pulmonary artery.

Cardiomyopathies and Anesthesia

■ INTRODUCTION

Cardiomyopathies are a group of diseases of unknown etiology that affect the cardiac muscles (myocardium). It is unrelated to the usual causes of heart disease such as the coronary artery disease, cardiac valvular dysfunction, essential hypertension, etc. It is common to all cardiomyopathies that they lead to a progressive life-threatening congestive heart failure. Though, it is of unknown etiology, still some probable causes for these myopathies are defined. These are: idiopathic, ischemic, infective (viral and bacterial), toxic (alcohol), systemic diseases (muscular dystrophy, collagen vascular diseases, sarcoidosis, myxedema, thyrotoxicosis, and pheochromocytoma), infiltrative (amyloidosis and hemochromatosis), nutritional, and genetic (familial) **(Box 1)**. The cardiomyopathies are classified on pathological basis into: (1) Idiopathic dilated cardiomyopathy (IDC), (2) Hypertrophic (obstructive) cardiomyopathy (HOCM), and (3) Restrictive cardiomyopathy. They can all be diagnosed by echocardiography.

■ IDIOPATHIC DILATED CARDIOMYOPATHY

In this type of cardiomyopathy, there is gradual decrease in the contractile force of the left or right ventricle, resulting in

systolic failure. It is characterized by: (1) the left ventricular (LV) or biventricular dilatation (although in early stages there may be no discernable dilatation), (2) impaired myocardial contractility, (3) decreased cardiac output (CO), and (4) increased ventricular end-diastolic filling pressure and volume. Among these, the ventricular dilatation is the most distinguishing morphological feature of IDC **(Fig. 1)**. The ventricular cardiac dysrhythmias and sudden death are common in patients with IDC. *Peripartum cardiomyopathy* is usually of this form and is specifically associated with late pregnancy or the first 6 months of puerperium. But, most often it is manifested in the period of first 1–6 weeks after delivery.

The clinical course of IDC is unpredictable, although most deaths occur within 3 years of the diagnosis of IDC, due to the progressive congestive heart failure. There are many *etiologies of IDC* such as alcohol, drugs, vitamin deficiencies, etc., but the *most common cause of IDC is ischemic heart disease (IHD)*. The *most common problems* encountered with IDC are heart failure, arrhythmias, and emboli from the

BOX 1: Etiology of cardiomyopathies.

- Idiopathic
- Infective—bacterial and viral
- Ischemic
- Toxic—drugs, alcohol, and poisons
- Nutritional
- Infiltrative—amyloidosis, metastasis, and hemochromatosis
- Thyrotoxicosis
- Myxedema
- Sarcoidosis
- Muscular dystrophy
- Collagen disease
- Genetic or familial

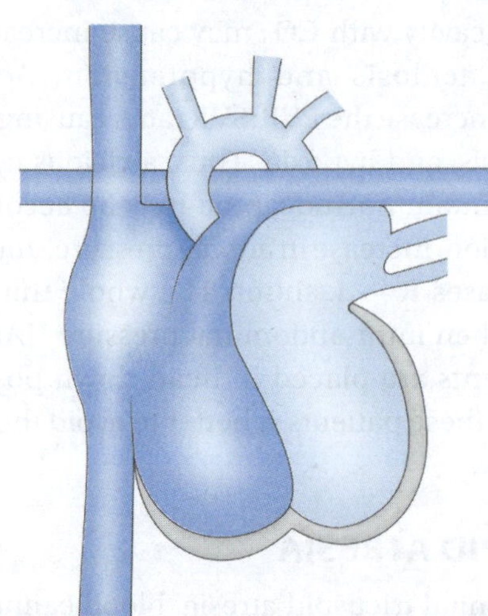

Fig. 1: Idiopathic dilated cardiomyopathy.

left side of cardiac cavities. Thus, they are treated with the combinations of diuretics, angiotensin-converting enzyme (ACE) inhibitors or angiotensin receptor blockers (ARBs), vasodilators, anticoagulants, and antiarrhythmic agents.

In IDC, there is marked reduction in the ejection fraction of left ventricle and it is most often <0.4 (i.e., 40%) when the heart failure supervenes. So, the most common initial manifestation of IDC is the congestive heart failure. Though the children and elders are also affected, but the most patients with IDC are first seen between 30 and 50 years of life. The hemodynamic abnormalities that predict a poor prognosis of IDC include: (1) ejection fraction <0.25, (2) left ventricular end-diastolic dilatation (LVEDD), (3) hypokinetic LV wall on echocardiography, (4) pulmonary capillary wedge pressure (PCWP) >20 mm Hg, (5) cardiac index (CI) <2.5 L/min/m^2, (6) systemic hypotension, and (7) pulmonary hypertension, and (8) increased central venous pressure (CVP).

The chest radiograph may show the evidences of cardiac enlargement, involving all the four cardiac chambers. The electrocardiogram (ECG) investigation characteristically shows the evidence of left ventricular hypertrophy (LVH), ST- and T-wave abnormalities, and bundle branch block. Different types of cardiac arrhythmias are also common in IDC. Systemic embolization in IDC is not uncommon. It reflects the formation of mural thrombus in dilated and hypokinetic left cardiac chamber.

The *preanesthetic management of IDC* includes general supportive measures which consist of adequate rest, weight control, controlled physical activity, and abstinence from tobacco-alcohol, etc. The vasodilator therapy by ACE-inhibitors, hydralazine, and isosorbide dinitrate is the standard initial treatment. It helps by reducing the myocardial workload for the patients with symptomatic LV dysfunction due to IDC. Patients with IDC are at increased risk for systemic or pulmonary embolism. As blood stasis occurs in the hypocontractile ventricle, so it leads to the activation of coagulation process. Hence, long-term anticoagulant therapy should be started in patient with IDC. Usually, warfarin is the drug of choice for long-term anticoagulation and is often adjusted to prolong the prothrombin time to an international normalized ratio (INR) of 2–3.

The risk of embolization is greatest in patients who are suffering from severe ventricular dysfunction, previous history of embolism, atrial fibrillation (AF), and present echocardiographic evidence of thrombus, etc. Digitalis effectively controls the symptoms of congestive heart failure in patients with IDC. Other inotropes such as amrinone, milrinone, or enoximone do not predictably improve the exercise tolerance like digitalis, when administered alone or in combination with digitalis.

During anesthetic management of a patient with IDC, the goals are:

- Prevention of increased LV afterload by controlling blood pressure (BP) and systemic vascular resistance (SVR)
- Avoidance of drug-induced myocardial depression
- Maintenance of normovolemia and preload.

During the *induction of anesthesia* thiopentone, propofol, etc., should be used cautiously, avoiding the myocardial depression. During the *maintenance of anesthesia,* myocardial depression, caused by the volatile anesthetic agents, must also be considered against the vasodilating properties of newer volatile anesthetic agents which are desirable. Opioids are associated with benign effects on cardiac contractility. So, it can be used judiciously. However, the use of N_2O with opioids may result in unexpected depression of myocardial contractility and pulmonary vasoconstriction. So, an anesthetist must justify himself regarding the use of N_2O in the cases of IDC, according to the merit of individual patient. Skeletal muscle paralysis should be provided by the nondepolarizing muscle relaxants which do not release histamine and lack significant cardiovascular effects. Tachycardia should be controlled by β1-antagonist such as esmolol, but keeping in mind the potential of these drugs to cause cardiac depression and severe bradycardia.

The *perioperative monitoring of patient,* suffering from IDC, will depend on the extent of the surgery and the severity of the disease. For the determination of cardiac filling pressure and CO, pulmonary artery catheterization is necessary. It will guide the intravenous infusion of fluid and blood. It will also help in the early recognition of volume overload and the need for inotropic support or the administration of peripheral vasodilating drugs. On venous pressure tracings, a prominent "A" wave reflects the decreased ventricular compliance and a prominent "V" wave indicates the functional incompetence of tricuspid or mitral valve, which is due to the cardiac dilatation. The intra-operative hypotension can be treated by vasopressor such as the ephedrine or phenylephrine. The ephedrine provides some degree of β stimulation, whereas phenylephrine produces α stimulation which evokes adverse increase in LV afterload, owing to the increased SVR.

In selected IDC patients, the regional anesthesia (RA) may also be an alternative to general anesthesia (GA), but caution is indicated to avoid an abrupt onset of blockade of sympathetic nervous system and sudden severe reduction of preload and afterload. The epidural anesthesia by a catheter produces the slow changes in preload and afterload and may meet the goals of the management of IDC.

HYPERTROPHIC OBSTRUCTIVE CARDIOMYOPATHY

Hypertrophic obstructive cardiomyopathy is an autosomal dominant inherited condition in which there is often massive asymmetrical ventricular hypertrophy and impaired diastolic function, i.e., decreased ventricular diastolic filling, causing the reduction of CO. It affects the patients of all ages. The excessive muscle bulk of LV wall also obstructs its outflow tract causing obstruction during systole. This HOCM is the most common form of cardiomyopathy with a prevalence of approximately 100 per 100,000 individual. In HOCM, the hypertrophy and the fibrosis of cardiac muscle mostly affects the septum, but may involve the whole left ventricle **(Fig. 2)**. Echocardiography reveals a large variation in the location and the extent of this ventricular muscular hypertrophy and fibrosis. Due to the ventricular muscular hypertrophy, there is also resistance to the inflow and therefore, the diastolic failure is the main problem. The hypertrophy of interventriculars septum may also cause dynamic LV outflow tract obstruction. But, even in the presence of severe LV outflow tract obstruction, ejection fraction is usually >0.8 (80%), reflecting the hypercontractile condition of heart (myocardium).

Hypertrophic obstructive cardiomyopathy presents a great diversity of morphological, functional, and clinical features. Some patients remain asymptomatic throughout their life with HOCM. Some have symptoms that extend from dyspnea, exercise intolerance, palpitation, and chest pain to severe CHF. In some patients, sudden death can occur particularly during exercise. The cause of this sudden death in HOCM is ventricular tachydysrhythmias such as ventricular tachycardia (VT) and ventricular fibrillation (VF). The symptoms and signs of HOCM are similar to those of aortic stenosis (AS). The marked LVH also makes the patient particularly vulnerable to myocardial ischemia. Clinically, the HOCM is detected by the murmur of dynamic

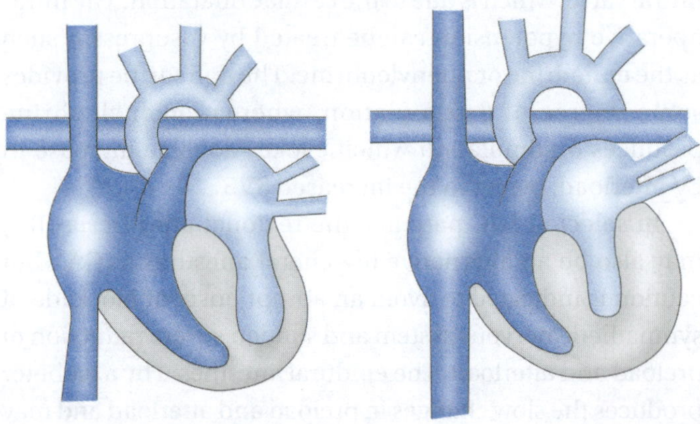

Fig. 2: Hypertrophic obstructive cardiomyopathy.

LV outflow tract obstruction in late systole. Its explanation is like that. Symptomatic patients frequently have a thickened intraventricular septum (IVS) of 20–30 mm. During systole, the anterior leaflet of mitral valve abuts the interventricular septum, producing obstruction and a late systolic murmur.

The diagnosis of HOCM is made by ECG, X-ray, and echocardiography. But, suspicions always should be raised by: (1) family history, (2) heaving or double apex, and (3) an aortic systolic murmur, but without a slow rising pulse like AS. The ECG and chest radiograph are usually abnormal and may show the features of massive LVH. The ECG usually also depict wide varieties of abnormal pattern such as pseudoinfarct, deep T-wave inversion, etc. In ECG, the massive hypertrophy of IVS presents abnormal Q-wave, mimicking myocardial infarction.

The *echocardiography is usually diagnostic*. However, diagnosis may be difficult, when the other causes of LV are present. When the ratio of septal and LV free wall thickness exceed 1.3:1, then the *diagnosis of hypertrophic cardiomyopathy should be considered*. Echocardiography is also useful for estimating the pressure gradient across LV outflow tract.

Cardiac catheterization may also demonstrate the presence of elevated left ventricular end-diastolic pressure (LVEDP) as a consequence of reduced LV compliance. The reduced LV compliance also produces the increased height of "A" waves during venous pressure tracing. It may exceed 30 mm Hg. If severe LV outflow obstruction is present, then there is demonstrable high-pressure gradient between the LV and aorta. Systemic thromboembolism is a very common complication of AF which is very commonly found in a patient presenting with HOCM.

Sudden death is an established complication of hypertrophic cardiomyopathy. The risk factors for this sudden death in HOCM are: (1) recurrent syncope, (2) exercise-induced hypotension, (3) marked increase in LV wall thickness, (4) multiple episodes of nonsustained VT (found in ambulatory ECG monitoring), (5) a history of previous cardiac arrest or sustained VT, and (6) an adverse family history. The patients with above mentioned three or more risk factors are thought to be at the high risk of sudden death, when they suffer from HOCM. Indeed, the HOCM is the most common cause of sudden death in young athletes and ventricular arrhythmia are thought to be responsible for many of such deaths in HOCM.

Anesthetic Management of HOCM

Though, the pharmacological therapy to improve the diastolic ventricular filling and to decrease the myocardial ischemia (which is due to the massive muscular hypertrophy)

is the primary goal of perianesthetic management for HOCM patient, still there is no treatment that is definitely known to improve the prognosis. The β-blockers and the heart rate (HR) limiting calcium antagonists (e.g., verapamil) have been used extensively to treat the HOCM preoperatively. It can also help to relieve the angina and to increase the exercise tolerance, by decreasing the HR with consequent prolongation of diastole and increased passive ventricular filling. But, there is no evidence that the β-blockers and verapamil will protect patients with HOCM from sudden death. Arrhythmias (mainly VF) are common in such patients and often respond to treatment with amiodarone. The control of arrhythmias in HOCM is very important, because it causes the rapid clinical deterioration by decreasing the diastolic ventricular filling and CO.

The dual chamber pacing and surgery are useful in selected HOCM patients, particularly those with outflow tract obstruction, due to massive ventricular muscular hypertrophy. The surgical reduction of the outflow tract obstruction is usually achieved by removing a small amount of cardiac muscle tissue from the ventricular septum. Surgery abolishes or greatly decreases the LV outflow obstruction in most patients. *Digoxin and vasodilator may increase the outflow tract obstruction and should be avoided or used with caution only in failure.* This is because many of these patients have diastolic dysfunction and require relatively high filling pressures to achieve adequate ventricular diastolic filling.

The intraoperative events that cause increased myocardial contractility are not desirable. Because, these events may also increase the LV outflow tract obstruction. So, the use of β-stimulant to increase myocardial contractility should be restricted (only in special situation). Anesthesia and surgery on patients, suffering previously from unrecognized (undiagnosed) HOCM, may manifest perioperatively as sudden unexpected hypotension. The administration of atropine in HOCM patient is questionable, as tachycardia could increase LV outflow obstruction and reduce LV diastolic filling by reducing the diastolic filling time. On the other hand, the use of scopolamine produces a desirable sedation and no increase in HR. Sedation is important, because it reduces the activation of sympathetic nervous system and LV outflow tract obstruction.

As the reduction of intravascular fluid volume causes the decrease in ventricular filling and subsequent decrease in CO, so the expansion of intravascular fluid volume during the preoperative period is useful to maintain the intraoperative stroke volume.

During the induction of anesthesia by inducing agents, the possibility of sudden decrease of SVR should be kept in mind, because it will increase the outflow tract obstruction and reduce the CO. On the other hand, the ketamine is not the likely choice as it stimulates the sympathetic system and increases the myocardial contraction (thus outflow obstruction). The activation of sympathetic system during laryngoscopy and intubation should be minimized by any cost by different procedures which are described before due to the same reasons.

The volatile anesthetic agents which cause the reduction of myocardial contractility, but do not decrease the SVR, are the ideal for HOCM patient. So, in such patient halothane is the ideal. But, there is no such evidence that volatile anesthetic agents, other than halothane, are detrimental for such patients. As opioids do not produce myocardial depression, so they are likely the choice for the maintenance of anesthesia. But, the opioid and N_2O combination cannot be used, because it produces the myocardial depression and increases the SVR.

The nondepolarizing muscle relaxants, with minimum effects on cardiovascular system, are the choice. In this regard, the pancuronium associated with increased HR, is not desirable. Intraoperative hypotension may be due to decreased preload or afterload or both. It should be monitored correctly by invasive method such as intra-arterial cannulation, pulmonary artery catheterization, or transesophageal echocardiography. Hypovolemia or vasodilatation can precipitate the myocardial ischemia and rapid decompensation. So, it should be avoided by any cost. When hypotension occurs, then drugs with predominantly α-adrenergic activity such as phenylephrine in the dose of 50–100 mg IV or metaraminol are useful for normalizing the systemic BP. Drugs with predominantly β-adrenergic agonist activity such as ephedrine, dopamine, or dobutamine are not recommended. Because these drugs cause increase in myocardial contractility and HR. Thus, they can increase the LV outflow tract obstruction. Intraoperative persistent increased systemic hypertension can also be treated by the gradual increase in the concentration of volatile anesthetic agents. But, the vasodilators such as nitroprusside, nitroglycerine, etc. should not be used, as the decreased SVR produced by them can accentuate the LV outflow tract obstruction.

The factors that increase the outflow tract obstruction in HOCM are: increased myocardial contractility (β-adrenergic stimulation, digitalis), tachycardia, decreased preload (hypovolemia, vasodilators such as nitroglycerine and nitroprusside), and decreased afterload (hypotension, vasodilators, and hypovolemia).

The factors that decrease the outflow tract obstruction in HOCM are: decreased myocardial contractility (β-adrenergic blocker, volatile anesthetics-halothane, and calcium channel blockers); increased preload (hypervolemia and bradycardia); and increased afterload (β-adrenergic stimulation and hypervolemia).

■ RESTRICTIVE CARDIOMYOPATHY

Among all the cardiomyopathies, it is the least common form. In this rare condition, the ventricular diastolic filling is impaired, because the walls of the ventricles become "stiff". Amyloidosis is the *most common cause* of stiff ventricle and the restrictive cardiomyopathy. However, the other causes of restrictive cardiomyopathy are: (i) glycogen storage disease, (ii) perimyocytic fibrosis, (iii) familial, etc. The increased stiffness of ventricular myocardium causes pressure within the ventricles to be increased precipitously, with only small volume of filling. Therefore, there is impaired ventricular filling, but no apparent diastolic dysfunction. The systolic function of ventricle usually remains normal. The diagnosis of restrictive cardiomyopathy is generally considered in patients, presenting with congestive heart failure, but there is no evidence of cardiomegaly or systolic dysfunction or hypertrophy.

The clinical presentation of restrictive cardiomyopathy is like constrictive pericarditis. Both the hearts (left and right) are affected equally. So, it may cause the symptoms and signs of right and/or LV failure. The diagnosis of restrictive cardiomyopathy is very difficult and may require investigations like complex Doppler echocardiograph, computed tomography (CT) scan, magnetic resonance imaging (MRI), or endomyocardial biopsy. It is usually diagnosed by the method of exclusion. It also must be differentiated from the age-related changes in ventricular diastolic compliance. The treatment of restrictive cardio-myopathy is symptomatic, but the prognosis is usually poor. AF is common in patient with restrictive cardiomyopathy. Angina pectoris does not usually occur in such patients.

The anesthetic management of patients with restrictive cardiomyopathy includes the same principles which are described for patients with other myopathies, usually those which are associated with ventricular diastolic dysfunction. AF is common in restrictive cardiomyopathy and by removing the artial contributing part to the ventricular filling, it may worsen the exiting diastolic dysfunction of LV with severe reduction of CO. So, the maintenance of normal sinus rhythm is very important. It can be achieved by digitalis or amiodarone or β-blockers or cardioversion or by pace making.

At the one hand, as the stroke volume tends to be fixed in the presence of restrictive cardiomyopathy, so the normal maintenance of venous return and intravascular fluid volume is essential for maintaining the normal CO. On the other hand, this form of myopathy is usually associated with pulmonary and systemic venous congestion which should be treated with diuretics. However, this diuretic may further decrease the ventricular filling pressure and CO. So, it should be used very cautiously. Anticoagulation with warfarin is likely with the aim to reduce the risk of embolic complications. The presence of anticoagulation and fixed CO may influence the decision of RA. The intraoperative monitoring is like that of other cardiomyopathies.

Pulmonary Diseases and Anesthesia

INTRODUCTION

The successful anesthetic management of patients with pulmonary (respiratory) diseases depends on: (1) the *accurate assessment* of the nature of pulmonary diseases, (2) the *extent* of the functional impairment of lungs due to these diseases, and (3) the *appreciation of the effects* of surgery and anesthesia on that already impaired pulmonary function of these patients. All these factors are interrelated and among these, the assessment of pulmonary function, before the anesthesia and surgery, is most important for the successful anesthetic management. This is because on it (the assessment of pulmonary function) depends the future anesthetic plan of action. Again, the proper assessment of functional impairment of lungs depends on: (1) the careful history, (2) the careful examination of the patient, and (3) the additional pulmonary functional tests, along with computerized tomography (CT) scan and magnetic resonance imaging (MRI).

EFFECTS OF ANESTHESIA AND SURGERY ON PULMONARY FUNCTIONS

Effects of Anesthesia on Pulmonary Functions

Anesthesia affects the pulmonary functions in the following ways:

- In a normal patient, general anesthesia (GA) induces the *reduction of functional residual capacity (FRC)* by about 450 mL (15–20% reduction). The normal value of FRC in a healthy individual is near about 3,000 mL. This reduction of FRC is due to the loss of the tone of respiratory muscles, such as the diaphragm and intercostal muscles. In a morbidly obese patient, this reduction of FRC may be up to 50% of the normal value in an *anesthetized, supine,* healthy individual. On the other hand, ketamine does not reduce the muscle tone and consequently FRC is not reduced so much. Contrary, it is maintained at the preanesthetic level.

- In normal situation, anesthesia *decreases both the tidal volume and the lung compliance*. This is due to the movement of diaphragm cranially and the movement of rib cage inwardly. The airway resistance also increases slightly, after GA due to these causes.

- Closing volume or closing capacity (CC) is the lung volume at which the closure of small airways begins. In a healthy unanesthetized patient CC < FRC. But under GA *CC > FRC* and the airway closure with air trapping occur, before the lung volume reaches its FRC value. This is more common in elderly, smokers, and those with underlying lung diseases. Due to this premature airway closure and air trapping (due to CC > FRC) there is decreased partial pressure of arterial oxygen ($\downarrow PaO_2$), increased partial pressure of arterial carbon dioxide ($\uparrow PaCO_2$), and mismatch ventilation–perfusion (V/Q) ratio.

- Intubation *reduces the dead space (Vd)* nearly to half of its normal value by circumventing the upper airway. But the *alveolar Vd rises* from 50 to about 70 mL.

- In over 80% of subjects, intubation causes *atelectasis* in the dependent portion of the lungs. As a result, the 10% of pulmonary blood flow is shunted through these areas of low V/Q ratio, resulting in *hypoxia* and *hypercarbia*.

- In anesthesia, the ventilatory response to hypoxia and hypercarbia is blunted and the acute response to this hypoxia and acidemia is almost abolished by anesthetic vapors at a concentration of as low as 0.1 MAC (minimum alveolar concentration).

- Most of these adverse effects, induced by anesthesia, usually improve within few hours, postoperatively. But they are more marked and improvement is delayed in patients with lung diseases. After surgery, they may last for several days.

Effects of Surgery on Pulmonary Functions

Surgery affects the respiratory functions in three ways and these are: (1) type of surgery, (2) site of surgery, and (3) existing pulmonary disease.

- The site of surgery has major implications on the respiratory functions and the incidences of pulmonary complications. For example, the lower abdominal surgery is associated with pulmonary complication only in 2–5% of cases. But these incidences of pulmonary complications in upper abdominal surgery go up to about 20–40%. These incidences are further higher in thoracic surgery and it is because following the thoracic and upper abdominal surgery, there are (1) shallow respiration, (2) inability to cough effectively, and (3) the reduction of lung volumes. All these factors lead to the poor entry of air in the basal portions of lung and sputum retention. Thus, this produces atelectasis and/or infection. The incidences and the severity of these complications can be reduced by (1) effective multimodal and opioid-sparing postoperative analgesia, (2) early mobilization, (3) pulmonary exercise, and (4) physiotherapy.
- Patients with already underlying pulmonary diseases are at the increased risk of developing pulmonary complications during and after surgery. The complications can be minimized, if the underlying pulmonary conditions are identified and optimally controlled preoperatively.

■ PREOPERATIVE EVALUATION

History of Pulmonary Diseases

For the assessment of pulmonary function, proper history of patient, regarding the previous pulmonary diseases, is very important. In history, the six cardinal symptoms of respiratory diseases, which are commonly asked for, are: *cough, sputum, hemoptysis, dyspnea, wheeze, and chest pain.*

Dyspnea

Now, among these six cardinal symptoms, the detailed history regarding the *dyspnea* provides the best assessment for the functional impairment of lung. So, some specific questions are required to elicit the extent to which the activity is limited by dyspnea. Dyspnea at rest or during minor activities clearly indicates severe pulmonary and cardiac disease. Again, for evaluating a patient with dyspnea, one should first determine the duration over which the symptoms have become manifested. When it develops in *acute form* over a period of hours, then the patients can have acute diseases, affecting the airways or lung parenchyma, such as acute asthma, acute pulmonary edema, or acute bacterial

infection (pneumonia). In other causes of acute dyspnea, the patient can have acute diseases affecting the pleural space or the pulmonary vasculature, such as the pneumothorax or pulmonary embolism or the acute cardiac causes.

The *subacute* presentation of dyspnea, over days or weeks, suggests the exacerbation of a preexisting airway disease, such as chronic asthma or chronic bronchitis. It may also be due to the slowly progressing inflammatory process of lung parenchyma (infective or noninfective) or slowly progressing pleural diseases, such as the pleural effusion from the varieties of possible causes or chronic cardiac disease.

The *chronic* presentation of dyspnea, over months or years, often indicates chronic obstructive lung disease (COLD) or chronic cardiac disease. Chronic disease of airways such as COLD and asthma are characterized by periodic exacerbations and remissions of symptoms. So the patients have severe symptoms, interspersed with periods in which the symptoms are minimal or absent. Ideally, in such a situation anesthesia is given and surgery is performed when the patient is optimally controlled. Any respiratory symptoms suggestive of cardiac diseases, such as orthopnea and paroxysmal nocturnal dyspnea also should be noted. Dyspnea can be graded using Roizen's classification. Undiagnosed dyspnea of grade II or above should be investigated further **(Table 1)**.

Cough and Sputum

Among other cardinal symptoms, after dyspnea, *cough* always indicates the presence of an active lung disease, but it does not help in differential diagnosis. The presence of other symptoms, accompanying with cough, always suggests the airway diseases and may be seen in asthma, chronic bronchitis, pneumonitis, etc. A productive cough with expectoration of *purulent sputum* always indicates an active infection of lung. The chronic copious sputum production may indicate bronchiectasis.

TABLE 1: Roizen's classification of dyspnea.	
Grades	**Features**
Grade 0	No dyspnea while walking at normal space on the ground level
Grade I	Taking time the patient can walk as far as he likes without dyspnea
Grade II	Patient can move only few corners of street without dyspnea
Grade III	Dyspnea on mild exertion, i.e., after walking a few steps
Grade IV	Dyspnea at rest

Hemoptysis

Hemoptysis can originate from the pathology of airways, lung parenchyma, or pulmonary vasculatures. The disease may be inflammatory, such as bronchitis, bronchiectasis, cystic fibrosis, or neoplastic such as bronchogenic carcinoma. The hemoptysis may also be due to localized pathologies, such as pneumonia, lung abscess, tuberculosis, or due to diffused pathologies such as Good pasture's syndrome and idiopathic pulmonary hemosiderosis. The vascular diseases which are potentially associated with hemoptysis, include pulmonary thromboembolic disease or pulmonary arteriovenous malformation.

Chest Pain

It is another common respiratory symptom other than dyspnea, cough, and hemoptysis. It is usually due to the involvement of parietal pleura, not lung parenchyma (involvement of lung parenchyma does not produce any pain). So, this chest pain is often referred to as the pleuritic pain and is accentuated by respiratory movement. The common causes of this pleuritic pain are inflammatory disorders or neoplasm of pleura. Again, the inflammatory disorders of pleura may be due to (1) the pleura itself, such as pleuritis, or (2) lung parenchymal disorders that extend up to the pleural surface, such as pneumonia and pulmonary infarction.

History of Smoking

A *history of smoking* and a history of occupational exposure to dust or fumes may suggest pulmonary pathology. The smoking history should include: the number of years and the intensity of smoking. The cigarette smoke contains highly additive nicotine and other 4,700 chemical compounds. Among these, 43 chemical compounds are known to be carcinogenic. The long-term smoking causes serious underlying problems, such as COLD, ischemic heart disease (IHD), vascular diseases, and lung neoplasm.

In smokers, the mucus is produced in large quantities from respiratory tract, but is cleared less efficiently due to the impaired mucociliary function of the airway epithelium. In such patients, the airways remain hyperreactive and there is impairment of both the cell-mediated and humoral immunity. These changes make the smokers more susceptible to respiratory complications, during anesthesia and also to postoperative atelectasis or pneumonia. The coexisting obesity with lung diseases also increases these pulmonary complications.

Increased airway irritability by smoking or dust increases cough, laryngospasm, and early desaturation of hemoglobin during induction of anesthesia by volatile anesthetic agents, especially isoflurane. This can be avoided by using less irritant

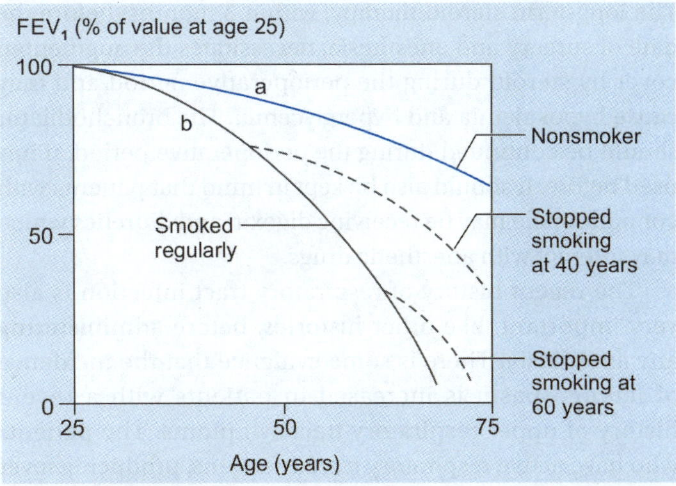

Fig. 1: Graphical representation of decline in forced expiratory volume in first 1 second (FEV$_1$) annually in susceptible smokers. The (line-a) at the top shows the normal decline of FEV$_1$ with age, in a nonsmoker. The (line-b) represents the smokers. When smoking is stopped, then the subsequent decline of FEV$_1$ is similar to that in healthy nonsmokers, represented by dotted line.

volatile anesthetic agents such as sevoflurane or halothane or intravenous (IV) agent such as propofol or deepening the anesthesia slowly, when the volatile anesthetic agents are used. During the maintenance of anesthesia by spontaneous respiration through endotracheal tube (ETT) or laryngeal mask airway (LMA), it may be troublesome due to airway irritation **(Fig. 1)**.

Now, if the patient is not a smoker, then the duration of cessation of smoking should also be enquired. Before anesthesia and surgery, the minimum 8 weeks of abstinence from smoking is required to decrease the morbidity from respiratory complications to a rate which is similar to that of nonsmokers. In very resistance cases, if it is not possible to stop smoking, then the patient can get benefit by restraining from smoking, for at least 10 hours, before surgery and anesthesia. During this period, the effects of nicotine, i.e., activation of sympathoadrenergic system, with raised coronary vascular resistance, will wear off. The carboxyhemoglobin, which may reach 5–15% in heavy smokers, will also fall during this period of abstinence. Carboxyhemoglobin reduces the O$_2$ carrying capacity of blood by shifting the O$_2$–Hb dissociation curb toward the left. Again, the carboxyhemoglobin has similar absorption spectrum to O$_2$–Hb. This will cause the pulse oximeter to give a falsely high O$_2$ saturation reading. The risk of lung cancer falls progressively, with increased interval, following the discontinuation of smoking. The loss of lung function, above the expected age-related decline, also ceases with the discontinuation of smoking.

A detailed drug history of a patient with pulmonary diseases, going for surgery and anesthesia, is important.

The long-term steroid therapy, within 3 months, before the date of surgery and anesthesia, necessitates the augmented cover by steroid during the perioperative period and may cause hypokalemia and hyperglycemia. The bronchodilator should be continued during the perioperative period, if it is used before. It should also be kept in mind that patients with cor pulmonale may be receiving digoxin and diuretics which may interact with anesthetic drugs.

The recent history of respiratory tract infection is also very important, like other histories, before administering any anesthesia. There is some evidence that the incidence of laryngospasm is increased in patients with a recent history of upper respiratory tract symptoms. The patients who have active respiratory tract infections, producing fever and cough, and with or without chest signs on auscultation, should not undergo elective surgery under GA. This is because it is associated with increased perioperative risk of pulmonary complications. But the adult patients with simple coryza are not at the significantly increased risk of developing perioperative pulmonary problems, unless they have preexisting respiratory diseases or are having major abdominal and thoracic surgery, compared with asymptomatic patients. The children, with symptoms of acute or recent upper respiratory tract infection (URTI), are more likely to suffer from more incidences of laryngospasm, ronchi, creps, and postoperative hypoxemia [peripheral oxygen saturation (SPO$_2$) <93%]. This is more marked when intubation is performed.

Examination of Respiratory System

For the assessment of lung condition and pulmonary function, like history, the physical examination of respiratory system is also very important. A full physical examination of patient is done with the aim of detecting (1) the signs of airway obstruction, or (2) increased work of breathing, or (3) active infection, or (4) any evidence of heart failure because all these can be treated preoperatively. The full physical examination of respiratory system of a patient includes: *inspection, palpation, percussion, and auscultation of respiratory system.* But among these examinations, the auscultation is most important. During auscultation, both the quality and the intensity of breath sounds, in both the lungs, should be looked for the presence of any extra or adventitious sounds.

Normal breath sound is heard through stethoscope at the periphery of lungs. These are described as vesicular. In it (the vesicular sound), the inspiration part is louder and longer than expiration. When the transmission of sound is improved through a consolidated part of lung, then the resulting bronchial breath sound is more tubular in quality

and is characterized by more pronounced expiratory phase. The primary adventitious or abnormal sounds that can be heard by stethoscope, during auscultation, include *crackles (rales), wheezes, and rhonchi.* The *crackles* represent the sound which is created when the alveoli and the small airways open and close during respiration. Therefore, often they are associated with interstitial lung disease, microatelectasis, or filling of alveoli by liquid.

Wheezes, which are generally more prominent during expiration than inspiration, reflect the oscillation of the walls of airways that occurs when there is an obstruction of airflow. Thus, it is produced by bronchospasm, airway edema, collapse, or intraluminal obstruction by neoplasm or secretions, etc. *Rhonchi* is the term, applied to the sounds, which is created when there is free liquid in the lumen of airway. The interaction between the free liquid in the lumen of airway and the moving air through it creates a high-pitched vibratory rhonchi sound. Other adventitious sounds, during the auscultation of lung, include pleural *friction rubs* and stridor. The gritty sound, which is produced by pleural friction, indicates inflamed pleural surfaces rubbing against each other. It is heard both during the inspiratory and expiratory phases of respiratory cycle. *Stridor* represents the flow of air through a narrowed upper airway which occurs primarily during inspiration.

After the meticulous examination of respiratory system, a careful general physical examination of the whole body of the patient, waiting for anesthesia, is also mandatory. This is because a number of systemic diseases, such as systemic lupus erythematosus, scleroderma, and rheumatoid arthritis may affect the respiratory system. So, they may be associated with pulmonary complications, even though their primary clinical manifestations and physical findings are not related to lungs. On the contrary, the other diseases that most affect the respiratory system, such as sarcoidosis, can have findings on physical examinations with other systems which are not related to the respiratory system. So, they have findings which are not related to the lungs, such as the ocular findings (uveitis, conjunctival granuloma) and the skin findings (erythema nodosum, cutaneous granulomas).

Investigations

X-ray

To evaluate the respiratory system of a patient, who is presented for anesthesia and surgery, with the history of pulmonary diseases, the chest radiograph is often the initial and the most important diagnostic procedure. This is because it can provide the initial evidence of pulmonary disease in patients, even who are still free of respiratory symptoms at present. The example of this is the accidental finding of one or more nodules or a big mass, when the chest X-ray is performed due to reasons, other than the evaluation of respiratory symptoms. The radiographic findings, even in the absence of respiratory symptoms, often indicate a localized disease affecting the local airways or a discrete disease affecting the whole pulmonary parenchyma. One or more nodules or a large mass may suggest intrathoracic malignancy. But they can also be the manifestation of a current or previous infective process. On the other hand, the patients with diffuse parenchymal lung disease, evidenced by radiographic examination, may be free of symptoms, as is sometimes seen in the cases with pulmonary sarcoidosis.

A localized opacity, involving the lung parenchyma, is usually characterized by having an alveolar or a nodular pattern. In contrast, the increased radiolucency can be localized, as occurs with a cyst or bulla, or generalized as seen with emphysema. The chest radiograph is also particularly useful for the detection of pleural disease. An abnormal picture of hila and/or mediastinum structure can suggest a mass or enlargement of lymph nodes. The patients with respiratory symptoms, but with a normal chest X-ray, most commonly have the diseases of airway. This is happened in asthma, chronic obstructive pulmonary disease (COPD) or interstitial lung disease, etc. The chest X-ray is also normal in respiratory symptoms, when there is disorder of respiratory pump mechanism, i.e., chest wall, and neuromuscular apparatus, controlling the movement of chest wall. Here, the pulmonary function test is helpful for diagnosis.

The preoperative chest X-ray is a poor indicator for the functional impairment of lungs. But still it is important for several following reasons, for the preoperative evaluation of respiratory system:

- It helps as baseline to assess the postoperative radiographs.
- It helps to discover any localized disease of lungs and pleura which are not symptom-producing and are not detected on clinical examination, such as a small neoplasm, a small collapse or consolidation, not symptom producing small effusion, etc.
- To reveal the underlying generalized lung disease in patients, presenting with acute pulmonary symptoms such as pulmonary fibrosis and emphysema

Computerized Tomography Scan of Thorax

For the proper diagnosis of pulmonary diseases, which have tremendous impact on the mode and the result of anesthesia, the preoperative CT offers several advantages over the routine chest X-ray. It is better for characterizing the tissue densities which helps in distinguishing the subtle differences between the adjacent structures and providing the accurate assessment of the size and the character of the lesions. It is particularly valuable in (1) assessing the hilar and mediastinal structures and their diseases, (2) identifying the diseases adjacent to the chest wall or spine, (3) identifying the areas of fat bodies (pulmonary fat embolism) in lungs, and (4) the calcification of pulmonary nodules. For the diagnosis, assessment, and staging of malignant mediastinal diseases, CT is the most important tool among all. By the use of contrast material, CT also makes it possible to distinguish the vascular from nonvascular structures. Helical CT scanning, which is more informative than conventional CT, allows the collection of continuous data over a large volume of lung tissue, during a single breath-holding maneuver. With high-resolution CT (HRCT) the thickness of individual cross-sectional images is approximately 1–2 mm, rather than the usual 10 mm. The images in HRCT are reconstructed by using high spatial resolution algorithms. The details, that can be seen in HRCT scan, allow better recognition of any subtle parenchymal and airway diseases, such as bronchiectasis, emphysema, and diffuse parenchymal diseases.

Magnetic Resonance Imaging Scan of Thorax

The MRI provides less described view of airways and pulmonary parenchyma than CT. So, the role of MRI in the evaluation of pulmonary diseases is less well defined. But the MRI has certain advantages over CT in certain clinical circumstances (pulmonary diseases). For example, by MRI the vascular structures can be easily distinguished from the nonvascular structures, without the need of contrast media. The flowing blood does not produce any signal on MRI. So, the vessels appear as hollow tubular structures in MRI. This feature is helpful in determining, whether the abnormal hilar or mediastinal structures are of vascular origin or not. For the diagnosis of aortic lesions, such as aneurysm or aortic dissection, MRI is extremely helpful. The another advantage of MRI over CT is that it can be reconstructed in sagittal, coronal, and transverse plane, whereas CT is constructed only in transverse plane.

Other radiological investigations, except the X-ray, CT, and MRI, for the accurate diagnosis of pulmonary diseases are: *scintigraphic imaging* and *pulmonary angiography.* In *scintigraphic imaging,* the radioactive isotopes, such as the (1) albumin macroaggregates, labeled with technetium 99 m, or (2) radiolabeled xenon gas, are administered either through the IV or inhalational route, respectively. It is most commonly used in ventilation–perfusion lung scanning (V/Q scan), and for the evaluation of pulmonary embolism. The IV isotopes demonstrate the *distribution of blood flow,* whereas the inhaled isotope demonstrates the *distribution of ventilation*. Thus, a perfusion–ventilation mismatch is constructed.

One such example is the pulmonary embolism where there is defect in perfusion, but there is no defect in ventilation. Another common use of such radioisotope scan is for the diagnosis of impaired lung function which is being considered for lung resection. The distribution of isotope also can be used to assess the regional distribution of blood flow and ventilation. The pulmonary arterial system can also be visualized by *pulmonary angiography*, in which radiopaque contrast media is injected into the pulmonary artery through a catheter which is previously threaded. The pulmonary angiography demonstrates the intravascular clot (pulmonary embolism), either as filling defect in the lumen of vessel (filling defect sign), or as an abrupt termination of a vessel (cutoff sign). In patients, with abnormal chest radiograph, this test is often difficult to interpret.

The ultrasound (USG) imaging is not useful for the evaluation of pulmonary parenchymal diseases because the USG energy is rapidly dissipated by air, present in lungs. USG is only helpful for the detection and localization of pleural fluid and as a guide for the placement of a needle for thoracocentesis.

Measurement of Diffusing Capacity or Gas Transfer Factor of Lung for Carbon Monoxide

The transfer factor or diffusing capacity of lung is the *measurement of lung's ability to transfer the gases* from its alveoli into blood. This test utilizes the uptake of carbon monoxide (CO), by a single breath, from a 0.3% mixture of it, in air. This gas is chosen for the measurement of transfer factor of lungs because it combines very rapidly with Hb and provides a true estimation of the diffusion or transfer of gases across the alveolar–capillary membrane. The diffusing capacity or the transfer factor of lungs is reduced in patients with diseases which principally affect the alveoli, such as fibrosis, alveolitis, and emphysema. The transfer coefficient is the measurement of diffusing capacity, expressed per volume of ventilated lung, during a single breath test. This is useful to confirm that a low diffusing capacity is due to alveolar disease, rather than maldistribution of ventilation. The high values of diffusing capacity may be seen in alveolar hemorrhage.

The measurement of H^+ ion concentration, PaO_2, $PaCO_2$, and bicarbonate concentration in arterial blood is also essential in assessing (1) the respiratory function of lungs, (2) the degree and the type of respiratory failure, and (3) the overall acid–base status of patient. A preoperative baseline provides a guideline for the further intraoperative and postoperative management of patient. It should be measured in any patient who is suffering from mild-to-severe dyspnea on minimal exertion. CO_2 retention will be detected and the efficiency of oxygenation is assessed. A resting $PaCO_2$ >6 kPa suggests pulmonary complications and pending ventilatory failure.

Pulmonary Function Tests

From the anesthetic point of view, the pulmonary function tests (PFTs) are very helpful for the determination of pulmonary functional reserve which deteriorates rapidly due to the different pulmonary airways and lung parenchymal diseases and the effect of bronchodilators on these diseases. So, the pulmonary function tests are discussed in detail in a separate chapter. But few parameters of it are discussed here which are peak flow rate, spirometry, and flow–volume (*F–V*) loops **(Table 2)**.

Peak flow rate: For the evaluation of airway obstruction, the measurement of airway resistance is specific and sensitive. But, the measurement of airway resistance is not easy and is very cumbersome. So, the airway obstruction is commonly evaluated by the measurement of maximal forced expiration or maximal mid-expiratory flow rate (MMEFR). The simplest of such measurement is the peak expiratory flow rate (PEFR). This is conveniently measured by a variable orifice flow meter at bedside. The main *disadvantage of this peak flow value* is that it is highly dependent on the personal effort and subject's cooperation. So, the result varies significantly. However, as the variation of measurement in the same subject is surprisingly low, so the *PEFR* is fairly a reproducible test of airway function. A single result of PEFR has no value. So, the serial measurement of it only indicates the deterioration. The PEFR of <200 L/min indicates that the effective coughing is difficult and pulmonary complications rate are high **(Fig. 2)**.

TABLE 2: Patterns of abnormal ventilatory capacity in spirometry.			
	Asthma	*Emphysema*	*Lung fibrosis*
FEV$_1$	↓	↓	↓
VC	↓	↓	↓
FEV$_1$/VC	↓	↓	N
TLCO	N	↓	↓
KCO	N	↓	↓
TLC	↑	↑	↓
RV	↑	↑	↓

↓ = Decreased, N = Normal, ↑ = Increased
(FEV$_1$: forced expiratory volume in first 1 second; KCO: transfer coefficient for CO; RV: residual volume; TLC: total lung capacity; TLCO: gas transfer factor of lung for carbon monoxide; VC: vital capacity)

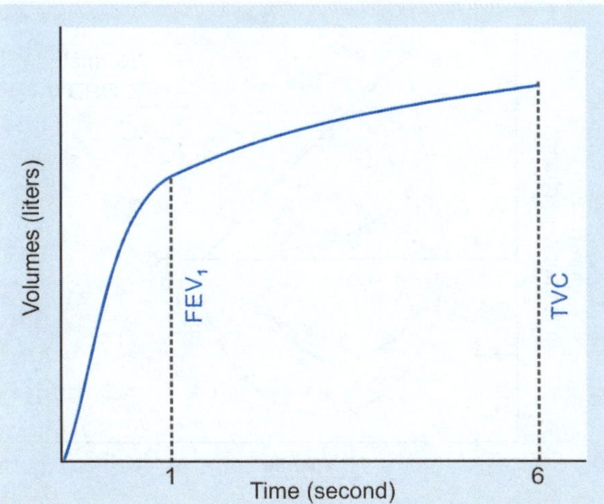

Fig. 2: This graph represents the peak expiratory flow rate demonstrating the forced expiratory volume in first 1 second (FEV₁) and total vital capacity (TVC), the next part of expiration.

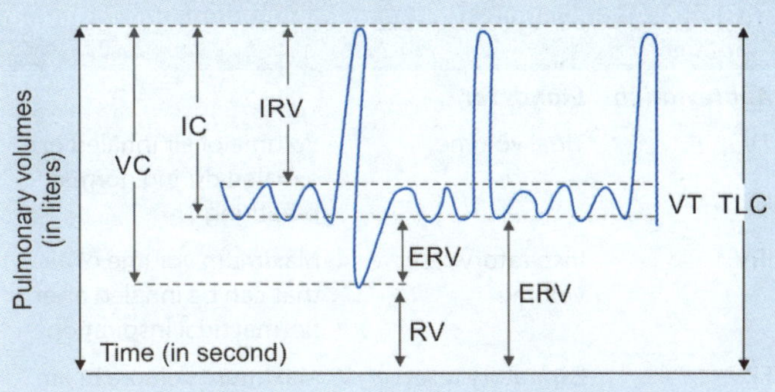

Fig. 3: Schematic diagram of normal spirogram showing different pulmonary volumes and capacities. (IC: inspiratory capacity; ERV: expiratory reserve volume; IRV: inspiratory reserve volume; RV: residual volume; TLC: total lung capacity; VC: vital capacity; VT: tidal volume)

The another extensively used indirect evaluation of airway obstruction is forced expiratory volume in first 1 second (FEV₁). It is the fraction of vital capacity (VC) which is expired *during the first 1 second of a forced expiration*. So, it is also called as the *timed vital capacity*. The VC is the largest amount of air that can be expired after a maximal inspiratory effort. So, the FEV₁ is measured frequently clinically, as the index of pulmonary function and gives a useful information, about the strength of the respiratory muscle. The FEV₁ also gives additional information because the VC may be normal, but the FEV₁ reduces in diseases, such as the airway obstruction (e.g., asthma) in which the airway resistance is increased by bronchial constriction.

Spirometry: Simple spirometry should be a routine procedure and is carried out by all the doctors, when assessing a patient who is breathless. It has been widely used to assess the functional reserve of lungs and to assess the magnitude of risks in patients who are suffering from significant pulmonary diseases and is scheduled for major surgery and anesthesia. It can also be used as a bedside method, using a device of bellow or in any investigating center, using a sophisticated instrument. In spirometer, different pulmonary volumes are studied by recording graphically the changes of the volume and capacities of lungs, under different conditions of respiration. This graphical recording of the different volumes and capacities of lungs is called the spirogram which is represented in **Figure 3**.

The different abbreviations, used in PFT, by spirometer are also shown in **Table 3**. All the present results of spirometry are compared with the predicted normal values which are based on age, sex, height, and ethnic group.

Normally, the forced vital capacity (FVC) is measured along with FEV₁ and the ratio of FEV₁/FVC is measured as percentage. Normally the FEV₁/FVC ratio is >70%. But when it is >70%, it indicates airflow obstruction. In obstructive symptoms, the reversibility, using the inhaled short-acting β₂-adrenoreceptor agonists (e.g., salbutamol or terbutaline), also can be tested. Full reversibility is diagnostic of asthma. If time permits and the patient has undertreated obstructive disease, then a course of steroids (prednisolone 20–40 mg daily for 7 days) should be assessed for effectiveness **(Fig. 3 and Table 3)**.

Recently, the evidences suggest that spirometry does not always predict the perioperative pulmonary complications, even in patients with severe COPD. Only the specific subgroups may be benefited by preoperative spirometry, such as (1) those with unclear diagnosis or those with equivocal clinical and radiological findings and (2) those where functional impairment of lungs cannot be assessed due to extreme disability.

There are no spirometric values which should be considered as prohibitive for anesthesia and surgery. Despite poor preoperative spirometry result, many series of patients, undergoing thoracic and major nonthoracic surgery, are being increasingly reported. A FEV₁ of <1,000 mL indicates that the postoperative coughing and the clearance of secretions will be poor and will increase the likelihood of respiratory support for a brief period, following major surgery.

F–V loop: Sometimes, there is no clinical evidence of bronchial asthma, COPD, etc., but the findings of reduced peak flow rate and reduced FEV₁ are present. This indicates the presence of upper airway obstruction, such as in larynx, pharynx, or trachea. In such a situation, the F–V loop is helpful

TABLE 3: Abbreviations used in pulmonary function testing in spirometer.

Abbreviation	Stands for	
TV	Tidal volume	Volume of air inhaled or exhaled during normal breathing
IRV	Inspiratory reserve volume	Maximum volume of air that can be inhaled after a normal tidal inspiration
ERV	Expiratory reserve volume	Maximum volume of air that can be exhaled after a normal tidal expiration
VC	Vital capacity	Maximum volume of air that can be exhaled after a forced inspiration, i.e., VC = TV + IRV + ERV
RV	Residual volume	Volume of air that remains in lungs after ERV (maximum expiration)
IVC or IC	Inspiratory vital capacity/inspiratory capacity	Maximum volume of air that can be inspired after reaching the end of a normal, quiet expiration, i.e. IVC = TV + IRV
FEV$_1$	Forced expiratory volume in first 1 second	Volume of air exhaled in first 1 second during complete forced expiration
FVC	Forced vital capacity	The amount of air that an individual is able to forcibly exhale from his/her lungs after taking the deepest breath they can
PEF	Peak (maximum) expiratory flow	The volume of air that can forcefully be expelled from lungs in one quick exhalation
TLC	Total lung capacity	The volume of air in the lungs after the maximum effort of inspiration. TLC = RV + IVC, or TLC = FRC + IC
FRC	Functional residual capacity	Volume of air that remains in lungs after a normal tidal expiration
TLCO	Gas transfer factor of lung for carbon monoxide	TLCO refers to the transfer capacity of lung for the uptake of carbon monoxide (CO). It also refers to the diffusion capacity for CO and also refers the extent to which the O$_2$ passes from the air sacs of lungs into the blood

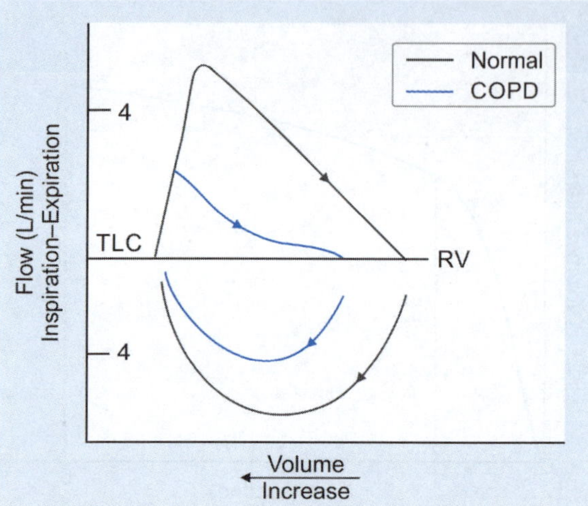

Fig. 4: Schematic flow–volume curve in a normal subject and in a patient with chronic obstructive pulmonary disease (COPD). (RV: residual volume; TLC: total lung capacity)

in differentiating between the upper airway obstruction in pharynx, larynx, or trachea (extrinsic obstruction) and the diffuse airway obstruction such as in asthma and COPD (intrinsic obstruction). In addition, they also provide useful data about the severity of the diffuse airway obstruction and the restrictive pulmonary diseases. The F–V loop not only helps in suspecting upper airway obstruction, but may also help to localize the site and the nature of obstruction **(Fig. 4)**.

In *F–V* loops, the flow and the volume are plotted on an X and Y axis respectively. The several characteristic patterns of *F–V* loop have been described, among which few are discussed below. In fixed airway obstruction, such as a growth in larynx, no significant change in airway diameter occurs during inspiration and expiration. As a result, the inspiratory and expiratory phase shows a plateau of constant flow, over the effort-dependent portion of vital capacity, in variable upper airway obstruction (extrathoracic), such as in vocal cord paralysis, pharyngeal muscle weakness, and chronic neuromuscular disorders. The inspiratory and expiratory phases are not equal. In upper airway obstruction, the period of inspiration is reduced more than the expiratory period which is reflected in loop.

This is because during forced inspiration the negative transmural pressure inside the airway tends to collapse the airway with increasing effort and reduce the inspiratory flow. But during expiration, the positive pressure in the upper airway tries to reduce the obstruction. So, the expiratory flow is not reduced and may even be normal. In variable airway obstruction (intrathoracic), such as tumor in trachea and major bronchi, the expiration becomes longer and plateau usually occurs. This is because during expiration compressed airway lumen assumes its minimal size at the area of lesions. But the inspiratory portion of F–V loop may be quite normal. In diffuse airway obstruction the F–V loop takes a characteristic appearance which is shown in **Figure 4**.

PREDICTING PERIOPERATIVE PULMONARY COMPLICATIONS

The multiple large and rigorous studies, identifying the risk factors for perioperative pulmonary complications, are still lacking, though the comparison of large prospective studies to identify the pulmonary risk factors are performed. This is because to make comparison between the studies on pulmonary function is very difficult. Still, some risk factors are identified **(Box 1)** and the incidence of perioperative complications can be reduced, if these patients are treated properly preoperatively.

Formerly, the spirometry was considered as an important tool for the assessment of risk factors. But recent evidence suggests that it does not properly predict the risk of perioperative pulmonary complications.

GENERAL PRINCIPLE FOR POSTOPERATIVE CARE IN PULMONARY DISEASE

The postoperative care of all patients, with pulmonary diseases, can be guided by the following principles.

Early Mobilization

Early mobilization is the cornerstone of postoperative management for a patient, suffering from respiratory diseases. It reduces the incidences of pulmonary thromboembolic manifestations. Lung performance, FRC, and clearance of secretions are also improved, when the patient is sitting or standing, in comparison to supine and prone position.

Therefore, it should not be used alone to determine the risks. The general scoring systems, such as American Society of Anesthesiologists (ASA) grading system, Goldman Cardiac Risk Index, and Charlson Comorbidity Index which

assess the overall comorbidity are also the best predictors for possible pulmonary complications. The abnormal chest findings on clinical examination and in X-ray reflect significant lung disease and are independent predictors of pulmonary complications.

Physiotherapy

As a part of pulmonary physiotherapy, the incentive spirometry and breathing exercise helps to clear the bronchial secretions and thus reduce the risks of atelectasis and its pulmonary complications.

Oxygen Therapy

In patients with lung disease, the dose (of anesthetic drugs)-dependent depression of respiratory function and the dose-dependent depression of the sensitivity of central chemoreceptors to the stimulatory effect of CO_2 on ventilation can occur for up to 72 hours postoperatively. It is mostly found at night. So, supplemental O_2 should be delivered for at least this period of time. The COPD patients chronically retain CO_2. Therefore, they depend on hypoxemia for their main ventilatory drive due to the downregulation of central chemoreceptors to CO_2. Hence, O_2 therapy should be controlled and guided by adequate monitoring, such as blood gas analysis. A preoperative data of PaO_2, SaO_2, and $PaCO_2$ are essential to establish a realistic ventilation target for each patient. During O_2 therapy, it must be humidified to help sputum clearance and physiotherapy.

Fluid Balance

Patients with lung diseases are at increased risk of fluid overload and pulmonary edema. This is caused by dilated and hypertrophied right ventricle, due to commonly associated pulmonary hypertension, with pulmonary disease. Thus, it may mechanically compromise the function of left ventricle, leading to pulmonary edema. So, a high index of suspicion, regarding the overload of fluid, leading to pulmonary edema, should be maintained clinically. The reading of CVP, as a guidance of fluid therapy, is misleading in the presence of pulmonary hypertension.

Pain Management

Good analgesia without sedation is very essential for the best postoperative management of patients, suffering from pulmonary diseases. This properly titrated postoperative analgesia helps by maintaining the early mobilization, increasing the compliance of physiotherapy, increasing the proper respiratory function, and minimizing the cardiac stress with heart diseases. The patients with respiratory diseases are best benefited by local or regional analgesia. It helps by avoiding the sedative and respiratory depressive

---

BOX 1: Risk factors to predict the perioperative pulmonary complications.

- Increased age >60 years
- Symptoms of chronic bronchitis
- Smoking within 8 weeks
- Body mass index >30
- Abnormal clinical findings in chest
- Abnormal finding in chest X-ray
- History of pulmonary malignancy
- P_aCO_2 >6 kPa
- Upper abdominal and thoracic surgery

($PaCO_2$: partial pressure of arterial carbon dioxide)

effect of narcotics. The risk–benefit ratio of opioid-based analgesia and regional analgesia should be weighted, against each other. The paracetamol and other nonsteroidal anti-inflammatory drugs (NSAIDs) are not absolutely contraindicated in pulmonary airway disease. They should be used, where possible.

Regular Clinical Review

Regular clinical review always allows early detection of respiratory deterioration and resolution of problem.

INDIVIDUAL PULMONARY DISEASE AND ANESTHETIC MANAGEMENT

Bronchial Asthma

Etiology and Pathology

Bronchial asthma is primarily the disease of small airways. It is characterized by the reversible obstruction of airflow, resulting from bronchial smooth muscle contraction, edema, and increased secretion due to the increased responsiveness of tracheobronchial tree to a number of stimuli. All the aspects of pulmonary functions are virtually compromised, during an acute attack of it. This disease is manifested clinically by paroxysms of dyspnea, cough, and wheeze, following a generalized narrowing as well as the inflammatory changes of air passages. As it is an episodic disease, so an acute exacerbation is interspersed with symptom-free periods. Usually, most of the acute attacks of bronchial asthma are mild and last for few hours. Sometimes, it becomes much more serious with severe obstruction, when this condition is called as the *status asthmaticus*. However during symptom-free phase, the patient may also experience some degree of airways obstruction daily. So, the asthma is classified as *acute* or *chronic*. Chronic asthma is again classified as *intermittent* and *persistent*. Now, persistent asthma is further classified as mild, moderate, and severe.

Bronchial asthma is the most common chronic obstructive pulmonary airway disease and is one of the leading causes of death in our country. The high mortality from bronchial asthma is due to the ineffective or inadequate treatment leading to gradual irreversible changes of the airways. Bronchial asthma occurs at all ages, but more common at early life. About one half of the cases develop before the age of 10 years and another one-third of the cases develop before the age of 40 years. In childhood when the incidence is very high, the male–female ratio is 2:1 and it gradually equalizes at the age of 30 years. (1) The presence of symptoms in childhood, (2) cough which wakes the patient at night, (3) diurnal variation, (4) specific trigger factors (especially allergic), (5) absence of smoking history, and (6) response to previous treatment, etc., may all be helpful

in differentiating bronchial asthma from COPD (now called COLD).

From the etiological point of view, the bronchial asthma is a heterogeneous disease. It can be described under two broad headings (i.e., types of asthma): *allergic* (extrinsic and attacks related to environmental exposure) and *idiosyncratic* (intrinsic and attacks not related to environmental exposure). In allergic type of bronchial asthma, patients should have (1) personal/or family history of allergic disease such as rhinitis, urticaria, and eczema, (2) ↑level of immunoglobulin E (IgE), (3) positive skin reaction to intradermal antigen test, and (4) positive response to provocative tests, involving specific antigens by inhalation, etc. On the other hand, in idiosyncratic variety no such positive history or test will be present. However, these classifications are imperfect and were used in past because many patients show the features of both forms.

In general, the bronchial asthma, that has its onset in early life, falls in the allergic group. The allergic asthma is dependent on an IgE response, controlled by T- and B-lymphocytes. It is activated by the interaction of antigen with the mast cells-bound IgE molecules. Most of the allergens that provoke the *seasonal form of bronchial asthma* are airborne. To induce a state of sensitivity (first reaction in the body), the allergens must be reasonably abundant for the considerable period of time. Once the sensitization of body has occurred, then the patient can exhibit exquisite hyperresponsiveness, so that the next exposure to the minute amounts of the offending agents can produce significant exacerbations of the disease. This allergic variety of asthma is most often observed in children and young adults and is usually seasonal. A *nonseasonal form of bronchial asthma* may result from the allergy to feathers, animal dander, dust mites, molds, and other antigens that are present continuously in the environment. From the above discussion, it is clear that the inhaled antigens cause an antigen–antibody (AG–AB) reactions on the surface of the bronchial mast cells and provoke an acute episode of asthma.

In the idiosyncratic group of bronchial asthma: (1) there is no personal or family history, (2) the level of IgE is not elevated, and (3) the skin test to antigen is negative. So, this group does not depend on immunological mechanism (AG–AB reaction) for its manifestation. The *initial insult* in this idiosyncratic group of asthma is usually the common cold or upper respiratory tract illness, leading to the paroxysms of wheeze and dyspnea. The bronchial asthma that develops late in life, usually falls in this group. Again, this idiosyncratic group cannot be confused with the group where the symptoms of bronchospasm superimposed on chronic bronchitis or bronchiectasis. On the other hand, in practice there are many patients that do not fit clearly into any of the abovementioned groups, and they are classified as mixed group.

Though, the basic mechanism is still unknown, but the main denomination of pathophysiology of bronchial asthma or bronchospasm is nonspecific hyperirritability of tracheobronchial tree and its neural control pathways (overactivity of parasympathetic system). The intensity of this hyperactivity of bronchial tree is directly proportional with the intensity of the symptoms and the aggressiveness of therapy. Following a viral infection of respiratory tract, the reactivity of airway rises and remains elevated for many weeks, even after recovery from infection, though seemingly trivial. This is very important from the anesthetic point of view. In this hyperactivity period, any exposure to antigen or chemical irritants (those also who have no history of bronchial asthma) cause bronchospasm.

The most popular hypothesis of bronchial asthma, now, is that of airway inflammation with increased number of mast cells, eosinophils, lymphocytes, neutrophils, and epithelial cells. This is because even when the acute episode of bronchial asthma is in remission, still the bronchial biopsy reveals large infiltration of mucosa by inflammatory cells and epithelial shedding. But, if this increased number of inflammatory cells and inflammation is the effect of Ag–Ab reaction (for allergic group) is still unknown because increased cellularity and elevated capillary density (i.e., findings of inflammatory process) are the most ubiquitous findings, even in asymptomatic group of patients. In idiosyncratic group of patients, inflammation is the effect of asthma. However, bronchospasm during anaphylactic reaction should not be confused with idiosyncratic asthma.

For the pathogenesis of asthma, the abovementioned inflammatory cells (mast cell, eosinophil, macrophage, lymphocyte, and neutrophil) and chemical mediators [histamine, bradykinin, leukotrienes (LTs)-C/D/E, prostaglandins E_2 and $F_2\alpha$, platelet-activating factors (PAFs)] which are released from these inflammatory cells (mainly by the degranulation of mast cells), play an important role, causing *inflammatory reaction.* This inflammatory reaction involves mucous production, bronchospasm, vascular congestion, and edema formation. These chemical mediators, then, attract more and more eosinophils, platelets, and polymorph nuclear leukocytes to the site of reaction by their chemotactic effects. Thus these infiltrating cells, the resident macrophages, and the airway epithelial cells produce additional mediators in *vicious cycle* and cause *immediate and delayed cellular phase reaction.*

The vagal afferents in bronchial tree are sensitive to histamine and multiple noxious stimuli, including cold air, inhaled irritants, and instrumentation (e.g., tracheal intubation). The *reflex vagal activation* results in bronchoconstriction, which is mediated by an increase in intracellular cyclic guanosine monophosphate (cGMP). The local inflammatory reaction exposes the nerve endings and initiates a neurogenic inflammatory pathway, converting primary local event into a generalized reaction by reflex mechanism. This is an alternative explanation of bronchial asthma, due to the *abnormal function of autonomic nervous system*. This hypothesis is supported by the increased expiratory airflow obstruction in patients with bronchial asthma, being treated with β-agonist, suggesting the presence of an imbalance between the excitatory and the inhibitory neural output.

It is likely that the chemical mediators, released from the mast cells, interact with the autonomic nervous system. Some chemical mediators can stimulate the airway's irritant receptors to trigger the reflex bronchoconstriction (*neurogenic bronchoconstriction*) while the other mediators sensitize the bronchial smooth muscles to the effects of acetylcholine (ACh) (*chemical bronchoconstriction*). In addition, the stimulation of muscarinic receptors facilitates the release of mediator from the mast cells by its degranulation, providing another positive feedback loop for sustained inflammation and bronchoconstriction. The stimuli that interact with airway responsiveness and incite acute episodes of bronchial asthma can be grouped into seven major categories and these are: allergenic, pharmacologic, environmental, occupational, infective, exercise-related, and emotional.

The allergenic factors, as the etiology of bronchial asthma, are already discussed. Among the pharmacological allergic factors, the important drugs that are commonly associated with the induction of the episodes of bronchial asthma are aspirin, tartrazine (coloring agent in food products), sulfiting agents (sodium and potassium metabisulfite/bisulfite, used as preservative in food preparation), beta adrenergic antagonist, etc. It is important to recognize that the drug-induced bronchial asthma is often associated with greater morbidity and sometimes with mortality. There is a great deal of cross-reactivity between the aspirin and other NSAIDs, such as ibuprofen, fenoprofen, indomethacin, and phenylbutazone.

The exact mechanism by which the aspirin and other drugs produce bronchospasm is still unknown. But the probable explanation is the generation of LTs which act as a chemical mediator for aspirin or other drugs. This is proved by the inhibition of LT synthesis or receptor activity, during the treatment of this type of problem. On the other hand, paracetamol (acetaminophen), sodium salicylate, and propoxyphene are well tolerated by these aspirin-sensitive group of patients. On exposure to even a small amount of aspirin, the sensitive individual develops ocular and nasal congestion and often acute severe airway obstruction. The aspirin-induced hypersensitivity usually starts with perineal vasomotor rhinitis that is followed by hyperplastic rhino sinusitis with nasal polyp. Progressive asthma then appears.

Several sulfiting agents such as potassium metabisulfite and sodium and potassium bisulfite used in the different food and pharmacological industries as preservatives, also can produce acute airways obstruction in sensitive individuals. Patients become sensitized, after their first exposure to these chemical agents. Then, after subsequent exposures, patients develop acute bronchial asthma. These subsequent exposures to the different sulfiting agents also usually follow by the ingestion of food and beverages (which also contain different sulfiting agents), such as shellfish, wine, salad, and fruit preparations. Some topical ophthalmic solutions, IV glucocorticoids preparations and bronchodilator solutions for inhalation also contain some sulfiting agents which produce bronchospasm.

The environmental causes of bronchial asthma are usually due to pollen (airborne antigen) and atmospheric pollutants such as ozone, nitrogen dioxide, and sulfur dioxide. This environmental cause of bronchial asthma can be treated by mast cells stabilizing drugs. The occupation-related bronchial asthma is due to the exposure to a large number of compounds, used in different types of industrial process. *Respiratory infection* is also an important stimuli to evoke exacerbation of bronchial asthma. Among the infections, viruses such as syncytial virus, rhino virus, influenza, and parainfluenza virus, are the predominant pathogens. Simple colonization of viruses do not cause bronchial asthma, but attacks of asthma occur when the symptoms of respiratory tract infection are present. The mechanism of virus-induced exacerbation of bronchial asthma is due to the production of T-cell derived cytokines that help in the infiltration of inflammatory cells into the already susceptible airways.

Exercise also precipitates acute onset of bronchial asthma by provoking bronchospasm to some extent in asthmatic patient. When such patients are followed for sufficient periods, then it is found that they often develop recurring episodes of airway obstruction which is independent of exercise. So, onset of exercise-induced bronchial asthma may be the first manifestation of the later full blown asthmatic syndrome. The exercise-induced asthma is not due to the contraction of smooth muscles, but is due to the *obstruction* produced by (1) the thermal-induced hyperemia and (2) the engorgement of the microvasculature structure of bronchial wall.

Pathophysiology

The hallmarks of the pathophysiology of bronchial asthma are: (1) vascular congestion, (2) edema of tracheobronchial

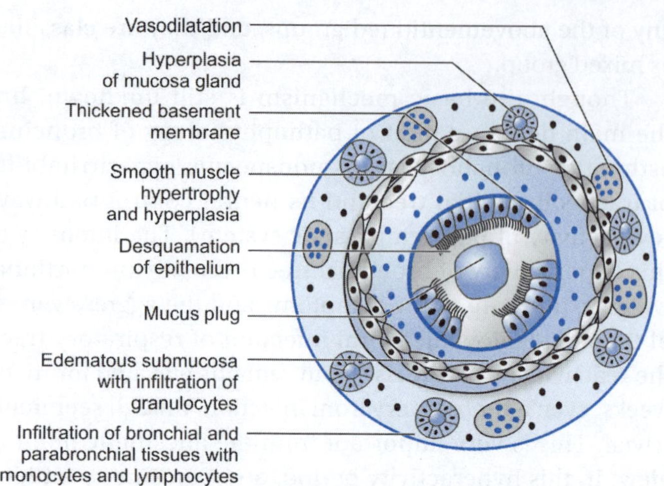

Fig. 5: Changes in bronchial wall during asthma.

wall, (3) thickening of mucous membrane, (4) reduction of airway diameter due to the contraction of smooth muscles, (5) copious tenacious secretions and plugging of airways (mainly the small airways), (6) hypertrophy of bronchial smooth muscle, (7) hyperplasia of mucosal and submucosal vessels, (8) eosinophilic infiltration of bronchial wall, and (9) shedding of surface epithelium **(Fig. 5)**. All these pathological changes lead to (1) increased airway resistance, (2) decreased forced expiratory volume, (3) decreased flow rates, (4) increased work of breathing, (5) hyperinflation of lungs and thorax, (6) decreased elastic recoil, (7) altered V/Q ratio, and (8) altered arterial blood gas concentration.

When the FVC of an asthmatic patient, with acute episode, goes below or becomes equal to the 50% of its normal value, then the FEV_1 comes down to 30% or less of its predicted value, and the maximum mid-expiratory flow rates are reduced to 20% or less of its expected value, then he or she presents for therapy. In acutely ill patient, with status asthmaticus, the residual volume (RV) frequently approaches 400% of its normal value and FRC becomes double (100% increase). The *F–V* loop of asthma shows a characteristic downward scooping of the expiratory limb of the loop **(Fig. 6)**. Where the inhaled and exhaled portion of a *F–V* loop becomes flat, then it helps to distinguish the wheezing, caused by upper airway obstruction such as foreign body, tracheal stenosis, mediastinal tumor, etc., from bronchial asthma. During moderate-to-severe attacks of bronchial asthma, the FRC may increase as much as up to 1–2 L, whereas the total lung capacity (TLC) usually remains within its normal range.

The mild bronchial asthma is usually accompanied by normal arterial O_2 and CO_2 tension because tachypnea and hyperventilation, which are observed during a mild asthmatic attack, do not reflect the compensatory phase of arterial hypoxemia but rather reflect the neural reflexes of lung that cause the tachypnea and hyperventilation.

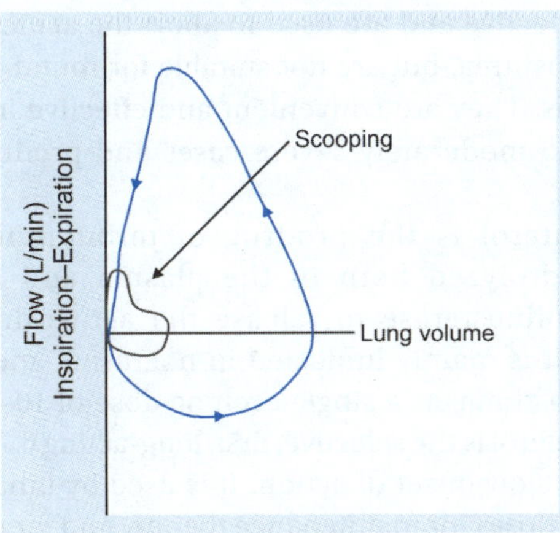

Fig. 6: Flow–volume curve of a normal (blue line) and an asthmatic (black line) individual.

During the moderate-to-severe form of attack, the abnormal blood gas analysis is the universal finding. This is associated with hypoxia, hypocapnia (due to hyperventilation), and *respiratory alkalosis* (due to hypocapnia). After that, as the severity of obstruction to expiratory airflow increases, then the associated gradual V/Q mismatching may result in PaO_2 <60 mm Hg (*hypoxia*) *but normocapnia*, while breathing room air. This is followed by compensatory hyperventilation which results in *hypocapnia and normal PaO_2*.

Then, gradually when this hypocapnia again comes to normal level or PCO_2 goes above normal level, due to the failure of excretion of CO_2, it indicates severe airway obstruction and the patient will no longer be able to maintain the work of breathing, proceeding to impending respiratory failure. The $PaCO_2$ is likely to increase when the FEV_1 is <25% of its predicted value and indicates impending respiratory failure. Equally, the presence of *metabolic acidosis* in the setting of acute bronchial asthma signifies *severe hypoxia,* due to acute obstruction. Cyanosis is very uncommon and is a late sign of bronchial asthma. Clinically, this hypoxia can go undetected. So, clinical indication should not be relied upon with any confidence. Therefore, in any acute asthmatic condition, with suspected alveolar hypoventilation, arterial blood gas tension must be measured.

Drugs for Bronchial Asthma

The drugs, used for treatment of bronchial asthma, are classified as:

- *Bronchodilators:*
  - *Adrenergic stimulants (β_2-sympathomimetics):* Epinephrine, salbutamol (albuterol), terbutaline, bambuterol, salmeterol, formoterol, ephedrine
  - Methylxanthines: Theophylline, aminophylline, etophylline, doxophylline, acebrophylline
  - Anticholinergics: Atropine, ipratropium, tiotropium

- *LT antagonists:* Montelukast, zafirlukast
- *Mast cell stabilizers:* Sodium cromoglycate, nedocromil, ketotifen
- *Corticosteroids:*
  - *Systemic:* Hydrocortisone, prednisolone, and others
  - *Inhalational:* Beclomethasone, budesonide, fluticasone, flunisolide, ciclesonide, triamcinolone
- *Anti-IgE antibody:* Omalizumab.

β_2-sympathomimetics: This group of drugs causes bronchodilatation through their agonistic action on adrenergic β_2-receptor and the activation of G-protein. This results in the increased formation of cyclic adenosine monophosphate (cAMP) in bronchial muscle cell, leading to the relaxation of it. This increased cAMP in mast cells also reduces AG:AB reaction which inhibits the release of chemical mediators, responsible for smooth muscle contraction. The sympathomimetic agents which are in widespread clinical use for bronchial asthma are listed previously. Among these, the epinephrine is the mainstay of treatment for reversible airway obstruction, but should be reserved for very refractory cases and used cautiously in hypertensive patients, cardiac patients and in those patients who are receiving digitalis. They are the fastest acting bronchodilators when inhaled.

Epinephrine (adrenaline) is both the α ($\alpha_1 + \alpha_2$) and β ($\beta_1 + \beta_2$) agonistic agent and causes prompt, but short-lasting bronchodilatation. The duration of action of epinephrine is only 30–90 minutes and is effective only when is administered by inhalational or by parenteral routes. The α-action (weakly bronchoconstrictor) of it is masked by its predominant β_2-mediated action. As the epinephrine is not a selective β_2 agonist, so it has considerable chronotropic and inotropic cardiac (β_1) actions also. The inhalation of adrenaline may also afford additional benefit by producing mucosal decongestion (α-action). The usual parenteral dose of epinephrine in the management of acute bronchial asthma is 0.3–0.5 mL of 1:1000 solution, *administered subcutaneously.*

Another catecholamine, such as isoprenaline, is also used for the management of bronchial asthma. It is devoid of α-activity and has both $\beta_1 + \beta_2$ activity. It is also a very potent bronchodilator and is usually administered in acute asthmatic patient as 1:200 solution by *inhalation.* Then, in 1960, sudden deaths among the asthmatics were increased markedly when the isoprenaline was used subsequently in this dose. This is because the inhalation of several doses of isoprenaline in succession, during the escalation of symptom and respiratory acidosis, results in cardiac arrhythmia and asystole. Then, death rate has dropped, following the restriction of this inhaler (isoprenaline) and

TABLE 4: Comparison of β_1 and β_2 activity of commonly used bronchodilators.

Drugs	β-adrenergic activity	
	β_1	β_2
Epinephrine	+ + + +	+ +
Albuterol (salbutamol)	+	+ + +
Bambuterol	+	+ + +
Formoterol	+	+ + + +
Salmeterol	+	+ + + +
Terbutalin	+	+ + + +

the development of more selective β_2 agonists which have replaced isoprenaline.

Other than epinephrine (adrenaline) and isoprenaline, the other drugs in this group are highly selective for the β_2-receptors of respiratory tract and are virtually devoid of any significant cardiac (β_1) effects, except at high doses **(Table 4)**. Their major side effect is tremor. They are active by all the routes of administration. Their peculiar chemical structure allows them to bypass the metabolic processes which degrades the catecholamines in liver when used through oral route. So, their effects are long-lasting (4–6 hours) than catecholamines.

The differences in potency and the duration of action among these agents can be eliminated by adjusting their doses and/or their administration schedules. Inhalation is the preferred route of administration of this group of drugs because through this route, it further increases the bronchial selectivity of the action of these drugs and allows the maximal bronchodilatation with fewer systemic side effects. This is also true during the treatment of severe acute airway obstruction and making the IV therapy obsolete during emergency. The IV administration of β_2-selective agonistic agent such as terbutaline and salbutamol offers no advantages over the inhalational routes.

Both the salbutamol and terbutaline are highly selective β_2-agonists. So, the cardiac side effects of these two agents are less prominent. Bronchial (β_2) selectivity of these agents is further increased by inhaling these drugs. Muscle tremor, caused by the salbutamol and terbutaline, is their dose-related side effect. Palpitation, restlessness, nervousness, throat irritation, and ankle edema may also occur. Salbutamol and terbutaline undergo presystemic metabolism in gut wall. So, the oral bioavailability of this drug is only 50% through their oral route. They are longer-acting. Inhaled salbutamol and terbutaline are currently the most popular drugs for the management of acute bronchial asthma. By inhalation, the peak bronchodilatation effect produced with these agents, occurs within 5–10 minutes, and lasts up to 2–4 hours. So,

they are effective and are used to abort the acute attack of bronchial asthma, but are not suitable for round-the-clock prophylaxis. They are convenient and effective in most of the mild-to-moderately severe cases and produce fewer side effects.

Bambuterol is the prodrug of terbutaline and is slowly hydrolyzed both in the plasma and lungs by pseudocholinesterase to release the active drugs over 24 hours. It is mainly indicated in nocturnal and chronic bronchial asthma, as a single evening dose of 10–20 mg by oral. Salmeterol is the selective, first, long-acting β_2-agonistic agent with slow onset of action. It is used by inhalation as twice daily doses for maintenance therapy and for nocturnal asthma, but not for acute symptoms. It is more lipophilic than salbutamol which probably accounts for its longer duration of action.

The regular use of inhaled sympathomimetics β_2-agonists does not reduce bronchial hyperactivity, but may even worsen it. Regular use also down regulates the bronchial β_2-receptors. This may be responsible for the gradually diminished responsiveness, seen after the long-term use of these drugs. Hence, it is felt that the use of β_2-agonist inhalers should be restricted to the symptomatic relief of wheezing.

Salmeterol is the recently introduced long-acting (9–12 hours) congener of salbutamol and selective β_2-agonist with slow onset of action (30 minutes). As it is long-acting (12 hours), so it is effective in producing sustained symptomatic relief. Therefore, it is used as twice daily dose for the maintenance of therapy and for nocturnal and exercise-induced asthma, but not for acute symptoms. It should not be used as a rescue drug for breakthrough symptoms. In addition, its long half-life means that administration of extra doses can cause cumulative side effects.

Methylxanthines: The drugs, used from this group of agent, for the acute cases of bronchial asthma, are theophylline and aminophylline. Theophylline and its various salts are bronchodilators of medium potency and work through an undefined mechanism. The probable explanations for their mechanism of action are: (1) release of Ca^{2+} from sarcoplasmic reticulum (SR), especially in cardiac and skeletal muscles, (2) inhibition of phosphodiesterase (PDE) which degrades cAMP, resulting in its (cAMP) increased concentration, and (3) blocking the action of adenosine which contracts the smooth muscles. Action (1) of theophylline is exerted only at concentration, which is much higher than the therapeutic plasma concentration of theophylline. The action of theophylline, exerted by (2) and (3) mechanism in the therapeutic plasma concentration of it, contributes to bronchodilatation. However, the pulmonary effects of methylxanthines seem much more complex and these are (including the inhibition of PDE and adenosine) catecholamine release, blockade of histamine release, and diaphragmatic stimulation.

Before the era of salbutamol, the theophylline and its compounds have been extensively used in bronchial asthma. But now it is not considered as the first line of drugs anymore. Theophylline is one of the three naturally occurring methylated xanthine alkaloids, such as caffeine, theophylline, and theobromine which are present in tea leaves, coffee seeds, and cocoa. The therapeutic plasma concentration of theophylline traditionally have been thought to lie between 10 and 20 µg/mL. But some schools recommend a lower therapeutic plasma concentration, ranging between 5 and 15 µg/mL to avoid its toxicity.

The dose required to achieve the desired therapeutic level and to reduce the toxicity of methylxanthines varies widely from patient to patient. This is due to the differences in the metabolism of theophylline in different patients. Theophylline clearance and thus its dosage requirement are decreased substantially in neonates, elderly, and those who are suffering with acute and chronic hepatic dysfunction, cardiac decompensation, cor pulmonale, and febrile illness. On the other hand, theophylline clearance increases in children. In addition, a number of important drug interactions can alter the theophylline metabolism. The clearance of methylxanthines (theophylline) also fall with the concurrent use of erythromycin, other macrolide antibiotics, quinolone antibiotics, cimetidine, etc. Clearance of theophylline also increases with the use of cigarettes, marijuana, phenobarbital, phenytoin, and other drugs that induce microsomal enzymes of liver. At therapeutic concentration, the t½ of theophylline in adults is 7–12 hours. Children eliminate it much faster with t½, 3–5 hours, but for the elderly t½ is >12 hours. In premature neonates and infants the t½ of theophylline extends from 24 to 36 hours. Long-acting theophylline compounds are also available for maintenance of therapy and are usually given once or twice per day **(Fig. 7)**.

The dose of this group of drug is adjusted on the basis of clinical response and the measurement of serum concentration. Now, the effectiveness or the role of aminophylline in the management of acute asthma is in debate. Still, in severe asthma it is used as infusion perioperatively. Both aminophylline and theophylline are available for IV use. The recommended IV dose of theophylline is 6 mg/kg as loading, followed by an infusion of 1 mg/kg/h for the next 12 hours and then 0.8 mg/kg/h thereafter. For older, heart failure, liver disease, and cor pulmonale patients the IV loading dose remains the same, but the maintenance dose is reduced to between 0.1 and 0.5 mg/kg/h. Sometimes, for patients who are already

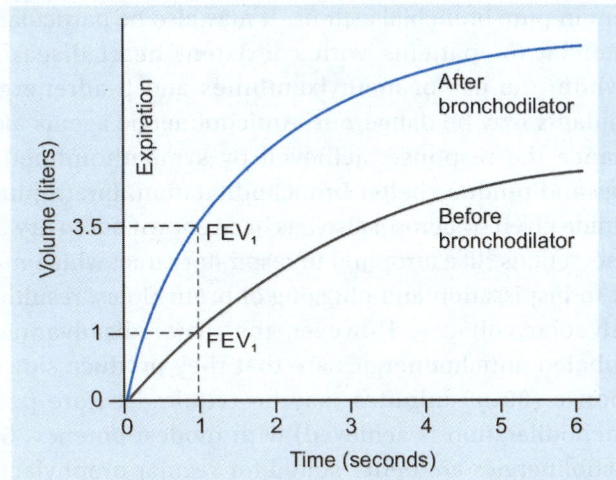

Fig. 7: Schematic representation of change in forced expiratory volume in first 1 second (FEV₁) before (black line) and after (blue line) administration of bronchodilator.

receiving theophylline, the loading dose is frequently withheld.

The most common side effects of aminophylline and theophylline are nervousness, nausea, vomiting, anorexia, and headache. At plasma levels of theophylline greater than 30 µg/mL, there is risk of seizures and cardiac arrhythmias. Very rapid IV injections of methylxanthines cause precordial pain, syncope, and even sudden death and these are due to marked fall in blood pressure (BP), ventricular arrhythmias or asystole. Theophylline has been found to reduce the frequency and duration of episodes of apnea that occur in some preterm infants in the first few weeks of life. So, for premature neonates, to prevent or to abolish the episode of apnea closely monitored IV treatment by theophylline or aminophylline is employed for 1–3 weeks.

Anticholinergic agents: The anticholinergic drugs, such as atropine sulfate produces bronchodilatation and blocks reflex bronchoconstriction in patients with bronchial asthma. It acts by blocking the cholinergic constrictor tone of vagus. But its use is limited by its systemic side effects and less effectiveness than sympathomimetic agents. However, after the introduction of nonabsorbable quaternary ammonium congener, such as atropine methyl nitrate, ipratropium bromide, and tiotropium, the anticholinergic agent has been found to be both (1) effective in the management of chronic bronchial asthma and (2) free of untoward anticholinergic side effects. The bronchoconstriction in patients of asthmatic bronchitis, COPD, and psychogenic asthma responds better than pure bronchial asthma to these anticholinergic agents because reflex vagal activity is an important factor, causing bronchoconstriction and increased secretion, in chronic bronchitis and COPD, but to a lesser extent in pure bronchial asthma. It may also be particularly beneficial for patients with coexistent heart diseases, in whom the use of methylxanthines and β-adrenergic stimulants may be dangerous. Anticholinergic agents also enhance the response, achieved by sympathomimetics drugs and produce better bronchodilatation. Ipratropium bromide given by aerosol also has been shown not to dry up the secretions (like atropine) in respiratory tract which may lead to inspissation and plugging of bronchioles, resulting in alveolar collapse. However, the major disadvantage of inhaled anticholinergics are that they produce slower response (60–90 minutes may be required before peak bronchodilatation is achieved) with modest potency. So, anticholinergics are better suited for regular prophylactic use than for control of an acute attack.

Glucocorticoids: They are not bronchodilators. But they act by: (1) reducing bronchial hyperirritability, (2) reducing mucosal edema, (3) stabilizing the cell membrane of inflammatory cells, and (4) suppressing inflammatory response, produced by AG:AB reaction or other stimuli. The indications of glucocorticoids in asthma are: (1) when severe airway obstruction is not resolving or is worsening, despite intense optimal bronchodilator therapy, (2) in chronic diseases when there has been failure of a previously optimal regimen with frequent recurrences of symptoms and increasing severity, and (3) to restore the responsiveness of sympathomimetics, once resistance to them has developed **(Fact file I)**.

The glucocorticoid molecule penetrates the cell membrane and binds to the glucocorticoid receptor (GR)

which is a protein in nature and normally resides in the cytoplasm of cell. These GRs are practically distributed in all the cells and made up of 800 amino acids. The GR has a steroid-binding domain, near to its carboxy terminus and a DNA-binding domain, having two 'zinc finger', at its mid region. Each zinc finger is made up of a loop of amino acids with chelated zinc ion. Normally, the GR remains in cytoplasm in association with three proteins such as heat shock protein 90 (HSP90), HSP70, and immunophillin (IP) **(Fig. 8)**.

These proteins (HSP and IP) have inhibitory influence on GR and prevent its dimerization. The binding of steroid molecule to GR dissociates these three complex proteins from GR and the dimerization region of GR is exposed. Thus, the dimerization of two GR with one glucocorticoid molecule occurs. Now, the dimer (a molecule or molecular complex, consisting of two identical molecules, linked

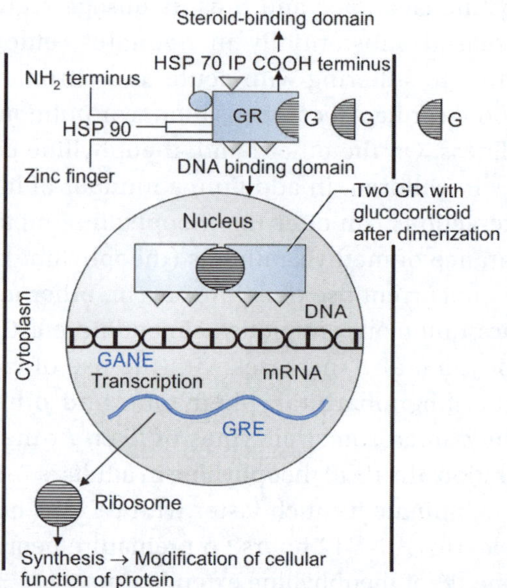

Fig. 8: The glucocorticosteroid (G) molecule first penetrates the cell membrane. Then, it binds to its glucocorticoid receptor (GR). Normally, the GR resides in the cytoplasm in association with three another complex proteins, named: heat shock protein 90 (HSP90), HSP70, and immunophillin (IP). The GR has two domains, one is the steroid-binding domain near its carboxy terminus. Another is the DNA-binding domain, having two zinc fingers at its middle. The binding of G to GR dissociates the complex proteins (HSP90, HSP70, etc.) from GR and thus removes the inhibitory influences of these complex proteins on GR. Thus a dimerization region present on the GR is exposed and helps in the dimerization of two GRs. Then, the steroid molecule-bound dimer of receptor (G + GR) translocates into the nucleus and interacts with a specific DNA sequence which is called as the glucocorticoid responsive elements (GREs). Then, the expression of the genes in DNA is altered. This results in the promotion or suppression of their transcription and the production of specific mRNA. The specific mRNA, thus produced, is directed to the ribosome and gives direction for the specific pattern of protein synthesis which ultimately modifies the cell function.

FACT FILE I

At cellular level the glucocorticoids act by the following mechanisms:

1. Induction of synthesis of lipocortins in macrophages, endothelial cells, and fibroblasts → ↑ in lipocortins inhibits phospholipase A_2 → decreases synthesis of prostaglandins, LTs, and PAF.

2. Negative regulation of genes for the synthesis of cytokines in macrophages, endothelial cells and lymphocytes → decreased production of IL-1, 2, 3, 6; TNFα, GM-CSF, γ-interferon → inhibition of fibroblast. (IL: interleukin; TNF: tumor necrosis factor; GM-CSF: granulocyte macrophage colony-stimulating factor)

3. Complement function is inhibited.

4. Decreased production of ELAM (endothelial leukocyte adhesion molecule) and ICAM (intracellular adhesion molecule) causing the suppression of adhesion and the localization of leucocytes.

5. Inhibition of the IgE-mediated release of histamine and LT–C_4 from basophil by which AG:AB reaction is inhibited.

6. Inhibition of the production of collagenase and the prevention of tissue destruction

togcthcr) of two GR with steroid molecules translocates within the nucleus of the cell and interacts with a specific sequence or region of DNA which is called as the glucocorticoid responsive elements (GREs). These are the regulatory regions of an appropriate gene of DNA. Thus, the expressions of these genes are consequently altered, resulting in the promotion or suppression of their transcription. The specific mRNA, thus produced (transcribed) from these genes (whose expression is altered), is directed to the ribosomes. Now, in the ribosome the messages, carried by these mRNA, are translated for a specific pattern of protein synthesis, which in turn modifies the functions of cell.

Thus, in summary we can say that the corticosteroid molecules penetrate the cells and bind to its highly specific cytoplasmic GR protein → a structural change occurs in these steroid receptor complex → allows its migration into the nucleus and bindings to specific sites on DNA → transcription of specific mRNA → regulation of protein synthesis → alterations of function of cells. This process takes at least 30–60 minutes. So, effects of steroids are not immediate and once the appropriate proteins are synthesized, then the effects persist much longer **(Fig. 8)**.

All the natural and synthetic corticosteroids, except the deoxycorticosterone acetate (DOCA), are effective by oral route. The water soluble esters of corticosteroid, e.g., hydrocortisone hemisuccinate, dexamethasone sodium phosphate, methyl prednisolone, etc., can be given through IV or intramuscular (IM) The IV hydrocortisone or methylprednisolone is used acutely for severe attacks, followed by tapering doses of oral prednisolone. They act rapidly and achieve high concentration in tissue fluids. The insoluble esters of corticosteroid, e.g., hydrocortisone acetate, triamcinolone acetonide, etc. cannot be injected through IV. They are slowly absorbed from IM absorption site and produce more prolonged effects **(Fig. 9)**.

The chemical structures of different natural and synthetic glucocorticoids are depicted in **Figure 9**. Among all the glucocorticoids, the *hydrocortisone* (the naturally occurring glucocorticoids and the daily rate of its synthesis is 10 mg/day) undergoes high fast pass metabolism in liver. So, it has low oral:parenteral activity ratio and is mainly used through IV route, whereas the oral bioavailability of other synthetic corticosteroids is high. The hydrocortisone acts rapidly, but it has short duration of action (t½ <12 hours). In status asthmaticus, the dose of it is 100 mg IV as bolus, plus 100 mg 8 hourly by infusion. The *prednisolone* is four times more potent and more selective glucocorticoid than hydrocortisone, but it cannot be used through IV route. While *methylprednisolone* (Solu-Medrol) is available for slow IV use for its strong anti-inflammatory action. Doses of different glucocorticoids are listed in **Table 5**.

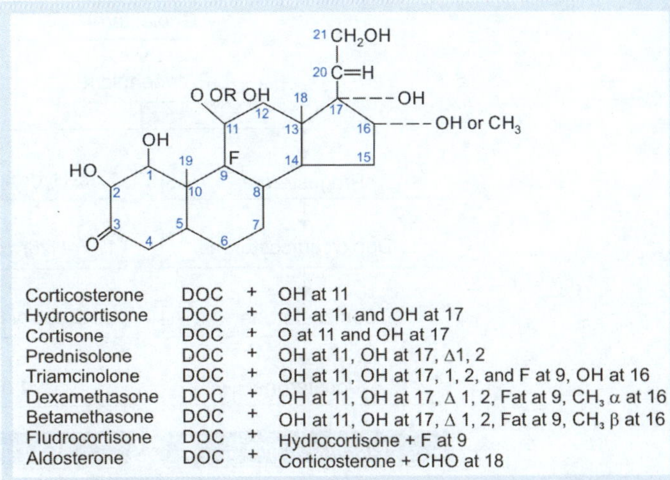

Fig. 9: Chemical structure of corticosteroid; black-lined structure is deoxycorticosterone (DOC); important substitutions which yield other compounds are shown by blue color.

TABLE 5: Equivalent doses of glucocorticoids.	
Glucocorticoids	*Dose (mg)*
Betamethasone	3
Dexamethasone	3
Methylprednisolone	16
Triamcinolone	16
Prednisolone	20
Hydrocortisone	80
Cortisone acetate	100

The *triamcinolone* is more potent and a selective glucocorticoid than prednisolone, but IV preparation of it is not available. It is used only by oral, IM, or intra-articular route. The *dexamethasone* is also a potent and selective glucocorticoid without fluid retention and hypertensive action (i.e., the mineralocorticoid actions). It is a long-acting (t½ >36 hours) glucocorticoid and its IV preparation is also available. As it has no fluid retention property, so it is used for the management of cerebral edema like betamethasone. The *betamethasone* is also available as IV preparation. Its action is like dexamethasone, but is long-acting (t½ >36 hours). The *fludrocortisone* is a potent mineralocorticoid with some glucocorticoid activity. The DOCA has only mineralocorticoid activity. The *beclomethasone, fluticasone, triamcinolone, ciclesonide, and budesonide* are used by inhalation as spray in bronchial asthma patient. They have high topical potency and reduce airway reactivity. The realization that bronchial asthma is primarily an inflammatory disease which accentuates with time. So, the availability of inhaled steroids, that are less hazardous in long-term use, have led to more extensive use of such glucocorticoids in chronic bronchial asthma **(Fig. 10)**.

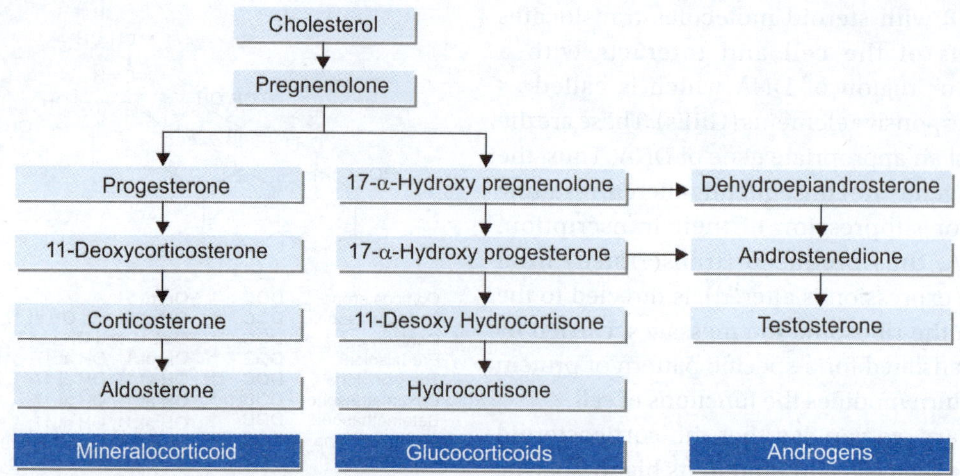

Fig. 10: Activity of glucocorticoids in chronic bronchial.

It should be emphasized that the effects of steroid in acute bronchial asthma are not immediate and their effects may not be seen for 6 hours or more, after its initial administration. Also, the correct dose of it in acute situations is a matter of debate. The available data indicates that the very high doses of glucocorticoids do not offer any advantage over their more conventional doses. So, the recommended dose of methylprednisolone in acute asthma is 40–60 mg through IV after every 6 hours. Since, the IV and oral administration produce the same effects, so the prednisolone in the dose of 60 mg, after every 6 hours orally, can be used instead of IV In UK, the acute bronchial asthma is treated with prednisolone in the dose of 30–40 mg once daily orally.

For bronchial asthma, the corticosteroids can also be used through inhalation route, and this inhalation route for the administration of corticosteroids is preferred than its oral administration because it is associated with less systemic side effects than its oral administration. The inhaled corticosteroids have direct anti-inflammatory action on bronchial mucosa and thus decrease the airway hyperresponsiveness. This decrease in airway hyperresponsiveness is not maximum, until the treatment has passed several months. The corticosteroids which are used through inhalation are: beclomethasone, fluticasone, budesonide, ciclesonide, etc.

Anesthetic Management

The anesthetic management of a patient with bronchial asthma requires an exhaustive understanding of the pathophysiology of this disease and the pharmacology of the drugs, being used for the management of it, which are already discussed. There is also evidence that the frequency of perioperative bronchospasm and laryngospasm is common in patients with the history of bronchial asthma, but when there are no symptoms before induction, whereas the symptomatic bronchial asthma patients, those have the signs of asthma just before the induction of anesthesia, are at increased risk for morbidity and mortality.

Perioperative assessment: The purposes for proper preoperative anesthetic assessment of a bronchial asthma patient are: (1) to determine the severity and the recent course of this disease, (2) to assess the degree of respiratory dysfunction, (3) to assess the efficacy of preoperative treatment and whether the patient is in optimal condition or not, and (4) to formulate the proper anesthetic plan. Patients with poorly controlled asthma at the time of anesthesia induction have a greater risk of perioperative complication rates. Conversely, well controlled asthma has not been shown to be a risk factor for intraoperative and postoperative complications.

To formulate the proper anesthetic plan, preoperative information should be obtained regarding (1) the frequency and the severity of attacks, (2) the history of drug, and (3) the recent episode of respiratory tract infection. Acute recent viral respiratory tract infection increases the bronchial reactivity and increases the incidence of intraoperative bronchospasm and laryngospasm. Physical examination of chest may be normal, though a forced expiration may provoke some end expiratory wheeze. Signs of cardiac and respiratory failure may or may not be present.

In addition to the routine tests, such as complete blood count, coagulation screening, urine analysis, and electrocardiogram (ECG), sometimes special attention should also be paid to the pulmonary function tests, arterial blood gas analysis, and X-ray of chest. The comparison of recent chest X-ray with the previous one is often useful to evaluate any further change during this recent disease process or not. A chest radiograph identifies (1) air trapping, (2) hyperinflated lungs resulting in flattened diaphragm, (3) a small appearing heart, and (4) a hyperlucent lung field.

In pulmonary function tests, the timed vital capacity (FEV_1) curve and *F–V* loop give the most valuable information regarding: (1) the degree of airway obstruction and (2) the degree of reversibility of obstruction with bronchodilators. The pulmonary function tests show the reduction in FVC, FEV_1, FEF (25–75%) and PEFR. The FEF at 25–75% is defined as the forced expiratory flow rate at 25–75% of FVC. The FEV_1 is a relative crude indicator of small airway obstruction compared to PEFR. The normal value of PEFR is 600–650 L/min in adult male and 450–500 L/min in adult female. Comparisons with previous measurements are invaluable. The values of FEV_1 are normally >3L for men and 2L for women. The FEV_1/FVC ratio should normally be >70%. An FEV_1, FEV_1/FVC or PEFR value, <50% of normal, are indicative of moderate-to-severe bronchial asthma.

A single peak flow reading can be helpful for preoperative assessment of a bronchial asthma patient. But the serial measurement is more helpful than a single result. The response to bronchodilators should also be measured. When the peak flow rate is >80% of the predicted value with minimal symptoms, then bronchial asthma is considered as mild and patient requires little extra treatment prior to surgery. The results of peak flow rate and spirometry should always be compared with their predicted values based on the age, sex, and height. Anesthesia should not be given for elective surgery, when the patient's asthma is less than optimally controlled. Viral infections are potent triggers of bronchospasm. So, postponement of elective surgery is considered with symptomatic URTI **(Table 6)**.

Depending upon the spirometric pulmonary functional impairment and arterial blood gas level, the bronchial asthma has been classified into five grades **(Table 6)**.

The preoperative blood gas analysis may be helpful, in providing a baseline, for the further management of asthma patients. Hypoxia and hypercarbia are seen only in patients with very severe asthma. In X-ray of chest, the hyperinflation, increased lung markings, and peribronchial thickening are the common radiological findings. It also helps to detect the presence of certain complications such as pneumonia, emphysema, and cyst.

Preoperative preparation and premedication: The proper preoperative preparation helps to reduce the perioperative morbidity and mortality in bronchial asthma patients. Preoperative chest physiotherapy, systemic hydration, appropriate antibiotics, and appropriate bronchodilator therapy are some of the important points which may improve the reversible components of bronchial asthma and may reduce the intraoperative and postoperative complications. The elective surgery should not be undertaken unless and until the bronchial asthma is well controlled. The incidence of perioperative bronchospasm and laryngospasm in asthmatic patients, undergoing routine surgery, is <2%, especially if they continue their routine medication. The frequency of complications is increased in patients over 50 years and in those with active disease.

The asthmatic patients with active bronchospasm, presenting for emergency surgery, should be treated aggressively. Supplemental O_2, nebulized β_2-agonists and anticholinergics, and IV glucocorticoids can dramatically improve lung function in a few hours. Arterial blood gases may be useful in evaluating the severity and adequacy of treatment. Hypoxemia and hypercapnia are typically of moderate or severe disease, even slight hypercapnia is indicative of severe air trapping and may be a sign of impending respiratory failure.

The bronchodilator drugs, used to treat bronchial asthma, should be continued at the time of premedication. Salbutamol and ipratropium/tiotropium should be changed to its nebulized form. In typical IM doses, the anticholinergics are not effective in preventing the reflex bronchospasm, following intubation. The cromoglycate, used as mast cells stabilizer preoperatively, can be continued safely during perioperative period, as it does not interact adversely with any drugs used during anesthesia. LT inhibitors can also be continued as preoperative medication and must restart when patient is taking oral medications postoperatively.

Exogenous corticosteroids should be continued or supplemented (if stopped before) before anesthesia for major surgery to combat the hypothalamic-pituitary-adrenal suppression which is likely in patient taking long term oral corticosteroids and to control the hyperreactivity of tracheobronchial tree to different anesthetic drugs. It is found that hypothalamic-pituitary-adrenal suppression is unlikely as a result of long-term inhaled corticosteroids. The preoperative supplementation of steroid (if stopped before) is considered, only when the previous daily dose of prednisolone is >10 mg or inhaled beclomethasone is

TABLE 6: Classification of the severity of bronchial asthma.

Severity of asthma	PaO_2 (mm Hg)	$PaCO_2$ (mm Hg)	FEV_1 (% predicted)
Normal patient	>60	<40	>80%
Mild asthma	>60	<40	65–80%
Moderate asthma	>60	<45	50–64%
Severe asthma	<60	>50	35–49%
Status asthmaticus	<60	>50	<35%

(FEV_1: forced expiratory volume in first 1 second; $PaCO_2$: partial pressure of arterial carbon dioxide; PaO_2: partial pressure of arterial oxygen)

>1.5 mg/day. Preoperatively, the oral prednisolone should be converted to IV hydrocortisone (1 mg prednisolone is equivalent to 5 mg hydrocortisone). When the preoperative FEV_1 is <80% of its normal value, then a preoperative course of oral corticosteroids must be used, even if the patient does not get steroid before.

The opioids have a number of actions on airway. They release histamine and other vasoactive substances from mast cells and produce bronchoconstriction. They also increase the bronchial smooth muscle reactivity, due to increase in vagal nerve activity. So, the clinical use of opioids in asthmatic patients is controversial. But there is no evidence that opioids, especially the newer synthetic opioids used in appropriate doses for preanesthetic medication or before intubation, stimulate the release of vasoactive substances from mast cells (histamine, LT, PAF) and produce bronchoconstriction. Moreover, they help to increase the depth of anesthesia which is mandatory for anesthetic management of asthmatic patients and tilt the balance in favor of the use of opioids as premedicants or during induction and before intubation. On the other hand, they depress the ventilating efforts and suppress the ventilating responses to hypoxia and hypercarbia, but not in premedicant doses. So, newer opioids are safe in bronchial asthmatics in premedication doses.

The use of anticholinergic drugs in the perioperative period is also controversial and should be individualized, remembering that these drugs can increase the viscosity of secretions and make it difficult to remove, causing the plugging of small airways and alveolar collapse. On the other hand, they decrease the airway resistance by inhibiting the postganglionic cholinergic receptors. Hence, the use of anticholinergic agents such as atropine and glycopyrrolate depends on the balance between their merits and demerits. The use of H_2 receptor blocker, as premedicant to increase the gastric pH in bronchial asthma patient, is also controversial because histamine mediates bronchoconstriction through their H_1 receptor and mediates bronchodilatation through their H_2 receptor. So, the H_2 receptor blocker can potentiate the H_1 receptor-induced bronchospasm. But in clinical practice it has no effect.

Anxiety may precipitate an acute attack of bronchial asthma. Benzodiazepines (BZDs) act on gamma-aminobutyric acid (GABA) receptors, present in the airway and attenuate this reflex-mediated bronchoconstriction. They also relax the airway smooth muscles directly. Therefore, perioperative BZDs are used to provide anxiolysis, but keeping in mind that in acutely ill patients the risk of depressing alveolar ventilation by BZD is greater and respiratory arrest has been reported to occur shortly after their use. Admittedly, most of the individuals are anxious and frightened, but experience has been shown that they can be calmed equally well by the presence and the reassurances of physician, without using BZDs. Hence, the preoperative use of BZD will depend on anesthetist's choice. It should also be kept in mind that a large number of asthmatic patients react adversely to aspirin or any NSAID. So, NSAIDs should be used cautiously, during the postoperative period, for the treatment of surgical pain.

Intraoperative management: Normally, the surgical and anesthetic stimuli that do not evoke bronchoconstriction in the absence of bronchial asthma may precipitate the life-threatening bronchospasm in patients with the history of bronchial asthma. For example, intubation (mechanical stimulus) can precipitate bronchoconstriction easily in asthmatic patient, if the bronchial reflexes are not obtunded properly by deepening anesthesia.

Different drugs (chemical stimuli), used in anesthesia, can also increase the airway reactivity and precipitate bronchospasm which is not found in normal patient. So, the goal, during the induction and the maintenance of anesthesia in patients with bronchial asthma is to depress the airway reflexes sufficiently by increasing the depth of anesthesia and by avoiding the drugs which can precipitate bronchoconstriction, if not absolutely necessary or to balance between the prevalence of bronchoconstriction and its beneficial effect.

The most critical time for asthmatic patients, who are undergoing anesthesia, is the instrumentation of airways. GA with noninvasive ventilation will circumvent this problem, but neither eliminates the possibility of bronchospasm. However, some clinicians believe that high spinal anesthesia may aggravate the bronchoconstriction by blocking the sympathetic tone to the lower airways (T1–T4) and allowing unopposed parasympathetic activity. The pain, emotional stress, or stimulation during light GA can precipitate bronchospasm. Drugs, often associated with histamine release such as atracurium and morphine, should be avoided or are given very slowly when used.

Regional anesthesia: Regional anesthesia (RA) is an attractive alternative procedure for the patients of bronchial asthma when the operative site is superficial, lower abdominal or on the extremities. This is because it avoids the instrumentation of airways (intubation) and the use of multiple drugs, which may precipitate bronchospasm. For the bronchial asthma patients, the RAs, such as the low spinal, low epidural or caudal are preferred for the surgeries on perineum, lower extremities, pelvis, or intraperitoneal and extraperitoneal organs restricting below umbilicus. This is because in such anesthesia complication rates are less in asthmatic patients, whereas the respiratory complications are quite common with high RA (block up to T_6–T_4 dermatome) like GA in bronchial asthma patient. So, the surgeries, requiring high RA are not alternative to GA. This is because high RA paralyzes the normal and the accessory respiratory muscles in an already compromised patient, necessitating artificial ventilation, where the GA has great advantage. High RA is also not possible without sedation which will further jeopardize the already compromised ventilation process. So, in such circumstances, significant differences will not be observed in asthmatic patients anesthetized with high RA and those undergoing GA by ketamine, cisatracurium, and isoflurane or sevoflurane. Nevertheless, it must be kept in mind that failed RA and the subsequent need to induce GA is always a possibility.

General anesthesia: During GA, in a bronchial asthma patient, the choice of inducing agent is less important, if adequate depth of anesthesia is achieved before intubation or surgical stimulation. In such patients, the induction should be done up to a deeper plane and tracheal intubation should be done under this deeper plane of anesthesia, because the patient may develop laryngospasm and bronchospasm in lighter plane of anesthesia. The cuff of an ETT should be placed just below the cord, but not touching it and without irritating the carina. Also the patient should be extubated at deeper plane of anesthesia avoiding any coughing and bucking (resisting) on ETT. However, the risk of aspiration, airway obstruction, and hypoventilation, due to extubation at deeper plane of anesthesia, should be weighed against its benefits.

For GA, induction is most often accomplished by IV injection of short-acting inducing drugs, such as thiopentone, propofol, etomidate, BZD, or ketamine. But the effects of barbiturates (thiopentone) on bronchial smooth muscles varied from relaxation to no effect to constriction. Some evidences also support that thiopentone produces a dose-dependent constriction of airways by releasing histamine. Some schools again thought that if thiopentone, at all, does not cause bronchospasm, but it fails to adequately suppress the upper airway reflexes and so the airway instrumentation can trigger bronchospasm.

On the other hand, propofol relaxes the airway smooth muscle (bronchodilation). But the mechanism of this bronchodilating effect of propofol is not known. The incidences of wheezing are significantly lower in asthmatic patients, induced with propofol than with barbiturates. Even, the respiratory airway resistance, following tracheal intubation, in healthy patients is lower after induction with propofol than after induction with thiopentone. So, based on these observations, it can be concluded that propofol is the agent of choice for induction of anesthesia in patients with bronchial asthma who are hemodynamically stable.

The hemodynamically unstable patient can be induced by adequate dose of BZD.

Ketamine depresses the neural airway reflex pathways and directly relaxes the bronchial smooth muscles (bronchodilation) by reducing the intracellular concentration of calcium. The catecholamines, released by ketamine, have also bronchodilating effect. Again ketamine has also been used successfully to decrease the airway resistance and to treat the status asthmaticus. So, alternatively ketamine can be used for induction of patients who are actively wheezing. Ketamine should probably not be used in patients with high theophylline levels, as the combined actions of the two drugs might precipitate seizure activity. Some generic formulation of induction agents which are available in market contain metabisulfites as preservatives and the presence of these metabisulfites causes bronchospasm in patients with hyperactive airways. So, an anesthetist should be careful of these generic formulations. The reflex bronchospasm can be blunted before intubation and after induction by an additional dose of IV inducing agent, ventilating the patient with 2 or 3 MAC sevoflurane for few minutes or administering IV or intratracheal lignocaine (1–2 mg/kg). But, one has to keep in mind that intratracheal lignocaine may initiate bronchospasm. Different substances influencing the tone of bronchial muscles are listed in **Box 2**.

After hypnosis and unconsciousness, established by IV inducing agents, it is better to ventilate the patient's lungs with gas mixtures [nitrous oxide (N_2O) and O_2], containing

---

BOX 2: Substances influencing bronchial smooth muscle tone.

Bronchodilatation:
- β_2-sympathomimetics: Salbutamol, terbutaline, isoprenaline, adrenaline, ephedrine, etc.
- Xanthine derivatives: Aminophylline, theophylline, caffeine, etc.
- Volatile anesthetics: Halothane, isoflurane, sevoflurane, ether, etc.
- Nitrites: Amyl nitrite, glyceryl trinitrate
- Prostaglandin (PG) E_1 and E_2:
- Muscarinic cholinergic receptor blockers: Atropine, glycopyrrolate, etc.

Bronchoconstriction:
- Muscarinic cholinomimetics
  - Anticholinesterases: Neostigmine, pyridostigmine, physostigmine, edrophonium, etc.
  - Choline esters and alkaloids: Pilocarpine, carbachol, methachol, etc.
- β_2-adrenergic blockers: Atenolol, propranolol, etc.
- Autacoids: Histamine, 5-HT, kinins, PG-$F_2\alpha$, etc.
  - Histamine releasing drugs: Pancuronium, atracurium, morphine, thiopentone, etc.
  - Allergic reactions
  - Carcinoid tumors
  - PG administration

volatile anesthetic agents. The goal is to further produce a deeper plane of anesthesia that depresses the hyperactive airway reflexes sufficiently and permit tracheal intubation without precipitating laryngospasm and bronchospasm. Otherwise, bronchospasm will be precipitated, if tracheal intubation is done without establishing sufficient depth of anesthesia. It is often assumed that any volatile anesthetic agent, at comparable doses, is equally effective producing bronchodilatation. The lesser pungency of halothane and sevoflurane (compared with isoflurane and desflurane) may make coughing less likely, as coughing may trigger bronchospasm. On the other hand, halothane is not ideal, as it sensitizes the myocardium to catecholamines which usually remain at high level in asthmatic patients, causing arrhythmias. Again, it is also known that the effect of sevoflurane on the airways resembles those of halothane and isoflurane. So, at conclusion, considering all aspects, it is thought that sevoflurane is the more suitable agent in patients with bronchial asthma. However, some schools thought that halothane has the maximum bronchodilating effect and is more potent than sevoflurane. So, it is the best suitable agent in asthma patient, producing deeper plane of anesthesia easily and maximum bronchodilatation. The mechanism of bronchodilating effect of volatile anesthetic agents is due to their direct effects on airway smooth muscles. This is explained by the fact that they block the intracellular calcium influx, impair calcium release from the SR, and disrupt the mechanism that sensitizes the myofilament contractile system to calcium. Except bronchodilatation, they (halothane and sevoflurane) also attenuate the responses of bronchial smooth muscle to bronchoconstricting stimuli. This action is due to the alteration (decrease) of the liberation of ACh and the depression of ganglionic transmission in vagal pathway.

An alternative technique to the administration of volatile anesthetic agents which suppress the airway reflexes before the use of muscle relaxant, laryngoscopy, and tracheal intubation may be the use of IV injection of lignocaine. Lignocaine in the dose of 1–1.5 mg/kg through IV, administered 2–3 minutes before the administration of muscle relaxant, laryngoscopy, and tracheal intubation is helpful for preventing reflex bronchoconstriction. The IV lignocaine antagonizes both the reflexes and antigen-induced bronchospasm in hyperreactive airway. It also relaxes the smooth muscles of airways in higher concentration. But the spray of lignocaine over the larynx and vocal cords, before intubation, has both the advantages and disadvantages. The beneficial effect (advantage) is surface anesthesia, produced by lignocaine, blocks the stimuli from the laryngoscopy and intubation. But the disadvantage is that lignocaine spray itself produces bronchospasm, by placing the solution like foreign body into a hyperactive airway of asthmatic patients which is not found in normal individuals. However, the clinical evidences show that at good level of anesthesia, lignocaine spray does not initiate bronchospasm.

The skeletal muscle relaxation, for the intubation and maintenance of anesthesia, is often obtained by nondepolarizing muscle relaxants. The selection of nondepolarizing muscle relaxant, for the bronchial asthma patient, depends mainly on the property of the release of histamine by these drugs. Drugs which release minimum amount of histamine or none are preferred for bronchial asthma patients. Nondepolarizing neuromuscular blocking drugs which cause histamine release should be avoided and they are listed in the table. After tracheal intubation, it is sometimes very difficult to differentiate insufficient muscular paralysis from bronchospasm as a cause of decreased lung compliance (increased peak airway pressure). This can be helped by adding additional dose of muscle relaxant **(Table 7)**.

Succinylcholine also causes the release of histamine, but to a lesser extent. Hence, there is no evidence that this drug is associated with increased airway resistance when administered in patients with bronchial asthma. Reversal of neuromuscular blockade by neostigmine and other cholinesterase inhibitor could theoretically cause bronchospasm. However, when administered with the adequate doses of anticholinergic drugs, such as atropine or glycopyrrolate, then neostigmine does not significantly change the airway resistance. Sugammadex avoids the issue of increasing the concentration of ACh, but few cases of allergic reaction to sugammadex have been reported.

Intraoperatively, the desired level of PaO_2 and end-tidal CO_2 ($ETCO_2$) tension is best maintained by mechanical

TABLE 7: Benzylisoquinoline and steroidal compounds.

Muscle relaxants	Doses causing release of histamine
A. *Benzylisoquinoline compounds*	
d-Tubocurarine	$0.6 \times ED_{95}$
Metocurine	$2 \times ED_{95}$
Doxacurium	$4 \times ED_{95}$
Mivacurium	$3 \times ED_{95}$
Atracurium	$2.5 \times ED_{95}$
Cisatracurium	None
B. *Steroidal compounds*	
Pancuronium	Minimum
Vecuronium	None
Pipecuronium	None
Rocuronium	None

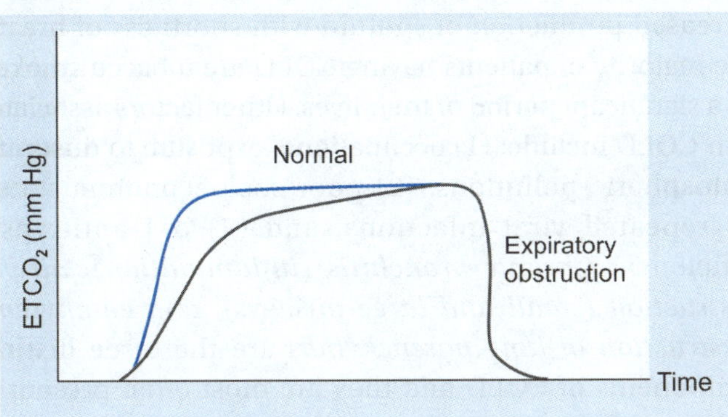

Fig. 11: Capnograph of a normal patient (blue line) compared with expiratory airway obstruction patient (black line). (ETCO$_2$: end-tidal carbon dioxide)

ventilation. Ventilation should be controlled with warmed humidified anesthetic gases, whenever possible. The airflow obstruction during expiration, due to bronchospasm, is apparent on capnography, as a delayed rise of ETCO$_2$ value **(Fig. 11)**. The severity of obstruction is generally inversely related to the rate of the rise in ETCO$_2$ tension. For mechanical ventilation, in asthma patient, a low inspiratory flow rate is used. It provides the optimal distribution of ventilation against perfusion. Severe bronchospasm is manifested by rising peak inspiratory pressures and incomplete exhalation. In the past, tidal volumes of 10–12 mL/kg with ventilatory rates of 8–10 breaths/min were considered desirable. However, currently, minimizing the tidal volume (<10 mL/kg) with prolongation of expiratory time may allow the more uniform distribution of gas flow to both the lungs and may help to avoid air trapping during expiration. This is because during expiration, sufficient time should be given to prevent air trapping in alveoli, in the presence of expiratory air flow obstruction, which is a characteristic of bronchial asthma. Positive end-expiratory pressure (PEEP) is not ideal for an asthma patient, as it may impair exhalation in the presence of narrowed airways.

Humidification and warming of inspired gases is vital. Nevertheless, it must be appreciated that sometimes humidification, as produced by ultrasonic nebulizers and pneumatic aerosols, can produce bronchospasm. The liberal use of IV fluid is mandatory during perioperative period in bronchial asthma patient because it helps adequate hydration and ensures the presence of less viscous secretions which can be expelled more easily. For the patients with history of bronchial asthma, it is prudent to remove the ETT, while the anesthesia is still in deep level. It avoids hyperreactive airway reflexes, causing bronchospasm during extubation. If there is risk of gastric aspiration, then extubation should be done, when the patient is awake, but there is chance of reflex bronchospasm. However, it can be managed by continuous IV infusions of lignocaine in the dose of 1–3 mg/kg/h.

Intraoperative bronchospasm: When bronchospasm occurs during intraoperative anesthetic period, then it should be differentiated from other conditions which also reduce the pulmonary compliance and mimic bronchospasm. For example, the conditions which mimic the intraoperative bronchospasm are: (1) mechanical obstruction of tracheal tube due to kinking, secretions, etc., (2) endobronchial intubation, (3) pulmonary edema, (4) pulmonary aspiration, (5) pulmonary embolism, (6) pneumothorax, and (7) during spontaneous respiration, active expiratory efforts by patient due to inadequate depth of anesthesia.

When the diagnosis of intraoperative bronchospasm is established, then the priority should be given to increase the depth of anesthesia by increasing the inspired concentration of volatile anesthetic agents. IV agents such as ketamine, propofol, and lignocaine may also be useful to increase the depth of anesthesia. Then, the conditions which are mimicking the acute bronchospasm should be searched for and treatment should be instituted according to the cause.

If it is confirmed that there is definite bronchospasm, then β$_2$-agonist should be nebulized through ETT, keeping in mind that the requirement is more due to the decreased efficiency of the drug delivery system to lungs, compared to unanesthetized ambulatory patients. In extreme circumstances, the inhaled β$_2$-agonists are ineffective due to inadequate tidal volume. In such circumstances, the IV adrenergic agonists such as epinephrine may be necessary. The IV aminophylline does not provide any additional benefit over halothane. Further, it may produce dysrhythmias that may accompany severe bronchospasm. The parenteral corticosteroid may be administered, but it takes several hours (3–4 hours) to exert its effect. The parameters of mechanical ventilation should be adjusted accordingly, to prevent gas trapping and barotrauma, by minimizing the airway pressure and prolonging the expiration.

Postoperative management: The postoperative respiration status of a bronchial asthma patient must be monitored very carefully. Venturi mask with fraction of inspired oxygen (FiO$_2$) of 0.24–0.40 should be used for oxygen therapy, during the immediate postoperative period. Regional nerve blocks and transcutaneous electrical nerve stimulation (TENS) may be used to provide postoperative analgesia, without using narcotics and depressing respiration. Following the major abdominal or thoracic surgeries, good pain control is important and for that epidural analgesia (not anesthesia) is frequently the best choice, provided the widespread intercostal block is avoided. The narcotics for analgesia should be used very carefully for postoperative bronchial asthma patient because respiratory depression may further compromise the airway. Morphine is contraindicated due to their histamine release property. Pethidine is safer than morphine and can be used in patient-controlled analgesia (PCA). Fentanyl or its congeners may be the better choice. Ideally, the NSAIDs are to be avoided, though the precipitation of bronchospasm due to the production of LTs is not very common (only 5–10% cases). But they can be used, if they have been tolerated before. If there is increasing dyspnea and wheezing after surgery, then other conditions such as left ventricular failure (LVF), pulmonary embolism, and fluid overload which may mimic bronchospasm should also be considered.

Drugs which are considered safe for bronchial asthma patients are:

- *Inducing agents:* Propofol, ketamine, midazolam
- *Narcotics:* Pethidine, fentanyl, sufentanil, etc.
- *Muscle relaxants:* Succinylcholine, vecuronium, rocuronium, pancuronium, etc.,
- *Volatile agents:* Halothane, isoflurane, sevoflurane

Prophylaxis for perioperative bronchospasm can be instituted by the following measures:

- Continued bronchial asthma pharmacotherapy up to the time of anesthesia and surgery
- Inhalation of β_2-agonists before induction
- Corticosteroid replacement therapy
- Preoperative anxiolysis
- Prefer RA, if possible
- Tracheal intubation at deeper plane of anesthesia but never at light plane
- Avoid anesthetic agents, which increase the airway reactivity.

Emergency surgery: The bronchial asthmatic patient, waiting for emergency surgery, is a two-way sword. This is because patients are presented usually with full stomach. So, one way of the sword is that intubation in light plane of anesthesia or awake intubation to prevent pulmonary aspiration triggers bronchospasm. Second, if anesthesia is deepened to prevent the reflex-initiated bronchospasm, then there is higher risk of pulmonary aspiration. So, an anesthetist has to balance between these two and the intensity of the emergency of surgery. Furthermore, there is often insufficient time to optimize the bronchodilatation and corticoid therapy prior to surgery. So, RA is always preferred, if the site of surgery suits properly and permits in such situations.

CHRONIC OBSTRUCTIVE LUNG DISEASE OR CHRONIC OBSTRUCTIVE PULMONARY DISEASE

The symptoms of COLD usually start after the age of about 55 years. The most common symptom of it is breathlessness. But there is often a combination of cough, wheeze, and increased production of sputum with shortness of breath. The majority of patients having COLD are tobacco smokers for a significant period of their lives. Other factors associated with COLD include: (1) occupational exposure to dusts and atmospheric pollutions, (2) poor socioeconomic status, (3) repeated viral infections, and (4) α-1-antitrypsin deficiency. *Chronic bronchitis (inflammation), airway obstruction (small and large airways), and emphysema (destruction of lung parenchyma)* are the three distinct components of COLD and they are most often present in different combinations. Among these three pathologies, the chronic bronchitis progressively leads to chronic obstructive bronchitis with extra addition of obstruction to airflow which is not fully reversible. *Chronic obstructive bronchitis* is also termed as chronic *asthmatic* bronchitis and when it is developed, then COLD consists of two components, i.e., *chronic asthmatic bronchitis* and *emphysema*. In the early part of this disease process of COLD, this obstruction is reversible and is due to bronchospasm and this bronchospasm can be improved by the administration of bronchodilators.

The *chronic bronchitis* is defined as a condition where there is excessive tracheobronchial mucus production for at least 3 months of a year and for >2 consecutive years, due to the inflammation of airways, (but at this phase there is no bronchoconstriction and obstruction). The chronic bronchitis has two parts: *hypersecretion of mucus and inflammatory changes in mucous membrane. Chronic obstructive bronchitis* which is the second phase of COLD is also defined as the condition, where there is both the excessive secretion of mucus and inflammation due to *chronic bronchitis* and *obstruction* due to bronchospasm, and experience both the *dyspnea and wheezing*. Such patients are also said to have chronic asthmatic bronchitis as there is both the picture of chronic bronchitis (secretion and inflammation) and asthma (obstruction). Chronic asthmatic bronchitis is characterized by partial reversibility of bronchial (air flow) obstruction with bronchodilator and abatement of inflammation. This group of patients also shows the hyperresponsiveness of airway to nonspecific stimuli, like bronchial asthma patients. So, confusion may persist between the chronic bronchitis with obstruction (chronic asthmatic bronchitis) and those of pure bronchial asthma who also may have chronic airways obstruction with inflammation.

Thus, the difference between the two is that patients with chronic asthmatic bronchitis have a long history of sputum production and cough (i.e., only bronchitis part at beginning) with a later onset of wheezing (asthmatic part), whereas the chronic bronchial asthma patients with chronic obstruction will first give a long history of wheezing with later onset of chronic productive cough. Emphysema which is the third component of COLD is defined as the permanent, abnormal distension of air spaces (alveoli) distal to the terminal bronchiole with destruction of alveolar septa. So, COLD = chronic obstructive bronchitis or chronic asthmatic bronchitis (chronic bronchitis + asthma) + emphysema.

The patients, suffering from COLD, with predominant emphysema is thin, tachypneic, and breathless at rest. They are described as *"pink puffer"*. Though, they are hypoxic, but CO_2 retention usually does not develop. Hypercapnia develops only as a late or terminal event, whereas the patients suffering from COLD with predominant chronic bronchitis are frequently overweight with marked peripheral edema, poor respiratory effort, and CO_2 retention. They are described as *"blue bloater"*. These two classical stereotyped pictures of "pink puffer" and "blue bloater" are relatively infrequent, as the majority of patients have a combination of these two features. In *"pink puffers"* which is associated with emphysema, PaO_2 is usually higher than 65 mm Hg, though they are hypoxic and $PaCO_2$ is normal to slightly decrease, whereas in *"blue bloaters"* which is associated with bronchitis, the PaO_2 is usually lower than 65 mm Hg and $PaCO_2$ is increased to >45 mm Hg. With advancing disease, both the "pink puffers" and "blue bloaters" will lead to the maldistribution of both the ventilation and pulmonary blood flow, resulting in the areas of low V/Q ratio (intrapulmonary shunt) and as well as areas of high V/Q ratios (Vd).

Pathology of Bronchitis and Emphysema of COLD

The usual findings of chronic bronchitis of COLD are: (1) the hypertrophy of mucus producing glands, (2) the increase in the number of goblet cells, (3) the reduction in the number of ciliated cells, and (4) the increase in the number of neutrophil, lymphocyte, and plasma cells in the mucosa and submucosa layer of the large cartilaginous airways (i.e., up to the terminal bronchioles) **(Fig. 12)**. So, it is characterized by the (1) hypersecretion of mucus fluid, (2) less secretion of serous fluid, and (3) inflammatory changes in bronchi. This causes daily cough and large production of sputum. On the other hand, due to the loss of ciliated epithelium and decrease of serous secretion, a large quantity of viscid mucus secretion becomes difficult to eliminate. Thus, there is always a tendency of the retention of secretion in the airway, which encourages the bacterial growth. So, a vicious cycle may set up which leads to chronic bronchitis. This vicious cycle is as follows: increased and retention of secretion → bacterial growth → repeated attack of infection and inflammation → repeated attack of chronic bronchitis.

Thus, with repeated acute exacerbation of inflammation and with increasing retention of secretion, there is gradual spread of chronic inflammatory changes along

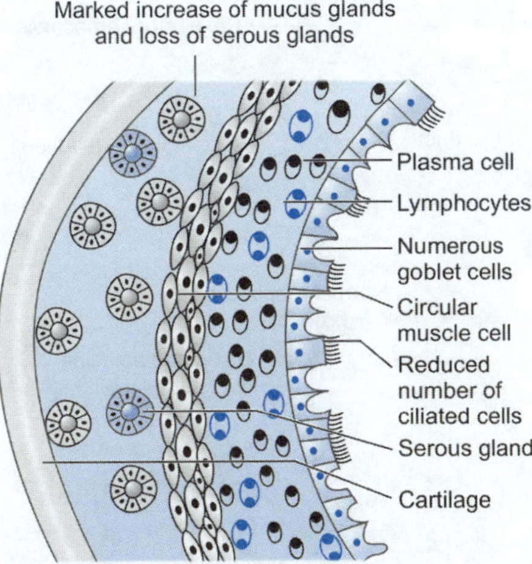

Fig. 12: The microscopic picture of airways of patient suffering from chronic obstructive lung disease (COLD).

the wall of bronchial tree and more and more damage is encouraged. When the terminal bronchioles are affected, then more serious changes take place. These are: seepage and retention of exudate in alveoli → leading to bacterial alveolar infection → leading to the patches of pneumonia during acute exacerbations. All these factors, with the lack of ciliary function, make the airway difficult to get rid of exudate which hinders the resolution. Then, healing takes place by the organization of fibrosis, causing the obliteration of small alveoli and bronchioles and leading to obstruction during expiration. Thus, emphysema develops. This chronic bronchitis is most common in industrial areas, where rainfall is high. In its serious form, it usually occurs in males over the age of 40, but the onset can be dated many years earlier. The prognosis of chronic bronchitis is poor. The death often occurs within 5 years, after the first episode of acute respiratory failure.

Emphysema is a condition where there is permanent increase in the size of air spaces (alveoli), distal to the terminal bronchiole. In emphysema, with the increase in the size of airspaces, there are also destructive changes in the walls of air spaces. Usually emphysema is of two types: alveolar or *centrilobular emphysema* and *panacinar emphysema* **(Figs. 13 and 14)**. In centrilobular emphysema, there is no increase in the volume of lungs. The distension and destruction are mainly limited to respiratory bronchioles with relatively less changes in the acinus (alveoli) at periphery. So, there is little radiological evidence of emphysema because the alveolar tissue is normal. These changes are also extremely common in normal lungs of persons who are above the age of 50. In panacinar emphysema, where the process is extensive, then in such situation the distension eventually spreads to involve the respiratory bronchiole and the whole acinus. Thus, the whole lungs become distended with definite radiological findings.

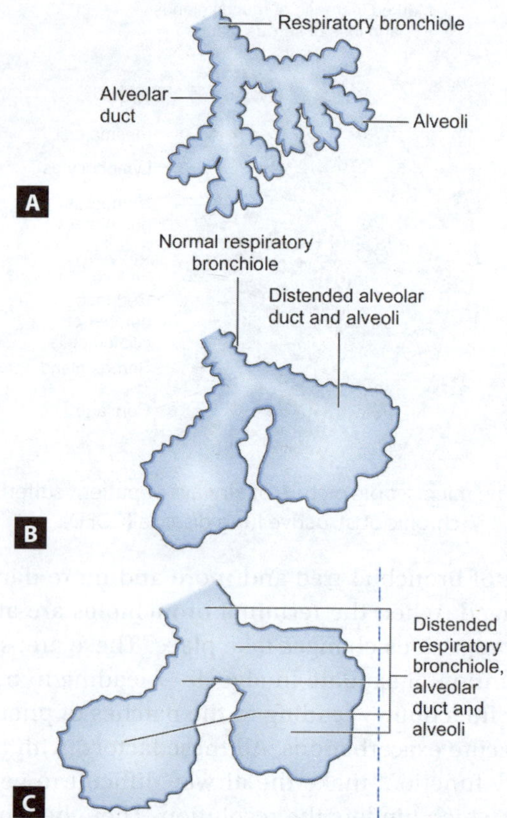

Figs. 13A to C: (A) Normal lung parenchyma; (B) alveolar emphysema; (C) panacinar emphysema.

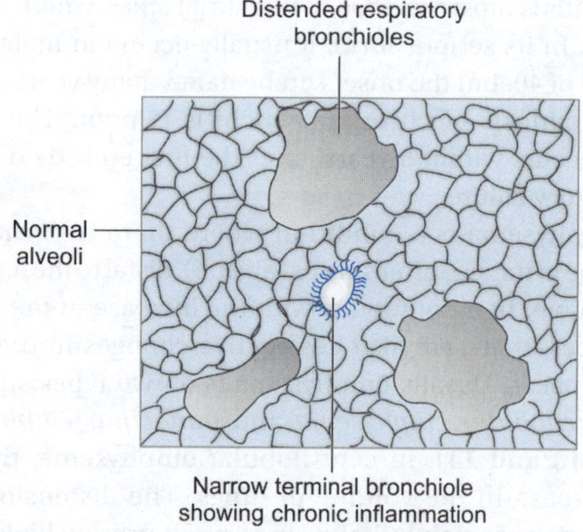

Fig. 14: Centrilobular emphysema; chronic inflammation of the terminal bronchioles is an important feature. In this type of lesion, there is little radiological evidence of emphysema because the alveolar tissue is normal for a considerable time.

Pathophysiology of COLD

In COLD patients, initially both the chronic bronchitis and emphysema can exist without any evidence of obstruction in airways. But later by the time, when a patient begins to

experience dyspnea, as a result of these processes, then obstruction is always demonstrable. Thus, when the two processes (bronchitis with obstruction and emphysema) are combined, then one process may dominate over the other. The therapeutic improvement of this condition depends on (1) the extent of inflammatory process, (2) the quantitative presence of secretions, and () the severity of bronchospasm. Both the chronic bronchitis and emphysema result in airways narrowing. The airways narrowing in chronic bronchitis is due to inflammation, secretions, hyperactive reflexes, etc. But the loss of elastic recoil of the lung in emphysema accounts for a decrease in airway caliber through the loss of radial traction on airways. In both these situations (i.e., chronic bronchitis and emphysema) the narrowing of airways (obstruction) is often associated with (1) an increase in the resistance of airways and (2) a diminution of maximal expiratory flow rates.

Mechanism of Diminution of Expiratory Flow Rate in COLD

During expiration, the failure to increase the flow rate by augmented (forced) expiratory effort results from the dynamic compression and the closer of airways. This can be described by a point named *equal pressure point (EPP)*. During expiration, the pressure head that helps to move the air from alveoli to mouth is provided by the intra-alveolar pressure (P_{alv}). At any fixed state of the dynamic process of respiration and at any given lung volume the P_{alv} is the sum of distending negative intrapleural pressure (P_{pl}) and recoiling pulmonary elastic recoiling pressure (P_{el}). At the end of inspiration, when there is no flow of air, then the P_{alv} becomes zero, i.e., becomes equal to the pressure of atmosphere at the level of mouth. At that condition, P_{pl} is maximum subatmospheric (i.e., maximum negative) but equal to and counterbalances the P_{el} (which is always positive).

During expiration, due to the passive reduction of thoracic volume, P_{pl} gradually becomes less negative and P_{alv} rises. Now, this increased alveolar pressure head gradually decreases along the airway and finally reaches to zero (atmospheric pressure) at the level of the mouth. When this pressure head is gradually decreasing along the airway from alveoli toward mouth, then at some point on the airway, the intraluminal pressure comes to a level that is equal to the surrounding P_{pl}. *This point is called as the equal pressure point and airways start to collapse at this level.*

During normal expiration, the P_{pl} does not usually become equal to the intraluminal pressure at any point throughout the airway from alveoli to mouth and the EPP never develops and the closure of airways usually does not occur. But during forceful expiration, P_{pl} rises and sometimes may become positive. P_{alv} also rises with forceful expiration, but it gradually comes down (decreases) along the airway toward the mouth and at mouth it becomes zero, i.e., equal to the atmospheric pressure. *Along the airway, when the intraluminal pressure is gradually coming down, then at some point, situated anywhere on the airway between the alveoli and the mouth, the P_{pl} becomes greater than the intraluminal pressure and EPP develops and airways start to close at that site.* If the EPP falls on the airway where cartilages are present, i.e., proximal to the eleventh generation of airways, then this airway will not collapse. But if the EPP falls on the airway, where there is absence of cartilages, i.e., distal to the 11th generation of airway, then only these airways are vulnerable to collapse. However, EPP is not a fixed point on airway, but a dynamic one. It changes according to different conditions such as P_{pl}, P_{alv}, force of expiration, and compliance of airway **(Figs. 15A to C)**.

In normal lungs, the airway usually does not close and if closes it occurs first at the basal portion of lungs and in the small airways of 0.5–0.9 mm of diameter. In normal healthy lungs, airway does not collapse at the end of expiration because from the beginning to the end of expiration, due to the increase in pressure in pleural cavity, the P_{pl} gradually becomes more negative to less negative, but still remains subatmospheric (or negative). During forceful expiration airways closer occurs first in the basal region because the difference between the distending P_{pl} and elastic recoil P_{el} becomes positive here, due to positive P_{pl} in forced expiration.

The early or premature airway closer and the reduction of expiratory flow rate, with air trapping in alveoli, occurs with slight active (forceful) expiration in patients, suffering from emphysema, bronchitis, bronchial asthma, and interstitial edema. In these four conditions, airway resistance is increased which causes a quick and larger decrease of pressure gradient from alveoli toward the mouth. Therefore, it causes potential negative intraluminal and P_{pl} pressure gradient and early collapse of airways with shifting of EPP more toward the alveoli. In addition, the structural integrity of airways is diminished due to chronic inflammation and scarring which also causes the early closure of airways, with the shifting of EPP toward alveoli, at high lung volumes in the abovementioned diseases. Thus, FRC is increased.

In COLD patients, the RV and FRC are almost always higher than normal. Normal FRC is the volume at which the inward elastic recoil force of lung is balanced by the outward distending force of chest wall or P_{pl}. So, the loss of inward elastic recoil property of lung in emphysema results in higher FRC. Again, prolongation of expiration, due to obstruction

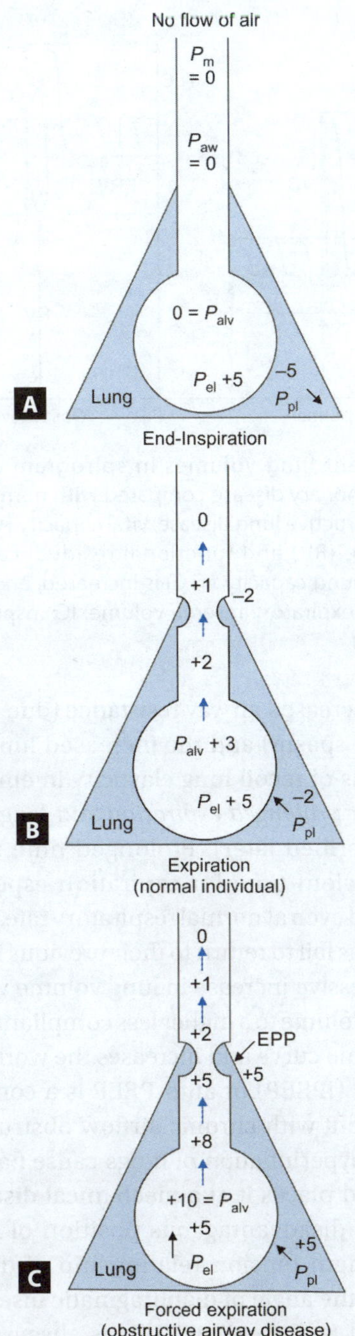

Figs. 15A to C: The concept of equal pressure point (EPP); also it tries to explain the mechanism of diminution of expiratory flow during forced expiration. (A) end of inspiration; (B) expiration in normal individual; (C) forced expiration in obstructive pulmonary disease. (P_{alv}: intra-alveolar pressure; P_{el}: pulmonary elastic recoiling pressure; P_m: pressure at mouth; P_{pl}: intrapleural pressure; P_{aw}: airway pressure)

and initiation of inspiration before the respiratory system reaches its static balance point during expiration, causes dynamic increase in FRC. With the increase of RV and FRC, due to decreased elastic recoil of lung, the TLC also increases **(Fig. 16)**.

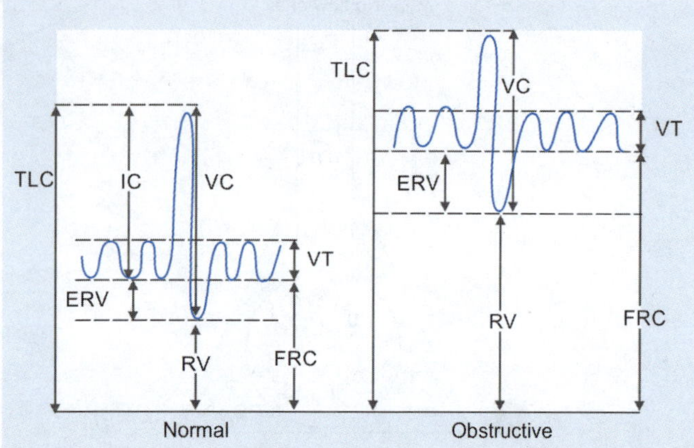

Fig. 16: Different lung volumes in spirogram during chronic obstructive pulmonary disease compared with normal values. In the presence of obstructive lung disease, vital capacity (VC) is decreased, residual volume (RV) and functional residual capacity (FRC) is increased, total lung capacity (TLC) is increased, and RV/TLC ratio is increased. (ERV: expiratory reserve volume; IC: inspiratory capacity; VT: tidal volume)

TABLE 8: Classification of chronic obstructive lung disease (COLD).

Severity	Spirometry	Symptoms
Mild COLD	FEV_1 60–80% of normal	Cough ± breathlessness on exertion
Moderate COLD	FEV_1 40–60% of normal	Cough + Breathlessness on exertion, ± Wheeze, ± sputum
Severe COLD	FEV1 <40% of normal	Prominent cough, wheeze, and breathlessness

(FEV_1: forced expiratory volume in first 1 second)

Both the increased airway resistance (due to mechanical obstruction in spasm) and the increased lung compliance (due to the loss of recoil lung elasticity in emphysema) are responsible for *prolonged expiration* and *long time constant* (which is described later). Prolonged time for expiration signify insufficient time for expiration especially during tachypnea, and even at normal respiratory rate. So, after every expiration lungs fail to return to their previous FRC. Thus this leads to progressive increase in lung volume which, in turn, push the tidal volume to a higher less compliant portion of the pressure–volume curve and increases the work of breathing. Intrinsic PEEP (iPEEP) or auto-PEEP is a common finding in such a patient with chronic airflow obstructive disease. Additionally, hyperinflation of lungs cause flattening of the diaphragm and places it at a mechanical disadvantageous position. This disadvantageous position of diaphragm is due to the length tension relationship of diaphragmatic muscle fibers, the angle of diaphragmatic insertion with the lower ribs and Laplace's law. This is always presented as mismatched V/Q ratio. When these mismatches are severe, then the impairment of gas exchange is reflected in the abnormalities of arterial blood gases.

There are some regions of lungs that are deficit in perfusion in relation to ventilation and it increases the wasted ventilation. Alternatively, there are some regions of lungs that have deficit of ventilation in relation to perfusion and it increases the wasted perfusion. Thus, in chronic bronchitis with obstruction and emphysema, there is increase in both the wasted ventilation and wasted perfusion. The resultant effect of this wasted ventilation and wasted perfusion is different for different patients. Some patients at the cost of extremely high effort of breathing and chronic dyspnea maintain a strikingly increased minute volume which results both in a normal to low $PaCO_2$ and a relatively high arterial PaO_2, despite high Vd/VT and high alveolar oxygen pressure (P_AO_2)–PaO_2 difference respectively. Other patients show only modest increase in minute volume and effort of breathings with less dyspnea, which results in high $PaCO_2$ and severely depressed PaO_2. The explanation behind this patient to patient difference is that the patients who maintain low $PaCO_2$ levels are of highly responsive type and have increased ventilatory drive in response to their high blood gas values. Those who chronically maintain high $PaCO_2$ and low PaO_2 levels have a diminished ventilatory drive in relation to their more severely deranged blood gas values **(Table 8)**.

Chronic obstructive lung disease is often associated with mild-to-severe pulmonary hypertension. Pulmonary hypertension is due to the reduction of total cross-sectional area of pulmonary vasculature. This can be attributed to anatomical changes and constriction of vascular smooth muscle in pulmonary arteries and arterioles as well as destruction of alveolar septa with loss of capillaries. The most important is constriction of the pulmonary capillaries in response to alveolar hypoxia and this vasoconstriction is reversible which depends upon the alveolar PO_2.

According to the arterial blood gas analysis, the COLD patients are divided into "pink puffers" where PaO_2 is usually higher than 65 mm Hg and $PaCO_2$ is normal to slightly decreased and "blue bloaters" where PaO_2 is usually lower than 65 mm Hg and $PaCO_2$ is chronically increased to >45 mm Hg. "Pink puffers" individuals are typically thin build, free of signs of right heart failure, and are usually found to have severe emphysema. On the other hand, "blue bloaters" typically exhibit excessive cough and sputum production, frequent respiratory tract infections and recurrent episodes of cor pulmonale. In "pink puffers", emphysema component predominates over bronchitis with obstruction component, whereas the blue boaters individual more often meet the criteria of chronic bronchitis with obstruction than emphysema. But the common denominator in all these patients is chronic cigarette smoking.

The "blue bloater" patients usually develop pulmonary hypertension due to arterial hypoxemia and respiratory acidosis which evoke pulmonary vasoconstriction. In response to chronic pulmonary hypertension, right ventricular hypertrophy and cor pulmonale is developed. Later on, right ventricular failure results with jugular venous congestion, peripheral edema, systemic venous hypertension, etc. So, they are referred to as "blue bloater" syndrome.

Patients with COLD who are characterized as "pink puffers" experience emphysematous lung destruction, leading to the loss of pulmonary capillaries, as a result of destroyed alveolar walls. The subsequent loss of pulmonary capillary vascular bed is manifested as the decreased diffusing capacity, although the PaO_2 is typically only mildly depressed, such that pulmonary vasoconstriction is minimal and cor pulmonale develops only rarely in these patients. When dyspneic, these patients with emphysema, often purse their lips to delay the closure of their small airways, which accounts for the term "pink puffers".

What is Time Constant?

It is defined as the time taken by the alveoli to reach its final volume if the initial gas flow rate is maintained throughout the inflation. Usually the normal inspiratory time is 1–1.5 second. A long inspiratory time increases the mean intrathoracic pressure and reduces the venous return with reduction of cardiac output. On the other hand, short inspiratory time causes poor distribution of the inspired gases throughout the lungs.

If the airway leading to an alveoli is narrowed and the resistance is increased, then the alveoli will still reach the same volume when inflated at same pressure. But it will take longer time to reach the final volume. Again if the wall of the alveoli is stiffened and compliance is decreased, then the alveoli will also take longer time to reach the final volume when inflated at same pressure. Thus the time constant depends on the resistance and compliance of the system and the relation is:

Resistance × compliance = Time constant

Typical values of resistance and compliance for an anaesthetized patient are 10 cmH_2O/L and 50 mL/cmH_2O (or 0.05 L/cmH_2O). So, the normal time constant is 10 × 0.05 = 0.5 second.

An increase in resistance and decrease in compliance result in longer time constant. Usually 94% of the final volume of lungs reaches within the three time constants due to different types of alveoli. This scattering of time constant is exaggerated in some forms of lung diseases such as asthma and emphysema. In such circumstances a short inspiratory

TABLE 9: Difference between pure chronic bronchitis and emphysema [component of chronic obstructive lung disease (COLD)].

Features	Chronic bronchitis	Emphysema
Airway obstruction (mechanism)	Due to mucus or inflammation	Nil
Cough	Frequent	Very less frequent
Dyspnea	Less frequent	More frequent
Sputum	Copious	Scanty
PaO_2	Markedly decrease (blue bloater)	Less decrease (pink puffer)
$PaCO_2$	Often elevated (> 40 mm Hg)	Usually normal or hypo (<40 mm Hg)
FEV_1	Decrease	Decrease
TLCO	Normal	Decrease
RV and TLC	↑RV, but normal TLC	↑RV and ↑TLC
Hematocrit	Increase	Normal
Elastic recoil	Normal	Decrease
Airway resistance	Increase	Normal to slightly elevated
Chest radiograph	Increased lung markings	Hyperinflation
Cor pulmonale	Early manifested	Late manifested
Prognosis	Poor	Good

(FEV_1: forced expiratory volume in first 1 second; PaO_2: partial pressure of arterial oxygen; $PaCO_2$: partial pressure of arterial carbon dioxide; RV: residual volume; TLC: total lung capacity; TLCO: gas transfer factor of lung for carbon monoxide)

time will result in poor ventilation of those zones of lung having a long time constant. Thus there will be a resulting increase in V/Q mismatch **(Table 9)**.

Anesthetic Management of COLD

The anesthetic management of patients, suffering from COLD and waiting for surgery, include:

- Proper preoperative evaluation of pulmonary function: by good history taking, clinical examination, investigations, and PFTs.
- Treatment of COLD in preoperative period to optimize the pulmonary function.
- Intraoperative management aimed at minimizing pulmonary complications and minimizing residual depressant effects of anesthetic drugs on respiration postoperatively.
- Postoperative pain control and pulmonary care by physiotherapy to reduce the pulmonary complications.

Preoperative Evaluation

The preoperative evaluation of patients with COLD is based on the recognition that the perioperative pulmonary complications are of predictable risks, with increased morbidity and mortality due to pneumonia, atelectasis, bronchospasm, acute respiratory failure requiring mechanical ventilation, etc. So, the history, clinical examination, investigations, and PFT including blood gas analysis of patients, suffering from COLD, provide a more accurate assessment for predictable risks which are likelihood to occur as perioperative pulmonary complications.

The history and clinical examinations are more important than PFT and blood gas analysis for the assessment of pulmonary risks and its complications. With regard to history, (1) the history of recent changes in dyspnea, (2) expectoration of sputum, (3) wheezing, (4) exercise intolerance, (5) chronic cough, (6) unexplained dyspnea, etc., are very important, and are directly related to increased mortality, due to pulmonary complications. Decreased breath sound, wheezing, and prolonged expiratory phase on clinical examination also predict increased risk of perioperative pulmonary complications. However, the values of PFTs, done as routinely for the preoperative evaluation of perioperative risks, is in doubt. Usually, the PFT is taken as a reference point during the management and optimization of pulmonary function in perioperative period, but not as a means to assess the risk. The preoperative lung function tests are also useful tools for assessing the lung functions and the responses to the therapy. But these tests do not provide the predictive information as to the likelihood of the rate of pulmonary complications.

Regarding the X-ray, chest radiograph should be reviewed carefully. The presence of bullous changes should be noted. Many patients have concomitant cardiac disease and should also receive a careful cardiovascular evaluation.

Regarding PFTs, the patients with FEV_1 <50% of predicted value (1.2–1.5 L) usually have dyspnea on exertion, whereas those with FEV_1 <25% of predicted value (<1 L) typically have dyspnea in mild activity. The latter finding is often associated with CO_2 retention and pulmonary hypertension. However, the value of PFTs, done as a routine preoperative evaluation of perioperative pulmonary risks, is in doubt. *Usually, PFT is taken as reference point, during the management and optimization of pulmonary function in perioperative period, but not as a means to assess the risks.* Pre-operative pulmonary function tests (PFTs) are also useful tools for assessing the lung functions and responses to the therapy. But these tests do not provide predictive information as to the likelihood of the rate of postoperative pulmonary complications. This is because patients defined as high risk by PFT (FEV_1<50% of predicted value, FEV_1/FVC <65%, and $PaCO_2$ >45 mm Hg)

can undergo surgery with acceptable risks for perioperative pulmonary complications. *The potential risk factors of patients with COLD for the development of perioperative pulmonary complications are: smoking, operative site, anesthetic drugs, advanced age, poor general health, etc.*

In contrast to asthma, only limited improvement in respiratory function may be seen after a short period of intensive preoperative preparation. The preoperative preparation of patients with COLD is aimed at (1) correcting the hypoxemia, (2) relieving bronchospasm, (3) reducing secretion, and (4) treating infection may decrease the incidences of perioperative pulmonary complications.

Smoking increases the perioperative pulmonary complications manyfold in a patient who is suffering from COLD. So, the cessation of smoking before operation is advised strictly. Although the sufficient time, required for the reversible changes to occur, after the cessation of smoking, is not correctly known. The operative site is also the most important predictor for perioperative pulmonary complications. The upper abdominal and thoracic surgery create the greatest risks for pulmonary complications. The perioperative pulmonary complications are less likely to occur, following the operations outside the thorax and the abdomen. The duration of surgery is also an important factor for the development of pulmonary complications. The duration of surgery >3 hours increases the risks for pulmonary complications. Anesthetic drugs and surgical trauma disrupt the normal activity of respiratory muscles, causing persistent decrease in FRC and VC with atelectasis that can last for several days after surgery, leading to increased pulmonary complications.

Preoperative Preparations

The preoperative preparations of patients suffering from COLD include:

- Stoppage of smoking
- Treatment of expiratory outflow obstruction such as bronchospasm
- Eradication of bacterial infection
- Physiotherapy, regarding lung volume expansion maneuvers.

To stop the cigarette smoking is strongly recommended for patients before undergoing elective surgery, as the risk of postoperative pulmonary complications predictably increases manyfold with smoking. Till now the optimal period of abstinence from smoking, before any elective surgery, is not clearly known. But it is clear that even a brief period of abstinence from smoking improves the oxygen carrying capacity of arterial blood. This is because the adverse effects of CO on O_2 carrying capacity of Hb and the adverse effects of nicotine on cardiovascular system (CVS) are short-lived. The sympathomimetic effects of nicotine on CVS are transient, lasting for only 20–30 minutes. The elimination half-life of CO is 4–6 hours. So, the smoke-free intervals of at least 12 hours could result in substantial decrease in carbomonoxyhemoglobin levels. Experimentally, it is seen that 12 hours abstinence from smoking increases P_{50} value of Hb (the PO_2 at which Hb is 50% saturated) from 22 to 26 mm Hg and the plasma levels of carbomonoxyhemoglobin decreases from 6 to 1%. The increased levels of carbomonoxyhemoglobin in blood can cause the pulse oximeter to falsely overestimate the SPO_2 level. Cigarette smoking also causes the hypersecretion of mucus, impairment of mucociliary transport activity and the narrowing of smaller airways. So, the abstinence from smoking definitely decreases the sputum production, and improves the ciliary action and smaller airway function. But these actions of recovery occur slowly over a period of weeks, after cigarette smoking is stopped. Only the effects of smoking on COHb (carboxy-hemoglobin) improves faster with short-term abstinence. It is found that when the abstinence from cigarette smoking in longer than 8 weeks, then the incidence of postoperative pulmonary complications decreases significantly.

Smoking also interferes the function of immune system and increases the incidence of postoperative pulmonary infections after anesthesia and surgery. The return of normal immune function may require at least 6 weeks of abstinence from smoking. Smoking also stimulates the hepatic enzymes which increases the postoperative analgesic requirement. Like immune response, 6–8 weeks of abstinence from smoking makes return of the hepatic enzyme to normal level. The cessation of smoking helps to diminish the symptoms of chronic bronchitis. It also helps to eliminate the accelerated loss of lung functions observed in those who continue to smoke. For preoperative preparation of COLD patients, chronic administration of O_2 (2 L/min for few hours per day) is recommended if the PaO_2 is <55 mm Hg (the goal is to achieve PaO_2 between 60 and 80 mm Hg), the hematocrit is >55% or there is evidence of cor pulmonale. Relief of arterial hypoxemia by administration of O_2 is very effective than any drug in decreasing pulmonary vascular resistance and preventing excessive erythrocytosis with associates increase in blood viscosity.

Preoperative administration of broad-spectrum antibiotics is seriously indicated, if there are acute episodes of worsening of clinical symptoms, which is marked by increased dyspnea, excessive purulent sputum production, wheezing, etc. Vaccinations against influenza and possibly pneumococcus may be beneficial. If the exacerbations of COLD is due to the viral infections of upper respiratory tract, then preoperative antibiotic treatment will not be helpful.

Drug induced diuresis may be considered for patients with cor pulmonale and right ventricular failure (peripheral edema). Diuretic induced chloride depletion may also result in hypochloremic metabolic alkalosis that depresses the ventilatory drive and may aggravate the chronic retention of CO_2.

Another mainstay for the preoperative preparation of patients, suffering from COLD, is bronchodilatation. Though it causes only a small increase in FEV_1 in patients with COLD, but these drugs reduce the symptoms of dyspnea. Bronchodilators such as mainly β_2-agonist improves exercise tolerance, though there is little improvement in spirometric measurements. The β_2-agonist also decreases the exacerbation of infections by reducing the adhesiveness of bacteria, such as *Haemophilus influenzae* with epithelial cells. But the anticholinergics are more effective in the treatment of COLD than this β_2-agonist which is more effective in the treatment of bronchial asthma.

Another important risk reduction strategy, during the preoperative preparation of patient suffering from COLD, to decrease the incidence of postoperative pulmonary complications, is to initiate the patient's education, regarding the lung volume expansion manoeuvers. The prophylactic lung volume expansion maneuvers such as the deep breathing exercise, incentive spirometry, chest physiotherapy, positive pressure breathing techniques, etc., are of proven benefit for preventing the postoperative pulmonary complications in high-risk patients. This physiotherapy of chest facilitates the removal of secretions from airways, reduces the risk of atelectasis, and increases the pulmonary functions. The institution of preoperative lung expansion manoeuvers definitely decreases the incidence of perioperative pulmonary complications than if education begins after surgery. The measurement of FRC is the most important lung volume parameter during postoperative period that provides a specific goal for therapy. The positive pressure breathing technique may be of two types: intermittent or continuous. Both are effective in reducing the incidences of perioperative pulmonary complications, but its cost has resulted in its decreased uses. The continuous positive airway pressure (CPAP) is usually reserved for very sick patients who are unable for intermittent positive pressure breathing (IPPB). Another type of positive pressure breathing, such as nasal positive airway pressure, also minimizes the postoperative reduction of lung volume, the incidences of atelectasis and acute respiratory failure.

Intraoperative Management

There is no specific drugs or specific anesthetic techniques for the better management of patients suffering from COLD. During the management of patients, suffering from COLD, always it should be kept in our mind that these patients are highly susceptible to the development of acute respiratory failure, during an intraoperative and postoperative period. Among the general and RA, the RA is the most desired method. But unfortunately it is only restricted to the surgeries of lower abdomen and upper or lower extremities. This is because the high RA affecting the dermatomes above T10 level, required for upper abdominal or thoracic surgeries, paralyses the more and more intercostal and accessory respiratory muscles and impairs the ventilation, leading to decreased lung volume, ineffective cough, dyspnea, retention of secretion, etc., in a patient whose respiratory system is already compromised.

General anesthesia is the usual choice for upper abdominal and intrathoracic operations which are associated with higher incidences of pulmonary complications. There is some debates or controversies between the incidences of pulmonary complications and the duration of anesthesia. But the general agreement is that the operation and anesthesia, lasting for longer than 3 hours, are more likely to be associated with higher pulmonary complications. So, where there is chance of postoperative respiratory failure, tracheal intubation and mechanical ventilation should be continued postoperatively. Alternatively, postoperative epidural analgesia (not anesthesia) by narcotics or local anesthetic agents permit a pain-free breathing which allows the early tracheal extubation and decreased systemic analgesic requirement with their associated depressant effects on ventilation and consciousness.

When GA is applied, then preoxygenation prior to induction is mandatory and it prevents the rapid oxygen desaturation that is often seen in these patients. Volatile anesthetic agents, proper humidification of inspired gases, and mechanical ventilation are the cornerstones of anesthetic technique. The intraoperative use of volatile anesthetic agents is more preferable than narcotics, because the patients are able to eliminate these drugs rapidly through their lungs and thus minimizes the early postoperative residual respiratory depression and pulmonary complications. Moreover, the volatile anesthetic agents cause bronchodilatation which has a distinct advantage over narcotics. The narcotics or opioids are less useful for COLD patients because of their direct prolonged postoperative depression effect on ventilation. Unfortunately, the use of bronchodilating anesthetics improves only the reversible component of airflow obstruction and significant expiratory obstruction may still present.

Expiratory airflow limitation, especially under positive pressure ventilation, may lead to (1) air trapping, (2) dynamic hyperinflation, and (3) elevated iPEEP. Dynamic hyperinflation may result in volume trauma of lungs,

hemodynamic instability, hypercapnia, and acidosis. Now, this trapping of air into lungs can be prevented by: (1) allowing more time to exhale decreasing respiratory rate and decreasing inspiratory to expiratory (I:E) ratio, (2) allowing permissive hypercapnia, (3) applying low level of extrinsic PEEP or avoiding it, and aggressively treating bronchospasm.

The COLD patients are often associated with emphysema. So, one should use N_2O carefully because it will diffuse into the pulmonary bullae, which are commonly associated with emphysema, and can lead to their enlargement and rupture, resulting in the development of tension pneumothorax during anesthesia. The another disadvantage of administration of N_2O in patients suffering from COLD is that it limits the concentration of inspired O_2. The inhaled volatile anesthetic agents attenuate hypoxic pulmonary vasoconstriction. This hypoxic pulmonary vasoconstriction is beneficial for maintenance of arterial oxygenation in nonanesthetized patient by shifting the blood from hypoxic to nonhypoxic zone. But as the volatile anesthetic agents attenuates this hypoxic pulmonary vasoconstriction, so its beneficial effect is lost and thus increase the degree of right to left intrapulmonary shunt. So, increased inspired concentration of O_2 is necessary to offset this anesthesia-induced pulmonary changes, which can be hindered by the use of N_2O.

Intubation which bypasses nearly the entire natural airway humidification system and the *high flows of dry anesthetics gases* from anesthetic machine both greatly intensify the need for the humidification of dry inspired gases to prevent the drying of secretions in airways. The systemic dehydration, due to inadequate fluid administration, during the perioperative period, also can increase the excessive drying of secretions in the airways, despite proper humidification of inspired gases, delivered from anesthetic machine.

Controlled ventilation is useful for COLD patients receiving GA. During controlled ventilation, large tidal volume (10–15 mL/kg) combined with slow inspiratory flow rates and low breathing rates (<10 breaths/min) maintains the optimum V/Q ratio. *Low breathing (respiratory) rates help by:*

- Allowing complete expiration and preventing air trapping which is characteristic of COLD patients
- Preventing hyperventilation which causes more reduction of $PaCO_2$
- Increasing venous return
- Reducing the likelihood of turbulent flow in airways.

The PEEP should not be incorporated in any ventilatory mode in COLD patients because it affects the expiratory flow. But large tidal volume, slow inspiratory flow, and low breathing rates act as alternative to and as effective as PEEP. If any time high positive airway pressure is required to provide adequate ventilation and proper oxygenation of blood, then pulmonary barotrauma and rupture of emphysematous bullae should be kept in mind. During spontaneous ventilation of COLD patients, ventilatory depression by volatile anesthetic agents should be observed carefully because depression of respiration, produced by narcotics and other anesthetic agents, are more sensitive than normal individual. So, whatever may be the ventilatory mode, arterial blood gases, pH, SPO_2 and $ETCO_2$ should be maintained at normal level.

The risk of pulmonary complication is often viewed as less, following surgery, performed under RA. But RA technique that produces sensory block above T_7 to T_{10} level are not recommended, as this high level of central neuraxial block leads to decrease in expiratory reserve volume. In turn, this decreased expiratory reserve volume causes the impairment of cough which leads to the reduction in the clearance of secretions from airways. Also block above T_7 to T_{10} level produces a feeling of suffocation and uneasiness, requiring sedation which further depresses the respiration. But different types of nerve blocks, field blocks, infiltration anesthesia, etc., carry much lesser risks than epidural or spinal anesthesia. Nevertheless, the RA remains a useful selections in patients with COLD, only when large doses of sedative drugs are not given because such patients are extremely sensitive to the ventilatory depressant effects of sedative agents.

Although, the pulse oximetry accurately detects significant arterial desaturation, but the direct measurement of arterial O_2 tension by blood gas analysis may be necessary to detect the more fine changes in intrapulmonary shunting. Moreover, the measurement of arterial CO_2 tension can guide the ventilation because the increased Vd widens the normal arterial to $ETCO_2$ gradient.

Postoperative Care

The *aim of postoperative care* for the patients, suffering from COLD, is to reduce the incidences and the severity of postoperative pulmonary complications. This can be achieved by lung volume expansion exercise, analgesia preferably by neuraxial approach and mechanical ventilation, if needed for respiratory failure. It is stated previously that the postoperative complications are greatest following upper abdominal and intrathoracic surgery. This is documented from the data that following upper abdominal surgery, the VC decreases about 40% from its preoperative value on the first postoperative day, which does not return to its preoperative level for next 10–15 days and FRC does not decrease to normal level in first 24 hours.

Astonishingly, it is also found that complete analgesia does not restore VC and FRC to the preoperative levels which suggests that surgical trauma is the main determinant factor for this diminution of VC and increase of FRC. Altered VC and

FRC are the main responsible factors for the decrease in PaO_2 and increase in $PaCO_2$ in the immediate postoperative period than the depression of ventilation by narcotics, inhalational anesthetics, anesthesia-induced impair regional hypoxic pulmonary vasoconstriction, and anesthesia-induced diminution of ventilatory responses to CO_2 and hypoxia. The incidences of postoperative pulmonary complications, however, is dramatically less after laparoscopic cholecystectomy than after open cholecystectomy.

■ BRONCHIECTASIS

Bronchiectasis is a chronic suppurative airway disease, characterized with airway obstruction, during expiration like COLD and focal or diffuse abnormal permanent dilatation of bronchi. It is either congenital, caused by genetic factors, e.g., cystic fibrosis or acquired, following the damage to lower respiratory tract, especially during severe early childhood infection. Most patients suffering from bronchiectasis have a chronic productive cough which may present throughout the year, despite the widespread availability of broad-spectrum antibiotics. In bronchiectasis, there is frequently a component of asthma associated with chronic inflammatory changes in the airways. It often affects the lungs at the segmental or sub-segmental level. The focal bronchiectasis involves the airways, supplying a limited region of pulmonary parenchyma, but diffuse bronchiectasis involves a wide area of lungs **(Figs. 17A and B)**.

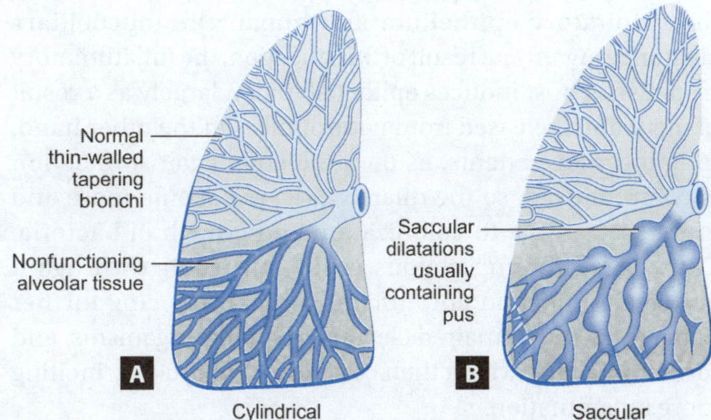

Figs. 17A and B: Bronchiectasis means a permanent dilatation of one or more bronchi. The main bronchi up to fourth division possess large supporting cartilage rings. So, bronchiectasis only affects the bronchi beyond this point. Two main anatomical varieties of bronchiectasis are described. But these may have similar causes and frequently both are found in the same lung. (A) This type of bronchiectasis is almost always found in the lower lobes. The bronchi are grossly dilated throughout their whole length. Intervening lung tissue is much reduced and much of it is fibrosed. (B) In this type of bronchiectasis, as the name suggests, the dilatations of bronchi tend to be more localized and exaggerated. They are roughly rounded and may be single or multiple.

The dilatation of bronchi is due to the destructive (destruction of cartilage, muscles and elastic tissue) and inflammatory changes, mainly of the walls of medium sized airways. Thus, the dilated airways frequently contain the pools of thick, purulent material, while the distal portion of it is often occluded by these secretions and is replaced by fibrous tissue. The lung parenchyma, supplied by the affected airways, also contains varying combinations of fibrosis, emphysema, pneumonia, and atelectasis. The affected bronchial wall becomes highly inflamed and vascular with associated enlargement of bronchial arteries, causing sometimes severe hemoptysis.

The etiology of bronchiectasis may vary from:
- Infective → by microorganisms
- Noninfective → due to exposure to toxic substances
- Obstructive → due to foreign bodies
- Impaired host defense mechanism → due to Ig disorders, causing pan-hypogammaglobulinemia
- Ciliary dysfunction → primary ciliary dyskinesia, Kartagener syndrome, and cystic fibrosis.

Whatever may be the etiology of bronchiectasis, the infection of airways by microorganisms is the cornerstone of its pathology. Once the disease process is established, the bacterial infection can be difficult or impossible to eradicate. *Pseudomonas aeruginosa* is the most common pathogen that may be present for many years and may be associated with intermittent exacerbations of respiratory symptoms. At the pathological site within the lungs, the microorganisms produce pigments, proteases and other toxins that injure the respiratory epithelium and impair the mucociliary clearance. Again as a result of this infection, the inflammatory response of host induces epithelial injury, largely as a result of mediators, released from neutrophils. On the other hand, in Ig disorder patients, as the protection against infection is compromised, so the dilated airways become more and more susceptible to colonization and growth of bacteria. Thus, a reinforcing vicious cycle can result with again and again infection and inflammation, producing further damage, further impaired clearance of microorganisms, and further infection which then completes the cycle by inciting more inflammation.

Anesthetic management of patients with bronchiectasis invokes the same principles, as outlined for patients with COLD. Prior to elective surgery, status of pulmonary function of patients should be optimized by appropriate therapy.

Preoperative therapy for bronchiectasis includes:
- Elimination of identifiable underlying causes
- Improving the clearance of tracheo-bronchial secretions
- Control of infections, particularly during acute exacerbations
- Reversal of airflow obstruction.

Appropriate treatment for bronchiectasis should be instituted, when a treatable cause is found. For example:
- If cause is the foreign body, it should be removed.
- Acute infection should be controlled by antibiotics, guided by Gram's stain and culture of sputum.
- Treatment of hypogammaglobulinemia by Ig
- Treatment of tuberculosis with antitubercular agents and allergic bronchopulmonary aspergillosis (ABPA) with glucocorticoids.

In bronchiectasis, due to cystic fibrosis, there is also malabsorption syndrome and it is due to pancreatic insufficiency. So, appropriate advice, regarding the diet and pancreatic supplements are essential. In cystic fibrosis induced bronchiectasis, the secretions are typically copious and thick and contribute to the symptoms. *Chest physiotherapy* by chest percussion, vibrations, or postural drainage frequently help the patients with copious secretions. *Mucolytic agents* to produce thin secretions and to allow better clearance are controversial.

Antibiotics have very important role in the preoperative management of bronchiectasis. But which antibiotics should be given and the frequency and the duration of administration of these antibiotic are not well established. When the patients present with frequent exacerbation of infection, characterized by an increase in quantity and purulence of sputum, then antibiotics are only commonly used. Although the antibiotic should be chosen by the culture and Gram's stain of sputum, but an empiric coverage is often given initially. When *P. aeruginosa* is suspected, then the appropriate treatment is oral quinolone or parenteral aminoglycosides or third generation cephalosporin. In patients with chronic purulent sputum, despite short course of appropriate antibiotic therapy, more prolonged course or intermittent, but regular courses of a single or rotating simple antibiotics have been used.

Bronchodilators are particularly useful in bronchiectasis patients, associated with airway hyperreactivity and reversible airflow obstruction. It improves the obstruction and also aids the clearance of secretions. The intraoperative anesthetic management of bronchiectasis is same as COLD. But only the especial point is that double lumen endobronchial tube may be used in severe cases and it is to prevent the spillage of purulent sputum, into the normal areas of lungs.

■ RESTRICTIVE LUNG DISEASES

The restrictive lung diseases (RLDs) are the conditions where the TLC is reduced. It may be of two types: *intrinsic and extrinsic*. In the *intrinsic variety* of restrictive lung disease (IRLD), there is alterations of the elastic properties of lungs, causing the lungs to be stiffed. Again IRLD may be of *acute* and *chronic*. The example of acute IRLDs are: ARDS, pulmonary edema, aspiration pneumonitis, etc. The examples of chronic IRLDs are: sarcoidosis, silicosis, asbestosis, eosinophilic granuloma, extensive pulmonary fibrosis, etc. Initially in chronic IRLD, there is an inflammatory reaction, in response to different stimuli, which is centered on alveoli, impairing gas exchange. Then, over a period of time, which can vary from days to years, collagen fibers are formed in and around these alveoli, causing more marked impairment of gas exchange and a smaller, stiffer lung. Then, pulmonary fibrosis is the final response of lung (elastic fiber → collagen fiber → fibrosis). The causes of these stimuli include those which are associated with autoimmune disorders (e.g., rheumatoid arthritis, scleroderma), inhaled dusts (e.g., asbestosis), or ingested substances, especially drugs (e.g., amiodarone, chemotherapy agents, etc.). Allergic response to inhaled substances can also cause fibrosis and chronic IRLD, if the exposure is prolonged.

The *extrinsic variety* of restrictive lung disease (ERLD) reflects the disorders of chest wall (obesity, flail chest, deformity such as severe kyphoscoliosis, etc.); pleura (pleural effusions, pneumothorax, etc.), mediastinum (mediastinal mass), etc. Intra-abdominal pressure changes, producing significant splinting of the diaphragm and small group of neuromuscular disorders where lung movement is restricted from outside are also the examples of ERLD.

The pathology of RLDs are:

- In RLD, the vital capacity is decreased (normal VC is 70 mL/kg). But in contrast to obstructive lung disease *the expiratory flow rate remains normal in RLD*. So, the FEV_1 remains normal and the ratio of FEV_1:FVC is preserved in restrictive lung disease. While in obstructive lung disease the ratio of FEV_1:FVC is reduced.
- The patients with restrictive lung disease, like obstructive lung disease, also complain of dyspnea, reflecting the increased work of breathing which is necessary to expand the poorly compliant lung.
- Tidal volume decreases in restrictive lung disease. So, to compensate this reduced tidal volume, the respiratory rate increases. Despite the increase in respiratory rate, the alveolar ventilation remains low which produces proportionate increase in $PaCO_2$ and decrease in PaO_2 **(Fig. 18)**.
- In RLD, resulting hypercarbia and associated hypoxia, due to hypoventilation, cause vasoconstrictive pulmonary hypertension and cor pulmonale.
- The intrinsic and extrinsic varieties of restrictive lung disease can be differentiated from each other by the measurement of elastic properties of lungs. Elastic

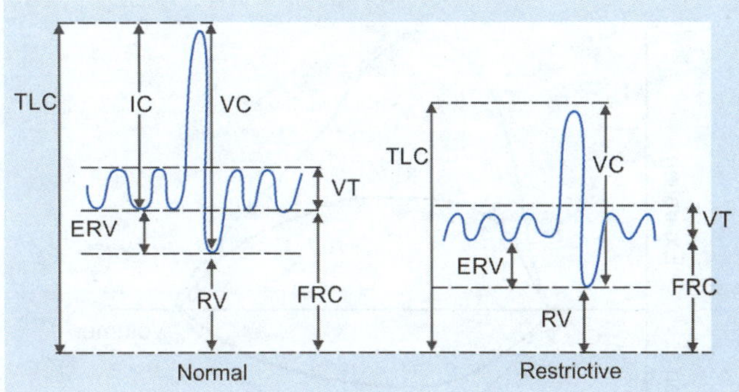

Fig. 18: Lung volumes in restrictive lung disease compared with normal values; in the presence of restrictive lung disease total lung capacity (TLC), functional residual capacity (FRC), residual volume (RV), and vital capacity (VC) are all decreased. (ERV: expiratory reserve volume; IC: inspiratory capacity; VT: tidal volume)

properties of lungs can be quantitated by measuring the lung compliance which is defined as the change in volume of lung per unit change in pressure. The compliance of normal lung is 0.1–0.2 L/cmH_2O, whereas in patients with intrinsic restrictive lung disease, the compliance comes down to as low as 0.02 L/cmH_2O. The *F–V* curves are shifted downward and to the right in patients with increased lung stiffness **(Figs. 19 and 20)**.

The anesthetic management of restrictive lung diseases includes: (1) preoperative diagnosis, (2) the assessment of the severity of the impairment of lung function, and (3) the treatment of reversible components. A preoperative history of dyspnea that limits the day-to-day activity and that can be referred to restrictive lung disease may be taken as an indication for the performance of PFTs and the measurement of arterial blood gases, in addition to the routine investigations, such as X-ray, and CT-scan, for the diagnosis of RLD. Restrictive lung diseases should be differentiated from obstructive lung diseases by the analysis of PFTs and *F–V* loop. If the VC is reduced to <15 mL/kg (where normal value is 70 mL/kg) and the resting $PaCO_2$ rises than normal, then there is more chances of developing exaggerated perioperative pulmonary complications.

Like COLD and bronchiectasis, the preoperative preparations of RLD also include: (1) the eradication of pulmonary infection, (2) the improvement of sputum clearance, (3) the treatment of cardiac dysfunction, (4) the exercise to improve the strength of breathing muscles, and (5) other specific treatments, such as the drainage of pleural effusion and management of pneumothorax. If there is mediastinal tumor, then the size and the degree of tracheal compression by the tumor should be assessed by CT scan or MRI. The prediction of tracheal compression by tumor mass is a useful assessment for difficult airway

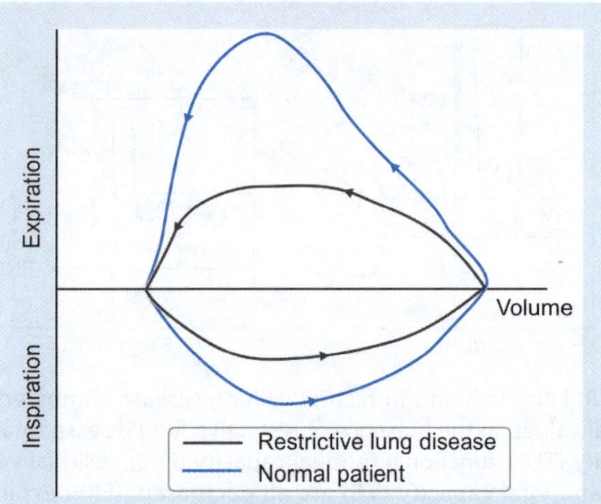

Fig. 19: Schematic representation of flow–volume loop in a normal patient (blue line) and in the presence of a restrictive lung disease (black line).

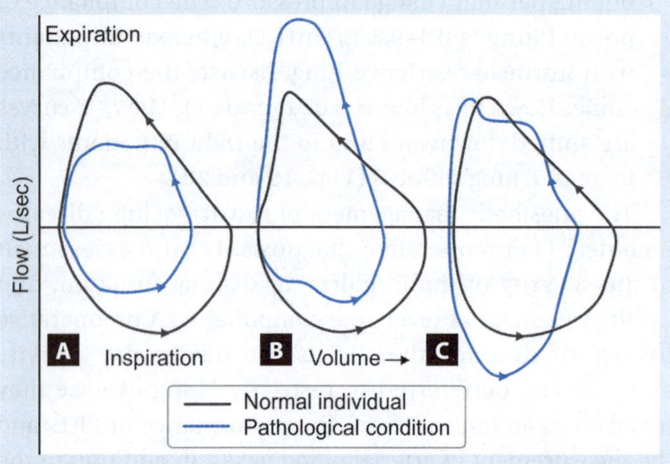

Figs. 20A to C: Different flow–volume loops in different conditions. (A) Represents flow–volume loop in *fixed* obstruction; (B) represents variable extrathoracic obstruction; (C) represents variable intrathoracic obstruction.

management. So, in such circumstances flexible fiberoptic laryngoscope/bronchoscope, under topical anesthesia, is a good preoperative method for evaluating the airway obstruction. A number of asymptomatic patients have developed unexpected airway obstruction during anesthesia without any previous warning.

Without bronchospasm, the only presence of restrictive lung disease does not influence the choice of drugs for the induction and the maintenance of anesthesia. During the induction and maintenance of anesthesia, a high index of suspicion for the presence of pneumothorax and the need to avoid or continue with N_2O must be assessed. Intraoperative controlled ventilation is prudent for the optimal oxygenation of patients with RLD, due to their poorly compliant lungs and sometimes high inflation pressure is needed to inflate the low compliant lungs. RA is suitable for lower abdominal operations or surgeries on extremities, but sensory block should be kept below the T_7 to T_{10} level, above which level the regional block is associated with impairment of the respiratory muscle activity which is necessary to maintain acceptable amount of ventilation and oxygenation. Tracheal tube must not be removed until the patients have obtained established criteria for extubation. Postoperative respiratory depression should be avoided by proper selection of intraoperative narcotics and sedative drugs. Postoperative pain is best managed by epidural analgesia.

LUNG CYST

These are fluid or air-filled cyst, located in the pulmonary parenchyma or adjacent to the tracheobronchial tree. They may be asymptomatic or may be the site of recurrent pulmonary infections or may be the cause of life-threatening airways obstruction. The *anesthetic interests of the lung cyst are:* the cautious use of N_2O and the use of positive pressure ventilation. N_2O usually diffuses into the cyst and causes its expansion, leading to the rupture and life-threatening respiratory/cardiovascular decompensation, due to pneumothorax. The institution of positive pressure ventilation may have a ball value effect, causing the expansion of cyst and the compression of lung parenchyma or the rupture of cyst, leading to pneumothorax. Despite all these concerns, the clinical experience confirms that N_2O, muscle relaxant induced skeletal paralysis, and intermittent positive pressure ventilation (IPPV) may all safely be utilized in patients with lung cyst.

Liver Diseases and Anesthesia

■ INTRODUCTION

Liver is the *largest gland* of our body. It consists of both an *exocrine* (or excretory) and an *endocrine* (or secretory) part. The exocrine part of liver excretes bile, which is conveyed through its biliary passages into duodenum. On the other hand, the endocrine part of liver liberates some useful chemical substances, such as glucose (from glycogen), ketone bodies, fatty acids, plasma proteins (except immuno-globulins), and heparin directly into blood. In addition, cholesterol, which is secreted by the liver, presents the cyclopentanoperhydrophenanthrene nucleus (structure) for the synthesis of different steroid hormones. Liver is also involved in the metabolism of all nutritional substances of our body, such as carbohydrates, proteins, fats, vitamins, and minerals. These metabolic activities dissipate much heat and thus the liver subserves as an important organ for the regulation of temperature of our body.

The liver is a wedge-shaped organ with a broad base, directed toward the right, and a narrow apex, directed toward the left. It occupies the whole of right hypochondrium, the upper part of epigastrium, and a part of left hypochondrium up to the left lateral plane. The weight of a liver in an adult person is approximately 1.4–1.8 kg (average 1.5 kg) and that of in a newborn is approximately 150 g. It is relatively larger in children than an adult. This is due to its increased hematopoietic function, during fetal life, and occupies about two-fifths of its whole abdomen. The weight of a liver represents 2% of total body weight of an adult and almost 5% of total body weight of a neonate. The liver is a highly vascular organ and so also acts as a reservoir of blood. When it is ruptured, then bleeding continues. Hepatic veins are unable to collapse, as these are directly attached to the plate of liver cells. The liver cells undergo rapid mitosis and regeneration, when a part of this organ is removed or damaged. Surgical removal of two-thirds of a liver may be compatible with life. But, the disorganized growth of liver cells, during regeneration, after degeneration or removal of a part of it or in cirrhosis, is detrimental and culminates into portal hypertension.

Patients with liver diseases, undergoing anesthesia and surgery, face a number of significant intraoperative and postoperative complications. This is because the liver diseases alter the patient's response to anesthesia and surgery in many ways, which is discussed later. Thus, it is important to understand: (1) the basic applied anatomy and physiology of liver, (2) factors which alter the hepatic blood flow, (3) the details of liver functions, (4) altered pharmacokinetics and pharmacodynamics of anesthetic drugs due to liver disease, etc. for proper perioperative management of these groups of patients.

■ MACRO- AND MICROANATOMY OF LIVER

The outer surface of liver is lined by a serous coat and this is derived from visceral peritoneum. Beneath this serous coat, there lies a thin layer of connective tissue, which is known as *Glisson's capsule*. It encloses the entire liver beneath the visceral peritoneal layer of it (liver). The Glisson's capsule also extends into the interior of liver as numerous branching septa. The radicles or the branches of portal vein, hepatic artery, and bile duct run together along these septa, ensheathed by this Glisson's capsule, in the form of *portal triads* (also called portal canals or portal tracts). On the other hand, the *hepatic veins* and their tributaries, which are named as the central vein and from where the hepatic vein starts, draw the blood from liver to the inferior vena cava (IVC) and run independently. They are not ensheathed by the Glisson's capsule, but these are surrounded by the laminas of hepatic cells.

Conventionally, the liver is imagined to be composed of a regular hexagonal mass of liver cells, which are called as the *hepatic lobules* and these are measured about 1 mm in width. These hexagonal lobules are arranged around a central vein

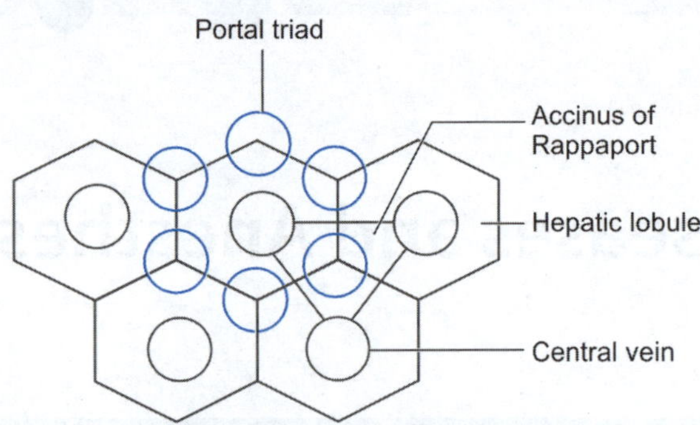

Fig. 1: Schematic anatomy of liver.

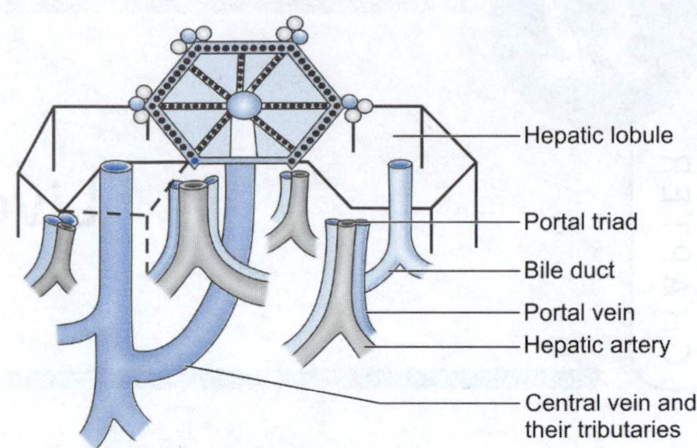

Fig. 2: Vascular anatomy of liver.

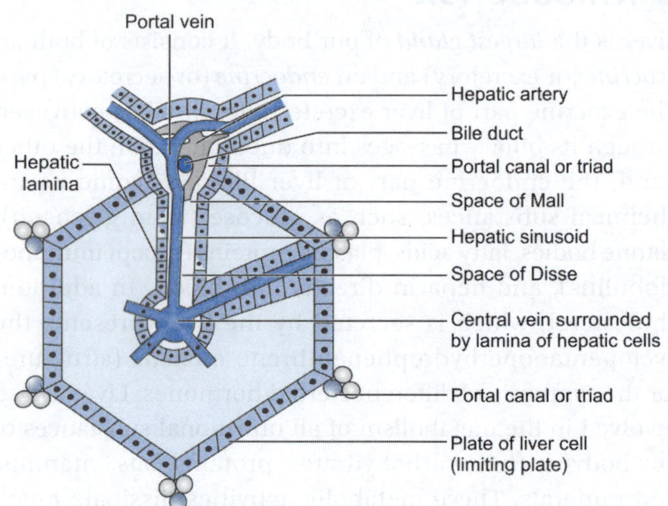

Fig. 3: Structures of hepatic lobules.

with portal tracts at their peripheral six corners. The *central vein*, which is a tributary of hepatic vein, occupies the central position of each of these hexagonal hepatic lobules. The *portal triads* or portal canals, covered by Glisson's capsule, are found in the interlobular spaces, i.e., at the meeting place of three adjacent liver lobules. Therefore, in a typical case, six portal triads or portal canals are found at the six corners of each hexagonal liver lobule (**Fig. 1**).

The liver cells are arranged as the multiple sheets or plates, and these multiple sheets or plates radiate outward from the central vein. These sheets or plates of hepatic cells are called as the hepatic laminae. At the periphery of each hexagonal hepatic lobule, these multiple hepatic laminae (sheets or plates), which are radiating from central vein, are joined together with one another by another plate of liver cells, which is called the *limiting plate*. The spaces between the multiple sheets of hepatic cells, radiating from central vein, are known as the *hepatic lacunae* which are occupied by *hepatic sinusoids*. These hepatic sinusoids receive the mixture of blood from both the portal vein (coming from intestine) and hepatic artery (branch of celiac artery, coming from aorta). The *limiting plates*, which surround or make the periphery of each hexagonal hepatic lobule, present numerous perforations. Through these perforations, the branches of portal vein and hepatic artery pass and open into the hepatic sinusoids (**Figs. 2 and 3**).

Then, after providing nutrition and O_2 to the liver cells, the blood of hepatic sinusoids drains into the central veins. Next, the central veins from the adjacent hexagonal hepatic lobules join together to form the hepatic veins and finally drain into the IVC. Truly speaking, each hexagonal liver lobule, centered around a central vein, is neither a structural, nor a functional unit of liver. It is in fact an *independent venous unit* and includes the area of liver whose venous blood drains into a particular central vein.

The walls of sinusoids (or hepatic lacunae) are also fenestrated and communicate with one another by some holes, through which the blood passes freely among the sinusoids within a hepatic lobule. The walls of the sinusoids are also lined by flattened endothelial cells. Some stellate-shaped *Kupffer's cells*, derived from bone marrow, are attached to these endothelial cells. These Kupffer's cells are actually mobile macrophages and are capable of engulfing foreign particles, bacteria and denatured proteins, etc. They also scavenge the breakdown products of red blood cells (RBCs) and have an important role in the metabolism of drugs and their intermediary metabolites. Along with these Kupffer's cells, there are also some cells, which are *highly mobile lymphocytes*. They act as defense against the viruses, other infective agents, and tumor cells (**Fig. 4**).

At the peripheral end of hepatic sinusoids, i.e., at the periphery of each hexagonal hepatic lobule, from where the hepatic arterioles and portal venules enter the hepatic sinusoids, there the pressure of portal venule is about 8–10 mm Hg and that of hepatic arteriole is about 90 mm Hg. Whereas, the central hepatic veins maintain a constant

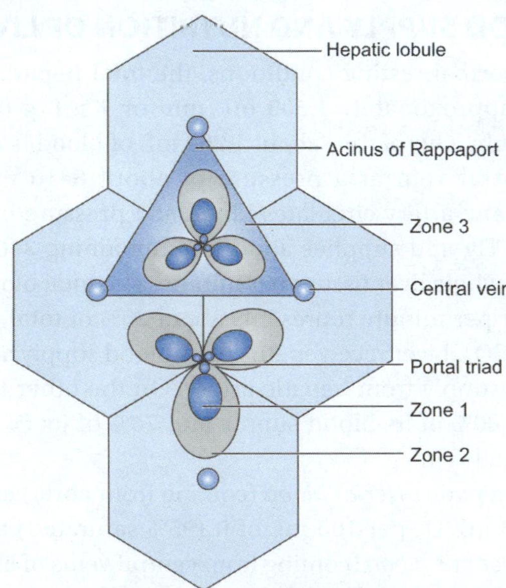

Fig. 4: Structural unit of liver.

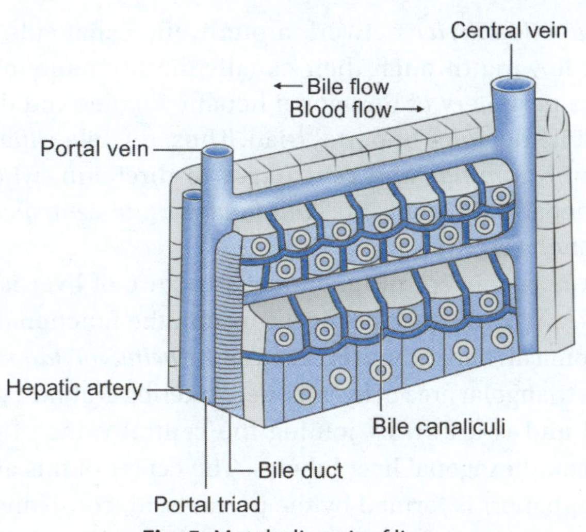

Fig. 5: Metabolic unit of liver.

pressure of about 5 mm Hg or less. In spite of this pressure difference, between the portal vein (10 mm Hg) and hepatic artery (90 mm Hg), the sinusoids convey a mixture of blood from both the vessels. This is because the sinusoids act as a huge vascular reservoir, like a mass of sponge, with intersinusoidal communication through multiple fenestrations and damp down the gradient of vascular pressure between the hepatic arterioles and portal venules. Thus, any disease of liver, reducing the capacity of this damping down of the gradient of vascular pressure of this vascular sponge, produces portal hypertension. Thereafter, any small changes in venous pressure (in central and hepatic vein) result in massive transudation of fluid as lymph and subsequent leakage of it through the outer surface of hepatic capsule into the peritoneal cavity. This fluid contains 80–90% of protein.

The walls of the sinusoids which are made by hepatic lamina (sheets or plates of liver cells) are covered by endothelial cells. Between the endothelial cells and the hepatic cells of lamina, there exists a potential space which is known as the *space of Disse*. This space of Disse is filled with plasma and chylomicrons which percolate from the blood of the sinusoids into this space of Disse and then enter the liver cells. The liver cells manufacture plasma proteins (except immunoglobulin) and these are delivered directly into this space of Disse and then into the blood of sinusoids. Moreover, chylomicrons are taken up by the liver cells from the space of Disse and are converted into lipoproteins. These are then again subsequently delivered into the circulating blood of sinusoids through the space of Disse.

The space of Disse also contains the *Ito cells*. These Ito cells secrete a collagenous matrix, named proteoglycans.

It provides growth factor for the regeneration of damaged liver cells and their subsequent reorganization as hepatic laminae. It also replaces the defunct liver cells with collagen fibers (as found in cirrhosis) and store the fat-soluble vitamin A in their lipid vesicles.

Between the Glisson's capsule of portal triad and the plate of hepatic cells, surrounding the Glisson's capsule, there exists another set of potential space, which is called as the *space of Mall*. At the periphery of hexagonal liver lobules, the space of Disse is continuous with the space of Mall. The lymphatics of liver begin first in this space of Mall as blind radicles. During excess accumulation of plasma in this space of Disse, it is reabsorbed by the lymphatics of the space of Mall **(Fig. 3)**.

The individual liver cell is roughly cuboidal in shape and presents six surfaces. Out of these six surfaces, two surfaces are related to the blood of sinusoids and the remaining four surfaces are surrounded by the polygonal network of *bile canaliculi* **(Fig. 5)**. Actually, these bile canaliculi are not any separate channels, but they are formed by the separation of plasma membranes of two adjacent liver cells. Numerous *microvilli* project into the walls of these bile canaliculi from liver cells and increase the surface area of these canaliculi, through which the liver cells can secrete more bile. The liver cells take up the *lipid-soluble (water insoluble) unconjugated serum bilirubin* from the blood of sinusoids through the space of Disse and then deliver the *water-soluble conjugated bilirubin glucuronide* into the bile of biliary canaliculi with the help of a conjugating enzyme named *UDP glucuronyl transferase (UGT)*. The borders around the biliary canaliculi are sealed by the tight junctions of the cell membrane between the adjacent hepatocytes and prevent the bile to re-enter into the hepatic cells from the bile canaliculi and hepatic sinusoids. Thus, this forms the *blood–bile barrier* network around bile canaliculi. Bile, after flowing through their canaliculi, ultimately passes to the periphery of hexagonal hepatic lobules and drains into bile ductules of portal triad. Thus, the bile canaliculi are *intralaminar* and *centrifugal* in direction, whereas the hepatic sinusoids are *interlaminar* and *centripetal* in direction **(Fig. 3)**.

A new concept of functional structure of liver is now in use. According to this new concept, the functional (not anatomical) hepatic unit is called as the *acinus of Rappaport*. It is a triangular area of liver tissue, centering around a portal triad and is drawn by joining the central veins of three adjacent hexagonal liver lobules. The center of this acinus of Rappaport is formed by the portal triad, consisting of a branch of portal vein, hepatic arteriole, biliary ductule, nerve fiber, and lymphatics. The area of this acinus of Rappaport gets its nutrition and O_2 from the radicles of portal vein and hepatic arterioles. Bile is collected in the bile ductule of this aforesaid portal triad. Blood flows perpendicularly from portal triad through sinusoids into central vein. Each of these transverse vessels and ductules forms the backbone, which provides nutrition to and collect the bile from a unit area of liver parenchyma which is known as the acinus of Rappaport. This acinus of Rappaport forms the metabolic unit of liver.

In terms of supply of O_2 and other nutrients, an acinus of Rapport is subdivided into three zones. The most inner zone *(zone-1)*, which is situated just around the portal triad, receives the blood with highest O_2 saturation and shows maximum metabolic activity. It is thought to be involved in protein anabolism and catabolism. The intermediate zone *(zone-2)* being intermediate in position is moderately oxygenated. The outer zone *(zone-3)*, which is situated close to the central vein, is least oxygenated and is most susceptible to hypoxic injury. This zone-3 is responsible for drug biotransformation **(Fig. 6)**.

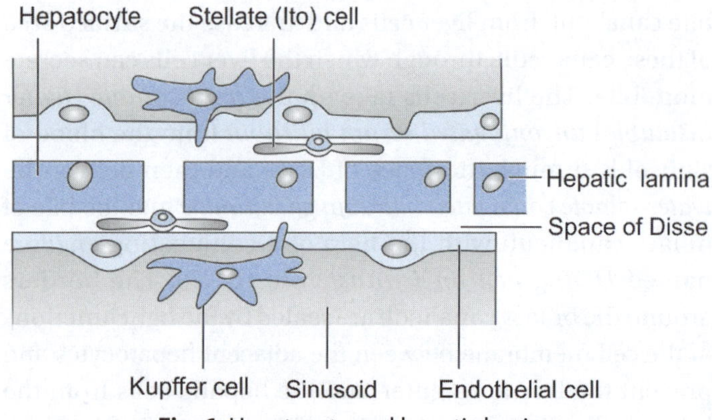

Fig. 6: Hepatocyte and hepatic lamina.

■ BLOOD SUPPLY AND NUTRITION OF LIVER

Under normal resting conditions, the total hepatic blood flow is approximately 1,500 mL/min or 1 mL/g (of liver tissue)/min. Out of this, about 1,200 mL of blood is derived from portal vein at a pressure of about 8–10 mm Hg. The hepatic artery circulates blood at a pressure of about 100 mm Hg and supplies about the remaining 300 mL of blood to whole liver tissues per minute. The total blood flow in a liver per minute represents about 25% of total cardiac output (CO). Liver receives 20% of its blood supply and 30% of its O_2 supply from hepatic artery. On the other hand, it receives 80% of its blood supply and 70% of its O_2 supply from portal vein.

The hepatic *arterial blood* (coming from aorta) contains about 19 mL O_2 per 100 mL of it (95% saturated) and the *hepatic venous blood* (coming from central veins of liver and draining into IVC) contains about 13.4 mL O_2 per 100 mL of it. So, the difference between the hepatic arteriovenous oxygen content is about 5.6 mL/100 mL. The *portal venous blood* (coming from intestine) contains about 17 mL O_2/100 mL of it (85% saturated) and so the difference between the O_2 content of portal vein and hepatic vein is about 3.6 mL per 100 mL of their blood. Hence, 300 mL of hepatic arterial blood supplies $3 \times 5.6 = 16.8$ mL O_2 per minute to the liver tissues. Likewise, 1,200 mL of portal venous blood supplies $12 \times 3.6 = 43.2$ mL O_2 per minute to the liver tissues. Thus, the total O_2 usage by liver is $43.2 + 16.8 = 60$ mL per minute, of which about 70% is supplied by hepatic portal system and 30% is supplied by hepatic arterial system. Before entering the liver, the hepatic artery and portal vein divide into their principal right and left branches.

Within the liver, these main (principal) branches of hepatic artery and portal vein further divide and subdivide to form their segmental and interlobular branches which ultimately run through the portal canals or triads. The further ramifications of these interlobular branches of hepatic artery and portal vein in the portal triads open into the hepatic sinusoids. These hepatic sinusoids are actually the hepatic capillaries, bounded by two hepatic laminae (sheet of hepatic cells). In this sinusoids, the branches of hepatic artery and portal vein drain. Thus, the hepatic arterial blood, coming from aorta, mixes with the portal venous blood, coming from intestine, into these sinusoids. There are no anastomoses among the tributaries of hepatic artery, and hence, the branch of each hepatic artery is an end artery.

The flow of blood through hepatic artery is dependent on (regulated by) the metabolic demand of liver cells under autoregulation. While the flow of blood through portal vein is dependent on (regulated by) the amount of blood flow through gastrointestinal tract and spleen. The hepatic artery has α_1-adrenergic, β_1-adrenergic, D_1-dopaminergic, and M_1-cholinergic receptors. The portal vein has only α_1-adrenergic and D_1-dopaminergic receptors. Among these, only the α_1-adrenergic is vasoconstricting receptor and the others are vasodilator receptors. Hence, sympathetic stimulation will result in vasoconstriction of hepatic artery and mesenteric vessels, resulting in reduced hepatic blood flow. As the stimulation of β_1-adrenergic receptor causes vasodilation, therefore, β-*blockers will reduce the hepatic blood flow and portal hypertension.*

VENOUS DRAINAGE, DRAINAGE, AND NERVE SUPPLY OF LIVER

The blood of hepatic sinusoids drains into central veins (interlobular veins), which then subsequently join to form the sublobular veins. These sublobular veins, then, again reunite to form hepatic veins which ultimately drain directly into IVC *(interlobular veins → sublobular veins → hepatic veins → IVC).*

The lymph of liver is rich in protein. The lymphatics of liver begin blindly around the portal triads in the spaces of Mall. Probably, the liver lobules are devoid of lymph capillaries and the interstitial fluid of lobules reaches the lymphatic radicles via the spaces of Disse and spaces of Mall. In obstruction of hepatic veins, the flow of liver lymph increases. The lymphatic network of liver consists of two sets—*superficial* and *deep*. The superficial lymphatic network runs on the surface of liver, beneath visceral peritoneum and terminates into the caval, hepatic, paracardial, and celiac lymph nodes. The deep lymphatic network partly ends in the nodes around the end of IVC and partly in the hepatic nodes.

The liver receives its nerve supply from hepatic plexus. It enters the liver through porta hepatis and contains both the *sympathetic* and *parasympathetic* fibers. The sympathetic fibers are derived from the branches of celiac plexus and the parasympathetic fibers are derived from both the right and left vagus and right phrenic nerve.

REGULATION OF LIVER BLOOD FLOW

Liver blood flow is regulated by two mechanisms—intrinsic and extrinsic.

Intrinsic Mechanism of Regulation

The intrinsic mechanism for the regulation of the flow of blood through liver does not depend on the nerves or any other blood-borne vasoactive compounds. It is operated mainly by three mechanisms and these are: (1) autoregulation, (2) metabolic regulation, and (3) hepatic arterial buffer response.

Autoregulation of Hepatic Blood Flow

It causes the local regulation of blood flow through liver and maintains a constant pressure in hepatic artery and its branches, in spite of wide range of its (pressure) change. This is also called as the local pressure–flow autoregulation. It is probably performed by hepatic arterial vasoconstriction and dilatation and is due to the myogenic response of arterial smooth muscle to stretch, imposed by increased arterial pressure. It is mainly found in metabolically active (i.e., postprandial) liver, but not in fasted liver. Unfortunately, as anesthesia and surgery are performed under fasting condition, so the pressure–flow autoregulation does not exist in this situation. However, this pressure–flow autoregulation is not evidenced in portal venous system. Instead, there exists a linear pressure–flow relationship, which means when the pressure in portal vein increases then the flow of blood through it also increases and vice versa.

Metabolic Control

Here, the metabolic factors, but not the pressure on the wall of the vessels of liver, regulate hepatic blood flow. In this mechanism, both the portal venous flow and hepatic arterial flow are controlled by the changes in the composition of blood, flowing within them, due to metabolism. These factors include the changes of blood partial pressure of oxygen (PO_2), partial pressure of carbon dioxide (PCO_2), pH, and osmolarity. By this mechanism, liver blood flow is increased during hypoxemia, hypercarbia, decreased pH (acidosis), postprandial hyperosmolar state (hyperglycemia), etc. and vice versa.

Hepatic Arterial and Portal Buffer (Reciprocal) Response

Here, the flow of blood through one system compensates the flow of blood through other system. Thus, when the flow through portal vein decreases then the flow through hepatic artery increases and maintains the total hepatic blood flow at constant level. This is called as the *buffer response or reciprocal response*. This *reciprocal mechanism* or relationship between the flow through hepatic artery and portal vein tends to maintain a constant supply of O_2 to liver which is essential for the function of hepatocytes (liver cells). Thus, when the portal venous flow decreases, then the hepatic arterial resistance also decreases by dilatation and hepatic arterial flow increases and vice versa. It is postulated that this is due to the locally produced adenosine.

Extrinsic Mechanism of Regulation

The extrinsic mechanism for the regulation of liver blood flow depends on both the neural and hormonal factors.

Neural Control

The sympathetic and parasympathetic nerves, which supply the liver, through hepatic plexus, terminate on the arterioles and venules of hepatic vessels. The stimulation of this *sympathetic* nervous system reduces the flow of blood through liver and expels near about 500 mL of blood into systemic circulation, immediately from liver. The liver in this way represents a *major reservoir of whole blood*, during emergency. But, the *parasympathetic* innervation influences the *regional distribution* of blood flow within liver by exerting their effects on perisinusoidal sphincters, rather than by affecting the total blood flow in liver.

Hormonal Control

The hepatic arterial bed has both α- and β-adrenergic receptors, whereas the portal vasculature has only α-adrenergic receptors. So, epinephrine, norepinephrine, and other catecholamines, administered exogenously, induce vasoconstriction of arterioles via α-receptors, which is partially compensated by vasodilation of arterioles, mediated by β-receptors. Dopamine has little effect on liver vasculature due to the absence of dopamine receptors on them. Vasopressin also induces marked splanchnic vasoconstriction in liver and intestine. Consequently, there is reduction in venous flow through portal system and reduction in resistance in portal vasculature, occurring after vasopressin administration. Thus, the vasopressin becomes very effective in alleviating the portal hypertension.

■ EFFECTS OF ANESTHESIA ON LIVER BLOOD FLOW

Anesthesia markedly alters the flow of blood through liver. It is due to the effects of: (1) individual anesthetic agents, (2) types of anesthesia, (3) mode of ventilation, and (4) type of surgery. Most of the anesthetic agents, which reduce BP and CO, decrease liver blood flow. However, among all the volatile anesthetic agents, halothane is the most significant. In contrast, isoflurane increases hepatic blood flow at the inspired concentration of 1 or 2 MAC (minimum alveolar concentration). During general anesthesia, as the resistance in splanchnic vascular increases, so the flow of blood through liver decreases. The application of positive end-expiratory pressure (PEEP) further decreases the hepatic blood flow by increasing the systemic and subsequently the hepatic venous pressure.

Regional anesthesia definitely decreases blood flow through liver, but it depends on the extent or the height of block. This is because the higher level of regional block is associated with more hypotension, and more hypotension is associated with more reduction of liver blood flow.

For example, the sensory block up to T_4 level reduces the hepatic blood flow up to 20%. But, this is not significant and runs parallel to the decrease of mean arterial pressure (MAP). It is also found that up to 40% reduction of MAP, there is no significant change of blood flow through liver, as there is contribution from both the portal and hepatic vascular system. Moreover, the reduction of MAP by >40% ensues the ischemic insult on liver. Among the types of surgery, upper abdominal surgery causes the maximum reduction of hepatic blood flow.

Thus, in conclusion, it can be said that although all the forms of anesthesia decrease liver blood flow, but simultaneously the O_2 requirements by liver also decrease. So, anoxic injury does not routinely occur during general or regional anesthesia.

■ FUNCTIONS OF LIVER

The liver acts as a well-equipped biochemical laboratory where (1) practically the metabolism of all nutritional substances such as carbohydrates, fats, proteins, vitamins, minerals, etc. is taken place, (2) multiple chemical substances (proteins, fats, carbohydrates, enzymes, hormones, etc.) are synthesized, (3) multiple toxic substances are detoxified, and (4) heat is produced. So, its functions are numerous which are briefly summarized here.

In Connection with the Constituents of Blood and its Circulation

- Red blood cell formation in fetal life
- Red blood cell destruction in adult life
- The pressure in portal vein is 10 mm Hg. The pressure in hepatic sinusoids is 2–3 mm Hg. So, the low resistance of hepatic sinusoids allows relatively large volume of blood to flow through portal vein. Any small changes in hepatic venous pressure, thus, can result in large changes in hepatic blood volume present within it (liver). Hence, liver acts as storehouse of blood and releases it during emergency and regulation of blood volume. During hemorrhage, a decrease in hepatic venous pressure shifts blood from hepatic veins and sinusoids into central venous circulation and augments circulating blood volume.
- In relation with blood clotting, (1) virtually all the coagulation factors, *except* the factor VIII and von Willebrand factor, which are protein in nature, are synthesized in liver; (2) Mast cells of liver produce heparin and prevent intravascular clotting; (3) The liver also produces other anticoagulant factors (protein C, protein S, and antithrombin III). Vascular endothelial cells synthesize coagulation factor VIII, the level of which

is therefore usually maintained in chronic liver disease. Vitamin K is the necessary cofactor in the synthesis of prothrombin (factor II) and factors VII, IX, and X. The liver also synthesizes plasma (pseudo) cholinesterase, an enzyme that hydrolyzes esters, including ester local anesthetics and some muscle relaxants, including succinylcholine.

- It helps in immune mechanism through its (liver's) reticuloendothelial (RE) system.
- It transfers blood from portal to systemic circulation.
- It manufactures all the plasma proteins (except immunoglobulins or globulins). These include albumin, α_1-antitrypsin and other proteases/elastases, transport proteins (transferrin, haptoglobin, and ceruloplasmin), complements, α_1-acid glycoprotein, C-reactive protein, and serum amyloid A. Albumin, the most abundant plasma protein, is responsible for maintaining a normal plasma oncotic pressure and is the principal binding and transport protein for fatty acids and a large number of hormones and drugs. Consequently, the changes in albumin concentration can affect the concentration of pharmacologically active, unbound fraction of many drugs.
- It stores iron, copper, and other hematinic factors, which help in the formation of red cells and hemoglobin.

Synthesis of Bile

Bile with their different constituents (bile salts, bile pigments, cholesterol, phospholipids, and other substances) is synthesized and excreted continuously from liver. Then, it is stored in gallbladder. *Cholesterol* is synthesized in liver from active acetate and is also excreted from liver. *Bile acids* such as cholic acid, deoxycholic acid, and lithocholic acid, which have been considered to be the derivatives of cholesterol, are synthesized in liver. These bile acids in conjugation with *glycine* and *taurine* form the compounds such as glycocholic acid, glycodeoxycholic acid, taurocholic acid, and taurodeoxycholic acid. *Bile salts* are the Na salts of these taurocholic acids and glycocholic acids, and have very important function during the process of digestion and absorption of fat and absorption of fat-soluble vitamins, such as A, D, E, and K.

This function is performed by emulsification of ingested fat and concurrent production of greater surface area, which enables the lipase and other fat-metabolizing enzymes to act more efficiently **(Box 1)**. Absorption of fat is helped by the formation of micelle formation. In our body, the stores of vitamin K are limited. So, in the absence of bile, vitamin K will not be absorbed and the deficiency of this vitamin K will be manifested as a coagulopathy due to the impaired

BOX 1: Synthesis of ketone bodies.

Fatty acid oxidation
↓
Acetyl-CoA
↓ ← Acetyl-CoA
Acetoacetyl-CoA
↓ ← Liver
Acetoacetic acid
↓ ← Reduced
β-hydroxybutyric acid
↓ ← Decarboxylation
Acetone

Note: It has been observed that acetyl-CoA produced during fatty acid oxidation condenses with oxaloacetic acid for oxidation through TCA (or citric acid) cycle. But the formation of oxaloacetic acid is depressed when glucose supply is restricted (starvation) or glucose metabolism is impaired (diabetes). In this condition, acetyl-CoA cannot be properly metabolized through citric acid cycle. Thus, acetyl-CoA condenses to form acetoacetyl-CoA, which next in the liver produces acetoacetic acid. Then, this acetoacetic acid forms β-hydroxybutyric acid which next, after decarboxylation, forms acetone. This acetoacetic acid, acetone, and β-hydroxybutyric acid are called ketone bodies. (CoA: coenzyme A; TCA: tricarboxylic acid)

formation of vitamin K-dependent coagulation factors, such as factors II (prothrombin), VII, IX, and X.

Bile pigments, named the biliverdin and bilirubin, are the breakdown products of hemoglobin, and are formed in RE system, present in the various parts of our body. Bone marrow, liver, and spleen have been considered to be the principal parts of this RE system and so are the principal sites for the formation of bile pigments. These bile pigments are insoluble in water. So, these are then carried to the liver and are conjugated to water-soluble bile pigments (bilirubin glucuronide), which are then next excreted through bile and is responsible for the normal color of stool.

In Relation with Carbohydrate Metabolism (Fig. 7)

Liver is immensely related to carbohydrate metabolism in the following ways:
- It converts nonglucose monosaccharides such as galactose, fructose, mannose, etc. to glucose and glycogen.
- It converts lactic acid, pyruvic acid, and glycerol to glucose and glycogen.
- It stores carbohydrates in the form of glycogen by glycogenesis, and when the blood sugar tends to be low then it mobilizes this glycogen by glycogenolysis and produces glucose.
- It takes an important part in the regulation of blood sugar. Most of the glucose, absorbed following a meal, is normally stored as glycogen, which only the liver and

muscle are able to store in significant amounts. When this glycogen storage capacity is exceeded, excess glucose is converted into fat. Insulin enhances glycogen synthesis and epinephrine and glucagon enhance glycogenolysis. Daily glucose consumption rate is near about 150 g/day and the hepatic glycogen store is normally depleted after 24 hours of fasting. After this period of fasting, gluconeogenesis is necessary to provide an uninterrupted supply of glucose for other organs.

- It is the site of neoglucogenesis. The liver and kidney are unique in their capacity to form glucose from lactate, pyruvate, amino acids (mainly alanine), and glycerol (derived from fat metabolism). The hepatic neoglucogenesis is vital in the maintenance of normal blood glucose level. Glucocorticoids, catecholamines, glucagon, and thyroid hormones greatly enhance this gluconeogenesis, whereas the insulin inhibits.

- It manufactures fats from carbohydrates and proteins. When the store of carbohydrate is saturated, then the liver converts the excess ingested carbohydrate and protein into fat. The fatty acids, thus formed, can be used immediately for fuel, or stored in adipose tissue or liver for later consumption. Nearly, all the cells utilize fatty acids, derived from ingested fat in foods or synthesized from intermediary metabolites of carbohydrates and proteins, as an energy source. Only the RBC and renal medulla are limited (obligatory) to glucose utilization. Nerve cells normally utilize only glucose, but after a few days of starvation, the neurons can switch over to ketone bodies, the breakdown product of fatty acid that has been synthesized by liver as a source of energy.

- Glucose is metabolized here aerobically through tricarboxylic acid (TCA) cycle and anaerobically through glycolysis [Embden–Meyerhof (EM) pathway] to produce adenosine triphosphate (ATP). Other alternative pathway for glucose metabolism, such as hexose monophosphate (HMP) shunt (phosphogluconate pathway), is also performed in liver and adipose tissue. This gluconate pathway produces ATP as energy and nicotinamide adenine dinucleotide phosphate (NADPH) which is needed for fatty acid synthesis.

- In liver, glucuronic acid is formed from *uridine diphosphate glucose* (UDPG). First, UDPG is converted to *UDP-glucuronic acid* by the help of *UDPG-dehydrogenase* enzyme. Then, this UDP-glucuronic acid is broken down into *glucuronic acid* and UDP by the help of *UDP-glucuronidase* enzyme. Now, this glucuronic acid plays an important role in the conjugation of bilirubin (**Fig. 8**).

- *Alcohol metabolism:* The liver is the main site for alcohol metabolism. In this, an enzyme, named *alcohol dehydrogenase*, catabolizes the ethyl alcohol

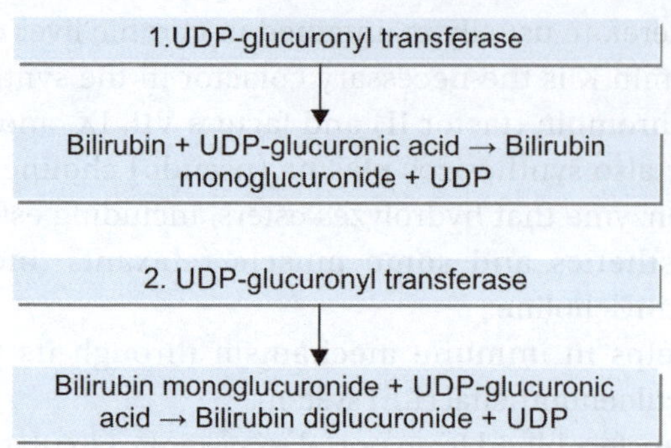

Fig. 7: Schematic diagram showing the conjugation of bilirubin by liver. (UDP: uridine diphosphate)

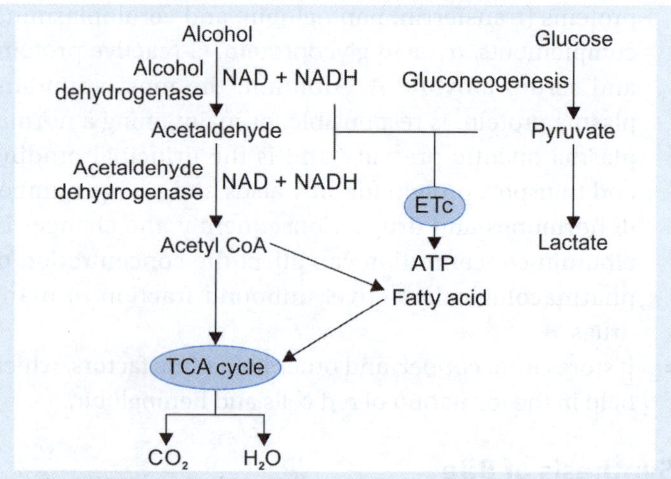

Fig. 8: Schematic representation of metabolism of alcohol in liver. (ATP: adenosine triphosphate; NADH: nicotinamide adenine dinucleotide hydrogen)

to acetaldehyde. Then, acetaldehyde dehydrogenase enzyme, which is present in the liver, converts this acetaldehyde to acetyl-CoA. Then, acetyl-CoA may be oxidized to CO_2 and H_2O through TCA cycle or is converted to other biochemical compounds, including fatty acids. When ethyl alcohol is converted to acetaldehyde and thereafter to acetyl-CoA, then NAD acts as cofactor, i.e., hydrogen acceptor in this reaction, and forms NADH. Thus, the ATP is generated during the oxidation of this NADH by the electron transport chain (ETC) and provides energy for the synthesis of fatty acids. Thus, the reduced NADH ($NADH^+ + H^+ = NADH$), which is produced during the metabolism of alcohol, can alter the intracellular NADH/NAD ratio appreciably. In turn, this altered NADH/NAD ratio can affect the multiple numbers of important intracellular metabolic reactions that use these two cofactors (NADH and NAD). The high level of NADH favors the formation of lactate from pyruvate, accounting for the lactic acidosis. This diminishes the concentration

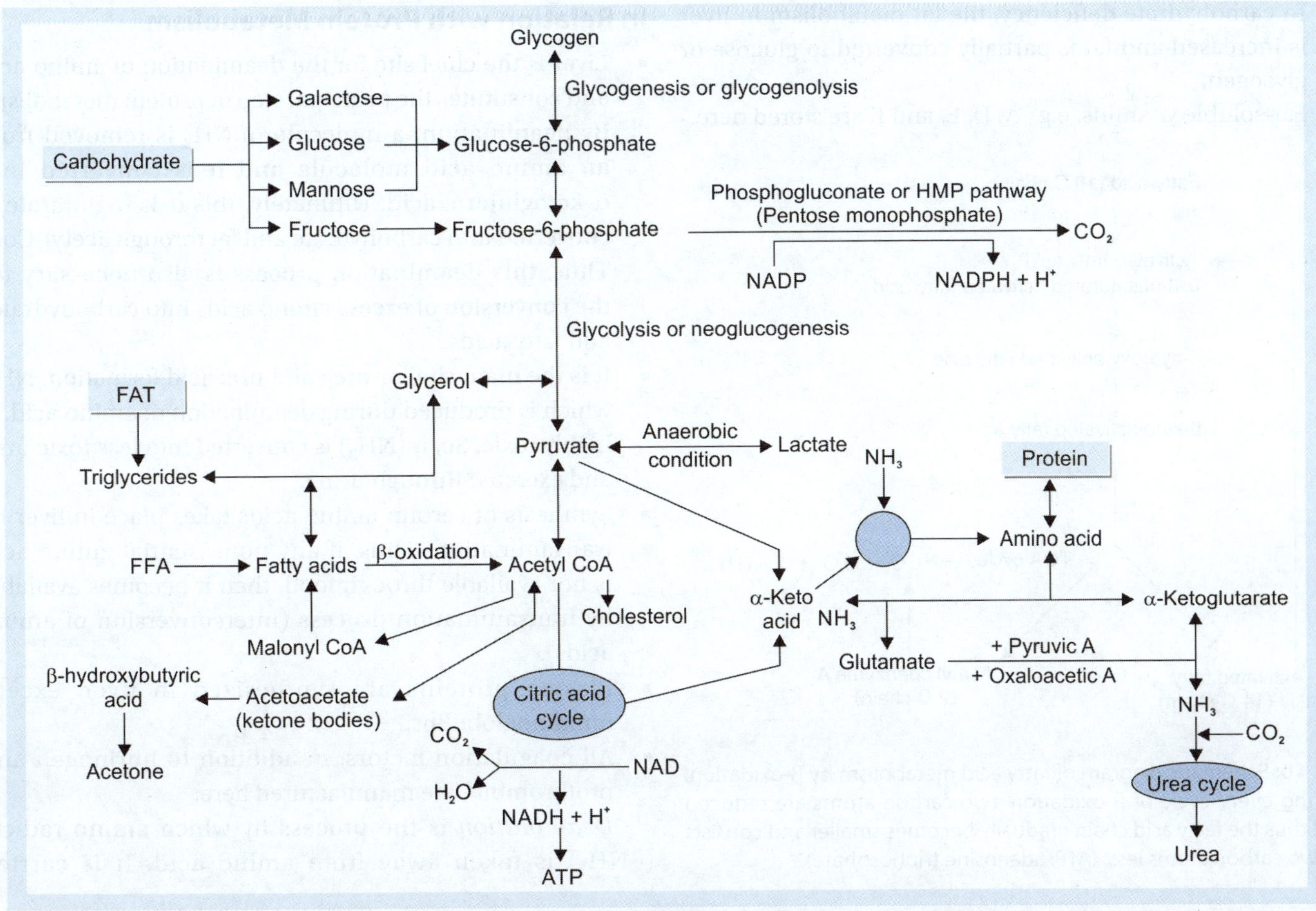

Fig. 9: Carbohydrate and fat metabolism in liver. (ATP: adenosine triphosphate; CoA: coenzyme A; FFA: free fatty acid; NADPH: nicotinamide adenine dinucleotide phosphate)

of pyruvate and thus inhibits gluconeogenesis. In severe cases, when liver glycogen is depleted due to less intake of carbohydrate and is no longer available for glycogenolysis, then this will result in hypoglycemia **(Fig. 9)**. Under the influence of alcohol, the hepatic microsomes help in the esterification of fatty acids to triglycerides, rather than phospholipids. So, the direct effect of alcohol may be alcoholic fatty liver which is due to increased hepatic fat synthesis, as well as decreased hepatic fatty acid oxidation.

In Relation with Fat Metabolism (Fig. 7)

The liver is related to fat metabolism by the following ways:

- It stores fats.
- It helps in the oxidation of fat, releasing energy in the form of ATP through TCA cycle. Fats (triglycerides) are first hydrolyzed into fatty acids and glycerol. These fatty acids are then converted into acetyl coenzyme A (acetyl-CoA), which is then oxidized via citric acid cycle to produce ATP.

- It is the site for synthesis of cholesterol and phospholipid from acetate (acetyl-CoA).
- It is the site for synthesis of phospholipids.
- It is the site for synthesis of fats from carbohydrates and proteins **(Fig. 10)**.
- It is the site for ketone body formation. In the presence of excess acetyl-CoA and in the absence of oxaloacetate (in the absence of TCA cycle or carbohydrate metabolism), acetoacetic acid (one of ketone bodies) is formed. The acetoacetate, released from hepatocytes, serves as an alternative energy source for some cells, which utilize ketone bodies for their energy, by reconversion into acetyl-CoA.
- The unused free fatty acids (FFAs), which are released from fat depot, are converted to triglycerides and other lipids in liver. These are then metabolized to meet energy requirement when necessary **(Fig. 11)**.
- The glycerol is oxidized in liver via the pathway of carbohydrate metabolism.

- In carbohydrate deficiency, the fat metabolism in liver is increased and fat is partially converted to glucose or glycogen.
- Fat-soluble vitamins, e.g., A, D, E, and K are stored here.

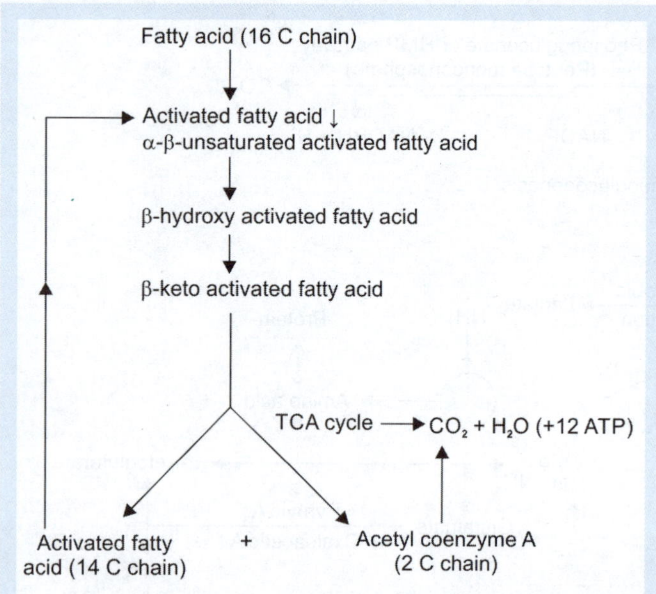

Fig. 10: Schematic diagram of fatty acid metabolism by β-oxidation. During every cycle of β-oxidation, two carbon atoms are reduced and thus the fatty acid chain gradually becomes smaller and consists of two carbon atoms less. (ATP: adenosine triphosphate)

In Relation with Protein Metabolism

- Liver is the chief site for the deamination of amino acid and constitutes the principal step of protein metabolism. By deamination, a molecule of NH_3 is removed from an amino acid molecule and it is converted into α-ketoglutaric acid. Ultimately, this α-ketoglutarate is converted into carbohydrate and fat through acetyl-CoA. Thus, this deamination process is also necessary for the conversion of excess amino acids into carbohydrates and fatty acids.
- It is the main site for urea and uric acid formation. NH_3, which is produced during deamination of amino acid, is highly toxic. So, it (NH_3) is converted into less toxic urea and excreted through urine.
- Synthesis of certain amino acids takes place in liver by transamination. Thus, if any nonessential amino acid is not available through food, then it becomes available by transamination process (interconversion of amino acids).
- Plasma proteins are synthesized in liver, except immunoglobulins.
- All coagulation factors, in addition to fibrinogen and prothrombin, are manufactured here.

Deamination is the process by which amino radicle (−NH₂) is taken away from amino acid. It is carried

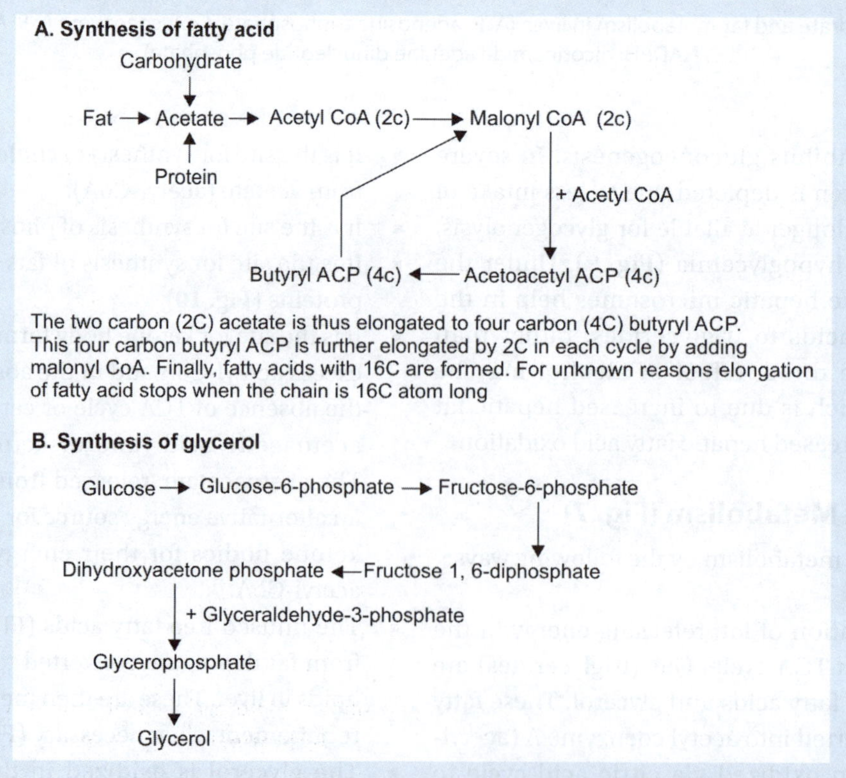

Fig. 11: Synthesis of fat (triglycerides = fatty acid + glycerol).

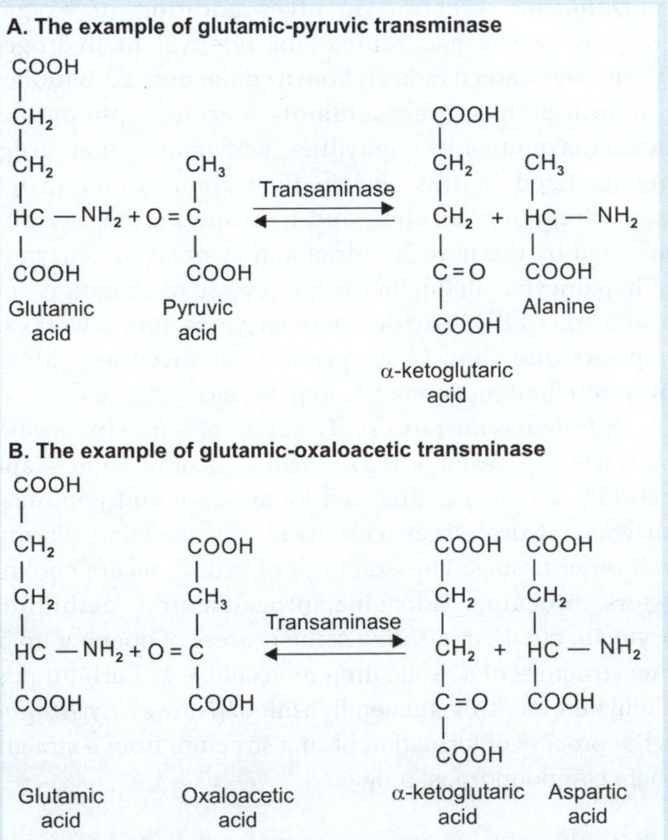

A. The example of glutamic-pyruvic transminase

$$\underset{\substack{\text{Glutamic} \\ \text{acid}}}{\overset{\begin{array}{c}\text{COOH}\\|\\\text{CH}_2\\|\\\text{CH}_2\\|\\\text{HC}-\text{NH}_2\\|\\\text{COOH}\end{array}}{}} + \underset{\substack{\text{Pyruvic} \\ \text{acid}}}{\overset{\begin{array}{c}\text{CH}_3\\|\\\text{O}=\text{C}\\|\\\text{COOH}\end{array}}{}} \underset{\text{Transaminase}}{\rightleftharpoons} \underset{\substack{\alpha\text{-ketoglutaric} \\ \text{acid}}}{\overset{\begin{array}{c}\text{COOH}\\|\\\text{CH}_2\\|\\\text{CH}_2\\|\\\text{C}=\text{O}\\|\\\text{COOH}\end{array}}{}} + \underset{\text{Alanine}}{\overset{\begin{array}{c}\text{CH}_3\\|\\\text{HC}-\text{NH}_2\\|\\\text{COOH}\end{array}}{}}$$

B. The example of glutamic-oxaloacetic transminase

$$\underset{\substack{\text{Glutamic} \\ \text{acid}}}{\overset{\begin{array}{c}\text{COOH}\\|\\\text{CH}_2\\|\\\text{CH}_2\\|\\\text{HC}-\text{NH}_2\\|\\\text{COOH}\end{array}}{}} + \underset{\substack{\text{Oxaloacetic} \\ \text{acid}}}{\overset{\begin{array}{c}\text{COOH}\\|\\\text{CH}_3\\|\\\text{O}=\text{C}\\|\\\text{COOH}\end{array}}{}} \underset{\text{Transaminase}}{\rightleftharpoons} \underset{\substack{\alpha\text{-ketoglutaric} \\ \text{acid}}}{\overset{\begin{array}{c}\text{COOH}\\|\\\text{CH}_2\\|\\\text{CH}_2\\|\\\text{C}=\text{O}\\|\\\text{COOH}\end{array}}{}} + \underset{\substack{\text{Aspartic} \\ \text{acid}}}{\overset{\begin{array}{c}\text{COOH}\\|\\\text{CH}_2\\|\\\text{HC}-\text{NH}_2\\|\\\text{COOH}\end{array}}{}}$$

Transaminase is recently referred to as aminotransferase. Transamination is reversible and combined process which is made up of deamination and amination. In most cases, there is transfer of amino group from amino acid to keto acid which is derived from either amino acid, carbohydrate and fat

Fig. 12: Transamination or deamination.

out chiefly in liver with the help of an enzyme, named *deaminase*. Deamination may also take place by the enzyme *transaminase*, which transfers the amino group from amino acid to a keto acid, converting the latter into an amino acid and the former into a keto acid. By this deamination process, the amino acid molecule is broken down into two parts—(1) a nitrogenous part (ammonia, NH_3) and (2) a nonnitrogenous part (α-keto acid) **(Fig. 12)**.

The nitrogenous part of an amino acid has the following fate:
- *Formation of urea:* Most of the NH_3, under normal condition, is converted to urea by K-H or ornithine cycle in liver. During this formation of urea, two molecules of NH_3 and one molecule of CO_2 are combined. About the 80% of total urinary nitrogen is found in this form of urea. Urea is mainly formed in liver.
- *Formation of ammonium salt:* A small part of ammonia combines with acids (such as sulfuric acid, phosphoric acid, etc.) other than carbonic acid in renal tubules and appears in urine in the form of ammonium salts, such

as ammonium phosphate, ammonium sulfate, urate, etc. It is obvious, therefore, that the amount of ammonium salts which will be formed will not depend upon the amount of ammonia, but on the relative proportion of acids or bases in the body. In acidosis, more ammonia is needed to neutralize the excess acids and so there will be proportionate increase in the formation of ammonium salts. In alkalosis, opposite changes will occur **(Fig. 12)**.
- *Ammonia may also be used* for the synthesis of some simple amino acids, such as glycine, alanine, etc. by transamination process and also for the amination of α-ketoglutaric acid to give glutamine.
- *Ammonia may also be used* for the synthesis of various nitrogenous substances such as creatine, purine, uric acid, pyrimidine, lecithine, etc.

The non-nitrogenous part of an amino acid has the following fate:
- Some will have the fate of carbohydrate. So, these amino acids increase the sugar level in blood. For this reason, in a diabetic subject, about 60% of food protein is converted into sugar. These amino acids are called the *antiketogenic amino acids*. Because, they act as carbohydrate in our body and prevent the formation of ketone bodies. They are also called the glucogenic amino acid. Glycine, alanine, serine, cysteine, arginine, lysine, valine, histidine, etc. belong to this group.
- Some undergo the fate of fats. These amino acids are broken down in our body as fatty acids, from which the ketone bodies are formed. These amino acids are therefore known as the *ketogenic amino acids*. It is known that in a diabetic subject, about 40% of proteins are converted into ketone bodies. Phenylalanine, tyrosine, isoleucine, etc. fall in this group **(Box 1)**.
- The sulfur and phosphorous, derived from the non-nitrogenous part of amino acids, are converted into various sulfur and phosphorous compounds and are excreted through urine.

Excretory Function of Liver

- The cholesterol and bile pigments are excreted from liver through bile.
- Various toxins, bacteria, and drugs are also excreted by liver through bile.

In Relation with the Metabolism of Vitamin and Other Miscellaneous Factors

- Liver manufactures prothrombin with the help of vitamin K.
- It forms vitamin A from carotene and is an important storage site for vitamin A, D, E, and K.

- The liver is the principal storage organ of vitamin B_{12}. Therefore, in any hepatocellular disease, the uptake and storage of vitamin B_{12} by this liver tissue is decreased.
- Chronic liver disease is always associated with folic acid deficiency. It is known that the liver converts folate to its active form → tetrahydrofolate. The tetrahydrofolate is the storage form of folic acid. In liver disease, this enzymatic transformation of tetrahydrofolate becomes impossible and thus folic acid is excreted through urine.
- The liver plays a major role in hormone, vitamin, and mineral metabolism. It is an important site for the conversion of thyroxine (T_4) into more active triiodothyronine (T_3). The liver is also the major site for degradation of thyroid hormone, insulin, steroid hormones (estrogen, aldosterone, and cortisol), glucagon, and antidiuretic hormone (ADH).

Detoxicating and Protective Functions of Liver

Liver is the principal site for the biotransformation of different toxic substances. They are either produced in our body during metabolism or taken along with food. Again, the liver converts some nonpolar compounds (lipid-soluble) to polar compounds (water-soluble) so that they are not reabsorbed by renal tubules, after filtration through glomerulus, and are thus excreted through urine. But, many water-soluble drugs such as streptomycin, neostigmine, and others are not biotransformed by liver and are filtered by glomerulus and are excreted unchanged through urine. Though the primary site of drug metabolism is liver, still other sites are also available for drug biotransformation. These are kidney, intestine, lungs and plasma, etc. The biotransformation reaction of drug can be classified into nonsynthetic or phase-I reaction and synthetic or phase-II reaction.

Nonsynthetic or Phase-I Reaction

This is also called the functionalization reaction. In this phase, the metabolites become either active (mostly) or inactive. The activation of metabolites is caused by the introduction of carbonyl, epoxide, or hydroxyl group into the parent compound. This phase-I reaction involves *oxidation, reduction, hydrolysis, deamination, dealkylation, sulfoxidation, cyclization, and/or decyclization. Oxidation* is the most common form of reaction in this phase, accounting for >90% of all the reactions. It (oxidation) is catalyzed by the *cytochrome P-450 enzyme system* of hepatocytes (liver cells) and to a lesser extent by the mixed function of *other enzymes, named oxidase*, present in hepatocytes. Many of the reduction pathways in liver are also catalyzed by the cytochrome P-450 enzyme system of hepatocytes.

Oxidation reaction involves addition of oxygen (negatively charged radical) or removal of hydrogen (positively charged radical) from a compound. Barbiturates, phenothiazines, paracetamol, steroids, phenytoin, benzodiazepines, theophylline, and many other drugs are oxidized in this way in liver. Some other drugs, e.g., adrenaline, alcohol, and mercaptopurine, are also oxidized by the mitochondrial and cytoplasmic enzymes of hepatocytes. Reduction is the reverse of oxidation and also involves P-450 cytochrome enzymes. But, it works in opposite direction. Drugs primarily reduced are chloral hydrate, chloramphenicol, halothane, etc.

Hydrolysis is the process of cleavage of a drug (molecule) by water, e.g., ester + H_2O = acid + alcohol amides and peptides are also hydrolyzed by amidase and peptidase enzymes. Hydrolysis also occurs in liver, intestine, plasma, and other tissues. The examples of hydrolysis are choline esters, procaine, lidocaine, procainamide, pethidine, oxytocin, etc. *Decyclization* is the process of opening up of ring structure of a cyclic drug molecule, e.g., barbiturates, phenytoin, etc. This is generally a minor pathway. *Cyclization* is the process of formation of ring structure from a straight chain compound, e.g., proguanil.

Synthetic or Phase-II Reaction

This phase of metabolism involves the conjugation of drugs or substrates, derived from the phase-I metabolism, to form a polar, highly ionized, organic substances, which are easily excreted through urine or bile. Conjugation reactions require high energy. This phase-II reactions include: (1) *conjugation of substances with glucuronide, sulfate, taurine, glycine, glutathione, etc., and* (2) *acetylation, methylation, etc.*

Glucuronide conjugation is the most common form of phase-II reactions. Compounds are easily conjugated with glucuronic acid, which is derived from glucose in liver. The common drugs which undergo this glucuronide conjugation are—chloramphenicol, aspirin, phenacetin, morphine, metronidazole, etc. Not only the drugs, but also many endogenous substrates such as bilirubin, steroidal hormones, and thyroxine also undergo transformation (conjugation) through this pathway.

After conjugation, these glucuronide compounds are excreted through bile and can also be hydrolyzed by bacteria in gut. Then, the liberated drug is reabsorbed and undergoes enterohepatic circulation and its action is then prolonged, e.g., phenolphthalein, oral contraceptives, etc. Some compounds are also conjugated with the help of acetyl coenzyme-A. This is called as the *acetylation*. The examples of this acetylation type of conjugation are—sulfonamides, isoniazid, PAS, hydralazine, etc. Multiple genes control the synthesis of acetyltransferase enzyme which is needed for this acetylation reaction, and the rate of this acetylation shows genetic polymorphism. Amines and phenols are conjugated by methyl group which is donated by methionine and cysteine. This is called as the *methylation*. The examples of this methyl conjugation are—adrenaline, histamine, and nicotinic acid. The chloramphenicol, adrenal hormones, and sex steroids undergo *sulfate conjugation*.

Some enzyme systems, such as *cytochrome P-450*, can be induced by exposure to drugs, such as ethanol, barbiturates, ketamine, and perhaps benzodiazepines. This results in increased tolerance to the effects of these drugs. In contrast, some drugs such as cimetidine and chloramphenicol inhibit this enzyme system and prolong the effects of these and other drugs. Some drugs, such as lidocaine, morphine, verapamil, labetalol, and propranolol, have very high rate of their hepatic extraction from circulation and this extraction of these agents from circulation by liver depends on hepatic blood flow. As a result, decrease in metabolic clearance of these agents reflects reduced hepatic blood flow rather than the dysfunction of liver.

Function of Liver in Maintaining Body Temperature

Liver produces large amount of heat from the metabolism of carbohydrate, protein, and fat and thus takes part in controlling our body temperature.

Function of Liver in Hormone Metabolism

Liver metabolizes the circulating hormones of adrenal gland (cortical and all sex hormones) both by reduction and conjugation reactions. The steroid hormones such as estrogen, cortisol, and testosterone are insoluble. Their solubility is increased and made excretable, after being conjugated with glucuronic acid and sulfuric acid in liver. The liver normally extracts about 97% of delivered aldosterone and inactivates it. The inactivation of insulin, glucagon, ADH, and other hormones also occurs here. In liver disease, the levels of all these hormones are increased.

■ CLASSIFICATION OF LIVER DISEASES

No single classification for all the types of liver diseases is entirely satisfactory. Because, in many instances, the etiology and the pathogenic mechanism of liver diseases are obscure. As a consequence, one finds an abundance of nomenclatures and labels, applied to the same hepatic disorders. For example, some individuals use the term "hepatitis" to imply the viral infection, whereas, others use it simply to mean the evidence of hepatic inflammation.

Similarly, the frequently used words such as acute, subacute, and chronic are also ambiguous. Chronicity is referred to the continuation or recurrence of the disease, whereas, the active is referred to evidence of the full presence or perpetuation of disease. This is most easily identified by the elevation of serum transaminase and by the degree of hepatocellular necrosis on biopsy. As there are many difficulties involved in defining the etiology of many types of liver diseases, so in most instances, the disease process is best defined and described by the examination of the morphologic character of the lesion. Therefore, a morphologic classification of liver diseases is outlined in **Box 2**, which appears at present the more practical than one based on etiology.

BOX 2: Classification of liver diseases.

- *Parenchymal:*
  - *Hepatitis (viral, drug induced, toxic, ischemic):*
    - Acute
    - Chronic (persistent or active)
  - *Cirrhosis:*
    - Alcoholic (portal and nutritional)
    - Postnecrotic, biliary
    - Hemochromatosis
    - Rare type (Wilson's disease, galactosemia, cystic fibrosis of pancreas, and α-antitrypsin deficiency)
  - *Infiltration:*
    - Glycogen
    - Fat
    - Amyloid
    - Lymphoma
    - Leukemia
    - Granuloma
  - *Space-occupying lesion:*
    - Hepatocellular carcinoma
    - Metastatic tumor
    - Abscess
    - Cyst
    - Gummas
- *Functional disorder associated with jaundice (hereditary or acquired):*
  - Gilbert's syndrome
  - Crigler–Najjar syndrome
  - Dubin–Johnson and Rotor syndromes
  - Cholestasis of pregnancy
  - Benign recurrent cholestasis
- *Hepatobiliary:*
  - Extrahepatic biliary obstruction (by stone, stricture)
  - Cholangitis (septic, primary biliary cirrhosis, drug, toxic)
- *Vascular:*
  - Chronic passive congestion and cardiac cirrhosis
  - Hepatic vein thrombosis (Budd–Chiari syndrome)
  - Portal vein thrombosis
  - Pylephlebitis
  - Arteriovenous malformations
  - Veno-occlusive disease

■ LIVER FUNCTION TESTS

The liver has enormous capability to regenerate. So, it has a large functional reserve. Therefore, the liver disease in an individual does not become clinically apparent, till it is well advanced. In addition, liver function tests (LFTs), which reflect the intracellular contents in circulation, may be abnormal in the presence of relatively normal functions of liver. Many disease processes of liver may lead to severe impairment of certain liver functions, while others remain entirely unaffected. Since, as no battery of tests is universally applicable, so those most appropriate to a given clinical problem must be selected. Also, their potential value and risk should be considered and the results are interpreted in relation to clinical findings. Thus, LFTs are only the crude indicators of real hepatic state and should always be correlated with its clinical picture. One isolated biochemical abnormality is insignificant. Tests should be done serially in order to evaluate the course of disease process. The abnormal LFTs may also be due to the effect of some systemic diseases of liver (e.g., chronic heart failure, malignancy, etc.) and this also must be taken into consideration, while deciding on anesthetic plan.

Usually, the liver function tests are carried out both for the screening and the identification of the specific type of liver disease, with the aim of—(1) detecting intrinsic hepatocellular damage, (2) detecting cholestasis, (3) detecting and differentiating between the types and causes of jaundice, (4) assessing synthetic functions of liver, and also (5) diagnosing primary carcinoma **(Fig. 13)**.

Plasma Bilirubin Estimation

Bilirubin is the degradation product of the heme part of hemoglobin (Hb). It is derived from Hb, after the breakdown of aging erythrocytes in mononuclear phagocytic system (MPS) or reticuloendothelial system (RES). The bilirubin is a yellow pigment, which is oxidized again to a green pigment, named biliverdin. According to some, biliverdin is formed first from heme and later by reduction, it (biliverdin) forms bilirubin. This unconjugated bilirubin (or indirect bilirubin) is bound to serum albumin, because it is insoluble in aqueous solution (water) at physiological pH. So, it (unconjugated bilirubin) cannot be excreted by glomerular filtration through urine, as it is bound with albumin.

On reaching the liver cells, via the blood of its sinusoids, the albumin is dissociated from bilirubin and free bilirubin enters the liver cells, where it is bound to a cytoplasmic protein, named *ligandin*. This cytoplasmic liver cell protein, ligandin, then assists in the transfer of bilirubin to the endoplasmic reticulum (ER) of liver cell for conjugation. In the ER of liver cell, bilirubin is conjugated with glucuronic

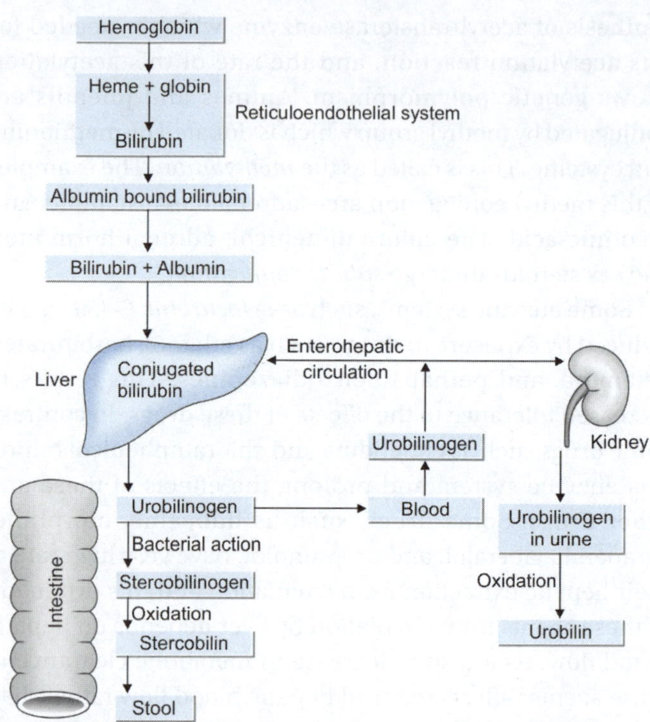

Fig. 13: Pathway of bilirubin formation and excretion.

acid, which is catalyzed by an enzyme, named glucuronosyl-transferase. Then, this conjugated *bilirubin glucuronide* (or direct bilirubin), which is water-soluble, is actively transported to the bile into biliary canaliculi from liver cells. A small amount of conjugated bilirubin (bilirubin glucuronide) escapes back into blood of sinusoids from these liver cells. Therefore, the total amount of plasma bilirubin, circulating into blood, normally includes—(1) free unconjugated bilirubin which enters the blood from RES and is bound to albumin and on their way to liver cells for conjugation, and (2) a small amount of conjugated bilirubin which is escaping back into the blood from liver cells. The normal value of total plasma bilirubin is 0.2–0.8 mg/dL. Out of which, the level of conjugated bilirubin is 0.00–0.2 mg/dL and the level of unconjugated bilirubin is 0.2–0.6 mg/dL.

The conjugated bilirubin imparts the brilliant yellow color to the bile. Most of the conjugated bilirubin passes via the bile duct into intestine. In the intestinal lumen, then, most of the conjugated bilirubin glucuronides are again deconjugated by intestinal bacteria and form the colorless *urobilinogen*. This urobilinogen and the residues of some intact pigment (conjugated bilirubin) are then largely excreted through feces as *stercobilinogen* and *stercobilin*, which are responsible for the brown color of stool. Some of this urobilinogen are reabsorbed from intestine and excreted through urine, as it is conjugated and water-soluble. Some are also returned back to the liver.

The complete obstruction of bile duct blocks the excretion of conjugated bilirubin from the liver into the gut and results in the disappearance of urobilinogen and stercobilinogen from the urine and stool. Thus, the assessment of urobilinogen in a freshly collected 2-hour urine specimen may distinguish the biliary tract obstruction from the parenchymal dysfunction of liver. But, this test has largely been superseded by other methods. In complete bile duct obstruction, as the pressure in bile canaliculi is increased, so the conjugated bilirubin from the bile canaliculi flows back through liver cells into the blood of sinusoids and then enters the systemic circulation. So, the level of conjugated bilirubin in blood becomes very high.

The disorders of bilirubin metabolism can be divided into five major categories: (1) increased pigment production (increased production of unconjugated bilirubin) in RE system, (2) reduced hepatic uptake of this unconjugated bilirubin, (3) impaired hepatic conjugation of this unconjugated bilirubin in liver cells, (4) decreased excretion of conjugated pigment from the liver cells into bile, (5) decreased passage of conjugated bilirubin and bile from liver to intestine. However, the last four points can be clubbed under the heading of *impaired excretion of bilirubin*. The first three disorders of bilirubin metabolism are associated predominantly with *unconjugated hyperbilirubinemia* and *no bilirubinuria*. The fourth and fifth groups of disorders are associated predominantly with *conjugated hyperbilirubinemia and bilirubinuria* **(Box 3)**.

Now, the increased plasma concentration of unconjugated bilirubin may be due to increased production, e.g., hemolysis (category I) or reduced liver uptake, e.g., Gilbert's syndrome (category II) or reduced conjugation of unconjugated bilirubin within the liver cells, e.g.,

Crigler–Najjar syndrome (category III) or those in whom both the mechanisms operate. In hemolytic anemia, due to unconjugated bilirubin, jaundice appears only when the rate of bilirubin production exceeds the amount that can be conjugated and removed by a normal liver which has an enormous reserve. In most cases of uncomplicated hemolytic states, the mean serum unconjugated bilirubin (or indirect) level will be in the range of 3–4 mg/dL. Rarely, higher levels may be seen, if the hemolysis is associated with fever, sepsis, hypoxemia, etc., or if the ability of the liver to handle the pigment load is compromised (i.e., when hemolytic disease is associated with liver disease).

Jaundice, due to increased pigment production, may also be seen as the consequences of large-tissue infarction (e.g., pulmonary infarcts) or the large collection of blood in tissues (hematoma). If hypotension or hypoxemia supervenes, then this jaundice usually becomes more pronounced and the resulting impairment of liver function may lead to significant increase in level of serum unconjugated bilirubin. Except in early infancy, the elevation of this serum unconjugated bilirubin levels is not harmful. Rather, the prognosis depends on the hemolytic process itself than the level of unconjugated bilirubin. However, in neonatal state and infancy, the unconjugated bilirubin levels above 20 mg/dL may lead to kernicterus. This is due to the deposition of this water-insoluble (fat-soluble) bilirubin into the lipid-rich basal ganglia of brain, as the blood–brain barrier is not well developed in neonates and infants like adults.

Currently, there are three syndromes such as *Gilbert's syndrome, Crigler–Najjar-II syndrome, and Crigler–Najjar-I syndrome*, which fall in the category of hereditary glucuronosyl transferase (*bilirubin-UDP-glucuronosyltransferase*) enzyme deficiency disorders. In these disorders, there is impairment of conjugation of bilirubin by the liver parenchymal cells. These three syndromes reflect progressive decrease in the activity of glucuronosyltransferase enzyme and thus may be the part of a spectrum of a single disease, i.e., from minimal deficiency to complete absence of glucuronosyltransferase enzyme (Gilbert's is the mild, Crigler–Najjar II is the moderate, and Crigler–Najjar I is the severe form). These three syndromes are characterized by unconjugated hyper-bilirubinemia, normal liver function tests, and no overt or clinically recognizable hemolysis. The liver cells, during liver biopsy, usually appear normal by light microscope.

Normally, between the 2nd and 5th days of life, almost every neonate shows some transient mild unconjugated hyperbilirubinemia. During intrauterine period, the placenta serves to clear this unconjugated bilirubin from the fetus. But, after birth, neonates detoxify the pigments themselves by their liver. However, at this stage, the hepatic enzyme, named glucuronosyltransferase, remains immature. As a result, the

---

BOX 3: Mechanisms producing jaundice.

- *Increased production of bilirubin:*
  - Hemolysis
- *Impaired excretion of bilirubin:*
  - *Congenital (nonhemolytic hyperbilirubinemia):*
    - Gilbert's syndrome
    - Crigler–Najjar type I and type II
    - Dubin–Johnson syndrome
    - Rotor's syndrome
  - *Hepatocellular jaundice:*
    - Acute parenchymal liver disease
    - Chronic parenchymal liver disease
- *Cholestasis or obstruction:*
  - Stone in CBD
  - Stricture of CBD
  - Cirrhosis
  - Pregnancy

(CBD: common bile duct)

unconjugated hyperbilirubinemia develops (usually not exceeding 5 mg/dL). Within several days to weeks after birth, the activity of this glucuronosyltransferase enzyme increases and concomitantly the serum unconjugated bilirubin level returns to normal. In infants with erythroblastosis (a superimposed hemolytic process), the excessive pigment (unconjugated bilirubin) load leads to more pronounced jaundice and unconjugated bilirubin level may go up to 20 mg/dL or above. Neonatal jaundice is not present at the time of delivery. If jaundice is present at birth, then other causes must be considered.

During neonatal period, if unconjugated bilirubin level exceeds 20 mg/dL, then the patient usually develops kernicterus (bilirubin encephalopathy) and eventually dies. This condition results from the deposition of unconjugated bilirubin in the lipid-rich basal ganglia (as unconjugated bilirubin is fat-soluble and not water-soluble). The current therapeutic approach of this unconjugated hyperbilirubinemia is phototherapy, in which the strong white or blue light leads to the photoisomerization of nonwater-soluble bilirubin to its water-soluble isomers that are rapidly excreted through bile, without prior need for conjugation. Another novel approach involves decreasing the production of bilirubin from heme by the inhibitors, such as heme oxygenase. Synthetic protoporphyrins, such as tin protoporphyrin, also have been administered successfully to the patients with neonatal unconjugated hyperbilirubinemia, causing the marked reduction in the level of serum bilirubin with no major side effects.

In jaundice, due to primary or parenchymal liver disease, the plasma usually exhibits an elevated level of both conjugated and unconjugated bilirubin, but urine contains only the water-soluble conjugated bilirubin. The relative proportion of these two pigments is highly variable. Such serum bilirubin pigment pattern (elevation of both unconjugated and conjugated bilirubin) is also seen with extrahepatic biliary obstruction. One cannot differentiate the intrahepatic and extrahepatic causes of jaundice only by the levels of unconjugated and conjugated bilirubin in serum, but from the prehepatic causes of jaundice (e.g., hemolytic jaundice). Thus, the main purpose of the initial fractionation of serum bilirubin is to distinguish the hepatic parenchymal and biliary obstructive diseases from the prehepatic disorders which are associated predominantly with unconjugated hyperbilirubinemia **(Table 1)**.

In many familial hepatic abnormalities, such as *Dubin–Johnson syndrome* (autosomal inheritance), the jaundice is largely due to the increase in *conjugated bilirubin*. Functionally, in Dubin–Johnson syndrome, there exists a defect in the excretion of conjugated bilirubin into biliary canaliculi from the liver cells, after its conjugation into

TABLE 1: Abnormalities shown by tests of liver function.

Test	Type of liver disease	
	Obstructive	Parenchymal
AST and ALT (SGOT and SGPT)	↑	↑ to ↑↑↑
Alkaline phosphatase	↑↑↑	↑
Albumin	N	↓ to ↓↓↓
Prothrombin time	N to ↑	↑ to ↑↑↑
Bilirubin	N to ↑↑↑	N to ↑↑↑
γ-glutamyl transpeptidase (GGT)	↑↑↑	N to ↑↑↑
5'-nucleotidase	T to ↑↑↑	N to ↑

Note: Correctable with parenteral vitamin K, if elevated.
N = normal, ↑ = elevated, ↓ = decreased

(ALT: alanine aminotransferase; AST: aspartate aminotransferase; SGOT: serum glutamic oxaloacetic transaminase; SGPT: serum glutamic pyruvic transaminase)

liver cells (at cellular levels). But, there is no defect in the conjugation process of unconjugated bilirubin into liver cells. So, the bilirubin after conjugation flows back from the liver cells into blood, due to the defect in its excretion into biliary canaliculi. Other familial defects in hepatic excretory function, where *conjugated hyperbilirubinemia* occurs, are *Rotor syndrome* (actually this syndrome is due to the impairment of storage capacity), benign recurrent intrahepatic cholestasis, recurrent jaundice during pregnancy, etc.

The acquired defects of hepatic excretory function at cellular level, where conjugated hyperbilirubinemia occurs, are drug-induced cholestasis (e.g., use of oral contraceptives), hepatitis, and cirrhosis. Hepatitis and cirrhosis are the most common disorders, associated with jaundice due to conjugates hyperbilirubinemia. When the liver cells are damaged as in viral hepatitis, then there is often impairment in all the three major hepatic phases of bilirubin metabolism, namely uptake, conjugation, and excretion. This is due to the impairment of the function of liver cells. So, there is also little increase in the level of serum unconjugated bilirubin. The acquired defects of biliary excretory function at extrahepatic level may be due to stones, tumors, or strictures in biliary tree. The clinical pictures of this obstructive jaundice are quite similar to that of intrahepatic cholestasis, with pronounced elevation of serum-conjugated bilirubin.

Serum Enzyme Assays

A number of serum enzymes have been used to assess the hepatocellular functions. But, none can truly assess these processes (hepatocellular functions) definitely and especially all have their inherent limitations in sensitivity and specificity. On the other hand, the elevation of these enzymes may also be seen in association with other nonhepatic disorders. Nevertheless, with proper and careful interpretations, a number of serum enzymes provide important clinical tools regarding the assessment of liver functions. These enzymes are discussed here.

Aminotransferase (Transaminase)

As an indicator of hepatocellular function, the assays of many serum enzymes have been proposed. But, among these, the activities of AST (aspartate aminotransferase, previously called SGOT) and ALT (alanine aminotransferase, previously called SGPT) enzyme have been proven to be the most useful. In contrast to ALT, which is found primarily in liver, the AST is also present in many tissues, including heart, skeletal muscle, kidney, and brain. Thus, AST is somewhat less specific, as an indicator of liver function, than ALT.

In a hepatocyte, the ALT is found exclusively in its cytoplasm, while the different isoenzymes of AST exist in both mitochondria and cell cytoplasm. The normal level of AST and ALT in serum is 35 U/L. The source of this normal serum AST and ALT level is still unclear. Although the elevated serum level of AST or ALT may also be observed in a variety of nonhepatic disease, notably in myocardial infarction and skeletal muscle disorders, but these disorders *can usually be distinguished clinically* from liver disease. In contrast, uremia may also lead to a false low aminotransferase value.

The absolute or a single level of aminotransferase correlates poorly with the severity of liver disease or its prognosis. Only the serial determination of the value of these enzymes is usually most useful. On the other hand, the very high level of these enzymes suggests the development of cholangitis with resultant hepatic cell necrosis. The modest elevation of the level of transaminases occurs in alcoholic hepatitis. Minimal elevation of AST and ALT is found in association with the biliary tract obstruction. In general, the serum AST and ALT levels are parallel with each other. But, there are some exceptions, e.g., in alcoholic hepatitis where the AST/ALT >2.

Alkaline Phosphatase

Alkaline phosphatase (AP) is a plasma membrane-derived enzyme of uncertain physiological function. It hydrolyzes the synthetic phosphate esters at pH 9. The human serum contains the several isoforms of it and the different techniques for the assessment of these different isoforms of AP have been developed that utilize different substrates. Serum AP usually arises from multiple sources, such as the bone, intestine, liver, and placenta. In the absence of intestine and bone disease or pregnancy (placenta), the elevated levels of AP reflect impaired biliary tract function. In liver diseases, the increased level of AP is due to the increased synthesis of this enzyme by hepatocytes and biliary tract epithelium, or due to the regurgitation of this enzyme by biliary tract obstruction. The probable explanation of it is that the bile acids play an important role both in inducing the synthesis and promoting the solubility of this membrane-associated enzyme activity.

Slight-to-moderate rise of AP level occurs in parenchymal liver disorders, such as in hepatitis and cirrhosis of liver. But, very high level of it is found in infiltrative hepatic parenchymal disorders, e.g., mycobacterial infection of liver. However, *consistently and striking increase* in AP level, which is 10 times greater than normal value (normal value is 30–120 U/L), occurs with the extrahepatic biliary tract (mechanical) obstruction or with intrahepatic (functional) cholestasis (as in drug-induced cholestasis or primary biliary cirrhosis). Conversely, it is unusual for the serum AP to remain normal when there is obstructive jaundice. On the other hand, a normal AP level argues strongly against the presence of cholestasis or obstruction.

In metastatic or infiltrative liver diseases, such as in leukemia, lymphoma, and sarcoidosis, the AP level is usually mildly elevated. Sometimes, the AP level is also elevated in nonhepatic disorders, most commonly in some bone disorder, such as in Paget's disease, osteomalacia, bone metastasis, etc. and sometimes with malignancy. Several methods can distinguish different isoenzymes of AP of different origins. For example, in contrast to that of AP, which is derived from bone, the hepatic isoenzyme of AP is stable on treatment with heat (56°C for 15 minutes). These isoenzymes can also be distinguished by electrophoresis. But, this is not practical for the diagnosis of specific diseases, because the parallel determination of serum 5'-neucleotidase helps in diagnosis. An increase of both 5'-neucleotidase and AP diagnoses hepatobiliary disease.

5-Nucleotidase Estimation

It is an enzyme, which catalyzes the hydrolysis of phosphate at the position 5 of a pentose component of a nucleotide. The enzyme, 5-nucleotides, is widely distributed in all tissues, but the hepatobiliary disease is especially associated with higher elevation of this enzyme. The normal plasma value of this nucleotide enzyme is 1–18 U/L. The principal importance of this 5-nucleotidase measurement is to confirm the hepatic origin of an elevated AP level in children or pregnant women or in those settings where the coincidental bone disease may be present. In the contrary, the lack of the elevation of 5-nucleotides always does not exclude the hepatic source of elevated serum AP level.

Estimation of Gamma-Glutamyl Transpeptidase

The gamma-glutamyl transpeptidase (GGT) plays a major role in amino acid transport. It also catalyzes the transfer of a γ-glutamyl group from a peptide, such as glutathione to other amino acids. It is distributed in various tissues, as well as in hepatobiliary system. In liver disease, the plasma level of GGT correlates well with that of AP levels and is the most sensitive indicator of biliary tract disease. GGT levels are also elevated in pancreatic, cardiac, renal, and pulmonary disorders, as well as in diabetes and alcoholism. So, the overall lack of the specificity of GGT has constrained its usefulness.

Estimation of Serum Proteins

Extensive liver cell damage or injury leads to decreased blood levels of albumin, prothrombin, fibrinogen, and other serum proteins, which are exclusively synthesized by the hepatocytes. So, in contrast to the measurement of serum enzymes which reflects directly the liver cell injury, the estimation of serum proteins also reflects the synthetic dysfunctions of liver cells.

During the interpretation of the level of serum proteins in hepatic diseases, there are three important principles:
1. The decreased level of serum proteins, synthesized by liver, is neither early nor a sensitive indicator for liver disease. This is because of the huge hepatic reserve and the prolonged half-life of serum proteins.
2. The decreased level in serum protein is not specific for any liver disease, because there are many other factors, which also cause the decreased level of serum proteins, such as nutritional deficiency, malabsorption, and others.
3. The decreased level of serum proteins is of little value in the differential diagnosis of different liver diseases.

Albumin and Globulin

The normal serum value of albumin ranges from 35 to 55 g/L (3.5–5.5 g/dL) and it is the most important protein, synthesized by the liver. The half-life of albumin is 14–20 days and its daily turnover rate is <5%. Moreover, there is a substantial power of reserve for the synthesis of albumin by hepatocytes. Thus, adequate synthesis of albumin may continue, though there is extensive hepatocellular injury. So, albumin estimation is not a good indicator for *acute and mild* hepatocellular injury. But, the value of albumin <2.5 g/dL indicates better the *chronic* liver disease. On the other hand, low serum level of albumin is also influenced by (or indicative for) a variety of nonhepatic factors, such as nutritional status (severe malnutrition), hormonal factors, kidney diseases

(nephrotic syndrome), and intestinal disease (protein losing enteropathy), which are not associated with the defective synthesis of albumin by liver, due to hepatic dysfunction. Still, the reduction of serum albumin level provides an excellent indicator of chronic liver disease (provided other systems remain free of diseases).

Serum globulins are a heterogeneous group of proteins (α, β, γ, etc.), which are synthesized in varieties of tissues. The normal serum globulin level is 20–35 g/L. It is often elevated in association with chronic liver disease, e.g., cirrhosis, hepatitis, fatty liver, etc. This reflects increased stimulation for the synthesis of immunoglobulin by peripheral RE system, due to the shunting of antigens which bypass the liver and are not cleared by hepatic *Kupffer cells*. There are many other nonhepatic conditions where globulin levels are also elevated. The albumin/globulin ratio has no such physiological significance.

Clotting Factors and Prothrombin Time

Virtually all the coagulation factors **(Table 2)**, which are protein in nature, are synthesized by liver and require the presence of vitamin K as cofactor for their synthesis (coagulation factors V, XII, and XIII do not need vitamin K as cofactor for their synthesis). Like serum proteins, these coagulation factors are also normally present in plasma in excess concentration. So, impaired coagulation is usually seen only in severe and prolonged liver disease. Impaired

TABLE 2: Numerical system for international nomenclature of blood coagulation factors and their half-life in hours within bracket.

Clotting factor	Synonym
I	Fibrinogen (100 hours)
II	Prothrombin (80 hours)
III	Tissue thromboplastin
IV	Calcium
V	Labile factor (18 hours)
VI	Proaccelerin (6 hours)
VII	Stable or proconvertin factor (6 hours)
VIII	Antihemophilic factor (AHF) (10 hours)
IX	Christmas factor (24 hours)
X	Stuart factor (50 hours)
XI	Plasma thromboplastin antecedent (PTA) factor (25 hours)
XII	Hageman factor or surface factor (60 hours)
XIII	Laki–Lorand factor (LLF) or fibrin stabilizing factor (90 hours)

coagulation can most efficiently be determined by one-stage prothrombin time (PT). The PT measures the rate of conversion of prothrombin to thrombin in the presence of thromboplastin plus calcium and requires the integrity of other vitamin K-dependent clotting factors. The vitamin K-dependent clotting factors are—factor II, VII, IX, and X.

The normal PT ranges between 11 and 14 seconds. The PT measures the activity of fibrinogen (factor I), prothrombin (factor II), and factors V, VII, and X, i.e., the activity or integrity of extrinsic pathway. The prolongation of PT >3–4 seconds from control [which usually corresponds to an international normalized ratio (INR) value >1.5] is considered significant and reflects liver dysfunction and coagulopathy. But, it cannot reflect the degree of hepatic dysfunction or coagulopathy. Because, in hepatic dysfunction, with the reduced synthesis of coagulation factors, there is also reduced synthesis of anticoagulation factors, such as protein C, protein S, and antithrombin III. The function of fibrinolytic system, which also prevents coagulation-like anticoagulation factors, does not depend on hepatic function. The relative short half-life of factor VII (4–6 hours) makes the PT useful in evaluating hepatic synthetic function of patients in an acute liver disease, but not in chronic liver diseases. Further, only 20–30% of normal coagulation factor activity is required for normal coagulation. Hence, the prolongation of PT usually reflects either severe liver disease or vitamin K deficiency, not the early and moderate liver disease or vitamin K deficiency. The INR is designed to reflect warfarin activity, but not the liver function. This is of great clinical importance as a prolonged INR, after a major surgery like liver surgery, may result in venous thromboembolic prophylaxis, being withheld until the INR normalizes. This may leave the patient at increased risk for a pulmonary embolus.

Two in vitro tests aPTT (activated partial thromboplastin time) and PT are employed for testing the integrity of intrinsic, extrinsic, and common pathways of coagulation cascade. The results are interpreted as given in **Table 3**.

Now, the patients are increasingly treated with factor Xa inhibitors, such as *apixaban* and *rivaroxaban*, for the prevention of thrombosis. Direct assays of anti-factor Xa activity may be employed to monitor their effects. The direct thrombin inhibitor *dabigatran* is also currently prescribed for prophylaxis.

Thus, PT depends on sufficient intestinal uptake of vitamin K and normal machinery for the synthesis of clotting factors by liver. The absorption of vitamin K requires adequate dietary intake, normal function of intestinal mucosa, and normal biliary secretions (as vitamin K is a fat-soluble vitamin). As the coagulation factors are of shorter half-life than that of serum proteins, so the PT may be an early indicator than serum albumin level in hepatic injury. In both

TABLE 3: Results of the integrity of intrinsic, extrinsic, and common pathways of coagulation cascade.

	PT	aPTT
Defect in intrinsic coagulation pathway	Normal	Prolonged
Defect in extrinsic coagulation pathway	Prolonged	Normal
Defect in common coagulation pathway	Prolonged	Prolonged

(aPTT: activated partial thromboplastin time; PT: prothrombin time)

TABLE 4: Coagulation test abnormalities.

	PT	aPTT	TT	Fibrinogen
Severe liver disease	↑	↑	N or ↑	N or ↓
Vitamin K deficiency	↑↑	↑	N	N
Heparin therapy	↑	↑↑	↑	N
Warfarin therapy	↑↑	↑	N	N
Hemophilia:				
• Factor VIII deficiency	N	↑	N	N
• Factor IX deficiency	N	↑	N	N
Factor VII deficiency	↑↑	N	N	N
Factor XIII deficiency	N	N	N	N
DIC	↑↑	↑↑	↑↑	↓↓

(DIC: disseminated intravascular coagulation; PT: prothrombin time; aPTT: activated partial thromboplastin time; TT: thromboplastin time; N: normal)

acute and chronic hepatocellular injury, an increase in PT serves as an ominous prognostic sign. As vitamin K is a fat-soluble vitamin, so the prolongation of PT can also result from vitamin K malabsorption which may occur with cholestasis, due to biliary tract disease or due to malabsorption syndrome for any cause (e.g., pancreatic insufficiency, steatorrhea, etc.). Poor dietary intake, antibiotic therapy, and use of warfarin type of anticoagulants are the additional causes of prolonged PT, owing to the deficiency of active vitamin K. This process can be distinguished from the failure of hepatic synthesis by demonstrating the normalization of PT (within 24–48 hours) after parenteral injection of vitamin K. The partial thromboplastin time (aPTT), which reflects the activity of fibrinogen, prothrombin, and clotting factors such as V, VIII, IX, X, XI, and XII, may also be prolonged in severe liver disease. Before any surgical procedure on patient, with liver disease including liver biopsy, clotting functions should always be assessed in all of them. Different diseases affecting the coagulation process can be assessed by estimating the aPTT, PT, TT, and plasma fibrinogen level which is shown in **Table 4**.

Viscoelastic Coagulation Monitoring

This is a special type of monitoring, by which we can perform real-time assessment of coagulation status. It includes thromboelastography (TEG), rotation thromboelastometry (ROETM), and Sonoclot analysis (SCA). The principle of these tests is that by assessing the viscoelastic properties of whole blood, we assess the total coagulation status of blood. By these tests, the total effect of balance (i) between the procoagulant and anticoagulant systems, (ii) between the profibrinolytic and antifibrinolytic systems, and (iii) the resultant clot tensile strength is obtained. Therefore, precise management of hemostatic therapy becomes possible. The information which is obtained by these tests is: (1) the rate of clot formation, (2) the strength of clot, (3) the impact of clot lysis, (4) the presence or absence of disseminated intravascular coagulation (DIC), (5) the effect of heparin and other anticoagulants on blood coagulation, and (6) the effect of platelet function and its inhibition. The viscoelastic coagulation monitoring is particularly helpful when assessing the coagulation and thromboembolic risk of the patient who has a prolonged INR due to severe liver dysfunction.

Blood Ammonia Estimation

Liver is the major site for amino acid or protein metabolism and their interconversions. It synthesizes proteins from amino acids, supplied from dietary source or supplied from metabolic turnover of endogenous proteins (primarily from muscle). The dietary amino acids enter the liver through portal vein and the amino acids from breakdown of endogenous proteins enter the liver through hepatic artery. In liver, these amino acids undergo deamination, transamination, and other metabolic processes. In liver diseases, the disruption of this normal amino acid metabolism pathway leads to the elevated plasma amino acid concentrations (levels).

Liver handles the amino acids by two major reactions—transamination and oxidative deamination (**Fig. 14**). In transamination, after transferring the NH_3 radicle, the amino acid enters the citric acid cycle. But, in oxidative deamination, amino acids are converted to keto acids and ammonia. This ammonia is very toxic product of nitrogen (protein) metabolism. So, it is converted to urea by Krebs–Henseleit or ornithine cycle (**Fig. 15**). In normal condition, the value of this whole blood ammonia varies between *45 and 65 mmol/L (80–110 mg/dL)*. So, the estimation of this NH_3 is of very clinical importance in a patient with severe liver disease. In advanced liver disease, urea synthesis is often depressed, leading to an accumulation of NH_3 in blood. This is sometimes associated with the significant reduction of blood urea nitrogen (BUN) level, which is an

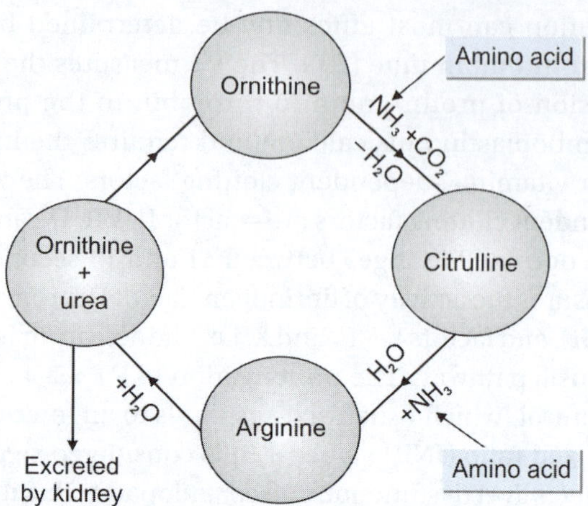

Fig. 14: Formation of urea by Krebs–Henseleit or ornithine cycle. In this cycle, one molecule of CO_2 (carbonic acid) and two molecules of NH_3 are neutralized.

ominous sign of liver failure. Urea is mostly excreted by kidney. The 25% of formed urea is also diffused into the lumen of intestine from blood, where it is again converted to NH_3 by bacterial enzyme, named urease. The intestinal production of ammonia also occurs from the bacterial action on unabsorbed amino acids and also from bacterial actions on proteins, which are derived from the diet, from the exfoliated cells of intestine, or from any free blood in gastrointestinal (GI) tract. The NH_3 from this GI tract is reabsorbed and transported to liver by portal system and again converted to urea. Kidney also produces the varying amounts of ammonia. The contribution of gut and kidney in ammonia synthesis has important implications in the management of hyperammonemic state, frequently seen in patients with advanced liver disease. Hyperammonemia usually leads to hepatic encephalopathy.

EFFECTS OF ANESTHESIA ON HEPATIC FUNCTION

Anesthesia influences the hepatic function by multiple ways and these are: (1) anesthetic procedure, (2) drugs used in and for anesthesia, (3) types of previous hepatic disease, and (4) type of surgery for which anesthesia is given.

- During both general and regional anesthesia, the hepatic blood flow is usually decreased. This is due to: (1) both direct and indirect effect of anesthetic agents, (2) type of ventilation that is employed, and (3) type of anesthesia that is being performed. Most of the anesthetic agents reduce CO and thus reduce hepatic blood flow. Regional anesthesia also reduces the hepatic blood flow by same mechanism ($\downarrow$ in venous return → $\downarrow$ in CO → $\downarrow$BP → $\downarrow$ hepatic blood flow). Controlled positive-pressure ventilation with high mean airway pressure reduces

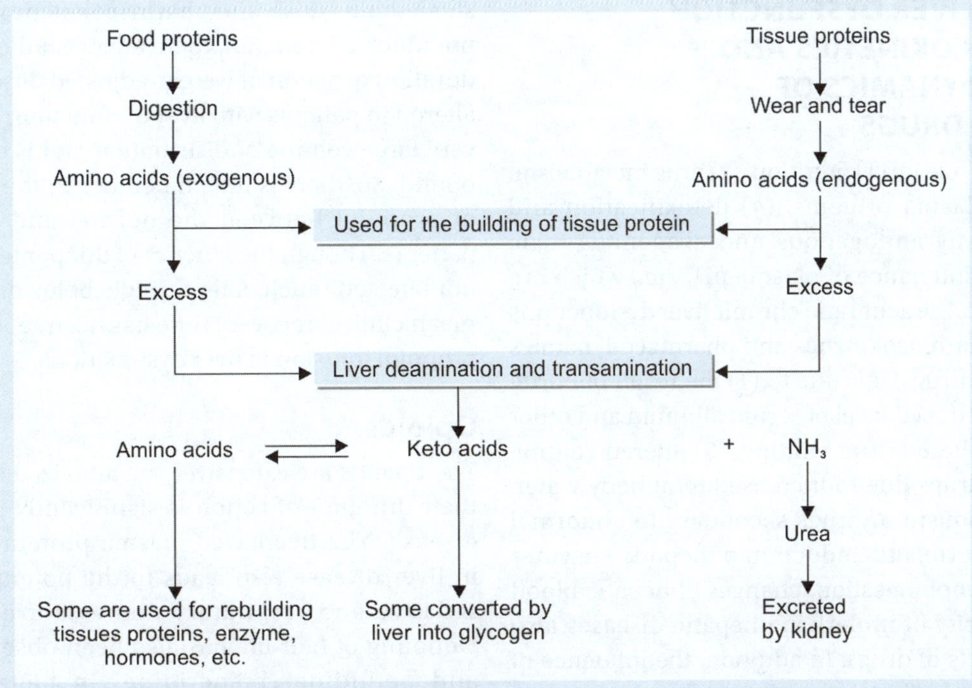

Fig. 15: Synthesis of proteins and amino acids in liver.

venous return and CO, leading to ↓ in hepatic blood flow. In positive-pressure ventilation, increased hepatic venous pressure also leads to reduced hepatic blood flow. PEEP further accentuates these effects.

- Surgical procedures near the liver can reduce the hepatic blood flow up to 50–60%. However, the mechanisms for this reduction of hepatic blood flow are not clear. But, the most likely explanations are—sympathetic activation, direct compression on portal and hepatic vessels, and local reflexes.
- The α_1-adrenergic agonists, β_2-adrenergic blockers, H_2-receptor blockers, and vasopressin reduce hepatic blood flow. Infusion of dopamine in the dose of 0.5–1.0 µg/kg/min increases hepatic blood flow.
- An endocrine stress response, secondary to fasting and surgical trauma, has profound effects on the metabolic functions of liver. These effects are characterized by elevated circulating level of catecholamines, glucagon, and cortisol, resulting in mobilization of carbohydrate store from liver, causing hyperglycemia. This neuro-endocrine response can be blunted by regional anesthesia, deep general anesthesia, or pharmacological blockade of sympathetic system.
- When the LFTs are abnormal postoperatively, the usual cause is underlying liver disease or the surgical procedure itself. The persistent abnormalities in liver tests may be indicative of viral hepatitis, sepsis, or surgical complications. Postoperative jaundice can result from a variety of factors, but the most common

BOX 4: Causes of postoperative jaundice.

- *Prehepatic causes (increased bilirubin production):*
  - Resorption of hematoma
  - *Hemolytic transfusion:*
    - Breakdown of aged RBC
    - Mismatch transfusion
- *Hepatic (hepatocellular dysfunction):*
  - Pre-existing liver disease
  - Ischemic injury to liver
  - Drug induced
  - Halothane
  - Intrahepatic cholestasis
- *Posthepatic (biliary obstruction):*
  - Postoperative pancreatitis
  - Postoperative cholecystitis
  - Bile duct injury
  - Retained CBD stone

(CBD: common bile duct; RBC: red blood cell)

cause is the overproduction of bilirubin, because of resorption of a large hematoma or red cell breakdown following transfusion. However, all the other causes for postoperative jaundice, given in **Box 4**, should also be considered. Correct diagnosis requires a careful review of preoperative liver function and a careful review of intra- and postoperative events, such as prolonged hypotension, hypoxia, transfusions, and drug exposure. Sevoflurane, isoflurane, and desflurane have minimal, if any, direct adverse effect upon hepatocytes.

EFFECTS OF LIVER DYSFUNCTION ON PHARMACOKINETICS AND PHARMACODYNAMICS OF ANESTHETIC DRUGS

Liver plays a critical role in: (1) nutrition, (2) drug metabolism, (3) synthesis of plasma proteins, (4) detoxification and elimination of many endogenous and exogenous toxic substances, (5) maintenance of plasma pH, etc., which are described before. So, the acute and chronic liver dysfunctions usually alter the pharmacokinetics and pharmacodynamics of many anesthetic drugs. It is due to (1) the result of portal hypertension, (2) reduced level of serum albumin and other proteins, causing altered drug binding, (3) altered volume of distribution of drugs due to increased total body water, (4) reduced metabolism of drugs secondary to abnormal function of hepatocyte, etc. Induction of hepatic enzymes due to chronic alcohol ingestion, changes of hepatic blood flow, and the severity of underlying hepatic diseases also influences the effects of drugs. In addition, the influence of liver disease differs for elimination of enteral and parenteral group of drugs. Portal hypertension causes the reduction in portal venous blood flow to liver and hence the drugs given by the oral route will have prolonged half-life.

The clearance of drugs by liver is dependent on its availability to liver cells, which in turn is dependent on liver blood flow. So, the metabolism of drugs, such as lignocaine and pethidine which have high-clearance ratio, is affected more than the drugs such as benzodiazepines (BDZ) which have low-clearance ratio. On the other hand, these drugs are more affected by altered protein binding, intrinsic hepatic clearance, and metabolism.

Premedicants

The advent of daycare anesthesia has virtually reduced the number of patients who are routinely subjected to premedication. The trend is now either no premedications or oral administration of short-acting benzodiazepines in very small doses. The recovery time and the elimination kinetics of sedative dose of a benzodiazepine are prolonged in patients with liver dysfunction. It is due to reduced protein-binding capacity and reduced metabolism of BZD in liver disease. Therefore, these drugs should be used with caution, when repeated intramuscular (IM) injections or continuous infusions are required. However, their effects may be reversed by flumazenil.

Intravenous Inducing Agents

Most intravenous inducing agents undergo extensive hepatic metabolism. However, studies suggest that after a single bolus dose, the pharmacokinetics of these agents is not much altered. But, there are no studies showing that the duration of action of weight-adjusted dose of thiopentone is altered in patients with liver dysfunction. The propofol has a very large volume of distribution and is extensively protein bound. So, there is little difference in the pharmacokinetics of propofol between the normal and liver dysfunction patients. Though the kinetics of thiopentone and propofol is not affected much, after a single bolus dose, but prolonged mean clinical recovery time has been reported, mainly after propofol infusion in liver dysfunction.

Opioids

The opioids are extensively metabolized by liver. Therefore, their duration of action is significantly prolonged in liver disease. The decreased plasma protein-binding capacity in liver disease also leads to the potentially exaggerated sedative and respiratory depressant effects of opioids. Doubling of half-life has also been observed in morphine and pethidine (meperidine) in hepatic dysfunction. Therefore, it is recommended to increase the administration interval by 1.5–2-folds for this group of drugs. In addition, the decreased clearance of norpethidine (normeperidine) in patients with advanced liver disease may precipitate neurotoxicity more commonly. The fentanyl and sufentanil are highly lipid-soluble synthetic opioids and are extensively metabolized in liver. However, their single-dose pharmacokinetics is not much altered in liver diseases. But, continuous infusion or repeated dosing may prolong their effect. Unlike these drugs, the half-life of alfentanil is almost doubled in patients with cirrhosis of liver, which can lead to its prolonged duration of action and enhanced effects of it. The remifentanil is rapidly hydrolyzed in plasma by tissue esterase, leading to rapid recovery, which is independent of the dose and the duration of infusion of remifentanil. So, the available data indicates that its elimination is unaltered in patients with severe liver disease or in those undergoing liver transplantation.

Muscle Relaxants

Suxamethonium and mivacurium are the substrates of plasma cholinesterase enzyme for hydrolysis. Plasma cholinesterase is synthesized in liver. So, the low-plasma cholinesterase concentration in liver dysfunction may prolong the half-life of succinylcholine and mivacurium. However, the reduction of plasma cholinesterase level is such that, even in fulminant hepatic failure (FHF), the action of succinylcholine is unlikely to be prolonged significantly. But, care should be taken, if mivacurium or succinylcholine is administered by infusion.

The nondepolarizing muscle relaxants are highly water soluble (e.g., d-tubocurarine, gallamine and pancuronium atracurium, vecuronium, rocuronium, etc.) and are, therefore, easily excreted through urine. However, increased volume of distribution in patients with liver disease leads to an apparent resistance to these agents with prolonged elimination. The modern steroid-based drugs (muscle relaxants), such as vecuronium and rocuronium, show little alteration in their pharmacokinetics in a jaundiced patient. However, the atracurium and cisatracurium undergo organ-independent elimination by ester hydrolysis and spontaneous Hoffman degradation in plasma. So, they have no change in elimination half-life or clinical duration of action, even in patients with both hepatic and renal failure. But, many of the newer nondepolarizing drugs are given by infusion and their effect may be unpredictable in patients with hepatic disease. So, the careful monitoring of neuromuscular function should be carried out with a nerve stimulator during anesthesia when muscle relaxants are used, especially by infusion in liver dysfunction patients.

PREOPERATIVE EVALUATION AND ANESTHETIC RISK ASSESSMENT OF PATIENT WITH LIVER DYSFUNCTION

Liver diseases can alter the responses of patients to anesthesia and surgery in many ways. So, it is important to understand (1) the applied anatomy and physiology of liver, and (2) the factors altering the hepatic blood flow, the liver functions, and the pharmacokinetics and pharmacodynamics of anesthetic drugs, etc. for the proper perioperative management of these patients. But, the complex functions of liver, the effects of perioperative stress and strain on liver function, and the unpredictable effect of drugs in patients with liver disease have made the preanesthetic evaluation and the risk assessment of a patient suffering from liver disease challenging. The perioperative risk assessment of a patient, suffering from liver disease, should take into account the type of liver disease, the degree of hepatic impairment, and the intrinsic surgical risk associated with this procedure. Patients with liver disease undergoing nonhepatic surgery and anesthesia face significant postoperative complications also.

For the assessment of anesthetic risk, liver disease can be graded (according to Child's classification which is modified by Pugh) on the basis of the impairment of synthetic functions of liver, mainly plasma albumin (measured by plasma albumin level) and prothrombin (measured by PT). *Mild hepatic disease* consists of positive clinical history and evidence of liver pathology, coupled with normal plasma albumin and PT. Other tests of hepatic function, such as

TABLE 5: Spectrum of liver disease.

Early stage	*Late stage*
1. Inflammatory response in liver usually predominates	Fibrotic response in liver usually predominates
2. Drug resistance is often observed	Drug sensitivity is often observed
3. No portal hypertension is observed	Portal hypertension is the dominant feature
4. Major laboratory abnormalities are elevated enzymes such as aminotransferase	Major laboratory abnormalities are disorders of hepatic synthetic functions such as albumin, prothrombin time, and others

Note: Bilirubin level in plasma is elevated in both the stages.

aminotransferase, may be elevated. *Moderate liver disease* consists of plasma albumin level of at least 3 g/dL and PT is not >2.5 seconds. *Severe liver disease* is defined as when albumin level falls below 3 g/dL and PT is above 2.5 seconds. The perioperative risk assessment of patient according to the type of liver disease is described below under the heading of asymptomatic and symptomatic patients and under the heading of early and late stage of liver disease **(Table 5)**.

Asymptomatic Patients

Asymptomatic patients, with the abnormalities of standard liver enzyme tests including AST, ALT, and AP, occur in 0.1–4% of general population. This incidence may be as high as 36% in patients with the history of daily alcohol consumption and drug abuse. Minor elevations of these enzymes, less than twice of the normal value in asymptomatic patients who have normal serum bilirubin and INR level, do not warrant additional testing before anesthesia and surgery. On the other hand, the larger elevations of transaminases, during routine preoperative investigations, signify a subclinical acute process of liver dysfunction, such as viral hepatitis or an acute on a chronic disorder such as chronic hepatitis. So, they require additional analysis, starting from the careful history and physical examination of patient to the history of previous surgeries, jaundice, blood transfusion, use of alcohol and other recreational drugs, sexual history, etc.

Careful attention should also be paid to the other systemic effects of liver disease including pruritus, excessive bleeding after minor trauma, abdominal distention, weight gain (due to accumulation of fluid), etc. Physical examination should also focus on the signs of liver disease, such as icterus, pallor, hepatomegaly, splenomegaly, testicular atrophy, palmar erythema, spider nevi, and gynecomastia. Further investigations should also be carried out to assess the hepatic functions, such as coagulation profile, electrolytes, and liver enzymes. The AST/ALT ratio may also be helpful in distinguishing between the viral and alcohol-related hepatitis. Alcohol tends to preferentially damage the mitochondria of hepatocyte, therefore causing much elevation in AST which is usually greater than twice of ALT values. In contrast, a decrease in this ratio is more consistent with a diagnosis of viral hepatitis. Elevated AP with abnormal bilirubin and GGT indicates hepatobiliary disease. Asymptomatic patients with significant abnormal liver function should have elective surgery postponed and are further investigated to reassess the perioperative risks.

Symptomatic Patients with Acute and Chronic Hepatic Diseases

Patients with acute liver disease or hepatic failure rarely represent for anesthesia and surgery. This is because mortality rate is very high and is near about 10–100% in this group of patients. Acute hepatic failure, during postanesthetic period, is due to the decompensation of previously apparent well patients with chronic liver disease. Paradoxically, hyperacute hepatic failure (encephalopathy within 7 days) has the best prognosis.

Some causes of acute liver disease (or failure) presenting for surgery and anesthesia are:

- *Acute viral hepatitis:* Type A to G, *Cytomegalovirus,* herpes simplex virus, Epstein–Barr virus, and Coxsackievirus, etc.
- *Acute hepatitis due to drugs:* Alcohol, halothane, paracetamol excess, idiosyncratic reactions, etc.
- *Acute hepatitis due to toxins:* Alcohol, carbon tetrachloride, mushrooms poison, etc.
- *Acute hepatitis due to miscellaneous causes:* Acute fatty infiltration of pregnancy, HELLP (hemolysis, elevated liver enzymes, and low platelets) syndrome, Wilson's disease, Reye's syndrome, etc.

Some causes of chronic hepatic diseases presenting for surgery and anesthesia are:

- *Cirrhosis:* The most common cause of chronic liver disease, presenting for anesthesia and surgery, is cirrhosis. Cirrhosis can be acquired, such as due to alcohol, viral hepatitis, drugs, secondary biliary disease, etc. or cirrhosis can be inherited such as due to primary biliary cirrhosis, hemochromatosis, Wilson's disease, galactosemia, and sickle cell disease.
- *Chronic hepatitis:* It is also widespread. It is defined as any hepatitis, lasting longer than 6 months, as evidenced by elevated serum aminotransferase. In evaluating patients for chronic hepatitis, laboratory test results may show only

BOX 5: Drugs associated with hepatitis.

- *Toxic substances:* Alcohol, paracetamol, salicylates, tetracycline, and vinyl chloride
- *Idiosyncratic:* Halothane, phenytoin, rifampin, sulfonamides, and indomethacin
- *Both toxic and idiosyncratic:* Isoniazid, methyldopa, Na valproate, and amiodarone
- *Cholestatic:* Chlorpromazine, oral contraceptive, cyclosporine, erythromycin, and methimazole

a mild elevation in serum aminotransferase activity and often correlate poorly with disease activity. The causes of chronic hepatitis are—viruses, alcohol, autoimmune, metabolic, and drugs (isoniazid and methyldopa). Both immunological factors and a genetic predisposition may be responsible in most cases. Evidence of cirrhosis is either present initially or eventually develops in 20–50% of patients.

Chronic hepatitis B develops in 3% of those infected by acute HBV (hepatitis B virus) infection. It is widespread in Far East, Africa, and infects 300 million people worldwide. Other high-risk groups for chronic HBV infection include—homosexuals, IV drug abusers, hemophiliacs, hemodialysis patients, etc. Chronic HBV infection may progress to cirrhosis or hepatocellular carcinoma. Chronic hepatitis develops in 75% of those infected by acute HCV (hepatitis C virus) infection. Risk groups for hepatitis C virus infection are similar to that of hepatitis B and cirrhosis or hepatocellular carcinoma can develop. Patients without chronic hepatitis B or C infection usually have a favorable response to immunosuppressants and are treated with long-term corticosteroid therapy with or without azathioprine.

Drug-induced chronic hepatitis can result from—(1) direct, dose-dependent toxic effect of a drug or its metabolites, or (2) idiosyncratic drug reaction, or (3) combination of these two causes. The clinical course of a drug-induced chronic hepatitis often resembles chronic viral hepatitis, making its diagnosis difficult. Ingestion of acetaminophen (paracetamol) of 25 gram or more usually results in fatal fulminant hepatotoxicity. The common drugs causing hepatitis are mentioned in **Box 5**.

INDIVIDUAL LIVER DISEASES AND ANESTHESIA

Hepatitis

Usually, hepatitis patients present in two ways—*acute* and *chronic.*

1. *Acute hepatitis* is usually the result of a viral infection. It may be due to the drug reaction or due to the exposure of liver to hepatotoxin **(Box 6)**. Acute hepatitis represents

BOX 6: Causes of hepatitis.

- *Viral infections:*
  - Hepatitis A virus
  - Hepatitis E virus
  - Hepatitis B virus
  - Herpes simplex virus
  - Hepatitis C virus
  - *Cytomegalovirus (CMV)*
  - Hepatitis D virus
  - Epstein–Barr virus (EBV)
- *Toxins:*
  - Alcohol
  - Drugs, e.g., methyldopa, isoniazid, halothane, amiodarone, and herbal drugs
- *Miscellaneous:*
  - Wilson's disease
  - Hemochromatosis
  - Autoimmune hepatitis
  - α_1-antitrypsin deficiency

it as an acute hepatocellular injury, with a variable degree of cellular necrosis. The clinical manifestations of acute hepatitis depend on the severity of inflammatory reaction and the necrosis of hepatic cells. Mild inflammatory reaction may represent merely as the asymptomatic elevation of serum transaminase level; whereas, hepatic necrosis represents as the acute FHF.

An acute hepatitis patient, viral or drug-induced, should always be taken seriously for anesthesia. So, an accurate diagnosis of the cause of hepatitis is exceedingly important during preanesthetic investigations. Here, we will mainly discuss the *acute viral hepatitis*. There are two points, of serious concern, in a patient suffering from acute viral hepatitis and who may require surgery and anesthesia. These two points are:

i. The combination of surgery, anesthesia, and acute viral hepatitis is associated with high-mortality rate. The available data indicates that the perioperative mortality rate ranges from 10 to 100%, if a patient with acute viral hepatitis requires surgery and anesthesia. Thus, a disease of low-to-moderate mortality is converted by the surgery and anesthesia to one of high mortality.

ii. Hepatitis B and C can be highly contagious via parenteral inoculation to the operating theater personnel. However, the exact time of surgery and anesthesia, which is safe after an acute attack of viral hepatitis, is still unknown. It is usually said that surgery is permissible some 30 days after the liver function studies have returned to normal. It is prudent to postpone the elective surgery in the acute phase

of hepatitis and wait for the level of transaminases to return to the normal ranges. In case of hepatitis B and C, there should be sufficient time to ensure that the patient does not enter into the phase of chronic persistent or chronic active hepatitis. A jaundiced patient waiting for anesthesia and surgery should be differentiated between acute viral hepatitis and posthepatic biliary obstruction as a cause of jaundice where in one condition, early surgery is necessary and in one condition where early surgery and anesthesia are associated with high-mortality rate.

There are five principal hepatitis viruses: A, B, C (older nomenclature of C is non-A/non-B), D, and E (enteric non-A and non-B). Hepatitis A and E are the classic oral–fecal, food-borne hepatitis with low-mortality rate and do not progress to chronic hepatitis. Hepatitis B and C are transmitted primarily by percutaneously and by contact with body fluids. They have higher mortality rate and can progress to chronicity. Hepatitis D is unique, in that, it may be transmitted by either route and requires the presence of HBV in the host to be infective.

Acute viral hepatitis due to hepatitis virus A and E usually resolves spontaneously, without entering in chronic hepatitis phase. The chronic phase of this viral hepatitis may be either *chronic persistent hepatitis, chronic lobular hepatitis,* or *chronic active hepatitis.* Chronic persistent hepatitis and chronic lobular hepatitis are mild nonprogressive disease. In most cases, these are due to either hepatitis B or C viruses. This chronic persistent and lobular viral hepatitis may be due to some unknown reasons and are slow to resolve, at times taking as long as 18 months. Then, these patients eventually do resolve and the prognosis is generally favorable. Since, these patients are eventually cleared of liver disease, usually within a year, so it is prudent to defer the elective surgery until their liver function studies become normal, for at least 1 month. If emergency surgery is required, then the risk in these patients is probably not increased (but there is no data to confirm this point).

2. *Chronic active hepatitis* has also been termed as chronic aggressive hepatitis. It is produced by hepatitis B and C viruses and progresses in most patients to cirrhosis and hepatic failure. Patients with chronic active hepatitis will eventually die of liver failure within 2–10 years, unless other causes of death supervene. The bilirubin level increases and aminotransferase levels fluctuate between 200 and 800 U/L. There will be elevated PT and hypoalbuminemia. Purely elective surgery is not wise in chronic active hepatitis and it falls within the domain of severe hepatic impairment.

Alcoholic Liver Disease (Alcoholic Hepatitis)

Patients with alcoholic liver disease or alcoholic hepatitis tend to have increased postoperative complications, such as poor wound healing, infections, delirium, and bleeding. Alcoholic hepatitis similar to other forms of liver disease or hepatitis runs as continuum and the severity of perioperative complications depends upon the severity of liver pathology. The end result of alcoholic hepatitis is cirrhosis. Patients with alcoholic fatty liver tolerate surgery well, while those with cirrhosis have increased postoperative morbidity and mortality. Asymptomatic alcoholic hepatitis produces some hepatomegaly with minimal alterations of liver functions tests. Mild alcoholic hepatitis adds mild jaundice with liver tenderness. Some acute alcoholic hepatitis adds increasing jaundice, fever, leukocytosis, and elevated PT. If patient is considered to have mild alcoholic hepatitis, evidenced by slightly elevated aminotransferase, lactate dehydrogenase, AP, and mildly elevated bilirubin with little or no change in PT, then the patient should be advised to abstain from alcohol to improve liver functions and then elective surgery and anesthesia can be proceeded with.

Cirrhosis

Boxes 6 and 7 illustrate the polarization of the spectrum of liver disease. A chronic inflammatory process of liver, initiated either by viral infections or by toxins (alcohol) or due to any other causes given in **Boxes 6 and 7**, produces an inflammatory response in hepatocytes. After a variable period of time, this chronic inflammation of liver tissues is replaced by scar tissues (fibrosis), leading to cirrhosis. Cirrhosis is then the end-stage of chronic liver inflammatory disease, which is characterized by severe fibrosis and the irregular nodular regenerations of the remaining liver parenchyma. The bundles of scar tissue infringe on the hepatic sinusoidal space, increasing their pressure. This increased sinusoidal pressure is transmitted to the low-pressure, high-flow portal venous system and in turn increases its pressure (portal hypertension). As a result, this increased pressure forces portal blood out of the liver. The blood is then diverted through other vessels, such as gastric and esophageal veins where there is communication between the portal and systemic circulation, producing esophageal varices. Therefore, increased portal venous pressure causes portal hypertension and other stigmata of it.

Patients with cirrhosis have altered and reduced hepatic blood flow that further worsens the liver functions and decreases the metabolism of commonly administered drugs. Associated with cirrhosis of liver, they have also nutritional disorders, ascites, coagulopathy, renal dysfunctions, and high risk of developing encephalopathy **(Box 7)**. There is no question that patients with advanced liver disease are at severe risk, if they require major surgery and anesthesia. The risks of surgery in these patients correlate well with the *Child's classification* of risk assessment. This classification is not only applied in cirrhotic patient, but also in other liver dysfunction. In this classification, there are five factors, affecting mortality and influencing the grading. These are ascites, albumin, bilirubin, encephalopathy, and nutritional status. However, this Child's classification is modified by Pugh who added PT as another risk factor. Prolongation of PT >2.5 seconds from control implies increased anesthetic risk and if >4.0 seconds, it implies severe risk. The levels of AST and ALT are not included in this list of risk factors, because the elevation of these plasma enzymes always does not imply acute hepatic injury. For each factor, score between 1 and 3 is allotted and usually three classes, such as A, B, and C, are described. The perioperative mortality rate in groups A, B, and C is respectively about <30%, 40%, and >90% **(Table 6)**.

BOX 7: Causes of cirrhosis of liver.

- Any cause of chronic hepatitis
- Primary biliary cirrhosis
- Secondary biliary cirrhosis (stones and strictures)
- Alcohol
- Wilson's disease
- Hemochromatosis
- Cystic fibrosis
- α_1-antitrypsin deficiency

TABLE 6: Child's classification (modified by Pugh) of risk for cirrhotic patients undergoing major surgery.

	Group A	Group B	Group C
Serum bilirubin (mg/dL)	<2	2–3	>3
Serum albumin (g/dL)	>4	3–4	<3
Ascites	None	Controlled	Poorly controlled
Neurological disorder	None	Minimal	Advanced
Nutritional status	Excellent	Good	Poor
Prothrombin time (seconds)	<2.5	2–4	>4
Surgical risk	Good	Moderate	Poor
Mortality risk	<10%	30%	>40%
For the factors of group A → 1 point each			
For the factors of group B → 2 point each			
For the factors of Group C → 3 point each			
Grading:			
Grade 5–6: Less risk (30% mortality)			
Grade 7–9: Moderate risk (40% mortality)			
Grade 10–15: High risk (90% mortality)			

The major causes of mortality in perioperative period in the patients with cirrhosis of liver or liver dysfunction are—sepsis, renal failure, bleeding, hepatic failure, and hepatic encephalopathy. However, this score is simple, but lacks linearity. Because, it does not take into account any specific underlying disease process. Although three of these factors such as ascites, encephalopathy, and nutritional status are purely subjective, but this score still remains a useful tool for preanesthetic assessment of patients with cirrhosis.

ANESTHETIC MANAGEMENT OF PATIENT WITH LIVER DISEASE AND JAUNDICE

The most common liver disease, encountered during anesthesia, is *inflammatory hepatitis (alcohol or virus) leading to cirrhosis.* If these patients require anesthesia during an acute attack of hepatitis, mortality can be extremely high. Among them, some patients with chronic hepatitis may remain *in some stages of progression to cirrhosis and portal hypertension,* which require anesthesia for nonhepatic surgical events. Sometimes, many patients present for surgery with acute biliary tract obstruction and jaundice (e.g., stone in CBD) without any hepatitis. The *pathognomonic features of advanced jaundice,* due to hepatitis or posthepatic obstruction or due to other causes which frequently anesthetists encounter and manage, *are hyperdynamic circulation, hypoxemia, metabolic alkalosis, clotting abnormalities, altered hepatic blood flow, cirrhosis, ascites, renal impairment, hepatic encephalopathy, and altered drug handling.*

Hyperdynamic Circulation

The striking features of a patient with advanced liver disease, with or without jaundice, are decreased systemic vascular resistance (SVR) and increased CO, resulting in bounding pulse. The increase in CO is proportional to decrease in SVR, which is again proportional to the severity of liver disease. But, if tense ascites is present, then CO will decrease due to the reduction of preload and pressure on IVC, and it will not improve until paracentesis is done. The decreased vascular resistance, in hepatic diseased patient, is due to arteriolar vasodilatation.

The blood pressure tends to be normal or may even be a bit lower. So, hypertension is very unusual in a patient suffering from jaundice. The atherosclerotic changes in vascular system are generally minimum or absent in liver dysfunction patient, because the deficiency of cholesterol and abnormal lipid metabolism are responsible for this. However, the tragedy is—despite having increased CO in jaundiced patient, many patients have the overt signs of underlying cardiomyopathy due to jaundice. So, the low-peripheral resistance of a liver dysfunction patient exerts a protective effect on left ventricular function. Thus, an abrupt return of vascular resistance to normal values, due to any cause, can unmask the acute left ventricular decompensation.

The cardiac glycosides are not of any benefit to cardiomyopathy in liver dysfunction patient. On the other hand, the plasma level of catecholamines is increased, indicating heightened sympathetic tone (compensatory mechanism) to compensate the blunted baroreceptor reflexes, which occur in jaundice. These appear to be due to decreased number of adrenergic receptors by downregulation in hepatic dysfunction. So, there is a rightward shift of dose-response curve, in contrast to normal patient, causing increased dose requirement of pressure-raising drugs. Thus, for the planning of anesthetic management, several considerations, regarding the cardiovascular system in liver dysfunction or jaundiced patients, should be kept in mind.

Drugs such as isoflurane and sevoflurane, which depress myocardial contractility, are not absolutely contraindicated in liver dysfunction patient, but should be used with great care. Since the decreased peripheral resistance seems to be somewhat of compensatory safeguard, so correction or normalization of this variable may not be in patient's interest. If catecholamines or pressure-raising agents are used, then the dose should be more than of normal patients. This is because of the downward regulation and the decreased number of adrenergic receptors.

Liver disease causes various types of shunts, such as from cutaneous spider angioma to portal and systemic arteriovenous shunts. These shunts, in combination with reduced SVR and increased extracellular fluid due to activated renin–angiotensin system, increase the CO often by 50%. In contrast, some alcoholics may have decreased CO, secondary to cardiomyopathy.

Hypoxemia

In a jaundiced or liver disease patient, arterial hypoxemia is common. This arterial hypoxemia is primarily due to the mismatch between the diffusion and perfusion in lungs. So, the partial pressure of arterial oxygen usually remains <70 mm Hg. This diffusion–perfusion mismatch in lungs is due to increased intrapulmonary shunts and again this is because of the dilatation of precapillary or capillary beds of lungs. This hypoxemia is further exacerbated in upright position, because gravity further increases blood flow toward the bases of lung where perfusion is greater than ventilation, causing more mismatch between diffusion and perfusion. This peculiar hypoxemia can also be due to true pulmonary shunts. The incidences of pleural effusion are more common in jaundice or may develop frequently in

<table>
<tr><td>

BOX 8: Effects of liver dysfunction on respiratory system.

- Decreased alveolar ventilation
- *Hypoxemia:* Hepatopulmonary syndrome (intrapulmonary shunting)
- *Pulmonary hypertension:* PPS, hypercapnia, and acidosis
- *Pulmonary aspiration:* Gastroesophageal reflux
- Require postoperative ventilatory support

</td><td>

BOX 9: Effects of liver dysfunction on hematology.

- *Blood loss:* Varicose vein, peptic ulcer
- *Anemia:* Chronic illness, hemolysis
- *Platelets:* Dysfunction, ↓ number
- Coagulation abnormality
- Fibrinolysis
- Blood and blood products should be ready for management

</td></tr>
</table>

postoperative period, especially if the abdominal right upper quadrant surgery has been performed. Lung infections are also common in a liver disease patient **(Box 8)**.

From the anesthetic point of view, hypoxemia is never allowed for the fear of hepatic cell necrosis in liver compromised patients for any reason. So, always a high-inspired O_2 concentration (FiO_2) should be employed during anesthesia on patients suffering from hepatic dysfunction. Sometimes, the splinting of diaphragm by ascites causing a decrease in PaO_2 cannot be improved by increasing this FiO_2. However, then this should be managed by diuretics or paracentesis. Pulmonary problems should be resolved in preoperative phase by: (1) stopping smoking, (2) giving appropriate antibiotics for lung infections, (3) paracentesis, (4) physiotherapy, etc. For moderate-to-major surgeries, the anesthetist should also consider the placement of an indwelling arterial catheter for perioperative blood gas analysis.

Metabolic Alkalosis

Patients, with liver dysfunction and jaundice, often have metabolic alkalosis and ↓ in plasma K^+ level (compensatory). The explanation of this metabolic alkalosis is like that in liver dysfunction, the aldosterone level remains high. This hormone causes excessive renal absorption of Na^+ in exchange of excess secretion of potassium and H^+ loss in DT and CT and renal retention of ammonia, causing azotemia. This K^+ loss is of particular importance, if the patient is under diuretic therapy preoperatively especially. So, an anesthetist must be careful about potassium replacement in hepatic failure patient. Failure to replace potassium perioperatively can lead to cardiac arrhythmias. Increased plasma ammonia can cause difficulty in reversing the neuromuscular block.

Clotting and Bleeding Abnormalities (Box 9)

As liver is the site for synthesis of vitamin K-dependent clotting factors such as II, V, VII, and X, so their levels are reduced in hepatic disease. Thus, the *PT* which measures the activities of these clotting factors and *extrinsic pathway* are increased. The aPTT which measures the activities of II, V, VIII, IX, X, XI, and XII clotting factors and *intrinsic pathway* are also increased. Thus, they provide an excellent

assessment for the risk of surgery. So, vitamin K should always be given parenterally for at least 72 hours, before surgery when the PT is increased. When the PT is >2.5 seconds, in a patient facing a major surgery, then the fresh frozen plasma (FFP) is probably indicated. Still, if there is persistent hepatic dysfunction, then repeated doses of FFP may be required. The rational approach in bleeding disorder in a jaundiced patient is to administer 2–6 U of FFP at 6–12-hour interval in an attempt to bring the PT to 2–3 seconds of control. If surgery progresses with enough bleeding, then FFP requirement certainly increases. If correction of PT is not obtained, even after what would seem to be adequate by recommended FFP therapy, then there may probably exist fibrinogen degradation product (FDP) in circulation. As factor VII has a half-life of only 4–8 hours, so the response to FFP measured by PT may not be long lasting.

The disorders of bleeding also develop in patients with liver diseases, due to the absolute deficiency in number and quality of platelets. The redistribution (sequestration) of platelet into spleen is also considered to be the most important factor, leading to absolute thrombocytopenia in liver compromised patient. The platelet infusions may be indicated when platelet count is <40,000–50,000/mm^3 of blood. Platelet function is best assessed by bleeding time. There would appear to be no problem in insertion of an epidural catheter, if the PT has been corrected to 2–3 seconds of control value and the platelet count is kept >40,000/mm^3, with normal bleeding time.

Hepatic Blood Flow

The total hepatic blood flow is the result of flow through hepatic artery plus the flow through portal vein. Among these, the portal venous flow is responsible for the 70% of total O_2 supply to liver. Buffer responses autoregulate this total hepatic blood flow, i.e., when blood pressure drops due to any reason (e.g., hemorrhage), then blood flow through the portal venous system drops first, due to low-pressure system. Then, due to the dilation of hepatic artery, blood flow through it again increases, so as to keep the total hepatic blood flow within normal limits. Again, the liver cells have unique property to increase its extraction of O_2 from blood when the blood flow through liver drops.

Both the general and regional anesthesia cause the reduction of hepatic blood flow and it is generally parallel with the drop of systemic blood pressure and CO. So, it seems that BP is the major determinant factor of blood flow through liver. So, during anesthesia on a liver dysfunction patient, mean arterial blood pressure should be maintained strictly within its normal range. During inhalational anesthesia at equal anesthetic concentrations, halothane compromises hepatic blood flow to a maximum extent than other inhalational agents. This is due to the absence or attenuation of buffer response during inhalational anesthesia, as the hepatic artery does not dilate in response to decreased portal venous blood flow and hypotension by volatile agents. However, the isoflurane and sevoflurane produce the lesser reduction of hepatic blood flow than halothane. Hepatic blood flow is best preserved during anesthesia, if there is proper maintenance of CO and BP. Interestingly, the intravenous anesthesia by newer synthetic opioids and propofol is considered to be the best technique in this regard. But, the patients with compromised liver functions respond poorly to opioids due to their (opioids) decreased clearance and increased central nervous system (CNS) susceptibility. Thus, a high dose of fentanyl or sufentanil is rarely an option for anesthesia in patients with poor liver function.

Except anesthetic agents, other factors that alter the hepatic blood flow are controlled ventilation, hypocapnia, and surgical intervention. Controlled ventilation, particularly PEEP, can cause up to 30% reduction in hepatic blood flow. Hypocapnia is also associated with a significant reduction in hepatic blood flow. This is due to the increase in hepatic arterial vasoconstriction and simultaneously the increase in vascular resistance. So, the end-tidal carbon dioxide ($ETCO_2$) tension should be kept as near-normal level as possible. The surgical maneuvers, especially in upper abdomen, decrease the splanchnic and total hepatic blood flow to a greater extent and even more than the general anesthetic agents. So, during surgical maneuvers, care should be taken to avoid undue pressure and strain on the supplying vessels to liver by manual traction, packs, retractors, etc.

Ascites

The presence of ascites with liver disease indicates advanced pathology and carries bad prognosis. So, the preoperative amelioration of ascites considerably improves the surgical prognosis. Hence, forced sodium and water excretion by diuretics is the cornerstone of preoperative therapy for ascites. Spironolactone is a weak diuretic and acts by inhibiting the action of aldosterone at distal and collecting renal tubule. It inhibits Na^+ reabsorption at distal renal tubule, but spares K^+ (potassium-sparing diuretic). Thus, conservation of K^+ is helpful in a jaundiced patient who has hypokalemia, due to increased aldosterone level.

The dose of spironolactone required to induce diuresis is proportional to plasma aldosterone concentration. Like spironolactone, other K^+-sparing and distal tubular acting diuretics, such as the triamterene or amiloride, are also the drugs of choice. The frusemide is not well tolerated in patients with ascites, cirrhosis, or other liver dysfunctions, because it prevents the reabsorption of both Na^+ and K^+ at proximal tubule. So, though natriuresis induced by frusemide is helpful, but hypokalemia is not helpful for liver dysfunction or jaundiced patient. Hypokalemia produces a dangerous situation in liver disease. So, the K^+ level should always be monitored and maintained strictly within its normal level. Following an aggressive diuretic therapy, an anesthetist will often find low-serum Na^+ level in patients scheduled for surgery. This is probably without hazard, if the sodium is not <130 mmol/L.

In some patients, diuresis cannot be initiated, despite the maximal dose of diuretic agents (e.g., 400 mg of spironolactone) which act on distal renal tubule. This is because of the avid proximal tubular sodium reabsorption. Then, more potent and proximally acting diuretics (frusemide, thiazide, etc.) can be added cautiously to this regimen. In such situation, spironolactone plus frusemide (20–80 mg/day) is usually sufficient to initiate a diuresis in most patients. However, such aggressive therapy must be used with great caution to avoid plasma volume depletion, azotemia, and hypokalemia which may lead to encephalopathy.

Except diuresis, paracentesis may also be employed successfully to reduce ascites. Paracentesis is considered as complementary to diuretic therapy and makes the patient definitely comfortable. Ascites can also be controlled by peritoneovenous shunts, which move the ascetic fluid into vascular compartments, causing overexpansion of vascular volume, ↑CO, ↑ renal blood flow, ↑ excretion of Na^+ and water. More recently, transjugular intrahepatic portosystemic shunting (TIPS) has been used effectively to control refractory ascites and may improve the postoperative outcome in these patients.

Renal Impairment (Box 10)

There are varieties of changes in renal function, induced by advanced liver disease. Among these, the hepatorenal syndrome and acute tubular necrosis are most common. These are due to the increased renin–angiotensin activation, which produces excessive sodium and water retention. The hepatorenal syndrome is a unique pathological condition of kidney which is seen only in advanced liver disease. It is a functional renal failure, occurs spontaneously and more

BOX 10: Renal effect due to liver dysfunction.

- Water overload
- Hypernatremia
- Hyperkalemia
- Circulatory decompensation
- Edema and ascites
- Hepatorenal syndrome

commonly due to the fluid shifts, particularly in patients with obstructive jaundice. However, the kidney is normal histologically and functions normally following a liver transplantation or if this kidney is transplanted into a healthy recipient. All the pathological changes, seen in ascites (renal sodium and water retention and plasma volume expansion), are present in an extreme form in this hepatorenal syndrome. So, the maintenance of adequate urine output by fluids and diuretics is the mainstay for the prevention of this syndrome. It is a serious complication in patients associated with cirrhosis and ascites. It is characterized by worsening azotemia with avid Na$^+$ and water retention and oliguria in the absence of identifiable specific causes of renal dysfunction. Once the renal failure occurs due to any cause in the presence of cirrhosis, then the mortality is usually 100%.

The exact cause of this syndrome is not fully known. But, the altered renal hemodynamic appears to be the probable explanation. The kidneys are structurally intact and renal biopsy is also normal. This risk for hepatorenal syndrome is great, if the serum bilirubin levels are high and there is also endotoxemia from infected bile. The hallmark of this hepatorenal syndrome is intense sodium retention, oliguria, hypotension, and intense azotemia. The patient hardly excretes any Na$^+$. The onset of this syndrome is very rapid. Urine analysis reveals little sodium (<10 mmol/L). Sometimes, in severe liver dysfunction, patients can also develop acute oliguric renal failure due to hemorrhage, hypotension, etc. This oliguric renal failure can be differentiated from the hepatorenal syndrome as urinary sodium is >30 mmol/L in oliguric renal failure. *The diagnostic criteria for hepatorenal syndrome are*—(1) urinary sodium <10 mmol/L, (2) urine: plasma osmolarity ratio and creatinine ratios >1, and (3) presence of chronic liver disease and ascites.

The anesthetic management of this problem includes adequate preoperative evaluation of fluid, electrolyte, and renal status. Urinary output is measured by continuous bladder catheterization. Central venous pressure (CVP) measurement is strongly advised during extensive operative procedure to guide fluid therapy. The most important factor predisposing to renal failure in the presence of hyperbilirubinemia is hypovolemia. Therefore, patients should not be allowed to be dehydrated in any situation. The intravenous fluid (0.9% normal saline) should be used liberally, though there is fluid overload, to ensure moderate-to-high CVP and urine output of 1 mL/kg/h or 50 mL/h (in adult). If, despite hydration, the urine output is low, then 20% mannitol, administered intravenously, is the treatment of choice. The dose of mannitol is 0.5 g/kg over 30 minutes.

A suitable antibiotic should be given preoperatively along with premedication, if there is endotoxemia. As there is activation of aldosterone–renin–angiotensin system, so these patients are avid Na$^+$ retainers. Hence, Na$^+$-containing IV fluids should be administered cautiously, during perioperative period. The use of nephrotoxic drugs, such as nonsteroidal anti-inflammatory drugs (NSAIDs) and gentamicin, in repeated doses should be avoided. The worsening of hepatorenal failure may result in death, despite hemofiltration or dialysis and can only be corrected by liver transplantation.

Hepatic Encephalopathy

Sometimes, the hepatic encephalopathy is seen in individuals with severe liver disease. It is characterized by—(1) decrease in consciousness, (2) fluctuating neurological signs, (3) flapping tremor, and (4) distinctive electroencephalogram (EEG) changes. This occurs in hyperacute (within 7 days), acute (7–28 days), and subacute (28 days to 6 months) hepatic failure. This classification does not include FHF, where encephalopathy developed within 8 weeks of severe illness. In severe cases of hepatic encephalopathy, irreversible coma and death may occur. Generally, this is a lethal syndrome with >90% mortality rate.

In hepatic encephalopathy, there are two issues of interest to an anesthetist. First is the high level of ammonia which is most often incriminated in the pathogenesis of hepatic encephalopathy. Second is the excessive concentration of gamma-aminobutyric acid (GABA) which is an inhibitory neurotransmitter in CNS and is responsible for reduced level of consciousness. In severe liver dysfunction, due to intrahepatic and the extrahepatic shunting of portal venous blood into systemic circulation, liver is largely bypassed. As a result of this shunting process, various toxic substances, mainly NH$_3$, absorbed from intestine are not detoxified by the liver and lead to elevated blood ammonia level, causing metabolic abnormalities in CNS. The salient point for an anesthetist, regarding hepatic encephalopathy, is hyperventilation, producing respiratory alkalosis which strongly helps in the conversion of ammonium ion (NH$_4^+$) to ammonia (NH$_3$). Ammonia (NH$_3$ not the ammonium ion NH$_4^+$) is the form that can cross the blood–brain barrier and cause or exacerbate encephalopathy **(Table 7)**.

TABLE 7: Grades of hepatic encephalopathy.

Grade 0	Alert and oriented
Grade I	Drowsy and oriented
Grade II	Drowsy and disoriented
Grade III	Stupor and restlessness
Grade IV	Coma—nonresponsive to deep pain

The increased level of GABA in CNS reflects the failure of liver to extract precursor amino acid which synthesizes GABA in brain or to remove GABA which is produced in intestine. It has been also recognized that benzodiazepine receptors (BZD) are closely associated with GABA receptor and also facilitate GABA transmission. Thus, BZD sometimes can precipitate hepatic encephalopathy or coma. This finding can be substantiated by the fact that the injection of flumazenil ameliorates the symptoms of clinical coma and EEG changes in a high percentage of cases. Thus, the clinical information to an anesthetist is that CNS depressant drugs such as sedatives (BZD), narcotics, and barbiturates, which are related to GABA receptors, may precipitate hepatic encephalopathy and coma. The mechanisms behind this increased CNS susceptibility to these drugs, which may be amplified by other altered drug-handling phenomenon, are ↓ biotransformation, ↓ albumin binding, etc. in liver diseases. So, large doses of these drugs should be avoided in late stages of liver dysfunction. Thus, a typical high dose of narcotic technique used for cardiac anesthesia has no role in liver disease and may be detrimental. In such situations, inhalational anesthetics have no limitation and are favored.

Other factors which can precipitate hepatic encephalopathy are—GI bleeding, azotemia, hypokalemia (directly stimulating ammonia production by kidney), hyponatremia, hypoxia, infection, surgery, etc. In severe encephalopathy, the decreased level of consciousness may compromise the airway and intubation may be required if cerebral edema develops.

Cirrhosis

Before surgery and anesthesia, cirrhotic patients may be benefited from increased aggressive preoperative treatment for coagulopathy, ascites, and encephalopathy, which are usually associated with cirrhosis. Patients with cirrhosis develop coagulopathy as a result of decreased synthesis and shortened half-life of vitamin K-dependent coagulation factors and abnormalities (both qualitative and quantitative) of platelets. Vitamin K administration normally corrects the prolongation of PT. However, it is not effective, when the decreased synthesis of coagulation factors is due to nutritional deficiency. In these cases, the FFP infusion usually brings the PT to normal. If this also fails, then cryoprecipitate is helpful to reduce the PT within 3 seconds to normal.

Cirrhosis is the most common cause of portal hypertension. In cirrhosis, the vascular bed in liver is distorted and the blood flow through it is mechanically obstructed. So, the normal portal venous pressure which is about 7 mm Hg is raised up to 50 mm Hg. As the portal venous system lacks valves, so the resistance at any level between the right side of heart and the splanchnic vessels of intestine results in retrograde transmission of this elevated pressure. Hence, this high pressure in portal venous system facilitates the retrograde flow of blood from the present high-pressure portal venous system to the low-pressure systemic venous system. The major sites of this collateral flow of blood between the portal and systemic venous system involve the veins around rectum (hemorrhoids), cardioesophageal junction (esophageal gastric varices), retroperitoneal space, and falciform ligament. Therefore, the major clinical manifestations of portal hypertension include—hemorrhage from the gastroesophageal varices, bleeding piles, splenomegaly with hypersplenic activity, ascites, and hepatic encephalopathy.

Cirrhosis is thought to be a major risk factor for patients undergoing nonhepatic surgery. Elective surgery is contraindicated in Child–Pugh class C patients. Surgery should also be avoided in patients with severe hypoalbuminemia, evidence of infection and encephalopathy. Alternatives to surgery should be considered, as it is associated with high-mortality rate.

PREOPERATIVE LABORATORY INVESTIGATION (BOX 11)

The following preoperative laboratory investigations should be done, before anesthesia and surgery, for the liver dysfunction patients:

- *Full blood count and studies of clotting profile:* Among these, the PT is the best marker of liver dysfunctions.
- *Tests for electrolytes, urea, and creatinine:* The urea level in blood is falsely low due to decreased hepatic production. Hypokalemia and metabolic alkalosis are not uncommon and are usually due to vomiting. Concomitant hypomagnesemia may be present in chronic alcoholics and predisposes to cardiac arrhythmias.
- *Tests for blood glucose level:* The hepatic stores of glucose and glycogen are often affected. Patients frequently suffer from hypoglycemia.
- *Liver function tests (LFTs):* LFTs must always be interpreted against each careful history and thorough examination of that particular patient. The liver has large reserve of its functional capacity and can often

BOX 11: Preoperative preparation for liver dysfunction patients.

- Restore and maintain normal blood volume
- Correct electrolyte imbalance, if any
- Maintain normal glucose level
- Correct coagulopathy with FFP and platelets
- Use vitamin K, according to the laboratory test
- Use DDAVP and aminocaproic acid as necessary
- Optimize the patient's nutritional and medical status
- Ascites if massive—abdominal paracentesis is preferred Otherwise, treated with Na^+ and water restriction and diuretics Rate of reduction of ascetic fluid should be 0.5 kg of body weight per day
- Administration of thiamine to patients experiencing acute withdrawal of alcohol and prophylaxis for delirium and tremors.
- Prevent hepatorenal syndrome by avoiding dehydration, avoiding nephrotoxic drugs such as aminoglycosides and NSAID, using dopamine infusions, using powerful diuretics, avoiding renal contrast, paracentesis of tense ascites, etc
- Iatrogenic factors, precipitating encephalopathy should be used cautiously like injudicious use of sedatives like BDZ, opioids, etc.
- Lactulose and neomycin should be used to limit bacterial toxins

(BDZ: benzodiazepine; FFP: fresh frozen plasma; NSAID: nonsteroidal anti-inflammatory drug)

withstand considerable damage before LFTs become deranged. On the other hand, serum liver functions tests are rarely specific. So, only the serial measurements of LFTs are useful and indicate trends. Among the liver function tests, PT, albumin level, and bilirubin level are the most sensitive markers. It is important not to give the FFP, unless there is active bleeding before the LFTs are performed. Because, it will alter the PT which is an excellent guide to overall liver functions. The PT is the best indicator of hepatic synthetic function. Persistent prolongation of PT >15 seconds (INR >1.5) following administration of vitamin K is indicative of severe hepatic dysfunction. Hypoalbuminemia is usually not present, except in protracted cases, with severe malnutrition or when chronic liver disease is present.

The AST and ALT (liver transaminases) are sensitive markers and can even indicate mild liver damage. But, they have no role in mortality prediction. Although the levels of transaminases increase in liver diseases, but it may also decrease in severe liver disease. The elevation of serum transaminases does not necessarily correlate with the amount of hepatic necrosis. The serum ALT level is generally higher than that of AST, except in alcoholic hepatitis, where the reverse occurs. AP is increased with biliary obstruction. Antinuclear antibody is present in 75% of patients with chronic active hepatitis. Smooth muscle antibody is present in nearly all the cases of primary biliary cirrhosis. α-fetoprotein is a marker of hepatoma.

- *Imaging techniques:* Ultrasound is the main initial investigation of obstructive jaundice. Other useful investigations include endoscopic retrograde cholangiopancreatography (ERCP), computed tomography (CT), magnetic resonance imaging (MRI), and CT- or MRI-guided cholangiograms.
- Arterial blood gases
- Urine analysis
- Hepatitis screening.

■ SOME PERIOPERATIVE CONSIDERATIONS

During anesthesia of patients, suffering from liver diseases, there are some principles or guidelines. These guidelines are given below. H_2 antagonists or proton pump inhibitors should be routinely used preoperatively in liver dysfunction patients. Rapid sequence induction of anesthesia will reduce the risks of gastric aspiration. Hepatic blood flow is often altered during anesthesia and surgery. This is due to the effect of anesthetic drugs, positive pressure ventilation, PEEP, and surgical technique. In most cases, anesthesia reduces liver blood flow, particularly if halothane is used. However, isoflurane actually seems to improve the hepatic blood flow. Sevoflurane is also a preferred volatile agent for liver disease. Regional techniques can be used as long as coagulation is not much deranged and it should also be remembered that all the local anesthetics are metabolized by liver.

■ POSTOPERATIVE JAUNDICE

The occurrence of postoperative jaundice is a problem of increasing incidence. It is, perhaps, seen more frequently now than in earlier years. This is because many patients are now undergoing more major surgical procedures and survive too. The incidence of postoperative jaundice varies from 1% of all the patients undergoing abdominal surgery to 17% of all the patients undergoing major surgery. Although the postoperative jaundice is relatively common, but the significant postoperative liver dysfunction is relatively rare. This rare postoperative liver dysfunction has varied etiology and often resolves without treatment. It should be remembered that hepatitis due to volatile anesthetic agents is extremely rare and is largely diagnosis of exclusion.

The causes for post-operative jaundice are given in **Box 12** and there are three major pathological mechanisms for postoperative jaundice. These are—(1) postoperative increased pigment load, (2) postoperative impaired hepatocellular function, and (3) postoperative intrahepatic/posthepatic obstruction of bile flow. Most of the etiologies for postoperative jaundice become apparent within 3 weeks

BOX 12: Causes of postoperative liver dysfunction or jaundice.

- *Bilirubin overload (hemolysis):*
  - Blood transfusion
  - Hematoma reabsorption
  - *Hemolytic anemia:*
    - Sickle cell anemia, G6PD deficiency, mismatched transfusion, etc.
- *Hepatocellular injury:*
  - Exacerbation of preexisting liver disease
  - Hepatic ischemia due to hypovolemia, hypotension, and cardiac failure
  - Septicemia
  - Hypoxia
  - Viral hepatitis
  - Drug induced (halothane and antibiotics)
- *Cholestasis (obstruction):*
  - *Intrahepatic:*
    - Benign, infective, drug induced, pregnancy, etc.
  - *Extrahepatic:* Retained stone in bile duct, postoperative cholecystitis, bile duct injury, pancreatitis, etc.

(G6PD: glucose-6-phosphate dehydrogenase)

after surgery and can be classified as mild or severe, if the serum bilirubin is <4 mg/dL or greater.

Increased pigment load occurs as a result of hemolysis following blood transfusions, drugs (which sometimes induce hemolysis), and also from reabsorption of blood from extravascular space. Approximately 10% of stored whole blood undergoes hemolysis within 24 hours of transfusion. Each 0.5 L of stored blood yields 7.5 g of hemoglobin, which is then converted to 250 mg of bilirubin. Multiple blood transfusions may, therefore, limit the ability of liver to conjugate and excrete this bilirubin load, i.e., reserve of liver function.

Hepatocellular damage and impaired hepatocellular functions postoperatively are caused by nonanesthetic drugs used during anesthesia, anesthetic agents (mainly halothane), ischemia due to hypotension, sepsis and viral hepatitis, etc. With lesser degree of hypotension and hypoxemia, morphological changes may be slight, but significant impairment of function may occur in severe hypotension and hypoxemia. Prior shock or hypotension plus pigment overload may produce significant liver dysfunction and jaundice. Extensive sepsis also can produce jaundice of cholestatic type. Concurrent renal impairment due to hypotension and hypoxemia may also enhance the degree of liver dysfunction and jaundice, and this is because of decreased renal excretion of conjugated bilirubin. Drug-induced hepatotoxicity is primarily due to idiosyncratic reactions or alterations in bile flow by drug, resulting in cholestasis.

The *extrahepatic obstruction to the flow of bile*, due to the surgical damage of biliary passage or stones within it, causing postoperative jaundice, needs to be considered and may be excluded by ultrasonography. Benign postoperative intrahepatic cholestasis mimics biliary obstruction and usually occurs after major surgery associated with hypotension, hypoxemia, or multiple transfusions.

GUIDELINE FOR ANESTHESIA ON PATIENTS WITH DECOMPENSATED LIVER FUNCTION

An anesthetist should always show a considerable degree of latitude, when making a mind to administer anesthesia on patients with advanced liver disease. The choice of drugs and the monitoring of patients, during the anesthesia of such patients, suffering from liver dysfunction, mainly depend upon the severity of liver disease, the type of surgery, and the experience of anesthetist. The surgical procedures can be divided into two groups: (1) the surgery on diseased liver to correct the dysfunction of it (liver) and (2) the extrahepatic surgery not related to liver and its biliary passage with liver dysfunction but not for the correction of this hepatic dysfunction. The extent of surgery on liver may vary from a simple liver biopsy to a major liver transplantation. Whereas, the extrahepatic surgery with liver dysfunction includes different general surgical procedures on other organs, except liver, with jaundice or asymptomatic carrier state of hepatitis and various surgeries to correct the complication which is developed due to liver dysfunction, e.g., making portacaval shunts, transesophageal ligation of varices, etc.

The type of anesthesia in liver dysfunction can be divided into regional and general. The regional anesthesia plays a significant role in patients with liver disease. The main limitation of regional anesthesia in liver dysfunction is clotting and bleeding abnormalities, causing hematoma in epidural space or bleeding in subarachnoid space. Otherwise, it is very safe, if it fits well with the type of surgery, i.e., lower extremities, obstetric and gynecological operations (lower abdomen), or some upper abdominal surgeries such as cholecystectomy. Now, mastectomy and other cardiac and thoracic surgeries also can be done by cervical or thoracic epidural anesthesia. Different types of nerves and plexus blocks, such as brachial or cervical plexus block, are also very safe for liver dysfunction patients. Clotting and bleeding abnormalities of patients with liver disease should be corrected before administering anesthesia, especially regional anesthesia. Otherwise, it is sheer madness to operate upon them.

If regional anesthesia is selected as the ultimate choice, then the guidelines for the detection of clotting and bleeding abnormalities are (1) PT must be <2.5 seconds of control value, (2) platelet count should be >40,000/mm^3, (3) bleeding time which measures the both platelet quantity (number) and quality should not be >12 minutes. If bleeding and clotting parameters are within these guidelines, then spinal, epidural, and other regional blocks, with continuous catheter technique for postoperative pain control, can be employed safely after major surgeries.

During the administration of GA, utmost care should be taken by an anesthetist when he uses the CNS depressant drugs like sedatives, narcotics, etc. for induction. Large doses of them always should be avoided in liver dysfunction patients. So, the titrating doses of these drugs are mandatory. Regarding premedication, none to small amount is suggested, according to the severity of liver dysfunction and the physical status of patient. If premedication is needed at all, the drugs handled by phase-II biotransformation such as morphine, lorazepam, or oxazepam are recommended.

Glycopyrrolate is preferred to atropine, as it does not cross the blood–brain barrier. Regarding induction, the preferred inducing agent is propofol. Thiopentone also can be used safely. Regarding the neuromuscular block, many anesthetists still use succinylcholine during elective surgery for intubation on liver dysfunction patients. This is because there is only theoretical speculation that the action of succinylcholine can be prolonged due to the deficiency of plasma cholinesterase in patients with liver disease. But, it is true and seems clinically insignificant, because the action of succinylcholine rarely becomes prolonged and causes any problem of overwhelming magnitude. Vecuronium, cisatracurium, and atracurium are ideal muscle relaxants for patients with liver dysfunction. Vecuronium is used for longer surgical procedures and atracurium is used for shorter ones. Isoflurane and sevoflurane are the backbones of anesthetic regimens for patients with liver disease, but doses should always be adjusted so as not to depress much the cardiovascular system. N$_2$O does not produce any injury to hepatocytes and can be used safely even in severe liver dysfunction patients, if there is no contraindication, e.g., bowel distension, middle ear surgery, etc. The small doses of opioids play an important role in anesthetic regimen by reducing the need of inhalational anesthetic agents, particularly if there is hypovolemia and central pump failure. But, larger doses of opioids should always be avoided in liver dysfunction patients. There is no contraindication for the use of neostigmine for the reversal of neuromuscular block and it responds well as normal fashion in patients with liver dysfunction.

The monitoring of liver dysfunction patients during perianesthetic period includes all the standard monitoring procedures, depending on the gravity of surgical procedures and the physical status of patient. The PT, aPTT, platelet count, and hematocrit values are required periodically. The other standard monitors include pulse oximeter, ECG, ETCO$_2$, HR, BP, etc. Urine output should always be monitored with a catheter. Invasive monitors such as intra-arterial catheter, CVP, Swan–Ganz catheter, and TEE are also indicated, depending on the clinical circumstances. The coronary vasoconstriction, caused by vasopressin, which is used to control variceal hemorrhage, can be reversed by conventional doses of nitroglycerin. Somatostatin can be used instead of vasopressin and causes less coronary vasoconstriction. Where there is concern about renal perfusion, then dopamine drip in the dose of 1–2 µg/kg/min may be of immense value.

■ HALOTHANE AND HEPATOTOXICITY

The liver dysfunction produced by halothane is called as the halothane-associated hepatitis (HAH). This HAH is defined (though the definition is unsatisfactory) as the appearance of liver damage within 28 days of halothane exposure in a person in whom the other known causes for liver disease have been excluded. Two syndromes are recognized in HAH or halothane-induced liver dysfunction: (1) the first is associated with the transient rise of the values of liver function tests and has low morbidity. This occurs often after the initial (first) exposure to halothane. (2) The second is associated with repeated exposure to halothane and there is high rise of values of liver function tests. It has an "immune" mechanism with the development of FHF and is associated with high-mortality rate. However, this FHF is rare with an incidence of 1 in 35,000 after halothane anesthesia.

Halothane-induced liver dysfunction may be due to—(1) the direct effect of drug on hepatocytes itself or (2) the effect of the metabolites of drug on hepatocytes (*metabolic cause*) or (3) an immune reaction following repeated exposure to halothane (*immunological cause*). The indirect cause for liver dysfunction, after halothane exposure, is due to hypotension, diminished liver blood flow, and subsequent reduced hepatic O$_2$ availability. These also appear to be of genetic susceptibility for halothane-induced hepatotoxicity as shown by *in vitro* test.

The metabolic cause for liver dysfunction, induced by halothane, is due to the metabolites, produced by the metabolism of halothane in hepatocytes. Up to 20–40% of halothane is metabolized in human liver. Whereas, 2–8% of enflurane, 1% of isoflurane, and 0.2% of sevoflurane are metabolized in liver. The metabolism of halothane in liver takes two pathways: one is the *oxidative pathway* and another is the *reductive pathway*. The metabolites of reductive pathways do not produce any injury to hepatocytes. But, the metabolites of oxidative pathway bind to liver microsome, which contains cytochrome P-450 system and induces hepatotoxicity. The chance of metabolic reaction, causing hepatotoxicity by volatile agents, is thought to be related to the amount it is metabolized.

As for example, only 2–8% of administered enflurane is metabolized. It should therefore cause 10 times fewer reactions than halothane. On the other hand, only 1% isoflurane is metabolized. There is, therefore, only a theoretical risk for the reaction to isoflurane and indeed there have been only a few case reports of isoflurane-induced hepatotoxicity. So, isoflurane is considered much safe for use in patients at risk of hepatic failure. Sevoflurane and desflurane also appear to be much safe in liver failure.

The immunological mechanism of hepatitis, particularly for fulminant type of hepatic failure (FHF), is evidenced or proved by the presence of antibodies to the metabolites of halothane in the sera of patients, suffering from FHF, after exposure to halothane and these are present in 70% of such patient. These antibodies against halothane have not been found in patients with HAH of other etiologies. It is also not found in patients exposed to halothane, but without developing FHF. The antibody is not directed against the reductive metabolites of halothane, but only against a particular oxidative metabolic compound of halothane, such as trifluoroacetyl halide (TFH). These are IgG type of antibodies and react with the cell surface of hepatocytes, making them susceptible to antibody-dependent cell-mediated toxicity. The halothane is a small molecule and it itself is unlikely to be immunoreactive. It is postulated that the binding of oxidative metabolite of halothane, i.e., TFH to liver cytochrome, which acts as a hapten, induces a hypersensitivity reaction. FHF, which carries a high-mortality rate, is particularly due to immune reaction, following repeated exposure. Any time interval between two exposures is not considered safe, because the mechanism of FHF is immunological and any exposure after the first could trigger an immunological response.

The HAH is usually present in two forms. *One is characterized* by moderate elevation of liver transaminase and transient mild jaundice with low morbidity and no mortality. *Another is characterized* by development of FHF with high mortality and is associated with repeated exposure to halothane (or isoflurane, enflurane, sevoflurane due to cross sensitivity).

Thyroid Diseases and Anesthesia

INTRODUCTION

The hypothalamus, pituitary, and thyroid gland, by making an axis are involved in the regulation of various cellular activity in our body. In this axis, as the target organ, the thyroid gland is very important. The different forms of thyroid diseases are very common in our country and it affects 5–10% of total general population. Among them, the females are more affected than male. The thyroid gland is not so essential for life. But, its absence causes the impairment of multiple cellular activities (or metabolism) and as a consequence produce several defects, such as the slowing of both physical and mental growth, the reduction of cardiac rate and contractility, the poor resistance to cold, etc. In children, mental retardation and dwarfism are manifested in the absence of thyroid hormone. In the contrary, excess thyroid secretions lead to nervousness, body wasting, tremor, tachycardia, excess heat production, etc.

The thyroid hormones are synthesized in our thyroid gland from *iodine* and an essential amino acid, named tyrosine. After absorption from gastrointestinal (GI) tract, the dietary iodine (I_2) is converted to iodide (I^-) and actively transported to thyroid gland. The thyroid gland has also the special capacity of abstracting iodide from circulating blood. In the thyroid gland, this iodide is again oxidized to iodine by *peroxidase enzyme* and combines with tyrosine to form monoiodotyrosine (MIT) and diiodotyrosine (DIT). In thyroid gland, these two compounds are again coupled to form triiodothyronine (T_3) and tetraiodothyronine or thyroxine (T_4). The last two compounds are released from thyroid gland and are called as the thyroid hormones. But, the T_4 is formed in far excess in amount than T_3. After their formation, within the thyroid gland, the T_4 and T_3 are immediately attached or conjugated to *thyroglobulin*, which is also a specific protein, secreted by thyroid cells. This conjugating material, i.e., thyroglobulin is popularly known as the *colloid substance* and it is in this form the T_4 and T_3 is

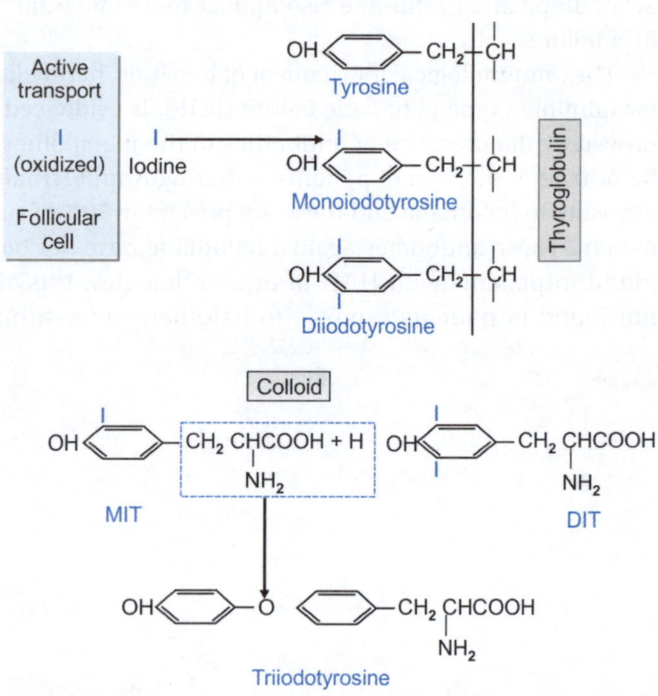

Fig. 1: Synthesis of thyroid hormones.

stored in the acini of thyroid gland. When required by the body, this conjugation breaks and large amount of T_4 with little amount of T_3 is liberated into circulation **(Fig. 1)**.

PHYSIOLOGY

The thyroid gland predominantly secretes two hormones named tetraiodothyronine or thyroxine (T_4) and a small amount of triiodothyronine (T_3). But, about 85% of this small amount of circulating T_3 at periphery is again also produced from T_4 by the process of monodeiodination in other peripheral tissues such as the muscles, liver, kidney, etc. *In vivo, the* T_3 is more potent than T_4 and metabolically is more active. While T_4 is probably metabolically inactive and may be regarded as the prohormone of T_3. The 99% of circulating

T_4 and T_3 are bound to a special transport protein in plasma called the thyroxine-binding globulin (TBG). The remaining small fraction of circulating thyroid hormones remains as unbound or free form and diffuses into tissues to exert their metabolic function.

It is possible to measure the total, bound (with TBG), and unbound (free) fraction of thyroid hormones, i.e., of T_4 and T_3 in plasma. But, the advantage of the measurement of free hormone is that they are not influenced by the changes in the concentration of TBG or plasma protein. For example, during pregnancy, the TBG level is increased and with it the total T_4 and T_3 level may be increased. But, the level of free thyroid hormone may remain normal.

The production of thyroid hormones from thyroid gland is stimulated by another hormone named thyroid-stimulating hormone (TSH). This TSH is released (secreted) from anterior pituitary in response to another thyrotropin-releasing hormone (TRH), secreted from hypothalamus. A circadian rhythm for the secretion of TSH is also found with its peak effect at 0100 hours and 1100 hours of the day. But, this circadian variation of the secretion of TSH is small and does not influence the timing of blood sampling for the assessment of thyroid function. There is some negative feedback response of thyroid hormones on the secretion of TSH from anterior pituitary and on the secretion of TRH from hypothalamus. So, when the plasma concentrations of T_4 and T_3 are raised in primary hyperthyroidism, then the level of both the TSH and TRH is reduced (**Table 1 and Fact file I**). Similarly, when the plasma concentrations of T_4 and T_3 are decreased in primary hypothyroidism, then the level of both the TSH and TRH is raised. In subclinical hyper- and hypothyroidism, the T_4 and T_3 levels remain normal, but the TSH level is suppressed or raised. This is because the anterior pituitary is very sensitive to the minor changes of the level of thyroid hormone in blood and keeps the level of T_4 and T_3 within their normal range *(compensatory stage)*.

The three major forms of thyroid diseases that are frequently encountered in our clinical practice by an anesthetist are hyperthyroidism, hypothyroidism, and goiter. Although no age group is exempted from thyroid disease, but the patients most likely to be affected are middle aged and female. In addition, the increasing tendency to screen the population and ready access to accurate tests of thyroid functions has led to the identification of many patients with abnormal result who are either asymptomatic or with nonspecific complaints such as tiredness, more sleep, weight gain, etc.

FACT FILE I

The thyroid gland secretes three hormones: (1) thyroxine (T_4), (2) triiodothyronine (T_3), and (3) calcitonin. The first two are secreted by the follicular cells of thyroid gland and have the same biological activity. So, they are termed as thyroid hormones. While the last one is secreted by the interfollicular cells and its biological activity is entirely different from thyroid hormone. It takes part in Ca^{2+} metabolism.

Both the T_4 and T_3 are iodine-containing derivative of a chemical compound named thyronine which is produced by the condensation of two molecules of amino acid called tyrosine. The total body content of iodine (I_2) obtained from food product is 40–50 mg. Out of this, one-fourth is present in thyroid gland. The concentration of iodine in blood is low (0.2–0.4 µg/dL). But the thyroid follicular cells have an active transport process and concentrate it in the gland. This trapping of I_2 in the gland is stimulated by TSH and exceed the gradient of >100-fold between the plasma and gland. The total iodine content of a thyroid gland also regulates the uptake of it by the gland. Little store of iodine stimulate and the large store inhibits the uptake of iodine by the gland. This iodine concentrating ability is also found in other organs such as salivary gland, skin, intestine, gastric mucosa, placenta, breast, etc. But their uptake of iodine is not regulated by TSH.

Dietary iodine is first absorbed by the GI tract. Then, it is converted to iodide ion (I^-) and actively transported to the thyroid gland. After trapping of iodide (I^-) by the follicular cells of thyroid gland, it is further oxidized to iodine (I_2). Then, it combines avidly with the tyrosine residue of thyroglobulin, and form MIT and DIT. Then, the pairs of iodinated tyrosine residues couple together to form T_4 and T_3. Normally, much more T_4 is formed than T_3. But, during the iodine deficiency, relatively more T_3 (active form) is formed. The thyroid hormones are synthesized and also stored as colloid in the cavity of thyroid follicle, (but not in the cells of follicle) as a part of thyroglobulin molecule. Thyroglobulin is glycoprotein in nature and is also synthesized by the thyroid follicular cells. Then, the thyroglobulin is transported from the cells into the cavity of follicle, where MIT, DIT, and by further coupling T_3 and T_4 are formed. During the release of thyroid hormones, colloid is taken back into the follicular cells from the cavity by endocytosis and broken down into T_4, T_3, DIT, and MIT. The T_4 and T_3 so released from thyroglobulin is secreted into the circulation, while the MIT and DIT residues are deiodinated and the released iodine is reutilized. The uptake of colloid and breaking down of it is stimulated by TSH. The resting thyroid gland has follicles, distended the cavity with colloid and the cells are flat or cubical. While the TSH-stimulated gland has columnar cells and colloid virtually disappears from the cavity.

TABLE 1: Patterns of thyroid function tests in different thyroid diseases.

Thyroid disease	T_3	T_4	TSH
1. Hyperthyroidism (Graves' disease)	H	h	L
2. T_3 hyperthyroidism	H	N	L
3. Subclinical hyperthyroidism	N	N	L
4. Primary hypothyroidism	L	L	h
5. Subclinical hypothyroidism	N	N	h
6. Secondary hypothyroidism	L	L	L
7. Secondary hyperthyroidism	h	h	h

■ HYPERTHYROIDISM

In over 90% of patients, the principal cause of hyperthyroidism is Graves' disease. The other causes of hyperthyroidism are multinodular goiter, thyroiditis, some drugs, etc. which are displayed in **Box 1**. The most common symptoms of hyperthyroidism are loss of weight, heat intolerance, palpitation, cardiac arrhythmia, tremor, muscle weakness, diarrhea, hyperactive reflexes, nervousness, etc. which are also displayed in **Box 2**. A fine tremor, exophthalmos, or goiter may be noted, particularly when the cause is Graves' disease. The new onset of atrial fibrillation is a classic presentation of hyperthyroidism. Although the diagnosis of this disease, i.e., hyperthyroidism can usually be made clinically, but still it is important to confirm this disease by laboratory tests such as by measuring the levels of circulating thyroid hormones and TSH.

The serum T_4 and T_3 level are elevated and TSH level is reduced in the majority of patients. But, the T_4 is at the upper part of normal range and T_3 is only raised in 5% of hyperthyroidism patient. This special condition is called the T_3 thyrotoxicosis and is found particularly in those who are suffering from recurrent hyperthyroidism or following thyroid surgery or after a course of antithyroid drugs. Other tests which are also performed to establish the etiology of hyperthyroidism include: (i) the estimation of TRAb (TSH receptor antibody) which is elevated in Graves' disease, (ii) isotope scanning, etc. The diagnosis of hyperthyroidism during pregnancy is very difficult. This is because, in pregnancy estrogen-induced increase in TBG results in increased total protein bound T_4 and T_3 level.

The symptoms and signs of hyperthyroidism reflect the excessive effect of T_4 and T_3 hormone on the cellular activity, particularly its metabolism which are also listed in **Box 2**. It mainly increases the carbohydrate and fat metabolism. Thus, the thyroid hormone determines mainly the growth and the metabolic rate of our body. But, from the anesthetic point of view, the important thoughts are that the hyperthyroidism-induced increase in metabolic rate is associated with an increase in O_2 consumption and CO_2 production which indirectly increases the minute ventilation. The cardiac contractility and heart rate (HR) are also increased. This is due to the alteration in the physiology of adrenergic receptor and other internal proteins or receptors by increased circulating level of thyroid hormones, as opposed to the increased level of plasma catecholamines **(Box 2)**.

The patients suffering from hyperthyroidism are usually treated by antithyroid drugs, inorganic iodine, β-adrenergic antagonist, radioactive iodine, and/or surgical removal of thyroid gland. During the period of the treatment of hyperthyroidism, patients are continuously monitored by the measurement of plasma TSH level which indicates if hypothyroidism is developing or not and the plasma T_4 level which indicates if hyperthyroidism is developing or not.

The commonly used drugs for the medical management of hyperthyroidism are: (i) antithyroid drugs such as carbimazole, methimazole, propylthiouracil, etc. (ii) iodine containing compounds such as potassium iodide, Lugol's solution of iodine, etc. (iii) lithium, and (iv) glucocorticoids. The other modes of treatment of hyperthyroidism are: use of radioactive iodine and surgery **(Table 2)**.

As antithyroid agent, the thiourea derivatives are first discovered in 1940. Subsequently, the methyl and propyl-thiouracil derivatives and the thioimidazole derivatives such as the methimazole and carbimazole were discovered and found to be safe and effective for the treatment of

---

BOX 1: Causes of hyperthyroidism.

Thyroid overactivity:
- Graves' disease
- Toxic multinodular goiter
- Solitary toxic adenoma
- Hashimoto's thyroiditis
- Thyroid cancer
- TSH-secreting pituitary tumor

Extrathyroidal:
- Administration of thyroid hormones (iatrogenic)
- Ectopic thyroid tissue
- Choriocarcinoma and hydatid form mole

BOX 2: Clinical features of hyperthyroidism.

- Goiter—diffuse or nodular
- Weight loss, diarrhea, nausea, and vomiting
- Tachycardia, atrial fibrillation, angina, and heart failure
- Tremor, nervousness, anxiety, hyper-reflexia, and myopathy
- Heat intolerance, fatigue, exophthalmos, and other eye signs

---

TABLE 2: Mechanism of action of antithyroid drugs.

	Drugs	Mechanism of action
A.	Antithyroid drugs propylthiouracil carbimazole methimazole	Inhibits the thyroid hormone synthesis
B.	β-adrenergic agonist esmolol, propranolol	Impairs the peripheral action of T_4 and T_3
C.	Iodine compounds, potassium iodide, Lugol's solution	Inhibits the release of T_4 and T_3
D.	Lithium	Inhibits the release of T_4 and T_3
E.	Glucocorticoids	Immunosuppressive action. Impair the peripheral action of T_4 and T_3

hyperthyroidism. All these antithyroid drugs bind to thyroid peroxidase enzyme and inhibit the iodination of tyrosine residue of thyroglobulin. Thus, they inhibit the production of MIT and DIT. They also stop the coupling of iodotyrosine residue of MIT and DIT to form T_3 and T_4. Thus, the thyroid colloid is gradually depleted of thyroid hormones (i.e., T_4 and T_3) overtime and blood levels of T_3 and T_4 are reduced. However, they do not interfere with the trapping of iodine by thyroid gland from plasma and do not modify the action of T_3 and T_4 on the peripheral tissues or on pituitary gland. The antithyroid drugs also do not affect the release of T_3 and T_4 from thyroid gland which are already synthesized in the cell. Hence, their effects are not apparent, till the thyroid gland is adequately depleted of its hormone content. Propylthiouracil also inhibits the peripheral conversion of T_4 to T_3. In India only carbimazole is available and routinely used. But, it acts largely by getting converted into methimazole by the peripheral tissues **(Table 3)**.

Though iodine is a constituent and as well as help in the formation of thyroid hormones, but still it is the fastest acting thyroid inhibitor. All the facets of thyroid function seem to be affected by iodine. But, the most important function of it is the inhibition of the release of thyroid hormone from the follicular cells of thyroid gland which has already been synthesized there. The endocytosis of colloid and subsequently the proteolysis process of thyroglobulin (with the attached MIT, DIT, T_3, and T_4) which helps in the release of thyroid hormones, comes to a halt. Thus, the enlarged gland slowly shrinks, and then, it becomes firm and less vascular.

With the daily administration of iodine, the thyroid status starts to return to normal slowly and the peak effects are seen within 10–15 days after the commencement of iodine therapy. After that, a phenomenon named as the *"thyroid escape"* may occur spontaneously and thyrotoxicosis may return with greater severity. So, this group of drugs,

i.e., iodine is only used temporarily for the preoperative preparation of thyrotoxic patient before thyroidectomy. It is generally given for 10 days, just before surgery with an aim to make the gland firm, less vascular and easier to operate on. Though the iodine itself lowers the thyroid status, but it cannot be solely relied upon to attain euthyroidism which is done by the concomitant use of carbimazole before starting iodine. Propranolol may be given additionally for the control of symptoms of hyperthyroidism, especially tachycardia, before anesthesia and surgery, if needed **(Fact file II)**. These β-adrenergic antagonists actually do not affect the function of thyroid gland and act only symptomatically. They also decrease the peripheral conversion of T_4 to T_3.

The commonly used radioactive isotope of iodine for the treatment of hyperthyroidism is I^{131} (other isotopes are I^{127}, I^{125}, etc.). Its half-life is 8 days and emits both the γ-rays and as well as β-particles. The former are useful for tracer studies, as they traverse the tissues and can be monitored by a counter. While the later are utilized for their destructive effect on thyroid cells. After administration, the radioactive I^{131} is actively concentrated by the thyroid gland, incorporated in their colloid and then emits radiation from the cavity within the follicles. The β-particles penetrate only the 0.5–2.0 mm of tissues. Thus, the thyroid follicular cells are affected from within the gland and undergo pyknosis and necrosis. Then, these necrosed tissues undergo fibrosis when a sufficiently large dose of I^{131} has been administered, without damage to the neighboring tissues. Hence, with the careful selected doses of radioactive I^{131} iodine, it is possible to achieve the partial pharmacological ablation of thyroid gland without surgery. It is used as sodium salt of I^{131} which is dissolved in water and taken orally. The response of radioactive iodine

TABLE 3: Differences between propylthiouracil and carbimazole.	
Carbimazole	**Propylthiouracil**
More potent (three times)	Less potent
Plasma half-life: 6–10 hours	Plasma half-life: 1–2 hours
Less plasma protein bound	High plasma protein bound
Large amount crosses the placenta	Little amount crosses the placenta
Duration of action: 12–24 hours	Duration of action: 4–8 hours
So single daily dose is used	Multiple daily doses are used
Produces active metabolic—methimazole	No active metabolite
Does not inhibit the peripheral conversions of T_4 and T_3	Can inhibit the peripheral conversion of T_4 to T_3

FACT FILE II

Advantages and disadvantages of antithyroid drugs over surgery and I^{131}:

- *Advantages:*
  - Can be used in young adults and children
  - No surgical risk such as injury of nerve, parathyroid gland, hematoma, and airway obstruction
  - No anesthetic risk
  - Used in pregnancy
- *Disadvantages:*
  - Prolonged treatment is needed
  - Release rate is high
  - Not applicable in psychiatric patient
  - Drug toxicity can occur

Thyroidectomy and I^{131} are contraindicated during pregnancy. Propylthiouracil is preferred than carbimazole during pregnancy. This is because its greater protein-binding capacity allows less transfer to the fetus and less chance of fetal hypothyroidism and goiter caused by antithyroid drugs. Due to the same reason, it is also preferred in the nursing mother after delivery.

FACT FILE III

Advantages and disadvantages of radioactive I^{131}:
- *Advantages:*
  - Treatment is simple, inexpensive, and outpatient procedure
  - No surgical and anesthetic risk
  - Cure is permanent
- *Disadvantages:*
  - Delayed response
  - Contraindicated during pregnancy
  - Not suitable for young patients
  - More likely to develop hypothyroidism and needs lifelong T_4 treatment

I^{131} is the treatment of choice after 35–40 years of age and if chronic heart failure, angina, or any other contraindication to surgery is present. In some center, the cut-off age for the treatment of hyperthyroidism by radioactive iodine has been lowered to 25 years.

is slow. Its action starts after 2 weeks of its administration and gradually increases to reach a peak effect at 3 months. The common indications for the use of I^{131} are: (i) patient above 45 years of age, (ii) recurrence of hyperthyroidism after surgery, (iii) hypersensitive or refractory to antithyroid drugs, and (iv) patients unfit for surgery **(Fact file III)**.

For the surgical management of hyperthyroidism, two types of surgeries are advocated. These are (i) subtotal thyroidectomy, and (ii) excision of only toxic nodule. Subtotal thyroidectomy is rarely used as an alternative to medical therapy, but is typically reserved for patients with large toxic multinodular goiter or solitary toxic adenoma. Graves' disease is usually treated with so called antithyroid drugs and radioactive iodine. The surgical treatment for hyperthyroidism is only indicated, when (i) there is large goiter, causing tracheal compression and cosmetic concerns and (ii) medical or radioiodine therapy have failed. Any patient with hyperthyroidism, scheduled for surgery, should be rendered first euthyroid by drugs, before anesthesia. This is because the toxic patients should not be dealt as such, for the fear of the development of thyroid crisis, during surgery and anesthesia. Therefore, the principles of preparation of a hyperthyroid patient before surgery and anesthesia are as follows:

- *Patients suffering from mild hyperthyroidism:* They are usually treated by only iodine preparation 14 days before operation. For this purpose, Lugol's iodine (10%) is used in the dose of five drops three times per day.
- *Patients suffering from severe hyperthyroidism:* They are usually treated by carbimazole. But, it takes long time, usually 8–12 weeks to make the patient euthyroid. However, within this treatment the size and the vascularity of gland increase and make the operation very difficult.

Some surgeons, therefore, stop or reduce the dose of antithyroid drug 14 days prior to surgery and for these 14 days they administer only iodine with the idea that iodine will cause the diminution of the size and the vascularity of thyroid gland. While this is true, but others do not favor the use of iodine, since it causes an increased friability of the gland which proves troublesome during operation.

- *During an emergency,* patients also can be prepared for surgery in <1 hour by IV administration of esmolol or propranolol.

The common complications of thyroid surgery, which may concern an anesthetist are: damage to the recurrent laryngeal nerve, airway obstruction, postoperative bleeding, thyroid crisis (thyroid storm), and postoperative hypoparathyroidism. The most common nerve, liable to damage during thyroid surgery, is the adductor fibers of recurrent laryngeal nerve. When this type of nerve damage is unilateral, then it is characterized by the paralysis of vocal cord of one side which assumes an intermediate position and produce a hoarseness of voice. Whereas, the bilateral injury of this nerve causes the paralysis of vocal cords on both sides which can then collapse together, producing aphonia, stridor, apnea, and total airway obstruction during inspiration.

Airway obstruction is also a common complication, following thyroid surgery. It may be due to (i) the adducting malfunction of vocal cords, caused by the recurrent laryngeal nerve injury of both sides, described above, (ii) the collapse of trachea for tracheomalacia, reflecting the weakness of tracheal ring, due to the chronic pressure from goiter, or (iii) the hematoma formation at surgical site, causing tracheal compression. This emergency condition, caused by the hematoma at operative site, is promptly treated by the removal of surgical stitches and the evacuation of blood clot or reintubation.

Another complication, followed by thyroid surgery and is important from the anesthetic point of view, is thyroid crisis (thyroid storm). It is a medical emergency situation and is characterized by tachycardia, hyperthermia, dehydration, tremor, congestive heart failure, shock, altered consciousness (e.g., agitation, delirium, and coma), etc. It can occur intraoperatively or 6–20 hours postoperatively. When the thyroid crisis occurs intraoperatively, then it mimics the malignant hyperpyrexia. But, unlike malignant hyperthermia, thyroid crisis is not associated with muscle rigidity, raised creatinine kinase, metabolic (lactic) acidosis, and respiratory acidosis. It generally occurs, when the patient is not properly made euthyroid prior to surgery. This condition usually results from the sudden entry of huge quantity of thyroid hormones into circulation due

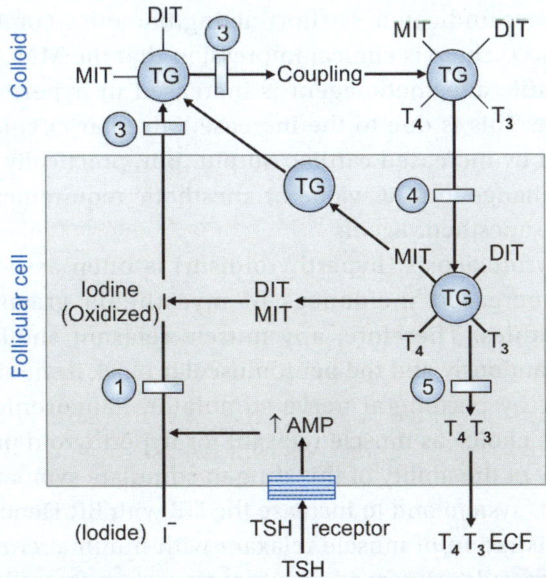

Fig. 2: The pathways of synthesis and secretion of thyroid hormones and the different sites of action of antithyroid drugs such as 1 = Potassium perchlorate, 2 and 3 = Carbimazole and propylthiouracil, 4 = Lithium, 5 = Iodide.
(DIT: diiodotyrosine; MIT: monoiodotyrosine; TG: thyroglobulin)

to (i) the pumping out of thyroid hormone from the gland by manipulation during surgery and (ii) the absorption of thyroxine (T_4) from the raw cut surface of thyroid gland **(Fig. 2)**.

The immediate treatment of thyroid crisis is very important and lifesaving. It includes:

- Sedation by morphine, or pethidine, or benzodiazepine
- Control of hyperpyrexia by infusion of IV cooled crystalloid solution, continuous ice sponging, air conditioning of room, etc.
- Control of severe tachycardia by propranolol or continuous infusion of esmolol until the HR comes down to <100 per minute
- Control of cardiac failure by digitalis
- Control of hypotension by IV fluid and glucocorticoids (100–200 mg every 8 hours) from the coexisting adrenal gland suppression
- Control of increased plasma T_4 and T_3 level by potassium iodide (1 g IV over 12 hours), which will block the release of T_4 and T_3 from thyroid gland and propylthiouracil (200–600 mg every 6 hours orally or by nasogastric tube) which will inhibit the extrathyroidal conversion of T_4 to T_3.

Hypoparathyroidism, causing tetany due to hypocalcemia, may also occur following thyroidal surgery. It results from either the removal of parathyroid glands with thyroid tissues or the impairment of blood supply to the parathyroid glands during thyroid surgery. If two of the four parathyroid glands remain intact, then the tetany will not develop. If damage to all the parathyroid glands occur during thyroid surgery, then the symptoms of hypoparathyroidism typically develop within 24–72 hours after operation. But, it may manifest as early as 1–4 hours postoperatively. The laryngeal muscles are most sensitive to hypocalcemia. So, inspiratory stridor which gradually leads to laryngospasm may be the first manifestation of surgically induced hypoparathyroidism. The treatment of this emergency condition consists of prompt administration of calcium (as calcium gluconate) through intravenous route until the laryngeal spasm or laryngeal stridor ceases.

ANESTHETIC MANAGEMENT OF HYPERTHYROIDISM

When surgery is indicated, due to any reason (on thyroid or any other organ than thyroid) on a patient, suffering from hyperthyroidism, then it should be deferred, until a euthyroid state is achieved. This can be performed by some preoperative preparation which are discussed before. Usually, it is the dictum that all the drugs used to maintain the euthyroid state should be continued throughout the perioperative period. During emergency, when the surgery cannot be deferred and there is a state of hyperthyroidism, then the hyperdynamic cardiovascular system has been controlled by continued IV infusion of esmolol in the dose of 100–300 µg/kg/min. The poor control of hyperthyroidism and surgery may precipitate life-threatening condition, like thyroid crisis.

Preoperative Medication and Preparation

The proper evaluation of a hyperthyroid patient, prior to surgery, is the corner stone of anesthetic management of it. Among these, the full thyroid function tests, the assessment of cardiovascular system, and the assessment of airway are most vital. The patient should have normal T_4 and T_3 concentration and should not have resting tachycardia. Antithyroid medications and β-adrenergic antagonists are continued through the morning of surgery. Administration of propylthiouracil and methimazole is particularly important, because of their relatively short half-lives. Incompletely treated hyperthyroid patients may be hypovolemic and prone to an exaggerated hypotensive response to induction of anesthesia.

For the evaluation of airway, other than clinical examination, the CT scan or MRI is also very helpful. This is especially applicable for large goiter or thyroid masses to rule out its extension into mediastinum. Such extension may mandate sternotomy for complete resection. Benzodiazepine is the choice of agent for sedation as preoperative medication and should be used judiciously. It will reduce both the anxiety and HR. The use of anticholinergic agent as premedicant is not always the choice, because it contributes to the increased HR. But, it is also not always absolutely contraindicated and where possible the glycopyrrolate is preferred than atropine.

Induction and Maintenance of Anesthesia

Among all the inducing agent for hyperthyroid patient, thiopentone is the most choiced agent. Because, its thiourea structure provides some antithyroid activity. However, it is also unlikely that a significant antithyroid effect can be produced by an induction dose of thiopentone. Propofol also can be used for the induction of anesthesia in hyperthyroid patient. But, ketamine is never used, except in some special situation like hypotension, shock, etc. where it is only indicated. This is because, it can stimulate the sympathetic nervous system and increase the HR, SVR, BP, etc. Other drugs, that also stimulate the sympathetic nervous system, should also be avoided because of the possibility of exaggerated elevation in HR and BP. Before the use of any muscle relaxant, the depolarizing or nondepolarizing agents for tracheal intubation, the possible obstruction of airway by a huge goiter and failed intubation should be kept in mind. Otherwise, their use is not contraindicated in hyperthyroid state, provided they do not affect the cardiovascular system.

Throughout the whole perioperative period, the hyperthyroid patient should be monitored for its full cardiovascular function and body temperature. The patient should be kept with 15–20° head raised position. It will help by increasing the venous drainage and reducing the blood loss from operative site. But, it may increase the chance of venous air embolism. Patient's eyes should be well covered, because exophthalmos in Graves' disease may increase the chance of corneal injury. The adequate depth of anesthesia during intraoperative period must be achieved to prevent the exaggerated sympathetic response due to laryngoscopy, intubation, and surgical stimulation which is already present in hyperthyroid patient and to avoid tachycardia, hypertension, and ventricular arrhythmias. Hyperthyroidism does not increase anesthetic requirements, that is, there is no increase in minimum alveolar concentration (MAC) of inhalational anesthetic agents. Among the volatile anesthetic agents isoflurane, sevoflurane, and desflurane are the attractive choice for the maintenance of anesthesia with adequate depth. This offsets the increased response of sympathetic nervous system due to surgical stimulation and also not sensitize the heart to catecholamines. An alternative choice to volatile anesthetic agents, where

it is contraindicated, is short-acting narcotics combined with N_2O. There is clinical impression that the MAC value of volatile anesthetic agent is increased in hyperthyroid patient. This is due to the increased alveolar circulation, caused by increased cardiac output. But, practically there is no change in MAC value or anesthetic requirements of volatile anesthetic agents.

Thyrotoxicosis (hyperthyroidism) is often associated with increased incidences of myasthenia gravis and myopathies. Therefore, any muscle relaxant should be used cautiously and the neuromuscular block is monitored closely by peripheral nerve stimulator. Pancuronium is not the choice as muscle relaxant for hyperthyroid patient in view of the ability of this drug to stimulate sympathetic nervous system and to increase the HR with BP. Hence, the administration of muscle relaxant with minimal effect on cardiovascular system is always preferred for hyperthyroid patient. The antagonism of neuromuscular blockade by anticholinesterase, combined with anticholinergic agent, in hyperthyroid patient introduces a great concern regarding the drug-induced tachycardia. So, it should be controlled by using glycopyrrolate which has less chronotropic effect than atropine and by using β-blocker.

The management of hypotension, due to any cause during surgery, should be treated by the cautious use of sympathomimetic agents with the possibility of exaggerated responses in a hyperthyroid patient. For these reasons, the use of decreased dose of phenylephrine is more logical than ephedrine. This is because, the former is direct acting and does not act in part by releasing some endogenous catecholamine like the later. During the immediate and delayed postoperative period, the patient should be closely monitored for any thyroid crisis, recurrent laryngeal nerve injury causing respiratory difficulty, airway obstruction by the formation of hematoma at surgical site, hypoparathyroidism, etc. which are specific to thyroid surgery. The management of this complications are discussed before.

■ HYPOTHYROIDISM

It is a condition where the body tissues are exposed to the decreased circulating concentration of thyroid hormones, such as T_4 and T_3. It may be the end result of number of diseases of thyroid gland (primary hypothyroidism), or it may be secondary to pituitary failure (secondary pituitary hypothyroidism) or hypothalamic failure (secondary hypothalamic hypothyroidism). The syndrome of adult hypothyroidism is also known as *myxedema*. But, sometimes this term is used mainly to refer specifically skin changes in hypothyroidism. However, when hypothyroidism is present since birth or before it during intrauterine life, then this hypothyroidism is called as the *cretinism* (a condition of marked physical and mental retardation).

The prevalence of hypothyroidism in general population is 1:100. But, if the subclinical hypothyroidism (characterized by normal T_4 and raised TSH) is included, then this prevalence rate may rise to 1:500. The females are more affected from hypothyroidism than male and the male female ratio is 1:6. There are many causes of hypothyroidism and these are displayed in the **Box 3**. Among these, (i) the spontaneous atrophic hypothyroidism, (ii) thyroid failure following the use of I^{131}, or (iii) surgical removal of thyroid gland for hyperthyroidism, and (iv) the hypothyroidism due to Hashimoto's thyroiditis account for about 90% of cases in those parts of the country which are not significantly iodine deficient.

The clinical features of hypothyroidism depend on the duration and the severity of it. Because, the complete thyroid failure may develop over months and even years insidiously. The main consequence of hypothyroidism is the infiltration of body tissues by many substances such as mucopolysaccharide, hyaluronic acid, and chondroitin sulfate, etc. causing thickening of it. Thus, there is development of low-pitched voice, poor hearing, slurred speech, large tongue, and compression of median nerve at wrist, etc. The infiltration of dermis by the previously described substances gives rise to a nonpitting edema or myxedema which is most marked on the skin of hands, feet, and eyelids. There is also periorbital puffiness which is often a striking feature of hypothyroidism. When this is combined with facial pallor due to vasoconstriction or anemia and parchment paper like lip, then the clinical diagnosis of hypothyroidism is simple. But, most of the cases of hypothyroidism are not so obvious. However, sometimes the diagnosis of hypothyroidism is possibly entertained in the middle-aged woman by complain of tiredness (lethargy), muscle fatigue, constipation, weight gain, cold intolerance, depression, hypoactive reflexes, carpal tunnel syndrome, etc., which provides an opportunity for early treatment, otherwise missed. In advanced cases, HR, myocardial contractility, stroke volume, and cardiac output are all decreased, and extremities are cool and mottled because of peripheral vasoconstriction. In more advanced cases, pleural, abdominal, and pericardial effusions are common.

In the most common form of hypothyroidism such as primary hypothyroidism, there is low serum T_4 and a high serum TSH level. The serum T_3 level is not important for hypothyroidism, so it is not measured. Other nonspecific biochemical abnormalities of hypothyroidism include: (i) elevation of enzyme lactate dehydrogenase (LDH), (ii) elevation of creatine kinase, (iii) raised cholesterol level, (iv) raised triglyceride concentration, (v) low Na^+ concentration, etc. In severe prolonged hypothyroidism, the ECG shows sinus bradycardia, low voltage complexes, and ST- and T-wave abnormalities. In rare secondary hypothyroidism, there is both low T_4 and TSH level. The treatment of hypothyroidism consists of the oral administration of thyroid hormone T_4. The optimal therapy of hypothyroidism is characterized by the disappearance of all the symptoms, and the normal level of T_4 and TSH.

Anesthetic Management of Hypothyroidism

In our day-to-day practice, the likely presence of undiagnosed subclinical hypothyroidism in many patients who undergo uneventful anesthesia and the lack of increased morbidity and mortality during anesthesia of diagnosed mild hypothyroid patient indicates that there is no reason for delaying elective surgery in these patients. It also indicates that the patients suffering from mild to moderate hypothyroidism are not extra sensitive to inhaled anesthetic agents and opioids and have no prolonged recovery time or do not experience increased cardiovascular complications. So, elective anesthesia and surgery should not preferably be deferred in patient suffering from *mild to moderate hypothyroidism*. However, this is not applicable for the patients suffering from *severe hypothyroidism* with some present complications, due to it, such as pericardial effusion, severe bradycardia, hypotension, etc. provided the surgery is not emergency. *Symptomatic hypothyroid patients* should receive minimal preoperative sedation, because they are prone to drug-induced respiratory depression. In addition, they may fail to respond to hypoxia with increased minute ventilation.

Most patients suffering from hypothyroidism usually receive thyroid hormone replacement therapy and are in euthyroid state during elective surgery and anesthesia. So, they must continue it preoperatively and at morning on the day of anesthesia. The serum T_4 is a long-acting agent and its half-life is 7–8 days. So, its scheduled morning dose

---

BOX 3: Causes of hypothyroidism.

Primary:
- Spontaneous atrophy of gland
- Hashimoto's thyroiditis congenital
- Excess iodine (inhibits release)
- Dietary iodine deficiency
- Previous subtotal thyroidectomy
- Previous radioiodine therapy
- Antithyroid medications

Secondary:
- Hypothalamic dysfunction
- Anterior pituitary dysfunction

on the day of surgery is optional. Whereas, T_3 is a short-acting drug and its half-life is 1–2 days. Therefore, a patient must not omit its usual morning dose of T_3 on the day of surgery and anesthesia.

Hypothyroid patients are more prone to respiratory depression in response to sedatives and narcotics. They also fail to response to hypoxia by increasing the rate and depth of respiration, i.e., minute ventilation. So, they usually do not require much sedation as preoperative medication. Regarding the anticholinergic agents, these are helpful to counter the usually present sinus bradycardia and for this purpose atropine is preferred than glycopyrrolate. Hypothyroid patients usually suffered from increased gastric emptying times (i.e., delayed process of gastric emptying). So, the premedications for hypothyroid patients by H_2 histamine antagonist and prokinetic agent, such as metoclopramide, are very essential. Theoretically, myocardial ischemia may be worsened by thyroid hormone replacement therapy. Because, it increases the myocardial O_2 demand, due to its inotropic and chronotropic effects on myocardium. But, the recent available data shows that the symptoms of angina pectoris actually is decreased with thyroid hormone replacement therapy. So, a controversy may condense regarding the use of thyroid hormone from outside as a preoperative medication in such patient.

The induction of anesthesia of a hypothyroid patient can be performed by the usual inducing agents such as thiopentone, propofol, ketamine, benzodiazepine, etc. But, it depends on the severity of the disease and the presence of associated complications. This is because hypothyroid patients are more susceptible to hypotensive effect of inducing agents, as there is blunted baroreceptor reflex, diminished intravascular volume, and reduced cardiac output. Therefore, ketamine or etomidate is frequently recommended as the choice of inducing agent for severe hypothyroid patient and in myxedema coma. Benzodiazepine is also a good choice as inducing agent in severely ill patient. Sometimes, the possibility of coexistent congestive heart failure and adrenal insufficiency should be taken into account in cases of refractory hypotension in a hypothyroid patient. Other potential coexisting conditions include hypoglycemia, anemia, hyponatremia, difficult intubation (because of large tongue), and hypothermia [due to low basal metabolic rate (BMR)].

Theoretically, the decreased cardiac output may speed up the induction of anesthesia by inhalation anesthetic agents and decrease in its MAC valve. But, practically the MAC value of inhalation anesthetic agents does not truly decrease in hypothyroid patient. In such patient, tracheal intubation can be facilitated by muscle relaxation produced

by succinylcholine or any nondepolarizing agent. But, it will have to keep in mind that the coexisting skeletal muscle weakness may be present in association with hypothyroidism and may potentiate the action of muscle relaxant. Other potential problems which should be kept in mind during the induction and intubation of a hypothyroid patient include large tongue, compression of trachea by large goiter, anemia, hypoglycemia, hypothermia due to low BMR, hyponatremia, etc.

The maintenance of anesthesia for a hypothyroid patient is usually achieved by using the mixture of N_2O and O_2 which is supplemented by short-acting narcotics or volatile anesthetic agent. However, the excessive volatile anesthetic agent is not recommended, because it may cause the excessive cardiac depression and peripheral vasodilatation, causing abrupt decrease in systemic blood pressure. Therefore, adequate muscle relaxation by the judicious use of neuromuscular blocker (NMB) and minimum use of intravenous and inhalation anesthetic agent is the appropriate goal for the management of severe hypothyroid patient. Among the NMB agents, pancuronium is preferred for hypothyroid patients due to its cardiovascular stimulating effect. On the other hand, the short- and intermediate-acting NMB agents are also preferred. This is because, they are less likely to produce prolonged neuromuscular blockade, as the reduced skeletal muscular activity is associated with hypothyroidism. The controlled ventilation is preferred than spontaneous ventilation in hypothyroid patient, because they are more prone to hypoventilation and hypoxia in response to anesthetic drugs. On the other hand, hypothyroid patients are more vulnerable to less production of CO_2 due to decreased BMR. This when again is associated with mechanical ventilation, then it causes more decreased $PaCO_2$ and subsequently low $ETCO_2$ value.

The aim of perioperative monitoring of a hypothyroid patient is directed to the prompt recognition of any exaggerated depression of cardiovascular system and the early detection of onset of hypothermia. So, the continuous monitoring of BP (noninvasive or invasive according to the gravity of necessity), HR, ECG, temperature, $ETCO_2$ etc. is mandatory. In addition, the glucose solution, used as intravenous fluid, should contain Na^+ to decrease the incidence of hyponatremia because the hypothyroidism is usually associated with the later. In the face of hypothermia, which is common in hypothyroidism, the body temperature is maintained (i) by increasing the temperature of operation theater (OT), (ii) by using a warming device placed under the patient, (iii) by warning the inhaled anesthetic gases, and (iv) by intravenous fluid by warmer, etc.

The perioperative hypotension of a hypothyroid patient is treated mainly by IV fluid, sympathomimetic agents, and glucocorticoids. Regarding the sympathomimetic agents, the α-adrenergic agonist, such as the phenylephrine could adversely increase the systemic vascular resistance in the presence of a failed heart with limited reserve that cannot reliably increase its contractility. On the other hand, β-adrenergic agonist may precipitate cardiac arrhythmias. Therefore, a useful approach for the management of hypotension in a hypothyroid patient is small dose of IV ephedrine (2.5–5 mg) while continuously monitoring the cardiovascular system (CVS). The possibility of acute adrenal insufficiency is thought, when there is persistent hypotension, despite adequate treatment with IV fluid and sympathomimetic agents. Then, glucocorticoids should be used.

Antagonism of nondepolarizing neuromuscular blockade by anticholinesterase, combined with anti-cholinergic agent, usually does not pose any extra hazard to hypothyroid patients. But, recovery from general anesthesia and extubation may be delayed in such patient. This is due to hypothermia, respiratory depression or slow drug biotransformation in hypothyroid patients. Patients should remain intubated until they respond appropriately and the body temperature is near 37°C. Hypothyroid patients often require prolonged ventilation because they are at increased vulnerability to respiratory depression. Despite all these facts, comparing patients who have mild- to-moderate hypothyroidism, with euthyroid patients, fails to demonstrate any significant difference in respect to (i) the incidence of cardiac dysrhythmias, (ii) the time to tracheal extubation, (iii) the need for vasopressor, (iv) hypothermia, and (v) the need for postoperative ventilatory support.

Myxedema Coma

This is a rare and acute presentation of hypothyroidism in which there is loss of deep tendon reflexes, hypoventilation, hypothermia, cardiovascular collapse, coma, and death. Body temperature may be as low as 25°C and the convulsions are not uncommon. Myxedema coma is a medical emergency condition. Sepsis and exposure to cold may be an initiating factor of it. However, the treatment should be started before the biochemical confirmation of this medical emergency condition is established. For this situation, the T_4 is not usually available for parenteral use. Instead, the T_3 is given as an intravenous bolus in the dose of 20 µg. It exerts its physiological effect within 6 hours and is repeated 8 hourly until there is definite clinical improvement. This administration of IV T_3 should be accompanied with the administration of cortisol, if the adrenal insufficiency

FACT FILE IV

Graves' disease:
It accounts for 70–80% of the cases of hyperthyroidism. It is distinguished from the other forms of hyperthyroidism by the presence of diffuse thyroid enlargement, ophthalmopathy, and pretibial myxedema (rare). It most commonly affects the 30–50 years age group of people. However, it may occur at any age, but unusual before puberty. It mostly affects the women, but the cause of this predilection toward the woman is still unknown. In Graves' disease, the hyperthyroidism results from the increased production of immunoglobulin G (IgG) antibodies directed against the TSH receptor present on the thyroid follicles which stimulate the receptor. This produces marked T4 and T3 secretion and enlargement of thyroid gland (goiter). However, due to the feedback effects of T4 and T3, the plasma TSH level is low.

Another hallmark of this disease is exophthalmos. It occurs in 50% of patients suffering from Graves' disease and often precedes the development of hyperthyroidism. The cause of this ophthalmic manifestation is still properly not known. But the probable explanation is that there is cytokine-mediated proliferation of fibroblasts which secrete hydrophilic glycosaminoglycans. This results in increased interstitial fluid content which combined with chronic inflammatory cell infiltration causes marked swelling of the orbital tissues and increased retrobulbar pressure. The other antithyroid antibodies which are present in Graves' disease also include the antibodies to thyroglobulin and thyroid peroxidase. In Hashimoto's thyroiditis, the autoimmune antibodies ultimately destroy the thyroid gland. But, during the early stage of inflammation of gland, it causes excess thyroid hormone secretion and thyrotoxicosis.

is suspected. In responders, there is gradual rise of body temperature within 24 hours. After 48–72 hours, it is possible to start substitution by oral thyroxine. The other measures of management in myxedema coma include slow rewarming, intravenous fluid, high flow of O_2, broad-spectrum antibiotics, etc. During fluid replacement, it is important to remember that these patients may be vulnerable to water intoxication and hyponatremia. Occasionally, assisted ventilation may be necessary (**Fact file IV**).

Hashimoto's Thyroiditis

It is an autoimmune disease. Hence, it is also known as autoimmune thyroiditis. In 90% of patients, with this disease, antibody against thyroid peroxidase is present in the serum. This condition is also not infrequently associated with other autoimmune diseases, such as autoimmune gastritis, pernicious anemia, myasthenia gravis, etc. This is the most common cause of goitrous hypothyroidism. It is typically found in the age between 20 and 60 years. They are usually old women who present with small or moderately sized diffuse goiter. At this stage, it may be impossible to differentiate

Hashimoto's thyroiditis from simple goiter by palpation alone. Usually, this disease runs in two stages. At first, there is moderate and uniform enlargement of gland with soft to firm feel. Then, usually it turns hard and nodular which depends on the relative degree of lymphocytic infiltration, fibrosis, and follicular cell hyperplasia of the gland. The thyroid function is usually low. But, in some patients, the level of serum T_4 is normal and the serum TSH is normal or raised. These patients are at increased risk of developing hypothyroidism in future. Hypothyroid state which is common for this disease is treated by thyroxine therapy. It also helps to shrink the goiter. The dose of thyroxine should be sufficient to suppress the serum TSH to an undetectable level without inducing hyperthyroidism.

Psychiatric Diseases, its Pharmacology and Anesthesia

INTRODUCTION

The term *"psyche"* means *mental process*. So, the *"psychiatric disorders"* mean the *disorders in mental process* (mental disorders). The term *"mental disorders"* encompasses a broad range of conditions which are characterized by abnormal patterns of behavior with psychological signs and symptoms that result from mental dysfunction. Mental disorders are highly prevalent in medical practice, although they are frequently ignored or untreated. They may present either as a primary disorder or as a comorbid condition. Approximately 20% of people in UK suffer from psychiatric diseases and apparently 1% of them will have a major disorder. The important considerations during anesthetic management of a patient with psychiatric diseases are:

- The psychotropic drugs that the patients are taking, may have potential serious interactions with the anesthetic agents.
- As the patients are frequently depressed, so they have little understanding or appreciation of the course of anesthesia.
- Patients suffering from psychiatric diseases may have associated copathology as the consequences of frequent alcohol or drug abuse by them.
- Psychiatric patients who require electroconvulsive therapy (ECT) may require repeated anesthesia.
- History taking from a psychiatric patient is very difficult. So, the relatives or caregivers of this patient may need to be present during preoperative assessment. The consent for surgery or anesthesia can only be given by a competent relative (not always blood related), though the majority of patients with psychiatric disorders can give consent themselves normally.
- Psychiatric patients are often surprisingly healthy, strong, muscular, and may become suddenly aggressive by unfamiliar faces or surroundings.

- Adequate sedative premedication should always be considered and adequate personnel should always be present during the induction and emergence from anesthesia of such patients.
- Many patients are on long-term medication and this should be continued throughout the perioperative period, whenever possible and have definite effect on anesthesia.

During the last 50 years, psychiatric treatment has witnessed many major changes, due to the advent of many specific drugs for specific illness. It has also changed the trend from custodial care of patient toward the restoring of individual patient in his own place in the community. Before 1952, the aim of psychiatric treatment was to quieten and sedate the agitated and violent patients. But, the introduction of chlorpromazine (CPZ) in that year had changed the situation and most schizophrenics could now be rehabilitated to their own productive life. Next, in the year of 1957–1958 came the tricyclic antidepressants (TCAs) and monoamine oxidase (MAO) inhibitors which successfully covered another group of psychiatric patients. Then, after 1980 many novel antipsychotics and antidepressants have been introduced. After that, the development of meprobamate and chlordiazepoxide has proved that anxiety could easily be tackled without producing any marked sedation. Now, the goal of treatment of psychiatric patient has been more realized by the development of benzodiazepine (BDZ) in 1960. Buspirone is a recent significant addition.

CLASSIFICATION OF PSYCHIATRIC DISEASES

Like any growing branch of medicine, the psychiatric illnesses have also seen the rapid changes in its classification. This is only to keep up with the growing research data and to deal with the changing epidemiology, symptomatology, prognostic factors, treatment methods, and new theories for the causation of psychiatric disorders. Now, all the principal types of psychiatric disorders are classified as: (1) psychosis, (2) affective or mood disorder, and (3) neuroses.

Psychosis

These are severe mental illnesses, characterized by serious distortion of thought, severe distortion of behavior, incapacity to recognize the reality and wrong perception (delusions and hallucination), and misconception. This psychotic patient is unable to meet the ordinary demands of life. Psychosis can be classified again into two disorders: (i) cognitive disorder, and (ii) functional disorder.

- *Cognitive disorder (organic brain syndrome):* This cognitive psychotic disorder is also known as organic brain syndrome. Because, it is always associated with some form of organic brain lesions. It may occur both in acute and chronic form. The prominent features of this cognitive psychotic disorder are: confusion, disorientation, defective memory, false believe, and disorganized behavior, etc. The examples of this disorder are *delirium* and *dementia*. Some toxic, traumatic, or pathological basis can often be found for this disorder.
- *Functional disorder:* Here, no underlying definitive organic cause or pathology in brain can often be found for this disorder. Memory and orientation are mostly retained, but the emotions, thought, and behavior are seriously altered. This disorder is again classified into *schizophrenia* and *paranoid states.*
  - *Schizophrenia (split mind):* It is also known as the hallucination state. Schizophrenia is thought to result from an excess of dopaminergic activity in brain. It is characterized by inability to think coherently. There is also splitting (separation) of perception and interpretation from reality (hallucination). Its prevalence rate normally varies between 2 and 4 per 1,000 normal population. Schizophrenia is characterized by the presence of any one of the Schneider's first rank symptoms in the absence of any physical or organic disease. Schneider's first rank symptoms include hallucination, delusional, disorganized behavior, disorganized thought, insertion of thoughts, somatic passivity, feelings, etc. Chronic schizophrenia is characterized by the presence of "negative symptoms" such as withdrawal, catatonic disturbances, and lack of emotion. It commonly begins in late adolescence of either sex and is found in any social group. In the acute phase, patients may be highly delusional and/or aggressive and may not be able to give informed consent. Controlled schizophrenics may be completely lucid and rational, but care must be taken to ensure that

their medication is continued where and when possible. As some chronic schizophrenics have predominantly negative symptoms and it is difficult to communicate with them, so history cannot be taken from them.

  - *Paranoid states:* It is characterized by the loss of insight into abnormality and false believes. This is also called the delusion disorder. This disorder is characterized by:
    - Persistent delusions of persecution (being persecuted against), grandeur (inflated self-esteem), and jealousy
    - Absence of hallucination
    - Personality disturbances
    - No underlying organic causes
    - Absence of schizophrenia and mood disorder.

Affective or Mood Disorder

The primary symptom of affective disorder is the change in mood. It may be manifested as mania and depression.

- *Mania:* It is characterized by the elation, hyperactivity, uncontrollable thought and uncontrolled speech. It may be associated with violent behavior.
- *Depression:* It is characterized by the sadness, guilty, physical slowing, mental slowing, melancholia, self-destructive idea, etc. Affective disorder may be bipolar (manic and depressive) with cyclically alternating manic and depressive phases. It may also be polar (manic or depression) with a waxing and waning of any single disorder.

Neuroses

This disorder represents the largest proportion of all the psychiatric illness, attending psychiatric outpatients department (75%). These are less serious condition. Here, ability to comprehend reality is not lost, though sometimes patient may undergo extreme suffering. In these disorders, catecholamine levels may be very high or the patient may suffer from hyperventilation. These patients require only a great deal of reassurance, but no drug. Premedication is often required to smooth the induction for these patients. Depending on the predominant feature, it may be classified as anxiety, phobic states, obsessive-compulsive disorder, and hysterical disorder.

- *Anxiety:* It is an unpleasant emotional state or thought for the future life.
- *Phobic states:* These are characterized by fear for unknown or some known specific objects, person, or situation.

- *Obsessive-compulsive disorder:* It is defined as abnormality of thought or behavior where the patient has limited ability to overcome, even on voluntary effort.
- *Hysterical disorder:* It is a drama like symptom, resembling serious physical illness. But, it is situational and always in the presence of others. The patient does not pretend and actually undergoes the symptoms against his or her will, though the basis is only psychic and not physical.

MULTIAXIAL CLASSIFICATION OF PSYCHIATRIC DISORDERS

Labeling a patient with a diagnosis of psychiatric disorder is not enough. This degrades the patient just as a diseased individual in hospital, but does not give any direct attention to the whole individual in a society. So, a recent classification is adopted by American Psychiatric Association (APA) in DSM-IV (Diagnostic and Statistical Manual-IV). This method of classification helps in more holistic assessment of a patient as a whole human. In this system, an individual patient is diagnosed on five axes.

Axis-I: Presence or absence of any major mental disorders (clinical psychiatric diagnosis).

Axis-II: Presence or absence of any underlying developmental and personality disorders.

Axis-III: Presence or absence of general medical disorders.

Axis-IV: Presence or absence of psychological and environmental or social problems (psychosocial disorder.

Axis-V: Overall rating of general psychological functions.

PSYCHOPHARMACOLOGY AND ANESTHETIC DRUGS INTERACTION

Till the recent years, the exact pathophysiology of many psychiatric illnesses is not clear. But, some ideas have been formed. As for example, dopaminergic overactivity in the limbic system may be involved in schizophrenia and mania. On the other hand, the monoaminergic (NE, 5-HT) deficit may underlie the depression disorder. So, the treatment of psychiatric diseases is empirical, symptom oriented, and not disease specific. However, this empirical and symptom-oriented management is highly effective in many situations. The drugs which are used for psychiatric diseases and have a significant effect on higher mental functions are also called *psychoactive* or *psychotropic drugs* (**Fact file I**). The psychotropic drugs can be classified as follows:

- *Antipsychotic drugs:* They are useful in all types of psychosis, especially schizophrenia. They are also called the *neuroleptics, major tranquilizers, or antischizophrenic drugs.*

FACT FILE I

Tranquilizer is an old term. It means "a drug which reduces the mental tension and produces the calmness, without inducing sleep or depressing mental facilities". This term is confusing and should not be used any more. Its division into major and minor tranquilizers is also not justified. Because the "minor tranquilizers" are not less important drugs. They are more frequently prescribed and carry higher abuse liability than the "major tranquilizers". Instead of tranquilizer, the newer terms such as sedative and hypnotic are more commonly used. Sedative is a drug that subdues the excitement and produces the calmness without inducing sleep, though drowsiness may be produced. Sedation also refers to the decreased responsiveness of central nervous system (CNS) to any level of stimulation. It is associated with some decrease in motor activity and reduction of formation of idea, but does not induce sleep. Whereas hypnotic is a drug that induces and/or maintain sleep (similar to normal arousable sleep). This should not be confused with "hypnosis" which means a transition like state where the subject becomes passive and highly suggestible. Both sedatives and hypnotics are more or less general CNS depressants with different time action and dose action relationship. Those with quicker onset, shorter duration, and steeper dose-response curve are referred to as the hypnotics. Whereas, more slowly acting drugs with flatter dose-response curve are referred to as the sedatives. However, there is considerable overlap. A hypnotic at lower doses may act as sedative and a sedative in higher dose may act as hypnotic.

- *Antianxiety drugs:* These are also called anxiolytic, sedative or minor tranquilizer. They are useful for anxiety and phobic states.
- *Drugs for affective disorder:* The drugs in this group is again classified as: (*i*) *antidepressant drugs and* (*ii*) *antimanic or mood stabilizing drugs.*
- *Psychomimetics or hallucinogens:* Now, they are seldom used therapeutically to produce psychosis like states. But, the majority of them are the drugs of abuse.

ANTIPSYCHOTIC DRUGS

The antipsychotic drugs are those agents which are used for the treatment of psychoses or psychotic symptoms. These are also known as the *major tranquilizers, neuroleptics, or antischizophrenic* drugs. But, the term antipsychotic is the most appropriate. These drugs have salutary effect on psychosis.

Classification of Antischizophrenic Drugs

- *Phenothiazines (**Fig. 1**):*
  - *Aliphatic side chain:* Chlorpromazine and triflupromazine.
  - *Piperidine side chain:* Thioridazine.
  - *Piperazine side chain:* Fluphenazine and trifluoperazine.

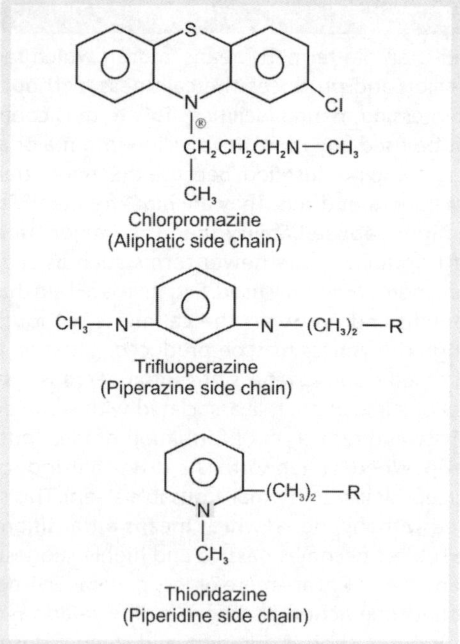

Fig. 1: Structure of various phenothiazines.

- *Butyrophenones:* Trifluperidol, haloperidol, penfluridol, and droperidol.
- *Thioxanthenes:* Flupenthixol, chlorprothixene, and thiothixene.
- *Miscellaneous:* Pimozide, molindone, and loxapine.
- *Atypical:* Risperidone and clozapine.

The pharmacological and mechanism of action of all these drugs in this antipsychotic group is more or less same, as that of CPZ. So, the pharmacology of CPZ is described here as the prototype of all these antipsychotic drugs. However, they only differ from each other in their varying degree of actions.

Mechanism of Action

The first-generation antischizophrenic drugs had strong dopamine (DA) antagonistic effects, leading to extrapyramidal side effects (e.g., muscle rigidity and progression to tardive dyskinesia). The third-generation of drugs has less DA antagonism and reduced extrapyramidal effects. The exact mechanism of action of all these antipsychotic drugs is still unknown. But, most probably, one of the major mechanisms of action of these agents is their *antidopaminergic activity*. The dopaminergic projections in the temporal and prefrontal areas constitute the limbic system of brain and are responsible for the psychological state of an individual. Also the dopaminergic projection in the mesocortical areas is probably responsible for the emotional reactions of an individual. Therefore, the overactivity of this dopaminergic pathway is responsible for

psychiatric illness. All the antipsychotic drugs have potent dopamine D_2 receptor blocking action and act at these areas. So, the antipsychotic potency of these agents has shown good correlation with their affinity and blocking property (ability) to this dopamine D_2 receptor. The phenothiazines and thioxanthenes also block the D_1, D_3, and D_4 receptors. Clozapine has weak D_2 blocking action, but is selective for D_4 receptors and also has significant 5-HT_2 and α_1-blocking action.

The side effects of these antischizophrenic drugs include orthostatic hypotension, acute dystonic reactions, and parkinsonism like manifestations. The risperidone and clozapine have little extrapyramidal activity. But, the latter is associated with a significant incidence of granulocytopenia. The *extrapyramidal symptoms (EPS)*, caused by this group of drugs, are due to the blockade of these D_2 receptors by them, situated in the EPS (basal ganglia). *Antiemetic action* of these groups of drugs is also due to the D_2 receptor blockade action of them in CTZ area. The *sedation*, produced by these agents, is caused by their adrenergic blockade action which is maximum for CPZ and thioridazine.

Pharmacological Action

These antipsychotic groups of drugs reduce irrational behavior, agitation, and aggressiveness of patient. They control the psychotic symptomatology. The disturbed thinking of patient is also corrected and the disturbed behaviors of patients are gradually normalized. Difficulties in attention and concentration are slowly corrected. Anxiety is relieved. Hyperactivity, hallucination, and delusions are suppressed.

All the phenothiazines, thioxanthenes, and butyrophenones have the same antipsychotic effects. But, the potency among them differs in terms of their equieffective doses. The aliphatic and the piperidine side-chained phenothiazines (CPZ, triflupromazine, and thioridazine) have low antipsychotic potency than that of piperazine side-chained phenothiazines (trifluoperazine), but produce more sedation and cause the greater potentiation of hypnotics and opioids. The sedative effect of these antipsychotic drugs is produced immediately, while the antipsychotic effect takes weeks to develop **(Table 1)**.

In normal individuals, the antipsychotic drugs also produce indifference to the surroundings, paucity of thought, psychomotor slowing, emotional quietening, reduction in initiative and tendency to go off to sleep from which the subject is easily arousable. Spontaneous movements are minimized, but the slurring of speech, ataxia, or motor incoordination does not occur. This has been referred to as the "neuroleptic syndrome" and is quite different

TABLE 1: Comparative properties of antipsychotic drugs.

Drugs and doses (in mg)	Sedation	Extrapyramidal	Hypotension	Antiemetic
Chlorpromazine (100–800)	S	M	S	M
Thioridazine (100–400)	S	L	S	N
Triflupromazine (50–200)	S	S	M	S
Fluphenazine (1–10)	L	S	L	S
Trifluoperazine (2–20)	L	S	L	S
Thioproperazine (5–30)	L	S	L	M
Trifluperidol (1–8)	L	S	L	S
Haloperidol (2–12)	L	S	L	S
Flupenthixol (3–15)	L	S	L	L
Chlorprothixene (50–400)	S	M	M	M
Molindone (50–150)	L	M	N	N
Pimozide (2–6)	M	S	L	L
Loxapine (20–100)	L	S	M	L
Risperidone (2–12)	L	N	L	N
Clozapine (25–300)	L	N	L	N

Note: S = strong, M = moderate, L = less, N = Nil

from the sedative actions of barbiturates, BDZ, and other similar drugs. These effects are appreciated as "neutral", but "unpleasant" by most of the normal individuals.

The performance and the intelligence of patients are relatively unaffected by this group of drugs, but vigilance is impaired. However, they lower the seizure threshold and can precipitate fits in untreated epileptics. Like sedatives and hypnotics, the medullary respiratory and other vital centers are not affected by these agents, except at very high doses. They have potent *antiemetic action* which is exerted through their action on the center of CTZ. But, they are ineffective in motion sickness.

All the neuroleptics also have the varying degree of α-*adrenergic blocking activity*. This may be graded as CPZ > triflupromazine > thioridazine > fluphenazine > haloperidol > trifluoperazine > clozapine > pimozide. Thus, it is concluded that the more potent compounds have lower propensity for α-adrenergic blocking activity. All the neuroleptics also have *anticholinergic property* in varying degree. The gradation of anticholinergic property is like that thioridazine > chlorpromazine > triflupromazine > trifluoperazine = haloperidol. The phenothiazines also have weak H_1 antihistaminic and antiserotonin (anti-5-HT) actions as well **(Fact file II)**.

The neuroleptics produce orthostatic *hypotension* by central as well as by peripheral blocking action of sympathetic tone. The hypotensive action is more marked after parenteral administration of this agent. It is roughly

FACT FILE II

The antipsychotic drugs most likely exert their effects by inhibiting the binding of dopamine at their postsynaptic receptors. So, they have an array of effect in overdose such as neuroendocrine, autonomic, cardiac, and ophthalmic, etc. But, still their therapeutic index is high and the overdose effects are rarely irreversible and serious. The most troublesome (but not serious) side effects of antipsychotic drugs are parkinsonism and dystonia. 50–70% of patients receiving antipsychotic drugs manifest some form of EPS. It gradually diminishes after 2–3 months of initiation of treatment. Acute dystonia, manifested by the contraction of skeletal muscles of mouth, neck, tongue, etc., is treated by diphenhydramine 25–50 mg through IV.

parallel to the α-adrenergic blocking property of this group of drugs. This is accentuated by hypovolemia. Reflex tachycardia accompanies this hypotension. For the side effects of antipsychotic drugs see the **Table 2**.

The release of ACTH, in response to stress, is diminished by the use of these drugs. So, corticosteroid levels fail to increase under circumstances of stress. High doses of CPZ directly depress the heart and produce some *electrocardiogram (ECG) changes*. These changes are increased PR interval, QT prolongation, widening of QRS complex, and T-wave suppression. CPZ also exerts some antiarrhythmic action and probably it is due to some membrane stabilization property of it. However, arrhythmias may still occur in overdose of these agents especially with thioridazine.

TABLE 2: Side effects of antipsychotic drugs.

Cardiovascular system	• Hypotension • Tachycardia • ↑PR interval • ↑QT interval
CNS	• Sedation • Extrapyramidal symptoms (dystonia, parkinsonism) • Cognitive impairment • Seizure
ANS	• Blurred vision • Urinary retention
GI	• ↓ Bowel motility • Cholestatic jaundice
Ophthalmic	• Opacities of lens and cornea • ↑IOP
Hematology	• Agranulocytosis • Leukopenia
Endocrine	• Weight gain • Amenorrhea • Galactorrhea

(ANS: autonomic nervous system; CNS: central nervous system; GI: gastrointestinal)

Most of the antipsychotic agents have narrow therapeutic window. It means, if the blood level of any of these agents is below than the lower limit of this window, then the drug is ineffective and if the blood level is higher than the upper limit of this window, then there is toxicity. Or in other ward, it means the gap (difference) between the maximum and minimum concentration of the drug for their therapeutic action is small.

All the antipsychotic agents are highly lipophilic and highly protein bound in nature. So, the half-life of all the antipsychotics is long and theoretically a single dose, administration per day, is enough to produce sustained therapeutic blood levels throughout the whole day. Once the drug is withdrawn, it may remain in the body for many days to many months.

Drug Interactions (Anesthetic Implications)

As all the neuroleptic agents have central sedative properties, so they potentiate the actions of all the CNS depressing agents, like hypnotics, anxiolytics (sedative), alcohol, opioids, antihistaminics, and analgesics. Therefore, the symptoms due to the overdose of these CNS depressing agents may easily occur and the requirements of other CNS depressing anesthetic drugs should be decreased. As all the antipsychotic agents have the potent DA receptor blocking action, so they block the actions of levodopa and

other DA agonists which are used in parkinsonism. So, the doses of drugs used in parkinsonism should be increased. The central anticholinergic effects of all the antipsychotic agents are additive with those of atropine and hyoscine. So, the glycopyrrolate is the preferred antisialagogue, where the antipsychotic drugs are used. The α-adrenoreceptor blockade action of antipsychotic agents also aggravates the hypotensive effect of anesthetic and other α-adrenoreceptor blocking agents.

This may be an important consideration during the management of anesthesia. This is particularly true with acute blood loss or regional anesthesia, as the compensatory sympathetic nervous system-mediated vasoconstriction is attenuated by the antipsychotic drug-induced α-adrenergic blockade. The seizures may occur often with clozapine than with other antipsychotic agents. When considering general anesthesia (GA), especially administering succinylcholine, then the patients with the history of neuroleptic malignant syndrome (NMS) are more vulnerable to develop malignant hyperthermia due to the common pathology.

Neuroleptic malignant syndrome: It is a life-threatening (mortality rate is 20–30%) and rare complication of antipsychotic therapy and may occur hours or weeks after drug administration. Meperidine and metoclopramide can also precipitate this disorder. The mechanism is related to DA blockade in basal ganglia and hypothalamus and impairment of thermoregulation. In its most severe form, the presentation is similar to that of malignant hyperthermia. Muscle rigidity, hyperthermia, rhabdomyolysis, autonomic instability, and altered consciousness are seen. Creatine kinase level is often elevated. Death usually results from kidney failure or arrhythmias. Treatment begins with the stopping of responsible drug and initiating supportive care. Dantrolene and bromocriptine are usually used. But, there is no strong evidence for their consistent efficacy. Differential diagnosis of NMS includes serotonin syndrome, malignant hyperthermia, malignant catatonia, and some other acute intoxications.

◼ ANTIANXIETY DRUGS

Anxiety is an emotional state which is associated with uneasiness, discomfort, and fear about some defined or undefined objects. The antianxiety drugs are also called the minor tranquilizers or anxiolytics. They are all ill-defined, mild CNS depressants without interfering the normal mental or physical functions. This group of antianxiety drugs differs markedly from the antipsychotic group of drugs and more closely resembles to the sedatives or hypnotics. Anxiety is very unpleasant in nature and some degree of it is always part and parcel of life. Treatment of anxiety is always not necessary. But, it is needed when anxiety is disproportionate to the situation or excessive.

Characteristic of Antianxiety Drugs

- They cannot control thought disorder of schizophrenia.
- They do not produce extrapyramidal side effects.
- They have anticonvulsant property and produce skeletal muscle relaxation.
- They produce physical dependence.
- They carry abuse liability.

Classification of Antianxiety Drugs

- *Benzodiazepines:* Chlordiazepoxide, diazepam, oxazepam, alprazolam, lorazepam, temazepam, and midazolam.
- *Azapirones:* Buspirone and gepirone.
- *Other sedatives:* Meprobamate and hydroxyzine.
- *β-blocker:* Propranolol **(Fig. 2)**.

Benzodiazepines

All the BZDs have the selective taming effect and suppress the induced aggression. They have slow onset and prolonged duration of action and relieve anxiety at low doses without producing major global CNS depression. In contrast to barbiturates, BZDs are more selective for limbic system. They have also been proved to be clinically better for the improvement in both the quality and quantity of anxiety and stress-related symptoms. However, they have very little effect on the other body systems. Withdrawal syndrome is milder and delayed due to their long half-life. They reduce nightmare and have been found to be relatively save, even in gross overdoses. They have least cardiovascular and respiratory depression effect at their antianxiety doses.

The BZDs act through their BZD receptors which is a part of the gamma-aminobutyric acid type A (GABA$_A$) (which is discussed in Chapter 14) receptors and so facilitates the

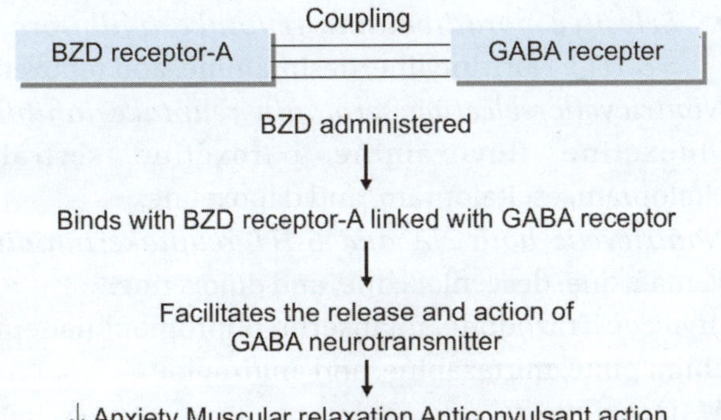

Fig. 2: Probable mechanism of action of benzodiazepine (BZD). (GABA: γ-aminobutyric acid)

release and action of major inhibitory neurotransmitter, such as GABA. Thus, it produces antianxiety, muscular relaxation, and anticonvulsant action **(Fig. 2)**. Among all the BZDs, the most commonly used agents in anesthesia practice are midazolam, alprazolam, lorazepam, midazolam, diazepam, and temazepam.

Azapirones (Buspirone)

Azapirones are a new class of non-BZD, antianxiety agents and buspirone is the first member of all the azapirone group of drugs. The characteristics of buspirone are that it does not produce any sedation or functional impairment and does not act through BZD or GABA receptors. It has no muscle relaxant or anticonvulsant property and does not produce any physical dependence.

The mechanism of action of buspirone is not exactly known. But, the probable explanation is that it acts by selective partial agonistic action on 5-HT$_{1A}$ receptors. It has no antipsychotic or extrapyramidal effects. Buspirone relieves only mild to moderate anxiety, but is ineffective in severe cases. The therapeutic effects of buspirone develop slowly over 2 weeks. Occasionally, a mild mood elevating action of buspirone has also been noted and it is due to the facilitation of central noradrenergic system.

Buspirone is rapidly absorbed through oral route and undergoes extensive hepatic first pass metabolism. Hence, the oral bioavailability of it is only <5%. It may cause rise in blood pressure (BP) in patients on MAO inhibitors (MAOIs). But, it does not potentiate the action of CNS depressants such as BDZ and barbiturates.

■ DRUGS FOR AFFECTIVE DISORDER

Affective disorders are also called the mood disorders and the two extremes of this pathological state are depression and mania. So, the classification of drugs used in this disorder is similarly divided into antidepressants (mood elevators) and antimanias (mood stabilizer). Antidepressant agents again are of two types, i.e., (1) TCAs and (20 MAOIs. The main antimanic agents are lithium.

Antidepressant

It is well established that depression is due to the deficiency of DA, norepinephrine, 5-HT, or altered receptor activities. Up to 50% patients with major depression hypersecret cortisol and have abnormal circadian secretion. Antidepressants are those psychiatric drugs which are used for the treatment of depressive illness. They are also called the mood elevators. All these drugs act by elevating DA, norepinephrine, and 5-HT at receptor level. The first antidepressant to be discovered was imipramine in 1958.

It is different from phenothiazines only by a replacement of a sulfur atom with an ethylene linkage. Due to this small structural difference, imipramine was no longer effective as an antipsychotic agent instead was quite beneficial in depressed patients. Since 1958, the number of antidepressants discovered has been gradually increasing.

The mechanism of action of imipramine (tricyclic compound) is to inhibit the noradrenaline (NA) and 5-HT reuptake by the presynaptic neurons at nerve terminal, and thus increasing the concentration of NA and/or 5-HT at their receptor site on the past synaptic membrane. So, the tricyclic compounds are also called the monoamine reuptake inhibitors (MARIs); as a large number of congeners of imipramine or tricyclic compound were soon added, so they are collectively called the tricyclic antidepressants (TCAs). But, it includes very few tricyclic compounds in structure as well. Some of these compounds have relatively greater inhibition on NA reuptake than 5-HT or greater inhibition on 5-HT reuptake than NA. Most significant development in this subject in the past 15 years is the introduction of highly selective serotonin reuptake inhibitor (SSRI) and also some atypical antidepressants. Most of the TCA compounds do not inhibit DA reuptake, except maprotiline and bupropion. Moreover, amphetamine and cocaine (which are not antidepressants, but CNS stimulants) are strong inhibitors of DA uptake. So, at the end, it can be summarized that the inhibition of DA reuptake correlates with the stimulant action of CNS and is not involved in antidepressant action whereas the inhibition of NA and 5-HT reuptake is associated with antidepressant action, but not correlates with CNS stimulant action. The inhibition of 5-HT reuptake is also responsible for sedation.

On the other hand, MAOIs act on the MAO. It is a mitochondrial enzyme and is responsible for the degradation of NA, DA, and 5-HT after their reuptake at nerve terminal. Thus, MAOIs allow NA, DA, and 5-HT to accumulate in their respective nerve terminal in the brain and periphery. Two isoenzyme forms of MAO have been identified. These are MAO-A and MAO-B. The MAO-A preferentially deaminates 5-HT, adrenaline, and NA, whereas the MAO-B preferentially deaminates all the nonpolar aromatic amines such as phenylethylamine, etc. The tyramine and DA are deaminated by both. Their distribution also differs. Both these isoenzymes are present in neural and nonneural tissues with a preponderance of MAO-A enzyme in the brain and MAO-B enzyme in the liver and lungs. MAOIs inhibit both these MAO enzyme and thus the resultant increased amine level (NA, DA, and 5-HT) in brain is probably responsible for their antidepressant action. Older MAOIs are nonselective (inhibiting both MAO-A and MAO-B isoenzyme) and

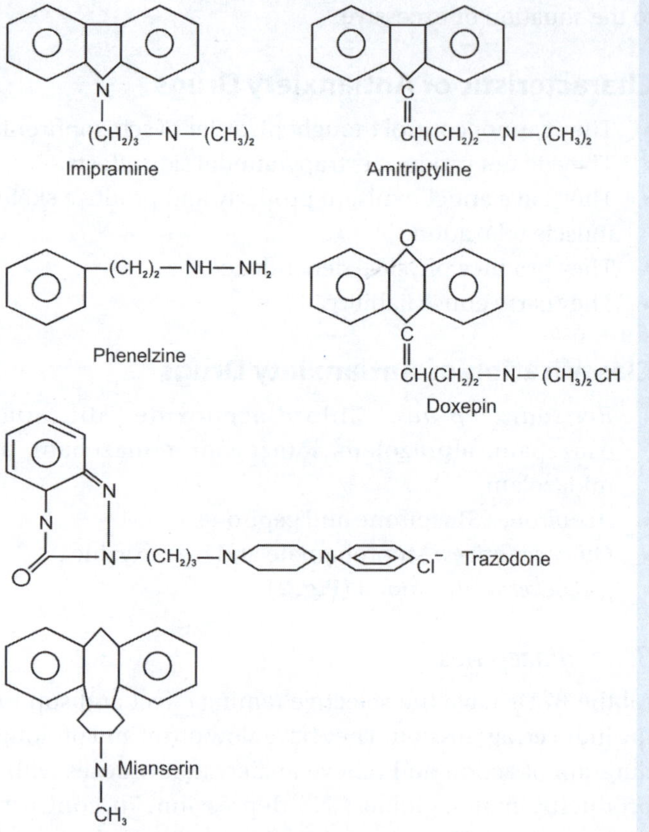

Fig. 3: Structural formula of some commonly used antidepressant.

irreversible. However, the newer types of MAOIs are selective for the MAO-A isoenzyme and cause their reversible inhibition (reversible inhibitor of monoamine oxidase type A or RIMA) **(Fig. 3)**.

Classification of Antidepressant Agents

- *Tricyclic antidepressants and related compounds:*
  - *Both noradrenaline and serotonin reuptake inhibitors:* Imipramine, trimipramine, amitriptyline, clomipramine, doxepin, and dothiepin.
  - *Selective noradrenaline reuptake inhibitors (NA > 5-HT):* Nortriptyline, desipramine, and reboxetine.
- *Nontricyclic selective serotonin reuptake inhibitors:* Fluoxetine, fluvoxamine, paroxetine, sertraline, citalopram, escitalopram, and dapoxetine.
- *Nontricyclic both NA and 5-HT reuptake inhibitors:* Venlafaxine, desvenlafaxine, and duloxetine.
- *Atypical:* Trazodone, mianserin, bupropion, tianeptine, amineptine, mirtazapine, and amoxapine.
- *MAO inhibitors:*
  - *Nonselective inhibitors:* Phenelzine, isocarboxazid, and tranylcypromine.

- *Selective inhibitors:*
  - *Selegiline (deprenyl):* Selective MAO-B inhibitors.
  - *Moclobemide and clorgyline:* Selective MAO-A inhibitors.

Pharmacological Action of TCA

The tricyclic antidepressants are used for the treatment of depression and chronic pain syndromes. The older TCAs inhibit the reuptake of both the monoamines (NA and 5-HT) and also block the variety of other receptors such as muscarinic, α-adrenergic, histamine (H_1), 5-HT_2, and occasionally dopamine (D_2). So, they have properties which include α-antagonistic, anticholinergic, antidopaminergic, and antihistaminic. However, the relative potencies to block these receptors differ among different compounds. The newer SSRIs and atypical TCAs interact with (block) fewer receptors and have more specific spectrum of action. So, they produce fewer side effects. The action of imipramine is described as prototype of all the TCAs and their related compounds **(Fig. 4)**.

In depressed patients, the TCA gradually elevates the mood. Patients become more communicative and start to take interest about their own surroundings. Thus, the TCAs are only antidepressants, but not euphoriants. They produce sedation, but this sedative property varies among different compounds. Most TCAs are potent anticholinergic and cause dry mouth, blurring of vision, constipation, and urinary hesitancy. The tolerance to this anticholinergic effect of TCAs develops gradually, but antidepressant action is maintained. They also potentiate the action of exogenous catecholamines. All the TCAs cause tachycardia and it is due to their anticholinergic and NA potentiating actions. Postural hypotension caused by TCAs is due to their inhibition of cardiovascular reflexes and α-blocking effect. The effects of TCA on cardiovascular system (CVS) are common and prominent. It occurs at therapeutic concentration of TCAs and may be dangerous in overdose. ECG changes due to TCAs are: T-wave suppression or inversion (most consistent changes), prolongation of PR interval, and widening of QRS complex. Arrhythmias may occur in the overdose of TCAs. It is due to the interference in intraventricular conduction and NA potentiating action combined with Ach blocking actions. The SSRI and atypical antidepressants are safer in this regard, but tolerance to these atypical antidepressants is higher and develops quickly. Increased appetite and weight gain is noted with most TCAs and trazodone, but not with SSRI and bupropion. Seizure threshold is lowered and fits may precipitate by TCAs. Cardiac arrhythmias induced by TCAs (especially in patients with ischemic heart disease) may be responsible for sudden death in these patients **(Fact file III)**.

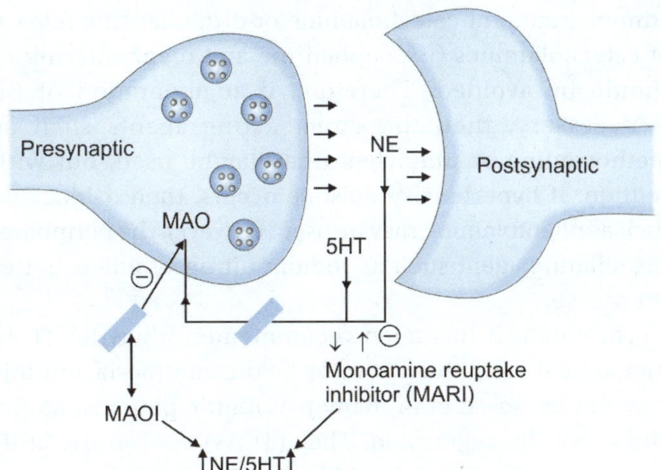

Fig. 4: Mechanism of action of antidepressant. (MAOI: monoamine oxidase inhibitor)

FACT FILE III

Tricyclic antidepressants and cardiovascular system:
In addition to producing anticholinergic effect and sedation, TCAs may cause CVS abnormalities. It includes arrhythmias and orthostatic hypotension. The TCA compounds try to slow the both ventricular and atrial depolarization. This is manifested as increased PR interval, QT interval, and wide QRS complex. These changes are benign and gradually disappear with continued therapy, in the absence of excessive plasma concentration. So, the previous thought that TCAs increase the risk of cardiac arrhythmias, is not now correct in the absence of overdose. In the presence of coexisting cardiac dysfunction, such as heart block, prolonged QT interval, etc. there may be increased risk. So, sometimes when the TCA therapy is contraindicated, due to patient's bad cardiac status, then electroconvulsive therapy (ECT) may be advised.

Anesthetic Implications and Drug Interaction between the Anesthetic Agents and TCAs

The interactions of TCAs with anesthetic drugs are common and generally predictable. The increased concentration of catecholamines at central sites by TCA may lead to the increased requirements of anesthetic agents and exaggerated response to endogenous or exogenous catecholamines. Similarly, the increased concentration of NA at postsynaptic sites in peripheral sympathetic nervous system is responsible for the increased systemic BP. This possibility for hypertensive crisis is maximum between the first 14 and 21 days during the acute treatment with TCA for acute depression. Whereas, the subsequent chronic management by TCA is associated with downregulation of receptors and decreased risk of hypertensive crisis, even after the administration of sympathomimetic agents. The threshold for ventricular dysrhythmias may also be lowered during chronic management by TCA. Still where possible, administration of catecholamine or drugs causing release of catecholamines (e.g., ephedrine and mephentermine) should be avoided. Therefore, if augmentation of BP is necessary, then the direct acting agents such as methoxamine or phenylephrine may be used, but with caution. If hypertensive episode occurs, then α-blockers such as phentolamine may be used. However, the peripheral vasodilating agent such as sodium nitroprusside is better alternative.

Although, it has been recommended that the TCAs should be discontinued 2 weeks before anesthesia, but this may not be possible in many psychiatric patients, as the illness will be aggravated. They (TCAs) abolish the anti-hypertensive action of clonidine by preventing their transport (reuptake) into adrenergic neurons. They potentiate the effect of other CNS depressants including alcohol and antihistamines. By their anticholinergic property, they (TCAs) delay gastric emptying. The centrally acting anticholinergic drugs (atropine, hyoscine, not glycopyrrolate) should be avoided as premedication for the patients taking TCAs, because their additive effect may precipitate confusion postoperatively, especially in the elderly. Dangerous hypertensive crisis with excitement and hallucination may occur, if MAOIs are used with TCAs.

Selective Serotonin Reuptake Inhibitors

This group of drugs was first introduced in 1987 and is now the most commonly prescribed antidepressant agents. They are highly selective for the inhibition of 5-HT reuptake at the presynaptic nerve terminal and are considerably less toxic than TCAs. The CVS side effects of it are very rare. Bradycardia has occasionally been reported. In patients with coronary artery disease, SSRI may precipitate coronary artery vasoconstriction. Nausea, vomiting, and diarrhea are the common side effects of SSRI due to the inhibition of 5-HT reuptake in GI tract. Platelet aggregation may occasionally be inspired. "Serotonin syndrome" may sometimes be precipitated by the addition of drugs such as MAOIs, TCAs, pethidine, or pentazocine, etc. with SSRI. It is due to the increased concentration of 5-HT at synaptic levels in brainstem and spinal cord. This syndrome consists of confusion, agitation, rigidity, autonomic instability, arrhythmias, and sometimes coma. The treatment of these symptoms is supportive. The acute withdrawal of SSRI, after its use for many years, may precipitate a syndrome of anxiety, agitation, and increased sweating. Unlike TCA, the SSRI lacks anticholinergic effects and do not generally affect cardiac conduction. They also do not cause postural hypotension or delayed conduction of cardiac impulses. The SSRI does not reduce the seizure threshold level.

Among the SSRI, fluoxetine is the potent inhibitor of certain cytochrome P_{450} enzymes. Hence, it may increase the plasma concentration of drug that depends on hepatic clearance. So, the addition of fluoxetine to TCA may result in three- to fivefold increase in plasma concentration of TCA. This mechanism may also be responsible for "serotonin syndrome".

Pharmacological Actions of MAOI

Monoamine oxidase inhibitors are the toxic psycho-pharmacological agents. So, the nonselective MAOIs are rarely used nowadays. However, the selective MAO-A inhibitors possess antidepressant property and is still used now in some countries. They are indicated in patients suffering from major depression, not responding to TCAs and in whom ECT is contraindicated or is refused. In contrast to TCAs, the MAOIs have negligible anticholinergic effects and do not sensitize the heart to cardiac arrhythmogenic effects of epinephrine. Orthostatic hypotension is the most common side effect, observed in patients, being treated with MAOIs. The mechanism for this orthostatic hypotension is unknown, but it may reflect the accumulation of some false neurotransmitters such as octopamine (also known as norsynephrine, chemically it is related to norepinephrine) which are less potent than norepinephrine.

Anesthetic Implication and Drug Interaction of MAOI

Certain varieties of cheese, beer, wines, pickled meat, and fish, etc. contain large quantities of tyramine and dopa. They are the precursors of norepinephrine (NE or NA). In MAO inhibited patients, these indirectly acting sympathomimetic amines escape degradation in intestinal wall and liver during their absorption. Then, reaching into systemic circulation, they displace the large amount of NA from transmitter-loaded adrenergic nerve endings, causing hypertensive crisis. This is called the "cheese reaction". It can be treated by IV injection of rapidly acting α-blocker, e.g., phentolamine, prazosin, or CPZ or directly acting vasodilators. Certain cold and cough preparations also contain some indirectly acting sympathomimetic amines (which act by stimulating the release of NE), e.g., ephedrine which causes in hypertension. So, any indirectly acting sympathomimetic agent, such as ephedrine and metaraminol, which may potentiate the hypertension, leading to crisis should be avoided. Excitement and hypertension also occur due to the increase in biological t½ of DA and NA that are produced from levodopa. The action of barbiturates, alcohol, opioids, and antihistamines is also intensified and prolonged by MAOIs.

The interaction between MAOIs and pethidine is also important, though uncommon. In this reaction, high fever, sweating, excitation, restlessness, rigidity, hypertension, delirium, convulsion, and severe respiratory depression with coma may occur. So, morphine appears to be the safe in this purpose. Other opiates which can safely be used with MAOIs include fentanyl, alfentanil, and remifentanil. The most accepted explanation of the reaction between MAOIs and pethidine is MAOIs retard the hydrolysis of pethidine, but not its demethylation. Thus, excess of norpethidine (normally a minor metabolite, but increase when hydrolysis is inhibited) is produced by the demethylation of pethidine which has profound excitatory action. The other possible explanation of this reaction is mass discharge from sympathetic nervous system, caused by the excess opioid and increased CNS concentration of 5-HT (secondary to blockade of 5-HT uptake). These hypertensive responses may be eliminated by the withdrawal of MAOIs, 2 weeks before anesthesia or by avoiding the administration of pethidine. But, like TCA, this also may not always be practical in the psychiatric patients, because the withdrawal of these agents (MAOIs) so long before surgery and anesthesia will produce recurrence of depression in more severe form. So, it is no longer recommended that these drugs (MAOIs) should be stopped 2 weeks preoperatively, but, care should be taken to avoid interaction with anesthetic drugs **(Fig. 5)**.

Benzodiazepines are most acceptable for preoperative treatment of anxiety in this group of patients. The induction of anesthesia in these patients can safely be performed with drugs like thiopentone and propofol. But, it will have to be kept in mind that the CNS depression effects and the depression of ventilation may be exaggerated. Ketamine is exception to this as it stimulates the sympathetic system. N_2O combined with volatile anesthetic agent is acceptable for the maintenance of anesthesia in patients taking MAOIs. But, halothane is not preferred as it may cause cardiac arrhythmia. Anesthetic requirement in these patients, taking MAOIs, is usually increased due to the increased level of catecholamines in their CNS. The spinal and epidural anesthesia is acceptable in this group of patients. But, hypotension and subsequent administration of vasopressors may put direction in favor of GA. If vasopressor is needed, then direct acting agent such as phenylephrine is the choice,

though ephedrine can be used with no apparent adverse effects. But, the doses of vasopressors should be reduced to minimize the likelihood of an exaggerated hypertensive response. The choice of nondepolarizing muscle relaxant is not influenced by MAOI with the possible exception of pancuronium. Pancuronium should be avoided in patients taking MAOIs, as it releases the stored adrenaline. Tranylcypromine is the most hazardous among all the MAOIs, due to its stimulant action. Phenelzine has been shown to decrease the pseudocholinesterase concentration and so there have been isolated reports of prolonged action of suxamethonium. This appears to be unique to phenelzine.

The new generation of selective MAO-A inhibitors such as RIMA (reversible inhibitors of monoamine oxidase-A) are now being increasingly used. They are of short half-life, well tolerated, have anticholinergic effects and do not cause postural hypotension. They have no central excitatory side effects, no interactions with TCAs, and a clinically insignificant response to ingesting tyramine. RIMA may still cause an excitatory response to pethidine. So, pethidine should be avoided in patients taking RIMA. Indirectly acting sympathomimetics (e.g., ephedrine, metaraminol) should also not be used with RIMA. Selegiline is a selective MAO-B inhibitor, used in the treatment of Parkinson's disease. Interactions of it with anesthetic agents are fewer than with the MAO-A inhibitors. Still, pethidine is best avoided and vasopressor should be used with care with MAO-B inhibitors.

Postoperative pain management is influenced by the interaction between MAOIs and opioids. If they are needed, then morphine and fentanyl is the drug of choice. But, the dose should be titrated according to the necessity to achieve desired analgesia. On the other hand, alternative to opioids is the nonsteroidal anti-inflammatory drug (NSAID) (nonopioid analgesics), peripheral nerve block, or transcutaneous electrical nerve stimulation (TENS). In such circumstances, the use of opioids through spinal or epidural route is not well studied.

Antimanic Agents

Mania is an autosomal dominant disease with variable penetrance among the off springs. It is manifested by inflated self-esteem, flight of ideas, short attention, decreased sleep, increased verbalization, etc. Lithium is the mainstay of antimanic treatment. Alternative treatment is the *carbamazepine or sodium valproate*.

Lithium

It is a small monovalent cation (Li^+) and is the drug of choice in the management of bipolar manic-depressive illness (MDI). It is extensively used at the centers where its serum levels

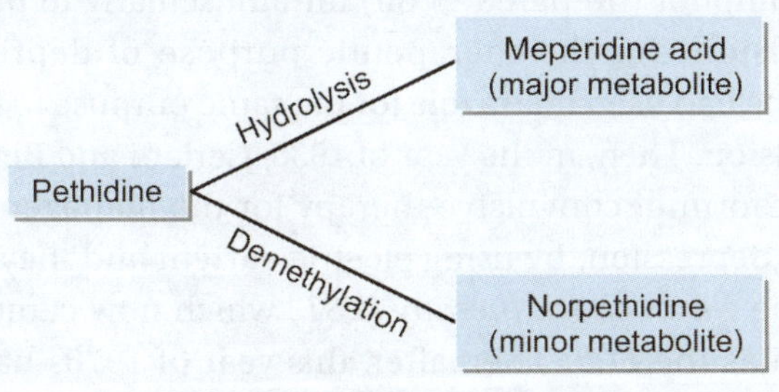

Fig. 5: Metabolism of pethidine.

can be measured accurately. Practically, it has no effect on normal individuals and is neither sedative nor euphoriant. On prolonged administration, it acts as a mood stabilizer in patients suffering from MDI. However, the mechanism of action of lithium is still not exactly known. Therefore, the probable explanations regarding the mechanism of action of lithium are:

- As the lithium (Li^+) resembles sodium ion (Na^+), so it penetrates through the voltage sensitive Na^+ channel and accumulates inside the cell, causing partial depolarization. Hence, Li^+ replaces body Na^+ and is equally distributed inside and outside of the cell. Thus, it affects the ionic movement across the cell membrane (mainly the brain cells) and modify the transmission of impulses, impairing the resting membrane potential (RMP) and the action potential of nerve cells.
- It decreases the release of NA and DA in brain without affecting the release of 5-HT. Thus, it may correct the imbalance in the turnover of brain monoamines.
- Li^+ inhibits the hydrolysis of inositol phosphate. Thus, it results in the reduction of the supply of free inositol for the regeneration of membrane phosphatidylinositol which is the source of inositol triphosphate (IP) and diacylglycerol (DAG). Thus, the hyperactivity of neurons, which is responsible for manic states, is reduced as the supply of inositol from extracellular sources is meager.

However, the hypothesis (i) and (ii) cannot explain why Li^+ has no effect on normal people, those are not suffering from MDI. Only hypothesis (iii) can explain this.

Li^+ is efficiently absorbed from stomach after its oral administration. It has a very low therapeutic window. So, as the margin of safety is narrow, therefore, the monitoring of serum Li^+ concentration is essential for its optimal therapy. Hence, the use of (Li^+), without monitoring its serum levels, is associated with unaccepted toxicity of lithium or no therapeutic effect. The therapeutic serum concentration of Li^+ for acute mania varies between 1 and 12 mEq/L. But, for prophylaxis, this level may fall to 0.6–0.8 mEq/L. The monitoring of serum lithium (Li^+) concentration by flame photometry usually 12 hours after its last oral dose is recommended. Because, it decreases the likelihood of its toxicity.

The toxicity of Li^+ occurs, when the serum concentration of it exceeds than 2 mEq/L. These Li^+ toxicities are manifested as skeletal muscle weakness, ataxia, sedation, widening of QRS complexes, atrioventricular (AV) block, hypotension, and seizures, etc. Lithium treatment can also cause hypothyroidism and vasopressin-resistant diabetes insipidus like syndrome (polyuria, polydipsia). The toxicity of lithium is also made worse by sodium depletion and dehydration.

Li^+ ion is handled in our body by kidney in the same way as that of Na^+ ion. So, most of the filtered Li^+ is reabsorbed from proximal convoluted tubule and is inversely related to the concentration of Na^+ ion in glomerular filtrate and its reabsorption through proximal convoluted tubule. Therefore, the loop diuretics and thiazides increases the concentration of serum lithium (Li^+) by enhancing the excretion of Na^+ and increasing the reabsorption of Li^+ by kidney. Hence, lithium toxicity is occurred in hyponatremic states, when there is intense attempt of renal conservation (reabsorption) of sodium and consequently the absence of Na^+ intense the absorption of lithium. When Na^+ is restricted then a large fraction of filtered Li^+ is also reabsorbed and vice versa. So, the IV administration of sodium-containing solution or osmotic diuretics favors the renal excretion of sodium and lithium in patients who show the evidences of lithium toxicity.

Anesthetic Implications

During preoperative evaluation of manic patients, especially those who are under lithium treatment, the search for any evidence of lithium toxicity is an important consideration and recently measured serum lithium concentration should be reviewed. In the perioperative period, Na^+-containing solution should be administered intravenously and judiciously to reduce the serum Li^+ level. Loop and thiazide diuretics should not be used or used very cautiously in patients receiving lithium. Monitoring of these patients by ECG for evidence of lithium-induced changes is useful to recognize the toxicity. Li^+ potentiates the sedative effect of intravenous and inhaled anesthetic agents and, therefore, their dose should be reduced. As lithium tends to act as an imperfect Na^+ ion, so potentiation of both depolarizing and nondepolarizing muscle relaxants occurs in patients receiving lithium and hence close monitoring of neuromuscular function is necessary. Lithium is contra-indicated in sick sinus syndrome.

Anesthesia and Electroconvulsive Therapy

For the first time, in the year of 1934, Von Meduna used 25% camphor (prepared in oil) intramuscularly to produce convulsions for the therapeutic purpose of depression. Later, he had used metrazole for the same purpose to induce convulsion. Then, in the year of 1938, Cerletti and Bini used a safer form of convulsive therapy for the management of severe depression, by using electric current and they called it as the *electroshock therapy (EST)* which now came to be known as the *ECT*. Thereafter, this year of 1970s had also saw a widespread criticism of ECT, restricting the use of it

BOX 1: Side effects of electroconvulsive therapy (ECT).

- Parasympathetic stimulation
- Bradycardia
- Hypotension
- Sympathetic stimulation
- Tachycardia
- Hypertension
- Dysrhythmias (cardiac)
- ↑Myocardial O_2 consumption
- ↑Cerebral blood flow
- ↑Intracranial pressure
- ↑Cerebral O_2 consumption
- ↑Intragastric pressure
- ↑Intraocular pressure

and making some modifications. However, following this modifications, now the ECT technique has become the much safer mode of treatment for severe psychiatric diseases which are unresponsive to the drugs or when the patient becomes acutely suicidal.

Some physiological effects of ECT are (Box 1):

- *Cardiovascular effect:* Immediate cardiovascular effects of ECT are bradycardia and hypotension. It is due to the immediate parasympathetic stimulation following ECT. After 1 minute of this parasympathetic stimulation, there is again sympathetic stimulation which is characterized by tachycardia, hypertension, dysrhythmias, increased myocardial O_2 consumption, etc.
- *Cerebral effect:* The important cerebral effects following ECT are increased cerebral blood flow, increased intracranial pressure (ICP), increased cerebral O_2 consumption, etc.
- *Others:* Other than cardiovascular and cerebral effects, increase in intragastric pressure, increase in intraocular pressure (IOP), etc. occur following ECT.

The contraindications of ECT are:

- *Absolute:* Recent myocardial infarction, recent cardio-vascular accident (CVA), ↑ICP due to intracranial mass lesion.
- *Relative:* Uncontrolled angina, congestive cardiac failure, severe pulmonary diseases, pheochromocytoma, severe hypertension, severe osteoporosis, major bone fractures, glaucoma, retinal detachment, etc. The pretreatment or preanesthetic assessment of patient waiting for ECT consists of (i) informed consent, (ii) detailed medical and psychiatric history, (iii) general and systemic physical examination, (iv) routine laboratory investigation on the light of history and examination, (v) ECG and plasma pseudocholinesterase level, (vi) examination of funds oculi (to rule out papilledema), etc.

So, some important points regarding the preoperative assessment of patients before ECT are:

- ECT is usually carried out in elderly patients who have a variety of coexisting diseases. So, an anesthetist must be very careful.
- The majority of patients are taking psychiatric drugs which have the potential to interact with anesthetic agents, used during GA for ECT.
- Patients are mostly noncooperative. So, histories are not reliable, even regarding the preoperative fasting.
- Sedative premedication, before ECT, is not always indicated, as it prolongs the recovery.
- ECT is a repeated procedure. So, previous anesthetic note should be studied carefully to see the effect of anesthesia on previous ECT.

The exact mechanism of action of ECT is still unclear. But one hypothesis states that ECT possibly affects the catecholamine pathways between the diencephalon (site of seizure generation) and limbic system (responsible for mood disorder), involving hypothalamus which is responsible for severe psychiatric illness. The previous concept of the therapeutic benefit of ECT on psychiatric illness depends on the production of generalized tonic-clonic seizures. But, that is not correct. Because, now it is established that the therapeutic efficacy of ECT is related to the amount of electric current passing through the brain, but not on the production of tonic-clonic seizures. The electrical stimulus given during ECT produces grand mal seizure which consists of brief tonic phase followed by long clonic phase. The electroencephalography (EEG) changes during ECT is similar to that of spontaneous grand mal seizure and typically 8–10 ECT is necessary which show 80% favorable response.

The techniques used for the administration of ECT are of two types: (1) direct ECT and (2) modified ECT. In direct technique, ECT is given in the absence of muscular relaxation and GA. This is infrequently used now. In the later technique, ECT is now modified to reduce or avoid generalized tonic-clonic seizure by drug-induced muscular relaxation and GA.

General anesthesia is usually administered to ensure the patient's safety and comfort during ECT. Patients are fasted as in GA. Sedative premedications are usually not used, because it prolongs the period of recovery following ECT. Anticholinergic (atropine or glycopyrrolate) is given before induction of anesthesia or delivery of electric current. This is to decrease the oral secretions and to prevent the vagal stimulation during ECT which can cause severe bradycardia or even cardiac arrest. Bradyarrhythmias are also particularly common during stimulus titration where subconvulsive stimuli are used to determine the seizure threshold. Centrally acting anticholinergic drugs such as atropine may have synergistic effects with central and peripheral anticholinergic effects of TCA which the patients are already taking and manifests as delirium and confusion during postanesthetic period. For this reason, glycopyrrolate is preferred to atropine when ECT is administered to patients being treated with TCA. Sympathetic stimulation during ECT in patients with cardiovascular disease may be undesirable. So, high rise of BP and tachycardia during intubation and electric current therapy can be controlled by esmolol (50–200 µg/kg/min) or nitroglycerin or nitroprusside. Monitoring of ECG is useful for recognizing ECT-induced cardiac dysrhythmias.

For induction during ECT, the commonly used inducing agents are thiopentone, propofol, or methohexital. However, among these, methohexital is the inducing agent of choice and is used most commonly in the dose of 0.5–1 mg/kg through IV. Thiopentone has no advantage over methohexital and may be associated with longer recovery time, but it can be used. The prior treatment of patients with TCAs or MAOIs could enhance the sedative effects of thiopentone. Propofol in the dose of 1–2 mg/kg is now also the agent of choice, giving rapid onset and recovery. Like thiopentone, ketamine, and etomidate have also been successfully used for induction of GA in ECT.

The use of muscle relaxants in ECT has virtually eliminated the potentially dangerous skeletal muscle contractions by the stimulation of electric current and the fracture of bone that can be produced by seizure activity. Succinylcholine in a dose of 0.3–0.5 mg/kg through IV route is the most commonly used muscle relaxant for ECT. This lower dose of succinylcholine is particularly selected, because it helps in sufficient visual confirmation of seizure activity during ECT. When it is not possible to visualize the seizure activity due to higher doses of muscle relaxants, then the most reliable method to confirm electrically induced seizure activity is the EEG. Alternatively, one limb can be isolated from the effect of muscle relaxant by applying tourniquet before its administration to see the seizure activity. Low dose of mivacurium (0.08 mg/kg) has also been tried. But although the recovery in case of mivacurium was found to be good, still seizure modification was inadequate. Therefore, if mivacurium is used, the dose should be at least 0.15 mg/kg and reversal will probably be necessary. Longer acting muscle relaxing agents are not generally suitable for ECT.

Provided, there are no risks for aspiration, then the airway and arterial oxygenation can normally be maintained with an oral airway and mask, unless muscle relaxants are used. Ventilatory support and the delivery of supplemental O_2 by mask and intermittent positive-pressure ventilation (IPPV) are recommended both before the production of seizure and until the effects of succinylcholine or mivacurium have been dissipated. After the induction of anesthesia (but before application of ECT stimulation), hyperventilation of patient's lungs by bag and mask lowers the seizure threshold and prolongs the duration of seizure. Thus, it increases the effectiveness of ECT. When the limbs become flaccid by muscle relaxant, then a rubber "bite block" is inserted into the mouth, between the teeth, before electrical stimulation is applied. This will prevent the damage to lips, tongue, and teeth during convulsion by electrical stimulation which is given after induction and muscular paralysis by muscle relaxant. During seizure, artificial ventilation with O_2 is continued to avoid arterial desaturation, until adequate spontaneous ventilation has returned.

The denitrogenation of patient's lung, by 100% O_2, before the production of convulsion by ECT, decreases the likelihood of arterial hypoxemia, if it becomes difficult or impossible to support the ventilation in the presence of seizure-induced skeletal muscle contractions. After ECT, the patients should be recovered in lateral position by trained nursing staff, with equipment available immediately, for the treatment of any emergency. Furthermore, it is important to keep in the mind of an anesthetist that apnea may last for 2–3 minutes following ECT, requiring ventilation, even in the absence of succinylcholine. The monitoring of arterial O_2 saturation by pulse oximetry is mandatory to guide the need for supplemental O_2 and mechanical ventilation for patients undergoing ECT. It is confirmed that ECT does not increase the succinylcholine-induced release of potassium. But, the monitoring of succinylcholine-induced neuromuscular blockade by peripheral nerve stimulator is also sometimes necessary, because repeated anesthesia is given by it for ECT. The use of peripheral nerve stimulator may help to identify the degree of blockade by succinylcholine with previously unrecognized atypical cholinesterase enzyme. It is also possible to establish the dose of anesthetic inducing drug and succinylcholine that will produce the most predictable and desirable effects in each patient.

Special attention should also be given to the patients with permanent pacemaker, waiting for ECT. But, fortunately most pacemakers have inbuilt safety measures, such as a shield, which are not affected by electrical currents, necessary to produce seizures. During the ECT of a patient with pacemaker, an external magnate should always be kept ready for converting the pacemaker mode to a synchronous nondemand mode, if the malfunctioning of pacemaker occurs in response to the externally delivered electrical current. The continuous monitoring of cardiac activity by ECG and peripheral arterial pulses by palpation is very important for uninterrupted function of artificial cardiac pacemaker.

Obstetrics Analgesia and Anesthesia

■ INTRODUCTION

The anesthetic care during all obstetric procedures [from normal vaginal delivery to cesarean section (CS) to other obstetrical surgeries] usually accounts for approximately 10–15% of total anesthetic procedures. Always, as an obstetric anesthetist, we should keep in our mind that the patients (obviously female), who enter the obstetric wing of a hospital, may potentially require any type of anesthetic care, either for labor analgesia or for CS which may be an emergency or maybe a planned one or other obstetric procedures such as the manual separation of placenta and cesarean hysterectomy. Hence, anesthesiologists those are in duty at an obstetric unit of a hospital should be cautious about the relevant history of all parturient patients after their admission. This history will include (1) the present and past medical, surgical, and obstetrics history, (2) the parity of patient, (3) the age of patient, and (4) the duration of pregnancy, etc. The patient should also be examined previously with the potential idea of future planned or emergency surgery. These preanesthetic examinations of a patient include (1) a general survey with special attention to blood pressure (BP), (2) airway assessment, (3) an examination of the spinal cord for regional anesthesia (RA), etc.

Regardless of the time of last oral intake, all obstetric patients should be considered to have a full stomach. So, they are all at the increased risk of pulmonary aspiration, if surgery is at all needed. Therefore, those patients who are especially at high possibility of operative delivery should take nothing per mouth, during the progress of labor. On the other hand, if the labor is uncomplicated, then a small amount of clear fluid can be provided, during prolonged labor. However, if there is any doubt, then the prophylactic oral administration of 0.3 M sodium citrate, at every 2–3 hours intervals, will help to maintain the gastric pH above 2.5 and will decrease the chances of aspiration pneumonitis.

This prophylaxis against aspiration pneumonitis also can be taken by oral or parenteral use of H_2 blocker/proton pump inhibitor (PPI) and metoclopramide in high-risk patients who are expected to receive general anesthesia (GA). The PPIs/H_2 blockers will reduce both the volume of gastric secretion and pH after its administration. But it has no effect on gastric contents which is already present.

On the other hand, metoclopramide reduces the gastric volume which is already present, by accelerating gastric emptying. But it cannot increase gastric pH. Contrary, it increases the tone of lower esophageal sphincter and reduces the incidences of gastric regurgitation. All the parturient patients should be placed in 15° left lateral position by a wedge, placed under their right hip to avoid inferior vena caval compression by gravid uterus and the reduction of preload.

The majorities of obstetric patients are in child-bearing age and therefore are healthy. So, they are considered to be at very less anesthetic risk. But certain changes in their body, due to pregnancy, such as pregnancy-induced hypertension (PIH), preeclamptic toxemia (PET), excessive weight gain, edema, and certain other medical diseases, which are aggravated by pregnancy, increase the obstetric anesthetic risk. The obstetric maternal mortality rate is calculated as the number of maternal death divided by the number of live birth. Recently, this rate has decreased tremendously and now approximately this number has touched to 6–12 per 100,000 live births.

The principal causes of maternal death associated with live birth are pulmonary embolism (20%), PIH (20%), sepsis (15%), cardiomyopathy (10%), hemorrhage (5%), cerebrovascular accident (4%), anesthesia (3%), and other medical condition (20%). On the other hand, the most common cause, among these aforementioned causes of maternal morbidity, which are encountered during obstetric practice, is severe hemorrhage and severe preeclampsia. Anesthesia itself accounts for approximately 2–4% of total obstetric maternal death. The anesthetic risk factors for this maternal death include age over 35 years, multiple pregnancies, black patients, PIH, previous postpartum hemorrhage (PPH), emergency lower uterine cesarean section (LUCS), etc. Among the anesthetic causes the most maternal deaths occur during or after LUCS. Recently this figure has been reduced, due to the frequent use of RA than GA.

PHYSIOLOGICAL CHANGES DURING PREGNANCY

Before any discussion, regarding anesthesia and analgesia in obstetrics, every clinician (anesthetist) should have profound knowledge, about the changes, which occur during the whole period of pregnancy and delivery. This is because pregnancy affects virtually all the organs of a female body and brings about multiple changes which alter the usual responses to anesthesia and analgesia and its related drugs. Many of these changes are physiological and appear to be adaptive and useful to the mother in tolerating the stresses of pregnancy, labor, and delivery. These changes occur due to mechanical and hormonal influences and are appeared to be useful to meet the increased demands of placenta, uterus, and fetus, and to tolerate (meet) the increased stress, that occurred during pregnancy, labor, and delivery. For example, during the whole period of pregnancy (280 days calculated from the first day of the last menstrual period) the uterus itself increases in weight from 30 to 1,000 g which has profound implications on anesthesia that is discussed later.

Changes in Cardiovascular System

The changes in the cardiovascular system (CVS) that occur during pregnancy, serve two functions. These are (1) to maintain increased uteroplacental circulation which is necessary to continue a pregnancy, and (2) to maintain the increased exchange of O_2, CO_2, nutrients, and other waste products between the mother and fetus.

The maternal blood volume increases by about 40% during the whole period of pregnancy. But the plasma volume increases (55%) in excess than that of the red cell volume (45%). Therefore, it apparently reduces the concentration of hemoglobin (Hb) and produces dilutional anemia in pregnancy which is physiological in nature. This dilution of blood reduces its viscosity and causes better perfusion (circulation) in tissues, which thus offsets the side effects of anemia, by increasing the delivery of O_2 to tissues. This drawback of physiological anemia is further offset by an increase in cardiac output (CO) and the shifting of the O_2-Hb dissociation curve toward the right. The blood volume increases by about 1,000–1,500 mL at term (total blood

TABLE 1: Cardiovascular changes during pregnancy.

Parameters	Changes
Blood volume	+35%
Plasma volume	+55%
Red blood cell (RBC) volume	+45%
Heart rate	+10–15%
Stroke volume	+25–30%
Cardiac output	+35–40%
Systolic pressure	−5 to 10 mm Hg
Diastolic pressure	−15 to 20 mm Hg
Systemic vascular resistance (SVR)	−15 to 20%

(+) = increase, (−) = decrease

volume reaches about 90 mL/kg) and this will allow a woman to tolerate the blood loss, during her delivery which is near about 400–500 mL in vaginal delivery, and 800–1,000 mL during CS. However, this increased blood volume returns to normal 1–2 weeks after delivery **(Table 1)**.

During pregnancy cardiac output also increases by about 40%. This increase in cardiac output is due to both the increase in heart rate (20%) and stroke volume (30%). The increased stroke volume is again due to myocardial hypertrophy and enlargement of cardiac chambers. *However, the pulmonary, central venous, and pulmonary occlusion pressure remains unchanged.* Most of these changes in cardiac output are observed during the first trimester and to a lesser extent during the second trimester of pregnancy. In the third trimester, the cardiac output does not appreciably increases, except during the process of labor and delivery. The greatest increase in cardiac output is seen during labor and immediately after delivery. Cardiac output then often does not return to normal until 2 weeks after delivery.

After 28 weeks of pregnancy, the cardiac output decreases in the supine position. This is due to the compression of inferior vena cava by gravid uterus and the impairment of venous return to the heart. This is called the *supine hypotension syndrome* and is found in 20% of patient. This syndrome is characterized by dizziness, restlessness, hypotension, pallor, sweating, nausea and vomiting, etc., when the patient lies directly on her back. Turning the patient on her side typically improves these symptoms. So, a pregnant patient with >28 weeks gestation should never be placed supine. Better, she should be placed in left lateral position and this can be performed by placing a wedge (>15°) under her right hip.

The Trendelenburg position of patient due to any cause also increases this compression on inferior vena cava and the risk of supine hypotension syndrome. The abdominal aorta is also compressed by gravid uterus when the woman lies in the supine position. This results in decreased circulation in femoral artery and more importantly the uteroplacental blood flow. This reduction in uteroplacental blood flow, produced by aortocaval compression, causes decreased cardiac output (due to reduction of preload), decreased uterine arterial perfusion (due to compression of aorta), increased uterine venous pressure (due to vena caval compression) and increased sympathetic tone. All these factors (changes) result in fetal hypoxia and acidosis.

During the process of labor, the contraction of uterus relieves this compression on inferior vena cava, but increases the compression on aorta. However, these problems of aortocaval compression will be grossly aggravated, following sympathetic blockade, during subarachnoid or epidural anesthesia. Therefore, the strict avoidance of supine position and adequate intravenous (IV) fluid to increase preload are the very essential part of any technique of RA.

Due to the elevation of diaphragm by an enlarged gravid uterus, the heart is also displaced upward, laterally, and forward. This results in (1) the appearance of a normal heart to an enlarged heart on a plain chest X-ray and (2) also the left axis deviation and T-wave changes in an electrocardiogram (ECG). Thus, the usual changes in ECG during pregnancy show the flattened T-waves or Q-waves in lead III as well as the innocent depression of the ST segment. Sinus tachycardia, premature ventricular contractions, or bouts of paroxysmal atrial tachycardia are also more common in pregnancy. In the first trimester of pregnancy, systemic vascular resistance (SVR) is reduced substantially. It decreases both the diastolic and systolic BP, but the reduction of diastolic BP is more than systolic BP. This decrease of SVR is maximum at the middle of the second trimester. Then, it passes through a plateau or slight increase for the remaining part of pregnancy. During pregnancy, the central venous pressure, pulmonary artery pressure, and pulmonary capillary wedge pressure are all usually remaining unchanged.

The physical examination of a pregnant patient often reveals (1) an exaggerated splitting of first heart sound, (2) an audible third heart sound, and (3) a soft systolic ejection flow murmur (grade I and II). Chronic partial obstruction of inferior vena cava (IVC) in the third trimester of pregnancy predisposes to venous stasis and edema of lower extremities. Further, this compression of IVC below the diaphragm distends and increases the blood flow through the paravertebral venous plexuses, including the epidural venous plexuses.

Respiratory System (Table 2)

With the progressive enlargement of uterus, diaphragm is gradually elevated upward in the thorax which is about 4–5 cm

TABLE 2: Respiratory changes during pregnancy.

Parameters	Changes
O_2 consumption	+20–50%
Respiratory rate	+15%
Tidal volume	+40%
IRV	+20%
Alveolar ventilation	+70%
PaO_2	+10%
Minute ventilation	+50%
Airway resistance	−35%
Total compliance	−30%
Residual volume	−20%
FRC	−20%
Closing capacity	Unchanged
Vital capacity	Unchanged

(FRC: functional residual capacity; IRV: inspiratory reserve volume; PaO_2: arterial partial pressure of oxygen)

in height. This reduces the volume of lungs. But usually, it is compensated by an increase in both the anteroposterior and transverse diameter of thoracic cavity, due to the hormone-induced relaxation of costal ligaments. This explains why thoracic breathing is favored over abdominal breathing in pregnancy. In pregnancy, O_2 consumption is increased by 20%. Therefore, to meet this increased need (demand) of O_2, the minute and alveolar ventilation is also increased by 50 and 70%, respectively. This is again due to the increase in both tidal volume and respiratory rate.

In pregnancy, the vital capacity (VC) and closing capacity (CC) remain unaltered, but the functional residual capacity (FRC) is reduced by 20%. This is principally due to the reduction in expiratory reserve volume, as the result of larger than normal tidal volume. Therefore, CC exceeds FRC in 50% of pregnant women and early closure of the airway occurs with normal tidal volume (during normal respiration). This is again more usual when the patient lies in the supine position and so atelectasis with hypoxemia occurs more readily in this position. This phenomenon along with increased O_2 consumption explains the cause of rapid O_2 desaturation during the period of apnea, and explains why preoxygenation with 100% O_2 prior to the induction of GA is mandatory to avoid hypoxia in pregnant woman. However, FRC returns to normal within 48 hours after delivery.

Due to the increase in ventilation, partial pressure of carbon dioxide ($PaCO_2$) decreases up to 25–30 mm Hg, causing respiratory alkalosis. This is compensated by the decrease in plasma HCO_3^- level. The pregnancy-induced respiratory alkalosis reduces the unloading of O_2 at the tissue level. But this is compensated by an increase in arterial partial pressure of oxygen (PaO_2) due to hyperventilation, an increase in 2,3-diphosphoglycerate (2,3-DPG) level which decreases the affinity O_2 to Hb (P_{50} of maternal Hb increases from 27 to 30 mm Hg), and increase in cardiac output which enhances the delivery of O_2 to tissues.

Pregnancy is associated with decreased airway resistance and pulmonary compliance. The anatomical dead space usually remains unaltered in pregnancy, but the physiological dead space and intrapulmonary shunt increase gradually as the pregnancy advances. The flow–volume loops of the lungs are unaffected by pregnancy. A chest X-ray during pregnancy often reveals prominent vascular markings and it is due to increased pulmonary blood volume increased pulmonary circulation and raised diaphragm.

During pregnancy, capillary dilatation, and edema of mucous membrane occurs throughout the respiratory tract. This easily predisposes the upper airway to trauma, bleeding, and obstruction. Hence, a small endotracheal (ET) tube than the calculated one and gentle laryngoscopy is essential during the administration of GA in pregnancy.

Central Nervous System

The pregnancy has also profound effects on the central nervous system (CNS), but the actual mechanism of which is still not known. However, probably it is due to the high concentration of progesterone, associated with pregnancy. It decreases the dose of inhaled anesthetic agents. The minimum alveolar concentration (MAC) value of all the volatile anesthetic agents is decreased by up to 40% in pregnancy which again returns to normal on the third day, after delivery. Like volatile anesthetic agents, local anesthetic (LA) agents also show higher sensitivity to neurons during pregnancy. Therefore, less amount of LA agents (30% reduction) is required during RA (spinal or epidural) to produce the same level of analgesia and anesthesia. This event can be explained by two mechanisms (1) *hormonal* and (2) *mechanical*. The hormonal effect is mediated by progesterone and β-endorphin which make the nervous tissue more sensitive to LA agents. During the whole period of pregnancy, there is a 20 times increase in the level of progesterone and there is also a surge of β-endorphin levels during labor and delivery.

The mechanical effect, causing a reduced dose of LA agent during spinal or epidural anesthesia, is due to the obstruction of inferior vena cava by gravid uterus. This causes the distention of epidural venous plexus. Therefore, the volume of the potential epidural space and subarachnoid space are reduced. This enhances the more cephalad spread of the same volume of LA agents during both the spinal and epidural anesthesia in pregnant than nonpregnant

state and needs the reduced doses of the drug (LA agent). The bearing down during labor further accentuates all these effects. The term minimum local analgesic concentration (MLAC) is used in obstetric analgesia and anesthesia to compare the relative potencies of local anesthetic agents. The MLAC is defined as the local analgesic concentration, leading to satisfactory analgesia in 50% of patients (EC_{50}).

Gastrointestinal Effects

Pregnancy places parturient women at higher risk for regurgitation and pulmonary aspiration. This is due to the hormonal and mechanical effects. The hormonal effect, responsible for higher risk to regurgitation, is due to the higher level of progesterone and gastrin, secreted from placenta. This high level of progesterone decreases the tone of lower gastroesophageal sphincter and increases the chance of regurgitation. On the other hand, gastrin increases the secretion of HCl in the stomach. The enlarged gravid uterus displaces the stomach upward and anteriorly. This again promotes the incompetence of lower gastroesophageal sphincter. Thus, the aforementioned three factors (progesterone, gastrin, and upward displacement of stomach) increase the risk for severe aspiration pneumonitis during GA in pregnancy. Nearly, all the pregnant patients have gastric pH <2.5, and the residual volume of gastric secretion is >25 mL. Thus, it has also a profound effect on causing pulmonary complications.

The effect of pregnancy on gastric emptying time is in controversial. It is particularly delayed following the administration of opiates for labor analgesia. Otherwise, gastric emptying takes place at widely variable rates during pregnancy. Anticholinergic agents delay this gastric emptying and reduce the tone of lower gastroesophageal sphincter. Contrary, prokinetic agents like metoclopramide usually speed up gastric emptying but is unable to reverse the effects of opiate and anticholinergic agent. However, the spinal and epidural anesthesia does not affect the gastric emptying time. It is the loss of tone of lower gastroesophageal sphincter and not the rise of intra-abdominal or intragastric pressure which is responsible for the high incidences of gastroesophageal reflux (heartburn) and esophagitis, occurring during pregnancy. However, the intragastric pressure remains unchanged throughout the pregnancy.

Hematological Changes (Table 3)

The maternal blood volume increases markedly during pregnancy. This increase in blood volume results from both the increase in plasma and erythrocyte volume. The usual pattern is that there is an initial increase in plasma volume and this is followed by an increase in the volume

TABLE 3: Hematological changes during pregnancy.

Parameters	Changes
Plasma volume	+40%
Red cell volume	+20%
Total blood volume	+45%
Hematocrit	−15%
Plasma albumin	−15%
Plasma globulin	+50%
Plasma fibrinogen	+50%
Plasma cholinesterase	−30%

of circulating erythrocytes, due to increased erythropoiesis. But the increase in plasma volume is much more than the increase in the volume of erythrocytes. So, the concentration of Hb apparently (falsely) decreases during pregnancy, due to the dilutional effect. The average Hb concentration at term is 12 g/dL, as compared to the level of 13 g/dL for nonpregnant women. The Hb concentration below 11 g/dL, especially in late pregnancy, is suggestive of an abnormal process. The blood leucocyte count varies considerably during normal pregnancy. Usually, it ranges from 5,000 to 12,000/mm^3 of blood. But during labor and early puerperium, it may become markedly elevated, attaining levels of 25,000/mm^3.

Pregnancy is a hypercoagulable state and it is beneficial in limiting the loss of blood during delivery. This is because; the plasma levels of several coagulation factors are increased during pregnancy. The concentration of plasma fibrinogen (factor I) increases by about 50%. The normal value of it ranges between 200 and 400 mg/dL (average 300 mg/dL). In pregnancy, it increases to an average value of 450 mg/dL (ranges between 300 and 600 mg/dL). The other clotting factors, and activation of which are increased appreciably during pregnancy are factors VII, VIII, IX, X, and XII. But the level of factor II (prothrombin) does not increase or increases only slightly during pregnancy, whereas the clotting factors XI and XIII are decreased during pregnancy. However, the prothrombin time and partial thromboplastin time (PTT) are both shortened slightly as pregnancy progresses.

Although some investigators have described a moderate decrease (10%) in the number of platelets, but still there is some controversy regarding this fact. This is because clotting time does not differ significantly between normal pregnant and nonpregnant women. Pregnancy is associated with the lower levels of antithrombin III and an increased level of plasminogen (profibrinolysin). Plasmin is called fibrinolysin and accelerated action of this fibrinolysin is observed in the third trimester of pregnancy. In spite of dilutional anemia, leukocytosis (up to 20,000/mm^3 or μL) is usually encountered during the third trimester of pregnancy.

Renal Changes

Apparently, the kidney increases in size slightly during pregnancy. Glomerular filtration rate (GFR) and renal blood flow (RBF) increase up to 50% during early pregnancy. This elevated GFR has been found to persist up to term, whereas the RBF decreases toward the nonpregnant value during the third trimester of pregnancy. Pregnancy is associated with increased renin and aldosterone secretion which subsequently promotes increased Na$^+$ and water retention. This causes the increased circulating volume of blood during pregnancy. During pregnancy, the concentration of creatinine and urea in plasma decreases up to the levels of 0.5–0.6 and 8–9 mg/dL, respectively as a consequence of increased GFR. Sometimes, the urea concentration during pregnancy may be as low as to suggest impaired hepatic synthesis, which often occurs with severe liver disease. So, creatinine clearance is the most useful test for renal function, during pregnancy.

The glycosuria, which is often found during pregnancy, is not necessarily always taken as an abnormal finding. The appreciable increase in glomerular filtration rate, together with the impaired renal tubular reabsorption capacity for glucose, is responsible for this huge amount of filtered glucose to pass through urine, causing glycosuria in pregnancy. Even though glycosuria is common during pregnancy, still the possibility of diabetes mellitus, which has separate implications on pregnancy, cannot be ignored. Proteinuria does not occur normally during pregnancy, except occasionally a mild one (<300 mg/dL) during or soon after vigorous labor. If not the result of contamination during collection, blood cells in urine during pregnancy indicate the disease, somewhere in the urinary tract. Plasma osmolality decreases by 8–10 mOsm/kg.

Hepatic Changes

During pregnancy, there are no distinct changes in the size and the morphology of liver. The overall hepatic function remains unchanged throughout the whole period of pregnancy, except for a minor increase in serum transaminases and lactic dehydrogenase levels in plasma, during the third trimester. The total alkaline phosphatase activity in serum approximately becomes double during normal pregnancy and commonly reaches a level that would be considered abnormal in a nonpregnant woman. Much of this increase in serum alkaline phosphatase level is due to the secretion of it from placenta. Pregnancy is associated with a decrease in plasma albumin level, showing it to average 3 g/dL, compared with 4–6 g/dL in nonpregnant women. This probably is due to expanded plasma volume. But globulin level in plasma increases in pregnancy and results in a decrease in albumin to globulin ratio, similar to that found in certain hepatic diseases. There is also a 30% reduction in serum (pseudo) cholinesterase activity in pregnancy. But rarely, it is associated with the prolonged action of succinylcholine. This decreased activity of pseudocholinesterase persists up to 6 weeks after delivery. But the breakdown of mivacurium by pseudocholinesterase does not appreciably alter during pregnancy.

The high level of progesterone during pregnancy appears to inhibit the release of cholecystokinin, resulting in incomplete emptying of the gallbladder. The latter, together with altered bile acid composition, can predispose to the formation of cholesterol gallstones, during pregnancy.

Metabolic Changes

In response to the rapidly growing fetus and placenta and their increasing metabolic demands, the pregnant woman undergoes some metabolic changes that are numerous and intensed. This is because of the altered carbohydrate, fat, and protein metabolism that favors fetal growth and development. The first and foremost metabolic changes that occur in pregnancy is weight gain of the mother. This large increase in maternal body weight during pregnancy is the result of metabolic alterations, especially retention of water, and the deposition of fat and protein. The average total gain of body weight in a pregnant woman during the whole period of pregnancy is about 11 kg and the minimum amount of extra water that an average pregnant woman could be expected to retain is about 6.5 L. The total accumulation of protein throughout the whole pregnancy is 1 kg, out of which 500 g is needed for the development of the fetus and placenta and another 500 g is required for the development of rest such as the uterus (as contractile protein), plasma protein, and Hb.

The pregnancy is potentially a diabetogenic process. So, an already present diabetes mellitus in a woman will be aggravated or a subclinical asymptomatic individual becomes an overt one when she becomes pregnant. The diabetogenic effect of pregnancy is principally due to the lactogen, secreted from placenta, which is called the *placental lactogen*. It opposes the action of insulin and produces or aggravates the diabetes mellitus. Thus, the ability of placental lactogen to oppose the action of insulin leads to increased maternal secretion of insulin. Therefore, the hyperplasia of the beta cells of pancreas will occur in response to increased demand for insulin secretions. The placental lactogen also promotes lipolysis which brings about an increase in the level of plasma-free fatty acid. These plasma-free fatty acids will provide an alternative source for energy other than glucose in the mother. Hence, in pregnancy, starvation will induce much more intense ketonemia and ketonuria.

The plasma lipid level increases appreciably during the later half of pregnancy. This increased level of plasma lipid involves the total lipids, esterified and nonesterified cholesterol, phospholipids, neutral fat, lipoproteins, etc.

PLACENTAL EXCHANGE INCLUDING RESPIRATORY GASES

Exchange of respiratory gases and different other nutrients and wastes between the fetal and maternal circulation through the placenta occurs by one of the six mechanisms.

These mechanisms are:

1. *Diffusion:* Respiratory gases (O_2 and CO_2), anesthetic gases, and small ions are exchanged by diffusion between the fetal and maternal blood through the placenta. Most anesthetic drugs, used through IV have molecular weights well under 1,000 and so also can readily diffuse through the placenta.

   At term, the fetal O_2 consumption is near about 7 mL/kg/min. The normal PaO_2 of fetal blood in placenta is 30–35 mm Hg. The fetal Hb has a higher affinity for O_2 (the fetal O_2 dissociation curve is shifted to the left) than the affinity of mother Hb to O_2 (the mother O_2 dissociation curve is shifted to the right). This helps the diffusion O_2 from mother to fetus. In addition, fetal Hb concentration is usually 15 g/dL, compared to mother's Hb concentration of 12 g/dL and it also helps in diffusion of O_2 from mother to fetus.

   Carbon dioxide readily diffuses across the placenta. Maternal hyperventilation increases the gradient for the transfer of CO_2 from the fetus into mother. Fetal Hb has less affinity for CO_2 than that of adult form of Hb.

2. *Osmotic process and hydrostatic pressure (bulk flow):* Water only moves between fetus and mother through the placenta by this osmotic process under hydrostatic pressure.

3. *Facilitated diffusion:* Glucose mainly enters the fetal circulation from maternal circulation through the placenta by this process. In this process, glucose is transported with the help of a transporter molecule from higher to lower concentration, without any consumption of energy.

4. *Active transport:* In this process, amino acids, vitamins, fatty acids, and some ions (Ca^{2+} and PO_4^{2-}) are transported from maternal to fetal circulation with the help of transporter molecules and energy.

5. *Vesicular transport:* It is also called pinocytosis. Large molecules, such as immunoglobulins are transported by this process. Fe also enters the fetal circulation by this process, with the help of ferritin and transferrin.

6. *Breaks:* There are some discontinuations (breaks) in fetal and maternal membranes and through these breaks maternal and fetal blood mixes with each other. This is probably responsible for Rhesus (Rh) sensitization.

■ UTEROPLACENTAL CIRCULATION

The delivery of most of the substances, essential for the growth and the metabolism of the fetus and placenta as well as the removal of most of the metabolic wastes from them, depends upon adequate perfusion through uterus and placenta. This is called the uteroplacental circulation and in turn it depends upon the blood flow through uterus by uterine and ovarian arteries and veins, and through the placenta by umbilical arteries and veins. There is a progressive increase in uteroplacental blood flow throughout the pregnancy. It represents about 10% of total cardiac output or 500 mL/min in late pregnancy. Among these, 80% of the flow goes to placental circulation and the rest goes to the growing myometrium of uterus.

During pregnancy, due to the maximum dilatation of uterine vasculature, its autoregulation is lost. Then, the blood flow through uteroplacental circulation is directly proportional to the difference between the uterine arterial and venous pressure, and inversely proportional to the uterine vascular resistance. During this autoregulation, the uterine arteries are under the control of neural mechanisms which are mediated by mainly α-adrenergic receptors and to a lesser extent by β-adrenergic receptors. Therefore, the α-adrenergic agonistic agents will cause uterine vasoconstriction and will decrease the uteroplacental blood flow. Examples of some of these α-adrenergic agonists are adrenaline, noradrenaline, phenylephrine, mephentermine, etc. As the β-receptors are sparse on uterine vasculature, therefore, the predominant β-adrenergic agonists such as the ephedrine do not decrease much the uteroplacental blood flow. Hence, it is the traditional vasopressor of choice to treat hypotension during obstetric regional analgesia and anesthesia but does not cause less fetal acidosis than phenylephrine. However, practically many clinical studies suggest that the predominant α-adrenergic agonists (phenylephrine), though constrict the uteroplacental vasculature, still are associated with less fetal acidosis than ephedrine, and are more effective in treating hypotension in pregnant patients during central neuraxial block (CNB). This is because they maintain adequate uterine blood flow, by maintaining systemic blood pressure and a good pressure gradient, provided excessive vasoconstriction is avoided.

The three major factors which decrease the uteroplacental blood flow during pregnancy are (1) systemic hypotension by decreasing the difference between the uterine arterial and venous pressure, (2) uterine vasoconstriction by increasing the uterine vascular resistance, and (3) uterine contraction by decreasing the difference between the uterine arterial and venous pressure, by elevating the uterine venous pressure. The intense uterine contraction decreases the uteroplacental blood flow by compressing the uterine vessels, as they traverse through the myometrium and also by elevating uterine venous pressure. Hypertonic uterine contractions by oxytocin infusion or due to other causes can critically reduce this uteroplacental blood flow and compromise the fetus.

Uterine blood flow is not usually significantly affected by respiratory gas tension, but in extreme hypocapnia when $PaCO_2$ goes <20 mm Hg, then uteroplacental circulation is reduced and causes fetal hypoxemia and acidosis.

Effects of Anesthetic Agents on Uteroplacental Blood Flow

More or less, all the anesthetic agents affect uteroplacental blood flow (UPBF) by acting directly or indirectly. Among the intravenous anesthetic agents, thiopentone, benzodiazepines (BZDs), and propofol reduce the UPBF. This is due to the indirect effect of systemic hypotension, produced by these agents in high doses, but the clinical-inducing doses of these groups of drugs do not produce any alteration in UPBF, if the systemic BP is maintained within normal level. However, a small inadequate dose of these inducing agents may reduce the UPBF and it is due to the stimulation of the sympathetic system, during laryngoscopy. The injection of ketamine causes the activation of sympathoadrenal axis and may reduce the UPBF by vasoconstriction. But the increase in BP by ketamine counteracts the effect of vasoconstriction and ultimately the UPBF remains the same. This explanation is applicable when the dose of ketamine is kept below 1–1.5 mg/kg of body weight, but when the dose of this ketamine is increased to >2–3 mg/kg of body weight, then it causes the hypertonic contraction of uterus and drastically reduces the UPBF.

The effects of volatile anesthetic agents on UPBF also depend upon the interactions between the effect of these agents on systemic BP and direct uteroplacental vasodilatation with uterine myometrial relaxation produced by them. In clinical doses (around the value of 1 MAC) they produce maximum uteroplacental vasodilatation and uterine relaxation than the systemic reduction of BP. Therefore, in these doses, the UPBF does not decrease, but rather increases till systemic BP falls to a greater extent. The N_2O has a negligible effect on UPBF. Regional anesthesia (central neuraxial block) does not directly affect the UPBF, provided the systemic BP is maintained. In severe hypotension, the UPBF is proportional to the fall of BP.

In preeclampsia, the RA has a very beneficial effect on UPBF and this is due to the reduction of uterine vasoconstriction by cutting down the sympathetic supply to it, but again this beneficial effect on UPBF is maintained up to a certain level of hypotension, below which the uterine and placental circulation is severely compromised. The use of the recommended dose of epinephrine with LA agent, during CNB, is not contraindicated for obstetric analgesia and anesthesia. Because, the intravascular uptake of epinephrine from epidural space is so small that it only produces the β-adrenergic effects and dilates the uterine vessels, instead of vasoconstriction.

Transfer of Anesthetic Agents through the Placenta

Most of the drugs, used during anesthesia, can cross the barrier of placenta, except the muscle relaxants. Because, they (muscle relaxants) are highly ionized and so their transfer through the placenta is impaired, due to this high ionization, causing minimum or no effect on the fetus. The transfer of any anesthetic agent through the placenta depends on multiple factors such as their (1) route of administration, (2) total dose, (3) method of administration (single-shot large, multiple small boluses, continuous infusion, etc.), and (4) the timing of administration. However, though the effect of anesthetic agents on the fetus depends on the aforementioned factors (placental transfer) but still the maturity of fetal organs (liver and brain) plays a major role. For example, giving a drug many hours before delivery is least likely to produce any fetal effect after delivery. Similarly, administration of a single IV bolus dose of any anesthetic agent, during uterine contraction and just prior to the delivery of baby, also produce a minimum concentration of it in fetus. The effects of any anesthetic agent on the fetus is evaluated by observing its (1) heart rate variability, (2) intrapartum acid–base status, (3) Apgar score, and (4) neurobehavioral status, during the postpartum period.

All the opiates cross the barrier of placenta very easily, but the newborns are most sensitive to morphine, regarding the respiratory depression effect of it, than any other opiates. The maximum respiratory depressions effect of meperidine occurs 1–4 hours after its administration. Its respiratory depression effect is higher than other opiates but still less than that of morphine. Fentanyl readily crosses the placental barrier but produces minimal respiratory depression effects, if the dose of it is kept below 1 μg/kg of body weight. Remifentanil also crosses the placental barrier, readily like fentanyl, but its fetal blood concentration is generally half than that of mother. This is probably due to rapid metabolism of it (remifentanil) in the neonate and placenta. Butorphanol and nalbuphine produce less respiratory depression than morphine and pethidine (meperidine), but they have a significant depressed neurobehavioral effect on the fetus.

The commonly used intravenous inducing agents in GA, such as thiopentone, propofol, ketamine and BZDs, can readily cross the barrier of placental. But except BZDs, the other agents in their usual induction doses, do not cause any significant effect on the fetus (provided the baby is delivered within 10 minutes of their administration), due to their characteristic distribution, metabolism, and placental uptake. Only the BZDs, in their induction doses, have a profound effect on the fetus, regarding respiratory depression and neurobehavioral effects. All the inhalational anesthetic agents freely cross the placenta, but they produce minimal fetal depression, if their dose is kept below the value of 1 MAC and is used for <10 minutes before the delivery.

The LA agents also freely cross the barrier of placenta, but it depends on three factors such as the pK value of this agent, maternal and fetal pH, and the degree of protein binding of this LA agents. The bupivacaine and ropivacaine are more protein bound than lignocaine. So, these LA agents diffuse poorly across the placenta and cause their lower levels in fetal blood than lignocaine. Fetal acidosis causes a higher concentration of LA agent in their blood. This is because H^+ binds with the nonionized form of LA agents and causes the trapping of it on the fetal side of placenta. Chloroprocaine has the least placental transfer because it is rapidly hydrolyzed by plasma cholinesterase, present in maternal circulation. Other drugs, which are frequently used during anesthesia such as ranitidine, metoclopramide, atropine, antihistamine, phenothiazines, β-blocker, and vasodilators can readily cross the placenta. But glycopyrrolate cannot, because it is an ionized quaternary ammonium structure. The pK is the dissociation constant. When the solution is acid, then this pK is called as the pKa. It determines the strength of an acid. A lower pKa value denotes a more powerful acid and vice versa. The difference between the pKa and pH is that the pKa indicates whether an acid is strong or weak, but the pH indicates whether a system is acidic or alkaline.

EFFECTS OF ANESTHETIC AGENTS ON UTERINE ACTIVITY

Intravenous anesthetic agents such as thiopentone, propofol, and BZDs have no effect on uterine contraction (myometrium). Opiates minimally decrease the uterine muscular activity. Ketamine in the dose of >2 mg/kg through IV increases uterine contraction. Below this dose, it has also little or no effect on uterine contraction. All the volatile anesthetic agents such as halothane, isoflurane, sevoflurane, desflurane, etc., decrease uterine muscular activity equally at equipment doses and cause dose-dependent myometrial relaxation. Thus, they produce uterine atony and increase postpartum blood loss, but at concentration <0.7 MAC (low doses), they do not interfere the action of oxytocin on myometrium. The N_2O has no effect on uterine activity. Uterine myometrium also contains both α- and β-adrenergic receptors which respectively produce muscular contraction and relaxation. Therefore, the α-adrenergic agonistic agents such as phenylephrine, mephentermine, and ephedrine augment uterine contraction. But this effect is found only in higher doses, whereas the β-adrenergic agonistic agents such as salbutamol and ritodrine produce uterine relaxation and are used to treat (stop) premature labor.

Regional anesthesia has little effect on uterine contraction. Therefore, it does not affect the course of labor by causing uterine atony. However, in a normal *anesthetic dose* of LA agents, it (RA) prolongs the labor or increases the incidences of CS by preventing the rotation of fetal presenting parts on pelvic floor by relaxing the muscles of pelvic floor and preventing bearing down due to the relaxation (paralysis) of abdominal muscles. *Regional analgesia*, using the combination of a low dose of a local anesthetic agent such as bupivacaine 0.125% or 0.062% and a low dose of an opiate such as fentanyl 5 µg/mL does not prolong the course of labor and does not increase the chances of instrumental delivery or CS. But when the higher concentrations of LA agents are used, it prolongs the labor by only affecting its second stage. This is an indirect effect and is due to the loss of Ferguson reflex, due to motor weakness and impairs the expulsive or bears down effort. This is not the direct effect of RA on the course of labor.

Intravenous fluid loading, crystalloid or colloid, is often used to reduce the severity and the incidences of hypotension following an epidural obstetric analgesia and/or anesthesia. The prophylactic infusion of phenylephrine, started at the time of anesthetic injection in epidural space is also most effective in preventing postepidural hypotension. However, the analgesic dose of LA agents in epidural space for *obstetric analgesia* is usually not associated with postepidural hypotension. Practically, moreover, it is found that this fluid loading to reduce this post-CNB hypotension in a euvolemic patient does not reduce the incidences of hypotension, but reduces the endogenous secretion of oxytocin from the pituitary and decreases uterine contraction.

Uterine muscle has both α-1 and β-2 adrenergic receptors. Epinephrine has both α and β receptor action. But in low concentrations, the β action of epinephrine predominates over its α action. Therefore, LA agent containing epinephrine, used for obstetric RA, may produce the prolongation of labor, as it is used in very low concentration, producing only β effect. But clinically the prolongation of labor is generally not observed, as it is used in very low concentrations, e.g., 1:200,000–1:400,000 dilution. Large doses of α-adrenergic agents such as phenylephrine cause both uterine arterial constriction and myometrial contraction. But small doses of it (40 µg) increase uterine blood flow by raising arterial blood pressure. In contrast, ephedrine has little effect on uterine contraction.

Prostaglandin F2α (carboprost tromethamine), a synthetic analog of prostaglandin F2 stimulates myometrial contraction and is used to control refractory PPH. It is used in the initial dose of 0.25 mg by intramuscular (IM) and may be repeated at 30–60 minutes intervals to a maximum of 2 mg. Its common side effects are nausea, vomiting, bronchoconstriction, diarrhea, etc. So, it is contraindicated in asthma. Prostaglandin E1 (cytotec and rectal suppository) or E2 (dinoprostone and vaginal suppository) is also sometimes used and has no bronchoconstriction effect.

Magnesium is used in obstetrics to stop or to prevent eclamptic seizures and as a tocolytic agent (to cause myometrial relaxation and to prevent premature labor). For this purpose, it is usually administered first as 4 g loading dose over 20 minutes, followed by a 2 g/h infusion. The therapeutic concentration of magnesium is considered to be 6–8 mg/dL. The side effects of this magnesium are muscle weakness, hypotension, sedation, heart block, etc. Mg in this dose usually also intensifies the neuromuscular blocking effect of nondepolarizing muscle relaxants.

■ CONSEQUENCES OF PAIN DURING LABOR

Pain is a noxious and unpleasant stimulus. It produces great fear and anxiety, which again aggravates this pain. Thus, a vicious cycle sets up. Pain during labor causes the reduction of uterine blood flow, ↓FHR, ↓fetal oxygenation, fetal acidosis, etc. All these are mediated by the activation of sympathoadrenal axis of mother. So, painful labor is associated with increased maternal plasma cortisol and catecholamine levels which are responsible for this reduction in uteroplacental blood flow (**Fig. 1**). Thus, the effective relief of pain during labor reduces the plasma concentration of cortisol and catecholamine with their bad effects. This relief of pain also prevents the development of metabolic acidosis in mother by reducing the rate of the rise of plasma lactate, and pyruvate in the mother, and decreasing the consumption of O_2 in mother up to 15%.

With the activation of sympathoadrenal axis in mother, the pain during labor also produces hyperventilation and hypocapnia (alkalosis) in mother. This alkalosis causes the reduction in uteroplacental blood flow and even tetany in some parturient patients. This respiratory alkalosis further impairs fetomaternal gas exchange by shifting the O_2-Hb dissociation curve toward the left. Thus, fetal PaO_2 may fall producing fetal acidosis.

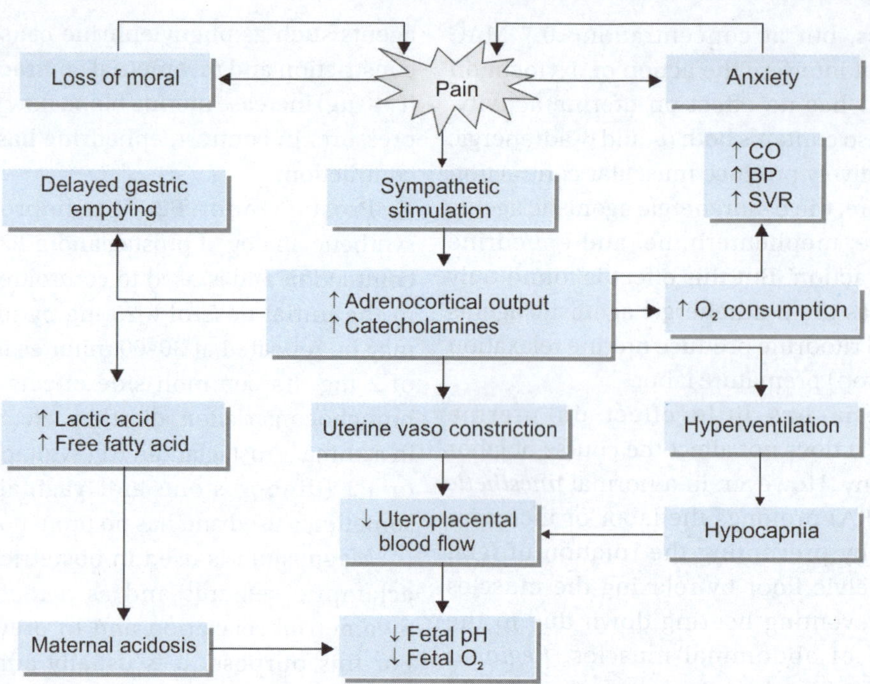

Fig. 1: Effect of pain on mother and fetus. (BP: blood pressure; CO: cardiac output; SVR: systemic vascular resistance)

■ PAIN PATHWAYS IN LABOR

Pain during the First Stage of Labor

Pain, during the first stage of labor **(Table 4)**, is due to the contraction, stretching, distortion, tearing, and possibly the ischemia of uterine tissues. It is also due to the simultaneous dilatation of the cervix with the stretching of the lower uterine segment. The intensity of pain, during the first stage of labor, increases progressively with the rising of the strength of myometrial contraction and the stretching of the lower segment of the uterus and cervix. These painful stimuli are transmitted through A-delta and C afferent fibers, accompanying the sympathetic pathway. It passes gradually through the pelvic and the inferior, middle, and superior hypogastric plexus → lumbar sympathetic chain → the white rami of T_{10} to L_1 spinal nerves → posterior root of these spinal nerves → T_{10} to L_1 segment of spinal cord (posterior horn of gray matter). During the early part of the first stage of labor, only the nerve roots of T_{11} and T_{12} spinal segments are involved. But as the intensity of uterine contraction increases, then gradually the T_{10} and L_1 nerve roots with their corresponding spinal segments are recruited.

Backache is a frequent complaint during the progress of labor. It is caused by one of these two mechanisms which are explained here. The pain, originating from the uterus or cervix, may be referred to the cutaneous branches of the posterior divisions of T_{10} to L_1 spinal nerves which migrate caudally for an appreciable distance before they innervate the skin, overlying the vertebral column. For example, the posterior cutaneous branches of T_{11} spinal nerve supply the skin overlying the L_3 and L_4 vertebrae. The pain, which is found in association with the fetal malpresentation or the unusual shape of sacrum, is due to the pressure on periuterine tissues and is referred to the L_5 and S_1 segments of the spinal cord which is felt as very low back pain.

Pain Pathways during the Second Stage of Labor

The onset of perineal pain at the end of the first stage of labor signals the beginning of fetal descent and the onset of the second stage of labor. In the second stage of labor, pain is mainly caused by the distention and the stretching of pelvic structures and perineum. This is due to the descent of fetal presenting part. This is also added to the pain of uterine contraction of the first stage of labor. Once the cervical dilatation is complete, the pain induced by uterine contraction may become less intense. The pain, initiated by uterine contraction, is continued to be referred to the T_{10} to L_1 dermatomes. But the pain produced by the stretching and pressure exerted on the intrapelvic structure including the pelvic floor (levator ani), bladder, urethra, and rectum is referred to the sacral segment. With the above manifestation, the direct pressure on the root of the lumbosacral plexus by the fetal presenting part is also manifested as a pain that is felt low on the back or on the inner side of the thighs. The pain in the second stage, produced by the compression

TABLE 4: Pain pathway and site of pain during labor.

Site of origin	Pathway	Site of pain
Uterus and cervix	• Afferent fibers which accompany the sympathetic pathway to the T_{10} to L_1 spinal segments • Dorsal rami of T_{10} to L_1 spinal nerves. This is referred to cutaneous branches of posterior divisions	• Whole abdomen and groin • Middle of back
Pressure by the presenting part of fetus on periuterine tissue	Lumbosacral plexus	Low back and thigh
Bladder, urethra, and rectum	Pudendal nerve ($S_{2,3,4}$)	Referred to perineum and sacrum
Vagina	Pudendal nerve ($S_{2,3,4}$)	Perineum
Perineum	• Pudendal nerve ($S_{2,3,4}$) • Genitofemoral nerve ($L_{1,2}$) • Ilioinguinal nerve (L_1) • Postcutaneous nerve of thigh ($S_{2,3}$)	Perineum

and stretching of perineal tissues, is transmitted through the pudendal nerve (S_2, S_3, and S_4), posterior cutaneous nerve of thigh (S_2 and S_3), genitofemoral nerve (L_1 and L_2), and ilioinguinal nerve (L_1) to the lumbosacral area, perineal area, gluteal region, and the inner sides of thigh, as the labor progresses **(Table 4)**.

During the first stage of labor, an epidural block in which the level of anesthesia is limited only to the T_{11} and T_{12} segment of the spinal cord (in a very early stage) and later is extended to the T_{10} and L_1 spinal segment is sufficient to provide excellent pain relief. While the neural blockade of sacral segment is not necessary for the relief of pain in the first stage of labor. Premature blockade of sacral segment in the early stage of labor can result in the loss of stimulating effect of Ferguson's reflex which initiates more contraction and helps in the rotation of fetal presenting part. Thus, the premature blockade of sacral segment causes more incidences of instrumental delivery and CS.

■ ANALGESIA FOR VAGINAL DELIVERY

Pain during vaginal delivery can be alleviated by different processes. These are mentioned here:

- Psychological and nonpharmacological techniques (no use of drugs)
- Pharmacological technique (use of drugs)
- Nerve block technique: Both central neuraxial block and peripheral nerve block.

Psychological and Nonpharmacological Technique

In this technique, exhaustive counseling of mother is done from 6 weeks before delivery, regarding the normal anatomy of the reproductive system, physiology of pregnancy, physiology of normal delivery and postpartum advice, etc. By this psychological counseling, pain during the process of

labor and vaginal delivery can be reduced by preconditioning the cerebral cortical activity of patients. Usually, a fear from an unknown or previous unpleasant experience aggravates the pain of labor. Thus, the removal of this fear by proper counseling helps to reduce this pain. The patient concentrates her mind away from the process of delivery and tries to relax herself. This distraction of mind from the process of normal delivery inhibits all the incoming painful stimulus from uterus and thus subsequently reduces the sensation of pain, associated with the uterine contraction.

Some common psychological techniques, used to reduce this labor pain are Lamaze, Doula, Dick–Read, Leboyer, and Bradley, etc. Among these, the Lamaze technique for the relief of labor pain is the most popular. In this technique, the patient is trained to take deep breaths (inspiration) at the beginning of each uterine contraction. This is followed by gentle slow expiration until the uterine contraction ends. Other psychological techniques used to reduce this labor pain are hypnosis, mesmerism, acupuncture, transcutaneous electrical nerve stimulation (TENS), etc. But the success of all these techniques varies from patient to patient and frequently needs a combination of some of these techniques or the addition of some new forms of pain relieving methods.

Pharmacological Technique

Nearly all the opioids and nonopioid analgesics and sedatives can be used to alleviate the labor pain, but all these agents relieve this labor pain to a certain extent and have their own advantages and disadvantages. They all cross the placenta and affect the fetus.

Opioids

Opioids are the most commonly used agents for the relief of labor pain. But fetal depression (respiratory, neurobehavioral, and movements) only allows the use of these agents at the early stage of labor. They are also used where RA techniques are not possible and not used. Among the opioids, the most commonly used agents are meperidine, morphine, fentanyl, butorphanol, nalbuphine, etc., and they produce more or less comparably equal pain relief. But the choice of drug, for clinical use, depends on their potential side effects, desired onset of action, duration of action, and the familiarity of these agents by an anesthetist. The main drawbacks of the use of opioids for the relief of labor pain are fetal respiratory depression, fetal respiratory acidosis, an abnormal neurobehavioral pattern of the fetus, loss of beat-to-beat variability of fetal heart rate, decreased fetal movement, ↓Apgar score, ↓oxygen saturation (SPO_2) of the fetus, maternal respiratory depression, maternal nausea and vomiting, maternal delayed gastric emptying, etc. The loss of beat-to-beat variability of fetal heart rate and decreased fetal movement by opioids also make the intrauterine monitoring of fetal well-being during the course of labor difficult.

Though morphine is the gold standard of all opioid analgesics, still it is not commonly used in the practice of obstetric analgesia. This is because it appears to cause more respiratory depression of the fetus than any other opioids in their equipotent analgesic doses. The other drawbacks of morphine are delayed onset of action and prolonged duration of action. Hence, due to these draw backs of morphine, the most commonly used opioid in the practice of obstetric analgesia is meperidine (pethidine). The peak effect of it occurs 10–20 minutes after its IV administration and 1–3 hours after its IM administration. The usual IV dose of meperidine for obstetric analgesia is 10–25 mg and IM dose is 25–50 mg, usually up to a total of 100 mg. The duration of action of meperidine of this dose is 2–4 hours. Therefore, meperidine is given during the early stage of labor, when the delivery is not expected at least within 4 hours after its administration.

The fentanyl is also used to relieve labor pain through IV or IM route and the usual dose is 25–50 and 50–100 µg respectively. After IV administration the peak effect of fentanyl occurs within 2–4 minutes after its administration and the duration of action lasts for 40–60 minutes. This duration of action of fentanyl will be more prolonged if multiple doses are used. It is found that the aforementioned doses of fentanyl do not cause neonatal respiratory depression, ↓Apgar score, adverse effects on neonatal neurobehavioral score, and adverse effects on umbilical cord blood gas analysis. So, it is concluded that fentanyl may be used as analgesic to reduce labor pain, as an alternative to either RA or GA. Another two commonly used opioids for obstetric analgesia are *butorphanol* and *nalbuphine*. They are synthetic agonists and antagonist opioids in nature. The analgesic dose of butorphanol and nalbuphine is 1–2

and 10–20 mg IM or IV respectively which is equivalent to 10 mg of morphine, 100 mg of meperidine, and 100 µg of fentanyl in respect to respiratory depression. But the advantage of these two drugs is that increasing the doses of them does not produce more respiratory depression with cumulative action (ceiling effect). On the other hand, large doses of these two compounds may produce excessive sedation, dizziness, somnolence, etc., which may be problematic.

Benzodiazepines

Benzodiazepines are also used in the practice of obstetric analgesia. The indications are to reduce anxiety, as anticonvulsants in eclampsia, as an adjunct to opioids, and as a premedicant for CS. Among all the BZDs, the commonly used agents in obstetric analgesia and anesthesia are diazepam, lorazepam, midazolam, etc., and they all cross the placental barrier readily. Within 1 minute after their IV administration, the maternal and fetal plasma concentration of all these BZDs approximately becomes equal. The use of BZDs in obstetric practice has also many advantages and disadvantages like opioids. The advantages of the use of BZDs for obstetric analgesia are the reduction of maternal anxiety and subsequently its consequences such as ↑catecholamines and ↓uteroplacental circulation due to constriction of uterine artery, fetal acidosis, etc. It also reduces the requirements of opioids (if it is used to alleviate labor pain) and cuts down its complication. But the disadvantages for the use of BZD are found mainly on the fetus. These are fetal respiratory depression, hypotonia, lethargy, hypothermia, depressed feeding, ↓SPO_2, etc. These adverse effects of BZDs are found, when the unusual large nonobstetric doses of them are used for obstetrics analgesia and anesthesia. But the small doses of BZDs have minimal effects on the fetus and neonates, though beat-to-beat variability is markedly decreased even in small doses.

Lorazepam does not offer any extra advantages over diazepam for the practice of obstetric analgesia and anesthesia, except that only <1% of it (lorazepam) is transformed to other pharmacologically active metabolites. If the total maternal dose of diazepam, during labor, exceeds than 20–25 mg, then the drug itself and its pharmacologically active metabolites persist above its therapeutic level for about at least 1 week. The usual nonobstetric doses of lorazepam (1–2 mg) are associated with adverse effects on neonates. The advantage of midazolam over the other BZDs is that it is a water-soluble and rapid onset and short duration of action.

Another usual drawback, for the use of BZD, in obstetric practice, is the anterograde amnesia of mother, produced by it. But all the mothers desire to recall the birth of their baby and it is highly pleasure to them. So, anterograde amnesia, produced by BZD, is an unwanted effect in obstetric practice, though it (amnesia) is highly desirable in other surgical patients.

Ketamine Hydrochloride

Ketamine is also used in obstetric practice to reduce labor pain, because it has a strong analgesic effect, even though in very low doses (0.1–0.25 mg/kg). But in higher doses (1 mg/kg), it causes induction of anesthesia. In very low doses it produces only analgesia without any effect of sedation or unconsciousness. In both aforementioned doses, ketamine does not affect the uterine blood flow, fetal Apgar score, and uterine muscle tone. But in higher doses than 2 mg/kg, ketamine can produce hypertonic uterine contraction. The main drawback of use of ketamine in obstetric practice is its unpleasant effect of hallucination which some obstetricians do not like. But this hallucination is usually not found in very low doses which are used in obstetric analgesia, but not in anesthesia.

Phenothiazine Derivatives and Hydroxyzine

Among all the phenothiazine derivatives, *promethazine* is the most commonly used agent in the practice of obstetric analgesia. Other phenothiazine derivatives which are also used in obstetric analgesia practice are chlorpromazine, prochlorperazine, etc., but they are not popular, because all of them possess high α-adrenergic blocking activity and frequently cause hypotension. *Hydroxyzine* is not a phenothiazine derivative, but it has similar properties of ataraxia (a state of detached serenity, without the depression of mental faculties or impairment of consciousness) like promethazine. So, it is frequently used in combination with promethazine and meperidine. However, both these drugs reduce the requirement of opioids, and the anxiety, nausea, and vomiting of mother. Also, they do not appreciably produce neonatal depression. These are the advantages of promethazine and hydroxyzine. The principal disadvantage of hydroxyzine is that the IV preparation of it is not available. So, it is administered only through IM route, causing its delayed onset and prolonged action. The usual dose of promethazine and hydroxyzine used for obstetric analgesia and anesthesia are 25–50 mg and 50–100 mg IM respectively.

Barbiturates

The short and medium-acting barbiturates such as pentobarbital (Nembutal), secobarbital (Seconal), amobarbital (Amytal), etc., are not used now in obstetric practice to reduce anxiety and labor pain, because they cause prolonged depression on neonates, even with smaller doses that do not cause maternal depression clinically.

Nonsteroidal anti-inflammatory drugs (NSAIDs) such as *ketorolac* is not recommended to relieve labor pain because it suppresses uterine contractions (antiprostaglandin) and promotes the premature closure of ductus arteriosus.

Inhaled Analgesic

The inhalation of different volatile anesthetic agents is also a popular method for the alleviation of labor pain. Through this inhalation (pulmonary) route, different inhaled anesthetic agents are administered alone in subanesthetic concentration, only to reduce the labor pain, but without any loss of consciousness or as supplementation to regional or local anesthesia. This form of relief of labor pain should not be confused with inhalational anesthesia where the patient losses her consciousness with the loss of protective laryngeal reflexes. With this technique, patient remains conscious and cooperative with the presence of full laryngeal reflexes, while she enjoys the analgesic effect of inhalational agents. Usually, the volatile pharmacological agent is administered either by patient herself or by an anesthetist via a face mask in an intermittent or continuous way. However, the main disadvantage of this method is that as the inhalational anesthetic agents are used in a subanesthetic concentration, so this method does not always provide an adequate amount of pain relief. Hence, it is usually used, as an adjunct to, other methods of pain relief.

The commonly used inhaled anesthetic agents are N_2O and O_2 mixture (50:50 = N_2O:O_2 mixture is called Entonox), desflurane (0.2%), isoflurane (0.25%), enflurane (0.2%), etc. Entonox has been used for many years to relieve the labor pain as a sole analgesic agent or as an adjunct to other systemic or regional analgesic techniques, but truly speaking, and is unfortunate to say that, the analgesia provided by 50% N_2O alone is not reliable. The maximum analgesic effect of N_2O occurs within 30–60 seconds after the starting of its inhalation. It is, therefore, advised that patients should start to inhale the gas at the early onset of uterine contraction and discontinue it after peak uterine contraction if intermittent method is applied. During the use of Entonox, the lack of proper availability and use of scavenging system, put the labor room staff at an unnecessary risk to the exposure against the excessive level of N_2O, over a prolonged period.

The subanesthetic concentration of other volatile anesthetic agents such as desflurane, isoflurane, enflurane, etc., has also successfully been used to provide labor analgesia, and their effectiveness also appears to be comparable to that of N_2O. Aforementioned dose of these volatile anesthetic agents are not fixed. It depends on the response of patient. If the patient becomes drowsy, noncooperative, confused and gradually progresses to unconsciousness, then the inspired concentration of volatile anesthetic agents should be lowered quickly. The major risk of this method of obstetric analgesia and anesthesia is accidental anesthetic overdose, producing unconsciousness. So, a trained person must remain in continuous verbal contact with the patient and will monitor the consciousness.

Nerve Block

Two types of nerve block are used to relieve the labor pain for vaginal delivery. These are (1) peripheral nerve block and (2) central neuraxial block.

Peripheral Nerve Block (Pudendal Nerve Block, Paracervical Block, and Perineal Infiltration)

Among the peripheral nerve block for obstetric analgesia and anesthesia, the *pudendal nerve block* is most commonly used. This is often combined with local infiltration of subcutaneous tissue of the perineum by local anesthetic agents if other forms of anesthesia are not previously applied or is inadequate. Thus, it provides complete perineal anesthesia only for the second stage of labor. The pudendal nerve is derived from S_{2-4} spinal nerve roots and provides sensory innervation to the vulva, the lower part of vagina, and perineum. It also provides motor innervation to the perineal muscles. The pudendal nerve can easily be blocked through the transvaginal route by depositing 10 mL of LA agents behind the sacrospinous ligament on each side, following a negative needle aspiration. This nerve block provides adequate local anesthesia only for the second stage of vaginal delivery, outlet forceps manipulation, episiotomy, and its repair, etc., but it does not provide adequate analgesia for midforceps manipulation, repair of upper vaginal laceration, exploration of the uterine cavity, etc. The pudendal nerve block is associated with low incidences of complication, but high incidences of failure rate. For pudendal nerve block, it is better to use a needle guide to limit the depth of the entry of the needle behind the sacrospinous ligament and to protect the fetus and vagina from the needle. The other potential complications of this pudendal block are intravascular injection, retroperitoneal hematoma, and retropsoas, and subgluteal abscess.

Another technique of peripheral nerve block for obstetric analgesia and anesthesia is the *paracervical block*. In this technique, the paracervical ganglion (or Fran Kenhausen's ganglion) which transmits all the visceral sensory nerve fibers from the uterus, cervix, and upper vagina, is blocked. So, this technique provides pain relief for the later part of the first stage of labor and the first part of the second stage of labor. The paracervical ganglion is situated lateral and posterior to the junction of cervix and the body of uterus.

Hence, for this technique, LA agent is deposited through the vaginal route at the outside of the fornix of vagina, and lateral to the cervix of uterus. However, this block does not affect the somatosensory fibers carrying pain sensation from lower vagina, perineum, and vulva. Therefore, it does not afford any pain relief during the second stage of labor. On the other hand, it does not adversely affect the dilatation of cervix and the progress of labor.

Recently, this paracervical plexus block is not used for obstetric analgesia and anesthesia. This is because it is associated with a high rate of fetal bradycardia, fetal acidosis, decreased fetal oxygen saturation, and increased likelihood of fetal depression. However, the probable explanation for these complications of paracervical block is the close proximity of injection site to the uterine artery which results in (1) uterine arterial vasoconstriction, (2) uteroplacental insufficiency, and (3) high levels of LA agent in fetal circulation. The fetal bradycardia usually develops within 5–10 minutes, after this paracervical injection and it lasts for another 10–30 minutes.

Central Neuraxial Block

Recently, the CNB is the most commonly used technique for obstetric analgesia and anesthesia. Compared to pharmacological methods and GA, this technique of obstetric analgesia and anesthesia is less likely to produce drug-induced depression of the fetus and aspiration pneumonitis of mother. It also provides relief in labor pain, while allowing the patient to remain fully awake and to participate actively in labor and delivery by performing the bearing down action. Central neuraxial block is also associated with lower levels of catecholamines in maternal circulation which is also beneficial to the fetus. The most common forms of CNB for obstetric analgesia and/or anesthesia are lumbar epidural, caudal epidural, subarachnoid, and different combinations of these techniques such as combined spinal and epidural by LA agent alone or opioid alone or mixture of LA agent and opioid with their different concentrations. Though, LA agents and opioids alone can provide adequate labor analgesia and/or anesthesia, still the combination of these two agents at different very low concentrations is most popular. This is because the synergistic effect, due to the combination of these two types of agents, decreases the individual dose requirement with few or nil maternal and fetal side-effects if these agents are used alone.

Lumbar epidural anesthesia–analgesia for vaginal delivery: This is the most commonly used RA and analgesia technique to relieve pain in all the stages of labor. It can be provided by a single-shot injection or by a continuous technique using a catheter. The continuous epidural anesthesia and analgesia technique by catheter provide the greater flexibility than a single-shot epidural technique. For this obstetric analgesia and/or anesthesia, the epidural catheter is placed at lumbar region and only *analgesia* is achieved when the patient wants it during at any stage of labor. But it is often advantageous, if the catheter is placed (1) in the early stage of labor, evaluated by her obstetrician, (2) when the patient is comfortable, and (3) can be positioned easily for the introduction of a catheter. Moreover, if emergency LUCS is needed at any time during the progress of labor, then it can be converted into epidural *anesthesia* and again this can be extended for postoperative analgesia. A more conservative approach for the commencement of this lumbar epidural labor analgesia (recommended by some obstetricians) is to wait, till the labor is well established, which is characterized by (1) regular uterine contraction at 3–4 minutes interval and each contraction is lasting for 1 minute, (2) minimum cervical dilatation of 3–4 cm, (3) no fetal distress, and (4) there is engagement of fetal presenting parts. Lumbar epidural *analgesia* by a low dose of opioid or mixture of a low dose of opioid and LA agent or low dose of LA agent alone (1) does not increase the rate of operative delivery, (2) has no or little effect on the progress of labor, (3) does not need oxytocin augmentation, and (4) does not need operative delivery (forceps or CS).

For lumbar obstetric epidural anesthesia–analgesia, the optimal interspinous space is L_{2-3} or L_{3-4} which is used by maximum anesthetists. This is because these spaces help to achieve the level of analgesia with a minimum amount of LA drug or opioid, extending between T_{10} to S_5 dermatomes. For this procedure, any position of the patient, i.e., lying or sitting can be used. But the sitting position of patient is more helpful for identifying the midline in obese patient. Sitting position also helps for better sacral spread of analgesia, if lumbar epidural is given at the second stage of labor. One disadvantage of this sitting position for epidural block is that as in this position, there is more cerebrospinal fluid (CSF) pressure, so there are increased incidences of unintentional dural puncture.

Most anesthetists prefer midline approach, while some favor the paramedian approach for this epidural placement of a catheter. The incidence of a wet tap (dural puncture) during lumbar epidural procedure varies in between 0.2 and 10%, depending upon the skill of the anesthetist. If an unintentional wet tap occurs, then the clinician has two choices (1) he can try again at another one segment higher or lower intervertebral space or (2) he can put the epidural catheter in this subarachnoid space and may convert the continuous epidural to continuous spinal anesthesia– analgesia. For the detection of epidural space by the loss of resistance technique, usually, air or normal saline is used,

but the amount of air, injected into the epidural space, should be as little as possible, probably <3–5 mL. This is because the injection of a large amount of air into epidural space is associated with headache, and unilateral or patchy anesthesia–analgesia (due to air the LA solution cannot spread uniformly in epidural space).

For obstetric epidural anesthesia and/or analgesia, the commonly used drugs to relieve labor pain are local anesthetic agents in different concentrations, with or without in combination with opioids, but the addition of opioid to LA agent for *epidural analgesia* has dramatically changed the practice of obstetric analgesia. Because, when the two are combined, then very low concentrations of both LA agent and opioid can be used with excellent effect and with minimum side effects of each. These two agents such as the LA agent and opioid have synergistic effects on each other, due to their separate sites of action. The opioids act on opiate receptors, situated at the dorsal horn cells of the spinal cord, while the LA agents act directly on the neuronal axons of nerve roots. Therefore, this synergistic effect helps to reduce the concentration and doses of these two agents. Therefore, the incidences of side effects of both the LA agents and opioids are reduced. For example, *hypotension*, due to chemical sympathectomy, and *motor block*, due to the block of conduction of motor nerve fibers, which are common adverse effects of LA agents in higher concentration in epidural space, are *absent* in lower concentration of these agents. Therefore, the patient can help herself in the second stage of labor, by bearing down and accelerating the normal vaginal delivery. In some, very low concentration of bupivacaine such as 0.062–0.125% with either fentanyl in the dose of 2–3 µg/mL or sufentanil in the dose of 0.3–0.5 µg/mL is used. In general, the lower the concentration of LA agent, the greater the concentration of opioid that is required. The very low LA mixture (bupivacaine 0.062%) generally does not produce a motor block. So, the patients even can walk during the first stage of labor, because in this very lower concentration, bupivacaine can only block the sensory fibers, sparing the motor. So, this is called the *"walking or mobile epidural".*

Similarly nausea, vomiting, and respiratory depression, which are the common side effects of opioids, are also absent in very low doses of opioids in epidural space. When the *opioid is omitted* from the mixture of opioid and LA agent, administered in epidural space, then the higher concentration of LA agent, such as bupivacaine in the concentration of 0.25–0.5% or ropivacaine in the concentration of 0.2% is needed to obtain the same obstetric analgesia and anesthetic effect. Then, this high concentration of LA agent will reduce the normal pelvic muscle tone by blocking the motor nerve which normally helps in the rotation and engagement of fetal presenting parts, and thus will impair the normal vaginal delivery. This higher concentration of LA agent will also paralyze the abdominal muscles and will impair the mother's ability to bear down as the labor progress.

Among the LA agents, bupivacaine, levobupivacaine, and ropivacaine are the drug of choice for *obstetric analgesia* by most of the anesthetists. Bupivacaine is chosen for *obstetric analgesia*, because (1) it produces optimal clinical effect in very low concentration, (2) it has a long duration of action, (3) there is an apparent lack of tachyphylaxis by bupivacaine, and (4) high protein bound characteristic of bupivacaine causes its less placental transfer. But the main disadvantage of bupivacaine is its cardiotoxicity effect. Bupivacaine is also very effective only for sensory block, without any motor block, in concentration as low as 0.125% or 0.0625% when it is combined with opioids *for early labor*. But some higher concentrations of bupivacaine such as 0.125% with opioids or 0.25% alone without opioids are needed for the *later stages of labor*. The concentration of 0.5% bupivacaine is only reserved for use during CS which causes both the sensory and motor block producing *obstetric anesthesia*. Ropivacaine is a newer amide local anesthetic agent with near similar structure and pharmacodynamics like bupivacaine. It is the first levo isomer (levo isomer of bupivacaine is levobupivacaine) LA agent to be marketed. It is less soluble than bupivacaine. Therefore, it is less potent. The cardiotoxic effect of ropivacaine appears to be intermediate in position between those of lignocaine and bupivacaine. Unlike bupivacaine, progesterone does not appear to enhance the cardiotoxicity of ropivacaine. Clinically, only for obstetric analgesia, to alleviate labor pain, it is used in the concentration of 0.2% only. It is now thought that the reduced toxic effect and reduced motor block effect, produced by ropivacaine, is due to its low potency.

Levobupivacaine is now used to provide epidural labor (obstetric) analgesia. It is the levo isomer of bupivacaine. The normally marketed bupivacaine contains mixture of R-enantiomer (racemic bupivacaine) and S-enantiomer (levobupivacaine). It is confirmed that levobupivacaine is long-acting and possess more safety profile than the normally marketed racemic mixture of bupivacaine. The lethal dose of levobupivacaine is 1.5–2 times higher than that of its racemic mixture, i.e., bupivacaine. The usual concentration of levobupivacaine, used in clinical practice, is 0.25–0.5%.

The addition of epinephrine to this LA agent, during epidural anesthesia–analgesia, to relieve labor pain is a controversial topic. It is known to all that epinephrine reduces the systemic absorption of LA agent and subsequently reduces the toxicity of LA agents and prolongs its duration of action. Therefore, epinephrine can (1) increase the total dose of LA agent, without increasing its toxicity, (2) provides a longer duration of action, and (3) intensifies the sensory

and motor block. But all these advantages of epinephrine, by adding to LA agent, are unnecessary during continuous epidural analgesia by catheter technique for vaginal delivery. This is because the small amount of LA drug in the form of low concentration is used for *epidural analgesia* to relieve labor pain in vaginal delivery, as a motor block is not needed, and the prolonged or indefinite period of action of LA agent is obtained by catheter without adding epinephrine. The only advantage of adding epinephrine to an LA agent for epidural anesthesia–analgesia to relieve labor pain is that it (epinephrine) acts as a marker in test dose, during the testing of inadvertent placement of a catheter into the blood vessels. The other disadvantage of epinephrine is its β-adrenergic receptor action which decreases uterine contraction and unnecessarily prolongs the duration of labor. On the contrary, many anesthetists prefer epinephrine in the concentration of 1:200,000–1:400,000 with LA agents for *epidural anesthesia* and postoperative analgesia, during CS, where *large amounts of drugs* in the form of *higher concentrations* are used to obtain profound both motor and sensory block.

Like LA agents, opioids are also not used alone clinically for *epidural labor analgesia*, because opioids alone frequently do not provide satisfactory and complete results. On the other hand, high doses of opioids are also needed when used alone for obstetric analgesia and these high doses have many adverse effects such as (1) maternal and fetal respiratory depression, (2) nausea and vomiting of the mother, and (3) loss of beat-to-beat fetal heart rate variability. So, the combination of LA agent in low concentration and opioids in low doses has now become very popular for *obstetric analgesia and/or anesthesia*. Among the opioids, the most commonly used agents are fentanyl and sufentanil in the doses of 25–50 and 10–20 µg respectively. The most significant advantage of this combination of LA agent and opioid in low doses is the striking lack of motor blockade, which allow a mother to experience a pain free, nonparalyzed, pleasant vaginal delivery. Till now the maximal total dose of fentanyl and sufentanil, when used continuously by a catheter through the epidural route, is not clear. But some believe that the maximum dose of sufentanil in continuous epidural should not exceed beyond 30–50 µg. For fentanyl, this maximum dose may go up to 200–300 µg.

After the successful placement of the epidural catheter a preliminary test dose is mandatory. This test dose helps to diagnose if there is any unintentional subarachnoid or intravascular placement of needle or catheter. For this test dose, 2–3 mL of local anesthetic agent with 1:200,000 epinephrine as a marker is used. This test dose of LA agent should be given at the interval, between two uterine contractions. This will help to reduce the false positive (+)

sign of intravascular injection of marker, (i.e., epinephrine), manifested by tachycardia which can also occur due to painful uterine contraction, if it (the test dose) is given during the period of contraction. This test dose will also help to diagnose the unintentional subarachnoid placement of the needle or catheter by extensive block like spinal anesthesia, instead of epidural block, with this small amount of LA drug, used in this test dose.

After 5–10 minutes of the test dose, the principal mixture of LA agent and opioid can be administered through an epidural catheter or needle by three methods. *The first choice* is the administration of a bolus 10 mL mixture of local anesthetic agent and opioid, in two incremental doses (5 mL each) at an interval of 1–2 minutes. This initial mixture usually contains 0.0625–0.125% bupivacaine or 0.1–0.2% ropivacaine with 10–20 μg sufentanil or 50–100 μg fentanyl. This will achieve sensory block, extending upward up to dermatomes of T_{10} level, if the catheter is placed through L_2 to L_3 interspinous space in lateral horizontal lying down position and then the patient is put in the supine position. After the first bolus dose patient should be monitored continuously by BP, heart rate, SPO_2 level, etc., for the first 30–40 minutes or until the patient becomes stable. This bolus dose can be repeated several times according to the need, till the total process of vaginal delivery is completed. Epinephrine in concentrations of 1:400,000–1:800,000 can also be added with LA solution to prolong analgesia with fewer additional doses.

The *second choice* is, instead of repeated bolus injection, continuous infusion of a mixture of local anesthetic agents and opioids at the rate of 10–15 mL/h. The mixture may contain bupivacaine (0.0625–0.125%) or ropivacaine (0.1–0.2%) with fentanyl (1–2 μg/mL) or sufentanil (0.2–0.4 μg/mL). Later, this dose should be adjusted according to the response of patient and the progress of labor.

The *third choice* is the patient's control epidural analgesia (PCEA). In this method, the patient itself administered the mixture of drug (i.e., LA agent and opioid) through epidural catheter. There are different PCEA settings that can be changed by the patient himself according to her response. But a typical setting is 5 mL/h as *basal* infusion rate and 5 mL as *bolus* at 10–20 minutes lockout intervals. Thus, within an hour 20–30 mL of 0.125% bupivacaine and 50 kg of fentanyl may be administered. The great advantage of PCEA is that the total drug requirement is less and patient's satisfaction is greater in this method. The drug and its concentration, used in PCEA, is same as mentioned earlier. For the relief of pain, during the second stage of labor, the sensory block should be extended below the S_{2-4} levels of dermatomes. For this, the drug should be administered in semirecumbent or sitting

position of the patient through an epidural catheter which will reduce the total dose of LA agent.

Caudal epidural anesthesia and/or analgesia for vaginal delivery: Caudal epidural block is also administered to relieve labor pain, during any stage of it, but it is usually accomplished only when the labor is well-progressed and is in the second stage. To relieve labor pain, during the first stage of labor, i.e., to extend the sensory block up to the T_{10} level through caudal epidural route, large volume of LA agent is required. So, this epidural route is usually not used to relieve labor pain, during its first stage. It is performed on patient, positioned either prone or lying on their sides. For caudal epidural block coccyx is always used as landmark and then for next successful result the sacral cornu and the sacrococcygeal ligament, covering the sacral hiatus is palpated. After the successful placement of an epidural needle into sacral canal, through sacral hiatus, the rectal and vaginal examination is mandatory. This is because it will exclude the possibilities of accidental puncture of fetal presenting part by the epidural needle and its subsequent sequelae. Through this epidural needle epidural catheter can also be passed into sacral canal for continuous caudal block. A test dose of LA agent mixed with epinephrine is also mandatory to use through needle or catheter because it is also possible to enter the needle or catheter in an epidural vessel or dural sac which ends at S_1 or S_2 vertebral level, producing spinal anesthesia. The volume of LA agent and opioid mixture to provide *labor analgesia* (not anesthesia) through sacral route during the *first stage of labor* should extend up to the T_{10} level of dermatome. Therefore, the volume of drug will be very high through this sacral route, which varies from 10 to 20 mL, in the first bolus dose. The subsequent doses of drug to maintain labor analgesia is also very high which is about 15 mL for every sitting. Hence, if one wants to achieve up to T_{10} level of block through sacral route with smaller volume of drugs, then the patient should be placed in head down position.

The lumbar epidural route to relieve labor pain is preferred than caudal route because:

- The level of analgesia, extending between T_{10} to L_1 dermatomes, which is necessary to relief pain, during the first stage of labor, can be achieved easily through lumbar route and spare the block of sacral dermatomes which is not desired for the first stage of labor.
- Less amount of drug is required through lumbar route than caudal route for labor analgesia, during the whole process of delivery through vagina.
- In epidural obstetric analgesia through route, lumbar pelvic muscles retain their tones. This will help in the

rotation of fetal presenting part and normal vaginal delivery.

- The placement of lumbar epidural needle is technically easier than caudal procedure, though in the previous technique, there is more chance of dural puncture. On the contrary, the advantage of caudal epidural analgesia, placed just before vaginal delivery, if it is not placed before, over lumbar epidural analgesia is that the onset of perineal analgesia and muscle relaxation is quicker in the previous one.

Subarachnoid anesthesia–analgesia for vaginal delivery: The subarachnoid block is not so popular to relieve labor pain for vaginal delivery, but it has some definite indications, advantages, and disadvantages. *It is particularly indicated* in a very distress (from pain) parturient patient, where the placement of an epidural catheter is very difficult or impossible. In such circumstances, a single-shot subarachnoid anesthesia–analgesia produced by any LA agent alone or any opioid alone or their mixture is very useful for emergency instrumental vaginal delivery in patient who does not have epidural catheter before, but the *disadvantage* of this technique is that it does not provide the flexibility of an epidural catheter. The *other problem of subarachnoid anesthesia–analgesia to relieve labor pain* is that it is very difficult to titrate the dose and concentration of LA agent or opioid by which we can get only the sensory block (labor analgesia), where motor block is not at all desirable for first and the second stage of labor. Motor block (muscular paralysis) will hinder the rotation of presenting parts of the fetus and the patient cannot bear down the fetus which is very essential for vaginal delivery.

Another advantage of a single-shot subarachnoid injection of LA agent alone or opioid alone or their mixture is that unlike epidural, it provides effective and rapid onset of labor analgesia and anesthesia (both motor and sensory block). If *only opioid alone is given in subarachnoid space* to relieve labor pain then it needs a very small dose than the only opioid given in epidural space (though this dose is greater than when used with LA agent). This is because it (opioid) directly acts on the dorsal horn cells of spinal cord, without usual systemic effects of narcotics. Thus, only intrathecal opioids have the potential advantage (unlike only narcotics through epidural space which needs larger doses and may have a systemic effect) of providing effective and safe labor analgesia with no motor and sympathetic block. Hence, there is no hypotension, no adverse effects on uterine contraction, and no maternal and fetal respiratory depression (due to small doses). So, this technique of using opioids alone in subarachnoid space to relieve the labor pain is *especially indicated* in patients with cardiac disease

who require adequate analgesia without motor block and hypotension. Thus, it will prevent the potentially dangerous increase in heart rate and myocardial O_2 consumption associated with painful labor.

But for obstetric analgesia only opioid through intrathecal route needs a relatively larger dose in comparison to the mixture of LA agent and opioid in intrathecal space and this relatively higher dose of only opioid in intrathecal space has a high risk of side effects which is most frequently respiratory depression.

The *continuous subarachnoid anesthesia–analgesia to relieve labor pain* by using the conventional epidural catheter in subarachnoid space (but not the microcatheter which is specially designed for continuous spinal anesthesia) is also considered in cases of accidental (during attempt of continuous epidural) or deliberate dural puncture for high-risk patients. But surprisingly due to unknown reasons the incidence of PDPH is very low in this continuous spinal labor analgesia and anesthesia, using a conventional epidural needle and catheter, during its accidental or deliberate dural puncture. In 1980, the spinal microcatheter was first introduced for continuous spinal (subarachnoid) anesthesia. Then, it quickly gained popularity because of the fast onset of block, convenience, and low incidence of PDPH, but it causes high incidences of cauda equina syndrome because of the improper mixing of local anesthetic agents of relatively higher concentration with CSF than that of used for epidural space (anesthesia). This is again also due to the less production of turbulence, (which is normally produced) during the injection of the drug within the intrathecal space through microcatheter. Hence, there is controversy regarding the use of microcatheter for continuous subarachnoid analgesia–anesthesia.

To relieve labor pain through subarachnoid route for vaginal delivery, the commonly used LA agents are hyperbaric lignocaine (25–50 mg or 0.5–1 mL of 5% hyperbaric lignocaine), or bupivacaine (5–10 mg or 1–2 mL of 0.5% hyperbaric bupivacaine), or tetracaine (4–5 mg). This dose provides both analgesia and anesthesia (both motor and sensory block) extending from T_{10} to S_5 dermatomes. But small doses of hyperbaric LA agents such as lignocaine (15–20 mg), bupivacaine (2–5 mg), and tetracaine (3 mg), administered in subarachnoid space in a sitting position, provide only sacral anesthesia and analgesia (saddle block) which is sometimes helpful only during the second stage of labor.

For *only subarachnoid labor analgesia (only sensory block)* the commonly used opioids and their dose when used alone or with LA agents are morphine (0.1–0.5 mg), meperidine (10–20 mg), fentanyl (10–25 µg), and sufentanil

(5–10 µg). When morphine is used alone without LA agent, the onset of its analgesic action is unfortunately slow, taking 40–60 minutes and lasting for 24 hours. The side effects of intrathecal morphine are usually more frequent and these include dizziness, pruritus, nausea, vomiting, drowsiness, retention of urine, respiratory depression, etc. So, for obstetric analgesia, intrathecal morphine alone is not used. Pruritus produced by intrathecal morphine can be lessened by the use of IV naloxone in the dose of 0.4–0.8 mg, followed by infusion of it in the dose of 0.4 mg/h. But this naloxone does not affect the analgesia caused by intrathecal narcotics. Increasing the subarachnoid dose of morphine from 0.25 to 1 mg does not prolong the analgesia, but instead increases the complications. Intrathecal 25 µg fentanyl alone also provides labor analgesia within 5 minutes and lasts for 1–2 hours. When it is used, mixing with LA agent, then the dose of fentanyl should not be reduced. The intrathecal 10 µg sufentanil alone also provides labor analgesia within 5 minutes and this action lasts for 3 hours. The onset of action of intrathecal 10 mg meperidine is 10 minutes and it lasts for approximately 2–4 hours. However, intrathecal opioids only do not provide adequate analgesia for episiotomy or for the use of forceps. Therefore, it needs supplemental anesthesia by mixing opioids with LA agents. The addition of 0.2 mg epinephrine to intrathecal opioids does not prolong the duration of pain relief, but it decreases the severity and the incidences of pruritus, while increases the incidences of nausea and vomiting. Hypotension, followed by the administration of intrathecal opioids to relieve labor pain, may be due to the resultant analgesia and decreased circulating level of catecholamine.

Combined spinal-epidural analgesia to relieve labor pain: This technique is also widely used now to provide the optimum and prolonged analgesia to relieve labor pain and if necessary anesthesia in obstetric practice. By this method, we obtain the benefits and remove the disadvantages of each technique such as spinal and epidural. It offers rapid onset, and effective analgesia, minimum risk of toxicity of LA agent and opioids, and minimally impaired or no motor block. The rapid onset of action performed by the spinal part of CSE overcomes the disadvantage of delayed onset of action by epidural part of it. This delayed onset of action by epidural part of CSE may sometimes be thought as incomplete or patchy analgesia, causing an unnecessary increase in the dose of LA agent and subsequent motor blockade. Furthermore, this method makes it possible to prolong the duration of analgesia as necessary by the use of epidural catheter which cannot be obtained from the spinal part of it. Patients found greater satisfaction with CSE than the only continuous epidural analgesia. This is perhaps because of

rapid onset and a greater feeling of self-control by patient. In addition, if an operative delivery is necessary, then the same epidural catheter may be used to provide operative obstetric anesthesia. The onset of action of analgesia in CES is almost immediate due to its spinal component. The duration of this spinal analgesia lasts for 2–3 hours but depends on which opioid (alone) or which mixture of opioid and LA agent is used. The addition of isobaric bupivacaine to the opioids in the subarachnoid space during CSE produces a greater density of sensory blockade and minimum or nil motor blockade. Conventionally in subarachnoid space 25 µg fentanyl or 10 µg of sufentanil is used only for spinal analgesia. But 15 µg fentanyl or 5 µg sufentanil produces the same effect when either of these agents is mixed with isobaric bupivacaine and is injected in the subarachnoid space. Another potential advantage of a CSE technique for obstetric analgesia is that it may be associated with the significantly reduced duration of the first stage of labor. On the other hand, the use of continuous epidural infusion by dilute LA agent such as 0.0625–0.125% bupivacaine plus opioid such as fentanyl 15 µg provides only sensory analgesia without any motor block which may permit many obstetric patients to ambulate during labor. Then it is termed "walking epidural". This is because any form of central neuraxial block or analgesia where there is no motor block is termed like that. But before ambulation, every patient should be assessed carefully for the maternal and fetal well-being and also the adequate motor function of the mother.

GENERAL ANESTHESIA FOR VAGINAL DELIVERY

To relieve pain during labor, GA is usually avoided for normal vaginal delivery. This is because of the increased risk of gastric aspiration into the lungs in an unprepared patient and the complete absence of mother's cooperation which is very part and parcel of a normal vaginal delivery. But sometimes it (GA during vaginal delivery) is necessary in the following emergency situations such as (1) acute fetal distress requiring immediate expulsion of baby, (2) instrumental vaginal delivery, (3) manual removal of retained placenta, (4) tetanic uterine contraction, (5) replacement of inverted uterus, (6) psychiatric patients who become sudden uncontrollable, etc., and (7) where the epidural catheter is not in place before. If the epidural catheter is in place before for labor analgesia, then obstetric RA (muscular paralysis) is rapidly instituted through this catheter, instead of obstetric analgesia (sensory block).

If a sudden decision of GA for vaginal delivery is taken, then the important previous medical histories of patient are quickly taken and a nasogastric or orogastric tube is put into the stomach to aspirate the gastric contents, provided the patient is not properly prepared. After that, this tube is removed. This is followed by quick preoxygenation of patient by 100% O_2 for 3–5 minutes or 4 full breaths of 100% O_2, while monitors are applied by an assistant. Once all possible monitors are applied and the obstetrician is ready, then rapid sequence induction is instituted, applying cricoid pressure when the patient becomes unconscious and reflexes are lost. For rapid induction, the commonly used drugs are thiopentone (4–5 mg/kg), propofol (1–2 mg/kg), or ketamine (1 mg/kg, used only if there is hypovolemia or hypotension) which is followed by succinylcholine (1–1.5 mg/kg). The fasciculation, produced by succinylcholine, is usually not prevented by the use of a small dose of nondepolarizing agent. Because most pregnant patients usually do not fasciculate and moreover this fasciculation does not appear to promote regurgitation, as the increased intragastric pressure, caused by fasciculation, is matched by a similar increase in the tone of gastroesophageal sphincter by succinylcholine.

After successful intubation with a 7 or 7.5 endotracheal (ET) tube, the patient is ventilated by 100 O_2 and 1–2 MAC of any potent volatile anesthetic agent. After the action of succinylcholine is over, if skeletal muscle relaxation is needed, then any short-acting to intermediate-acting nondepolarizing muscle relaxing agent is used. Once fetus and placenta are delivered, then N_2O and opioids are added or propofol infusion is started to avoid recall. Simultaneously, the concentration of volatile anesthetic agent is reduced to 0.5 MAC or discontinued and oxytocin infusion is started at the rate of 10–20 U/L in IV fluid. At the end of the surgical procedure, the action of nondepolarizing muscle relaxant is reversed by anticholinesterase and the patient is extubated, while the reflexes are fully returned.

■ ANESTHESIA FOR CESAREAN SECTION

There are lots of medical and obstetric indications for CS which are done under RA or GA, but the choice between these two types of anesthesia (RA or GA) is determined by multiple factors which include the indications for CS, the severity of urgency, the skill of anesthetist, patient's preference, surgeon's preference, etc. However, now, RA is most frequently preferred than GA for excessively long umbilical cords (ELUCs) because the later (general anesthesia) is mostly associated with increased maternal mortality and morbidity, but recently many studies have shown that the morbidity and mortality in these two types of anesthesia is equal. Death or severe maternal morbidity in RA is mainly due to severe hypotension, or epidural hematoma, or sepsis of the spinal cord. Death or severe maternal morbidity

associated with GA is mainly due to airway problems, failed intubation, failed ventilation, aspiration pneumonitis, pulmonary edema, etc.

The advantages of GA over RA for CS are (1) very reliable, (2) rapid onset, (3) better control of airway, (4) better control of ventilation, (5) less incidences of severe hypotension, and (6) better management of patient in the face of severe bleeding such as in placenta previa, accidental hemorrhage, etc., whereas *the advantage of RA over GA are* (1) minimal risk to pulmonary aspiration, (2) less neonatal depression due to minimal or no exposure of the fetus to potentially depressant general anesthetic drugs, (3) provide a better option for postoperative analgesia, and (4) pleasant experience by mother during the birth of her child.

After taking decision for RA in CS, the next question that is arose is whether spinal or epidural. Except for few special indications for each technique, usually, the decision between the spinal or epidural anesthesia depends on the physician's preference. *Continuous epidural anesthesia allows* (1) slow, better, and prolonged control of sympathetic, sensory, and motor block which is very helpful for severely ill patient, (2) prolonged surgery, and (3) postoperative analgesia. Contrary, the *spinal anesthesia* has a more rapid onset, is easier to perform, and produce more intense motor, sensory, and sympathetic block, and because of a small dose of LA agent it does not have the potential for serious drug toxicity.

Now, at the end of the discussion, we can say that whatever may be the type of RA (epidural or spinal), patients should always be prepared for GA because at any time during the process of applying RA, it (general anesthesia) may be needed. Though, the principal disadvantage of GA is drug-induced fetal depression, but the present technique of it limits the dose of intravenous-inducing agent and reduces fetal depression. Clinically, it (fetal depression) is not significant in GA, if the delivery of the fetus can be done within 10 minutes of the induction of GA. On the contrary, whatever may be the type of anesthesia such as regional or general, if the baby is delivered within 3 minutes of uterine incision, then there is a better Apgar score.

Regional Anesthesia for Cesarean Section

The CS, performed under RA (spinal or epidural), requires sensory block up to the level of T_7 dermatomes. Therefore, it blocks more than half of the sympathetic outflow (this is because a sympathetic block is always two dermatomes above the sensory block, so here the sympathetic block is up to T5 spinal segment) and causes high incidences of severe hypotension. So, patients during CS must receive 500–1,000 mL of crystalloid intravenous fluid (usually Ringer's lactate) prior to CNB. But a small volume of IV administration of colloid is more effective than a huge volume of crystalloid. Whatever may be, the prophylactic IV administration of fluid (crystalloid or colloid) does not consistently prevent hypotension, induced by medical sympathectomy in RA. Therefore, if hypotension still persists in spite of adequate preload, then 10 mg IV ephedrine should be used to maintain the systolic BP above 100 mm Hg, or MAP should not be reduced <20% of the previous one. Instead of ephedrine, 25–100 µg of IV phenylephrine can also be used safely. Some anesthesiologists use the ephedrine or phenylephrine prophylactically, i.e., 1 minute before administering the LA agent in epidural or subarachnoid space, to avoid the immediate precipitous fall of BP, after instituting the regional block which sometimes can cause cardiac arrest.

This prophylactic measure (administration of ephedrine or phenylephrine 1 minute prior to the administration of LA drug in neuraxial space) is more applicable in spinal anesthesia than epidural because the onset of action of spinal block is very fast, but it may produce severe hypertension, if the severity of the proposed hypotension is not properly titrated with the doses of pressure rising agent and given at the proper time which is matched with the peak level of hypotension. Therefore, many anesthetists do not like it. Slight 10–15° head down position of patient reduces the chances of hypotension by encouraging venous drainage and increasing the preload, but it does not increase the extension of the sensory and sympathetic block by allowing more cranial flow of LA agent. During continuous epidural anesthesia, by using a catheter for CS, if there is an unintentional dural puncture, then it can be converted to continuous spinal anesthesia by advancing the epidural catheter through this needle in subarachnoid space. If during the first attempt of epidural anesthesia, there is an unintentional dural puncture, then another attempt through the spaces above or below the previous one is again tried.

The *commonly used drugs for spinal anesthesia in CS are:* Lignocaine (50–100 mg), bupivacaine (10–15 mg), or tetracaine (5–10 mg), but 0.1 mg epinephrine can also be used with this LA agent for spinal anesthesia which enhances the quality of the block and prolongs the duration of action of it. The addition of 25 µg fentanyl or 10 µg sufentanil or 0.2 mg morphine with the LA agent enhances the intensity of block and prolongs the duration of action without adversely affecting the neonatal outcome.

The *commonly used drugs for epidural anesthesia in CS are:* About 15–20 mL of 2% lignocaine or 0.5% bupivacaine, or 3% chloroprocaine. Similar to spinal block, addition of 50–100 µg of fentanyl or 10–20 µg of sufentanil, or 5 mg of morphine, etc., with the LA agents will greatly enhance the density of block and will prolong the duration of the action

of it, without adversely affecting the neonatal outcome. For epidural anesthesia, 15–20 mL of the recommended initial volume of the drug is not injected quickly as bolus. It is injected slowly in 5 mL incremental doses at 1–2 minute intervals. If due to any reasons, sensory levels recede and pain develops, then LA agent is further added through catheter in 5 mL incremental doses to maintain a sensory block up to T_7 level. Patchy epidural blocks due to some unknown reasons is usually treated by small doses of IV ketamine, prior to the delivery of the baby, but after the delivery of baby, it is managed by the adequate doses of opioids, propofol, etc. However, if the pain remains intolerable, in spite of these aforementioned measures then it necessities GA with ET intubation.

General Anesthesia for Cesarean Section

In recent decades, the use of GA for CS has declined dramatically, but still, it is used in some circumstances, where the *RA is contraindicated* such as (1) when the patient refuses to give consent, (2) coagulopathy, (3) local sepsis, (4) systemic infection, and (5) anesthesiologist has failed to provide RA, due to some technical difficulties or there is no time to institute RA, for example, during life-threatening severe maternal hemorrhage, life-threatening fetal compromise, etc. Several recent studies also have found that the maternal death rate, associated with properly managed RA has dramatically declined, but not in GA. Therefore, the difference in the rate of maternal mortality between the RA and GA has increased to 16 times. *There are no absolute contraindications for GA in CS like RA.* But there are certain conditions such as malignant hyperthermia and very difficult airway where the modified general anesthetic technique is required. The two principal problems associated with GA for CS are (1) *failed intubations* and (2) *pulmonary aspiration of gastric contents.*

Failed Intubations

The most common causes of maternal death, related to GA during CS, are *failed intubations with concomitant, failure to ventilate by mask, or failure to recognize esophageal intubation.* On the other hand, the common causes of failed intubation in obstetric patients, compared to nonobstetric surgical patients are weight gain, edema of airway, large breasts obstructing the manipulation of handle of laryngoscope, short neck (due to edema), etc. Therefore, this *anticipation of a difficult airway* and its subsequent difficult intubation will help to reduce the incidences of severe maternal hypoxemia and death during GA. Hence, the careful assessment of airway, before instituting GA for CS, is very crucial and from this airway assessment, the anticipation of difficult intubation may help to reduce this failed intubation catastrophe.

Among all the methods of evaluation of airway, the Mallampati classification is the most useful predictor. It has been found that the airway of Mallampati class IV, protruding maxillary incisions, short neck, mandibular recession, etc., are associated with the greatest risk for failed intubation. Hence, a simple examination of oropharynx, neck, mandible, dentition, etc., often helps to predict which patient will produce a problem or not. The patient who has a normal airway before pregnancy becomes problematic during this pregnancy. Again, it has been demonstrated that pregnancy is associated with some changes in the maternal airway. So, all the patients must have a repeat airway assessment before induction of anesthesia for CS, though the patient is examined initially. Last, it may be said that the experience of an anesthetist is the key factor for this general anesthesia (GA) related maternal mortality.

Because, in one vast study in a big teaching hospital, it is found that most cases of failed intubation has occurred when patients are cared for by a less experienced anesthetist.

Anticipating difficult intubation, varieties of laryngoscope blades, ET tubes of different sizes, stylets, bougies, classic laryngeal mask airway (LMA), intubating LMA (Fastrach), fiber optic laryngoscope, Combitube, kit for cricothyrotomy and tracheostomy, etc., should be made ready. The proper positioning of head and neck may facilitate tracheal intubation in difficult cases. These manipulations are flexion of cervical spine, elevation of shoulder and extension of atlantooccipital joint, etc. When this difficult intubation is anticipated, then the anesthesiologist must have a clear plan and obviously mother's life will get priority over the fetus **(Flowchart 1)**. After failed intubation, if mask ventilation is possible, then different methods of intubation should be tried. Or in the absence of fetal distress, a patient can be awakened and later an awaked intubation by infiltration of LA agents can be tried. If mask ventilation is not possible or not adequate, then other methods of ventilation by using LMA, Combitube, etc., are also tried. But still, if ventilation is not adequate then cricothyrotomy or tracheostomy or awakening of the patient can be tried to save the mother's life.

Pulmonary Aspiration of Gastric Contents

Another important cause of maternal death, related to GA during CS, is the pulmonary aspiration of gastric contents. Therefore, the increase of gastric pH and the decrease

Flowchart 1: Algorithm for difficult intubation in obstetric practice.

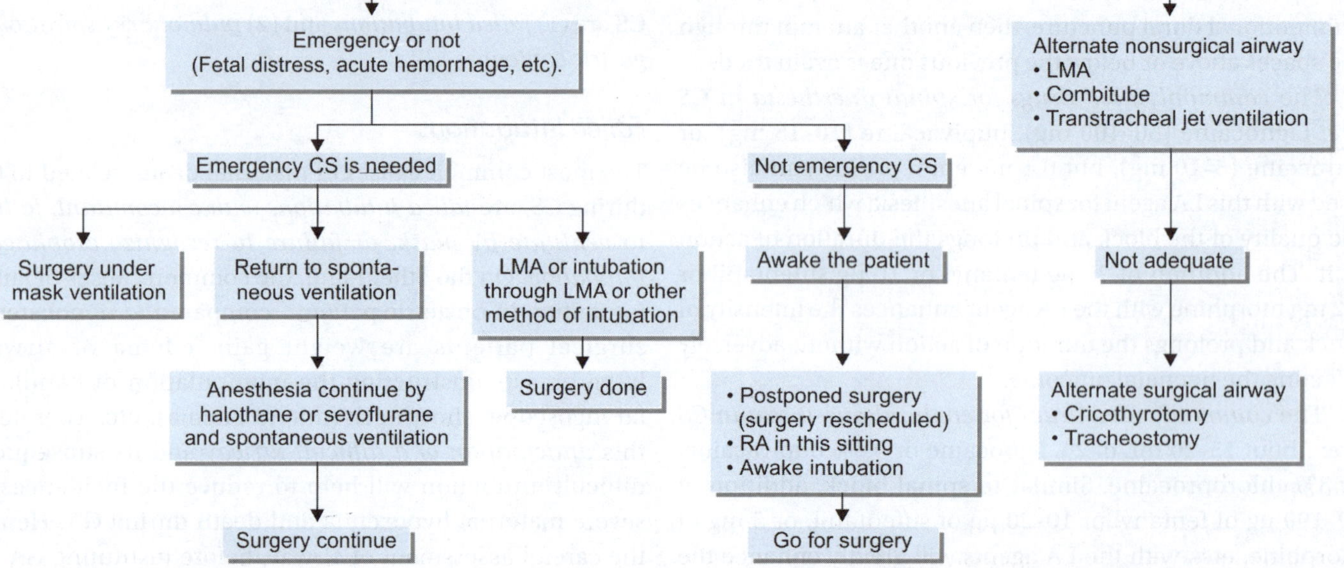

(CS: cesarean section; GA: general anesthesia; LMA: laryngeal mask airway; RA: regional anesthesia)

of its volume in a labor patient is the prime importance for an anesthetist. However, both of these effects can be accomplished by the following methods. Generally, gastric pH can be raised by the routine use of antacids prior to the induction of anesthesia, but the use of antacids does not reduce the risk of pulmonary aspiration. Although antacids increase gastric pH, but as most of them contain a suspension of particulate matter, so they may produce a severe pulmonary reaction, if they are aspirated. So, instead of nonclear antacid, a clear antacid such as 0.3 M sodium citrate is used. The advantage of both these types of antacids (clear and nonclear antacids) is that they act immediately, but the disadvantage is that they immediately increase the volume of gastric content after their use.

Except for antacids, gastric acidity and the volume of gastric content also can be decreased by using an H_2 receptor blocker (ranitidine), or a proton pump inhibitor (omeprazole, pantoprazole, etc.), but both of these drugs do not act immediately like antacids. Therefore, at least 1–2 hours of interval, after their oral administration, or 45–60 minutes of interval after their IV or IM administration, is required. It should also be kept in mind that both these drugs cannot change the pH and volume of gastric contents which are already secreted into the stomach.

Metoclopramide is another prokinetic agent that increases the emptying of the stomach and raises the tone of lower gastroesophageal sphincter. Thus, it reduces the gastric volume (but does not change the gastric pH) and decreases the subsequent chances of aspiration of gastric contents by regurgitation or vomiting. On the other hand, it does not raise the gastric pH and has no adverse effects on the fetus or neonates.

To prevent pulmonary aspiration of gastric content, the use of invasive positive pressure ventilation (IPPV) before intubation should also be avoided. Because it can inflate the stomach by air and thus can make the patient more vulnerable to regurgitation and pulmonary aspiration of gastric contents. Another mechanical way to reduce this risk of pulmonary aspiration of gastric contents is the Sellick maneuver (cricoid pressure) which occludes the esophagus. Finally, the risk of pulmonary aspiration of gastric contents can also be minimized by intubating the trachea with an ET tube and extubating the patient only after she is fully awake with a good return of laryngeal reflexes. **Box 1** shows some strategies to reduce maternal mortality in obstetric general anesthesia.

The steps of general anesthesia in CS are like that:
- Taking of history and airway assessment meticulously.
- Proper preparation of patient by oral antacid or H_2 blocker or proton pump inhibitor and metoclopramide.

BOX 1: Some strategies to reduce maternal mortality in obstetric anesthesia.

- Less experienced anesthetists should not take sole responsibility for obstetric anesthesia
- The anesthetist must have a skilled helper, irrespective of his or her experience
- Antacid does not give full protection against Mendelson syndrome. Therefore H_2 blocker or proton pump inhibitor (PPI) and prokinetic agent are mandatory
- Cricoid pressure must be applied
- Failed intubation drills should be exercised by all obstetric anesthetists
- No matter how urgent the obstetric anesthesia, history, and monitoring must not be neglected
- Epidural labor analgesia should be supervised by a skilled person and an anesthetist should be available immediately in an emergency

- The patient is placed supine with 15° left uterine displacement by putting a wedge under her right buttock.
- Starting of IV infusion by a large bore cannula.
- Preoxygenation by 100% O_2 with high flow rate (>6 L/min) for 3–5 minutes. Four full vital capacity breaths of 100% O_2 is also adequate for denitrogenation.
- Monitors are applied
- The patient is prepared by antiseptic dressing over abdomen and is draped.
- The surgeon is ready to begin surgery and an assistant of anesthetist is also ready to apply cricoid pressure.
- Rapid sequence induction and muscular paralysis is performed, by using thiopentone (4–5 mg/kg) or propofol (1–2 mg/kg) or ketamine (1 mg/kg, in hypovolemic or asthmatic patient) and succinylcholine (1–1.5 mg/kg). Defasciculation is not necessary in CS.
- Trachea is intubated by a properly sized ET tube and the cuff is inflated. Cricoid pressure is maintained till trachea is sealed off. Proper placement of the ET tube is confirmed by capnography.
- Maternal $PaCO_2$ below 25 mm Hg by hyperventilation is avoided. Because it can reduce the uterine blood flow by vasoconstriction and subsequently fetal acidosis. Hyperventilation also causes the leftward shift of maternal O_2-Hb dissociation curve and decreases the O_2 availability to fetus.
- Respiration is maintained by IPPV using 50:50 N_2O:O_2 mixture with any potent volatile anesthetic agent in low concentration (0.5% halothane or 0.75% isoflurane or 1% sevoflurane or 3% desflurane). This low concentration of volatile anesthetic agent helps to produce amnesia and does not cause excessive uterine relaxation or impair uterine contraction by oxytocin.

- Nondepolarizing muscle relaxants of intermediate duration of action such as rocuronium, atracurium, cisatracurium, or mivacurium are used when necessary.
- The 20–30 units of oxytocin per liter of IV fluid are infused after the neonate is delivered. Then, the umbilical cord is clamped and placenta is removed.
- Anesthesia is deepened by increasing the percentage of N_2O in the inspired gas mixture by up to 70% and by further adding narcotics, BZDs, or propofol.
- If there is hypotonicity of uterine muscle, then the halogenated volatile anesthetic agent should be discontinued.
- If there is still relaxation of uterine musculature, then 0.2 mg methylergometrine or 0.25 mg of 15 methyl prostaglandin F2α may also be given by IM or IV.
- At the end of surgery, the effect of muscle relaxant is reversed by anticholinesterase (neostigmine) with anticholinergic (glycopyrrolate) and extubated when there is full return of laryngeal reflexes.

ACID ASPIRATION OR MENDELSON'S SYNDROME

In 1946, Mendelson had first described a syndrome in which gastric contents had been regurgitated and aspired into the lungs and initiated a series of characteristic pulmonary signs and symptoms constituting a syndrome. So, now, it (this syndrome) bears his name. The morbidity and mortality of this syndrome are very high and it depends upon the volume, nature, acidity (pH), and the nature of the distribution of aspirated material into the lungs. If the aspiration of gastric contents is of sufficient quantity or solid, then it will cause asphyxia, due to airway obstruction. Otherwise, if the gastric content is of very low pH (<2.5), though is of a small amount (as small as 25 mL), it will cause serious pulmonary reaction and death without producing asphyxia. It has been found that the 60% of obstetric patients at term have >40 mL of gastric juice and its pH is <2.5 in an empty stomach.

The pathophysiological consequences and the clinical picture of this syndrome, following the aspiration of gastric acids, fit with acute respiratory distress syndrome (ARDS), but this ARDS may also develop due to other causes. These other causes are pulmonary injury by other substances, except acid, which enters through the airway or by indirect blood-borne insult to lungs **(Box 2)**. Some severe form of this syndrome may develop immediately and patient collapsed, but sometimes the symptoms, following the aspiration of a little to moderate amount of liquid gastric contents with low pH, may become apparent slowly over 6–8 hours, after the aspiration.

After the aspiration of gastric acid content into lungs, there is severe inflammation of pulmonary tissue and

BOX 2: Conditions predisposing to acute respiratory distress syndrome (ARDS).

Direct through airway:
- Aspiration of gastric contents
- Toxic gases
- Near drowning

Indirect by blood-borne:
- Severe sepsis
- Multiple trauma
- Anaphylaxis
- Pancreatitis
- Drugs
- Amniotic fluid and fat embolism

simultaneously there is also release of large number of mediators which include cytokines (such as tumor necrosis factor, interleukins 1 and 6, platelet activation factor), prostaglandins, leukotrienes, lysosomal enzymes, etc. These mediators trigger a complex interaction between the endothelial cells, platelets, coagulation pathways, and white blood cell (WBC) which become activated and damage the vascular endothelium. Then, the fluid and cells pass across this damaged endothelium, from blood vessels into the interstitial space, causing pulmonary edema and further tissue inflammation. Thus, a vicious cycle of endothelial injury, intravascular coagulation, microvascular occlusion, tissue damage, and the further release of inflammatory mediators sets up. Patient often suffers from cough, tachypnea, wheezing, rhonchi, hypoxia, and all the other features of pulmonary edema. *The criteria defining ARDS are* (1) hypoxemia which is defined as PaO_2 <200 mm Hg, (2) chest radiograph showing diffuse bilateral infiltration, (3) absence of raised left atrial pressure—pulmonary arterial wedge pressure (PAWP) <15 mm Hg, and (4) impaired lung compliance.

The term ARDS is often limited to patients, who are requiring ventilatory support. But the less severe forms of ARDS is conventionally referred to as acute lung injury (ALI). The suction through an endotracheal tube, which reveals bile-stained fluid, is often diagnostic. While over a longer term, serial chest X-rays, and serial arterial blood gas estimations will reveal progressive changes.

The management of this Mendelson's syndrome is very difficult. It includes proper arterial oxygenation by ventilation through an ET tube, suction through an ET tube, correction of blood volume and acid–base balance, steroids, antibiotics, etc., and adequate monitoring in intensive care unit (ICU). As prevention is better than cure, so an anesthetist will always try to take measures which will prevent to develop it. This is described in **Box 3**.

BOX 3: Measures to avoid acid aspiration.

- *Decreasing the acidity of gastric fluid:*
  - Use of antacid to neutralize the existing acid
  - Use of H_2 blocker/PPI to stop the secretion of acid and to elevate pH
- *Decreasing the volume of gastric fluid:*
  - By restricting oral intake
  - By increasing the emptying of stomach by metoclopramide
  - By decreasing gastric secretion
  - By physical means suction through a large bore tube
- *Preventing the regurgitation of gastric secretion:*
  - Increase in intragastric pressure should be avoided
  - Increase in tone of lower gastroesophageal sphincter
  - Induction in an upright position
- *Preventing the aspiration of regurgitant material:*
  - By applying cricoid pressure.
  - By suction
  - By induction in the Trendelenburg position
- *Avoiding GA:*
  - RA avoids gastric aspiration
- *Avoiding difficult intubation:*
  - By proper assessment of the airway
  - By appointing a skilled anesthetist

(GA: general anesthesia; PPI: proton pump inhibitor; RA: regional anesthesia)

PREECLAMPSIA, ECLAMPSIA, AND ANESTHESIA

Preeclampsia is also termed pregnancy-induced hypertension (PIH). *Hypertension in pregnancy may be due to* (1) PIH or (2) chronic essential hypertension, existing before pregnancy or (3) recent development of essential hypertension, during this pregnancy or (4) chronic hypertension with superimposed preeclampsia. Preeclampsia complicates up to 8–10% of all pregnancies and is the most common difficult condition, encountered by an anesthetist during his/her practice of obstetric anesthesia, where otherwise a previously healthy patient suddenly becomes severely ill.

The classic triad of preeclampsia are hypertension, proteinuria (>500 mg/day), and edema (hand and face). Hypertension in preeclampsia is usually defined as systolic and diastolic BP above than 140 mm Hg and 90 mm Hg respectively, or persistent increase in systolic and diastolic BP by 30 mm Hg and 15 mm Hg respectively above the normal baseline value, on two occasions at least 4 hours apart after the 20th week of gestation in a woman with previous normal BP. *The other characteristic features of preeclampsia are* (1) hypertension occurring after 20 weeks of gestation and resolving within 48 hours after delivery or developing in the early postpartum period and returning to normal within 3 months of delivery, (2) oliguria and proteinuria >300 mg/day, (3) serum and urine creatinine concentration ratio >0.09 and urine protein/creatinine ratio >0.3, (4) headache

with visual disturbances, (5) increased level of liver enzymes, (6) ↑lactate dehydrogenase, ↑thrombocytopenia, ↑hemolysis, and (7) disseminated intravascular coagulation (DIC).

When convulsions occur in preeclampsia, then this condition is called *eclampsia,* where the prognosis of both mother and fetus worsens. But now, it is less common in modern obstetric practice. Severe PIH contributes about 30–40% of maternal death and 15–20% of perinatal death. *The principal causes of maternal death in preeclampsia are* stroke, pulmonary edema, and hepatic necrosis or rupture or failure, and a combination of these complications. There are some predisposing factors for preeclampsia. These are a family history of preeclampsia, chronic renal disease, chronic hypertension, multiple gestation, age >40 years, diabetes, etc.

Hemolysis, elevated liver enzymes and low platelets (HELLP) syndrome, found in preeclampsia, is a pathological condition that is characterized by (1) hemolysis (H), (2) elevated liver enzymes (EL), and (3) low platelet count (LP). This represents a severe form of preeclampsia with the aforementioned signs. It occurs in 20% of pregnant patients who develop severe preeclampsia with many of its manifestations, occurring in postpartum period. Its severity ranges from a mild self-limiting condition to a fulminant process, leading to multiorgan failure. No signs and symptoms of this syndrome (HELLP) are diagnostic, because all these signs and symptoms are found in patients with severe preeclampsia–eclampsia, but without HELLP syndrome.

Preeclampsia may be classified as *mild or severe* according to the severity of symptoms and signs which are demonstrated in **Table 5**. Assuming, there is no presence of any coagulopathy, then hemostasis is not usually a problem unless the platelet count is decreased below 40,000/mm³ in preeclampsia. In such circumstances, RA is contraindicated. This abnormal platelet count usually returns to normal within 72 hours of the delivery of the fetus. But this thrombocytopenia may persist for longer periods.

Preeclampsia is the disease of theories, as the precise cause of it is still unknown, in spite of extensive research. It is mainly associated with (1) *abnormal activities of trophoblastic cells* and (2) *vascular endothelial dysfunction of placenta.* Thus, it leads to the maladaptation of maternal spiral arteries and is particularly found in women with vascular disorders. The secondary pathology in preeclampsia is also linked to an *immunological basis* and *endothelial dysfunction (vascular hyper-reactivity),* causing *excessive activation of coagulation.* This is due to the abnormal metabolism of prostaglandin.

This preeclamptic patient has (1) increased production of TXA_2 (thromboxane A_2) which is a potent vasoconstrictor and helps in platelet aggregation and (2) decreased

TABLE 5: Classification of preeclampsia.

	Mild	*Severe*
Systolic pressure	<160 mm Hg	>160 mm Hg
Diastolic pressure	<110 mm Hg	>110 mm Hg
Urine output	>500 mL/24 h	<500 mL/24 h
Urinary protein	<5 g/24 h	>5 g/24 h
Platelet count	>100,000/mm^3	<100,000/mm^3
Pulmonary edema	Absent	Present
Headache (CNS symptoms and signs)	Absent	Present
Epigastric pain	Absent	Present
Visual disturbance	Absent	Present
HELLP syndrome	Absent	Present
Serum creatinine	<1.1 mg/dL	>1.1 mg/dL

(CNS: central nervous system; HELLP: hemolysis, elevated liver enzymes, and low platelets)

TABLE 6: Complications of preeclampsia and eclampsia.

CVS	Hypertension, ↓ intravascular volume, ↑ vascular resistance, ↓ cardiac output, heart failure, and stroke
RS	Airway edema and pulmonary edema
Kidney	↓ GFR, oliguria, proteinuria, and renal failure
NS	Hyperexcitability, convulsions, headache, visual disturbance, intracranial hemorrhage, and cerebral edema
Liver	Elevated liver enzymes, impaired functions, hematoma, and rupture of blood vessels
Hematology	Thrombocytopenia, coagulopathy, microangiopathic hemolysis, platelet dysfunction, and prolonged PTT

(CVS: cardiovascular system; GFR: glomerular filtration rate; NS: nervous system; PTT: partial thromboplastin time; RS: respiratory system)

production of PGI_2 (prostacyclin) which is a potent vasodilator and reduces platelet aggregation. Another mechanism of action of endothelial dysfunction is decreased production of nitric oxide (NO) which is a potent vasodilator and increased production of endothelin-1 which is a potent vasoconstrictor. Thus, marked endothelial immunological injury due to its hyper-reactivity leads to widespread systemic manifestation as well as reduced placental perfusion.

The systemic manifestation of preeclampsia includes generalized edema with special importance to airway, ↑SVR, ↓intravascular volume, hyperdynamic circulation, decreased GFR, ↑uric acid, liver dysfunction, pulmonary edema, etc., **(Table 6)**. The pulmonary edema in preeclampsia is due to (1) high left atrial and pulmonary capillary wedge pressure, (2) low plasma colloid and osmotic pressure, and (3) increased pulmonary capillary permeability. Increased levels of uric acid in preeclampsia result from decreased renal excretion, tissue ischemia, and oxidative stress. Acute renal failure is rare in preeclampsia but is mostly associated with HELLP syndrome. Liver dysfunction is also mostly associated with HELLP syndrome. Cardiac output in preeclampsia may be high, normal, or low depending on the severity of increased SVR, the severity of decreased intravascular volume, and the degree of hyperdynamic cardiac function (contractility).

The immediate delivery of fetus and placenta is the definitive and principal way of treatment for severe preeclampsia and all eclampsia during the life-threatening condition of mother at any stage of gestation. Otherwise (i.e., when there is no life-threatening condition to mother), the aim of the treatment of preeclampsia is to control hypertension and to prevent convulsions. The drugs used to treat severe hypertension in preeclampsia

TABLE 7: Pharmacology of labetalol and hydralazine.

	Labetalol	*Hydralazine*
Mode of action	Slight α blocker mainly β blocker	Direct vasodilatation
Dose	10–20 mg IV	5–10 mg IV
Maintenance	20–160 mg/h	2–20 mg/h
Speed of onset	Quick	Gradual
Tachycardia	Absent	Present

are repeated doses of hydralazine (5 mg IV), and labetalol (5–10 mg IV). The other agents used during an emergency are nitroglycerine, Na-nitroprusside, and esmolol. The nitroprusside is helpful only for a short-term basis because the prolonged infusion of it is associated with increased risk of cyanide toxicity. The Ca^{2+} channel blockers are usually not used to control hypertension in preeclampsia because they are contraindicated in pregnancy. It is recommended that corticosteroid may be given, if the fetus is viable and 33 weeks of gestation and less **(Table 7)**.

$MgSO_4$ is the agent of choice to control the convulsions of eclampsia and to prevent of recurrent eclamptic fits. It is effective in >50% of patients, without serious maternal morbidity. Another beneficial effect of $MgSO_4$ is that it causes vasodilatation and decreases SVR, causing increased cardiac output. The initial bolus dose of $MgSO_4$ is 4 g and is administered through IV slowly over 10 minutes. This is followed by infusion at the rate of 1–3 g/h. The $MgSO_4$ has a low therapeutic index with serum Mg^{2+} level between 4 and 6 mEq/L, being safe and effective. It is excreted through kidney. Therefore, in the presence of renal failure, the dose of $MgSO_4$ should be reduced and guided by serum magnesium level. During the use of $MgSO_4$, the level of plasma Mg should be monitored carefully in conjunction with the clinical signs which include respiratory depression and decreased tendon reflex, indicating the toxicity of Mg. If the toxicity of $MgSO_4$ occurs, then 10 mL of 10% calcium gluconate is given through IV slowly which counteracts the side effect of Mg. Invasive arterial and central venous monitoring are indicated in patients with severe hypertension, pulmonary edema, refractory oliguria, or combination of these.

Anesthetic Consideration during Preeclampsia and Eclampsia

For *mild preeclampsia*, standard anesthetic practice is sufficient. The first step during the anesthetic management of a *severe preeclamptic or an eclamptic* patient includes detailed history taking regarding the severity of the condition, the degree of systemic involvement, fluid status, airway assessment, cardiovascular status, renal condition, coagulation status, etc. It also includes complete blood count, liver function tests, renal function tests, platelet count, coagulation profile, etc. But routine coagulation screening is not recommended by all clinicians, except the presence or suspected of coagulopathy clinically. Central neuraxial block is contraindicated in the presence of coagulopathy or low platelet count ($<100,000/mm^3$). But some anesthetists take this lower count of platelet as $70,000/mm^3$ for contraindication of CNB. However, a platelet count as low as $50,000/\mu L$ may be acceptable in selected cases, particularly when the count has been stable and global coagulation, as measured by *thrombelastography* testing, is normal.

Preeclampsia–eclampsia is associated with exaggerated Na^+ and water retention, but still it is characterized by decreased intravascular volume (hypovolemia). This is due to the shift of fluid and protein in the interstitial space from intravascular compartment. Thus, the intravascular fluid volume is inversely proportional to the severity of hypertension in preeclampsia and eclampsia. So, the measurement of central venous pressure (CVP) in the presence of severe preeclampsia–eclampsia will be a false guide. Therefore, before any mode of anesthesia, patient should be hydrated properly by intravenous infusion. This will improve maternal tissue perfusion, will increase cardiac index, will decrease SVR, and will increase GFR, etc.

Regarding the mode of anesthesia in preeclampsia–eclampsia, it is found that any form of anesthesia (RA or GA) is equally safe if they are properly conducted with extra caution. But there should be some choice, as both these modes of anesthesia have their own advantages and disadvantages. But in the absence of coagulopathy, the *first choice of anesthesia* for most patients with preeclampsia–eclampsia during the process of labor, vaginal delivery and CS is continuous epidural analgesia and anesthesia. It offers the advantage of gradual onset of sympathetic blockade, gradual hypotension, cardiovascular stability, due to gradual compensation with the passing of time, and no neonatal depression that can be caused by general anesthetic drugs. The reduction of hypertension and the diminution of vasospasm (due to sympathetic block and decreased catecholamine secretion), caused by RA, will improve uteroplacental blood flow, provided severe hypotension is avoided and adequate IV fluid is used to correct hypovolemias. The RA also reduces the risk of upward exaggerated hemodynamic alterations, associated with intubation and extubation of GA and airway complications. On the other hand, if CNB is badly managed, then it is frequently associated with extensive sympatholysis and profound hypotension (if not controlled) which may lead to decreased cardiac output, decreased uteroplacental blood flow, and in extreme conditions even fetal and maternal cardiac arrest. This is more likely with single-shot spinal anesthesia if severe hypotension is not corrected immediately. Hence, even though the single-shot spinal block is considered acceptable by many anesthetists, but is still taken by others to be relatively contraindicated for women with severe preeclampsia–eclampsia. *However, multiple recent studies have suggested that the magnitude of the decline of maternal BP after spinal and epidural block appears to be similar.* Hence, spinal block is not contraindicated and can easily be instituted on a severe preeclampsia patient undergoing CS.

Hypotension induced by CNB can easily be avoided by meticulous attention, use of IV colloid infusion, and/or use of vasopressor (ephedrine 5 mg) in a titratable fashion, because preeclamptic patients tend to be very sensitive to these agents. It is also true that hypotension associated with CNB can easily be controlled than the exaggerated surge of hypertension in GA during laryngoscopy, intubation, and extubation which can only be controlled by appropriate treatment with labetalol, nitroglycerine, nitroprusside, hydralazine, trimethaphan, etc. In GA, the risk of failed intubation also should be weighed against the risk of hypotension, when deciding between GA and RA for CS of the patient who is suffering from severe preeclampsia–eclampsia. If GA is instituted on a preeclamptic–eclamptic patient receiving $MgSO_4$, then anesthetist should be careful regarding the use of muscle relaxant—depolarizing and nondepolarizing. This is because the action of both will be potentiated by $MgSO_4$. Hence, the use of muscle relaxants in a patient receiving $MgSO_4$ should be guided by the peripheral nerve stimulator. $MgSO_4$ also blocks the release of catecholamines after sympathetic stimulations and blunts the response of vasoconstrictors. Therefore, there is also more chance of severe hypotension after CNB in a patient receiving $MgSO_4$.

The patients with Mg toxicity, manifested by hyporeflexia, excessive sedation, blurred vision, respiratory compromise, and cardiac depression are treated with IV Ca-gluconate. All the preeclamptic and eclamptic patients associated with severe hypertension, pulmonary edema, refractory oliguria, receiving IV vasodilators, etc., should be monitored by intra-arterial BP, CVP, pulmonary capillary wedge pressure (PCWP), etc.

OBSTETRIC HEMORRHAGE AND ANESTHESIA

Obstetric hemorrhage is one of the leading causes of maternal morbidity and mortality, necessitating immediate anesthesia and surgical intervention. The common causes of this obstetric hemorrhage are placenta previa, abruptio placentae, uterine inversion, uterine rupture, and uterine atony. Placenta previa and abruptio placentae account for about 0.5 and 1–2% of total pregnancies, respectively.

In placenta previa, the placenta is situated on lower uterine segment, covering internal os which may be complete or partial. The complete placenta previa is more dangerous than partial one, regarding the severity of vaginal bleeding. Placenta previa usually presents as painless vaginal bleeding and stops spontaneously in mild cases, when it is a partial one, but severe bleeding can occur at any time and usually it occurs in complete placenta previa, covering completely the internal os. During severe vaginal bleeding there are two problems (1) on the one hand the life of mother and (2) on the another hand the life of the fetus. If the duration of pregnancy is <37 weeks and the bleeding is mild to moderate, then conservative management may be allowed by bed rest and close observation, whereas the definitive management of obstetric hemorrhage for any cause after 37 weeks of gestation is CS.

In abruptio placentae, there is premature separation of placenta causing painful bleeding which may be revealed through vagina or concealed. Occasionally, the blood may extend into the myometrium which is called the couvelaire uterus. Any vaginal bleeding of a pregnant woman is assumed to have placenta previa, until proved otherwise. The actual diagnosis is performed by ultrasound. Uterine rupture is another cause of obstetric hemorrhage causing emergency. It is relatively uncommon and can occur as a result of dehiscence of a previous scar on the uterus or due to any intrauterine manipulation or due to very prolonged labor. It can present as acute fetal distress, frank hemorrhage, loss of uterine tone, or severe hypotension with occult bleeding into the peritoneal cavity.

In all the acute obstetric hemorrhage the mother should be assessed first about its hemodynamic status.

If the bleeding is mild to moderate, resuscitation by fluid is adequate and the condition of patient is stable when decision for surgery is taken, then RA may be considered. Otherwise, acute bleeding or a patient with unstable hemodynamic status may require surgical intervention under GA. All these patients should be tackled with at least two large bore (16 or 18G) intravenous catheter. Intravascular volume deficit must be replaced vigorously. A central venous line is especially useful for monitoring of preload and rapid transfusion. Two units of whole blood should be immediately available.

The choice between the regional and general anesthesia during surgery to tackle obstetric hemorrhage depends upon the urgency for delivery and maternal hemodynamic stability. In such situation close communication is very necessary with the concerned surgical team regarding about the mother, fetus, or both who are in immediate danger requiring GA or there is time to safely administer RA. If epidural catheter is already in place for painless labor (labor analgesia), then severe hypotension due to massive bleeding and delay in establishing adequate anesthesia by further adding anesthetic dose of LA agent through this epidural route may prohibit its use.

In acute emergency if GA is decided, then adequate preoxygenation is quickly achieved by four full breaths of 100% O_2, while possible necessary monitors are being applied during this period of preoxygenation. For induction instead of thiopentone and propofol, ketamine in the dose of 1 mg/kg is used for hypotension. Other steps for emergency CS are also taken which will help in prevention to develop aspiration pneumonitis (Mendelson's syndrome) and will also help to develop proper ventilation with adequate oxygenation if failed intubation occurs. Continuous precise fetal monitoring is very essential, because it may help by avoiding the unnecessary GA as emergency for acute fetal distress, diagnosed by imprecise monitoring. Otherwise extra time may be allowed to institute RA. For example, in most of the cases the fetal distress is diagnosed by fetal heart rate variability, but it has high false positive result and may land in GA showing acute distress, giving no time for RA. Hence, careful interpretation of other parameters such as fetal pulse oximeter or fetal scalp pH is necessary which may change the mode of anesthesia.

In abruptio placentae, RA is contraindicated if there is coagulopathy, particularly following fetal demise. This coagulopathy is due to activation of circulating fibrinolysin (plasminogen) and the release of tissue thromboplastin. This may precipitate DIC which is characterized by low fibrinogen level, low platelet count, and high fibrinogen degradation product. Fibrinogen level is mildly reduced with level between 150 and 250 mg/dL in moderate abruptio placentae. But in severe one the fibrinogen level may go below 150 mg/dL.

Anesthesia in Laparoscopic Surgery

■ INTRODUCTION

Due to the development of better surgical equipment and anesthetic facilities and also due to the increased knowledge and the understanding of the anatomy and pathophysiology of different diseases, the different surgical procedures gradually also have improved, i.e., become less invasive. Thus, it (less invasive surgical procedure) (i) reduces the trauma to the patient, (ii) causes less blood loss, (iii) causes less postoperative pain, (iv) causes early recovery, (v) causes the reduction of morbidity and mortality, (vi) causes short hospital stay, and consequently (vii) causes the reductions in healthcare costs by the concept of *"minimally invasive or endoscopic surgery".*

The endoscopic procedures had first started in early 1970's for various gynecological operations (for both diagnosis and treatment). Then, it soon becomes *very popular* among the gynecologists only. But, during this period, it was *not very popular* among the general surgeons, until 1987, when, laparoscopic cholecystectomy was first described in late 1980's by Philippe Mouret in France. After that, gradually, it became a very well-established technique for cholecystectomy in that country (France). Then, very soon this technique was accepted by surgeons all over the world and now >90% of all cholecystectomies are done by laparoscopic procedure with (i) less postoperative pain, (ii) reduced hospital stay, (iii) reduced cost, and (iv) earlier return to home for work. During that period *acute cholecystitis, obesity, and previous intra-abdominal surgeries* were considered as the contraindications for cholecystectomy by laparoscopic procedure. But, these are now no longer considered as contraindications, like before, for laparoscopic cholecystectomy and the laparoscopic procedure has become quite safe in the hands of experienced surgeons in these conditions which were taken as contraindications previously. Subsequently, many other new intra-abdominal and extra-abdominal laparoscopic or endoscopic surgical techniques have been developed such as (i) gastrointestinal surgeries (surgeries on esophagus, vagotomy, appendisectomy, fundoplication, colonic surgeries, gastric surgeries, splenic surgeries, hepatic surgeries, etc.), (ii) gynecological surgeries (hysterectomy and others), (iii) urological surgeries (nephrectomy, cystectomy, prostatectomy, etc.), (iv) hernia repair, (v) testicular surgeries, etc.

So, these new minimum invasive endoscopic surgical techniques have created new interests to anesthetists with separate anesthetic considerations for the management of such patients. Gradually, the list of these surgical procedures, which are now commonly performed endoscopically, has grown rapidly. The laparoscopic surgical techniques which are included in this list are now extending from intraperitoneal to transabdominal preperitoneal to totally extraperitoneal procedures. For example, a laparoscopic fundoplication procedure which is performed as antireflux surgery, proves a very cost-effective technique for patients, suffering from gastroesophageal reflux and on long-term medical management.

The pathophysiological changes due to (i) pneumo-peritoneum, (ii) different patient's position (required during laparoscopic surgeries), (iii) long duration of some laparoscopic surgeries, (iv) risk of some unsuspected visceral injury, (v) difficulty in evaluating the amount of blood loss during surgery, and (vi) some other factors, etc. make the anesthesia for laparoscopic surgery a potentially high-risk procedure. Young healthy women are the largest group of patients who are undergoing the different gynecological and different surgical (mainly cholecystectomy) laparoscopic surgery. Usually, they are associated with minor to moderate cardiorespiratory changes which are of little concern to an anesthetist. But, older patients with known or latent coexisting systemic diseases, waiting for endoscopic surgery, are prone to more risk, necessitating intensive care and thorough knowledge of pathophysiological changes, associated with laparoscopic surgery.

Compared with the open laparotomy, the major advantages of laparoscopic surgery are: (i) reduced tissue trauma (as less surgical exposure), (ii) reduced wound size, (iii) reduced postoperative pain due to small wound, (iv) reduced incidence of postoperative ileus, (v) earlier mobilization of patients, (vi) shorter hospital stay, (vii) improved postoperative respiratory function, etc. For example, following open cholecystectomy, due to postoperative pain, the forced vital capacity (FVC) is reduced by approximately 50% and this change is still evident up to 72 hours postoperatively. Contrary, following laparoscopic cholecystectomy, the FVC is reduced by approximately only 30% and becomes normal within 24 hours postoperatively.

On the other hand, technically the laparoscopic surgery differs from the open laparotomy by the following points:

- Laparoscopic surgery needs gravitational displacement of abdominal viscera from the site of operation by Trendelenburg or anti-Trendelenburg position.
- It (laparoscopic procedure) needs pneumoperitoneum which separates the abdominal wall from viscera. For pneumoperitoneum the upper limit of intra-abdominal pressure (IAP) is 15–20 mm Hg. Modern pneumoperitoneum-producing equipment has the ability to maintain continuously this upper limit of IAP automatically. Older laparoscopic equipment, which may not have this automatic adjustment for upper limit, can deliver uncontrolled gas flows, producing a very high IAP (sometimes >40 mm Hg).
- It needs decompression of abdominal viscera, especially the stomach by nasogastric tube and the bladder by urinary catheter to prevent their injury during the insertion of trocar, before producing pneumoperitoneum.

PATHOPHYSIOLOGICAL CHANGES OF RESPIRATORY AND CVS DURING LAPAROSCOPY

Two systems of our body are mainly affected during laparoscopic surgery. These are *respiratory system (RS) and cardiovascular system (CVS)*.

Changes in Respiratory System during Laparoscopy

The insufflation of CO_2 (current routine practice) into peritoneal cavity to create pneumoperitoneum for laparoscopic surgery results in ventilatory and respiratory changes in patients. Due to pneumoperitoneum, the resulting increase in IAP displaces the diaphragm upward

and causes (i) a decrease in the compliance of both chest wall and lungs, (ii) an increase in airway resistance, and (iii) an increase in peak inspiratory pressure. There is also (iv) an increase in the risk of gastric regurgitation during pneumoperitoneum due to increase in IAP.

The compliance of lung is reduced to 30–50%, but the shape of the pressure-volume loop of it does not change. Once the pneumoperitoneum is created up to the surgeon's desired level and IAP is kept constant, then this lung compliance is not further affected or reduced, after reaching its upper limit, either by the subsequent patient tilting or by the increase of minute ventilation which may be required to avoid intraoperative hypercapnia. That means the compliance of lung decreases and becomes fixed at a given increased IAP. Then, further decrease or deterioration of compliance cannot be detected by increasing IAP. After that point, if there is any deterioration of lung's compliance, then it will be only due to the pathology of lungs and other causes, but not due to the increase in IAP. Therefore, continuous compliance and pressure-volume loop monitoring are helpful in diagnosing any secondary complication, resulting from increased airway pressure due to the bronchospasm, changes in muscle relaxation, endobronchial intubation, pneumothorax, etc. which are responsible for further decrease in the compliance of lungs after it becomes fixed at certain given IAP **(Fact file I)**.

The elevation of diaphragm and subsequently the increased intrathoracic pressure also causes (1) diminished functional residual capacity (FRC), (2) increased ventilation-perfusion mismatch (preferential ventilation of nondependent areas of lungs can be associated with intrapulmonary shunting and hypoxemia), (3) increased physiological dead space, and (4) increased intrapulmonary shunt, contributing to decrease in arterial oxygenation. Such changes would also favor to the development of atelectasis of lungs. But, these changes are generally not found or minimally found in normal healthy individuals. On the contrary, (i) in obese patients, (ii) in respiratory disabled patients, or (iii) in patients with cardiovascular problems, these changes may be more significant.

FACT FILE I

- Pneumoperitoneum → ↑IAP → ↑elevation of diaphragm → ↓compliance of lung → ↑airway resistance and ↑air way peak pressure → ↓FRC → ↑V/Q mismatch, ↑shunt, ↑dead space, and ↑atelectasis → ↑hypoxia (↓PaO_2) and ↑$PaCO_2$.
- Pneumoperitoneum →↑IAP and ↑elevation of diaphragm → compression of venous capacitance vessel, ↑intrathoracic pressure, compression of arterial resistance vessel (↑SVR) → ↓venous return → ↓CO → ↑sympathetic neurohormonal response → ↑SVR → ↓CO → vicious cycle.

Due to increased systemic absorption of highly soluble CO_2 by the vasculature of peritoneum, arterial CO_2 tension ($PaCO_2$) increases. It reaches a plateau value at 15–30 minutes, after the beginning of the insufflation of peritoneal cavity by CO_2 under general anesthesia and this is found *only in anesthetized patient with spontaneous ventilation* and in head-down (Trendelenburg) or head-up tilting position. But, during laparoscopy under local anesthesia, where the patient is not under GA, then $PaCO_2$ remains unchanged or remains normal. It is due to the compensatory increase in minute ventilation (hyperventilation) by the stimulation of the respiratory center by hypercapnia in a nonanesthetized person. In such condition, compensatory hyperventilation in unanesthetized patient is achieved by increasing the respiratory rate, rather than by increasing the tidal volume.

Usually, the mechanical factor (decreased tidal volume) is compensated by the increase in respiratory rate (in unanesthetized under local anesthesia patient), or by controlled ventilation (in anesthetized paralyzed patient), except in anesthetized spontaneously ventilated patient, where both the increase in respiratory rate and tidal volume is jeopardized. This is because if laparoscopy is performed under general anesthesia with spontaneous ventilation, the compensatory hyperventilation is not achieved. This is again due to the anesthesia induced depression of respiratory center, causing the reduction of both respiratory rate and tidal volume. As it takes 15–30 minutes for $PaCO_2$ to reach a plateau value, after the starting of pneumoperitoneum by CO_2, so the GA with spontaneous respiration can be considered only for short laparoscopic procedures with low IAPs.

Like local anesthesia, *during laparoscopy under regional anesthesia (RA)*, $PaCO_2$ remains also unaltered due to the absence of ventilatory depressant effects, provided the level of block (muscular paralysis) is not much high up. For the monitoring of $PaCO_2$ and oxygen saturation, the capnography and oximetry are the two reliable devices for a healthy patient. But, in sick patients (ASA III-IV), $ETCO_2$ tension is not always reliable, because $PaCO_2$ and $ETCO_2$ tension gradient increases due to the inadequate capacity of the excretion of CO_2 through alveoli. So, for the higher risk patients, preoperative pulmonary function tests and intraoperative arterial blood gas sampling are recommended as preoperative assessment and as a guide line for intraoperative monitoring of patient, respectively.

The increase in $PaCO_2$ during pneumoperitoneum by CO_2 gas is due to (Box 1):

- The increased absorption of CO_2 from peritoneal cavity, because of its high diffusibility and large absorption area (the rate of absorption of any gas from peritoneal cavity

BOX 1: Causes of ↑$PaCO_2$ during laparoscopy surgery.

- Increased physiological dead space and V/Q mismatch
  - Steep head-down position
  - Abdominal distension
  - Reduced cardiac output
  - Reduced ventilation
- Absorption of CO_2 through peritoneal cavity
- Depression of respiration by anesthetic drug in a spontaneous ventilated patient
- Increased metabolism for stress due to inadequate anesthesia
- Accidental events such as:
  - Capnothorax
  - CO_2 emphysema
  - CO_2 embolism
  - Change of position of endotracheal (ET) tube

depends on its diffusibility, the area of its absorption, and the perfusions of absorptive walls).

- The impairment of pulmonary ventilation and perfusion ratio by mechanical factors such as abdominal distension, elevated diaphragm, patient's position, and the depression of ventilation by sedative premedication, and anesthetic drugs.
- Accidental events such as CO_2 emphysema, capnothorax (pneumothorax by CO_2), CO_2 embolism, etc.

The $PaCO_2$ does not increase, if the other gases like N_2O, helium, O_2, etc. are used for pneumoperitoneum instead of CO_2 which indicates that the absorption of gases through peritoneal cavity plays a vital role for the increase in $PaCO_2$ rather than the impaired mechanical ventilatory factors, due to ↑IAP, in healthy patients. This is because, in healthy patient the mechanical factors responsible for ↑$PaCO_2$ is compensated by hyperventilation in unanesthetized patient or controlled ventilation by IPPV in anesthetized patient, except in anesthetized patients with spontaneous respiration. Whereas, in cardiorespiratory compromised patients, both the increased absorption of CO_2 and compromised ventilation factors to excrete excess CO_2 play vital role (mechanical factor cannot be compensated) for ↑$PaCO_2$.

Hemodynamic Changes during Laparoscopy

The hemodynamic changes, observed during laparoscopic surgery, result from the combined effects of (i) anesthesia, (ii) ↑$PaCO_2$ due to increased CO_2 absorption from peritoneal cavity, (iii) ↑IAP due to pneumoperitoneum, (iv) patient's position, (v) intravascular volume status, and (vi) the preexisting cardiorespiratory status of patient **(Fig. 1)**. The insufflation of peritoneal cavity, raising IAP higher than 10–12 mm Hg (the 12 mm Hg of abdominal pressure is the

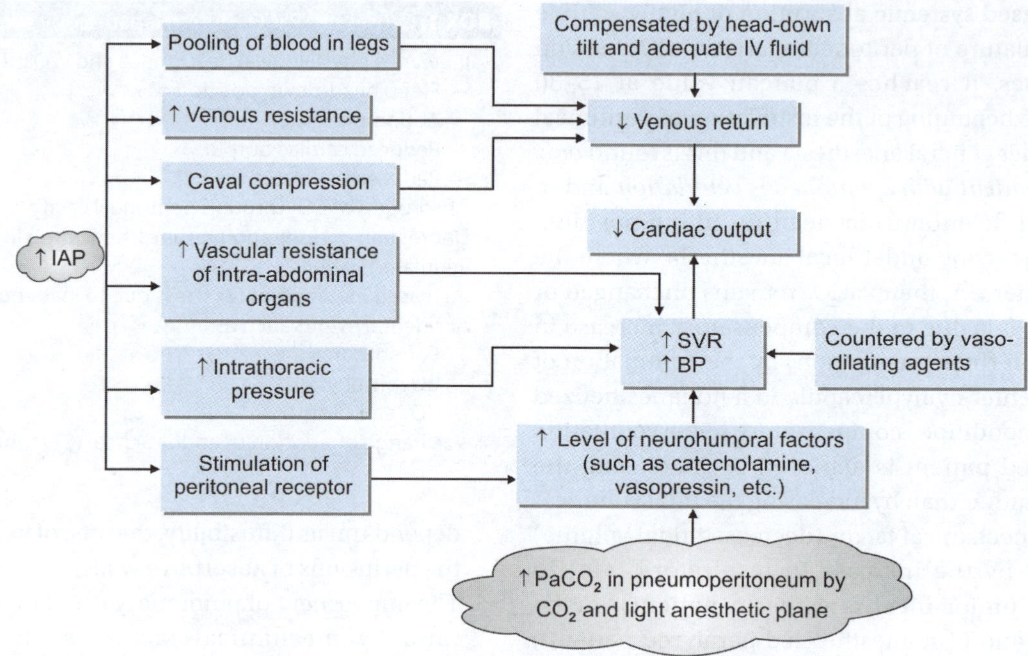

Fig. 1: Effect of increased IAP, due to pneumoperitoneum, and patient's position on CVS. (BP: blood pressure; CVS: cardiovascular system; IAP: intra-abdominal pressure; SVR: systemic vascular resistance)

threshold pressure and up to that level it has minimal effects on hemodynamic function), causes major hemodynamic alterations and these are characterized by: (i) ↓in cardiac output, (ii) increased systemic vascular resistance (↑SVR), (iii) increased pulmonary vascular resistance (↑PVR), (iv) increased mean arterial pressure (MAP) (as the ↑SVR> ↓CO), and (v) pulmonary hypertension.

Cardiac output is reduced by 10–30%, whether the patient was placed in head-down or head-up position and this is well tolerated by a healthy patient. The causes of this reduction of cardiac output are: (i) the pooling of blood into legs due to increased IAP, (ii) reduced venous return, due to the compression on inferior vena cava (IVC) and the compression on both the venous capacitance system and the arterial resistance vessels (this compressive mechanical effect on the venous system will involve in the reduction of venous return to the heart and on arterial resistance vessels will cause increase in SVR), and (iii) decreased venous return due to increased intrathoracic pressure (↓preload).

All these abovementioned factors lead to the reduced venous return to the heart and this reduced venous return to the heart will cause the reduction in left ventricular end-diastolic volume (preload) and reduced cardiac output. But, paradoxically, central venous pressure (CVP) and pulmonary capillary wedge pressure (PCWP) rises due to the increased intrathoracic pressure, in spite of the reduction of preload. So, in pneumoperitoneum the measurement of right atrial pressure and pulmonary arterial pressure, which is generally taken as the cardiac (left ventricle) filling pressure, cannot be the proper guide for the left ventricular end-diastolic pressure and cardiac output.

Following pneumoperitoneum, due to these mechanical factors, the filling pressure (but not the filling volume) of both the right and the left side of the heart will substantially increase. The decreased cardiac output associated with the pneumoperitoneum and ↑IAP is also associated with decreased stroke index, since heart rate is not significantly affected. Normally, the cardiac index is reduced to 30% from the baseline when the patient is kept in anti-Trendelenburg position and is further reduced to 50% by starting of pneumoperitoneum in this position, provided the laparoscopy surgery is done in head-up tilt position. Then, the cardiac index gradually comes to normal within 10 minutes after the completion of insufflation. The magnitude of this reduction of CI is directly proportional to this increased IAP, caused by insufflation.

The pneumoperitoneum and ↑IAP is associated with ↑SVR (afterload) and ↑MAP. The increase in MAP reflects the increase in afterload with an associated *deterioration in CI*. The magnitude of this reduction of CI is directly proportional to the insufflation pressure (or IAP). The threshold of intraperitoneal pressure that had minimum effect on hemodynamic function is 12 mm Hg. The *causes of ↑SVR*, due to pneumoperitoneum, are: (i) the compression of intra-abdominal aorta and arterioles by raised IAP (mechanical factors) and (ii) the release of neurohormonal factors such as catecholamines, prostaglandins, renin-angiotensin, and vasopressin, etc. due to the mechanical stimulation of peritoneal receptor, caused by its stretching due to pneumoperitoneum.

Within a physiological limit, a normal heart can tolerate this increase in afterload and ↓in CO. But, the patients with cardiac diseases cannot tolerate this ↑in afterload and ↓in CO. The ↑SVR in pneumoperitoneum is also due to the reflexly increased sympathetic activity in response to the reduced cardiac output. This is proved by the fact that SVR decreases in Trendelenburg position which tries to increase the venous return and CO and increases in head-up position, which tries to decrease the venous return and CO. The increased SVR or afterload can be corrected by vasodilating agents like isoflurane, nitroglycerine, nitroprusside, nicardipine, α_2-agonist (clonidine or dexmedetomidine), etc.

The magnitude of the cardiovascular response due to pneumoperitoneum (↑IAP) is directly proportional to the insufflation pressure. So, to avoid any cardiovascular response, IAP should be kept below 12 mm Hg. On the other hand, most of the anesthetic agents depress the myocardium and further reduce the cardiac output. Head-up tilt further deteriorates these parameters (↑SVR and ↓CO).

Increased intra-abdominal pressure (↑IAP) also results in venous stasis in lower limbs which predisposes to the development of thromboembolic complications. Increased IAP decreases renal plasma flow, glomerular filtration rate (GFR), and urine output. ↑IAP also leads to decreased blood flow in all intra-abdominal organs, except adrenal gland. Mesenteric blood flow, blood flow in intestinal mucosa, and splenic blood flow are also decreased. Thus, the ischemia in intestinal mucosal results in decreased intestinal mucosal pH and may delay the return of normal bowel function.

The hemodynamic changes due to pneumoperitoneum (↑IAP) are well tolerated in healthy patients, as is suggested by the normal arterial O_2 saturation and normal plasma lactate level, observed during laparoscopic procedures. But this tolerance might be different in patients with impaired cardiac function, anemia, or hypovolemia. Therefore, IV nitroglycerine, IV nicardipine, or IV dobutamine, etc. are used to manage these hemodynamic changes (↑SVR, ↑MAP, and ↓CO), induced by ↑IAP in selected patients with heart disease. In these patients, the preoperative preload is also augmented by the judicious use of IV fluid that offsets the hemodynamic effect of pneumoperitoneum, i.e., the reduction of preload and the subsequent reduction of cardiac output.

Steps to prevent hemodynamic changes due to pneumoperitoneum during laparoscopy:
Several measures can be taken during laparoscopic surgery to prevent the hemodynamic changes, caused mainly by the pneumoperitoneum and head-down or head-up position of patient. These are as follows:

- Premedication with α_2-adrenergic agonist such as clonidine or dexmedetomidine (more selective α_2 agonist)
- Use of anesthetic agents having least hemodynamic effects such as fentanyl/alfentanil/sufentanil, isoflurane/sevoflurane, vecuronium, etc.
- Maintenance of proper plane of anesthesia
- Increasing circulating blood volume by infusing crystalloid solution at the rate of 7–8 mL/kg before inducing pneumoperitoneum
- Considering the gasless laparoscopy
- Slow insufflation of CO_2 for pneumoperitoneum (at the rate of 1 lit/min) which will allow adequate time for compensation.
- Maintaining low IAP, maximum up to 10 mm Hg
- Head-up tilt after insufflation
- Considering the vasodilating drugs like nitroglycerine, nicardipine nitroprusside, etc. for the prevention of hemodynamic changes associated with pneumoperitoneum, i.e., ↑SVR.

■ PROBLEMS DURING LAPAROSCOPY

Problems Due to Hypercarbia (↑$PaCO_2$)

The mild hypercarbia ($PaCO_2$ is between 45 and 50 mm Hg) has little impact on hemodynamic system. However, the increased $PaCO_2$ from 55 to 70 mm Hg has direct *myocardial depressant* and *vasodilating effect*. At the cellular level, it has both (i) depressant effect on myocardial contractility and (ii) stimulant effect on myocardial irritability and arrhythmogenicity. Hypercarbia also increases the responsiveness of blood vessels to catecholamines. It also causes vasodilatation, especially on venous side, leading to peripheral pooling of blood, decreased venous return, and decreased cardiac output. However, exception exists in pulmonary vessels which undergo vasoconstriction in the response to ↑$PaCO_2$. This effect of ↑$PaCO_2$ on pulmonary vessels is due to indirect acidosis rather than direct hypercarbia. But, the local effect of $PaCO_2$ on pulmonary vessels is over shadowed by its systemic effects or the effects of ↑$PaCO_2$ on the central nervous system.

Hence, the net effect of CVS in response to ↑$PaCO_2$ usually are: ↓cardiac output (after an initial increase), ↓stroke volume, ↓heart rate, ↓force of myocardial contraction, ↑blood pressure, ↑CVP, vasoconstriction of pulmonary vessels, ↑peripheral vascular resistance, and cardiac arrhythmias. Respiratory acidosis also increases sympathetic outflow resulting cardiac arrhythmia, especially in the presence of halogenated anesthetic agents such as halothane, isoflurane, and sevoflurane. Among these, the halothane is most notorious. Bradycardia and other cardiac arrhythmias may also occur from increased vagal reflexes (stimulation) and it is due to peritoneal stretching during the insufflation of peritoneal cavity.

In summary, (i) the insufflation of gas into the peritoneal cavity which is followed by the stretching of peritoneum, followed by the raised IAP and (ii) altered patient's position cause a range of clinical responses. These are:

- *Sympathetic response:* Hypertension, tachycardia, and ↑SVR. These are treated by increasing the dose of volatiles, short-acting opioids (fentanyl, sufentanil, and remifentanil), vasodilators, and/or β blocker.
- *CVS response:* CVS depression with fall in cardiac output leads to hypotension, tachycardia, or bradycardia. This is treated by fluids, vasodilators, and/or inotropes.
- *Vagal response (stimulation): Asystole,* sinus bradycardia, nodal rhythm, hypotension, etc. This can be treated by vagolytics.

Problems Related to Patient's Position

For the laparoscopic surgeries, the patient is positioned, with his head-down or lithotomy position (for pelvic or inframesocolic surgery), or his head up (for supramesocolic surgery). These altered positions of patients working synergistically with ↑IAP are responsible for the development of different pathophysiological changes during laparoscopy. *These pathophysiological changes associated with the head-up or head-down position of the patient are also influenced by:* (i) the extent of the tilt, (ii) the intravascular volume status, (iii) the age of the patient, (iv) the drugs administered for anesthesia, (v) the associated cardiac diseases, and (vi) the type of ventilation techniques. The changes in RS and CVS due to head-down position are same as that due to ↑IAP, but only in exaggerated form. On the other hand, the changes in the respiratory and CVS due to head-up position are opposite to the changes due to ↑IAP and favor improved pulmonary dynamics.

In head-down position, the FRC, total lung volume, FVC, and the compliance of lung all decreases which facilitate the development of atelectasis, intrapulmonary shunt, hypoxia, and hypercarbia. Further, in head-down tilting position, there is also increase in central blood volume and decrease in vital capacity and all of these are due to the raised diaphragm and the diminution of diaphragmatic excursion. Thus, the changes due to the head-down position of patient are *unfavorable* for RS. In healthy patient these changes in RS are minimally seen, but are more marked in obese and elderly patient. In the contrary, the changes due to the head-up position of patient are *favorable* for the RS.

When the head-down tilting position of patient does not increase >15°, then the shifting of blood from peripheral to central compartment is too small to induce any clinically significant hemodynamic changes. *In normal healthy subject,* the isolated increased hydrostatic pressure associated with head-down position results in increased venous return, ↑CVP, and ↑CO whereas, isolated ↑IAP due to pneumoperitoneum causes ↑venous return, ↑CVP, and ↓CO. So, during laparoscopic surgery, both Trendelenburg (head down) position and pneumoperitoneum (↑IAP) together produces ↑↑CVP, ↑↑PCWP, and ↓↑CO. These changes are tolerated well by healthy patient, but not by patients with low cardiopulmonary reserve. Isolated (only) reverse Trendelenburg position causes ↓preload, ↓CVP, ↓MAP, and ↓CO (↑IAP also causes ↓preload though CVP paradoxically increases ↑MAP and ↓CO). So, during laparoscopic surgery, anti-Trendelenburg position with pneumoperitoneum together causes ↓↓preload, ↓↑CVP, ↓↑MAP, and ↓↓CO. The steeper will be the upward tilt, the greater will be the fall in CO.

If there is any intraoperative hypoxia during laparoscopic surgery, then the causes may be:

- Hypoventilations due to pneumoperitoneum, head-down position, inadequate ventilation during IPPV, etc.
- Ventilation-perfusion mismatch due to reduced FRC, atelectasis, endobronchial intubation, extraperitoneal gas insufflation, bowel distension, pulmonary aspiration, and rarely pneumothorax.
- Reduced cardiac output due to IVC compression, arrhythmias, hemorrhage, myocardial depression, venous gas embolism, and extraperitoneal gas.

So, the patient should be tilted very slowly and progressively, avoiding sudden respiratory and hemodynamic changes. Further, the position of endotracheal (ET) tube should be checked after every change in the position of patient. Moreover, the mask ventilation may inflate the stomach. So, it should be aspirated by a nasogastric tube before the introduction of trocar and cannula to prevent gastric perforation.

CONTRAINDICATIONS OF LAPAROSCOPIC SURGERY

There is no absolute contraindication for laparoscopic surgery. Therefore, all the contraindications to laparoscopic surgery are relative. For example, when the physiological effects arising from the insufflation of CO_2 into abdominal (peritoneal) cavity under pressure are combined with the effects, arising from the various positioning of patients, then they have some major impacts on cardiopulmonary function, particularly in the American Society of Anesthesiology

(ASA) grade III and IV and are contraindicated. But, the recent report of *"gas less laparoscopy"* using an abdominal wall lifting device may obviate the requirement of pneumoperitoneum and allow safe laparoscopy for these ASA grade III and IV patients. Successful laparoscopic procedures also have now been carried out on patients who are anticoagulated, morbidly obese, or pregnant which are previously contraindicated. Even the different literatures now confirm that laparoscopy cholecystectomy (LC) can be safely be performed in all the trimesters of pregnancy with no increase in fetal and maternal morbidity. The available data suggest that the efficacy and the safety during LC in pregnancy can be increased by using the open Hasson technique for intraperitoneal instrumentation. *This safety can also be increased by:*

- Limiting the IAP during pneumoperitoneum in pregnancy
- Ensuring adequate maternal oxygenation and normocapnia by proper ventilation
- Using appropriate maternal and fetal monitoring
- Using active antithromboembolism measures
- Preventing abdominal aorta and inferior vena caval compression by tilting the patient on left side.

Acute cholecystitis, despite concerns about technical difficulties due to associated edema, inflammation, and necrosis, etc., is no longer considered as contraindication to laparoscopic cholecystectomy, which was taken as contraindication previously. Any previous intra-abdominal surgery was initially taken as contraindication for laparoscopic surgery, but they are now considered safe in experienced hand. There is considerable controversy regarding the appropriateness of laparoscopic surgery for the treatment of known malignant disease. For example, laparoscopic cholecystectomy in known gallbladder malignancy is controversial. Fit and young patients tolerate the physiological changes well and definitely are not contraindicated. But the elderly patients of ASA III and IV status with cardiac and pulmonary disease have more marked and deleterious responses to laparoscopy, but still they are not contraindicated. Contrary, they should be thoroughly reviewed and their medical condition is optimized preoperatively and should have a surgeon well experienced in this procedure.

COMPLICATIONS OF LAPAROSCOPIC SURGERIES

Surgical Complications

The unusual and unexpected vascular trauma and hemorrhagic shock is responsible for >30% of all the major complications in laparoscopic surgeries. The blood vessels of

FACT FILE II

i. Laparoscopic surgery provides lots of benefits which include less trauma, less pain, quick recovery, less pulmonary complications, less hospital stay, less cost, etc.

ii. Pneumoperitoneum causes cardiorespiratory changes. $PaCO_2$ increases due to absorption of CO_2 through peritoneal cavity when CO_2 is used for pneumoperitoneum.

iii. In sick patients (ASA III and IV), these cardiorespiratory changes due to IAP and head-down tilt is further accentuated by ↑$PaCO_2$.

iv. Hence, better knowledge, regarding the pathophysiology of these hemodynamic changes, allow successful anesthetic management of sick patients by optimizing preload and using vasodilating agents.

v. Gasless laparoscopy is theoretically helpful, but technically it is very difficult.

vi. Alternative to CO_2, other inert gases such as argon, helium, and N_2O seem to reduce the hemodynamic changes, due to ↑$PaCO_2$ but do not reduce hemodynamic changes, due to mechanical effect of pneumoperitoneum.

vii. The death rate in laparoscopic surgery is 0.1–1 per 1,000 cases. The incidence of both visceral injury and hemorrhagic complications is 2–5 per 1,000 cases. This is favorable when compared with open surgery.

viii. No anesthetic technique is superior to other. But, GA with controlled ventilation is safest for operative laparoscopy.

anterior abdominal wall, peritoneal cavity, or retroperitoneal space may be punctured by the Veress needle or by the trocar and cannula. Near the level of umbilicus, both the medial vessels (superficial and inferior epigastric) and lateral vessels (superficial and deep circumflex iliac) are at this increased risk of injury. But, we will have to keep in mind that the blood loss in the anterior abdominal wall and retroperitoneal space may be considerable in amount before its detection than the blood loss into peritoneal cavity. The retroperitoneal hematoma can develop insidiously and result in significant amount of blood loss without major intraperitoneal effusion, leading to delayed diagnosis. Other than injury of blood vessels, another important complication of endoscopic surgery is trauma to any abdominal visceral which may lead to peritonitis, subdiaphragmatic abscess, and septic shock. The accidental fulguration of intestine by electrocautery has also been associated with bowel burns and bowel gas explosions (**Fact file II**).

The examples of other complications resulting from endoscopic surgeries are: hepatic and splenic rupture by Veress needle/trocar and cannula, avulsions of band arising from previous adhesions, omentum disruption, or herniation at trocar insertion site, etc. To avoid these abovementioned injuries, caused by the blind Veress needle or trocar insertions, "Hasson" mini laparotomy technique has also been advocated for the creation of pneumoperitoneum.

In this technique, a mini laparotomy incision is primarily made, through which a trocar is inserted under direct visual guidance to create pneumoperitoneum.

It is very important to mention that all the abovementioned complications of endoscopic procedure are surgery related. But, the anesthesiologist must be aware of all these surgical complications and also the timing of their occurrence. Because, they should be prepared to respond promptly to these adverse situations.

Respiratory Complications

The use of pressurized gas during the creation of pneumoperitoneum introduces the possibility of extravasation of this used gas, along the tissue planes, resulting in subcutaneous or retroperitoneal emphysema. This may prolong the surgery or cause its abandonment. The subcutaneous emphysema occurs when the tip of the Veress needle does not enter the peritoneal cavity before the insufflation of gas. This produces the accumulation of insufflating gas in between the fascia's sheath and peritoneum or in the plane of subcutaneous tissue of anterior abdominal wall. The incidences of these complications are near about 0.4–2% and are most common. If the insufflating gas is CO_2 then the extraperitoneal accumulation of this gas (CO_2) may cause quick absorption of it than the intraperitoneal insufflation and may be the cause of sudden rise in $PaCO_2$ and $ETCO_2$ tension.

If the pressure used to inflate the peritoneal cavity by gas is too high, then this gas may be forced out through some *occasionally present congenital foramina (patent pleuroperitoneal canal) in diaphragm*, causing pneumothorax, pneumopericardium, or pneumomediastinum. These complications occur primarily on the right side of the thorax and are usually reduced within 30–60 minutes after deflation. The insufflated gas from peritoneal cavity also may track around the aortic and esophageal hiatuses of diaphragm into the mediastinum and then may rupture into pleural space. Commonly, these weak points or defects in diaphragm occur at pleuroperitoneal hiatus or foramen of Bochdalek.

Sometimes, these complications remain undiagnosed and pneumomediastinum or pneumothorax may become life threatening. The subcutaneous emphysema over the chest wall, neck, and face should also alert the anesthetist regarding the possibility of these dreaded complications. The intraoperative diagnosis of these complications can be confirmed by the presence of increased airway pressure, hemodynamic instability, and O_2 desaturation. If the patient is hemodynamically unstable and there is clinical evidence of pneumothorax, then abdominal insufflation should be stopped immediately. The diagnosis of pneumothorax should be confirmed by chest radiograph and immediate decompression of thorax should be done by putting a tube into pleural cavity. Once the chest decompression is in a satisfactory position, then the abdomen can be insufflated again by gas and the procedure can be continued, if the patient remains stable.

The gas embolism is the most feared complication of endoscopic surgery which may lead to hypoxemia, pulmonary hypertension, pulmonary edema, and cardiovascular collapse. The causes of this gas embolism are: (i) the Veress needle or the trocar and cannula may enter directly into the vessel or (ii) the gas may be forced into the vessels through some open sinuses of surgical site by high IAP. Unlike the air embolism in CO_2 embolism, there is no bronchoconstriction, but only the end tidal CO_2 tension may increase transiently.

Sometimes, inadvertently, the ET intubation may be converted into endobronchial intubation by the cephalad shift of the diaphragm, along with the cephalad shift of intra-abdominal organs, due to the ↑IAP, due to the intraperitoneal insufflation and head-down position of patient. So, the ET tube should be firmly taped and its cuff should lie well above the carina. Therefore, it should be re-checked after pneumoperitoneum and after any further change in patient's position.

The ↑IAP decreases the *risk of regurgitation* (by increasing the tone of lower esophageal sphincteric) and head-down position further reduces the risk of *aspiration* of these regurgitated material (if regurgitation occur) into the lungs. Still, the preoperative administration of H_2 receptor blocker or proton pump inhibitor is recommended, since the risk of regurgitation and aspiration persists in high-risk patients.

Cardiovascular Complications

There are high incidences of cardiac arrhythmias, during laparoscopic surgeries. However, hypercapnia is the major cause of it (cardiac arrhythmias). The other precipitating factors for these cardiac arrhythmias during laparoscopic surgeries are: hypoxia, hemodynamic changes, and vagal reflexes (resulting from sudden stretching of peritoneum due to pneumoperitoneum). In the light plane of anesthesia, this intense vagal stimulation may cause severe bradycardia, cardiac arrhythmias, and even asystole. The high incidences (27%) of this vagal stimulation have been reported in the spontaneously breathing patients under halothane anesthesia. However, these incidences of cardiac arrhythmias may be reduced to 5% in mechanically ventilated patients and when the peritoneal insufflation is done with

N_2O, rather than CO_2. Therefore, mechanical ventilation and adequate depth of anesthesia, by the use of isoflurane/sevoflurane, etc., are recommended to reduce the incidences of cardiac arrhythmia during laparoscopic surgeries. This cardiac arrhythmia may also be the first sign of gas embolism. The cardiac arrhythmias occurring during the early part of CO_2 insufflation (when $PaCO_2$ is at normal level) is mainly due to vagal stimulation, caused by rapid hemodynamic changes and rapid rise of IAP. So, these arrhythmias are quickly treated by the stoppage of insufflation, injection of atropine (for bradycardia), and deepening of anesthesia, only after recovery of heart rate from bradycardia.

Nerve Injury

Sometimes nerve injury is a potential complication during laparoscopic surgery in head-down and lithotomy position. The commonly inflicted nerves are brachial plexus and common peroneal. The nerves of brachial plexus are commonly injured due to the overextension of arm. So, prevention of overextension of arm and cautious use of shoulder braces can reduce the incidence of brachial plexus injury. Common peroneal nerve is highly vulnerable during prolonged lithotomy position and so care should be taken during the positioning of patient in lithotomy position. Lower extremity compartment syndrome is also reported after prolonged lithotomy position.

ALTERNATIVES TO CO_2 PNEUMOPERITONEUM

Besides CO_2, pneumoperitoneum can also be produced by using air, O_2, N_2O, and N_2. *But, CO_2 is generally preferred and at present it is the most commonly used gas for laparoscopy.* This is because of its (i) greater solubility in blood (so the risk of gas embolism is reduced), (ii) rapid elimination by lungs, (iii) ready availability, (iv) low cost, and (v) noninflammability during electrocautery which is part and parcel of laparoscopic surgery. Therefore, during laparoscopy surgery to produce pneumoperitoneum and to avoid the disadvantages of CO_2, the N_2O also can be used for the insufflation of peritoneal cavity. But, the *disadvantage of N_2O* is that it is inflammable during electrocautery. However, the other advantage of N_2O to produce pneumoperitoneum is that it does not increase the size of CO_2 bubble in blood. Other alternative approach for pneumoperitoneum in laparoscopy is the use of inert gases or even gasless laparoscopy.

Inert Gases

Among the inert gases, only the argon and helium have been used to cause pneumoperitoneum instead of CO_2 during laparoscopy. The only advantage of inert gases is that it avoids the increase in $PaCO_2$, secondary to CO_2 absorption through peritoneum. But, the inert gases cannot avoid the pulmonary and hemodynamic changes due to ↑IAP. On the contrary, the main disadvantage of the use of inert gases is their low blood solubility and decreased safety in the event of gas embolism.

Gasless Laparoscopy

The peritoneal cavity can also be expanded by elevating the anterior abdominal wall by using a fan-shaped retractor instead of using any gas. Thus, it avoids the hemodynamic and respiratory changes, due to the increased IAP and the use of CO_2, especially in the patients with cardiorespiratory compromisation. But, the gasless laparoscopic procedure compromises the surgical exposure and increases the technical difficulty. Therefore, combining the abdominal wall lifting with fan-shaped retractor with low pressure CO_2 pneumoperitoneum (5 mm Hg) might improve the surgical exposure and will reduce the bad effect of high IAP due to CO_2 pneumoperitoneum on RS and CVS. The other advantage of gasless laparoscopy is that it is associated with the less incidence of postoperative nausea and vomiting (PONV) and the less incidence of metastasis of malignancy at the site of laparoscopic port.

LAPAROSCOPY DURING PREGNANCY AND CHILDREN

The most common surgeries that are performed by laparoscopy during pregnancy are appendisectomy and cholecystectomy. During laparoscopic surgery in pregnancy, the important points that should be kept in mind are the following:

- Any abdominal surgery (endoscopic or not) during pregnancy increases the risk of miscarriage and premature labor and this is maximum before 12th week of pregnancy and after 24th week of pregnancy. So, the laparoscopic surgery performed between 12 and 23 weeks of pregnancy has the minimum risk for miscarriage and preterm labor and also provides adequate intra-abdominal working space for endoscopy.
- The laparoscopy has the special risk of directly hitting and damaging the gravid uterus. This can be avoided by selecting the alternative sites for the entry of Veress needles and trocar cannula.
- Open laparoscopy can also be used to avoid damaging uterus.
- The pneumoperitoneum produced by CO_2 can induce significant fetal acidosis. So, the maternal $PaCO_2$ should always be monitored closely and is maintained at normal levels. Hence, the mechanical ventilation should be

adjusted correctly to maintain a physiological maternal alkalosis.

- The tocolytic agents should be used routinely during laparoscopy with pregnancy to arrest the preterm labor.
- Fetal monitoring is must during laparoscopy by transvaginal USG.
- The IAP during pneumoperitoneum in the state of pregnancy should be limited between 8 and 10 mm Hg. The gasless laparoscopy is an alternative to avoid the potential side effects of pneumoperitoneum by CO_2 and elevated IAP during pregnancy. Operation in a left lateral position is a safeguard against supine hypotension syndrome which is often found during pregnancy.
- Laparoscopy during pregnancy under epidural anesthesia reduces the hazards of anesthetic drugs on the fetus and the course of pregnancy.

The diagnosis of acute appendicitis during the course of pregnancy continues to be a great problem for clinicians despite the significant advances in surgery over the past few decades. In 20% of patients with appendicitis, the diagnosis is missed clinically. On the other hand, the appendix is normal in 15–40% of cases when they are undergoing emergency surgery for suspected appendicitis. Now, more and more laparoscopy-guided surgery is performed in children and the most common indication of these laparoscopy-guided surgeries is appendisectomy. But, data concerning the hemodynamic changes and ventilatory tolerance produced by pneumoperitoneum in children is inadequate. Due to the increased ratio of peritoneal surface area to body weight in children, the absorption of CO_2 in CO_2 - pneumoperitoneum is intense and faster in children. But, for brief laparoscopic procedure, the $ETCO_2$ tension rises slightly and in such situation no increase in ventilation is required. Otherwise, for laparoscopic surgeries of prolonged duration in children, ventilation should be increased to keep $ETCO_2$ at normal level.

In a recent randomized study, it is seen that the laparoscopic appendisectomy does not actually improve the postoperative recovery and analgesia in children. The laparoscopic appendisectomy technique is associated with longer duration of surgery, but the shorter duration of stay in hospital. Therefore, there is no difference in terms of time, to return to normal activity, compared with conventional open surgery.

■ ANESTHETIC PROCEDURE

Any standard anesthetic technique, such as LA, RA, or GA, if properly adapted according to the need for laparoscopic surgery, does not play any major role in patient's outcome. But, GA with ET intubation and controlled ventilation is considered as the *safest technique for any long laparoscopic*

surgical procedure. During pneumoperitoneum, the CO_2 which is absorbed through peritoneum, increases the $PaCO_2$ and thus makes the tracheal intubation and artificial ventilation very necessary. During laparoscopic surgeries, general anesthesia followed by ET intubation and artificial ventilation is also chosen, because under LA or RA patients feel great discomfort, due to the creation of pneumoperitoneum and due to the extent of Trendelenburg position, necessary for the laparoscopic procedures.

In general, the local or regional anesthetic technique is not recommended for upper abdominal and long laparoscopic surgeries. The reason behind it is explained above. However, the choice of anesthetic agents, for the induction and maintenance of GA are not important, except that cardiodepressant agents should be avoided. There is higher incidence of PONV after laparoscopic surgery, especially following gynecological procedures. So, an antiemetic agent should be given prophylactically routinely in all the cases of laparoscopic surgeries.

As the pneumoperitoneum needs the increment of minute ventilation by 15–25%, so it can be achieved by increasing the respiratory rate rather than the tidal volume, which avoids much alveolar inflation and reduces the risk of pneumothorax (by rupturing the emphysematous bullae). This principle of ventilation is more applicable for chronic obstructive pulmonary disease (COPD) and emphysematous patients. Therefore, whatever may be the technique of ventilation, the tension of $ETCO_2$ should be maintained at approximately 35 mm Hg. The N_2O used for the maintenance of anesthesia is not contraindicated for any laparoscopic surgery. But, it is better to avoid in laparoscopic intestinal and colonic surgery. However, IAP should be monitored closely and is not allowed to exceed maximally above 15 mm Hg in any condition.

Theoretically, profound skeletal muscle relaxation is not necessary for laparoscopic surgery. But, inadequate muscle relaxation may intensely increase IAP without adequate pneumoperitoneum and will reduce the working space. Reversely, adequate muscle relaxation will provide adequate working space without much increase in IAP.

The use of LMA, as an alternative to ET tube in laparoscopic surgery, has both the advantages and disadvantages. *The advantages of LMA in laparoscopic surgery are:* less laryngeal irritation, less postoperative cough, easy to insert, etc. which are discussed in appropriate airway chapter. *The disadvantages of LMA in laparoscopic surgery are:* (i) It cannot protect the airway from the aspiration of gastric contents and (ii) controlled ventilation is sometimes difficult when the airway pressure exceeds 20 cmH$_2$O due to the decreased thoracopulmonary compliance and due to pneumoperitoneum. So, the use of LMA for laparoscopic surgery is limited, only to the healthy and thin patients, for both spontaneous or controlled ventilation. The GA with spontaneous respiration, without LMA or intubation, should be used only for short procedures with low IAP and slight degrees of head-down tilt.

The laparoscopic surgeries performed under local anesthesia include very short, precise, and gentle surgical procedure such as tubal ligation, some diagnostic procedures, some investigation during infertility management, etc. The laparoscopic surgery, done under LA, provides several advantages. These are: fewer hemodynamic changes, early diagnosis of complication, early recovery, reduced PONV, and the avoidance of the complications of GA. But, the success of endoscopic surgery under LA, depends on the relaxation and cooperativeness of patient, quality of trained OT staff, skill of surgeon, and as low as possible of IAP.

During laparoscopy under local anesthesia patients usually suffer from discomfort due to pneumoperitoneum and so may necessitate IV sedation. But, sedation and pneumoperitoneum both usually produce early O_2 desaturation and so care should be taken for it. Regional anesthesia (spinal and epidural) for laparoscopic surgeries share the same advantages and disadvantages like LA, but it may be applied for surgical procedures which are longer than that can be done under LA, but shorter than that which need GA. Whereas very long laparoscopic surgical cases should be done under GA, rather than RA. The RA provides better muscle relaxation and so less sedation is needed (than LA) without major impairment of ventilation. The surgical stress related to metabolic responses is also reduced in RA which is a great advantage of it than GA. The hemodynamic effects of pneumoperitoneum under RA are still being studied. So, (i) the patient's cooperation, (ii) experienced surgeon, (iii) less increase in IAP, and (iv) moderate head-up or head-down tilt position are the key factors for the success of laparoscopic surgeries under RA.

Laser Surgery and Anesthesia

■ INTRODUCTION AND PHYSICS

The full form of the word "laser" is *light amplification by stimulated emission of radiation*. In simple form, it can be said that laser provides a huge quantity of energy in the form of light or photon particles which can be transferred very rapidly to a remote and a very specific location to destroy the tissue by heat and vaporization. Actually, the visual light is an electromagnetic wave with *combined electrical and magnetic properties*. It propagates at a speed of 299,792,458 m/s. *Thus, ordinary light is a form of radiant energy that spans in the middle range of the whole spectrum of electromagnetic wave.* It is released as photon particles and travels as wave. This was the explanation of Maxwell about light in 1864. The wavelength of visible light ranges between 385 and 760 nanometer (nm). The light below this wavelength is called the *ultraviolet rays* and the light above this wavelength is called the *infrared rays*.

Subsequently, Max Plank had also said that if a light only of blue in color and of certain wavelength falls on a specific metal, then it emits some electrons from the metal at a rate which is proportional to the brightness of the light. After that, in 1905, Einstein, by his quantum mechanics explained that the electromagnetic radiation or wave of normal light which consists of photons have properties of both the particle (mass) and the energy (wave). Einstein also said that the emission of electrons from a specific metal, as a result of this fall of blue light, is independent of the number of photons present in the falling light. But, energy is the key factor for the emission of electrons from metal, i.e., only photons of high energy with high frequency wave can provide this energy which is necessary to stimulate this electron emission from metal. On the other hand, the lower energy photons in falling light, even arriving in large numbers at a given time, cannot emit electrons from this specific metal. *These findings results in the development of laser.*

The electrons usually encircle the nucleus of an atom in many orbits and each orbit has its specific energy level with a fixed number of electrons. If an electron moves from one orbit to another, i.e., from higher to lower or lower to higher orbit, then it absorbs or emits an amount of energy which is exactly equal to the difference in energy between these two adjacent orbits. When an energy particle or a photon falls from outside on an atom, then the electron of lower energy orbit absorbs it and jumps to the outer next orbit of higher energy. This phenomenon is called the *stimulated absorption* and the new state of this atom is called the *stimulated state*. Similarly, when an electron from an orbit of higher energy enters into the next inner orbit of lower energy, then it emits some energy or photon. This phenomenon is called the *spontaneous emission* and the new state of this atom is called the *emission state*.

A third situation, predicted by Einstein in 1917, is the stimulated emission which is the combination of previously mentioned both the stimulated and emission states of an atom. Here, if a photon or energy particle of a particular wavelength colloids with an atom which is ready, from previously, for a spontaneous emission (i.e., having an electron already in the higher energy orbit and ready to enter in lower energy orbit with emission of energy or photon) then *two photons or energy waves* will come out from this atom (one that is falling on the atom and the other by the mechanism of spontaneous emission). Thus, the emitted two photons will have the *identical wavelength, phase, and directions*. This phenomenon is called the *stimulated emission*.

The energy differences among the different orbits are specific in different atoms. Thus, the emission and absorption spectra of energy of an atom is very specific, like the fingerprint for this atom and hence is used for atom's chemical identification. Normally, in the state of thermodynamic equilibrium, the electrons of an atom usually lie in the orbit of lowest available energy. So, *the key for the formation of laser* is to pump up (put) the electrons from the orbit of lower energy to the orbit of higher energy (stimulated state) where they will wait for an external photon to collide and start a chain reaction (or amplification) of stimulated emission, i.e., when one photon will collide with an stimulated atom, then two photons will come out (emission), which again falls on another atom lying in already stimulated state. Thus, four photons will come out which again fall on another stimulated atom and this type of chain (amplification) reaction will go on repeatedly.

The technology for previous pumping up of electron from the orbit of lower energy to orbit of higher energy in an atom of a material (which is known as the *laser medium*) and to achieve stimulated state of an atom was introduced in 1958. Then later, a method was also developed by placing the laser medium between two parallel reflecting mirrors, so that *stimulated emitting photons* could traverse the medium by repeatedly striking the more and more atom of this laser medium which are already in the stimulated state and emitting more and more photon and thus maximizing the number of stimulated emission **(Fig. 1)**.

Now, this amplified photons or light energy that is radiated (coming out) by the mechanism of stimulated emission (laser light) differs from the ordinary light in that the laser light consists of the waves of photons that have very well defined wavelength of narrowband. Whereas, the ordinary light consists of the waves of photons of wide wavelength and less defined. The laser light has no dispersion. It is confined and propagated as a very narrow beam. Whereas, the ordinary light spread out in all directions from the point of its source. All the waves of photons (or energy) of laser light always remain in the same phase, whereas the waves of ordinary light remain in different phases. This property of laser is called the coherent, i.e., all the peaks of the waves of energy or photon move synchronously at the same direction and same amplitude. Another property of laser is that it is monochromatic, i.e., all the waves are of same wavelength. Thus, these three characteristics allow the laser: (1) to generate intense light beam, (2) to send such light beam efficiently and accurately at distance places through lenses, and (3) to deliver intense energy on a very small target site.

So, to produce laser, we need three things: (i) the laser medium containing the atoms whose electrons could be capable of creating the laser light, (ii) an energy source to pump and excite (stimulate) the electrons of the atom of laser medium from the orbit of lower energy to the orbit of higher energy, and (iii) two resonating mirrors to amplify the amount of liberated photons and to create the chain reaction.

Three types of laser medium are used practically. These are: (i) *Gaseous laser medium,* for example CO_2, argon, krypton, helium, neon, etc. (ii) *Liquid laser medium* such as some dyes and semiconductors, and (iii) *Solid laser medium* such as chromium, neodymium, holmium, and synthetic crystals known as YAG (yttrium aluminum garnet) **(Table 1)**. According to the mode of delivery of light beam, laser also can be classified into *intermittent, short, and long or continuous.* The gas laser produces either a continuous or intermittent pulsed beam. But, the solid laser medium always produces intermittent pulsed beam. The continuous wave of CO_2 laser produces radiation, having a wavelength of 10 μm. It is strongly absorbed by water and damages tissue surfaces up to the depth of 200 μm. For this reason, the CO_2 laser is suitable for removing any superficial lesions, for example,

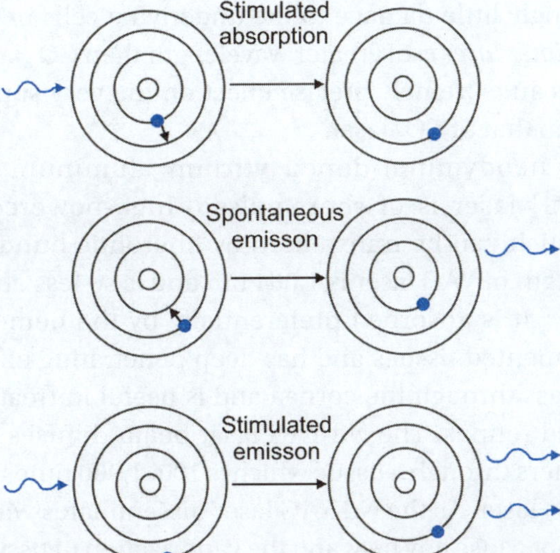

Fig. 1: Interaction of photon with electron. Stimulated absorption: Here a photon strikes an electron and transfers its energy to this electron. This transferred energy pushes the electron into a higher orbit. Spontaneous emission: Here an electron is pushed from higher energy orbit to lower energy orbit. Thus, it loses some energy which is emitted as photon. Stimulated emission: Here, an incoming photon interact with an electron that is already pushed in a high energy orbit before by some energy, with the result that two photons or energy particles leave the electron and it is pushed back in the lower orbit.

TABLE 1: Different types of laser and their wavelength and color.		
Laser type	*Color*	*Wavelength (nm)*
Argon	Blue/green	488–515
CO_2	Far-infrared	10,600
Helium-neon	Red	633
Dye	Blue to red	360–670
Ruby	Red	694
Nd-YAG	Near infrared	1,064
(Nd-YAG: neodymium-doped yttrium aluminum garnet)		

the removal of a small growth from the vocal cords or larynx. For the energy source, which is used to pump and excite the electrons from the orbit of lower energy to the orbit of higher energy in the atoms of a laser medium, usually the xenon flash lamp (for solid laser medium) or high electrical power (for gaseous laser medium) is used. As lasers mediums are not very efficient in converting electrical energy into light energy, so they require a large power supply (for example, a laser with 10 W output requires a 1,000 W of current).

After the emission of laser, usually a light guide is used which directs the laser beam to the surgical site. But, now the development of fiberoptic bundles provides a convenient and flexible way to deliver the laser light to a distant surgical site. At the end of this light guide or the fiberoptic bundle, there is a lens which focuses the laser light to a minimum size (sometimes the spot size is 30 µm or 0.03 mm), creating a very high density of power or energy over a small area. In operating microscope, the laser light is focused on the tissue by the lenses of microscope.

CLINICAL APPLICATION AND BIOLOGICAL EFFECTS OF LASER

So long, we have learnt that the laser is nothing but an intensely amplified number of photon particles or energy, directed at a very small pinpoint area. Actually, it does not increase the energy of a particular photon, but simply places or concentrated the more photons or energy particles at a given place and time than the ordinary light sources. This high density of power or energy, delivered at the very small target site, produces enormous heat at the rate of many thousand calories per second (approximately 2,500 calories/s). This causes rapid vaporization of any tissue or material and except metals. So, to remove the tissues (by heat and vaporization) laser is used as a scalpel, allowing highly precise microsurgery, to perform in a confined or difficult to reach sites. Laser also causes electrocoagulation. So, the laser surgeries are relatively dry, providing a near instantaneously sealed small blood vessels and lymphatics, even in the presence of clotting abnormalities. In summary, the advantages of using laser include: less bleeding, ability to coagulate small blood vessels, maintenance of sterile operating conditions, less tissue handling and reaction, increased precision of dissection, and preservation of surrounding normal tissues.

Normally, water is the main constituent of tissues, and any living tissue is a complex aqueous solution, containing varieties of molecules **(Fig. 2)**. The amount of the absorption of laser energy in this water of living tissue (the mechanism of action of laser on tissues) depends on the wavelength of this laser light. The larger will be the wavelength, the more will

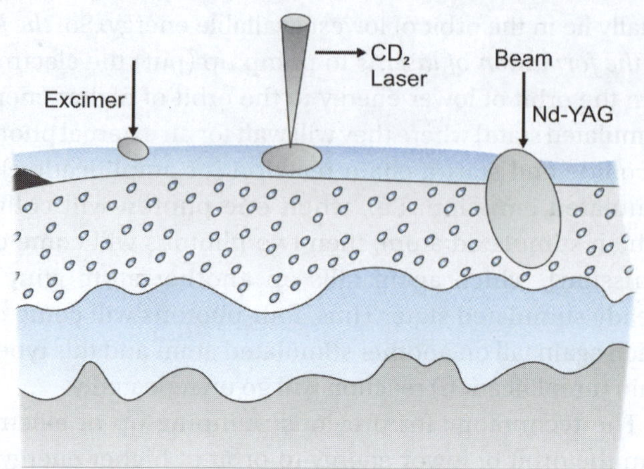

Fig. 2: Laser beam of different wavelength causes different patterns of tissue destruction. The actual tissue destruction by laser light depends on both the laser parameters and tissue factors. The laser parameters are: power density, duration, and wavelength. The tissue factors are: absorption, scatter, thermal conductivity, and local circulation.
(Nd-YAG: neodymium-doped yttrium aluminum garnet)

be the absorption of laser light energy into the water of the tissues and more will be the production of heat for the vaporization of tissues. The CO_2 laser (10,600 nm wavelength) is completely absorbed by water. So, after the falling of CO_2 laser on tissues, it cannot penetrate or pass, except for a few superficial cell layers of the tissues. Thus, only these surface tissues or cell layers are heated and vaporized with surprisingly little damage to the underlying cells or tissues. The *excimer laser* is of greater wavelength than CO_2 laser and so it has an extremely precise effect on the very superficial cells than that of CO_2 laser.

The neodymium-doped yttrium aluminum garnet (Nd-YAG) laser is of short pulsed, high-powered glass laser which can be transmitted by fiberoptic bundle. The wavelength of YAG laser is 1,064 nm and is so less absorbed by water. It is absorbed preferentially by the hemoglobin and pigmented tissues and has deep penetrating effect. So, it can pass through the cornea and is useful in treating the detached retinas. The Nd-YAG laser beam diffuses several millimeters through a tissue which is 100–1,000 times greater than CO_2 laser. As the Nd-YAG laser disseminates widely, so it does not cause any heat and the vaporization of tissues, but produces thermal coagulation.

Some lasers, such as the ruby laser has wavelength of 694 nm (very small). So, it is also poorly absorbed by tissues, except by the cells, containing dark pigments. The *argon* (wavelength 514,488 nm) and *krypton* (wavelength 476,521,568 nm) gas lasers is transmitted through water, though they have large wavelength (so it passes through cornea), but is intensely absorbed by Hb. It has the ability to

FACT FILE I

Laser light striking the tissue surface may be:

i. *Reflected:* Reflection of laser rays from the shiny surfaces may damage the eyes of any person in the vicinity.

ii. *Transmitted:* Laser light which is transmitted through superficial tissues to the deeper layers of variable depth is partially determined by the wavelength.

iii. *Scattered:* After striking the tissue surface, some laser light scatters. Shorter wavelength induces greater scattering.

iv. *Absorbed:* After falling most of the laser rays are absorbed by the tissues. This produces the clinical effect by converting the absorbed light into heat. Organic tissues contain various substances capable of absorbing light. Each substance has a particular absorption spectrum which is determined by its chemical structure. Laser light which has the frequencies close to the absorption spectrum of the tissue will be most effective for that tissue.

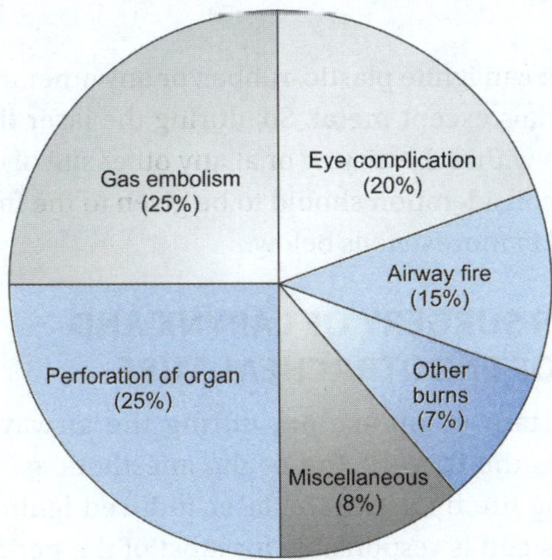

Fig. 3: Types and percentage of laser injury.

penetrate skin or ocular structures and selectively coagulates the vascular or pigmented regions (so, it is also useful in treating detached retinas) **(Fact file I)**.

HAZARDS OR RISKS OF LASER SURGERY

There are five main risks or hazards of laser surgery. These are **(Fig. 3)**:

1. Atmospheric pollution
2. Perforation of great vessels or structures
3. Gas embolism
4. Energy transfer at wrong location
5. Fire.

Atmosphric Pollution

An important problem during laser surgery is the pollution of environment of OT. This is due to the excessive smoke produced during vaporization of tissues. The plumes of smoke and fine particles produced during the vaporization of tissues by laser energy may be transported and deposited in the distant tissues, especially during laryngeal surgery. Here, the smoke and fine particles can be deposited in the alveoli, causing bronchitis, increased tracheobronchial secretion, interstitial pneumonia, inflammation and reduced mucociliary clearance, etc. CO_2 laser produces smoke maximally, whereas Nd-YAG laser (contact probe) produces much less. However, the effective method of preventing this dissemination of smoke is immediate sucking of it from the surgical site. Many operation theater (OT) personals may find the odor of this smoke very objectionable and complain of headache, nausea vomiting, and irritation due to inhalation of this smoke **(Fig. 3)**.

Perforation of Great Vessels or Structures

Sometimes the desired depth of tissue penetration by laser beam cannot be controlled. Thus, it may cause perforation of the structure (if it is hollow) or may cause damage to the other tissues and great vessels underneath the said tissue. Vessels >5 mm are not coagulable by laser energy and may cause profuse bleeding. With Nd-YAG laser, it is impossible immediately to assess the depth of injury, until the necrosis of tissues becomes maximal, several days after the laser surgery.

Gas Embolism

The tip of the contact probe of Nd-YAG laser contains a gas as coolant. During hysteroscopic surgery by Nd-YAG laser, if this coolant gas of the probe accidentally leaks and inflates the uterine cavity, then fatal gas embolism may occur. So, the liquid coolant in the laser probe is strongly recommended during the hysteroscopic surgery. If a coolant gas has to be used, then CO_2 is preferred. Because, it produces less damage, following embolization than either N_2 or air. Venous gas embolism has also been reported during the section of tumor by Nd-YAG laser in the trachea and during the various types of laparoscopic and endoscopic procedures by it.

Energy Transfer at Wrong Location

The misdirected laser energy may perforate any hollow viscous or a large blood vessel, situated by the side of the operative site. For example, laser-induced pneumothorax has been reported following a laryngeal procedure. Similarly, pressing the laser control trigger at a wrong time and at wrong site also can precipitate tragic scenarios, including the ignition of surgical drapes or burning of an endotracheal (ET) tube, during an airway surgery.

Fire

Laser light can ignite plastic, rubber, or any other inflammable materials except metal. So, during the laser therapy of any lesion within the airway or at any other site of our body, a careful consideration should to be given to the fire. This is discussed in more details below.

LASER SURGERY OF LARYNX AND FIRE OF ENDOTRACHEAL TUBE

An important complication, during the airway surgery by laser, is the ET tube fire or the anesthetic gas mixture is catching fire by itself. The laser-induced ignition of ET tube or its cuff is responsible for most of the perioperative complications (40%) of laryngeal laser surgery. This is followed by postoperative laryngeal web (20%) and laser-related facial burns (10%). *Fire, during the laryngeal laser surgery, is due to* (i) the proximity of ET tube to surgical sites around the larynx where laser is used, (ii) the use of high energy, delivered by laser light during laryngeal laser surgery, and also (iii) the presence of other hydrocarbon materials including plastic, rubber, other polyvinyl chloride (PVC) material and even tissue, except ET tube, which also can catch fire and burn easily, especially in an O_2-enriched atmosphere.

The CO_2 laser beam can penetrate an ET tube and ignite fire, which would then be supported by O_2 and N_2O gas mixture, present within the tube. Usually, the most fires are located on the outer surface of ET tube, causing the local thermal tissue destruction. But, sometimes, the fire can catch the innerside of tube, without recognition from outside, and produces a *blow torch-like flame*. This is due to the flow of O_2-enriched gas mixture through the tube. In such situation, ventilation further blows the hot smoke and toxic products of combustion in the fashion of blow torch-like flame, down to the distal pulmonary parenchyma, causing serious damage to the distal lung parenchyma. Again, the perforation of ET tube or the puncture of the cuff of ET tube by laser beam causes the O_2-enriched gas to flood the operative site and increases the chance of a devastating fire.

So, the ET tube fire, due to laser, can be the result from the following:

- Direct ignition of ET tube by laser
- Indirect ignition of ET tube from reflected laser light
- Incandescent particles of tissue, blown from the surgical site
- Ignition of cottonoids (cotton like) or gauze pieces by laser.

So, to reduce the incidence of fire of ET tube, two things can be done.

1. Reduction of the inflammability of ET tube by different methods
2. Removal of inflammable ET tube (if used in the absence of noninflammable tube) from the airway by using *Venturi jet ventilation procedure* by a metallic cannula or *apneic anesthesia technique* with intermittent ventilation.

Reduction of the Inflammability of ET tube

The inflammability of ET tube can be reduced by changing the material by which it is made or by adopting some procedures which will prevent the catching of fire of conventional inflammable tube made of PVC, red rubber or silicon, etc. The ideal properties of a laser safe ET tube, which will not catch fire, should be the following:

- Noninflammable
- Malleable
- Thin walled
- Disposable
- Soft, pliable, and low pressure cuff
- Inexpensive
- Electrically nonconductive
- Impervious to laser beam of multiple wavelength of **(Fact file II)**.

Only the metal ET tube is 100% resistant to fire, caused by laser energy. But the ET tubes which are made up of *only metal* have many disadvantages. Because, *it cannot maintain the mechanical property* of the conventionally used PVC, silicon, and red rubber tube. So, the ET tube made up of materials, other than the metal and conventionally used materials, such as the PVC, red rubber, or silicon, are tried which are less inflammable. But, like PVC, silicon and red rubber ET tube, they also provide fuel for the potential airway fire during the microlaryngeal laser surgery, though with less incidence and less severity. So, the different types of ET tubes made up of *different materials*, other than

FACT FILE II

Thin plastic endotracheal tube cuff is extremely susceptible to laser energy. Simple puncture of the cuff by misdirected laser beam is more common than combustion. Then this unrecognized cuff puncture may lead to enrichment of the area, surrounding surgical site and ET tube, with O_2. This increases the likelihood of catastrophic airway fire. Practically, the laser-resistant ET tube cuff which maintains its mechanical properties necessary to minimize the tracheal trauma is not available. Sometimes, it is recommended to fill the cuff with colored saline which clearly identifies the puncture and also helps off the fire. The cuff should be placed as far distal as possible in the trachea from the laser surgical site. Surgeon should completely cover the visible part of the cuff with moist cotton plugs during the laser surgery. The cotton tails attached to the plugs should be replaced by uninsulated wire.

conventional PVC, silicon, and red rubber, are used and *different methods* are also employed to prevent fire during the administration of anesthesia in laser surgery. These are:

- The conventional red rubber ET tube protected usually by adhesive aluminum or copper foil. This type of ET tube is most widely used for the airway laser surgery.
- The conventional PVC ET tube which is most susceptible to fire can also be protected like above.
- Silicon ET tubes are less inflammable with laser beam. It also can be protected like above.
- Norton (metal of stainless steel) ET tube
- Oswal–Hunton (metal) ET tube is completely resistant to fire but it is of enormous cost. So, it is rarely used.
- Xomed laser-shield ET tube
- Mallinckrodt Laser-Flex ET tube
- Bivona "Foam Cuff" laser ET tube.

Red Rubber and PVC Endotracheal Tube, Wrapped with Metal Tape

Red rubber and PVC ET tubes are highly inflammable to laser energy. But this high inflammability can be reduced by adapting different methods. Among these the most popular approach is by wrapping the red rubber or PVC ET tube with metallized foil or tape. Three types of foil or tape have been used (i) *aluminum foil, (ii) copper foil, and (iii) plastic tape thinly coated with metal on one side*. All these foils and tapes have adhesive coating on one side. These tape and foil are widely available from retail electronics, arts and crafts, or building supplying shops. *Lead foil* is similar in appearance with adhesive coating on one side, but is very toxic and should never be used in the airway **(Fig. 4)**.

These tapes, though give protection to the shaft of the tube from laser energy, *but do not provide any protection to the cuff from fire* as the cuff is not included within the wrapping. If the wrapping of ET tube is the chosen method for laser protection, then the *technique for wrapping* is also important in ensuring the protection from both the (i) ignition of fire and (ii) foil or tape-induced mucosal abrasions. It is often helpful to first sparingly paint the tube with a medical adhesive such as benzoin. Then, the one end of the tape should be cut and wrapping is begun, by aligning the *cut end of the tape* with the junction of the tube and the proximal end of the cuff. After that wrapping is done in a spiral fashion with 30–50% overlapping between the layers. The wrapping of ET tube with metal foil or metal coating tape should also include the inflation pilot tube and should be continued until just short of the pilot balloon, with care taken not to wrinkle the tape at any point which may cause abrasions of the tracheal mucosa **(Fact file III)**.

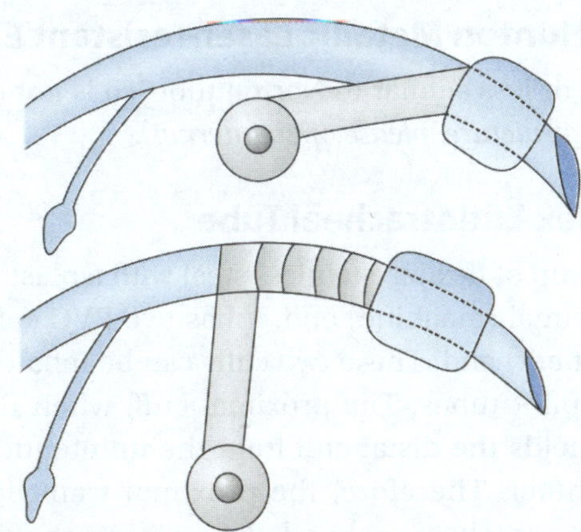

Fig. 4: The method of wrapping of endotracheal tube by metal foil.

Laser-resistant ET tubes are usually bulkier and more rigid than conventional tubes. So, they are more liable to produce mucosal abrasions and require particular care. Surgeons must be particular that laser energy should not reflect from the smooth metal surfaces of any surgical instrument or metal ET tube and is directed at other sensitive structures.

Norton Metallic Laser-resistant ET Tube

It is a metal ET tube without any cuff, and is made up of spirally winded stainless steel (see its picture from internet). Sometimes, a separate cuff may be placed at the distal end of this tube. The exterior of the tube has a matte or sand blast (rough) finish. This decreases the reflection of laser beam and hence the indirect incidences of fire, caused by reflected laser beam. The tube is of thick walled. The roughness of the exterior of the tube can cause damage to the mucosal surface of the airway. The wall thickness is also considered as a disadvantage, since a smaller caliber tube (with further reduction of inner diameter) is usually selected in laryngeal laser surgery. This is because it will allow the surgeon a better exposure. The ET tube large external diameter (thick) and its stiffness or rigidity (as made of metal especially which is not spirally winded) makes the surgical exposure and the positioning of an operating laryngoscope difficult. The Norton tube also may not be airtight into the trachea and it is due to the absence of its cuff. This could cause the contamination of surgical field with the anesthetic gases which is back flowed and have a high concentration of O_2 and thus increases the chances of combustion (catching of fire) of tissues by laser energy. During the use of this type of metal ET tube, the ventilation of patient may also be impaired by the leak at the site of the larynx and it is due to the absence of cuff of this type of tube (*For pictures of this ET tube, please open internet*).

Oswal–Hunton Metallic Laser-resistant ET Tube

It is more or less similar to Norton tube, so is not discussed further (*For picture, please open internet*).

Laser-Flex Endotracheal Tube

It is made up of flexible stainless steel with a plastic adapter at its proximal (machine) end. It has two PVC cuffs on the distal (patient) end. These two cuffs can be inflated via two separate pilot tubes. The proximal cuff, when filled with saline, shields the distal cuff from the unintentional laser beam contact. Therefore, the proximal water-filled cuff allows for a tracheal seal and also protects the distal cuff (*For picture of this tube please open internet*).

Xomed Laser-Shield Endotracheal Tube

It is a fabricated ET tube, made up of a nonreflective silicone elastomer, with an outer layer coated by finely divided aluminum powder. This aluminized powder layer also extends over the inflatable cuff. It is designed to offer protection from CO_2 laser at a power setting below 25 W and at focal diameters of <0.8 mm in the pulsed mode only. The tube can, however, be penetrated and perforated by CO_2 laser, if sufficient energy is used. The cuff of this ET tube is very thin and is easily punctured by CO_2 laser. The penetration and the ignition of Xomed tube by laser beam required higher energy than either red rubber or PVC tubes. However, the prohibitive cost and the possibility of silica ash (if set on fire) which cause an extensive damage to the lungs than the PVC or red rubber ET tube (if they caught fire) are points against the use of Xomed tube (**Fact file IV**) (*For picture of this ET tube, please open internet*).

Bivona "Foam Cuff" Laser Endotracheal Tube

This ET tube features (i) a metal aluminum spiral tube in core, (ii) which is covered with silicone from outside, and (iii) a cuff made of foam. The *"foam cuff"* consists of polymethane sponge with a silicone envelope. The tube is inserted initially, after aspirating all the air out of the foam cuff and it is squeezed. Then, once the tube is inserted, the pilot tube is simply left open to the air. The cuff inflates automatically without air having to be injected. The inflation of the foam cuff with saline solution is however recommended for CO_2 laser surgery. The pilot tube runs along the outside of the wall of the main tube and is marked in black, so that it can be positioned away from the laser beam. A distinct advantage of this ET tube is that the foam cuff will still remain inflated, even when it gets struck by the laser beam. This feature allows continued invasive positive pressure ventilation (IPPV) and also causes separation of anesthetic gases, enriched with O_2, from the surgical site which catch fire (*For picture of this tube, please open internet*).

Type of Ventilation when Endotracheal tube is not used for the Reduction of the Incidence of Fire

Venturi Jet Ventilation by Metallic Cannula

This is a very simplest form of ventilation, avoiding the use of ET tube and thus subsequently reducing the risk of ET tube fire altogether. This procedure involves the use of a jet of O_2 in high pressure and subsequently the entertainment of it (jet of O_2) by atmospheric air. The metallic injector or cannula, used for O_2 jet, is placed into the lumen of a rigid laryngoscope or bronchoscope, which are placed in the larynx and are open at both ends and permits the entrainment of O_2 with air during inspiration and escape of CO_2 during expiration, while the patient is in muscle relaxant. This system is safe and reduces the chance of barotrauma producing pneumothorax. Intravenous anesthesia is usually employed to ensure an adequate depth of anesthesia during this Venturi jet ventilation, as only the O_2 and air without any gaseous anesthetic mixture is used for ventilation. In such situation, the depth of anesthesia is very important, because it prevents the patient from moving and coughing during the surgical procedures using laser. So, a suitable muscle relaxant should be used and the depth of neuromuscular transmission is monitored with a nerve stimulator.

Apneic Anesthesia Technique with Intermittent Ventilation

The need for an alternative technique of ventilation for laryngeal laser surgery was felt because of the shortcomings (mentioned later) of the conventional technique of ventilation by ET tube and the Venturi jet ventilation by metallic cannula. Thus, the apneic anesthetic technique, with intermittent ventilation, provides a good alternative, as it allows the intermittent withdrawal and insertion of ET tube and permits unhindered surgery by laser in the interval. In this procedure, the muscle relaxant must be used to

FACT FILE IV

It has been found that during laser resection of tumor, carbon monoxide is evolved in the smoke. Patients undergoing laser resection of an airway tumor by Venturi jet ventilation can absorb this carbon monoxide through lungs. This CO may result in false overestimation of arterial O_2 saturation in pulse oximetry. Jet ventilation without ET tube usually provides adequate ventilation without introducing large obstacles or inflammable material at the surgical field. This is a great advantage. But the potential disadvantages of it include barotrauma, pneumothorax, gastric distension, only dependence on IV anesthetic agents, applicable only for compliant lungs.

maintain the adequate depth of anesthesia. The withdrawal of ET tube connotes the apneic phase.

Laser surgery is done in the apnea period, in between two ventilatory spells through ET tube, by reinserting it. Such an approach totally eliminates the risks of airway fire, barotrauma, and other complications associated with ET tube and eliminates the disadvantages of jet ventilation by metallic cannula (as enriched O_2 environment around the surgical site causes fire), besides providing a clear and unobstructed view of the laser site to the surgeon. But, hypoxia, hypercarbia during apneic phase, and their associated complications are the inherent dangers of this technique. However, these risks are largely held in check by the alertness of concerned anesthetist, judicial use of monitors and their interpretations, along with in-depth understanding of the physiology of respiration.

In this type of anesthesia, the ET tube is removed intermittently and surgery is done after removal of the tube. Then, again ET tube is reinserted and ventilation is resumed when SPO_2 falls. This insertion and removal of ET tube is done in cyclical manner. Before removing the tube N_2O is switched off and the patient is ventilated with 100% O_2 with isoflurane mixture in order to achieve a high PaO_2, although an SPO_2 is of 100%. Sevoflurane is not generally used in this procedure, because it is very short acting and the adequate depth of anesthesia cannot be maintained for the desired period. Halothane is also not used as it is phasing out due to its propensity causing arrhythmia. Supplemental doses of thiopentone and muscle relaxant are given when required. After induction, intubation, and placement of operating bronchoscope or microlaryngoscope as a first step of this apneic anesthetic technique, the ET tube is gently withdrawn without disturbing the position of microlaryngoscope. This marks the beginning of the first apnea phase. The surgeon now starts excising the lesion with laser which is now clearly visible and accessible to him, because of no hindrance by the ET tube or metallic cannula for O_2 jet. Also there is no risk of fire, since there is no combustible material and O_2-rich anesthetic mixture at the surgical site. The ET tube is reintroduced after the apneic phase through the suspension of laryngoscope and ventilation is again resumed when there is:

- Sliding down of SPO_2 to 93% (allowing for an after drop to 90%)
- Apneic period beyond 7 minutes
- Any severe arrhythmias or obvious ST-segment changes
- Extremes of heart rate (HR) and blood pressure (BP)
- Compulsory stoppage of surgery at intervals to allow the laserized area to cool and also to allow the suction and evacuation for clearing off the excessive smoke and charred tissue that accumulates.
- Completion of laser excision.

At the end of first and subsequent apneic phase, ET tube is further reintroduced. Thus resumption of ventilation is done with 100% O_2 and hyperventilation is performed for first few seconds in order to correct the arterial desaturation and to wash off the accumulated CO_2. This is followed by ventilation of patient with O_2 and isoflurane mixture till SPO_2 reaches 100% and $ETCO_2$ comes down to 30 mm Hg. The ET tube is then again withdrawn and the next episode of apnea and surgery begins. Thus, these cycles of ventilation - apnea - ventilation will continue, till the surgeon achieves a satisfactory clearance of the disease. Toward the end of the surgery, isoflurane is switched off. Satisfactory SPO_2 and $ETCO_2$ level is achieved with ventilation. Then, the patient should receive steroid, as prophylaxis against the postoperative laryngeal edema. The microlaryngoscope is removed and the patient is intubated with normal size conventional oral-cuffed ET tube. Then, the neuromuscular block is reversed by neostigmine with atropine sulfate and the patient is extubated **(Fact file V)**.

No ET tube is safe for (resistant to) laser, except metal. The ET tubes of all the materials, except metal, are in fact

FACT FILE V

As ET tubes of any material such as PVC or red rubber or silicone (except metal) are not resistant to laser so protection of tube from fire by laser should be given at first. Initially, the protection of tube by wrapping it with moistened muslin or dental acrylic was tried. But problem is that when the muslin is dried, it becomes highly inflammable by the laser. On the other hand, the dental acrylic makes the tube hard and rough (outer surface) and may cause trauma to the mucous surface of larynx. So, the best approach to the problem of fire by laser is by wrapping the nonmetallic tube (PVC, red rubber and silicone) with metallized foil tape. The metallized foil tapes, which are in use are of aluminum and copper with adhesive on one side. But these metallized foil tapes do not provide protection to the cuff of the tube and is not 100% resistant to all types of laser. So, now Mercel laser guard tape (approved by FDA) consisting of an adhesive metal foil laminated on a synthetic sponge surface is used and provides protection against most of the lasers. But it cannot protect the cuff. There is another ET tube (FDA approved) which uses integral laser-resistant metal coating during the manufacture of the tube.

Laser-resistant cuff that will maintain the mechanical properties and also will minimize the tracheal trauma is not yet available. The air-filled ET tube cuff is highly susceptible to misdirected laser. Simple puncture is more common than fire of the cuff. Unrecognized cuff puncture causes leaking and enrichment of the ventilating O_2 around the surgical site and hence more likelihood of airway fire. So, to prevent the cuff injury, it should be placed in the trachea as distal as possible from the surgical site and the visible portion should be moistened by cotton pledgets continuously by surgeon. Many authors recommend filling of the cuff with saline, colored with methylene blue which will help to detect the rupture of cuff.

quite vulnerable to fire and this vulnerability of different types of tubes (red rubber, PVC, and silicone) depends on the type of laser. For CO_2 laser, the PVC tube is most vulnerable and then red rubber and silicone tube. But, the red rubber tube produces more toxic combustion products than the PVC tubes. The silicone tube is most resistant to ignition than the other two varieties, but produces copious white silica ash, if it catches fire, suggesting the potential for late development of silicosis. For Nd-YAG laser PVC tube is resistant (in vitro) as it is transparent. But, during practical use any coating of mucus and blood on PVC tube will absorb laser energy and does not make it safe, catching fire.

■ AIRWAY FIRE PROTOCOL

The incidence of ET tube fire, during the laser assisted airway surgery, is estimated to be in the range of 0.14–1.5%. During the laser surgeries, surgeons also should take the responsibility to prevent fire. They should set the laser power as low as possible (10–15 W) and use the noncontinuous mode. They must always use wet gauzes to protect the nontarget tissue in the surgical field and the cuff of ET tube from their damage by laser beam. Between the repeated pulses of laser, sufficient time should be allowed to disperse the heat. Nitrous oxide and oxygen mixture is known to support the combustion. So, the FiO_2 should be kept as low as possible as the patient's O_2 saturation of hemoglobin permits (usually between 0.25 and 0.3). Some anesthetists avoid the use of N_2O and use air/O_2 mixture. Alternatively, helium/O_2 mixture can be used.

Whatever the type of ET tube is used, the cuff should be inflated with sterile saline to which methylene blue may be added. This is because the methylene blue will help to detect the cuff rupture easily by a misdirected laser beam. Also, the cuff of the ET tube should be placed as far distally as possible, so that it is out of the line of the target of laser.

Though, the sudden airway fire and explosion usually incapacitate all the operating room staff temporarily, still the surgeon and anesthetist must act quickly, decisively, and in a very coordinated fashion. Usually, the surgeon detects the fire first. So, he should stop the laser, as soon as he will detect the fire and inform the anesthetist immediately. The anesthetist will also immediately stop the ventilation, will disconnect the circuit from the anesthetic machine and will extubate. Before extubation, pharynx should be flushed with water. So, as a source of water, a 50 mL syringe, filled with cold saline, should always be immediately available. These maneuvers will remove the flame and will stop the flow of O_2-enriched gas to the burning site.

After extubation, the flaming tube should be dipped into a bucket of water which should always be available in OT during laser surgery. Then, ventilation should be done with 100% O_2 by mask. After that, direct laryngoscopy and rigid bronchoscopy should be performed to assess the damage and to remove all the debris. If the fire is of interior blow torch type, then the fiberoptic assessment of distal bronchial damage (if available) and gentle bronchial lavage is necessary. If the airway damage is severe and artificial ventilation is needed for the proper management of complication, then patient should be reintubated for ventilator management or tracheostomy should be done.

Pulmonary damage, due to the heat or smoke inhalation, also necessitates prolonged intubation and mechanical ventilation. The pulmonary damage from the heat and/or smoke inhalation should be assessed by taking repeated arterial blood gas samples and repeated chest radiographs. Late complications from airway fire include the formation of granulation tissue or stenosis in the larynx and/or trachea. So, a brief course of high dose of steroids may be helpful. Fortunately, in most of the cases, small fire involves the exterior of the ET tube and does not cause appreciable damage to local tissues.

In case of difficult airway, leading to difficult intubation during the induction of anesthesia, the tube should not be removed immediately. Because, there is further fear of difficult reintubation or failed intubation and hypoxia. Here, all the abovementioned steps should be taken immediately to stop the fire and *the patient is not extubated*. Instead, the tube and the trachea should be flushed with water. After flushing and extinguishing the fire, a tube exchanger is inserted through the lumen of the previous tube and then the burn tube is removed. Then, another fresh ET tube is inserted over the tube exchanger.

■ LASER SAFETY PROTOCOL

In every hospital, where laser is used for different surgical procedure, should have a laser safety protocol. This protocol is described here:

- A designated trained laser safety officer must be present continuously in OT, when a laser machine is in use. An indicator light must be displayed outside the OT, when the laser is in play.
- Laser light is usually reflected off from the shiny exterior smooth surfaces metal instruments and metal ET tubes, like a mirror. So, all the surgical metal instrument and tubes, used during laser surgery, should have matt exterior surfaces, rather than shiny.
- The eye is the most susceptible part of our body for injury by laser. So, all the operating room personnel must use safety glasses. These should have side shields which will protect the lateral aspect of eye. If an anesthetized

patient is scheduled to receive laser therapy, close to the eyes, then a protective metallic eye cover with exterior matt finish should be applied. Otherwise, the eye should be taped closed and covered with moist swabs.

- Damage to the skin of patient, by laser beam, can also occur. But, it depends on the type of laser in use. The OT personnel do not normally need to protect their skin from the damage, caused by laser. Because, they will be able to move away from the path of a misdirected laser beam. However, this is not possible for an anesthetized patient. So, the anesthetized patients must have all the exposed skin, covered with drapes, except the surgical site. The drapes should be made of absorbable material and not plastic which is potentially highly combustible to laser. Plastic drape is much more combustible than the canvas type drapes. So, it should be avoided. Tissues adjacent to the surgical site should be protected with moistened gauzes or swabs.

- Some fluids, used for skin preparation during surgery, also are highly inflammable. So, these should not be used during laser surgery.
- Efficient smoke evacuation system must be maintained, close to the surgical site. Because, laser surgery is associated with the production of large amount of smoke.
- During the laryngeal laser surgery, the conventional ET tube, made of PVC or red rubber, should be avoided, if possible, in fear of fire and ventilation is maintained by Venturi principle. If in any circumstances, the use of an ET tube cannot be avoided, then the specially prepared nonflammable laser tubes are used or tracheal tube protector, such as metal foil or metalized tape, can be wrapped around the conventional tubes which are discussed earlier.
- All the airway fire protocols should be maintained.

Anesthesia for ENT Surgery

INTRODUCTION

The patients who have undergone ear, nose, and throat (ENT) surgery are usually young and healthy adult. But the patients, who have approached for laryngeal operation, are usually older. Previously most of the operations in ENT department were done as indoor cases. But, now-a-days, most of the ENT operations are performed as day cases, *under local anesthesia (LA) or under fast-track general anesthesia (GA).* Thereby, the need for inpatient admission for ENT surgeries has been reduced and also the workload on ENT anesthetic department has been lowered.

The children and young adults are apprehensive. So, if they are chosen for ENT surgeries *under LA,* then they require *extensive reassurance and exhaustive counseling* or they need GA. Some of them may have an atopic history (history of allergy) which influences the anesthetic technique, if GA is required. The older patients, who are waiting for laryngeal operations, usually have hypertension, ischemic heart disease (IHD), and other coexisting diseases. So, they require proper extensive perioperative care, as most of the laryngeal operations are done under GA.

During ENT operations under GA, two things should be taken into mind by an anesthetist. *These are (i) smooth anesthesia, (ii) clear airway, (iii) provision for bloodless field for microsurgery, and (iv) prevention of aspiration of blood and surgical debris during and after operation.* Because, most of the ENT operations are now done under microscope. So, the very smooth and deep anesthesia is needed which will help to avoid coughing, straining, bucking, etc. that usually occurs under light anesthesia and causes venous congestion and increases bleeding and spoils the goal of microsurgery under a high powerful microscope.

Operations on nose and throat, *but not ears,* involve the airway, and both the surgeon and the anesthetist work on this airway, fighting with each other for their working site and causing the complete or partial obstruction of airway. The complete obstruction of airway is a life-threatening condition. The partial obstruction of airway leads to hypoxemia and hypercapnia. So, the maintenance of clear airway by an anesthetist is very crucial for ENT surgeries. During all the ENT surgical procedures, the patient's eye should be protected from corneal abrasions.

GENERAL PRINCIPLES

An anesthetist during the preparation of patients scheduled for ENT operations under GA, will be concerned with the following particular problems:

- The provision for satisfactory pulmonary ventilation while permitting adequate surgical access for the nose and throat surgeries, because the airway is shared by both the surgeons and the anesthetist in such surgeries.
- The prevention of aspiration of blood, pus, or other materials into the lungs during nose and throat surgeries
- The provision of good operating conditions for microsurgery of the ear and larynx
- Care of patients undergoing major surgery of the head and neck
- Maintenance of the airway in upper respiratory tract obstruction—partial or complete.

Sharing of Airway

Problems arise when the same airway is shared by both the anesthetists and the surgeons. But, these problems are usually solved by the following ways. For nasal operations, this problem is solved by passing an oral endotracheal (ET) tube through mouth. Then, the surgeon usually approaches the nose from the patient's right hand side. So, it will be helpful, if the anesthetist shifts the ET tube toward the left side of patient's mouth.

For oral operations, e.g., tonsillectomy, where the surgeon uses mouth gag and tongue blade, etc., then this airway problem is solved by the anesthetist by passing a nasal ET tube through nose which will give a clear oral surgical field to surgeon without compromising the airway.

But, sometimes, this nasal intubation is difficult, due to the presence of some nasal obstruction or is undesirable in small children or if postnasal space is required during surgery. Then, in that situation, an adequate surgical exposure and an unobstructed airway can also be provided by an anesthetist by the presence of an oral ET tube with the use of Doughty's modifications of Boyle–Davis mouth gag (here a tongue blade is added and the ET tube is held within the slot of tongue blade). In this modification of Boyle–Davis gag, the ET tube lies comfortably within the slot of the tongue plate of Boyle–Davis gag and does not obstruct the surgeon's view and also provides a clear airway. However, sometimes the ET tube is also compressed by the tongue plate of Boyle–Davis gag which is detected during intermittent positive pressure ventilation (IPPV) by the decrease in compliance of lungs and the increase in inflation pressure (peak inspiratory pressure) or in spontaneously breathing patients by the decreased movement of reservoir bag. Then, this difficulty also can be corrected by using a long metallic special connector with the larger portion of it inside the tube. This will prevent the compression and subsequently the obstruction of ET tube.

Prevention of Aspiration

In oral, laryngeal, and nasal surgery, not only the restoration of clear airway, but also the protection of airway from aspiration during and after anesthesia (if intubated or nonintubated) and the quick restoration of postoperative protective laryngeal reflexes after extubation should also be in the forefront of an anesthetist's mind.

Although, a cuffed ET tube provides a good intraoperative protection from aspiration, still it is possible for the blood to collect in a pool, above the cuff, and may enter the lungs when the cuff of ET tube is deflated, either deliberately at the end of operation for extubation or accidentally anytime. Therefore, it is a very usual practice to insert a well lubricated gauze pack into the laryngopharynx or around the laryngeal inlet above the cuff of the ET tube, before any nasal or oral operations is started.

For the quick restoration of postoperative protective laryngeal reflexes, the following measures are usually taken. It is generally agreed that the preoperative medications with long-acting opioid drugs has a prolonged depressant effect on the laryngeal protective reflexes. So, better, it should not be used, where the quick return of reflexes are desired. But, the use of narcotics in ENT surgeries is not absolutely contraindicated. It depends on anesthetist's judgment. For example, the newer short-acting opioids, like fentanyl and its congeners, especially remifentanil can be used safely.

Again, the local anesthetic agents applied topically either in the form of spray or gel may also reduce the integrity of laryngeal protective reflexes and should be avoided.

However, this is also not absolutely contraindicated. As a whole, the conduct of GA should obviously be designed in such a fashion that it will ensure the rapid return of swallowing and cough reflexes (i.e., protective laryngeal reflexes) at the end of each ENT surgical procedure. There is little objective evidence of the superiority of any particular anesthetic technique in this respect. So, an anesthetist must apply his or her own judgment and assessment for any preferable method for that particular case, but will ensure that the depth of anesthesia will not be very light intraoperatively causing cough, ↑BP, ↑HR, increased bleeding at operative site, etc. which is very troublesome, especially during microsurgery.

Postoperatively, the likelihood of aspiration is also reduced, if the patient is placed in lateral position with head tilted slightly down. At the end of every ENT surgery, the pharynx should be sucked out completely under direct vision and there should be evidence that the reflex activity of larynx has returned adequately before the ET tube is removed. The partial incompetence of laryngeal closure reflex may persist for 2 hours after extubation, even after a relatively short duration of anesthesia. So, the practice of maintaining this lateral position and avoiding the fluid intake for 2 hours postoperatively after an ENT surgery is important. It should also be borne in mind of an anesthetist that a progressive impairment of protective laryngeal reflexes occurs with the advancement of age.

PREOPERATIVE EVALUATION AND AIRWAY ASSESSMENT

Since, anesthesia in ENT surgeries is very challenging, so the proper preoperative evaluation and the proper preoperative airway assessment of every patient by proper history taking, clinical examination, and investigation are very vital.

History

- Many preparations of antihistamines and certain other medications which are used rampantly in patients suffering from common cold may contain aspirin. So, a special attention should be given to the platelet function tests and coagulation profiles preoperatively in these patients.
- Polyps and other causes of nasal obstructions, for which the patients come for nasal surgery, may make the ventilation by mask very difficult. Hence, clinical examination for the above causes and airway assessment for obstruction in these patients is mandatory.
- Stridor is a common ENT problem. So, it requires direct laryngoscopy or bronchoscopy for preoperative airway evaluation of patient. Age of onset, cause, and the

position of patient that make the stridor better or worse should be evaluated well preoperatively. Along with this stridor, some other symptoms such as wheeze, cyanosis, chest retraction, nasal flare, etc. which indicate some form of airway obstruction, should also be carefully noted preoperatively.

- Patients with long-standing history of stridor, hemoptysis, or hoarseness of voice are usually booked for diagnosis by endoscopy or are booked for major surgery (when diagnosis is confirmed beforehand and it is usually malignancy). These patients are usually elderly with significant comorbidity. For example, chronic obstructive pulmonary disease (COPD), CVS disorders, anemia, alcoholism, smoking, etc. remain the commonly associated problems with these patients. So, the assessment of all these risks in these groups of patients, preoperatively, is very important for better perioperative management.
- Endocarditis from recurrent streptococcal bacteremia, due to infected tonsil or due to other infected focus in the body such as in ear, throat, or nose is not uncommon in patients, especially children, scheduled for ENT surgeries with cardiac valvular disease. So, during the anesthesia of ENT surgery, anesthetist should be careful about it.
- Prolonged preoperative airway obstruction presented for ENT surgery, especially in children, causes chronic hypoxemia, hypercarbia, etc. which may lead to cor pulmonale. So, all these also should be taken into consideration before anesthesia during preanesthetic evaluation. Along with cor pulmonale right ventricular hypertrophy, cardiomegaly, pulmonary artery hypertension, ventricular dysfunction, cardiac arrhythmia, etc. are also some possible complications of these patients who are suffering from chronic airway obstruction. So, proper evaluation of these patients by an anesthetist before being put up for ENT surgery is very vital.
- Enlarged tongue or tonsil and/or adenoid make a patient more prone to obstructive sleep apnea (OSA) syndrome. These syndromes consist of periods of absent (obstructed) nasal and oral airflow during sleep, despite continuing respiratory effort. This is at least partly due to the backward movement of tongue and pharyngeal wall collapse (glossoptosis) secondary to the impaired normal coordinated contraction of pharyngeal and hypopharyngeal muscles. These OSA patients are at increased risk of airway obstruction, especially during the induction and recovery phase of anesthesia. So, vigorous clinical monitoring, use of different airway devices (nasopharyngeal or Guedel oropharyngeal airway) or carrying out induction and recovery in sitting or lateral position, etc. may minimize this risk of OSA syndrome and can reduce the complications due to airway obstruction.

- Most patients who are scheduled for ENT surgeries such as tonsillectomy, adenoidectomy, or myringotomy with tube insertion, etc. are usually children, present with repeated chronic upper respiratory tract infection (URTI). But, here, the repeated postponement of surgery due to this repeated chronic URTI is not recommended or desirable, since the removal of the infected focus is important to resolve this chronic URTI in the presence of it (chronic URTI).

Airway Assessment

Before bringing the patient to operation theater (OT), an anesthetist must try to ensure whether problems will precipitate or not from airway. So, the preoperative airway assessment should start from the history of any previous airway diseases such as abscess, tumor, infection, trauma, presence of postirradiation or postsurgical scarring, or any postoperative difficulty of airway from the record of previous anesthesia, etc. After taking history, the proper assessment of airway is now next done by the physical examination of patient. *These physical examinations include* (i) the general appearance of any gross deformities of head and neck, obesity, etc. (ii) the observation of the type of breathing—stridor, mouth breathing, wheezing, etc. (iii) the inspection of mouth and chin—extent of opening of mouth, loose teeth, size of tonsil, size and mobility of tongue, micrognathia, Mallampati score, etc. (iv) the inspection of nose—nasal obstruction, mucosal congestion, deviated nasal septum, etc. (v) the inspection of neck and larynx—short neck, position of trachea, mobility of cervical spine, mobility of atlanto-occipital joint, thyromental distance, goiter, etc. Indirect laryngoscopy can be carried out before surgery for extra information of the airway. If it is needed, the help of computed tomography (CT) scan and magnetic resonance imaging (MRI) may be taken for this proper assessment of airway. *If there is any substantial doubt about the airway, then one has to consider special technique for intubation such as awake intubation, intubation by accessory devices such as fiber-optic intubation or performing a tracheostomy under LA before induction of anesthesia.*

■ PREOPERATIVE MEDICATION

Narcotics or Opioids

The *disadvantages* of the use of opioids, as premedicant in ENT surgeries, have already been mentioned in previous discussion. These disadvantages of opioid are also compounded by the fact that the operations on the middle and inner ear may themselves be associated with nausea and vomiting, which may be exaggerated by these narcotics or opioids used during premedication. Keeping all these facts in mind, *it is still justified* to use narcotic analgesics, where it is necessary such as (i) to relieve severe pain, if present, preoperatively, (ii) to maintain an intraoperative stable hemodynamic condition, and (iii) for the preparation of major ENT surgeries such as for malignancy.

Sedatives and Tranquillizers

Among the sedatives and tranquillizers, *the benzodiazepines are the most widely used drugs* and are also very effective in relieving anxiety when given by mouth preoperatively. They produce both the sedation and amnesia effect. The commonly used benzodiazepines are diazepam, lorazepam, alprazolam, and midazolam. In children, trimeprazine and promethazine are also very popular drugs for premedication. It provides *sedative, antiemetic, antisialagogue, and amnestic effects*. It is always worthy by re-emphasizing that the frequent preanesthetic visits to an anesthetist's clinic by patient and his relatives are associated with the reduced incidences of nervousness and apprehension. Thus, it also reduces the dose of preoperative sedatives as premedication.

Anticholinergic

Although, there are some objections to the routine use of atropine before anesthesia, but ENT surgeons find it very helpful to have a dry mucous membrane, when they are operating on the nose and throat. This may only be achieved by the use of atropine or glycopyrrolate preoperatively by IV route. But, before the induction and the institution of an IV route, in case of a children, IM route is the only option. If atropine is contraindicated or tachycardia is not desired, then glycopyrrolate is the best alternative or perhaps is the first choice. It (glycopyrrolate) works more effectively and persistently when given by IM rather than IV 30 minutes to 1 hour before surgery and may prove helpful by minimizing secretions, thereby facilitating airway visualization. Intravenous administration of atropine or glycopyrrolate at the time of induction is not seen to be so effective.

Antiemetic

Although, there may be an increased incidence of nausea and vomiting, after aural (ear) operations, still it is questionable whether the routine use of antiemetic drugs in such operations is justifiable or not. This is because many patients may be subjected to unnecessary antiemetic therapy. Therefore, it may be reasonable to prescribe them only when the patient complains of previous postoperative vomiting, although there is no such drug that can guarantee

any success. The drugs, which are successful in the treatment of motion sickness, are likely to be successful antiemetic after operation on ear such as cyclizine and prochlorperazine (stemetil).

■ ANESTHETIC AGENTS

Inducing Agents

Any inducing agent that is used for the induction of anesthesia in other discipline of surgery, can be used for ENT surgeries. So, it does not need any special discussions.

Muscle Relaxants

Cuffed ET intubation is needed for most of the ENT surgeries, where GA is applied. But, this should be performed with the background in mind of obstructed airway and the possibilities of difficult intubation. So, obviously, suxamethonium is the choice to facilitate intubation, where the possible difficulty of it is anticipated. But, the choice of relaxants for the next part of operation after intubation and reversal from suxamethonium is influenced by the expected duration of the next part of operation. For shorter surgical procedures, supplementary doses of suxamethonium may be given by intermittent bolus doses or by infusion of it. If operation is longer than 30 minutes duration, then a nondepolarizing muscle relaxant is preferable. On the other hand, full muscular relaxation is not an absolute prerequisite for ENT surgeries. So, anesthesia can be maintained by volatile anesthetics and spontaneous ventilation after intubation and reversal from suxamethonium.

Nitrous Oxide

Like other surgeries, N_2O also plays an integral part in the anesthetic gas mixture used for the majority of ENT operations. But, for the middle ear surgeries, its use has a definite disadvantage. Since, N_2O is 34 times more soluble than nitrogen in blood, so during N_2O anesthesia, one N_2 molecule leaving from the air cavities of our body are replaced by 34 number of N_2O molecules. Therefore, if the cavities are not distensible (e.g., middle ear), then there will be a constant rise in pressure in it; which may reach maximum after 30–40 minutes of the commencement of the inhalation of N_2O. At the end of surgery, when the N_2O is withdrawn, then it takes also a similar time for the pressure to return to normal. Hence, during certain types of tympanoplasty, this variation of pressures may cause the instability of graft (dislodgment of graft). So, if the N_2O is used, then it should be turned off some 30–40 minutes before the expected completion of surgery.

Alternatively, N_2O should be omitted altogether and anesthesia should be maintained with volatile agents, O_2, and air (which should be used in place of O_2/N_2O gas mixtures). However, recently, the surgical techniques have been improved and modified over the years, so that an increase in middle air pressure has no longer effect on tympanoplasty graft and does not influence the result of surgical procedure. It is, therefore, no longer necessary to turn off N_2O before the end of surgical and anesthetic procedure.

Halothane and Other Volatile Anesthetic Agents in ENT Surgeries

Like other surgeries, halothane is also the most commonly used volatile anesthetic agent in ENT surgeries, both during controlled and spontaneous ventilation. Whereas, the most ENT surgeons wish to use adrenaline as topical or local injectable form for vasoconstriction which makes the field dry. But, it is well-established that adrenaline in the presence of halothane may induce different types of cardiac arrhythmias, even ventricular fibrillation. So, to balance between the use and the nonuse of adrenaline, the present dictum is that adrenaline can be used safely with halothane, provided there are limits to its concentration and dose used for a given period, and hypoxia and hypercarbia are avoided, or the two drugs should never be used simultaneously, i.e., when adrenaline is used halothane should be turned off. Alternatively the surgeon should be aware of the properties of other vasoconstrictors such as octapressin (felypressin), ornithine-8-vasopressin (POR-8), etc. which are more compatible with halothane. Otherwise, other volatile anesthetic agents such as sevoflurane, isoflurane, etc. are the better choice than halothane in the presence of adrenaline, as they maintain a good hemodynamic stability and there is less chance of arrhythmia.

Anesthetic Circuits

The anesthetist must keep himself out of surgeon's way during ENT surgeries. So, it is very inconvenient to use an equipment with an expiratory valve close to the patient which may need frequent adjustment. Hence, this would preclude the use of Mapleson A circuit, Ruben valve, or a miniature ventilator. So, it indicates the use of a circle system in adult or T-piece arrangement in children. However, the Bain anesthetic circuit which is a coaxial system with expiratory valve on bag mount, is particularly useful in these conditions.

Induced Hypotension

Now, most of the ENT surgeries are performed with the help of a microscope. So, it is argued that even a small amount of blood would be magnified under the operating microscope and this will make the microsurgery difficult and does not allow the surgeon to take the necessary decision for a successful outcome. Hence, in order to minimize the bleeding (especially during microscopic surgery), it has long been advocated that one should induce deliberate hypotension aiming at mean arterial blood pressure (BP) around 60–65 mm Hg. This can be achieved by using drugs such as sodium nitroprusside, nitroglycerine, hydralazine, β-blockers, etc. On the other hand, this induced hypotension has a potentially harmful effect on cochlear blood flow during otological surgeries. Autoregulation is also lost during controlled hypotension.

Experienced practitioners (anesthetists) have used hypotensive techniques for many years with impressive safety. But, even when adequate precautions are taken, still controlled hypotension is not free of complications. These complications, however uncommon, may become major problems involving the heart and central nervous system (CNS). So, the goal of induced hypotension should be diminished bleeding without the CVS and CNS complications, rather than an absolutely bloodless field. Again, newer reports say that there is no correlation between the BP and the quality (i.e., dryness) of operative field. So, the individual anesthetist and surgeon vary in their views and their desirability.

An anesthetist should not practice, unnecessarily, the hypotensive technique on his patients and also the surgical colleagues should not force to practice it against the anesthetists will. For those anesthetists who are unwilling or insufficiently experienced to use the hypotensive method, a modified hypotensive technique can be achieved. This is based on the clear airway, controlled ventilation with halothane, absence of straining, use of topical vasoconstrictors, and moderate degree (15°) of head-up tilt. Another best way to reduce the surgical bleeding during microscopic surgery is (usually) to combine the use of opioids with isoflurane or sevoflurane in a N_2O/O_2 or air/O_2 gas mixture. This is titrated to maintain a systolic BP at around 90 mm Hg (not the mean arterial pressure at 50–55 mm Hg). The total intravenous anesthesia with propofol, as the main agent, can also be used. The advantages of using propofol for ear operations are its lower incidence of postoperative nausea and vomiting (PONV), the reduction of BP without a compensatory increase in heart rate (HR), and the preservation of autoregulation of inner ear blood flow during controlled hypotension and its excellent recovery profile.

Blood Loss

Blood loss in most ENT operations is small with obvious exception for the major head and neck surgeries, especially for malignancy. For example, in the majority of adenotonsillectomy operation in children, the blood loss is <10% of the estimated total blood volume of our body. Sometimes, up to 20% of the estimated total blood volume of our body may be lost during operation. So, in such circumstances, if the postoperative hemorrhage (if occur) is added to this loss, then blood transfusion should be given to this patient. An experienced anesthetist usually can estimate the amount of intraoperative blood loss by visual impression. But, if there is any doubt, then it is a simple matter to get some estimation of blood loss by weighing swab and measuring of contents of suction bottle.

Laryngeal Mask Airway

Now, instead of ET tube, the laryngeal mask airway (LMA) has been used for many types of ENT surgeries. But, to justify its use, the anesthetist must be able to explain that it has some advantages over the traditional use of an ET tube for that particular case (surgery). After the introduction of a flexible reinforced version, LMA is now gradually becoming very popular in ENT surgery. This flexible reinforced version of LMA has many advantages in comparison to standard classic LMA. These advantages which make the flexible reinforced LMA more useful in ENT surgeries are (i) it is more resistant to kinking and obstruction caused by oropharyngeal instruments (e.g., mouth gag), (ii) it is less likely to be displaced during the movement of head and neck, and (iii) it can be connected to a breathing system from any angle.

Gradually, the LMA itself is becoming an important anesthetic tool in ENT surgery, because it can be inserted blindly without the need of muscle relaxant in a spontaneously ventilating patient, where there is any chance of difficulty or failed intubation. The another advantage of LMA over the ET tube during ENT surgery is that coughing which increases the risk of rebleeding or displacement of grafts after ear surgery can be avoided. This is because, the LMA is better tolerated and associated with less coughing in comparison to ET tube. The another advantage of LMA over ET tube is that in case of an expected prolonged recovery, following a major surgery of head and neck, the trachea can be extubated in deep plane of anesthesia and then a LMA can be inserted further to maintain the patient's airway during the prolonged recovery period. This technique will also help to reduce the incidence of postoperative coughing and subsequently bleeding.

■ INDIVIDUAL SURGERY

Tonsillectomy

The age of most of the patients scheduled for tonsillectomy operations are <15 years and most of these children attend hospital on the day of surgery. So, before the day of admission during the routine preoperative anesthetic evaluation of these children, special emphasis should be given on checking for the loose tooth, recent ingestion of aspirin, and the determination of coagulation profile. As discussed before, the use of premedication is also a debatable matter in tonsillectomy operation. Because, some anesthetists like them and some do not. If premedication is given, it is administered most conveniently to the younger children as syrup of trimeprazine (1.5 mg/kg) or promethazine (1 mg/kg) or diazepam (0.2 mg/kg), or midazolam, and atropine (0.02 mg/kg) orally.

The aims of different techniques of anesthesia for elective tonsillectomy are:

- To provide deep anesthesia that prevents reflex tachycardia arising from surgical stimuli in light plane of anesthesia and cardiac arrhythmias. This is because, one of the important intraoperative complication in tonsillectomy is arrhythmias which is caused by the increased levels of endogenous epinephrine (catecholamine) from light GA and sensitization of myocardium to this catecholamine.
- To provide adequate muscle relaxation which will allow easy placement of mouth gag.
- To prevent bucking, coughing, or straining
- Rapid recovery to consciousness and also rapid return of protective airway reflexes.

Most of the children, who are presented for tonsillectomy surgery, are younger enough and allow an intravenous induction of anesthesia. But, in some children with poor venous access, inhalation induction may be preferred followed by IV access. Oral or nasal intubation is facilitated by succinylcholine or performed under deep inhalational anesthesia by halothane, sevoflurane, or isoflurane.

Anesthesia for tonsillectomy is usually maintained by using N_2O, nondepolarizing muscle relaxants, and narcotics with or without volatile anesthetic agents. A topical spray of 4% lignocaine on tonsillar operative area or infiltration of 2% lignocaine at surgical site will help to decrease general anesthetic requirements, the incidence of arrhythmias, and postoperative stridor and laryngospasm. Blood loss should be replaced, if it exceeds 10% of circulating blood volume.

Tracheal extubation is performed with patient's head slightly down in lateral position, and after complete suction which ensures that the pharynx and larynx is free from blood, secretions, and any tissue debris. Extubation may be done either under deep anesthesia or when the patient is fully awake. When "extubation is done under deep anesthesia" to prevent cough, vomiting, laryngospasm, etc. then the anesthetist must continue to take the responsibility of protecting the airway after extubation too. Commonly, the trachea is extubated in the operating room, when the patient is awake and the protective airway reflexes have come back. It results in some cough and laryngospasm which usually do not interfere with the surgical closure of tonsillar bed. Sometimes IV lignocaine (1 mg/kg) may be used to decrease this laryngospasm after extubation.

After extubation, patient should be observed for any bleeding and for any airway obstruction in recovery room for at least 90 minutes in tonsillar position (i.e., on one side, with the head slightly down). This is because it will allow the blood or secretions to drain out rather than to flow back into larynx through vocal cords. Then, the pharynx should be rechecked directly by laryngoscope for bleeding before the discharge from recovery room.

The incidences of nausea and vomiting can be as high as 70% during the first 24 hours after tonsillectomy. Although, the postoperative bleeding is the most serious complication, but the persistent vomiting and poor oral intake are the most common cause for the readmission of patient after discharge. To reduce the incidences of post-tonsillectomy (postoperative) vomiting, it is important to modify some anesthetic techniques and also to develop some recovery protocol such as (i) the avoidance of narcotics as postoperative analgesic, (ii) the emptying of stomach from blood by suction, (iii) the administration of antiemetic regimen, (iv) the proper hydration, (v) never force early oral food or fluid intake, etc.

The use of LMA in tonsillectomy is very difficult, because the Boyle–Davis gag cannot be placed in position, if LMA is used and the obstruction to the airway occurs more frequently. Also the LMA cannot protect the larynx from the regurgitation and the aspiration of stomach content during operation. It also cannot protect from the aspiration of blood coming from operating site.

■ ADENOIDECTOMY

The adenoidectomy surgery is usually combined with tonsillectomy or examination under anesthesia (EUA) of ear (for pediatric group of patient). In the absence of tonsillectomy operation, the only adenoidectomy surgery is usually performed as a day case procedure. For this surgery, oral tracheal intubation is must and is performed under deep inhalation anesthesia or is facilitated by the use of succinylcholine. Nasal intubation is not done for adenoidectomy operation as it obliterates the surgical space. After oral intubation, the Boyle–Davis mouth gag is inserted into oral cavity and the adenoid is curetted. Then, the nasopharynx or postnasal space is tightly packed by gauzes to achieve hemostasis for 3 minutes. Next, after the removal of this pack, when proper hemostasis is achieved

(if hemostasis is not achieved, nasopharynx should be packed again), then only the patient is extubated and is turned to tonsillar position.

Peritonsillar Abscess

It is usually drained and/or decompressed by giving incision or doing needle aspiration under LA. GA with intubation is only applied in pediatric age group of patients or uncooperative patients. In peritonsillar abscess, the risks of GA include difficult intubation, because the respiratory tract is already partially obstructed due to inflammation, edema, and abscess itself. Intubation may cause further obstruction because difficult intubation produces further (i) edema, (ii) traumatic rupture of abscess, and (iii) subsequent spilling of pus into an unprotected airway before intubation. On the other hand, difficult intubation in peritonsillar abscess may be due to distorted anatomy, edema, and trismus (masseter muscle spasm). If difficult intubation is anticipated, then the following three methods can be adopted: (i) Awake intubation under local block, (ii) Intubation with inhalational anesthesia with spontaneous respiration, (iii) Elective tracheostomy. Sometimes, planning of intubation and GA for drainage of a peritonsillar abscess may include the preoperative partial decompression of abscess by needle aspiration. It will help to minimize the risk of rupture of abscess and aspiration of pus during subsequent intubation.

Bleeding Tonsil after Tonsillectomy

The management of bleeding tonsil after tonsillectomy is a great challenge to an anesthetist. The incidence of this postoperative bleeding that actually requires resurgery is near about 0.3% and usually occurs within 6 hours of primary surgery. The problems which an anesthetist faces during the handling of such patients are unsuspected hypovolemia, full stomach (due to blood or food), and airway obstruction by blood. So, before sending the patient again to OT, the following things should be done: (i) blood loss should be assessed which is usually underestimated, (ii) no premedication should be given, (iii) coagulation profile should be rechecked, (iv) blood should be grouped, crossmatched, and kept ready for transfusion, and (v) patient should be properly hydrated by IV fluids.

By nasogastric tube, blood should be sucked from stomach before reinduction of anesthesia. Rapid sequence induction with cricoid pressure and head slightly down in lateral tilted position is followed to prevent the aspiration of blood which is continuously oozing out. During induction and intubation of GA, an assistant must be available who will continuously suck blood from the pharynx.

Like elective tonsillectomy, extubation should also be done when the patient is fully awake and the protective airway reflexes have returned.

ANESTHESIA FOR MINOR SURGERY SUCH AS ENDOSCOPY AND MICROSURGERY OF LARYNX

Endoscopy of upper airway includes (i) laryngoscopy for any diagnostic or operative procedures on larynx, (ii) microlaryngoscopy which means laryngoscopy for diagnostic and operative purposes, aided by an operating microscope for conditions like vocal cord cyst, polyp, upper airway papillomatosis, etc., (iii) esophagoscopy, (iv) bronchoscopy, etc. Any laryngeal endoscopic procedure may or may not be accompanied by laser surgery. *Patients presenting for laryngeal endoscopic surgery are often evaluated preoperatively for* stridor, hoarseness of voice, hemoptysis, etc. with which the patients are usually presented. The possible causes of these symptoms are tumor on vocal cord, foreign body aspiration, upper airway papillomatosis, trauma to trachea, tracheal stenosis, vocal cord dysfunctions, etc. which have tremendous implication on subsequent intubation and GA. For better review of these patients, anesthetist can also stake the help of X-rays, CT, MRI, ultrasound, etc.

The operating microscope has revolutionized the treatment of operative laryngeal disorder. At the same time, a wide variety of anesthetic techniques have evolved for these microlaryngeal and laryngeal endoscopic surgeries. But, the *common aims of all these anesthetic techniques are* (i) to provide the surgeon a clear, immobile view, (ii) to provide adequate space for work to surgeon, (iii) adequate relaxation of masseter muscle for the introduction of suspension laryngoscope, (iv) to provide good ventilation and oxygenation for patient, (iv) to protect the trachea from aspiration, (v) cardiovascular stability despite rapidly varying levels of surgical stimulation, and (v) rapid awakening with quick return of protective airway (laryngeal) reflexes.

Patients coming for microlaryngoscopy (endoscopy) or microsurgery of larynx have varieties of upper airway pathology which extends from a minimum to severe one, for examples, a small lesion on vocal cord (carcinoma in situ, polyp, etc.), or a large potentially obstructive lesion above the glottis (such as papillomatosis) or a large friable subglottic tumor that will completely obstruct the glottic opening. So, according to the pathology, preoperative decision about tracheal intubation or different modes of ventilation and anesthetic management is taken on.

Only light premedication by benzodiazepines is desirable or advisable for rapid reawakening from the brief laryngeal endoscopic or microsurgical procedures. Antisialagogue is must to facilitate the drying up of oral secretions. Small dose of narcotics may also be helpful. If there is any doubt about the airway (regarding ET intubation or ventilation) preoperatively, then direct laryngoscopic examination should be performed (after topical laryngeal block) in the awake patient to assess the difficulty of any mask ventilation or intubation.

As previously said, although varieties of anesthetic techniques have been developed to satisfy the requirements of adequate pulmonary ventilation and oxygenation and unimpeded surgical view for microlaryngeal surgery, but a few among them are used practically.

- *Technique 1:* The most popular anesthetic technique, among them, is the use of *Coplan's or Mallinckrodt* microlaryngoscopy tube (a type of ET tube). Actually, the standard ET tubes of smaller diameters are designed for pediatric patients and therefore too short for the adult trachea. These standard pediatric ET tubes have low volume cuff and will exert increased pressure against tracheal mucosa. So, the Coplan's and Mallinckrodt ET tube have been designed which are actually pediatric ET tube, but of adult length. They are narrow (5 mm ID), but long tube (31 cm) and constructed of hard plastic (stiffer than conventional ET tube of same diameter, so less prone to compression) with a 10 mL cuff volume (high volume and low pressure cuff). These tubes can be passed either orally or nasally. The small diameter of this tube does not impede the surgeon's view and allows a good surgical access to the larynx by surgeon.

- Of all the pathological conditions of larynx, asking for microsurgery, in 95% of cases, the pathology is situated on the anterior two-thirds of vocal cord or the anterior commissure. Only in 5% cases, the pathology involves the posterior two-thirds of vocal cord or the posterior commissure. Hence, this narrow tube does not obscure the anterior commissure. The posterior commissure can be inspected by moving the tube aside. Adequate ventilation and oxygenation can be maintained in adults by controlled ventilation through this narrow ET tube and the cuff of the tube also protects the trachea from contamination by blood or tissue debris. These narrow ET tubes also allow a variety of GA regimens, even for an indefinite period of surgery. At the end of the surgical procedure, the pharynx and larynx is cleared by suction under direct vision. Then, the muscle relaxants are antagonized and tracheal extubation is performed in lateral position. Oxygen is administered to minimize the risk of hypoxemia, if laryngeal stridor occurs **(Fact file I)**.

FACT FILE I

The anesthetic goal for endoscopy include (i) adequate ventilation and oxygenation during surgical manipulation of airway, (ii) profound muscle paralysis to provide good relaxation of masseter muscle for introduction of suspension laryngoscope, (iii) an immobile surgical field, and (iv) a good cardiovascular stability during the period of rapidly varying surgical stimulation. Several methods have been successfully used during endoscopy to provide adequate ventilation and oxygenation. But, most commonly the patients are intubated by a small diameter ET tube such as 4–6 mm of ID. However, unfortunately the ET tubes of these sizes are designed for pediatric group of patients. Therefore, they tend to be too short for adult trachea. Hence, a special type of ET tube called microlaryngeal tracheal (MLT) tube is commonly used whose size varies from 4 to 6 mm ID. The other characteristics of this tube are: the same length as an adult tube, has high volume low pressure cuff, and more stiffer (less prone to compression) than a regular tracheal tube. The advantages of intubation for endoscopy or microlaryngo surgery are: better ventilation and oxygenation, protection from pulmonary aspiration, ability to administer inhalational anesthetics, provide unlimited time for surgery, continuous monitoring of $ETCO_2$.

In some cases, the intubation may interfere the surgeon's performance such as when the lesion involves the posterior commissure of vocal cord. In such circumstances, a simple alternative is insufflation of high flows of O_2 through a small catheter placed in the trachea. These patients are usually not paralyzed by neuromuscular blocker (NMB). This is because, though oxygenation is maintained for brief periods in patients with good lung function, but it is inadequate for longer periods unless the patient is allowed to breathe spontaneously.

Another possibility for ventilation and oxygenation for endoscopy and microlaryngeal surgery is the intermitted—apnea technique in which alternate apnea and ventilation with 100% O_2 by face mask or tracheal tube is performed. In this technique full muscle relaxant is used and the surgeon acts during the apneic period.

Another sophisticated technique for endoscopy or microlaryngo surgery involves jet ventilator by connecting a jet ventilator to the side effect of the laryngoscope. During inspiration O_2 under high pressure is directed through the glottic opening and entrains room into the lungs by venturi effect. Expiration is passive and patients are kept under spontaneous respiration. Therefore, it is crucial to monitor the movement of patient's chest wall (as there is no breathing bag) and to allow the sufficient time for expiration to avoid air trapping and barotrauma.

A variation of this abovementioned technique is high-frequency jet ventilation where muscle relaxant is used. It utilizes a small cannula or tube in the trachea, through which gas is injected 100–300 times per minute. In this technique, capnography will tend to greatly underestimate the $PaCO_2$. This is due to constant dilution of alveolar gases by O_2. In all the abovementioned technique such as insufflation by high flow of O_2, intermittent apnea, jet ventilation, and high-frequency jet ventilation (except standard anesthetic technique using Coplan's microlaryngoscopy tube (MLT) or stand and (ET tube) need continuous intravenous anesthetic.

■ *Technique 2:* Another method of anesthesia for microlaryngeal surgery is *jet ventilation via laryngoscope side port or by a separate metal cannula* using venturi entrainment effect of air. This jet ventilation method provides both anesthesia and ventilation without the use of an ET tube. This venturi injector technique, to achieve the artificial ventilation, was first used in bronchoscopy and was then subsequently adopted for laryngeal (diagnostic and short therapeutic) procedures. In this procedure, a thin 16 G cannula is introduced into the trachea either by the oral, nasal, or transtracheal route through cricothyroid membrane, just below the cricoid cartilage. Then, during inspiration (1–2 seconds), intermittent jet of O_2 passed down the cannula will entrain the sufficient amount of air through the glottis to provide adequate pulmonary ventilation. With the lungs of average compliance, this is true, even if the glottis tends to close reflexly or becomes partially obstructed during inspiration.

If the glottis is open (by muscle relaxant), then additional air will be entrained, and a given tidal volume will be achieved more quickly. In this method, it is not easy to measure the tidal volume directly, but a rough clinical assessment of tidal volume by the observation of chest movement can be made. If there is some degree of glottic obstruction, then a longer expiratory phase (normal duration of expiration 4–5 seconds) will be observed. However, the failure to allow for the adequate deflation of lungs may increase the risk of pneumothorax. This method of anesthesia is also applicable in children. But, for the pediatric group of patients, it is essential to use more smaller bore cannula and lower inflating pressure.

Similar anesthetic techniques using ventilating laryngoscope also have been described. Here, the cannula is incorporated into the blade of laryngoscope. So, the surgeon has an unobstructed view of larynx. During inspiration (1–2 seconds), a high pressure (30–50 psi) jet of O_2 is directed through the glottic opening and entrains a mixture of O_2 and room air into the lungs (venture effect). Expiration (4–6 seconds) is passive. During this jet ventilation, the movement of chest wall should be monitored and sufficient expiration time should be allowed in order to avoid air trapping and barotrauma. Capnography will not provide an accurate estimate of $ETCO_2$ during jet ventilation due to constant and sizable dilution of alveolar air. As the jet of O_2 is applied above the vocal cords, so it is difficult to control the direction of gas flow. Hence, here the alignment of laryngoscope blade with the tracheal axis is essential. Also, the vocal cords need to be relaxed fully and any pathological condition in the airway must not be so large as to obstruct the airflow into trachea.

It has also been observed that blood and biopsy material may be blown into the lungs by this jet ventilation technique. This is the main disadvantage, if the jet ventilation is applied above the level of vocal cord or above the level of surgical site.

- *Technique 3:* Another method of ventilation for microlaryngeal surgery is the apneic oxygenation technique where a period of ventilation is followed by a period of apnea when the ET tube is taken out and it is again followed by intubation and ventilation, thus repeating this cycle again and again. It is found that ventilation of lungs by 100% O_2 (not jet) by ET tube can provide adequate oxygenation in apneic patient (i.e., when the ventilation is not done) for the certain period of time after the elimination of body N_2. But, the limiting time factor for apnea, from the clinical point of view, is the rate of rise of arterial PCO_2. This may be reduced slightly by using higher flow rates of gas such as 10 L/min. In practice, it is not advisable to prolong the surgical procedure for >10 minutes. So, it is a suitable method for a brief therapeutic and diagnostic microlaryngeal surgical procedure (It is further discussed in LASER Chapter).
- *Technique 4:* It is another simple alternative method. Here, high flow of O_2 through a small catheter placed in the trachea is instituted. Although oxygenation may be maintained in patients with good lung function, but ventilation will be inadequate for longer procedures, unless the patient is allowed to breathe spontaneously.

Intraoperative good muscle relaxation is an essential part of anesthetic management for the microsurgery of larynx. This can be achieved by intermittent boluses or infusion of nondepolarizing muscle relaxant of intermittent duration (e.g., cisatracurium, rocuronium, and vecuronium) or infusion by succinylcholine. Rapid recovery is important, as endoscopy is often an outpatient procedure. As the profound muscle relaxation is often required, until the very end of microsurgical procedure, so microsurgical endoscopy remains one of the few remaining indications for succinylcholine infusion. The use of sugammadex to reverse the profound degree of neuromuscular blockade produced by rocuronium or vecuronium is an alternative approach.

Technique of Anesthesia for Microlaryngeal Surgery

The use of injector technique (*jet ventilation*) or a *small (narrow) endotracheal tube* (microlaryngeal ET tube), allows a surgeon for more time for the leisurely examination of the larynx and microsurgery which is not possible by *apneic oxygenation technique*. In addition, many things such as the teaching and photography may be done without being pressed for time by the above two techniques. Anesthesia is provided by an intravenous-inducing agent. This is followed by suxamethonium and the chosen technique and equipment which is then put into place. A few minutes of preoxygenation before induction of anesthesia help to provide a favorable alveolar-arterial O_2 tension gradient. Further doses of suxamethonium are given when it is required to maintain the apnea.

During jet ventilation, if jets of O_2 only are used for ventilation, then it is important to give supplementary doses of IV induction agent (e.g., propofol). Otherwise, the patient may awake during the procedure and experiences the terror of being paralyzed, but awake (feeling of drowning) and may also hear remarks of OT personals. In children, microlaryngoscopy is performed by using spontaneous respiration via an oral tracheal tube which is one size smaller than that is used normally. The larynx should be sprayed with measured quantity of lignocaine in an attempt to prevent postoperative laryngospasm.

During these endoscopic laryngeal procedures, the HR and BP of patient often fluctuate markedly for two reasons. (1) Most of these patients are elderly and have long history of tobacco smoking and alcohol abuse that predisposes them to cardiovascular disease. In addition, these endoscopic surgeries are a series of physiologically stressful laryngoscopic procedures and interventions with rise of HR and BP followed by varying periods of minimal surgical stimulation with lowering of HR and BP. (2) Attempting to maintain a constant level of anesthesia invariably results in alternating intervals of hypertension and hypotension. This is usually tackled by providing a modest baseline level of anesthesia which is supplemented with short-acting anesthetics (propofol, remifentanil, etc.) or sympatholytic agents (esmolol, labetalol, etc.) or both as needed during the period of increased stimulation. Alternatively, some anesthetists provide regional nerve block (glossopharyngeal nerve and superior laryngeal nerve) to minimize these intraoperative swings in HR and BP.

■ HEAD AND NECK CANCER SURGERY

Preoperative Consideration

These surgeries usually include laryngectomy, pharyngectomy, glossectomy, hemimandibulectomy, laryngo-esophagectomy, radical neck dissection, etc. and these are done for the malignancy of larynx, pharynx, tongue, etc. Airway obstruction is the major perianesthetic problem in this group of surgery. An endoscopic examination following induction of anesthesia often precedes these surgical procedures. *Timing of tracheostomy* depends on surgical planning and the extent of patient's preoperative airway compromise. All these surgical procedures are of long duration and substantial blood loss.

Alcohol, smoking, and old age are the etiological factors of all these malignancies which may also influence the course of anesthesia. So, anesthetist has to frequently face the patients who are elderly, having bronchitis, emphysema, COPD, diabetes, chronic cardiovascular diseases (hypertension and IHD), etc. If the tumor interferes with proper eating, then weight loss, malnutrition, anemia, dehydration, and electrolyte imbalance can also be significant and an anesthetist has to face all these problems. So, all these patients are properly evaluated and treated as representing difficult ET intubation and with potential problems in airway management preoperatively. Respiratory functions should be assessed preoperatively by pulmonary function test. But, this is difficult to measure accurately, if there is any airway obstruction. Chest physiotherapy should always be prescribed, as it aids the clearance of secretions pre- and postoperatively. These operations are often prolonged and associated with considerable blood loss necessitating generous preoperative provisions of compatible blood.

Intraoperative Consideration

Induction and Intubation

In these types of surgeries, the management of airway may be complicated by abnormal airway anatomy, an airway obstructing lesion, and preoperative radiation therapy that has fibrosed, immobilized, and distorted the patient's airway. This complicated management of airway is tackled by (i) the avoidance of intravenous induction in favor of *awake fiber-optic* laryngoscopy and intubation under slight sedation and LA (in cooperative patient), or fiber-optic intubation following an *inhalational induction* maintaining spontaneous ventilation (in uncooperative patient). Another way of intubation is like that IV inducing agent is given very slowly, till consciousness is lost. Then, patient's lung is inflated using face mask and bag. If it is possible, then it will indicate that the patient will not go to *"not to ventilate and not to intubate condition"*. Then, only succinylcholine is given to facilitate intubation. If not, face mask ventilation is continued till spontaneous respiration is returned. Then, anesthesia is deepened with volatile agent and intubation is tried with fiber-optic method. (ii) Elective tracheostomy under LA, prior to induction of GA, is often a prudent option. In any such cases (cancer surgeries of head and neck), appropriate equipment and qualified personnel must always be available for emergency tracheostomy.

If elective tracheostomy is not decided and *the patients are scheduled for tracheostomy* after intubation, then respiratory obstruction is also suspected. In these groups of surgeries before tracheostomy, ET intubation is done by the following way. Narcotic and sedative premedications should be avoided. All the patients should have preoperative assessment of airway by flexible nasal or oral endoscope to know the magnitude of obstruction of larynx (previously said) which have a great implication during induction and intubation. If there is a possibility of complete mechanical obstruction and failed intubation after muscular paralysis, then an inhalational technique should also be used for intubation. All these volatile anesthetic agents dilate the bronchi, depress the airway reflexes, and permit the use of higher concentration of O_2. If the inhalational technique results in possibility of severe obstruction, then an awake ET intubation should also be tried.

Tracheostomy: Immediately prior to surgical entry into trachea, the ET tube and hypopharynx should be sucked properly to avoid the risk of aspiration of blood and secretion into lungs. If electrocautery is used during surgical dissection (entry) of trachea, then FiO_2 should be lowered to 30% or less to avoid the risk of fire. Better, a surgeon should not use cautery, when he will enter the trachea. After dissection up to trachea, the cuff of ET tube is deflated to avoid its perforation by scalpel. The, the ET tube is withdrawn slightly and the tracheal wall is transected, so that the tip of ET tube is immediately cephalad to the incision. Next, a sterile cuffed tracheostomy tube is placed into trachea, the cuff is inflated, and the tracheostomy tube is connected to a sterile breathing circuit. Now, the correct position of tracheostomy tube is confirmed by capnography and bilateral chest auscultation and the original ET tube is removed.

If elective tracheostomy is not decided and *also the patients are not scheduled for tracheostomy after intubation,* then ET intubation is done by the abovementioned methods and the tube is not removed and the surgery is preceded following ET intubation.

Maintenance of Anesthesia

During the dissection of neck, thyroidectomy, parotidectomy, etc. the surgeon may request the anesthetist to avoid to use the NMBs. Because, it will help the surgeons to identify the nerves (facial, vagus, spinal accessory, etc.) by their direct stimulation and to facilitate their preservation. For direct nerve stimulation, ET tube integrated with nerve monitoring system also can be used. In such situation, succinylcholine can be used to facilitate only the intubation.

Intraoperative-induced hypotension is often used to reduce the blood loss during surgical dissection of neck tissue. But, it is not without risk in debilitated patients and it may be unnecessary and dangerous too in these groups of patients. Therefore, alternatively moderate hypotension by deep halothane or other volatile anesthetic agent and 10–15° tilt (head-up) is sufficient (to produce this moderate hypotension) and diminish the intraoperative blood loss, instead of restoring deliberate induced hypotension.

The intraoperative surgical manipulation of carotid sinus during the dissection of neck tissue may elicit a strong vagal reflex (cardiovascular instability) that can cause severe bradycardia, hypotension, arrhythmia, or even cardiac arrest. If this is persistent, then the infiltration of this carotid sinus with local anesthetic agent or IV atropine may be an effective treatment. Trauma to the right stellate ganglion and cervical autonomic nervous system during laryngeal surgery can also prolong the QT interval and lower the threshold for ventricular fibrillation. But, its incidences are low. Still, like carotid sinus, the stellate ganglion should also be protected by infiltration of local anesthetic agent. Bilateral neck dissection may result in postoperative hypertension and loss of hypoxic drive due to the denervation of carotid sinuses and carotid bodies. Like neurosurgery, opened neck veins may also create the possibility of air emboli during major laryngeal surgery. All these major surgeries are associated with substantial amount of blood loss. But, the decision regarding blood transfusion must balance between the patient's immediate surgical risk and the possibility of increased cancer recurrence rate resulting from transfusion-induced immunosuppression.

When the larynx and the trachea have been dissected free from the surrounding tissues to divide the trachea, then it is important to check, whether a second sterile cuffed tracheostomy tube, catheter mount, and a compatible connector, which will attach the tracheostomy tube with anesthetic machine, are included in the surgical instrument trolley or not. Before the division of trachea, patient is ventilated with 100% O_2 for 2 minutes. Then, the previous ET tube is withdrawn from the larynx, and the trachea is divided. The withdrawn of the ET tube should not be full. It should be withdrawn only above the proposed line of incision on trachea. Next, a second tracheal tube is rapidly placed through the opened end of the trachea. After this, the second tracheal tube is connected to the anesthetic circuit and secured firmly. This tube should be positioned carefully within the shortened trachea to prevent inadvertent one-lung anesthesia. The previous oral ET tube, having been withdrawn above the incision line on trachea, is left in place until the new airway is secured. In cases of difficulty, it can be remanipulated into the trachea, so that the cuff lies distal to the incision.

At the end of the surgery, the patients should be reversed completely from the neuromuscular block and the tracheal tube is changed for tracheostomy tube. When a patient with previous tracheostomy presents for anesthesia, a cuffed tube should be inserted before induction of anesthesia and anesthesia is maintained through this tracheostomy route.

Monitoring during Anesthesia

As all these cancer surgeries are associated with (i) substantial amount of blood loss, (ii) coexisting morbidities, due to old age, and (iii) long duration, so they need extensive monitoring. For this extensive monitoring, arterial cannulation is performed for invasive BP monitoring and frequent laboratory analyses. Before the institution of central venous line in internal jugular vein (IJV) or subclavian vein, surgeon should always be consulted if it will interfere the surgical procedure or not. As an alternative site, antecubital and femoral veins can be used. All these central lines should not be placed on the arm of operated site. During intra-arterial BP monitoring, transducer should be placed at the level of external auditory meatus to determine the cerebral circulation. A forced air warming blanket should always be used to maintain normal body temperature, as hypothermia is common occurrence in such major surgeries.

During the head and neck cancer surgeries, intraoperative nerve monitorings are now frequently used by surgeons to preserve nerves such as facial, superior laryngeal, recurrent laryngeal, vagus, cranial accessory, etc. So, the surgeons frequently request the anesthetists to use ET tube integrated with nerve monitoring system (Medtronic Xomed NIM endotracheal tube) and not to use NMBs, except succinylcholine for intubation.

ANESTHESIA FOR NASAL AND SINUS SURGERIES

The common nasal and sinus surgeries are polypectomy, septoplasty, rhinoplasty, endoscopic sinus surgery, Caldwell–Luc operation (maxillary sinusotomy), etc. The main preoperative considerations during nasal and sinus surgeries are (i) considerable degree of nasal obstruction, caused by polyps, deviated septum, or mucosal congestion. This will lead to difficult face mask ventilation, particularly if combined with other causes of difficult ventilation, e.g., obesity, maxillofacial deformities, etc. (ii) Nasal polyps are often associated with allergic disorders such as asthma, allergic to aspirin, etc. and they should not be given any nonsteroidal anti-inflammatory drug (NSAID) for postoperative analgesia. (iii) Nasal polyps are a common feature of cystic fibrosis. (iv) Because of rich vascular supply of nasal mucosa during preoperative evaluation of patient, question should include regarding the medication use such as aspirin, clopidogrel, and any history of bleeding problem.

All the operations on nose and sinuses have one common feature, i.e., they involve surgery on a very vascular structure (mucous membrane of nose and sinuses). In 1942, Moffatt had first described the method of topical anesthesia for nasal surgeries using cocaine. Cocaine is the first discovered local anesthetic agent with the intense vasoconstrictive properties. There are *three advantages of this local anesthetic method* for nasal and sinus surgeries by cocaine for its vasoconstrictive property. These are (i) minimal patient's discomfort from pain during operation due to LA by cocaine, (ii) shrinkage of blood vessels of mucous membrane due to vasoconstrictive effect of cocaine, and (iii) blood less surgical field. But, cocaine is known to have sympathomimetic side effects and sensitizes the myocardium to epinephrine by blocking its reuptake at synaptic level. So, the major cardiovascular complications (such as the VT, VF, MI, etc.) are also reported, even after the use of topical cocaine, especially when it is combined with the use topical epinephrine or with the use of halothane. So, this lead to the question whether cocaine still has a role in nasal surgery or not. Because, studies have shown that lignocaine with epinephrine and/or oxymetazoline are good effective alternatives to the cocaine and so cocaine is obsolete now.

Still, if one wants to use cocaine topically, the dose will be 4% solution or less (without addition of epinephrine) with a maximum dose of 1.5 mg/kg or a total dose of 160 mg. However, now, most of the nasal operations are done under LA using various local anesthetic agents (lignocaine or bupivacaine or ropivacaine) mixed with some vasoconstrictor (adrenaline) **(Fact file II)**. However, when the epinephrine is used, the maximum concentration of it should not exceed 1:100,000 or 10 µg/mL. Further, the epinephrine of lower concentration is also acceptable, because no differences were found in the degree of vasoconstriction with the use of epinephrine at concentration as low as 1:400,000 (2.5 µg/mL). The concentration and the total dose of epinephrine should be kept as low as possible, because it is known that the combined use of volatile anesthetic agents during GA (especially halothane) and epinephrine can induce cardiac arrhythmias.

By blocking the sphenopalatine ganglion, most of the sensory supply to the nose (including the anterior ethmoidal nerve) can be blocked. But, only the columella part of the nose is not affected by this method (sphenopalatine ganglion block) and requires a separate injection. Indications and contraindication of LA and/or GA for nasal and ear surgeries are like ophthalmic anesthesia and are discussed in details in "ophthalmic anesthesia" Chapter.

Most of the nasal surgical procedures such as septoplasty, removal of polyp, reduction of fractured nasal bones, etc. are often carried out safely under LA by using the infiltration of tissue by local anesthetic agents combined with or without sedations. However, potentially serious complications may arise, if the patient moves during endoscopic sinus surgery. These serious complications may

FACT FILE II

Most nasal surgeries can be performed satisfactorily under local infiltration of anesthesia with or without sedation. The nasal septum and the lateral wall of the nose get their sensory innervation by anterior ethmoidal and sphenopalatine nerves. Both these nerves can be blocked by topical application of LA agent by packing the nose with gauze or cotton swab soaked with local anesthetic agent. Supplementation of this topical anesthesia by submucosal injection (infiltration) of LA agent is often required. This topical anesthetic agent should be allowed to remain in place for at least 10 minutes before surgery. Sometimes, in addition to this topical application, local infiltration of LA agent in the submucosal level is often required. This is mainly found, particularly if scar tissue is present from prior surgery. The use of epinephrine containing LA solution or cocaine solution (usually a 4% or 10% solution) will shrink the nasal mucosa and reduce the intraoperative blood loss. The disadvantage of cocaine is that it is very rapidly absorbed and may cause detrimental cardiovascular effects. GA is needed for nasal surgeries when the topical or local infiltration block is inadequate, producing discomfort, or when the pediatric and psychiatric patients are met.

include entering the intracranial space, blindness due to entry into the orbital cavity, damage to the internal carotid artery, etc. So, the paralysis of patients is advised when the risk of complications from movement is high. Thus, GA is recommended for these types of endoscopic surgeries, where the chances of movement are high such as mainly in pediatric and psychiatric group of patients. However, GA for these endoscopic nasal surgeries has been revolutionized by the introduction of LMA. In the presence of nasal packing, difficulty in maintaining airway is almost completely eliminated by leaving the LMA in place postoperatively, until the patient himself rejects it spontaneously in the recovery room.

Because of the proximity of surgical field, it is important to cover the patient's eye to avoid corneal abrasion. One exception to this is the endoscopic sinus surgery, when the surgeon may wish to check periodically the eye movement, because of the close proximity of sinuses and orbit. Nonetheless, the eyes should remain protected, until the surgeon is ready to observe them. Therefore, under LA, there is every chance of the movement of the patient and the chance of the injury of orbit. On the other hand, under GA the surgeon cannot observe the movement of the eyeball and cannot determine if any injury in orbit is occurred or not.

The GA for nasal surgeries may be maintained by using either spontaneous or controlled ventilation. However, during GA of nasal surgeries, whatever the type of tube is used (ET or LMA) and whatever the spontaneous or controlled ventilation are chosen, the posterior pharynx should be packed with gauze, so that the blood, pus, or debris will not contaminate the larynx and at the time of extubation may not lead to coughing and/or laryngospasm. The techniques to minimize the intraoperative blood loss and its collection include topical vasoconstriction with cocaine or epinephrine containing local anesthetic agent, maintaining a slightly head-up position and providing a mild degree of controlled hypotension. After surgery, the packs are removed, the pharynx is cleared, and the patient is turned in lateral tonsillar position. It is safer to extubate the patient while he/she is completely awake. Sometimes, after nasal surgery, but before extubation, blood may collect at the back of the soft palate.

Therefore, in the immediate postoperative period following extubation, these clots may dislodge from its site (the back of the soft palate) and fall into the glottis leading to complete airway obstruction. This clot is called as the *"coroner's clot"*. So, the reduction of bleeding by using topically applied vasoconstrictive drugs, head-up position by 15–20° which will provide a mild degree of hypotension, and good suctioning before extubation, will help to reduce the incidences of this problem.

■ ANESTHESIA FOR EAR SURGERIES

The ear gets its sensory supply by four nerves, these are (i) the auriculotemporal nerve, (ii) the great auricular nerve, (iii) the auricular branch of vagus nerve, and (iv) the tympanic nerve (**Fig. 1**). The *auriculotemporal nerve* is the branch of the mandibular division of trigeminal nerve. It supplies the anterior wall and roof of external auditory meatus. It can be blocked by infiltrating the 3 mL of local anesthetic agent into the anterior wall of external auditory meatus. The *greater auricular nerve* is the branch of cervical plexus. It supplies the middle and lower aspect of auricle and a small part of the external auditory meatus. The *auricular branch of vagus nerve* supplies the concha and the external auditory meatus. These two nerves, i.e., the great auricular and the auricular branch of vagus can be blocked by infiltrating the 3 mL of local anesthetic agent, posterior to the external auditory meatus. The *tympanic nerve* is the branch of glossopharyngeal nerve and supplies the tympanic cavity. It can be blocked by the instillation of 4% lignocaine into the middle ear.

The frequently performed ear surgeries are stapedectomy or stapedotomy, tympanoplasty, mastoidectomy, myringotomy with the insertion of tympanostomy tube, etc. Most of the ear surgeries can be performed both under LA with or without sedation and under GA. The operations such as premeatal operations, stapedectomy, uncomplicated middle ear surgeries (of <2 hours duration), etc. are

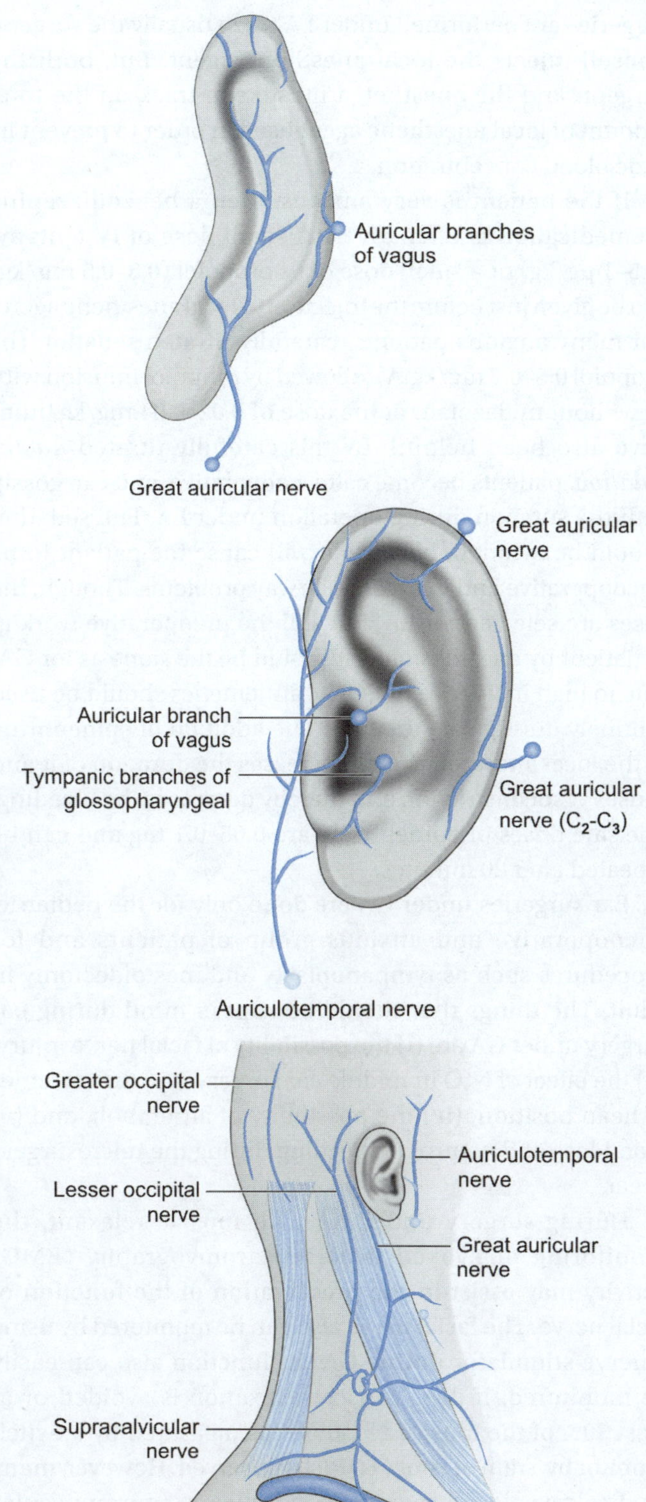

Fig. 1: This figure depicts the sensory supply of ear. The sensory supply of ear is carried by auriculotemporal, great auricular, auricular branch of vagus, and tympanic nerve.

usually performed under LA. The GA is needed only when the patient is noncooperative or for pediatric age group of patients or the surgeries for malignancy. When ear surgeries are performed under LA, then usually the surgeon himself injects the local anesthetic agent. But, both the surgeon and the anesthetist must keep track on the total amount of local anesthetic agent used in order to prevent its toxic blood concentration.

If the patient is very anxious, then a benzodiazepine premedication is often given. A small dose of IV fentanyl (0.5–1 µg/kg) or a small dose of IV propofol (0.3–0.5 mg/kg) can be given just before the injection of local anesthetic agent. For many anxious patients, carefully titrated sedation (by propofol 0.5–0.7 mg/kg IV, followed by propofol infusion with or without midazolam at the dose of 0.02–0.04 mg/kg/min) have also been helpful. By this carefully titrated *awake sedation*, patients become calm, cooperative, and can gossip with the surgeon during operation under LA. Full sedation should be avoided, because it will cause the patient to be uncooperative and may cause airway problems. Though, the cases are selected for LA, but still the preoperative workup of patient by anesthesiologist should be the same as for GA. Due to high incidence of PONV, antiemetics should be used routinely during ear surgeries. The addition of epinephrine to the local anesthetic agent increases the duration of it and causes vasoconstriction and thereby decreases the bleeding. The safe doses of epinephrine are 0.05–0.1 mg and can be repeated after 20 minutes.

Ear surgeries under GA are done only for the pediatric, uncooperative and anxious group of patients and for procedures such as tympanoplasty and mastoidectomy in adult. The things that should be kept in mind during ear surgery under GA are (i) the possibility of facial nerve injury, (ii) the effect of N_2O in middle ear surgery, (iii) the extremes of head position, (iv) the possibility of air emboli, and (v) blood loss and control of bleeding during the microsurgery of ear.

During surgery under GA with muscle relaxant, the monitoring of evoked facial electromyography (EMG) activity may assist in the preservation of the function of facial nerve. The facial nerve also can be monitored by using a nerve stimulator during GA. Its function also can easily be monitored, if deep muscle relaxation is avoided or at least 30% of the muscle response [as measured by a twitch monitor by Train of Four (TOF)] is preserved. However, many studies revealed that despite significant neuromuscular block, as measured by no response state on the stimulation of ulnar nerve, facial nerve activity could still be detected on electrical stimulation.

The middle ear like the other cavities (e.g., sinuses) of our body is a closed air containing space. It is connected to the environment by eustachian tube (whereas the sinuses are connected with environment through ostium). During N_2O

anesthesia, N_2O enters the cavity 34 times rapidly than N_2 exits (absorbed by blood) the cavity (as N_2O is 34 times more soluble in blood than N_2, blood gas coefficient of N_2 being 0.013 and N_2O 0.46). This results in the increase in volume and pressure of air in the middle ear. As a result, there is bulging of ear drum and lifting of the tympanic membrane which causes the disruption of graft in tympanoplasty surgery.

Normally, the changes in middle ear pressure caused by N_2O are well tolerated as a result of passive venting through the eustachian tube. But, the patients with the history of chronic ear problems such as otitis media, sinusitis, etc. often suffer from obstructed eustachian tube and may suffer from hearing loss or tympanic membrane rupture on rare occasion from N_2O anesthesia. In eustachian tube block, the middle ear pressure can rise up to 375 mm H_2O within 30 minutes of the starting of N_2O inhalation. In addition, after discontinuation of N_2O, the gas is rapidly absorbed in blood than N_2 which enters in the cavity causing marked reduction of the volume and negative pressure in the middle ear. Sometimes, this negative pressure in the middle ear becomes so great that it causes serious otitis, disarticulation of stapes, impaired hearing, etc. However, during tympanoplasty, the middle ear is open to the atmosphere and there is no buildup of pressure in the middle ear cavity.

Finally, it can be concluded that fluctuation of middle ear pressure during N_2O anesthesia causes problems (is also a cause for PONV) only in susceptible persons, i.e., those with the previous eustachian tube block due to otological surgery, acute or chronic otitis media, sinusitis, URTI, adenoids etc. There is also no evidence of interference in graft placement or outcome of surgical procedure in type 1 tympanoplasty if N_2O is used in <50% concentration. But it is better to avoid possibilities of complications. So, anesthetist should limit the concentration of N_2O to 50% and discontinue N_2O 15 to 20 minutes before the closure of middle ear. The subsequent decrease of middle ear cavity pressure to subatmospheric level can be avoided by flushing the middle ear cavity with air prior to closure of the tympanic membrane. During ear surgery under GA, an anesthetist should be careful about the extreme positions of neck such as extreme extension or rotation which may cause injury to the cervical spine, brachial plexus, etc. Patients with limited carotid artery supply to the brain are especially vulnerable to further decrease in flow from exaggerated neck position. Also, in patients with Down syndrome or with rheumatoid arthritis, the extreme rotation of neck should be avoided because of the risk of C_1-C_2 subluxation.

As with any form of microsurgery, even tiny amounts of blood can obscure the operating field during the microsurgery in ear. Control of bleeding during microsurgery of ear under local or GA can be done (i) by maintaining 10–15° head-up tilt position which will increase the venous drainage and will decrease the venous bleeding. Thus, they will create a relatively dry operative field and help in microsurgery of ear. (ii) The infiltration of operative area by local anesthetic agent, mixed with adrenaline (epinephrine), is also helpful for controlling the bleeding and helps in postoperative analgesia. But, the total dose of adrenaline should be limited to 0.1 mg (20 mL of 1:200,000 solution in which 1 mL contains 5 µg adrenaline) which can be repeated after 20 minutes. This is also a safe practice in a well-ventilated (normocapnic) patient who is given halothane anesthesia. Isoflurane and sevoflurane does not sensitize the myocardium to catecholamines to the same extent as does the halothane and hence are more safe. The topical application of epinephrine in ear is also helpful to reduce bleeding from operating site and to make a dry operative field. But, the higher concentrations of adrenaline like 1:50,000 need not provide any additional vasoconstrictive effects. (iii) Because, coughing on ET tube during emergence (particularly during neck movement associated with head bandaging) will increase venous pressure and may cause bleeding and increased middle ear pressure, deep extubation is often utilized.

Laryngeal mask airway is used in major ear surgery, but the anesthetist must be aware that if the airway is lost during the procedure, as a result of the movement of head, then the operation may have to be abandoned. The preservation of facial nerve is an important factor during some ear surgeries such as the resection of glomus tumor, acoustic neuroma, etc. During such surgeries, the intraoperative muscular paralysis by NMBs will make the identification of facial nerve difficult by direct nerve stimulation. Hence, during some ear surgeries, intraoperative paralysis should not be employed unless requested by the surgeon. As the inner ear is intimately involved with the sense of balance, so ear surgery may cause postoperative dizziness (vertigo) and PONV. Hence, the induction and maintenance of anesthesia during middle ear surgery by propofol has been shown to decrease PONV. Prophylaxis by dexamethasone, prior to induction and a 5-HT3 blocker prior to emergence will also be helpful. After middle or inner ear surgery during postoperative period the patient should be closely assessed for vertigo and is closely monitored for balance during walking in order to minimize the fall.

▌MAXILLOFACIAL RECONSTRUCTION AND ORTHOGNATHIC SURGERY

These are the major surgeries and are usually performed for (i) the fractures of mandible or maxilla, (ii) the radical cancer surgeries (mandibulectomy, maxillectomy, block resection of lymph nodes in neck, etc.), (iii) the correction of severe developmental malformation of face and orthognathic procedures for skeletal malocclusion (LeFort osteotomies, mandibular osteotomies, etc.). The main problems of these major surgical procedures during anesthesia are *maintenance of airway and blood loss*. In these types of surgeries, the airway challenge will start from mask ventilation to intubation to intraoperative ventilation to extubation and the maintenance of airway in postoperative period. All these problems are due to the improper fitting of mask, micrognathia, retrognathia, problem in neck mobility, dental pathology, macroglossia, abnormal jaw opening, wiring between maxilla and mandible, postoperative tissue edema around the airway, etc. If there are any anticipated signs for difficult mask ventilation or ET intubation, then the airway should be secured by fiber-optic oral or nasal intubation or tracheostomy with LA and cautious sedation before the induction of GA. If nasal intubation is chosen, then preformed nasal Ring-Adair-Elwyn (RAE) tube is preferred and is directed cephalad over the patient's forehead.

All the maxillofacial reconstructive and orthognathic surgeries involve the *substantial amount of blood loss*. Hence, three strategies are taken to minimize this blood loss and these three strategies are (i) slight head-up position, (ii) controlled ventilation, and (iii) the local infiltration of epinephrine solutions. A pharyngeal pack at the oral and laryngeal level is often placed tightly to minimize the amount of blood and other surgical debris, reaching the larynx and trachea and an anesthetist will not forged to remove this pack at the end of the surgery, but before the jaws are closed by wire. All the vital monitoring according to the extensiveness of surgery are attached, for example, central venous pressure monitoring, invasive BP monitoring through intra-arterial line, capnography, ECG, etc. If the head-up tilt is used, then it is must that the transducer for measuring the intra-arterial BP should be zeroed at the level of external auditory meatus (brain) in order to most accurately determine the cerebral perfusion pressure. In the setting of head-up tilt, an anesthetist must also be alert to the increased risk of venous air embolism.

In all the ENT surgeries, the main problem is that because of the proximity of airway to the surgical sites, the positioning of surgical team and the positioning of patient's head remain far away from the anesthesia providers. Hence, there is an increased risk of critical intraoperative airway problems such as (i) ET tube displacement, (ii) disconnection of ET tube from breathing circuit, (iii) kinking of ET tube, (iv) perforation of ET cuff by surgical instrument, etc. There are more chances of these above risks during the major maxillofacial and orthognathic surgeries. Therefore, to detect these problems, intraoperative monitoring of $ETCO_2$, peak inspiratory pressure, and breath sounds via an esophageal stethoscope assume greater importance in such cases. As the operative site is near the airway, so the use of electrocautery and laser also increases the risk of fire. There is another great problem during these major maxillofacial surgeries and this is profound postoperative tissue edema involving the structures around the airway after extubation. So, patient should be closely observed after extubation and perhaps kept intubated. In such uncertain situations, extubation may be performed over an ET tube exchanger. The advantage of this ET tube exchanger is that it facilitates reintubation and provides oxygenation in the setting of immediate postextubation airway obstruction. In addition, anesthetic team should be prepared for emergency tracheostomy or cricothyrotomy in postoperative period for any emergency airway obstruction threatening life. Patients with intermaxillary fixation (maxillomandibular wiring) must have appropriate wire cutting tools and suction apparatus by his/her bed side continuously, because of vomiting or other airway emergencies.

Anesthesia for Geriatric Patients

INTRODUCTION

There is no precise definition for the terms named *elderly, geriatric, old, or aged*. There is also no specific clinical marker for the geriatric group of population (in the society) from which we can stamp that this patient is elderly or aged or in geriatric group. This is because aging is a continuous process. So, the determination of age at which the people are considered elderly also remains arbitrary. But, still, it is generally agreed for the administrative and epidemiological purposes that the patients aged >65 years are considered as *geriatric or elderly*. However, some specific classifications of *geriatric population* are persons in-between 65 and 74 years of age are called the *"elderly"*, persons in-between 75 and 84 years of age are called the *"aged"*, and those above 85 years of age are called the *"very old"*.

Age itself is an independent single factor for the increased morbidity and mortality of an individual in a society. It (age) is also an important independent factor for a number of diseases, i.e., injuries, hospitalization, and adverse drug reactions which occur predominantly in this higher age group of patients. It itself has also been shown to be an independent predictor for perioperative outcome. As, all over the world, the geriatric population is now on its rise, so the India is also not lagging behind of this fact that increased number of geriatric patients are coming for surgery in this country also. So, the anesthesiologists are now going to encounter increased number of elderly patients in operation theater (OT), intensive care unit (ICU), high-dependency unit (HDU), etc. Therefore, it is mandatory to understand precisely the pathophysiological changes which occur with age and to evaluate its effect on anesthetic risk. Thus, equipped with proper knowledge, an anesthesiologist will be in a better position to take a good perioperative care of these geriatric groups of patients.

The medical specialty of geriatric cases (geriatric medicine), such as the *geriatric medicine* has, therefore, become increasingly important and is gradually now developing in recent years in all the countries. The geriatric medicine is not only concerned with the prolonging the lives of elderly people. But, it is much more concerned with keeping the old people young. Similarly, the surgery on the elderly should be comprised not only the possibilities of treating an illness by operation, but also it includes an assessment of the patient's ability to withstand the surgery and benefit from it. The modern development in anesthesia has made surgical procedures, which was previously deemed unfit due to age, now become feasible. But, this must not obscure the dangers of postoperative period that will throw an additional strain on their cardiovascular and respiratory systems which the aged patient may not be able to sustain. On the other hand, the general view is that all the surgeries in the very old are "unwarranted interference" and cannot be justified, especially if it does not improve the quality of life and cannot bring comfort for the remaining months or years of patient's life.

Aging is defined as a progressive physiological process that produces measurable changes in the structure and the function of tissues and organs. Till now, the *mechanism of this aging* is not yet clearly understood. But, it is postulated that the decreased production of cellular energy, due to the deterioration of mitochondrial function (mainly in cardiac and neural tissues), plays a fundamental role in the age-related decline of the functions of tissues or organs. The aging is a natural, inevitable, and a biological phenomenon of every cellular structure. However, the onset and the rate of progress of this age-related changes vary with every individual, depending on few known and many unknown variables. The biological age (the decrease of production of cellular energy with passing of time) of a person is not identical with his or her chronological age.

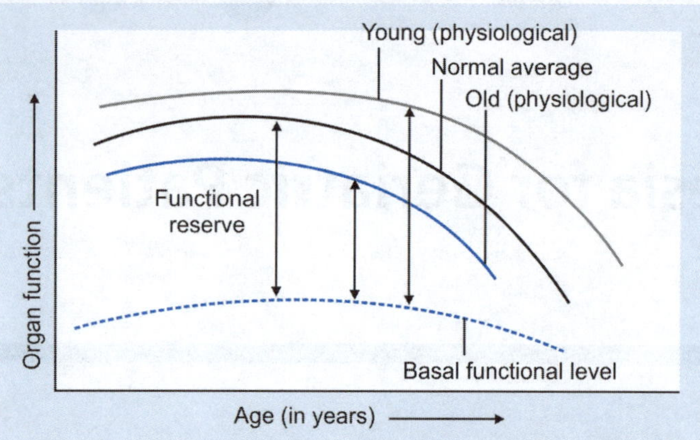

Fig. 1: When there is lesser rate of decline of functional reserve, then this geriatric person is called "physiological young". Contrary, when there is greater rate of decline of functional reserve, then this geriatric person is called "physiological old". They have significant different functional reserve. Functional reserve is the difference between the maximum (unbroken lines black for average, grey for young, and blue for old) and the basal level of function (broken line).

Aging appears to be a universal phenomenon. It is characterized by degenerative changes involving both the structures and the functions of tissues. It is not a linear progress as it was earlier thought. The decrement of the functions of tissues, due to the process of aging in most organs, are now believed to be relatively subtle, up to the middle past of adult life and then the progress of it (aging process) is faster after 70s. The elderly persons who maintain a greater average functional capacity than the others are referred to as the *physiologically young* and when the function declines early, they are often referred to as the *physiologically old* **(Fig. 1)**. The difference between these twos (the maximum level of organ function and the basal level of organ function) is the functional reserve of an organ system. In healthy geriatric patients, the maximum level of organ function is higher than its basal level of organ function at his or her all ages. This functional reserve of organs is able to meet the additional demands of O_2, cardiac output, CO_2 elimination, or protein synthesis imposed by the trauma, surgery, or disease.

In fact, good anesthetic management of geriatric patients depends upon an exhaustive understanding of the normal changes in anatomy, physiology, and responses to pharmacological agents that occur due to aging. Moreover, there are many similarities between the elderly and pediatric patients and these are: (i) Decreased ability to increase heart rate (HR) in response to hypovolemia, hypotension, and hypoxia due to decrease autonomic responsiveness, (ii) Decreased lung compliance, (iii) Decreased arterial O_2 tension, (iv) Impaired ability to cough, (v) Decreased renal tubular function, and (vi) Increased susceptibility to hypothermia.

Physiological and Pathological Changes Associated with Aging

Perhaps, the chronological aging (age in number of years) of a person only wrinkles the skin. But, the worry, doubt, fear, anxiety, self-distrust, etc. wrinkle the soul (biological aging) as the chronological age of a person progresses. With the current continuation of the decline in fertility and increase in life expectancy, the current population of the world will be aged much faster in the next half-century than the previous one. For example, the total population of the elderly persons in the world is supposed to grow 3.5 times in 75 years, from 2.5 billion in 1950 to 8.46 billion in 2025 (projected). The world population of 60 years old and above will increase sixfold from 201 million (in 1950) to 12 billion in 2025 (projected).

In this period, the fastest growing age group will be 80 years and above. Most astonishingly, this population will increase from 13 million (in 1950) to 137 million in 2025. We are further concerned with the fact that in many developed countries the two-thirds of their hospital beds are occupied by the aged person, of which 50% need surgery. As the age advances, the physiological functions of their body get compromised. The degenerative changes in all the tissues become are more common. But, their history is always not reliable. So, hospital notes sometimes become formidable. With this, the body's mechanism of drug handling gets altered, leading to ever increasing problems to anesthesiologist during the administration of anesthesia. So, it will be worthwhile to recapitulate the physiological changes and the altered mechanism of drug handling in these elderly age groups of patients.

Cardiovascular Function

It is very important to distinguish between the changes that occur normally due to aging and the changes that occur due to the pathology of diseases, common in geriatric population. As for example, atherosclerosis is a pathological process. It is not present in healthy elderly patients. On the other hand, a reduction in arterial elasticity caused by the fibrosis of tunica media of blood vessels is a part of the normal aging process. The geriatric surgical groups of patients have the higher incidences (50–60%) of the overt and/or subclinical cardiovascular diseases. These cardiovascular diseases mainly include hypertension, ischemic heart disease, cardiac conduction abnormalities, myocardial wall motion abnormalities, etc. The coronary disease has been found even in the completely symptom-free octogenarian.

More than half of all the mortality in this geriatric population is due to these cardiovascular disorders. With increased age, the ventricular compliance gradually decreases and it is due to the gradual increase in (i) ventricular wall thickness, (ii) myocardial fibrosis, and (iii) valvular calcification. Thus, due to this increased stiffness of cardiac chambers (reduction of compliance) the hemodynamic function of an elderly heart runs within a narrow range of end-diastolic pressure and its subsequent narrow range of end-diastolic volume. Hence, they become volume dependent (preload) and easily become volume intolerant.

With increased age, the elastic fibers of blood vessels also show the thickening and fragmentation. This change of elastic fibers of blood vessels, along with the progressive arteriosclerotic changes in arterial wall, makes the arterial tree narrow and less distensible. So, this causes the rise in blood pressure (BP) (due to nondistensibility), rise in pulse pressure, and impaired vascular compensation during blood loss (as the vessels fails to contract properly). With increased age, this gradual narrowing, and the stiffness of the wall of blood vessels also causes the ↑in systemic vascular resistance (SVR) and ↑in diastolic pressure. This increase in SVR and diastolic pressure causes increased impedance to the ejection of stroke volume and elevated systolic pressure associated with that given stroke volume. Thus, this increase in afterload (SVR) further increases the ventricular work load, which again increases the wall thickness and stiffness of ventricle, with the further decrease in diastolic ventricular filling and cardiac output (a vicious cycle). Due to this impedance of ejection, cardiac index (CI) also progressively decreases with age (linear relationship). Age imposes a ceiling on the increase of cardiac output as a person grows from childhood. It becomes maximum at the middle of a life and then it decreases approximately 1% per year, starting from the middle of adulthood.

As the age advances, so due to the decrease in ventricular end-diastolic volume (due to the stiffness and the hypertrophy of ventricular wall), the ventricular diastolic filling and subsequently the CO now depends on atrial contraction. Hence, the loss of sinus rhythm or atrial contraction (e.g., atrial flutter and fibrillation) produces severely compromised CO in elderly patients. In the elderly persons, the hemodynamic insufficiency due to diastolic ventricular dysfunction is more common than that of young adults. In children and young adults, the CO increases by tachycardia and β-adrenergic agonistic action. But, in the elderly or aged persons, during the increased demand, the CO can only be increased by increasing the left ventricular end-diastolic volume in response to the augmented preload (by IV fluid or by prolonged filling time by reduction of heart

rate) which compensate for slow heart rate (as the heart rate decreases with age). This increase in cardiac output is associated with little enhancement of ejection fraction. Here, the mechanical compensatory mechanism by increasing the preload predominates over the compensatory mechanism by increasing the heart rate, caused by the adrenoreceptor activation or baroreflex activity. So, due to the limited baroreceptor reflex mediated ability to increase the heart rate, hypotension can be frequent and severe during both the intraoperative and postoperative period in the older surgical patients. Thus, Frank–Sterling principle with increased O_2 demand works in elderly heart.

Only the loss of arterial elasticity (*not narrowing* due to atherosclerosis) causes normal diastolic BP, but increase in systolic BP and widens the pulse pressure while, the *narrowing of arterial wall* with loss of elasticity causes both ↑systolic, ↑diastolic pressure and ↓pulse pressure. Now, the reduction of this pulse pressure decreases the coronary artery perfusion and next the narrowing of coronary artery, due to the atherosclerosis in aging process, further decreases the coronary flow. So, hypotension is usually badly tolerated by the aged persons. Due to same reasons, blood flow to the kidneys and brain is also reduced with age with impaired autoregulation. The physiological response to cardiovascular disturbance may be also blunted with advanced age, due to reduced baroreceptor sensitivity and impaired autonomic function.

In geriatric group of patients, the functional capacity of <4 metabolic equivalents (METs) is associated with potential adverse outcome. In geriatric population, due to decreased sensitivity of adrenergic receptors, there is reduction in heart rate. Maximal heart rate declines by approximately 1 beat/min/year of age over 50. In elderly patients, the fibrosis of conduction system and the loss of the cells of sinoatrial node (SA) node increase the incidences of dysrhythmias, particularly atrial fibrillation and flutter.

Some elderly individuals will present for anesthesia and surgery with *previously undetected conditions* that require preoperative treatment. These are arrhythmia, congestive heart failure (CHF), myocardial ischemia, etc. All the elderly patients should undergo echocardiographic evaluation before anesthesia and surgery. In this investigation, many patients are found with diastolic ventricular dysfunction or systolic ventricular dysfunction. This diastolic ventricular dysfunction should not be confused with the diastolic heart failure. In diastolic dysfunction, the ventricle becomes less compliant and inhibits diastolic ventricular filling and consequently ventricular diastolic filling pressure is increased. Marked diastolic dysfunction may be seen with systemic hypertension, coronary artery disease, cardiomyopathies, valvular heart diseases, etc. all of which are more common in older than younger patients. Patients may be asymptomatic or complain of exercise intolerance, dyspnea, cough, or fatigue. The elderly patients with diastolic dysfunction may poorly tolerate perioperative fluid administration, resulting in elevated left ventricular end-diastolic pressure and pulmonary congestion.

Pulmonary Function

With advancing age, there are also changes both in the chest wall and lung parenchyma. In lung parenchyma, the quality of elastin deteriorates with age (but the total quantity of elastic tissue does not decrease). This results in the progressive loss of lung recoiling effect, after inspiration and decrease in the tethering property (pulling outward) of it (elastin fiber) which is normally helpful for the patency of small airways and homogeneous distribution of inspired gases. Thus, the lungs become more voluminous (alveoli become large), less compliant (due to the loss of recoiling or elastic property), and the patency of airways is impaired (airways close early during expiration). Therefore, the residual volume (RV), functional residual capacity (FRC), and closing capacity (CC) are all increased with aging. Even in normal persons, CC exceeds FRC (CC > FRC) at the age of 45 years (below 45 years this does not occur) in supine position and at the age of 65 years in sitting position. When this happens, i.e., some airways close during the part of a normal tidal breathing, then there will be mismatched ventilation and perfusion with $\downarrow$PaO$_2$.

The breakdown of alveolar septa (due to the reduction of tethering property of elastin fibers) with increasing age also causes the merging of small alveoli into a large alveoli and reduces the total alveolar gas exchanging surface area. So, the lung becomes emphysematous and dead space (both anatomic and alveolar or physiological) increases. As the lungs become emphysematous and the recoiling property is lost, so the RV of lung increases at the expense of expiratory reserve volume ($\downarrow$ERV). At the same time, FRC increases at the expense of vital capacity ($\downarrow$VC) also.

The anatomical dead space increases because, the diameter of larynx and trachea increases with age. So, a large ET-tube is needed for an older patient. The calcification, fibrosis, and osteoarthritic changes of chest wall also reduce the movement and the compliance of it (chest wall). This results in increased work of breathing, decreased FEV$_1$, and decreased tidal volume. Thus V$_D$/V$_T$ ratio increases with age, causing also V/Q mismatch, arterial hypoxemia, and reduction of CO$_2$ elimination. The rhonchi are fairly common in elderly patients without underlying pulmonary disease, but crepitations are usually a sign of incipient

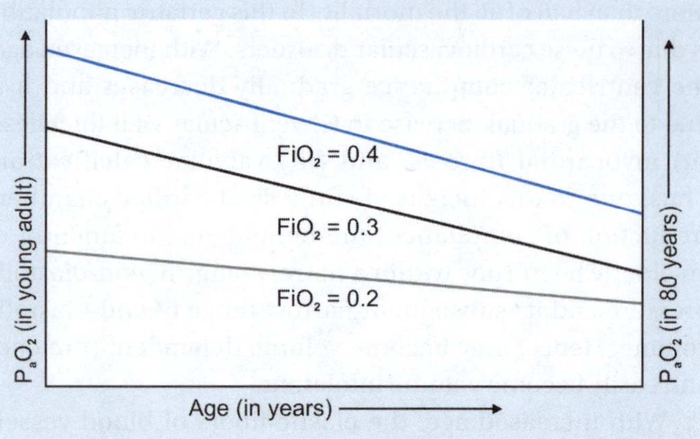

Fig. 2: The decrease in arterial O$_2$ tension with age at different inspired O$_2$ concentration (FiO$_2$).

pneumonia or CHF (**Fig. 2**). Many patients also present with obstructive and restrictive lung diseases. In patients who have no intrinsic pulmonary disease, gas exchange is unaffected by aging.

It is advisable, whenever possible, to have a preoperative chest X-ray in all the elderly patients. Atelectasis, pulmonary embolism, and chest infection are all more common in the elderly patients. The later, in part, is due to the ineffective mucociliary activity for advanced age. The P$_A$O$_2$ and PaO$_2$ decrease with age (P$_A$O$_2$ = 100 – age/4 mm Hg). The geriatric persons also have a markedly decreased ventilatory response to hypercapnia and hypoxia. The elderly has further increased incidence of sleep apnea which make them more susceptible to hypoxemia in recovery room.

Renal Function

Like all the other organs, the kidney also becomes aged with time. So, among all the geriatric patients who undergo surgery, 30% have kidney dysfunction. Also, the acute renal failure is responsible for one-fifth of total perioperative death in geriatric population. The prevalence of renal disease, among the geriatric group of patient, not only increases the perioperative risk for acute renal failure in them, but also affects the duration of action (pharmacokinetic) of many anesthetic and its adjuvant drugs. With aging, the renal tissue mass is also atrophied, the total number of nephrons decrease, fatty tissue accumulates, and interstitial renal fibrosis occurs. About the 20% of the total renal tissue mass is lost by the eighth decade and more than one-third of the glomeruli with their tubule disappear by the 85 years of age.

With increased age, the renal mass (both glomerular number and tubular length) decreases gradually. With this decreased renal mass, the renal blood flow (RBF) also decreases (10% per decade) along with the decrease of glomerular filtration rate (GFR) with increased age.

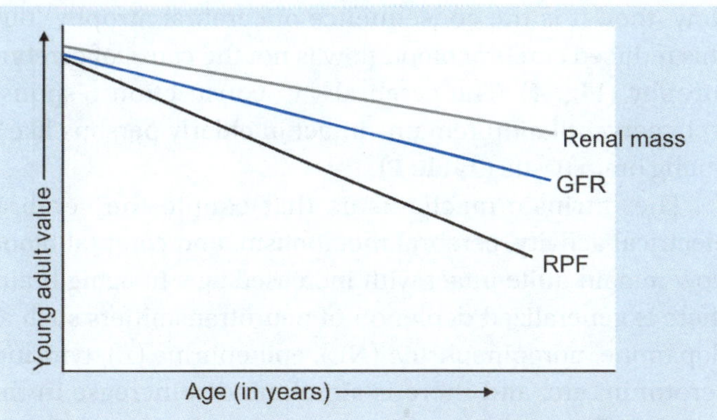

Fig. 3: The effect of age on renal function such as renal plasma flow (RPF), glomerular filtration rate (GFR), and renal mass in man.

This decrease of RBF is about one-half of that of a young adult. The rate of the decrease of GFR is 7–8 mL/min/1.7 m^2/day. This decrease of GFR and RBF is more acute than the decrease of renal tissue mass. This is because the renal vasculature is compromised preferentially with age **(Fig. 3)**. The active tubular secretion and the reabsorption of drugs and other solutes are also reduced with age. Thus, the elimination half-life of virtually every anesthetic drug is prolonged in elderly patients, especially in those with preexisting renal dysfunction.

The excretion of free water load is also markedly delayed in elderly people. Creatinine clearance also declines, but the serum creatinine level does not rise, as the creatinine load on the kidney also decreases, due to the reduction of the skeletal muscle mass with increasing age. So, a modest rise in serum creatinine level in elderly persons may represent a significant renal impairment. Tubular functions are also impaired with reduced renal concentrating ability and reduced free water clearance. The fluid balance in elderly patient is more critical. Because, the compensatory responses to both the fluid loading and dehydration are impaired. Although, the renal function deteriorates with the advancement of age, still the residual function remains sufficient to avoid the gross uremia, if the demands are basal.

The other changes in renal function in geriatric patients are (i) ↓responsiveness to antidiuretic hormone (ADH) and aldosterone, (ii) ↓reabsorption of filtered glucose by renal tubules (glycosuria), (iii) ↓ability to conserve or excrete Na^+ (impaired Na^+ handling), and (iv) ↓ in concentrating and diluting capacity of urine and functional hypoaldosteronism. This impaired Na^+ handling makes the elderly patient more prone to both the dehydration and fluid overload.

In older age, the reduction of lean body mass decreases the total body stores of K^+ and thus predisposes to hypokalemia. This is further complicated by the common use of diuretics in the elderly population. Therefore, due to the limited renal functional reserve, the geriatric patients require meticulous calculation and the monitoring of fluid and electrolyte balance during the perioperative period. But, no fluid replacement protocol is appropriate for this group of patient. Acute renal failure is usually responsible for at least (approximately) one-fifth of perioperative mortality in elderly surgical patients. This age-related change in renal function has important pharmacokinetic consequences, causing the prolonged elimination half-life of anesthetic drugs and its metabolites, which require renal route for their clearance.

Hepatic Function

With the advancement of age, the size of hepatic tissue, hepatic blood flow, and hepatic function decreases. This loss of hepatic function with the advancement of age is quantitative and not qualitative (i.e., the quality of hepatocellular enzymatic function does not decline). This is because, normally, as much as 40–50% of total hepatic tissue may involute by the age of 80 years. Thus, there is progressive redistribution of perfusion (blood flow), away from the hepatic splanchnic vascular bed, to the other organs, due to the atrophy of it (liver). Hence, this quantitative loss of hepatic tissue plays a major role in the age-related decline of anesthetic drug clearance.

The duration of clinical effect of anesthetic agents may be further prolonged, if their primary or secondary metabolites take the renal route for their elimination, instead of the drug itself. On the other hand, as the quality of hepatocellular function does not decline, so the microsomal and nonmicrosomal enzyme activity of hepatic cells appears to be well preserved. But, the hepatic synthesis of plasma cholinesterase is deficient in many elderly men. The hepatic capacity for protein synthesis is significantly reduced by the eighth decade of life. But, still, this reduction of protein synthesis can meet the requirements for normal coagulation process due to the previous huge reserve. Due to the present limited hepatic functional reserve, the elderly persons produce many postoperative complications and so require supportive therapy and intensive care.

Nervous System (Central, Peripheral, and Autonomic)

With increased age, the brain itself also undergoes definite structural and functional changes. The age itself reduces the size and the weight of the brain. The average weight of a brain of an 80-year-old person is approximately 20% less than that of a 30-year-old person. This very rapid decrease of the weight of brain tissue occurs after the sixth decade of life. At the same time, there is also a compensatory increase in cerebrospinal fluid (CSF) volume. So, the aging normally produces a low pressure hydrocephalus. Normally, the supportive glial cells constitute about almost one-half of a total brain mass and this reduction of brain size reflects the minimal atrophy of glial cells, but mainly the reduction of the number of neurons in brain. This neuronal loss of brain is prominent in cerebral cortex, particularly the frontal lobes. The average rate of this neuronal loss in an aging brain tissue is approximately about 55,000 per day. However, among these neurons, the neurons which are responsible for the synthesis of neurotransmitters undergo the greatest degree of age-related attrition. The neurons lose the complexity of their dendritic tree and the number of synapses. The synthesis of neurotransmitters [serotonergic, adrenergic, and γ-aminobutyric acid (GABA)] is reduced. The number of astrocytes and microglial cells increase.

With increased age, the intelligence does not decline. The storage, integration, and consequently the processing of information which is responsible for language skills, esthetic skill, and personality remain also intact. However, on the other hand, the short-term memory, visual reaction time, and auditory reaction time, etc. that require rapid retrieval of information and immediate processing gradually decreases. With aging, the cerebrovascular diseases are common and confusion is more likely during both the pre- and postoperative period. In elderly, the autoregulation of cerebral blood flow (perfusion) in response to the changes in arterial BP is still maintained. Therefore, aging is not associated with inadequate cerebral perfusion with the change of BP. If there is any decrease in cerebral blood flow, then it is the consequence of cerebral atrophy. But, this reduced cerebral blood flow is not the cause of cerebral atrophy **(Fig. 4)**. The cerebral vasoconstriction response to hyperventilation remains intact in elderly persons like a young brain tissue **(Table 1)**.

The intrinsic mechanisms that couple the cerebral electrical activity, cerebral metabolism, and cerebral blood flow remain quite intact with increased age. In aging brain, there is generalized depletion of neurotransmitters such as dopamine, norepinephrine (NE), epinephrine (E), tyrosine, serotonin, etc. and there is simultaneous increase in the activity of enzymes such as monoamine oxidase (MAO) and catechol-O-methyltransferase (COMT) which are responsible for the breakdown of these neurotransmitters. One of the examples of this deficiency of neurotransmitter

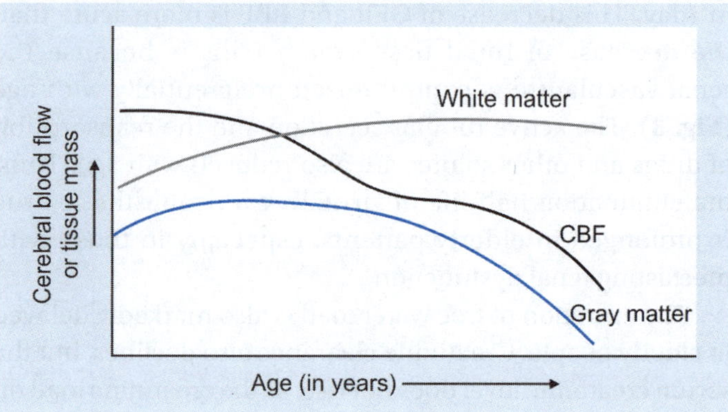

Fig. 4: The relation between the increased age and the change in brain tissue mass and cerebral blood flow (CBF).

System	Anatomic changes	Functional changes
TABLE 1: The summary of anatomical and functional changes due to aging.		
Body composition	↓Skeletal muscle mass ↓Lean tissue ↓Relative	↑Drug effect ↓Metabolism and heat production ↓Resting cardiac output
CVS	↓β-adrenergic responsiveness ↓Vascular elasticity ↓Ventricular hypertrophy	↓Cardiac and arterial compliance ↓Maximal heart rate and CO ↓Pulse pressure
Nervous system	↓Neuronal tissue mass ↓Central neurotransmitter activity, degeneration	↓Neural plasticity ↓Anesthetic requirement Impaired (↓↑) autonomic homeostasis
Pulmonary system	↑Thoracic stiffness ↓Lung recoil ↓Alveolar surface area	↓Vital capacity, ↑RV, ↑FRC, ↑CC, ↑Work of breathing, ↑Dead space, ↑V/Q mismatch ↓Efficiency of gas exchange
Blood and immune system	Thymic involution Reabsorption of bone marrow	↓Immune competence ↓Hematopoietic reserve
Renal/hepatic system	↓Tissue mass ↓Vascularity and perfusion	↓Drug clearance, ↓GFR, ↓Plasma flow ↓Ability to withstand salt and water loads

(CC: closing capacity; CVS: cardiovascular system; FRC: functional residual capacity; GFR: glomerular filtration rate; RV: residual volume)

is Alzheimer's disease, where there is deficiency of acetylcholine in cerebral cortex. The affinity of these neurotransmitters to their receptors is also diminished and it is due to the reduction of the number of receptors. In aging brain, the upregulation (increase in the number of receptor in response to the reduction in neurotransmitter secretion) is less vigorous than in young population. The central nervous system (CNS) "plasticity" (the ability to reroute the neural pathways) to compensate the neural injuries is less marked and less complete in aged person than that of a young. Therefore, recovery from neural injury (e.g., after stroke, accident, etc.) in geriatric patient is slow and incomplete.

The dose requirements of inhalational anesthetics [minimum alveolar concentration (MAC)] for general anesthesia (GA) are reduced. The administration of a given volume of epidural local anesthetic tends to result in more extensive spread in elderly patients. A longer duration of action should be expected from a given dose of spinal local anesthetic.

In the elderly persons, at peripheral nervous system, there is also a great reduction of both the velocity and the amplitude of electrical transmission of impulses through both the afferent (sensory) and efferent (motor) pathways. In old age, different degenerative changes in sensory receptors also occur and the threshold for the perception of sensory stimulus such as touch, pain, temperature, smell, vision, hearing, etc. will increases. Hence, the impairment of cortical transmission will delay the onset of voluntary motor activity. But, the skeletal muscles do not undergo any degenerative changes with age. With increased age, the number and the density of motor end plate also decreases. So, to compensate this, there is both the thickening and the spreading of the existing postjunctional membrane, beyond the usual areas of motor end plate, will occur with the increase in the number of cholinergic receptors at the end plates and surrounding areas. However, the sensitivity to nondepolarizing muscle relaxants does not decrease significantly with age. Alternatively, the sensitivity to succinylcholine is increased in some elderly persons. It is due to the reduced plasma cholinesterase enzyme concentrations and not due to the changes in neuromuscular junction itself with age.

With increased age, the plasma level of NE increases gradually, though there is regular attrition of neurons in the pathways of sympathoadrenal system. But, clinically, the increased effect of this increased level of NE is not always found due to the reduction of the autonomic end-organ responsiveness with age. With increased age, there is also significant impairment of the ability of the β-adrenergic agonist to stimulate the β-receptors, causing the less positive inotropic and chronotropic actions. The probable mechanisms of this reduction in the action of β-adrenergic agonists are (i) the attrition of receptors, (ii) the reduced affinity of neurotransmitter toward the receptors, and (iii) the impairment of adenylyl cyclase activation, due to the decreased cell membrane fluidity. The autonomic reflexes maintaining the cardiovascular homeostasis also decrease progressively with age. So, the BP is less well maintained in a steady state level in adverse situations (i.e., in hypotension or hypertension) in an elderly patient than a young. Hence, the anesthetic agents (such as β-blockers, etc.) and the anesthetic techniques (spinal or epidural) that block the sympathetic system cause more hypotension in an elder than a young.

Currently, much work has been done to determine whether the surgery and anesthesia make any harm to the brain or not and it is found that up to 30% of patients develop postoperative cognitive dysfunction (POCD). Unlike delirium, which is a clinical diagnosis (a confusional state), this POCD is diagnosed by some neurobehavioral testing. The etiology of POCD is likely multifactorial and includes drug effects, pain, hypothermia, metabolic disturbances, etc. Elderly patients are particularly sensitive to the centrally acting anticholinergic agents, such as atropine and scopolamine.

Hemopoietic Function

The age has little effect on red blood cell (RBC), white blood cell (WBC), and platelet count. The hypercoagulability of blood and subsequently the thrombosis in vessels is not directly related to the process of aging. The age, actually, indirectly enhances this platelet mediated hemostasis (hypercoagulability and increased intravascular thrombosis). The common observation of the ecchymotic lesions on the skin of the extremities of many elderly individuals is the result of age-related increase in the fragility of cutaneous blood vessels. The volume of bone marrow and also the mass and the volume of spleen, responsible for hemopoiesis, reduce in size with age. So, the anemia cannot be corrected easily in the elderly patients, though clinically significant anemia is not the physiological process of aging. Although, the volume of bone marrow, spleen, and the other hemopoietic reserved tissues are reduced with age, but the effect of aging is rarely enough to alter the day-to-day hemostasis or the acute hematologic responses to accidental injury or mild stress.

With age the anatomical involution of thymus occurs (that begins at young adulthood) and causes a decrease in the immune responsiveness in elderly. With the quantitative age-related change in thymic mass, there is also a progressive change in thymic composition. Thus, both these quantitative and qualitative changes of thymus play a central role in the reduction of adaptive immune system, primarily the T-lymphocyte-mediated responses. So, the elderly are particularly predisposed to streptococcal pneumonia, meningitis, and septicemia. The infection or sepsis is notoriously occult in geriatric surgical patients. It is the second only cause after cardiac failure for the increased perioperative morbidity and mortality related to age. Erythropoietin levels remain generally normal in elderly persons, but may be depressed easily by infection.

Body Composition, Drug Distribution, and Metabolism

After the 60 years of age, the body weight decreases rapidly and the chemical composition of body also changes. Throughout this whole path, extending from the young adulthood, through the middle age to the old age, a person generally gain 12 kg of adipose tissue, but lose about 8 kg of skeletal muscle mass. When this loss of muscle mass and the atrophy of central organs is combined with the loss of subcutaneous fat, then it produces a significant fall in the total body weight in an aged person. The age-related changes in body composition are universal, progressive, and irreversible. This change is due to the steady increase in the ratio of lipid to aqueous tissues (i.e., lipid fraction increases and water fraction decreases) and results in the increase in lipid fraction of total body mass which acts as the reservoir for anesthetic and other lipid soluble drugs. This total body fat increment is more profound in woman than man. Thus, this significant reduction of the intracellular and interstitial water reflects the attrition of the metabolically active tissues. Diminished thirst, poor diet and the use of diuretics to treat the age-related hypertension also make the intracellular and interstitial dehydration a more common finding during the preoperative examination of the elderly patients.

Glucose intolerance is almost universal among the elderly patients. The cause of this glucose intolerance at this age is due to the insulin antagonism and the impairment of insulin function, but is not due to the decreased secretion of insulin. The reduction of lean body mass that provides the storage for carbohydrate is also an explanation for the intolerance to carbohydrate. So, the loss of skeletal muscle mass is also associated with the progressive impairment of ability to handle an intravenous glucose challenge.

In elderly, the basal resting metabolism is reduced by 10–15% and it is in parallel with the reduction of the lean tissue mass. So, the rate of production of body heat gradually declines. Simultaneously, there is also age-related impairment of thermosensitivity and also the impairment of autonomic thermoregulation which in combination increase the risk of inadvertent hypothermia, especially in cold environment in OT. The intraoperative decrease in the core body temperature is almost 1°C per hour which is about twice that observed in young adults under similar circumstances. So, the core body temperature of geriatric patients frequently falls during the intraoperative and postoperative period.

In a similar manner to the reduction of intracellular and interstitial water volume, the plasma volume which is the major determinant of the β-phase (molecular aspect of drug distribution from plasma to other compartment) of the pharmacokinetics of drugs is also reduced. So, the doses of drugs based on body weight show higher concentration than expected in blood and explain the increased sensitivity to drugs in elders. Ultimately, with increased age, the pharmacology of different drugs is changed and this is described in **Table 2**.

Most of the drugs, which are used in anesthesia, are metabolized in liver (small amount is metabolized in extra hepatic tissue) before their elimination and a very small amount of them is eliminated in intact form through the bile or urine. Therefore, with age as the hepatic blood flow and the hepatic mass is reduced, so the clearance of these drugs also declines. Therefore, there is a growing interest in replacing the pharmacokinetic parameters, which are derived from the multicompartmental models, by a more complex but realistic analysis, such as the context-sensitive pharmacokinetics. This context sensitive pharmacokinetics of anesthetic drug definitely show the difference between the elderly and the younger populations. The MAC is the minimum alveolar concentration (in volumes percent) of a volatile anesthetic agent at 1 atmospheric pressure that prevents the movement of the 50% of population to a standard given stimulus. For the inhalational anesthetic agents, the anesthetic requirement is typically quantified by MAC. Whereas for the intravenous agents, the anesthetic requirement is typically quantified by ED_{50} which is required to abolish the response to a given standard stimulus in the 50% of subjects. With increasing age, both the MAC or ED_{50} requirement decreases progressively with increased sensitivity to many anesthetic agents, especially the CNS depressant drugs. The MAC decreases steadily with age (4–5% per decade after 40 years of age, for example, the MAC of isoflurane is approximately 0.92 at 80 years of age).

The diazepam has the elimination half-life of 20 hours at 20 years of age and 85 hours in 80 years of age. The plasma concentration of midazolam required to prevent the responses against verbal command in an 80-year-old person is only 25% of that required in a 40-year-old proving the increased sensitivity of brain to benzodiazepines with increased age. The MAC decreases with age proving the increased sensitivity of inhalational anesthetic agents in elderly. The MAC values of halothane are 0.84, 0.76, and 0.64 at 25, 42, and 81 years of age, respectively. While the

TABLE 2: Effects of aging on pharmacology of anesthesia related drugs.

Drugs	Cause	Pharmacology
Inducing agents • Propofol • Thiopentone	CNS changes Decreased volume of distribution	• ↑drug effect • ↓dose requirement
Benzodiazepines • Diazepam • Midazolam	CNS changes ↓Liver and renal mass ↓Blood flow of liver and kidney	• ↓dose requirement • ↑drug effect
Opiates • Morphine • Fentanyl	↓Volume of distribution ↓Hepatic and renal blood flow CNS changes	• ↑drug effect • ↓dose requirement
Volatile anesthetics • Halothane • Sevoflurane • Isoflurane	CNS changes	• ↑drug effect • ↓dose requirement
Muscle relaxants • Succinylcholine	↓Plasma cholinesterase	• ↓dose requirement
Nondepolarizing agent	• Neurogenic atrophy • Decreased renal and hepatic function	• ↓dose requirement • ↑drug effect

MAC values of isoflurane are 1.28, 1.15, and 1.05 at 26, 44, and 64 years of age, respectively. Therefore, the incidence of awareness during anesthesia is a rare occurrence in elderly.

The plasma proteins are often reduced resulting in the reduced protein binding of drugs and its metabolites in the elderly. Thereby, there is every chance of increasing the levels of free (not protein bound) anesthetic drug and its possible toxic effects in the geriatric group of patients. About 15–20% decrease in the plasma albumin concentration leads to the decreased binding and the increased bioavailability of intravenous induction agents. Study has shown that there is 44% decrease in thiopentone requirement in elderly persons compared to a young adult as up to 80% of this drug is albumin bound. On the other hand, the brain sensitivity to thiopentone does not reduce with age. This also explains the increased response of thiopentone in geriatric patients.

Though, the propofol has a decreased (15–30%) dose requirement in elderly patient, still the rapid clear headed recovery is not observed in them. In spite of the increased incidences of hypotension and apnea, the propofol is not contraindicated in elderly patients, if not judiciously administered. The cardiovascular stimulatory effects of ketamine are retained in the elderly age group of patients. Thus, this effect makes this agent very useful in high risk patients, but with cautious use in ischemic heart disease. However, the ketamine's hallucinogenic effects are not more marked in the elderly.

The regional anesthesia (RA) provides a desirable alternative to GA for the geriatric group of patients, as the maintenance of intraoperative consciousness in the former (RA) permits the prompt recognition of angina pectoris and the acute changes in cerebral function, if any occurs, during the intraoperative period. The RA is associated with less postoperative confusion compared to the patients receiving GA. Apart from the decreased operative blood loss, the lowered incidences of postoperative deep vein thrombosis in RA, following a hip surgery, have been observed in elderly patients and it is a great advantage in RA. The another advantage of RA over the GA in elderly patients is less respiratory problems in postoperative period.

The limb and plexus nerve blocks are also ideal for the surgery performed on extremity in elderly. Still, in patients with severe cardiovascular disease, GA is a better alternative. One review had concluded that the RA may reduce the mortality in 1 month, but both the RA and GA appear to produce comparable (similar) results for long-term mortality. Like most other drugs, the dose requirements for RA are significantly less in elderly. During spinal anesthesia, the level of subarachnoid analgesia is usually two segments higher in elderly patients which may even be unpredictable due to the higher specific gravity of CSF in this age group. There is also decreased segmental dose requirement of the local anesthetic agent during the epidural analgesia in elderly. This may also reflect the decreased volume of epidural space in elderly patients due to the arteriosclerotic changes of vertebral column. Though, the hypotension is more frequent, but the postspinal headache is less in geriatric group of patients.

ANESTHETIC MANAGEMENT AND PERIOPERATIVE RISK OF GERIATRIC PATIENTS

Preoperative Assessment

To improve the quality of geriatric anesthetic care, extensive preoperative assessment of elderly patients waiting for surgery is very essential and for this a check list is prepared by American Geriatric Society which is given here.

> *Checklist for the optimal preoperative assessment of geriatric patients:*
> - Patient's cognitive ability and capacity to understand the anticipated surgery should be assessed.
> - Depression of patient should be screened.
> - Patient's risk factor for developing postoperative delirium should be identified.
> - Alcohol and other substances on which patient has developed dependence should be screened.
> - According to the American College of Cardiology, preoperative patient's cardiac evaluation is must.
> - Patient's risk factor for the development of postoperative pulmonary complications should be identified.
> - Functional status and history of fall should be documented.
> - Baseline frailty score of patient should be determined.
> - Nutritional status of patient should be assessed.
> - Determine the patient's family and social support system
> - Appropriate preoperative diagnostic tests should be performed.

A cognitive assessment of patient is usually done by "Mini-Cog" examination (collect it from internet) who do not have a history of dementia or cognitive impairment. In addition to this (cognitive assessment) depression screening should also be conducted. Frailty reflects a decrease in functional reserve capacity and an inability to respond to the physiological challenges, presented by the stress of surgery. Frailty is assessed by using a scoring system which is given **(Table 3)**. This scoring system is based on 5 criteria and the patients are divided into 3 categories. The 5 criteria are: unintentional weight loss, poor hand grip strength, self reported exhaustion, slow walking speed, and low physical activity. The patient is given 1 point for each criterion. Score 0–1 = not frail; score 2–3 = intermediate frail; score 4–5 = frail.

Regarding history, the elderly patients are frequently treated with β-blockers. This should be continued perioperatively, if patients are taking such medications chronically. Otherwise, there will be β-blocker withdrawal symptoms. Elderly patients are also frequently treated with oral hypoglycemic agents, angiotensin-converting enzyme inhibitors (ACEIs), angiotensin receptor blockers (ARBs), antiplatelet agents, statins, and anticoagulants. Hence, anesthetist should be careful regarding the interactions of these drugs with anesthetic agents.

Anesthetic Technique

For the anesthetic management of elderly patients, there is no specific technique or specific anesthetic agent which can reduce the perioperative risk or mortality in this group of patients. There is no difference in the outcome between the GA and RA when they are applied correctly on elderly for the same surgery. Though, the RA has many advantages over the GA, but the hypotension is more commonly seen in elderly patients, undergoing the spinal/epidural anesthesia. This is due to the impaired autonomic function and reduced compliance of arterial tree in geriatric group of patients. Conversely, the rates of intravenous fluid administration that would be modest for young adults may precipitate CHF and pulmonary edema in the elderly patients.

General anesthesia may be the best for those who require the precise control of BP and heart rate. During the procedure of GA, measures to prevent perioperative hypoxia in elderly patients include a longer preoxygenation period prior to induction, increased inspired O_2 concentration (FiO_2), positive end-expiratory pressure (PEEP), and pulmonary toilet. Aspiration pneumonia is a potentially life-threatening complication in elderly patients. Ventilatory impairment in the recovery room is more common in elderly than younger patients. Factors associated with an increased risk of postoperative pulmonary complications include older age, COPD, sleep apnea, malnutrition, and abdominal, or thoracic surgical incision.

The RA for hip fracture may reduce the mortality at 1 month, but the RA and GA appear to produce comparable (similar) results for long-term mortality. Under both RA and GA, the overall perioperative morbidity and mortality rate is same between the healthy, fit, octogenarians and young adults, undergoing the similar surgical procedures. Only very debilitated and sickly older patients are particularly prone to perioperative complications.

The three major risk factors that appear to determine the mortality rates for the geriatric group of patients are: (1) the operative site, (2) the need (indication) to perform surgery on an emergency basis, and (3) the physical status of patient at the time of surgery. When the elderly patients are undergoing emergency surgery, then the mortality rate rises many fold. It is due to (i) the inadequate preoperative

TABLE 3: *Frailty score.*	
Criteria	**Definition**
Shrinkage	Unintentional weight loss > last 10 years
Weakness	Decreased grip strength
Low physical activity	Low energy expenditure
Exhaustion	Poor energy and endurance
Slowness	Slow walking

evaluation and the preparation of elderly patient and (ii) the nature of surgical lesion and its acute consequences, such as the hemorrhage, dehydration, ischemia, acidosis, etc. on the already critically reduced organ's reserve. The infection and sepsis are the two major important causes of death in the elderly patients, despite the vigorous, IV antibiotic therapy. This is due to the age-related reduction of immune response. The operative site is also an important determining factor for mortality rate in elderly patients. The superficial surgeries as for example cataract surgery, skin biopsy, superficial excision, etc. under local anesthesia have much lesser risk than a surgical entry into any major body cavity. The mortality risk for herniorrhaphy, transurethral prostatectomy, etc. lies in between the abovementioned two categories of surgery. The preoperative physical status of the elderly patients clearly correlates well with the perioperative mortality.

The age was previously misunderstood as the factor of increased mortality. But, now it has been properly evaluated that the age-related disease causing the poor physical status is the most important determinant factor for mortality rate and not the age itself. For example, the one-half of the elderly surgical patients have hypertension which have widespread effects on multiple organs causing decreased reserve and thus increase the risk of anesthesia despite continuing therapy. The significant portions of geriatric patients also have coronary artery, metabolic (most common is diabetes mellitus), pulmonary, renal, and hepatic diseases with ill effects on multiple organs and reduce the reserve in every systems. Preoperative malnutrition or hypoalbuminemia or the development of negative protein balance may also have predictive value on the rate of surgical and anesthetic mortality for the elderly patients. The metabolic response of elderly patients to tissues injury is sluggish. The ability to ambulate properly after surgery is also the fundamental determinants of uncomplicated surgical recovery. But, these cannot be achieved in older adults, simply by giving the injection of growth hormone or increasing the parenteral protein replacement.

Though, there is no specific or best anesthetic agent or technique especially for the elderly patients, still a satisfactory and uncomplicated anesthetic course can be carried out by (i) a proper and good preoperative evaluation and preparation of patient, (ii) a proper anesthetic plan, and (iii) vigilant monitoring fitting with the physical status of patient and the type and site of surgery. In old age, the arm-brain circulation time is increased and the dose requirements for the induction agents are drastically reduced. So, during induction, the anesthetic drugs should be titrated very slowly against the effect. Due to the loss of functional reserve of all the organs, the anesthetic agents which have cardiodepressant effects and reduces cardiac output (e.g., volatile anesthetic and others) should be used very cautiously. The RA (causing pharmacological sympathectomy) is also less well tolerated in the elderly patients who have already reduced the circulating blood volume due to the age-related physiological changes. From the beginning of young adulthood, the MAC (for inhalational agents) and ED_{50} value (equivalent to MAC for noninhalational agents) decline linearly with increasing age. Typically, an 80-year-old patient requires only two-thirds to three-fourths of the anesthetic dose which is needed to produce similar effects in a young adult. This reduction in MAC and ED_{50} with age probably reflects the fundamental neurophysiological changes in the brain (reduced neuron density and reduced concentration of brain neurotransmitter) due to aging. The amount of anesthetic requirement may be a quantifiable measure of the functional reserve of the central nervous system. This reduction of the requirement of intravenous anesthetic agents (due to $\downarrow ED_{50}$) is similar to that observed for inhalational agents (due to $\downarrow MAC$). This is simply due to the result of higher than expected initial plasma concentration of these drugs, during the early phases of their redistribution, from plasma to body tissues. This may be again due to the exaggerated age-related early or alpha phase of pharmacokinetic changes, rather than the pharmacodynamic changes.

The classic two or three compartment models, used for the pharmacokinetic analysis of intravenous anesthetic agents, is also less predictable for elder subjects. The dosage of opioids and benzodiazepines should be reduced due to the age-related changes in pharmacokinetics and pharmacodynamics of these drugs, for example, the increased sensitivity of cerebral cortex (pharmacokinetic) and reduced elimination (pharmacodynamic) of fentanyl, etc. As remifentanil, atracurium, and cisatracurium do not depend on organ-based elimination, so their clinical effects in elderly patients are prompt and predictable.

The dose of nondepolarizing muscle relaxants is same or slightly increased in elders than younger. But, their duration of actions is prolonged due to the decreased rate of their clearance. The pharmacodynamic change of muscle relaxant reflects the quality and the quantity of the dynamics of cholinergic nicotinic receptor at neuromuscular junction, but not the skeletal muscle mass itself. The upregulation of these nicotinic receptors appears to offset the declining prejunctional acetylcholine mobilization in elderly patients.

Though the dose of anticholinesterase, to reverse the effect of muscle relaxant, is same in elderly and younger patients, but the incidence of arrhythmias, produced by these drugs, is higher in elderly, especially who have cardiovascular diseases. For any given level of preexisting neuromuscular blockade, the choice of reversal agent is determined by the speed and the completeness of recovery of neuromuscular transmission, but not by the patient's age. In the elderly, the action of all the drugs becomes prolonged, if they require hepatic or renal biotransformation for their elimination. The elderly patients, due to their loss of muscle mass and impaired thermoregulations, are more prone to perioperative hypothermia. So, the body heat should be conserved aggressively by fluid warmer or body warming devices, whenever possible, to avoid the cardiovascular and metabolic stress, due to shivering with already diminished reserve.

Though the function of central nervous system return quickly and completely after GA, still the neurological examination shows abnormality up to 60 minutes after recovery. The residual central nervous system dysfunction in subtle (subclinical) form, after GA, is unique for geriatric population. In 25% of cases, there is memory deficit and impaired spatial and verbal cognition, even up to 7 days postoperatively. All these are due to the increased volume of distribution, reduced drug clearance, delayed transfer of drugs among the compartments, and the combination of these factors. For the older patients, the postoperative delirium, disorientation, and acute brain syndrome are common and it is due to the disorder of metabolic states such as the hyper- or hypoglycemia, hypoxia, hypercarbia, fluid and electrolyte imbalance, prolonged anesthetic effects, etc. It also may be the expression of subclinical age-related neurological disease.

The intraoperative gross central nervous system injury can happen from cerebral embolism, cerebral hemorrhage, or cerebral ischemia. In postoperative period, such major injuries are distinguishable from residual central nervous system dysfunction or residual anesthetic effect by their severity, focal nature, and the absence of conspicuous improvement in first few hours after anesthesia. Reduced responsiveness of protective airway reflexes in elderly patients need routine protection against regurgitation and aspiration of gastric contents. All the elderly patients should be administered O_2 postoperatively to compensate for the inevitable decrease in PaO_2 due to the loss of body reserve.

Obesity and Anesthesia

■ INTRODUCTION

The obesity is defined as an abnormal growth of adipose tissue. It may be due to the enlargement of the size of fat cells *(hypertrophic obesity)* or due to the increase in the number of fat cells *(hyperplastic obesity)* or even the combination of both. It is the consequence of an interaction between the environmental forces (excess energy intake) and the individual genetic makeup. The genes, which are responsible for fat metabolism, try to enhance the storage of fat and do not cause obesity where food is limited and energy expenditure is high. But, these genes will cause an increased risk of obesity when food is abundant and energy expenditure is less or reduced.

The term "obesity" is derived from the Latin word "obesus" which means "fattened by eating". This is due to the excessive net energy intake in excess of net energy expenditure. This excess energy intake is laid down on the various parts of our body as fat resulting in obesity. The modern life-styles and the better standards of living have been in the way of contributing increased prevalence of obesity. So, the obesity is taken as a chronic disease and is gradually becoming widespread and is posing a serious risk in the development of noninsulin-dependent diabetes mellitus (NIDDM), hypertension, ischemic heart diseases (IHDs), peripheral vascular disease, gallstones, osteoarthritis, etc. which cause increased risk for anesthesia and mortality. Hence, the undernutrition and the malnutrition are the problems of developing countries, while the obesity is the bane of developed countries.

The total body fat and its distribution in a person are affected by his or her gender, age, degree of physical activity, and number of drugs used. In both men and women, body fat increases with age. In lean young healthy men, the body fat is usually <20% of his body weight and may rise with age to >25%. In young women, this total body fat is usually around 30% of her body weight and increases gradually to

>35% in older women. At all ages after puberty, the women accumulate more fat than men. Sometimes, the term obesity is frequently used synonymously with "overweight" from the aspect of risk factors. But, the term *"overweight"* means an "excess average weight for a given sex", as per height and age. Overweight is usually due to obesity, but can arise from other causes also, such as abnormal muscle development or fluid retention **(Fact file I)**.

FACT FILE I

There are *four processes* which are involved in the regulation of food intake. These are (i) olfactory and gustatory factors which can stimulate or inhibit the intake of food according to its appetizing property, (ii) release of gastrointestinal hormones such as cholecystokinin and gastrin-releasing peptide, (iii) gastrointestinal distension, and (iv) the activation of thermogenic component of efferent sympathetic nervous system. All these factors work together to induce satisfaction and do not produce new arousal for seeking food, till the next blood glucose level dips.

Excessive energy, taken as food, is stored in our body as fat. To maintain the normal body fat, dietary nutrients should be oxidized in proportion by which they are taken through diet. Among the ingested carbohydrate, fat, and protein, the intake of carbohydrate approximates the body stores of it. While the intake of fat and protein constitutes a small fraction of stored quantities of these nutrients. Therefore, as the daily intake of carbohydrate nearly equals to the body store of it, so the carbohydrate store in our body is more vulnerable to the changes in our dietary carbohydrate than its fat or protein content. The respiratory quotient (RQ) of fat (0.7) is less than that of carbohydrate (1). Hence, if the percentage of dietary fat increases, the RQ should be declined to maintain the body weight stable. But, if RQ does not decline (which normally occurs in obese patient) the body continues to oxidize the carbohydrate store and must replace these by eating more food to obtain carbohydrate or synthesize endogenous glucose from protein stores. This adjustment strongly depends on the genetic determinants.

If the carbohydrate oxidation is reduced or not available, then the oxidation of fat increases to provide energy and lower the RQ. If the body is unable to reduce carbohydrate oxidation, then

Contd...

Contd...

the compensatory mechanism is elevated increasing intake of carbohydrate food with increasing fat storage and obesity.

Estimated total energy need = BMR × Activity factor

For low or sedentary activity, the activity factor is 1.3, for intermediate activity such as regular exercise the activity factor is 1.5, and for high activity the activity factor is 1.7.

The estimation of basal metabolic rate (BMR):
- **For women:**
  - *15–30 years* = (LBW × 0.0621 + 2.0357) × 240 kcal/day
  - *30–60 years* = (LBW × 0.0342 + 3.5377) × 240 kcal/day
- **For men:**
  - *15–30 years* = (LBW × 0.063 + 2.8957) × 240 kcal/day
  - *30–60 years* = (LBW × 0.0484 + 3.6534) × 240 kcal/day
  - LBW = Lean body weight

Daily energy requirement (calculated):
- At rest : 2,000 kcal (8.4 MJ)
- Light work : 2,700 kcal (11.3 MJ)
- Heavy work : 3,500 kcal (14.6 MJ)

The regional maldistribution of fat also has profound influence on health risks. For example, only increased deposit of fat around visceras or abdomen (visceral and abdominal fat) correlate well with the risks for heart disease, diabetes, atherosclerosis, and hypertension, etc. For estimating or measuring the total or regional deposit of body fat, there are several techniques which are listed in **Table 1**. Among these, the *dual energy X-ray absorptiometry* provides the *best method for the assessment of total body fat, but not the regional body fat.* The regional body fat can only be measured accurately by magnetic resonance imaging (MRI) or computed tomography (CT)-scan. But, for practical purposes, the waist circumference or sagittal diameter of it is the *most useful* parameter for the estimation of regional fat in our body. The ratio of waist circumference to hip circumference is also *widely used* to measure or estimate the regional fat distribution but is not so accurate. For the estimation of total body fat X-ray absorptiometry, CT-scan, MRI, etc. are *highly accurate*, but such measurements may not be clinically feasible **(Table 1)**.

The body weight, though, is not an accurate measurement of excess body fat, but still it is a widely used *index of obesity*. In epidemiological studies, it is conventional to accept that the deviation of +2 SD (standard deviation) from the median weight for that height, as the cutoff point for obesity. So, the overweight or obesity can be defined from the tables of standard height and weight. On the other hand, the ideal body weight (Broca index) can also be estimated from the height (cm) by deduction of 100 from it. For example, if a person's height is 160 cm, then his ideal body weight should be 160–100 = 60 kg. A person is said to be obese when his or her actual body weight exceeds this

TABLE 1: Methods of estimating body fat and its distribution.

Method	Accuracy	Ease of use	Estimation of regional fat
Weight and height	High	Easy	No
Waist circumferences	Moderate	Easy	Yes
Skinfold	Low	Easy	Yes
Density			
• Immersion	High	Moderate	No
• Plethysmograph	High	Difficult	No
Ultrasound	Moderate	Moderate	Yes
Potassium isotope	High	Difficult	No
Heavy water	High	Moderate	No
Bioelectric impedance	High	Easy	No
Total body electrical conductivity	High	Moderate	No
Computed tomography	High	Difficult	Yes
MRI	Difficult	High	Yes
Neutron activation	Difficult	High	No

TABLE 2: Body mass index according to weight.

Weight	BMI [Wt (kg)/height^2]
Underweight	<18.5
Normal	18.5–24.9
Overweight	25–29.9
Obese	30–39.9
Extremely obese	>40

ideal body weight by >20%. However, the most widely used formula for relating height and weight in a person is the *body mass index (BMI)* which is calculated by weight (kg) divided by height (meter) in square [i.e., BMI = mass (kg)/height^2 (m)]. A BMI between 20 and 25 kg/m^2 is considered usually as a *good weight* for most individual. A BMI of 25–30 kg/m^2 is considered as *overweight*, but with low risk for associated serious medical complications. Those with BMI of >30 kg/m^2, >35 kg/m^2, and >55 kg/m^2 are respectively considered as *obese, morbidly obese,* and *super morbidly obese.* Weight gain confers increased health risk, even if the BMI does not excess 25 kg/m^2 **(Table 2)**.

The height of an 80 kg weight patient is 1.7 m. Therefore, his/her BMI = 80 kg/1.7^2 = 80/2.89 = 27.68 kg/m^2.

The height of a patient is 1.8 m and his body weight is 70 kg. Therefore, his BMI = 70 kg/1.8^2 = 70/3.24 = 21.60 kg/m^2.

In a woman, a weight gain of >5 kg is associated with an increased risks of diabetes and heart disease. In a man, any weight gain after age of 25 years appears to carry increased health risks **(Fig. 1)**.

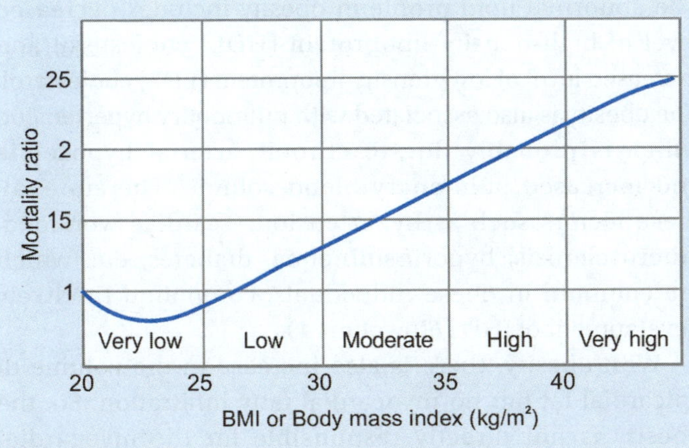

Fig. 1: The relationship between the BMI and the overall mortality rate. At BMI >20 kg/m^2, but <25 kg/m^2, there is decrease in mortality.

Another method of assessing the total body fat is the measurement of subcutaneous fat by measuring the thickness of skin fold. It is a rapid and noninvasive method and several varieties of calipers are available for this purpose. This measurement is taken at the four sites of our body such as at mid triceps, biceps, subscapular, and suprailiac regions and the sum of these measurements should be <40 mm in boys and should be <50 mm in girls. Unfortunately, any standards of this subcutaneous fat for the determination of obesity do not exist. Further, in extreme obesity, these measurements of subcutaneous fat may be impossible. Another main drawback of this skinfold measurements for assessing the total body fat is their poor repeatability.

It is now also well recognized that in addition to the amount of excess fat, present in an obese individual, the anatomical distribution of this fat has an important bearing on health risk. The *central or android type of distribution of fat,* which is more common in men, manifests as abdominal obesity. In contrast, the *peripheral or gynecoid type of distribution of fat,* which is more common in females, manifests as the deposition of fat mainly around the hips, buttocks, and thighs. The central adipose tissue is more metabolically active than the fat deposited at periphery. Here, the obese individuals who have a more central distribution of body fat, tend to suffer more from metabolic complications such as dyslipidemias, glucose intolerance, diabetes mellitus, IHD, heart failure, and stroke, etc. As the abdominal fat is more easily mobilized, so the men also tend to lose their body weight more readily than women.

When the triglycerides are deposited in fat cells then the cells initially increase in size until a maximum limit is reached at which point the cells divide. The moderate degree of obesity (BMI <40 kg/m^2) is likely to result from an increase in the size of fat cells, whereas the extreme degree of obesity

FACT FILE II

There are three known predictors which control the future weight gain. These are (i) low metabolic rate, (ii) high RQ indicating high carbohydrate oxidation and the need to eat more to replace this carbohydrate, and (iii) insulin resistance. The regulation of food intake is controlled by feedback system with afferent and efferent signals. Factors that increase hunger include decrease in blood glucose level, an increase in gastric contractions or abdominal uneasiness. These peripheral signals are integrated by neurotransmitters in the brain to regulate food intake. Several neurotransmitters increase or decrease the food intake. In addition, some neurotransmitters are specific modulators for the intake of specific food such as fat, carbohydrate, and protein. Thus, decrease or increase of intake of carbohydrate, fat, and protein occur as a major response to specific neurotransmitter which are controlled by the genetic code of this individual.

BOX 1: Some specific causes of weight gain.

Genetic:
Prader–Willi syndrome, Laurence–Biedl syndrome, etc.

Endocrine factors:
Hypothyroidism, insulinoma, and Cushing's syndrome

Drugs used:
Phenothiazines, tricyclic antidepressants, sulfonylurea, oral contraceptive, glucocorticoids, and antiepileptic (valproate)

(BMI >40 kg/m^2) is likely to result from the proliferation of fat cells **(Fact file II)**.

FAT CELLS AND OBESITY

The fat cells not only store the fat, but also secrete some enzymes named lipoprotein lipase. This enzyme hydrolyzes the triglycerides of very low-density lipoprotein (VLDL) and chylomicrons. They also produce some complements like D$_2$, C3b, cytokines, etc. (such as angiotensinogen, leptin, and lactate), and metabolize glucose to provide glycerol-3-phosphate for synthesis of triglyceride. The fat cells also synthesize long-chain fatty acids when there is abundance of diet **(Box 1)**.

PHYSIOLOGICAL CHANGES ASSOCIATED WITH OBESITY

The obesity is associated with certain physiological changes that have important anesthetic implications. Because, obese individuals handle drugs differently than their normal counterparts, as the pharmacokinetic and the pharmacodynamic of drugs are changed in obese patients. So, the understanding of these physiological and pharmacological changes associated with obesity is very essential for the proper management of anesthesia on such patients presenting for surgery either to reduce the obesity (gastric bypass, vertical banded gastroplasty, uvulopalatopharyngoplasty, liposuction, etc.) or for other diseases.

Cardiovascular System

The metabolic rate of an individual is proportional to his or her body weight. So, in obese person, this increased metabolic rate is associated with ↑O_2 demand, ↑CO_2 production, and ↑ alveolar ventilation. Hence, the obesity is associated with the increased work load on heart for ↑ circulation and hypervolemia (to perfuse additional fat stores), leading to the development of hypertension. The obesity is also associated with the increase in absolute blood volume, although this is lower than normal in relation to the body mass (occasionally 45 mL/kg). Increased extracellular fluid volume resulting in hypervolemia and increased cardiac output is estimated to increase by 0.1 L/min for each kilogram of weight gain. Each kilogram (kg) of body fat contains extra 3,000 meters of blood vessels. Mild to moderate degree of systemic hypertension is seen in 50–60% of obese patients, while severe hypertension is present in 5–10% of obese patients (mechanism being unclear).

The probable hypotheses for this hypertension in obese patients are (i) obesity is associated with increased insulin resistance and hyperinsulinemia which enhance Na^+ reabsorption from the renal tubules, (ii) obesity causes increased sympathetic outflow, promoting arterial vasoconstriction, and (iii) the enhancement of pressure activity (or sensitivity) of norepinephrine and angiotensin II in obesity.

The obesity is also associated with the increased risk of sudden death, and this is probably due to sudden cardiac arrhythmia. It is also associated with an increased risk of atherosclerosis, probably due to abnormal lipid profile.

The abnormal lipid profile in obesity includes decreased level of high-density lipoprotein (HDL) cholesterol and increased level of low-density lipoprotein (LDL) cholesterol. The obesity is also associated with pulmonary hypertension which is probably due to chronic arterial hypoxemia and increased pulmonary blood volume. Therefore, all these factors such as hypertension, ↑cardiac workload, atherosclerosis, hyperinsulinemia, diabetes, etc. which are common in obese individuals, compound the likely development of IHD **(Flowchart 1)**.

With obesity, there is also increase in the volume of epicardial fat but no myocardial fatty infiltration. So, the obesity is not directly responsible for the myocardial weakness and heart failure, but indirectly responsible for all these ailments. Hence, the obesity-induced cardiomyopathy is mainly due to hypertension, IHD, hypervolemia, ventricular dysfunction and these are responsible for heart failure. Left ventricular (LV) hypertrophy and its dysfunction demonstrated by echocardiography is the characteristic of obesity. The obesity-induced changes in cardiovascular system reduce its (cardiovascular) reserve and limit its exercise tolerance. The morbidly obese patients tolerate exercise poorly. This is because the increase in cardiac output, necessary for exercise, is achieved only by increasing the heart rate, but without an increase in stroke volume or ejection fraction, i.e., without an increased myocardial contractility in obesity due to cardiomyopathy. On changing position from sitting to supine, the obesity is also associated with higher increase in pulmonary capillary wedge pressure (PCWP) and mean pulmonary arterial pressure.

Respiratory System

Moderate obesity, in the absence of any underlying pulmonary disease, has little effect on respiratory function. Whereas, in severely obese individuals, the obstructive sleep

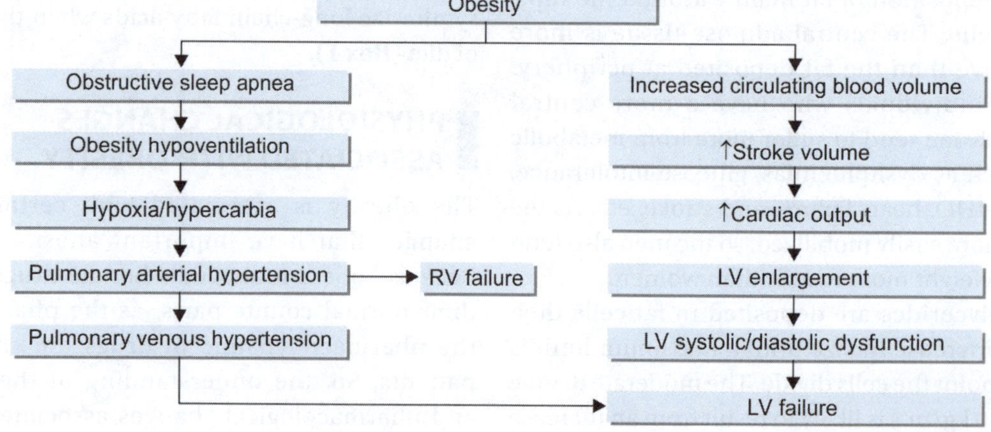

Flowchart 1: Obesity-induced cardiomyopathy and association of obesity with congestive heart failure.

(LV: left ventricular; RV: right ventricular)

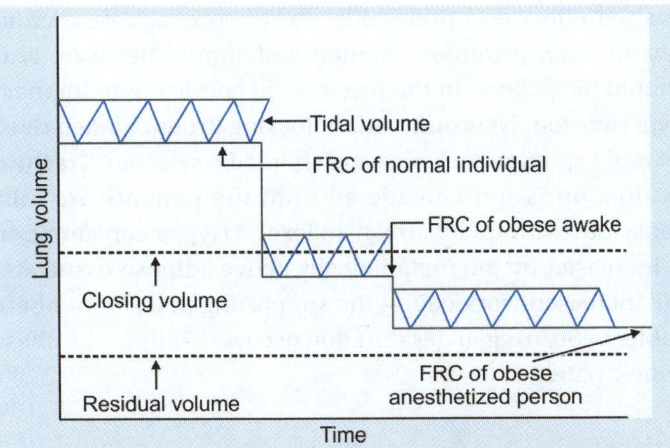

Fig. 2: The effect of severe obesity on functional residual capacity (FRC) during awake and anesthetized condition which result in (i) small airway closure, (ii) ventilation perfusion mismatch, and (iii) impaired arterial oxygenation.

apnea (OSA) syndrome is a potentially serious problem. This is because the increased BMI is associated with exponential decrease in respiratory compliance. In extreme cases, this respiratory compliance can fall up to 30% of its predicted value. The reason for this decrease in respiratory compliance is due to the twofold accumulation of fat in and around the chest wall, leading to the reduction of chest wall compliance and due to the increased pulmonary blood volume, resulting in the decrease in lung compliance and splinting of diaphragm (increased abdominal mass forces the diaphragm cephalad, yielding lung volumes suggestive of restrictive lung disease). The reduction of this lung volume is accentuated by the supine and Trendelenburg position.

The reduction of this total respiratory compliance (both chest wall and lungs) is in turn associated with a decrease in functional residual capacity (FRC) and encroachment of this decreased FRC on closing volume which causes impairment of gas exchange (V/Q mismatch) **(Fig. 2)**. Therefore, the increase in intrapulmonary shunt and the increase in alveolar-to-arterial oxygen tension difference, which are evident as arterial hypoxemia, are more worsened during the induction of anesthesia of an obese person. So, always a high inspired O_2 concentration is required during the induction of anesthesia and during the whole perioperative period in highly obese patients to combat this arterial hypoxemia. The reduced FRC associated with morbid obesity can be increased by administering positive end-expiratory pressure (PEEP) or large sustained manual inflation. But, the use of PEEP does improve this arterial O_2 tension (PaO_2) at the expense of cardiac output ($\downarrow CO$) and oxygen delivery to tissues is improved **(Fact file III)**.

Obesity also imposes a restrictive ventilation defect. This is due to the extra weight, added to the thoracic cage and the abdominal wall impeding motion of the diaphragm, especially in supine position. This results in decrease of functional residual capacity (FRC), expiratory reserve volume (ERV), and total lung capacity. FRC declines exponentially with increasing BMI. FRC may be decreased to such a point that small airway closure occurs within the tidal volume resulting in a ventilation-perfusion mismatch (shunt and arterial hypoxemia). Further, induction of anesthesia in an obese individual results in 50% decrease in FRC as compared to 20% decrease in a nonobese individual.

Sleep Apnea

Sleep apnea is defined as an intermittent cessation of airflow to lungs through the nose and mouth during sleep. By convention, an apnea of at least 10 seconds duration is considered important. But, in most of the patients these sleep apneas are of 20–30 seconds duration and also may be as long as 2–3 minutes.

The sleep apnea, which is a type of respiratory dysfunction, is a serious consequence of obesity. The cessation of breathing during apnea may be either due to the occlusion of airway (obstructive sleep apnea or OSA) or absence of respiratory effort (central sleep apnea), or a combination of these two factors (mixed sleep apnea). Approximately, the 5% of morbidly obese patients present with the features of OSA characterized by the episodes of apnea or hypopnea during sleep. Failure to recognize and appropriately treat these conditions may lead to sometimes serious cardiovascular complications and increased mortality rate.

The hypopnea is a term which is defined as the 50% reduction in airflow through airways and is sufficient to cause a decrease in arterial O_2 saturation. More than 10–15 apneas per hour or >30 apneas per night is significant in OSA. It is also important to say that the clinical sequelae of OSA, such as the hypoxemia, hypercarbia, systemic and pulmonary hypertension, cardiac arrhythmias, right ventricular failure, and polycythemia, etc. are more important than the frequency and duration of apnea. All such patients usually always show some evidences of sustained daytime hypoxemia in addition to the nocturnal ventilatory disturbance usually as a result of reduced ventilatory drive and/or diffuse airway obstruction. The most of these patients are obese and sleepy and are, therefore, said to have the Pickwickian syndrome.

The apnea occurs when the pharyngeal airway collapses (obstructive) due to the relaxation of their pharyngeal muscles during sleep and/or there is no central drive (central) for respiration. However, both these mechanisms for apnea are also responsible for apnea during anesthesia in obese patients. In an obese individual, the local accumulation of fat in tracheopharyngeal area or the compression of pharynx by the superficial fat masses of neck also predisposes to airway collapse. (In nonobese patient with OSA, the adenotonsillar hypertrophy, craniofacial skeletal abnormalities, such as retrognathia and macroglossia, etc. are taken as responsible for airway closure during sleep).

Normally, the patency of pharyngeal airway is maintained by the action of dilator pharyngeal muscles. During sleep, the tone of these dilator muscles is reduced and the airway becomes narrowed, causing turbulent air flow, and snoring (due to the high frequency vibration of the palatal and pharyngeal soft tissues), and obstruction. The resulting hypoxia and hypercarbia from this airway obstruction causes the arousal of individual which in turn again restores the upper airway tone. The individual, then, falls asleep again and the cycles are repeated. The predisposing factors for this sleep apnea during anesthesia of an obese patient are (i) the degree of obesity (BMI >30), (ii) middle age, (iii) male, and (iv) anesthetic drugs depressing the respiratory center and muscle tone.

Disturbed sleep at night in OSA patients leads to daytime somnolence and inability to concentrate the mind. Obese individuals with OSA gradually develop features of chronic hypoxia and hypercarbia in the form of polycythemia, pulmonary hypertension right heart failure, and respiratory acidosis. An extreme form of OSA is the obesity hypoventilation syndrome (OHS) which initially results in the desensitization of respiratory centers to hypercarbia (limited to sleep) manifesting as the central apneic events (apnea without respiratory efforts). Eventually, the patients with OHS present with type II respiratory failure with increasing dependency on the hypoxic drive for maintaining ventilation.

The anesthetic management of a patient with the history of OSA poses significant risks. These patients are highly sensitive to all the anesthetic drugs causing upper airway obstruction or apnea even in minimum doses. So, sedatives (benzodiazepine) or opioids should be used very cautiously in the perioperative period. The upper airway abnormalities due to decreased anatomical space (due to accumulation of fat), accommodating the large tongue and displacing it anteriorly, cause great difficulty in the exposure of glottic opening during direct laryngoscopy. When awake, these obese patients compensate this compromising airway anatomy by increasing their craniocervical angulation which increases the space between the mandible and the cervical spine and elongates the tongue and soft tissues of neck.

This postural compensation is lost, when these obese patients are rendered unconscious or paralyzed. So, all the anesthetic drugs should be titrated to get their just desired effect and preferably short-acting agents such as sevoflurane, propofol, remifentanil should be used. N_2O should be avoided in the presence of coexisting pulmonary hypertension. Neuromuscular blocking drugs characterized by rapid spontaneous recovery should be selected. Tracheal extubation is not considered until the patients are fully conscious with intact airway reflexes. Oxygen consumption is increased by the metabolically active adipose tissue and the increased workload of the supporting muscles in obese subjects. So, oxygen desaturation occurs rapidly in the obese apneic patients.

Others

Very frequently, obesity is associated with glucose intolerance and diabetes. This is due to the increased resistance of insulin by the presence of increased adipose tissue. So, the hyperinsulinemia is a uniform feature of obesity and its level is directly related to the degree of obesity. Thus, NIDDM commonly coexists in obese individuals. Reversely, NIDDM is almost nonexistent in an individual with a BMI below 22 kg/m^2. Still, in obese patients with NIDDM, the catabolic response to surgery may necessitate the use of exogenous insulin during the perioperative period.

The obese patients are also more prone to gallbladder and biliary tract diseases due to the increased excretion of cholesterol through their hepatobiliary system. The amount of cholesterol synthesized in our body per day is increased by about 20 mg for each kilogram increment of adipose tissue. So that a 10 kg increase in adipose tissue mass increases the daily cholesterol production and excretion by an amount, which is comparable to the cholesterol, present in one egg. On the other hand, obesity is usually associated with abnormal liver function tests and fatty liver infiltration. So, the volatile anesthetic agents should be used cautiously.

The incidence of deep vein thrombosis (DVT) is almost double in obese patients than in nonobese patients. This is due to the effects of polycythemia increased abdominal pressure and prolonged immobilization. This obesity also increases gastric volumes raises intra-abdominal pressure and increases the incidence of hiatus hernia which poses a significant risk for aspiration.

■ INFLUENCE OF OBESITY ON THE PHARMACOKINETIC OF DRUGS

The pharmacokinetic of drugs used in anesthesia practice is changed due to the changes in pathophysiology associated with obesity. The volume of distribution of drugs in obese individual is influenced by (i) the increase in blood volume and cardiac output, (ii) the decrease in total body water content (fat contains less water), and (iii) the lipid solubility of drug. Despite the occasional presence of liver dysfunction, the hepatic clearance of drugs is not usually altered in obese individuals. The renal clearance of drugs is increased due to the increased renal blood flow and glomerular filtration rate (GFR) in obese. For a desired concentration of drugs in plasma, two factors operate in obesity. One is the increased plasma volume in obesity which decreases the drug concentration in plasma and the other is the less blood flow in adipose tissue which increases the plasma drug concentration. So, the actual plasma concentration for a given bolus inducing dose of a drug is difficult to predict. It would, therefore, be wise to calculate the initial loading dose of a drug on the basis of "ideal body weight" (lean body mass) than the actual present body weight.

Subsequently, the further (repeated) doses of a drug should be adjusted according to the pharmacological response of patient to the initial dose of this drug. Repeated injection or infusion of drugs, particularly the lipophilic group, could result in a cumulative effect and hence a prolonged response. It is due to the gradual storage of drugs (mainly lipophilic) into depot fat and later its subsequent release from it (depot fat) into systemic circulation as the plasma concentration of drug declines. It should be kept in mind that just as the increased fat depot in obesity increases the storage of drugs, but poor total blood supply to adipose tissues also limits the delivery of drugs to it (blood in adipose tissue). So, multiple factors playing on the pharmacokinetics of a drug make the calculations of its plasma concentration composite and difficult.

ANESTHETIC MANAGEMENT OF OBESE PATIENT

Regional Anesthesia versus General Anesthesia

Bony landmarks are likely to be obscured in obese patients. So, the spinal and epidural anesthesia is technically very difficult in such group of patients. As compared to a nonobese individual, in obese the requirement of local anesthetic agents for spinal and epidural anesthesia is 20% lower. This is due to the reduced volume of epidural space and this is again because of the fatty infiltration and vascular engorgement in it (in this epidural space). But, the advantages of regional technique over the general anesthesia (GA) in obese individual include the avoidance of difficulties related to the securing of airway, perioperative hypoxemia, ventilation, and pulmonary complications. The regional anesthetic techniques also provide good postoperative pain relief and hence the use of drugs for postoperative pain relief, such as the opioids that may depress respiration, can be avoided.

Preoperative Assessment

A detailed preoperative assessment of an obese patient is routinely performed before the induction of anesthesia which includes mainly the air passage, respiratory system, and cardiovascular system. The difficulties in mask ventilation and tracheal intubation should always be anticipated in obese patients and this is because of the unique anatomical features in them such as (i) big-fat face and cheeks, (ii) short neck, (iii) large tongue, (iv) restricted mouth opening, (v) little airway space due to excessive palatal and pharyngeal soft tissue, (vi) high and anteriorly placed larynx, (vii) limitations of the movement of cervical spine, and (viii) restriction of the atlanto-occipital flexion and extension due to the accumulation of fat in neck, etc.

A BMI of 45 kg/m^2 is associated with 13% risk of difficult intubation. Although, the inspection of previous anesthetic records might provide some evidences of previous difficulties during intubation, but one should bear in mind that an uneventful previous anesthesia may not be relevant any longer in this present case and it is due to the further accumulation of fat and weight gain during this interval. Preoperatively, an airway is usually assessed clinically by different measurements and scoring systems, and by some the investigation such as X-ray, MRI of soft tissues, CT-scan, etc. and also by referral to an otolaryngologist for the direct and indirect laryngoscopy which helps in a more complete evaluation of airway. It is also useful to assess the airway in both erect and supine positions.

With an airway assessment, the venous access and the risk of aspiration in an obese patient also should be assessed. If any difficult intubation is anticipated by any clinical scoring system or radiological investigations, then the possibilities of awake intubation, fiberoptic-aided intubation, cricothyroid puncture with jet ventilation, tracheostomy, and the provision for postoperative ventilation should always be kept in mind and make ready. In addition to the airway assessment, the preoperative assessment of patient should also include the complete blood count (CBC), chest X-ray, supine and upright blood gases, lung function tests, and overnight oximetry, etc. according to the merits and demerits of each case. The patients with symptoms suggestive of OSA should also be evaluated by polysomnography and their condition is optimized with preoperative noninvasive ventilation, such as continuous positive airway pressure (CPAP) and bilevel positive airway pressure (BIPAP). The possibility of other endocrine disorders associated with obesity (such as thyroid) or mistaken for obesity (such as Cushing's disease where the diurnal variations in plasma cortisol and the concentration of urinary free cortisol is abnormal) should also be considered and is evaluated if necessary **(Table 3)**.

TABLE 3: Medical and surgical risk factors associated with obesity.	
CVS	• Systemic hypertension • Ischemic heart disease • Cardiomegaly • Congestive heart failure • Deep vein thrombosis • Peripheral vascular diseases • Pulmonary hypertension • Pulmonary embolism • Cerebrovascular accident • Sudden death
Respiratory system	• Obstructive sleep apnea • Restrictive lung disease • Hypoventilation syndrome
GI system	• Gallstones • Fatty liver • Inguinal hernia • Hiatus hernia
Endocrine	• Diabetes mellitus • Hypothyroidism • Cushing's syndrome

(CVS: cardiovascular system; GI: gastrointestinal)

Like respiratory system, the cardiovascular system also should be evaluated properly before anesthesia of an obese patient. The severity of the impairment of cardiovascular system may be underestimated by clinical evaluation only before anesthesia in obese patients. So, echocardiogram may be frequently asked for to get information about the left ventricular function and other associated cardiac abnormalities (e.g., ventricular hypertrophy, cardiomegaly, cardiomyopathy, etc.). But, echocardiography may be technically difficult in an obese patient and it is due to the inability to obtain a proper acoustic window because of the fat. Rapid weight gain, preoperatively, due to edema may indicate worsening cardiac failure and it can be mistaken for obesity. In such circumstances, the cardiac performance may deteriorate quickly following induction and tracheal intubation or due to many other reasons during anesthesia. So, an anesthesiologist must always be prepared with a selection of inotropes, vasodilators, and other drugs. The preoperative electrocardiogram (ECG) is mandatory for obese patients. But, the overlying excessive adipose tissue may result in low voltage complexes in ECG, masking any ventricular hypertrophy that might be present.

Premedication

In obese patients, the opiates and sedative drugs as premedication should be used very cautiously and in a titrating dose. This is because, with the same degree of sedation, there is more chance of airway obstruction in

obese than in nonobese patients. But, the degree of central respiratory depression is same for the same doses of drug in both the obese and nonobese patients. The premedication in obese patients should be given orally or intravenously. The intramuscular route for delivery of drugs in obese patients is associated with unpredictable pharmacokinetics and frequently the drug is deposited mainly into subcutaneous fat.

So, this route should be avoided, especially in obese patients. The antisialagogue should be used routinely in obese patients as there is more chance of difficult intubation in obese patients and with it the increased secretions make it more difficult. The obese patients are traditionally presumed to be at the increased risk for pulmonary aspiration (probably due to increased intra-abdominal pressure, delayed gastric emptying, and increased incidence of hiatus hernia) during the induction of anesthesia and intubation. But there is no supporting evidence for this notion. So, perhaps a group of anesthetists thought that the greater risk of pulmonary aspiration is potentially related to the technical difficulty during tracheal intubation. Hence, as prophylaxis a combination of H_2 receptor blocker (ranitidine 150 mg) or proton pump inhibitor (omeprazole) and a prokinetic agent (metoclopramide 10 mg) should be administered orally 12 hours and 2 hours before surgery to reduce the risk of aspiration. In addition, some anesthesiologists also advocate the administration of 30 mL of 0.3 M sodium citrate orally just before the induction of anesthesia. The advantages and disadvantages of the administration of sodium citrate just before the induction and intubation are discussed earlier.

The morbidly obese patients are more likely to develop DVT. Because, they are likely to be less ambulant during the postoperative period. So, a low dose of subcutaneous heparin should be given as prophylaxis in the preoperative period and continued into the postoperative period, until the patient is fully mobile. Other measures like pneumatic leggings, a graded compression stockings, etc. are also useful in reducing the incidences of DVT in obese patients.

Induction of Anesthesia

The induction of anesthesia is very tricky in an obese patient. Always an experienced assistant or a second anesthetist should be available by the side of principal anesthetist during the induction of anesthesia and intubation, apprehending difficult intubation, difficult ventilation, and other airway-related problems. On the other hand, tracheal intubation and invasive positive pressure ventilation (IPPV) is very essential for oxygenation in the morbidly obese patients as spontaneous respiration is very difficult and sometimes becomes impossible too. The intubation may be warranted for all except the briefest procedures due to the risk of aspiration. *Therefore, risk of aspiration and hypoventilation are the two main indications for routine intubation of obese patients for very short surgical cases.*

Invasive positive pressure ventilation is often necessary because there is increased work of breathing and tendency to hypoventilation in spontaneous respiration. The choices among the awake intubation, intubation under inhalational anesthesia or intubation after muscle paralysis depends on the experience of anesthesiologist and his preoperative evaluation regarding the anticipated difficulties of intubation. Some authors recommend awake intubation when the actual body weight is >175% of the average body weight. The presence of features, suggesting significant OSA, may also indicate the possible difficulties with bag and mask ventilation.

Another approach for intubation in obese patient is by direct laryngoscopy under topical and infiltration anesthesia. If laryngeal structures cannot be visualized, then fiberoptic intubation is probably a safe option. Blind nasal intubation with spontaneous ventilation can also be tried, but practically it is very difficult (not practiced frequently) and trouble-some as nasal bleeding might cause further deterioration of an already difficult airway.

Apart from different techniques of intubation, the rapid sequence induction and intubation using succinylcholine following an adequate period of preoxygenation and deep sedation is essential. The low FRC associated with obesity means that there is rapid decrease in arterial oxygen tension during direct laryngoscopy and tracheal intubation. The risk of quick arterial oxygen desaturation emphasizes the importance of maximizing the oxygen content into the lungs before initiating direct laryngoscopy and also emphasizes the importance of monitoring of the arterial oxygen saturation continuously by pulse oximetry.

The anesthetist should be well prepared with full range of aids for tracheal intubation such as the short-handled laryngoscope, polio blade laryngoscope, McCoy laryngoscope, gum elastic boogies, laryngeal mask airway (LMA), etc., anticipating difficult intubation. The equipment for emergency cricothyrotomy always should also be kept ready and capnograph must be available to confirm the correct placement of endotracheal (ET) tube as the auscultation of breath sounds is difficult. The obese patient will require ventilation with high inspired O_2 fraction (FiO_2), particularly in lithotomy, or Trendelenburg, or prone position and the addition of PEEP to maintain adequate arterial oxygen tension.

Maintenance of Anesthesia

There is nothing special for the maintenance of anesthesia in obese patients. Use of sevoflurane and propofol during intraoperative period helps in rapid induction and recovery from anesthesia in such group of patients. Though, it is often stated that the obese individuals have prolonged induction and awake slowly from GA by volatile anesthetics than nonobese individuals. But, the same does not happen in actual practice, if the short-acting agents are used in very titrating doses. N_2O is frequently used for maintenance of anesthesia in obese patients because of its rapid elimination and quick recovery. But, the frequent need for increased oxygen concentration in the inspired anesthetic gas mixture may sometimes limit the usefulness of the administration of N_2O. Controlled ventilation using large tidal volume is often used in an attempt to improve oxygenation in obese individual, but the adverse effects of it on cardiac output and subsequently less tissue oxygen delivery must be borne in mind.

Theoretically, greater fat stores increases the volume of distribution for lipid soluble drugs, for example, benzodiazepines, opioids, etc., relative to lean person of same body weight. So, they will need increased dose and their action will be prolonged. The water soluble drugs, for example, the neuromuscular blockers (NMBs) have small volume of distribution, which are minimally increased by body fat. Therefore, the dosing of water soluble drugs should be based on the ideal body weight to avoid over dosage. Obese patients typically require 20–25% less local anesthetic per blocked segment because of epidural fat and distended epidural veins. Continuous epidural anesthesia has the usual advantages of providing surgical anesthesia and postoperative pain relief, decreasing respiratory complications in postoperative period. Regional nerve block combined with multimodal pain control has the additional advantage as the prophylaxis of DVT.

For noninvasive blood pressure monitoring, the width of sphygmomanometer cuff should be of appropriate size (width will be 20% greater than the diameter of arm) which is usually not available in operation theater (OT). To get an intravenous line is extremely difficult for a very obese patient. Invasive blood pressure monitoring may be required, if necessary. An arterial line allows accurate monitoring of arterial blood pressure and frequent blood gas analysis. Central venous pressure monitoring is desirable, as it helps in better assessment of cardiac functions in obese patients. The obese patients with cardiac failure may get benefit from the use of pulmonary artery catheter. The fluid balance may be difficult to assess clinically and increased blood loss is common in obese patients due to difficult surgical conditions.

Postoperative Care

The incidence of postoperative mortality of obese patients is twice than that of nonobese patients. Because, respiratory failure is a major postoperative complication for morbidly obese patients. Pulmonary atelectasis is common and lung capacities remain in decreased state for at least 5 days after abdominal surgery in obese patients. So, to optimize the FRC and closing capacity ratio, ideally the obese patients are recovered in a head up or semisitting position (since this position is best for respiratory mechanics) and extubation is done when (i) the patient is fully awake, (ii) reflexes are recovered fully, and (iii) until there is no doubt that an adequate airway and tidal volume will be maintained by reversal of NMB. Postoperative ventilation is sometimes required in obese patients who are suffering from coexisting cardiorespiratory diseases and especially in those who have undergone prolonged surgery.

It is mandatory that the obese patients should be monitored intensively for hypoxemia, especially with the history of OSA syndrome and humidified oxygen should be given regularly during postoperative period including during transportation OT to recovery room. Obese patients with the history of OSA syndrome may also benefit from nocturnal nasal CPAP. The episodes of OSA are most frequent during rapid eye movement (REM) sleep. But, the incidence of it is relatively low in initial postoperative period, and is common between the third to fifth postoperative nights. The hazards of OSA may, therefore, be worst a few days after surgery. This has great implications for the duration of postoperative monitoring by oximetry and oxygen therapy. The maximum decrease in PaO_2 occurs typically at second and third days postoperatively. Regular physiotherapy should be administered postoperatively for obese patients.

Frequently a question arises, if the obese patients should be taken as outpatient basis or not. And its answer is like that morbidly obese and OSA patients may be candidates for outpatient surgery, provided they are adequately monitored and assessed postoperatively before discharge and provided the surgical procedure will not require large doses of opioids for postoperative pain control.

Ophthalmic Anesthesia

■ ANATOMY

Osteology

Our two eyeballs lie in two bony cavities called *orbits*. It is situated in the sagittal plane of skull and on the either side of the root of nose. Each orbit is pyramidal or a truncated pear in shape, with its base lying anteriorly and apex posteriorly, directed toward the optic canal. The optic canal forms the stalk of this pear. Each orbit is made up of seven bones. The orbit develops around the eyeball. So, nearly 1 mm behind the anterior margin of orbit lies the widest diameter of it (orbit) that corresponds with the equator of the eyeball.

The seven bones which take part in the formation of bony orbit are—frontal, maxilla, zygomatic, lacrimal, ethmoid, palatine, and sphenoid bone. Each orbital cavity has a (i) roof, (ii) floor, (iii) medial wall, and (iv) lateral wall. All these four walls of orbital cavity are directed forward laterally and slightly downward, diverging anteriorly. The roof, floor, and the lateral wall of an orbit are more or less triangular in shape, but the medial wall is oblong.

The medial wall of each orbit lies in the sagittal plane of head and is in parallel with the medial wall of the contralateral orbit. The lateral wall of an orbit forms a 90° angle with the lateral wall of contralateral orbit. The medial and the lateral walls of each orbit make a 45° angle when they meet posteriorly with each other **(Fig. 3)**. The apex of an orbit, including the optic foramen, lies in the same sagittal plane as the medial wall of the orbit. The anterior end of the medial wall of orbit lies about 20 mm in front than that of the lateral wall of orbit. The eyeball occupies the frontal half of each orbit, and projects anteriorly beyond the anterior margin of it. When the eye is fixed in primary gaze, then the visual axis lies in the sagittal plane. The anatomical axis of each orbit diverges from the visual axis by 23° **(Fig. 3)**.

The orbit lies beneath the anterior cranial fossa and above the maxillary sinus. The medial wall of the orbit separates it from the ethmoidal sinuses and the middle meatus of the nose. The lateral wall of the orbit separates it (orbit) from the middle cranial fossa posteriorly and from the muscular temporal fossa anteriorly. The anterior margin of each orbit is known as the orbital rim. It forms a protective buttress for all vital structures, held within the orbit, and comprises of three robust bones such as zygomatic, frontal, and maxillary bones. This orbital rim forms the rounded rectangular base of the pear-shaped orbital pyramid which tapers posteriorly to form a tight apex and is made up of the greater and lesser wings of sphenoid bones. The greatest diameter of an orbit is the part which is situated immediately inside the anterior margin of it. The volume of an adult orbit is about 30 mL, while that of an average-sized globe is 6.5 mL. The typical dimensions of an orbit at the level of its anterior rim (margin) are 35 mm vertically and 40 mm horizontally. The depth of an orbit, measured from the inferior orbital rim (margin) to the optic foramen, ranges from 42 to 54 mm. The lateral orbital rim lies 12–18 mm behind the level of cornea, allowing the exposure of the globe at its equator laterally. Medially, the orbital margin breaks its continuity at lacrimal fossa.

The *anterior orbital margin* of an orbit consists of superior, lateral, inferior, and medial parts (margins). The superior orbital margin is formed entirely by the orbital arch of frontal bone. It is sharp at its lateral two-thirds and rounded at its medial one-third. At the junction of these two parts of superior orbital margin lies a notch, called the supraorbital notch, and through this notch supraorbital nerves and vessels pass. Sometimes, this notch is converted into a foramen or into a canal by a periosteal ligament which ossifies in about 20% of cases. Another small foramen, named supraciliary canal, is also found near this supraorbital notch. It transmits a nutrient artery and a branch of supraorbital nerve to frontal sinus. About 6 mm medial to this supraorbital notch, there is another notch called the Notch of Arnold which transmits the medial branches of supraorbital nerve and vessels. Just medial to it (i.e., 10 mm medial to this supraorbital notch) lies the supratrochlear notch which transmits the supratrochlear nerves and vessels. The *lateral orbital margin* is formed by the zygomatic process of frontal bone above and the frontal process of zygomatic bone below. It is the strongest portion of orbital outlet (anterior orbital margin). Just outside the lateral orbital margin, but below the frontozygomatic suture, there is a tubercle, called the zygomatic or molar tubercle. The *inferior orbital margin* is formed by the zygomatic bone laterally and the maxillary bone medially, usually in equal parts. The suture between the two is frequently marked by a tubercle which can be felt on palpation. The infraorbital foramen lies about 4 mm below this tubercle and transmits the intraorbital nerves and vessels. The *medial orbital margin* is formed by the frontal bone above and the frontal process of maxilla below. The medial margin of orbit is indistinct in its lower part. In this indistinct part of medial orbital margin, it presents a double contour, forming *lacrimal fossa* for lacrimal sac. The anterior margin of lacrimal fossa or the anterior lacrimal crest lies on the frontal process of maxilla and the posterior margin of lacrimal fossa or the posterior lacrimal crest lies on lacrimal bone. At the junction of medial and superior orbital margins, a tubercle is present which is called as the *lacrimal tubercle*. The orbital septum is attached to the entire medial orbital margin (**Fig. 1**).

The *roof of an orbit* is formed anteriorly by the orbital plate of frontal bone and posteriorly by the thick lesser wing of sphenoid bone. A *fossa for the lodgment lacrimal gland* is located on this orbital roof, anteriorly and laterally. The *trochlear fossa* is a small dimple (depression) which is located on the roof, 5 mm behind the anterior margin on its medial side and lodges a *cartilaginous trochlear pulley*, through which passes the tendon of superior oblique muscle. The roof of the orbit is separated from its lateral wall, anteriorly by zygomaticofrontal suture and posteriorly by *superior orbital fissure*. The roof of the orbit is separated from its medial wall by a suture which are situated between the orbital plate of frontal bone above and the ethmoid, lacrimal, and maxilla below (from posterior to anterior). In the frontoethmoidal sutures, there are two foramina, anterior and posterior, through which passes the anterior and posterior ethmoidal vessels and nerves. Superior to the roof of the orbit and in the anterior cranial fossa lies the frontal lobe of brain. Inferior to the roof of this orbit lies the frontal nerve, levator palpebrae superioris (LPS) muscle, superior rectus muscle, superior oblique muscle, supraorbital artery, trochlear nerve, and lacrimal gland. The optic foramen lies at the apex of this roof of orbit. A prominent tubercle on the sphenoidal part of this orbital roof gives origin to the extrinsic muscles of eyeball (**Fig. 2**).

The *floor of an orbit* is formed by three bones— zygomatic bone laterally, maxillary bone medially, and a

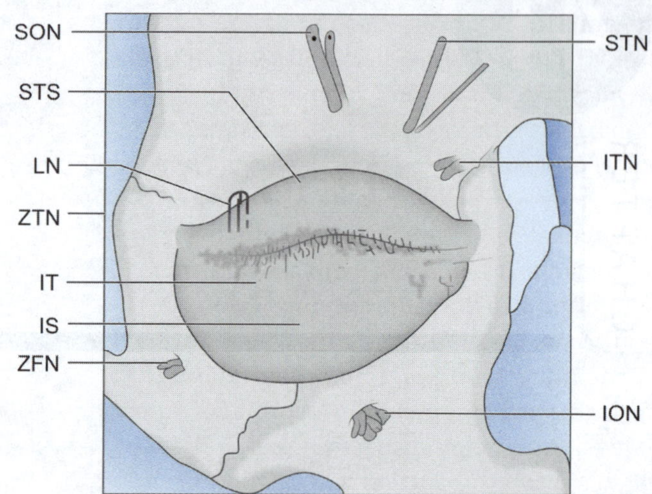

Fig. 1: The dissection of orbit from front. Orbicularis oculi muscle has been removed. (ION: infraorbital nerve and artery; IS: inferior septum; IT: inferior tarsal plate; ITN: infratrochlear nerve and artery; LN: lacrimal nerve and artery; SON: supraorbital nerve and artery; STN: supratrochlear nerve and artery; STS: superior tarsal plate and septum; ZFN: zygomaticofacial nerve and artery; ZTN: zygomaticotemporal nerve and artery)

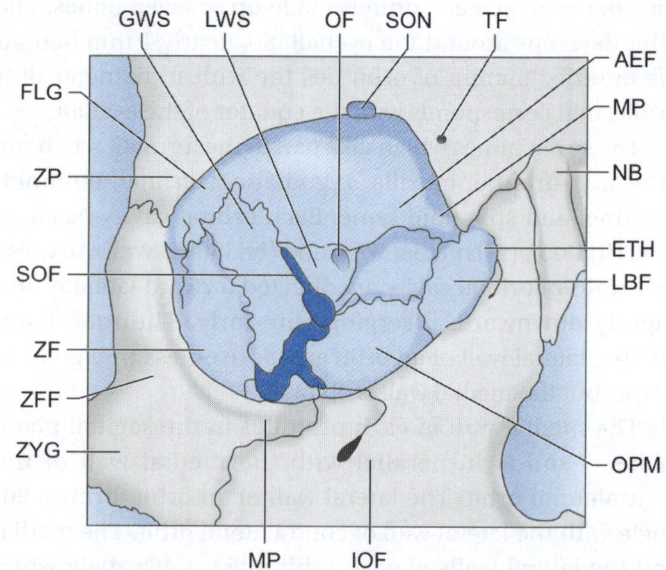

Fig. 2: The right orbit. (AEF: anterior ethmoidal foramen; ETH: ethmoid bone; FLG: fossa for lacrimal gland; GWS: greater wing of sphenoid; IOF: inferior orbital foramen; LBF: lacrimal bone and fossa; LWS: lesser wing of sphenoid; MP: maxillary process; NB: nasal bone; OF: optic foramen; OPM: orbital plate of maxilla; SOF: superior orbital fissure; SON: supraorbital notch; TF: trochlear foramen; ZF: zygomatic foramen; ZFF: zygomatic facial foramen; ZP: zygomatic process; ZYG: zygomatic bone)

small portion of palatine bone posteriorly. The infraorbital fissure (posteriorly) and its canal (anteriorly) extend forward from the apex of the orbit to its floor. This *infraorbital canal* which transmits infraorbital vessels and nerves finally exits anteriorly at infraorbital foramen. It is situated 1 cm inferior to the middle point of the inferior orbital margin. The *nasolacrimal canal*, which is 12 mm in length, lies in the maxillary bone. It commences anteromedially from the floor of orbit and passes vertically downward into the nasal cavity. It passes the *nasolacrimal duct* and drains tears from conjunctival sac into the inferior meatus of nose. In the extreme anteromedial angle of orbital floor and just behind the inferior orbital margin and lateral to the nasolacrimal canal, there lies a fossa that gives origin to the inferior oblique muscle. Superiorly, this floor of orbit is related to inferior rectus muscle, inferior oblique muscle and the nerve to an inferior oblique. Inferiorly this floor of orbit is related to maxillary antrum and palatine air cells. Anteriorly the floor and the lateral wall are continuous with each other while posteriorly the floor is separated from the lateral wall by *inferior orbital fissure* **(Fig. 3)**.

The *medial wall of an orbit* is more or less quadrangular in shape and comprises of four bones—most anteriorly the frontal process of maxilla, followed by the lacrimal, ethmoid, and lesser wing of sphenoid (from anterior to posterior). The *lacrimal fossa,* which measures about 15 × 5 mm in size and houses the lacrimal sac, is situated on the medial wall of orbit and is bounded by the anterior and posterior lacrimal crests. The *anterior lacrimal crest* is formed by the frontal process of maxilla and the *posterior lacrimal crest* is formed by the lacrimal bone itself. Besides lacrimal sac, the fossa also lodges lacrimal fascia, some areolar tissue containing the plexus of veins, and some fibers of orbicularis oculi muscle which is known as the Horner's muscle. The lacrimal fossa which contains the nasolacrimal sac continues below with nasolacrimal canal and contains the nasolacrimal duct. The anterior lacrimal crest extends inferiorly to join with the lower orbital margin and forms an elevation called the *lacrimal tubercle*. The posterior lacrimal crest extends superiorly to join with the superior rim. The ethmoidal bone is the thinnest and the weakest part of orbit and is called as the *lamina papyracea*. The two medial walls of orbit of both sides are almost parallel. The medial wall of orbit is related medially to the anterior, middle, and posterior ethmoidal sinuses, middle meatus of nose, and sphenoidal air sinuses. The superior oblique muscle, the medial rectus muscle, the nasociliary nerve, and the terminal part of ophthalmic artery run along the lateral surface of this medial wall of orbit **(Fig. 4)**.

The *lateral wall of orbit* is made up of zygomatic bone (anterior one-third) and the greater wing of sphenoid bone (posterior two-thirds). The superior and inferior orbital fissures separate the posterior portion of this lateral wall of orbit from the roof and the floor of it (orbit), respectively.

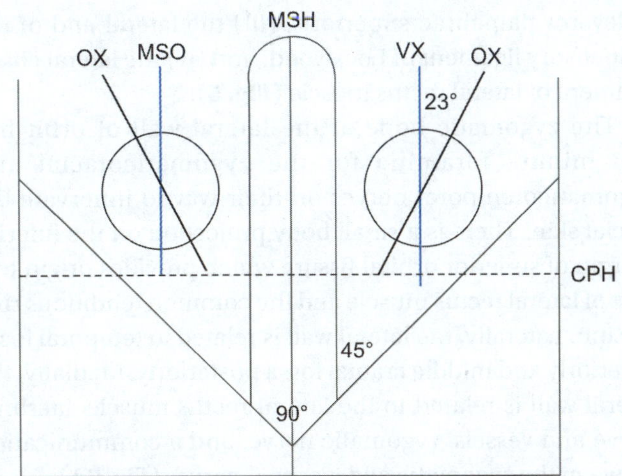

Fig. 3: The planes of head and orbital. (CPH: coronal plane of head; MSH: midsagittal plane of head; MSO: midsagittal plane of orbit; OX: orbital axis; VX: visual axis)

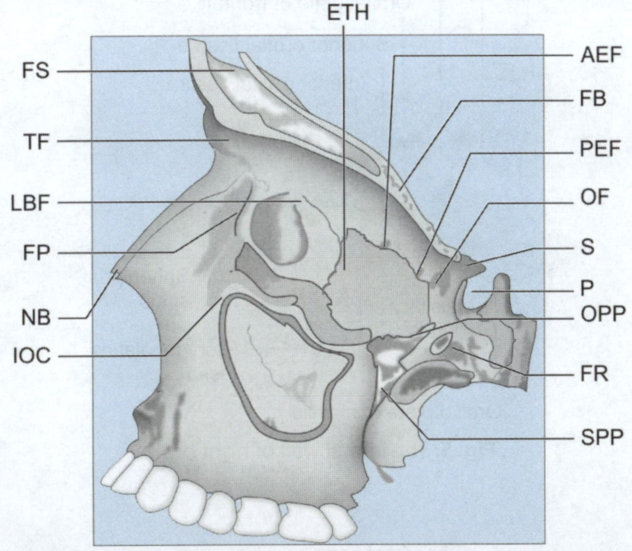

Fig. 4: Medial wall of the orbit. (AEF: anterior ethmoidal foramen; ETH: ethmoid bone; FB: frontal bone; FP: frontal process; FR: foramen of rotundum; FS: frontal sinus; IOC: infraorbital canal; LBF: lacrimal bone and fossa; NB: nasal bone; OF: optic foramen; P: pituitary; PEF: posterior ethmoidal foramen; OPP: orbital process of palatine; S: sphenoid; SPP: sphenoid process of palatine; TF: trochlear foramen)

It (the lateral wall) is triangular in shape with its base lying anteriorly. The greater wing of sphenoid bone, which forms the posterior two-thirds of this lateral wall of orbit, separates the superior from inferior orbital fissure. On this lateral wall of orbit a prominence, called the lateral orbital *tubercle of Whitnall*, is situated 4 mm behind the midpoint of lateral orbital margin and 10 mm below the zygomaticofrontal suture. This tubercle of Whitnall gives attachment to (i) the lateral palpebral raphe, (ii) the lateral horn of the tendon of levator palpebrae superioris, (iii) the lateral end of the suspensory ligament of Lockwood, and (iv) the lateral check ligament of lateral rectus muscle **(Fig. 5)**.

The zygomatic bone at the lateral wall of orbit has two minute foramina for the zygomaticofacial and zygomaticotemporal nerves on their way to innervate the fascial skin. There is a small bony projection on the inferior margin of superior orbital fissure which provides origin to a part of lateral rectus muscle and the common tendinous ring of Zinn. Laterally, the lateral wall is related to temporal fossa anteriorly and middle cranial fossa posteriorly. Medially, the lateral wall is related to the lateral rectus muscle, lacrimal nerve and vessels, zygomatic nerve, and a communication between the zygomatic and lacrimal nerves **(Fig. 6A)**.

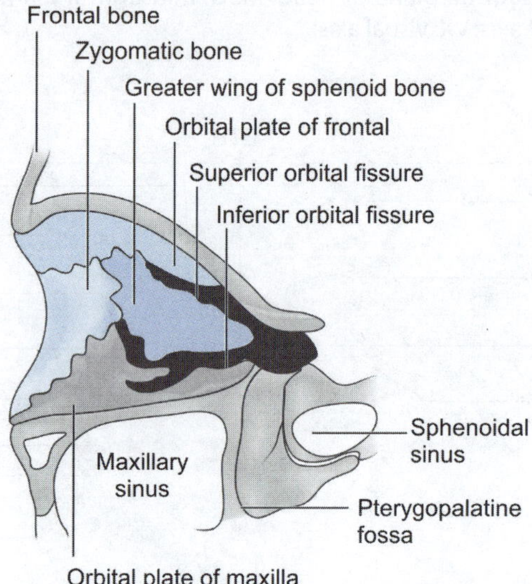

Fig. 5: The lateral wall of right orbit.

The *superior orbital fissure* is the gap, situated between the greater and the lesser wings of sphenoid bone. It lies between the roof and the lateral wall of orbit. The frontal bone forms the lateral boundary of this fissure. It is comma or retort shaped because it is wider at its medial end and narrower at its lateral end. At the junction of these two parts (wider part and narrower part) of superior orbital fissure, there lies a spine which gives *origin to the lateral rectus muscle*. Its medial end is separated from the optic foramen by the posterior root of the lesser wing of sphenoid bone. The anterolateral part of this fissure is closed by dura mater so that no structure can pass through it. However, its posteromedial part communicates with the middle cranial fossa, allowing the passage of nerves and vessels between the cranial cavity and eyeball. The *annulus tendineus communis*, spans over this superior orbital fissure and divides this fissure into *three parts*—(1) the upper or lateral part transmit the trochlear, frontal and lacrimal nerves, and the superior ophthalmic vein, (2) the middle part transmits the superior divisions of oculomotor nerve, nasociliary nerve, the sympathetic root of ciliary ganglion, the inferior division of oculomotor nerve, and abducent nerve. It is also called as the oculomotor foramen, and (3) the inferior part transmits only the ophthalmic vein **(Fig. 6B)**.

The *inferior orbital fissure* lies between the lateral wall and the floor of orbit. It connects the orbital cavity with the inferotemporal fossa in front and the pterygopalatine fossa behind. It is bounded anteriorly by the maxilla and posteriorly by the greater wing of sphenoid bone. It is separated from the posterior end of superior orbital fissure by a bridge of bone extending from the greater wing of sphenoid.

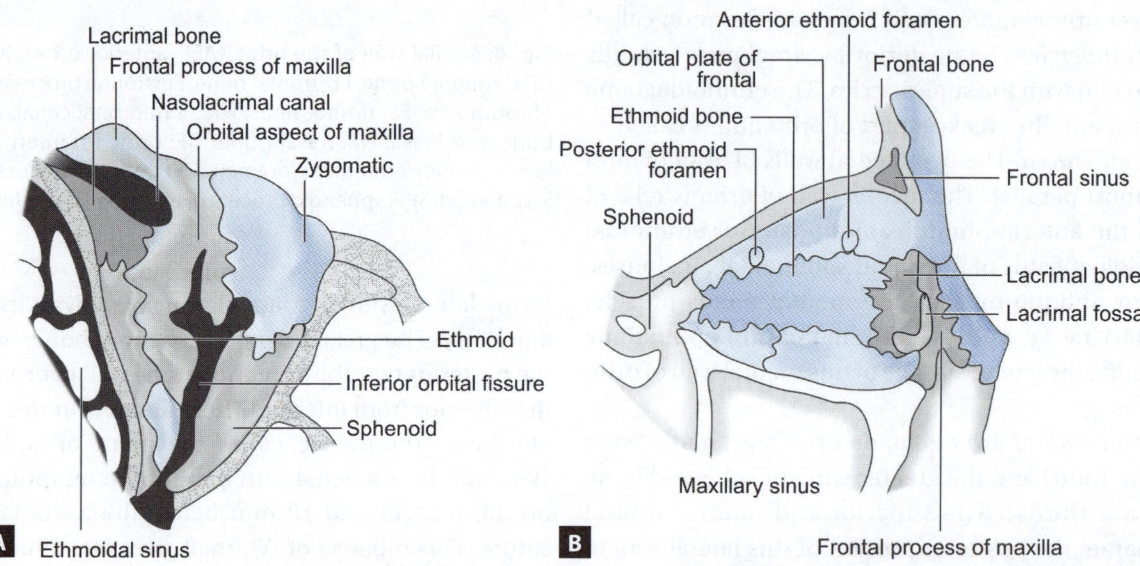

Figs. 6A and B: (A) The floor of right orbit and (B) The medial wall of right orbit.

Both the fissures are covered by a periorbital membrane and the Muller's muscle. The inferior orbital fissure transmits— (i) the infraorbital nerve, (ii) the zygomatic nerve, (iii) the branches from pterygopalatine ganglion, and (iv) a communication between the inferior ophthalmic vein and pterygoid venous plexus **(Fig. 7)**.

The *optic foramen* is actually a canal which is formed by the union of the two roots of lesser wing of sphenoid bone with its body. The optic canal, starting from the optic foramen, makes a communication between the apex of the orbit and the middle cranial fossa. This optic canal is about 10 mm in length and 5 mm in breadth. It transmits the optic nerve and along with it the meninges, the ophthalmic artery and few twigs of sympathetic plexus along the artery. At this optic canal, the dura mater splits into two layers—the inner layer forms the sheath of optic nerve, while the outer layer continues with the periosteum of orbit. The common tendinous ring is also attached to the infraoptic tubercle which is an elevation present inferolateral to the optic foramen. The posterior ethmoidal air sinuses are situated just medial to this optic canal.

The anterior and posterior ethmoidal foramen and its canals are situated at the junction of roof and medial wall of orbit and form a communication between the orbit and anterior cranial fossa. The anterior ethmoidal canal transmits the anterior ethmoidal nerve and vessels, while the posterior ethmoidal canal transmits the posterior ethmoidal vessels and nerve.

Orbital Connective Tissue

Orbital Periosteum

The periosteum of orbital bone is known as the *periorbita* and it lines the bones of orbit loosely. So, it can easily be stripped off from underlying orbital bones. It is thickened along the anterior orbital margin and is called as the *arcus marginalis*. Along the anterior orbital margin, it is continuous with the periosteum of facial bones and with the orbital septum circumferentially. Posteriorly at the apex of the orbit, this periorbita is continuous through the optic canal with the periosteum of the cranial bones (pericranium) and also with the dural sheath of optic nerve **(Fig. 8)**.

Here, it provides origin to the four rectus muscles from a *common ring-like area*. Anteriorly, it encloses the *lacrimal sac* in its fossa and then passes down with nasolacrimal duct to become continuous with the periosteum of the inferior meatus of the nasal cavity. Posteriorly, it forms a dense membrane, covering the superior orbital fissure. Some fine lamellae of this periorbita (periosteum of orbital bones) divide the orbital fat into many lobules and form a covering for the nerves and vessels. The orbital septum is a strong membranous sheet which is attached to the anterior margin of the orbit and is continuous with the facial periosteum and the periosteum (periorbita) of the orbit. It defines the anatomical anterior border of the orbit. On the nasal side, it is attached with both the anterior and the posterior lacrimal crests. Its central attachments are in the upper and lower eyelids and lie deep to the orbicularis oculi muscle **(Fig. 9)**.

Tenon's Capsule

In **Figure 9**, the Tenon's capsule or bulbar fascia is a thick fibrous membrane-like structure which envelops the eyeball.

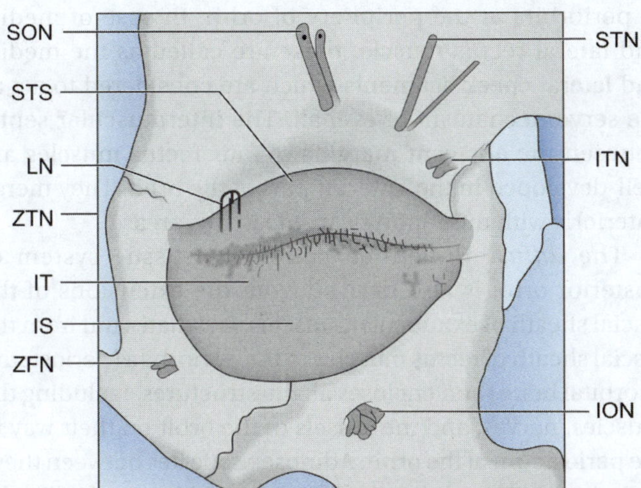

Fig. 7: The apex of orbit, fissures, vessels, and nerves. (ION: infraorbital nerve and artery; IS: inferior septum; IT: inferior tarsal plate; ITN: infratrochlear nerve and artery; LN: lacrimal nerve and artery; SON: supraorbital nerve and artery; STN: supratrochlear nerve and artery; STS: superior tarsal plate and septum; ZFN: zygomaticofacial nerve and artery; ZTN: zygomaticotemporal nerve and artery)

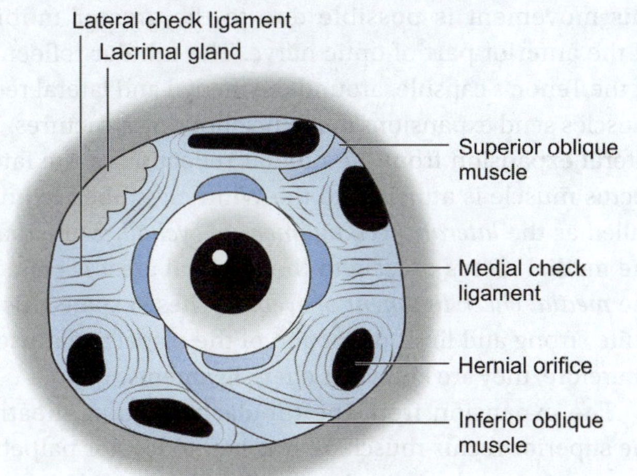

Fig. 8: The connective tissue diaphragm of orbit with the hernial orifices. It is situated just anterior to the equator of globe. The eyelids and orbital septum are removed.

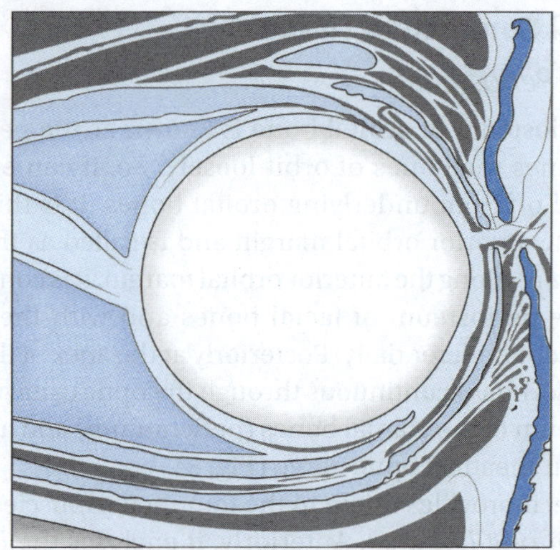

Fig. 9: The display of connective tissue (white lines) around the structures into orbit.

It extends from the corneal limbus anteriorly to the optic nerve posteriorly where it blends with the meninges of optic nerve. Posteriorly, it comes in contact with orbital fat and is pierced by ciliary nerves with their accompanying arteries. Anteriorly, it merges with subconjunctival connective tissue and is pierced by the tendons of six extraocular muscles (the four rectus muscles pierce this Tenon's capsule behind the equator of eyeball, while the two oblique muscles pierce it anterior to the equator of eyeball) prior to their insertion on sclera. At the site of the insertion of the tendons of these extraocular muscles, the Tenon's capsule sends tubular reflection (projection) around these tendons so as to clothe them like a glove and allows the unrestricted control of the movement of these muscles within this capsule.

The globe rotates around its central axis within the smooth inner lining of this Tenon's capsule. However, this movement is possible due to the greater mobility of the anterior part of optic nerve. The tubular reflections of the Tenon's capsule, around the medial and lateral rectus muscles send expansions to the neighboring structures. The lateral expansion from the tubular reflection of the lateral rectus muscle is attached to the Whitnall's tubercle and is called as the *lateral check ligament of eyeball,* while that of the medial rectus muscle to the lacrimal crest is called as the *medial check ligament of eyeball.* These expansions are quite strong and limit the action of the respective muscles. Therefore, they are known as check ligaments.

The expansion from the tubular reflection sheath of the superior rectus muscle is attached to levator palpebrae superioris muscle through a band and that of the inferior rectus muscle is inserted between the tarsal plate and the orbicularis oculi muscle of lower lid. The expansions from the reflection sheaths of superior oblique and inferior oblique muscles are attached to the trochlea and to the lateral part of the floor of the orbit, respectively. The expansions from the fascial sheaths of inferior rectus and inferior oblique muscles also extend posteriorly and are joined by the expansions from the lateral and medial rectus muscles to form a sling on which the eyeball rests. It provides an effective support to eyeball and is so known as the *suspensory ligament of Lockwood.* All these fibrous expansions, from the reflection covering of muscles, are attached to conjunctiva, thereby preventing its folding during their action. The intermuscular septa between the adjacent margins of four rectus muscles which divide the orbital space into intraconal and extraconal area are well-developed in the anterior part of orbit. They merge with Tenon's capsule in this area.

Diffuse Connective Tissue System of Orbit

The diffuse connective tissue system of orbit is divided into two parts—(1) The clearly defined, supporting, connective tissue system of anterior orbit and (2) the diffuse, ill-defined, connective tissue system of posterior orbit.

The *clearly defined,* supporting, connective tissue system in the anterior part of the orbit consists of a diaphragm which extends out from the Tenon's capsule and the globe of the eyeball to the periorbita just behind the orbital margin. The some condensation of these connective tissues above and below the globe, form the suspensory ligaments which are known as the *ligaments of Whitnall and Lockwood,* respectively. They support the globe and limit its displacement. The several sheets of connective tissue also fan out from the respective muscle sheaths (which is formed by the reflection of Tenon's capsule) to be attached to periorbita at the periphery of orbit. In case of medial and lateral rectus muscle, these are called as the medial and lateral check ligaments which are considered to act as the servomechanism of eyeball. The intermuscular septa, between the adjacent margins of four rectus muscles are well-developed in the anterior part of the orbit. They merge anteriorly with the Tenon's capsule in this area.

The *diffuse ill*-defined connective tissue system of posterior orbit is also derived from the extensions of the fascial sheath of extraocular muscles. It radiates out from the fascial sheath of rectus muscles to the periorbita (periosteum of orbital bone) and encloses all the structures, including the muscles, nerves, and the vessels of the orbit on their way to the periosteum of the orbit. Adipose tissue lies between these radiations of fascial sheath **(Figs. 10 and Fig. 11)**. Unlike the anterior orbit, posteriorly the intermuscular septa are less well-developed, particularly at the inferotemporal quadrant of the orbit where almost none exists. Of the rectus muscles, only the medial rectus is significantly separated from its adjacent bony orbital wall by a fat compartment.

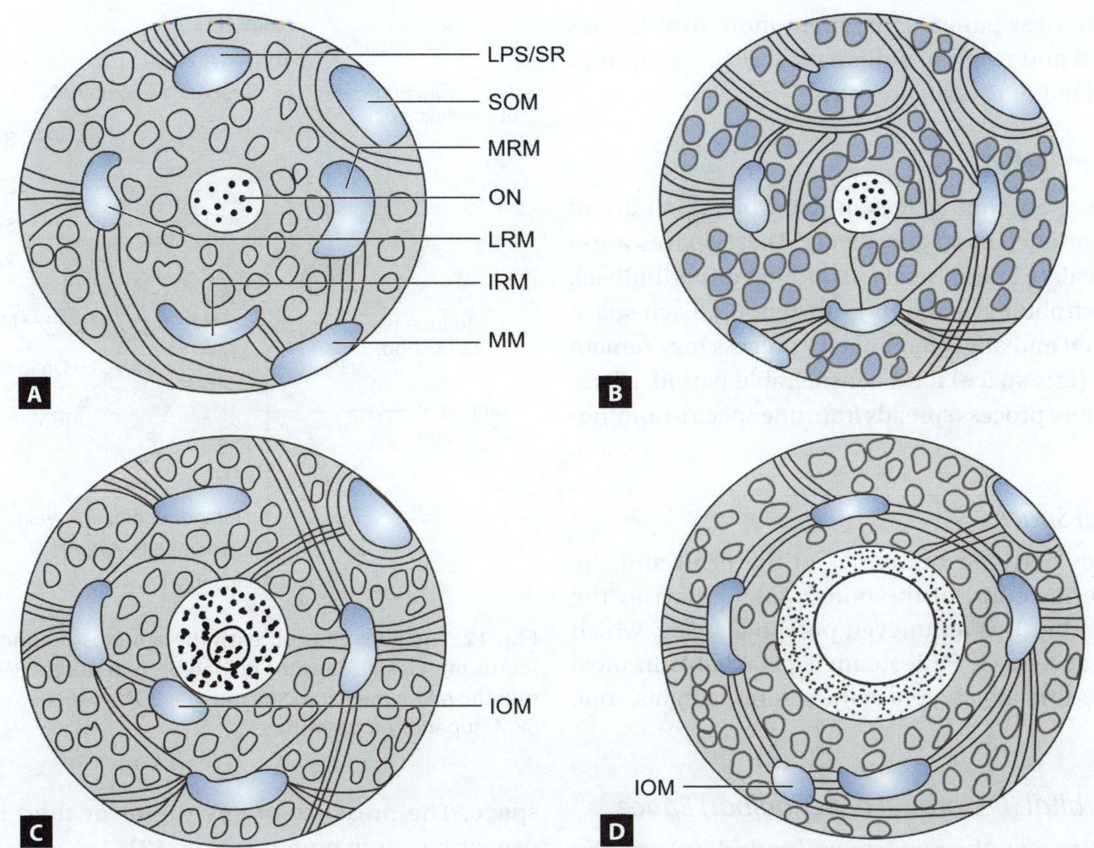

Figs. 10A to D: Extraocular muscles and the connective tissue system, in different coronal sections of the orbit. (A) Coronal section at the apex of orbit; (B) Coronal section of orbit at the posterior pole of globe; (C) Coronal section of orbit, midway between the posterior pole and the equator of globe; and (D) Coronal section at the equator of the globe. (IRM: inferior rectus muscle; LPS: levator palpebrae superioris; LRM: lateral rectus muscle; MM: Muller's muscle; MRM: medial rectus muscle; ON: optic nerve; SR: superior rectus; SOM: superior oblique muscles)

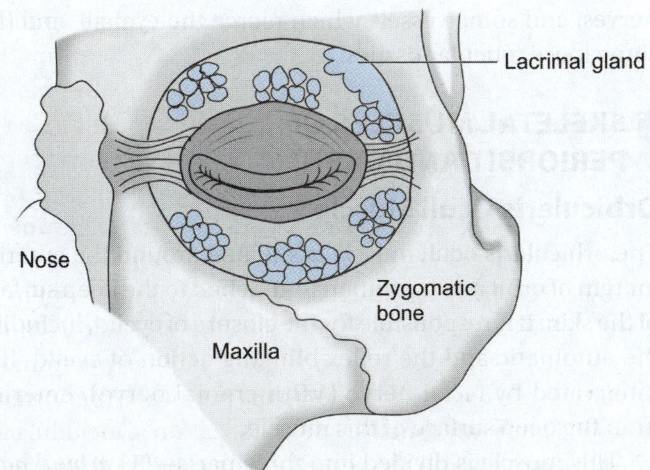

Fig. 11: The pads of orbital fat, coming out of different apertures, present in connective tissue system of left orbit.

The connective tissue around the medial rectus muscle exhibits connections or extensions to the orbital floor and roof. At the level of the equator, a condensation of connective tissue of the medial rectus extends nasally to the medial orbital wall. This is called the medial check ligament. The medial compartment opens anteriorly above and below the medial check ligament as two hernial orifices in the connective tissue diaphragm that surrounds the globe. Thus local anesthetic (LA) agent, deposited in the medial orbital compartment by injection will spread through these orifices to the orbital septum into the upper and lower eyelids. This spread of local anesthetic agent in the upper and lower eyelids is in this tissue plane which is deep to the orbicularis oculi muscle and where the fine terminal motor branches of VIIth cranial nerve lie. So, they are readily blocked.

The quality of these connective tissues among the different individuals varies. The quality deteriorates with increasing age and thus the weaker connective tissues are more permeable to local anesthetic agents injected into the midorbit. So, the critical concentrations of drug to block the oculomotor nerve near the apex are more easily attained in the elderly as compared to young adults. Similarly, orbital hemorrhage in the elderly which drains in the anterior orbit, causing black eye, may be of less important than a similar bleeding in younger patients, in whom more firm tissues may trap blood and result in a dramatic loss of vision from the unrelieved building up of pressure.

Spaces in the Orbit

Surgically, there are four spaces in the orbit which are of immense importance to an anesthetist. These spaces are—(i) subperiosteal, (ii) peripheral (periorbital or peribulbar), (iii) central (retrobulbar), and (iv) sub-Tenon's. Each space is self-contained and any inflammatory process may remain confined in it (this space) for a considerable period. Then, this inflammatory process spreads from one space to another space.

Subperiosteal Space

This space lies between the bones of the orbit and the periorbita (periosteum) of the bones, taking part in the formation of orbit. It is an uneven potential space, which is obliterated at sutures. Periosteum is detachable in most parts, except its firm attachment at the sutures margins, roof, and fissures.

Peripheral Orbital (Periorbital or Peribulbar) Space

It is the area between the periosteum (periorbita) and the extraocular muscles with their fascial expansions extending between them, forming more or less a continuous circular space. This space is limited anteriorly by the check ligaments and posteriorly by the approximation of common tendinous ring with the periosteum, at optic foramen. This periorbital space contains—(i) the lacrimal gland, (ii) the branches of trigeminal (frontal, lacrimal, infraorbital, and nasociliary) and trochlear nerves, (iii) the lacrimal and infraorbital vessels, and (iv) the ophthalmic vein. The collection of fluid in this space may extend through the orbital septum and lead to the edema of eyelids **(Fig. 11)**.

Central (Retrobulbar) Space

It is a cone-shaped area which is situated behind the eyeball and is enclosed by the four rectus muscles and their fascial expansions in between them. Anteriorly the space is limited by the posterior aspect of eyeball, laterally by the rectus muscles and their fascial sheaths and posteriorly by the common tendinous origin of the extraocular muscles at the apex of the orbit. This space contains—(i) the optic nerve and its meningeal coverings, (ii) the superior and inferior divisions of oculomotor nerve, (iii) abducent nerve, (iv) ophthalmic artery, (v) superior ophthalmic vein, and (vi) the nasociliary nerve. The last three structures pass to the peripheral surgical space from this central retrobulbar space, after piercing the medial aspect of this retrobulbar

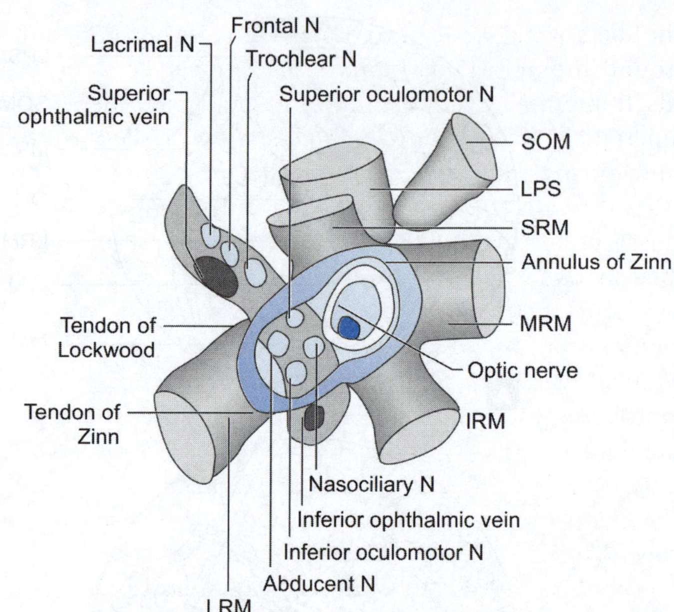

Fig. 12: The apex of orbit with the annulus of Zinn. (IRM: inferior rectus muscle; LPS: levator palpebrae superioris; LRM: lateral rectus muscle; MRM: medial rectus muscle; SOM: superior oblique muscle; SRM: superior rectus muscle)

space. The presence of any tumor or fluid in this space usually results in proptosis **(Fig. 12)**.

Sub-Tenon's Space

It lies between the Tenon's capsule and the sclera and forms a potential space around the globe. It contains—(i) the insertions of the tendons of extraocular muscles, (ii) some nerves, and some vessels which pierce the eyeball, and (iii) some loose reticular tissues.

SKELETAL MUSCLES OF PERIORBIT AND ORBIT

Orbicularis Oculi Muscle

The orbicularis oculi muscle is situated around the anterior margin of orbit and is intimately attached to the deep surface of the skin. It is responsible for the closure of eyelid, including the automatic and the reflex blinking action of eyelid. It is innervated by facial nerve (VIIth cranial nerve), entering from the deep surface of this muscle.

This muscle is divided into three parts—(1) *orbital part,* (2) *preseptal part, and* (3) *pretarsal part.* The last two parts of this muscle together are called as the *palpebral part* of this muscle.

The *orbital part* of this muscle originates from—(i) the medial third of the upper and lower orbital margins, (ii) medial palpebral ligaments, (iii) the maxillary process of frontal bones, and (iv) the frontal process of maxilla.

The fibers of this muscle are arranged in a concentric manner, around the anterior orbital margin, and covers the eye lids. It intermixes with the brow muscle (levator palpebrae superioris) and frontalis. *This orbital part of orbicularis oculi muscle helps in the firm closure of eyelid.*

The *palpebral part* (preseptal and pretarsal) of this muscle originates from the medial palpebral ligament and its adjacent bone. Then, it passes over the septal and tarsal area and forms the lateral palpebral raphe by merging with the septum orbitale and finally gets attached to the tubercle of Whitnall. The *pretarsal part* of this orbicularis oculi muscle contributes to form more or less the entire thickness of eyelid margin. The follicles of eyelashes, the glands of Moll, and the meibomian ducts traverse the pretarsal part of this muscle. *The palpebral part of orbicularis oculi muscle helps in the smooth and gentle closure of eyelids during blinking.*

The third part of this orbicularis oculi muscle which is known as *pars lacrimalis* is attached to the posterior lacrimal crest and the lacrimal fascia. It helps in the dilatation of lacrimal sac and thus facilitates the drainage of tear by *tear pump mechanism.*

Extraocular Muscles

These extraocular muscles of orbit are involved in the movement of eyeball and its adnexa. They may be divided into three broad groups:
1. The extrinsic muscles of eyeball
2. The striated muscles of eye lid
3. The nonstriated muscles of eye lid.

Extrinsic Muscles of Eyeball

These extrinsic muscles of eyeball are comprised of *four recti* and *one superior* and *one inferior oblique* muscle **(Fig. 13)**. These four recti, with their average 40–42 mm of length, have a common origin from a tendinous ring (annulus of Zinn)

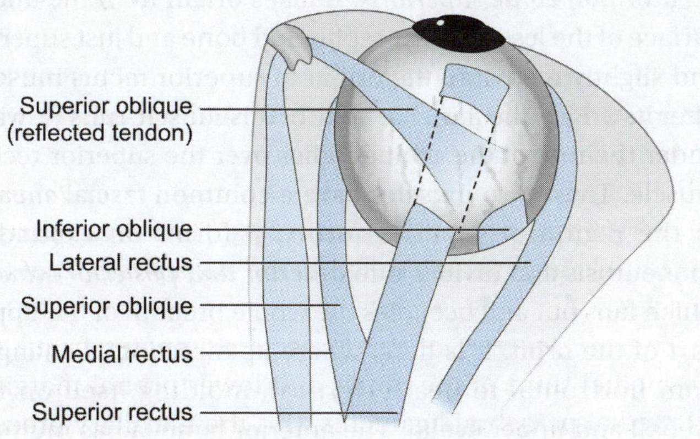

Fig. 13: The extraocular muscles of the eyeball.

which is attached to the sphenoid bone at the apex of the orbit. This tendinous ring encircles the optic foramen and the medial end of the superior orbital fissure. This annulus ring forms the apex of the intraconal (retrobulbar) space whose base is formed by the Tenon's capsule, covering the posterior surface of the eyeball.

This intraconal (retrobulbar) space is now no longer considered as a closed compartment which was originally thought. But, because of its intimate relationship with the optic, oculomotor, sensory, and autonomic nerves, this intraconal space is important for understanding and mastering the ophthalmic regional anesthesia. These four rectus muscles of eyeball run forward, after their origin from their tendinous ring, close to the optic foramen and are then inserted on the sclera, *anterior to the equator* of eyeball. Their muscle bellies are replaced, before their insertion, by a tendon near the globe. The superior and inferior oblique muscles are inserted obliquely in the posterosuperior and posteroinferior quadrant of globe, respectively, *behind the equator* and are almost lateral to the mid vertical plane.

Superior rectus muscle: It takes origin from the upper part of the tendinous ring (annulus of Zinn), from the lateral side of the optic foramen and from the optic nerve sheath. It is inserted on the sclera, 7.7 mm behind the limbus, by a tendon. At its origin, this muscle is related *inferiorly* to the dural sheath and the optic nerve, *superiorly* to the levator palpebrae superioris muscle and frontal nerve, *medially* to the medial rectus muscle and *laterally* to the lateral rectus muscle, lacrimal artery, and lacrimal nerve. The levator palpebrae superioris muscle remains above the superior rectus muscle throughout its course. Between the superior rectus muscle and the optic nerve lie some orbital fat, the ophthalmic artery, and the nasociliary nerve. In the anterior part of its course, the tendon of superior oblique muscle runs between the superior rectus muscle and the globe. The superior rectus muscle is supplied by the superior division of *oculomotor nerve* which enters the muscle from its undersurface at the junction of its middle and posterior-third.

Inferior rectus muscle: It arises only from the lower part of the tendinous ring (annulus of Zinn). It is the shortest of all the rectus muscles of orbit. It passes forward along the floor of the orbit and is inserted on the sclera at its inferior aspect, approximately 6.5 mm posterior from the limbus. The optic nerve, orbital fat, the inferior divisions of oculomotor nerve and the eyeball lie *above* this inferior rectus muscle. The floor of the orbit, maxillary sinus and the infra orbital vessels and nerves lie *below* it. The nerve to the inferior oblique muscle and the lateral rectus muscle itself form the *lateral relation* of this muscle. The inferior oblique muscle crosses the orbit below this inferior rectus muscle and the fibrous sheath of these two muscles blend at this crossing. The inferior rectus muscle is also attached to lower lid by some fascial expansion of its sheath. It is supplied by a branch from the inferior division of *oculomotor nerve* which enters the muscle from its bulbar surface.

Medial rectus muscle: It takes origin from the medial part of the tendinous ring (annulus of Zinn) and from the sheath of optic nerve. It is the strongest and the thickest of all the extrinsic muscles of eyeball. After its origin, it runs forward along the medial wall of the orbit and is inserted on the sclera at its medial aspect, 5.5 mm behind the limbus. The superior oblique muscle runs from the posterior to the anterior part of the orbit *along the upper border of* this medial rectus muscle. The ophthalmic artery and its branches, the ethmoidal nerve, and the infratrochlear nerve run between these two muscles from the posterior to the anterior part of the orbit. The floor of the orbit lies *below the lower border* of this medial rectus muscle. The orbital plate of ethmoid bone and the ethmoidal air cells are placed *medial* to this muscle, while the central orbital fat lies laterally. The medial rectus muscle is supplied by a branch from the inferior division of *oculomotor nerve* from its lateral surface.

Lateral rectus muscle: It arises from the lateral part of the tendinous ring (annulus of Zinn). Then, this muscle runs forward and laterally between the eyeball and the lateral wall of the orbital. It is inserted on the sclera at its lateral aspect 6.5 mm behind the limbus. The lacrimal gland, the lacrimal nerve, and the lacrimal artery lie above the upper border of this lateral rectus muscle. The floor of the orbit and the tendon of inferior oblique muscles form the lower relations of this muscle. Laterally, it lies directly on periosteum. It is supplied by *VIth cranial (abducent) nerve* which enters the muscle from its medial aspect.

Superior oblique muscle: It takes *origin* from the body of the sphenoid bone, just above and medial to the optic foramen. It is the longest and the thinnest of all the extrinsic muscles of the eyeball. After origin, it runs forward between the roof and the medial wall of the orbit, and between the superior and medial rectus. Then, just behind the anterior orbital margin, it becomes a rounded tendon which passes through a pulley, called the *trochlea*. After that the superior oblique muscle runs downward, backward and laterally at an angle of about 55°, underneath the superior rectus muscle and fans out before its *insertion* on the posterior superior quadrant of sclera. The superior oblique muscle has two distinct parts. A direct muscular part which is about 40 mm in length and extends from its origin up to trochlea, and a tendinous reflected part which is about 20 mm in length and runs from the trochlea to its insertion. It is supplied by trochlear (IVth cranial) nerve.

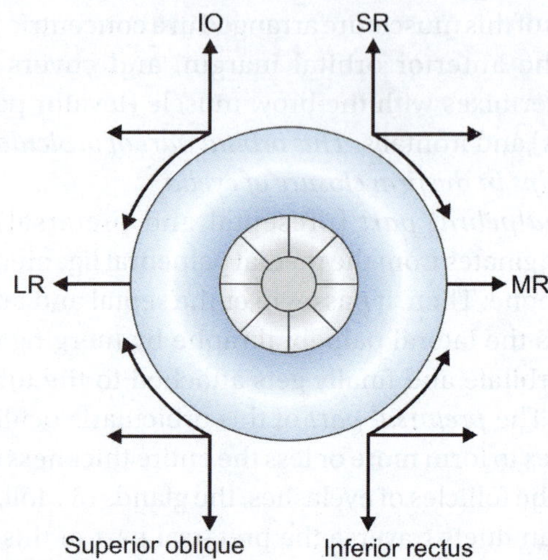

Fig. 14: The actions of extraocular muscles of right eye. (IO: inferior oblique; IR: inferior rectus; LR: lateral rectus; MR: medial rectus; SO: superior oblique; SR: superior rectus)

Inferior oblique muscle: It is the only extrinsic muscle of eyeball which does not take origin from the annulus of Zinn. It *arises* from a rough area (small depression) situated on the orbital plate of maxilla, just lateral to lacrimal fossa. Then, it runs backward and laterally, passing between the inferior rectus muscle and the floor of the orbit and curves around the eyeball to lie underneath the lower border of lateral rectus. It is *inserted* on the posterolateral quadrant of sclera, underneath the lateral rectus muscle. This muscle is innervated by the inferior division of *oculomotor nerve* **(Fig. 14)**.

Muscles of Eye lids

The levator palpebrae superioris and the *superior palpebral muscles* elevate the upper eyelid. The tendinous palpebral expansion of inferior rectus and the *inferior palpebral muscle* retract the lower eyelid. The orbicularis oculi helps in the closure of eyelids **(Fig. 13)**.

Levator palpebrae superioris: It takes origin from the under surface of the lesser wing of sphenoid bone and just superior and slightly medial to the origin of superior rectus muscle. After its origin, the thin, flat belly of this muscle runs forward under the roof of the orbit and lies over the superior rectus muscle. These two muscles have a common fascial sheath. In the region of superior fornix, it forms an expanded aponeurosis and divides into *anterior and posterior lamella* which fans out and occupies the whole breadth of the upper part of the orbit. It is here, where its direction is changed from horizontal to nearly vertical, molding itself on the eyeball and upper eyelid. The anterior lamella has multiple diffuse terminal attachments which is described underneath. While the posterior lamella which is known as the *sympathetic muscle of Muller* is inserted on the superior border of the tarsal plate.

The insertion of the anterior lamella of levator palpebrae superioris:

- The bulk of these fibers passes through the muscle fibers of orbicularis oculi and gets inserted into the skin of upper eyelid, at and below the upper palpebral sulcus.
- Some fibers are attached to the front and the lower parts of tarsal plate.
- The fascial sheath of the muscle is also attached to the conjunctiva of superior fornix.
- The two horns of levator aponeurosis get attached to the orbital bones, at the midpoint of lateral and medial orbital margin. The lateral horn is stronger than the medial horn. The lateral horn divides the lacrimal gland into its orbital and palpebral portions, and supports the gland against the orbital roof. The medial horn is attached to the frontolacrimal suture medial to the palpebral ligament.

The roof of the orbit, the trochlear nerve, the frontal nerves, and the supraorbital vessels lie above this levator palpebrae superioris muscle. The trochlear nerve crosses this levator muscle near its origin from lateral to medial side. Similarly, the frontal nerve crosses it obliquely from lateral to medial. The superior rectus muscle and the eyeball lie below this muscle. The muscle is supplied by the superior division of oculomotor nerve. The sympathetic fibers carrying through the oculomotor nerve supply; the nonstriated superior and inferior palpebral muscles along the respective divisions of oculomotor nerve.

Nonstriated muscles of orbit: A group of the nonstriated muscles of the orbit almost completely envelop the eyeball. It has *superior, inferior, and medial palpebral parts.* The superior palpebral part of this muscle is also known as the *superior palpebral muscle of Muller.* This muscle arises from the inferior aspect of levator palpebrae superioris at the level of the superior fornix in the form of a wide band and runs a near vertical course to be inserted on the upper edge of the superior tarsal plate. The inferior palpebral part is also known as the *inferior palpebral muscle of Muller* and passes from the bulbar surface of the inferior rectus muscle to the lower margin of the lower tarsal plate. The fibers of these muscles spread out mostly as a fascia, lying between the inferior rectus muscle and the inferior oblique muscle. These muscles are innervated by the *sympathetic nerve.* The superior palpebral muscle *elevates the upper lid* and the inferior palpebral muscle *retracts the lower lid.* So, the irritation of sympathetic nerve results in the retraction of both the eyelids.

NERVES OF THE EYE, ORBIT, AND PERIORBIT

The cranial nerve IInd (optic), IIIrd (oculomotor), IVth (trochlear), Vth (trigeminal), VIth (abducent), and VIIth (facial) are responsible for the sight, motor function, sensation, and autonomic control of the eyeball and the ocular region of the face. So, they are called as the nerves of the eyeball, orbit, and periorbita.

Optic Nerve

Strictly speaking, the optic nerve is not a cranial nerve, rather it is considered as the extension of brain. Because, unlike of the other cranial nerves it carries meningeal coverings over it from the cranial cavity. The outer meningeal covering of optic nerve is nothing but the extension of dura, and blends anteriorly with the sclera **(Fig. 15)**. The middle and inner coverings of optic nerve are also the continuation of the cerebral arachnoid and pia mater. Like the meninges, the subdural and the subarachnoid space also extend around the optic nerve and separate the three sheaths of the optic nerve from each other. From the optic chiasma to retina the total length of an optic nerve is approximately 5 cm. Anatomically, the optic nerve is divided into four parts—(1) intracranial, (2) intracanalicular, (3) intraorbital, and (4) intraocular. The *intracranial portion of optic nerve* extends from optic chiasma to the cranial end of optic canal and is approximately 1 cm in length **(Figs. 16A and B)**.

The anterior cerebral artery and the frontal lobe of the brain lie superior to it. As the optic nerve emerges from the cavernous sinus, the internal carotid artery lies lateral to it. The *intracanalicular portion of optic nerve* is only 5–6 mm in length and lies in the optic canal. As the dural sheath is tightly adhered to the periosteum of this canal, so this portion of optic nerve is completely rigid. The *intraorbital*

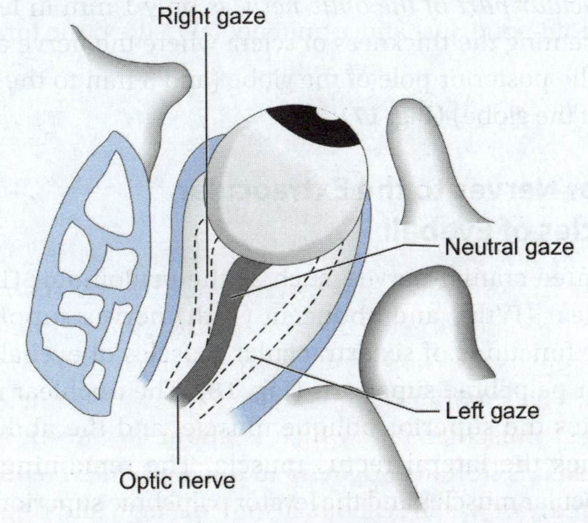

Fig. 15: Transverse section of right orbit, showing the different positions of optic nerve, during neutral, right, and left gaze.

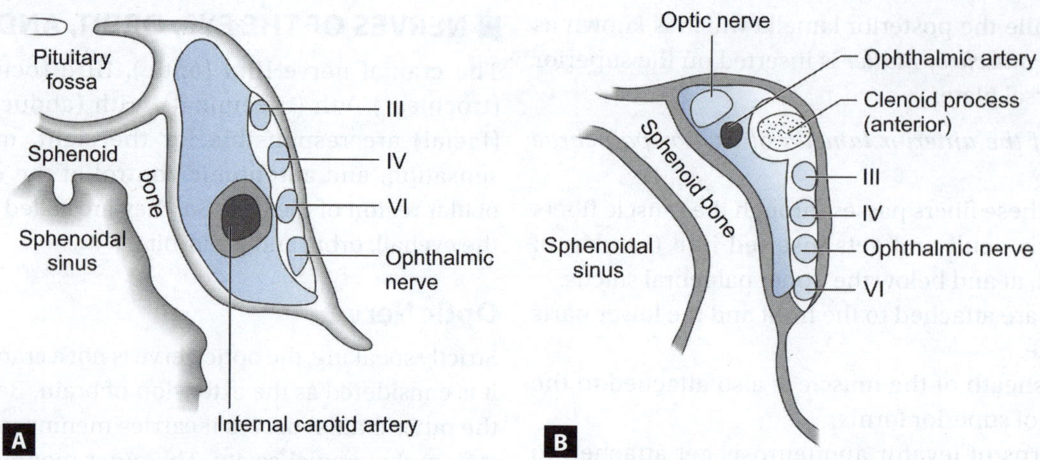

Figs. 16A and B: The cavernous sinus and different other nerves and arteries on its lateral wall. (A) The coronal section at the level of pituitary fossa and (B) The coronal section at the level of anterior clinoid process.

portion of optic nerve extends from the optic foramen to the posterior surface of the eyeball, 3 mm on its nasal side. It is 3 cm in length. But the distance from the optic foramen to the eyeball is only 2.5 cm. So, this portion of optic nerve is loose, lax, and tortuous. This tortuosity of this portion of optic nerve permits the free movement of globe in its all positions, without detrimenting its function.

The dural sheath of optic nerve fuses anteriorly with the sclera and posteriorly with the periorbita (periosteum) at the optic foramen. The cerebrospinal fluid (CSF) flows freely under this dural and subarachnoid sheath around the optic nerve and is in continuity with the CSF of midbrain. In *primary gaze position,* the intraorbital portion of optic nerve is closer to the medial than the lateral rectus muscle and assumes a tortuous course between the posterior pole of the globe and optic foramen. In *abduction and upward gaze,* the optic nerve becomes straight. In *abduction and downward gaze* the optic nerve takes a S-shaped curve. The *intraocular part of the optic nerve* is only 1 mm in length, representing the thickness of sclera where the nerve enters near the posterior pole of the globe (and 3 mm to the nasal side of the globe) **(Fig. 17).**

Motor Nerves to the Extraocular Muscles of Eyeball

The three cranial nerves, such as the oculomotor (IIIrd), trochlear (IVth), and abducent (VIth) nerves supply the motor functions of six extraocular muscles of eyeball and levator palpebrae superioris **(Fig. 18)**. The trochlear nerve supplies the superior oblique muscle, and the abducent supplies the lateral rectus muscle. The remaining four extraocular muscles and the levator palpebrae superioris are supplied by the oculomotor nerve. *The oculomotor nerve also carries the parasympathetic fibers for the sphincter muscles of*

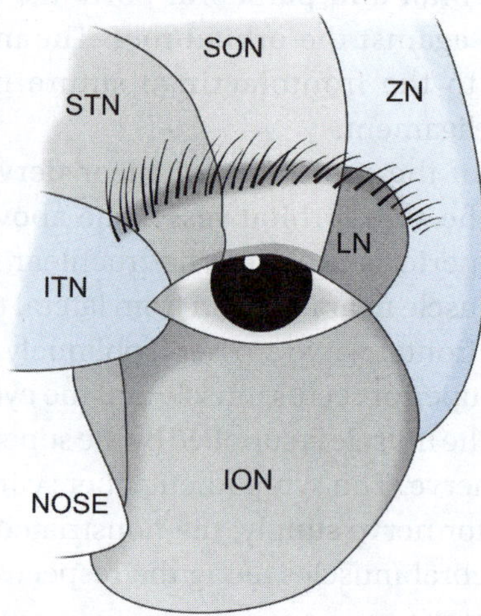

Fig. 17: The cutaneous nerve supply of periorbital region. (ION: infraorbital nerve; ITN: infratrochlear nerve; LN: lacrimal nerve; SON: supraorbital nerve; STN: supratrochlear nerve; ZN: zygomatic nerve)

iris and ciliary muscles. The dilator muscles of iris are supplied by sympathetic fibers carried by the nasociliary nerve. The motor nerve to the four rectus muscles and the inferior oblique muscle enter their respective muscle from within the muscle cone. Whereas, the trochlear nerve remains outside the cone and enters its supplying muscle, named the superior oblique through its superolateral edge, remaining outside the muscle cone. This anatomic difference explains the cause of delayed onset of akinesia of this muscle (superior oblique muscle), following a small volume of intraconal local anesthetic injection.

Oculomotor Nerve

It supplies all the extraocular muscles, except the superior oblique and lateral rectus muscle. It also supplies the

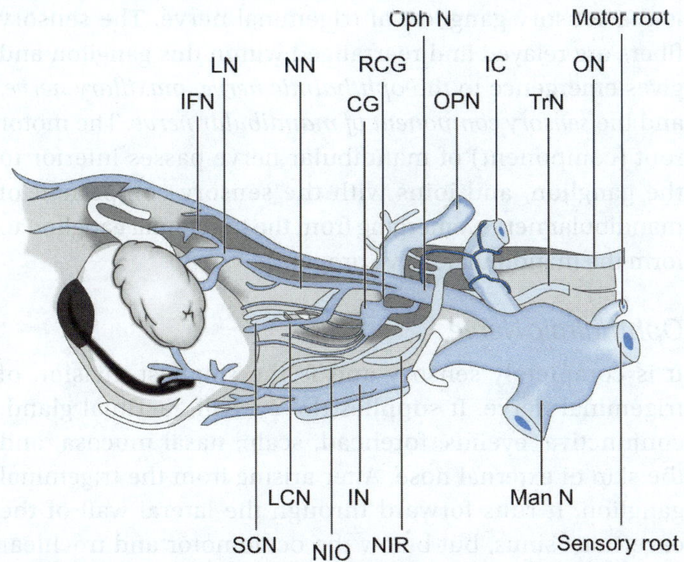

Fig. 18: Nerves within the orbit. (CG: ciliary ganglion; IC: internal carotid artery; IFN: infratrochlear nerve; IN: infraorbital nerve; LCN: long ciliary nerve; LN: lacrimal nerve; Man N: mandibular nerve; NIR: nerve to inferior rectus; NIO: nerve to inferior oblique; NN: nasociliary nerve; ON: oculomotor nerve; Oph N: ophthalmic nerve; OPN: optic nerve; RCG: ramus to ciliary ganglion; SCN: short ciliary nerves)

parasympathetic fibers to sphincter pupillae and ciliary muscles which are intraocular. So, the functional components of oculomotor nerve are as follows:

- Somatic efferent (motor) for the movement of eyeball
- General visceral efferent for the accommodation and the contraction of pupil (these fibers come from Edinger–Westphal nucleus)
- General somatic afferent for the proprioceptive impulses from the muscles of eyeball.

The oculomotor nerve emerges from the interpeduncular sulcus, present on the ventral surface of the brainstem, by 15–20 rootlets which then quickly coalesce into a single trunk. It then passes between the posterior cerebral and superior cerebellar arteries and traverses through the lateral wall of the cavernous sinus, but above the trochlear nerve. It divides here into the superior and inferior branches, and then these two divisions enter into the intraconal space of orbit through the intermediate part (oculomotor foramen) of superior orbital fissure. The nasociliary nerve and the sympathetic twig to the ciliary ganglion now lie between these two divisions of oculomotor nerve, and the abducent nerve lies lateral to them.

In the intraconal space, the superior division of oculomotor nerve now runs lateral to the optic nerve and supplies the superior rectus and levator palpebrae superioris muscle. In the intraconal space, the inferior division of oculomotor nerve divides again mainly into three branches

such as—(1) the nerve to the medial rectus muscle, (2) the nerve to the inferior rectus muscle, and (3) the nerve to the inferior oblique muscle. The nerve to the medial rectus muscle passes inferior to the optic nerve. The nerve to inferior rectus passes downward and enters the muscle from its upper aspect. The nerve to the inferior oblique passes in between the inferior rectus and the lateral rectus muscle and supplies the inferior oblique muscle from its posterior border. It also gives a thick branch to the ciliary ganglion. This branch carries the preganglionic parasympathetic fibers to ciliary muscles and sphincter pupillae.

Trochlear Nerve

The trochlear or IVth cranial IVth cranial nerve is the longest and the thinnest of all the cranial nerves. It first exits from the dorsum of brain stem. Then, it winds around the brain stem and traverses along the lateral wall of the cavernous sinus, inferior to the oculomotor nerve. After that it, enters the orbit through the superior orbital fissure, outside of the annulus of Zinn. In the orbit, it passes forward along its roof (but outside of the intraconal space) and supplies the superior oblique muscle from its orbital surface **(Figure 18)**. As the motor supply of superior oblique muscle is from the outside of the cone of four rectus muscles, so there may be some retained activity of superior oblique muscle (intorsion), following a small volume of intraconal local anesthetic injection in the procedure of retrobulbar block. The functional components of trochlear nerve are—(i) the somatic efferent (motor) to the superior oblique muscle for the movement of eyeball, and (ii) the somatic afferent for the proprioceptive impulses from the superior oblique muscle. In the cavernous sinus, these fibers carrying the proprioceptive impulses, leave the trochlear nerve and join with the ophthalmic division of trigeminal nerve. These fibers, then, relay into the mesencephalic nucleus of trigeminal nerve.

Abducent Nerve

The abducent nerve is designated as the VIth cranial nerve and supplies the lateral rectus muscle only. It emerges from the central nervous system (CNS) at the groove which is situated between the medulla and the pons (pontomedullary junction). Then, it ascends on brainstem and makes a sharp bend over the petrous part of temporal bone. After that, it enters the cavernous sinus where it lies between the internal carotid artery medially and the trigeminal ganglion laterally. In the lateral wall of the cavernous sinus, the abducent nerve lies inferior to the oculomotor and trochlear nerves, but internal carotid artery lies superomedial to it. During its intracavernous course, the abducent nerve is joined by some branches from sympathetic nerve which supplies the dilator pupillae. Then, the abducent nerve enters the intraconal space of the orbit through the superior orbital fissure, but within the common tendinous ring, lying inferolateral to oculomotor and nasociliary nerve. It supplies only the lateral rectus muscle from its ocular surface (**Fig. 19**).

Trigeminal Nerve

The trigeminal nerve is the Vth and the largest cranial nerve. It is the nerve of the first brachial arch. The functional components of this trigeminal nerve are—(i) general somatic afferent fibers which carries the sensation from the eyeball, lacrimal gland, conjunctiva, whole face, anterior half of scalp, auricle, oral cavities, and nasal cavities, (ii) somatic efferent fibers carrying motor to the muscles of mastication, tensor veli palatini, tensor tympani, mylohyoid, and the anterior belly of digastric muscle.

It arises from the ventral surface of the pons by two roots—a small motor root (the motor component of the mandibular nerve) and a larger sensory root. These two roots, then, run forward toward a notch which is situated at the upper margin of the petrous part of temporal bone. After crossing the superior border of the petrous part of temporal bone, the two roots then enter the middle cranial fossa to join trigeminal ganglion. This trigeminal Gasserian ganglion

is the sensory ganglion of trigeminal nerve. The sensory fibers are relayed and rearranged within this ganglion and gives emergence to the *ophthalmic nerve, maxillary nerve,* and the *sensory component of mandibular nerve*. The motor root (component) of mandibular nerve passes inferior to the ganglion, and joins with the sensory component of mandibular nerve, emerging from the trigeminal ganglion to form the mandibular nerve proper.

Ophthalmic Nerve

It is completely sensory and is the smallest division of trigeminal nerve. It supplies the eyeball, lacrimal gland, conjunctiva, eyelids, forehead, scalp, nasal mucosa, and the skin of external nose. After arising from the trigeminal ganglion, it runs forward through the lateral wall of the cavernous sinus, but below the oculomotor and trochlear nerve. In the front of the cavernous sinus, the ophthalmic nerve then divides into three branches such as the *lacrimal, frontal, and nasociliary nerve* which ultimately run forward and enter the orbit separately through superior orbital fissure. The lacrimal and frontal nerves pass outside of the annulus of Zinn and the nasociliary nerve passes through the annulus of Zinn of superior orbital fissure (**Fig. 20**).

The *lacrimal nerve* enters the orbit as the lateral most structure through superior orbital fissure. Then, it runs forward along the upper border of the lateral rectus muscle and enters the posterior border of lacrimal gland. Besides

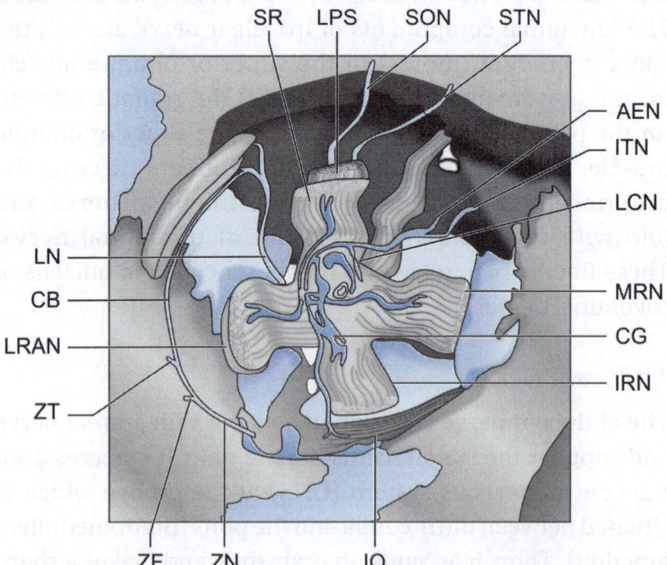

Fig. 19: Orbital nerves from the front. (AEN: anterior ethmoidal nerve; CB: communicating branch; CG: ciliary ganglion; IO: inferior oblique; IRN: inferior rectus and its nerve; ITN: infratrochlear nerve; LCN: long ciliary nerve; LPS: levator palpebrae superioris; LRAN: lateral rectus and abducent nerve; LN: lacrimal nerve; MRN: medial rectus and its nerve; SON: superior orbital nerve; SR: superior rectus; ZF: zygomaticofacial nerve; ZN: zygomatic nerve; ZT: zygomaticotemporal nerve)

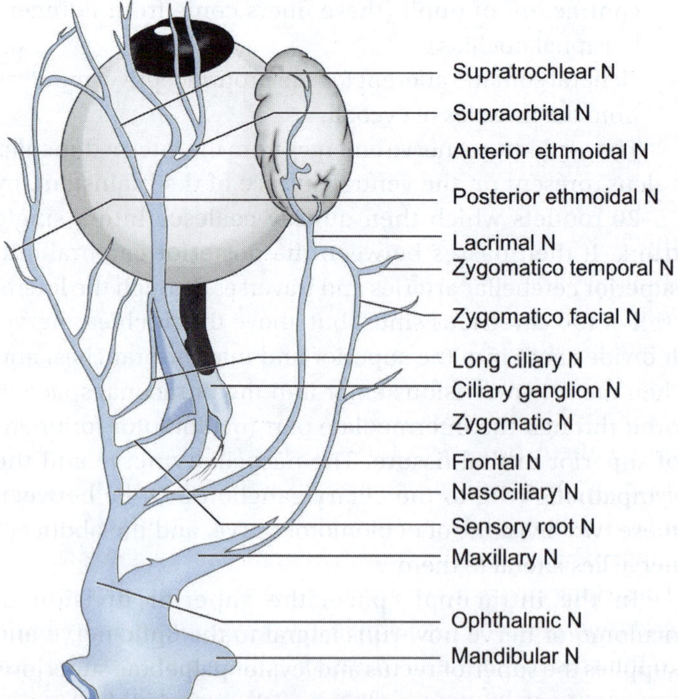

Fig. 20: Nerves within the orbit (view from above).

supplying the secretomotor fibers to lacrimal gland, it also innervates the most lateral part of the skin of upper eyelid and adjacent conjunctiva. This lacrimal nerve also receives a branch from zygomaticotemporal nerve. This branch carries the postganglionic parasympathetic fibers which are secretomotor to the lacrimal gland. The origin of these preganglionic parasympathetic (secretomotor) fibers to the lacrimal gland is from the *lacrimatory nucleus*, which is situated in the lower part of the pons.

These secretomotor fibers, arising from this lacrimatory nucleus first run through the *nervous intermedius part of facial nerve*. Then, they run through the *greater petrosal branch of facial nerve* and joins with the *deep petrosal nerve* to form the *nerve of pterygoid canal*. Here, the fibers make connection with the postganglionic fibers in the *pterygopalatine ganglion*. Then, the postganglionic fibers arising from the pterygopalatine ganglion enter the *maxillary nerve* and passes through its *zygomatic branch* and then its *zygomaticotemporal branch to join the lacrimal nerve*.

The *frontal nerve*, like the lacrimal nerve, as a branch of the ophthalmic division of trigeminal nerve, enters the orbit through supraorbital fissure above the annular tendon and traverses between the levator palpebrae superioris and the roof of the orbit. At the midway between the apex and the anterior margin of orbit, it divides into two branches—*supraorbital* and *supratrochlear*. The supratrochlear nerve runs anteromedially above the trochlea and supplies the skin of the upper medial part of the upper eyelid, medial conjunctiva, and the skin of the scalp. The supraorbital nerve passes forward and emerges at the front of orbit, either through the supraorbital foramen (20%) or through the supraorbital notch (80%). It provides sensation to the rest of the forehead, the anterior two-thirds of the scalp, the skin of the upper central part of the eyelid and adjacent conjunctiva. Thus, the peripheral conjunctival sensation is mediated via the lacrimal and frontal nerves, both of which do not course through the intraconal space. *So, sometimes incomplete conjunctival anesthesia may result from a small volume of intraconal local anesthetic injection.*

The *nasociliary branch* of the ophthalmic division of trigeminal nerve passes through the annulus of Zinn and enters the orbit. Then, it enters the intraconal space and sends a communicating branch to the ciliary ganglion. As it (nasociliary nerve) passes over the optic nerve, the long ciliary nerves (three or four in number) are given off from it. These long ciliary nerves accompany the short ciliary nerves and then pierce the sclera close to optic nerve. In addition to the afferent sensation from iris, ciliary body, cornea, and the central bulbar conjunctiva, these nerves also carry the sympathetic motor fibers to the dilator pupillae muscle.

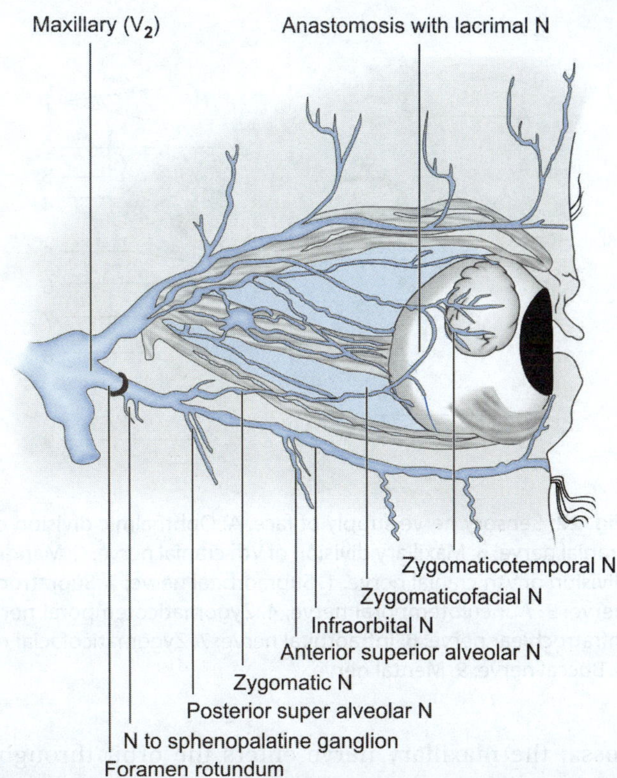

Fig. 21: Nerves within the orbit (view from lateral side).

After passing over the optic nerve, the nasociliary nerve runs along the medial orbital wall of the orbit in close relation with ophthalmic artery. Here, it gives off the *anterior and posterior ethmoidal branches* which pass through their respective foramina on the medial orbital wall of the orbit and supply the mucosa of the ethmoidal sinuses and the lateral wall of the nasal cavity. The most anterior division of nasociliary nerve is the *infratrochlear nerve*. It runs along the superior border of the medial rectus muscle and penetrates the orbital septum to innervate the skin of the lateral side of external nose, the skin of the medial side of lower eyelid, the adjacent conjunctiva, and also the lacrimal sac **(Fig. 21)**.

Maxillary Nerve

The *maxillary nerve* is the second division of trigeminal nerve (ophthalmic nerve is the first division of trigeminal nerve). It is *completely a sensory nerve* **(Fig. 22)**, supplying the middle portion of face, anterior temporal region, lower eye lid, and upper lip. It also supplies the sensation to upper gums and teeth, the mucous membrane of the upper mouth, nasopharynx, and maxillary sinuses. After emerging from trigeminal ganglia, it runs forward through the lateral wall of the cavernous sinus. Then, it exits from the cranial cavity through the *foramen rotundum* and enters the *pterygopalatine fossa*. Here, it sends the branches to pterygopalatine ganglion. After crossing the pterygopalatine

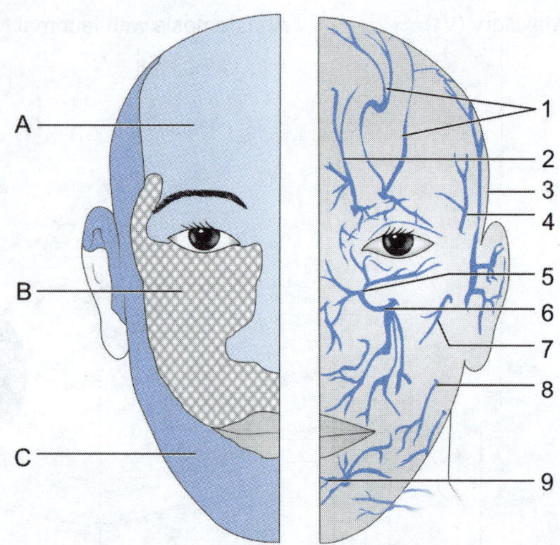

Fig. 22: Sensory nerve supply of face. A: Ophthalmic division of Vth cranial nerve; B: Maxillary division of Vth cranial nerve; C: Mandibular division of Vth cranial nerve. 1. Supraorbital nerve; 2. Supratrochlear nerve; 3. Auriculotemporal nerve; 4. Zygomaticotemporal nerve; 5. Infratrochlear nerve; 6. Infraorbital nerve; 7. Zygomaticofacial nerve; 8. Buccal nerve; 9. Mental nerve.

fossa, the maxillary nerve enters the orbit through the infraorbital fissure, where it is known as the *infraorbital nerve.*

Passing anteriorly from the posterior, this nerve lies in the infraorbital groove. Then, it runs through the infraorbital canal to reach the front of the face, where it comes out from the infraorbital foramen which is situated 1 cm below the midpoint of the infraorbital rim. The infraorbital nerve supplies the skin of the lower eyelid, nose, the upper lip, and the central part of the face. In the pterygopalatine fossa, the maxillary nerve gives off its *zygomatic branch.* This branch then enters the orbit through the infraorbital fissure and divides into *zygomaticofacial and zygomaticotemporal nerves.* The former exits the orbit through a foramen bearing the same name and supplies the skin overlying the malar bone. The later also travels a short distance along the lateral orbital wall. Then, it also exits the orbit through a foramen, bearing the same name, and innervates the skin of anterior temporal region.

The preganglionic parasympathetic secretomotor fibers to the lacrimal gland emerge from the brainstem with the facial nerve. Then, it is transferred to the trigeminal nerve by a complex pathway and travels through the maxillary nerve. It relays in another peripheral ganglion of the parasympathetic system, named the sphenopalatine ganglion. This ganglion lies in the pterygopalatine fossa. From the ganglion, the postganglionic parasympathetic fibers reach the lacrimal gland, via the interconnections between the zygomaticotemporal and lacrimal nerve.

There is a great anatomical proximity of the central and peripheral orbital nerves, with their shared innervating adipose tissue compartments and the skin. This explains easily the widespread area of peripheral sensory block, associated with the intraorbital regional anesthesia. The spread of intraorbital regional anesthetic block to the frontal nerve complex in superior orbit and the maxillary nerve complex in inferior orbit results in a unilateral loss of sensation, which extends from near the occiput above to the upper lip below, and from the midline of nose to the anterior temporal region laterally, including the anesthesia of the mucosa of the upper mouth and teeth and the nasal cavity. So, patients usually experience unilateral nasal stiffness or nasal block, and feel that their nose is running.

Mandibular Nerve

The detailed anatomy of mandibular nerve has no direct importance to an ophthalmic anesthetist. So, it will not be discussed here in detail.

Facial Nerve

It is the VIIth cranial nerve and is the nerve for second brachial arch. Among all the functional components of facial nerve, only the efferent (motor) component of it for the facial muscles is of main interest to an ophthalmic anesthetist. The functional components of facial nerve are (**Figure 23**):

- Efferent (motor) fibers for all the facial muscles of face
- General *visceral parasympathetic* efferent fibers for the submandibular and sublingual salivary glands and also for the lacrimal, nasal, palatine, and pharyngeal glands
- Special *visceral afferent* fibers for taste sensations from the presulcal area of tongue (anterior two-thirds) and palate
- General *somatic afferent* fibers from the concha of auricle.

The facial nerve originates from the pons. Then, it exits from the base of the skull through stylomastoid foramen in close proximity to the glossopharyngeal, vagus, and spinal accessory nerves which are emerging from the jugular foramen. Here, the whole branchiomotor component of the facial nerve comes out, except the fibers going to stapedius muscle. The landmark of this stylomastoid foramen is 2 cm deep and medial to the anterior border of mastoid process. So, the block of this facial nerve at this level results in a complete hemifacial akinesia and the spread of injected local anesthetic agent to the other adjacent major cranial nerves.

After its exits from stylomastoid foramen, the facial nerve first crosses the styloid process of temporal bone. Then, it passes under the external auditory meatus and enters the substance of parotid gland through its posterior border. At

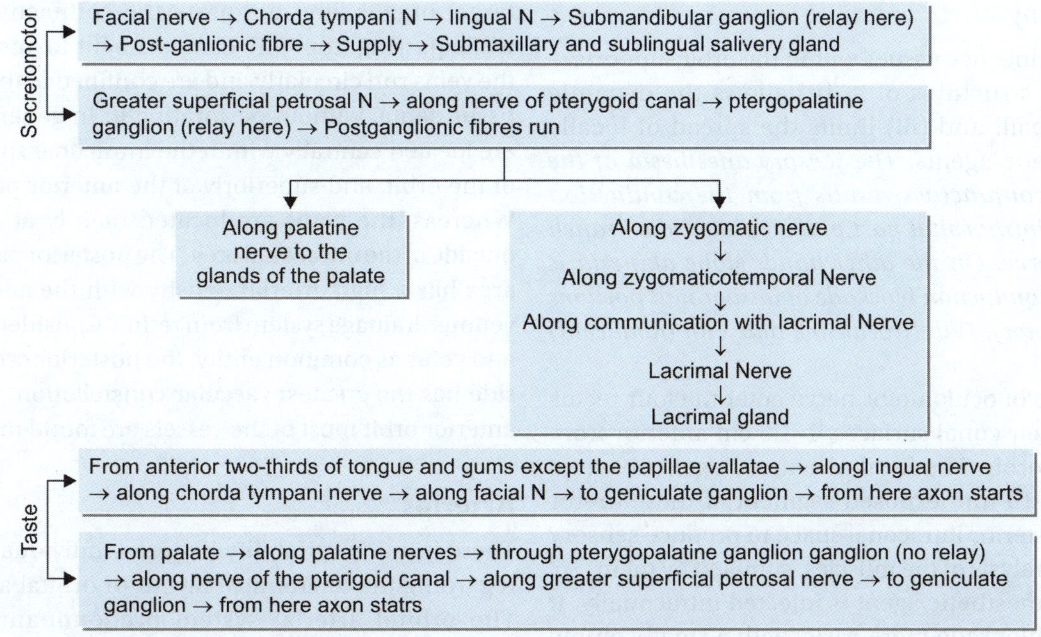

Fig. 23: Fibers carrying the secretmotor and special sense (taste) component of facial nerve.

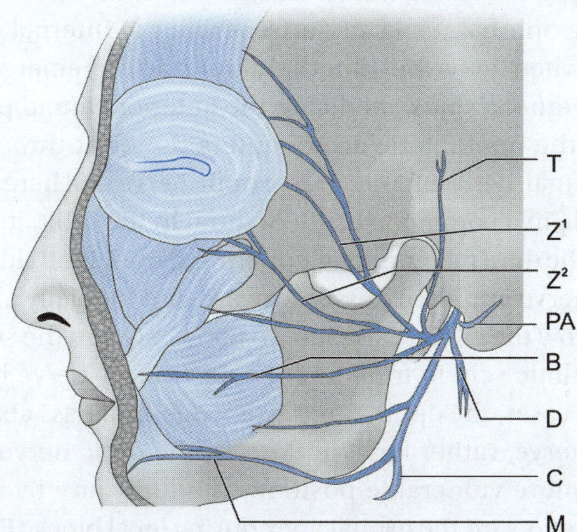

Fig. 24: The branches of facial nerve. (B: buccal branch; C: cervical branch; D: branch to posterior belly of digastric and stylohyoid; M: mandibular branch; PA: posterior auricular branch; T: temporal branch; Z¹ and Z²: upper and lower zygomatic branch)

this level, the facial nerve supplies the occipitalis, auricularis posterior, auricularis superior (through its posterior auricular branch), stylohyoid, and the posterior belly of digastric muscles. Inside the parotid gland the facial nerve divides first into two main divisions and then subsequently divides into several branches such as the *temporal, zygomatic, buccal, mandibular, and cervical branches* (**Fig. 24**). However, the pattern of this breakup and distribution of the branches of facial nerve within the parotid gland varies greatly between individuals.

The *temporal branch* supplies the intrinsic muscles on the lateral surface of the auricle and the auricularis anterior, auricularis superior, frontalis, orbicularis oculi, and corrugator muscles. The *zygomatic branch* supplies the orbicularis oculi. The *buccal branch* supplies the buccinator, the small muscles of nose, levator anguli oris, levator labii superioris, and zygomaticus major. The *mandibular branch* supplies the depressor anguli oris, depressor labii inferioris, and mentalis muscle. The *cervical branch* supplies only the platysma muscle.

The fibers, carrying the secretomotor and the special sense (taste) component of facial nerve are discussed in **Figure 23**. The efferent or motor components of facial nerve, which hold the interest of an ophthalmic anesthetist, are the upper branches of facial nerve such as the temporal and zygomatic branches. This is because they innervate the forehead and the eyebrow musculature (*frontalis muscle*) and the *three components of orbicularis oculi muscles*. It is also important to remember that all the facial muscles, which are supplied by the facial nerve, are innervated from their deep surfaces. So, the block of these terminal fibers of facial nerve depends on the technique of block. This is because if the local anesthetic drugs are injected superficial to the facial muscles, then they may not spread to their deep surfaces effectively. So, this will frequently cause the poor abolition of their muscles action. Usually, the orbital rim, the zygomatic arch, the mastoid process, and the temporomandibular joint form the important bony landmarks which are used for the peripheral facial nerve blocks (**Fig. 24**).

Applied Anatomy

The matrix of connective tissues within the orbit supports— (i) the different structures of it, (ii) allows the dynamic function of eyeball, and (iii) limits the spread of locally injected anesthetic agents. *The sensory anesthesia of the globe and the conjunctiva results from the conduction blockade of the intraorbital part of the ophthalmic branch of trigeminal nerve. On the other hand, globe akinesia is achieved by the conduction blockade of intraorbital portions of IIIrd (oculomotor), IVth (trochlear), and VIth (abducent) cranial nerves.*

The branches of oculomotor nerve enter the four rectus muscles from their conal surfaces, 1–1.5 cm anterior from the apex of the orbit. The local anesthetic agents have to reach at least 5–10 mm exposed segment of these motor nerves in the posterior intraconal space to produce sensory block and the paralysis of the muscles, supplied by them. So, when the local anesthetic agent is injected intraconally, it achieves motor blockade more easily with a small volume of drug than when an extraconal method is used. The motor branch of the oculomotor nerve which supplies the inferior oblique runs a long intraconal course. Therefore, it is most easily blocked by intraconal injection. On the other hand, the trochlear nerve which runs a short intraconal course, but a long extraconal course before entering the muscle at its superolateral edge, is most resistant to the intraconal local anesthetic injection.

The autonomic nerves and the sensory nerves have a longer course within the orbit from their point of entry through the apex to globe and other supplying structures than that of the motor nerves. So, the local anesthetic agents have a greater access to these sensory and autonomic nerves and produce a faster block than their motor component. The corneal and perilimbal sensation is mediated through the nasociliary nerve which lies within the cone of the extraocular muscles. So, the intraconal injection of local anesthetic agent effectively produces anesthesia of cornea and conjunctiva immediately surrounding it. The lacrimal, frontal, and infraorbital nerves, supplying the peripheral conjunctiva, run outside the muscle cone. So, the surgical pain may be experienced in this area, following a solely intraconal block.

■ BLOOD VESSELS OF EYE AND ORBIT

Generally, in our body the arteries and veins travel together. But, in orbit the path of the arteries and the veins behave differently. They run independently according to their anatomical distribution. The veins of the orbit do not accompany their corresponding arterial system and vice versa, but rather take their own course and direction. The arteries of the orbit radiate from its apex toward their target organs, and perforate the connective tissue septa while passing from one compartment to another. Whereas, the veins run circularly and are confined to these connective tissue septa, without perforating it. In general, the arteries are located centrally within the intraconal space at the apex of the orbit, and superiorly at the anterior part of the orbit. Whereas, the veins are located mainly at the periphery, outside of the intraconal area. The posterior part of intraconal area has a high arterial density with the addition of some venous drainage system from retina. Considering the arteries and veins as common entity, the posterior orbit on its lateral side has the greatest vascular constellation, whereas in the anterior orbit most of the vessels are found medially.

Arteries

There is much variability between individual to individual, regarding the anatomical layout of orbital arterial system. The orbital arterial system predominantly consists of *ophthalmic artery* which is the branch of the *internal carotid artery.* There are also variations in the contributions of supplying orbital arterial system from *external carotid artery*.

The ophthalmic artery arises from the internal carotid artery when this vessel (internal carotid artery) emerges from the cavernous sinus, medial to the anterior clinoid process. Then, the ophthalmic artery enters the orbit through the optic canal, lying inferolateral to optic nerve and here both of them lie in a common sheath of dura. In the orbit, it pierces out of the dura mater, and winds around the lateral side of the optic nerve and then passes forward and medially above it, but below the ciliary ganglion (in 80%) between the superior ophthalmic vein in front and the nasociliary nerve behind. In 20% cases, the ophthalmic artery does not pass above the optic nerve, rather lies underneath the optic nerve which is the more vulnerable position of it for injury by needle, directed toward the orbital apex during local block **(Fig. 25)**.

When the ophthalmic artery lies below the optic nerve, then it gives off its first branch, called the *central retinal artery.* It pierces the dural sheath of optic nerve, usually from its inferomedial aspect and 1–2.5 cm posterior to the globe, to reach the center of the optic nerve. This tiny vital artery then runs forward within the core of the optic nerve and emerges at optic disk where it divides into multiple retinal arteries, supplying the retina. When the ophthalmic artery turns around and reaches above the optic nerve, then it gives off the second branch, named the *lacrimal artery.* The lacrimal artery passes forward along the upper border of the lateral rectus muscle and terminates as *superior and inferior lateral palpebral arteries* for the upper and lower eyelid, respectively. These superior and inferior lateral palpebral arteries anastomose with the superior and inferior medial

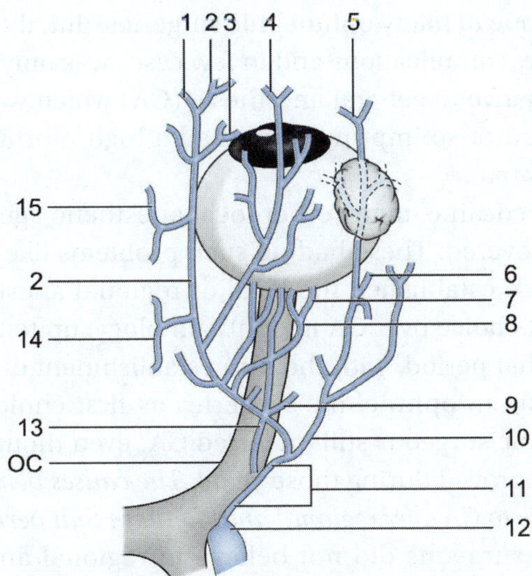

Fig. 25: Arterial supply within orbit. (1: dorsal nasal artery; 2: supratrochlear artery; 3: medial palpebral artery; 4: supraorbital artery; 5: lateral palpebral branch; 6: zygomatic branch; 7: long and short posterior arteries; 8: muscular branch of lacrimal artery; 9: muscular branches of ophthalmic artery; 10: lacrimal artery; 11: ophthalmic artery; 12: internal carotid artery; OC: optic canal; 13: central retinal artery; 14: posterior ethmoidal artery; 15: anterior ethmoidal artery)

palpebral arteries. In its course, the lacrimal artery gives of multiple branches such as the muscular, zygomatic, and recurrent meningeal arteries and branches to the lacrimal gland. The recurrent meningeal branch passes back through the superior orbital fissure, and anastomoses with the middle meningeal artery.

When the ophthalmic artery turns nasally above the optic nerve, it gives off some muscular branches to the rectus muscles, and the *long and short posterior ciliary arteries.* These long and short posterior ciliary arteries enter the globe after piercing the sclera in association with the long and short ciliary nerves, close to optic nerve. The long posterior ciliary arteries usually are two in number. They course forward within the globe, deep to sclera and supply the anterior part of uveal tract. The multiple short posterior ciliary arteries also pierce the sclera like the long posterior ciliary artery, and supply the choroidal coat of the eye and the ciliary body. The *anterior ciliary arteries* arise from the different muscular arterial branches, and enter the globe close to limbus. They supply the anterior parts of the uveal tract.

The ophthalmic artery then reaches the medial wall of the orbit and passes forward along this wall between the medial rectus and the superior oblique muscles. At the medial end of the upper eyelid, the ophthalmic artery divides into two terminal branches, which are named as the *supratrochlear* (sometimes called the frontal artery), and

dorsal nasal artery. After the ciliary arteries are given off, when the ophthalmic artery touches the medial wall of the orbit, it gives off a branch, named the *supraorbital artery.* This branch courses forward with the nerves of same name. After the supraorbital artery, the ophthalmic artery while passing along the medial wall of the orbit, gives off the following branches—*posterior ethmoidal artery, anterior ethmoidal artery, and the superior and inferior medial palpebral artery.* The anterior and posterior ethmoidal arteries, as they exit through their respective foramina, anchor the ophthalmic artery to the medial wall of orbit.

During regional anesthesia, any needle should not be introduced into this posterior 1.5 cm from the orbital apex. This is because the large vessels are located there which may be the potential sources of any vision-threatening bleeding. This area also contains vital structures, such as the optic nerve and the origins of extraocular muscle which are tightly packed there and may be subjected to any serious damage due to any bleeding or due to direct injury from needle tip.

There are, however, three adipose tissue compartments in the anterior and midorbital area, which are relatively avascular and are so the preferred sites for local anesthetic injection. These compartments are: the *inferotemporal, superotemporal, and medial.* The superotemporal space extends from the sagittal plane of lateral limbus, close to the roof and about 3 cm behind the orbital rim. In the medial space the needle entry point should be at the extreme medial end of the palpebral fissure on the nasal side of the caruncle. The needle should be directed up to the maximum distance of 2.5 cm in transverse plane and 5° medial to the direct sagittal plane. *The superonasal quadrant should be avoided as an injection site,* because it contains the end arteries of ophthalmic artery, a large venous connection between the facial angular vein and the superior orbital vein, and the trochlear mechanism of superior oblique muscle. The transconjunctival injection is less likely to produce significant ecchymosis in comparison to transcutaneous route.

Veins

The two principal veins that drain the blood from eyeball and other orbital structures are—(1) *the superior ophthalmic vein* and (2) *the inferior ophthalmic vein.* Among these two, the former is the most constant structure. The superior ophthalmic vein is formed by the *confluence of the major tributaries of the superior orbital vein, supratrochlear vein and the angular facial vein.* The angular facial vein descends lateral to the nose, with the angular artery. It is subcutaneous and is often visible as a blue ridge, until it pierces the orbicularis oculi muscle. This vein complicates the surgical approaches to the lacrimal sac. It (the angular vein) is continuous with the facial vein and communicates freely with the cavernous sinus through the superior ophthalmic vein.

After its formation, the *superior ophthalmic vein* runs backward along the medial boarder of the superior rectus muscle, from where it enters the intraconal space. Within the conal space, it runs further backward and laterally in a hammock-like structure of the connective tissue septa which is suspended under the superior rectus muscle, between it (superior rectus muscle) and the optic nerve. It (superior ophthalmic vein) again exits the intraconal space at the lateral border of the superior rectus muscle. Here, it runs backward in the direction of the superior orbital fissure, through which it gains access to the cavernous sinus above the annulus. During its course, it (superior ophthalmic vein) accompanies the ophthalmic artery and receives the tributaries that correspond with the branches of the accompanying artery.

The *inferior ophthalmic vein* which is also called the inferior orbital vein begins at the floor of the orbit and collects the blood from the inferior orbital muscles, lacrimal sac, and lower eyelid. It drains in the cavernous sinus either directly or after joining with the superior ophthalmic vein. It communicates with the pterygoid venous plexus through the inferior orbital fissure.

The other veins of the orbit and globe are the—vortex vein, central retinal vein, middle ophthalmic vein, and medial ophthalmic vein. The vortex veins are usually four or more in number. The superomedial vortex veins drain into the first part of the superior ophthalmic vein; while the superolateral vortex veins enter its third part. The inferior vortex veins join to form the inferior venous plexus. The central retinal vein leaves the optic sheath and joins the network of venules from the sheath. It drains usually in the superior ophthalmic vein. The middle ophthalmic vein arises near the lateral side of the medial rectus. It drains in the inferior venous network and joins the confluence of the superior ophthalmic vein with the cavernous sinus.

◼ REGIONAL VERSUS GENERAL ANESTHESIA

The term *"regional anesthesia* (RA)*"* signifies the conduction block of a *specific nerve or a group of nerves* of a region by local anesthetic agents. Whereas, the term *"local anesthesia"* should be restricted to the technique of infiltration of local anesthetic agent in *an area of local tissue* resulting in the blockade of only the *nerve endings in that area*. On the other hand, the term *"topical anesthesia"* implies to the action of local anesthetic agents, when it is applied on the surface of an epithelial tissue.

After the discovery of cocaine, as a local anesthetic agent, the topical and regional anesthesia had become the cornerstone of many ophthalmic surgeries. But, the cocaine had many complications and in few cases was only taken as an alternative to general anesthesia (GA) which was at that time also not so improved and had a high morbidity and mortality rate.

After cocaine, many other local anesthetic agents were also discovered. These had no such problems like cocaine, and hence established the local or regional anesthesia as their first choice over GA in ophthalmology, up to the 1950. During that period, with the firm establishment of regional anesthesia in ophthalmic surgeries as first choice, some ophthalmic surgeons still preferred GA, even though it was not so improved during those years. *The causes behind their preference to GA over regional anesthesia in that period are—* (i) some surgeons did not believe in regional anesthesia as the local anesthetic agents had just been developed, (ii) some surgeons were not mentally prepared to wait for the local anesthetic agent to act, (iii) some surgeons thought that postoperative results were better with GA than RA, and (iv) simply, some surgeons did not like to operate on a conscious patient.

Then, in between 1950 and 1960, a swing back to GA from regional anesthesia for most of the ophthalmic surgeries had again occurred. This is because, during that period, improved anesthetic drugs, machines, and techniques for GA became available. During that period, surgeons were also comfortable to perform ophthalmic surgeries under GA, as the ophthalmic surgical techniques were not so improved, matching with the regional anesthesia and surgical complication rates were high under RA. But, in the last part of that century and over the last two decades, regional anesthesia has again been supplanting GA for many ophthalmic surgical procedures. This is because the surgical techniques were improved with the help of modern surgical equipment of higher technology. Thus, the average surgical time for cataract extraction and other complicated surgical procedures has markedly decreased and this may be one of the causes for preferring regional anesthesia over GA, recently. This surgical improvement, in combination with the efficient scheduling of operation time and the predominant use of out-patient surgical facilities has made a high volume of patients-turnover possible. So, this form of practice again dictates itself to the regional anesthesia techniques, prohibiting GA, for most of the ophthalmic surgeries, except in certain special cases.

Stress of patients is a common and almost unavoidable factor, during the *perioperative period* of ophthalmic surgeries, performed *under RA*. It is associated with the release of catecholamines, cortisol and glucose in circulation, and this is evidenced by the signs of tachycardia, hypertension and elevated blood glucose level. The increased plasma level of catecholamines in patients, undergoing ophthalmic surgery under RA, resulted primarily from the *endogenous sources* and sometimes secondarily (less important) from the *exogenous sources.* It is found that, as an exogenous source, the 10 mL of local anesthetic solution containing 1:200,000 epinephrine (5 µg/mL) causes no untoward clinical effect. It is also found that the entry of a patient into operating area for regional anesthesia is the most significant stress factor than the performance of block (RA) itself.

So, for the perioperative management of a patient, who is scheduled for ophthalmic surgery under RA, *adequate counseling* during the first meeting of him (patient) with a hospital personal is extremely important for the successful attenuation of this stress. This can be *performed efficiently* by repeated reassurance, preoperative visit with an anesthetist, booklet, video, tape, etc. Many patients appreciate music as their distraction, before giving block. The simple act of a staff member, i.e., holding the hand of a patient during regional anesthesia and surgery, has a considerable calming effect. In extreme cases, judicious use of benzodiazepine (midazolam) orally or intravenously may be useful to reduce this stress response. But, in an ambulatory setting (day case surgery) the use of preoperative sedative medications should be such that it allows the patients to be discharged promptly after the completion of surgery **(Box 1)**.

For a small percentage of elderly patients, who are benefited from preoperative sedation, fine judgment is required to select the correct drug and dosage of any sedative agent which are to produce only the calming effect, but the patient will remain alert and cooperative without any respiratory depression. The advantages of regional anesthesia over GA can be negated rapidly with the excessive use of sedation. The combination of regional anesthesia with heavy sedation may produce a less satisfactory outcome than the either methods on their own.

The time, spent by an anesthetist for establishing a good rapport with the patient, is more effective in removing anxiety than depending on the pharmacological methods. To perform regional anesthesia efficiently and successfully, anesthetist must have certain personality traits and good communication skills. This enables him or her to gain the trust of patients rapidly. This will also educate the patients, regarding the experiences that they have to face during operation. Thus, properly treated and prepared patients, scheduled for ophthalmic surgery under RA, will have a minimal anxiety and have a low incidence of perioperative complications. Sometimes, the absence of such a skill in an anesthetist may force him to take the decision in favor of GA.

There is also of a widespread opinion that patients do better under regional anesthesia than GA. But, scientifically it is very hard to prove, except in some specific cases. Multiple, major, retrospective, and prospective non-randomized studies have failed to favor one method of anesthesia over the other. On the other hand, the cataract surgeries which constitute the main bulk of ophthalmic surgeries are more frequently performed on the elderly patients. The more elderly a patient, the higher is the intrinsic risk of death. This should be added to the risk of death which is associated with clinical intervention. The elderly patients are associated with multiple systemic diseases, such as hypertension, coronary arterial disease, chronic obstructive pulmonary disease (COPD), diabetes mellitus, obesity, etc. These are also added to the operative risk and present additional challenges to the operating team, mainly anesthetist. It is also demonstrated that the rate of complications correlates well with the number of associated diseases, rather than the age of the patient.

All the patients, scheduled for ophthalmic surgery under GA or RA, require proper preoperative assessment and preparation. They also need an open discussion regarding the risks and complications of anesthesia and surgery which is based on a thorough history and physical examination. The whole system requires cooperation among the patients, their relatives, their family doctors, surgeons, and anesthetists. A list of medications, currently taken by the patients is also required. Because, it ensures that essential therapy can be continued through the time of surgery and potential drug interaction can also be anticipated. Necessary preoperative

---

BOX 1: Respective advantages of regional and general anesthesia (GA). Advantages of one type of anesthesia are the disadvantages for another type and vice versa.

- *Regional anesthesia (RA):*
  - Simple technique
  - Early recovery
  - Less hospital stay
  - Early discharge
  - Quick turnover
  - Less expensive
  - Better postoperative analgesia
  - Avoidance of oculocardiac reflex
  - No loss of control of patient
  - Less physiological change
  - Absence of respiratory depression
  - Full mental status retained
  - No risk of malignant hyperthermia
- *General anesthesia:*
  - Complete control of patient
  - Risk of globe perforation is nil
  - Risk of intraorbital hemorrhage is nil
  - Risks of myotoxicity, nerve injury are nil
  - Risk of allergy to local anesthetic agent is nil
  - Applicable to all ages
  - Preferable for teaching of surgery methods for trainees

laboratory and radiological investigations should be done, only when these are indicated, and appropriate for that particular patient or according to American Society of Anesthesiologists (ASA) guidelines. Whatever is the method of anesthesia, regional or general, every effort should be made to have the patients in best possible medical condition prior to surgery. Most ophthalmic surgeries are nonemergency. Therefore, the date of surgery should usually be postponed, until the medical status of each patient becomes optimal.

The decision, whether general or regional anesthesia should be selected, is based on the consensus among the team members who are involved in this surgery and anesthesia, including the patient. The choice of anesthetic technique is usually predicted by the team's previous experience for that type of surgery on a particular group of patient in that institution (**Box 2**).

Whether regional anesthesia or GA, the skill of application of the anesthetic technique is more important for patient's morbidity and mortality than any academic discussion of the merits or demerits of these two anesthetic techniques, i.e., regional anesthesia and GA. However, a high standard perioperative monitoring and anesthetic skill must be maintained for both the forms of anesthesia. Usually, it is a common practice to select sick patients for RA, because they are unfit for GA. But, it should be kept in mind that regional anesthesia should be an alternative to GA for the more fit and healthy patients, and regional anesthesia should always not be considered as an alternative means of anesthesia for operating on unfit patients. This is because unfit patients do not cooperate well, even under regional anesthesia for prolonged periods. Thus, the tragedy is that the patients who are unfit for GA cannot be selected under RA, and vice-versa.

Before selecting the patients for GA, few things can be tried or followed which may help to perform surgery under regional anesthesia instead of GA. For example, in the management of patients with mild to moderate degrees of senile dementia or mental retardation, who are presented for ophthalmic surgeries under RA, a family member can hold hands with the patient and give verbal support in the operating room. It also acts in same fashion in the presence of any language barrier, where communication with the patient becomes impossible which results in the choice of GA. In such situations, a family member can be recruited to interpret the language.

When a patient with slight tremor of head is scheduled for ophthalmic surgery under RA, then intravenous sedation in titrable doses can control this Parkinsonian head tremor effectively. Incomplete block can be best managed by further supplementation of anesthetic drug. Because operation in the presence of partial regional anesthesia or block failure

BOX 2: Contraindication to RA and GA with decreasing order of importance from absolute contraindication at the top of the table. Contraindications of RA are indications to GA and vice versa.

- *Contraindications for RA:*
  - Refusal of informed consent by the patient
  - Surgeon preference for GA
  - Surgery on open eye injury
  - Prolonged surgery (>2 hours)
  - Children up to the age of early teens
  - Unsuitable psychological status:
    - Psychiatric disorders
    - Uncooperative patient
  - Mental retardation
  - Senile dementia
  - Communication barrier:
    - Language
    - Deafness
  - Head tremor or movement:
    - Parkinsonism
    - Tardive dyskinesia
  - Inability to lie flat:
    - Severe arthritis
    - Respiratory diseases
    - Cardiac diseases
  - Claustrophobia
  - Previous complication from RA
  - High myopia
  - Inexperience of anesthetist on RA
  - True allergy to local anesthetic agent
  - Patients on anticoagulants
  - Needle phobia
  - Intractable cough
- *Contraindications for GA:*
  - Refusal of informed consent by the patient
  - Severe medical condition, ASA III or IV
  - History of difficult airway
  - History of serious adverse effect from previous GA
  - History of malignant hyperthermia
  - Muscle diseases:
    - Dystrophia myotonica
    - Myasthenia gravis
  - Hemoglobinopathies
  - COPD
  - History of porphyria
  - History of atypical pseudocholinesterase

(COPD: chronic obstructive pulmonary disease; GA: general anesthesia; RA: regional anesthesia)

puts the patients in a severe unpleasant and stressful experience. Use of IV sedation which is not up to the level of GA and is used to cover the block failure or partial block is hazardous and inappropriate. In such situations, full GA with all precautions and monitoring should be the real answer.

In the past, when the ophthalmic surgeries were performed under conventional GA, then it was the traditional domain of an anesthetist, while the local regional block was the domain of an ophthalmologist. The ophthalmologists were also considerably reluctant to permit anesthetists to perform the orbital regional anesthesia. This is because; they believed that only the physicians of their own discipline had the necessary elaborate anatomical and technical knowledge to avoid serious ophthalmic complications during regional block. But, for the last two decades, a change has been under way, due to many reported or unreported deaths, during regional anesthesia by ophthalmologists. So, at present in many developed and under developed countries, the idea to improve the care of patient, by increasing the involvement of an anesthetist, including the administration of regional block by them, has been given official sanction.

The various commonly used methods of regional anesthesia for ophthalmic surgeries are all completely blind procedures. So, multiple serious complications have been reported, following regional anesthesia by efficient persons of both the disciplines (surgeon and anesthetist). It does not depend on the person of any particular discipline who is administering the block. It depends on the good knowledge of the anatomy of orbit and anesthetic technique. On the other hand, there is an obvious added disadvantage when an ophthalmic surgeon act both as an anesthetist and surgeon together, with giving a complete attention to patient's medical condition during surgery under RA, especially in the absence of an anesthetist who can continuously monitor the patient. He can never give his undivided attention to the general condition of a patient which an anesthetist can. Moreover, in the event of an emergency and serious cardiopulmonary complication, anesthetists are more familiar with these complications and can perform better and more efficient cardiopulmonary resuscitative measures can be taken than their surgical colleagues. There is also no inherent reason why an anesthetist who is proficient in various regional anesthesia outside the orbit should not become efficient in ophthalmic cases, too.

TECHNIQUES OF REGIONAL ANESTHESIA FOR OPHTHALMIC SURGERIES

History of Ophthalmic Anesthesia

The history of anesthesia for ophthalmic surgery dates back to over 2,500 years from present date. The earliest authentic writings on this subject were those of *Susruta* who was an ancient Indian surgeon. He first described cataract surgery by couching, around 600 BC. Couching is nothing but pushing back the lens into the vitreous cavity by a blunt pressure on eyeball. He also outlined the use of inhalational anesthesia for this method, but the name of this inhalational agent was not known and also described aseptic techniques. Later, Egyptian and Assyrian surgeons had

described the use of *carotid artery compression* to produce the transient unconsciousness by cerebral ischemia, under which couching was performed. In the first century of AD, *Dioscorides* had produced a soporific sponge from an extract of mandrake, boiled in wine, and was used to produce unconsciousness.

After that, 1,200 years had passed without any advancement in the science of ophthalmic surgery and anesthesia. Then, in 13th century, a Spanish alchemist had described a liquid which was produced by the mixture of sulfuric acid and alcohol to make the patient unconscious, after inhalation of this liquid. He called this mixture as *"sweet vitriol"*. But, in 1730, this substance was renamed as *ether*. However, during this period, nobody except this alchemist knew the anesthetic property of this compound. In 1818, Faraday had discovered its anesthetic effects accidentally. Up to that period, all the ophthalmic surgeries, mainly the cataract were done under GA, produced by the excessive consumption of alcohol, opium, etc. In 1855, *Gaedcke* had first extracted crude alkaloid from the leaves of cocoa plant. Then, 5 years later, it was purified and named as *cocaine* by *Niemann*. He noted that cocaine numbed the nerves of tongue and deprived it from the feeling of taste. Then, 25 years later, in 1884, *Koller* in collaboration with *Sigmund Freud* had first used cocaine, as the topical anesthetic agent, for minor surgeries only on conjunctiva. However, News of this discovery rapidly spread across the whole world. Then, in New York City an ophthalmologist, named *Dr Herman Knapp* had used cocaine in all the type of ophthalmic surgeries, by injecting it into the orbital cavity and published his work in December of same year. This publication also included his own work on retrobulbar injection of cocaine. He had done this for the painless enucleation of an eyeball. But, subsequently serious toxic effects and death were experienced by the other surgeons with the use of cocaine which was injected in large doses into the orbital cavity for nerve blocks, particularly in general surgery. This had deterred other ophthalmologists from using cocaine for regional anesthesia in ophthalmic surgeries, until well up to the 20th century. But, topical anesthesia using cocaine continued, apparently successfully, for minor conjunctival surgical procedures and all the other ophthalmic surgeries were done under GA.

During the early part of twentieth century, adrenaline (in 1901) and procaine (in 1905) were discovered. After that, various and much safer regional anesthetic techniques *were developed in general surgery* which was accomplished with larger doses of local anesthetic agents, other than cocaine. But, unfortunately this was not introduced into ophthalmological practice for many years. Then, in 1914,

Van Lint had first reported his classical facial nerve block technique, using procaine. This (facial nerve block) removed the problem of suddenly high rise of intraocular pressure (IOP) by the forceful contraction of orbicularis oculi muscle, during ophthalmic surgery. This akinesia (paralysis) of facial muscles were commonly used, as an adjuvant to *topical anesthesia* for corneal and conjunctival surgeries and was in routine practice, until 1930. Later, *retrobulbar techniques* in conjunction with the facial nerve block for ophthalmic regional anesthesia, using procaine, became wide spread instead of topical ophthalmic anesthesia. Although, this retrobulbar block, using cocaine as local anesthetic agent, was first done in 1884 by Knapp, but he *failed to popularize* this method, until 1930.

From 1934 to 1964, *Atkinson* published many articles on regional anesthesia for ophthalmic surgeries. At this time, hyaluronidase was not available. He used only procaine and adrenaline. In 1936, he convinced all the ophthalmologists that for the best results, the injection should be given within the muscle cone and just posterior to the globe. Atkinson also advocated that the *inferotemporal quadrant* is relatively avascular and the safe route for the introduction of needle into the orbit for regional block. During his period, many other persons such as *Lowenstein, Swan, Gifford,* and *O'Brien* also worked on this retrobulbar (intraconal) block by using procaine with different size, length, and position of needle and also with the different volume of local anesthetic drugs. Then came the peribulbar method which was also described long ago, in 1914, by Allen. But, this technique did not come into common ophthalmic practice, until 1986.

The whole scenario of this ophthalmic regional anesthesia practice was changed dramatically, after the synthesis of *lignocaine* by Lofgren and Lundqvist, in 1943, and after the introduction of hyaluronidase around 1956. Lignocaine was first used clinically, after its synthesis by Gordh, in 1947. Then, with the introduction of *mepivacaine*, in 1957, and *bupivacaine,* in 1963, the stage was rightly set for dependable clinical ophthalmic regional anesthesia practice to cover a wide range of ophthalmic surgical procedures and to provide a greatly improved postoperative analgesia.

Practical Management and Patient Preparation for Regional Anesthesia

An anesthetist, who is totally, devoting his practice on ophthalmic regional anesthesia, should have a thorough knowledge regarding—(i) the anatomy of the orbit and eyeball, (ii) the physiology of eye, and (iii) the pharmacology of the ocular and local anesthetic drugs. It will enormously help him to prevent any criticism and opposition from any ophthalmologist, during any complication which may occur, during the administration of RA. The anesthetist, who also wants to engage himself in this type of work, is always encouraged to meet (visit) and to observe the work, performed in some highly specialized ophthalmic centers, operated by qualified personnel (anesthetists) with wide experience and vast knowledge on this subject. The goal of each such practitioner (ophthalmic anesthetist) is to build up an experimental database by himself, from which later increasingly good judgment may result.

During ophthalmic operations, the required anesthetic technique (RA or GA) is mainly dictated by the—(i) the type of surgery, (ii) the surgeon's particular preference to the type of anesthesia for that surgery, and (iii) the wishes of patient. So, a good understanding between the anesthetist and the ophthalmologist's preference, to the type of anesthesia for this surgery, is essential. For example, some surgeons quarrel for complete akinesia, while some surgeons do not want complete akinesia during cataract extraction. Again, it is not absolutely necessary or desirable in all such (cataract extraction) cases. The achievement of complete akinesia demands a higher volume of injected local anesthetic agent, which may increase the intraorbital and subsequently the intraoccular pressure. This may also be of great disadvantage to some surgeons. Again, most surgeons may prefer globe hypotony during cataract extraction. But, some surgeons may not prefer it and there may be certain situations where this becomes undesirable.

On the other hand, ophthalmic surgeons who are operating under regional anesthesia must know how to deal with an awaked patient on an operating table. It is unwise for an ophthalmic surgeon to ask repeatedly whether the patient is feeling pain or not. If the achievement of complete motor akinesia (paralysis) is used as the yard stick of effectiveness of block, then pain will not be experienced. This is because motor fibers are blocked only after the block of sensory fibers. In such situations, the appreciation of touch and tissue movement by the patient (proprioceptive sensation) may be interpreted wrongly as pain in nervous patients.

If the local anesthesia is not adequate, then it is usually not difficult to recognize it (patient is getting pain) by an anesthetist. But, if it is not, i.e., when the block is very good and the patient is not getting pain, and then it is a very bad practice to take suggestion from the patient. Again, it will make the patient feel that the surgeon does not have the required confidence on the surgery and anesthesia. The surgeon, who knows better and trusts a carefully selected anesthetic team by himself, should start the operation without any confusion. At the same time, he should be aware of any significant nonverbal responses from the side of patient, due to pain.

Most of the patients presenting for ophthalmic surgery are at the extremes of age. Again, the majority of eye surgeries consist of cataract extraction and they are performed as day-cases under local or topical anesthesia. As most of the patients are elderly, so they have many serious systemic diseases. Hence, the preoperative assessment and the preoperative preparation of patient, undergoing ophthalmic surgery under regional anesthesia, is same as that of GA. On the other hand, in many centers, the patients undergoing cataract extraction under regional anesthesia do not warrant routine investigations. But, more stress is given on the psychological aspect of the patients for preoperative preparation. All the patients should receive a careful explanation of the anesthetic and surgical procedure that lies ahead on the day of surgery.

Whatever may be the type of surgery and anesthesia (even topical), an informed consent from every patient is mandatory. During the period of preanesthetic examination, preparation, and taking consent, the patients should be given the opportunity to ask questions and to receive answers, regarding the anesthetic and surgical procedure. Routine premedication may or may not be indicated in all the cases. Care should be taken during the application of sedative premedication on very elderly patients. Oral sedation may produce pleasure in some patients, but some may complain of vertigo and dislike it. But, as a whole, the use of short acting oral benzodiazepines, as premedication, is beneficial for most of the patients.

The preoperative fasting protocol for regional anesthesia (RA) is similar to that of GA. Clear fluid may be given 3 hours before sending the patient to anesthesia room. But, some clinics or hospitals maintain their own fasting protocol for regional anesthesia, required for ophthalmic surgeries. They do not routinely make starve such patients and provide a light meal 2–3 hours before operation, thinking that it is less disruptive (trouble producing) for the elderly population and also facilitates better diabetic control. Regular medications, taken by the patients during the preoperative period, should be continued up to and also on the day of surgery, including antihypertensives, antidiabetics, anticoagulants, anti-inflamatory, antiasthamatic drugs, etc. Prophylactic antibiotic are generally not considered necessary for patients with cardiac lesions, undergoing routine anterior chamber (cataract) surgery. In patients receiving anticoagulant therapy, international normalized ratio (INR) should be kept <2.5. Whenever required, the anticoagulant therapy should be adjusted to reduce the INR <2.5. If this is considered inappropriate, e.g., in patients with artificial heart valve, then the relative risks of GA must be considered. An alternative option is to use sub-Tenon's approach or just topical anesthesia.

Preoperatively, the axial length of an eyeball should always be measured in all cases. In severe myopic patients (axial length >26 mm) the globe often has a long anteroposterior diameter (sausage-shaped eyeball). This increases the likelihood of globe perforation during regional anesthesia which is diagnosed by—(i) sudden pain during injection, (ii) loss of vision, (iii) poor red reflex, or (iv) vitreous hemorrhage. So, where the axial length is >26 mm, then a single medial canthus injection, sub-Tenon's approach, topical anesthesia or GA should be considered. Hearing aids and dentures in patients are left in place during RA.

It is a very good practice to set up a venous line routinely for all patients. Though, it is not a part of a planned routine intravenous therapy, but will be helpful in the event of an unplanned emergency intervention, calling for intravenous therapy. Good record keeping of every patient is essential. This includes medical history, the health status of patient, the type and length of surgical procedure, surgical complications, anesthetic procedure, and patient's reaction to it, etc. Anesthetic record will include—the name of used anesthetic drugs, its volume, its concentration, sites of injection, increased intraorbital pressure due to injection, decompression procedures, etc.

The parameters of all the vital signs of patient should also be measured and recorded. A full proof system for the checking of all the drugs and equipment in anesthetic room and operating theater is essential. It will help to avoid dangerous errors and damage to the patients, particularly during emergency. It will also help in the smooth and safe functioning of whole unit in operating suit. Personal or self-confidence of an anesthetist is also acquired with the repeated use (performance) of different regional anesthetic techniques and tackling their complications. This inturn will help the patients to be more stable, reassured, and less dependent on sedative premedicant drugs.

The history of claustrophobia is also very important. Because, many patients undergoing ophthalmic surgery are covered to some degree with surgical drapes which encroach on their nose and face. In such circumstances, alternative draping techniques or light intravenous sedation will be helpful. In extreme situations, good sedation or GA is indicated.

No patient should be left unattended in anesthesia room and OT. The engagement of all patients with light conversation by both the anesthetist and surgeon during both the administration of anesthesia and surgery is considered a good practice. Patients should be encouraged to express any difficulties on their part. By doing so, they act as their own monitor and are more reliable than any electronic gadget. While a surgeon is working with a particular patient, then conversation with a staff or an anesthetist or with another surgeon regarding other patients is inappropriate. This is because operating patient thought that he or she is not getting proper attention, as they are under RA.

Most of the patients undergoing ophthalmic surgery are elderly. They are frequently suffering from arthritis, spondylitis, kyphosis, osteoporosis, etc., which are sometimes painful. So, it is frequently impossible for them to accommodate on the especially made ophthalmic operating table for prolonged period which have little or no head rest. Hence, the intraoperative posture of a patient is very important for RA. Ophthalmic surgeons usually prefer the patient's head in a horizontal plane under the microscope. But, the peculiar ophthalmic table with little or no head rest makes it difficult for elderly patients to accommodate their head in this horizontal plane. This can be achieved by necessary number of pillows under the occiput on OT table.

Types of Surgeries which can be Undertaken under Regional Anesthesia

Usually, the type of surgery is not an important factor for the selection of regional or GA. Any type of surgery, except a few, can be performed under any type of anesthesia. But, most of the ophthalmic surgeries are performed under RA, except a few where intraorbital injection is contraindicated or topical cornea-conjunctival anesthesia is not appropriate, or regional anesthesia cannot be provided due to patients health factors such as ASA III and ASA IV group of patients. The regional anesthesia is also not applicable for ophthalmic surgeries in pediatric, psychiatric, cerebral palsy group of patients, etc., whose long list are enumerated in **Boxes 1 and 2**.

The long lists of surgeries which can be performed safely using regional anesthesia are—cataract extraction with or without intraocular lens implantation, corneal transplantations, trabeculectomy, strabismus repair, lid surgeries, oculoplastic surgeries, vitreoretinal surgeries, etc. But the main limitation of regional anesthesia is its fixed time frame. The duration of operations, extending beyond 2–2.5 hours, tend to be rather difficult under RA. This difficulty is more applicable for conscious elderly patients who have cervical spondylosis or increased frequency of micturition due to enlarged prostate, or any other cause for which he is unable to lie supine for prolonged period.

For regional anesthesia a wide range of local anesthetic drugs are now available, with which the duration of safe therapeutic time-window usually can be predictably planned. For example, 10 mL of 2% lignocaine with 1:200,000 adrenaline and 7.5 turbidity units of hyaluronidase per mL will produce a dependable 60–90 minutes of therapeutic

time-window for complete akinesia. For surgical procedures, lasting for 2–3 hours, such as vitreoretinal surgeries, long acting agents such as bupivacaine, ropivacaine, and etidocaine should be the agent of choice. Because, both of these agents produce a therapeutic time-window for about 2–3 hours.

Retrobulbar or Intraconal Block

"Retrobulbar" or "intraconal" are two clinically interchangeable words, because both usually signify the same space. But the *'retrobulbar'* is a more vague term, as it indicates the any space with in the orbit, but behind the globe (or bulb) and may not be within the geometric confines of four rectus muscles. Whereas, the term *intraconal block* exactly signifies that the needle tip and the injection placement is within that space which is confined by the four rectus muscles. On the other hand, when the needle tip is placed and the local anesthetic agent is deposited within the orbit, but not within the geometric cone formed of four rectus muscles, then it is called as the *peribulbar or periconal or periocular block*. This peribulbar block may be posterior or anterior to the equator of globe. When the peribulbar block is placed posterior to the equator of globe, then it is called as the *posterior peribulbar or periconal block* and when the peribulbar block is placed anterior to the equator of globe, then it is called as the *anterior peribulbar block*. The intraconal area is always posterior to the globe. So, there is no need to mention the word "posterior" during its use, i.e., the word "posterior retrobulbar" is never used. On the contrary, during the use of name "peribulbar" we can fix the word posterior with it ("posterior peribulbar"), as there is also a peribulbar space anterior to the equator of globe **(Fig. 26)**.

Contents of intraconal and extraconal compartment are enumerated in **Box 3**. During the intraconal or retrobulbar block, a straight needle with different lengths and sizes (discussed later), mounted on a syringe containing the chosen anesthetic mixture, is introduced within the orbit either transconjunctivally or transcutaneously. This site for the introduction of needle is through the inferotemporal quadrant of orbit which commences at the junction of lateral one-third and medial two-thirds of inferior orbital margin. The safety of this retrobulbar block mainly depends on the proximity of the needle tip to the orbital wall at the time of first entry and until the globe equator is passed. Initially, the inferotemporal orbital margin is palpated by the finger of left hand (for right handed person) and its (finger) relationship to the globe is noted, including the orientation of the equator of globe with the lateral orbital margin.

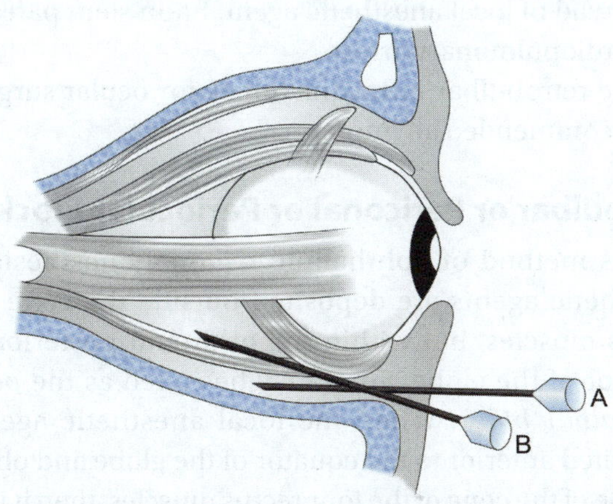

Fig. 26: Transcutaneous approach of intraconal block through inferotemporal space. In position A, the path of the needle is followed close to the orbital floor, until the equator of globe is crossed. Then, in position B the angle of direction of the movement of needle is changed upward and medially, and is advanced to enter the intraconal space, posterior to globe.

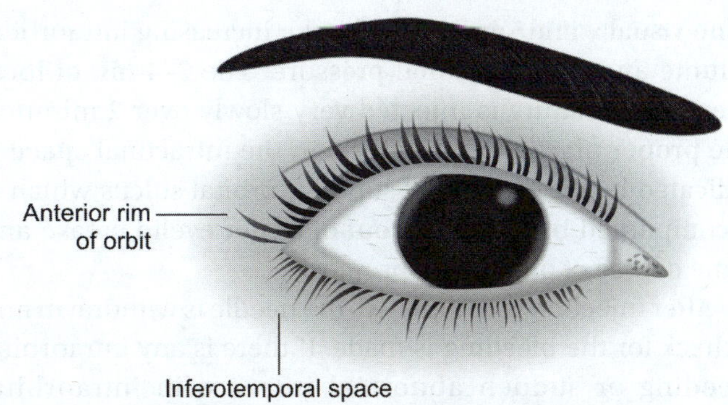

Fig. 27: The inferotemporal space which is wide and recommended for the entry site of needle for regional block.

> **BOX 3:** Contents of intraconal and extraconal compartment.
>
> - Contents of intraconal compartment:
>   - Fat
>   - Cranial nerves—optic nerve, oculomotor nerve and its branches, and abducent nerve
>   - Nasociliary branch of ophthalmic nerve
>   - Ciliary ganglion
>   - Ophthalmic artery
> - Contents of extraconal compartment:
>   - Fat
>   - Cranial nerves—trochlear nerve, lacrimal and frontal branch of ophthalmic nerve
>   - Lacrimal gland

When the *transconjunctival route* is chosen for this retrobulbar block through the inferotemporal quadrant, then the tip of the needle enters the orbit just behind the lower tarsal plate at inferior orbital rim. But, if the *transcutaneous route* is used, then the lower lid is not retracted and the needle entry point would be inferior to the lower tarsal plate. The needle runs first parallel and close to the orbital floor with slight medial direction. In this direction when the needle tip crosses the equator of the globe, then the angle of the direction of this needle tip is adjusted upward, medially, and posteriorly, as if the tip enters the cone of four rectus muscles, posterior to the globe. After crossing the equator, for this direction, the needle tip should be aimed at an imaginary point behind the globe on the axis, formed by the center of the pupil and the macula in primary gaze position. During this advancement of needle in retrobulbar space, great care should also be taken to avoid crossing the midsagittal plane

of globe. During either transconjunctival or transcutaneous route, the tip of the needle should always run inferior to the lower border of the lateral rectus muscle, till it crosses the equator of the globe. During this advancement of needle, the globe should also be observed continuously to detect any rotation or movement that may indicate the fixation of needle tip into sclera **(Fig. 27)**.

The needle then enters the intraconal space by piercing the intermuscular septum, just inferior to the lower border of the lateral rectus muscle. During the advancement of needle, the continuous observation of the relationship between the shaft and the hub junction of needle and the plane of iris usually establishes an appropriate depth of insertion of needle within the orbit.

The inferotemporal space for retrobulbar or peribulbar block is chosen for three reasons because:

- It is relatively most avascular. The other two low vascular areas are superotemporal and medial compartment.
- The lateral orbital rim is set back from the line of the equator of globe at the inferotemporal region.
- The space between the globe and orbital rim for the placement of needle in deeper orbital structures is widest here.

To avoid the trauma to the inferior oblique muscle or its supplying motor nerve, the needle placed through the inferotemporal space should be lateral to the sagittal plane of lateral limbus. During injection, the deposition of local anesthetic agents, directly into any of the extraocular muscles, should be diligently avoided. Otherwise, direct muscle injury from the needle prick and the myotoxicity from local anesthetic agent may result in a prolonged diplopia which may even become permanent.

Following negative aspiration test of blood, the injection is performed, confirming the absence of abnormal resistance during the pushing of drugs or the presence of atypical discomfort. If anyone is suspected, then the needle tip should be relocated. While injecting the drug, monitoring should be done visually and/or digitally for the increasing intraorbital volume and the intraconal pressure. The 3–4 mL of local anesthetic mixture is injected very slowly over 2 minutes. The proper placement of needle in the intraconal space is indicated by the bulging of superior orbital sulcus which is accompanied by the filling out of upper eyelid crease and some degree of ptosis with proptosis.

After injection is completed, the needle is withdrawn and a check for the bleeding is made. If there is any intraorbital bleeding or sudden abnormal increase in intraorbital pressure, then immediate digital compression over the eyeball should be instituted to minimize any potential complication from high intraorbital pressure which has built up in the orbit. During the introduction of needle into orbit, no attempt is made to contact with the bone of orbital floor. This is because the tip of the needle may enter the infraorbital canal or fissure resulting in unpleasant infraorbital nerve paresthesia **(Fig. 28)**.

Following injection, a period of gentle message or decompression of eyeball by "pinky" for about 2–5 minutes is done. Then, the effectiveness of this block is assessed by checking the globe movements (paralysis of extraocular muscles), the activity of levator palpebrae superioris, and the function of orbicularis oculi. If there is any ineffective block, then it can be completed by supplementation. The supplementing injections are—*medial periconal injection* and/or *superotemporal periconal injection* (which are discussed later).

The complications of retrobulbar intraconal block are:
- Globe perforation (0.1–7%)
- Intravascular injection
- Intraorbital hemorrhage (1%)
- Penetration and injection within the optic nerve sheath (0.3%) with resulting optic nerve damage, subarachnoid

spread of local anesthetic agent, brain stem paresis, and cardiopulmonary arrest.

So, the retrobulbar intraconal block for ocular surgeries is not recommended anymore.

Peribulbar or Periconal or Periocular Block

In this method of ophthalmic regional anesthesia, local anesthetic agents are deposited outside the cone of four rectus muscles, but within the orbit and posterior to the equator of the globe. So, it may be called as the *posterior peribulbar block.* When the local anesthetic agents are deposited anterior to the equator of the globe and obviously outside of the cone of the four rectus muscles, then it is called as the *anterior peribulbar block* **(Fig. 29)**.

The peribulbar or periconal block was first described, as early as in 1914, by Allen. But, it came into common practice only, in 1986. Davis and Mandel first published papers on this method of peribulbar block. They used two routes: one below and one above the globe. Both the routes were chosen at the inferior and superior orbital margins respectively, through the inferotemporal and the superotemporal quadrant of the orbit up to the depth of 3.5 cm, where near about 10 mL of local anesthetic solution was injected. Through both the routes, the needles were directed to the floor or the roof of the orbit respectively, but not to the axis joining the center of the pupil and the macula. Then, Bloomberg did more work on this peribulbar block. He entered the orbit only through inferotemporal route and the needle was directed to the floor

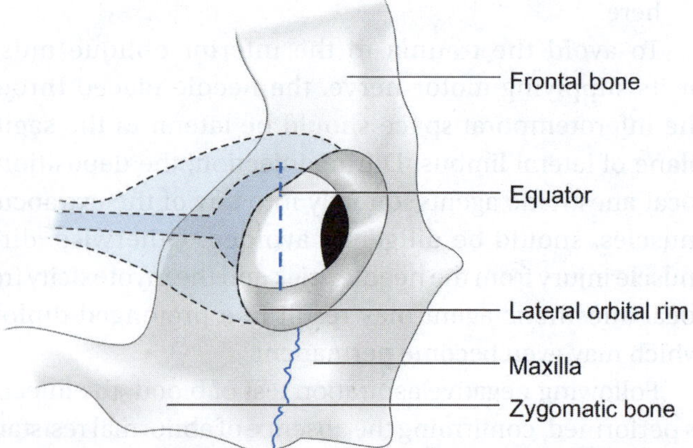

Fig. 28: The lateral orbital margin which is set back in line with the globe of equator. Thus, it makes the inferotemporal approach as the route of choice for regional block.

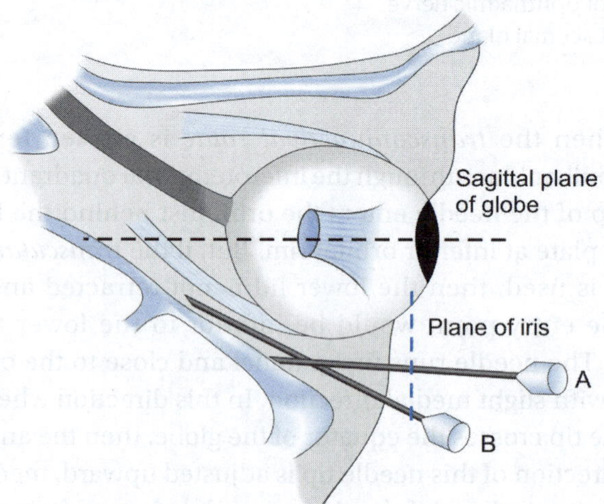

Fig. 29: Transcutaneous approach for periconal block through inferotemporal space. (A) A needle of 24G width and 24 mm long enters the orbit close to the floor of orbit. (B) The needle then passes backward in sagittal plane parallel to orbital floor. It crosses the equator of globe up to a depth when the needle hub junction reaches the plane of iris. This technique is equally applicable for transconjunctival route.

of the orbit. Then, the needle was directed slightly medial (20°) and cephalad (10°) and 5–10 mL of local anesthetic drug was deposited. In this method, there was a controversy, regarding the failure rate and the incidences of subsequent supplemental block. In some studies, only 5% patients required supplemental upper superotemporal quadrant injection to achieve complete globe akinesia, while many studies reported up to 50% failure rate.

At that time, many other techniques of peribulbar block were also tried, using different routes (*inferotemporal, superotemporal, medial periconal, etc.*) at a time in different permutation and combination, using the needle of different lengths and sizes. They have wide variations in their results. Among all these permutation and combinations, three-needle technique is the best, requiring only 5% supplementation through the medial periconal route. *This three-needle-technique consists of*—(i) a preliminary subcutaneous or subpalpebral conjunctival (lower) infiltration of local anesthetic agent which is followed by, (ii) a second infratemporal periconal injection, and (iii) lastly a superotemporal periconal injection. But, whichever the peribulbar technique is used, it is important to note that there is insufficient space between the lateral rectus and the lateral wall of the orbit and the inferior rectus and the inferior wall of the orbit. So, true periconal block is very difficult or may be theoretical in inferotemporal quadrant.

After the introduction of periconal block, many variations of this technique have developed which have already been discussed. But, the *difference between the peribulbar and the retrobulbar block* is that in peribulbar block—(i) the onset of akinesia is considerably slower, ii) the volume of local anesthetic agent requirement is greater, and iii) the supplementation rate is higher. In both the retrobulbar and peribulbar block the young patients are more resistant to the total akinesia and the analgesia of the globe and the peribulbar tissues than the elderly. This is because the more dense connective tissues in the young patients hinder the access of the local anesthetic solution to the sensory and motor nerves, which are situated both in the intraconal and periconal spaces, there will be more resistance the effect of the local anesthetic solution.

The *advantages of peribulbar* technique are—(i) the less risk of perforation to the globe, (ii) the less risk of injury to the optic nerve, (iii) the less risk of injury to the vessels of orbit, and (iv) the less pain on injection. The *disadvantages of peribulbar* technique are—slow onset, and increased likelihood of ecchymosis.

There are three main routes for peribulbar block:
- Inferotemporal peribulbar block (most commonly used)
- Medial peribulbar block
- Superotemporal peribulbar block.

Types of Needles

There are volume of discussion, regarding the types of needles, used for regional anesthesia in ophthalmology. But, the traditional teaching favors the use of a dull tipped needle, with intermediate size (gauge). It has the advantage of pushing the blood vessels aside, rather than traumatizing (penetrating) them and the tissue planes are more accurately felt. This is because the more the needle will be thick (blunt), the less it will pierce the blood vessels and different resistance will be felt when this needle will pass through the different tissues of different densities. There is also a common believe among the ophthalmologists, though it is not true, that it is more difficult to penetrate the globe and the optic nerve sheath with a blunt or dull tipped needle. But, multiple studies have shown that the penetration or perforation of eyeball by a dull tipped needle (if it occurs) causes more serious damage than when a fine or sharp (i.e., of higher gauge) needle is used.

Thus, it questions the arguments which advocate the use of blunt tipped needle. Any needle, blunt or sharp tipped, when is advanced blindly within the orbit, has the potential for causing serious complications such as globe perforation, optic nerve injury, and retrobulbar hemorrhage. Therefore, any serious practitioner of ophthalmic regional anesthesia must keep a thorough knowledge of the anatomy and the contents of the orbit, rather than the choosing of blunt or sharp tipped needle. It is also found that the pain and the tactile discrimination is progressively reduced by decreasing the width of the, i.e., by increasing the gauge (size) of the needle. This is because; the increased resistance caused by a blunt needle is no more appreciated here, due to the increased preload at the tip of the fine needle.

Special attention should also be paid to the length of any needle which enters beyond the orbital rim (margin). However, at any circumstance, the intraorbital distance of 31 mm as measured from the orbital rim should never be exceeded. During the medial direction of needle, which advances from the inferotemporal entry point, the direction should be such that the midsagittal plane of eyeball should never be crossed. All the needles placed periconally or intraconally should be oriented tangentially with the beveled opening, facing toward the globe.

The force, required to inject the local anesthetic agent at a given rate, through a given needle, mounted on a larger syringe, is more than a smaller syringe. This is because; larger syringe has a greater plunger cross-sectional area than a smaller one. So, a change in resistance, while injecting the 10 mL of drug is more easily felt by the injecting finger when smaller size syringes are used. Here, the fingers serve as a transducer. It relays information to the sensory cortex of an anesthesiologist. The ability to detect the changes in resistance during the injection of local anesthetic solution, (more or less easily), is very important for the avoidance of complications.

Facial Nerve Block

Before the era of the retrobulbar and peribulbar block, the techniques of combining the corneoconjunctival topical anesthesia by cocaine with transcutaneous VIIth cranial nerve block was in vogue. The facial nerve block causes the paralysis of orbicularis oculi muscle and prevents the squeezing or the movements of eyelids. During that period, various methods of VIIth cranial nerve block were introduced by Van Lint, Wright, O'Brien, Atkinson, Nabath and Rehman, and Spaeth, etc. But, among these, the Van Lint is the most distal and the Nabath and Rehman is the most proximal site of block for facial nerve, after its emergence from the base of the skull through stylomastoid foramen. In Van Lint block, the local anesthetic drug is injected directly deep to the muscle of orbicularis oculi and close to the bone at the lateral angle of the eye. The Nadbath technique blocks the facial nerve, at its exit level from stylomastoid foramen, under the external auditory canal, in close proximity to vagus and glossopharyngeal nerves. This block is not recommended, because it has been associated with vocal cord paralysis, laryngospasm, dysphagia, and respiratory distress.

Before the days of hyaluronidase and the development of decompression devices, a small volume retrobular block with facial nerve paralysis at the stylomastoid foramen was the only choice for most of the ophthalmic surgeries under regional anesthesia. But, with the discovery of hyaluronidase and the decompression devices, the peribulbar block allows the injection of large amount of local anesthetic agent into orbit. It has been observed that an effective spread of this adequate (large) amount of local anesthetic agent from the orbit through the orbital septum under the orbicularis oculi muscle, causes the akinesia of orbicularis oculi muscle, which makes the block of VIIth cranial nerve at the level of stylomastoid foramen unnecessary. The local anesthetic drug spreads out from the orbit with the help of hyaluronidase into the deep plane of orbicularis oculi muscle and abolishes the activity of lid closure by blocking the terminal divisions of VIIth cranial nerve, entering the muscle from its deep surface. Thus, in the technique of peribulbar block, using hyaluronidase and large amount of local anesthetic agent, in vast majority of cases sufficient blockade of lid closure activity of orbicularis oculi muscle is achieved.

Hence, the painful transcutaneous VIIth cranial nerve block at the level of the stylomastoid foramen through the sensitive facial skin, along with its serious complications which are described above, are avoided and found to be unnecessary. So, the historical and traditional concept of—(i) globe akinesia and anesthesia by retrobulbar injection and (ii) orbicularis muscle akinesia by the direct separate intervention of VIIth cranial nerve, after its emergence from the skull at sternomastoid foramen level, is not needed now. In an occasion, patient who exhibits strong recruitment of more peripheral fibers of orbicularis oculi muscle and/or exhibits excessive use of brow musculature, then only supplemental transcutaneous blocking of orbicularis oculi by Van Lint method may be necessary.

COMBINED RETROBULBAR (INTRACONAL) AND PERIBULBAR (PERICONAL) METHOD

The multiple distinct techniques of the injection of local anesthetic agent for the regional anesthesia of orbit were studied. From these, it was determined that a method of combining an initial intraconal (best through inferotemporal route) injection with a secondary supplemental periconal (best medialpericonal) injection is most suited for the ophthalmic regional anesthesia for the rapid turnover in day case ophthalmic practice. Alternatively, a technique with solely periconal placement of local anesthetic agent for the ophthalmic regional anesthesia may be a more prudent practice for the relatively *inexperienced anesthetic practitioner.*

This combined method (retrobulbar plus peribulbar) consists of a preliminary injection of local anesthetic mixture, diluted with balanced salt solution, at subjunctional or subcutaneous level by a 30G needle to anesthetize the local area. It is followed by two full strength local anesthetic injections in retrobulbar and peribulbar space. The *first* is an *inferotemporal intraconal* injection and the *second* is a *medial periconal* injection. The rationale behind this three-needle-technique is to provide effective (i.e., low supplementation rate) and safe (low complication rate) local anesthesia and akinesia according to the requirements. This method is virtually pain free. As a result preoperative and intraoperative sedation are usually not necessary, except a good rapport and assurance to the patient. This no-sedation approach avoids the problem of patients, falling into a deep sleep during surgery and awakening precipitously with potential detrimental effects on surgery in hand.

Inferolateral (inferotemporal) Periconal Block

This is the most commonly used technique for the peribulbar or periconal block. Sometimes, it is supplemented with the medial and/or superotemporal periconal block. This is because a single inferolateral injection is often inadequate and may not be predictable for complete anesthesia (sensory loss and akinesia) of globe.

After the proper examination of patient, an IV line is accessed and the monitoring is started as a standard rule. If mild sedation is indicated, then it is administered by midazolam (0.5–1.5 mg) and/or fentanyl (50 µg) or sufentanil (150 µg). Topical local anesthetic drops are instilled into the conjunctival sac to anesthetize the palpebral conjunctiva. For this purpose, 1% amethocaine or 2% xylocaine is sufficient, but it may cloud the cornea. So, 0.4% oxybuprocaine or 0.5% proxymetacaine may be the better alternative. This topical anesthesia of conjunctiva is only necessary for the transconjunctival route of inferotemporal periconal block. The junction of medial two-thirds and lateral one-third of the inferior orbital rim is palpated by the finger of nondominant hand and a groove is felt at the junction of the maxilla and zygoma. Just lateral to this point and 1 mm above the orbital margin, a standard hypodermic needle (25G and 25 mm), mounted on a 10 mL syringe is inserted and passed slowly backward, perpendicular to all the planes. The entry of the needle can be either subcutaneous or transconjunctival (by retraction the lower lid). If the needle tip touches the bone, then it is redirected slightly superomedially to follow the orbital floor once more, i.e., at a 10° angle with the transverse plane. Then, the he needle is advanced further, till the tip of it reaches the level of the posterior pole of the globe (i.e., until the hub of the needle reaches the plane of iris).

The globe should be observed carefully for any sign of rotation during the insertion of the needle into the orbit, indicating the contact of the needle with the scleral (globe). In such situation, every temptation to wriggle the needle to confirm the scleral engagement should be avoided. Because, this may increase the risk of hemorrhage, if the perforation of globe occurs. After proper positioning of the needle and aspiration, 6–8 mL of local anesthetic agent is injected slowly and at the same time the globe should be palpated with other hand to assess the tension. If the globe becomes tensed or proptosed or the upper eye lid droops, then the injection should be stopped. Because, this likely indicates the retrobulbar injection, requiring much smaller volume of local anesthetic agent. After the completion of injection, the needle is slowly withdrawn and a small volume of local anesthetic solution is deposited under the orbicularis oculi muscle of lower lid when the needle is withdrawn. Then, digital massage or a compression device (Hanon's balloon) should be applied to dissipate the local anesthetic solution within the orbital tissue, which quickly normalizes the IOP. The block is assessed after 5 to 10 minutes and a second injection is repeated, if a greater degree of akinesia and analgesia is required. In modern ophthalmic practice, a completely akinetic eye is less often required and a second injection doubles the risk of complication. So, the required

extent of block should be discussed with the surgeon beforehand.

The larger volume of local anesthetic drug, which is required for peribulbar block, tends to cause proptosis and a temporary increase in IOP. However, in the intact globe this has no significance. But, it becomes problematic when the globe is opened for surgery. After the dissipation of the local anesthetic drug in the surrounding orbital tissue with the passing of time, the raised IOP usually disappears. Alternatively, digital massage by the fingers or the application of Hanon's balloon on the eyeball helps in the dissipation of local anesthetic drug. The Hanon's balloon is a type of tamponade which is applied on the eyeball at a set pressure of 25 mm Hg. This compresses the eyeball and transiently increases the IOP further. During compression, the volume of blood and aqueous within the eyeball is reduced. After the release of tamponade, the "empty" eye becomes hypotonic and remains so for about 15 minutes, until the blood and aqueous volumes are reestablished.

Medial Periconal Block

Here, the local anesthetic agent is administered (injected) into the compartment, containing a large amount of fat, situated on the nasal side of the medial rectus muscle. This block has distinct advantages, due to the relative avascularity of this region and the peculiar arrangement of connective tissue in this area. The local anesthetic mixture, injected into this area, spreads to the orbital apex posteriorly, but its spread is restricted laterally by the intraconal compartment. Subsequently, the local anesthetic drug spreads anteriorly through the two hernial orifices which are situated above and below the medial check ligament of the connective tissue diaphragm that surrounds the globe just near its equator. The drug also passes through the orbital septum into the upper and lower eyelid in the tissue plane, deep to the orbicularis oculi muscle. Here, the fine terminal motor branches of VIIth cranial nerve are readily blocked.

Superiorly, the access of local anesthetic agent to the motor nerve supply of superior oblique, superior rectus and levator complex is also facilitated. The injection of local anesthetic agent in this space also promotes the spread of the drug to the lacrimal and frontal nerves and the peripheral conjunctiva. Thus, it effectively abolishes the intraoperative discomfort which is sometimes observed in the low-volume, solely intraconal technique.

The entry point of the needle for this medial periconal block is a small depression, immediately medial to the caruncle. The caruncle is a specialized portion of conjunctiva which occupies the extreme medial end of the palpebral fissure. The caruncle lies medial to the sagittal plane of the medial equator of globe in almost all patients. So, there is no chance of perforation of sclera by a needle, when it enters the orbit through this point. The needle should be passed in transverse plane, directed toward the midline of the skull at occiput.

This medial compartment of the orbit is 5–10 mm wide anteriorly at the equator of the globe, and 3–5 mm wide at the posterior surface of the eye. Then, it rapidly becomes narrower as the medial rectus muscle reaches its bony origin posteriorly. The needle must avoid the penetration of the medial rectus muscle, because the injection of local anesthetic agent directly into any rectus muscle could result in myotoxicity with resultant prolonged paralysis or paresis of this muscle. If there is any doubt, then the needle tip should hit the periosteum of the medial wall of orbit, and then should be withdrawn slightly to redirect it with a lesser medial inclination. This allows the needle tip to be free in the fatty tissue of medial compartment. If the above mentioned guidelines are obeyed, then the entry of needle into the medial rectus muscle directly will not occur.

After the proper placement of needle, a volume of 2–4 mL of drug is injected into this space (medial compartment of the orbit). This volume of drug will depend on the degree of supplementation block required, aiming at not to impede the desired goal of intraocular hypotomy. The residual activity of extraocular muscles, which persists even after the initial inferotemporal intraconal block, is effectively abolished within 3–5 minutes in most cases, following the medial compartmental supplementation block.

Though, this compartment is relatively avascular, but it contains a portion of superior ophthalmic vein, anterior ethmoidal artery, and the supra and infra trochlear arteries. But, they lie above the point of the needle entry. These vessels are traumatized, if the needle enters through the superonasal quadrant of the orbit. In such situation, the incidences of bleeding by a 30G width and 31 mm long needle are negligible and always minor in nature. As a whole, the medial periconal block is an effective and safe method of supplementation of the primary inferotemporal block. It is painless because, the needle entry point which is innervated by the nasociliary nerve, lies inside the cone of the rectus muscles and is relatively well-blocked by the previous inferotemporal intraconal injection.

Superotemporal Periconal Block

It mainly affects the superior rectus and levator palpebrae superioris muscle. Even after the primary inferotemporal block, sometimes the activities of these muscles are retained. The explanation of this failure is that the injection of local anesthetic agent, through the inferotemporal route, does not reach in sufficient quantities to the branches

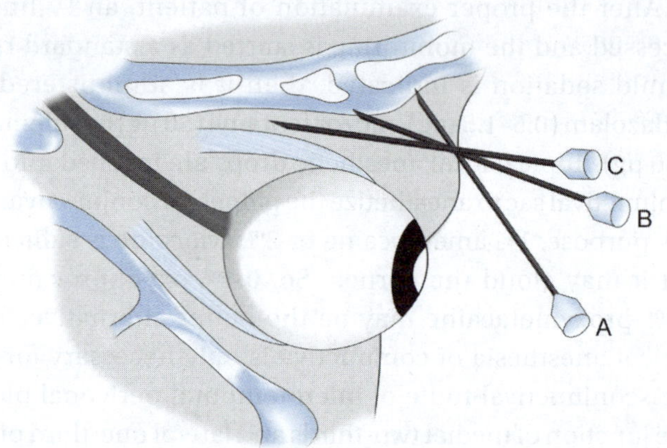

Fig. 30: The superotemporal periconal block. The needle is inserted through the superotemporal route and is advanced toward the roof of orbit (A). Then, the needle tip walks along the periorbit of the orbit in a curved line fashion (B), until the needle tip is at a depth of 24–30 mm (C). At this point injection is made with usual precautions. It is superotemporal block.

of the oculomotor nerve which supplies these muscles. Such a situation may arise, because the connective tissue hammock for the superior ophthalmic vein is usually well-developed in some individuals. This is partially permeable to local anesthetic agent and prevents it from accessing the nerve in the central core of this compartment. So, by this superotemporal block, the access of local anesthetic agent to the nerve, supplying these muscles such as superior rectus and levator palpebrae superioris, from aforementioned is possible.

The point of entry of needle for this block is the superior orbital margin and 3–4 mm lateral to the sagittal plane of the lateral limbus. Thus, this relatively avascular area lies between lacrimal vessels on the temporal side and the supraorbital vessels on the medial side. The needle is inserted tangentially from above the globe which is directed toward the roof of the orbit. After making the first bony contact with the orbital roof, the needle is then redirected 5° degree medially. Then, it is further advanced posteriorly till the depth of 31 mm from the superior orbital margin is reached. Following negative aspiration test, the 3–4 mL of local anesthetic solution is injected in this position, with the aim of not increasing the intraorbital pressure excessively. This superotemporal supplemental block is needed only in 5–10% cases **(Fig. 30)**.

RECENTLY DEVELOPED REGIONAL ANESTHETIC TECHNIQUES FOR OPHTHALMIC SURGERIES

The large incision cataract surgery, constituting the main bulk of all ophthalmic operations and done in the past, requires complete paralysis of all the extraocular muscles (or akinesia) including orbicularis oculi to avoid the loss of globe contents by muscular contraction during surgery. But, the recent small-incision, closed-system surgical technique for cataract extraction does not require complete akinesia or paralysis of all the extra occur muscles. Rather, it may require only surface anesthesia which is solely confined to the surface of the anterior part of eyeball. So, the concept of alternative nonakinetic methods of regional anesthesia for cataract extraction surgery has been introduced. These are:

- Subconjunctival injection of local anesthetic agent
- Sub-Tenon's block
- Topical corneoconjunctival anesthesia.

But these newer methods of regional anesthesia are not universally applicable to all the patients for cataract surgery. This is because of the—(i) different patient's temperament, (ii) different lens pathology, and (iii) personal variations of skill among the surgeons.

Subconjunctival Block

In this subconjunctival block (first technique) a small amount of local anesthetic agent is injected under the conjunctiva, near the superior limbus and this technique is used mainly for the anterior segmental surgery. This technique is also combined with the intracameral injection of a preservative free lignocaine (Xylocard). But, in these subconjunctival and topical corneoconjunctival techniques (described below) which is combined with or without intracameral injections of local anesthetic agent, anesthesia is not as complete as with the standard intraorbital blocks. The iris and the ciliary body retain their sensation and the akinesia of the extraocular muscles is not a feature. So, many ophthalmologists do not prefer this technique. Because, the avoidance of the intraconal or periconal block for the fear of complications allows exposure to the greater risk of performing intraocular surgery in the presence of extraocular muscle activity.

Sub-Tenon's Block

The sub-Tenon's block was first introduced by Swan, in 1956, and was then used extensively after 1960. At that time, he had suggested that this sub-Tenon's block produces better iris and anterior segment anesthesia than a subconjunctival injection. But, the eyeball mobility is usually retained which depends on the volume of local anesthetic drug. Subsequently this technique gained popularity as an easy, safe, and effective alternative to the retrobulbar and peribulbar anesthesia. It has the advantages of avoiding the entry of a needle blindly into the orbit and so has no appreciable risks of complications which are discussed later.

This technique involves the dissection of a space beneath the Tenon's capsule and passing a blunt curved cannula (Southampton's cannula) into this space, beyond the equator of eyeball, to deposit the local anesthetic agent there. It effectively blocks the ciliary ganglion with the long and short ciliary nerves. If larger volumes of local anesthetic agent are deposited more posteriorly, then it may also block the motor nerves and the extraconal branches of ophthalmic and maxillary nerves. Thus, this large volume of local anesthetic agent produces the complete anesthesia of eyeball. During this procedure, first the conjunctiva is anesthetized by topical anesthesia. This is followed by a small incision on conjunctiva at the inferolateral quadrant of the globe which is then dissected up to the plane between the sclera and the Tenon's capsule.

Here, the Tenon's capsule is recognized by its white, avascular structure, easily distinguished from the vascular sclera. Then, a blunt curved Southampton's cannula is passed backward beyond the equator through this incision and 3–5 mL of local anesthetic solution is deposited there. If the cannula is placed subconjunctivally, then an attempt to push the local anesthetic agent shall immediately make it apparent by chemosis. Following the deposition of local anesthetic solution, beneath the Tenon's capsule by the cannula, the local anesthetic agent will spread mainly into the anterior intraconal space and produces anesthesia.

The degree of akinesia of the extraocular muscles, produced by this sub-Tenon's injection, is proportional to the volume of local anesthetic solution. The peripheral orbital anesthesia, such as the peripheral conjunctiva, eye lids, orbicularis oculi, etc., is usually incomplete by this block. So, supplemental local anesthetic injection may sometimes be necessary to achieve the patient comfort or to complete the surgery. Intravenous sedation is often used during surgery, following this method of anesthesia. Sub-Tenon's block can be used safely in patients where the axial length of the globe is >26 mm and intraorbital block is more risky. It is also the block of choice in anticoagulated patients, since any bleeding point can be cauterized directly in such anesthetic procedure. It may be more easily performed by the surgeon, though it is now being increasingly performed by anesthesiologist too.

Topical (Surface) Anesthesia

Throughout the whole 19th century and the first few decades of 20th century, cocaine was the only available local anesthetic agent. At that period, it was only used for retrobulbar injection in ophthalmic surgeries and for conduction block (local anesthesia) in different minor general surgeries. But, due to its high toxicity, cocaine was abandoned from retrobulbar injection. Then, it was used solely for topical corneoconjunctival anesthesia, albeit without the advantages of modern surgical technology which was not developed during that period.

However, the history is repeating itself. So, after the cocaine, many good local anesthetic agents have been synthesized with the more development of sophisticated technology for cataract extraction by a very small sclerocorneal incision. Therefore, reintroduced by Fichman, topical anesthesia by newer local anesthetic agents is now again being commonly used (now gaining popularity) for cataract extraction (history is repeating itself).

For cataract surgery, under topical corneoconjunctival anesthesia, the critical selection of subjects (patients) is important and there must be a continuous and open dialog between the surgeon and the patient throughout the operation. This is because as the eyeball of the patient is not paralyzed, so surgeons have to verbally guide the position of eyeball of patient continuously. This topical corneoconjunctival anesthesia is most applicable for only cataract extraction by phacoemulsification with or without foldable lens in very cooperative patients.

For topical corneoconjunctival anesthesia, the most commonly used drugs are 0.5% bupivacaine and 2% lignocaine. They are very effective, but may produce stinging sensation initially and cloud the cornea. So, the newly developed local anesthetic agents such as the 0.4% oxyprocaine and 0.5% proxymetacaine are considered superior. This topical corneoconjunctival anesthetic method cannot be used in patients with language barrier, deafness, dementia, and obviously in children. The dense or trauma-induced cataracts, small pupils failing to dilate, macular degeneration, etc., cannot be managed with this type of topical corneoconjunctival anesthesia alone. They are best managed with the other forms of intraorbital regional anesthesia.

The clear advantages of topical corneoconjunctival anesthesia are:

- Appeal for no-needle procedure
- Avoidance of complications caused by intraorbital injection
- Early visual rehabilitation, especially in patients with only one-sighted eye
- Suitability for patients on anticoagulant medication
- The patient's ability to look at any direction directed by the surgeon, which facilitates the surgery also.

Junior surgeons still do not prefer this technique and are happier to perform surgery under akinetic block-anesthesia, as they are less experienced, regarding the use of topical conreoconjuctional anesthesia. Patients having cataract

BOX 4: Qualities in a surgeon required to select topical anesthesia.

- Senior surgeons
- Vast experiences regarding scleral tunnel and intracapsular phacoemulsification
- Good communication skill of surgeon with the patient
- Appropriate mental makeup to perform the surgery under topical anesthesia
- Willingness to talk continuously with their patients during the surgical procedures, are most suited for this anesthetic technique

surgery under topical corneoconjunctival anesthesia, require more psychological preparation and oral anxiolytic premedication. The topical agent best suited for this method is 2% lignocaine without preservative. Unlike cataract extraction under intraorbital regional anesthesia, here is no reduction of optic nerve function in topical anesthesia. Hence, an awareness of the brightness of the light of microscope may be disturbing enough to some patients. However, this problem can usually be overcome by starting with reduced illumination from the light of microscope and then bringing it up gradually. The iris and the ciliary muscles retain their sensation. So, the intraoperative use of intracameral miotic agents may precipitate discomfort from ciliary muscle spasm. This can also be prevented by intracameral injection of local anesthetic agent, or by avoiding the touching of iris by operating instruments **(Box 4)**.

RECENT GUIDELINES FOR ANESTHETIST IN OPHTHALMIC SURGERY

In 1993, the Royal College of Anaesthetists and the College of Ophthalmologists published certain guidelines on the roles and the responsibilities of anesthesiologists, during ophthalmic surgery, under local (regional) and topical anesthesia. These guidelines said that the presence of an anesthesiologist is mandatory to monitor the general condition of the patient throughout the operation and to give resuscitation, as and when required. In addition, it was also recommended that the anesthesiologist should be whole responsible for—(i) providing the sedation when necessary, (ii) administering the local anesthesia or block, and (iii) providing the IV access. These recommendations are also applied to simple infiltration anesthesia for extraocular surgery also.

In 2001, these above guidelines were updated with further certain recommendations. These are as follows:

- Local anesthesia can also be administered by appropriately trained staff, but an anesthetist must be present

- Surgeons may administer topical, subconjunctival or sub-Tenon's anesthesia, but an anesthetist must be present
- An anesthetist must be available, when surgery is performed under retrobulbar or peribulbar anesthesia
- An anesthetist must be present and have sole responsibility, if sedation is required.

SPECIFIC SURGICAL PROCEDURES AND MODIFICATION OF REGIONAL ANESTHESIA

Today, though most of the ophthalmic surgeries are performed under regional anesthesia and follow a generalized rule, still some specific ophthalmic surgical procedures may need certain modifications of this regional anesthetic technique, according to their necessity. For example, secondary intraocular lens implantation in aphakic patients requires more surgical time than that of a standard cataract extraction and intraocular lens implantation procedure. So, it warrants for the selection of more long acting local anesthetic agents.

Trabeculectomy usually needs complete akinesia and complete sensory anesthesia of globe. So, topical anesthesia has no place in such type of surgery. For trabeculectomy operation, the intraconal or periconal block is the ideal RA. But, sub-Tenon's block may be an alternative to this intraconal and periconal anesthesia for trabeculectomy. If there is presence of any bleb of previous trabeculectomy operation, then no external pressure for intraorbital decompression, after retro or peribulbar block, should be used. Cataract surgery may be combined with trabeculectomy or trabeculectomy may be designed alone to reduce the IOP in glaucoma. But, in the management of only glaucoma by trabeculectomy, the orbital decompression devices are, after interconal block, best omitted. During the surgery of glaucoma, instead of intra operative control of IOP, the normal IOP is usually achieved by—(i) careful preoperative control of higher IOP (by acetazolamide and/or topical β-blocker), (ii) perioperative induction of osmotic diuresis with mannitol, (iii) using low volume of local anesthetic agents for intraorbital block, incorporating hyaluronidase in anesthetic mixture and allowing sufficient time (at least 15 minutes) to pass between the completion of the block and the commencement of surgery.

The strabismus (squint) surgery usually requires full akinesia (paralysis) of extraocular muscles and deep sensory anesthesia of globe by intraconal and/or periconal block. But, many other methods of regional anesthesia have also been described, including sub-Tenon, topical, or nonakinetic periconal block for squint surgery.

For refractive keratoplasty procedures, including Excimer laser keratectomy, topical surface anesthesia by 2% lignocaine is sufficient. But, these surgical procedures are associated with moderate postoperative discomfort or pain for 24–36 hours. So, this can be postoperatively managed by conjunctival instillations of topical nonsteroidal anti-inflammatory drugs (NSAIDs) preparation, combined with the use of bandage contact lens.

For corneal grafting, the regional anesthetic technique requires a dependable therapeutic time window of 1–2 hours with full akinesia and sensory anesthesia of eyeball, including both the lids. So, intraconal and/or periconal block with a large volume of long acting anesthetic agents is the choice for this type of surgery. Large volume of anesthetic agents results in an increased intraorbital and subsequently increased IOP. This can be reduced by preoperative induction of osmotic diuresis by mannitol. An orbital decompression device is also used to reduce the intraocular pressure. By the use of hyaluronidase and by giving sufficient time between the completion of block and the commencement of surgery, ocular hypotony can be produced.

Epikeratophakia and keratomileusis require a long therapeutic window of 2–2.5 hours with full globe akinesia and sensory anesthesia, including both the eyelid. In both these cases, the moderately potent systemic analgesics are also required postoperatively for about 48 hours. So, appropriate agents should be used with proper postoperative care. During regional anesthesia for these types of surgeries, anesthesiologist should avoid the production of conjunctival chemosis, if possible.

Photocoagulation is done with argon laser and it is very painful in an unanesthetized eye. At the same time the slight globe movement may momentarily expose the relatively healthy part of retina to iatrogenic injury. So, complete akinetic orbital regional anesthesia is required for patient's safety and also for surgeon's comfort. Hence, intraconal and/or periconal block is used for this type of surgery. But, some surgeons prefer sub-Tenon's technique also. Oculoplastic surgeries are also commonly performed under regional anesthesia and the principles are same, as those for other ophthalmic regional anesthesia in general. However, in oculoplastic surgeries higher concentration of adrenaline is used with the mixture of local anesthetic agent to reduce bleeding.

For vitreoretinal surgery under regional anesthesia a more prolonged therapeutic time window is necessary. So, intraconal and/or periconal block by a sufficient amount of long-acting local anesthetic agent is advocated. Adrenaline is also usually used to prolong the duration of action of the local anesthetic agent and to reduce the blood concentration of it, as the large amount of drug is used. The duration of the planned surgery in itself may dictate in favor of GA or a combined regional anesthesia and intravenous sedation technique in the interest of patient's comfort.

COMPLICATIONS OF ORBITAL REGIONAL ANESTHESIA

The complications of orbital regional anesthesia may be acute or delayed in onset. Again, it may be systemic or is only confined to the orbit and its contents. The complications of this orbital regional anesthesia may also range from a trivial one to something serious, such as the death of a patient. The orbital regional anesthetic complications are sometimes directly related to local anesthetic drugs or may be due to the technique of the administration of local anesthetic agent. The orbital regional anesthesia, sometimes, indirectly invites the complications, resulting from sedative or narcotic drugs and from GA, but only if they are combined with the previous one in case of inadequate or failed block.

In many centers, patients sometimes receive sedative or narcotic drugs to facilitate the incomplete regional anesthetic technique, or to supplement inadequate psychological preparation of patient. But, these sedatives or narcotics are often unnecessary. Because, intravenous medications are only rarely required, if the patients are psychologically properly prepared and the depth of regional anesthesia is adequate. Thus, the side-effects and the complications related to the use and the misuse of these sedatives, narcotics, or general anesthetic drugs are minimized. The most appropriate management of an inadequate block (regional anesthesia) is supplementation of it by further injection of local anesthetic agent, rather than the suppression of reflex reactivity with systemic medications such as sedatives and narcotics.

In the past and before the firm establishment of peribulbar technique for better ophthalmic regional anesthesia with the help of hyaluronidase, the desired goal of complete global and adnexal anesthesia with akinesia and concurrent global hypotony is achieved only by a *two injection method* which is described underneath and had become the traditionally accepted technique. This two injection method was combining—(1) the deposition of a small volume of local anesthetic agent near the apex of orbit (retrobulbar) with (2) the block of VIIth cranial nerve at some point along its extracranial path. But, recently, the introduction of hyaluronidase, peribulbar block, and orbital decompression devices allow a larger volume of local anesthetic drug, to be injected into orbital cavity for complete block. This avoids the necessity to block the VIIth cranial nerve, because an adequate volume of drug spreads through the orbital septum to paralyze the orbicularis oculi muscle.

However, as larger volumes of drugs are used, it is easy to understand the mechanisms, causing complications in ophthalmic regional anesthesia due to this local anesthetic agent.

Safe regional anesthesia can be accomplished by both the intraconal and periconal techniques. But, serious complications can arise from both the techniques, if carried out incorrectly. So, it cannot be said that one technique is better than the other. Although, there are definite description of both the intraconal and periconal techniques for orbital RA, but recently multiple exhaustive studies have failed to find out any evidence of a closed "cone," consisting of four rectus muscles and their interconnecting intermuscular septa, thus creating a distinct cone-like compartments in the posterior part of globe. So, it can be concluded that the concept of discrete intraconal and periconal compartments are erroneous **(Box 5)**.

The advancement of the needle by an anesthetist, within the confines of orbital cavity for regional ophthalmic anesthesia, essentially is a *blind procedure*. So, it has the

---

BOX 5: Complications of ophthalmic regional anesthesia.

- *Globe perforation:* It causes trauma to retina or choroid. Diagnosed by hypotomy of globe, intravitreal hemorrhage, retinal detachment, retinal tear at the point of perforation, loss of vision, etc.
- *Venous hemorrhage:* It is caused by the puncture of any orbital vein. Diagnosed by retrobulbar hematoma which progresses slowly than arterial hemorrhage. Hematoma produces proptosis, tight globe, subconjunctival hemorrhage, ecchymosis, etc.
- *Arterial hemorrhage:* It is caused by the puncture of any orbital artery. Produces same picture like venous hemorrhage, but very rapidly progressing (acute)
- *Optic nerve injury:* It is caused by direct needle injury to the nerve or ischemic compression by hematoma. Diagnosed by optic atrophy, optic nerve head swelling, visual field defects, permanent loss of vision, etc.
- *Intravascular injection:* It is caused by direct injection of LA agent in vein or artery. Produces increased systemic levels of local anesthetic or cerebral levels of LA. Diagnosed by dizziness, drowsiness, confusion, twitching, convulsion, unconsciousness, hypotension, bradycardia, apnea, coma, and cardiac arrest
- *Deposition of LA agent in subarachnoid space:* It is caused by needle penetration of optic nerve sheath and direct spread of LA agent in the central CSF. Diagnosed by vertigo, deafness, aphasia, facial palsy shivering, convulsion, hemiplegia, paraplegia, quadriplegia, loss of consciousness, apnea, hypotension, bradycardia, and cardiac arrest
- *Oculocardiac reflex:* It is caused by dull or blunt needle and rapid injection of drug in a fixed orbital space. Diagnosed by bradycardia, hypotension, loss of consciousness, and cardiac arrest

(CSF: cerebrospinal fluid; LA: local anesthetic)

potential of serious complications. Therefore, the perception of the changes of tissue planes, during the advancement of needle through these planes of tissue is very important for safe regional anesthesia. But, it is an *acquired skill which requires experience* and continuous practice to reduce the rate of complications. The traditional teaching of placing a needle intraconally through inferotemporal route with the globe elevated and adducted, i.e., "up and in" position (Atkinson technique) *has largely been abandoned now*. Because, in this position the optic nerve is brought easily closer to tip of the injecting needle and the macular area is further exposed to the damage. So, the penetration of the optic nerve sheath, optic nerve trauma and globe penetration by the needle may result more frequently in this position of the globe. Further, the posterior pole of the globe is more endangered, particularly in the ovoid shaped globes of myopic patients in such "up and in" position. *But, many of the serious complications can be avoided by having the patients eyes, directed in the primary gaze position,* during the placement of the needle and subsequent injection. However, this has been substantiated by computed tomography (CT)-scanning and magnetic resonance imaging (MRI).

Special attention should also be paid to the length and the direction of the needle which enters the orbital cavity beyond its margin. Longer needles which is >31 mm may reach the orbital apex, where the vessels are numerous and of larger diameters. Again, at the apex, the optic nerve and the vessels are less mobile. So, the retrobulbar hemorrhage or optic nerve trauma may result more frequently, if the needle tip approaches more toward the apex of the orbit. Thus, while it is possible to get a beautiful block with a small volume of drug, if it is injected at the apex of the orbit, but the risks of the injury to the vessels and nerves increase manifold. *So, a distance of 31 mm within the orbit, as measured from the orbital margin, should never be crossed.*

Also, a needle which is advanced from the inferotemporal entry site should not be allowed to pass the midsagittal plane of eyeball. All the needles used for intraconal and/or periconal injection should also be directed obliquely against the globe, with the beveled opening facing the eyeball. This tangential or oblique alignment of needle is most easily achieved through the transcutaneous route, by putting a finger between the globe and the inferior orbital margin of the orbit, over the lower eyelid than transconjunctival route. This is because the finger pushes the globe upward and makes a better room for the needle in inferotemporal quadrant.

The finger also helps—(i) to assess the size of the globe, (ii) to assess the distance of the equator from the inferior orbital margin, and (iii) guide the direction of needle tangentially. If a tangentially aligned needle touches the sclera, still globe penetration is less likely to occur than when a needle approaches to sclera at an acute angle. Having placed the needle at a desired depth, if there is an increased resistance, which is more than expected during pushing the drug, then it is imperative to reposition the tip of the needle first, rather than inject against this resistance.

The blocking of the main trunk of facial nerve, after its exit from stylomastoid foramen, may be associated with the unilateral blocking of vagus, glossopharyngeal, and spinal accessary nerve which are also coming out from the base of the skull through jugular foramen, near the stylomastoid foramen. This may cause the difficulty in swallowing and respiratory distress. So, for the facial nerve block at the stylomastoid foramen, it is wise not to go deeper than the recommended 12 mm depth from the skin and to avoid hyaluronidase. Thus, *bilateral facial nerve block at the stylomastoid foramen should never be allowed.* Another vital structure near the stylomastoid foramen is the internal carotid artery which can also be injured by the deeper placement of the needle.

There is a communication or a continuation of the subarachnoid space, surrounding the optic nerve, with that of the chiasma and the subarachnoid space which surrounds the pons and midbrain. The dural sheath at the apex of the orbit and along the optic nerve is not impervious to the local anesthetic agents. So, the local anesthetic agents, deposited in the orbital cavity, can easily diffuse into the subarachnoid space which surround the optic nerve. This is evidenced by the incidences of temporary ipsilateral amaurosis (loss of vision, especially that occurring without apparent lesion of the eye), following intraorbital block. The studies of cortical visual evoked potential also indicate the temporary suppression of optic nerve conduction which is greater with intraconal blockade, than with the periconal block. All these points favor the theory of the absorption of local anesthetic agents into the CSF, bathing the optic nerve and extension of it to the CNS with the brainstem anesthesia following intraorbital block.

This was explained and was first published in mid-1980s, although there was previous knowledge of this meningeal pathway. About 4–5% of patients, undergoing cataract extraction under regional anesthesia, generate emergency calls for an anesthetist. Among these, the direct cerebral spread of local anesthetic agent from the orbit is very important. The effect of spread of the local anesthetic agent into the CNS, during the intraconal or periconal block, *depends on*—(i) the amount of the drug entering the CNS and (ii) the specific area of CNS to which it has spread. Usually, the patient describes the symptoms about 2–3 minutes after the intraorbital injection. Frequently, the peak is reached at about 10–15 minutes and resolves over 1–2 hours.

The clinical picture of the spread of local anesthetic agent into the CNS is protean and *produces the signs and symptoms* which vary from mild confusion to marked shivering or convulsions. The clinical pictures may also show the bilateral brainstem nerve palsies, including the hemi or para or even quadriplegia and with or without loss of consciousness. In extreme cases, the clinical picture shows apnea with marked cardiovascular instability. As this is a potential complication, which may occur in any intraorbital block, so the patients should not be covered with the drapes for surgery, until 20 minutes have passed, after the completion of the block. Otherwise, the identification and corrective treatment may be dangerously delayed and serious sequelae including death could obviously result.

The central spread of the local anesthetic agent *should be suspected,* if there is onset of any of the following signs and symptoms, such as—mental confusion, signs of extraocular paresis or amaurosis of the contralateral eye, shivering, convulsion, nausea or vomiting, dysphagia, sudden changes in the vital cardiovascular signs, dyspnea, or respiratory depression, etc. The *treatment of this serious complication* includes—ventilatory support with oxygen, intravenous fluid, pharmacological circulatory support with vagolytics, and vasopressors and anticonvulsants with close vital sign monitoring.

The traditional Atkinson's technique, with elevated and adducted globe during the placement of the needle into the inferotemporal space, increases the chances of cerebral spread of local anesthetic agent. Because, this position places the optic nerve with its subarachnoid space in close ploximity to the advancing needle. On the other hand, "down and out" position of the globe advocated by some anesthetist, where the optic nerve is less vulnerable has the disadvantage of bringing the approaching inferotemporal needle into the field of vision of the patient. So this may be frightening to the patient. However, the "down and in" position of the globe which places the anterior part of the optic nerve in a safer position in the intraconal space and the needle is away from the field of vision of the patient, is more acceptable to avoid this complication.

Whatever may be the reason, the avoidance of the deep penetration of the orbit by needle during any technique, is the key factor for both to prevent the cerebral spread of the local anesthetic agent and to avoid the other serious complications of regional anesthesia. The maximum penetration of the needle from the orbital rim should not be >31 mm. The modern regional anesthetic techniques avoid the deep orbital placement of the needle and advocate the accurate site of injection at the limited orbital depth, using the increased volume of the local anesthetic drug in order to achieve the critical blocking concentration at the apex.

The true incidences of scleral penetration (only the entry wound is present) and perforation (both the entry and exit wound are present) are not known, because most of the cases are not reported. So, the reported incidence ranges from none in a series of 3,000 peribulbar (periconal) anesthesia to 1 in a series of 10,000 combined peri- and intraconal anesthesia to 3 in a series of 3,000 intraconal block. But, it is definite that the incidences are higher in both the myopic patients and intraconal block. The myopic patients with posterior staphyloma are particularly at higher risk. The patients, presenting for retinal detachment and radial keratotomy, also have higher propensity of scleral perforation due to large globe, like myopes. Recessed eyes, tight lower eyelids, small orbital cavity, etc., are also more challenging situations and are at an increased risk of scleral penetration. In such situations, periconal (peribulbar) needle placement may be safer than the intraconal placement of needle.

When someone does not believe in the difference between the periconal (peribulbar) and intraconal (retrobulbar) block, they just try to direct the needle tip toward the orbital floor during the placement of the needle through the inferotemporal route and the orbital roof during the superotemporal route to avoid this complication. A safe prerequisite to perform the regional anesthesia of orbit is to know the exact axial length of the eyeball prior to the block. This warns one about the higher risks in larger than average sizes of eyes.

In cataract surgery the precise axial length of the eyeball is usually available *from the biometry* which is done to calculate the power of the intraocular lens. But, in other than cataract procedures, where the axial length is not precisely known, then the close attention to the diopter power of patient's spectacles or contact lenses will provide the valuable clues to the dimensions of the globe. The ultrasonography (USG) of eyeball, with suspected staphyloma and high myopia, is also effective in reducing this complication rates. In such situations, it is prudent to perform periconal method and/or intraconal injection (if it is absolutely necessary) with patient's gaze directed downward and outward or to opt for GA.

Though the incidences of the penetration or the perforation of eyeball caused by thick blunt needles is low, but it results in more serious and permanent damage to the eyeball than when such injuries result from the use of fine disposable ones. Fine disposable needles which are less painful for the patient have been proved to be relatively safe than the blunt needles in respect to the postpenetration management. About >50% of all the iatrogenic globe perforations go unsuspected at the time of their occurrence. The event of perforation may be suspected if there is *hypotomy, vitreous hemorrhage, poor red reflex from the retina,* etc. Patients may complain of marked pain during the occurrence of perforation, particularly if the local anesthetic agent is injected intraocularly. Fundoscopy confirms the diagnosis. Globe perforation, involving only the retinal tears with minimum blood in vitreous, can be managed with laser photocoagulation, cryotherapy, or sometimes by close observation only. When much blood is present in the vitreous cavity, then emergency vitrectomy may be indicated. Without surgical intervention, this severe vitreous hemorrhage frequently leads to the proliferative vitreoretinopathy and the subsequent detachment of the retina, where prompt surgical treatment is indicated. Actually, the appropriate management of scleral penetration and perforation is complex **(Box 6)**.

The *intraorbital bleeding* is another common complication of ophthalmic regional anesthesia. It may be manifested as *retrobulbar hemorrhage, peribulbar hemorrhage, subconjunctival hemorrhage, lid ecchymoses, etc.* The retrobulbar or peribulbar hemorrhage varies in severity. It may be small enough and go unrecognized or is severe enough which results in the loss of vision, due to the tamponade effect of the small nutrient vessels of the optic nerve. This explains those cases of profound visual loss,

where the findings of retinal vascular occlusion were not seen, but late optic atrophy had developed. This loss of vision may also occur due to the tamponade of central retinal artery from massive retrobulbar or peribulbar hemorrhage.

Some retrobulbar hemorrhage are of venous origin and spread slowly. Whereas, the arterial hemorrhage produces the rapid and tight orbital swelling, marked proptosis, immobility of globe, massive blood staining of lids and conjunctiva, etc. Due to the increased intraorbital pressure from arterial bleeding, the serious impairment of the vascular supply to the retina and globe may result. The anterior orbital hemorrhage, subconjunctival bleeding and lid ecchymoses are also the most disconcerning sequelae of the intraconal (retrobulbar) or periconal (peribulbar) anesthesia. These commonly cause the patient and his family to make complain. Nevertheless, even if bruising occurs, then the patients and the accompanying person should be informed. In such circumstances reassurance should be given to them that the surgical outcome will not be affected at all and the bruising will clear away spontaneously within a few days.

The anterior orbit has less vessels than the posterior orbit. *Three anterior orbital locations are relatively avascular.* These are the *inferotemporal, superotemporal, and the nasal side of medial rectus muscle.* So, by using the fine needles and confining the needle prick within these three locations and not going beyond 31 mm from the orbital rim posteriorly, we can reduce the incidences and the severity of intraorbital bleeding. If it occurs, it may be minimized by constant vigilance for any sign of bleeding immediately following needle withdrawal and by rapid application of digital pressure with a gauge pad, applied to the closed lids. The other management of retrobulbar hemorrhage are osmotic diuresis and lateral canthotomy, which allows the drainage of the blood and the decompression of the orbit. So, the surgeons should be informed immediately and the pulsation of the central retinal artery should be assessed. The superonasal area should be avoided for needle insertion, because the complex trochlear mechanism of the superior oblique muscles is located there.

The *prolonged malfunction of the extraocular muscle* may also sometimes occur, after the regional anesthesia of orbit. Among these, the *diplopia* and *ptosis* are common which may last for 24–48 hours postoperatively, when the long acting local anesthetic agents have been used in higher concentration and in large volume. When these persist for long period and fail to recover, then it may give the evidences of the toxic changes of muscles by local anesthetic agents. Where the recovery is delayed for >6 weeks, then the 25% of this toxic change becomes permanent. It is indeed pathetic, when a patient who has come for a perfect optical result, ends up with the devastating diplopia, because the eyes are misaligned. Local anesthetic agents containing hyaluronidase and/or adrenaline may be more myotoxic than the plain local anesthetic solutions. The higher the concentration of the local anesthetic agents is more likely to result in a more intense myotoxicity. Another common cause of prolonged malfunction of extraocular muscles is the *direct intramuscular injection* of local anesthetic agent of any concentration.

Ptosis is also a very common complication after ophthalmic RA. This postoperative ptosis is of multifactorial origin. Among these, the injection of the local anesthetic agent, directly into the levator palpebrae superioris muscle, plays an important role. The toxic damage of muscle fibers from local anesthetic agent which is not injected directly into the muscle may also account for many cases of transient and permanent ptosis **(Box 7)**.

Most postoperative ptosis also occurs in the patients in whom the levator aponeurotic apparatus was already in pathological condition beforehand and the regional anesthesia only serves to accelerate the preexisting condition. The preexisting degenerative conditions of the aponeurosis of levator palpebrae superioris muscle which usually accelerate the postanesthetic ptosis include: the disinsertion in tarsal plate, the dehiscence, and the rarefaction of the aponeurosis. Many of these lids, with the above mentioned pathologies, would have become ptotic, even if surgery and regional anesthesia had not been performed. The regional anesthesia has just accelerated the preexisting pathological process. A low incidence of postoperative ptosis is seen in surgeries which are done under GA than with local anesthesia. Surgical correction of such postoperative ptosis is done, when there is only interference with the vision. But, it should be delayed for 6 months, until a self-correction up to a certain limit occurs and a stable state has been reached. So, it is very prudent and should be a routine practice to check the positions of eyelid margins above the central cornea, before embarking on surgery and is documented with photography, if needed. Patients also should be informed beforehand about the possibility of ptosis which may be temporary or permanent after surgery. Written consent for surgery acknowledging this complication of ptosis should also be taken.

The exposure of anesthetized cornea and subsequently its abrasion are also very common complications of

ophthalmic regional anesthesia. This abrasion is seen as a dull nonreflective patch or as a positive area by fluorescein staining. So, care must be taken to protect the anesthetized cornea by occlusive dressing, during the whole perioperative period. An occlusive dressing should be used, after anesthesia, to keep the eyelids shut, until their full function and reflexes have recovered. The time of recovery for this full function of eyelid will depend on the duration of the action of the chosen anesthetic drug. On the other hand, a prolonged patch can provide a moist atmosphere beneath the gauge, as an ideal culture medium for the organisms to grow. That's why some experienced surgeons do not use patch over the eye postoperatively, especially after small wound phacoemulsification cataract extraction with foldable intraocular lens implantation, under solely topical anesthesia.

But, the safety of this decision from the point of view of the risks of superficial corneal damage would depend on the degree of the recovery from anesthesia. After recovery from anesthesia, corneal abrasion (if it occurs) is manifested as pain, foreign body sensation, tearing, conjunctivitis, and photophobia. Pain is also made worse by blinking. The management of corneal abrasion consists of covering the eye with an antibiotic eye ointment. But, topical applications of anesthetic drops and steroids over the cornea to reduce pain are contraindicated, because they impair the healing of wound.

■ OCULOCARDIAC REFLEX

Oculocardiac reflex (OCR) is a *trigeminal-vagal reflex* which is manifested by cardiac arrhythmias such as bradycardia, nodal rhythm, ectopic beats, ventricular fibrillation, asystole, etc., in response to vagal stimulation. Although the most common manifestation of this reflex is sinus bradycardia, but virtually any cardiac dysrhythmia, such as nodal, junctional, atrial, or any serious ventricular arrhythmia may occur. This oculocardiac reflex was first described by Aschner and Dagini by two simultaneous, but independent reports, in 1908. *The impulses for this OCR usually arise from the stretch and pressure receptors which are present throughout the globe and the orbit. The afferent pathway of this reflex first goes through the long and the short ciliary nerves to the ciliary ganglion. Then, it passes to the Gasserian (trigeminal) ganglion along the ophthalmic division of the trigeminal nerve (the Vth cranial nerve). Ultimately, these afferent pathways terminate at the main trigeminal sensory nucleus which is situated on the floor of the fourth ventricle. From this central nucleus, then, the efferent pathway comes down by the vagus nerve and ends at the cardiovascular center, respiratory center and vomiting center, causing the negative ionotropic*

BOX 7: Some factors responsible for muscle damage and ptosis.

- Pressure applied to the globe and upper lid
- Edema of the eyelid
- Traction on the superior rectus muscle complex
- Pressure exerted by the lid speculum
- Prolonged postoperative patching

effects, negative chronotropic effects, conduction defects, vomiting, sinus arrest, and/or respiratory arrest. So, the term "oculocardiac reflex" should be changed to "oculomedullary reflex", consisting of oculocardiac, oculorespiratory, and oculoemetic reflexes.

The OCR may be triggered by many factors such as the pressure on eyeball, traction on extraocular muscles, orbital hematoma or many others. The traction on medial rectus muscle produces the more marked effects than the traction on the other muscles. This reflex seems to be most active in children. So, the OCR occurs most often during the strabismus surgery in children. But, it may also occur occasionally during retinal surgery or at the time of injection of intraorbital block.

The reported incidence of OCR varies considerably from 30 to 90%. Because, it depends on the intensity of observation and the definition of arrhythmias. The transient cardiac arrest may occur as frequently as 1 in 2,000 cases of strabismus surgery. The force and the type of stimulus usually influence the incidences of OCR. The more acute, stronger, and sustained will be the stimulus and the more sensitive will be the patient, the more likely is the OCR to occur. Therefore, the electrocardiogram (ECG) should always be monitored continuously during ophthalmic surgery. The OCR ceases when the stimulus (from pressure or traction) ends. So, the surgeon and anesthesiologist should not hesitate to communicate with each other, during any procedure, involving the possibility of an OCR.

The intramuscular atropine or glycopyrrolate, as premedication, are not very effective in preventing this oculocardiac reflex, compared to their intravenous administration. The atropine in the dose of 0.02 mg/kg through IV prior to the surgery will reduce the incidences of OCR by 5–15%. The intravenous glycopyrrolate in the dose of 0.01 mg/kg, is preferred than atropine, as it causes less tachycardia. Hypercarbia increases the sensitivity to this reflex, and an anesthetic technique such as controlled ventilation, rather than spontaneous ventilation, might be preferred.

The first step of treating the OCR is to stop the production of stimulus by surgeon, before the arrhythmia progresses to sinus arrest. Fortunately, the repeated and the sustained stimulation usually cause the OCR to become fatigue. If the arrhythmias still persist after stopping the production of stimulus, then treatment with atropine (20 µg/kg IV) and injection of local anesthetic agent into the eye muscle may be necessary. If the patient still remains sensitive to the manipulations of extraocular muscles, then the anesthesiologist should check the adequacy of the depth of GA, the existence of normocarbia and the

gentleness of surgical manipulation. If the dysrhythmia is fast or ventricular in origin, then surgery should be stopped immediately. Then, we should wait for the return of normal rhythm, before giving atropine; otherwise it (atropine) may provoke ventricular tachycardia or fibrillation.

■ INTRAOCULAR PRESSURE AND ANESTHESIA

Intraocular pressure helps to maintain the shape and the optical properties of eye. During the day to day normal activities, the temporary variations of IOP, within its normal ranges, are normally well tolerated. For example, the blinking of eyes raises the IOP by 5 mm Hg and the squeezing (forced contraction of orbicularis oculi muscle) of eyes may transiently increase the IOP >50 mm Hg. However, even the brief episodes of increased IOP in patients with underlying low pressure in ophthalmic artery (e.g., from systemic hypotension, arteriosclerotic involvement of retinal artery) may cause the retinal ischemia and damage.

The IOP is the result of a dynamic balance between (i) the production of aqueous humor by the ciliary body in the posterior chamber of the eyeball and (ii) its eventual elimination by episcleral venous system via the spaces of Fontana and the canal of Schlemm at iridocorneal angle. So, the most important factors which influence the IOP are— (i) the production and the movement of aqueous humor, (ii) the changes in the choroidal blood volume, (iii) the central venous pressure, and (iv) the extraocular muscular tone. The normal IOP is approximately 15–20 mm Hg.

The ciliary body lies behind the root of the iris and consists of two parts. The posterior muscular part is called the *pars plana*. The muscle in this part (pars plana) has *three important functions*—(i) the most important of which is to relax the suspensory ligament of lens. Thus, the lens becomes more spherical and allows the accommodation of near vision, (ii) Secondly; it exerts tension on the scleral spur. This widens the spaces in trabecular meshwork and thus facilitates the drainage of aqueous humor, (iii) A third and minor action of this muscle is as the dilator of iris. The pars plana is the favored site for sclerotomies through which the insertion of instruments into the eyeball is done during vitreoretinal surgery. The anterior part of this ciliary body is thrown into about 70–80 folds and is called as the *pars plicata*. Here, the stroma is highly vascular and is richly supplied by fenestrated capillaries. It is from these folds the aqueous humor is secreted. The aqueous humor is produced at a rate of about 2 µL/min.

After secretion, this aqueous humor circulates freely from the posterior chamber into the anterior chamber of eyeball, around the free margin of the iris. If there is any increase in the venous pressure, or decrease in the cross sectional area of this spaces of Fontana, then there is increase in the resistance to the outflow of aqueous humor which increases the IOP. Mydriatic drugs relax the ciliary muscles and close the iridocorneal angle at Fontana's spaces. Thereby, they increase the IOP. Coughing, straining, airway obstruction, Trendelenburg position, and Valsalva maneuvers, etc., significantly increase the central venous pressure (CVP). Thus, they decrease the outflow of the aqueous humor from the Schlemm's canal into the episcleral venous system and increase the IOP. Due to the aforementioned factors, along with the increase in CVP and decrease in the drainage of aqueous humor, there is also increase in choroidal blood volume, causing the increased IOP.

The uveal tract is the intermediate vascular coat of globe, lying in between the sclera and retina. It consists of choroid, ciliary body, and iris. The choroid coat is present in the posterior 5/6th of eyeball and is juxtaposed to sclera. It extends forward up to the ora serrata of retina. It is chocolate-brown in color and is highly vascular. Choroid is being fed by the branches of short posterior ciliary arteries and is drained by a venous network which ultimately converges into four or five vortex veins. This vortex veins, then, pierce the sclera 5–8 mm posterior to the equator of globe. One of these is located at the lateral border of inferior rectus muscle and 5 mm posterior to the equator. It may be the common source of intraorbital bleeding, during the inferotemporal needle placement. The choroid is responsible for the nutrition of the outer layer of retina. The inner layer of retina receives its blood supply from the central retinal artery. The vascularity of choroid layer increases with systemic venous congestion, arterial hypertension, hypoxia, and hypercarbia. The sclera and the choroid are loosely adherent and are separated by a potential suprachoroidal space which may fill with blood during an expulsive or suprachoroidal hemorrhage. This is a dreaded surgical complication.

The choroidal blood flow or its volume affects the IOP significantly. But, it is usually autoregulated over a wide range of systemic blood pressure to keep the IOP stable. The sudden increase in systolic blood pressure causes a transient increase in choroidal blood volume and IOP. Hypotension (systolic blood pressure <90 mm Hg) reduces the choroidal volume and subsequently decreases the IOP. During an open eye surgery, the IOP usually remains lower than normal. But, a sudden increase in choroidal blood volume can force the vitreous gel forward into anterior chamber and also cause the prolapse of iris. Any cause which increases the CVP; increases the choroidal blood volume and its pressure and thus elevates the IOP **(Table 1)**.

The choroidal circulation, choroidal pressure, and subsequently the IOP are also sensitive to the changes of the partial pressure of oxygen. So, hypoxia increases the

TABLE 1: Physiological factors affecting IOP (intra-ocular pressure).

Factors	*IOP*
Central venous pressure • Increased • Decreased	 • ↑↑↑ • ↓↓↓
Arterial blood pressure • Increased • Decreased	 • ↑ • ↓
PaO_2 • Increased • Decreased	 • 0 • ↑
$PaCO_2$ • Increased • Decreased	 • ↑↑ • ↓↓

TABLE 2: Anesthetic agents affecting IOP.

Drugs	*Effects on IOP*
Intravenous anesthetics • Thiopentone • Propofol • Ketamine • Benzodiazepines • Opioids	 • ↓↓ • ↓↓ • ↑ • ↓ • ↓
Inhaled anesthetics • NO • Volatile agents	 • ↓ • ↓↓
Muscle relaxant • Succinylcholine • Nondepolarizing	 • ↑↑ • ↓

choroidal circulation and its volume by vasodilatation and increases the IOP. Respiratory acidosis and hypercarbia also increases the choroidal blood flow by vasodilatation and, therefore, elevates the IOP. Hypocarbia decreases IOP through the vasoconstriction of the choroidal blood vessels, and decrease in the formation of aqueous humor through the reduced carbonic anhydrase activity.

The IOP is also controlled by CNS through the neurovascularly-mediated responses and extraocular muscle tone. These are usually depressed by barbiturates, volatile inhaled anesthetic agents, and nondepolarizing muscle relaxants **(Table 2)**. It is also found that IOP is more directly related to CVP than the arterial pressure. So, a slight head up tilt during any intraocular surgery reduces the IOP, due to any cause. The external pressure on the eyeball initially increases the IOP. But, this increased IOP promotes increased outflow of aqueous humor and thus returns IOP toward normal **(Fig. 31)**.

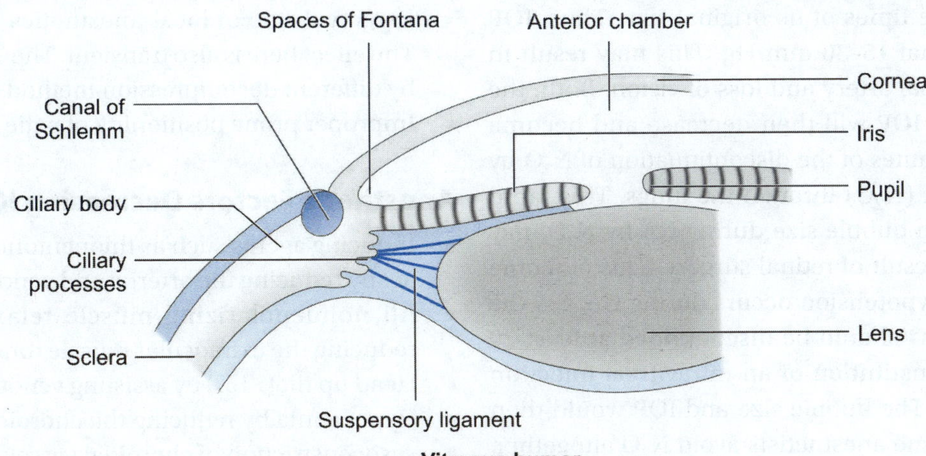

Fig. 31: Circulation of aqueous humor.

In general, the most anesthetic agents, except ketamine and succinylcholine, (i) relax the extraocular muscle tone, (ii) depress the CNS, (iii) improve the outflow of aqueous humor, (iv) lower the venous and arterial pressure, and thus reduce the IOP. Ketamine raises the arterial blood pressure and does not relax the extraocular muscles. So, it does not reduce the IOP, rather it increases IOP. The inducing agents such as thiopentone and propofol also lower IOP by depressing the CNS and improving the outflow of aqueous humor. Antisialagogues, such as atropine and glycopyrrolate, given as premedication through IV or any other route have no significant effect on IOP, even in patients with glaucoma. However, when these drugs are applied topically on eye, they cause mydriasis, increase IOP and precipitate or worsen angle closure glaucoma. Similarly, neostigmine and atropine combination, which are used intravenously to reverse the nondepolarizing muscle relaxants, do not significantly alter IOP. But, when neostigmine is used topically, it reduces IOP. On the other hand, laryngoscopy and intubation or extubation elevate the IOP. However, the mechanism of it is not clear, but is probably related to sympathetic cardiovascular responses to tracheal intubation or extubation.

Several attempts have been advocated to attenuate the IOP response, related to laryngoscopy and intubation or extubation. These are: pretreatment with IV lignocaine, narcotics, and β-blockers. The oral administration of any centrally acting antihypertensive drug, such as, clonidine in the dose of 5 µg/kg of body weight and given 2 hours before the induction of anesthesia will blunt the IOP response to intubation. Benzodiazepines, administered intravenously, reduce the IOP, but not when administered orally. On the other hand, narcotics do not decrease the IOP, even in glaucoma. The effect of ketamine on IOP is controversial. Early studies show an increase in IOP after an IV administration of ketamine. But when ketamine is used after premedication with BDZ, then IOP does not elevate.

All the nondepolarizing muscle relaxants lower the IOP. But, succinylcholine increase IOP 5–10 mm Hg for 5–10 minutes (transient) after its administration, due to prolonged contracture of extraocular muscles. This is because, the cells of extraocular muscles contain multiple neuromuscular junctions, and depolarization of these cells by succinylcholine causes prolonged contracture. However, in studies of hundreds of patients with open eye injuries, no patient experienced extrusion of ocular contents after the administration of succinylcholine. Therefore, practically succinylcholine is not contraindicated in cases of open eye injuries, though theoretically. Nevertheless, dogmatism often wins the statistical data and so ophthalmic surgeon request not to administer during open globe surgeries. The resulting transient increase in IOP may have several effects. It will cause false higher measurements of IOP during EUA in glaucoma patients, potentially leading to unnecessary surgery. Prolonged contracture of extraocular muscles may result in an abnormal "forced duction test" (it is test utilized in strabismus surgery to evaluate the cause of extraocular muscle imbalance and to determine the type of surgical correction).

During retinal surgery, the ophthalmologists, sometimes, inject gases into vitreal cavity to tamponade the retina. The gases commonly used for this purpose are C_3F_8 (octafluoropropane) and SF_6 (sulfur hexafluoride). They are inert, very insoluble in water, and are so poorly diffusible. N_2O is 117 times more diffusible than SF_6 and so it enters into the gas bubble of SF_6, present in retina very rapidly. Therefore, if administration of N_2O is continued after injection of C_3F_8 or SF_6 gas into the vitreal cavity, then the size of these injected gas bubbles rapidly increases and becomes about three times of its original size. Thus, IOP increases from normal 15–30 mm Hg. This may result in the occlusion of retinal artery and loss of vision. Both, the bubble size and the IOP will then decrease and become normal within 15 minutes of the discontinuation of N_2O by 90% elimination of it (N_2O) through the lungs. This rapid and wide variation in bubble size during GA by N_2O may adversely affect the result of retinal surgery. This outcome is more affected, if hypotension occurs during GA. So, the administration of N_2O should be discontinued at least 20 minutes before the institution of an intravitreal injection of C_3F_8 or SF_6 gases. The bubble size and IOP would then remain stable. So, some anesthetists avoid N_2O altogether, when the intravitreal injection of gas is planned. The SF_6 gas remains in vitreal cavity for at least 10 days. Other gases remain in the vitreal cavity for as long as 20–30 days. So, N_2O should always be avoided in any patient, returning for retinal resurgery, within 3–4 weeks of undergoing intravitreal injection of gases. Patients with intravitreal gas bubbles may also risk ocular damage, during air travel. This is because, if patients having intraocular air volumes of only 0.25 cc, were subjected to pressures, simulating that inside a commercial airplane, there would be an average rise of IOP by 40 mm Hg. This will again decrease to lower than normal, after return to preflight pressures.

Factors Affecting Intraocular Pressure

These are analogous to the factors, affecting ICP (intracranial pressure). The factors which affect the IOP are:
- Head up or down position
- Volume of aqueous humor, determined by the balance of production and drainage
- The tone of extraocular muscles
- Choroidal blood volume, determined by the balance of arterial flow and venous drainage
- *Mannitol and acetazolamide:* Mannitol in the dose of 0.5–1.0 g/kg IV reduces the IOP by withdrawing fluid from the vitreous. Acetazolamide in the dose of 500 mg orally or IV reduces the IOP by reducing the production of aqueous by ciliary body
- Anesthetic factors

Anesthetic Factors Increasing IOP

- External compressions on globe by face mask which is applied tightly.
- Laryngoscopy—through pressure response or from straining in an inadequately relaxed patient.
- Suxamethonium—through its effect on extraocular muscles.

- Large volume of local anesthetics placed in the orbit. The effect here is also transient. The ↑IOP can be reduced by different decompression method
- Improper prone positioning of patient.

Anesthetic Factors Decreasing IOP

- Inducing agents such as thiopentone and propofol. They act by reducing the arterial and venous pressure
- All nondepolarizing muscle relaxants. They act by reducing the extraocular muscle tone
- Head up tilt (>15°) by assisting venous drainage
- Hypocapnia by reducing the choroidal blood volume by vasoconstriction of choroidal vessels.

Systemic Effects of Ophthalmic Drugs

Topically applied eye drops are systemically absorbed by the vessels of conjunctiva and the mucosa of nasolacrimal duct and nose. The rate of absorption of drugs through this mucosa is intermediate between that of intravenous and subcutaneous injection. For example, one drop of 10% phenylephrine contains near about 5 mg of drug (1 drop = ±1/20 mL). Now one can easily compare this dose with the IV dose of phenylephrine (0.05–0.1 mg) which is used to treat hypotension in an adult patient.

Echothiophate (an irreversible cholinesterase inhibitor) is often used in the treatment of glaucoma. Topical use of it leads to its systemic absorption and an inhibition of plasma cholinesterase activity. Therefore, echothiophate will prolong the duration of the action of succinylcholine, because it (succinylcholine) is metabolized by cholinesterase enzyme.

Epinephrine eye drop can cause hypertension, tachycardia, ventricular arrhythmia, etc. But, direct instillation of epinephrine into the anterior chamber of eyeball has not been associated with these cardiovascular complications.

Timolol (a nonselective β adrenergic antagonist) is used frequently in glaucoma to reduce IOP by decreasing the production of aqueous humor. Topically used timolol, after its absorption through conjunctiva and nasal and nasolacrimal mucosa, often causes reduced HR. In rare cases, it has been associated with atropine resistant bradycardia, hypotension, and bronchospasm, during GA.

■ RETINOPATHY OF PREMATURITY

As the neonatal care has been improved due to the advancement of technology, so more and more premature infants now survive. Therefore, the incidence of retinopathy of prematurity is gradually increasing. It has a complex cause with many etiologies. Previously, it was thought that the retinopathy of prematurity (ROP) was only associated with hyperoxic conditions during neonatal care. But, the full term nonhyperoxic neonates and infants can also have this condition just like premature infants who have never had O_2 therapy. So, it is decided that ROP may also be associated with factors such as hypoxia, hypocarbia, hypercarbia, sepsis, apnea, etc., other than hypoxia. The ROP still occurs, despite the efforts in the neonatal intensive care unit to control and monitor the O_2 delivery. ROP also occurs even when the capillary PO_2 is kept between 35 and 40 mm Hg and PaO_2 is maintained between 50 and 70 mm Hg in premature infants. So, the problem for the anesthetists who is giving GA to a premature infant is to balance the risk between the hypoxic damage and prolonged exposure to high O_2 concentration, causing ROP. Although, there is no convincing evidence that ROP has always occurred solely because of high O_2 concentration, given during anesthesia, still prolonged exposure to high intraoperative concentration of O_2 is best avoided during the period of retinal immaturity, i.e., until 8 months of age. PaO_2 is maintained between 60 and 90 mm Hg by keeping SPO_2 in pulse oximetry between 90 and 95%.

GENERAL ANESTHESIA FOR OPHTHALMIC SURGERY

The list of indications of GA for ophthalmic surgery has been tabled before. The main aim of GA in ophthalmic surgery is to minimize the increase in IOP and keeps the patient motionless, while maintaining cardiovascular stability. But, deep anesthesia should be avoided as the main population in ophthalmic surgery is likely to be elderly with several comorbidities. General anesthesia is provided, unless there are overwhelming risks. Then, the patients and their attendants are informed about the risks and GA is provided only if they accept them. Always a risk-benefit ratio has to be calculated, keeping in mind that ophthalmic surgeries are not life-saving. The preoperative assessment and preparation for GA in the patients scheduled for ophthalmic surgeries follow the same guidelines as GA for other surgeries.

A Standard Technique of General Anesthesia Which is Usually followed for Ophthalmic Surgeries

The choice between local anesthetic and GA should be made jointly by the patient, anesthesiologist, and surgeon. The patient may refuse local anesthetic due to—(i) fear of awake during operation, (ii) fear of injection for local anesthetic at eye, (iii) unpleasant memory of a previous eye block, and (iv) local eye procedure. General anesthesia is indicated in children and uncooperative patients, because even a small head movement may cause serious complications during eye microsurgery.

Premedications

About 99% of ophthalmic surgeries are done as outdoor basis. So, sedative premedication may delay the discharge procedure. On the other hand, patients are often elderly or children. Elderly patients are usually associated with hypertension, coronary artery disease, diabetes, etc., and pediatric patients will obviously cry continuously, if kept in empty stomach for long time, demanding premedication. Hence, after careful consideration of patient's medical status, premedication (sedation) should be administered with caution.

- During ophthalmic surgery, the choice of induction depends more on patient's medical condition than on eye diseases, with one exception, i.e., ruptured globe. Usually, intravenous induction is done by propofol or thiopentone. Ketamine is used, only if properly indicated. For surgery on an open eye injury, the key to anesthesia is smooth induction. Especially, coughing should be avoided during induction and intubation by any cost. It is achieved by deep level of anesthesia and profound paralysis. The IOP response to laryngoscopy and intubation can be moderated by prior administration of IV lignocaine (1.5 mg/kg), or esmolol (0.5–1.5 mg/kg).

- Nondepolarizing muscle relaxants are preferred. Many patients with open globe injury have full stomach and require a rapid sequence induction and intubation to avoid aspiration. Succinylcholine can be used, only if it is properly indicated. Despite theoretical concerns, succinylcholine does not increase the likelihood of vitreous loss with open eye injuries.

- Airway is maintained by endotracheal tube (ET) tube or laryngeal mask airway (LMA). Eye surgery often necessitates the positioning of anesthetist away from the patient's airway, making the close monitoring of patient by pulse oximetry and capnography mandatary. ET tube kinking, breathing circuit disconnection and unintentional extubation may be more likely, because the surgeon works very close to airway. Kinking and obstruction of ET tube can be minimized by using preformed oral Ring–Adair–Elwyn (RAE) ET. In contrast to most other type of pediatric surgery, the body temperature of pediatric patients may rise during ophthalmic surgery, because of head-to-toe draping and minimum body surface exposure. So, the end-tidal carbon dioxide ($ETCO_2$) analysis helps to differentiate this situation from malignant hyperthermia.

- Ventilation is maintained by intermittent positive pressure ventilation (IPPV) or spontaneous ventilation. Analgesia is provided with fentanyl/alfentanil/sufentanil/remifentanil, etc.
- Maintenance of anesthesia is by O_2 with air/N_2O/propofol infusion by target control infusion (TCI)/volatile inhalational agents. N_2O should be avoided in vitreoretinal surgeries, especially if SF_6 or C_3F_8 gases are used.
- The pain and stress evoked by eye surgery are considerably less than other general surgical procedures. So, lighter plane of anesthesia is adequate, if the movement of patient is not so potentially catastrophic. The lack of cardiovascular stimulation, inherent to most of the eye procedures, combined with the need for adequate anesthetic depth to prevent the movement of patient, can result in hypotension in elderly individuals. This problem is usually avoided by ensuring adequate intravenous hydration and by administering small doses of IV vasoconstrictors. Judicious administration of nondepolarizing muscle relaxants, to avoid patient movement, is better in such circumstances in order to allow the reduced depth of GA.
- Use of glycopyrrolate as antisialagogue is preferred in ophthalmic surgeries. It reduces the volume of saliva which often produces cough, laryngospasm, etc.
- Airway should be secured properly, as the intraoperative emergency access to the airway is limited by the surgical drapes, instrument trolleys, and other equipment, overlying in this area. Most importantly, there prevails a low threshold for moving everyone out of the way to inspect the airway, when some problem is suspected.
- Which is the better or safe for ophthalmic surgeries—an ET tube or a LMA? This is a potent question which is often asked. Unless contraindicated, the LMA is ideal for ophthalmic surgeries, as it avoids laryngoscopy with the consequent adverse effects of it on IOP. It produces minimal stimulation once is *in situ* and permits a lighter anesthesia. The quality of emergence is also better than ET tube and very smooth in case of LMA. About 10% of lignocaine is usually sprayed in larynx during endotracheal intubation. But unfortunately, its effect is very short lived and so may no longer be effective during extubation. Extubation of ET tube in a deep plane or administration of a bolus dose of IV lignocaine (1 mg/kg) or propofol (0.5 mg/kg/min) just before extubation are some of the methods which are often opted for smooth extubation. It is better, not to lighten the plane of anesthesia, before the completion of surgery and the removal of typical sticking drapes used in ophthalmic surgeries. If a peribulbar block is not used, drape removal may well be the most stimulating part of the procedure. During extubation emergence hypertension and a concomitant rise in IOP can be managed by the use of IV lignocaine and/or β-blocker.
- Choice between the IPPV and spontaneous ventilation is another important question in ophthalmic surgeries. For minor and extraocular surgeries, the spontaneous ventilation is acceptable. Controlled ventilation or IPPV has a number of advantages in intraocular and other major ophthalmic surgeries. It allows a more precise control of CO_2, reducing IOP, and desensitizing the oculomedullary (oculocardiac) reflex. It also allows the benefits of a balanced anesthesia technique. IPPV by LMA is also uneventful. But, high pressure (>15 cm of H2O) with risk of gastric insufflation should be avoided. CO_2 wave-form should always be monitored. Any change in the waveform usually heralds a change in ventilation, before it is clinically apparent (malpositioned LMA, inadequate muscle relaxation, etc.). Nerve stimulators should be routinely used for ophthalmic surgeries, because coughing and gagging are less well tolerated by ophthalmic surgeons, than their colleagues of other surgical streams.
- If local block is used as a supplement to GA, it should be administered only after induction. However, since the principal benefit of a local block is the avoidance of GA. But when it is used in addition to GA. Then the risk-benefit ratio is now altered. So, it may no longer be justified now. But, many anesthesiologists still use a local block in addition to GA, especially in ophthalmic surgeries, because it allows a very good control of patients even with lesser anesthetic drugs and most importantly it provides better postoperative analgesia.

Kidney Diseases and Anesthesia

■ INTRODUCTION

The kidneys are a pair of essential excretory and endocrine organs which (1) form urine, (2) eliminate nitrogenous waste products from blood, produced during protein metabolism, (3) maintain electrolyte and water balance of our body, (4) eliminate toxins, (5) secrete hormones, including renin and erythropoietin, and (6) synthesize the active form of vitamin D. In the kidney, the fluid, resembling plasma, is ultra-filtered through the capillaries of glomeruli and is collected in Bowman's capsule. Then, this fluid (glomerular filtrate) passes down the renal tubule, and its volume and composition are gradually reduced and changed by the reabsorption of water and by the secretion and absorption of K^+, H^+, Ca^{2+}, HCO_3^-, PO_4^{2-}, Cl^-, urea, and other substances.

The composition of this glomerular filtrate while passing through the renal tubule is also altered by the process of tubular reabsorption and secretion of different other solutes to form finally the urine whose composition may vary according to circumstances. Many homeostatic mechanisms try to maintain the compositions of plasma or extracellular fluid (ECF) normal by changing the composition of urine. In addition, the kidneys also secrete the renin for autoregulation of RBF and blood pressure (BP), erythropoietin for the maturation of red blood cells (RBCs), and 1,25-dihydroxycholecalciferol for the control of calcium metabolism, which may modify the action of parathyroid hormone (PTH).

Thus, the kidneys also subserve the function of endocrine organs. The other endocrine part of the kidney includes the interstitial tissue of medulla. These interstitial cells are also called the "type I medullary interstitial cell". They secrete prostaglandin (PG), predominantly prostaglandin E2 (PGE_2). The PGE_2 is also secreted by the cells of the collecting duct (CD). Prostacyclin (PGI_2) and other PGs are also secreted by the afferent arterioles and glomeruli. They maintain the internal homeostasis of the kidney.

■ STRUCTURE OF KIDNEY

The structure of kidney can be studied under two headings—macroscopic and microscopic.

Macroscopic Structure of Kidney

On coronal section, macroscopically, the kidney presents two parts: (1) The inner renal sinus and (2) the outer renal substance itself. The *outer renal substance* itself again consists of two parts: (1) The *inner medulla* and (2) the *outer cortex* (**Fig. 1**).

Medulla

In coronal section, the renal medulla presents 8–18 striated, pale, and conical masses which are called the *renal pyramids.* Each of these renal pyramids has a base directed toward the cortex and an apex projected into the renal sinus. The part of the apex of renal pyramid that projects into the renal sinus is called the *renal papilla.* Each renal papilla of renal pyramid is perforated by 16–20 ducts of Bellini. The renal sinus, which receives renal papilla, is called the calyx minor. As a rule,

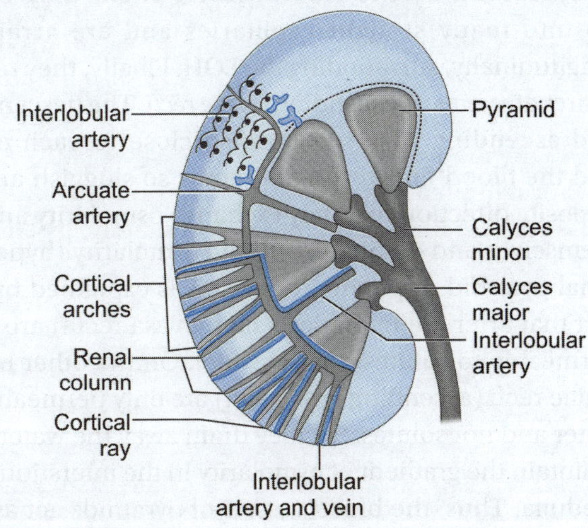

Fig. 1: Macroscopic structure of kidney in coronal section.

only one calyx minor receives one to three renal papillae. Each renal pyramid, capped with the adjoining part of the renal cortex on its outer surface, forms the individual *lobe of kidney*. There are many striations on each pyramid which are due to the following factors:

- *Long loops of Henle (LOH) of the juxtamedullary glomeruli with their long descending and ascending limbs:* These long renal tubules are derived from glomeruli which are situated in cortex but nearer to the medulla (juxtamedullary glomeruli), and their long renal tubules are plunged into the substance of pyramids. Among these, the longest loops even extend close to the renal papilla. The short LOH, which are derived from the most superficial cortical nephrons, do not extend up to the medulla, or if they do extend, they reach only close to the basal zone (base) of pyramid. These U-shaped long LOH of the juxtamedullary glomeruli with their vasa recta (blood vessels) act as a countercurrent osmotic multiplier system and are responsible for maintaining the graded osmolarity of the interstitial fluid of renal pyramids or parenchyma. The apexes of these pyramids are hypertonic, whereas the bodies of them are isotonic, and the bases of the pyramids are hypotonic to plasma.
- *Collecting tubules (CTs) and ducts of Bellini:* The area from the base to the apex of the pyramids are traversed by the CTs and the ducts of Bellini. When the CDs and the ducts of Bellini pass through the hypertonic apical zone of pyramid, the urine becomes concentrated and hypertonic and is ultimately collected in the minor calyces.
- *Arteriole recti and venae recti:* These vessels are also called the vasa recta. *Arteriole recti* are the wide bored straight vessels (arterioles). They arise from the efferent glomerular arterioles of juxtamedullary glomeruli and descend by the side of LOH. Then, they break up into many straight capillaries and are arranged longitudinally, surrounding the LOH. Finally, they return to arcuate veins as ascending *venae recti*. The descending and ascending vasa recta are so close to each other and the blood flow through them is so sluggish and in opposite direction that they exchange osmolarity among themselves and do not disturb the osmolarity (hyper) of renal pyramid or parenchyma. This is explained by the fact that arteriole recti (descending vasa recta) are only permeable to solutes but not water. On the other hand, venae recti (ascending vasa recta) are only permeable to water and not solutes. So, they drain away the water and maintain the gradient of osmolarity in the interstitium of medulla. Thus, the blood vessels of pyramids act as the countercurrent osmotic exchanger.

Cortex

The outer portion of the renal substance, situated above the renal medulla, is called the renal cortex. This renal cortex is granular in appearance (not striated) and consists of *cortical arches* and *renal columns*.

- *Cortical arches* are the area of cortex which intervene between the bases of the pyramids and the surface of the kidney. Each cortical arch again consists of numerous *cortical rays* and *smooth parts* in between them. Each cortical ray is a narrow conical (triangular) mass, like the small pyramid. The apex of each cortical ray is directed toward the surface of kidney, and the base is continuous with the striations of the pyramid. Each cortical ray is occupied by CTs and the commencement of duct of Bellini. The *interlobular blood vessels* pass outward along each side of these cortical rays.

The convoluted smooth or plain part of cortex is the area that intervenes between the two adjacent cortical rays. It is occupied by nephrons which consist of renal corpuscles and renal tubules with different convoluted parts of them, up to collecting tubules (CTs). The renal corpuscles and their renal tubules are arranged into 13 or more superimposed layers in these smooth parts between the two cortical rays. The nephrons, which are situated in the superficial portions of renal cortex, are called *cortical nephrons* and their glomeruli are called *cortical glomeruli.* The renal tubules of these cortical nephrons are short, and the capillaries around them remain confined within the cortex.

On the other hand, the nephrons which are situated in the cortex but close to the medulla are called *juxtamedullary nephrons*, and their glomeruli are called *juxtamedullary glomeruli.* Their corresponding LOH are long and extend into the pyramid of medulla with the straight capillaries (vasa recta) around them.

- The *renal columns* of cortex are the areas that intervene between two adjacent areas of cortical arches. These areas of renal column also extend into medulla between two pyramids. It contains nil or few renal corpuscles and is traversed mainly by the *interlobar blood vessels*.

Blood Supply of Kidney

Each kidney is supplied by a renal artery, which is a branch of the abdominal aorta. Each renal artery, after its direct origin from aorta, reaches the hilum of the respective kidney and divides first into *anterior and posterior trunks*. The anterior trunk again subdivides into four *segmental arteries* and the posterior trunk continues as a separate segmental artery (i.e., therefore, there are five segmental arteries, supplying the kidney). These segmental arteries again divide into *lobar branches* which further divide into *interlobar branches*.

These interlobar arteries then pierce the substance of kidney and run through the renal columns in between the two adjacent renal pyramids. At the junction of the renal cortex and medulla, these interlobar arteries divide again dichotomously into *arcuate arteries* and run as an arch, over the base of the pyramids. These arcuate arteries do not anastomose with one another and act as the *end arteries*. From these arcuate arteries, numerous *interlobular arteries* arise and run outward toward the surface of the kidney, through the cortex by the sides of the cortical rays. Then, the extreme terminal branches of the interlobular arteries ramify beneath the renal capsule to form a subcapsular plexus **(Fig. 2)**.

Each interlobular artery, when it runs through the cortex by the sides of the cortical rays, gives origin to a number of *afferent glomerular arterioles* from their sides at different directions. Each afferent glomerular arteriole, then, forms a glomerular capillary plexus in Bowman's capsule. Next, the *efferent glomerular arterioles* arise from these glomerular capillary plexuses, and they are somewhat narrower in diameter than their corresponding afferent arterioles. The efferent arterioles, after their origin from the glomeruli of the superficial zone of renal cortex, break up into the *multiple peritubular plexus* around their corresponding renal tubules. However, they are usually confined within the cortex. The efferent arterioles arising from the glomeruli, which are situated in the superficial part of the renal cortex, do not go deep into the medulla and do not take part in the countercurrent multiplier system. Blood from these cortical peritubular arterial plexuses then empties into the *interlobular veins*, which again drain into the *arcuate vein* and finally drain into the *inferior vena cava*, after

passing successively through the arcuate, *interlobar, lobar, segmental,* and *renal veins*, which corresponds with the arteries.

About 15% of afferent arterioles, arising from the interlobular arteries, form the glomerular capillary plexus in juxtamedullary glomeruli. These juxtamedullary glomeruli are larger and lesser in function than the superficial cortical glomeruli. The diameter of the efferent arteriole, arising from these juxtamedullary glomerular capillary plexuses, is either equal to or slightly larger than their corresponding afferent arteriole and goes deep straight into the renal pyramids. These straight arterioles, which are the continuation of the efferent arterioles of the juxtamedullary glomerular capillary plexus, divide further into 20 or more straight arterial branches (vasa recta) and later break up into capillary plexus (peritubular capillaries) around the renal tubules, which also arise from the corresponding juxtamedullary glomeruli and go deep into the renal medulla.

These peritubular capillary plexuses, then, return to the arcuate veins at the corticomedullary junction by forming some straight veins. These straight arterioles, which arise from these efferent arterioles of the juxtamedullary glomerular capillaries, are called the *descending vasa recta*. The straight venules arising from the peritubular plexus drain into the arcuate veins and are called the *ascending vasa recta*. In medulla, these straight vessels and their divisions run parallel to one another and with the renal tubules. Thus, these straight vascular patterns with renal tubules, arising from juxtamedullary glomeruli, form the structural basis of the countercurrent multiplier system of renal pyramid. This is because the endothelial linings of the glomerular capillary plexus, cortical peritubular capillaries, and ascending vasa recta are fenestrated and permeable to water, but not permeable to solute. On the other hand, the endothelial lining of descending vasa recta is not fenestrated and is lined by the continuous endothelial cells. So, it is not permeable to water but permeable to solute.

Nerve Supply of Kidney

The kidneys are supplied by both the sympathetic and the parasympathetic nerves. The *sympathetic preganglionic efferent* innervation of the kidney comes from the lateral horn of lower three thoracic and upper one or two lumbar segments of the spinal cord. The *postganglionic efferent sympathetic* fibers are then derived from the sympathetic chain and pass through the celiac and renal plexuses. The sympathetic fibers are distributed primarily to (1) the afferent and efferent arterioles, (2) the proximal tubule (PT) and distal tubule (DT), and (3) the juxtaglomerular (JG) cells. In addition, the sympathetic fibers also deeply enter

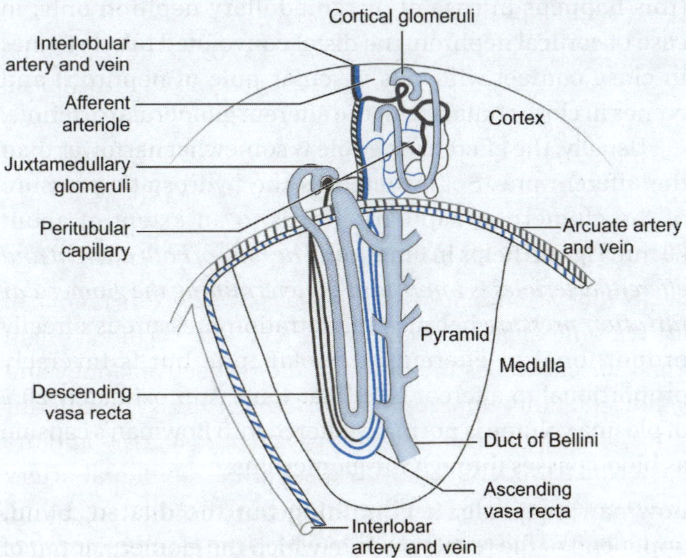

Fig. 2: Microscopic structure of kidney.

into the renal parenchyma and supply the thick ascending limb of LOH. The *afferent sympathetic* fibers, carrying the nociceptive pain sensation from kidney, also run parallel to the efferent sympathetic fibers and enter the lower thoracic and upper lumbar segment of the spinal cord, through their respective dorsal nerve roots. Some renal afferent sympathetic fibers mediate a reflex called the *renorenal reflex*. The function of this reflex is to decrease the activity of efferent nerve and subsequently to increase the excretion of Na$^+$ and water in one kidney, in response to the increase in ureteral pressure in another kidney. Both the kidneys also get the *parasympathetic innervation* from the vagus nerve, but its function is uncertain.

Microscopic Structure of Kidney

The kidney is composed of numerous nephrons, and these nephrons are the functional and structural unit of kidney. These nephrons consist of closely packed glomeruli and their tortuous uriniferous or renal tubules, which are held together by the connecting tissue stroma. A nephron, consisting of glomeruli and its renal tubule, is divided physiologically into two parts: A *secreting part*, which is developed from *the metanephros*, and a *collecting part*, which is developed from the *ureteric bud*. The secreting part of a nephron includes renal corpuscle (glomerulus) and renal tubule up to distal renal tubule and the collecting part of a nephron includes the CTs and the ducts of Bellini.

Nephron

The total number of nephrons in each human kidney is near about 1–1.3 million and forms the structural and functional unit of it. The size of each kidney is determined largely by the number of nephrons they contain. The total length of each nephron varies between 5 and 5.5 cm and consists of two parts: (1) Renal corpuscles (or glomerulus) for filtration and (2) renal tubules for selective reabsorption and secretion. The nephrons are classified under two broad groups and these are cortical nephrons (85%) and juxtamedullary nephrons (15%). The cortical nephrons are primarily responsible for the absorption of Na$^+$, and the juxtamedullary nephrons are primarily responsible for the reabsorption of water by the countercurrent mechanism.

Renal corpuscles (glomeruli): The renal corpuscle or glomerulus is also called *Malpighian body*, and it consists of (1) a plexus of capillaries (called glomerular capillary plexus or plexus of glomerular capillary) and (2) Bowman's capsule into which this capillary plexus invaginates. The renal corpuscles are 200 µm in diameter. They are mainly located in the cortical arches and a few in the renal columns.

Glomerular capillary plexus: It is a lobulated tuft of the capillary plexus and is formed by an afferent and a slightly narrower efferent arteriole. This tuft of capillary plexus projects into Bowman's capsule and is invested by the visceral layer of it (Bowmen's capsule). About 50 intercommunicating lobules are present in each glomerular capillary plexus, and each lobule consists of few capillary loops which are virtually suspended into the capsular space by a mesentery, derived from the visceral layer of Bowman's capsule. This mesentery for capillary loop contains some *mesangial cells*, which are both *phagocytic* and *contractile* in nature. This mesentery also contains some acellular matrix. The contractility of these mesangial cells is due to their cytoplasmic content of some myosin-like filaments and angiotensin II receptors at their surface. Hence, the mesangial cells contract, reducing the glomerular filtration, in response to angiotensin II, vasopressin, norepinephrine, histamine, endothelin, thromboxane A$_2$, leukotrienes, prostaglandin F$_2$ (PGF$_2$), and platelet-activating factor. They (the mesangial cells) relax, thereby increasing glomerular filtration, in response to atrial natriuretic peptide (ANP), PGE$_2$, and dopaminergic agonists. This suggests that they have an immense role in the control of blood flow through the loops of glomerular capillary. They also take part in (1) the regulation of glomerular filtration, (2) the secretion of various tubular substances, and (3) the formation of *immune complexes*. These mesangial cells are involved in the production of immune-related glomerular disease.

In each renal corpuscle, the afferent and efferent glomerular arterioles, at their entry and exit sites of glomeruli, are approximated to each other and form the vascular pole of the nephron. The *thick* ascending limb of the LOH returns to this vascular pole of the corresponding mother nephron (this happens in case of juxtamedullary nephron only; in case of cortical nephron, the distal convoluted tubule comes in close contact with this vascular pole of nephron) and comes in close contact with the afferent glomerular arteriole.

Usually, the efferent arteriole is somewhat narrower than the afferent one. So, it increases the hydrostatic pressure of the glomerular capillary plexus to an extent of about 60 mm Hg and helps in filtration. *The tone of both afferent and efferent arterioles is important in determining the glomerular filtration pressure* because the filtration pressure is directly proportional to efferent arteriolar tone but is inversely proportional to afferent arteriolar tone. Approximately 20% of plasma volume is normally filtered into Bowman's capsule as blood passes through the glomerulus.

Bowman's capsule: It is nothing but the dilated, blind, upper end of the renal tubule in which the glomerular tuft of capillaries invaginates. Thus, Bowman's capsule consists of

(1) a parietal layer, (2) a visceral layer in which the glomerular capillary plexus invaginates, and (3) a capsular space which is filled with glomerular filtrate. The parietal layer of Bowman's capsule is made by a single continuous layer of flattened epithelium, resting on a basement membrane. On the other hand, the visceral layer of Bowman's capsule is made up of a single *discontinuous* layer of large polyhedral cells, resting on a basement membrane, which interdigitate tightly with one another, leaving relatively small filtration slits of approximately 25 nm and rest on a basement membrane. These large polyhedral cells are called the "podocytes". From the cell body of these podocytes, numerous major processes pass outward parallel to the basement membrane. Then each major process gives rise to a number of minor processes which are attached to the basement membrane by their expanded *foot plates* or pedicles. These foot plates of the minor processes of podocytes overlap on one another to form a diaphragm with numerous slits. Therefore, when viewed from the capsular space, the podocyte cells present as the stellate appearance **(Fig. 3)**.

Thus, glomerular endothelial cells are separated from the epithelial cells of Bowman's capsule only by their fused basement membranes, and the structures intervening between the blood of the glomerular capillaries and the intracapsular space of Bowman's capsule from within outward are as follows **(Fig. 4)**:

- The fenestrated flattened endothelial layer of capillaries with numerous pores. Here, the pore size is about 160 Å (70–100 nm).
- A continuous but porous basement membrane upon which rests the flat capillary endothelial cells. The thickness of this basement membrane is about 0.33 µm. It is formed by the interlacement of fine reticular fibers, which are held together by some amorphous materials. The average pore size of the basement membrane is about 110 Å.
- The fenestrated layer of podocytes with its processes and foot plates. The pores within this layer are arranged like a zip fastener between the cell processes or foot plates. The diameter of pores in this layer is about 70 Å (25 nm).

The glomerular basement membrane, which is situated between the capillary endothelium and the podocytes, acts as a true membrane for ultrafiltration. It allows the filtration of water with simple solutes of low molecular weight which are present in the plasma. Therefore, the glomerular filtrate consists essentially of true plasma minus macromolecules of proteins, droplets of lipid, and blood cells. The constituents of plasma, which are of 68,000 molecular weight or above, are held back in plasma by this basement membrane and are not filtered. It is also postulated that filtration through the structures intervening between the blood of glomerular

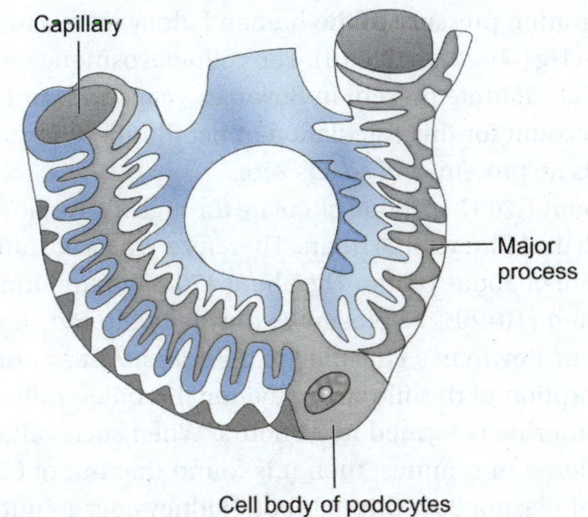

Fig. 3: Podocytes or glomerular epithelial cells lining the visceral layer of Bowman's capsule.

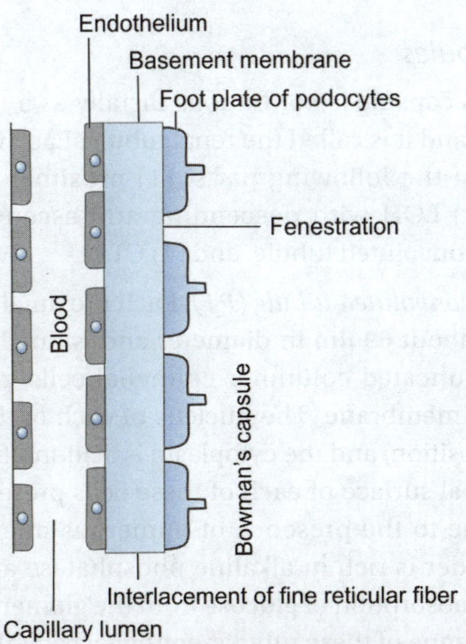

Fig. 4: Structures intervening between the blood of glomerular capillaries and the intracapsular space of Bowman's capsule.

capillaries and Bowman's capsular space, is governed by an electrostatic force. As for example, the matrix of the basement membrane, which acts as a filtration barrier, is negatively charged due to the presence of acidic glycoproteins, and this opposes the passage of negatively charged molecules of blood, such as albumin.

The diameter of each renal corpuscle (glomerulus) is about 0.2 mm, and the total surface area for filtration of all the glomeruli of both kidneys averages about 1.5 m^2. The net glomerular filtration pressure in each renal corpuscle is equal to the glomerular capillary BP (60 mm Hg) minus the colloid osmotic pressure of plasma (32 mm Hg) and Bowman capsular hydrostatic pressure (18 mm Hg). Therefore, the net filtration pressure of the human kidney comes to about 10 mm Hg ($60 - 32 - 18 = 10$). The colloidal osmotic pressure of the ultrafiltrate present in Bowman's capsule is not taken into account for this calculation of net filtration pressure as there is no protein, and so it is zero.

About 1,700 L of blood circulate through all the glomeruli of both the kidneys in 24 hours. Therefore, with a net filtration pressure of about 10 mm Hg, about 170 L of ultrafiltrate are collected (10–20% of plasma is normally filtered) into the space of Bowman's capsular in 24 hours. After abundant reabsorption of this filtrate by the renal tubules, only about 1.5 L of urine is formed in 24 hours. When such values are considered in minutes, then it is found that out of 650 mL normal plasma flow through both kidneys per minute, the glomerular filtration rate (GFR) comes to about only 125 mL/min. Therefore, the filtration coefficient at the filtration pressure of 1 mm Hg is about 12.5 mL.

Renal Tubules

Bowman's capsule is continuous distally as a thin tubular structure, and it is called the renal tubule. Each renal tubule consists of the following parts: (1) proximal convoluted tubule, (2) LOH with descending and ascending limbs, (3) distal convoluted tubule, and (4) CT.

Proximal convoluted tubule (PT): Each proximal convoluted tubule is about 69 µm in diameter and is lined by a single layer of truncated columnar epithelial cells, resting on a basement membrane. The nucleus of each of these cells is basal in position, and the cytoplasm is acidophilic in nature. The luminal surface of each of these cells presents a brush border due to the presence of numerous microvilli. This brush border is rich in alkaline phosphatase and helps in the active absorption of glucose from the glomerular filtrate. The basal zone of these tubular epithelial cells also presents numerous cytoplasmic infoldings. The mitochondria in each cell are arranged radially at the basal zone of these cells in between these cytoplasmic infoldings.

Close to the apical zone, near the luminal surface, the tubular cells are connected to one another by tight junction, but the rest of the lateral surfaces of these tubular columnar cells of PT are separated by the intercellular clefts. The cytoplasm of these tubular cells contains acid phosphatase (in membrane-bound lysosomes), which helps in the hydrolysis of low-molecular-weight proteins into amino acids, when the former is absorbed directly from the glomerular filtrate, through these tubular cells of PT, by pinocytosis. The cytoplasm of tubular cells also contains a number of enzymes such as cytochrome oxidase, succinic dehydrogenase, acid phosphatase, and glucose-6-phosphatase, which suggests active transport of some ions and small molecules from the tubular lumen into the peritubular capillary plexus against their concentration gradients through these cells **(Fact file I)**.

The PTs allow the active reabsorption of sodium (Na^+) and then subsequently the reabsorption of potassium (K^+), chloride (Cl^-), calcium (Ca^{2+}), bicarbonate (HCO_3^-), phosphate, glucose, and amino acids, etc., along with this reabsorption of Na^+. Here, the water is absorbed passively as a solvent (with solutes) along the osmotic gradients through some specialized water channels present on the apical surface of these tubular cells of PT. These water channels are composed of membrane protein which are called aquaporin-I. So, it is known as the obligatory reabsorption of water. Thus, about 60–70% of glomerular filtrate is absorbed from PTs. During the absorption and passing through PT, although the volume of the glomerular filtrate is reduced, it remains isotonic to the blood or plasma. After the absorption from tubular lumen into the cell of PT, the absorption of Na^+ then actively takes place at the basal zone of these cells of PT by some active Na^+-K^+-ATPase (sodium–potassium adenosine triphosphatase) pump, which is present on the capillary (basal) side of the cell membrane of these cells. The energy for this action is derived from the adenosine triphosphate (ATP) of mitochondria of these proximal tubular cells. As a result, more sodium with water, as a solvent, rush passively into the cytoplasm of proximal tubular columnar cells from tubular lumen to replenish the loss within the cell **(Fig. 5)**.

FACT FILE I

Regulation of Na⁺ reabsorption
In renal tubule, the reabsorption of Na^+ plays a major role in the reabsorption and secretion of other ions such as H^+, K^+, Cl^-, SO_4^{2-}, PO_4^{2-}, HCO_3^-, glucose, amino acids, organic acids, and other substances across its wall. For this, various pumps, cotransporter, antitransporter (or exchanger), channels, etc., are involved. At the capillary side of tubular cells, Na^+ is actively pumped out of the cell by the Na^+-K^+-ATPase system, which extrudes $3Na^+$ in exchange of $2K^+$. Then, subsequently Na^+ moves from the tubular lumen into the tubular epithelial cell by cotransporter or antiporter system in PT, thick portion of the ascending limb of LOH, DT, and CD. The tubular cells are connected by tight junctions at their luminal end, but there is space between the cells along the rest of their lateral border. Most of the Na^+ is actively transported into these spaces through the cell and then into the capillary. The remaining portion of Na^+ is transported through the capillary side of tubular cells and then in the capillary blood. Principally, Na^+ is reabsorbed at the luminal surface of tubular cells by Na^+-H^+ antitransporter at PT, Na^+-K^+-Cl^- cotransporter at the thick ascending limb of LOH, Na^+-Cl^- cotransporter at DT and ENaC (epithelial sodium channel) in CD. This ENaC or Na^+ channel is the site for action of aldosterone and homeostatic adjustment of Na^+ balance.

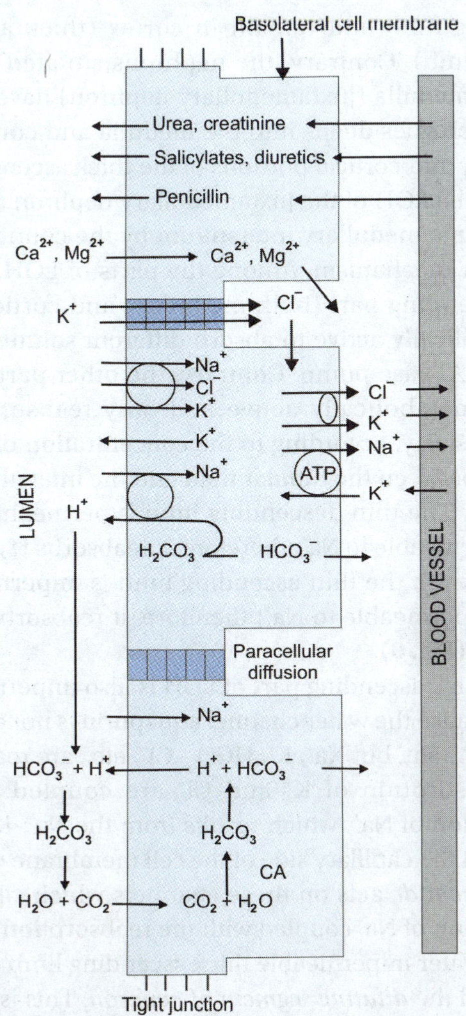

Fig. 5: Mechanism of secretion and absorption in proximal tubular cells. (ATP: adenosine triphosphate)

The fluid entering the PT from Bowman's capsule has a composition similar to that of plasma, except for the absence of protein. But as the PT is considered to be the bulk reabsorber of glomerular filtrate, it is responsible for reducing the volume of glomerular filtrate by approximately 65%. 70% of filtered sodium and chloride, 90% of filtered calcium bicarbonate and magnesium, and 100% of filtered glucose, phosphate, and amino acids are all reabsorbed within the proximal convoluted tubule. The main ion to be reabsorbed in PT is Na⁺, on which the reabsorption of other ions depends.

Sodium is reabsorbed through proximal tubular cells both passively and actively. The passive reabsorption of sodium from the tubular lumen through the luminal surface of tubular cells occurs by two gradients: Chemical and electrical. In the passive reabsorption process by the chemical (or concentration) gradient, the intracellular Na⁺ concentration in the proximal tubular cells is 12–13 mmol/L which is considerably less than the concentration of Na⁺ in the tubular fluid which is about 140 mmol/L and creates a chemical (or concentration) gradient for the reabsorption of it. Therefore, the Na⁺ travels down the chemical (or concentration) gradient from tubular lumen into proximal tubular cells. In the passive reabsorption process by the electrical gradient, the electrical potential difference between the tubular cells and the lumen acts, which is –70 mV. This creates an electrical gradient for the positively charged sodium ions to travel from the lumen into the cells. Angiotensin II and norepinephrine enhance the reabsorption of Na⁺ in the early PT. In contrast, dopamine and fenoldopam decrease the proximal reabsorption of Na⁺ via the activation of D₁ receptor.

It is already stated that after the entry of Na⁺ into the cells of PT by a passive chemical or electrical gradient, it is actively pumped out of the proximal tubular cell through their basal surfaces into the peritubular capillaries by the Na⁺–K⁺-ATPase pump. But in the PT, this reabsorption of Na⁺ is facilitated by angiotensin II and norepinephrine, while fenoldopam and dopamine inhibit it. Thus, the Na⁺–K⁺-ATPase system, situated at the capillary side of the cell membrane of proximal tubular cells, provides energy indirectly for the reabsorption of most other solutes through the luminal end of these cell membranes. The net loss of intracellular +ve charges due to the absorption of Na⁺ from the proximal tubular cells into the capillary blood also favors the absorption of other cations such as K⁺, Ca²⁺, and Mg²⁺ from the tubular lumen into the proximal tubular cells.

At the luminal side of the cell membrane of proximal tubular cells, the reabsorption of Na⁺ is coupled with the secretion of H⁺ by the counter or antitransporter system. This secretion of H⁺ into the proximal tubular lumen again helps in 90% reabsorption of filtered HCO₃⁻ from the lumen of PT into its cells. Chloride (Cl⁻) is also absorbed actively from the cells of PT into capillary blood by the K⁺–Cl⁻ cotransporter system situated at the capillary side of the cell membrane of proximal tubular cells. As a result, the further absorption of Cl⁻ from the tubular lumen into the proximal tubular cells occurs passively, following its concentration gradient. But, unlike other solutes, Cl⁻ also traverses through the tight junction between the two adjacent proximal tubular cells. Most of the other substances also first traverse through the luminal side of proximal tubular cells and then cross the cell membrane at their basolateral side to enter the renal interstitium, before entering the peritubular capillaries. The low-molecular-weight proteins, which are filtered by glomeruli, are normally reabsorbed by proximal tubular epithelial cells and are metabolized intracellularly.

Other than reabsorption, the PT is also capable of secreting some organic cations and anions. These organic cations are trimethoprim, pyrimethamine, cimetidine, creatinine, quinidine, etc., and the organic anions are urea, salicylate, penicillin, cephalosporins, keto acids, diuretics, etc. But they share the same pumping mechanisms and the secretion of one interferes the secretion of other. These pumps also play a major role in the excretion of many circulating toxins and X-ray dyes. As the organic cations use the same pump for their secretion, the excretion of creatinine is inhibited by trimethoprim, pyrimethamine, etc., leading to an increase in the serum creatinine level **(Fact file II)**.

Loop of Henle: The LOH is the part of a nephron which is situated next to the PT. It is directly responsible for maintaining a hypertonic medullary interstitium and indirectly responsible for concentrating urine by helping the CT. Only 25–30% of ultrafiltrate, formed in Bowman's capsule, normally reaches the LOH, where 15–20% of the filtered Na^+ load is again reabsorbed. The LOH consists of three parts: (1) The thin descending limb, (2) the thin ascending limb, and (3) the thick ascending limb. The thick ascending limb is again subdivided into two parts: (1) *Thick medullary portion* and (2) *thick cortical portion*. These divisions are only for the juxtamedullary nephrons.

The nephrons, situated in the renal cortex (cortical nephron), have the LOH of small length and does not contain the thin ascending limb. They have only thick ascending limb and remain in cortex (thick ascending cortical limb). Contrary, the nephrons situated in cortex near the medulla (juxtamedullary nephron) have the long LOH which goes deeps into the medulla and contains the medullary and cortical portions of the thick ascending limb of LOH. The LOH of the juxtamedullary nephron maintains a hypertonic medullary interstitium by the countercurrent multiplier mechanism. Among the parts of LOH, only the thick ascending part (both medullary and cortical parts) is metabolically active to absorb different solutes and has a Na^+–K^+-ATPase pump. Contrary, the other parts of LOH are not metabolically active and only reabsorb Na^+ or water passively, according to the concentration or osmotic gradient between the tubular fluid and the interstitial tissue of kidney. The thin descending limb is permeable to H_2O and impermeable to Na^+; therefore, it reabsorbs H_2O but not Na^+. However, the thin ascending limb is impermeable to H_2O and permeable to Na^+; therefore, it reabsorbs Na^+ but not water **(Fig. 6)**.

The thick ascending part of LOH is also impermeable to water because the water channel aquaporin is not expressed in this segment, but Na^+, K^+, HCO_3^-, Cl^-, etc., are reabsorbed. The reabsorption of K^+ and Cl^- are coupled with the reabsorption of Na^+, which results from the Na^+–K^+-ATPase activity on the capillary side of the cell membrane of tubular cells. *Frusemide* acts on these channels which couple this reabsorption of Na^+ coupled with the reabsorption of K^+ and Cl^-. The water impermeable thick ascending limb of LOH is also called the *diluting segment of nephron*. This is because, as the Na^+ and other solutes are reabsorbed from this segment of tubular lumen, so only water remains in this part of tubular fluid and reduces the osmolality of tubular fluid. As a result,

---

FACT FILE II

Regulation of K^+ reabsorption and excretion

The maximum portion of filtered K^+ in the glomerular filtrate is reabsorbed in PT, though some K^+ is also secreted in this portion of renal tubule. But the net result is the maximum absorption of K^+. The thin descending limb of LOH is not permeable to K^+, whereas the thin ascending limb of LOH is permeable to K^+ like Na^+. In this thin descending and ascending limb of LOH, there is no Na^+–K^+-ATPase pump. So, in this portion of renal tubule, reabsorption or secretion of K^+ depends on the concentration gradient between the interstitium and the tubular fluid. The thick ascending limb of LOH also absorbs and secretes K^+, but the net effect is more absorption than secretion. As a whole, in the absence of any complicating factors or diseases, the amount of reabsorption of K^+ is equal to the amount of K^+ filtered, and the amount of K^+ secreted is approximately equal to the amount of K^+ intake. Thus, the K^+ balance of our body is maintained. The rate of the secretion of K^+ is parallel to the rate of the flow of tubular fluid through the distal portion of nephron. Because, with rapid flow, there is less opportunity for the tubular K^+ concentration to rise to a value that stops further secretion. In the CD, Na^+ is reabsorbed and K^+ is secreted, but there is no fixed one for one exchange and also much of the K^+ movement is passive. As Na^+ is reabsorbed in association with secretion of H^+, there is competition between the secretion of K^+ and H^+ for the absorption of Na^+. The secretion of K^+ is decreased, when the quantity of Na^+ reaching the DT is reduced or when the secretion of H^+ is increased.

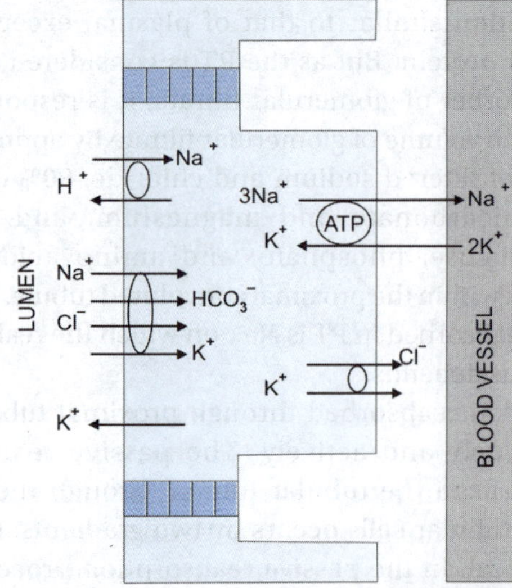

Fig. 6: Mechanism of secretion and reabsorption in the thick ascending limb of loop of Henle (LOH). (ATP: adenosine triphosphate)

the fluid flowing out of the thick ascending part of LOH is hypotonic (100–200 mOsm/L), and the renal interstitium surrounding the LOH is, therefore, hypertonic. Hence, a *countercurrent multiplier mechanism* is established such that both the tubular fluid and the medullary interstitium become increasingly hypertonic with increasing depth into the medulla. The concentration of urea also increases from outer to inner medulla and contributes to this graded hypertonicity. This countercurrent mechanism includes the LOH, cortical and medullary CT, and adjacent capillaries (vasa recta). The thick ascending LOH is also an important site for Ca^{2+} and Mg^{2+} reabsorption, and *PTH* augments Ca^{2+} absorption at this location.

Like the cells of the PT, as the Na^+ is reabsorbed actively into capillary blood through the capillary side of the cell membrane of the tubular cells by ATPase activity, the Na^+ from the lumen is further absorbed into the cells through the cell membrane of the luminal side. This is coupled with the secretion of H^+ into the lumen by the Na^+–H^+ antiporter system, which helps in the absorption of Na^+ and excretion of H^+. Another important symporter system, which is present on the luminal side of cell membrane, couples the reabsorption of K^+, Cl^-, and HCO_3^- along with the reabsorption of Na^+.

This is the major site of action of thiazide loop diuretics which inhibit the reabsorption of Na^+ along with water at the thick ascending limb of LOH. As the concentration of K^+ in the tubular lumen of this segment is much lower than that of Na^+ and Cl^-, there is a need for K^+ to be recycled in this segment. It means K^+ should be secreted in the tubular lumen of this segment and reabsorbed. Ca^{2+} and Mg^{2+} are also reabsorbed from this thick ascending limb of LOH. At this segment of renal tubule, the reabsorption of Ca^{2+} is controlled by PTH. The fluid leaving the thick ascending limb of LOH is hypotonic whose osmolality varies between 100 and 200 mmol/L.

On the other hand, the interstitial tissue of kidney, surrounding the tip of the LOH, is hypertonic. Therefore, a countercurrent multiplier mechanism is established between the tubular fluid in LOH and the interstitial tissue of kidney, which increases gradually with the increase of the depth of medulla from cortex. This countercurrent mechanism includes the CTs, LOH, and their capillaries. This LOH accounts for another 15% reabsorption of glomerular filtrate.

Distal (convoluted) tubules: This portion of renal tubule lies next to the cortical portion of the thick ascending limb of LOH. The tubular cells in this portion are tightly attached to each other and maintain a relative impermeability to both water and Na^+. The DT receives hypo-osmolar fluid from the thick ascending portion of LOH and slightly modifies its composition **(Fig. 7)**.

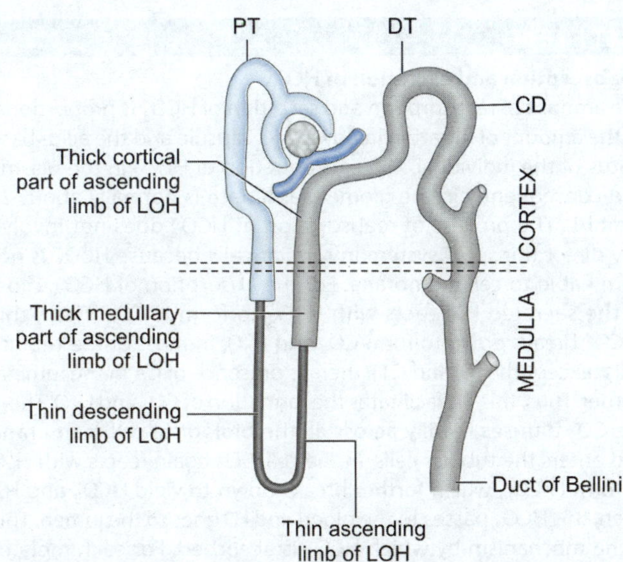

Fig. 7: Nephron. (CD: collecting duct; DT: distal tubule; LOH: loop of Henle; PT: proximal tubule)

This segment has less capacity for Na^+ reabsorption than the segments proximal to it, but it shows considerable capacity to adapt it in the face of increased Na^+ load passing from its proximal part of nephron. This portion of renal tubule accounts for about 5% reabsorption of glomerular filtrate, according to its necessity. This reabsorption includes Na^+, K^+, Cl^-, Ca^{2+}, etc. Like the other parts of the nephron, the reabsorption of Na^+ in this part is also associated with Na^+–K^+-ATPase activity on the capillary side of its tubular cells.

But, on the luminal side of these tubular cells, Na^+ is absorbed from the lumen by the concentration gradient, created by the absorption of it in capillary blood by the Na^+–K^+-ATPase system, and Cl^- is reabsorbed by the Na^+–Cl^- cotransporter (carrier) system. The thiazide diuretics act on this Na^+–Cl^- carrier system. The amount of reabsorption of Na^+ in this segment of renal tubule is directly proportional to the amount of Na^+ delivered in this part of tubule from LOH. This latter portion of DT is referred to as the connecting segment. In this connecting DT portion of renal tubule, the reabsorption of Na^+ and Ca^{2+} is controlled by aldosterone and PTH, respectively **(Fact file III)**.

Collecting tubule or duct: This portion of renal tubule can also be divided into *cortical and medullary portions*, which normally accounts for the reabsorption of the last 13–15% of glomerular filtrate and finally form and modify the composition of urine. The cortical portion of CT has two types of cells. These are *principal cells (P cells) and intercalated cells (I cells)*. The P cells primarily reabsorb Na^+ and secrete K^+ with the help of aldosterone, whereas the intercalated cells (or I cells) are responsible for acid–base regulation by secreting H^+ ion. Aldosterone enhances the Na^+–K^+-ATPase activity on the capillary side of the P cells in this part of nephron and

FACT FILE III

Reabsorption and excretion of HCO_3^-

The amount of reabsorption and secretion of HCO_3^- is proportional to the amount of filtration in Bowman's capsule and the acid–base status of the individual. The concentration of HCO_3^- in the plasma and consequently in the glomerular filtrate is normally about 24 mmol/L. The process of reabsorption of HCO_3^- does not involve any direct transport system in tubular cells because HCO_3^- is not permeable to cell membrane. For the absorption of HCO_3^-, most of the secreted H^+ reacts with HCO_3^- to form H_2CO_3. Then, this H_2CO_3 breaks down to form CO_2 and H_2O. In most of the tubular cells (except the DT and CT), there is presence of CA in the luminal border. Thus, this CA facilitates the formation of CO_2 and H_2O. Then, the CO_2 diffuses readily across all the biological cell membrane and enters the tubular cells. In the cell, CO_2 again reacts with H_2O to form H_2CO_3, which further breaks down to yield HCO_3^- and H^+. Then, this HCO_3^- passes to the blood and H^+ goes to the lumen. This is the mechanism by which HCO_3^- is absorbed. For each mole of HCO_3^- removed from the tubular fluid, one mole of HCO_3^- diffuses from the tubular cells into the blood, but these two HCO_3^- ions are not the same. In acidosis, when the plasma HCO_3^- concentration is low, then all the filtered HCO_3^- is reabsorbed through tubule by the use of secreted H^+ ion. The excess of H^+ ion after neutralization of HCO_3^- is excreted through urine, and the urine becomes acidic. The excess of H^+ also reacts with NH_3 and forms NH_4^+, which is excreted through urine. But in alkalosis, when the plasma HCO_3^- concentration is high above the normal level, then some filtered HCO_3^- appears in the urine after neutralization of all the H^+, and the urine becomes alkaline. The normal HCO_3^- level in plasma is 24–27 mmol/L.

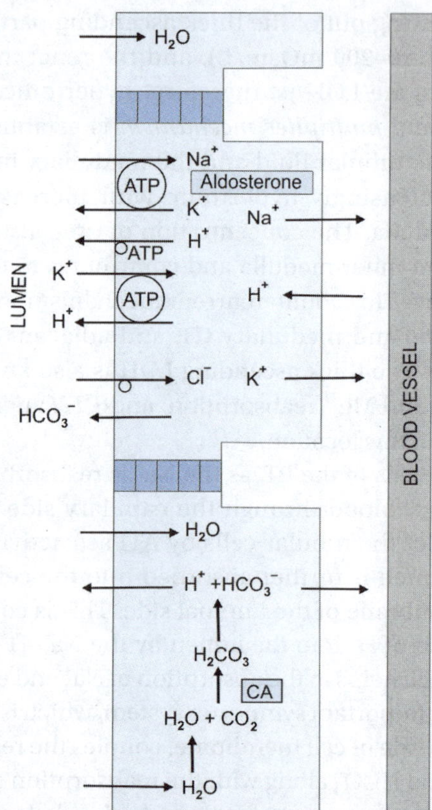

Fig. 8: Mechanism of secretion and reabsorption in the cortical portion of the collecting tubule (CT). (ATP: adenosine triphosphate; CA: carbonic anhydrase)

increases the active reabsorption of Na^+. Subsequently, there is increased passive reabsorption of Na^+ at the luminal side of the tubular P cells with the subsequent indirect secretion of K^+ into the tubular fluid by increasing the number of open K^+ and Na^+ channels on the luminal membrane of P cells in this segment of renal tubule.

Aldosterone also enhances the H^+-secreting ATPase activity on the luminal border of I (intercalated) cells and increases the secretion of H^+. Unlike PT, the secretion of H^+ in this part of renal tubule (CT) is nondependent of reabsorption of Na^+. Because in this part of renal tubule, most of the H^+ is secreted actively by an ATPase-driven proton pump, where aldosterone acts and increases or decreases its secretion. So, hyperaldosteronism is associated with alkalosis. These I cells are like the parietal cells of stomach and contain an abundant carbonic anhydrase (CA) enzyme, which also helps in the formation of H^+. These I cells additionally also have a luminal H^+–K^+-ATPase pump, which secretes H^+ in the exchange of absorption of K^+. As these I cells help in the regulation of acid–base balance, they also have anion exchange protein (such as Cl^-–HCO_3^- exchanger), which is capable of preventing the reabsorption of HCO_3^- in exchange of Cl^- in response to large alkaline loads. With Cl^-, Na^+ and water are also absorbed, but the absorption of water is in excess than Na^+ and makes the tubular fluid from hypo-osmolar to iso-osmolar **(Fig. 8)**.

The medullary portion of CT runs down through the hypertonic interstitial tissues of medulla and joins with other CT to form the duct of Bellini, which empties at the tip of the pyramid. This medullary portion of CT is the principal site of the action of antidiuretic hormone (ADH) or arginine vasopressin (AVP). Therefore, permeability of water in this portion of CT is entirely dependent on the presence of ADH. This ADH acts through the V_2 subtypes of ADH or vasopressin (V) receptors which are situated on the basolateral membrane of tubular cells in CD. Activation of these V_2 receptors increases cyclic adenosine monophosphate (cAMP) formation intracellularly → activation of protein kinase A → increased exocytosis of "aquaporin 2" water channel through the apical membrane of tubular cells at CD → more aqueous channels get inserted into the apical membrane of tubular cells → increased absorption of water. Dehydration increases ADH secretion and increases the permeability of the luminal surface of this portion of CT to water.

As a result, more and more water is reabsorbed, and concentrated urine is formed whose osmolality can increase up to 1,400 mOsm/L. On the contrary, proper hydration inhibits the secretion of ADH and permeability of this portion of CT to water is lost. This results in nonabsorption of water and the formation of diluted urine whose osmolality varies between 100 and 200 mOsm/L. In the absence of ADH (diabetes insipidus), the osmolality of urine may come down to 30 mOsm/L. This medullary portion of CT also contains P and I cells. Like the cortical portion, P cells here also regulate the reabsorption of Na^+ with the help of aldosterone and I cells regulate the acid–base balance by secreting H^+ in the form of titrable acids of phosphates ($H_2PO_4^-$) and ammonium ions (NH_4^+).

Urea contributes to the establishment of osmotic gradient in the medullary interstitial tissues. Thus, it helps to form a concentrated urine in the CD. The mechanism is like that the fluid entering the proximal part of DT is hypo-osmolal (100 mOsm/L). Then, in the CT, the osmolality of tubular fluid returns to that of plasma (300 mOsm/L) due to the absorption of water by ADH. But, unlike the contents of PT, the solute component of DT largely consists of urea, creatinine, and other excreted compounds. In the presence of ADH, water moves out of the CT, and the tubular fluid becomes hypertonic and the urea becomes highly concentrated in urine. In the presence of ADH, the innermost part of medullary CT becomes permeable to urea also. Thus, urea then diffuses out deeply into the medullary interstitial tissues, and subsequently, the amount of urea in the urine varies with the amount of urea filtered. Now, the urea that diffuses out deeply into the medullary interstitial tissues of kidney establishes a high osmotic gradient in the medullary interstitial tissues and draws the water from the lumen of CT and the urine becomes concentrated. This in turn varies with the dietary intake of protein. Therefore, a high protein diet increases the ability of the kidney to concentrate the urine **(Table 1)**.

Juxtaglomerular Apparatus or Complex

The renal tubule, after making a sharp bend at LOH, ascends upward and its thick ascending part reaches again near to its own glomerulus from which this renal tubule arises. Here, the renal tubule rests between its afferent and efferent arterioles, forming juxtaglomerular apparatus (JGA). Thus, the JGA is formed by (1) the afferent arteriole, (2) efferent arteriole, (3) renal tubule (thick ascending limb of LOH or DT), and (4) some intervening tissues, resting between them. In this junction or JGA, the smooth muscle cells of afferent arterioles are modified and are called the *JG cells*. The epithelial cells of renal tubule (thick ascending part of LOH) in this junction are also modified and are called the *macula densa*. The specialized mesangial cells, entangled

TABLE 1: Functional divisions of nephron.

Glomerulus	Ultrafiltration
Proximal tubule • Absorption • Secretion	 • Water, sodium, potassium, chloride, bicarbonate, calcium, magnesium, phosphates, urea, uric acid, glucose, protein, amino acid • Ammonia products, some anions and cations
Loop of Henle • Absorption • Secretion	 • Water, sodium, potassium, chloride, calcium, magnesium • Nil
Distal tubule • Absorption • Secretion	 • Water, sodium, potassium, chloride, bicarbonate, calcium • Hydrogen ion, potassium, calcium
Collecting duct • Absorption • Secretion	 • Water, sodium, potassium, chloride, bicarbonate • Hydrogen ion, potassium, ammonia products
Juxtaglomerular apparatus	Secretion of renin

between the afferent arteriole, efferent arteriole, and renal tubules, also take part in the formation of JGA and are called the Lacis cells. Thus, the JGA consists of (1) granular JG cells of afferent arteriole, (2) macula densa cells of the thick ascending limb of LOH or DT, and (3) nongranular interstitial cells of Lacis. The JGA is thought to be related to some way in the controlling of circulating blood volume, BP, RBF, GFR, salt balance, and erythropoiesis **(Fig. 9)**.

The JG cells are deeply innervated by the sympathetic nervous system and contain baroreceptors. So, they respond to the changes in pressure of afferent arteriole and regulate the flow of blood through the glomerulus and subsequently GFR. These JG cells also contain an enzyme, named renin. The secretion of this renin is determined by the degree of stretching of afferent arteriole, Na^+ concentration of macula densa cells, and β-adrenergic stimulation. After the release of renin in response to hypotension, it acts on a special circulating protein in bloodstream named angiotensinogen, which is synthesized by the liver. By the action of renin, this angiotensinogen is converted to inert angiotensin I (decapeptide) which is then rapidly converted to angiotensin II (octapeptide) in the lungs by the angiotensin converting enzyme (ACE). This angiotensin II plays a major role in (1) the secretion of aldosterone, (2) the control of BP, (3) the control of RBF, and (4) the formation of adequate volume of urine.

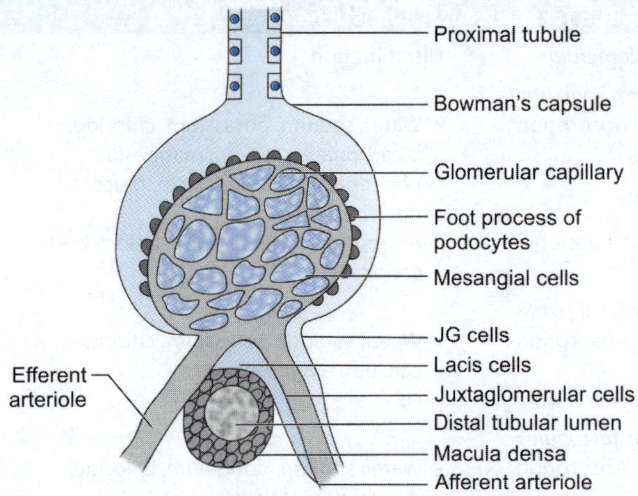

Fig. 9: Juxtaglomerular (JG) apparatus.

The angiotensin II is also formed locally in the tissues of kidney (intrarenal angiotensin II), and there is presence of angiotensin II receptors which controls the absorption of Na⁺ through renal tubules, other than aldosterone. This is found in PT. The proximal renal tubular cells have ACE as well as angiotensin II receptor. Here, in PT, intrarenal formation of angiotensin II enhances Na⁺ reabsorption. Except kidneys and lungs, there are also other extrarenal sites where renin and angiotensin II are synthesized and secreted locally. These are vascular endothelium, brain tissue, and adrenal gland. Angiotensin II modulates the tone of afferent and efferent arterioles and subsequently maintains the RBF and GFR. It is also known that under hypoxic state or following hemorrhage, a hormone named erythropoietin is formed in blood by the interaction of renal erythropoietin factor (REF) with plasma globulin. This erythropoietin stimulates the process of erythropoiesis. This REF is secreted by the JG cells.

The cells of macula densa appear to have chemoreceptor function. They sense the concentration of NaCl in the fluid of tubular lumen of the thick ascending limb of LOH or DT and regulate the secretion of aldosterone from adrenal gland which in turn regulate the reabsorption of Na⁺. However, the function of Lacis cells is still unknown **(Fact files IV to VII)**.

■ RENAL CIRCULATION OR RENAL BLOOD FLOW

The kidneys are the only organs where the consumption of O_2 is determined by its own blood flow (O_2 supply), in contrast to other organs where the blood flow (supply of O_2) is determined by the consumption of O_2 by that organ. In kidney, there are two sets of capillaries: *Glomerular and peritubular*, with their separate distinct functions. In contrast to glomerular capillaries, which perform the job

FACT FILE IV

Excretion of water through urine

Every day, normally about 150–180 L of fluid is ultrafiltered through all the glomeruli of both kidneys. But the average daily urine formation varies between 1 and 1.5 L. In an adverse situation, this volume of urine may come down to 500 mL or may go up to 23 L (diabetes insipidus). On the other hand, the same load of solute is excreted in 24 hours within this varying volume of urine with varying osmolality, which varies from 1,400 to 30 mOsm/L. Normally, among this ultrafiltrate, 87% of water is reabsorbed mandatorily. The reabsorption of the remaining 23% of water varies without affecting the excretion of the total solute. When the urine is concentrated, the water is reabsorbed in excess of solute. On the other hand, when it is diluted, water is lost in excess of solute. The key regulator of this water absorption and excretion through renal tubules is ADH (vasopressin), which acts on the CD.

In PT, water moves out of the tubule along with the osmotic gradient, which is set up by the active transport of solutes, and thus, isotonicity of the remaining fluid in the tubule is maintained. Therefore, the tubular fluid passing at the end of PT is isotonic or isoosmotic. About 65% of filtered water and 65% of filtered solute are absorbed in PT. In the thin descending and ascending limbs of LOH, there is no system of pump for active transport of Na⁺. The thin descending limb of LOH is permeable to water only, whereas the thin ascending limb of LOH is permeable to Na⁺ only. On the other hand, there is graded increase in the osmolality of interstitium of renal medulla from the outer cortex to the tip of pyramid. Therefore, the fluid flowing down the descending limb of LOH gradually becomes hypertonic as water moves out of this part of renal tubule into hypertonic interstitium. Then, this hypertonic fluid gradually becomes hypotonic as it flows up the thin ascending limb of LOH, because in this portion only Na⁺ moves out, leaving water in the tubule.

In the thick ascending part of the limb of LOH, an active Na⁺ transport system is present and is also impermeable to water. Therefore, fluid passing up the thick ascending limb of LOH gradually becomes more dilute, and when it reaches the top, it becomes maximum hypotonic in relation to plasma. During passing through the LOH, 15% of filtered water is now removed. So, approximately, next 20% of filtered water now enters the DT. DT is less permeable to water but more permeable to solutes. So, continuous removal of solute in excess of water from DT further dilutes the fluid in this segment of nephron. Only 5% of filtered water is removed in this segment.

The CD has two portions—cortical and medullary. The cortical portion of CD receives hypotonic fluid from DT. The vasopressin or ADH, secreting from the posterior pituitary, acts on this portion of renal tubule, that is, CD. In the presence of enough vasopressin, maximum antidiuretics occurs. Therefore, maximum amount of water now moves out of this hypotonic fluid in the cortical portion of CD and enters into the interstitium of cortex. Thus, here the tubular fluid becomes isotonic. In this fashion, 10% of filtered fluid is removed in the cortical portion of CD. Next, the isotonic fluid enters the medullary portion of CD. Here, an additional 3.5% or more water from the filtered tubular fluid is reabsorbed into the hypertonic interstitium of medulla and producees concentrated urine. In a human being, the osmolality of urine may reach 1,400 mOsm/L which is five times greater than that of plasma with total 99.5% of filtered water being absorbed.

In the absence of ADH or vasopressin (AVP), CD is impermeable to water. The fluid in CD, therefore, remains hypotonic and a large amount of tubular fluid flows into the renal pelvis. In such circumstances, the urine osmolality in human beings may be as low as 30 mOsm/L.

FACT FILE V

Excretion of H$^+$ and acidification of urine

The cells of the PT, thick ascending limb of LOH, DT, and CD secrete H$^+$, like the cells of the gastric gland. This secretion of H$^+$ primarily involves the Na$^+$–H$^+$ antiporter system situated on the luminal side of cell membrane of the tubular cells. This Na$^+$–H$^+$ antiporter system acts as secondary to Na$^+$–K$^+$-ATPase system on the capillary end of tubular cells, which lowers the intracellular Na$^+$ concentration and allows subsequent entry of Na$^+$ from the tubular lumen coupled with extrusion of H$^+$. This H$^+$ comes from the intracellular dissociation of H$_2$CO$_3$, which is formed by the reaction of CO$_2$ and H$_2$O. The HCO$_3^-$ formed from the dissociation of H$_2$CO$_3$ diffuses back into the interstitial fluid. Thus, for each H$^+$ secreted, one Na$^+$ and one HCO$_3^-$ enter the interstitial fluid and are preserved in the body.

In respiratory acidosis, there is more CO$_2$ in the body, which produces more H$_2$CO$_3$ and more H$^+$ and HCO$_3^-$. This means more H$^+$ is excreted through urine and urine becomes acidic. The excess HCO$_3^-$ produced from excess CO$_2$ is preserved in body and produces compensatory metabolic alkalosis. In respiratory alkalosis, the reverse occurs. There is less CO$_2$ due to more washout through lungs. This leads to less H$_2$CO$_3$ and subsequently less H$^+$ and HCO$_3^-$, which leads to less excretion of H$^+$ and urine becomes alkaline (metabolic acidosis). In metabolic acidosis, there is more formation of H$^+$ in the body. So, there is more excretion of H$^+$ through urine and urine becomes acidic. Subsequently, due to more H$^+$, there is more consumption of HCO$_3^-$ and more formation of CO$_2$ and H$_2$O. This excess CO$_2$ is excreted through lungs (compensatory metabolic alkalosis). On the contrary, in metabolic alkalosis (e.g., vomiting), the reverse occurs. There is less H$^+$ or more HCO$_3^-$ in the body. Therefore, the body tries to preserve the H$^+$ and less excretion of it. Thus, urine becomes alkaline. Due to less H$^+$, there is less consumption of HCO$_3^-$ and less formation of CO$_2$. This causes less excretion of CO$_2$ through lungs (compensatory respiratory acidosis).

The amount of H$^+$ secreted in the tubular fluid depends on its pH. If the pH of tubular fluid is 4.5, that is, an H$^+$ concentration in it is 1,000 times more than that of the plasma, then the secretion of H$^+$ stops. Thus, the pH of urine, which goes up to its maximum, is 4.5. This is normally reached in the CDs. If there is no buffer in the renal tubules which neutralize the H$^+$, then pH will rise rapidly and the secretion of H$^+$ will stop. There are three important buffers in tubular fluid which remove the free H$^+$ and permit more H$^+$ to be secreted. These are HCO$_3^-$ forming CO$_2$ and H$_2$O, H$_2$PO$_4^-$ forming H$_3$PO$_4$, and NH$_3$ forming NH$_4^+$. Among these, HCO$_3^-$ is the most important, which maximum neutralizes the H$^+$. This is because the concentration of HCO$_3^-$ in plasma and subsequently in glomerular filtrate is normally about 24 mEq/L, whereas that of phosphate is only 1.5 mEq/L. The secreted H$^+$ reacts with dibasic phosphate (H$_2$PO$_4^-$) to form a monobasic phosphate (H$_2$PO$_4^-$). This happens to the greatest extent in the DTs and CDs because it is here that the phosphate which escapes proximal reabsorption is greatly concentrated by the reabsorption of water. The reaction of H$^+$ and NH$_3$ occurs maximally in the PT and DT.

Each H$^+$ that reacts with the abovementioned buffer, such as H$_2$PO$_4^-$ and NH$_3$ constitutes or is called the titrable acidity of urine because this is measured by determining the amount of alkali needed to change the urinary pH to 7.4, which is the pH of the glomerular filtrate or plasma. However, it does not measure the HCO$_3^-$ part because it is converted to CO$_2$ and H$_2$O. It measures the other two fractions of acid secreted.

FACT FILE VI

Secretion of ammonia

The multiple reactions in renal tubular cells produce NH$_4^+$. Among these, the principal reaction is conversion of glutamine to *glutamate* with the production of one molecule of NH$_4^+$. This reaction is catalyzed by glutaminase enzyme which is abundant in renal tubular cells. Glutamate is again converted to α-*keto glutamate* by the help of enzyme glutamic dehydrogenase enzyme, when more NH$_4^+$ is produced. Subsequently, metabolism of α-keto glutamate utilizes 2H$^+$ and makes free 2HCO$_3^-$ ions. In the tubular cells, NH$_4^+$ remains in equilibrium with NH$_3$ and H$^+$. The pK value of this equilibrium is 9. So, in acidosis, this equilibrium shifts toward NH$_3$ and therefore more NH3 is produced from NH$_4^+$4

Then this NH$_3$ enters the tubular fluid, because NH$_3$ is lipid soluble and diffuses across the cell membrane down its concentration gradient. In the tubular fluid, it reacts with H$^+$ and forms nonabsorbable NH$_4^+$ which remains in urine. Thus, excretion of NH$_4^+$ causes further removal of H$^+$ from the tubular fluid and consequently further enhancement of secretion of H$^+$.

$$\text{Glutamine} \xrightarrow{\textit{Glutaminase}} \text{Glutamate} + NH_4^+$$

$$\text{Glutamate} \xrightarrow{\textit{Glutamic}} \text{α-ketoglutarate} + NH_4^+ \text{ dehydrogenase}$$

$$NH_4^+ \leftrightarrow NH_3 + H^+$$

FACT FILE VII

The medullary concentration of solutes and osmolality (1,400 mOsm/L) is very high. This is because (1) the ascending limb of the LOH actively reabsorbs Na$^+$ and Cl$^-$, but not water into the interstitial tissue of its medulla, and (2) the large amount of urea enters the deeper part of renal medulla from the CD. This is because the cortical and the outer medullary parts of the CD are the sites of passive diffusion of water but impermeable to urea. So, the urea gradually becomes concentrated in the CD of the deeper medulla, which is permeable to it and moves passively down its concentration gradient. Again, the high concentration of urea, Na$^+$, and Cl$^-$ in the deeper medulla are not washed out because blood flow in this portion (medulla) is low (minimum), and the configuration of capillaries (vasa recta) allows *countercurrent exchange*. Thus, all these factors cause the gradual increase of tonicity from outer cortex to medulla.

of filtration, the peritubular capillaries perform the job of reabsorption. Both the kidneys receive 20–25% of total cardiac output as their blood supply. This results in total 1–1.5 L/min of blood flow through both the kidneys. There is much discrepancy regarding the flow of blood, delivery of O$_2$, and the consumption of O$_2$ between the renal cortex and the medulla. Approximately 80% of the total blood flow of each kidney goes to its outer cortical nephrons in superficial cortex and only 15% reach the juxtamedullary nephron in the juxtamedullary cortex. The medulla of kidney receives only the remaining 5% of total RBF.

TABLE 2: Distribution of renal blood flow (RBF) between its medulla and cortex.

	Medulla	Cortex
Blood flow (mL/min/g)	0.05	5
% of RBF	5	95
PO_2 (mm Hg)	10	50
O_2 extraction ratio	0.8	0.2

The average O_2 tension in the medulla of kidney is about 10–15 mm Hg, whereas the average O_2 tension in renal cortex is 50 mm Hg. This indicates that renal cortex has high blood flow but extracts little O_2 than medulla. On the other hand, renal medulla has low blood flow but extracts more O_2 than cortex. This is because the renal cortex is metabolically less active than its medulla as it is concerned mainly with the filtration function whereas the renal medulla is metabolically more active than cortex as it is mainly concerned with the reabsorption of more solute and water to maintain a high osmotic gradient in the interstitial tissues of kidney and to concentrate urine, respectively **(Table 2)**.

Therefore, severe hypoxia and necrosis will develop first in the renal medulla, sparing the cortex, during compromised circulation. Thus, in conclusion, we can say that the kidney is such an organ where its O_2 consumption is primarily determined by its blood flow, but not by its metabolic activity or O_2 demand whereas, in other organs, the blood flow is primarily determined by its O_2 demand which again depends on its metabolic activity (previously said). In an adverse condition, the sympathoadrenal response tries to redistribute the flow of blood from the cortex of kidney to its medulla by cortical vasoconstriction, mediated by the increased level of catecholamines and angiotensin II.

When the systemic mean arterial pressure (MAP) is 100 mm Hg, then the glomerular capillary pressure at the afferent arteriole is about 40 mm Hg. This pressure further drops to only 1–2 mm Hg at its efferent end of the arteriole, after the blood flows through glomerular capillaries (i.e., the MAP at the efferent end of the arteriole is 38 mm Hg). Then, it drops much at peritubular capillaries and comes down to about 10 mm Hg. Therefore, the pressure gradient of glomerular capillary which is more or less similar to that of the afferent arteriole is about 40% of mean systemic BP.

Regulation of Renal Blood Flow

The flow of blood through the kidney is regulated by few very complex mechanisms that are interplayed by several factors such as the autoregulation (intrinsic), tubule-glomerular feedback mechanism (reflex), different hormones, and nerves.

Intrinsic Autoregulation of RBF

The RBF usually remains autoregulated between the systemic MAPs of 80 and 200 mm Hg. It means that within this range of MAP, the RBF remains the same. Beyond this range of MAP, the RBF becomes pressure dependent, that is, when the MAP goes below 80 mm Hg, the RBF is reduced, and when MAP goes above 200 mm Hg, the RBF is increased. This is due to the changes in renal vascular resistance, in response to the changes in pressure within this value (when pressure increases, the resistance increases and the flow is reduced, and when the pressure falls, the resistance falls and the flow is increased) and keeps the RBF relatively constant. This type of autoregulation is also seen in other organs, such as the brain, liver, and heart, and several factors contribute to it.

This autoregulation is also present in a denervated, isolated, well-perfused, and transplanted kidney. But it can be prevented by the administration of drugs, which paralyze the vascular smooth muscles. Thus, it indicates that this autoregulation is an intrinsic myogenic response of afferent arterioles (vasoconstriction and dilatation) to the changes in BP which keeps the RBF constant. This intrinsic myogenic response to regulate the RBF is nothing but the direct contractile response of the smooth muscles of the afferent arteriole to stretch, mediated by the baroreceptors.

Nitric oxide (NO) may also be involved in this intrinsic autoregulation of RBF. The RBF is generally decreased or autoregulation fails, when this MAP falls below 80 mm Hg or rises above 200 mm Hg. Outside this limit, this autoregulation of RBF becomes pressure dependent, that is, when the pressure increases, the RBF increases and vice versa. Glomerular capillary pressure and subsequently the filtration pressure gradient come down to zero and filtration ceases, when the MAP falls to 40–50 mm Hg **(Fact file VIII)**.

FACT FILE VIII

The release of renin from JGA is controlled by several mechanisms. A reduction in renal artery perfusion pressure stimulates the baroreceptors in afferent arterioles. Then, subsequent stimulation of the sympathetic nerve and increased circulating catecholamines act on α and β adrenergic receptors on the afferent arteriole which produces vasoconstriction and simultaneously causes release of renin. The cells of medulla densa also sense the increased concentration of Na^+ in the tubular fluid and triggers the release of renin from the afferent arteriole in hypotension. Thus, this tubule-glomerular reflex appears to play a role in modulating GFR, during normal and abnormal renal function through feedback loop. Hence, renin secretion is stimulated by actual hypovolemia (hemorrhage, diuresis, Na^+ loss, etc.) and relative hypovolemia or decreased perfusion (heart failure, IPPV, sepsis, etc.).

Regulation of Renal Blood Flow by Tubule-glomerular Feedback Mechanism

This tubule-glomerular feedback reflex is also very important to maintain the renal circulation (blood flow) and subsequently the GFR, over a wide range of variation of perfusion pressure. Although the mechanism of this reflex is very poorly understood, the macula densa cell is still thought to be responsible for controlling this reflex by changing the tone of the smooth muscles of the afferent arteriole and subsequently the RBF and the pressure gradient of the glomerular capillary. This tubule-glomerular reflex is nothing but the changes of RBF and GFR with the changes in the flow of fluid through the renal tubules, mainly through the thick ascending limb of the LOH and DT. The increase in tubular flow through the thick ascending limb of LOH or DT reduces RBF and GFR, whereas the decrease in tubular flow increases the RBF and GFR. Thus, it is completely a compensatory mechanism.

During hypotension, when the thick ascending limb of the LOH becomes ischemic, then the reabsorption of NaCl through this part of renal tubule ceases, and the delivery of NaCl to the macula densa cells is decreased. This causes the increased release of renin and angiotensin II from afferent arteriole and triggers the arteriolar constriction and decreases GFR. During overhydration, the reverse occurs. Thus, the tubulo-glomerular reflex mechanism induces oliguria, conserves intravascular volume, and protects the organism from dehydration. Another probable mechanism of tubule-glomerular reflex is the local release of adenosine in response to volume expansion of thick ascending part of LOH. It inhibits the release of renin and dilates the afferent glomerular arteriole. In dehydration, the release of adenosine is inhibited and the secretion of renin is increased, which causes the constriction of afferent arteriole and decrease of GFR. In overhydration, the opposite effect occurs and GFR is increased.

Hormonal Regulation

For this type of autoregulation, two important hormones, named renin and angiotensin II, come into play for actions. During any circumstances, such as in hypotension, surgical stress, trauma, and severe sepsis, there is stimulation of the sympathetic system and secretion of these two hormones (first renin and then conversion of renin to angiotensin), which causes the constriction of afferent arteriolar and the reduction of RBF with the reduction of GFR. Thus, they preserve ECF volume. Both the afferent and efferent arterioles are constricted, but because the efferent arterioles are smaller, their resistance becomes greater than that of afferent arterioles, and therefore, GFR (though minimum),

FACT FILE IX

Two mutually dependent but opposing neurohormonal systems are present in the kidney, which control the BP, intravascular volume, and concentration of salt with water homeostasis by a complex set of interactions. Among these, the renin–angiotensin II–aldosterone–ADH system acts against the hypovolemia and hypotension by promoting vasoconstriction (renin and angiotensin) and salt and water retention (aldosterone and ADH). On the other hand, another system including bradykinins, some PGs, and ANP protect against hypervolemia and hypertension by producing vasodilatation and excretion of salt and water.

tends to be preserved. This autoregulation can also be carried out by adrenal hormones and catecholamines such as epinephrine and norepinephrine and by aldosterone. The angiotensin-induced secretion of vasoconstrictive PGF_2 is also responsible for this autoregulation. The inhibition of the synthesis of this PGF_2 by nonsteroidal anti-inflammatory drugs (NSAIDs) can, thus, block this autoregulation (**Fact file IX**).

The renal synthesis of some vasodilating PGs, such as PGE_2 and PGI_2, are also some important renal protective factors and play important protective mechanisms, during the period of systemic hypotension and renal ischemia. Another local hormone named ANP (atrial natriuretic peptide) is also secreted from arterial myocytes. It is a direct smooth muscle dilator and antagonizes the vasoconstrictive action of epinephrine, norepinephrine, and angiotensin II. It preferentially constricts the efferent arterioles and dilates the afferent arterioles. It, thus, effectively increases GFR and protects the kidney during hypotension. ANP also inhibits the release of aldosterone, induced by renin and angiotensin II and its (aldosterone) action on renal tubules (**Flowchart 1**).

Neuronal Regulation

The sympathetic system innervates the JG cells through their β_1-receptors. It also innervates the afferent and efferent arterioles of renal vasculature through their α_1- and α_2-receptors. However, both these receptors mediate vasoconstriction and are responsible for stress-induced reduction in GFR. The action of sympathetic nerves on JG cells, mediated by β_1-receptors, causes the increased secretion of renin. The PT and DT and the thick ascending limb of LOH are thickly innervated by sympathetic nerves. Here, the α_1-receptor is responsible for the reabsorption of Na^+ in PTs whereas the α_2-receptors inhibit the reabsorption of Na^+ and promote the excretion of H_2O. There are also D_1 and D_2 receptors in kidney. The activation of D_1 receptor directly dilates the afferent arterioles. Whereas, the activation of D_2 receptors, situated on the presynaptic

Flowchart 1: Neurohormonal regulation of renal function.

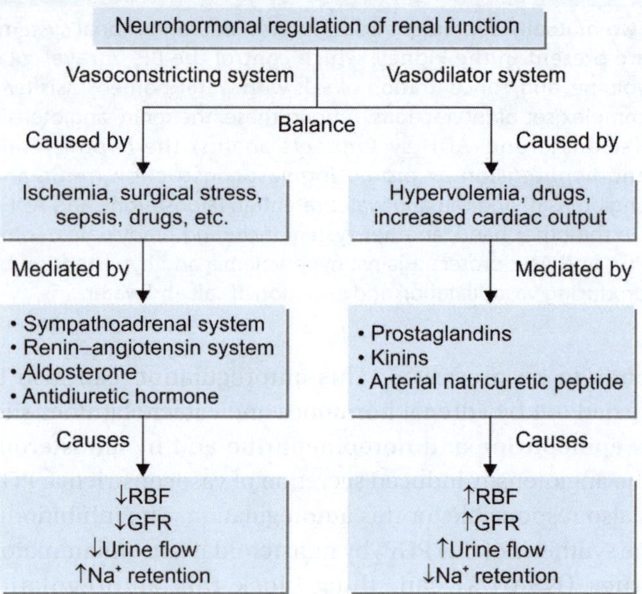

(GFR: glomerular filtration rate; RBF: renal blood flow)

FACT FILE X

Mild adrenergic stimulation, during the initial stage of hormonal and neural autoregulation of RBF, causes the activation of α-receptor and produces only preferential glomerular efferent arteriolar constriction. This preserves the filtration fraction and GFR, still in the face of hypotension and decreased RBF. This α-adrenergic stimulation occurs through the renin–angiotensin system. Therefore, the importance of this protective mechanism is lost and GFR is reduced, if an ACE inhibitor is used in patients with hypotension, renal insufficiency, and renal artery stenosis. Contrary, severe α-adrenergic stimulation (late stage of hormonal and neural autoregulation) causes predominant constriction of afferent arteriole and decreases GFR with RBF. This can be opposed by α-adrenergic blockade.

membrane of postganglionic neuron, inhibits the release of norepinephrine and indirectly dilates the afferent arterioles. Thus, the dopamine (acting on both the D_1 and D_2 receptors) and fenoldopam (acting only on D_1 receptor) cause the dilatation of afferent glomerular arteriole and increase GFR **(Fact file X)**.

Measurement of Renal Blood Flow

Renal blood flow can be measured by indicator dilution technique, radiolabeled tracers, Doppler USG, electromagnetic procedure, or some other types of flowmeter. It can also be measured by applying the Fick principle. For Fick principle, a nontoxic substance that is completely cleared by the kidney and not metabolized, stored, or produced by the body or kidney and does not itself affect the RBF is

used. By Fick method, first renal plasma flow (RPF) is measured, and then from it RBF is calculated. This is because the kidney ultrafilters the plasma, and RPF is equal to the amount of substance removed from plasma per unit of time divided by the renal arteriovenous concentration difference of that substance. Therefore, $RPF = [U] \times V/[A] - [V]$. Here, $[U]$ is the urinary concentration of substance which is used to measure the RBF, V is the urinary flow rate or volume of urine formed in a unit of time, $[A]$ is the arterial plasma concentration of that substance, and $[V]$ is the renal venous plasma concentration of that substance.

Renal plasma flow is measured by using PAH (para-aminohippuric acid) through the intravenous (IV) route. PAH is used to measure RPF because it is physiologically inert, nontoxic, filtered completely at the glomerulus, secreted through the renal tubule, and eliminated completely from the plasma by single passage through kidney, making the concentration of PAH in renal venous blood to nil (renal arterial and venous concentration difference of PAH is zero). When PAH is infused at low doses, 99.9% of it is removed by a single circulation through kidney. It, therefore, becomes easy to calculate the RPF by dividing the amount of PAH in urine ($[PAH]_U$) × urine volume in 1 minute by the plasma PAH level ($[PAH]_P$), ignoring its level in renal venous blood. Peripheral venous plasma can be used for plasma PAH level because its (PAH) concentration is essentially identical to that in arterial plasma, reaching the kidney. Thus, the value obtained is called the effective renal plasma flow (ERPF) which does not need to measure the renal venous plasma PAH level. Therefore, $ERPF = [PAH]_U \times V_U/[PAH]_P$, where $[PAH]_U$ is the urine PAH level, V_U is the volume of urine, and $[PAH]_P$ is the plasma PAH level. This also indicates the clearance of PAH like the clearance of insulin and creatinine. In human, the average ERPF value is 700 mL/min.

Example:

Urinary concentration of PAH or $[PAH]_U$ is 14.4 mg/mL

Urine output or V_U is 1 mL/min

Plasma concentration of PAH or $[PAH]_P$ is 0.02 mg/mL

Therefore, $ERPF = 14.4 \times 1/0.02 = 720$ mL/min

This ERPF can be converted to actual RPF.

This can be done by: ERPF/excretion ratio of PAH

$= 720/0.9$ (excretion ratio of PAH is 0.9)

$= 800$ mL/min

Therefore, the actual RPF = 800 mL/min.

RBF is calculated from RPF from the following formula:

$RBF = RPF \div (1 - \text{Hematocrit value})$

$= 800 \div (1 - 0.45)$ [normal hematocrit value is 45%]

$= 800 \div 0.55$

$= 1,454.5$ mL/min

Therefore, RBF is 1,454.5 mL/min.

GLOMERULAR FILTRATION

Usually, both the kidneys receive the total blood flow of about 1.2–1.3 L/min (1.2 to 1.3 × 60 × 24 = 1,720 to 1,872 L/day), which is about 25% of our cardiac output per minute. But out of this, only 125 mL/min or 7.5 L/h or 180 L/day of fluid is filtered by the capillaries of glomerulus. However, again, out of this total 180 L of fluid, which is filtered in a day, 178 L/day of fluid is reabsorbed in renal tubules and only 1–2 L/day of urine is formed. Therefore, 99% or more of glomerular filtrate is reabsorbed in renal tubules. It is estimated that to clear the nitrogenous waste products from our body, produced during metabolism throughout the whole day, at least 400–500 mL of urine per day is required to be formed mandatorily. For the reabsorption of glomerular filtrate in renal tubules, the countercurrent multiplier exchanger system is a critical component that helps the kidney's ability to excrete or conserve (reabsorb) the salt and water (filtrate). The Na^+ and water reabsorption by kidney depend on the hypertonicity of the renal medullary interstitial tissue, which again depends on the maintenance of normal RBF. The major hormonal factors determining the conservation or the loss of filtered Na^+ and water are aldosterone, ADH, ANP, and renal PGs. At the filtration rate of 125 mL/min, the kidney filters an amount of fluid which is about 4 times of our total body water, 15 times of our total ECF volume, and 60 times of our total plasma volume per day.

Like the capillaries of the other parts of our body, the filtration in glomerular capillary is also governed by four capital forces opposing to each other. These capital four forces are (1) hydrostatic pressure in glomerular capillary (C_H), (2) oncotic pressure in glomerular capillary (C_{ON}), (3) hydrostatic pressure in Bowman's capsule (B_H), and (4) oncotic pressure in Bowman's capsule (B_{ON}). Therefore, the effective glomerular filtration pressure is: $(C_H - B_H) - (C_{ON} - B_{ON})$ and GFR $= K_f [(C_H - B_H) - (C_{ON} - B_{ON})]$, where K_f is the glomerular ultrafiltration coefficient.

The K_f depends mainly on four factors. These factors are (1) the permeability of glomerular capillary, (2) the electric charge of filtrate substances, (3) the size of filtration pore, and (4) the size of capillary bed. Therefore, GFR depends upon these abovementioned factors which determine the filtration coefficient and the hydrostatic and the oncotic pressure of glomerular capillary and Bowman's capsular fluid **(Box 1)**.

Capillary permeability is different in the different parts of our body. The permeability of glomerular capillary is 40–50 times more than that of the skeletal muscles. The substances with their molecular diameter of <4 nm are freely filtered out through the glomerular capillary whereas the substances with a molecular diameter of >8 nm are not at all filtered out.

BOX 1: Factors affecting glomerular filtration rate (GFR).

- *Changes in hydrostatic pressure of glomerular capillary*
  - Changes in systemic blood pressure
  - Contraction of afferent or efferent arteriole
- *Changes in oncotic pressure of glomerular capillary*
  - Hypoproteinemia
  - Dehydration
- *Changes in hydrostatic pressure of Bowman's capsule*
  - Obstruction in urinary passage
- *Changes in oncotic pressure of Bowman's capsule*
  - Oncotic pressure in Bowman's capsule is negligible as the ultrafiltrate does not contain any protein or very minimum amount
- *Changes in permeability coefficient*
  - Changes in surface area for effective filtration
  - Changes in permeability of glomerular capillary
- *Changes in renal blood flow*

Therefore, filtration of substances with molecular diameter between 4 and 8 nm is inversely proportional to their molecular size.

The GFR also depends on the electric charge of filtered substances. The wall of the glomerular capillary (or filtered membrane) itself is negatively charged and it is due to the presence of sialoprotein (a special type of protein). So, this –ve charge of capillary bed repels the –ve charged substances in blood and reduces their filtration. Hence, the filtration of –ve charged substances of 4 nm molecular diameter is more or less half than that of the neutral charged substances of the same molecular diameter.

On the contrary, the filtration of +ve charged substances of 7 nm molecular diameter is greater than the neutral and –ve charged substances of the same molecular diameter. This probably explains why the normally –ve charged albumin with a molecular diameter of 6–7 nm has a concentration of only 0.1–0.2% of its plasma concentration in the glomerular filtrate. This is far less than the expected higher concentration of albumin in the glomerular filtrate, calculated on the basis of their molecular diameter alone. The total amount of protein in urine is usually <100 mg/day. However, most of this is not filtered but comes from the shed tubular cells. In nephritis, the –ve charge of the glomerular capillary bed is lost, and then albuminuria can occur without any increase in the size of pores of filtration membrane.

The sizes of filtration pores, present on the filtration membrane of the capillary bed, depend on the contraction and relaxation of mesangial cell. The increase in contraction of these mesangial cells decreases the size of the filtration pores and K_f (glomerular filtration coefficient). Many agents such as angiotensin II, epinephrine, norepinephrine, vasopressin, thromboxane A_2, PGF_2, and leukotrienes also induce the contraction of these mesangial cells and decrease filtration by reducing the size of the filtration pores whereas the ANP, dopamine, PGE_2, etc., relax these mesangial cells and increase the size of the pores with an increased rate of filtration.

The hydrostatic and the oncotic pressure of glomerular capillary blood and Bowman's capsular fluid also alter the GFR. The afferent glomerular arterioles are short and arise directly from the interlobular arteries. Further, in the downstream, the efferent arterioles also have the relatively high resistance. Therefore, the hydrostatic pressure in glomerular capillary is much higher than that of other capillaries in the other parts of our body. This glomerular capillary hydrostatic pressure, which is the main filtration pressure here, is opposed by the hydrostatic pressure in Bowman's capsule. This is further opposed by the oncotic pressure gradient across the glomerular capillary bed, that is, $C_{ON} - B_{ON}$. Usually, the BON is negligible as there is no protein in the capsular filtrate. So, the equation of GFR can be rewritten as: GFR = $K_f [(C_H - B_H) - C_{ON}]$.

The net filtration pressure at the afferent end of the glomerular capillary is 16 mm Hg. But it gradually falls to zero, and a filtration equilibrium is reached at the efferent end of the glomerular capillary. This is due to the gradual leaving of fluid and other solutes, except protein from the capillary bed; therefore, there is a gradual increase in the oncotic pressure of the capillary blood due to the increased concentration of serum protein, while the blood passes through the glomerular capillary from afferent to efferent end.

Due to the autoregulation, by changing the renal vascular resistance, the nature tries to stabilize this net hydrostatic filtration pressure to a normal level. But when the MAP drops below this autoregulatory range, the GFR falls sharply. The GFR is maintained when the efferent arteriolar constriction is greater than afferent arteriolar constriction. But the constriction of both the arterioles decreases the GFR **(Table 3)**.

TABLE 3: Net filtration pressure at the afferent and efferent ends of the glomerular capillary.

Net filtration pressure = $C_H - B_H - C_{ON}$
C_H = Hydrostatic pressure in glomerular capillary, B_H = Plasma oncotic pressure in glomerular capillary, C_{ON} = Hydrostatic pressure in Bowman's capsule

	Afferent end (mm Hg)	Efferent end (mm Hg)
C_H	45	44
B_H	−10	−10
C_{ON}	−25	−34
Net filtration pressure	10	0

Measurement of Glomerular Filtration Rate

The normal value of GFR varies between 120 and 130 mL/min. It is usually about 20% of RBF (this RBF is again 25% of cardiac output). The GFR is usually measured by inulin or creatinine. The creatinine is a breakdown product of phosphocreatine, which is normally present in the muscles whereas inulin is a fructose polysaccharide with a molecular weight of 5,200. The measurement of GFR by inulin or creatinine is also called the *inulin or creatinine clearance rate*, respectively. The concept of clearance is frequently used in measurement of RBF and GFR. The renal clearance of a substance is defined as the volume of blood that is completely cleared of that substance per unit of time (usually per minute). For clearance, three substances are used and these are PAH, inulin, and creatinine. The PAH clearance is taken as RBF. But, the clearance of inulin and creatinine are taken as GFR. Because, the PAH is cleared from blood by both filtration at glomeruli and secretion at renal tubules after a single passage of blood through renal circulation (RBF). Whereas, inulin/creatinine is only filtered through glomeruli for its single pass clearance from RBF.

Inulin is completely filtered out by the glomerular capillary bed, and it is neither secreted nor reabsorbed by the renal tubules. Therefore, the use of inulin gives very accurate result of GFR (or inulin clearance rate) whereas the use of creatinine to measure the GFR (creatinine clearance rate) tends to overestimate the result because though it (creatinine) is completely (freely) filtered out of the glomerular capillary, a small amount of it is secreted through the renal tubule. In addition, the determination of plasma creatinine is inaccurate at a low plasma creatinine level. This is because the method used to estimate plasma creatinine also measures the small amount of other plasma constituents, such as chromogens. In spite of this, creatinine clearance is frequently measured in patients to estimate the GFR accurately. This is because (1) it is more practical, (2) it is easy, and (3) the value matches quite well the value of GFR, measured by inulin. This is also true, because although $U_{CR} \times V$ is high as a result of tubular secretion, the value of P_{CR} is also high as a result of nonspecific chromogens. Therefore, the two errors cancel each other. Hence, the measurement of endogenous creatinine clearance (from outside creatinine is not injected) is a worthwhile index of renal function. The creatinine clearance (C_{CR}) is measured by the following formula, like that of RBF by PAH: $C_{CR} = U_{CR} \times V/P_{CR}$ (U_{CR}: creatinine concentration in urine; V: urinary flow rate; P_{CR}: creatinine concentration in plasma).

Example:

$$U_{CR} = 35 \text{ mg/mL}, \quad V = 0.9 \text{ mL/min}, \quad P_{CR} = 0.25 \text{ mg/mL}$$

Therefore, $C_{CR} = 35 \times 0.9/0.25 = 126 \text{ mL/min}$

The ratio of GFR to RPF is called the filtration fraction and is usually 20%.

■ ASSESSMENT OF RENAL FUNCTIONS

Generally, the kidney performs three principal functions in our body. These are (1) excretion of potentially toxic and nontoxic metabolic end products, (2) regulation of water and electrolyte balance, and (3) production of hormones. The direct assessment of all these renal functions is practically impossible, and also simultaneously direct online evaluation of these renal functions is limited. Most of the renal functions are, therefore, assessed indirectly. Furthermore, these assessments of direct renal functions are not simple and are very expensive. On the other hand, the readily available tests fail to accurately reflect the status of kidney in a large percentage of patients, especially in elderly, malnourished, and dehydrated individuals.

The kidneys perform their functions through glomerulus and renal tubules. So, the renal functions are mainly divided into two groups: Glomerular functions and tubular functions. But this classification is arbitrary because in any renal diseases, both these functions are impaired simultaneously. On the contrary and fortunately, any standard test performed for renal functions evaluates both the glomerular and the tubular functions. Furthermore, it is also important to remember that most of the renal function tests are insensitive to detect the early renal dysfunction. Therefore, the subsequent serial results are more helpful than a single result **(Box 2)**.

The most common tests for renal function are urine analysis, measurement of blood urea nitrogen (BUN) in plasma, estimation of serum creatinine level, creatinine clearance (GFR), etc. Many other IV tests, urography, renal ultrasound, renal magnetic resonance imaging (MRI), renal computed tomography (CT), renal biopsy, etc., may also be performed to diagnose the renal pathology, responsible for renal dysfunction.

Urine Analysis

The information from urine analysis should be interpreted very cautiously to assess the renal function because there are many flaws. The urine analysis includes (1) the measurement of urine output, (2) the measurement of urinary osmolality and specific gravity, and (3) the microscopical examination of urine.

The estimation of urine output is an indirect parameter for the assessment of renal function. This is because many prerenal factors directly and profoundly affect the output of urine, without the presence of any renal dysfunction. For example, *oliguria* due to severe systemic hypotension and subsequently due to reduced renal perfusion, without any renal parenchymal dysfunction or any obstruction at anywhere on the passage of the urine, on one hand, and *polyuria* due to the central diabetes insipidus, without any impairment of the renal function on the other side, make it obvious that urine output does not always specifically reflect the renal function. This is more true intraoperatively when several other factors, such as the increased secretion of ADH, aldosterone, catecholamines, angiotensin, etc., due to stress, affect or decrease the output of urine with normal renal function.

Still, the measurement of urine output, as a primary indicator of renal function, is important in certain situations, where the anuria can develop due to some parenchymal diseases of kidney or due to impaired RBF for any cause that may lead to renal dysfunction. The evidence of formation of urine, regardless of its amount, suggests that there is adequate blood flow to the kidney. The intraoperative oliguria does not always indicate the impaired renal function, and if is not due to impaired renal function, it does not correlate (if the cause is prerenal) with the increased BUN and creatinine level or decreased creatinine clearance. The level of nitrogenous waste in blood depends on its production and its clearance through the kidney. On the other hand, the renal clearance depends on RBF and glomerular filtration. In the circumstances of reduced RBF, the kidney will maximally concentrate the glomerular ultrafiltrate, so that at least (minimally) 400–500 mL of urine should be excreted, which is obligatorily required to clear the daily nitrogenous waste **(Table 4)**.

During the analysis of urine, the measurement of the specific gravity and the osmolality of urine are also used as an important parameter to assess renal function. This indicates the tubular function only, that is, the concentration capacity of renal tubules. In specific gravity, the mass of 1 mL of urine

---

BOX 2: Tests used to evaluate renal function.

Glomerular function
- Blood urea nitrogen (BUN) (normal value: 10–20 mg/dL)
- Plasma creatinine level (normal value: 0.5–1.5 mg/dL)
- GFR or creatinine clearance (normal value: 120–130 mL/min)
- Proteinuria (normal value: <100 mg/day)

Renal tubular function
- Urine osmolality (normal value: 30–140 mOsm/L)
- Urine specific gravity (normal value: 1.003–1.030)
- Excretion of Na^+ through urine (normal value: <40 mmol/L)
- Renal glycosuria, cellular cast, urinary lysozyme

TABLE 4: Difference in urinary indices of patients with oliguria due to prerenal, renal, and physiological causes.

Indices	Renal causes	Prerenal causes	Physiological causes
Urinary osmolality (mOsm/kg)	200–300	>450	>700
Urine/plasma osmolality	<1.5	>2	>2.5
Urinary Na$^+$ concentration (mmol/L)	>40	<20	<10
Fractional Na$^+$ excretion (%)	>1	<1	<0.5
Urine and plasma creatinine ratio	<20	>40	>60
Specific gravity of urine	1.010–1.015	>1.015	>1.024
Urine and plasma urea ratio	>3 (rarely >10)	>20	>100

is compared to the mass of 1 mL of distilled water whereas in osmolality, the number of osmotically active particles in solution (urine) is measured. Usually, the force of osmolality governs the movement of fluid throughout the body and also in kidney. Therefore, the measurement of osmolality of urine is more superior to the measurement of specific gravity as a test of renal function.

In poor renal perfusion, due to reduced circulation (prerenal azotemia), the kidneys try to concentrate the urine. Therefore, its osmolality and specific gravity may go up above 500 mOsm/kg of H_2O and 1.003, respectively whereas, in acute tubular necrosis (ATN) (renal tubular dysfunction), urine osmolality and specific gravity may go below 350 mOsm/kg of H_2O and 1.001, respectively. Thus, it makes an important guideline to differentiate the causes of low urine output due to *renal causes* from *prerenal causes*. Still, the measurement of the osmolality and the specific gravity of urine is nonspecific for the diagnosis of renal dysfunction because there are many other factors which affect the osmolality and specific gravity of urine, other than renal dysfunction. These are the presence of protein, glucose, mannitol, dextrose, antibiotics, etc., in the urine and the use of diuretics, etc.

Hematuria, which is defined as more than two RBC per high-power field of centrifuged urine, indicates glomerular diseases or trauma to the kidney, ureter, lower urinary tract, etc. If the urine test is positive for blood, but there is no RBC, then it indicates the presence of free hemoglobin in urine (hemoglobinuria). Urine, normally, may contain hyaline or granular cast, but the presence of cellular cast in urine confirms the pathological condition of the kidney. Trace proteinuria may be a normal finding whereas 3 to 4+ proteinuria suggests glomerular disease as the proteins are not prevented from filtration. The patients, without renal disease, may excrete up to 100 mg of protein per day, but a greater amount may be present after heavy exercise or after prolonged standing. Massive proteinuria with protein content above 500–700 mg/day is always abnormal and

BOX 3: Factors that influence the result of renal function.

- Variable protein intake
- Dehydration
- Degree of catabolism
- GI bleeding
- Skeletal muscle mass
- Advanced age
- Timing of measurement of urine volume

(GI: gastrointestinal)

indicates severe glomerular damage. However, proteinuria may also be due to (1) the failure of tubular reabsorption of a small amount of protein that is normally filtered, (2) the abnormally increased concentration of normal plasma protein, and (3) the presence of abnormal plasma proteins which are excreted through urine. Pyuria indicates infection at any level of the genitourinary system.

The measurement of urinary pH may assist in the diagnosis of some acid–base disturbances in our body. But the determination of pH from a single sample of urine has no value. The presence of glycosuria without hyperglycemia suggests proximal tubular damage. The normal urinary lysozyme level is <1.9 mg/mL. The urinary level of it >5 mg/mL indicates significant renal tubular disease **(Box 3)**.

Estimation of Blood Urea Nitrogen

The primary source of urea in our body is the liver. During protein catabolism, NH_3 is produced from the deamination of amino acids. But this NH_3 is very toxic, so our body converts this ammonia into urea in the liver: $2NH_3 + CO_2 \rightarrow H_2N\text{-}CO\text{-}NH_2 + H_2O$. Therefore, BUN is directly proportional to protein catabolism. The normal concentration of BUN is 10–20 mg/dL. Like urine analysis, the estimation of BUN is a commonly performed test to assess the renal function, mainly GFR. With GFR, the level of BUN is indirectly proportional. The level of BUN >50–60 mg/dL indicates renal disease, unless proved otherwise or protein catabolism is normal and constant. But the abnormalities in the level of BUN indicates the renal dysfunction which is already advanced. This is the limitation of the test.

The other limitations of this test to assess renal function are as the urea is filtered and then is partially reabsorbed and is partially secreted, so the level of BUN is not always a sensitive index for GFR or renal dysfunction. The level of BUN is falsely elevated during low circulatory states, such as in congestive heart failure and dehydration. This is due to the increased reabsorption of filtered urea for renal hypoperfusion, caused by congestive heart failure and dehydration. The reabsorption of urea is greater, approximately 60% of the filtered load, when urinary flow is low and only about 40% when this flow is high. There are other multiple nonrenal conditions, where the BUN level is increased. These are high protein diet, gastrointestinal (GI) bleeding, large hematoma, increased tissue breakdown, high protein catabolic state of body such as sepsis, fever, starvation, and steroid therapy (due to increased protein catabolism). On the other hand, the BUN level may remain within normal range despite significant reduction in GFR, if there is liver disease which causes decreased synthesis of urea.

Estimation of Plasma Creatinine

Like BUN, the plasma creatinine level is also measured to assess the renal function (*mainly GFR*). In a normal individual, daily a constant amount of creatinine (20–25 mg/kg/day) is produced (nonenzymatically) in his or her body from creatine phosphate, present in the muscle. It is only excreted by glomerular filtration through kidney, without any reabsorption and secretion through renal tubules. As the muscle mass of an individual is relatively constant, its daily production is also constant. Therefore, the measurement of the serum creatinine level is a better index than the measurement of BUN to assess the renal function or GFR. The normal serum creatinine level of a healthy adult with normal muscle mass is 0.8–1.3 mg/dL. Therefore, a very muscular individual may have a falsely high plasma creatinine level, though GFR is normal. On the other hand, an individual with low muscular mass may have a falsely normal creatinine value, despite significant reduction of GFR. Thus, like BUN, an increased plasma creatinine level is also a late sign of renal dysfunction. This is because GFR must often be reduced as much as 50%, before the elevation of creatinine concentration and to reach the abnormal level.

Further, this is more true for the individuals with reduced muscle mass who already has a low creatinine value. As creatinine is the product of skeletal muscle's protein catabolism, it is formed at a lower rate in elderly and women than young and male persons. Consequently, the plasma creatinine level does not accurately reflect the magnitude

of loss of nephron because creatinine production is *directly* proportional to muscle mass and *indirectly* proportional to nephron loss. Therefore, many chronically ill, wasted, elderly patients may have a plasma creatinine value in the normal range, though there is reduced renal concentrating ability and GFR. The utility of a *single* serum creatinine measurement as an indicator of GFR is less valued in critically ill patients than in healthy ambulatory patients because, in critically ill patients, the production of creatinine is frequently changed due to change in catabolism of muscle mass and the volume of distribution of creatinine.

Measurement of Creatinine Clearance

The excretion or filtration of creatinine from plasma by glomeruli (the amount of plasma cleared from creatinine by glomeruli) measures or reflects the ability of glomeruli to filter it (GFR). This is called creatinine clearance or GFR. It gives more useful result than the only plasma creatinine value to quantify the renal reserve. It also provides the *most accurate method* available for clinically assessing the kidney function.

From the only plasma creatinine level (without measuring the urinary concentration of it, which is needed to measure the creatinine clearance rate or GFR as described before), the creatinine clearance rate can also be measured with reasonable accuracy by the following formula:

$$\text{Creatinine clearance} = [(140 - \text{Age}) \times \text{Body weight in kg}] \div [72 \times \text{Plasma creatinine value}]$$

But the precise measurement of creatinine clearance (using the formula $C_{CR} = U_{CR} \times V/P_{CR}$) requires the collection of urine samples for a fixed time, say 24 hours or 2 hours. The 24-hour urine collection gives more accurate results than its 2-hour collection. This is because the changing hydration of a patient invalidates the result, calculated from the short-term collection of urine volume (2 hours), which varies greatly. On the other hand, for a patient with acute renal failure, a test that requires 24-hour collection of urine is often impractical.

Hence, at present the determination of 2-hour creatinine clearance rate is done routinely instead of 24 hours, and it is reasonably accurate and easier to perform. The *mild impairment of kidney function* generally results in creatinine clearance rate (GFR) of 40–60 mL/min. The clearances of creatinine between 25 and 40 mL/min indicates the *moderate impairment of kidney function* and nearly always causes symptoms. The creatinine clearance rate <25 mL/min indicates an *overt kidney failure*.

During the end-stage kidney disease, other than filtration, there is also the secretion of creatinine through PT for its excretion by urine. As a result, with declining kidney

FACT FILE XI

Creatinine (anhydride of creatinine) is mostly formed from the breakdown of creatine phosphate, which is present in muscles. This process is not catalyzed by any enzymes and is irreversible. It is formed within the muscle itself. So, liver diseases do not affect the blood creatinine level. It is considered as a waste product and serves practically no function in our body. It is a nonthreshold substance and is filtered completely by glomeruli. A small amount of creatinine is also secreted by the renal tubular cells and is passed through urine. Its excretion is not related to exogenous food protein. The normal plasma value of creatinine is 0.7–2 mg/dL. This level is very constant and is considered to be pathological, when its value increases above 2 mg/dL in plasma. Usually about 1.2–2 g of creatinine is excreted in 24-hour urine. This amount is remarkably constant for a particular individual. It is related to muscle bulk and is higher in muscular persons. Creatinine excretion increases in fevers, starvation, carbohydrate-free diet, and diabetes mellitus where the breakdown of muscle mass is increased.

Creatinine represents the waste products of creatine metabolism. It arises in the body (muscle) from creatine during the spontaneous breakdown of creatine phosphate. Therefore, the creatinine level increases during excessive muscle destruction, releasing creatine or due to failure of creatine being properly phosphorylated. So, creatinine excretion is independent of exogenous food protein and is considered as an index of endogenous protein metabolism. Due to any inborn metabolic disorders, creatine does not convert to creatinine and appears in urine. This is known as creatinuria. Usually, a small amount of creatine is excreted through urine along with creatinine. But it gradually disappears as the maturity advances.

function, the creatinine clearance rate (GFR) progressively overestimates the true GFR. Moreover, with progressive damage of kidney, there is compensatory hyperfiltration in the remaining nephrons and increases the GFR or at least does not allow the decrease of GFR. It is, therefore, important to look for the other signs of deteriorating kidney function, such as hypertension, proteinuria, or abnormalities of urine sediment.

Creatinine clearance may also be used to differentiate the prerenal azotemia from ATN or renal azotemia. In the postoperative period, a creatinine clearance value which is <25 mL/min, measuring over 2 hours, appears to be a good and early predictor of impaired renal function **(Fact file XI)**.

BUN: Creatinine Ratio

The normal plasma level of BUN is 10–20 mg/dL, and the normal plasma creatinine level is 0.8–1.5 mg/dL. Hence, under a normal condition, the ratio of BUN to creatinine varies widely. But under a pathological condition, this ratio of 10:1 is taken as the normal upper limit. In low renal tubular flow rates, due to hypotension and decreased renal perfusion, the reabsorption of urea is enhanced. But the filtration of creatinine is not enhanced. Hence, the ratio of BUN to serum creatinine is elevated to >10:1. This BUN:creatinine ratio >15:1 is therefore seen in volume depletion and low renal perfusion (congestive heart failure, nephrotic syndrome, cirrhosis of liver, etc.). An increase in protein catabolism also increases this ratio.

Miscellaneous Tests

Except the abovementioned tests, there are other tests that may be used to take an overview about the renal functions. Among these, some are not so reliable, but only few are very promising. For example, the urine–plasma creatinine ratio and the urine–plasma urea ratio (or index) were initially introduced as very promising methods for evaluation of patients with suspected ATN or renal dysfunction. But subsequently these tests show their lack of reliability and have more prognostic than diagnostic value.

The concentrating capacity of renal tubules also can be assessed by measuring the urinary Na^+ concentration and fractional excretion of Na^+ (FENa). If these two values go above 40 mEq/L and 1, respectively, then it indicates ATN. On the contrary, in hypotension, ADH-induced increased Na^+ reabsorption leads to a decrease in urinary Na^+ concentration <20 mEq/L and FENa <1 in prerenal azotemia, which indicates the fallacy of this test. Some other tests of tubular function, such as concentrating ability, ability to excrete water load, and ability to excrete acid through kidney, are valuable in some circumstances.

More accurate measurement of GFR is now most easily undertaken by ascertaining the clearance of ^{51}Cr-labeled EDTA. This has largely replaced the estimation of inulin and creatinine clearance in clinical practice.

ANESTHESIA, SURGERY, AND RENAL FUNCTION

Any anesthesia and surgery have enormous impact on renal function. This enormous impact of anesthesia and surgery on renal function can be caused *directly or indirectly*, affecting the renal physiology, due to the changes in the levels of different hormones, electrolytes, body water, cardiac output, RBF, pH, etc., associated with anesthesia and surgery.

Surgical Effects on Renal Function

Surgery affects the kidney function by two ways: Indirect and direct. *Indirectly*, surgery affects the renal function by physiological changes associated with the neuroendocrine stress response to surgery. Increased sympathetic tone commonly occurs in the perioperative period as a result of anxiety, pain, light anesthesia, and surgical stimulation.

Increased sympathetic activity increases the renal vascular resistance and activates the several hormonal systems, reducing the RBF, GFR, and urine output.

Directly, certain surgical procedures can significantly alter the physiology of kidney. During laparoscopic surgeries, produced pneumoperitoneum creates an abdominal compartment syndrome like state. The increased intra-abdominal pressure often produces oliguria or anuria that is proportional to insufflation pressure. Mechanisms include the compression on renal parenchyma, inferior vena cava, and renal vein → decreased cardiac output → increased sympathetic activity → increase in plasma level of renin, aldosterone, and ADH. Abdominal compartment syndrome can also be precipitated by a number of comorbid problems, with similar adverse effects on kidney function via the same mechanisms. Other surgical procedures that can deteriorate kidney functions and may also increase the risk of acute kidney injury (AKI) are Cardiopulmonary bypass, during cross clamping of aorta, aortic dissection near renal artery, etc.

In many minor invasive or noninvasive diagnostic surgical procedures, where radiocontrast dyes are used in the perioperative period, these radiocontrast agents can adversely affect the renal functions, especially in the presence of preexisting renal diseases. The mechanisms of renal injury in these settings are vasoconstriction, direct tubular injury, drug-induced immunological and inflammatory responses, and renal microvascular and tubular obstruction caused by radiocontrast dyes. This type of renal injury, inflicted by a radiocontrast agent, is treated or can be prevented by proper IV hydration and pretreatment with *N*-acetylcysteine. This *N*-acetylcysteine is used in the dose of 600 mg orally every 12 hourly and 4 doses, administered before the administration of contrast dye, and has been shown to decrease the risk of radiocontrast agent-induced acute renal injury in patients with preexisting renal dysfunction. The protective action of acetylcysteine is due to free radical scavenging or sulfhydryl donor reducing properties of it. The *N*-acetylcysteine has not been shown to be protective in the perioperative setting, except in patients who receive radiocontrast dyes. Further, fenoldopam, mannitol, loop diuretics, and renal dose of dopamine, etc., cannot help to protect this radiocontrast agent-induced acute renal injury.

Anesthesia Effects on Renal Function

In general, anesthesia results in the decrease of RBF and subsequently results in the deterioration of renal function, due to decreased GFR by the decrease of RBF. The likely mechanism of this deterioration of renal function, induced by anesthesia, includes the loss of renal autoregulation, increased neurohormonal factors (ADH, vasopressin, renin, angiotensin), and increased neuroendocrine response. This in turn decreases the excretion of nitrogenous wastes, electrolytes, H⁺, anesthetic, and other drugs and causes the conservation of body fluid. The decreased excretion of anesthetic and other drugs lead to the prolongation of their effect. On the other hand, anesthetic agents also affect the renal function directly. This is mainly applicable for the volatile anesthetic agents, such as methoxyflurane which produces many nephrotoxic metabolites in our body after its administration. The IV anesthetic agents have minimal direct effects on kidney. They deteriorate the renal function indirectly by reducing the RBF. Among the anesthetic agents which are mostly concerned about the renal function are IV anesthetic agents, inhalational anesthetic agents, NSAIDs, and muscle relaxants and their reversal.

Anesthetic Agents

Intravenous Anesthetic Agents

In patients with impaired renal functions, the central nervous system (CNS) depressant effects of IV anesthetic agents are exaggerated. This is because they are mostly protein (albumin) bound, and in renal dysfunction as the level of albumin is reduced, most of the drug remains in an unbound free form and their actions are exaggerated. In addition, the renal dysfunction is frequently associated with acidosis, which increases the unionized form of drug as their pK value acts usually at the physiological range of plasma. The unionized form of these IV drugs is more lipid soluble. Therefore, it causes higher drug concentration in CNS. Hence, thiopentone, which remains as 15% unbound free and unionized form in a normal individual, increases to 30% in chronic renal failure. Therefore, the induction and the maintenance dose of thiopentone should be reduced in uremic patients.

On the other hand, as the metabolism of thiopentone in liver remains unchanged in renal dysfunction patient, the amount of it which is necessary to produce and maintain anesthesia is reduced. This same consideration is also true for methohexitone, another inducing agent, although the metabolism of it in liver plays a slight greater role in termination of its therapeutic effect than thiopentone. On the other hand, the reversal of the effect of ultra-short-acting barbiturate, such as thiopentone, depends only on their redistribution and hepatic metabolism, but very little or nil on the elimination through kidney. Therefore, the recovery from thiopentone in a renal dysfunction patient is not affected.

However, it is surprising that in a renal dysfunction patient, the pharmacodynamics and pharmacokinetics of a new IV anesthetic agent, such as propofol, do not change and are very safe to use. Ketamine should be avoided in a renal failure patient because it causes an exaggerated reaction to coexisting hypertension and tachycardia, if they are already present. However, ketamine is reported to minimally affect the renal function directly. It also tries to preserve the renal function during hemorrhage and hypovolemia. Agents with α-adrenergic blocking activity may prevent catecholamine-induced redistribution of RBF by autoregulation. For the benzodiazepines (BZDs), the increased free fraction of these drugs, due to decreased protein binding, also increases their CNS sensitivity. Further, due to the impairment of excretion, caused by renal dysfunction, there is accumulation of active metabolites of some long-acting BZD, such as diazepam, lorazepam, and oxazepam, which prolongs their clinical effect.

For narcotics, the same is true as that of barbiturates and BZDs. As the protein-binding capacity is reduced in a renal dysfunctional patient, the unbound level of morphine and its active metabolites, such as morphine-6-glucuronide (nontoxic) in plasma, increases and predisposes the patient to more and prolonged respiratory depression. Meperidine (pethidine) has a toxic metabolite, named normeperidine (norpethidine). So, it is not recommended for use by repeated bolus doses or through infusion in a renal failure patient, due to gradual accumulation of these toxic metabolites, which are excreted through kidney. The pharmacokinetic and pharmacodynamic effects of alfentanil and fentanyl are appeared to be unaffected by renal dysfunction. Further, fentanyl has short half-life and its metabolites are inactive. So, these agents are a good choice in a patient with renal disease.

Drugs with antidopaminergic activity such as metoclo-pramide and phenothiazines may impair the renal response of dopamine, when it (dopamine) is used as protection for the kidney. The inhibition of the synthesis local renal PGs, which have a renal vasodilating property, by the use of any NSAID or ketorolac has a profound deleterious effect on kidney function. Hence, the use of NSAIDs is not recom-mended in patients with renal dysfunction. This is especially important in patients with a high level of angiotensin II and norepinephrine, which causes renal vasoconstriction. Thus, it attenuates the renal protective response and decreases GFR, producing or exaggerating renal dysfunction. ACE inhibitors also block the protective effect of angiotensin II which is locally produced and causes additional reduction in GFR during anesthesia. Thus, it potentiates the detrimental effect of the anesthetic agent on renal perfusion.

Volatile Anesthetic Agents

Indirectly, the volatile anesthetic agents affect the renal function by eliminating the renal autoregulation and reducing the RBF and GFR, with decreased urine output. All these hemodynamic changes, produced by the volatile anesthetic agents, are dose dependent and can be attenuated by adequate preoperative hydration which probably helps to maintain better renal perfusion.

On the other hand, the volatile anesthetic agents also *directly* affect the renal functions by their nephrotoxic metabolites, which are formed by the liver and excreted through the kidney. Though 99% of volatile anesthetic agents are excreted through lungs, still to some extent all the inhaled anesthetics are biotransformed to nephrotoxic metabolites, during their metabolism in liver. The impaired renal function does not alter the pharmacodynamics and pharmacokinetic effect of any volatile anesthetic agents, but these agents affect the function of kidney. So, from the point of view of selecting a volatile anesthetic agent, one should be careful regarding the effect of the agent on kidney which may make further deterioration of its function than the effect of renal dysfunction on the hemodynamic and pharmacodynamic effects of that agent.

All the modern volatile anesthetic agents, such as methoxyflurane, enflurane, halothane, isoflurane, sevoflurane, and desflurane, are halogenated compounds, containing mainly fluorine. These fluorinated volatile anesthetic compounds produce inorganic fluorides as their metabolites, which are nephrotoxic. This inorganic fluoride-induced nephrotoxicity depends on the type of volatile agent used and the duration of its exposure. The threshold level of nephrotoxicity of these inorganic fluorides is 50 µM/L. The amount of inorganic fluoride, below this level, does not produce nephrotoxicity. However, in impaired renal function, the methoxyflurane is absolutely contraindicated because it is extensively biotransformed into inorganic fluoride and oxalic acid during its metabolism into liver, and these metabolites of methoxyflurane are extremely nephrotoxic.

This inorganic fluoride-induced nephrotoxicity, caused by volatile agents, includes an inability to concentrate the urine in response to ADH, leading to polyuria, hypernatremia, and increased serum osmolality. The other halogenated volatile agents are also metabolized in our body, during their use to inorganic fluoride, but their levels remain below their nephrotoxic threshold level. For example, after 3–4 hours of use of enflurane, the inorganic fluoride level in the plasma is about 20 ± 5 µM/L, which is far below the nephrotoxic threshold level.

Again, obesity is associated with the production of a higher level of inorganic fluorides, following enflurane anesthesia whereas the plasma fluoride level, after the use of isoflurane and halothane, increases to only 3–4 and 1–2 µM/L, respectively. Therefore, the use of isoflurane and halothane is a better alternative in a renal failure patient.

A recently introduced volatile anesthetic agent is desflurane. It is highly volatile and its boiling point is 19°C (near the room temperature). But it is very stable in soda lime and also resists degradation by the liver. So, the mean inorganic fluoride concentration, after 1 hour exposure of desflurane, at the dose of 1 MAC, is only 1 μM/L or less.

On the other hand, sevoflurane is very unstable in soda lime which decomposes it. It is also biotransformed into liver. So, after prolonged exposure to sevoflurane, the level of nephrotoxic inorganic fluoride may reach up to 50 μM/L. But still there is no report of any gross change of renal function in humans, after its prolonged use.

As previously noted, compound A, a breakdown product of sevoflurane in soda lime, causes acute kidney injury in laboratory animals. Low fresh gas flow rates (<2 L/min) promote its accumulation in the breathing circuit of the anesthesia machine. However, no clinical study has detected renal injury in human as a consequence of sevoflurane anesthesia. But, still, some authorities recommend a fresh gas flow rate of >2 L/min with sevoflurane to minimize the risk of this theoretical problem.

Muscle Relaxant

The level of plasma cholinesterase is reduced in a severe renal dysfunction patient. But this value is rarely so low to cause prolonged action of succinylcholine. Therefore, it can be used without difficulty in a patient with decreased or absent renal function. Succinylcholine is metabolized by plasma (pseudo) cholinesterase to nontoxic succinic acid and choline. The metabolic precursor of these two compounds is succinylmonocholine, which is excreted through the kidney. Hence, prolonged use of succinylcholine by infusions or repeated bolus doses of it should be avoided in patient with renal failure. The use of succinylcholine is associated with the transient rise of plasma K^+ level to 0.5–0.7 mEq/L. This rise may be as great as 5–7 mEq/L in burn, trauma, or neurologically injured patient. In renal failure patients, the level of plasma K^+ also remains high.

Hence, the use of succinylcholine in a renal failure patient with this high level of plasma K^+ can cause cardiovascular collapse. So, the use of succinylcholine in a severe renal failure patient is not advisable, unless the patient has undergone dialysis within 24 hours prior to anesthesia and surgery. Still, succinylcholine is the agent of choice for rapid-sequence induction and intubation for difficult airway (as its onset of action is not delayed and the duration of action is not prolonged in a renal dysfunction patient), if the plasma K^+ level permits. In the majority of patients with renal failure, a single dose of succinylcholine is considered safe, provided the serum K^+ level is <5 mEq/L.

The two nondepolarizing muscle relaxants, such as atracurium and its derivative cisatracurium, are broken down in plasma by enzymatic ester hydrolysis and by nonenzymatic alkaline degradation (Hofmann elimination) to their inactive products. Therefore, they are not dependent on renal excretion for their termination of action. Hence, the indices of these two muscle relaxants, such as the onset of action, the duration of action, and the recovery from their action are the same in a patient with normal and with severely impaired renal function. So, they appear to be the neuromuscular blocking agent of choice for renal failure patients. Severe renal dysfunction does not prolong the neuromuscular blocking effect of these two agents, even when it is given by constant infusion over several days. Laudanosine is one of the important metabolic end products of atracurium and cisatracurium and it may cause convulsion. This laudanosine is excreted through kidney. But, fortunately, the risk of convulsion from the accumulation of laudanosine in a renal failure patient, after the continuous infusion of atracurium or cisatracurium in an intensive care unit (ICU), has not been reported.

Vecuronium is another nondepolarizing muscle relaxant that is 70–80% metabolized in liver, and the remaining 20–30% is excreted as an original compound through kidney. Hence, in patients with renal failure, the normal intubation and the maintenance doses of vecuronium should be reduced, and the intermittent dosing interval should also be increased. One of the metabolites of vecuronium is 3-desacetyl vecuronium, and it is pharmacologically active and is excreted through kidney. Hence, the continuous infusion of vecuronium is not recommended in a renal failure patient in fear of accumulation of this active metabolite.

Another short-acting nondepolarizing muscle relaxant is mivacurium which is metabolized by plasma cholinesterase, but slowly than succinylcholine. Therefore, as the level of plasma cholinesterase is reduced in impaired renal function or after dialysis, its duration of action is prolonged by another 10–15 minutes in two such conditions. But the use of this drug in a renal failure patient is not a contraindication. This agent can be used cautiously with lower doses in a state of renal failure. The clearance of rocuronium is not changed in a renal failure patient, but its elimination half-life is increased. This is due to the increase in its volume of distribution in a renal dysfunction patient. Therefore, there is somewhat longer duration of action of rocuronium in renal failure.

Other long-acting nondepolarizing muscle relaxants, such as pancuronium, doxacurium, and pipecuronium, show their reduced clearance rate, increased elimination half-life, and prolonged duration of action in patients with renal disease. Therefore, if possible, these agents should be avoided or can be used with lower doses and a longer dosing interval in renal failure patients. The use of any neuromuscular blocking agent in the presence of renal dysfunction should be monitored by a nerve stimulator.

The anticholinesterases, such as neostigmine, edrophonium, and physostigmine, are excreted mainly through the kidneys. Among these, 50% of neostigmine and 70% of edrophonium and physostigmine are excreted unchanged through urine. So, in renal dysfunction, their actions are exaggerated and prolonged, but this is matched with the exaggerated and prolonged action of neuromuscular blocking agents.

Anesthetic Procedures

Before operation, it is not always possible to become sure whether the patient has any renal disease or not. The best way to know the presence or absence of renal disease is past medical history. The physical findings are often minimum, until the renal disease is far advanced. This is because until approximately 50% of renal function is lost, the laboratory results remain within normal limits, except the creatinine clearance. Patients with this 50% loss of renal function are said to have decreased renal reserve and their anesthetic management is the same as that of the patients with normal renal functions **(Box 4)**.

For renal dysfunction, two terms are used. These are *Renal insufficiency* and *renal failure*. The renal insufficiency is characterized by mild anemia, mild azotemia, and slight decrease in urine concentration ability. During anesthesia of these categories of patients, attention is paid to avoid the conditions which may further deteriorate their renal function. On the other hand, renal failure is said to be present, when the patients have hypocalcemia, hypernatremia, hyperphosphatemia, hyperchloremia, hyperkalemia, progressive anemia, and loss of urinary concentrating or diluting ability. In these renal failure groups of patients, the plasma creatinine value and the plasma creatinine clearance rate vary between 3.5 and 4 mg/dL and 15 and

20 mL/min, respectively. They are also unable to adapt the rapid changes in fluid balance. Hence, they run the risk of becoming acutely hypovolemic or fluid overload, and the clinical condition of these patients is uncertain. The aim of the anesthetic management of these categories of patients is directed at avoiding of the further deterioration of renal function, which will cause them to become grossly uremic and require hemodialysis.

Drugs which are excreted through the kidney should completely be avoided or if required at all, they should be given very cautiously in decreased doses or at prolonged intervals. If the patients lack significant medical history, focusing on renal disease and its function, then the routine preoperative blood tests and urine analysis for screening of the status of renal function are sufficient for early identification of renal disease or its dysfunction.

During screening, if the renal dysfunction is thought to be present, then more precise methods for assessing the degree of deterioration of renal function are necessary. Therefore, the routine laboratory tests, useful for preoperative evaluation of renal functions, are as follows: Urine analysis (including output, appearance, pH, specific gravity, protein content, etc.), blood tests (including hemoglobin percentage (Hb%), coagulation profile, electrolytes, pH, BUN, creatinine, etc.), electrocardiogram (ECG), chest X-ray, etc. If necessary, other renal function tests, such as the creatinine clearance rate and GFR, should also be measured. Among these, many are described before and those which are not described before are mentioned below.

Hematocrit

Anemia is a common finding for renal diseases and the severity of it (anemia) depends on the depth of renal dysfunction. It is due to the decreased production of erythropoietin (erythropoiesis-stimulating factor). The hematocrit value running in between 25 and 30% is appeared to be well tolerated and does not always need blood transfusion because it (blood transfusion) is associated with unnecessary several disadvantages, such as volume overload, hyperkalemia, and viral infections. If this hematocrit value is thought not to be justified for the proposed surgery or is poorly tolerated, due to some systemic diseases, such as cardiac disease, then blood transfusion should not be withheld **(Table 5)**.

Coagulation Profile

Hemorrhagic episodes remain the major risk factor, contributing to the morbidity and mortality, associated with anemia in a renal dysfunction patient. Prothrombin time (PT) and partial thromboplastin time (PTT) remain usually

---

BOX 4: Manifestations of renal dysfunction.

- Hyperkalemia
- Hyponatremia
- Hypocalcemia
- Hyperchloremia
- Hyperphosphatemia
- Metabolic acidosis
- Anemia
- Coagulopathies
- Unpredictable intravascular fluid volume status
- Hypertension
- Congestive heart failure

TABLE 5: Treatment of coagulopathy due to renal failure.

Drug	Dose	Onset of action	Peak effect	Duration of action
Cryoprecipitate	10–15 units IV over 15–30 minutes	<1–2 hours	6–12 hours	12–24 hours
Desmopressin	0.3–0.6 µg/kg IV or SC	<1–2 hours	2–4 hours	4–8 hours
Estrogen	0.6 mg/kg/day	6 hours	6–7 days	15 days

(IV: intravenous; SC: subcutaneous)

normal in such a patient, though they have an increased tendency to bleed. Hence, the bleeding time (BT) is the best screening test for this group of patients that correlates well with the tendency to bleed in a renal dysfunction patient. The treatment of the uremic bleeding patient usually includes the administration of cryoprecipitate plasma, which provides the factor VIII or the administration of desmopressin (1-desamino-8-D-arginine vasopressin or DDAVP). The DDAVP is an analog of ADH and increases the circulating level of factor VIII. Thus, it decreases the bleeding disorder.

The maximal effect of desmopressin is found within 2–4 hours, after its administration, and lasts for 6–8 hours. It acts by increasing the binding capacity of the platelet membrane receptor with factor VIII and making a more active complex. Although cryoprecipitate plasma and desmopressin can correct BT and the surgical procedures can be performed without excessive bleeding in a renal failure patient, the effects of both these drugs last only for few hours. Therefore, if a prolonged effect is desired, then conjugated estrogen may be given in the dose of 0.6 mg/kg/day through the IV route. The repeated daily administration of estrogen for 5 days decreases the BT within 6 hours and this lasts for 15 days. The administration of erythropoietin also decreases BT. It probably acts by increasing the erythropoiesis, which acts like blood transfusion.

Electrolytes and Acid–base Status

As a preoperative checkup, the plasma Na^+, K^+, HCO_3^-, pH, BUN, and creatinine level of a patient, suffering from renal dysfunction, should be checked routinely. If the plasma Na^+ level is <125 mmol/L, K^+ level is >5.5 mmol/L, and both are associated with hypoalbuminemia and acidosis, then the patient should be put under hemodialysis to control all these parameters, before induction of anesthesia. Among these, the plasma K^+ concentration is most important. So, though, if dialysis is performed 24 hours before surgery, then the plasma K^+ level should still be checked just before induction of anesthesia. This is because the plasma K^+ level is changed very rapidly than that of other electrolytes in plasma.

In emergency circumstances, if dialysis cannot be instituted immediately before anesthesia and surgery, then the plasma K^+ level can be controlled by administration of IV glucose with insulin. Hyperventilation, after induction and intubation, may also decrease the plasma K^+ level by about 0.5 mmol/L for every 10 mm Hg reduction of $PaCO_2$ level. The renal dysfunction is also associated with acidosis (low HCO_3^- level). So, control of this acidosis by IV administration of bicarbonate also controls the plasma K^+ level. But to control this acidosis and hyperkalemia, bicarbonate should be infused very slowly, keeping in mind that its rapid administration may precipitate the overt symptoms of hypocalcemia.

If the serum bicarbonate level is very low, that is, between 12 and 15 mmol/L, then the anion gap acidosis, for example ketoacidosis, should be thought. In renal dysfunction, as the GFR is reduced, the filtration of glucose is also reduced. Therefore, the control of plasma glucose level, especially in a diabetic patient, is very difficult. Furthermore, an increase in the plasma glucose level causes an increase in the plasma K^+ level. If the plasma BUN level goes >100 mg/dL, then dialysis should be performed 12–24 hours before any anesthesia and surgery. It will help to remove the waste products and excess fluid. It will also help to control the plasma K^+ and Na^+ levels and acidosis **(Table 6)**.

Electrocardiogram and Chest X-ray

Renal dysfunction is associated with electrolytes imbalance, mainly K^+ and Na^+. Therefore, ECG in patients with renal failure often reveals conduction abnormalities and arrhythmias. Hence, continuous perioperative ECG monitoring is mandatory, during anesthesia of a renal failure patient. A preanesthetic chest radiograph also should always be obtained in a patient, suffering from renal dysfunction because renal failure is commonly associated with pulmonary infection, congestion, edema, pleural or pericardial effusion, etc.

Premedication

For premedication, before any anesthesia and surgery, in a renal dysfunction patient, BZDs are the most commonly

TABLE 6: Management of hyperkalemia.

Type of treatment	Dose	Onset of action	Mechanism of action	Side effects
• Sodium bicarbonate	• Na^+ 50–100 mmol IV	• Rapid	• Shifting of K^+ into cells	• Na^+ overload
• Glucose and insulin	• 50 mL of 50% glucose solution with 10 units soluble insulin	• 6–8 hours	• Shifting of K^+ into cells	• Hypo- or hyperglycemia
• Calcium gluconate	• 10–20 mL of 10% solution IV	• Rapid	• Directly antagonize the effects of K^+ on heart	• Arrhythmia
• Dialysis		• According to severity of renal dysfunction	• Directly remove K^+ from the body	• Require vascular access
• Ion exchange		• According to severity of renal dysfunction	• Directly remove K^+ from the body	• Na^+ overload

(IV: intravenous)

used agents for sedation and anxiolysis. But caution must be exercised by reducing their dose and avoiding its repeated administration, as they may cause excessive and prolonged sedation. Other premedicants, such as H2 blocker (ranitidine) or proton-pump inhibitor (omeprazole) and prokinetic agent (metoclopramide), may be used safely in a renal dysfunction patient. But their doses should also be reduced appropriately. On the other hand, the use of these agents is mandatory in renal dysfunction patients because the gastric emptying time is delayed in uremia. The patients who are already under chronic steroid therapy should receive steroid preoperatively and in higher doses than the previous one. This is because the long-term use of steroid impairs the stress response, and therefore higher doses of it are needed. The doses of anticholinergic agents, such as atropine and glycopyrrolate, should also be reduced accordingly, as they are partially excreted through urine.

Monitoring

The routine monitoring devices, which are used for other patients, should also be applied here to renal dysfunction patients. Among these, the ECG is very important to detect the conduction abnormalities and arrhythmias, which are commonly associated with hyperkalemia, found in renal failure patients. The BP cuff should not be used on the same extremity on which the arteriovenous fistula for dialysis is performed. This is because a fistula can be blocked by thrombosis, during the inflation of cuff. Special monitoring techniques such as intra-arterial BP monitoring, central venous pressure (CVP) monitoring, and pulmonary arterial pressure monitoring are needed according to the severity of renal dysfunction and the extent of surgery. A peripheral nerve stimulator may also be useful to avoid the excessive dose of muscle relaxant with prolonged neuromuscular blockade.

Induction of Anesthesia

The commonly used inducing agents, such as thiopentone and propofol, have a hypotensive effect which may be exaggerated in patients, suffering from renal dysfunction. So, an anesthetist must be careful about it, and the incidence of severe hypotension can be reduced by reducing the doses of these abovementioned inducing agents and maintaining an adequate intravascular volume status, prior to induction. In this regard, ketamine is safe and is the agent of choice in a severely ill patient, provided there is no hypertension which is commonly associated with renal dysfunction. The rapid-sequence induction and intubation are preferred in a severe renal failure patient because delayed gastric emptying and the risk of aspiration are high in renal failure patients. If the succinylcholine is contraindicated due to hyperkalemia, then a quick acting nondepolarizing muscle relaxant that does not depend on the kidney for its clearance may be used. But, unfortunately, such an ideal agent is not available. Therefore, atracurium, cisatracurium, rocuronium, mivacurium, etc., are the better choices. The laryngoscopy should be brief because the prolonged apnea and hypoxia may lead to respiratory acidosis which may aggravate the existing hyperkalemia. After intubation, slight hyperventilation is preferred, because it can correct acidosis and subsequent hyperkalemia, if these are present.

Maintenance of Anesthesia

After induction and intubation, the general anesthesia is maintained by N_2O and volatile anesthetic agents. Among the volatile anesthetic agents, methoxyflurane and enflurane are contraindicated, and sevoflurane is best avoided in patients with impaired renal function, the cause of which is discussed before. Therefore, isoflurane and halothane are the agents of choice as volatile anesthetic agents in such patients. Opioids such as fentanyl, sufentanil, and remifentanil can be used safely in conjugation with volatile anesthetic agents. During the maintenance of anesthesia, slight hyperventilation is better, the reason of which has also been discussed earlier. On the other hand, excessive hyperventilation is not desirable which is more applicable in anemic patients only. This is because respiratory alkalosis, resulting from hyperventilation, may shift the O_2 dissociation curve toward left and thus affect the O_2 unloading in tissues.

During artificial mechanical ventilation, the intrathoracic pressure should be maintained at the optimum level by appropriately adjusting the respiratory rate, tidal volume, and inspiratory-to-expiratory (I:E) ratio. Otherwise, the increased intrathoracic pressure may decrease the cardiac output and further deteriorate the renal function by decreasing the perfusion in kidney. The intraoperative severe hypertension can be controlled by infusion of nitroglycerine and nitroprusside. Cyanide toxicity following prolonged infusion of nitroprusside is unlikely in patients suffering from renal failure. This is due to the decreased excretion of thiosulfate through kidney, which facilitates the conversion of cyanide to thiocyanate.

During the maintenance of general anesthesia, the intraoperative monitoring of renal function is important. This can be performed by measuring the urine output. Oliguria or anuria should be recognized promptly and treated immediately, which may thus avoid the development of acute renal failure. If there is any suspicion of intraoperative acute renal failure, then rapid infusion of 500 mL of normal saline as bolus and a small dose of frusemide (0.1–0.2 mg/kg), if intravascular volume is adequate, are effective. Still, if the urine output does not increase, then the intravascular volume status and cardiac output are monitored by invasive monitoring, such as CVP and pulmonary wedge arterial pressure (PWAP). Once the filling pressure is optimized by IV fluid and the urine output does not increase by frusemide, then dopamine in the dose of 1–2 µg/kg/min is used to increase the RBF and urine output. Sometimes, severe hypotension refractory to adequate intravascular volume repletion may occur in severe renal failure and dialysis patients, which is due to autonomic dysfunction. This is generally treated by increasing the dose of dopamine (5 µg/kg/min), which increases the cardiac function and RBF or by administering noradrenaline **(Flowchart 2)**.

Postoperative Care

The postoperative care of patients, suffering from renal dysfunction, is similar to that of other patients, except some special points. Hyper- or hypokalemia usually occurs

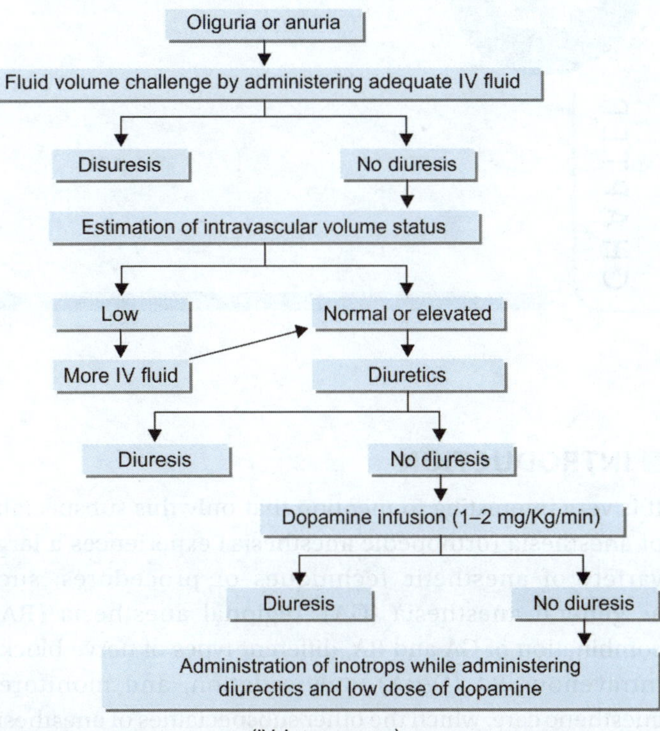

Flowchart 2: Management of oliguria in renal dysfunction.

during the first 24 hours of the postoperative period in renal failure patients, which depends on the severity of failure. So, the electrolytes level should be checked routinely in the recovery room and measures should be taken accordingly. Continuous ECG monitoring is essential for the detection of any conduction abnormalities in heart and arrhythmias, which is common due to electrolyte disturbances, during the first 24 hours of the postoperative period, in a renal dysfunction patient. Patient-controlled analgesia (PCA) using fentanyl is the best method of postoperative analgesia, for patients with impaired renal function. The regional analgesic technique is very helpful for postoperative analgesia, if the coagulation profile remains within the normal limit. If a patient with a history of impaired renal function shows skeletal muscular weakness, then the partial reversal of the action of muscle relaxant should be thought. So, the neuromuscular conduction should be monitored by nerve stimulator and, if necessary, the additional dose of anticholinesterase with an anticholinergic agent can be administered. The postoperative renal failure patient may suffer from hypertension or hypotension. Hence, the BP should be monitored closely and the recovery room sister should be informed, regarding the site of the AV fistula, used for dialysis, to avoid the inadvertent placement of BP cuff on the same extremity.

Orthopedic Anesthesia

■ INTRODUCTION

It is very interesting to mention that only this subspecialty of anesthesia (orthopedic anesthesia) experiences a large variety of anesthetic techniques or procedures, such as general anesthesia (GA), regional anesthesia (RA), combination of GA and RA, different types of nerve blocks, intravenous RA (IVRA), only sedation, and monitored anesthetic care, which the other subspecialties of anesthesia do not. Also, this orthopedic anesthesia encompasses a wide range of patients, extending from a child with congenital skeletal deformities requiring surgery and anesthesia to a young adult with multiple trauma or fractures due to accident or while playing to a very old person with multiorgan problems coming in with fractured neck, femur, etc.

The degree of surgical complexity also varies, from minor surgical manipulation of a joint that has limited mobility due to scars, fibrosis, adhesions, etc., to minor finger surgery, to major surgery such as joint replacement, to very major surgery such as hemipelvectomy. There is also huge advancement in orthopedic surgical techniques, which is gradually making it a lesser and lesser invasive procedure, and this is due to the development of computed tomography (CT) scan, magnetic resonance imaging (MRI), and computer and their guided surgery. This causes only overnight stays or the same-day discharge of the patient. Earlier, after surgery, they were kept admitted for many days. All these above-mentioned factors have great implications for anesthesia.

The other peculiarities of orthopedic surgeries that anesthetists have to face are (1) the different positions of the patient to facilitate surgery, which has many implications on the patients and subsequently on the anesthesia technique; (2) the use of tourniquet, which has many complications, though it also has many advantages; (3) the use of orthopedic cement and its many advantages and bad consequences; (4) the venous, fat, and air embolism, which are very common for orthopedic surgery; and (5) the amount of blood loss, which may vary from few drops to 2 L or more, and blood transfusion-related complications. So, different types of techniques are adapted to reduce this blood loss during major orthopedic surgery, such as induced hypotension, hemodilution, and cell saver technique, which have their own intrinsic complications and have to be tackled by an anesthetist.

It is also very interesting to note that some orthopedic surgeries are very simple and of short duration, while some are very long and complex in nature, requiring extensive monitoring, such as intraarterial pressure monitoring, central venous pressure (CVP) monitoring, and transe-sophageal echocardiography (TEE). Therefore, the rate of perioperative morbidity and mortality in orthopedic surgeries varies greatly and is different from other surgical disciplines.

Some patients seeking orthopedic surgery also have rheumatoid arthritis, ankylosing spondylitis, etc., affecting the cervical, thoracic, and lumbar spinal vertebrae along with the other bony joints of their body. These patients may also have instability of cervical spine or atlantoaxial joint, which can make airway management difficult **(Box 1)**. In rheumatoid arthritis, the damage of the atlantoaxial joint is due to the erosion of the ligaments around the odontoid process of C2 vertebra by rheumatoid involvement. So, an iatrogenic acute subluxation of this joint between C1 and C2 vertebrae may occur, by the flexion of the neck, during intubation, and it may result in cervical cord compression or sudden death. Hence, during anesthetic management

---

BOX 1: Causes of atlantoaxial instability.

- Down's syndrome
- Adult rheumatoid arthritis
- Juvenile rheumatoid arthritis
- Ankylosing spondylitis
- Fractured cervical spine
- Morquio disease (mucopolysaccharidosis)

of these types of patients, previous diagnosis of this type of ailment is essential, and all the precautions should be taken to prevent the flexion of neck and maintain the stability of cervical spine. Therefore, orthopedic anesthesia sometimes demands a high degree of skilled airway management facility, requiring fiberoptic laryngoscope, flexible bronchoscope, intubating laryngeal mask airway (LMA), and all other accessories to prevent the movement of cervical spine during intubation.

Ankylosing spondylitis is more common in men than in women, and it involves the ossification of ligaments of joints at their attachment to the bones. Progressive ankylosing spondylitis also involves the cartilages of joint and intervertebral disk, with the diminution of their spaces. Thus, the vertebral column gradually becomes fused, making lumbar epidural or spinal anesthesia difficult or impossible. Due to the ankylosing spondylosis, sometimes the positioning of the patient also becomes very painful and difficult while he/she is awake for central neuraxial block.

Similarly, when the patient is suffering from severe ankylosis of shoulder joint, then there is also a choice between the axillary and the interscalene routes of brachial plexus block for the RA of the upper extremity. The difficulty of positioning the patient or extremities may also arise from fractures, joint deformities, or unstable vertebrae, which influence the mode of anesthesia. Sometimes, it is very helpful to exercise the position preoperatively while the patient is awake.

Arthritis and ankylosis, affecting the temporomandibular joint, may also restrict the opening of mouth and may cause the visualization of larynx difficult. These diseases may also affect the cricoarytenoid joint and may leave the vocal cord with limited mobility and restricted glottic opening. Therefore, all these may produce difficulty during tracheal intubation. On the other hand, as both rheumatoid arthritis and ankylosis spondylitis are systemic diseases, they may also affect the different organs or systems of our body, other than bones and joints, causing different diseases. These are cardiac valvular lesions, ischemic heart disease (IHD), pericarditis, pulmonary interstitial fibrosis, etc. **(Table 1)**. However, these patients also have an impaired immune system, wasted musculature, and underlying hypermetabolic state, which will contribute to an increased rate of postoperative infections and other complications.

Many patients admitted for orthopedic surgeries have a history of corticosteroid therapy in the recent past. Therefore, it has become routine for many anesthetists to administer a large dose of glucocorticoids on the day of surgery, with the aim of avoiding the risk of acute adrenal insufficiency during the perioperative period. But many anesthetists oppose this view, and their arguments are as follows: (1) Acute adrenal

TABLE 1: Systemic manifestations of rheumatoid arthritis.

System	Manifestations
Cardiovascular system (CVS)	Pericardial effusion, conduction defects, myocarditis, valvular defects, coronary arteritis, etc.
Respiratory system	Interstitial pulmonary fibrosis, pleural effusion, etc.
Others	Anemia, thrombocytopenia, adrenal insufficiency, impaired immune system, etc.

insufficiency, causing unwanted hypotension, is rare and can be better treated after it occurs than taking prophylactic measures. (2) Preoperative large doses of corticosteroids may impair wound healing and immune function. Thus, it causes more harm to patients than good. (3) The previous history of steroid therapy does not always predict the occurrence of adrenocortical deficiency, and thus it is impossible to select the patient who should receive the prophylactic steroid therapy without prior testing of adrenal response. (4) The daily dose of corticosteroids is sufficient unless the severity of surgical stress warrants larger doses.

SOME SPECIFIC PROBLEMS RELATED TO ORTHOPEDIC SURGERIES AND ANESTHESIA

As discussed previously, orthopedic surgeries have some specific problems that are not found in other subspecialties of surgical discipline. So, anesthetists have to face these problems, only or more frequently, during orthopedic anesthesia. These problems specific to orthopedic surgery and anesthesia are tourniquet, bone cement, embolism, deep vein thrombosis (DVT), blood loss, position of the patient, etc.

Tourniquet (Pneumatic or Elastic)

Tourniquet is frequently used in orthopedic surgeries, around the upper and lower extremities, to reduce or eliminate intraoperative blood loss and to provide a clear surgical field. Though it is very useful, it is not completely devoid of problems (complications) because it produces many changes in body such as hemodynamic changes, metabolic alterations, embolic manifestations [arterial thromboembolism and pulmonary embolism (PE)], pain, and neurological damage (permanent peripheral nerve damage), which are detrimental to patients. When the tourniquet is applied and inflated above systolic pressure to get a bloodless, dry surgical field, then the distal tissue is cut off from its oxygen (O_2) supply. So, within 8–10 minutes of the application of tourniquet, the partial pressure of O_2 in the mitochondria of the cells of ischemic tissue falls to zero, and anaerobic metabolism begins. Thus, the number of stored nicotinamide adenine dinucleotide (NAD) and creatine phosphate in the cells of ischemic tissues decreases and is completely depleted within 60 minutes. Hence, the pH of tissues, distal to tourniquet rapidly falls to <6. Thereafter, due to the prolonged application of tourniquet, the developed cellular hypoxia and acidosis will cause the release of myoglobin from muscle tissue (rhabdomyolysis) and the release of intracellular enzymes and K^+ from the tissue cells into circulation (hyperkalemia). Subsequently, the endothelial integrity of blood vessels is also lost. This is due to the release of thromboxane, and tissue edema supervenes. Gradually, after that, the ischemic portion of extremities becomes cool and approaches room temperature.

The application of tourniquet is also associated with some hemodynamic changes in the body. This is due to the exsanguination of limb before the application and inflation of tourniquet, which causes a sudden shift of a large volume of blood from the peripheral compartment into the central compartment. But, usually, in a healthy adult patient, this sudden shifting of the huge amount of blood from the peripheral to the central compartment does not produce any significant hemodynamic effect, except for a small increase in CVP and arterial pressure. However, patients with poor ventricular compliance and diastolic dysfunction and with extensive varicose veins, where the tourniquet is applied over these limbs, may experience a considerable increase in pulmonary and systemic artery pressure.

Also, the bilateral application of tourniquet at a time and the exsanguination of both the limbs before its application may cause the shift of the huge amount of blood, resulting in a higher rise of CVP and systemic blood pressure (BP). This may not sometimes be tolerated in healthy patients, causing congestive cardiac failure. For the proper function of a tourniquet, the inflation pressure within it should be raised to about 50–100 mm Hg above the present mean arterial BP. This is needed to block arterial flow. Then, the BP of a patient may increase after surgical incision or due to any cause during the intraoperative period. Therefore, the BP measured during the preinduction period of the patient is not always a reliable guide to set the pressure of tourniquet during the intraoperative period. Hence, the tourniquet inflating pressure should be changed according to the intraoperative BP of the patient. The time of application of tourniquet and the periodic pressure within it should be noted on the anesthetic record. Like all other medical devices, the pneumatic tourniquet also requires regular preoperative periodic checkup and calibration.

For the proper functioning of a tourniquet, the width of the cuff (tourniquet) should be more than half the diameter of limb because it will improve the transmission of cuff pressure to deeper tissues and occlude the artery better. For the good functioning of tourniquet, it should also be placed over a smoothly applied cotton padding around the limb. This will prevent the damage of the underlying skin caused by a tourniquet. It will have to be kept in mind that the antiseptic solution, used to prepare the skin of surgical site, should not spread under the tourniquet. Otherwise, it may cause chemical burns to the skin underlying the tourniquet.

Within 30 minutes of inflating the tourniquet, the conduction of impulses through nerves (afferent and efferent) also ceases, which may also contribute to anesthesia at the surgical site, other than the action of anesthetic agents on the central nervous system (CNS). Due to tourniquet, as the extremity is isolated from central circulation and becomes cool, so it (tourniquet) also reduces the sensation of extremity. The neurological and vascular problems arise when the tourniquet is inflated for a prolonged period (>2 hours) or when excessive inflation pressure is applied.

After the speculated time (still even if the surgery is not completed) or when the surgery is over (before the speculated time), the tourniquet is deflated, and the ischemic limb is again reperfused from itself, resulting in reduction of CVP and arterial BP. Sometimes, this reduction of systemic BP becomes excessive and may result in cardiac arrest. The other contributing factors for this cardiac arrest, associated with the tourniquet, may be due to the excessive loss of blood from the surgical site or the circulatory effects of metabolites (e.g., thromboxane) from the ischemic limb after the deflation of the tourniquet. The washout of accumulated metabolic wastes from the ischemic limb into general circulation also increases partial pressure of carbon dioxide in the arterial blood ($PaCO_2$), end-tidal carbon dioxide ($ETCO_2$), serum lactate, and serum K^+ levels. These metabolites can increase minute ventilation in a spontaneously ventilated patient. Tourniquet-induced ischemia of the lower extremity may lead to the development of DVT. TEE can detect subclinical PE (miliary emboli in the right atrium and right ventricle), following tourniquet deflation, even in minor cases such as diagnostic knee arthroscopy.

Some patients, after receiving spinal, epidural, or IVRA or brachial plexus block, feel pain at the site of the application of tourniquet before the effect of anesthesia recedes from the site of tourniquet, where it is applied (tested by pinprick). This pain occurs inconsistently during the intraoperative period and occurs at intervals. Similarly, some patients undergoing GA also feel pain after the inflation of the tourniquet. This *special tourniquet pain* is reflected by the sudden unexplained intraoperative hypertension after 1 hour of the application of tourniquet. The mechanism of this tourniquet pain is not exactly known. Still, the probable explanation is that is the unmyelinated, slow-conducting fine sympathetic

C nerve fibers which are relatively resistant to local anesthetic (LA) agents and carry this pain sensation. However, this is an explanation only for RA. The explanation for this tourniquet pain in GA is given below. But this argument for tourniquet pain in lower limbs during RA is sometimes contradicted by the observation that he tourniquet pain from the lower extremity is still experienced despite the blockade up to the level of T4 spinal segment, and stellate ganglion block also cannot ameliorate this pain in the upper extremity.

The management of intraoperative hypertension, due to this pain from tourniquet (tourniquet pain) during GA, is very difficult. This is because attempts to relieve this pain with IV narcotics and increasing the dose of inhaled anesthetics are not always successful. This pain can only be relieved by deflating the tourniquet for 10–15 minutes and then reinflating it again. Thus, this correlates well with the relief of pain with the correction of cellular acidosis and also explains another mechanism of this *tourniquet pain* in GA. The uncontrolled intraoperative hypertension, due to tourniquet pain, which cannot be managed by increasing the dose of narcotics and inhaled anesthetics, can usually be managed by vasodilator agents such as IV nitroprusside, nitroglycerine, or nifedipine. This tourniquet pain, under spinal or epidural anesthesia, sometimes becomes so severe that the patient may need supplemental analgesia or light GA, despite the regional block being adequate for surgical incision.

Now, after multiple studies, it is also observed that the tourniquet pain is mainly related to the quality or intensity of neural block rather than the level of block. This is confirmed by the observation that tourniquet pain can also be relieved during continuous regional block by: (1) increasing the density of block, (2) increasing the concentration of LA agent, (3) adding some opioids to LA agent, or (4) adding bicarbonate to LA agent, which increases the fraction of the drug present as free base. It is also found that hypobaric and isobaric spinal techniques result in a lower incidence of tourniquet pain than the hyperbaric technique, even when the drugs, their doses, and their blocking dermatome levels are same.

Bone (methacrylate) Cement

Chemically, bone cement is a complex *polymethyl-methacrylate* compound and is frequently used in joint arthroplasty. It acts only by making strong binding between the metallic prosthetic device and the cancellous or the medullary part of the patient's bone (bone cement interdigitates within the interstices of bone and strongly binds the prosthetic device with the patient's bone). It also acts as a space filler and improves the fitting of the implanted

prosthetic device into the marrow cavity of the bone. However, the quality of interface between the cement and the bone will improve if there is no layer of blood covering the bone surface when the cement is applied. So, some anesthetists use hypotensive anesthesia during the use of cement. But it (hypotensive anesthesia) has some disadvantages that are described below and are not routinely used.

The mixing of solid methyl-methacrylate polymer powder with the liquid methyl-methacrylate monomer causes the polymerization and crosslinking of polymer chain and produces this polymethyl-methacrylate compound, which is known as bone cement. This is an exothermic reaction and leads to the hardening and the expansion of cement substance. During the preparation and hardening of this bone cement, a strong pungent vapor is given off, which produces some air pollution in an operating theater. This exothermic reaction may also cause some risk of thermal injury to the patient's tissues.

The major concern regarding the use of bone cement during joint arthroplasty is the pulmonary and cardiovascular responses of a patient to this bone cement. These cardiopulmonary responses of a patient are (1) increased pulmonary vascular resistance (PVR), (2) development of pulmonary hypertension, (3) reduced cardiac output, (4) hypotension, (5) cardiac arrhythmias, and (6) even cardiac arrest. These cardiovascular responses of a patient, during the use of bone cement, may be due to the indirect and/or direct effect of cement. However, the indirect effect is more important than the direct effect of cement. The indirect effect of cement is due to the embolization of bone marrow into the right side of the heart, and the direct effect of bone cement is due to the toxic effect of the cement itself. In the indirect effect, as the cement improves the fitting between the prosthetic device and the walls of the marrow cavity, it increases the intramedullary pressure (>500 mm Hg). This is because, during the curing of cement in the marrow cavity, it expands in volume. Thus, it forces out the remaining bone marrow contents, fat, cement, and air into the bloodstream (venous channels) and produces the catastrophic PE of bone marrow, fat, cement, and air with the above-mentioned complications.

It is proved by TEE, which shows the continuous raining of echogenic substances (pieces of bone marrow) in the right side of the heart, after the application of cement. Sometimes, a few large emboli may be observed in the right side of the heart, completely obstructing the right ventricular outflow tract and leading to (1) acute right-sided heart failure, (2) reduced cardiac output, (3) hypotension, and (4) cardiac arrest. The small emboli of bone marrow traverse the right ventricle and embolize into the lung. These may increase pulmonary artery pressure and intrapulmonary shunt. In patients with patent foramen ovale, these emboli may pass into the systemic circulation through this foramen ovale and cause systemic embolic manifestations, such as infarction and stroke.

This is also proved by the fact that the insertion of the stem of femoral prosthesis into the marrow cavity of femur increases the intramedullary pressure >1 atmospheric pressure and produces more entry of medullary contents into the bloodstream than the only act of cementing of acetabular prosthesis, which is shown by echocardiography. It is also found that the emboli during the prosthesis of hip are larger in size than the other joint arthroplasties, such as knee. In patients undergoing total knee replacement surgery, this reaction is not observed until the tourniquet is deflated, which also proves the above explanation. However, this entry of bone marrow contents into the circulation is not so severe during other orthopedic surgeries using bone cement, such as surgeries on the proximal humerus. Also, these reactions are not as common or as severe in prostheses where the cement is not used. This increase in intramedullary pressure by bone cement not only causes the embolization of bone marrow contents but also causes the embolization of fat and air into the femoral venous channels.

The direct toxic effect of bone cement on the cardio-vascular system (CVS) of the patient is due to the direct vasodilating and decreased systemic vascular resistance ($\downarrow$BP) effect of the monomer component of bone cement. It also releases thromboplastin, which triggers the aggregation of platelet. It also helps in the formation of micro thrombus in the lungs. Thus, it causes cardiovascular instability. *Nevertheless, most patients experience no adverse response to the application of bone cement.*

Therefore, the clinical symptoms (manifestations) of bone cement implantation are due to its indirect embolic effect on the lungs and direct toxic effect on CVS, all of which include pulmonary hypertension, hypoxia, hypotension, decreased cardiac output, cardiac arrhythmias, and even cardiac arrest. As most of the incidences of hypotension, after the use of cement, usually result from impaired left ventricular filling, due to PE and increased PVR, the previous existing hypovolemia will further impair the left ventricular filling and aggravate the hypotension, leading to cardiac arrest. Hence, the management of the cardiovascular responses of bone cement includes (1) increasing fraction of inspired oxygen (FiO_2), (2) maintaining euvolemia before the use of cement, (3) continuous monitoring of BP, and (4) the use of vasopressors if necessary.

The other measures which can also prevent the cardiovascular responses to bone cement during the joint arthroplasty are: (1) using of a plug previously into the marrow cavity of the femoral shaft that will limit the distal spread of cement into the femur, (2) waiting for the cement to become more viscous before its insertion, (3) making a vent hole in distal femur that will decrease the intramedullary pressure, (4) employing the vacuum drainage of marrow substances from the proximal femur during riming, (5) performing high-pressure lavage into the distal femoral shaft that will remove the debris, or (6) adopting some other procedures where cement is not necessary.

Another major drawback of the use of bone cement during arthroplastic surgery is the delayed gradual loosening of prosthesis, and it is due to the breakage of cement into small pieces over the years in the marrow cavity. In cement-less arthroplastic surgeries, the natural bone grows slowly and fits the implants tightly. So, cementless arthroplasty lasts longer and is advantageous for the younger and active group of patients, where healthy, active bone will be formed although the full recovery is slow and prolonged. Therefore, bone cement is preferred for arthroplastic surgery where the chance of active healthy bone formation is less, such as in older (>80 years) and less active patients who are suffering from osteoporosis or other diseases. Hence, the use of bone cement depends on the patient's status, surgical technique, and the type of joint to be replaced. In modern practice, the articular surface is made up of plastic, ceramic, or metal.

Fat Embolism

Fat embolism means the appearance of fat globules in the bloodstream. Some degree of fat embolism probably occurs with all long bone fractures. This incidence of fat embolism is as high as 90% for the victims of major trauma. But, the majority of cases remains subclinical and are only detected by active investigations of serum or urine for the evidence of macroscopic fat globules. However, an association between the age and the incidence of fat embolism may be seen. Its incidence is low in very young group of patients and much higher in very old subjects. When fat embolism is manifested clinically, then it is known as fat embolic syndrome (FES). However, the actual incidence of FES is rare (1–2%), but it is fatal with a high mortality rate (10–20%) when it occurs. It classically presents as a *triad* of pulmonary symptoms (dyspnea), CNS symptoms (confusions), and cutaneous symptoms (petechial hemorrhage), such as dyspnea, confusion, and cutaneous petechiae. But the clinical diagnosis of FES is based on its major or minor criteria, as described in **Table 2**. It usually appears within 72 hours, following a major orthopedic surgery or trauma. This syndrome can also be seen, following cardiopulmonary resuscitation (CPR), parenteral feeding with lipid infusion,

TABLE 2: Diagnostic criteria of fat embolism.

Major criteria	Minor criteria
PaO_2 <60 mm Hg	Tachycardia (HR >120/m)
↑ PVR	Fat in urine
↑ Pulmonary artery pressure	Fat in sputum
Pulmonary edema	Emboli in fundoscopic examination
Petechial hemorrhage	Thrombocytopenia

(HR: heart rate; PaO_2: partial pressure of oxygen; PVR: pulmonary vascular resistance)

and liposuction. A full-blown FES has cutaneous, CNS, pulmonary, and hemodynamic manifestations, with less clinical effects on the other organs, depending on the site of embolic events.

Till now, two theories have been advanced for the pathogenesis of fat embolism. Among them, the most widely accepted theory for the etiology of fat embolism is mechanical tissue trauma, which forces out the fat globules (released by the disruption of fat cells) into the circulation through some tears in medullary vessels. This is proved by the fact that malignancy of long bones causes higher incidences of fat or marrow embolism. This is because the enlarged venous sinuses, caused by the malignant tumor, permit greater access of fat globules into the circulation. Another alternative theory for this fat embolism is that the circulating fat globules in vessels result from the aggregation of increased circulating free fatty acid (FFA) molecules. This is due to changes in the metabolism of FFA following trauma or surgery.

Regardless of these theories and the sources of fat globules (thrombus) in circulation, the *clinical manifestation of fat embolism*, which is known as FES, is due to the result of the deposition of these fat particles in different organs as well as due to the activation of some enzymes (particularly lipase) that leads to (1) capillary damage, (2) endothelial leakage, and (3) the release of many vasoactive substances, such as prostaglandins and vasoactive amines. Ultimately, all these lead to cutaneous manifestations (petechial hemorrhage, mainly over the neck, back, chest, and trunk), pulmonary manifestations [acute respiratory distress syndrome (ARDS)], CNS manifestations (confusion, agitation, stupor, coma, etc., and these CNS manifestations are due to capillary damage of cerebral circulation and cerebral edema), CVS manifestations (due to pulmonary manifestation caused by fat embolus in pulmonary vasculature), ophthalmic manifestations (retinal exudate due to capillary leakage which is seen by fundoscopic examination as cotton wool), etc. It must also be considered that for the systemic

manifestations of fat embolism, there must be a patent foramen ovale or intrapulmonary shunt that bypasses the pulmonary filtration system and contributes to the passage of fat globules directly into the systemic circulation from venous circulation.

The first step for the diagnosis of early FES needs a suspicious mind of high index. So, during anesthesia for patients with higher risk and increased chances of FES, attention should be focused on the early signs and symptoms of FES and on the alterations of normal physiology that indicate that the fat embolism is occurring. The signs of pulmonary fat embolism during GA include ↓$ETCO_2$, ↑$PaCO_2$, ↑pulmonary arterial pressure, ↓cardiac output, hypotension, etc., which are like the PE of bone marrow substance, during the use of bone cement in arthroplasty. For the diagnosis of cutaneous involvement of FES, petechial hemorrhage on the chest, upper extremities, axillae, and conjunctiva can be obvious. It can further be confirmed by retinal fundoscopic examination if cotton wool exudates are found. The clinical diagnosis of pulmonary involvement of FES may range from mild hypoxia with normal chest findings to moderate hypoxia with wheezing, crepitation, secretion, etc., to a full-blown picture of ARDS. The diagnosis of cardiovascular involvement of FES depends on the stage of its evolution. An early CVS finding, when an early FES is evolving, is only nonspecific tachycardia and right heart electrocardiogram (ECG) changes, which may later progress to severe hypotension, cyanosis, and left ventricular failure. Later, disseminated intravascular coagulation (DIC) can result. Fat embolism to any specific part of the brain can cause seizure activity and predict serious FES. Coma can evolve from ischemia, hypoxia, and embolism in any key area of brain stem.

There is no specific laboratory test which absolutely confirms the diagnosis of FES. Serum lipase activity may be elevated in the majority of FES cases, but it bears no relationship to the severity of disease process. A large number of cases of fat embolism will be detected by the presence of fat globules in their sputum, serum, or urine. But this test is too sensitive to be used as an indicator of serious FES. Different coagulation abnormalities, as a part of DIC, may be present in FES. There is general agreement that an unexplained low PaO_2 (<60 mm Hg), which is not linked to other pathology, is highly suggestive of FES. Patients with (A-a) O_2 tension gradients > 100 mm Hg represent a high probability of severe FES. It is also reported that bronchial lavage has both diagnostic and therapeutic values in FES.

The first step in the treatment of clinically manifested fat embolism (FES) is to minimize the factors which contribute to this process, such as decreased manipulation of fractures, decreased reaming of the medullary canal, and early immobilization of fractured long bones (early stabilization of fractures decreases the likelihood of fat embolism). The second step in the treatment for this disease process is supportive, which is designed to decrease the impact of changes due to fat emboli. This includes support to pulmonary system and CVS, as necessary. The support to the pulmonary system will be the key factor for the survival of a patient with severe FES. The principal objective of this pulmonary support is adequate oxygenation to tissues, particularly the CVS, CNS, and other end organs. This is accomplished by maintaining optimum cardiac output and adjusting ventilation to achieve best possible O_2 delivery to the tissues, with the lowest possible FiO_2 to avoid the injury to the pulmonary parenchyma from high FiO_2 for a prolonged period (O_2 toxicity). This mandates the optimum positive end-expiratory pressure (PEEP) and the best mode for mechanical ventilation required for this patient.

The defects in the coagulation system must be treated based on the accurate assessment of the step of defects. For example, thrombocytopenia is treated by platelets. The decreased labile clotting factor or factor V (this factor is necessary for the conversion of prothrombin into thrombin and is used up during clotting) is managed by fresh frozen plasma. The decreased fibrin level is maintained by pooled cryoprecipitate. The clinical situation where the laboratory results have long return intervals can also be managed by thromboelastogram (TEG) and Sonoclot (SC) devices, which can provide accurate information and direct therapy. As the pathology of FES mainly involves the inflammatory reaction in the lungs and other tissues, it is rational to use high doses of steroids for their profound anti-inflammatory property and to decrease the release of tissue-activating factors from cellular injury (vasoactive substances). But the role of corticosteroid in high doses for the management of FES is not supported by any randomized clinical trials. Previously, for the management of FES, ethyl alcohol was used with an aim to decrease the activity of lipase. But now its use has been abandoned as it had no effect. Similarly, dextran and heparin were used previously to consolidate the fat, but recently, these treatments have also been found to be ineffective and abandoned. Further, they may contribute to the instability of the coagulation system.

Deep Vein Thrombosis

Pulmonary embolism, originating from the clots of the deep venous system by the process of thrombosis (DVT), may be the leading cause of morbidity and mortality following major trauma or orthopedic surgeries on pelvis and lower extremities. The incidences of DVT are usually determined by a number of factors. These are advanced age (>60 years),

prolonged bed rest or immobility, obesity, use of pneumatic tourniquet, prolonged surgery (>30 minutes), surgery on pelvis or lower extremities, prior history of DVT or PE, malignancy, etc. Decreased fibrinolysis or the release of plasminogen activating factors, secondary to the inflated tourniquet, is also a cause of tourniquet-related DVT.

The risk of both DVT and subsequently its embolism from the immobilization of the patient increases with the duration of this immobilization. The risk of both DVT and embolism from the upper extremity is very uncommon and is only related to trauma, but not surgeries. The use of oral contraceptive pills among young woman patients also doubles the normal low incidence rate of DVT. The incidences of DVT in the lower extremity following orthopedic surgery, using tourniquet and without any prophylactic measures, vary between 40 and 60%. This is demonstrated by a venogram. These incidences are more higher in pelvic fractures, and this is due to the direct trauma of pelvic venous structures whereas the incidence of clinically significant PE following hip surgery is only 20–30%, among which only 1–2% becomes fatal. Although the clinical detection of DVT most often occurs between the third and the fifth day of surgery, many clots are present in the subclinical stage from earlier. This can only be detected by radiolabeled fibrinogen immediately after the surgical procedure. The likely major pathophysiological mechanism of DVT includes venous stasis and decreased fibrinolytic activity, leading to a hypercoagulating state, which is further influenced by hormone related to pain or surgical stress. These facts comprise the triad of DVT, which includes (1) the changes in the constitution of blood, (2) the change in the vessel wall, and (3) the change in the flow of blood. Therefore, the prophylaxis of DVT acts at any of these steps.

Like fat embolism, the diagnosis of DVT is also triggered by a high index of suspicion among patients in high-risk groups. The first step in the diagnosis of DVT is clinical examination. Unfortunately, the diagnosis of DVT by clinical examination alone may frequently overlook the presence of thrombosis, which is sufficient to cause embolization and morbidity. So, other more accurate methods for the diagnosis of DVT have gradually evolved. *The gold standard for the diagnosis of DVT is a contrast venogram.* This is only performed by the cannulation of the distal vein in the involved limb and then the injection of contrast dye into that cannulated vein to get the radiological picture of that venous system. A contrast venogram has a very high detection and very low false-negative rate.

But its invasive nature, high cost, patient's discomfort, difficulty during cannulation, and sometimes the chance of contrast media to cause thromboembolic disease itself lead to the search for ultrasound techniques for the diagnosis of DVT. The ultrasound technique diagnoses the presence of thrombi noninvasively by detecting the altered flow of blood in the venous system. Unfortunately, however, in an ultrasound technique, the false-negative rate is very high. This is because of the absence of a preoperative baseline study to compare with this postoperative picture and if the study is not performed by the same specialist pre- and postoperatively, and also especially if the patient is obese.

Next, the radioactive fibrinogen study for the diagnosis of DVT also has high false-negative and false-positive rates. Another technique for this diagnosis of DVT, such as impedance plethysmography, also has a high detection but a low false-negative rate. But technically, it is not very simple for clinical application. Therefore, in specialized centers performing major orthopedic surgeries and when the suspicion is very high, the combined approach of clinical examination, ultrasonography, and venography is usually performed.

The prophylaxis for DVT is certainly more appealing than the treatment of it and its sequelae, such as PE, cerebral embolism, and coronary embolism. This is because the institution of postoperative therapy in an established case of DVT with full doses of heparin may increase bleeding at the surgical site and, therefore, morbidity by the formation of hematoma at the operative site and in the spinal or epidural space. The treatment of an established case of DVT also increases the chances of postoperative infection, the length of hospitalization, the cost, etc. Therefore, the prophylaxis for DVT has immense importance than its treatment. The prophylaxis of DVT is performed by interfering with the steps that lead to thromboembolic manifestation. These include physical measures, antithrombotic drugs, and some modifications of surgical and anesthetic techniques.

Among the physical measures, the compressive elastic stocking or the intermittent compressive pneumatic stocking is most effective. This is because they more readily simulate normal muscular contraction, which helps in venous pumping from lower extremities. These should be applied prior to surgical preparation and also during the surgical procedure. The old electrical stimulation and the contraction of calf muscles for the prophylaxis of DVT have proved to be no more effective than simple intermittent compression of calf muscles. In the postoperative period, the most effective prophylactic physical measure for DVT is the as early as possible ambulation after orthopedic surgery.

Many antithrombotic drugs that interact with the coagulation cascade have been used for the prophylaxis of DVT. These drugs are various concentrations of high molecular weight dextran, antiplatelet agents, aspirin, coumarin, heparin, and recently low-molecular-weight heparin (LMWH). The dextran acts by decreasing the activity of platelets and interfering with the deposition of fibrin. Despite its initial enthusiastic report, dextran is now used very rarely for the prevention of DVT and not at all for its treatment. The aspirin acts by preventing the adhesion of platelets at the injured site of the vessel wall. It is given orally or rectally. It is not so effective in preventing the formation of thrombus because the concentration of aspirin necessary to achieve the antiplatelet activity for antithrombotic effect increases the intraoperative blood loss and causes a higher incidence of wound hematoma formation postoperatively. However, among the antiplatelet agents, only dipyridamole is used as prophylaxis for DVT. It acts in the same way as aspirin or other prostaglandin synthetase inhibitor and has the same disadvantage as aspirin, which is discussed above.

Coumarin (warfarin) is the most commonly used drug for the prophylaxis of DVT in high-risk patients. It is usually used in the evening following surgery or the next morning. The therapeutic endpoint of the administration of coumarin (warfarin) is increasing the prothrombin time (PT) by 50% over its control value. The use of coumarin preoperatively is now abandoned because it also increases intraoperative bleeding. When DVT occurs in spite of the use of coumarin, then heparin is started as an acute course. Later, coumarin is reinstated for maintenance.

The heparin acts by activating plasma antithrombin III. At low concentrations of heparin, the factor Xa-mediated conversion of prothrombin to thrombin is selectively affected (antithrombin activity). The anticoagulant action of heparin is exerted mainly by the inhibition of factor Xa as well as by the inhibition of thrombin (IIa)-mediated conversion of fibrinogen to fibrin. For the treatment of DVT or pulmonary and systemic embolism, such as cerebral embolism and coronary embolism, the full anticoagulating dose of heparin is used. But this is too dangerous for the prophylaxis of DVT. This is because of the fear of excessive bleeding, formation of hematoma, and other hemorrhagic events, elsewhere in the body. So, the idea of a low dose of heparin has evolved. It is administered in the dose of 5,000 units, every 8 hourly, through the subcutaneous route, which only interferes with the formation of a clot at the site of the injured vessel. In the majority of cases, the PT or activated partial thromboplastin time (aPTT) is not prolonged. But as the result is not absolutely guaranteed, it may raise a concern in spinal and epidural blocks, and most of the anesthetists feel that the evaluation of PT/aPTT is mandatory prior to performing any central neuraxial block, even in a patient receiving low doses of subcutaneous heparin as prophylaxis.

Refined heparin preparations, containing only the smaller molecules of it, which is called LMWH, have less effect on the function of platelets than the standard heparin. So, they have the same antithrombotic activity but have less direct effect on the coagulation activity, providing effective DVT prophylaxis with a decreased risk of postoperative bleeding and hematoma formation. The PT or aPTT is also not prolonged by LMWH. Therefore, unless the patients present any exceptionally high risk that demands anticoagulant treatment preoperatively, then all these anticoagulants should be started a few hours after surgery only to prevent excessive intraoperative surgical bleeding and prophylaxis of DVT.

Though it is generally agreed that preoperative full anticoagulation or fibrinolytic therapy provides an unacceptable high risk for spinal or epidural hematoma formation following RA, there is still some controversy regarding the danger of patients who receive the low dose of anticoagulation preparation as prophylaxis preoperatively and undergo RA—spinal or epidural. However, it is agreed that the placement of the spinal or epidural needle or catheter should generally not be undertaken within 8–10 hours after the administration of the last dose of unfractionated heparin through the subcutaneous route or within 12–24 hours of LMWH. The concomitant use of the antiplatelet agent with heparin may further increase the risk for spinal or epidural hematoma formation. It is also interesting to mention that RA with continuous postoperative analgesia can mask the signs and symptoms of an expanding hematoma, resulting in cord compression (back pain, muscular weakness, etc.) and thus delaying the diagnosis and treatment.

It is an established fact that there are less incidences of DVT among patients undergoing orthopedic surgeries of the pelvis or lower extremities under spinal or epidural anesthesia compared to GA. There is also more reduction in the incidences of DVT when the regional anesthetic technique is extended postoperatively as a continuous epidural infusion for postoperative analgesia. However, the method of detecting DVT must be the same, with either venogram or radio-labeled fibrinogen uptake. The probable theories about this decrease in the thromboembolic manifestation associated with RA are that it improves blood flow in microcirculation due to the effect of sympathectomy, as venous stasis is a known cause of DVT.

Another probable theory is that the pain or stress response inhibits fibrinolysis activity, and thus, RA, by relieving pain, is associated with an increase in fibrinolytic activity and a reduction in the incidences of DVT. Some works have also established that there is an increase in DVT when blood loss is higher. Therefore, as RA is known to decrease blood loss, it also causes a decrease in the incidences of DVT.

Blood Loss

The major orthopedic surgeries are associated with a significant amount of blood loss. But the blood loss during orthopedic surgeries is somewhat different from blood loss in other specialties of surgery. This is because in a major orthopedic surgery, a large amount of blood is lost from the raw surfaces of bones and muscles. This limits the surgeon's ability to control it directly and allows much of the shed blood to escape the method of retrieval by the suction catheter and gauze sponges, and it also continues after the closure of surgical wound. It is also proved by radioisotope studies that the actual amount of blood loss in major orthopedic surgeries is 50% higher than the amount which is estimated clinically. Thus, surgeons and anesthetists always underestimate blood loss during major orthopedic surgeries.

There are also many factors that increase the loss of blood during orthopedic surgeries. These are (1) previous surgeries, (2) large area of raw bones, (3) proximal site of operation where a tourniquet cannot be applied, (4) presence of infection at the operative site, (5) previous radiation at the operative site, (6) surgeon's technique, etc. The reduction of blood loss during orthopedic surgeries has many benefits to the patients. It reduces the exposure of the patient to donated blood (homologous banked blood) and the transmission of fatal viral diseases, such as hepatitis and human immunodeficiency virus (HIV), as well as protozoal diseases, such as malaria and syphilis. The use of donated blood may have other harmful effects, which can also be reduced by decreasing blood loss. The intraoperative decrease in blood loss also causes a reduction in postoperative infections, improved surgical results, better binding of cement to the bone, etc.

There are different methods by which the intraoperative blood loss and/or the donation of homologous banked blood during the orthopedic surgeries can be reduced. These may begin with the use of a tourniquet, preservation of normothermia, intraoperative hemodilution, etc., and end with the predonation of autologous blood, induced hypotension, conduction anesthesia, use of cell saver, progressive use of erythropoietin, use of an antifibrinolytic agent, etc. In practice, the combination of several of these modalities is most effective in reducing the blood loss and subsequently reducing the incidence of homologous blood transfusion. Cell savers are expensive and have certain risks. So, they are used selectively in the operating room for major orthopedic and spinal surgery.

Antifibrinolytic drugs, such as tranexamic acid and aprotinin, and postoperative cell salvage are probably best used when the expected blood loss exceeds 2 L. But it is warranted in a minor procedure due to the risks of aprotinin. It acts by inhibiting the fibrinolytic pathway and intrinsic coagulation pathway by decreasing the activation of plasminogen. Thus, it reduces intraoperative blood loss. However, it is usually reserved for high-risk cases (coagulopathies), revision arthroplasty, or bilateral hip arthroplasty. This is because it has a high propensity to produce immunological sensitization. However, the use of aprotinin does not increase the incidence of DVT or PE.

A pneumatic tourniquet, placed proximal to the site of surgery on extremities and inflated to occlude arterial blood flow at the operative site, eliminates intraoperative blood loss. But significant loss of blood will occur postoperatively when the tourniquet is removed. So, some surgeons routinely deflate or remove the tourniquet before closing the wound to control postoperative bleeding. Another method for this reduction of intraoperative blood loss is to avoid hypothermia. This is based on the finding that mild hypothermia (35°C) is associated with an average increase of 500 mL of blood loss during a single total hip arthroplasty.

Hemodilution and the maintenance of normal blood volume, with the normal BP, of a patient undergoing orthopedic surgery, by administering the cell-free fluids such as saline, starch solution, and albumin solution, etc., is also a common method of managing blood loss (not to reduce blood loss) and reducing the use of banked blood (homologous transfusions). When the patient's hemoglobin concentration falls between 6 and 7 g/dL, the anesthesiologists must determine whether the risk to the patient, due to inadequate oxygenation caused by anemia (due to blood loss), will justify the transfusion of blood on not.

The transfusion of banked (homologous) blood can be replaced by the more safer autologous blood transfusion. This can be arranged by collecting the blood from the surgical field or that donated by the patient and preserving it preoperatively. This autologous transfusion of blood will remove the adverse effects of homologous transfusion for which the intraoperative reduction of blood loss is attempted. Recently, much attention has been directed at the use of synthetic erythropoietin factor to increase the red cell mass of patients preoperatively. It is used in the dose of 600 IU/kg subcutaneously, weekly beginning 3 weeks before surgery. It increases the red cell mass by enhancing its production of it, by stimulating the division and maturation of megaloblasts in the bone marrow. Therefore, it increases the number of collected autologous blood units and reduces the amount of homologous blood transfusion.

During orthopedic surgeries, under RA or GA, the intraoperative loss of blood from the raw oozing surfaces of bones and muscles can also be reduced by induced hypotension. This can be achieved by high spinal or epidural anesthesia or by using sodium nitroprusside and nitroglycerine during GA, and maintaining the BP at a lower level, such as mean arterial pressure (MAP) at 60–70 mm Hg. But many patients scheduled for orthopedic surgeries are old

enough and may present relative contraindications to this type of hypotensive anesthesia. High RA increases a patient's discomfort, which can be ameliorated by combining it with GA. So, it is now suggested that the combination of high-level spinal or epidural anesthesia with GA is safer and may be applied as a method of choice for reducing the loss of blood during orthopedic surgeries.

Positioning of Patient

For different orthopedic surgeries, different positions of the patient are needed. Further, these different positioning of patients places them at a risk of varieties of injuries, but mostly the nerves get injured by compression. Therefore, an anesthetist must be aware of it and try to prevent their occurrences. This does not occur in an awake patient because an awake patient will not tolerate this compressive nerve injury for a long time, as the pain and restlessness caused by the ischemia of nerve will trigger the patient to correct his position spontaneously. But in a sedated or an anesthetized patient, this is not possible. So, different nerves and other structures, such as blood vessels, skin, and muscles, become liable to injury during anesthesia. If a patient incurs a nerve injury during anesthesia and surgery, then the anesthetist will be held responsible for it, whether this injury is related to the position, the surgery itself, or other causes.

The principal cause of brachial plexus injury under GA is stretching **(Fig. 1)**. This is due to (1) the hypermobility of the upper extremity, (2) the long course of the nerves into the plexus, (3) the extreme mobility of the neck, and (4) some points of fixation of nerves within this plexus during its formation. When the patient's arm is constantly held for a long time in an excessively abducted position, with flexion and rotation of the neck to the contralateral side, then it puts the brachial plexus under stretching and subsequent

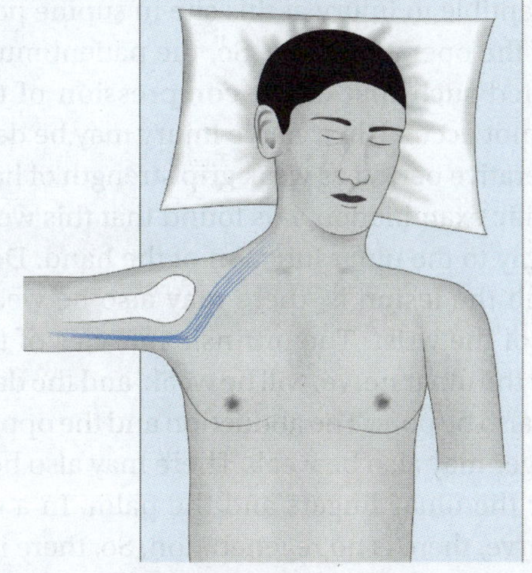

Fig. 1: Stretching of brachial plexus due to the excessive abduction of arm and the flexion and rotation of neck.

ischemia. Here, the head of the humerus acts as a pivotal point against which the stretching of nerves occurs. In another circumstance, if the humerus is allowed to fall posteriorly against the trunk, which is in supine position, then it also causes excessive stretching of nerves into the brachial plexus and leads to injury **(Fig. 2)**. When the patient is kept in a lateral position, then the brachial plexus is also at the risk of injury for both the dependent and the nondependent limbs, with more risk to the previous one. This is because in a dependent limb, the brachial plexus is compressed between two bony structures, i.e., the rib cage and the head of the humerus.

So, in order to avoid this compression injury of brachial plexus, the weight of the patient's thorax must be kept off the humerus and a roll of foam or towel of proper size should be placed in the axilla. The vascular integrity of the dependent arm should also be checked by a pulse oximeter. But it does not always guarantee the integrity of the brachial plexus. In prone position, there is more danger to the ipsilateral brachial plexus if the patient's head is rotated toward the contralateral side, placing the brachial plexus under stretch at its origin. In the postoperative period, the diagnosis of brachial plexus injury is first suspected if the patient has unusual pain in neck and upper arm on the first postoperative day. This pain may be accompanied by numbness and loss of motor function. It can affect the entire brachial plexus (C_5 to T_1), but commonly it involves only the upper roots (C_5 to C_7, Erb's palsy) with the involvement of the upper arm and forearm, and less commonly the lower roots (C_8 to T_1) with the involvement of hand.

Just immediately above elbow, the ulnar nerve is situated very superficially in olecranon notch. So, the direct compression at this place can render the ulnar nerve ischemic, and after prolonged ischemia, neuropraxia of the ulnar nerve can occur. For a patient under GA, the ulnar nerve is highly susceptible to injury at this site in supine position by the edge of the operating table. So, the patient must always be positioned such that direct compression of the ulnar nerve does not occur. Ulnar nerve injury may be detected in the postoperative period as weak grip strength of hand.

By specific examination, it is found that this weakness is localized only to the ulnar function of the hand. Depending on how high the lesion is, there may also be weakness of the flexors of the wrist. The intrinsic muscles of the hand, supplied by the ulnar nerve, will be weak, and the dexterity of fingers will also be poor. The abduction and the opposition of the fifth finger may also be weak. There may also be sensory deficit over the ulnar fingers and the palm. In a complete lesion of nerve, there is no regeneration. So, there is wasting and the contracture of intrinsic muscles, resulting in claw hand **(Fig. 3)**.

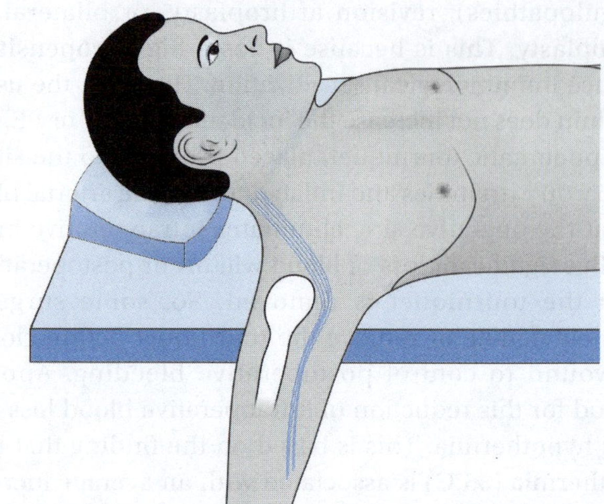

Fig. 2: Stretching of brachial plexus due to the hanging of hand below the table.

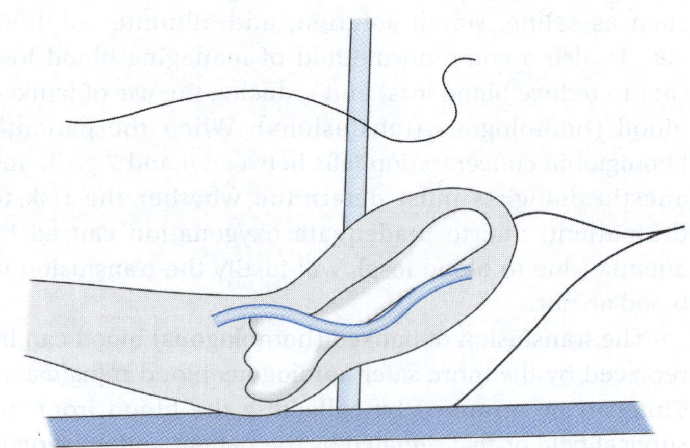

Fig. 3: Compression of radial nerve.

The saphenous nerve is very superficially situated at the medial side of the upper part of leg, below knee. So, this nerve is also more susceptible to injury at this site by compression when the patient is positioned in lithotomy by some devices **(Fig. 4)** for the immobilization of the knee during arthroscopy. This compression injury of the saphenous nerve produces only sensory loss over the distribution of this nerve on the medial side of leg and foot. The saphenous nerve of the dependent leg is also at risk from pressure injury when the patient is kept in a lateral position for a prolonged period.

Normally, in supine position, the sciatic nerve is protected from compression injury by the muscles of the buttock. However, in supine position, especially in thin and malnourished patients or due to any position of buttock over the edge of a positioning device, compression injury of the sciatic nerve can result. The incorrect application of the

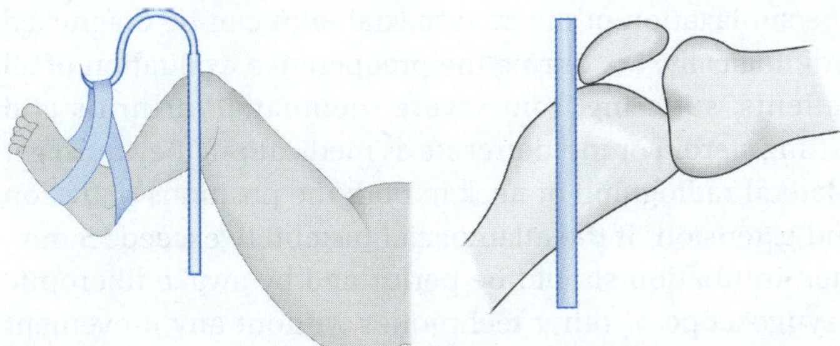

Fig. 4: Compression of the saphenous nerve on the medial side of the leg below knee by iron stand.

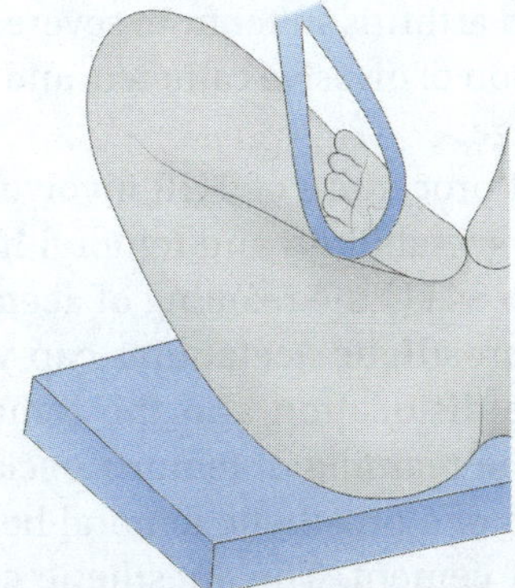

Fig. 5: Compression of common peroneal nerve over the head of fibula.

TABLE 3: Problems faced by an anesthetist during prone position of a patient.	
Airway	• Dislodgement of ET tube • Kinking of ET tube
Nerves	• Stretching or compression of brachial plexus • Compression of ulnar nerve • Compression of common peroneal nerve • Gross hyperextension or hyperflexion of neck • External pressure on eyes • Excessive rotation of neck
Others	• Kinking or obstruction of blood vessels • Excessive lordosis

(ET: endotracheal)

lateral position of patient can also put the sciatic nerve of the dependent side liable to injury by the edge of the operating table or by any positioning devices or other irregular surfaces due to direct compressions over the lateral gluteal surfaces. Intramuscular injection in the buttock should be performed in the superior and medial location to minimize the possibility of intraneural injection of the sciatic nerve, as it emerges from pyriformis. Trauma to the branches of the sciatic nerve is also possible. For example, the common peroneal nerve is very superficial and is highly liable to injury by direct pressure as it sweeps around the head of the fibula, just below the joint line of knee **(Fig. 5)**. This occurs in the dependent leg when the patient is kept for a prolonged period in lateral position or during lithotomy position when the leg is kept medial to the stand, which is erected to hold the leg in hanging position.

When the sciatic nerve injury occurs, then (1) all the muscles below the knee will be paralyzed or become weak and (2) numbness of the anterolateral part of the calf and foot, except the saphenous area, will also occur. When the injury of the common peroneal nerve occurs, then loss of dorsiflexion of ankle (foot drop), accompanied by loss of sensation on the anterolateral side of the calf and the medial planter side of foot will occur. The injury to the deep

peroneal nerve also involves foot drop and the numbness (loss of sensation) of the dorsum of the foot. The injury to the posterior tibial nerve will result in the numbness (loss of sensation) of the plantar surface of the foot, toes, and the lateral edge of the foot, combined with weakened plantar flexion.

Of all the positions chosen for orthopedic surgery, the prone position is least physiological for a patient under anesthesia **(Table 3)**. The prone position brings most of the challenges to an anesthetist, depending on the types of surgery and the mode of anesthesia selected. GA presents different issues from RA and LA with or without sedation. There is a definite problem for ventilation and excessive surgical bleeding in prone position. In addition to the increased risk of injury to the nerve, the prone position may also precipitate an increased risk of injury to the muscle and skin also. The direct prolonged contact of bed with the body during the prone position is sometimes associated with an isolated lesion of different terminal branches of the facial nerve, brachial plexus, femoral, and other nerves by pressure. Different positioning devices that facilitate prone position can also injure the different nerves or their branches. Curved frames that allow the abdomen to hang freely may also give direct pressure on the lower abdomen. But care should be taken to avoid direct pressure to ilioinguinal and iliohypogastric nerves in the region of iliac crest.

The use of a tourniquet is also a risk factor for nerve injury. So, the proper size of the cuff, the proper placement of it, the proper padding, and the duration of cuff inflation are all important considerations. The inflation of a tourniquet for >2 hours increases the risk of ischemic injury to the underlying muscles and nerves. However, the nerve of the upper extremity is more sensitive to injury by a tourniquet than that of the lower extremity.

When the fractured table is used for some orthopedic surgeries with the patient in a supine position, then all the risks of injury arising from the supine position will persist, and other extra risks to this type of table will also be added. The purpose of the fractured operating table is to immobilize the patient's lower extremities and also to allow for some rotation and traction of the leg, which will facilitate the surgery. After anesthesia, the patient is shifted from a regular bed to the fractured table. The trunk and hips are placed in a supine position, and the legs hang freely, supported by heels. Longitudinal traction is applied, and countertraction is indirectly imposed at a fixed post placed between the patient's leg. Thus, the potential injury to the lower extremities can occur from traction and countertraction or due to other positions caused by the fractured table. The post is placed at the perineum. So, the external genitalia, especially of a male, are at an increased risk of injury from the compression by post.

INDIVIDUAL ORTHOPEDIC SURGERY

Total Hip Replacement or Arthroplasty

Most of the patients who are advised for total hip replacement (THR) surgery usually suffer from osteoarthritis, rheumatoid arthritis, avascular necrosis of the bones of hip joint, etc., and it is for these disease processes that they are advised for such surgery. Osteoarthritis is a degenerative process that affects not only the bones of hip joint for which the patient is put for surgery, but also the articular surfaces of bones of other joints. But, among all these joints, the hip and knee are mostly affected. The bones of vertebral column are also affected by osteoarthritis. So, making different positions of the patient during THR surgeries, as well as the positioning of the neck during intubations, is very difficult, which is important to an anesthetist. This is because excessive movement of the vertebrae during the positioning of the patient or intubation can cause nerve root compression or disk prolapse.

Unlike osteoarthritis, rheumatoid arthritis is an immune-mediated disease which also affects the synovial membrane of joints, in addition to the articular surfaces of bones. It affects multiple joints including the hip, knee, vertebrae, shoulder, and some small joints of hands and legs. It becomes a concern to an anesthetist when it involves the cervical vertebra and temporomandibular joint. When the cervical vertebrae are involved, it causes the sublaxation of the atlantoaxial joint. The sublaxation of the atlantoaxial joint is important to an anesthetist because during the flexion of neck for intubation, the odontoid process may protrude into the foramen of magnum and can compress the spinal cord or brainstem, causing serious injury or death.

The rheumatoid arthritis is also a concern to an anesthetist because it may produce difficulty in intubation due to the involvement of the temporomandibular joint.

The sublaxation of the atlantoaxial joint can be diagnosed radiologically. So, during the preoperative evaluation of all patients, suffering from severe rheumatoid arthritis and getting steroid or methotrexate as medication, they must get a lateral radiograph of neck in both the positions of flexion and extension. If the atlantoaxial instability exceeds 5 mm, then intubation should be performed by awake fiberoptic laryngoscope or other techniques without any movement of the neck. The rheumatoid arthritis also has multiple systemic involvement, affecting the immune, hematology, pulmonary, and cardiovascular systems, which have immense implications on anesthesia. Sometimes, patients with rheumatoid arthritis suffer from severe deformities that make the insertion of invasive catheters and even gaining an IV line a challenge.

The surgical procedure of THR involves the prosthetic replacement of acetabulum and femoral head. It includes procedures such as (1) the reaming of acetabulum and the insertion of a prosthetic acetabular cap with or without cement, (2) the dislocation and the removal of femoral head, and (3) the reaming of femur's neck and shaft, and (4) the insertion of a prosthetic femoral head into its shaft with or without cement. The anesthetic consideration of THR involves the general principles of orthopedic surgeries, which are discussed under the heading of "introduction" and "specific problems related to orthopedic surgery" in the first part of this chapter. Among these, the three potential life-threatening complications of THR are intra- and postoperative hemorrhage, bone cement implantation syndrome, and DVT.

Total hip replacement is a major surgical procedure and takes 2–3 hours of intraoperative time. The expected perioperative blood loss during THR is 1–1.5 L, and the position of the patient to facilitate the surgery is lateral (more common) or supine. To maintain this lateral position of a patient, an anesthetist must discuss with the surgeon the proper placement of anterior pelvic brace. Because if it is placed too far caudally, it will exert much pressure on the femoral triangle of the dependent leg of the patient, causing venous or arterial obstruction. On the other hand, if it is placed too far cranially, it will also press the patient's abdomen too forcefully and can limit the movement of the diaphragm, causing the impairment of respiration. The THR surgery is particularly amenable to RA with slight sedation or full GA. But this anesthetic technique may be influenced by the patient's wishes and his medical status. In RA, the postdural puncture headache is very rare with 25G needle, as the procedure mainly involves the older age group of patients.

As THR is a major surgery and may involve many complications, the intraoperative monitoring of the patient by an invasive arterial line, TEE, $ETCO_2$, etc., may be considered. These are more applicable for revision arthroplasty, following a failed prior surgery, bilateral hip arthroplasty, or very sick patients. But unless the patient is at a particular risk due to severe illness, intraoperative monitoring by measuring BP with an arm cuff (NIBP), saturation of peripheral oxygen (SPO_2), and measuring the urine output with a bladder catheter are usually sufficient for the CVS.

The embolic phenomenon most frequently occurs during the insertion of femoral prosthesis or at the end of surgery when the hip is relocated. This is because, during the relocation of leg, emboli formed by the contents of bone marrow are dislodged from the previously obstructed femoral vein. More emboli occur in patients when the cement is used for THR than when it is not used. Therefore, uncemented THR is preferred for patients at higher risk of FES. The measures taken to avoid the embolic manifestations include (1) Omitting the use of cement, (2) high-pressure washout of femoral canal to remove debris (potential for microemboli), and (3) drilling a venting hole in the distal part of femur to relieve intramedullary pressure. Increased pulmonary artery pressure at the time of cementing is a usual finding during THR surgery. So, many anesthetists increase the FiO_2 prior to cementing. Careful maintenance of blood volume at the time of the placement of prosthesis and hip relocation attenuates the chance of a decrease in BP due to bone marrow emboli. Severe hypotension during THR reflects large emboli in the pulmonary artery, causing the large increase in PVR, decreased cardiac output, and resultant right heart failure. Severe hypotension during the THR also reflects the severe reaction from cement. So, immediate inotropic support is recommended. As DVT is prevalent after THR, all the measures to prevent this complication should be taken when managing the THR. This has been already discussed before, and among these, RA is important. So, the THR should better be performed under spinal or epidural block.

Blood loss in THR is expected to be large and may increase to about 2 L or above in case of revision of a prior arthroplasty (repeat arthroplasty). It depends on many factors such as the surgical technique, the skill of surgeon, and the type of prosthesis chosen. These losses of blood can be reduced by deliberately inducing controlled hypotension. So, a combination of RA (like continuous lumbar epidural or single shot spinal with or without narcotic) with an anesthetic level up to the T4 dermatome and light GA could be employed. With MAP, maintaining at 60–70 mm Hg, the intraoperative blood loss can be reduced to <300–500 mL.

Thus, by providing dry surgical field, controlled hypotension also improves the results of THR, using cement, and shortens the duration of surgery. If deliberate hypotension is contraindicated due to any reason, then deliberate hemodilution and/or preoperative preservation of autologous blood unit can prevent the intraoperative transfusion of banked blood. The preoperative administration of recombinant human erythropoietin represents another alternative for perioperative allogeneic blood transfusion. The maintenance of normal body temperature is also another means to reduce intraoperative blood loss. The preoperative insertion of an epidural catheter and diluted LA solution, with or without opiates, greatly facilitates postoperative pain management in THR. This may extend for up to 48–72 hours.

The THR of both sides at the same sitting is a longer and more invasive procedure than the THR of one side. So, they are associated with more hemodynamic changes, particularly if cement is used. Therefore, in such a situation, consideration should be given to direct arterial pressure monitoring, access to a large-bore venous system for quick transfusion, and other full hemodynamic monitoring, especially in an elderly frail patient. The amount of blood loss may go above 2 L. It can safely be performed in one anesthetic sitting if there is no significant PE of bone marrow contents after the insertion of the first femoral component. The monitoring of pulmonary artery pressure may indicate pulmonary embolization by a rise in pulmonary artery pressure and fall in cardiac output. The normal pulmonary artery pressure is 200 dyne $\times$ s $\times$ cm^{-5}. If it rises above normal, then the plan for surgery of the contralateral side should be postponed. Recently, a synthetic prosthetic system is available that does not require cement, and therefore cementless hip arthroplasty of both sides at one sitting does not require the monitoring of pulmonary artery pressure.

Hip Fracture

Usually, there are two types of hip fracture: Intracapsular and extracapsular. The intracapsular fracture is again of two types: Subcapital and transcervical. The extracapsular fracture is again of three types: At the base of femoral neck, intertrochanteric, and subtrochanteric **(Fig. 6)**. In general, the intracapsular fracture is associated with a lesser amount of blood loss (400 mL) than the extracapsular fracture (800 mL). Most of the patients coming with hip fracture for surgery and anesthesia are aged, frail, and suffering from many concomitant systemic diseases, such as osteoporosis, IHD, chronic obstructive pulmonary disease (COPD), hypertension, diabetes mellitus, cerebral vascular diseases, and psychiatric disorders. In such a group of patients, the most common cause of this hip fracture is indirect trauma due to the fall. But occasionally young patients may also present with hip fracture, and this is mainly due to direct accidental trauma.

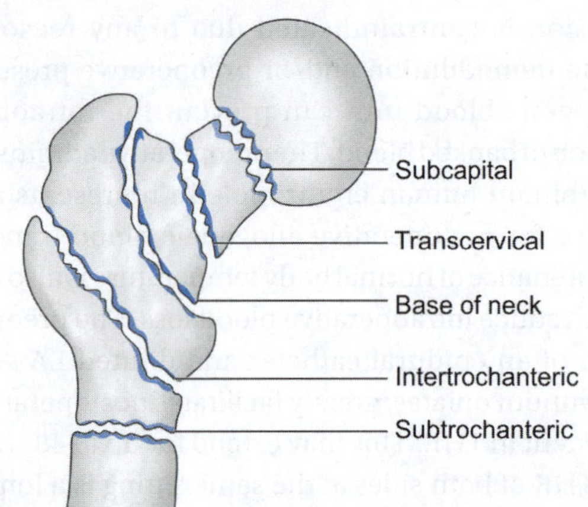

Fig. 6: Different types of fracture of the head of femur.

The patients presenting with hip fracture are often severely dehydrated. This is because of (1) occult blood loss at the site of fracture, (2) use of diuretics in case of a hypertensive patient, (3) inadequate oral intake in psychiatric patients, (4) delayed rescue after accident and trauma, etc. They also present with a false normal or borderline normal hematocrit value and it is due to dehydration and hemoconcentration or actual anemia due to occult blood loss. It is also very important to know the cause of fall or cause of accident, which may be brain stroke, myocardial infarction (MI), cardiac arrhythmia, etc., resulting in hip fracture. All these have an immense effect on anesthesia.

Generally, the operative decision for a hip fracture is taken in the hope of getting the older patient out of the bed as quickly as possible in order to reduce the bad effects of prolonged staying in bed. These bad effects, due to the prolonged staying in bed, include the bed sore, pneumonia, thromboembolic manifestation, etc. However, any emergency surgery for hip fracture is not undertaken and is usually performed after 1 or 2 days, during which period the patient is treated for the concomitant diseases and is also prepared for surgery. However, more delay in surgery does not increase the mortality, but increase only the morbidity, which are mainly related to the lungs and skin.

Sometimes, during the preoperative evaluation of a patient, the examination of mental status of the patient is very important. This is because (1) the dementia patients are not suitable for RA, (2) mental illness is associated with delayed recovery and increased mortality, (3) they cannot be communicated during the perioperative period, and (4) others that are discussed in the chapter of "Psychiatric diseases and anesthesia." The hip fractured patients are more likely to be hypoxemic than expected for their age. This may probably be due to the result of occult fat embolism. Many studies have reported that the rate of mortality, following

hip fracture, may vary from 10 to 15% during the admission of patient in hospital and 20 to 25% at the end of 1 year. The significant predicting factors for this mortality include old age >85 years, pulmonary complications, infection, depressed mental function, etc.

The choice between GA and RA for fractured hip surgery is also extensively studied and is tilted toward the latter (RA) like other orthopedic surgeries. This is because RA is associated with (1) decreased thromboembolic manifestation, (2) induced hypotension facilitating surgery, (3) reduced blood loss, (4) postoperative analgesia, (5) more prompt return to a preoperative mental state, (6) lower mortality rate in the early postoperative period, etc. However, in recent studies, it has been found that the mortality rates after 1–2 months, following RA or GA, are more or less the same. There is also a general impression that RA is less associated with postoperative confusion and mental impairment than GA, but it is only in the absence of previous psychiatric disease and if excessive sedation is not used perioperatively. However, recent studies do not confirm it and show that both types of anesthesia (general and regional) produce the same postoperative confusion and mental impairment.

The postoperative confusion correlates best with (1) the presence of preoperative confusion, (2) the presence of preoperative hypoxemia, and (3) the use of drugs with anticholinergic effects, but not on the mode of anesthesia. The mode of anesthesia in fractured hip also depends on the type of surgery, which varies from close reduction with surface traction to open reduction with different types of internal fixation, such as cannulated screw fixation, intramedullary gamma nail, and extramedullary sliding screw and plates, according to the site of fracture, degree of displacement, and patient's status.

Total Knee Arthroplasty

The anesthetic consideration of total knee arthroplasty (TKA) is more or less similar to that of THR surgery. RA offers several advantages to the patients undergoing such surgery and is therefore preferred. The usual position of a patient for TKA is supine, and a tourniquet is commonly used to reduce blood loss. So, there are more chances of DVT and other thromboembolic manifestations than THR, and prophylactic measures do not seem to reduce the incidences of these problems. When the TKA, using cement, is performed under a tourniquet, then the syndrome of $\uparrow$PVR, $\downarrow$CO, systemic hypotension, etc., which are usually found after the use of cement, is delayed until the tourniquet is deflated at the end of surgery. Otherwise, when a tourniquet is not used, then this syndrome may begin immediately after the insertion of prosthesis. The patient may suffer from the combined effects of embolism arising from cement, blood clot, fat or marrow debris, and blood loss. This can be diagnosed by TEE, which shows emboli in the right ventricle, increased pulmonary artery pressure, hypotension, and hypoxemia. The large emboli, >5 mm, produces fatal consequences and is more commonly associated with a tourniquet. So, the vital signs of the patient should be monitored continuously in the perioperative period, especially after the insertion of prosthesis or deflation of the tourniquet (when the bone cement is used), and the patient is treated with O_2, fluid, and pressure agents as required. The sick patients or with cardiovascular diseases who might not be able to compensate adequately for these events during TKA should be monitored extensively by the invasive method, and ventilators should be kept ready at hand.

Recently, many studies have shown that the complication rate and initial recovery of knee movement are better when TKA is performed without a tourniquet. The expected blood loss in a single TKA is about 1–1.5 L. The use of a tourniquet reduces this intraoperative blood loss, but may be the same after deflation of the tourniquet. Deliberate hypotension reduces the perioperative blood loss but may increase the incidence of PE.

The surgical insult caused by a single TKA is usually tolerated by most of the healthy patients who do not have serious pulmonary and cardiovascular diseases. On the other hand, bilateral TKA in one sitting is associated with double the amount of blood loss, requiring subsequent blood transfusion and double the risk of PE. Therefore, the decision of TKA in both legs in one sitting will depend on the patient's health status, invasiveness of monitoring, and the outcome of surgery of one leg. It is better to stage the bilateral TKA procedure into two when performed in one sitting so that the second part does not begin until it is seen that there is no complication after the first phase of the TKA procedure.

The postoperative pain following TKA is more severe than THR. Therefore, effective postoperative analgesia is very essential for early physical rehabilitation after TKA. This will, in turn, prevent joint adhesions and will increase its movement. The noncooperative patients will not do exercise even with good postoperative analgesia. So, there should be a balance between the pain control and a cooperative patient willing to exercise. The preoperative placement of an epidural catheter is the best way for postoperative pain management and physiotherapy. For this, a 0.2% ropivacaine infusion at a rate of 10 mL/h will provide good analgesia with minimum motor blockade. Alternatively, the placement of an indwelling catheter into the femoral sheath may be performed for postoperative analgesia. Through this catheter, 0.2% ropivacaine or 0.25% bupivacaine can be infused continuously at a rate of 5–10 mL/h for good analgesia with minimum motor block.

Knee Arthroscopy

The arthroscopic surgeries have revolutionized orthopedic surgery. They can be performed on many joints, such as hip, knee, shoulder, ankle, elbow, and wrist. The joint arthroscopies are usually performed as outpatient procedures. The surgeries of knee joint that can be done through arthroscopy include menisectomy, ligament repairs, replacement of cruciate ligaments, removal of loose foreign bodies from knee joint, etc. The typical patients undergoing knee arthroscopic surgeries are young, healthy adults, usually athletes. However, they are also performed on aged persons with multiple medical problems. All forms of anesthesia, on an outpatient basis, are suitable for knee arthroscopic surgery. So, the anesthesia may vary from GA to spinal anesthesia using a fine pencil-point needle, to combined spinal epidural anesthesia, to peripheral nerve block (femoral block), to periarticular or intraarticular injection, employing LA solution with or without adjuvants combined with IV sedation, etc. The least invasive and least prolonged procedures are performed with the intraarticular injection of LA solution. The absorption of an LA agent from the joint surface is slow, and the addition of epinephrine in this LA solution will further decrease its absorption. Therefore, the concentration of the LA agent in the blood will always be minimum, and 30 mL of 0.5% bupivacaine with or without epinephrine is safe. If bloodless field is required for arthroscopic surgery, then a tourniquet should be applied, and the mode of anesthesia should also be changed accordingly.

Comparing between spinal and epidural neuraxial anesthetic techniques, on the basis of patient satisfaction and success, has shown that both are equal. However, for ambulatory surgery, the time of discharge following neuraxial anesthesia is prolonged compared with GA.

Hip Arthroscopy

Recently, as an alternative to open arthrotomy, hip arthroscopy is also gradually gaining popularity after knee arthroscopy. It is a minimally invasive procedure used for a variety of surgical indications on hip, such as femoroacetabular impingement (FAI), acetabular labral tears, loose bodies, and osteoarthritis.

Computer-Assisted Minimally Invasive Arthroplasty

Minimally invasive surgical procedures, assisted by computer [computer-assisted surgery (CAS)], are gradually coming in front to (1) improve the surgical outcomes, (2) cause less pain, and (3) promote early rehabilitation. In such hi-tech surgeries, the computer software is upgraded to accurately reconstruct three-dimensional images of bone and soft tissues of joints based on the radiographs, fluoroscopy, CT/MRI data, etc. Tracking devices are attached to the target bones and the instruments used during surgery. The navigation system utilizes optical cameras and infrared light-emitting diodes to sense their positions. Thus, CAS allows the placement of implants accurately through a small incision on joint, repairs the damaged ligaments of joints, and causes the reduction of tissues. In computer-assisted hip arthroplasty, the lateral approach utilizes a single incision with the patient in a lateral position, while the anterior approach utilizes two small incisions (one for acetabular component and another for femoral component) with the patient in supine position.

Closed Treatment of Fracture, Joint Manipulation, and Reduction of Dislocation

The management of these groups of patients is more or less similar. As the procedures are very brief, GA is often preferred than regional techniques. The regional anesthetic techniques are chosen for elderly patients with multiple medical problems and full stomach. For example, the reduction of Colles fracture in an elderly patient can be achieved by IVRA or brachial plexus block. If GA is chosen, then violent fasciculation by succinylcholine, which may disturb some fractures, should be avoided. Whatever may be the type of anesthesia, profound muscle relaxation is mandatory. This will allow the surgeon to distinguish between the limitations of joint movement due to an anatomical cause or muscle guarding. Thus, short-acting IV anesthetic agents and a small dose of succinylcholine are effective. If the surgical lesions permit, then the intraarticular injection of LA may provide some postoperative analgesia after joint manipulation.

Revision Hip Arthroplasty

Sometimes, a previously performed hip arthroplasty needs revision due to the malfunctioning of the hip joint, and it is called the revision arthroplasty. It is associated with much greater blood loss than the initial procedure. But this blood loss depends on multiple factors, including the skill and the experience of the surgeon. However, this huge blood loss can be reduced if we use RA (spinal or epidural, preferably continuous epidural) instead of GA for revision hip arthroplasty. Due to some unknown reason (cause is still not known), it has been seen in multiple studies that at equal MAP, blood loss in RA is less in comparison to GA. To reduce the homologous perioperative blood transfusion and to increase the autologous blood transfusion, preoperative

autologous blood donation and intraoperative blood salvage are encouraged. The preoperative administration of iron, vitamin K, vitamin B_{12}, etc., is also encouraged to treat anemia. To facilitate autologous blood transfusion by collecting the patient's own blood and to combat intraoperative blood loss by increasing hematocrit, the recombinant human erythropoietin (600 IU/kg subcutaneously weekly) is also started 21 days before surgery. Maintaining normal body temperature during revision arthroplasty also reduces the intraoperative blood loss.

Surgery on Upper Extremity

The orthopedic surgical procedures on upper extremity, requiring anesthesia, range from simple fracture reduction (Colles wrist fracture) to nerve entrapment syndrome (carpal tunnel syndrome) to disorders of shoulder (subacromial impingement and rotator cuff tears) to many autoimmune or degenerative joint diseases.

Shoulder Surgery

Shoulder operations may be closed (arthroscopic) or opened and are performed in a lateral lying position (less common) or in a sitting "beach chair" position (more common). Both GA and RA may be employed for the surgeries on shoulder with their own advantages and disadvantages that are discussed many times before. Here, we will discuss some special points. The "beach chair" position is associated with some problems which are Decreased cerebral perfusion, blindness, stroke, and even brain death. So, during anesthesia and surgery in beach chair position, BP should be monitored at the level of the brain. For this monitoring of BP, if a noninvasive method is decided, then the BP cuff should be applied on the upper arm, but not on the leg calf. Because the systolic BP reading from the leg calf will show 40 mm Hg higher than that of brachial reading. Further, if the surgeon wants controlled hypotension, then intraarterial BP monitoring should be employed, and the transducer should be kept at the level of the external meatus of ear (at the level of brain stem).

Brachial plexus block through the interscalene approach, with or without the placement of a catheter for continuous effect, is ideally suited for surgical procedures on shoulder. The advantages and disadvantages of supraclavicular, infraclavicular, and axillary approaches for brachial plexus block for shoulder surgery are discussed in full detail in Chapter 23 (Peripheral Nerve Block). Even when GA is employed, brachial plexus block can still be used to supplement this GA for effective postoperative analgesia. Alternatively, at the end of surgery, the surgeon may also place a catheter at the subacromial region to provide continuous infusion of an LA agent for postoperative analgesia. However, the direct placement of a catheter into the glenohumeral joint for bupivacaine infusion is not recommended. Because several studies have shown that it is associated with glenohumeral chondrolysis.

Distal Upper Extremity Surgeries

These operations are usually performed on an outpatient basis. The common position of the patient for these operations is supine, and a tourniquet is used. In most cases, the operative arm is abducted at a 90° angle and is kept on a hand table. However, the exception to this rule often involves some surgeries around the elbow, and certain operations may require the patient, be in a lateral or even in prone position. Minor soft-tissue operations of short duration, performed on hands, are usually done with local infiltration anesthesia or by IVRA (Bier block) or by brachial plexus block. The limiting factor of IVRA is tourniquet intolerance after a fixed time.

If the operations on the upper extremity involve the joints and/or take >1 hour and are more invasive, then the brachial plexus block is the first choice. The approach for this brachial plexus block will depend on the planned surgical site and the location of the tourniquet (if used). The brachial plexus block does not anesthetize the intercostobrachial nerve, which is a branch of the dorsal rami of T1 or T2 spinal nerve. Hence, the area extending over the medial side of the upper arm, supplied by this intercostobrachial nerve, remains unaffected and a tourniquet cannot be applied over the upper arm. Therefore, if the tourniquet is applied to the upper arm, then this nerve should be blocked by a separate local subcutaneous infiltration method.

The continuous brachial plexus block, by placing a catheter in close proximity to the nerves of this plexus, is also performed for inpatients and some selected outpatients for postoperative analgesia, facilitating physiotherapy.

Anesthesia for Surgeries on Genitourinary Tract

■ INTRODUCTION

Surgeries on genitourinary tract vary from a simple outpatient cystoscopy to complicated radical cystectomy and nephrectomy for renal cell carcinoma (RCC) with vena caval thrombosis. About 15–20% of all anesthetic procedures are undertaken for surgeries on genitourinary tract. With the drastic revolution in technology and introduction of fiberoptic instrument, the complicated surgical procedures on genitourinary tract have now become common and less invasive or noninvasive. Patients undergoing genitourinary tract surgeries may be of any age, but are usually elderly with multiple and coexisting medical disorders including kidney dysfunction. Thus, making anesthesia for them is more challenging. The effect of anesthesia on kidney function has been discussed in Chapter 42. Now, in this chapter, we have discussed only the anesthetic management of common genital urological surgeries.

The commonly used lithotomy position, for the approach through transurethral route, for the surgeries on genitourinary tract, makes the anesthetic procedures complicated. Further, with this lithotomy position, steep head-down (Trendelenburg) position makes the anesthetic procedure more complicated. (i) The proper and meticulous preoperative evaluation and the proper optimization of patients, (ii) the understanding of surgical procedures and estimating the approximate time for surgery, (iii) good perioperative management and proper postoperative rehabilitation help the anesthesiologist to formulate the best anesthetic plan and allow more patients with coexisting diseases to be considered acceptable candidates for kidney transplantation, extensive tumor debulking surgery, and reconstructive genitourinary procedures.

The anesthetic plan for all the surgeries on genitourinary tract mainly depends on the spinal level of innervation of that surgical area **(Table 1)**. The motor supply of the bladder is by parasympathetic nerves. The sensation for the fullness

TABLE 1: Level of regional anesthesia required for the surgeries of different structures of genitourinary tract.

Urethra		S_2–S_4
Bladder	Dome	T_{11}-L_2
	Urethra	S_2–S_4
Ureter		T_{10}
Prostate		T_{11}–L_2 and S_2–S_4

and the stretching sensation from bladder are carried by afferent parasympathetic fibers. The sympathetic fibers carry the pain, touch, and temperature sensations from the bladder. Pain from the ureter and kidney is felt in the low back area, flanks, scrotal, labial, and ilioinguinal areas, i.e., along the innervation of 10th thoracic spinal nerve mainly, but also extending second lumbar (L_2) spinal segment. The nerves from the lumbosacral area innervate the prostate. Some important genitourinary procedures will be discussed now to help the further understanding of this subject.

■ CYSTOSCOPY

One of the most commonly performed surgical procedures on genitourinary tract is cystoscopy. The introduction of *flexible* fiberoptic scope has made this procedure very easy to perform now.

Indications

Cystoscopy is done for both diagnostic and therapeutic purposes. Urinary tract obstruction, hematuria, renal stone, transurethral resection of bladder tumor (TURBT), placement or manipulation of ureteric stent, extraction or laser lithotripsy of kidney stone, recurrent pain at the suprapubic region or along the line of ureter, and recurrent urinary tract infection are the common indications for this cystoscopy. Following a thorough cystoscopy, in this same sitting, bladder tumor biopsies and its resection, renal stones extraction, and placement of ureteric stents, etc. are also done through this same cystoscope. Retrograde pyelograms are also performed through a cystoscope.

For surgeries on genitourinary tract, the mode of anesthesia depends on (i) the age of patient, (ii) the gender of patient, and (iii) the purpose of cystoscopy. For example, (a) General anesthesia (GA) is usually employed on pediatric patients, (b) Topical anesthesia using lignocaine gel is usually employed on female patient for *only* diagnostic cystoscopy because of short urethra, (iii) On the other hand, GA or regional anesthesia (RA) is employed for all therapeutic cystoscopy such as taking biopsies, cauterization, manipulation of ureteral catheters, etc. on female patients, (iv) Male patients generally require general or regional anesthesia both for diagnostic and therapeutic cystoscopy due to long urethra.

Position of Patient

The most commonly used position of patients for the surgical procedures (cystoscopy) on genitourinary tract is lithotomy, which may be accompanied by Trendelenburg (head-down) posture also. Tis lithotomy and head-down position have their own implications on anesthesia. The improper positioning of patient for cystoscopy may also cause severe iatrogenic complications, such as pressure sore, nerve injury, and compartment syndrome, etc. For this lithotomy position, the patient should lie in supine and the straps, holders, and stirrups (or supports), etc. will hold the legs in position. These supports, where the leg or foot comes in contact with hard objects, should be properly padded to prevent the injuries of nerve of lower extremities.

The legs should hang freely. If these supports are not properly padded, then the pressure of strap on the lateral side of the leg at fibular neck will cause injury to the common peroneal nerve with loss of dorsiflexion of foot. The pressure of the straps medially on the leg will injure the saphenous nerve causing numbness along the medial side of the calf. The obturator and the femoral nerves may be damaged by the too much flexion of thigh. The extreme flexion of thigh may also damage the sciatic nerve due to overstretching. The most common nerve injuries directly associated with this lithotomy position is lumbosacral plexus. Prolonged lithotomy position may often present with a compartmental syndrome of inferior extremities with rhabdomyolysis.

There is chance to injury of brachial plexus, if the upper extremities are inappropriately positioned, i.e., shoulder is hyperextended or extremely abducted. When the patient's arm is tucked by the side of operating table, then caution must be exercised to prevent the injury of fingers, from being caught between the middle and lower section of operating table, when the lower section is raised or lowered. To prevent this injury of fingers, some anesthetists completely cover the patient's hands and fingers by protective padding.

Other than nerve injuries, the various physiological changes are also associated with this lithotomy and head-down position, which makes the work of anesthesiologist more demanding. The elevation of legs drains blood immediately from the periphery into the central circulation and increases CO along with MAP. Congestive cardiac failure may precipitate or exaggerate in low cardiac reserve patients, as the raising of legs suddenly increase venous return and preload. The lowering of legs similarly suddenly decreases the venous return, preload, CO, and blood pressure without giving time for compensation. This hypotension is further increased by regional or general anesthesia due to vasodilatation. So, blood pressure measurement and its continuous monitoring is essential before and after keeping the patient in lithotomy position. Lung atelectasis and hypoxia are common after lithotomy position, as the functional residual capacity of patient decreases, which is further aggravated by steep Trendelenburg position (30–45° head down).

Anesthesia for Cystoscopy

The age of the patient, its gender, and the indications for cystoscopy decides the plan of anesthesia. Cystoscopy in children is always performed under GA. Short urethra in females may allow the cystoscopic procedure to be performed under topical anesthesia, with viscous lignocaine, with or without sedation, *but only for diagnostic purposes*. However, all the cystoscopic procedures for *therapeutic purposes* on female patients are preferred under GA, not under topical anesthesia. In males, all the cystoscopic procedures for diagnostic as well as for therapeutic purposes are done under general or regional anesthesia.

In an outpatient setting, GA is preferred than RA by most anesthesiologists for diagnostic cystoscopy or for brief therapeutic cystoscopic procedures due to short duration (about 15–30 minutes). Patients are usually very apprehensive and so they too prefer GA. In such situations, laryngeal mask airway (LMA) is usually used for the management of airway. Oxygen saturation is closely monitored in all the patients, especially in obese, elderly, and low cardiopulmonary reserve patients, as they are placed in lithotomy and as well as in Trendelenburg position.

Regional anesthesia may also be opted for the therapeutic cystoscopic procedures. Either spinal or epidural anesthesia may be performed, though most anesthesiologists choose spinal anesthesia than epidural anesthesia, as the later takes longer time for its onset of action, whereas spinal anesthesia takes just few minutes for its onset of action. All the cystoscopic procedures can be done with a sensory block maximum up to T_{10} spinal level. Most anesthesiologists believe that the local anesthetic agent used for regional block (spinal or epidural) should be well "fixed" with nervous tissues before putting the patient in lithotomy position, otherwise the drug may spread in cephalad direction and may raise the level of block with the likelihood of severe hypotension. But, there is no such substantial clinical evidence to prove this. Because, multiple studies have failed to demonstrate that the immediate elevation of legs into lithotomy position following the administration of hyperbaric spinal anesthesia, either increase the dermatomal extent of anesthesia to a clinically significant degree or increase the likelihood of severe hypotension.

Obturator reflex is not abolished by regional anesthesia. Muscle paralysis by GA is needed to block this obturator reflex (electrocautery on the lateral wall of bladder stimulates the obturator nerve, which causes the external rotation and adduction of thigh).

TRANSURETHRAL RESECTION OF THE PROSTATE

Benign prostatic enlargement or hypertrophy (BPH) frequently leads to urinary bladder neck obstruction in male older than 65 years of age. So, to remove this obstruction, transurethral prostatectomy (TURP) is the most commonly adopted operative procedure for either benign or malignant hypertrophy of prostate in elderly men.

Indications

The principal indication for TURP is BHP in elderly male patients. Other than BHP, the indications for TURP in male patients are obstructive uropathy, recurrent episodes of urinary retention, hematuria, and recurrent urinary tract infections, etc. TURP is preferred in patients with a prostate gland volume <45–50 mL. Prostate with larger volumes require alternative approaches such as suprapubic prostatectomy or peroneal prostatectomy. TURP is also the procedure of choice and helps to relieve urinary obstruction in male patients with prostatic carcinoma who are not the candidate (unfit) for radical prostatectomy.

Position of Patient

The usual position of patient for TURP is lithotomy with their head slightly down.

Anesthesia for TURP

Most of the patients undergoing TURP are elderly and have coexisting pulmonary, cardiac, or renal diseases. But, no wonder, despite advanced age and prevalence of significant comorbidity, the perioperative mortality and morbidity for TURP are <1% even today. The proper preoperative evaluation and the optimization of patient presenting for TURP is an utmost importance to an anesthesiologist. Spinal anesthesia is the choice for most of the anesthesiologists, though the other forms of regional anesthesia, like epidural block may be opted for too. Block up to T_{10} sensory level is enough to make the patient, surgeon, and anesthesiologist comfortable. Regional anesthesia is contraindicated, only when there is the possibility of lumbar metastasis of prostatic cancer and then GA is preferred.

When compared to GA, the RA has some advantages during TURP **(Box 1)**. These advantages of RA are: (i) It reduces the incidences of postoperative venous thrombosis. (ii) It less likely masks the signs and symptoms of TURP syndrome. Hence, early diagnosis and treatment of TURP syndrome is possible in RA. Acute hyponatremia from TURP syndrome may delay or prevent emergence from GA. (iii) It less likely masks the signs and symptoms of bladder perforation. However, multiple clinical studies have failed to show any difference in blood loss, postoperative cognitive function, and mortality between RA and GA.

All the vital monitorings are must for the TURP surgical procedure **(Box 2)**. In awake or moderately sedated patients,

---

BOX 1: Comparison of regional anesthesia over GA in TURP.

- Regional anesthesia does not mask the signs and symptoms of TURP syndrome, unlike GA
- Regional anesthesia does not mask the signs and symptoms of bladder perforation, unlike GA
- Regional anesthesia decreases the incidence of postoperative venous thrombosis
- Reversal and recovery from general anesthesia may be delayed due to hyponatremia, caused by TURP syndrome
- GA is preferred in cases of lumbar metastasis from prostate cancer

(GA: general anesthesia; TURP: transurethral resection of the prostate)

BOX 2: Essential intraoperative and early postoperative monitoring for patients undergoing transurethral resection of the prostate (TURP).

- *Mental status:* Any alteration of mental status detects early signs of TURP syndrome and bladder perforation
- *Arterial oxygen saturation:* Any decrease in SPO_2 detects pulmonary edema due to fluid overload
- *Temperature:* To detect hypothermia
- *Electrocardiogram (ECG):* To detect ischemic changes
- Blood chemistry: Hemodilution may decrease the hematocrit values.
- *Blood loss:* Larger prostatic volume (>45 mL) and longer operative procedures (>1.5 hours) may require blood transfusion, as controlling prostatic bleeding is often difficult. So, blood should be crossmatched and arranged.

the periodic evaluation of mental status is the best monitor for the detection of the early signs of bladder perforation and TURP syndrome. Due to the use of irrigating solution, it is very difficult to assess the blood loss during TURP procedure. So, an anesthetist has relied on the clinical signs of hypovolemia. Due to hemodilution, due to the absorption of irrigating fluid, always there is some transient decrease in hematocrit value during postoperative period. But, that does not indicate excessive blood loss. Very few patients need intraoperative blood transfusion. Usual blood loss during TURP is 4–5 mL/min of resection (total 300–400 mL). Therefore, prolonged surgical procedure will increase blood loss.

TURP Procedures

In this procedure, an especial type cystoscope, which is more precisely called the resectoscope, is introduced through urethra and is advanced up to the prostatic urethra. It has both the cutting and coagulating monopolar wire loop at its tip. By flowing a cutting current through this monopolar electrical loop, the hypertrophic prostatic tissue is resected and is removed from its enlarged lobes under continuous irrigation and direct visualization of surgical site. Continuous irrigation is used, because it distends the bladder, removes the resected materials, and clears the field of surgery.

Complications of TURP

Because of the especial characteristics of prostate and as a large amount of irrigation fluid is often used, so the TURP is associated with many serious complications. Here, some of these major complications of TURP are mentioned here:

- *More common, but less serious:* Failure to void, clot retention, uncontrolled acute hematuria, chronic hematuria, and urinary tract obstruction.
- *Less common, but more serious:* TURP syndrome, bladder perforation, septicemia, hypothermia, coagulopathy [disseminated intravascular coagulation (DIC)], and rarely death due to myocardial infarction, renal failure, or pulmonary edema.

Recently, instead of old monopolar TURP method, different other TURP methods are used for prostatic resection in BHP. These include: low voltage bipolar TURP, laser and radiofrequency ablation, and cryotherapy, etc. The advantage of this low voltage bipolar TURP is that it uses isotonic saline as irrigating fluid and thus avoids TURP syndrome with the exception of persisting risk of fluid overload. Another advantage of this low voltage bipolar TURP is that this procedure simultaneously cauterizes as it resects. So, it decreases the risk of clot retention.

TURP Syndrome

The prostate has a dense network of large venous sinuses around it. During the transurethral resection, these venous sinuses open up and cause the absorption of irrigating fluid into the systemic circulation. This results in a set of manifestations, which is commonly referred to as the TURP syndrome. It may become evident intraoperatively or in early postoperative period. The principal symptoms and signs of TURP syndrome are headache, restless, confusion, cyanosis, dyspnea, arrhythmia, hypotension, seizure, or a combination of these. If this TURP syndrome is not treated instantaneously with utmost care, then fatality is not uncommon. The amount of irrigating fluid, which is absorbed and produces manifestations, depends on a number of factors and these are listed in **Box 3**.

The irrigating fluid should be nonelectrolytic because electrolyte solutions will disperse the electrocautery current passing through the loop of the wire. Visibility is best with water, but it is not used for irrigation, because a large amount of it is absorbed through prostatic open sinuses and can cause severe water intoxication and the lysis of red blood cell (RBC) (due to its hypotonicity) following its absorption. The use of water as irrigating fluid is generally restricted to TURBTs only. So, to increase the osmolality of the irrigating fluid the mannitol, glycine, sorbitol, urea, etc. also have been added to water. But, one has to be careful about that these solutes and their metabolites should be nontoxic and will be easily excretable **(Boxes 4 and 5)**.

For monopolar TURP, slightly hypotonic nonelectrolyte irrigating solutions, such as 1.5% glycine or a mixture of 2.7% sorbitol and 0.54% mannitol are most commonly used.

BOX 3: Factors on which the absorption of irrigating fluid depends.

- The duration of surgical procedure
- The type, nature, and amount of fluid used for irrigation
- Amount of irrigating fluid absorbed through prostatic veins
- The hydrostatic pressure of irrigating fluid
- The number, size, and pressure in venous channels which are opened up in prostate during transurethral resection of the prostate (TURP)
- The volume of prostate resected
- The skill of surgeon

BOX 4: Common irrigating fluids used for transurethral resection of the prostate (TURP).

- Plain water
- Glycine solution (1.5%—230 mOsm/L)
- Mixture of sorbitol (2.7%) and mannitol (0.54%—195 mOsm/L)
- Sorbitol solution (3.3%)
- Mannitol solution (3%)
- Dextrose solution (2.5–4%)
- Urea solution (1%)

> **BOX 5:** Characteristics of an ideal irrigating fluid in transurethral resection of the prostate (TURP).
>
> It should be isotonic
> It should be nonhemolytic
> It should be nontoxic
> It should be nonelectrolytic
> It should allow clear visibility
> It should not affect the osmolality
> It should be rapidly metabolized
> It should be an osmotic diuretic

> **BOX 6:** Common clinical manifestations of TURP syndrome.
>
> - *CNS manifestations:* Restlessness, confusion, anxiety, agitation, nausea, disorientation, visual disturbance, seizure, and coma
> - *CVS manifestations:* Increased CVP, bradycardia, anginal pain, ischemic changes in ECG, hypotension, congestive cardiac failure, cyanosis, arrhythmia, etc
> - *Respiratory symptoms:* Dyspnea, pulmonary congestion, and pulmonary edema
>
> (CNS: central nervous system; CVP: central venous pressure; CVS: cardiovascular system; ECG: electrocardiogram; TURP: transurethral resection of the prostate)

> **BOX 7:** Major physiological changes in transurethral resection of the prostate (TURP) syndrome.
>
> - Circulatory fluid overload
>   - Congestive heart failure
>   - Pulmonary edema
>   - Hypotension
>   - Water intoxication
> - Hypo-osmolality and hypotonicity
> - Hyponatremia—from all irrigating fluid
> - Hemolysis
> - Solute toxicity
>   - Hyperglycinemia—from glycine solution
>   - Hyperammonemia—from glycine solution
>   - Hyperglycemia—from sorbitol or dextrose solution
>   - Intravascular fluid volume expansion from mannitol solution

The less commonly used irrigating solutions are 3.3% sorbitol, 3% mannitol, 2.5–4% dextrose, and 1% urea. However, all these fluids are hypotonic and significant amount of them can be absorbed. The factors influencing the amount of irrigating fluid which will be absorbed depend on the volume of prostate resected, the duration of resection, the amount of irrigating fluid used, the pressure of irrigating fluid, etc.

Due to the intravascular absorption of large amount of nonelectrolytic hypotonic irrigating fluid, *hyponatremia* and *hypoosmolality of blood* occurs. The central nervous system (CNS) symptoms of TURP syndrome are usually due to this hyponatremia causing cerebral edema and metabolic encephalopathy. The clinical manifestations of hyponatremia appear only when the concentration of serum Na^+ falls below the 120 mEq/L. When the serum Na^+ level goes below the 100 mEq/L (marked hypotonicity), then intravascular hemolysis may also result.

To increase osmolality against plasma, glycine is commonly added into the irrigating fluid used for TURP. Hence, *hyperglycinemia* (↑plasma glycine level) due to intravascular absorption of this glycine containing irrigating fluid is also responsible for most of the CNS symptoms of TURP syndrome **(Box 6)**. Visual disturbances such as transient blindness have also been reported due to this hyperglycinemia, but the vision usually returns back to normal within 24 hours. The normal plasma glycine level is about 12–15 mg/L and it may increase to 900–1,000 mg/L

after TURP syndrome. The CNS symptoms for glycine is because, it acts as an inhibitory neurotransmitter in CNS. It also acts on the retinal receptors as inhibitory agent to cause transient blindness. Glycine also causes cerebral edema.

Ammonia is the metabolic product of glycine. So, *hyperammonemia* following the hyperglycinemia causes the phenomenon of seizure and coma in TURP patients by increasing the concentration of neurotoxic substances (ammonia) in brain. The normal level of ammonia in blood is 5–50 µmol/L and it may exceed 100–150 µmol/L in TURP syndrome patients. Dextrose or sorbitol in irrigating fluid may cause hyperglycemia. Mannitol does not undergo any metabolism in our body. It causes osmotic diuresis, increases fluid overload, and may cause congestive cardiac failure or pulmonary edema **(Box 7)**.

The absorption of irrigating fluid may be intravascular or extravascular. The intravascular absorption of irrigating fluid occurs, when the hydrostatic pressure of irrigating fluid (the height of irrigating fluid above the open venous channels of prostate) is more than the pressure inside the venous sinusoids of prostate. The extravascular absorption of irrigating fluid occurs, only when the prostatic capsule is perforated during surgery and it affects the hemostasis.

Treatment of TURP syndrome: The treatment of TURP syndrome depends on its early detection and the severity of symptoms. The patients should be closely monitored for TURP syndrome. Investigations should be done immediately to evaluate the severity of TURP syndrome. Electrocardiogram (ECG) should be done immediately. Blood glucose, urea, creatinine, glycine, ammonia, and electrolyte level (mainly Na^+) should be evaluated immediately. Fluid overload is managed by the restriction of fluid and IV administration of furosemide. *Hyponatremia* should be corrected to prevent its CNS manifestations with *hypertonic saline solution (3% or 5%)* in patients with normal renal function. The amount

TABLE 2: Signs and symptoms of hyponatremia.

Serum Na⁺ level	Manifestations
Between 125–135 mEq/L	Usually asymptomatic or mild symptoms, such as nausea, vomiting, and weakness
Below 120–125 mEq/L	Lethargy, confusion, etc.
Below 120 mEq/L	Ventricular fibrillation, seizure, coma, and death

and the rate of infusion of this hypertonic saline solution to correct hyponatremia to a safe level, patient's plasma concentration of Na^+ should be measured frequently. In patients with renal failure, *dialysis* should be started. Hyponatremia creates acute hypotonicity and in such circumstances, our aim should be to shift the fluid from intracellular compartment to extracellular compartment. This will help to decrease cerebral edema. But, one should be careful that rapid correction of hyponatremia may cause circulatory overload, cerebral hemorrhage, or cerebral demyelination. The rate at which hypertonic saline solution is given should not be >100 mL/hour and the requirement for the amount of hypertonic saline solution depends on the level of hyponatremia **(Table 2)**.

The seizure activity due to hyponatremia can be corrected by diazepam (2–5 mg), or midazolam (2–4 mg), or thiopentone (75–100 mg), or phenytoin (10–20 mg/kg) by their slow IV administration. Lasix may be given to correct fluid overload. Transient blindness may evaluated by an ophthalmologist, but it is usually self-limiting. Hyperglycemia and hyperammonemia do not require any specific treatment. Hypoxemia should be avoided at any cost. Endotracheal (ET) intubation may be advised in very severe cases with coma, mainly to avoid aspiration and to maintain SPO_2.

The dreaded complications of TURP syndrome may be avoided by decreasing the time for prostate resection (maximum 1 hour), by consultation with surgeon. The procedure should be performed under spinal anesthesia rather than GA for early detection and management of symptoms. Hypotension due to spinal anesthesia *should not be corrected* with large volume of hypotonic IV fluid, instead vasopressors should be used. The 0.9% saline solution is considered the best for IV infusion during TURP.

Bladder Rupture or Perforation

Bladder rupture or perforation may be caused by over-distention of bladder with irrigating fluid or by direct injury to bladder wall by fiberoptic resectoscope. In most of the cases, this perforation of bladder is *extraperitoneal* and an *awake patient* complains of supra- or retropubic, inguinal or periumbilical pain, accompanied by diaphoresis, nausea, and vomiting, etc. The poor return of irrigating fluid during surgical procedure signals the extraperitoneal perforation of bladder. In awake patient, the *intraperitoneal perforation* of bladder presents with hypotension, bradycardia, generalized abdominal pain, and acute abdominal symptoms. In *anesthetized patient* (general or regional), the sudden acute hypotension and vagally-mediated bradycardia are the most important signals for the perforation or rupture of bladder.

Hemorrhage and Coagulopathy

Diffuse uncontrollable bleeding is often seen during TURP and is sought to manage aggressively. This uncontrollable bleeding may be due to the development of coagulopathy. The causes for this coagulopathy are (i) During TURP, thromboplastin is released from prostate and enters into the circulation and causes disseminated intravascular coagulopathy (DIC) leading to nonstop bleeding. (ii) The absorption of irrigating fluid often causes the dilutional thrombocytopenia and excessive bleeding. (iii) Primary fibrinolysis, caused by the metastatic carcinoma of prostate due to the release of fibrinolytic enzymes from cancer cells, causes the coagulopathy and hence profuse hemorrhage. Laboratory tests confirm this diagnosis of DIC, or any other coagulopathy and the help of a hematologist is also sought for. Heparin, replacement of clotting factors, and infusion of platelets are used to treat DIC. Primary fibrinolysis is treated with epsilon-aminocaproic acid (EACA) in the dose of 5 g stat through IV and is repeated at the dose of 1 g/hour through IV.

Bacteremia and Septicemia

The prostate is a common site for bacterial colonization and chronic infection. The opening up of the prostatic venous sinuses and the surgical procedure on prostate causes these bacteria to escape into the circulation leading to bacteremia and septicemia. Even, septic shock may result, if this bacteremia is neglected. Fever, rigor, and tachycardia are the common symptoms of this bacteremia and septicemia. The antibiotics like third- or fourth-generation cephalosporin, piperacillin, levofloxacin, gentamycin, etc., preferred by most surgeons are prophylactically given before TURP to avoid this complication.

Hypothermia

(i) The large volume of irrigating fluids used for TURP and (ii) the large volume of intravenous fluids given to correct the hypotension of spinal or epidural anesthesia at room temperature causes acute hypothermia. This often leads to the rigor during postoperative period. But, this should be avoided at any cost because it may dislodge the hemostatic clots at the resection site that is formed and thus will increase the chances of acute postoperative hemorrhage. Hence, all the fluids, whether irrigating or intravenous, should be heated to body temperature before their use to prevent hypothermia.

■ LITHOTRIPSY

Within these past few years, the treatment of kidney, ureter, and bladder stone has been changed drastically from open surgical procedures to less invasive procedures to noninvasive procedures. These *less invasive procedures* are intracorporeal shock wave lithotripsy (laser and electromagnetic), percutaneous, and laparoscopic nephrolithotomy. The *noninvasive procedures* are cystoscopy, flexible ureteroscopy, medical expulsive therapy (MET), and extracorporeal shock wave lithotripsy (ESWL). The less invasive surgical procedures are applied for the larger and impacted stones. The noninvasive procedures are applied for the stones of 4 mm to 2 cm in diameter.

In shock wave lithotripsy (intracorporeal or extracorporeal), the high energy shock waves (sound waves) are generated and focused on the stone, causing it to be fragmented. For this generation of high energy shock waves in ESWL, the *electrohydraulic, electromagnetic,* or *piezoelectric methods* are used. For the generation of shock waves in *intracorporeal lithotripsy,* the *laser and electromagnetic methods* are used. These shock wave generators are enclosed in a water-filled casing (container) and comes in contact with the patient via a conducting gel on a plastic membrane.

During ESWL, with older electrohydraulic unit, the patient is placed in a hydraulic chair and immersed in a heated water bath which conducts the shock waves to the patient. The modern lithotripters (shock wave generators) generate shock waves either *electromagnetically or from piezoelectric crystals.* In *electromagnetic machine,* the vibration of a metallic plate in front of an electromagnet produces the shock waves. In *piezoelectric machine,* the change in the external dimensions of some ceramic crystals with the application of electric current result in the generation of shock waves.

After focusing the shock waves on stone, the change in the acoustic impedance at tissue-stone interface creates the shear and tear forces on the stone, fragmenting it sufficiently to allow its passage in small pieces down the urinary tract. Ureteral stents are often placed prior to the procedure. The contraindications to the lithotripsy procedure or ESWL include (i) the inability to position the patient, so that lung and intestine are away from the focus of shock (sound) waves,

(ii) urinary obstruction below the stone, (iii) untreated infection, (iv) a bleeding diathesis, and (v) pregnancy. The presence of nearby aortic aneurysm or an orthopedic prosthetic device is a relative contraindication.

Indications of Lithotripsy

Stones in urinary bladder and in the lower part of ureters are removed by intracorporeal lithotripsy. This intracorporeal lithotripsy may be laser lithotripsy or electrohydraulic lithotripsy. The intracorporeal laser lithotripsy uses a holmium-YAG laser. Stones in the upper part of the ureters and kidney are removed by ESWL or percutaneous nephrolithotomy. Percutaneous nephrolithotomy is used to remove big (>2 cm), impacted, and hard stones such as cysteine stones, uric acid stones, and calcium oxalate monohydrate stones. It is similar to ureteroscopy and the approach is through percutaneous sheath over kidney with the patient in prone position.

Mechanism of Lithotripsy

Extracorporeal shock wave lithotripsy comprises a lithotripter. A lithotripter has (i) a spark plug, which is the energy or shockwave generator; (ii) a reflector; (iii) a concentrator; and (iv) either a fluoroscope or a ultrasonogram for viewing the stone. A water bath or a conducting gel attaches the generator to the patient. The spark plug produces the waves of energy repeatedly and this energy vaporizes the water in water bath, thus creates an external shock wave (sound waves) there. As the acoustic density of tissue and water is same, then these shock waves travel from the water bath into the tissue of patient's body, without any damage to the tissue or loss of energy. When these extracorporeal shock waves meet a stone, then this acoustic density changes (between the tissues and stone) and energy is released. As these shock waves pass through the stone and leaves it to enter the tissue again, then the energy is released again. This double power (energy) breaks the stone into fragments and then the small pieces are washed down the urinary tract. Ureteral stents placed preoperatively with the help of a cystoscope allows larger stones to pass through without damaging the tissue.

There are three types of shock wave generators used in ESWL **(Table 3)**. In older electrohydraulic lithotripters, the patient is submerged in a hot water bath placed on a hydraulic chair. The patient was so placed in this hydraulic water bath with the help of two image intensifiers, that an underwater spark plug (energy generator) was the first focus of an elliptical reflector, while the stone was the second focus. Modern lithotripters generate energy using electromagnetic waves or from piezoelectric crystals.

TABLE 3: Extracorporeal shock wave generator used in extracorporeal shock wave lithotripsy (ESWL).

Type	Model
Electrohydraulic generator • With tube • Tubeless	 • Dornier HM3 • Dornier MFL5000
Electromagnetic generator	Dornier Doli, Compact Delta, Sigma, Siemens, Lithostar, Storz Modulith
Piezoelectric generator	Wolf Piezolith

In electromagnetic energy generators, a metallic plate is placed in front of an electromagnet, the vibration of which produces shock waves. In piezoelectric lithotripters electric current is passed through ceramic crystals and shock waves are produced when their external dimensions change. Both the electromagnetic and the piezoelectric generators are put in a case, filled with water and a plastic membrane or conducting gel couples it to the patient. These newer lithotripters have facilities for both ultrasonography and fluoroscopy for the localization of stones.

Anesthesia for Lithotripsy

Anesthetic consideration for cystoscopy guided bladder stone removal, ureteroscopy, stone manipulation, and laser lithotripsy, etc. is similar to that (anesthetic consideration) for cystoscopic procedures described earlier. Only the ESWL requires special consideration, particularly when the older lithotripters requiring the patient to be immersed in water are used.

Extracorporeal shock wave lithotripsy by an older electrohydraulic lithotripter using warm water bath (36–37°C) was painful. Because, in these older electrohydraulic lithotripter high voltage (high intensity) shock waves were required to pass through the patient and the pain is felt from the dissipation of the small amount of energy from skin when the shock waves enter the body through skin. The pain is therefore localized to the skin and is proportional to the shock wave intensity. So, the regional or general anesthesia was preferred for this older ESWL lithotripsy. Now, the newer ESWL lithotripters use low voltage (low intensity) shock waves. These are coupled directly to the skin and are painless and can be performed even with light sedation.

Continuous epidural anesthesia for ESWL was the procedure of choice for most of the anesthesiologists previously. Kidney is supplied between T_{10} and L_2 spinal segment. So, a sensory block up to T_6 level was sufficient for ESWL. Fentanyl can be used epidurally for better analgesia. Light intravenous sedation with oxygen supplementation through a face mask or nasal catheter also can be given.

During the insertion of epidural needle and catheter for continuous epidural anesthesia, air should not be put into the epidural space (for testing the loss-of-resistance feeling). Instead, saline should be used. Because, air in the epidural space can dissipate the shock waves and may promote injury to the neural tissue. Further, foam tapes should be avoided for the fixing of (to secure) epidural catheter, as this type of tapes will dissipate the energy, when the shock waves will come in their path causing tissue damage.

Instead of epidural as the regional block the spinal anesthesia can also be used satisfactorily. But, it offers less control over the upper limit of sensory level and is not suitable for an uncertain duration of surgery. Hence, epidural anesthesia is usually preferred for ESWL procedure. Spinal anesthesia for lithotripsy is also avoided, because the postdural puncture headache is common due to the sitting position of patient in hydraulic chair after spinal block. A loading volume of 1,200–1,500 mL of lactated Ringers solution is given to the patient intravenously before-hand to prevent the postural hypotension during the positioning of patient after regional anesthesia. Further, 1,500–2,000 mL of lactated Ringers solution is given along with a diuretic intraoperatively to increase the flow of urine and to wash out the fragmented stone, clots, and debris. However, less and calculated fluid should be given to patients with low cardiac reserve.

In RA, diaphragmatic movement cannot be controlled by anesthetist. Hence, the movement of diaphragm during the spontaneous respiration of patient may move the stone in and away from the direction of shock waves, and thus may prolong the surgical procedure. So, the patient is asked to take shallow breaths, but that is not always practical, especially when light sedation is administered along with RA to calm the patient. Hence, GA is preferred by some anesthesiologists, especially when the electrohydraulic lithotripters with water bath is used.

For GA, the ET intubation with muscle relaxation is preferred, but placing an anesthetized intubated patient on a hydraulic chair and the raising and lowering him to submerge in a water bath carries its own risks. The newer methods of ESWL require low voltage shock waves and can be done under sedation, avoiding all these complications. In most of the cases of new ESWL, propofol infusion with midazolam and some opioid analgesic is often sufficient.

Monitoring is important in ESWL. Standard monitoring is applied for GA, or RA, or conscious sedation, and deep sedation. ECG leads should be attached with some water-proof dressing. Oxygen saturation should be noted and the temperature of water bath is maintained. Pulse and blood pressure monitoring is mandatory for each patient. Still, with R wave synchronized shocks, supraventricular tachycardia may occur. So, anesthetists must be careful.

Complications of Lithotripsy

Placing a patient in a heated water bath (36–37°C) causes vasodilatation and transient hypotension. In water bath, the hydrostatic pressure of water on inferior extremity and abdomen causes the redistribution of the venous blood of this area toward centrally. Thus, the preload is increased and central venous pressure (CVP) and pulmonary capillary wedge pressure (PCWP) is raised. The stroke volume increases, the cardiac output increases, but the heart rate remains the same. Subsequently, the systemic vascular resistance (SVR) rises and the cardiac output falls. This increase in venous return can cause congestive cardiac failure in patients with poor cardiac reserve. Moreover, the increase in intrathoracic blood volume reduces the FRC and may predispose some patients to hypoxemia. Along with the decrease of FRC, the hydrostatic pressure of water on the chest wall of patient also decreases the vital capacity and tidal volume. Thus, the work of respiration is increased.

The shock waves of ESWL can damage the parts of a permanent pacemaker or internal cardiac defibrillator (ICD). Thus, it can precipitates arrhythmia in these patients. If the shock waves are synchronized with the R wave of ECG and better if the shock waves are timed 20 ms (millisecond) after the R wave corresponding with the ventricular refractory period of cardiac cycle, then the arrhythmias may be avoided. However, the multiple studies have shown that asynchronous delivery of shock waves may be safe in patients without heart disease.

Contraindications and Special Considerations of Lithotripsy

Pregnancy is complete contraindication for ESWL. Coagulopathies and anticoagulant therapies are relative contraindications for ESWL. The aortic aneurysms in abdomen, especially with calcification and any orthopedic prosthesis should be kept away from the path of shock waves. An obesity is a problem for ESWL due to mechanical factors. The temperature of water in water bath may affect the body temperature. The lungs and intestine should be kept away from the path of shock waves as air tissue interfaces can dissipate energy and cause tissue damage. Chronic infection and the obstruction of urinary tract below the level of stone is a contraindication for ESWL. Ecchymosis, hematoma, and blistering or the bruising of skin are common at the site of

treatment. The development of perinephric hematoma has also been observed.

 ## ANESTHESIA FOR NONCANCER SURGERIES ON KIDNEY AND UPPER URETER

The surgeries on kidney and upper ureter usually include partial and total nephrectomy, nephrolithotomy, removal of stone from renal pelvis and upper ureter, pyeloplasty, live donor nephrectomy, etc. All these surgical procedures can be approached through transperitoneal and retroperitoneal route and the laparoscopic procedures are increasingly being used for these urological surgeries. Because, laparoscopy provides some advantages over the conventional open surgical procedures and these include less perioperative pain, shorter hospital stay, rapid convalescence, and rapid return to work. Anesthetic management of these patients for laparoscopic procedures is similar to that for other laparoscopic procedures **(Table 4)**.

Open surgical procedures for these abovementioned noncancer surgeries are often carried out in "kidney rest" or lateral flexed position. With full lateral position, the nondependent leg is fully extended and the dependent leg is fully flexed. The operating table is then extended to achieve the maximum separation between the costal margin and iliac crest on operated side. Next, the kidney rest component of operation theater (OT) table is raised to elevate the iliac crest of operated side and to improve the surgical exposure. An axillary rest is placed beneath the dependent part of the upper chest to minimize the risk of brachial plexus injury.

In nonlaparoscopic open surgical procedures, the flexed lateral position of the patient has great implication on its respiratory and cardiovascular system. FRC is reduced in dependent lung, but it increases in nondependent lung. Hence, in anesthetized patient with controlled ventilation, the dependent lung receives lesser ventilation, but receives greater blood flow. On the other hand, the nondependent lung receives greater ventilation, but receives lesser blood flow. Therefore, the lateral position on kidney rest will cause ventilation/perfusion mismatch, increased dead

TABLE 4: Other common surgeries of the genitourinary tract.	
Name of surgery	**Disease**
Laparoscopic procedures	• Pyeloplasty • Partial nephrectomy
Nephrectomy	Renal cancer
Radical prostatectomy	For adenocarcinoma of prostrate
Cystectomy	For bladder cancer
Orchiectomy	For testicular cancer
Renal transplantation	

space ventilation (in nondependent lung), shunt-induced hypoxemia, increased end tidal CO_2 tension, and atelectasis. Extended position of OT table cause venous pooling leading to decrease in preload, and CO and anesthesia-induced hypotension.

The ET tube may be displaced during the positioning of patient in lateral position. So, after the final lateral positioning of patient and prior to skin preparation and surgical draping, the proper position of ET tube should be verified and confirmed. Because of the potential for large blood loss and a limited access to the major blood vessels in lateral flexed position, the intravenous line should be secured properly before the positioning of patient. In lateral position on kidney rest, there is always a chance of pneumothorax as the result of surgical entry into pleural space.

ANESTHESIA FOR SURGERIES OF UROLOGICAL MALIGNANCIES

Following radical surgical resection, the excellent survival rates now have resulted in the increase in the number surgeries for bladder, prostatic, and renal cancer. Now, many surgeries for urological malignancies, e.g., radical prostatectomy, cystectomy, pelvic node dissection, nephrectomy, etc. are also performed by pelvic and abdominal laparoscopic procedure due to the accelerated and less complicated recovery with smaller and less painful incision. Recently, robotic-assisted technology has increasingly been applied to these surgical procedures for urogenital malignancies.

Many urological surgeries for malignancy are performed with the patient in supine and hyperextended position. Because, this position of patient facilitates the exposure of pelvis during pelvic lymph node dissection, retropubic prostatectomy, or cystectomy, etc. For this supine and hyperextended position, the patient is kept in supine with his iliac crest over the break of operating table. Then, the table is gradually extended such that the distance between the subcostal margin and the iliac crest becomes maximum. The operating table is also tilted head down, as if the operative field becomes horizontal.

Bladder Cancer

Preoperative Consideration

Second to prostate adenocarcinoma, the transitional cell carcinoma of bladder is the most common malignancy of male genitourinary tract. The average age for bladder cancer is 60–70 and the male to female ratio is 3:1. There is good correlation between the cigarette smoking and bladder cancer. So, it coexists with coronary artery disease and chronic pulmonary obstructive disease. If the kidney disease coexists with bladder cancer, then it is only due to age related or secondary to urinary tract obstruction. The surgeries which are usually performed for bladder cancer are TURBT, radical cystectomy, urinary diversion, etc. The TURBT is usually done for low grade, noninvasive bladder tumors via cystoscope. Some patients receive preoperative radiation to shrink the tumor before radical cystectomy. Urinary diversion is usually performed immediately following cystectomy.

Intraoperative Consideration

Transurethral resection of bladder tumors: The two important anesthetic implications related to TURBT are (i) In contrast to TURP, the TURBT is more commonly performed under GA and neuromuscular blocked by muscle relaxant. Because, if RA and GA without muscle relaxant are administered, then the use of cautery resectoscope may result in the stimulation of obturator nerve causing the adduction of legs (the laterally located tumors may lie in proximity to obturator nerve). (ii) Unlike TURP, the TURBT is rarely associated with the absorption of significant amounts of irrigating solution.

Radical cystectomy: The surgery radical cystectomy includes (i) the removal of all anterior pelvic organs, (ii) pelvic node dissection, and (iii) urinary diversion. As the anterior pelvic organs in male the bladder, prostate, and seminal vesicles are removed and in female the bladder, uterus, cervix, part of anterior vaginal vault, and ovaries are removed. Radical cystectomy is associated with high perioperative morbidity and mortality, especially in elderly patient population. But, now with the development newer surgical and anesthetic technology, the rate for this morbidity and mortality after radical cystectomy has been reduced. Further, the robot-assisted radical cystectomy is associated with reduced perioperative complications, less blood loss and blood transfusion, and shorter hospital stay.

General anesthesia with ET intubation and use of muscle relaxant provides optimal operating conditions. The duration of radical cystectomy may vary from 6 to 8 hours according to centers and surgical skill. In extreme good centers, this duration for radical cystectomy may come down to 4 hours and blood transfusion is frequently utilized. Controlled hypotensive anesthesia is frequently shouted for radical cystectomy. Because, it reduces blood loss, reduces transfusion requirement and improves surgical visualization. But, the reduction of mean arterial pressure (MAP) below 70–65 mm Hg is frequently associated with increased risk of acute kidney injury and stroke.

Continuous epidural anesthesia can also be choiced for radical cystectomy. Because, it will provide induced hypotension, will decrease general anesthetic requirements and will facilitate postoperative analgesia. Using noninvasive cardiac output monitoring, optimized intraoperative fluid administration may decrease blood transfusion, postoperative complications, and hospital stay. As it is a major surgery and is usually performed on elderly patients, so all vital monitorings are provided. Like all lengthy operative procedures, here the risk of hypothermia is also minimized by the use of forced air warming blanket and intravenous fluid warming.

Urinary diversion: Following radical cystectomy, urinary diversion is usually performed immediately. Urinary diversion means implanting the ureters into a segment of bowel. The selected segment of bowel is either left in situ such as in ureterosigmoidostomy or the segment of bowel is divided with intact blood supply through mesentery and is attached to a cutaneous stoma or urethra.

During this urinary diversion, the aim of an anesthetist should be the patient will be well hydrated, but the urine output will be low (brisk) once the ureters are opened. Plus, if RA is provided, then unopposed parasympathetic activity, due to sympathetic blocked, will produce contracted, hyperactive bowel that makes urinary diversion into bowel difficult. Administration of glycopyrrolate and papaverine may solve this problem. Significant metabolic disturbances may be produced due to prolonged contact of urine with bowel mucosa after urinary diversion into bowel. When the ureters are transplanted in jejunum, then hyponatremia, hypochloremia, hyperkalemia, and metabolic acidosis occur. On the other hand, when the ureters are implanted in ileum and colon, then hyperchloremic metabolic acidosis occurs. However, the use of temporary ureteral stents and the maintenance of high urinary output will help to alleviate this problem during early postoperative period.

Prostatic Cancer

Preoperative Considerations

The most common carcinoma of prostate is adenocarcinoma. After lung cancer, prostate cancer is the second most common cause of cancer death in men older than 60 years. The extensiveness of surgeries for prostate cancer varies from (i) simple taking transrectal ultrasound (USG)-guided biopsy from prostate to (ii) cryoablation to (iii) radical prostatectomy with lymph node dissection to (iv) salvage prostatectomy following failure of radiation therapy to (v) bilateral orchiectomy for hormonal therapy. The type of surgery depends on the age of patient, the grade and stage of malignancy, the concentration of prostate specific antigen (PSA), and the presence of medical comorbidity. The staging of prostate cancer is based on the Gleason score of biopsy specimen and the migration of tumor cells determined by MRI and bone scan.

Intraoperative Consideration

Here, we will only discuss the anesthetic implication of radical prostatectomy with pelvic lymph node dissection. The radical prostatectomy is usually performed through retropubic route and it may be open or robot-assisted laparoscopic.

Open radical retropubic prostatectomy: It can be performed both under GA and continuous epidural anesthesia under deep sedation. But, GA is always preferred. Because, patients typically do not tolerate RA without deep sedation as this operation is always performed in supine hyperextended Trendelenburg position. If RA is selected, it requires sensory block up to T6 level. The open radical retropubic prostatectomy is usually performed along with pelvic node dissection. For this purpose, a lower midline abdominal incision is given and en block prostate is removed along with seminal vesicle, ejaculatory ducts, and a part of bladder neck. Following bladder neck removal, the remaining portion of bladder is anastomosed directly with urethra over an indwelling urinary catheter. Then, surgeons usually ask anesthetists to administer indigo carmine intravenously to visualize the ureters and this dye always cause hypertension or hypotension.

This extensive surgical procedure is always associated with significant intraoperative blood loss and transfusion of blood. However, the amount of this intraoperative blood loss varies considerably from case to case and from center to center, with mean value ranging between 500 and 700 mL to 1,000 mL. Because, the factors influencing blood loss include the size of prostate, the duration of surgery, the skill of surgeon, and others. All the vital monitors are employed for the monitoring of these patients. Most centers use direct arterial blood pressure monitoring and CVP monitoring. Other centers routinely use noninvasive cardiac output monitoring (FloTrac or LiDCO). The risk of hypothermia should be minimized by utilizing a forced air warming blanket and an intravenous fluid warmer.

To enhance recovery, the postoperative care should be standard varying according to coexisting medical disease. The important postoperative complications following this open radical prostatectomy with pelvic node dissection are hemorrhage, deep vein thrombosis (DVT), obturator nerve injury, urinary incontinence and impotence, injury to rectum and ureter, etc. To prevent DVT, warfarin or fractionated heparin is used routinely. Extensive surgical dissection around the pelvic veins increases the risk for intraoperative venous air embolism and postoperative thromboembolic complications. For postoperative analgesia, standard protocol led by each institution should be followed.

Robot-assisted laparoscopic radical prostatectomy: Like open radical prostatectomy, the laparoscopic prostatectomy is usually also accompanied with pelvic lymph node dissection. In most of the developed countries, now these laparoscopic prostatectomies with pelvic node dissection are performed by robotic assistance. Most of these laparoscopic surgeries are performed in steep (>30°) Trendelenburg position of patient. Therefore, this steep Trendelenburg position of patient, duration of surgery, abdominal distention due to inflation of gas, and desirability to increase minute ventilation to prevent hypoxia, etc. dictate to use GA with ET intubation and muscle relaxant as routine. Continuous epidural can be added with GA to reduce the doses of general anesthetic agents and postoperative analgesia. RA alone is not decided for this type of surgery. During GA, the N_2O is usually avoided to prevent bowel distention. When compared to open retropubic radical prostatectomy, the advantages of robot-assisted laparoscopic radical prostatectomy are (i) though it is associated with longer surgical time, but it causes less blood loss and fewer blood transfusions, (ii) it causes lower postoperative pain score and lower opioid requirement, (iii) it is associated with less postoperative nausea and vomiting, and (iv) it causes shorter hospital stay.

Intraoperative monitoring during surgery and post-operative monitoring, and postoperative analgesia after robot-assisted radical laparoscopic prostatectomy is similar to that of open radical prostatectomy and according to institutional protocol. But, postoperative epidural analgesia is not so warranted, because of relatively low postoperative pain scores and because patients may be discharged 24 hours after surgery. Some complications which are special for these type of surgeries are (i) the steep Trendelenburg position of patient maintained for prolonged period leads to head and neck tissue edema and increased intraocular pressure, (ii) upper airway edema and postextubation respiratory distress, (iii) postoperative visual loss involving ischemic optic neuropathy or retinal detachment, and (iv) brachial plexus injury, etc. From time to time, surgeon should be alarmed about the length of time during which this steep Trendelenburg position of patient is maintained.

Kidney Cancer

Preoperative Considerations

Renal cell carcinoma is the most common (90%) cancer of all kidney cancers. About 9 out of 10 kidney cancers are RCC. It is also called renal cell cancer or renal cell adenocarcinoma. Its peak incidence is in between fifth and sixth decade of life

and 2:1 is its male to female ratio. Most of the time, it remains as asymptomatic. It becomes symptomatic when the tumor grows to a considerable size and the classical symptoms (classical triad) are hematuria, pain, and palpable mass. Commonly, it is discovered accidentally during the course of investigation for other unrelated medical problems, for example during MRI performed for evaluation of back pain.

Renal cell carcinoma is frequently associated with erythrocytosis, hypercalcemia, hypertension, and non-metastatic hepatic dysfunction and these are together called paraneoplastic syndrome. One peculiarity of RCC is that the tumor cells extend into renal vein and subsequently into inferior vena cava (IVC) as thrombus. In extreme cases, this thrombus of tumor cells extends into right atrium through IVC. According to this extension of tumor cells along the venous line, Mayo has classified the venous thrombus invasion of RCC into four levels.

Tumors confined to kidney only are treated by open or laparoscopic partial or total nephrectomy or by percutaneous cryoablation or by radiofrequency ablation. Tumors extending out of kidney are treated by palliative surgery (debulking of mass). Before any plan for surgery, staging of renal tumor by CT and MRI scan and arteriogram is mandatory.

The preoperative anesthetic evaluation of patient before the surgery of kidney cancer include (i) tumor staging, (ii) kidney function tests, and (iii) tests according to coexisting systemic diseases. Preexisting kidney function impairment depends upon the tumor size of affected kidney and coexisting systemic disorders such as hypertension, diabetes, ischemic heart disease (IHD), etc. For RCC, smoking is an important predisposing factor. Hence, these patients have high incidences of underlying coronary artery disease and chronic obstructive pulmonary disease.

Intraoperative Considerations

Radical nephrectomy: In radical nephrectomy, the kidney, adrenal gland, and perinephric fat are removed en block with their surrounding fascia (fascia Gerota). For this surgery, most of the time GA with ET intubation and muscle relaxant in combination with continuous epidural block are used. Operation is carried out via an anterior subcostal, flank, and midline incision (rarely). So, patient is positioned according to this incision. Some centers also utilized thoracoabdominal approach, particularly for larger tumors and when tumor thrombus is present.

These tumors of RCC become very vascular. So, the surgeries on RCC have great potential for huge blood loss. Hence, anesthetist must be sure of an intravenous line and blood transfusion. Radical nephrectomy for large tumor and tumor thrombus extension need extensive monitoring by indwelling peripheral arterial catheter, transesophageal echocardiography (TEE), esophageal Doppler, or peripheral pulse wave analysis (FloTrac/Vigileo). Because of the potential for acute kidney injury and postoperative kidney dysfunction of contralateral kidney by reflex vasoconstriction, intraoperative hypotension is not induced or if is needed, it is induced only for a brief period to reduce blood loss. Hypothermia should be avoided by monitoring core temperature, warming intravenous fluid, and using forced air warming blanket. For open nephrectomy, the subcostal, flank, or midline incisions are very painful. So, in such circumstances, epidural analgesia is very helpful and accelerates convalescence.

Radical nephrectomy with excision of tumor thrombus: Here, though there is extensive metastasis of tumor cells as a thrombus along the venous line, still surgery significantly prolongs and improves the quality of life. Because, this metastasis regresses after the resection of primary tumor. A preoperative TEE is done to determine the uppermost margin of the extension of tumor thrombus, i.e., if the uppermost margin of the tumor thrombus extends up to the diaphragm, or above the diaphragm, or into the right atrium, or cross the tricuspid valve. A preoperative ventilation-perfusion scan is also done to detect any preexisting pulmonary embolization of tumor thrombus. An increased CVP is typical with significant venous obstruction.

Anesthetic management of this surgery is actually challenging. Because, there is a great potential for major blood loss, associated with this operation. The complete obstruction of IVC by tumor thrombus will also markedly increase the intraoperative blood loss, because there are dilated venous collaterals around the primary tumor. Plus, the presence of large thrombus (level II, level III, and level IV) complicates the anesthetic management. Hence, the problems associated with massive blood transfusion should be anticipated and all the measures related to it have to be taken. Central venous catheterization should be performed cautiously to prevent the dislodgment and embolization of tumor thrombus.

There is high risk of catastrophic intraoperative pulmonary embolization of tumor and this is heralded by sudden supraventricular arrhythmias, arterial hypoxemia, and profound hypotension. All these can be diagnosed by intraoperative TEE. In this surgery, cardiopulmonary bypass should be ready for use, if the surgeon fails to pull back the tumor thrombus from right atrium into vena cava. In such situation, heparinization and hypothermia will further increase surgical blood loss.

Day-case Anesthesia

INTRODUCTION

The day-case anesthesia is also termed as "the outpatient anesthesia" or "ambulatory anesthesia". This day-case or outpatient or ambulatory anesthesia is the subspecialty of anesthesiology that deals with the preoperative, intraoperative, and postoperative anesthetic care of patients undergoing (i) admission, (ii) same day surgical procedure under anesthesia, and (iii) discharge from the surgical unit within 24 hours after this surgical and anesthetic procedure. *Office-based anesthesia* refers to the delivery of anesthesia in a practitioner's chamber that has a procedural suit incorporated into its design. Office-based anesthesia is frequently administered to patients undergoing cosmetic surgery or dental procedure.

Over the last few decades, the day-case surgery and according to the need of this day-case surgery, the day-case anesthesia has also grown up at an exponential rate. It is mainly (i) due to the major development of sophisticated surgical equipment advocating more and more minimal invasive surgery and (ii) due to the development of newer ultrashort-acting anesthetic drugs which help in quick recovery. A day-case (or an outpatient) surgery and anesthesia is one which is performed on a patient who is admitted only (i) for the investigation under anesthesia, (ii) for the minor examination under anesthesia, (iii) for the operation on a planned nonresident basis, and (iv) who nonetheless requires any overnight indoor facilities for recovery.

Today, almost 60% of all the elective surgeries and anesthesia are performed at the day-case (outpatient) surgical and anesthesia setting unit in the form of general anesthesia (GA), local anesthesia (LA), or monitored anesthetic care (MAC). In USA and UK, over 80% of all the elective surgeries are performed as an outpatient (day case) basis and this is likely to increase more and more in near future, in response to the economic pressures on healthcare market.

For day-case surgery and anesthesia, while the surgical procedure is same, but the anesthesia and the nursing care are significantly different one, if the same is performed at the inpatient setting. In day-case surgical unit, the anesthesiologists are mainly responsible for evaluating, screening, informing, and preparing the patients both by physiologically and psychologically. Specialized skills are required for this day-case anesthesia, because the patients are discharged to their home soon after their operation.

So, at conclusion, we may say that to achieve a pain-free ambulatory day-case patient, it requires a skillful patient selection criteria, experienced anesthetists, and skilled surgeons working coordinately in a day-case surgery and anesthesia unit. The day-case surgery and anesthesia unit is also termed as "the cost-effective quality care unit." This is because, the costs for anesthesia and surgical procedures are much less in such setting than when the same procedure is performed as the inpatient setting without sacrificing quality. The costs in a day-case anesthesia unit can be minimized without sacrificing quality by (i) the proper preoperative screening, (ii) the unnecessary cancellation of surgery, (iii) decreasing the room turn over times, (iv) decreasing the stays in postanesthesia care unit (PACU), and (v) reducing the unanticipated readmission and staffing.

The cost of surgery and anesthesia as day-case basis has been estimated to be about 25–75% less than the similar inpatient procedures. The day-case surgery and anesthesia also offers a wide variety of other advantages to all the parties involving patients, surgeons, and insurance companies. Patients and their relatives experience less disruption to their personal lives and can rapidly return to their daily activities. Patients are also able to recover at home in familiar surroundings. Thus, it provides an additional psychological benefit. There is also a reduced risk of complications such as wound infections (from other patients), deep venous thrombosis, pulmonary embolism, paralytic ileus, and pneumonia (nosocomial), etc.

PATIENT SELECTION

The selection of patients for day-case surgery and anesthesia is the most important point, if the maximum use of resources and the smooth running of a day-case unit is to be made. Only, the proper preanesthetic planning will minimize (i) the unexpected cancellation of surgery or (ii) unnecessary postoperative readmissions. It will also allow for easy access to the department of inpatient services of the day-case individual when necessary due to emergency. The *selection criteria of patients* for day-case anesthesia and surgery should include (i) the overall medical health of the patient [American Society of Anesthesiologists (ASA) physical status], (ii) the age of the patient, (iii) social factors, (v) the extensiveness of surgical procedure, (vi) the limitations of surgical facility, and (vii) the limitations of healthcare providers.

Normally, the patients of ASA I and II status included in the day-case surgical and anesthesia unit. For example: (i) normal healthy patient with or without minor systemic diseases, not interfering with the surgical and anesthetic procedures or (ii) medical conditions that are well controlled by previous therapy such as the hypertension or noninsulin-dependent diabetes, etc. But, gradually the increasing numbers of medically stable ASA III patients are now included in the day-case surgical and anesthesia unit, (i) due to the use of more and more local and topical anesthesia and (ii) due to the more and more use of minimally invasive (endoscopic) surgical procedures.

Also it is important to notice that some ASA III patients do better in a day-case environment, rather than an inpatient environment, e.g., chemotherapy patients, stable diabetics, etc. But patients with significant cardiovascular or respiratory diseases, insulin-dependent diabetes or those with gross obesity, etc. are not suitable for day-case anesthesia. The stable asthmatics are suitable for day-case surgery and anesthesia. Whereas, the frequent hospitalization, oral steroid therapy, and poor control of symptoms in bronchial asthma suggest the unsuitability of these patients for day-case unit. The stable epileptics on medications are suitable for day-case surgery and anesthesia, but propofol should be avoided, if they have a driving license. Undiagnosed hypertensive disease and uncontrolled atrial fibrillation should be re-evaluated on the day of surgery and anesthesia for their suitability as day case.

Recently in USA, the patients of status ASA IV are also included in the day-case surgery and anesthesia. It is based on the findings that (i) there is no obvious relationship between the ASA physical status and the rate of major morbidity or mortality after day-case surgery and anesthesia, (ii) It is also found that those with preexisting disease have the same

> **BOX 1:** Common day-case surgical procedures.
>
> - *General surgery:* Superficial biopsy, abscess drainage, hernia repair, hemorrhoidectomy, laparoscopic cholecystectomy, varicose vein surgery, anal fistula repair, muscle biopsy, etc.
> - *Gynecology:* Superficial biopsy, dilatation and curettage, tubal ligation, polypectomy, hysteroscopy, and Bartholin cystectomy.
> - *Orthopedics:* Close reduction, biopsy, arthroscopy, anterior cruciate ligament repair, amputation, carpal tunnel release, excision of ganglion, removal of screw and plate, etc.
> - *Urology:* Circumcision, orchidectomy, cystoscopy, lithotripsy, prostate biopsy, orchidopexy, urethral dilatation, etc.
> - *Ophthalmology:* Cataract extraction, squint surgery, enucleation, ptosis surgery, chalazion excision, pterygium, etc.
> - *ENT:* Tonsillectomy, adenoidectomy, tympanoplasty, rhinoplasty, polypectomy, myringotomy, mastoidectomy, removal of foreign body, etc.
> - *Plastic surgery:* Cleft lip repair, skin graft, scar excision, basal cell cancer excision, mammoplasty, etc.
> - *Miscellaneous:* Angioplasty, laser treatment, esophageal dilatation, bone marrow aspiration, and lumbar puncture.

complication rate as healthy patients, (iii) There is also no significant relationship between the effect for preexisting disease and the incidences of perioperative complications in the day-case surgery and anesthesia, (iv) Major morbidity occurs less often in the day-case surgical population than in the age and gender-matched population, not having the day-case surgery and anesthesia. So, now a wide variety of surgical and anesthetic procedures can be performed as day-case basis **(Box 1)**.

Ultimately, the surgeon and anesthesia provider will identify the patients for whom the day-case surgery and anesthesia is likely to provide benefits (e.g., convenience, reduced costs, and charges, etc.) that outweigh the risks (e.g., the lack of immediate availability of all hospital indoor services during any emergency). Factors considered in selecting the patients for day-case anesthetic procedure include (i) present systemic illness and their current management, (ii) airway management problems, (iii) sleep apnea, (iv) morbid obesity, (v) previous adverse anesthetic outcomes, (vi) allergies, and (vii) patient's social network (availability of someone to be responsive to the patient in any emergency). Patient with difficult airways should probably not be a candidate for office-based surgical and anesthetic procedures. Because, they may be appropriately cared for in a well-equipped and fully staffed ambulatory/outpatient surgery center. The important considerations for such patients include the availability of difficult airway equipment such as an intubating laryngeal mask airway and video laryngoscope, the availability of additional experienced anesthesia providers, and someone capable of performing emergency tracheostomy/cricothyroidotomy.

An anesthesiologist must know which preexisting medical conditions may precipitate specific intraoperative or postoperative adverse events for that patient. Likewise, anesthetic procedures suitable for ambulatory surgery should have (i) a minimal risk of perioperative hemorrhage, (ii) airway compromise, and (iii) no particular requirement for specialized postoperative care. Based on risk identification, the anesthetist should be able to reduce the likelihood of unforeseen adverse events and smooth functioning of outpatient anesthetic unit.

The duration of surgical procedure also has no impact on day-case surgical and anesthesia unit, as long as the postoperative physiological impairment of patient is at an acceptable level. There is great controversy on correlation between the duration of surgical procedure and anesthesia with its recovery time. In one study, it is found that there is no correlation between the duration of anesthesia and the recovery time. In another study, longer anesthetic procedure is associated with longer recovery time and higher incidence of postoperative nausea and vomiting (PONV) necessitating patient's readmission in hospital and overnight observation. So, the general rule is that operations lasting for >60–90 minutes and those are associated with increased risk of postoperative pain, hemorrhage, excessive fluid shifts, and prolonged immobility, should not be performed in day-case unit. However, recently many oral, plastic, general, gynecological, and orthopedic surgical procedures lasting for 2–4 hours are now being routinely performed successfully in many day-case surgical and anesthetic unit in USA.

Some day-case surgical and anesthetic centers question about the extremes of age (<6 months and >70 years) for the selection of their patients. The causes are being (i) the recovery of the fine motor and cognitive functions are slower in older patients and (ii) the preterm infants who are <48 weeks of postconceptual age are at an increased risk for apneic episodes after anesthesia. But, the age alone should not be considered as a deterrent factor for the selection of patients for day-case surgery and anesthesia.

Still, the infants <60 weeks postconceptual age (gestational plus postnatal age) should not be considered suitable for the day-case surgery and anesthesia and postanesthetic apnea monitoring for at least 12–24 hours has been recommended for them. However, now, in many centers of developed countries, there is no upper age limit for day-case anesthesia. Because, there physiological fitness for surgery and anesthesia is considered first rather than the chronological age. This is based on the findings that there is no increase in morbidity with increasing age, when only the age factor is considered.

However, special attention must be paid to the *discharge criteria* for that group of patient from day-case unit, because recovery of fine motor function and cognitive skills, following GA or sedation is slower in the elderly. Children are usually well suited for the day-case surgery and anesthesia unit. This is because those who are treated on a same day basis have less psychological disturbances than those who are admitted on the day before and discharged on the day after the surgery.

In some day-care surgical and anesthetic units, the severely obese patients are not selected. The upper limit of body mass index (BMI) for day-case anesthesia is 30–34 [BMI = weight (in kg)/height in meter^2]. Moderate obesity itself does not preclude them from day-case surgery and anesthesia, but does cause unpredictable problems in terms of the length of surgery and anesthesia. BMI alone is not always considered as the ideal tool for assessing the fitness for day-care surgery and anesthesia.

Obese patients in a day-case unit should be scheduled for surgery at mid-morning which will allow the time for preoperative antacid therapy to work and will also allow adequate time for recovery. It will also have to remember that obesity may cause many problems to the surgeons or anesthetist which will force them to treat these patients as indoor basis.

A limit is also set for the distance from the hospital to the patient's home during the selection of patients for day-case anesthesia and surgery. A responsible adult must be present at home with the patient during the first 24 hours after day-case surgery and anesthesia. All the patients must be escorted to home during the postoperative period by a responsible and a well-informed adult. All the patients should be adequately supervised during their recovery at home for a minimum period of 24 hours. Similarly, all the patients must have suitable home conditions with adequate toilet facility and a telephone for advice during an emergency. The patient should also live within 1 hour traveling distance from the hospital.

Patients with obstructive sleep apnea (OSA) are at increased risk of postoperative respiratory complications such as prolonged airway obstruction and apnea, particularly if they receive opioids postoperatively. The identification and assessment of OSA, which is described below, for predicting the probability of these complications can aid in the preoperative assessment. An anesthesiologist may be the first physician to detect the presence or risk of sleep apnea. The preoperative initiation of continuous positive airway pressure (CPAP) may reduce the incidence of postoperative cardiac complications. The avoidance of respiratory depression by the use of opioid sparing multimodal analgesia, neuraxial, and regional anesthetic technique is likewise suggested when appropriate.

In addition to usual discharge criteria, the ASA also recommends that the patients at increased risk of OSA not

BOX 2: Identification and assessment of obstructive sleep apnea (OSA) by clinical signs and symptoms.

- *Physical characteristics:*
  - BMI is >35 kg/m^2
  - Neck circumference is >17 inches
  - Presence of anatomical nasal obstruction
  - Tonsils nearly touching the midline
- *Airway obstruction during sleep:*
  - Frequent snoring
  - Pauses in breathing during sleep
  - Awakens from sleep with chocking sensation
  - Frequent arousals from sleep
- *Somnolence (sleepiness):*
  - Frequent fatigue and sleepiness, despite adequate sleep
  - Falls asleep easily in a nonstimulating condition such as watching TV, reading, etc.

If a patient has signs and symptoms in two or more of the above categories, then there is significant probability of moderate OSA. If one or more of the above-mentioned signs and symptoms is severely abnormal, then there is probability of severe OSA.

Actually, *OSA scoring* is done by apnea and hypopnea index (AHI). (i) AHI 0–5 = no OSA, (ii) AHI 6–20 = mild OSA, (iii) AHI 21–40 = moderate OSA, and (iv) AHI >40 = severe OSA

to be discharged to an unmonitored setting, until they are no longer at risk for perioperative respiratory depression. The identification and assessment of obstructive sleep apnea (OSA) by clinical signs and symptoms are described in **Box 2**. These ASA recommendations are (i) Return of SpO$_2$ to base-line level when breathing room air prior to discharge, (ii) Observation of respiratory function in unstimulated patient such as when sleeping, (iii) If frequently hypoxia is developed postoperatively, then noninvasive positive pressure ventilation (NIPPV) such as CPAP is considered, and (iv) Prolonged postoperative observation to ensure that the patient with OSA are not at increased risk from postoperative respiratory depression compared with non-OSA patient.

STOP–BANG questionnaire for screening of patients to determine the risk of OSA

S = Snoring. Does the patient snore loudly?
T = Tiredness. Does the patient feel sleepy during daytime?
O = Observed apnea. If anybody has observed stoppage of breathing during the sleeping of patient
P = Pressure. If the patient has hypertension
B = BMI >35 kg/m^2
A = Age >50 years
N = Neck circumference >40 cm
G = Male gender

The ASA guidelines recommend that if a patient presents with a pacemaker or ICD and electrocautery is employed on them, then they should not leave a monitored setting,

until the device is interrogated. However, it is believed that this ASA recommendation is overly conservative, if bipolar cautery is used at a distance of >15 cm from the device or if unipolar cautery is used below the umbilicus and the ground pad is on the leg. Likewise, if an implantable cardioverter defibrillator (ICD) is present and there is anticipated electromagnetic interference the device's antitachycardia feature should be inhibited perioperatively. An external defibrillation capability should always be available whenever the ICDs antitachycardia feature is inactivated.

■ SURGICAL PROCEDURES

There is a long list of surgical procedures from the different disciplines of medicine which can be performed at a day-case surgical and anesthesia unit. But, always it should be kept in mind that the procedures, in which the postoperative surgical and anesthetic complications are likely to occur should be performed as an inpatient basis. The surgical procedures, necessitating excessive fluid infusion or blood transfusion, should be handled in the hospital's indoor patient setting. The operative procedures, requiring prolonged immobilization and parenteral analgesic therapy, are not ideally suited for the outpatient unit.

PREOPERATIVE VISIT, ASSESSMENT AND PREPARATION OF PATIENTS FOR DAY-CASE SURGERY AND ANESTHESIA

It is already said that the preoperative patient selection is the cornerstone of running a day-case anesthesia and surgery unit. So, for this selection, the preoperative visit of a patient to the day-case anesthetic unit is important. The preoperative visit of a patient to a day-case anesthetic unit has two parts: (1) preoperative assessment and (2) preoperative preparation. The preoperative preparation of patient again consists of pharmacological preparation, nonpharmacological preparation, and preparation by information **(Box 3)**.

Preoperative Visit and Assessment

The preoperative assessment is the part of a preoperative preparation of patient before coming to the day-case anesthetic unit of a hospital on the day of surgery. The practice of not preparing the patients, prior to the day of anesthesia and surgery, can result in unnecessary delays, last minute cancellation and inadequate patient management and its flow. So, the starting point of a day-case anesthetic process is the proper preoperative assessment of patient for the day on surgery. Preoperative visit and assessment has also some public educative value, because anesthetist may present

BOX 3: The components of preoperative visit.
- *Preoperative assessment:*
  - History
  - Physical examination
  - Laboratory investigations
- *Nonpharmacological preparation:*
  - Preparation by information
  - Counseling for stress and anxiety reduction
  - Counseling for reduction of pain
- *Pharmacological preparation:*
  - Anxiolysis
  - Amnesia
  - Antisialagogue
  - Antiemetic
  - Analgesia
  - Prevention for aspiration pneumonitis

(describe) different anesthetic procedures and its related risks and complications to the patient and its relatives.

During the preoperative assessment of patient, the time required for taking history can be shortened by the use of preanesthetic questionnaire. By that questionnaire, information is usually obtained regarding the patient's present medical problems, previous operations, drug, and family history, etc. and as well as it also provides a general review of the patient. The use of computerized questionnaire, prior to the preoperative examination of patient by anesthetist, is more time saving and efficient. The modern computerized questionnaires are more accurate in listing the positive and negative information than a physician's interview. This also can be used correctly to predict the need for the necessary preoperative laboratory testing. This approach has been shown to reduce the number of laboratory tests and results in considerable cost savings. In the near future, interactive screening process will almost certainly become available over the Internet.

However, sometimes, it is not always possible (or practical) to examine all the patients in the preanesthetic day-case unit, regardless of their medical conditions, prior to anesthesia and surgery. So, many day-case institutions find alternative ways to achieve these same goals. Such alternative is, surgeons are asked to screen their own patients at their initial office visit prior to fixing the date of surgery. Patients who are of physical status like ASA I or II and who do not require any special laboratory testing or are not overly anxious about the surgery, can be seen by the anesthesiologist on the day of anesthesia and surgery. During this screening of patient by surgeon, if the surgeon feels that the patient is suffering from any disease which should be cared by anesthetist, then this patient should be referred to on duty anesthetist for preoperative checkup and required investigations.

The preoperative laboratory investigation component should be tailored according to the need of the patient, past history of diseases, type of surgery, and the skills or preferences of anesthesiologist. Preoperative list of testing should also be based on the patient's age, history, and examinations. The laboratory examinations should not be a lengthy screening procedures. Because, it does not always provide benefit to the patient, anesthetist, surgeon, hospital, or society. Indiscriminate laboratory testing also produces a large number of false positive, false negative, or random abnormal results and among them most of which are ignored by the anesthesiologist. On the other hand, general physicians may treat these borderline or false positive abnormalities which can lead to patient's harm without any benefit.

It is reported in a study that >60% of the routinely ordered preoperative laboratory investigation could be eliminated, if these are tailored solely, according to their correct indication. It is also known that only 0.2% of abnormalities, which are reported, might have influence on the perioperative anesthetic care. The elimination of these unnecessary tests results in cost savings. It is also deplorable that some preoperative tests, which are frequently ordered, are not recommended at all, while others which are not ordered, though they are recommended. So, it is recommended that no laboratory tests are needed for active healthy male patients, below the age of 40 without any history of previous medical disease and undergoing superficial day-case (outdoor) surgical procedures such as biopsy, herniorrhaphy, circumcision, cataract, dacryocystorhinostomy (DCR), dacryocystectomy (DCT), etc. For the female patients in this age group (i.e., childbearing age) only Hb or hematocrit estimation should be done. The estimation of hemoglobin or hematocrit value is also appropriate for children under the age of 5 years. The patients with an unexpected Hb concentration of <10 g/dL should undergo further evaluation, prior to the elective day-case surgery and anesthesia, because low Hb concentration may be associated with many diseases that could influence the perioperative mortality and morbidity. Patients with chronic diseases such as diabetes, hypertension, chronic obstructive pulmonary disease (COPD), etc. will require additional laboratory investigations according to the severity of diseases (**Fact file I**).

Preoperative Preparations

The preoperative patient preparations of patients have a great impact on the smooth functioning of a day-case (outpatient) surgical and anesthetic departments. This is because, if the selected patients are not prepared properly, then they might result in unexpected cancellation and great

FACT FILE I

In summary, the following preoperative investigations for day-case surgery and anesthesia should be performed when appropriate. These are:

- Full blood count (FBC) only for patients with the possibility of anemia, e.g., bleeding piles, menorrhagia, childbearing age, etc.
- Sickle cell test in all patients of Afro–Caribbean origin
- Serum electrolytes and creatinine in patients on diuretics
- Blood sugar in patients who are diabetic
- Electrocardiogram (ECG) in all male patients over the age of 40 years and women over 50 years of age and younger patients if they have a history of cardiac disease or signs of hypertension, dysrhythmias, diabetes, etc.
- X-rays only for the patients with COPD, breathlessness, history of severe chest and cardiac disease or for all patients over 70 years of age. Very few patients, waiting for day-case surgery and anesthesia, need a preoperative chest radiograph.

After the preoperative visit in anesthetist's room, patients must visit the hospital's business office for financial interview to familiarize himself and his party with the center, and to complete all the paper works including the consent form, which will effectively prepare the patient for outpatient surgery on the schedule day. This is because outpatients usually dislike to wait for long time on that day before surgery.

chaos. As for example, blood pressure (BP) and blood sugar can go up in unprepared hypertensive and diabetic patient, leading to the cancellation of surgery and so on so forth. Besides control of medical disorders, from which the patient is suffering, the main aim of preoperative preparation of a day-case anesthetic department is also the alleviation of the anxiety of patient. Always a significant amount of anxiety is present among all the patients waiting for surgery. Hence, this increased anxiety further increases the release of stress hormone and thus increases the anesthetic requirement, resulting in prolonged recovery time. The high level of anxiety can also be associated with other adverse outcomes such as the increased incidence of tachycardia, increased BP, emesis, etc. Again, for day-case anesthesia, the surgical patients are not given any sedative premedications, because of the fear of prolonged recovery. So, to relieve this anxiety, the patients must be prepared preoperatively by strong assurance. This is called the *nonpharmacological* and *informative methods* of preanesthetic preparation.

The pharmacological methods to reduce anxiety are only applied when it is absolutely necessary. This excessive anxiety may later precipitate many behavioral problems in patients, especially in pediatric group of patients after surgery. These behavioral problems are aggression, regression, eating and sleeping disturbances, fears, angers, bed-wetting, increased dependency, etc. One of the key points to reduce this anxiety of a child is to allow the parents in anesthesia room who will support their child during the induction of anesthesia. This will help in relieving child's anxiety and producing smooth induction of anesthesia. Similarly, the parents should be allowed to meet their child in the recovery room as soon as possible. It will also help to reduce the separation anxiety.

Nonpharmacological and Informative Method for Preoperative Preparation of Patient in a Day-case Unit

An important and first step of nonpharmacological and informative method for preoperative preparation of patient is to visit the anesthetist's room by patient and its relatives. The rationality behind this nonpharmacological preoperative preparation of patient is that the information received by the patients in the anesthetist's room will help them to build expectation and will encourage for cognitive control over the surgical events. A meeting among the anesthetist, patient, and his family member is more effective to reduce the anxiety than the preoperative benzodiazepines, barbiturates, or any sedatives. Among the information, only the perioperative events such as general plan for anesthesia and surgery, benefits of relaxation, discussion of postoperative pain, hospital stay, etc. should be given. This type of preparation of patient by information will be beneficial, because this reduces uncertainty and subsequently anxiety. The patients may feel better having more control over the situation due to the more clearly defined expectations. This will help in reducing the psychological stress factors which is associated with the increased incidences of emesis.

These information can be given in the form of booklets or audiovisuals. Relaxation training is also given to reduce the anxiety and postoperative pain successfully. These methods are economical and have no side effects which is the drawback of drugs or any medications. Patient's motivation and acceptance becomes high in nonpharmacological method than pharmacological one. Overall, a well-informed patient recovers faster and better and he/she experiences less pain. The proper preoperative anesthetic preparations should also include verbal and written instructions regarding the time of arrival, place of surgery, fasting instructions, postoperative advice, limitations of driving abilities after anesthesia, and the need for a responsible adult to escort and accompany the patient, while returning back to home.

Pharmacological Method for Preoperative Preparation of Patient in a Day-case Unit

For the preoperative pharmacological preparation of patients, the use of drug as premedication for day-case anesthesia is controversial. But, this is not saying about the drugs which are taken preoperatively for medical disorders. The aim of premedications in a day-case anesthetic department is like that of the indoor patients, i.e., anxiolysis, sedation, analgesia, amnesia, vagolysis, antiemesis, and the prevention of aspiration pneumonia. But, the problem is that the use of sedatives, hypnotics, analgesics, etc. prolongs the recovery time (some studies say) and causes more PONV which are very important concerns for a day-case (outpatient) anesthesia. Also the prolonged amnesia of patient is not always desired in the day-case anesthesia setting. But, recently many other studies have shown that the use of sedative premedication does not delay the recovery and discharge of patients, although the coordination and the reaction time may be impaired up to 6–12 hours. Hence, the judicious use of sedatives as preoperative medication can be extremely beneficial for some day-case patients without increasing morbidity. But, we will have to keep in mind that the choice of agents and the timing of premedication for day-case patients requires different considerations than inpatients with special attention to the specific needs of the patient and the pharmacokinetic and the pharmacodynamic properties of used drugs. So, in conclusion, it can be said that the proper choice of premedication drugs with its correct dose and timing balanced with the need of the patient, actually (i) will facilitate the discharge of patient, (ii) will reduce the anesthetic requirement, and (iii) will reduce the degree of postoperative emesis.

Among the sedatives and hypnotics, now, barbiturates are not used as premedicant. This is because of their prolonged postoperative recovery time. So, now, benzodiazepines and among them only the short-acting benzodiazepines are the drug of choice. So, the oral midazolam in the dose of 0.05 mg/kg with a little undiluted sweet fruit juice (due to severe bitterness of the oral preparation of midazolam) is used in day-case setting due to its short elimination half-life and lack of significant side effects. The rapid onset of action of midazolam than other benzodiazepine and its water solubility offer a number of advantages for day-case anesthesia and surgery. This agent (midazolam) may also be given through IM 30–40 minutes before surgery or preferably through IV before induction. Midazolam (1–2 mg) given through IV, prior to the induction of GA, reduces the anxiety and increases amnesia without prolonging the recovery room stay. It may be associated with impaired postoperative psychomotor skills. Midazolam given orally has been reported to be highly effective for adults, as well as for children, although larger doses of it are required because of its first pass metabolism in liver. The intranasal and rectal midazolam are also highly effective routes for its administration, if the child tolerates them.

Temazepam in the dose of 10–20 mg in adult has also been reported to be an important oral premedicant for day-case anesthesia. Lorazepam, like diazepam due to its long duration of action is not in choice for day cases. If the patient expresses severe anxiety in preoperative visit, then benzodiazepines can be given in a titrable fashion (in the evening at home and in the morning before leaving home). On the day of surgery after admission, if severe anxiety is apparent in patient, then IV midazolam is the drug which is most often administered.

For children, chloral hydrate (40 mg/kg orally) is reported to increase the calmness and make asleep before the induction of anesthesia compared with midazolam (0.05 mg/kg orally), alprazolam (0.005 mg/kg PO), and placebo. As premedication, the injection of ketamine (2 mg/kg) given through IM to uncooperative children, also permits smooth inhalation induction by halothane or sevoflurane after 2–3 minutes of its administration. Although early recovery time is unaffected, but home discharge may be delayed by an average of 30–40 minutes after ketamine premedication.

The nonselective α_2-agonist such as clonidine and highly selective α_2-agonist such as dexmedetomidine has also been proved to be useful adjunctive, as premedication for day-case anesthesia. Because, they cause (i) the sedation, (ii) the potentiation of the effects of other anesthetic agents, and (iii) the attenuation of the sympathoadrenal stimulation during the intubation and surgery. In addition, dexmedetomidine also has analgesic and anxiolytic property and reduce the plasma stress hormone level. But, still the hemodynamic effects of these drugs limit their use as the primary anesthetic agent and may prove to be valuable as adjunctive to other premedicants.

As premedication, the opioid analgesics are not so much helpful to reduce the anxiety and to produce the sedation. This is because there are other better and specific drugs for these purposes (to reduce anxiety and to produce sedation), except when the patients present with painful conditions. In these circumstances (i.e., in painful condition), the preoperative opioid analgesics, as premedicants, are beneficial for (i) the acute control of preoperative pain and anxiety, (ii) decreasing the requirements of anesthetic drugs, and (iii) providing the postoperative relief of pain. But, the drawback of opioids, as premedicant, are that it is associated with more PONV and slow gastric emptying time. Therefore, it should not be used (i) in patients who are very obese, very old, and fragile, and (ii) in patients with COPD, etc.

The PONV is another common problem for day-case anesthesia. Because, it can delay the discharge and may result in unplanned postoperative hospital readmission for repeated vomiting. So, its management should be started preoperatively. There are multiple causes of PONV such as age, gender, menstrual cycle, pregnancy, previous history of nausea and vomiting, anxiety, obesity, anesthetic agents, type of surgery (laparoscopy, ear surgery, etc.), postoperative pain, movement, hypotension, etc. The incidence of PONV is very low in infants and gradually increases with adulthood. It is true that any single drug is not effective in preventing PONV in all conditions. So, a combination of two or three drugs is more successful. Droperidol, an active antagonist of dopamine receptor (D_2), is highly effective against PONV. But, the full doses of droperidol as premedication may result in dyskinesia, restlessness, and dysphoria which may persist for up to 24 hours after surgery. So, these drawbacks limit the use of droperidol, as a routine antiemetic premedicant, for day-case anesthesia. But, the droperidol in low doses is as effective as higher doses in preventing PONV without delaying recovery. Thus, lowest effective dose (judged by anesthetist) of droperidol is recommended as premedicant for the prophylaxis of PONV.

The metoclopramide is another antidopaminergic antiemetic agent (i.e., block the dopamine receptors) which has also gastrokinetic effects and facilitates both the gastric and small bowel motility. It has some antagonistic effect on 5-HT3 receptor also. It is postulated that the metoclopramide is more effective in opioid-induced vomiting and especially if it is given at the end of anesthesia with or without any other antiemetics. But, the drawback of metoclopramide is that it causes extrapyramidal side effects, drowsiness, dry mouth, or urinary retention.

The ondansetron, granisetron, and tropisetron are the other $5\text{-}HT_3$ receptor antagonists. They are also effective in preventing both the nausea and vomiting, both when is administered alone or in combination with ranitidine and/or metoclopramide. The smaller doses (1 mg) of ondansetron also appear to be effective as prophylaxis for nausea and vomiting. It is especially effective in cytotoxic drug-induced vomiting and has no extrapyramidal side effects like metoclopramide.

The anticholinergic drugs such as atropine and glycopyrrolate are also used for premedication, as they are antisialagogues and vagolytic agent. They also have central antiemetic effects. But, some anesthetists do not use them, because the modern intravenous and inhalational anesthetic agents are not irritant to the airways and also the postoperative dry mouth is very unpleasant for the patients. They also do not like tachycardia caused by atropine or glycopyrrolate. When the antihistamines are used as antiemetics, then they act on the vomiting center by inhibiting the histamine and vestibular pathways. They also cause the drowsiness and prolong recovery time. Extrapyramidal side effects are also commonly associated with these drugs. So, antihistamines are not used routinely in outpatients anesthesia department.

Benzodiazepines, especially lorazepam also have antiemetic properties. In pediatric population, lorazepam is as effective as droperidol in reducing postoperative nausea and vomiting.

An another important aspect for the preoperative preparation of patient for day-care anesthesia is the reduction of the risk of pulmonary aspiration. This can be achieved by reducing the volume and increasing the pH of gastric contents. The incidence of pulmonary aspiration in day-care surgical patients is very low. It is only 1 in 40,000 and mortality rate is 0.00002. However, several studies have found that 50–60% of day-care patients would be defined as theoretically "high risk" for aspiration pneumonitis by the traditional criteria, where the gastric volume is >25 mL, with pH <2.5, despite an overnight fast. It has also been suggested that all the patients receiving GA by mask or laryngeal mask airway (LMA) should be protected against the pulmonary aspiration. So, the reduction of the volume of gastric contents and the increase of the pH of it should be done and this can be achieved by fasting and medication (metoclopramide and H_2 blocker).

However, the prolonged fasting does not always guarantee an empty stomach (i.e., does not reduce the residual volume which is always present in the stomach) at the time of induction and so the risk of aspiration always persists. Again the prolonged fasting (conventional fasting, i.e., 6–8 hours) causes moderate-to-severe hunger and thirst which may contribute significantly to the preoperative anxiety. On the other hand, the half-life of a clear fluid in stomach is about 11 minutes which justify that prolonged fasting is unnecessary. So, the ingestion of 150 mL of water, tea, coffee, apple juice, or orange juice (3 mL/kg), as late as 2–3 hours before anesthesia and surgery, has no significant effect on residual gastric volume and pH. Instead, it decreases the gastric volume, thirst and hunger (especially in children), and anxiety (mainly children's parents). There are also data to suggest that the intake of oral fluids may dilute the already present, concentrated gastric secretions and actually stimulate the gastric emptying. So, the prolonged fasting, causing discomfort to the day-case patients and without any apparent benefit, is not recommended now.

Thus, the starvation instructions for the day-case patients will be like that (i) for the patients of morning list—no solid food after midnight and free clear fluids up to 6.30 hours, (ii) for the patients of afternoon list—no solid food after 6.30 hours and free clear fluids up to 11.30 hours. Preoperative verbal and written instructions are important so that milky drinks are avoided. Only the patients, suspected or known to be at risk for delayed gastric emptying (e.g., diabetes, hiatus hernia, gastroesophageal reflux, gastric outlet obstruction, etc.) should be considered for prolonged fasting. The H_2 receptor antagonist such as ranitidine and its congeners or proton pump inhibitor (PPI) and its congeners are effective both in increasing the gastric pH and decreasing the gastric volume by inhibiting the gastric acid secretion, though they have no influence on the volume and the pH of gastric secretion which is already present in stomach. Ranitidine is given either orally or parenterally with peak effect occurring within 2 hours. Compared to fasting without ranitidine, patients who receive coffee or orange juice with oral ranitidine, 2–3 hours prior to the induction of anesthesia have lower residual gastric volumes, higher pH values, and decreased incidence of thirst. It has been suggested that all the patients who receive GA by mask should be protected by H_2 blocker from pulmonary injury by gastric acid component.

The use of metoclopramide in combination with an H_2 blocking drugs increase the gastric pH and decrease the residual gastric volume by increasing the gastric emptying time. However, the metoclopramide also offers an additional advantage by increasing the lower esophageal sphincter tone and thus reducing the chance of regurgitation and aspiration of gastric contents. The molar sodium citrate (0.3 M, 30 mL), a nonparticulate oral antacid is effective by directly raising the gastric pH (less effective than H_2 blocker), but it increases the gastric volume. This drug can only be useful in combination with metoclopramide when the prophylaxis against pulmonary aspiration is desired, but only little time is available prior to the operation, as the onset of action of sodium citrate is immediate.

Actually, there is no evidence of any increase in regurgitation and aspiration in day-case anesthesia. So, the routine use of H_2 blocker, metoclopramide or molar sodium citrate is probably unnecessary. However, in those with a history of regurgitation, ranitidine (300 mg orally) or omeprazole (40 mg orally) with metoclopramide is appropriate. The ASA task force on preoperative fasting has recommended no routine use of gastric acid secretion blockers, antiemetics, antacids, gastrointestinal stimulants, anticholinergics, or combinations of these medications for patients who have no apparent increased risk for pulmonary aspiration.

Non-steroidal anti-inflammatory drugs (NSAIDs), e.g., diclofenac in the dose of 50–100 mg, given orally or rectally or IM, reach its peak effect after 1–2 hours of its administration and are a useful adjunct to preoperative medication with very few side effects. But, the slow release oral preparations of it does not reach the plasma steady state concentrations, until after several doses, and are thus not useful for early analgesia during postoperative period.

ORGANIZATION OF A DAY-CASE ANESTHESIA UNIT

The day-case anesthesia unit is usually of three types:

1. A day-case unit within the hospital main complex, but with separate operation theater (OT) complex, ward, and staff (including surgeon and anesthetist) for day cases.
2. A day-case unit with separate ward, but using the hospital's main OT complex (No separate OT complex for day-case surgeries and anesthesia).
3. A day-case unit remote from the main hospital complex with separate building, OT complex, ward, and staff including surgeon and anesthetist.

Ideally, the day-case surgical and anesthesia unit should have a separate building, but not be far away from the main hospital complex. It should be situated by the side of the main inpatient department and its OT complex. The ward area of it should be nearby of its own OT to reduce the transport time of patients, particularly when the multiple short operative procedures are to be performed. This arrangement also enables the parents to accompany their children to the anesthetic room, when it is desired.

The ideal separate day-case surgical and anesthesia unit which is situated in a separate building, adjacent to the main hospital complex, must have its separate admission area, an anesthesia room, an operating theater, and a fully equipped recovery room. An admission area will include (i) a reception area, (ii) an examination and treatment room, (iii) a nurse's station, (iv) a lavatory, and (v) a discharge area. The anesthesia room should be fully equipped too. It (anesthesia room) should be large enough to allow the free access of an anesthetist around the patient's trolley to permit the use of both local and GA. There should be good arrangements for lighting, scavenging, piped gases, suction equipment, anesthetic machine and all the types of standard monitoring equipment with all emergency drugs.

The hazards and risks of GA in a day-case surgery and anesthesia unit are not less than that of an inpatient surgery and anesthesia unit. Indeed, they may be greater and the facilities should be like an inpatient anesthesia room. An OT for day-case surgery and anesthesia unit should be of the same specification, as the main inpatient's OT complex. There is always some possibility of a minor surgery developing unexpectedly into a major operation and so this demands that the theater should be well equipped to deal with any eventuality. Like the main inpatient recovery unit, the day-case recovery room should also be well equipped and staffed properly for the safe recovery of patients after GA.

On the day of anesthesia and surgery, patients should be admitted in the day-case ward with adequate time for history taking and examination (if not done before).

The results of prescribed investigations should be available during preoperative examination and it is noted. Patients should receive an identity tag with the name and necessary information printed on it. The surgeon should ensure that the indication for surgery is still present, as there may be a long gap between the first clinical examination and the day of surgery. The consent form should be signed, if not already done during the outpatient appointment. The names should be entered in the nursing record and the operation site should be marked. A pregnancy test for the women of vulnerable age should be performed, if there is any risk of pregnancy.

Technique of Anesthesia

There is no any separate special technique for day-case (outpatient) anesthetic procedure. The intraoperative anesthetic management in the day-case patient undergoing surgery is aimed at providing (i) rapid emergence, (ii) good postoperative analgesia, (iii) minimal postoperative PONV, and (iv) rapid return to fitness for discharge, while creating acceptable operating conditions. Often these goals compete with each other.

General, local, or regional anesthesia (RA), which are generally used for indoor patients, can be administered safely to day-case patients. But, the choice of technique is tailored made and should be determined by the (i) surgical requirements, (ii) anesthetic consideration, (iii) patient's physical status, and (iv) preference by surgeon or anesthetist. The ideal general anesthetic technique for day cases should include rapid and smooth induction, followed by adequate intraoperative amnesia, analgesia, and muscle relaxation, i.e., good surgical condition and good recovery without any side effects. The day-case anesthesia delivery system requires the same basic care, safety, and efficiency as an inpatient anesthesia including the same basic monitoring equipment such as ECG, BP, pulse oximeter, capnography, temperature, etc. The EEG-based monitoring of the depth of anesthesia helps to titrate the hypnotic and sedative effect of anesthetic agents and thus reduces their (anesthetic agents) dose and helps in rapid recovery.

Although inhalational anesthesia with sevoflurane may speed emergence compared with total intravenous anesthesia (TIVA), the likelihood of PONV may be greater, if an additional prophylactic drug is not administered. Numerous studies have shown how RA can speed discharge time compared with GA in the ambulatory population in part by potentially reducing the incidence of PONV and the need for opioid analgesia. The N_2O increases the likelihood of PONV. But, this effect can be overcome by adding a prophylactic agent. Moreover, multimodal perioperative analgesia can be approached using a variety of drugs including local anesthetics, paracetamol, and other NSAIDs to reduce the use of opioids which contribute to PONV risk.

General Anesthesia

It is the most widely choiced anesthetic technique in day-case department by surgeons, anesthetists, and patients. For GA, there is no special separate anesthetic technique for outpatients. But, there are a vast array of pharmacologically active anesthetic drugs. So, when they are combined at different concentration in a rational manner and carefully titrated, then they can produce the desired general anesthetic condition for day-case patients with an acceptable cost and recovery profile. The aim of GA in day-case department is to deliver it (GA) safely with minimum side effects and rapid recovery. For surgical procedures under GA, lasting less than 15–20 minutes, and those can be done by only inhalational anesthesia with spontaneous mask ventilation with minimum blood loss (for example, circumcision, abscess drainage, gynecological dilatation, and curettage), do not require any IV administration of fluid. This is because perioperative fasting, even for the periods of 10–15 hours, do not usually result in hypoglycemia in healthy individual who is >5 years old and adult. However, for longer periods or circumstances, where the patient has been without oral intake for an excessive period of time (>10–15 hours), an intravenous line is essential for the maintenance of fluid balance and glucose hemostasis as well as facilitating the administration of intravenous anesthetic and emergency drugs during the perioperative period. But, this dictum is not always followed in many developed countries. Therefore, any minor procedure even under topical or local block, intravenous line is procured with all standard monitoring.

The choice of an inducing agent for GA depends upon the requirement of patient's condition and the preference of anesthetist. But, the aim of selecting any inducing agent in day-case anesthesia is rapid and smooth induction and good immediate recovery with minimal postoperative sequelae, and a rapid return to street fitness. Several agents such as the propofol, thiopentone, methohexital, etomidate, or any benzodiazepine have been used successfully for the induction of anesthesia in a surgical day-case unit. But, the *propofol* has replaced all due to its favorable recovery profile for day-case anesthesia. One of the main advantages of propofol is the easy and rapidity with which the patients recover from its (propofol) effects. Patients are usually of clear headed and have the lower incidences of PONV after recovery, when propofol is used as an inducing agent. The induction of anesthesia with propofol is associated with a greater decrease in BP and heart rate than with either thiopentone or methohexital. It is used in elderly patients with reduced doses. Pain on injection of propofol can be significant. But, this may be reduced by the addition of lignocaine with propofol using a large vein or by cooling the propofol to 4°C.

Thiopentone is also characterized by rapid induction without significant side effects. But, the psychomotor recovery is sometimes delayed and the prolonged subjective feelings of tiredness and drowsiness by patients receiving thiopentone are the drawbacks to its use in day-case anesthesia. *Methohexital* is associated with slightly shorter awakening and recovery times than that of thiopentone. But, the pharmacokinetic property of it makes its administrations possible only by continuous infusion. The recovery of fine motor skills from methohexital is not completed, until 8–10 hours is passed after induction by it. It may also cause pain on IV injection, involuntary muscle movements, and hiccup. But, the use of small doses of rapid-acting opioids (fentanyl, sufentanil, and remifentanil) can minimize these side effects of methohexital without prolonging its recovery. Among the *benzodiazepines*, midazolam (0.2–0.4 mg/kg, through IV) only can be used as an inducing agent for day-case anesthesia (where propofol and thiopental is not indicated), but its onset of action is slow and recovery is prolonged than that of propofol and thiopentone whereas, the onset of action of midazolam and the recovery from it is quicker than that of other benzodiazepines. Compared to propofol, recovery after flumazenil antagonized midazolam anesthesia is still significantly slower.

For day-case anesthesia, the inhalational induction by halothane or sevoflurane is also an alternative to intravenous induction, where the intravenous access is very difficult or contraindicated. This inhalational induction should not normally be used for patients with symptom of gastroesophageal reflux or where there is chance of gastric regurgitation and aspiration. In children, inhalational induction is a very useful alternative to the standard intravenous induction techniques which is usually adapted in adult patients. But, unfortunately, the induction of anesthesia by inhalation is more time consuming and many children object to face mask due to the apprehension and the pungent smell of inhaled volatile anesthetic agents. However, this problem can be reduced by the use of single breath induction technique. Traditionally, volatile anesthetic agents are considered as better than intravenous agents for the maintenance of anesthesia. But, there is little or no basis for this justification. On the other hand, the combination of intravenous agents for induction and inhalation agents for the maintenance of anesthesia for very short procedures is associated with long recovery time than inhalation agents alone.

For the maintenance of anesthesia, the combination of O_2 and N_2O mixed with minimum concentration of volatile anesthetic agents is the most popular technique in day-case anesthesia department. The extreme slow solubility of N_2O (0.46) causes rapid onset and also rapid recovery from its central nervous system (CNS) effects and makes it a valuable adjunct for combination with other volatile or intravenous anesthetic agents. Thus, it also reduces the requirement of other anesthetic agents and helps in early recovery. But, the use of N_2O for the maintenance of anesthesia has been shown to increase the risk of PONV (by increasing the pressure in middle ear and thus stimulating the vestibular system) and this incidence is more when N_2O is combined with other volatile anesthetic agents or opioid analgesics. However, the minimum concentration of it reduces the requirement of volatile or opioid agents and reduces the incidence of PONV. In many developed countries, this N_2O is not used now and it has become obsolete. But still the use of N_2O is standard practice in other developing nations.

For the maintenance of day-case anesthesia, the three commonly used volatile anesthetic agents are (1) halothane, (2) isoflurane, and (3) sevoflurane. Among these, halothane and sevoflurane are also used for induction as both are nonirritant to the airway. But, sevoflurane has the advantages of more rapid induction and recovery with minimal cardiovascular side effects than halothane. However, sevoflurane causes more PONV than propofol, but less than the other volatile anesthetic agents. Isoflurane is not used for the induction of anesthesia, as it is irritant to the airways, but the recovery of anesthesia from isoflurane is faster than halothane and produces more stable cardiovascular effect than halothane. Ventricular arrhythmias are more likely to occur during halothane anesthesia. Desflurane also provides stable CVS condition, like isoflurane, and helps in quick recovery, as its blood solubility (0.42) is less than N_2O. But, it possesses airway irritant property and may cause breath holding, laryngospasm, apnea, etc. like isoflurane.

The opioid and nonopioid analgesics are also frequently administered in the immediate preinduction period and during the maintenance of GA. They may reduce the dose of sedative and hypnotic agents for induction and thus help in early recovery. The morphine and meperidine are not popular analgesic for day-case anesthesia. The more potent, rapid, short-acting, narcotic analgesics such as fentanyl (1–4 µg/kg), sufentanil (0.25–0.5 µg/kg), and remifentanil are popular for day-case anesthesia and are used to attenuate effectively the cardiovascular responses to laryngoscopy and intubation. They are also useful supplements to the inhaled anesthetic agents during the maintenance of anesthesia.

Some studies have demonstrated improved intraoperative conditions and a more rapid recovery from anesthesia when fentanyl or one of its newer congeners were administered as a part of N_2O, narcotic and relaxant (balanced) technique. Remifentanil is a pure μ-opioid receptor agonist and is metabolized by esterase enzyme. Its biological half-life is only 3–5 minutes regardless of its total dose and the duration of infusion. It has no accumulation property even after its prolonged infusion. So, remifentanil has become very useful in providing profound analgesia for day-case surgery and anesthesia without effecting (prolonging) recovery. However, its short duration of action is a definite disadvantage, if significant and prolonged postoperative analgesia is needed.

The choice of opioid analgesic usually depends on the desired duration of its effect. If a strong analgesic effect is needed for a brief period, then this is achieved by bolus administration of fentanyl, sufentanil, alfentanil, or remifentanil. For a short surgical procedure, the addition of fentanyl (50–100 μg) does not much affect the recovery from a propofol, N_2O, and muscle relaxant combination technique without increasing PONV. In these circumstances, the alfentanil and remifentanil would have slight advantage. But, fentanyl is the better choice, if analgesia is needed to maintain postoperatively. If a strong analgesic effect is needed by repeated bolus injections or continuous infusion, then remifentanil, fentanyl, or sufentanil are the best choice. If patients require moderate analgesia for 2–3 hours or more, then an injection of morphine is a reasonable alternative to multiple bolus dose of fentanyl, sufentanil, or remifentanil.

The newer techniques such as the target controlled infusion (TCI) of propofol with or without the ultra-rapid-acting opioid such as remifentanil or the use of sevoflurane may confer some advantages. But, these have to be balanced against the cost of these agents. The TCI of propofol is an intravenous technique for the maintenance of intraoperative hypnosis. It takes into account the patient's weight (kg) and the desired drug concentration in blood (μg/mL). An initial target plasma concentration of 4–6 μg/mL for propofol is often set and then adjusted appropriately. Subsequently, the infusion rate is calculated by a computer within the pump according to the concentration of drug in blood.

The anesthesia for day-case surgery requires a variety of airway management techniques. This is because of the wide varieties of surgical procedures which are performed in the day-case surgical unit. In all these surgical cases, a clear airway is the fundamental requirement for safe anesthesia. The endotracheal (ET) intubation causes the higher incidences of airway-related complications such as sore throat, croup, hoarseness, etc., and a greater morbidity during and after surgery. Thus, ET intubation is not essential or desirable for all the day cases GA and surgical procedures. For day-case anesthesia of small duration, simple face mask

with Guedel airway is sufficient and is commonly used. Spontaneous ventilation via face mask does not result in significant hypercarbia or acidosis for the brief surgical and anesthetic procedures. Thus, by avoiding laryngoscopy and intubation, the amount of anesthetic drugs that is required for intubation, is reduced and a faster recovery with fewer postoperative side effects may be anticipated. So, some anesthetists have chosen not to intubate a selected group of low-risk patients.

Instead of face mask and ET tube (i.e., where face mask is not appropriate and ET intubation is not desired), alternatively LMA also can be used for both the adults and children. Longer procedures may necessitate the use of ET tube. Thus, it is suggested that LMA is better than face mask for unobstructed spontaneous ventilation, but inferior to ET tube for the management of airway. It can be positioned without direct visualization of larynx and neuromuscular block. Patient is allowed to breathe spontaneously throughout the procedure and anesthesia is maintained continuously by volatile anesthetic agents by attaching LMA with anesthetic machine or by TIVA.

Compared to anesthesia with face mask and simple pharyngeal airway, the patients of the LMA group did not have any increased requirements of anesthetic agents. The *other advantages of LMA* are (i) it offers a hands free approach to airway management allowing the anesthetist to complete other tasks, (ii) there is decrease in hemodynamic changes during both induction and emergence, (iii) reduced work of breathing compared with the use of ET tube and spontaneous respiration, and (iv) if necessary controlled ventilation also can be performed, but up to a maximum airway pressure of 15–20 cmH_2O. The *disadvantage of LMA* is that it cannot protect the airway from gastric aspiration and hence it should not be used in patients with high risk of regurgitation, aspiration, and upper airway bleeding. Another disadvantage of LMA is that when greater airway pressure is needed for ventilation then there is chance of gastric dilatation and subsequent regurgitation and aspiration of gastric contents.

Although few ambulatory or day-case procedures require a secure airway by ET tube, but patients undergoing laparoscopy are often intubated. This is because gas insufflation and the head-down position are believed to increase the risk of regurgitation and hypoventilation. But, in some units, the patients undergoing small laparoscopic surgery are not intubated. These centers report that the spontaneous ventilation via face mask or LMA in the head-down position does not result in significant hypercapnia or acidosis in nonobese patients and not it is associated with reflux of gastric contents. Thus, by avoiding laryngoscopy and intubation for laparoscopic surgery requiring brief period, the amount of anesthetic drugs can be decreased and there is faster recovery with fewer and minor side effects.

For ET intubation during day-case anesthesia, the choice of muscle relaxant depends on the anticipated duration of surgery. Many day-case surgical and anesthetic procedures that can be carried out by face mask and without intubation do not require any muscle relaxant. The conditions where face mask or LMA cannot be used and intubation is needed, only then muscle relaxant is used to facilitate the tracheal intubation and to optimize the surgical condition. In addition, the use of muscle relaxant decreases the other anesthetic requirements and shortens the recovery time.

Before the introduction of atracurium, mivacurium, and vecuronium, the depolarizing agent succinylcholine was the most popular muscle relaxant for day-case anesthesia, both for intubation and maintenance, by infusion or repeated doses (only for short procedures). But, as the succinylcholine causes a lot of problems such as hyperkalemia, arrhythmia, malignant hyperpyrexia, severe muscle pain, etc. so it is now abandoned from modern anesthesia except in certain few indicated cases for day-case anesthesia. Therefore, with the availability of many short-acting nondepolarizing muscle relaxants such as atracurium, vecuronium, and mivacurium, the prompt reversal of neuromuscular blockade can be achieved after 15–30 minutes of brief surgical procedures.

Atracurium, vecuronium, and mivacurium are metabolized through their distinctly different pathways. As atracurium and mivacurium release histamine, it should not be used in certain cases. Mivacurium has the shortest duration of action and hence is the ideal for outpatient anesthesia. But, as it undergoes hydrolysis by plasma cholinesterase, so a small number of patients may suffer from prolonged muscle paralysis like succinylcholine and this is because of plasma cholinesterase deficiency. After the use of recommended tracheal intubating dose of atracurium or vecuronium, the duration of action (to 95% spontaneous recovery) is roughly 1 hour. Rocuronium may have great role in outpatient anesthesia like succinylcholine, as it has a more rapid onset of action than any of the other nondepolarizing muscle relaxants providing intubating conditions within 30–60 seconds. However, it has a longer duration of action, similar to that of vecuronium. Recently, the stereoisomer of atracurium and cisatracurium has been introduced with similar duration of action to that of atracurium, but without the side effects of histamine release **(Fact file II)**.

Regional Anesthesia

Regional anesthesia (spinal or epidural) offers *many advantages over GA* in day-case surgical and anesthesia unit such as (i) less nausea, vomiting, dizziness, lethargy,

FACT FILE II

In summary, total intravenous anesthesia with propofol is widely used for short outpatient surgery and anesthesia. Inhalation of O_2-enriched air will also allow omission of N_2O. Propofol induction with maintenance by isoflurane/sevoflurane is an alternative. Incremental fentanyl (2–4 µg/kg) is often used in divided doses. Whenever possible LMA should be used avoiding intubation, muscle relaxants, and reversal agents. LMA for gynecological laparoscopy and armored LMA for wisdom teeth extraction and many nasal operations can be used safely in many circumstances. Antiemetics are not indicated routinely, but should be reserved for the treatment of any PONV or as prophylaxis in those with a history of PONV. Proper hydration reduces the postoperative morbidity such as thirst, dizziness, drowsiness, etc. It is found that a patient who receives 20 mL/kg IV fluid instead of 2 mL/kg has less postoperative morbidity. However, this postoperative morbidity also can be reduced by using heated humidifiers, heat, and moisture exchangers, etc., which conserve heat and decrease the fluid loss.

etc., (ii) no side effects of tracheal intubation, (iii) better postoperative analgesia, (iv) minimal postanesthetic nursing care, and (v) decreased recovery time. Still, its use is limited in day-case (outpatient) anesthesia unit due to the occurrence of unacceptable incidences of postdural puncture headache (PDPH) and lignocaine-induced transient radicular irritation (TRI). The actual lack of good alternative to lignocaine for its short duration of action without the risk of TRI (incidence is 16–20%) has been the subject of recent controversy. Typically, the pain of TRI begins within 24 hours after the lignocaine induced spinal anesthesia and lasts for approximately 2 days. The 5% hyperbaric lignocaine has the highest incidence of TRI. This is amenable to treatment by rest and oral analgesics. The bupivacaine is not associated with TRI. But, it is not the agent of first choice in a day-case anesthesia unit, because it is long acting. Now, there is an open debate, whether RA is truly safer than GA in a day-case anesthesia unit or not. Only the caudal epidural block may be useful in adult for day-case anesthesia without any debate.

During the caudal epidural block, the use of diluted solutions of LA agent (0.125% bupivacaine) with the addition of preservative free opiates, or ketamine 0.5 mg/kg, or clonidine 1 µg/kg, etc. may prolong the duration of analgesia for up to 24 hours without any loss of motor function. In the caudal epidural block, patient should also be warned about the ambulation difficulties. The caudal epidural anesthesia or analgesia is usually employed for anorectal, scrotal, penile, inguinal, and some gynecological surgical procedures involving only the lower part of vagina and perineum. This caudal epidural technique is associated with (i) nil or fewer hemodynamic changes, (ii) no incidences of PDPH, (iii) no urinary retention, and (iv) provide faster recovery when compared with spinal or lumbar epidural anesthesia for the same procedures.

The PDPH after spinal anesthesia should always be differentiated from the other causes headache rather than regional anesthesia. These are neurological, vascular, musculoskeletal, metabolic, etc., such as migraine, rapid expansion of brain tumor, intracranial hemorrhage, withdrawal of caffeine, hypoglycemia, etc. There are different treatment modalities which will relieve the symptoms of PDPH. But, the prophylaxis for PDPH is always better than treating it which has been discussed earlier. The intake of excessive water does not decrease the severity of PDPH, as it does not increase the production of cerebrospinal fluid (CSF). The intake of caffeine may sometimes treat mild PDPH. The activity of outpatients should not be limited with mild PDPH.

In children, regional block is performed immediately after the induction of GA. It can (i) reduce the requirement of general anesthetic drugs, (ii) provide postoperative analgesia, and (iii) allow more rapid recovery from GA due to the lesser amount of general anesthetic drugs (which are essential for day-case anesthesia). Caudal epidural anesthesia is an effective technique for children undergoing surgical procedures on lower abdomen, perineum, and lower extremity. The combined or individual ilioinguinal and iliohypogastric nerve block or caudal epidural anesthesia reduce the pain following herniotomy and herniorrhaphy. Postcircumcision pain can be reduced by the block of the dorsal nerve of penis or the subcutaneous ring block of penis or by the application of topical local anesthetic ointment over the surgical site.

The peripheral nerve block is one of the first and excellent choice of anesthesia for day-case patients. For the operations on hand or arm, the brachial plexus block is the unique. But, the axillary approach for this brachial plexus block is preferred than the supraclavicular approach. Because, in supraclavicular approach of brachial plexus block, the risk for the production of pneumothorax is more which may become apparent only after discharge. The infraclavicular and axillary approaches for brachial plexus block are preferred for surgery on the elbow, forearm, and hand. While the interscalene approach for brachial plexus block is more commonly used for shoulder surgery. The coracoid technique for infraclavicular approach of brachial plexus block has been shown to be very effective. This technique avoids the important neurovascular structures in the neck and minimizes the risk of pneumothorax also. If brachial plexus block is used with GA, then the diluted solution of LA agent (0.25% bupivacaine) is used to minimize the motor block. During the use of brachial plexus block,

without GA, one must take into account the time of onset of block during the planning of surgical list. Otherwise, it will make unnecessary delay and at the end of the day the list may remain incomplete. Peripheral nerve block is also useful for day-case surgery on legs.

The "3-in-1" type of regional anesthetic technique (obturator, femoral, and lateral femoral cutaneous nerve block by one injection) is useful for any type of day-case knee surgery (such as knee arthroscopy) with excellent postoperative analgesia and a high degree of patient acceptance. The sciatic nerve block in popliteal fossa may also be used successfully for the different surgical procedures on lower leg and foot in 92% of patients, where the supplemental regional anesthesia is required only in 5% of cases and GA only in 3% of cases. Different nerve blocks at the level of ankle are also simple and effective for surgeries on foot at day-case unit. There are other types of peripheral nerve block which can be used safely as day-case anesthesia.

The intravenous regional anesthesia (Bier's block) may also be used successfully for upper and lower extremity surgery as day-case procedure. This block is generally considered safe, when it is performed by clinicians, who are familiar with this technique and with the safe doses of LA agent. The most commonly used drug in Bier's block is 40–50 mL of 0.5% lignocaine, using a double tourniquet with cuff pressures of 250 mm Hg or 100 mm Hg above the systolic BP. Ketorolac and clonidine can also be used with lignocaine which improve the quality of regional anesthesia and analgesia. The intravenous regional anesthesia of leg requires a larger volume of solutions and higher cuff pressures, so it is not frequently used.

The local infiltration of operative site by the diluted solutions of local anesthetic agent is also the simplest and safest technique of regional anesthesia for the day-case patients. The day-case arthroscopy of knee is commonly performed under infiltration LA. Different ophthalmic surgeries are also performed by peribulbar or retrobulbar type of infiltration anesthesia as day cases. Now, cataract surgeries are also done under topical anesthesia as day-case surgery. Inguinal hernia repair can be performed by individual ilioinguinal and iliohypogastric nerve block and local infiltration of the surgical site. A combination of local infiltration and intercostal nerve blocks can also be used for day-case lithotripsy. There are many other surgical examples which are performed under RA, but cannot be listed fully here.

The infiltration of local anesthetic agent at the surgical sites is often associated with significant discomfort. So, the use of sedation and analgesics (conscious sedation) during the infiltration of local anesthetic agent is popular. But, with the local anesthetic agent, only the short-acting sedative drugs will increase the tolerability of local infiltration block. It is also noted that the sedation is a poor adjunct to an imperfect local anesthetic block. However, the judicious use of intermittent midazolam or propofol infusions (TCI 1–1.5 µg/mL) can provide good amnesia with fewer postoperative side effects.

Regional anesthesia is widely used in Europe and North America for day-case surgery and anesthesia. The timing and planning of RA in a day-case unit are important. Because, the regional blocks take a longer time to wear off compared with GA. So, the discharge of patient may be delayed. For spinal block, 25 or 26-gauge pencil-tipped needle and 0.25% heavy bupivacaine (1:1 diluted 0.5% heavy bupivacaine by sterile saline) are used. This gives a similar onset of anesthesia with shorter discharge time (4 hours vs. 6 hours). The epidural procedures (except caudal) are less suitable for day-case anesthesia.

Usually, RA is performed early on the day which will allow the maximum time for recovery before the discharge and safe ambulation of patient. However, sometimes, it is reasonable to discharge the patients with still persisting plexus blocks. This is applicable only to the brachial, lumbar, and sacral plexus block, but not to the spinal and epidural anesthesia. This will allow the benefit of prolonged postoperative analgesia at home without any motor involvement. In such circumstances, the patients need special instructions for the care of anesthetized part of their body, so as to avoid any inadvertent damage. For example, this would include a sling for patients with brachial plexus blocks.

Recovery and Discharge

Before discharge, proper recovery from anesthesia (GA or RA) is an important aspect of day-case anesthesia. So, it (recovery from anesthesia) should be assessed properly. If the assessment is not correct and the patients are discharged without full recovery from anesthesia, then catastrophy can occur. The assessment of patient's recovery from anesthesia is divided into three phases: (1) early, (2) intermediate, and (3) late **(Table 1)**.

The *early recovery phase* extends from the completion of surgery and the end of anesthesia to the awakening and the returning of patient to orientation. Endotracheal tube is extubated in this phase and the patient is monitored vigilantly. After that, the patient is transported to PACU-1 without unattended. During this early recovery phase in PACU-1, the patient may undergo many rapid physiological changes and so close observation of patient is important. This first postanesthetic care unit should be provided with continuous monitoring of BP, heart rate, respiratory rate,

TABLE 1: Stages of recovery.

Stage of recovery	Clinical definition
Early recovery	Awakening and recovery of vital reflexes
Intermediate recovery	Immediate clinical recovery and home readiness
Late recovery	Full clinical and psychological recovery

temperature, ECG, SPO$_2$, etc. In this phase, the patients especially the pediatric population are routinely given O$_2$. When the patient is sufficiently awake with stable vital signs and responsive to commands, then only he is signed out to the care of recovery room staff. The patients who have received (i) monitored anesthetic care, or (ii) only intravenous sedation in minimum doses, or (iii) regional anesthesia, may not always require supplemental O$_2$. Patient should be monitored in PACU-1 until he or she is completely awake, oriented, and their vital signs are stable and adequate pain relief is achieved. Once the above criteria are achieved and the patient is able to maintain a semisitting position, then the patient is only shifted to the second phase of postanesthetic care unit, i.e., PACU-II.

This *intermediate recovery phase* extends from the admission in PACU-II to discharge from this unit. In this recovery phase, patient should be able to sit alone without any support. Gradually, he starts to walk and takes oral fluids and should have minimum pain. This second phase of recovery involves lower nursing dependency and the patient is not attached to any monitoring system any more. Proper anesthetic technique, high quality postoperative analgesic care and prophylaxis of PONV have major impact on the duration of this intermediate recovery phase. Prolonged intermediate recovery phase will fail to discharge the patient in time and will increase the cost of patient's hospital visit. At the end of this phase, patient will be able to walk unaided, tolerate oral fluids without vomiting, has minimal pain, and is ready to be discharged from the hospital. Patient's family can participate in this phase of recovery, when the criteria for "home readiness" are achieved and patient is discharged.

The last and *late recovery phase* starts with the patient's return to his or her home and continues until the full functional recovery is achieved. Most anesthesia-related postoperative side effects such as pain, nausea, vomiting, dizziness, headache, myalgia, etc. usually resolve within first 24 hours after operation. In this period, the patient should be advised to refrain from activities such as driving a car, operating machines, and drinking alcohol. However, the recovery from surgery itself has the highest impact on patient's full functional recovery. During discharge, a responsible person should be present to escort the patient to home and both the responsible person and the patient should be given the verbal and written discharge instructions. In some hospitals, patient's general practitioner is communicated over telephonic helpline and is made aware of the operation, performed and the requirement for postoperative follow-up.

Discharge Criteria

Following a GA, it is very difficult to determine when it is safe to discharge a patient from a day-case unit. So, the accurate assessment of the complete recovery of cognitive, sensory, and psychomotor function is important. Because, it will help in determining the appropriate time for discharge. Varieties of tests have been advised to assess the recovery from sensory, motor, and cognitive function, but there is currently no standardized discharge criterion. The main principles on which basis the patients are discharged from day-case unit are (i) they must have stable vital signs, (ii) there is no significant nausea, vomiting, and pain, (iii) they are fully oriented and are able to sit and walk unaided. Some tests which are used to assess the *recovery of cognitive functions,* they are: processing (mental arithmetic and reaction time); integration (critical fashion flicker test), memory (digit span), and learning (word lists). The tests to assess the *recovery of sensory functions* are: stimulus detection, auditing perception, and Maddox wing test. The tests to assess the *recovery of psychomotor* functions are: choice reaction time, the post box test, the Trieger dot test, etc.

Although these cognitive, sensory, and psychomotor tests can provide adequate information, which are sometimes useful in developing practical discharge criteria, but most of these tests are too complex and time consuming to use. So, some simple tests for memory and sensorimotor coordination appear to be the most useful indices of recovery. The Bender–Gestalt Track tracer test is a very reliable, valid, objective, noninvasive, and inexpensive test to assess the postoperative recovery that can be easily performed in <60 seconds.

Many scoring systems have been devised to facilitate timely and safe PACU discharge and assess home readiness after ambulatory surgery. Among these *Aldrete scoring system* is followed most and it includes: activity, respiration, circulation, consciousness, and O_2 saturation **(Table 2)**.

The discharge criteria after spinal and epidural anesthesia are different from GA. It should include the return of normal sensation, muscle strength, and proprioception as well as the return of the functions of sympathetic nervous system.

TABLE 2: Modified Aldrete scoring system for determining when patients are ready for discharge from the postanesthesia care (PACU).

Activity: Able to move voluntarily or on command	
• Four extremities	2
• Two extremities	1
• Zero extremities	0
Respiration:	
• Able to deep breathe and cough freely	2
• Dyspnea and shallow breathing	1
• Apneic	0
Circulation:	
• BP ± 20 mm Hg from preanesthetic level	2
• BP ± 20–50 mm Hg from preanesthetic level	1
• BP ± 50 mm Hg from preanesthetic level	0
Consciousness:	
• Fully awake	2
• Arousable on calling	1
• Not responding	0
O_2 saturation:	
• On room air SPO_2 is >90%	2
• With O_2 supplementation SPO_2 is >90%	1
• With O_2 supplementation SPO_2 is <90%	0

A score of >9 is required for discharge from PACU, but not for home.

After regional anesthesia, motor and sensory functions return before the return of the function of sympathetic nervous system. So, some investigators suggest that patients can safely be discharged, when the decrease between the two successive orthostatic mean arterial pressure (MAP) is <10% of the preanesthetic level, which indicates the return of sympathetic function. Prior to ambulation and discharge, patients should also have (i) normal perianal (S_{4-5}) sensation, (ii) the ability to plantar flex the foot, and (iii) the proprioception of big toe which indicates the free of lowest spinal segment from the effect of local anesthetic agent.

"Home discharge" Criteria

- Stable vital signs for >30 minutes
- After the operation, there are no new signs and symptoms of complications.
- No active bleeding
- No nausea or vomiting for >30 minutes
- Able to void, able to dress, and able to walk without assistance
- Fully awake and no loss of orientation to person, time, and place
- Minimal dizziness after sitting for >10 minutes
- Pain controllable with oral analgesics, no excessive pain

- Intact neurocirculatory function without the evidence of swelling or impaired circulation after extremity surgery
- Able to eat and drink
- Patient must be discharged by both anesthetist and surgeon or by their designate. For postoperative period written instructions are given including a contact place and person.

Specific Discharge Criteria

- *Spinal:*
  - Full recovery of motor power and proprioception
  - Passed urine
  - Full recovery of autonomic nervous system
- *Brachial plexus block:*
  - Some regression of motor block
  - Understanding of protection of partially blocked limb
- *Lower limb block:*
  - Some regression of motor block
  - Adequate mobility demonstrated on crutches
  - Understanding of protection of partially blocked limb.

Postoperative Analgesia

Pain control is an important factor for determining when a patient can be discharged after surgery and anesthesia from a day-case unit. So, the pain must be treated rapidly and effectively in order to minimize the delay of discharge. The excessive postoperative pain is usually due to surgery-related causes, but not due to anesthetic causes. But, the provision for good postoperative analgesia is primarily the responsibility of an anesthetist. An anesthetist can do a little for the number of patients requiring readmission for surgical complications, but can play a major role in reducing the readmissions caused by pain and vomiting. The postoperative pain control should be started from pre- or intraoperative period by supplementing any technique of anesthesia with (i) NSAID, (ii) short-acting opioid analgesics, and (iii) local/regional block intraoperatively.

Any type of NSAID can be used, but recently ketorolac is very useful for postoperative analgesia in day-case surgery. It is a potent peripherally acting injectable analgesic associated with few CNS side effects. Caudal block, using 0.125–0.25% bupivacaine also provides excellent postoperative analgesia in herniorrhaphy, anal operations, perianal operation, hypospadias, circumcision, orchidopexy, etc. In caudal block, care should also be taken that the skeletal muscular strength of lower extremities should not be compromised. Other than caudal block, there are many other types of nerve block by which postoperative analgesic can be provided, matching with the day-case anesthetic unit.

Postoperative Admission

The reasons for not discharging the patient at time on the day of surgery and overnight admission are:

- Unexpected surgical or anesthetic complications requiring more close postoperative observation
- Unexpectedly more extensive surgery
- Do not fulfill the discharge criteria before the schedule closure of day-case surgical and anesthesia unit
- Uncontrolled pain and/or PONV
- Inadequate social circumstances at the home of patient

The overall incidence of complicated and not to be in discharged condition, after a surgical procedure, in a day-case unit is only 0.5–2%. Among these, the gynecology and urology day-case department have the highest readmission rates. The surgical causes for postoperative readmission are 3–5 times greater than that of anesthetic causes. The most common anesthetic causes for postoperative readmission are: inadequate recovery, nausea, vomiting, and postoperative pain. The anesthesia-related complications, responsible for readmission, are more frequent with GA than with local or RA with or without sedation. The surgical reasons for readmission include bleeding, extensive surgery, perforated viscus (it is the singular form of viscera), etc. which needs further treatment.

Anesthesia at Remote Location and for Radiodiagnosis and Radiotherapy

■ INTRODUCTION

The delivery of anesthetic care for bronchoscopy, gastrointestinal endoscopy, cardiac catheterization, cardiac electrophysiological investigations, electroconvulsive therapy, lithotripsy, dental surgeries, radiological diagnostic, and radiological therapeutic procedures, etc. in a room which is not originally designed for such a work (anesthesia) and is located far away from the main operation theater (OT) complex of the hospital *is called the anesthesia at remote location*. It is also called the off-site anesthesia or nonoperating room anesthesia or NORA **(Box 1)**. For NORA, the same basic standards for anesthesia care must be met, regardless of the location for the delivery of anesthetic care. Furthermore, the challenges for unfamiliar environments

---

BOX 1: Common locations for NORA.

- *Radiology:*
  - CT scan
  - MRI scan
  - PET scan
  - Vascular radiology
  - Neurointerventional radiology
- Radiation therapy
- *Invasive cardiology suit:*
  - Cardiac catheterization
  - Electrophysiological investigation
  - Cardioversion
- *Endoscopy unit:*
  - Bronchoscopy
  - Gastrointestinal endoscopy
- *Psychiatry:*
  - Electroconvulsive therapy
- *Urology:*
  - Lithotripsy
- Dental surgery

(CT: computed tomography; MRI: magnetic resonance imaging; NORA: nonoperating room anesthesia; PET: positron emission tomography)

---

require advance planning for the off-site anesthesia provider. In contrast to the patients undergoing ambulatory surgery, these patients for NORA are frequently among the sickest of inpatients.

The potential problems for an anesthesiologist providing a good anesthetic care for the patients in such remote locations are (i) poor physical layout of anesthetic machine, anesthetic monitoring equipment, gas supply unit, suction apparatus, emergency drugs, etc. and so subsequently providing poor facility for anesthesia at remote area; (ii) presence of unfamiliar and outdated anesthetic equipment in such areas, because those which are not usually used in main OTs, are dumped at such remote area in most of the institutions; (iii) working with personnel who are less familiar with the anesthetic aspects of patient's care; and (iv) remoteness from available intensive critical help during dire emergency.

The basic principles for NORA can be broadly classified into three categories:

1. *Patient factors:* They include comorbidity, airway assessment, fasting status, and monitoring
2. *Environment factors:* They include anesthesia equipment, emergency equipment, and magnetic and radiation hazards
3. *Procedure-related aspects:* They include duration of procedure, level of discomfort, patient position, and surgical support.

A few years ago, very few investigations in the department of radiology does require any form of anesthesia. But, now due to the development of many modern noninvasive radiodiagnostic and radiotherapeutic procedures and due to the development of fast track ambulatory outpatient anesthesia; there is an increasing demand, both by the patient and the radiologist for the use of anesthesia in the department of radiology. Therefore, any form of anesthesia, i.c., from conscious sedation to monitored anesthetic care (MAC) to deep sedation to general anesthesia (GA) with various levels of consciousness (continuum of depth of sedation ranging from minimal sedation to GA), is now used, according to the necessity of patient, at such remote area.

Among them, the most common form of anesthesia is *conscious sedation* or MAC and it is such a state that where a sedated patient can respond appropriately to verbal command and other stimuli **(Box 2)**. In conscious sedation, the patient can maintain the patency of airway independently by himself and retain his own protective airway reflexes. Deep sedation is a state in which the patient is not easily aroused and their airway reflexes with patency are lost. This deep sedation is more akin to GA and outside the OT it (deep sedation) is a challenge to an anesthetist **(Table 1)**. This is because the environment of a radiological department creates a unique problem to an anesthetist and the whole anesthesia procedure which will be discussed later. But, instead of all these problems, an anesthetist must attempt to provide service as good as the main OT complex without compromising the standards, safety, and the comforts of patients.

The American Society of Anesthesiologists (ASA) standards required for basic anesthetic monitoring at the areas of remote location are:

- A qualified anesthetist must be present there continuously.

> **BOX 2:** Monitored anesthetic care (MAC).
>
> Monitored anesthetic care has been described as a specific anesthesia service for diagnostic or therapeutic procedures, performed under local anesthesia (LA) along with sedation and analgesia, titrated to a level that preserves spontaneous breathing and airway reflexes. MAC essentially comprises three basic components: (i) conscious sedation, (ii) measures to allay patient's anxiety, (iii) effective pain control. MAC results in less physiological disturbances and a more rapid recovery than general anesthesia (GA). The MAC is suitable for day care and off-site surgical procedures as it helps in fast tracking.

- A continuous source for O_2 should always be available there. During anesthesia, patient's oxygenation should be measured continuously by monitoring the inspired O_2 concentration (FiO_2) and patient's SpO_2.
- Adequacy of ventilation should always be evaluated continuously by clinical examination of patient and expired gas analysis for $ETCO_2$ tension.
- Disconnection alarms must be used with mechanical ventilators.
- Circulatory status should always be evaluated by continuous display of electrocardiogram (ECG) and by frequent determination of noninvasive arterial blood pressure (BP) and heart rate.
- ET tube positioning must be verified by frequent auscultation of chest with stethoscope or by continuous measurement of $ETCO_2$ tension.
- There should be readily available equipment to measure the patient's temperature continuously.
- There should have a complete arrangement (emergency cart, defibrillator, and drugs) for the management of a situation like "cardiac arrest" with cardiopulmonary resuscitation (CPR).
- There must have a suction apparatus and a waste gas scavenging system.
- There should be safe electrical outlets, good illumination, battery backup, and a good communication system between the anesthetist, radiologist, and assistant personal.
- There should be sufficient space for anesthesia personnel, equipment, and others.
- There should be adequate facility for postanesthetic management.

▌ INDICATIONS FOR ANESTHESIA IN RADIOLOGY DEPARTMENT

The common indications for any type of anesthesia (MAC to conscious sedation to deep sedation to GA) for radiodiagnosis and radiotherapy at remote locations are:

TABLE 1: Continuum of depth of sedation, ranging from minimal sedation to general anesthesia.

Type	Level	Airway	Responsiveness	Ventilation	CVS
Minimal	1	Unaffected	Response to verbal stimulation	Normal	Normal
Moderate	2	Intervention may or may not required	Response to tactile stimulation, not to verbal stimulation	Depressed, but adequate	Slightly depressed
Deep	3	Simple intervention (Guedel airway) is sufficient	Response to painful stimulus only	Depressed and inadequate, only O_2 supplementation	Moderately depressed
General anesthesia	4	LMA or ET tube is required	No response to painful stimulus	Manual ventilation is required	Manipulation required

(CVS: cardiovascular system; ET: endotracheal; LMA: laryngeal mask airway)

- Neonates, infants, or uncooperative children.
- Older children or adults with psychological, behavioral, or movement disorders.
- Many interventional procedures performed under computed tomography (CT) or magnetic resonance imaging (MRI) guidance, requiring analgesia, sedation, or anesthesia.
- For certain investigations in already intubated patients who is receiving intensive care in intensive care unit (ICU).

HAZARDS IN RADIOLOGY DEPARTMENT AND GENERAL CONSIDERATIONS

The hazards which the anesthetists have to face in the radiology department while providing their anesthesia service can be divided into two main headings: (i) the environment and (ii) the adverse reactions resulting from contrast media.

Environmental Hazards

Poor Visibility

The poor visibility, due to darkness, which is an immense necessary for a radiology unit, makes a great difficulty to the anesthetists for their work. The radiological investigations are usually done under dark surroundings and the anesthetist may then have obviously great problems in delivering good anesthesia by observing the patients and monitoring the anesthetic machines in this dark vicinity. Again, when an anesthetist is asked to move away from the patient during X-ray exposure then it adds further problems. This problem can be solved by only illuminating anesthetic machines and the monitoring devices and using audible alarm systems. So, the use of a shaded angle lamp to illuminate the anesthetic

machine's area and the some part of the patient, while minimally or nil interfering the radiologist's ability to see a picture clearly on the image intensifier, is very helpful.

Electrical Hazards

Usually, in a radiology department, the high voltage apparatuses are used and they often cause the malfunctioning of the sophisticated electronic gadgets used for delivering anesthesia and monitoring the patient. Unfortunately, it is also often necessary to use an earth lead attached to the patient in order to obtain a reasonably interference free electrical recording of an ECG. So, if there is any small leakage of current from any of these high voltage radiological equipment which surround the patient, then the danger of the patient through this earth lead is clear, especially if a central intravenous line is present. The leakage of current of few microamperes in these circumstances may also precipitate cardiac arrhythmias. But, recently, several monitors have been developed which can be used successfully without any outside interference by high voltage radiological equipment.

Radiation Hazards

X-ray is a form of electromagnetic radiation with a wavelength varying between 0.01 – 10 nm, corresponding to frequencies in the range of 3×10 to the power 16 – 3×10 to the power 19 Hz and energies in the range of 100. They are shorter in wavelength than UV rays and longer than gamma rays. This is usually generated by impinging a stream of electron beam on certain metals **(Figs. 1A and B)**. The biological effects or hazards of this ionic radiation are caused by the ionization of tissue cells. This ionization of tissue cells occurs when electrons travel through the tissues and causes physicochemical changes in the molecules of cells. The two types of potentially harmful physicochemical changes due

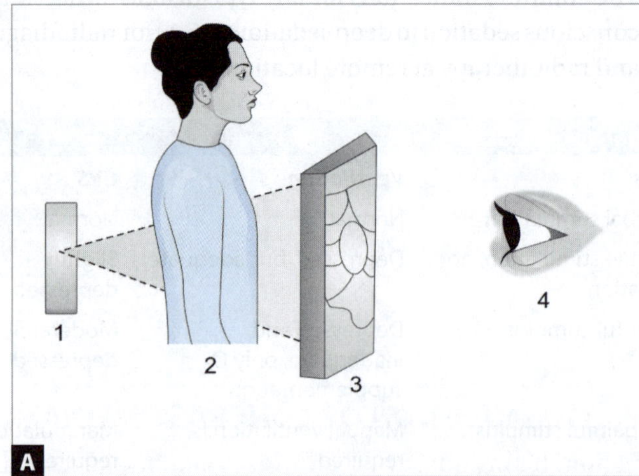

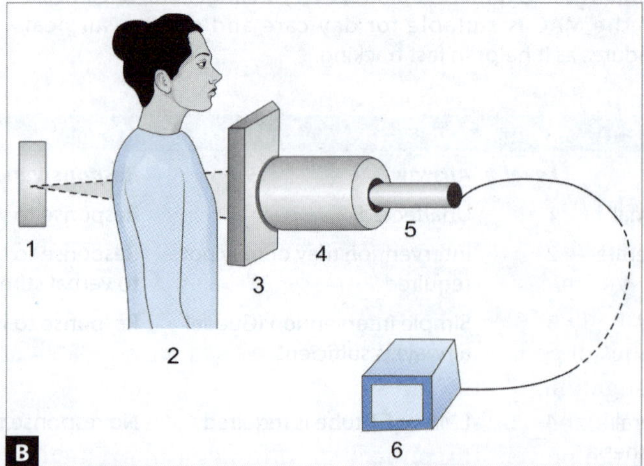

Figs. 1A and B: (A) Simple screening by X-ray; 1 = Tube, 2 = Patient, 3 = Fluorescent screen, 4 = Radiologist; (B) Screening with image intensifier and TV link; 1 = Tube, 2 = Patient, 3 = Fluorescent screen, 4 = Image intensifier, 5 = Camera, 6 = Monitor.

to ionization occur. These are: (i) *somatic effects*, causing skin burn, dermatitis, leukemia, etc. and (ii) *genetic effects*, resulting in fetal abnormality due to the damage of gonadal cells. The maximum permissible limits of radiation (dose) for an occupationally exposed person is 50 mSV (millisievert) per year or 10 mSV × age for lifetime cumulative dose and 0.5 mSV per month for a pregnant woman. So, an anesthetist, who is frequently called upon in radiology department to anesthetize patients, should be cautious of this radiation hazard and must avoid staying in the immediate vicinity of patient during radiological exposure.

The X-rays travel in straight line and the intensity of radiation diminishes in direct proportion to the square of the distance from its source. So, an anesthetist should stand outside the direct line of radiation and as far away as possible from the source of radiation as circumstances permit. They also wear protective clothing such as lead apron, thyroid shield, etc. which are helpful in absorbing radiation and preventing exposure to it. This radiation exposure can also be reduced by employing moveable lead metal (Pb) lined glass screens, between the source of radiation and the anesthetist and by many other innovative techniques, such as allowing the monitoring of patient (to be conducted) away from the patient's immediate contact by the use of microphones and close circuit television, etc. It is very important to mention that the greatest source of radiation is usually from the fluoroscopy and digital subtraction angiography screen. The chances of ionizing radiation from a CT scanner are relatively low, because here the X-rays are highly focused.

Space Problem

Radiology rooms are so crowded with huge radiological equipment that little space is left for the anesthetic persons, anesthetic apparatuses, and monitors. So, some compromise has to be made between the radiological and anesthetic equipment and the available space. So, an anesthetist should spend adequate time to be familiar with this new environment. Sometimes due to space crisis, access to the patient also becomes difficult and dangerous during emergency.

Patient Movement

Sometimes, during radiotherapy or radiological investigation, an anesthetized patient moves away a distance of several feet from an anesthetist and its machine and varieties of patient's positions are also used for radiological investigation. So, the anesthetic circuits should be much long, flexible, light weight, and tightly anchored to the patient to prevent disconnections during this movement of patient. Therefore, Mapleson D or F anesthetic circuit has been proved to be very successful and it is because of their

length, simplicity, and lightness in these circumstances. Further, the length of the Mapleson D and F circuit may be easily adjusted to suit the varying distances of movement involved.

Miscellaneous

Truly speaking, anesthetic equipment, used in the department of radiology is often the oldest in the hospital as previously said. This is because the older anesthetic machines with features that do not meet with the recent standards, are usually relegated from the main modern OT complex to the remote area such as the radiology unit for anesthesia. But, the practice of using these obsolete equipment in remote locations, such as in the radiology unit, should be condemned. The more tragedy is that it is again often disconnected and moved away to a corner of the radiology room when they are not in use for long period. Also the modern monitoring equipment at least ECG, SPO$_2$, and ETCO$_2$ are not readily available in remote area.

So, an anesthetist must be very vigilant in checking the anesthetic machines before every use though it is once upon a time. Empty gas cylinders should be replaced as soon as it becomes empty. All the anesthetic and emergency drugs, spare laryngoscope, batteries, suction machine, and other routine equipment for anesthesia should be present before delivering anesthesia and should be checked by anesthetist himself. Often the preparations of patients scheduled for radiological investigation and therapy are inadequate for anesthesia. Anesthetic assistance is not up to the mark in remote area and the communication between the radiologist, radiotherapist, and the anesthetist is poor. Recovery rooms too are often nonexistent in such situation.

So, the modern radiology rooms have been designed and built by matching with the up-to-date anesthetic requirements. These include O$_2$ and anesthetic gas supply through pipeline, wall mounted suction unit, properly placed modern anesthetic machine with ventilator and monitor, and an anesthetic supply cart fully equipped with all types of drugs, airway adjuncts, laryngoscope, syringes, etc. Within easy reach, the fully monitoring stack should be placed which can be viewed through a window from outside the scan room. Now, some modern scanners have close circuit television which images the patients in control room as they lie within the tube and allow the constant observation of continuing chest wall movement of patient.

ADVERSE REACTION RESULTING FROM THE INJECTION OF CONTRAST MEDIA

Though the quality of contrast media, used for radiodiagnosis, has considerably improved in recent years, still their injection may involve a definite morbidity and mortality. The radio-opacity of contrast media is due to its high atomic number which helps to absorb X-ray. This high atomic number of contrast media is due to its containing iodine (atomic number of iodine is 53). The examples of oldest contrast media are meglumine, iothalamate, diatrizoate, metrizoate, etc. These are toxic, ionized, and hyperosmolar. The high osmolarity of these older contrast media is responsible for many of the bad hemodynamic responses of patients. The osmolarity of these old contrast media is usually 4–5 times higher than that of the blood. Sometimes, it is eight times higher than that of the serum. So, occasionally, gross hypervolemia may result from the injections of large amount of these older agents resulting in depressed myocardial contractility and pulmonary edema.

Hence, recently the nonionized, highly iodinated, water-soluble contrast media which have much lower osmolarity are increasingly used despite their high cost. The examples of these newer agents are iohexol, iopamidol, iopromide, and ioversol. The use of these newer agents as contrast media is associated with much lower incidences and severity of adverse effects. They are typically used in the concentrations which are equivalent to 300–320 mg of iodine per milliliter. The volume of contrast media required for radiodiagnosis varies with the preparation of contrast media, type of investigation, age of the patient, and the total body weight of the patient. But, it may be used maximally up to 150 mL. For example, for the CT of head of an adult patient 50–100 mL, for the CT of whole body of an adult 100–150 mL, for aortography of an adult 100 mL, for urography 2–3 mL/kg, and for child 10+ 2 mL/kg is used.

The adverse effects encountered with these contrast media include nausea and vomiting, hypertension, hypotension, bradycardia, bronchospasm, various arrhythmias, pulmonary edema, and even ventricular fibrillation, or cardiac arrest. Most organs or systems are affected, but the cardiovascular system (CVS) and respiratory system (RS) are potentially at greatest risk. The adverse reactions usually occur within the first 5–10 minutes following the injection of contrast media. So, it is advised to keep the patient under close observation for first 20 minutes following injection. These iodine-containing contrast media occasionally also trigger allergic reactions (iodine sensitivity) and rarely anaphylaxis. These agents may cause renal failure in patients who are dehydrated or have impaired renal function.

So, the adequate hydration should be ensured in patients who have been starved for prolonged period for GA. Lactic acidosis can be precipitated in patients taking biguanides (metformin) and so these oral hypoglycemic agents should be stopped 48 hours before the administration of contrast media. Disseminated intravascular coagulation (DIC) also can follow severe hypotensive shock after the intravenous injection of these contrast media. The incidences of these complications and the severity of it depend on (i) the agents which are used, (ii) the type of investigations which are performed, (iii) the total dose and the speed of injection, and (iv) the most importantly—patient susceptibility. Hypotension induced by contrast media's reaction can render the patient unconscious. Convulsions have been reported in patients with a history of epilepsy. Renal failure is a well-documented complication with the use of contrast media, particularly in patients with preexisting renal disease.

The patients who have experience of mild previous reaction to contrast media have higher incidences of potentially severe reactions (anaphylaxis), if they are exposed to these agents again. Pretesting appears to be of little value in the prediction of these reactions that are truly anaphylactic. The increased prevalence and the severity of reaction caused by contrast media can be reduced by the pretreatment of patient with prednisolone and diphenhydramine (antihistamine). The mechanisms of these adverse drug reactions are often unclear. Some of these adverse effects are immunologically based. But, this is not universal. So, the treatment of complications due to contrast media is directed at the specific components of patient's reaction. For example: (i) the shock and hypotension is treated by fluid and vasopressor, (ii) bronchospasm is treated by bronchodilator, (iii) bradycardia is treated by atropine, (iv) anaphylaxis is treated by steroid, O_2, adrenaline, etc.

PREANESTHETIC MANAGEMENT OF PATIENTS UNDERGOING X-RAY INVESTIGATIONS UNDER GENERAL ANESTHESIA

The preanesthetic management consisting of the assessment and the preparation of patients before any type of anesthesia in radiology department is often neglected. This is because, unfortunately, many radiological studies have been wrongly regarded as minor procedures where anesthesia and sedation are given with little importance. But, clearly this is not true, particularly in those patients who are of greater anesthetic risk due to their age and coexisting medical conditions such as coronary artery disease, respiratory disease, diabetes, obesity, etc. for which radiological investigations are ordered.

Again unfortunately, the attitude such as "he is only going for X-ray" prevails among all the staff of radiology department and is not correct for any patient who is going for X-ray under GA. Patients usually come at the morning on the day of investigation. They remain very much anxious, because it may be his or her first experience of anesthesia. Again the huge radiological equipment and its surroundings are frightening to them. Also the patient may be anxious about what the X-ray investigation may reveal and about the prospects of subsequent surgery depending on the radiological report. The anticipation of all these result in anxiety that is normally felt by the patients, and a brief explanation of the anesthetic procedure before any anesthesia by the anesthetist does much to allay the patient's fear, while establishing a rapport prior to anesthesia.

The patients presenting in radiology department are frequently old. They have frequently cardiovascular diseases and because of the association with cigarette smoking also they have the respiratory problems. So, for these patients, the careful control of blood gases is required during their cerebral and cardiac angiography. For some radiological procedures, precise manipulation of the depth of anesthesia is needed which may finish suddenly, once satisfactory films have been taken after a prolonged trial. Yet the patient must be deeply anesthetized during the injection of contrast media to avoid reflex movement. Such brief movements may be of little inconvenience to a surgeon. But, it may easily ruin an X-ray film which may result in multiple X-ray exposure, with the patient is repeatedly receiving unnecessary radiation and dangerously large doses of contrast media. So, if the patient has to be managed in such circumstances, then a high standard preanesthetic check-up and investigations should be maintained. This includes full clinical examination and all the necessary investigations including routine Hb%, blood film, urine, chest X-ray ECG, and not infrequently pulmonary function tests according to the patient's history and examination. A normal clotting time is preferred, because of the danger of hemorrhage from a relatively large puncture on the wall of blood vessels, left by the radiologist's needle, especially if the Seldinger technique is used.

For many arteriography procedures, a preoperative ECG is essential. This is because of the presence of generalized cardiovascular disease. The patients undergoing carotid angiography may present problems with a raised intracranial pressure (ICP) due to trauma or due to the presence of a space occupying lesion for which radiography is done. In these patients, vomiting, dehydration, and consequent electrolyte disturbances due to ↑ICP indicate the need for serum electrolyte investigation. Renal failure patients presenting for renal angiography require full investigations too. The pediatric patients undergoing any sorts of echocardiography under sedation or GA require a detailed examination and investigations of CVS prior to radiography.

INDIVIDUAL ANESTHETIC MANAGEMENT IN RADIOLOGY DEPARTMENT

The common procedures for which anesthetic department is called upon to anesthetize the patients in radiology department are angiography, CT, MRI, Doppler and echocardiography, and other noninvasive procedures. Recently, many invasive radiological procedures are also done quite frequently under anesthesia. The patients are usually children or uncooperative adult who are suffering from psychiatric diseases, cerebral palsy, Down syndrome, etc. Patients scheduled for elective scan are rarely normal. So, the indications for anesthesia for scanning and the nature of the underlying pathology such as developmental delay, epilepsy, malignancy, psychiatric, and movement disorders, etc. should be checked properly. Several "syndromes" with their manifestations on RS and CVS are also not uncommon. The presence of pain and lengthy radiological procedures may also be an indication for anesthesia in adult, advised for radiological investigation. The patients those are brought from ICU for radiological investigation may be noncooperative and critically ill too.

The principal aim of anesthesia during the radio-diagnostic or radiotherapeutic procedures is to keep the patient just motionless. So, the radiological studies do not demand deep level of anesthesia as the surgical stimulus is not so intense. Therefore, all the types of anesthesia ranging from MAC to conscious sedation to GA may be applied. However, most of the times conscious sedation is sufficient to alter the perception of pain and anxiety and will keep the patient motionless, while maintaining protective airway reflexes and the ability to respond appropriately to verbal commands.

The benzodiazepines and opioids are frequently used for this MAC or conscious sedation. Among the benzodiazepines, the midazolam is mostly preferred due to its some definite advantages such as (i) water solubility, (ii) minimum discomfort during intravenous injection, (iii) no adverse effects on cerebral metabolism and cerebral blood flow, (iv) shorter half-life, and (v) lack of its active metabolites. In clinical doses, generally, the midazolam does not produce any significant cardiovascular depression.

Then, among the opioids, the commonly used opioid is fentanyl (1–2 µg/kg). But, the combination of midazolam and fentanyl can produce significant respiratory and cardiovascular depression. However, the higher doses of fentanyl can result in chest wall rigidity. Tachyphylaxis to propofol and ketamine have been reported.

Computed Tomography or CT Scanning

As the name implies, it provides a series of computer-integrated tomographic axial slices of different parts of our body. The CT produces a two-dimensional, cross-sectional, transverse images by rotating an X-ray beam around the area which is to be examined. A typical CT scan comprises 20 such transverse sections. It is usually used for the investigation of brain, thorax, and abdomen. It has also proved to be valuable in studies of vascular malformation and tumor. Each image is produced by the computer integration of differences in the absorption coefficient of radiation between the different normal and abnormal tissues. The image of the structure under investigation is generated by X-ray and the brightness of each area is proportional to the radiation absorption value of that tissue which is later integrated by computer. Sometimes, contrast medium is also used orally or through parenteral route in conjunction with CT scan to enhance the quality of image. This is called contrast CT. In this situation such as when contrast medium is used orally and if GA is needed, then there is higher risk of aspiration. So, in such circumstances, the patient should be always intubated.

During CT scan, the patient is moved slowly inside a dark tunnel and a gantry rotates around the whole body of the patient to cut the transverse slices of image **(Fig. 2)**. Every cutting slice is produced by a single rotation of gantry and thus multiple series of slices are made by several rotation of gantry at interval of 7 mm. The interval of slices can be decreased or increased depending on the diagnostic information sought. The first-generation scanners took 4–5 minutes for cutting every slice of image. But, the newer generation takes only 2–4 seconds. The older CT machines scan the slices in a series of discrete steps. While the modern spiral CTs acquire only image data by a single continuous pass and later they constitute the image. In modern machines, individual scan takes few seconds (2–4 seconds) and a complete study may require only 5–10 minutes. Unlike MRI, in CT scanning, the environment does not restrict the use of conventional type of

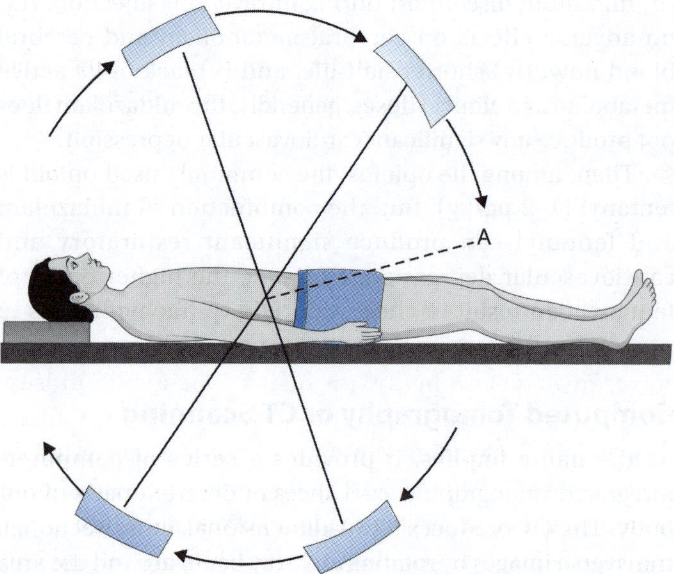

Fig. 2: Computer-integrated tomography. A is the pivotal point of bar connecting tube and films.

anesthetic equipment and monitoring. But, the space is often limited. So, compact anesthetic machines and monitors are more practical.

The CT scan is a painless noninvasive procedure. So, it does not need any anesthesia for adults. Only children, uncooperative individual, and psychiatric patients need anesthesia to keep them motionless. Sometimes, critical patients, who are brought from ICU for CT scan, needs supervision by anesthetist. GA is usually not needed for them. Sedation is sometimes needed and is sufficient for them. Only light anesthesia producing immobility and lack of awareness is required.

A variety of general anesthetic technique can be used for CT scan by applying inhalation or intravenous agents with spontaneous or controlled ventilation (respiration). But, the final choice should be determined by the equipment available and the patient's needs, e.g., only maintenance of clear airway, control of raised ICP, respiratory support, etc. If there is any anticipated problem regarding the clear airway due to felled back tongue under sedation and patient's head is inaccessible during CT scan, then this airway can be cleared by laryngeal mask airway (LMA), provided the patient does not require intermittent positive pressure ventilation (IPPV) or airway protection from aspiration. If intubation is needed for any cause, then every effort should be made to reduce the ICP (especially if the CT is being done for intracranial space occupying lesion) by hyperventilation causing hypocapnia and by avoiding the use of volatile anesthetics agents.

The anesthetists may have to adopt their own techniques depending on whether the patient is an elective one or an emergency trauma victim with ongoing blood loss. These latter patients must be treated, as if they have full stomach and therefore, sedation is not an option. These patients should be scanned in fully awake condition or be intubated following a rapid sequence induction and intubation, if GA is needed. Before laryngoscope and intubation, cervical spine (if fractured) should be stabilized. During the extreme flexion of head (required for the examination of posterior cranial fossa), kinking and disconnection of tube should be cared for.

The positioning of patient and the movement of gantry during the whole radiological procedure may also cause the kinking or disconnection of anesthetic circuit. Cannulas, catheters, drains, and even the endotracheal (ET) tubes can be pulled out during the transfer or movement of patient through the scanner. The radiographer should be asked for how far the table will move. There should be always checking that IV lines and breathing circuit have not been snagged with other equipment. The CT scanning generates the potentially harmful ionizing radiation. So, it is preferable for the anesthetist to monitor the patient from the outside of scanning room. In this circumstance, the patient can also be monitored visually through a lead glass window that is supplemented, if necessary by closed circuit television.

If the anesthetist observes the patient from his control room, then the monitor's alarm should be a visual one that can be easily seen from the control room. But, if it is necessary for an anesthetist to remain near the patient, then the wearing of appropriate radiation protection gown is advisable. During the scanning of thorax and abdomen, to reduce the artifacts caused by respiratory movement, the patient may require brief periods of apnea or breathe holding. To achieve this, both the paralyzed or spontaneously breathing patients should be ventilated manually and their lungs are held standstill in inspiration phase for few seconds. Patient of ICU requiring CT scans should be managed like any inter-ICU transfer with full monitoring and ventilatory support during transfer.

Magnetic Resonance Imaging

It is not based on ionizing radiation. It depends on magnetic field and radiofrequency (RF) pulses for the production of images. In MRI machine, there is a large magnet in the form of a tube capable of accepting the whole length of a human body and creating a huge magnetic field around it. This magnet is approximately 2 m in length and 500 kg in weight. Within this magnetic tube RF transmitting coils, which transmit radiomagnetic waves, are also incorporated surrounding the patient. These RF transmitting coils transmit RF waves of certain length. These coils also act as a receiver to detect the reflected RF waves from the patient and construct an image.

Magnetic resonance imaging is based on the fact that some atoms which contain unpaired protons or neutrons in their nucleus and simultaneously unpaired electrons in their outer orbit have the potential to act as magnetic dipoles. This property of atom is possessed by the following paramagnetic elements such as ^{1}H, ^{13}C, ^{23}Na, etc. and therefore, they behave like tiny magnets. In this purpose, hydrogen atoms of body, which contain a single proton in its nucleus and a single electron in its outer orbit, are particularly suitable for acting as a tiny magnet and produce an MRI image, since they are normally present in vast numbers in our body tissues. Normally, the hydrogen atoms (which is equivalent to a proton) of our body tissue are arranged in a random haphazard fashion. But, the use of a strong external magnetic field will force a proportion of these atoms to align in a new magnetic axis (parallel or antiparallel to the applied magnetic field) from their previous random orientation **(Figs. 3A and B)**. The power of external magnetic field used in MRI for clinical practice ranges from 0.15 to 1.5 Texla (1,500–15,000

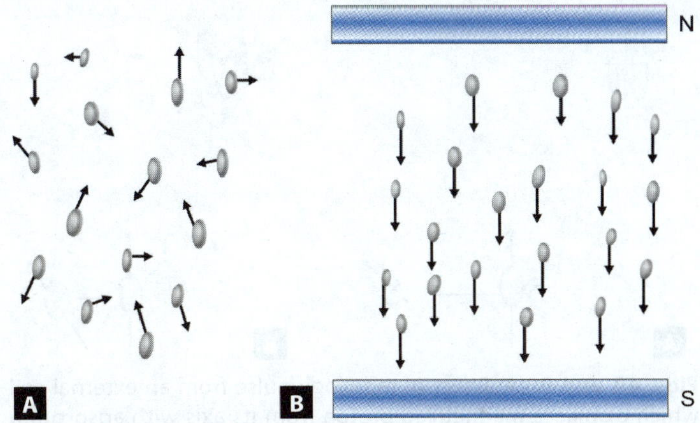

Figs. 3A and B: Mechanism of magnetic resonance imaging (MRI). (A) Protons behaving like tiny bar magnets are oriented randomly; (B) Alignment of protons when immersed in a strong external magnetic field.

Gauss) as compared with that of the earth's magnetic field which is only 0.5 Gauss.

In addition to the large and costly magnet required for MRI, the machine also uses pulses of RF waves. These RF waves are generated by RF transmitting coils that closely surround (incorporated within the magnetic tube) the patient. These RF waves are essential to excite and detect the magnetized aligned hydrogen protons. The pulsed RF wave displaces the nuclei or protons of hydrogen atom from their new parallel or antiparallel position which was produced by external strong magnetic force. Then again the nuclei or protons return to their previous parallel or antiparallel position produced by the external magnetic force immediately after the pulse ceases. At the same time, some energy is released from the tissue as a radio-signal which is detected by the same RF transmitting coils used for the transmission of RF waves. Since, the returned radiosignal is proportional to the concentration of tissue protons (hydrogen atoms), so it forms the basis for a digital record of the total proton content of the tissues by a highly sophisticated computer **(Figs. 4A and B)**.

The computer creates cross-sectional or three-dimensional images from this minute returned radiosignal which is generated when the hydrogen atoms are flipped in and out of the parallel or antiparallel alignment by a powerful magnetic field with high RF magnetic pulses. Then using a similar technique which is used in CT, the returning radiosignal (captured by RF coils) is converted by the computer of MRI into an analog image presented on a cathode ray tube in varying shades of black and white.

The radiosignal received by the RF transmitting coil during this MRI scanning is of very low electrical intensity and so is easily subjected to interference by any electronic

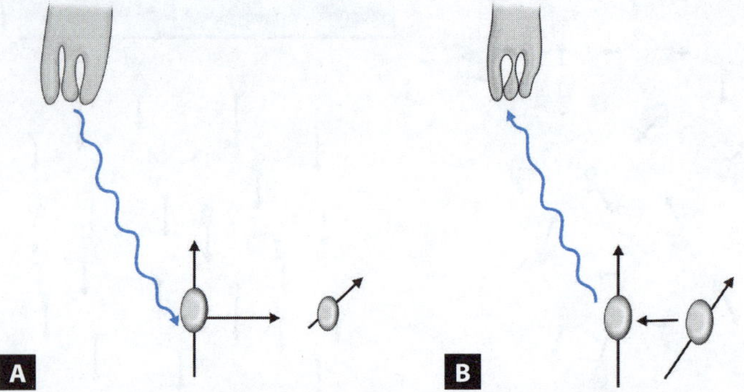

Figs. 4A and B: (A) Effect of radiology pulse from an external coil which displaces magnetized proton from its axis with absorption of energy; (B) Return of magnetized proton to its former axis with release of energy as radiofrequency pulse which can be registered by receiving coil and quantified.

equipment or anesthetic monitoring device. For this reason, the MRI scanning area is completely enclosed by a RF shield which is incorporated usually into the fabric (painting) of MRI imaging suite. The prevention of interference of MRI scanning from anesthetic monitors is usually made by using isolated power sources or battery, some filters and sometimes enclosing the anesthetic monitor in its own small RF shield. The provisions for both safe anesthesia and good MRI image requires specialized anesthetic equipment and careful organization. Unlike CT, it is not possible to take simply the standard conventional anesthetic machines and monitors to the MRI room.

Anesthetic procedure in an MRI suite creates several problems: (i) some arise from the effects of magnetic fields of MRI scanners on anesthetic equipment and (ii) some from the effects of anesthetic equipment on the magnetic field of MRI scanner. The MRI image quality is superior to CT scan. It can differentiate clearly between the white and gray matter of brain which is not possible by CT scan. Again, unlike the CT scan which gives picture only in transverse section, the MRI can display the images in transverse, sagittal, coronal, and oblique planes. Unlike CT scan, it is also capable of detecting diseases in the posterior fossa. MRI provides vascular picture without the need of intravenous contrast media. It requires very little patient preparation. As MRI is not an ionizing radiation, so it does not produce biologically deleterious effects on patients and other personals present in this room and is noninvasive. MRI also permits evaluations of blood flow, cerebrospinal fluid (CSF) flow, contraction, and relaxation of organs, etc. Calcium does not emit signals in MRI. This lack of signal from calcium, however, prevents the MRI from detecting any pathological calcification in soft tissue tumor and pathological changes in cortical bone.

Another disadvantage of MRI over CT scan is that a relatively long time is required to obtain images. Individual

MRI scans may take up to 20 minutes and an entire examination may take not <1 hour. The other disadvantages of MRI are that very obese patient cannot be examined in this narrow magnetic tunnel and body surface absorb the RF energy causing increased body temperature. But, it is usually unlikely that the patient's temperature will increase by >1°C.

Anesthesia and monitoring of patient in MRI suite poses several unique problems. These are:

- Need to exclude all the ferromagnetic components from the surrounding of patient
- Limited patient's access and poor visibility of patient in the MRI tunnel
- Low image quality of MRI due to disturbed RF waves caused by anesthetic electric equipment
- Interference and malfunctioning of anesthetic monitoring equipment due to high magnetic field of MRI.

Patient acceptance of MRI is generally high. Most adults and small babies (recently well fed and wrapped) tolerate the procedure without sedation. Sedation may be required only in older children and in adults who cannot cooperate. This *sedation* may be conscious sedation or deep sedation akin to GA. *Conscious sedation* can be defined as a medically controlled state of depressed consciousness which allow the protective reflexes of airway to be maintained and retains the patient's ability to maintain a patent airway independently. It also permits an appropriate response of the patient to physical stimulation or verbal command. Whereas *deep sedation* can be defined as a medically controlled state of depressed consciousness which may be accompanied by a partial or complete loss of protective airway reflexes, inability to maintain a patent airway independently and inability to respond purposefully to physical stimulation or verbal command. GA is more or less close to deep sedation. *GA is defined* as a medically controlled state of unconsciousness accompanied by a loss of protective airway reflexes including the inability to maintain a patent airway independently and the inability to respond purposefully to physical stimulation or verbal command.

Sedation (usually for pediatric group) is usually ensured by chloral hydrate (50 mg/kg orally) or midazolam (0.3–0.5 mg/kg orally) or diazepam (0.1 mg/kg orally). For adult, sedation can be maintained by thiopentone or propofol. For each of these groups of patients, the requirement of anesthesia for MRI scan is only immobility.

In order to obtain high quality images, patients need to remain immobile within the confined space of magnetic core for at least 20 minutes. Complex scan may take much longer time. So, though, most of the patients tolerate the procedure without sedation, still a large number of patients near about 3% of healthy adults are unable to do this without adjuvant sedation or GA.

Magnetic resonance imaging (MRI) scanner is very noisy and a patient has to lie for a long time on a thin table in a dark confined space made by the tube within this high noise. This can cause claustrophobia or anxiety even in adults necessitating sometimes sedation or anesthesia. The MRI has two implications on anesthesia: (i) inaccessibility of an anesthetized patient to an anesthetist when the body enters totally into the scanner magnetic tunnel and (ii) malfunctioning of anesthetic ferromagnetic monitors in the strong magnetic field of MRI. Within the MRI tunnel except conscious sedation in deep sedation (only if it is needed), the manual control of the airway of a patient is impossible. So, tracheal intubation or LMA is essential to clear the airway of an anesthetized patient from falling tongue. If the indication of scanning under GA is for suspected raised ICP or if GA is indicated in a patient with a potentially full stomach, then intubation with positive pressure ventilation is required. The effect of increasing the length of expiratory limb of Ayre's T-piece has been studied on ventilation. Different studies have shown that with 10 m long breathing circuit, there is only minimal decrease in tidal volume as a result of circuit compliance. So, it dictates that remote ventilation from outside the scanner room can be performed by using the long Bain circuit or Mapleson D circuit when the patient is within the MRI room and the anesthetic machine is outside the MRI room.

The maintenance of anesthesia by volatile anesthetic agents or propofol infusion have both been employed. However, with the latter, the dose adjustment can be unpredictable, because the infusion pump may malfunction in the strong magnetic field. The use of LMA is gaining popularity in MRI setting, where intubation is not absolutely indicated and is used for only better maintenance of airway. As there is no risk of ionic radiation in MRI, so the anesthetist can observe the patient from both the ends of the MRI tunnel and can take out the patient quickly, if necessary. Due to intense magnetic field, the anesthetic monitoring equipment also does not work properly. Reversely, the ferromagnetic anesthetic monitoring equipment distorts the magnetic field sufficiently and degrades the image. It is also likely that the ferromagnetic anesthetic monitoring equipment are propelled toward the scanner machine and may cause a significant accident, if it makes contact with the patient or staff at a certain speed.

The MRI room or suite can be laid out in two fashions for anesthesia. If the majority of anesthetic equipment needs to be kept inside the radiology room, then the MRI compatible instrument should be used. But, usually most of the time, the anesthetic machine and the monitoring equipment are kept outside the room and long MRI compatible (shielded or nonferromagnetic) anesthetic circuits, ECG cables, SpO$_2$ cables, etc. are used and they lead to the patient from outside the room. The disadvantage of this approach includes the need for extra-long monitoring cables, breathing tubes and other connections which frequently cause disconnection and leak.

Another common approach is to induce anesthesia in the induction area, adjacent to MRI suite, but outside the magnetic field using conventional anesthetic equipment with the patient on a nonferromagnetic table or trolley, made of aluminum or stainless steel (MRI compatible). Then, this table is transported with the patient after induction into the MRI room where the maintenance of anesthesia and monitoring are continued using MRI compatible anesthetic machine and monitoring devices. The portable anesthetic machine constructed of nonmagnetic material, aluminum gas cylinders, and MRI compatible O$_2$ analyzer also are used in MRI suite. Consideration also needs to be given to IV fluid stands, gas cylinders, ventilators, stethoscope, etc. Standard batteries of laryngoscope should be replaced with nonmagnetic lithium batteries, if it is used in MRI suite.

Laryngeal mask airways without metal spring in the pilot tube valve (armored) should also be available. The heart rate and respiratory rate can be monitored with an esophageal stethoscope. If the patient is allowed to breathe spontaneously, then the movement of the reservoir bag may also be used as an index of ventilation. The metallic tubing connectors for noninvasive automated arterial pressure monitor should be replaced by nonmetallic connectors. But, the extended length of tube from the BP cuff to its base unit is associated with some damping of signal. Invasive monitoring is also possible. But in order to minimize damping, the transducer must be kept as close to the patient as the magnetic field will allow. If the transducer is kept within the 0.5 mT line, close to the patient, then to avoid the damping of RF, the use of filter will limit the interference **(Fact file I)**.

Patients fitted with a demand cardiac pacemaker should not be exposed to MRI. This is because the induced electrical currents within the pacemaker by huge magnetic field may be mistaken for the natural activity of heart and may inhibit the pacemaker output, even in the absence of normal cardiac electrical activity. Other potential problems of the cardiac pacemaker due to MRI include (i) possible reed switch closure or damage, (ii) automatic switch over to an asynchronous mode, and (iii) changes of program, etc.

Intracranial metallic vascular clips may be dislodged from the blood vessels due to magnetic induction of clips during the procedure of MRI. Malfunctioning of shunts, wire spiral of ET tube, automatic implantable cardiac defibrillators, and implanted biologic pumps are also other dangers. Metallic objects such as scissors, stethoscope, BP instrument,

FACT FILE I

Specific problem and its solution during anesthesia and monitoring of a patient in a MRI suite is like that:
- Pulse oximeter must have the fiberoptic signal-linking facilities between the monitor and the sensor, RF filter, and ECG-locking device.
- ECG must have a RF filter for its proper functioning and its leads should be placed as close as possible to the center of the magnetic field.
- The metal connection of BP cuff and pipes should be changed to plastic one for the noninvasive monitoring of BP.
- The side stream capnography functions satisfactorily in MRI unit, but the length of this sampling tube may cause significant delay in signal transduction.
- The precordial or esophageal stethoscope does not function well. This is because of the noise created by the scanner during its operation.
- The temperature probe should have a RF filter for its proper functioning in MRI unit.

It is also to be remembered that anesthesia monitoring units which function satisfactorily in one MRI unit, produce problems in another MRI suite. This is due to the differences in RF and magnetic field strength, employed by two MRI system. Some centers permit the patient to breathe spontaneously during anesthesia. But controlled ventilation by neuromuscular blockade is preferred. This is because it not only provides satisfactory gas exchange, but also avoid excessive head, neck, chest, and abdominal movement that may interfere the imaging process.

cylinder opener, laryngoscope, etc. which are brought in the vicinity of MRI magnet can literally fly into it and may cause severe injury to the patient and the bystanders.

Electric motors (e.g., in syringe infusion pump) may run erratically and administer wrong doses of drug to the patient. Also any information stored on magnetic media of credit card, bank cards, cassette tape, floppy disk, etc. will be erased by demagnetization. The magnetic field decreases as distance from the scanner increases. Places beyond the 0.5 mT boundary line or outside of the scanning room can be considered safe. During scanning, the noise level may sometimes reach 95 decibel. So, ear plugs should be worn, even for anesthetized patients to avoid the damage of cochlea. Devices made from stainless steel which is not ferromagnetic can be taken into the scan room. Even weakly ferromagnetic objects such as the metallic make up on face or tattoos can distort the image, or be heated by the powerful magnetic field of the MRI machine to a point, which can cause burn.

In complying with the minimum perianesthetic monitoring standards, a balance must be made between (i) the loss of MRI image quality due to the electromagnetic interference from different anesthetic and monitoring equipment and (ii) the degradation of monitor signal quality as the result of the powerful magnetic field of MRI. There are several monitoring systems that are nonferromagnetic and, therefore, are compatible for their use in MRI room. Central capnography is not possible to use in MRI room, because within magnetic field the sampling unit of central capnography will tend to be overheated and would grossly distort the image. Side stream capnography should be used, but it necessitates a long sampling tube to keep the monitor beyond the MRI room or 0.5 mT line.

The long ECG cable can cause the reduction of the quality of both the monitor and scan signals. So, the telemetric ECG is very useful in an attempt to circumvent this problem which is now available commercially. A liquid crystal display for cardiac monitoring should be used to avoid the distortion of cathode ray tracing by the magnet of MRI machine. Recently, surgeries like laparotomies and craniotomies are being carried out with the intermittent MRI picture to allow the accurate tumor resection. In such condition, scanners are horseshoe-shaped in design like the C arm X-ray with one side open to allow the access to the patient. Here, all the same precautions and principles are applied like the nonoperative MRI, except the titanium instruments are used.

Angiography

For angiography, an arterial catheter is passed directly into the arterial lumen and a contrast medium is injected into the artery that produces image and is viewed by a conventional cut film radiography or by digital subtraction angiography. The arteries of viscera and lower extremities may be approached via the femoral artery, although arterial occlusive disease may require translumbar approach to reach the aorta. It is an invasive technique, so the development of CT scan and MRI has now reduced the use of this type of invasive angiography. Also the advent of spiral and double helical CT scanner allows the whole vascular territories to be mapped out within 30 seconds. Regarding the angiography, MRI produces superior images than CT scanning including three-dimensional pictures and is also sensitive to the detection of flow.

Most of the angiographies are done under local anesthesia (LA) with or without mild sedation. This is because the gaining of vascular access and the injection of contrast media into the vessels may result in patient's discomfort. So, some patients may get benefit from the judicious administration of analgesics and sedatives. The indications for GA in angiography are same as for CT scan and MRI.

The *disadvantage of GA* for angiography is it prolongs the time taken for investigation, and increases the cost and the risk associated with GA. In GA, the another disadvantage is that patient will not be able to react to untoward reactions due to radiocontrast medium, while under LA a conscious patient can describe symptoms and allow the procedure to be stopped immediately. Usually, the patients undergoing arteriography to determine the extent of vascular occlusive disease have a higher incidence of serious comorbid conditions such as diabetes mellitus, coronary heart disease, hypertension, renal disease, etc. So, appropriate monitoring and precautions should be taken when applying sedation and anesthesia for angiography or CT or MRI scan in this group of patients.

Cerebral Angiography

Cerebral angiography is usually done for the diagnosis of arteriovenous malformations, aneurysms or tumors, etc. in the brain where radiopaque contrast medium is given in the carotid artery and a plane or a digital X-ray is taken. It is mostly done under LA. The indications for GA in cerebral angiography are same as that of CT scan or MRI. But, most of the patients scheduled for cerebral angiography have increased ICP. So, all the measures have to be taken to prevent the rise of ICP, if the patient requires GA. Smooth induction for GA should be instituted avoiding coughing, bucking, straining, etc., and permitting BP to be well maintained. It is reasonable to employ a technique of controlled ventilation avoiding the use of volatile anesthetic agents as they increase the ICP. Hyperventilation produces hypocapnia and it is useful for the reduction of ICP. So, during the maintenance of anesthesia, the reduction of $PaCO_2$ by hyperventilation causes vasoconstriction of cerebral vessels resulting in slow cerebral circulation and increased transit time of contrast medium which will improve the delineation of small vascular lesions. Sometimes, transient hypotension, bradycardia, or asystole may occur during cerebral angiography due to contrast dye injection. Acute cerebral edema has also been reported following the injection of contrast media due to the hyperosmolarity of dye and also due to the changes in permeability of endothelium of blood-brain barrier. Other complications of cerebral angiography are hemorrhage which is due to the rupture of lesion or vessel and ischemia which is due to thromboembolism or vasospasm.

Coronary Angiography

Coronary vasculature is visualized by injecting a radiopaque contrast media into the ostium of any coronary artery. Thus, it helps in (i) the determination of anatomy of coronary artery, (ii) in the detection of the presence and the location of any stenosis, and (iii) in the detection of coronary vasospasm. Thus, the information obtained from coronary angiography dictate further treatment ranging from simple medical therapy for myocardial ischemia to angioplasty during angiography to coronary artery bypass graft (CABG). Though, the CT and MRI help in the diagnosis of coronary

arterial disease, but still coronary angiography is the "gold standard" method for the diagnosis of coronary arterial disease. During coronary angiography, some interventional procedure can also be performed to improve the coronary blood flow.

During coronary angiography, LA is provided at the site of the introduction of arterial catheter which is either around the femoral artery or the brachial artery. Under LA, coronary angiography is usually performed by passing a catheter via the femoral artery in a retrograde fashion to the aortic root. Then, for selective angiography, contrast medium is injected into the ostia of each coronary artery. During coronary angiography, every patient should have an intravenous cannula for the administration of emergency medicines (if needed), analgesics, or sedation. For analgesia, usually fentanyl and for sedation usually midazolam are helpful in reducing the discomfort during injection of contrast media and in maintaining the motionless supine position of patient during long procedures. Any benzodiazepines, given IV slowly, provide adequate sedation for most of the cases. However, sometimes, this fentanyl and midazolam are supplemented with propofol. Standard anesthetic monitoring protocol is used during the whole procedure of angiography including the continuous monitoring of SpO_2, heart rate, respiratory rate, ECG, arterial BP (by directly transduced from arterial introducer), etc. The infusion of glyceryl trinitrate (GTN) should be readily available for administration, if the patient develops myocardial ischemia. Supplemental O_2 should be administered to every patient via face mask or nasal cannula. The complications of coronary angiography are more common in the patients with severe coronary artery disease and it includes arrhythmias, heart failure, and strokes. Local bleeding and hematoma at the site of catheter introduction are the surgical complications. Arrhythmias are not uncommon and are both due to the direct stimulation of myocardium by catheter and following the injection of contrast media. Bradycardia is also common as the nonspecific ECG changes. Left heart failure is easily induced which is due to the rapid rise in left ventricular end-diastolic volume and pressure caused by the injection of contrast media in bolus. Myocardial infarction has been noted in 0.5% of patients during coronary angiography. Thorough proper preoperative examination, correction of preexisting arrhythmias where possible, and good control of the serum electrolytes clearly minimizes the potential dangers during coronary angiography.

Interventional Transvascular Coronary Arterial Procedure

Once the presence and the location of any coronary arterial block or stenosis are confirmed, then a variety of methods or interventional procedures can be employed to improve the myocardial blood flow directly. Heparin is used prior to any angiography and interventional therapeutic procedures. One of the methods or interventional coronary arterial procedure is the percutaneous transluminal coronary angioplasty (PTCA). Here, the stenosed or blocked area of coronary artery is traversed by a balloon-tipped catheter which is introduced through the femoral artery. The balloon is then inflated to dilate the area of stenosis and to remove the block which will increase the coronary blood flow. During balloon inflation, transient coronary artery occlusion can occur. So, patient's hemodynamic status must be closely monitored.

Other interventional coronary arterial procedures are placement of coronary stents, removal of atheromatous plaque, extracorporeal circulation, etc. Extracorporeal circulation is usually established in patients who are not otherwise candidates for CABG surgery such as those with unacceptably poor ventricular function. It is performed via the femoral artery and vein following GA and systemic heparinization. The coronary atherotomy may be performed using atherotomy catheter or excimer lasers. During all these procedures, different types of ventricular arrhythmias can be precipitated and these hemodynamically unstable arrhythmias can be treated with lignocaine or cardioversion. The rupture of coronary artery during these interventional transvascular coronary arterial procedure may result in pericardial tamponed and is treated by emergency pericardiocentesis.

The other complications of interventional coronary angiography are: (i) coronary artery dissection, (ii) coronary artery vascular spasm due to the dysfunction of coronary artery endothelium, and (iii) intra-arterial thrombus formation. Once, the thrombus is formed, then the intracoronary injection of urokinase or streptokinase may dissolve this thrombus. Sometimes, acute coronary artery occlusion does not respond to transluminal treatment in cardiac catheterization laboratory. Then, it may require emergency CABG. The spectrum of treatment, provided in the cardiac catheterization laboratory, is now constantly changing. Various combinations of the above described procedures and some new procedures may be performed on individual patient. But, it depends on the severity and the location of the lesions and the frequency of practice performed at each individual institution.

Cardiac Catheterization

The cardiac catheterization is nothing but the placement of a catheter into great vessels or into the chambers of heart through a transvenous or transarterial route. It helps in: (i) the determination of cardiac anatomy, (ii) the determination

of valvular anatomy, (iii) the determination of pulmonary vascular anatomy, (iv) the measurement of pressure in different cardiac chambers and major blood vessels, (v) the injection of contrast media for radiological visualization of various vascular structures, (vi) the injection of indicator dye with distal sampling for flow determination (using Fick principle), (vii) blood sampling for the measurement of O_2 and CO_2 tension to detect the presence and the location of shunts, etc.

The right side of the heart is accessed via the femoral, brachial, cephalic, or internal jugular vein and the left side of the heart is accessed via the femoral, brachial artery, or radial artery. Although, all the above mentioned parameters can be measured by echo and Doppler cardiography, still the cardiac catheterization is the "gold standard" technique. For the measurement of flow and pressure from different cardiac chambers and subsequently to measure the shunt (by the difference in O_2 tension), a steady state preanesthetic cardiovascular and respiratory function is necessary. Any change in the flow and pressure in any cardiac chamber due to anesthetic procedure may result in incorrect result (for the measurement of shunt). So, the arterial O_2 and CO_2 tension should be strictly maintained at preanesthetic levels or should not change (if abnormal for that patient) by any anesthetic technique or by giving (administering) O_2. These constraints make the anesthetic management extremely difficult for cardiac catheterization.

The cardiac catheterization in adults is done under LA and/or sedation, produced by midazolam and/or fentanyl and if necessary with propofol. It is frequently performed in conjunction with coronary angiography. The O_2 is administered only when the O_2 saturation falls below the level of baseline and care must be taken to maintain the previous arterial blood gas level, if the dishunts or pulmonary hemodynamics are to be measured. GA is sometimes required for the placement of aortic stents which are increasingly performed by cardiologists in the cardiac catheterization laboratory. Recently, specially built hybrid surgical suites enable both the open and catheter-based vascular repairs. Increasingly, patients for transcatheter aortic valve replacement are managed with LA and sedation, rather than GA. Institutional protocols and patient characteristics determine the GA/sedation management of these patients. GA is frequently administered to the patients in neurointerventional suite for the treatment of cerebral aneurysms and ischemic strokes.

The complications of cardiac catheterization are similar to that of coronary angiography, because catheter is placed within the cardiac chambers. So, the supraventricular and ventricular arrhythmias are very common during this procedure. Hence, an anesthetist must be ready to deal with these acute hemodynamic and/or respiratory instability in patients who may have severe valvular and myocardial dysfunction. Fortunately, however, these cardiac arrhythmias are usually resolved with immediate withdrawal of catheter. Sometimes IV medication, vagal maneuvers, or cardioversion may be necessary to terminate these arrhythmias. Other than different cardiac arrhythmias, the other complications of cardiac catheterization are perforation of cardiac chambers, perforation of great vessels, bleeding, hematoma formation, aortic dissection, embolic phenomenon, etc.

Patients requiring electrophysiological procedures for catheter-mediated arrhythmia ablation often need GA. Such patients may have both systolic and diastolic heart failure leading to potential hemodynamic difficulties perioperatively. Other patients require sedation for the placement of ICDs. Once placed, the device will be tested by inducing ventricular fibrillation. During this testing, deeper level of sedation are required, as the defibrillation shock can be frightening and very uncomfortable.

Likewise, anesthesia staff is called upon to provide anesthesia for cardioversion of patients in atrial fibrillation. These patients usually have associated cardiac diseases and require brief IV anesthetic agents to facilitate cardioversion. Often, a TEE is performed prior to cardioversion to rule out clot in the left atrial appendage. In such cases, anesthesia staff may also provide sedation for this procedure. Determination as to whether a patient needs sedation or GA with or without intubation is dependent upon the routine assessment of patient.

Only children require GA for cardiac catheterization. The children requiring cardiac catheterization usually suffer from different types of congenital heart diseases and often present with cyanosis, dyspnea, heart failure, etc. These congenital cardiac anomalies may vary from simple atrial septal defect to complex cardiac defects with shunts at various levels, as for example hypoplastic left heart syndrome with severe ventricular dysfunction, etc. The pediatric patients suffering from congenital heart disease may also have coexisting noncardiac congenital anomalies. So, only when an experienced cardiac anesthetist is readily available, then it has now become the custom in many institutions to employ GA on children for cardiac catheterization. During the procedure of cardiac catheterization, the aim of an anesthetist is to maintain a steady circulatory state. This may require considerable preoperative preparation of patient in close conjunction with cardiac physicians, surgeons, and radiologists. Oxygen, digitalis, and diuretic therapy, together with the correction of electrolyte imbalance and acidosis, should be carried out before cardiac catheterization when

possible. Some infants may be seriously ill and may present with cardiac failure as potential surgical emergencies.

During cardiac catheterization, an ideal anesthetic technique (i) should not produce any myocardial depression, (ii) should avoid any hypertension/hypotension and tachycardia, (iii) must preserve normal O_2 tension and maintain normocapnia [to avoid alterations in pulmonary vascular resistance (PVR)] while maintaining respiration on air. Even in cyanotic patients, supplemental O_2 is not administered unless O_2 saturation falls below the baseline level. Spontaneous respiration with volatile anesthetic agents may not be suitable for patients with significant myocardial disease. Controlled ventilation is essential using room air, as long as O_2 saturation does not fall below critical level. Controlled ventilation avoids the increase in $PaCO_2$ which is frequently found in spontaneous respiration. As an alternative to volatile anesthetic agents, patients can be managed with total intravenous anesthesia (TIVA) using various combination of opioids, midazolam, propofol, and ketamine. During the procedure of cardiac catheterization, repeated blood gas analysis is essential, because the metabolic acidosis may be the initial sign of low cardiac output state due to myocardial depression. Even, a mild degree of metabolic acidosis should be treated in critically ill patients by inotropic therapy. Initially, there was some reluctance in many centers for administering GA and this is because of the disturbances of normal cardiopulmonary physiology during GA. Sudden cardiorespiratory failure may occur during cardiac catheterization. Contrast medium in the coronary circulation may cause profound transient changes in the ECG. Therefore, continuous ECG and invasive arterial pressure monitoring should be used to allow rapid assessment of arrhythmias and hypotension for critically ill patients.

Patients often require GA and tight BP control to facilitate the coiling and embolization of cerebral aneurysms, arteriovenous malformations, or stenting and clot removal for acute strokes. Patients taken to radiology department for the relief of portal hypertension via the creation of a transjugular intrahepatic portosystemic shunt (TIPS) are frequently intravascular volume depleted with profound ascites, and are at increased risk of esophageal variceal bleeding and aspiration. GA with intubation is preferred for the management of TIPS procedure.

Anesthesia providers are at times called to deliver anesthesia in ICU for bedside tracheostomy or emergency chest and abdominal exploration in patients who are considered too critically ill to tolerate transport to the OT room. In such cases, the anesthesia staff generally employ the ICU ventilator and monitors. Intravenous anesthetic agents are typically used along with muscle relaxants. When performing anesthesia for bedside tracheostomy, it is important that the ET tube should be withdrawn from trachea, until the $ETCO_2$ is measured from the newly placed tracheostomy tube.

■ ANESTHESIA FOR RADIOTHERAPY

The indications and the process of management of MAC or conscious sedation or GA for pediatric or adult group of patients for radiotherapy are same as that of radiodiagnosis, for example, CT, MRI, angiography, etc. Radiotherapy in children is usually performed under GA. As the patient had received anesthesia recently for a diagnostic procedure and then will require anesthesia more than once for radiotherapy, so, the halothane should be avoided. It is also, therefore, desirable to avoid repeated invasive procedures as far as possible and to keep the anesthetic technique as simple as possible. During anesthesia in radiotherapy, anesthetist may be exposed to radiation repeatedly. So, proper precautions should be taken by anesthetist.

The children usually undergo radiotherapy for variety of reasons, as for example: Wilms tumor, retinoblastoma, acute leukemia, etc. The implications of radiotherapy on anesthesia are (i) as during radiotherapy, high doses of radiation (X-ray or any other) are administered by linear accelerator, so all the staffs should remain outside the room leaving the anesthetized patient alone; (ii) as the radiotherapy needs repeated doses for several weeks, so the anesthesia is also given repeatedly; (iii) the anesthetized child must remain alone and motionless for a short period of time in the radiotherapy room. For that period clinical monitoring should continue and is observed by a close circuit television from the control room; (iv) As the radiotherapy is arranged on an outpatient basis, so the recovery should be fast; (v) Patient's physical status may remain compromised before and it is due to malignant disease which has immense impact on GA; (vi) With in the therapeutic radiology department, there should have facilities and monitors that must satisfy or exceed the current standards, promulgated by the ASA.

The actual process of radiotherapy is of very short duration, i.e., for only 30–60 seconds. But, a considerable longer period of anesthesia is required, i.e., for 20–30 minutes, for radiotherapy. Because, before the treatment begins, the field which is to be irradiated is plotted and marked, so that the X-ray can be accurately focused on the marked site for radiation, without damaging the surrounding structures. During that period, the child has to be remained motionless.

There is no pain in radiotherapy. So, the aim of anesthesia for radiotherapy is only to keep the patient motionless for a few minutes. This can be achieved by oral sedation. But, heavy oral sedation delays recovery time. Injection of ketamine, through IV or IM route is also helpful to keep the baby motionless, provided the patient does not have intracranial lesion. A need to increase the dose of ketamine gradually with successive radiation treatment (tachyphylaxis) may be observed. Intravenous propofol infusion can also be used satisfactorily for the children. Similarly, the increasing dose requirements have also been noted with propofol (tachyphylaxis). If airway control is difficult during anesthesia, then LMA can be instituted and anesthesia can be given by a combination of N_2O, O_2, and volatile anesthetic agents. In most of the cases, LMA is sufficient and ET intubation is rarely necessary. No analgesia is required and relatively light plane of anesthesia is maintained which allows rapid emergence and recovery. The monitoring of patient under GA during radiotherapy is only done by seeing the movement of bag and by seeing the screens of different monitor through the close circuit camera from control room. A microphone can help to hear the sound of different monitors and also the saturation dictated by the pitch of pulse oximeter.

Neuromuscular and Muscular Diseases and Anesthesia

INTRODUCTION

The neuromuscular diseases are the disorders that adversely affect the function of muscles due to the abnormalities of their neuromuscular junction. On the other hand, the muscular diseases are the disorders that adversely affect the function of muscles due to the abnormalities of the muscle fiber itself. However, in some books, the neuromuscular diseases are defined as the disorders that adversely affect the function of muscle due to the abnormalities of muscle itself, nerve, and neuromuscular junction. They are presented in operation theater (OT) or in nonoperating areas (i) for any diagnostic studies, (ii) for the treatment of these diseases or their complications, and (iii) for surgical management of other disorders associated with these diseases. Anesthetic providers also have to tackle the patients, suffering from these diseases in emergency department, intensive care unit, and in-hospital ward.

All the neuromuscular and muscular diseases usually manifest with some obvious clinical symptoms and signs which are mainly related to the skeletal muscles. But, many patients with some *occult state* of many of these disorders without any symptoms and signs may also be presented for anesthesia and is very important to an anesthetist, because they may cause many unwarranted complications during perioperative period. The most common neuromuscular diseases which an anesthetist usually encounters during perioperative period are *myasthenia gravis* and *Lambert–Eaton myasthenic syndrome (LEMS)*. Other than neuromuscular diseases, the muscular diseases which are commonly encountered by an anesthetist during perioperative period are initially divided under three broad headings such as (1) *muscular dystrophies*, (2) *myotonia*, and (3) *dyskalemic (hypokalemic) familial periodic paralysis*, the subclassification of which will be discussed later. The diseases of nerve affecting the function of muscle are amyotrophic lateral sclerosis, poliomyelitis, Guillain–Barré syndrome, etc.

All these neuromuscular and muscular diseases cause diminished muscle strength and increased sensitivity to neuromuscular blocking agent, which predispose the patients to respiratory failure, pulmonary aspiration, and slow recovery postoperatively. So, thorough understanding of all these neuromuscular and muscular disorders and their potential interactions with various anesthetic agents is very crucial for an anesthetist to avoid any morbidity and mortality of patients. All these neuromuscular diseases are associated with cardiovascular involvement including cardiomyopathies and dysrhythmias.

Paraneoplastic syndromes are immune-mediated diseases which are associated with an underlying cancer and where the organ or tissue dysfunction due to this cancer occurs distant from this primary cancer. Myasthenia gravis is often considered as a paraneoplastic syndrome. Because, it is an autoimmune disorder, associated with thymus hyperplasia or tumor. Other neurological or neuromuscular paraneoplastic syndromes include LEMS, limbic encephalitis, neuromyotonia, myotonic dystrophy, polymyositis, etc.

NEUROMUSCULAR DISEASES

Myasthenia Gravis

It is an acquired chronic autoimmune neuromuscular disorder and is characterized by the weakness of different skeletal muscles due to the decrease in the number and the functioning of nicotinic ACh receptors at their motor endplate. This decrease in the number and the function of nicotinic ACh receptors at the motor endplate is due the complement mediated destruction or inactivation of it (nicotinic receptor) by circulating antibodies which are formed against these receptors **(Figs. 1A and B)**. However, the cause of the origin of these ACh receptor antibodies is still unknown, but the thymus gland is suspected as the culprit. This is due to the close association of the presence of thymus

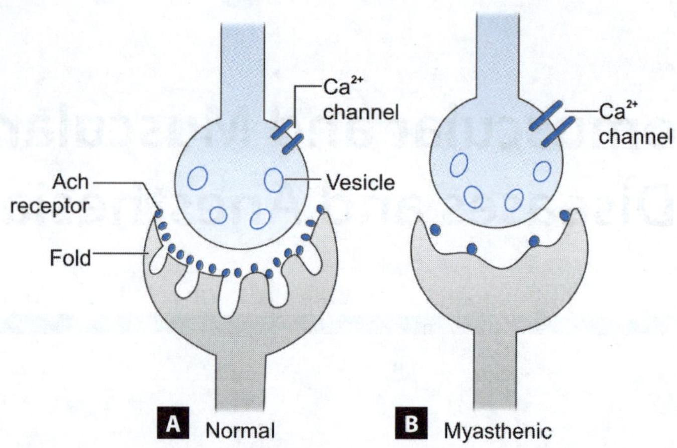

Figs. 1A and B: The normal (A) and myasthenia gravis affected (B) neuromuscular junction. In comparison to normal the myasthenic neuromuscular junction has shallow synaptic fold, few acetylcholine receptors and widened synaptic gap.

TABLE 1: Classification of myasthenia gravis.	
Class I	Weakness limited only to extraocular muscles
Class IIA	A mild weakness to skeletal muscles other than extraocular muscles—mainly the bulbar muscles. Respiratory muscles are spared
Class IIB	Respiratory muscles are involved
Class III	Moderate weakness of skeletal muscles with rapid deterioration
Class IV	Acute onset or severe weakness of skeletal muscles. Tracheal intubation and ventilation may be needed

gland abnormalities (thymoma and thymic lymphoid follicular hyperplasia) with the disease of myasthenia gravis. This is because the muscle like cells (myeloid cells) which also bear ACh receptors on their surface are present within the thymus gland and may serve as the source of autoantigen and trigger the autoimmune reaction within the thymus gland, producing ACh receptor antibody. The immunoglobulin G (IgG) antibody against these ACh receptors is not present in all the cases, but is found in 80–90% of patients with generalized myasthenia gravis and in 50–70% of patients with ocular myasthenia gravis.

Myasthenia gravis is not a rare disease, having a prevalence of at least 1 out of 7,500 general population. It affects the individuals of all the age groups. But, the women are affected more frequently (3:2) and at early ages than men. So, the females are affected mainly in their third decades of life and the males are affected mainly in the third and sixth decades of their life (two peaks). The women with myasthenia gravis also experience increased muscular weakness in the last trimester of pregnancy and in the early postpartum period. The babies of myasthenic mothers may also show transient myasthenia for at least 1–3 weeks after their delivery. This is due to the transplacental transfer of ACh receptors antibody, necessitating sometimes control ventilation in neonate.

The disease myasthenia gravis usually runs in relapsing (exacerbation) and remitting (remission) courses, especially during the early courses of this disease. The myasthenic patients also have the increased incidences of association with several other medical disorders. For example, 10–20% of patients who are suffering from myasthenia gravis

are associated with the presence of *thymoma*. Whereas, the 60–70% of patients with myasthenia gravis develop the *hyperplasia of thymus gland*. The other autoimmune disorders which are also present in association with the myasthenia gravis in remaining 10% of patients are *rheumatoid arthritis, hypothyroidism, thyroiditis, Graves' disease, systemic lupus erythematosus, skin diseases, family history of autoimmune disorder, etc.* Pernicious anemia occurs more commonly in patients with myasthenia gravis than in those without that (myasthenia gravis). The myasthenia gravis may also be more commonly associated with myocardiopathy and myocarditis which may result in atrial fibrillation and heart block.

The cardinal features of myasthenia gravis are the gradual increased weakness and easy fatigability of skeletal muscles, but without any loss of tendon reflexes or any impairment of sensation or any deficit of other neurological functions. The strength of skeletal muscle is maintained at normal level in well-rested patients (after the patient taking rest) and their atrophy is unlikely. These weakness and fatigability of skeletal muscles is characterized by its gradual deterioration during repeated use and may improve following rest and sleep. The exacerbations and the remissions of this muscular weakness usually occur, particularly during the first few years after the onset of this disease. Then, these remissions and exacerbations rarely occur and muscular weakness becomes a permanent feature **(Table 1)** for the classification of myasthenia gravis disease.

The weakness of skeletal muscles affected by myasthenia gravis is asymmetrical confined to one group of muscles or generalized. The distribution of this skeletal muscular weakness in myasthenia gravis has a characteristic pattern. The cranial muscles such as the muscles of lids and extraocular muscles are involved most early. So, the ptosis and diplopia are the *most common initial manifestation* of myasthenia gravis. Then, the difficulty in swallowing may occur and it is due to the result of weakness of the muscles of tongue, palate, pharynx larynx, etc. giving rise to nasal regurgitation or aspiration of food, if the cough is ineffectual. This also causes dysarthria (difficulty in speak) and difficulty in clearing the secretion from mouth, pharynx, and larynx.

Any limb muscle may be affected in this disease, but it is often the proximal part of the upper limb such as the muscle of shoulder girdle which is affected *most commonly* and may be asymmetrical on both sides. So, the patient is unable to work above the shoulder level such as the combing of hair without taking frequent rest. The weakness of pharyngeal and laryngeal muscles during the chewing and speaking is most noticeable after their prolonged use as in chewing meat or delivery of continuous speech during teaching. In severe form of this myasthenia gravis disease, if the respiratory muscles become very weak and require respiratory assistance, then the patient is said to be in *myasthenic crisis*. The infection, stress, electrolyte imbalance, pregnancy, surgery, etc. often cause the exacerbation of this disease and may lead to myasthenic crisis. Some drugs such as aminoglycosides, penicillamine, and ciprofloxacin usually exacerbate the neuromuscular blockade and should be avoided in patients with myasthenia gravis.

The clinical diagnosis of myasthenia gravis is suspected on the basis of the history of the weakness and the easy fatigability of the skeletal muscles in their typical distribution pattern described above. This suspicion about diagnosis should always be confirmed before the treatment of myasthenia gravis is undertaken. Because (i) the other treatable conditions such as drugs, hyperthyroidism, Graves' disease, botulism, intracranial mass compressing cranial nerves, etc. may cause muscular weakness and closely resemble myasthenia gravis, (ii) the definite treatment of myasthenia gravis may involve surgery, and (iii) erroneously the prolonged use of drugs for the treatment myasthenia gravis has adverse side effects.

For the clinical diagnosis of myasthenia gravis, the IV injection of edrophonium (a short-acting anticholinesterase whose onset of action is only 30 seconds and duration of action is only 5 minutes) is taken as a very valuable diagnostic aid which is known as the *Tensilon test*. The whole procedure of this test is divided into two parts. In the first part 2 mg of edrophonium is given initially through IV route. Then, if definite improvement (examiner should focus on one or more group of weak muscles and evaluate their strength objectively) of any muscle strength is occurred, then the test is considered as positive and terminated. If there is no change or improvement of muscle strength, then the patient is again given additional 8 mg of edrophonium through IV route **(Box 1)**.

This Tensilon test is divided in two parts, because the maximum test procedures become positive by the initial

<table>
<tr><td colspan="2" style="background:#2e6da4;color:white">BOX 1: Diagnosis of myasthenia gravis.</td></tr>
</table>

BOX 1: Diagnosis of myasthenia gravis.

- *History:*
  - Weakness of muscle with characteristic distribution
  - Ptosis and diplopia
  - Fatigue of muscle due to repeated activity
  - Muscle weakness improves by rest
  - Effects of treatment
- *Physical examination:*
  - Absence of other neurological defects, ptosis, and diplopia
  - Quantitative testing of muscle strength
  - Forward arm abduction time (<5 minutes)
- *Laboratory tests:*
  - *ACh receptor antibody:* If positive, then diagnosis is confirmed, 80% positive in generalized myasthenia, 50% positive in ocular myasthenia, and negative result does not exclude myasthenia
  - *Tensilon test:* Highly probable of myasthenia, if test is unequivocally positive
  - *Repetitive nerve stimulation:* Decrement of 20% at 3 Hz highly probable of diagnosis
  - *CT and MRI:* To exclude intracranial lesion

small dose of edrophonium and does not need the second large dose. Some patients react to this anticholinesterase by subsequent large doses with many adverse effects such as increased salivation, nausea, vomiting, diarrhea, muscular fasciculation throughout the whole body and rarely syncope. So, the second large dose is omitted if not needed and atropine (0.6 mg) should be given with edrophonium or be kept at hand for IV administration if these symptoms become troublesome.

Instead of edrophonium, another long-acting anticholinesterase agent such as neostigmine (1 mg) can also be used. However, the advantage of this long-acting anticholinesterase is that it better permits more time for the detailed evaluation of muscle power. Sometimes, false positive test occurs with the other neurological disorders such as amyotropic lateral sclerosis. Sometimes false negative or equivocal result may also occur. In such circumstances, the neostigmine is more helpful than edrophonium by giving more time for the evaluation of muscle power. However, virtually in all the instances, it is desirable to carry out the further testing to establish *(confirm)* the diagnosis of myasthenia gravis and these investigations are electromyography (EMG), estimation of ACh receptor antibody, etc. The presence of positive antiskeletal muscle antibodies suggest the presence of thymoma, but all the patients should have a thoracic computed tomography (CT) to exclude this condition which may not be visible on plain radiographic examination. Screening for other autoimmune disorders, particularly thyroid disease, is also important.

The *principles of the treatment* of myasthenia gravis are (i) to maximize the activity of ACh neurotransmitter which acts on the remaining functional nicotinic ACh receptor at the motor end plate by reducing the activity of cholinesterase enzyme which destroys the ACh transmitter by administering anticholinesterase agent, and (ii) to abolish or limit the immunological attack on ACh receptor at the motor endplate by surgical thymectomy, immunosuppression (corticosteroids, azathioprine, and cyclosporine), and short-term immunotherapy (plasma exchange, administration of immunoglobulin, and monoclonal antibody). Among all these methods, the administration of anticholinesterase agent is the first line of treatment for the mild-to-moderate cases of myasthenia gravis and for this *oral pyridostigmine* is the most widely used agent in the dose of 30–120 mg 6 hourly producing an effect in 30 minutes and peak effect at 120 minutes after its administration. During the clinical use of this anticholinesterase agent, the muscarinic cholinergic effect of pyridostigmine (or any anticholinesterase) such as excessive salivation, diarrheas, intestinal colic, etc. is controlled by the subsequent use of propantheline with pyridostigmine in the dose of 15 mg or as required.

However, the dose and the schedule of pyridostigmine should be tailored according to the patient's response, but the maximum dose rarely exceed 120 mg at the interval of every 3 hours. It produces fewer side effects than the other anticholinesterase such as neostigmine and 60 mg oral pyridostigmine is equivalent to 2 mg of it through IM or IV route. Higher doses may precipitate *cholinergic crisis* by producing excessive muscarinic effect (salivation, vomiting, intestinal colic, etc.) and muscular paralysis by blocking the motor endplate. This cholinergic crisis is characterized by fasciculation, accentuation of skeletal muscular weakness or muscular paralysis, bradycardia, pallor, sweating, salivation, bronchospasm, miosis, etc. This should be distinguished from severe muscular weakness due to the exacerbation of myasthenia gravis (myasthenic crisis) by the clinical features and if necessary by the injection of a small dose of edrophonium.

Although the anticholinesterase agent makes benefit for most of the myasthenic patients, but their effects gradually wane after prolonged treatment and improvements become incomplete. So, *thymectomy* is the next alternative for the management of myasthenia gravis. But, the actual mechanism of action of thymectomy (surgical removal of thymus) in the treatment of myasthenia gravis is still unknown. However, there is definite improvement in the clinical symptoms and there is decrease in the level of ACh receptor antibody reducing the dose of immunosuppressive agents or completely eliminating the need for continuing medical treatment. It should be performed in the early stages

of this disease leading to a better overall prognosis whether a thymoma is present or not. It should also be performed as soon as possible in any antibody positive patient with symptoms not only confined to the extraocular muscles and unless the disease has been established for >7 years. Generally, the myasthenic patients between the ages of puberty and about 50 years are the best candidates for the surgical removal of thymus.

Before thymectomy for the treatment of myasthenia gravis, all the patients should always be prepared preoperatively to optimize the strength of muscle, especially of the respiratory muscles. For example, if the patient's vital capacity is <2 L, then plasmapheresis must be performed before surgery to improve the strength of respiratory muscles. But, the immunosuppressive drugs should not be continued (if started) before operation for the possible increased risk of postoperative infection. Endoscopic thymectomy through a small cervical incision is preferred than median sternotomy, because it is associated with smaller incision, less chance of infection, and less postoperative pain. The benefit of thymectomy on myasthenia gravis is not immediate and is typically delayed for months to years.

Drugs Used Most Frequently To Treat Myasthenia Gravis		
Drugs	*Mode of action*	*Risks*
Pyridostigmine	Acetylcholinesterase inhibition	Cholinergic crisis
Prednisolone	Immunomodulation	Cushingoid appearance
Azathioprine	Suppression of B- and T-cells	Hepatotoxicity, leukopenia
Methotrexate	Inhibition of folate metabolism	Hepatotoxicity, leukopenia
Tacrolimuss	Suppression of T- and NK cells	Nephro- and hepatotoxicity
Cyclosporine	Suppression of T- and NK cells	Kidney toxicity
Mycophenolate mofetil	Suppression of B- and T-cells	Leukopenia
Rituximab	Suppression of B cells	Leukoencephalopathy
Immunoglobulin	Neutralization of antibodies	Allergic reaction

Immunosuppression by using glucocorticoids, azathioprine, mycophenolate mofetil, cyclosporine, and other immunosuppressive drugs (methotrexate and cyclophosphamide) are effective in nearly all the patients with myasthenia gravis, where the weakness of skeletal muscle is not adequately controlled by anticholinesterase drug. The choice of these drugs should be guided by their relative risks and benefits in individual patient.

But, corticosteroids are the most commonly used immunosuppressive agents for the treatment of myasthenia gravis. The improvement of muscle power by corticosteroid is commonly preceded by a marked exacerbations of myasthenic symptoms. So, the treatment should be initiated in hospital and then is continued at home for months or years. They are also associated with the greatest likelihood of adverse side effects.

The indication for the use of immunoglobulin and plasmapheresis in the treatment of myasthenia gravis is more or less same, i.e., to produce rapid improvement for brief period during myasthenic crisis and to quickly prepare the patient before any surgery. But, their mechanism of action is different. In plasmapheresis, the antibodies against ACh receptor are removed from patient's circulation. Whereas the mechanism of action of immunoglobulin are not known, because it has no consistent effect on the amount of measurable circulating ACh receptor antibody.

Anesthetic Management

The patients with myasthenia gravis may present for thymectomy, which is related to the treatment of this disease or the patients with myasthenia gravis may present for other surgical procedures, which are not related to the treatment of myasthenia gravis such as the obstetric surgery, general surgery, urological surgery, etc. In all these cases, the patient's medical condition, mainly the muscular strength, should be optimized prior to surgery. So, the myasthenic patients should carefully be evaluated preoperatively giving focus on the affected muscle groups recent course of disease, present history of drug therapy, and other consisting illness. Patients with bulbar (pharynx, larynx, face, tongue, etc.) muscular and respiratory muscular involvement are at increased risk for postoperative respiratory complications and pulmonary aspiration. So, the proper preoperative preparation of myasthenic patients with immunoglobulin, plasmapheresis, metoclopramide, and H_2 blocker may decrease these risks.

During the preoperative preparation of myasthenic patients, the continuation of anticholinesterase agents, which was started before, is controversial and should be individualized. The potential problems regarding the preoperative treatment of myasthenic patients by anticholinesterase agent include the possible drug interaction between it and the other anesthetic agents, (i) mainly the muscle relaxants (described later), (ii) the increased vagal reflexes by anticholinesterase, and (iii) the possibility of disruption of bowel anastomosis due to hyperperistalsis caused by anticholinesterase during bowel surgery. On the other hand, patient's muscle power may deteriorate rapidly, if the anticholinesterase agents are withheld preoperatively.

The patients with myasthenia gravis are very sensitive to the impairment of respiratory function during perioperative period and it is due to the weakness or paralysis of respiratory muscles. So, as preoperative medication, the drugs such as opioids, benzodiazepines, and other similar sedative agents should be used with caution, or is completely omitted, if the circumstances permit. It is already said that the myasthenic patients are at increased risk for postoperative respiratory failure due to muscular weakness or paralysis. So, the *preoperative criteria* that are predictive for the need of postoperative ventilatory support following trans-sternal thymectomy or any major surgery in myasthenic patients are (i) the duration of disease for >6 years, (ii) the presence of some concomitant lung diseases, (iii) the dose of preoperative pyridostigmine is >750 mg/day, (iv) the peak inspiratory pressure is >20 cmH$_2$O, and (v) the preoperative vital capacity is <4 mL/kg. However, these criteria are less relevant to the endoscopic transcervical thymectomy, because these less invasive surgical procedures have a respiratory sparing effect.

Except thymectomy, in other surgical procedures, where the myasthenia gravis is present as coexistent disease, then the regional (epidural or spinal) anesthesia is preferred than general anesthesia (GA). Because, it avoids the potential problems of increased neuromuscular blocking effect with respiratory depression of muscle relaxant during the postoperative period in GA. However, excessive high spinal level of motor blockade can also result in hypoventilation in regional anesthesia (RA) and also should be avoided. During GA, the induction in myasthenic patients is usually accomplished by all the standard short-acting intravenous-inducing anesthetic agents, but in small doses, keeping in mind that the relaxation effect of these inducing drugs on weak respiratory, laryngeal, and pharyngeal muscles may be accentuated in such group of patients.

Sometimes, tracheal intubation can also be performed without further addition of neuromuscular blocking agent in such patients by taking the advantage of muscular weakness of such disease and the muscular relaxing effect of intra-venous and volatile anesthetic agents used during the induction of anesthesia. The only volatile anesthetic agent-based anesthesia is usually sometimes satisfactory for intubation in some myasthenic patients. Because, in myasthenic patients the deep anesthesia produced by volatile anesthetic agents provide sufficient muscle relaxation for tracheal intubation and intraoperative procedures. So, many anesthetists try to avoid muscle relaxants and use only volatile anesthetic agents in patients suffering from myasthenia gravis.

The response of succinylcholine in myasthenic patients is unpredictable. The patients may show (i) a relative *resistance* or (ii) *higher sensitivity* and a prolonged effect or (iii) an *unusual phase II block* in response to succinylcholine. The mechanism by which the myasthenic patients are resistant to succinylcholine are not known, but the reduced number of ACh receptor at the motor end plate may be the possible explanation of it. On the other hand, the anticholinesterase agents such as pyridostigmine not only inhibit the true cholinesterase at the motor endplate, but also inhibit the plasma cholinesterase enzyme causing the possibility of higher sensitivity and prolonged effects of succinylcholine. In contrast to succinylcholine, the myasthenic patients always show high sensitivity to nondepolarizing muscle relaxant and it is due to the decrease in total number of functional ACh receptors.

The balance between the number of functional and nonfunctional ACh receptors determine the degree of the sensitivity of myasthenic patients to the non-depolarizing muscle relaxing agents. Sometimes, the small dose of nondepolarizing agent, desired to attenuate the succinylcholine-induced fasciculation, may produce adequate muscle relaxation for intubation. So, if non-depolarizing agents are required, then the small doses of a relatively short-acting agent such as cisatracurium and mivacurium are preferred. The potency of atracurium is increased two times in mild-to-moderate myasthenic patients compared to normal individual.

As the mivacurium is eliminated rapidly, so it can be titrated easily to achieve the desired level of muscular paral-ysis with confidence that this can be reversed predictably at the end of surgery. During the whole intraoperative period, the neuromuscular blocking effect of muscle relaxant should closely be monitored by peripheral nerve stimulator and at the end of surgery the ventilatory function should carefully be evaluated prior to extubation and this is to avoid any postoperative pulmonary complications. Theoretically, the anticholinesterase drugs, which are usually taken by the patients during preoperative period, may antagonize and decrease the sensitivity of nondepolarizing agents. But practically this does not happen. Conversely, the preoperative corticosteroid therapy may produce resistance to neuromuscular blocking effect of nondepolarizing agents.

The monitoring of neuromuscular blocking effect at the wrist or elbow by a peripheral nerve stimulator may over- or underestimate the degree of neuromuscular blockade caused by muscle relaxant in patients with myasthenia gravis. So, it is better to monitor the neuromuscular blocking effect of a muscle relaxant at the level of orbicularis oculi muscle which is most commonly affected in myasthenic

patient to avoid any complication. Intraoperative anesthesia is usually maintained by N_2O and volatile anesthetic agents which decrease the dose of muscle relaxants or completely eliminate the need for their use. However, if it is absolutely necessary to use the nondepolarizing agents, then their initial dose should be reduced to at least half or two-thirds of the usual dose and the response is observed by nerve stimulator. At the end of surgery, it is wise not to extubate, until the patient shows an adequate functional ability for ventilation. It is very interesting in myasthenic patients that the strength of the skeletal muscles often seem adequate during the early postoperative period, but only deteriorate a few hours later.

Lambert–Eaton Myasthenic Syndrome

There are other many conditions like myasthenia gravis, which also presents with muscle weakness due to transmission defect at motor endplate. The most common of these is the LEMS which is also an autoimmune disease producing *antibodies against the presynaptic voltage-gated Ca^{2+} channels* and reducing the quantal release of ACh at motor endplate. This is in contrast to myasthenia gravis which is not due to the defect in quantitative release of ACh, but it is due to the defect in nicotinic ACh receptor where the released ACh acts. In a high percentage of cases, this condition is usually associated with an underlying malignancy, mainly the small cell carcinoma of lungs where these small carcinoma cells express the identical voltage-gated Ca^{2+} channels, serving as a trigger antigen for the autoimmune response. Otherwise, LEMS is also seen with other occult cases of malignancy or as an idiopathic autoimmune disease **(Table 2)**.

As it is an autoimmune disease, so LEMS is also associated with dry mouth, male impotence, and other manifestations of autoimmune dysfunction, like myasthenia gravis. The cardinal differences (the other differences are tabled) between the LEMS and myasthenia gravis are that in the former there is absence of tendon reflexes and the muscle weakness improves with repeated contraction. So, this condition is diagnosed electrophysiologically by the presence of post-tetanic potentiation of motor response after the stimulation of nerve fiber at the rate of 20–30 per second and the investigations are directed toward the detection of underlying malignancy. In contrast to MG, the muscle weakness in LEMS does not improve by anticholinesterase drugs.

The 3,4-diaminopyridine (DAP) and guanidine hydro-chloride are two drugs which increase the presynaptic release of ACh. So, they can be used in LEMS to improve the muscle power (contraction). But, the use of guanidine for the

TABLE 2: Comparison between myasthenia gravis and myasthenic syndrome.

	Myasthenia gravis	*Myasthenic syndrome*
Gender	Females > males	Males > females
Associated pathology	Thymoma, thymus hyperplasia	Small cell carcinoma of lungs
Manifestation	• Ocular, bulbar, facial muscles are more commonly affected • Arms > legs • Exercise worsens strength • No muscle pain • Tendon reflex normal	• Not common • Legs > arms • Exercise improves power • Muscle pain • Tendon reflex absent
Response to muscle relaxant	• Resistant to succinylcholine • Sensitive to nondepolarizing agent • Good response to anticholinesterase	• Sensitive to succinylcholine • Sensitive to nondepolarizing agent • Poor response to anticholinesterase

treatment of LEMS is limited due to its hepatotoxic effect. So, the DAP is only used for the treatment of LEMS in most of the countries. Like myasthenia gravis, the most patients with LEMS also improve with immunosuppression and/or plasmapheresis by decreasing the level of antibodies against Ca^{2+} channel. The anticholinesterase agents which are effective in the management of myasthenia gravis do not produce any improvement of muscle strength in myasthenic syndrome.

Unlike myasthenia gravis, the patients with myasthenic syndrome are *sensitive to both the succinylcholine and nondepolarizing neuromuscular blocking agents.* So, the potential presence of undiagnosed myasthenic syndrome and the subsequent reduction of the dose of muscle relaxant always should be kept in mind during the anesthetic management of patients with known malignancies or during the anesthetic management of patients for the diagnosis of malignancy by bronchoscopy, mediastinoscopy, exploratory thoracotomy for suspected lung cancer, etc. The response of other anesthetic drugs such as the opioids, benzodiazepines, IV inducing agents, and volatile anesthetic agents etc., and the intraoperative monitoring in myasthenic syndrome during the anesthetic management of it is similar to that of myasthenia gravis. The postoperative management of myasthenic syndrome is also similar to that of myasthenia gravis.

■ MUSCULAR DISEASES

Other than the disorders at neuromuscular junction, the skeletal muscles itself is also subjected to a range of disorders with limited spectrum of symptoms and signs. These are initially classified as (i) *muscular dystrophy,* (ii) *myotonia (dystonia),* and (iii) *dyskalemic (hypo- or hyperkalemic) familial periodic paralysis.* Muscular dystrophies are a heterogeneous group of hereditary diseases of skeletal muscles. It is characterized by painless degeneration and atrophy of voluntary muscles. So, there is symmetrical progressive weakness and wasting of skeletal muscles, but with intact sensation and reflexes indicating the normal skeletal muscle innervation (nerve supply). The main pathology of muscular dystrophy is the *increased permeability of muscle cell fibers, leading to necrosis, degeneration, and fibrosis.* The muscular dystrophy is again of different types and according to decreased frequency, these are (i) *Duchenne muscular dystrophy, (ii) Becker muscular dystrophy, (iii) myotonic dystrophy, (iv) Limb–Girdle dystrophy, (v) facioscapulohumeral dystrophy, etc.*

Muscular Dystrophy

Duchenne Muscular Dystrophy

It is also known as the pseudohypertrophic muscular dystrophy and is the most common form among others. It is caused by the mutation of gene, which is responsible for the production of normal *dystrophin.* Actually, the dystrophin is a protein compound and is localized to the inner surface of the sarcolemma of muscle fiber. With another glycoprotein molecule, it forms a *dystrophin glycoprotein complex* and confers stability to the sarcolemma. In the absence of this dystrophin protein, the sarcolemma of muscle cells (fibers) become weak and more permeable leading to tear and a cascade of events causing the death of muscle fibers and necrosis. This chain of events occurs repeatedly during the whole life of a patient suffering from Duchenne muscular dystrophy.

The incidence of this type of muscular dystrophy varies between 2 and 3 per 10,000 life-births. It is an X-linked recessive disorder. So, the males are affected almost exclusively and the females are usually become carrier. It is present from birth, but becomes apparent between the 3 and 6 years of life, when the children fall frequently on ground due to muscle weakness while playing with their friends. The running, jumping, hopping, and climbing up the stair are invariably abnormal. By the age of 6 years, this muscle weakness will become obvious and is characterized by using hands to climb up himself when a child tries to get up from floor (Gower's maneuver) after fall. In younger children, the muscles, particularly of the calves, are usually enlarged and it is due to true compensatory muscular hypertrophy, due to over use. But, later the affected muscles become apparently larger as a result of fatty infiltration and this accounts for the designation of this disorder as pseudohypertrophy.

The involvement of legs in this disease is more frequent and severe than that of arm. After that, there is a steady deterioration of the strength of many other skeletal muscles and along with the fixed contractures of joints are developed. By the age of 12 years, most of the patients are confined to a wheelchair and it is due to the weakness of the large group of muscles and contracture of many joints. Progressively, scoliosis, and kyphoscoliosis are also often developed which may be associated with pain. This is due to the unopposed action of antagonistic group of muscles against the affected weak dystrophic groups of muscles in the body. Thus, gradually the severe chest deformity associated with scoliosis is developed which impair the pulmonary function that is already previously diminished by muscle weakness. The skeletal muscle atrophy can also predispose to long bone fractures. In this disorder, the intellectual impairment is also common, but generally nonprogressive. In patients with muscular dystrophy, the degeneration of respiratory muscles also interferes the mechanism of effective coughing and thus causes the retention of secretion and frequent pulmonary infection.

Then, gradually by the age of 20 years, the patients are predisposed to serious and sometimes fatal pulmonary infection leading to death. The other causes of death in this muscular disorder include the aspiration of food and acute gastric dilatation. The degenerative changes of cardiac muscles are also common in patients with muscular dystrophy. This results in dilated or hypertrophic cardiomyopathy. Mitral regurgitation may also accompany with muscular dystrophy in 25% cases and this is due to the dysfunction of papillary muscles in ventricle. The characteristic electrocardiogram (ECG) changes associated with this muscular dystrophy are short PR interval, tall R-wave in V1, and deep Q-wave in precordial leads. Cardiac failure is also an important cause of death in patients suffering from this type of muscular dystrophy which usually occurs between 15 and 25 years of age.

The level of serum creatine phosphokinase (CK) are invariably elevated and reach between 10 and 100 times of the normal value. This reflects the increased permeability and necrosis of muscle fibers. The female carriers often also have high plasma CK levels, though there is no manifestation of this disease. In affected male child, the increased level of CK is found at birth. But, it declines later with the progress of the disease and it is due to the loss of muscle mass. The EMG

of patients suffering from this type of muscular dystrophy demonstrates the features of typical myopathy. The diagnosis of Duchenne muscular dystrophy is only confirmed by muscle biopsy showing the necrosis, degeneration, fibrosis, and subsequently some regeneration of muscle fibers.

The connective tissues replace the lost muscle fibers. The definite diagnosis of Duchenne muscular dystrophy can only be established on the basis of the determination of the *amount and alteration in the size of dystrophin molecule* (present on the sarcolemma of muscle cell) by the western blot analysis of muscle specimen taken for biopsy, or analysis of deoxyribonucleic acid (DNA) on peripheral blood leukocytes showing the deletion and duplication of dystrophin gene. Actually, there is no treatment in this disease, but prednisolone in the dose of 0.5–1 mg/kg/day has been shown to delay significantly the progress of this disease. However, this is only for 2–3 years.

Becker Muscular Dystrophy

Like Duchenne muscular dystrophy, the Becker muscular dystrophy is also an *X-linked recessive disorder* with almost same manifestations, but in less severe and delayed form. So, it is often also called the benign form of *pseudohypertrophic muscular dystrophy*. It is less frequent than Duchenne and the incidence rate is about 3 per 100,000 male life births. Till recently, it is not known whether these two diseases, such as the Duchenne and Becker muscular dystrophy, are the genetically two distinct disorders or not. Like Duchenne, it is also thought to be due to the point mutation or the deletion of dystrophin gene, which is located on X-chromosome, leading to the defect in the production of the dystrophin protein in the sarcolemma of muscle fiber. But, the amount of mutation and deletion varies.

The onset of symptoms in Becker muscular dystrophy occurs usually around 10 years of age, although it may delay to third or fourth decade of life and progress very slowly. The proximal muscles, especially of the lower limbs, are first involved and as the disease progresses, then the weakness spreads to other muscles and becomes more generalized. By definition, the patient suffering from Becker muscular dystrophy can ambulate beyond the age of 15 years which is not possible in Duchenne and this is the clinical distinction between the Duchenne and Becker muscular dystrophy. Mental retardation may be seen in Becker dystrophy, but is not as common and severe as in Duchenne.

Cardiac involvement may also occur in this type of dystrophy leading to heart failure. Though, the life expectancy in Becker muscular dystrophy is reduced than normal, still the most patients reach the fourth or fifth decade of life and some may survive up to the seventh decade of their life.

During the diagnosis of Becker dystrophy, the findings from serum CK measurement, EMG, and muscle biopsy closely resemble with those of Duchenne dystrophy. But, still the definite diagnosis of Becker muscular dystrophy requires the western blot analysis of muscle tissue, taken by biopsy, demonstrating the dystrophin gene of reduced amount and of abnormal size.

Limb-girdle Muscular Dystrophy

It also represents a heterogeneous group of more than one muscular disorders which are further classified by the analysis of molecular genetics. In this group of dystrophy, each disorder is slowly progressive and benign. The muscular weakness in this type of dystrophy affects both the male and female group of patients with onset varying from second to fifth decades of life. Mainly the muscles of shoulder girdle or hip girdle or both are involved in this disease. So, it is named like that. The distribution of the weakness of muscles and the rate of progress of this disease vary from family to family. The respiratory insufficiency from the weakness of dia-phragm may occur in this type of dystrophy. In some patients, the involvement of cardiac muscle may also result in congestive heart failure or arrhythmia. Intellectual function remains usually normal in this type of muscular disorder. The plasma CK levels are usually elevated. The EMG findings and muscle biopsy represent the characteristic changes in limb girdle dystrophy.

Myotonic Dystrophy (or Dystrophia Myotonica)

It is the most common form of muscular dystrophy in adults (not childhood) and is a multisystem disorder involving many organs other than muscles. The incidence of this disorder varies between 10 and 15 per 100,000 live births and both the males and females are affected. It is an autosomal transmitted disease and is caused by the expansion of a trinucleotide repeat on chromosome 19. The diagnosis of this myotonic dystrophy is now possible by measuring this repeat by sequencing the chromosome.

This myotonic dystrophy usually manifests between the second and third decades of life. During the early stage of this disease process, myotonia (slowing of relaxation after the contraction of muscle, for example, slow relaxation of hand grip following forced voluntary closure) but not weakness is the main manifestation. But, as the disease progresses, the weakness and the atrophy of muscles become more evident. This weakness and the atrophy of muscles usually affect the cranial group of muscle such as the facial, temporalis, masseter, etc. and result in the typical appearance of face which is known as the "hatched face". As opposed to the other muscular dystrophies, the distal muscles are more

involved than proximal muscles in myotonic dystrophy. So, the weakness of wrist extensors, finger extensors and intrinsic hand muscles impair the function of hand. The weakness of ankle dorsi flexor may cause foot drop. The involvement of the muscles of tongue, palate, and pharynx produce dysarthria of speech, nasal voice, and swallowing problems. Some patients have weakness of diaphragm and intercostal muscles, resulting in respiratory in sufficiency. Congenital myotonic dystrophy is rare, and represents a more severe form of this disease and occurs approximately in 25% of infants of affected mothers. It is characterized by severe facial and bulbar weakness and neonatal respiratory insufficiency.

Cardiac disturbances occur in most of the patients with myotonic dystrophy. The ECG abnormalities include different types of conduction defects or heart block. Mitral valve prolapse occurs commonly in myotonic dystrophy patients. As in myotonic dystrophy the multiple organ or systems are affected, so it is associated with premature frontal baldness, presenile cataract, multiple endocrine dysfunction (such as thyroid, adrenal, pancreatic, and gonadal insufficiency) decreased esophageal and colonic motility, etc. Uterine atony can prolong labor and will increase the chances of retained placenta.

The diagnosis of myotonic dystrophy can usually be made on the basis of clinical findings. The serum CK level may be normal or mildly elevated. The evidence of myotonia in this type of muscular dystrophy by EMG will readily be found in most cases. Usually, the severity of myotonia in patients suffering from myotonic dystrophy is mild and rarely warrants any treatment.

But, if the treatment is required, then it is undertaken by membrane stabilizing agents such as phenytoin, quinidine, or procainamide. Among these the phenytoin is the pre-ferred agent, whereas the quinidine and procainamide has the cardiac adverse effects, precipitating or worsening conduction defect. The insertion of cardiac pacemaker may be considered in some patients, suffering from myotonic dystrophy with unexplained syncope or major conduction abnormalities with evidence of second-degree heart block or trifascicular block with marked prolongation of PR interval.

Facioscapulohumeral Dystrophy

It is an autosomal dominant disorder, due to the deletion of gene at locus q35 of DNA in chromosome 4. It affects both the males and females and the incidence varies between 1 and 3 per 100,000 live births. The patients usually present with muscular weakness in the second and third decade of life and as the name signifies the weakness is confined primarily to the muscles of face and shoulder girdle. So, there is inability to smile, whistle, fully close the eyes, or elevate the arms. The scapular winging becomes apparent with attempts to abduction or forward movement of arm. The muscles of lower limbs are rarely affected and the respiratory muscles are usually spared. Cardiac involvement is also rare in this disease. The serum CK level may be normal or mildly elevated. The EMG usually indicates myopathic pattern. The muscle biopsy also shows the features of myopathy.

Anesthetic Management

Anesthetic management of Duchenne and Becker muscular dystrophy: The patients, with these two diseases of muscular dystrophy, usually come for anesthesia to do muscle biopsy for the diagnosis or for the correction of progressive orthopedic deformities, caused by these two diseases, or for other surgical causes, unrelated to these muscular dystrophies. Unlike myasthenia gravis, the anesthetic management of patients associated with these two types of muscular dystrophies is complicated not only for the presence of muscle weakness and paralysis, but also for the presence of associated cardiopulmonary complications due to the presence of these diseases. In these groups of patients, the hypomotility of gastrointestinal (GI) tract may delay gastric emptying. So, this GI hypomotility further in the presence of weak laryngeal reflexes and respiratory muscular weakness increases the risk of pulmonary aspiration. So, some definite preoperative and intraoperative measures should be taken to avoid this complications. Any sedative or opioid as preoperative medication should also be avoided due to the same reasons.

Succinylcholine should also be avoided in these groups of patients and this is because of the fear of rhabdomyolysis, hyperkalemia, malignant hyperthermia, and subsequent cardiac arrest. In some patients, sudden ventricular fibrillation leading to cardiac arrest during the induction of anesthesia and intubation using succinylcholine has been proved later to have these types of muscular dystrophies. Patients with these two types of muscular dystrophies also usually exhibit higher sensitivity to the nondepolarizing muscle relaxant. Malignant hyperthermia has also been observed in these groups of patients when succinylcholine and volatile anesthetic agents are administered. So, RA is always preferred for these groups of patients to avoid these unique risks of GA related to these muscular dystrophies. The intraoperative monitoring during anesthesia of these patients is directed to the early detection of malignant hyperthermia, hyperkalemia, and cardiac arrhythmia. In the postoperative periods, the need for temporary mechanical ventilation for these patients, due to the weakness of respiratory muscles should always be kept in mind.

Anesthetic management of myotonic dystrophy: The anesthetic management of patients suffering from myotonic dystrophy becomes frequently complicated and it is due to the commonly presence of patient's pulmonary and cardiac abnormalities and altered response of these patients to a number of anesthetic medicines. It is presumed that the asymptomatic patients with myotonic dystrophy also have some degree of cardiomyopathy which may alter the course of anesthesia. The patients of myotonic dystrophy become very sensitive to sedatives and opioids. So, any small doses of it can cause sudden and prolonged apnea. Hence, these should be avoided (if possible) as premedicant and should be used in small doses during the induction of anesthesia. Succinylcholine is not used in these patients, because prolonged skeletal muscle contraction triggered by it may occur. So, the trismus and the contraction of laryngeal muscles can prevent the opening of mouth and may make the intubation difficult. The rigidity of chest wall also may make the ventilation difficult or impossible. Conversely, the response of these myotonic dystrophic patients to nondepolarizing agents is normal. But, the reversal of neuromuscular blockade by neostigmine can aggravate this myotonia. This is due to the facilitation of depolarization at neuromuscular junction by anticholinesterase. Hence, the short-acting nondepolarizing agent not requiring reversal such as cisatracurium, mivacurium, etc. are preferred.

There is also a theoretical concern that these patients are susceptible to malignant hyperthermia. Intraoperative maintenance of body temperature and postoperative avoidance of shivering are important for these groups of patients, because cold may induce myotonia. Although, the intraoperative high concentration of volatile anesthetic agents may abolish myotonic contraction, but it is associated with postoperative shivering and myotonic contraction in postoperative room. In such situations, a small dose of meperidine (pethidine) can often prevent such shivering and perhaps the myotonic contraction. So, due to these above-mentioned complications, GA should be avoided in known myotonic dystrophic patients, if not absolutely indicated. Therefore, preoperative diagnosis of myotonic dystrophy is very vital to an anesthetist. But, the patients with this disease may be undiagnosed before or he may not divulge intentionally the information preoperatively. Sometimes, the diagnosis of myotonic dystrophy comes to light when the patient suffers from prolonged apnea or myotonia after GA.

Myotonia

It is defined as a type of muscular disorder where tonic spasm of a single muscle or a group of muscles occur and it is probably due to the repeated depolarization of muscle cells (fibers) causing contraction, stiffness, and impaired relaxation of it. In this disease, the skeletal muscles are only involved, but the other organs or systems are not affected like myotonic dystrophy. There is no cardiac involvement in this disease like muscular dystrophy. This disease of myotonia does not progress. So, it does not result in decreased life expectancy. However, in contrary, the myotonic dystrophy (described before) is associated with myotonia and other systemic manifestations and muscle weakness. In myotonia, there is usually no weakness of muscle, rather the muscles are very well developed, due to constant muscular contraction.

In myotonia, the contraction of muscles is painless. But, still, it disables the patients by interfering the movement of extremities and ambulation. In myotonia, the stiffness of muscle is often exaggerated by cold, but is characteristically reduced by repeated muscular exercise. The flaccid muscular paralysis in myotonia may be produced by warming the muscles. The EMG is normal at room temperature, but typical myotonic discharges start, when the muscles are cooled.

Principally, there are two types of myotonia such as (i) *myotonia congenita* and (ii) *paramyotonia congenita*. The myotonia congenita is caused by the mutation of gene on chromosome 7 at locus q35, resulting in defects of the function of chloride channels. It has both autosomal dominant and recessive variant. On the other hand, the paramyotonia congenita is due to the defect of gene on chromosome 17 and is very rare autosomal dominant disorder. The defect of Na^+ channel is associated with this disease and is characterized by paradoxical myotonia, i.e., the myotonia which worsens with repeated muscular activity. So, it is named as paramyotonia congenita. In myotonia, the stiffness or contraction of muscles are alleviated by quinine, phenytoin, or mexiletine. Other medications that have been used in the treatment of myotonia include prednisolone, dantrolene, tocainide, etc.

The anesthetic management of myotonia is complicated by the abnormal responses of patients to muscle relaxants. The nondepolarizing muscle relaxant paradoxically causes the generalized contraction of muscles such as trismus, contraction of vocal cord, etc. leading to difficult intubation and ventilation. Intraoperative hypothermia may also lead to muscular contraction in myotonia patients. This disease does not cause malignant hyperthermia. Infiltration of muscles with local anesthetic solutions (diluted) at operative field reduces the myotonic contraction.

Dyskalemic Familial Periodic Paralysis

This is a spectrum of muscular disorders characterized by the intermittent acute attack of weakness or paralysis of the skeletal muscles of limbs. Peculiarly, it does not affect the respiratory muscles including the cranial and thoracic musculature like muscular dystrophy. This periodic attack usually lasts for few hours (usually 1 hour, but can last several

days) and each frequent attack may lead to progressive long-term muscular weakness in some patients. This weakness or paralysis of muscles are due to the loss of the excitability of muscle fibers. This is again due to the incomplete (partial) depolarization of resting muscle potential, because of either decrease in K^+ conductance or increase in Na^+ conductance due to the defect in the channels of some ions (present on cell membrane) such as Ca^{2+}, Na^+, or K^+ etc. However, both are associated with fluid and electrolyte disturbances.

This whole spectrum of diseases (muscular disorders) is classified into (i) primary genetic or congenital and (ii) secondary or acquired form. The primary genetic form of this dyskalemic familial periodic paralysis is inherited as an *autosomal dominant traits,* but has a number of mosaic variants, resulting in different manifestations in different families. The genetic or inherited form of this muscular disorder is due to the mutation of gene, responsible for the voltage-gated Ca^{2+}, Na^+, or K^+ channels. *The inherited defect in voltage-gated Ca^{2+} channels is typically associated with low serum K^+ level during the periodic attack of weakness or paralysis. On the other hand, the inherited defect in Na^+ channels is typically associated with the increased serum K^+ level during the attack of periodic weakness or paralysis.* So, both these defects result in hypokalemia, hyperkalemia, or normokalemia associated with nonexcitable muscle membrane causing weakness or paralysis of muscle. This spectrum of diseases is classified according to the clinical manifestations, but not according to the defect of ion channels. This is because (i) it is useful as a guide to the prognosis and therapy, and (ii) defect in same channel may cause different clinical pictures and defect in different channels may have same clinical picture.

Secondary hypokalemic and hyperkalemic paralysis can also occur, if there is loss of K^+ through GI tract or retention of K^+ due to kidney disease, respectively. The associated muscular weakness is at times episodic and the plasma K^+ levels in secondary hypo- or hyperkalemic paralysis are much lower or higher than the genetic variants of hypo- or hyperkalemic periodic paralysis. The plasma potassium level that exceeds 7 mEq/L between the episodes of weakness suggests a secondary form of hyperkalemic periodic paralysis.

Hypokalemic Form of Familial Periodic Paralysis (Ca^{2+} Channel Abnormality)

This disease is due to the defect of voltage-gated Ca^{2+} channel and the mechanism of this disease is unrelated to the defect of ion channel at neuromuscular junction. It is the most common form of familial periodic paralysis and is sometimes associated with hyperthyroidism. It may present at any decade of life between the childhood to adulthood and as the time progresses the frequency of attack increases, although it may subside at later life. The episodes of attack of the weakness or paralysis of muscle are most common in the morning, lasting for 3–4 hours, but it may last for whole day. This episode of muscular weakness or paralysis is precipitated by heavy exercise or high carbohydrate diet and is characterized by low serum K^+ level.

On the contrary, the mild exercise actually prevents it. There may be ECG changes consistent with low serum K^+ level. The onset (presence) of unexpected skeletal muscular weakness at the postoperative period may suspect familial periodic hypokalemic paralysis which is with or without additive action from the trailing effects of nondepolarizing muscle relaxants used during anesthesia and surgery. The diagnosis of this disease is usually made from patient's history, family history, EMG and ECG changes, etc. The weakness of skeletal muscle provoked by the infusion of glucose and insulin *confirms the diagnosis of this type of familial hypokalemic periodic paralysis.* Barium blocks the K^+ channel. So, consumption of large amount of barium for any diagnostic purposes may precipitate this hypokalemic familial periodic paralysis. The secondary acquired form of hypokalemic paralysis caused by the loss of K^+ through kidney and GI tract may also develop and should not be confused with primary genetic cause. An acute attack of this disease is treated with 5–10 g of potassium through oral route but without glucose. This is because the uptake of glucose by cells may increase hypokalemia and weakness. During the treatment of this periodic familial paralysis of hypokalemic form, the administration of K^+ through IV route is not recommended, because it may lead to sudden unwanted hyperkalemia.

The anesthetic considerations of this hypokalemic periodic paralysis include the avoidance of factors which trigger the hypokalemic attacks. These are heavy exercise, cold environment, heavy carbohydrate diet, etc. So, the carbohydrate diet should be avoided 24 hours before surgery in such patients suffering from this disease. The drugs known to cause hypokalemia by shifting K^+ into the cell such as β-blocker, insulin, etc. should also be avoided. The IV glucose infusion should also be avoided. As succinylcholine increases the serum K^+ level, so it is suitable for this group of patients. In patients with periodic weakness or paralysis, the response of nondepolarizing muscle relaxant is unpredictable. Therefore, the short-acting nondepolarizing

agents are preferred and the neuromuscular function should be carefully monitored by nerve stimulator. In the intraoperative period, if the diuresis is needed due to any cause, then K^+ losing diuresis should be avoided for the fear of hypokalemia. Hence, the infusion of mannitol is a better alternative. The RA can safely be applied on these patients.

Hyperkalemic Form of Familial Periodic Paralysis (Na⁺ Channel Abnormality)

It is due to the defect of voltage-gated Na^+ channel and the muscular weakness or paralysis is triggered by the abnormal activation of these Na^+ channels with prolonged depolarization like depolarizing muscle relaxant (succinylcholine) which causes prolonged depolarization at the motor endplate. So, Na^+ with water flow into the cells and K^+ comes out of the cell causing hyponatremia, hyperkalemia, and hemoconcentration. It is manifested during the early childhood of life usually at the morning and these attacks are shorter and more frequent than the hypokalemic one. This muscular weakness and paralysis is worse during the rest after heavy exercise, but mild exercise prevents it. During periodic attacks, the serum K^+ level rises above 5–6 mEq/L. But, remains normal in between the attacks. Hypothermia, hypoglycemia, glucocorticoids, pregnancy, etc. aggravates this condition. The diagnosis of this disease is usually made from patient's history, family history, serum K^+ level during attack, EMG, etc. The skeletal muscle weakness in response to the oral administration of K^+ confirms the presence of hyperkalemic form of periodic paralysis.

The anesthetic management of hyperkalemic periodic paralysis includes the avoidance of factors which increase the hyperkalemic attacks or to take the measures which will decrease the serum K^+ level. So, perioperative voluntary K^+ depletion by furosemide-induced diuresis is very important and succinylcholine is contraindicated, as it is associated with hyperkalemia. The potassium (K^+)-containing solutions or the potassium-releasing drugs should always be avoided in the perioperative period during the anesthetic management of such patients. Carbohydrate depletion during fasting should always be managed by glucose-containing IV solutions.

The frequent monitoring of serum K^+ concentration is indicated during the perioperative course of anesthesia. Careful ECG monitoring is indicated to detect cardiac arrhythmias associated with hyperkalemia. Hypothermia and shivering trigger the hyperkalemia. So, the maintenance of body temperature during the perioperative period is very important.

Malignant Hyperthermia

INTRODUCTION

The term malignant hyperthermia (MH) refers to a rare (1: 15,000 in pediatric patients and 1: 40,000 in adult patients) genetic hypermetabolic clinical syndrome (disease of muscle) which is characterized by rapidly increased body temperature (as great as 1°C/5 min), cellular metabolism, O_2 consumption, $\uparrow CO_2$ production, metabolic and respiratory acidosis, lactate production, muscular rigidity, sympathetic activity, and high mortality. This results from an acute uncontrolled increase in skeletal muscle metabolism that may proceed to severe rhabdomyolysis. It is also defined as a pharmacogenetic disease, because the susceptible patients have a genetic predisposition for the development of this syndrome and are not manifested, until they are exposed to some triggering pharmacological agents such as mainly the volatile anesthetic agents and succinylcholine (SCh). There are also many other pharmacological agents which trigger this syndrome. It is also an example of subclinical myopathy that becomes unmasked after the exposure to triggering factors.

However, SCh is less frequently used in modern anesthesia practice and about half of the cases of last decade were associated with halogenated volatile anesthetic agents as the only triggering agent. Hence, whether the SCh is a triggering agent, in the absence of a volatile anesthetic agent, is now under controversy. Nearly ±50% of patients who experience an episode of MH have had at least one previous uneventful exposure to anesthesia, during which they have received a recognized triggering agent.

Although, the onset of clinical features of this disease is acute and rapid after the exposure to volatile anesthetic agents and SCh, but occasionally it (MH) may present more than an hour after the emergence from anesthesia and rarely may occur without exposure to known triggering agents **(Box 1)**. Most cases have been reported in young males, and few have been reported in elderly, and almost none have been reported in infants. However, all the ages and both the sexes may be affected. The incidence of MH varies greatly from country to country and within a same country among its different localities, reflecting varying gene pool.

There is no doubt that this syndrome had been responsible for many anesthetic deaths from the middle of 19th century to the middle of 20th century, since the introduction of ether, chloroform, and SCh. But, during that period nobody knew about this syndrome. Among these incidences, the few remarkable examples are: between 1915 and 1925 one family experienced three anesthetic deaths from MH, featuring muscular rigidity and hyperpyrexia. In 1960, Denborough and Lovell described a 21-year-old Australian who was suffering from an open leg fracture and was more anxious about anesthesia than surgery, because 10 of his relatives had died due to anesthesia before. This had given a very good description of anesthetic reaction, leading to death and its inheritance as an autosomal dominant character. Later, this anesthetic reaction was described as MH. However, actually the genetic inheritance of MH, which has been confirmed recently is more complex than this simple straight forward autosomal dominant variety. It may be autosomal recessive, multifactorial, or unclassified.

In 1966, Wilson had first used the term MH in his book. In the past, death related to anesthesia was not uncommon

---

BOX 1: Agents known to trigger malignant hyperthermia (MH).

- *Volatile anesthetic agents:*
  - Halothane
  - Methoxyflurane
  - Enflurane
  - Isoflurane
  - Desflurane
  - Sevoflurane
  - Ether
- *Depolarizing muscle relaxant:*
  - Succinylcholine

and the causes of these deaths were multiple including MH. So, this relatively rare cause of death, only due to MH during anesthesia, was not given any importance and was not recognized. But, after that, when the anesthesia has become progressively safer, then the high mortality due to MH has become more and more significant. During earlier period, the mortality rate due to MH was 70–80%. But, with earlier diagnosis, increased awareness among anesthetist, and improvement in monitoring this mortality rate due to MH had dropped significantly to 25%. Then, in 1979 with the advent of dantrolene, this mortality rate due to MH has further dropped to 5%. When the volatile agents and SCh are considered as the principal cause, then the overall estimated incidence of MH in UK population is approximately 1 in 8,000.

ETIOLOGY

Normally, during muscular contraction, the wave of depolarization moves from the endplate of muscle fiber to the sarcoplasmic reticulum (SR) which is present within the cell, through the T-tubules of sarcolemma (the cell membrane of muscle cell). The end of these T-tubules, which come in contact with the SR, possesses the voltage-gated Ca^{2+} channel of type I. These are labeled as dihydropyridine receptors (DHPRs). Through these Ca^{2+} channels or DHPR small amount of Ca^{2+} first enter into the muscle cell from the extracellular fluid (ECF) in response to the T-tubular depolarization. The part of the SR, which comes in contact with T-tubules, also contains the *ryanodine receptors (RYRs or RyR1)*. These are also known as the Ca^{2+} efflux channel or foot plate protein and connect between the DHPR of T-tubules and SR. With the wave of depolarization and the intracellular entry of small amount of Ca^{2+} from ECF through DHPR, these receptors of T-tubules (i.e., DHPR) make coupling with the RyR (or RyR1) of SR and transfers the wave of depolarization from T-tubules to SR, resulting in the release of huge amount of Ca^{2+} from SR. Thus, the free ionized intracellular Ca^{2+} level within the muscle cell fiber rises from 10^{-7} M to about $10^{-5} \times$ 5 M due to the depolarization of SR. Then, this increase in intracellular Ca^{2+} removes the inhibition of troponin from the contractile elements of muscle cell, causing muscular contraction. After that, when this contraction of muscle is over, then the multiple intracellular Ca^{2+} pumps, situated on the SR and mitochondria, rapidly transfers the free intracellular Ca^{2+} back into the SR, causing the relaxation of muscle. This increased intracellular concentration of Ca^{2+} also stimulates the multiple intracellular functions such as metabolism, heat production, enzyme secretion, hormone secretion, etc.

Now, there is a general agreement that the MH is due to the defect or abnormal properties of these RyR1 causing

FACT FILE I

Malignant hyperthermia susceptible skeletal muscle differs from normal muscle in that it is always closer to the loss of the control of Ca^{2+} concentration within the muscle fiber. It also involves a generalized alteration in cellular or subcellular membrane permeability. This is an excitation contraction (EC) coupling defect, resulting from the alteration (mutation) in gene encoded for RyR1. It is a heterogeneous disorder, having 30 mutations in *RyR1* gene. The evaluation of affected families is guided by the (1) measurements of circulating creatine kinase (CK), (2) *in vitro drug-induced contracture test,* and (3) genetic testing of deoxyribonucleic acid (DNA) samples.

increased release of intracellular Ca^{2+} from SR. Now, this sudden release of Ca^{2+} from SR removes the inhibition of troponin, leading to intense and sustained contraction of muscles and marked increase in intracellular metabolism. It is very well known that Ca^{2+} is an important ion, controlling the different functions of cell. So, the loss of this hemostasis of Ca^{2+} causes many abnormal metabolisms within the cells which depend not only on the RyR, but also on the other organelle of cells such as the T-tubules, DHPR, inositol phosphate, oxidation-reduction activity, etc. So, this explains why the different chemical agents such as SCh, halothane, etc. trigger the same MH and there is strong evidence of heterogeneity of this syndrome **(Fact file I)**.

GENETICS

Ryanodine (RyR1) receptor is the largest known receptor in our body and is 4–5 times larger than that of ACh receptor. In MH, the properties of these RyR1 receptors are altered due to its *genetic mutation* and these alterations due to its genetic mutation include: increased rate of Ca^{2+} release from SR, changes in the patterns of binding of RyR1 receptor with DHPR and the effects of Ca^{2+} on this binding and the increased sensitivity of RyR1 to caffeine which is also known to cause the increased release of Ca^{2+} from SR. It is proved that the muscles of an individual, susceptible to MH, are more sensitive to caffeine. Most of the patients with an episode of MH have relatives who have had a similar episode or have an abnormal *halothane-caffeine contracture* test. The complexity of genetic inheritance patterns in a family reflects the fact that this MH is associated with a *variety of this genetic mutation of RyR1 gene.*

Ryanodine is a toxic plant alkaloid. It was first extracted by Rogers and his coworkers from a plant named *Ryania speciosa*. It acts on these RyR (from where these receptors get this name) and has profound poisonous effect producing rigidity of skeletal muscle. Later, it was purified and radiolabeled and extensively used in the research of MH. The research to establish the relationship between *RyR* gene and MH gets its fuel with the subsequent identification of link between the mutation of *RyR* gene and MH. There are three forms of RyR (such as RyR1, RyR2, and RyR3) and for these three forms of RyR, there are three types of genes. But, among these only the mutation of *RyR1* gene has been linked to MH. The gene of RyR1 which is responsible for MH, is located on human chromosome 19, which is also the genetic coding site of the Ca^{2+} release channel of SR.

At the beginning of the research on MH, the identification of *HAL* genes in pig which is responsible for the similar MH syndrome in pig (but not identical and is known as the porcine stress syndrome) is the first step. Then, subsequently the identification and localization of *RyR1* genes on human chromosome 19 at q13-13.2 position and transportation of *HAL* gene at that place had stimulated intense research of this subject. Gradually, it was found that the gene responsible for MH is not only situated on chromosome 19, but is also situated on the chromosome 1 and 7, and also possibly on the chromosome 3, 5, and 17. These many genes are also responsible for the various subunits of DHPR which forms the triadic junction complex with the RyR at the SR. Over the next past 20 years, with the revolution in the technique of molecular biology, it has also been possible to study the susceptibility of a family to MH, using DNA markers of known chromosomal location.

In swine, a single genetic mutation of *RyR* gene is responsible for all the cases of MH. But, in human, a series of different mutations or even a lack of any mutation of this *RyR* gene indicates the heterogeneous character of genetic basis of human MH.

◼ CLINICAL FEATURES

The onset of clinical symptoms for this MH syndrome may be (1) acute and rapid when volatile anesthetic agents and/or SCh are used in full doses or (2) may be delayed for several hours when the inhalational agents have been used in low concentration to prevent the only patient's awareness during anesthesia and sometimes not become evident, until the patient enters the recovery room. But, once the reaction or pathology for MH is initiated, then the next course of it cannot be stopped by the discontinuation of these triggering factors (SCh and inhalational agents) and will must progress to a full-blown picture. However, the reaction of MH does never start, after the discontinuation of triggering factors.

The affected person had undergone tremendous increase in muscle rigidity and cellular metabolism, after the onset of this MH, due to the exposure to volatile anesthetic agents and/or SCh. This leads to the intense production of heat (body temperature may exceed 108°F), increased production of CO_2 ($PaCO_2$ may exceed 100 mm Hg), reduced mixed venous O_2 saturation, and increased plasma lactate level. This causes *metabolic and respiratory acidosis marked base deficit,* and altered acid-base balance. So, the plasma pH may be <7.0. The increase in temperature is the cardinal feature of MH, because muscle is the pathological site of this disease which constitutes about 40–45% of total body weight. Another important feature of MH is MMS (*masseter muscle spasm*) or whole-body muscle rigidity **(Box 2)**.

Associated with this muscular rigidity, there is also increased permeability of muscle cell membrane causing increased level of serum K⁺, CK, and serum myoglobin level, leading to hypermagnesemia, *hyperkalemia, myoglobinemia,* and *myoglobinuria* with dark urine. Sometimes moderate-to-severe form of rhabdomyolysis may also occur during an acute episode of MH. But, milder form of it occurs more often than realized and it would have to keep in an anesthetist's mind. Due to the false identification of myoglobin for hemoglobin, the myoglobinuria can be misdiagnosed as hemolysis, when a massive shifting of fluid occurs, during an episode of MH. With the onset of MH, there is hypertension which may be rapidly followed by hypotension, if cardiac depression occurs. When the peak serum CK levels (the maximum is usually measured at 12–18 hours after anesthesia) exceed 20,000 IU/L, then the diagnosis of MH is strongly suspected. It should be kept in the mind of an anesthetist that the administration of SCh in some normal patients without MH may cause serum myoglobin and CK levels to increase markedly.

In exception to other muscles of body, the only masseter and lateral pterygoid muscles contain the slow tonic fibers. So, they sometimes response abnormally to SCh with contracture or spasm, when the other muscles become flaccid. This abnormal response of masseter muscle may or may not be a part of MH syndrome. It may occur separately. This spasm of jaw muscles cannot be altered by pretreatment with the defasciculating dose of nondepolarizing muscle relaxant. It can be graded as tight jaw, rigid jaw, and very rigid jaw. When the spasm of these jaw muscles is very severe which is designated as "very rigid jaw" (impossible to open mouth) and especially prolonged, then this condition is designated as a separate syndrome, named masseter muscle spasm (MMS) and greatly increases the risk of MH **(Fact file II)**.

This MMS or severe form of masseter spasm caused by SCh is entirely considered as pathological and its causes may include MH, myotonia, or other pathological situations. In the absence of family history, the first indication of susceptibility of an individual to MH is this exaggerated response of masseter muscle to a depolarizing muscle relaxing agent. When this MMS is associated with the rigidity of other body muscles, then the chance of MH is absolute. In such circumstances, anesthesia should be stopped immediately and the treatment for MH should be started.

BOX 2: Signs of malignant hyperthermia (MH).

- *Markedly increased metabolism:* (1) $\uparrow CO_2$ production, (2) $\uparrow O_2$ consumption, (3) $\downarrow$ mixed venous O_2 tension, (4) cyanosis, and (5) metabolic acidosis
- *Hyperthermia:* (1) High fever and (2) sweating
- *Muscle damage:* (1) Generalized rigidity, (2) masseter spasm, (3) $\uparrow$ serum CK level, (4) hypernatremia, (5) hyperkalemia, (6) hypermagnesemia, (7) hyperphosphatemia, (8) myoglobinemia, and (9) myoglobinuria
- *Increased sympathetic activity:* (1) Tachycardia, (2) hypertension, and (3) arrhythmias

FACT FILE II

The evaluation of affected families is guided by the measurement of circulating creatine phosphokinase (CK) and subsequently by the analysis of drug-induced (caffeine and halothane) contracture in muscle biopsy specimen in laboratory. The measurement of plasma CK also provides a basic screening test for MH, because it reflects the stability of muscle cell membrane which is disturbed in MH. It is elevated to 70–80% in affected people. When the plasma CK value is elevated in a close relative of a susceptible person, then this relative is also considered as susceptible to MH, and requiring contracture testing. On the other hand, the CK value remains normal in the susceptible patients on several occasions. In the same way, isolated CK elevations in normal asymptomatic individual are seldom associated with positive contracture test. So, in such circumstances, it has no predictable value and muscle biopsy is necessary for contracture study. The contracture study also becomes positive in patients who are suffering from myopathies and not related to MH in any way. Dantrolene should not be given to patient before muscle biopsy, because it may mask the contracture test.

When the MMS is appeared alone without other manifestations, then the chance of MH is 30%. But, when it is associated with the rigidity and damage of other muscles which is evidenced by the increased plasma level of CK and myoglobinuria, then this chance of MH, associated with MMS, is increased to 70–80%. The true response of jaw muscles to SCh in MH, as opposed to the only exaggerated response of rigidity of jaw muscles to SCh, is that the former is associated with metabolic stimulation and the consequences of the loss of the integrity of sarcolemma, leading to hyperkalemia and myoglobinemia. When the clinical signs of MH such as the $\uparrow ETCO_2$, tachycardia, muscle rigidity, temperature, etc. suggest this syndrome, then the diagnosis of MH is not strong, unless more than one abnormal sign is noted. When there is a single suggestive adverse sign, then the diagnosis is usually not MH. If the patient suffering from MH is carefully monitored during the perioperative period, then one or more abnormalities will always be detected. A postoperative pyrexia occurring after a normal intraoperative and immediate postoperative period is not always an indication of MH.

Other than MMS, the increased sympathetic activity, due to increased cellular metabolism, may frequently be the first sign of MH. This increased sympathetic activity causes tachycardia, sweating, hypertension, tachypnea, hypoxia, etc. With metabolic exhaustion, the cellular permeability may also increase in MH. It may cause generalized edema including cerebral edema. As MH progresses to disseminated intravascular coagulation (DIC) (due to cellular destruction), so cardiac failure and renal failure may also develop. Hyperkalemia, due to increased cellular permeability and acidosis, may also cause cardiac arrhythmia, even asystole.

■ DIAGNOSIS OF MALIGNANT HYPERTHERMIA

In the absence of specific drug, such as dantrolene, the treatment of MH is difficult. But, the diagnosis of it during intraoperative period (however, not in postoperative period) is more difficult than its treatment. This is because: (1) The MH is a disorder of cellular metabolism and so the early signs and symptoms of it are masked or become subtle during the course of anesthesia; (2) The diagnosis of MH is also difficult, because the onset of it may sometimes be delayed, until the patient is recovered from anesthesia; (3) During the course of anesthesia, the effects of different anesthetic drugs on different systems of body may also complicate and confuse the signs of MH and make the diagnosis of it difficult; (4) Much of the problem in diagnosing the MH also arises from its variable presentation.

When the hyperthermia is taken as the important diagnostic point, then this syndrome of MH should also be differentiated from other disorders which have same manifestations such as hyperthermia and increased muscular rigidity and confuse the diagnosis of MH. These include: heat stroke, preoperative atropine, septicemia, hyperthyroidism, pheochromocytoma, neuroleptic malignant syndrome (NMS), pontine hemorrhage, etc. However, the differentiating point is that these above-mentioned disorders, confusing the diagnosis of MH, are not associated with the other clinical and laboratory evidence of MH **(Box 3)**.

The most early and sensitive indicator for the intraoperative diagnosis of MH is the measurement of $ETCO_2$ tension (which usually becomes double or triple in MH) at the constant rate of ventilation, without any change of its course (mode). This is because, if the ventilation is increased with the increase of $ETCO_2$ tension, then the $ETCO_2$ tension will remain same and the diagnosis of MH will be masked and delayed. However, the other causes, increasing the tension of $ETCO_2$ should also be ruled out, such as the stuck valve, exhausted soda lime, inadequate fresh gas flow,

BOX 3: Differential diagnosis of hyperthermia in the intraoperative and immediate postoperative period.

- Malignant hyperthermia
- Thyroid storm
- Pheochromocytoma
- Sepsis
- Drug-induced hyperthermia (atropine)
- Serotonin syndrome
- Iatrogenic hyperthermia
- Brainstem/hypothalamic injury (pontine hemorrhage)
- Neuroleptic malignant syndrome
- Transfusion reaction
- Hypercarbia due to CO_2 insufflation in laparoscopy

BOX 4: Classification of drugs according to their potentiality for triggering MH.

Unsafe:
- All volatile anesthetic agents
- Succinylcholine
- Decamethonium

Probably safe:
- Tricyclic antidepressants
- Monoamine oxidase inhibitors
- Phenothiazines
- Haloperidol

Safe:
- Benzodiazepines
- Propofol
- Ketamine and opiates
- Barbiturates
- Metoclopramide
- Atropine and glycopyrrolate
- Nondepolarizing muscle relaxants
- All local anesthetics
- Epinephrine and norepinephrine
- Nitrous oxide
- Neostigmine

inappropriate breathing circuit, etc. In general, MH is not expected in any patient when general anesthesia (GA) is administered with the help of barbiturates, propofol, N_2O, opiates, benzodiazepines, and nondepolarizing muscle relaxants. On the other hand, when GA is administered with the help of volatile anesthetic agents and depolarizing agent such as SCh, then the chance of occurrence of MH should always be kept in mind of an anesthetist and will start to suspect it when the patient will develop undue tachycardia, tachypnea, increased body temperature, cyanosis, arrhythmia, rigidity of muscle, sweating, molting of skin, etc. Then, the diagnosis of MH should be confirmed by the subsequent evaluation of serum pH, hyperkalemia, arterial blood gases, myoglobinuria, etc.

For the diagnosis of MH, the level of O_2 and CO_2 tension in arterial blood is less important than that of the central venous blood, as it is the disease of increased cellular metabolism, and the $ETCO_2$ and central venous CO_2 level are the more accurate reflection of whole-body CO_2 stores. In normal condition, the level of CO_2 in venous blood is only 5 mm Hg higher than that of the arterial blood. But, in MH, this difference will exceed this normal value. The upper limit of venous PCO_2 and PO_2 is suggested as 55 mm Hg and 35 mm Hg respectively, provided the arterial PO_2 is higher than 100 mm Hg. If venous PCO_2 is >60 mm Hg and base deficit is more than –5 to –7 mEq/L, then the diagnosis of MH is confirmed. So, from this above discussion it is found that the most important monitoring devices for the early detection of MH are capnography, pulse oximeter, blood gas analysis, and ECG. But, the most appropriate prerequisite for the early diagnosis of MH is an appropriate suspicious mind of an anesthetist.

TRIGGERING FACTORS AND DIAGNOSIS OF SUSCEPTIBILITY

There are many factors which trigger the onset of MH in human being. But, among these, the volatile anesthetic agents and depolarizing agent, such as SCh, are prime triggering agents. Again, among the volatile anesthetic agents, the halothane is the most potent, while the desflurane and sevoflurane are the less potent triggering agent, causing gradual onset of MH. The onset of MH may be explosive, if SCh is concomitantly used with volatile anesthetic agents and muscular rigidity is developed within 5 minutes. The response of susceptible patients to the triggering agents, such as SCh, may be different. It may be only muscular contracture or only increased permeability of muscle cells, causing hyperkalemia and myoglobinuria or increased cellular metabolism, in association with the muscular contracture and increased permeability. It is most unlikely that N_2O acts as a triggering factor, because previously it has been used safely and repeatedly in a susceptible individual patient without any evidence of MH.

The nondepolarizing muscle relaxant is not a triggering agent for MH. Rather, they block or at least attenuate the effects of SCh and volatile anesthetic agents, causing MH. Propofol is not a triggering factor for MH. On the other hand, it stabilizes the cell membrane of MH affected muscle cells and has opposite effects to those of volatile anesthetic agents. Like propofol, the other intravenous anesthetic agents such as thiopentone, benzodiazepines, opioids, ketamine also have no triggering effect, causing MH. Previously, it was believed that the amide group of local anesthetic agents, such as the lignocaine and others, also may trigger MH. But, later it was proved that they are safe for patients who are susceptible to MH **(Box 4)**.

The predictability of the onset of MH in susceptible persons are not always correct. Because, many affected persons have previously experienced the exposure to the triggering factors without the onset of MH. So, from this history, we cannot say that this patient is not susceptible to MH, during the present course of anesthesia. On the other hand, many patients suffer from MH during anesthesia without any exposure to known triggering factors. So, from this history, we also always cannot predict which patient will develop MH, even if the triggering agents are not used. All these events dictate that the exact mechanism of the triggering of MH by triggering factors during anesthesia is still unresolved.

Recently, the two *in vitro* tests were described to diagnose the preanesthetic susceptibility of an individual to MH. These are the open muscle biopsy and the exposure of some strips of living muscles to halothane and caffeine, producing abnormal contracture response to these two agents. This later test is also known as the *in vitro contracture test* (IVCT) and offers 93% specificity and 99% sensitivity. This IVCT test have 10–20% false positive rate, but the false negative rate is close to zero. Very few centers worldwide perform this test, and there are only two such centers remaining in the USA. More commonly and much more conveniently, genetic testing of patients and their first-degree relatives is performed. This IVCT test is not offered to children who are below 10 years of age as screening for susceptibility to MH, because in children, this test may yield more false negative result.

After a patient is diagnosed as susceptible to MH syndrome by IVCT, then a DNA testing for the mutation of gene, responsible for MH, from muscle biopsy should follow. If one is detected as positive, then the other relatives of this person with that mutation are considered to have susceptibility to MH syndrome and do not need IVCT. The result of the use of DNA screening test from biopsied muscle for the diagnosis of susceptibility to MH is not always straight forward. This is due to the marked heterogeneity and the lack of orderly mutations in many families. However, all these tests to diagnose the susceptibility to MH, is invasive and destructive. So, recently a noninvasive nuclear magnetic resonance test probably has the greatest promise to diagnose the susceptibility for MH. There are also many diseases which make the individual more susceptible to MH. Among these, the myopathies are most important. For example, Duchenne muscular dystrophy may result in an episode of MH, after the exposure to any triggering factors, despite normal contracture testing. Patients with occult myopathies of any type may also have the potentiality to develop rapidly this disastrous anesthetic event. Other muscular disorders

FACT FILE III

The muscular rigidity, which occurs during the onset of MH and is known as contracture, is not the normal contraction of it which is the usual form of muscle movement. The process of muscular contraction is reversible, brief, and is due to the propagated wave of depolarization. On the other hand, the process of contracture is irreversible, nonpropagated, and prolonged. In laboratory, the degree of contracture of cut muscle fibers are used to study the various aspects of MH under the strict guidance of European or North American protocol, with different concentration of caffeine and halothane which vary between these protocols.

that have inconsistent association with MH include myotonia, NMS, sudden infant death syndrome (SIDS), etc. **(Fact file III)**.

All the patients who are suspected to develop MH are referred to higher medical centers which are recognized to tackle this type of patients for anesthesia and surgery. Because, due to any reason the surgery should not be denied to these group of patients, only for the fear of uncapability to manage a case of MH, if it develops. The key to safe anesthesia for this type of patient is to avoid the use of triggering factors, mainly SCh and volatile anesthetic agents. So, the regional anesthesia (RA) is the best option to these individuals who are susceptible to MH as local anesthetic agents do not trigger it. If GA is required, then it is best provided by barbiturates, propofol, benzodiazepine, N_2O, opiates, and nondepolarizing muscle relaxant only. Hence, the routine use of total intravenous anesthesia (TIVA) to deliver GA in these patients, who are susceptible to MH, is more straightforward. However, when a patient who is susceptible to MH is presented with difficult airway, then they are truly exposed to greater risk. This is because, in such circumstances, either a rapid sequence intubation by SCh or inhalation technique for intubation by volatile anesthetic agents (due to the fear of failed intubation and failed ventilation, if nondepolarizing muscle relaxants is used) cannot be used.

Theoretically, to deliver GA on a MH susceptible patient, a dedicated vapor-free anesthetic machine is ideal. But, if this is not available, then both the machine and the ventilator are made ready to use for these susceptible patients by removing all the vaporizers from machine and flushing the ventilator with maximum flow of O_2 for at least 30 minutes. As volatile anesthetic agents are absorbed by the rubber or plastic, so new breathing circuit and face mask should be used mandatorily. If all these preventive measures are taken meticulously and all the well-known triggering factors are avoided, then the prophylactic use of dantrolene to avoid the onset of MH is not recommended or required.

TREATMENT FOR MALIGNANT HYPERTHERMIA

The treatment of an MH episode is directed at terminating the pathology of it and treating the complications such as hyperthermia and acidosis. The mortality rate for MH, even with prompt treatment, ranges from 5 to 30%. If the patient survives the initial presentation, then the acute kidney failure and DIC can rapidly ensue. The other complications of MH include cerebral edema with seizures and hepatic failure. Most MH deaths are due to DIC and organ failure due to the delayed or no treatment with dantrolene **(Box 5)**.

The key point for the treatment of MH, after its development, is the immediate discontinuation of all the triggering factors, as soon as it is diagnosed or suspected. This can be accomplished by quick turning off the vaporizer, and by quick and total eliminating of all volatile anesthetic agents from the body of patient by hyperventilation and by changing the anesthetic circuit. Because, even a trace amount of volatile anesthetic released from sodalime, breathing tubes, and breathing bags may be detrimental. If the episode of MH is diagnosed as a fulminate one (venous PCO_2 is above 90 mm Hg, base deficit is <5 mEq/L and the rate of increase of temperature is 1°C/15 min), then an aggressive therapy should be started immediately to save the life of this patient.

Dantrolene is the specific drug for the treatment of MH. Its safety and efficacy mandate its immediate use in this potential life-threatening situation. It rapidly halts the increase in cellular metabolism and make possible to return back the level of catecholamine and K^+ to normal. The dantrolene acts by inhibiting the release of Ca^{2+} from SR, but does not affect the uptake of it by SR and mitochondria. The site of action of dantrolene is at the level of RyR1 receptor by binding with it and interrupts the transmission of impulses from DHPR to RyR1 receptor. Thus, it decreases the resting level of intracellular Ca^{2+}. In the past, it was used in neuromuscular disorders with better results which are due to the increased intracellular Ca^{2+} level from any cause. Then, this gives the idea of using dantrolene in MH. It is used in the dose of 2–2.5 mg/kg through intravenous route and in fulminate case this dose may be repeated after every 5 minutes up to the maximum dose of 10 mg/kg.

Dantrolene is available now as orange colored powder in vial. Each vial of it contains 20 mg of dantrolene sodium, 3 g of mannitol, and NaOH each. It is reconstituted prior to the use by mixing it with 60 mL of water. The pH of this preparation is 9–10 and this is due to the presence of NaOH. The high pH of this reconstituted solution (or high alkalinity) helps the dantrolene to dissolve in water. The mannitol is added in this preparation to make the solution isotonic. It is not dissolved by 5% dextrose solution, because it may lead to the salting out effect, with greater difficulty in dissolving. If it does not dissolve immediately into water, producing a clear yellow to yellow orange color solution, then it should be heated under tap water or autoclaved for few minutes.

During extreme emergency, it can be administered through the filter of blood transfusion set without worrying about the crystals of dantrolene. In some fulminant cases of MH, the cardiac output falls rapidly. So, it should be given while adequate cardiac output and muscle perfusion is still present. The half-life of dantrolene is 6 hours. So, it can be repeated after every 6 hours in several doses for 24–48 hours to prevent relapse (MH can recur within 24 hours of an initial episode). If there is no recurrence of MH, it can then be discontinued. To save the life during very emergency for the rapid initial dose, the reconstitution of the "conventional" dantrolene is unavoidably time consuming. Hence, a new more costly formulation is available in which 250 mg can be constituted in 5 mL, making it an attractive option for the initial dose of dantrolene, given as an emergency treatment when the MH is first diagnosed.

Following the administration of dantrolene, most of the patients promptly revert to normal acid-base status and no further pharmacological treatment is necessary. The most serious complication, following the acute administration of dantrolene is generalized muscle weakness that may result in respiratory insufficiency. Dantrolene can cause phlebitis in small peripheral veins and should be given through a central venous line if it is available. Dantrolene is a relatively safe drug that is also used to decrease temperature in patients with "thyroid storm" and "neuroleptic malignant syndrome".

Though the administration of dantrolene is the key to therapy of MH, but still the use of other symptomatic therapy to control the body temperature, acid-base balance, and renal perfusion, etc. which are developed with the onset of MH which is also very important. But, during this symptomatic therapy of MH, an anesthetist should always keep a notion

---

BOX 5: Protocol for immediate treatment of malignant hyperthermia (MH).

- Discontinue volatile anesthetic agent and SCh. Inform the surgeon. Immediate call for help.
- As soon as possible administer dantrolene IV in the dose of 2.5 mg/kg and repeat it after 6 hours
- Institute cooling measures
- Counter metabolic acidosis by IV bicarbonate
- Counter hyperkalemia by IV glucose (25–50 g) and insulin (10–20 units)
- If needed administer antiarrhythmic agent
- Monitor $ETCO_2$, electrolytes, blood gases, creatine kinase, serum myoglobin, core temperature, urine output and its color, and coagulation status

in his mind that this supportive therapy will not be able to stop the uncontrolled increased metabolism mayhem within the muscle cells or the actual pathology of MH. So, he or she will not be much preoccupied or busy with such supporting symptomatic works, neglecting the prime factor in therapy. Hence, active cooling is not a prominent feature. Usually, hyperthermia is tried to control by applying ice sponging all over the whole body and putting ice pack over the axilla and groin, IV infusion of refrigerated crystalloid solution, peritoneal lavage with sterile-iced fluids and in extreme cases blood heat exchanger with pump oxygenerator, where this facility is available. The cooling of body only prevents the potentially harmful effect of hyperthermia on other cellular function but it does not stop the pathology of hyperthermia. During cooling, it will also have to keep in mind that cooling causes peripheral vasoconstriction which prevents further heat loss and may produce sudden inadvertent hypothermia. So, the cooling should be halted when the body temperature comes down to 38–39°C. In such circumstances, adequate intravascular fluid load is only the answer. The IV methylprednisolone in the dose of 10 mg/kg is also effective vasodilator and has been shown to reduce muscular contracture **(Fact file IV)**.

After the discontinuation of volatile anesthetic agent (if the patient develops MH), the patient should be hyperventilated with 100% O_2 to counter the effects of uncontrolled CO_2 production and increased O_2 consumption. This will also help to increase the elimination of volatile anesthetic agents from patient's body. Due to hypermetabolism, excessive lactate is also formed by the

---

FACT FILE IV

The anesthetist will response according to the degree of tightness of jaw, due to masseter spasm, during the induction of anesthesia and intubation after the administration of SCh and/or volatile anesthetic agents. If the mouth is impossible to open and the jaw is very tight, then the anesthetic procedure should be halted immediately and the patient should be monitored closely for impending MH. The therapy including the use of dantrolene should be started immediately, if there is any suggestion of the onset of MH. On the other hand, if the jaw is moderately tight and the anesthetist has any suspicion of the onset of MH in his mind, then there are two options. First, if the facilities for subsequent monitoring and management of MH (if it occurs) are available, then the anesthetist can proceed the anesthetic procedure slowly and cautiously with nontriggering agents, still the onset of MH is confirmed. Second, the anesthetist can halt the procedure, if he thinks that this medical center is not well equipped to tackle such cases. Patients who are suffering from fever may have exaggerated reaction to SCh and increased tightness of jaw. So, the patients who develop trismus under the influence of SCh and volatile anesthetic agents should be screened for the susceptibility to MH.

---

skeletal muscle which may result in recurrent metabolic acidosis. This is further corrected by titrating with intravenous sodium bicarbonate at the dose of 2–4 mEq/kg, recognizing that this treatment will worsen the hypercarbia. Thus, hyperventilation with 100% O_2 is needed to remove this additional CO_2 load also. Antiarrhythmic agents, vasopressors, and inotropes should be administered, if indicated. Ca^{2+} channel blockers should not be given to the patients, receiving dantrolene, because this combination appears to promote hyperkalemia. Furosemide may be used to establish diuresis and prevent acute kidney failure which may develop as a consequence of myoglobinuria. Dantrolene contains a considerable amount of mannitol. Thus, furosemide or bumetanide should be used in preference to mannitol for diuresis.

The serum K^+ level should be measured frequently, since the onset of MH. If there is alarming hyperkalemia, then it should be treated immediately, but slowly. The best way of treating mild-to-moderate hyperkalemia is the reversal of MH by the proper doses of dantrolene. Otherwise, it is corrected by the infusion of dextrose with insulin or ion exchange or hemodialysis (only in refractory case). To correct hyperkalemia, IV calcium can be used, but only when there is impending life-threatening arrhythmia. This is because the influx of extracellular Ca^{2+} may further trigger MH response.

Malignant hyperthermia is associated with myoglobinemia. This may block the renal tubules, leading to renal failure. So, it is essential to maintain the normal urine output at any cost. Hence, all the patients, suffering from MH, should be catheterized and diuresis is ensured by mannitol or furosemide. Dopamine is also used to increase the renal blood flow which subsequently will increase the urine output in acute phase of illness to prevent renal failure. Myoglobinuria can usually be detected by coca color urine in first voided specimen. But, the increased level of CK due to muscle damage, which is diagnostic of myoglobinemia and subsequently MH, takes 24 hours to develop. However, it is obvious that significant amount of myoglobinemia should have to be developed, before myoglobinuria has to be detected. Ultimately, DIC develops in a severe fulminating case of MH. It is due to the tissue damage, release of thromboplastin and intravascular hemolysis. It is treated according to the standard lines of treatment.

MANAGEMENT OF PATIENTS SUSCEPTIBLE TO MALIGNANT HYPERTHERMIA

Before anesthesia and surgery, an anesthetist must discuss this special anesthetic problems with the patient who is susceptible to MH and with his or her relatives. This will make the patient very anxious. So, with the discussion of this problem an anesthetist will also assure the patient and his or her party with the confidence that maximum care will be taken to avoid this problem and if problem occurs then the appropriate management of international standard with best drugs, knowledge, and skill will also be taken. Hence, the patient will enter the operation theater (OT) in relaxed mind with full confidence that he or she will not die.

If a particular surgery can be performed under RA, then it should be performed under this technique as RA is very safe for the MH susceptible patients. However, if GA is required, then it should be delivered by benzodiazepines, propofol, barbiturates, ketamine, N_2O, opioids, nondepolarizing muscle relaxant, neostigmine, atropine, and glycopyrrolate. However, at any cost, volatile anesthetic agents and depolarizing muscle relaxant should be avoided in any concentration, even in the presence of dantrolene. Some susceptible patients develop hypermetabolic state, despite all these precautions. Then, these patients should be treated by dantrolene and usually they respond. So, the present consensus is that the preoperative use of dantrolene as a prophylactic measure to MH is superfluous in susceptible patients and the avoidance of triggering factors and the only use of nontriggering agents are the sufficient for the anesthetic management of MH susceptible patients. But, if any anesthetist wants to use preoperative dantrolene, then it should be given in the dose of 2 mg/kg through IV just before the induction of anesthesia. In obstetric susceptible patients, this prophylactic dose of dantrolene is given, after the cord is clamped. This is because if dantrolene is administered before the cord is clamped, then the cord blood level of dantrolene may approach to 60–70% of the patient's plasma level which may result in floppy child.

How do you differentiate malignant hyperthermia from other causes of hyperthermia and hypercarbia?

- In current practice, the most common condition confused with MH is hypercarbia from CO_2 insufflation for laparoscopy. This condition can result in unexpected increase in $ETCO_2$ with accompanying tachycardia. But, there will be no hyperthermia.
- Anesthesia and surgery can precipitate thyroid storm in undiagnosed or poorly controlled hyperthyroid patient. All the signs of thyroid storm are like MH. But, in contrast to MH, hypokalemia is very common in thyroid storm and it generally develops postoperatively.
- Pheochromocytoma is associated with dramatic increase in heart rate (HR) and blood pressure (BP), but not an increase in CO_2 production and $ETCO_2$ tension or temperature. Here, cardiac arrhythmias and ischemia are more prominent. Rarely, such patients may have hyperthermia.
- Sepsis shares several characteristics with MH, including fever, tachycardia, metabolic acidosis, etc. So, it can be difficult to differentiate from MH, if there is no obvious primary site for infection.
- Drug-induced hyperthermia may be encountered in the perioperative period. In these cases, the drugs appear to markedly increase the activity of serotonin in brain, causing hyperthermia, shivering, hyper-reflexia, confusion, etc. The drug combination associated with this serotonin syndrome includes monoamine oxidase inhibitors (MAOIs) and meperidine.
- Iatrogenic hyperthermia is also a possibility, particularly in pediatric patients. The common sources of excessive heat in the operating room include humidifiers on ventilators, warming blanket, heat lamps, etc.
- Injuries to the brainstem, hypothalamus, or nearby regions can be associated with marked hyperthermia and they can be differentiated from MH by the history of trauma.

Neurosurgery and Anesthesia

■ INTRODUCTION

Usually, all the neurosurgeries and its related anesthesia are relatively high-risk procedures. The patients, who are undergone the neurosurgical procedures, present many problems to an anesthesiologist. This is because: (1) the anesthetic agents may have profound effects on cerebral metabolism, cerebral blood flow (CBF), the dynamics of cerebrospinal fluid (CSF), cerebral blood volume (CBV), and pressure (intracranial pressure or ICP), and (2) the soft brain tissue is positioned (kept) in a hard bony skull which acts as a rigid closed box and its (brain tissue) function depends mainly on the ICP, which subsequently depends on the cerebral circulation and the dynamics of CSF, within this closed bony cavity, other than the effect of anesthesia. (3) The diseases, for which the patients are presented for neurosurgeries, itself interfere this cerebral circulation and dynamics of CSF with the fluctuation of ICP that predisposes to cerebral ischemia and, therefore, cerebral damage. For example, an intracranial space occupying lesion (SOL) causes increased ICP and as the lesion grows the danger increases due to the increase of ICP. The other examples are: (1) the patients who are presented for neurosurgeries for subarachnoid hemorrhage (SAH), may suffer from cerebral vascular spasm and subsequently cerebral ischemia and infarction. (2) The patients with pituitary diseases, who are presented for neurosurgery, usually suffer from endocrine disorders that increase the risk of anesthesia during surgery. Anesthetic drugs also have powerful effects on ICP, as they also have immense effects on cerebral circulation and dynamics of CSF.

So, during the anesthesia of neurosurgical procedures, an anesthesiologist needs profound knowledge regarding the physiology of central nervous system (CNS) including the cerebral metabolism, CBF, dynamics of CSF, intracranial volume, ICP, and the effects of anesthetic agents on this physiology of CNS. Hence, the goal of this chapter is to provide adequate information to an anesthesiologist for his or her rational approach during anesthetic management of intracranial, spinal, or any other neurosurgical procedures.

■ CEREBRAL PHYSIOLOGY

Cerebral Metabolism

The brain has tremendously high rate of O_2 consumption and energy utilization reflecting its high metabolic rate. But, it has a very limited energy storage capacity. Hence, due to the absence of significant energy reserves, the interruption of cerebral perfusion (O_2 supply) usually results in unconsciousness within 10 seconds. Therefore, if the CBF is not re-established within 3–8 minutes, then irreversible cerebral damages occur. It is found that the 60% of total cerebral energy utilization is needed (i) to maintain the electrophysiological function of brain such as the depolarization-repolarization activity of nerve cells which is shown in electroencephalography (EEG) and (ii) for the synthesis, transport, and reuptake of neurotransmitter by nerve cells. Another 40% of the total cerebral energy utilization is used to maintain the normal homeostatic activities of the nerve cells of brain including maintaining the integrity of cell membrane (i.e., basic functions of cell).

The adult human brain weighs about 1,350 g which represents approximately 2% of total body weight. At rest, for the production of energy, the human brain consumes O_2 at an average rate of 3.5 mL/100 g of brain tissue/min. Therefore, the whole human brain consumes O_2 at the rate of 47 mL/min ($13.5 \times 3.5 = 47$). This represents the 20% of total body O_2 consumption (250 mL) in a minute. The cerebral metabolic O_2 consumption rate ($CMRO_2$) is maximum at the gray matter of cerebral cortex and it is parallel with the electrical activity of it (gray matter of cerebral cortex).

The neuronal cells of brain mainly utilize glucose aerobically, as their substrate, to produce energy in the form of adenosine triphosphate (ATP). Normally, the rate of utilization of glucose by brain tissue is about 5 mg/100 mg of brain tissue/min. But, during starvation, ketone bodies such as β-hydroxy butyric acid, acetoacetic acid, and acetone also become the substrate for brain tissue for energy production. In the absence of supply of O_2 lactic acid is formed as a result of anaerobic glycolysis with the little production of energy. Therefore, for the proper function of brain, and for this the continuous supply of huge amount of energy in the form of adequate ATP, continuous supply of two things are needed—glucose and O_2 through the circulation of blood. Hence, the failure of adequate supply of any one of these two substances, i.e., glucose (in hypoglycemia) and O_2 (in hypoxia) will cause a devastating damage to the brain. The interruption of supply of O_2 through circulation for 10 seconds in brain results in unconsciousness. If this supply of O_2 cannot be re-established within 3–5 minutes, then irreversible brain damage occurs, as the energy store in neuronal tissue in the form of ATP is very limited. On the contrary, hyperglycemia (explained later) and hyperbaric O_2 (by vasoconstriction) will also cause global or focal hypoxic brain injury by producing cerebral acidosis and cellular injury.

Cerebral Blood Flow

Previously, it is described that energy expenditure by brain tissue is parallel to the cerebral metabolic rate (CMR). This CMR is also parallel (or directly proportional) to CBF. For example, motor activity of a limb is associated with the rapid increase in regional cerebral blood flow (rCBF) of the corresponding motor cortex. Similarly, the visual activity is associated with an increase in rCBF of the corresponding occipital visual cortex. The normal approximate value of CBF in a healthy adult is 50 mL/100 g of brain tissue/min. Among these, as the gray matter is metabolically more active, so here the CBF is estimated to be about 30 mL/100 g of tissue/min. But, as the white matter of brain is metabolically less active, so the CBF in this region is estimated to be only 20 mL/100 g of tissue/min. This total CBF including gray matter and white matter is estimated to about 675 mL/min (13.5 × 50 = 675) which is 12–15% of or a total cardiac output. The CBF has a critical value, below which level the function of brain deteriorates. For example, when the CBF has fallen to approximately 20 mL/100 g of tissue/min, then the evidence of ischemia of brain in EEG begins to appear. At CBF level of approximately 15 mL/100 g of tissue/min the cortical EEG becomes isoelectric. However, when the CBF is reduced below 10 mL/100 g of tissue/min, then the irreversible damage of brain occurs.

There are various methods to measure the CBF directly and these are positron emission tomography (PET), xenon washout method, and computed tomography (CT) perfusion scans. However, these methods cannot be used for the bedside monitoring of CBF. So, in clinical settings, the indirect methods are used to estimate the CBF and to estimate the delivery of O_2 to brain tissues. Now, these indirect methods are:

- *Measurement of the velocity of CBF by Doppler method:* By placing the ultrasound probe over temporal area, the velocity of blood flowing through middle cerebral artery and extracranial internal carotid artery is measured. Normally, the velocity between these two arteries is equal and is 55 cm/second. The velocity of CBF in middle cerebral artery >120 cm/second (which is 2–3 times higher than extracranial internal carotid artery) indicates cerebral artery vasospasm, following SAH or hyperemic blood flow.
- *Infrared spectroscopy:* It reflects cerebral venous O_2 saturation and decreased O_2 saturation of cerebral venous blood which indicates impaired cerebral O_2 delivery, provided the extraction of O_2 by cerebral tissues is constant.
- *Brain tissue oximetry:* It measures the tension of O_2 in brain tissue through the placement of a bolt with Clark O_2 electrode. The normal O_2 tension of brain tissue varies between 20 and 50 mm Hg. This tension of O_2 in brain tissues <10 mm Hg indicates brain ischemia.

Regulation of CBF

There are some elaborate mechanisms in brain for the regulation of CBF. These include chemical, myogenic (auto), neurogenic, and some other extrinsic mechanisms.

Chemical mechanism of CBF: The chemical mechanism for the regulation of CBF includes the changes in CMR, and subsequently its $PaCO_2$ and PaO_2. It is already stated that the increased neuronal activity in brain results in the increased cerebral metabolism and this increase in CMR is associated with well-matched proportional increase in CBF. For this (increase in CBF), a variety of metabolic byproducts has been considered to act as intermediaries to increase this CBF. These include: H^+ concentration, extracellular K^+ and/or Ca^{2+} concentration, thromboxane, certain prostaglandins, adenosine, etc.

Cerebral blood flow also changes directly with the changes in $PaCO_2$ **(Fig. 1)**. But, this changing effect of CBF is greatest within the normal range of physiological changes in $PaCO_2$, i.e., between 30 and 70 mm Hg. Within this normal range of changes in $PaCO_2$, (i) the CBF changes by 1–2 mL/100 g of brain tissue/min for each 1 mm Hg change in $PaCO_2$ and (ii) the CBV changes by 0.05 mL/100 g of brain per 1 mm Hg change in $PaCO_2$. This response is attenuated (blunted), when the $PaCO_2$ falls below the 25 mm Hg.

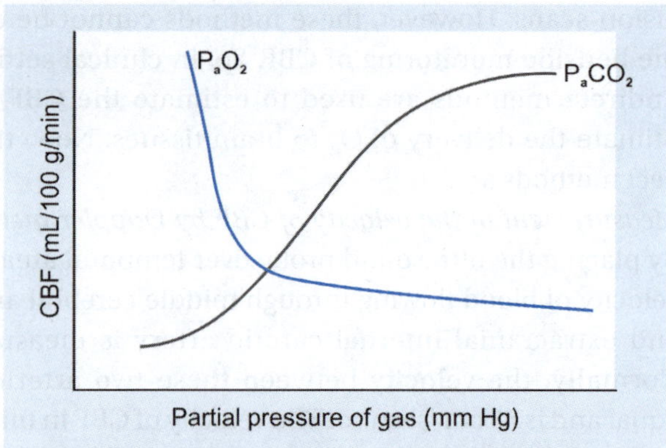

Fig. 1: Relationship of cerebral blood flow (CBF) with arterial O$_2$ tension (blue line) and arterial CO$_2$ tension (gray line).

This change in CBF, caused by the changes in PaCO$_2$ is due to the changes in *pH of extracellular fluid (ECF) (or CSF)* of brain, but *not due to the changes in intracellular H$^+$* concentration which increases in metabolic acidosis. This is because H$^+$ cannot readily cross the blood-brain barriers (BBBs). So, this change in PaCO$_2$ causes the free CO$_2$ to diffuse freely across the cerebrovascular endothelium. Thus, the acute metabolic acidosis which is mainly concerned with the increase in H$^+$ concentration (intracellular) has little effect than the respiratory acidosis (where CO$_2$ level is mainly increased) on CBF.

After 6–8 hours, this elevated CBF returns to normal in spite of the elevation of PaCO$_2$. This is because the pH of ECF of brain gradually normalizes due to the adjustment of plasma HCO$_3^-$ level. Similarly, the reduction in PaCO$_2$ reduces the CBF. But, several investigations indicate that in normal subjects ischemia will not occur at PaCO$_2$ above 20 mm Hg. However, the physiological alterations of brain function, as evidenced by EEG and metabolic abnormalities, are observed when the PaCO$_2$ is reduced below 15 mm Hg by hyperventilation. So, there is little benefit in terms of improvement of ICP, rather it causes harm, if PaCO$_2$ is reduced lesser than 20–25 mm Hg.

Like the PaCO$_2$, the PaO$_2$ has not much effect on CBF. The changes in PaO$_2$ between 60 and 300 mm Hg have little influence on it (CBF). But, when PaO$_2$ falls below 60 mm Hg, then this CBF increases rapidly. However, this mechanism of vasodilatation, caused by hypoxia, is not exactly known. But, the probable mechanism of this hypoxia-induced vasodilatation is neurogenic effect which is initiated by peripheral chemoreceptor and direct hypoxic effects on vascular smooth muscles mediated by lactic acidosis.

Myogenic mechanism or Autoregulation of CBF: Over a wide range of change in mean arterial pressure (MAP), the CBF is maintained automatically by changing the resistance of cerebral vessels (constriction or dilatation) intrinsically. This is called the myogenic mechanism or the autoregulation of CBF. In normal human beings, the range of MAP within which the CBF is maintained by autoregulation at its constant level is 60–160 mm Hg. Above and below this level of MAP, the CBF is not autoregulated and becomes pressure dependent and changes (CBF reduces or increases with the reduction or increase of MAP) accordingly in linear fashion. The difference between the MAP and ICP is known as the cerebral perfusion pressure (CPP), i.e., MAP – ICP = CPP which determines the rate of diffusion of substrates into the brain tissue from vessels. The normal value of CPP is 80 – 100 mm Hg. Normally, the value of ICP is <10 mm Hg. So, the CPP is primarily dependent on MAP. The moderate to severe increase in ICP (>30 mm Hg) can compromise CPP and CBF, even in the presence of normal MAP. The patients with CPP value of <50 mm Hg often show the slowing of EEG, whereas those with CPP value varying between 25–40 mm Hg typically have a flat EEG.

When the MAP goes above 160 mm Hg and the autoregulation fails, then the ICP also rises and CPP falls. The increased MAP, beyond its autoregulation range, can disrupt the BBB. This may result in intracranial hemorrhage and cerebral edema.

The exact mechanism of this autoregulation (myogenic mechanism) of CBF is not known. But, still, it is postulated that the intrinsic characteristic of the smooth muscle of cerebral blood vessel is responsible for this myogenic autoregulation of CBF. Another theory is also put forward for this myogenic autoregulation of CBF. This is known as the *metabolic mechanism.* This theory explains that cerebral metabolic demand determines the cerebral arteriolar tone and CBF. Thus, when the brain tissue demands more metabolic need, then the cerebral vessels dilate and CBF increases and *vice versa.* So, it is also known as the myogenic regulation. This autoregulation or myogenic reflex of CBF is influenced by various pathological processes such as intracranial tumors, head injury, many disease processes of cerebral vessels, SAH, volatile anesthetic agents, vasodilators, etc. This myogenic or autoregulation of CBF is not a fixed one. If a person suffers from chronic essential hypertension for long time, then this autoregulation curve with its upper and lower end shifts to the right. It means the CBF is maintained at higher level of upper and lower range of MAP **(Fig. 2)**.

Neurogenic mechanism for the regulation of CBF: There is strong evidence for extensive innervation of cerebral vessels. These are sympathetic (vasoconstrictive), parasympathetic (vasodilator), serotonergic, vasoactive intestinal peptidergic (VIP), etc. But, the density of innervation decreases with the decrease of vessel's size. So, the neurogenic mechanism

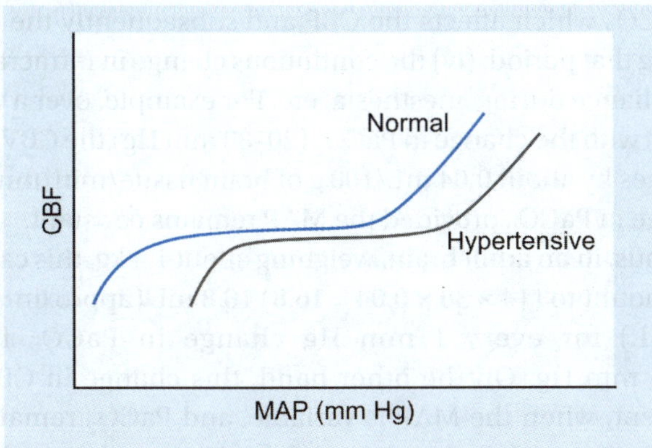

Fig. 2: Autoregulation curve of cerebral blood flow (CBF) in normal (blue line) and hypertensive (gray line) subject. In hypertension, it is shifted to the right.

for the regulation of CBF exists only on the large cerebral vessels. The exact functional significance of this neurogenic regulation of CBF is not known. But, still it may play an important role in some pathological states. For example, in hemorrhagic shock the increased sympathetic activity causes the lowering of CBF by vasoconstriction at a given MAP than which is found when hypotension is produced by sympatholytic agents. This is probably because during shock the vasoconstrictive effect caused by sympathetic overactivity shifts the lower end of autoregulation curve of CBF to the right. The sympathetic and parasympathetic innervation may also play a vital role in regulating CBF during stroke and brain injury.

Some extrinsic mechanisms or factors for the regulation of CBF

Temperature: The CMR and subsequently the CBF immensely depend on the temperature of cerebral tissue. It is found that the CMR and CBF decrease by 5–6% for every 1°C reduction of temperature (hypothermia) of brain. So, the CMR and CBF fall to 50% of its original value for the reduction of the temperature of brain from normal 37°C to 27°C. Then, with the further reduction of temperature of brain to 20°C, the EEG (which signifies the electrophysiological activity of brain), becomes isoelectric with the further reduction of CMR and CBF. With the further reduction of the temperature of brain, from 20°C to downward, the CMR will also further decrease with the further decrease of CBF. This is because hypothermia causes decrease in CMR which is associated with both the electrophysiological function and the maintenance of common basic cellular functions. The reduction of temperature up to 20°C is responsible for the reduction of CMR which is associated with cerebral electrical activity and the reduction of temperature below 20°C is responsible for the reduction of CMR which is associated with basic cellular activities.

In contrast, the anesthetic agents (with the deepening of anesthesia by increasing the dose of them) reduce the CMR which is only associated with the electrophysiological function of brain and is evidenced by only EEG. So, after the EEG becomes isoelectric, with the further increase in the dose of anesthetic agents, the CMR and subsequently the CBF will not reduce further. With the reduction of temperature from 27°C to 17°C, there is further 50% reduction in CMR and CBF. Therefore, it probably accounts for the brain's tolerance to total circulatory arrest for moderate periods at this level of hypothermia.

Hyperthermia has the opposite effect to hypothermia or cerebral physiology. Between 37 and 42°C, both the CMR and CBF increase (for every 10°C increase in temperature, the CMR doubles). But, above 42°C the CMR again begins to fall. This indicates that 42°C is the threshold level for the toxic effect of hyperthermia and this is due to the neuronal cell damage resulting from the degradation of protein (enzymes of cell) due to heat.

Viscosity: One of the single most important determining factors for the viscosity of blood is the hematocrit value of it. So, the effect of viscosity of blood on CBF is estimated from the angle of hematocrit level. The viscosity of blood or the hematocrit level of it has some influence on CBF. But, this is not found within the normal range of hematocrit value (33–45%) in a healthy adult individual. But, beyond this range, the changes in CBF due to the changes in hematocrit value are more substantial. A decrease in hematocrit value (anemia) improves the CBF. This is due to the decrease in the viscosity of blood. On the other hand, simultaneously, it also reduces the O_2 carrying capacity of blood to brain. But, practically this occurs after getting the maximum benefit from the increased blood flow to brain, due to the decreased level of hematocrit and viscosity. Thus, the anemia can potentially impair O_2 delivery in brain, but below a certain level of hematocrit value, where the maximum beneficial effect from the increase in CBF due to anemia has already been taken.

The reduction of hematocrit (anemia) or viscosity increases the CBF by reducing the vascular resistance (i.e., by vasodilatation) in response to low O_2 carrying capacity in blood. This effect of the reduction of viscosity on CBF is more important in the case of focal cerebral ischemia, where local vasodilatation in response to low O_2 delivery is maximum. In this setting, the reduction of viscosity produced by hemodilution results in increased CBF in the ischemic territory of brain. It is also evidenced from different studies that the optimum delivery of O_2 to brain in anemia can occur at hematocrit value of 30%. Increased hematocrit and viscosity in polycythemia has opposite effect and reduce CBF.

Vasoactive drugs: Many vasoactive drugs such as systemic vasodilators, sympathetic agonists and antagonist, etc. which are used rampantly in anesthetic practice, have some definite effects on CBF. The *systemic vasodilators* which are used for induced hypotension during anesthesia practice such as Na-nitroprusside, nitroglycerine, calcium channel blockers, etc. cause cerebral vasodilatation and increase CBF or maintain it at prehypotensive level up to a certain value of the reduction of MAP. If the hypotension is induced slowly by these agents, then ICP does not rise due to increased CBF. This is probably explained by the shifting of the CSF and venous blood (as compensatory mechanism) when the changes in the increase of CBF occur very slowly. Otherwise, vasodilator drugs will cause increased CBF and increased ICP.

The *sympathetic α1 agonists* do not increase CBF, though they cause acute increase in MAP. This is probably due to the presence of autoregulation and intact BBB. In defective BBB or in the absence of autoregulation, these α1 agonists may increase CBF and ICP tremendously. In cases of β *agonists,* it is found that in low doses they have little direct effect on CBF. But, in higher doses they definitely increase CMR coupling with increased CBF. The β *blockers* probably have no effect on CBF or reduce it with the reduction of CMR. However, the level of circulating plasma catecholamines at the time of the administration of β blockers and the status of BBB may influence the effects of these agents on CBF. There is unlikely to have side effects of these agents on patients with intracranial pathology, other than the secondary changes due to reduction in CPP caused by decrease in CBF.

The effect of *dopamine* on CBF is very interesting. In lower doses (2–6 µg/kg/min), it probably causes the dilatation of cerebral vessels and increases CBF. But, there is possibility of vasoconstriction and reduction of CBF in higher doses (6–20 µg/kg/min). In doses lesser than 2 µg/kg/min dopamine also causes cerebral vasoconstriction.

▎ EFFECTS OF ANESTHETIC AGENTS ON CEREBRAL PHYSIOLOGY

Except ketamine, all the anesthetic agents reduce the electrical activity of CNS and subsequently its energy consumption. Therefore, they increase the amount of energy, stored in the form of ATP, adenosine diphosphate (ADP), and phosphocreatine. However, this study of effects of anesthetic agents on cerebral physiology is difficult. This is because, it is often complicated by many factors during the procedure of surgery and anesthesia such as (i) the continuous change in MAP due to sympathetic overactivity during surgery and anesthesia due to stimuli, (ii) the concomitant use of many other drugs during anesthesia, (iii) the continuous change

in $PaCO_2$ which affects the CBF and subsequently the CBV during that period, (iv) the continuous change in intracranial compliance during anesthesia, etc. For example, over a wide range, with the change in $PaCO_2$ (20–80 mm Hg) the CBV also changes by about 0.04 mL/100 g of brain tissue/min/mm Hg change in $PaCO_2$ provided the MAP remains constant.

Thus, in an adult brain, weighing about 1.4 kg, this can be an amount to $(14 \times 30 \times 0.04 = 16.8)$ 16.8 mL (approximately 17 mL) for every 1 mm Hg change in $PaCO_2$ from 25–55 mm Hg. On the other hand, this change in CBV is different, when the MAP is variable, and $PaCO_2$ remains a constant factor. It is already stated that autoregulation serves to prevent the MAP-related change in CBF and CBV. In the face of rising MAP, the cerebral blood vessels constrict to maintain a constant CBF and thus CBV decreases to normal and *vice versa* (compensatory mechanism). But, when this autoregulation is impaired by anesthetic agents or its upper and lower limit (150 mm Hg and 50 mm Hg) is exceeded, then the CBF and CBV increase or decrease as the MAP increases or decreases.

Intravenous Anesthetic Agents

Barbiturates

They produce a dose-dependent reduction in CMR and CBF. With the onset of anesthesia, this reduction of CMR and CBF is 30%. But, with the deepening of anesthesia, by gradually increasing the doses of barbiturates, when the EEG becomes isoelectric, then this reduction of CMR and CBF touches to 50%. However, the further increase in the dose of barbiturates beyond this point had no effect on CMR, CBF, and CBV. This is because barbiturates only cause the reduction in the component of cerebral metabolism (CMR) which is related only to the neurophysiological activity of brain, but not the component of cerebral metabolism which is related to the basic cellular activity such as ion transport, etc. which is responsible for the maintenance of the integrity of cell membrane. This is in contrast to hypothermia where both the CMR and CBF are reduced, still beyond the point of isoelectric EEG (described before) **(Fig. 3)**.

The reduction of CMR by barbiturates is greater than that of CBF. So, there is always some store of metabolic energy during barbiturate anesthesia as supply (CBF) exceeds the demand (CMR). Barbiturates also cause the constriction of smooth muscles of cerebral blood vessels and are the cause of the reduction of CBF along with the reduction of CMR (this mechanism is separate from the reduction of CBF when CMR is reduced due to hypothermia or other causes). But, this is found in normal brain tissue. In ischemic brain tissue, barbiturate causes the dilatation of vascular smooth muscle and diverts the blood flow from normal to the ischemic area

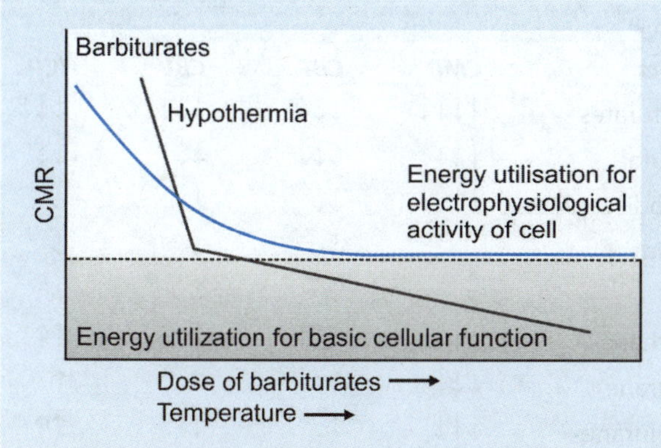

Fig. 3: The effects of barbiturates (blue line) with its increasing dose and the effects of gradual lowering of temperature or hypothermia (gray line) on CMR. The maximum reduction of CMR that occurs with the increased dose of barbiturate, result in silent EEG. At this point, the energy utilization by cell for electrophysiological activity comes to zero. But, the energy utilization for basic cellular activity remains unchanged which is only reduced by hypothermia. (CMR: cerebral metabolic rate; EEG: electroencephalography)

of brain which is helpful. It is known as the *reverse steal or Robin Hood phenomenon*. So, the ischemic areas of brain get maximum amount of blood supply during barbiturate anesthesia.

Other than the reduction of ICP, by reducing CBF during neurosurgeries, the barbiturates also help by facilitating the dynamics of CSF. It helps in the absorption of CSF. So, the ICP is further reduced and protects the brain from damage by increased ICP and the reduction of CPP. The barbiturates also have the anticonvulsant property. Thus, it prevents convulsion and reduces CMR along with the reduction of CBF and ICP (convulsion is associated with increased CMR, CBF, and ICP) causing decrease in the chance of ischemia of brain.

Propofol

Like barbiturates, the propofol also reduces the CMR and CBF. These reductions of CMR and CBF, caused by propofol, are approximately 30 and 50%, respectively. Hence, it shows that there is more reduction of CBF than CMR, in propofol anesthesia, which is unlike to barbiturates. Thus, it is also helpful in neurosurgery by reducing ICP and protecting the brain from ischemia. Though, the propofol causes chorea form and dystonic movements, but it has also significant anticonvulsant property like barbiturates. So, it also protects the brain from ischemic injury during convulsion. However, both the autoregulation and the CO_2 responsiveness to CBF appear to be preserved during the administration of propofol.

The short elimination half-life of propofol makes it a useful (most common) inducing agent for neuroanesthesia. Propofol infusion is commonly used for the maintenance of total intravenous anesthesia (TIVA) in patients at risk of intracranial hypertension.

Benzodiazepines

Like propofol and barbiturates, the benzodiazepines (BZDs) also cause the reduction of CBF and CMR. But, the extent of this reduction of CMR and CBF is probably intermediate in position, lying in between the narcotics (minimal) and barbiturates (maximum). For example, 15 mg diazepam reduces CMR and CBF to 25% of its original value, provided respiratory depression and increase in $PaCO_2$ do not occur. The BZDs also have useful anticonvulsant properties. Midazolam is the BZD of choice in neuroanesthesia, because of its short half-life. Midazolam, used as an induction agent, may cause decrease in blood pressure (BP) and CPP and may result in prolonged emergence.

Narcotics

They have minimal reduction effect on CMR and CBF in normal unstimulated patients. So, they cannot decrease CMR and CBF, especially if there is any factor, which increases the ↑$PaCO_2$ and ↑MAP. The CO_2 responsiveness and autoregulation to CBF remain unaffected by narcotics. Regarding the effect of narcotics on ICP, it is found that morphine and fentanyl reduce ICP by reducing the CMR, CBF, CBV, and CSF pressure. But, it is found that sufentanil and alfentanil sometimes increase ICP.

Ketamine

Among all the intravenous anesthetic agents, ketamine is the only one, which increases the CMR and subsequently the CBF (50–60%) by dilating the cerebral vessels. Thus, it increases the ICP also. It selectively activates the limbic structure and the area of reticular formation of brain, while it selectively depresses the cortical area of brain. Seizure, caused by ketamine, further increases ICP by increasing CMR, CBF, CBV, and CSF volume. So, it is not beneficial for neurosurgery. Hyperventilation can reduce the elevation of ICP caused ketamine, because CO_2 responsiveness to CBF remains intact by it.

Therefore, in conclusion we can say that ketamine administration does not increase ICP in neurologically impaired patients under controlled ventilation with the concomitant use of propofol and/or BZD. Further, the ketamine offers some neuroprotective effect, according to some investigators. Their explanation is like that during brain injury there is increased level of NMDA receptors and as the ketamine blocks these NMDA receptors, so it protects the brain from the toxic effect of NMDA receptors. Though, theoretically it is said that ketamine increases ICP, still it has been used now in many centers in brain injured patients without any deleterious effects on ICP.

Inhalational Anesthetic Agents

Volatile Agents

The pattern of influence of volatile anesthetic agents on cerebral physiology is strikingly different from that of the intravenous anesthetic agents. *Here, the reduction of CBF, caused by the volatile anesthetic agents, does not follow the foot print of the reduction of CMR caused by the intravenous anesthetic agents.* All the volatile anesthetic drugs dilate the cerebral blood vessels (in contrast to barbiturates and propofol which constrict these vessels). Thus, they all increase the CBF and CBV, while simultaneously they produce dose-related reduction in CMR. Hence, all the volatile anesthetic agents increase ICP, especially in patients with reduced intracranial compliance. Regarding the effects of volatile agents on CBF, CBV, and ICP, the halothane is the most potent and isoflurane is least potent agent. The influence of the newer volatile anesthetic drugs such as sevoflurane and desflurane on cerebral physiology is more or less similar to that of isoflurane. For example, halothane increases CBF up to 200%, compared to 20%, produced by isoflurane at the equivalent dose of minimum alveolar concentration (MAC) and similar reduction of BP. Regarding the reduction of CMR, isoflurane produces the greatest maximal depression (up to 50% reduction), whereas it has the least effect (<20% reduction). Hence, isoflurane causes maximum reduction of CMR and minimum increase in CBF.

On the other hand, halothane produces relatively homogenous changes in CBF in brain. Therefore, the CBF is globally increased and CMR is globally decreased by halothane. In contrast, these changes (reduction of CMR and increase of CBF) caused by isoflurane are more heterogeneous resulting on increase in CBF in subcortical and hind brain structures than the structures of neocortex. However, for the CMR the reverse is true for isoflurane causing greater reduction in neocortex than that in subcortex and hind brain. All these data dictate that isoflurane is preferred in neurosurgery, if volatile anesthetic agents are at all used in the setting of impaired (decrease) intracranial compliance. But, that does not indicate that halothane is completely contraindicated in these circumstances. It is clearly demonstrated that halothane can safely be used in such circumstances, if only $PaCO_2$ is maintained at normal level by hypo- or hyperventilation, the explanation of which is described as follows **(Table 1)**.

TABLE 1: Effects of anesthetic agents on cerebral physiology.

Agents	CMR	CBF	CBV	ICP
Barbiturates	↓↓↓↓	↓↓↓	↓↓↓↓	↓↓↓
Propofol	↓↓↓	↓↓↓	↓↓	↓↓
Benzodiazepines	↓↓	↓↓	↓	↓
Opioids	↓	↓	↓	↓
N_2O	↓	↓	↓	↓
Halothane	↓↓	↑↑↑↑	↑↑↑	↑↑↑
Isoflurane	↓↓↓	↑	↑	↑
Sevoflurane	↓↓↓	↑	↑	↑↑
Desflurane	↓↓↓	↑	↑	↑↑
Ketamine	↑	↑↑↑	↑↑	↑↑↑

(CBF: cerebral blood flow; CBV: cerebral blood volume; CMR: cerebral metabolic rate; ICP: intracranial pressure)

All these volatile anesthetic agents abolish the autoregulation mechanism of CBF in response to increase or decrease in MAP. So, the changes in CBF do not run in parallel to the changes in MAP. But, after few hours, the increased CBV due to increased CBF returns to normal due to some other compensatory mechanism. However, this time course, needed for this compensation, is dependent on the magnitude of the initial elevation of CBF. It is already previously stated that the reduction of CMR, caused by volatile anesthetic agents, is not similar to that of hypothermia. In hypothermia, the CMR is further reduced after the EEG becomes isoelectric which is not found in volatile agents and intravenous anesthetic agents. CO_2 responsiveness to the changes for CBF is well preserved during anesthesia by all the volatile anesthetic agents. Therefore, hyper- or hypoventilation can control the CBF, CBV, and ICP when anesthesia is provided by volatile anesthetic agents.

From the above discussion, it is learnt that the volatile anesthetic agents cause the uncoupling of normal relationship between the CBF and CMR, i.e., reduce the CMR, but increase the CBF. So, this aspect of the influence of volatile anesthetics on cerebral physiology is beneficial by preventing ischemia, especially during the use of isoflurane in neurosurgery. But, this beneficial effect is off set by the steal phenomenon caused by these volatile anesthetic agents. This steal phenomenon explains that the volatile anesthetic agents though dilate the vessels of normal brain tissue, but do not dilate the vessels of ischemic area which are already maximally dilated due to ischemia. So, the ultimate result is the starved ischemic area due to the stealing (diversion) of blood to the normal healthy area from the ischemic area of the brain. Further, they increase ICP, especially in patients with decreased intracranial compliance, causing further damage to the brain.

Nitrous Oxide

Nitrous oxide causes the vasodilatation of cerebral vessels. This vasodilating effect of N_2O is clinically more significance during neurosurgery in patients who have reduced intracranial compliance. Hence, the available data till now unequivocally suggest that N_2O produces substantial increase in CBF, CBV, and ICP when used alone in neurosurgeries. For example, when N_2O is used alone during the removal of intracranial tumors, then ICP may rise from the mean value of 10–13 mm Hg to 30–40 mm Hg. But, the magnitude of this effect varies considerably, according to the presence or absence of other anesthetic agents such as intravenous or volatile. When N_2O is used in combination with intravenous anesthetic agents such as thiopentone, propofol, BZDs, etc. then the vasodilating property of N_2O is completely inhibited or attenuated. So, there is no increase in CBF and ICP. Again, during neurosurgery, the combination of N_2O and narcotics also has the similar effects. On the contrary, when N_2O is used in combination with volatile anesthetic agents, then substantial increase in CBF, CBV, and ICP is occurred. So, the present status, regarding the use of N_2O in neurosurgery, is that till now there is no strong adequate evidence to prohibit its use. Hence, N_2O is now widely used in neurosurgery, but in circumstances, where ICP is persistently elevated causing tight surgical field, then N_2O should be taken as the responsible factor for this and avoided.

Muscle Relaxants

Depolarizing Agents

In a lightly anesthetized patient, succinylcholine is found to produce the elevation of ICP. This is possibly due to the result of cerebral activation, caused by the afferent impulses to the brain from muscle spindle during its fasciculation. So, this elevation of ICP is found to be maximum after 1–3 minutes of the administration of succinylcholine and return to base line after 8–10 minutes. Thus, this succinylcholine-induced elevation of ICP can be attenuated by deepening the induction of anesthesia and preventing the fasciculation, by using a small defasciculating dose of nondepolarizing agent. Hence, its use need not be viewed as contraindication in neurosurgery with elevated ICP, where the rapid achievement of skeletal muscle paralysis and intubation by succinylcholine is justified, due to any cause such as difficult airway. Little hazard should follow its use, if it is administered with proper control of MAP, $PaCO_2$, depth of anesthesia, and using the method of defasciculation.

Nondepolarizing Agents

These agents cannot penetrate the BBB. So, they have no direct effect on cerebral vasculatures. The only indirect effect of it on CBF is via the release of histamine by these agents. Histamine decreases MAP by systemic vasodilatation and increases ICP by cerebral vasodilatation. Thus, it can result in the reduction of CPP. Among the nondepolarizing agents, tubocurarine is the most notorious for the release of maximum amount of histamine. But, the commonly used nondepolarizing agents in clinical anesthesia such as atracurium, mivacurium, rocuronium, vecuronium, etc. release histamine in lesser quantities. So, their use in neurosurgeries with elevated ICP is clinically inconsequent, unless they are administered in large doses which are necessary to achieve rapid intubating condition. The nondepolarizing agents, which increase MAP such as pancuronium may elevate the ICP. But, this is only possible when the rise of this MAP is abrupt and autoregulation is disrupted by the disease processes of CNS for which the surgeries are shouted. On the other hand, the nondepolarizing agents can reduce ICP by decreasing the impedance of cerebral venous outflow by preventing the coughing and straining. In most of the cases, during neurosurgery, the increase in ICP following the administration of muscle relaxants, laryngoscopy, and intubation is due to the hypertensive response for light plain of anesthesia.

■ CEREBROSPINAL FLUID

A clear, colorless, transparent, and modified tissue fluid fills all the ventricles and the cisterns of brain, and the whole subarachnoid space, bathing the total CNS (both brain and spinal cord). This is called the CSF. The major functions of CSF are (i) to protect the CNS from trauma, (ii) to clear the waste from CNS, and (iii) to maintain the physiology of brain. The CNS is devoid of lymphatic supply. So, in CNS the CSF replaces the lymph. In a healthy adult human, the volume of CSF is about 150 mL. It is continuously formed and absorbed. The normal rate of the production of CSF in a healthy adult is about 500 mL/day or 20 mL/hour or 0.3 mL/minute. About 60–70% of CSF is produced by the choroid plexus of lateral ventricles. The remaining 30% of CSF is secreted directly from the ependymal cells, lining all the ventricles. Yet a smaller quantity of CSF is formed by the fluid, leaking into the surrounding of perivascular space from cerebral vessels (BBB leakage). The production of CSF is independent of ICP and every day, it is totally exchanged for three times **(Fact file I)**.

After its formation from two lateral ventricles (right and left) of brain, the CSF first passes through the respective foramina of Monro (right and left intraventricular foramina) to the third ventricle which is situated in the midline of brain. Then, it flows through the aqueduct of Sylvius. This aqueduct of Sylvius is a fluid-filled channel which runs through the midbrain and connects the third ventricle with the fourth

FACT FILE I

Protective function of CSF

The meninges and CSF protect the brain. The dura mater is the outermost layer of three meninges and is located directly underneath the bones of skull and vertebral column. It is made up of fibrous connective tissue and is thick, tough, and inextensible. The dura mater consists of two layers: (1) endosteal layer and (2) meningeal layer. The endosteal layer of dura mater lines the inner surface of the bones of cranium as periosteum. Within the cranial cavity, the endosteal layer and the meningeal layer of this dura mater are adhered together and cannot be separated, except at the site of sagittal, transverse, sigmoid, and other intracranial sinuses.

In the vertebral column, the endosteal and the meningeal layer of dura mater are not adhered together. In the vertebral column, the endosteal layer of dura mater also lines the inner surface of the vertebral bone as their periosteum, but the meningeal layer of dura mater remains separated from its endosteal layer by a potential space which is known as the *epidural space*. At the level of the foramen magnum, these two layers of vertebral dura mater are fused and run in the cranial cavity as a single layer of dura mater except at the sites of sinuses. So, the epidural space extends above up to the level of foramen magnum and does not extend into the cranial cavity. There is a thin potential space between dura and arachnoid mater which is known as the *subdural space*. It contains a thin film of fluid. Thus, the arachnoid mater is held with the dura mater by surface tension of this thin layer of fluid. Below the arachnoid mater lies the pia mater and the space between these arachnoid and pia mater is known as *subarachnoid space* which is filled with CSF. The pia mater remains adhered with the nerve tissue of brain. The brain with its pia mater covering hangs or floats within the CSF filled subarachnoid space supported by blood vessels, nerve roots, and multiple fine fibrous arachnoid trabeculae which pass from arachnoid mater to the pia mater through subarachnoid space.

The brain weighs about 1,400 g in air. But, when it floats in CSF, then it has net weight of only 50 g. The buoyancy (floating effect) of this organ (brain) in CSF is due to the flimsy attachment between the brain and the arachnoid layer through the blood vessels, nerve roots, and arachnoid trabeculae which suspend the brain in CSF very effectively. When the head receives a blow, then the brain moves. But, this motion of brain is gently checked by the CSF cushion and these connections between the brain and the arachnoid layer (blood vessels, nerve roots, and arachnoid trabeculae).

The leaking of CSF after lumbar puncture causes severe headache. This is because, after the removal of more CSF the floating effect of brain in CSF lost. So, it hangs more by the vessels and nerve roots and traction on them stimulates pain fibers.

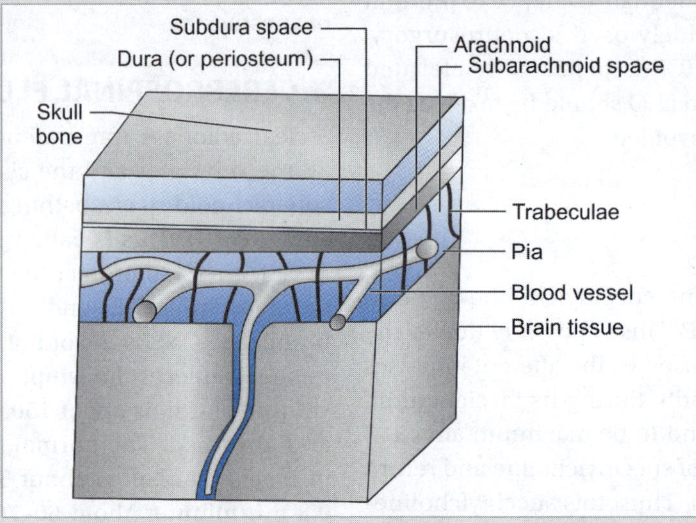

Different layer from skull bone to brain

ventricle. Now, the CSF enters the fourth ventricle of brain situated in medulla. After that, from the fourth ventricle, the CSF passes through three foramina to the cerebral subarachnoid space. These three foramina are (i) a central one, named the *foramen of Magendie* (also called median aperture) which ends directly into *cisterna magna* and (ii) two lateral ones, named the *foramen of Luschka* which end into *cisterna pontis* which is situated at the basal aspect of brain stem. From the fourth ventricle the CSF also passes into the central canal of spinal cord **(Fig. 4)**. The ciliary movement of ependymal cells, which lines the ventricles and spinal canal, helps in the circulation of CSF.

From the subarachnoid space, the CSF is absorbed through arachnoid villi which are projected into the veins (sinuses) of cranial cavity. These arachnoid villi are formed by the fusion of arachnoid membrane and the endothelium of venous sinuses. The projections of arachnoid villi act as valves and permit the bulk direct flow of CSF into the blood of venous sinuses. This bulk direct flow of CSF through these villi accounts for about 500 mL/day. In addition, a small amount of CSF is also being absorbed by direct diffusion into the cerebral blood vessels and at the nerve root sleeves by meningeal lymphatics. The large amount of CSF accumulates when the reabsorption capacity of these arachnoid villi is

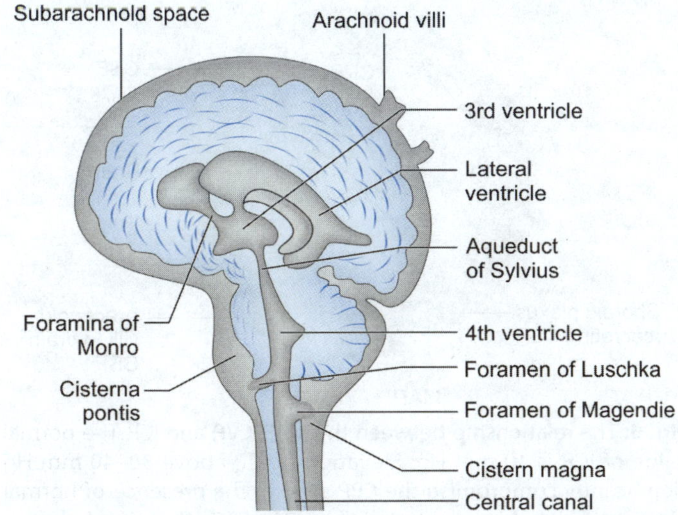

Fig. 4: The passage for the flow of cerebrospinal fluid (CSF).

<table>
<tr><td>

FACT FILE II

Blood-brain barrier

The cerebral vessels have a number of unique anatomical features. In the capillary wall of choroid plexus, there are gaps (65°A) between the *endothelial cells* which are like the capillaries of other tissues in our body. But, the *epithelial cells* of the choroid plexus of ventricle that separate the blood in capillaries from CSF are connected to one another by tight junctions. However, in the capillaries of other portion of brain, there are tight junction between the endothelial cells (the gap is only 8°A) and limit the passages of substances through this endothelial junction. As a result, large molecules such as protein and most ions are prevented from entering the brain's interstitial space. This unique limited exchange of substances into the brain tissue itself is referred to as the *blood-brain barrier*. But, some physiologist use this term only to refer to the barrier in the capillary wall of brain tissue and use the term blood CSF barrier to refer to the barrier in the choroid epithelium. However, the barrier is similar and it seems more appropriate to use the term "blood-brain barrier" to refer to both the barriers. There is little evidence that anesthetic agents alter the function of this BBB in most of the circumstances. But, it has been repeatedly demonstrated that the acute hypertension can breach this barrier.

Multiple transport system (active and carrier mediated) are present in the capillary endothelial cells. Water, CO_2, and O_2 can penetrate the brain easily. So, do the lipid soluble free forms of many substances including anesthetic drugs, whereas their protein bound form and all proteins do not. The easy penetration of CO_2 in contrast to slow penetration of H^+ and HCO^{-3} has definite physiologic significance in the regulation of respiration. Glucose is the major source of energy for nerve cells. Its passive transport through BBB is slow. But, its transport through the walls of brain capillaries by the glucose transporter GLUT1 is rapid. The brain contains two forms of GLUT1 such as GLUT1, 55K and GLUT1,45K. Both are encoded by the same gene. Infants with congenital deficiency of GLUT1 develop low CSF glucose concentration in the presence of normal plasma glucose. So, they have seizures and delayed development.

Another important transporter in the cerebral capillaries is Na^+-K^+-$2Cl^-$ transporter. It helps to keep the brain K^+ concentration low. In addition, there are specific transporter system for each several organic acids, thyroid hormone, choline, nucleic acids, etc.

</td></tr>
</table>

impaired. Then this is called the *external or communicating hydrocephalus*. On the other hand, when there is obstruction at the foramina of Luschka and Magendie or within the ventricular system, then there is also accumulation of CSF proximal to this block and ventricles are distended. Then, this is called the *internal or noncommunicating hydrocephalus*.

The components of CSF are essentially same as that of ECF of brain. Its formation involves the active secretion of Na^+ from choroid plexuses along with water and is isotonic with plasma, though the concentration of K^+, bicarbonate and glucose is low in CSF than plasma. In comparison to plasma, the protein content of CSF is very low and this protein is only due to the small leak of it in perivascular fluid, other than some pathological conditions, when the protein content in CSF becomes very highs. The normal CSF pressure which normally reflects the ICP varies between 110 and 130 mm H2O. The absorption of CSF which takes place largely in the cranial venous sinuses is proportional to this pressure and inversely proportional to the cerebral venous pressure which is again proportional to the central venous pressure (CVP). At a pressure (ICP) of 110 mm H$_2$O secretion and absorption of CSF are equal. But below a pressure of approximately 65 mm H2O, the absorption of CSF stops. The CSF pressure rises on standing, coughing, sneezing, crying, etc. Compressing of internal jugular vein also increases the CSF pressure by inhibiting its flow in the intracranial venous sinuses. It is known as the Queckenstedt's sign. Acetazolamide (carboxyanhydrase inhibitor), diuretics, corticosteroids, vasoconstrictor, etc., decrease the pressure of CSF by attenuating its secretion **(Fact file II)**.

The intracranial compliance is determined by measuring the changes of ICP in response to the changes in intracranial volume which depends on the volume of three components such as brain, blood, and CSF. Normally, a small increase in the volume of any one component is initially well compensated and ICP does not rise. Then, a point is reached after which a small further increase in the volume of any one component will produce a precipitous rise in ICP. The compensatory mechanisms which initially prevents in the rise of ICP are (i) an initial displacement of CSF from the cranial cavity to the spinal compartment, (ii) an increase in CSF absorption, (iii) a decrease in CSF production, and (iv) a decrease in total CBV (primarily venous) **(Fig. 5)**.

■ INTRACRANIAL PRESSURE

The nerve tissue of brain, the blood vessels supplying it, and the intracranial part of CSF are all situated in a rigid bony cranial cavity, named as the skull. In an adult cranial cavity,

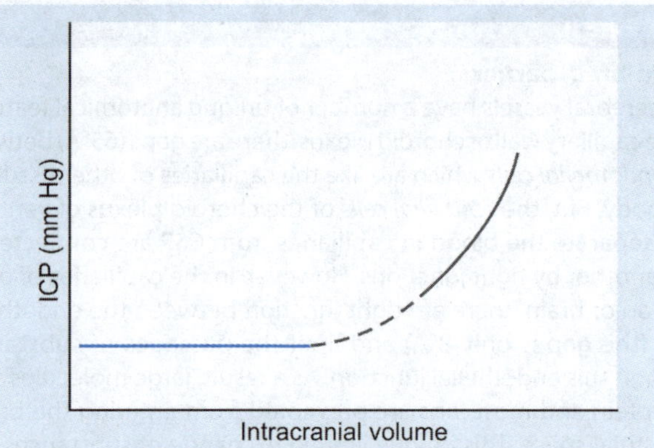

Fig. 5: Cerebral compliance curve. Dotted part of the curve signifies the onset of cerebral ischemia (focal ischemia). Then the continuous grey part of the curve signifies global ischemia. In the initial part of the curve (blue line) ICP increases slightly though bulk of brain tissue expands. This buffering is due to the reduction of other intracranial volumes, usually CSF. The rate of increase of ICP is determined by the rate of expansion of intracranial mass, the compliance of CSF space, and resistance to CSF absorption. (CSF: cerebrospinal fluid; ICP: intracranial pressure)

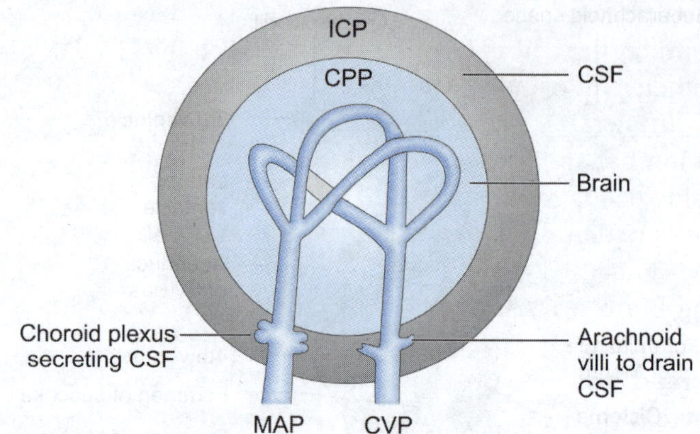

Fig. 6: The relationship between the MAP, CVP, and ICP. The normal value of ICP is 10 mm Hg. Elevation of ICP above 30–40 mm Hg significantly compromise the CPP even in the presence of normal MAP. The CPP below 50 mm Hg shows the EEG. When it is between 20 and 40 mm Hg, EEG becomes flat. CPP below 20 mm Hg cause irreversible brain damage. (CPP: cerebral perfusion pressure; CSF: cerebrospinal fluid; CVP: central venous pressure; EEG: electroencephalography; ICP: intracranial pressure; MAP: mean arterial pressure)

the brain usually weighs about 1,400 g, at any moment the volume of blood is 75 mL and the volume of intracranial part of CSF is 75 mL. They constitute about 80%, 12%, and 8% of the total volume of cranial cavity, respectively. Among these, the nerve tissue and the CSF component is incompressible and the blood component is compressible. It is postulated that at any time the total volume of nerve tissue, blood, and CSF in any cranial cavity will remain constant at a certain ICP. This is known as the *Monro-Kellie doctrine.* Therefore, any increase in the volume of any one component must be offset by an equivalent decrease in the volume of another component in cranial cavity *to keep the ICP constant* or to prevent the rise of it. Otherwise, the ICP will rise. As the blood is the only compressible component in a cranial cavity (CSF is partially compressible), so any increase or decrease of ICP, due to increase in the volume of nerve and CSF component, then the main burden will come on CBV and *vice versa,* i.e., any change in CBV promptly causes a similar change in ICP.

In a closed cranial cavity the ICP, MAP, and CVP interplay within themselves to determine the pressure which help to diffuse the different nutrient substances and gases from blood into nerve tissue. This diffusion pressure in the tissue of brain (nerves) is known as the CPP. Normally, this CPP varies between 80 and 100 mm Hg. This CPP is the difference between the MAP and ICP or CVP *which will be the greater.* Due to any condition when CVP exceeds ICP, then CPP will be the difference between MAP and CVP. Thus the CPP = MAP – ICP, or CPP = MAP – CVP. So, any elevation of ICP (due to increase in the volume of brain, blood, or CSF) will

tremendously reduce the CPP and will impair the cerebral function, due to the impairment of the diffusion of nutrients and O_2 into brain. Increase in CVP also will decrease CPP *by increasing ICP* **(Fig. 6)**.

Conventionally, the pressure measured in CSF from lateral ventricle (at supratentorial level) or over the cortex is considered as ICP. This was first introduced by Lundberg in 1960 and still remains as the gold standard technique for the measurement of ICP with which the other techniques are compared. In this technique of the measurement of ICP, a small catheter or a needle is introduced into the CSF of lateral ventricles and is connected to an external standard pressure transducer. This transducer always should be zeroed and calibrated and monitored with the currently available electronic display system. During the measurement of ICP, the zero reference point of the transducer is important, because CSF pressure is very position dependent. So, a standard practice is to calibrate the pressure transducer at the level of external auditory meatus and to correct the difference in height between the level of heart and the head when calculating CPP.

This method of measuring ICP is an invasive one and the complications of this technique are infection, hematoma formation, injury to nerve tissues during the passage of catheter through brain, etc. Sometimes a large mass, hematoma, severe brain swelling, etc. may distort the cavity of ventricle and make the introduction of catheter into it very difficult. So, the other less invasive techniques for the measurement of ICP was thought and these include the threading of a hollow bolt into the skull above a small supracortical dural opening, the placement of a subdural catheter, intracranially implanted transducer, etc.

In lateral recumbent position, the CSF pressure measured at lumbar spinal level very closely approximates with the value of supratentorial ICP. The intracranial compliance is measured by determining the changes in ICP in response to the changes in every unit of intracranial volume. Normally, the brain tissue outside the cranial cavity is very much compliant, but this complacency is lost when it is put in a rigid box, like the skull, for protection. So, the initial increase in the volume of brain is well compensated without increasing ICP. But, when this compensatory mechanism is lost or exhausted quickly (as there is no scope for much expansion of brain due to rigid bony skull) then further slight increase in the volume of brain tissue will cause precipitous increase in ICP **(Fig. 5)**.

There are four compensatory or buffering mechanisms which prevent the increase in ICP during the increase in intracranial volume of brain (nerve tissue). These are: (i) decrease in CSF production, (ii) increase in CSF absorption, (iii) displacement of CSF from cranial cavity into spinal compartment, and (iv) decrease in CBF and CBV. The major causes of increase in intracranial volume and increase in ICP are cerebral edema due to any trauma, intracranial hemorrhage (extradural, subdural, subarachnoid, and within the brain tissue), expansion of CSF or CBV, and growing intracranial mass. The location and the expansion rate of these lesions are the determining factors for the rate of rise of ICP and the rate and the degree of abovementioned compensatory buffering mechanism.

So, a lesion situated on the pathways of CSF flow causes a rise in ICP proximal to the block at an accelerated rate by blocking the flow of CSF. Obliteration of CSF pathway can also block the transmission of pressure along the craniospinal axis. So, in this situation the measurement of CSF pressure at the lumbar spinal level does not reflect the actual change in ICP.

Increased ICP causing ischemia and damage of nervous tissue is the end result of a number of different cerebral pathology. The normal value of ICP at supine position is 10–15 mm Hg. If there is sustained elevation of ICP over 20 mm Hg, then it is called intracranial hypertension. Although according to definition the elevation of ICP >20 mm Hg indicates a pathological states, but it does not always indicate that this high ICP impairs the function and viability of CNS. Because, the impairment of function and the viability of CNS depend directly on the type of pathological process, but not on the intensity of the rise of ICP. The increased ICP impairs the function and viability of nerve tissue indirectly by jeopardizing the CBF to nerve tissue. It is also often found that

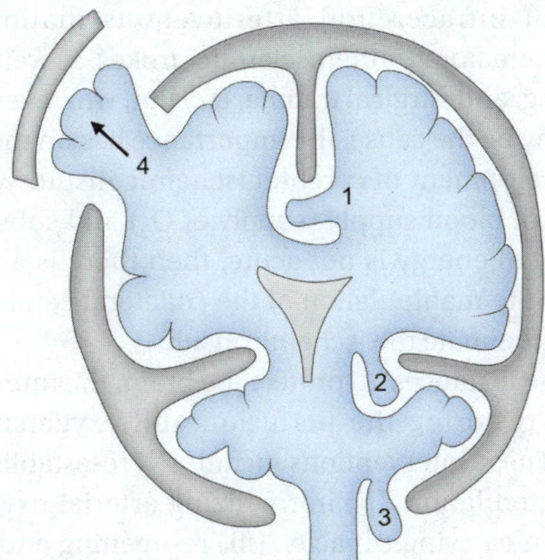

Fig. 7: Different herniation site of brain: (1) Under the falx cerebri, (2) Through the tentorium cerebelli, (3) Through the foramen magnum, and (4) Through the defect in skull.

during normal coughing, vomiting, straining, etc., the ICP goes well above 30 mm Hg without any cerebral dysfunction. With high sustained elevation of ICP, there is vascular compression, regional ischemia, and/or intracranial tissue shift which are called herniation of brain. This herniation of brain occurs through one of these four sites such as through any defect in the bony skull, under the falx cerebri, through foramen magnum, and through tentorium cerebelli **(Fig. 7)**.

METHODS OF REDUCTION OF ICP OR STRATEGIES FOR THE PROTECTION OF BRAIN

The strategies for the protection of brain are theoretically most effective, if it is started before the onset of ischemia of brain. But, practically this is always not possible, due to many socioeconomic reasons. There are different types of injury to brain such as trauma, hemorrhage, thrombosis, infarction, vascular spasm, intracranial mass, etc. But, the ultimate insult of all these injuries is the increase of ICP causing the reduction of CBF and the ischemia of brain which stops the function of it (brain). The ischemia involves a process when the supply of energy falls short below the demand of it. In the presence of ischemia, the intracellular environment deteriorates (by the increase in intracellular Ca^{2+} and decrease in intracellular pH), cell membrane damages, and the accumulation of free radicals occur that further aggravate the insult of ischemia. The ischemic brain injury is usually classified as the complete (global) and incomplete (focal) one. The best example of complete (global) ischemia is cardiac arrest and acute respiratory failure due to drowning, asphyxia, etc. The best examples of incomplete (focal) ischemia are local intracerebral thromboembolism, rupture of intracerebral arteriovenous malformation, subdural hematoma, atherosclerotic strokes, as well as blunt, penetrating, and surgical trauma, etc. But, whatever (focal or global) may be the cause, the importance lies on the rapidity of the development of cerebral ischemic insult. Where the occlusion of blood supply (supply of O_2) and subsequently the supply of energy is not acute, then there is a potential period for the manipulation of the collateral cerebral blood supply to attenuate the ischemic insult.

In some instances, to protect the brain, the interventions aimed at restoring the perfusion and oxygenation, are possible. These interventions include: (i) re-establishing the effective circulation, (ii) normalizing arterial oxygenation and oxygen carrying capacity, (iii) re-opening and stenting an occluded vessels. With focal ischemia, the brain tissue surrounding the severely damaged area (ischemic penumbra) may suffer marked functional impairment, but still remain viable. Such areas are thought to have very marginal perfusion (<15 mL/100 g/min). But, if further injury can be limited and a normal flow can be rapidly restored, then these areas may recover completely. When these interventions are not applicable or available, then emphasis must be on limiting the extent of brain injury.

Whether the ischemic insult is focal or global, the *goal for the protection of brain from ischemia are* (i) the optimization of CPP by reducing ICP, (ii) the reduction of cellular metabolic rate of brain tissue by different methods, and (iii) the reduction of the action of mediators which cause further cellular injury. *There are different methods which help to reduce the ICP.* These are: (i) cerebral dehydration by using osmotic and loop diuretics, (ii) the use of corticosteroids, (iii) hyperventilation, (iv) the reduction of cerebral venous pressure, (v) the drainage of CSF, (vi) surgical decompression, and (vii) the use of some drugs which increase the cerebral vascular resistance and reduce the CBF. For the protection of brain, the CMR can be reduced by hypothermia by anesthetic agents and by some other specific adjustments. To block the action of different mediators which may cause further cellular injury, the corticosteroid is the main stay of treatment.

Reduction of ICP

The aim of the reduction of ICP is to protect the brain and the methods which are applied to protect the brain, works by the reduction of ICP. So, the reduction of ICP and the protection of brain are the two facets of a single thing. The ICP is reduced by different agents or methods. These are described here.

Osmotic Diuretics

Among the osmotic diuretics, the most commonly used drug is 20% mannitol and is used in the dose of 0.25–1 g/kg (average 0.5 g/kg) of body weight. It is an inert osmotic agent and preferentially removes more water from brain than other tissues. This is because intact BBB impedes the diffusion of mannitol into the nerve tissue of brain, maintaining a strong osmotic diffusion gradient between the nerve tissue and the blood in vessel and withdrawing more water from nerve tissues. The decompression action of mannitol on ICP occurs within 10–15 minutes, after its administration, and is independent of its diuretic action. The renal excretion of mannitol and subsequently the osmotic diuresis produced by it occurs within 20 minutes after its administration. This also causes systemic dehydration which also helps to keep the ICP low.

Mannitol also reduces ICP by decreasing the formation of CSF. However, with larger doses and after repeated administration of mannitol, great abnormality in plasma osmolality and electrolyte balance and excessive intravascular volume depletion may occur. Other complications caused by mannitol are congestive heart failure and rebound increase in ICP. The congestive heart failure, caused by mannitol, is due to the transient initial intravascular hypervolemia (before onset of diuresis) produced by mannitol, as it draws the fluid from extracellular compartment to the intravascular compartment. In pathological conditions, when BBB is disrupted, then mannitol itself enters the nerve tissues of brain rapidly (mannitol penetrates the BBB very slowly under normal circumstances) and potentially can draw water back from the circulation into the brain tissue, causing cerebral edema and rebound increase in ICP, when the plasma concentration of mannitol declines. This rebound increase in ICP can be prevented by restricting the replacement of intravascular volume to about two-thirds of that lost during osmotic diuresis caused by mannitol. Mannitol sometimes also causes the transient increase in ICP. This is due to the hyperosmolarity induced dilatation of cerebral and extra cerebral vascular smooth muscles (**Fact file III**).

Mannitol is contraindicated prior to the surgical opening of cranium in patients suffering from ruptured cerebral aneurysm, rupture arteriovenous malformation, and sub- or extradural hematoma. Because, in such circumstances, the osmotic agents (such as the mannitol) entered the collected blood (hematoma) and encourage the further expansion of this hematoma (intra- or extracerebral) and the shrinkage of healthy brain tissue. In aged patients, this sudden shrinkage of brain may rupture the fragile veins, entering into the sagittal sinus from dura mater, causing further subdural hematoma. The prolonged use of mannitol combined with loop diuretics and fluid restriction may also cause the state of systemic hyperosmolality and electrolyte depletion. The upper limit of hyperosmolality of plasma is 320 mOsm/L, where beyond this level renal and neurological dysfunction may occur.

FACT FILE III

Cerebral edema

It is defined as the increase in water content of brain and is due to the loss of function of BBB. It occurs in three forms —(1) vasogenic, (2) nonvasogenic, and (3) interstitial. The vasogenic cerebral edema is most common. It refers to a type of cerebral edema where the BBB is disrupted (cf. cytotoxic cerebral edema where the BBB remains intact). This vasogenic edema is an extracellular edema and mainly affects the white matter via the leakage of fluid from capillaries. The causes of this vascular defect in BBB are trauma, acute hypertension, inflammation, and endothelial destructive (or vasoactive) substances such as histamine, bradykinin, free radicals, exciting factors, neurotransmitters, arachidonic acids, etc. releasing from tumor cells. In the pathogenesis of cerebral edema, once the plasma constituents cross the BBB, it draws more water from capillaries and produces more swelling. Corticosteroids and Ca^{2+} channel blocker are helpful to reduce this cerebral edema. Steroids act directly on the capillary endothelial cells by inhibiting the activity of phospholipase A2 which results in decrease in the concentration of lipoxygenase. Ca^{2+} channel blockers act by inhibiting the effect of Ca^{2+} which increase the permeability of capillary endothelium in hypertension.

In nonvasogenic cerebral edema, the integrity of BBB remains intact. The probable explanations of this type of nonvasogenic cerebral edema are (i) increase in the osmolality of brain than that of plasma and (ii) toxin. The most common representations of cerebral edema where brain osmolality increases than plasma osmolality and water is drawn within the brain parenchyma are water intoxication and rapid reduction of blood glucose level during the treatment of nonketosis hyperglycemic coma. The examples of nonvasogenic cerebral edema, where the toxins are the cause, are hepatic encephalopathy, hypoxia, cardiac arrest, different drugs and poisons, etc. The example of interstitial cerebral edema is obstructive hydrocephalus, where the over distended ventricles rupture and allow the CSF to enter into the parenchyma of brain.

The clinical manifestation of cerebral edema is due to the increased ICP. There are no pathognomonic signs and symptoms of increased ICP. The common signs and symptoms of cerebral edema (↑ICP) are nausea, vomiting, headache, papilledema, unilateral dilatation of pupil, paralysis of abducent, and oculomotor nerve, etc. In extreme cases, there is abnormal ventilatory pattern and loss of consciousness. In such situation, clinical examination does not always determine the severity of cerebral edema. So, it is assessed by measuring the ICP directly by measuring the CSF pressure.

The severity and the location of cerebral edema are also assessed by CT scan or magnetic resonance imaging (MRI). The management of cerebral edema depends on the pathophysiology of it and several approaches are taken simultaneously. This is because different antiedema measures act synergistically due to their different mechanism of action. For example, (i) to reduce the formation of vasogenic cerebral edema, steroid is used to decrease the permeability of BBB and (ii) to reduce the formation of nonvasogenic cerebral edema, BP is controlled to reduce the hydrostatic pressure which drives the fluid across the capillary wall into the tissue interstitial space. Another example is, to increase the reabsorption of edema fluid into the capillary, the osmotic pressure of blood is increased by mannitol.

Loop Diuretics

Among the loop diuretics, the commonly used agent to reduce ICP is furosemide. It reduces the ICP by three mechanisms: (i) diuresis mediated dehydration of brain, like all other tissues, (ii) the reduction of the formation of CSF, and (iii) the improved cellular water transport. Its action on brain tissue starts 30–45 minutes after its intravenous administration. It does not have the problems on CVS such as congestive failure which is inherent to osmotic diuretics. Hence, it is the agent of choice to reduce ICP in patient suffering from congestive heart failure. In extreme cases, the combination of osmotic and loop diuretics is indicated, but it is at the cost of severe intravascular volume and electrolyte depletion. So, the use of these combination is only restricted to patients, where there is no preexisting renal diseases and electrolyte disturbances.

Corticosteroids

These agents are more frequently used to reduce the ICP, which are mainly related to cerebral ischemia and cerebral edema. The probable mechanisms of action of steroids to reduce ICP are: brain dehydration, inhibition of lysosome, and phospholipase A2 activity, improvement of the action of BBB, etc. Some thought that the role of corticosteroids to improve the cerebral compliance is still not definitely established. But, the general dictum is that the steroids should be used, because if it does not do any good, it does not do any harm. The main drawback of steroids is that it takes hours to be effective in lowering ICP. The side effects during the use of steroids in neurosurgeries are: hyperglycemia, glycosuria, increased chance of infection, gastrointestinal (GI) bleeding, electrolyte imbalance, etc.

Hyperventilation

In previous discussion, it is already stated that the lowering of $PaCO_2$ has beneficial effect on cerebral insult. It provides this beneficial effect by increasing the cerebral vascular resistance by vasoconstriction and thus reducing CBF, CBV, and ICP. The reduction of $PaCO_2$ up to 25–30 mm Hg by hyperventilation has maximum beneficial effect on ICP with minimum risk of cerebral ischemia. However, this positive effect of hyperventilation acts till the responsiveness of CO_2 to vascular smooth muscle remains intact. When this reactivity is impaired (such as during anesthesia), then hypocapnia may be ineffective in reducing the elevated ICP. To control the increased ICP, hyperventilation should be initiated as early as possible. Hence, in conscious and cooperative patients with increased ICP, hyperventilation is instituted by asking him to take deep and quick repeated breath before induction of anesthesia during preoxygenation. But, if this is not possible, then hyperventilation is immediately started after induction and intubation. So, the intubation and hyperventilation is mandatory to reduce ICP in patients with score 7 or less in Glasgow Coma Scale.

Reduction of Cerebral Venous Pressure

When there is impairment of cerebral venous drainage, then the cerebral venous pressure is increased. This increased cerebral venous pressure is associated with increased CBV and increased ICP. So, always during neurosurgeries, attempts are made to reduce ICP by removing the factors which impede the venous drainage from brain. Hence, most neurosurgeons prefer to raise the position of head above the level of chest and avoid any flexion or rotation of neck that impede cerebral venous outflow and cause increased ICP and increased tissue bulk of brain. It is obvious that osmotic diuretics, loop diuretics, hyperventilation, etc. are ineffective in reducing ICP, if the cerebral venous drainage is not properly maintained. So, a simple change in head position, which impedes the cerebral venous drainage, can immediately achieve the desired goal.

Increase in central venous pressure also increases ICP by obstructing the cerebral venous drainage. This is observed in positive end-expiratory pressure (PEEP) or any other mode of ventilation, where there is potential to increase the intrathoracic pressure, causing increased central venous pressure. So, if PEEP is required to improve arterial oxygenation, then the rise in PaO_2 is against the proper cerebral venous drainage and its sequelae. Hence, these two opposite factors have to be balanced. Muscle relaxants can reduce this elevated ICP by decreasing the resistance to mechanical ventilation and intrathoracic pressure, which impedes the cerebral venous outflow.

Drugs Increasing Cerebral Vascular Resistance

Increase in cerebral vascular resistance, by vasoconstriction, acutely reduces ICP by reducing CBF and CBV. The pharmacological agents causing this effect are propofol, thiopentone, etomidate, lignocaine, etc. However, these drugs receive their best application during induction and maintenance of anesthesia, but not in nonanesthetized patient. Hyperventilation also reduces ICP by constricting the vessels. But the difference is that these pharmacological agents require coupling between the decrease in CMR caused by these agents and subsequent reduction of CBF, CBV, and ICP, which is not seen during the reduction of ICP by hyperventilation. Reduction of ICP by hyperventilation does not decrease CMR, but only constrict the blood vessel and reduce CBF. So, it is not beneficial to nerve cells.

Drainage of CSF

The drainage of CSF is a definite method and instantly controls the raised ICP by creating a sufficient operative space. This is performed by transdural ventricular CSF tap, prior to dural opening, especially when the brain is tight. This is applicable for large supratentorial masses and for decompressing the hydrocephalus, secondary to posterior fossa tumors. Excessive drainage of CSF through spinal route is also useful for surgery of pituitary lesion, intracerebral aneurysms, intracranial arteriovenous malformation, repair of skull defects, etc. This is performed by the introduction of a malleable needle, connected with a catheter, into the lumbar subarachnoid space following induction of anesthesia. The successful chronic control of high ICP, due to hydrocephalus, can also be obtained by implanting CSF shunts.

Reduction of Secretion of CSF

The reduction of the secretion of CSF is another method for reducing ICP. Approximately, about 50% CSF production can be inhibited by acetazolamide. But, this effect is transient and has only been used clinically during the acute elevation of ICP in chronic hydrocephalus.

Surgical Decompression

There are two types of surgical decompression—(1) internal and (2) external. The internal surgical decompression includes complete or partial removal of intracranial tissues or masses. Besides reducing ICP, the internal surgical decompression can also stop the shifting of brain tissue that is associated with herniation. External surgical decompression includes the removal of a portion of skull. But, in contrast to internal decompression, this external decompression may exaggerate the shifting of brain tissue, while still reduce the ICP. For this reason, the external surgical decompression is usually performed only as a last step in the sequence of treating persistent intracranial hypertension (↑ICP).

Protection of Brain

Hypothermia

Hypothermia is justifiably and firmly established as the principal cerebral protective measure in the face of any circulatory arrest. This protective effect of hypothermia is largely due to the reduction of CMR which enhances the cerebral tolerance to the episode of both focal and global ischemia. Indeed, severe hypothermia is often applied for up to 1–1.5 hours, in the face of total circulatory arrest with the little evidence of the impairment of neurological function. Hypothermia not only reduces CMR, but also subsequently reduces CBF, CBV, and CSF secretion rate along with the reduction of ICP. However, this reduction of ICP is more expeditiously accomplished by pharmacological agents and the use of hypothermia to reduce ICP is practiced rarely. The pharmacological agents reduce (60%) only that component of CMR which is only associated with the electrical activity of neural cells, measured by EEG, whereas the hypothermia causes the reduction of CMR which is responsible for both the electrical (60%) and basal cellular activity (40%). Therefore, hypothermia causes the continued decrease in metabolic requirement of nerve cells even after the complete electrical silence of it. A large number of studies have demonstrated that even a mild degree of hypothermia (33–35°C) can also offer substantial protection of brain, as evidenced by histologically. But, cardiac arrhythmias and a number of other complications, related to hypothermia, may occur if the temperature goes below 28°C. Whenever hypothermia technique is employed to protect the brain, then the use of muscle relaxant and other drugs, that centrally suppress shivering, may need mechanical ventilation (**Fact file IV**).

Anesthetic Agents

Previously, it is already stated that some anesthetic agents have protective effect on brain. Among these, the barbiturates, propofol, etomidate, and isoflurane are the most remarkable. With gradual increasing doses, they reduce CMR and produce electrical silence. Thus, they eliminate metabolic cost for electrical activity in brain cells. But, like hypothermia, they cannot eliminate the metabolic cost for basal cellular activity of the neuronal cells of brain. It is also true that like hypothermia these anesthetic agents are not protective against global ischemia. Furthermore, their protective effect on brain is not uniform. They are helpful only for focal ischemia. Other than reduction of CMR, the other mechanisms for the protection of brain, caused by these anesthetic agents, are: blockade of Na^+ channel, inhibition of free radical formation, and inhibition of Ca^{2+} influx, etc. They also protect the brain by reducing ICP by constricting the cerebral vessels and decreasing the CBF and CBV.

Specific Adjustments

Among the specific adjustments, which have protective value on brain from ischemic insult, the Ca^{2+} channel blockers are very important. Further, among the Ca^{2+} channel blockers, the nimodipine and nicardipine have been shown to have better neurological outcome (better protective effect on brain), if they are administered following stroke or SAH. But, unfortunately it is not used throughout the whole world uniformly, because still there is some controversy about its positive outcome and nonavailability of parenteral form of

FACT FILE IV

Pathophysiology of cerebral ischemia

The brain has very low energy (ATP) storage capacity, but has very high rate of utilization of it. So, it is very vulnerable to injury (or ischemia) in the face of the interruption of the supply of energy in the form of substrates, such as glucose and O_2. In the pathology of the ischemic injury of the brain, calcium (Ca^{2+}) plays a most vital role. All the cellular functions are controlled or mediated by the intracellular Ca^{2+} and its concentration is strictly maintained. Calcium enters the cell through the voltage-gated and neurotransmitter-gated calcium channel. It is also released from the intracellular storage site such as endoplasmic reticulum (ER) and mitochondria by the action of inositol triphosphate (IP) which is generated by the action of neurotransmitter and the receptor, present on the cell surface (membrane). This intracytoplasmic input of Ca^{2+} is balanced in a narrow range by the extrusion of it from the cytoplasm. This extrusion of Ca^{2+} from the cytoplasm is energy dependent and the processes are: resequestration in ER and mitochondria, extrusion from the cell and the inhibition of process that helps to release it from the intracellular storage site.

In ischemia, there is failure of supply of energy (ATP). So, all the energy dependent extrusion processes which help to bring out the Ca^{2+} from cytoplasm are stopped in the absence of ATP. On the other hand, cerebral ischemia causes the excessive release of neurotransmitter in the synaptic cleft which activates the influx of Ca^{2+} into the cell through receptor. Thus, in cerebral ischemia the concentration of intraneuronal Ca^{2+} increases tremendously and overactivate the various intracellular enzymatic processes such as lipases, proteases, nucleases, etc. Thus, the overactivation of this enzymatic processes causes the structural damage of cell and the release of free fatty acid such as the arachidonic acid from cell membrane. Then, this arachidonic acid forms the various prostaglandins and leukotrienes with the help of cyclo-oxygenase and lipoxygenase pathways respectively. Now, these prostaglandins and leukotrienes bring out all the effects such as vasodilatation, vasoconstriction, change in membrane permeability, chemotaxis, etc., all of which contribute to the evolution of ischemic insult of neuronal cell of brain tissue.

In the failure of the supply of O_2 (ischemia), lactic acid is formed by the process of anaerobic glycolysis and intracellular pH is decreased. This decrease in intracellular pH further deteriorates the intracellular environment and causes the injury of neuronal cells. The excessive presence of glucose into the cell stimulates the anaerobic glycolysis and aggravates the lactic acidosis and also increases the neuronal injury. So, the infusion of glucose solution is not advised in neurosurgery. Thus, lactate formation is an additional element of pathophysiology of cerebral ischemia.

these agents. Other agents that have protective effect on brain from ischemic insult are: dextromethorphan, magnesium, dexmedetomidine, etc. Methylprednisolone also has been shown to reduce neurological deficit following spinal cord injury.

Other Measures

There are also many other measures which protect the brain and reduce the neurological deficit following injury of it.

The hematocrit value should be maintained in-between 30 and 35% for the optimum delivery of O_2 to brain tissue. An elevated hematocrit value will reduce CBF, because of increased viscosity effect due to elevated hematocrit. The lowering of hematocrit value below this optimum level also does not prove effective. Arterial O_2 tension also should be maintained at normal level. The maintenance of high normal CPP is also very important. This is achieved by maintaining normal or slightly elevated MAP and avoiding the increase in CVP and ICP. Measures designed to improve CBF is also very important. This is because small increase in CBF has the potential to prolong the survival time of nerve cells.

Hyperglycemia aggravates the neurological injury following a complete or incomplete ischemia of brain. So, in the presence of cerebral ischemia, the withholding of the intravenous infusion of glucose-containing solution is a standard practice. The plasma glucose level should be maintained below 150–180 mg/dL. Still, it is in controversy that glucose elevation associated with brain injury may be the result of stress caused by cerebral insult (either traumatic or ischemic) or hyperglycemia itself. Hypercapnia and hypocapnia always should be avoided, because both have adverse effects on cerebral injury (ischemia). Hypercapnia has the potential to worsen the intracellular pH and causes intracerebral steal. On the other hand, hypocapnia has not generally been proved to be effective in laboratory and clinical setting in spite of the favorable inverse steal (Robin Hood) effect.

EFFECT OF ANESTHESIA ON ELECTROPHYSIOLOGICAL MONITORING DURING NEUROSURGICAL PROCEDURES

During the neurosurgical procedures, electrophysiological monitoring is frequently used to assess the functional integrity of CNS. Now, the most commonly used monitor for neurosurgical procedures is evoked potential. Electroencephalography (EEG) is less commonly used now. The proper interpretation of these monitoring critically depends on the knowledge regarding the effect of anesthesia and anesthetic agents on these monitorings.

Electroencephalography

It is a useful monitoring for assessing the adequacy of cerebral perfusion during carotid endarterectomy (CEA) and for assessing the depth of anesthesia. The EEG changes can simply be described as either activation (high frequency and low-voltage activity) or depression (low frequency and high-voltage activity). EEG activation is seen in light anesthesia and surgical stimulation, whereas EEG depression is seen in deep anesthesia and cerebral compromise. Most anesthetics

TABLE 2: EEG changes during anesthesia.

Activation	Depression
• Volatile anesthetic agents (<1 MAC)	• Volatile anesthetic agents (>1 MAC)
• Barbiturates (small doses)	• Barbiturates
• BZDs (small doses)	• Propofol
• N_2O	• Opioids
• Ketamine	• Hypothermia
• Sensory stimulation	• Marked hypoxia
• Early hypoxia	• Marked hypercapnia
• Mild hypercapnia	• Hypocapnia

(BZDs: benzodiazepines; MAC: minimum alveolar concentration)

produce activation at their subanesthetic doses followed by dose-dependent depression of EEG **(Table 2)**.

Evoked Potentials

The interpretation of evoked potential (EP) is more complicated than that of EEG. The EPs have the period of poststimulus latency and this latency is of three types: (1) short, (2) intermediate, and (3) long. In general, the EPs of short latency, which are raised from nerve stimulated or brain stem, are least affected by anesthetic agents, whereas the EPs of long and intermediate latency, which are raised from cortex, are affected by even subanesthetic levels of most agents. The visual evoked potentials are most affected by anesthetics, whereas the brainstem auditory evoked potentials are least affected.

The somatosensory EPs assess the integrity of the dorsal columns of spinal cord and sensory cortex. It is useful during the resection of tumors from spinal cord, instrumentation of carotid artery, and aortic surgery. On the other hand, motor EPs assess the anterior part (anterior columns) of spinal cord and are useful for assessing the adequacy of perfusion of spinal cord during aortic surgery. The brainstem auditory EPs assess the integrity of 8th cranial nerve and the auditory pathways above the pons and are used for the surgeries in posterior cranial fossa. The visual EPs are used to assess the integrity of optic nerve and occipital cortex during the resection of large pituitary tumors.

The intravenous anesthetic agents in their clinical doses generally have less marked effects on EPs than that of volatile agents. In high doses, they decrease amplitude and increase latency.

ELECTIVE NON-NEUROSURGICAL PROCEDURES AFTER A STROKE

After a stroke, *the loss of normal vasomotor responses to $PaCO_2$ and MAP (autoregulation)* in the early postinsult period is very common. In case of a small infarct, this temporary loss of vasomotor response usually persists for 2 weeks, though it may last beyond that period, depending on the location and the size of infarct. The CBF undergoes marked changes following a stroke and the area of both high and low blood flow in brain occurs. This is apparent for 2–4 weeks. Abnormality in the function of BBB is also found following a stroke which is evidenced by the accumulation of contrast agent in brain used for CT scan. This is also apparent for approximately 4 weeks in the postinsult period in case of small infarction.

However, the histological resolution is not complete for several months and years, following a stroke which depends on the size and the location of the insult. So, there is no definite statement (conclusion) as to how long the elective non-neurosurgical procedures should be deferred following a stroke. But, a general agreement is that in case of a small infarct a 6-week interval can give some assurances of likely recovery of CO_2 responsiveness, autoregulation MAP and integrity of BBB, though in large infarction this interval may extend up to 6 months. So, at the end, conclusion is that (i) it seems reasonable to defer any elective surgery for at least 6 weeks after a small infarction, or (ii) surgery is performed after 6 weeks from the point at which a stable neurosurgical state has been achieved in case of large infarct.

DIFFERENT POSITIONING OF PATIENT DURING NEUROSURGERY

Only for neurosurgeries, different peculiar positions of patients are required to facilitate the surgical procedures. Among these, the supine, prone, lateral, and sitting position with their many modifications to a specific procedure are commonly encountered. Certain neurosurgical procedures are long. Hence, some complications may occur only due to these prolonged abnormal position of patient and these (complications due to peculiar positioning) should be prevented by taking proper care, e.g., good padding of pressure point, avoiding hyperflexion or hyperextension of head, neck, and extremities, etc. During neurosurgical procedures, due to prolonged immobilization of patient in abnormal position, the incidence of thromboembolism is also very high which can be lowered by the intraoperative use of pneumatic venous compressive devices on legs and taking other measures.

Supine Position

This position is indicated for frontal, parietal, temporal, or sometimes occipital incision with the head rotated to one or other side. This rotation of head can impair cerebral venous drainage by obstructing the jugular venous system due to twisting. So, slight reverse Trendelenburg position (10–20°) with modest shoulder lift promotes better cerebral venous drainage. In supine position, the head is kept at midline without rotating to any side during trans-sphenoidal approach for pituitary and bifrontal craniotomy. For anterior approach to cervical spinal cord, this supine position is also used with moderate head traction. In all neurosurgeries, especially for frontal incision, the eyes should be closed and covered properly with thick pad to prevent the antiseptic solution, used for the preparation of skin, to come in contact with the eyes.

Lateral Position

This position is used for some special surgeries on spinal cord, and during some surgeries on lateral and posterior cranial fossa. It may be an alternative to supine or prone position and *vice versa*. The main disadvantage of this position is to maintain the stability of patient's trunk, exactly in this position for prolonged period, because the body is usually inclined automatically due to its weight toward front or backward. So, sometimes vacuum mattress is used which greatly helps to maintain the patient's body in this position.

Prone Position

This position is used especially for the surgeries on posterior cranial fossa and for the posterior approach of spinal cord. Before positioning to prone, the induction of anesthesia and the intubation of patient are done in supine position. Then, the patient is turned to prone position carefully with required additional personal. During this positioning from supine to prone, the major problem is the maintenance of basic cardiovascular monitoring. because all the monitoring systems require long cables from the patient's site of attachment to the display modulus which make complicate this rotation of patient (from supine to prone) through 180° arc. Frequently, they are detached from the patient end or be entangled with each other or give incorrect result due to the movement of patient with continuous buzzing of alarm which distracts the attention of anesthetist from patient in respect to tube position, ventilation, oxygenation, stability of CVS, etc. The positioning of an anesthetized patient also may cause circulatory instability. So, the total blackout of monitoring during this positioning of patient is also not desirable. Hence, if it occurs then only palpation of peripheral pulses by an anesthetist during the turning of patient from supine to prone can provide a continuous qualitative assessment of cardiovascular status. The electrocardiography (ECG) contact pads are positioned on the patient's back or side so that patient will not lie on them after positioning.

In prone position, if the endotracheal (ET) tube comes out of trachea, then it is very difficult to reintubate and sometimes it becomes impossible. So, hundred percent full proof fixation of ET tube after intubation in supine position is of paramount importance when neurosurgery is done on prone patient. This full proof fixation of tube is again complicated by the inability to use a circumferential tie around the neck which is the location of surgery. So, sometimes to avoid difficulties during the turning of patient from supine to prone, awake tracheal intubation in prone position is tried under combination of good local anesthesia of airway and judicious selection and titration of narcotics or sedatives. Currently, this technique is kept reserved only for severely obese patients which cannot be turned from supine to prone after anesthesia.

After turning the anesthetized patient from supine to prone position, the head should be kept on a horseshoe shaped rest or on a depression at the head end of the operating table or on a customized disposable head holder. There are many options of supporting the trunk of patient in prone position according to the need of planned operation. First, firm supports are applied under the chest and pelvis leaving the abdomen free. Second, for lumbar spine surgery, the surgeon needs support and fixation of lumbar spine which can be offered by Wilson frame. But, whatever may be the support, the compression on abdomen by faulty position should be avoided. Otherwise, the diaphragm will be pushed more toward the thoracic cavity and it will result in increased central venous pressure causing the impairment of cerebral venous drainage and engorged epidural veins. Ultimately, all these will complicate the neurosurgery.

A dreaded complication of prone position during neurosurgery is blindness. This is due to the retinal ischemia caused by prolonged compression on eyeball in prone position. This may be catalyzed by low arterial BP and impaired cerebral venous drainage which will reduce the retinal blood flow and will encourage retinal venous thrombosis. Other pressure points that have to be cared in prone position, like eyes, are the breasts, genitalia, knees, iliac crest, etc.

Sitting Position

The indications for sitting position in neurosurgery include the lesions in posterior cranial fossa (infratentorial lesions) and posterior cervical spine. However, its use is now diminishing gradually due to the potential serious complications caused by this position, and the presence of alternative position, permitting to perform the abovementioned neurosurgeries. The two major hazards which are confronted by patients in sitting position are: (i) the abnormal distribution of intravascular fluid volume, cardiac

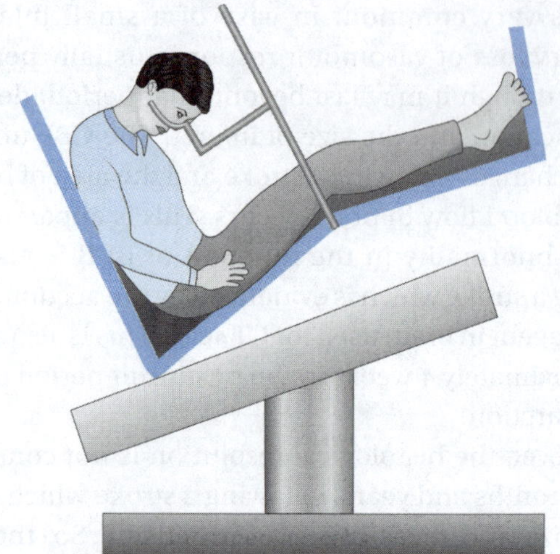

Fig. 8: Sitting position of a patient with the head rested on a holder.

filling pressure, and CPP, due to the influence of gravity, and (ii) the pulmonary and/or systemic air embolism due to the venous air entrainment, due to gravity. *Thus, the potential complications caused by sitting position are the venous air embolism (VAE), pneumoencephalus, circulatory instability, quadriplegia, etc.* But, the sitting position of patient has also *many advantages* which facilitate the neurosurgical procedures. These are: better access to midline lesion, low ICP, better venous drainage, better drainage of blood from surgical field by gravity facilitating surgery rather than collecting it at the operating site, better drainage of CSF by gravity, less blood loss requiring less blood transfusion, etc. Though, its use is gradually diminishing, but it is still used in some centers and some recently developed new neurosurgical procedures find its usefulness **(Fig. 8)**.

Actually, the term sitting position is a misnomer, because the properly done position is nothing but a modified recumbent position, where the legs are kept as high as possible promoting better systemic venous drainage (preload) and circulatory stability. Recently, many modifications are also done of sitting position which permits the lowering of head when necessary without taking the patient out of the head holder and not disturbing the continuation of surgery. This is important, because it is not always possible to alter the conventional sitting position in the middle of surgery without disturbing it, if VAE is suspected and this will allow precious moments to pass without appropriate treatment is instituted. In sitting position, some degree of head flexion is mandatory for better visualization of surgical site and easy access to the posterior cranial and spinal structures. But, the excessive flexion of head has also many disadvantages and should be avoided, maintaining at least a finger breath's distance between the patient's sternum and chin.

Venous Air Embolism

Venous air embolism occurs when a vein is opened to air and its intraluminal pressure (venous intraluminal pressure) is subatmospheric. Therefore, during neurosurgery, in sitting position, as the head is positioned above the level of the heart, so an open vein into air and negative intravenous pressure, relative to the atmospheric pressure, promotes the entry of air into the cerebral venous system causing VAE. The vertical distance between the head and the heart varies between 20 and 60 cm in different position (sitting or nonsitting) of patient during the different neurosurgical procedures. Hence, the VAE occurs in any position of head (sitting or nonsitting) during neurosurgery. But, its incidence is maximum during sitting position. The incidence of VAE varies as 25, 18, 15, and 10% in sitting, lateral, supine, and prone position, respectively. However, this incidence rate is calculated when the central venous catheter is used for air aspiration to diagnose VAE. But, when the Doppler, transesophageal echocardiography (TEE), and other more sensitive monitoring methods are used to diagnose VAE, then the incidence of VAE is increased enormously. For example, this incidence is increased to 50% when Doppler is used to diagnose VAE in suboccipital craniotomy. So, the use of more sensitive monitoring system, like Doppler, for early diagnosis of VAE also decreases the occurrence of clinically significant VAE (this is because diagnosis of VAE at subclinical level make the anesthetist prompt to take the steps which will prevent the progress of VAE from subclinical stage to a clinically significant stage), but increases the reported rate of incidence. Poor surgical technique also increases the incidence of VAE. So, the incidence and the danger of VAE can be reduced only with good monitoring, better surgical and anesthetic techniques, and early good communication between the surgeon and anesthetist.

Though VAE occurs at any time during craniotomy in any position, but the peak incidence and the peak occurrence time of it is during the sitting position and during the exposure of bony venous sinusoids at the time of dissection of bone and skin muscles. The maximum incidences of VAE occur, when the major dural sinuses are opened in sitting position. Once air embolism has occurred, the factors which influence the severity are: (i) the volume of air that enters the venous system, (ii) the rate of entry of air into venous sinuses, (iii) the pressure of the right side of heart, (iv) the presence or absence of right-to-left intracardiac shunt, e.g., patent foramen ovale or ventricular septal defect (VSD), (v) cardiac contractility, and (vi) the presence or absence of N_2O. The presence of right-to-left intracardiac shunt is important because it can facilitate the entry of air into arterial circulation from venous circulation. This is called the *paradoxical air embolism.*

The entry of large amount of air within a short period in venous system causes foaming of blood within the heart. This leads to mechanical obstruction to right ventricular outflow (obstruction to left ventricular outflow occurs if there is patent foramen ovale or VSD) and reflex pulmonary vasoconstriction resulting in increased pulmonary arterial pressure (PAP) and decreased venous return to the left side of the heart. Thus, the effective pumping action of the left side of the heart is interrupted (cardiac output falls) resulting in cardiovascular collapse.

The entry of small amount of air into venous system has little clinical significance and is well tolerated by most patients. It is absorbed at pulmonary level with little increase of PAP by reflex mechanism with the release of vasoactive substances which constrict the pulmonary arterial tone. However, the presence of any preexisting cardiac and pulmonary disease enhances the adverse effects of VAE and relatively small amount of air may produce marked hemodynamic changes. N_2O by diffusing into air bubbles and increasing their volume can markedly accentuate the effects of even small amounts of entrained air. The lethal volume of venous air in experimental animals, receiving N_2O anesthesia is reduced to one-third to one-half that of control animals, not receiving N_2O.

But, with the entry of more and more air into venous system and during the absorption of it at pulmonary level, the PAP gradually rises coming to a plateau or equilibrium when the entry of air and its maximum absorption capacity by lungs become equal. Crossing this equilibrium causes further increase in pulmonary arterial spasm, increase in PAP, increase in intrapulmonary shunt, decrease in left ventricular output, and ultimately cardiovascular collapse. The increase in intrapulmonary shunt leads to increase in dead space ventilation (areas with normal ventilation, but decreased perfusion), decline in $ETCO_2$ excretion, decrease in $ETCO_2$ tension, and decrease in arterial O_2 saturation. Thus, the measurement of $ETCO_2$ tension gives an opportunity to detect VAE. The diagnosis of VAE is confirmed by blood gas analysis which shows the increased difference in tension between $ETCO_2$ and arterial CO_2 tension, in the absence of any recent change in controlled ventilation. Hypoxemia is the late feature of VAE and is mainly secondary to great increase in intrapulmonary shunt. Paradoxical air embolism can result in a stroke or coronary occlusion, which may be apparent only postoperatively. It is more likely to occur in patients when the intracardiac right-to-left shunt is reversed due to high PAP.

The use of N_2O as an anesthetic gas increases the size of intravenous air bubble, because it (N_2O) is 34 times more soluble in blood than N_2 and rapidly diffuses in the air bubbles of venous system. Hence, it is suggested that avoidance of N_2O during neurosurgery enhances the safety, especially in sitting position or N_2O should be used only when the sensitive monitor to detect VAE is used and during any suspicion of VAE ventilation with 100% O_2 is immediately instituted, stopping N_2O. With the confirmed diagnosis of VAE, attempts are also made to aspirate air from the right side of the heart by central venous catheter which is already placed there for intraoperative monitoring of CVS. But, there is only limited evidence that this influences outcomes after the occurrence of VAE. The cardiovascular drugs are administered as required to support the circulation. To prevent further entry of air in the venous system, the elevation of central venous pressure by elevating airway pressure is not always suggested. This is because, it may further reduce the venous return to the heart and may aggravate the cardiovascular instability.

The rapid inflation of antigravity G-suit may provide transient cardiovascular support during this critical period by increasing the venous pressure and venous return. After that, still, if the stability of cardiovascular system is not attained quickly, then the patient is repositioned to supine and cardiopulmonary resuscitation is started as required. The further entry of air into venous system at surgical site can also be prevented by (i) lowering the head, (ii) increasing the cerebral venous pressure by applying compression on internal jugular vein (unilateral or bilateral), (iii) packing the wound with mop, and (iv) flushing the surgical site with sterile saline.

So, as soon as the VAE is suspected or diagnosed, then the surgeon should be quickly informed and he will immediately flood the operation site with saline **(Box 1)**. Neck compression is also given to occlude the neck veins. This will prevent further air embolism and will cause venous bleeding from the operative site which will allow the surgeon to detect and seal the point at which the air is entering. A central venous catheter should always be placed during neurosurgery in sitting position, because it will help to aspirate air easily, if the abovementioned simple methods fail to prevent large amount of air entering the venous system. It is found that the catheter placed in superior vena cava is more helpful to aspirate air than it is placed in the right atrium.

The most sensitive detectors to diagnose VAE should be available. Detecting even a small amount of venous air emboli is important, because it allows surgeon to control the entry site, before the additional air is entrained. Currently, the most sensitive method in detect the VAE is the TEE and precordial Doppler sonography technique where the probe is placed at right sternal edge, between the 3rd and 4th intercostal space. By Doppler method air bubbles as small as 0.25 mL can also be detected. The TEE has the

BOX 1: Protocol to treat VAE.

- Surgeon should be immediately informed, so that he can flood the surgical field with saline or pack it with wet gauzes and apply bone wax to the skull edges, until the air entry site is identified and occluded
- N_2O should be immediately stopped and the patient is ventilated only by 100% O_2
- If central venous catheter is present, then it should be aspirated in an attempt to retrieve the entrained air
- Vasopressor, antiarrhythmic drugs, etc. should be given to manage hypotension and cardiovascular instability
- Adequate fluid should be given to increase CVP
- Bilateral jugular venous compression may slow or stop air entrainment by increasing intracranial venous pressure. It causes back bleeding which may help the surgeon to identify the entry point of air
- Some anesthetists advocate PEEP to increase cerebral venous pressure and prevent the further entrainment of air
- If the previously listed measures are failed, then the patient is positioned head-down and the wound is closed quickly
- Persistent circulatory arrest necessitates to make the patient supine and to start resuscitation efforts using advanced life support algorithms

(CVP: central venous pressure; PEEP: positive end-expiratory pressure; VAE: venous air embolism)

added benefit of detecting the volume of air bubbles and any transarterial passage through a patent intracardiac shunt. The changes in $ETCO_2$ tension and $PaCO_2$ are less sensitive, but are important monitors that can detect VAE before overt clinical signs are precipitated. VAE causes a sudden decrease in $ETCO_2$ tension, but decrease of it can also be seen with hemodynamic changes unrelated to VAE, such as decreased cardiac output. A reappearance or increase in N_2 in expired gases may also be seen with VAE. The changes in BP and heart sounds ("mill wheel" murmur) are late manifestations of VAE.

However, the main disadvantages of Doppler in detecting VAE are that its signal is interrupted by the radiofrequency signal of diathermy. Hence, during the peak time of occurrence of VAE, i.e., during the muscle incision and bone work, the diathermy is also in full use for this muscle incision and bone work. So, it will interfere the work of Doppler which is necessary to work at the same time to detect VAE. But the good news is that the newer model of Doppler is now provided with some special filters which are able to reject the diathermy signal and are capable to work without interference.

Pneumoencephalus (Pneumocephalus)

It is another complication of neurosurgery, when after dural closure, air remains trapped inside the skull, then it acts as an intracranial mass lesion. Some degree of pneumoencephalus always occurs after neurosurgery in any position. But, it is found maximum in sitting position (3–4 times higher than prone and park bench position). During neurosurgery, in sitting position, after opening the dura, the CSF drains away from the intracranial space and air enters into the cranial cavity, like an inverted pop bottle. The air in pneumoencephalus, which causes the mass effect after the closer of craniotomy wound, may be asymptomatic or symptomatic (depending on the amount of air) producing headache, lethargy, confusion, impaired memory, etc. The huge amount of air in pneumoencephalus may also cause the shifting of brain tissue along the midline. In the absence of severe symptoms or extensive brain shifting, the patient with pneumoencephalus is usually managed conservatively, because the symptoms are commonly nonprogressive and resolve after few days in postoperative period. However, the breathing of 100% O_2 helps to absorb air and tries to resolve pneumoencephalus quickly.

Postoperatively, the air in pneumoencephalus can be detected both by CT scan and plain X-ray. In the postoperative period, if there is expansion of brain due to cerebral edema (caused by surgical trauma), then the air pocket will be pressurized and may exaggerate the mass effect. Sometimes, due to the development of tension pneumoencephalus, like the tension pneumothorax, high pressure may be built-up in the air cavity. The tension pneumoencephalus is suspected in patients who shows progressive deterioration of cerebral function or do not awaken following surgery.

N_2O anesthesia is not contraindicated and can safely be continued until neurosurgery is completed, provided there is no VAE. This is because, during surgery, with open dura, equilibration of N_2O with intracranial air occurs and does not increase ICP. Rather, when the dura is closed at the end of surgery, then the faster reabsorption of N_2O than air reduce the ICP or counter the rise of ICP caused by brain expansion (cerebral edema) postoperatively.

Cardiovascular Instability

Cardiovascular instability evidenced by hypotension is another complication of sitting position during neurosurgery. It may be mild (when reduction of BP varies between 20 and 30 mm Hg) or moderate (when reduction of BP is >50 mm Hg) and their incidences are 30% and 5%, respectively. So, the preoperative history, indicating coronary artery disease, heart failure, and cerebrovascular occlusive disease, etc. are contraindication for sitting position during neurosurgery. There are many measures which can prevent the incidences of this hypotension. These are: (i) slow changes in position from supine to sitting, titrated with the changes in BP, (ii) use of

vasopressor, (iii) optimum preoperative hydration, (iv) the wrapping of legs with elastic bandages to counteract the gravitational shifting of intravascular blood volume into lower extremities, and (v) use of antigravity compression device (G-suit). When the pins are applied from the head holder to make the head steady in sitting position, then the abrupt elevation of arterial BP occurs and this is due to the stimulus arising from the application of pin on head. The infiltration of the site of pin prick by local anesthetic agent or the addition of the bolus doses of IV anesthetic agent, just before application of pin, blunt this response of hypertension. However, some anesthetists apply the pins from head holder to keep the head steady, just prior to arrange the patient in sitting position and tries to counteract the hypertension, caused by pinprick by hypotension caused by immediate sitting posture.

■ MONITORING DURING NEUROANESTHESIA

Extensive monitoring during neuroanesthesia is very important for better outcome, because neurosurgery is frequently complicated by (i) rapid and large amount of blood loss, (ii) different positions of patient, required for surgery, has different special complications, (iii) surgeries, especially those in the posterior fossa, may involve cardiovascular instability, hypotension, etc. So, all the patients undergoing neurosurgery need: (i) a large bore intravenous cannula for rapid transfusion of crystalloid, colloid, or blood, (ii) arterial cannulation for beat-to-beat monitoring of arterial BP, (iii) central venous cannulation for the measurement of central venous pressure and diagnosis of VAE, and (iv) the placement of ventricular, intraparenchymal, and subdural placement of devices by neurosurgeon for the measurement of ICP from where CPP can be derived, etc.

For the correct measurement of CPP, the pressure transducer for the measurement of ICP *should be placed at the level of the base of the skull (external auditory meatus) and should be zeroed to the same reference level as the arterial pressure transducer.* In sitting position, the intra-arterial pressure transducer which measures the MAP should also be placed at the level of the base of the skull (at the level of external auditory meatus, instead of at the level of right atrium) to know accurately the arterial pressure by which the blood is forced into the brain and to facilitate the calculation of CPP. The importance of the accurate measurement of CPP is that as little as 5–10 mm Hg difference in pressure below the critical ischemic threshold value may cause the brain damage, if maintained for prolonged period.

The central venous catheter (i) provides the measurement of intravascular volume status, (ii) diagnoses air embolism, and (iii) evacuates the intravascular air bubble. The use of internal jugular vein for central venous catheterization is theoretically problematic, because a large bore catheter may interfere the venous drainage from brain resulting the elevation of ICP. Hence, the external jugular, subclavian, or other peripheral veins may be the suitable insertion sites for central venous catheterization. A bladder catheter is necessary, because of the use of diuretics, the long duration of most neurosurgical procedures, and the utility of bladder catheterization in guiding the fluid therapy and measuring the core body temperature.

In addition to the abovementioned monitorings, the measurement of SPO_2, core temperature (preferably nasopharyngeal or esophageal), and $ETCO_2$ tension are also mandatory during neurosurgery. The measurement of O_2 saturation is very important, because the patients undergoing neurosurgical procedures are more sensitive to the arterial hypoxemia and it causes brain swelling (edema) from hypoxemia-induced hyperemia. Moreover, many of the conditions, for which the neurosurgeries are shouted, are related to the focal cerebral ischemia to which the addition of slight degree of hypoxemia causes more danger.

As it is previously stated that the control of $PaCO_2$ is one of the factor of improving the quality of neuroanesthesia, so the measurement of $ETCO_2$ tension is of immense importance. It helps to set accurately the levels of ventilation and to monitor the occurrence of VAE. The $ETCO_2$ measurement alone cannot be relied upon for the precise regulation of mechanical ventilation. The arterial to $ETCO_2$ gradient must be determined. At the beginning of surgery, the difference between the $PETCO_2$ and $PaCO_2$ is measured from capnography and blood gas analysis and then it is repeated throughout the whole intraoperative procedures intermittently. Normally, this difference varies between 2 and 5 mm Hg.

The neuromuscular function should be monitored on the unaffected side of the patients with hemiparesis, because the *twitch response is often abnormally resistant on the affected side*. The monitoring of the response of visual evoked potential may be useful in preventing the optic nerve damage during the resection of large pituitary tumors.

The measurement of body core temperature is also important, because most of the neurosurgical procedures are prolonged, and these prolonged surgeries are associated with large fall in body temperature. This hypothermia causes postoperative shivering producing (i) hypoxemia, (ii) increased intrathoracic pressure, (iii) ventilatory impairment, etc. The measurement of oxygen saturation (SPO_2) from internal jugular vein also provides a useful guide to the occurrence of the global cerebral ischemia. The normal range of SPO_2 value in the blood of internal jugular

vein varies in-between 55% and 85%. However, the values above this range indicate hyperemia and the values below this range indicate hypoxemia that is the demand of O_2 is greater than the supply of it.

For the monitoring of VAE, the Doppler technique has already been described. *But, the TEE is 10 times more sensitive than Doppler technique in detecting the VAE.* This is because it provides the visual representation of air bubble in the right and the left side of the heart. It also can detect patent foramen ovale and VSD by detecting air in the left side of the heart. But, the *disadvantage of TEE* is lack of specificity. This is because it can detect fat and blood emboli and cannot differentiate them from air.

Attempts are also taken for the electrophysiological monitoring of brain, by the analysis of EEG and evoked potential, to assess the functional integrity of CNS. But, the proper application of these monitoring system depends on the specific area from where the signal is picked up or monitoring is done and the recognition of the anesthesia-induced changes of this area (depth- and dose-related changes and changes related to physiological variables such as BP, body temperature, and respiratory gas tension).

Electroencephalography is very helpful for assessing the adequacy of cerebral perfusion and the depth of anesthesia, especially during controlled hypotension in neurosurgery and in CEA. The changes in EEG are described as either depression or activation. The *EEG depression is manifested* by high-voltage and low-frequency curve and found in deep anesthesia or cerebral damage, whereas the *EEG activation is manifested* by low-voltage and high-frequency curve, and is found in light anesthesia or surgical stimulation. Most of the inhalational and intravenous anesthetic agents cause initial cerebral activation followed by dose-dependent depression of EEG. This is called the biphasic pattern of changes in EEG. With the further increase of doses, all these anesthetic agents produce *burst suppression* with or without changes in EEG to isoelectric level (electrical silence). With the high doses, the *desflurane and sevoflurane* produce burst suppression, but not the electrical silence, whereas the *isoflurane* causes isoelectric EEG. The *barbiturates and propofol* produce both burst suppression and isoelectric EEG at high doses, whereas *opioids* cause only monophasic dose-dependent EEG changes, i.e., depression. Ketamine only causes activation of EEG which consists of rhythmic high-amplitude theta activity. With the increase in dose of ketamine, this theta waves are replaced by high-amplitude gamma and low-amplitude beta waves.

Evoking the response of a nerve either motor or sensory after giving a stimulus is called the evoked potential. Analysis of this evoked potential for monitoring of nervous system is more complicated than EEG which does not need any stimulus to brain for its evoking (and recording) and is the difference between the two. All the evoked potentials have the latency period, which are classified as short, intermediate, and long. The evoked potential of *intermediate- and long-latency period* arises from the cortex, whereas the evoked potential of *short-latency period* arises from the brain stem, spinal cord, and spinal nerves. These short-latency evoked potentials are least affected by anesthetic agents, while the intermediate- and long-latency evoked potentials are affected even by the subanesthetic doses of inhalational and intravenous anesthetic agents. But, the *evoked potential with long-latency period cannot be measured during the intraoperative period.* So, the short- and intermediate-latency evoked potentials are only used during the intraoperative monitoring of neuroanesthesia.

There are *two types of evoked potentials—(1) sensory and (2) motor.* The sensory evoked potential is again of two types—(1) *somatosensory* (general sensation) and (2) *special* (auditory and visual). The motor evoked potential is best useful to assess the adequacy of function of spinal cord during aortic surgery, whereas the somatosensory evoked potential is best useful to assess the functional integrity of sensory cortex and dorsal spinal columns, carrying the sensory nerve fibers during the surgeries on spine and aorta. Among the visual and auditory, the visual evoked potential is easily affected by anesthetic agents, whereas the auditory evoked potential is the least and last to be affected. The visual evoked potential is usually used to monitor the upper brain stem and optic nerve during surgery on large pituitary tumors. The auditory evoked potential is used to monitor the 8th cranial nerve during the surgery in posterior cranial fossa.

All the anesthetic agents, intravenous and inhalational, depress (decrease in amplitude and increase in latency) both the motor and sensory evoked potential. But, the effect of volatile agents on evoked potential is greater than that of intravenous agents. However, among the intravenous anesthetic agents, the barbiturates do not depress the evoked potential even when the EEG becomes isoelectric. Opioids depress the evoked potential by increasing the period latency, but not decreasing the amplitude.

ANESTHETIC MANAGEMENT OF NEUROSURGERIES

Anesthesia for the neurosurgery or for the diagnosis of different neuropathological conditions may be required in operation theater (OT) or in the imaging room for CT scan, MRI, or X-ray. Usually, these patients are very sick. So, the proper assessment of these patients for the fitness of anesthesia is very important. In addition, many special risk factors arising from the neuropathological diseases for which the surgery or radiodiagnosis and anesthesia is shouted, must be evaluated as if the appropriate anesthetic procedure can be under taken. The most common neuropathological condition for which neuroanesthesia and neurosurgery are shouted is the intracranial mass, requiring craniotomy. It may be congenital or acquired. The acquired variety may be again noninfective or infective (cyst or abscess), neoplastic (benign or malignant and primary or secondary), vascular (aneurysm, hematoma, and arteriovenous malformation), etc. The primary neoplastic tumor may arise from the supporting tissues (meningioma, schwannoma, or choroidal papilloma), ependymal cells (ependymoma), glial cells (astrocytoma, oligodendroglioma, and glioblastoma), or pituitary gland (pituitary adenoma) of brain. Astrocytoma, medulloblastoma, and medulloblastoma are the most common primary brain tumor in children, whereas the most common acquired primary brain tumors in adult are meningioma, glioblastoma, pituitary adenoma, etc. The secondary metastatic brain tumor is also common in adult and their primary sites are lungs and colon. Astrocytoma is typically a benign slow growing tumor in any cerebral hemisphere and medulloblastoma most often arise from cerebellum.

The signs and symptoms of patients with intracranial mass or any SOL, presenting for neuroanesthesia and surgery, depends on the location and the growth rate of this mass or this SOL and the rate of increase of ICP. A benign slow growing tumor may be asymptomatic for long periods, whereas a rapidly growing tumor presents with lot of symptoms and signs within a short period, before anesthesia and surgery. Increased ICP is the most likely explanation for signs and symptoms, caused by a brain tumor. So, the *common symptoms of intracranial mass* are headache, nausea and vomiting, convulsions, focal neurological deficit, mental changes, disturbances of consciousness, etc. The *supratentorial lesions* usually relate to the cerebral hemisphere dysfunction and present as hemiplegia, convulsions, spatial disorientation, aphasia, dysphagia, etc., whereas the *infratentorial lesions* rapidly cause obstructive hydrocephalus and intracranial hypertension. Cerebellar dysfunction such as ataxia, nystagmus, dysarthria, and brainstem compression, manifested by cranial nerve palsies and abnormalities in respiratory pattern, localize the lesions at *posterior fossa* in infratentorial area.

Preoperative Assessment and Premedication

The preoperative evaluation of a patient with intracranial mass, presented for neurosurgery and anesthesia, is

TABLE 3: Glasgow coma scale.

Sign	Evaluation	Score
Eye opening	Spontaneous	4
	To speech	3
	To pain	2
	Nil	1
Verbal response	Oriented	5
	Confused conversion	4
	Only few inappropriate words	3
	Few sounds	2
	Nil	1
Motor response	Obey command	6
	Localize pain	5
	Withdrawal response	4
	Flexion response	3
	Extension response	2
	Nil	1

primarily directed toward the assessment of the presence or absence of increased ICP and the assessment of neurological status, using general and neurological examinations which consist of the documentation of the patient's present level of consciousness, any cranial nerve dysfunction, any other gross focal neurological deficit, the presence or absence of vomiting, mydriasis, papilledema, bradycardia, breathing disturbances, etc. **(Table 3)**. This examination (assessment) of patient should also be repeated in OT, just prior to the induction of anesthesia. This is because any changes in the patient's neurological status can occur overnight and/ or precipitated by premedication. When the spinal surgery is planned, then the preoperative neurological assessment should be focused on the function of the structures which is controlled by the segment of spinal cord that is involved in surgical procedure.

The neurosurgical patients are often dehydrated, hyperglycemic, and have the history of convulsions. Among the factors which contribute to this dehydration include: decreased fluid intake due to the reduced level of consciousness, use of diuretics (osmotic and loop) to reduce ICP, iatrogenic restriction of water input to reduce cerebral edema, neuroendocrine abnormalities, etc. Patients are often hyperglycemic because steroids are used in high doses to reduce ICP by decreasing brain edema. So, the history of preoperative medication should mainly be focused on the use of diuretics, corticosteroids, and the anticonvulsant medications. Laboratory investigations are also should be directed to rule out any electrolyte disturbances, caused by diuretics or hyperglycemia, induced by corticosteroid.

Radiological investigations such as CT scan, MRI, and X-ray, etc. must be reviewed to find out any shifting of brain tissue along the midline, the size of ventricle, and the presence or absence of cerebral edema. The supratentorial lesions are usually presented to an anesthetist with the problem, related to increased ICP, due to cerebral edema, whereas the infratentorial lesions are presented to an anesthetist with the problems related to (i) the different surgical positioning of patient (prone or sitting) during surgery, (ii) the proximity of surgical site to the vital brainstem structures, involved in circulatory and respiratory controls, and (iii) hydrocephalus.

Premedication before neurosurgery depends on the level of consciousness of patient. Usually, heavy sedation with or without narcotics is not appropriate in this group of patients. This is because respiratory depression causes increase in $PaCO_2$ which may produce cerebral vasodilatation and further increase in ICP. But, many patients who have no impairment in the level of consciousness are very apprehensive at the thought of having a neurosurgery and are associated with the increased level of plasma catecholamines. This causes undue hypertension which is obviously dangerous in respect to rupture of an unclipped aneurysm. So, for these groups of patients premedication with proper sedation is appropriate. This is provided by oral BZDs in titrating doses. Patients who are waiting for spinal surgery due to disk prolapse suffer from acute pain. In this group of patients, the use of strong analgesic (narcotic or non-narcotic) as premedicant is very valuable.

Induction and Intubation

Induction and intubation are an art in neuroanesthesia, because these patients are presented with the elevated ICP and compromised cerebral compliance. The aim of an anesthetist during induction and intubation in neuroanesthesia is to prevent the elevation of ICP at any cost by maintaining the arterial BP at normal level and controlling ventilation to maintain $PaCO_2$ between 30 and 35 mm Hg. Arterial hypertension during induction and intubation increases CBF, CBV, and ICP. Thus, it decreases the CPP and promotes cerebral ischemia and edema. However, excessive reduction of MAP also decreases CPP and impairs cerebral function. Some neurosurgical conditions, for which anesthesia and surgery are shouted such as SAH from ruptured aneurysm and head injury, etc., produce local cerebral ischemia by vasospasm. So, in such circumstances hypotension should be avoided to prevent further increase in ischemia. During induction, the position of patient should be such that the drainage of blood from cerebral veins should not be obstructed.

Before induction of anesthesia, all the measures (described before) are taken to reduce ICP, if it is already elevated. At all the stages of induction and intubation procedure, the hypoxia, hypercarbia, and vasodilation should also be avoided at any cost. For induction in neuroanesthesia, the most commonly used agents are thiopentone, propofol, and etomidate. Thiopentone and propofol are very useful for this purpose, because both these agents reduce CMR with resultant reduction in CBF and ICP, particularly when a SOL with increased ICP is present. Etomidate also reduces CMR, like thiopentone and propofol, but gives better cardiovascular stability. However, it is associated with greater rise in MAP during laryngoscopy and intubation than the other two inducing agents. All the cooperative and conscious patients are asked to hyperventilate for hypocapnia during preoxygenation before the induction of anesthesia. After induction, the patient is also hyperventilated manually by mask and bag and this can also easily be done with the help of neuromuscular blocking agent which will facilitate later in intubation and will prevent coughing, bucking, and straining, etc., all of which will abruptly increase ICP.

In neuroanesthesia, the intubation is usually performed by nondepolarizing muscle relaxant. Among these, vecuronium, cisatracurium, rocuronium, etc. provide the greater hemodynamic stability. Preoperative neurological impairment frequently leads to muscle wasting. When this degenerative process of muscle is of recent onset or is chronically progressive, then the use of succinylcholine for intubation is contraindicated. In such circumstances, the depolarizing agent causes the development of severe hyperkalemia and its related arrhythmia. Succinylcholine may also increase ICP during fasciculation. So, it is not generally used in neuroanesthesia. But, succinylcholine is the agent of choice in neuroanesthesia when there is probability of difficult intubation or risk of aspiration. Intubation should always be attempted, when the peak effect of muscle relaxant is reached and the muscular relaxation is complete and maximum. Otherwise coughing, bucking, straining, etc. resulting from premature attempts of intubation prior to the establishment of deep muscular relaxation, will cause increased ICP, due to marked pressure response and increased intrathoracic pressure which impedes the cerebral venous drainage. Laryngoscopy and intubation is associated with acute surge of sympathetic overactivity causing acute hypertension and increased ICP. This acute pressure response during laryngoscopy and intubation presents an obvious extra risk to neurosurgical patients with an arterial weakness such as in aneurysm or arteriovenous malformation for hemorrhage. There is also a great danger for patients with vascular tumor. This is because with the acute rise of BP during intubation, the bulk of the tumor also rises causing increase in ICP. Indeed, there is also likely to be an increase in ICP in patients in whom there is no vascular

tumor. This is because the rapidity of the pressure response due to intubation exceeds the ability of cerebral circulation to be autoregulated **(Fact file V)**.

FACT FILE V

There are many causes for the SAH and among these causes the subarachnoid rupture of intracranial aneurysm (75–80%), rupture of arteriovenous malformation (5%), idiopathic (15%), and the rupture of vascular tumors account for the majority. Following SAH the neurological status of a patient is classified by Hunt–Hess gradation. This is as follows:
- Grade I: Minimum headache, slight nuchal rigidity, or asymptomatic.
- Grade II: Moderate to severe headache and nuchal rigidity, cranial nerve palsy (often oculomotor).
- Grade III: Drowsiness, confusion, and focal neurological deficit.
- Grade IV: Stupor, hemiparesis, and early decerebrate rigidity.
- Grade V: Deep coma.

The rebleeding (principal cause of death) after the spontaneous stoppage of primary bleeding from ruptured aneurysm and cerebral vasospasm (principal cause of ischemia) are the two devastating early complications of SAH following the rupture of an aneurysm. So, for grades I to IV, the early clipping by surgical intervention within the 72 hours of the initial rupture of aneurysm is the management of choice. But, unfortunately this early treatment is technically more difficult due to the edema of tissue and there is less time to stabilize the patient with concomitant medical conditions. If the early intervention is not possible, then the surgery is often delayed till the risk of maximum vasospasm has decreased. A number of aneurysms are currently treated by endovascular coiling and these patients are very sick with greater number of medical comorbidities.

Cerebral vasospasm, following SAH due to ruptured aneurysm or other reasons, is the cause of delayed cerebral ischemia. It can present as neurological continuum form drowsiness to stroke. The etiology of this cerebral vasospasm following SAH is believed to be due to the presence of blood in subarachnoid space around the circle of Willis in the basal cisterns. So, the blood clot should be removed at the time of clipping of a ruptured aneurysm to decrease the incidences of this vasospasm. The signs and symptoms of vasospasm are usually seen in 40% of patients after 5–15 days following the rupture of an aneurysm. Angiography most early demonstrates vasospasm and surgery is delayed, if it is suspected.

The cerebral vasospasm following SAH is usually treated by hypertensive and hypervolemic hemodilution. This hypervolemia is achieved by intravenous infusion of crystalloid or colloid solution, maintaining CVP between 8 and 12 mm Hg and pulmonary capillary wedge pressure (PCWP) between 18 and 20 mm Hg. This hypervolemia will result in hemodilution with ideal hematocrit value between 27% and 30%. This reduces the viscosity of blood and improves the microcirculation of brain. After the clipping of aneurysm, vasopressor (dopamine) is used to induce hypertension maintaining MAP at 20–30 mm Hg above the baseline systolic pressure. This will also counteract cerebral vasospasm and improve circulation. Calcium channel blockers (nimodipine and nicardipine) have also been found to decrease the vasospasm, if they are started within 4 days of SAH. They are not affective, if the vasospasm is already established.

So, this pressure response, related to laryngoscopy and intubation, should be attenuated at any cost and is usually achieved by the use of any short-acting opioids such as fentanyl in the dose of 2–3 µg/kg or any of its congener just prior to induction and intubation. Other measures which attenuate this intubation-related pressure response are the use of β-blockers (esmolol 0.5–1 µg/kg) or lignocaine (0.5–1 mg/kg IV 90 seconds before intubation), or deepening the anesthesia with the additional dose of thiopentone or propofol. This intubation-related pressure response can also be attenuated by hyperventilation with low dose (<1 MAC) of isoflurane and sevoflurane. Due to the potentially deleterious effect on CBF and ICP, the vasodilators such as nitroprusside, calcium channel blockers, nitroglycerine, etc. should generally be avoided, till the dura is opened. The transient hypotension due to any cause during induction and intubation or during the course of anesthesia is generally treated by incremental doses of vasopressors (noradrenaline, phenylephrine, or ephedrine) rather than intravenous fluids.

Maintenance of Anesthesia

During the maintenance of neuroanesthesia, an anesthetist must concentrate his mind on some important factors which will help him to provide a good quality of anesthesia and avoid many complications. These are: (i) the maintenance of stable arterial BP (no hypertension and no hypotension), (ii) the avoidance of factors that lead to increased ICP (such as hypoxia, hypercarbia, vasodilatation, and cerebral venous obstruction), (iii) the maintenance of adequate CPP, (iv) the reduction of the total volume of brain (cerebral swelling), and (v) the avoidance of cerebral ischemia, etc. Now, to provide good quality neuroanesthesia by maintaining these abovementioned factors, a deep plane of anesthesia is required, sometimes with induced hypotension and hypothermia. But, on the other hand, after surgery rapid recovery of consciousness is essential, so that the level of response can properly be assessed to know the functional integrity of CNS. So, during neuroanesthesia it is essential to balance between these two factors such as the deep anesthesia, but quick recovery.

After opening the skull and dura (the most painful part of neurosurgery), the part of neurosurgery which is only confined within the brain matter itself is painless, unless the dura is stretched during the handling of brain tissue which is most likely to occur near the points of dural attachment. During neurosurgery, the only painful part is the initial craniotomy which includes the cutting of skin, the reflecting of galea aponeurotica, the drilling of bar holes and the stripping of dura or periosteum from the bones. The another painful part of neurosurgery is when the head is held by a head clamp in which pins (mounted in this frame of the clamp) are fixed into the outer table of the skull. This pain can be ameliorated by giving appropriate analgesic just before the pins are applied or infiltrating the skin by local anesthetic agent. Hence, in neurosurgery, even though the period of pain stimulus is fairly limited, still the neuromuscular blocking agents are used judiciously to maintain the deep plain of anesthesia. This is because: (i) it helps to prevent any slight intraoperative movements, coughing, bucking, and straining, etc. which increases the ICP; (ii) it helps to reduce the dose of anesthetic agents and quick recovery, (iii) it helps in proper ventilation and reduction of ICP, etc.

Neuroanesthesia is usually prolonged and lasts for several hours. It is frequently maintained by N_2O, opioids (fentanyl or any of its congener) and nondepolarizing muscle relaxant, without using volatile anesthetic agent. During the maintenance of neuroanesthesia, the airways, venous access, and monitoring lines, etc. should be well secured (fixed) in such a way that an anesthetist can completely rely on it up to the end of surgery, as the clinical monitoring is not possible intraoperatively, due to the inaccessibility of the upper portion of patient. Normally, during neuroanesthesia an armored ET tube is used to avoid its kinking, due to the different positions of patient. It is fixed in such a fashion that the fixation tape or rope does not produce any pressure on the vein of head and neck and will leave the cerebral venous drainage free. Many anesthetists like to support the ET tube by oropharyngeal pack, especially if the prone or sitting position is chosen. The placement of tube is also very critical, because if it is placed too close to the carina, then slight flexion of patient's head and neck to facilitate the surgery will cause the tube to be advanced into any of the main bronchus—right or left. On the other hand, if it is placed too close to the vocal cord, then slight extension of patient's head and neck will cause the tube to come out of the trachea **(Fact file VI)**.

The intraoperative part of neuroanesthesia is maintained by hyperventilation, keeping the $PaCO_2$ between 30 and 35 mm Hg, the cause of which is discussed before. But, the lowering of $PaCO_2$ below 25 mm Hg by more and more hyperventilation provides a little additional benefit. Rather, it causes some disadvantages by shifting the O_2-Hb dissociation curve to the left which offsets (prevents) the release of O_2 from Hb to tissues. Thus, it causes tissue hypoxia. Hypocapnia also causes cerebral vasoconstriction and cerebral ischemia. Wrong ventilating patterns such as PEEP or rapid and small tidal volume ventilation should be avoided. This is because, they cause high mean airway pressure which has adverse effect on ICP by increasing CVP. But, in severely hypoxic patients, due to lung pathology, PEEP is used to maintain the arterial oxygen tension at

FACT FILE VI

With the opening of skull by craniotomy, the ICP falls to the atmospheric pressure. But, if the factors which were responsible for the increased volume of brain, due to increased ICP, are still remain active, then it will be difficult for a surgeon to retract the swelled up brain into cranial cavity during surgery. Sometimes, the surgery becomes impossible or increased pressure on edematous brain by retractor cause neuronal damage. Moreover, if the swelling of brain is marked, then part of it protrudes through the dural incision and the tight edges of dura will impair the CBF causing cerebral infarction. It is also true that if there is moderate swelling of brain, then the closure of dura at the end of surgery will be difficult, causing pressure underneath the dura by swelled brain which also results in cerebral infarction or sometimes the closure of dura becomes impossible.

Therefore, it is very important to prevent the increase in the volume of brain. This is possible by avoiding the factors (faulty) which help to increase the volume of brain (swelling of brain) and by using drugs which will reduce the swelling of brain, after it occurs. The faulty factors which cause the swelling of brain are:
- Poor cerebral venous drainage:
  - Head-down position
  - *Jugular venous obstruction:*
    - Intrathoracic pressure
    - Neck rotation
    - Tapes around neck
    - Bad ventilator setup
  - PEEP
- Hypercapnia and hypoxia
- Inadequate muscle relaxation
- Arterial hypertension.

normal level, which causes the vasoconstriction and the reduction of CBF, to save the life.

All the volatile anesthetic agents cause the cerebral vasodilatation and increase the CBF in different proportions. Thus, they increase the volume of brain tissue and are not used in neuroanesthesia. But, the isoflurane, sevoflurane, and desflurane are used by some anesthetist in low doses, below the value of 1 MAC, and it is to control sometimes the intraoperative persistent hypertension. In such circumstances, it is thought that the gradual increase in hypertension may cause more danger than this small dose of volatile agents. However, some anesthetists have opinion that volatile anesthetic agents can be used successfully, if hyperventilation is maintained at the same time. This is because, the increase in CBF, caused by volatile anesthetic agents, is counteracted (by the reduction of CBF, caused) by hyperventilation. Volatile anesthetic agents affect the reactivity of cerebral vessels to the changes in PaCO2. This effect is greater with isoflurane than sevoflurane. So, the decrease in ICP by hyperventilation is more successful in isoflurane anesthesia than in sevoflurane and desflurane anesthesia.

Blood loss in neurosurgery is usually <500 mL. But, sometimes during the handling of some vascular tumors such as the meningioma, aneurysm, arteriovenous malformation, etc., rapid extensive blood loss may occur. Therefore, the ability of an anesthetist to replace the blood which is lost and to control the arterial pressure is important. In neurosurgical patients, hyperglycemia is a common occurrence and this is due to the stress and the use of corticosteroids in high doses to reduce ICP. Hyperglycemia causes increase in ischemic brain injury. So, the intraoperative intravenous fluid management should be restricted to only glucose free isotonic crystalloid (normal saline) or colloid solution. But, the large amount of crystalloid solutions is avoided in neurosurgical patients, because it may precipitate severe brain edema. So, the amount of intraoperative fluid replacement by crystalloid solution should be below the calculated required value. Colloid solutions are generally used to restore the intravascular volume deficit, whereas the isotonic crystalloid solutions are used as a maintenance fluid. Urethral catheterization is essential during neuroanesthesia, because it helps to know that diuresis has developed after the use of osmotic diuresis and it also helps in intravascular fluid management.

Extubation and Emergence from Anesthesia

At the end of surgery, after the dressing of head and bandages are applied, the decision should be taken, if the patient remains intubated or is extubated, on the basis of the intactness of neurological function. If the decision is taken that the patient remains intubated, then more sedation and/or muscle relaxant is added. But, if the extubation is decided, then it is a hard task to an anesthetist, because it should be very smooth and at any cost coughing, bucking, or any other type of straining which may precipitate an intracranial hemorrhage or worsen the cerebral edema by increasing ICP should be avoided. When the surgical team is moved away from the side of the patient by completing everything, then the anesthetic team takes this site and the patient with the OT table is turned back to their original position. Then, all the monitoring and the IV lines are checked, and the oropharyngeal pack is removed if it is placed. After that anesthetic gases are turned off and attempts are made to have the patient breathe spontaneously by reversing the neuromuscular block. When this reverse is judged as complete and the patient is able to take full breathe, then a gentle laryngoscopy should be carried out, and the pharynx is cleared quickly from the secretion. After that the patient is extubated smoothly.

Some anesthetists use lignocaine (1–1.5 mg/kg through IV) or small dose of thiopentone (20–40 mg) or small dose of propofol (20–30 mg) 90 seconds before suctioning, in an attempt to suppress the coughing and bucking reflexes during extubation. Some anesthetists use esmolol, verapamil (0.1 mg/kg), and/or remifentanil (1 µg/kg) to attenuate the cardiovascular responses during extubation. After extubation, rapid awakening and rapid return of cerebral function is desirable, because it will help to assess the central neurological function. However, delayed awakening may occur and is due to the overdose of opioid or prolonged use of volatile anesthetic agents.

Postoperative pain after neurosurgery is less severe than the other form of surgeries. So, analgesics should be given very carefully and the overdose of it may confuse the neurological assessment of patient. However, some patients experience severe postoperative pain, especially those who have undergone frontal craniotomy. In such patients, adequate analgesia is needed to avoid exaggerated sympathetic activity. In the postoperative period, after neurosurgery, most of the patients are sent to intensive care unit (ICU) for close intensive monitoring of neurological, cardiovascular, and respiratory function. When the surgery is finished and craniotomy is closed, then some air is frequently left into cranial cavity. This is seen in all the type of scans or X-rays which are taken on the first postoperative day. Among these, two-thirds collections are judged as moderate or large. This incidence comes down to 70% at the end of first week following surgery. At the end of second postoperative week, 10% collection of air is judged to be moderate and large.

SOME SPECIAL NEUROSURGICAL PROCEDURES

Anesthesia for Stereotactic Surgery

The stereotactic neurosurgery is usually performed to treat the involuntary movement disorders, epilepsy, intractable pain, etc. It is also used to diagnose and treat the brain tumors which are located deep very deep. The stereotactic neurosurgeries are usually performed under local anesthesia for continuous evolution of patient. With local anesthesia, dexmedetomidine, or propofol can be used for sedation and amnesia. But, during sedation, we will have to keep in our mind that there should be no increase in $PaCO_2$, due to hypoventilation, resulting increased ICP. Then, there should be provisions for controlled ventilation. There should also be provision for general anesthesia (GA) during emergency craniotomy, if needed. But, it will be complicated by the platform and localizing frame that is attached to the patient's head for the procedure. During emergency, mask ventilation or introduction of laryngeal mask airway (LMA) or orotracheal intubation might be readily accomplished. For a patient whose head is already fixed in a stereotactic

frame, awake intubation by a fiber-optic bronchoscope or videolaryngoscope may be the safest approach when intubation is necessary.

Recently, functional neurosurgeries are increasingly performed and these are the removal of lesions, adjacent to speech and other vital brain centers. Sometimes, these patients are managed by managed by sleep—awake—sleep technique, with or without insertion of LMA or ET intubation. The idea behind this technique is patient should be awake and participate during cortical mapping to locate the key speech center such as Broca's area. Patient will only sleep during the painful part of surgical procedures, i.e., during the opening and closure of skull. During the asleep part of surgical procedure, LMA is employed to manage the airway. Local anesthetic infiltration of scalp may facilitate awake craniotomy.

During the insertion of stimulator, deep into the brain to control movements and other disorders through a burr hole under radiological guidance, patient should not be sedated, because microelectrode recording (MER) is obtained to know the correct placement of stimulator deep into brain structure and the effect the stimulation of this stimulator is noted. Sedation will adversely affect the MER potential and will not make possible the placement of stimulator at correct depth. However, dexmedetomidine can be used for conscious sedation.

Cerebral Aneurysm

The cerebral vascular aneurysms are usually located at the bifurcations of major cerebral vessels at the base of the brain (circle of Willis) and the rupture of it is the most common cause of nontraumatic intracranial hemorrhage. The cerebral aneurysms are diagnosed both in ruptured or unruptured condition. In ruptured aneurysm, the bleeding may be manifested as subarachnoid, epidural, or intracranial hemorrhage, and among all the causes of SAH the rupture of cerebral aneurysm in subarachnoid space is the most common. The aneurysm is usually manifested as a single one and of different sizes. But, only 10–20% of patients have more than one aneurysm and those which are larger than 5–7 mm in diameter are considered for elective surgical obliteration, if it is diagnosed in unruptured state.

The mortality rate following the rupture of a cerebral aneurysm is very high. Of those that survive from the initial acute insult of hemorrhage after the rupture of an aneurysm, about 10% subsequently die within 1 week and about next half of the survivors die within next 3 months, after the onset of rupture. Further, among these survivors, half of the patients have major neurological deficits. Despite successful surgical clipping of a ruptured aneurysm, one-third of the patients do not get back the preruptured quality of life. The major causes of this high rate of morbidity and mortality following a SAH from ruptured aneurysm are: (i) rebleeding, (ii) ischemic cerebral injury, (iii) infarction due to cerebral vasospasm which is the characteristic of SAH, and (iv) development of hydrocephalus, etc.

The cerebral vasospasm, following the rupture of an aneurysm in subarachnoid space, is probably due to the breakdown products of oxyhemoglobin which causes the scavenging of nitric oxide from the wall of blood vessels and thus block the vasodilating effect of it. The development of hydrocephalus, due to the rupture of a cerebral aneurysm in subarachnoid space, is caused by the interference of absorption of CSF by RBC. The cerebral vasospasm occurs in 25–30% of patients and is the major cause of morbidity and mortality, following the rupture of a cerebral aneurysm in subarachnoid space. So, the Ca^{2+} channel antagonists (nimodipine) are used to prevent this cerebral vasospasm and to reduce the morbidity and mortality of patient suffering from SAH, following a ruptured aneurysm **(Fig. 9)**.

Usually, most of the patients, suffering from aneurysm of cerebral vessels, present after rupture. But, before rupture the prodromal signs and symptoms of an undiagnosed aneurysm are: headache, third cranial nerve palsy (most common), visual field defect, convulsion, trigeminal neuralgia, hypothalamic-pituitary dysfunction, etc. These are due to the local compression of nerve tissues by an expanding aneurysm. The unruptured aneurysm is usually diagnosed incidentally by CT angiography, MRI angiography, or simple angiography. The treatment of unruptured intracranial aneurysm is elective surgical clipping, following craniotomy or obliteration of it by interventional radiology. These patients are usually of good health and aged between 40 and 50 years.

On the other hand, the ruptured aneurysm presents with acute signs and symptoms which depend on the amount of blood in subarachnoid space. Minor bleeding in the subarachnoid space presents only with slight nuchal rigidity, headache, and other minor signs of meningeal irritation. The transient increase in ICP in this type of SAH reduces the pressure gradient across the ruptured aneurysm and subarachnoid space and promotes the tamponed effect on bleeding. So, the bleeding from aneurysm is stopped and partial to complete neurological functional recovery may occur spontaneously with this type of SAH. However, more severe bleeding in subarachnoid space may lead to tremendous increase in ICP, herniation of brain, unconsciousness, and rapid demise.

All these are due to the rapid development of severe intracranial hypertension, precipitous fall in CPP and cerebral ischemia. These acutely comatose patients are managed in ICU by proper maintenance of airway, ventilation, oxygenation, etc. In this life-threatening condition, medical intracranial decompression therapy is instituted immediately which is followed by craniotomy, evacuation of clot and then control of bleeding by the clipping of ruptured aneurysm. However, the lowering of ICP by medical decompression therapy may increase the chance of rebleeding from a ruptured aneurysm by withdrawing the tamponed effect. But, it should be kept in mind that this chance of rebleeding should be balanced against the risk of death, caused by the extremely high ICP and ischemia of brain, if ICP is not reduced. So, the general opinion is that ICP should always be reduced by medical intracranial decompression, before the craniotomy, aimed for the clipping of aneurysm **(Fact file VII)**.

The aim of neurosurgery on patients, who survive the immediate insult, resulting from the acute intracranial bleeding due to ruptured aneurysm, is to exsanguinate the hemorrhage from the rupture site and the prevention of cerebral vasospasm. It is evident that cerebral vasospasm occurs in about 70% of SAH, due to the rupture of aneurysm, and cerebral ischemia and/or infarction of brain tissue, due to this cerebral vasospasm is responsible for the delayed neurological deficit. If the patient is conscious and ICP is normal, then he is sedated until the anesthesia is induced. This sedation will help to prevent the rebleeding from ruptured aneurysm by lowering BP. But, if the patient is not conscious, then obviously there is no question of sedation. During the intraoperative management of aneurysm, every attempts should be made to prevent the bleeding or rebleeding (if it is sealed) from the unruptured or ruptured aneurysm. So, the arterial BP should be controlled accurately. This is accomplished by avoiding the precipitous increase in arterial BP during laryngoscopy and intubation.

The rebleeding from a ruptured aneurysm may also be prevented by maintaining a low intra-aneurysmal to intracranial pressure gradient, but not much lowering the ICP which acts as a tamponed. The intraoperative severe hypotension (except when induced hypotension is decided) also should be avoided which will aggravate the cerebral ischemia, already caused by cerebral vasospasm. The patients with SAH (from ruptured aneurysm and increased ICP) are more prone to hypovolemia and hypotension. So, the liberalization of intake of IV fluid reduces the cerebral ischemia and mortality due to vasospasm without altering the risk of rebleeding. Thus, the restoration of adequate blood volume preoperatively is important, not only for the intraoperative cardiovascular stability, but also for the improvement of neurological function, prior to the neuroanesthesia and surgery.

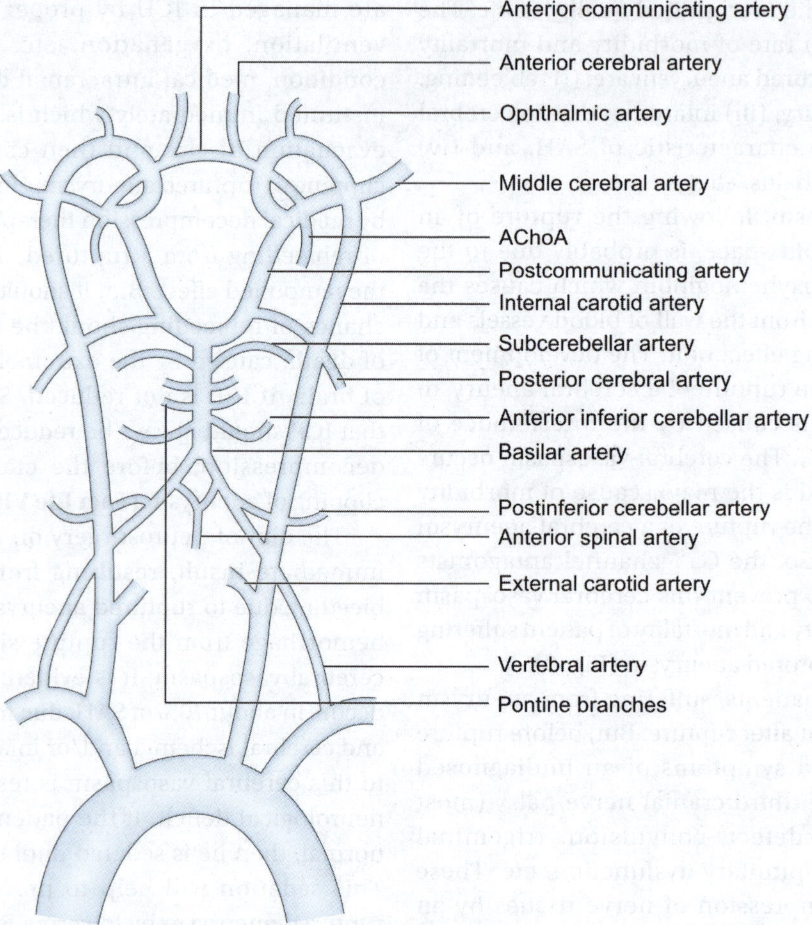

Fig. 9: Cerebral arteries.

FACT FILE VII

Arterial supply of brain

The principal arterial flow to the brain in human is by four arteries: two internal carotid arteries and two vertebral arteries. The two vertebral arteries join together at the lower border of pons to form the basilar artery. At the base of the brain, the branches of these four main arteries are interconnected forming an arterial circle named the *circle of Willis*. These interconnection between the branches of four main arteries helps to equalize the pressure in the arteries of two sides. The internal carotid artery, the basilar artery, and the vertebral artery give the following branches at the base of the brain.
- *Internal carotid artery:* Ophthalmic artery, anterior cerebral artery, middle cerebral artery, posterior communicating artery, and anterior choroidal artery.
- *Basilar artery:* Pontine artery, labyrinthine artery, anterior inferior cerebellar artery, superior cerebellar artery, and posterior cerebral artery.
- *Vertebral artery:* Meningeal artery, anterior spinal artery, posterior spinal artery, posterior inferior cerebellar artery, and medullary artery.

Substances injected into one carotid artery are distributed *almost exclusively* to the cerebral hemisphere on the same side. This is due to the equal pressure on both sides. Even when, the anastomotic channels are present in this circuit, do not permit a very large flow between the two sides. So, the obstruction in one carotid artery often causes ischemia on the same side. There are precapillary anastomoses between the cerebral arterioles. But, flow through these collateral channels is generally insufficient to maintain the circulation and to prevent the infarction when a cerebral artery is occluded.

During preoperative assessment, before neurosurgery and anesthesia, for the control of bleeding from ruptured aneurysm by clipping, in addition to the neurological finding, the evaluation of patient should also include the search for other coexisting diseases that may be contraindication for the institution of elective hypotension in the intraoperative period which will facilitate the surgery. The preoperative presence of severe hypertension, renal dysfunction, cardiac diseases, etc. may be contraindication to the induced hypotension. The SAH from ruptured aneurysm are also commonly associated with sympathetic overactivity with abnormalities in ECG and arrhythmia. So, these do not necessarily always reflect the underlying cardiac diseases and do not prevent the institution of induced hypotension.

The reduction of MAP in induced hypotension decreases the bleeding from ruptured aneurysm. Thus, it reduces the blood loss, improves the visualization of bleeding site from ruptured aneurysm, and facilitates the surgical clipping. Hence, the elective-induced hypotension, but not up to that level which will cause cerebral ischemia, is useful for aneurysmal surgery. But, it is not without danger, because it may cause ischemic damage to the brain and other organs. It has been suggested that the MAP should not be reduced >50 mm Hg from the preexisting MAP level. This is because chronic arterial hypertension shifts the hypotensive threshold level for autoregulation of CBF to the right. So, the maximum lower limit of this reduction of BP, to which a hypertensive patient can tolerate, without producing any cerebral ischemia, is adjusted upward. In addition to recognizing the lower limit of autoregulation, it is also important to understand that this autoregulation takes time. Thus, the slow and controlled induced hypotension is safer than the rapid induction of hypotension.

Sometimes, more profound-induced hypotension is required, than it is recommended, for the facilitation of aneurysmal surgery. In such situation, when more profound hypotension is used, then their duration should be restricted as less as possible to reduce the ischemic damage of brain tissue. Recently, the induced hypotension has fallen into disuse. This is because the patients with cerebral vasospasm, due to SAH, have disorder in autoregulation to CBF causing the reduction of CPP and ischemia of brain. So, induced hypotension in such patients further aggravates this ischemia. During surgery, the pressure exerted by the retractors further decreases the local CPP and aggravates the ischemia of brain. So, moderate hypotension combined with intermittent unilateral or bilateral manual carotid artery compression better facilitates the surgery by reducing the intracranial bleeding dramatically. Thus, it avoids the dangers of induced hypotension. Further, the combination of slightly head up position and use of isoflurane in low doses (<1 MAC) enhances the effects of any of the commonly used hypotensive agents and is better than induced hypotension.

Recently, due to some technical improvements and introduction of temporary vascular clips, it has enabled the surgeons to cut down blood flow temporarily to the surgical site during aneurysmal surgery without applying induced hypotension. On the contrary, the arterial BP of patient is kept at normal or at slightly higher level to protect cerebral perfusion during aneurysmal clipping. During prolonged vascular occlusion or excessive hypotension,

the administration of thiopentone and mild hypothermia may protect the brain from ischemia. Rarely, for surgery on aneurysm, arising from large basilar artery, total hypothermic circulatory arrest is used.

Carotid Endarterectomy

Carotid artery stenosis may be symptomatic or asymptomatic. Asymptomatic carotid stenosis, diagnosed accidentally by bruits during auscultation with stethoscope, is heard in 5–10% of general population. The complications of carotid artery stenosis are mainly transient ischemic attack (TIA) and stroke. The CEA is the surgical treatment of both symptomatic and asymptomatic carotid artery stenosis when its lumen's diameter is <70% of normal (1.5 cm). Asymptomatic patients (diagnosed by bruits) are also treated, because they have also the high incidence rate of TIA and stroke than the patient who are without bruits.

Stenosis in carotid artery also induces autoregulation in CBF. So, in an effort to autoregulate, the CBF beyond the obstruction, due to the drop of pressure and due to stenosis, the cerebral vasculatures dilate. As the degree of stenosis progresses, the cerebral vasculature dilates maximally to a point, beyond which they lose the ability of autoregulation. Then, with the further progress of stenosis, the CBF will become passive and arterial pressure dependent without autoregulation. So, it is important to maintain the intraoperative arterial BP in a patient, during CEA operation, because they have no autoregulation to counter the anesthesia-induced hypotension. The normal CBF inhuman is 50–60 mL/100 g of tissue/min (15% of cardiac output) and the requirement of O_2 for cerebral metabolism is 3–4 mL/100 g of tissue/min (20% of whole body O_2 consumption). The reduction of CBF at which level the cerebral ischemia occurs (that is evidenced by EEG) is termed as the "critical rCBF" and it is 18–20 mL/100 g of tissue/min. The surgery of CEA does not cause much fluid shift. So, the introduction of pulmonary artery catheter is not necessary, if not otherwise indicated for other causes such as the pulmonary hypertension, low ventricular function, etc. However, intra-arterial pressure monitoring is mandatory during CEA to maintain autoregulation-deprived and pressure-dependent CBF.

During CEA operation, the stump pressure which is measured immediately cephalad to the carotid cross-clamp does not always provide the reliable information regarding the status of cerebral perfusion, because it is found that the brain in some patients, with stump pressure <50–60 mm Hg, are adequately perfused, whereas the brain in some patients with adequate stump pressure have suffered from cerebral ischemia. So, in CEA, the intraoperative monitoring by evoked potential to judge the integrity of cerebral function, jugular venous, or transconjunctival O_2 saturation to know the hypoxia at nerve tissue level, trans-Doppler, echocardiography, etc. provides better method of monitoring of cerebral perfusion. Although, EEG is a highly selective and early indicator of global cortical ischemia, but it is not applicable in CEA operation. So, no data shows that monitoring by EEG during CEA operation result in better outcome.

The CEA can be performed under both regional and general anesthesia and these two procedures have both the advantages and disadvantages. But, the ultimate choice between the RA and GA depends on the patient's stability, surgeon and patient's preference, and the surgeon and anesthetist's experience. The main advantage of doing CEA under RA is the ability to evaluate the adequacy of cerebral perfusion by continuous neurological assessment in an awake cooperative patient. But, the disadvantage of RA is that if the patient develops cerebral ischemia, then he or she may lead to disorientation, inadequate ventilation, hypoxia, and disturbed surgical field. In such setting, immediate rescue induction, followed by ET intubation and institution of GA, which provides maximum cerebral protection, may prove difficult. The advantages of GA are good control of airway, a quiet undisturbed operation field, and ability to provide maximum cerebral protection if ischemia develops. But, the main disadvantages of GA are the loss of continuous neurological evaluation like of an awake patient (**Fact file VIII**).

ANESTHESIA FOR SPINE SURGERY

Indications

Spine surgery is mostly performed to relief compression on spinal cord or nerve roots secondary to (1) trauma, (2) degenerative changes, (3) intervertebral disk prolapse, and (4) osteophytic bone within spinal canal or intervertebral foramen in spondylosis, etc. Spondylosis more commonly affects the lower cervical spine than the lumbar spine and the prolapse of intervertebral disk more commonly affects at 4th and 5th lumbar or 5th and 6th cervical level. The other indications of spinal surgery are: (i) to correct deformities (scoliosis), (ii) to fuse spine if is disrupted by trauma, (iii) to resect tumor of neoplastic origin or vascular malformations, and (iv) to drain abscess or hematoma.

Preoperative Management

Other than general, the preoperative evaluation mainly focuses on (i) the restriction of neck movements due to the presence of collar or traction or other devices and

FACT FILE VIII

A. Modulation of arginine-NO-GMP system is the central to the changes in cerebral vascular tone caused by several processes. NO which is responsible for vasodilatation, caused by Na-nitroprusside, is the mediator of cerebral vasodilatation, caused by hypercapnia, ↑CMR, volatile agents, and neurogenic stimulation.

B. In normal subject, the initial increase in CBV does not result in significant elevation of ICP. This is because, there is general tendency for compensatory adjustment by other intracranial compartment such as the translocation of venous blood to extracranial vessels, the shifting of CSF from cranium to spinal space.

C. Hyperventilation has circulatory side effects, requiring consideration. The shallow rapid positive pressure ventilation actually increases mean airway pressure which impedes cerebral venous drainage and increase ICP. Similarly, PEEP elevates ICP and reduces mean arterial pressure (MAP), whereas the ventilation with long expiratory periods results in low mean airway pressure and ↓ICP, during hyperventilation. Hypocapnia (↓$PaCO_2$) has no effect on CSF secretion and absorption. Besides, reducing ICP, extreme alkalosis caused by hyperventilation impairs the dissociation of O_2 from Hb at tissue level by shifting the curve to left. Respiratory alkalosis also increases O_2 consumption and in the presence of pulmonary shunting this can reduce arterial oxygenation. Hypocapnia also reduces coronary blood flow. Hypocapnia also lowers inotropic sympathetic influence on heart and reduce arterial BP and CPP.

(ii) any other anatomical abnormalities of neck which may complicate the airway management. With these, any neurological deformities should also be documented. Patients with unstable cervical spine should be managed by either awake fiber-optic intubation or after induction by in-line stabilization.

Intraoperative Management

Spinal surgery is usually complicated by (i) potential large amount of blood loss, (ii) excessive distraction of cord can injure it or nerve roots, (iii) transthoracic approach of spine requires one lung ventilation, and (iv) anterior or posterior approach to spine may require the patient to be positioned in the middle of surgery.

Positioning

Most of the surgical procedures on spine are carried out in the prone position of patient. But, for the anterior approach of cervical spine, the patient is positioned supine and in this position of patient, anesthetic management is comparatively easier. However, it (anterior approach of cervical spine) carries increased risk for injury to trachea, esophagus, recurrent laryngeal nerve, carotid artery, jugular vein, and sympathetic chain, etc. Occasionally, other than prone and supine position, lateral and sitting positions are also used.

Following induction and intubation in supine position, patient is turned to prone, if the spine is approached from posterior. Then, the head may be turned to any one side or remains down on a cushioned holder. When the head remains down, then care must be taken to avoid corneal abrasions or retinal ischemia from pressure on globe. Care also must be taken to avoid pressure injuries on genitalia, breasts, chin, forehead, etc. Abdomen should hang free to facilitate ventilation and chest should rest on parallel rolls made of sponge or foam or gel, etc. (chest rolls). The arms should be tucked by the side of the patient in a comfortable position.

Turning the patient prone is a critical maneuver and the adverse effects are: (i) hypotension, (ii) abdominal compression, leading to impairment of venous return and engorged epidural veins, causing excessive intraoperative blood loss, (iii) airway and facial edema in head down position, and (iv) inadvertent extubation. If it is determined that spine will be approached from posterior in prone

position of patient, then after intubation in supine position, the ET tube should be fixed in 100% confidence, because reintubation in prone position is extremely difficult.

Monitoring

All the standard monitors should be attached such as oximeter, capnography, ECG, noninvasive blood pressure (NIBP), temperature, etc. If there is preexisting cardiac disease or major blood loss is anticipated, then intra-arterial pressure monitor should be considered, prior to positioning the patient prone. During spinal surgery, it requires the ability to detect spinal cord injury intraoperatively. It is achieved by continuous monitoring of somatosensory evoked potential and motor evoked potential. These monitoring techniques require substitution of propofol, opioid, or ketamine infusions for deep level of volatile anesthetics and avoidance of neuromuscular paralysis. Alternatively, to detect intraoperative spinal cord injury, wake-up technique may be employed, using N_2O, narcotic or TIVA which will allow the testing of motor function after awaking the patient in the middle of surgery. Once motor function is tested, patient's anesthesia is again deepened.

Blood Transfusion

HISTORY

The first historical attempt of blood transfusion was described by Stefano Infessura in 15th century (1492). The patient was Pope Innocent VIII who sank into coma. The blood of three boys was infused into the dying pope through mouth, as the concept of human blood circulation and the method for intravenous access did not exist at that time. In 17th century, Harvey's experiment on the circulation of blood had begun and the successful experiments on blood transfusion between the animals were done. However, the successive attempts in transfusion between humans continued to have fatal results.

The actual science of blood transfusion dates back to the first decades of 19th century with the discovery of blood groups (A, B, AB, and O). During that early period, some blood from donor was mixed with some blood of recipient before transfusion, as an early form of crossmatching. In 1818, Dr James Blundell, a British obstetrician had performed the first successful blood transfusion of human blood for the treatment of PPH.

Then, in 1901, Karl Landsteiner had discovered that the clumping of blood during the mixing of donor and recipient blood, before blood transfusion, is an immunological reaction and it occurs when the blood of recipient contains antibodies against the donor blood group antigen. Hence, the work of Karl Landsteiner had made it possible to determine (not discover) the blood group of donor and recipient which paved the way for safe blood transfusion. For that discovery, he was awarded the Nobel Prize in medicine in 1930. Next, in 1940, another breakthrough was done, when K Landsteiner, A Wiener, and P Levine had discovered the Rhesus blood group system.

Before 1910, the blood transfusion had to be made directly from donor to recipient before the blood coagulates. In 1910, it was discovered that by adding anticoagulant and refrigerating the blood, it was possible to store it for some days. Hence, it opens the idea of blood bank. The first nondirect (stored) blood transfusion was performed on March 27, 1914 by a Belgian doctor named Albert Hustin. He used Na citrate as coagulant. In 1943, JF Loutit and PL Mollison had introduced the acid citrate dextrose (ACD) solution which permitted the transfusion of greater volume of blood and allowed its long-term storage in freeze at 4°C. On January 1 of 1916, the first stored and cooled blood transfusion was performed.

Dr Oswald Hope Robertson, a medical researcher and US army officer, is credited for establishing the first blood bank, while serving in France during World War I. Though, it was the World War II that had provided the main impetus for the using stored and cooled blood from blood banks. In the post-World War era, many blood banks were set up across the USA and several other countries including the Britain.

In late 1930s and early 1940s, the research of Charles R Drew had led to the discovery that the blood could be separated into blood plasma and red blood cells (RBCs) and that plasma could be frozen separately. The blood stored in this way lasted longer and was less likely to become contaminated.

As early as 1943, it was observed that some patients had developed "post-transfusion hepatitis". The increasing use of blood also saw an increase in the incidences of hepatitis. But, little was known about its causative agent. Then, in 1970 the hepatitis B virus (HBV) and in 1980 the human immunodeficiency virus (HIV) were identified. In 1985, the first blood screening test to detect the probable presence of HIV was licensed and implemented by blood banks in the USA. The testing of donor blood for HIV-1 and HIV-2 antibodies was implemented in 1992. In 1996, the testing of donated blood for the HIV p24 antigen began.

On the 7th April of 1948, the World Health Organization (WHO) was established. Its objective is the attainment of the highest possible level of health by the all people of world. Its head quarter is situated at Geneva in Switzerland. WHO is involved in setting up an expert advisory panel on blood transfusion medicine developing a global database for blood safety, evaluating test kits for HIV, HBV, or hepatitis C virus (HCV) and purchasing reagents for blood transfusion services in bulk.

From 1950 to 1970, stem cell transplantation was tried at the Fred Hutchinson Cancer Research Center under the guidance of E Donnall Thomas. Later, his work was recognized and he got the Nobel Prize in Medicine. The work of Thomas had showed that the bone marrow cells infused intravenously could repopulate the bone marrow and can produce the new blood cells. The first physician to perform a successful human bone marrow transplant was Robert A Good at the University of Minnesota in 1968.

In 1979, a new anticoagulant preservative named CPDA-1 was prepared which can extend the shelf life of whole blood and RBCs to 35 days. In 1983, the newly introduced blood additive solution had resulted in extending the shelf life of RBC to 42 days. The "World Blood Donor Day" is an annual event and it is held in each year on 14th June. This day creates an awareness for the importance of voluntary blood donation and encourages the more people to become regular blood donors. It also celebrates and thanks all those who voluntarily donate their blood without any reward. In1942, the first blood bank was established in India at Calcutta. Next, during World War II, in-between 1943 and 1945, blood banks were established at Pune, Bombay, and Lucknow. In-between 1946 and 1950, in postwar period another 20 blood banks were established in premier medical institutions. In-between 1951 and 1970, 300 blood banks were established in medical colleges and large hospitals.

COMPOSITION OF BLOOD

An adult human has about 5–6 L of blood. It is roughly about 80% (80 mL/kg) of total body weight. The infants and children have comparatively lower volume of blood, proportionate to their body size. The composition of blood is highly complex consisting of liquid component plasma and solid component blood cells. This plasma component accounts for 55% and the cell component accounts for 45% of total blood volume. The plasma is the extracellular substance in which the cell components of blood [RBC, white blood cell (WBC), platelets, etc.] are suspended. The normal pH of blood is 7.40 (slightly alkaline) and specific gravity is 1,050–1,060.

The composition of blood is like that:

- *Blood cells (45%):*
  - RBCs
  - *WBCs:*
    - *Granulocytes:* Neutrophil (60–70% of total WBC), eosinophil (1–4% of total WBC), basophil (0–1% of total WBC)
    - *Agranulocytes:* Lymphocyte and monocyte
  - Platelets (1.5–4 lacs per mm^3)
- *Plasma (55%):*
  - Water (92%)
  - *Solid (8%):*
    - *Inorganic:*
      - *Anion:* Cl^-, HCO_3^-, PO_4^{3-}, and SO_4^{2-}
      - *Cation:* Na^+, K^+, Ca^{2+}, and Mg^{2+}
    - Organic:
    - Colloids:
      - Plasma proteins (albumin 4.5–5.5 g%, globulin 1.5–2.5 g%, fibrinogen 0.2–0.4 g%, prothrombin 0.1 g%).
      - Plasma lipids (chylomicron, very low-density lipoprotein (VLDL), low-density lipoprotein (LDL), high-density lipoprotein (HDL), free fatty acid (FFA), etc.)
    - *Crystalloids:* Glucose, urea, uric acid, etc.
- *Miscellaneous:* Hormones, enzymes, coagulating factors (except fibrinogen), and many other chemicals

If a sample of blood is allowed to coagulate, then a straw-colored fluid is separated which is called the serum. Therefore, Serum = Plasma – Fibrinogen and other clotting factors.

PREPARATION OF BLOOD COMPONENTS FOR TRANSFUSION

Blood may be transfused as whole (blood) or as one of its components. The transfusion of a single component of blood means the transfusion of only that portion of blood which is needed by the patient for a specific condition or disease, rather than the whole blood. The single blood components which are used for transfusion are packed RBCs, white cells (granulocyte concentrate), platelet-rich plasma, platelet concentrate, cryoprecipitate, cryosupernatant, albumin, immunoglobulin, coagulation factors (factor VIII concentrate, factor IX concentrate, and Rh immunoglobulin), etc.

The transformation of whole blood or its components is usually supportive means for hemostasis or for the deficiencies of certain component or factor. The blood components are obtained from blood by apheresis (a technique by which a particular substance or component is removed from the blood) or recombinant technique. If the blood is treated to prevent its clotting and is permitted to stand in a container, then the RBCs which weigh more than the other components of blood will settle to the bottom of the container and the plasma will remain at the top and the WBCs with platelets will remain suspended between the plasma and RBCs. Now, the platelet-rich plasma is removed and placed into a sterile container which can be used to prepare the platelet preparation, plasma protein preparations such as albumin, immunoglobulin [intravenous immuno-globulin (IVIG)], and clotting factors. The components, particularly the clotting factors and platelets deteriorate within hours of donation. It is necessary to separate, process, and store the components of blood within the 6–12 hours of donation.

PREPARATIONS FROM BLOOD CELLS

Preparation of RBC Components

Packed red blood cells: It is the most recognizable and most commonly transfused components of whole blood. The average volume of a unit of packed red blood cell (PRBC) is approximately 250 mL. A unit of PRBC is collected in an anticoagulant preservative solution such as CPDA-1, Adsol, Nutricel, Optisol, etc. The shelf life of RBC in these solutions is 35 days at 4°C. The RBCs can be stored at 4°C for 42 days with dextrose and adenine-saline solutions (AS-1, AS-3, and AS-5) or SAGM solution (saline, adenine, glucose, and mannitol solution). The RBCs are capable of (i) transmitting cytomegalovirus (CMV), (ii) mediating graft versus host reaction, and (iii) causing febrile, nonhemolytic reaction. Hence, for the recipient patients who at particular risk from these complications, the use of CMV-reduced preparation of RBCs, gamma-irradiated preparation of RBCs, and leukoreduced preparation of RBCs should be considered.

Deglycerolized red blood cells: During this preparation of RBCs, the PRBCs are progressively washed in a bath of propylene glycol. Then, this product is freezed. This technique is used for the long-term storage of some rare units of RBC. The glycerol is used to protect the cells during freezing. This preparation of deglycerolized RBC is stored at 1–4°C for only 24 hours and at – 65°C for 10 years. Before use, this preparation is first thawed and washed to remove the glycerol.

Washed RBCs: This preparation of RBC is produced by washing the RBC by 1–2 L of saline manually or by an automated cell washer. This RBC preparation has a hematocrit value of 70–80% and is depleted of 99% plasma proteins and 85% of WBC. The washing of RBC also removes cytokines that cause febrile illness. The sole indication for washed RBCs in adults is to prevent the recurrent or severe allergic reactions when the specific allergen is not identified. This product is indicated in patients with clinically significant antibodies to IgA, when the blood from IgA deficient donor is not available.

Leukocyte-reduced red blood cells: The cellular blood components that contain less than a known and accepted range of leukocytes are considered as the leukocyte-reduced blood components. The leukocyte-reduced red blood cells (LR-RBCs) are defined as the cells containing $<5 \times 10^6$ leukocytes per unit. The reduction of leukocytes of transfused RBCs has been suggested as the way to reduce the toxicity of RBC transfusion. The leukocyte reduction filters remove >99.9% of the leukocytes. The LR-RBCs are effective in the prevention of the transmission of CMV or alloimmunization and in patients with a history of multiple febrile nonhemolytic transfusion reactions (FNHTRs).

Irradiated RBCs: The irradiation is used to reduce the risk of transmission of HBV, HIV, CMV, graft-versus-host reaction (GVHR), etc. Only the cellular components of blood are irradiated. The fresh frozen plasma (FFP), cryoprecipitate, and purified clotting factors do not need to be irradiated to prevent the transmission. The irradiated RBCs are indicated in bone marrow transplant recipients, congenital cellular immunodeficiency syndrome, intrauterine transfusion, premature newborn, neonatal exchange transfusion, granulocyte transfusion, Hodgkin's and non-Hodgkin's lymphoma, etc.

Preparation of Granulocyte (Neutrophil) Component

The granulocytes (neutrophil, eosinophil, and basophil) make up a very small part of blood volume, normally only about 1%. Neutropenia is present, whenever the total WBC count is <1000/μL. The life span of neutrophil is 18–36 hours. The granulocytes are collected by leukopheresis from an ABO and Rh compatible donor. Since, there are a large number of red cells in granulocyte concentrate preparation, so the compatibility testing must be performed between the donor and recipient sample. The preparation of granulocyte concentrate should always be irradiated to prevent the GVHR. The granulocytes have a very short shelf life. So, they should be transfused within 12 hours of its collection. If this is not possible, the storage should be done at room temperature for no longer than 24 hours. After the initiation of granulocyte therapy, it is generally continued once daily, until the infection clears or the neutrophil count begins to recover.

The indications for granulocyte transfusion are (i) absolute neutrophil count $<0.2 \times 10/L$ (200/μL), (ii) neonates with bacterial sepsis, and (iii) abnormal neutrophil function.

Preparation of Platelet Component

The normal platelet count in blood is 250,000/mm^3. Platelet count <50,000/mm^3 suggests thrombocytopenia which is the cause of bleeding. The dramatic reduction of the count of platelet in blood which is <20,000/mm^3 may be associated with the high risk of bleeding and death. The platelets are also labeled with ABO and Rh group like the RBC. Because, the ABO compatible platelets are preferred, but the crossmatching is not needed, as the concentrate platelet preparation contains only small amount of red cells. The risk of viral transmission is the same, as that for any unit of blood transfusion.

Platelets are normally supplied in a single 50 mL bag containing an adult dose of platelets (>240 × 10^9/L). Each platelet concentrate also provides fresh plasma, some WBCs, and few RBCs. Platelets are stored at room temperature of 20°C (not in a fridge) for 5 days. The life span of platelets is 5–7 days. The viability of platelets is lost when they are stored at 4°C for longer than 24 hours. The platelets should be infused within 30 minutes and the duration of this infusion should not exceed than 4 hours. The platelets are transfused in volumes of 0.1 unit/kg or 10 mL/kg. The infusion of one unit of platelets produces a rise of platelet count, ranging from 5,000 to 10,000. The measurement of platelet count should be performed 3 hours after transfusion. The six units of platelets are required to ensure an adequate hemostasis. Always use a fresh transfusion set for platelets. Do not transfuse platelets through a standard filter directly after the transfusion of red cells because the platelets will get caught up in fibrin strands or debris, etc.

The indications for platelet transfusion are (i) Idiopathic thrombocytopenic purpura (ITP)—avoid platelet transfusion in thrombotic thrombocytopenic purpura (TTP) where platelet transfusion may actually worsen the thrombosis. (ii) Reduced platelet production by the bone marrow in aplastic or hypoplastic anemia or myelodysplastic anemia. (iii) In leukemia, lymphoma, carcinoma, sarcoma, patients under chemotherapy, and whose platelet count is <20,000/μL. (iv) A patient who receives 10–15 units of whole blood or packed red cells requires platelet transfusion. (v) Patients who are scheduled for invasive procedures such as biopsy, thoracocentesis, lumbar puncture, epidural anesthesia, etc. but their platelet count is <50,000/μL. (vi) Patients suffering from major blood loss, particularly during cardiac surgery with prolonged bypass. (vii) Patients with leukemia are the largest single group receiving platelet transfusion, and (viii) Disseminated intravascular coagulation (DIC) where the consumption of platelets and clotting factors is very high.

The contraindications of platelet transfusion are: Platelet transfusion should not be given simply in response to a given blood count. The underlying mechanism causing thrombocytopenia and the clinical risks of thrombocytopenia must be considered. The transfusion of platelet is contraindicated in patients with hemolytic uremic syndrome (HUS) or heparin-induced thrombocytopenia (HIT) or TTP.

Preparations from Plasma

Fresh Plasma

Fresh plasma is a natural product. It is prepared from donated blood. It is poor in platelets and is infused within 6 hours of collection. The use of fresh plasma seems promising in the reduction of mortality, mainly due to septicemia among the babies with neonatal tetanus. The infusion of fresh plasma is also helpful to stop bleeding after surgery, dental procedures, or any injury with bleeding disorders. These conditions include hemophilia and von Willebrand disease.

Fresh Frozen Plasma

It is prepared from whole blood. One unit of FFP is the plasma which is taken from a unit of whole blood. After separation from whole blood, the plasma is frozen to –40°C within 6 hours of its collection and can be stored for 10 years from the date of its collection. The FFP contains all the coagulation factors in normal concentrations. It is free of RBCs, leukocytes, and platelets. It must be ABO compatible. During the transfusion of FFP, the Rh factor need not be considered. Since, there are no RBC and leukocyte, so plasma does not carry the risk of the transmission of CMV and host-versus-graft disease (HVGD).

Fresh frozen plasma is *indicated for use* in (i) bleeding caused by vitamin K deficiency, (ii) urgent reversal of anticoagulant therapy (warfarin causes the deficiency of vitamin-dependent coagulation factors II, VII, IX, and X), (iii) acquired or inherited coagulopathy except hemophilia and von Willebrand disease [low blood clotting factors, international normalized ratio (INR) > 1.5], and (iv) bleeding due to DIC. (v) It is also indicated for the treatment of congenital deficiencies of single clotting factors, when this specific concentrate is not available. (vi) It may also be used as the replacement fluid in plasma exchange. (vii) It should be used to treat the increased microvascular bleeding or to correct the demonstrated significant abnormalities in prothrombin time (PT) or partial thromboplastin time (PTT). Two units of FFP should be given, if the PT values exceed 1.5 times of control. Each unit in an adult will increase the clotting protein levels by 10%. (viii) As the liver ordinarily synthesizes coagulation factors, so the patients with hepatic disease need plasma, if they are actively bleeding. (ix) To prime the extracorporeal membrane oxygenation (ECMO) circuit, regardless of the results of blood clotting assays, FFP can be used.

The crossmatching is not required for the transfusion of FFP. But, the plasma must be blood group specific.

The preparation time for the transfusion of FFP is about 30 minutes, because it is stored frozen. Once thawed, it should be transfused within 4 hours. Because, there is progressive loss of labile coagulation factors. The dose of FFP is generally 12–15 mL/kg every 12 hours. The recommended infusion rate of this thawed FFP is one unit over 30 minutes to an uncompromised adult. In cardiac compromised patient, in elderly patients, and in very small babies, this transfusion rate of plasma should not exceed 2–4 mL/kg/hour **(Table 1)**.

Cryoprecipitate

Cryoprecipitate means a substance which is precipitated from a solution, especially from blood, at low temperature. In medicine, it is an extract which is rich in blood clotting factors, and is obtained as a residue when the frozen blood plasma is thawed. It is a frozen blood product, prepared from plasma. To create cryoprecipitate, the FFP is thawed first to 1–6°C. Then, it is centrifuged and the precipitate is collected. The precipitate is next resuspended in a small amount of residual plasma and is then refrozen (-18°C) for storage for a maximum period of 1 year. The cryoprecipitate is rich in fibrinogen, factor VIII, von Willebrand factor, and factor XIII. One unit of cryoprecipitate derived from one unit of whole blood or 250 mL of plasma contains 80–100 units of factor VIII, 150–250 mg of fibrinogen, 50–100 units of factor XIII, and 50–60 mg of fibronectin. When required the cryoprecipitate is thawed in a 37°C-water bath and issued in individual bags. Once thawed, it must be kept at room temperature and should be used within 4–6 hours.

At present, the transfusion of cryoprecipitate is indicated for hypofibrinogenemia, von Willebrand disease, hemophilia A, factor XIII deficiency, and management of bleeding related to thrombolytic therapy. It should not be used to prepare fibrin glue or to treat sepsis. It may be used for temporary treatment of bleeding tendency in uremia. When the fibrinogen value is <80 mg%, then 1–2 units of cryoprecipitate per 10 kg of body weight is administered to maintain the fibrinogen concentration at 6–100 mg%.

The adult therapeutic dose is two pools of five or one unit per 5–10 kg of body weight depending on the degree of fibrinogen deficiency. For the older children, the typical dose is 5–10 mL/kg. Response should be monitored by repeated coagulation tests. The transfusion of cryoprecipitate has the same risk of transmitting blood-borne pathogens such as HIV, hepatitis B and C, as the other blood components. On the other hand, the factor concentrates are subjected to viral inactivation steps for HIV, hepatitis B and C, and become much safer products for transfusion.

Albumin Preparation

Albumin is prepared for medical use by fractionating it from the large pools of plasma of healthy donors and then heating it to inactivate disease causing agents. This albumin preparation is often used in the treatment of malnourished patients for nutritional supplementation of proteins. The albumin is also helpful in the treatment of burns.

Immunoglobulin Preparations

Immunoglobulins function as antibodies. So, they play an essential role in the body's immune system. They are glycoprotein in nature and are divided into five major classes such as immunoglobulin G (IgG), IgA, IgM, IgD, and IgE. These immunoglobulins are produced by the plasma cells and lymphocytes (B-lymphocytes or B-cells) in response to an immunogen. Any disease that harms the development or function of B-cells will cause the decrease in the amount of antibodies produced. The immunoglobulins prepared in special concentrated form are used to provide the immediate short-term protection against disease or from developing the serious complications from disease. The immunoglobulins are collected from the pooled blood. To prepare a single injection 3 L of whole blood is required **(Box 1)**.

Immunoglobulins are administered both intravenously and intramuscularly. The normal *nonspecific* human immunoglobulin preparations for hepatitis A, measles, polio, mumps, and rubella, and *specific* immunoglobulin preparations for hepatitis B, rabies, and varicella zoster are available for

TABLE 1: Differences between FFP and cryoprecipitate.

	FFP	*Cryoprecipitate*
Volume	250–300 mL	10–20 mL
Time to prepare	30 minutes	30 minutes
Fibrinogen	700–800 mg	150–250 mg
Other coagulation factors	All including factor II, VII, VIII, IX, X, XI, and vWF	Factors VIII, XIII, and vWF

(FFP: fresh frozen plasma; vWF: von Willebrand factor)

BOX 1: Some immunoglobulin preparations.

- *Human immunoglobulin:* Used to prevent and treat hepatitis A, measles, rubella, polio, yellow fever, etc.
- *Hepatitis B immunoglobulin (HBIG):* Used to prevent and treat hepatitis B
- *Tetanus immunoglobulin:* Used to prevent and treat tetanus
- *Rabies immunoglobulin:* Used to prevent and treat rabies
- *RhD immunoglobulin:* Given to Rh negative mother to prevent hemolytic disease of the newborn in future pregnancies

intramuscular use. The recommendations for the routine use of IVIG include the conditions such as multifocal motor neuropathy, chronic lymphocytic lymphoma, chronic inflammatory demyelinating polyneuropathy, Kawasaki disease, acquired hypogammaglobulinemia, hemolytic diseases of newborn, and ITP, etc. The mechanism of the action of IVIG is that it acts as an immunosuppressant and is found to help to reduce the symptoms of autoimmune diseases that exhibit the excessive inflammation in our body.

Concentrated Products of Blood Components

Concentrated products of clotting factor VIII and IX, anticlotting factor antithrombin III, etc. are prepared *directly from human plasma* to treat hemophilia A and B, von Willebrand disease, venous thromboembolic disorders, etc. The factor VIII concentrate is used to treat hemophilia A and von Willebrand disease. It is cell free and is administered without any regard to the ABO and Rh status of patient and donor. It can be stored at 35–45°C up to 2 years. But, it should be infused within 4 hours of preparation (reconstitution) to reduce the risk of bacterial growth. The half-life of circulating factor VIII is 10–12 hours. Hence, the transfusion of factor VIII may need to be repeated after every 12–24 hours to maintain a hemostatic level. Following surgery, it is necessary to maintain a hemostatic level for up to 2 weeks to prevent the delayed bleeding and to promote the wound healing in the hemophilic patient.

The factor IX concentrate is used to treat hemophilia B. It is refrigerated at 1–4°C. The infusion of factor IX is repeated after every 12 hours or until the symptoms resolve. After 1990s, the pharmaceutical companies began to use *recombinant technology* to synthesize the clotting factor VIII, clotting factor IX, clotting factor VIIa, antithrombin III, α1-proteinase inhibitor, etc. in concentrated form.

■ APHERESIS

This is a medical technology where the blood of a donor or a patient is passed through an appropriate filter of a machine, called the apheresis machine that filters (separates) out one particular component of blood and then returns back the remainder to the circulation. A volunteer donor will undergo apheresis to supply the specific components of blood to the patients or a patient will undergo apheresis to remove a toxic component from his or her blood. An apheresis donor may receive emergency requests to donate for a patient to whom the donor is matched. The forms of apheresis include:

- *Plasmapheresis:* To harvest plasma
- *Leukapheresis:* To harvest leukocytes
- *Granulocytapheresis (GCAP):* To harvest granulocytes (neutrophils, eosinophils, and basophils)
- *Erythroapheresis:* To harvest erythrocytes
- *Plateletpheresis:* To harvest platelets.

Plasmapheresis is a process in which the plasma is separated from the blood cells by a cell separator and the cells are returned. The therapeutic plasmapheresis has found widespread clinical application in autoimmune, hematologic, renal, metabolic, and neurological disorders. The plasmapheresis is indicated in the following conditions such as myasthenia gravis, Guillain–Barré syndrome, Waldenstrom's macroglobulinemia, Goodpasture's syndrome, Paraproteinemia, etc.

Leukapheresis is a clinical procedure in which the leukocytes are separated from a sample of blood. It is a specific type of apheresis. It is used to decrease the count of WBC and obtain WBCs for later transplant. Ordinarily, the leukapheresis is done in patients with acute myeloid leukemia (AML) or in the accelerated phases of chronic myeloid leukemia (CML) when the blast count exceeds $100,000/mm^3$ or when the rapidly rising blast counts are higher than $50,000/mm^3$. It is a part of a novel form of immunotherapy, called the chimeric antigen receptor (CAR) T-cell therapy.

Erythroapheresis is used in newborn polycythemia vera, paroxysmal nocturnal hemoglobinuria, arsenic poisoning, etc. Plateletpheresis is the most common means for supplying the human leukocyte antigen (HLA)-matched platelets to patients who become HLA sensitized and requires platelets from a single donor whose HLA type matches with that patient.

■ PLASMA EXCHANGE

In plasma exchange, usually 40 mL/kg of plasma is removed. Then, this plasma is replaced by fluid, consisting of two-thirds of human albumin solution and one-third of normal saline. It is given in the dose of 10–15 mL/kg where there is risk of bleeding due to the depletion of clotting proteins. The therapeutic plasma exchange combined with other medical treatment is indicated in the conditions like Guillain–Barré syndrome, myasthenia gravis, TTP, peripheral neuropathy associated with monoclonal gammopathy, hyperviscosity syndrome (e.g., myeloma, Waldenstrom's macroglobulinemia, etc.), familial hyper-cholesterolemia, etc.

■ TRANSFUSION COMPLICATIONS

The administration of blood and its products is safe, successful, and lifesaving, but not without its "price". These adverse reactions following the transfusion of blood or its components are due to immunologic, infectious, chemical, and physical. All these adverse reactions are subdivided into three types such as (i) acute severe (life-threatening) reactions, (ii) acute minor reactions, (iii) delayed reactions,

---

BOX 2: Complications due to blood transfusion.

Acute severe (life-threatening reactions):
- Acute hemolysis (acute hemolytic transfusion reaction)
- Anaphylaxis
- Septicemia
- Transfusion related acute lung injury
- Congestive heart failure
- Air embolism

Acute minor reactions:
- Fever (febrile nonhemorrhagic transfusion reaction)
- Allergic reaction to protein IgA
- Thrombophlebitis

Delayed reactions:
- Delayed hemolysis (delayed hemolytic transfusion reaction)
- Graft-versus-host disease (GVHD)

Transmission of infections:
- *Viral:* Hepatitis A/B/C, HIV, CMV, EB virus, West Nile virus
- *Bacterial:* Trypanosomiasis, *Salmonella*, *Brucella*
- *Parasitic:* Malaria, *Toxoplasma*, babesiosis
- *Immune sensitization:* Rh-D antigen

Massive transfusion:
- Coagulopathy
- Hypothermia
- Hypocalcemia (citrate toxicity)
- Hyperkalemia
- Lactic acidosis
- Congestive failure

(CMV: cytomegalovirus; EB virus: Epstein–Barr virus; HIV: human immunodeficiency virus; IgA: Immunoglobulin A)

(iv) transmission of infection, and (v) massive transfusion reaction **(Box 2)**.

Acute Hemolytic Transfusion Reaction

Acute hemolytic transfusion reaction (AHTR) is the leading cause of death associated with transfusion. Usually, it is due to the accidental transfusion of ABO incompatible RBCs, plasma, and platelets. It is due to an accelerated destruction of RBCs in a transfused recipient occurring during or within 24 hours after a blood transfusion. The destruction of RBCs results from an interaction between the existing antibodies in the recipient and the antigen in transfused RBCs or the existing antibodies in the transfused blood and the antigens in the recipient's RBCs.

This AHTR is characterized by the sudden onset of fever, chills, chest pain, low back pain, hypotension, and dyspnea and may result in severe complications such as renal failure and DIC. *Vigorous supportive care is important for the treatment of AHTR and these are:*
- Stop the transfusion immediately
- Generous fluid replacement with saline (100–200 mL/h) and diuretics to support the urine output above 100 mL/hour to prevent acute renal failure

- Vasopressor such as dopamine, or dobutamine, or noradrenaline may be required according to the necessity to raise the blood pressure.
- If massive hemolysis has already occurred, then hyperkalemia is likely to occur. Then, intensive cardiac and electrolyte monitoring in ICU and acute hemodialysis and other managements according to the necessity are required.
- Obtain a blood sample for a direct antiglobulin test and for a plasma free hemoglobin level
- Cautious heparinization (10 U/kg/hour) for the next 12–24 hours may prevent DIC, if it has not already occurred.
- Consider the alkalization of urine with bicarbonate (1 mEq/kg) through IV, until the urine pH = 7.5–9.0.
- To maintain the O_2 and C_2O level in blood, according to the necessity, artificial ventilation should be started.

Allergic or Anaphylactic Transfusion Reactions

These are among the most common transfusion reaction to occur. These are not due to the antigen and antibody reaction related to the ABO blood group system (mismatched transfusion). These may occur from the presence of allergy causing antigens (other than ABO and Rh system) within the donor's blood, or transfusion of antibodies from a donor who has allergies followed by antigen exposure in recipient. These reactions are almost and always due to the presence of class specific IgG and anti-IgA antibodies in patients who are IgA deficient. It may be due to the infusion of whole blood, or plasma, or packed red cells, or platelets, or granulocytes, or cryoprecipitate, or gamma globulin.

The onset of allergic reaction is manifested as (i) edema of lips, tongue, uvula, and conjunctiva; (ii) maculopapular rash, pruritus, and urticaria; (iii) generalized flushing and erythema; (iv) tachycardia, hypotension, angioedema, and respiratory distress, etc. Shock may occur within few seconds to few minutes following the initiation of transfusion. This anaphylactic reaction can be classified as *mild, moderate, and severe* **(Table 2)**. This anaphylactic reaction is not generally seen or may be less severe following the administration of normal serum albumin, plasma protein fraction, or concentrated coagulation factors.

The treatment of the allergic transfusion reactions consists of the following steps:
- Immediate cessation of transfusion
- Maintenance of airway and oxygenation, if necessary
- Maintenance of blood pressure and blood volume with saline or others, if necessary
- Antihistaminics and hydrocortisone

TABLE 2: Gradation of anaphylactic reactions.	
Mild	Rash, urticaria, pruritus, flushing, etc.
Moderate	• Wheeze (bronchospasm), angioedema, but the blood pressure is normal and there is no respiratory compromise. There may or may not be an associated rash or urticaria
Severe	• Severe breathing problems (bronchospasm, stridor), angioedema, hypotension requiring immediate intervention • Anaphylaxis

- Administration of adrenaline (0.3–0.5 mL of 1:1,000 solution) subcutaneously in moderate and severe cases.
- Vasopressors if necessary.

If the symptoms are only mild, then the patient may be treated with an antihistamine and if the symptoms completely disappear and the patient feels well, the transfusion may be restarted. A mild allergic transfusion reaction during transfusion usually does not progress to a more severe anaphylactic reaction after the infusion of additional product from the same unit. If the symptoms are more than mild, the transfusion should not be restarted.

Prevention of Allergic Transfusion Reactions

To prevent the allergic transfusion reaction, it is possible to use the patient's own blood for transfusion. This is referred to as the *autologous transfusion.* The patient's own blood is collected and washed to produce the concentrated RBCs (PRBCs). There are multiple ways to wash the RBCs. The two main methods that are used to wash the cells are (1) *centrifugation* or (2) *filtration*. There is no evidence that the antihistamine premedication prevents the allergic transfusion reactions, although these drugs can mitigate the symptoms, once they occur.

Transfusion-Related Acute Lung Injury

It is caused by the interaction between the recipient's leukocytes and preexisting donor antileukocyte antibodies. This results in the activation of complements and increased pulmonary vascular permeability. In addition, the multiple mediators of inflammation (that is formed while the blood is in storage) also contribute in this reaction. The symptoms for this reaction may vary from mild to life-threatening form. The life-threatening situation includes the rapid onset of the shortness of breath, severe hypoxemia, tachycardia, hypotension, cyanosis, and noncardiogenic pulmonary edema. The treatment of this reaction consists of fluids, oxygen, ventilation, and others according to needs.

Transfusion-Associated Graft-Versus-Host Disease

There is a small but significant risk for transfusion-associated graft-versus-host disease (TA-GVHD) in persons receiving blood from relatives, because of similar genetic makeup. Though the incidence of TA-GVHD is rare, but is a fatal condition and has no effective treatment. Normally, the donor lymphocytes are recognized as being the foreign and are destroyed. In some situations, when the donor is immunocompromised or when the donor is homozygous and the recipient is heterozygous for an HLA haplotype, then these defense mechanisms may fail resulting in GVHD. All the units of blood should undergo gamma irradiation to destroy any WBCs that could cause TA-GVHD. This adds significantly to the cost of blood processing and these units must be discarded, if not used within 24 hours.

Delayed Hemolytic Transfusion Reaction

This reaction is the consequence of rapid formation of irregular antibodies against the erythrocytes. The production of these antibodies proceeds so rapidly that the reduction of the level of Hb occurs. The delayed hemolytic transfusion reaction (DHTR) is seen generally 2–10 days after transfusion. Unlike AHTR, the most patients with DHTR are either asymptomatic or present with mild symptoms such as low-grade fever and jaundice. Occasionally, the patients may present with anemia and hemoglobinuria. The preferred therapy is IVIG in high doses (400–500 mg/kg/day for 5 days). The high doses of corticosteroid are also useful.

Febrile Nonhemolytic Transfusion Reaction

This febrile nonhemolytic transfusion reaction is caused by the alloantibodies that present in the recipient's plasma against the antigens and in the donor leukocytes and/or platelets. The clinical manifestations of this reaction include fever associated with chills, tachycardia, and mild dyspnea within 1–6 hours after the transfusion of whole blood, red cells, or platelets. Platelet transfusion is associated with the higher risk of FNHTR. Any significant increase in temperature ($>1°C$ or $2°F$) occurring during transfusion must be taken seriously and should not be ignored. Fever during or shortly after transfusion can also be caused by the hemolysis of RBCs by antibodies against the RBC or through the bacterial contamination of blood. Fever may be the first manifestation of life-threatening reaction in acute hemolysis, transfusion-associated sepsis or transfusion-related acute lung injury. The administration of antipyretics and corticosteroid is recommended for FNHTR in patients with chill and rigor.

Transmission of Bacterial and Viral Infections

Bacterial Infections

The blood is an excellent culture medium for the growth of bacteria. The transmission of infection is the second most common complication of blood transfusion. The bacterial contamination of a blood unit usually occurs during its collection, processing, pooling of components, and transfusion. Then, the refrigeration of blood after its collection limits the growth of the bacteria in it and does not create any problem except transient mild bacteremia. But, few gram-negative bacterial species such as the *Yersinia*, *Serratia*, and *Pseudomonas* grow well at 1–4°C and may produce a dangerous level of endotoxins and bacteremia leading to septicemia and death.

The *risk of transmitting syphilis* through blood transfusion is extremely rare. Because, the storing of blood at 1–4°C for >96 hours leads the death of spirochetes.

Viral infections

- *Human immunodeficiency virus:* The advent of HIV has posed a challenge to the service of blood transfusion. However, the risk of transmission of HIV through blood transfusion has almost been completely eradicated by the compulsory screening test of donor's blood for HIV [by enzyme-linked immunosorbent assay (ELISA) or reverse transcription polymerase chain reaction (RT-PCR)].
- *Hepatitis B virus:* HBV infection is also a challenge to the service of blood transfusion. But, this challenge is taken by compulsory screening test of donor's blood for hepatitis B surface antigen (HBsAg) by ELISA or rapid chromatography card test. However, the use of HBc antibody (antibody against hepatitis B core antigen) test may exclude many healthy donors.
- *Hepatitis C virus:* Like HIV and HBV, the prevention of the transmission of HCV is a great challenge to the service of blood transfusion. Hence, the compulsory screening of donor's blood for HCV has almost completely eradicated this risk of transmission of this virus.
- *Cytomegalovirus:* Cytomegalovirus belongs to the herpes group of virus and is rarely transmitted by blood transfusion. The CMV infection is usually mild, but it becomes serious or fatal in those who are immunocompromised, particularly low birth weight infants and bone marrow and organ transplant patients. Once a person is infected with CMV, it stays there for whole life. If a patient is at high risk of getting CMV infection through blood transfusion, then the blood that tests negative for CMV should be transfused. Alternatively, leukoreduced transfusion can be given.

Parasitic Infection

Malaria: It is a potentially serious complication of blood transfusion that transmitted easily through the infected RBCs. The malaria parasites survive in the RBCs that have been stored up to 1 week at 4°C. Many donors are unaware that they have malaria which may be latent and transmissible for a number of years. The prospective donors must be asked about malaria. The screening of donated blood for the evidence of malaria is not without its problems. The examination of blood films is still the basis for diagnosing acute malaria. The screening of donated blood for specific antimalarial immunoglobulin provides an effective means of minimizing the risk of transmission of malaria. In severe falciparum malaria with hyperparasitemia, the exchange transfusion may be tried in patients who are severely ill and not responding adequately to the antimalarial therapy.

COLLECTION OF BLOOD AND ANTICOAGULANTS

The collection of blood and the blood transfusion service (blood bank) is an essential component for a healthcare system. Blood is a very scarce resource, as it is obtained only through the donation of healthy individuals. The establishment of blood bank had taken place first in 1915, when Richardson of Mount Sinai Hospital of New York had first initiated the use of sodium citrate as an anticoagulant. Then, 2 years later, after the introduction of citrate glucose solution by Francis and Turner, the storage of blood in container for several days had started. It increases the supply of blood and facilitates the sharing of resources among the blood banks.

The collection of blood requires the proportional adjustment of anticoagulant in the collection bag. As the anticoagulant maintains a reasonable amount of pH, so it provides a higher degree of red cells survival rate and O_2 delivery. The following types of anticoagulants are used for the storing of whole blood.

Acid Citrate Dextrose

The introduction of sodium citrate as an anticoagulant was a major advance in the storage of human blood and it later made possible the creation of blood bank. The first citrated blood adding dextrose was introduced in 1915. It was demonstrated that the ACD solution at 4°C increases the 70% survival of RBC for 21 days. The use of ACD anticoagulant results in a significant improvement in 2,3-diphosphoglycerate (2,3-DPG) with no significant loss in the concentration of adenosine triphosphate (ATP). The citrate anticoagulates the blood by chelating the Ca^{2+}.

Citrate Phosphate Dextrose

The citrate phosphate dextrose (CPD) solution was introduced in 1957 as anticoagulants and is much superior to the ACD. It is stored at 4°C for different periods and treated with a solution containing the pyruvate, inosine, phosphate, and adenine to increase the ATP and 2, 3-DPG level in RBC and to maintain the normal P_{50} level for up to 21 days.

Citrate Phosphate Dextrose Adenine

The citrate phosphate dextrose adenine (CPDA) solution differs from CPD solution as it has 1.25 times higher the dextrose concentration and 17.3 mg of adenine per 63 mL of its solution. The pH of this CPDA solution varies in-between 5.5 and 6.0 and this pH helps in maintaining the function of Hb and the viability of red cells with extended storage for >35 days. According to the concentration of adenine, this CPDA solution (anticoagulant) may be of three types such as (1) CPDA-1, (2) CPDA-2, and (3) CPDA-3. The ATP concentration in RBC is better maintained throughout the storage of 42 days in CPDA-2 and CPDA-3 solution than CPDA-1 solution.

Additive Solution (AS-1, AS-3, AS-5)

It is an extended storage preservative solution, consisting of the varying amounts of dextrose, sodium chloride, mannitol, trisodium citrate, citric acid, and sodium phosphate or phosphate buffer. The AS-3 solution may be used safely for the small volume of RBC transfusion in high-risk patients.

Saline, Adenine, Glucose, and Mannitol Solution

It is the modified formulation of CPDA solution for the storage of whole blood and red cells. It (i) maintains the concentration of 2,3-DPG (nutrition source) and ATP level in RBCs, (ii) adjusts the osmotic pressure, and (iii) supports the integrity of the membrane of red cells to avoid hemolysis. The new SAGM-1 and SAGM-2 solutions support the survival of RBCs for >42 days.

Blood storage temperature: The quality of stored blood containing the RBCs is highly temperature dependent. It should be cooled within 30–60 minutes after collection and if this cooling is delayed for 6 hours, then it exhibits a substantial loss of 2,3-DPG in red cells. After transfusion, the onset of the recovery of 2,3-DPG takes about 4 hours and may take several hours and days to reach its normal value, even if the temperature is brought to normal. The proper storage of the whole blood and its components at particular temperature is very essential. The blood is perfectly preserved at a temperature of 1–4°C. The transfusion of blood should be started within the 30 minutes of removal from the blood bank refrigerator.

■ CHANGES IN STORED BLOOD

Gradually, the collection, storage, and the transfusion of blood have progressed to a specialty and have improved the ability to store the blood in liquid state. The collected blood has its limited shelf life and gradually deteriorates its quality day by day. The storage technique has been improved and has extended the storage period up to 42 days. The transfusion of blood, older than 14–21 days, may lead to the greater incidences of multiorgan failure.

Changes in Red Blood Cells

After storage, there is metabolic, biochemical, oxidative, and molecular changes in RBCs which may lead to the irreversible damage and harmful consequences in recipient. Due to storage, there is accumulation of lactate and chloride in RBCs and they have a markedly increased osmotic fragility. The membrane Na-K-ATPase activity is inhibited and the ATP level in RBC is decreased to 50%. The P_{50} level within the RBC also progressively decreases following the storage. The stored RBCs have a volume of 5–8% greater than that of the normal cells.

Due to the loss of endogenous antioxidants due to the storage, there is oxidative injury of the cytoskeleton proteins and membrane phospholipids of RBCs. These lead to the changes in RBC shape from discoid to globular (spherocytes). Now, these deformed RBCs can either block the capillaries or reduce the microcirculation resulting in the overall diminished O_2 delivery to the organs. Due to the storage, there is increased conversion of Hb to met-Hb which is incapable of binding with O_2 leading to decreased delivery of O_2 to the organs. RBC adhesion also increases with the duration of storage which causes capillary slugging and obstruction, thereby predisposing the patient to tissue ischemia and decreased O_2 delivery. The RBCs stored for >14 days cannot release the sufficient O_2 to make the blood transfusion efficacious.

The storage of blood in ACD anticoagulant solution gradually depletes the red cells from its 2,3-DPG and increases the affinity of Hb for O_2. Hence, the storage of blood leads the reduced delivery of O_2 to the tissues. The adequate level of 2,3-DPG is not maintained beyond the 10 days of storage of blood.

Changes in White Blood Cells

The life span of WBC (the average life span of WBC is 42 days) in blood is shortened after its storage. Hence, as the WBCs die, they release the varieties of inflammatory mediators such as interleukins (ILs), tumor necrosis factor-α (TNF-α), and other cytokines which are toxic to the cells. The concentration of these mediators and factors (cytokines) become significant after about the 14 days of storage of blood. So, the prestorage leukoreduction is now the standard practice in many countries to minimize this storage lesion of WBCs. These inflammatory cytokines accumulated in blood that stored at 4°C are considered to be the cause of *febrile nonhemolytic transfusion reaction* following blood transfusion.

Changes in Platelets

After the storage of blood, the impairment of platelet function is due to hypothermia. After 3 hours of storage at 4°C, the viability of platelets is reduced to 60%. This viability of platelets is further reduced to only 12% after 24 hours and 2% after 48 hours of storage at 4°C. There is virtually no platelet function when the blood is stored at 4°C for longer than 24 hours.

Changes in Clotting Factors

The stored blood contains all the coagulation factors, but the concentration of factor V and factor VIII are reduced after 2 days. The presence of even minute clots in the stored blood causes the more marked decrease of these two factors. However, the activities of factors such as I, II, IX, XII, and XIII remain for longer time.

Changes in Ions

The storage of RBCs resulted in the rise of K^+ and the fall of Na^+, Cl^-, and pH. The problem of using aged blood includes *hypocalcemia* due to the binding of Ca^{2+} with citrate and *hyperkalemia*. For hyperkalemia, the potassium levels in stored blood increase by approximately 1 mEq/L/day and it is due to the passive leakage of K^+ out of the RBCs into plasma and cell lysis. The concentration of K^+ peaks at about 30 mEq/L in whole blood and 90 mEq/L in packed red cells after 21 days of storage. After the transfusion of blood, this K^+ is diluted in the blood of recipient and is excreted through urine. After the storage of blood, ammonia increases three times and hyperbilirubinemia occurs due to the breakdown of RBCs.

Changes in pH

The pH of blood falls (becomes acidic) after its storage and the rate of this fall of pH is 0.1 per week. After 3 weeks of storage, the pH of blood becomes 4.0. The development of acidosis due to the storage of blood is due to the citric acid in anticoagulant and due to the accumulation of CO_2, lactic acid, and pyruvic acid from the metabolism of RBCs. Most of the drop of pH is due to the accumulation of CO which cannot escape from the stored blood.

Free Hemoglobin

Free Hb in the storage blood due to the gradual hemolysis of RBCs increases throughout the whole period of storage.

Microaggregate Formation

The stored blood contains lots of microaggregates and becomes responsible for the pathogenesis of posttraumatic pulmonary insufficiency.

■ PLASMA SUBSTITUTES

Immediately after World War II, the search was intensified for some type of macromolecular substances (plasma substitutes) that could be given to maintain plasma volume until the whole blood was available. These plasma substitutes are liquids that are used to replace the blood plasma. These substances only replace the volume of blood, but do not enhance the O_2 carrying capacity of blood. The restoration of macro- and microcirculatory perfusion and the prevention of its deleterious consequences such as organ dysfunction and multiorgan failure in shock are the primary goal of volume therapy. Plasma substitutes are used as short-term measures to treat the massive hemorrhage until the blood is available.

These plasma substitutes are colloid in nature. They shift the fluid from extravascular space into intravascular space by exerting an osmotic effect and maintain blood pressure. They can be stockpiled without refrigeration and do not pose limitations related to the blood group of recipient.

Plasma Substitutes and Its Mechanism of Action

Properties of an Ideal Plasma Substitute Colloid Solution

- It should be nontoxic.
- It will remain only in intravascular compartment.
- It should be iso-oncotic with plasma and of low viscosity.
- It will not cause any electrolyte and acid-base disturbance.
- It will have long shelf life and will be nonexpensive.
- It will not need any special storage system.
- It will not interfere with blood grouping, crossmatching, or agglutination.
- It will not interference with hemostasis, coagulation, or organ function, even with repeated administration.
- It will not promote any bacterial, viral, or protozoal infections.
- It will be nonpyrogenic, nonallergenic, and nonantigenic.
- It should be metabolized or excreted and not stored in the body.

Natural Colloids

Albumin: Among all the colloid solutions used clinically, serum albumin is the "gold standard" to maintain the plasma oncotic pressure. The molecular weight (MW) of albumin is 69,000 Da. It represents about 60% of plasma protein by weight and accounts for about 80% of the total plasma oncotic pressure. The 5% albumin is isotonic with plasma. It increases the blood volume by an amount approximately equal to the volume of albumin infused. However, the 25% albumin expands the intravascular volume approximately five times in 30–60 minutes. Albumin is transfused at the rate of 1 g/kg of body weight, and 1–2 mL/min. Albumin has several theoretical and biological benefits including drug binding and antioxidant. The 5% and 25% albumin are valuable in severe blood loss, bleeding disorders, burns, acute liver failure, nephritis, malnutrition, ascites, hyperbilirubinemia, hypoproteinemia, etc.

Albumin can be stored for 3 years. It is used with caution in hypertensive patients, because of the risk of pulmonary edema. Albumin may induce severe anaphylactic reaction.

Synthetic Colloids

Synthetic colloidal plasma substitutes can be divided into the products, based on dextran, starch, and gelatin. These solutions are safe with respect to the effects on coagulation, platelets, RE system, renal function, etc.

Dextran: Dextran colloid is a complex, nonprotein, branched, polysaccharide, made of many glucose molecules joined into chains of varying lengths. It is synthesized from sucrose by certain lactic acid bacteria. The MW of dextran varies in-between 10,000 and 150,000. It has similar intravascular effect (increases plasma oncotic pressure) like that of albumin. The dextran-40 produces a powerful oncotic effect leading to intravascular volume expansion of 750 mL within first hour and 1,050 mL within 2 hours. The total dose of dextran should not exceed 20 mL/kg during the initial 24 hours. The half-life of low-MW dextran is 4–6 hours. Approximately, 50–70% of infused dextran is excreted unchanged through urine within 24 hours and the remaining 30% is retained in body for several more days. The dextran solutions are available either in 0.9% normal saline or 5% dextrose as 6 and 10% solution.

The indications for the use of dextran are (i) to improve the local circulation in various conditions, especially peripheral vascular occlusion or reconstruction, (ii) plasma volume expansion during hypovolemic shock due to surgery and trauma, (iii) prophylaxis of postoperative and post-traumatic thromboembolism.

Some precautions should be taken during the infusion of dextran. It can interfere with blood grouping, crossmatching, and biochemical tests. Therefore, blood sample should be taken before starting the infusion. It should be avoided in patients with cardiac diseases, renal impairment, congenital coagulation disorders (hemophilia and von Willebrand disease), or acquired defects (thrombocytopenia) and patients receiving antithrombotic agents. Dextran is not an anticoagulant, but its antithrombotic effects are (i) due to the hemodilution of blood and (ii) due to the temporary change in the function of factor VIII. Dextran dramatically impairs hemostasis and fibrinolysis. However, in doses <20 mL/kg/day, clinical bleeding is usually not encountered.

Dextran promotes the release of histamine causing anaphylaxis in 1–5% of cases. This is manifested by tachycardia, unexplained hypotension, urticaria, broncho-spasm, etc. This anaphylactic reaction is due to the antibodies against dextran.

Gelatin: The gelatin-based plasma substitutes are denatured collagens and thus contain the complex mixture of proteins. Gelatin is prepared by the hydrolysis of collagen from various animal sources. It is sterile and pyrogen free. There is no infection risk from the product, if it is stored and administered correctly. It contains no preservatives and has a recommended shelf life of 3 years when stored at temperatures <30°C. It does not need refrigeration. The solutions of gelatin form gel at about 20°C. Therefore, it cannot be used in cool or temperate climates. The gelatin solutions probably do not contribute significantly to nutrition. Their only place in medical therapy is to restore the circulating blood volume.

The MW of gelatin ranges from 5,000 to 50,000 with an average of 35,000. Therefore, the effect of gelatin on blood volume expansion is limited and the duration of this effect does not exceed >2 hours. It is used in the doses up to 50 mL/kg. Gelatin is rapidly excreted through kidney and it appears to be almost devoid of significant damaging effect on the kidney. The commercially commonly used gelatins are Haemaccel and Gelofusine. Their MWs are 35,000 and 30,000 respectively. Polygeline is supplied as 3.5% solution with electrolytes (Na^+ = 145, K^+ = 5.1, Ca^{2+} = 6.25, Cl^- = 145 m. mole/L). The gelatin solution directly stimulates the release of histamine and may initiate severe anaphylactic reaction.

Hydroxyethyl starch: The hydroxyethyl starch (HES) is a nonionic derivative of starch. It is a powerful synthetic colloid derived from the waxy portion of corn. It is composed almost entirely of amylopectin which is a branched chain polyglucose resembling glycogen. It is used to maintain, replace, or expand the volume of plasma prophylactically or therapeutically in hypovolemic or circulatory shock such as in surgery, trauma, sepsis, and burns.

The MW of HES ranges from 10,000 to 3,000,000 Da with an osmolality of 309 mOsm/L. It exerts oncotic pressure near about 66 mm Hg. The smaller molecules of HES with MW <50,000 will be readily excreted through urine with plasma half-life of approximately 24–36 hours. A varying portion of HES will tend to accumulate in the RE tissue as well as in the skin and even in the nerves. Hence, pruritus may occur and may even persist for several months, after HES administration. This risk of tissue accumulation is greater in the presence of renal failure, so that the use of HES is not recommended in anuric renal failure.

The commercial preparations of HES are available according to the MW namely Hestar-450 (high-MW, available as 10% solution) and Pentastarch-200 (low-MW, available as 3%, 6%, and 10% solution). Both the starches with low- and high-MW are effective as 5% albumin when used for volume replacement. Anaphylactic reaction occurs in about 0.09% of cases with 10% HES. The allergic potential of HES is seven times lower than that of gelatin and dextran. Blood coagulation is impaired by high-MW HES associated with increased postoperative blood loss. The HES is prohibited in patients with impaired hemostasis due to congenital coagulation disorder (hemophilia and vWD) or acquired defect (thrombocytopenia). The serum amylase levels can be elevated after hetastarch.

Diabetes Mellitus and Anesthesia

■ INTRODUCTION

The word "diabetes" literally means "to go through" ("dia" means "*through*" and "betes" means "*to go*"), because this disease causes the loss of body weight, as if the *body mass is going through urine*. The word "mellitus" means "*sweet*" and is attached to the nomenclature of this disease as the urine of the patient suffering from this disease is sweet in taste due to the presence of sugar. The disease, diabetes mellitus (DM), is known from the very ancient time. In 400 BC, the Charaka had given a vivid description of this disease in his treatise as "*madhumeha*" (sweet urine).

The disease, diabetes mellitus, is a metabolic disorder characterized by hyperglycemia, glycosuria, negative nitrogen balance, hyperlipidemia, and ketonemia (sometimes). It is due to the absolute or relative deficiency of insulin hormone. The relative deficiency of insulin hormone means the increase in the resistance of insulin or the decrease in the responsiveness of insulin. The number of patients suffering from DM is growing throughout the whole world and it is due to the rise in type 2 DM.

The main systemic pathological changes in DM are due to the *nonenzymatic glycosylation of tissue protein* due to the persistent high rise of blood sugar. This leads to the formation and accumulation of abnormal protein that leads to the decrease in elastance of tissue and the tensile strength of wound healing. The persistent elevation of glucose also increases the *synthesis of macroglobulin by liver*. Therefore, there is increase in the viscosity of blood. Along with the nonenzymatic glycosylation of protein, there is also *increase in the production and accumulation of nondiffusible large molecule, i.e., sorbitol* (a reduced form of glucose) in the cells leading intracellular swelling.

All these biochemical changes lead to a widespread pathological changes that is characterized by (i) the increase in the matrix of vessel wall, (ii) the thickening of capillary basement membrane, (iii) the narrowing of vessel lumen,

and (iv) the cellular proliferation resulting in (a) generalized atherosclerosis, (b) sclerosis of glomerular capillaries, (c) retinopathy, (d) neuropathy, (e) nephropathy, and (f) peripheral vascular insufficiency (diffuse microvascular lesion, macrovascular lesion, and end-organ dysfunction).

■ CLASSIFICATION OF DIABETES MELLITUS

The DM can be classified as follows:

- *Type 1 diabetes mellitus:* It is also known as the insulin-dependent diabetes mellitus (IDDM) or juvenile-onset diabetes mellitus (JOD). This type 1 DM is characterized by low or very low level of insulin and the individuals tend to be young and nonobese. They are more prone to the development of ketosis (ketoacidosis). It has low genetic predisposition. The pathology behind this type 1 DM is the destruction of the β-cells of pancreatic islets. The cause of this destruction of β-cells of pancreas is autoimmune. Because, the antibodies against these β-cells are detectable in the majority of cases and are associated with the other autoimmune diseases, such as Graves' disease, Hashimoto's thyroiditis, Addison's disease, myasthenia gravis, etc. In some cases, no antibodies can be detected. These are taken as idiopathic.
- *Type 2 diabetes mellitus:* This is also known as the noninsulin-dependent diabetes mellitus (NIDDM) or maturity-onset diabetes (MOD). Most of the diabetes patients (90%) belong to this type of DM. Here, the circulating insulin level is normal, or high, but low relative to the blood glucose level. In this type of DM, no β-cell antibody can be demonstrated and has high genetic predisposition. There is no loss or the moderate loss of β-cell population. The causes for this type 2 DM are:

  - *Abnormality of glucose receptor on β-cell:* Due to the abnormality of the β-cells of pancreas, there is impairment of the secretion of insulin in response to even high blood glucose level. Therefore, there is relative β-cell or insulin deficiency (β-cell failure, not loss).

- *Reduction of the sensitivity of insulin receptors to insulin:* This is also known as insulin resistance. Due to the reduction of the sensitivity of insulin receptor, which is present on the peripheral cell of tissues, insulin cannot act. This leads to increased secretion of insulin (hyperinsulinemia) as compensatory mechanism and finally there is downregulation of insulin receptors (number of insulin receptor is reduced due to high insulin level). Now, this hyperinsulinemia causes the proliferation of cells leading to angiopathy and accelerated cardiovascular diseases. This insulin resistance is particularly found at the level of liver, muscle, and fat.

  Patient's age does not allow a firm distinction between the type 1 and type 2 DM, because the type 1 DM with ketosis can even develop in an elder person and the type 2 DM in an overnourished child. Normally, the individuals suffering from type 2 DM tend to be overweight, relatively resistant to ketoacidosis, and susceptible to the development of hyperglycemic hyperosmolar nonketotic state. Some examples of genetic influence on type 2 DM are defective glucokinase enzyme. The mutation of this enzyme produces the relative insulin deficiency by increasing the threshold for glucose-induced insulin secretion. This mutation is at the hepatocyte nuclear factor 1 alpha (HNF-1α) gene. These patients respond to sulfonylurea. When there is mutation of HNF-1β gene then insulin is required.

- *Diabetic prone states:* This group includes (a) impaired fasting glycemia (IFG), (b) impaired glucose tolerance test, and (c) gestational DM.

- *Secondary diabetes mellitus:* This group includes individuals suffering from DM due to other causes such as (a) drug induced (β-blockers and steroids), (b) endocrinopathies (acromegaly, Cushing syndrome, thyrotoxicosis, etc.), (c) pancreatic diseases (pancreatitis, cystic fibrosis, etc.).

IMPAIRED GLUCOSE TOLERANCE, IMPAIRED FASTING GLYCEMIA, AND METABOLIC SYNDROME

As per World Health Organization (WHO) recommendation, in a *normal person the level of fasting glucose level is* 70–110 mg/dL and the postprandial glucose level is below 140 mg/dL. According to WHO, the person who has fasting blood sugar level >126 mg/dL and postprandial blood sugar

level is >140 mg/dL are called the diabetic. But, recently the revised upper limit for the normal person for the fasting glucose level is <100 mg/dL. Those who have fasting glucose level >100 mg/dL are suspicious and are checked periodically. The persons who have fasting blood glucose level between 110 and 126 mg/dL and postprandial blood glucose level between 140 and 200 mg/dL are called the *impaired glucose tolerance.*

These individuals are diagnosed by *oral glucose tolerance test* (OGTT). This OGTT also diagnoses the alimentary glycosuria, renal glycosuria, and IFG. In this IFG, the fasting plasma glucose level is above the normal, but below the fasting diabetic level, i.e., between 110 and 126 mg/dL. However, in this group, the postprandial level is within normal limits (i.e., <140 mg/dL). These persons need no immediate treatment, but are to be kept under constant vigilance. In *alimentary glycosuria,* the fasting and postprandial blood glucose level are normal. But, a high rise of blood glucose level is found after taking food. This is due to the increased absorption of glucose from intestine. It is found in patients after gastrectomy and hyperthyroidism.

In *renal glycosuria,* the blood glucose levels (fasting and postprandial) are within normal limits, but the glucose appears within urine. The normal renal threshold for glucose is 175–180 mg/dL. That is up to this blood glucose level, glucose will not appears in urine and all the filtered glucose will be absorbed by the renal tubules. If the blood glucose rises above this level, then the glucose starts to appear in urine. But, when the renal threshold value is lowered in renal glycosuria due to defective renal tubular glucose reabsorption and due to the abnormal sodium-glucose transport protein 2 (SGLT-2) carrier protein, then the glucose starts to appear in urine, despite the normal blood glucose value. This renal glycosuria occurs in Fanconi's syndrome due to renal tubular transport defect. In Fanconi syndrome along with glycosuria, there is amino aciduria and phosphaturia.

When the impaired glucose tolerance (fasting blood sugar >110 mg/dL and postprandial <140 mg/dL) is associated with some other features such as hyperinsulinemia (insulin resistance), normal blood glucose level, elevated waist circumference (for men >90 cm, for women >80 cm), elevated triglycerides (>150 mg/dL), reduced high-density lipoprotein (HDL) cholesterol (for men <40 mg/dL, for women <50 mg/dL), elevated blood pressure (>130/85 mm Hg), elevated fasting glucose (>100 mg/dL), coagulation abnormality, and hyperuricemia, then this is called the metabolic syndrome (MetS).

The patients with MetS are at the increased risk of the development of type 2 DM and coronary artery disease. Due to insulin resistance, the following things happen: (i) due to the absence of glucose metabolism, the increased hydrolysis (metabolism) of stored fats (triglycerides) will elevates the plasma free fatty acid (FFA) level, (ii) due to the reduced glucose uptake by cells and its utilization, there is reduced glycogen storage in the liver and muscle cells, (iii) due to the compensatory hyperinsulinemia, there is downregulation of insulin receptor potentiated by the inherent defects within target cells.

METABOLIC DERANGEMENTS IN DIABETES MELLITUS

The insulin has immense role in carbohydrate, lipid, and protein metabolism. In the absence of insulin, all these metabolisms are reversed.

- *Derangements in carbohydrate metabolism:* The deficiency of insulin causes the reduced uptake of glucose by the cells. Within the cells, the insulin-dependent enzymes responsible for carbohydrate metabolism become inactive in the absence of insulin. So, subsequently the intracellular metabolism of glucose is halted. Therefore, the net effect is the inhibition of glycolysis and the stimulation of neoglucogenesis leading to hyperglycemia.
- *Derangements in lipid metabolism:* In the absence of glycolysis, energy is derived from fat. So, first the triglycerides in depot fat is hydrolyzed and there is high FFA level in plasma. This leads to fatty liver. The increased availability of FFA leads to the increased breakdown of it and increased level of acetyl-CoA. But, this acetyl-CoA cannot be efficiently oxidized through the tricarboxylic acid (TCA) cycle due to the nonavailability of oxaloacetate. Because, the oxaloacetate is directed to the gluconeogenesis which is stimulated in the absence of insulin. Therefore, there is accumulation of acetyl-CoA and this excess acetyl-CoA leads to the ketone body formation and ketogenesis.
- *Derangements of protein metabolism:* In the impairment of glucose metabolism or glycolysis, the energy is derived from protein. So, there is increased breakdown of protein (muscle wasting) and increased amino acid (AA) level in blood. The increased amino acid level in blood provides the substrate for gluconeogenesis.

INSULIN

In 1869, Langerhans had first identified the β-cells in the islets of pancreas. The word "insulin" is derived from a Latin word "insula" which means islet (island). In 1921, Banting and Best first extracted insulin from pancreas. Before that, in 1889, von Mering and Minkowski had proved that pancreas is responsible for the maintenance of blood glucose level by producing experimental diabetes after pancreatectomy on animal. In 1926, Abel had first produced the pure crystallized form of insulin. In 1956, the full amino acid sequence of insulin is worked out by Sanger. The molecular weight of insulin is 6,000. It has two polypeptide chains: A and B. The A chain has 21 amino acids and the B chain has 30 amino acids. These two chains are joined together by two disulfide bonds between the A7–B7 and A20–B19 amino acids. In A chain, between its 6th and 11th amino acid, there is an intrachain disulfide bond.

Insulin was first synthesized by ribosome as a large precursor single-chain peptide called the preproinsulin (110 amino acids). It is next converted to proinsulin after the removal of 24 amino acids by endoplasmic reticulum (ER). Then, it is transported to the Golgi body where the connecting C-protein (35 amino acids) is cleaved away and insulin is formed. Now, both these C-protein and insulin is stored as granules in cells. The insulin is packed in granules as form of hexamer with two zinc (Zn) ions and one calcium ion. When the insulin is secreted, C-peptide is also secreted along with it. So, the measurement of C-peptide is taken as the index of the rate of the secretion of insulin.

Regulation of Insulin Secretion

The secretion of insulin from pancreas is regulated by chemical, hormonal, and neural mechanism.

Chemical Mechanism

Glucose, different gastrointestinal (GI) hormones, proteins, and amino acids act as stimulant for the secretion of insulin. Among these, the glucose is the major stimulant. The glucose induces the secretion of insulin in two phases (biphasic). After the ingestion of food, a brief pulse of insulin secretion occurs within 2 minutes. This is the first phase and this insulin was synthesized previously and was stored in the β-cells of pancreas. This first phase of insulin secretion is followed by a delayed, but more sustained second phase of insulin secretion and its immediate release. The pancreatic β-cells have glucose sensing mechanism. This is nothing but the entry of glucose into β-cells through glucose transporter 2 (GLUT2) receptor (transporter) situated on the cell membrane of β-cells. After the entry, this glucose is now oxidized and adenosine triphosphate (ATP) is formed. As the more glucose will enter, the more ATP will be formed. Now, these ATPs stimulate the *ATP-binding cassette protein* which is referred to as the *sulfonylurea receptor (SUR)*. These SURs inhibit the ATP sensitive K^+ channel (K^+ATP) resulting in the depolarization of β-cells of pancreas. This increases intracellular Ca^{2+} availability and the release of insulin stored in granules.

The secretion of insulin is also enhanced by other GI hormones such as secretin, pancreozymine, gastrin, etc. After taking food, the levels of these hormones are increased. Among the amino acids, the leucine and arginine are potent stimulant for the secretion of insulin.

Glucose, given orally, acts as a better stimulant for the secretion of insulin than it is given IV. This is due to the production of chemical signals, called the *incretins* from the specialized cells in GI tract which act on the β-cells of pancreas and causes the secretion of insulin. Among these, two hormones are most important. These are *glucose-dependent insulinotropic polypeptide (GIP) and glucagon-like peptide 1 (GLP-1)*. These incretins have a very short half-life and have their receptors on the β-cells for their action. The newer oral drugs which are now developed to treat DM either stimulate or inhibit these incretin hormones.

Hormonal Mechanism

A number of hormones such as the glucagon, somatostatin, growth hormone, corticosteroids, thyroid hormones, etc. also modify the release of insulin in response to glucose. Among these, the intraislet paracrine system is very important. In the endocrine part of pancreas, the β-cells are most abundant and constitute the core of the islets. The α-cells and the δ-cells constituting the 25% and 10% of the islet cell mass respectively surround the core of β-cells. Some pancreatic polypeptide (PP) cells interspersed the α-cells and δ-cells as well. The α-cells secrete glucagon, the δ-cells secrete somatostatin, and the PP cells secrete PP, which increase the secretion of glucagon from α-cells. Somatostatin inhibits the secretion of both insulin and glucagon. Glucagon stimulates the secretion of both insulin and somatostatin. Insulin inhibits the secretion of glucagon.

Nervous Mechanism

The islets of pancreas are richly supplied by sympathetic and parasympathetic (vagus) nervous system. Parasympathetic stimulation causes increased insulin secretion through acetylcholine (Ach)-muscarinic receptor which acts on intracellular IP_3/diacylglycerol (DAG) and Ca^{2+} pathway. The activation of adrenergic α_2-receptor decreases insulin secretion and the activation of β_2-receptor increase insulin secretion through adenylyl cyclase pathway. The primary site for the regulation of insulin secretion through nervous mechanism is hypothalamus. The stimulation of ventrolateral nuclei of hypothalamus evokes the release of insulin and the stimulation of ventromedial nuclei of hypothalamus inhibits the release of insulin. This nervous mechanism governs both the basal as well as evoked insulin release.

■ MECHANISM OF ACTION OF INSULIN

Insulin acts on specific receptor (insulin receptor) located on the cell membrane of all tissue cells. But, their density is very high on liver, fat, and muscle cells. In obesity, the number of receptors on target cells is decreased and this tissue becomes resistant to insulin (type 2 DM). It (insulin receptor) is a glycoprotein and has four subunits: two α- and two β-units. The β-subunit is long and traverses the cell membrane. The one end of the β-subunit lies outside the cell membrane and here the α subunit is attached with the β-subunit.

Insulin binds with α-subunit. The another end of β-subunit is exposed in the cytoplasm and is associated with the tyrosine kinase activity. The two β-subunit is linked by disulfide bond. When the insulin is attached with α-subunit, then the tyrosine kinase at the cytoplasmic end of β-subunit is activated leading to autophosphorylation of β-subunit. This subsequently phosphorylates another molecule named insulin receptor substrates (IRSs). Then, a cascade of phosphorylation and dephosphorylation are set in motion which results in the stimulation and inhibition of enzymes involved in the metabolism of carbohydrates, proteins, and fats.

Insulin also acts at the transcription level regulating the synthesis of >100 proteins including glucose transporter 4 (GLUT4) protein. Thus, insulin helps in the entry of glucose into the cells through GLUT4 transporter.

■ METABOLIC ACTIONS OF INSULIN

Insulin activates and inhibits many intracellular enzymes involved in the metabolism of carbohydrates, lipids, and proteins. Thus it helps in (i) glycolysis (liberation of energy from glucose), (ii) inhibits gluconeogenesis, (iii) promotes glycogen deposition, (iv) favors lipogenesis, (v) inhibits lipolysis, (vi) decreases ketogenesis, (vii) favors protein synthesis, and (viii) inhibits catabolism of proteins.

Carbohydrate Metabolism

- *Glycolysis is favored by the stimulation of following enzymes:*
  - Translocase
  - Glucokinase
  - Phosphofructokinase
  - Pyruvate kinase
- *Gluconeogenesis is depressed by the inhibition of following enzymes:*
  - Pyruvate carboxylase
  - Phosphoenolpyruvate carboxykinase
  - Fructose 1, 6-bisphosphatase
  - Glucose 6-phosphatase

- *Glycogen deposition is promoted by:*
  - Activation of glycogen synthase
  - Inhibition of glycogen phosphorylase.

Lipid Metabolism

- Lipolysis is inhibited by the inhibition of hormone-sensitive lipase enzyme
- *Lipogenesis is stimulated by the stimulation of following enzymes:*
  - Glucose-6-phosphate dehydrogenase
  - Acetyl-CoA carboxylase
  - Glycerol kinase
- Cholesterol synthesis is enhanced by the stimulation of hydroxymethylglutaryl (HMG) CoA reductase enzyme.

Protein Metabolism

- Protein catabolism is inhibited by the inhibition of transaminase enzyme.
- Protein synthesis is favored by the stimulation of ribonucleic acid (RNA) polymerase enzyme and ribosome assembly.

■ PREPARATIONS OF INSULIN

As the insulin is peptide in nature, so it cannot be given orally. Because, it gets degraded in GI tract. Previously, the insulin was prepared from pork and beef pancreas and contains >10,000 ppm of other proteins of pancreas of these animals which are potentially highly antigenic. Hence, these types of insulins are no longer produced and these older commercial preparations of insulin are replaced by (i) highly purified beef and pork insulin, (ii) recombinant human insulin, and (iii) insulin analogs.

Highly Purified Beef and Pork Insulin

These are called the *monocomponent (MC) insulin.* It contains contaminated tissue proteins <10 ppm. Hence, they are more stable, less antigenic, cause less insulin resistance, and less injection site lipodystrophy. Beef insulin is more antigenic than pork insulin. So, beef insulin is not used. However, the MC pork insulin is antigenically more or less similar to that of the recombinant insulin. According to the onset and duration of action, the MC pork insulin is of three types **(Table 1):**

1. *Regular or soluble insulin (pork insulin):* Its pH is neutral. It contains little amount of zinc than ultralente and semilente insulin. So, the insulin molecules aggregate around zinc atoms and form a hexamer. After subcutaneous (SC) injection of this soluble preparation, the insulin molecules are slowly released from the hexamer structure of zinc and insulin and then

TABLE 1: Types of insulin preparation and its analogs.

Type	Appearance	Onset of action (hour)	Peak (hour)	Duration of action (hour)
Rapid acting:				
• Insulin lispro	Clear	0.2–0.3	1–2	3–5
• Insulin aspart	Clear	0.2–0.3	1–2	3–5
• Insulin glulisine	Clear	0.3–0.4	1–2	3–5
Short acting:				
Regular insulin	Clear	0.5–1	2–3	6–8
Intermediate acting:				
• Lente insulin	Cloudy	1–2	8–10	12–24
• NPH insulin	Cloudy	1–2	8–10	12–24
Long acting:				
• Insulin glargine	Clear	2–4	No peak	24
• Insulin detemir	Clear	2–4	No peak	24
• Insulin degludec	Clear	3–5	No peak	48

pass into the circulation. The peak action of the regular soluble insulin starts after 2–3 hours of injection and this action lasts for 6–8 hours. Generally, it is injected 1 hour before meal and creates a mismatch between the need and the availability of insulin. Hence, it results in early postprandial hyperglycemia and late hypoglycemia. However, it is not slow acting, when injected IV because the insulin hexamer dissociates rapidly in plasma.

2. *Lente insulin (pork):* It is a mixture of ultralente and semilente insulin in the ratio of (7:3). The ultra- and semilente insulin are nothing but the different types of insulin zinc preparation depending on the amount of zinc and the pH of the solution. In ultralente preparation, the insulin-zinc complex produces larger particles, insoluble in water and they are long-acting. Whereas, in the semilente preparation, the insulin-zinc complex produces smaller particles, amorphous and is short acting. In lente insulin (7:3 mixture of ultralente and semilente insulin), the onset of action and duration of action is intermediate.

3. *Isophane insulin (neutral protamine Hagedorn or NPH insulin):* Here, the insulin is complexed with protamine (a basic protein) and make it (soluble insulin) insoluble. Here, the protamine is added with insulin in such an amount that all the insulin molecules make complexes with protamine and there is no any free form of protamine and insulin. The pH of protamine insulin is neutral. After SC injection of such insoluble form, insulin is slowly released from the site of injection and becomes longer acting. It is mostly combined with regular insulin at the ratio of 70:30 (70% isophane insulin and 30% regular

insulin) or 50:50. This is called the Mixtard insulin. It is injected through SC route twice daily, before breakfast and before dinner.

4. *Protamine zinc insulin:* Here, the protamine is added in excess amount with insulin zinc preparation, so that the complexed insulin releases insulin very slowly from the site of injection. It is rarely used now.

Human Insulin (Recombinant)

These are prepared by recombinant DNA technology. It has the same amino acid sequences with the natural human insulin. Like the highly purified pork insulin, it is prepared in three forms such as human regular insulin, human lente insulin, and human isophane insulin. The human Mixtard insulin contains the mixture of human soluble (regular) insulin (30%) and human isophane insulin (70%) or 50:50 ratio.

Human lente insulin is no longer prepared in USA now. It is proved that the human insulin is not superior to pork MC insulin. The only indication for the transfer from the purified pork MC insulin to the human insulin is allergy to the pork insulin. However, it is unwise to transfer from one species to another species of insulin preparation without any good reason.

Insulin Analogs

These insulins are also produced by recombinant DNA technology like human insulin. Here, intentionally the amino acid sequences of the natural human insulin are slightly changed. As a result, the pharmacokinetic effects (onset and duration of action) of these recombinant analog insulins become tailored made with same pharmacodynamic (pharmacological) effects like natural insulin.

Insulin Lispro

In this recombinant analog type of insulin, the proline and lysine amino acid at the 28th and 29th position in the β-chain is reversed. Pharmacokinetically, it is very quick and short acting. It is injected subcutaneously, immediately before (0–15 minutes) or after meal and the peak action is obtained within about half to 1 hour after injection. Hence, it offers good control over the postmeal hyperglycemia. So, the doses of lispro insulin can be adjusted according to the quantity of meal and is taken 2–3 times per day.

Insulin Aspart

Here, in the β-chain of natural human insulin, at the position of 28, the proline is replaced by aspartic acid. Its time action profile (pharmacokinetic property) is similar to that of insulin lispro. But, its advantage over lispro is that insulin aspart more closely mimics with the "physiological pattern of insulin release from the pancreas" after meal.

Insulin Glulisine

It is another rapidly acting insulin analog. Here, in the β-chain of natural human insulin at the position of 23 and 29 the asparagine and lysine is replaced by the lysine and glutamic amino acid, respectively. However, all other pharmacokinetic properties of it are similar to insulin lispro.

Insulin Glargine

In this recombinant insulin analog, at the carboxy terminus of β-chain two additional arginine amino acid residues are added and at the 21 position of α chain the asparagine amino acid is replaced by glycine amino acid. It is soluble at pH 4, but precipitates at body pH. Hence, after SC injection a depot is created at the site of injection and then this depot insulin dissociates slowly from this site of depot to enter the circulation. Therefore, the onset of action of this glargine insulin is very slow and no peak effect is reached (peak less insulin). Thus, it always provides a background of a basal low blood level of insulin for 24 hours. So, the fasting and interdigestive blood glucose level is effectively lowered. But, it cannot control the postmeal hyperglycemia which is usually controlled by lispro and aspart insulin. It is given at bed time with the low incidence of midnight hypoglycemia. Because of acidic pH, it cannot be mixed with any other preparation of insulin and it must be injected separately once daily dose through SC route.

Insulin Detemir

This insulin analog is prepared by attaching a fatty acid with the lysine amino acid, presents at the 29th position in the β-chain of insulin. As a result, after SC injection, it binds with the albumin at the injection site and from there the free insulin is released slowly. Its pattern of action (pharmacokinetic) is similar to that of glargine insulin and is given once daily dose.

Insulin Degludec

It is a very ultra-long-acting new insulin analog. Its plasma glucose lowering effect lasts for near about 40 hours and like insulin glargine, it also provide a basal low plasma insulin level. So, an alternate day regimen has been tried, but the result is not so satisfactory. So, it is given as once daily dose with intermittent injection of rapid-acting aspart insulin.

■ ORAL HYPOGLYCEMIC AGENTS

The drug of choice for any type of DM is insulin. But, the main disadvantage of insulin is that till now any preparation of it cannot be given orally. It is used only by injection. So, the orally active agents to reduce the level of blood glucose have always been sought. There are many orally active hypoglycemic agents and they act by different mechanisms. This is very important to an anesthesiologist. According to the mechanism of action, the orally active hypoglycemic agents are classified in the following way.

Classification of Oral Hypoglycemic Agents (Table 2)

Increase Insulin Secretion

- *Sulfonylurea:*
  - *First generation:* Tolbutamide
  - *Second generation:* Glibenclamide, glipizide, gliclazide, and glimepiride
- *Meglitinide analog:* Repaglinide and nateglinide
- *Glucagon-like peptide 1 receptor agonist:* Exenatide and liraglutide
- *Dipeptidyl peptidase 4 (DPP4) inhibitors:* Sitagliptin, vildagliptin, saxagliptin, teneligliptin, and linagliptin.

Overcome Insulin Resistance

- *Biguanide:* Metformin
- *Thiazolidinediones:* Pioglitazone and rosiglitazone

Miscellaneous

- *α-glucosidase inhibitors:* Acarbose and voglibose
- *SGLT-2 inhibitors:* Dapagliflozin, empagliflozin, and canagliflozin

Sulfonylureas

They all act by blocking the ATP-assisted K^+ channel (K^+-ATP channel), resulting depolarization and the secretion of insulin from the β-cells of pancreas. It reduces the level of blood glucose in type 2 DM and even in normal subject. It has no action on type 1 DM, as there is no functioning β-cells (β-cells are destroyed by antibodies) or on pancreatectomy patient. For the function of sulfonylurea, at least 30% β-cells should be present. All the first-generation sulfonylureas are discontinued except tolbutamide. This is also infrequently used now. The second-generation sulfonylureas are 100 times more potent than first generation.

Repaglinide

They act like sulfonylureas on sulfonylurea receptor (SUR) and block the ATP-dependent K^+ channel. Thus, it prevents the hyperpolarization leading to the depolarization of the β-cells of pancreas and release of insulin. Its onset of action is very fast and the duration of action is very short. It is

TABLE 2: Oral hypoglycemic drugs and their uses.

Drug	t1/2 (hour)	Duration of action (hour)	Daily dose	Doses per day
Tolbutamide	6	6–8	0.5–3 g	2–3
Glibenclamide	2–4	24	2.5–15 mg	1–2
Glipizide	3–5	12	5–20 mg	1–2
Gliclazide	10–20	18–24	40–240 mg	1–2
Glimepiride	6–8	24	1–6 mg	1–2
Repaglinide	1	4–6	1–8 mg	3–4
Nateglinide	1–2	2–4	180–480 mg	3–4
Sitagliptin	12–24	24	100 mg	1
Vildagliptin	2–4	12–24	50–100 mg	1–2
Metformin	2–3	6–8	0.5–2.5 g	1–2
Pioglitazone	3–5	24	15–45 mg	1

administered before each meal to control the postprandial hyperglycemia. The dose should be omitted if meal is skipped. Its indications for use are some selected cases of type 2 DM who suffer from severe postprandial hyperglycemia.

Nateglinide

Its mechanism of action is similar to that of repaglinide, but its onset of action is more fast (15 minutes) and duration of action is more short (4 hours) than that of repaglinide.

Glucagon-like Peptide 1 Receptor Agonists

Incretins are the local hormones. They are secreted from the gut in response to the ingestion of glucose and stimulate the β-cells of pancreas to secret insulin. Among all the incretins, the GLP-1 is an important incretin and it promotes the release of insulin from the β-cells of pancreas. But, this GLP-1 cannot be used clinically. Because, it is rapidly degraded by an enzyme, named DPP4 enzyme, presents in the gut mucosa, liver, kidney, etc. Hence, clinically the synthetic GLP-1 analogs, such as *exenatide and liraglutide*, which are DPP4 resistant, are used to promote the release of insulin from the β-cells of pancreas. However, they are inactive orally and are always used through SC route. The main adverse effect of these two GLP-1 receptor agonists is acute pancreatitis. *Albiglutide* and *dulaglutide* are very long-acting GLP-1 analogs and are injected once weekly.

Dipeptidyl Peptidase 4 Inhibitors

The DPP4 is an enzyme which is normally present in the gut mucosa. It breaks the endogenously secreted GLP-1 from the gut which is an incretin and helps in the release of insulin from the β-cells of pancreas. Now, if we inhibit this

DPP4 enzyme, then the GLP-1 incretin will accumulate and will release insulin from the β-cells of pancreas. This is the mechanism of action of DPP4 inhibitors. Now, these groups of drugs are now available worldwide. The clinical efficacy of all the members of DPP4 inhibitors are more or less same and are used as the first line of oral hypoglycemic agent. All they have long duration of action (24 hours) and are used as once daily dose. Now, the clinically used DPP4 inhibitors are *sitagliptin, vildagliptin, and saxagliptin, teneligliptin.*

Biguanide

There are two biguanides: (1) phenformin and (2) metformin. Among these, phenformin is withdrawn from clinical use throughout the whole world including India. So, only *metformin* is now in clinical use. The mechanism of action of biguanide is somewhat different from the previous group of drugs. It does not increase the secretion of insulin. It only potentiates the insulin-mediated action by activating the adenosine monophosphate (AMP)-dependent protein kinase (AMPK) at the cytoplasmic end of the β-unit of insulin receptor. Thus, it overcomes the insulin resistance. It reduces the blood sugar by (i) suppressing the hepatic gluconeogenesis, (ii) increasing the insulin-mediated glucose uptake, (iii) promoting the peripheral glucose metabolism through anaerobic glycolysis, etc. As it does not help in insulin release, so it does not cause hypoglycemia in nondiabetic person and in diabetic individual also. Metformin promotes anaerobic glycolysis. So, the lactic acid level is increased. But, this lactic acidosis is very rare. Alcohol ingestion can precipitate lactic acidosis.

Pioglitazone

It is completely a separate class of drug. It does not release insulin. It acts at DNA level. It acts as selective agonist for nuclear peroxisome proliferator-activated receptor-γ (PPAR-γ) which is expressed mainly in fat and muscle cells and thus enhances the transcription of several insulin responsive genes. Hence, the glitazones tend to reverse the insulin resistance by enhancing the expression (synthesis) and translocation of GLUT4 receptor (protein) and thus the entry of glucose into fat and muscle cells. Hepatic neoglucogenesis is suppressed. The activation of gene regulating fatty acid metabolism contributes to the insulin sensitizing (overcoming resistance) action of it. In addition, the pioglitazone lowers serum triglyceride level and raises HDL level without much changes in low-density lipoprotein (LDL) level. As it does not increase insulin level, so it is not used in type 1 DM. The pioglitazone is primarily used to supplement the sulfonylureas or metformin in case of insulin

resistance. It may be used as monotherapy along with diet and exercise in mild cases. Some cases of liver dysfunction and congestive heart failure (CHF) have been reported during the use of this drug. So, in such circumstances, it is better not to use this drug. All the pharmacological actions and adverse effects of *rosiglitazone* are similar to that of pioglitazone.

Acarbose and Voglibose

The α-glucosidase is the final enzyme for the digestion of carbohydrate on the brush border of small intestine. The acarbose and voglibose inhibit this enzyme and decreases the digestion and absorption of polysaccharides. Thus, the postprandial hyperglycemia is reduced without significant increase in the secretion of insulin. It does not cause hypoglycemia during its monotherapy. The small fraction of the dose is absorbed. The main disadvantage of acarbose is flatulence, abdominal discomfort, and loose stool. This is due to the fermentation of unabsorbed carbohydrate.

SGLT2 Inhibitors

Practically, all the glucose are filtered at glomerulus and are again reabsorbed in proximal tubules (PTs) by sodium-glucose cotransporter 2 (SGLT2). All the gliflozins (*dapagliflozin, empagliflozin, canagliflozin*, etc.) block these SGLT2 and glucose is not absorbed in the PT of nephron. Hence, the glucose will be excreted through urine and the blood glucose will be lowered. The drawbacks of all the gliflozins are that they cause glycosuria, predisposing to ↑urinary frequency, ↑electrolyte imbalance, ↑urinary tract infection (UTI), ↑genital infection, etc.

◼ ANESTHESIA

The number of patients suffering from DM and presenting for anesthesia and different types of surgeries are gradually increasing. This is mainly due to the increase in the number of patients suffering from type 2 DM not type 1 DM. The type of surgeries may vary from minor day-case surgery requiring only topical anesthesia [such as extracapsular cataract extraction by phacoemulsification and intraocular lens (IOL) implantation] to infiltration block to spinal or epidural block to prolonged complicated cardiac and neurosurgery requiring postoperative intense ICU management. Hence, according to the type of surgery, the mode of anesthesia also should be tailor made. Therefore, according to this tailor made mode of anesthesia, the perioperative blood sugar control also should be more or less intensified. The patients suffering from type 2 DM do not benefit much from tight perioperative control of blood sugar unless they need intensive care. The type 1 DM needs the tight control of blood sugar perioperatively by insulin only.

The major risk factors for DM undergoing anesthesia and surgery are the end-organ damage causing: (i) cardiovascular dysfunction, (ii) renal insufficiency, (iii) neuropathies, (iv) autonomic dysfunction, (v) inadequate granulocyte production, (vi) infection, (vii) poor wound healing, etc. The preoperative proper investigations of these systems (cardiac, pulmonary, renal, and nervous) and the measurement of HbA1c in blood may help in identifying those patients who are at greater risk, increased complications, and worse postoperative outcome.

The preoperative chest radiograph in diabetic patient is must. It may likely to uncover the cardiac enlargement, pulmonary vascular congestion, or pleural effusion. In preoperative ECG, the diabetics have the increased incidences of ST segment T-wave abnormalities (coronary ischemia). The echocardiography may show the different abnormalities of (i) cardiac wall motion, (ii) ejection fraction, (iii) cardiac systolic and diastolic function, etc. due to coronary ischemia and microangiopathy. The diabetic autonomy neuropathy may limit the cardiac ability to compensate for intravascular volume changes. It may also predispose the patient to cardiovascular instability (postinduction hypotension, sudden cardiac death, cardiac dysrhythmia, QT abnormalities, absence of beat-to-beat variation, etc.). This autonomic dysfunction also contributes to delay in gastric emptying, vomiting, diarrhea (gastroparesis), etc. So, the proper preoperative preparation of diabetic patients by fasting (which may predispose hypoglycemia), metoclopramide, and H_2 blocker or proton pump inhibitor (PPI) is very important.

Renal dysfunction in diabetic patient is manifested by proteinuria and elevated serum creatinine level. So, it should be evaluated properly through investigation of urine and blood. As the uncontrolled chronic hyperglycemia leads to glycosylation of tissue protein, so it limits the mobility of joints by glycosylating the collagen proteins which is predominant in joints. Hence, during the preoperative anesthetic evaluation of patient, the adequate movement of temporomandibular joint, adequate cervical spine mobility should be evaluated which will anticipate difficult tracheal intubation.

The DM causes accelerated aging. Thus, the anesthetic risks involved in diabetes are similar to those for someone who are much older than age. The regional anesthesia (spinal and epidural) are not contraindicated in diabetic patients who have well controlled preoperative blood sugar level diagnosed by HbA1c level. But, the following consideration should be kept in mind that local anesthetic (LA) requirement is less and risk of nerve injury is high.

In addition, the combination of epinephrine with LA agents may cause even the greater risk for ischemic nerve injury in diabetes.

The nosocomial infection rates can be reduced by perioperative tight control of blood glucose. The long standing, but well-controlled DM does not appear as important cause for any complication. But, the different end-organ dysfunction due to previous less controlled diabetes is important cause for complications. The perioperative tight control of blood glucose has definite benefit on certain cases, such as pregnant diabetic, diabetic undergoing cardiopulmonary bypass, those who have global central nervous system (CNS) ischemia, and those patients who require the postoperative care in ICU, and patients suffering from type 1 DM.

But, the perioperative tight control provides the little benefit to other group of patients who do not need intensive care in ICU. In these groups of patients, the primary aim of perioperative blood sugar management should be to avoid the hypoglycemia. However, although the tight control of blood sugar is unnecessary for these nonintense groups, but the unnecessary poor control of blood sugar above 180–200 mg/dL also carries the risk causing hyperosmolarity, infection, poor wound healing, etc.

Due to the dependency of brain on glucose, both the hyper- and hypoglycemia worsen the neurological outcome following an episode of cerebral ischemia. During anesthesia, the main focus of an anesthetist should be on the different types of end-organ dysfunction. Because, the diabetes and blood sugar level itself do not appear as an important issue (except ketoacidosis, hyperosmolar nonketotic coma, and hypoglycemia), provided if there is no end-organ diseases such as macrovascular diseases (coronary artery diseases, cerebral vascular diseases, peripheral vascular diseases, etc.), microvascular diseases (retinopathy, nephropathy, etc.), and nervous system diseases (autonomic nervous system neuropathy, peripheral neuropathy, etc.). The causes of end-organ dysfunction due to the prolonged uncontrolled diabetes are discussed before. The long-term tight control of blood sugar prevents this end-organ dysfunction.

The infection accounts for the two-thirds of postoperative complications and 20% of perioperative deaths in diabetic patients. Many factors make the diabetic patients vulnerable to infection such as alteration in leukocyte's functions including ↓chemotaxis, ↓phagocytic activity, ↓intracellular killing of bacteria, etc. Keeping blood glucose level around 150 mg/dL appears to maintain the ability of immunoglobulin to precipitate or neutralize the antigen. If the blood glucose level is kept below 200 mg/dL, then the phagocytic function of granulocytes is improved and the intracellular killing of bacteria is restored to normal level.

Many diabetic patients require emergency surgery following the accident or trauma and they have significant metabolic decompensation. In such circumstances, very little time is available for the stabilization of patient. But, this little time is sufficient to correct the fluid volume, electrolyte and pH, but not the blood sugar. If there is ketosis, then it is futile to delay the surgery in an attempt to eliminate the ketosis completely. Because, if the surgery is delayed, then the underlying causes will lead to the further metabolic deterioration. The intraoperative cardiac arrhythmia and hypotension, resulting from ketoacidosis, will be reduced, the intravascular volume depletion and hypokalemia are at least partially treated.

During the immediate reduction of blood sugar, the regular or lispro insulin is given IV in bolus doses and then by continuous infusion. The first bolus dose of insulin varies between 10 and 20 units. This depends on the present blood sugar level of patient and anesthetist's experience. The infusion rate of insulin per hour is determined easily by dividing the last blood glucose level by 150. During this emergency control of blood glucose level, the total amount of insulin administered is less important than the regular monitoring of blood glucose level, pH, and serum electrolyte level. The maximum permissible level of the reduction of blood glucose is 70–100 mg/hour, regardless of the dose of insulin. In the initial phase, the IV fluid obviously should not contain any glucose. When the blood glucose level will come down to around 200 mg/dL, then the IV fluid includes 5% dextrose with insulin.

The amount of fluid required for the resuscitation of patient will depend on the amount of loss, the acuteness of loss, and the cardiovascular status of patient. If there is no acute loss of fluid, then the one-third of total fluid deficit is corrected during the first 6–8 hours and the remaining two-thirds is corrected over the next 24 hours. Generally, there is hyponatremia and this is fictitious due to hyperglycemia or hypertriglyceridemia. The plasma Na^+ concentration decreases by about 1–6 mEq/L for every 100 mg/dL increase in blood glucose level. The degree of acidosis is determined blood pH, PCO_2, HCO_3^- level, and anion gap. The increase in anion gap >16 mEq/L is due to ketone bodies in ketoacidosis or lactic acid in lactic acidosis or increased organic acid due to renal insufficiency.

The diabetic ketoacidosis (DKA) can easily be distinguished from lactic acidosis. The lactic acidosis is easily identified by the elevated plasma lactate (>6 mmol/L) and the absence of ketone bodies in urine and plasma. But, they can coexist when both the lactate and ketone level in plasma will be high. In only DKA, the only ketone bodies and the blood sugar level in plasma will be high. The lactate level in plasma will be below 6 mmol/L. In starvation ketoacidosis,

the blood sugar level will not be high, rather low normal, but the ketone bodies will be high. In alcoholic ketoacidosis, there is history of recent consumption of alcohol. Such patient has disproportionate increase in β-hydroxybutyrate compared to acetoacetate.

The most important electrolyte disturbance in DKA is the total body deficit of K^+. But, there is no hypokalemia in serum. Instead, there is hyperkalemia. With the start of the treatment by insulin, the serum K^+ level declines rapidly due to its intracellular shifting resulting in the further lowering of serum K^+ level. So, during the management of DKA, aggressive K^+ replacement therapy is required with insulin. K^+ moves into the cell with insulin and correct the total body K^+. Because, though there is hyperkalemia, still there is intracellular K^+ deficit. In DKA, the total body K^+ deficit is due to the increased excretion of it through urine. This is because, there is increased delivery of Na^+ to the distal renal tubules that accompanies volume expansion. In DKA, there is also the deficiency of phosphorus and it is approximately 1 mmol/kg of body weight. The deficiency of phosphorus is due to the increased tissue catabolism and increased urinary loss. This phosphorus deficiency causes organ dysfunction and muscular weakness. The replacement of phosphorus is needed, if the plasma concentration decreases below 1 mg/dL.

The principal key for the perioperative blood glucose control is to set a clear goal. Then, an anesthetist must frequently monitor the blood glucose and adjust the therapy to reach this goal. The tight control of perioperative blood glucose does not give any benefit for the type 2 diabetic patients, unless they need intensive care in ICU. The tight control of blood sugar during the perioperative period has a definite benefit in type 1 DM, pregnancy, expected CNS insult, and some other types of complicated surgeries.

Basically, there are two regimens for the perioperative control of blood sugar, though there are many protocols made by the anesthetist yourself from their own experiences.

1. *Nontight control regimen* for day case or other simple surgeries when the ICU care is not expected, no excessive fluid or blood loss, no end-organ dysfunction, and there is previous chronic good control of blood sugar. In this regimen, the patient should be given nothing per mouth after midnight. The time of surgery should be fixed on the next day morning. On the next day morning, the blood sugar is checked and 5% dextrose is started through IV infusion at a rate of 125 mL/hour/ 70 kg of body weight. After starting the IV infusion, half of the usual morning dose of insulin is given through the subcutaneous route. Usually, the NPH insulin is used. The intraoperative hyperglycemia (180–200 mg/dL) is treated by the intravenous regular or lispro or aspart insulin according to the sliding scale, and supplemental

dextrose is administered if the patient becomes hypoglycemic (<70 mg/dL). One unit of regular insulin lowers the blood glucose 30 g/dL.

An alternative method against this subcutaneous NPH insulin is the continuous infusion of regular or lispro insulin. The advantage of this technique is the better control of blood sugar than the subcutaneous NPH insulin. Here, the 250 units of regular or lispro or aspart insulin is added in 250 mL of normal saline and infusion is started at the rate of 1–2 unit/hour (or blood glucose level/150 = unit of insulin/hour) through a separate line. The general target for intraoperative blood sugar level should be <180–200 mg/dL. It will be better if blood sugar is maintained between 120 and 150 mg/dL. It will be prudent if 20 mEq of KCl is added to each liter of fluid. Because, insulin causes the intracellular shift of K^+ and hypokalemia in the face of total body K^+ deficit.

If the intraoperative fluid loss is within the normal range (no fluid imbalance), then the rate of infusion will be the same, i.e., 125 mL/hour/70 kg of body weight. At the end of the operation and anesthesia, the blood glucose is checked. In the recovery room, the blood glucose level should be monitored on sliding scale.

2. *Tight control regimen when the postoperative ICU care is expected:* Here the aim of this regimen is to keep the blood sugar between 70 and 120 mg/dL. Because, it will improve the wound healing, prevent wound infection, improve neurological outcome if there is any CNS ischemic insult, and improve weaning from ventilators, etc. Like the previous regimen, the patient should be given nothing per mouth after midnight. On the next day morning, blood glucose level is checked. An IV line is instituted and 5% dextrose is started at the rate of 50 mL/hour/70 kg of body weight. A piggy bag infusion of regular insulin containing 50 units in 250 mL of 0.9% normal saline is attached with dextrose IV line through infusion pump. Before attaching this insulin line with dextrose line, the insulin line should be flushed with insulin and dextrose mixture solution and discarded the flushing solution. This approach will saturate the insulin-binding site of plastic tubing. Then, the insulin infusion is started at the rate (unit/hour) which is calculated by dividing the blood sugar level by 150. In this regimen, repeated blood glucose level is measured after every 2–4 hours and the insulin infusion rate is adjusted accordingly. The intraoperative fluid and electrolytes are managed by the administration of nondextrose-containing fluid.

Many patients take oral hypoglycemic agent preoperatively instead of insulin. These groups of patients are maximum, and in such cases, the drug should be continued till the day before surgery and in intraoperative period the blood sugar is controlled by insulin. Some anesthetists stop sulfonylurea and metformin 24–48 hours before surgery, as they are long acting. Some anesthesiologists switch over from oral hypoglycemic agent to insulin preoperatively. Because, the stress of surgery causes the elevation of blood sugar, due to the elevation of catecholamines, glucocorticoids, growth hormone, etc. and inflammatory mediators such as the tumor necrosis factor (TNF) and interleukins (ILs). This is more prudent, except in some very minor surgical procedures where the oral drug can be resumed very quickly. However, the key to any management regimen is to monitor the blood glucose level frequently and always an anesthetist will keep in his mind that there is great variation from patient to patient. The patients with type 1 DM need blood glucose management every hour, while the patients with type 2 DM need the monitoring after every 2–4 hours. The whole thing will depend upon the total situation.

During postoperative period, the patients should also be closely monitored by frequent blood sugar measurement, till the IV fluid is omitted, and the patient resumes oral diet. If the large volume of lactate containing IV fluid has been administered intraoperatively, then the blood sugar will rise after 24–48 hours postoperatively.

There are three life-threatening acute complications of DM which may occur during the perioperative period and their management is anesthetist's responsibility. These life-threatening complications are DKA, hyperosmolar nonketotic hyperglycemic coma, and hypoglycemia.

Diabetic Ketoacidosis

Diabetic ketoacidosis generally occurs in type 1 DM (IDDM), but less frequently in type 2 DM. The predisposing factors for DKA are infections, trauma, stress, inadequate dose of insulin, etc. The signs and symptoms of DKA are vomiting, osmotic diuresis, ketonuria, dehydration, acidosis, hyperosmolarity of blood, hypotension, shock, tachycardia, hyperventilation, and the impairment of consciousness. The two main pathologies leading to these conditions are hyperglycemia and ketosis. The mechanisms of DKA are like that:

- Hyperglycemia → glycosuria → osmotic diuresis → loss of electrolytes (Na^+, K^+, Ca^{2+}, and Mg^{2+}) and water → dehydration → hypotension, shock, and tachycardia
- Ketosis → vomiting → dehydration → hypotension
- Acidosis → due to ketone bodies → shifting of K^+ from cells to intercellular and vascular compartment → intracellular K^+ depletion
- Vomiting + osmotic diuresis + hyperventilation → dehydration
- Dehydration + hyperglycemia → hyperosmolarity of blood → intracellular dehydration → impairment of consciousness

- Impairment of consciousness is due to intracellular dehydration and impairment of glucose entry into brain cell due to the lack of insulin.

The principal treatment of DKA includes IV fluid, insulin, KCl, Na-bicarbonate, and the removal of cause. As the DKA is a life-threatening condition, so according to severity, the promptness of management should be matched. The IV fluid is very essential to correct dehydration. Normal saline is started initially at a rate of 1–2 L/hour. Then, according to the condition of patient (BP, HR, renal perfusion, etc.), the rate of infusion is slowed to 0.5 L/hours to 0.5 L/4 hours. When the blood glucose level will fall to 200 mg/dL then IV 5% glucose will be started. Because, the blood glucose usually falls before ketone bodies are completely cleared from circulation. Also, the glucose is required to restore the depleted glycogen from liver.

Along with the beginning of IV fluid insulin therapy is started. First a bolus dose of 0.1–0.2 unit/kg of regular insulin is given through IV route. This is followed by 0.1–0.2 unit/kg/hour infusion. The expected fall of blood glucose level is 10% of pretreatment value per hour and will indicate adequate response. Sometimes, due to the resistance of insulin, there is no response. In such circumstances, insulin infusion rate should be doubled. Usually, within 4–6 hours the blood glucose level reaches to 200–300 mg/dL and then insulin infusion rate should be halved. This should be continued till the consciousness is regained. After that, the routine subcutaneous insulin is reinstituted.

As it is previously said that in DKA there is depletion of total body K^+ due its loss through urine. But, still there is normal to high serum K^+ level due to the shifting of it from intracellular space. So, with the start of insulin therapy, K^+ moves into the cell and there is severe hypokalemia. So, with the institution of insulin therapy, K^+ is given in the form of KCl at the rate of 10–20 mEq/hour. And this should be monitored by serial serum K^+ measurement and ECG.

There is some controversy regarding the use of $NaHCO_3$ to correct the acidosis. Because, this acidosis in DKA is automatically corrected if the ketosis and blood glucose level is corrected. The only indication for its use is if the blood pH is <7.1 and is not corrected by hyperventilation and insulin therapy. The infusion of bicarbonate is continued slowly till the blood pH rises above 7.2.

Hyperosmolar (Nonketotic Hyperglycemic) Coma

It occurs mainly in type 2 DM and the exact cause of it is still obscure. But, the probable mechanism of it is that the uncontrolled glycosuria produces the osmotic diuresis resulting in dehydration and hemoconcentration. The urine output gradually falls. The blood sugar gradually rises (>800 mg/dL) and the plasma osmolarity elevates (>350 mOsm/L). This leads to coma and death if the patient is not treated vigorously. The principal of treatment is more or less same as DKA. But, the faster fluid therapy is instituted to reduce the osmolarity. Like type 1 DM, as the insulin deficiency is not so prominent, so the ketone body formation and acidosis is not so problem. The main problem is elevated plasma osmolarity. Despite intensive therapy, the mortality in hyperosmolar coma remains high.

Textbook of
Anesthesia
for Postgraduates

Complimentary Slides

Available complimentary PPTs for easy understanding of the following topics:

- Anesthetic Machine
- Anesthetic Delivery System
- Anesthetic Instruments
- Vaporizers
- Capnography
- Oxygen
- ECG
- Local Anesthetic Agents
- Intravenous Anesthetics
- Inhalational Anesthetics
- Muscle Relaxants
- Mechanical Ventilation

To access the PPTs, simply scan this QR code.

Textbook of
Anesthesia
for Postgraduates

Second Edition

VOLUME 1

TK Agasti
MBBS (Kol) DGO (Kol) DA (Kol) MD (Guj)

Consultant Anesthetist
Zenith Super Specialist Hospital
Midland Multidisciplinary Hospital
Disha Eye Hospital
Kolkata, West Bengal, India

Foreword
Atul Prabhakar Kulkarni

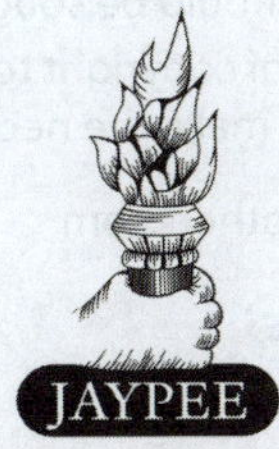

JAYPEE BROTHERS MEDICAL PUBLISHERS
The Health Sciences Publisher
New Delhi | London

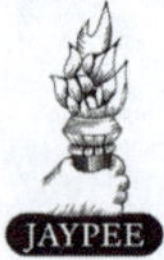

Jaypee Brothers Medical Publishers (P) Ltd

Headquarters

Jaypee Brothers Medical Publishers (P) Ltd
EMCA House, 23/23-B
Ansari Road, Daryaganj
New Delhi 110 002, India
Landline: +91-11-23272143, +91-11-23272703
+91-11-23282021, +91-11-23245672
Email: jaypee@jaypeebrothers.com

Corporate Office

Jaypee Brothers Medical Publishers (P) Ltd
4838/24, Ansari Road, Daryaganj
New Delhi 110 002, India
Phone: +91-11-43574357
Fax: +91-11-43574314
Email: jaypee@jaypeebrothers.com

Overseas Office

JP Medical Ltd.
83, Victoria Street, London
SW1H 0HW (UK)
Phone: +44 20 3170 8910
Fax: +44 (0)20 3008 6180
Email: info@jpmedpub.com

Website: www.jaypeebrothers.com
Website: www.jaypeedigital.com

© 2024, Jaypee Brothers Medical Publishers

The views and opinions expressed in this book are solely those of the original contributor(s)/author(s) and do not necessarily represent those of editor(s) or publisher of the book.

All rights reserved. No part of this publication may be reproduced, stored or transmitted in any form or by any means, electronic, mechanical, photocopying, recording or otherwise, without the prior permission in writing of the publishers.

All brand names and product names used in this book are trade names, service marks, trademarks or registered trademarks of their respective owners. The publisher is not associated with any product or vendor mentioned in this book.

Medical knowledge and practice change constantly. This book is designed to provide accurate, authoritative information about the subject matter in question. However, readers are advised to check the most current information available on procedures included and check information from the manufacturer of each product to be administered, to verify the recommended dose, formula, method and duration of administration, adverse effects and contraindications. It is the responsibility of the practitioner to take all appropriate safety precautions. Neither the publisher nor the author(s)/editor(s) assume any liability for any injury and/or damage to persons or property arising from or related to use of material in this book.

This book is sold on the understanding that the publisher is not engaged in providing professional medical services. If such advice or services are required, the services of a competent medical professional should be sought.

Every effort has been made where necessary to contact holders of copyright to obtain permission to reproduce copyright material. If any have been inadvertently overlooked, the publisher will be pleased to make the necessary arrangements at the first opportunity.

Inquiries for bulk sales may be solicited at: jaypee@jaypeebrothers.com

Textbook of Anesthesia for Postgraduates (2 Volumes)

First Edition: 2011
Second Edition: **2024**

ISBN: 978-93-5696-265-1

Printed in India at Rajkamal Electric Press, Kundli, Haryana.

Dedicated to
My loving father and mother

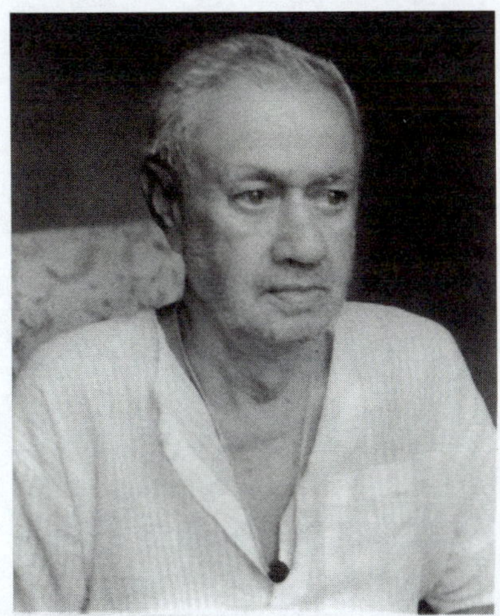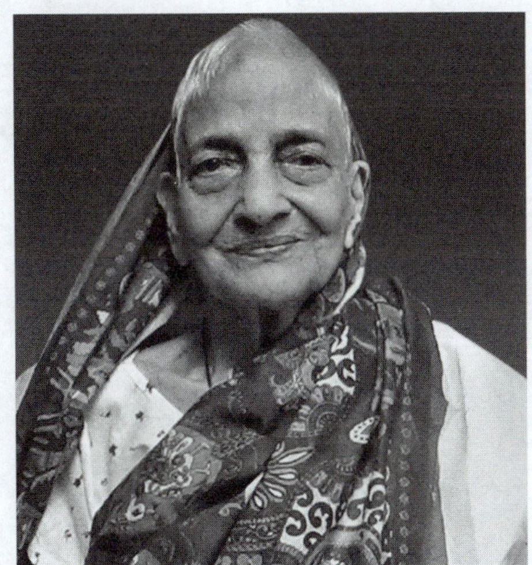

Late Shri Anil Kumar Agasti   **Late Usha Rani Agasti**

Thou hast made me endless, such is thy pleasure.
This frail vessel thou emptiest again and again, and fillest it ever with fresh life.

আমারে তুমি অশেষ করেছ
এমনি লীলা তব।
ফুরায়ে ফেলে আবার ভরেছ
জীবন নব নব।

—*Rabindra Nath Tagore*

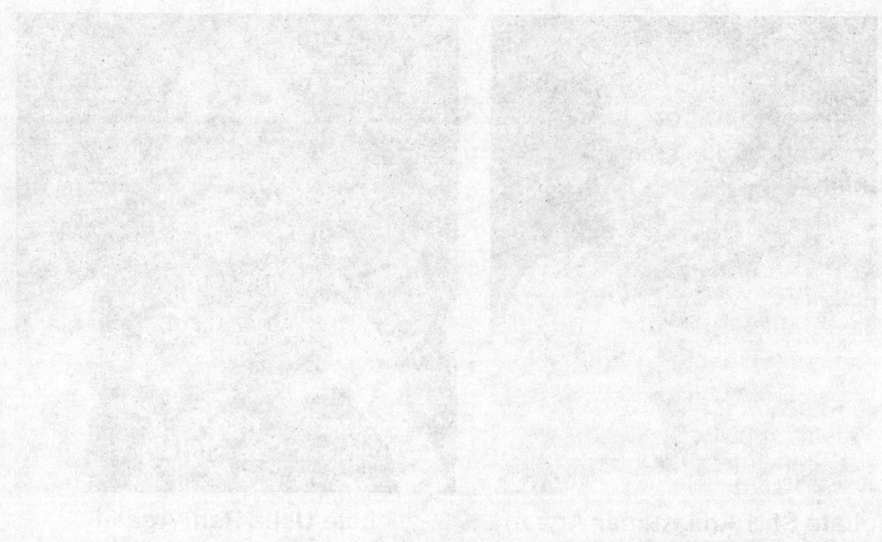

Foreword

It is a great pleasure with which I write this foreword to the *Textbook of Anesthesia for Postgraduates.* John Steinbeck, the great American Nobel Prize winning writer, said "I guess there are never enough books." There are many books on anesthesia, some short, some tiringly long. Contrary to what people often say; what can you write about the same old subject; I believe that a new book always bring out a fresh perspective. Each new book makes us see the same subject in a different light and reading a new book is like meeting a new person for the first time. Each book carries its own personality, along with subtle nuanced differences.

I am happy to see that *Textbook of Anesthesia for Postgraduates* covers all topics of relevance to the postgraduate students. It discusses the fundamental principles of physiology and describes anesthesia delivery systems and other relevant anesthetic equipment succinctly. All physiological principles are covered briefly without cluttering the minds of the readers with too many details. The anesthesia management in a succinct manner with relevant anatomy, pertinent physiology and with regional anesthesia where relevant, and general anesthesia. A separate chapter covers blood and component transfusion, along with techniques such as apheresis, plasma exchange and complications of transfusion. The book thus manages to a bird's eye view of anesthetic management.

I wish all the best to this new endeavor and hope readers like it as much as I do.

Atul Prabhakar Kulkarni
MD (Anesthesiology) FISCCM PGDHHM FICCM
Professor and Head
Department of Critical Care Medicine
Tata Memorial Centre
Mumbai, Maharashtra, India

Preface to the Second Edition

The subject, anesthesiology, is mainly studied at the level of postgraduate, after passing MBBS, without giving much emphasis, during the course of undergraduate. But, this interesting branch of medical science involves the extensive knowledge of all preclinical and clinical subjects. When this knowledge is incorporated with some special knowledge of patient's condition during trauma, pain, severe medical illness, surgery, and how a patient is kept unconscious during surgery without any or minimum alteration of body physiology, then a new subject called "anesthesiology" is evolved.

Specialization in this subject of anesthesiology does not involve the specialization on a single organ such as skin, eye, heart, etc., or a single system such as gastrointestinal system, nervous system, urinary system, etc. Moreover, this subject of anesthesiology incorporates knowledge of many diseases and the effect of surgery and anesthesia on these diseases and handles many cardiotoxic and nephrotoxic drugs which are not used by the specialists of other disciplines of medical science. It also involves multiple sophisticated and complicated machines and equipment for the delivery of anesthesia and monitoring of patients during the surgery and anesthesia and also during the recovery of an already very sick patient from anesthesia after surgery which cannot be imagined in the other subjects of medicine. Further, this subject of anesthesiology is gradually becoming very vast, as the equipment, used in other discipline of medicine, are also gradually incorporating in this subject, such as USG machine for nerve block and intravenous or intra-arterial cannulation and different models of ICU ventilators in critical care medicine, etc. An anesthesiologist also must have to keep adequate knowledge regarding all the advancement of other disciplines of medicine.

There are many books which help the students during the study of postgraduate course in anesthesiology. But still the students require the help of many preclinical and clinical books of anatomy, physiology, pharmacology, medicine, etc. for the meticulous understanding of this subject of anesthesiology. So, during the study of postgraduate course of anesthesiology, referring to too many books on preclinical and clinical subjects makes the students confuse, irritation and helplessness. Therefore, in this book, an earnest attempt has been made to fill all the gaps, so that the postgraduate students of anesthesiology course do not have to go through other preclinical and clinical books.

There is no end for knowledge. So, as the provider of knowledge, no book can be complete. If an author shifts toward more completeness of his or her book, then its volume increases tremendously which may also be irritating and troublesome to many students. So, there should be a compromise between the information provided by a book and the volume of this book. Every new book gives some new information and so I also have tried my level best to provide these new information in my book which will help the students without going through many books, I think.

I have added two new chapters such as (i) blood transfusion, and (ii) diabetes mellitus and anesthesia in the second edition of this book. I have tried my level best to correct the mistakes which were found in the first edition of my book. But, still, despite my best intention, I fear that errors will be found in this edition also. So, I apologize to my readers for that. I will be grateful to my readers, who will help to improve this edition. I make an earnest request to all my readers to e-mail me at *agastitusar@gmail.com* if they find any error in this edition of the book. Any suggestion from any reader is also welcome at this e-mail address. I will also be grateful to my readers, if they go through Internet for better pictures and videos which is not possible to incorporate all these in one book.

There is nothing more to write. So, at the end, thanking all, I am starting my second voyage.

TK Agasti
agastitusar@gmail.com

Preface to the First Edition

The anaesthesiology is a subject which is mainly studied at the postgraduate level, after passing MBBS, without giving much emphasis during the undergraduate course. But, this interesting branch of medical science involves the knowledge of all preclinical and clinical subjects just like the branch of medicine of medical science. When this knowledge is incorporated with some special knowledge of patient's condition during trauma, pain, severe medical illness, surgery and anaesthesia, then a new subject called anaesthesiology is evolved.

Just like specialising on the subject of medicine, the specialisation in this subject of anaesthesiology also does not involve a single organ such as skin, eye, heart, etc. or a single system such as gastrointestinal system, nervous system, etc. Moreover, this subject of anaesthesiology links many disease processes with surgery and handles many cardiotoxic drugs which are not used by the specialists of other disciplines of medical science. It also involves multiple sophisticated and complicated machines and equipments for the delivery of anaesthesia, monitoring of patients during surgery and also during recovery of already very sick patients which cannot be imagined in other subject of medicines.

Moreover, this subject of anaesthesiology is very vast. It is linked with all the disciplines of medical science and also infiltrates the other specialities like critical care, trauma, pain management, intensive care, etc. This branch of medical science has also changed drastically during the last few years in terms of technology, for maximum safety of patients. All these lead to extreme work load, necessity of advanced knowledge and intense responsibilities of anaesthesiologist.

There are many books which helps the students during the study of postgraduate course in anaesthesiology. But still the students are required to take the help of many preclinical and clinical books of anatomy, physiology, pharmacology, medicine, etc. for meticulous understanding. So referring to too many books confuses the students causing irritation and even helplessness. Hence, in this book an earnest attempt has been made to fill all the gaps so that students do not have to go through other preclinical and clinical books.

There is no end to knowledge. So as the provider of knowledge, no book can be complete. If an author shift towards the more completeness of a book, then its volume increase tremendously which may also be irritating and troublesome to many students. So, there should be a compromise between the information provided and the volume of book. Every new book gives some new information and I have tried my level best to collect all these information in my book which helps the students without going through many books, I think.

Many chapters are also lacking in this edition of my book which I commit to provide in the subsequent editions. So, I am regretful to my readers. I think there are many mistakes in this first edition of my book which is very obvious. For this I also apologise to my readers. I make an earnest appeal to all my readers to communicate with me regarding any mistake in my book and/or suggestions, if they have any.

At the end there is nothing more to write. So, thanking all, I start my first voyage towards the deep and vast ocean of knowledge of all readers of my book.

TK Agasti
agastitusar@gmail.com

Acknowledgments

I am extremely grateful to all my colleagues who consistently inspire me to write a book on anesthesiology which must cover the anatomy, physiology, pharmacology, medicine, and the historical aspects of all the chapters which are lacking in most of the commonly available books on anesthesiology. I am greatly indebted to my wife, Dr Bidisha Agasti and to my son, Tamoghna Agasti who constantly inspire me to write a book which is get rid of complex scientific experiments and their inferences that make the students very tired and confused. I am paying my sincere and boundless thank to Dr Debasish Bhattacharya, Director of Disha Eye Hospital at Barrackpore, Kolkata and Dr Tapan Kundu, Director of Zenith Super Specialist Hospital at Dunlop, Kolkata, West Bengal, for being my friend, philosopher, and guide. I will also take the opportunity to thank to Dr Samar Basak, a world-famous ophthalmologist for being my inspiration.

Finally, I am grateful to all my patients who had submitted themselves for anesthesia and permitted me to learn the subject of anesthesiology. At last, I am also grateful to M/s Jaypee Brothers Medical Publishers (P) Ltd, New Delhi, for publishing this book in a very presentable manner in a very short time.

TK Agasti
agastitusar@gmail.com

Contents

Anesthetic Machine

■ INTRODUCTION

The Boyle's anesthetic machine is a continuous flow type of anesthetic equipment which is used for the administration of inhalational anesthesia and artificial ventilation. It receives gas supply from different gas supply units, consisting of *cylinders* or *pipelines*. These gas supply units and the machine have different control systems to regulate the flow of gases to the machine and to its flow meter, by reducing their pressure to the desired safe level. The Boyle's anesthetic machine also has vaporizers that vaporizes the volatile anesthetic agents and finally delivers a gas mixture to the breathing circuit.

It was introduced first by HEG Boyle (Henry Edmund Gaskin Boyle), in 1917. After that, it was modified at different times, by different persons, and different companies which are discussed in more details in "Inhalation Anesthesia" Chapter 15. Now, it has become more modernized by attaching (i) all essential monitors (capnograph, pulse oximeter, oxygen analyzer in fresh gas flow, anesthetic gas analyzer, spirometer, airway pressure monitor, etc.), (ii) all essential alarms (oxygen failure alarm, ventilator alarms, multimonitor's alarms, etc.), (iii) ventilators, (iv) suction port, (v) auxiliary O_2 source, (vi) provision for closed and semiclosed circuits, (vii) scavenging system, (viii) multiple storage drawers for equipment, and (ix) electric plugs integrated as a single unit.

The anesthetic machine, invented by HEG Boyle in 1917, is actually the modification of American Gwathmey apparatus of 1912. The Boyle's apparatus was first commercially made by Coxeter and sons. It was later acquired by the British Oxygen Company (BOC). "Boyle" is the trade name of BOC. It was named so to respect the inventor. However, HEG Boyle was not the pioneer in manufacturing of anesthetic machine. Two other great men had done excellent work before him. One was James Taylor Gwathmey who was practicing in New York and invented the Gwathmey machine in 1912. Later, Geoffrey Marshal had developed a machine during the First World War in 1914, based on the Gwathmey machine. Boyle had developed his machine from Gwathmey's basic model in 1917 and presented his invention to the Royal Society of Medicine in London in 1918. Even though Marshal had developed his machine much before Boyle, but he presented his machine before the medical community, much later than Boyle. So all the credit goes to the Boyle.

- *In 1921:* Waters to-and-fro absorption apparatus was introduced.
- *In 1927:* Flow meter for carbon dioxide was included. The volatile controls were of the lever type and the familiar back bar made its first appearance.
- *In 1930:* The plunger of the vaporizer had appeared.
- *In 1930:* The circle absorption system was introduced by Brain Sword.
- *In 1933:* Dry bobbin flow meter was introduced.
- *In 1952:* The pin index safety system (PISS) was introduced by Woodbridge.
- *In 1958:* The Bodok seal was introduced.

Also, the Boyle's anesthetic machine have become more extremely sophisticated by incorporating (1) many built in safety features and (2) one or more microprocessors that can integrate, enhance, and automatically monitor all the components of machine. These microprocessors of ventilators, now, also provide option for (i) many sophisticated ventilatory modes, (ii) automated record keeping, and (iii) networking with the local or remote computer monitors for information and advice and as well as with hospital information system. So, it (Boyle's anesthetic machine) has evolved from *Boyle's basic* to *Boyle's major* and now it is called the *anesthetic workstation* (**Figs. 1A to C**). Due to this extreme sophistication, lots of adverse outcomes are now coming in front, related to the malfunction of machine. This is mainly because of the nonfamiliarity of an extremely sophisticated anesthetic machine or workstation with the anesthetist. So, these preventable adverse outcomes, resulting many mishaps, can easily be avoided by increasing the familiarity of machine with the anesthetists through proper education, training, and proper checking of the function of machine previously before administering anesthesia (**Fact file I**).

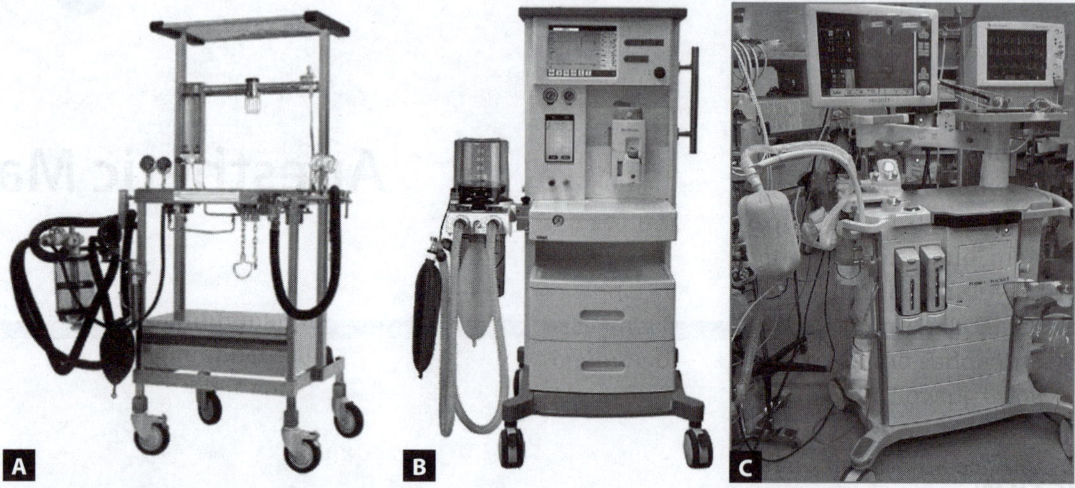

Figs. 1A to C: (A) Boyle's minor anesthetic machine; (B) Boyle's major; and (C) Anesthesia workstation-2.

FACT FILE I

The safety features of modern anesthetic machine or system are:

1. Color-coded cylinders, color-coded pipelines, color-coded hoses, noninterchangeable screw thread (NIST) system, or DISS for connection of color-coded hose pipe to machine from pipeline for central gas supply system and pin index system for cylinders. All these prevent wrong fitting of central supply pipelines and cylinders with machine
2. Color-coded pressure gauges for different gases
3. First stage and second stage pressure regulators
4. When O_2 pressure will be low, the supply of N_2O to patient will be cut off
5. O_2 and N_2O ratio monitor and controller, called hypoxic guard or fail safe valve, stops or decreases flow of other gases, if O_2 pressure falls
6. *Safety features of flow meter:* (i) Color-coded knobs for different gases, (ii) color-coded, more fluted, larger, and protruded O_2 knob, (iii) O_2 tube at the extreme right (downstream) of rotameter, (iv) O_2 and N_2O (or other gases) ratio proportioning system, (v) florescent back panel of rotameter for visualization in dark, (vi) rotameters are hand calibrated to minimize errors, and (vii) rotameters are antistatic to prevent sticking of bobbin to tube
7. *Safety features of vaporizers:* (i) Color-coded markings (chemical formula and name of agent), mentioned on each vaporizer, (ii) color-coded control dial knob, (iii) color-coded filling system, specific for each agent (red → halothane, purple → isoflurane, yellow → sevoflurane and blue → desflurane), (iv) interlock devices which prevent more than one vaporizer to be turned on at the same time, (v) temperature compensated, (vi) flow compensated (increased flow of fresh gas through rotameter does not increase the concentration of agent coming out of vaporizer at a certain setting of control dial, and (vii) not affected by back pressure (pumping effect)
8. *Pressure relief valve:* It opens when there is excessive pressure in machine

9. Oxygen flush can deliver high flow of O_2 during emergency
10. Inspired O_2 concentration (FiO_2) monitor or analyzer detects final delivered concentration of O_2 to the patient
11. Oxygen supply failure audible alarm
12. Alarm during disconnection of ventilator
13. Flow sensor detects ventilatory failure, disconnection, extubation, bronchospasm, etc.
14. *One way check valve:* It is placed before machine's single gas outlet to prevent back-flow effect during positive pressure ventilation
15. The anesthetic machine using central gas pipeline should have at least one O_2 cylinder in reserve
16. Antistatic rubber tyres to prevent current flow

A *modern anesthetic machine consists* of the following *basic components:* (i) multiple gas supplying unit through pipelines or cylinders, (ii) multiple pressure gauges, (iii) first and second stages reducing valves or pressure regulators, (iv) flow meters (rotameter), (v) vaporizers, (vi) common gas outlet, (vii) ventilators, (viii) (closed) circle breathing system, (ix) multimonitors, and (x) miscellaneous, such as emergency O_2 flush, nonreturn pressure relief valve, O_2 supply failure alarm, anesthetic gas analyzing unit, hypoxic guard, suction apparatus, waste scavenging system, etc. **(Fact file II).**

The whole anesthetic machine is divided into two parts: (1) pneumatic parts, and (2) electric or electronic parts. The different pneumatic parts of Boyle's anesthetic machine work on different pressures. So, the whole pneumatic division of an anesthetic machine is again divided into three parts:

1. *High-pressure system:* It extends *from* gas cylinders or pipelines and its entry point *to* first stage pressure reducing valve *through* pin index system or diameter index safety system (DISS). It includes: (i) hanger yoke

FACT FILE II

The components of an anesthetic workstation are:

1. Provision for the secondary (auxiliary) source for the supply of gases in the event of failure of primary source
2. Provision for safe and accurate delivery of anesthetic gases and vapors by electronic rotameter and Aladin agent specific color-coded cassette vaporizers
3. Provision for inbuilt breathing system with circle absorber (using Amsorb or lithium hydroxide) and its related circuits
4. Provision for any respiratory support of patient by sophisticated automatic ventilators with full range of ventilatory modes according to patient's need
5. Provision for monitoring the full range of patient's physiological parameters (pulse oximeter, respiratory rate, capnograph, FiO_2, tidal volume, airway pressure, different pressure–volume curves, pressure–flow curve, etc. with display
6. Provision for monitoring the full range of function and settings of all the components of machine with audio and visual alarm
7. Provision for automatic record keeping
8. Provision for online access to information through internet for expert decision
9. Provision for appropriate connection to an anesthetic gas scavenging system
10. Provision for suction vacuum system with regulator.
11. Provision for auxiliary O_2 flow meter with supplemental O_2 supply
12. Storage facility for items of everyday use

assembly, (ii) DISS or noninterchangeable screw thread (NIST), (iii) cylinder and pipeline pressure gauge, (iv) check valve or first stage pressure regulator (pressure reducing valve), and (v) emergency O_2 flush.

2. *Intermediate-pressure system:* It extends from first stage pressure reducing valve to flow control knobs of rotameter, through second stage pressure reducing valve. It includes: (i) second stage pressure reducing valve (present in some machine) which reduces gas pressure to 15–30 psi, (ii) oxygen failure audio alarm, (iii) fail-safe valve which either cutoff or proportionately decreases the flow of N_2O and other gases with the decrease flow O_2, and (iv) flow control valve in rotameter.

3. *Low-pressure system:* It extends downstream from the flow control knobs of rotameter to common gas outlet. It includes: (i) rotameter (flow meter assembly), (ii) hypoxic prevention devices, (iii) vaporizers and their mounting devices, (iv) unidirectional check valve which prevents the pumping effect, and (v) common gas outlet.

■ GAS SUPPLY UNIT

Pipeline

Now, in a big hospital or nursing home, the supply of gases such as O_2, N_2O, compressed air, etc., through pipelines to many anesthetic machines situated at different operation theater (OT) or to multiple ventilators situated in intensive care unit (ICU), critical care unit (CCU), high-dependency care unit (HDU), etc., from a central source is a common feature. The advantages of supplying gases, through these pipelines from a central source to multiple points, are that it is easy, convenience, economic, and avoid frequent changing of cylinders. There is also less chances of explosion and increased patient's safety. But, the high initial cost is the only disadvantages of it. The pipeline system for the delivery of gases to anesthetic machines or ventilators consist of (i) a central supplying storage unit, using tank or concentrator or cylinders for O_2, only cylinders for N_2O and cylinders or compressor for compressed air and (ii) distributing pipelines with their multiple outlets, located at their multiple points of use, far away from central source. The supplying pipeline is made up of *high quality copper alloy* which *prevents the decomposition of gases* and has *bacteriostatic property*. The usual pressure of gases, kept in pipeline, is about 375–400 kP (kilo Pascal) or 55–58 psi (pound per square inch) or 3.74 kg/cm^2 (1 kP = 0.145 psi and 1 kg/cm^2 = 14.7 psi). However, the size (diameter) of the pipeline differs according to the demand of the different unit of the hospital. The pipes of 42 mm diameter are usually used for leaving the central supply unit and the smaller diameter tubes of 15 mm diameter are used, after repeated branching. They also have specific international color code, according to the gas, they carry, for example: *Oxygen* → white, *Nitrous oxide* → blue, *Air* → black, *Vacuum* → yellow.

The network of central pipelines ultimately terminate in the OT, ICU, CCU, HDU, and/or ward at their terminal outlet which is mounted on the wall **(Fig. 2)** or suspended from ceiling, as arm or gas column. These terminal outlets of pipeline, at their point of use, is easily identified (i) by their specific color code, (ii) by their specific shape, and (iii) by the name of gas stamped on them. They accept the matched and quick connect/disconnect "Schrader" probe, attached with a flexible color code hose, which ultimately connect the terminal outlet of the central pipeline to the anesthetic machine or ventilator **(Fig. 3)**.

The anesthetic machine end of these color-coded hoses may be connected with the machine (i) permanently by a screw and thread system where the screw and thread is gas specific and not interchangeable, known as *NIST* system, or (ii) temporarily through the usual yoke assembly with a specific pin index system. It (pin index system) is located on the metal yoke bar of anesthetic machine, where the cylinders are usually attached. The previously described NIST system of connection on the anesthetic machine, which attaches the hosepipe from the terminal outlet of pipeline to the anesthetic machine, is also known as the DISS where a hose

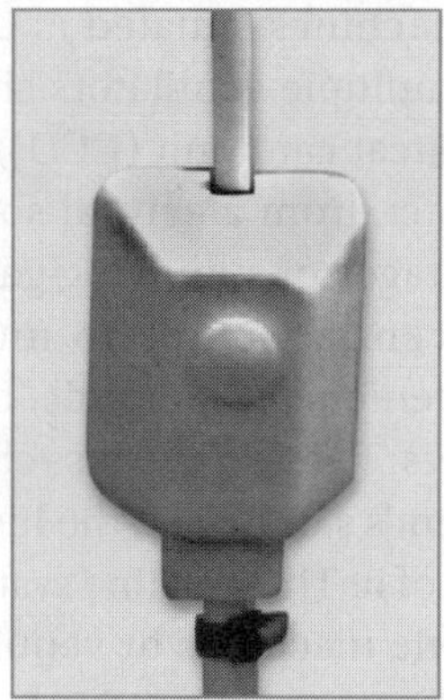

Fig. 2: Wall mounted outlet in operation theater (OT) from the central oxygen pipeline.

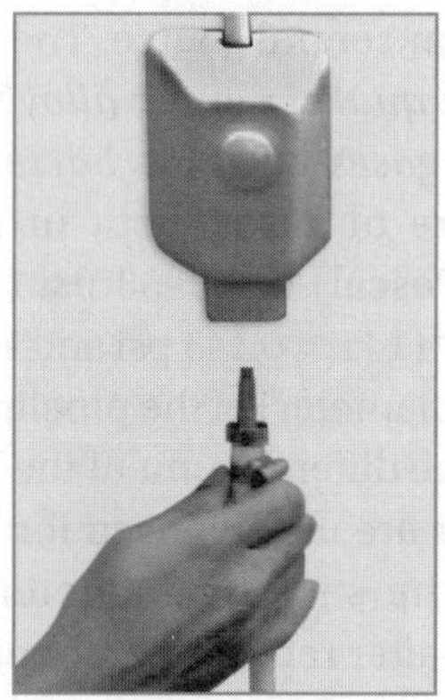

Fig. 3: Flexible color-coded Schrader probe.

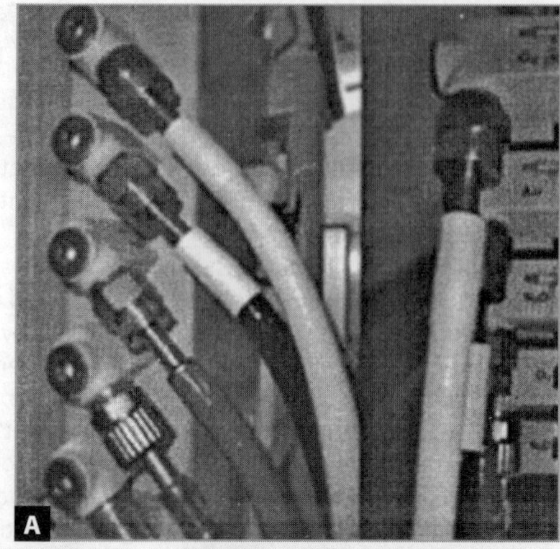

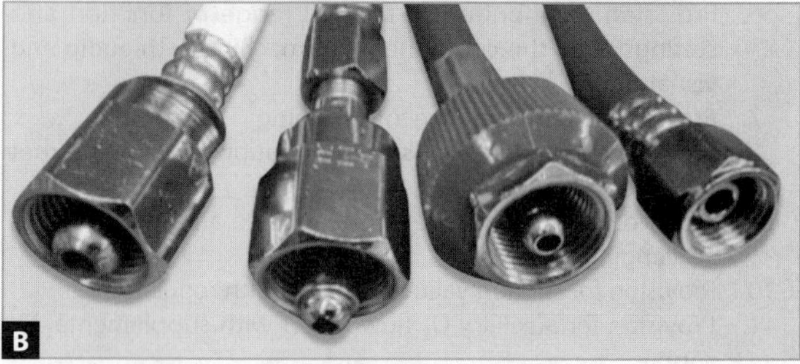

Figs. 4A and B: (A) Hoses with Diameter Index Safety System (DISS) attached with anesthetic machine; (B) Open hoses with DISS.

pipe of a particular diameter for O_2, N_2O, air, and suction line can only be connected to the coupler of that gas, present on anesthetic machine **(Figs. 4A and B)**. But, the disadvantage in this system is that there is delay in connection with this system. So, the quick connect/disconnect "Schrader" couplers are preferred, where its other end is connected to the machine through a pin index system.

At the central gas supplying room, from where the pipelines are distributed, there should have a low-pressure alarm system which will detect the failure of supply of gases through pipeline, due to empty cylinder. A reserve bank of cylinders should be available, if primary supply from cylinders, through pipeline, fails. An anesthetist is only responsible for the supply of gases, *from* the terminal outlet of pipeline *to* the anesthetic machine, in the OT or ICU or HDU. While, the engineering department will be responsible for the supply of gases through the gas pipelines, behind the wall of OT, ICU, HDU, etc. There is also the risk of rupture or fire in pipeline, carrying O_2 under high pressure, from the central source of supply to the machine, due to worn out or damage of it. So, for the maintenance and to avoid any mishap, the pipelines should be tested from time to time, according to the guidelines, laid by the international or national committee. Some examples of such tests are: tug test to detect wrong connection, single hose test to detect cross connection, etc.

The *central sources of gases* which are distributed by the pipeline may be (i) *For O_2:* Liquid O_2 in storage tank or O_2 cylinders arranged in manifold or O_2 concentrator, (ii) *For N_2O:* N_2O cylinders arranged in manifold, and (iii) *For compressed air:* Compressed air cylinders arranged in manifold or air compressor machine.

In *oxygen storage tank,* the O_2 is stored as liquid between $-160°$ to $-170°C$ temperature at a pressure of about 5–10 atmosphere. The capacity of this O_2 storage tank varies according to the need of hospital. The 1 mL of this liquid O_2 at this temperature and pressure gives 840 mL of O_2 as gas at the normal atmospheric temperature ($15°C$) and pressure. Therefore, it (liquid O_2) is very advantageous by storing large amount of O_2 in a small container. Actually, the O_2 storage tank acts as huge thermo flask. It is made up of double layer steel, with vacuum in between them. The inner sides of these two steel layers are lined by a chemical, named perlite. The vacuum between these two steel layers acts as an insulator and maintain the temperature of the inside of the tank. During the use of tank, the evaporation of liquid O_2 requires

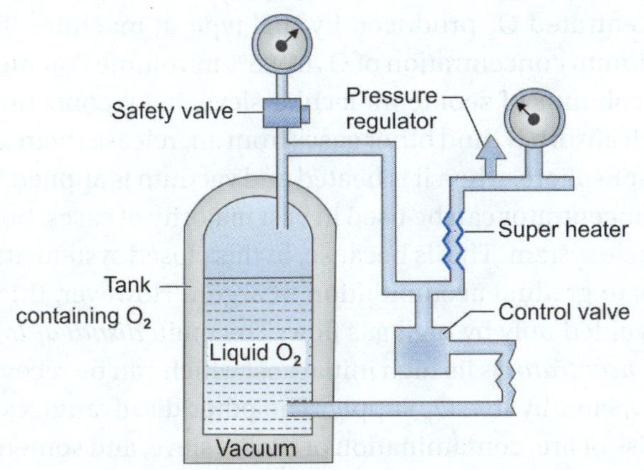

Fig. 5: The schematic diagram of O_2 tank, containing liquid O_2.

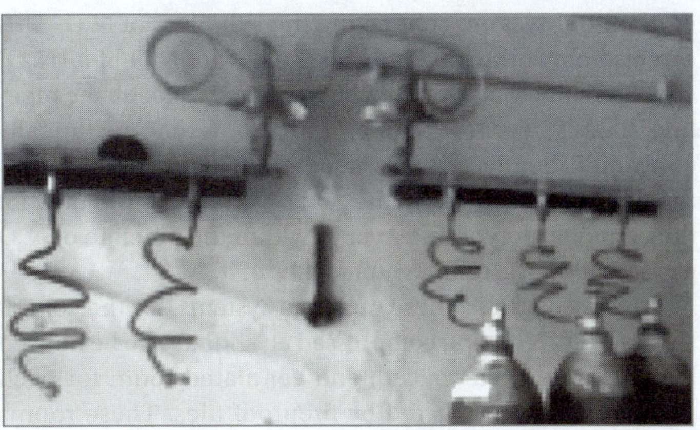

Fig. 6: Cylinder manifold.

heat, which is known as the latent heat of evaporation. It is taken from the remaining liquid O_2 stored in the tank. Thus, it helps to maintain such low temperature of the remaining liquid portion of O_2 inside the tank. By a coiled copper tubing, the cold O_2 gas which comes out from tank is warmed for use **(Fig. 5)**.

Then, a pressure regulator allows the gas to enter the pipelines with pressure at 375–400 kP or 55–58 psi. There is also a safety valve on O_2 storage tank which will allow the gas to escape in environment, only during emergency, when the excessive pressure builds up inside the tank, during no use or under (less) demand of use of O_2. During excessive use of O_2 the control valve, which is usually kept closed, is opened and it allows the liquid O_2 to pass through an uninsulated coils of copper tube. Thus, during this excessive use, the passage of liquid O_2 through this uninsulated copper tube, allow it (O_2) to evaporate within the tube and can supply more O_2 as gas. The storage O_2 tank usually rests on a weighing balance. It measures the mass of liquid O_2 in tank and thus gives an idea of the total contents of the tank.

A *differential pressure gauge* is also used which measures the difference of pressure between the liquid O_2 at the bottom and the gaseous O_2 at the top of the tank and gives an idea of the total contents of both the liquid and gaseous O_2 in a tank. This is because, as the liquid O_2 evaporates, its mass and pressure at the bottom decreases. So, by measuring this difference in pressure between the bottom and the top, the actual contents of the tank are calculated. At one atmospheric pressure and 15°C temperature, 1 L of liquid O_2 gives 842 L of gaseous O_2. When the supplying tanks of hospital become empty, then liquid O_2 is pumped into the tank, from an outside O_2 tanker, by a cryogenic hose assembly. During this process of filling, the spillage of cryogenic liquid O_2 on the handling person can cause frost bite, cold burns, and hypothermia. The reserve bank

of cylinders should always be kept ready when O_2 is used from a storage tank particularly in case of sudden accidental failure. The O_2 tank should always be housed away from the main hospital building, due to fire hazard.

Other than storage tank, multiple O_2, N_2O, and air cylinders, arranged in *manifold system,* is also used in a small hospital or nursing home, as a central source for the supply of O_2, N_2O, and compressed air **(Fig. 6)**. In this system, large bulk cylinders (usually type H with pressure of 2,000 psi or 137 kg/cm² for O_2 and 760 psi for N_2O, the cylinder mounted on anesthesia machine is usually type E) are used and divided into two groups which alternately supply the gases in pipeline. The number and the size of cylinders in each group depend on the expected demand of gas, used by this hospital. All the cylinders of each group are connected to a common pipeline through a nonreturn valve and a pressure gauge. Then, this common pipeline from each group, in turn is connected with the distributing pipeline system through a check valve and a pressure regulator.

In each group of manifold system, all the cylinders are opened at the same time and allow them to empty equally at the same time. When all the cylinders of one group become empty, then the manifold system allows the supply to change over automatically to another group of cylinders. This automatic changeover, from one group to another group of cylinders, is achieved through a pressure sensitive automatic device that also activates an electric audio signal to alert staff. At the same time, the exhausted groups of cylinders are turned off automatically. All the exhausted cylinders of previous group are, then, should be replaced by fresh full cylinders immediately.

The *manifold system, for the supply of N_2O,* may be cooled to very low temperature, due to their latent heat of vaporization. So, the water vapor of atmosphere may condense or even freeze on the outer surface of the pipeline of manifold system, connecting the cylinders of N_2O. This can also block the pipeline and the flow of N_2O, if it (N_2O) contains some water vapor which will freeze inside the pipeline, at this very low temperature. So, a thermostatically controlled heater may be needed, at the outlet of N_2O manifold system, to warm the gas at 47°C, which will prevent the condensation of water vapor within the pipeline of N_2O gas and allow the uninterrupted flow of it.

Like the O_2 tank, these manifold systems, for the central supply of O_2, N_2O, and compressed air should also be housed in a separate, well-spaced, and ventilated room for each gas, which is constructed by fireproof tiles. These rooms should be located away from the main hospital building and on the ground floor for the easy access of transport trucks. This room which is used to store tank or manifold system of cylinders should not be used as general store room for the other empty and full cylinders which are not in use. All the empty cylinders should be removed immediately after they are exhausted.

Like the manifold system, the *motor-driven air compressor* for the central supply of air, the *motor-driven O_2 concentrator* for the central supply of O_2, and the *central vacuum plant* should also be located there, but in separate room. The central vacuum pipeline should be provided with color code, separate pressure gauge, and high and low-pressure signal device.

The *compressed oil-free medical air* which is cleaned by filters and is also supplied in hospital through pipelines to run many power-driven tools in ICU, CCU, HDU, OT, and for other clinical uses is also supplied at pressure of 400 kP or 55 psi. They may be supplied from manifold system consisting of large cylinders, containing compressed air or more economically by a motor driven air compressor. The anesthetic machines and the blender of most intensive care ventilators accept this air connection from this 400 kP or 55 psi outlet of compressed air pipeline.

The *O_2 concentrator* is a machine or device which extracts O_2 from air by differential absorption method and, then, supplies it. They become a small one which is designed to supply O_2 only for a single anesthetic machine or a single ventilator. Otherwise, it can be large enough to supply adequate O_2 through pipeline system. The small O_2 concentrators are of lightweight, portable, and can be used at remote location or for domestic purpose. In this O_2 concentrator machine, there is a compressor which first filters air from atmosphere and then compressed it. After that, this compressed air is exposed to multiple columns of zeolite (hydrated aluminum silicate of alkaline earth metal) molecular sieve, at a certain pressure, which retain N_2 and other unwanted components of air, except the O_2 and argon. Hence, the argon cannot be separated from the concentrated O_2 produced by this type of machine. Thus, maximum concentration of O_2 by 95% in volume is achieved. The columns of zeolite molecular sieve, in O_2 concentrator, which absorb N_2 and other gases from air, release them again in atmosphere, when it is heated and vacuum is applied. This O_2 concentrator can be used in vast majority of cases, but not in circle system. This is because, in this closed system, its use leads to gradual accumulation of argon. However, this can be avoided only by high gas flow. The main *disadvantage of O_2 concentrator* is its high initial cost which can be recovered easily, later by free O_2 supply. The other disadvantages of it are risk of fire, contamination of zeolite sieve, and sometimes malfunction.

Cylinder

Boyle's anesthetic machine is equipped with O_2 and N_2O gas cylinders, which are used, when there is no provision for pipeline supply of gases or during emergency when the pipeline supply of gases have failed. These gas cylinders are made up of light weight seamless *molybdenum steel*, designed to withstand intense internal pressure when gases are stored in gaseous (in case of O_2) or liquid form (in case of N_2O) under high pressure. Some of the newer cylinder contains *chromium* alloy to decrease the weight of cylinder. The cylinders, which are used in MRI unit, are made up of *aluminum* (with aluminum anesthetic machine). However, the very large bulk cylinders are made of manganese steel. The very light weight cylinders of O_2 also can be made from aluminum alloy, with fiber glass covering, by epoxy resin matrix. These are used for domestic or transport purposes in ambulance or for mountaineering purposes **(Fig. 7)**.

The *cylinders, supplying a particular gas, are identified* (i) by their specific color code, (ii) by labeling of serial

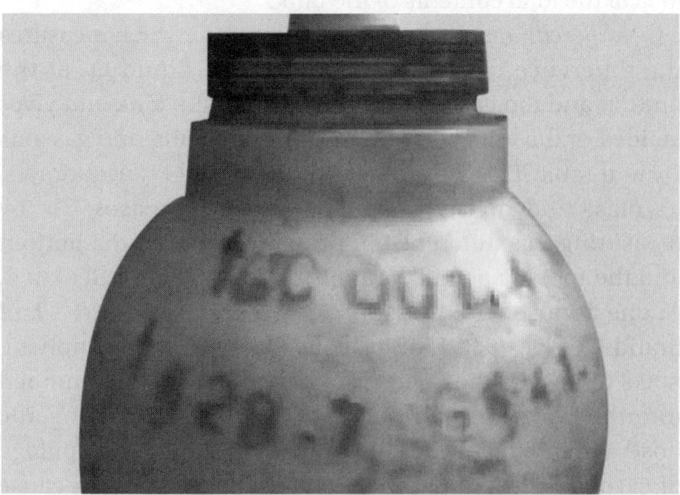

Fig. 7: Shoulder of a cylinder with engraved marking.

TABLE 1: Color coding of medical gas cylinders.

Name of gas	Color of body	Color of shoulder	Type of cylinder and pressure and capacity	Physical state in cylinder
N_2O	Blue	Blue	E, 760 psi, 1,590 L H, 760 psi, 15,800 L	Liquid Liquid
O_2	Black (UK) Green (USA)	White (UK) Green (USA)	E, 2,000 psi, 660 L H, 2,000 psi, 6,900 L	Gas Gas
CO_2	Gray	Gray	E, 750 psi, 1,590 L	Liquid
Air	Gray (UK) Yellow (USA)	Black and white (UK) Yellow (USA)	E, 2,000 psi, 625 L H, 2,000 psi, —	Gas Gas
Heliox	Black	Brown and white shoulders	E, 2,000 psi, — H, 2,000 psi, —	Gas Gas
Entonox	Blue	White	E, 2,000 psi, — H, 2,000 psi, —	Gas Liquid

number, capacity of cylinder, symbol of gas, tare weight (TW) (empty weight), date of hydraulic test, etc. stamped on their shoulder, and (iii) by plastic or paper collar, hanged from the neck of the cylinder. All the cylinders should be tested at every 5 years interval. In the past, different countries use different color-code system for their cylinders containing different gases and there was no pin index system. So, with time when this color of the cylinder is lost and the level is indistinguishable, then any interchange of N_2O and O_2 cylinder, during their attachment to the anesthetic machine, can lead to mortality. So, an international standard, which is given in **Table 1**, was laid out regarding the *color code and pin index system* (discussed later) by which the cylinders can easily be identified and cannot be interchanged, when they are attached to the anesthetic machine (i.e., it is practically impossible to attach any cylinder to wrong yokes). There are two international standard of color code, according to the school of UK and USA. However, in India, the UK standard is followed.

The cylinders are also manufactured in different sizes which are usually named by alphabet from A to L. Among these, the size A is the smallest and the size L is the largest one. The smallest sized A cylinder can hold 1.2 L of water and the largest sized L cylinder can hold 50 L of water. The cylinders, which are attached with the anesthetic machine, are usually of D and E size and the cylinders of size H or J are commonly used for the manifold system for central supply. The O_2 and N_2O cylinder of size D contains 400 L of O_2 and 940 L of N_2O respectively, whereas the O_2 and N_2O cylinder of size E contain 660 L and 1,590 L of O_2 and N_2O respectively. A full O_2 cylinder of any size at atmospheric pressure can deliver O_2 which is 130 times of its original capacity.

The O_2 is stored in a cylinder as a gas at a pressure of 2,000 psi and N_2O is stored in a cylinder as a liquid at a pressure of 750 psi. So, the cylinder which contains a gas in the form of liquid, such as in the case of N_2O and CO_2 is partially filled. This amount of partial filling of a cylinder is described as a term, named the *filling ratio* and it is defined as the weight of fluid in a cylinder divided by the weight of water required to fill the cylinder. The cylinders containing gases in liquid form are not filled up fully. This is because the partial filling of cylinders with liquid, such as in the case of N_2O and CO_2, reduces the risk of explosion, due to the sudden dangerous increase in pressure within the cylinder, due to increase in temperature of atmosphere or fire. So, in cold country, such as in UK, the filling ratio for N_2O and CO_2 cylinder is kept at 0.75, whereas in hot countries the filling ratio of these two types of cylinders is kept at 0.67.

Cylinders, containing only gas, during its emptying at constant temperature show a linear and proportional decrease in cylinder pressure. But, this does not happen in case of cylinder which is filled with gas as liquid, such as N_2O and CO_2. Here, initially the pressure inside the cylinder remains constant, because some amount of gas is produced by evaporation from liquid to replace the gas that is used. After that, once when all the liquid of N_2O has been evaporated to gaseous state, then the pressure in the cylinder starts to decrease with the process of emptying. So, the O_2 pressure gauge shows continuously the contents of a cylinder which is proportional to the gauge pressure. But, the N_2O pressure gauge does not show the actual content of the cylinder, till the whole liquid is completely evaporated to gas. During the emptying of such cylinder, containing gas as liquid, the temperature of it (cylinder) also decreases. This is because of the withdrawn of latent heat, for the vaporization of liquid within the cylinder, from the outside of cylinder from atmosphere, leading to the formation of ice on the outside of cylinder. As the pressure gauge of N_2O cylinder cannot tell the total content of it, so a full N_2O cylinder can only be identified by comparing the weight of it (full cylinder) with that of an empty one. Or in other way, a full cylinder will give a ringing sound, when a tap is made on the cylinder by a metal, while an empty cylinder will give a dull thud sound.

The cylinders are tested, after their manufacture, at regular intervals, usually of 5 years by:

- Visual inspection from outside or inside (endoscopic).
- Tensile test, where multiple strips of a cylinder are cut longitudinally and stretched, till they are elongated with a yield point which is not being <15 tons/square inch.
- Flattening test, where one cylinder is kept in between two compression blocks and pressure is applied to flatten it, till the distance of these two blocks becomes six times of the thickness of the cylinder wall, without crack.
- Bend test, where a strip of 25 mm width is cut from the cylinder wall and equally divided into four strips. These strips are then bend inward, till the inner edge is apart, proving cylinder wall will not develop any crack.
- Impact test, where three longitudinal and three transverse strips are cut from a cylinder wall and struck by mechanical hammer, with mean energy, needed to produce a crack. It should not be <5 lbs for transverse strip and 10 lbs for longitudinal strip.
- Pressure or hydraulic or water jacket test, where the cylinder is subjected to high pressure which is >50% of their normal working pressure without damage.

All these tests are usually done for at least one, out of every 100 cylinders. The gases and vapors should be free of water vapor when they are stored in cylinders, because water vapor may freeze and block the exit port of cylinder when the temperature of cylinder valve decreases tremendously on opening. All the cylinders, after filled with gas, should be stored in a dry, well ventilated and fireproof room, and are not subjected to extremes of heat. They should not be stored near flammable materials like grease or oil, etc., or near any source of direct heat or fire.

A cylinder has four parts such as (1) body, (2) shoulder, (3) neck, and (4) valve **(Fig. 8)**. The size of the body of a cylinder varies according to the designations which are named as A to L. The body of a cylinder is painted according to the color code. The upper part of the body of a cylinder begins to be narrow which is called the *shoulder*. The shoulder, then, suddenly becomes narrow. This is called the *neck*. The shoulder and the neck of a cylinder are also painted according to the color code which may be the same with the body or not. The neck ends in a tapered screw thread into which the *valve* of a cylinder is fitted. This tapered screw thread end of the neck, (between the neck and the valve of a cylinder), is sealed by a special material, with low melting point, which melts if the cylinder is exposed to excessive heat suddenly, and allows the contents of the cylinder to

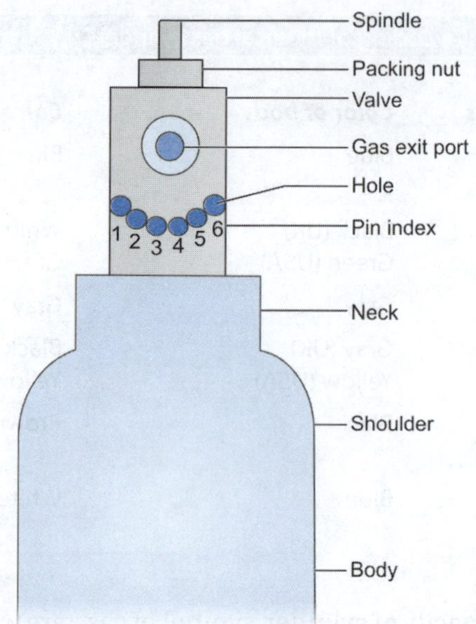

Fig. 8: The different parts of a cylinder and different combination of pin index. Gas exit port accommodates the yoke nipple and the hole accommodates the pine of pin index system.

escape, avoiding the risk of explosion. There is a plastic disk around the neck whose color and shape indicates the year when the cylinder was last examined. The marks engraved on the shoulder of a cylinder are: date of last test performed, test pressure, chemical formula of the contents of this cylinder, and TW (weight of empty cylinder) **(Fig. 7)**. Every cylinder should also have a paper and plastic printed level which is attached on the body or will hang from the neck. This will show: cylinder size code, specification of contents (which include name, chemical symbol, pharmaceutical formula, proportion of gases in a gas mixture), batch number, maximum cylinder pressure in bars, nominal cylinder contents in liter, filling and expiry date, direction of use, hazard and safety instruction, storage, handling precaution, etc.

At the top, every cylinder is fitted with a valve which is known as the cylinder valve. Several types of cylinder valves, like *flush type, bull nosed, straight type, angle type*, etc., are available **(Figs. 9 and 10)**. But, the noninterchangeable flush type of valve, with pin index system which is commonly used to attach a cylinder at the yoke bar of anesthetic machine, will be discussed here. It (valve) is screwed into the neck of a cylinder via a threaded connection which is sealed by a special material with low melting point. This cylinder valve is made of brass and plated with chromium or nickel which allows the rapid dissipation of heat, if it is generated due to compression during filling.

The chemical formula of gas, by which the cylinder is filled up, is engraved on its valve. The valve seals the contents of a cylinder and it (valve) is used to start, regulate, and stop the

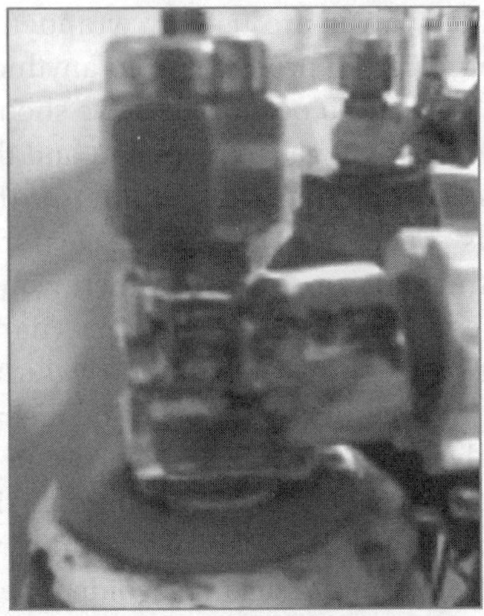

Fig. 9: Bull nose type of cylinder valve.

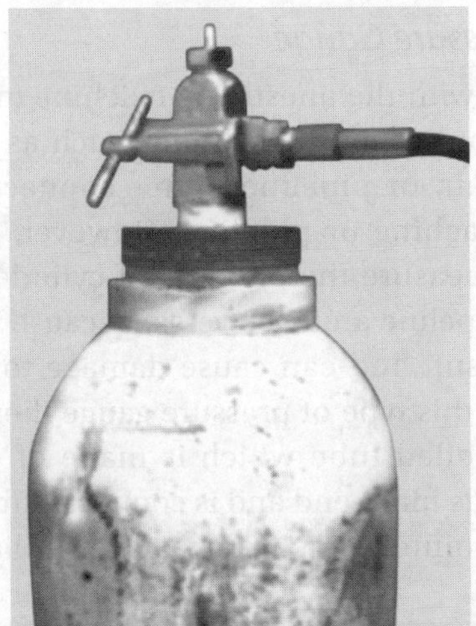

Fig. 10: CO_2 cylinder with flush type cylinder valve.

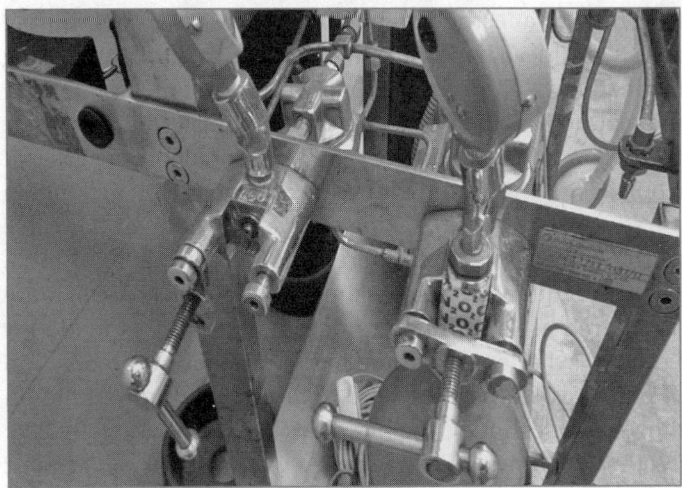

Fig. 11: Hanger yoke assembly.

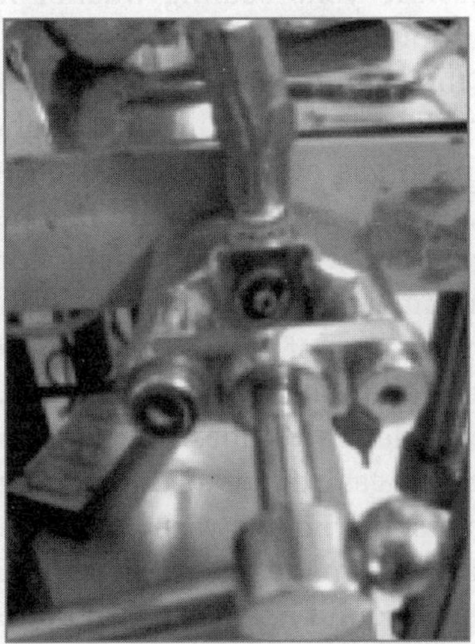

Fig. 12: Pin index system (yoke assemble).

flow of gas from the cylinder by a spindle which is described below. On the top of the cylinder valve, there is an on/off stem or spindle, with packing nut. When this stem is turned on with a spanner, then it allows the gas to flow through the outlet, situated on the valve. In modern modification, the top of the valve is so designed that the on and off of cylinder can be done by the manual turning of the stem or spindle with the packing nut simple by hand, without the need of a spanner. There is an outlet (exit) hole of gas and another two holes, below the gas outlet hole, at the one side of the cylinder valve, which fits with the yoke assembly of Boyle's machine, through a specific noninterchangeable pin index system, consisting of a nipple and two pins.

Yoke Assembly

Hanger yoke assembly is that part of the machine where the cylinders get fitted with the machine **(Fig. 11)**. It (1) supports and orients the cylinders, (2) provides a gas tight seal between the cylinders and machine, and (iii) ensures unidirectional gas flow. A hanger yoke assembly consists of: (i) the *body* which produces the main frame work from where the cylinders hang, (ii) *retaining screw*, (iii) pin index pins (one nipple and two pins), (iv) a gas seal (*Bodok seal*) to prevent the leak between the cylinder and the yoke, (v) *yoke plug* which prevents the leaking of gas through nipple if a cylinder is not attached to that pin index assembly, (vi) a *filter*, and (vii) a *check valve* assembly (It is a unidirectional valve allowing an unidirectional flow of gas into machine from cylinder. It also prevents the transfilling of gas from full to empty cylinder) **(Fig. 8 and Fig. 12)**.

Pin index system is a very important safety mechanism of an anesthetic machine. It prevents the wrong fitting of one agent-specific gas cylinder at the position determined for another agent-specific gas cylinder. It is a part of yoke assembly of anesthetic machine. It consists of one nipple and two pins. These two pins are 4 mm and 6 mm long respectively. The nipple of pin index system enters into the exit hole of the valve and the two pins enter into their corresponding holes on the valve, present below the gas exit whole (**Fig. 8**). The pin index system is made by making an arc (a part of a circle), taking the gas exit hole on the valve as the center. The circumference of this arc is 9/16 inch. Then, six equidistant points are made on this arc which are numbered as 1–6. Another additional point 7 is made for Entonox cylinder. According to the number of the position of pin on yoke assembly and their corresponding hole on the valve of cylinder, the pin index are like that: $O_2 \rightarrow 2, 5$; $N_2O \rightarrow 3, 5$; Air $\rightarrow 1, 5$; Nitrogen $\rightarrow 1, 4$; Entonox $\rightarrow 7$; Heliox *(a low density gas mixture of helium and oxygen)* $\rightarrow 2, 4$; and $C_2O \rightarrow 2, 6$.

A compressible yoke sealing washer named *Bodok seal* (**Fig. 13**) should be placed in between the anesthetic machine and the cylinder valve. It is a specialized washer that has the crucial role of ensuring an air tight seal between a regulator and a gas cylinder. It is used extensively in breathing equipment and anesthetic machines. This will make a gas tight joint, when the cylinder is connected to the anesthetic machine at its yoke assembly. If the yoke nipple is damaged or the pins of yoke assembly and the holes of cylinder valve are not aligned properly (i.e., pin index of a particular cylinder valve does not match with the yoke assembly), then the gas exit port of the cylinder valve will not seal tightly against the Bodok washer and the gas will leak. The Bodok washer is made of carbon impregnated rubber with a metal ring around it. It is 2.4 mm thick and only one seal (Bodok washer) is allowed in between the cylinder valve and yoke assembly to fit the cylinder without leak. The excessive tightening of the screw of yoke assembly to press the cylinder valve against this seal may also damage it.

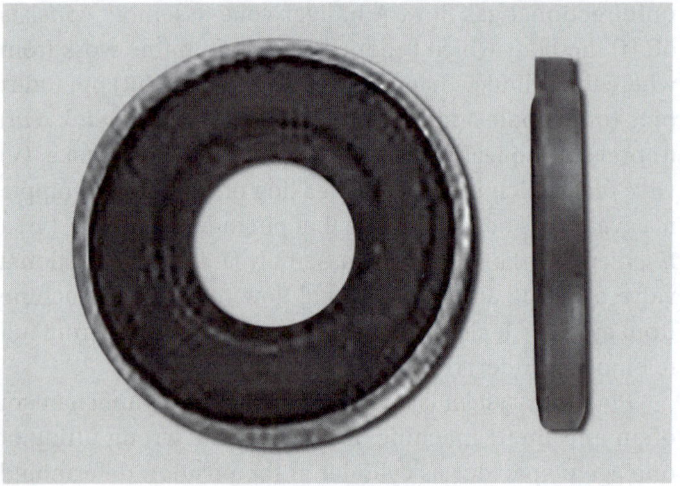

Fig. 13: Bodok seal.

The cylinder valves are usually wrapped by a plastic covering, after filling, to protect it from anything which can enter the exit port and block it. The valve should be slightly opened, allowing some gas to come out and then is closed again, before connecting the cylinder with anesthetic machine. This procedure will usually clean dust, oil, and grease from the exit port of valve which would otherwise enter the anesthetic machine and may damage it. The cylinder valve should be turned on slowly during use, when it is attached to the anesthetic machine, because it (slow opening of valve) prevents the sudden rise in the pressure and temperature of gas while flowing through the machine's pipeline. During the closure of cylinder valve, over-tightening of valve should also be avoided, because it may damage the seal between the valve and the neck of cylinder (**Fact file III**).

Bourdon Pressure Gauge

It is attached with the anesthetic machine to measure the pressure of gas within the cylinder, such as O_2, N_2O, and compressed air, or pipelines, after connecting with the anesthetic machine or pipeline. However, one which is designed to measure the pressure of cylinder, should not be used for pipeline and vice versa, because it may lead to inaccurate result and can cause damage to the pressure gauge. Inside this type of pressure gauge there is a robust, but flexible coiled tube which is made of copper alloy. It is closed at its inner end and is connected through a lever to a needle pointer which moves over a dial, indicating

FACT FILE III

Machine inlets

Most anesthetic machines have three separate inlets each for O_2, N_2O, and air. Some machines also have a 4th inlet for CO_2, helium or heliox. However, the compact models of machine lack the air inlet. These inlets of machine which are connected with the pipelines are separated from the inlet of machine which are connected with the cylinder. So, the machines have separate pressure gauges, each at pipelines inlet and cylinder inlet to measure their respective pressure. However, there are many machines which (we commonly use in our country) have no separate inlets for the pipeline and cylinder and the pipeline supply is attached at the inlet of machine where the cylinders are attached. In the machines where there is separate inlet for pipeline (and cylinder), a color-coded hose pipe is used to connect the outlet of pipeline to the anesthetic machine through a noninterchangeable DISS that prevents incorrect hose attachment. At this connection, a filter is attached which helps to filter the gas and a one way check valve is attached which prevents the retrograde flow of gas in the pipeline. At the cylinder inlet of machine, the cylinders are attached to the machine through a yoke assembly that utilizes pin index safety system (PISS) to prevent the wrong connection of cylinders. The yoke assembly includes PISS, a washer, a gas filter, and a check valve that prevents retrograde gas flow. In some machines, there have an extra O_2 or air inlet which is used to drive the ventilator.

pressure. The other end of this coiled tube is opened to gas supply line, coming from the cylinder or pipeline (**Figs. 14 and 15**).

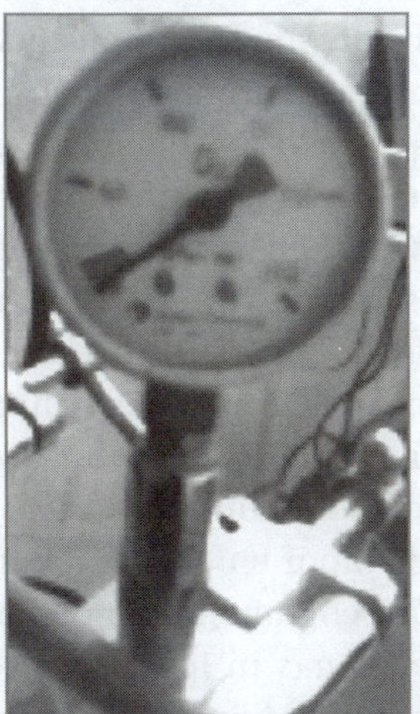

Fig. 14: Bourdon pressure gauge.

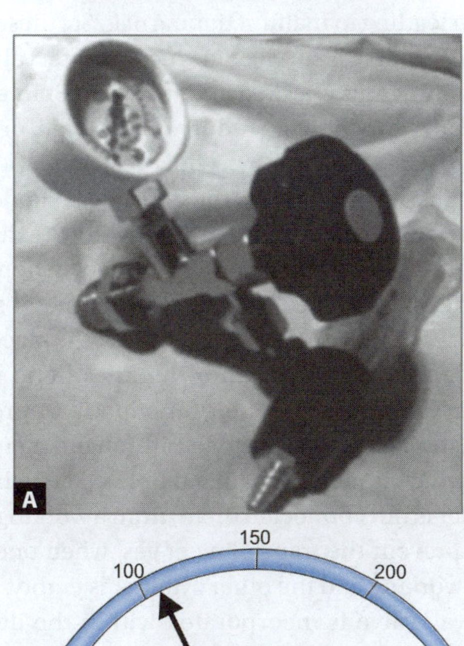

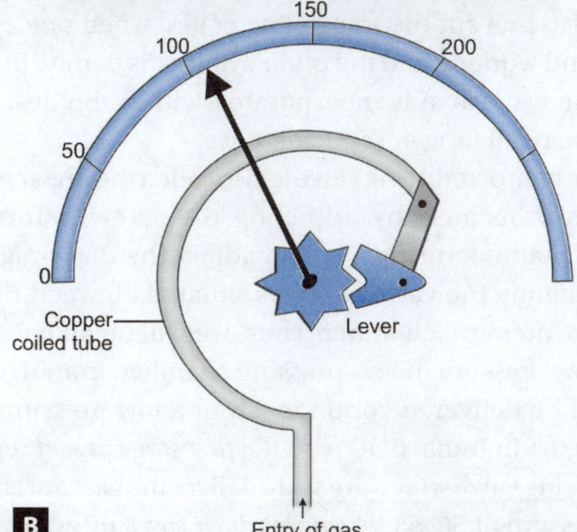

Figs. 15A and B: (A) Bourdon pressure gauge; and (B) The mechanism of action of Bourdon pressure gauge.

After turning on the valve and opening the cylinder, the gas under high pressure first starts to flow into this coiled copper tube of pressure gauge and causes it to uncoil or straight out. Then, this movement of the tube, during uncoiling, causes the needle pointer to move on dial and indicates pressure of gas inside the cylinder or pipeline. Each pressure gauge is calibrated for a particular gas and its dial is color-coded. It bears the name and symbol of gas, for which types of gas cylinder or pipeline, it is used. At the front, every pressure gauge is protected by a cover of heavy fiber glass. So, in case of any breakage of coiled copper tube, the gas escapes from behind, rather than the front. The measured pressure in the pressure gauge is depicted in different unit, such as kP or lbs/square inch (pound per square inch or psi) or kg/cm^2 or bar, etc. When the central pipeline for O_2 supply is connected to the anesthetic machine, then the pressure gauge at the connection shows 4 bars or 60 psi pressure.

Heliox cylinder contains the mixture of 79% helium and 21% oxygen. This gas mixture is mainly used in upper airway obstruction and is stored in cylinder whose body is black color, representing O_2, with brown and white shoulder (brown representing helium). *Entonox cylinder* contains the mixture of 50% nitrous oxide and 50% oxygen. This gas mixture is used to produce analgesia during labor and is stored in cylinder whose body is blue color (blue representing N_2O) and shoulder is white color (white representing O_2).

Reducing Valve or Pressure Regulator

The gases are usually presented to anesthetic machine under different high pressure from different types of cylinders or pipelines. So, it is needed to pass these gases from these high-pressure sources, through a single or multiple pressure reducing valves or pressure regulators, which are placed between the cylinder or pipelines and the rest of the components of an anesthetic machine and which will decrease their high variable pressure to a safe constant operating pressure, before reaching the gas to flow meter. These reducing valves allow a delicate control of gas flow through flow meter and also protect the different sophisticated component of anesthetic machine against the sudden surges of high pressure of gases and their damage. Further, in the absence of these reducing valves, when the pressure of a cylinder decreases with use, then in order to maintain the supply of gases to a patient at a constant flow and pressure, continuous adjustment of flow meter is required. These pressure reducing valves or regulators which are attached in the machine after the pipeline entry point reduce the pipeline pressure from 55 psi to 45 psi. The pressure regulators which are attached after the direct attachment of cylinder with the machine reduce the pressure of cylinder from 2,000 psi to 45 psi and 760 psi to 45 psi in case of O_2 and N_2O respectively. After the reduction of cylinder or pipeline pressure to 45 psi, it is further reduced to 15–30 psi by second stage (group) pressure reducing valves **(Fig. 16)**. Then, the gases enter the rotameter with this 15–30 psi pressure.

In this type of pressure regulator or reducing valve, there are two chambers, such as (1) a high-pressure chamber and (2) a low-pressure chamber **(Fig. 17)**. These two chambers are connected through a gap which is guarded by a small valve. The high-pressure chamber gets its gasflow, through its inlet, directly from cylinder or pipeline. The small valve, intervening between the high and low-pressure chamber, is attached to a diaphragm which is again attached to a spring through which the pressure regulator can be adjusted to get

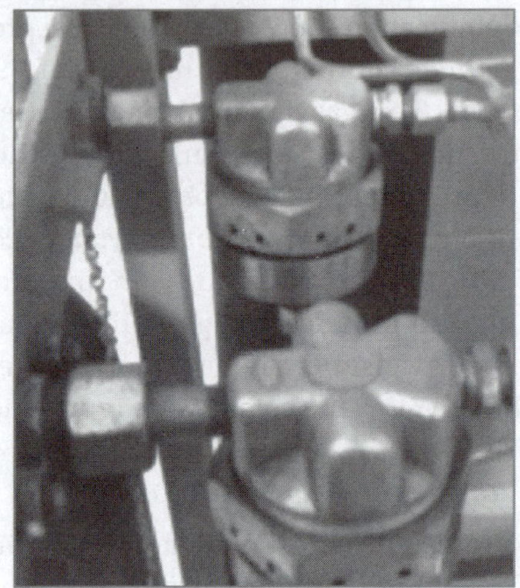

Fig. 16: Reducing valve.

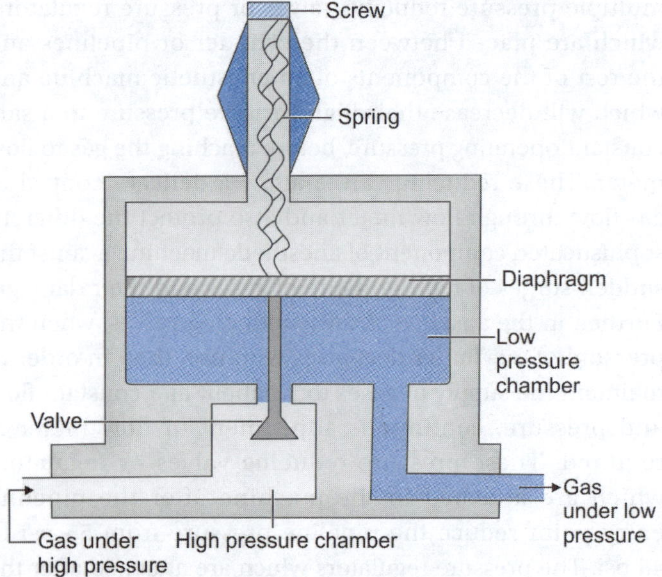

Fig. 17: The mechanism of action of reducing valve.

the supply of gas flow at a desired constant low pressure, set by the engineer. After entering the gas into the high-pressure chamber, directly from a cylinder or pipeline, the force exerted by the gas, under high pressure tries to close the gap, guarded by the small valve and decrease the gas flow to low-pressure chamber from the high-pressure chamber. On the other hand, the opposite opening force, exerted by the spring and the diaphragm, tries to open the small valve. Then, a balance is reached between these two forces, leading to a constant fixed opening or gap. Then, this constant fixed opening will allow a constant flow of gas, under a fixed desired pressure, to low-pressure chamber from high-pressure chamber and ultimately the gas passes out.

If the gas in cylinder contains water vapor, then, when the gas with water vapor enters the low-pressure chamber from high-pressure chamber, then due to the loss of heat due to expansion of gas in low-pressure chamber, there are chances of ice formation inside the regulator, causing malfunctioning of it. There are also the chances of rupture of diaphragm leading to malfunctioning of it. So, these pressure regulators should be serviced at regular intervals and the rubber diaphragm is checked and renewed. Before entering the machine, the control (reduction) of high pressure in pipeline is also achieved by a flow restrictor (a separate type of device which controls the flow of gas) and a second stage pressure regulator. If there is only flow restrictor and no pressure regulator for pipeline, then, when there is some change in pipeline pressure, the flow meter should be adjusted accordingly. A *one way valve* is also placed within the cylinder supply line within the anesthetic machine, next to the inlet of yoke. Their function is to prevent the back flow and loss or leakage of gas through an empty yoke assembly which is consists of one nipple and two index pins (if a cylinder is not connected there) from a working cylinder. They also prevent the transfilling of gas, when one cylinder is full and working and the other cylinder is empty. Recently, this one way valve is incorporated within the design of a pressure regulating or reducing valve.

This type of reducing valve is also called the *preset pressure regulator,* because by adjusting the screw beforehand, during manufacturing, we can adjust the diaphragm and subsequently the valve which is situated between the high and low-pressure chamber. Thus, we will be able to keep a fixed low pressure in low-pressure chamber, from which the gas will be delivered continuously at a low pressure to the flow meter. In India, BOC uses the *first stage* preset regulator or reducing valve which are set to deliver the gases at constant low pressure of *50–55 lbs/square inch (psi)*, by adjusting the screw and thus subsequently adjusting the inside diaphragm and valve of regulator. At the *second stage*, this pressure is further reduced to *15–30 psi* by the second stage pressure regulators. Gases from this second stage reducing valves reach the rotameter where the flow is further regulated the flow control knob. Finally, the gas mixture is delivered at the common outlet of the machine at a pressure of *5–8 psi*. There is another type of preset pressure regulator which is called the Adam's valve. These are used in many anesthetic machines **(Fact file IV)**.

The pressure regulators are so adjusted that the anesthetic machine can use the gas both from the pipelines and cylinders. *The anesthetic machine always uses the gas from the sources that have higher pressure.* So, the exit pressure level of the reducing valves, present in the pipelines, is set at higher level than that of the reducing valves, present in the cylinder lines and the machine preferably uses the pipeline gas, if both the cylinders and pipelines are opened. But, when the gases from the pipeline are being used, the cylinders should be closed. This is because, if both the cylinders and the pipelines are opened, then the machine will always use the gas from the pipeline source that has higher pressure. But, sometimes if the pipeline pressure drops below that supplied (or set) by cylinder and its valve is open, then some gas will be withdrawn from the cylinder. Thus, gradually the cylinder will be exhausted without the knowledge of anesthetist and then it will not help during emergency.

Flow Meter

It is incorporated into the Boyle's anesthetic apparatus to regulate and to measure the flow of gases, such as O_2, N_2O, and air, which are passing through it (Boyle's machine). The control and the measure of the flow of gases, through an anesthetic machine, can be done by mechanical or electronic method **(Figs. 18 and 19)**. The flow meter, which is used in anesthetic machine and measures the flow of gases mechanically, is also known as the rotameter **(Fig. 20)**. It consists of flow control valves, flow meter tubes, rotating bobbins within the tubes, and a common manifold (channel) at the top of the tubes where all the tubes join. For the rotating bobbins, this type of flow meter is known as the rotameter. The other types of flow meter which are used in industry are: Waterside, Heidbrink, Connell, Foregger, etc. type of flow meter. The flow meter, used in anesthetic machine, consists of a series of especially designed glass tube (Thorpe tube), with rotating bobbin inside it, to measure the flow of individual gases in the flow meter. This bobbin or float is made of aluminum. The Thorpe tubes are placed within a *chromium-plated* metal casing. In front of this casing, there is a transparent plastic window which helps in clear reading and protection of flow meter tube, from damage and dust.

FACT FILE IV

After passing through the Bourdon pressure gauge and check valve the gases from pipeline and cylinder passes through a common pathway to the flow meter. The pressure regulator situated on the cylinder supply line is so adjusted that in this common pathway the gas pressure coming from the cylinder is always lower than the gas pressure coming from the pipeline. So, it allows the machine to use preferentially the gas from pipeline, still if the cylinder is left open (unless the pipeline pressure drops below the gasline pressure coming from cylinder attached with machine). A high-pressure relief valve is also sometimes provided in some machines distal to pressure regulator. It sets open when the supply pressure from cylinder or pipeline exceeds the machine's maximum safety limit in case of failure of pressure regulator. Some machines also use a second stage pressure regulator, instead of this relief to drop both the pipeline and cylinder pressure in case of the failure of first one. This is known as two-stage pressure regulation. This two-stage pressure regulation is also needed for an auxiliary O_2 flow meter, to drive gas to power the pneumatic ventilators, or for the O_2 flush mechanism. The pressure in the supply of O_2 is reduced more than that of N_2O. This differential reduction of pressure between these two gases is important for the proper functioning of N_2O/O_2 flow linkage safety device, i.e., in the failure of the supply of O_2, the N_2O will not also flow. This safety device senses the pressure of O_2 through a small piloting pressure line that is derived directly from gas inlet or second regulator. If the pressure in this pilot line falls below a threshold level, it shuts off the valve preventing the flow of N_2O. Modern machines also uses some proportioning safety devices (discusses in text) with the pressure of this threshold shut off valve which proportionately reduces the flow of N_2O gas when the flow of O_2 reduces below 25% in total gas mixture. All machines also have an O_2 supply low-pressure sensor that activates an electric alarm or a gas whistle when the inlet gas pressure of O_2 goes below the threshold value. The gas lines proximal to the controlling knob of flow valve of rotameter are considered as the high-pressure circuit and the gas lines distal to it up to the common gas outlet are considered as the low-pressure circuit of machine.

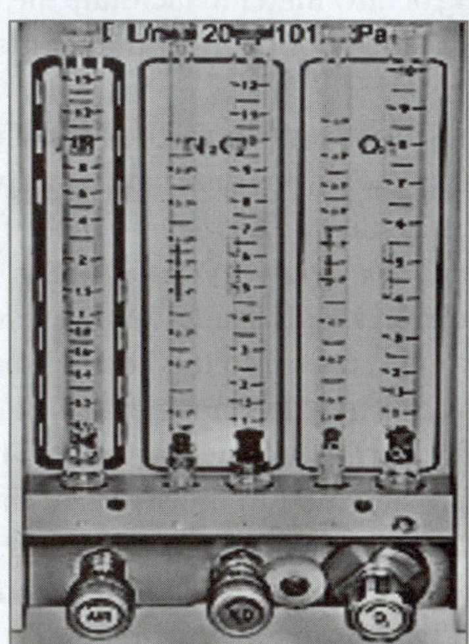

Fig. 18: Mechanical rotameter.

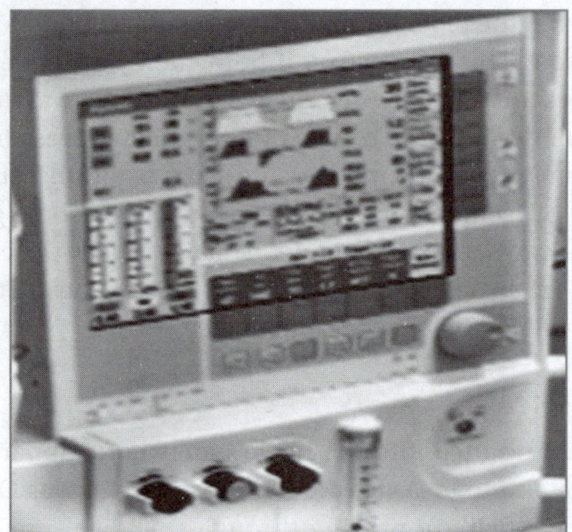

Fig. 19: Electronic flow meter.

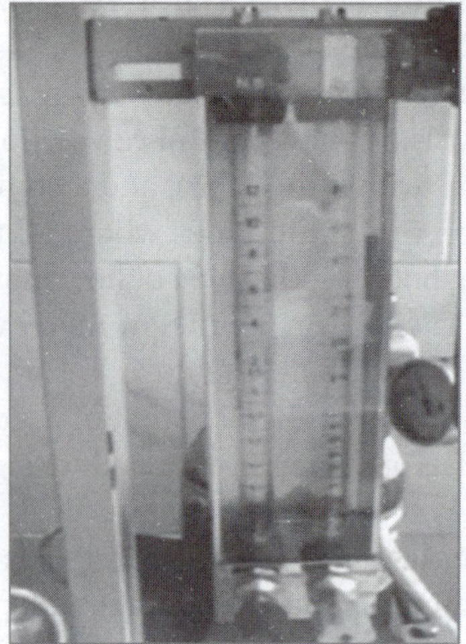

Fig. 20: Flow meter (rotameter).

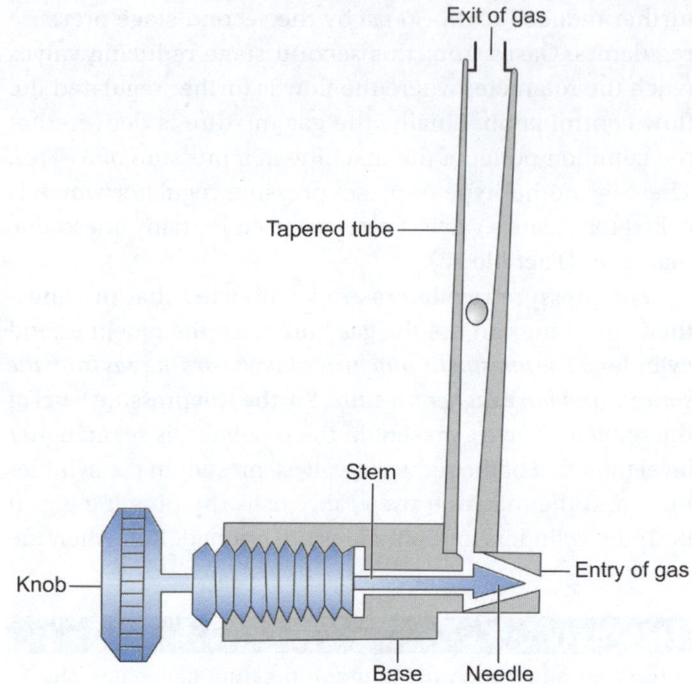

Fig. 21: The parts of a flow control valve and the Thorpe tubes of flow meter.

A detachable *radiolucent plate* is also provided at the back of the metal casing of flow meter to facilitate the observation of a working and rotating bobbin within the tube during use in a darkened OT.

The flow control valves control the flow of gases, through the tubes of flow meter, by the manual adjustment of its (valves) knobs. It is situated at the base of the flow meter and consists of *knob, stem, body, and needle* (**Fig. 21**). The body of the flow control valve is made up of brass. The stem of the adjusting knob screws into the body of this flow control valves and ends as a needle. The needle is placed at the site of the inflow of gas to the tube of flow meter. The flow control knobs, which are attached to the stems of the flow control valve, are labeled (chemical formula of gas is embedded on each knob) and color-coded for their respective gases. This color coding of knob is like that *white* for O_2, *blue* for N_2O, and *black* for air. In some design, the O_2 control knob is

more fluted, larger, and has a longer stem (more prominent or protruded toward the anesthetist) than the other stems and knobs, used for the other gases. So, this O_2 knob makes it easily recognizable and acts as one of the safety measures of rotameter or machine. In some designs, a special device known as the *flow control knob guard* is attached to the flow meter to protect against the accidental adjustment of flow meters by hand movement, due to other causes.

The Thorpe tubes of flow meter are especially made of tapered glass tube, with a rotating bobbin inside it. They are set strictly in vertical position on the body of flow control valve, because inclined position of tube gives incorrect reading, by causing friction of bobbin on the wall of the tube and thus producing resistance during the flow of gas. Each tube is individually calibrated at room temperature and one atmospheric pressure for that gas, which flows through it, giving accuracy of about ±99.9% in measuring the rate of flow of gases. For the flows below 2 L/min, the measuring units are mL/min and for the flows above it, the measuring units are L/min. The rotating bobbin or ball in the flow meter tubes, which shows us the rate of gas flow through it, is made of light aluminum. They are held floating within the tube by the gas, flowing around it, through the gap between the tubes wall and bobbin. During floating, the effect of gravity on the bobbin is counteracted by the flow of gas. When the bobbin is lifted by the flow of gas, then the upward pressure caused by the gas (some portion of the gas passes away by the side of the bobbin and some portion of the gas gives upward pressure on the bobbin) and the weight of the bobbin is in equilibrium at that height of the bobbin, showing the rate of flow of gas (by the upper margin of the bobbin).

The flow meter tubes are tapered in such a fashion that the clearance or gap between the bobbin and the wall of the tube gradually widens from the bottom to the top **(Figs. 22A and B)**. *So, at low flow rate, the clearance between the bobbin and the wall of the Thorpe tube (the orifice of tube) is longer and narrower, acting as a tube and at these circumstances the gas flow is laminar, governed by the viscosity of gas. On the other hand, at high flow rate, the clearance between the bobbin and the wall of the tube is wider and shorter, acting as an orifice.* Thus, under these circumstances the flow is turbulent and governed by the density of gas. So, each flow meter is calibrated for its specific gas, according to its density and viscosity.

The flow meter can give inaccurate result, if the bobbin sticks to the wall of the tube due to dirt, from contaminated gas supply and/or due to static electricity, caused by continuous friction, arising from the rotating bobbin during floating. The problem of dirt can be eliminated, by using the filter at the gas inlet site of anesthetic machine and the problem of static electricity can be solved, by making the bobbin of antistatic material or applying some antistatic spray over it or coating the tubes interior with a conductive substance which grounds the whole flow meter system and reduces the effect of static electricity. At the upper margin of the bobbin, there are many cuts or slits (flutes) at the sides. So, when the gas flows by the side of it, these flutes cause the bobbin to rotate. There is a radiolucent dot on the bobbin and it indicates that the bobbin is rotating and is not stuck to the wall of the tube. There are two bobbin stops which are made of spring and are situated at the extreme either ends

(top and bottom) of the Thorpe tube. It always ensures the visibility of bobbin during operation at the extremes of flow.

According to the shape and size, the different types of bobbins are also used in flow meter, such as ball, H float, skirted bobbin, and nonskirted bobbin **(Fig. 23)**. But, usually the ball and the skirted bobbin are commonly used in anesthetic machine. To know the gas flow per minute through rotameter, the reading of flow meter is taken from the top of the bobbin. But, when a ball is used instead of bobbin, then the reading is generally taken from the midpoint of the ball. When very low flow is required such as in circle breathing system, then an arrangement of two flow meter tubes for each gas which are attached in series in rotameter are used for the fine adjustment of flow. But these two tubes are controlled by single flow control valve and knob.

The O_2 tube of a flow meter is kept at the extreme right of all the gas tubes **(Figs. 24 and 25)**, because when it is placed at extreme left of all the tubes, then if any crack develops in a flow meter distal (downstream) to it, then O_2 may leak through this distal crack and may deliver hypoxic mixture (as the O_2 is already leaked out) to the patient. So, to avoid this problem, O_2 is the last to be added to the gas mixture and is finally delivered to the back bar of anesthetic machine. During mechanical ventilation, pressure rises at the common gas outlet when the bag is compressed by ventilator or manually. This is transmitted back to the gas in the tube of flow meter above the bobbin which results in the drop of it during inspiration and inaccurate reading.

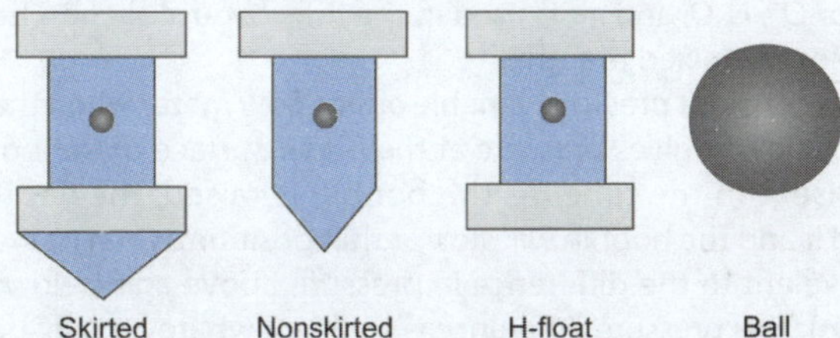

Fig. 23: Different types of bobbin used in rotameter.

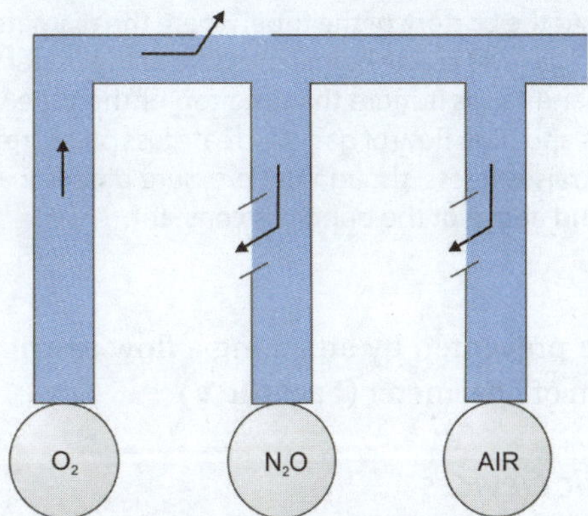

Fig. 24: How the O_2 will leak from cracks at different sites, if its tube is placed at extreme left.

Figs. 22A and B: (A) The route of flow of gases through the tubes of flow meter; and (B) Gap between the bobbin and tube wall increases as bobbin goes up.

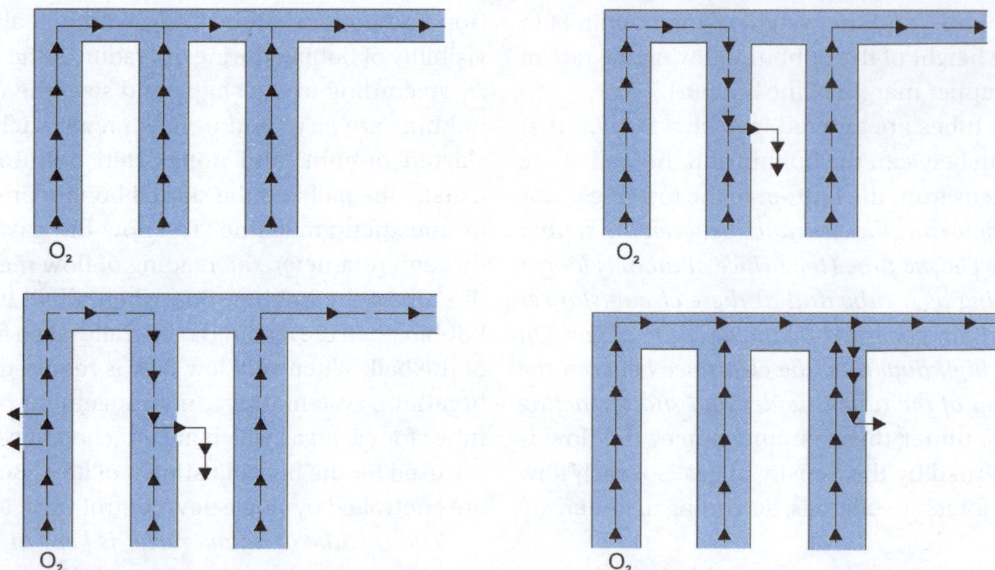

Fig. 25: The problems are shown, if the O_2 tube is kept at extreme left. So, in modern anesthetic machine, the O_2 tube is kept at extreme right.

FACT FILE V

The flow meters of anesthetic machines are classified either as a *constant pressure variable orifice* flow meter which are commonly used (and is already described in text) or an electronic flow meter. In an electronic flow meter, the amount of pressure drop, caused by a flow restrictor, is the principle for the measurement of gas flow and the amount of flow is displayed digitally and/or graphically on screen. In such circumstances, a backup conventional auxiliary O_2 flow meter is also provided for emergency. In anesthetic machine where electronic flow meter is used, there is separate flow meter each for O_2, N_2O, and air is used in the flow control section before the gases are mixed together.

In the constant pressure variable orifice flow meter when the gas starts to flow, it gives pressure at the under surface of the bobbin and raise it in the tube. As the bobbin is raised, the gas flows around it and the bobbin will stop at that position, when its weight is equivalent to the difference in pressure above and below of it (bobbin). This pressure difference is constant whatever may be the rate of flow and the position of the bobbin in the tube. However, it depends on the cross-sectional area of the tube and the weight of the bobbin. At the bottom of the tube, where the diameter is small, a low flow of gas will create higher pressure at the under surface of the bobbin and raises it more than the top of the tube where the tube widens and high flow of gas will create less pressure under the bobbin and raises it less, though the pressure difference between the below and above of the bobbin is constant.

This can be prevented by attaching a flow restrictor at the downstream of flow meter (**Fact file V**).

Antihypoxic Devices

There are many devices which are incorporated in the modern anesthetic machine to stop the flow of N_2O in the absence of the flow of O_2 or there should be a minimum 25% concentration of O_2 in the delivered gas mixture to patient or the machine will give audible alarm when the O_2 pressure drops in the pipeline of anesthetic machine. These antihypoxic devices are consist of hypoxic guard and O_2 failure alarm. This hypoxic guard device maintains a minimum 25% flow of O_2 in the delivered gas mixture or when the O_2 flow is reduced to or below the 25% of total flow, then the N_2O flow will be automatically reduced. It works by mechanical, pneumatic, or electronic principle. In mechanical method (principle) the N_2O and O_2 flow control valves in rotameter are linked together by a chain. This chain relays the movement of O_2 knob to the N_2O knob. So, when the O_2 flow control knob is turned to reduce the flow of this gas (O_2), then the chain link will also move and reduce the flow of N_2O, as if always a minimum 25% of O_2 mixture can reach to the patients or without the flow of O_2, the N_2O will not flow alone.

The O_2 flow control knob in rotameter can be independently opened further. But, it cannot be closed below a setting that will produce <25% O_2 in the gas mixture, if N_2O is used. In *pneumatic method* (principle), there is a special type of valve, known as the ratio mixer valve, where the O_2 is exerting pressure on the one side of the diaphragm and N_2O on the other side. Thus, when there is increased flow of N_2O, then it will also cause increased flow of O_2 maintaining a minimum 25% concentration of it. But, when the flow of O_2 is only increased, the flow of N_2O will not increase. In *electronic device*, a paramagnetic O_2 analyzer is used to analyze the mixture of gases which are sampled continuously. Then, if due to any reason, the O_2 concentration falls below 25% in

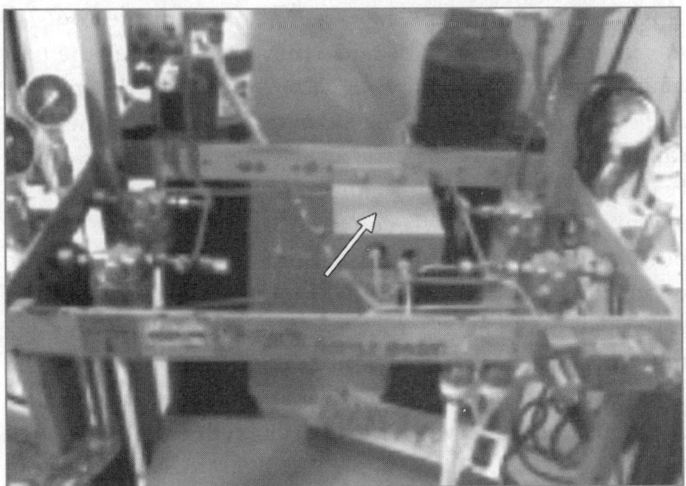

Fig. 26: Oxygen failure alarm.

the inspired gas mixture, then the flow of N_2O will also be stopped and give an alarm.

In O_2 supply failure *alarm,* when the pressure in the pipeline of machine, carrying only O_2 drops below a certain fixed level, then the O_2 is directed through a whistle to produce a sound causing alarm **(Fig. 26)**. This alarm is activated only when the pressure of O_2 in the machine gas pipeline falls below 200 kP. This alarm cannot be switched off unless the O_2 supply is restored.

Vaporizers

A vaporizer is a device, by which a controlled amount of vapor of a volatile anesthetic agent, after vaporizing it from its liquid, is added to the mixture of fresh gas flow, coming from rotameter (flow meter). The material by which a vaporizer should be made must have high specific heat and high thermal conductivity. As the Copper possesses these properties, the vaporizers are made up of copper. Initially, all the types of vaporizers are divided under two broad headings: (1) variable bypass vaporizers, and (2) measured flow vaporizers.

In *variable bypass vaporizers* (*variable bypass means by rotating the dial knob, it can be decided how much fresh gas will bypass the vaporizer and how much gas will pass through the chamber of vaporizer*), the fresh gas flow is first splitted into two, so that only a small portion of it passes through the vaporizers and then, when it passes over the liquid volatile anesthetic agent in the vaporizing chamber, it (fresh gas flow) becomes saturated with the vapor of this volatile anesthetic agent. Then, it leaves the vaporizer and mix with the remaining fresh gas flow that has gone through the bypass. Therefore, the final desired concentration of volatile anesthetic agent is achieved, by *varying the splitting ratio,* between the bypass gas and the gas that enters the

vaporizing chamber of a vaporizer, using an adjustable valve (regulating dial). For example, when the dial knob of vaporizer is set at 5% concentration, then most of the fresh gas will pass through the vaporizer and when the dial knob is set at 0.1% concentration, then most of the fresh gas will bypass the vaporizer, i.e., the amount of fresh gas bypassing the vaporizer is variable, set by dial knob.

On the other hand, some vaporizers can be designed so that, it heats the volatile anesthetic liquid to a temperature above its boiling point and make it a gaseous state in the chamber of vaporizer which is then allowed to leave the vaporizer in calculated amount (measured), controlled by regulating dial, to mix with the fresh gas flow, in achieving the desired concentration of it. These are known as the *measured flow vaporizers.* The example of this measured flow vaporizer is TEC-6, TEC-6 plus, D-TEC, where desflurane is only used. Another example of measured flow vaporizer is *Aladin cassette vaporizer* which is used to deliver all the volatile anesthetic agents, requiring just the insertion of color-coded cassette of each agent.

The variable bypass vaporizers are again divided into two types, such as (1) *the draw (or blow) over vaporizers, and (2) the plenum vaporizers (theoretically plenum vaporizer is a type of partial blow-over vaporizer, because the fresh gas blow over the wicks which are soaked by volatile anesthetic liquid. Here, the fresh gas does not directly blow over the surface of the anesthetic liquid. So, somebody does not consider it as the blow-over vaporizer).* In the simple *draw-over or blow-over vaporizers,* a portion of the fresh gas flow, regulated by the controlled knob or dial, is allowed to simply flow over the liquid volatile anesthetic agent and to pick up the vapor of this agent (*in bubble through vaporizer the fresh gas is bubbled through the liquid of volatile anesthetic agent, e.g., copper kettle vaporizer. The ether bottle vaporizer which was used previously in Boyle's machine can be used both as blow over and bubble through vaporizer, because when the plunger is above the anesthetic liquid, then the fresh gas blow over the liquid and when the plunger is dipped into the anesthetic liquid, then the fresh gas is bubbled through the anesthetic liquid*). The older Goldman halothane vaporizer, ether bottle vaporizer, etc. are of variable bypass plus the blow over type vaporizers and of low resistance and the anesthetic vapor, leaving these old vaporizers, is not fully saturated with the vapor of liquid anesthetic agent.

The splitting valve, which divides the gas flow to the vaporizers and to the bypass channel, is of wide bore (so of low resistance) and works over a wide range of fresh gas flow rates. This type of vaporizer is also known as *"inside the circuit"* vaporizer, because being of low resistance and having no unidirectional valve, it acts as a continuous component of the circuit of an anesthetic machine. As these old blow-over

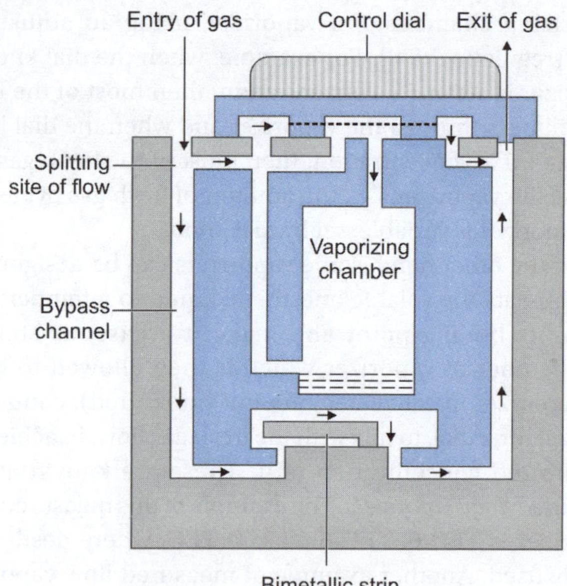

Fig. 27: TEC-5 plenum vaporizer.

vaporizers have no unidirectional valve, so they are affected by *pumping (back pressure)* effect. On the other hand, the modern TEC-5 or TEC-7 vaporizers are called the plenum (which means high resistance due to *narrow splitting valve and unidirectional flow*) vaporizer and the carrier gas which enters the vaporizing chamber of the vaporizer, is made to be fully saturated by the vapor of volatile anesthetic agent, present in the vaporizer, and is partially pressurized (*but not heated, like TEC-6 or Aladin. Cause of this partially pressurized is described later*) so that it is rather forced to mix with the bypass fresh gas flow than it simply blows over the surface of the volatile liquid anesthetic agent in vaporizing chamber, taking the unsaturated vapor of it, like the draw-over vaporizer **(Fig. 27)**.

The vaporizing chambers of the plenum vaporizers act as a partially pressurized chamber, containing fully saturated vapor of volatile anesthetic agent during its working time (i.e., when the vaporizer is kept on and fresh gas start to flow through vaporizer), from where the continuous flow of gas, fully saturated with anesthetic agent comes out. This is made possible by increasing the capacity of vaporization of liquid volatile anesthetic agents to a very high level, by adding wicks and baffles inside the vaporizing chamber, and by restricting the exit of gas from the chamber by control valve than the vaporizing capacity of vaporizer (*TEC-6 and Aladin vaporizers are fully pressurized, even though fresh gas does not start to flow through it, because, by electrically heating the liquid anesthetic, vapor is previously produced in these vaporizers*). Due to the presence of unidirectional valve, these plenum vaporizers are not affected by pumping (back pressure) effect, during positive pressure ventilation.

These plenum vaporizers are also called the *"outside the circuit"* vaporizers, because they do not act as the part of anesthetic circuit, due to *high resistance and the splitting valve is of narrow bore*. They also do not act over the wide range of flow rate, like the draw-over vaporizers. So, it (vaporizer) needs to be calibrated very accurately. The examples of the draw-over vaporizers are: Boyle's ether bottle vaporizer, Goldman vaporizer, Oxford miniature vaporizer (OMV), Epstein-Macintosh-Oxford (EMO) vaporizer, and TEC-3 vaporizer. The TEC-3 vaporizer is a draw-over vaporizer but temperature compensated. The examples of plenum vaporizers are: all the temperature compensated (TEC) vaporizers of Datex Ohmeda series such as TEC-4, TEC-5, TEC-7, and Drager vaporizer, such as the 19 and 2000 series. These different models or the different types of plenum vaporizers differ among themselves only by their interior design, regarding the arrangement of baffles and wicks, to increase their capacity of vaporization, made by different companies, to remove some technical disadvantages of previous one. But, their basic mechanism of action is same. The old model plenum TEC-3 vaporizer is out of market now. At present, the commonly used model of plenum vaporizers are TEC-5 and TEC-7 of Datex Ohmeda series and Drager vaporizer of 19 and 2000 series. The Aladin vaporizer, which is discussed in more details in Chapter 15, is another example of plenum vaporizer where vaporization is controlled by electronic method. The TEC-6 vaporizer, which is developed to use only the desflurane, is also an example of measured flow vaporizer. TEC-6 and Aladin vaporizer are not the plenum type (partial blow over) vaporizer. They are heated (electronically) and pressurized vaporizers.

All the plenum vaporizers are temperature compensated. It means, with the cooling of volatile anesthetic agent during vaporization, the delivered vapor concentration of volatile anesthetic agent does not reduce. This is achieved by controlling the splitting ratio of fresh gas flow, before entering the vaporizer by a temperature sensitive bimetallic strip. It is made of two strips of metal, with different coefficients of thermal expansion, bonded together. It allows more flow into the vaporizing chamber by bending, as the temperature decreases and vice versa **(Fig. 28)**. This bimetallic strip or temperature sensitive valve is located in the vaporization chamber in TEC-2 model, whereas in the TEC-3, TEC-4, and TEC-5 model it is situated outside the vaporization chamber **(Fact file VI)**.

All the variable bypass plenum vaporizers are flow compensated and its explanation is described below. Before, entering the vaporizer, the fresh gas flow is splitted into two streams. The main larger stream of the gas flows through the bypass channel and the smaller narrow stream of gas flows through the vaporizing chamber of vaporizer. After

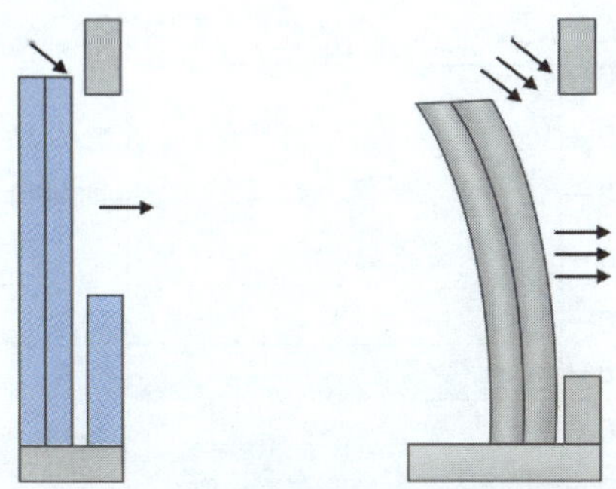

Fig. 28: The mechanism of action of bimetallic strip, causing thermocompensation of vaporizer.

FACT FILE VI

The vaporizers where the volatile anesthetic agents are vaporized by heating it electrically, such as TEC-6 desflurane vaporizers or where there is an electronically regulated flow control valve located at the outlet of vaporizing chamber but vaporization is done by conventional blowing the gas over the volatile liquid anesthetic agent like other variable bypass vaporizers, such as Aladin cassette vaporizers are called the electronic vaporizers.

The boiling point of desflurane is 22°C. Thus, it boils almost at room temperature. So, its vapor pressure is very high which is near about 681 mm Hg at 20°C (halothane = 243°C, isoflurane = 240°C, sevoflurane = 160°C). Again the potency of it is near about 1/5th than that of other volatile anesthetic agent. Hence, all these characteristic of desflurane presents a unique delivery problem of it and is solved by the development of TEC-6 vaporizer where only desflurane is used. In this vaporizer, there is a reservoir containing desflurane which is heated electrically to 39°C to vaporize it. So, this reservoir always contains the dense vapor of desflurane at the pressure of 2 atmosphere. On the other hand, no fresh gas from flow meter is allowed to flow over the desflurane for vaporization of it through bypass channel, like other variable bypass vaporizers. Rather, the measured amount of pure vapor of desflurane is allowed to flow from the reservoir which is regulated by a control dial and to mix with the fresh gas flow coming from flow meter to make the desired delivered concentration of it. Thus, it maintains a desired constant concentration of desflurane over a wide range of fresh gas flow rates.

In Aladin cassette vaporizer, the volatile liquid anesthetic agent is also vaporized by heating it electrically, like TEC-6 vaporizer. Here, like other conventional plenum vaporizer, the fresh gas flow from flow meter is divided which is regulated by control dial and a portion of it is allowed to flow through the vaporizing chamber to vaporize the anesthetic liquid. However, this vaporization is conducted into an agent-specific color-coded cassette (Aladin cassette). The anesthetic machine accept one cassette at a time and recognize this cassette through magnetic leveling. Unlike the traditional vaporizers, here the liquid anesthetic agents cannot escape from it during handling and so it can be carried in any position.

vaporization, this narrow stream of gas flow comes out of the vaporizing chamber with the fully saturated volatile anesthetic agent and reunit with the main larger stream of

the fresh gas flow. This splitting of gas flow, before entering the vaporizer, is controlled by a regulating dial which dictate how much gas will enter the vaporizing chamber. The vaporizing chamber of a plenum vaporizer is such designed that the gas, leaving it, is always fully saturated with vapor of volatile liquid anesthetic agent, before it joins with the gas of bypass stream, whatever may be the amount of fresh gas flow into the vaporizing chamber. So, this is called the flow compensated vaporizer.

This is achieved by increasing the surface area of contact between the gas, entering the vaporizing chamber and the volatile liquid anesthetic agent by adding wicks, soaked by the agent and making a series of baffles. Thus, *whatever may be the rate of fresh gas flow,* through the vaporizing chamber, the delivered concentration of anesthetic agent can be controlled by both controlling the flow of gas, entering the vaporizing chamber (under a certain dial setting the portion of gas entering the vaporizing chamber does not vary with the rate of fresh gas flow) and controlling the rejoining of gas, fully saturated with anesthetic agent, with the main gas flow by the controlling dial. Thus, the delivered concentration of volatile anesthetic agent will not be influenced by the rate of fresh gas flow, through vaporizer, like the draw-over vaporizer, such as Goldman vaporizer, ether vaporizer, etc. In modern designs, the anesthetic concentration of volatile anesthetic agent, supplied by the vaporizer, is independent of gas flow through vaporizing chamber between 0.5 and 15 L/min. Hence, they are flow compensated. But, the changing of composition of gas from 70% N_2O to 100% O_2 may increase the concentration of anesthetic agent, due to the greater solubility of N_2O in volatile liquid anesthetic agents.

In comparison to the flow compensated vaporizers, the draw-over vaporizers are not flow compensated, because under a certain dial setting the portion of gas entering the vaporizing chamber varies with the rate of fresh gas flow, and the gas coming out from the vaporizing chamber is not fully saturated. Thus, the rejoining of gas mixed with variable concentration of anesthetic agent to the main gas flow is not controlled. During vaporization, due to the loss of latent heat for vaporization, the cooling of anesthetic agent occurs and makes it less volatile, reducing vaporization. So, in order to compensate this heat loss two measures are taken. One, the vaporizer is made up of such material which has high density, high specific heat, and high thermal conductivity, such as copper. So, it acts as heat reservoir and readily gives heat to the cooled anesthetic agent, maintaining its temperature and its vaporization nearly constant. Two, a temperature sensitive valve, made of bimetallic strip, allows more flow into the vaporizing chamber by bending, as the temperature of volatile anesthetic agent decreases and vice versa.

All the modern vaporizers are agent specific. So, the filling of them (vaporizers) with wrong agents (volatile liquid anesthetics) should be avoided. For example, the filling of vaporizer, which is specific for halothane, by sevoflurane would lead to anesthetic concentration in *under doses and vice versa.* This is because the vapor pressure of halothane at one atmospheric pressure and 20°C is 243 mm Hg, whereas the same of sevoflurane is 160 mm Hg. So, if sevoflurane is used in halothane TEC-7 or TEC-5 vaporizer, it will cause near about 40% lesser amount of anesthetic concentration to be released and vice versa. So, the modern TEC-5 and TEC-7 vaporizers (TEC-4 is also obsolete now) are equipped with (i) the agent-specific filling ports and (ii) the color-coded agent-specific filling devices, to prevent the use of wrong agent in wrong vaporizer.

In older vaporizers, during invasive positive pressure ventilation (IPPV), there may be transient reversal (backflow) of the flow of fresh gas and the pressure into vaporizer, through the bypass channel and it will lead to the delivery of unpredictable concentration of anesthetic agent. This is known as the *pumping effect* which is more pronounced with low gas flow. Hence, in modern vaporizers some changes, in the design of the vaporizer and the placement of a one way check valve, limit the occurrence of this problem. During transport or due to any reason, if the vaporizers are tilted excessively, then the anesthetic agent may spill over and flood the bypass channel of vaporizer. Then, this may lead to sudden delivery of dangerously high concentration of anesthetic agent when first used. So, during handling of it, when not attached to machine, excessive tilting of vaporizer should be avoided.

Ventilator

For IPPV, during anesthesia, all the modern anesthetic machines are now equipped with ventilators which are of bag in bottle type in most of the cases. They have mainly the continuous mandatory ventilation (CMV) mode for ventilation. But, some have the facilities to provide other few more modes for ventilation, such as the synchronized intermittent mandatory ventilation (SIMV), continuous positive airway pressure (CPAP), bilevel positive airway pressure (BiPAP), and positive end-expiratory pressure (PEEP), etc. This is because more and more critically ill patients are now entering in OT for surgical interference. Hence, the distinction between the ICU ventilators which are more sophisticated and anesthetic ventilators which are more simple, is gradually becoming blurred.

From the designing aspect, all the ventilators are divided into two groups: (1) double circuit system ventilators (bag in bottle type of ventilators), and (2) piston type ventilators.

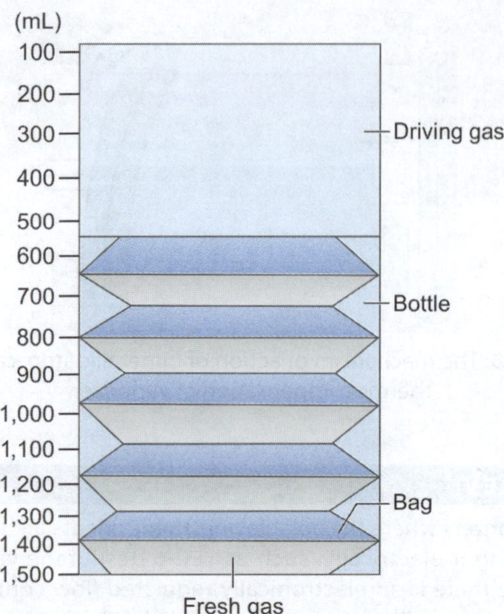

Fig. 29: The mechanism of action of a bag in bottle type of ventilator.

Traditionally, the ventilators which are incorporated in anesthetic machine, are of *bag in bottle type* (**Fig. 29**). As they have two circuits (one is to drive the ventilators and another is to ventilate the patient), so they are also called the *double circuit system ventilators*. These ventilators are driven pneumatically by compressed air or O_2 from pipeline or cylinder. But, their control panel is driven by the electric current. The newer machines also incorporate microprocessor and sophisticated precise pressure and flow sensors to achieve the multiple ventilatory modes (like the ICU ventilators), accurate tidal volumes, and enhanced safety features. In the *piston design ventilators*, the bellow is substituted by piston and is driven by electric power, with no or minimal pneumatic (compressed air or O_2) power. The major advantage of this piston ventilator is its ability to deliver the accurate tidal volume to patient, with very poor lung compliance and to very small patients.

These bags in bottle type of anesthetic ventilators have mainly two basic components: (1) a driving unit, and (2) a control unit. The driving unit consists of a chamber (bottle) with tidal volume marks, ranging from 0 to 1,500 mL and *an ascending or descending type of bellow* (bag), receiving fresh gas flow within it (**Figs. 30A and B**). In pediatric version, the tidal volume marks on the chamber, ranges from 0 to 400 mL, whereas in the adult version the tidal volume marks on the chamber, ranges from 100 to 1,500 mL. The control unit of the ventilator contains varieties of controlling knobs, varieties of display system on screen and varieties of alarms. The controlling knobs include the knob controlling the respiratory rate, tidal volume, airway pressure, inspiratory/

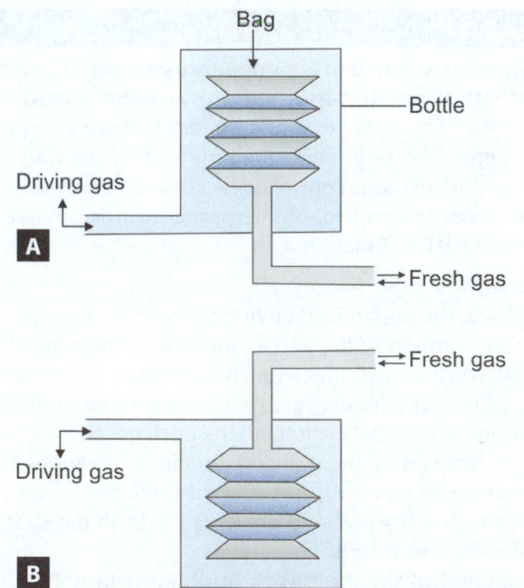

Figs. 30A and B: (A) Ascending; and (B) Descending type of bag in bottle ventilator.

expiratory (I/E) ratio, power supply, etc., to regulate the IPPV of patient during anesthesia.

In these types of bag in bottle ventilators, the compressed air or O_2 is used, as the driving pressure. On entering the driving chamber (bottle) of ventilator, this driving gas forces the bellows down, in case of the ascending type of bag in bottle ventilator and delivers the fresh anesthetic gas mixture to the patient which was accommodated inside the bellow, during the previous expiratory phase of respiratory cycle. The volume of driving gas, entering the chamber (bottle), is always equal to the tidal volume and remains completely separated from the fresh gas flow which enters inside the bellow. Then, during expiration the bellow again ascends, due to the flow of fresh gas, mixed with expired gas from patient within it (bellow) and the driving gas from chamber comes out. A ventilator's flow control valve regulates the flow of driving gas into the pressurizing chamber (bottle).

This flow control valve is controlled by ventilator setting in the control panel. The ventilators with its microprocessor also utilize the feedbacks from the flow and pressure sensors and control this flow control valve. If O_2 is used for pneumatic power, then it will be consumed at a rate, at least, equal to the minute ventilation of the patient. Therefore, a large amount of O_2 will be consumed, if the ventilator is driven by O_2. Hence, some anesthetic machines reduce this huge consumption of O_2 by incorporating a venture device that draws in room air to provide air plus O_2 pneumatic power.

There are another type of ventilator where the below is of descending type. Here, during expiration the gas is sucked from the patient into bellow by a weight, placed at the base of it (bellow). So, the probable advantage of this type of descending bellow in ventilator is the absence of expiratory resistance. This advantage is not available in ventilator with ascending bellow, because it is claimed that the pressure, required to fill the bellow, both by the fresh gas from machine and the expired gas from patient, adds some expiratory resistance to the patient and may prevent complete exhalation. Therefore, it is claimed that the ascending bellow provides a degree of PEEP (2–4 cmH$_2$O) which may otherwise be beneficial.

The another advantage of ascending bellow is that it collapses to an empty position and remains stationary at that empty position, if there is any leak in the bag or disconnection of circuit, whereas in the descending design of bellow, it automatically hangs down to fully expanded position, even if there is any leak or disconnection of circuit and may continue to move almost normally. In such condition, the driving gas would also be able to enter the bellow through the leak and dilute the anesthetic gas mixture within it which is not possible in ascending variety.

The arrangement in descending bellow also allows the driving control unit to be placed above the bellow in free standing version. So, the bellow of it could be placed on the lower shelf of an anesthetic machine, with the controls panel easily at hand. However, the descending bellow is now no longer popular **(Fact file VII to IX)**.

In the anesthetic machine, there is a bag or ventilator switch (change over). When, it is turned toward the bag, then the ventilator is cut off (excluded) from the common gas out let of machine and now the fresh gas flows from the common gas outlet toward the manual breathing bag of anesthetic machine and its breathing circuit with adjustable pressure-limiting (APL) valve. In such circumstances, the manual bag ventilation can be done or the patient can be allowed for spontaneous ventilation. When the bag or ventilator changeover is turned toward the ventilator, then the manual breathing bag, anesthetic breathing circuit, and APL valve is cut off from the common gas out let of anesthetic machine and the fresh gas flows from the common gas outlet of the anesthetic machine into the ventilator circuit. In such circumstances, manual bag ventilation or spontaneous ventilation is not possible.

The ventilator contains its own pressure relief (pop off) valve which is also called the spill valve. It is pneumatically closed by driving gas during inspiration, so that +ve pressure can be generated. During expiration, the spill valve is no longer closed and the driving (pressurizing) gas is vented out through spill valve, as there is no flow of driving gas. During expiration, the expired gas flows through patient's circuit from the patient into ventilator bag (bellow), along with the fresh gas and when the bellow is completely filled

FACT FILE VII

Other than the bellows in bottle which is squeezed pneumatically it may be inflated or deflated without bottle by a piston that is powered by gas and is attached to the bellow by a lever. The advantage of this principle is that it removes the potential danger of mixing between the driving gas which is situated outside the bellow and the patient's gas which is situated inside the bellow. Another advantage of this principle is that the piston may be driven by a smaller quantity of gas from cylinder. So, it is very valuable where there is scarcity of gas. The Manley Servovent and Oxford Mark 2 ventilators work on this principle. The bellows may also be moved mechanically by motor and suitable levers and gears. The speed of motor can be changed to produce the varieties of flows both during inspiration and expiration. This principle is used in the Drager E series of ventilators. In some ventilators, the bellows are not used, instead a long wide bore hose pipe is substituted. In this method, the driving gas is directly pushed into the breathing system with the fresh gas by ventilator, but it does not mixed with the fresh gas due to long length of hose pipe. The example of ventilator working on this principle is Penlon Nuffield 200 series.

FACT FILE VIII

There are now many major advances in the working principles of ventilator which are used in intensive care unit and also anesthetic ventilator. Among these, the two most important parts are electronic flow valve and microprocessor. In an electronic flow valve, first current is allowed to pass through a wire coil (solenoid) to produce a magnetic field which moves the ferromagnetic piston and closes and open the valve with the help of a spring. The movement of the valve depends on the flow of current and thus controls the movement of driving gas by corresponding amount of closing and opening of it. As this valve is used in high-pressure gas pathways, so the little movement of valve is enough to control the flow of driving gas very quickly varying between 1 and 120 L/min. The response time of this type of solenoid valve is only 5 ms and is very compact to be fitted easily in a small equipment.

The microprocessor part of a ventilator controls the electrical signal to the electronic flow valve of it. They are usually programmed to provide a wide variety of ventilatory modes and response. Most of the ventilators now work on this principle but they only differ according the user display, variable programming, and the quality of components.

FACT FILE IX

Description of function of a commonly used bag, in a bottle type of anesthetic ventilator, attached with anesthetic machine.

This represents a model of a pneumatically driven bag in bottle type of ventilator, with an arrangement of ascending bellows. There, the driving gas is controlled by electronic flow valve, which is again under the control of microprocessor to provide a wide range of ventilatory function.

Inspiratory

In this phase, the pressurized driving gas (not the fresh gas flow) is first passed through a filter and a regulator to enter the electronic flow valve which is held shut when not in use. Then, the gas passes to the bottle that contains an arrangement of ascending bellow and compresses the bellow forcing the fresh gas to flow through a wide bore hose into a breathing system for inspiration of patient. This driving gas also supplies a small pneumatic valve which closes the expiratory port and prevents the fresh gas destined for inspiration from escaping.

The passing of driving gas through electronic flow valve is controlled by a microprocessor which receives information from the ventilator setting of front panel by anesthetist, fresh gas flow through the anesthetic machine, and inspiratory flow to the patient. Thus, the changes in these flows will also change the flow of driving gas through the electronic flow valve and consecutively control the tidal volume which depends on the force on the bag caused by driving gas.

Expiratory valve

At the end of the time cycled inspiratory phase the microprocessor instructs the electronic flow valve to close and a second valve to open. Thus, the driving gas passes away to the atmosphere from bottle through second valve and causes its pressure to fall to zero. This allows the exhaled gas from patient mainly from dead space and fresh gas to enter the bellow. If Bain circuit is used then this exhaled gas comes from the patient through the wider external tube which is attached to the input of ventilator. When the bellow becomes full and its pressure is raised above the atmosphere, then the expiratory port opens and expired gas from alveoli containing CO_2 escapes to the atmosphere through output channel. At the same time the driving gas leaving the bellow also passes out through the output channel.

---

up, then the excess gas is directed to scavenging system, through spill valve. Therefore, during inspiration the spill valve of ventilator is completely closed and no gas comes out through this valve. On the other hand, during expiration both the driving (pressurizing) gas and the patient's expired gas come out. Sticking of this valve can result in abnormally elevated airway pressure during exhalation.

Peak inspiratory pressure (PIP) is the maximum pressure (cmH_2O) in the breathing ventilatory circuit during inspiration. It is measured at the beginning of inspiration and provides an idea regarding the dynamic compliance of lungs. Plateau inspiratory pressure is the pressure which is measured during inspiratory pause (at the end of inspiration when gas flow stops). It mirrors the static compliance. Without any lung disease, during normal ventilation of a patient, the PIP is equal to or slightly greater than plateau pressure. An increase in both pressures commonly indicates either decrease in lung compliance of patient or increase in tidal volume setting in ventilator. *The causes for decrease in lung compliance are:* pulmonary edema, Trendelenburg position, pleural effusion, endobronchial intubation, tension pneumothorax, abdominal packing, ascites, etc. *An increase in PIP, without any change in plateau pressure indicates an increase in airway resistance or increase in inspiratory gas flow rate. The causes of increase in airway resistance are:* bronchospasm, bronchial secretions, blocking of ET tube, airway compression, kinking of tube, etc. Hence, the shape of breathing circuit pressure waveform can provide many important information and so, now many anesthesia machines itself (not ventilator) graphically or numerically display the breathing circuit pressure.

Miscellaneous

Nonreturn pressure relief valve: It is situated on the back bar of an anesthetic machine, after the vaporizer or at the common gas outlet. Here, it acts as nonreturn valve and helps to prevent the effect of back pressure on the vaporizers or flow meter (rotameter) during positive pressure ventilation by ventilator or by manual. Another advantage of it is that it also opens when the back bar pressure exceeds 30 kP and acts as pressure relief safety valve **(Fig. 31)**.

Emergency O_2 flush: It is presented in the anesthetic machine as nonlocking button. When it is pressed with the thumb of a hand, then only pure O_2 at the flow rate of 30–70 L/min is supplied to the patient from the common outlet of anesthetic machine bypassing the flow meter and vaporizers **(Fig. 32)**. It is also used to flush the breathing circuit or to rapidly refill the breathing bag. It should not be activated when the minute volume divider ventilator is in use. Injudicious use of this emergency O_2 flush may dilute the anesthetic gases and may cause inadequate depth of anesthesia and awareness. Moreover, inappropriate use of flush valve may result in backflow of gases into pressure circuit, causing malfunction of machine. It may also cause barotrauma, when the patient is connected to a completely closed breathing circuit, through an endotracheal tube (ET), because when the O_2 flush valve is activated, it will supply O_2 to breathing circuit at a line pressure of 45–55 psi.

Common gas outlet and O_2 analyzer: All the anesthetic machines have only one common outlet to patient, supplying fresh anesthetic gases, mixed with O_2 to breathing circuit, in contrast to multiple inlets which supply different gases to the machine. The modern machines are equipped with devices which measure the flow of gases to patient, through this common outlet and gives signal during the detachment of this outlet from the breathing circuit. In some modern machines, the antidisconnect retaining device is also used to prevent the accidental detachment of breathing circuit from machine.

It is fundamental to monitor the inspired O_2 concentration (FiO$_2$) or partial pressure of it (O_2) in the fresh mixture, delivered to the patient. Without an O_2 analyzer, which measures the inspired O_2 concentration, an anesthetic

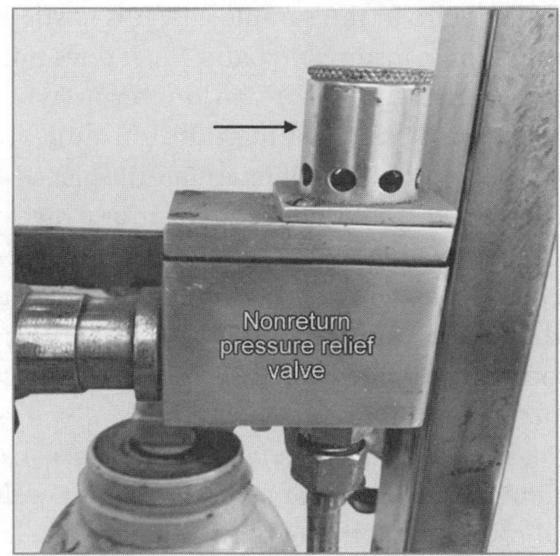

Fig. 31: Nonreturn pressure relief valve.

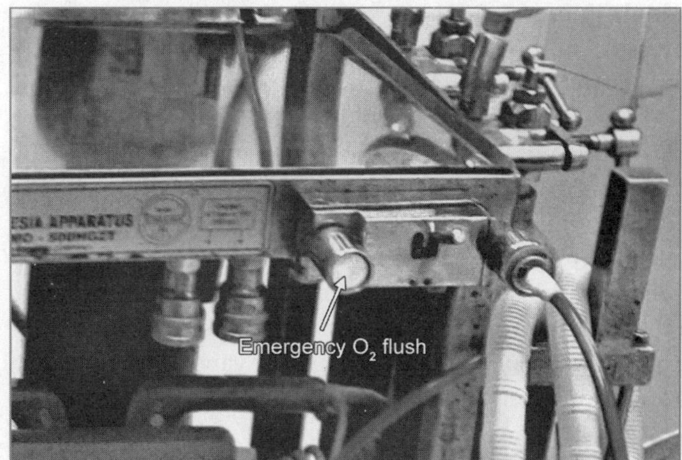

Fig. 32: Emergency O$_2$ flush.

machine is always incomplete and general anesthesia (GA) should never be administered. It is placed in the inspiratory or expiratory limb, if close circuit is used. Otherwise, if the circuit has one limb, then it should be placed at the patient's end of it. But, it should not be placed at the fresh gasline. It should be kept in mind that due to O_2 consumption by patient, the partial pressure of O_2 in expiratory limb is slightly lower than that of the inspiratory limb. An audible alarm can be set for high and low concentration of inspired O_2 such as 40% and 28% respectively.

Three types of O_2 analyzers, which measures FiO$_2$ are used in modern anesthetic machine. These are: *paramagnetic*, or *fuel cell (or galvanic)*, or *Clark electrode (polarographic)*. The *paramagnetic sensor* works on the principle that only O_2 will be attracted by the magnetic field, whereas the other gases will be repelled. This attraction and repulsion of individual gas depends on their concentration and partial pressure in the sample gas. It is costly than the others and has no consumable parts. So, it does not require frequent replacement. Therefore, on long term it is less costly. Its response time is very fast than the galvanic and Clark electrode O_2 analyzers. It can differentiate the partial pressure of O_2 between the inspired and expired air, as it measures the inspired and expired O_2 concentration simultaneously, on breath by breath basis. However, this paramagnetic analyzer is affected by water vapor in sample gas. Therefore, a water tap is incorporated in the design. Another advantage of this paramagnetic sensor is its self-calibrating.

The *galvanic* and *polarographic sensor* is also called the electrochemical sensor, because both of them contain the anode and cathode electrodes, embedded in an electrolyte gel, which is separated from the gas sample by an O_2 permeable membrane. After diffusing through the membrane, O_2 reacts with the electrode in the gel and produces a current which is proportional to the concentration and partial pressure of it (O_2) in the sample gas. Thus, they measure the partial pressure of O_2 as percentage. These galvanic and polarographic O_2 analyzers have slow response time (20–30 seconds), because they are dependent on membrane diffusion of O_2. These sensors have limited life span to about 1 year. This is because of the exhaustion of material (electrolyte gel) in it, due to continuous exposure to O_2. It needs regular service and calibration is achieved by using 100% O_2 and room air (21% O_2). It reads only inspiratory or expiratory O_2 concentration and water vapor does not affect its performance.

N₂O and other inhalation anesthetic agent concentration analyzer: The measurement of inspired and end-tidal concentration of N_2O and the concentration of other inhalational anesthetic agents are very important, mainly when the circle system is used. This is because the expired inhalational anesthetic agents are recirculated and are added to the fresh gas flows which is also carrying the volatile anesthetic agents. So, when the circle system is used, the ultimate inspired concentration of inhalational anesthetic agents is different from the setting of vaporizer, especially during low flow. Hence, the modern analyzers can assure the inspired concentration of all the inhalational anesthetic agents such as N_2O, halothane, isoflurane, sevoflurane, and desflurane. The principles by which the concentration of inhalational anesthetic agents are measured are: infrared technique, ultraviolet ray absorption technique, mass spectrometry, Raman spectroscopy, Piezo electric quartz crystal oscillation technique, etc.

In infrared technique, a light of wavelength of 4.6 nm is used for N_2O. On the other hand, an infrared light of wavelength of 8–9 nm is used for the other volatile anesthetic agents. This is to avoid interference from the methane and alcohol that happens at the lower 3.5 nm wavelength. Some infrared analyzers are not agent specific. These must be programmed by the user for specific agent being administered. Incorrect programming result in incorrect result. In piezoelectric oscillation technique, a lipophilic-coated piezoelectric quartz crystal is used which undergoes continuous changes in its frequency of oscillation when lipid soluble inhalational anesthetic agent is exposed to it. This change in the frequency of oscillation is directly proportional to the concentration of agent. Mass spectrometer is used to analyze the inhalational anesthetic agents on breath to breath basis. In this technique, the principle of action is to change the particles of sample gas by bombardment on them with electron beam and then to separate the components arising from this bombardment by a magnet into different spectrum according to their specific mass: charge ratio. The relative concentration of ion in a spectrum of a specific mass: charge ratio is determined by the concentration of a particular agent in gas mixture **(Table 2)**.

Measurement of tidal and minute volume: During GA, the measurement of tidal volume and from it the measurement of minute volume is very critical which the anesthetic machine performs by Wright spirometer (respirometer), hot-wire anemometer, ultrasonic flow sensor, and pneumotachograph. These are used in all the modern sophisticated anesthetic machines to measure the exhaled tidal volume by attaching them in breathing circuit near the exhalation valve. Some machines measure the inspiratory tidal volume by attaching these just distal to the inspiratory valve. However, in the latest model of Datex Ohmeda machine, these are attached near the Y-connection of patient to measure the actual delivered and exhaled tidal volume.

In Wright respirometer, there is a rotating vane which is surrounded by multiple slits and this vane is attached to a pointer on a dial. When the gas passes through it (vane), then the slits which surround the vane, create a circular

TABLE 2: Various methods used to analyze gases.			
Methods	*O_2*	*CO_2*	*N_2O*	*Volatile agents*
Infrared	–	+	+	+
Galvanic	+	–	–	–
Polarography	+	–	–	–
Paramagnetic	+	–	–	–
Raman Spectroscopy	+	+	+	+
Mass Spectrometry	+	+	+	+
Piezoelectric Oscillation	–	–	–	+

flow and rotate the vane with pointer on front dial. The vane does 150 revolutions for each liter of gas passing through it. This is the mechanical method to measure the tidal volume by Wright spirometer (respirometer). In clinical use, the respirometer reads accurately the tidal volume within the range of 4–24 L/min of airflow. A minimum airflow of 2 L/min is required for the respirometer to function accurately. A pediatric version of spirometer is also now available which can measure the tidal volume in the range of 15–200 mL/breath. A sophisticated version of this Wright spirometer uses the reflection of light technique (photoelectric method) to measure the tidal volume more accurately. Other modification of this Wright spirometer is the use of semiconductive device, where the tidal volume is measured from the changes in magnetic field during gas flow and converting it electronically.

The hot-wire anemometer is used in Drager Fabius anesthetic machine to measure the tidal volume. Here, electrically heated fine platinum wires are used. The cooling effect of these wires by increasing gas flow through it causes a change in electrical resistance which is proportion to the gas flow and is determined by the current needed to maintain a constant wire temperature. In ultrasonic flow sensors an upstream and downstream ultrasonic beams are passed at an angle from where the shift of Doppler frequency is measure which is proportional to the flow of gas or tidal volume. In pneumotachograph, the parallel bundles of tubes of small diameter in a chamber or a mesh screen is used which provide resistance to airflow and drop of pressure. This drop of pressure across the resistance is sensed by a differential pressure transducer and is proportional to the flow rate. Thus, calculation of flow rate over time measures the tidal volume. Moreover analysis of this volume, pressure, and time relationship will give us the potential valuable information about lungs and airway mechanics.

CIRCUIT PRESSURE

To measure the breathing circuit pressure, somewhere in between the inspiratory and expiratory unidirectional valve, different types of pressure gauge or electronic sensor is always used. However, the exact location of pressure sensor depends on the model of anesthetic machine. If the pressure sensor is placed at the Y-connection, then the most accurate measurement of both the inspiratory and expiratory pressure can be obtained, because as close as possible to the patient, the breathing circuit pressure will be measured, it will reflect the patient's airway pressure. A rise in circuit pressure (equivalent to patient's airway pressure) indicates ↓ in pulmonary compliance of patient, or ↑ in tidal volume which is set in the machine, or obstruction in circuit/trachea/

airway of patient. On the other hand, a drop in the pressure of circuit indicates ↑ (improvement) in the compliance of lungs of the patient, or ↓ in tidal volume setting in machine, or any leak in circuit or its detachment. If the circuit pressure is measured at the level of CO_2 absorber, it will not mirror the actual airway pressure of the patient.

HUMIDIFIERS

Humidity of gas means the amount (in mg) of water in the form of vapor in 1 L of this gas. It may be absolute or relative. The absolute humidity means the maximum amount (in mg) of water that can be hold by 1 L of gas at a particular temperature. The relative humidity means the ratio of amount of water now present in 1 L of gas to the maximum amount of water that can be hold in 1 L of gas at a particular temperature. Relative humidity is 100% means the gas is fully saturated with the water vapor or it (gas) contains the maximum amount of water in 1 L of this gas at that particular temperature or the relative humidity touches the number of absolute humidity. Another point we will have to keep in our mind that as the temperature of a gas will increase, its ability to hold the amount of water vapor will also increase or the number of absolute humidity will increase and vice versa.

The gases which are supplied to the patients from anesthetic machine are much below the body temperature and are little or not humidified at all. These gases are, therefore, warmed to body temperature and humidified with water (vapor) by the upper respiratory tract during mask ventilation. Tracheal intubation and high (cool) fresh gas flow bypass this normal humidification system of upper respiratory tract and exposes the lower respiratory tract to take this burden (to increase the temperature of fresh gases and to humidify it).

Therefore, prolonged anesthesia following tracheal intubation leads to prolonged humidification of gases by the lower respiratory tract, causing dehydration and drying of its mucosa, less secretion, altered ciliary activity, etc., resulting inspissation of secretion, atelectasis, and even ventilation/perfusion mismatch, particularly in patients with underlying lung diseases. Body heat is lost, as gases are warmed and further when the body water is vaporized to humidify the gases, it takes temperature from the body. The heat of vaporization of water is 560 cal/g of water and this heat loss accounts for about 10% of total intraoperative heat loss from body. However, this is not so significant for short surgical procedures (<½ to 1 hours). But, it has prominent effect on pediatric and elderly patients and the patients with severe underlying lung disease.

The device by which the dry inhaled anesthetic gases are humidified (addition of water vapor) is known as humidifier.

They also increase the temperature of cold inhaled anesthetic gases to body temperature. So, this device is called the heat and moisture exchanger (HME). This humidification and warming of dry cold anesthetic gases, supplied from cylinders or pipeline (pipeline gases attain room temperature when they pass through pipes) can be done by passive and active methods.

Passive Humidification or Humidifier

Here the device is very simple. It does not add heat and water vapor to the inhaled dry and cold anesthetic gases from itself. Rather, it contains a hygroscopic material that traps exhaled water vapor and heat from the patient and released them during subsequent inhalation. According to the design, they may substantially increase the apparatus dead space (>60 mL) which can cause significant rebreathing and increase in EtCO$_2$. It also significantly increases the breathing circuit resistance and work of breathing during spontaneous respiration. Also, excessive saturation of an HME with water or secretion can obstruct the breathing circuit. Some such passive humidifier devices also act as effective bacterial and viral filters and are important for ventilating patients with respiratory infections or compromised immune system.

Active Humidification or Humidifiers

Active humidifier is more effective than a passive one, because it preserves more water and heat. Active humidifier is again of four types: (1) pass over, (2) bubble through, (3) wick, and (4) vapor phase. In pass over active humidifier, the inhaled gases are passed over the surface of water, contained in a chamber. In bubble through active humidifier, the inhaled gases are bubbled through water. In wick active humidifier, the inhaled gases are passed through water saturated wick. In vapor phase humidifier, the inhaled gases are mixed with vaporized water. Among these, the vapor phase humidifier is best, because it is a thermostatically controlled heated humidifiers and heat helps in more vaporization of water plus increasing temperature of gas increases the capacity of inhaled gas to hold more water vapor.

But, the heated humidifier has some disadvantages. These are: (i) more chances of thermal lung injury (so, the temperature of inhaled gases should not exceed body temperature), (ii) nosocomial infection, (iii) increase airway resistance from excess water condensation in the breathing circuit, (iv) interference of flow meter function, (v) does not filter micro-organisms, and lastly (vi) increased chances of circuit disconnection. However, active humidifier is very valuable in children, as it helps to prevent both hypothermia and plugging of small tracheal tube by dried secretions.

■ WASTE GAS SCAVENGER

Continuously different types of gases are released into OT from breathing circuit through APL valve or from ventilator through its spill valve. Hence, this causes heavy pollution of the operating room environment with anesthetic gases and poses a great health hazard to the OT personnel. But, still there is no general consensus to define the safe level of exposure to the anesthetic agents. However, the International Committee for Occupational Safety and Health recommends limiting maximally the room concentration of N$_2$O to 25 ppm and halogenated agents to 2 ppm. The reduction of the concentration of the anesthetic gases below this maximum limiting level is possible only with properly functioning waste gas scavenging (WGS) system which scavenges the anesthetic gases that are vented out from the breathing circuit through APL; valve or ventilator spill valve, without spilling in OT.

To scavenge the waste gases, both the APL and ventilator spill valves are connected to a hose which leads to scavenging system and this scavenging system may be inside the machine or an external attachment. The pressure immediately downstream to WGS system should be kept between 0.5 and 3.5 cmH$_2$O. The WGS system may be described as either open or closed. In open WGS system, it is opened directly to the outside environment and usually requires no pressure relief valve. In contrast, a closed WGS system is closed to outside environment and required –ve or +ve pressure relief valve. The –ve pressure relief valve protect the patient from the –ve pressure of vacuum system and the +ve pressure relief valve protect the patient from an obstruction in the disposal tubing.

WGS system also can be classified as passive scavenging and active scavenging. When the outlet of scavenging system is a direct line to the outside through a ventilation duct, beyond any point of recirculation, then it is called the passive scavenging. On the other hand, when the outlet of scavenging system is connected to hospital vacuum system, then it is called the active scavenging. The vacuum control valve of an active scavenging system should be adjusted to allow the evacuation of 10–15 L of waste gas per minute. This rate is adequate for the periods of high fresh gas flow (i.e., induction and emergence) and minimizes the risk of transmitting –ve pressure to the breathing circuit, during lower flow conditions (maintenance of anesthesia). In some machine, there is both active and passive scavenging.

■ SOME KEY POINTS

- Medical grade O$_2$ is 99–99.5% pure oxygen. It is manufactured by fractional distillation of liquid air.

- H cylinders are used in two separate banks, connected by manifold with an automatic cross over feature. Only one bank is utilized at a time. The pressure in H cylinders is 2,000 psi. The manifold system contains reducing valve. It reduces the cylinder pressure of 2,000 psi to the line pressure of 55 psi. When all the cylinders of one bank are exhausted, then the responsibility of uninterrupted supply of O_2 and other gases is automatically switched over to another bank by an automatic switch.

- Some important pressure unit conversions are: 1 kP = 0.145 psi (pound per square inch) = 0.01 bar = 7.5 mm Hg = 10 cm of water = 0.1013 atmosphere = 1 $kg/m/s^2$.

- Liquid O_2 is stored always below its critical temperature of –119°C, because gases can be liquefied by pressure, only if stored below their critical temperature.

- Most anesthetic machines accommodate D and E size cylinder, though A–E size cylinders can be attached with anesthetic machine by PISS.

- At 2,000 psi pressure and 20°C temperature, the cylinders contain 660 L of O_2 and at 1,000 psi pressure and 20°C it is approximately half full and contains 330 L of O_2.

- As a safety feature, the oxygen E cylinders have a plug, made from Wood's metal. This metallurgical alloy has a low melting point and allows the dissipation of pressure in a fire when the intracylinder pressure tremendously rises due to the expansion of gas in the cylinder due to excessive heat. Otherwise, the fire might heat the cylinder to the point of explosion.

- The pressure relief valve is designed to rupture at 3,300 psi. It is well below the pressure which an E cylinder can withstand and it is >5,000 psi. Hence, the pressure relief valve prevents the overfilling of cylinder.

- The critical temperature of N_2O is 36.5°C which is above the room temperature. So, in normal room temperature (<36.5°C), the N_2O can be kept liquefied without any extreme freezing system. Further, the N_2O is not an ideal gas and is easily compressible. Its transformation into gaseous phase is not accompanied by a great rise in cylinder pressure. In spite of it, like the O_2 cylinder, all the E cylinders of N_2O are equipped with Wood's metal plug to prevent explosion under the conditions of unexpectedly high gas pressure, for example unintentional overfilling or during fire.

- All the N_2O cylinders, even its smaller size, also contain N_2O in its liquid state. Therefore, the volume of N_2O, remaining in cylinder is not proportional to cylinder pressure. If the liquid N_2O is kept at a constant temperature (20°C), it will vaporize at the same rate at which it is consumed and will maintain a constant pressure (745 psi), until all the N_2O is exhausted.

- The only reliable way to determine the residual volume of N_2O in a cylinder is to weigh the cylinder. For this reason, the TW or the empty weight of cylinder, containing liquefied N_2O is often stamped on the shoulder of the cylinder. The pressure gauge of a N_2O cylinder should not exceed 745 psi at 20°C. A higher reading implies gauge malfunction, tank overfill (liquid fill), or a cylinder containing a gas other than N_2O.

- The popularity of N_2O and the unnecessary use of N_2O in high concentration are gradually declining. Hence, the use of air is becoming more frequent in anesthesia practice. The air in the cylinder should be of medical grade and is obtained by blending O_2 and N_2. The critical temperature of air is –140.6°C. So, it (air) exists as gas in cylinder and its pressure falls in proportion to the amount of air in cylinder. Dehumidified, but unsterile air also can be provided into hospital pipeline system by compression pumps.

- N_2 gas is not administered to the patients. But, the compressed N_2 gas is used in OT to drive the operating room equipment, such as the saws, drills, and surgical hand pieces. In an operating room, the N_2 gas supply system includes either the use of single H type cylinder or central pipeline system by multiple H cylinders, connected through manifold or compressor driven central pipeline supply.

- Unlike N_2 gas, the CO_2 is administered to patients, because it is required to insufflate the body cavities, during the laparoscopic or robotic surgeries. It is odorless, colorless, noninflammable, and slightly acidic gas. For the supply of compressed CO_2 gas in OT, large M type cylinders or L and K cylinders are used. These cylinders share a common size orifice and thread with O_2 cylinder and can be inadvertently interchanged.

- When the medical gases are supplied from their central supply sources to the OT through the network of pipes, then these pipes are so sized that the pressure drop across the whole system never exceeds 5 psi. These gas pipes are usually constructed by seamless copper tubing. These gas pipes appear in the OT, as hose drops or gas columns or articulating arm. The color-coded hose pipes connect these outlets of pipeline in OT with anesthetic and other equipment.

- Quick coupler mechanism which varies in design with different manufacturers connects one end of the hose to the appropriate pipeline gas outlet in OT. The end of the hose connects to the anesthetic machine through a noninterchangeable DISS or PISS that prevents incorrect hose attachment.

- The E cylinders of O_2, N_2O, and air are attached directly to the anesthetic machine through PISS to discourage incorrect cylinder attachment. In PISS, there are two holes in the cylinder valve and these holes mate with their corresponding pins on the yoke bar of anesthetic machine. The relative positioning of the pins and holes is different and unique for each gas and this constitutes PISS.

- The functioning of central medical gas supply sources and pipeline system are constantly monitored by indicator light and audible alarm to warn to change over for secondary gas sources, abnormally high pipeline pressure (pressure regulator malfunction) and abnormally low pipeline pressure (supply depletion).

- The monitoring of FiO_2 does not reflect the O_2 concentration, distal to its monitoring port. Thus, it should not be used as reference to the O_2 concentration within distal devices, such as ET tubes.

- The anesthetic workstation-related adverse outcome are rarely due to device malfunction or failure. Rather, the misuse of anesthetic workstation is three times more prevalent for anesthetic adverse outcome. The misuse of anesthetic workstation includes: errors in its preparation, improper maintenance, and improper deployment of device. The preventable anesthetic mishaps are frequently traced to (i) operator's lack of familiarity with the equipment, (ii) an operator's failure to verify the function of machine, prior to its use, or (iii) both.

- Now the modern anesthetic workstation has four gas inlets, such as: O_2, N_2O, and air. The 4th gas inlet is for helium/heliox/C_2O or NO. The separate gas inlets are provided for the primary pipeline gas supply that passes through the walls of hospital and secondary cylinder gas supply. The anesthetic machine or workstation, therefore, has two gas inlet pressure gauges for each gas: one for pipeline pressure and another for cylinder pressure.

- The noninterchangeability of DISS is achieved by making the bore diameter of the body and that of the connection nipple, specific for each supplied gas. In this DISS, a filter helps to trap the debris from the wall supply and a one-way check valve prevents the retrograde flow of gases into the pipeline supply.

- Many modern anesthetic machines have an extra oxygen (pneumatic) power outlet which is used to drive the ventilator or to provide an auxiliary O_2 flow meter.

- The pressure of H type cylinder, used in manifold is ±2,000 psi. In pipeline, this cylinder pressure is reduced to ±55 psi. This 50–55 psi pressure is delivered to the anesthetic machine.

- The gas cylinders are color-coded for specific gases to allow for easy identification. In North America, the following color coding scheme for the cylinders is used: O_2 = green, N_2O = blue, CO_2 = gray, Air = yellow, helium = brown, N_2 = black. In UK, O_2 = white, air = black and white.

- When anesthetic machine uses gas supply from pipeline, then E type of cylinders are attached to machine for back-up supply of high-pressure source of medical gases. The pressure of gas, supplied from the cylinder to anesthetic machine is 45 psi.

- At 20°C, a full E cylinder contains 600 L of O_2 at a pressure of 2,000 psi and 1,590 L of N_2O at 745 psi.

- The pipelines supply the gases to anesthetic machine relatively at constant pressure. But, the high and variable gas pressure in cylinders makes flow control to machine difficult and potentially dangerous. Hence, anesthetic machine utilizes a pressure regulator to reduce the cylinder gas pressure to 45–47 psi and gets gas supply at constant pressure, like pipeline and makes flow control of gas in machine easy. This 45–47 psi pressure is slightly lower than the pipeline supply and allows preferential use of pipeline supply, even if cylinder is left open and unless the pipeline pressure drops below 45 psi. After passing through pressure gauges and check valves, the pipeline gases share a common pathway with cylinder gases.

- A pressure relief valve is provided for each gas and it is set to open when the supply pressure exceeds the machine's maximum safety limit pressure which is 95–110 psi and it happens due to both the pipeline and cylinder regulator failure.

- *Oxygen supply failure protection devices:* In modern anesthetic machine, O_2 can pass directly to rotameter through flow control knob. But, the N_2O and other gases must first pass through safety devices before reaching rotameter. This safety device permits the flow of N_2O and other gases, only if there is sufficient O_2 pressure in the safety device. Thus, this safety device prevents the accidental delivery of N_2O and other gases in the event of O_2 supply failure. This safety device senses the O_2 pressure via a small piloting pressure line that is derived from the O_2 line going to rotameter. If the pressure in the pilot line falls below a threshold value (20 psi), then the shut off value in the safety device close and the flow of N_2O and other gases is stopped. This is called the threshold shut off safety device. But, now the modern anesthetic machine uses a proportioning safety device. Here, the flow of N_2O and other gases proportionately reduces with the reduction of pressure in O_2 pipeline and their flow is completely shut off or stopped when the O_2 pressure goes below 10 psi.

- O_2 from the common inlet pathway, in addition to supplying the rotameter through flow control knob, is used to pressurize the safety device, O_2 flush valve, ventilator power outlet, and low-pressure sensor that activates alarm sound.

- After reducing the pressure to safe level (±50 psi), each gas is allowed to pass through flow control knob (valve) and flow meter (rotameter). Then, these gases mix with each other and enter the vaporizer. Next, the total gas mixture along with the gases of volatile anesthetic agent from vaporizer exits from the machine through its common gas outlet. The gas lines, proximal to the flow control knob, are considered as the high-pressure circuit of machine. And the gas lines, distal to the flow control knob (valve), extending up to the common gas outlet are called the low-pressure circuit of the machine.

- As a safety feature, the O_2 knob is usually color-coded, fluted, larger, and protruded than the other knobs. So, this touch and color coding makes the O_2 knob more difficult to turn wrong off or on.

- Flow control knob (valve) controls the gas entry into flow meter by its needle valve. The flow meter of an anesthetic machine is classified as either of rotameter which provides constant pressure with variable orifice or electronic. In rotameter, a ball or a bobbin or a float is used as indicator and during the flow of gas its weight is supported by the pressure below its lower surface which depends on the amount of flow of gas. Near the bottom of Thorpe's tube, where the diameter of the tube is narrow, a low flow of gas will create a sufficient pressure under the rotating bobbin to raise it in the tube and little amount of gas will pass surrounding the bobbin. Next, with the increase of flow of gas, as the bobbin rises, the orifice of the tube also widens and allows the more gas to flow around the bobbin. But, at that position the pressure under the lower surface of bobbin is same as before and is equivalent to its weight. With the more flow of gases, the pressure underneath the bobbin does not increase, because the extra flow of gas passes by the side of the bobbin. Therefore, the flow rate of gases or the position of bobbin in Thorpe tube varies depending on the bobbin's weight and the orifice diameter (variable orifice), but the pressure under the bobbin remains constant which is equivalent to bobbin's weight (constant pressure).

- Some flow meters have two glass tubes for each gas. Among these, the narrower tube is for the low flows and the wider tube is for the high flows. These two tubes are arranged in series and are controlled by one pin valve.

- Some anesthetic machines have electronic flow meter and measure the flow of gas electronically. In such circumstances, an auxiliary conventional flow meter is also provided. In some models, the conventional flow meter (rotameter) is used, but its gas flow through Thorpe's tube is measured electronically and this measurement is displayed digitally or graphically or by both. In these machines, each gas has a separate electronic flow measurement device. The amount of pressure drop, caused by a flow restrictor, is the basis for the measurement of gas flow rate in electronic flow meter. The electronic flow meter is required, if the gas flow rate data is needed to be recorded automatically by computerized anesthesia recording systems in anesthesia workstation.

CHECKING OF ANESTHESIA MACHINE AND CIRCUITS

Before administering anesthesia, comprehensive manual tests (checking) of machine must be performed to avoid any mishap. But, many of the modern sophisticated machines provide a series of automatic self-checking systems. These checking should begin from the high-pressure system up to the breathing circuits.

- *Checking of high-pressure system:* (i) O_2 cylinders are opened and we will have to be sure that all the cylinders are at least half filled (>1,000 psi), (ii) we will have to check that all the hoses for central supply unit are appropriately connected with the machine and the reading in the O_2 pressure gauge of central supply unit is at least ±55 psi.

- *Checking of low-pressure system:* (i) We will have to be sure that gases are flowing smoothly in rotameter, (ii) without opening O_2 knob and not allowing the flow of O_2 gas through the O_2 tube of flow meter, we will turn on the N_2O knob in rotameter. Thus, we will see the integrity of the O_2 and N_2O proportioning system and fail save valve. Anesthetic machine should not allow the flow of N_2O, without the flow of O_2.

- *Tests to detect leaks in low flow system:*
  - *Positive pressure test:* First the flow of O_2 through rotameter is opened and subsequently the common outlet of the machine is occluded by the hand. Now, we will have to observe the position of bobbin in the flow meter tube. If there is no leak, then due to back pressure, the height of the bobbin should drop. It should again bounce back to normal, if the occlusion is released. However, if the machine has a back pressure control valve, then this test is invalid. In modern machines, a back pressure control valve is usually installed just before the common machine

outlet to prevent the back pressure effect of positive pressure ventilation on vaporizer output.

- *Negative pressure test:* All the inlet flows of machine are closed and a suction bulb is attached to the single common outlet of the machine. Then, this suction bulb is kept on squeezing, till it collapses completely. Therefore, it will generate a negative pressure in the machine. Now, if there is any leak at anywhere in the machine, then air will be sucked in and the air bulb will be inflated automatically. On the other hand, if there is no leakage at anywhere in the machine, the collapsed bulb will still remain in collapsed stage. If the bulb remains in collapsed stage >10 seconds, then it should be considered that there is no leak. Now, the same test is done by opening the each vaporizer, as there may be leakage in vaporizer. Unlike the positive pressure test, this negative pressure test can be performed, even if there is a back pressure control valve, attached to machine. Therefore, the negative pressure test is the most sensitive of all the tests to detect leak. So, this test is called the universal leak test and it can detect the leak as low as 30 mL.

Anatomy and Physiology of Respiratory System

INTRODUCTION

An anesthesiologist must acquires an extensive knowledge, regarding the anatomy and physiology of respiratory system, before taking any care of his patients in operating room, high-dependency unit (HDU), and intensive care unit. This is because mastery on anatomy and physiology of respiratory system is the principal prerequisite to understand the mechanism of gas exchange that occurs during anesthesia, surgery, and in different disease processes of patients in operation theater (OT) and in intensive care unit. From anatomical point of view, the respiratory system is made up of a gas exchanging organ (lungs) and a pumping system that ventilates this gas exchanging organ (lungs). This pumping system is again consists of chest wall, respiratory muscles, and some areas in brain, tracts, and nerves that connect the brain with these respiratory muscles and control the contraction of these muscle. The lung is again consists of lung parenchyma and its conducting part, including trachea, bronchus, bronchioles, alveolar ducts, and alveoli, through which air enters the lung.

TRACHEA

The trachea is a membranocartilaginous structure. It extends downward as a continuation of larynx from the lower margin of cricoid cartilage.

Course and Measurement

The trachea, as a continuation of larynx, begins at a level which lies opposite to the lower border of C6 vertebra or the lower border of cricoid cartilage. It then passes downward to end opposite to the sternal angle by dividing into right and left principal bronchus. This bifurcation of trachea or the beginning of principal bronchus corresponds with the lower border of T4 vertebra in supine position or T6 vertebra in standing position of an adult person. But, in newborn the trachea bifurcates at higher level, opposite to the T3 vertebra.

The length of an adult trachea is about 10–12 cm. The external diameter of a trachea is about 2 cm in an adult male and 1.5 cm in an adult female. The internal diameter of trachea is approximately 12 mm in an adult. In newborn, the internal diameter of trachea is only 3 mm, which persists up to third year of life. Thereafter, the lumen increases by about 1 mm for each year up to 12th year, after which it remains fairly constant. So, this knowledge is very important for an anesthetist in selecting the size of an endotracheal (ET) tube, during intubation in children. In children, the trachea is deeply placed and more movable, whereas in adult it is superficial and more fixed. Moreover, in children the left brachiocephalic vein and the summit of the arch of aorta crosses trachea at higher level than an adult near suprasternal notch. So, low tracheostomy is risky in children than adult.

The trachea moves with flexion and extension of head (neck) and with respiration. With deep inspiration, the trachea moves 2.5 cm downward and during expiration this same length is moved upwards. The extension of head and neck which is an ideal position to maintain an unobstructed airway in an anesthetized patient, usually increase the length of trachea by about 20–30%. In some clinical situation, where a patient is intubated with head in flexed position and the tip of ET tube just passes beyond the vocal cords, then the subsequent extension or hyperextension of head and neck may withdraw the tube above cords.

Structure of Trachea

The trachea consists of a number of posteriorly incomplete C-shaped cartilaginous rings. They form the anterior and the lateral walls of trachea. On the posterior surface, the two free ends of these incomplete C-shaped cartilaginous rings are connected by a strong fibroelastic membrane and involuntary muscles, named trachealis.

The posteriorly incomplete C-shaped tracheal cartilaginous rings are made up of hyaline cartilage. The total number of these C-shaped cartilaginous rings varies in between 16 and 20 in an adult. Among all these C-shaped cartilaginous rings, the first is the broadest and the last is triangular in shape which is called *carina*. It hooks upward from the lower margin of trachea and then surrounds the commencement of two bronchi. The carina represents a ridge in the interior of tracheal bifurcation and acts as a guide for the surgeons during bronchoscopy or other endoscopic examination of trachea or bronchi. The tracheal lumen narrows slightly as it progresses toward carina. The cricoid cartilage is the narrowest part of trachea, with an average diameter of 17 mm in men and 13 mm in women. Starting from carina, trachea divides 23 times dichotomously (each branch divides into two smaller branches) and ends at *alveolar sac* after forming 23 generations. With each generation, the number of airways is approximately doubled. At the end *each alveolar sac gives 17 alveoli.*

The mucous membrane of upper respiratory tract, at the level of carina, is most sensitive and is associated with maximum cough reflex. So, the carina is often considered to act as the last line of defense, causing the expulsion of aspirated foreign body by violent cough. As the C-shaped cartilaginous ring of trachea is deficient posteriorly, so it allows the expansion of esophagus during the deglutition and the passing of food through esophagus. The air pressure in trachea is negative in relation to atmosphere during inspiration. Therefore, the positive pressure from outside might collapse the trachea. In order to avoid this, by nature, the tracheal wall is composed of elastic and rigid cartilaginous rings and thus maintains the potency of lumen of it. For this purpose, the cartilage cells are nature's best choice than bone cells. Because, the cartilage requires no separate blood supply and they get nutrition only by diffusion from the nearest capillary plexus.

The interior of trachea is lined by *pseudostratified ciliated columnar epithelium*, resting on a basement membrane, with numerous serous and mucous glands. The epithelial cells are arranged in single layer with different heights and different nuclear positions. Hence, this layer shows apparent stratification under light microscope and is so called as pseudostratified. The taller cells in this pseudostratified epithelium present cilia and each cell supports about 270 cilia. The electron microscope shows that each cilium contains 11 microtubules. Among these microtubules, two microtubules are situated at center and the other nine microtubules are situated at periphery, surrounding the center. The mucous, secreted by the goblet cells of mucous glands of the columnar epithelium of trachea entrap dust, other foreign particles, and bacteria. Then, these entrapped

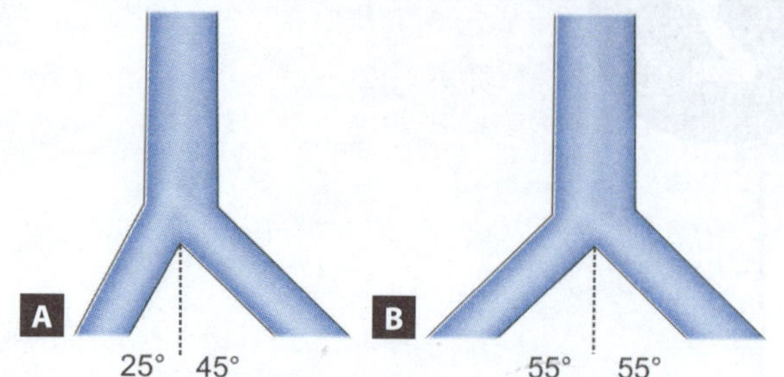

Figs. 1A and B: Angle of main bronchi:
(A) In adult; (B) In children.

particles are swayed by the ciliary beats toward the upper part of trachea and larynx. Then, they are expelled out of larynx by cough reflexes. Thus, the mucous membrane helps in defensive mechanism for respiratory passage by acting as a mucociliary barrier. The *cilia in airway epithelium are present as far as up to the terminal bronchiole* where they give way to squamous cells without cilia **(Figs. 1A and B)**.

The serous glands, mucosal glands, and the cartilages are also present up to the beginning of the preterminal or terminal bronchioles. The bronchioles <1 mm in diameter do not have cartilages in their walls. As the bronchioles are traced distally, it is found that the cartilaginous rings recede gradually and are replaced by some irregular cartilaginous plates (not rings) which present sporadically, until the diameter of bronchiole comes down to 0.6 mm and then they (cartilaginous plates) disappear completely. The loss of cartilaginous support causes the patency of smaller airways to become dependent on the radial out ward traction, caused by the elastic recoil property of surrounding lung tissues. If we progress more downward, continuously along the bronchial tree, then it is also found that the tubular outline of bronchial wall start to change. Gradually, small projections appear from the airways in all directions and gradually the number of these small projections increases. Now, these areas of airways with these projections are termed as the respiratory bronchiole and these small projections are called as the alveolar ducts, which lead to alveolar sacs. On an average, each alveolar sac gives 17 alveoli. The walls of the bronchioles contain more smooth muscle than that of bronchi. Of which the *largest amount of muscles, relative to the thickness of its wall, is present in terminal bronchioles.* Smooth muscles are found in the walls of all airways down up to the level of alveolar duct and are most abundant in terminal bronchioles. On the contrary, the trachea and bronchi have cartilages in their walls, but contain relatively little smooth muscles.

■ BRONCHUS

The trachea bifurcates into two main (principle) bronchi: (1) right and (2) left. Then, each of these two main bronchi enters their corresponding lung through their hilum. After that, each bronchus again divides and subdivides into successive smaller and smaller bronchi and finally produce terminal respiratory bronchioles which merge with the alveolar sacs and ultimately terminate into alveoli which constitute the lung parenchyma.

Right Principle Bronchus

The right principle bronchus passes downward and toward right from the bifurcation of trachea and makes an angle of 25° with the midline. While, the left principle bronchus makes an angle of 45° with the midline. But, in children under the age of 3 years, the angulation of two main bronchi with midline at carina is equal on both sides and this is 55°. Right bronchus enters the hilum of right lung at the level of 5th thoracic vertebra (T5). It is wider, shorter, and more vertical than that of the left. The length of the extrapulmonary part of right bronchus is about 2.5 cm. Therefore, the distance from the carina of tracheal to the origin of right upper lobe bronchus (i.e., the first division of right principal bronchus) is an average 2.5 cm. It is wider than that of the left one, because it supplies the more voluminous right lung than that of the left lung. It is more vertical than left one, because the trachea at its bifurcation deviates more toward right side. So, a foreign body in trachea is usually aspirated into right lung. However, the short length of right bronchus makes the approach to the lumen of it more difficult when it is required during thoracic anesthesia **(Fig. 2)**.

Within the right lung, first this right principal (or primary) bronchus divides into three secondary or lobar bronchi to supply the each lobe of right lung (right lung has three lobes). Then, again, each of these three secondary or lobar bronchi subdivides into segmental or tertiary bronchus. Thus, there are 10 segmental or tertiary bronchi in right lung. The areas of lung supplied by these tertiary or segmental bronchi are known as the bronchopulmonary segments which act as a functionally *independent respiratory district or unit*. So, there are 10 bronchopulmonary segments in right lung.

These 10 bronchopulmonary segments, supplied by 10 tertiary or segmental bronchi, in right lung are:

- *Upper lobe:* Apical, anterior, and posterior
- *Middle lobe:* Medial and lateral
- *Lower lobe:* Apical, anterior basal, posterior basal, medial basal, and lateral basal.

Each bronchopulmonary segment is wedge-in-shape with their base is directed toward the surface of lung. These segments are separated from one another by intersegment areolar septa which prevent the spread of infection from one segment to another. The branches of pulmonary artery (carrying deoxygenated blood) follow the segmental

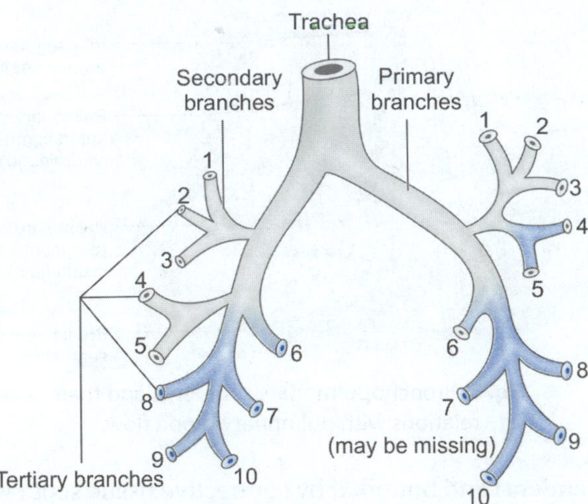

Fig. 2: Distribution of tertiary bronchi in right and left lungs.

Upper lobe (of both lungs):
1. Apical bronchus
2. Posterior bronchus
3. Anterior bronchus
4. Superior lingular bronchus (only for left upper lobe)
5. Inferior lingular bronchus (only for left upper lobe)

Middle lobe (of right lung):	*Middle lobe (of left lung):*
4. Lateral bronchus	Absent
5. Medial bronchus	

Lower lobe (of both lungs):	
6. Apical bronchus	6. Apical bronchus
7. Medial basal (cardiac)	7. Medial basal (sometimes missed)
8. Anterior basal bronchus	8. Anterior basal bronchus
9. Lateral basal bronchus	9. Lateral basal bronchus
10. Posterior basal bronchus	10. Posterior basal bronchus

or tertiary bronchi and are segmental in distribution. Whereas, the tributaries of pulmonary vein (carrying oxygenated blood) run through the intersegmental septa and are intersegmental in drainage. Thus, the area of lung drained by an intersegmental tributary of pulmonary vein is known as the *bronchovascular unit* which includes a number of *bronchopulmonary segments*. Hence, the surgical resection of a bronchopulmonary segment produces profuse hemorrhage **(Fig. 3)**.

Now, the tertiary or segmental bronchus further divides and subdivides and then finally ends into smaller branches which enter into the *lung lobules* through their apices. These smaller divisions of bronchus which enter the lung lobules are called as the *preterminal bronchioles* (15th order of division). Thus, a preterminal bronchiole is the part of conducting system (zone) of airway which supplies a lung lobule. *A preterminal bronchiole is intralobular and is devoid of cartilages and glands*. The lung lobules are self-contained

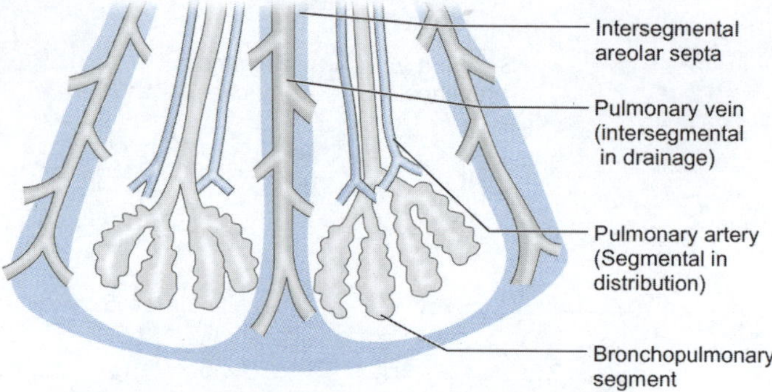

Fig. 3: Bronchopulmonary segments and their relations with pulmonary blood flow.

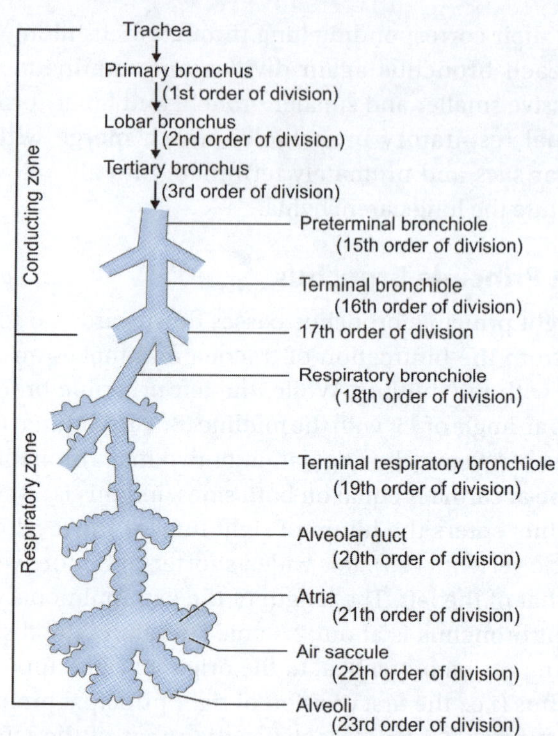

Fig. 4: Acinus (or primary lobule) is a subunit of pulmonary tissue consisting of respiratory bronchiole, alveolar ducts, atria, and alveoli. Intercommunications exist between acini. Thus disease can spread from acinus to acinus. But functional deficiency in any part of one acinus can be compensated by bypass mechanisms via these anastomotic channels. Secondary or lung lobule is the unit of pulmonary tissue served by a preterminal bronchiole. They are self-contained and bounded by connective tissue septa. It has no anastomotic connections with other lobules.

(dependent) and bounded by connective tissue septa which have no anastomotic connections with the other adjacent lobules. In every lung lobules, each preterminal bronchiole then divides into 3–7 *terminal bronchioles*. After that each *terminal bronchiole* (16th order of division) again subdivides dichotomously by three successive orders (17th, 18th, and 19th order of division) into *respiratory bronchioles* and the last order of these respiratory bronchioles is termed as the *terminal respiratory bronchioles* (19th order of division). Each terminal respiratory bronchiole, then, terminates by branching into 2–11 *alveolar ducts* (20th order of division). The alveolar ducts are cone-shaped and thin-walled tubes with squamous epithelial lining. The number of alveolar ducts in each lung is about 2 million. Each alveolar duct, then, further divides or ends by branching into 2–4 *atria* (21st order of division). Next, numerous *air saccules (alveolar sacs)* open off from these atria (22nd order of division). The total number of air saccules (alveolar sacs) in each lung is about 4 million. Ultimately, each air saccule gives rise to 15–30 *alveoli* (23rd order of division) **(Fig. 4)**.

About up to 16 orders of division of respiratory passage take place from principal bronchus to terminal bronchioles. *Among these, from 4th order of division to 19th order of divisions are called as bronchioles.* The last seven orders of division (17th to 23rd) occur after terminal bronchiole to alveoli (three orders for respiratory bronchioles and next four orders from alveolar duct to alveoli). The total number of terminal bronchioles in each human lung is about 33,000. Each terminal bronchiole subdivides into respiratory bronchiole under three orders. Respiratory bronchioles exhibit alveolar out-pockets from their side walls. Last order of respiratory bronchioles is termed as terminal respiratory bronchiole. The total number of terminal respiratory bronchioles in each human lung is about 260,000.

Therefore, the total 23 (16 + 7) orders of division are encountered from principal bronchus to alveoli. The total number of alveoli in each lung is estimated to be about 150 million. Hence, the total number of alveoli in both the lungs

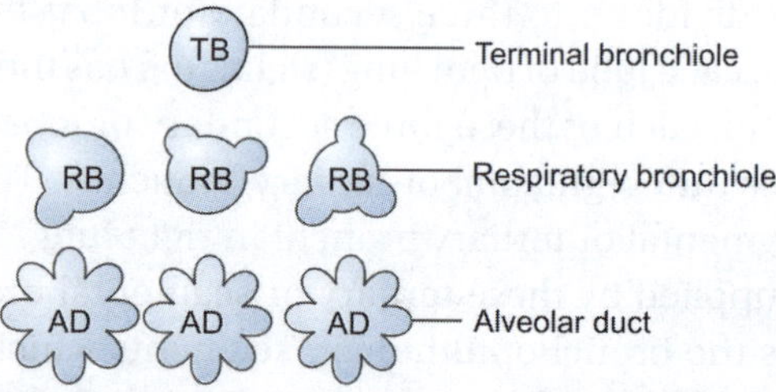

Fig. 5: A definitive flow of air is maintained up to the terminal bronchiole. Beyond this point the actual flow of air stops and air movement is affected by diffusion. One terminal bronchiole (TB) gives rise to 3–5 respiratory bronchiole (RB), and diameter of each RB = diameter of TB. Each RB gives rise to several alveolar duct (AD) of similar diameter to RB.

of an adult is about 300–500 million. All these alveoli of both the lungs together represent the total surface area (for gas exchange) of about 70–100 square meters. The total number of alveoli in both the lungs of a newborn is about 20 million and by about 8 years, after birth, the adult number of alveoli is reached **(Fig. 5)**.

The area of lung supplied by one terminal respiratory bronchiole (19th order of division) is known to take part in gaseous exchange. So, from the functional point of view the area of lung, supplied by one terminal respiratory bronchiole, is known as the functional pulmonary unit or functional lung unit. Thus, one functional lung unit consists of one terminal respiratory bronchiole, four successive orders of dichotomous subdivision of terminal respiratory bronchioles into alveolar duct (20th order of division), atria (21st order of division), air saccules (alveolar sacs), and alveoli (23rd of division). Each functional lung unit or functional pulmonary unit is also called as acinus. Intercommunications exist between two adjacent acini or functional lung units and also between adjacent acini and respiratory bronchioles. Thus, the disease can spread from one acinus to another acinus and functional deficiency in any part of an acinus (functional lung unit) can be compensated by bypass mechanism via these anastomotic channels to another acinus.

Respiratory bronchioles (17th order of division) and air passages distal to it are lined by simple squamous epithelium resting on a basement membrane and surrounded externally by intense pulmonary capillary plexus. *But, lymphatic plexus is absent from terminal bronchioles and distal to it.* The part of bronchial tree extending from trachea up to terminal bronchiole, i.e., the first 16 order of divisions of air passage is called as the *conducting zone* and does not take part in gas exchange. This part of air passage is lined by ciliated columnar epithelium proximally and later by ciliated cuboidal epithelium. The part of respiratory passage, extending from terminal bronchioles to alveoli, i.e., the distal seven order of divisions of air passage is called as the *respiratory zone* and take part in gas exchange, because it is lined by squamous epithelium. Glands and cartilages are present up to the beginning of preterminal bronchioles. *These multiple divisions of respiratory passages greatly increase the total cross-sectional area of airways from 2.5 cm² in trachea to 11,800 cm² in alveoli. So the velocity of air flow in small airways declines from very rapidly to a small value* (**Fig. 6**).

Thus, the divisions and subdivisions of respiratory passage from trachea to alveoli may be summarized as follows:

- *Conducting zone:*
  - Principal bronchus (1st order of division)
  - Secondary or lobar bronchi (2nd order of division)
  - Tertiary or segmental bronchi (3rd order of division)
  - Preterminal bronchioles (15th order of division)
  - Terminal bronchioles (16th order of division)
- *Respiratory zone:*
  - Primary respiratory bronchioles (17th order of division)
  - Respiratory bronchioles (18th order of division)

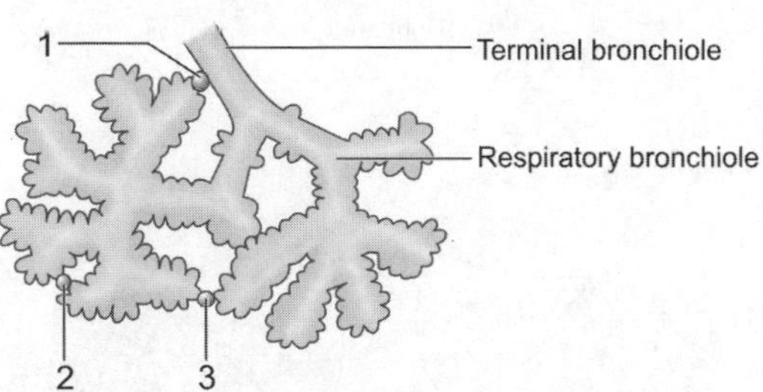

Fig. 6: Anatomical intercommunicating channels in acinus. These exist at three levels: (1) Between one or more atria and the related terminal bronchiole; (2) Between the alveoli of atria of same respiratory bronchiole; (3) Between the alveoli of adjacent respiratory bronchioles. These alveolar connections are known as the pores of Kohn.

  - Terminal respiratory bronchioles (19th order of division)
  - Alveolar ducts (20th order of division)
  - Atria (21st order of division)
  - Air saccules or alveolar sacs (22nd order of division)
  - Alveoli (total 23 order of division)

17th, 18th, and 19th order of divisions are together called *respiratory bronchioles.*

Left Principle Bronchus

The left principal or primary bronchus is longer, narrower, and more oblique than that of the right one. The length of its extrapulmonary part is about 5 cm. It makes an angle of 45° with trachea at midline (at carina) and passes downward and toward slightly left, below the arch of aorta. It then enters the left lung through its hilum at the level of 6th thoracic vertebra (T6).

Then, the left principal or primary bronchus divides only into upper and lower secondary or lobar bronchus to supply the respective lobe of left lung. Because, the left lung is divided only into two lobes (whereas the right principal on primary bronchus divides into three secondary or lobar bronchus). After that the left upper secondary or lobar bronchus again divides into five tertiary or segmental bronchi: apical, anterior, posterior, upper lingular, and (5) lower lingular. The lower secondary lobar bronchus divide into four or five tertiary or segmental bronchi: apical, medial basal (*may be missing*), lateral basal, anterior basal, and posterior basal (**Fig. 7**).

So, the nine or ten bronchopulmonary segments of left lung, supplied by the tertiary or segmental bronchi are:

- *Upper lobe:* Apical, anterior, posterior, upper lingular, and lower lingular.
- *Lower lobe:* Apical, medial basal (*may be missing*), lateral basal, anterior basal, and posterior basal.

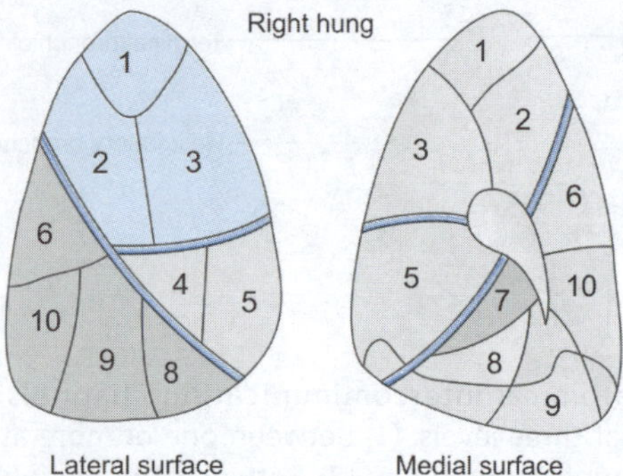

Fig. 7: Bronchopulmonary segments of right lung: (1) Apical segment of upper lobe; (2) Posterior segment of upper lobe; (3) Anterior segment of upper lobe; (4) Lateral segment of middle lobe; (5) Medial segment of middle lobe; (6) Apical segment of lower lobe; (7) Medial basal segment of lower lobe; (8) Anterior basal segment of lower lobe; (9) Lateral basal segment of lower lobe; (10) Posterior basal segment of lower lobe.

Structure of Bronchus (Both Right and Left)

As discussed before, after entering into the lung, a principal bronchus divides successively into secondary (lobar), tertiary (segmental), and numerous subtertiary branches up to the alveoli. All these branches of bronchi run into interlobular septa, accompanied by their corresponding branches of pulmonary arteries, pulmonary veins, and bronchial vessels, till the preterminal bronchioles is reached when it leaves the interlobular septa and enters into the pulmonary or *lung lobule* through its apex. *Actually, the smaller branches of bronchi which leave interlobular septa and enter into lung lobules are generally known as the bronchioles. A bronchiole is intralobular (not interlobular) and is devoid of cartilages and glands (Fig. 8).*

Structurally, a bronchus consists of from outside to inward:

- Fibroelastic coat
- Irregular plates of hyaline cartilages
- Involuntary bronchial muscles which are helical in arrangements, and run in opposite directions, winding like a shoelace pattern
- Mucous membrane which is *ciliated columnar* in nature and provided with goblet cells, mucous glands, and numerous serous glands. Ultrastructurally, 10 types of cells are present in the epithelial layer of mucous membrane of tracheobronchial tree. Among them, the important cells are: *ciliated columnar cells, serous cells, goblet cells, cells with brush border, intermediate cells, Clara cells, macrophages, mast cells, and argentaffin cells.*

In the bronchial mucous membrane, the ciliated columnar cells are abundant in number and their cilia are wrapped by low viscous or more serous fluid, with their tip projected into it. This serous fluid is secreted by the serous cells and the mucous is secreted by the goblet cells.

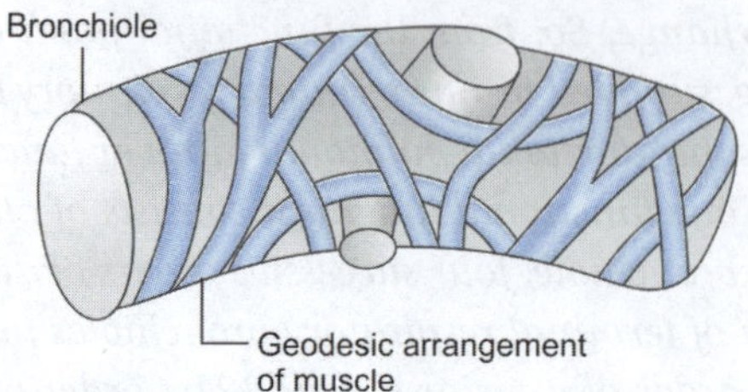

Fig. 8: The arrangement of muscle fibers on a bronchiole: The principal aim of this arrangement of muscles fibers in bronchiole is to permit the alterations of the length and width of airway tube during the various phases of respiration. So, this type of arrangement of muscle fibers on airway is of great importance. This arrangement of muscle fiber on airway is known as the "geodesic network". A geodesic line is defined as the shortest distance between two points on a curved surface. Therefore, a geodesic pattern is the ideal method of withstanding or producing maximum pressures in a tubular structure without any tendency of being slipped of fibers along the surface of the tube.

The brush cells are absorptive in functions. The intermediate cells are somewhat undifferentiated and probably help in the regeneration of ciliated or secretory cells. The *clara cells* are nonciliated and are concerned with the secretion of some amount of surfactant. The *argentaffin cells* belong to the diffuse endocrine system of amine precursor uptake and decarboxylation (APUD) cells and secrete serotonin or histamine in response to chemical or nervous stimuli.

Applied Anatomy

- The breath sound over the apex of right lung is more and distinctly audible than the left one. Because, the trachea comes in more close contact with the apex of right lung than that of the left.
- Since the right principal (primary) bronchus is shorter, wider and more vertical than the left bronchus, so a foreign body is more likely to be aspirated into right lung.
- *The apical tertiary segment of lower lobe (in supine position) and the posterior tertiary segment of upper lobe (lying on side) are the more common sites for lung abscess on both sides. Because, these segments are most dependent part of lungs in recumbent position. In such condition, the patient is advised to lie in prone position which allows the infected material from these segments to accumulate in principal bronchi and on carina and subsequently this purulent material is expectorated out by stimulating cough reflex (Figs. 9A and B).*

Such natural drainage, by adopting different postures, may have some drawbacks. For example, pus from the apical segment of lower lobe may trickle in prone position, through the opening of middle lobe bronchus. Because, the mouths of two bronchi are facing here each other. In order to avoid such incidence, the segmental resection of apical segment

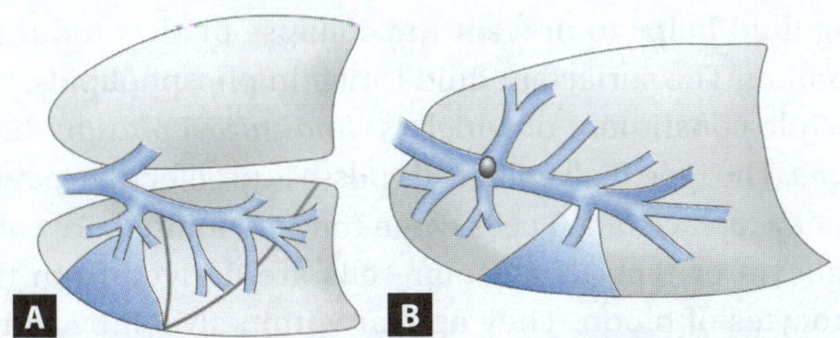

Figs. 9A and B: Relationship between the posture and the common site of lung abscess. (A) When a patient lies on his side, then the common site of lung abscess is the posterior segment of his right upper lobe. Because, inhaled materials easily collect in this bronchopulmonary segment; (B) When a patient lies on his back, then the common site of lung abscess is the apical segment of his right lower lobe.

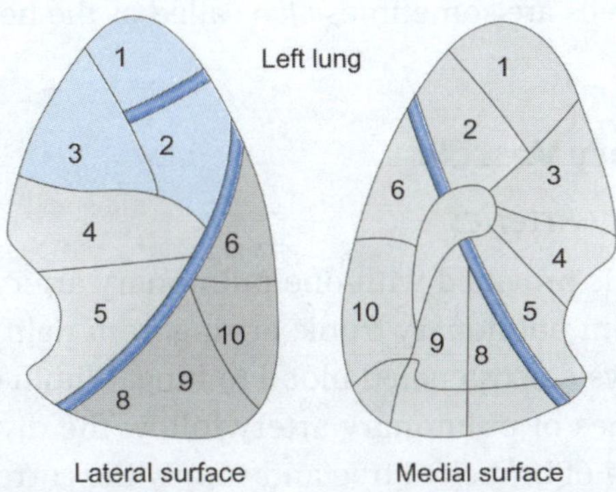

Fig. 10: Bronchopulmonary segments of left lung: (1) Apical segment of upper lobe; (2) Posterior segment of upper lobe; (3) Anterior segment of upper lobe; (4) Superior lingular segment; (5) Inferior lingular segment; (6) Apical segment of lower lobe; (7) Medial basal segment of lower lobe (may be missing); (8) Anterior basal segment of lower lobe; (9) Lateral basal segment of lower lobe; (10) Posterior basal segment of lower lobe.

of lower lobe should be done. *The apical segment of lower lobe is most frequently involved in aspiration pneumonia (Mendelson's syndrome).*

- *The posterior segment of right upper lobe is the most frequent site for tuberculosis.*
- The patency of middle lobe bronchus of both lungs is particularly vulnerable to lymph gland swelling. Because they are closely related to tracheobronchial group of glands **(Fig. 10)**.

■ LUNGS

Lung Parenchyma

Actually, the lungs have more a space than an organ. It is composed of (from outside inward) serous coat, subserous coat, and pulmonary substance or parenchyma itself. The serous coat invests the entire lung, except hilum and is derived from pulmonary pleura. The subserous coat consists

of thin elastic fibroareolar tissue and invests the whole lung under its serous coat. It again projects into the interior of lung through its hilum, as numerous fibroelastic septa, and divides and subdivides the whole lung. The smallest spaces between these septa are called the lung lobules. Each lung lobule is provided with one preterminal bronchiole and about 20,000 lobules are present in each lung.

Though, the *lobule* is the *anatomical pulmonary unit of lung,* but the alveoli are the functional or physiological unit of lungs. However, on the other hand, gas exchange occurs not only at the level of alveoli, but also occurs at the level of respiratory bronchioles, alveolar ducts, atria, and air saccules (alveolar sacs). So, the area of lung supplied by terminal respiratory bronchiole (19th order of division) is actually the *functional pulmonary unit.* Hence, from the functional aspects the exact anatomical differences between these structures such as alveoli, air saccules, atria, alveolar ducts, etc. are not of great importance.

The pulmonary alveoli are polygonal or polyhedral in shapes and are packed very tightly within lung lobule. Alveolar size is a function of both gravity and lung volume. In upright position, the largest alveoli are present at the pulmonary apex, whereas the smallest are present at the pulmonary base. With inspiration, these discrepancies in alveolar size are diminished. On an average, each alveolus is about 200–300 µm in diameter at functional residual capacity (FRC) level and is surrounded by about 1,800 capillary segments. The total length of pulmonary capillary bed of both the lungs measures about 1,500 miles and contains about 70–150 mL of blood at any moment. Each alveolus is lined by thin squamous epithelial cells with an insoluble thin film of lipoprotein, called surfactant spreading over it. The average thickness of this thin film of surfactant is 50Å in human being **(Fig. 11)**.

Many structures intervene between the air in alveoli and the blood in pulmonary capillaries and constitute the *pulmonary air-blood barrier (or alveolar capillary membrane)* through which gaseous exchange takes place. These structures are:

- The flattened epithelial cells of alveoli which is about 0.05 µm thick.
- The basement membrane upon which these alveolar epithelial cells rest.
- The basement membrane of capillary endothelium on which the capillary endothelial cells rest. At some places, these two basement membranes are fused, while in other places these two membranes are separated by an interval which is occupied by some undifferentiated mesenchyme cells or leukocytes.
- The flattened endothelial cells of capillaries.

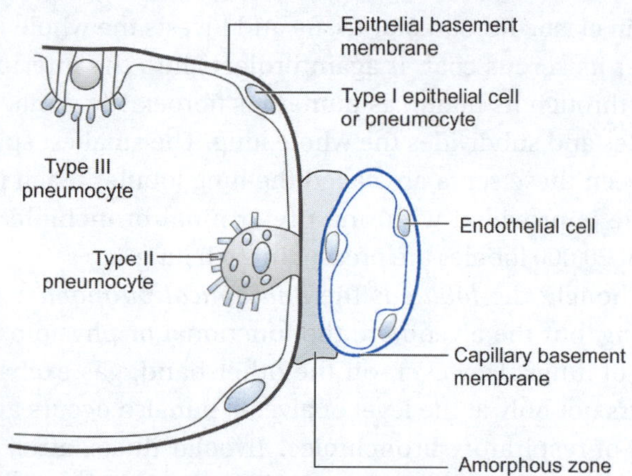

Fig. 11: The histology of alveolus. The type I pneumocytes are extremely thin and their nucleus is situated at the angle of alveolus. Its thin cytoplasmic extension lines (covers) most of the alveolar surface and helps in exchange of gases. The type II granular pneumocytes project into the cavity of alveoli and are covered by microvilli. They produce surfactant and are essentially reserved cells which undergo hyperplasia, when the type I pneumocytes are injured. Type III pneumocytes are pyramidal in shape with thick microvilli and contain filaments extending through the cell body. It resembles the chemoreceptor cells and has phagocytic property.

The *total thickness of this pulmonary air-blood barrier is about 0.2–0.5 µm.* The air surface of alveoli is corrugated. This is due to the presence of capillaries and various subcellular structures. The alveoli share their walls with their neighboring alveoli and constitute an interalveolar septum between the two. Sometimes, there are some gaps in this septum which are called as the alveolar pores. Thus, there is direct connection between two alveoli through these pores.

There are three types of cells that line alveoli and form the alveolar wall. These are type I alveolar cells or membranous pneumocytes, type II alveolar cells or granular pneumocytes and type III alveolar cells or alveolar phagocytes. The type I alveolar cells are simple squamous epithelial cells and are connected with each other by tight junctions. These tight junctions are important in preventing the passage of large oncotically active molecules, such as albumin into alveolus from capillary. They (type I pneumocytes) make up to 90% of alveolar surface area and take part in gaseous exchange. The nucleus of these cells is situated at any one angle of it and a thin cytoplasmic extension lines most of the alveolar surface. The type II pneumocytes or alveolar cells are round shaped, contain many inclusion (or lamellar) bodies and project into alveoli. They are covered by microvilli. The type II pneumocytes are more numerous than type I pneumocytes, but because of their shape, they only occupy <10% of alveolar surface area. They secret surfactant (present in lamellar bodies) which by reducing the surface tension of alveolar

living fluid helps to prevent the collapse of alveoli during expiration. The surfactant fluid is rich in phospholipids, the principle constituent of which is *dipalmitoyl phosphatidyl choline.* The type II alveolar cells possess proliferative power and may replace type I cells when they are injured. Alveolar phagocyte or type III alveolar cells are derived from the monocytes of blood. They appear within alveoli by active migration from capillary blood through air blood barrier. These cells phagocyte the bacteria, dust particles and other debris materials which enter the alveoli. Then, they move toward the bronchioles where the phagocytized materials with the cells are eliminated by coughing. In congestive heart failure, these alveolar phagocytes engulf the extravasated red blood cells and produce brick red or pink color sputum. So, these cells are sometimes also called as the heart failure cells.

Pulmonary Vessels

Pulmonary Arteries

Each lung is provided with one pulmonary artery which is derived from pulmonary trunk, arising from right ventricle, and conveys deoxygenated blood to lung. Within each lung the branches of pulmonary artery follow the division and subdivision of bronchial tree and supply the corresponding bronchopulmonary segments by forming capillary plexus around the alveoli. So, the pulmonary arteries are segmental in distribution. Usually, they supply the deoxygenated blood to alveolar capillary plexus and nutrition to the respiratory part (not conducting part) of lung. Although, the flows through systemic and pulmonary circulations are equal, but the lower pulmonary vascular resistance results in pulmonary arterial pressure lower than those in systemic vessels. As a result, the pulmonary arteries have thinner walls than systemic arteries with less smooth muscles. The branches of pulmonary and bronchial arteries anastomose with each other around the intrapulmonary part of bronchi and bronchioles, but they have different vascular pressure. This direct communication between bronchial and pulmonary circulation is normally insignificant, but may become important in certain pathological states. For example, during stenosis, embolism, or any obstruction of pulmonary artery, the bronchial artery supplies nutrition to the respiratory part of lung.

Pulmonary Veins

Each lung presents two pulmonary veins: upper and lower and so there are total four pulmonary veins. The upper pulmonary vein of right lung drains the blood from upper and middle lobes. While the upper pulmonary vein of left lung drains the blood only from upper lobe. The lower pulmonary vein drains the blood from lower lobe of respective lung. The pulmonary vein begins from capillary plexus around the alveoli and terminates directly into left atrium. In the peripheral part of lung, the pulmonary veins are intersegmental in position (whereas pulmonary arteries are segmental in distribution) and receive blood from adjacent of bronchopulmonary segments. The pulmonary veins do not convey 100% oxygenated blood from alveoli to left atrium. Because, it receives some deoxygenated blood from deep bronchial veins.

Bronchial Arteries

Usually, they are three in number: two on left side and one on right side. The two left bronchial arteries supplying left lung arise from thoracic aorta (left side of heart) and the single right bronchial artery supplying right lung arises either from an intercostal artery or from upper left bronchial artery (left side of heart). In addition to these three main bronchial arteries, there are also other many smaller bronchial arteries. This bronchial circulation provides a small amount of blood flow (<3–4% of cardiac output).

On entering the lung through hilum, the bronchial arteries make themselves embedded in the connective tissue layer around the bronchus and then run along the divisions and subdivisions of bronchial tree, until the distal end of terminal bronchiole is reached. Up to this level of terminal bronchiole, by multiple branches, the bronchial arteries supply O_2 and nutrition to the wall of the conducting part of airways and then ultimately drain through bronchial veins into azygos, hemiazygos, or intercostal veins.

After reaching terminal bronchiole, the terminal part of bronchial arteries start to break into multiple branches and produce a distinct set of capillary plexus around the respiratory bronchioles. Gradually, this capillary plexus fuses with the plexuses that is formed around the alveolar duct, atria, alveolar sacs, and alveoli by the branches of pulmonary artery and ultimately drain through pulmonary veins. Some branches of bronchial artery form plexuses around the airways below the level of terminal bronchiole and ultimately drain directly into pulmonary vein through bronchopulmonary vein. *They constitute the true shunt* **(Fig. 12)**. Below the level of terminal bronchioles, regarding the supply of O_2 and nutrition, the lung tissues are supported by a combination of alveolar gas, pulmonary circulation, and bronchial circulation.

Bronchial Veins

The bronchial veins consist of two systems: (1) superficial and (2) deep. The superficial bronchial veins drain blood

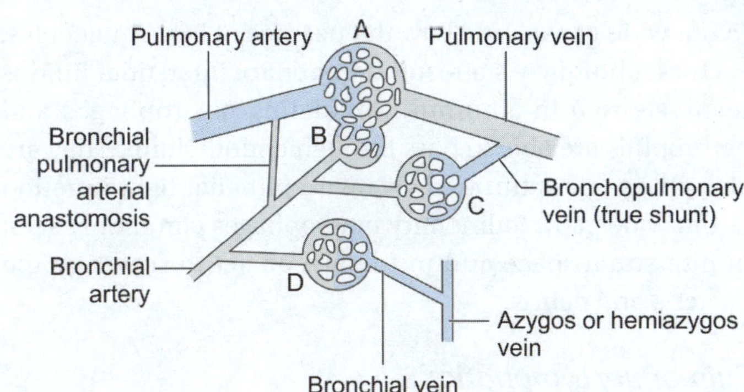

Fig. 12: Relationship between the bronchial and pulmonary circulation. (A) Represents the pulmonary capillary network around the alveoli, atrium, alveolar duct, and respiratory bronchiole (gas exchanging part). It is supplied by the pulmonary artery and drained by the pulmonary vein; (B) Represents the bronchial capillary network which joins with pulmonary capillary network (A) and drains through the pulmonary vein; (C) Represents the capillary network around the bronchi which do not communicate with pulmonary capillary. These vessels form the bronchopulmonary veins and empty into the pulmonary veins (true shunt); (D) Represents the bronchial capillary network around the lobar and segmental bronchi (conducting airway). These networks form true bronchial veins which drain into the azygos, hemiazygos or intercostal veins.

from pleura and the conducting part of bronchi. From right lung, the superficial bronchial veins drain into azygos vein, whereas from left lung they drain into hemiazygos and left superior intercostal vein. The deep bronchial veins receive blood from respiratory part of bronchi and terminate into one of pulmonary veins. *Thus, the superficial bronchial veins drain into right heart and the deep bronchial veins drain into left heart (true shunt).*

Therefore, the lungs get its nutrition from two sources: (i) *the conducting part of respiratory passage*, up to the beginning of respiratory bronchiole or the distal end of terminal bronchiole is supplied by bronchial arteries and (ii) *the respiratory part* is supplied by pulmonary arteries via the pulmonary capillary plexus.

Pulmonary capillaries: Pulmonary capillaries are incorporated into the walls of alveoli. The average diameter of these capillaries is about 10 µm and is just enough to allow to pass a single red cell. Because of relatively low pressure in pulmonary circulation, the amount of blood flowing through a given capillary network is affected by both gravity and alveolar size. At the apex of lung, the alveoli are large and have small capillary cross-sectional area. Hence, at the apex of lung, there is increased resistance and low blood to flow. On the other hand, at the base of the lung, the alveoli are smaller in size, having large capillary cross-sectional area. Hence, at the base of the lung there is less resistance and large amount of blood to flow. Like alveolar epithelium, the capillary endothelial cells do not form so tight junctions

(5 nm wide gaps) and allow the passage of large molecules, such as albumin. As a result, pulmonary interstitial fluid is relatively rich in albumin. Circulating macrophages and neutrophils are able to pass through endothelium. They are also able to pass through alveolar epithelial tight junction (1 nm wide gap). Pulmonary macrophages commonly seen in interstitial space and inside alveoli act to scavenge the bacteria and debris.

Pulmonary Lymphatics

Pulmonary lymphatic channels originate from the interstitial spaces of terminal bronchioles and its above larger airways and run close to bronchial arteries. The interstitial spaces around the alveoli are continuous with the peribronchial and perivascular interstitial spaces of larger airways, starting from terminal bronchioles. So, the fluids, proteins (mainly albumin), cells, etc. that have entered the alveolar interstitial space are returned back to blood via peribronchial and perivascular interstitial spaces of larger airways and lymphatic channels. Because of large endothelial junctional gap, the pulmonary lymph has a relatively high protein contents and total pulmonary lymph flow may be as much as 20 mL/hour. Large lymphatic vessels travel upward alongside the airways, forming trachea-bronchial chain of lymph nodes. The lymphatic drainage channels from both lungs communicate along the trachea.

Innervation of Lungs

The lungs are innervated by both sympathetic and para-sympathetic nerves. The postganglionic sympathetic fibers are derived from first to fourth thoracic ganglia, inferior cervical ganglion, and sometimes from middle cervical ganglion of sympathetic chain. The parasympathetic supply of lungs is derived from vagus and joins with sympathetic fibers to from posterior pulmonary plexus, behind the roots of lungs. The fibers from these posterior plexus also pass in front of the roots of lungs and again form the anterior pulmonary plexus.

The pulmonary nervous plexuses (posterior and anterior) divide into two: periarterial and peribronchial plexus. The peribronchial plexus again divides into two: extrachondrial and intrachondrial plexus, in relation to cartilaginous ring. On reaching the noncartilaginous part of bronchial tree, these two nervous plexuses again reunite and continue distally as single plexus. For parasympathetic system, the peripheral ganglia are found at the level of bronchial tree. The short postganglionic parasympathetic fibers arise from these peripheral parasympathetic ganglia and supply their target structures. The parasympathetic vagus (not sympathetic) nerve provides sensory innervation to the trachea-bronchial tree of lung. Both the sympathetic and parasympathetic autonomic innervation of lung supply the bronchial smooth muscles, glands, vessels, etc. The parasympathetic vagal activity mediates bronchoconstriction and increased bronchial secretion via parasympathetic (cholinergic) muscarinic receptors. Sympathetic activity mediates bronchodilatation and decreased secretion via adrenergic β2 receptors. Both α- and β-adrenergic receptors are present in pulmonary vasculature. But, the sympathetic system normally has little effect on pulmonary vascular tone. The sympathetic α_1 activity causes vasoconstriction and sympathetic β_2 activity causes vasodilation. Parasympathetic vasodilatation activity also seems to be mediated via the release of N_2O.

Diaphragm is innervated by somatic phrenic nerve, arising from C3, C4, and C5 nerve roots. Unilateral phrenic nerve palsy reduces about 25% pulmonary function. Bilateral phrenic nerve paralysis causes the severe impairment of pulmonary function. But, the activity of accessory muscle may maintain adequate ventilation and continue life, in the presence of bilateral phrenic nerve paralysis. The intercostal muscles are innervated by their respective thoracic intercostal nerves. The cervical cord injury above the level of C5 is incompatible with spontaneous ventilation. Because, both the phrenic and intercostal nerves are affected.

■ MECHANISM OF RESPIRATION

Introduction

The respiration is divided into two processes: inspiration and expiration. Among these, in natural spontaneous respiration, the inspiration is defined as active and the expiration is defined as passive process. In a quiet resting state of breathing, with 20 respiratory rate per minute, the inspiration persists for about 1 second and the expiration persists for about 2–3 seconds. So, in an adult, the normal respiratory rate varies in-between 16 and 20 per minute and the inspiratory: expiratory ratio varies in-between 1:2 or 1:3. In *infant*, this respiratory rate ranges in-between 30 and 40 per minute and in *children* it ranges in-between 25 and 30 per minute. The inspiration involves the expansion of chest cavity by (i) the downward movement of diaphragm, so as to increase the longitudinal length of it (chest cavity) and (ii) the elevation of ribs by the contraction of intercostal muscles, so as to increase in anteroposterior and transverse diameter of chest cavity. As the expiration is a passive process, so it involves all the reverse movement which occurs during inspiration. Thus, the respiration is accompanied by respiratory muscles which again are controlled by the respiratory center.

Respiratory Muscles

The respiratory muscles themselves have no inherent rhythmicity for their contraction. But, they contract at certain intervals by motor impulses, originating from respiratory centers, situated at cortex (voluntary), midbrain, medulla, and pons in brain, and travelling through phrenic and intercostal nerves. Diaphragm is a large, dome-shaped sheet of muscle and separates the thoracic cavity from abdominal cavity. *It is the principal muscle of inspiration* that take part in quiet breathing. But, it is not absolutely essential for breathing. Because, in absence of it, other muscles also can take the responsibility of it (inspiration). The contraction of diaphragm increases all the three diameters (vertical, anteroposterior, and transverse) of thorax and helps in inspiration **(Figs. 13A to C)**.

On the other hand, it (diaphragm) is the only inspiratory muscle in neonates and infants. Because, all the ribs at this age are horizontal and the movements of ribs by the contraction of intercostal muscles in neonates and infants cannot increase the diameter of thorax. The oblique direction of ribs appears after the age of second year. Hence, the respiration below second year is predominantly abdominal in type, depending only on diaphragm. Again, the diaphragm is very essential for the maintenance of respiration, during anesthesia under spontaneous respiration. Because, the intercostal muscles are paralyzed and become inactive early than diaphragm during anesthesia. Besides these, during the paralysis of intercostal muscle, due to any disease or during thoracic spinal and epidural anesthesia, only the diaphragm can maintain basic respiration. This diaphragmatic respiration is known as the abdominal type of respiration.

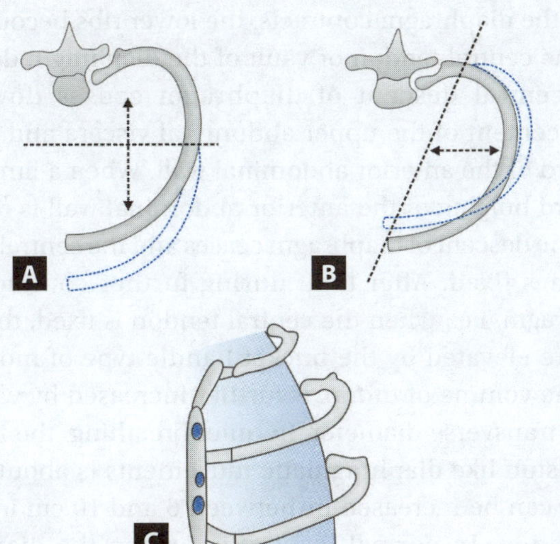

Figs. 13A to C: (A) Pump-handle type of movement; (B) Bucket-handle type of movement; (C) Ribs and their movements at manubriosternal joint.

The diaphragm is supplied by phrenic nerve which takes origin from cervical spinal cord by the anterior roots of 3rd, 4th, and 5th cervical spinal nerve. So, during high central neuroaxial block such as thoracic epidural, where the level of anesthesia extends below the level of cervical segments, but affect the whole thoracic segment of spinal cord and all intercostal muscles, then the respiration also can be maintained only by diaphragm. This is because maximum intercostal muscles become paralyzed in such condition.

The intercostal muscles move the ribs and thus help in inspiration and expiration with diaphragm. *Among them, the external intercostal muscles elevate the ribs and cause active inspiration, while the internal intercostal muscles depress the ribs and cause active expiration.* However, we will have to keep in mind that the external intercostal muscles may take part in normal active inspiration, but the internal intercostal muscle does not take part in normal passive expiration.

The external intercostal muscles run obliquely *downward and forward* from the lower border of upper ribs to the upper border of lower ribs. So, when they contract they elevate the lower ribs. This pushes the sternum outward and increases the anteroposterior diameter of thoracic cavity. In this movement, the transverse diameter of thoracic cavity also increases along with the anteroposterior diameter of thorax, but to a lesser extent. On the other hand, the internal intercostal muscles run obliquely *downward and posteriorly* from the lower border of upper ribs to the upper border of lower ribs. Therefore, the contraction of these muscles cause the downward pull on rib cage which is opposite to the movement of inspiration and thus produce expiration.

During inspiration, the movements of upper six ribs by the contraction of external intercostal muscles increase mostly the anteroposterior diameter of thorax. Whereas, during inspiration, the movements of lower ribs by the contraction of external intercostal muscles widen mainly the transverse diameter of thorax. The electromyographic (EMG) studies of intercostal muscles suggest that the lower intercostal muscles are active in quiet breathing and the upper intercostal muscles are only involved progressively during deep expiration. Increase in 1 cm of circumference of thorax during inspiration allows about 200 mL of air to flow into lungs.

The *scalene group of muscles* and the *sternocleidomastoid* muscles are active only during *deep and active inspiration*. The scalene group of muscle elevates the first and second ribs, while the sternomastoid muscle elevates the clavicle. In quiet respiration, the first and second ribs and the clavicle remain fixed and do not take part in respiration. The pectoral group of muscle and serratus muscle also helps in only forced inspiration. It works only when the bones of upper limbs are fixed. The erector spinae muscles make the thoracic part of vertebral column straight and help it to act as a pivot, against which the other muscles can act and bones can move. Thus, it also facilitates the spreading of lower ribs, with widening of infrasternal angle and so help in deep inspiration. The quadratus lumborum muscle fixes the last rib and helps in the action of diaphragm during deep inspiration. The other accessory muscles that take part in decreasing the resistance of air flow and help in *active inspiration* are the mylohyoid, digastric, alae nasai, platysma, chick muscles, levator palati, laryngeal muscles, tongue muscles, posterior neck muscles, etc. During muscular exercise, when ventilation increases manifold, then all the accessory muscles of inspiration, including the trapezius and back muscles also take part in action.

It is previously said that *normal expiration* is a passive process and it is due to the elastic recoil property of lungs and thoracic cage. So, during inspiration, some potential energy is gained due to the contraction of inspiratory muscle and during *quite expiration* this stored energy, gained by inspiratory muscles, is released from these muscles by the elastic recoil property of lungs and thoracic cage and expiration is performed. But, only few muscles come into active action during *forced expiration*. These are the flat muscles of anterior abdominal wall (external and internal oblique, transversus abdominis, rectus abdominis, etc.), latissimus dorsi, and internal intercostal muscles. The contraction of flat muscles of anterior abdominal wall aids in active expiration by pulling the rib cage downward. The muscles of anterior abdominal wall also compress the abdomen and increase intraabdominal pressure. Thus, it displaces the diaphragm upward and the volume of thoracic cavity is diminished, causing expiration. In normal breathing, they are practically inactive, but during coughing, sneezing, etc., they become highly active. The latissimus dorsi also reduces thoracic volume by compressing the thorax from behind.

The anteroposterior diameter of thorax is increased by the elevation of ribs, mainly from 2nd to 6th. An oblique axis passes through the costovertebral and costotransverse joints of the neck of the ribs of one side and the costochondral junction of the ribs of opposite site. When the ribs move around this axis, then the anteroposterior diameter of thorax is increased. This is caused by the contraction of external intercostal muscles of one side and the internal intercostal muscles of opposite side due to their same fiber direction. This movement of ribs is called as the *pump-handle type of movement*. In this type of movement, the body of sternum moves forward during the elevation of ribs (at sternomanubrial joint) during inspiration and swings backward during expiration. The first rib and manubrium sterni form a rigid unit and do not move in quiet breathing,

except during forced inspiration. The 2nd to 6th ribs sloped downward and forward with their cartilages. So, their elevation cause forward and upward movement of the body of sternum and increase the anteroposterior diameter of thorax.

The 7th to 10th ribs is sloped downward and forward, but their cartilages are directed upward and medially to join the body of sternum. So, the movement of these ribs around this oblique axis causes the backward movement of sternal body at sternomanubrial joint and diminishes anteroposterior diameter. Therefore, two opposite forces work together at sternomanubrial joint. Movement of upper ribs produces forward movement and movement of lower ribs produces backward movement. Thus, this explains the formation of sternal angle at the junction between manubrium and body of the sternum.

The transverse diameter of thoracic cavity is increased by two methods: active and passive. Active process is observed between 7th and 10th ribs. Here, the movement of ribs takes place around an axis which passes through the costovertebral and the costosternal joint of same side. Movement of these ribs around this axis causes the elevation of the middle portion of ribs, resembling bucket handle type of movement and increase the transverse diameter of thorax. Movement of 2nd to 6th ribs around the oblique axis which increases the anteroposterior diameter also increases the transverse diameter of thorax passively. This passive increase of transverse diameter is facilitated by the curved nature of articular surfaces of costotransverse joint.

The vertical diameter of thorax increases due to up and down piston like movement of diaphragm. It also helps to increase the transverse diameter. Initially during inspiration when the diaphragm contracts, the lower ribs become fixed and the central tendon or vault of the diaphragm descents. This central descent of diaphragm causes downward displacement of the upper abdominal viscera and bulging forward of the anterior abdominal wall. When a limit of the forward bulging of the anterior abdominal wall is reached, then the descent of diaphragm ceases and the central tendon becomes fixed. After that, during further contraction of diaphragm, i.e., when the central tendon is fixed, the lower ribs are elevated by the bucket handle type of movement and the volume of thorax is further increased by widening of the transverse diameter. In quiet breathing, the range of this piston like diaphragmatic movements is about 1.5 cm which can be increased in-between 6 and 10 cm in forced respiration. In normal respiration, when the diaphragm descends about 1.5 cm, the thoracic volume is increased by about 400 cc. Normally, out of 500 cc of tidal air, 400 cc is due to this 1.5 cm movement of diaphragm.

Summary

The lungs can be inflated or deflated by two ways:

1. By downward and upward movement of the diaphragm which increases or decreases the volume of chest cavity and subsequently the volume of lungs.
2. By elevation and depression of the ribs which increases and decreases the anteroposterior and transverse diameter of the chest cavity and subsequently the volume of lungs.

The normal quiet breathing is almost entirely accomplished by only the movement of diaphragm. During inspiration, the diaphragm contracts and increases the volume of lungs, the mechanism of which is described before and air is rushed in. During expiration the diaphragm simply relaxes. Thus, due to the elastic recoil property of the lungs, chest wall and abdominal structures all compress the lungs and air is rushed out.

But, during heavy or active breathing, the second method of the expansion of lungs by the movement of rib cage comes into play. In natural resting position, the ribs are slanted downward. But, when the rib cage is elevated by the muscular contraction, then the ribs project forward and upward directly. Thus, the sternum also moves upward and forward away from the spine, increasing the anteroposterior diameter of thoracic cavity. With the forward elevation of the ribs, there is also buckle handle type of movement of ribs which increase the transverse diameter of rib cage. Therefore, the muscles that elevate the chest cage are called the muscles of inspiration and the muscles that depress the chest cage are called the muscles of expiration. So, the muscles of inspiration are: external intercostal (main inspiratory muscles), sternocleidomastoid (by lifting the sternum upward), anterior serratus (by lifting many of the ribs where it is attached), and scalene muscles (by lifting the first two ribs). The last three muscles are called the helping inspiratory muscles. The muscles of expiration are: abdominal recti (by pulling downward the lower ribs and at the same time with other abdominal muscles by compressing the abdominal contents upward against the diaphragm) and internal intercostal (by pulling the ribs downward due to the downward and backward direction of their attachment).

Intrathoracic and Intrapulmonary Pressure

Under normal resting condition, when there is no inspiration or expiration, then the *intrathoracic pressure*, more precisely called as the *intrapleural pressure* is subatmospheric and measures about –2 mm Hg. In similar condition, the *intra-alveolar* or *intrapulmonary pressure* is zero, i.e., equal to atmospheric pressure.

The chest wall and the lung are covered by a thin layer of membrane which is known as the parietal and visceral pleura, respectively. These two layers of pleura are separated by a thin layer of fluid, which is called the pleural fluid and it lubricates the movement of visceral pleura, covering the lungs, on parietal pleura covering the inner side of chest cavity. The pressure within the space, between these two pleura, is called the *intrapleural pressure*. Theoretically, this intrapleural pressure is –8 to –10 mm Hg. This negative intrapleural pressure is caused by the more rapid absorption of pleural fluid by lymphatic and by the capillaries of visceral pleura, since such lymphatic and blood capillaries are belonged to low pressure pulmonary circulatory system. On the other hand, the value of pressure on pleural surface, due to the contact between the visceral and parietal pleura is about +6 mm Hg. So, the resultant practical intrapleural pressure, which we measure, is the theoretical negative intrapleural pressure due to the absorption of fluid plus the positive intrapleural contact pressure, i.e., –8 + (+ 6) or –2 mm Hg. But, this value is an average one. Actually, the intrapleural pressure at the base of lungs which is normally about –2 mm Hg at the start of inspiration, decreases to about –6 mm Hg at the end of inspiration in quite breathing. Strong inspiratory efforts may increase this negative intrapleural pressure to the values as low as –30 mm Hg or more, producing the corresponding greater degrees of lung inflation (**Figs. 14A and B**).

Such negative intrapleural pressure, which helps the lungs to inflate, allows the visceral and parietal pleura to come in close contact with each other, as if they are glued together. But, the presence of thin intrapleural fluid allows the free movement of these two pleura when the chest contracts and expands. The lungs tissues possess an inherent elastic property to recoil from the chest wall, but this

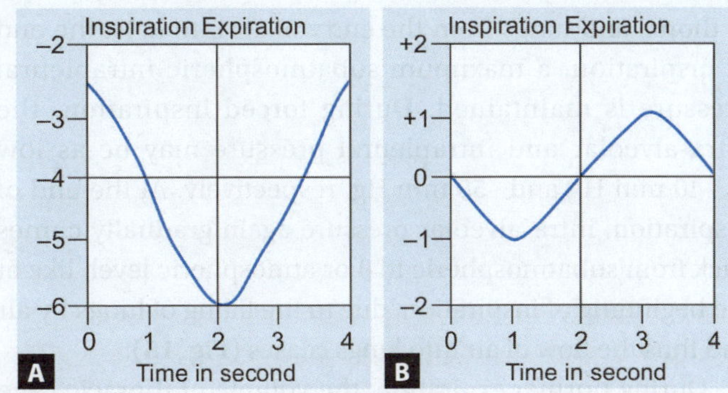

Figs. 14A and B: (A) It is the graphical representation of changes in intrathoracic or intrapleural pressure during respiration (inspiration and expiration); (B) The graphical representation of changes in intrapulmonary or intra-alveolar pressure during respiration (inspiration and expiration).

negative intrapleural pressure prevents this recoiling. Thus, the intrapleural pressure being subatmospheric keeps the lungs in apposition with chest wall and make it partially inflated. But, if the chest wall is opened to atmosphere, the lungs will collapse due to its inward recoiling elastic property and due to the absence of subatmospheric intrapleural pressure. On the other hand, if the lungs lose their recoil property or elasticity, it remains in inflated or expanded condition and becomes barrel shaped. It is estimated that the one-third of inward recoiling elastic force of lungs is derived from the stretched elastic fibers within it such as elastin, collagen, etc. and two-thirds from the surface tension of fluid, lining the alveoli.

At rest, when there is no inspiration or expiration the intrapulmonary or intra-alveolar pressure is maintained at 0 mm Hg (i.e., same as atmospheric pressure or 760 mm Hg). So, at this condition no air enters in or comes out of lungs. During inspiration, as lungs expand due to more and more subatmospheric intrapleural pressure which is again due to the expansion of chest wall, then the intra-alveolar or intrapulmonary pressure gradually falls and an alveolar-upper airway pressure gradient is established, causing air to rush into lungs. Thus, during inspiration the intra-alveolar pressure gradually falls from 0 mm Hg to about –2 or –6 mm Hg (at that time intrapleural pressure also falls from –2 mm Hg to –6 mm Hg or –10 mm Hg or more). During deep inspiration, this intrapleural pressure becomes more subatmospheric and this is due to the active contraction of inspiratory muscles. That active contraction of inspiratory muscles try to create more negative intrapleural pressure and subsequently more negative intra-alveolar pressure to overcome the different resistances, such as (i) the elastic recoil of lung, (ii) the frictional resistance due to the deformation of tissues of lungs and thorax, and (iii) the frictional airway resistance which prevents the expansion of thorax and lungs from the entry of air into it. At the end of inspiration, a maximum subatmospheric intrapleural pressure is maintained. During forced inspiration, the intra-alveolar and intrapleural pressure may be as low as –40 mm Hg and –50 mm Hg, respectively. At the end of inspiration, intra-alveolar pressure again gradually comes back from subatmospheric to 0 or atmospheric level, like at the beginning of inspiration, due to the filling of lungs by air and thus the flow of air into lungs ceases **(Fig. 15)**.

During normal expiration, the volume of thoracic cage and the volume of lung decreases passively, due to the inward elastic recoiling property of lung parenchyma and chest wall tissues. Thus, the intra-alveolar or intrapulmonary pressure rises above the atmospheric level. It generally goes up to

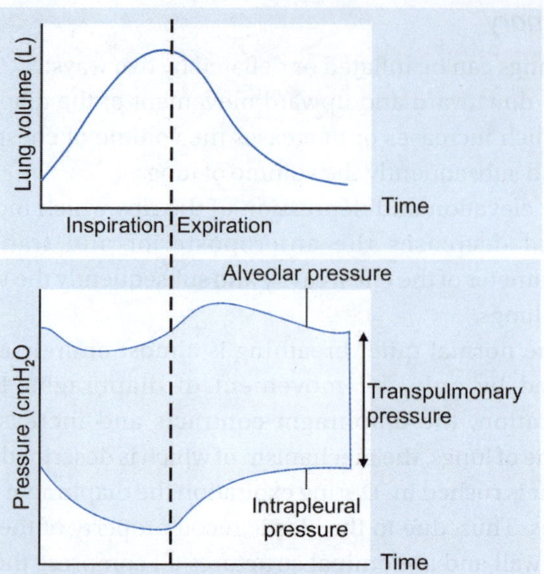

Fig. 15: Changes in alveolar pressure, intrapleural pressure, transpulmonary pressure, and lung volumes during normal inspiration and expiration. Transpulmonary pressure = alveolar pressure – intrapleural pressure ($P_{transpulmonary} = P_{alveolar} - P_{intrapleural}$) and Transthoracic pressure = atmospheric pressure – intrapleural pressure ($P_{transthoracic} = P_{atmospheric} - P_{intrapleural}$)

+3 or +4 mm Hg and permits the exit of air from lungs. At that time, the intrapleural pressure also comes back from –6 mm Hg to –2 mm Hg, but always remains –ve (subatmospheric). When the forced expiratory efforts are made with closed glottis, such as during muscular exercise, defecation or micturition, etc., then the intrapleural pressure becomes +ve (+10 to +40 mm Hg) and the intrapulmonary pressure may also go up from +10 mm Hg to +40 mm Hg or more. In coughing and sneezing, the intrapulmonary pressure may also go far above the normal level and may be +100 mm Hg with glottis closed. At the end of expiration, when air stops to exit, then the intra-alveolar pressure again gradually comes down to atmospheric or zero level.

Thus, it is to be noted that during normal inspiration and expiration the changes of pressure within lungs (or intra-alveolar pressure) goes both above and below the "0" line or atmospheric pressure. But, the pressure changes in pleura (i.e., intrapleural pressure) always remain below the "0" line or subatmospheric level (i.e., negative) and pressure level in the abdomen always remain above the "0" line (i.e., positive). The difference between the intra-alveolar pressure and the intrapleural pressure is called the transpulmonary pressure. Actually, it is the pressure difference between the inside and the outside of lungs and is equivalent to the elastic forces of lungs that tend to collapse it at the each moment of respiration.

The physical principles that determine the respiration are the production of pressure gradient between the interior of lungs (alveoli) and the atmosphere. According to physical laws, the air will flow from a higher pressure head to a lower one. During inspiration, the intra-alveolar pressure falls below the atmospheric one and so the air rushes in. But, during expiration, the intra-alveolar pressure goes above the atmospheric pressure level and the air goes out. Thus, the normal breathing is called the *negative pressure breathing*. But, if the atmospheric pressure is raised above the intra-alveolar pressure to push the air into the lungs during inspiration, and the pressure outside the mouth is lowered below the atmospheric pressure to bring out the air from alveoli, then this type of respiration is called the *positive pressure breathing* which is used during general anesthesia with complete muscular paralysis.

Compliance of Lungs

The compliance is usually defined as a stretching force that is needed to stretch or inflate the lungs. This is opposite to elastic force that tries to collapse the lungs. It is measured as the change of volume of lungs, during expansion of it, for each unit increase of transpulmonary pressure. The average total compliance of both the lungs together, in an adult human being, is about 200 mL/cmH$_2$O (or 0.2 L/cmH$_2$O) transpulmonary pressure. It means that for increase in every cmH$_2$O of transpulmonary pressure, the total volume of both the lungs will expand to 200 mL. Therefore, the compliance of single lung is 100 mL/cmH$_2$O (or 0.1 L/cmH$_2$O). During this discussion, we will not any confusion between the *compliance of chest wall* and the compliance of lungs.

Usually, the compliance of lungs is represented diagrammatically by two curves. Among these, one is called the inspiratory compliance curve and the other is called the expiratory compliance curve. While the entire diagram (area in between these two curves) represents the total compliance of lungs.

It is previously explained that the compliance, which is usually defined as the stretching force, is opposite to the elastic forces (or elasticity). So, the compliance of lungs is best understood and calculated from it (elasticity). On the other hand, the elasticity has two components: (i) the elasticity caused by the lung tissue or parenchyma itself, and (ii) the elasticity, caused by the surface tension of fluid, lining the inside of alveoli. The elastic forces (elasticity) of lung parenchyma are caused by the interwoven elastin and collagen fibers, situated in the parenchyma of lungs. In completely collapsed lungs these fibers are in completely contracted state. Thus, when the lungs expand, then these fibers become stretched and thereby exert an elastic (inward contraction) forces which prevent the expansion **(Fig. 16)**.

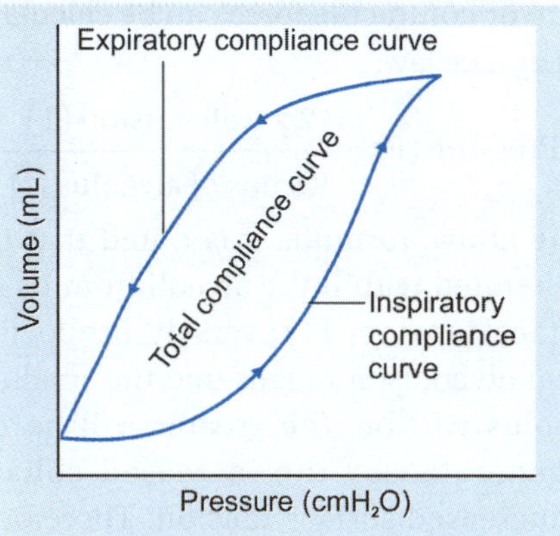

Fig. 16: Two compliance curves of lung.

The elasticity caused by the surface tension of fluid, lining the alveoli is more interesting. On the inner side of alveolar wall, there is always some thin layer of fluid. So, when the lungs are filled with air, there is always an interface between the fluid and the air in alveoli. This fluid and the air interface in alveoli are responsible for this surface tension of alveoli which tries to collapse the alveoli and subsequently the lungs. This is because, when a fluid has a surface with air then the fluid molecules, on this interface with air, have a strong force of attraction for one another. This is called the surface tension. As a result, the fluid surface, toward the air, always tries to contract and takes the smallest spherical shape. Thus, the alveoli with their fluid surface try to collapse, forcing the air out of the lungs. This elastic force caused by this fluid-air surface tension in alveoli is two-thirds of total lung elasticity. On the other hand, the tissue elasticity due to the stretching of elastin and collagen fibers represents only about one-third of total lung elasticity.

The surfactant is a surface active chemical agent which greatly reduces the surface tension of liquid. This chemical agent or surfactant is present in the fluid lining the alveoli and subsequently reduces the surface tension of fluid lining the alveoli and subsequently reduces the contractile elastic force of lungs, due to surface tension (not due to elastin and collagen fibers of lung parenchyma). In the absence of this surfactant, the surface tension in alveoli and subsequently the collapsing forces of alveoli due to this surface tension will increase tremendously and then, it is not possible to inflate the lungs. This chemical agent or surfactant is a complex mixture of many phospholipids, proteins, and ions. Among these components, the most important components are: dipalmitoylphosphatidylcholine (DPPC), apoproteins, and calcium ions. They act by not completely dissolving in fluid, lining the alveoli, but remain spread over the surface of fluid that lines the inner side of alveoli.

Due to this surface tension, alveoli tend to collapse. Thus, an increased level of pressure is generated within the alveoli.

This pressure or contractile force can be calculated from the formula of Laplace law:

$$\text{Pressure (P)} = \frac{2 \times \text{wall tension (T)}}{\text{Radius of alveolus (r)}}$$

From the above formula, it is noted that the pressure which is generated within the alveoli from its contraction, due to surface tension, is inversely proportional to the radius of that alveolus. It means that the smaller the radius of the alveolus will be, the greater will be the alveolar pressure, generated by the increased collapsing force due to the increased surface tension. Therefore, when the size of the alveoli will decrease during expiration, then the pressure tending to collapse or collapsing force will increase and thus a vicious cycle will be established. But, in practical this does not occur, because as the alveoli are coated with surfactant which reduces the surface tension and as the alveoli decrease in size during expiration, so the amount of surfactant per unit area of alveolar surface will also increase and reduces the surface tension more than the expected. Thus, the action of surfactant will be more efficient when the alveoli will decrease in size. Therefore, contrary to Laplace's law, the smaller alveoli can be inflated more easily than a larger one in the presence of surfactant. If there is no surfactant, then the larger alveoli would tend to inflate further, at the expense of smaller ones which collapses readily in the absence of surfactant.

The radius of a normal adult alveoli is 100 μm. The normal value of surface tension in such alveoli, created by the lining fluid with normal amount of surfactant, varies between 5 and 30 dynes/cm. Then, the intra-alveolar pressure is calculated to 4 cmH_2O. In newborn, the radius of alveoli is 50 μm which is half than that of an adult. In such situation, pressure generated by collapsing alveoli due to the surface tension, will be doubled, with normal amount of surfactant. This is more significant in premature newborn where the radius of alveoli is more or less one quarter than that of an adult person. Here, the pressure inside the alveoli, due to its collapse, increases to fourfold. Further, many premature newborn has little or no surfactant in their alveoli. So, their lungs have extreme tendency to collapse which is sometimes as great as eight times than that of a normal adult person. This explains why such patients need high positive pressure ventilation.

■ RESPIRATORY CENTER AND ITS REGULATION

The normal rate of respiration in an adult healthy individual is about 14–18 per minute, with a tidal volume of about 500 mL. But the rate and depth of respiration, i.e., the total pulmonary ventilation per minute varies according to the requirements of the body.

The important functions of respiration are:

- To supply the adequate amount of O_2 and to eliminate CO_2.
- To regulate H^+ ion concentration of blood.
- To maintain the temperature of our body.
- To excrete volatile substances such as ammonia, ketone bodies, alcohol, water vapor, etc. from our body.
- To help in circulation. During inspiration the intrathoracic pressure falls and intra-abdominal pressure rises. This is one of the most important factors that help in the return of venous blood to heart and lymph in the circulation.

Whenever these requirements increase, then the respiration is stimulated. For example, when the metabolic rate increases due to any cause, then the necessity for supplying more oxygen and the necessity for eliminating more CO_2 will also rise. In this condition, blood will tend to become more acid and heat production will be more. So, to maintain these factors at their normal level, respiration will also have to be stimulated. This is also found in muscular exercise, when the pulmonary ventilation rises enormously. On the other hand, during sleep the metabolic requirements are low; hence, the respiration is also depressed. As a whole, it can be stated that the total pulmonary ventilation is directly proportional to the metabolic need of our body. Since, as the rate and depth of respiration can be accurately adjusted according to the body needs, so it is necessary that there must be an efficient mechanism for its regulation.

The spontaneous respiration is produced by the rhythmic discharge of impulses from some motor neurons (higher respiratory center) which are situated in the brain and that innervate the respiratory muscles through the cervical and thoracic segment of spinal cord. These rhythmic discharges of impulses from the respiratory centers that produce spontaneous respiration are regulated by the alternations of the arterial PO_2, PCO_2, and H^+ concentration (chemical regulation). Again this chemical control of breathing is supplemented by a number of other nonchemical stimuli (nervous regulations) that also have influences on it **(Fig. 17)**.

Usually, there are two separate neural mechanisms which regulate the respiration. Among these, one is responsible for the voluntary control and the other is responsible for the automatic rhythmical control of respiration. The center for voluntary control of respiration is located in the cerebral cortex and sends impulses directly to the respiratory motor neurons (not the respiratory center) supplying the diaphragm and the intercostal muscles, situated in the spinal cord (cervical and thoracic segment) via the corticospinal tracts. On the other hand, the automatic rhythmical control of respiration is driven by a group pacemaker cells situated in

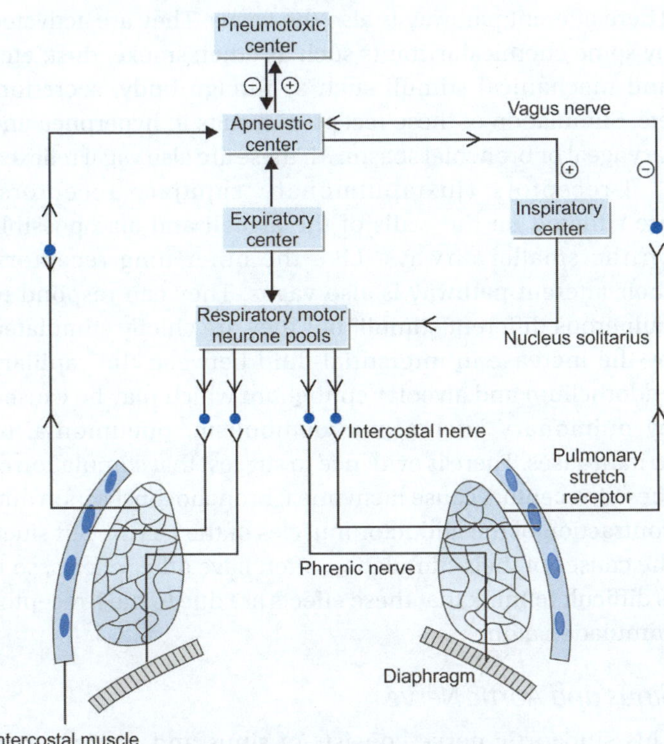

Fig. 17: Diagrammatic representation of central respiratory mechanism.

the brainstem, medulla, and pons which are called together as the respiratory center. Impulses from these cells activate rhythmically the motor neurons in the cervical and thoracic segment of the spinal cord that innervate the inspiratory muscles. Those in the cervical segment of spinal cord activate the diaphragm via the phrenic nerves and those in the thoracic segment of spinal cord activate the external and internal intercostal muscles.

The motor neurons to the expiratory muscles are inhibited, when the motor neurons, those supplying the inspiratory muscles, are activated and vice versa. This is called the reciprocal innervation of RC. Thus, the mechanism of regulating the respiration has been arbitrarily divided into three parts: (1) respiratory center, (2) nervous regulation, and (3) chemical regulation.

Respiratory Center

It has been suggested that there are certain collection of nerve cells in brainstem, medulla, and pons (although they do not form any discrete structure) that control the respiratory movements of chest wall and diaphragm automatically without any interruption. These collections of nerve cells together are called the respiratory center which under normal circumstances generate the rhythm of impulses (breathing) and organize the respiration. However, this organization of respiratory center is very complex and

includes several subcenters. These subcenters on each side consists of inspiratory center, pneumotaxic center, apneustic center, and expiratory center which are located at the various level of brainstem, medulla, and pons.

These respiratory subcenters are bilateral in situation and control the respiratory muscles of ipsilateral and contralateral side simultaneously. They (respiratory subcenters) also freely communicate with each other. Connections exist within the similarly acting centers of the opposite sides and within the oppositely acting centers of the same side. For example, an impulse that stimulates one center will inhibit the others and vice versa. But the center of one side controls the respiratory muscles of the same side. Thus, the respiratory center of right side is connected to the spinal motor neurons of phrenic and intercostal nerves, supplying the muscles of respiration of the right side.

Though, there is much uncertainty regarding the actual site of the origin of impulses for respiratory rhythmicity, but still it is generally thought that there is an inherent rhythmicity in the certain groups of respiratory neurons in the brainstem which is modified by other afferent inputs. At present, the established theory is that first the primary inspiratory drive comes from the apneustic center to the inspiratory center. Then, the inspiration starts with the increasing activity of this inspiratory center. During inspiration, the tonic impulses from the apneustic center also excite the pneumotaxic center to send, in turn, the inhibitory impulses from pneumotaxic center to the apneustic center. At the height of inspiration, the inhibitory impulses from the pneumotaxic center, as well as inhibitory impulses from the pulmonary stretch receptors through vagus depress the apneustic center. Thus, inspiration is ceased and the expiration starts passively. Expiration is normally a passive process during quiet breathing. But, it becomes active during exercise. During expiration, the same inhibitory effects on the apneustic center from pneumotaxic center are no longer present and so inspiration starts again. Thus, this process is repeated again and again and respiration (active inspiration and passive expiration) goes on spontaneously. It is probable that the medullary inspiratory center is not under direct control of pneumotaxic center, but it is under the direct control of pontine apneustic center. With the inhibition of the inspiratory center, the expiratory center starts functioning, keeping in mind that in quiet breathing expiration is passive. The expiratory center functions actively only during active expiration, but not during quite breathing.

Summary

- The activity of two feedback mechanism such as the inhibitory vagal afferent impulses from the pulmonary stretch receptors and the negative impulses from the pneumotaxic centers have got probably no direct inhibitory control upon the inspiratory center or direct stimulating effect upon the expiratory center.

- The apneustic center probably sends tonic discharges simultaneously to the inspiratory center and to the pneumotoxic center
- The inspiratory center discharges impulses to the spinal motor neurons supplying the respiratory muscles for normal inspiratory efforts
- The pneumotaxic center in its turn discharges inhibitory impulses to apneustic center
- The apneustic center, being inhibited by the inhibitory impulses from the vagus and also from the pneumotaxic center, ceases to stimulate the inspiratory center.
- The inspiratory center ceases its activity and expiration follows passively.

Nervous Regulation

In nervous regulation of respiration, the respiratory centers are regulated by few reflexes conducted through different nerves and centers. These are described here.

Vagus Nerve

The rhythm and the depth of respiration are controlled by the reflexes, originating from the lungs itself and the impulses for this reflex pass through the vagus nerve. This reflex is called the Hering–Breuer reflex. This is an inflation reflex and the pulmonary stretch receptors are responsible for this. These receptors are uncapsulated and are found in the smooth muscle of the airway without an end organ. They are generally believed to be responsible for signaling the changes of mechanical state of the lungs to the brain. During inspiration, the stretching of pulmonary tissue send inhibitory impulses to the apneustic center which subsequently for this inhibitory impulses fails to send stimulatory impulses to inspiratory center. When inspiration is going on, then due to the gradual increase in the volume of lungs more and more inhibitory impulses pass to the apneustic center and at the maximum inhibition of apneustic center inspiration stops. Then, passive expiration starts and the inhibitory impulses to the inspiratory center gradually wane. When these inhibitory impulses over the inspiratory center completely wane or totally withdrawn during expiration, then inspiration again starts.

The afferent nerve endings, responding to both the mechanical and chemical factors, regulating the respiration, also have been described. They are situated on the epithelium of airways and extend from the trachea to the respiratory bronchioles. They are concentrated mainly at the carina and at the points of branching of bronchial tree.

There afferent pathway is also the vagus. They are activated by some chemical irritants such as ether, smoke, dust, etc., and mechanical stimuli such as foreign body, secretion, etc. Stimulation of these receptors results in hyperpnea and laryngeal or bronchial spasm. All these are also vagal reflexes.

J-receptors (juxtapulmonary capillary receptors) are situated on the walls of the alveoli and also possibly on the smaller airways. Like the other lung receptors, their afferent pathway is also vagus. They can respond to numerous different stimuli, but they are chiefly stimulated by the increase in interstitial fluid between the capillary endothelium and alveolar epithelium which may be caused by pulmonary edema, microembolism, pneumonia, or irritant gases. There is evidence to suggest that stimulation of these J-receptors cause tachypnea, bronchoconstriction and contraction of the adductor muscles of the larynx. But since the causes of their stimulation often have other effects, so it is difficult to think that these effects are due to the J-receptor stimulation alone.

Sinus and Aortic Nerve

This sinoaortic nerve consists of sinus and aortic nerve. The sinus nerve (afferent) arises from the carotid sinus (baroreceptor) and carotid body (chemoreceptor) and passes along the glossopharyngeal nerve to end in the medulla in close relation with the respiratory, cardiac, and vasomotor center. On the other hand, the aortic nerve (afferent) arises from aortic arch (baroreceptor) and aortic body (chemoreceptor) and passes along the vagus nerve to end in the medulla in close relation with the respiratory, cardiac, and vasomotor center. So, they regulate the respiration during the changes of blood pressure, arterial CO_2 and O_2 tension, and H^+ concentration.

CO_2 excess will stimulate the respiration by reflexly acting through the carotid and aortic bodies. Alteration of H^+ concentration due to any other causes such as in metabolic acidosis or alkalosis other than changes in CO_2 concentration will also act in the same way as CO_2. Oxygen lack will also stimulate the respiration by reflexly acting through the carotid and aortic bodies. But its direct action on the respiratory center is depression of respiration. Rise of blood pressure will also depress the respiration, but fall of blood pressure will stimulate the respiration. They act through the baroreceptors such as the carotid sinus and the aortic arch.

Impulses from Higher Centers

Certain and several parts of the cerebral cortex, hypothalamus, limbic systems, vasomotor center, and other parts of the brain also reflexly alter and regulate the respiration through respiratory center.

Other Factors

There are certain other factors which also affect the respiratory centers reflexly. These are cough, yawning, hiccough, sneezing, and other reflexes arising from the body surface and viscera (such as thermoreceptor, pain receptor, touch receptors, etc. also affect respiration). Reflexes arising from the muscles and joints increase pulmonary ventilation during exercise and are partly due to the impulses originating from the active muscles and joints.

Chemical Regulation

The respiratory centers are highly sensitive to the alterations of chemical composition of the blood. Changes in the CO_2 tension, O_2 tension, and H^+ ion concentration of blood alter the pulmonary ventilation profoundly. In any case, the main purpose is to adjust the respiration in such way that it may be able to meet the demands of the body adequately during emergency. The effects of these changes are briefly summarized below.

The chemical regulatory mechanism adjust ventilation in such a way that the alveolar PCO_2 is normally held constant, the excess H^+ in the blood are combated, and arterial PO_2 is raised, when it falls to a potentially dangerous level. The respiratory minute volume is proportionate to the metabolic rate, but the link between the metabolism and the ventilation is CO_2, but not O_2. The link between metabolism and ventilation is established by the receptors in the carotid and aortic bodies which are stimulated by the rise in arterial PCO_2 or H^+ concentration or decline in PO_2.

Effects of Changes in CO_2 Tension

The arterial PCO_2 is normally maintained at 40 mm Hg (between 35 and 45 mm Hg), because the respiratory center is extremely sensitive to the slight alteration in arterial CO_2 tension. A slight rise of CO_2 concentration in inspired air increases respiration enormously. Respiration increases at first in depth and then in rate and last by both. Thus, the total pulmonary ventilation is raised. The degree of stimulation of respiration shows a quantitative relationship with the increase of CO_2 tension. The total pulmonary ventilation is so nicely adjusted that the alveolar CO_2 tension which is proportional to the arterial CO_2 tension (if there is no abnormality in the diffusion of CO_2 at the level of alveoli) remains more or less constant. This reflex works maximally up to the inspired CO_2 concentration of 5%. But, if the percentage of CO_2 concentration in inspired air goes above 5%, then this adjustment fails and consequently the alveolar CO_2 content (concentration) rises. So, the breathing of air containing up to 5% CO_2 will not do any harm, although the respiration will be stimulated. But, if the inspired CO_2 content

is raised further, then the alveolar CO_2 tension will rise in spite of hyperventilation. This will lead to the accumulation of CO_2 in the blood and thereby will cause the toxic effects of CO_2, i.e., CO_2 narcosis (headache, confusion, and coma).

The CO_2 acts on respiratory center both (i) by directly (centrally mediated) acting on it and (ii) by reflexly or indirectly acting through the carotid and aortic bodies (reflex mediated). During anesthesia, the threshold level of arterial CO_2 tension which stimulates the respiratory center increases. Thus, in anesthetized condition respiratory center becomes insensitive to CO_2 and not stimulated even in high CO_2 tension (hypercapnia).

Effect of Changes in H^+ Concentration

The changes of H^+ ion concentration in blood also alter the pulmonary ventilation. During metabolic acidosis, the respiration rises (is stimulated) and during metabolic alkalosis, it falls (is inhibited). The purpose of this change in respiration, according to the changes in $[H^+]$, is briefly stated as follows:

During acidosis, due to only metabolic causes, respiration increases and more and more CO_2 is eliminated from the alveoli. This lowers the alveolar CO_2 tension below the normal. Consequently, more and more CO_2 comes out of the bloodstream into the alveoli which is formed by the reaction between H^+ and HCO^- ions. Thus, the concentration of H^+ ion in blood is lowered and the metabolic acidosis is compensated. On the other hand, during metabolic alkalosis, respiration is depressed → less and less CO_2 is washed out → alveolar CO_2 tension increases → less CO_2 diffuses out of the blood → more CO_2 accumulates in bloodstream → increase in H^+ ion concentration of blood → combat alkalosis. Thus, blood reaction is maintained by the adjustment of pulmonary ventilation during metabolic acidosis and alkalosis. But, this is applicable only to metabolic causes (metabolic acidosis or alkalosis). In respiratory acidosis and alkalosis, this is not applicable, because here, the lungs or respiratory system does not act as compensatory organ. Because they themselves are the cause of respiratory acidosis and alkalosis.

The mode of action of H^+ ion in regulating respiration is same as CO_2. So, as the mechanism of action of CO_2 and H^+ ion in regulating respiration is same, therefore, it is thought that the action of CO_2 is not due to its own effect, but due to the associated change in H^+ ion concentration. There is controversy that whether it is the intracellular H^+ or CO_2 which regulates the activity of respiratory center. CO_2 is more easily diffusible through the cell membrane than H^+ ion. So, it is probable that CO_2 diffuses inside the respiratory neurons which are carried here by blood from the different body tissues and inside the cell with the help of carbonic anhydrase; this CO_2 is changed to H_2CO_3. Then, this intracellular H_2CO_3 is ionized and H^+ ions are liberated. Now, the intracellular H^+ ions are supposed to be the sole factor, regulating the rhythmical activity of respiratory center.

$$CO_2 + H_2O \leftrightarrow H + CO_3 \leftrightarrow H^+ + HCO_3^-$$

Effect of Changes of Oxygen Tension

The effect of the changes of O_2 tension on respiratory center can be described under two headings: (1) the effects of oxygen lack and (2) the effect of oxygen excess. Oxygen lack acts on the respiratory center reflexly through the carotid and aortic chemoreceptors and it is stimulating in effect. But, the direct effect of O_2 lack on the respiratory center is depression. The effects of oxygen lack on respiratory center will vary according to the severity and the rapidity with which the lack of O_2 is produced. If severe oxygen lack is produced very rapidly, then the results will be disastrous. Here, we will discuss only the effects of the gradual reduction of oxygen concentration or tension (pressure). It is seen that the O_2 tension in inspired air can be reduced to 13% without any appreciable change in respiration and any discomfort on the part of the subject. But, with the further reduction (>13%) of O_2 concentration in inspired air, respiration starts rising with a feeling of uneasiness. This shows that the respiratory apparatus is much less sensitive to oxygen lack (hypoxia) than to CO_2 excess (hypercapnia).

On the other hand, we can say that the arterial CO_2 tension is the strongest stimulus in adjusting respiration. Oxygen lack or hypoxia will be stimulus, only when it is sufficiently reduced. In many circumstances, hypoxia and hypercapnia exist together and they act synergistically. When they act separately in different circumstances, then the effect, including the blood pH, is also different. If the O_2 lack is gradual as in high altitude, it stimulates the breathing. Thus, the alveolar and the arterial CO_2 tension fall and alkalosis is produced which got depressing effect on respiration. But, the excess of alkalis are excreted by the kidney and alkalosis is combated.

It is previously stated that the reflex effect of hypoxia, acting through the carotid and aortic chemoreceptors, is to stimulate the respiratory center. But, the direct effect of it on respiratory center is depression. However, as the reflex effect is dominant, so the respiration is found to increase. The 60% oxygen mixture can be breathed continuously for any length of time without any distress or ill effect. The 75% O_2 mixture can be tolerated for several days, after which some ill effects may appear. Pure oxygen (100%) at 1 atmospheric pressure can be breathed for few hours without any ill effects. But when the oxygen pressure is raised to several atmospheres, the patient develops convulsions and dies rapidly. Human beings develop bad effects in <1 hour (fainting, fall of BP, etc.), if they are exposed to oxygen at 4 atmospheric pressure.

Breath-holding

Respiration can voluntarily be inhibited for some time which is ordinarily called breath-holding. But, eventually this voluntary control of breathing cannot be performed for unlimited period and the automatic onset of breathing is overridden. The point at which the breathing can no longer be voluntarily inhibited is called the *"breaking point"*. However, this breaking is due to the rise in arterial PCO_2 and the fall in arterial PO_2. Individuals can hold their breath longer after the removal of their carotid bodies. Breathing 100% O_2 before breath-holding raises arterial PO_2 initially, so that the breaking point is delayed. The same is true for hyperventilation with room air, because CO_2 is blown off and arterial PCO_2 is lower than normal at the beginning of breath-holding. Reflex stimulations and mechanical factors also appear to influence the length of breaking point. Psychological factors also play an important role and subjects can hold their breath longer, when they are told that their performance is very good than when they are not.

■ METABOLIC FUNCTIONS OF LUNG

Except the gas exchange and chemical control of blood, the lungs have also many metabolic functions. For example, lung is the major site for the inactivation of 5 HT, bradykinin (a potent endothelium-dependent vasodilator and mild diuretic which also causes the contraction of nonvascular smooth muscle in bronchus and gut, increased vascular permeability and involved in mechanism of pain), and noradrenaline. Near about 30% of these compounds are metabolized during their single passage through lungs. But, this is not applicable for adrenaline. This metabolic function of lung is very selective. This is because, >90% of prostaglandin E1 (PGE1), PGE2, prostaglandin F_2 (PGF2) are metabolized during the single passage of these compounds through lungs. Whereas, the prostaglandin A1 (PGA1), PGA2, and prostacyclin are not metabolized by lungs.

There are different converting enzymes in the endothelial cells, present at the wall of pulmonary capillary. They catalyze the angiotensin-I (A-I) to angiotensin-II (A-II) which is a very potent vasoconstrictor. Lungs also secrete certain substances like SRS-A (slow reacting substance of anaphylaxis) and histamine during anaphylaxis. Prostacyclin, a potent vasodilator, and an inhibitor of platelet aggregation are also secreted by lungs. Its generation at the lungs is stimulated by A-II, hyperventilation, and some other peptides. Hyperventilation acts by the stretching of lung tissues.

Pulmonary Physiology Related to Anesthesia

PULMONARY CIRCULATION

Physiological Anatomy

Lungs get its blood supply from two sources: (i) *pulmonary arteries*, arising from pulmonary trunk, which again originate from right ventricle and carry deoxygenated blood and (ii) *bronchial arteries*, arising from aorta, which again originate from left ventricle and carry oxygenated blood. The pulmonary trunk arises from right ventricle and *is only 5 cm in length*. Shortly after arising from right ventricle, it divides into right and left main branches (right and left pulmonary artery) that supply the right and left lungs, respectively. The wall of pulmonary artery is thin, elastic, and distensible. But, the cross-section of it is like that of aorta. Through this pulmonary trunk (artery), the total output of right ventricle which is same as that of left ventricle passes to both the lungs. The right and left main branches of pulmonary trunk, i.e., right and left pulmonary arteries, after arising from pulmonary trunk, next break-up into multiple branches and finally break into arterioles and capillaries, forming a very rich network around the alveoli of lungs.

The branches of pulmonary arteries are short and all the branches of it, even the arterioles and capillaries, have larger diameters than their systemic counterpart. *Thus, the three properties of it (pulmonary arteries) such as (i) wide diameter, (ii) thin wall, and (iii) higher distensibility give the pulmonary arterial system a large compliance (elasticity or distensibility) which is near about 7 mL/mm Hg.* However, the total compliance of this whole pulmonary arterial system is similar to that of entire systemic arterial system, though the former is of much lower volume than the later. Thus, it (higher compliance) allows the pulmonary arterial system to accommodate the total output of right ventricle which is similar to that of left ventricle or systemic circulation, though of low volume. Like the pulmonary arteries, pulmonary veins are also short and the main pulmonary veins are four in number. They drain into left atrium.

The pulmonary arteries carry nutrition and deoxygenated blood to alveoli. Alternatively, bronchial arteries carry oxygenated blood and nutrition to bronchial tree and some supporting tissues of lungs (parenchyma). The bronchial arteries arise from aorta. Then, it breaks up into capillaries around bronchial trees and few around alveoli. The capillaries of bronchial arteries which are formed around the alveoli, ultimately join with the capillaries around the alveoli which are formed from pulmonary artery and subsequently drain into pulmonary vein. On the other hand, the capillaries of bronchial arteries which are formed around the bronchial tree, drain into systemic venous system through bronchial and azygous veins. Bronchial artery carries about 1–2% of cardiac output (CO). So, *the deoxygenated blood of bronchial veins which drain in the oxygenated blood of pulmonary vein also carry 1–2% of CO. Thus, the left ventricular output is 1–2% greater than that of right ventricle and contains 1–2% deoxygenated blood. This is called the intrapulmonary true shunt.* Thus, the nutrition and O_2 supply to pulmonary tissues comes from both deoxygenated blood through pulmonary artery and as well as from oxygenated blood through bronchial artery.

Total Blood Volume in Pulmonary Circulation

Like the output of left ventricle, the output of right ventricle is 5 L/min. Therefore, approximately 5 L of blood circulates per minute through both the lungs together. However, actually the total blood flow per minute through both the lungs is the sum of right ventricular output per minute plus the total blood flow per minute through bronchial arteries from aorta. *But, at any moment, both the lungs, together, contain approximately 450–500 mL of blood and it is called pulmonary blood volume.* It is about 9% of total blood volume of our body. Of this total pulmonary blood volume, *only about 70 mL of blood remains in pulmonary capillary of each lung (140 mL in both lungs) at any moment and undergoes gaseous exchange.* The remainder is divided equally to fill the pulmonary arteries and veins. *At alveolar level, this small 70 mL of pulmonary capillary blood forms a sheet of 50–100 m² area and one red cell thick.* On the other hand, the total amount of blood flow through pulmonary circulation in a minute passes through a sheet of 100–200 m² area.

The total amount (volume) of blood flow through pulmonary circulation varies under different physiological and pathological conditions. These variations in the quantities of pulmonary blood flow, under different physiological and pathological conditions, may change from as little as half of normal value to twice of it, but with little change in pressure as a result of passive dilatation of thin-walled pulmonary vessels and some recruitment of collapsed pulmonary vessels. During inspiration, both the intrapleural and intra-alveolar pressure falls. Therefore, more blood flows through lungs. This is also facilitated by the elongation of capillaries due to stretching and their dilatation due to negative pressure during inspiration. Thus, during inspiration lungs hold 10% more of total pulmonary blood volume. During expiration, the reverse occurs. If high pressure builds up into lungs during expiration such as in coughing, playing trumpet, applying intermittent positive pressure ventilation (IPPV) and positive end-expiratory pressure (PEEP) with high pressure, etc., then as much as 250 mL of blood can be expelled out from pulmonary circulation into systemic circulation. On the other hand, during hemorrhage the loss of blood from systemic circulation can be compensated by the shift of blood from lungs (pulmonary circulation) into systemic circulation. A shift in posture from erect to supine also increases pulmonary blood volume up to 30%. Similarly, change in posture from supine to erect has the opposite effect. The changes in systemic capacitance (venous blood volume) also influence the pulmonary blood volume. For example, systemic vasoconstriction shifts the blood from systemic to pulmonary circulation whereas, systemic vasodilation causes pulmonary to systemic redistribution. Thus, lungs act as a reservoir for systemic circulation and vice versa.

If there is any pathology on the left side of heart causing obstruction to blood flow, then it also causes the collection of huge amount of blood in pulmonary circulation. Sometimes, it may increases up to 100%, causing large increase in pulmonary vascular pressure. But, as the volume of systemic circulatory bed is nine times greater than that of pulmonary circulation, so a small amount of shift of blood from systemic circulation to pulmonary circulation has greater effect on it with mild or no effect on previous one (systemic circulation).

In influencing pulmonary vascular tone, local factors are more important than the influence of autonomic supply. *Hypoxia is the most powerful stimulus for pulmonary vasoconstriction.* This is opposite to the systemic effect of hypoxia, where it dilates the vessels. Both the pulmonary arterial (mixed venous) and alveolar hypoxia induce pulmonary vasoconstriction. But, the alveolar hypoxia is more powerful stimulus. On the other hand, hyperoxia has little effect on pulmonary vasculature. Hypoxia-induced pulmonary vasoconstriction is either due to direct effect on pulmonary vessels or increased production of vasoconstrictor leukotrienes (LTs) relative to vasodilator prostaglandins (PGs). Inhibition of NO production also may play a role in hypoxic pulmonary vasoconstriction. Hypoxic pulmonary vasoconstriction has an important physiological (compensatory) role in reducing intrapulmonary shunting and preventing hypoxemia. Hypercapnia and acidosis have pulmonary vasoconstrictor effect. Whereas, hypocapnia has pulmonary vasodilatation effect, the opposite of what occurs in systemic circulation.

Pressure in Pulmonary Circulatory System

The right side of heart and pulmonary circulatory system is a low pressure system than the left side of heart and systemic circulatory system. The different level of pressure at the different parts of the path from superior vena cava to aorta is shown in the **Table 1**. In human being, the systolic pressure of right ventricle averages to about 25 mm Hg. So, subsequently the systolic pressure in pulmonary artery is also about 25 mm Hg. But, the diastolic pressure in right ventricle suddenly comes down to 0 or 1 mm Hg whereas the diastolic pressure in pulmonary artery does not fall precipitously to this value. Because, due to closure of pulmonary valve, blood from pulmonary artery does not go back to right ventricle and pulmonary artery does not become empty immediately. So, the diastolic pressure in pulmonary artery falls slowly to around 8–10 mm Hg, as blood flows away from pulmonary artery to its smaller branches and the capillaries of lungs. Thus, the mean pulmonary arterial pressure results in 15 mm Hg, whereas the mean pressure in right ventricle remains at 25 mm Hg **(Fig. 1)**.

The mean hydrostatic pressure in pulmonary capillary is about 8 mm Hg whereas, the mean hydrostatic pressure in major pulmonary veins and left atrium varies between as low as 1 mm Hg to as high as 5 mm Hg according to the position of body. So, the average pressure in pulmonary veins and left atrium (LA) is about 2 mm Hg in recumbence position.

Clinically, it is not feasible to measure the pulmonary venous and LA pressure directly in human being. This is because it is not possible to pass a catheter directly through the right side of heart into pulmonary veins and LA (i.e., the left side of heart) through pulmonary capillary. So, we try to measure the pressure of the left side of heart indirectly with moderate accuracy by wedging a balloon, situated at the tip

TABLE 1: The systolic and diastolic pressure of different areas from superior vena cava to aorta.

Place	Pressure (mm Hg)	
	Systolic	Diastolic
Superior vena cava	0.5	0.0
Right atrium	5.0	0–1
Right ventricle	20–25	0–1
Pulmonary trunk	15–25	8–15
Pulmonary artery	15	
Pulmonary capillary (wedge)	8	
Pulmonary vein	5	1
Left atrium	10	5
Left ventricle	90–140	60–90
Aorta	120	80

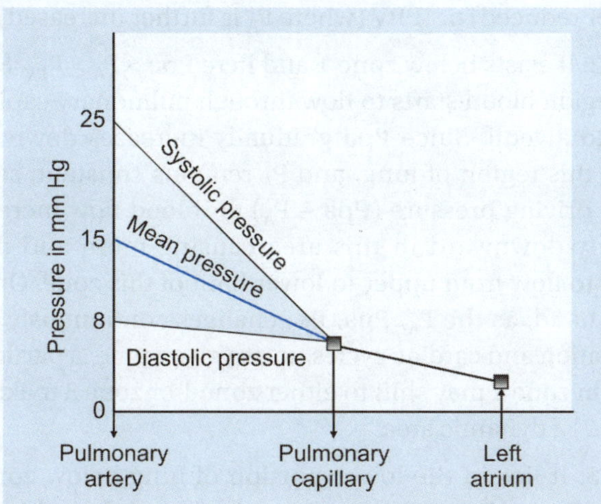

Fig. 1: The pressure of pulmonary artery, pulmonary capillary, and left atrium.

of a catheter which is introduced into pulmonary capillary (but actually this is not pulmonary capillary, it is the smallest branch of pulmonary artery), as far as possible, by passing it through large systemic veins [like internal jugular vein (IJV), subclavian vein, etc.], right atrium (RA), right ventricle, and PA. After wedging of balloon in the smallest branch of pulmonary artery, blood flow is stopped in this vessel and then the tip of the catheter, with an aperture at its tip, directly communicates with the venous side of pulmonary circulatory system and LA beyond the balloon's tip. Thus, the tip of the catheter senses the pressure in this smallest branch of pulmonary artery which is proportional to pulmonary venous system and LA. This is called the *pulmonary capillary wedge pressure (PCWP)*, which is clinically taken as pulmonary venous and LA pressure and is about 5 mm Hg. This PCWP is usually 2–3 mm Hg greater than that of actual LA pressure.

Distribution of Pulmonary Blood Flow

The distribution of pulmonary blood flow (perfusion) into lungs is not uniform. It is different at different areas. This is because lung tries to accomplish adequate (maximum) oxygenation of blood which is the most important function of it. So, to achieve this (maximum oxygenation of blood), blood has to be distributed (perfused) more to those areas of lungs where the alveoli are better ventilated and vice versa. Thus, the distribution of pulmonary circulation to the different areas of lungs is governed (controlled) by the following mechanisms or principles. These principles are described here.

Effect of Alveolar O_2 Tension on Local Pulmonary Blood Flow

This is a very unique feature of lungs. *When the O_2 concentration into alveoli decreases below 70% (or the O_2 tension in alveolar air goes <70 mm Hg), then the local blood vessels in pulmonary tissue constrict and pulmonary vascular resistance (PVR) increases locally.* This causes the shifting of blood to other parts of lungs, where it is well ventilated and try to compensate the hypoxia. This increase in PVR at less ventilated area of lungs may be six-fold in extreme hypoxia. This is opposite to the effect, found in systemic circulation where hypoxia causes vasodilatation, decrease in vascular resistance, and increase in circulation. But, the mechanism of pulmonary vasoconstriction in response to hypoxia is not clearly known. The probable theory is that the local pulmonary vasoconstriction is accomplished by some chemical substances secreted by hypoxic epithelial cells.

Effect of Hydrostatic Pressure Gradient on Pulmonary Blood Flow

Another important factor which causes different amount of blood flow (different perfusion) through different areas of lungs is the hydrostatic pressure gradient. *The principle is that the area of lung enjoying more hydrostatic pressure will receive more blood supply (better perfusion) and vice versa.* The hydrostatic pressure is nothing but the weight of blood column in a blood vessel. The difference in height between the highest (top) and the lowest point (bottom) of lung is 30 cm in upright position. This different in height between two different parts of a lung causes a difference in hydrostatic pressure in pulmonary artery at apex and at base of a lung and it is about 23 mm Hg, however taking into account that the pressure in pulmonary artery at the level of heart is zero. This can be explained in another way that in a standing person, the pulmonary arterial pressure at the top of the lung is about 15 mm Hg less (–15 mm Hg) than the pulmonary arterial pressure at the level of the heart and the pulmonary arterial pressure at the base of the lung is about 8 mm Hg higher (+8 mm Hg) than that at the level of the heart. Thus, the difference of hydrostatic pressure in pulmonary artery between the apex and the base of the lung is 8 – (–15) or 23 mm Hg. *This also can be calculated in another way that the pulmonary arterial pressure increases or decreases by about 1 cmH₂O (along with pulmonary arterial blood flow or pulmonary perfusion) per centimeter of change in vertical distance of a lung.* This change of hydrostatic pressure in pulmonary artery is due to the influence of gravity on the distribution of pulmonary circulation and is important because this (pulmonary circulation) is a low pressure system.

Effect of Cardiac Output and Exercise on Distribution of Pulmonary Blood Flow

Actually, CO and exercise exert their effect on total amount of pulmonary blood flow, but not on the local distribution of it in lungs. This is because, heavy exercise and increased CO increase pulmonary blood flow near about 5–7 times, but with very little increase in pulmonary arterial hydrostatic pressure. This increased blood flow in lungs caused by exercise and increased CO is accomplished by increasing the number of opened capillaries and distending it. These two changes in pulmonary vasculature decrease PVR. So, there is little or no increase in pulmonary arterial hydrostatic pressure and no change in local distribution of blood flow in lung despite total increase in blood flow in lungs **(Fig. 2)**.

Effect of Alveolar Pressure and Pulmonary Venous Pressure on Local Distribution of Pulmonary Blood Flow

The increased alveolar pressure and pulmonary venous pressure decreases pulmonary blood flow. On the other hand, the local distribution of pulmonary blood flow in different parts of lungs not only depends on pulmonary alveolar pressure and pulmonary venous pressure, but also on the interaction between pulmonary capillary (hydrostatic) pressure (Ppa), alveolar pressure (P_A), and pulmonary venous (hydrostatic) pressure (P_{PV}). Thus, lungs can be divided into four zones according to P_A, Ppa, P_{PV}, and P_{ISF}:

Zone 1: In this region, $P_A > Ppa > P_{PV}$ and this region is situated at the apex of the lungs. Thus, at this area, as the alveolar pressure (P_A), outside the vessels, is greater than the pulmonary capillary pressure (Ppa), so no blood flow will occur through the wall of these alveoli and no gaseous exchange will take place. Hence, this region (zone 1) acts as an alveolar dead space. Normally, in physiological condition, no or little area of zone 1 exists. But, it greatly exists or increases in oligemic (hypovolemic) shock (where Ppa is further reduced) or IPPV (where P_A is further increased).

Zone 2: It exists below zone 1 and here $Ppa > P_A > P_{PV}$. So, in this region blood starts to flow through pulmonary capillary around alveoli. Since Ppa gradually increases downward along this region of lung, and P_A remains constant, so the mean driving pressure (Ppa – P_A) for blood flow increases linearly downward in this area causing more and more blood to flow from upper to lower limit of this zone. On the other hand, as the P_A, Ppa, P_{PV} changes continuously with respiration and cardiac cycles, so at a given time, a particular point in zone 2 may shift to either zone 1 or zone 3 making it (zone 2) a dynamic area.

Zone 3: It lies in the lower portion of lung below zone 2, where $Ppa > P_{PV} > P_A$. So, here the blood flow depends on pulmonary arteriovenous pressure difference (Ppa – P_{PV}), but not on Ppa – P_A difference. As in this region, the pulmonary vascular pressure (Ppa – P_{PV}) always exceeds alveolar pressure (P_A), so the vessels remain permanently open and blood flows continuously, not depending on alveolar pressure (P_A), during inspiration and expiration. If we go further downward along this zone 3, then we will see that gravity will cause the increase in both Ppa and P_{PV} but at the same rate, so that the driving pressure (Ppa – P_{PV}) remains unchanged. On the other hand, the pressure outside the vessels, i.e., pleural pressure (P_{Pl}) increases from above downward, but at a rate lesser than that of Ppa and P_{PV}. So, the transpulmonary distending pressure (i.e., Ppa – P_{Pl} and $P_{PV} – P_{Pl}$) increases gradually downward along this zone 3. Hence, the radii of vessels increase, vascular resistance decreases, and blood flow further increases from upper to lower limit of this zone.

Zone 4: Normally, a small amount of fluid flows into pulmonary interstitial space (IS) from pulmonary

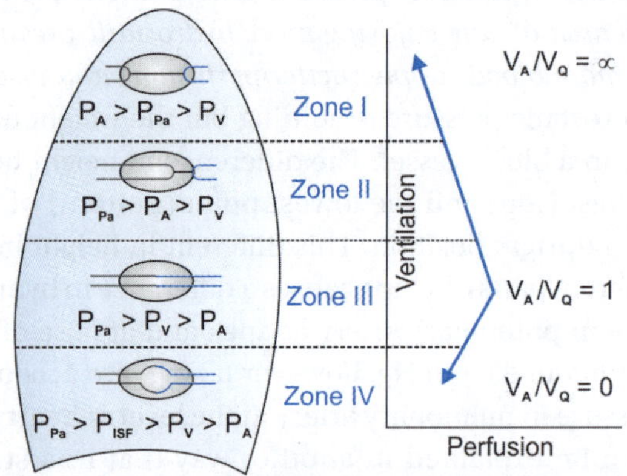

Fig. 2: The difference of distribution between ventilation and perfusion and V_A/V_Q ratio at different parts of the lung.

intravascular space and is cleared immediately and adequately by lymphatics. But, when the pulmonary vascular pressure is very high such as in volume overload, pulmonary hypertension, pulmonary embolism, mitral stenosis etc., then excessive amount of fluid transudates into interstitial compartment which cannot be cleared by lymphatic. Thus, the expansion of pulmonary IS by fluid causes increased pulmonary interstitial pressure (PISF) and exceeds P_{PV}. Hence, at the base of the lung a zone is created where Ppa > P_{ISF} > P_{PV} > P_A. This is called the zone 4. In this zone, the flow of blood through pulmonary capillaries is governed by the Ppa – P_{ISF} value, which is less than the Ppa – P_{PV} value. Therefore, in zone 4 blood flow is less than zone 3. Again as PISF increase in zone 4, it causes vascular compression and increased vascular resistance which further decreases blood flow in this region.

Throughout the whole lung, from above downward, when Ppa and P_{PV} increases gradually, but without any increase in P_A then three things happen:

1. If both Ppa and P_{PV} increase from low to moderate range, then recruitment of more alveoli is the principle. So, zone 1 will become zone 2 and zone 2 will become zone 3 and so on.
2. If Ppa and P_{PV} increase from moderate to high range, then the distention of vessels is the principle. So, the vessels of zone 3 will dilate and blood flow will increase. Thus, the area of zone 3 will increase.
3. If Ppa and P_{PV} increase from high to very high ranges, then the zone 3 vessels will become so dilated that they leak fluid and transudation occurs. Thus, zone 3 vessels converted to zone 4 vessels.

Dynamics of Pulmonary Capillary Circulation

After entering into lung parenchyma and making multiple division and subdivision, the pulmonary arteries form pulmonary capillaries which line the alveolar walls. So, finally the alveolar walls are surrounded by so many capillaries that they lie side by side touching with one another, as if the alveolar wall is bathed by a sheet of blood flow. Therefore, the alveolar gas is separated from this pulmonary capillary blood by a number of anatomical layers. From capillary side, these layers are: (i) endothelial layer of pulmonary capillary, (ii) basement membrane of this endothelial layer on which the capillary endothelial cells rest, (iii) IS, (iv) basement membrane on which the alveolar epithelial cells rest, and (v) the layer of alveolar epithelial cells (type I pneumocytes) on this basement membrane. The IS lying between the basement membrane of endothelial (capillary) and epithelial (alveolus) cells contains some connective tissues which make lung parenchyma. These connective tissues are made of elastic

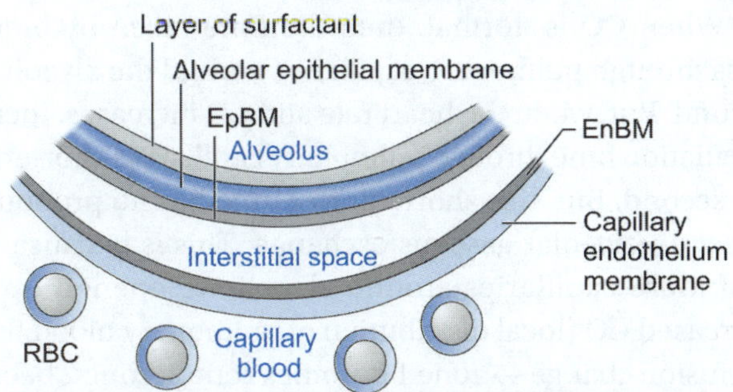

Fig. 3: This is a schematic diagram of structures intervening between the alveolar air and capillary blood. (EnBM: Endothelial basement membrane; EpBM: epithelial basement membrane; RBC: red blood cell)

fibers, tissue fibrils, fibroblasts, and macrophages, and are continuous with the connective tissues around the airways and blood vessels of lungs. Thus, the IS which surrounds the alveoli (perialveolar space) is continuous with the IS which surrounds the airways and its associated vessels. Because, both the spaces contain the same connective tissues of lung. Lymphatics start in this IS at the level of terminal bronchiole and flow upward toward the larger bronchi and trachea. But, it is absent downward (distally) beyond it (terminal bronchioles) toward alveoli **(Fig. 3)**.

The endothelial and epithelial cells are not tightly attached with one another. There are multiple holes at their junctions which provide potential path for the fluid to move from capillaries into IS and finally from IS into alveoli and vice versa. The holes between the endothelial cells of pulmonary capillary are relatively larger than that of epithelial cells of alveoli and are therefore termed as "loose". On the other hand, the holes between the epithelial cells of alveoli are smaller and therefore are termed as "tight". The pulmonary capillary permeability (K) is thus the expression of the sizes of these holes and its subsequent function.

During the development of lungs, the airways and blood vessels, as a bud of tissues, first grow into the pleural cavity at the level of hilum with a connective tissues sheath (lung parenchyma) around them. The growth of this connective tissue sheath then ends at the level of the terminal bronchiole and there it become continuous with the connective tissues of IS between the alveolar epithelium and capillary endothelium. Thus, the potential space around the airways and its vessels, containing connective tissues, is continuous with the IS between the alveolar epithelium and capillary endothelium containing same connective tissues. The pressure in this IS is negative and progressively increases from distal to proximal, i.e., from alveoli to bronchiole to bronchi. This negative interstitial pressure in connective tissues surrounding the vessels, bronchi, bronchioles, and alveoli exerts a radial outward force of traction which tends to hold them open and increases their diameter.

When CO is normal, then the time taken by blood to pass through pulmonary capillaries around the alveoli is 0.8 second. But, when the heart rate and CO increases, then this circulation time through pulmonary capillary is shortened to 0.3 second. But, this shortening of time has no pronounced effect on alveolar gaseous exchange. This is because more and more capillaries around alveoli are opened up with increased CO (local distribution of pulmonary blood flow or perfusion change → zone 1 becomes zone 2, zone 2 becomes zone 3, etc.) and within the fraction of a second blood can takes up O_2 and gets out its CO_2.

The dynamics of pulmonary capillary circulation and the exchange of gas and fluid between the pulmonary capillaries and alveoli are qualitatively same, as that of the systemic capillary circulation. But, they differ only quantitatively.

The difference between the dynamics of pulmonary and systemic capillary circulation is:

- The mean pulmonary capillary hydrostatic pressure (PCHP) is 7 mm Hg (the mean left atrial pressure is 2 mm Hg and the mean pulmonary arterial pressure is 15 mm Hg), whereas the mean systemic capillary hydrostatic pressure is 17 mm Hg.
- The interstitial fluid pressure (or hydrostatic pressure in IS) in lungs is negative and is about –8 mm Hg, whereas the interstitial fluid pressure in peripheral tissues is not so negative, rather positive.
- The colloidal oncotic pressure of pulmonary capillary due to the presence of plasma protein is about 28 mm Hg and this is equal to that of systemic capillary. The pulmonary capillaries are loose. So, protein molecules continuously come out into IS around the alveoli from capillary. Therefore, a colloidal oncotic pressure is formed in this space which is about 14 mm Hg. This is approximately one-half of the colloidal oncotic pressure of IS in peripheral tissues.

Thus, the net forces governing transcapillary fluid movement in IS of lung tissue can be calculated as follows. This net force (F) is equal to the difference between the PCHP (P_{in}) and interstitial hydrostatic pressure (P_{out}) and between the capillary colloidal oncotic pressure (O_{in}) and interstitial colloidal oncotic pressure (O_{out}). The P_{in} pushed the fluid out of capillary into IS, but P_{out} opposes this force. On the other hand, O_{out} draws the fluid in capillary from IS, but O_{out} opposes this force.

So, $F = K\{(P_{in} - P_{out}) - \sigma(O_{in} - O_{out})\}$; here K is the filtration coefficient and is related to total capillary surface area, and σ is the permeability coefficient of capillary endothelium. When, the value of σ is one, then it indicates endothelium is completely impermeable to albumin and zero value of σ indicates free passage of albumin and other particles.

Normally, the pulmonary endothelium is partially permeable to albumin. So, the interstitial albumin concentration is one-half of that of plasma. Therefore, O_{out} must be about 14 mm Hg (one half of that of plasma). Therefore, $F = \{7 - (-8)\} - (28-14) = 15 - 14 = +1$.

This net force (F) which governed the movement of fluid from pulmonary capillary to IS and subsequently into alveoli can also be calculated from another angle.

i. The forces which tries to move or push the fluid from pulmonary capillary into IS are:
   Capillary hydrostatic pressure = 7 mm Hg
   IS oncotic pressure = 14 mm Hg
   Negative IS hydrostatic pressure = –8 mm Hg
   So, the total outward force which pushes the fluid from pulmonary capillary into IS = 7 + 14 + 8 = 29 mm Hg

ii. The forces which try to draw the fluid from IS into pulmonary capillary [i.e., the opposite force to (i)] is only: Plasma colloidal oncotic pressure = 28 mm Hg

Thus, the total outward filtration pressure from capillary to IS is: Total outward driving force (29 mm Hg) – Total inward driving force (28 mm Hg) = 1 mm Hg. Therefore, the net outward driving force (F) = +1 mm Hg.

So, this slight positive outward filtration pressure continuously causes the movement of small amount of fluid from the pulmonary capillaries into the IS and subsequently from IS to alveoli. Then, part of this fluid evaporates through the alveoli and the remaining part is pumped back into the circulation through the pulmonary lymphatic system. This also explains why the alveolar surface remains always dry and there is constant lymphatic flow which is about approximately 500 mL/day (10–20 mL/hour). Again, when the extra fluid appears in the alveoli from exogenous source then it will simply be sucked into the IS of lung, mechanically through the openings between the alveolar epithelial cells. This excess fluid is then further carried out through pulmonary lymphatic into circulation. Thus, under normal situations, the alveoli are kept constantly dry except that a small amount of fluid which sips from epithelial cells on their alveolar surface to keep them moist.

Pulmonary Edema

The pulmonary edema is regarded as an exaggeration of this pulmonary capillary dynamics. It occurs when the amount of transudation of fluid in IS is more than its reabsorption capacity, through lymphatics and gradually accumulates in IS, i.e., when the safety and reserve factors, which are described later, fail. The alveolar epithelial membrane is usually impermeable to albumin, but permeable to water and gases. Thus, when fluid accumulates in IS, then it also moves from IS to inside of alveoli and produces the full picture of pulmonary edema. So, the mechanism of formation of pulmonary edema is same as that of formation of systemic edema, elsewhere in our body. The most common factors which play important roles in the formation of pulmonary edema are the following.

Factors Playing Important Roles in Pulmonary Edema

Increased pulmonary capillary hydrostatic pressure: It may be due to any cause such as pulmonary hypertension, left ventricular failure (LVF), fluid overload, disease of mitral valve, etc. All these factors will cause the rapid increase in pulmonary venous hydrostatic pressure and subsequently the PCHP producing flooding of IS and alveoli with fluid. *When the pulmonary artery pressure rises above 30 mm Hg, then it is called the pulmonary hypertension.* Increase in PCHP again can be due to four mechanisms.

Increase in pulmonary blood flow: It occurs when a left (L) to right (R) shunt is present, e.g., ventricular septal defect (VSD), atrial septal defect (ASD), etc., In these conditions, blood flow through lungs or right ventricular output increases three times or more than that of left ventricular output. If these states persist for few years, then PVR begins to rise due to some structural changes in pulmonary vessels. Thus, the pulmonary artery pressure rises further. Eventually, if the pressure on the right side of the heart exceed than that on the left side, then this left-to-right shunt is reversed and subsequently a right-to-left shunt with central cyanosis appears.

Increase in left atrial pressure: It is due to aortic or mitral valve disease or LVF which increases left atrial pressure with dilatation and/or hypertrophy. Thus, subsequently the back pressure from left atrium into pulmonary vasculature causes pulmonary arterial hypertension.

Rise in pulmonary vascular resistance: It occurs in massive pulmonary embolism and in some lung diseases [such as in chronic bronchitis, chronic obstructive pulmonary disease (COPD), emphysema, etc.]. In chronic lung diseases, pulmonary hypertension is due to the combination of chronic hypoxia and obliteration of some pulmonary vascular bed by disease process itself.

Overtransfusion: Excessive IV transfusion of any fluid may lead to increased PCHP and pulmonary edema.

Increased pulmonary capillary permeability: It is due to some chemical injury of pulmonary capillary membrane caused by bacterial endotoxin (septicemia), breathing toxic gases, acute respiratory distress syndrome (ARDS), acute lung injury (ALI), etc. In each of these cases, there is rapid leakage of both plasma protein and fluid out of capillaries into both IS and alveoli. This further increases O_{out} and subsequently the effective or net filtration pressure (F). Thus, a vicious cycle sets up to produce pulmonary edema.

Diminished pulmonary capillary colloidal oncotic pressure: It is very unlikely that it can be the cause of pulmonary edema in clinical situations, but it can intensify the already set process initiated by other causes.

Pulmonary lymphatic obstruction: It is unlikely to be the primary cause of pulmonary edema, but might be an important secondary factor.

Extremely negative pleural pressure: Normally, the negative intrapleural pressure is subsequently transmitted to peribronchial, perivascular, and IS space. So, this negative (or subatmospheric) IS hydrostatic pressure (P_{out}) promotes the slow loss of fluid into this space across the capillary endothelial holes by suction. But if due to any cause, sudden extremely negative intrapleural and subsequently sudden excessive negative IS hydrostatic pressure is developed, then there is excessive accumulation fluid in IS across the endothelium (exceeding absorption by lymph) and will cause pulmonary edema. The causes of excessive negative intrapleural pressure producing pulmonary edema are vigorous spontaneous respiration against an obstructed airway. This may be due to upper airway mass, severe laryngospasm, severe inflammation and edema of upper airway, vocal cord paralysis, strangulation, vigorous pleural suction (e.g., thoracocentesis), etc.

Neurogenic pulmonary edema: It occurs in patients with head injury or other intracranial pathology. It is thought to be due to intense centrally mediated pulmonary vasoconstriction by sympathetic stimulation caused by central nervous system (CNS) injury. Hypoxia has no role as an etiological factor in this type of pulmonary edema and administration of O_2 does not help to restore the nonpermeability of this type of injured and leaky capillary membrane.

Thus, the causes of pulmonary edema are divided under two broad headings: *(i) hemodynamic or cardiogenic pulmonary edema and (ii) noncardiogenic pulmonary edema.* In the former, there is increase in PCHP due to cardiac problems causing increase in net filtration pressure across the capillary membrane. But, in later, there is increase in permeability of capillary membrane without any increase in pulmonary hydrostatic pressure due to noncardiogenic causes. The difference between these two etiologies (cardiogenic and noncardiogenic pulmonary edema) can often be diagnosed by measuring pulmonary artery occlusion pressure (PAOP which is also called pulmonary capillary wedge pressure or PCWP) and the protein content of edema fluid. If the PAOP is >18 mm Hg, then it indicates that increased hydrostatic pressure is the cause of pulmonary edema and vice versa. And, if the protein content in the fluid of pulmonary edema is high, then increased permeability without any increase in hydrostatic pressure of pulmonary capillary is the cause of pulmonary edema.

The normal value of left atrial pressure is 1–5 mm Hg. In healthy individual, it never rises above +6 mm Hg even during heavy exercise. This small change in left atrial pressure even during strenuous exercise has virtually no effect on the hemodynamics of pulmonary circulation. This is because, it merely expands the existing capillaries and does not open up more capillaries, so that the blood flows easily and causes better oxygenation without increasing the capillary hydrostatic pressure. But, when the left heart fails, then blood begins to accumulate in left atrium. As a result, the left atrial pressure may rise from its normal value to 30–40 mm Hg. The initial rise of pressure up to 7 mm Hg in left atrium has very little effect on pulmonary circulation. But, when this pressure rises above 7 or 8 mm Hg, then there is equal and parallel increase in pulmonary arterial pressure. When the left atrial pressure rises above 30 mm Hg, then pulmonary edema is likely to develop.

Pulmonary Reserve and Safety Factors

There are some pulmonary reserve and safety factors which prevent the formation of pulmonary edema, when there is mild-to-moderate changes, but not severe, in pulmonary capillary hydrostatic pressure (PCHP) occurs. It is found experimentally that PCHP must rises to a higher value, which is at least equal to the colloidal oncotic pressure of plasma before significant pulmonary edema occurs. In human being, the normal plasma colloid oncotic pressure is 28 mm Hg. Therefore, one can expect that PCHP must increases from its normal level of 7–8 mm Hg to >28 mm Hg to cause pulmonary edema. This is called the reserve factor for the development of pulmonary edema. Thus, the reserve factor against the development of pulmonary edema is 28 – 7 = 21 mm Hg increase in PCHP.

On the other hand, if PCHP gradually elevated over a prolonged period, at least >2 weeks, then the lungs become more resistant to pulmonary edema due to starting of compensatory mechanism. This is because the lymph vessels increase their capability of carrying more fluid away from IS as much as 10-fold. Therefore, in chronic MS, PCHP is frequently measured to 40–50 mm Hg without any development of pulmonary edema. This is the maximum safety factor of pulmonary edema.

If PCHP rises rapidly, even slightly above its safety level, then pulmonary edema ensures within an hour. The development of pulmonary edema depends on the speed of the increase of PCHP above its safety level (**Box 1**).

Stages of Pulmonary Edema

Pulmonary edema is considered as an exaggeration of the dynamics of pulmonary capillary fluid exchange, which continuously operates under normal physiological condition within its reserve. So, pulmonary edema develops in stages when this reserve is gradually burnt out. These stages are:

Stage I: In this first phase, the excessive accumulation of fluid in IS is not totally countered or compensated by increased flow of lymphatic which may go up to 10 times. Thus, fluid gradually accumulate in IS and lungs become stiff (↓compliance). So, at this initial phase, patient only becomes tachypneic due to gradual decrease of pulmonary compliance. Hence, this initial phase is only called the interstitial pulmonary edema and is only diagnosed by chest X-ray which shows the increased interstitial markings and peribronchial cuffing.

Stage II: In this phase, the fluid begins to reach and fill the alveoli in addition to IS, but being *only confined to the angles between the adjacent septa.*

Stage III: In this phase, the flooding of alveoli with capillary fluid occurs and many alveoli are completely filled with fluid containing no air. Initially, this is most prominent only at the *dependent portion of lungs*, but later it spreads *throughout the whole lungs*. So, this phase is called the alveolar flooding phase. Blood flows through this wall of fluid-filled alveoli without any gas exchange and causes large increase in intrapulmonary shunt (however, these are not true shunt). So, hypocapnia (due to hyperventilation of the nonaffected parts of lung) and hypoxia (due to intrapulmonary shunting of blood without any gaseous exchange) are the characteristic of this stage.

Stage IV: Finally, the flooding of alveoli with edema fluid is of *sufficient magnitude*. Now, it spreads all over the lungs and also spills over into the airway as froth. This is frequently pink in color, because of the rupture of capillaries and increased diapedesis of erythrocytes into alveoli. In this final stage of pulmonary edema, gaseous exchange is severely compromised. So, progressive hypercapnia and severe hypoxemia will follow due to both airway obstruction and massive intrapulmonary shunting.

■ ALVEOLAR VENTILATION (V_A)

Alveolar ventilation is defined as the part of total ventilation which takes part in gaseous exchange, i.e., oxygenation of blood and excretion of CO_2 through lungs. It is a part of minute volume ventilation (MVV) and is so calculated as L/min. We know that the minute ventilation (volume) is the total inspired volume of gas (ventilation) in 1 minute. So, the MVV = Tidal volume (V_T) × Respiratory rate (f). How the variation in respiratory rate and tidal volume affect the MVV is shown in **Table 2**.

All the inspired gases (minute volume) do not reach alveoli and do not take part in the process of gaseous exchange (ventilation). So, some air remains in airway and later exhaled with expired alveolar gas. Hence, the part of minute ventilation which remains in airway without taking part in gaseous exchange is known as the dead space (V_D) ventilation. Therefore, the alveolar ventilation (V_A) is defined as a part of volume of inspired gases in one minute (minute ventilation) which only takes part in gaseous exchange. *Thus, Alveolar ventilation (V_A) = {Tidal volume (V_T) – Dead space (V_D)} × Respiratory rate (f) or $V_A = (V_T - V_D) × f$. The dead space (V_D) in lungs is actually the sum of space (or amount of gases) of conducting zone of airways (anatomical dead space) and the volume of alveoli that are not perfused, but only ventilated (alveolar dead space). So, this V_D is called physiological dead space.*

The normal value of alveolar ventilation is 3.5–4.5 L/minute or 2–2.4 L/minute/m^2 of body surface area in adult. From the above equation, we can easily say that *alveolar ventilation depends on three factors such as (1) tidal volume, (2) dead space, and (3) respiratory rate.* When the tidal volume decreases or dead space increases or respiratory rate decreases, then alveolar ventilation drastically falls.

But, fortunately in healthy adult, the dead space decreases with decrease of tidal volume, so that the effect on alveolar ventilation is lessened. *Hyperventilation (increase in alveolar ventilation) is not a very effective way of increasing alveolar PO_2 (or preventing hypoxia) as effective for washing out of CO_2 (or preventing hypercarbia). But, hypoventilation is potentially a disastrous cause of hypoxia than hypercarbia.* On the other hand, a small rise in alveolar CO_2 concentration due to hypoventilation will further produce a fall in alveolar O_2 tension, unless extra O_2 is added to inspired air. So, in a patient under anesthesia with spontaneous respiration, any reduction of V_A due to any changes in respiratory rate, tidal volume, dead space, and anesthesia induced any changes such as V_D/V_T ratio, compliance, functional residual capacity/closing capacity (FRC/CC) relationship, work of breathing, etc., will cause severe arterial hypoxemia **(Fig. 4)**. Thus, it is always advisable to administer a minimum 33% of O_2 with all the anesthetic gas mixtures to prevent hypoxia during anesthesia. We know that alveolar ventilation (V_A) is not distributed evenly throughout whole lungs. The right lung is better ventilated than that of left and the *lower dependent area of lung gets more ventilation than its upper apical area.* This is due to the gravity-induced gradient of transpulmonary distending pressure which decreases from above downward and allows the more potentiality (if necessary) of distention of alveoli at the lower dependent area of lung, which is *now* less distended and smaller in size.

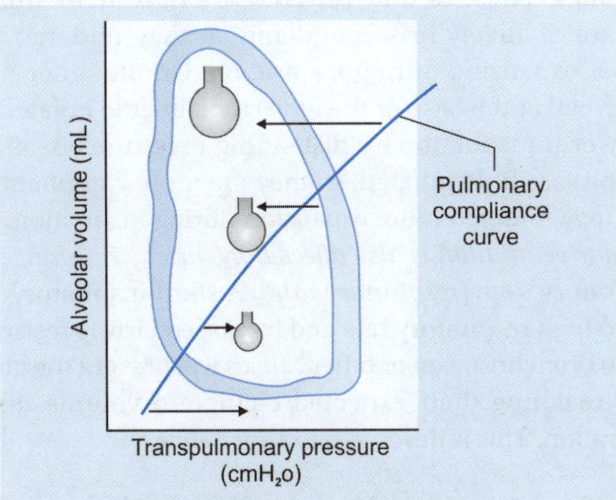

Fig. 4: As the intrapleural pressure relatively increases from top to the bottom of the lung, so the alveolar volume decreases from apex to the base of the lung. The caliber of air passages also decreases from apex to the base of the lung. The blue line represents the transpulmonary pressure and alveolar volume curve. The less compliant and already distended large alveoli at the apex of the lung are situated at the flat upper portion of the curve. Whereas the most compliant, small alveoli (now not distended, but can be distended) at the base of the lung are situated at the steep lower portion of the curve and receive the largest share of tidal volume.

TABLE 2: Effect of variations of respiratory rate (f) and depth (tidal volume) on alveolar ventilation.

	A	B
Tidal volume (mL)	400	200
Dead space (mL)	150	150
Respiratory rate (per minute)	20	40
Minute volume (in liter)	8	8
Alveolar ventilation (in liter)	(400–150) × 20 = 5	(200–150) × 40 = 2

Distribution of Alveolar Ventilation (V$_A$)

Truly, the lung is a viscoelastic structure. Within its visceral pleural sac, lung is situated just like a gel within a plastic bag. When lung is not within its chest wall, then gravity causes this plastic bag (visceral pleura) filled with gel (lung) to bulge outward at the bottom and inward at the top. But, within the chest wall, the present shape of the lung is maintained by relatively more negative intrapleural (transpulmonary) pressure at the top than the bottom of pleural cavity. *So, the intrapleural pressure (PPl) at the bottom of chest cavity is relatively more positive (i.e., less negative) than the top of it. This intrapleural pressure increases (becomes less negative) from top to the bottom of chest cavity at the rate of 0.25 cmH$_2$O/cm of height (or 1 cmH$_2$O per 3 cm of height). The height of an upright lung is 30 cm. Thus, the intrapleural pressure (P$_{Pl}$) increases by 30 cm × 0.25 cmH$_2$O/cm = 7.5 cmH$_2$O from apex to the bottom of the lung. But, the intra-alveolar pressure (P$_A$) remains same throughout the whole lung from top to the bottom of it. Thus, the transpulmonary distending pressure (P$_A$ – P$_{Pl}$) is greater at apex than the bottom of lung.*

This difference in transpulmonary pressure, which helps to distend the alveoli, has placed the different sized alveoli of different areas of lungs at different points on the *pulmonary compliance curve*. So, the alveoli in the upper part of lung (at apex) remain in maximally inflated state and become relatively noncompliant and this is due to the higher transpulmonary distending pressure at the apex of the lungs. Thus, as they (alveoli) are maximally inflated and are relatively less compliant, so they undergo little further expansion during inspiration. On the other hand, the alveoli at the base of the lungs remain little inflated due to lower transpulmonary distending pressure. So, as they (alveoli) are little inflated, so they are more compliant and later may undergo more expansion during inspiration. *This alveolar ventilation is also affected by airway resistance and inspiratory time (respiratory rate).* A short inspiratory time due to high respiratory rate and increased airway resistance due to bronchospasm or other causes will prevent the alveoli from reaching their expected change in volume during inspiration. This is described further below.

Time Constant and Alveolar Ventilation

The inflation of alveoli or alveolar ventilation depends on a time constant (T). It is defined as time (in second) which the alveoli would take to reach its final volume, provided adequate gas flow rate is maintained throughout its inflation. *This time constant again depends on (i) the resistance in airways to the flow of air and (ii) the compliance of lung.* This is calculated as Time constant = Airway resistance × Compliance.

In normal lung, the compliance is 0.1 L/cmH$_2$O and resistance is 2 cmH$_2$O/L/s. So, the time constant is 0.2 second. Increase in airway resistance and decrease in compliance of lungs give rise to longer time constant. It means, the alveoli will take a long time for a given volume of inflation. In such condition, short inspiratory time during tachypnea will result in poor ventilation of those zones of lung, where the alveoli have long time constant due to increase in resistance and decrease in compliance. As a result there will be increase in V$_A$/Q mismatch.

Normally, the resistance and compliance is not uniform throughout the whole lung. The compliance of normal functioning individual alveoli differs from the apex of a lung to its bottom. Again, normally the resistance of individual airway differs widely, depending on their length and its caliber. Therefore, varieties of alveoli with different time constant for their inflation will exist throughout the whole lung. Thus, the regional variations in resistance and compliance of different alveoli with different time constant not only impair the alveolar filling, but will also cause asynchrony. So, during inspiration as some alveoli may continue to fill, while others are completely empty or completely filled.

Ventilation (V$_A$)/Perfusion (Q) Ratio or V$_A$/Q

Pulmonary blood flow (perfusion) is not uniform from the apex to the base of a lung. According to body position, dependent areas of lung receive higher blood flow than the nondependent areas. This is due to (i) the effect of gravitational force which is 1 cmH$_2$O/cm of lung height and (ii) the normal low pressure system of pulmonary circulation which allow the gravity to exert a significant effect on the amount of pulmonary blood flow. Also, in vivo, the perfusion scanning of a normal lung has shown a typical *"onion-like" layering distribution of perfusion* (pulmonary blood flow) with reduced flow at the periphery and an increased flow at the hilum of a lung. On the other hand, in contrast to pulmonary blood flow (perfusion) and its pressure (perfusion pressure), the alveolar ventilation (V$_A$) and its distending pressure remain relatively constant from periphery to the hilum of a lung. But, it (V$_A$) increases from top to the bottom of a lung.

So, according to the interplay, between alveolar distending pressure (P$_A$), pressure at the arterial end of pulmonary capillary (Ppa), pressure at the venous end of pulmonary capillary (P$_{PV}$), and pressure at the IS of alveolar wall (P$_{ISF}$), lung is divided into four zones (zone-1/2/3/4) which is described before. Now, here we will discuss the alveolar ventilation and perfusion (blood flow) relationship at the different areas of a lung.

V_A/Q ratio expresses the amount of alveolar ventilation (V_A) against the amount of perfusion or blood flow (Q) at any given regions of lungs at any certain time (moment). Ventilation and perfusion is not same at different areas of a lung. Therefore, V_A/Q ratio is not same at the different parts of a lung. Hence, the lungs are usually divided into four zones in reference to different V_A/Q ratio. We know from previous discussions regarding the distribution of perfusion and ventilation that both of them increase linearly from above downward in normal upright position of lung, but not in same proportion. Perfusion increases more rapidly than ventilation, while the distance is going down from apex to the bottom of lungs. *Thus, the V_A/Q ratio also decreases gradually from apex to the bottom of lungs. Normally, the total alveolar ventilation is approximately 4 L/min and total pulmonary perfusion is about 5 L/min. So, an average V_A/Q ratio of lung is about 0.8. But, it can range from zero (no ventilation, only perfusion at the bottom of lung) to infinity (only ventilation, but no perfusion at the apex of lung where ventilation is going wasted). Thus, the zero V_A/Q ratio refers to true pulmonary shunt and infinity V_A/Q ratio refers to alveolar dead space. Usually, in a normal healthy lung V_A/Q ratio at its different area ranges between 3.3 and 0.63 with major area remaining close to the value of 1.0. The apex of a lung is less perfused in relation to their ventilation ($V_A/Q >1$ and near about 3.3), whereas the base of a lung is somewhat overperfused in relation to their ventilation ($V_A/Q <1$ and near about 0.63). Thus, the bottom of a lung is relatively hypoxic and hypercarbic compared to the top of a lung, where ventilation is going wasted* **(Fig. 5)**.

The importance of V_A/Q ratio is that it tells us the efficiency with which a lung unit works, i.e., absorb O_2 and eliminate CO_2. The low V_A/Q ratio of one part of a lung is compensated by the high V_A/Q ratio of another part of a lung. But, practically this does not happen, because less oxygenation of one part of a lung is not compensated by better oxygenation of other part of lung, like excretion of CO_2. This is explained in further details below. Thus, an unequal V_A/Q ratio has different effect on arterial O_2 and CO_2 tension (PaO_2 and PaCO_2). The blood passing through highly perfused, but underventilated alveoli, which are present at the base of a lung, tends to retain CO_2, and cannot take up adequate O_2. So, the blood passing through this area is hypoxic and hypercarbic. On the other hand, the blood passing through over ventilated, but less perfused alveoli, present at the top of a lung gives up excess CO_2 as a compensatory of underventilated alveoli, but cannot take up increased amount of O_2 as a compensatory for underventilated alveoli. *This is due to the flatness of the upper part of O_2 dissociation curve (pulmonary end-capillary blood is usually already maximally saturated with O_2) and less solubility of O_2 than CO_2 in blood (CO_2 is 20 times more*

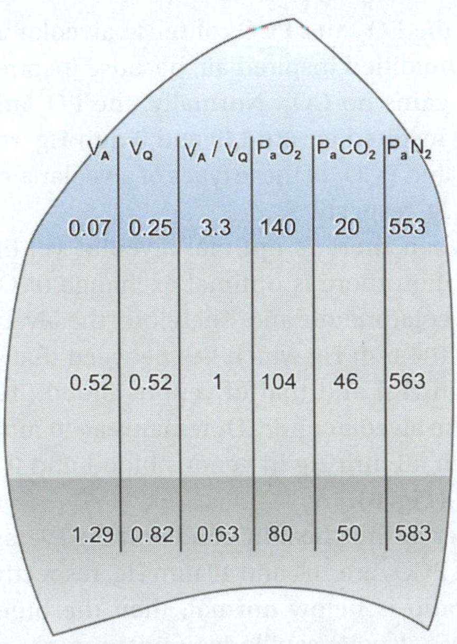

Fig. 5: The regional differences of alveolar ventilation (V_A), perfusion (Q), and V_A/Q ratio. This figure also compares the top with the bottom of a lung which has low ventilation (V_A), high perfusion (Q), and low V_A/Q ratio. This bottom area is relatively more hypoxic and more hypercarbic.

TABLE 3: Diffusion coefficient of different gases.

Gases	Diffusion coefficient
O_2	1
N_2	0.53
CO_2	20.3
He	0.95
CO	0.81

soluble in blood than O_2). Thus, due to uneven V_A/Q ratio the gradient between P_ACO_2 and $PaCO_2$ remains small (so, the P_ACO_2 or $ETCO_2$ can be considered as equivalent to $PaCO_2$), but the gradient between P_AO_2 and PaO_2 remains high **(Table 3)**.

The concept of alveoli of zero and infinity V_A/Q ratio with the concept of physiological shunt (here $V_A = 0$) and physiological dead space (here $Q = 0$).

The alveoli of zero V_A/Q ratio means, there is no (zero) alveolar ventilation (V_A), but there is presence of adequate perfusion. So, the air which is already present within this type of alveoli will come in equilibrium with PO_2 and PCO_2 of venous blood without getting further O_2 from air and without excreting CO_2. Normally, the PO_2 and PCO_2 of venous blood are 40 and 46 mm Hg, respectively. Therefore, the PO_2 and PCO_2 of air of these types of alveoli with zero V_A/Q ratio will be 40 and 46 mm Hg, respectively.

The alveoli of infinity V_A/Q ratio means, there is only presence of ventilation in these alveoli but no perfusion.

Therefore, the PO_2 and PCO_2 of these alveolar air become equal to humidified inspired air, because inspired air loses no O_2 and gains no CO_2. Normally, the PO_2 and PCO_2 of humidified inspired air are 149 and 0 mm Hg, respectively. So, the PO_2 and PCO_2 of these types of alveolar air will be 149 and 0 mm Hg, respectively.

Now, when there is optimal alveolar ventilation and perfusion, then there is optimal exchange of O_2 and CO_2 through alveolar membrane. Therefore, the alveolar air PO_2 remains at 104 mm Hg which lies between that of inspired air (149 mm Hg) and that of venous blood (40 mm Hg). Similarly, the alveolar air PCO_2 remains at 40 mm Hg which lies between 46 mm Hg in venous blood and 0 mm Hg in inspired air **(Fig. 6)**.

So, under normal healthy condition the average alveolar air PO_2 and PCO_2 are 104 and 40 mm Hg, respectively. When the V_A/Q ratio is below normal, then the blood flowing through these alveolar capillaries is not properly oxygenated. Therefore, a portion of venous blood that does not undergo any gaseous exchange through alveolar capillaries due to less ventilation returns back to systemic circulation. *This is called the shunted blood and the total quantity of shunted blood per minute in normal physiological conditions is called the physiological shunt.* The greater the physiological shunt, the greater the amount of blood fails to be oxygenated, while passing through lungs. This physiological shunt is measured by analyzing the concentration of O_2 in both mixed venous blood and arterial blood and calculating CO. From these values, the physiological shunt is obtained by the formula here:

$$\frac{\text{Physiological shunt}}{\text{Cardiac output}} = \frac{\begin{array}{c}\text{(Normal concentration of} \\ O_2 \text{ in arterial blood) – (Measured} \\ \text{concentration } O_2 \text{ in arterial blood)}\end{array}}{\begin{array}{c}\text{(Normal concentration of } O_2 \text{ in arterial} \\ \text{blood) – (Measured concentration} \\ O_2 \text{ in mixed venous blood)}\end{array}}$$

This physiological shunt is also called the venous admixture (Q_S). This venous admixture is defined as the amount of mixed venous blood on right side of heart that is added (mixed) with the fully oxygenated pulmonary end capillary blood without any gaseous exchange at alveolar level to account for the difference in O_2 tension between the systemic arterial and pulmonary end capillary blood. Pulmonary end capillary blood is considered to have the same O_2 concentration as alveolar gas. The venous admixture is usually expressed as a fraction of total CO (Q_S/Q_T). The venous admixture in normal individuals is typically <5%. This physiological shunt or venous admixture is usually expressed as a fraction of total CO and is calculated clinically by obtaining a sample of mixed venous blood from pulmonary artery catheter and by arterial blood gas measurement **(Fig. 7)**.

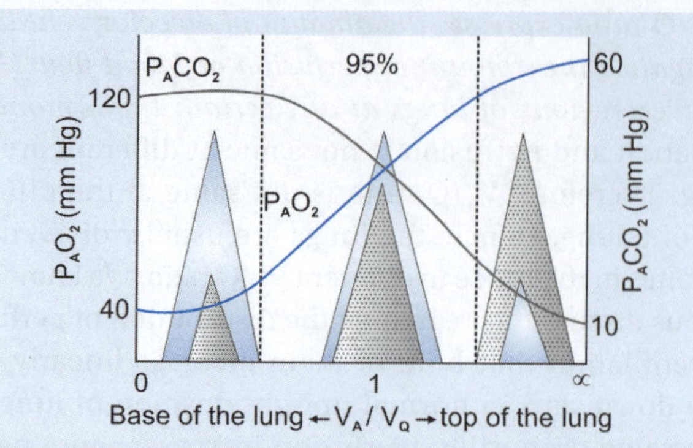

Fig. 6: Distribution of V_A/Q ratio at different parts of lungs. Blue non-dotted triangle is the perfusion and grey dotted triangle is the ventilation. 95% of the lung volume has matched ventilation and perfusion ratio.

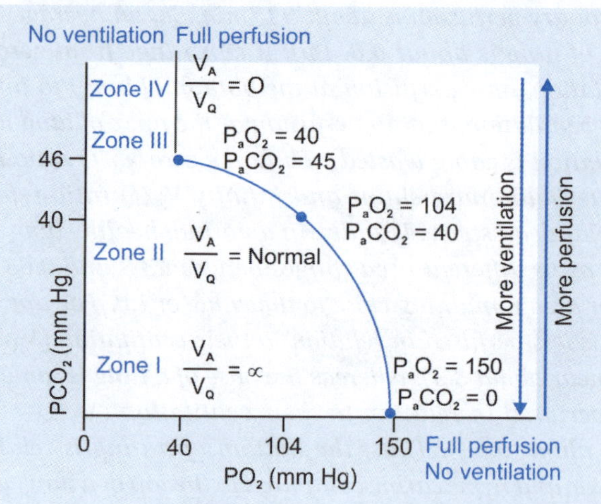

Fig. 7: V_a/V_Q curve.

When the V_A/Q ratio is above normal, then there is far more available O_2 in alveoli than can be transported away by flowing blood. Thus, some of alveolar ventilation is wasted. When this wasted alveolar ventilation is summed up with the wasted ventilation of anatomical dead space, then we will get the physiological dead space. This physiological dead space can be measured by analyzing the tidal volume and PO_2 and PCO_2 in arterial blood and expired air, respectively. From these values, physiological (total) dead space is obtained by the formula here:

$$\frac{\text{Physiological dead space (VD)}}{\text{Tidal volume (VT)}} = \frac{\begin{array}{c}\text{[Arterial CO}_2 \text{ tension (PaCO}_2\text{)] –} \\ \text{[CO}_2 \text{ tension in expired air (PECO}_2\text{)]}\end{array}}{\text{Arterial CO}_2 \text{ tension (PaCO}_2\text{)}}$$

This above equation is also called the Bohr equation. In this equation, we can place $PACO_2$ instead of $PaCO_2$ because in normal healthy adult $PACO_2$ is usually equivalent to $PaCO_2$. In chronic obstructive lung disease, there are both the features of obstruction of small airways and emphysema. The alveoli beyond the obstruction are not ventilated with uncompromised perfusion. So, the V_A/Q ratio approaches to zero. On the other hand, in emphysematous part of lung, most of the ventilation is wasted because of inadequate blood flow. So, the V_A/Q ratio approaches to infinity. Thus in COPD, some area of lungs show excessive physiologic shunt and some areas show excessive physiologic dead space. So, both of these conditions produce severe V_A/Q mismatch and seriously impair the effectiveness of lung's function.

ALVEOLAR OXYGEN TENSION (P_AO_2), PULMONARY END CAPILLARY OXYGEN TENSION (PCO_2), ARTERIAL OXYGEN TENSION (PAO_2), MIXED VENOUS OXYGEN TENSION

Alveolar Oxygen Tension (P_AO_2)

When a gas is kept in a container, it gives pressure on the surfaces of its walls. Thus, the pressure or tension of a gas in this container is due to the multiple impacts or bombardment of its (gas) moving molecules against the surfaces of this container. Hence, in case of a mixture of gases, the total pressure exerted by this gas mixture on container's wall is the summed up forces of impact of all the molecules of different gases against the container's surface at any given moment. This means the pressure, exerted by a single gas component of a mixture of gases, is the fraction of total pressure, exerted by this gas mixture. *This is called the partial pressure of that component gas in a gas mixture and it is directly proportional to the concentration of this component gas in this total mixture.* In atmospheric air, there are mainly two gases N_2 and O_2 and their respective proportion or concentration is 79% and 21%, respectively (The actual composition of air is 78.62% N_2, 20.84% O_2, 0.04% CO_2, and 0.5% H_2O). The total pressure of atmospheric air at sea level is about 760 mm Hg. Thus, it is clear from the previous discussion that partial pressure (which for individual gas in a mixture of gases is called the partial pressure) contributed by each gas, out of this total 760 mm Hg pressure, in air at sea level is directly proportional to their individual concentration. *So, in air at sea level, 79% of 760 mm Hg pressure (760 × 0.79 = 600.4), i.e., 600 mm Hg pressure is exerted by N_2 and 21% of 760 mm Hg pressure (760 × 0.21 = 159.6), i.e., 160 mm Hg pressure is contributed by O_2. Thus, the partial pressure of N_2 in air is 600 mm Hg, the partial pressure O_2 in air is 160 mm Hg at sea level and the total pressure of air, exerted by both N_2 and O_2 at sea level is 600 + 160 = 760 mm Hg* (as other gases which are present in the air are in very minimal concentration, so here, they are deliberately omitted from this calculation for easy understanding). The partial pressure of individual gases in a gas mixture is designated as PO_2, PN_2, PH_2O, etc. *The general formula for calculation of partial pressure of a component gas (let O_2) in its mixture, i.e., PiO_2 (partial pressure of O_2 in inspired gas mixture) = P_B (barometric pressure at that level) × FiO_2 (fractional concentration of O_2 in gas mixture). Let, a mixture of 33% O_2 and 67% N_2O is given to a patient through an anesthetic machine. Therefore, the partial pressure of O_2 in this anesthetic gas mixture is 760 × 0.33 = 760 × 33/100 = 250.8 mm Hg.*

When air, containing little or no water vapor is breathed in, then it is immediately humidified in our respiratory passage by water vapor, evaporating from the surfaces of airway. Therefore, the partial pressure exerted by these water molecules in inspired air is called the partial pressure of water vapor (PH_2O). The quantity of evaporation of water from the surfaces of respiratory passages and its concentration in inspired air depends on our body temperature. At normal body temperature of 37°C, the concentration of water vapor in air entering alveoli is 6.2%. *Therefore, the water vapor pressure at 37°C in inspired air entering alveoli is 6.2% of 760 mm Hg or 47 mm Hg.* This is constant as our normal body temperature, i.e., 37°C is constant at normal condition. *So, the partial pressure of N_2 and O_2 in inspired air entering alveoli after full humidification at 37°C in air passage will come down to 564 and 149 mm Hg respectively, after addition of 6.2% of water vapor (564 mm Hg N_2 + 149 mm Hg O_2 + 47 mm Hg H_2O = 760 mm Hg humidified inspired air).*

O_2 is continuously absorbed from alveoli into blood and then new O_2 is continuously breathed (entered) into alveoli from atmosphere. When more and more O_2 is absorbed into blood from alveoli (e.g., during exercise) and less new O_2 enters in alveoli (e.g., respiratory depression, high altitude, etc.) then the lower will be the concentration and partial pressure of O_2 in alveoli ($\downarrow P_AO_2$). Alternatively, when less O_2 is absorbed into blood from alveoli (e.g., at rest) or the higher of its concentration is in inspired air (e.g., during O_2 therapy), then higher will be its concentration and partial pressure in alveoli ($\uparrow P_AO_2$). Further, in alveoli the inspired gases will be mixed with CO_2, which diffuses out from blood into alveoli. Therefore, the concentration and subsequent partial pressure of O_2 in alveoli is controlled by (i) the rate of absorption of O_2 in blood from alveoli, (ii) the rate of entry of new O_2 into alveoli, and (iii) CO_2 tension in alveoli which is equivalent to arterial CO_2 tension ($PaCO_2$). Hence, the partial pressure or tension of O_2 in alveoli (P_AO_2) can be calculated by the following formula: $P_AO_2 = P_IO_2 - PaCO_2/RQ$. Here, RQ = respiratory quotient, P_IO_2 = inspired O_2 tension, and $PaCO_2$ = arterial CO_2 tension which is equivalent to the alveolar CO_2 tension (P_ACO_2). RQ is usually not measured. From this equation, we can say that increase in $PaCO_2$ (>75 mm Hg) readily produce hypoxia (<PaO_2) at room air, but not at high inspired O_2 concentration.

When air enters the body from atmosphere, it rapidly becomes saturated at 37°C (i.e., body temperature) with water vapor in airways and reaches alveoli, where it is mixed with CO_2. This CO_2 comes in alveoli from pulmonary artery (venous blood). The partial pressure of water vapor and CO_2 in alveoli at 37°C is 47 mm Hg and 40 mm Hg, respectively. So, the next 673 mm Hg (760 – 47 – 40 = 673 mm Hg) accounts for the combined partial pressure of N_2 and O_2. The partial pressure of N_2 in air of alveoli is 569 mm Hg. Therefore, the partial pressure of O in air of alveoli ($P_A O_2$) = 673 – 569 = 104 mm Hg.

Thus, the P_AO_2 is 104 mm Hg when a normal healthy adult person breaths atmospheric air at sea level. But if the patient breaths only 100% O_2, then the alveolar gas contains only O_2, CO_2, and water vapor, and no N_2.

In such situations: $P_AO_2 = P_iO_2 - PaCO_2 - PH_2O = 760 - 40 - 47 = 673$ mm Hg (RQ is usually not measured).

Another simple method of estimating P_AO_2 (in mm Hg) is to multiply the percentage of inspired O_2 concentration by 6.7. Thus, at 40% of FiO_2, the P_AO_2 is $6.7 \times 40 = 268$ mm Hg and at 100% FiO_2, the P_AO_2 is $6.7 \times 100 = 670$ mm Hg at normal atmospheric pressure (i.e., at 760 mm Hg pressure).

Pulmonary End Capillary O$_2$ Tension or Pulmonary Venous O$_2$ Tension Entering Left Atrium

Oxygen passes from alveoli into pulmonary capillaries by passive diffusion and then oxygenates the blood (hemoglobin). Therefore, at the end of this diffusion, the pulmonary end capillary O_2 tension (PCO_2) rises and becomes more or less equal to that of alveoli (P_AO_2). Therefore, $P_AO_2 - PCO_2$ gradient (alveolar – capillary O_2 tension gradient) is normally insignificant. But, if there is any impairment of diffusion of O_2 across the alveolar capillary membrane (respiratory membrane), then $P_AO_2 - PCO_2$ gradient will increase. *The diffusion of O_2 from alveoli into blood through pulmonary capillary membrane depends on many factors and these factors are:*

- The rate of diffusion of O_2 across the alveolar capillary membrane
- The pulmonary capillary blood volume or flow
- The transit time (time taken by blood to pass through pulmonary capillary)
- The capacity of binding of O_2 with Hb.

Rate of Diffusion of O$_2$ Across the Respiratory or Alveolar Capillary Membrane

This again depends on the following factors:
- The thickness of respiratory membrane (from alveolar epithelium to capillary endothelium)
- The total surface area of respiratory membrane
- The diffusion coefficient of gases (here O_2)
- The difference of partial pressure of gases (here O_2) between the alveoli and capillary (mixed venous blood).

Thickness of respiratory membrane: The O_2 diffuses from alveoli into red blood cell (RBC) through different layers or membranes which constitute the respiratory or alveolar capillary membrane. These layers are (i) layer of fluid, lining the alveolus and containing surfactant, (ii) alveolar epithelium, composed of thin epithelial cells, (iii) an epithelial basement membrane, (iv) a thin IS between the alveolar epithelial basement membrane and capillary endothelial basement membrane, (v) capillary endothelial basement membrane, and (vi) capillary endothelium, composed of thin endothelial cells. The average *thickness of this respiratory membrane is 0.4–0.6 µm.* Sometimes, it is as thin as 0.2 µm. This extreme thinness of respiratory membrane facilitates the diffusion of O_2 from alveoli to blood and CO_2 from blood to alveoli, because the rate of diffusion of gases through a membrane is inversely proportional to the thickness of it. Any factor that increases the thickness of respiratory membrane such as edema, fibrosis, deposition of substances in membrane, etc., significantly interferes the diffusion of gases (here O_2) across this respiratory membrane.

Total surface area of respiratory membrane: Like thickness, the surface area through which a gas diffuse also modulates the rate of diffusion of it and they are directly proportional. Hence, the large surface area of alveoli also greatly facilitates the diffusion of O_2 through respiratory membrane. *The total surface area of respiratory membrane is about 70 m^2 (range varies between 50 and 100 m^2) in a normal healthy adult male.* The total quantity of blood present in alveolar capillaries, at a given moment, is 60–140 mL (average 70 mL) and this small amount of blood is spread over such a big surface area. So, it is easily understood, how O_2 is easily diffused from alveolar air into pulmonary capillary blood through this such huge surface area. When this surface area for diffusion is reduced such as in emphysema, then the diffusion is significantly impaired. In emphysema, the alveoli are coalesced due to rupture of their wall and new alveoli are formed. This new alveoli are larger than the original one, but the total surface area of respiratory membrane is greatly reduced.

TABLE 4: Solubility coefficient of different gases.	
Gases	**Solubility coefficient**
O_2	0.024
N_2	0.012
CO_2	0.57
He	0.008
CO	0.018

TABLE 5: Partial pressure of gases (mm Hg) in the different inspired and expired air.				
Gases	**Atmospheric air**	**Humidified air**	**Alveolar air**	**Expired air**
N_2	597 (80%)	563	563	566 (74.4%)
O_2	159 (20%)	150	150	120 (15.7%)
H_2O	4	47	40	27 (3.5%)
CO_2	–	–	47	47 (6.1%)
Total pressure (mm Hg)	760	760	760	760

Diffusion coefficient of gases: The capacity for diffusion (diffusion capacity) of gases through a respiratory membrane is expressed as their diffusion coefficient. Because, the amount of diffusion of gases from alveoli to capillary blood is dictated by the diffusion coefficient of that gases. It depends (i) directly on the *solubility of gases* in water and (ii) inversely on the square root of their *molecular weight* (mw). Further, the solubility of individual gas in water depends on (i) their *partial pressure* in their gaseous phase at one side of membrane and (ii) their *concentration* (expressed in volume of gas dissolved in each volume of water) on the other side of membrane. This relation is expressed as the solubility coefficient in water at body temperature for individual gases. On the other hand, the solubility determines the partial pressure of gas in its liquid phase which again dictates the net diffusion of it between its gaseous and liquid phase. *Thus the solubility coefficient can be calculated from the Henry's law, which is expressed as: Solubility coefficient = Concentration of dissolved gas ÷ partial pressure* (**Table 4**).

From this solubility coefficient table, it is found that CO_2 is 20 times more soluble in water than O_2 and O_2 is two times more soluble in water than N_2. So, for a given partial pressure, CO_2 diffuses 20 times more rapidly out from capillary blood to alveoli than O_2 from alveoli to capillary blood and O_2 diffuses two times more rapidly than N_2. from alveoli to capillary blood. Therefore, C_2O diffuses out 20×2 = 40 times more rapidly than N_2 from blood to alveoli.

The diffusing capacity of O_2 is expressed as DLO_2. This $DLO_2 = O_2$ uptake$/(P_AO_2 - PCO_2)$. Here, PCO_2 cannot be measured accurately. So, the diffusion capacity of carbon monoxide (CO) or DLCO is measured to assess the transfer of gases across the alveolar capillary membrane. Because, CO has a very high affinity for Hb and there is little or no CO in pulmonary capillary blood, so that when it is administered at low concentration, then the capillary CO tension can be considered zero ($P_cCO = 0$). Therefore, DLCO = CO uptake$/P_ACO$. The reduction in DLCO implies that there is an impediment in the transfer of gases across the alveolar capillary membrane due to its destruction.

Difference in partial pressure of gases between alveoli and capillary: There are some types of gas molecules which are physically or chemically attracted to water molecules, while others are repelled. This attraction property of gas molecules to water molecule is called solubility. The more solubility of a gas means more molecules of this gas are attracted to water molecules and dissolved within it without building up excess pressure within its aqueous solution. The partial pressure of a gas in its aqueous solution is expressed by its number of free molecules in water which is not dissolved. Alternatively, in the case of those that are not readily attached to water molecules, are repelled and make an impact or make a force on the surface or membrane. Thus, they develop a pressure on the surface with fewer dissolved molecules. So, the water solubility of a gas is inversely proportional with the development of partial pressure which means increased water solubility decreases the partial pressure exerted by this gas (**Table 5**).

Now, it is clear from previous discussion that after dissolving in water or body tissues, every gas exerts pressure on the surface of a membrane according to their solubility in water or body tissues. This is because every dissolved gas molecule moves randomly and has kinetic energy. When a mixture of gases exerts a pressure, then the individual pressure exerted by individual gases are called the partial pressure of these gases. Again this partial pressure of a gas in a liquid phase depends on their concentration in liquid and the solubility coefficient of that gas (Henry's law) in this liquid.

There is difference between the partial pressure of gases in alveoli and the partial pressure of gases in capillary blood. The partial pressure of a gas means the total number of molecule of a particular gas striking on a unit area of surface in a unit time either as gaseous phase (gas in alveoli) or as liquid phase (gas in capillary blood). Therefore, the difference in partial pressure represents the net tendency for these gas molecules to move through a membrane to any of their phase. So, when the partial pressure of any gas (as for example O_2) in alveoli is greater than the partial pressure of

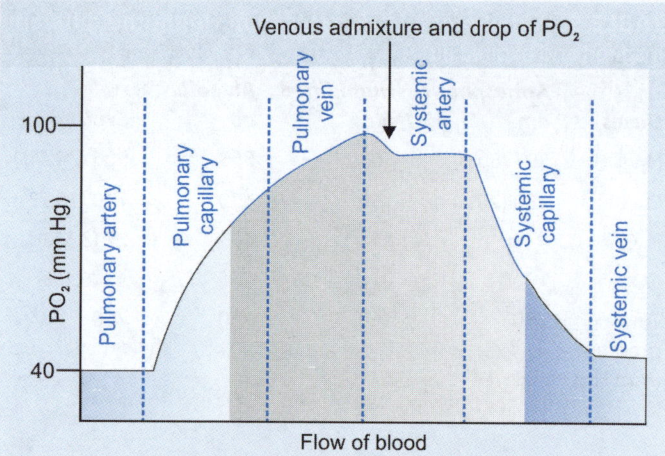

Fig. 8: The changes in PO$_2$ while blood is flowing through systemic vein, to right ventricle, to pulmonary artery, to pulmonary capillary, to left ventricle, to systemic artery, to systemic capillary, and again to systemic vein.

gas in blood, then the net diffusion from alveoli into blood occurs. Similarly, when the partial pressure of any gas (as for example CO_2) in blood is greater than the partial pressure of it in alveoli, then net diffusion from blood into alveoli occurs **(Fig. 8)**.

Pulmonary Capillary Blood Volume or Flow

The pulmonary capillary blood volume, especially the volume of red cells which are able to take O$_2$ and release CO_2 is also a very important factor for the amount of diffusion of O$_2$ and CO_2 between the alveoli and capillary. Thus, anemic patients tend to have low diffusion factor and a polycythemia patients have a higher one.

Pulmonary Capillary Transit Time

The pulmonary capillary transit time (the time taken by blood to pass through alveolar capillary), which also have great impact on the diffusion of O$_2$ from alveoli to capillary blood, can be estimated by dividing the pulmonary capillary blood volume (70 mL) by CO (5,000 mL/min). Thus, the normal capillary transit time is 70 mL ÷ 5,000 mL/min = 0.014 minutes = 0.84 seconds. But, the majority of diffusion of O$_2$ from alveoli to capillary occurs within first one-third (0.3 second) of this transit time. Thus, virtually a complete equilibrium of O$_2$ tension, between the alveolus and pulmonary capillary blood has been established at the venous end of capillary within this small 0.3 second time, providing a large safety of margin (0.5 second). So, during exercise almost complete equilibrium of O$_2$ still occurs, though the transit time may be reduced to two-thirds of this 0.3 second time, i.e., 0.1 second.

Capacity of Binding of O$_2$ with Hb

The rate of binding of O$_2$ with Hb also appears to be a rate limiting factor for diffusion of O$_2$ from alveolus to capillary. This is further discussed elsewhere. Binding of O$_2$ to Hb seems to be the principal rate limiting factor in the transfer of O$_2$ from alveoli to blood.

Arterial O$_2$ Tension (PaO$_2$)

When breathing air, the tension of O$_2$ (PO$_2$) in the air of alveoli averages to about 104 mm Hg (discussed before), whereas the PO$_2$ in mixed venous blood, entering the pulmonary capillary at its arterial end, averages only about 40 mm Hg. Therefore, the initial pressure difference which cause the O$_2$ to diffuse into pulmonary capillary from alveoli is 104 − 40 = 64 mm Hg. **(Fig. 9)**.

After diffusion from alveoli into capillary blood, the O$_2$ build up a tension in it (blood) and this oxygen tension (PO$_2$) gradually reaches an equilibrium. Thus, the PO$_2$ of blood that enter left atrium, through pulmonary veins from the venous end of pulmonary capillary, is also like that of alveolar PO$_2$ and averages about 104 mm Hg. But, the blood coming from lungs to heart with PO$_2$ of 104 mm Hg constitute 98% of CO **(Fig. 10)**.

Another 2% of CO comes from bronchial vein which is not oxygenated. Normally, 2% of CO passes from aorta through bronchial circulation and supplies mainly the deep tissues of lungs. This blood is not exposed to alveolar air for oxygenation and comes back through bronchial vein to left atrium with PO$_2$ about 40 mm Hg which is similar to that of systemic venous system. This deoxygenated blood flow is called the shunt (true) flow. When this deoxygenated shunted blood (PO$_2$ = 40 mm Hg) combines with oxygenated blood of pulmonary vein (PO$_2$ = 104 mm Hg) in left atrium, then this mixed blood is called the *venous admixture with arterial blood* and PO$_2$ in left atrial and left ventricular blood *(mixed arterial O$_2$ tension)* comes down to 97 mm Hg from 104 mm Hg. Then, this venous admixture arterial blood that enters the left side of heart is pumped out into aorta with mixed arterial PO$_2$ of about 97 mm Hg. *This is the actual systemic arterial O$_2$ tension (PaO$_2$).* Then, when this oxygenated arterial blood (actually venous admixture blood) with PO$_2$ of 97 mm Hg passes through different tissues, then the PO$_2$ comes down in stages at different site which is shown in figure as "O$_2$ cascade" in "O$_2$ and CO_2" (Chapter 4).

Alveolar and Arterial O$_2$ Tension Difference (P$_A$O$_2$ – PaO$_2$)

When a patient is breathing air at normal atmospheric pressure (760 mm Hg) in sea level at 37°C temperature, then normal P$_A$O$_2$ is 104 mm Hg and PaO$_2$ is 97 mm Hg.

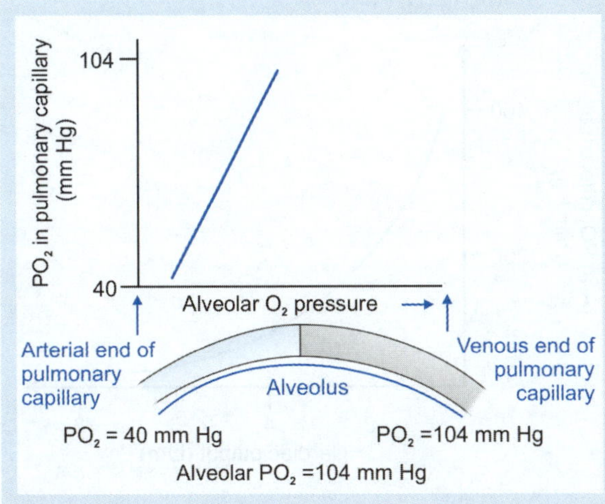

Fig. 9: Diffusion of O$_2$ from alveolar air into the pulmonary capillary blood.

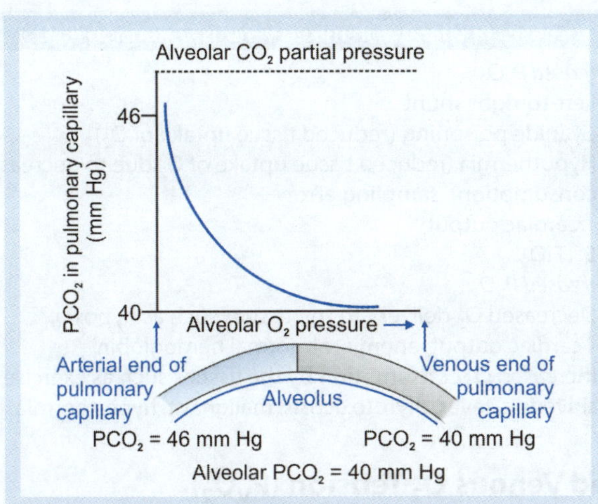

Fig. 10: Diffusion of CO$_2$ from pulmonary capillary blood into the alveolar air.

So, the normal alveolar to arterial O$_2$ tension difference (P$_A$O$_2$ – PaO$_2$ or A–a oxygen tension gradient) is 104 – 97 = 7 mm Hg, and usually it lies below 15 mm Hg. But, it may vary between 5 and 25 mm Hg, and this A–a gradient increases progressively with increase of age up to 20–30 mm Hg. This is due to progressive increase in CC in relation to FRC with increased age. From age, the PaO$_2$ can be calculated by the following formula: PaO$_2$ = 102 – age/3.

The P$_A$O$_2$ – PaO$_2$ or the A–a gradient is the most common mechanism of hypoxemia. The A–a gradient for O$_2$ depends on (i) V$_A$/Q ratio, (ii) shunt and (iii) mixed venous O$_2$ tension (not mixed arterial O$_2$ tension). It is directly proportional to V$_A$/Q mismatch and shunt and inversely proportional to mixed venous O$_2$ tension. Thus, the P$_A$O$_2$ – PaO$_2$ difference is influenced by the following factors.

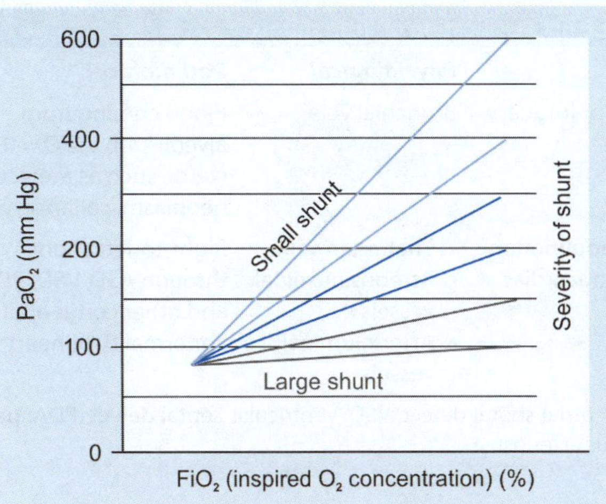

Fig. 11: The effect of various concentration of inspired O$_2$ concentration on arterial O$_2$ tension (PaO$_2$) with various amount of shunt. In case of very large shunt, there is very little benefit with increasing inspired O$_2$ concentration.

V/Q ratio: From the aspect of ideal V$_A$/Q ratio, no alveoli are ideal. Some are overventilated or some are overperfused (overcirculated). So, the blood from different parts of lungs after passing through alveolar capillaries and after taking part in gaseous exchange with different PO$_2$ mixes at the venous end of pulmonary capillary and flows through pulmonary vein to left atrium. There, final arterial PO$_2$, i.e., mixed arterial PO$_2$ (mixed PaO$_2$) is definitely lower than P$_A$O$_2$. Therefore, more V$_A$/Q mismatch results in more P$_A$O$_2$ – PaO$_2$ difference or more A–a oxygen tension gradient.

Shunt: The blood which passes through alveoli (better say lungs), but without any gaseous exchange, is called the shunted blood. As more and more blood passes through such shunts and mixes with oxygenated blood coming from different alveoli with different V$_A$/Q ratio at the left side of the heart, then P$_A$O$_2$ – PaO$_2$ difference will increase. *These shunts can be classified into two: (1) true and (2) false shunts.* True shunts are those that do not pass through alveolar capillary or not through lungs at all. They are also called the *anatomical or true shunt.* The examples of anatomical or true shunts are bronchial circulatory system, reverse ASD, reverse VSD, reverse patent ductus arteriosus (PDA), etc. False shunts are those that pass through alveolar capillary, but due to different pathological condition they cannot take part in gaseous exchange. They are also called the *physiological or false shunt* and indicate mainly the zero V$_A$/Q zones of lungs **(Fig. 11)**.

The venous admixture (admixture of venous or deoxygenated blood with oxygenated or arterial blood) or shunt causes reduction in arterial O$_2$ content (tension) and increase in arterial CO$_2$ content (tension). Further, due to the

TABLE 6: Classification of "true shunts".

Site	Physiological	Pathological
Intrapulmonary	Bronchial vein	Blood coming from alveoli with $V_A/Q = 0$ (zero), such as atelectasis, neoplasm, collapse, etc.
Extrapulmonary or intracardiac	• Thebesian veins • Arteriosinusoidal vessels • Arterioluminal vessels	Right-to-left shunt through ASD, VSD, PDA, and other congenital abnormality of heart

(ASD: atrial septal defect; VSD: ventricular septal defect; PDA: patent ductus arteriosus)

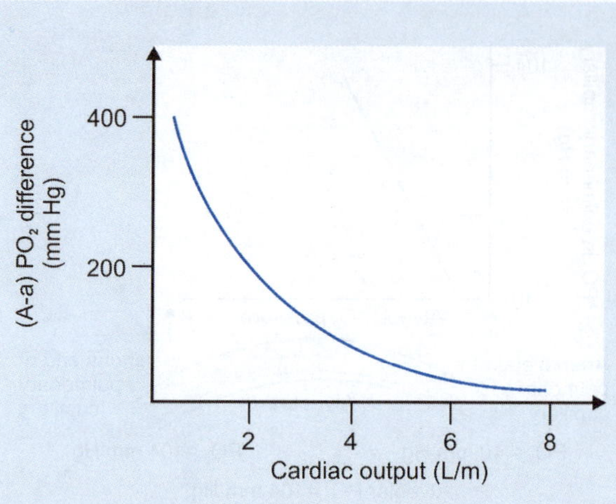

Fig. 12: The relationship between cardiac output and (A–a) PO$_2$ difference due to venous admixture. As cardiac output increases (A–a) PO$_2$ decreases and (A–a) PO$_2$ rises steeply at low cardiac output.

*shape of O$_2$ and CO$_2$ dissociation curve, a small reduction of O$_2$ content is reflected as a large reduction in arterial PO$_2$ (about 7 mm Hg), whereas a small increase in CO$_2$ content is reflected by only a small increase in arterial PCO$_2$ (<1 mm Hg). The arterial PO$_2$ is, therefore, best indication for the amount of venous admixture or shunt than arterial PCO$_2$. So, the high P$_A$O$_2$ – PaO$_2$ difference is due to V$_A$/Q mismatch or true shunt and can be detected only by giving the subject 100% O$_2$ to breath. If there is small or no increase in arterial PO$_2$, then the P$_A$O$_2$ – PaO$_2$ difference or hypoxemia is due to true shunt. Up to the presence of 50% shunt, changes of FiO$_2$ have virtually no effect on PaO$_2$ (**Table 6**).*

Venous admixture and O$_2$ tension in mixed venous blood: When blood passes through different organs or tissues of our body, then the extraction of O$_2$ from blood by these different organs or tissues depends on the rate of metabolism of these tissues and the fraction of CO, supplied to these tissues. So, the partial pressure (tension) of O$_2$ in venous blood coming from different tissues is different. Now, when these venous blood coming from different organs or tissues with different PO$_2$ reach at the right side of heart, then they mix and produce a mixed venous blood with a given O$_2$ tension in this mixed venous blood. The causes which reduce the O$_2$ tension in this mixed venous blood (P$_V$O$_2$), such as increased metabolism and low CO, increases the P$_A$O$_2$ – PaO$_2$ difference. Low CO tends to increase the effect of V$_A$/Q mismatch and subsequently its effect on shunt and ultimately their effects on PaO$_2$ and P$_V$O$_2$. On the other hand, low CO reduces the venous admixture secondary to the increased pulmonary vasoconstriction due to lower mixed venous O$_2$ tension (compensatory phenomenon) **(Fig. 12 and Box 2)**.

Concentration of Hb also has an effect on O$_2$ tension of mixed venous blood and subsequently on A–a oxygen gradient. Low Hb concentration can depress mixed venous PO$_2$ and increase the gradient between A–a oxygen tension.

BOX 2: Causes of changes in mixed venous O$_2$ tension (P$_V$O$_2$).

- *Increased P$_V$O$_2$:*
  - Left-to-right shunt
  - Cyanide poisoning (reduced tissue uptake of O$_2$)
  - Hypothermia (reduced tissue uptake of O$_2$ due to decreased consumption), sampling error
  - ↑Cardiac output
  - 5 ↑FiO$_2$
- *Decreased P$_V$O$_2$:*
  - Decreased O$_2$ delivery to the tissues such as hypoxia, ↓cardiac output, anemia, abnormal hemoglobin
  - Increased O$_2$ consumption by the tissues such as exercise, shivering, fever, thyrotoxicosis, malignant, hyperthermia, etc.

Mixed Venous O$_2$ Tension (P$_V$O$_2$)

Mixed venous O$_2$ tension represents the overall balance between the total delivery and the total consumption of O$_2$. The normal value of it in a healthy adult is 40 mm Hg. A true mixed venous blood sample coming from different organs for the measurement of mixed venous O$_2$ tension should be obtained from SVC, IVC, and right heart. So, it should be obtained by pulmonary artery catheter. Other details regarding PVO$_2$ are described in previous paragraph. Like mixed venous O$_2$ tension, there is also *mixed venous CO$_2$ tension*. Its normal value is 46 mm Hg. It is the end result of mixing of blood coming from different tissues of varying metabolic activity (skin with lowest metabolic activity and heart with highest metabolic activity) at the right side of heart.

■ DEAD SPACE

When a person breaths, then all the air, taking during inspiration and entering into lungs does not take part in gaseous exchange. Some of the air reach the alveoli and take

BOX 3: Causes altering dead space.	
1. Age	1. Increase
2. Posture	2.
i. Standing	i. Increase
ii. Lying	ii. Decrease
3. Neck	3.
i. Extension	i. Increase
ii. Flexion	ii. Decrease
4. Artificial airway	4. Decrease
5. Intermittent positive pressure ventilation (IPPV)	5. Increase
6. Hypertension	6. Increase
7. Emphysema	7. Increase
8. Tracheostomy	8. Decrease
9. Anesthetic circuit	9. Increase
10. Face mask	10. Increase
11. Hypotension	11. Increase
12. Pulmonary emboli	12. Increase

TABLE 7: The causes for increase and decrease of anatomical dead space.	
Anatomical dead space increases in	Old age, neck extension, jaw protrusion, bronchodilators, increased lung volume, atropine (by bronchodilatation), anesthesia mask and circuit, intermittent positive pressure ventilation (IPPV), and positive end-expiratory pressure (PEEP)
Anatomical dead space decreases in	Intubation (nasal cavity is bypassed plus diameter of endotracheal (ET) tube is < airway diameter), tracheostomy (nasal cavity, pharynx, and larynx are bypassed), hyperventilation (decreasing lung volume), neck flexion, and bronchoconstrictors

part in gaseous exchange, but some simply fill the respiratory passages (airways) such as nose, nasopharynx, trachea, etc., where gas exchange does not occur. Thus, the part of inspired air which does not take part in gaseous exchange is called the dead space air. During expiration, this dead space air is expired first followed by the exit of air from alveoli that takes part in gaseous exchange and contain CO_2. Therefore, the dead space is very disadvantageous for gaseous exchange, i.e., oxygenation of blood and elimination of CO_2 and for removing the expiratory gases from lungs. Normally, two-thirds of each breath takes part in gaseous exchange and this portion (or volume) of breath is called alveolar ventilation. Whereas, the remaining one-third of each breath does not take part in gaseous exchange and this portion (or volume) of breath is called dead space or dead space ventilation **(Box 3)**.

The dead space is actually composed of two components: (1) *anatomical dead space* and (2) *alveolar dead space*. The sum of these two is referred to as *the total or physiological dead space. Normally, in healthy adult the anatomical and physiological dead space is nearly equal (because alveolar dead space is considered as zero) and is about 150 mL each.* This is because in a given healthy subject the anatomical dead space remains fixed and all the alveoli are functional with no alveolar dead space. But, in some persons, this physiological dead space may be as high as 10 times of anatomical dead space and it is due to the presence of some partial functioning or completely nonfunctioning alveoli in some parts of lungs which increases alveolar dead space.

Anatomical Dead Space

It is constituted by space occupied by air which is not participating in gaseous exchange. It is that portion of total or physiological dead space which occupies only the conducting path of respiratory passage (nose, pharynx, trachea, and bronchial tree up to terminal bronchioles). *It varies with the age, sex, and size of lung. Normally, in a healthy adult the approximate value of it (anatomical dead space) is 2 mL/kg or 150 mL. But in young women, it is as low as 100 mL and in old man it can rise as much as up to 200 mL. The anatomical dead space is reduced when the neck is flexed and tongue falls back (30 mL reduction). It also can be reduced by pneumonectomy, tracheostomy, etc. On the other hand, anatomical dead space is increased by the protrusion of jaw and extension of neck (40 mL increase). In supine position, the anatomical dead space is equal to total or physiological dead space as alveolar dead space becomes zero or negligible due to obliteration of zone 1 (in lying position perfusion is equal in all the parts of lung). But, in erect posture, the alveolar dead space increases from zero to 60 or 80 mL due to the creation of zone 1. So, physiological dead space also increases. The causes for increase and decrease of anatomical dead space are given in **Table 7**.*

Alveolar Dead Space

It is that portion of total or physiological dead space that occupy or ventilate the nonperfused (no or minimum blood circulation) alveoli. It is constituted by the volume of alveoli which are only ventilated but not perfused. So, in that portion of lung, ventilation (air entry) goes wasted. *It is 60–80 mL in standing position. It is zero in lying position (in lying position perfusion or circulation is equal in all parts of lung). It increases when zone 1 area increases such as in upright position, hypotension, low CO state, IPPV, PEEP, etc. It also increases in lung pathologies affecting diffusion at alveolar capillary membrane such as interstitial lung disease, pulmonary embolism, pulmonary edema, and ARDS.*

Total or Physiological Dead Space

As the total or physiological dead space is the sum of anatomical and alveolar dead space, so when any of the above two dead space increases, then the physiological or total dead space also increases. The examples are: old age, upright position, high respiratory rate (inspiratory time <0.5 second), administration of atropine, COPD, asthma, pulmonary embolism, hemorrhage, hypotension, etc.

Apparatus (Anesthesia) Dead Space

Anesthetic apparatus dead space is considered as anatomical dead space. All anesthetic circuits, masks, humidifiers, etc. increase anatomical dead space. It is the volume of gas that is present in any anesthetic apparatus between the patient and the point in anesthetic circuit where rebreathing of exhaled gases ceases to occur, for example: expiratory valve in Magill circuit, side arm in Ayre's T-piece, etc. The volume of apparatus (anesthetic) dead space in Magill system is 125 mL. So, it is very important for an anesthetized small children.

Anesthesia and Dead Space

- ET tube and tracheostomy decreases anatomical dead space by bypassing upper airway
- All inhalational anesthetic agents increase both the anatomical and alveolar dead space. Anatomical dead space is increased, because all these agents are bronchodilators. Alveolar dead space is increased, because of hypotension (decreased perfusion) produced by these agents.
- Positions during anesthesia, especially lateral position causes more ventilation in upper lung (nondependent lung) and more blood flow in lower lung (dependent lung), thereby increasing V/Q mismatch and hence alveolar dead space. Other positions such as Trendelenburg and lithotomy positions also cause V/Q mismatch.
- Anesthetic ventilation technique such as IPPV, PEEP, etc. increase both anatomical and alveolar dead space. Anatomical dead space is increased by increasing lung volume and alveolar dead space is increased, because of hypotension produced by IPPV and PEEP (increase in intrathoracic pressure produced by IPPV or PEEP decreases venous return, CO, and hence hypotension).

Dead Space and Alveolar Ventilation

Alveolar ventilation (V_A) is the major determining factor of alveolar O_2 and CO_2 tension which later subsequently determine the O_2 and CO_2 tension in blood. On the other hand, dead space (total or physiological) is the major determining factor of alveolar ventilation. So, it is easily understood how the dead space (total, V_D) controls the alveolar and arterial O_2 and CO_2 tension through alveolar ventilation from the formula: $V_A = (V_T - V_D) \times F$

$V_A = Alveolar\ ventilation, V_T = Tidal\ volume, V_D = Dead\ space, F = Respiratory\ rate.$

For a healthy adult person, if V_T = 450 mL (6 mL/kg), V_D = 150 mL and F = 12/min, then, V_A = (450–150) × 12 = 3,600 mL/min.

The dead space (total or physiological) to tidal volume ratio (V_D/V_T) also provides a useful expression of the efficiency of ventilation. Normal V_D/V_T ratio is 0.25 to 0.4. It averages to 0.3 which means dead space is 30% and ventilation is 70% of tidal volume. In patient with obstructive airway disease V_D/V_T ratio may increase to 0.6 or 0.7 (60 or 70%). It means dead space is increased to 60–70% and ventilation is reduced to 40–30% of total tidal volume, or ventilation which is grossly inefficient. V_D/V_T ratio also increases with age which can be roughly estimated from formula: $V_D/V_T = 33 + Age/3\%$.

This is due to the more vascular obliteration with age. The V_D/V_T ratio also can be derived by the Bohr equation:

$$\frac{V_D}{V_T} = \frac{(P_A CO_2 - P_E CO_2)}{(P_A CO_2)}$$

$P_A CO_2$ = alveolar CO_2 tension, $P_E CO_2$ = expired CO_2 tension. In normal healthy adult, $P_A CO_2$ is equivalent to $PaCO_2$ and $P_E CO_2$ is the average measured over several minutes. So, this equation is useful clinically, because we can measure the V_D from this equation. For example, $P_A CO_2$ = 40 mm Hg, $P_E CO_2$ = 28 mm Hg and V_T = 500 ml. So, V_D/V_T = (40 – 28)/40 = 12/40 or V_D = 12/40 × 500 = 150 mL.

■ RESISTANCE OF BREATHING

During respiration, i.e., inspiration and expiration, the chest wall and lungs move out and in and the air flows in and out through airways. But, this movement of chest wall with lungs and with them the flow of air through airways is always associated with some impedance. This impedance is called the resistance. This is due to *friction* (i) during the movement, between the tissues of chest wall and lungs, and (ii) during the flow of air, between the air and its passage. Generally, this resistance is overcome, by creating a *pressure gradient,* between the atmosphere and alveoli which is accomplished by *work of breathing. Thus, the resistance is defined as the unit change of pressure gradient (accomplished by work of breathing) causing unit volume of air to flow (**Box 4**).*

The type of resistance is divided under two broad headings: (A) elastic resistance and (B) nonelastic resistance. The elastic resistance is imparted by (due to): (i) the elastic recoil property of lungs and chest wall and also by (ii) the surface tension acting at the air fluid interface in alveoli. Elastic resistance is measured in terms of compliance as the compliance is opposite to elastic resistance, contributed both by elastic recoil property of lungs and chest wall and

BOX 4: Components and its percentage that constitute the resistance of breathing.

- Elastic resistance (65%)
- *Nonelastic resistance:*
  - Airway frictional resistance (28%)
  - Viscous nonelastic resistance such as bones, muscles, etc., (7%)

BOX 5: Causes of elastic and non-elastic resistance of thorax.

- *Elastic resistance:*
  - Elastic recoil property of lungs
  - Elastic recoil property of chest wall
  - Surface tension in alveoli at air fluid interface
- *Nonelastic resistance:*
  - Friction of air in air passage
  - Friction among tissues such as bones and muscles.

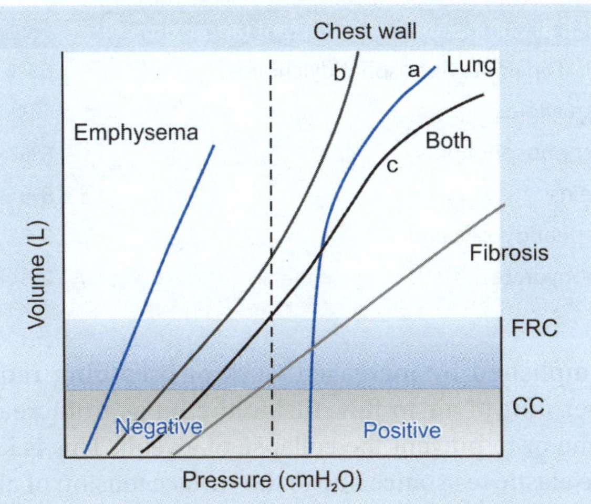

Fig. 13: The compliance or pressure volume relationship of lung (line-a), chest wall (line-b) and both together (line-c).

alveolar surface tension. *On the other hand, the nonelastic resistance is imparted (i) by the friction of air in air passage during its flow through it and (ii) by the friction among tissues during the movement of nonelastic part of lungs and chest wall such as bones, muscles, etc. (Box 5).*

The work of breathing, performed by respiratory muscles, is done during inspiration and it is necessary to develop pressure gradient to overcome elastic resistance for the flow of air into alveoli. It is stored during inspiration as potential energy, and is subsequently used during expiration which is passive whereas, the work of breathing, necessary to overcome the nonelastic resistance for the flow of air into alveoli, is expressed as heat.

Elastic Resistance

From previous discussion, it is now clear that elastic resistance is due to (i) the *elastic recoiling property of lung tissues which have tendency to collapse,* (ii) the elastic *recoiling property of soft tissues of chest wall which have tendency to expand outward and (iii) the surface tension in alveoli.* The collapsing elastic recoiling property of lung is proved by when the pleural space is exposed to atmosphere, the lungs collapse completely, and all the gases within it (lung) is expelled. On the other hand, the outward expanding elastic recoiling property of chest wall is proved by when the pleural space is exposed to atmosphere, the chest wall usually expands about 1 L in adults. Again the elastic recoiling property of lungs is due to their high content of elastin and collagen fibers and even more important, the surface tension forces in alveoli. On the other hand, the elastic recoil property of chest wall is due to (i) their structural components that resist deformation and (ii) chest wall muscle tone. Clinically,

the elastic resistance of lung, offered by these elastin and collagen fibers, cannot be measured directly and individually. Similarly, the only measurement of elastic resistance, offered by the surface tension of alveoli, is not so helpful clinically. Therefore, *the whole elastic resistance is measured indirectly by the compliance* **(Fig. 13)**.

Elastic Resistance due to the Elastic Recoiling Property of Lung Tissues and Soft Tissues of Chest Wall

The total elastic resistance of lungs and chest wall are calculated together indirectly by compliance. Because, compliance is opposite to resistance, i.e., compliance = 1/resistance (or vice versa) and it is also reproduced, like the resistance, by pressure volume curve. *If the lungs are affected by fibrosis (e.g., interstitial pulmonary fibrosis) where the elastin and collagen fibers are replaced by fibrous tissues, then the elastic resistance will increase and the compliance will decrease. Thus, the lungs will become stiff and the pressure volume curve will shift downward and toward right. On the other hand, in emphysema the total mass of elastin and collagen fibers are reduced and the recoiling property of lungs is lost. Thus, it becomes voluminous and the elastic resistance will decrease with the increase of compliance. So, the pressure-volume curve will shift upward and toward left.*

Elastic Resistance due to Surface Tension

Another important factor affecting the elastic resistance of lung is alveolar surface tension which is due to the gas (air)-fluid interface present in alveoli. This surface tension or force tries to reduce the gas-fluid interfacing area and favors alveolar collapse. Thus, it increases the pressure gradient

TABLE 8: Composition of surfactant (approximate).	
DPPC (Dipalmitoylphosphatidylcholine)	65%
Neutral lipids	12%
Other phospholipids	8%
Proteins	8%
Phosphatidyl glycerol	5%
Carbohydrate	2%

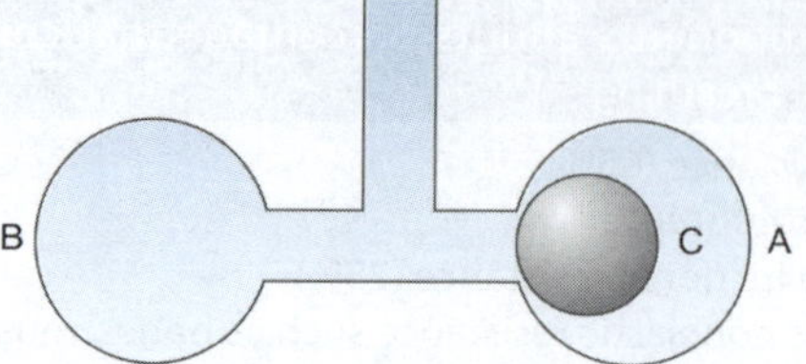

Fig. 14: According to Laplace law P = 2T/R.

Story 1: The two alveoli A and B are of same size, but alveoli A have no surfactant. The radius of alveoli A is 0.5 cm and surface tension is 10 dynes/cm, whereas the radius of alveoli B is 0.5 cm and surface tension is 5 dynes/cm due to the presence of surfactant. Then, the intra-alveolar pressure of alveoli A will be P = 2 × 10/0.5 = 40 dynes/cm². The intra-alveolar pressure of alveoli B with surfactant of same radius will be P = 2 × 5/0.5 = 20 dynes/cm². So, due to high pressure in alveoli A, the air will flow from it to alveoli B and gradually the alveoli A will reduce in size. On the other hand, alveoli B will increase in size. Hence, in this story alveoli A needs surfactant to reduce the intra-alveolar pressure.

Story 2: The two alveoli C and B of different radius, but of same surface tension. The radius of alveoli C is 0.2 cm and surface tension is 5 dynes/cm, whereas the radius of alveoli B is 0.5 cm and surface tension is 5 dynes/cm. Then the pressure within alveoli C will be P = 2 × 5/0.2 = 50 dynes/cm². While the pressure within alveoli B will be P = 2 × 5/0.5 = 20 dynes/cm². So the smaller alveoli C will drain in alveoli B and will reduce in size. Hence, in this story alveoli C needs more surfactant than B, though surface tension is same, because its radius is small.

Story 3: In the presence of surfactant the smaller alveoli will have less surface tension due to crowding of the surfactant molecule in a small space. For example, there are two alveoli C and B. The radius of alveoli C is 0.2 cm and surface tension is 1 dynes/cm, whereas, the radius of alveoli B is 0.5 cm and surface tension is 5 dynes/cm. Then, the pressure within alveoli C will be P = 2 × 1/0.2 = 10 dynes/cm² whereas, the pressure within alveoli B is 20 dynes/cm². Thus, the gas will flow from alveoli B to alveoli C, until the two alveoli reach to equal size and volume become stable.

accomplished by increased work of breathing required for per unit of air to flow inside the lungs to increase its volume or to prevent the collapse of alveoli. This is known as the elastic resistance due to the surface tension of alveoli. If the lung is filled with saline, then surface tension will become zero due to the absence of air-fluid interface. In such condition, the elastic resistance will measure only the soft tissue elastic resistance of lungs and chest wall. Whereas, the elastic resistance obtained from alveoli filled with air, measures both the soft tissue elastic resistance of lungs and chest wall and the elastic resistance due to surface tension of alveoli **(Table 8 and Fig. 14)**.

Normally, the elastic resistance due to the surface tension of alveoli is reduced by the presence of surfactant. In the absence of surfactant, the alveoli will collapse due to increased surface tension, producing increased inward retraction force, especially during expiration, when the alveoli are gradually becoming smaller. This is because when the alveoli are gradually becoming more and more small, then the surface tension in alveoli gradually increases, following the Laplace law. This is because as the fluid molecules, present on the surface of alveoli, come more and more close with the reduction of the diameter of alveoli during expiration, then the attraction force between these fluid molecules increases. This surface tension has theoretically two disadvantages:

1. Smaller alveoli have greater surface tension and have more tendency to collapse than a larger alveoli. So, each small alveolus will progressively discharge its air into a large one and ultimately a gigantic alveolus would be left.
2. The retractile forces of lung due to increased surface tension should increase as the lung volume gradually decreases. So, the lung volume will decrease in vicious manner and ultimately it will completely collapse.

This above phenomenon can be explained by the *Laplace law*. According to the *Laplace law: P = 2T/r*. Here, P is the pressure at inside of alveolus which increases or decreases according to the size of alveolus and again it depends on surface tension. T is the surface tension and r is the radius of alveoli. From Laplace law, it is easily understood that smaller alveoli with smaller radius (r) have increased intra-alveolar

pressure (P) which indicates its collapsing nature due to increased inward retraction force or increased surface tension (T). On the other hand, we can say that the collapse of alveoli is more likely when the surface tension increases or alveolar size decreases. Thus, the alveolar collapse (for that intra-alveolar pressure or P) is directly proportional to surface tension (T) and inversely proportional to the radius of alveolus (r).

Moreover, within the alveolus the ability of surfactant to reduce surface tension is directly proportional to its concentration. So, when the alveoli become smaller during expiration or due to any cause, the concentration of surfactant on the lining fluid of alveoli will be increased and the surface tension will be more effectively reduced offsetting the increased surface tension due to the reduction of the size of alveoli. Alternatively, when the alveoli are over distended, the concentration of surfactant on the lining fluid of alveoli is reduced and the surface tension is less effectively reduced.

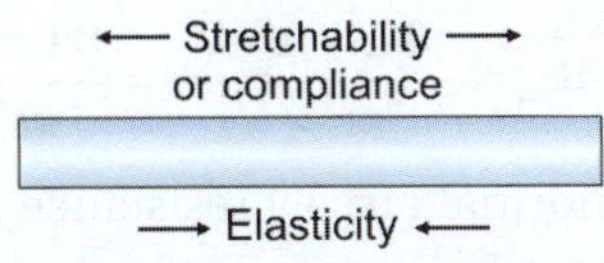

Fig. 15: Compliance.

Thus, a balance is reached when larger alveoli are prevented from overdistention and smaller alveoli are prevented from collapse.

Compliance

Compliance is also termed as "stretch-ability (inflate-ability)". In character, it is opposite to elasticity (retract-ability or contract-ability) which is described before. Elasticity tries to squeeze (or deflate) the lungs and chest wall, and offers resistance for air to flow into lungs. Whereas, it (this elasticity) is countered by the stretch-ability of both lungs and chest wall which is called the compliance. Thus, the elastic resistance which prevents the air to flow into lungs is measured indirectly in the form of stretch-ability or compliance which facilitates the air to flow into lungs **(Fig. 15)**.

For air to flow into lungs, a pressure gradient must have to be developed which will help to overcome the elastic and nonelastic resistance of lungs and chest wall. *So, the compliance (C) is defined as the unit change in volume of lung for unit change in developed pressure and is calculated by dividing the total change in volume (ΔV) of lung by the total distending pressure (ΔP) which causes this change. Whereas, the resistance is defined as the total changes in distending pressure divided by the total changes in the volume of lungs.* Thus, C (L/cmH$_2$O) = ΔV (in L)/ΔP (cmH$_2$O) and R = $\Delta P/\Delta V$ or 1/C

Compliance is usually measured under static condition, i.e., at equilibrium during a particular moment and at that moment airway resistance is zero as air flow is stopped. *Dynamic lung compliance (Cdyn)* is measured during rhythmic breathing and is also dependent on airway resistance.

Compliance may be calculated individually by taking only the compliance of chest wall (Cw) or the compliance of lung (C$_L$) component separately or both together (C$_T$). So, the equation of compliance for individual component can be represented as:

- C$_L$ in L/cmH$_2$O = Change in lung volume/change in transpulmonary pressure = ΔV in L/transpulmonary pressure gradient or (P$_A$ – P$_{Pl}$) cmH$_2$O [P$_A$ = alveolar pressure, P$_{Pl}$ = intrapleural pressure]
- C$_W$ in L/cmH$_2$O = Change in chest volume/Change in transthoracic or transmural pressure = ΔV L/transmural pressure gradient or (P$_{Pl}$ – P$_{atmos}$) cmH$_2$O [P$_{atmos}$ = atmospheric pressure] **(Figs. 16A to C)**.

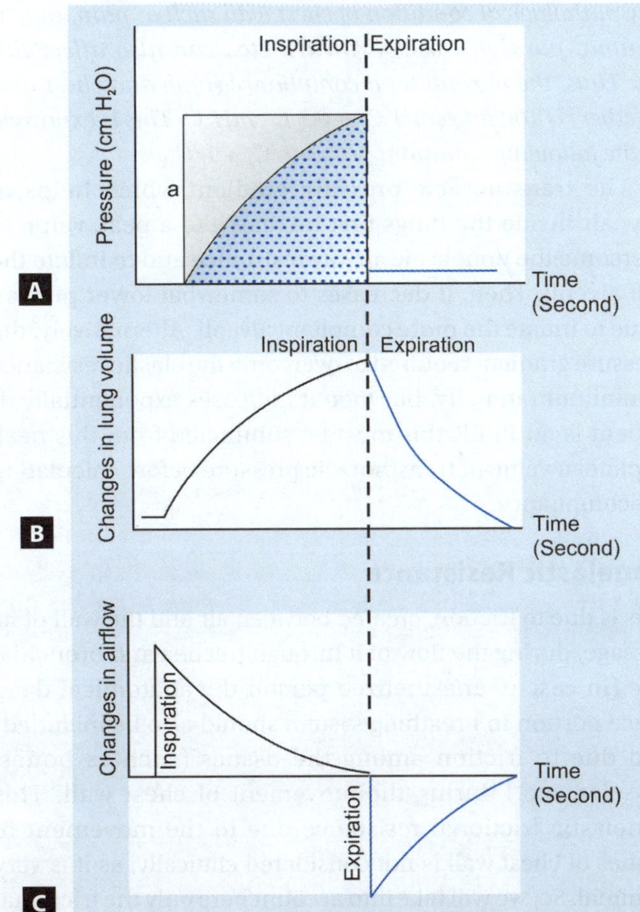

Figs. 16A to C: Figure A represents the graphic changes in intrapulmonary pressure during intermittent positive pressure ventilation (IPPV) when a constant pressure is applied (square wave). Line a represents the sudden rise of intrapulmonary pressure produced by a pressure gradient to overcome the both elastic and nonelastic airway resistance. Among these, the dotted area represents the nonelastic airway resistance and the non-dotted area represents the elastic resistance. The pressure gradient to overcome the nonelastic resistance is maximum initially and then decreases exponentially. Whereas, the pressure gradient requires to overcome the elastic resistance is minimum initially and then increases exponentially. Alveolar filling ceases when the pressure from elastic forces balance the applied pressure. Expiration is passive and intrapulmonary pressure suddenly comes down to zero level with the ending of inspiration and initiation of expiration. Figures B and C show the changes in lung volume and airflow respectively which correspond to the Figure A.

Thus C$_T$ L/cmH$_2$O = ΔV L/transthoracic pressure gradient or (P$_A$ – P$_{atmos}$) cmH$_2$O [C$_T$ is the total compliance].

$$\text{Raw (cmH}_2\text{O/L/s)} = \frac{\text{P(cmH}_2\text{O)V}}{\text{(L/s)}}$$

The normal C$_L$ value is 200 mL/cmH$_2$O or 0.2 L/cmH$_2$O. Any pathological condition of lungs such as pulmonary edema, atelectasis, emphysema, etc., can affect this C$_L$. The normal C$_W$ value is also 200 mL/cmH$_2$O or 0.2 L/cmH$_2$O.

Any pathological condition of chest wall such as pain, injury, trauma, paralysis, osteoarthritis, etc., can also affect this C_W. Thus, the normal total compliance (lung and chest wall together) is 100 mL/cmH_2O or 0.1 L/cmH_2O. This is expressed by the following equation: $1/C_T = 1/C_L + 1/C_W$

The transthoracic pressure gradient which helps to flow air inside the lungs first increases to a peak value to overcome the nonelastic airway resistance and to inflate the stiff alveoli. Then, it decreases to somewhat lower plateau value to inflate the more compliant alveoli. Alternatively, the pressure gradient required to overcome the elastic resistance is minimum initially, but then it increases exponentially. If patient is on PEEP, this must be subtracted from this peak or plateau value of transthoracic pressure before calculating the compliance.

Nonelastic Resistance

This is due to friction, created between air and the wall of its passage, during the flow of it through trachea and bronchial tree (in case of anesthetized person the anatomical dead space portion in breathing system should also be included) and due to friction among the tissues (such as bones, muscles, etc.) during the movement of chest wall. This nonelastic frictional resistance due to the movement of tissues of chest wall is not considered clinically, as it is very minimal. So, we will take into account here only the frictional resistance due to the flow of air through tracheobronchial tree. Usually, there are three patterns of airflow: (1) laminar flow, (2) turbulent flow, and (3) orifice flow.

The laminar flow occurs in tubes where its sides are parallel. It can be thought as concentric cylinders of gases, flowing at different velocities and this velocity is greatest at center and lowest at periphery. The *resistance to air flow (laminar or turbulent) is not constant. It increases in proportion (direct) to gas flow. Moreover, it directly proportional to gas density and inversely proportional to the fifth power of the radius of tube. As a result turbulent flow is extremely sensitive to radius of airways.*

For an air to flow, a pressure gradient has to be developed and during this flow of air due to friction between the air and its wall resistance is developed. So, the relationship between the developed pressure gradient (P), airway resistance (R_{aw}) and the rate of flow of air or the change in the volume of lungs can be calculated from an equation. This equation is:
Flow = Pressure gradient/Resistances or

Resistance = Pressure gradient/Flow

According to Poiseuille's law:

Pressure gradient (P) = Flow (V) × 8 length of tube (L) × viscosity (μ)/π × radius⁴ (r^4). Therefore, resistance (R_{aw}) will be:

$$R_{aw} = \frac{8\,L \times \mu \times V}{\pi r^4 \times V} = \frac{8\,L \times \mu}{\pi r^4}$$

The value of normal airway resistance is 0.5–2 cmH_2O/L/s. When the flow of air exceeds the *critical velocity*, then the laminar flow becomes turbulent. The important feature of this *turbulent flow* is that the drop of pressure during the flow of air along the airway is not directly proportional to the flow rate, but is proportional to the square of it. Therefore, the pressure increases much more than the increase in flow. So, the resistance in turbulent flow will also increase much more than the laminar flow and is proportional to the gas flow which is opposite to the laminar flow. Therefore, in the turbulent flow the equation of Poiseuille's law is:

$$\text{Pressure gradient} = \frac{V^2 \times \text{Gas density}}{r^5}$$

Therefore, during turbulent flow the resistance (R_w) = P/V

$$\text{or, } R_{aw} = \frac{V^2 \times \text{Gas density}}{r^5 \times V} = \frac{V \times \text{Gas density}}{r^5}$$

So, the nonelastic airway resistance in turbulent flow is directly proportional to the amount of flow (V) and the density of gas and is inversely proportional to the fifth power of the radius (r^5). Therefore, the turbulent flow is extremely sensitive to the airway caliber **(Table 9)**.

The turbulence air flow generally occurs (i) during high gas flow, (ii) at the sharp angles of airways, and (iii) during the certain changes in airway diameter. Whether the flow will be turbulent or laminar, usually depends on Reynolds number. The equation of Reynolds number is:

$$\text{Reynolds number} = \frac{\text{Linear velocity} \times \text{Diameter} \times \text{Gas density}}{\text{Gas viscosity}}$$

If the Reynolds number is below 1,000, then the flow of gas will be laminar. Whereas, if Reynolds number is above, 1500, then the flow of gas will be turbulent. The gases with low density/viscosity ratio have less Reynolds number and produce the laminar flow. Thus, they reduce the airway resistance. For example, helium (He) and O_2 mixture has least density/viscosity ratio and less likely to cause turbulent flow with reducing airway resistance. So, it is useful clinically during severe turbulent flow caused by the upper airway obstruction.

TABLE 9: Density/viscosity ratio of O_2, N_2O, and He.

Gases	Density	Viscosity	Density/Viscosity
O_2	1.11	1.11	1.0
N_2O and O_2 (60:40)	1.41	0.89	1.49
He and O_2 (80:20)	0.33	1.08	0.31

The orifice flow occurs when it meets a severe constriction. The equation for orifice flow is equal to the turbulent flow. So, here the drop of pressure or the gradient is proportional to the square of flow rate and gas density replaces its viscosity. As density is used as a numerator in the equation of resistance of gas flow, so it is easily understood why the low density gas such as helium diminishes the resistance to flow. It diminishes the flow of resistance three-fold as compared to air in severe obstruction.

The orifice flow occurs in larynx. Whereas the turbulent flow is mainly confined to trachea, main bronchi, and other secondary and tertiary bronchi during most of the respiratory cycle. On the other hand, laminar flow is found in airway whose diameter is below 1 mm (<1 mm). This is because though the division and subdivision of airways below the principal, segmental, and tertiary bronchi reduce the individual diameter, but the total cross-sectional area of airway increases due to this branching. Thus, the resistance to air flow in large bronchi is low because of their large diameter and also the resistance in small bronchi is low because of their large total cross-sectional area. So, the velocity of air flow also decreases causing laminar flow. But during bronchoconstriction, the diameters of smaller bronchi and bronchioles reach such a critical level that the laminar flow is converted to turbulent flow with increase of resistance.

WORK OF BREATHING

Ventilation is the main function of lungs. So, for ventilation air has to enter into it. But, three resistance factors have to be overcome for entry of air into lungs. These are: (i) elastic recoiling resistance of chest wall and lungs (elastic resistance), (ii) frictional resistance due to flow of air into airways (nonelastic resistance), and (iii) tissue frictional resistance (nonelastic resistance). So, for breathing work has to be done by respiratory muscles to overcome all these three resistance by stretching the elastic tissues of lungs and chest wall (elastic resistance work) and by moving the nonelastic tissues such as bones and muscles of chest wall (viscous resistance work) and thus by creating a pressure gradient which helps to move the air through airways overcoming frictional resistance from air and airways (airway frictional resistance work). Thus, the total work of breathing, done by inspiratory muscles against all these resistance during inspiration is stored as potential energy in these muscles. Later, it is used passively during expiration to expel the gases. So, the overcoming of expiratory resistance in normal individual is nonactive (used from stored energy) as the entire expiratory cycle is passive. But, this is not applicable in obstructive airway diseases, where expiration is also active.

The increased inspiratory resistance is overcome by the increased effort of inspiratory muscles. But, when the expiratory resistance increases, then the lung volume also increases as a compensatory phenomenon to such a level that tidal volume (VT) reaches to FRC level. Thus, the greater energy stored at a higher lung volume, by more active contraction of inspiratory muscles, tries to overcome the added expiratory resistance. Except that excess expiratory resistance also stimulates the expiratory muscles to work more **(Figs. 17A and B)**.

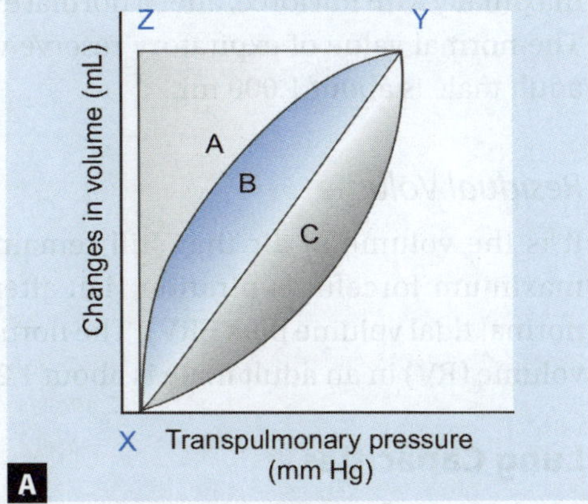

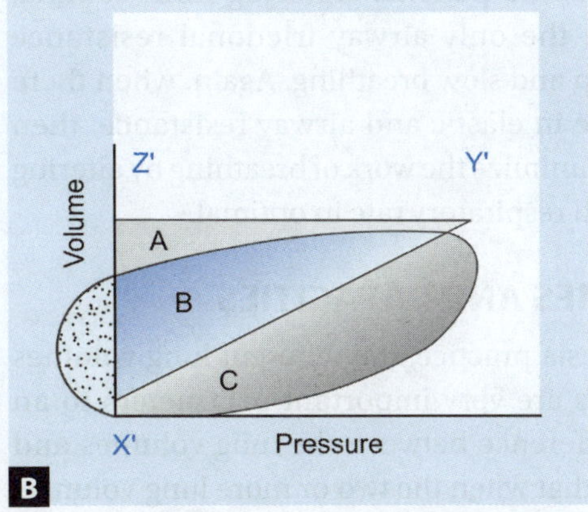

Figs. 17A and B: Pressure and volume curve or the compliance of lung. Figure A is for the normal patient and Figure B is for the anesthetized patient. In Figure A, the XY line indicates compliance which is about 100 mL/cmH$_2$O. In Figure B the X 'Y' line indicates compliance which is about 50 mL/cmH$_2$O. Figure A is the picture of highly compliant, small, dependent alveoli situated at the base of the lung. Whereas Figure B is the picture of less compliant, medium-sized alveoli situated normally in the middle of the lung. The dimensions of pressure multiplied by volume are the work of breathing. In the picture, the total area shown by A, B, and C represents the total work of breathing. The blue area B represents the inspiratory work necessary to overcome the airflow resistance during inspiration. The triangle XYZ represents the fraction of total inspiratory work which is necessary to overcome the elastic resistance. The area C represents the passive expiratory work. In Figure B, the dotted area represents the active expiratory work necessary to overcome the airflow resistance during forced expiration.

We know: Work = Force × Distance. But, Force = Pressure × Area and Distance = Volume/Area. Thus, Work = Pressure × Volume. So, the respiratory work (g × cm) can be expressed as the product of pressure (g/cm^2) and volume (cm^3).

During optimum conditions, in a normal healthy adult, the respiratory muscles work only with 10% efficiency and 90% energy is dissipated as heat due to elastic and airway frictional resistance. For that, only 2–3% of total O_2 consumption of body is used. But, it can raise up to 50%, if the patient suffers from pulmonary diseases. The estimated total work for quite breathing in a healthy adult ranges from 0.3 to 0.8 kg/m/minute.

When the work of breathing is increased by increasing only the depth of respiration, but not the rate of respiration, then the work done only against nonelastic airway resistance will increase. On the other hand, when the work of breathing is increased by increasing the respiratory rate, then the work done only against the airway frictional resistance will increase. Thus, when these two phenomenons are summed up, then there is optimal increase in the depth and frequency of respiration, where the total increase in work of breathing is minimal. This phenomenon can be explained by another way. The increased work required to overcome increased elastic resistance is accomplished by not increasing tidal volume (V_T) or depth of respiration, but by increasing the rate of respiration. Whereas the increased work required to overcome increased airway frictional resistance is accomplished by not increasing the respiratory rate, but by increasing the depth of respiration. So, patients suffering from pulmonary edema, interstitial fibrosis, etc., where elastic resistance increases favor rapid and shallow breathing. Whereas, the patients suffering from asthma, COPD, etc., where the only airway frictional resistance increases favor deep and slow breathing. Again, when there is both the increase in elastic and airway resistance, then the patient tries to minimize the work of breathing by altering the tidal volume and respiratory rate in optimal.

■ LUNG VOLUMES AND CAPACITIES

For clinical anesthesia practice, the different lung volumes and lung capacities are very important parameters to an anesthetist. The difference between the lung volumes and lung capacities are that when the two or more lung volumes are combined together, then we get the lung capacities. There are four basic lung volumes which are usually measured. Then, from these four basic lung volumes, the different lung capacities are computed. As for examples, the sum of these four basic lung volumes which are described below is equal to the maximum capacity of lung, i.e., the total lung capacity (TLC) to which both the lungs can be maximally inflated.

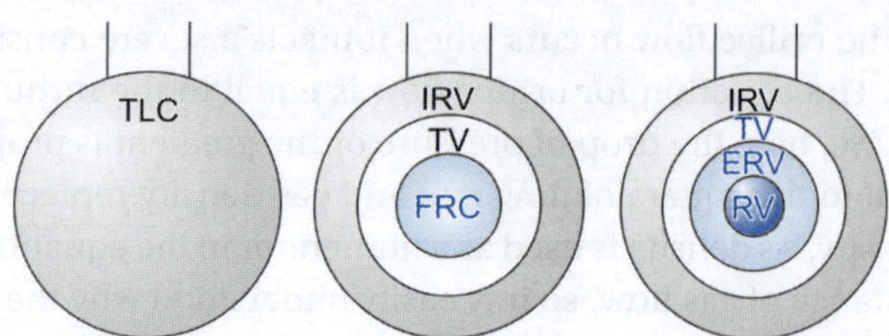

Fig. 18: Different lung volumes. (ERV: expiratory reserve volume; IRV: inspiratory reserve volume; RV: residual volume; TLC: total lung capacity: TV: tidal volume)

The simple method of studying different lung volumes is called the spirometry and the instrument is called the spirometer **(Fig. 18)**.

Lung Volumes

Tidal Volume (V$_T$)

It is the volume of air which is inspired or expired during each normal breathing. The normal value of inspiratory or expiratory tidal volume (V_T) in an adult male is about 500 mL.

Inspiratory Reserve Volume

It is the maximum extra volume of air that can be inspired with full force, *after* a normal inspired tidal volume. The normal value of inspiratory reserve volume (IRV) in an adult male is about 3,000 mL.

Expiratory Reserve Volume

Similar to IRV, it is the extra volume of air that can be expired maximally with full force, after a normal expired tidal volume. The normal value of expiratory reserve volume (ERV) in an adult male is about 1,000 mL.

Residual Volume

It is the volume of air that still remains in lungs, after a maximum forceful expiration (i.e. after the expiration of normal tidal volume plus ERV). The normal value of residual volume (RV) in an adult male is about 1,200 mL **(Fig. 19)**.

Lung Capacities

Inspiratory Capacity

It is the inspiratory tidal volume plus the IRV (i.e., IC = inspiratory V_T + IRV) after a normal expiration. So, it is the amount of air that a person can forcefully maximally inspire after a normal expiration. The normal value of inspiratory capacity (IC) in an adult male is about 3,500 mL (500 mL +3,000 mL).

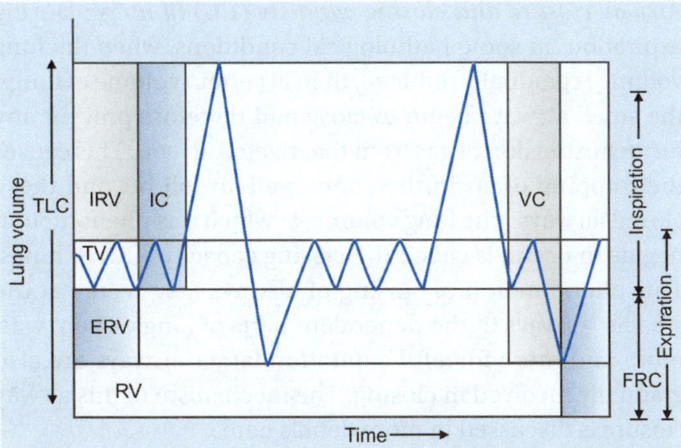

Fig. 19: The graphical representation of different lung volumes. (ERV: expiratory reserve volume; FRC: functional residual capacity; IC: inspiratory capacity; IRV: inspiratory reserve volume; RV: residual volume; TLC: total lung capacity; TV: tidal volume; VC: vital capacity)

Functional Residual Capacity

It is the volume of air which is equal to ERV plus RV (i.e., FRC = ERV + RV). So, the FRC is the amount of air that remains in lungs after a normal tidal expiration or at the beginning of normal tidal inspiration. The normal value of FRC in an adult male is about 2,200 mL (1,000 mL + 1,200 mL). It is a very important parameter for lung function test in clinical anesthesia practice, because its value markedly changes in different types of pulmonary diseases. So, it is often desired to measure this parameter. The FRC cannot be measured directly from spirometer, because RV cannot be measured directly, as it never be expired on spirometer for its measurement. But, this volume (RV) constitutes near about half of FRC. So, to measure FRC, spirometer is used indirectly by (i) applying N_2 washout method, (ii) helium wash out (or dilution) method, or (iii) body plethysmograph. *The significance of FRC parameter is that it indicates a volume of lung at the end of normal tidal expiration, where the inward elastic recoil property of lung becomes equivalent to or is balanced by the outward stretching forces on lung, which is called the compliance of lung. The outward stretching forces on lungs include negative intrapleural pressure and outward elastic recoil force of chest wall.* The FRC also defines a volume of lung from where, in normal breathing, inspiratory tidal volume starts to take place. There are multiple factors which affect this FRC. These are:

- *Height, sex, and age:* FRC is directly proportional to height. Female has 10% less FRC value than male. Pregnancy is associated with tremendous reduction of FRC. The relation between the age and FRC is discussed later under the heading of CC.
- *Posture:* FRC is reduced in supine or prone from upright position. This is due to the reduction of chest compliance in lying-down condition, as the diaphragm is pushed upward by abdominal viscera. Up to 30° change in inclination from upright 90° position, there is no change in FRC. But, it occurs maximally between 60 and 90° downward inclination from upright position.
- *Obesity:* Obesity is inversely proportional to FRC. This is because, it directly reduces the chest wall compliance and indirectly reduces the lung compliance. Height is also an important determining factor of FRC and is also directly proportional.
- *Lung diseases:* Any pulmonary disease which affect the compliance of lung or chest wall or both (characteristic of restrictive pulmonary disorder) are associated with low FRC.
- *Anesthesia:* Induction of anesthesia also reduces FRC. It is due to both decrease in compliance and increase in elastic recoil property of lung in anesthesia during both spontaneous respiration and IPPV.
- *Postoperative period:* FRC is also reduced in post-operative period due to abdominal distention, pneumoperitoneum, spasm of abdominal and thoracic muscles due to pain, etc.
- *PEEP:* Positive end-expiratory pressure always increases FRC and is an important mode of management in different lung diseases where FRC < CC.
- *Diaphragmatic tone:* Normally, the diaphragmatic tone contributes for a part of FRC. Decreased diaphragmatic tone is responsible for decreased FRC. This is evident during phrenic nerve paralysis.

During expiration, the lung is reduced in volume and there comes a point at which some small airways begin to close. This volume of lung when the small airways begin to close during forceful expiration is called the CC. On the other hand, the closing volume (CV) is the volume of lung when all the airways are closed during forceful expiration. Then, the remaining volume of the lung is the residual volume. So CC = CV + RV **(Figs. 20 and 21)**.

Vital Capacity

Vital capacity (VC) is a frequently measured clinical index of pulmonary function test. It is the largest amount of air that can be expired after a maximal inspiratory effort. It equals to the IRV plus V_T plus ERV. The normal value of VC in an adult male is about 4,500 mL/or 60–70 mL/kg. The fraction of VC which is expired in the first 1 second during forced expiration is also an important parameter for lung function test and gives additional information. This is designated as FEVI and is called the timed VC. For example, in some disease where

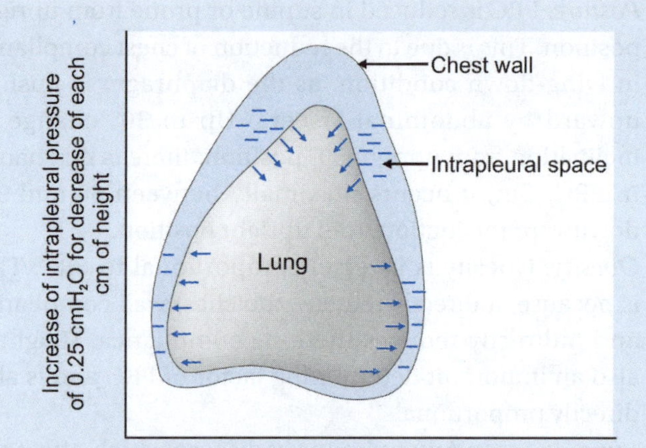

Fig. 20: Lung is a viscoelastic structure, like gel. So, it tends to collapse from chest wall and tries to take a globular shape. Due to this gel like property of lung tissue, the top of the lung collapses inward and the base of the lung tries to spread outward. Thus, a relatively more negative pressure is created at the apex of intrapleural space and a relatively less negative pressure is created at the base of intrapleural space. So, the intrapleural pressure increases (becomes less negative) from top to bottom of the lung by 0.25 cmH₂O per cm of decrease of height.

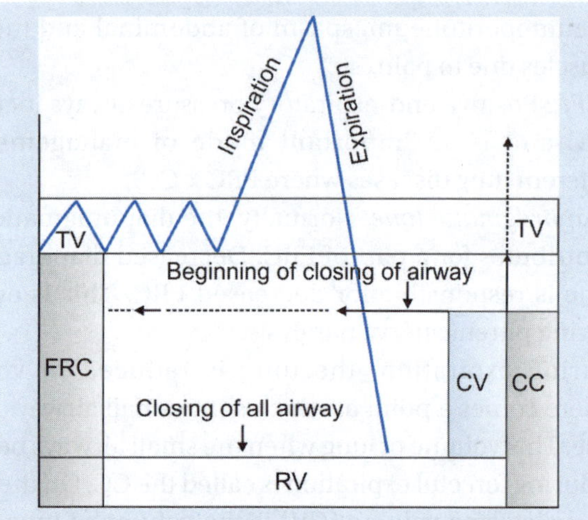

Fig. 21: The relationship between the functional residual capacity (FRC), closing capacity (CC), and closing volume (CV). (RV: residual volume; TV: tidal volume)

airway resistance is increased such as in asthma, COPD, etc., VC may be normal, but the FEVI is reduced. It gives a useful information about the strength of respiratory muscles. In addition to the body height, weight, posture, etc., VC is also dependent on the chest and the lung compliance.

Total Lung Capacity

It is defined as the maximum volume of lungs which can be inflated with the greatest possible effort. It equals to the VC + RV. The normal value of TLC in an adult male is about 6,000 mL **(Fig. 21)**.

Airway closure and closing capacity (CC) of lungs: During expiration, in some pathological conditions, when the lung volume is gradually reduced, then at certain volume of lungs, the small airways begin to close and therefore prevent any further expulsion of gas from that related alveoli. This causes the trapping of air in the concerned alveoli beyond these closed airways. The lung volume, at which this phenomenon begins to occur, is called the closing capacity (CC) of lungs. This phenomenon of closing of airways first occurs at the smaller airways in the dependent parts of lungs. Then, with more and more forceful expiration larger airways are also gradually involved in closing. The mechanism of this airway closure is discussed in more details here.

The lung is made of a viscoelastic tissue. So, it tries to take the globular shape within the chest wall. Thus, the apex of the lungs collapse inward and the bottom of the lungs spread outward. So, a negative intrapleural pressure is created at the apex of the lung and a relatively positive (less negative than the apex) intrapleural pressure is created at the base of the lung. Hence, normally the intrapleural pressure increases from above downward (though both are negative) by 0.25 cmH₂O for each centimeter of change in the height of the lung. This intensity of negative intrapleural pressure determines the regional alveolar size and the regional difference in the compliance and the ventilation of alveoli **(Fig. 20)**.

At normal resting end expiratory volume of lung (or FRC), the gradient (difference) between these two distending transpulmonary and transmural pressure is –5 cmH₂O. This negative gradient (outward direction) of pressure makes the airway patent at the end of tidal expiration. During inspiration, this pressure gradient increases more to –7 cmH₂O which causes the more dilatation (patency) of airway and entry of air into alveoli. Then, after inspiration, expiration starts and it is passive. During expiration, the intra-alveolar pressure is increased and this is due to the elastic recoil property of lungs and the passive inward movement of chest wall. So, air comes out and the gradient between the transpulmonary and transmural pressure increases (becomes less negative) to –3 cmH₂O. But, still, as this pressure gradient is still negative, so it still favors the patency of small noncartilaginous airway. But, during forced expiration in a normal lung, this pressure gradient increases far above the atmospheric pressure and is transferred to the alveoli and the small airways which tries to expel the air from alveoli, but closes the airways. Actually, during expiration the intra-alveolar pressure is 2 cmH₂O higher than this pressure gradient due to the addition of elastic recoil property of alveolar septa. During exhalation of air through airways, the intraluminal pressure in airways gradually comes down along the length of airways from alveoli to bronchi. Along the airway from alveoli to bronchi, at a point where this pressure gradient becomes greater than the airway intraluminal pressure, then the airway closes. This point is called the *equal pressure point (EPP)*. When this EPP falls on the airways which are distal to the 11th generation of division and have no cartilages, then they close during expiration at certain lung volume. But, when this EPP falls on airways which are proximal to the 11th generation of division and have cartilages, then they (airways) are held open by these cartilages. The progressive movement of EPP from larger to smaller airways depends on the lung volumes and the force of expiration. When the lung volume decreases more and more or the expiration becomes more and more powerful, then the EPP moves progressively from smaller to larger airways and more and more airways close. The volume of lung at which the smaller noncartilaginous airways begin to close in the dependent areas of lungs is called the *CC* of lung. *Residual volume is also included in this CC.*

The CC is measured by the single breath N_2-washout technique. In this process during breathing of normal air, the individual will slowly expire up to RV. Then, he will slowly take a single breath of 100% O_2 up to his maximum inhalation which will be held for few seconds and after that it will be expired slowly. During expiration, the N_2 concentration and the volume of expired air is measured and recorded serially. Thus, a characteristics curve is obtained. This curve has four phases: Phase (I) dead space gas, Phase (II) mixed dead space and alveolar gas, Phase (III) mixed alveolar gas from all the alveoli, and a phase (IV) at which there is sudden increase in concentration of N_2. The CC is the volume at which phase IV begins **(Fig. 22)**.

The explanation is as follows. During inspiration, the oxygen is preferentially distributed to the smaller alveoli at the dependent part of the lungs. This is due to the shape of the alveolar compliance curve which causes a larger change in the volume of smaller alveoli at the bottom of the lungs than the larger one at the apex of it. Therefore, N_2 will be more diluted by O_2 in the smaller alveoli at the bottom of the lung. During expiration, the initial exhaled gas (phase I) is the gas that filled the anatomical dead space and consequently contains no N_2. This is followed by a mixture of dead space and alveolar gas (phase II) which contains N_2. So, N_2 concentration will suddenly increase in this phase. Then in next phase, the gas other than in dead space which has already been expelled in previous phase is expelled, containing gases coming from all the alveoli of lungs. This indicates phase III. Here, the N_2 concentration remains constant and maintains a plateau level, as the expired air is coming from all the alveoli without any closer of the airway. This phase will continue until the point at which airway closure begins. At this moment, the N_2 concentration suddenly again increases and the phase IV

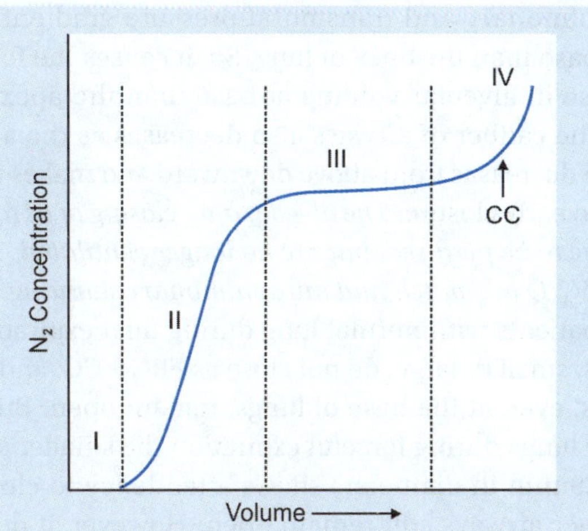

Fig. 22: Nitrogen washout technique for measuring the closing capacity (CC), functional residual capacity (FRC), and dead space. First patient will take a deep breath of pure O_2 (100%). Then he will exhale steadily while the N_2 concentration in the expired air is continuously measured and a graph is prepared. Initially in phase I, the expired gas does not contain any N_2 as it comes from the anatomical dead space. This is followed by phase II which contains the mixture of dead space gas and alveolar gas. Here, the concentration of N_2 in expired gas rises steadily as more and more alveolar gas containing N_2 is expired. Then comes the phase III where the concentration of N_2 in expired air takes a plateau level. This is because the expired gas in this phase contains only the alveolar gas which comes from all types of alveoli from top to the bottom of lungs and contains an average fixed concentration of N_2. Phase III terminates at CC and is followed by phase IV during which the N_2 content of the expired gas increases suddenly. CC is the lung volume [above residual volume (RV)] when the airways in the lower dependent parts of the lungs begin to close. The gas in the upper portion of lung is richer in N_2 than the gas in the lower dependent portion. This is because the alveoli in the upper portion of lung are more distend and less compliant at the start of the inspiration of O_2. So, they undergo less ventilated and subsequently, the N_2 in them is less diluted by O_2. Therefore, the expired gas in phase IV comes mainly from upper part of the lungs containing more N_2 as the airways in the lower part of the lung closes. Phase III has a slight positive slope even before phase IV. This indicates that even during phase III, there is gradual increase in the portion of the expired gas which comes from the relatively N_2-rich upper part of the lung. The volume of the dead space is the volume of gas expired from beginning of expiration to the mid portion of phase II.

begins. The volume of lung at the beginning of phase IV is the CC. This is because the expulsion of gases from the smaller airways ceases and exhalation is continued from those areas of lungs (i.e., apex of lung) where the nitrogen concentration is higher due to the less dilution by O_2. Instead of N_2, other tracer gases such as argon, helium, [133]xenon, etc., also may be used in a similar way.

Thus, the lung volume above the residual volume at which these small airways begin to close is called the CC. It usually starts at the dependent part of lungs, because the distending transpulmonary and transmural pressure gradient is less at the base than the apex of lung. So, it causes the four-fold decrease in alveolar volume at base than the apex of the lung. The caliber of airways also decreases as the alveolar volume decreases from above downward and makes it more prone to early closure. *The alveoli, after closing of its airways, continue to be perfused, but are no longer ventilated. Thus, it causes V_A/Q mismatch and intrapulmonary shunting.*

In patients with normal lung during tidal expiration the airways, small or large, do not close as FRC > CC, and all the airways, even at the base of lungs, remain open. But, with normal lungs during forceful expiration the smaller airways (0.5–.0.9 mm in diameter) shows a tendency to close and the larger airways still remain open. However, it does not produce any impact on PaO_2 or $PaCO_2$. Now, if due to any reason CC increases above FRC or FRC goes much below the CC level, then more and more airways close and causes hypoxia and hypercarbia.

Closing capacity is normally well below FRC. But, it rises steadily with age. This increase of CC above FRC with increase in age is responsible for the normal age-related decline in arterial O_2 tension. At an average age of 44 years, CC is equal to FRC in supine position. Then, at an average age of 66 years, the CC is equal to or exceeds FRC in upright position in most individuals. Unlike FRC, the CC is unaffected by posture. The CC also approaches or exceeds FRC in morbidly obese patients.

In patients with emphysema, bronchitis, asthma, pulmonary edema, etc., the early airway closer occurs with mild active expiration, and at higher lung volumes. In all these conditions, the airway resistance also increases. This causes larger pressure decrease along the airways from alveoli to larger bronchi. Thus, it creates a potential for positive intrapulmonary and intra-airway pressure gradient which causes early closing of airways and trapping of air in alveoli. Moreover, the structural integrity of airways is lost due to inflammation and scaring during the disease process. Therefore, these airways are easily collapsed or closed at higher lung volumes and low pressure gradient **(Fig. 23)**.

In emphysema, the airways are poorly supported (or stretched) due to the loss of lung parenchyma and the intraluminal pressure becomes quickly negative. So, the EPP shifts close to the alveolus. Therefore, with only a mild forced expiration the airway closes early. Thus, the use of PEEP or CPAP in an emphysematous patient maintains the intraluminal pressure and prevents the airway collapse. In asthma, due to bronchospasm the middle-sized airways are narrowed. During forced expiration they are further narrowed by positive intrapulmonary intraluminal pressure gradient. Thus PEEP or CPAP is also important to maintain the airway in asthma patient.

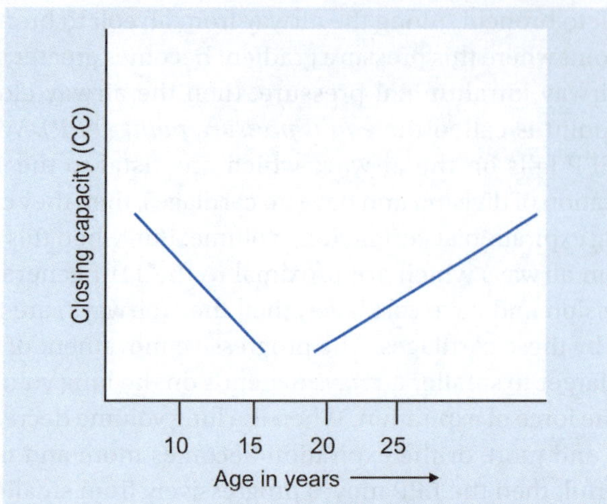

Fig. 23: The relationship between the age in years and the closing capacity in normal subject.

Closing capacity is also expressed as the percentage of TLC. It is obtained by adding CV with the residual volume. In healthy individual, CC is normally well below FRC. But it rises steadily with age and is the probable explanation for the normal age-related decline in PaO_2. At the age of 60 years, CC = FRC in upright position, but CC > FRC in supine position. On the other hand, at the age of 40 years CC < FRC in upright position but CC = FRC in supine position. Thus, in subject with normal lung CC becomes equal to FRC in age of 60 years in upright position and in the age of 40 years in supine position. CC is minimum at teenage between 15 and 20 years. Before 15 years and after 20 years CC continues to increase and tries to touch the FRC. Except age and position, smoking and obesity also affect CC. They decrease FRC and increase CC.

Relationship between FRC and CC: The FRC and CC relationship is very important than the consideration of FRC and CC separately. Because this relationship will determine, whether a given lung unit will remain in normal, atelectatic, or in low V_A/Q ratio state. FRC is the normal resting *end-expiratory lung volume* whereas CC is the *expiratory lung volume when airways begin to close during expiration.* In normal situation, FRC > CC. It means during normal expiration, after the end of inspiration of tidal volume, when lung volume is gradually decreasing then FRC does not reduced to CC level, where airways start to close. But, this may happen, even in normal lungs when the patient tries to expire forcefully and FRC goes below the level of CC. So, in normal healthy patient with expiration of tidal volume small airways and alveoli remain open during both inspiratory and expiratory phase and help in adequate gas exchange with normal V_A/Q ratio **(Figs. 24A to C)**.

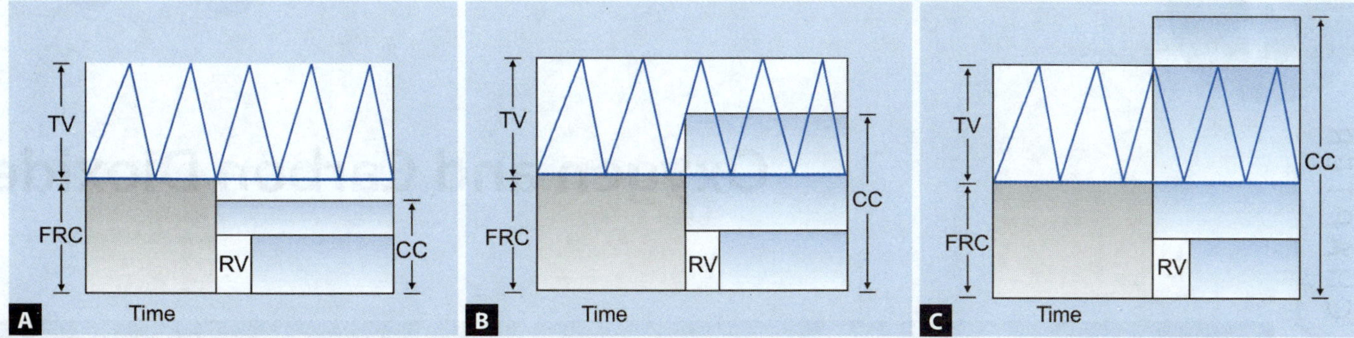

Figs. 24A to C: These three figures show the relationship between FRC and CC, which result in normal to low V_A/V_Q ratio (ventilation perfusion ratio) causing atelectasis. FRC is the percentage of total lung capacity (TLC) that exists at the end of normal (tidal) expiration. Normally (in Figure A), the closing capacity remains below the FRC level and the alveoli open and empty fully, before the airway closes or the airway does not close before the end of expiration. Increase in CC above FRC means airway closes before full exhalation during normal inspiration and expiration. When CC rises up to the middle level of tidal volume (TV) (in Figure B), then alveoli open and close partially and tidal volume is reduced to half. When CC level rises above the level of TV (in Figure C), then alveoli never open and atelectasis results. (CC: closing capacity; FRC: functional residual capacity; RV: residual volume)

In pathological condition, FRC can decrease relative to CC or the CC can increase relative to FRC, thus changing the equation FRC > CC to CC = FRC or CC > FRC. So, in such condition, before the completion of expiration up to its tidal level or before reaching the volume of FRC, the airways start to close, i.e., CC volume reaches. Thus, during the entire period of inspiration, the airways remain open and air enters the alveoli. But, during the middle of expiration, when FRC goes below the level CC (as the level of CC is increased) or before reaching the full tidal volume, airways start to close. This causes the stoppage of ventilation and the stoppage of gas exchange and makes these areas of lungs of low V_A/Q ratio. If the value of CC lies in between the upper and lower limit of tidal volume, then as the lung volume increases during inspiration, some previously closed airways (which occur during the previous expiration) will open for a short time. Then, when during expiration lung volume recedes and FRC once again goes below the CC (but within the range of tidal volume), the airways close. Thus, during the closing and opening of airways at expiration and inspiration, they will open for short period with less time in participating for fresh gas exchange, causing low V_A/Q ratio with hypoxemia.

In severe pathological conditions, when the value of CC rises above the level of the upper limit of inspiratory tidal volume, then the equation will be CC >> FRC, i.e., the level of CC at much higher level than FRC. In such situation, as the CC always lies above the upper limit of tidal inspiratory volume, so no airway will open even during normal inspiration. Thus, all the alveoli will remain close both during inspiration and expiration. This condition is called atelectasis and will cause severe V_A/Q mismatch with severe hypoxemia and hypercapnia.

In condition when CC > FRC and if PEEP is applied to IPPV, then PEEP will increase the FRC above CC value and restore the normal FRC and CC relationship. Thus, no airway will close during expiration with normal tidal volume and no ventilation perfusion mismatch with hypoxemia will occur.

Oxygen and Carbon Dioxide

HISTORY

William Harvey of London (1538–1657) had first described circulation of blood in his book, named "deMotu Cordis". He was a student of Galileo. He had first observed the difference of color between arterial and venous blood. But, he was not able to give any reason regarding this difference in color and was unable to draw any firm conclusion about the function of lungs. Then, in-between 1665 and 1675, Robert Hooke, Robert Boyle, Richard Lower, and John Mayow of Oxford had made a understanding that certain components of air is absorbed by lungs and this process is necessary for both the maintenance of life and burning of substances. At that time, "phlogiston theory" was invoked for nearly 100 years. According to this theory, "phlogiston" was supposed to be a part of all the combustible substances and was liberated during their combustion or during an animal's respiration. When it is accumulated in excess as a result of combustion or by respiration in a closed container, then it prevents further chemical activity of life, causing the stoppage of combustion or respiration and death.

After that, *Joseph Priestly* had first prepared oxygen as gas from potassium nitrate in 1771, and was first given the credit for discovering oxygen. But, instead of oxygen, he called this gas as "dephlogisticated air". Because, he observed that this new gas was better than air for supporting respiration and combustion. He also supposed this, because it contained less "phlogiston". So, he called it as "dephlogisticated air".

Then, *Lavoisier* had first clarified the use of oxygen in the process of respiration and combustion of substances. Simultaneously, he also clarified the production of carbon dioxide during combustion of substances and respiration. He subsequently demonstrated that oxygen is absorbed by lungs and after metabolism in our body, it is eliminated as CO_2 and water. Later, he and Laplace had coined the term *oxygen* (oxy = acid, gene = producer) in 1779. They were also the first to compare the heat produced during respiration in animal with that produced during the combustion of carbon and showed the relationship between the oxygen used and carbon dioxide produced. But, later *Lavoisier* was executed by guillotine during French revolution.

Then, Von Liebig had showed, in 1851, that carbohydrates and fats were the substrates of metabolism in cell and not carbon itself. In 1850, French chemist, Boussingault also had first discovered that at a temperature of about 1,000°C, barium monoxide absorbs oxygen from air forming barium dioxide and again releases it at a more higher temperature. Then, this process made charmed and was patented by his pupils, named *Brin brother*, in 1880. After that, they had formed a company and their company eventually, then, became the *British oxygen*.

PROPERTIES OF OXYGEN

Oxygen is a tasteless, colorless, and odorless gas. The concentration of O_2 in atmospheric dry air at 760 mm Hg pressure is 20.95%. The molecular weight of oxygen is 32. In atmosphere, mainly O^{16} isotope of oxygen is present, but a small amount of O^{17} and O^{18} isotopes of it is also found. In one atmospheric pressure (760 mm Hg) and at –183°C temperature, the oxygen becomes liquid (boiling point of liquid oxygen) and in same atmospheric pressure (760 mm Hg) at –218°C temperature, it becomes solid (melting point of solid oxygen). The critical temperature of oxygen is –118°C. So, at temperature greater than this, oxygen exists as gas and cannot be liquefied by raising the pressure. The relative density (air = 1) of oxygen is 1.105. The solubility of O_2 in plasma at 37°C temperature is 0.003 mL/100 mL of blood.

The O_2 cannot be ignited itself, but it aids combustion of substances. So, substances often burn more vigorously or even explode in the presence of oxygen. Hence, explosion can occur due to the presence of grease on the valves of oxygen cylinder. Due to some unpaired electrons, in the outermost orbit of its atom, the oxygen molecules are attracted to the region of high-magnetic field and is so said it as the paramagnetic gas. Hence, this property of O_2 is utilized in some oxygen analyzers to measure the concentration of it in a mixture of gases.

■ PREPARATION OF OXYGEN

Commercially in large scale, the oxygen is prepared or manufactured by *fractional distillation of liquid air*. When this liquid air is gradually heated, then the more volatile nitrogen gas (boiling point at 760 mm Hg pressure is −196°C) is separated first, followed by oxygen (boiling point at 760 mm Hg pressure is −183°C). After that, gradually the other components of air are also separated, as required, one after another.

■ STORAGE OF OXYGEN

Oxygen is usually stored at high pressure as gas in cylinders or as liquid in insulated tanks. For large hospitals, the storage of O_2, as liquid form in an insulated tank, is much more economical. Tank with huge capacity of liquid oxygen is usually insulated by a high-vacuum shell to maintain the inside temperature of tank in-between −175 and −150°C. But, still there is continuous evaporation of some liquid O_2 present within the tank. This is due to the continuous absorption of small amount of heat from the surrounding, in spite of this vacuum insulation. So, if no oxygen is drawn off for long time from the tank, then this accumulated gas (O_2) within the tank should be vented out to the atmosphere. All the O_2 tanks or cylinders are guarded with a pressure regulator valve maintaining a constant supply of oxygen at constant pressure, from the tank or the cylinder into the hospital pipeline system.

The medical grade O_2 contains 99–99.5% pure form of it. In most of the small hospitals, the O_2 is stored in more than two separate banks of cylinders, consisting of the H type of cylinders. They are connected by manifolds and valves. The number of cylinders in one bank and the number of banks in one hospital depend on the anticipated daily demand of O_2 by this hospital. Only one bank is utilized at one time. The valves in manifold connection reduce the cylinder pressure to the given pressure of pipeline and supply gases at target points at this set pressure. A bank automatically switches to another bank when all the cylinders of a bank are emptied. In large hospitals, where the liquid O_2 is used in tanks, an additional smaller O_2 supply system of compressed O_2 cylinders or a bank of cylinders should be there, which can be used as reserve in emergency. Most of the anesthetic machines accommodate one or two E type of O_2 cylinder, in addition to pipeline connection, to guard against the hospital pipeline failure. Anesthesiologists must ensure the supply of O_2 from these cylinders, directly attached to anesthetic machine, before starting of any operation.

■ OXYGEN TRANSPORT IN BODY

The anesthetists are mainly concerned about the transport and delivery of O_2 from the air to the tissues at cellular level. The delivery of O_2 from the air to the cells at mitochondrial level is a continuous process and is occurred in four phases. These are: (1) the mechanical act of breathing by which air with O_2 reaches the alveoli, (2) the exchange of gas in alveoli by which O_2 passes from the air into the blood, (3) the oxygenated blood, then, is transported to the tissues by circulation, and finally (4) at the level of tissue, from capillaries O_2 enters into the cell and mitochondria.

Transport of Oxygen from Air to Alveoli

The mechanical act of breathing which transports the air with O_2 from the environment to alveoli is fully discussed in separate chapter. But, here, we will discuss only how the tension of oxygen (PO_2) in air falls gradually during its transport from environment to alveoli. When the O_2 reaches from atmosphere to the mitochondria of a cell through alveoli, then the tension of O_2 (PO_2) drops in steps. This is called as the *oxygen cascade*. The PO_2 drops in stages from 159 mm Hg in dry air of atmosphere to a very low level of 2 mm Hg in mitochondria. When the level of PO_2 in mitochondria falls below about 1–2 mm Hg, which is called as the *Pasteur point*, then the aerobic metabolism inside the cells stops. The partial pressure or tension of O_2 in inspired air (PiO_2) is about 20 kPa (kilopascal) or 159 mm Hg (1 kPa = 7.6 mm Hg). It is influenced by the barometric or atmospheric pressure (P_B) and the fractional concentration of oxygen (FiO_2) in air. The normal barometric pressure at sea level is known as one atmospheric pressure and is equivalent to 760 mm Hg, and in this condition, the normal concentration of oxygen or FiO_2 in air is 21% or 0.21. So, the equation of PiO_2 is: $PiO_2 = P_B \times FiO_2 = 760 \times 21/100 = 159$ mm Hg.

Then, the inspired air is saturated and diluted by water vapor after mixing with it, while it is passing through air passages to reach alveoli. So, it causes the reduction of PO_2, when it reaches the alveoli. The partial pressure of water vapor at 1 atmospheric pressure and body temperature (37°C) is 47 mm Hg. So, when the inspired air, saturated with water vapor, reaches the alveoli, then the PiO_2 comes down to 149 mm Hg, which is calculated by the following way: *PiO_2 (Sat) = $(P_B - PH_2O) \times FiO_2 = (760 - 47) \times 21/100 = 149.73$ mm Hg ≈ 149 mm Hg* (**Flowchart 1**).

Then, the inspired gas (air), containing oxygen and water vapor, is further diluted by addition of CO_2 and removal of

Flowchart 1: Oxygen cascade.

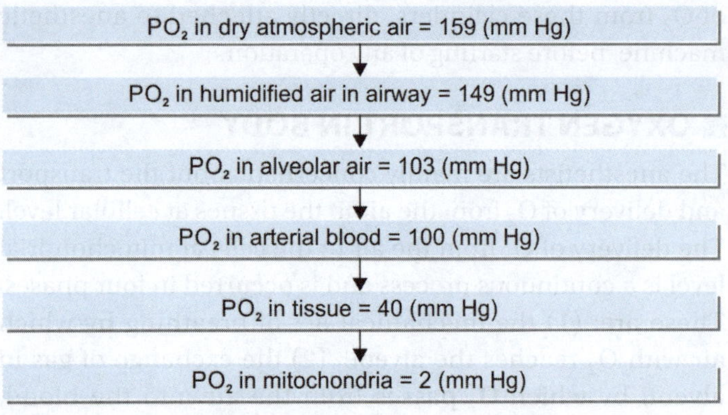

(PO$_2$: partial pressure of oxygen)

TABLE 1: Partial pressure of gases in alveoli during normal ventilation and hypoventilation with breathing air.

	Normal ventilation with PaCO$_2$ = 40 mm Hg	Hypoventilation with PaCO$_2$ = 100 mm Hg
O$_2$	103 mm Hg	43 mm Hg
N$_2$	570 mm Hg	570 mm Hg
CO$_2$	40 mm Hg	100 mm Hg
H$_2$O	47 mm Hg	47 mm Hg
Total	760 mm Hg	760 mm Hg

O$_2$ in alveolus. So, the *final alveolar oxygen tension* in alveoli (P$_A$O$_2$) can be estimated by *"alveolar gas equation"*. This alveolar gas equation is: $P_AO_2 = [FiO_2 (P_B - 47) - PaCO_2] \times F = [21/100 (760 - 47) - 46] \times F = 103.73\ F \approx 103$ (while it is taken as 103 mm Hg and F is ignored). Here, P$_A$O$_2$ = alveolar O$_2$ tension, FiO$_2$ = in air fractional inspired O$_2$ concentration, P$_B$ = barometric pressure, 47 is the vapor pressure of water at body temperature (37°C), PaCO$_2$ is the arterial CO$_2$ tension, and F is the respiratory exchange ratio. On the other way, the *final alveolar oxygen tension* also can be calculated by deducting the CO$_2$ tension in alveoli (which is equivalent to PaCO$_2$) from the inspired O$_2$ and water vapor tension in alveoli, i.e., 149 − 46 = 103 mm Hg.

From the above equation, it is estimated that the normal value for P$_A$O$_2$ is 103 mm Hg at sea level. This normal P$_A$O$_2$ will decrease with (1) increasing altitude or decreasing P$_B$, (2) increasing PACO$_2$, or (3) with decreasing FiO$_2$. So, a hypercapnic patient at high altitude would have a substantially lowered P$_A$O$_2$.

Exchange of Gases in Alveoli

The oxygen tension (PO$_2$) in blood, entering at the arterial end of pulmonary capillaries, coming from the right side of heart through pulmonary artery, is 40 mm Hg [oxygen saturation (SpO$_2$) is 75%]. Whereas, the PO$_2$ in alveolar air is 103 mm Hg. Thus, this pressure gradient helps the O$_2$ to enter into blood from alveolar air across the alveolar membrane. In the blood, O$_2$ first dissolves in plasma and then finally unites with hemoglobin (Hb) for its carriage to tissues. Thus, at the venous end of pulmonary capillaries, the PO$_2$ in blood is 103 mm Hg. In peripheral tissues, the tension of O$_2$ at the arterial side of capillary blood is about 100 mm Hg. The O$_2$ tension **(Table 1)** in the tissue is near about 40 mm Hg. When the arterial blood passes through the tissues, it carries about 20 mL of O$_2$ as oxyhemoglobin and about 0.3 mL of O$_2$ as physical solution in plasma per 100 mL of blood.

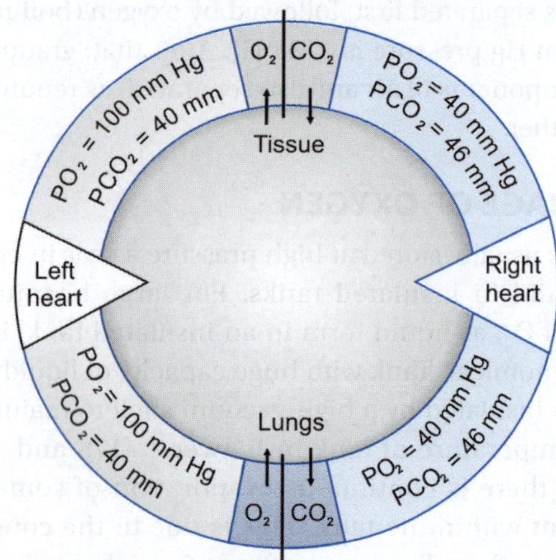

Fig. 1: Transport of O$_2$ in blood.

As the O$_2$ tension in tissue level is much lower, so the oxygen present as physical solution in plasma first passes from plasma to the tissues by diffusion. As a result, the O$_2$ tension in arterial plasma falls. So, the oxyhemoglobin in red blood cell (RBC), being exposed to low O$_2$ tension in plasma, dissociates and releases O$_2$ form Hb. Then, this O$_2$ from RBC enters into plasma and is carried as physically dissolved solution. Again, this physically dissolved O$_2$ leaves the bloodstream and enters the tissues. Thus, the portion of O$_2$ dissolved as physical solution in plasma remains always constant and this is measured as PO$_2$ in blood. About 30% of O$_2$ is liberated from blood to supply the tissues, when the tissue cells are in resting phase. This dissociation of oxygen from oxyhemoglobin in RBC depends upon: (1) the plasma O$_2$ tension, (2) the plasma CO$_2$ tension, (3) plasma H$^+$ concentration, (4) plasma electrolyte content, and (5) the temperature of blood and tissues **(Fig. 1)**.

The CO$_2$ tension and its content in tissues are much higher than that of its capillary blood. Due to this difference of pressure (tension), CO$_2$ diffuses from tissues into the blood of capillaries in tissues. Thus, CO$_2$ tension in tissue capillary blood rises, which also subsequently favors the dissociation of O_2 from oxyhemoglobin into the blood of tissue capillary and enters into tissues. As the increase in PCO_2 in tissue capillary blood favors the dissociation of O_2 from Hb, similarly the increase in PO_2 in tissues favors the dissociation of CO_2 from tissues. Hence, as a result of supply of O_2 to tissues from tissue capillary blood, the O_2 tension and O_2 content of tissue capillary blood fall.

Thus, at the venous end of capillaries in tissues, the O_2 tension of blood is about 40 mm Hg and O_2 content is about 14–15 mL as oxyhemoglobin and about 0.15 mL as physical solution per 100 mL of blood. Subsequently, when this systemic venous blood with PO_2 of about 40 mm Hg passes through the pulmonary capillaries into lungs, wherein the alveoli PO_2 is about 103 mm Hg, then O_2 again enters from alveoli into the systemic venous blood during passing through the pulmonary artery and capillaries. Therefore, O_2 tension (PO_2) rises and more oxy-Hb is formed in the red cells. Simultaneously, CO_2 diffuses out from the systemic venous blood of pulmonary artery into the alveolar air. CO_2 tension and H^+ concentration in the venous blood fall which also favor the entry of O_2 in the pulmonary capillary. The entry of O_2 in pulmonary capillary blood from alveoli also favors the exit of CO_2 from pulmonary capillary blood to alveoli.

Carbon dioxide is much more soluble in plasma than O_2. Hence, as a large amount of CO_2 remains in plasma as solution and diffuses out easily from pulmonary capillary into alveoli, so *hypercapnia ($\uparrow$ in $PaCO_2$) is rarely a problem in pulmonary fibrosis*, which is discussed in Chapter 3. *It does occur only when the alveolar ventilation is severely inadequate and there is much V_A/Q inequality. If, due to any cause, the $PaCO_2$ increases, other than the decrease in ventilation, then by increasing ventilation the extra CO_2 can easily be expired out. But, it accumulates when the ventilation is severely compromised. It is to be noted that in normal condition, the difference between P_ACO_2 and $PaCO_2$ is very small and alveolar ventilation (V_A) has a great impact on $PaCO_2$ and PaO_2. Doubling the V_A results in half of $PaCO_2$ and reducing the V_A to half results in a doubling of $PaCO_2$. Therefore, relationship between V_A and $PaCO_2$ is exponential. Similarly, if this change is entered into "alveolar gas equation", then also we will get the relationship between V_A and PaO_2. It can also be seen that hypoxemia develops rapidly than hypercarbia as V_A decreases. But, it can readily be corrected by a small increase in FiO_2 from 0.21 to 0.3. In summary, we can say that decrease in V_A readily produces hypoxemia than hypercarbia. But, increase in V_A readily corrects hypercarbia than hypoxia. Increase in inspired oxygen concentration (FiO_2) only readily corrects hypoxemia, but not hypercapnia.*

Transport of Oxygen by Blood

Oxygen from higher pressure in the alveolar air enters into the blood of pulmonary capillary, where PO_2 is low than blood. Hence, O_2 gets dissolved in plasma. As more and more O_2 gets dissolved, PO_2 in plasma will increase and then O_2 will enter inside the RBCs. In RBCs, this O_2 will combine with Hb to form HbO_2 (oxyhemoglobin). Thus, O_2 remains in blood as physical solution and also as oxyhemoglobin.

The amount of O_2 transported or delivered to the tissues by blood depends on—(1) the *blood flow (cardiac output)* and (2) the quantity of O_2 carried by blood (O_2 content). Again, the O_2 content carried by blood depends on—(1) the *rate of diffusion of O_2* or the oxygenation of blood in lungs (PaO_2 and SaO_2 where SaO_2 is the percentage of available binding sites of O_2 on Hb) and (2) *Hb content* (**Box 1**). On the other hand, oxygenation of blood or diffusion of O_2 in blood depends on the inspired and subsequently alveolar O_2 tension. The alveolar O_2 tension (P_AO_2), on the other hand, determines the arterial O_2 tension (PaO_2). The *alveolar and arterial O_2 tension difference (A-a) or gradient* is the simplest way of quantifying the pulmonary diffusion of O_2 from alveolar air into pulmonary capillary blood. Other determining factors of PaO_2 are *R-L shunt and pulmonary diffusion barriers*. We should consider these two factors during determination of PaO_2 only in pathological condition. *Oxygen is transported by blood: (1) as simple physical solution by dissolving oxygen in plasma, and (2) as oxyhemoglobin (HbO_2) combining with Hb.*

Carriage of O_2 by Simple Physical Solution Dissolving in Plasma

A very small proportion of total O_2 content of blood is carried as physically dissolved solution, i.e., 0.3 mL/100 mL of blood/100 mm Hg pressure (0.003 mL/100 mL of blood/1 mm Hg pressure). *But, this small quantity of O_2 is very important, because it alone reflects the tension of O_2 in blood (PO_2). On the other hand, the amount of O_2 present as HbO_2 does not determine PO_2. For example, in case of anemia, the HbO_2 is less, but the dissolved O_2 and PO_2 in arterial blood are normal.* This dissolved O_2 in plasma remains in equilibrium

BOX 1: Factors influencing the amount of O_2 delivered to tissues.

- Amount of O_2 delivered to tissues depends on—blood flow and O_2 content in blood
- O_2 content in blood depends on—Hb concentration and rate of diffusion of O_2
- Rate of diffusion of O_2 through alveolar wall depends on—(A-a) O_2 tension difference
- (A-a) O_2 tension difference depends on—R-L shunt and pulmonary diffusion barrier

with HbO_2. Hence, first when O_2 enters into bloodstream, it dissolves as physical solution in plasma. Then, from this plasma, the O_2 enters into RBC to attach with Hb. At tissue level, this plasma part of dissolved O_2 is first transferred to tissue cells and its position is then rapidly taken over (replaced) by O_2 liberated from Hb. In this way, the dissolved O_2 in plasma is responsible for movement of O_2. This dissolved O_2 in plasma assumes its practical importance in case of hyperbaric O_2 therapy. Here, the dissolved amount of O_2 in plasma can be increased by giving O_2 at a very high pressure (2 or 3 times of atmospheric pressure or $2-3 \times 760$ mm Hg) in the treatment of gas gangrene, acute CO poisoning, etc.

Carriage of O_2 by Attaching with Hb (as HbO_2)

Other than physical solution, O_2 is also carried by combining with Hb, which is present in the red cells. This combination of O_2 with Hb is called oxyhemoglobin, which is a loose and reversible compound. O_2 is quickly combined with Hb in the capillary of alveoli, where its tension is high and then is equally quickly dissociated from Hb in the capillary of tissues where its tension is low.

Hemoglobin is a chromoprotein and has four subunits. Each subunit **(Box 2)** contains one structure of heme, consisting of four pyrrole rings with one iron (Fe^{2+}) atom. One heme structure is attached with one α- or β-polypeptide chain of globin (a globin molecule consists of four polypeptide chains: 2α and 2β). So, a hemoglobin molecule contains four atoms of iron in ferrous form and its molecular weight is 68,000. Each atom of iron can reversibly combine with one molecule of O_2. As one Hb molecule contains four heme units and four iron atoms, so it reacts with four molecules of O_2 with formation of oxy-Hb (Hb_4O_8). Under physiological conditions, the reaction of Hb with O_2 takes place in four separate but simultaneous reactions: $Hb_4 + O_2 \rightarrow Hb_4O_2 + O_2 \rightarrow Hb_4O_4 + O_2 \rightarrow Hb_4O_6 + O_2 \rightarrow Hb_4O_8$. The attachment of first O_2 molecule is difficult, but then there is a conformational change in Hb molecule and subsequent O_2 molecules can attach easily. This is called as heme–heme reaction. Amount of O_2 present as HbO_2 depends not only on the amount of Hb, but also on the partial pressure of O_2 to which the blood is exposed and the other factors, such as PCO_2, $[H^+]$, temperature, and 2,3-diphosphoglycerate (2,3-DPG).

Oxygen content: The total oxygen content (in milliliter) in each 100 mL of blood is the total quantity of O_2 attached with Hb in red cells in 100 mL of blood plus the total quantity of O_2 dissolved in plasma in 100 mL of blood, that means the amount of O_2 transported per 100 ml of blood which is shown in **Table 2**. Average Hb level in an adult male is

BOX 2: Gradient of CO_2 and O_2 at tissue and pulmonary level.

At lungs:

A. Venous PCO_2 = 46 mm Hg
   Alveolar PCO_2 = 40 mm Hg

   Gradient of PCO_2 = 6 mm Hg

B. Venous PO_2 = 40 mm Hg
   Alveolar PO_2 = 103 mm Hg

   Gradient of PO_2 = 63 mm Hg

At tissue:

C. Arterial PO_2 = 100 mm Hg
   Tissue PO_2 = 40 mm Hg

   Gradient of PO_2 = 60 mm Hg

D. Arterial PCO_2 = 40 mm Hg
   Tissue PCO_2 = 46 mm Hg

   Gradient of PCO_2 = 6 mm Hg

(PCO_2: partial pressure of carbon dioxide; PO_2: partial pressure of oxygen)

TABLE 2: Transport of O_2 through blood.

Transport of O_2 by arterial blood	• As physical solution: 0.3 mL/100 mL of blood at PaO_2 of 100 mm Hg • As oxyhemoglobin: 20.85 mL/100 mL of blood at PaO_2 of 100 mm Hg • Total: 21.15 mL/100 mL of blood at PaO_2 of 100 mm Hg
Transport of O_2 by venous blood	• As physical solution: 0.12 mL/100 mL of blood at P_VO_2 of 40 mm Hg • As oxyhemoglobin: 15.63 mL/100 mL of blood at P_VO_2 of 40 mm Hg • Total: 15.75 mL/100 mL of blood at P_VO_2 of 40 mm Hg

about 15 g/100 mL and 1 g of fully oxygenated Hb contains maximal 1.39 mL of O_2 (in some book, it is written that 1 g of fully oxygenated Hb contains maximum 1.34 mL of O_2). At an arterial PO_2 of 100 mm Hg, Hb is 100% saturated. On the other hand, oxygen content as physically dissolved solution in plasma is 0.3 mL/100 mL of blood/100 mm Hg PaO_2 (0.003 mL/100 mL of blood/1 mm Hg pressure).

So, the total O_2 content in 100 mL of arterial blood at PO_2 of 100 mm Hg pressure is: as oxyhemoglobin + as physical solution.

$$= 1.39 \times Hb \times \% \text{ of saturation} + 0.003 \times PaO_2$$
$$= 1.39 \times 15 \times 1 + 0.003 \times 100$$
$$= 20.85 + 0.3$$
$$= 21.15 \text{ mL/100 mL}$$

Sometimes, this value is taken as average 20 mL/100 mL of arterial blood.

In the venous blood, PO_2 is 40 mm Hg and Hb is 75% saturated.

TABLE 3: Distribution of the amount of O_2 in arterial and venous blood.

Oxygen	Arterial blood	Venous blood
Amount of O_2 as physical solution in plasma	0.3 mL/100 mL	0.13 mL/100 mL
Tension of O_2	100 mm Hg	40 mm Hg
Amount of O_2 combined with Hb	21 mL/100 mL	15 mL/100 mL
Saturation of O_2	100%	75%

(Hb: hemoglobin)

So, O_2 content in 100 mL of venous blood at 40 mm Hg pressure.

$$= 1.39 \times Hb \times \% \text{ of saturation} + 0.003 \times P_VO_2$$
$$= 1.39 \times 15 \times 0.75 + 0.003 \times 40$$
$$= 15.63 + 0.12$$
$$= 15.75 \text{ mL/100 mL}$$

Therefore, tissue extracts only 21.15 – 15.75 = 5.4 mL (average 5 mL) of O_2 from every 100 mL of arterial blood, while it is passing through the tissue capillaries. Similarly, every 100 mL of blood while passing through lungs takes about 5.4 (average 5 mL) mL of O_2 (**Table 3**).

O_2 capacity of Hb: It is the maximum amount of O_2 that can combine with Hb in 100 mL of blood. If a sample of 100-mL blood contains 14 or 15 g Hb, then the O_2 capacity of that sample of blood is 14 or 15 × 1.39 = 19.4 or 20.8 mL.

Saturation of Hb by oxygen (oxygen saturation) at particular PO_2: It means the fraction of Hb in the form of HbO_2 out of total Hb in 100 mL of blood at a particular oxygen tension. This is calculated as follows: Present O_2 content/maximum O_2 capacity that can be content × 100. For example, in a sample of 100-mL blood there is 19 mL of O_2 at PO_2 of 100 mm Hg. But, it can combine with 20 mL of O_2 at maximum. Therefore, O_2 saturation of Hb in that sample is: Present O_2 content / maximum O_2 capacity × 100 = 19/20 × 100 = 95%. If in any blood sample, the O_2 cortent is 20 mL, which is equal to its maximum capacity, then O_2 saturation of Hb is: 20/20 × 100 = 100% saturated. This is the arterial blood. In venous blood, the O_2 content is 15 mL in 100 mL of blood. Therefore, O_2 saturation in venous blood is: 15/20 × 100 = 75%. On the other way, when blood contains 20 mL of O_2, then this blood is 100% saturated. Therefore, when a sample of blood is 75% saturated, then the O_2 content is: 20/100 × 75 = 15 mL.

Oxygen flux: The total amount of O_2 leaving the left ventricle per minute, when breathing air (with 21% O_2) at sea level (760 mm Hg pressure), has been termed as the oxygen flux. The normal oxygen content of arterial blood is 21.15 mL/100 mL or 211.5 mL/L. The normal cardiac output is 5 L/min.

So, oxygen flux = 5 × 211.5 mL/min = 1057.5 mL/min.

The O_2 content of venous blood is 15.75 mL/100 mL or 157.5 mL/L.

Therefore, the total amount of O_2 leaving the right ventricle = 5 × 157.5 = 787.5 mL/min.

Hence, 1057.5 – 787.5 = 270 mL of O_2 is used up by whole body, during cellular metabolism in every minute and this amount of O_2 is taken up from alveolar air in every minute.

Oxygen flux when Hb drops to 4 g/100 mL in anemia: This can be calculated by the following way:

The O_2 content of 100 mL arterial blood with 4 g of Hb/100 mL of blood

$$= 1.39 \times 4 \times 1 + 0.003 \times 100$$
$$= 5.56 + 0.3$$
$$= 5.86 \text{ mL/100 mL}$$
$$= 58.6 \text{ mL/L}$$

Therefore, O_2 flux = 5 × 58.6 mL/min = 293 mL/min. It indicates there will be no O_2 reserve.

Oxygen Delivery at Tissues

The mechanism of delivery of O_2 at tissue level has been discussed in this chapter before. But, here we will discuss only some extra points. Previously, it was stated that the amount of O_2 delivered to tissues depends on cardiac output and total oxygen content in blood. This overall flow rate of O_2 to tissues is called as O_2 delivery. With a normal cardiac output of 5 L/min and with normal O_2 content in blood (20 mL/100 mL of blood), the normal O_2 delivery to tissues is 1,000 mL/min or 1 L/min.

Cardiac output varies with the size of patient. So, cardiac output is commonly indexed to body surface area (BSA). This is called as the cardiac index (CI) and can be represented as: CI = CO/BSA (L/min/m^2) or CO = CI × BSA. So, O_2 delivery can be expressed as index: therefore O_2 delivery (index) = CO$_2$ × CO (mL/min) = CO$_2$ × CI × BSA (mL/min/m^2). In normal adult patient, the O_2 content = 20 mL/100 mL of blood, the CI = 3 L/min/m^2 and BSA = 10 m^2. So, the O_2 delivery index is 600 mL/min/m^2.

■ LACK OF OXYGEN OR HYPOXIA

The failure to receive adequate quantities of O_2 by tissues is called as *hypoxia*. Whereas, the total lack of O_2 is called as *anoxia* and it is used in more restricted sense. Less oxygen content in blood is termed as *hypoxemia*. The *asphyxia* is a condition, characterized by decreased O_2 and increased CO_2 (asphyxia = hypoxia + hypercapnia). It (asphyxia) is

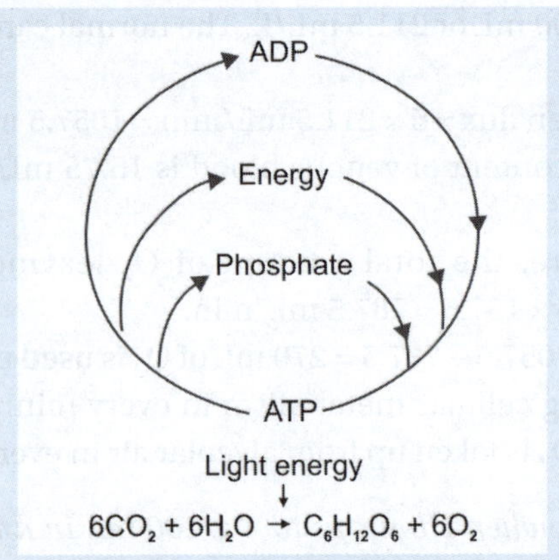

Fig. 2: Mechanism of formation of ATP. (ADP: adenosine diphosphate; ATP: adenosine triphosphate)

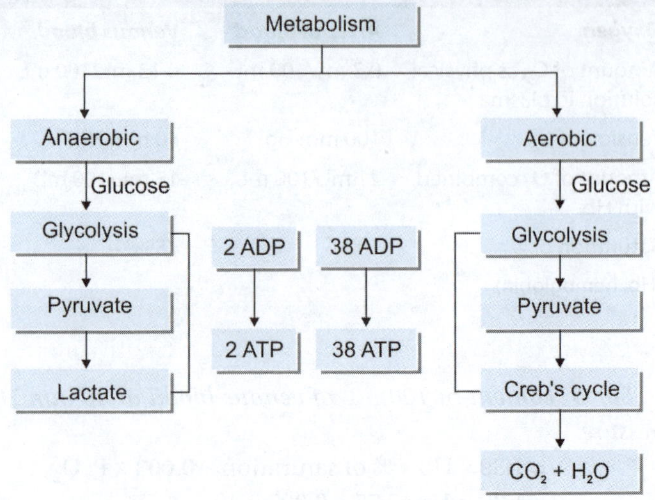

Flowchart 2: Difference between aerobic and anaerobic metabolism. (ADP: adenosine diphosphate; ATP: adenosine triphosphate)

discussed in more details, after hypoxia. It occurs mainly due to obstruction of airway such as strangulation and hanging. In conscious patient, there are certain regulatory mechanisms, which prevent the tissue to suffer from lack of oxygen (hypoxia). But, during the course of anesthesia, due to the lack of this regulatory mechanism, the hypoxia has a deleterious effect **(Fig. 2)**.

We get energy from the sun. Earth's atmosphere originally contains no O_2. But, during photosynthesis with the help of CO_2, plant absorbs this light energy in form of glucose and releases O_2 in atmosphere.

$$\text{Light energy}$$
$$\downarrow$$
$$6CO_2 + 6H_2O \rightarrow C_6H_{12}O_6 + 6O_2$$

But, within our cell, this reaction is reverse. The solar energy, which is incorporated into glucose, is released by oxidation with the help of oxygen and is used for cellular activity.

$$C_6H_{12}O_6 + 6O_2 \rightarrow 6CO_2 + 6H_2O + \text{Energy (heat)}$$

So, O_2 is very essential to maintain life. Some energy also can be obtained in absence of O_2 (anaerobic metabolism), but in terms of adenosine triphosphate (ATP) production, the anaerobic process is 1/19 as less efficient as aerobic process of metabolism. Because, during aerobic metabolism, one glucose molecule produces 38 ATP (recently it is said that one glucose molecule produces 32 ATP molecules), whereas in anaerobic process, only two ATP is produced from one glucose molecule. Again, lactic acid accumulation, as a result of anaerobic metabolism, will lead to metabolic acidosis. Then, when O_2 becomes available, this lactate can further be metabolized to CO_2 and H_2O with further ATP formation.

The hypoxia may result from various causes and according to the causes of hypoxia, it can be classified into five types: (1) hypoxic hypoxia, (2) anemic hypoxia, (3) stagnant hypoxia, (4) histotoxic hypoxia, and (5) conditions where P_{50} is low **(Flowchart 2)**.

Compensatory Changes due to Hypoxia

Compensatory changes take place, if the hypoxia is persistent and gradual. Because, body gets time to fight with deficiency of O_2. These compensatory changes are:

- Hypoxia stimulates respiratory center, leading to hyperventilation, with an aim to raise PaO_2. The role of hyperventilation in raising PaO_2 can be proved by the alveolar gas equation.
- Rise of BP and there is polycythemia with increased Hb concentration, leading to increased O_2 content of blood.
- Increase in 2,3-DPG content in RBCs, leading to increased delivery of O_2 to tissues.

Aim of these changes is to increase the O_2-carrying capacity in blood and also to increase the ability to release more O_2 at tissue level. Hypoxia, produced due to ventilator failure, also leads to accumulation of CO_2 into tissue. But, mild cases of ventilatory failure are not accompanied by hypercapnia ($\uparrow CO_2$). This is due to higher diffusivity of CO_2. This is also true for pulmonary edema or pneumoconiosis. So, initially these cases are pure hypoxias. Whereas, the chronic cases of gross ventilatory failure, e.g., asthma, chronic bronchitis, etc., actually lead to increase in $PaCO_2$ along with hypoxia. The immediate treatment of hypoxia is O_2 therapy. But in chronic cases, where there is hypercapnia ($\uparrow CO_2$), particularly where chronic airway obstruction is the cause, O_2 should be given with great care. Because, getting O_2 the ventilatory stimulation will be withdrawn and more CO_2 will be accumulated. In such situation, both O_2 therapy and assisted ventilation are needed.

Types of Hypoxia

Hypoxic Hypoxia

Here, the cause of hypoxia is defective oxygenation of blood in the alveoli of lungs. This results in incomplete saturation of hemoglobin by oxygen and less amount of O_2 is available in physically dissolved form, causing low-oxygen tension in arterial blood. Hypoxic hypoxia is produced in the following conditions.

Decreased partial pressure of O_2 in inspired gas (PiO$_2$↓): This is due to:

- Fall in fractional concentration of O_2 in inspired gas (FiO$_2$). This occurs during rebreathing or when the supplied gas is hypoxic in mixture (contains less O_2).
- Fall in barometric pressure, for example, at high altitude. At sea level, with 1 atmospheric pressure (760 mm Hg), the air contains 20–21% O_2 concentration and alveolar air contains 14% O_2 concentration. The remaining part of alveolar air is filled up by CO_2, N_2, and H_2O vapor. The total pressure, exerted by all these gases in alveoli, is same as the barometric pressure (760 mm Hg). So, the partial pressure of O_2 (PO$_2$) in alveoli is 14% of 760 mm Hg or about *106 mm Hg*. At an altitude of 5,500 meters or 18,000 feet, the barometric pressure is only 380 mm Hg. So, the partial pressure of O_2 in alveoli at this altitude will be 14% of 380 mm Hg, i.e., only about *50 mm Hg*. At Mount Everest, where barometric pressure is only 236 mm Hg, the alveolar PO$_2$ is only *40 mm Hg* (after saturated with water vapor at nasopharynx and adding CO_2 in alveoli). Thus, due to diminution of partial pressure of O_2 in alveoli, which is due to the reduction of barometric pressure at high altitude, less amount of O_2 will diffuse from alveoli into blood and as a result, there will be reduced tension of oxygen in blood.

Fink effect or diffusion hypoxia: At the end of anesthesia, which is carried out by N_2O and O_2, when the patient breaths room air, the N_2O will diffuse out from body tissues via venous blood into alveoli. Subsequently, the N_2 now being breathed with room air will fill the alveoli and diffuse back from alveolar air into tissue. Due to the higher solubility of N_2O than N_2, relatively small amount of N_2 will diffuse in from alveolar air into blood and restore tissue PN$_2$. But, much larger amount of N_2O than N_2 will diffuse out from tissues into alveoli and dilute (reduce) the alveolar O_2 concentration. Thus, it (N_2O) reduces alveolar PO$_2$ and produces hypoxia which is opposite to the phenomenon, occurring during the induction of anesthesia with N_2O–O_2 mixture. *This is called as diffusion hypoxia and is opposite to second gas effect* (**Fig. 3**).

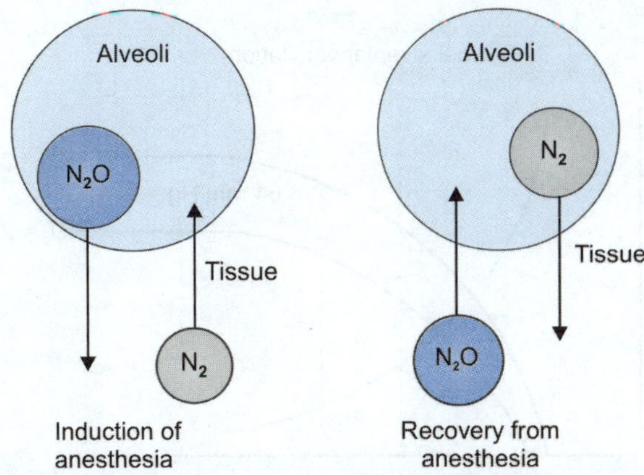

Fig. 3: The comparison between N_2O and N_2 regarding their speed and amount of entry and exit during induction and recovery from anesthesia.

Second gas effect: N_2O is more soluble in blood than N_2. So, during induction with N_2O, the volume of N_2O taken up by blood is much higher than the volume of N_2 entering the alveoli from tissue via blood. Therefore, the alveoli become gradually smaller and the partial concentration of remaining gases in alveoli increases. Now, if another inhalation anesthetic agent (e.g., halothane) is also given with N_2O, then the fractional concentration of this anesthetic gaseous agent will also increase. This phenomenon is called the *second gas effect*, and it increases the speed of induction by this anesthetic gaseous agent. In the early part of induction, the volume of N_2O absorbed from alveoli is in the order of 1 L/min. Although the volume of N_2O in alveoli has decreased, due to high absorption of it from alveoli into blood, but the concentration of it does not reduce to that same extent, because the volume of alveoli is also decreased.

- *Reduced alveolar ventilation:* Arterial O_2 tension (PaO$_2$) depends on alveolar O_2 tension (P$_A$O$_2$) which again depends on alveolar ventilation. The relationship between the alveolar ventilation (V$_A$) and alveolar PO$_2$ (P$_A$O$_2$) is hyperbolic. It indicates (**Fig. 4**) that a reduction in alveolar ventilation (V$_A$) of 2 L/min, i.e., from 6 to 4 L/min has little effect on P$_A$O$_2$. Whereas, the reduction of ventilation from 4 to 2 L/min has very marked effect on P$_A$O$_2$. Again, raising the inspired PO$_2$ by 64 mm Hg (achieved by increasing the FiO$_2$ from 0.21 to 0.3, i.e., 21 to 30%) results in a rise in P$_A$O$_2$ of same amount, like the reduction of ventilation from 4 to 2 L/min. Increase in O_2 consumption also shifts the V$_A$ and P$_A$O$_2$ relationship downward and toward the right. It means that what was previously a perfect adequate alveolar ventilation may be grossly inadequate now, if the oxygen consumption increases. For example, "halothane shake" is a common cause of increased O_2 consumption and hypoxic hypoxia that occurs in the early part of postoperative period.

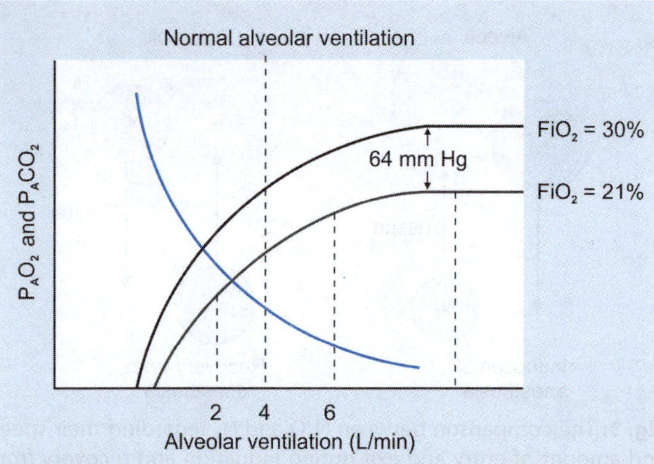

Fig. 4: The effect of the change of alveolar ventilation on alveolar O_2 tension (P_AO_2) drawn in black line and alveolar CO_2 tension (P_ACO_2) drawn in blue line. It also shows the effect of change of FiO_2 from 21 to 30% on P_AO_2. Doubling of V_A results in half of $PaCO_2$ and vice versa. The relationship between V_A and PaO_2 also shows that hypoxemia develops rapidly as V_A decreases. But, it can be readily corrected by a small increase in FiO_2. On the other hand, hyperventilation results in little increase in PaO_2. (FiO_2: fraction of inspired oxygen; $PaCO_2$: arterial CO_2 tension; V_A: alveolar ventilation)

- *Reduced diffusing capacity of O_2 across alveoli:* Due to thickening of alveolar capillary membrane for any cause, there is also impairment of diffusion of O_2 from alveolar gas across the alveolar and pulmonary capillary membrane into pulmonary capillary blood, causing hypoxia. The examples of such type of hypoxia are emphysema, pulmonary edema, pneumonia, interstitial fibrosis, etc.
- *Abnormalities of pulmonary mechanics:* Many abnormalities in pulmonary mechanics such as asthma, emphysema, pneumothorax, collapse, and obstruction in air passages also produce hypoxic hypoxia by reducing the ventilation or decreasing the FiO_2 or changing the V_A/Q ratio.
- *Venous admixture and shunt:* This refers to some conditions when blood passes directly from the venous side of circulation to the arterial side of circulation, i.e., from right side of heart to the left side of heart, without picking up any oxygen from lungs or passing through the zones of lung with low V_A/Q ratio, so that it is less oxygenated than normal. The examples of such direct communication between the right and the left side of heart are true shunt which is responsible for not picking up any oxygen from lungs. This takes place in patent ductus arteriosus (PDA), patent foramen ovale or ventricular septal defect (VSD), etc. with pulmonary hypertension where blood flows from right to left side of heart (true shunt).

Anemic Hypoxia

Here, the problem lies in the carrying of O_2 by blood to tissues, but not in the oxygenation or uptake of O_2 by Hb in alveoli. The characteristic of this anemic hypoxia is that the total O_2 content of arterial blood is reduced, but the partial pressure and the saturation of Hb by O_2 are normal. Therefore, the hemoglobin is fully saturated with O_2, but as the quantity of O_2-carrying Hb is low, so the total amount of O_2 carried by it is below normal. This is called as the anemic hypoxia. Anemic hypoxia will result from following.

Anemia: When the Hb concentration in blood becomes half, then the total O_2 content of blood is also reduced to half. But, the partial pressure of O_2 (which is due to dissolved O in plasma) in blood remains same. Thus, O_2 dissociation curve shifts to the left. But, for compensatory mechanism, anemia causes increase in 2,3-DPG level, therefore shifting again the oxygen dissociation curve to the right at its normal position and favor the unloading of O_2 to tissue. The shifting of O_2 dissociation curve toward left prevents the unloading of O_2 into tissues.

Carbon monoxide (CO) poisoning or carboxyhemoglobinemia (Fig. 5): As affinity of CO to hemoglobin is 250 times greater than that of O_2, so a small amount of CO will replace a substantial amount of O_2 from Hb and will produce large amount of carboxyhemoglobin. Therefore, little free hemoglobin will be available for carrying O_2. The other changes produced by carboxy-Hb are the shifting of O_2 dissociation curve to the left. The significance of this shifting of O_2 dissociation curve toward left is that it also unfavors the unloading of remaining O_2 to tissues. *The shift in oxygen dissociation curve of Hb is usually presented mathematically as changes in P_{50} value.* The P_{50} value is defined as the PO_2 at which Hb is 50% saturated. The normal value of P_{50} is 27 mm Hg. It means that at 27 mm Hg in O_2 tension, Hb is only 50% saturated. A shift to the left of O_2 dissociation curve lowers the P_{50} value, i.e., it indicates that at 50% saturation of Hb, the O_2 tension is <27 mm Hg. Similarly, a shift to the right of O_2 dissociation curve raises the P_{50} value, which indicates that at 50% saturation of Hb, the O_2 tension is >27 mm Hg. But, the changes in P_{50} have only a modest effect on the uptake of O_2 in the lungs. The main consequence of alterations of P_{50} is on the release of O_2 in tissues. A low P_{50} or shifting of O_2 dissociation curve to the left decreases the O_2 availability to tissues and, therefore, may lead to cellular hypoxia. Similarly, a high P_{50} value or shifting of O_2 dissociation curve to the right increases the O_2 availability to tissues. As the upper part of O_2 dissociation curve is flat, so the changes in PO_2 at this portion have relatively little effect on Hb saturation by oxygen and, therefore, the blood O_2 content. Whereas, over the lower more vertical part of the curve, the changes in PO_2

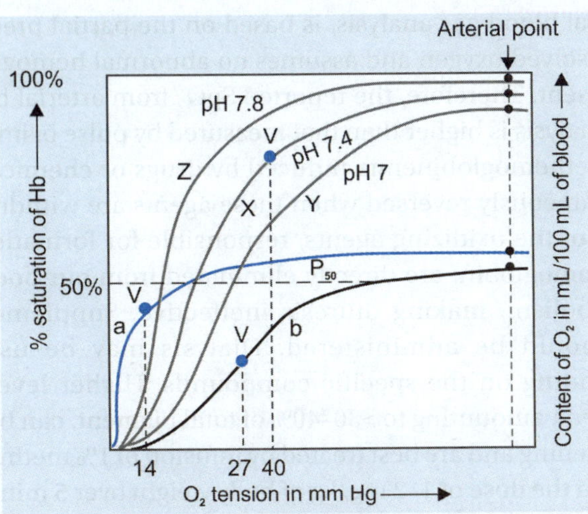

Fig. 5: Different O_2–Hb dissociation curves in different conditions, such as normal, acidosis (pH = 7), and alkalosis (pH = 7.8) (X, Y, and Z curves), CO poisoning (a), and anemia (b). (Hb: hemoglobin)

TABLE 4: Classification and causes of hypoxia.

Hypoxic hypoxia	↓FiO_2, ↓barometric pressure, ↓V_A, diffusion hypoxia, V/Q mismatch, pulmonary diffusion defect, R → L shunt
Anemic hypoxia	Anemia, copoisoning, methemoglobinemia, sulfhemoglobinemia
Stagnant hypoxia	↓cardiac output, MI, heart failure, dehydration
Histotoxic hypoxia	Cyanide poisoning
Low P_{50}	↑ pH, ↓ 2,3-DPG

(DPG: diphosphoglycerate; FiO_2: fraction of inspired oxygen; MI: myocardial infarction)

have a very marked effect on the percentage of saturation of oxy-Hb so the transfer of O_2 from Hb to tissues. These changes in O_2 dissociation curve are also very crucial to the survival of patient, following a massive blood transfusion. Another significance of the shifting of point P_{50} or O_2 dissociation curve is that in order to offload the same amount of O_2 to tissues, the venous PO_2 is also reduced to a much lower level. When the Hb level is 14.4 g/dL, the venous point is 40 mm Hg. In anemia (Hb = 7.2 g/dL), the venous point is 27 mm Hg. In 50% HbCO (Hb = 14.4 g/dL), the venous point is 14 mm Hg. So, although this shift of oxyhemoglobin dissociation curve has little effect on arterial O_2 content, but its effect on venous PO_2 is very significant. At a cerebral venous PO_2 of 14 mm Hg, the subject will be unconscious.

Coal gas has 10% CO as its content. Natural gas also contains trace amount of CO but does not cause CO poisoning. So, coal gas has been replaced by natural gas, which contains about 90% methane with only trace amounts of carbon monoxide. Carboxyhemoglobin level also goes up to 10% in cigarette smoking. Car exhaust and commercial paint removal, containing methylene chloride, cause also severe CO poisoning.

The treatment of CO poisoning consists of hyperbaric O_2 mixed with 5% CO_2, in order to shift the oxyhemoglobin dissociation curve to the right toward its normal position **(Table 4)**.

Methemoglobin and sulfhemoglobin: Methemoglobinemia is another important, but uncommon etiology for the development of cyanosis and anemic hypoxia, which demands prompt diagnosis and treatment. So, for quick evaluation, the history, physical examination, bedside diagnostic techniques, and laboratory confirmation are all important. But, in the absence of significant history, mild cyanosis can easily be missed in dark-skinned individuals during the preanesthetic checkup.

Actually, methemoglobinemia is a condition where the ferrous iron (Fe^{2+}) of hemoglobin complex is oxidized to ferric iron (Fe^{3+}). Usually, under normal conditions, methemoglobin ($HbFe^{3+}OH$) is continuously being formed into RBCs of a normal individual by the process of auto-oxidation. But, a continuous reduction mechanism maintains the methemoglobin levels in blood <1% of total hemoglobin. The most important mechanism for converting the methemoglobin back into normal hemoglobin is the enzymatic reduction by nicotinamide adenine dinucleotide hydrogen (NADH) cytochrome-b5 reductase enzyme. Other minor alternative pathways of methemoglobin reduction utilize the reduced form of nicotinamide adenine dinucleotide phosphate hydrogen (NADPH), which is generated by glucose-6-phosphate dehydrogenase (G6PD) enzyme in the pentose phosphate pathway. Glutathione and ascorbic acid also can reduce the methemoglobin to normal hemoglobin directly, but quantitatively are not very important.

The accumulation of large amounts of chocolate brown, reversibly oxidized methemoglobin in RBCs may be either inherited or acquired. The inherited condition producing methemoglobinemia is also due to two reasons: (1) a dominantly inherited abnormality in the synthesis of a special type of hemoglobin, called hemoglobin M, in which the structural lesion prevents the reduction of methemoglobin to hemoglobin and (2) a recessively inherited deficiency in the synthesis of enzyme methemoglobin reductase.

Thus, in summary, the congenital causes of methemoglobin anemia include—hemoglobin M disease in which there is globin chain mutation defect (autosomal dominant) and deficiency of enzyme such as NADH cytochrome-b5 reductase (autosomal recessive). Hereditary methemoglobinemia, once regarded as a homogeneous clinical entity, is now known that it is the result of at least 10 different mutations at three distinct gene loci: two at the locus coding for the α chain of hemoglobin, three at the locus that encodes the β chain of hemoglobin, and at least five at the NADH dehydrogenase locus. The acquired methemoglobinemia also can be caused by the exposure of hemoglobin to coal gas, car exhaust, smoking, and other oxidizing chemicals or drugs such as nitrites, xylocaine, prilocaine, phenacetin, acetanilide, and sulfonamide.

The irreversible formation of another hemoglobin, causing anemic hypoxia, is sulfhemoglobin. It has distinct abnormal spectral properties and results from the administration of drugs, particularly sulfonamides. This condition is called the sulfhemoglobinemia. The sulfhemoglobinemia also can be produced by other compounds that cause methemoglobinemia and these two conditions frequently coexist. Sulfhemoglobinemia produces marked cyanosis, but disappears spontaneously, as the cells containing abnormal pigment are gradually removed from circulation with the passing of time and further production is prevented.

As the methemoglobinemia results due oxidation of iron from its ferrous (Fe^{2+}) to its ferric (Fe^{3+}) state, so the concomitant oxidation of hemoglobin protein may cause its precipitation as Heinz bodies and resulted in hemolytic anemia. The methemoglobin (ferric hemoglobin) cannot carry oxygen and when present in excess, it results in functional anemia. It also shifts the oxygen dissociation curve to left and thus limits the release of oxygen to tissues. So, the symptoms of methemoglobinemia are due to hypoxia and anaerobic metabolism. In many cases, there are no clinical features, other than cyanosis. But, when the concentration of methemoglobin rises to 20–45%, then anoxic symptoms such as headache, fatigue, dyspnea, and lethargy may develop. There may also be alteration in the level of consciousness when methemoglobin level rises to 44–55%. Cardiac arrhythmias, circulatory collapse, seizures, and even death may occur at methemoglobin level of 70% or more.

The diagnosis of methemoglobinemia is based upon the presence of central cyanosis, unresponsive to oxygen therapy and decreased SpO_2 in presence of still normal PaO_2. Since, methemoglobin has an absorption characteristic similar to that of deoxyhemoglobin, so its presence in blood falsely lowers the saturation of Hb, as read on pulse oximeter. On the other hand, SpO_2 measured by pulse oximetry may be falsely normal. If co-oximetry is not available, methemoglobin levels can also be estimated by the difference between SpO_2, calculated from PaO_2 and that measured directly by blood gas analysis. The saturation of oxygen, reported on

arterial blood gas analysis, is based on the partial pressure of dissolved oxygen and assumes no abnormal hemoglobin is present. Therefore, the reported SpO_2 from arterial blood gas analysis is higher than that measured by pulse oximeter.

Methemoglobinemia induced by drugs or chemicals is spontaneously reversed when these agents are withdrawn. Most of the oxidizing agents, responsible for formation of methemoglobin, are directly eliminated from our body by metabolism, making diuresis ineffective. Supplemental O_2 should be administered. Dialysis may be useful, depending on the specific compounds. Higher levels of pigment, amounting to >30–40% of total pigment, can be life threatening and are best treated by infusion of 1% methylene blue in the dose of 1–2 mg/kg of body weight over 5 minutes. Cyanosis alone is not an indication for methylene blue therapy in methemoglobinemia. In patients with anemia or cardiovascular disease, where the manifestations of hypoxia are present, methylene blue treatment may be indicated at a lower level of methemoglobin. After methylene blue, if clinical response is not observed within 1 hour, then the dose may be repeated. A methemoglobin level of 40 g/L can be expected to decrease by half in 1–2 hour, after the beginning of treatment with methylene blue. However, as long as the oxidizing agent remains in our body, the methemoglobin will be generated and additional doses of methylene blue may be necessary. This methylene blue dye helps to combine the highly efficient NADP-linked methemoglobin-reducing system to methemoglobin and thus will result in rapid reduction of methemoglobin to hemoglobin in all patients, but not in G6PD-deficient patients.

The side effects of methylene blue that occur during the treatment of methemoglobinemia include precordial pain, dyspnea, restlessness, tremor, apprehension, and transient blue color of skin and urine. Methylene blue is contraindicated in patients with G6PD deficiency, because it can cause hemolysis. Exchange transfusion for the treatment of methemoglobinemia is only indicated when methemoglobin level is very high, the patient is refractory to the treatment by methylene blue, and the patient is deficient in G6PD enzyme. Although the methemoglobinemia due to methemoglobin reductase deficiency also responds to methylene blue treatment, but this chronic disorder is best treated by the daily oral administration of 1–2 g of ascorbic acid. Cyanosis due to hemoglobin M does not respond to any treatment, but is ordinarily a benign condition.

To conclude, low SpO_2 reading in the presence of normal PaO_2 suggests the possible presence of dyshemoglobin (methemoglobin or other abnormal Hb) which may affect the accuracy of pulse oximeter. This is because only two wavelengths of light are used in this device, one for oxy-Hb and another one is for deoxy-Hb or reduced Hb. The role

TABLE 5: The O_2 tension and O_2 saturation of arterial and venous blood, and the difference of arterio-venous O_2 tension in different types of hypoxia.

| | Arterial blood | | Venous blood | | A–V difference of O_2 |
	O_2 tension	O_2 saturation (%)	O_2 tension	O_2 saturation (%)	
Hypoxic hypoxia	↓	↓	↓↓	↓	Unchanged
Anemic hypoxia	Normal	↓	↓	↓	Unchanged
Stagnant hypoxia	Normal	Normal	↓↓	↓↓	Very high
Histotoxic hypoxia	Normal	Normal	↑	↑	Very low

of laboratory co-oximeter, which uses light of several wavelengths, can only identify and quantify the different types of dyshemoglobins. Thus, its role in such situations cannot be overemphasized.

Stagnant Hypoxia

This type of hypoxia occurs when there is decreased circulation in tissues or when the demand of O_2 at tissue level increases than the supply in it. Hence, it causes increased difference between the supply and demand of O_2 at tissue level. This hypocirculation of tissue is due to reduced cardiac output, peripheral vasoconstriction, trauma, arterial occlusion due to embolism or atheroma, etc.

Histotoxic Hypoxia

Here, the diffusion of O_2 at the level of alveoli and transport of it through blood to tissues are all right. But, the defect lies at the cellular mitochondrial level which impairs the utilization of O_2 by cells and produces hypoxia. In mitochondria when glucose is oxidized, H^+ is removed by NAD and becomes NADH. Then, this H^+ is passed down through the cytochrome enzymatic systems with formation of ATP and at the last, this H^+ reacts with O_2 to form H_2O. Thus, poisoning of this cytochrome enzyme system by cyanide, nitroprusside, etc. causes stoppage of this machine and makes unable the use of O_2, delivered to the tissues, causing the stoppage of aerobic metabolism and hypoxia within tissues, despite no deficiency of O_2 in cells. So, as the metabolism within the cells is stopped, therefore, CO_2 is not produced and O_2 is not utilized. Thus, reduced production of CO_2 by tissues causes fall in venous PCO_2 and subsequently reduced O_2 consumption rises mixed venous PO_2.

Condition where P_{50} is low, i.e., oxygen dissociation curve is shifted to the left: P_{50} is the partial pressure of O_2 at which Hb is 50% saturated. The normal value of P_{50} is 27 mm Hg, which means at PO_2 of 27 mm Hg hemoglobin is 50% saturated. Low P_{50} means the oxygen dissociation curve of Hb is shifted to left which means at low partial O_2 pressure (<27 mm Hg), Hb is 50% saturated or in other words at 50% saturation of Hb, it has low O_2 tension. For diffusion of O_2 at tissues, the

TABLE 6: Effects of chronic hypoxia.

CVS	↑Cardiac output, ↑BP, ↑HR, ↑sympathetic activity, cerebral vasodilatation, ↑SVR
RS	↑Ventilation, ↑PVR
Metabolism	↓Aerobic metabolism, ↓ATP formation, ↑anaerobic metabolism, ↑metabolic acidosis
Hemoglobin	Polycythemia, ↑viscosity of blood, cyanosis, reduced Hb is a better buffer
Organ failure	Depressed myocardium, unconsciousness

(ATP: adenosine triphosphate; BP: blood pressure; CVS: cardiovascular system; HR: heart rate; PVR: pulmonary vascular resistance; RS: respiratory system; SVR: systemic vascular resistance)

partial pressure of O_2 at tissue level must be lower than that of blood. But if partial pressure of O_2 at capillary level remains less, then O_2 will not flow from blood into tissue, leading to cellular hypoxia. The examples of low P_{50} value causing hypoxia are acidosis, hypothermia, electrolyte imbalance, etc. At the end of the discussion of the different types of hypoxia, the level of O_2 tension, O_2 saturation in arterial and venous blood and the arterial - venous O_2 tension difference is shown in **Table 5**.

Effects of Hypoxia

The effects of hypoxia or anoxia **(Table 6)** vary according to the severity and the rate of occurring of it. When the supply of oxygen is cut off very rapidly, then sudden loss of consciousness will occur. But, if the hypoxia develops gradually, such as in mountaineering, then the effects of it (hypoxia) on the different systems are as follows.

On Cardiovascular System

The hypoxia has profound effect on cardiovascular system (CVS). By direct effect, it causes systemic vasodilatation and fall of BP. These hypotension and hypoxia are compensated by hypoxia-induced ↑ sympathetic activity by peripheral baroreceptor and chemoreceptor stimulation. In the preliminary compensatory stage, due to the stimulating effect of hypoxia and hypotension on vasomotor and cardioaccelerator center, there is rise in heart rate, cardiac output, and blood pressure. Therefore, the splanchnic and cutaneous blood vessels constrict. Thus, a large amount of blood is shifted from nonvital organs to vital organs, such as the heart and brain, so that they may be supplied by adequate amount of oxygen. In nonanesthetized person, if hypoxia continues, then hypotension will no longer be compensated and heart rate will increase further. But, the force of cardiac contraction becomes gradually weaker, due to the weakness of cardiac muscles, caused by hypoxia ($\downarrow$ATP formation) and heart starts to fail. Then, CO and BP gradually go to zero and cardiac arrest will result. In anesthetized person, where there is no compensatory mechanism, this fall of BP and cardiac arrest will occur early. The prognosis of hypoxic cardiac arrest is extremely poor, because by the time, the heart is stopped as a result of hypoxia, there is always nearly irreversible brain damage, though hypoxia increases the blood flow to most organs, especially in brain.

On Respiratory System

It is seen that no alteration of respiration or breathing takes place till the O_2 content in inspired air is reduced to about 13–14%, when a slight increase in respiratory rate is seen. Later, if the O_2 content in inspired air is more and more reduced, then this respiration is gradually more and more stimulated. Thus, this increased ventilation tries to keep the arterial O_2 tension normal, but washes out excessive amount of CO_2 (diffusibility of CO_2 is $>O_2$). This excess excretion of CO_2 also favors better oxygenation. So, O_2 content of blood remains proportionately high, but the CO_2 tension falls ($\downarrow PaCO_2$). Then, gradually due to the low CO_2 tension, the reflex respiration is not further stimulated and dies down, causing again less ventilation and reduced oxygenation of blood with raised CO_2 tension ($\uparrow PaCO_2$). Consequently, respiration is again stimulated. In this way, respiration becomes alternately stimulated and depressed, resulting in what is known as the *periodic breathing*. The sequence of these events may be summarized as follows: lack of O_2 stimulates breathing $\rightarrow$ washes out more CO_2 $\rightarrow$ arterial CO_2 tension is lowered $\rightarrow$ respiration is depressed $\rightarrow$ CO_2 tension in blood is again raised $\rightarrow$ breathing is stimulated and so on. In this way, respiration goes on alternately waxing and waning during gradual increase in severity of hypoxia.

Thus, when the inspired O_2 concentration is reduced more and goes down below 15%, then cyanosis develops. The consciousness becomes dull and soon after this, the person becomes unconscious, due to the effects of hypoxia on higher centers.

But, when the lack of oxygen or hypoxia is very gradual, then the results are different. Because the compensatory changes are brought into play. It is best studied in subject, ascending slowly to higher altitudes. At higher altitude, the

percentage of composition of air is same as over the plane (O_2 is 20% and N_2 is 80%). But, due to less barometric pressure, the air is more rarified or much less condensed, so that each mL of such air will contain less number of molecules of oxygen and other gases, which causes less partial pressure of them than over the plane. The symptoms first appear at about 3,657 meters or 12,000 feet height, where the barometric pressure is two-thirds of 1 atmospheric pressure (760 mm Hg), i.e., about 500 mm Hg. At that height, the pressure of O_2 in air is 20% of 500 mm Hg, i.e., 100 mm Hg (at sea level, it is 20% of 760 mm Hg or 152 mm Hg). So, slight breathlessness and tendency to periodic breathing, especially during sleep, will appear. Nervous symptoms, which closely resemble of alcohol poisoning, will also appear. Gradually, all the other systems will be affected and the subject will get what is called as the *"altitude sickness" or "mountain sickness"*. The altitude sickness with mental depression, nausea, vomiting, etc. usually starts 8–12 hours after the exposure to that height and may even present for few days after descent from this high altitude. But, generally these effects pass off quickly. If the lack of oxygen is severe and the exposure is prolonged, then serious after effects may occur. For example, in hypoxia due to CO poisoning, even when the composition of blood has been restored to normal, still the subject may not regain consciousness for many hours. He may pass into coma and may die. Even if the patient becomes conscious and apparently be normal, still there may be bouts of convulsions at intervals, owing to the irritation of nervous systems. Even the paralysis of various parts of body may follow as a result of the damage of nerve cells. There may be complete dementia or just a temporary impairment of mind.

All these features point out that the hypoxia or anoxia devitalizes and injures the whole body. From such observations, Haldane has remarked that "hypoxia or anoxia not only stops the machine, but also wrecks the machinery". Hypoxia causes pulmonary arteriolar vasoconstriction and as a compensatory phenomenon shifts the blood from hypoxic to well-ventilated area of lungs, keeping the PaO_2 at normal. This is a beneficial effect for one lung intubation, lobar consolidation, etc. Chronic hypoxia due to intracardiac shunts, such as in reversed atrial septal defect (ASD), VSD, and PDA, causes total pulmonary arteriolar vasoconstriction and increases the right-sided pressure of heart with reversal of shunt and arteriolar desaturation. This is because chronic hypoxia causes irreversible increase in pulmonary vascular resistance (PVR) with pulmonary hypertension.

On Metabolism

In hypoxia, anaerobic metabolic path is switched on with formation of less ATP and accumulation of lactic acid (metabolic acidosis). The total mechanism is described here.

There is requirement of glucose for energy in all tissues. But, in some tissues such as brain and erythrocytes, the requirement of glucose is substantial (mandatory) and other tissues may get their energy from fatty acid and amino acid also, in the absence of glucose. Glycolysis is the **(Fig. 6)** major pathway of metabolism of glucose for energy and is found in all the cells. It is a unique pathway, because it can utilize oxygen, if available (aerobic), and it can also function in the absence of O_2 (anaerobic) if it is not available. Glycolysis is the principal route of glucose metabolism, leading to production of pyruvate which undergoes further oxidation in citric acid cycle through acetyl coenzyme A (acetyl-CoA) in the presence of O_2. Glycolysis also provides the main dependable pathway for the metabolism of fructose, galactose, and other substrates derived from diets. The crucial biological significance of glycolysis is its ability to provide ATP, still in the absence of O_2. So, it allows the skeletal muscle to perform glycolysis at very high levels when the aerobic oxidation becomes insufficient to survive anoxic episodes. Conversely, the heart muscle, which is adapted only for the aerobic performance, has both the relatively poor glycolytic ability and poor survival rate under conditions of ischemia.

Though it has been customary to separate carbohydrate metabolism into anaerobic and aerobic phases, but this distinction is arbitrary. Because the steps of reactions in glycolysis are the same as in the presence of oxygen or in its absence, except in extent and the end products. When the O_2 is not in supply, then reoxidation of NADH formed from NAD during glycolysis is impaired. Under these circumstances, NADH is only reoxidized during the reduction of pyruvate to lactate and the NAD so formed is used again at the step 5 of glycolytic pathway and allows further glycolysis to proceed. This reaction from pyruvate to lactate is catalyzed by lactate dehydrogenase. Thus, glycolysis also can take place under anaerobic condition. But, this has to be given price for its limited action, regarding the low amount of energy (only two ATPs) liberated per mole of glucose oxidized. Consequently, to provide a given amount of energy, more glucose must undergo glycolysis under anaerobic condition, as compared with aerobic conditions.

$$\text{Pyruvate} + \text{NADH} + \text{H}^+ \leftrightarrow \text{Lactate} + \text{NAD}^+$$

The reoxidation of NADH to NAD during lactate formation allows glycolysis to continue even in the absence of oxygen by regenerating sufficient NAD^+. Thus, tissues that function under hypoxic circumstances continue the glycolysis to produce lactate. This is particularly true for skeletal muscle, where the rate at which the organs perform work is not limited by its capacity for oxygenation. So, the additional quantities of lactate thus produced may be

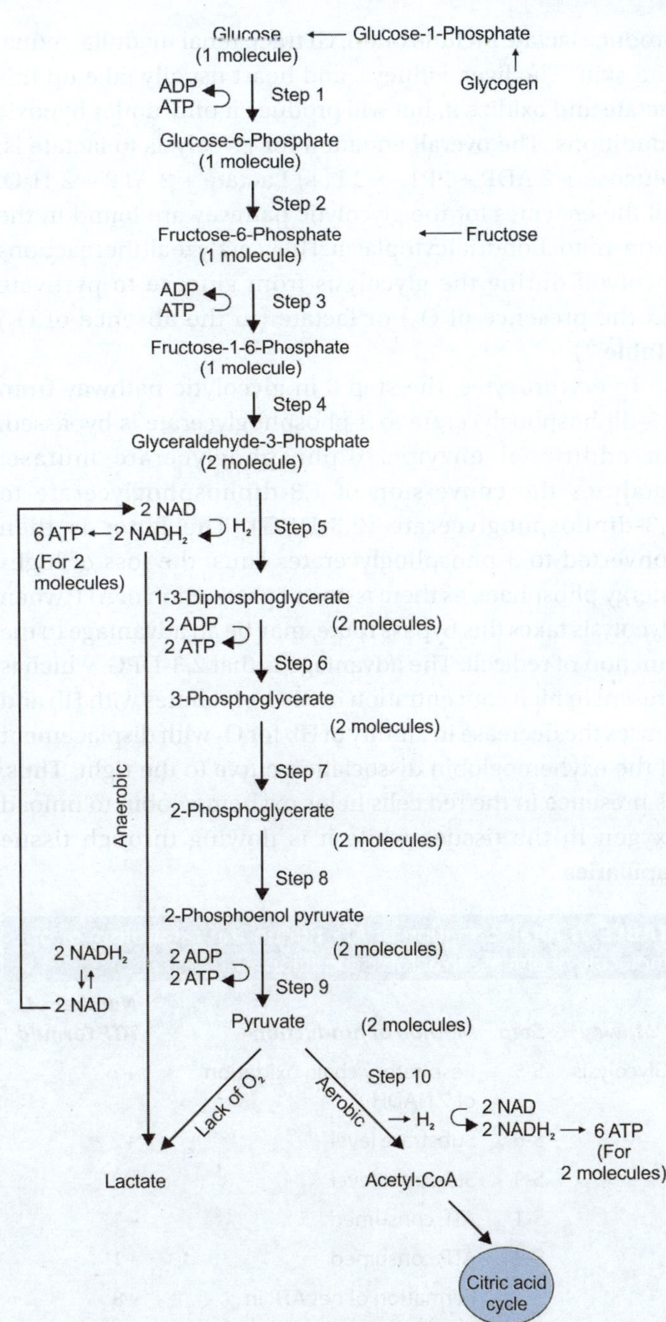

Fig. 6: Schematic representation of glycolysis. (ADP: adenosine diphosphate; ATP: adenosine triphosphate; CoA: coenzyme A; NADH: nicotinamide adenine dinucleotide hydrogen)

detected in the tissues and in the blood and urine. Glycolysis which occurs in erythrocytes even under aerobic conditions always terminates in lactate. Because the mitochondria that contain enzymatic machinery for aerobic oxidation of pyruvate through citric acid cycle are absent in RBC. The mammalian erythrocyte is unique, in that about 90% of its total energy requirement is provided by only the glycolysis. Besides skeletal muscle and erythrocytes, other tissues that normally derive most of their energy from glycolysis and produce lactate include brain, GI tract, renal medulla, retina, and skin. The liver, kidneys, and heart usually take up this lactate and oxidize it, but will produce it only under hypoxic conditions. The overall equation for glycolysis to lactate is: Glucose + 2 ADP + 2P1 → 2 L(+) Lactate + 2 ATP + 2 H_2O. All the enzymes for the glycolytic pathway are found in the extra-mitochondrial cytoplasm. They catalyze all the reactions involved during the glycolysis from glucose to pyruvate (in the presence of O_2) or lactate (in the absence of O_2) **(Table 7)**.

In erythrocytes, the step 6 in glycolytic pathway from 1,3-diphosphoglycerate to 3-phosphoglycerate is bypassed. An additional enzyme, diphosphoglycerate mutase, catalyzes the conversion of 1,3-diphosphoglycerate to 2,3-diphosphoglycerate (2,3-DPG). The latter is then converted to 3-phosphoglycerate. Thus, the loss of high-energy phosphate, as there is no net production of ATP when glycolysis takes this bypass route, may be an advantage to the function of red cell. The advantage is that 2,3-DPG, which is present in high concentration in RBC, combines with Hb and causes the decrease in affinity of Hb for O_2 with displacement of the oxyhemoglobin dissociation curve to the right. Thus, its presence in the red cells helps oxyhemoglobin to unload oxygen in the tissues while it is flowing through tissue capillaries.

Before the pyruvate can enter the citric acid cycle, it must be transported into the mitochondria. Within the mitochondria, the pyruvate is first decarboxylated to acetyl-CoA.

Pyruvate + NAD + CoA → Acetyl-CoA + NADH + H^+ + CO_2

The citric acid cycle, which is also known as the Krebs cycle or tricarboxylic acid (TCA) cycle, is a series of reactions in mitochondria. It brings about the catabolism of acetyl residues of acetyl-CoA liberating hydrogen ions which after oxidation while passing through cytochrome system lead to the release of most of the free energy in the form of ATP for tissue fuels. Thus, the major function of this citric acid cycle is to act as the final common pathway for the oxidation of substrates including carbohydrates, lipids, and proteins. This is because glucose, fatty acids, and many amino acids are all metabolized to acetyl-CoA, which can enter the citric acid cycle. It also plays a major role in gluconeogenesis, transamination, deamination, and lipogenesis. Several of these processes are carried out in many tissues, but the liver is the only tissue in which all the reactions occur to a significant extent **(Table 8)**.

Essentially, the citric acid cycle starts with the combination of a molecule of acetyl-CoA with a molecule of oxaloacetate of four carbon atoms, resulting in the formation of a citrate with six carbon atoms. Then, this follows a series of reactions, in the course of which two molecules of CO_2 are released and again oxaloacetate is regenerated. The citric acid cycle is an integral part of the metabolic process by which huge amount of free energy in the form of ATP is liberated. During the course of oxidation of acetyl-CoA in the citric acid cycle, reducing equivalents in the form of hydrogen or electrons are formed which are taken by NAD or FAD, forming NADH or FADH. These reducing equivalents then enter the respiratory chain, where large amounts of ATP are generated by the process of oxidative phosphorylation.

TABLE 7: Total formation of ATP during the catabolism of one molecule of glucose in aerobic condition.

Pathway	Step	Method of production	Number of ATP formed
Glycolysis	S-5	Respiratory chain oxidation of 2 NADH	+ 6
	S-6	Substrate level	+2
	S-9	Substrate level	+2
	S-1	ATP consumed	−1
	S-3	ATP consumed	−1
		Formation of net ATP in glycolysis	+8
Krebs cycle or Citric acid cycle	S-11	Oxidation of 2NADH	+6
	S-15	Oxidation of 2 NADH	+6
	S-17	Oxidation of 2 NADH	+6
	S-18	Substrate level	+2
	S-19	Oxidation of FADH2	+4
	S-21	Oxidation of 2 NADH	+6
		Formation of net ATP in Krebs cycle	+ 30

Note: Total formation of ATP molecules in aerobic condition from each molecules of glucose is 30 + 8 = 38.
(ATP: adenosine triphosphate; NADH: nicotinamide adenine dinucleotide hydrogen)

TABLE 8: Total formation of ATP during catabolism of one molecule of glucose in anaerobic condition.

Pathway	Step	Method of production	Number of ATP formed
Glycolysis	Step 6	Substrate level	+2
	Step 9	Substrate level	+2
	Step 1	ATP consumed	−1
	Step 3	ATP consumed	−1
Formation of net ATP in glycolysis in absence of Krebs cycle (in absence of O_2)			+2

Note: Formation of 2 molecules of NADH at step 5 is used for further metabolism of pyruvate to lactate in anaerobic condition.
(ATP: adenosine triphosphate; NADH: nicotinamide adenine dinucleotide hydrogen)

This process is aerobic, requiring O_2 as the final oxidant of the reducing equivalents. Therefore, absence (anoxia) or partial deficiency (hypoxia) of O_2 causes total or partial inhibition of the cycle.

The enzymes of this citric acid cycle are located in the mitochondrial matrix, either free or attached to the inner surface of the mitochondrial membrane. These enzymes facilitate also the transfer of reducing equivalents to the adjacent enzymes of the respiratory chain, situated also in the inner mitochondrial membrane.

When 1 mole of glucose is combusted in a calorimeter to CO_2 and H_2O, then approximately 2,780 kJ are liberated as heat. But, when this oxidation occurs in the tissues, then some of this energy is not lost immediately as heat, but is

"captured" as high-energy phosphate in ATP. Usually, 38 moles of ATP are generated per molecule of glucose when it is oxidized both by the glycolysis and citric acid cycle to CO_2 and H_2O. Assuming each high-energy bond in ATP to be equivalent to 30.5 kJ, then the total energy captured as ATP per mole of glucose oxidized is 1,159 kJ, which is approximately 41.7% of the energy of combustion or metabolism. Most of the ATP is formed as a consequence of oxidative phosphorylation through cytochrome system, resulting from the reoxidation of reduced coenzymes such as NADH and FADH by the respiratory chain. The remainder is generated by phosphorylation directly at the substrate level. **(Fig. 7).**

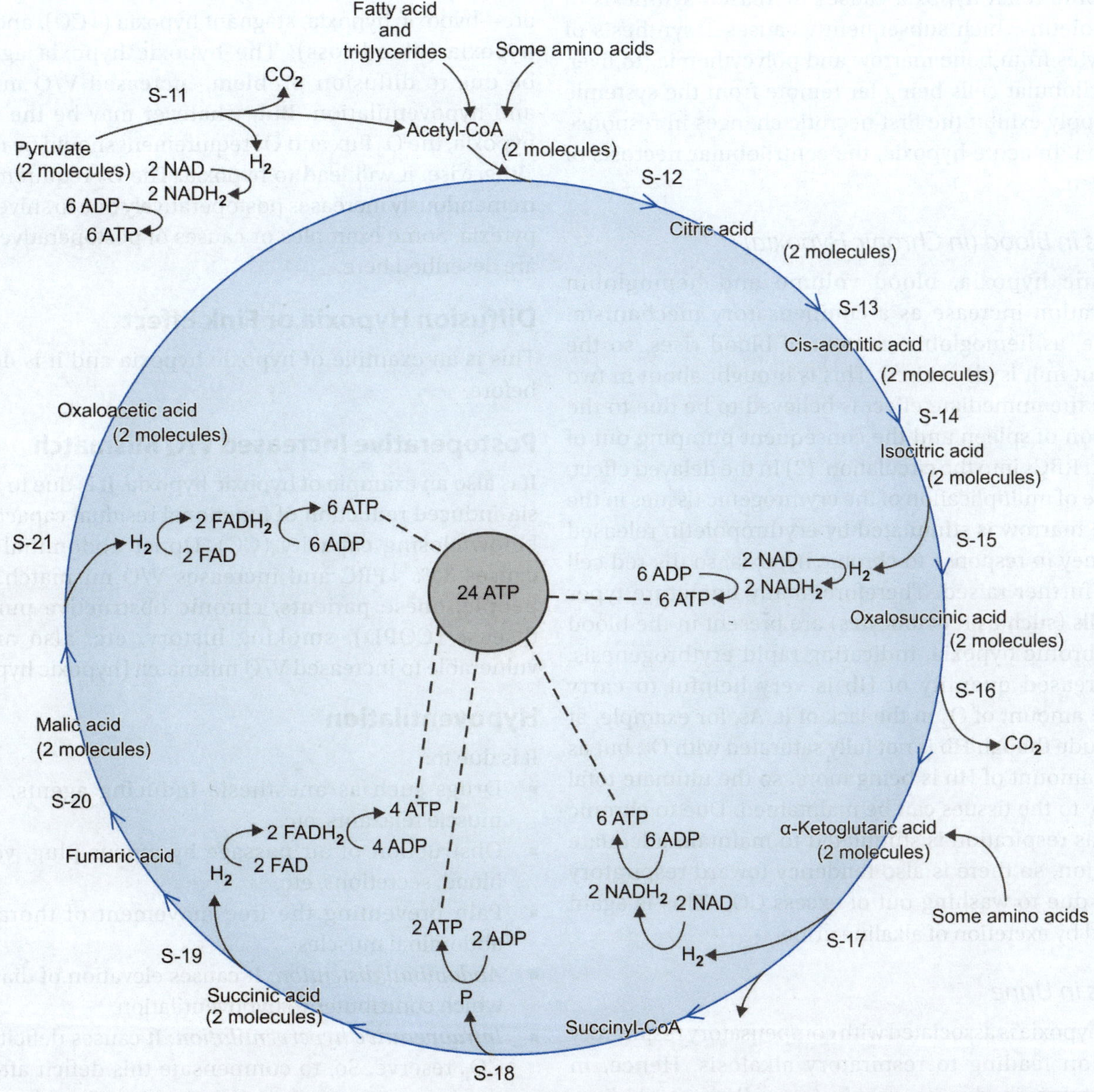

Fig. 7: Schematic representation of citric acid cycle (tricarboxylic acid cycle or TCA cycle). (ADP: adenosine diphosphate; ATP: adenosine triphosphate; CoA: coenzyme A; NADH: nicotinamide adenine dinucleotide hydrogen)

On Organs

Brain and retina are most sensitive to hypoxia. Due to the lack of O_2, the cerebral function gradually deteriorates like changes of mood to confusion to unconsciousness. If circulation stops, then the time taken for brain from stop of functioning to the extent of loss of consciousness is called the "survival time". Usually, the survival time is 0.5 minute. Whereas, the "revival time" is defined as the time beyond which the recovery of function of brain is not possible. Usually, the revival time of brain is 3 minutes. Spinal cord is also very sensitive to hypoxia, for example, clamping of aorta, occlusion of anterior spinal artery, etc. Kidney has survival times of 10 minutes. More prolonged hypoxia than this causes renal tubular necrosis, renal cortical necrosis, etc. Chronic renal hypoxia causes increased synthesis of erythropoietin which subsequently causes ↑ synthesis of erythrocytes from bone marrow and polycythemia. In liver, the centrilobular cells being far remote from the systemic blood supply exhibit the first necrotic changes in response to hypoxia. In acute hypoxia, the centrilobular necrosis of liver is seen.

Changes in Blood (in Chronic Hypoxia)

In chronic hypoxia, blood volume and hemoglobin concentration increase as a compensatory mechanism. Therefore, as hemoglobin content of blood rises, so the O_2 content in it is also raised. This is brought about in two ways: (1) the immediate effect is believed to be due to the contraction of spleen and the consequent pumping out of the stored RBCs into the circulation. (2) In the delayed effect, as the rate of multiplication of the erythrogenic tissues in the red bone marrow is stimulated by erythropoietin released from kidney in response to chronic hypoxia, so the red cell count is further raised. Therefore, many immature types of red cells (such as reticulocytes) are present in the blood during chronic hypoxia, indicating rapid erythrogenesis. This increased quantity of Hb is very helpful to carry adequate amount of O_2 in the lack of it. As, for example, at high altitude though Hb is not fully saturated with O_2, but as the total amount of Hb is being more, so the ultimate total O_2 supply to the tissues can be maintained. Due to chronic hypoxia as respiration is stimulated to maintain adequate oxygenation, so there is also tendency toward respiratory alkalosis due to washing out of excess CO_2. This is again combated by excretion of alkaline urine.

Changes in Urine

Chronic hypoxia is associated with compensatory respiratory stimulation leading to respiratory alkalosis. Hence, in chronic hypoxia due to respiratory alkalosis, kidney excretes alkaline urine as a compensatory mechanism. So, in urine, the urea content is increased and ammonium salt is decreased. In other words, the ammonia coefficient of urine falls. Therefore, there is less excretion of acid in urine. All these are attempts to combat respiratory alkalosis.

Delayed Changes

The red marrow proliferates as a result of hypoxia. The yellow marrow may be transformed into red marrow. This is due to an attempt to increase the O_2-carrying capacity by increasing the red cell production as a compensatory phenomenon. Vital capacity (VC) of lungs also increases in those people who live at higher altitude for long periods.

■ CAUSES OF POSTOPERATIVE HYPOXIA

Three types of hypoxia can occur postoperatively. These are—hypoxic hypoxia, stagnant hypoxia (↓CO), and anemic hypoxia (blood loss). The hypoxic hypoxia again may be due to diffusion problem, increased V/Q mismatch, and hypoventilation. But, whatever may be the cause of hypoxia, the O_2 flux and O_2 requirement should be matched. Otherwise, it will lead to hypoxia. The O_2 requirement also tremendously increases postoperatively due to shivering and pyrexia. Some examples or causes of postoperative hypoxia are described here.

Diffusion Hypoxia or Fink Effect

This is an example of hypoxic hypoxia and it is described before.

Postoperative Increased V/Q Mismatch

It is also an example of hypoxic hypoxia. It is due to anesthesia-induced reduction of functional residual capacity (FRC) below closing capacity (CC). Upper abdominal surgery causes 30% ↓FRC and increases V/Q mismatch. Elderly people, obese patients, chronic obstructive pulmonary disease (COPD), smoking history, etc. also are more vulnerable to increased V/Q mismatch (hypoxic hypoxia).

Hypoventilation

It is due to:
- Drugs such as anesthesia-inducing agents, opiates, muscle relaxants, etc.
- Obstruction of air passage by mucus plug, vomiting, blood, secretions, etc.
- Pain preventing the free movement of thoracic and abdominal muscles
- *Abdominal distention:* It causes elevation of diaphragm, which contributes to hypoventilation.
- *Intraoperative hyperventilation:* It causes deficit of body CO_2 reserve. So, to compensate this deficit after anesthesia, spontaneous ventilation is reduced producing hypoxia.

Reduction of Cardiac Output due to any Cause

It is an example of stagnant hypoxia. So, prolonged operation, thoracic and upper abdominal surgery, old age, previous lung diseases, heart diseases, huge blood loss, sickle cell disease, heavy sedation, inadequate recovery, hypotension, shivering, pyrexia, etc., where there is every possibility of hypoxia, need postoperative O_2 therapy by masks at the rate of 3–4 L/min to prevent this hypoxia. Increase in PVR by hypoxia may initiate R-L shunt through VSD, ASD, or PDA, if they are patent.

■ HYPOXIA AND ALTITUDE

As the altitude increases, subsequently then the atmospheric pressure and then the partial pressure of O_2 (not the concentration or percentage of O_2) in the inspired air is reduced. A list, depicted in **Table 9**, will show how the atmospheric pressure and subsequently the PO_2 in air will decrease with the increase of altitude.

Normally, when a person breaths air, he becomes unconscious, if the SpO_2 falls to 50% or below. Usually, this happens at 23,000 feet height. But, when this person breaths only O_2 instead of air, then this height goes up to 47,000 feet at which or above unconsciousness ensures in spite of inhalation of 100% O_2. The height at which the symptoms of altitude sickness actually start or the physiological changes manifest is not common to all. Generally, within 10,000 feet (3,000 meters) height, there is no necessity for additional O_2 to breathe. It has, however, been noticed that in most cases, breathing becomes labored at about 12,000 feet height. At about 18,000 feet heights, there is definite panting and other symptoms of altitude sickness appear. Additional O_2 is necessary from 10,000 to 34,000 feet height. It has been generally observed that beyond 22,000 feet, acclimatization sometimes fails and there is a steady deterioration of condition, advising to use O_2 supplementation. Pure O_2 is required from 34,000 to 42,000 feet height and pressure suit or pressure cabin becomes essential beyond 42,000 feet height.

TABLE 9: Partial pressure of O_2 in atmosphere at different height from sea level.

Height	Partial pressure of O_2 (PO_2)	Atmospheric pressure
At sea level	159 mm Hg (20% of 760 mm Hg)	760 mm Hg
5,000 feet	130 mm Hg	
10,000 feet	110 mm Hg (20% of 522 mm Hg)	522 mm Hg
15,000 feet	90 mm Hg	
20,000 feet	73 mm Hg (20% of 346 mm Hg)	346 mm Hg
30,000 feet	48 mm Hg	
50,000 feet	18 mm Hg (20% of 85 mm Hg)	85 mm Hg

Physiological Changes at High Altitude and Acclimatization

If a person is brought to high altitude sufficiently slowly (taking several weeks), then some changes occur in his body. This is called as acclimatization. Acclimatization as such means the process of adjustment in a new situation. The changes in acclimatization are directed against hypoxia. These changes are as follows:

- *Hyperventilation:* At high altitude, the physiological changes occur in following manner: High altitude → hypoxia → stimulation of peripheral chemoreceptor → hyperventilation → washout of CO_2 → ↓ $PaCO_2$ → *development of alkalosis* and respiration is inhibited → induces renal excretion of bicarbonate → production of alkaline urine → pH gets corrected and respiration starts again → allowing peripheral chemoreceptor to drive ventilation unopposed. In fact, washing out of CO_2 makes room for O_2 in the alveolar air and P_AO_2 increases. This helps the transfer of more O_2 to blood. Ventilation reaches maximum at 4th days and reaches to equilibrium over year if stays at high altitude for long time. When he again comes down to sea level, reverse reaction occurs which can be summarized as: ↑P_AO_2 → ↓peripheral chemoreceptor drive → ↓ ventilation → ↑ $PaCO_2$ →↑ brain PCO_2. As the pHs of cerebrospinal fluid (CSF) and extracellular fluid of brain are now lower than normal (since the bicarbonate concentration is still lower than normal), so ventilation is driven by an increased central drive which gradually declines as CSF bicarbonate reaccumulates and brings back the pH of brain to normal.
- *Polycythemia:* This is due to excess secretion of erythropoietin from kidney, as the effect of hypoxia. RBC count may be as high as 15 million/mm^3 and Hb may rise up to 19–20 g%. This helps to carry more O_2 in the face of less P_AO_2.
- *Changes in oxygen dissociation curve:* In presence of hypoxia, a shift of this curve to right occurs at tissue level due to increased 2,3-DPG level in RBCs. So, more oxygen will be delivered to tissues. When the blood is in pulmonary capillary, then comparatively more CO_2 will leave through the alveoli of lungs. This is due to low P_ACO_2, caused by associated hyperventilation. In lungs, the oxygen dissociation curve will be shifted to left, so more O_2 will be taken up, even in the presence of high 2,3-DPG in RBCs. Normally, at pulmonary level, the O_2 dissociation curve is shifted to left and at tissue level, this O_2 dissociation curve is shifted to right. But, in hypoxia, this shifting is exaggerated to take more O_2 from lungs and to deliver more O_2 to tissues.

- *Number of capillaries* in tissues also increases so that the intercapillary distance is decreased and even with low PaO_2, tissues can be supplied with enough O_2.
- *Maximum voluntary ventilation (MVV), VC,* etc. are increased due to the less viscosity of rarified air at high altitude.
- *Numbers of mitochondria* and mitochondrial enzymes are elevated, so that O_2 in tissues can be used more effectively.
- *Hypoxic pulmonary vasoconstriction (HPV)* also leads to pulmonary hypertension and right ventricular hypertrophy.
- *Hyperdynamic circulation* also results due to hypoxic stimulation of VMC (vasomotor center). This helps by increasing blood flow.

Sudden ascend to 10,000 feet height by an unacclimatized man leads to mountain sickness, which ranges from weakness and shortness of breath to pulmonary and cerebral edema. Prophylaxis of this can be taken by slow ascend or acetazolamide. Highest permanent habitation in the world is at about 16,000 feet height where P_AO_2 is only 45 mm Hg, requiring 40% inspired O_2 concentration to restore the sea level condition. There are many major cities at 6,000 feet height, where PO_2 in inspired air is only 118 mm Hg, which is equivalent to 16% O_2 in air at sea level and P_AO_2 to 75 mm Hg. At sea level, concentration and tension of O_2 in inspired air are 20–21% and 152–159 mm Hg, respectively. Alveolar O_2 tension (P_AO_2) with breathing air at sea level is 103 mm Hg.

High-altitude Pulmonary Edema

People staying at high altitude, even after acclimatization, show shortness of breath, cough, pink frothy sputum, etc. This is due to pulmonary edema. The cause of this edema is not only due to rise in pulmonary capillary pressure (pulmonary hypertension), but probably due to uneven vasoconstriction due to hypoxia.

■ OXYGEN EXCESS OR TOXICITY

The oxygen toxicity is a complex phenomenon. So, in spite of much investigations over many years, still it remains an enigma. Although, it is possible that high O_2 tension could affect many, but not all the organs and systems. It would also appear that certain organs or systems are more susceptible than others. It is thought that the organs and systems in our body, which are more susceptible to oxygen toxicity, are lungs, retina, brain, and cardiovascular system, etc. Oxygen toxicity is a potential complication, when FiO_2 of 0.6 or greater of it is given for >72 hours. The condition can be prevented in some cases by the use of positive end-expiratory pressure (PEEP), which allows FiO_2 values to keep below 0.6 for maintaining adequate PaO_2 instead of higher FiO_2 while primary therapy for the underlying pathological condition is instituted. There is, at present, no evidence that pulmonary oxygen toxicity develops in man at an inspired O_2 concentration (FiO_2) below 0.5, even with prolonged exposure. At inspired O_2 concentration of 0.5 (FiO_2 = 0.5), the damage occurs very slowly, if it at all happens and at O_2 pressure greater than 3 ATA, the pulmonary problem is overshadowed by the signs of central nervous system (CNS) toxicity, such as convulsions. The rate of development and the degree of damage to lungs appear to be proportional both—(1) to the concentration of oxygen and (2) to the duration of exposure. Thus, O_2 is safe within a narrow spectrum of partial pressure to maintain a life. It is lethal to life at partial pressure outside that ranges.

Pulmonary Effect

Prolonged inhalation of high concentration of O_2 is known to damage mainly the lungs. For the development of pulmonary O_2 toxicity, local alveolar than arterial O_2 tension is more important. Breathing 100% O_2 at 1 atmospheric pressure can cause discomfort and reduction in VC, after as little as 10 hours. But, the recovery of this decreased VC may take several days after the resumption of breathing of air. So, the administration of 100% O_2 for up to 10 hours at sea level with normal atmospheric pressure (760 mm Hg) can be considered safe. But, administration of >50–60% O_2 at sea level or at 1 atmospheric pressure for >24 hours may lead to O_2 toxicity and is undesirable.

Oxygen is irritant to the lungs and produces inflammation and congestion. This pulmonary O_2 toxicity is thought to be due to the generation of highly reactive metabolites of O_2 such as superoxide, activated hydroxyl ions, and hydrogen peroxide in the cells. These metabolites of oxygen are cytotoxic and cause damage to the cellular DNA, sulfhydryl proteins, and lipids of the alveolar epithelial cells. The O_2-mediated pulmonary injury produces a syndrome that is clinically and pathologically indistinguishable from acute respiratory distress syndrome (ARDS). In mild cases, the bronchopulmonary dysplasia and tracheobronchitis may also result.

The pulmonary oxygen toxicity shows—(1) increased capillary endothelial permeability, causing the accumulation of fluid in interstitial space, (2) depression of mucociliary transport function of airway, (3) inhibition of phagocytosis of alveolar macrophages, (4) changes in surfactant activity and its production. The exact highest concentration of O_2, which causes these lung damages, is still not known and it varies with—(1) individual sensitivity, (2) presence of concomitant previous lung diseases, and (3) the concentration and the duration of exposure to O_2. In intensive coronary care unit (ICCU), the FiO_2 should be kept as lower level as possible with optimum PaO_2.

If only O_2 remains in alveoli, it is quickly absorbed by pulmonary capillary and subsequently alveoli collapse. At sea level in healthy subject, the normal ventilation is maintained by small hypoxic drive. But, in severe COPD patient, the main ventilatory drive is severe hypoxia or low PaO_2. So, therapy by high concentration of O_2 in such pathological situations removes this respiratory drive causing ↓ ventilation →↑ PCO_2 → ↓ PaO_2 resulting respiratory arrest, arrhythmia, and cardiac arrest. In such patient, appropriate inspired O_2 concentration and ventilation are ensured by repeated blood gas analysis.

Cardiovascular System Effect

The effects of increased arterial O_2 concentration or tension causing O_2 toxicity of CVS are as like as administering peripheral vasoconstrictor, producing ↑ peripheral vascular resistance, ↑BP, and ↑HR.

Effect on Body N_2 Store

Inhalation of 100% O_2 causes rapid fall of arterial and body N_2 content. Blood is cleared of N_2 in few minutes, but brain tissue takes 20 minutes to clear its N_2 store. Whereas, the other tissues such as fat, muscle, and bone take few hours to clear their N_2 store. Thus, the inhalation of 100% O_2 is used to remove the air and N_2 from body cavities and to prevent air embolism. When a normal subject breaths 100% O_2, the different values of tension of different gases in blood in comparison to when breath air are given in **Table 10**.

From this **Table 10**, we can see that PvO_2 during breathing of 100% O_2 is slightly higher than that of when breathing air. This is because of the shape of O_2–Hb dissociation curve, characterized by its top part, which is virtually horizontal. The amount of O_2 carried by physical solution in plasma is negligible compared with that in combination with Hb. So, the O_2 content of arterial blood during the breathing of 100% O_2 is only slightly greater than that during breathing air. Therefore, there is very little difference between the

mixed venous O_2 content and the arterial O_2 content. This is because, as we are now operating on the steep part of the O_2 dissociation curve, where this small O_2 content difference is reflected by only a small PO_2 difference.

As the gases diffuse down along the gradient of their partial pressure at the level of alveoli and tissue, so the breathing of 100% O_2, containing no N_2, will enormously increase the rate of elimination of N_2 and other gases from different gaseous cavities within our body, such as pneumothorax, emphysematous bullae, and air embolism.

Central Nervous System

In CNS, the convulsions, similar to those of grand mal epilepsy, occur during oxygen toxicity.

Retrolental Fibroplasia

The retrolental fibroplasia (RLF) is the result of O_2 toxicity of retina and is caused by retinal vasoconstriction. Due to high PaO_2, the obliteration of most of the immature retinal vessels and the subsequent new vessel formation at the site of damage is the principal pathology of this disease. So, the RLF is also called as the proliferative retinopathy. Leakage of extravascular fluid from this new proliferation of blood vessels in retina also leads to vitreoretinal fibrosis, adhesions, and subsequent retinal detachment. RLF usually occurs in infants exposed to hyperoxia in the neonatal intensive care unit (NICU). It is related not to the FiO_2, but to an elevated retinal arterial PO_2. This is because high FiO_2 is not always related to high PaO_2 due to different lung pathology in neonates or prematurity, which prevents the diffusion of O_2 through alveoli. It is not known the actual threshold level of PaO_2, which is responsible for the development of this retinal damage. An umbilical arterial PO_2 of 60–90 mm Hg is associated with a very low incidence of RLF. It should be noted, however, that there are also many factors which are involved in the development of RLF in addition to retinal arterial hyperoxia.

Retrolental fibroplasia is recently termed as ROP (retinopathy of prematurity). It develops in 84% of premature infants born at ±28 weeks of gestational period. But, fortunately, it resolves in 80% of cases without any visual loss form retinal detachment and scarring. Risk of ROP increases not only with delivery at early gestational period (severity of prematurity), but also with the other comorbidities such as sepsis, ARDS, and others, which need management by ventilators with high FiO_2. In contrast to pulmonary toxicity, ROP correlates better with PaO_2 than P_AO_2. In-between 1940 and 1950s, ROP had reached an epidemic level. This was due to the administration of high O_2 concentration ($FiO_2 > 0.5$) in incubators. So, the recommended PaO_2 for premature

TABLE 10: Partial pressure of different gases in arterial and venous blood when breathing 100% O_2 and air.

Tension of gases in arterial and venous blood	Breathing 100% O_2 (mm Hg)	Breathing of air (mm Hg)
PaO_2	600	100
$PaCO_2$	40	40
PaN_2	0	569
PvO_2	50	40
$PvCO_2$	46	46
PvN_2	0	569

infants receiving O_2 is 50–80 mm Hg. But, if due to any cardiopulmonary reasons, a premature infant needs arterial O_2 saturation of 96–99%, then it should not be withheld in the fear of ROP.

■ OXYGEN DELIVERY SYSTEM

The O_2 can be delivered at different concentrations and at different atmospheric pressures by the different techniques such as nasal catheters, simple mask and pipe from oxygen cylinder, complicated anesthetic machine, heart lung machine, and O_2 pressure suit. But, here only, few bedside methods of O_2 delivery system have been discussed.

Nasal Catheters or Cannulas

This is the simplest bedside device for the delivery of O_2 to patients. It is available in all the sizes for adults, children, infants, and neonates. Two types of nasal cannulas are used—one is soft, plastic, blind ended with an over-the-ear head-elastic adjustment and the second is dual flow with under-the-chin variable adjustment. The FiO_2 during the use of these cannulas is unpredictable. It is determined by—the total O_2 flow, tidal volume, respiratory rate, and the nasopharyngeal volume of the patient, which acts as the O_2 reservoir during inspiration or during mouth breathing. Since, as the O_2 flows continuously through these catheters, so 80% of the delivered O_2 is wasted during expiration, which again depends on the rate of respiration. The FiO_2 increases by approximately 1–2% for each liter of O_2 flow during quite breathing. By the flow of 3–4 L/min, the FiO_2 can be increased up to 30–35%. Again by the flow of 5 L/min, the FiO_2 can be increased up to 40%. But the higher flow rate >5 L/min is poorly tolerated by patient. This is due to the discomfort as the gas jets into the nasal cavity and causes dry crusting of the nasal mucosa **(Table 11)**.

The advantages of nasal cannula are that it is comfortable, well tolerated, and allows the patient to speak, eat, drink, etc. during O_2 therapy. It is also nonclaustrophobic and allows long-term use. It also can be used by cannula fixed with spectacles frame for more convenience or cosmetic purpose. To avoid the wastage of O_2 during expiration, the cannulas fitted with inlet reservoir are also used by the patients who are receiving long-term O_2 therapy. This concept has resulted the development of reservoir device, with a valve, which stores the incoming O_2 during expiration, till the inspiration occurs.

Cannulas, providing O_2 to the patient, are connected to the flow meter and cylinders or pipeline through a humidifier and a small-bore tubing. Nowadays, the pediatric sized nasal cannulas are also available for pediatric patient and this use has become increasingly common. During reduced

TABLE 11: Different O_2 delivery system, O_2 flow rate, and FiO_2.

Delivery system	Flow rate (L/min)	FiO₂ (%)
Nasal cannula	2	25
	4	30
	6	40
Mask without reservoir	6	40
	8	50
Mask with reservoir	4	40
	6	50
Venturi mask	4	24
	6	28
	8	35
	10	40
	12	50

(FiO_2: fraction of inspired oxygen)

minute ventilation, due to any cause, the flow of O_2 through the cannulas should also be proportionately reduced. This generally requires a pressure-compensated flow meter, which accurately delivers O_2 flow <1–3 L/min and will reduce the wastage. With the pediatric sized cannulas when the O_2 flows at the rate of 0.25, 0.5, 0.75, or 1 L/min, then the FiO_2 reaches 35%, 45%, 60%, and 70%, respectively.

Oxygen Mask with or without Reservoir Bag

It is a simple, disposable, and transparent plastic device, which is placed over the face, covering both the nose and mouth. When it covers only the nose, then it is called as the nasal mask. The lower edge of the nasal mask rests on the upper lip surrounding the external nose only. The advantage of nasal mask over the cannula for delivery of O_2 is that it is not jetted into the nasal cavity like cannula and allows patient's comfort.

Both the nasal and the face masks are fastened to the patient's face by adjustable elastic headband. Some manufacturers provide a malleable metal nose bridge adjustment device for the proper fitting of mask at the root of the nose. When the O_2 masks are used, then the patients receive the mixture of O_2 and entrained room air, which enters through the leak between the mask and the face. In some masks, there have some small room air entrainment holes near the connection between the mask and the tubing which lead to the flow meter.

The body of the face mask actually acts as a reservoir for both the inspired O_2 and expired CO_2. So, a minimum O_2 flow of approximately 5 L/min is needed to avoid rebreathing during the use of face mask. The level of desired FiO_2 during the management of hypoxia with a face mask depends on the O_2 flow, mask volume, tidal volume, and the respiratory rate (pattern of ventilation) of patient. Usually, during normal breathing, the FiO_2 reaches 30–60%, when the O_2 flow varies between 5 and 10 L/min. The FiO_2 can be higher with low respiratory rate or increased tidal volume. Masks are used for patients who need high level of FiO_2 than nasal cannula and for a short period of time such as during patient transport, in the postanesthetic care unit, and in emergency department. But, it is not the device of choice for delivery of O_2 in patient who is suffering from severe hypoxemia, tachypnea, or unable to protect their airway from aspiration.

Sometimes, a plastic bag is attached to the face mask, which acts as a reservoir of O_2 during inspiration. These are called the reservoir face mask. These are more scientific than the usual cannula or only face mask without reservoir. The reservoir masks are again of two types: (1) the rebreathing reservoir mask and (2) the nonrebreathing reservoir mask. In rebreathing reservoir mask, the patient's expired air enters the bag and refills it. But usually, this expired gas comes from the patient's dead space and does not cause any significant rebreathing of CO_2. In nonrebreathing reservoir mask, a valve is used between the bag and the mask, which prevents rebreathing. The successful use of reservoir face mask needs sufficient flow of O_2, so that the bag is at least partially full during inspiration. Typically with O_2 flow of 5–10 L/min, the FiO_2 reaches between 40 and 60%. With flow of 15 L/min, the FiO_2 may approach 100%. So, this type of mask is indicated for severe hypoxemia, myocardial infarction (MI), or carbon monoxide poisoning, etc.

Venturi Masks

These masks are also called the air-entrainment mask or high airflow with oxygen entrainment (HAFOE) system. In this system, O_2 is directed by a small-bore tube in jet. Then, a large amount of air is entrained through the ports, which are present by the side of the small tube and mix with O_2. The final O_2 concentration depends on the ratio of air drawn in through the entrainment ports and the principal O_2 flow. The manufacturers have developed both the fixed and adjustable type of venturi mask, where the amount of air entrained in the mask can be adjusted or fixed. The venturi mask is used for patients whose hypoxemia cannot be controlled by nasal cannula or face mask. But, it is always advised to use the minimum flow of O_2 in the venturi mask. As a large amount of air entrains into mask, so the patients get adequate amount of flow for inspiration. Hence, patients with COPD who tend to hypoventilate with moderate FiO_2 are the best candidates for the venturi mask. As low flow of O_2 is used in venturi mask, so slight interruption of O_2 flow may cause

serious problem, resulting in hypoxemia and hypercarbia. On the other hand, if the entrainment ports are accidentally obstructed by any means, such as by bed sheet and patient's hands, then FiO_2 will suddenly increase due to getting pure O_2 without mixing with air.

Oxygen Hood

Many young infants and neonates do not tolerate appliances like nasal cannulas and masks over their faces, though different pediatric sizes of it are available. So, for them, the oxygen hood is the best alternative for short-term O_2 therapy. Actually, hood is ideal for newborns and inactive infants. While the nasal cannula, face mask, or venturi mask provides greater acceptability for mobile pediatric group of patients. Hoods can be of different sizes for different age group of pediatric patients. Some are simple plexiglass box. But, others have definite system for sealing the neck opening. There should be no attempt to completely seal the system, which can cause the accumulation of CO_2. So, to remove CO_2, the hood needs minimum flow of O_2 >7 L/min, but flows of 10–15 L/min are adequate for majority of patients.

■ HYPERBARIC OXYGEN

Hyperbaric condition is defined as the circumstance where the total environmental or atmospheric pressure is increased. Thus, the O_2 therapy at this hyperbaric condition is known as the hyperbaric oxygen. The higher will be the atmospheric pressure, the higher will be the PO_2 in air for a fixed concentration of it in air. This is because, at higher atmospheric pressure, there will be increased concentration of O_2 molecule in a given volume of air, which will increase the partial pressure of O_2. The higher will be the PO_2 in the inspired gas or air, the higher will be the alveolar PO_2 and arterial PO_2, provided the diffusion of O_2 through the alveolar membrane is normal. The relationship between the alveolar PO_2 and the arterial PO_2 is almost linear. The higher will be the arterial PO_2, the higher will be the amount of oxygen carried as physical solution in arterial blood. This is because the amount of O_2 carried as physical solution in blood only determines the arterial PO_2 or (PaO_2). But, the amount of O_2 carried by Hb which determines the SpO_2 will not increase.

At the sea level, the fresh air contains 21% O_2, the rest being mainly nitrogen. At the sea level, the barometric pressure (atmospheric pressure) is of 760 mm Hg and the partial pressure of O_2 in inspired air is thus 159 mm Hg, which is 21% of 760 mm Hg. When this air is inspired at 760 mm Hg, then during its passage through respiratory tract, it rapidly becomes saturated with water vapor at body temperature in the airway and on entering the alveoli it mixes with alveolar gases which contain expired CO_2.

The partial pressure of water vapor and CO_2 accounts for about 47 mm Hg and 40 mm Hg respectively of the total alveolar gaseous pressure which is 760 mm Hg and thus leaving pressure of 673 mm Hg as only for the combined pressures of nitrogen and oxygen in the inspired air. At 1 atmospheric pressure, air contains 78% N_2 and it comes down to 75% when reaches the alveoli. So, the partial pressure of N_2 in alveolar air is 75% of 760 mm Hg or 569 mm Hg. Thus, the partial pressure of O_2 in alveolar air or alveolar O_2 tension (P_AO_2) is 673 − 569 = 104 mm Hg. Thus when 100% O_2 alone is inspired, then nitrogen is displaced from the alveoli, leaving the whole 673 mm Hg partial pressure for only O_2. Thus, the alveolar O_2 pressure or tension can readily be calculated when breathing 100% O_2 at various ambient pressures from the following formula:

$$P_AO_2 = PiO_2 - PH_2O - PCO_2$$
$$= 760 - 47 - 40$$
$$= 673 \text{ mm Hg}$$

PiO_2 = Partial pressure of O_2 in inspired air at different atmospheric pressure

P_ACO_2 = Partial pressure of CO_2 in alveolar air (usually 40 mm Hg)

PH_2O = Partial pressure of water vapor in alveolar air (47 mm Hg at 37°C).

Table 12 shows the alveolar O_2 tension or pressure at different atmospheric pressure when pure or 100% O_2 is administered. The alveolar PO_2 is the principal determining factor of arterial PO_2. Normally, the difference between these two (O_2 tension in alveolar air and arterial blood) is small (2–4 mm Hg) and is mainly due to venous admixture.

Oxygen is carried in blood by chemical combination with Hb and as dissolved physical solution in plasma. 1 g of Hb combines with 1.34 mL of O_2 at one atmospheric pressure. Assuming hemoglobin concentration is of 14.6 g per 100 mL of blood, the amount of O_2, which can be carried as the chemical combination with Hb, will be 19.6 mL per 100 mL of blood. When breathing air at one atmospheric pressure, Hb is only 97% saturated with O_2. So, only 19 mL

of O_2 which is 97% of 19.6 mL is carried per 100 mL of blood. In a healthy individual when 100% O_2 is breathed at one atmospheric pressure, the Hb becomes fully saturated and carries maximum up to 19.6 mL of O_2. By increasing the atmospheric pressure, this amount of O_2 carried by Hb cannot be increased.

In equilibrium, the amount of physically dissolved oxygen in plasma is proportional to the partial pressure of O_2 in alveolus, which again depends on the atmospheric pressure. Normally, the plasma contains 0.003 mL O_2/100 mL blood/mm Hg arterial O_2 pressure. When breathing room air at an alveolar PO_2 of 104 mm Hg which corresponds to the arterial O_2 tension (PaO_2) of 100 mm Hg at equilibrium, then the amount of dissolved O_2 as physical solution mounts to 0.3 mL O_2 per 100 mL of blood. If the P_AO_2 rose to 673 mm Hg (when the patient breathed pure 100% oxygen at 1 atmospheric pressure) then the PaO_2 rises to 600 mm Hg and the amount of physically dissolved O_2 in plasma would be 1.8 mL per 100 mL of blood. If a subject breathes O_2 at 3 ATA, then the P_AO_2 will be 2,193 mm Hg and the arterial PO_2 will be 2,000 mm Hg. In this situation, the amount of physically dissolved O_2 would be 6 mL/100 mL of blood. Here, the dissolved O_2 would be sufficient to supply all the O_2 required for a resting man and venous blood would return to the lungs with Hb still fully saturated. It means that the amount of O_2 dissolved in plasma as physical solution is sufficient for the body need per minute and the O_2 attached with Hb remains intact.

Thus, at normal atmospheric pressure, the total O_2 content of arterial blood is largely dependent on the Hb content. But, when the hyperbaric O_2 is given, then the Hb cannot increase its O_2 load, because it is already fully saturated and in such circumstances as the P_AO_2 rises, so the O_2 content of plasma carried only by the physical solution increases.

When an individual is breathing room air, then his or her O_2 stores as the physically dissolved part in plasma are extremely limited and confined mainly to O_2 carried by Hb. However, O_2 stores in the dissolved form in plasma are considerably increased when the hyperbaric O_2 is given. At 3 ATA, O_2 is physically dissolved in body water, including plasma, to the extent of about 6 mL/100 mL. In a 70-kg adult, with 50 liters body water, this would create a potential high O_2 reservoir of 6 × 500 = 3,000 mL of O_2. So, such increase in O_2 store will theoretically allow the tissues to survive temporary anoxia for much longer periods which is not possible without hyperbaric O_2.

It was also stressed before that the tissue O_2 levels depend not only on the arterial O_2 tension, but also upon other factors, which are responsible for delivery of O_2 to tissues. These include hemoglobin, cardiac output, its distribution

TABLE 12: Different alveolar O_2 tension in relation to different atmospheric pressure.

Atmospheric pressure ATA	Alveolar PO_2 tension (P_AO_2) in mm Hg
1	673
2	1,438
3	2,193
4	2,953
5	3,713
6	4,473

in different tissue, and some transfer factors. The hyperbaric O_2 may also cause some physiological adjustments, which tend to offset the increase in tissue O_2 levels. For example, cerebral blood vessels may constrict in response to changes in CO_2 transport and thus limit the increase in cerebral tissue O_2 tension.

Today, the clinical applications of hyperbaric O_2 are only confined to some unusual disease processes, which include carbon monoxide poisoning, gas gangrene, congenital cardiac anomalies, peripheral vascular insufficiencies, and cancer therapy.

Carbon monoxide has considerably greater affinity for Hb than O_2. So, exposure of even low concentration of carbon monoxide (CO) to Hb rapidly leads to "anemic hypoxia", because this gas interferes with the ability of Hb to combine with O_2 and its transport. So, prompt institution of hyperbaric O_2 therapy has an important part to play in the management of carbon monoxide poisoning. O_2 therapy between 2 and 3 atmospheric pressure alleviates this situation in three ways: (1) it provides enough amount of physically dissolved O_2 in the plasma to keep the patient alive. (2) It causes the shift of the O_2 dissociation curve to the right—thus enabling the remaining oxyhemoglobin to give up more O_2 at tissue level. (3) It accelerates the rate of dissociation of carboxyhemoglobin twice than that achieved by conventional treatment with 5% CO_2 in 100% O_2 at normal (one) atmospheric pressure. The treatment by hyperbaric O_2 should be continued until the carboxyhemoglobin is no longer detectable in the blood by which time the consciousness will return, provided there has been no brain damage.

OXYGEN–HEMOGLOBIN DISSOCIATION CURVE

Hemoglobin is a big complex molecule, consisting of four heme parts and one globin part. Again, the each heme part of hemoglobin is formed by a divalent iron (Fe^{2+}) atom and four porphyrin (pyrrole) rings. In a hemoglobin molecule, as there are four heme subunits, so there are four divalent iron atoms in each Hb molecule. Only this divalent Fe^+ atom can combine with O_2 and each iron atom takes only one molecule of O_2. So, one Hb molecule can carry four O_2 molecules. The globin part of Hb consists of two α and two β subunits and these four subunits of globin are held together by weak bonds. Each heme unit is attached with one subunit of globin.

Each gram of Hb interacts and combines chemically with 1.39 mL of O_2. This interaction between Hb and O_2 to form oxy-Hb (HbO_2) occurs in four steps. However, this every step of interaction between Hb and O_2 to form HbO_2 brings some conformational changes in Hb and accelerates the next step. Thus, binding of first three molecules of O_2 with Hb greatly accelerates the binding of last fourth molecule of O_2 and is responsible for last 75–100% O_2 saturation of Hb, which is again responsible for the peculiar S-shaped line of oxy-Hb dissociation curve. After 90% saturation of Hb by O_2, the availability of receptors on Hb for binding of O_2 suddenly declines. Then, O_2 combines with Hb very slowly and saturation rises gradually up to 100%. After that, the SpO_2 of Hb does not rise further, as all the O_2-binding sites of a hemoglobin molecule are occupied with O_2 and are nothing left. But, only O_2 tension of blood can be raised indefinitely, without any limit, as the physically dissolved amount of it (O_2) in plasma, which depends on atmospheric pressure and is responsible for O_2 tension (PO_2) in blood, is increased **(Fig. 8)**.

The saturation of Hb by O_2 is defined as the percentage of oxy-Hb which is present at now (present amount of O_2 attached with Hb) against the total amount of Hb to be oxygenated (the total amount of O_2 can be attached by Hb, i.e., O_2 capacity of Hb). After the initial entry of O_2 into bloodstream, it first physically dissolves in plasma and produces a tension of O_2 in blood. Then, this O_2 enters in RBC to combine with Hb, producing oxyhemoglobin. But, this part of O_2, which combines with Hb, does not produce any oxygen tension in blood. Thus, Hb gradually becomes saturated with O_2 and in the vertical part of oxygen dissociation curve, the percentage of oxy-Hb (SpO_2 of Hb) rises sharply with less increase in O_2 tension in plasma (this less increase of O_2 tension in this vertical part of oxygen dissociation curve is due to gradual passing of O_2 from plasma to Hb). In last vertical part of oxygen dissociation curve, after 100% saturation of Hb by oxygen, O_2 is not taken further by Hb and it remains in plasma as in dissolving state.

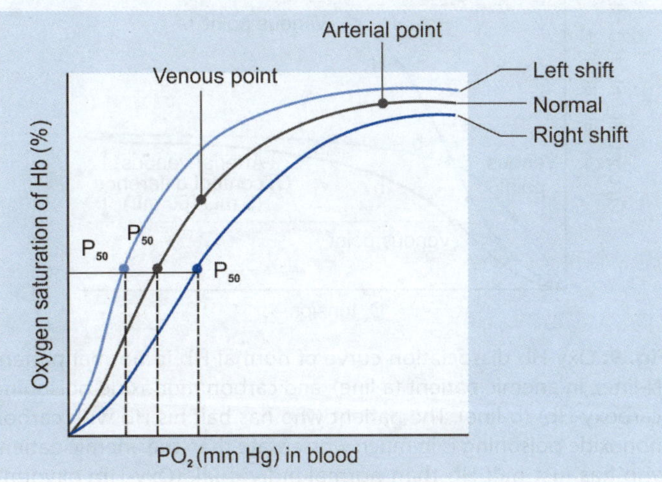

Fig. 8: O_2–Hb dissociation curve.

So, in that phase, the percentage of saturated oxy-Hb does not rise, but only the O_2 tension (PO_2) in blood increases **(Fig. 9)**.

Thus, the graphical representation of this whole event of relationship between the percentages of saturated oxy-Hb and the gradually developed tension of O_2 in blood (plasma) forms the oxygen–hemoglobin dissociation curve. *Actually, the O_2-Hb dissociation curve tells us: (1) the percentage of saturation of Hb by O_2, (2) the tension of O_2 in blood, (3) the total content of O_2 in blood, and (4) the availability of O_2 to tissues.* The O_2-Hb dissociation curve is an elongated S-shaped or sigmoid-shaped line and has mainly two slopes or parts: (1) the upper flat or near horizontal slope (part) and (2) the lower straight or near vertical slope (part). The vertical downward slope starts when the O_2 saturation of Hb or SpO_2 level comes down to 90% from 100%, which corresponds to arterial O_2 tension (PaO_2) of 60 mm Hg. After that, any slight fall of PaO_2 causes steep fall of O_2 saturation of Hb. This is due to large amount of O_2 uncombined from Hb for delivery to tissues, which increases greatly for a given slight decrease in arterial PO_2 from 60 mm Hg.

There are many factors, which can influence this O_2-Hb dissociation curve. But, among them, the important factors are: (1) CO_2 tension, (2) H^+ concentration (acidosis and alkalosis), (3) types of Hb, (4) body temperature, and (5) the concentration of 2,3-DPG (diphosphoglycerate) level. The influences of these above factors can be expressed by P_{50}. The P_{50} is defined as the O_2 tension (in mm Hg) at which Hb is 50% saturated. Normally, P_{50} value is 27 mm Hg. It means that at 50% saturation of Hb by oxygen, the O_2 tension

in blood reaches to 27 mm Hg. Increase or decrease of P_{50} value indicates shifting of O_2-Hb dissociation curve to the right or left. The P_{50} value <27 mm Hg describes the leftward shifting of curve which means that at 50% O_2 saturation of Hb, there is less tension of O_2 (<27 mm Hg) in blood. It also means that at this given O_2 tension (<27 mm Hg), Hb is still 50% saturated, which also means Hb has a higher affinity for O_2, leading to less release or unloading of O_2 at tissues, causing cellular hypoxia. *The principal causes of this leftward shifting of oxy-Hb dissociation curve are—alkalosis (metabolic or respiratory), hypothermia, abnormal forms of Hb (e.g., fetal-Hb, methemoglobin, carbomonoxy-Hb, etc.), and decrease of 2,3-DPG level.*

The P_{50} value > 27 mm Hg describes the shifting of O_2-Hb curve toward right. It means for the same 50% saturation of Hb, blood has higher O_2 tension (>27 mm Hg) or at any given PO_2, Hb is less saturated. It indicates Hb has low affinity for O_2 or more O_2 is present in plasma as dissolved state and will readily give up O_2 to tissues. *The principal causes of this rightward shifting of O_2-Hb dissociation curve are acidosis (metabolic or respiratory), hyperthermia, other hemoglobinopathies (thalassemia and sickle cell anemia), or the presence of other abnormal Hb and increased 2,3-DPG level* **(Fig. 10)**.

Acidosis and alkalosis control the O_2-Hb dissociation curve by controlling CO_2 tension or H^+ concentration in blood. An increase in plasma H^+ concentration or CO_2 tension decreases the affinity of O_2 to Hb and vice versa. This is called *Bohr effect.* When the blood flows through tissue capillaries, then the gradual increase of CO_2 tension in plasma shifts the O_2-Hb dissociation curve toward right and the affinity of Hb for O_2 is reduced, which facilitates the release of O_2 from Hb to tissues. Reversely, in pulmonary capillaries, the lowering

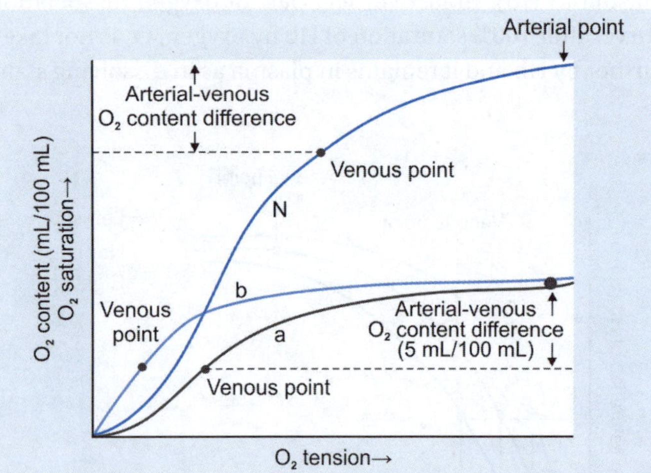

Fig. 9: Oxy-Hb dissociation curve of normal Hb in normal patient (N-line), in anemic patient (a-line), and carbon monoxide poisoning (carboxy-Hb) (b-line). The patient who has half his Hb with carbon monoxide poisoning is in much worse state than the anemic patient who has just half Hb than normal individual. (Oxy-Hb: oxygen–hemoglobin)

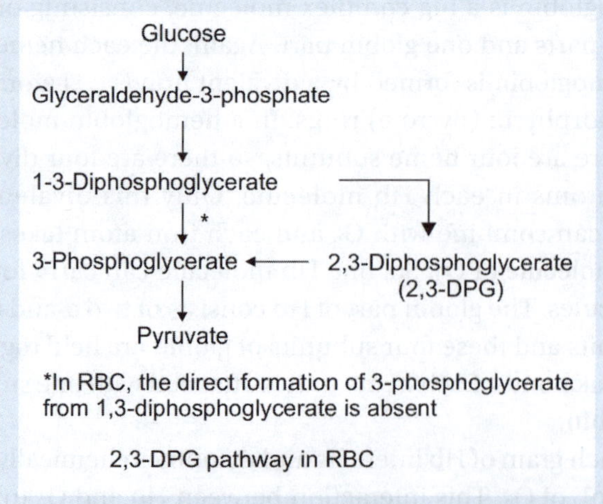

Fig. 10: The steps of synthesis of 2,3-DPG in RBC. (2,3-DPG: 2,3-diphosphoglycerate; RBC: red blood cell)

of CO_2 tension due to its gradual release in alveoli shifts the O_2-Hb dissociation curve toward left. Thus, the affinity of Hb for O_2 increases and facilitates the uptake of O_2 by Hb in alveoli. *Haldane effect* is described here.

Increased 2,3-DPG level in plasma shifts the O_2-Hb dissociation curve toward right and reduces the affinity of Hb for O_2 causing increased unloading of O_2 at tissues. This is because the 2,3-DPG has higher affinity toward Hb for binding than O_2. This plays an important compensatory role in patients with chronic hypoxia, anemia, and in blood transfusion. The 2,3-DPG is a byproduct of glycolytic pathway in RBC and accumulates within it only during anaerobic metabolism. Thus, it helps in hypoxic condition by increasing the supply of O_2 to (unloading of O_2) tissues through its effects on oxy-Hb dissociation curve. Under physiological condition, the glycolytic pathway in RBC runs in normal pathway and there is less formation of 2,3-DPG through alternate pathway. So, the effect of 2,3-DPG on this curve is minimum in aerobic condition.

Due to the use of ACD (acid citrate dextrose) as anticoagulant during collection of blood for transfusion, there is an immediate fall of 2,3-DPG level in RBC, after it is taken from human body and the O_2 dissociation curve of Hb in RBC shifts toward left. So, the recently transfused blood is reluctant to give up O_2 to tissues. Then, 2–3 days are required to recover the level of 2,3-DPG in RBC after transfusion. Whereas, the use of CPD as anticoagulant in stored blood delays the fall of 2,3-DPG level for 10 days, at which time the level is still near to normal in CPD blood **(Fact file I)**.

The abnormal hemoglobins, which have influences on O_2-Hb dissociation curve, are methemoglobin, sulfhemoglobin, fetal hemoglobin, sickle cell hemoglobin, hemoglobin C, hemoglobin E, etc. They prevent the carrying of O_2 by Hb and have their own O_2 saturation characteristics. The fetal-Hb has greater affinity for O_2 than adult Hb and shifts the dissociation curve toward left. Some chemicals such as carbon monoxide, cyanide, and nitric acid also combine with Hb at O_2-binding site and prevent the O_2 to combine with Hb. Thus, they all shift the O_2 saturation curve toward left. Carbon monoxide has 200–300 times more affinity for Hb than O_2 and combines with it forming carboxyhemoglobin. Thus, it decreases the O_2-carrying capacity of Hb by shifting the saturation curve toward left and impairs the release of O_2 to tissues.

The O_2 dissociation curve is also shifted toward right, during the rise of temperature (hyperthermia), like the fall of plasma pH (acidosis), showing the decreased affinity of Hb for O_2 and increased unloading of it at tissue level. Reverse effect is seen when the temperature is decreased (hypothermia).

FACT FILE I

2,3-DPG is very plentiful in RBC. It is formed from 3-phosphoglyceraldehyde as a product of glycolysis via the Embden–Meyerhof pathway. It is a highly charged anion and binds to the β-chain of deoxyhemoglobin, preventing binding of O_2 with Hb. One mole of deoxyhemoglobin binds to one mole of 2,3-DPG. The reaction is:
$HbO_2 + 2,3\text{-DPG} \leftrightarrow Hb\text{--}2,3\text{-DPG} + O_2$

In this equation, an increase in the concentration of 2,3-DPG shifts the reaction toward right, causing more O_2 to be liberated. Factors affecting the concentration of 2,3-DPG in RBC include pH. This is because acidosis inhibits red cell glycolysis and the formation of 2,3-DPG and vice versa. Exercise causes an increase in 2,3-DPG within 60 minutes. Therefore, much more O_2 is removed from each unit of blood, flowing through active tissues during exercise, which have low PO_2. Finally, at low PO_2, the O_2-Hb dissociation curve is steep and large amount of O_2 is liberated per unit drop of PO_2. Ascent to high altitude also causes a rise in 2,3-DPG level, with consequent increase in P_{50} and increase in availability of O_2 to tissues (increase unloading of O_2 at tissue level).

The affinity of fetal-Hb (Hb-F) for O_2 is greater than adult Hb. This facilitates the movement of O_2 from mother toward fetus. This is due to the poor binding of 2,3-DPG by the γ-polypeptide chain of globin part of Hb, which is the characteristic of Hb-F. Some abnormal Hb in adults have low P_{50} values and the resulting high O_2 affinity of these Hb causes enough tissue hypoxia to stimulate increased RBC formation, with resulting polycythemia. It is because these Hb do not bind to 2,3-DPG. The 2,3-DPG concentration in RBC is increased in anemia and in variety of diseases where there is chronic hypoxia. This facilitates the delivery of O_2 to the tissues by raising PO_2 at which O_2 is released in peripheral capillaries.

(2,3-DPG: 2,3-diphosphoglycerate; PO_2: partial pressure of oxygen; RBC: red blood cell)

Myoglobin is another iron-containing pigment, which resembles hemoglobin. It is present in muscle and its affinity for O_2 is much higher than Hb. So, the O_2-Hb dissociation curve of myoglobin shifts toward left and looks like rectangular hyperbola. O_2 from myoglobin is released, only when it is exposed to very low PO_2. *Summary: If the affinity of Hb toward O_2 is increased, then 50% O_2 saturation of Hb will occur at <27 mm Hg pressure ($\downarrow$P50) and the O_2 dissociation curve will shift toward left. On the contrary, if the affinity of Hb toward O_2 is decreased, then 50% saturation of Hb by O_2 will occur at >27 mm Hg pressure ($\uparrow$P50). This will lead to shifting of O_2 dissociation curve toward right.*

Bohr Effect and Haldane Effect

Increased CO_2 content of blood helps to release more O_2 from Hb into tissues. This is called Bohr effect. On the other hand, decreased O_2 content of blood helps to contain more CO_2 by blood at tissue level is called Haldane effect. The explanation of Bohr effect is like that increased CO_2 in blood produces increased amount of H^+ ($CO_2 + H_2O = H^+ + HCO_3^-$, by carbonic anhydrase. This carbonic anhydrase is present only in RBC, not in plasma) in RBC and the pH inside of RBC will decrease. This increased concentration of H^+ in RBC alters the configuration of Hb and affinity of O_2 to Hb is reduced. Therefore, O_2 is released to tissue. The explanation of Haldane effect is like that release of O_2 from Hb makes it (Hb) more acidic and then this acidic deoxygenated Hb acts as better acceptor of proton (H^+). Hence, the H^+ produced inside the RBC from CO_2 by hydration is taken up by Hb and CO_2 content of blood is increased.

Coefficient of O_2 Utilization

It indicates what percentage of arterial O_2 is used up from its total contents by a tissue. It is expressed by the following formula:

Coefficient of O_2 utilization =

$$\frac{O_2 \text{ taken up by the tissue}}{O_2 \text{ content of arterial blood}} \times 100$$

Normally, the arterial blood contains 19 mL and venous blood contains 14 mL of O_2 per 100 mL of blood. So, usually the arteriovenous difference of O_2 content is about 5 mL. Thus, the coefficient of O_2 utilization is $5 \times 100/19$ or 26%. The arteriovenous O_2 difference or the utilization coefficient of O_2 is directly proportional to the rate of tissue activity. In heavy exercise, this coefficient may increase up to 80%. Normally, in heart tissue, the arteriovenous O_2 difference or O_2 taken up by myocardium is 12 mL. So, the O_2 utilization coefficient of heart is $12 \times 100/19$ or 63%. During exercise, it further rises. Hence, the O_2 utilization coefficient is a true index of degree of tissue activity.

Effect of O_2-Hb Saturation (Dissociation) Curve on CO_2 Content and Its Transport

The deoxygenated Hb has 3.5 times greater affinity for CO_2 than the O_2-Hb (Haldane effect). So, when the blood passes through tissue capillaries and Hb gives up O_2 becoming deoxygenated, then this process of deoxygenation helps deoxygenated Hb to carry more CO_2. As a result, venous blood contains more CO_2 than arterial blood. Similarly, O_2-Hb has 3.5 times less affinity for CO_2, which helps it to give up CO_2 at pulmonary level. As a result, the arterial blood has less CO_2 than the venous blood. Hence, the combination of CO_2 with Hb depends on the O_2 status of it (Hb) and vice versa. It is called the Haldane effect. Thus, the deoxygenation at tissue level and oxygenation at pulmonary level help the Hb to combine with CO_2, transport of it, and release of CO_2 at lung. This is indicated by that the O_2-Hb dissociation curve shifts to the right at tissue level and shifts to the left at pulmonary level.

The Haldane effect can be explained by the following way. It also explains the acid–base behavior of Hb. At physiological pH, the Hb acts as buffer due to its high content of histidine. Moreover, at tissue capillary level, the removal of O_2 from Hb causes it to behave more like a base, $HbO_2 \leftrightarrow Hb + O_2$. So, it takes up more hydrogen ion which is formed from carbonic acid: $CO_2 + H_2O = H_2CO_3$. $H_2CO_3 = H^+ + HCO_3^-$, $Hb + H^+ = HbH^+$. Thus, by taking up H^+, the Hb shifts the CO_2 and bicarbonate equilibrium in favor of more bicarbonate formation or increased CO_2 content of blood.

$$HbO_2 + CO_2 + H_2O \leftrightarrow HbH^+ + HCO_3^- + O_2$$

This indicates that the deoxygenation of Hb increases the content and transport of CO_2 in venous blood as bicarbonate. Hence, the CO_2 content in venous blood increases, which is reflected as an increase in bicarbonate. In the lungs, the reverse occurs. Here, the combination of O_2 with Hb causes it to behave more like an acid and gives up hydrogen ion and shifts the CO_2–bicarbonate equilibrium in favor of more formation of CO_2, which is excreted through lungs.

$$HbH^+ + O_2 = HbO_2 + H^+$$
$$H^+ + HCO_3^- = H_2CO_3$$
$$H_2CO_3 = CO_2 + H_2O$$

In tissue: $HbO_2 + CO_2 + H_2O \leftrightarrow HbH^+ + HCO_3 + O_2$ and this released O_2 enter the tissue.

Hence, the total CO_2 content in blood decreases, which is reflected by decrease in HCO_3^- level.

■ CARBON DIOXIDE DISSOCIATION CURVE

Under different physiological and pathological conditions, the *CO_2 content* and its *(CO_2) tension* in blood vary. So, like O_2 dissociation curve, when these variations of CO_2 content and its tension in blood and the relationship between these variations are plotted in a graph, then it is called as the CO_2 dissociation curve **(Fig. 11)**. But, here the volume of CO_2 (CO_2 content) as percent is taken instead of saturation of CO_2 as percent. The CO_2 dissociation curve is shifted to right, when the saturation of Hb with O_2 is increased (opposite to O_2 dissociation curve) and the CO_2 dissociation curve is shifted to left, when the saturation of Hb with O_2 is decreased (opposite to O_2 dissociation curve). Therefore, the dissociation curve of CO_2 is shifted toward right in arterial blood and the dissociation curve of CO_2 is shifted toward left in venous blood.

Usually, the facts, which can be expressed from this CO_2-dissociation curve, are:

- At any given CO_2 tension, the reduced or deoxygenated Hb takes up larger amount of CO_2 than oxygenated Hb. So, in our body, the reduction or deoxygenation of Hb in tissue capillaries increases the degree of CO_2 uptake by blood from tissues.

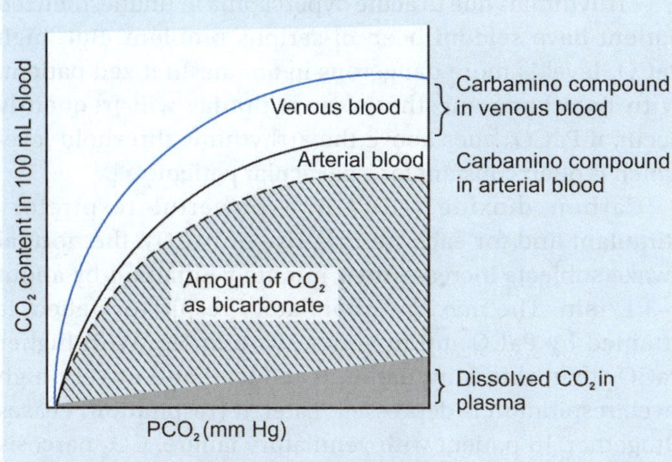

Fig. 11: CO_2 dissociation curve of arterial and venous blood. (PCO₂: partial pressure of carbon dioxide)

- Oxygenation of Hb causes the release of CO_2 from it and this happens in lungs. On the other hand, the deoxygenation of Hb causes the attachment of CO_2 with Hb (in the form of H^+) and this happens in tissues.
- As the CO_2 tension in blood is increased, the total amount of CO_2 taken up by blood also rises. On the other hand, as the CO_2 tension in blood falls, the total CO_2 content in blood also diminishes.

The factors which influence the O_2 dissociation curve also influence the CO_2 dissociation curve, but in opposite direction; that is, the factors which decrease the affinity of Hb for O_2 and shift the O_2 dissociation curve to the right also shift the CO_2 dissociation curve to the left and increase the affinity of Hb for CO_2.

CARBON DIOXIDE STORES

In our body, continuously the production, store, and the elimination of CO_2 are going on and in normal physiological condition, these three factors remain in an equilibrium. Usually, CO_2 is stored in our body in three forms: (1) as dissolved form in plasma, (2) as bicarbonate, and (3) as CO_2-Hb. The amount of total stored CO_2 in an adult is about 120 liters. It is stored in our body in three compartments, which are designated as rapid, intermediate, and slow compartment. The rapid compartment consists of highly vascular structures such as brain, heart, liver, and kidney. The intermediate compartment mainly consists of muscle tissues, and slow compartment consists of fat and bones. When there is imbalance between the production and elimination of CO_2, then there is also change in the total amount of CO_2 stored in our body and a new equilibrium is established. This usually takes a long time, near about 20–30 minutes (compared with O_2, which takes <3–5 minutes),

and it is due to the large capacity of intermediate and slow compartments. During equilibrium, the rate of rise of CO_2 tension in arterial blood is generally slower than its fall following acute change in ventilation.

HYPERCAPNIA AND HYPOCAPNIA

Hypercapnia refers to the accumulation of CO_2 in blood. This is indicated by an arterial CO_2 tension >6 kPa or end-tidal CO_2 tension >60 mm Hg. On the other hand, hypocapnia refers to the deficit of CO_2 in blood and is indicated by an arterial CO_2 tension <4 kPa or end-tidal CO_2 tension <40 mm Hg.

Causes of Hypercapnia

Common causes of hypercapnia during anesthesia are: (1) inadequate CO_2 removal or (2) excessive CO_2 production. Inadequate CO_2 removal is most commonly caused by— (i) hypoventilation and (ii) increased alveolar dead space. But, it may also result from—(iii) inadequate fresh gas flow or (iv) exhausted soda lime.

Hypoventilation

It is due to abnormal position of patient during surgery, increased airway resistance, decreased compliance of thorax and lungs, decreased respiratory drive due to anesthetic agents and sedatives, and mechanical hypoventilation during intermittent positive pressure ventilation (IPPV). The equipmental or technical causes of hypoventilation are obstruction, kinking, leak or disconnection, etc. at any part of the breathing circuit.

Increased Dead Space Ventilation

- It occurs when the pulmonary artery pressure drops due to hypotension. It increases the area of pulmonary zone. Thus, subsequently it increases the ventilation–perfusion mismatch and alveolar dead space ventilation.
- It also occurs when the airway pressure increases, which subsequently increases the area of pulmonary zone I. Thus, subsequently it increases the ventilation–perfusion mismatch and alveolar dead space ventilation.
- Pulmonary embolism, thrombosis, vascular obliteration, etc. also increase the amount of lung that is ventilated but underperfused. This also increases the dead space ventilation by increasing the ventilation–perfusion mismatch.
- Rapid short inspiration may be distributed preferentially to the more compliant alveoli, causing the less compliant alveoli or stiff alveoli are minimally ventilated. This is due to the short time constant of the less compliant alveoli. This also increases the dead space ventilation.

- Anesthesia apparatus also increases the total dead space by increasing the length of airway and by increasing the rebreathing of expired gas, which is equivalent to dead space ventilation. The order of increasing the rebreathing during spontaneous ventilation with Mapleson circuit is A, D, C, B and during controlled ventilation is D, B, C, A. There will be no rebreathing in circuit E (Ayre's T-piece) if the patient's duration of expiration is long enough permitting the complete washout of the expired gases for a given fresh gas flow, however, only if the fresh gas flow is greater than the peak inspiratory flow rate.

The effect of increased dead space can be countered by increasing the respiratory rate, for example, if minute volume of a patient is 10 L/min and V_D/V_T is 30%, then alveolar ventilation is 7 L/min. If due to any reason V_D/V_T is increased to 50%, then minute ventilation should be increased to 14 L/min to maintain the alveolar ventilation at 7 L/min.

Increased CO_2 Production

Fever, malignant hyperthermia, sepsis, shivering, hypertension, thyroid storm, increased release of catecholamines, etc. are the few of many causes of increased CO_2 production during anesthesia. In febrile patient, there is 13% increase in CO_2 production for each 1°C rise in temperature. Inadvertent or excessive CO_2 delivery from the anesthetic machine due to exhausted soda lime and the excessive absorption of CO_2 during laparoscopic procedure are also other causes of hypercapnia. They indirectly increase the CO_2 production.

Effect of Hypercapnia

In an awake normal patient, the progressive hypercapnia stimulates the sympathetic nervous system. It results in ↑BP, tachycardia, sweating, arrhythmias, and increased cerebral blood flow. This increased cerebral blood flow is dangerous for patients with ↑ICP (intracranial pressure) such as in brain tumor. As the anesthesia suppresses the autonomic responses, so these signs may not occur and are masked until CO_2 tension is markedly increased. The mechanism of effect of hypercapnia on CVS is same as hypoxia. So, like hypoxia, it acts both through direct effect on myocardium which is depression and through indirect reflex (through sympathetic neural and humoral) mechanism which is stimulation. But, the direct depression effect of myocardium by CO_2 is overshadowed by the indirect activation of myocardium by sympathetic nervous system. Hypercapnia, like hypoxemia, also increases the myocardial O_2 demand (due to tachycardia, early hypertension) and decreases the myocardial O_2 supply (due to late hypotension). With moderate-to-severe hypercapnia, hyperkinetic circulation also results. This is due to increased cardiac output and decreased systemic vascular resistance (SVR).

Arrhythmias due to acute hypercapnia in unanesthetized patient have seldom been of serious problem. But, high $PaCO_2$ level is more dangerous in an anesthetized patient. With halothane anesthesia, arrhythmias will frequently occur, if $PaCO_2$ goes above the arrhythmic threshold level which is often constant for a particular patient.

Carbon dioxide (CO_2) is a powerful respiratory stimulant and for each mm Hg rise of $PaCO_2$, the normal awake subjects increase their minute ventilation by about 2–3 L/min. The maximal stimulatory respiratory effect is attained by $PaCO_2$ up to about 100 mm Hg. With higher $PaCO_2$ than this, stimulation is reduced and at very high level, respiration is depressed. Later, it (respiration) ceases altogether. In patient with ventilatory failure, CO_2 narcosis occurs, when $PaCO_2$ rises between 90 and 120 mm Hg. This unconsciousness is due to fall in CSF pH at high $PaCO_2$ level. Chronic hypercapnia or respiratory acidosis results in compensatory increased resorption of bicarbonate by kidney, constituting secondary metabolic alkalosis. On the other hand, chronic hypocapnia causes the reverse. In each case, blood pH returns to normal value, but bicarbonate concentration departs further from normal and may exceed 40 mEq/L. Hypercapnia causes leakage of Ca^{2+} and K^+ from cells in plasma. So, it is also associated with hypercalcemia and hyperkalemia.

Causes of Hypocapnia

Causes of hypocapnia are opposite to hypercapnia. These are hyperventilation, decreased dead space ventilation (change from mask to ETT, decreased PEEP, increased pulmonary artery pressure, and decreased rebreathing), decreased CO_2 production (hypothermia and deep anesthesia), etc. Among these, the mechanical passive hyperventilation is the most common cause of hypocapnia.

Effect of Hypocapnia

Unintentional hyperventilation in association with decreased arterial CO_2 tension ($PaCO_2$) is the usual cause of hypocapnia during anesthesia. Hypocapnia produces respiratory alkalosis with decrease in serum potassium concentration. There are reductions in cerebral blood flow, cardiac output, and tissue O_2 delivery. There may also be delay in onset of spontaneous ventilation at the end of anesthesia.

Hypocapnia causes decrease in CO_2 by three mechanisms:

1. *First:* Increase in intrathoracic pressure by increasing ventilation causes hypocapnia and decreased CO_2 tension.
2. *Second:* Hypocapnia withdraws the sympathetic nervous system activity and thus decreases the inotropic state of heart.

3. *Third:* Hypocapnia can increase blood pH and thus decreases the ionized Ca^{2+} and in turn the inotropic state of heart. Hypocapnia with respiratory alkalosis shifts the oxy-Hb dissociation curve to the left, which increases Hb affinity for O_2 and thus impairing O_2 unloading at tissue level. Hypocapnia also increases the whole body O_2 consumption by increasing the pH-mediated uncoupling of oxidation from phosphorylation. The $PaCO_2$ of 20 mm Hg will increase tissue O_2 consumption by 30%. Hypocapnia causes VA/Q abnormalities by inhibiting the compensatory HPV.

■ TRANSPORT OF CO$_2$

Carbon dioxide (CO_2) is produced in tissues by metabolism. Then, it enters the bloodstream at tissue capillary level and is carried to lungs where it is liberated in alveolar air. The 100 mL of venous blood carries about 52 mL of CO_2, whereas 100 mL of arterial blood carries about 48 mL of CO_2. Therefore, the average normal arteriovenous difference of CO_2 content is about 4 mL per 100 mL of blood. In other word, each 100 mL of arterial blood, while passing through tissues, collects about 4 mL of CO_2. Similarly, each 100 mL of venous blood, while passing through lungs, also releases 4 mL of CO_2. So, the blood always carries a constant amount of CO_2 in the form of bicarbonates (or HCO_3^-), which is about 48 mL per 100 mL. This constitutes the alkali reserve, because CO_2 mainly remains in blood as H^+ and HCO_3^-. This H^+ is attached with Hb and forms H-Hb and HCO_3^- remains as $KHCO_3$.

Although much CO_2 is carried through blood, yet blood reaction does not become acid ($CO_2 + H_2O = H_2CO_3$). This proves that during CO_2 transport, some buffer systems in blood play a very important role to maintain the acid–base balance. The CO_2 is carried through blood in following forms **(Fig. 12)**.

As Physical Solution

Like dissolved O_2, the CO_2 also dissolves in plasma and remains as physical solution. Like the physical solution of O_2, this physical solution of CO_2 also provides the platform for transfer of CO_2. That means CO_2, entering into blood, first gets dissolved in plasma and then is converted to other forms (such as bicarbonates and carbamino compounds). Similarly, during release, CO_2 from other forms comes to this dissolved state in plasma, wherefrom CO_2 is released in the alveoli of lungs. The amount of dissolved CO_2 in plasma depends on the solubility of CO_2 in plasma and PCO_2 of plasma. The CO_2 present in this physical form is about 2.7 mL/100 mL in venous blood and is slightly less in arterial blood. This physical form of CO_2 is responsible for about

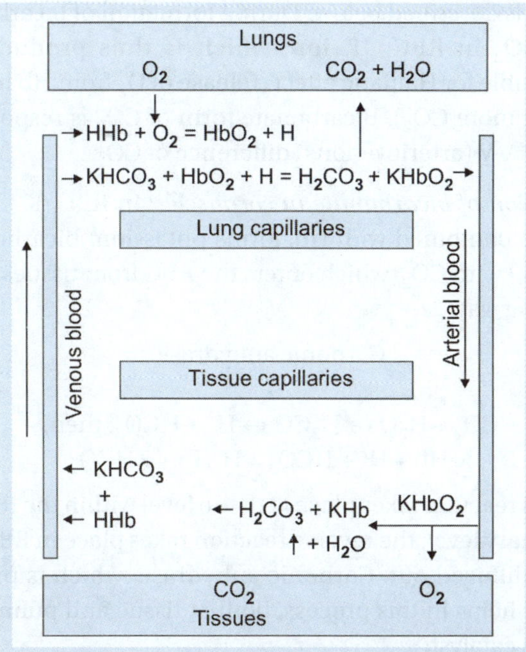

Fig. 12: Mechanism of entry and exit of O_2 and CO_2 at lung and tissue level.

10% of A-V (arteriovenous) difference of CO_2. This physical solution form of CO_2 represents a very small portion of total CO_2 carried in blood. The major portion of CO_2 is transported as bicarbonate and carbamino compound forms.

As Chemical Compounds

Two types of chemical compounds are formed from CO_2 in blood during its transport. These are:

1. *Bicarbonates:*
   - *As NaHCO$_3$ in plasma:* In arterial blood—33.1%, in venous blood—35.2%
   - *As KHCO$_3$ in red cells:* In arterial blood—9.8%, in venous blood—10.5%
2. *Carbamino compounds:*
   - Carbaminohemoglobin in red cells (in arterial blood—2%, in venous blood—2.6%)
   - Carbamino-proteins (with plasma proteins) in plasma (in arterial blood—1%, in venous blood—1.1%)

Carriage of CO$_2$ as Bicarbonate

Bicarbonate is another form by which CO_2 is transported through blood and in this form, major portion of CO_2 is transported. Another interesting part is that though maximum portion of bicarbonate is present in plasma, but it is formed in RBC. This is because RBC has the required enzyme, named carbonic anhydrase, for the synthesis of bicarbonate. Therefore, RBCs take major responsibility for transport of CO_2. How bicarbonates are produced in RBC and plasma is described below. During formation of bicarbonate from CO_2 in RBC, H^+ ion, which is thus produced, is responsible for Haldane effect (release of O_2 from Hb helps it to carry more CO_2). Bicarbonate form of CO_2 is responsible for 60% A–V (arteriovenous) difference of CO_2.

Formation of bicarbonate in corpuscles: In RBC, K^+, which remains combined with Hb, forms potassium bicarbonates ($KHCO_3$) with CO_2, which enters the RBC from tissues in the following way:

Carbonic anhydrase
↓

$$CO_2 + H_2O \leftrightarrow H_2CO \leftrightarrow H^+ + HCO_3^-; \text{ then,}$$
$$K\text{-}Hb + H^+ + HCO_3^- = H\text{-}Hb + KHCO_3$$

This reaction takes place at tissue level within the RBC. At pulmonary level, the reverse reaction takes place in RBC and CO_2 is diffused out. Carbonic anhydrase, which is present in RBC, helps in this process, both at tissue and pulmonary level, as catalyst.

Carbonic anhydrase: The rate of formation and breakdown of bicarbonates depends upon the rate of this primary reversible reaction: $CO_2 + H_2O \leftrightarrow H_2CO_3 \leftrightarrow H^+ + HCO_3^-$. This reaction is catalyst by carbonic anhydrase. In absence of carbonic anhydrase when water is exposed to CO_2, a period of about 15–30 minutes is required for this reaction to take place. Similarly, about the same time is required for the complete dissociation of CO_2 from its water solution (H_2CO_3). But, in our body, blood in tissue capillaries becomes saturated with CO_2 in about 1–2 seconds only and the same time is required for the release of CO_2 from blood in lungs. This is due to the existence of an enzyme, called carbonic anhydrase in RBC. It is protein in nature containing Zn and its action is inhibited by cyanide and acetazolamide. In blood, it is almost exclusively present in red cells. So, this reaction mainly takes place in RBC. All other tissues also contain it, but in traces. However, kidney, pancreas, and stomach contain considerable amounts.

Formation of bicarbonate in plasma:

- *By phosphate buffer:* Alkaline phosphates combine with carbonic acid and form sodium bicarbonate.

$$Na_2HPO_4 + H_2CO_3 \leftrightarrow NaH_2PO_4 + NaHCO_3$$

- *By plasma proteins:* The plasma proteins mostly remain combined with sodium (to be represented as Na-Pr.) and form bicarbonates in the following way:

$$Na\text{-}Pr. + H_2CO_3 = H\text{-}Pr. + NaHCO_3$$

- *Chloride shift or Hamburger phenomenon:* When the whole blood is saturated with CO_2, then the following changes are seen:

TABLE 13: CO_2 content in arterial and venous blood.

	Venous blood (mL/100 mL)	Arterial blood (mL/100 mL)
As dissolved CO_2	2.7	2.4
As bicarbonates	45.7	42.9
As carbamino compounds	3.7	3.0
Total CO_2 content	52.1	48.3

- The bicarbonate contents in plasma and red cells increase.
- The chloride content in plasma is diminished and that of red cell is increased.
- The total base (cations) in both plasma and red cells remains unchanged.
- The water content and the volume of red cells increase **(Table 13)**.

When CO_2 is removed from blood into alveoli, then reverse changes take place. From these observations, it is evident that when CO_2 enters the blood at tissue level, then chlorine of NaCl from plasma enters the red cells, while the base (Na^+) is left behind in plasma. When CO_2 escapes from blood at alveoli level, then chlorine again leaves the red cells, enters the plasma, and combines with base (Na^+). This alternate movement of chloride ion is called as the *chloride shift or Hamburger phenomenon*. This can be explained by the following way: CO_2 can pass through all biological membranes and it diffuses into capillaries from tissues very easily along the pressure gradient. Thereby, PCO_2 in plasma increases, so the CO_2 diffuses inside the RBC. The membrane of red cells is not permeable to basic ions (K^+, Na^+, etc.), but is permeable to anions (HCO^-, Cl^-, etc.). When CO_2 enters the bloodstream from tissues, then H_2CO_3 is formed in plasma. But, it is very little in amount in plasma and largely in RBCs, because red cells are rich in carbonic anhydrase enzyme and permeable to CO_2. The red cells contain 4–5 times more carbonic anhydrase than that of plasma. In RBC, the H_2CO_3 breaks to form H^+ and HCO_3^- ($CO_2 + H_2O = H_2CO_3 = H^+ + HCO_3^-$). This ensures continuous entry of CO_2 into RBCs. This H^+ is taken up by Hb, so the HCO_3^- concentration in RBC increases. Hence, HCO_3^- diffuses out to plasma down the concentration gradient. Now, to maintain the electrical neutrality inside the RBC, another negative ion (Cl^-) enters from plasma inside the RBCs, with the help of a membrane protein, called the band-3 protein. This phenomenon of entry of Cl^- into RBC, in exchange of HCO_3^-, is called as *chloride shift or Hamburger phenomenon*. This occurs in the capillaries of tissue.

In this process, even after equilibrium, some HCO_3^- remains inside the RBCs plus some Cl enters in it. So, the total electrolyte inside the RBC increases. Hence, there is increase in osmolarity inside of RBC and water is drawn within RBCs. Therefore, RBCs become slightly larger in venous blood and osmotic fragility of these RBCs is more than those of arterial blood. This is called *Hamburger effect*.

Reverse changes occur when the blood is in pulmonary capillaries. Here, the Hb in RBC is oxygenated. So, it releases H^+ and this H^+ reacts with HCO_3^- which is still present in small amount in RBC even after equilibrium (discussed before) to form CO_2. Now, this CO_2 gets out to alveolar air. Hence, the concentration of HCO_3^- in RBC decreases and more HCO_3^- enters in RBC from plasma to produce CO_2 and to get out in alveoli. Chloride ions, which entered in RBC during chloride shift, now come out of RBCs and this phenomenon is called as *reverse chloride shift*. This will reduce the osmotic pressure of red cells and water will come out. This will cause the volume of RBC to shrink and osmotic fragility to reduce. Hence, the RBC of venous blood is larger with increased osmotic fragility than that of arterial blood.

Carriage of CO₂ as Carbamino Compounds

Carbon dioxide (CO_2) is also carried as carbamino compounds in blood. In this process, the terminal or free NH_2 radicle of globin part of hemoglobin and that of other plasma proteins combines with one molecule of CO_2 (as free gas, but not as H_2CO_3) and forms carbamino compounds. It does not require the help of carbonic anhydrase enzyme. This reaction may be presented as: CO_2 + Pr. NH_2 ↔ Pr. NH. COOH. For transport of CO_2 in this form of carbamino compounds, the globin part of Hb contributes a lot due to its amount, which is higher than any other blood proteins. The carbamino compound formed by globin part of Hb is called as carbaminohemoglobin. About 3.7 mL of CO_2 is carried in this form per 100 mL of venous blood (2.6 mL in red cells and 1.1 mL in plasma) and 3 mL in arterial blood.

■ SUMMARY

Thus, it will be seen that CO_2 is carried out through blood in three forms. These are:

1. As physical solution (2.7 mL)
2. *As bicarbonates (45.7 mL):* Bicarbonates are formed in four ways by the reaction of H_2CO_3 with: (i) with Na-Pr, (ii) with Na_2HPO_4, (iii) with NaCl helped by "chloride shift", and (iv) with KHb. These (bicarbonates) are the chief forms in which CO_2 is carried in blood. It can explain about 90% of total CO_2 transport through blood, of which the major part is carried in plasma as $NaHCO_3$. A large part of this bicarbonate remains permanently in plasma and constitutes the so-called *alkali reserve* of blood.
3. *As carbamino compounds (3.7 mL):* These are chiefly formed in red cells (2.6 mL) from globin part of Hb and

only in traces in plasma (1.1 mL) from plasma protein. It constitutes about 5–10% of total CO_2 carriage and is responsible for a large part of normal arteriovenous difference.

The 100 mL of venous blood carries about 52 mL of CO_2. Out of this 52 mL of CO_2, 4 mL is given out through lungs and, therefore, 100 mL of arterial blood contains about 48 mL of CO_2. Out of 4 mL CO_2, which excreted through lungs, 2.4 mL is contributed by $-HCO_3^+$, 1.2 mL by carbamino compounds, and 0.4 mL from physical solution. From 100 mL of blood, 4 mL of CO_2 diffuses out through lungs and 5 liters of blood circulates through lungs per minute. Therefore, 200 mL of CO_2 ($4 \times 10 \times 5 = 200$ mL) is excreted through lungs per minute. Whereas, 250 mL of O_2 is entered through lungs per minute (per minute O_2 consumption by our body is 250 mL).

Interrelation between the carriage of oxygen and carriage of carbon dioxide: It has been found that reduced blood can take up more CO_2 than oxygenated blood. Also, blood containing less CO_2 **(Fig. 13)** will take up relatively more O_2. In other words, these two gases tend to displace each other. This is explained by the fact that oxyhemoglobin acts as a stronger acid (than H_2CO_3) and unites with more base. Reduced hemoglobin, on the other hand, is a weaker acid (than carbonic acid) and can unite with less base. Hence, oxygenation of Hb in the lungs makes it a stronger acid and unites with more base. The latter being taken from the bicarbonates (thus carbonic acid is formed from where CO_2 is liberated through lungs). On the other hand, reduced hemoglobin as in the tissues being weaker acid cannot hold its base and taken away by $-HCO_3$ to form bicarbonate. This $-HCO_3$ comes from carbonic acid, which is formed in the RBCs. In the RBC, carbonic acid is formed from CO_2, which comes from tissues with the help of carbonic anhydrase.

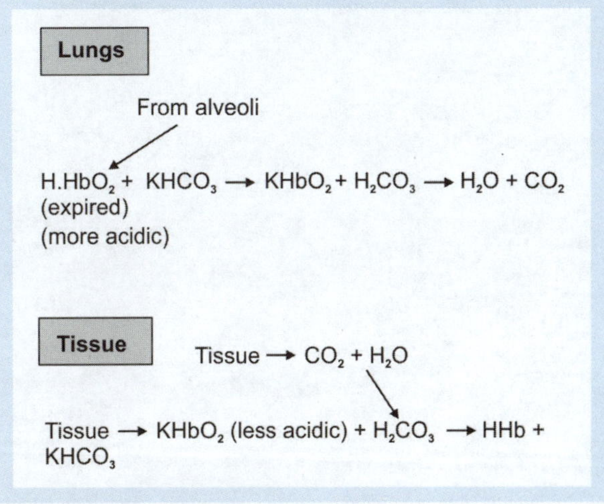

Fig. 13: The basic mechanism of transport of O_2 and CO_2 from lungs to tissues and tissues to lungs, respectively.

Factors that Determine the Intake of CO_2 from Tissues into Blood

The following factors are responsible for entry of CO_2 from tissues into bloodstream.

Pressure Gradient

In tissue capillaries, the tension of CO_2 at its arterial end is about 40 mm Hg. The tension of CO_2 in resting tissues is about 46 mm Hg. In active tissues, it may be much higher (about 63 mm Hg). Due to this difference of partial pressure, CO_2 diffuses out of the tissues and enters into capillaries.

Reduction (Deoxygenation) of Hemoglobin

Oxyhemoglobin is reduced (deoxygenated) in tissues, so that the base freed from the reduced hemoglobin is made available for fixing H_2CO_3. Thus, more and more amount of H_2CO_3 is formed from CO_2, which diffuses from tissues into blood.

With the Help of Hamburger Phenomenon

Chloride shift is also called as the Hamburger shift or phenomenon, named after Hartog Jakob Hamburger. This chloride shift refers to the exchange of bicarbonate and chloride across the membrane of RBCs and it is described before.

Carbamino Compounds are Formed

This is helped by increased CO_2 tension as well as reduction (deoxygenation) of oxyhemoglobin in tissue capillaries.

Factors Concerned in Liberation of CO_2 through Lungs

Since CO_2 is liberated through lungs, so it is obvious that in pulmonary vascular bed (capillary), the factors responsible for releasing CO_2 must be the reverse (opposite) of those that are operating in tissues.

Cardiovascular System (Anatomy and Physiology)

BRIEF ANATOMY OF A HEART

■ INTRODUCTION

The Greek name of heart is "card", from where we get the word "cardiac" and the Latin name of heart is "cor", from where we get the word "coronary". Heart is a hollow muscular and a somewhat conical structure. It is situated in the middle of mediastinum and is covered by pericardium. It is about the size of a clenched fist of a normal adult individual. In a healthy adult individual, a heart measures about 12 cm in its longitudinal diameter extending from apex to base, 6 cm in its anteroposterior diameter, and 9 cm in its widest transverse diameter. The transverse diameter of a heart should not be more than one-half of the transverse diameter of thorax. The weight of a heart varies from 250 g in a healthy adult female to 300 g in a healthy adult male.

The human heart is considered as two parallel pumps and is composed of four chambers: (1) right atrium, (2) right ventricles, (3) left atrium, and (4) left ventricles. The atria lie above and behind the ventricles. The two atria are separated from each other by interatrial septum. Similarly, the two ventricles are separated from each other by interventricular septum. The atrium and the ventricles are separated externally by coronary sulcus or atrioventricular (AV) groove. On the other hand, the two ventricles are also separated on the external surface by two grooves which are called the anterior and posterior interventricular groove. The anterior interventricular groove is situated on the sternocostal surface and the posterior interventricular group is situated on the diaphragmatic or the inferior surface of heart. They meet at the apex. The heart presents: apex, base, three surfaces, and three borders. The three surfaces are: (1) sternocostal, (2) diaphragmatic, and (3) left surfaces. The three borders are: (i) right, (ii) inferior, and (iii) left borders.

■ APEX OF HEART

It is a conical area of heart and is formed only by left ventricle. It is directed downward, forward and to the left. It is situated at 5th intercostal space, about 9 cm lateral to the midline and slightly below and medial to the left nipple (male). The apex is separated from anterior thoracic wall by the anterior part of left lung and pleura. The apex beat is defined as a forward thrust which is felt at left 5th intercostal space, just medial to midclavicular line or 9 cm lateral from the midsternal line during ventricular systole. It is due to the twisting of heart, due to the vortex like disposition of ventricular muscles, and close to the apex. In new born, the apex beat is usually felt at left 4th intercostal space, just lateral to the midclavicular line. But, after about 2 years, it reaches the adult position.

■ BASE OF HEART

The base or the posterior surface of heart is somewhat quadrilateral in outline and is the most fixed part of the heart. It is directed backward and to the right. It is formed by two atria, of which 2/3rd is formed by left atrium and 1/3rd is formed by right atrium. At the base of the heart, the superior vena cava (SVC) and the inferior vena cava (IVC) open into right atrium and the four pulmonary veins, two from each lung, open into left atrium. Between the base of the heart and the vertebral column there lies: the right and left bronchi, esophagus, and descending thoracic aorta. The distended left atrium in mitral stenosis may produce difficulty in swallowing due to esophageal compression. This is called the Ortner's syndrome (**Fig. 1**).

■ RIGHT BORDER OF HEART

It is rounded and convex in shape and is formed only by right atrium. It extends from the right side of the opening of SVC to that of the IVC. The right border of the heart separates

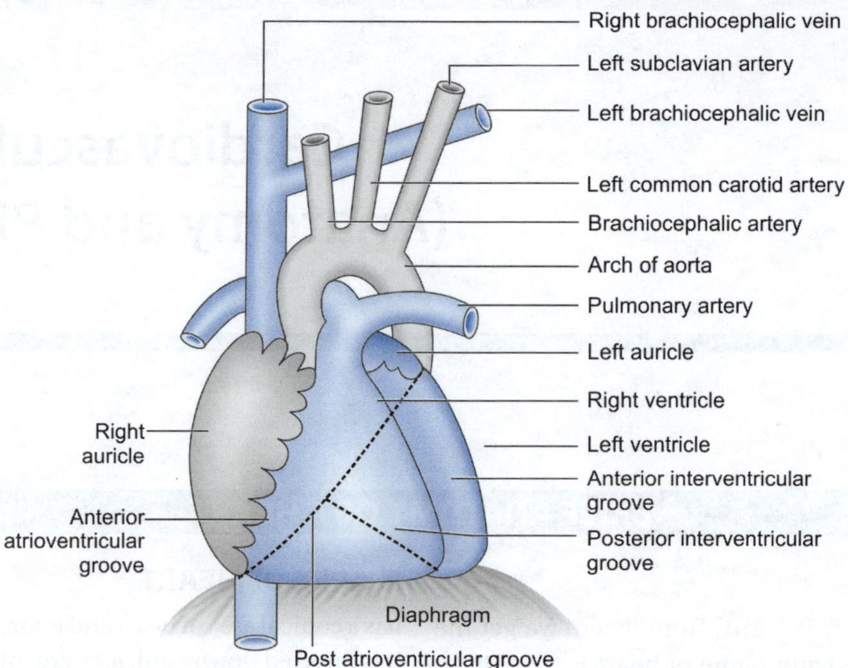

Fig. 1: The anterior surface of the heart.

the base it from its sternocostal surface. A shallow vertical groove, known as the sulcus terminals, accompanies the right border of the heart. It corresponds with an internal ridge, named crista terminalis in the interior of right atrium.

INFERIOR BORDER OF HEART

It is a sharp border and separates the sternocostal surface of heart from the diaphragmatic surface of it. It extends from the opening of IVC to the apex of the heart. This inferior border of heart is accompanied by the right marginal branch of right coronary artery and its corresponding vein. Close to the apex, it (inferior border of heart) presents a notch known as the incisura apicis cordis which gives passage to the anterior interventricular branch of left coronary artery.

LEFT BORDER OF HEART

It is an ill-defined, convex border. It separates the sternocostal surface of the heart from its left surface. It extends from the left auricle to the apex of the heart with convexity directed upward and to the left. This border is accompanied by the left marginal branch of left coronary artery and its corresponding vein.

Sternocostal Surface of Heart

It is directed forward, upward, and laterally toward the left. It is separated from the base of the heart by its right border, from the diaphragmatic surface of the heart by its inferior border, and from the left surface of the heart by its left border.

It lies against the posterior surface of the body of sternum and 3rd to 6th costal cartilages on both sides. This sternocostal surface is formed by the following parts of the heart such as:

- The anterior surface of right atrium and its auricle
- The anterior surface of right ventricle (2/3rd)
- A part of the anterior surface of left auricle
- The anterior surface of left ventricle (1/3rd)

This sternocostal surface of heart presents:

- The anterior part of AV groove which passes downward and to the right between the right atrium and right ventricle. The groove holds the trunk of right coronary artery and the anterior cardiac vein.
- The anterior interventricular groove which passes downward and parallel to the left border of the heart. It meets the inferior border of the heart at its apex. The groove holds the anterior interventricular branch of left coronary artery and great cardiac vein.

Diaphragmatic or Inferior Surface of Heart

It is a flat surface and rests on the central tendon and the left part of the musculature of diaphragm. It is formed by two ventricles, of which 2/3rd is formed by the left and 1/3rd is formed by the right ventricle. It is separated from the sternocostal surface by inferior border, from the base by the posterior part of AV groove and from the left surface by a less defined unnamed border which is the backward continuation of the inferior border of heart. The posterior interventricular groove runs forward along this surface and

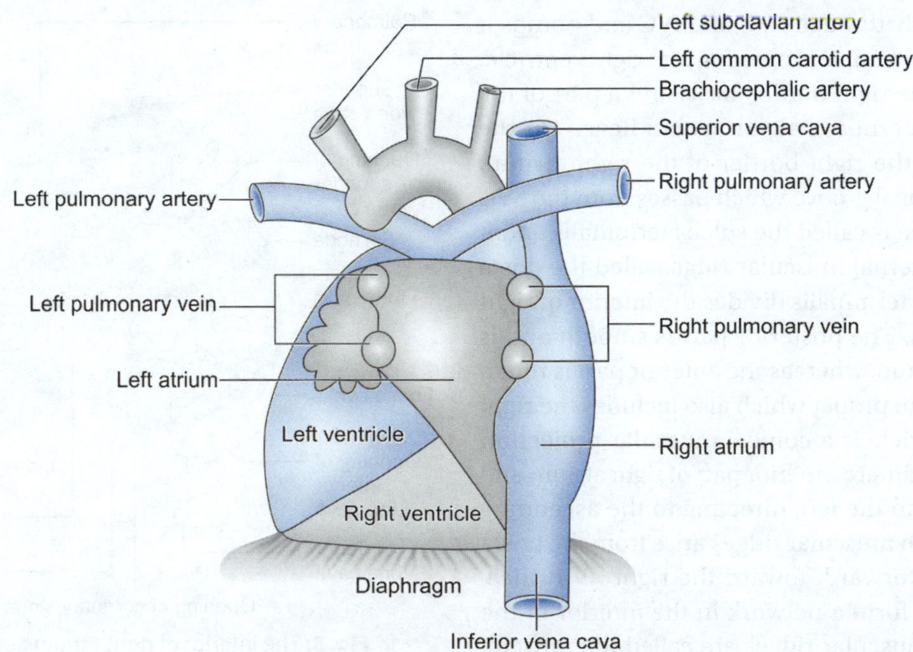

Fig. 2: The posterior surface of the heart.

meets with the anterior interventricular groove at the apex of the heart. This posterior interventricular groove lodges the posterior interventricular branch of right coronary artery and middle cardiac vein **(Fig. 2)**.

Left Surface of Heart

It is directed backward, upward, and to the left. It is formed mainly by the left ventricle and partly by the left atrium and its auricle. This lateral surface of the heart lies against the cardiac impression of the left lung. The left part of the AV groove lies in this surface and lodges the following structures:
- Trunk and the circumflex branch of left coronary artery
- Termination of the great cardiac vein
- Commencement of the coronary sinus.

Atrioventricular Groove

It is a C-shaped curve and is deficient in front due to the presence of the root of pulmonary trunk and aorta. It is divided into anterior and posterior part. The anterior part is again subdivided into right and left halves. The right part of the anterior AV groove runs downward and to the right between the right atrium and the right ventricle. It contains the trunk of right coronary artery. The left part of the anterior AV groove intervenes between the left auricle and the left ventricle. It lodges the trunk and the circumflex branch of the left coronary artery, the termination of the great cardiac vein and the commencement of the coronary sinus.

The posterior part of the AV groove intervenes between the base and the diaphragmatic surface of the heart.

It contains coronary sinus and the anastomoses between the right and left coronary arteries. The meeting point of the posterior interatrial groove, posterior interventricular groove, and posterior part of the right and left AV groove from opposite direction is known as the "crux" of the heart.

Some Points to Remember

- The apex of a heart is formed only by left ventricle.
- The base of a heart is formed only by two atria.
- The right border of a heart is formed only by right atrium.
- The diaphragmatic surface of a heart is formed by two ventricles.

One-third and Two-thirds Features of Heart

- *Base:* The 1/3rd of the base of a heart is formed by right atrium and 2/3rd by left atrium.
- *Diaphragmatic surface:* The 1/3rd of the diaphragmatic surface of a heart is formed by right ventricle and 2/3rd by left ventricle.
- *Sternocostal surface:* The 1/3rd of the sternocostal surface of a heart is formed by left ventricle and 2/3rd by right ventricle.
- *Entire heart:* The 1/3rd of the entire heart is right to the midline and 2/3rd is left to the midline.

■ CHAMBERS OF HEART

Right Atrium

The atria are thin walled, low pressure chambers, and served as the conduits of ventricle. The right atrium receives venous blood from whole body through SVC and IVC and pumps it out through right AV or tricuspid opening into right ventricle. Right atrium forms the right border, base, and a part of the anterior surface (or sternocostal surface) of heart. On the outer surface, along the right border of the right atrium, there is a shallow vertical groove which passes from the SVC to the IVC. This groove is called the sulcus terminalis and it corresponds to an internal muscular ridge called the crista terminalis. This crista terminalis divides the interior of right atrium into two parts. The posterior part is smooth and is called the sinus venarum, whereas the anterior part is rough and is called the atrium proper which also includes the right auricle. The right auricle is a conical muscular projection which arises from the anterosuperior part of right atrium and extends upward and to the left, directing to the ascending aorta. Multiple smooth muscular ridges arise from the crista terminalis and pass forward, toward the right AV orifice. Some of these ridges form a network in the interior of the right auricle. These muscular ridges are called the musculi pectinati. Thus, the right auricular appendage is a potential site for the formation of thrombi, which if dislodged, can result in pulmonary embolism. The opening of coronary sinus is situated between the opening of IVC and right AV orifice in the lower part of interatrial septum. Just above, the opening of coronary sinus lies the AV node. The sinoatrial (SA) node is situated at the upper part of sulcus terminalis. On the external surface, the right atrium is separated from right ventricle by right atrioventricular groove which contains the right coronary artery.

The right and left atrium is separated by a septum, called the interatrial septum. It is placed obliquely, so that the right atrium lies in front and to the right side of left atrium. The upper part of this septum is thicker than its lower part. The right side of this interatrial septum is characterized by the presence of fossa ovalis, annulus ovalis, and the AV node. The fossa ovalis is an oval depression in the lower part of the septum and the floor of this fossa is formed by septum primum. It represents foramen ovale during intrauterine life. The annulus ovalis is a sickle-shaped fold which surrounds the upper, anterior, and posterior margins of this fossa ovalis. It represents the lower free margin of septum secundum. The AV node is situated in the lower part of interatrial septum above the opening of coronary sinus **(Fig. 3)**.

The interatrial septum is developed from septum primum, septum intermedium, and septum secundum. The septum primum grows as a septum from the roof and the dorsal wall of the primitive single chamber of atrium. Then, like a curtain, it passes downward. During that period, another septum, named septum intermedium also grows from the below and passes upward. They do not unite and keep a gap between them. Thus, a foramen known

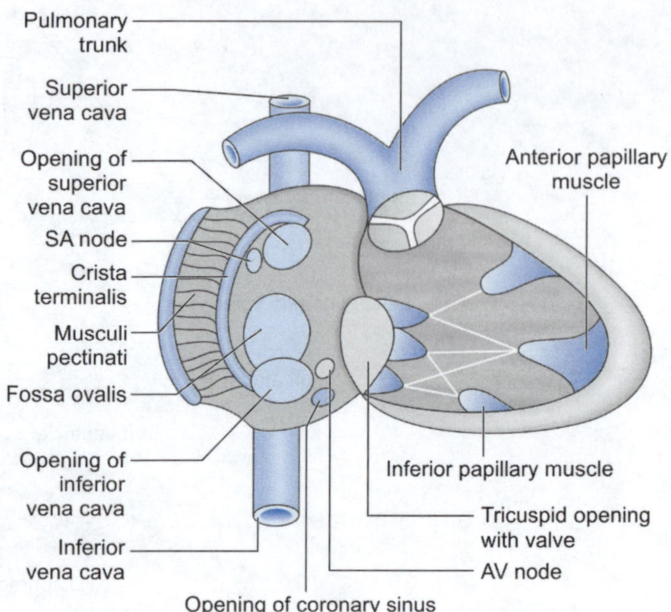

Fig. 3: The interior of right atrium and right ventricle.
(AV: atrioventricular; SA: sinoatrial)

as *"ostium primum"* is formed between the upper border of septum intermedium and the lower border of septum primum. Later, ostium primum is closed by the fusion of these two septa. Again, with the closure of ostium primum, the upper part of septum primum disintegrates forming a foramen known as the *"ostium secundum"*. Then, another septum, called the septum secundum also grows from above and passes downward with a sickle-shaped lower free margin. The lower margin of this septum secundum grows sufficiently to overlap the ostium secundum situated on the septum primum. Thus, a flap-like valvular opening, formed between the lower margin of septum secundum and the upper margin of ostium secundum of septum primum is known as the *"foramen ovale"*. The purpose of the development of septum secundum is to convert the ostium secundum into a valvular foramen ovale, so that it can regulate the flow of blood from the right to the left atrium, but not in opposite direction.

After birth, the intra-atrial pressure on both the sides of the atrium becomes equal and the foramen ovale is closed at first functionally and later anatomically by the fusion of the margins of septum primum and septum secundum. In about 20% of human heart, the foramen ovale is closed functionally, but anatomically it may remain patent which can be proved by passing a probe from the right to the left side of the heart.

Congenital atrial septal defects (ASD) are of the following types:
- *Probe patency of foramen ovale:* It occurs when the foramen is closed functionally, but remains patent anatomically. These subjects are considered as normal.

- *Persistent ostium secundum:* This is due to the incomplete development of septum secundum or extensive disintegration of septum primum, forming a large ostium secundum.
- *Persistent ostium primum:* This may appear as single defect or associated with the patent interventricular foramen.
- *Biventricular monoatrial heart:* This is due to complete failure of the septation of primitive single chamber of atrium.
- *Prenatal closure of foramen ovale:* This is a rare anomaly.

The opening of IVC in right atrium is guarded by a rudimentary valve. During intrauterine life, this valve guides the inferior vena caval blood, which is oxygenated and comes from placenta and the lower half of the body of fetus, to flow into left atrium through foramen ovale. The "intervenous tubercle of Lower" is a very small projection on the posterior wall of the atrium and situated just below the opening of SVC. During embryonic life, it directs the superior vena caval blood to the right ventricle which is deoxygenated and comes from the head and neck and upper extremities.

The right atrium proper communicates with right ventricle through right atrioventricular (tricuspid) orifice. This opening is oval in shape. It permits usually the tips of three fingers and is guarded by tricuspid valve. This area of right atrium proper is also known as the vestibule of tricuspid valve. The plane of atrioventricular orifice is almost vertical, so that blood flows almost horizontally from the right atrium to right ventricle.

Right Ventricle

It forms the whole inferior border, larger part (2/3rd) of anterior surface and a smaller part (1/3rd) of inferior surface of the heart. The wall of right ventricle is thinner than that of left ventricle and the ratio of thickness between the right and left ventricular wall is 1:3. But, in utero the ratio of RV: LV wall thickness is approximately 1:1. This is because, the right ventricular pressure or the pressure of the right side of the heart is greater or equal to the left side of the heart. After delivery, pulmonary vascular resistance rapidly decreases with the expansion of lungs and the systemic vascular resistance (SVR) increases rapidly with the loss of placenta. So, the right side of the heart becomes of low pressure system than that of the left side of the heart and undergoes less muscular hypertrophy than the left ventricle after birth. Therefore, over the first month of extrauterine life the RV: LV wall thickness ratio becomes 1:3 which is similar to that of an adult.

On cross section, the interior of right ventricle is semilunar, whereas, that of left ventricle is circular. This is because, the interventricular septum bulges with its convexity toward right ventricle due to increased left ventricular pressure than that of right ventricular pressure. The thickness of the muscular wall of right ventricle is 3–5 mm and that of the left ventricle is 8–12 mm.

The interior of right ventricle consists of two parts: the inflowing rough part or inflow tract or the ventricle proper and the outflowing smooth part or outflow tract. This outflow tract of right ventricle is also known as conus arteriosus or infundibulum (conical pouch formed from the upper and left angle of right ventricle). The inflow tract receives blood from right atrium and the outflow tract ejects the blood from right ventricle into pulmonary trunk. The conus arteriosus of right ventricle with its outflow orifice is situated in front, above and to the left side of the inflow tract. Therefore, the blood of inflow tract, during its ejection through outflow tract, bends roughly at an obtuse angle. The supraventricular crest intervenes between this inflow and outflow tract of right ventricle.

The right ventricle receives blood from right atrium through tricuspid orifice which is guarded by a tricuspid valve. Then, it ejects this blood into pulmonary trunk or artery through pulmonary orifice which is guarded by a pulmonary valve. The right AV or tricuspid orifice is oval in shape. It is oriented almost vertically, making an angle of 40° with sagittal plane. This tricuspid orifice is directed forward, downward, and to the left toward apex. This tricuspid valve has three cusps: (1) anterior, (2) medial, and (3) posterior and admits the tips of three fingers (8–11 cm^2). The chordae tendinae connect the free margins of these three cusps of tricuspid valve with the three papillary muscles and prevent the eversion of cusps toward atrium during right ventricular contraction. There are three papillary muscles and each papillary muscle is connected to the contiguous halves of two cusps. Of these three papillary muscles, anterior is the largest. The tricuspid valve is closed, during ventricular systole, by the apposition of the atrial surfaces of cusps near their serrated margins.

The pulmonary valve which guards the pulmonary orifice is also called the semilunar valve, because their cusps are semilunar in shape. It comprises three cusps such as anterior, right, and left. Normally, the pulmonic valve area is 4 cm^2 in size. Usually, the right ventricular pressure varies between 15–30 mm Hg during systole and 0–10 mm Hg during diastole, whereas the pulmonary artery pressure varies between 15–30 mm Hg during systole and 3–12 mm Hg during diastole, respectively.

Left Atrium

It forms the 2/3rd of base, the greater part of the upper border, part of the anterior and lateral surfaces, and a part of the left border of heart. The muscular wall of left atrium is thicker than that of right atrium and the thickness is being about 3 mm. Anterosuperiorly, the left atrium presents a conical projection which is called the left auricle. It projects upward and medially toward the root of pulmonary trunk. Most of the interior wall of left atrium is smooth. But, a network of musculi pectinati (muscular ridges) is found within the cavity of left auricle. It (left atrium) receives only oxygenated blood from lungs through four pulmonary veins, where the orifices are not guarded by any valve and pumps it (oxygenated blood) out to left ventricle through the bicuspid or mitral orifice which is guarded by bicuspid or mitral valve. The area of mitral valve is only 6–8 cm^2 and admits the tip of two fingers. The mitral valve has two cusps, a larger anterior and a smaller posterior. Hence, it is called the bicuspid valve. The cusps of mitral valve are smaller and thicker than those of tricuspid valve. There are two papillary muscles in left ventricle: anterior and posterior. Chordae tendinae from both these papillary muscles are attached to both the cusps of mitral valve. Both the right and left atrial pressure vary anywhere between 0 and 10 mm Hg. The clinical importance of left auricle are:

- It is a potential site for formation of thrombi which may dislodge at any time and can result in cerebral, renal, or any systemic embolism.
- During mitral valvotomy operation, amputation of the left auricle may injure the circumflex branch of left coronary artery.

Left Ventricle

It forms the apex, left border, left surface, and the 2/3rd of the inferior surface of heart. It is conical in shape, and circular on cross section. Its musculature is three times thicker than that of right ventricle. The muscular thickness of left ventricle is about 8–12 mm. The muscle of left ventricle is thin at its apex and at aortic vestibule the muscles of left ventricle are mostly replaced by fibrous tissue. The interior of left ventricle is similar to that of right ventricle. Thus, it consists of an inflow tract or ventricle proper and an outflow tract or aortic vestibule. The inflow tract of left ventricle consists of mitral valve complex and conducts blood from left atrium to the apex of left ventricle. The outflow tract is also called the aortic vestibule. It is smooth walled and ejects the blood into aorta through aortic orifice. The area of this aortic opening is only 3–4 cm^2 and is guarded by aortic valve, with three semilunar cusps. These semilunar cusps of aortic valve are named as posterior, right, and left. Opposite to these each cusp, the aortic wall is dilated and forms the aortic sinuses. The right and left coronary arteries arise from these right and left aortic sinuses, respectively. The opening of coronary

arteries in aortic sinuses is called the "coronary ostia". These aortic sinuses are significant, because they prevent the occlusion of coronary ostia.

The right and left ventricles are separated by the interventricular septum. It consists of a thin upper membranous part and a thick lower muscular part which forms the major portion of interventricular septum. It is placed obliquely backward and toward right and presents a convexity toward the right ventricle. Hence, on cross section the right ventricular cavity is semilunar and the left ventricular cavity is circular in outline. The attachment of intraventricular septum within the ventricle is indicated on the outer surface of heart by anterior and posterior interventricular grooves. The left branch of AV bundle first passes through the right side of the membranous part of interventricular septum and then appears on the left side by piercing it. On the right side of interventricular septum, the base of the septal leaflet of tricuspid valve extends from the muscular part of interventricular septum to the central region of the membranous part of it. As a result, the part of interventricular septum which is situated in front of the septal leaflet intervenes between the two ventricles. But, the portion behind the septal leaflet separates the right atrium from the aortic vestibule of left ventricle. This portion of interventricular septum is known as the atrioventricular septum.

The interventricular septum develops from three sources: ventricular septum proper (septum inferior), proximal bulbar septum, and septum intermedium. The primitive right and left ventricles develop as a single cavity. It lies between the common atrium on dorsal side and the bulbus cordis (bulb of the heart) on ventral side. From this single cavity of common atrium develops two atriums, whereas the bulbus cordis develops the outflow tract of two ventricles and the root of the pulmonary and aortic trunk. Therefore, for the complete separation of ventricle, it must be done in harmony with the septation of atrium, ventricle, and the proximal part of bulbus cordis. The ventricular septum proper or septum inferior grows from below from the floor of the primitive ventricle and passed upward. It presents a sickle-shaped margin with the concavity directed upward and backward. Again a septum develops which divides the bulbus cordis into right and left chambers. This is called the bulbar septum which grows downward and fuses with the upper margin of the ventricular septum proper. But, still a small gap remains between these two septa. The right part of bulbus cordis incorporates with right ventricle and forms the infundibulum part of it. Similarly, the left part of bulbus cordis forms the aortic vestibule of left ventricles. The small gap, which still remains after the fusion of previous two septa, is closed later by septum intermedium. Sometimes, this small gap is not closed and remains as ventricular septal defect (VSD). The part of the septum formed from septum intermedium persists in adults as the membranous part of interventricular septum.

When the septum intermedium is not developed, then it affects the membranous part of interventricular septum and may appear as single defect (VSD). Thus, it also complicates the Fallot's tetralogy. The Fallot's tetralogy includes: (1) pulmonary stenosis, (2) displacement of aortic orifice to right to override the ventricular septum, (3) patent interventricular foramen, and (4) the hypertrophy of right ventricle. The primary defect in Fallot's tetralogy lies in pulmonary stenosis which is due to the unequal division of bulbus cordis, so that the bulbar septum fails to fuse with ventricular septum. Sometimes, there is complete absence of interventricular septum. Then, this condition is known as the biatrial monoventricular heart. Normally, the left ventricular pressure varies between 100–140 mm Hg during systole and 3–12 mm Hg during diastole. The normal aortic pressure also varies between 100–140 and 60–40 mm Hg during systole and diastole, respectively.

CONDUCTING SYSTEM OF HEART

Normally, the atria and ventricles are separated by an eight-shaped fibrous ring. But, the fibrous tissue is not able to conduct electrical impulses, so this ring acts as an insulator between the atrium and ventricles. Hence, a conducting system is needed for the conduction of electrical impulses from the atrium to ventricles after its initiation in atrium. This conducting system is actually made up of specialized fine myocardial cells. These specialized fine myocardial cells which form the electrical conducting system of heart are completely striated and include the: SA node, AV node, junctional tissues, bundle of HIS (or AV bundle), right and left divisions of this bundle, their arborization under the endocardium (Purkinje fibers), and finally the terminal fibers which penetrate the ventricular musculature. Thus, this electrical conducting system of heart connect certain pace maker regions of heart with the ordinary working cardiac myocytes and speed up the wave of excitation to travel for the synchronous action of different chambers of the heart. The intrinsic rhythmic excitation of cardiac muscle fibers is regulated by some pace maker cells in heart and the rhythmicity of these pacemaker cells in turn is regulated by the nerve impulses from the vasomotor centers of brain stem which supply the heart **(Fig. 4)**.

The conducting tissue of heart is composed of three types of specialized myocardial cells: (1) nodal, (2) transitional, and (3) Purkinje myocytes. The nodal and transitional myocytes possesses high rates of rhythmical excitability, but their conduction velocity is slow. On the contrary, the Purkinje myocytes are blessed with maximal conduction velocity, but are less excitable. The Purkinje myocytes possesses a conduction velocity of 2–3 m/s, whereas the nodal and transitional myocytes conduct the impulses only at the rate of 0.6 m/s. The SA node of conducting system is mainly composed of highly rhythmic nodal myocyte cells, but few transitional and Purkinje myocytes are also present within it. On the other hand, the AV node is mainly composed of transitional myocyte cells and the Purkinje fibers are mainly composed of Purkinje myocyte cells.

Sinoatrial Node

The SA node was first discovered in 1907 by Keith and Flack. It is a horseshoe-shaped structure and is situated at the atriocaval junction on the upper part of sulcus terminalis. It extends downward along the sulcus terminalis for a distance of about 2 cm and measures about 20 mm × 5 mm × 2 mm in dimensions. It is developed from the right-sided embryological structure. So, there is a preponderance of right vagal innervation on it. The parasympathetic terminal

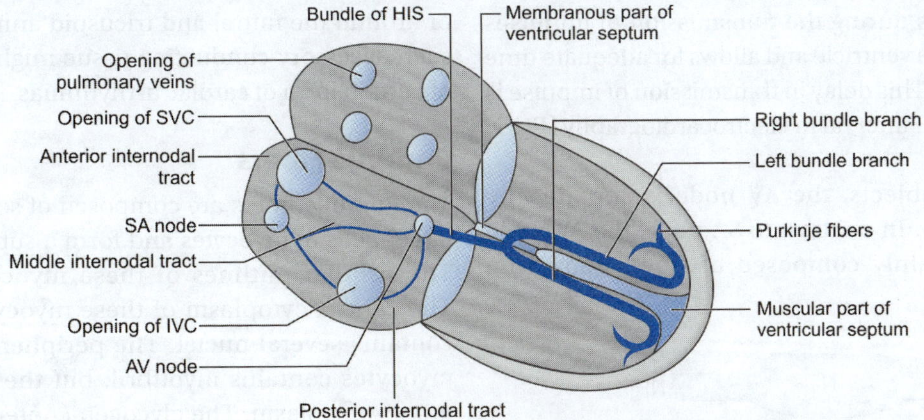

Fig. 4: The conducting system of heart. (AV: atrioventricular; IVC: inferior venacava; SA: sinoatrial; SVC: superior vena cava)

neurons of vagus are only numerous at the periphery of SA node, whereas the excitatory postganglionic sympathetic fibers are present in the center of it.

The discharge of impulses from SA node passes to AV node, through atrial muscular wall, via three bundles of fibers. These are the anterior internodal tract of Bachmann, the middle internodal tract of Wenckebach, and the posterior internodal tract of Thorel. Of these three tracts, probably the most important is the anterior internodal pathway which also conducts impulses directly to left atrium.

The central longitudinal axis of SA node is traversed and supplied by a nodal artery. In the majority of human population, it is derived from the right coronary artery. Possibly, the thickened adventitia of this nodal artery acts as baroreceptors. It monitors the aortic pressure and regulates the sinus rhythm by means of feedback. The SA node is composed of nodal myocytes (maximum quantity), transitional myocytes (less quantity) and Purkinje myocytes (least quantity). They are arranged circularly around the nodal artery from within outward.

Atrioventricular Node

Before the discovery of SA node, this node was discovered in 1906 by Tawara. It is a button-shaped structure, but smaller than SA node and measures about 20 mm × 10 mm × 2 mm in dimensions. It is situated on the lower and dorsal part of interatrial septum, just above the opening of coronary sinus. The AV node is embryologically originated from the left-sided structure of heart and is innervated, therefore, mainly by the left vagus nerve. The electrical impulses, originating from SA node converge on AV node through three internodal tracts which are described before. Microscopically, the AV node is divided into three discrete functional regions or zones. These are: (1) AN region which joins the atrial musculature with node; (2) N (nodal) or central region or AV node proper, and (3) NH region which joins the node to bundle of HIS. The AN and to a lesser extent the N region is responsible for the delay that occurs during the transmission of impulses from the atrium to the ventricle and allows for adequate time for the filling of later. This delay in transmission of impulse is responsible for the PR interval in electrocardiography (ECG) **(Fig. 5)**.

In 80–90% of subjects, the AV node is supplied by right coronary artery. In contrast to SA node, the AV node is essentially or mainly composed of slow conducting transitional myocytes, occasional nodal myocytes and covered by Purkinje myocytes which are in continuity with the AV bundle. Due to the rich population of this transitional myocytes, there is a conduction delay in the AV node.

Atrioventricular Bundle (Bundle of His)

It is the only muscular (myocytes) connection between the atrium and the ventricles which are separated by an eight-shaped nonconducting fibrous ring. The bundle of HIS begins at AV node as the continuation of it. It is enveloped by a vascular connective tissue sheath and crosses the right fibrous ring. Then, it descends along the posterior-inferior border and the right side of the membranous part of interventricular septum (subendocardially) and reach the upper medial part of the muscular interventricular septum. At the upper border of this muscular part of interventricular septum, it divides into right and left branches. Then, the left branch pierces the interventricular septum and reaches the left side of it.

Right Branch of Atrioventricular Bundle

It passes along the right side of the interventricular septum and reaches the anterior wall of the right ventricle where it terminates into Purkinje fibers.

Left Branch of Atrioventricular Bundle

It consists of 2–3 fascicules and passes subendocardially along the left side of the interventricular septum in an envelope of connective tissue sheath. Then, after traversing a course of 2–3 cm, it splits into anterior and posterior sheets to reach the base of the corresponding papillary muscles. Finally, it terminates into Purkinje fibers.

Sometimes the few fibers of conducting myocytes of the internodal tracts between the SA and AV node bypass the AV node and join straight with the common AV bundle. Many speculations appear about the existence of this accessory AV bundle in close proximity to the common AV bundle or around the mitral and tricuspid annuli. The presence of such accessory conducting tissue might explain the causes of certain form of cardiac arrhythmias.

Purkinje Fibers

The Purkinje fibers are composed of somewhat specialized larger cells of myocytes and form a subendocardial plexus. The cellular outlines of these myocytes are indistinct. The central cytoplasm of these myocytes is granular and contains several nuclei. The peripheral cytoplasm of the myocytes contains myofibril, but these are separated by more sarcoplasm. The glycogen content of Purkinje cell is very high.

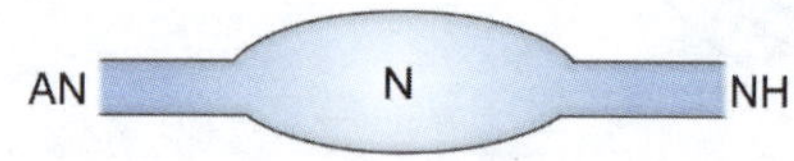

Fig. 5: The microscopic structure of atrioventricular (AV) node.

ARTERIES SUPPLYING HEART

The heart is supplied mostly by two coronary arteries such as the right and left. They arise from the root of ascending aorta and run in the corresponding atrioventricular groove or coronary sulcus. Only the inner 100 μm of endocardial surface of the myocardium of heart gets nutrition directly from the blood of cardiac chambers. Otherwise, the rest portion of myocardium gets its nutrition through coronary arteries. Anatomically, the coronary arteries are not the end arteries, because they anastomose with each other by their trunks, branches and subbranches, mostly at the precapillary level. But, functionally, however, they behave like end arteries, since most of the anastomoses remain impervious. Each coronary artery is actually a vasa vasorum of ascending aorta, because the heart is developed from the fusion of two primitive endothelial tubes, from where the great vessels are developed.

Right Coronary Artery

It is smaller than the left coronary artery. It arises from the right aortic sinus of ascending aorta, behind the right aortic cusp. It, then, passes forward and to the right and emerges on the surface of the heart between the root of pulmonary trunk and right auricle. It, then, runs downward along the right anterior AV groove or coronary sulcus up to the junction of right and inferior border of heart. Then, it winds round the inferior border of heart to reach the diaphragmatic surface of heart. After that, it runs backward and to the left through right posterior coronary sulcus to reach the postinterventricular group, where it gives a branch, named the postdescending artery (in 60% population) and terminate by anastomosing with left coronary artery. In 60% subjects, the terminal part of right coronary artery anastomoses with the circumflex branch of left coronary artery at the "crux of the heart" which is the meeting point of the posterior interatrial, posterior interventricular and the posterior part of atrioventricular grooves. In 20% cases, the right coronary artery traverses the entire posterior atrioventricular groove and reaches the left border of heart where it makes anastomosis with left coronary artery. In 10% cases, it directly reaches the apex of the heart through posterior interventricular groove instead of giving posterior descending artery and makes anastomosis with the anterior descending artery. In remaining 10% subjects, it is very short and reaches only up to the junction of the right and inferior border of the heart **(Fig. 6)**.

The branches of the right coronary artery are: (1) right conus artery, (2) right marginal artery, (3) posterior descending or interventricular artery, and (4) the multiple muscular branches to right atrium and right ventricle. The right conus artery is usually the first branch of right coronary

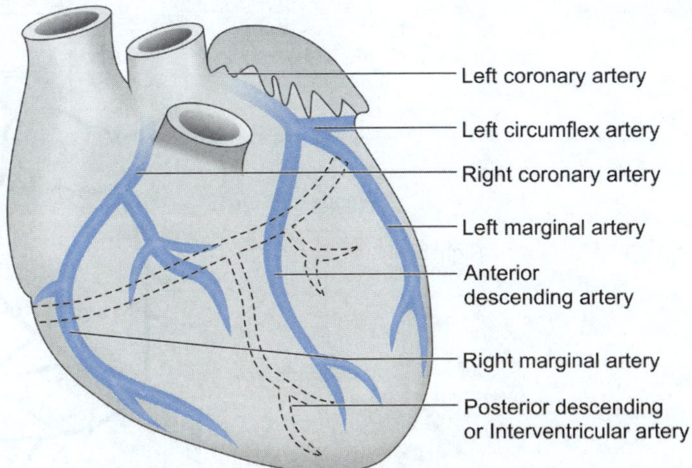

Fig. 6: Coronary arteries and their branches.

artery and supplies the infundibulum of right ventricle. Sometimes, it arises directly from the anterior aortic sinus and then it is called the *third coronary artery*. The right conus artery sometimes anastomoses in front of the aortic root with the same type of left conus artery, derived from the circumflex branch of left coronary artery. This anastomotic necklace, thus formed around the infundibulum, is known as the *annulus of Vieussens.*

The right marginal artery arises from right coronary artery at the junction of right border and the inferior border of heart. Then, it runs along the inferior border of heart toward the apex and supplies the adjoining surfaces of right ventricle. The atrial and ventricular branches or rami are the small arteries which arise from right coronary artery at right angles of it at fixed interval, while it passes through the right half of anterior and posterior atrioventricular group. The anterior ventricular branches supply the sternocostal surface and the posterior ventricular branches supply the diaphragmatic surface of right ventricle. Atrial rami (branches) are also grouped in anterior and posterior and supply the anterior and posterior wall of right atrium. Among the atrial rami, one large artery supplies the SA node which is called the *"sinoatrial nodal artery"*. In 65% cases, this SA nodal artery arises from the right coronary artery and in 35% subjects, it arises from the circumflex branch of left coronary artery **(Fig. 7)**.

In 60% cases, the posterior descending artery, or the posterior interventricular branch arises from right coronary artery near the crux and passes downward along the posterior interventricular groove toward apex. At the apex, it anastomoses with the anterior descending or anterior interventricular branch of left coronary artery. In 10% individuals, the posterior interventricular branch is derived as a continuation of left coronary artery. So, on the basis of

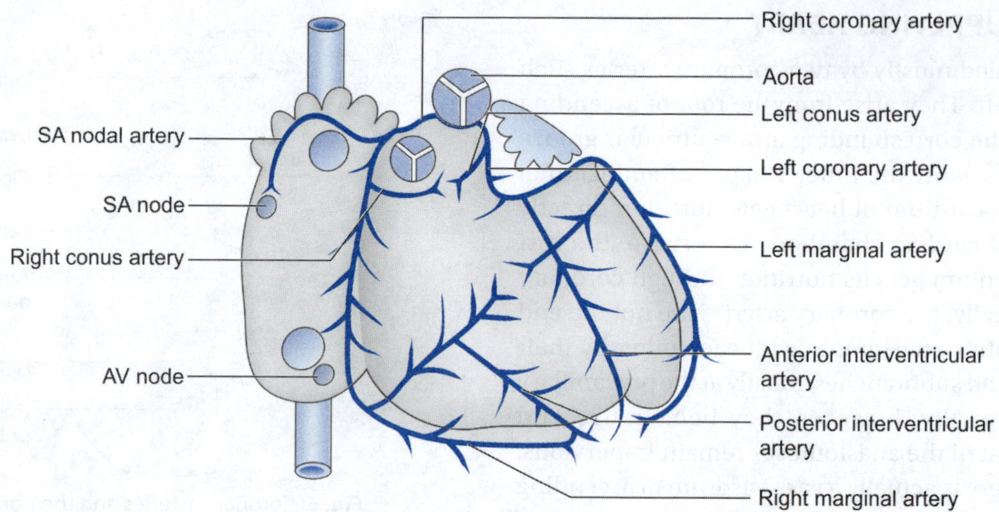

Fig. 7: Right and left coronary arteries with their branches. (AV: atrioventricular; SA: sinoatrial)

the origin of posterior interventricular branch from the right or left coronary artery, the *"right coronary predominance" or the "left coronary predominance of heart"* is described. It supplies the diaphragmatic surface of both the right and left ventricle and posteroinferior part (½) of the interventricular septum. The first septal branch of the posterior descending or posterior interventricular artery supplies the AV node. In 80–90% subjects, the AV nodal artery is derived from right coronary artery and in 10–20% cases it is derived left coronary artery.

Left Coronary Artery

It is larger than right coronary artery and arises from left aortic sinus, behind the left cusp of aortic valve. After arising from aorta, it first runs forward and to the left, between the pulmonary trunk and left auricle. Here, it gives off the anterior interventricular branch or anterior descending artery which runs downward toward apex through the anterior interventricular groove. While passing through the anterior interventricular groove, the anterior descending artery gives off multiple branches at right angle which supplies the sternocostal surface of both the ventricles and the anterior portion of interventricular septum. One such branch of anterior descending artery supplying the left ventricle is large and is called the *diagonal artery* which arises from the junction of anterior descending artery and the circumflex branch of left coronary artery. In such condition, the trunk of left coronary artery actually trifurcates. The septal branches of the anterior descending artery supply the anterior 2/3rd of interventricular septum. The rest posterior 1/3rd of interventricular septum is supplied by the posterior descending artery which is the branch of right coronary artery.

The further continuation of left coronary artery is sometimes called the *left circumflex artery*. After giving off the anterior interventricular branch, this left circumflex artery runs toward left in the left anterior ventricular groove or left coronary sulcus. Then, it winds round the left border of heart and continues through left coronary sulcus posteriorly. Near the posterior interventricular groove, this circumflex artery terminates by anastomosing with the right coronary artery. The circumflex artery lies close to the mitral valve and is usually damaged during mitral valve replacement surgery. While passing through the anterior and posterior AV groove, the circumflex artery gives of multiple branches, supplying the adjoining surfaces of left atrium and left ventricle. During winding round the left border of heart, it gives a prominent branch which follows the left border of heart toward the apex. It is called the *left marginal artery*. In coronary artery bypass graft (CABG) surgery, a vascular autograft is usually anastomosed with left marginal artery distal to the site of obstruction. Thus, the main branches of left coronary artery are: (1) anterior interventricular (anterior descending) artery, (2) left marginal (or obtuse marginal) artery, and (3) multiple atrial and ventricular muscular branches or rami.

Summary of Coronary Circulation

- The left coronary artery supplies: (a) the whole left atrium, (b) most of the left ventricle, except a strip along the posterior and inferior surface, and (c) the anterior 2/3rd of interventricular septum.
- The right coronary artery supplies: (a) the whole right atrium, (b) most of the right ventricle, except a strip along the anterior interventricular groove, (c) posterior 1/3rd of the interventricular septum, and (d) SA node and AV node in the majority of subjects.

- Sometimes left coronary artery arises from pulmonary trunk and produce left ventricular failure. Occasionally, it arises from anterior aortic sinus and undergoes a longer course behind the pulmonary trunk before dividing into its branches. In this anomaly, the main artery may be compressed between the aorta and pulmonary trunk after severe exercise and results in sudden cardiac death.
- The parasympathetic stimulation has negligible direct effect on coronary vessels. Sympathetic α-receptors (constrictor effect) are predominant over the epicardial segment of coronary vessels. But, sympathetic β-receptors (dilatation effect) are predominant over the intramuscular segment of coronary arteries. Therefore, sympathetic stimulation constricts the epicardial arteries and dilates the intramuscular arteries.
- The coronary arteries are the only vessels in our body, where the blood flows maximally during the diastole of cardiac cycle.
- Majority of people possesses "right coronary artery predominance" where the posterior interventricular or posterior descending artery is derived from right coronary artery. Minority of population has "left coronary artery predominance" where posterior descending artery extends as a continuation of the left coronary artery. These people are likely to be affected by coronary disease. This is because, the entire left ventricle and the interventricular septum are under the nutritional control of left coronary artery. So, the obstruction of latter may produce output failure for systemic circulation. Sometimes, on rare occasions, the posterior descending artery is derived from both the right and left coronary arteries. Individuals with such balanced type of coronary distribution are least affected by coronary disease.
- In subepicardial fat, potential communication exists between the branches of coronary arteries, the branches of internal thoracic artery and the branches of descending aorta such as pericardial, bronchial, phrenic, and esophageal artery. In slow obstruction of coronary arteries, these collateral channels dilate and maintain the nutrition of heart.
- Clinically, the occlusions of main coronary arteries and their major branches are located (1) within the first 2 cm of anterior descending artery, (2) and/or circumflex artery, or (3) proximal distal third of right coronary artery. Average frequencies of critical narrowing of three major arterial trunks are as follows: (a) anterior descending branch of left coronary artery (LAD) 40–50%, (b) right coronary artery (RA) 30–40%, and (c) (left coronary) circumflex artery 15–20%. Other infrequent locations of coronary artery occlusion are: (i) diagonal branches of

anterior descending artery, (ii) left marginal branch of circumflex artery, and (iii) trunk of left coronary artery.

- The total coronary circulation time is about 8 seconds. The volume of coronary blood flow is about 225 mL/min. It is about 5% of total cardiac output (CO) in resting condition. The flow of blood through coronary capillary falls during systole and rises during diastole. Blood flow through the subendocardial arterial plexuses falls almost to zero during systole. But, in diastole blood flow through the subendocardial arteries is greater than that of epicardial arteries. This explains why myocardial infarction in coronary occlusion involves first the sub-endocardial regions.
- The incomplete and spasmodic obstruction of coronary arteries is expressed as angina pectoris, where the subject complains of intense precordial pain, and which is occasionally referred along the left upper arm. In cardiac ischemia, due to vascular occlusion, CABG operation is advocated with promising results. It is now possible to dilate the obstructed coronary arteries with a balloon, introduced percutaneously [percutaneous transluminal coronary angioplasty (PCTA)] **(Fig. 8)**.

Venous Drainage of the Heart

Most of the venous blood from myocardium returns to heart through *great (anterior) cardiac vein* and *coronary sinus*. Both of them drain into right atrium. The coronary sinus conveys blood mainly from left coronary artery and the anterior cardiac vein conveys blood from right coronary artery. The coronary sinus is a wide channel. It is about 2–3 cm long and is situated in posterior AV groove. It receives 60% of venous blood from myocardium. It begins in the left part of post-AV

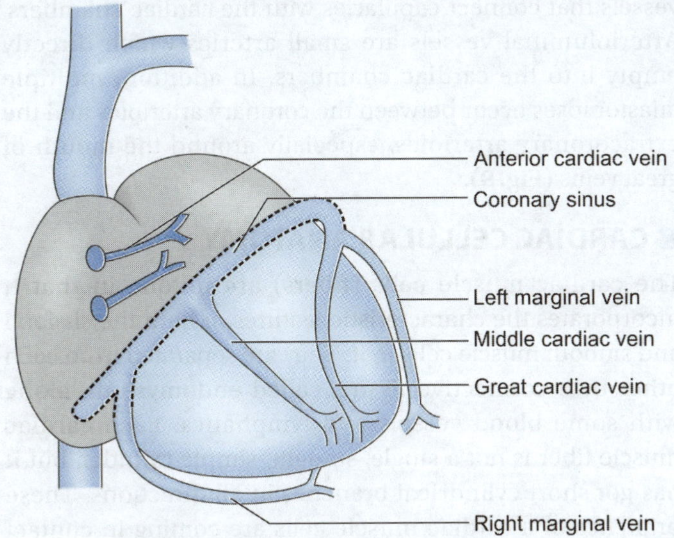

Fig. 8: The venous drainage of myocardium.

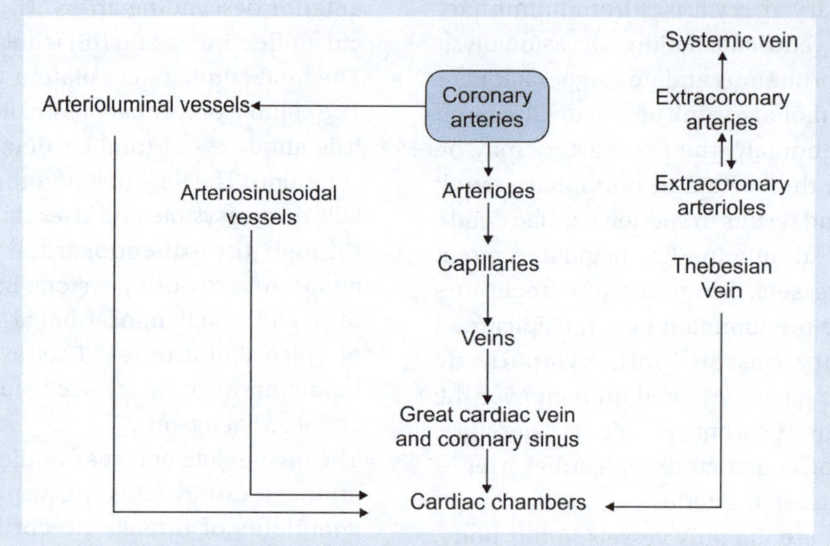

Fig. 9: Schematic diagram of venous drainage of heart.

groove, where it receives the great cardiac vein. Then, the sinus runs toward right and drains into right atrium between the opening of IVC and right atrioventricular orifice. Its main tributaries are: (1) great cardiac vein, (2) middle cardiac vein, (3) right marginal vein, and (4) left marginal vein. The great cardiac vein begins at the apex of the heart and passes upward along the anterior interventricular groove. Then, it winds with coronary sinus. The middle cardiac vein starts at the apex and runs upward along the posterior interventricular groove to join the coronary sinus. There are also other vessels which drain directly into any of the cardiac chamber. These vessels are: arteriosinusoidal, Thebesian, and arterioluminal vessels. The arteriosinusoidal vessels are capillary like sinusoidal channels which connect the arterioles with cardiac chambers. The Thebesian veins are vessels that connect capillaries with the cardiac chambers. Arterioluminal vessels are small arteries which directly empty into the cardiac chambers. In addition, multiple anastomoses occur between the coronary arterioles and the extracoronary arterioles, especially around the mouth of great veins **(Fig. 9)**.

■ CARDIAC CELLULAR ANATOMY

The cardiac muscle cells (fibers) are unique in that it incorporates the characteristic features of both the skeletal and smooth muscle cells in it. They are separated from each other by a connective tissue, called endomysium, along with some blood vessels and lymphatics. Each cardiac muscle fiber is not a single, straight, simple cylinder, but it has got short cylindrical branches in all directions. These branches of a cardiac muscle cells are coming in contact with that of the adjacent cardiac muscle cells and ultimately

form a three-dimensional network structure. Under light microscope these network of cardiac muscle cells appear as syncytium (cytoplasmic continuation in between the neighboring cells) which is also supported by the property of cardiac muscle that if one myocardial cell contracts, then all the muscle cells and the heart will contract as a whole. But, electron microscope (EM) reveals that the cytoplasm of each cardiac muscle cell is separated from other by an intercalated disc. So, heart muscle is not a structural, but functional syncytium, because the electrical resistance offered by the intercalated disk is very low and impulse passes easily, as if there is no barrier between the cytoplasm of two myocardial cells. Thus, when one cell is excited then this excitation process spreads easily and quickly across the intercalated disk to its neighboring cells and ultimately to all the cardiac muscle cells **(Fig. 10)**.

Impulse propagation in the heart depends on two factors such as the magnitude of depolarizing current (usually Na^+ current) and the geometry of electrical connection between two myocardial cells. Cardiac cells are long, thin branched, and are well attached at their longitudinal end or at their branched end with the next cell through a specialized gap junction protein, called the intercalated disk, whereas the lateral (transverse) gap junction protein are sparser. As a result, impulses which spread along the longitudinal axis of the cells are 2–3 times faster than that of the transverse axis of the cells. This "anisotropic" (direction dependent) conduction may be a factor in the generation of certain arrhythmias.

Each myocardial cell (fiber) is 100 µm in length and 15 µm in breadth. They are covered by an outer cell membrane, called the sarcolemma. It surrounds the numerous striated

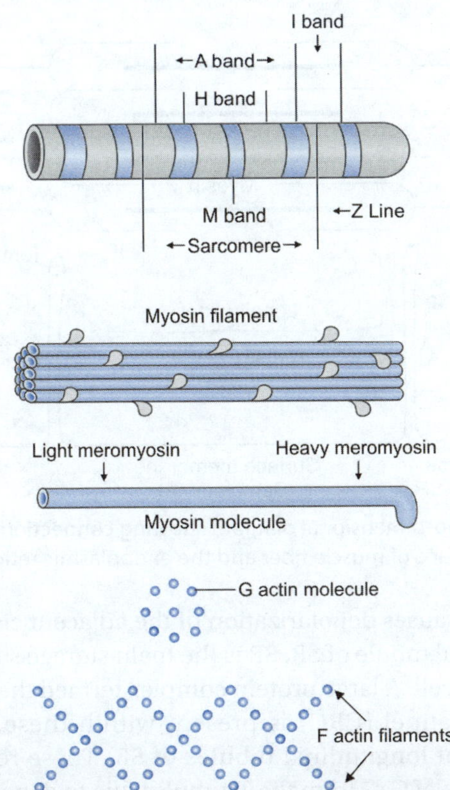

Fig. 10: Schematic diagram of a muscle fiber shown under polarized light, structure of myosin and actin myofilament.

myofibrils (myofilaments) which are present longitudinally in the cytoplasm of myocardial cell. Each myofibril consists of two contractile proteins: actin and myosin. They are interrupted at intervals of 1.2–2.5 µm by dark lines, known as Z-lines. The portion enclosed by two adjacent Z-lines of a myofibril is considered as the contractile unit and is named as the *sarcomere*. It extends about 2–3 µm in length. During each cardiac contraction, the myosin and actin filaments combine reversibly to form action-myosin complex. This interaction is the fundamental basis of muscular contraction.

Each cardiac muscle cell (fiber) consists of alternate light and dark bands. This dark band is shown as the doubly refractive (anisotropic) area when studied under polarized light. Hence, this dark band is named as the A-band. The light band is shown as mono refractive (isotropic) area under the polarized microscope. Hence, it is called the I-band. This I-band is bisected at the midpoint by the so called Z-line. At the Z-line, one cardiac muscle cell ends anatomically. Here, the cell membrane (sarcolemma) contains an extensive networks of interdigitating folds, and give attachment to the ends of individual actin filaments of two adjacent cells. These intercellular junctions are called the intercalated disk and are indicated by the Z-line. These intercalated disks form the tight connection with lowest resistance between the two adjacent myocardial cells

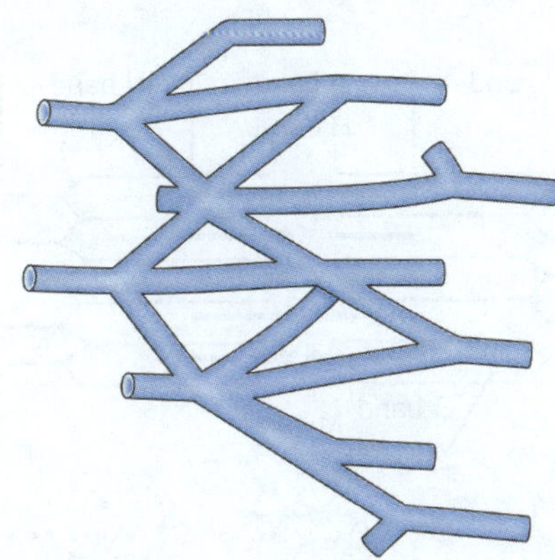

Fig. 11: Branched actin filaments or Z-filaments at Z-line.

and give attachment to the longitudinally arranged actin myofibrils. This also allows for tension to be transferred uniformly between the cells on that particular longitudinal axis. The EM reveals that intercalated disk or Z-line is made up of the cell membranes of two adjacent cells. A complex pattern of ridges and papillary projection of the cell membrane at each end of the cell fits into the corresponding grooves and pits of the other cell membrane which form an elaborately interdigitated junction or specialized cell-to-cell cohesion with intercellular space obliteration. These areas of the intercellular space obliteration are of low electrical resistance which helps in the rapid propagation of electrical impulses from cell to cell and throughout the whole mass of the heart through their branching and thus assisting the myocardium to behave as syncytium **(Fig. 11)**.

The light areas adjacent to the Z-line are made up of only thin actin filaments which are anchored to the Z-line. The actin filaments, before approaching the Z-line, appear to be branched into four fine diverging filaments, called the Z-filaments which ultimately anchored with Z-line.

The dark central A-band of each cardiac muscle cell is due to the interdigitation or overlapping of thick myosin and thin actin filaments. Again the central portion of this A-band is pale in color and called H-band. This is due to only the presence of myosin filaments and absence of actin filaments. At the mid-point of the H-band, there is also a narrow dark line which is called the M-band, where each myosin filament is thickened maximally. This myosin and actin filaments are overlapped at the peripheral dark portion of the A-band which is named as the O-band. Transverse section of the myofibrils at different levels of the A-band and I-band will give different representations **(Fig. 12)**.

Transection through the I-band will show the thin actin filaments only. Transverse section through the O-band will present both the thin actin and thick myosin filament and that at the H-band and M-band only myosin filament will be presented. In cross section at the O-band, the arrangements

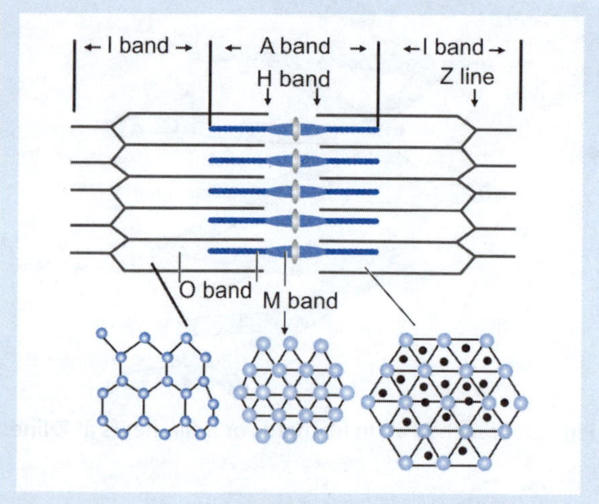

Fig. 12: Schematic diagram showing disposition of actin and myosin filament.

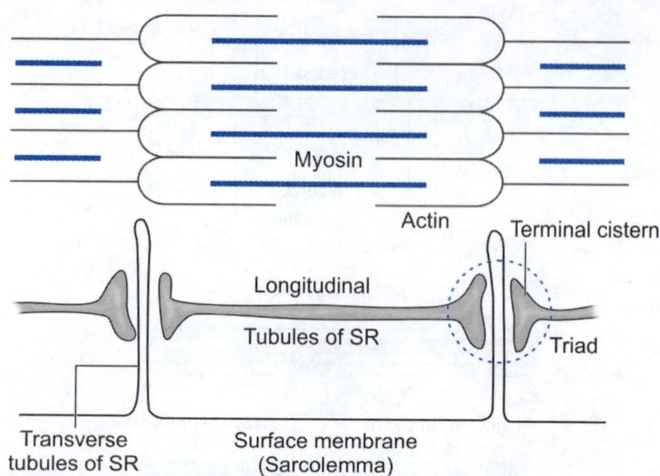

Fig. 13: Two-dimensional diagram showing connection between the surface of muscle fiber and the endoplasmic reticulum.

of the thin actin filaments appear in hexagonal shape with one myosin filament at the center. But again when the thick myosin filaments are considered then the myosin filaments are appeared forming triangles with one central actin filaments. But in the longitudinal section, each myosin filament is followed by two actin filaments. The thin actin filaments are also connected with each other longitudinally by means of still more thin S-filaments.

Under EM, within the myocardial cell the myofibrils or the myofilaments are seen to have surrounded by another longitudinal network of membranous tubular structure, called the sarcoplasmic reticulum (SR). This SR is identical with the endoplasmic reticulum of other cells, but with the difference that its membrane does not possess ribosomes. These longitudinal tubules of SR is dilated at their terminal end and called the "terminal cistern". In each myocardial cell, at the level of Z-line, a transverse invagination of the sarcolemma (plasma membrane) occurs. Thus, this results in extension of the extracellular space into the more central portion of the myocardial cells at the level of the Z-lines. These transverse invagination or tubules of sarcolemma are called T-tubules. Thus, at the level of each Z-line these T-tubules approximate with the longitudinal tubules of SR, but do not anastomose with each other. So, the term "triad" is used to describe this arrangement of the terminal dilatation of two longitudinal tubules (terminal cisterns) from opposite direction on each side of the transverse tubule **(Fig. 13)**.

The depolarization of sarcolemma causes the development of an action potential which is conducted through the transverse tubules (T-tubules) into the central portion of the cells snd causes a small pntracellular influx of Ca^{2+} from it. This small release of Ca^+ from the T-tubules occurs through the L-type of calcium channel which is situated in it. Then, the impulse which passes down the

T-tubules causes depolarization of the adjacent cisternae of longitudinal tubule of SR. SR is the main storage site for Ca^{2+} within the cell. A large protein complex termed the calcium-release channel (CRC) is present within these terminal cisternae of longitudinal tubules of SR. These respond to small influx of Ca^{2+} from the T-tubules due to depolarization of cell membrane and then subsequently release the large amounts of Ca^{2+} from the stored SR into myoplasm or sarcoplasm. This results in a sudden large increase in the intracellular Ca^{2+} concentrations from 10^{-7} M to 10^{-5} M. The short distance between the L-type Ca^{2+} channel in T-tubule and the foot process of the CRC in terminal cisternae of SR allows the Ca^{2+} entry from L channel to CRC channel and immediate release of huge amount of Ca^{2+} in cytoplasm from the later.

Ca^{2+} then diffuses from cytoplasm into the myofibrils or filaments and activates myosin. Myosin then splits adenosine triphosphate (ATP), yielding the necessary energy for the formation of the actomyosin complex for the contraction of muscle. After contraction, the Ca^{2+} again actively transported back into the cistern of longitudinal tubules of SR and relaxation occurs. This occurs through Ca/Mg ATPase pump which is embedded in the whole membrane of the longitudinal SR. After removal of Ca^{2+} from cytoplasm, the intracellular concentration of it is again restored to 10^{-7} M at diastole.

Like other cells, cardiac muscle cells or fibers also contain numerous mitochondria surrounded by myofibril, single nucleus, small Golgi apparatuses, and abundant cytoplasm.

Mechanism of Myocardial Contraction

Myofilaments or myofibrils are the contractile units of the cardiac muscle cells. They are of two types such as the thinner ones (50 Å in diameter) are called the actin filaments and the thicker ones (100 Å in diameter) are called the myosin filaments.

The molecular weight of actin myofibril is 43,000. With very high magnification under EM, it is found that each actin filament consists of two strands, arranged spirally. Each strand of actin filaments which are called fibrous actin or F-actin appears as beaded and seems to consist of globular subunits, called G-actin. The two strands or F-actin are entwined in a helix. Two complex proteins such as tropomyosin and troponin are interposed between this two thin strands (F-actin) of actin filaments. Molecular weight of tropomyosin is 70,000 and lies within the sulcus of two thin strands of actin filaments (F-actin). Troponin is also consists of three distinct polypeptides troponin T, troponin I, and troponin C and lies within the groove of two thin strands of actin filaments (F-actin) at regular interval. Each polypeptide of troponin fulfills different functions in the regulations of muscular contractions. Troponin T binds with the tropomyosin and forms a complex. Troponin I inhibits the reactions of actin with myosin filament. Troponin C binds Ca^{2+} and activates contractions by inhibiting troponin I. The binding of Ca^{2+} to troponin C is the triggering factor that initiates the chain of reaction causing conformational changes of actin and leads to the development of mechanical activity (like troponin C, calmodulin which is present in other nonmyocardial cells in place of troponin C also binds with Ca^{2+} and initiates the different enzymatic reactions in these cells) **(Fig. 14)**.

The thicker contractile element of myofibrils or myofilaments is called myosin. It consists of large asymmetrical molecules, consisting of two heavy chains and four light chains. The molecular weight of heavy chain and light chain is 220,000 and 20,000, respectively. Each myosin molecule consists of: (1) one globular head containing the activity of enzyme ATPase which hydrolyses ATP to provide energy and interacts with actin to form cross bridges, (2) one neck area, appears to be involved in the development of tension, and (3) one tail which helps to anchor one myosin molecule to another forming thick myosin filament. The head and neck portion of each myosin molecule is called the heavy meromyosin and tail or rod-like portion of it is called the light meromyosin. The thickness of the myosin filament is believed to be due to the parallel arrangement of myosin molecules in such a fashion that the globular heads project outward near the surface of the myosin filaments and the rod-like tail part takes its position in the smooth central portion of the myosin filament. The heads of myosin molecules are arranged in a radial pattern and each set of six head complete one revolution around the myosin filament within one 400 Å segment. Each head of the myosin molecule is pointed toward a separate actin filament and makes a

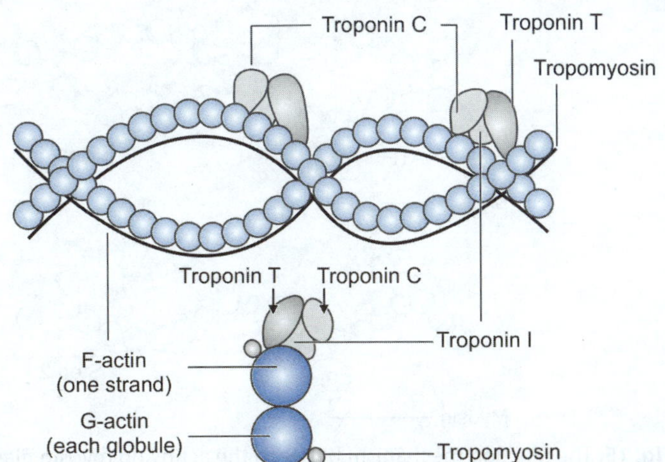

Fig. 14: The structure of actin filament. The backbone of each actin filament is two strands which are made up of actin monomers (G-actin). Each strand is called F-actin. Troponin complex which is made up of one molecule each of troponin C, troponin I, and troponin T are distributed at regular intervals along the actin filaments. Elongated tropomyosin molecule, which is another protein structure and is attached to the actin filaments, lies in the grooves between the two actin strands. A cross section of actin filaments at the level where troponin complexes are located shows the probable relationship between the actin, tropomyosin, and the three components of the troponin complex. The strength of the bond linking troponin I and actin varies. It depends on whether Ca^{2+} is bound to troponin C or not.

cross bridges during actin myosin complex formation and muscular contraction.

The impulse or the wave of depolarization is propagated from the sarcolemma (cell membrane) through the T-tubules into the interior of the cell. Then, the depolarization of the T-tubules cause the entry of small amount of Ca^{2+} from the extracellular space into the sarcoplasm. This small entry of Ca^{2+} occurs through the L-type of Ca^{2+} channel situated on the T-tubules and acts solely as a trigger to initiate the huge release of Ca^{2+} from the longitudinal tubules of SR. The Ca^{2+}-release channel on the "terminal cisterns" of the longitudinal tubules of SR is a huge protein molecule of molecular weight of 565,000 with foot process which lies in close proximity to the L-type of Ca^{2+} channel. The short distance between the L-type of Ca^{2+} channel in the T-tubular membrane and the foot process of Ca^{2+} channel on terminal cistern (CRC or calcium-release channel) allows the immediate entry of this small amount of Ca^{2+} in the SR and subsequent huge release of Ca^{2+} from the "terminal cistern" of it **(Fig. 15)**.

After release of Ca^{2+} and contraction of muscle, it again reaccumulates back in the longitudinal tubules of SR. This is accomplished by Ca/Mg-ATPase pump, embedded on the membrane of the longitudinal tubule of SR. So, the removal of free intracellular Ca^{2+} from the sarcoplasm back into

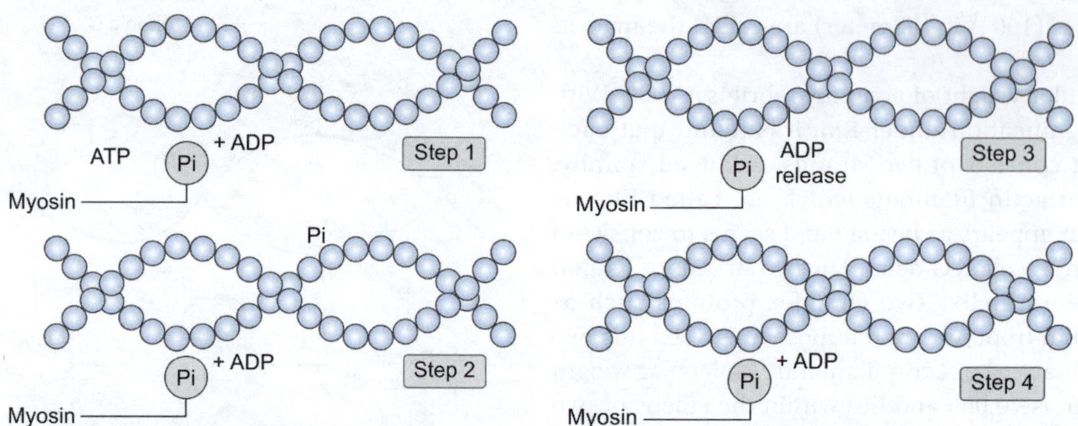

Fig. 15: The reaction mechanism between the actin and myosin filament is described in simplified form in four steps:

Step 1: On the head of the myosin filaments, there is an adenosine triphosphate (ATP) hydrolyzing site. After hydrolysis of myosin bound ATP at this site, energy is released. This is transferred to the myosin head and it is activated and energized. In a relaxed muscle the intracellular Ca^{2+} concentration is low and in this low Ca^{2+} concentration troponin and tropomyosin complex on the actin filaments do not allow the actin filaments to interact with the energized activated myosin head. Therefore, even though the myosin heads are energized, they cannot interact with actin filament.

Step 2: After depolarization, there is increased concentration of intracellular Ca^{2+}. Then, increased Ca^{2+} is attached with troponin C and makes some conformational changes of actin filaments. This conformational changes of actin filament causes binding of actin with the already energized myosin filaments and formation of cross bridges.

Step 3: After the attachment of head of the myosin with the actin filament energy is released from the head which causes changes in the angle of the attachment of the head of myosin filament and the rowing motion of cross bridges. This is called the power stroke which produces muscle contraction.

Step 4: Then the muscle returns to its resting state and the cycle ends when a new molecule of ATP binds with the myosin head and dissociates the cross bridges from the actin filaments. The contraction continues until Ca^{2+} is dissociated from the troponin C of the actin filament which causes the contractile proteins to return to the resting state. Thus, (i) binding of another ATP molecule which leads to the detachment of cross bridge, (ii) the cycle of hydrolysis of ATP, and (iii) reattachment of myosin head with formation of cross bridge with actin filament begin again.

longitudinal tubule of SR is an active and energy consuming process. Thus, the low sarcoplasmic Ca^{2+} concentration, i.e., 10^{-7} M from the high Ca^{2+} concentration, i.e., 10^{-5} M is restored by the tubule of the SR during diastole.

The activity of Ca^{2+} channel on the SR can be augmented by the cyclic adenosine monophosphate (cAMP)-dependent phosphorylation of an another SR protein called phospholamban. The β-adrenergic stimulation leads to the increase in phosphorylation of this phospholamban, causing increased Ca^{2+} channel activity and increase in concentration of Ca^{2+} in sarcoplasm and increased force of contraction.

In the resting state, the troponin I exerts an inhibitory effect on the actin filaments via tropomyosin and troponin T. But troponin C has an affinity for Ca^{2+} and binds calcium to its saturation point when the sarcoplasmic Ca^{2+} concentration rises to 10^{-5} M. Thus, when troponin C is

activated, it inhibits troponin I. As a result the inhibitory influence of the troponin-tropomyosin complex on actin is removed. Simultaneously, the rise in the Ca^{2+} concentration in the sarcoplasm activates the ATPase enzyme situated on the myosin head. This activated ATPase breaks the ATP to adenosine diphosphate (ADP) with the release of energy which energizes the myosin head and forms cross bridges with actin causing muscular contraction.

In summary, the mechanism of myocardial contraction and relaxation may be expressed as the following order.

- *Contraction:* Membrane depolarization → Ca^{2+} released from the SR → myosin ATPase is activated → cross bridges formed → actin slides along the myosin filaments → tension is developed.

- *Relaxation:* Ca^{2+} pumped back into SR → myosin ATPase is depressed → cross bridges broken → actin is pulled back to its resting state → tension disappears.

CARDIAC ELECTROPHYSIOLOGY

The flow of different charged ions across the cell membrane results in the appearance of different ionic currents such as the Na^+ current, K^+ current, Ca^+ current, etc. and these make up the cardiac action potential. The action potential of a cell is a highly integrated event. Changes in the flow of one ionic current almost inevitably produce stimulatory or inhibitory secondary changes on the flow of other ionic currents. The movements of ions across the cell membrane occur not only passively through the lipid bilayer of it, but also actively through the different specific ion channels and transporter systems, situated on it (cell membrane). These occur in response to either electrical or concentration gradient or both.

The contraction and relaxation of cardiac muscle are due to the event of action potential (like skeletal muscle and nerve fibers) which originates from the SA node and passes to the AV node through atrial muscle. This initiates the atrial contraction and relaxation. It then passes through the bundle of HIS and Purkinje fibers to the ventricular muscle and initiates the ventricular contraction and relaxation. The rapid alteration of electrical potential during depolarization of cardiac muscle cell differs little from that of the nerve fibers and skeletal muscle cells which is discussed later. But, the repolarization in cardiac muscle cell requires 400 ms. This is entirely different from the situation found in skeletal muscle cells and nerve fibers in which the total action potential including the depolarization and repolarization is completed within few milliseconds. Because of this long duration of action potential, due to the prolonged repolarization, the cardiac muscle cells cannot be further re-excited for few fraction of a second, even when the previous mechanical contraction is almost complete. Thus, the heart muscle cannot be tetanized like the skeletal muscle. This property of long refractory period ensues enough time for recovery of the cardiac muscle cells.

Action potential of heart is of two types. One is *"the fast response action potential"* which occurs in the cells of atrial muscle, ventricular muscle, and Purkinje fibers and second is *"the slow response action potential"* which occurs in the SA and AV node and is responsible for the automaticity or pace maker activity. The myocardial cells which have the characteristic of "fast response action potential" also possesses the pace maker activity. But, it is usually suppressed by the activity of myocardial cells (the cells of SA and AV node) which have the characteristic of "slow response action potential".

The differences between these two types of action potentials are discussed under different headings below.

■ RESTING MEMBRANE POTENTIAL

In slow response action potential, the resting membrane potential attains rarely more negative than –60 mV, whereas, in fast response action potential which is found in other cardiac muscle cells, except the SA and AV node, the resting membrane potential approximately goes down to –80 or –90 mV. In the type of slow response action potential, during the period of phase 4, the resting membrane potential spontaneously and progressively changes from –60 mV to approximately –40 mV which is the threshold value for excitation, and thereafter a fulminant upstroke of a full action potential or depolarization occurs. This slow ascent of membrane potential to a more positive value, i.e., from –60 mV to –40 mV, during the phase 4 of AP, characterizes the "pace maker" activity of the SA or AV node. This is due to the slow inward flow of sodium current in phase 4 through cell membrane of the SA and AV nodal cells. Initially, this inward Na^+ current only slightly exceeds the outward K^+ current. But, gradually the outward K^+ current stops allowing continuous inward Na^+ current to produce a progressively more positive or less negative membrane potential **(Fig. 16)**.

Once the resting membrane potential achieves a threshold level of –40 mV, then there occurs a very rapid rise of inward flow of Na^+ current and the depolarization part of action potential takes off. It indicates that the threshold level for excitation is achieved earliest in the SA nodal cell and the action potential, generated there, is conducted to the other cardiac cells. As other cardiac cells are latent pacemaker and the depolarization, arising from SA node, arrives there before their own diastolic depolarization in phase 4 and is reached to threshold level, so their automaticity is suppressed.

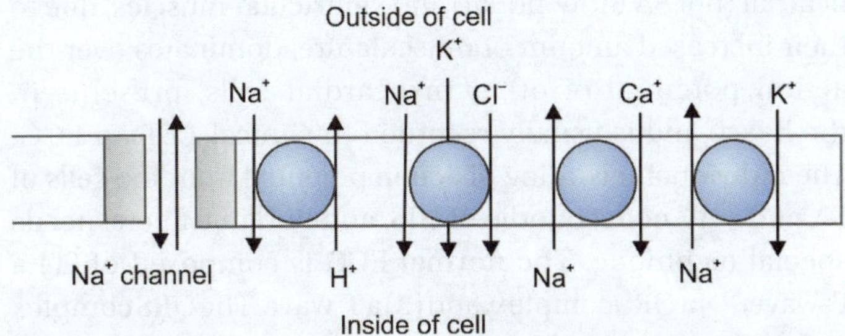

Fig. 16: Different types of Na^+ transport systems which act during the different phases of action potential. From left to right, these include: only Na^+ channel, Na^+-H^+ antiport exchange, Na^+-K^+ cotransport, Na^+-Ca^{2+} exchanger, and the Na^+-K^+ ATPase pump.

RATE OF RISE OF UPSTROKE IN ACTION POTENTIAL

In the slow response action potential of SA and AV nodal cell, there is slow depolarization phase, slow repolarization phase, and also the slow slope of diastolic depolarization phase (phase 4 of action potential). The peak of action potential in case of slow response is rounded, but uninterrupted. In atrial, ventricular, and Purkinje cells where the fast response action potential occurs, there the depolarization phase is very sharp and the peak is mostly pointed. Besides these, there is interrupted fall of repolarization and the upward slope of diastolic depolarization phase is absent (actually not absent, but depressed). Thus, in SA node dominated heart, the pace maker activity of the cells of atrial muscle, ventricular muscle, and Purkinje fibers are depressed due to the higher rhythmical activity of SA node. This is evident from the absence of the slope of slow diastolic depolarization phase in these groups of muscle fibers. But, if the transmembrane potential is recorded from isolated fibers of these groups of muscle cells, then the slope of slow diastolic depolarization (phase 4) is observed **(Fig. 17)**.

PROPAGATION AND VELOCITY OF AP

It is important to note that the conduction velocity of impulses through AV node is slow (0.2 m/s). Thus, it ensures an appreciable delay between the atrial and ventricular depolarization (contraction). This slow conduction of AV node is partly due to the small size (radius 7 μm) of the AV nodal cells, compared to the Purkinje cells (fibers) (radius 50 μm) which conduct the impulses at the rate of 4 m/s. It is also partly due to the fact that the amplitude of ionic currents, generated by the AV nodal fibers, is far less than those developed by the Purkinje fibers.

There is direct relationship between the transmembrane action potential, recorded from the individual cardiac muscle cells (SA node, atrium, AV node, ventricular muscle, and Purkinje fiber), and ECG. But, the total action potential of atrial (not SA or AV nodal) and ventricular muscles, due to their increased amount of musculature, dominates over the action potential of other myocardial cells, presents in the heart, and is usually recorded in clinical 12-lead ECG. The individual recording of action potential from the cells of SA node, AV node, bundle of HIS, and Purkinje fibers, needs special technique. The normal ECG is composed of (1) a P-wave, (2) a QRS complex, and (3) a T-wave. The QRS complex has often, but not always, three separate components: (i) the Q-wave, (ii) the R-wave, and (iii) the S-wave. The P-wave is caused by the electrical potentials when the atria depolarize and its contraction begins. The QRS complex is also caused by the generated electrical potentials when the

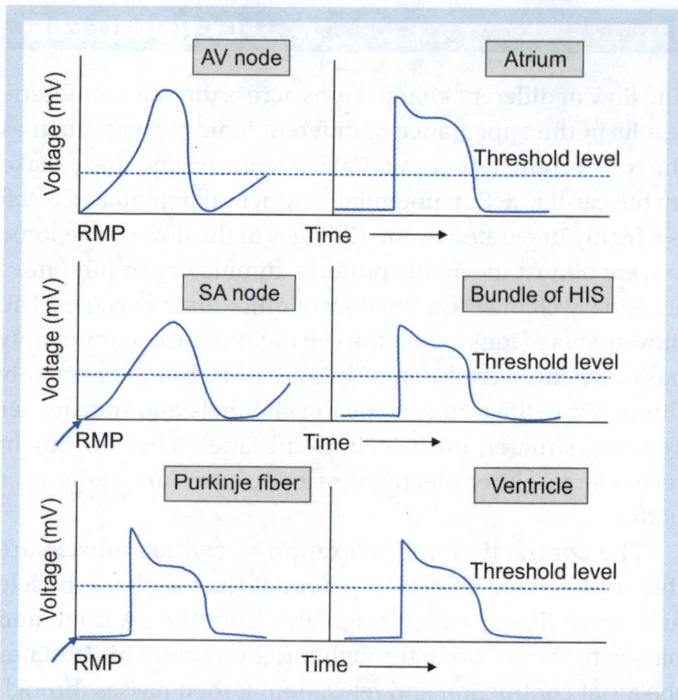

Fig. 17: Different configurations of action potential of different tissues (cells) of heart. The SA node has the steepest phase 4, showing a rapid spontaneous depolarization in diastole. So, it undergoes fast self-excitation and acts as pacemaker. Other tissues also undergo the phase 4 slow depolarization, but at a slower rate. So, they receive a propagated impulse from SA node, before their phase 4 of action potential reach the threshold level and they remain as latent pacemakers. Two types of action potentials are found in different cardiac tissues. These are slow and fast action potential. The slow action potential is characterized by: (i) shorter duration, (ii) phases 1, 2, and 3 of action potential are not clearly demarked, and (iii) low amplitude, rounded overshoot, initiation of action potential at lower threshold (less negative) level.

ventricle depolarizes and its contraction begins. Therefore, both the P-wave and the components of QRS complex are depolarization waves, whereas the T-wave is caused by the electrical potentials when the ventricles recover from the state of depolarization. This process normally occurs in ventricular muscle 0.25–0.35 seconds after its depolarization. So, the T-wave is known as the repolarization wave of ventricles. The repolarization of atrium falls within the duration of QRS complex. So, it cannot be seen in usual 12 leads ECG.

The cellular electrical properties of myocardium which can be assumed from the ECG are:

- *Heart rate:* It reflects the pace maker activity of sinus (SA) node and the P-wave reflects the whole atrial depolarization and the initiation of its contraction. The only depolarization of the cells of SA node (without the depolarization of atrial muscle) cannot be recorded by clinical ECG. The atria repolarize, which lasts for about 0.15–0.2

second, after the termination of its depolarization or P-wave. This also occurs approximately when the QRS complex is being recorded in the clinical ECG. Therefore, the atrial repolarization wave, known as the atrial T-wave, is usually obscured by the much larger QRS complex in ECG. For this reason, an atrial T-wave seldom is observed in a clinical ECG. Atrial depolarization and repolarization make atrial systole. This atrial systole is followed by atrial diastole which extends from the end of its repolarization (it cannot be seen in ECG as it is overshadowed by QRS complex) to the beginning of next P-wave.

- *PR interval:* It reflects the AV nodal conduction time, i.e., the time taken for the wave of atrial depolarization to cross the AV node from atrium to ventricle. This period is also called the PQ interval, if Q-wave is present. But, usually the Q-wave is likely to be absent and so it is termed as the PR interval.

- *QRS duration:* It reflects the time taken for the conduction of impulses to travel through the muscles of ventricle and the depolarization period of whole ventricle.

- *QT interval (Fig. 18):* It is the total duration of ventricular depolarization plus repolarization (T-wave in clinical ECG represents ventricular repolarization. Atrial or ventricular contraction includes their depolarization + repolarization), i.e., a full period of ventricular action potential or contraction. Among this (QT interval), the only QRS duration implies the time taken for the initiation of depolarization of different parts of ventricle to full ventricular depolarization. The ST segment implies the duration in which the whole ventricle stays in full depolarization state and the T-wave implies the full repolarization period of whole ventricle. Thus, the contraction of ventricle lasts almost entirely from the beginning of Q-wave (or R-wave, if Q-wave is absent) to the end of T-wave. The time interval in an ECG between the end of one T-wave and the beginning of next QRS wave corresponds with the phase 4 of action potential and ventricular diastole.

If we corresponds the action potential graph of ventricle and ECG, then we will find that the QRS wave will appear at the beginning of the action potential of ventricle or ventricular depolarization (or phase 0) and the T-wave will appear at the end of phase 3 of action potential. In between these waves and also after the T-waves no electrical potential difference will be recorded. This is because, there is no movement of impulse and its corresponding graph is recorded as isoelectric line in the ECG when the whole ventricular muscle is either completely depolarized (corresponding with the isoelectric line after the QRS complex) or completely repolarized (corresponding with the isoelectric line

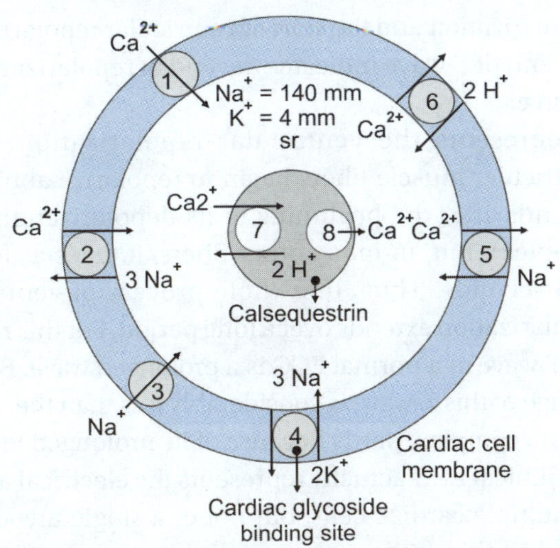

Fig. 18: The exchange of Na$^+$ and Ca^{2+} through sarcolemma during action potential of cardiac muscle cells. Na$^+$ and Ca^{2+} enter the cells during each cycle of depolarization. It triggers the release of larger amount of Ca^{2+} through Ca^{2+}-release channel (8), present in the sarcoplasmic reticulum (SR). The resulting tremendous increase in the concentration of intracellular Ca^{2+} interacts with troponin C. This interaction is responsible for the activation of cross bridge reactions between the actin and myosin filament. Thus, they form the cross bridges that result in sarcomere shortening. The electrochemical gradient for Na$^+$ and K$^+$ across the cell membrane is maintained by active adenosine triphosphate (ATP) consuming Na$^+$-K$^+$ ATPase pump (4). It extrudes Na$^+$ out of the cell. While the Na$^+$ is actively extruded by Na$^+$-K$^+$ ATPase pump, the bulk of cytosolic Ca^{2+} is pumped back again by the Ca^{2+} ATPase pump (7) in the SR. In the SR, Ca^{2+} is stored by binding with a protein, named calsequestrin. The remaining portion of intracellular Ca^{2+} is removed from the cell by either a plasma membrane-bound Ca^{2+}ATPase pump (6) or by a Na$^+$-Ca^{2+} cation exchange protein or channel (2 and 5). This cation protein exchanger (2 and 5) exchanges 3Na$^+$ in for every single Ca^{2+} out. The direction of this cation exchange is reversed briefly during depolarization. This is because, when the electrical gradient across the cell membrane is transiently reversed. The β-adrenergic receptor agonists and phosphodiesterase inhibitors activate the protein kinase (1) by increasing the intracellular cyclic adenosine monophosphate (cAMP) levels. This activated protein kinase (PK) enhances the contractile state by phosphorylating the target proteins including phospholamban and the α-subunit of L-type Ca^{2+} channel. 1 = Ca^{2+} channel, 2 = Na$^+$-Ca^{2+} exchange, 3 = Na$^+$ channel, 4 = Na$^+$-K$^+$ ATPase pump, 5 = Na$^+$-Ca^{2+} exchanger, 6 = Ca^{2+} ATPase pump, 7 = Ca^{2+} ATPase pump, 8 = Ca^{2+}-release channel.

after T-wave). Hence, only when a muscle mass is partly polarized (i.e., partly depolarized or partly repolarized) then the current will flow from one part of the atrium or ventricle to its another part. Therefore, current will also flow on the surface of the body to produce a graph in ECG. The beginning of QRS complex indicates start of ventricular depolarization. The QRS complex and ST segment indicates the whole duration of ventricular depolarization. The beginning of T-wave indicates end of depolarization and the start of ventricular repolarization. The end of T-wave indicates the end of repolarization.

- **T-wave:**

  It represents the ventricular repolarization. Some ventricular muscle fibers begin to repolarize about 0.20 seconds after the beginning of its depolarization (QRS complex). But, in many other fibers, it takes as long as 0.35 seconds. Thus, the whole process of ventricular repolarization extends over a long period. For this reason, the T-wave in a normal ECG is a prolonged wave. But, the voltage of this T-wave is considerably less than the voltage of QRS complex, partly because of its prolonged length.

  Clinical ECG actually represents the electrical activity of multiple cardiac cells, but not of a single myocardial cell. For this reason, the amplitude and the shape of the P, R, and T-waves of an ECG mostly dependent upon the amount of electrical activities, offered together by the group of these cardiac cells and also upon the different configuration of action potential of these cells than that of an individual one.

CARDIAC ACTION POTENTIAL

The whole action potential of cardiac tissues is divided into two stages: depolarization and repolarization or more **(Fig. 19)** scientifically into five phases, numbered as 0, 1, 2, 3, and 4. Among these, the phase 0 represents the depolarization and the phases 1, 2, and 3 represent repolarization. The heart remains in systole both at the stages of depolarization and repolarization, i.e., from phase 0 to phase 3. But, it remains in diastole only during phase 4. After repolarization, i.e., after phase 3 and in phase 4, the membrane potential comes down to its normal resting level. But, the ionic distribution of Na^+ and K^+ across the cell membrane remains in opposite state to that which is found in the resting state. So, in phase 4 of nonpace making cardiac cells, the opposite ionic distribution of Na^+ and K^+ comes back to its normal state without any change of the resting membrane potential which is achieved at the end of phase 3. But, this phase 4 is called the *"slow diastolic depolarization"* for the pace making myocardial cells, because, in this phase of pace making cells, the inside of the cell again starts to become slowly positive (i.e., depolarization) from normal resting membrane potential which is achieved at the end of the phase 3, though the ionic concentration of Na^+ and K^+ is opposite to the resting condition. This slow process of depolarization during diastole of heart is the characteristic of pacemaker activity of the SA or AV nodal cells and is absent in other cells than pace maker cells.

At rest, in the nonpace making myocardial cells, the membrane potential (resting membrane potential Vm) is

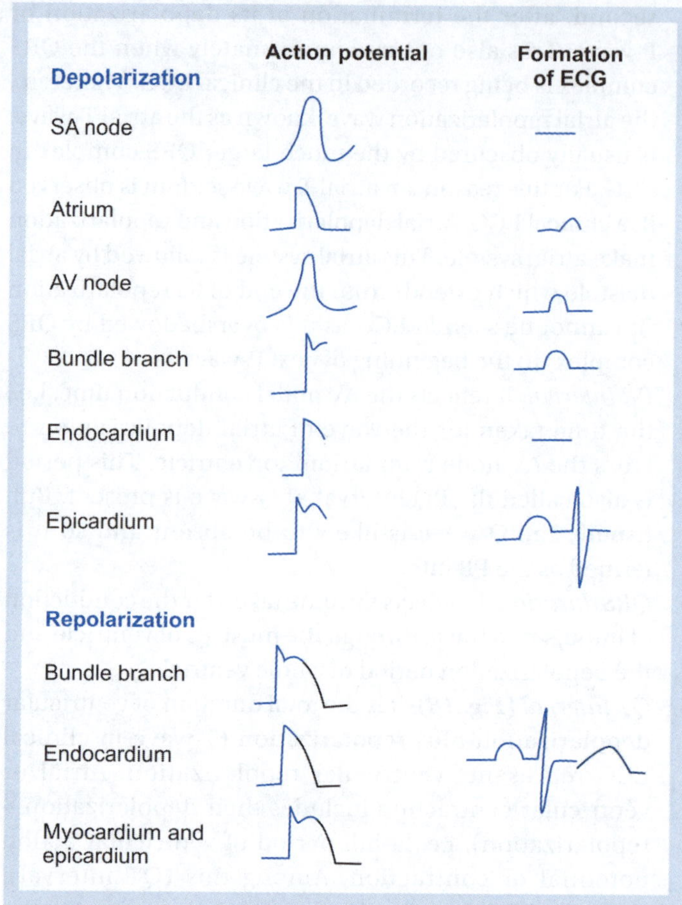

Fig. 19: The action potential and its subsequent ECG formation of different tissues of heart are shown. Red line indicated depolarization and blue line repolarization. (AV: atrioventricular; ECG: electrocardiogram; SA: sinoatrial)

maintained at the level of –60 mV to –70 mV, with negativity inside and positivity outside of the cell, like the resting nerve and muscle cells. This resting membrane potential or the electrical gradient between the inside and the outside of the cell is established by pumps, especially the Na^+-K^+ATPase pump, which extrudes the Na^+ from the cell and pushes the K^+ inside the cell and some fixed anionic charges which are present within the cells. Other Na^+ channels remain closed at this negative transmembrane potential and so no Na^+ does enter inside the normal resting myocardial cell through these Na^+ channels. Whereas, the other specific K^+ channel (inward rectifier K^+ channel) remains in an open conformation at this negative resting membrane potential and allows the normal cardiac cells to become permeable to K^+ from outside to inside at rest. This inward rectifier K^+ channel along with the Na^+-K^+ATPase pump maintains the intracellular K^+ concentration which is higher than the extracellular concentration of it. So, the concentration of K^+ in the extracellular space is the major determinant factor for the resting membrane potential.

For each individual ion, there is an equilibrium potential (Ex) after which there is no movement of ion across the cell membrane, still if the channels are open. For K^+ this value of equilibrium potential is –94 mV, i.e., at this voltage there is no net force which drives the K^+ into or out of the cells. The Na^+ channels which allow Na^+ to move along the gradient are closed at negative transmembrane potential. So, Na^+ does not enter into the normal resting cardiac cells **(Fig. 20)**.

The negative resting membrane potential will be maintained, until the resting state is not disturbed by the propagated impulse or the slow diastolic depolarization in phase 4. If there is any propagated impulse or the slow diastolic depolarization reaches the threshold level, then the resting membrane potential is changed fulminantly from –90 mV of nonpace making cells to the value of +30 mV, making the inside of the cell positive in respect to outside. This initial stage of action potential is called the depolarization or phase 0 and this is due to the sudden influx of Na^+ into the cell from outside, after the threshold level is reached and also due to some influx of Ca^{2+} into the cell from outside. The entry of Na^+ into the cell is operated through the voltage dependent double-gated fast Na^+ channel. In these channels, the outer m-gate (activation gate) remains closed and the inner h-gate remains open during resting state at the end of repolarization and become ready for depolarization **(Fig. 20A)**. When the stimulus is reached, outer m-gate then opens and Na^+ is allowed to flow in the cell along its concentration and electrostatic gradient **(Fig. 20B)**. As the membrane potential reaches +30 mV, then the inner h-gate (inactivation gate) closes preventing the further influx of Na^+ and marks the end of depolarization or phase 0 **(Fig. 20C)**.

Then, when repolarization starts, the upper m-gate closes. In this state, both the m- and h-gate is closed and is known as the closed and inactivated state of Na^+ channel **(Fig. 20D)**. During the repolarization of cell membrane, Na^+ channel also changes its conformation from closed and inactivated state to its close and activated state when the outer m-gate remains close, but the inner h-gate opens and makes the Na^+ channel ready for the next further depolarization. During depolarization, both the gates are again opened and Na^+ enters through this "open and activated" sodium channel. Thus, this cycle of closed and inactivated (D) → closed and activated (A) → open and activated (B) → open and inactivated (C) form of Na^+ channel repeats.

After depolarization, repolarization occurs in several steps and these are:

- There is an initial partial rapid repolarization or phase 1, where the membrane potential falls from +30 mV to + 10 mV.

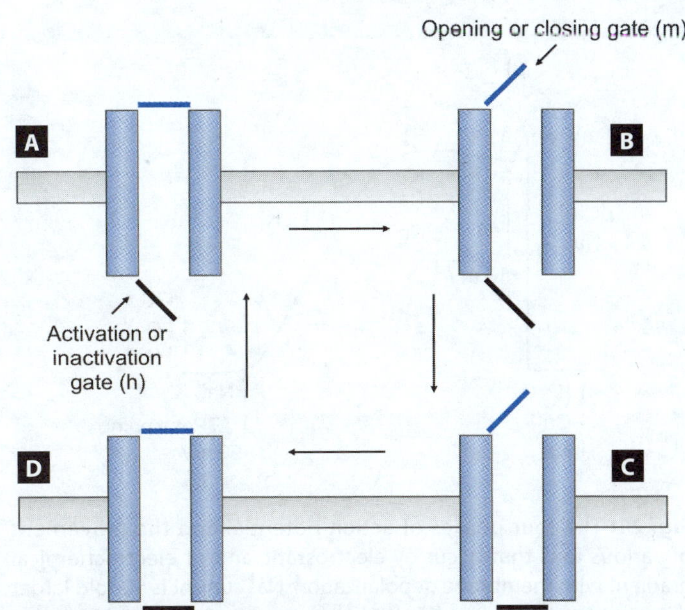

Figs. 20A to D: (A) Closed and activated channel but no current flows. (B) Open and activated channel with current flows. (C) Open but inactivated channel and no current flows. (D) Closed and inactivated channel—no current flows. Schematic diagram of dynamics of a voltage-dependent double gated fast Na^+ channel that occurs during action potential of a cardiac cycle. At resting stage the channel is initially closed, but activated, where the upper m-gate is closed, but the lower h-gate is opened. Then, depolarization causes the activation of channel which opens the upper m-gate and allows the entry of Na^+ into the cell. Subsequently, the time-dependent h-gate closes after a fixed time of few milliseconds and inactivates the channel and prevents the ion flow where the m-gate still remains open. Then, both the m-gate and h-gate is closed. This is followed by the removal of inactivation, which causes the opening of h-gate and the priming of Na^+ channel for voltage-sensitive activation.

- It is followed by a plateau or phase 2, in which the membrane potential falls slowly from +10 mV to –20 mV.
- Then, it is followed by a last stage or phase 3, where a relatively more rapid drop of membranes potential to the resting value of –90 mV (for nonpace making cells) or –60 mV (for pace making cells) is achieved from –20 mV **(Fig. 21)**.

After the cells are depolarized by inward Na^+ currents (phase 0), the K^+ channels transiently change their conformation and reach its open state. This results in an outward movement of K^+ or repolarization current which contributes to phase 1. The small notch of phase 1 is also associated with the flow of inward Ca^{2+} current which opposes the outward repolarizing K^+ current and is responsible for the shortness of this notch. The transient outward K^+ channels, like the Na^+ channels, then rapidly it is inactivated. After that, phase 2 starts and is dominated by the increased influx of Ca^{2+} through the L-type voltage-dependent Ca^{2+} channel and to a lesser extent by the influx of Na^+ through its slow channel

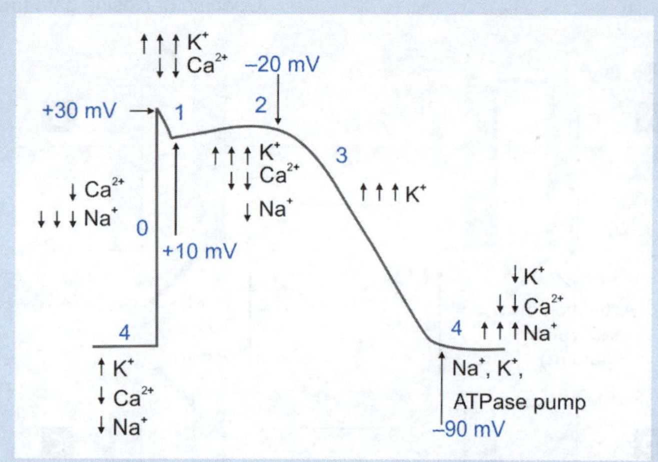

Fig. 21: The four phases of action potential and the movement of various ions that occur by electrostatic and/or electrochemical gradient with membrane depolarization. Na^+ current is 50-fold larger than any other current. Multiple types of Ca^{2+} current have also been identified. It is likely that each represents a different channel (proteins) and is responsible for the hemostasis of Ca^{2+}. Downward arrow indicates the influx of ions into the cell and the upward arrow indicates the efflux of ions out of the cell.

(not fast channel) and balance the still outward repolarizing K^+ current through the "delayed rectifier" K^+ channel (not the previous K^+ channel). In this stage, repolarizing (outward) K^+ current balance the depolarizing (inward) Ca^{2+} and Na^+ current and thus maintain a plateau of electrical gradient. The entry of Ca^{2+} into the cell triggers the further releases of Ca^{2+} from the intracellular SR and initiates the contractile process of muscle (myocardial) cells. Catecholamines such as epinephrine and norepinephrine increase this inward Ca^{2+} current and increase the contractile forces which is inhibited by Mg^{2+} and calcium channel blockers (dihydropyridines). After this phase 2, the phase 3 occurs, as with the passing of time, the outward K^+ current through the "delayed rectifier K^+" channel increases, while inward Ca^{2+} current inactivated. This result in a relatively rapid repolarization of cardiac cells (several hundred milliseconds after the initial Na^+ channel opens). Thus, the repolarizing outward K^+ current through the "delayed rectifier K^+" channel gradually lower the transmembrane potential to the resting state with the closure and the inactivation of slow Ca^{2+} and Na^+ channels. During this period, no further depolarization of cell take place and is, so, known as the absolute refractory period. Thus, at the end of repolarization, i.e., after phase 3, though the resting membrane potential is achieved, but the Na^+ and K^+ concentration in the intra- and extracellular fluid is opposite to the normal resting condition of the cell. Thus, the restoration of concentration of Na^+ and K^+ to their

pre-excitation level inside and outside of the cell occurs via an active transport system, called the Na^+/K^+ ATPase pump at a ratio of 6 Na^+ out for every 3 K^+ in. As a result, the act of pumping itself generates a net outward (repolarizing) current. There are also other channels through which K^+ enters the cells and maintains the pre-excitation intracellular K^+ concentration, balancing the excess extrusion of Na^+ by Na^+- K^+ ATPase pump. But, other Na^+ channels remain closed during the phase 4, except in the cell with the character of automaticity, where few Na^+ channels open and gradually Na^+ enters the cells causing the slow diastolic depolarization.

The homeostasis of intracellular Ca^{2+} which enters the cell during phase 2 is maintained by (1) Ca/Mg ATPase pump on SR, (2) Ca-ATPase pump on sarcolemma, and (3) Na^+-Ca^{2+} exchange mechanism on cell surface, which exchange three Na^+ in for each Ca^{2+} out from the cell. In phase 0 (depolarization), Na^+ enters and Ca^{2+} exits the cell and in phase 2 vice versa. This Na^+-Ca^{2+} exchange is not shown in the figure of action potential.

Finally, the phase 4 represents the period between the completion of repolarization and the initiation of depolarization for next action potential. During this period, K^+ continues to leak slowly from the cell along its concentration gradient. On reaching its most negative value, after repolarization, the membrane potential again gradually ascends to more positive value due to the gradual entry of Na^+ into cell and dropping of K^+ efflux from cell. When K^+ efflux stops and due to gradual entry of Na^+, the threshold transmembrane potential of approximately −40 mV is achieved, then spike action potential again takes off and a new cycle for action potential starts.

This phase 4 or slow progressive depolarization which occurs during diastole is called the slow diastolic depolarization. This phase is very important for generating automaticity or pace making activity and is the characteristic of cells of nodal tissue. Normally, the rate of rise of diastolic depolarization is 15–20 mV/second in SA node, whereas that of AV node and other cells are appreciably slower. In some cardiac cells, this phase is flat with maintaining the resting membrane potential fixed at −90 mV.

Acetylcholine (ACh) causes a threefold increase in the rate of loss of the positively charged K^+ from the cell with resulting more negativity of inside of the cell and thereby hyperpolarizes the cell. Atropine prevents this membrane action of ACh even though it is present. Vagus stimulation, like ACh, also abolishes the slow diastolic depolarization and indeed hyperpolarizes the cell and abolishes the spontaneous rhythm. Sympathetic stimulation increases the rate of diastolic depolarization and thus the rate of heart rate.

Different Types of Action Potential for Different Types of Cardiac Cells

In heart, there are different types of cardiac cells and therefore, there are different types of action potentials. This is due to the variability in the number of different ion channel (genes expressed), present on cell membrane, of individual cells. The cells of His–Purkinje system have action potential of very long duration. The atrial cells have action potential of short duration than that of His–Purkinje system. The cells of the SA and AV node display the phenomenon of spontaneous slow diastolic depolarization in phase 4 and thus the RMP spontaneously reach the threshold value for the regeneration of new action potentials. The cells of AV node, bundle of HIS and Purkinje system has also the slow diastolic depolarization phase in action potential and pace making activity. But, the rate of spontaneous firing is usually fastest in the SA nodal cells and serves as the natural pacemaker of the heart, suppressing the pace making activity of others.

Modern technique helps us to study the electrophysiological behavior of single ion channel protein and identify the channels that may be particularly responsible for the particular pathological condition. For example, mutation in the genes which is responsible for the encoding of repolarizing K^+ channel (both "transient outward" and "delayed rectifier") is responsible for the congenital long QT syndrome. Some K^+ channels remains quiescent when the intracellular ATP store is normal and they become active when ATP store is depleted. Such ATP-inhibited K^+ channel also sometimes is important to produce arrhythmia in myocardial ischemia. Most antiarrhythmic drugs affect more than one ion channel and thus usually exert multiple action which can be beneficial or harmful in individual patient **(Fig. 22)**.

■ NERVE SUPPLY OF HEART

The heart is supplied by both the parasympathetic and sympathetic nerve with their both afferent and efferent fibers and controls the different cardiac functions. Both these nerves fibers are also responsible for carrying cardiac pain sensation and different cardiac reflexes. To supply the heart, both the afferent and efferent fibers of sympathetic and parasympathetic nerves form the cardiac plexus, from where the heart derives its nerve supply. This cardiac plexus is formed by the interlacement of nerve fibers and nerve cells and is situated at the base of the heart. This plexus is consists of two parts: superficial and deep. The atria and the conducting system of heart are innervated by both the sympathetic and parasympathetic nerves. On the other hand, ventricular muscle is supplied only by the sympathetic nerves.

The afferent (sensory) nerves from the heart pass both through the parasympathetic and sympathetic nerves as follows:

- From the heart → through vagus and from the aortic arch → through aortic nerve. Both are parasympathetic.
- From the heart → through superior, middle, stellate and first four thoracic sympathetic ganglion → through white rami communicantes → through posterior nerve root and posterior dorsal ganglion → to the posterior horn cells.
- From the carotid sinus → through sinus nerve, a branch of glossopharyngeal nerve (parasympathetic).

The efferent (motor) nerves supplying the heart also run through both the parasympathetic (vagus) and sympathetic nerves as follows:

The efferent preganglionic fibers of parasympathetic (vagus) nerve, supplying the heart, arise from the nucleus ambiguous and from the dorsal nuclei of vagus in brain. They are situated on the floor of 4th ventricle in the medulla. After their origin, they descend downward as the vagus nerve. Then, the cardiac fibers separate from the main trunk of vagus nerve in the neck and proceed toward the heart to form the deep and superficial cardiac plexuses with the fibers from sympathetic nerve. After that, the parasympathetic fibers finally reach the atrial muscle where they make the synaptic connections with the cells in the peripheral parasympathetic ganglion, which are situated near the SA node and AV node. From the ganglion, postganglionic parasympathetic fibers arise and supply the SA and AV node and also extend between the atrial muscle fibers **(Fig. 23)**.

The efferent preganglionic sympathetic fibers start from the lateral horn cells of T_1 to T_5 or T_6 thoracic segments of spinal cord. These are called the spinal sympathetic cardiac

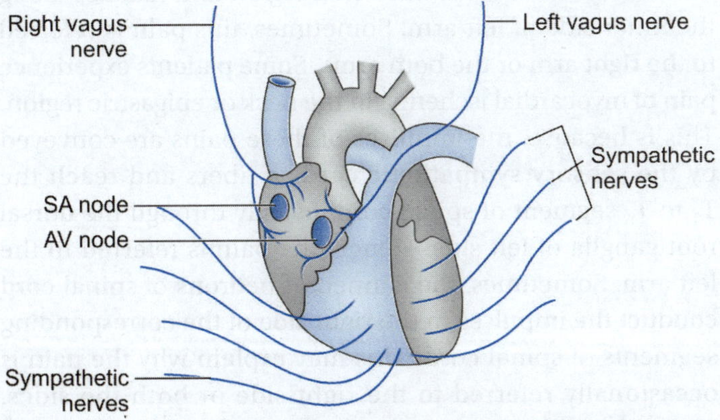

Fig. 22: Sympathetic and parasympathetic nerves supplying heart. (AV: atrioventricular; SA: sinoatrial)

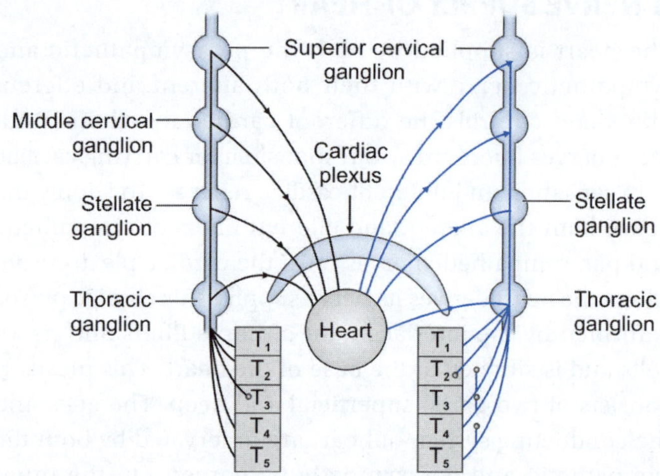

Fig. 23: Schematic diagram of sympathetic supply of heart. Red line indicates sympathetic motors (efferent) and green line indicates sympathetic sensory (afferent).

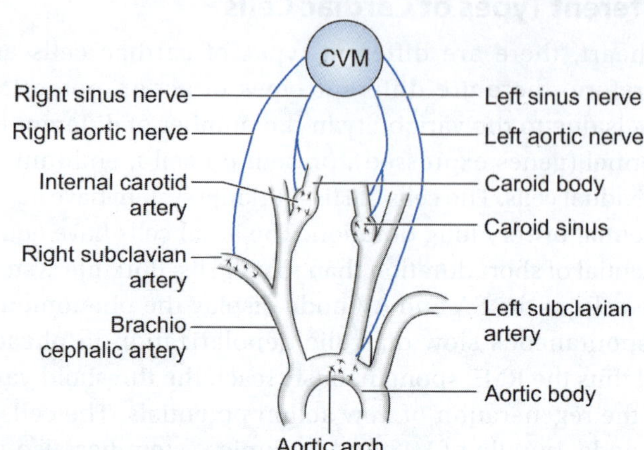

Fig. 24: The baroreceptors and chemoreceptors in the aorta and internal carotid artery with aortic and sinus nerves. (CVM: cardio-vascular medullary center)

centers. Preganglionic sympathetic fibers, then, enter the sympathetic chain after coming out via the ventral root of T_1 to T_5 spinal nerve and the white rami communicantes. After that these preganglionic fibers make synapses with the ganglionic cells situated in the superior, middle, and inferior cervical ganglia and the upper thoracic ganglia from where the postganglionic sympathetic fibers arise. In human beings, the last cervical ganglion and the first thoracic ganglion fuses together to form the stellate ganglion. Then, the postganglionic fibers, arising from the superior cervical, middle cervical, and stellate ganglion, pass directly to the heart and form the cardiac plexus.

Cardiac branches from the superior cervical sympathetic ganglion do not contain any afferent fibers. It contains only the efferent postganglionic sympathetic fibers. Otherwise, all the cardiac branches of vagus and sympathetic nerve contain both the afferent and efferent fibers. In contrast to vagus, the exact location of the higher cardiac sympathetic center in the brain is not yet fully known. Usually, the spinal sympathetic cardiac centers are controlled by the higher centers of brain like the cortex, thalamus, hypothalamus, etc.

The dorsal motor nucleus of vagus in the medulla is the cardioinhibitory center and it continuously transmits tonic inhibitory vagal impulses to the heart. It is because, this higher parasympathetic center gets direct connection from the afferent fibers, coming from the peripheral baroreceptors and chemoreceptors through the sinoaortic nerves. Reflex bradycardia during the rise of systemic blood pressure (BP) is due to the stimulation of this cardioinhibitory vagus center by the afferent impulses from baroreceptors. On the other hand, tachycardia during the fall of BP is due to the inhibition of this cardioinhibitory center, i.e., withdrawal

of vagal tone from this cardioinhibitory center. Under such condition, sympathetic cardiac center also take the upper hand secondarily **(Fig. 24)**.

As mentioned earlier, the SA node develops from the right-sided embryological structure. So, it receives innervation from the right vagus nerve (parasympathetic) and the right stellate ganglion (sympathetic). Similarly, also as the AV node is developed from the left-sided embryological structure, so it is supplied by the left vagus nerve (which produces variable degree of nodal conduction block) and the left stellate ganglion which have a greater effect on the contractility of heart. Thus, in general, the sympathetic and the parasympathetic supply via the left stellate ganglion and the left vagus nerve have a greater effect on the contractility of heart and the sympathetic and parasympathetic supply via the right stellate ganglion and the right vagus nerve have a greater effect on the heart rate.

The pain of angina pectoris or myocardial infarction is commonly felt at the retrosternal region and radiates along the inner side of left arm. Sometimes, this pain is referred to the right arm or the both arms. Some patients experience pain of myocardial ischemia in the neck or epigastric region. This is because, the impulses of these pains are conveyed by the sensory sympathetic cardiac fibers and reach the T_1 to T_5 segment of spinal cord, usually through the dorsal root ganglia of left side. Hence, the pain is referred to the left arm. Sometimes, the connector neurons of spinal cord conduct the impulses to the right side of the corresponding segments of spinal cord. This may explain why the pain is occasionally referred to the right side or both the sides. Since, the embryonic heart is initially located in the neck and later descends in the thorax, so it is not unlikely that the pain fibers for the heart reach from the upper cervical spinal segment via the sympathetic nerve. So, sometimes the pain is also felt in the neck region.

The parasympathetic efferent fibers work through cholinergic muscarinic (M_2) receptors and the sympathetic efferent fibers work through β-receptors on myocardial cells. The action of both the parasympathetic and sympathetic nerve balances each other. But, under normal resting condition in an adult, the parasympathetic tone predominates over the sympathetic tone. The efferent parasympathetic diminishes the heart rate and coronary blood flow (secondary effect). Larger branches of coronary arteries are predominantly supplied by sympathetic nerves, whereas the smaller branches are supplied by the vagus nerves. Sympathetic efferent increases the heart rate and cardiac output. It produces the vasodilatation of the intramuscular branches of coronary artery and vasoconstriction of the epicardial arteries.

There are three types of afferent receptors through which parasympathetic reflexes work. Type A receptor is supplied by the myelinated vagal afferent fibers and is responsible for the control of heart rate. Type B receptor is also supplied by the myelinated afferent vagal fibers and is responsive to atrial stretches and the changes in volume than heart rate. Type C receptors are also responsive to the changes in pressure. All the abovementioned receptors are located in the atrium. There are also receptors in the ventricle which are supplied by the myelinated vagal afferent fibers and are responsive to the changes in the rate of rise of ventricular pressure and send impulses at the onset of ventricular ejection.

The sympathetic fibers form an extensive plexus or network over the epicardium of heart and penetrate the myocardium along the various branches of coronary vessels. Sympathetic innervation on ventricle is more dense than atrium, whereas the parasympathetic innervation is more dense on atrium than ventricle.

Sympathetic neurotransmitter or agonist works through the β-adrenergic receptors which are located on the myocardial cell surface. The attachment of sympathetic agonist with the adrenergic β-receptor induces a conformational change of this receptor and permits the interaction of this receptor with the stimulatory G-proteins (Gs) at the inner site of the cell membrane. The G-proteins are in the family of heterotrimeric structure, and composed of α, β, and γ subunit. Binding of Gs protein with the receptor causes the dissociation of α-subunit from the remaining β–γ complex of G-protein, with the concomitant expenditure of guanosine triphosphate (GTP) to guanosine diphosphate (GDP). This broken α-subunit then stimulates the adenyl cyclase, located on the cytoplasmic side of cell membrane which hydrolyzed ATP to cAMP. Thus, the increase in

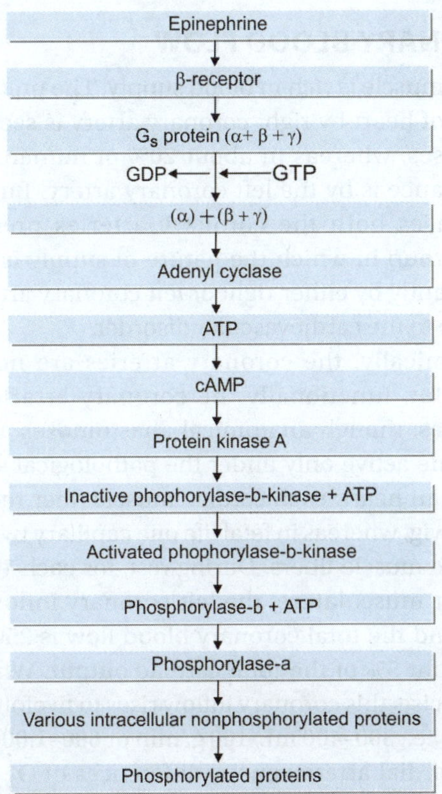

Flowchart 1: The mechanism of action of sympathetic agonist through its β-receptor.

(ATP: adenosine triphosphate; cAMP: cyclic adenosine monophosphate; GDP: guanosine diphosphate; GTP: guanosine triphosphate)

cAMP, in turn act on certain protein kinases (PKA) which phosphorylates the various intracellular proteins, especially those are related to SR and ultimately raise the intracellular Ca^{2+} concentration. The phosphorylation of many other functional proteins including troponin and phospholamban also helps to interact with Ca^{2+}, resulting in increased force of contraction **(Flowchart 1)**.

The parasympathetic stimulation works through the neurotransmitter named acetylcholine (ACh) which binds with muscarinic M_2 receptor, located on the myocardial cell membrane. The binding of ACh with M_2 receptor causes the conformational changes of this receptor and in turn allow the binding of receptor with the inhibitory Gi protein. This (binding of Gi protein with M_2 receptor) activates the Gi protein by dissociating the α-subunit from it. The activated Gi protein, then, inhibits adenyl cyclase leading to the decrease in cAMP synthesis and in turn inhibition of PKA and its sequelae described above.

Finally, the ACh released from the parasympathetic postganglionic nerve terminals that lie in close proximity to sympathetic postganglionic nerve terminals may also inhibit the release of norepinephrine and this in turn decrease the β-receptor stimulation and ultimately cAMP levels.

■ CORONARY BLOOD FLOW

The heart muscle is rich in blood supply. The predominance of supply of heart by right coronary artery is seen in about 50% of cases, whereas in about 20% of human heart, the predominance is by the left coronary artery. But, in about 30% of cases both the coronary arteries predominate. The last group in which the nature of supply is not made predominantly by either right or left coronary artery is least vulnerable to the cardiovascular disorder.

Anatomically, the coronary arteries are not the end arteries. But, functionally the coronary arteries are the end arteries, though anatomical anastomoses are present and become active only under the pathological state. In an adult human heart, each cardiac muscle fiber receives one capillary twig, whereas in fetal life one capillary twig supplies 4–6 cardiac muscle fibers. During rest, for each 100 g of left ventricular musculature, the left coronary inflow is 65–85 mL/min and the total coronary blood flow is 250 mL/min. This is about 5% of the total cardiac output. While during heavy exercise, this coronary inflow rises to fivefold than that of the rest, i.e., 300–400 mL/100 g/min or 800–1,000 mL/min. The myocardial arteriovenous differences of O_2 content at rest is also very high and is about 10–15 mL/100 mL of blood (desaturation is 70%). This signifies that the extraction of O_2 from arterial blood by the cardiac muscle is very high. Normally, the myocardial tissue extracts about 65–70% of O_2 supplied by the myocardial arterial blood. Thus, if the arterial O_2 content is 20 mL/100 mL of arterial blood, then the blood in the coronary sinus, which drains the blood from left ventricle, contains only 6–7 mL of O_2/100 mL of venous blood, even when the individual is at rest. The ratio of systolic coronary blood flow to diastolic coronary blood flow is approximately 0.22 at rest which is increased to 0.9 during exercise **(Flowchart 1)**.

■ CARDIAC CYCLE

The different phages of cardiac cycle of atrium and ventricle are shown in **Figure 25**. The two atriums of the heart contract and relax simultaneously in a cyclical fashion like two ventricles. But, when the atria contract, the ventricles relax and vice versa. The duration of systole and diastole of atrium is 0.1 second and 0.7 second, respectively, whereas the duration of systole and diastole of ventricle is 0.3 second and 0.5 second, respectively. However, though the atrium and ventricle have the separate cycle of function, but mainly the ventricular cycle will be considered here as the cardiac cycle and will determine the variations of coronary blood flow during the different phases of it. It starts at point A

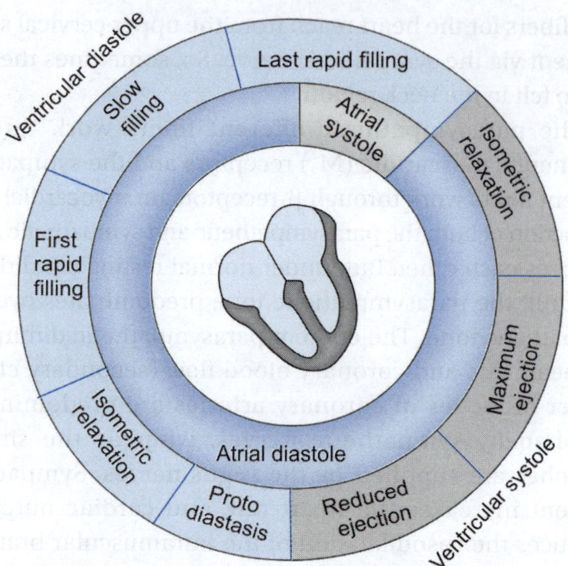

Fig. 25: The cardiac (atrial and ventricular) cycle.

(Fig. 26) and signifies the latter half of ventricular diastole with filling of blood from atrium. This blood comes to the atrium at its phase of diastole, during the time of previous ventricular systole. In the middle of ventricular diastole when the ventricular pressure goes below the atrium or atrial pressure exceeds than that of the ventricle, then the AV valves (tricuspid and mitral) open (point A) and blood enters the ventricular chamber. At this stage, both the atrium and the ventricle are in diastole and blood flows passively to ventricle from atrium which accounts for roughly 75% of the total ventricular filling. The rest of the ventricular filling is contributed by the active atrial contraction or atrial systole (point A') which begins with the depolarization of SA node and corresponds to the P-wave of ECG. Thus, the curve of ventricular filling, shown in **Figure 26** by the AB segment, depends on the compliance of ventricle and the venous return to the atrium. Passive ventricular filling will be hampered, if the ventricle and its wall becomes less compliant (such as muscular hypertrophy, fibrosis, and many other causes) and if there is hypovolemia. In these circumstances, atrial systole is very important to maintain adequate ventricular filling.

After the ventricular filling at its diastole, ventricular systole starts with the closure of tricuspid and mitral valve and corresponds to the R-wave on ECG and point B on the picture 5.26. The first part of ventricular systole is called the isovolumic or isometric contraction (shown in **Figure 26** by BC segment), where all the valves are closed and the intraventricular pressure rises sharply without any change in the intraventricular volume. In the second part of this ventricular systole, at the point when the developed pressure within the two ventricles exceed than that of the pulmonary artery and aorta (point C, **Fig. 26**), then the pulmonary and aortic valves open and allow the blood to flow into their respective circulations. This second portion of ventricular systole is called the ventricular ejection phase (shown in **Figure 26** as CE segment). It has an initial rapid phase (point C to D) or maximum ejection phase, characterized by maximal forward flow of blood. Then, it gradually tapers, because as the systole progresses (point D to E) the ejection phase is slowly reduces.

After systole, the ventricular diastole begins at the point E **(Fig. 26)** with the closure of pulmonary and aortic valve. This is due to the fall of intraventricular pressure below that of the aorta and pulmonary artery. The EA segment of ventricular diastole is called the isovolumetric or isometric relaxation phase, because, during this period the pulmonary and aortic valve closes, but the AV valve does not open and no flow of blood occurs into the ventricle from atrium. After the beginning of ventricular diastole as point E, the ventricular pressure continues to drop, until they fall below that of the right or left atria. At the point A of ventricular diastolic period, the AV valve (tricuspid and mitral) opens and blood starts to flow from the atrium to the ventricle. Thus, the ventricular filling commences and the cycles repeat themselves. This point E corresponds to the end of the T-wave on ECG.

During systole, the peak left ventricular pressure is about 120 mm Hg and the peak right ventricular pressure is about 25 mm Hg. At the end of the diastole, the volume of the ventricles is about 130 mL and it is called the *"end-diastolic ventricular volume"* (EDVV). About 50 mL of blood always remains in each ventricle after ejection at the end of its systole. This is called the *"end-systolic ventricular volume"* (ESVV). The percent of EDVV which is ejected with each stroke is called the "ejection fraction" and is about 65–85% in a normal healthy individual.

The cardiac muscle has unique property of depolarization and repolarization which is faster than that of any other muscles of our body. This is more prominent when the heart rate increases. The duration of ventricular systole decreases from 0.3 second at the heart rate of 75/min to 0.2 second at the heart rate of 200/min. This shortening is mainly due to the decrease in the duration of systolic ejection period. However, the duration of systole of a ventricle is much more fixed than that of its diastole. So, when the heart rate is increased, then the duration of diastole of a ventricle is shortened to a much greater extend, than that of its systole. For example, at a heart rate of 75/min, the duration of diastole is 0.5 second, whereas at a heart rate of 200/min, it (diastole) is only 0.1 second. This fact has important physiologic and clinical implications. This is because, it is only during diastole that the heart muscle rests and coronary blood flow to the subendocardial portions (which is most vulnerable to infarction) occurs. Furthermore, most of the ventricular filling occurs in diastole. Thus, up to the heart rate of about

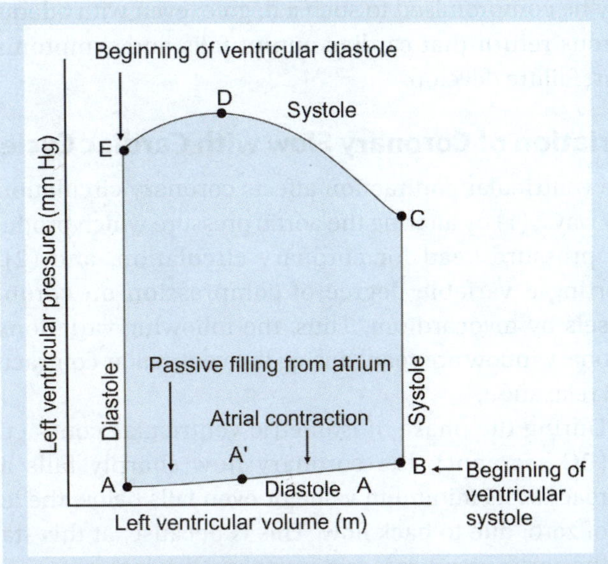

Fig. 26: The changes of left ventricular volume and pressure during different phases of cardiac cycle. (AA': atrial diastole; AB: ventricular diastole; A'B: atrial systole; BC: isometric ventricular contraction; CD: rapid ventricular ejection; CE: ventricular ejection phase; DE: slow ventricular ejection; EA: isometric relaxation of ventricular diastole; B point: beginning of ventricular systole and atrial diastole)

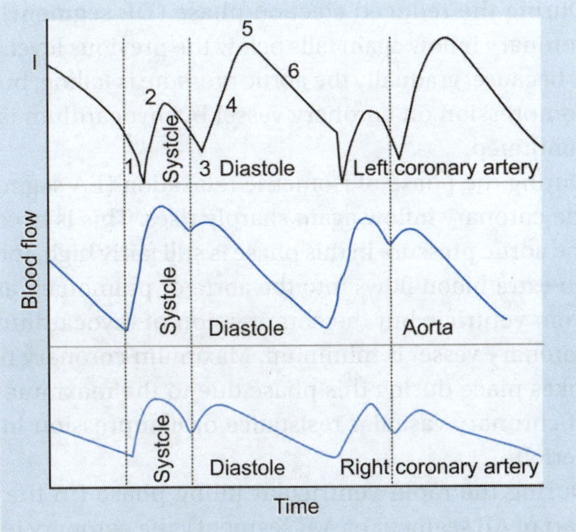

Fig. 27: The blood flow in the aorta, left coronary artery, and right coronary artery during the various phases of cardiac cycle. (1) Isometric ventricular contraction (BC segment of Fig. 26), (2) Maximum ejection phase (CD segment of Fig. 26), (3) Reduced ejection phase (DE segment of Fig. 26), (4) Isometric relaxation phase (EA segment of Fig. 26), (5) Rapid ventricular filling phase (1st part of AB segment of Fig. 26), and (6) Later part of diastole (second part of AB segment of Fig. 26).

180/min, the ventricular filling and **(Fig. 27)** cardiac output remain adequate, but as long as there is ample venous return. However, at very high heart rates (>180) ventricular filling may be compromised to such a degree, even with adequate venous return that cardiac output falls and symptoms of heart failure develop.

Variation of Coronary Flow with Cardiac Cycle

The ventricular contraction affects coronary circulation in two ways: (1) by altering the aortic pressure which produces the pressure head for coronary circulation, and (2) by exerting a variable degree of compression on coronary vessels by myocardium. Thus, the following variations of coronary inflow are seen, during the ventricular contraction and relaxation.

- During the phase of isometric ventricular contraction (BC segment), the coronary flow sharply falls and reaches its minimum value or even falls below the level of zero, due to back flow. This is because, at this stage, the aortic pressure is minimum and this is due to no flow of blood into aorta from ventricle and the subsequent compression on coronary vessels by myocardium is maximum.
- During the maximum ejection phase (CD segment), the coronary inflow rises sharply due to the sudden rise of aortic pressure. This is again due to the high aortic inflow which reaches its maximum, during this period.
- During the reduced ejection phase (DE segment), the coronary inflow again falls below the previous level. This is because, gradually the aortic pressure is falling, but the compression on coronary vessel by myocardium is still continued.
- During the phase of isometric relaxation (EA segment), the coronary inflow again sharply rises. This is because, the aortic pressure in this phase is still fairly high, though no extra blood flows into the aorta or pulmonary artery from ventricle but the compression of myocardium on coronary vessel is minimum. Maximum coronary filling takes place during this phase due to the maximum fall of coronary vascular resistance or compression in this period.
- During the rapid ventricular filling phase (in the first part of AB segment or AA′ segment), the coronary inflow again continues to rise, but slowly. This is because, the relaxation of myocardium continues and the vessels begin to open.
- During the later part of diastole (i.e., during the later part of AB segment or in the A′B segment), the coronary inflow again slowly diminishes. This is because, the aortic pressure is failing and the coronary vessels are stretched due to the gradual filling of heart and the consequent elongation of cardiac muscles **(Fact file I)**.

Nevertheless, from the above discussion, the conclusion can be drawn like that about 80% of the total coronary blood

So, greater coronary inflow takes place in diastole than systole due to the less compression of coronary vessels, during the relaxation of cardiac muscles and the diminution of intramural tension. The left coronary inflow during systole is affected much, as the pressure difference between the aorta and the left ventricle becomes −2 mm Hg. But the right coronary inflow, during systole, is not so much affected, as the pressure difference between the aorta and the right ventricle is 95 mm Hg.

flow occurs in diastole and this is because though during this period the mean aortic pressure head is low, than systole, but the true coronary vascular resistance caused by the myocardial compression on the vessels is still even lower.

During the ventricular isometric contraction phase, the blood flow through right coronary artery sharply falls and then rapidly rises again in the maximum ejection phase. Then, it again falls during the reduced ejection phase. During the isometric relaxation phase, the right coronary inflow rises again, but not so steeply high like the left coronary inflow.

In conclusion, it is said that the coronary blood flow is dependent on pressure gradient which is principally guided by the difference between the mean aortic pressure and the resistance of coronary arteries, due to the compression by ventricular musculature. The coronary blood flow through the left coronary artery is maximum during the period of early diastole, corresponding to the period of isovolumic ventricular relaxation which accompanied by the minimal coronary vascular compression by the myocardium. However, the coronary blood flow through the right coronary artery is maximum during the period of peak systole. This is because, the developed right intramyocardial pressure and consequently the vascular compression on right coronary artery by right ventricle are considerably less than the pulmonary arterial pressure and thus allows the anterograde flow of blood through right coronary artery during both systole and diastole of right ventricle **(Table 1)**.

Although the blood flow through left coronary artery, supplying the subendocardial portion of left ventricle, occurs only during diastole, but as the contractile force during systole is sufficiently dissipated from the more superficial portions of left ventricular myocardium, i.e., epicardium, so some blood flow in this region of left ventricle will also occur during systole, and therefore, throughout the whole cardiac cycle. Since, the ventricular diastole becomes more short, when the heart rate is high, so the left ventricular coronary flow is further reduced during tachycardia. Thus, as during both the systole and diastole, no blood flow occurs through the myocardium and the subendocardial portion of left ventricle during tachycardia, so this region is maximally

TABLE 1: Pressure in aorta, LCA, and RCA.

	Pressure in aorta (mm Hg)	Pressure in LV and LCA (mm Hg)	Pressure difference between aorta and LCA (mm Hg)
Systole	120	122	−2
Diastole	80	0	80
	Pressure in aorta (mm Hg)	Pressure in RV and RCA (mm Hg)	Pressure difference between aorta and RCA (mm Hg)
Systole	120	25	95
Diastole	80	0	80

(LCA: left coronary artery; LV: left ventricle; RCA: right coronary artery)

prone to ischemic damage and is the most common site of myocardial infarction.

Blood flow to the left ventricular musculature is further decreased in patients with stenotic aortic valves. This is because, in aortic stenosis, the pressure in the cavity of left ventricle must be much higher than that of the aorta to eject the blood. Consequently, the coronary vessels are severely compressed during systole and there is less development of pressure (**Fact file II**) head in the aorta for coronary flow due to the less ejection of blood into aorta. So, patients with this disease are particularly prone to develop symptoms of myocardial ischemic, (1) in part because of the compression of coronary arteries by the left ventricular musculature, (2) in part because of the myocardium requires more O_2 to expel blood through the stenotic aortic valve, and (3) in part because of the less coronary flow due to less ejection of blood into aorta. Coronary flow is also reduced when the aortic diastolic pressure is low. The rise in venous pressure, in condition such as congestive heart failure, also reduces the coronary flow, because it decreases the effective coronary perfusion pressure.

The difference between the minimum (resting) and the maximal coronary blood flow is termed as the "*coronary flow reserve*". Under normal circumstances, the myocardial wall pressure is highest near the endocardium and lowest near the epicardium. Thus, a coronary blood flow, with a gradual negative gradient, was seen to exist during the ventricular systole from epicardium to endocardium. So, the outer layers of ventricular wall receives a larger share of blood flow and innermost wall presumably receives no flow of blood at the peak of systole and thus make the endocardium relatively more sensitive to ischemia. Thus, the endocardial blood flow is greatly influenced by ventricular relaxation during diastole which decreases the myocardial wall pressure and enhances the coronary flow from epicardium to endocardium. So, the endocardium is more sensitive to pathological changes

FACT FILE II

Factors influencing the coronary circulation

- *Mean aortic pressure:* It is the chief motive force for driving the blood into coronary vessels. Any alteration of aortic pressure will, therefore, cause parallel changes in coronary circulation (blood flow).
- *Cardiac output:* Obviously, the coronary inflow is directly proportional to the cardiac output. Increased output raises coronary flow in two ways: (1) by raising the aortic pressure and (2) by the reflex inhibition of vagal vasoconstrictor tone.
- *Metabolic factors:* With increased metabolism of heart, the O_2 requirement, and subsequently the coronary circulation is also increased. There is a casual relationship between the myocardial metabolic activity, O_2 consumption, and coronary blood flow.
- *CO_2 and O_2:* If O_2 supply to the heart muscle is decreased, then the coronary flow is increased. But, if the supply of O_2 to myocardium is more than requirement, then the coronary circulation is decreased. Similarly, CO_2 stimulates the coronary flow. When the CO_2 concentration in blood is increased, then coronary flow is also increased in first stage in order to maintain the total O_2 requirement of cardiac muscle. If this state prevails further, the coronary flow is decreased abruptly and the heart stops in diastole.
- *Effects of ions:* K^+ in low concentration dilates the coronary vessels, whereas the K^+ in higher concentration constricts the coronary vessels. Ca^{2+} in therapeutic doses increases the coronary flow and O_2 consumption of cardiac muscle.
- *Polypeptides:* Angiotensin II is an active octapeptide, which causes arteriolar constriction of the skin, kidney, brain, and also in coronary vessels. Bradykinin is claimed to cause coronary vasodilatation but still its physiological role is not proved.
- *Adenine nucleotides:* It is discussed in the test.
- *Cardiac sympathetic and parasympathetic nerves:* Stimulation of the cardiac sympathetic fibers from the stellate ganglion produces increased coronary flow. This is mainly due to the release of norepinephrine, which causes coronary dilatation and increased coronary flow.
- *Heart rate:* When the heart rate is increased, then the minute cardiac output and aortic BP are also increased, but the stroke volume decreases. The phasic coronary blood flow and O_2 consumption per beat decrease, but the minute coronary flow and O_2 consumption per minute are increased. With the increase of heart rate, O_2 consumption of the heart muscle is increased and is maintained normally through increase of minute flow.
- *Pitressin or vasopressin:* It causes increased coronary resistance and diminution of coronary flow.
- *Temperature:* With rise of body temperature, body metabolism, and O_2 requirement is increased. Therefore, to meet this O_2 demand coronary flow also increases.
- *Viscerocardiac reflex:* The coronary flow is markedly decreased during visceral distention and it is often encountered in a patient with ischemic heart disease.
- *Anemia:* In anemia, the coronary flow is increased sharply in order to maintain the normal O_2 need of cardiac muscle.

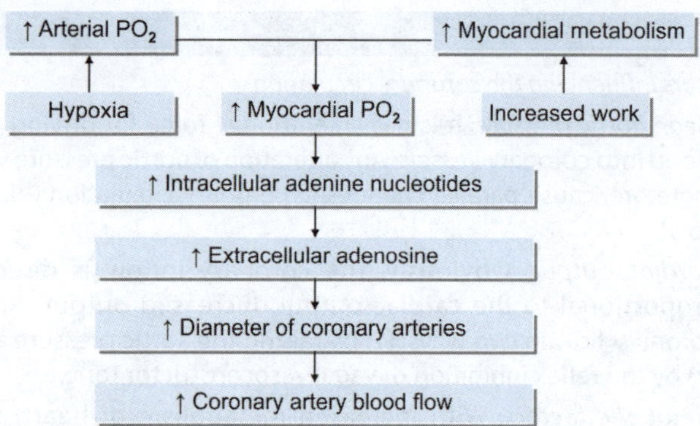

Fig. 28: The local mechanism of control of myocardial blood flow.

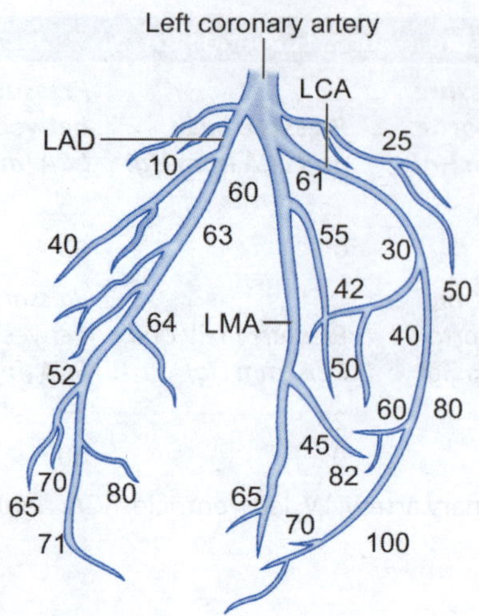

Fig. 29: The myocardial perfusion pattern following the injection of 133Xe into left main coronary artery. The numbers indicates the flow values in mL/100 g/min, measured by scintillation detector. (LAD: left anterior descending artery; LCA: left circumflex artery; LMA: left marginal artery)

like hypotension, coronary occlusion, hypertrophy, aortic stenosis, etc. **(Fig. 28).**

Regulation of Coronary Blood Flow

Like renal and cerebral arteries, the coronary arteries also have the autoregulation. This autoregulation maintains a constant coronary blood flow, within its normal perfusion pressure, ranging between 50 and 120 mm Hg and is independent of myocardial O$_2$ demand. Coronary perfusion pressure is defined as the difference between the diastolic aortic pressure and the left ventricular end-diastolic pressure. Sympathetic adrenergic stimulation causes the coronary artery dilation. This can be explained by the following way. Unopposed α_1-adrenergic stimulation produces coronary vasoconstriction and unopposed β-adrenergic stimulation causes coronary vasodilation. But, when the both act at the same time, then the β-receptor's vasodilating properties predominates over the α-receptor's vasoconstricting properties.

Sympathetic stimulation also increases coronary blood flow due to their stimulant effect on both cardiac contractile force and metabolism. But, the increase in coronary blood flow secondary to metabolic changes in heart is of far less quantitative significance than that caused by the increased discharge of impulse from sympathetic nerves and receptor stimulation which occur simultaneously.

The stimulation of parasympathetic muscarinic receptor also produces coronary vasodilation. Though vagus is not proven to supply the coronary vessels, but vagal stimulation, sufficient to cause cardiac arrest, does increase coronary flow. This effect is probably due to the lessened intramural tissue pressure and lessened extravascular resistance, caused by the reduction of force of contraction. There are other various chemical mediators which control the coronary vascular tone. These are O$_2$, CO$_2$, K$^+$, histamine, prostaglandins, and adenosine. Among these, adenosine is the most important chemical mediator which couples the coronary blood flow to the O$_2$ consumption and demand.

Adenosine arises from the adenine nucleotides (ATP and ADP) of myocardial cells which are disrupted by hypoxia. This nucleoside, adenosine, does traverse the myocardial cell membrane and gain access to the resistance vessels including the precapillary sphincters of coronary vascular system and causes dilation. Like adenosine, the ATP and ADP are equally potent vasodilator, but are not permeable to cell membrane. In the blood, adenosine is destructed by adenosine deaminase to inosine and hypoxanthine which has no vasodilating properties. Like cerebral circulation, coronary circulation is also conspicuous in manifesting self-control on vascular resistance (VR) which is affected by chemical rather than by nervous influences. Thus, with increase metabolism of heart, the O$_2$ requirement is increased and the circulation is greatly increased. Similarly, CO$_2$ also stimulates the coronary blood flow. For the increased coronary blood flow, this increased O$_2$ requirement acts through hypoxia and adenosine mechanism **(Fig. 29).**

Study of Coronary Blood Flow

The coronary blood flow has been viewed by angiography. It also can be measured by inserting a catheter into coronary sinus, and by taking blood sample and applying the Kety method on heart. A number of techniques, utilizing radionuclides, radioactive tracers, etc. that can be detected with radiation detectors over the chest, also have been used to study the regional blood flow in the heart. It detects the areas of ischemia and infarction, and also evaluates the ventricular function.

When radionuclide, such as thallium-201 (^{201}TI) is used, it is forced into the cardiac muscle cells by Na$^+$-K$^+$ ATPase pump and equilibrates with the intracellular K⁺ pool. For the first 10–15 minutes, after IV injection, thallium-201 distribution is directly proportional to the myocardial blood flow. Then, the areas of ischemia can be detected by their low uptake of thallium-201 in the myocardial tissues by special instrument. The uptake of this isotope by heart is often determined soon after exercise and again several hours later to bring out areas in which exertion leads to compromised flow. Conversely, radiopharmaceutical agent, such as technetium 99m pyrophosphate (⁹⁹ᵐTc-PyP) also can be used which is selectively taken up by the infarcted tissue by an incompletely understood mechanism and make the infarct area to stand out as "hot spots" on the computed tomography (CT) scans of chest. The coronary angiography also can be combined with the measurement of 133Xe washout technique to provide the detailed analysis of coronary blood flow. Radiopaque contrast medium is first injected into the coronary arteries and X-rays are used to outline their distribution. The angiographic camera is then replaced with a multiple crystal scintillation camera and ¹³³Xe washout is measured. An example of normal flow distribution, after injection in a left coronary artery, is shown in **Figure 29**.

■ MYOCARDIAL METABOLISM

To maintain the cell integrity by controlling the Na⁺, K⁺ ionic gradients across the cell membrane and for contraction of myocardium, energy is needed. Heart uses ATP and creatine phosphate as the source of this energy to perform this mechanical and chemical work such as contraction and ion transport. Substrates such as glucose, lactate, and fatty acids are usually used by the heart muscle to get its metabolic energy source of ATP. During fasting, the free fatty acids are the main substrate for the energy source of heart. When carbohydrates are used as energy source, the myocardial respiratory quotient (RQ) exceeds 0.9. But, fasting lowers the RQ to 0.7. This characterizes that fat is metabolized during fasting.

When cardiac muscles contract, the ATP is broken down to ADP and inorganic phosphate (Pin) is produced. But, ATP is again rapidly synthesized by the Lohmann reaction from creatine phosphate.

Lohman reaction:

Actomycin

ATP → ADP + Pin (energy)

Creatine phosphotransferase

ADP + CP → ATP + C (creatine)

When the heart is subjected to hypoxia, then the creatine phosphate concentration drops strikingly and the ATP/ADP **(Fig. 30)** ratio of the myocardium falls precipitously. The

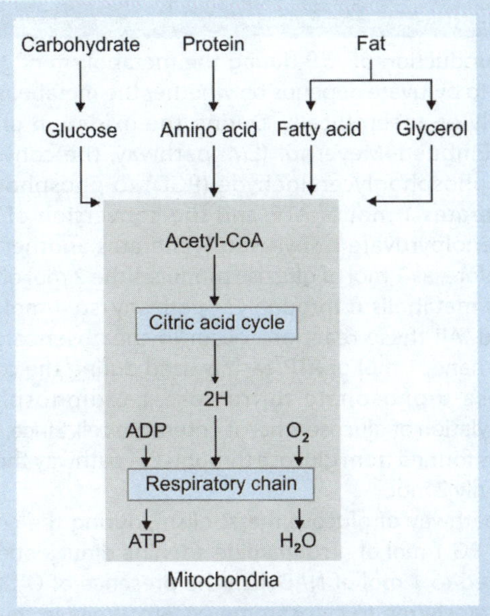

Fig. 30: The myocardial metabolism. (ADP: adenosine diphosphate; ATP: adenosine triphosphate; CoA: coenzyme A)

myocardial cells contain phosphorylase in an inactive form, i.e., phosphorylase-b. This inactive form can be activated by the cAMP to phosphorylase-a. The cAMP is formed from ATP by the enzyme adenyl cyclase which is again activated by adrenaline. Phosphorylase-a breaks down the glycogen to yield glucose-1-phosphate which is converted to glucose-6-phosphate. This compound is then broken down in myocardium by glycolysis to give pyruvic acid (in aerobic metabolism) which again enter the citric acid cycle to yield further energy by the synthesis of ATP (aerobic metabolism).

The inner membrane of mitochondria consists of multiple folds and contains multiple enzymes which are needed for the aerobic metabolism or the citric acid cycle. The mitochondria also contain cytochrome system which is involved in the electron transport and ATP formation. Thus, mitochondria and O₂ become the sources of continuous supply of energy in the form of ATP for continuous cardiac function **(Fact file III)**.

Glucose is metabolized by the glycolytic pathway to yield pyruvate. Then pyruvate is metabolized to lactate when O₂ supply is inadequate. But, if the supply of O₂ is adequate then pyruvate enters into the mitochondria for citric acid cycle. In the first step of citric acid cycle, this pyruvate is enzymatically transformed to *acetyl CoA* and NADH. The enzyme responsible for this transformation of pyruvate to acetyl-CoA is *pyruvate dehydrogenase* which is a highly step limiting regulated enzyme found in the inner mitochondrial membrane. Then, this one molecule acetyl-CoA in citric acid

FACT FILE III

The net production of ATP during the metabolism of glucose or glycogen to pyruvate depends on whether the metabolism occurs aerobically or anaerobically. During the oxidation of glucose, through Embden–Meyerhof (EM) pathway, the conversion of 1 mol of phosphoglyceraldehyde (PGD) to phosphoglycerate (PG) generates 1 mol of ATP, and the conversion of 1 mol of phosphoenolpyruvate to pyruvate generates another 1 mol of ATP. Therefore, as 1 mol of glucose produces the 2 mol of pyruvate during its metabolism through EM pathway, so 4 mol of ATP is generated. All these reactions occur in the absence of O_2. On the other hand, 1 mol of ATP each is used during the conversion of fructose-6-phosphate to fructose-1-6-diphosphate and phosphorylation of glucose when it enters the cell. Since, when the pyruvate is formed from glucose through EM pathway the net gain of ATP is only 2 mol.

In EM pathway of glucose metabolism, during the conversion of PGD to PG 1 mol of nicotinamide adenine dinucleotide (NAD^+) is converted to 1 mol of NADH. In the presence of O_2, this H^+ of NADH is transferred to cytochrome system. While in the absence of O_2, pyruvate accepts this hydrogen from NADH, forming NAD^+ and lactate, where this NAD^+ is again used for the conversion of PGD to PG. Thus, in absence of O_2 pyruvate cannot enter the citric acid cycle.

$$\text{Pyruvate} + NADH = \text{Lactate} + NAD^+$$

In this way, glucose metabolism with production of lactate and energy may continue for a while without O_2. During aerobic glucose metabolism (glycolysis), the net production of ATP is 19 times more than the two ATPs, formed under anaerobic conditions. Six ATPs are formed from two NADH (3 ATPs from one NADH, recent studies say 2.5 ATP from one NADH) by oxidation through flavoprotein-cytochrome system. These two NADHs are formed when 2 mol of PGD is converted to PG.

Then, six ATPs (recent studies say 5 ATP) are formed from the two NADHs which are produced when 2 mol of pyruvate is converted to acetyl-CoA for the pyruvate to enter into the citric acid cycle. After that 24 ATPs (recent studies say 20 ATPs) are formed from the citric acid cycle. Of these, 18 (recent studies say 15) are formed from the oxidation of six NADH, 4 (recent studies say 3) from the oxidation of two flavin adenine dinucleotide (FADH), and 2 from succinyl-CoA, when it is converted to succinate. This succinyl-CoA to succinate reaction actually produces GTP, but the GTP is converted to ATP. Thus the net production of ATP per mol of glucose metabolism aerobically by the EM pathway and the citric acid cycle is $2 + (2 \times 3) + (2 \times 3) + (2 \times 12) = 38$. (recent studies say 32 ATPs)

cycle is ultimately broken down to CO_2 and H_2O yielding 3NADH, 1FADH$_2$, and 1ATP. These NADH and FADH$_2$ then enter in the respiratory chain (cytochrome system) where they are oxidized by giving up H^+. This hydrogen atom is carried out by the cytochrome system or respiratory chain and at the end of the cytochrome system in the presence of O_2, this H^+ form water (aerobic metabolism). Thus, during the oxidation of one molecule of reduced coenzyme (NADH) via the respiratory chain (cytochrome system), metabolic

energy equivalent to 3ATP molecule (recent study says 2.5 molecules ATP) is generated.

Many steps
$$NAD, 2H + \tfrac{1}{2} O_2 \rightarrow NAD + H_2P + Pi$$
$$3\,ADP + 3\,Pi \rightarrow 3\,ATP$$

Thus, from each hydrogenated NAD molecule (i.e., NADH), three molecules of ATP are formed. In the absence of O_2, the transport of H^+ or electron will proceed only until all the coenzymes/cytochrome has been exhausted **(Fig. 31)**.

■ CARDIAC OUTPUT

The cardiac output is defined as the total amount of blood pumped out by each ventricle per minute. This is also called the minute volume. The stroke volume means the amount of blood pumped out by each ventricle during each stroke or beat. So, the minute volume or cardiac output is the stroke volume multiplied by the heart rate. As the volume of blood pumped out by the both sides of heart is same, so the cardiac output is to be multiplied by 2 to calculate the total quantity of blood pumped out by the whole heart in a minute. The ejection fraction of left ventricle is defined as the stroke volume divided by the left ventricular end-diastolic volume. It indicates the percentage of blood, ejected per ventricle per beat during its systole. The typical value for ejection fraction in a healthy adult male ranges from 60% to 70%. The values of ejection fraction <40% represent severe ventricular contractile dysfunction or severe reduction of ventricular preload.

In adults, the average stroke volume is about 70 mL and the minute volume or cardiac output is about 5–6 L/min. In other words, the total volume of blood present in the body is expelled by each ventricle in every minute. The cardiac output is not the same in all individuals and in all ages. It is shown that cardiac output increases approximately in proportion to the surface area of our body. So, the cardiac output is frequently stated in terms of cardiac index (CI). Thus, the CI is defined as the cardiac output per minute per square meter of body surface area. The average value of this CI in a healthy adult male is about 3.3 L/min/m^2 (the surface area of an average-sized adult male is about 1.7 m^2). Similarly, the stroke volume per square meter of body surface area is also known as the stroke volume index (SI). The average value of SI in a healthy adult male is about 47 mL/min/m^2.

Since, the venous return to the heart per minute should be the same as the minute output or cardiac output, so it follows that blood flow through all the tissues together per minute must also be the same as the cardiac output. In other words, 5 L of blood passes out per ventricle per minute, 5 L of blood flows through all the tissues per minute and the same

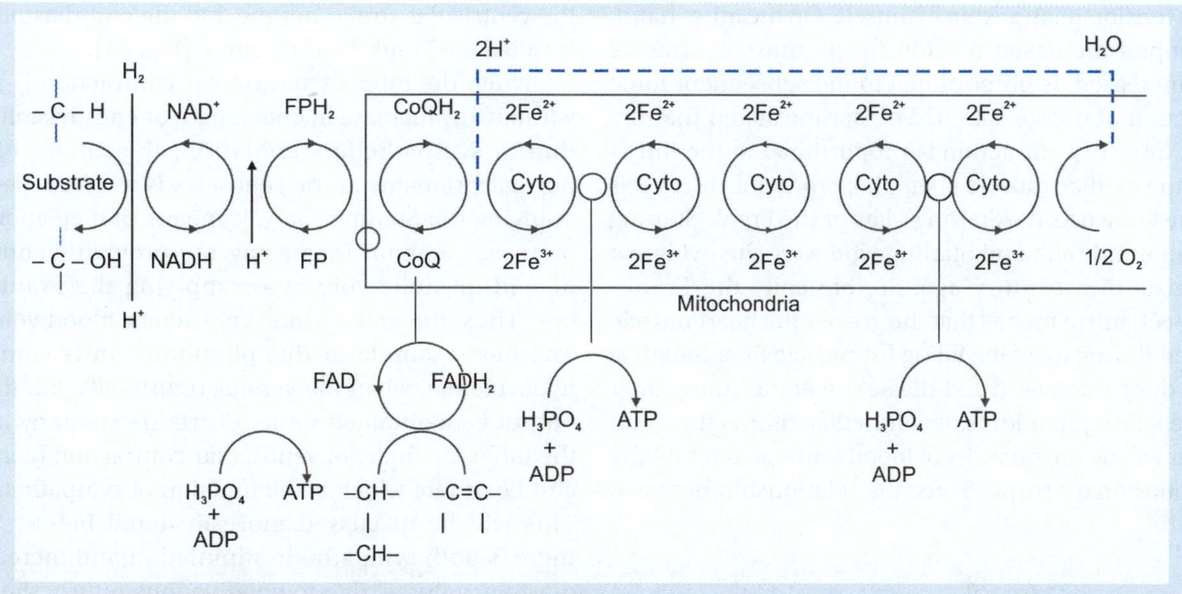

Fig. 31: Model of electron transport chain which is found within the mitochondrial matrix. Reducing substances such as NADH or $FADH_2$ usually enter at the two points of the respiratory chain. But, the synthesis of ATP occurs at three separate sites. At the end O_2 accepts electron (H^+) from cytochrome (cyt) and yields H_2O. Hydrogen (H^+) or electron flows through the chain of different cytochrome in steps from the more electronegative components to the more electropositive oxygen. When the substrates are oxidized via NAD linked dehydrogenase and the respiratory chain, 3 molecules of inorganic phosphate are incorporated into 3 molecules of ADP to form 3 molecules of ATP (recent studies say 2.5 molecules of ATP) per one-half molecule of O_2 consumed. For $FADH_2$ only 2 molecules of ATP (recent studies say 1.5 molecules of ATP) are formed. This reaction is called oxidative phosphorylation. (ADP: adenosine diphosphate; ATP: adenosine triphosphate; FAD: flavin adenine dinucleotide)

5 L of blood comes back to the heart to be distributed again to the different tissues per minute, such as kidney—1,300 mL/min; brain—700–800 mL/min; coronary arteries—200 mL/min; muscle—600–900 mL/min; liver—1,500 mL/min, etc. The total quantity of blood distributed in these organs does not exceed 4,500 mL/min. So, the remaining amount of blood is distributed to the skin, bones, gastrointestinal (GI) tract, and other less perfused tissues.

Cardiac reserve is defined as the capacity of heart which helps to generate the sufficient amount energy to expel a large quantity of blood above the basal level during emergency. Generally, the normal hearts expel about 5–6 L of blood per minute per ventricle. But during exercise, this amount may increase up to 30–40 L/min/ventricle **(Fig. 32)**.

Determinants of cardiac output

Cardiac output mainly depends on the following four factors. These are: *(1) preload, (2) force of cardiac contraction, (3) afterload, and (4) heart rate* **(Fig. 33)**.

Preload or Venous Return

The relationship between the length and tension of cardiac muscle is similar to that of a skeletal muscle. When the muscle is stretched or its length is increased, then the resultant developed tension, for next contraction, in the muscle

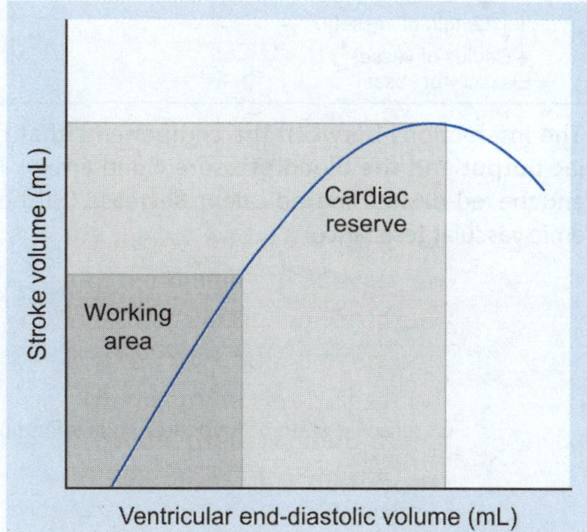

Fig. 32: Graphical representation of Starling's law of heart. When the end-diastolic volume (or the myocardial fiber length) is increased, then the ventricles contract more vigorously and stroke volume increases. The pink area shows the cardiac reserve area and the blue area is the normal functioning area. When the function of heart goes beyond the reserve range, then the stroke volume decreases and the relationship is reversed.

fiber also increases. But, this is up to a limit, because the developed tension in the muscle for subsequent contraction declines as the stretch becomes more extreme. This is called the length tension relationship of muscle. On the other hand, the developed increased tension in the muscle, after its length is increased, is proportional to the subsequent force of contraction of the muscle. Then, Starling stated that the energy or force of contraction is proportional to the initial length of the cardiac muscle fiber. This pronouncement has come to be known as the Starling's law or the Frank–Starling law, in honor of Frank and Starling who were the two great physiologists of a century ago. So, basically the Frank–Starling mechanism means that the greater the heart muscle is stretched during diastolic filling (or muscle fiber length is increased due to increased end-diastolic volume), the greater will be the subsequent force of ventricular contraction, and the greater will be the quantity of blood pumped out into the aorta or pulmonary trunk. Thus, the relationship between

the ventricular stroke volume and the end-diastolic volume is called the Frank–Starling curve **(Fig. 34)**.

When the force of ventricular contraction is increased without any increase in fiber length or end-diastolic volume, due to sympathetic stimulation, then more blood that normally remains in the ventricles is also expelled without applying the Starling's law. It means that ejection fraction increases without increasing the preload, venous return or end-diastolic volume or applying the Frank–Starling law. Thus, the end-systolic ventricular blood volume falls. The best example of this phenomenon is compensated hypovolemia, when the venous return falls, but the cardiac output is maintained up to a certain extent, by increasing the inherent ability of ventricular contraction (contractility) and heart rate which is the function of sympathetic system. This will be discussed more in detail below. So, when there is both sympathetic stimulation and increased end-diastolic volume, due to good venous return, then there is tremendous increase in cardiac output. This is simply due to the application of both Starling law and sympathetic stimulation **(Fig. 34)**.

Thus, the preload is defined as the end-diastolic fiber length or end-diastolic volume of ventricle. But, preload actually means the pressure within the ventricle at the end of its diastole for a given volume of blood which depends on the venous return or ventricular filling during diastole. Anything that increases or decreases the venous return will also increase or decrease the preload and the cardiac output accordingly. *These are: (1) intravascular volume status, (2) capacitance of venous system, and (3) ventricular compliance.*

There is pressure difference between the arterioles, capillaries, and venules. At the level of the heart, pressure at

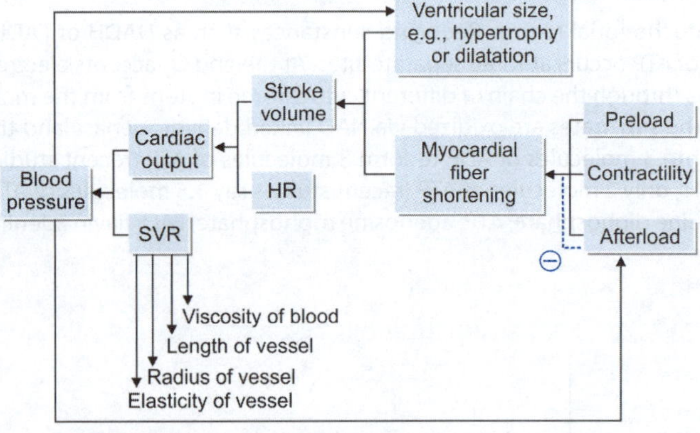

Fig. 33: The interactions between the components that regulate the cardiac output and the blood pressure. Solid arrows indicate increase and the red-dashed line indicates a decrease. (HR: heart rate; SVR: systemic vascular resistance)

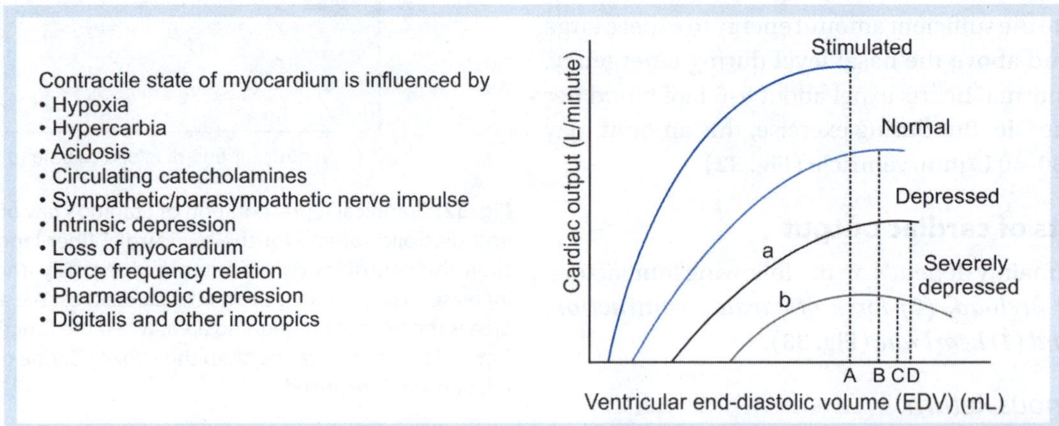

Fig. 34: The Frank–Starling curve and the effects of changes in myocardial contractility on this curve. The curve shifts downward and to the right (a and b line) as contractility is depressed. The factors influencing the myocardial contractility are summarized in the table. The vertical-dashed line ABCD indicates the portion of ventricular function curve, where the maximum contractility has been exceeded, and corresponds with the point on the descending limb of Frank–Starling curve.

the arteriolar end of a capillary loop is about 32 mm Hg and at the venous end of a capillary loop is about 12 mm Hg. So, the mean capillary pressure is about 25 mm Hg. Pressure in the great veins may vary from positive to negative. Venous dilatation, without any arteriolar dilatation or without any fall of general BP, will increase venous return and CO. But, the resultant effect may show no increase in BP due to the different reflex mechanism which tries to maintain the BP at normal level. On the other hand, arteriolar dilation definitely shows the decrease of BP or afterload, even though the cardiac output increases. On the contrary, arterial dilatation without venous dilatation will cause decrease in venous return and ⁻cardiac output and ↓BP. During both the arterial and venous dilatation, there is tremendous reduction of cardiac output and fall of BP which is seen in spinal and epidural anesthesia **(Fig. 35)**.

Vasomotor system control the pumping action of heart, the lumens of arterioles, the lumens of venules and thereby ultimately control the preload, cardiac output, and afterload. In shock, the intravascular volume status is altered definitely or relatively, affecting the preload, cardiac output, and afterload.

Force of Cardiac Contraction (Contractility of Heart)

Within the physiological limits, the heart pumps 70–80% of total blood that returns to it by the way of veins (ejection fraction). The amount of blood that returns to the heart accounts for the preload and is estimated by the EDVV or the initial length of muscle fibers of ventricle before its contraction. Cardiac output not only depends on this preload, but also on the inherent pumping action or the contractility of ventricle. So, this pumping action or the force of cardiac contraction is defined as the inherent isotropic or contractile ability of the heart. This is due to the balance between the parasympathetic and sympathetic activity on it. This contractility of myocardium will also exert a major influence on the stroke volume (or cardiac output) other than preload. This intrinsic contractile ability of heart that is controlled by sympathetic system, cannot be explained by the Frank–Starling mechanism which relates the best initial length of muscle fiber or end-diastolic volume with the subsequent force of contraction. So, it (Frank–Starling mechanism) is described previously under the heading of preload **(Fig. 36)**.

The best way to express the functional or contractile ability of ventricles is "ventricular function curve". It describes that as the intraventricular pressure increases by ventricular contraction due to sympathetic activity the respective ventricular output also increases. Thus, the ultimate force of cardiac contraction depends on the following factors:

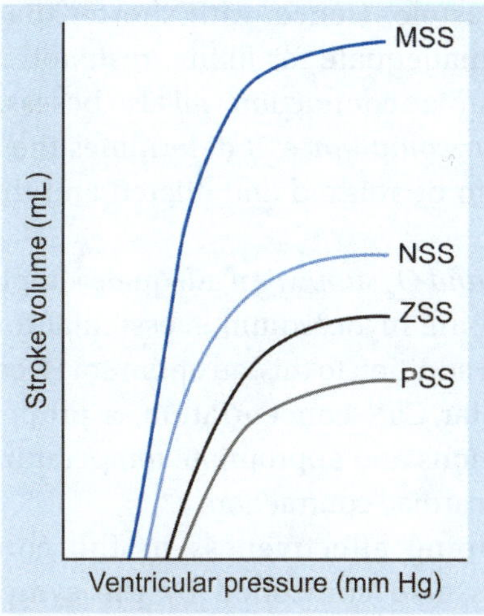

Fig. 35: The effect of different degree of sympathetic stimulation on the stroke volume. (MSS: maximum sympathetic stimulation; NSS: normal sympathetic stimulation; PSS: parasympathetic stimulation; ZSS: zero sympathetic stimulation)

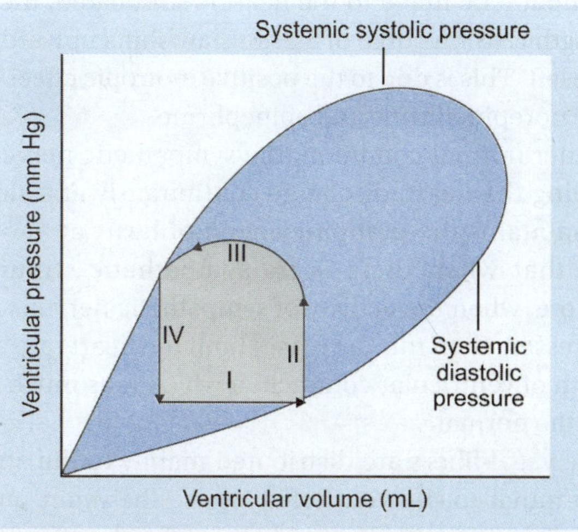

Fig. 36: The central square-shaped figure represents the relationship between the left ventricular volume and the left intraventricular pressure during diastole and systole. The outer-shaded area represents the work performed by the heart. I = Period of filling, II = Isovolumic contraction, III = Period of ejection, IV = Isovolumic relaxation.

- *The initial length of cardiac muscle fiber:* Within the physiological limits, greater the initial length, stronger will be the force of contraction (Starling's law). It is an inherent self-regulating mechanism that permits heart to adjust the changing end-diastolic volumes. It is obvious that the initial length of the muscle fiber of a ventricle is proportional to the degree of its filling which again depends on the venous return (preload).

- *The length of ventricular diastolic pause:* The filling, rest, and recovery of the heart muscle usually take place during diastole. Hence, with shorter diastolic period which is inadequate for filling, rest, and recovery, the force of cardiac contraction will also be less.

- *Ventricular compliance:* It determines the ability of the ventricle to be relaxed and dilated and thus the filling capacity.
- *Nutrition and O_2 supply:* An adequate supply of nutrition and O_2 to the myocardium is essential for its efficient activity. In addition to this, an optimum H^+ concentration, intracellular Ca^{2+} concentration, a proper balance of inorganic ions and appropriate temperature are needed for better cardiac contraction.
- The pumping effectiveness or the contractility of a heart is also controlled by the sympathetic and parasympathetic nerves. By sympathetic stimulation, the cardiac output often can be increased >100% (both by increasing the heart rate and force of contraction). By contrast, the cardiac output can be decreased to as low as zero by parasympathetic (vagal) stimulation. When the sympathetic nerve to the heart is stimulated, the whole length tension curve of Starling law shifts upward and to the left. This is due to the positive inotropic effect of both the norepinephrine and epinephrine.

Under normal condition, the sympathetic nerve fibers, supplying the heart, discharge continuously at a slow rate that maintains the pumping action of heart at about 30% above that when there is no sympathetic stimulation. Therefore, when the activity of sympathetic nervous system is depressed, then this decreases both the heart rate and the strength of ventricular contraction which is as much as 30% below the normal.

The vagal fibers are distributed mainly to the atria and not so much to the ventricles, where the main power of contractions of heart occurs. This explains the effect of vagal stimulation which is mainly to decrease the heart rate, rather than greatly to decrease the strength of cardiac contraction. Nevertheless, the great decrease in heart rate combined with a slight decrease in its contractile strength can decrease the ventricular pumping ability or cardiac output to 50% or more **(Fig. 37)**.

Afterload

The afterload of a ventricle is defined as the pressure in the principal arteries which are originating out from the ventricle and opposes its ejection. This afterload closely, but not exactly corresponds to the systolic pressure, described by the phase III curve of the volume pressure diagram. Sometimes, the afterload is loosely considered as the resistance in the vessels of circulation, rather than the pressure. But, it is incorrect. So, only the mean arterial BP is equivalent to the

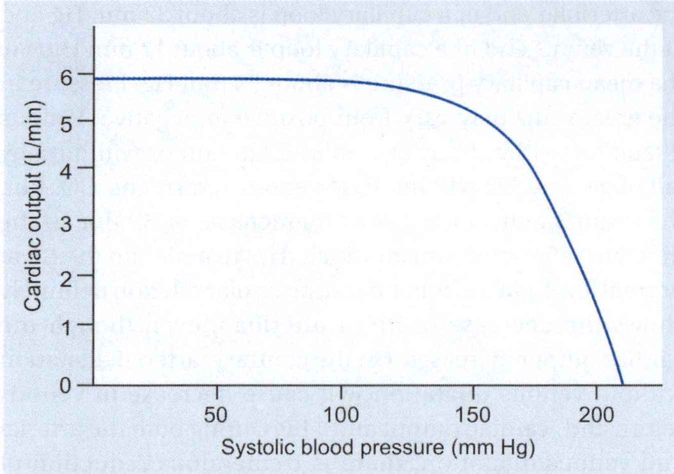

Fig. 37: The relationship between the systolic blood pressure and the cardiac output. When the blood pressure rises above 150 mm Hg the cardiac output falls significantly.

afterload and therefore, it may be defined as the force or pressure opposing the ventricular ejection (the unit of force is dyne or mm Hg whereas the unit of pressure is dyne/cm^2 or mm Hg/cm^2).

The importance of the concept of preload and afterload is that in many abnormal functional states of the heart or circulation, the intraventricular pressure during filling of it (i.e., the end-diastolic ventricular pressure or the preload which closely corresponds with end-diastolic volume) and the arterial pressure against which the ventricle must contract (i.e., the afterload) or both are severely altered from the normal.

Increasing the arterial pressure in aorta or afterload does not decrease the cardiac output, until the mean arterial pressure (MAP) rises above the approximately 160 mm Hg. In other words, during the normal function of heart at normal systolic arterial pressure (80–140 mm Hg), the cardiac output is determined almost entirely by the ease of flow of blood through the tissues which in turn controls the venous return of blood to the heart and cardiac contractility.

Total peripheral systemic resistance: It is also an extremely important factor for controlling the cardiac output. We know that the arterial pressure is equal to the cardiac output multiplied by the total peripheral systemic resistance. On the other hand, we can say that the cardiac output is equal to the arterial pressure divided by the total peripheral systemic resistance. Thus, under most normal circumstances, the cardiac output varies reciprocally with the changes in total peripheral resistance (PR). In **Figure 38**, when the PR is exactly normal, i.e., at the 100% mark, the cardiac output is also normal. Then, when the systemic resistance increases above the normal, then the cardiac output

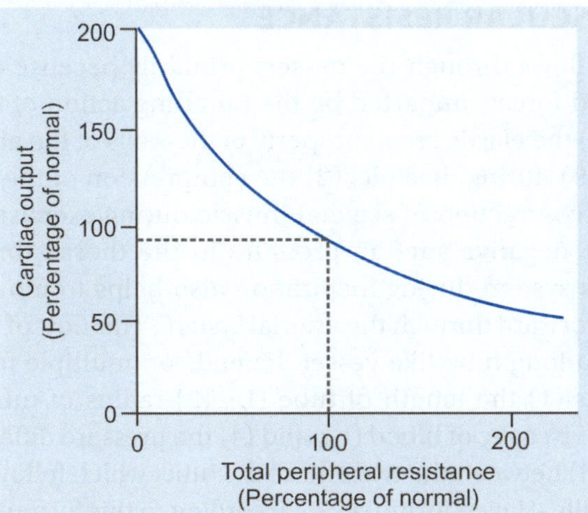

Fig. 38: The relationship between the total peripheral systemic resistance and the cardiac output which is reciprocal in nature. Here 100% is taken as normal.

gradually falls. Conversely, when the resistance decreases, the cardiac output increases.

Thus, one can easily understood this relationship by reconsidering one of the forms of Ohm's law as expressed by:

Cardiac output (or flow of current)

$$= \frac{\text{Arterial pressure (electromotive force)}}{\text{Total peripheral resistance (electrical resistance)}}$$

Heart Rate

Heart rate affects both the stroke volume and the minute volume. It affects the stroke volume by altering the period of diastole and there by altering the degree of ventricular filling (preload) and subsequently the force of contraction. Minute volume is equal to the heart rate multiplied by the stroke volume. So, the heart rate also affects the minute volume by altering one of the determinants of it. It should be noted that BP depends directly upon the minute volume or cardiac output and indirectly on the stroke volume (BP = CO × SVR) though there are also many other factors which determine the BP.

Venous return remaining constant, the rise of heart rate will reduce the diastolic pause and, therefore, the stroke volume. But, the product of stroke volume multiplied by heart rate (i.e., CO) may not fall, even it may rise above the resting value. Thus, minute volume (CO) and therefore, BP may rise, even if the stroke volume falls, provided the venous return is maintained. This happens with a moderate rise of heart rate, i.e., up to 160/min. If the heart rate becomes too high, then ventricular filling and the stroke volumes become so low that the minute output (CO) falls far below

the normal, though venous return is maintained. Thus, BP may drop and the subject may become unconscious. This happens in paroxysmal tachycardia, when the frequency of heart beat suddenly rises to 150–200/min. But, muscular exercise is an exception. Here, both the frequency of heart beat and the rate of venous return increases. Therefore, cardiac filling becomes more than the normal, even during the short diastolic period during exercise. Hence, both the stroke volume and the minute volume increase.

On the other hand, when the heart rate becomes very low (as in heart block or due to any other causes), then although the stroke volume is much higher than normal, yet due to the same reason, the total minute volume may fall. This is because, the product of heart rate and stroke volume which determines the cardiac output may be less than normal. But, with the moderate slowing of heart rate, the minute volume may not fall at all. In some instances, it may rise. Thus, alteration of the heart rate, on either side, i.e., not too high or not too low will generally raise the minute volume up to a certain extent. Beyond that limit, the minute volume or cardiac output will fall.

Measurement of Cardiac Output

In animal experiments, one can cannulate the aorta, pulmonary artery or any other great veins or arteries entering or exiting from the heart and thus can measure the cardiac output directly by using any type of flow meter (invasive method). But, noninvasively, cardiac output can be measured in experimental animal only by an electromagnetic flow meter placed on the root of the aorta or pulmonary artery. In human beings, the methods which are used to measure the cardiac output are: Doppler combined with echocardiography method, direct Fick principle method and indicator dilution method (a popular indicator dilution method is thermodilution method where the heat is used as an indicator).

Doppler and Echocardiography Combined Technique

The wall movement of cardiac chambers and also the other aspects of cardiac function can be evaluated by echo cardiography. It is a noninvasive technique and thus does not involve injections or insertion of catheter into any cardiac chamber or in any great vessel. In echo cardiography, the pulses of ultrasonic sound waves, commonly at a frequency of 2.25 MHz are made emitted from a transducer. This transducer also functions as a receiver to detect ultrasonic waves which is reflected back from the various parts of the heart. This reflections always changes whenever the acoustic impedance changes. Thus, when this recording of the changing echoes is placed against time on an oscilloscope, it provides a record of the movements of the wall, septum, and valves of different cardiac chambers during different phases of cardiac cycle. When this echo cardiography is combined with Doppler principle, then this combined method, can be used to measure the velocity and the volume of flow through the valves and thus cardiac output.

Fick Principle

Normally, 200 mL of O_2 is absorbed from the alveoli of lungs into the pulmonary blood in each minute. It is found that blood entering the right side of the heart has an O_2 content of 160 mL/L, whereas the blood leaving the left side of the heart has an O_2 content of 200 mL/L. From these data we can calculate that each liter of blood passing through the lungs absorbs 40 mL of O_2. Therefore, dividing this total quantity of O_2 absorbed into the blood from the lungs, i.e., 200 mL by the O_2 absorbed by per liter of blood (which is obtained by the arteriovenous O_2 difference), i.e. 40 mL, we can get the total amount of blood passing through the pulmonary circulation per minute which absorb this total amount of 200 mL O_2. Therefore, the total quantity of blood flowing through the lungs each minute is 200 mL/40 mL = 5 L. Thus, the cardiac output can be calculated by the following formula: Cardiac output (L/min) = Total amount of O_2 absorbed by the lungs (mL/min)/arteriovenous O_2 difference (mL/L of blood). This is the Fick principle.

In applying this Fick principle, for measuring the cardiac output in the human being, mixed venous blood is usually obtained by a catheter which is inserted through the brachial vein of the forearm, and passed through the subclavian vein, and then through the right atrium into the right ventricle or pulmonary artery finally. Systemic arterial blood can be obtained from any systemic artery of the body. The rate of O_2 absorption by the lungs is measured by the rate of disappearance of O_2 from the expired air, i.e., from the difference in O_2 concentration in the inspired and expired air, using any type of oxygen meter.

Indicator Dilution Technique

In this technique, a known amount of any substance, such as a dye or more commonly a radioactive isotope is injected into any vein of an arm and then the concentration of this indicator from the serial samples of arterial blood is determined. The output of the heart (i.e., cardiac output) is equal to the amount of indicator injected divided by its average concentration in arterial blood after a single circulation through the heart. The indicator must of course be a substance that stays in the blood stream during the test and has no harmful hemodynamics effects. A popular indicator dilution technique is a thermodilution technique, in which the cold saline is used as an indicator.

■ VASCULAR RESISTANCE

Blood flows through the vessels primarily because of the forward forces, imparted by the pumping action of heart. But, (1) the elastic recoil property of the walls of the arteries **(Fig. 39)** during diastole, (2) the compression of the veins by the contraction of skeletal muscle during exercise, and (3) the negative suction pressure in the thorax through venous system during inspiration also helps to move the blood forward through the arterial system. This flow of blood (F) in a long tube like vessel depends on multiple factors such as (1) the length of tube (L), (2) radius of tube (r), (3) the viscosity of blood (η), and (4) the pressure difference (PA–PB) between the two end of the tube, which follows the Poiseuille–Hagen formula. So, according to this formula:

$$F = (P_A - P_B) \times \frac{\pi}{8} \times \frac{1}{8} \times \frac{r^4}{8}$$

But, we know from Ohm's law that flow is equal to the pressure difference ($P_A - P_B$) divided by resistance (R).

Current (I) or flow (F)

$$= \frac{\text{Electromotive force (E) of pressure difference}}{\text{Resistance (R)}}$$

So, from here, we can calculate the resistance (R) as:

$$\frac{8\,\eta L}{\pi r^4}$$

The resistance to the flow of blood depends very slightly on the viscosity of blood, but mostly on the radius or diameter and the length of the vessels (principally of the arterioles, because they are more in length) **(Fig. 40)**.

Plasma is about 1.8 times more viscous than water, whereas the whole blood is 3–4 times more viscous than

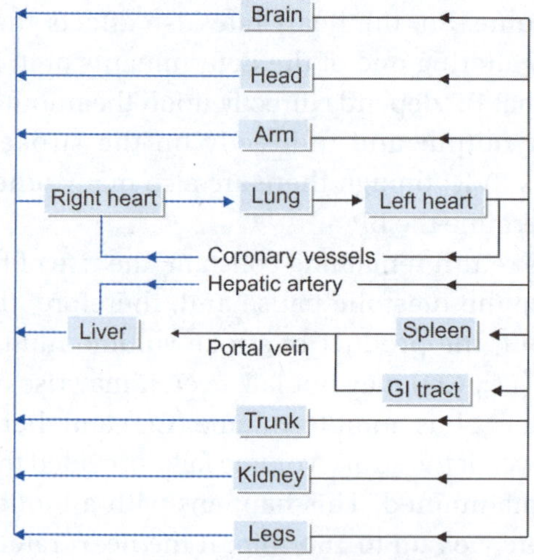

Fig. 39: Schematic diagram of different parallel (not in series) circuits of circulation.

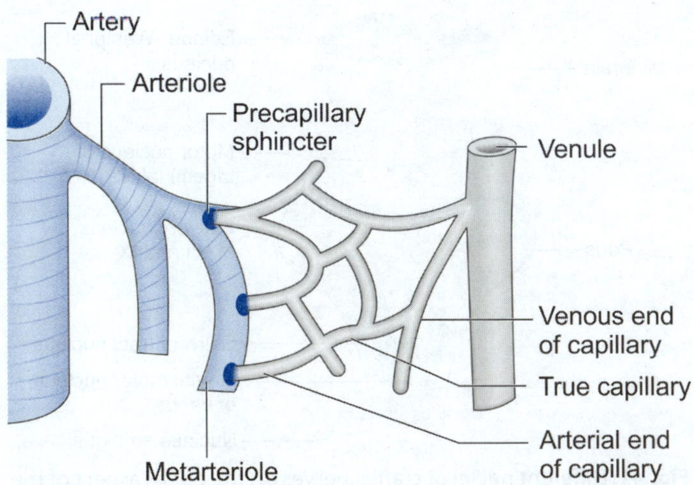

Fig. 40: The microcirculation. Arterioles give rise to metarterioles which give rise to capillary. The capillary drains into the venule. The walls of artery, arteriole, and venule contain relatively large amounts of smooth muscles. But the wall of metarteriole contains few smooth muscle and capillaries have no smooth muscle. The openings of the capillaries are guarded by muscular precapillary sphincters.

water. Thus viscosity depends mainly on the hematocrit value, i.e., percentage of the volume of blood occupied by the red blood cells. In large vessels, the increase in hematocrit causes appreciable increase in viscosity and therefore the resistance. However, in vessels smaller than 100 µm in diameter, i.e. arterioles, capillaries, and venules, etc., the change of viscosity due to per unit change of hematocrit has much less effect on resistance than it is in the large bore vessels of large diameter. This is due to the difference in nature of flow through the small vessels. Therefore, the net change in viscosity due to per unit change in hematocrit and its subsequent effect on total resistance is considerably smaller in the body as the smaller vessels occupy the larger portion of the total length of blood vessels. This is why the changes in hematocrit value have relatively little effect on the SVR, except when the changes are larger.

The flow of blood through each tissue or organ is regulated by the local chemical and/or the general neural and humoral mechanisms which causes dilatation and constriction of the vessels. The blood flows through the lungs without any change of the circuit. But, the systemic circulation is made up of numerous different circuits which are arranged in parallel. These arrangements permit wide variation in regional blood flow without changing the total systemic flow and resistance.

The walls of the aorta and other arteries of large diameter contain less amount of smooth muscles, but contain a relatively large amount of elastic tissues which are primarily located in the inner and external elastic laminas. They are stretched during systole and recoil on the blood column during diastole which is responsible for the forward motion and circulation of blood. On the other hand, the walls of the vessels of smaller diameter or arterioles contain less elastic tissue, but much more smooth muscle. These muscles are innervated by noradrenergic nerve fibers which function as constrictors, but in some instances they are innervated by cholinergic fibers which dilate the vessels. The arterioles are the major site of the resistance to blood flow and thus is the main determinant of the afterload, because this afterload is the BP which is obtained by multiplying the cardiac output with the resistance imparted by these arterioles, i.e., afterload or BP = CO × SVR.

The arterioles divide into smaller vessels which are sometimes called the metarterioles and these in turn feed into capillaries. In some vascular bed, these metarterioles are connected directly with venules through fare vessels. The true capillaries are an anastomosing network of side branches of this through fare vessel. The openings of the true capillaries are surrounded on their upstream side by some smooth muscles sphincter which is called the precapillary sphincters.

The true capillaries are about 5 µm in diameter at the arterial end and 9 µm in diameter at the venous end. When the sphincters are dilated then the diameter of the capillaries is just sufficient to permit a squeezed red blood cell through it. The total surface area of all the capillary walls in the body is near about 6,300 m^2 in an adult. The walls of the venules are only slightly thicker than those of the capillaries. The walls of the large veins are also thin and easily distended. They contain relatively little smooth muscle than the metarterioles. But, considerable venoconstriction can be produced by the activity of the noradrenergic nerves on the veins or by circulating vasoconstrictors such as endothelins, epinephrine, norepinephrine, etc. Variations in venous tone are very important in circulatory adjustments.

Blood always flows from the areas of high pressure to the areas of low pressure. The relationship between the mean flow, mean pressure, and the resistance in the blood vessels is analogous to the relationship between the flow of current (I), electromotive force (E), and the resistance (R) in an electrical circuit which is expressed as Ohm's law described before as I = E/R or the flow = Pressure/Resistance.

Thus, the flow of blood in any portion of the vascular system is equal to the effective perfusion pressure in that portion divided by the resistance. The effective perfusion pressure is the mean intraluminal pressure at the arterial end minus the mean intraluminal pressure at the venous end. The unit of resistance (pressure divided by flow) is expressed as dynes/s/cm.^{5} But to avoid the dealing of such complex units, resistance in the cardiovascular system is sometimes expressed as R units. This is obtained by dividing the pressure in mm Hg by flow in mL/sec. Thus, for example, when the mean aortic pressure is 90 mm Hg and the flow is

90 mL/sec, then the resistance is 90 mm Hg/90 mL/second = 1 R units.

When the blood is poured into any segment of the vena cava or other large distensible veins, then the pressure does not rise rapidly until the very large volumes of fluid are injected. So, the veins are called the blood reservoir. Normally veins remain in partially collapsed state. A large amount of blood can be added to the venous system before the veins become fully distended to the point where further increments in volume produce a large rise in venous pressure. The veins are, therefore, also called the capacitance vessels. On the other hand, the walls of the arterial system are not distensible. Therefore, the addition of little amount of blood in this system causes precipitous increase in pressure. So, the small arteries and the arterioles are referred to as the resistance vessels, because they are the principal site of producing BP and the PR.

At rest, at least about 50% of the total circulating blood volume remains in the systemic veins, 12% is in the cavities of heart, and 28% is in the low pressure pulmonary circulation. However, only 2% is in the aorta, 8% in the arteries, 1% in the arterioles, and 5% in the capillaries. When extra blood is administered by transfusion, then <1% of it is distributed in the arterial system (the high pressure system) and all of the rest is found in the systemic vein, pulmonary circulation and the cardiac chambers of low pressure system (i.e., the right side of the heart) other than the left ventricle.

■ CARDIAC REFLEXES

Cardiac reflexes are carried out by (1) afferent pathways, (2) vasomotor center (VMC), and (3) efferent pathways, lying within the sympathetic and parasympathetic nervous system, whose activities are further modified by the thalamus, hypothalamus, and some other higher centers.

Vasomotor Center

It is situated on the floor of 4th ventricle in the reticular formation. There are practically two areas in the vasomotor center. These are: (1) a pressure center and (2) a depressor center. The pressure center situated laterally and cranially which causes the rise of BP, whereas the depressor center is situated medially and caudally which causes the fall of BP. These are the completely physiological areas as there is no clear-cut anatomical separation between the pressure and depressor areas. In the intermediate region they overlap **(Fig. 41)**.

Sometimes, it is appropriate to use the term "medullary cardiovascular center" (MVC) instead of "vasomotor center", because it is recognized that the area contains both the neurons which excite and inhibit the thoracolumbar sympathetic center supplying the heart and blood vessels.

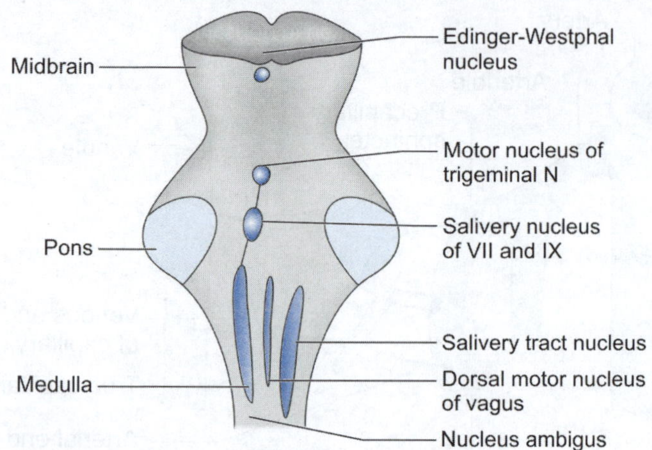

Fig. 41: Different nuclei of cranial nerves on the dorsal aspect of the brain stem, with nucleus of vagus nerve.

Within the VMC there lies (1) the nucleus of tractus solitarius which receives the sensory fibers, carrying general visceral sensations, through vagus and glossopharyngeal nerve, (2) the dorsal motor nucleus of vagus which supplies the motor to heart, lungs, esophagus, stomach, small intestine, and large intestine up to the right two-thirds of transverse colon, and (3) the nucleus ambiguus which contributes fibers to the glossopharyngeal and vagus nerves **(Fig. 42)**.

The depressor center is not the direct vasodilator center. This center causes the inhibition of sympathetic vasoconstrictor tone and thus indirectly dilates the vessel. The depressor center relays the inhibitory impulses to the pressure center. Pressure and depressure centers form the one functional physiological unit and it is defined as the VMC. The VMC discharges impulses which pass down the lateral white column of spinal cord through the cervical, thoracic, and lumbar segments and form the synaptic connection with the lateral horn cells of spinal cord (spinal sympathetic center) **(Fig. 43)**.

When BP rises, then the signals from the baroreceptors of carotid sinuses and aortic arch goes to the depressor center which in turn relays the inhibiting impulses to the pressure center, causing the slowing of heart rate and the dilatation of arterioles. Thus, the vasodilatation and the fall of BP is due to the inhibition of the vasoconstrictor effect of sympathetic (pressure reflex) system. On the other hand, the diminution of BP fails to stimulate the baroreceptor of carotid sinuses and aortic arch. Thus, the inhibitory impulses over the pressure center is withdrawn and BP is raised reflexly through the overactivity of sympathetic system.

Afferent Pathways

The afferent pathways, lying in the nerve fibers, start from the two sets of receptors that continuously carry the information

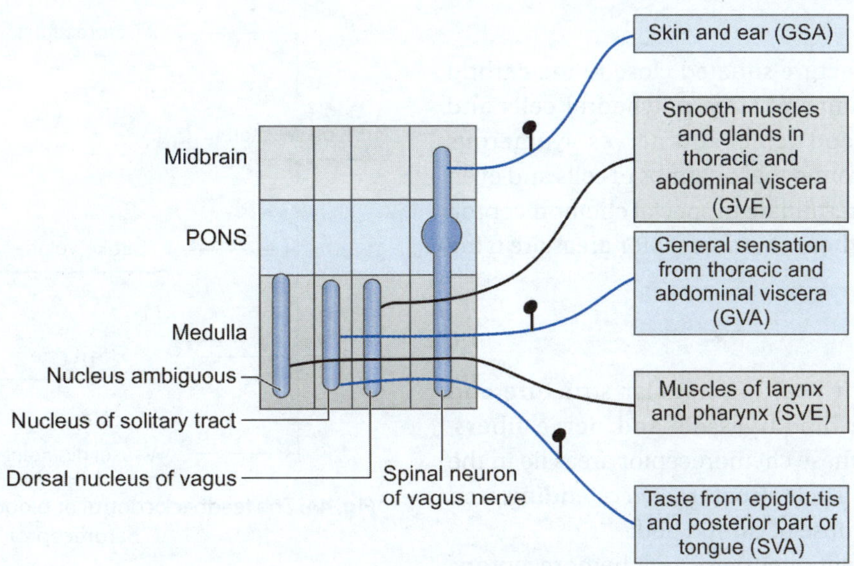

Fig. 42: Functional components of vagus nerve. (GSA: general somatic afferent; GVA: general visceral afferent; GVE: general visceral efferent; SVA: special visceral afferent; SVE: special visceral efferent)

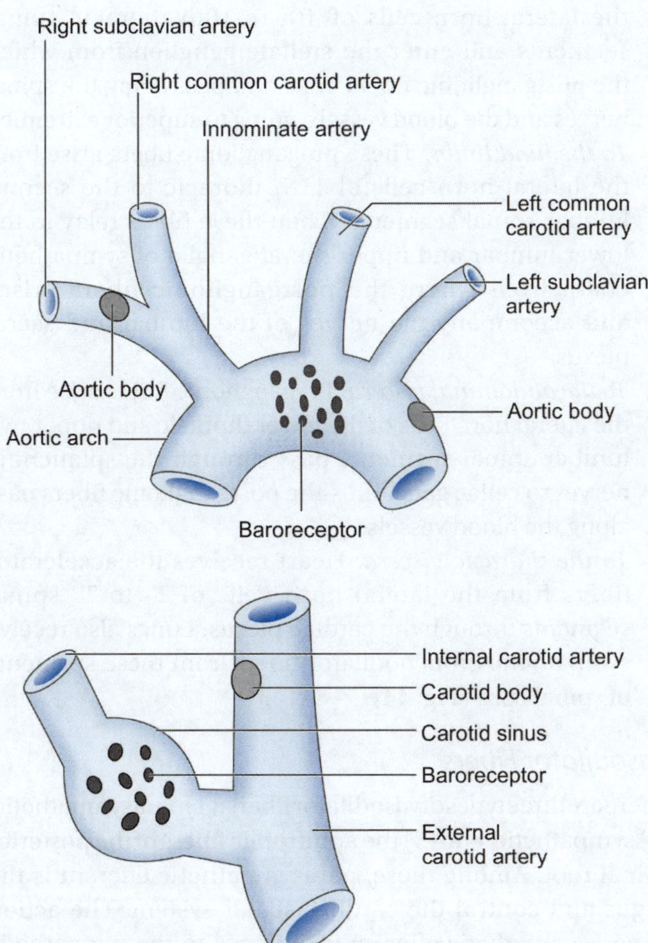

Fig. 43: The baroreceptors and chemoreceptors in the carotid sinus and aortic arch.

regarding the peripheral circulatory status to VMC. These sensory receptors are baroreceptors and chemoreceptors. The baroreceptors include the carotid sinus and aortic arch, whereas the chemoreceptors include the carotid body and aortic body.

Carotid Sinus

It is a dilatation at the root of internal carotid artery, often involving the common carotid artery. The wall of this carotid sinus is thin and is due to less amount muscle fibers in its tunica media layer. In the deeper part of adventitia, an extensive network of afferent nerve fibers is present. The nerve fibers end here as its free terminals. These are the pressure receptors and are sensitive to stretch, being stimulated by the rise of BP. The nerve arising from the carotid sinuses (baroreceptor) and carotid body (chemoreceptor) is purely afferent and is called the sinus nerve. It passes along the glossopharyngeal nerve and ends in the medulla.

Aortic Arch

The stretch receptor and afferent nerves, similar to those of carotid sinuses, are also present in the adventitia of aortic arch, the roots of the great vessel arising from aorta, and even in the adjoining parts of left ventricle. They serve the same function as that of carotid sinus. The nerve arising from the aortic arch (baroreceptor) and aortic body (chemoreceptor) is called the aortic nerve. It is purely afferent nerve and passes through the vagus to end in the medulla.

Carotid Body

It is a small nodular structure situated close to the carotid sinus. It consists of clumps of large polyhedral cells and richly supplied with blood vessel and nerves. Numerous afferent nerve fibers surround these clumps of cells and even the individual cells and terminate in special chemoreceptor. Afferent pathways from these chemoreceptor areas are lying in the sinus nerve.

Aortic Body

Like the carotid body, it is also a nodular structure and supplied richly by the blood vessels and nerve fibers. Afferent pathways from these chemoreceptor areas lie in the aortic nerve and vagus. Their structure, nerve ending, and functions are similar to those of carotid body.

Except these abovementioned baro- and chemoreceptors, there are also other baroreceptors and chemoreceptors which are distributed throughout the whole body. These baroreceptors are located in the right atrium, left ventricle, left atrium, at the junction of superior thyroid artery and common carotid artery, at the junction of subclavian artery and common carotid artery, throughout the common carotid artery, in-between the superior thyroid artery and subclavian artery, thoracic arch of aorta, and in central veins. The chemoreceptors are also located in the ventricular cavity and throughout the wall of whole blood vessels.

Efferent Pathways

Efferent pathways pass through the vagus and sympathetic nerves which control the cardiovascular system by modifying the cardiac activity and the lumen of blood vessels. These efferent pathways are divided into vasoconstrictor and vasodilatation fibers, carried by the different nerves.

Vasoconstrictor Fibers

These fibers pass mainly through the sympathetic outflow, extending from the lateral horn cells of first thoracic to the second lumbar segments of spinal cord and distributed in the following ways:

- *To the skin and muscle:* These fibers pass out through the gray rami communicantes, as the postganglionic sympathetic fibers, from all the ganglion of sympathetic chain. Then, these fibers run through the mixed spinal nerves and finally distributed over the whole body through the somatic motor and sensory nerves. The distribution is strictly unilateral and stops sharply at the midline.
- *To the head and neck:* These preganglionic fibers come from the lateral horn cells of first to fourth thoracic spinal segments. Then, these fibers enter the superior cervical

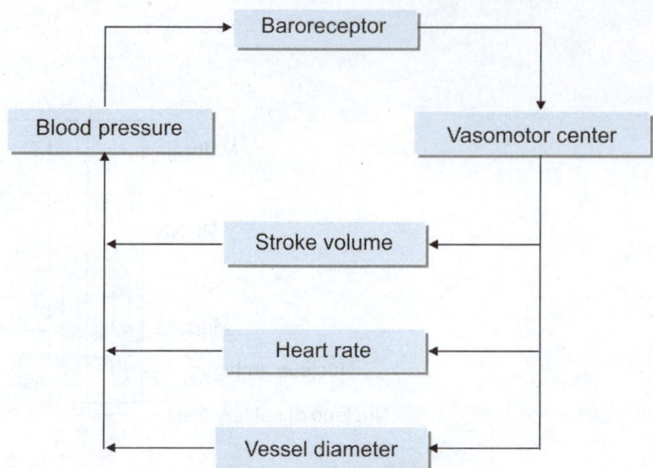

Fig. 44: The feedback control of blood pressure (BP) through baroreceptor.

ganglion from which the postganglionic fibers arise and pass along the carotid artery and its branches and along the spinal nerves of cervical plexus.

- *To the fore limbs:* These preganglionic fibers arise from the lateral horn cells of 4th to 10th thoracic spinal segments and enter the stellate ganglion from which the postganglionic fibers arise and pass along the spinal nerves and the blood vessels, going to superior extremity.
- *To the hind limbs:* These preganglionic fibers arise from the lateral horn cells of 11th thoracic to the second lumbar spinal segments. Then these fibers relay in the lower lumbar and upper sacral ganglia of sympathetic chain from where the postganglionic fibers arises and accompany the nerves of the lumbar and sacral plexus.
- *To the abdominal viscera:* Preganglionic fibers arise from the lateral horn cells of the lower thoracic and upper two lumbar spinal segments pass through the splanchnic nerves to celiac ganglion—the postganglionic fibers pass along the blood vessels.
- *To the thoracic viscera:* Heart receives the accelerator fibers from the lateral horn cells of T_1 to T_4 spinal segments through the cardiac plexus. Lungs also receive sympathetic bronchodilator fibers from these segments of spinal cord **(Fig. 44)**.

Vasodilator Fibers

There are three types of vasodilator fibers: (1) parasympathetic, (2) sympathetic, and (3) the antidromic fibers of the posterior spinal root. Among these, parasympathetic efferent is the vagus and control the cardiovascular system. The action of parasympathetic efferent is opposite to the sympathetic efferent. The sympathetic fibers are mostly vasoconstrictor in nature. But some sympathetic vasodilator fibers are also present. For instance, (1) the dilator fibers of the coronary vessels come through the sympathetic nerves, (2) some sympathetic dilator fibers also have been demonstrated in the peripheral nerves in human beings, (3) stimulation of the last anterior thoracic root produces dilatation of the vessels of kidney, (4) stimulation of the right splanchnic nerve sometimes cause vasodilatation and fall of BP.

Some common cardiac reflexes

Baroreceptor Reflex

This reflex controls the BP by both the circumferential and longitudinal stretching of baroreceptors, present in the carotid sinus and aortic arch. Increase in BP stimulates these two receptors and send impulses along the glossopharyngeal and vagus nerve to the depressor center, containing the nucleus of tractus solitarius, situated in the MVC. Inhibitory impulse, then, moves from the depressor center to the pressure center. Therefore, the response is decreased sympathetic activity and increased parasympathetic activity, causing the lowering of BP and decrease in heart rate. Typically, this reflex works in the range varying between the systolic BP of 170–50 mm Hg. When the systolic pressure falls below the 50 mm Hg, then this compensatory mechanism fails. In chronic or poorly controlled hypertensive patients, the upper set point of this reflex shifts upward.

Chemoreceptor Reflex

This reflex controls the arterial PO_2 and PCO_2 (pH status) via the chemoreceptors, and presents in the carotid and aortic bodies. Increased H^+ ($\uparrow PCO_2$) and hypoxia ($\downarrow PO_2$) stimulate these chemoreceptors and send impulses along the carotid branch of glossopharyngeal (nerve of Hering) and vagus nerve to the chemosensitive area of medulla. This area, then, stimulates the respiratory center and increase ventilation.

Bainbridge Reflex

This is actually a baroreflex which involves the stretch receptors, located in the right atrial wall and vena cava-atrial junction. Increase in right-sided filling pressure due to the increased intravascular volume stimulates these receptors and send impulses through the vagal afferent to inhibit the parasympathetic activity and increase the heart rate.

Bezold–Jarisch Reflex

Here, the mechanoreceptors, present in the left ventricular wall, respond to the noxious ventricular stimuli (e.g., myocardial ischemia), and send impulses along the unmyelinated vagal afferent fibers. Thus, it increases the parasympathetic tone, leading to vasodilatation, bradycardia, hypotension, and coronary artery dilatation.

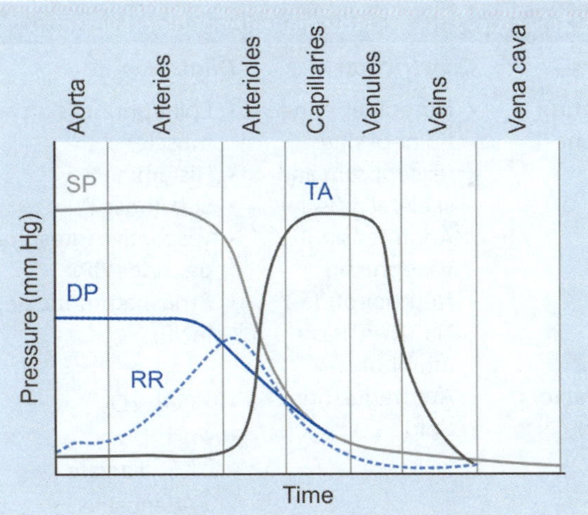

Fig. 45: The changes in systolic pressure (SP), diastolic pressure (DP), total cross-sectional area (TA), and resistance (RR) as the blood flows through the systemic circulation.

Valsalva Maneuver

If forced expiration against closed glottis is done, then it increases the intrathoracic pressure, decreases the venous return to heart, decreases CO and $\downarrow$BP. Now, this decrease in BP causes the stimulation of baroreceptor, sympathetic stimulation, and $\uparrow$HR with $\uparrow$BP. When glottis opens the reverse phenomenon occurs and heart rate decreases **(Fig. 45)**.

Cushing's Reflex

This reflex is manifested by increased HR, cardiac contractility and BP in response to increase intracranial pressure. It is the initial response of the reflex in an effort to increase the cerebral perfusion pressure. This is followed by reflex bradycardia mediated by baroreceptor within carotid sinus and aortic arch as a result of the increased peripheral vascular tone.

Oculocardiac Reflex

This is discussed in the Ophthalmic Anesthesia chapter, Chapter number 41.

■ CIRCULATION

An average adult has a blood volume of about 5–6 L in his circulation and it is more or less equal to the resting cardiac output. But, during heavy exercise this cardiac output may increase up to 25 L/min which indicates the increased (five times) circulation. The main purpose of this circulation is to supply adequate O_2, carbohydrate, fats, amino acids, hormones, immunological agents, etc. to the tissues and to remove the waste products of its metabolism. But, for this circulation only a little heart, weighing about 300 g, acts as

TABLE 2: Factors affecting the diameter of blood vessels.

Factors	Constriction	Dilatation
Circulating hormone	• Norepinephrine • Epinephrine (except skin and skeletal muscle) • Angiotensin-II • Vasopressin • Neuropeptide-Y • Na^+-K^+-ATPase inhibitor	• Epinephrine (skin and muscle) • Histamine • Substance P • Vasoactive intestinal peptide (VIP) • Atrial natriuretic peptide (ANP)
Local factors	• Autoregulation • Cold	• $\uparrow CO_2$, $\downarrow O_2$ • $\downarrow pH$ • $\uparrow K^+$, $\uparrow$Lactate • $\uparrow$Adenosine • Heat
Neural factors	• Sympathetic stimulation	• Sympathetic inhibition • Activation of cholinergic • Vasodilator fibers to skeletal muscle (sympathetic and parasympathetic)
Endothelial factors	• Endothelin • Thromboxane A2 • Serotonin	• Kinins • NO • Prostacyclin

a pump and is highly adequate. Still, no engineers have yet been able to develop such an efficient pump with long-term performance like it (heart) **(Table 2)**.

Heart provides energy for circulation. Its phasic ejection of blood into aorta produces a pressure into it and subsequently the pressure head or pressure gradient between aorta and peripheral capillary. This pressure head may be regarded as the cause of the flow of blood or may be regarded as the potential energy for circulation.

During spinal or epidural anesthesia, in the anesthetized portion of the body both the pressure gradient (E) and the resistance (R) is reduced. But, the ultimate flow (F) which depends on the relative ratio of E and R (according to the Ohm's law) is adequate even though the MAP is low. Whereas in the unanesthetized segment (i.e., in the upper part of the body during lumbar spinal or epidural anesthesia), resistance does not fall, even increases due to the compensatory elevated sympathetic activity in this portion of the body for the fall of systemic BP. Thus, the pressure head responsible for circulation in the unanesthetized segment severely falls due to the fall of MAP and thus blood flow (I) in this segment is tremendously jeopardized. So, BP should not be reduced below the 20–25% of its MAP to maintain adequate supply to the vital organs during central neuraxial block.

There are different values of resistance against the flow of blood in the different parts of our body. But to counter this variable resistance, exhibited in the different parts of our body, the pressure gradient must be adequate to maintain the circulation. Again, as the cardiac output is pulsatile, so the pressure head and the flow into the arteries from the heart are also pulsatile. This means that the peripheral arterial system at the capillary level should possess a system of low impedance which will convert this pulsatile flow into the continuous flow. This is because, the tissues themselves require a steady flow of blood through the capillaries, so as to benefit maximally from the diffusion between the blood and the tissues.

On the other hand, the resistance and subsequently the cardiac work can be lessened by increasing the radius of the vessels into which the blood is delivered. But, this will reduce the pressure gradient which requited for flow (circulation). While, on the other hand, adequate pressure gradient is required to provide an adequate flow. Alternatively, the cardiac work also can be reduced by considerably increasing the distensibility or stretching of the vascular system and this would decrease the pulsatile pressure and hence the impedance. However, such an increase in the distensibility of the vascular tree would prevent the immediate increase in cardiac output and arterial pressure which is needed in biological emergencies and may be of immense important for the survival of life. If the system took long time to inflate, then the urgent requirement for blood supply to the brain and the myocardium by increasing BP in emergencies circumstances could not be achieved, because for the pressure head available to such organs would rise too slowly, due to increased distensibility of the vessels **(Fig. 46)**.

So, some compromise should, then, have to be arrived. The arteries are distensible, but the arterioles convert the pulsatile ejection of heart into a steady flow to the tissue capillaries. The arterioles also offer resistance and step down the hydrostatic pressure within the capillaries. Veins have been equipped to serve as capacitance vessels. This is because, by appropriate variation of their diameter, the mobilization of blood to the heart is controlled in various circumstances.

The blood enters the right and left atrium at a pressure near about zero. The left ventricle pumps the blood into the aorta when the left intraventricular pressure reaches a peak value during its contraction phase (systole) which is about 120 mm Hg or so. During diastole the aortic pressure subsides to some 80 mm Hg. This is due to some elastic recoil property of arterial system and due to some resistance to the outflow offered by the peripheral arterioles. This combination of the elasticity and the resistance converts the pulsatile ejection flow of the heart into a steady outflow at capillary level.

So, the whole vascular system of our body can be described as consisting of:
- Windkessel vessels (arteries up to metarteriole level)
- Precapillary resistance vessels

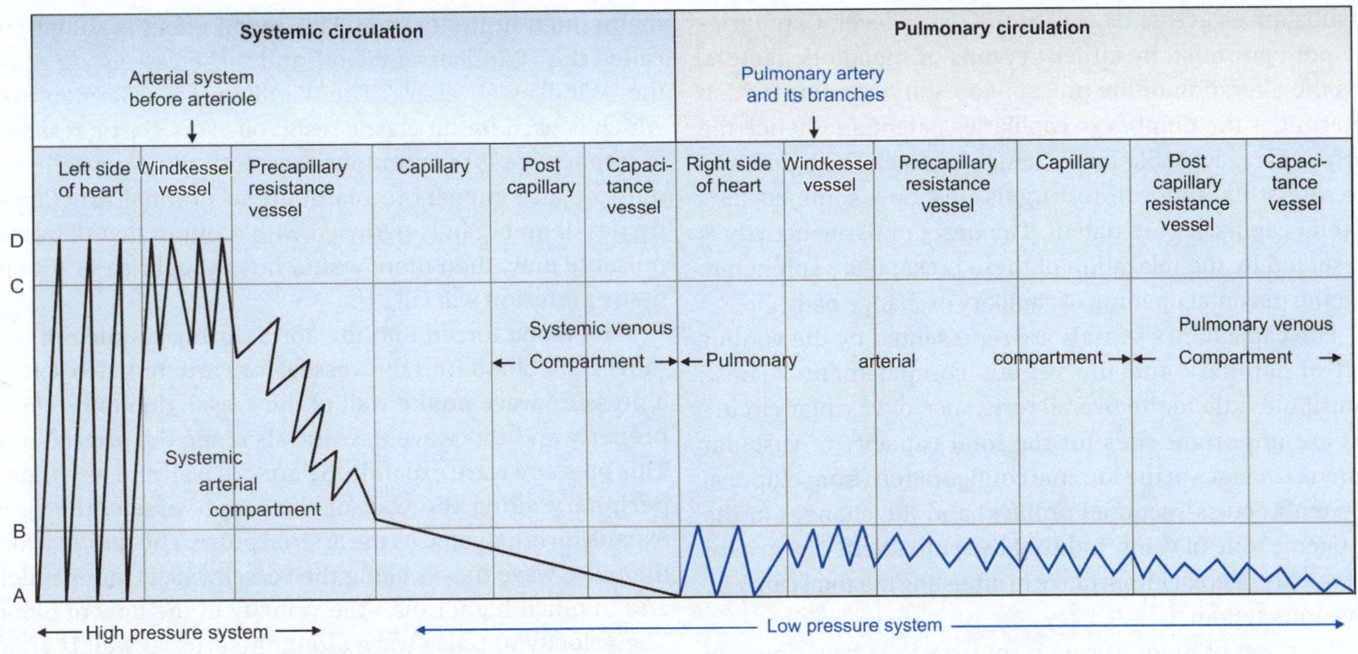

Fig. 46: Differential level of pressure in different systemic and pulmonary vessels.

- Precapillary sphincters
- Capillary
- Postcapillary resistance vessels
- Capacitance vessels (veins).

The concept of Windkessel vessels (Windkessel means "elastic reservoir", Windkessel vessels are those arteries which have high elasticity in their wall) is represented by the aorta and its large- and medium-sized branches which have high elastic (distensible) wall. Systolic ejection of blood into aorta from ventricle distends these vessels and renders the blood to flow forward continuously toward periphery. During diastole (when the ventricle is not ejecting blood into aorta) the elastic recoil of these vessels also sustains the pressure gradient and renders the blood to flow forward continuously to the periphery. This is because, the potential static energy, stored during cardiac contraction in the elastic tissue of the aorta and its large branches, is reconverted into kinetic energy for the circulation during diastolic phase. In disease process, the degenerative changes in the media of the large vessels cause a loss of this arterial elasticity. Thus, a high-pulse pressure results owing to the lack of this Windkessel effect.

The precapillary resistance vessels (arterioles) provide the majority of SVR. It exhibits an efficient local myogenic control of their own vascular radius and on this local myogenic tone is superimposed an extrinsic neural control, affected by the sympathetic constrictor nerves and the parasympathetic vasodilator nerve. Normally, these nerves discharge impulse at the frequency of 1 impulse per second, but the rate of discharge may be increased to 10–16 impulse per second in emergency circumstances (e.g., hemorrhage) and entirely suspended (e.g., in the skin vessels) during heat stress.

The blood vessels in muscles represent by far the most important site for PR. This is due to the high degree of basal sympathetic myogenic tone in these vessels. The blood flow in the muscle of a resting man is only 2·7 mL/100 g/min. However, during exercise this flow may increase up to 50–70 mL/100 g of muscle/min. This enormous increase in blood flow in muscles is achieved by the vasodilation of arterioles and the precapillary sphincters, caused by local metabolites, produced by active tissues. But, it is not due to the neural factors. In resting muscle, however, the influence of sympathetic constrictor nerves on precapillary sphincter is partly responsible for keeping the muscle blood flow at low level. In resting circumstances, the cutaneous vessels are also responsible for high regional resistance.

The precapillary sphincters, which are also a part of precapillary resistance vessels, are particularly important in determining the size of total capillary area. For example, any increase in the patency of these sphincters causes an enormous increase in the number of capillaries open. The radius of these precapillary sphincters is controlled both by the neurogenic factors (sympathetic and parasympathetic) and by the local concentration of tissue metabolites.

The capillaries consist of a single layer of endothelial cells, resting on a basement membrane. This allows the exchange of substances across its wall at the tissue level. Capillaries are not controlled by either nervous or metabolic factors. It is the alteration of the precapillary sphincter tone which determines the number of capillaries patent and hence the surface area, available for exchange between the blood and the interstitial fluid. In resting tissues, only some 20–25% of total capillaries are patent. The onset of tissue activity is presented by the relaxation of these precapillary sphincters and the maximal opening of capillary exchange bed.

The capacitance vessels are represented by the venous end of capillary and the venous compartments. These contribute little to the overall resistance of vascular circuit, but are important sites for the total capacity of vascular system. Changes in the luminal configuration (from elliptical to circular cross-sectional profiles) and the changes in the myogenic tone of veins, induced by sympathetic constrictor nerves, are of great importance in adjusting the total capacity of venous system.

Shunting of blood through some vessels occur only in few tissues, most notably in the skin. Such vessels bypass the capillaries and if patent they permit a rapid flow of blood. Their patency is controlled entirely by the sympathetic vasoconstrictor discharge. Thermal stress causes (via central nervous system) the abolition of such sympathetic discharge and the tremendous increase of cutaneous blood flow which allows the dissipation of heat from our body surface.

Windkessel Concept

The arterial system is a very complex network of elastic tubes which at its one end accepts the intermittent spurts of blood from the left ventricle of heart and at its other end, through its myriad of termination, passes the blood by a steady stream into the resistance vessels, which perfuse the organs and tissues of the body. Thus, the arterial system acts both as conduit and as cushion when delivering the blood with a minimum fall in pressure to peripheral tissue (conduit function) and by reducing the fluctuations of pressure imposed by the intermittent ventricular action (cushioning function). Thus, this complex network of tubes can be viewed as a simple system, at least as first approximation. This simple idea is the Windkessel concept. This concept is based on the elastic property of blood vessels. During systole, the elasticity of the great vessels causes dilatation. This dilatation reduces the BP, reduces the resistance of vessels, and reduces the cardiac work. It also tries to reduce the pulsatile flow of blood to a stream line nonpulsatile flow by absorbing the energy. But, during diastole, the recoiling property of this elastic tissue of blood vessels helps for the forward movement of blood during diastole and maintains the diastolic pressure. Thus, a continuous flow of blood is maintained in the tissues. This recoil effect is sometimes called the "Windkessel effect" and these vessels are called the "Windkessel vessels". The Windkessel is a German word which is used for an elastic reservoir. This elastic reservoir is responsible for continuous flow both during systole and diastole and appears to maintain an optimal function of tissues. If an organ is perfused with a pump that delivers a pulsatile flow, then there would be gradual rise in VR and tissue perfusion will fail.

The blood forced into the aorta during systole not only moves the blood into the vessels forward, but also sets up a pressure wave on the wall of the vessel, due to its elastic property and this wave now travels along the arterial wall. This pressure wave expands the arterial wall and as it travels periphery along the wall of the large vessels, then this expansion is palpated as the arterial pulse. The rate, at which the pulse wave travels along the vessel wall, is independent and of much higher than the velocity of the flow of blood. The velocity of pulse wave along the arterial wall is about 4 m/s in the aorta, 8 m/s in the large arteries, and 16 m/s in the small arteries. Whereas, the velocity of the flow of blood in aorta is 40 cm/s. Actually, the velocity of blood flow in aorta ranges from 120 cm/s during systole to negative value during diastole.

■ ARTERIAL BLOOD PRESSURE

The BP is defined as the lateral pressure which is exerted by the blood on the wall of the vessels, while flowing through it. There are four common terms regarding the BP.

- *Systolic pressure:* It is the maximum pressure in artery during the systole of the cardiac cycle of ventricle.
- *Diastolic pressure:* It is the minimum pressure in artery during the diastole of the cardiac cycle of ventricle.
- *Pulse pressure:* It is the difference between the systolic and the diastolic pressure.
- *Mean arterial pressure:* It is the average pressure throughout a single cardiac cycle of ventricle, i.e., during both systole and diastole. So, it depends on the duration of the cardiac cycle and indicates the arithmetic mean of the systolic and diastolic pressure throughout the ventricular cycle. Thus, as the systole is shorter than the diastole, so the mean pressure is slightly less than the value which is halfway between the systolic and diastolic pressure. It can actually be determined by integrating the area of pressure curve which is shown in the **Figure 47** by the shaded area. However, a close approximation to the MAP may be obtained by adding the diastolic pressure with one-third of pulse pressure.

The BP falls very slightly in the large- and medium-sized arteries, though their resistance is small. This is because, the flow of blood is high in these vessels due to low resistance.

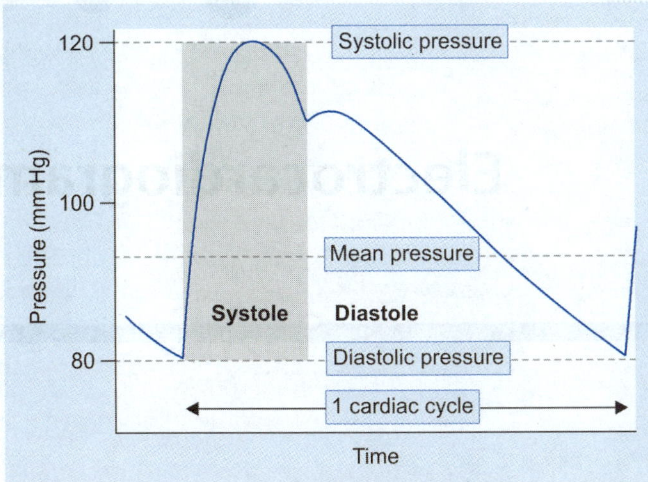

Fig. 47: This figure shows the graphical representation of mean arterial pressure (MAP).

But, it (BP) falls rapidly in the small arteries and arterioles, though they are the main sites of SVR against which the heart has to pump. Here, yet the resistance is high, but still the pressure is low. This is because, due to high resistance, flow of blood is low. The mean pressure at the end of arterioles is 30–38 mm Hg. Pulse pressure also declines rapidly to about 5 mm Hg at the end of the arterioles. The magnitude of the drop of pressure along the arterioles also varies considerably depending on whether they are constricted or dilated.

Thus, in summary, it is stated that the pressure in the aorta, brachial, and other large arteries in a young human adult rises to a peak value (systolic pressure) of about 120 mm Hg and falls to a minimum value (diastolic pressure) of about 70 mm Hg during each cardiac cycle. So, the arterial pressure is conventionally written as systolic pressure over diastolic pressure, e.g., 120/70 mm Hg. In SI unit, one millimeter of mercury equals 0.133 kPa. So, in this unit system, the value of arterial pressure is 16/9.3 kPa.

The height of systolic pressure indicates:
- The cardiac output
- The degree of pressure which the arterial walls have to withstand. Diastolic pressure is the measure of PR. It indicates the constant load against which heart has to work.
- The extent of work done by the heart

The height of the diastolic pressure indicates:
- The constant load against which heart has to work.
- The measure of PR.

The factors controlling the blood pressure: There are two main determining factors which can control the BP. These are: (1) cardiac output, and (2) SVR. So, any alteration of cardiac output and SVR will alter the BP according to Ohm's law. Cardiac output again depends on: (i) the venous return to heart, (ii) the force of myocardial contraction, (iii) the contractility (pumping action) of heart, (iv) the frequency of contraction or heart rate, and (v) the ventricular size. Venous return (preload) again depends on: (a) the blood volume and (b) the venous constriction or dilatation. Cardiac output depending on the factors such as cardiac contractility and the frequency of contraction or heart rate is already discussed previously under the heading of cardiac output. Ventricular size also determines the cardiac output. For example, a hypertrophied heart prevents proper diastolic filling and reduces the cardiac output.

Systemic vascular resistance is also an important determining factor of BP. The chief site of SVR in a vascular tree is the arterioles. SVR depends on: (i) the velocity of blood, (ii) the viscosity of blood, (iii) the elasticity of arterial walls, (iv) the radius of the lumen of vessels, and (v) the length of the vessel. For a given elasticity of arterial wall and the velocity of blood, the other factors responsible for SVR can be represented by Poiseuille's (Hagen–Poiseuille) law.

According to Poiseuille's law, the resistance in any blood vessels varies directly with the viscosity of blood and the length of blood vessel, and inversely with the fourth power of the radius of blood vessel. Thus, it can be represented by the formula:

$$R = 8\eta L/(\pi r^4)$$

Here R stands for the resistance to blood flow, η for the viscosity of blood, L for the length of blood vessel, r for the radius of blood vessel. The value of π is 3.14 and 8 is the Hagen's integration factor.

According to Ohm's law, the relationship between PR or SVR, cardiac output (CO), and BP is: (i) BP $\propto$ CO × PR, (ii) CO $\propto$ BP/PR, and (iii) PR $\propto$ BP/CO.

Electrocardiogram

INTRODUCTION

During each contraction of heart, an electrical impulse is generated in sinoatrial (SA) node. It is, then, simultaneously transmitted to atrioventricular (AV) node, bundle of His, two bundle branches, Purkinje fibers, ventricular muscle fibers, and lastly to the surrounding body tissues in which the heart is bathed in. Thus, an electrical impulse that is initiated in cardiac muscle is ultimately transmitted throughout our whole body. So, if two suitable electrodes (or leads) are placed on the surface of our body, opposite to the heart and are connected to a very sensitive galvanometer, with a recording device, then this electrical potential can easily be recorded. This *record (graph)* is called the *electrocardiogram (ECG)* and the *machine* by which this ECG is recorded is called the *electrocardiograph*. However, from our body surface area, this process of continuously making graphic records of this variation in electrical potential, caused by the electrical activity of heart muscles, is called the *electrocardiography*. Practically, the electrocardiograph is a sophisticated galvanometer where a sensitive electromagnet detects and records the changes of electrical potential, generated in our heart and transmitted throughout the whole body. Hence, for this detection of changes in cardiac electrical potential, two electrodes or leads (one +ve and another –ve) are needed. *So, the theoretical straight line, joining these two electrodes or leads, is called the lead axis. However, this should not be confused with the electrical axis of heart or cardiac axis.*

ELECTROCARDIOGRAPHIC PAPER

The electrocardiographic paper is divided into 1 mm small and 5 mm large squares, both horizontally and vertically. Therefore, within one large square, there are five small squares accommodated both horizontally and vertically. Hence, every large square is 5 mm in length, both vertically and horizontally **(Fig. 1)**

After every 15 large squares, there is a vertical line at the upper border of ECG paper. Horizontally, the squares measure the time in seconds and vertically they (squares) measure the amplitude of deflection in millivolt. *Conventionally, the ECG is always recorded at a paper speed of 5 large squares or 25 mm (25 small squares) per second. So, every small square of 1 mm measures a time of 1/25 seconds or 0.04 seconds and one large square is 0.2 seconds (0.4 × 5 = 0.2). Vertically, one small square measures a deflection of 1 mV.*

ELECTROGRAPHIC LEADS

An electrographic lead can be placed on our body surface in respect to any three-dimensional relationship of heart, such as frontal (coronal), sagittal, and horizontal. But practically, we use only 12 conventional leads in frontal and horizontal planes (six leads in frontal plane and six leads in horizontal plane). Other different types of leads which are used in different planes in special conditions are discussed later **(Fig. 2)**.

So, the leads can be classified according to the planes where they are situated. These are frontal plane leads, horizontal plane leads, and sagittal plane leads **(Fig. 3)**.

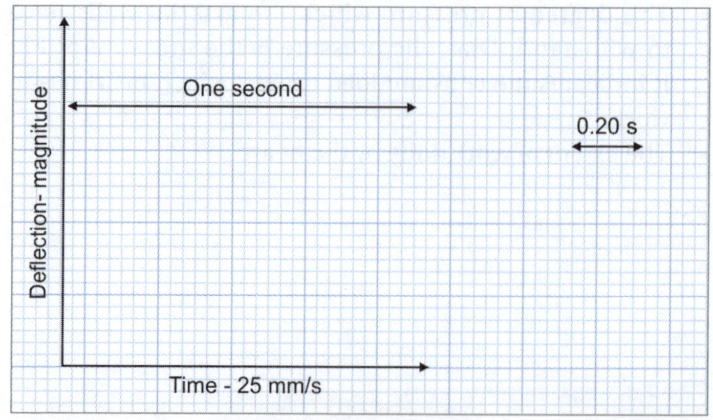

Fig. 1: An electrocardiograph paper with a time scale at a recording speed of 25 mm/second.

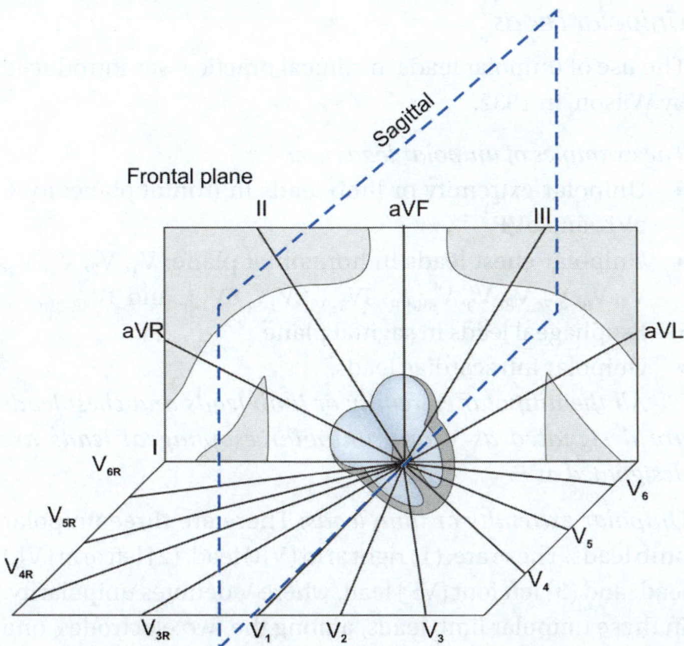

Fig. 2: The frontal (coronal) and the horizontal plane leads.

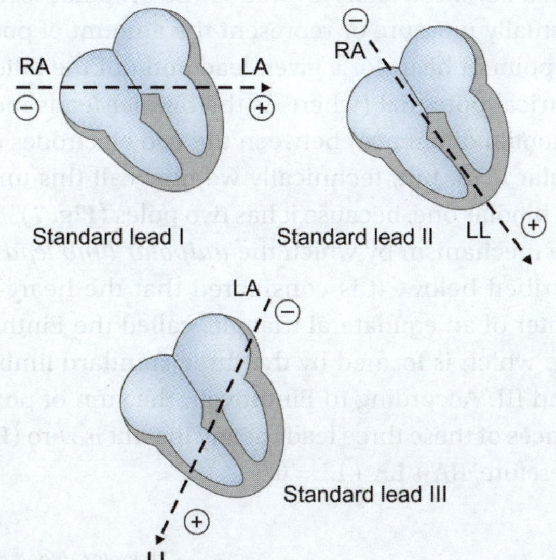

Fig. 3: Different arrangements of electrode placements, producing standard leads I, II, and III. The positive poles in standard leads I, II, and III are located respectively at the left arm (LA), right arm (RA), and left leg (LL).The three axes (plural of axis) formed by these three leads form a triangle. As the electrodes are situated at equidistant from the heart, so it is also considered that the axes are also situated equidistant from the heart and the heart is located at the center of the triangle, formed by these three axes. This equilateral triangle formed by these three axes is called the Einthoven's triangle.

Frontal (Coronal) Plane Leads

The frontal plane leads consist of standard leads I, II, III, and the leads aVR, aVL, and aVF. *These leads are oriented or*

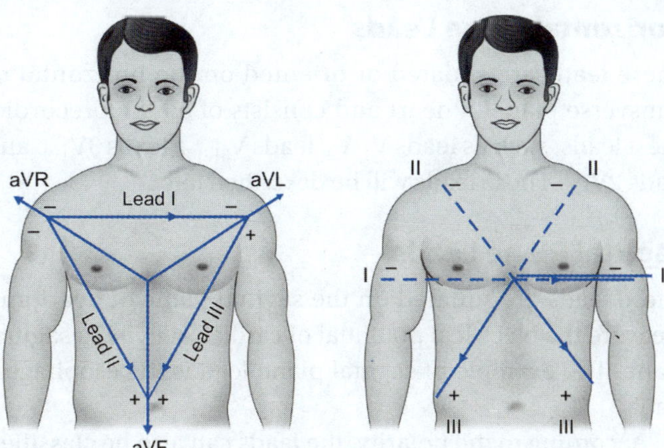

Fig. 4: Einthoven's triangle and the frontal plane bipolar leads.

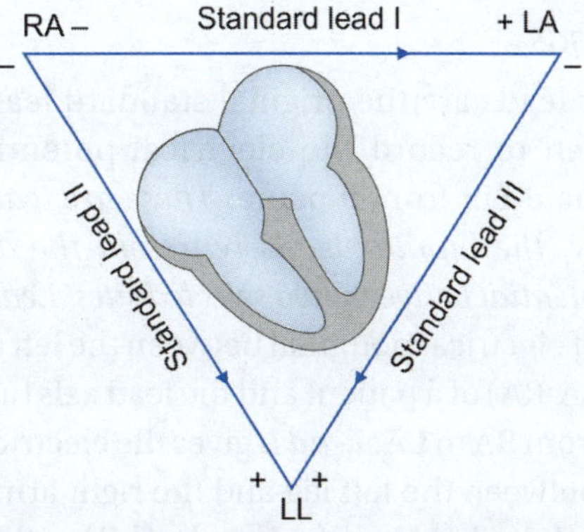

Fig. 5: Einthoven's triangle. (LA: left arm; LL: left leg; RA: right arm)

*situated on frontal or coronal plane of our body and looks at the heart from its sides (**Fig. 4**).*

The sides or angles from which these leads look at the heart depend upon the lead in question. *Thus, the lead aVR looks at the cavity of the heart from patient's right shoulder. Whereas, the lead aVL looks at the cavity of the heart from patient's left shoulder and the lead aVF looks directly at the heart from the foot end of patient* (**Fig. 5**).

In *standard lead I*, the lead axis is derived from the placement of positive (+ve) electrode (lead) on the left arm and negative (–ve) electrode (lead) on the right arm of the patient. In *standard lead II*, the lead axis is derived from the placement of positive (+ve) electrode (lead) on the left foot and negative (–ve) electrode on the right arm of the patient. In the *standard lead III*, the lead axis is derived from the placement of negative (–ve) electrode (lead) on the left arm and positive (+ve) electrode on the left foot of the patient. *These standard I, II, and III leads are also called the bipolar leads and are the original leads described by Einthoven. All the ECG machines also have a connection with the right leg of patient by an electrode and this acts as a ground wire and plays no role in the production of ECG.*

Horizontal Plane Leads

These leads are situated or oriented on the horizontal or transverse plane of heart and consists of all the precordial chest leads, such as leads V_1-V_9, leads V_{3R-9R}, leads $3V_{1-9}$, and leads $2V_{1-9}$. These leads will be described later.

Sagittal Plane Leads

These leads are situated on the sagittal plane of heart and measure the electrical potential of cardiac activity in sagittal plane. The example of sagittal plane lead is the esophageal lead.

According to the polarity, the leads can also be classified into two groups: (1) bipolar leads and (2) unipolar leads **(Figs. 6A and B)**.

Bipolar Leads

The bipolar leads are the original standard leads, selected by Einthoven to record the electrical potential of heart and are situated in frontal plane. *These are leads I, II, and III. Actually, the bipolar leads represent the difference of electrical potential between two selected sites. Lead I* gives the difference of electrical potential between the left arm and the right arm (LA-RA) of a patient and the lead axis (axis of lead I) is directed from RA to LA. *Lead II* gives the electrical potential difference between the left leg and the right arm (LL-RA) of a patient and the lead axis (axis of lead II) is directed from RA to LL. *Lead III* shows the potential difference between the left leg and the left arm (LL-LA), and the lead axis (axis of lead III) is directed from LA to LL.

The relationship of electrical potential between these three bipolar leads is expressed algebraically by Einthoven's equation. The equation states that Lead II = Lead I + Lead III, i.e., amplitude of any deflection in lead II is equivalent to the sum of the amplitude of deflections in lead I and II.

Unipolar Leads

The use of unipolar leads in clinical practice was introduced by Wilson, in 1932.

The examples of unipolar leads are:

- Unipolar extremity or limb leads in frontal plane: aVR, aVL, and aVF
- Unipolar chest leads in horizontal plane: V_1, V_2, V_3, V_4, V_5, V_6, V_7, V_8, V_9, V_{3R-9R}, $3V_{1-9}$, $2V_{1-9}$, $6V_{1-9}$, and $3V_{3R-9R}$.
- Esophageal leads in sagittal plane
- Unipolar intracardiac leads.

All the unipolar extremity or limb leads and chest leads are designated as V and unipolar esophageal leads are designated as E.

Unipolar extremity or limb leads: There are three unipolar limb leads. These are: (1) right arm (VR) lead, (2) left arm (VL) lead, and (3) left foot (VF) lead, where V denotes unipolarity. In these unipolar limb leads, among the two electrodes, one is an exploring electrode and acts as a positive end. The negative end of that lead is not actually negative, but is at "0" potential. So, these leads are called the unipolar leads and they actually measure or represent the amount of potential at that point of heart for a given lead and not the difference of electrical potential (where as the bipolar leads measure the potential difference) between the two electrodes of that particular lead. But, technically we may call this unipolar lead as bipolar one, because it has two poles **(Fig. 7)**.

The mechanism by which the *unipolar limb lead* works is described below. It is considered that the heart lies at the center of an equilateral triangle, called the Einthoven's triangle which is formed by the three standard limb leads I, II, and III. According to Einthoven, the sum of potential differences of these three leads at any instant is zero **(Fig. 8)**.

Therefore, RA + LA + LL = 0

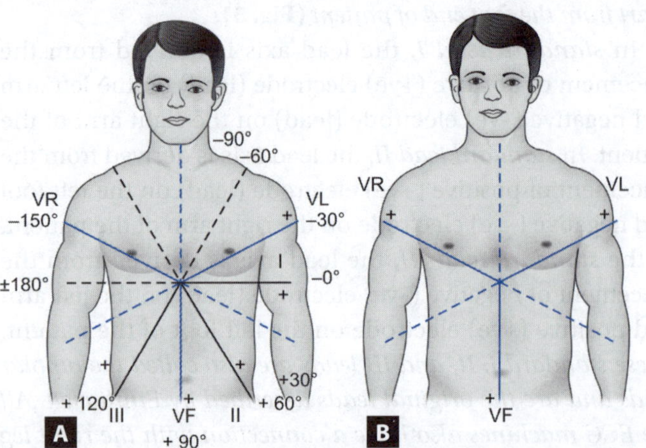

A

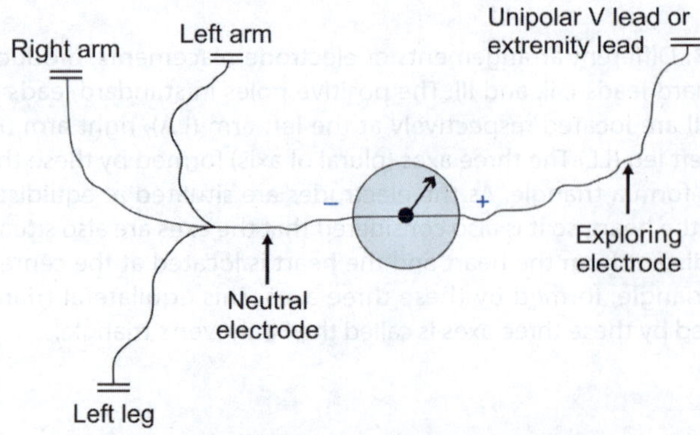

B

Figs. 6A and B: (A) Total frontal (coronal) plane leads both bipolar and unipolar limb leads and (B) Only frontal plane unipolar leads.

Fig. 7: Derivation of unipolar (chest and extremity) leads. The neutral limb is connected to the negative pole of galvanometer. The exploring electrode is connected to the positive pole of galvanometer.

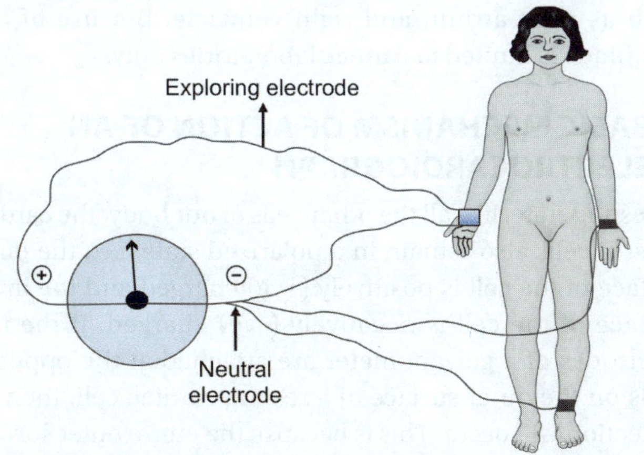

Fig. 8: Derivation of lead aVR. Here, the right arm has connections from both the neutral and the exploring electrodes.

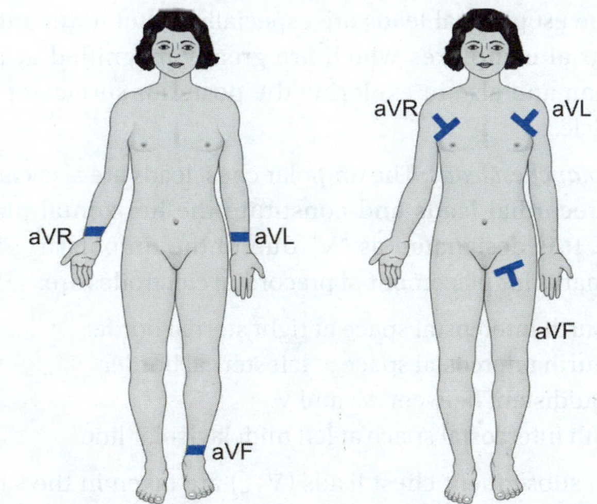

Fig. 9: Diagrammatic representation of unipolar extremity leads.

Hence, when these three leads are at first connected together and then finally to one end of a galvanometer and the other end of the galvanometer is attached to the exploring electrode (this is how the unipolar lead is formed), then unipolar limb lead will be formed and the machine will record the true potential of body tissue under that exploring electrode **(Fig. 9)**.

However, using the above technique, the electrical potential obtained by the exploring electrode of unipolar limb lead is of low voltage. This low voltage can be augmented by omitting the connection of neutral terminal to the limb which is being tested and allowing it to hang free. Then, the unipolar limb lead is called the augmented limb lead and designated as aVR, aVL, and aVF (where "a" stands for the word augmented) **(Fig. 10)**.

Lead aVR (or AVR) is the augmented ("a" or "A") unipolar (V) right arm (R) lead and is usually oriented toward the cavity of heart from right shoulder. So, all the deflections, such as the P, QRS, and T are normally negative in this lead. This is because the vector of electrical current, making all these waves, passes away from this lead. The lead aVL (AVL) is the augmented unipolar left arm lead and is oriented to the anterolateral or superior surface of heart from left shoulder. The lead aVF (AVF) is the augmented unipolar left leg lead and is oriented to the inferior surface of the heart from left leg.

Unipolar esophageal leads: The unipolar esophageal leads are taken from within esophagus at sagittal plane of heart and constitute the sagittal plane leads. A nasal catheter, which is threaded with a wire and having an electrode attached to its tip, is passed through the nares into esophagus. Using this as exploring terminal and zero potential at other terminal, a unipolar esophageal lead can be obtained. This is designated as E lead. The nomenclature of different types of esophageal lead is derived from the distance from the tip of the nares to the position of electrode in esophagus in centimeters.

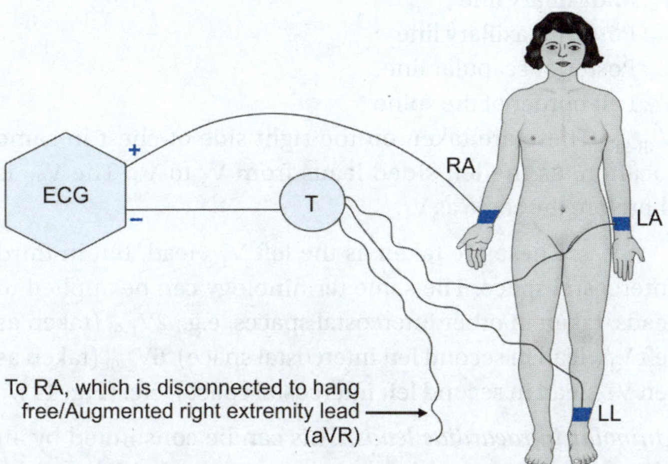

Fig. 10: Principle of augmented unipolar extremity leads. All modern electrocardiograph (ECG) machines are so designed that the augmented unipolar extremity leads can be taken with the same electrode attachment on the body which are used for the standard leads and chest leads by just turning the selector dial to aVR, aVL, and aVF. Unipolar (not augmented) chest leads are also taken by applying the electrodes on the chest to any desired position and turning the selector dial of the ECG machine to the V position. If a modern ECG machine is not available, an ECG machine that can record standard leads like I, II, and III can also be used to obtain the augmented extremity leads satisfactorily. To get this, one first constructs an indifferent electrode T by attaching RA, LA, and LL electrodes together and then to the negative pole of the machine. Then, the connection of the neutral terminal to the limb which is being tested, is disconnected and is allowed to hang free and the exploring positive side of the machine is attached to that limb. This will produce an augmented version of the unipolar limb leads.

Thus, E_{50} represents a unipolar esophageal lead, at a distance of 50 cm from nares. Lead $E_{40\text{-}50}$ usually reflects the posterior surface of left ventricle. Lead $E_{15\text{-}25}$ reflects the atrial area and $E_{25\text{-}35}$ reflects the region of AV groove.

The esophageal leads are especially useful in recording the atrial complexes which are greatly magnified at this location and also in exploring the posterior surface of left ventricle.

Unipolar chest leads: The unipolar chest leads are also called the precordial leads and constitute the horizontal plane leads. It is designated as "V" due to the unipolarity. The landmarks for placement of precordial electrodes are:

V_1: Fourth intercostal space at right sternal border
V_2: Fourth intercostal space at left sternal border
V_3: Equidistant between V_2 and V_4
V_4: Fifth intercostal space at left midclavicular line.

All subsequent chest leads (V_{5-9}) are taken in the same horizontal plane as V_4.

V_5: Anterior axillary line
V_6: Midaxillary line
V_7: Posterior axillary line
V_8: Posterior scapular line
V_9: Left border of the spine
V_{3R-9R}: These are taken on the right side of chest in same location, as the left-sided leads from V_3 to V_9. The V_{2R} is therefore the same as V_1.

$3V_{1-9}$: These are taken as the left V_{1-9} lead, but in third intercostal space. The same terminology can be applied to leads, taken in other intercostal spaces, e.g., $2V_{1-9}$, (taken as left V_{1-9} lead in second left intercostal space), $6V_{1-9}$, (taken as left V_{1-9} lead in second left intercostal space), etc. **(Fig. 11)**.

Unipolar intracardiac leads: This can be constituted by an electrode, contained in a cardiac catheter which can be passed to the various chambers of heart and the ECG can then be recorded from the various intracardiac chambers,

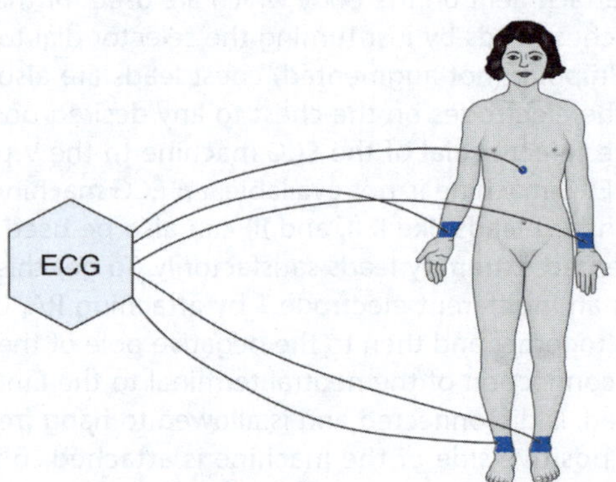

Fig. 11: Unipolar chest (precordial) leads in a modern electrocardiogram (ECG) equipment. It records the potential difference in horizontal plane, without being influenced by the actual potential from an indifferent electrode. The unipolar precordial lead does not record only the electrical potential from a small area of underlying myocardium, but also records all the electrical events of the entire cardiac cycle, as viewed from the selected lead site.

such as right atrium and right ventricle. But use of this technique is limited to cardiac laboratories only.

BASIC MECHANISM OF ACTION OF AN ELECTROCARDIOGRAPH

In resting state, like all the other cells of our body, the cardiac muscle cells also remain in a polarized state, i.e., the outer surface of the cell is positively (+ve) charged and the inner surface of the cell is negatively (–ve) charged. If the two electrodes of a galvanometer are attached at the opposite ends on the outer surface of a resting cardiac cell, then no deflection will occur. This is because the entire outer surface of the cardiac muscle cell has the same +ve charge and the measured potential difference will be zero **(Fig. 12)**.

But, when the muscle cell is stimulated or activated, then the surface of the stimulated portion of the cell becomes electrically negative (as the positive charges pass into the cell). This process is termed as the depolarization. Then, an impulse of this negative charge will progress along the outer surface of the cell toward its other end which is still positive **(Figs. 12 and 13)**.

When this impulse passes through many resting (polarized) cells of an organ, then those cells which are initially activated or depolarized will have negative charges on their surface, while those not yet activated will have

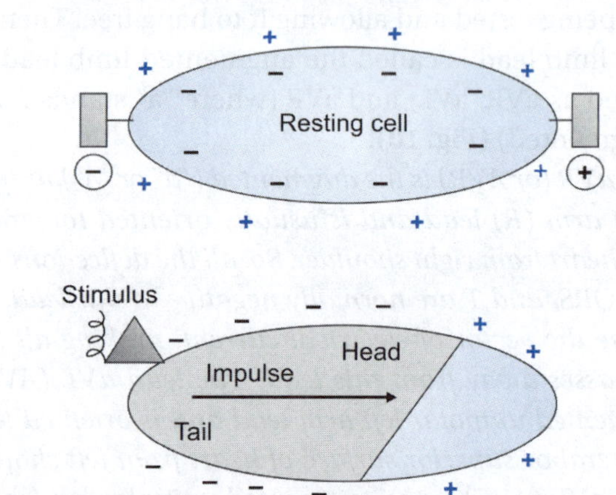

Fig. 12: This figure shows electrical potential of a resting and a stimulated muscle.

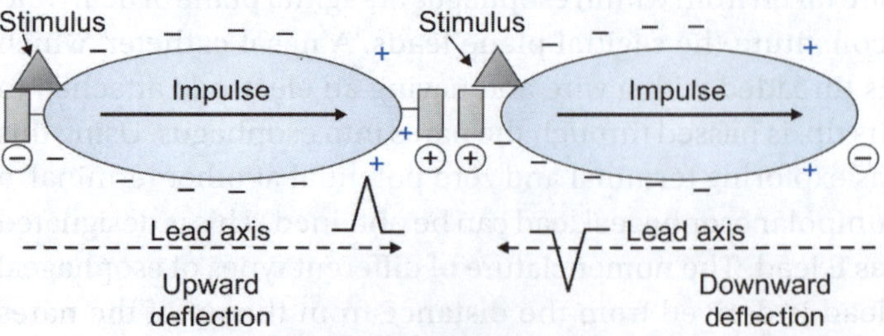

Fig. 13: Process of depolarization.

positive charges on their surface. Therefore, a sum-up potential difference of electrical charges will exist between the surface of the excitable cells and the surface of the adjacent nonexcited resting cells of the same organ. So, a current will flow from the depolarized area of this organ (heart) to the nondepolarized area of that organ.

Now, this flow of current will have a positive charged head and a negative charged tail. So, the positive pole of a bipolar lead or a unipolar lead, oriented toward the oncoming positive charged head, will record a positive or upward deflection. On the other hand, if the positive pole of a bipolar lead or a unipolar lead is oriented toward the receding negative charged tail-end of the flow of current, then it will record a negative or downward deflection in ECG (Fig. 13).

Therefore, the direction in which an impulse spreads through the muscle of heart and the position of the positive electrode of a lead in relation to the direction of the spread of impulse will determine the positive or negative deflection in ECG tracing. Thus, for example, an upright QRS complex in any particular lead means the flow of current during ventricular depolarization (i.e., the QRS vector) is directed toward the positive pole of that particular lead. Alternatively, if the QRS is inverted in any particular lead, it means that the QRS vector is directed away from the positive pole of that particular lead. This principle is also applied to all the electrocardiographic deflections, such as P, T, U, and the ST segment (if it is deviated).

If the positive electrodes of a lead are placed on the midportion of the passage of current (wave of depolarization), then the deflection will be biphasic, because the initial positive deflection will be upward due to the orientation of advancing positively charged head of flow of current toward the positive pole of electrode and the second negative deflection will be downward due to the orientation of negatively charged receding tail of current toward the positive pole of electrode **(Fig. 14)**.

On the other hand, if the two muscle mass is stimulated in the middle with the positive electrodes of lead oriented at either end of the muscle, then both the positive electrodes of lead will show positive deflection of depolarization of equal magnitude. This is because both the positive electrodes recognize the positively charged head of passing current **(Figs. 15 and 16)**.

If the two muscle masses are of markedly different sizes (analogous to the right and left ventricle) and are stimulated at a central point of their junction, then a large positive deflection will be produced by the positive electrode oriented over the larger muscle mass and a small positive deflection, followed by a deep negative deflection or an

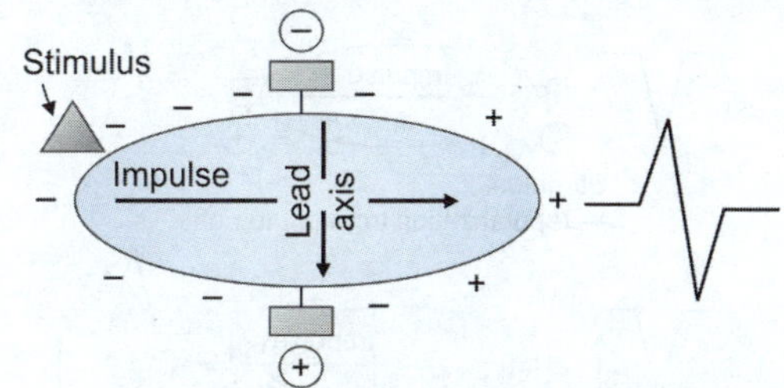

Fig. 14: Process of downward deflection.

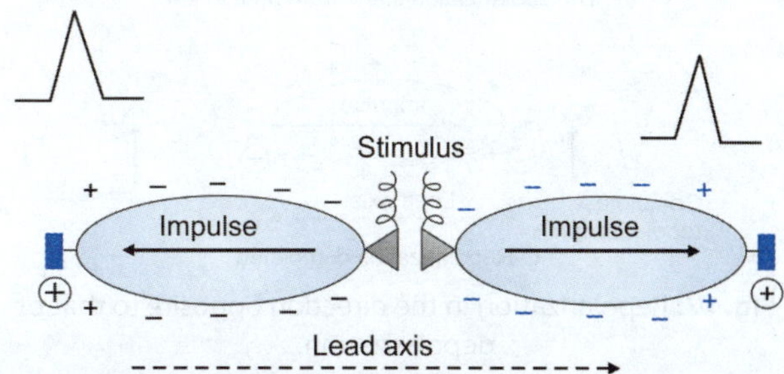

Fig. 15: Two muscle masses of equal size.

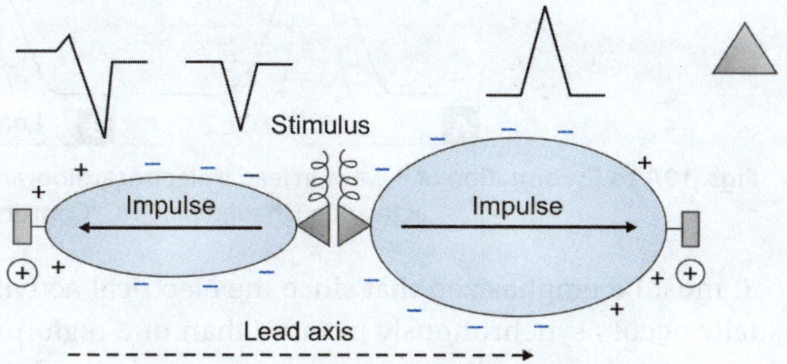

Fig. 16: Two muscle masses of different sizes.

entirely negative deflection will be produced by the positive electrode oriented over the small muscle mass. This is because the positive deflection due to the depolarization of smaller muscle mass will be masked by the negative deflection due to the depolarization of larger muscle mass and the electrode over the smaller muscle mass will partially or fully recognize the larger muscle mass **(Figs. 16 and 17)**.

The return of stimulated muscle mass to its resting state is known as repolarization. If repolarization occurs in the same direction as that of depolarization, then deflection on positive pole of galvanometer will be opposite to that of depolarization. But, if the repolarization occurs in the opposite direction to that of depolarization, then the deflection on positive pole of galvanometer will be same as that of depolarization. Since this flow of current is electromagnetic in nature like depolarization, so it has also a vector. Thus, it also possesses both magnitude and direction **(Fig. 18)**.

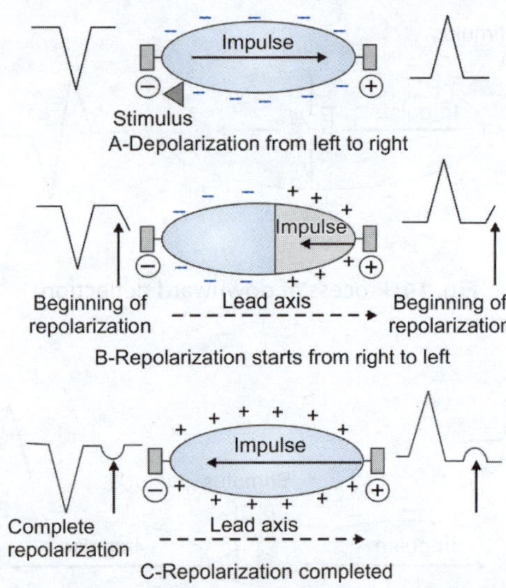

Fig. 17: Repolarization in the direction opposite to that of depolarization.

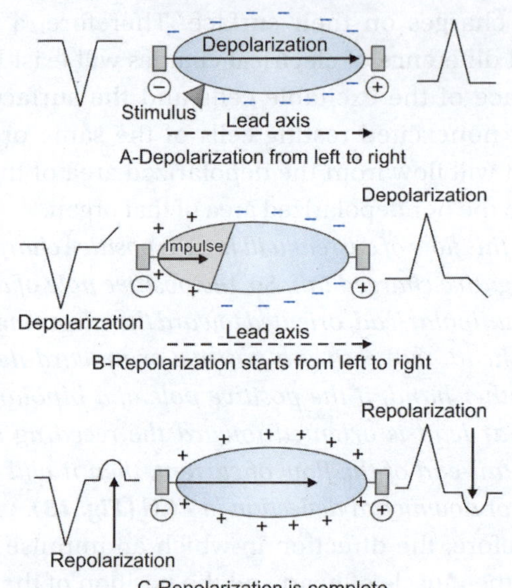

Fig. 18: Repolarization occurs in the same plane as depolarization.

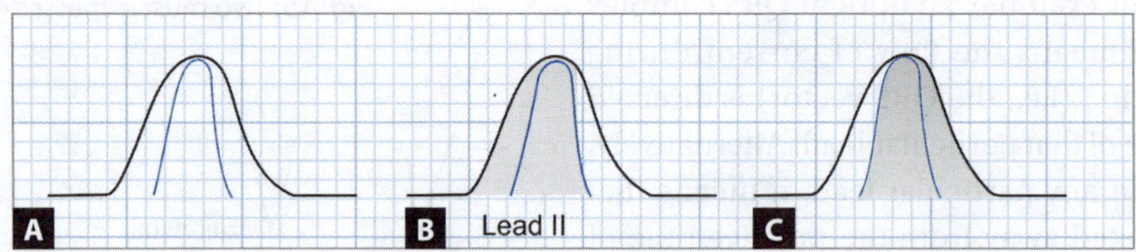

Figs. 19A to C: Formation of P-wave in lead II electrocardiogram (ECG): (A) A normal composite P-wave. (B) Contribution of right atrial activation (shaded part). (C) Contribution of left atrial activation (shaded part).

It must be emphasized that since the electrical activity usually occurs synchronously in more than one region of heart, so the electrocardiograph at any given moment reflects the resultant force of several small synchronous electrical activity, traveling in different directions.

GENESIS OF P-WAVE

The P-wave is the deflection in ECG, produced by atrial depolarization. The initial depolarization in heart begins in SA node. *But, this initial depolarization of SA node cannot be recorded in clinical ECG.* Then, the impulse generated from SA node traverses to AV node through three internodal pathways (Bachmann, Wenckebach, Thorel) and *depolarizes the whole atrium (both right and left), producing the whole atrial contraction and P-wave.* As the SA node is situated in right atrium, so the right atrial activation begins first which is followed by left atrial activation. Hence, the P-wave is a composite deflection of both the right and left atrial activation. The right atrial activation constitutes the ascending limb and the left atrial activation constitutes the descending limb of P-wave **(Figs. 19A to C)**. *There is no clear and normal range for P-wave height, but any P-wave over 2.5 mm (2.5 small squares) in height should arouse suspicion.*

*Normally, the width of P-wave is <0.08 seconds (two small squares). But, the maximum duration of P-wave is 0.11 seconds (**Figs. 20A to C**).*

Normally, the vector of P-wave (the direction of current, flowing from SA node to AV node) is oriented inferiorly (in the frontal plane) and to the left and slightly anterior (in the horizontal plane). Therefore, the polarity (upward or downward deflection) of P-wave in any given lead will depend on the relation of the positive electrode of that lead (axis of lead) to the direction of this vector (axis of P-wave). In the frontal plane, the P-wave vector (axis) is usually aligned or parallel to the direction (axis) of standard lead II. So, the P-wave is positive and best seen and studied in standard lead II **(Fig. 21)**.

In other leads of frontal plane, such as in lead I and lead aVF and in some leads of the horizontal planes, and in V3-V6 leads (in the horizontal plane, the P vector is directed leftward and anteriorly), the P vector (axis of P-wave) is directed toward the positive pole of these leads. So, in these abovementioned leads, the P-wave is upright. The normal axis of P-wave is directed in-between +45° to +65°, clockwise. Hence, an axis of P-wave of less than +45° is reflected as left axis deviation and a P-wave axis of greater than +70° is

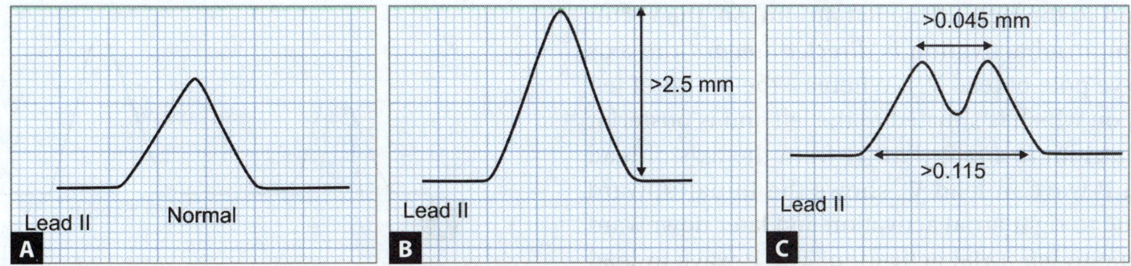

Figs. 20A to C: The figure shows: (A) Normal P-wave in lead II. (B) P-wave due to right atrial enlargement in lead II. (C) P-wave due to left atrial enlargement in lead II.

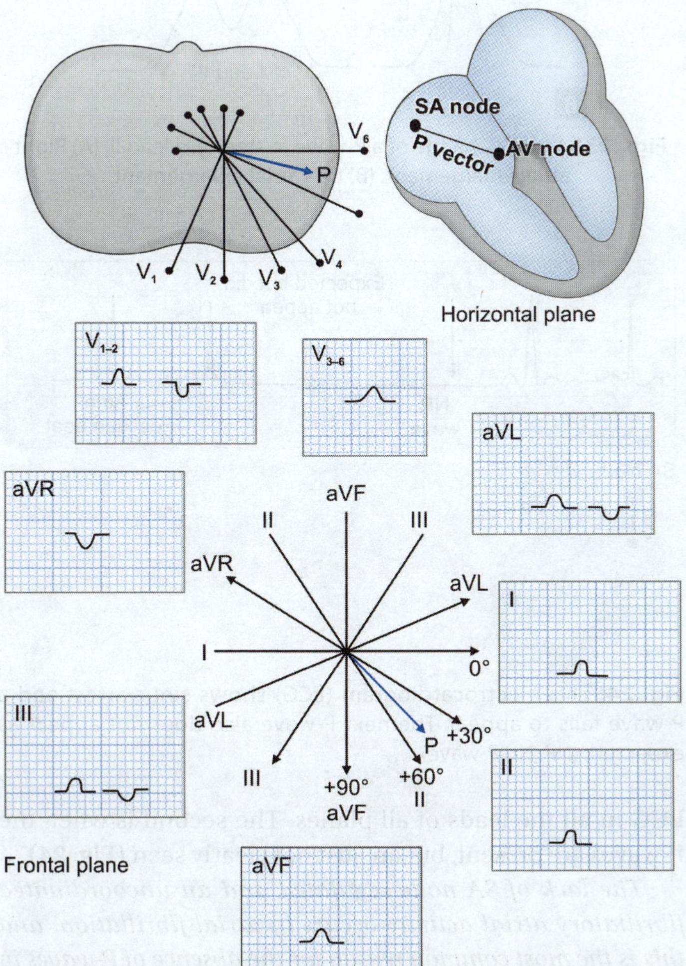

Fig. 21: Direction of normal P vector in frontal and horizontal planes. The normal P vector in frontal plane lies in-between 0° and +90°. So, a P vector in-between 0° and +30° will produce an inverted P-wave in lead III and a P vector past +60° will produce an inverted P-wave in lead aVL. The amount of clockwise or anticlockwise orientation (rotation) of P vector in horizontal plane will also determine whether the P-wave will be upright or inverted in lead V_1 to V_6. (AV: atrioventricular; SA: sinoatrial)

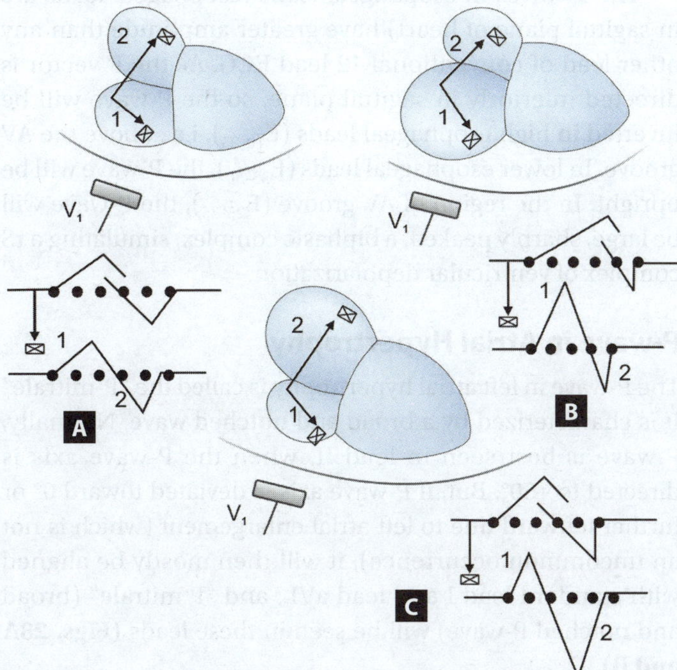

Figs. 22A to C: Figure A illustrates the normal activation of both the atria, (when they are normal in size), the P vector and its effects on V_1. **Figure B** illustrates the effect of right atrial enlargement in lead V_1. **Figure C** illustrates the effect of left atrial enlargement in lead V_1.

Alternatively, during right axis deviation of P-wave, when it is directed to the region of +80° to +90°, then it is most aligned to the lead aVF and so in this circumstances, it is best evaluated in this lead. In lead aVR, the P-wave is always inverted, as the direction of the vector (axis) of P-wave is always away from the direction of axis of this unipolar lead. The direction of this unipolar aVR lead is toward the right shoulder, because the positive pole of this lead is at right shoulder. In lead III, aVL, V_1, and V_2, the P-wave may be upright, biphasic, flat or inverted, according to the direction of the axis of these leads (according to the +ve pole of these axis) and the direction of the axis of P-wave **(Figs. 22A to C)**.

The P-wave in lead V_1 is usually biphasic, having an initial positive and a terminal negative deflection. The explanation for this biphasic P-wave in lead I and V_1 is as follows: the right atrium, with its SA node, which is activated first, is situated

reflected as right axis deviation. In left axis deviation, when the P-wave is directed toward the 0°, then it will be best aligned to the standard lead I and is best evaluated in this lead.

anteriorly and to the right of the left atrium. So, the vector (axis) of right atrial activation *is directed toward* the axis of lead V_1 (+ve pole of lead V_1). Whereas, the vector of left atrial activation which is situated to the left and is posterior to the right atrium *is directed away* from the axis of lead V_1.Thus, the P-wave in lead V_1 shows the initial upward deflection due to right atrial activation and later downward deflection due to left atrial activation. The P-wave in lead V_1 is thus a composite deflection of both the right and left atrial activation making it biphasic.

The P-waves in esophageal leads (esophageal leads are in sagittal plane of heart) have greater amplitude than any other lead of conventional 12 lead ECG. As the P vector is directed inferiorly in sagittal plane, so the P-wave will be inverted in high esophageal leads (E_{10-25}), i.e., above the AV groove. In lower esophageal leads (E_{35-50}), the P-wave will be upright. In the region of AV groove (E_{25-35}), the P-wave will be large, sharply peaked, a biphasic complex, simulating a rS complex of ventricular depolarization.

P-wave in Atrial Hypertrophy

The P-wave in left atrial hypertrophy is called the "P-mitrale". It is characterized by a broad and notched wave. Normally, P-wave is best seen in lead II, when the P-wave axis is directed to +50°. But, if P-wave axis is deviated toward 0° or further leftward due to left atrial enlargement (which is not an uncommon occurrence), it will then mostly be aligned with standard lead I and lead aVL, and "P mitrale" (broad and notched P-wave) will be seen in these leads **(Figs. 23A and B)**.

The broad P-wave, in left atrial hypertrophy, is due to the delayed activation of hypertrophied or enlarged left atrium (separation of right and left atrial component in the genesis of P-wave). In lead V_1, a wide, slurred, biphasic P-wave is characteristically seen in left atrial hypertrophy, where the downward component of P-wave is most prominent. Clinically, the left atrial enlargement is found in systemic hypertension, concomitant with left ventricular hypertrophy, mitral stenosis, mitral incompetence, etc. The right atrial hypertrophy is characterized by tall, slender, peaked P-waves, called "P-pulmonale" and is found in lead II, III, and lead aVF. Right atrial hypertrophy is found in chronic obstructive pulmonary diseases.

Completely Absent P-wave

There are two reasons for the P-wave to be absent from ECG. The first is when there is not a single coordinated full atrial contraction or activity, regulated by SA node, which is responsible for the formation of P-wave. Hence, as the P-waves are not being formed, so are completely absent from

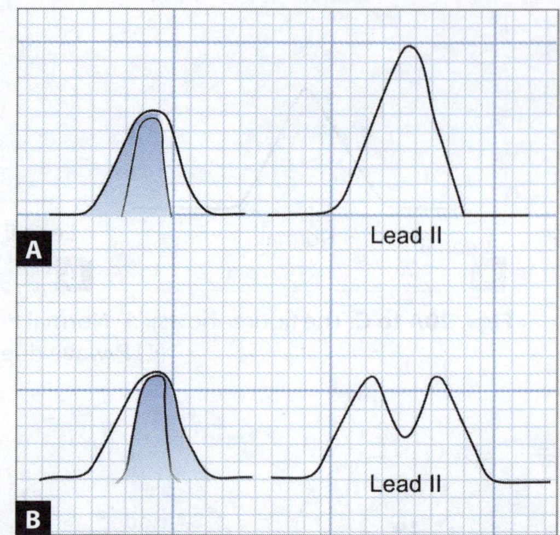

Figs. 23A and B: Change of a P-wave in standard lead II. (A) Right atrial enlargement. (B) Left atrial enlargement.

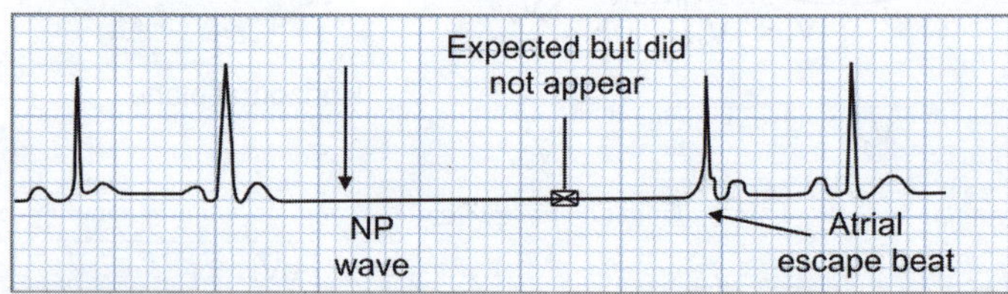

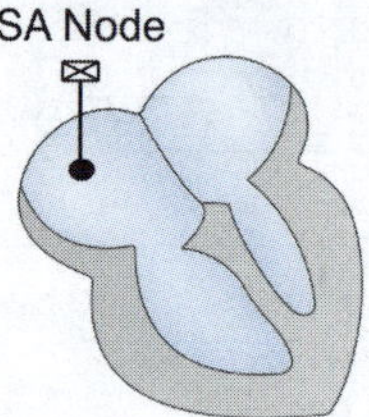

Fig. 24: This electrocardiogram (ECG) shows sinus arrest and a P-wave fails to appear. The next P-wave also does not appear as expected. (NP: No P-wave)

ECG in all the leads of all planes. The second is when the P-waves are present, but are just not clearly seen **(Fig. 24)**.

The lack of SA node regulated and an uncoordinated fibrillatory atrial activity occurs in atrial fibrillation, and this is the most common reason for the absence of P-waves in ECG of all the leads of all planes. In such situation, instead of a definite P-wave, the chaotic atrial activity produces a low-amplitude oscillatory or fibrillatory waves in ECG. These are called the fibrillatory or "f" waves. So, the atrial fibrillation can be recognized by (1) the absence of P-wave, (2) the presence of fibrillatory waves in the place of P-waves, and (3) the erratic formation of QRS complexes (irregular pulse). On the other hand, the configuration of QRS complexes is normal, unless there is concomitant bundle branch block. The ECG manifestation of atrial fibrillation is best seen in frontal (coronal) plane leads, especially standard leads II, III, and aVF. The fibrillatory or "f" waves are usually of negative

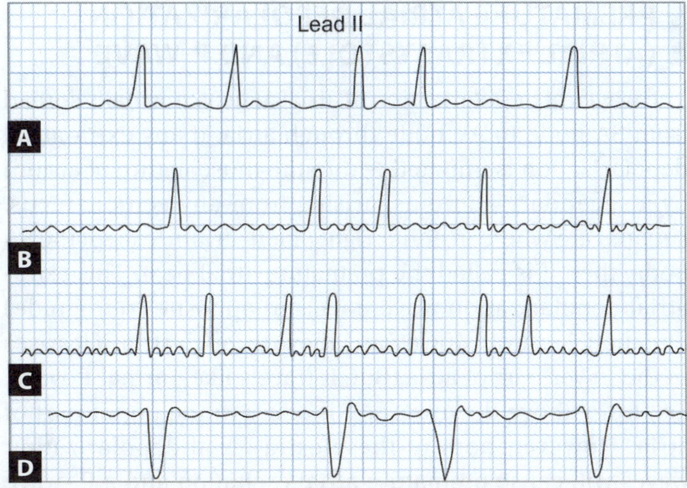

Figs. 25A to D: Electrocardiogram (ECG) tracings in lead II show the various manifestations of atrial fibrillation. (A) Long-standing atrial fibrillation, with a smooth slightly undulating baseline and slow irregular ventricular response, with narrow QRS complexes. (B) Coarser and more recent fibrillation with relatively slow ventricular response. Here, the baseline is irregular and ragged. (C) The same features as B, but with a rapid ventricular response with narrow QRS complexes. (D) Atrial fibrillation with complete atrioventricular (AV) block (broad QRS complexes).

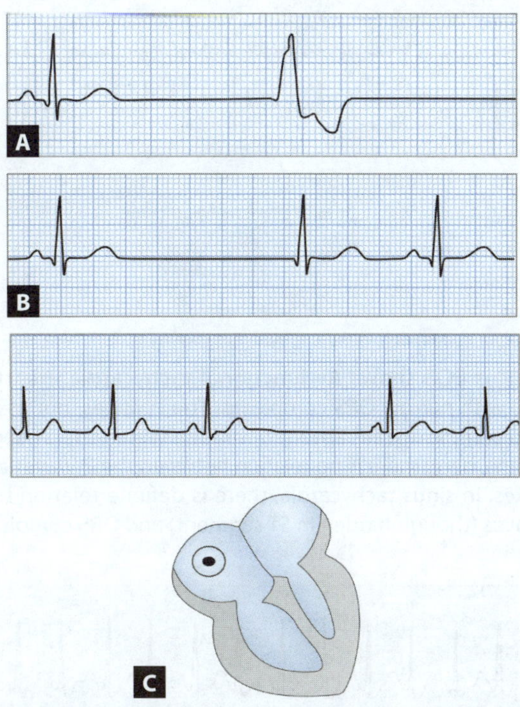

Figs. 26A to C: (A) Figure shows SA block with ventricular escape rhythm and (B) Shows SA block with escape junctional rhythm. (C) This ECG shows sinoatrial block. P-wave fails to appear at its predetermined place, but next P-wave appears where expected.

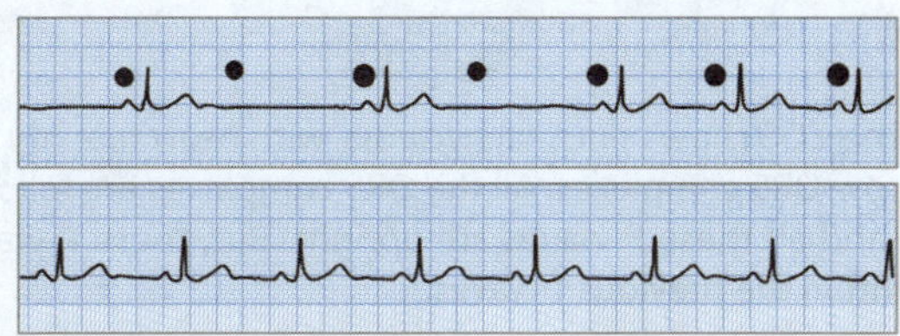

Fig. 27: This ECG shows SA exit block with 2:1 ratio, characterized by slow regular rhythm and HR becomes double after administration of atropine.

deflection in these leads, reflecting caudal to cranial atrial activation. In the horizontal lead V1, in contrast to the frontal plane leads, the P-wave usually shows an isoelectric feature or is usually masked by the f-waves (**Figs. 25A to D**).

The P-waves will also be completely absent if there is prolonged period of sinus arrest or SA block. In these conditions, the atrial activation does not occur, because SA node either fails to depolarize (sinus arrest) or fails to transmit the depolarization from the SA node to the atrial musculature (SA block). Either condition may cause ventricular asystole, but more commonly an escape AV junctional or escape ventricular rhythm occurs (**Fig. 26A and B**).

During a sinus arrest in ECG, the P-wave will suddenly fail to appear at its expected place, and there is a gap of variable length, until the sinus node fires again and again a P-wave appears or an escape ventricular beat takes over the responsibility. On the other hand, in SA block, the sinus node depolarizes normally (which cannot be recorded in ECG). But this impulse fails to reach the atria from depolarized SA node. So, it is also called an exit block. However, like the sinus arrest, the P-wave in exit block also fails to appear at its expected place, but the next one usually appears exactly where it is expected, without any gap (**Fig. 26C**).

Rarely, the SA exit block may occur at regular intervals, e.g., 2:1 ratio. This resembles the slow regular rhythm of sinus bradycardia. But, the diagnosis can only be established, when in contrast to the gradual acceleration of sinus bradycardia,

the sinus rate suddenly doubles with the effect of atropine (**Fig. 27**).

In SA block, neither the P-wave (atrial activity or contraction), nor the QRS complex (ventricular activity or contraction) is recorded at the moment of block. Whereas, in AV block, all the P-waves are recorded, but the P-waves of blocked beat is not followed by a QRS complex. SA exit block is found in the same conditions as in sinus bradycardia and is the result of an increased vagal tone. It occurs in normal high vagotonic persons, e.g., athletes. It can also be produced by pressure on carotid sinus or eyeball (during eye surgery) or other increased vagal reflexes (**Fig. 28**).

It is very mandatory for the P-waves to be present, except in certain conditions. But, sometimes is not evident in many ECG tracings. So, an ECG should be searched carefully

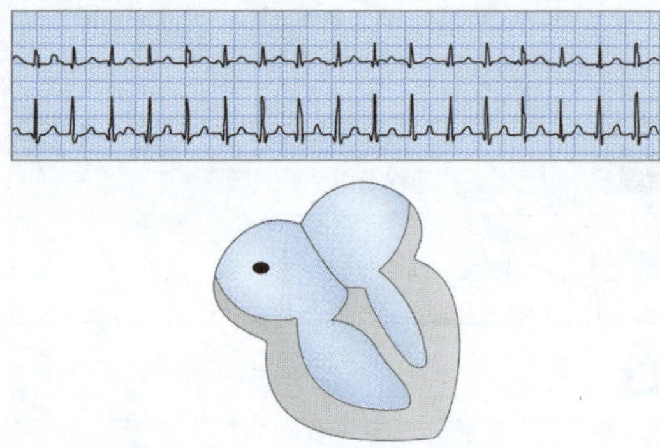

Fig-28: This ECG shows AV junctional tachycardia. Heart rate is 130/min, with narrow QRS complexes. The P-waves, not associated with QRS complexes, are absent or hidden within the ST segments. That means, here, there is no relation between the P-waves and QRS complexes. In sinus tachycardia, there is definite relation between the P-waves (though hidden in ST segment) and QRS complexes.

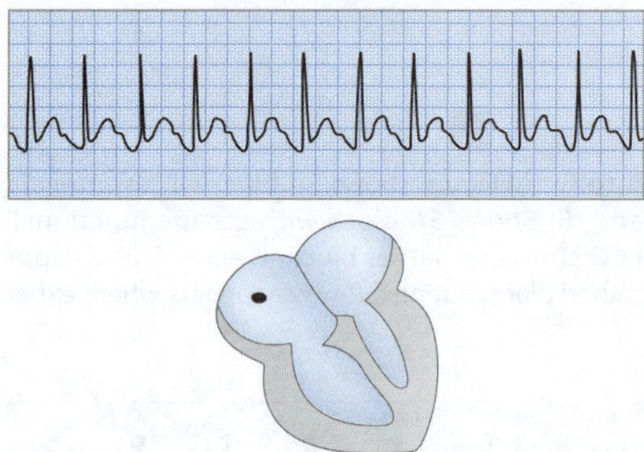

Fig. 29: This ECG shows sinus tachycardia, with heart rate of 150/min, with narrow QRS complexes. All the QRS complexes are followed by P-waves and all these P-waves are upright. But, these P-waves are hidden within the previous T-waves.

for evidence of P-wave, before concluding that they are absent. This is because the P-waves are often hidden by QRS complexes in any very severe tachycardia. For example, in *AV junctional tachycardia* with a heart rate (HR) of 130 beats/min, at a first glance the P-waves appear to be absent. On close inspection, they can just be seen, buried within the ST segment. Even in sinus tachycardia, at high rates the P-wave may be overlapped with the T-wave of previous beat, making it hard to identify **(Fig. 29)**.

In ventricular tachycardia, the retrograde (backward) conduction of ventricular impulses through AV node may cause each ventricular complex to be followed by an abnormal P-wave which may not be immediately obvious and may also be inverted. Even more importantly, the independent atrial activity from SA node can occur during ventricular tachycardia and these P-waves can be buried anywhere within the QRS complex. So, the evidences of independent atrial activity is a very useful clue in the differentiation of ventricular and supraventricular tachycardia.

PREMATURE ATRIAL DEPOLARIZATION (ATRIAL EXTRASYSTOLE) AND P-WAVE

The waves of depolarization of atrial activity normally spread from SA node to AV node through atria. If any extra-atrial depolarization is initiated within the musculature of atrium by a secondary stimulus, arising from any ectopic focus, situated anywhere in either right or left atrium, except the SA node, then it is called the premature atrial beat. This extra-atrial depolarization wave travels in opposite (retrograde) direction, i.e., from downward above through atria, if it arises in the lower part of atria. But, it travels like normal P-wave, i.e., from above downward, if it arises in the upper part of atria. However, both of these extra-atrial depolarization waves will cause premature atrial excitation and a P′-wave in ECG. *Simultaneously, it will also initiate a ventricular complex with normal QRS configuration because ventricular activity, caused by impulses, passing through AV node will produce normal QRS complexes, whereas the ventricular activity, caused by impulses, arising in ventricle below bundle of His will produce wide abnormal QRS complexes.*

From view point, for most of the positive electrode of different leads, this abnormal P-wave which is originating from the lower part of atrium, will show to *move away from them* (positive electrode), rather than to flow toward them and thus an inverted P′-waves (instead of an upright P-wave) will be produced in most of the leads **(Fig. 30)**. However, in aVR lead, this retrograde P′-wave will produce a positive deflection as it is *moved toward* the positive pole of this lead from lower part of atrium. Many abnormal sources of atrial activation which can thus cause retrograde depolarization and inverted P′-waves includes atrial ectopic, AV junctional rhythm, ventricular tachycardia, ventricular ectopic, etc. **(Fig. 31)**.

If an ectopic atrial stimulus arises from the upper end of atrium, then the resulting abnormal P′-wave will have the same normal direction and configuration like the normal P-wave. However, this premature atrial depolarization will usually depolarize the SA node, upsetting its rhythmicity. The next normal sinus impulse, therefore, will not occur as scheduled, because the SA node needs to pass through a complete recovery (repolarization) cycle, before it can

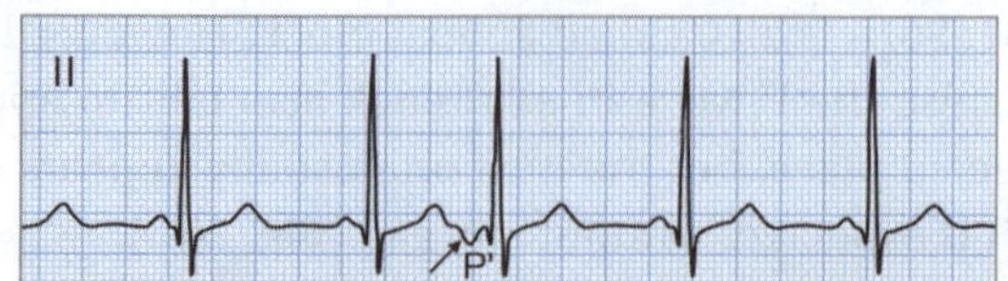

Fig. 30: This ECG shows premature atrial contraction (P′) with low atrial ectopic focus as it is inverted in lead II. This is the reverse of normal P-wave and indicates a low atrial ectopic focus, The QRS complexes are normal.

discharge again. The basic rhythm of SA node is thus disturbed and a pause will follow the ectopic atrial beat. This is called the *compensatory pause of SA node*. This pause is usually incomplete, i.e., it does not fully compensate for the prematurity of extrasystole. This means that, *the sum of the pre- and postectopic intervals (Y-Z) is less than the sum of two consecutive normal intervals (X-Y). We should compare these events with those occasioned by a ventricular extrasystole, when the sinus rhythm is not disturbed and where the compensatory pause is subsequently complete* (**Fig. 32**).

The unifocal atrial extrasystole tends to have a fixed coupling interval, i.e., the interval between the extrasystole and the preceding beat tends to be the same for all unifocal extrasystoles. This fixed coupling with atrial extrasystoles, however, is usually not as constant as that which occurs with ventricular extrasystoles. If an atrial extrasystole (which is conducted to the ventricle) occurs after every atrial normal systole conducted by sinus impulse, then it will result in *ventricular bigeminal* rhythm. If an atrial extrasystole is not conducted to the ventricle and occurs after every conducted sinus impulse, then it will result in an *atrial bigeminal* rhythm and a slow regular ventricular rhythm. Three or more consecutive atrial extrasystoles constitute a paroxysmal atrial tachycardia (**Fig. 33**).

Atrial premature beats may frequently occur in normal individuals. At times, it may occur secondary to stimulation, due to emotional disturbances, tobacco, tea, coffee, etc. Digitalis may also produce such an arrhythmia. Almost any form of organic heart disease, e.g., rheumatic heart disease, chronic coronary artery disease, hyperthyroidism, viral infection, etc., may be responsible for premature atrial beats and in such instances the atrial arrhythmia may be the precursor of paroxysmal atrial tachycardia and atrial fibrillation.

■ WANDERING ATRIAL PACEMAKER

In this type of atrial arrhythmia, normally some impulses arise from SA node, whereas the other ectopic impulses arise from the different ectopic sites of atrium. It may even be from the AV node. As a result, there will be variation of atrial rhythm, changing configuration of P′-wave (due to atrial activation from different ectopic foci) and changing in P′R interval (**Fig. 34**).

Normally, an inverted P-waves in aVR and an upright P-waves in aVF will be found from impulses arising at SA node or from ectopic focus (P′) arising at the upper portion of atrium, whereas an upright P′-wave in aVR and inverted P′-wave in aVF will be found from impulses arising from an ectopic focus situated in the lower portion of atrium or AV junction.

This type of atrial arrhythmia (wandering atrial pacemaker) may also occur in a normal individuals with increased vagal tone. Digitalis may be another important etiological factor for this. Various forms of organic heart diseases, e.g., acute rheumatic disease can also produce this type of arrhythmia.

■ PAROXYSMAL SUPRAVENTRICULAR (ATRIAL) TACHYCARDIA

It is due to rapid electrical discharges from a single or multiple ectopic atrial focus, causing regular and consecutive atrial extrasystoles. It is characterized by regular atrial rhythm at the rate of 160–220 beats/min. This atrial tachycardia differs from sinus tachycardia, as the impulses are generated from an ectopic focus, somewhere, within the atrial myocardium rather than sinus node (**Fig. 35**).

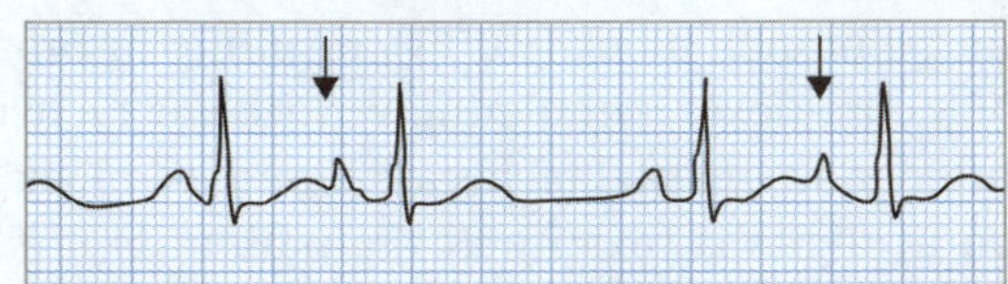

Fig. 31: This is an ECG of alternate atrial extra systole, marked by arrow.

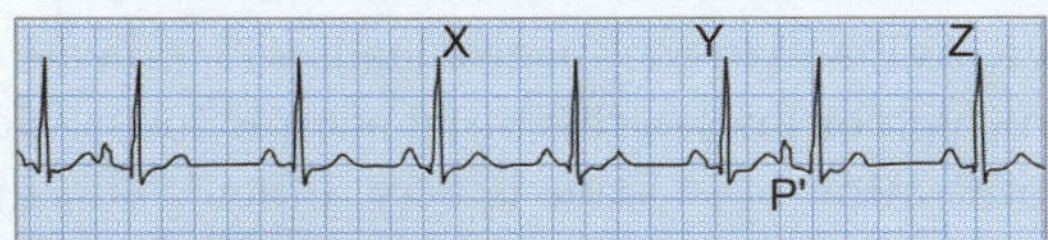

Fig. 32: This is an ECG of atrial extrasystole marked as P′ characterized by positive narrow pointed wave. The sum of pre and post ectopic interval (Y-Z) is less than sum of two consecutive normal sinus interval (X-Y).

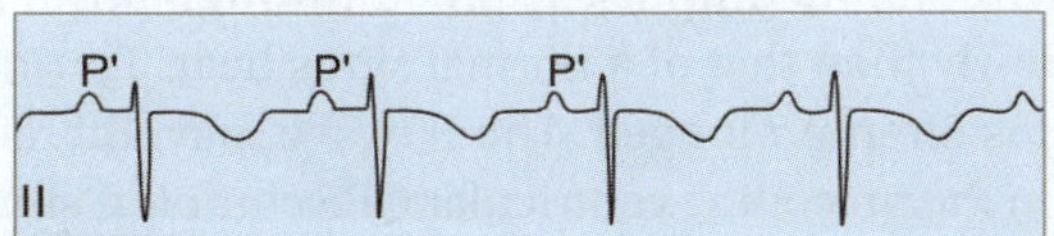

Fig. 33: This is an ECG of high atrial extrasystole. In lead II, upright P′ indicates that the atrial ectopic focus is high enough. The P′ is followed by normal QRS which indicates that the conduction is through the AV node and the Purkinje fibers of ventricle.

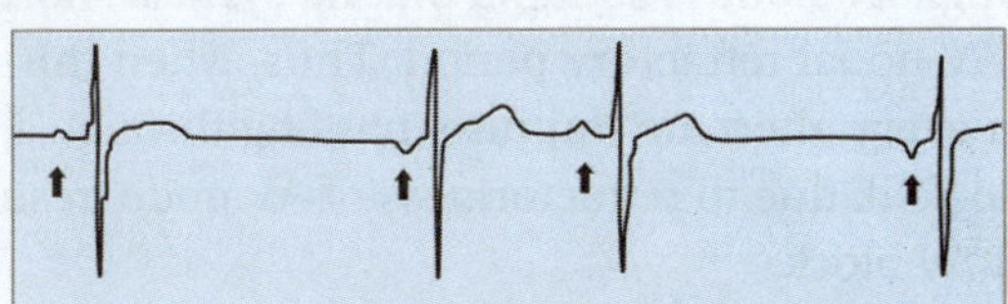

Fig. 34: This is an ECG of a wandering atrial pace maker with four P of different morphology. The rhythm is irregular. There is a marked variation in the morphology of P-waves, indicating varying atrial pacemakers.

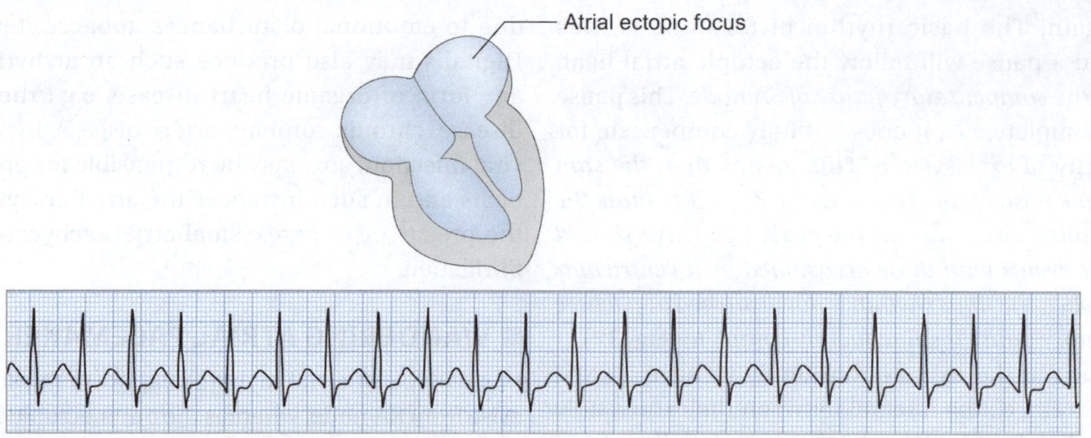

Fig. 35: This is an ECG of PSVT (atrial tachycardia), characterized by HR >160/ min, P-waves are not visible.

Some claim that re-entry mechanism is mainly responsible for this paroxysmal supraventricular tachycardia (PSVT), rather than the ectopic focus which simply fire repeatedly on its own. This re-entry mechanism may be localized within the sinus node, atrial muscle or the AV node, involving conduction in an anterograde direction through AV node or in retrograde direction through an AV bypass tract. Such a bypass tract may also conduct anterogradely, in which case the Wolff–Parkinson–White (WPW) syndrome is said to be present. When the bypass tract conducts only retrogradely, then it is termed as "concealed bypass tract" and in this case QRS complex is normal without any delta waves. In the absence of WPW syndrome (i.e., anterograde conduction through the bypass tract), the re-entry of impulses through AV node or through a concealed bypass tract constitutes for >90% of all PSVTs. This results in atrial rhythm with the following characteristic features: HR >100 beats/min and abnormally shaped P or P'-waves.

In most instances, there is 1:1 AV conduction. But, when the atrial rate goes above 200 beats/min, then the AV node struggles to keep up space with this rapid conduction of impulses and an AV block may precipitate. On reaching AV node, the atrial impulses may be conducted as follows:

- With a normal AV conduction, resulting in normal PR interval
- With first-degree AV block
- With second-degree AV block—the passing of impulses through AV node is so rapid that its cycle is shorter than the AV nodal refractory period. Thus, when this occurs, then every alternate impulse, passing through AV node is blocked, due to refractoriness of AV node, resulting in a 2:1 AV block.

The atrial tachycardia may also be associated with more complex form of second-degree AV block, e.g., 3:2 block. On reaching the ventricles, the atrial impulses may be conducted like normal intraventricular conduction which

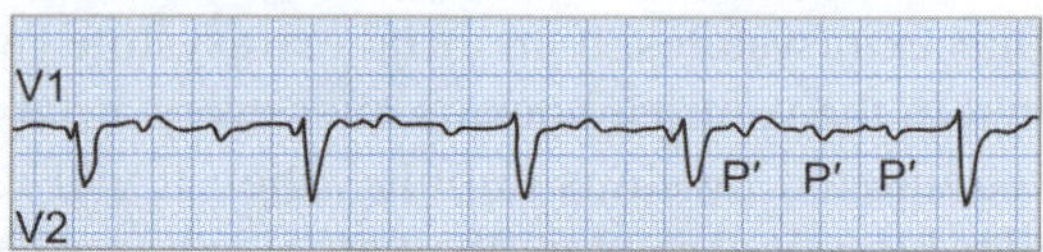

Fig. 36: This ECG shows extra-systolic atrial tachycardia, characterized by varying second degree AV block. The P'-waves are bizarre and the P'–P' interval measures 0.24 second, representing an atrial rate of 250/min. The AV conduction ratio varies between 2:1 and 3:1.

is manifested as rapid regular or irregular QRS complexes (if block is present) or with aberrant ventricular conduction in the presence of left bundle branch block (LBBB) or right bundle branch block (RBBB), resulting in broad and rapid QRS complexes, simulating ventricular tachycardia. The combination of atrial tachycardia and AV block is very common in digitalis toxicity. If the patient is not taking digitalis, then the probable causes of PSVT are: rheumatic heart disease, ischemic heart disease (IHD), sick sinus syndrome (SSS), cardiomyopathy etc. **(Fig. 36)**.

In atrial premature beats, the direction of P'-wave in leads aVR, aVF, and in esophageal leads will indicate the site of origin (high or low) of this atrial ectopic focus. However, the identification of P'-wave is very difficult and the P' to QRS relationship cannot be established with certainty. So, this rhythm is sometimes termed as *supraventricular tachycardia*, because the exact site of origin of these atrial ectopic focuses is not diagnosed and whatever may be the site of origin of ectopic focus, it is above the ventricle. In this type of arrhythmia, the impulses spread through atrial muscle more slowly than that of a normal sinus beat. Thus, the P'R interval is often prolonged. The P'-wave may, therefore, be buried in the preceding ventricular QRS complex, simulating an AV junctional tachycardia **(Fig. 37)**.

When a paroxysmal atrial tachycardia arises from an ectopic atrial focus, which is high in the atrium, then it produces normally directed P-waves. This may be

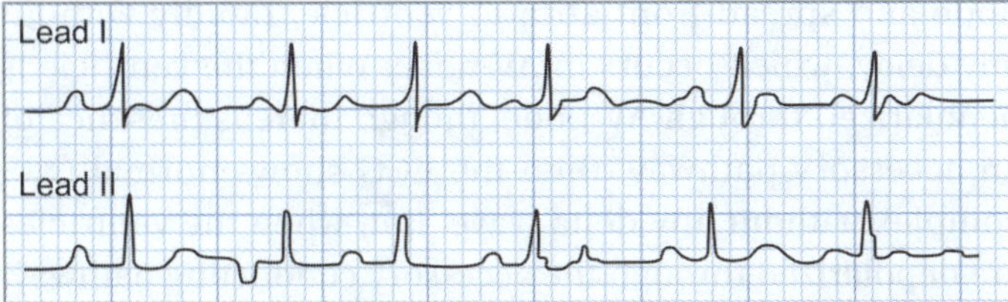

Fig. 37: This electrocardiogram (ECG) shows multifocal atrial tachycardia, where the ventricular rhythm is irregular. Each QRS is preceded by a P-wave which varies in configuration and direction. PR interval varies from beat to beat, and some of the P-waves do not activate the ventricles (blocked atrial beats).Therefore, this ECG tracing represents an atrial tachycardia, resulting from multiple atrial foci (wandering atrial pacemakers).

indistinguishable from a sinus tachycardia arising from SA node at rates of approximately 140–160 beats/min in one single ECG. A constant RR interval without any change with respiration will favor the diagnosis of paroxysmal atrial tachycardia. The response to carotid sinus pressure may also help in the diagnosis. In PSVT, this maneuver may abruptly terminate the attack, whereas in sinus tachycardia, there may be slow, gradual, and slight slowing of HR. If there is no response to carotid sinus pressure, then one must compare the pattern of P or (P′) waves of this tachycardia to the pattern, present during the previous regular sinus rhythm. If there is difference in the configuration of atrial complexes in these two tracings, then the diagnosis of paroxysmal atrial tachycardia is justified.

Paroxysmal supraventricular tachycardia occurs most commonly in normal individuals. It may show no clinical evidence of heart disease. It may occur even in relation to emotional trauma. The lesser common etiological factors of PSVT are rheumatic valvular disease, pulmonary embolism, cardiac surgery, thyrotoxicosis, coronary arterial disease, etc. It is the most common arrhythmia associated with WPW syndrome. Atrial tachycardia with AV block is a common manifestation of digitalis toxicity.

Mechanism of Paroxysmal Supraventricular Tachycardia

Several mechanisms are responsible for the production of paroxysmal supraventricular tachycardia or atrial tachycardia. These are explained below:

- *AV nodal re-entry tachycardia:* This is the most frequent mechanism for PSVT. In this circumstance, there is a functional longitudinal dissociation of AV node which results in a dual AV nodal pathway with different functional properties. This dual AV nodal pathway is designated each as "slow" and "fast" pathways. The "slow" pathway has a longer refractory period, and allows anterograde conduction of atrial impulse. The "fast"

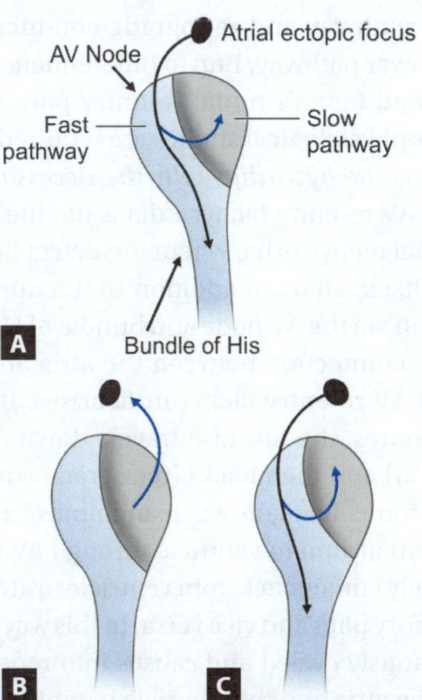

Figs. 38A to C: Mechanism of atrioventricular (AV) nodal re-entry tachycardia. In such situation, the AV node is divided into two parts (shaded or slow and unshaded or fast in the figure), according to the conducting and refractory characteristics of nodal tissues. (A) An impulse comes from the atrial ectopic beat and tries to pass both through the shaded and unshaded areas. But, due to the faster conduction property of unshaded part, the impulse first passes through it and depolarizes the ventricle. Passage of impulse through the shaded part is blocked due to its slow conduction property. (B) After a few milliseconds, when this shaded area is no more refractory, then few impulses from the unshaded area enter the shaded portion and pass back (through retrograde conduction) to the atrium, resulting in another atrial depolarization. Impulses from this second atrial depolarization again pass through the shaded and the unshaded areas and depolarize the ventricle (anterograde) and atrium (retrograde) like the previous manner. (C) Thus repeat re-entry of impulses in atria causes atrial tachycardia.

pathway has a shorter refractory period and prevents any anterograde conduction (**Figs. 38A to C**).

Thus atrial tachycardia is produced sequentially by:
- An ectopic atrial depolarization
- An anterograde conduction in one pathway (usually the "slow" one) which results in ventricular capture, because of an unidirectional anterograde block in the other pathway (usually the "fast" one).
- An retrograde conduction then occurs through the previously blocked (fast) pathway, resulting in another atrial depolarization, which in turn again activates the ventricle, like the previous one, which passes through the slower pathway.
- Thus, there is continuation of this re-entry circuit within the AV node, producing tachycardia. Less commonly the anterograde conduction occurs via the

faster pathway and retrograde conduction through the slower pathway. But, to differentiate between this slow and fast AV nodal re-entry pathways, special electrophysiological studies are required.

- *AV re-entry tachycardia with the accessory pathway:* Here, the AV re-entry tachycardia is not the same as that of AV nodal tachycardia, where the defect lies within the AV node itself. Here, in addition to the normal route of conduction via the AV node and bundle of His, there is an accessory connection between the atria and ventricles, for which AV re-entry tachycardia arises. By any one of the two routes, the impulse travels down (anterograde conduction) and then backs (retrograde conduction) by the other route. It means when an impulse anterogradely travels from atrium to ventricle through AV node, then it retrogradely comes back from ventricle to atrium through the accessory path and vice versa. In this way, the impulse is continuously cycled and causes into repeated activity of firing the atria and the ventricle in rapid succession.

The classic examples of PSVT with this mechanism are the pre-excitation syndrome, WPW syndrome, and Lown–Ganong–Levine syndrome.

Wolff–Parkinson–White Syndrome

In this condition, there is a strip of accessory conducting tissue that allows the electrical impulse to bypass the AV node and spread from atria to ventricle, rapidly without any delay, which occurs in AV node. When the ventricle is depolarized through AV node, though there is presence of an accessory pathway, then the ECG shows normal QRS complex without any delta wave. But, when the ventricles are depolarized through the accessory conducting pathway, then the ECG shows a very short PR interval, delta wave, and a broad QRS complex. This is because the accessory pathway has high conduction velocity rate than that of AV node. The ECG manifestation of WPW syndrome may differ from normal in the following ways **(Figs. 39A to D)**.

- *Sinus rhythm:* In sinus rhythm, with an accessory conducting system, the ventricles are partly depolarized through AV node and partly through accessory pathway. Thus, it produces an ECG with a short PR interval and a slurred, broad QRS complex. The characteristic slurring of the upstroke of QRS complex is known as *the delta wave*. The ECG depends on the degree of the proportion of electricity (impulses) passing down the accessory pathway (i.e., pre-excitation) and therefore the ECG appearances may vary a lot. Sometimes, the ECG may also look normal.

- *Orthodromic tachycardia:* This the most common form of tachycardia in WPW Syndrome. Here, the re-entry circuit passes anterogradely from atrium to ventricle, through the AV node and then comes back retrogradely

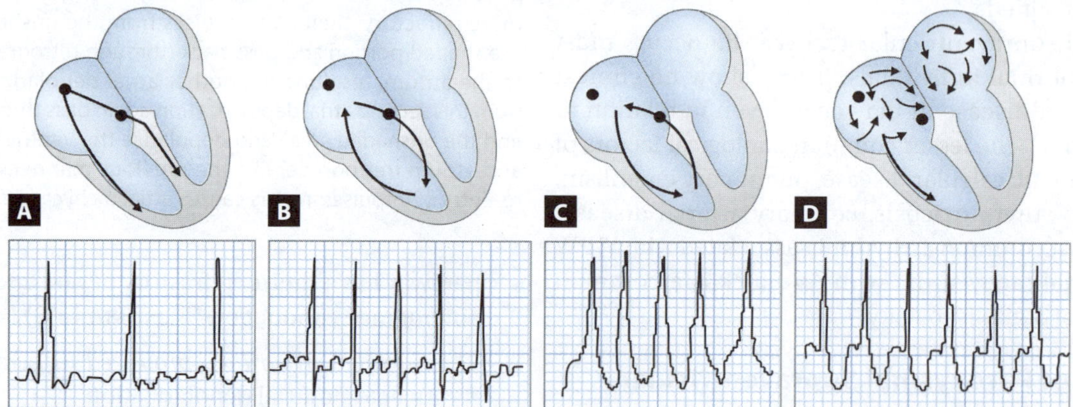

Figs. 39A to D: Mechanism of WPW syndrome. (A) Here, the cardiac rhythm is sinus, arising from SA node, without any tachycardia and the impulse passes through both the pathways (accessory and AV node). The ventricle is depolarized by impulses which pass partly through the accessory pathway and partly through AV node. The accessory pathway has faster conduction rate than the AV node and is responsible for short PR interval and also delta wave. The next part of QRS complex (after the delta wave) is as usual and is formed by the impulse coming through the AV node. The ultimate configuration of QRS complex depends upon the degree of pre-excitation, i.e., the proportion of impulse passing through the accessory pathway and normal AV node. Therefore, the appearance of ECG may vary a lot and it may look normal or abnormal. (B) This shows tachycardia with WPW syndrome. Here, the re-entry circuit passes through the AV node (anterograde) and comes back through the accessory pathway (retrograde or orthodromic). Thus, the ventricles are depolarized by normal AV nodal path and produces normal narrow QRS complex tachycardia without delta wave which is indistinguishable from other causes of SVT. (C) This also shows tachycardia with WPW syndrome. But, here the impulse first passes through accessory pathway and then comes back through AV node (retrograde or antidromic), after depolarizing the ventricle. As the ventricle is depolarized first by the accessory pathway, so it produces broad QRS complex tachycardia. (D) This shows atrial fibrillation associated with WPW syndrome, where the ventricle is depolarized by impulses passing through accessory pathway, producing broad QRS complex tachycardia. (AV: atrioventricular; ECG: electrocardiogram; WPW: Wolff–Parkinson–White)

FACT FILE I

Atrioventricular re-entry tachycardia

The accessory pathway is an extra connection between the atria and ventricles, which is anatomically separated from AV node. Accessory pathways make the patient susceptible to the episodes of *AV re-entry* tachycardia, with anterograde conduction via the AV node and retrograde conduction via the accessory pathway. In such circumstances, delta wave is not seen in ECG. In a variety of re-entry tachycardia, where the impulses take the opposite route, i.e., anterograde flow down the accessory pathway and retrograde flow up the AV node, which is very rare, then delta waves are seen (delta waves are seen when anterograde impulse passes through the accessory pathway). The *AV nodal re-entry* tachycardia is called when both the accessory pathway and normal AV pathway lie within the AV node, in which anterograde conduction usually occurs down the normal AV nodal tissue and returns retrogradely via the abnormal (accessory) AV nodal tissue.

Both the *AV re-entry and AV nodal re-entry* tachycardia have the following characteristics:
- Heart rate is 120–240 beats/min.
- There is one P-wave for every QRS complex, but P-waves are not always seen clearly.
- QRS complexes are regular, if there is no AV block.
- QRS complexes are narrow, if there is no conduction defect or bundle branch block.

  If there is a preexisting bundle branch block, then QRS complexes will be broad and re-entry tachycardia will be mistaken for VT. So, a previous ECG will be helpful in determining whether a bundle branch block existed before the tachycardia or not. In *AV re-entry* tachycardia, the inverted P-waves are often seen halfway between QRS complexes. Whereas in *AV nodal re-entry* tachycardia, the inverted P-waves are impossible to see, as they buried within the QRS complexes. Although the position of P-waves may help to distinguish between AV re-entry and AV nodal re-entry tachycardia, still an ECG in sinus rhythm is more helpful, as it may reveal a short PR interval or delta wave, suggesting WPW syndrome. Still, a definite diagnosis is very difficult and sometimes requires electrophysiological studies.

through accessory pathway. The ventricles are therefore depolarized in the normal way and produce a narrow QRS complex tachycardia that is not distinguishable from other forms of supraventricular tachycardia.

- *Antidromic tachycardia:* Here, the re-entry circuit passes anterogradely from the atrium to ventricle through accessory pathway, and then comes back retrogradely through AV node. The ventricles are then depolarized through accessory pathway producing a broad QRS complex tachycardia.
- *Atrial fibrillation:* In this rhythm, the ventricles are largely depolarized through the accessory pathway producing an irregular broad complex tachycardia (**Fact file I**).

Bradycardia Tachycardia (Brady-Tachy) Syndrome

It is one of the presentations of a group of disease, characterized by wide (potential) spectrum of disorder of rhythm such as SSS. It (SSS) is apparently a paradoxical association between a depressed conduction activity with hyperexcited conduction activity. But, the precise mechanism of this SS syndrome is not known.

Here, there is an abnormality of impulse formation and impulse conduction, involving both the SA node, AV node, and its appendages, such as bundle of His, right and left bundle branches, and Purkinje fibers. Bradycardia part of this SSS is due to sinus bradycardia, sinus arrest, or sinus block. This bradycardia may or may not be associated with conduction defects in AV node and its appendages and with or without adequate escape rhythm. The supraventricular tachyarrhythmia often emerges as an adequate escape rhythm in response to an episode of severe bradycardia, due to sinus arrest or sinus block. The supraventricular tachyarrhythmias may also be paroxysmal atrial tachycardia, atrial flutter, or atrial fibrillation. These tachyarrhythmias may manifest first or may precipitate as a compensatory response to a long pause, due to sinus arrest or block. The diagnosis of SSS is suspected when following the termination of tachyarrhythmias, there is a period of exceptionally very slow sinus rate, manifested as bradycardia which may be as slow as 25–35 beats/min for a short period. This tachyarrhythmia may ultimately establish as atrial fibrillation. The abnormal AV nodal conduction often become apparent when a patient with brady-tachy syndrome develops AF with AV nodal failure to conduct all the atrial impulses, leading to slow ventricular response.

The most common cause of brady-tachy syndrome or sick-sinus syndrome is the degeneration and fibrosis of the sinus node, AV node, and the conducting system. Other causes are IHD, drugs (digoxin, quinidine, and β-blockers), cardiomyopathy, amyloidosis, etc. The symptoms of brady-tachy syndrome are dizziness, fainting, or even syncope due to low cardiac output, caused by severe bradycardia. In addition to symptoms of bradycardia, patients may also experience episodes of supraventricular tachycardia.

The asymptomatic patients of brady-tachy syndrome do not require any treatment. Symptomatic patients may be considered for permanent pacemaker implantation. Medical therapy for tachycardia requires antiarrhythmic drugs which again worsens the phase of bradycardia. Therefore, pacing is also helpful to prevent this serious bradycardia and also permits medical therapy for tachycardia. The paroxysmal tachycardia, which arises as an escape rhythm to episodes of bradycardia, may also improve as a consequence of pacing.

Atrial Flutter

Atrial flutter (AF) is the manifestation of rapid and regular extrasystolic atrial excitation. It shares the same mechanism as paroxysmal atrial tachycardia, arising from an ectopic atrial focus or results from a continuous depolarization encircling the atrium through an accessory pathway, i.e., re-entry mechanism.

The ectopic atrial focus, producing AF, causes rapid electrical discharge from its ectopic site, similar to that of atrial extrasystole or PSVT (atrial tachycardia). But, this is not a well-accepted concept for atrial flutter. However, the re-entry mechanism can be described by the re-entry pathway which is situated within the atrium and does not involve the AV node. This is the most acceptable explanation for atrial flutter **(Fig. 40)**.

Other than mechanism of origin, the atrial flutter also differs from atrial tachycardia by its atrial rate (P-wave) which is higher in AF than atrial tachycardia and is usually 250–350 beats/min. The ventricular response to this rapid atrial activity depends upon the efficacy of conduction of impulses through AV node. The AV node cannot keep up space with such a high atrial rate and AV block occurs. Most commonly there is 2:1 block, where only alternate atrial impulses get through AV node to initiate a QRS complex. Though, 3:1, 4:1, 6:1, or variable other degrees of blocks are also seen. Thus, the ventricular rate is less than the atrial rate and is often 150, 100, or 75 beats/min according to the AV block, but is regular **(Figs. 41A and B)**.

We should always suspect atrial flutter with 2:1 block when a patient has a tachycardia with a regular ventricular

rate around 150 beats/min. Occasionally, every atrial impulse is conducted to ventricles with 1:1 response (i.e., without any block), resulting in a very fast, but regular ventricular rate.

The cardinal sign of atrial flutter in ECG is the presence of regular undulating waves, resulting in characteristic "sawtooth" appearance with prominent negative deflection in tracing. These manifestations are usually best seen in standard leads I, II, and aVF and chest lead V1. The T-wave is usually masked or deformed by flutter waves. In atrial flutter, the QRS complexes are normal, unless there is a coincidental bundle branch block **(Figs. 42A to D)**.

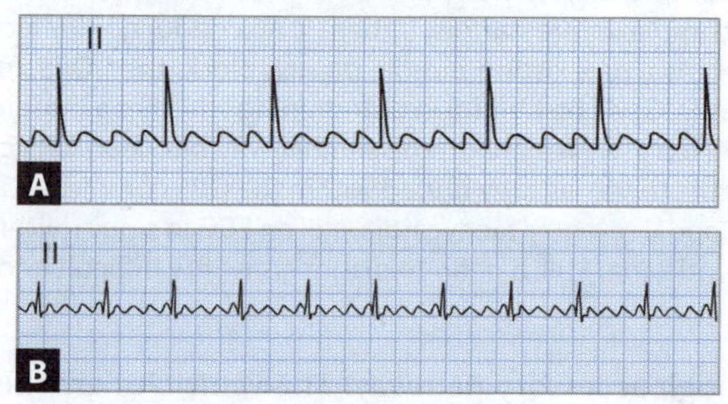

Figs. 41A and B: The figure A shows atrial flutter with 3:1 block and the figure B shows atrial flutter with 4:1 block.

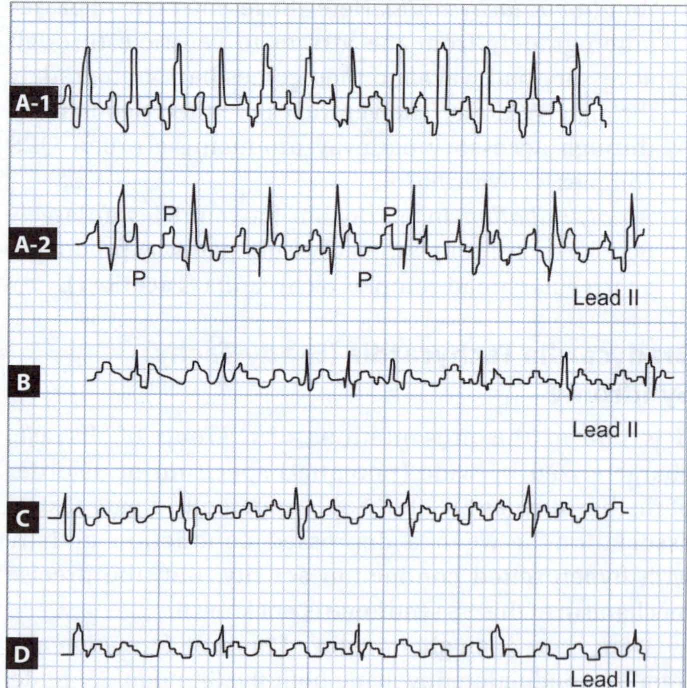

Figs. 42A to D: This electrocardiogram (ECG) shows various forms of atrial flutter. The key points of atrial fibrillation are rapid atrial rate, wide sawtooth deflection in the place of P-wave, and absent or barely noticeable baseline. (A-1) This shows atrial flutter with a 1:1 response. (A-2) This shows 2:1 response of atrial flutter after treatment with digitalis in same patient. (B) This shows atrial flutter with 2:1 response, but without treatment with digitalis. (C and D) This shows atrial flutter with 4:1 response.

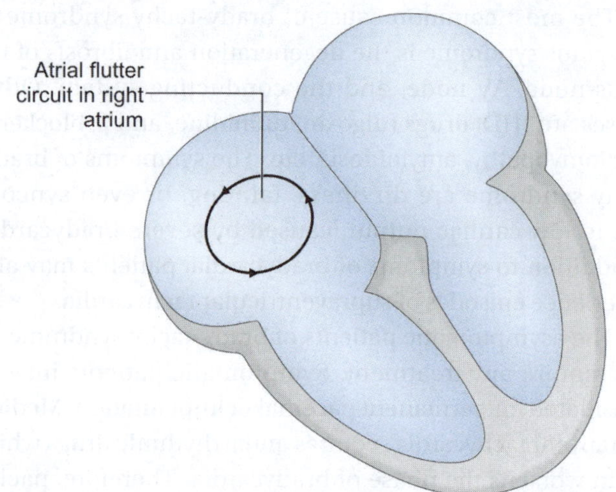

Fig. 40: Atrial flutter circuit. Its key point is the circuit of activity, which encircles in the right atrium continuously.

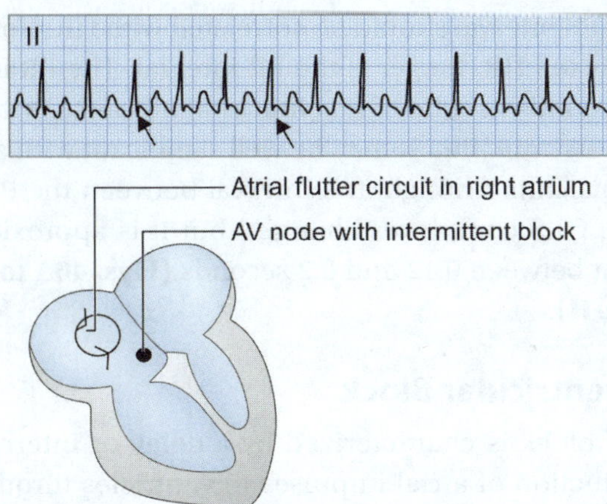

Fig. 43: This ECG shows atrial flutter with 2:1 block and is mistaken as 1:1 conduction. Because, one of the P-wave is buried in QRS complex (marked by arrow).

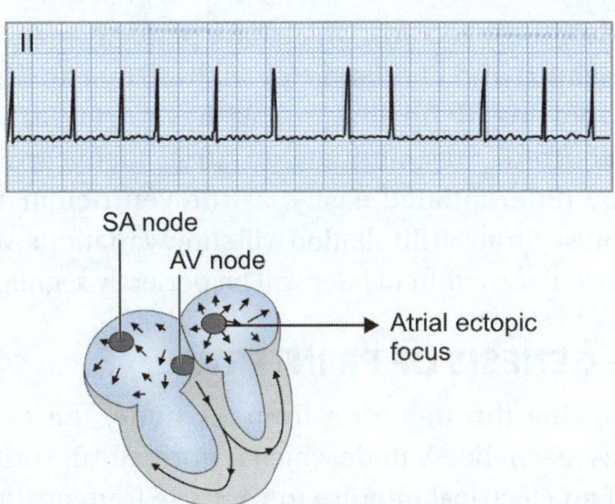

Fig. 44: This ECG shows atrial fibrillation. Due to the absence of definite atrial contraction, there is no P-wave and the ECG base line consists of low amplitude fibrillatory waves. As there is no fixed AV block, the ventricular rhythm (appearance of QRS complexes) is totally irregular. The P-waves are replaced by

The basic difference between atrial tachycardia and atrial flutter are the atrial rate, site of re-entry, presence and degree of AV block, and responses to therapy.

Sometimes, atrial flutter with 2:1 AV block may be mistaken as atrial tachycardia with 1:1 conduction (i.e., no block) or even regular sinus rhythm, because P-waves may be buried in QRS complexes **(Fig. 43)**. Atrial flutter may also be mistaken *the basic difference between the atrial flutter and fibrillation is that in fibrillation* due to rapid atrial rates many leads of the ECG will not clearly show the regularly recurring P′-waves, whereas in atrial flutter, P′-waves are regularly and clearly seen. If the ventricular response is irregular, then it will simulate an atrial fibrillation.

Atrial Fibrillation

Atrial fibrillation is more common than atrial flutter, affecting 5–10% of all elderly people. It may be permanent or paroxysmal, particularly in younger people. In atrial fibrillation, no P-waves are seen and the ECG base line consists of low amplitude fibrillatory waves. In atrial fibrillation, the excitation and recovery processes of atria are completely disorganized and chaotic. The whole atrium is functionally divided into numerous islands of tissue which are in a different chaotic electrical state and in various stages of excitation and recovery stage. These numerous excitatory wavelets or stimuli pass irregularly through the whole atria, without any effective atrial contraction. Normally, the human atrium can respond and contract regularly against stimulus, only up to a certain rate. This is usually in the range of 350 beats/min. But, at a rate faster than this, the atrium can no longer respond completely too each stimulus. So, a chaotic electrical disturbance, with asynchronous atrial depolarization and ineffective atrial contractions results in atrial fibrillation. In atrial fibrillation, the atrial activation is manifested in ECG, by an undulating baseline or by a more sharply inscribed atrial deflection of varying amplitude and frequency, ranging from 350 to 600 beats/min **(Fig. 44)**

The ventricular rhythm is totally irregular, because the majority of atrial impulses, reaching AV node, are blocked and it is because of the refractoriness of AV node at this high atrial rate. There is no fixed 2:1 or 3:1 or 4:1 AV block, like the atrial flutter. The AV node can only conduct some of these stimuli, because following the conduction of one such stimulus, it is refractory for a short period and impulses reaching the AV node, during this period, are blocked. Only occasional impulses meet the AV node, during its nonrefractory period and are conducted distally to activate the ventricles. This is called the "*concealed conduction*". Although, around 350–600 impulses reach the AV node in every minute, but only 120–180 of these will reach the ventricles to produce normal QRS complexes, provided there is no bundle brunch block.

In atrial fibrillation, in ECG the atrial deflections are recorded as irregular, chaotic, fibrillatory waves (F-wave) resulting in a ragged baseline. In ECG, there is no P-wave and irregularly irregular ventricular rhythm also will be seen. In long-standing cases of atrial fibrillation, the atrial deflections may be of a low amplitude and the ECG base line may be found almost as straight line, with minimum and smooth undulation of low amplitude. At times, the rhythm may alternate between the flutter and fibrillation in a single tracing. These are the borderline cases in which a precise differentiation between a flutter and fibrillation cannot be made. In such instances, the term "flutter-fibrillation" may be used. However, it is better to reserve the term "flutter" for those records, which have perfectly regular atrial depolarization and fibrillation for all those that are irregular.

A rapid atrial fibrillation, with ventricular rate of 200 beats/min, may simulate an atrial tachycardia. But, it can be differentiated easily, as the ventricular rhythm (radial pulse) in atrial fibrillation will show variations, whereas the ventricular rhythm in later will be perfectly regular.

■ THE GENESIS OF PR INTERVAL

After flowing through atria from SA node, the electrical impulses reach the AV node which is normally the only entry route of an electrical impulse to ventricle from atrium. This is because the rest of atrial myocardium is separated from ventricles by a nonconducting ring of fibrous tissue. The activation of AV node does not produce any obvious wave in ECG, like SA node. But, it does contribute to time interval between the P-wave (atrial contraction) and the subsequent Q or R wave, heralding the beginning of ventricular contraction. So, sometimes the PR interval is referred to as the PQ interval when a Q comes before a R-wave. By delaying the conduction from atrium to ventricle, the AV node acts as a safety mechanism which prevents the rapid atrial impulses from spreading to ventricles at the same rate **(Fig. 45)**.

So, the time taken for a depolarization wave to pass, after its origin from SA node, to ventricles across the atria and through AV node, is called the PR interval. This is measured from the beginning of P-wave to the beginning of R-wave and is normally between 0.12 and 0.2 seconds (maximally up to 0.22 seconds) or 3–5 small squares. Thus, it includes (1) the time required for atrial depolarization to travel from SA node to AV node (usually 0.03 second), (2) the time required for normal conduction delay in AV node (approximately 0.07 second), and (3) the time required for an impulse to pass through bundle of His and the bundle branches to ventricle.

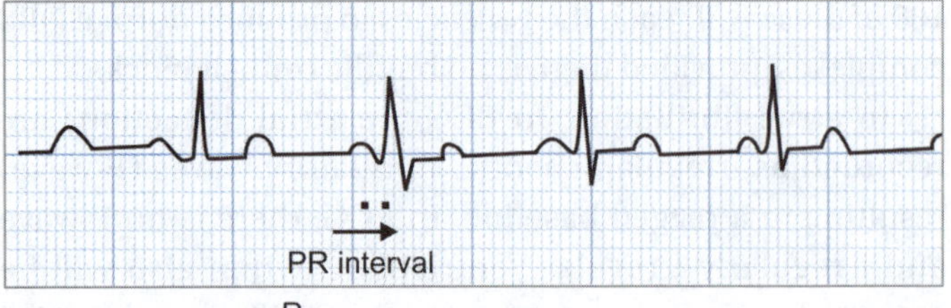

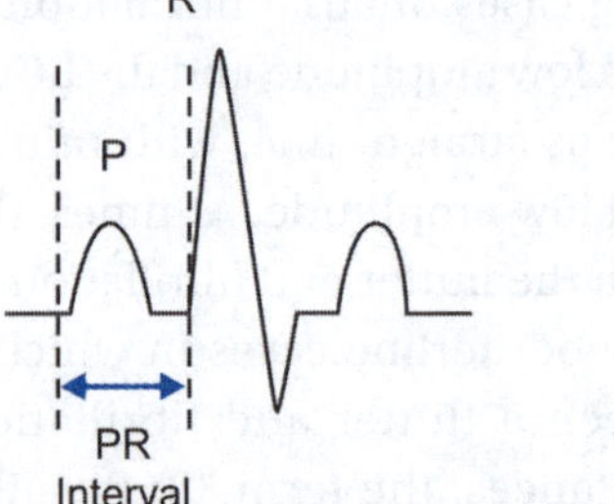

Fig. 45: PR interval. The normal interval is 0.12–0.20 seconds.

The PR interval should be correlated with HR. Normally, slower is the HR, longer is the PR interval. The PR interval of 0.2 seconds may be of no clinical significance, with a HR of 60 beats/min. But, it may be well significant with a HR of 100 beats/min. Though, the interval between the P-waves and the QRS complexes changes, but it is approximately constant between 0.12 and 0.2 seconds **(Figs. 46A to C and Fact file II)**.

Atrioventricular Block

The AV block is characterized by a delay or interruption in conduction of atrial impulses to ventricles through the specialized AV conduction system, such as the AV node, bundle of His or its bundle branches (right and left bundle branches). *The AV block can be classified into three degrees:*
1. In first-degree block, there is delay in conduction of impulses >0.2 second through AV node.
2. In second-degree block, there is intermittent or incomplete interruption of conduction of impulses through AV node.
3. In third-degree block, there is permanent or complete interruption of conduction of impulses through AV conduction system. The first- and second-degree heart block is called the *partial or incomplete heart block* and the third-degree heart block is called the complete AV block or *complete heart block.*

First-degree AV or Heart Block

In this condition, there is a disturbance or delay in conduction through AV node and bundle of His. This results in the prolongation of PR interval above its upper limit (>0.2 second), constituting the first-degree AV or heart block.

In first-degree AV block in ECG, all the P-waves are followed by QRS complexes. It is usually asymptomatic and in general does not progress to other degrees of heart block. Hence, no specific treatment is necessary for first-degree AV block in its own right, but needs close observation. It is not an indication for pacemaker implantation **(Fig. 47)**.

Second-degree AV or Heart Block

Second-degree AV or heart block is again classified into: (1) Mobitz type I (Wenckebach phenomenon) and (2) Mobitz type II block.
- *Mobitz type I of second-degree AV block:* Here, the PR interval gradually lengthens with each successive beat, until after several beats, usually 3–6 beats, when an atrial depolarization completely fails to pass to ventricle and fails to initiate a ventricular response, due to complete block of AV node and thus this beat is dropped. Hence, a long diastolic pause results. Then, this diastolic pause,

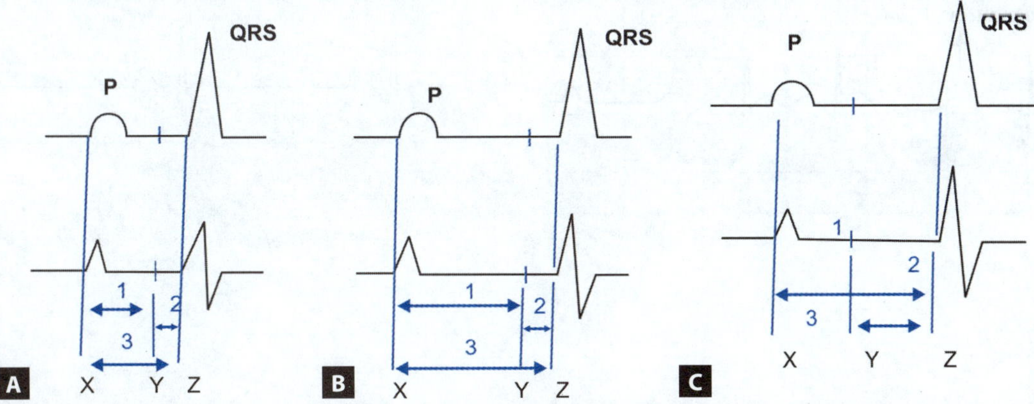

Figs. 46A to C: (A) This figure shows normal AV conduction. (B) This figure shows first-degree AV block. Here, 1 is prolonged, but 2 is normal. So, the 3 is also prolonged. Therefore, the block is proximal to Bundle of His in AV node. (C) This figure also shows first-degree AV block. Here, 1 is normal, but 2 is prolonged. So, the 3 is again prolonged. Therefore, the block is distal to Bundle of His in intraventricular conduction system. The QRS interval is prolonged (wide QRS complex), when there is block distal to Bundle of His.

FACT FILE II

Mechanism and the site of AV block

The AV block results either from a functional or pathological defect in atria, AV node, bundle of His or its bundle branches, causing delay in the relay or conduction of impulses through AV node. The functional block of AV node can occur as a result of increased vagal tone. The AV block produced by digitalis toxicity is also partly due to vagal stimulation. The PR interval can be subdivided into two segments as follows:

1. The time from the beginning of P-wave to the end of the depolarization of AV node. This is represented in the figure as XY interval.
2. The time from the end of AV node depolarization to the beginning of ventricular depolarization. This is represented in the figure as YZ interval. Therefore, the measurements of XY and YZ interval are of major clinical significance.

In the presence of first-degree AV block (prolonged PR interval) the block may be at the following sites:

- Above the bundle of His (therefore in AV node), giving a prolonged XY interval and a normal YZ interval
- Below the bundle of His (therefore in intraventricular conduction system), giving a normal XY interval, but a prolonged YZ interval
- A combination of both (1) and (2) with prolonged XY and YZ intervals. Even in the presence of a normal PR interval, either the XY or the YZ interval may be prolonged.

The bundle of His recordings, although not available as a routine clinical tool, have resulted in more clarification of the mechanism and sites of first, second, and third-degree AV block.

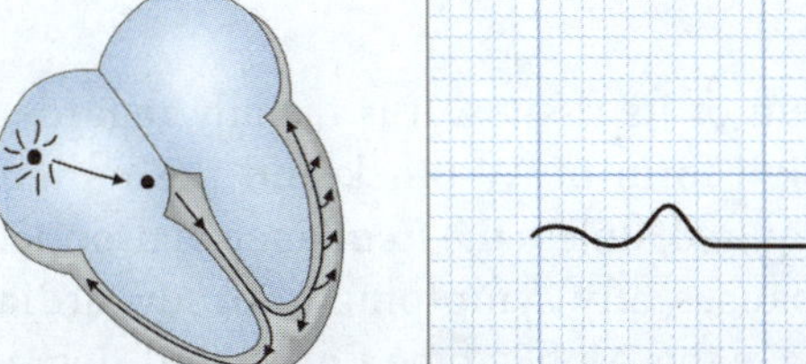

Fig. 47: This figure shows first-degree AV block or delay in conduction through AV node, Bundle of His or atria. This produces the lengthening of PR interval.

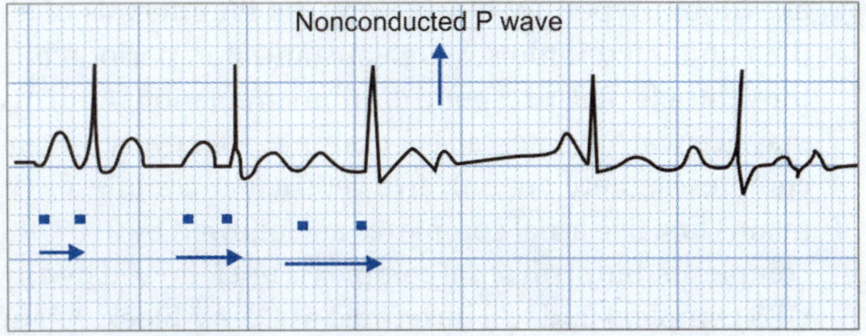

Fig. 48: Here, the electrocardiogram (ECG) shows Mobitz type I variety of second-degree AV block (Wenckebach phenomena). There is progressive lengthening of PR interval with intermittent failure of P-wave to be conducted to ventricle. Then, PR interval again resets to its normal and this cycle repeats again and again.

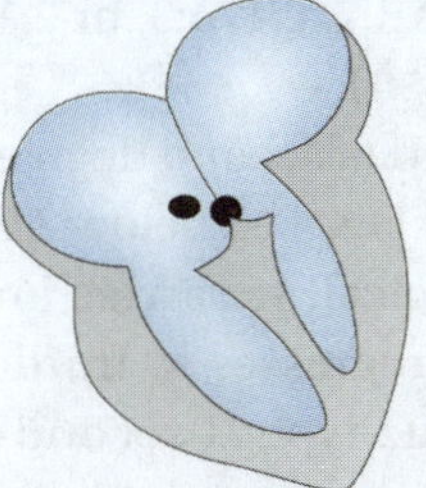

caused by this dropped beat, allows the conducting system to recover. Now, the PR interval again resets back to its normal and allows the atrial depolarization to be further conducted to ventricles. This sequence is then repeated. Here, the defect lies within the AV node **(Fig. 48)**.

The Mobitz type I AV block is thought to be as the result of abnormal conduction through AV node itself and can result simply from high vagal activity. So, it sometimes occurs even during sleep. It may also occur in any generalized disease

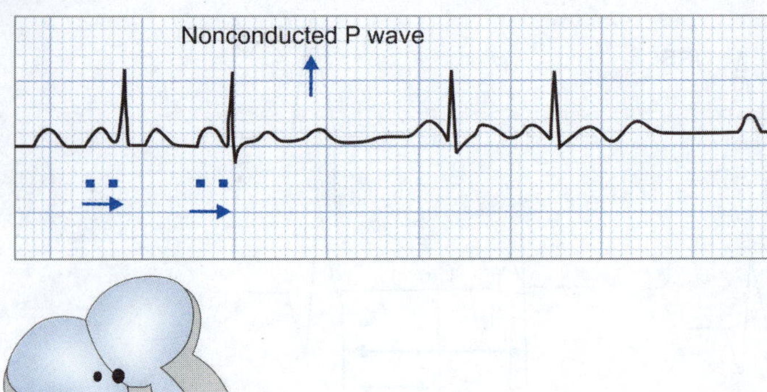

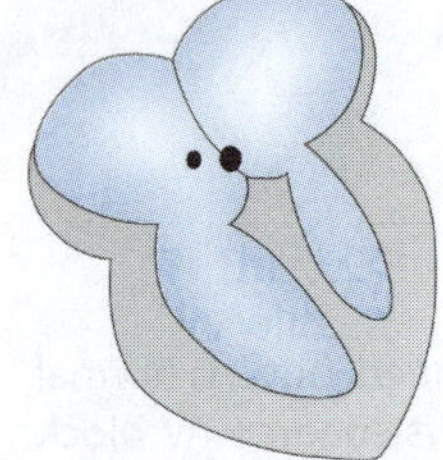

Fig. 49: This is an electrocardiogram (ECG) of Mobitz type II variety of second-degree AV block. It is characterized by a normal and constant PR interval, but occasional P-wave fails to be conducted.

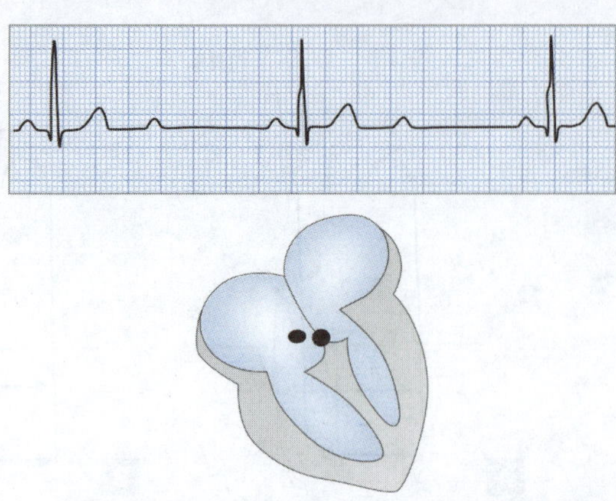

Fig. 50: This ECG shows 2:1 AV block, where alternate P-waves fail to be conducted to ventricle from atrium.

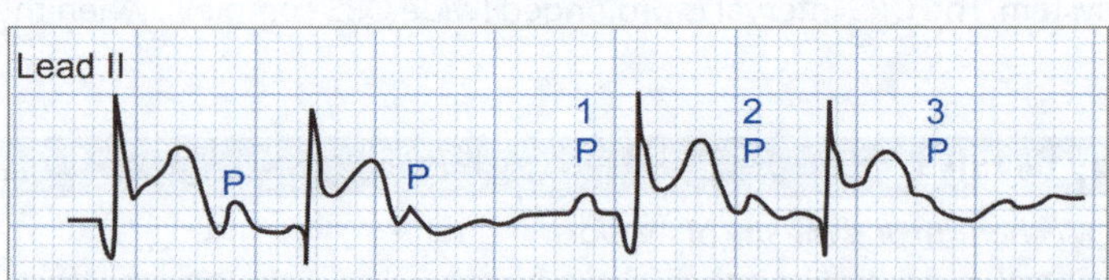

Fig. 51: This is an ECG of inferior wall MI in hyperactive phase, with 3:2 second-degree AV block of Wenckebach type (Mobitz type I). This is evidenced by tall R-wave, elevated ST segment and tall-wide T-wave. The first PR interval is normal, the second PR interval widens, and the third P-wave is not followed by a QRS complex. (AV: atrioventricular; ECG: electrocardiogram; MI: myocardial infarction)

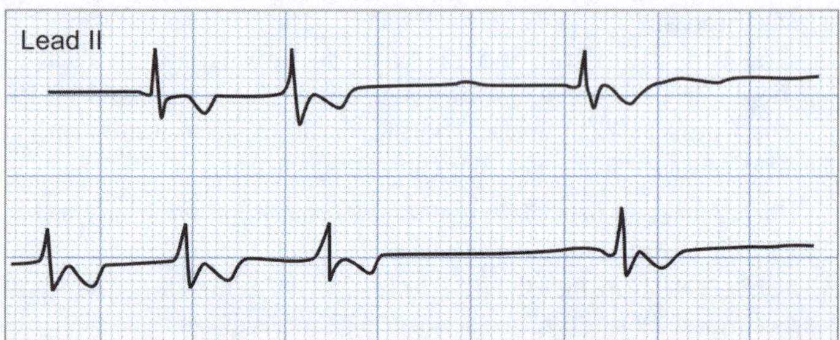

Fig. 52: This ECG shows Mobitz type II second-degree AV block. This is evidenced by irregularly dropped P-waves, resulting in successive 3:2, 2:1, 4:3, and 2:1 AV block. The PR interval is prolonged, but is same for all the conducted beats. (AV: atrioventricular; ECG: electrocardiogram)

of conducting system or its tissues. It is usually regarded as a relatively benign form of AV block and permanent pacemaker is not required, unless the frequency of dropped ventricular beats causes any symptomatic bradycardia. Patients, found to have this Mobitz type I of second-degree AV block prior to surgery, will usually require temporary pacing perioperatively.

- *Mobitz type II of second-degree AV block:* Here, there is no gradual progression or prolongation of PR interval, like Mobitz type I AV block. Here, the PR intervals of all the conducted impulses are constant. But, periodically the ventricles fail to respond to atrial stimulations and this may occur at any interval. For example, after every 6 atrial complexes, there are only five ventricular complexes (it means first five atrial complexes are followed by five QRS complexes, but sixth atrial complex is not followed by any QRS complex) and will be termed as 6:5 AV block. Again it may be of any combination, such as 3:2, 2:1, 4:3, or 2:1 AV Mobitz type II block **(Figs. 49 and 50)**.

The lesion in this form of Mobitz type II of second degree AV block is actually situated in bundle of His, i.e., below AV node and is always organic or pathological. It carries an adverse prognosis, since it frequently progresses to third-degree or complete AV block. So, Mobitz type II second-degree AV block is more serious than Mobitz type I AV block. It is also an indication for perioperative pacing **(Fig. 51)**.

2:1 Mobitz type II second-degree AV block is a special form of second-degree heart block (also termed as "second-degree constant block") in which alternate P-waves are not followed by QRS complexes. Regular sinus rhythm complicated by 3:2 AV block will result in a *ventricular bigeminal rhythm* **(Fig. 52)**.

Third-degree AV or Complete Heart Block

The third-degree AV block is characterized by the complete or permanent interruption of AV conduction. All the supraventricular impulses (sinus rhythm, atrial tachycardia, atrial fibrillation, etc.) are blocked to pass to ventricle at the level of AV conducting system. The ventricles are then activated by subsidiary ectopic foci, acting as a pacemaker for escape rhythm, situated on the AV node but below the level of block or within the ventricles **(Fig. 53)**.

The atrium is thus activated by one pacemaker (usually sinus or may be ectopic) and ventricle by another idioventricular pacemaker. Hence, the two rhythms, i.e., atrial and ventricular rhythms run independently and asynchronously.

The features of complete AV block are:

- P-wave has no relationship with QRS complex and if it is sinus in origin, then the rate is 60–80 beats/min. Any abnormal atrial rhythm can coexist with the third-degree heart block and so the P-wave may be abnormal or even absent.
- There is slow ventricular rate or QRS complex, usually in the range of 35–40 beats/min and it is not under vagal influence (since ventricles have no parasympathetic activity). It is thus not usually affected by exercise, emotions, or atropine.
- If the subsidiary pacemaker activity arises from AV node, below the block or bundle of His, then the configuration of QRS complex is normal (narrow) or near normal in shape (i.e., not wide).
- If the pacemaker is situated in ventricle, peripherally in the Purkinje fibers or in ventricular musculature, then the QRS complexes will be abnormal and broad. Sometimes, the ventricle may be under the control of 2 or 3 alternative pacemakers, arising from different foci, resulting in QRS complexes of different configurations.

A combination of bradycardia and broad QRS complexes should alert a suspicion of third-degree heart block. For the management of this type of complete block, temporary pacing is always indicated, regardless of patient's symptom, or hemodynamic state. Pacing is also necessary perioperatively for patients who are waiting for surgery.

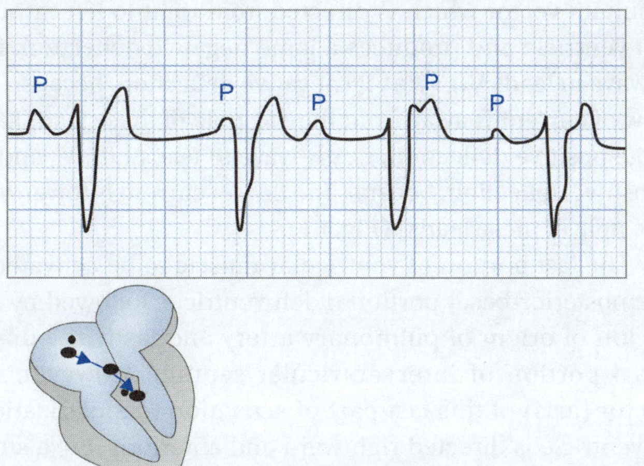

Fig. 53: This ECG shows third-degree AV or complete heart block. This is characterized by (i) no relation between P-waves and QRS complexes, (ii) broad QRS complexes, (iii) P-wave (atrial rate) is 86 beats/min and QRS complex (ventricular rate) is 50 beats/min. (AV: atrioventricular; ECG: electrocardiogram)

Atrioventricular Junctional Rhythm

This type of rhythm is also called the AV nodal rhythm, because here the impulse arises from AV node as an ectopic focus. The impulse then spreads upward into atrium and downward into ventricle. This usually produces an upright P′-wave in aVR and in high esophageal leads and an inverted P′-wave in lead II, aVF, and low esophageal leads. Thus, P′-wave is inverted in leads, where it is normally upright and vice versa **(Fig. 54)**.

The QRS complex is of normal configuration, as it arises from AV node and passes through normal conducting pathway. If the retrograde conduction to atria is faster than the anterograde conduction to ventricles, then P′-wave will precede the QRS complex. But, if the opposite occurs, then P′-wave will follow the QRS complex. On the other hand, if the conduction to atria and ventricles occurs at same rate, then the P′-wave will be hidden within the QRS complex **(Figs. 55 and 56)**.

These junctional beats may appear as escape beats when the sinus rate is very slow or as premature beats when an increased automaticity of the AV junction site develops. This increased automaticity of AV junction may be due to digitalis toxicity. The transient or permanent AV junctional rhythm may result from organic heart diseases like IHD, myocarditis, rheumatic heart disease, etc. The significance of these junctional beats or rhythm is similar to that of atrial premature beats. The escape beats are protective in nature as

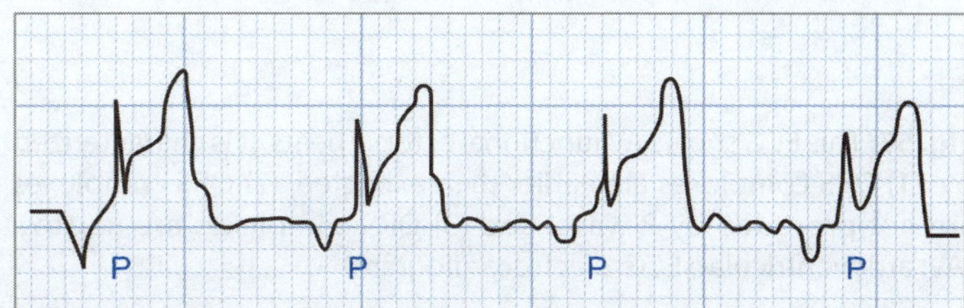

Fig. 54: This ECG illustrates the AV nodal rhythm with retrograde conduction to atria. So, an inverted P-wave precedes each QRS complex. (AV: atrioventricular; ECG: electrocardiogram)

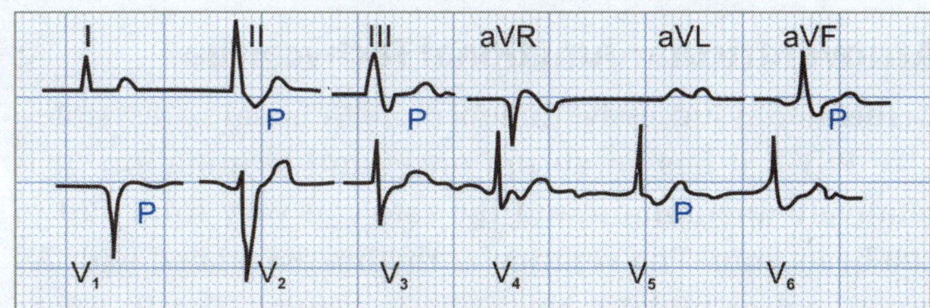

Fig. 55: This ECG shows AV nodal junctional rhythm with late retrograde conduction and activation of atria. Here, P-waves follow each QRS complex and are inverted. This inverted P-wave is seen in Lead II, III, aVF, V₄, and V₅. (AV: atrioventricular; ECG: electrocardiogram)

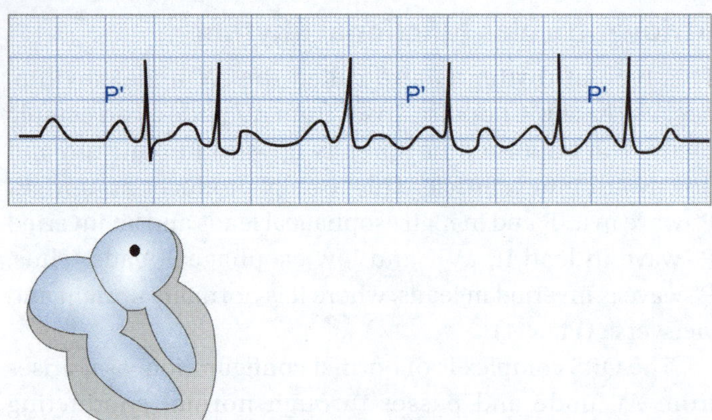

Fig. 56: This electrocardiogram (ECG) shows atrial ectopic beats. The key points are: (1) P-waves are earlier than expected and (2) P-waves are abnormally shaped.

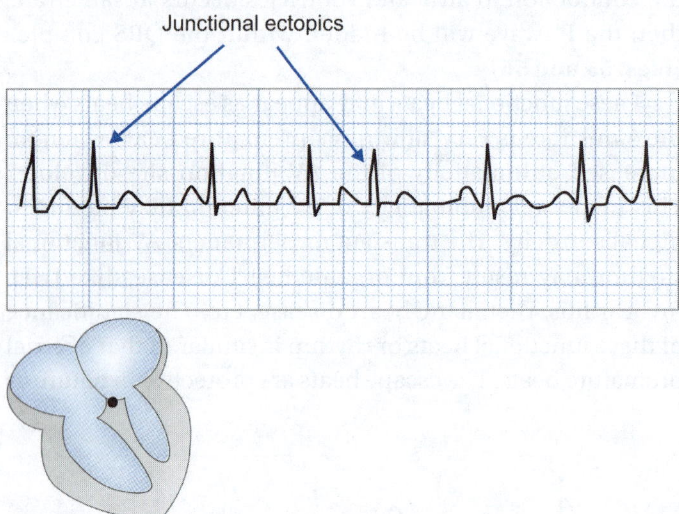

Fig. 57: This ECG shows AV junctional ectopic beats. It is characterized by: (1) QRS complexes are earlier than expected, (2) QRS complexes are not preceded by P-wave, and (3) QRS complexes are narrow. (AV: atrioventricular; ECG: electrocardiogram)

they represent a secondary pacemaker (to SA node) and take over the responsibility, when the primary pacemaker slows or fails **(Fig. 57)**.

Atrioventricular Junctional Tachycardia

It is defined as successive three or more AV nodal extrasystoles. Like PSVT, it has an abrupt onset and termination. It is relatively uncommon and the rate can vary from 120 to 200 beats/min. The ventricular rhythm associated with AV junctional or nodal tachycardia is regular. The P'-waves originating from AV junctional tissue may precede, be buried in, or follow the QRS complexes. The pattern of each QRS complex is identical to that of a junctional premature beat. With a rapid rate during tachycardia, it is impossible to identify any single P'-wave. Practically, one cannot differentiate the ECG pattern, produced by AV junctional tachycardia, from that produced by atrial tachycardia, arising from a low atrial ectopic focus. Therefore, the appropriate term such as supraventricular tachycardia is more applicable to AV junctional tachycardia and atrial tachycardia. The clinical significance of AV junctional tachycardia is similar to that of atrial tachycardia (supraventricular tachycardia) **(Figs. 58 and 59)**.

◼ GENESIS OF QRS COMPLEX

The activation or depolarization of ventricle is reflected by QRS complexes in an ECG tracing. The normal QRS complexes have different appearances in each of 12 ECG leads **(Fig. 60)**.

The activation of ventricle starts at the left side of interventricular septum in the bundle of His and then it spreads from left to right. This is called the septal force or septal vector (axis) of QRS complex, producing septal activation and is responsible for a small positive deflections or r-waves in V_1 and V_2 leads and a small negative deflections or q-waves in leads I, V_5, V_6, and aVL. As the amount of electrical activation is little at septum, so the amplitude of deflection is very small.

The activation of septum is then followed by the activation of free walls of both the ventricles. This can be represented by a large right-to-left force through the thick free walls of left ventricle, which occur simultaneously with a smaller opposing force directed from left to right through the thinner free wall of right ventricle. The larger right-to-left force of left ventricle dominates and counteracts the smaller left-to-right force of right ventricle. This results in an effective or net resultant vector which is directed from right to left through left ventricle and produces a large negative deflection, i.e., S-wave in leads V_1, V_2, aVR (negative deflection, because the flow of current is away from the +ve pole of these leads) and large positive deflection, i.e., R-wave in leads I, II, V_5 and V_6 (positive deflection, because the flow of current is toward the +ve pole of these leads) **(Fig. 61)**.

The last portion of ventricular muscle to be activated is the posterior-basal portion of left ventricle, followed by the region of origin of pulmonary artery and lastly the upper most portion of interventricular septum. However, the vector (axis) of this last part of activation (depolarization) of ventricle is directed rightward and anteriorly. So, a small positive deflection will be recorded in lead V_{1-2}, and a small negative deflection S will be recorded in leads I and V_{5-6}. Thus, the right oriented leads (V_1 and V_2) will therefore, normally reflect an rS or rSr complex, and the left oriented leads (V_5 and V_6) will reflect a qR, or qRs complex. Lead V_3 and V_4

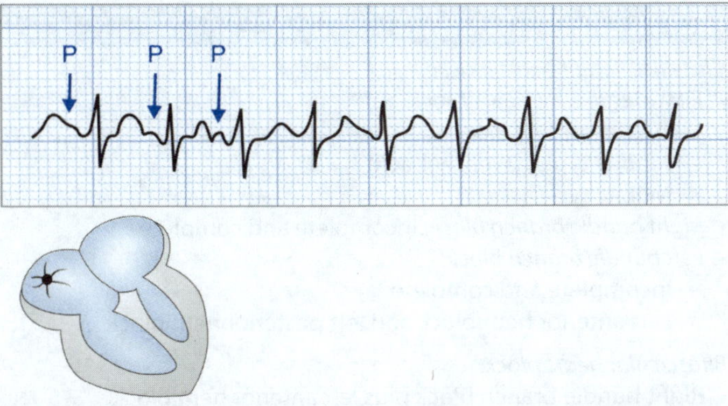

Fig. 58: This is an electrocardiogram (ECG) of sinus tachycardia. It is evidenced by narrow QRS complexes and P-waves are hidden within the previous T-waves.

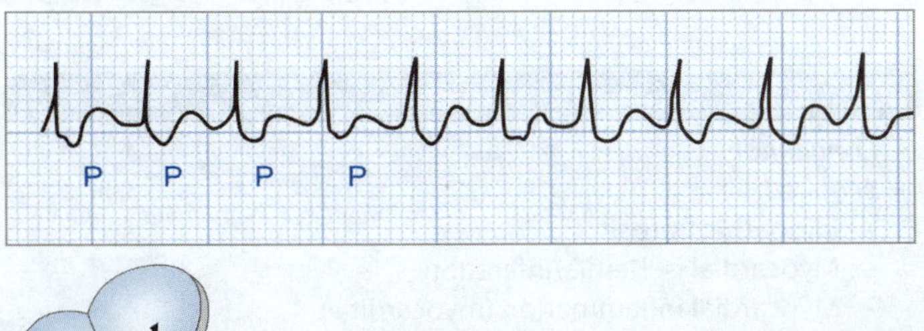

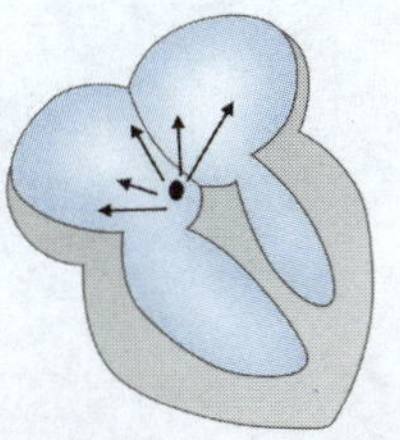

Fig. 59: This an ECG of AV junctional tachycardia. The key points are: (1) tachycardia, (2) narrow QRS complexes, (3) P-waves follow QRS complexes, and (4) P-waves are inverted in lead II. (AV: atrioventricular; ECG: electrocardiogram)

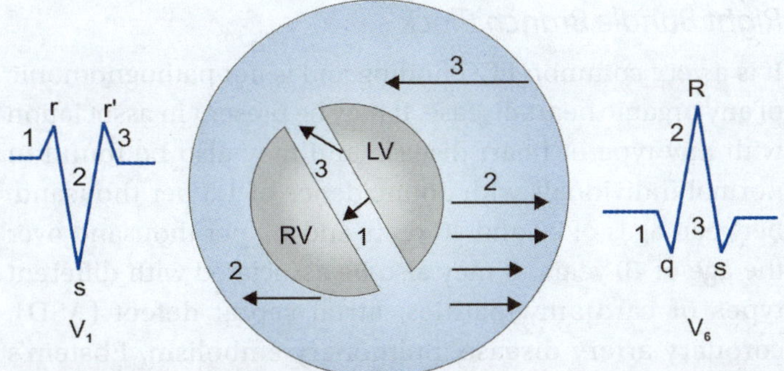

Fig. 60: Basic vector (axis) of ventricular depolarization and its effects on leads V_1 and V_6. 1= Septal activation. 2 = Activation of ventricular wall. 3 = Activation of posterior basal portion of left ventricle and the area of the origin of pulmonary artery. (LV: left ventricle; RV: right ventricle)

are the transitional leads and reflect the transition from rS complex to qR complex. The transition pattern is usually a RS complex. But, sometimes the pattern may be relatively

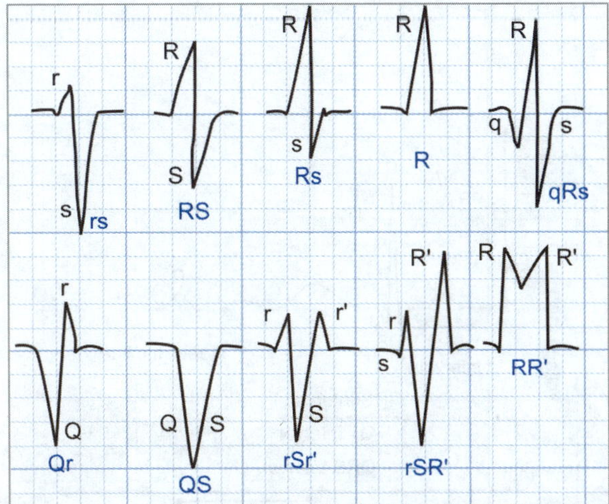

Fig. 61: This figure shows the various forms of QRS complexes and their nomenclatures.

bizarre and depends on the presence of clockwise or counter clockwise rotation of heart. So, the transition pattern should be ignored **(Fig. 61)**.

An initial downward deflection, after the P-wave, is called the Q-wave (small q is for a small downward deflection) and an initial upward deflection, after the P-wave, is called the R-wave (small r for a small upward deflection). After Q (downward deflection) and/or R (upward deflection), the next downward deflection is called the S-wave. After the S-wave the next positive deflection (second positive deflection of QRS complex) is called the R′ or r′ (r′ for a small amplitude deflection). These different nomenclatures of a QRS complex are given in the figure. The QRS interval is the measurement of total ventricular depolarization time. It is measured from the onset of Q-wave or R-wave (if there is no Q-wave) to the termination of S-wave or r′-wave. The upper limit of QRS interval is 0.12 seconds **(Fig. 62)**.

The ventricular activation time (VAT) is an indirect measurement of time which is taken for an impulse to traverse the whole thickness of left ventricular wall. It is measured from the beginning of QRS complex (or the beginning of Q or r-wave) to the peak of R or S-wave. The upper limit of VAT is 0.04 seconds.

Intraventricular Conduction Defects

The intraventricular conduction defect is the result of conduction abnormality through one or more divisions of ventricular conduction system which are distal to bundle of His. The anatomical structures for normal intraventricular conduction are (from the end of bundle of His to ventricular muscle fibers): (1) right bundle branch, (2) left bundle branch, (3) left anterior fascicle, (4) left posterior fascicle, (5) septal fibers from left bundle branch that enter the left

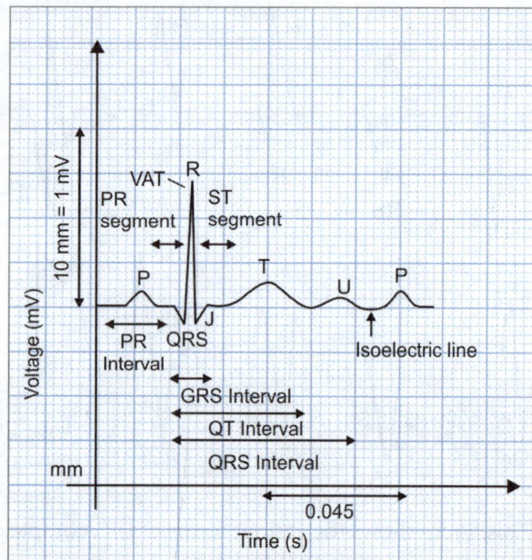

Fig. 62: A schematic diagram of ECG complexes, intervals, and segments. The graph is magnified for clarity and better understanding. (ECG: electrocardiogram; VAT: ventricular activation time)

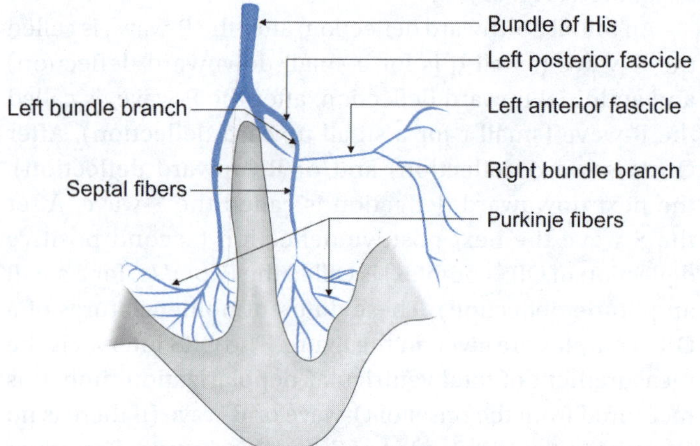

Fig. 63: Intraventricular conduction system.

septal myocardium, and (6) peripheral Purkinje fibers **(Fig. 63)**.

The severity of conduction defect may vary from delayed conduction through conducting pathway to total block. But, as the ECG cannot distinguish between the two, so it is better to use the term "conduction defect". The conduction defect is only an ECG diagnosis, but not a clinical diagnosis.

The classification of heart block is depicted in **Fact file III**.

The ECG criteria's for conduction defects (or blocks) of heart are:

- Abnormal QRS configuration due to abnormal spread of conduction through the conducting system of ventricle
- Prolongation of QRS interval, i.e., >0.12 second

FACT FILE III: Classification of heart block.

Classification of heart block:
- First-degree AV heart block
- *Second-degree AV block:*
  - Mobitz type I (Wenckebach)
  - Mobitz type II
- *Right bundle branch block:* Incomplete and complete
- *Left bundle branch block:*
  - Incomplete and complete
  - Left anterior hemiblock and left posterior hemiblock

Bifascicular heart block:
- Right bundle branch block plus left anterior hemiblock
- Right bundle branch block plus left posterior hemiblock
- Right or left bundle branch block with prolonged AV conduction

Third-degree (complete) heart block: Nodal and infranodal **(Box 1)**

BOX 1: Causes of complete heart block.

- *Congenital:*
- *Acquired:*
  - Idiopathic fibrosis
  - Myocardial ischemia/infarction
  - Myocardial inflammation (myocarditis)
  - Trauma (cardiac surgery)
  - Drugs such as digoxin and β-blockers

- Prolonged VAT
- The ST segment is depressed and the T-wave is inverted in leads that record abnormal R′-wave

In an incomplete block, all the above criteria should be present, except the QRS interval which is not >0.12 second.

Right Bundle Branch Block

It is a very common ECG finding and is not pathognomonic of any organic heart disease. It may be present in association with any type of heart disease and may also be found in normal individuals with an incidence of 1.5 per thousand, between ages of 20 and 40 years and 2.9 per thousand over the age of 40 years. It may also be associated with different types of cardiomyopathies, atrial septal defect (ASD), coronary artery disease, pulmonary embolism, Ebstein's anomaly, etc. **(Fact file IV).**

Mechanism: Here, the spread of excitation (depolarization) from SA node to AV node and then up to the bundle of His is normal. After that the septal activation occurs normally from left to right through bundle of His. In leads V_1 and V_2 as a result of normal septal activation which is oriented to the right and anteriorly (vector 1), a small positive r-wave will be recorded (because, positive pole of lead V_1 and V_2 is also oriented toward right and anterior). Since, the

FACT FILE IV: Causes of heart block.

Common causes of bundle branch block
- *RBBB:* Normal variant
  - Coronary artery disease, congenital heart disease (e.g., ASD)
  - Right ventricular hypertrophy or strain (e.g., pulmonary embolism)
  - Cardiomyopathy
  - Ebstein's anomaly
- *LBBB:* Coronary artery disease, hypertension, coarctation of aorta
  - Hypertrophic cardiomegaly
  - Aortic valve disease
  - Cardiomyopathy
  - Fibrosis of the conduction system

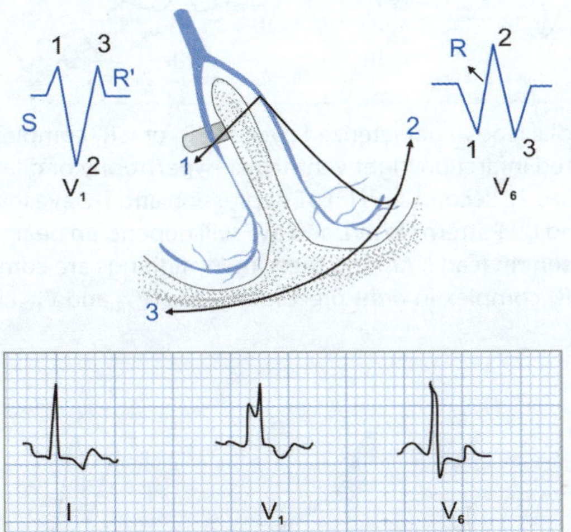

Fig. 64: This ECG shows RBBB. The key points are: (1) Broad QRS complexes, (2) R'-wave in lead V_1, and (3) S-wave in lead V_6. In RBBB, the QRS looks like "M" in lead V_1 and "W" in lead V_6. In figure, the vector-1 is due to septal activation, vector-2 is due to left ventricular activation, and vector-3 is due to right ventricular activation. (ECG: electrocardiogram; RBBB: right bundle branch block)

right bundle branch is blocked, so the excitation wave will next spread downward and left (vector 2) through the left bundle branch and left ventricular myocardium, resulting in a large negative S-wave in leads V_1 and V_2 (because, positive pole of V_1 and V_2 is oriented toward right and upward). The impulse will then pass around the apex of heart, upward and toward right (vector 3), bypassing the blocked right bundle branch, into right ventricular myocardium, producing a large positive R'-wave in leads V_1 and V_2. Thus, a typical pattern of rsR' will be found in leads V_1 and V_2 in RBBB. If the S-wave is small or absent, then the pattern will be RR'. The ST segment will be depressed and so the T-wave is inverted **(Fig. 64)**.

The T-wave is opposite in direction to the terminal QRS deflection. Thus, if the terminal deflection is R', for example, in lead V_1 and V_2, then the T-wave will be inverted. However,

the associated ST segment will show deflection which is slightly convex upward or sometimes minimally depressed. If, on the other hand, the terminal deflection is an S-wave, for example, in lead V_5 and V_6, then the T-wave will be upright. The associated ST segment will be slightly concave downward and at times is minimally elevated.

In lead V_5 and V_6, an initial small negative q-wave will be formed as a result of normal left-to-right septal activation (because, here the axis of depolarization or *vector 1* is oriented toward right, but the positive pole of leads are oriented toward left). This will be followed by large positive R-wave, resulting from a large left ventricular activation (because, here the axis of depolarization or *vector 2* is oriented toward left and the positive pole of leads are also oriented toward left). Then, this R-wave will be followed by large negative S-wave which results from the delayed large activation of right ventricle (because, here axis of depolarization or *vector 3* is oriented toward right and the positive pole of leads is oriented toward left). The ST segment is isoelectric and the T-wave is upright.

So, in RBBB the QRS complex will look like "M" in leads V_{1-2} and "W" in leads V_{5-6}. The characteristic feature of RBBB is a delayed electrical force of right ventricular depolarization, oriented to the right and anteriorly. This late right vector force produces a wide S-wave in lead-I, V5-6 and a wide R or R' (RSR' pattern) in lead aVR and V_{1-2}. The ST and T are opposite in direction to this late force of ventricular depolarization (R or R'-wave) in the precordial leads. *An initial q-wave will never be present in V_{1-2} leads in RBBB or an initial q-wave in V_{1-2} lead indicates it is not RBBB. Alternatively, an initial q-wave in V_{1-2} leads always indicates LBBB* **(Figs. 65A to C)**.

Incomplete RBBB: A delay, but not a complete stoppage of conduction of impulses, through right or left bundle branches manifests as an incomplete right and left bundle branch block. In case of incomplete RBBB, the conduction through right bundle branch is still possible, but is delayed. It is now increasingly clear that this slowed down conduction of impulses is not the only cause for the genesis of an incomplete RBBB. But, the increased length of right bundle branch may also play a significant role for relative conduction delay, where the conduction itself is not delayed. For example, an increased length of right bundle branch is responsible for longer time of conduction, producing relative delay and incomplete RBBB. This anatomical factor (increase in length), responsible for the cause of incomplete RBBB, is clearly significant when there is dilatation of right ventricle due to volume or diastolic overload. The causes of this right ventricular dilatation are: ASD, tricuspid insufficiency, chronic cor pulmonale, right ventricular hypertrophy, etc.

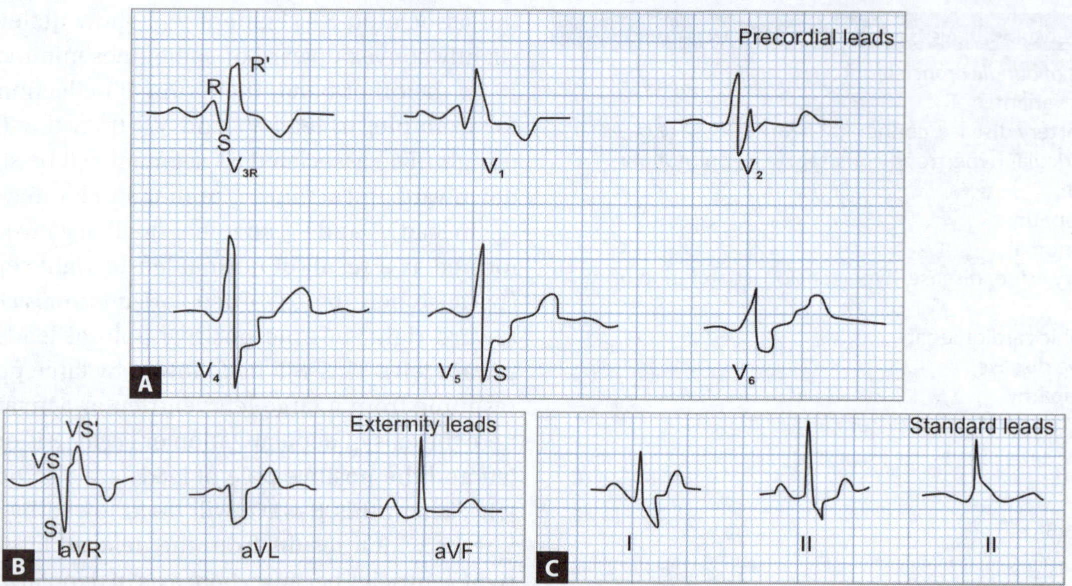

Figs. 65A to C: Summary of right bundle branch block (RBBB). (A) Depicts precordial leads, characterized by: (1) RSR$_1$ or rsR$_1$ complexes in V$_{3R}$ and V$_{1-2}$. An initial "q" wave is never present in these leads unless there is associated infarction, right ventricular hypertrophy or dilatation, or additional left ventricular fascicular block, (2) Wide S-wave in V$_{5-6}$, (3) QRS interval >0.12 second, and (4) ST depression and T-wave inversion in V$_{1-3}$; (B) Depicts extremity leads, characterized by: (1) Wide rsR$_1$ complex in aVR and (2) Patterns in aVL and aVF will depend on heart position; (C) Depicts standard leads, characterized by wide S-wave which is invariably present in lead I. Among these many findings are common but are not essential for the diagnosis. So, minimum criteria for RBBB diagnosis is rsR$_1$ complex in right precordial leads (V$_{3R}$ and V$_{1-2}$) with QRS interval >0.12 second and a wide S-wave in lead I.

The pattern of ECG in incomplete RBBB is similar to that of complete RBBB, except that the QRS interval is not >0.12 seconds. Sometimes, it is impossible to differentiate between the incomplete RBBB and normal QRS pattern in lead V$_1$ and V$_2$.

Left Bundle Branch Block

Complete LBBB always indicates some form of organic heart disease. It is commonly associated with ischemic heart, left ventricular hypertrophy due to a hypertensive heart, and aortic valvular diseases. But, it may occur with almost any form of heart disease. It is rarely seen in individuals, with no clinical evidence of an organic heart disease.

Mechanism: Here, the spread of excitation (vector) from SA node to AV node and through bundle of His is normal. Then, obviously, due to block in left bundle branch, the impulse cannot enter the left bundle system (the left side of septum). So, septal activation starts on the right side of heart and follows to the left, resulting in an initial vector oriented from the right to left (opposite to normal, septal activation occurs normally from left to right through bundle of His) **(Fig. 66)**.

Therefore, in leads V$_{1-2}$, an initial negative q-wave will (does not normally present in lead V$_{1-2}$) result which is due to septal activation from right to left (here, the negative q-wave is because the +ve pole of lead V$_1$ and V$_2$ is oriented toward right, but the axis of depolarization is right to left). Since, the

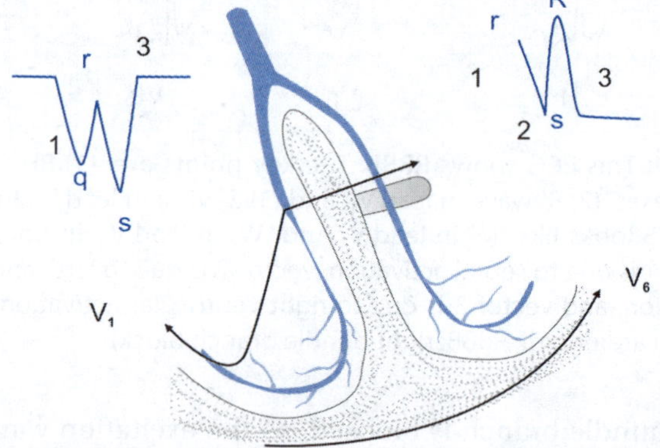

Fig. 66: This figure shows an ECG of a fully evolved LBBB. (ECG: electrocardiogram; LBBB: left bundle branch block)

left bundle branch is blocked, so the excitation wave, from bundle of His, next spreads down the right bundle branch to right ventricular myocardium, resulting in a positive "r" wave in V$_{1-2}$ leads. Because of the relative thinness of right ventricular wall, the amplitude of this "r" wave may or may not pass above the isoelectric line or may produce a positive notch in negative qS-wave in these V$_{1-2}$ precordial leads. The impulse, then, passes from right ventricular myocardium, around the blocked left bundle branch, into left ventricular myocardium and produces a deep wide S-wave (this negative S-wave in lead V$_1$ and V$_2$ is because, here the positive pole

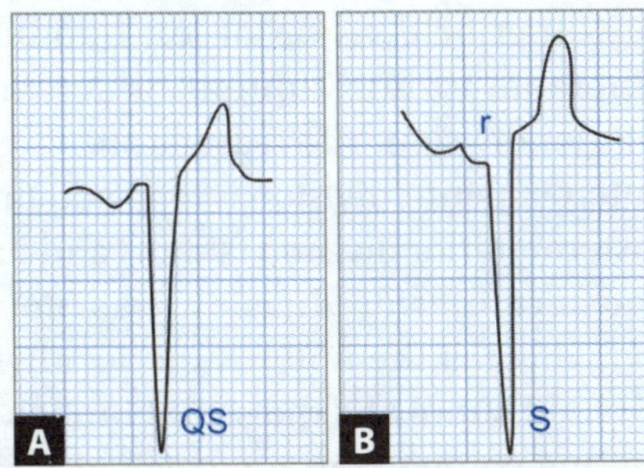

Figs. 67A and B: (A) ECG changes of LBBB in right ventricular cavity complex. (B) ECG changes of LBBB in left ventricular cavity complex. (ECG: electrocardiogram; LBBB: left bundle branch block)

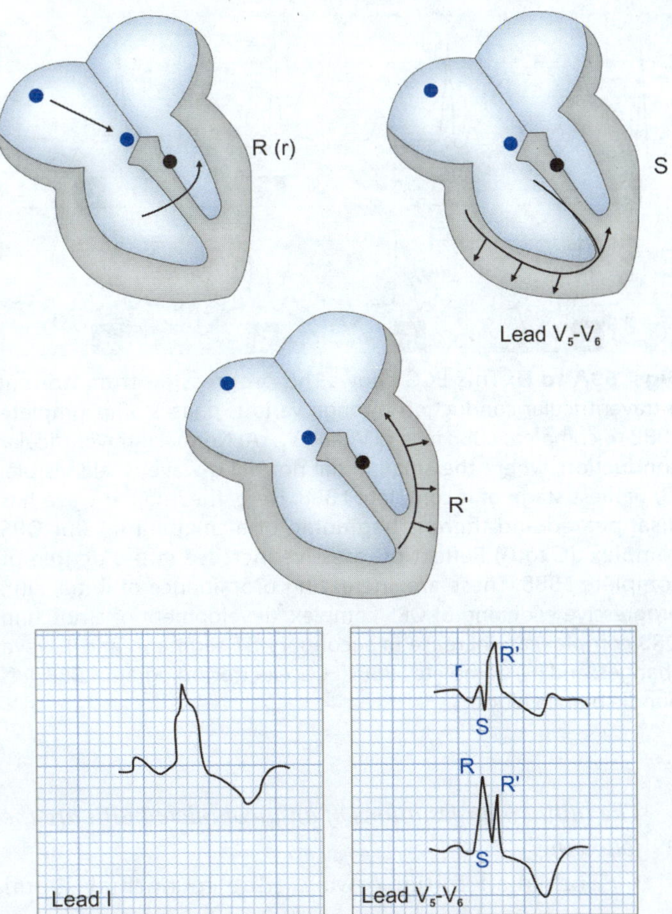

Fig. 68: ECG of LBBB in left epicardial complex. (ECG: electrocardiogram; LBBB: left bundle branch block)

of these leads are oriented toward right, but the axis of depolarization or vector is oriented toward left). *Thus, a typical W-pattern QRS complex will be developed in leads V$_{1-2}$. Occasionally, either a small q or r-wave cannot be recorded. Therefore, the QRS pattern will look like rs or QS complex. The ST segment may be elevated and T will be upright* **(Figs. 67A and B).**

In leads V$_{5-6}$ as a result of septal activation from right to left, a small initial positive r-wave will be recorded (here axis of depolarization is toward left and the +ve pole of leads V$_5$ and V$_6$ is also on left side. So, there is positive r-wave). The negative q-wave will not be formed (in normal ECG a negative q-wave is must in V$_{5-6}$ lead). This is followed by the activation of right ventricle and a negative deflection "S" wave in leads V$_5$ and V$_6$ (here the negative S-wave is because the + pole of leads V$_5$ and V$_6$ is on left side, but the axis of depolarization is toward the right). Because of the thinness of right ventricle, this small negative "S" wave may not go below the isoelectric line, but may merely produce a notch in the next positive R-wave. The impulse then passes around the blocked left bundle branch into left ventricle through its myocardium and produces a R′-wave. Thus, a typical pattern of rsR′ or RsR′ or a slurred and widened R-wave will be formed. The ST segments are usually depressed and T-waves are inverted (opposite the direction of last wave). So, in LBBB the QRS complex looks like "W" in V$_{1-2}$ leads and looks like "M" in V$_{5-6}$ leads **(Fig. 68).**

Thus, the characteristic feature of LBBB is the absence of normal septal q-wave in lead I and in left precordial leads V$_{5-6}$. Conduction delay is present through most of QRS vector, producing a broad and slurred R-wave or rsR′ or RSR′ complexes in lead I and V5-6. The QRS interval is >0.12 seconds.

Significance of LBBB is that it may be permanent or transient. Transient LBBB may occur during the course of myocardial infarction (MI), heart failure, acute myocarditis, and as a result of drug therapy (quinidine, procainamide, amiodarone, etc.). However, the permanent LBBB is always the result of some organic heart disease.

In the right ventricular cavity complex, the LBBB will produce a wide QS complex. This is because the septal activation is from right to left and the cavity will be negative throughout the ventricular depolarization. In left ventricular cavity complex, the initial septal depolarization is from right to left and will produce an initial small r-wave. Then, ventricular depolarization proceeding from endocardial to epicardial surfaces results in a larger negative deflection S-wave. The left ventricular cavity complex is therefore rS.

- *Incomplete LBBB:* In case of incomplete LBBB, the conduction of impulses through left bundle branch and its ramifications is still possible. But this is delayed. Hence, the type of ECG changes which occurs with incomplete LBBB will depend upon the degree of delay of conduction of impulses through the left bundle branch. The progressively increasing delay of conduction through the left bundle branch will result in a progressive sequence of ECG changes, leading to a complete block. Therefore, the all grades of incomplete LBBB are illustrated in **Figures 69A to H.**

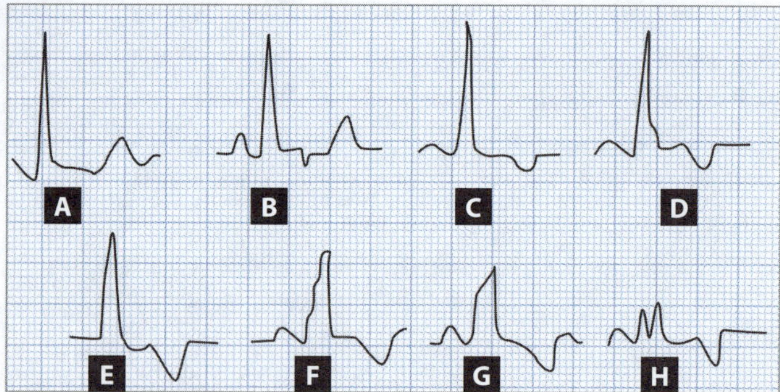

Figs. 69A to H: This ECG shows the progression from normal intraventricular conduction through various phases of incomplete LBBB to complete LBBB in lead V$_5$ and V$_6$. (A) Normal intraventricular conduction, where the small initial normal q-wave is still visible; (B) Earliest stage of incomplete LBBB. Here, the initial q-wave has disappeared and there is beginning of a small initial slur QRS complex; (C to G) Reflect progressive increase in the degree of complete LBBB. These are: increasing prominence of initial slur, progressive widening of QRS complex, development of a notch in QRS complex, an increase in secondary ST segment, and T-wave changes; and (H) Complete LBBB. (ECG: electrocardiogram; LBBB: left bundle branch block)

The initial manifestations of an incomplete LBBB are the following:

- The small initial q-wave (due to normal septal activation) of the normal qR complex in the left oriented leads, i.e., V5-6 and I disappears. This results in a single tall R-wave.
- The small initial r-wave (due to normal septal activation) of the normal rS complex in lead V$_{1-2}$ disappears. This results in a QS complex.
- With further progression, a slur appears on the upstroke of QRS complex. This slur becomes increasingly prominent and is accompanied by widening and an eventual notching of the QRS complex, until the fully developed manifestation of complete LBBB is attained. Such a manifestation is due to the increasing dominance of the right ventricular factors due to the increasing delay of conduction within the left bundle branch.

- *Fascicular block (hemiblock):* It is defined as a delay or interruption of conduction through one of the two major divisions or fasciculi of left bundle branch of bundle of His. The left bundle branch, after its origin from the bundle of His, divides immediately into two major divisions:
  1. *Anterosuperior division:* It passes anteriorly and superiorly
  2. *Posteroinferior division:* It passes posteriorly and inferiorly.

The anterosuperior division of left bundle branch is more vulnerable to interruption of activity than the posteroinferior division. The reasons are:

- The anterosuperior division is long and thin, whereas the posteroinferior division is short and thick.
- The posteroinferior division has double blood supply, whereas the anterosuperior division has a single blood supply by the septal branch of anterior descending coronary artery which also supplies the right bundle branch.

Thus, the anterosuperior division is more vulnerable to injury (ischemia, fibrosis, etc) and interruption of activity than the posteroinferior division. *This also explains the frequent association of RBBB with left anterior fasciculi or hemiblock.*

Left anterior fascicular or hemiblock: It is the delay or interruption of conduction through the anterosuperior division of left bundle branch. It may be due to fibrosis or infarction. The fibrosis may be due to coronary artery disease, cardiomyopathy, long-standing hypertension, long-standing chronic heart failure, etc.

When there is an interruption in conduction through anterosuperior division of left bundle branch, then the entire conduction from left bundle branch passes through its posteroinferior division, resulting in a mean QRS axis or vector in frontal plane, directed superiorly and to the left, i.e., left axis deviation (greater than –30°). Thus, the left axis deviation is the diagnostic criteria of left anterior hemiblock (LAHB) in ECG. There is no appreciable widening of QRS complex **(Fig. 70)**.

In LAHB, the first part of ventricle to be activated is the inferior septal region and the posterior region of free left ventricular wall, i.e., the posteroinferior region of left ventricle. Therefore, it results in an initial QRS forces to be directed toward right (q-wave in lead I) and inferiorly (r-wave in lead II, III, and aVF). This initial activation is followed by a delayed activation of the anterosuperior and the lateral region of the free left ventricular wall by anterior fascicle via the interconnecting Purkinje fibers, distal to the site of block. This results in a QRS vector oriented toward left (R-wave in lead I) and superiorly (S-wave in lead II, III, and aVF). Thus, a qR-wave in lead I and a rS-wave in lead II diagnose the left axis deviation and LAHB. But, other causes mimicking the left axis deviation should be excluded.

Therefore, LAHB causes the following modifications of QRS complex:

- A prominent QRS vector which is directed toward the right.
- Left QRS axis deviation
- Slight increase in QRS duration
- Increased magnitude of QRS deflection.

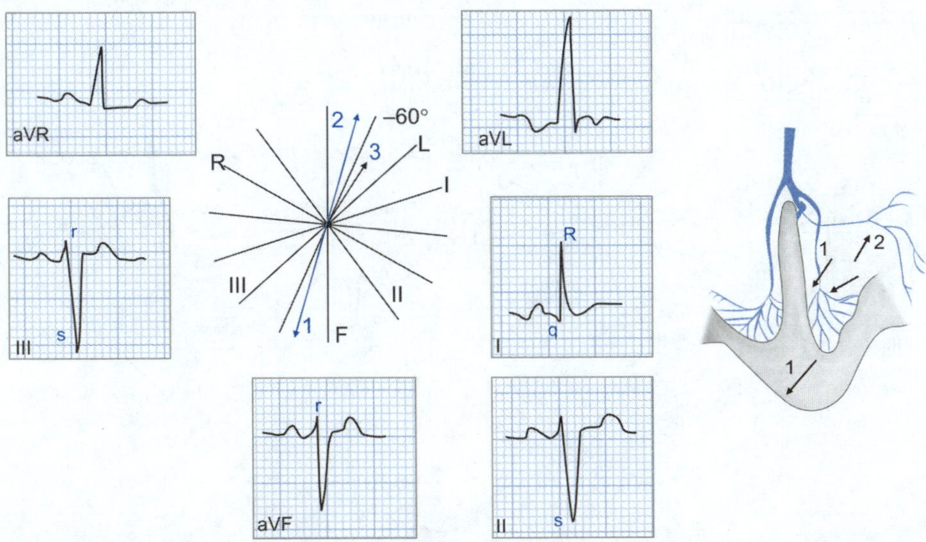

Fig. 70: This figure shows the left anterior fascicular or hemiblock. The initial QRS vector (1) is directed toward the right, causing q in lead I and inferiorly causing r in lead II, III, and aVF. The terminal QRS vector (2) is directed toward the left, causing R in lead I and superiorly causing S in lead II, III, and aVF. Thus, the resultant QRS frontal plane vector (3) is oriented to –60°.

The other causes of left axis deviation are:

- Myocardial infarction of inferior wall
- Pacing arising from the apex of right ventricle (right or left)
- WPW syndrome (some presentation)
- Ventricular ectopic beats (VEBs) arising from the apex of heart
- Some congenital heart diseases
- Coronary artery disease
- Left ventricular hypertrophy
- Pulmonary emphysema.

Left anterior hemiblock is the most common cause of left axis deviation and is most frequently due to fibrosis. This fibrosis may be due to chronic cardiac failure, chronic coronary insufficiency, or chronic left ventricular decompensation which occurs with chronic cardiomyopathy and long-standing systemic hypertension. In elderly patients, the LAHB may be due to subclinical coronary artery disease. When the LAHB is associated with congestive heart failure, then it usually indicates a long-standing heart disease.

The isolated LAHB in the absence of any overt cardiac disease does not necessarily imply an adverse prognosis or constitute a great risk factor. When LAHB is associated with RBBB (bifascicular block), then it usually indicates an adverse prognosis and may precede to complete heart block. *Bifascicular block in a patient with syncopal attacks is often a sufficient indication for permanent pacemaker implantation. Asymptomatic bifascicular block is not necessarily an indication for pacing.*

Left posterior fascicular or hemiblock: It is a very rare occurrence and results from the lesions in posterior fascicle of left bundle branch. In LPHB, the left ventricular conduction initially spreads through the anterior fascicle, resulting in a QRS vector oriented toward the left (r-wave in lead I) and superiorly (q-wave in lead II, III, and aVF). *So, the last part of anterior hemiblock is manifested first here.* Then, the posterior fascicule is activated via the interconnecting Purkinje fibers, distal to the site of block. This results in a vector, oriented toward right (S-wave in lead I) and inferiorly (R-wave in lead II, III, and aVF). *So, the first part of anterior hemiblock is manifested later here. Hence, the mean QRS axis in frontal plane is deviated toward right (right axis deviation)* **(Fig. 71)**.

There are other causes of right axis deviation, such as right ventricular hypertrophy and lateral MI, which can be excluded from left posterior hemiblock. Therefore, an ECG diagnosis of left posterior hemiblock can be made only by excluding the possibility of right ventricular hypertrophy and MI.

An easy workout for the determination of cardiac axis is:
- A predominantly positive QRS complex in both lead I and lead II indicates the normal axis.
- A predominantly positive QRS complex in lead I and a predominantly negative QRS complex in lead II indicates the left axis deviation.
- A predominantly negative QRS complex in lead I and a predominantly positive QRS complex in lead II indicates the right axis deviation.

Bilateral Bundle Branch Block

It indicates conduction defects in both the right and left bundle branch systems in different combinations. According to this combination they are classified as:

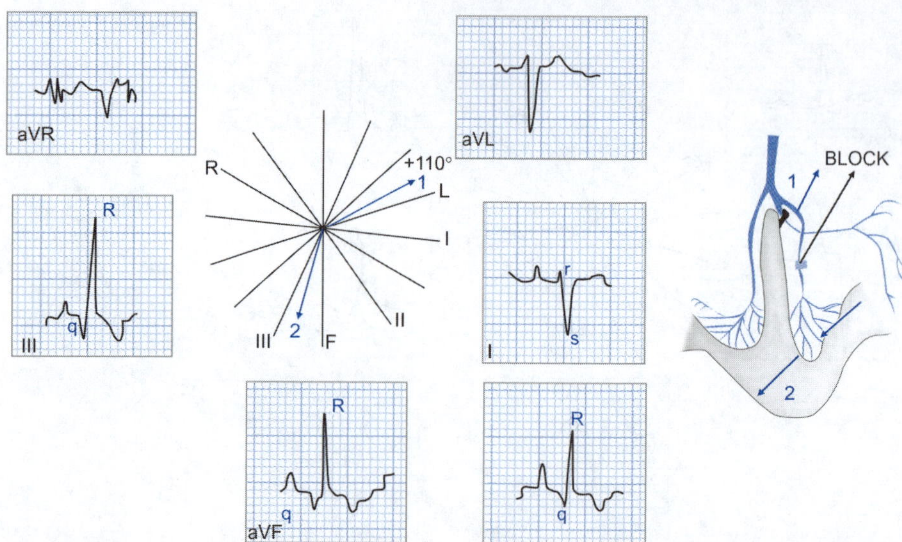

Fig. 71: This figure shows left posterior fascicular or hemiblock. The initial QRS vector (1) is directed toward left, causing r-wave in lead I and superiorly, causing q-wave in lead II, III, and aVF. The terminal QRS vector (2) is directed rightward, causing S-wave in lead I and inferiorly, causing R-wave in lead II, III, and aVF. Thus, the resultant QRS vector in frontal plane is oriented to +110°.

- RBBB with left anterior hemiblock or fascicular block
- RBBB with left posterior hemiblock or fascicular block
- Right or left bundle branch block with prolonged AV conduction (PR interval >0.20 seconds)
- RBBB with left anterior fascicular block and left posterior fascicular block. This means RBBB with complete LBBB or a complete heart block.

The bilateral bundle branch block is prognostically significant. Because, they greatly increase the probability of complete heart block. The most common cause of bilateral bundle branch block is a degenerative process that involves the upper part of intraventricular septum and the annulus structure of mitral and/or aortic valve, leading to fibrosis and calcification. The next common cause of this type of block is coronary artery disease. When bilateral bundle branch block is associated with MI, the prognosis is very poor. When RBBB is combined with left anterior or posterior hemiblock, it is termed as *bifascicular block*. It means two of the three main conducting pathways to ventricles are blocked. Again, if bifascicular block is combined with a first-degree AV block (long PR interval), then it is called the *trifascicular block*. Actually, trifascicular block means all the three fascicules (right bundle branch, left anterior and left posterior fascicules) of interventricular conducting system are blocked and it is not possible for a supraventricular impulse to activate the ventricle. So, it is a situation equivalent to third-degree or complete heart block with idioventricular rhythm. But, the term trifascicular block is not used as a nomenclature for complete heart block.

- *RBBB with LAHB:* This condition can be recognized easily in ECG by (1) typical finding of complete RBBB and (2) left axis deviation of QRS vector, greater than −30° in frontal plane. It is one of the most common types of bilateral bundle branch block or bifascicular block. There is a combination of both the features of RBBB and LAHB, i.e., (1) delayed terminal QRS forces, oriented toward the right and anteriorly, producing a wide S-waves in lead I, V_{5-6} with a wide RSR′-waves in V_1, V_2, and a W pattern QRS complex in lead V_{5-6}, and (2) left axis deviation, i.e., QRS vector in frontal plane is greater than −30° **(Fig. 72)**.
- *RBBB with LPHB:* This condition can be recognized in ECG by (1) the typical findings of complete RBBB and (2) the right axis deviation of QRS vector, greater than +110° in frontal plane. The RBBB alone does not produce such a higher degree of rightward axis deviation. As in isolated left posterior hemiblock, the right ventricular hypertrophy must be excluded, which is also responsible for right axis deviation **(Fig. 73)**.
- *Right bundle branch block with left anterior or posterior hemiblock with prolonged PR interval:* This is also termed as *trifascicular block*, but the term is not appropriate (actual meaning of trifascicular block has been explained previously). Again, this condition should not be included in bifascicular block, because only one bundle branch is affected and the prolonged PR interval is not due to the defect in bundle branch, but due to the defect in AV node.

Ventricular Arrhythmias

There are different forms of ventricular arrhythmias. These are:

- Ventricular premature (or extrasystole or ectopic) beats
- Ventricular tachycardia

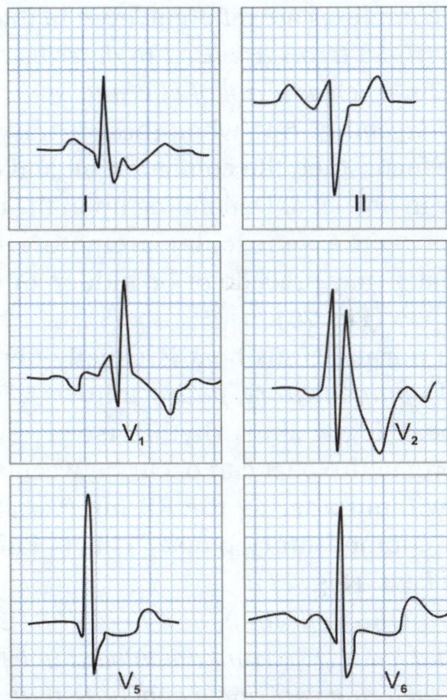

Fig. 72: This figure shows an ECG of bifascicular block (RBBB with left anterior hemiblock or LAHB). Here, the QRS pattern in V_{1-2} is rsR1 (M pattern) which indicates RBBB. There is also left axis deviation, because there is a predominant positive QRS complex in lead I and a predominant negative QRS complex in lead II. (ECG: electrocardiogram; LAHB: left anterior hemiblock; RBBB: right bundle branch block)

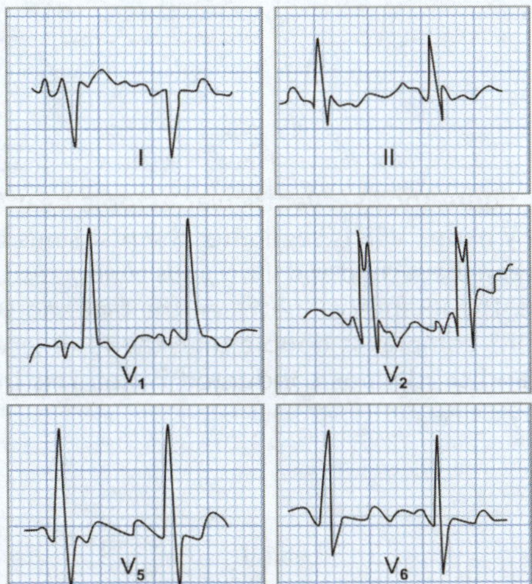

Fig. 73: This is an ECG of RBBB, with left posterior hemiblock (LPHB), a type of bifascicular block. The RBBB is evidenced by M-pattern or positive QRS complexes in lead V_{1-2}. Left posterior fascicular (hemi) block is evidenced by right axis deviation, because there is predominant negative QRS complex in lead I and predominant positive QRS complex in Lead II. (ECG: electrocardiogram; RBBB: right bundle branch block)

- Ventricular flutter and fibrillation
- Ventricular escape beat.

Ventricular Extrasystoles

This is due to premature depolarization and subsequent contraction of ventricles, due to the discharge of impulses from an ectopic focus, situated at any portion of ventricular myocardium. It is less common than supraventricular ectopic, but like it (supraventricular ectopic) the ventricular extrasystoles also may occur even in normal individual. Though, the ventricular premature beats are commonly seen in association with any form of organic heart disease, but are most common in IHD, infarction, myocarditis, digitalis toxicity, etc. Ventricular extrasystoles may also result from the effect of some drugs, e.g., catecholamines, halothane, digitalis, etc.

Mechanism or pathophysiology of ventricular extrasystole: The ventricular extrasystole results from an irritable extra focus, situated at any portion of ventricular myocardium. So, these impulses do not travel through the normal specialized conductive tissue, i.e., Purkinje fibers. Contrarily, these impulses travel through the ordinary ventricular muscle tissue (myocardial cells) which is a poor conducting medium. *As a result, the QRS complex is bizarre, widened, slurred,* or notched. This premature impulse activates both the right and left ventricles and a premature ventricular contraction occurs **(Fig. 74)**.

The regular SA nodal rhythm is not disturbed during ventricular extrasystoles, as the ectopic ventricular impulse does not penetrate the AV node and activates the atria or depolarizes the SA node. Again the regular sinus impulse, following the premature beat, will usually not be able to activate the ventricles, since the latter (ventricle) is still in refractory state from the previous premature contraction. Thus, the next sinus impulse will activate the ventricles only when the refractory period is over, provided another ventricular extrasystole does not occur within this time **(Fig. 75)**.

Therefore, the interval between the two successive sinus beat preceding and following the premature beat will be exactly twice of the regular sinus interval. The ventricular extrasystole is premature. It arises in ventricular diastolic period, caused by the preceding sinus beat. It is therefore recorded earlier than the next anticipated sinus beat.

The ventricular extrasystole fails to penetrate the AV node retrogradely. Thus, the SA node is protected from ectopic ventricular impulse and is not disturbed from its rhythmic function. Following an extrasystole, as the ventricles remain in a refractory stage, so the regular normal incoming impulses from SA node fails to initiate regular ventricular contraction. Hence, following an extrasystole, there is a time gap, during which the ventricle is waiting for impulses from SA node in normal a rhythm. This time gap following the extrasystole is called the *compensatory pause*. The interval between the ectopic beat and the previous sinus beat is called the *coupling interval*. It is constant for all extrasystoles, arising from same focus. This is because the extrasystole is anyway related to or forced by or precipitated by the previous sinus beat.

ECG pattern of ventricular extrasystole: The QRS complexes of ventricular extrasystoles are broad, bizarre, slurred, and notched in appearance. The ST segment and T-wave is directed opposite to the main deflection of ectopic QRS complex. When the ventricular extrasystoles arise from multiple ectopic foci, then the configuration and direction

of extra QRS complexes are different, even in the same lead. *Couplet and triplet terms are used to describe two or three successive VEBs, whereas a run of alternate sinus and ectopic beat is called bigeminy.* But, when these extrasystoles arise from a single focus, then the configuration and direction of them is same in one lead. Depending upon the relationship of timing between a ventricular premature beat and a P-wave, the later may precede or be hidden or even follow the QRS complex **(Fig. 76)**.

Since the normal sinus beat is usually not disturbed, hence a full *compensatory pause* follows a ventricular premature beat. If the sinus rhythm is very slow, then a ventricular premature beat can occur between two normal sinus beats without altering the RR interval and without producing a compensatory pause. This is known as the *"interpolated beat"* **(Fig. 77)**.

If the extra QRS deflection, due to a VEB, is upright in right precordial leads (V_{1-2}) and downward in left precordial leads (V_{5-6}), then one can safely conclude that this ectopic focus is situated in left ventricle. The reverse is true for the

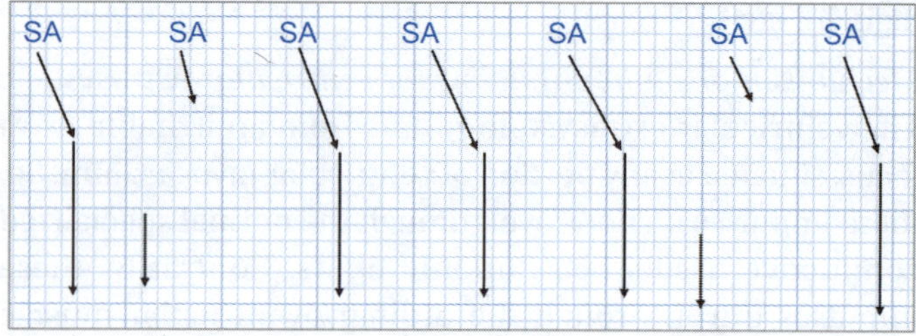

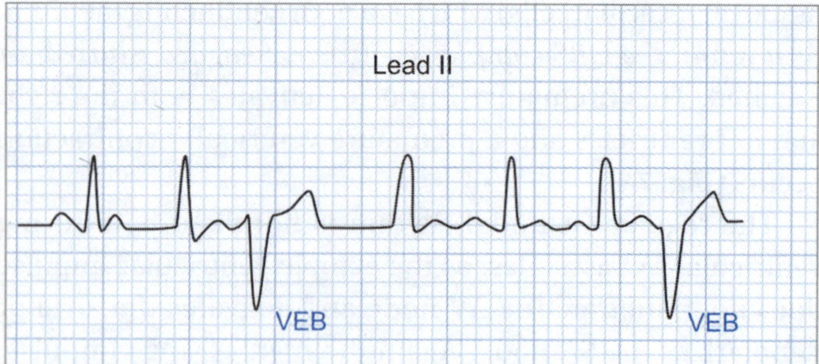

Fig. 74: Unifocal ventricular ectopic beats (VEBs). Two VEBs are seen in association with a regular sinus ventricular rhythm. Both VEBs are of same configuration and direction which indicates a same single focus of origin.

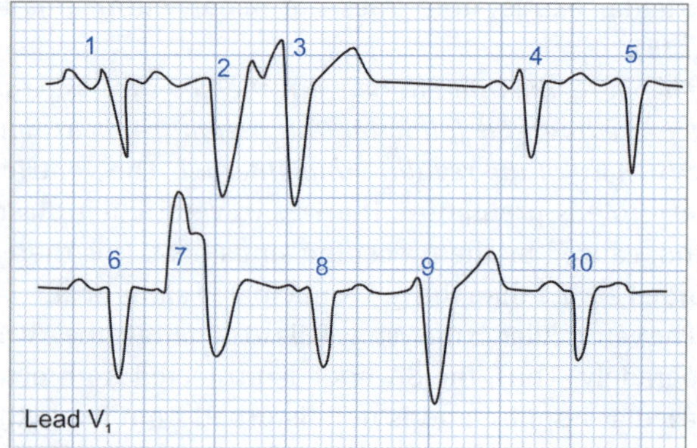

Fig. 75: Multifocal ventricular ectopic beats (VEBs) in lead V_1. Here, QRS complexes (1, 4, 5, 6, 8, and 10) are sinus conducted. Ectopic QRS complexes (2, 3, and 9) are oriented toward the left (deep S-wave in V_1), which indicates right ventricular origin. Ectopic QRS complex (7) is oriented toward right (tall R-wave in V_1) which indicates left ventricular origin.

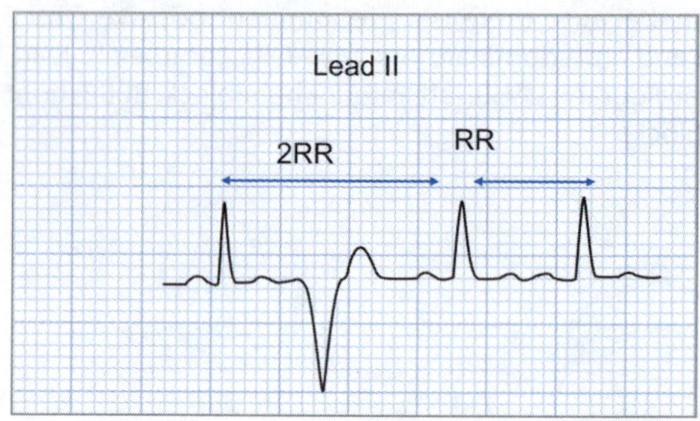

Fig. 76: This figure shows a ventricular ectopic beat (VEB) with a compensatory pause. VEB is seen after the first sinus beat. The RR interval between the second and third sinus conducted QRS complex is 0.8 second. The RR interval between the first and second sinus conducted QRS complex is double than the RR interval between the second and third sinus conducted beats. This indicates full compensatory pause.

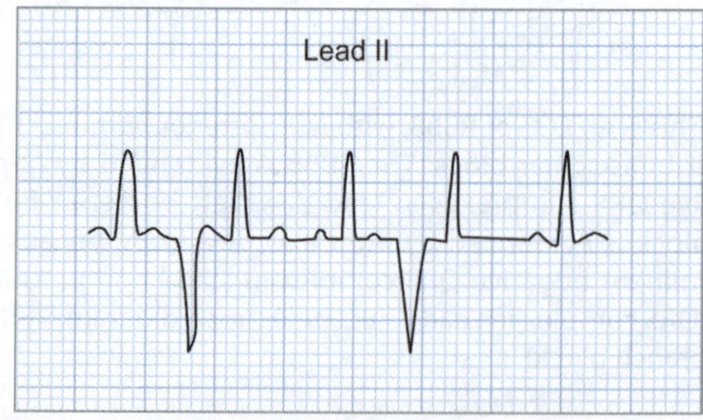

Fig. 77: This figure shows interpolated ventricular ectopic beats (VEBs). This VEB is seen after the first and third sinus beats, without any compensatory pause.

*right ventricular premature beats (**Figs. 78 and 79**). Thus, the left ventricular extrasystole mimics the QRS pattern of complete RBBB and right ventricular extrasystole mimics the QRS pattern of complete LBBB. The ventricular premature beats may occur in association with other arrhythmias also (**Figs. 80 and 81**).*

The premature ventricular contraction by ectopic beats produces a low stroke volume, because this ventricular contraction is ineffective. The pulse is, therefore, irregular

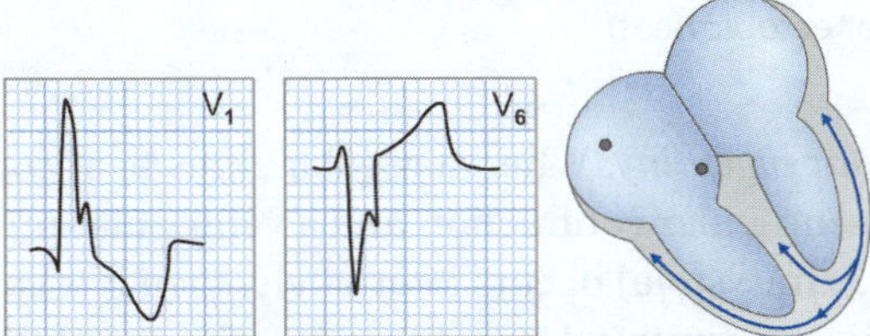

Fig. 78: Here, the ectopic ventricular focus is situated in left ventricle. So, the main spread of impulse is away from the positive electrode at V₆, causing a downward QRS deflection. On the other hand, this impulse spreads toward the positive electrode at V₁, causing an upward QRS deflection.

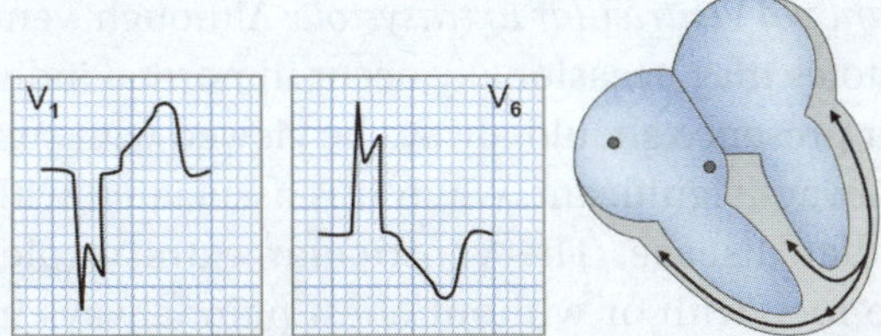

Fig. 79: Here, the ectopic ventricular focus is situated in right ventricle. So, the main spread of impulse is away from positive electrode at V₁, causing a downward QRS deflection. On the other hand, this impulse spreads toward the positive electrode at V₆, causing an upward QRS deflection.

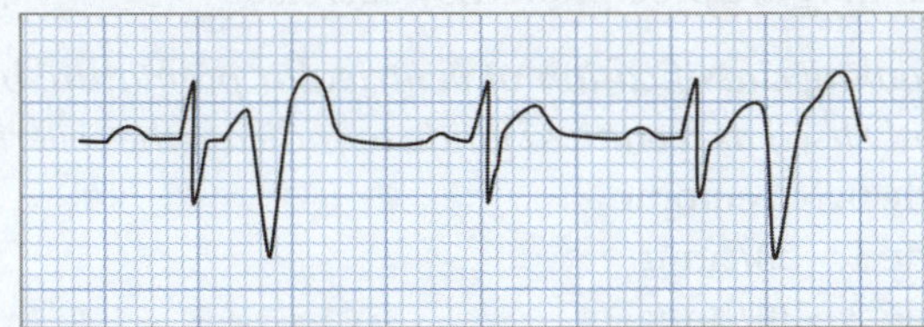

Fig. 80: This electrocardiogram (ECG) shows ventricular premature contractions, during a vulnerable period, i.e., before the completion of T-wave of the preceding beat (R on T phenomenon).

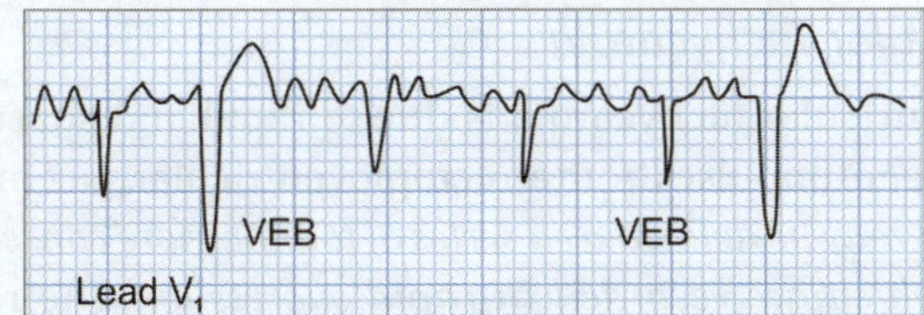

Fig. 81: This figure shows ventricular ectopic beats (VEBs) in association with atrial fibrillation.

with weak or missed beats (not-palpable). Patients are often asymptomatic, but may complain of an irregular heartbeat, missed beats, or abnormally strong beats. The significance of VEBs depends on the nature of underlying heart disease.

Ventricular ectopic beats may frequently found in normal people and their prevalence increases with age. VEBs are more prominent at rest in patients with otherwise normal hearts and tend to disappear with exercise. The outlook of these types of VEB is excellent and so treatment is unnecessary. Although a low dose β-blocker treatment is sometimes used to suppress the anxiety and palpitation. VEBs are sometimes a manifestation of subclinical heart disease. There is no evidence that such patients are merited by antiarrhythmic therapy. But, the discovery of frequent VEBs may prompt some general cardiac investigations.

Frequent VEBs are often observed during acute MI. But, they are of no prognostic significance and require no special treatment. However, persistent and frequent VEBs in patients, who have survived the acute phase of MI, are indicative of a poor outcome. Unfortunately, antiarrhythmic therapy does not improve and may even worsen the prognosis in these patients.

Ventricular ectopic beats are common in patients with heart failure and are associated with adverse prognosis. But, again, the outlook is not better, if they are only suppressed with antiarrhythmic drugs, without treating the underlying causes for heart failure. In such circumstances, the effective treatment of heart failure may abolish the ectopic beats. VEBs are also the feature of digoxin toxicity and may occur as escape beats in the presence of an underlying bradycardia. However, the treatment of VEBs should be directed according to their underlying causes.

R on T phenomenon: The QT interval approximates the refractory period of the action potential of cardiac (ventricular) myocytes. Ventricular extrasystoles usually occur after the T-waves of previous beat and before the next beat. Sometimes, the ventricular extrasystole starts at the upstroke or downstroke of T-wave of previous beat **(Figs. 80 and 82)**.

This portion of T-wave coincides with the *supernormal excitability period of action potential* of cardiac myocyte (mainly ventricular cells) and is very vulnerable for repetitive firing. So, such an ectopic beat is prone to initiate repetitive discharges of impulses, i.e., ventricular tachycardia or ventricular fibrillation (VF). *This phenomenon is called the R on T phenomenon and has serious clinical significance (Fig. 80).*

Supernormal excitability: The time period in action potential curve, during which no stimulus will be able to initiate another action potential, is known as the *absolute refractory*

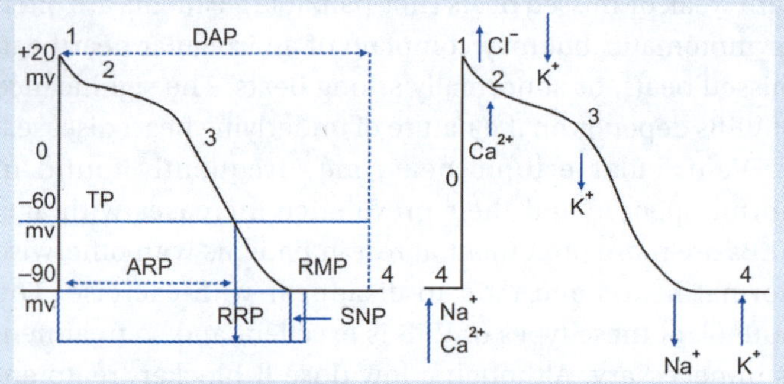

Fig. 82: Action potential (AP) of a cell of ventricular muscle. [ARP: absolute refractory period; DAP: duration of action potential; TP: threshold potential; RMP: resting membrane potential; RRP: relative refractory period; SNP: super normal period; 0 = depolarization phase; 1, 2, 3 = repolarization phase; 4 = diastolic phase. Depolarization + repolarization = ventricular systole (0 + 1 + 2 + 3 phase)].

Note: Action potential (AP) occurring cyclically is described below:

Phase 4 = Resting condition or diastole where the resting membrane potential (RMP) is -70 to -90 mV. This mainly depends on K^+ concentration, as it is more permeable than Na^+.

Phase 0 = Rapid depolarization phase, due to Na^+ and Ca^{2+} influx.

Phase 1 = Initial repolarization phase. It is due to influx of Cl^- and coming out of K^+.

Phase 2 = Plateau phase of repolarization, with slow influx of Ca^{2+} and coming out of K^+ from cells. The amount of entry of Ca^{2+} and exit of K^+ is same and balance each other. So, a plateau of electrical potential is maintained.

Phase 3 = Rapid repolarization phase. It is due to the efflux of K^+, causing rapid return of intracellular potential to -70 or -90 mv. It establishes the normal negative resting potential. But, the inside of cell is left with excess of Na^+ and deficit of K^+.

Phase 4 = The Na^+ goes out of cell in exchange of K^+, which enters the cell and maintains RMP. In resting state, the outside of the cell is positive while the inside of the cell is negative. This is called the polarized state (phase 4). When the outside of cell becomes negative and the inside of cell becomes positive, then this condition is called the depolarized state (phase 0). Again when the outside of the cell becomes positive and the inside of the cell becomes negative, but the intracellular and extracellular concentration of Na^+ and K^+ is opposite to that of normal, it is called the repolarized state (phases 1, 2, and 3). When the polarization of the cell remains same as repolarization, but the Na^+ and K^+ concentration becomes normal, it is called the polarized state.

period. This period includes phases 0, 1, 2, and a part of phase 3. Following this, there is a time period when only a strong stimulus can evoke a response of action potential. This is called the *relative (or effective) refractory period*. It begins when the transmembrane potential in phase 3 reaches the threshold potential level (about –60 mV) and ends just before the termination of phase 3. This is followed by a period of *supernormal excitability period* (terminal part of phase 3 and beginning of phase 4), when even a relatively weak stimulus can evoke a response.

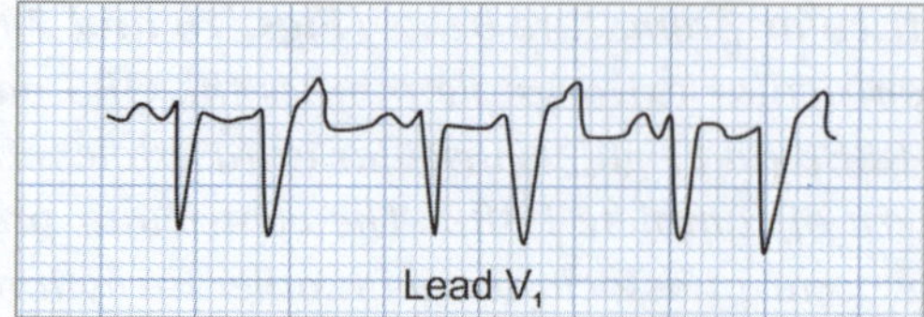

Fig. 83: This is an ECG of ventricular bigeminy. It is characterized by regular sinus rhythm and subsequently followed by a VEB, a pause, a sinus ventricular beat and then repetition of this sequence. The time interval between the sinus beat and the VEB is perfectly constant. This is called *fixed coupling*. The P-waves of sinus beat are buried in the QRS complex of each VEB (ECG: electrocardiogram; VEB: ventricular ectopic beat)

Ventricular bigeminy: When a regular sinus beat controlled normal ventricular contraction and a ventricular premature beat (or extrasystole) occurs alternately, then it is called the ventricular bigeminy. Here, there is a fixed coupling, i.e., there is a constant interval between a sinus beat controlled ventricular beat and a premature ventricular beat. This fixed coupling indicates that the sinus beat controls the VEB by re-entry mechanism, present in the ventricular myocardium **(Fig. 83)**.

Significance of Ventricular Extrasystole: Although, ventricular extrasystoles may occasionally occur in normal individuals, still their presence should always be viewed with suspicion. VEB is always significant, when it is associated with some myocardial disease. The ventricular extrasystoles from multiple foci, with or without chest pain, always indicate serious myocardial disease. Unifocal ventricular extrasystoles are usually indicative of cardiac diseases, (1) if they occur in persons over 40 years of age, (2) if they occur frequently, i.e., in crops or showers, (3) if they occur in association with other cardiac diseases, (4) if they occur in bigeminal rhythm, and (5) if they are precipitated by exercise.

The following classification of ventricular premature beats is commonly used as a clinical guide to indicate the severity:

- Grade 0: No ectopic
- Grade 1: <30/hour
- Grade 2: >30/hour
- Grade 3: Multiformed complexes
- Grade 4: Couplets of three or more (ventricular tachycardia)
- Grade 5: R on T phenomenon.

Ventricular Tachycardia

The ventricular tachycardia is due to rapid and successive discharge of impulses from an ectopic ventricular pacemaking focus. *It may be defined as a series of four or more consecutive VEBs which are recorded in rapid succession.* The rate of ventricular tachycardia usually varies in-between 140 and 220 beats/min. There are two principal forms of ventricular tachycardia. These are: (1) *idioventricular tachycardia* and (2) *extrasystolic ventricular tachycardia* **(Fig. 84)**.

The basic principle of idioventricular tachycardia is the development idioventricular rhythm, where there is complete heart block and there is increased escape ventricular rate. Actually, it is a severe form of accelerated ventricular rhythm. On the contrary, the extrasystolic ventricular tachycardia is not associated with complete heart block and impulses originating from SA node come to ventricle regularly. But, there is an increased automaticity of any ventricular tissue, making ectopic focus.

The ventricular tachycardia is also the result of re-entry mechanism within the ventricular myocardium, like supraventricular tachycardia. It is most commonly associated with a recently manifested acute MI. It may also occur in association with hypertensive and atherosclerotic heart diseases and certain drugs (digitalis, quinidine, etc.) intoxication. It also occurs in association with WPW syndrome. Ventricular tachycardia is a very serious condition and always indicates a serious heart disease. It should be treated successfully, otherwise mortality rate is very high.

ECG pattern of ventricular tachycardia: The ECG tracing of ventricular tachycardia is constituted by rapid succession of ventricular premature beats, where it may be impossible to separate the QRS complexes from ST segments and T-waves. However, the abnormal ventricular complexes are regular and the ECG tracing has the appearance of a series of regular, wide, and large undulations.

The normal sinus rhythm usually continues independently and passes to the ventricle (not in idioventricular tachycardia, but in extrasystolic ventricular tachycardia) with the ventricular tachycardia. But, the P-waves cannot be seen within the images of ventricular complexes. Ventricular tachycardia may occur independently with sinus rhythm or also in the presence of any atrial arrhythmia. But, it cannot be diagnosed without the use of esophageal leads or intracardiac monitoring. It has been assumed that ventricular tachycardia, originating from left ventricle, would result in ventricular complexes simulating RBBB and that ventricular tachycardia, originating in right ventricle would simulate LBBB.

The ventricular tachycardia differs from VF by its uniformity, constancy, and deflections of relatively large amplitude. The deflections of VF are small, completely chaotic, and irregular.

Torsades De Pointes: This is also called the *"multiform ventricular tachycardia or flutter"*. As the name signifies, it is polymorphic type of origin where the QRS complexes arise from multiventricular ectopic foci. Therefore, the QRS complexes vary from upright to inverted in direction and come in cyclic fashion. The sharp points of the QRS complexes may for a short period be directed upward, which is followed for a short period by a change in QRS contour, where the sharp points are directed downward. Hence, the term *"torsades de pointes" which means twisting or torsion of points* is applied. The most common cause of this situation is prolongation of ventricular repolarization and this is due to drug toxicity, such as quinidine and amiodarone **(Fig. 85)**.

Accelerated idioventricular rhythm: The heart has many potential pacemaking cells or tissues, such as SA node, AV node, atrial muscle, ventricular muscle, and special conducting tissues, like Purkinje fibers, etc. But, among these, only one pacemaking cell which has the highest rate of automaticity controls the HR. This is because the impulses, arising from the tissues with higher automaticity rate, reach the other potential pacemaker cells and abolish their discharges, before they have the time to mature and fire **(Fig. 86)**.

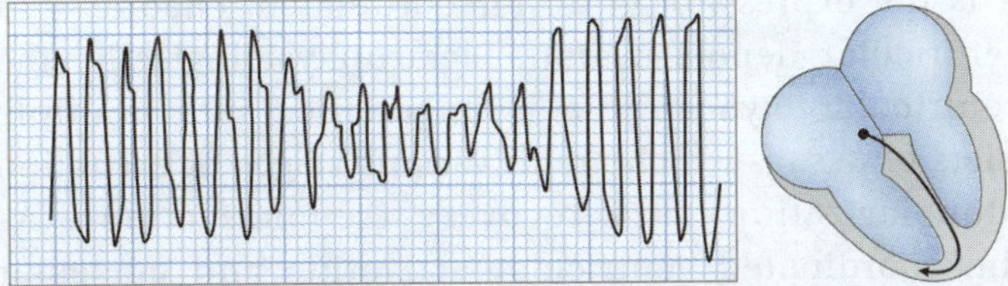

Fig. 85: This is an electrocardiogram (ECG) of torsades de pointes. The key points are: broad complex tachycardia and variations in QRS axis.

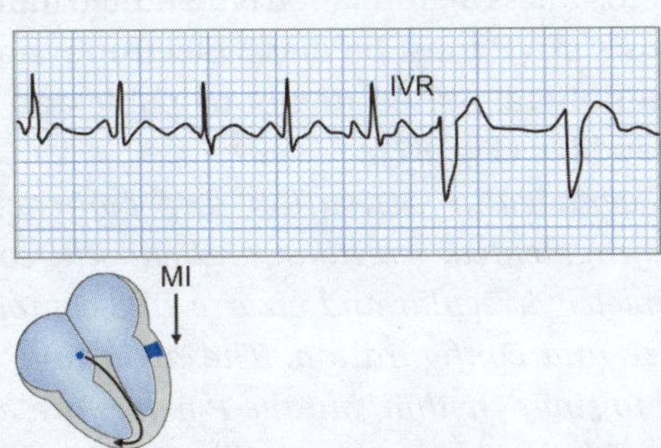

Fig. 86: This ECG shows onset of accelerated idioventricular rhythm, marked in the figure by IVR. It is idioventricular, because the QRS complexes are broad and it is accelerated because the rate is ±88/min. (ECG: electrocardiogram; IVR: idioventricular rhythm; MI: myocardial infarction)

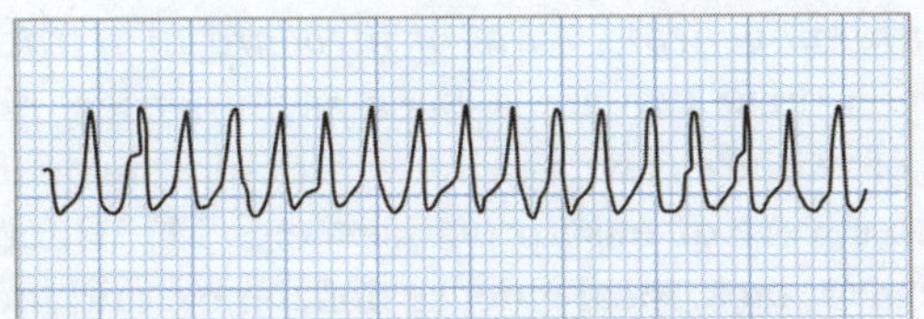

Fig. 84: This is an electrocardiogram (ECG) of ventricular tachycardia, characterized by repeated broad QRS complexes (broad complex ventricular tachycardia).

Therefore, the subsidiary pacemaker area gets some protection from the impulses of fastest pacemaker area. Under certain circumstances, the automaticity of these subsidiary pacemakers area becomes enhanced. For example, when the AV nodal discharge rate exceeds the sinus rate, then the AV nodal rhythm manifests as AV nodal tachycardia. Similarly, in a complete heart block when the ventricular myocardium acts as pacemaker and beats 30–40 times per minute, then it is called the *idioventricular rhythm*. When this idioventricular rhythm is enhanced due to any cause, then it is called the *idioventricular tachycardia* whose rate is usually 150–200 beats/min. The accelerated idioventricular rhythm is in-between these two conditions (idioventricular rhythm and idioventricular tachycardia) where HR varies between 60 and 100 beats/min. Here, the term tachycardia is not used, because the HR remains below 100 beats/min.

This condition is most commonly seen in association with acute MI. It is usually transient and may not require any therapy at all, especially if the hemodynamic status is stable. It is a much more benign abnormal ventricular rhythm than the slow idioventricular rhythm with complete heart block, or ventricular tachycardia with sinus activity. Therapy is not indicated initially, but close observation is needed for any clinical deterioration and then management is started.

Ventricular Flutter and Fibrillation

It is the expression of an uncoordinated, chaotic, and ventricular depolarization. Electrophysiologically, the ventricular myocardium is fragmented into multiple islets of tissues which are in various stages of excitation (depolarization) and recovery (repolarization). As the coordinated ventricular activation and muscular contractions are lost and the ventricular myocardium starts fibrillating, therefore the hemodynamic pumping action of heart ceases and death ensues, due to reduction of cardiac output to zero, unless defibrillation is instituted immediately. The diagnosis of VF must be made electrophysiologically, since the peripheral pulses are not palpable and the heart sound is inaudible **(Fig. 87)**.

As the ventricular activation and contractions are completely fragmented, irregular, and chaotic, so the ECG shows completely irregular and bizarre QRS complexes with varying size and configuration. The atria may continue to respond to sinus rhythm, but the P-waves are not visible without the aid of esophageal leads **(Fig. 88)**.

The factors that give rise to ventricular tachycardia may also be responsible for VF. Among them, the most important factor is MI and this explains many sudden deaths in this disease. It may also occur as the terminal manifestation

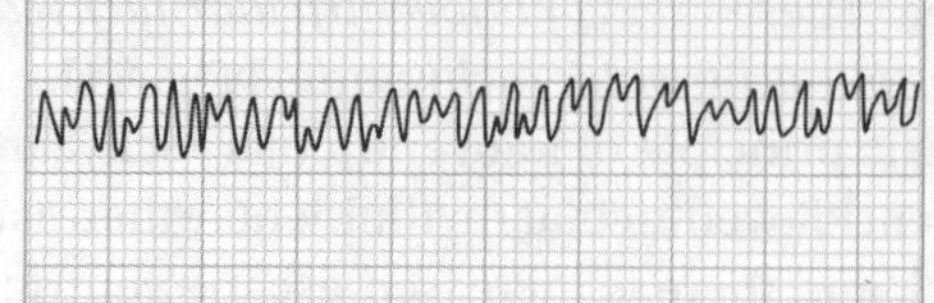

Fig. 87: This is an electrocardiogram (ECG) of ventricular fibrillation, characterized by chaotic ventricular activity.

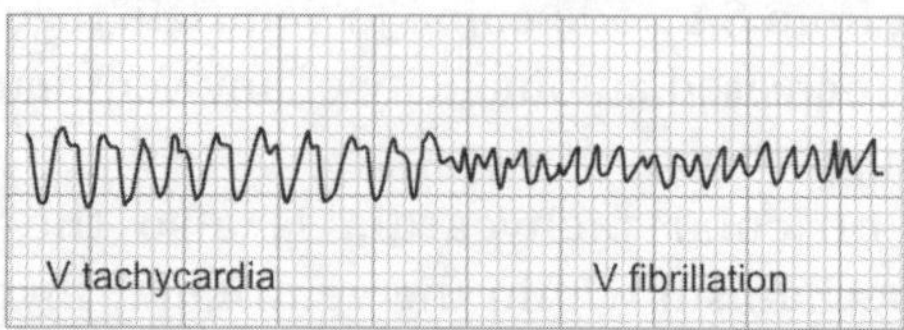

Fig. 88: This is an electrocardiogram (ECG) of ventricular fibrillation after ventricular tachycardia. The QRS complexes are more bizarre during the period of ventricular fibrillation and vary in size and configuration from beat to beat.

of many organic heart diseases and hypokalemia. It may also occur during surgical procedures, performed under general anesthesia (GA) where hypoxia is the most common precipitating factor. It occurs characteristically with hypothermia, when the body temperature drops below 28°C. The electrical shock may also produce VF. The VF can be classified into: (1) primary VF and (2) secondary VF.

The *primary VF* is defined as the VF that occurs in patients without any preexisting cardiac diseases, e.g., hypotension, (systolic pressure <80 mm Hg, due to blood loss), hypokalemia, heart failure, etc. It responds relatively well to electrical defibrillation and resuscitation is usually successful. The *secondary VF* is defined as the VF which occurs in patients with serious medical disorders in the presence of previous cardiac diseases (e.g., severe uncorrected hypotension, respiratory failure, cardiac failure, liver diseases, electrolyte imbalance, etc.). Resuscitation is usually unsuccessful in secondary VF.

Etiopathology of Ventricular Fibrillation: The development of ventricular flutter and VF is usually caused by the coincidence of the following two fundamental events and these are:

1. The development of advanced physiological asymmetry between two ventricular areas, as there is a *nonhomogeneous state of myocardial refractoriness* between these two areas. Such asymmetrical refractory state of two areas within the ventricular myocardium is due to severe disease processes, e.g., M1 which results in local O_2 lack, local glucose deficiency, and local ionic changes, such as Ca^{2+}, Na^+, and K^+.

2. The premature repetitive stimulation of ventricular myocardium which aggravates the out of phase state and

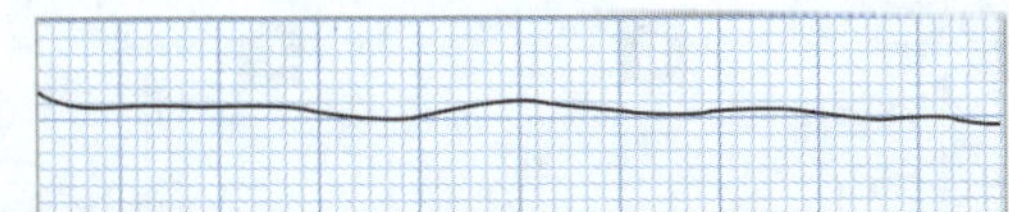

Fig. 89: This is an electrocardiogram (ECG) of an asystole, characterized by a "flat line" with no spontaneous atrial or ventricular activity.

precipitates fibrillation. The source of such premature rapid stimulation is ventricular extrasystoles with very short coupling interval. Ventricular extrasystoles with R on T phenomenon represent the most vulnerable type of ventricular excitability and precipitates ventricular flutter and VF.

Clinical significance and prognosis of ventricular fibrillation: Ventricular fibrillation is most serious among all the cardiac arrhythmias and should be treated promptly. The prompt treatment of patients with VF, which is commonly associated with MI in coronary care units, has largely reduced its mortality rate and this becomes possible by its immediate recognition. VF may occur in transient paroxysms and may be the cause of Stokes–Adams syndrome. Prognosis is very poor for such VF and recovery is rare, if arrhythmia continues for over 5 minutes. Prognosis is better when this arrhythmia occurs in operating room or in intensive care unit where immediate resuscitative measures including electrical defibrillation can be instituted immediately.

Clinically, VF cannot be differentiated from a ventricular standstill (asystole) **(Fig. 89)**, *because in both these conditions, there is no palpable or auscultatory evidence of cardiac action. So, it is essential to differentiate these two conditions electrocardiographically, since their treatment differs considerably. For example, ventricular standstill may respond to epinephrine, isoproterenol, atropine, or even electrical pacing, whereas the VF requires immediate electrical defibrillation.*

■ GENESIS OF ST SEGMENT AND T-WAVE

In ECG tracing, the point at which QRS complex ends and ST segment begins is called the J point or J junction. The portion of tracing from this J junction to the onset of T-wave is called the ST segment. The ST segment is usually an isoelectric line, but may vary from 0.5 to +2 mm in precordial leads. It is elevated or depressed in comparison to that portion of baseline which is situated between the termination of T-wave and the beginning of next P-wave. The ST segment usually merges smoothly and imperceptibly with the proximal limb of T-wave.

The ST segment and T-wave represents ventricular repolarization. As the normal ST segment is isoelectric, so

it does not manifest any axis. Only in abnormal conditions when the ST segment is deviated above or below the baseline, then it produces a measurable axis. The measurement of the deviation of the axis of ST segment is based on same principles as those used for the P, QRS, and T-wave axis. For this measurement of deviation of the axis of ST segment, the first step is to look out for the lead in which the ST segment is more or less isoelectric or equiphasic. Then, it is obvious that the axis of ST segment in this particular tracing is perpendicular to that lead. For example, if the ST segment is isoelectric, i.e., no deviation in lead aVR, then the ST segment axis is perpendicular to the lead aVR and/or is parallel to the lead III, where it is maximally deviated from the isoelectric line. Thus, the ST segment is parallel to the positive pole of that lead which is perpendicular to the isoelectric lead.

When the ST segment is deviated above or below the baseline, as a result of coronary artery disease, then in both horizontal and frontal plane, it is directed toward the surface of injury.

■ CORONARY INSUFFICIENCY

The impaired coronary blood flow into myocardium may be an established case (i.e., inadequate coronary blood flow both during rest and during increased demand) or may be a relative one (i.e., blood flow being adequate at rest, but inadequate when myocardial demand is increased such as in exercise) or may even be due to some additional transient factors (i.e., coronary vasospasm). In ECG, coronary artery disease may be reflected as the changes in QRS complex, ST segment, T-wave, and U-wave. Like before, these changes may be present at rest or may be precipitated by factors which induce transient myocardial ischemia, e.g., exercise.

Effects of Coronary Insufficiency on ECG

The QRS complexes represent the phase of depolarization of ventricle, while the ST segment and T-wave represent the repolarization process of ventricle. The effects of coronary insufficiency are reflected in both the depolarization and repolarization processes. But, the earliest changes are usually evident during repolarization, i.e., on the ST segment and T-wave. As a rule, the changes in depolarization, due to ischemia, tend to be permanent, whereas the initial changes in repolarization tend to be temporary **(Figs. 90A to E and 91)**.

Effects on QRS Complex

The effects of coronary insufficiency on QRS complexes are like the changes during depolarization and are permanent, e.g., LBBB, left axis deviation, etc.

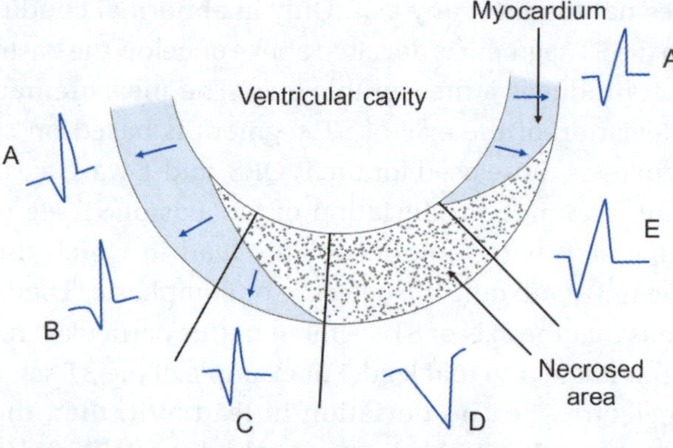

Figs. 90A to E: This diagram illustrates: (A) Normal endocardial to epicardial QRS activation. (B) Minimal subendocardial necrosis with slight change or unchanged QRS activation. (C) Significant subendocardial necrosis with diminished QRS activation, and a pathological Q-wave. (D) Total transmural necrosis with absent QRS activation and presence of Q-wave. (E) Subepicardial necrosis with diminished QRS activation.

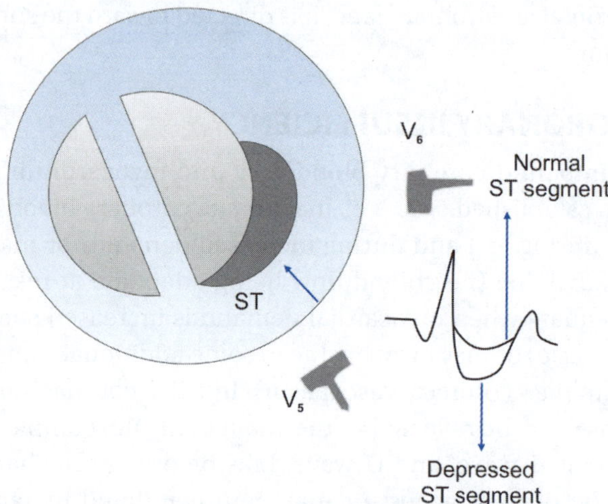

Fig. 91: This figure shows the basic principles of electrocardiogram (ECG) changes in subendocardial and subepicardial injury in angina pectoris. The subendocardial ischemia results in the shifting of ST segment toward the injured surface, i.e., toward the left ventricular cavity in lead aVR and away from the left ventricular cavity in precordial leads V1 to V6. Thus, it results in ST segment depression in leads V1 to V6 and elevation in lead aVR.

Effects on ST Segment

Coronary insufficiency may depress and alter the shape of ST segment. Occasionally, it may also present with transient elevation of ST segment. This is the manifestation of variant forms of angina pectoris such as Prinzmetal angina.

Effects on T-wave

The T-wave is the most unstable, but a significant component of an ECG recording. Certain nonspecific changes of this deflection may occur with hyperventilation, heavy meals, anxiety, etc. **(Figs. 92A to C)**.

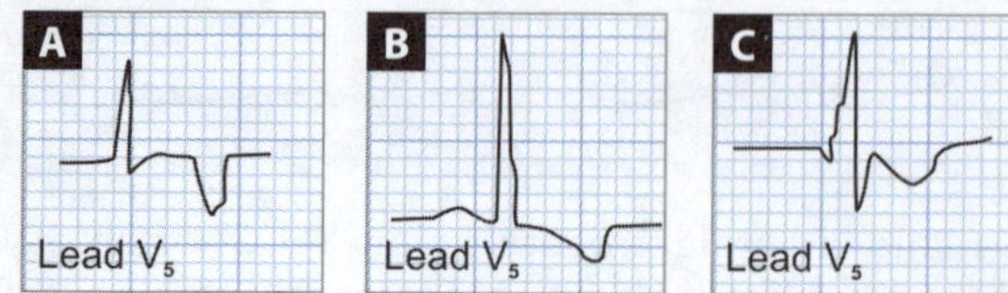

Figs. 92A to C: These electrocardiogram (ECG) show the ST segment and T-wave changes. (A) Coronary insufficiency. (B) The "strain" pattern associated with ventricular hypertrophy. (C) The effect of digitalis.

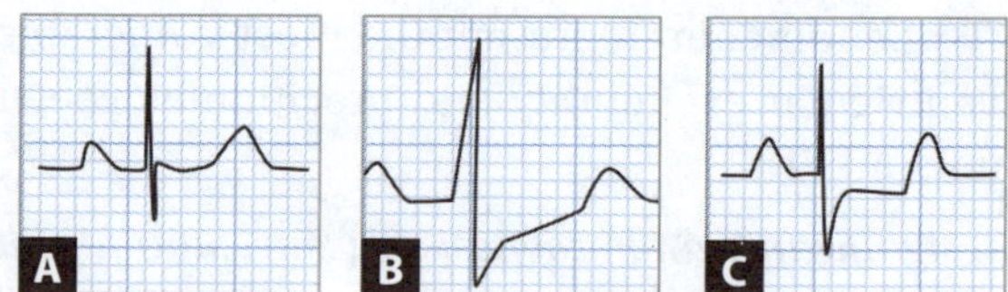

Figs. 93A to C: This electrocardiogram (ECG) shows: (A) Normal ST segment. (B) Junctional ST segment depression. (C) Plain ST segment depression.

Despite this, there are certain specific T-wave changes that are frequently suggestive of coronary insufficiency. The T-wave changes, associated with coronary insufficiency, have symmetrical limbs and a sharp pointed arrow-head vertex. The changes of T-wave configuration from other causes usually show asymmetrical limbs with a relatively blunt vertex or nadir. As a result of ST segment depression, the T-wave may be dragged downward, giving an appearance of inversion. This T-wave inversion is of slight to moderate degree. Occasionally, one may see a very deep T-wave inversion, simulating that seen in MI **(Figs. 93A to C)**.

Depression and Significance of Shape of ST Segment

Normally the ST segment merges gradually, smoothly, and imperceptibly with the ascending limb of T-wave, so that a separation between the two is difficult or impossible **(Fig. 94)**.

One of the earliest signs of coronary insufficiency is an alteration in the shape of ST segment, resulting in a sharp-angled ST-T junction. This produces a horizontal appearance in ST segment. A further evaluation of this effect is the depression of ST segment. The depression of the horizontal ST segment gives the appearance of plane depression. The ST segment may also have a sagging depression.

ST Segment Depression

The most significant criteria of ST segment change in coronary insufficiency is the depression of 1 mm or more of a point which is situated 0.08 seconds after the onset of ST segment

(J point). Clinically, the character of ST depression has major significance. The various types of ST segment depression are:

- *Down sloping ST segment:* There is ST depression which is 1 mm or more at J point. This finding has the *highest specificity* for the diagnosis of myocardial ischemia. The false positive incidence is <1–2%.
- *Horizontal ST segment:* There is ST depression of 1 mm or more at J point and then this ST segment continues horizontally in depressed condition, for 0.8 seconds. Although, such a finding has been considered the diagnostic of myocardial ischemia, but its false positive incidence is approximately 15–20%.
- *Slow upstroke of ST segment:* This is defined as ST depression of 1 mm or more at "J" point, with an upward sloping of ST segment, which is not >1 mV/second. The false positive incidence of this type of ST segment exceeds 40%.
- *Rapid upstroke of ST segment:* There is 1 mm or more ST depression at "J" point, but the ST segment goes rapidly upward and its slope exceeds 1 mV/second **(Figs. 95A to D)**.

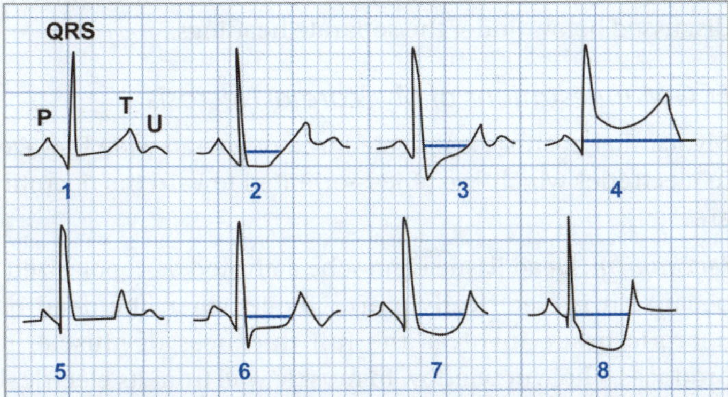

Fig. 94: This diagram illustrates: (1) Normal P-QRS-T-U complex, (2) Junctional depression, (3) Depression with upward sloping, (4) Elevation of ST segment and increase in T-wave amplitude, (5) Horizontal ST segment with sharp-angled ST-T junction, (6) Plain depression with U-wave inversion, (7) Sagging depression, and (8) Depression with downward sloping.

Mechanism of depression of ST segment: The transient myocardial ischemia, as manifested clinically by the classic form of angina pectoris, results in temporary subendocardial ischemia at the apical region of left ventricle. This injured surface faces the left ventricular cavity. The basic principles for the determination of the ST segment deviation are that the ST segment vector is always directed toward the surface of injury. Thus, +ve pole of a lead, oriented to this injured surface (in this case the left ventricular cavity), e.g., lead aVR will reflect the ischemia by *a raised ST segment* and an inverted T-wave. Positive pole of leads, facing the external surface, mainly leads V5 and V6 will reflect a *reciprocal ST segment depression.*

ST Segment Elevation

Uncommonly in response to ischemia, the ST segment elevation of >1 mm can develop. This is generally an evidence of severe transmural ischemia. This variant form of angina pectoris is due to the transient subepicardial ischemic injury. This condition manifests characteristically with transient elevation of ST segment in leads, which +ve pole is oriented toward the injured surface. This type of angina pectoris was first described by Prinzmetal and his associates, so it is named as "Prinzmetal angina".

Computer Analysis of ECG

Recently, computers are frequently used to measure accurately the amount of depression and elevation of ST segment and its slope in ECG records. It is definitely more correct than visual interpretation by an individual. Nowadays, a newer and better computer programs are being developed, which measure the ST segment depression or elevation in multiple leads and integrate it with the changes in voltage of R-wave, HR, at which these abnormalities appear, effect of exercise and the duration of such changes. The computer analysis improves the specificity and sensitivity of ECG recordings.

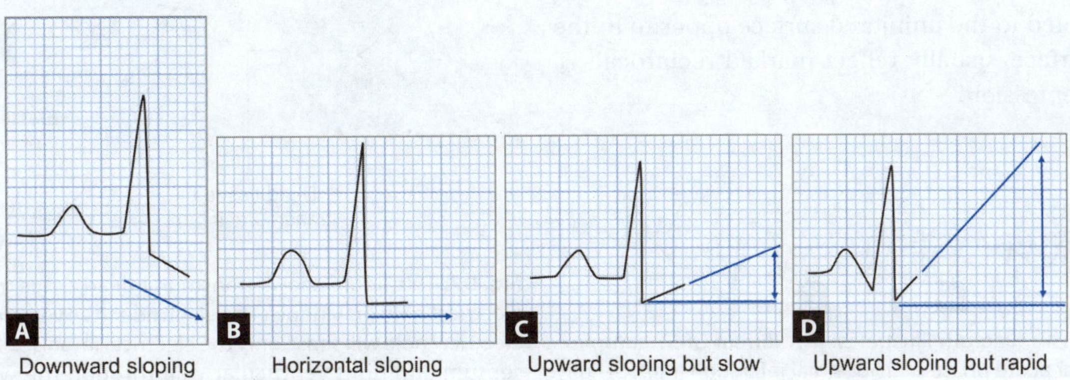

Figs. 95A to D: This figure shows different types of ST segment depression.

MYOCARDIAL INFARCTION AND ECG CHANGES

The site of MI is actually constituted (formed) by three pathological conditions, such as *necrosis, injury, and ischemia.* So, the different electrical charges in these three pathological areas are reflected at a time in ECG and help to constitute a *composite ECG picture of MI.* Again the MI passes through (*1*) *three phases and (2) has different sites of occurrence.* So, according to these three factors (pathological condition, different phases of evolution, and various sites) the ECG graph also changes. The ECG of MI also changes with the presence of concomitant arrhythmias, e.g., RBBB, LBBB, atrial arrhythmias, ventricular tachycardia, etc. The three phases, through which the MI passes, are: (1) *hyperacute phase, (2) fully evolved phase, and (3) phase of resolution.*

Hyperacute Phase

This hyperacute phase of MI occurs just after its acute onset and it should be distinguished from the next phase, i.e., the fully evolved phase. This hyperacute phase of MI is most important, because it is very critical from the prognostic point of view and also for the occurrence of complications, such as primary VF and death which is most likely to occur in this phase. So, the manifestation of hyperacute phase is an indication for intense vigilance and proper coronary care monitoring.

ECG Pattern

During the hyperacute phase of MI, the ECG is characterized by the following three principal changes in leads, whose +ve pole is oriented to the infarcted surface **(Figs. 96A to C)**.

- *Slope elevation of ST segment:* The ST segment is markedly elevated up to the apex of T-wave, which becomes widened and tall. The ST segment and the proximal limb of T-wave blends in such a smooth and imperceptible way that they (ST segment and the proximal limb of T-wave) cannot be identified separately. The +ve pole of leads oriented to the uninjured surface opposite to the injured surface, usually reflect marked reciprocal ST segment depression.

- *Tall and widened T-wave:* The T-wave becomes widened and is taller (height may even exceed that of R-wave). Its proximal limb blends with the elevated ST segment and the two components cannot be distinguished separately. The classical and pathological diagnostic Q-wave of MI does not develop, until the large amplitude of T-wave regresses.

- *Increased ventricular activation time:* This is due to the delay in onset of intrinsic deflection, i.e., the time from the beginning of QRS complex to the apex of R-wave (X-Y interval in the picture). This delay is due to the activation process of ventricular myocardium which takes a longer time to travel through the injured, but still viable infarcted region. This hyperacute phase of MI is analogous to the manifestations of a variant form of angina pectoris. But, in angina, it is transient and in MI it proceeds to the next fully evolved phase of MI.

Fully Evolved Phase of Acute MI

A fully evolved site of MI has usually three pathological areas, i.e., *(1) necrosis, (2) injury, and (3) ischemia.* Each area has separate distinguishable reflection in ECG which is discussed below under the separate headings.

ECG Manifestations of Myocardial Necrosis

Myocardial necrosis is reflected by a deep and wide Q-wave in electrodes which +ve pole is oriented toward the necrotic area.

Mechanism: Dead tissue cannot be activated or depolarized, because it is electrically inert. Hence, when the dead or necrotic tissue involves the full thickness of muscle, it produces a hole or window in muscle wall from its electrical sense (i.e., no electrical activity over this necrotic area). So, when a +pole of an electrode is placed over or oriented to this electrical hole (necrotic area), it reflects the activity of distant healthy muscle as seen through the window (hole) **(Fig. 97)**.

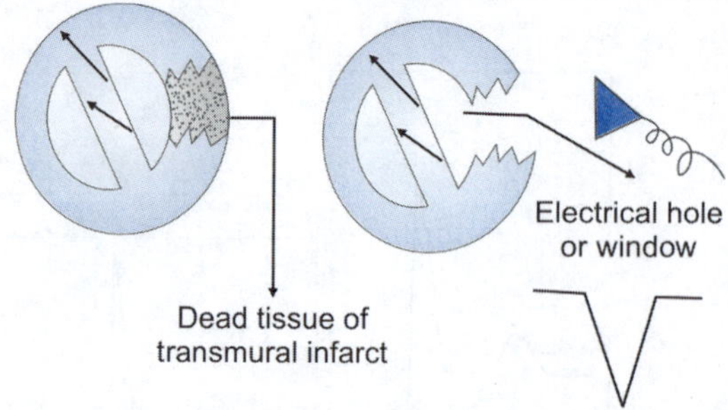

Fig. 97: This figure shows transmural dead tissue, representing the electrical hole or window. The electrode (its +ve pole) placed on this electrical hole will sense only the electrical impulse of interventricular septum and right ventricular wall through the window which is running away from the electrode and will produce a Q-wave.

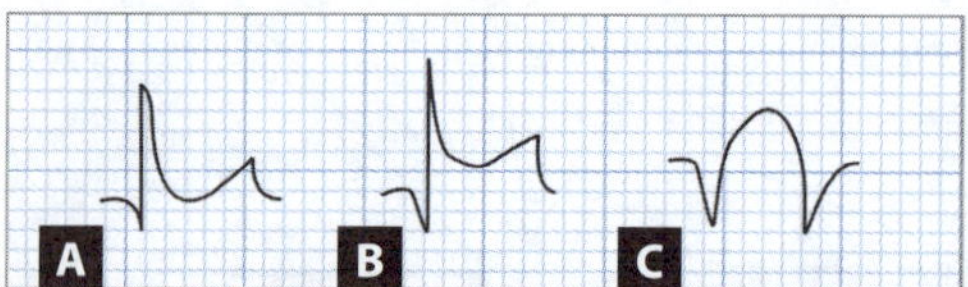

Figs. 96A to C: This diagram illustrates: (A) Normal QRST complex. (B) Hyperactive or acute phase of myocardial infarction (MI). (C) Fully evolved phase of MI.

Thus, a +ve pole of an electrode is placed over an area of dead muscle tissue of left ventricular wall, i.e. left precordial leads (V_{5-6}), it reflects the initial septal depolarization which is passing from the left toward right. So, as this electrical impulse passes away from the (+ve pole of) lead V_{5-6}, so this is reflected as a negative deflection in these leads. Then, this left precordial lead senses only the distant right ventricular depolarization which is again from the left toward right, due to the electrical impulses, passing through the muscle of right ventricle, in the absence of electrically active healthy normal left ventricular tissue. Thus, it produces a further negative deflection. Hence, this results in a broad deep Q-wave which is called the pathological Q-wave of MI. As there is no R-wave, so this Q-wave can be termed as the QS-wave.

ECG Manifestation of Myocardial Injury

In ECG, the myocardial injury is reflected by deviation (raised or depressed) of ST segment and this deviation is toward the surface of injured tissue. This is because as discussed previously, the current will flow from uninjured tissues to injured tissues, so the ST segment will be deviated toward the surface of injured tissue. Thus, if the injury is present dominantly on left epicardial surface then the ST segment is deviated toward the injured left epicardial surface. It means the current will pass from the uninjured tissue of the right side of the heart to the injured tissue on the left and leads oriented toward this epicardial surface (e.g., lead V6 in the diagram) will reflect a raised ST segment. On the contrary, a lead oriented toward the uninjured surface (e.g., lead aVR in diagram A) will reflect a depressed ST segment. With a dominant subendocardial injury a lead oriented to the injured subendocardial surface, e.g., lead aVR will reflect an elevated ST segment, whereas in subendocardial injury a lead oriented to the uninjured surface, e.g., lead V6 will reflect a depressed ST segment **(Fig. 98)**.

Since, as the myocardial injury in most MI is predominantly epicardial with some subendocardial "sparing" effect, so the manifestation presented electrocardiographically is an elevated ST segment in leads oriented to epicardial surface. Thus, the ST segment in the leads oriented over the injured epicardial surface in a fully evolved phase of infarction is coved or convex-shaped **(Figs. 99A and B)**.

ECG Manifestation of Myocardial Ischemia

The myocardial ischemia is reflected by an inverted T-wave (in reverse to the acute phase of MI, where the T-wave is upright and tall) in leads oriented to the ischemic surface. *This T-wave becomes inverted when Q-wave appears in the fully evolved phase of MI. This T-wave inversion may be due to many conditions. But, in myocardial ischemia it has certain characteristics, which tend to reflect their "ischemic"*

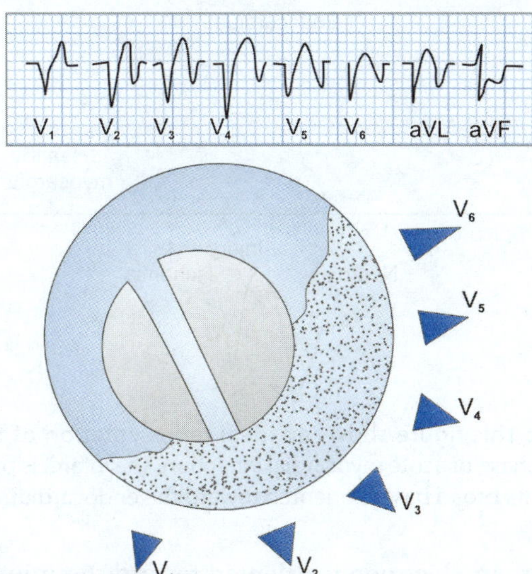

Fig. 98: This figure shows electrocardiogram (ECG) changes in acute extensive myocardial infarction.

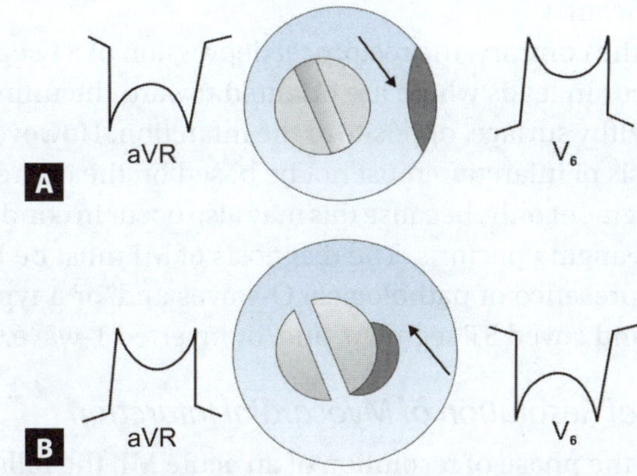

Figs. 99A and B: This figure shows deviation of ST segment in: (A) Subepicardial injury and (B) Subendocardial injury.

origin. These are usually "arrow headed", being peaked and symmetrical in appearance.

Total QRS pattern of fully evolved phase of MI: As mentioned previously, an infarcted area consists of a centrally situated necrotic tissue, surrounded by a zone of injured tissue which again is surrounded by a zone of ischemic myocardial tissue. So, a conventional electrode placed over the heart cannot pinpoint the individual injured tissue and so cannot reflect the electrical activity of that individual tissue of this infarcted area. *Again, as the leads are situated on body surface, i.e., some distance away from the heart and subserves a relatively large area, so such electrodes shall reflect all the three electrical patterns of these three types of tissues, such as (1) pathological Q-wave (for necrosed tissue), (2) raised and coved ST segment (for injured tissue), and (3) pointed inverted-symmetrical T-wave (for ischemic tissue). This is referred to as the typical infarction pattern* **(Fig. 100)**.

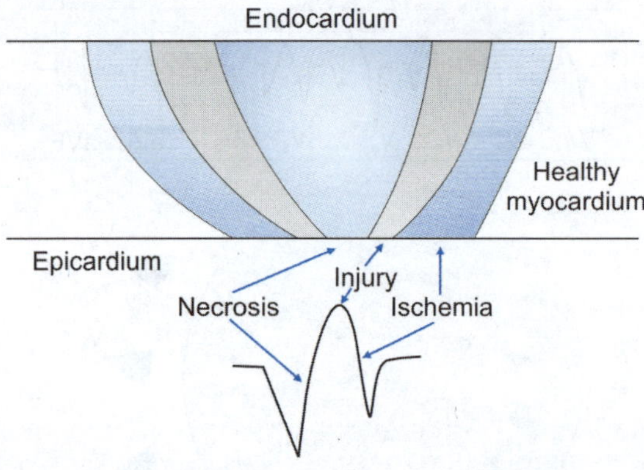

Fig. 100: This figure shows an ideal representation of the fully evolved phase of acute myocardial infarction. The infarct is pyramidal in shape. Its broad base is oriented toward the endocardium.

When an electrode is oriented toward the injured and ischemic tissue only, but not on the necrotic tissue, then it will record only the coved and raised ST segment and an inverted T-wave. The pathological Q-wave will be absent or insignificant.

On the contrary, the reciprocal depression of ST segment will occur in leads which are oriented toward the uninjured and healthy surface, opposite to the infarction. However, the diagnosis of infarction must not be based on the depression of ST segment only, because this may also occur in conditions such as angina pectoris. The diagnosis of MI must be based on the presence of pathological Q-waves and/or a typically raised and coved ST segment, and/or inverted T-wave.

Phase of Resolution of Myocardial Infarction

During the phase of resolution of an acute MI, the following ECG changes occur progressively:

- There is a gradual return of elevated ST segment to its baseline, over a few weeks.
- Simultaneously, there is an appearance of a tall symmetrical T-wave in leads, oriented to the uninjured surface.
- Then, over a few weeks, the abnormal T-waves gradually return to their normal configuration.
- The pattern, then, stabilizes into a residual state. In this state, the only evidence of previous MI is recognized by an abnormal Q-wave in leads, oriented to the infarcted area **(Figs. 101A and B)**.

■ SUMMARY

- *Acute infarction or hyperactive phase:* Slope elevation of ST segment, tall widened T-wave, and increased VAT.
- *Fully evolved phase:* Pathological Q-wave, coved and raised ST segment, and inverted symmetrical T-wave.
- *Old infarction:* Pathological Q-wave, but the ST segment and T-wave may be normal or equivocal.

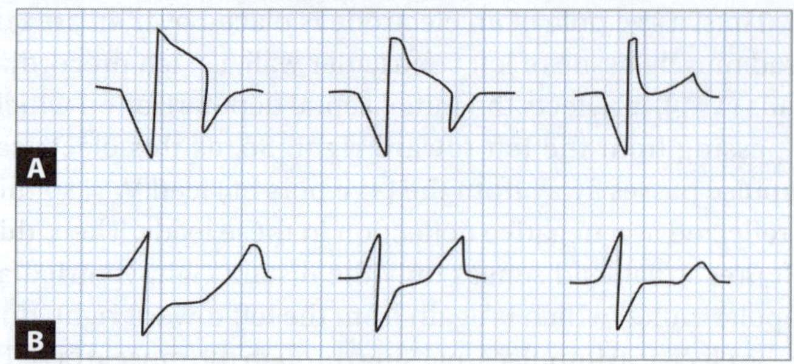

Figs. 101A and B: Resolution of MI. (A) When the lead is oriented toward injured surface and (B) When the lead is oriented toward uninjured surface.

Significance of Q-waves

Normal Q-waves (q)

The small "q" waves which indicates the initial activation of interventricular septum are normally present in left precordial leads (V4-6), lead aVL, and standard lead I with the heart in horizontal position and in left axis deviation. It is also present in standard leads II, III, and lead aVF with the heart in vertical position or right axis deviation.

The normal deep wide Q-wave or QS complex may normally be present in lead aVR and in lead V_1. This is because the positive poles of these leads are oriented toward the cavity or the basal region of heart, so that the ventricular activation process moves away from these leads.

Pathological Q-waves

The pathological Q-wave which is designated as capital letter has certain characteristics. These are:

- It should be wide >0.04 seconds in duration, i.e., one small square.
- It should be deep >4 mm, i.e., more than four small squares.
- Pathological Q-wave is associated with the great loss of height of subsequent R-wave and the Q: R ratio will be 25% or greater.
- Pathological Q-wave may appear in several leads where normal q-waves are not found. As for example, with anterolateral infarction, the pathological Q-waves will be present in standard lead I, lead aVL, and the lateral precordial leads V5-6. With inferior infarction, the Q-waves will be present in standard leads II, III, and aVF.
- The abovementioned characteristics of Q-wave must appear in leads which do not normally have deep and wide Q-wave (i.e., deep Q-wave does not indicates infarction, if it appears in lead aVR and possibly in lead V_1).

Q-waves and bundle branch block: In the presence of LBBB, the normal septal activation, representing q-waves, is absent in leads oriented to the left precordial leads, i.e., V5-6. Thus, in the presence of LBBB, the manifestations of any small q-wave in these precordial V5-6 leads, no matter how small, are always pathological and usually signifies MI. Alternatively, in the presence of LBBB, a deep Q or a QS complex in lead V_1, resembling a pathological Q-wave, does not necessarily signify an infarction. The significance of the appearance of q or s-waves in the presence of RBBB is same as in normal individuals.

Significance of Q-wave in standard lead III: It is common for lead III to record a Q-wave of 0.04 second duration and a Q: R ratio >25%. This is especially seen in normal ECG, with a mean frontal QRS axis between +30° and 0° (horizontal heart position). When this is seen as normal finding, lead aVF will not record an abnormal Q-wave. Therefore, the diagnosis of infarction must never be made on the basis of lead III tracings alone.

Further, pathological Q-waves are also present in lead III in conditions other than MI. These are acute pulmonary embolism, left posterior hemiblock, etc. The presence of a Q-wave in lead III is suggestive of MI, only if it carries the following criteria. They are:

- The duration of Q-wave must be of minimum 0.04 seconds
- The presence of any small q-wave in leads aVF and II along with lead III. The normal q-wave, present in lead III, sometimes disappears when the patient takes a deep inspiration. So, it is always suggested to take a deep inspiration, while recording a standard lead III ECG.

Localization of Infarcted Areas

Myocardial infarction occurs predominantly at anterior, inferior, and posterior walls of left ventricle according to the rate of incidences **(Fig. 102)**.

Anterior Wall Infarction (Fig. 103)

The anterior wall of left ventricle is oriented toward all the precordial leads, aVL, and standard lead I. Thus, an anterior wall infarction will be reflected by the presence of a typical infarction pattern of QRS complex and ST-T segment, such as pathological Q-wave, raised ST segment, and inverted T-wave in standard lead I, aVL, and all the precordial leads **(Fig. 104)**.

The anterior wall infarction is further subdivided into:

- *Extensive anterior wall infarction:* It is reflected by typical infarction pattern in all the precordial leads, standard lead I and lead aVL.
- *Anteroseptal wall infarction:* This indicates infarction across the interventricular septum. This is reflected by infarction pattern in leads V_{1-4}.

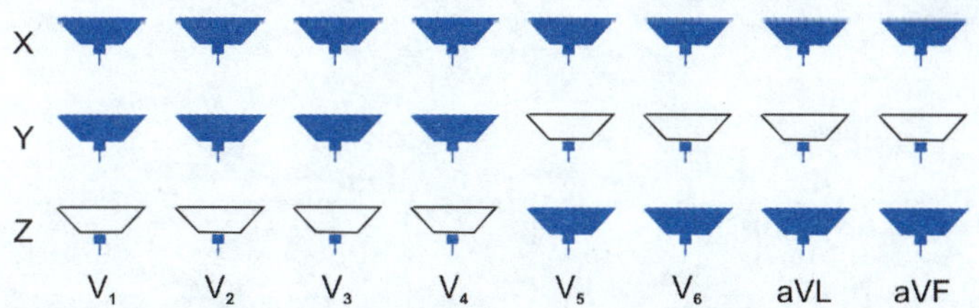

Fig. 102: Classification according to the extension of infarction. The black leads indicate the areas of infarction. (X) Extensive anterior infarction, (Y) Anteroseptal infarction, and (Z) Anterolateral infarction.

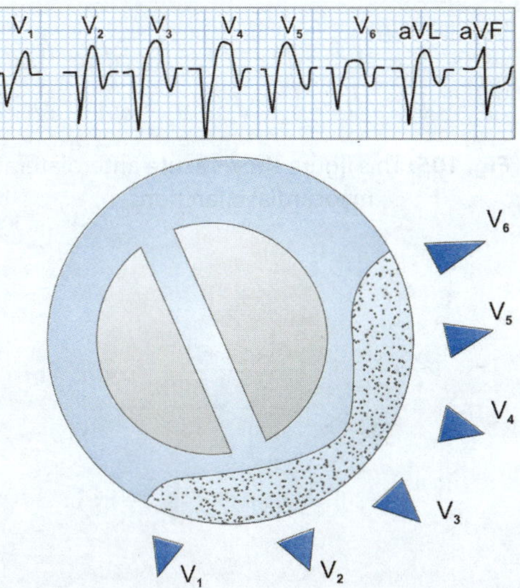

Fig. 103: This figure shows massive acute myocardial infarction (MI) (extensive as all the leads are involved). All leads from V1 to V6 show the fully evolved phase of MI, which indicates acute and extensive anterior myocardial infarction.

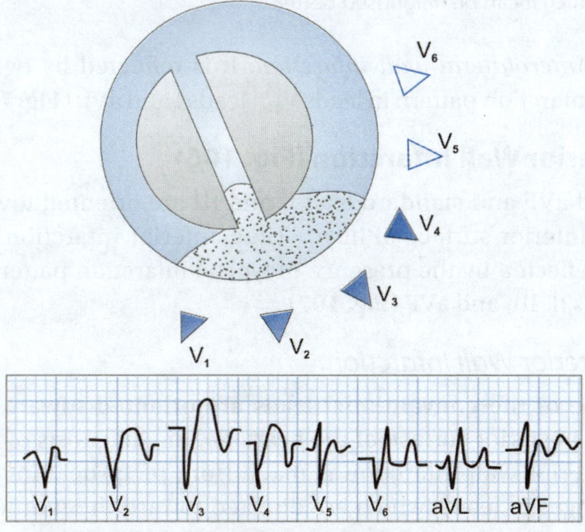

Fig. 104: This figure shows acute anteroseptal myocardial infarction.

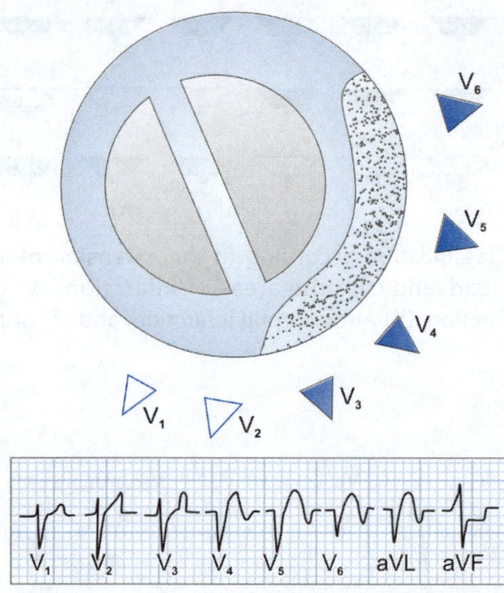

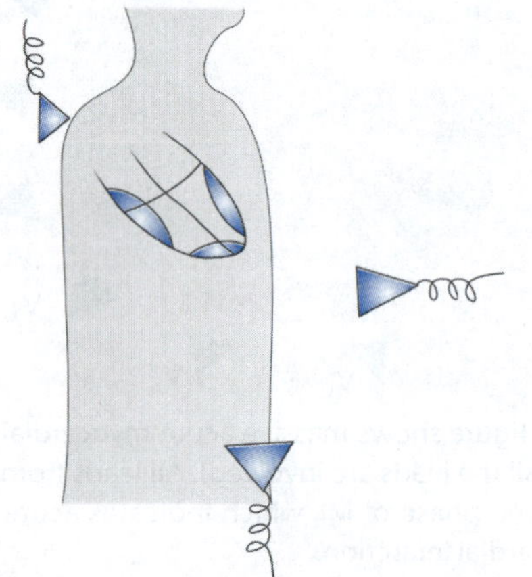

Fig. 105: This figure shows acute anterolateral myocardial infarction.

Fig. 106: This figure shows the location of inferior, anterior, and posterior acute myocardial infarction and the corresponding leads by which it can be diagnosed better.

- *Anterolateral wall infarction:* It is reflected by typical infarction pattern in leads V_{4-6}, leads I and aVL **(Fig. 105)**.

Inferior Wall Infarction (Fig. 106)

Lead aVF and standard lead II and III are oriented toward the inferior surface of heart. Thus, inferior infarction will be reflected by the presence of typical infarction pattern in leads II, III, and aVF **(Fig. 107)**.

Posterior Wall Infarction

None of the conventional leads are oriented toward the true posterior surface of the heart. So, the diagnosis of true posterior wall infarction is made from reciprocal inverse changes in leads, which are directed toward the uninjured anterior surface of the heart, i.e., lead V_{1-2} **(Figs. 108A and B)**.

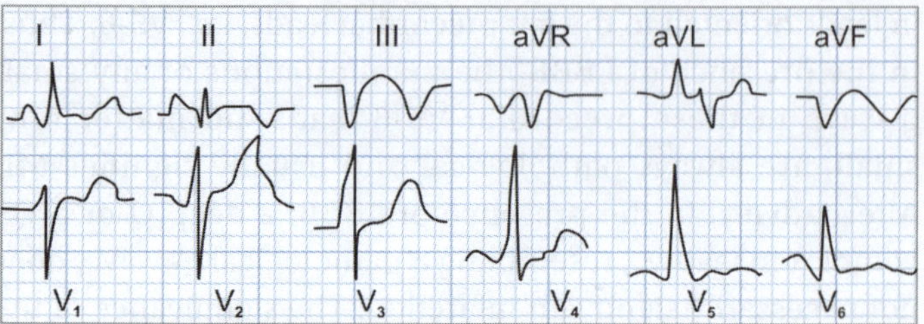

Fig. 107: This figure shows a fully evolved acute inferior MI. A typical infarction pattern in standard lead III and lead aVF indicate that the infarction is situated at the inferior wall of ventricle.

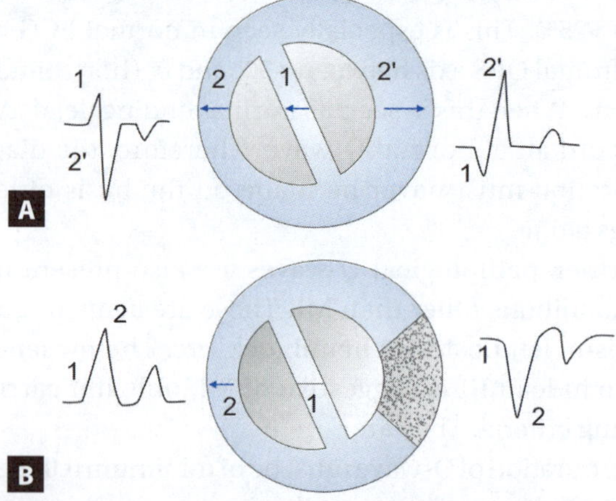

Figs. 108A and B: (A) The electrode is placed on left and right ventricle and there is no infarction. The subsequent normal electrocardiogram (ECG) shows the pattern which should be formed. (B) There is infarction in left ventricle and the second component (2') of left ventricular electrical impulse is absent. The subsequent ECG shows how it (ECG) is formed in respective electrodes.

■ CARDIAC AXIS AND NORMAL ECG

What is Cardiac Axis?

In simple term, the cardiac axis is defined as the general direction, according to which the vector of a wave of any depolarization and repolarization of different cardiac activity flows through the atria and ventricles, during different cardiac cycles. The cardiac axis is, therefore, conventionally referred to (or measured as) the angle of direction of flow of different electrical current, through the atria and ventricles and is measured in degree. The reference or zero point, for the measurement of this angle of direction, is taken as the horizontal line which looks at the heart from left. The angle of direction of the flow of electrical current which is situated below the horizontal **(Figs. 109 to 114)** line, is expressed as a positive number, i.e., *clockwise measurements are positive.* On the other hand, when the angle of direction of the flow of electrical current is above the horizontal line, then the angle is expressed as negative number, i.e. *anticlockwise measurements are negative.* Hence, the cardiac axis may be either +1° to +180° (clockwise) or –1° to –180° (anticlockwise).

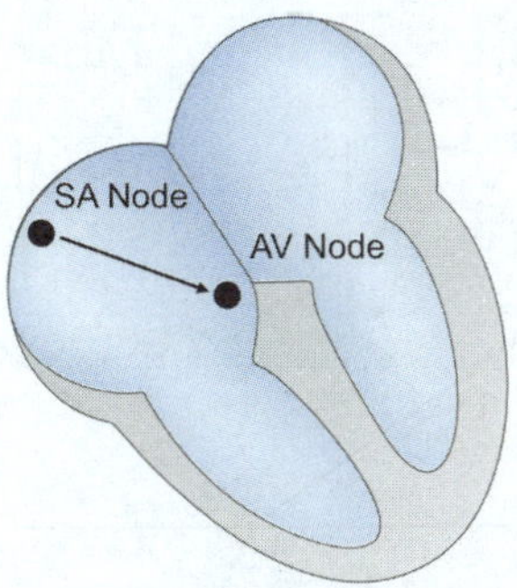

Fig. 109: Atrial activation. (AV: atrioventricular; SA: sinoatrial)

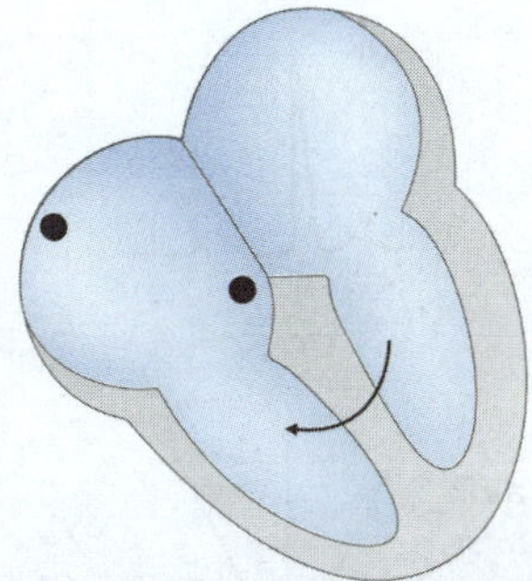

Fig. 110: Septal activation from left to right.

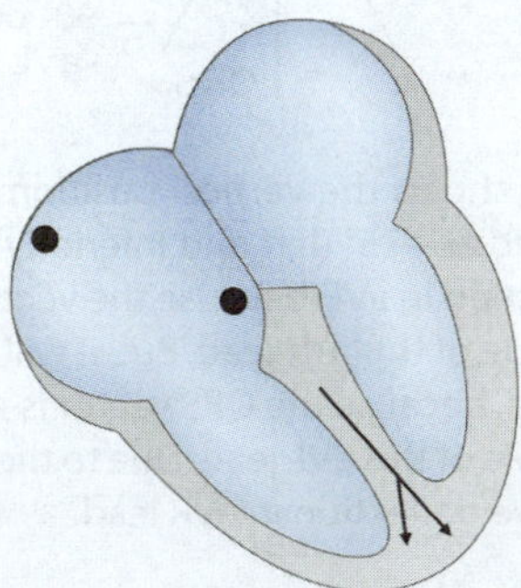

Fig. 111: Activation of the anteroseptal region of ventricular myocardium.

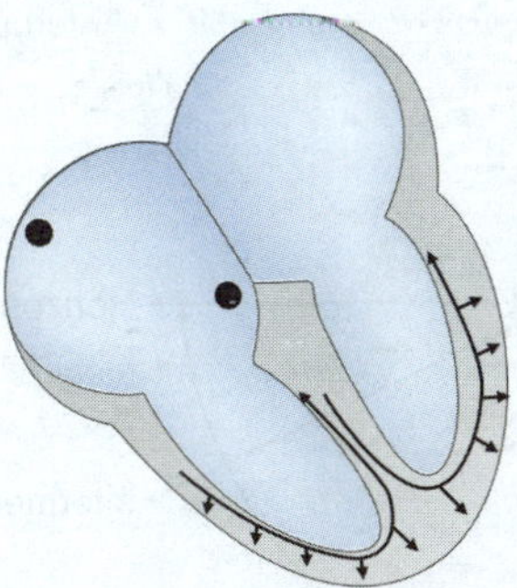

Fig. 112: Activation of the major portion of ventricular myocardium from endocardium to epicardial surface.

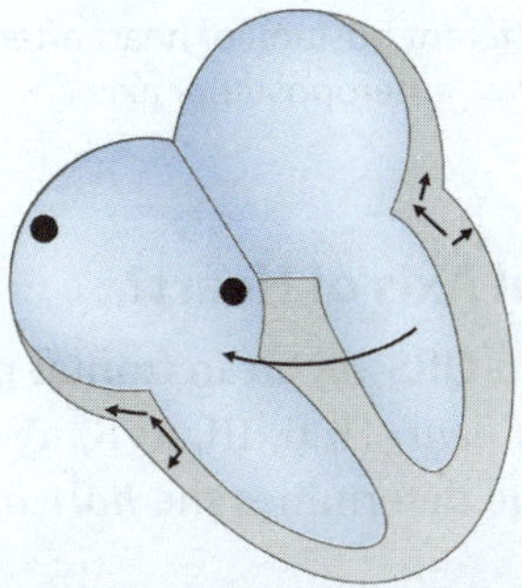

Fig. 113: Late activation of the posterobasal portion of left ventricle, and pulmonary conus, and the uppermost portion of interventricular septum.

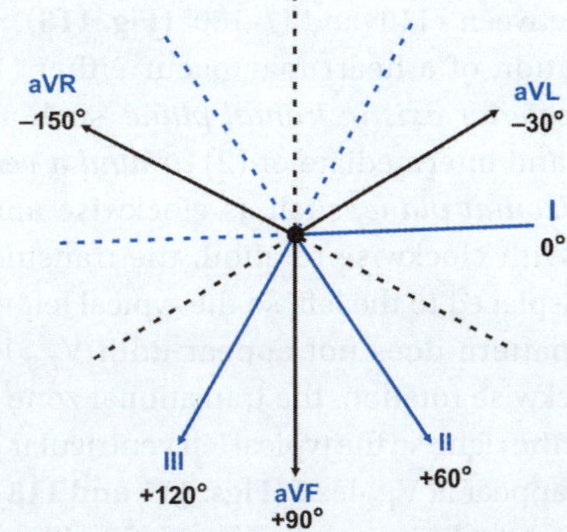

Fig. 114: Viewpoints of six limb leads in frontal plane, such as bipolar I, II, III, and unipolar aVR, aVF, and aVL. Each lead looks at the heart from different angles.

The six limb leads (three bipolar standard limb leads and three unipolar augmented limb leads) look at the heart from six different sides or viewpoints with different angles in frontal plane.

The different angles from which the different limb leads look at the heart in *frontal plane* are given in **Table 1**. The six conventional precordial leads look at the heart from six different view pointes from the anterior side of heart with different angles in *horizontal plane*. Thus, the axis or vectors of different depolarization and repolarization waves of heart in both the frontal and horizontal planes give an idea of the formation (or configuration) of different ECG complexes in all the 12 conventional leads.

TABLE 1: Limb leads and their angles of view.	
Limb leads	**Angles of view**
I	0
II	+60
aVF	+90
III	+120
aVR	−150
aVL	−30

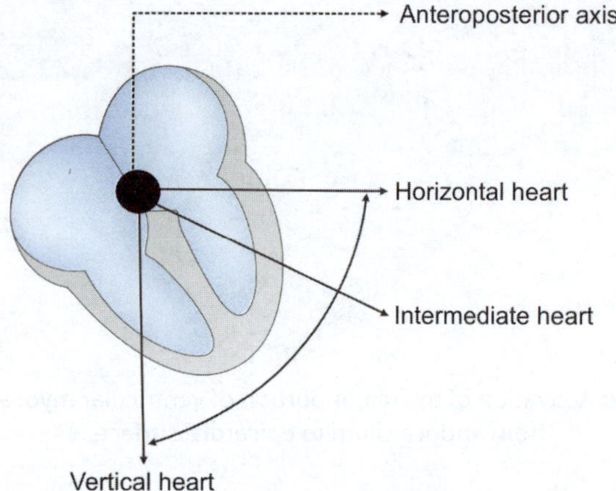

Fig. 115: Different position of heart after rotation in anteroposterior axis.

What is Normal Axis of Heart?

The angle of mean QRS vector in frontal plane determines the *frontal axis of heart* (I, II, III, aVR, aVL, and aVF), and in horizontal plane determines the *horizontal axis of heart* (V_{1-6}) **(Fig. 115)**.

In frontal plane, the normal axis of heart lies in-between –30° and +110°. Therefore, the *left axis deviation of heart* is defined as when the QRS vector (axis) lies between –30° and –90° and *right axis deviation* is defined as when the QRS vector lies between +110° and +/–180° **(Fig. 116)**.

The rotation of a heart may occur either (1) *around an anteroposterior axis in frontal plane*, such as vertical, horizontal, and intermediate or (2) *around a vertical long axis in horizontal plane*, such as clockwise and counter clockwise. With clockwise rotation, the transitional zone (V_3, V_4) is displaced to the left, so the typical left ventricular precordial pattern does not appear until V_{7-9} lead. With counter clockwise rotation, the transitional zone (V_3, V_4) is displaced to the right, so the typical left ventricular precordial pattern will appear at V_{1-2} lead **(Figs. 117 and 118)**.

The term "clockwise rotation" is defined by persistent S-waves in lead V_{5-6}, i.e., the configuration of lead V_{1-2} is seen in lead V_{5-6}. In counterclockwise rotation, the transitional zone is displaced to right, resulting in configuration of left ventricular epicardial complex is seen as early as in lead V_2 **(Figs. 119 and 120)**.

Within normal axis deviation in frontal (vertical) plane, around an anteroposterior axis, the axis between 0° and –30° represents a normal position of heart (horizontal, vertical, or intermediate) and within normal axis deviation in horizontal plane, around a vertical axis, the axis between +75° and +110° represents a normal position of heart (clockwise or counterclockwise) **(Fig. 121)**.

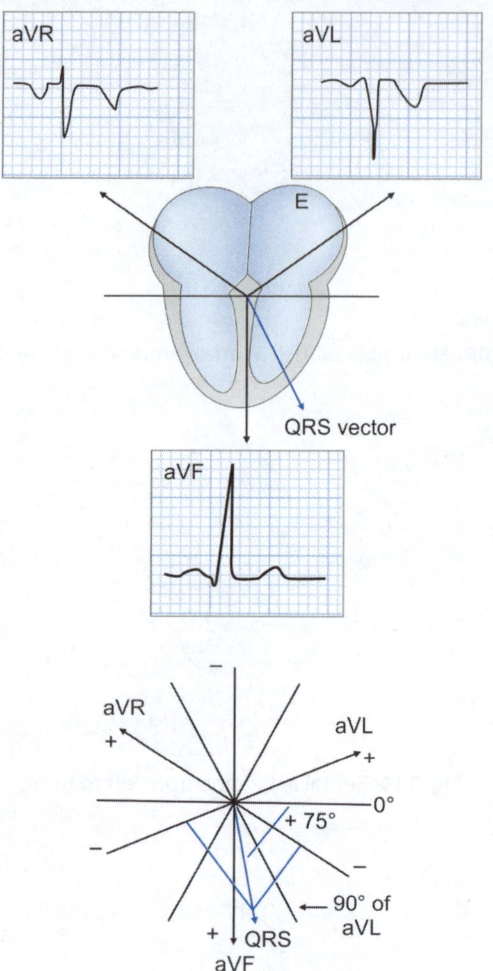

Fig. 116: This figure shows the vertical position of heart. The mean QRS vector is oriented at +75° (left and inferiorly). So, it will produce a positive QRS deflection in aVF, because the vector is situated within 90° of the positive pole of this aVF lead. But, it will produce a negative deflection in aVL lead, because the QRS vector is situated beyond the 90° of the positive pole of this aVL lead. Due to the same reason, it will also produce negative deflection in aVR lead.

Principles

The main principle of ECG is that when the electrical flow through myocardium is toward the positive pole of a lead, then it will cause a positive deflection in this lead in ECG. Similarly, a cardiac electrical flow away from the positive pole of a lead will cause a negative deflection in this lead in ECG **(Fig. 122)**.

Using this principle, now we will consider how lead II records ventricular depolarization. From lead II's point of view, the flow of current for the depolarization of atria and ventricles is entirely directed toward the positive pole of it (lead II) and so the P and QRS complexes are entirely positive in this lead. The lead aVL, however, will see the same flow of current at right angles to lead II and will record an isoelectric

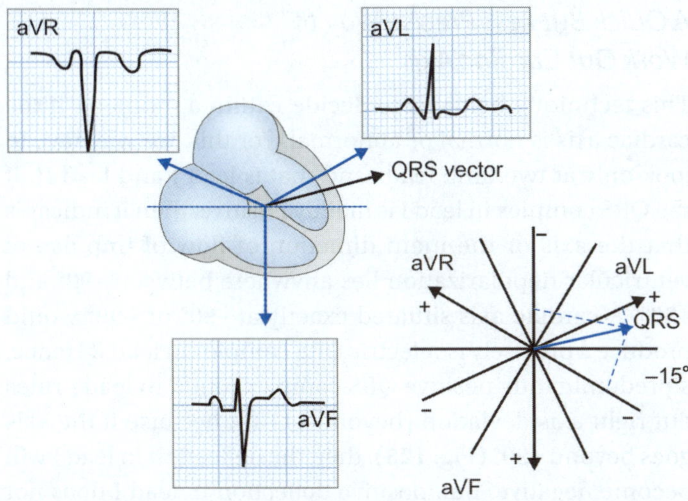

Fig. 117: This figure shows the horizontal position of heart. The QRS vector (axis of ventricular depolarization) is situated at −15°. Thus, it is oriented toward left and superiorly, more toward the positive pole of aVL leads. Due to same reasons, described in the vertical position of heart, this orientation of QRS vector will produce positive deflection in aVL and negative deflection in aVF and aVR leads.

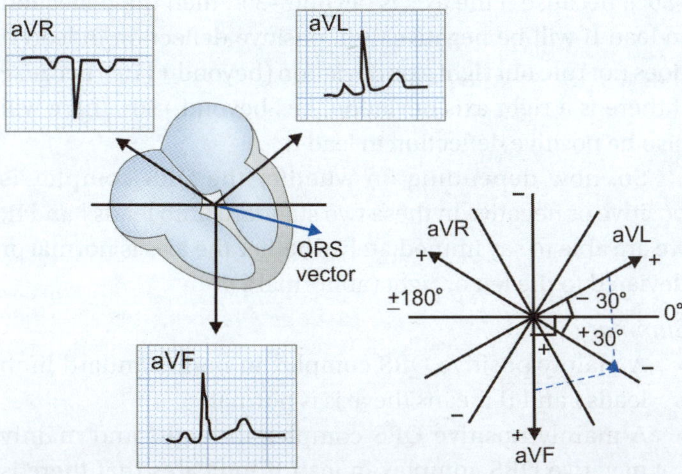

Fig. 118: The mean QRS vector is oriented toward the left and inferior at +30°. So, it is 60° away from both leads aVF and aVL that is midway between the positive poles of these two axes. Thus, it will produce a positive QRS deflection of equal magnitude in both aVL and aVF leads. The QRS deflection is positive in these two leads, because it lies within 90° of the positive poles of these two leads (aVL and aVF). Equal magnitude of deflection in aVL and aVF leads indicates that the heart is in intermediate position. Since the QRS vector is situated beyond the 90° of the positive pole of aVR lead, so it will produce a downward deflection in this lead.

or biphasic (equal upward and downward deflection) QRS complex. Because, if the current of heart flows at right angles to the +pole of a given lead, then the ECG complexes, which are analyzed by this lead, will be isoelectric or biphasic, i.e., the positive and negative deflections will be equal in magnitude and will cancel each other **(Fig. 123)**.

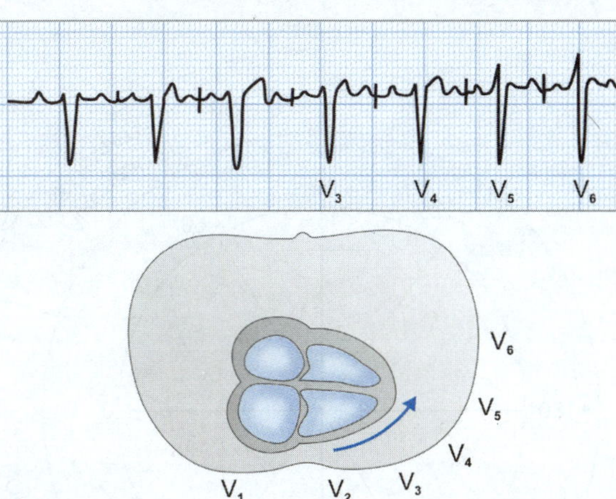

Fig. 119: This figure shows the clockwise rotation of heart: In precordial leads RS complex is still present in V_5 and V_6, indicating that a left ventricular epicardial complex has not yet been reached and clockwise rotation of heart.

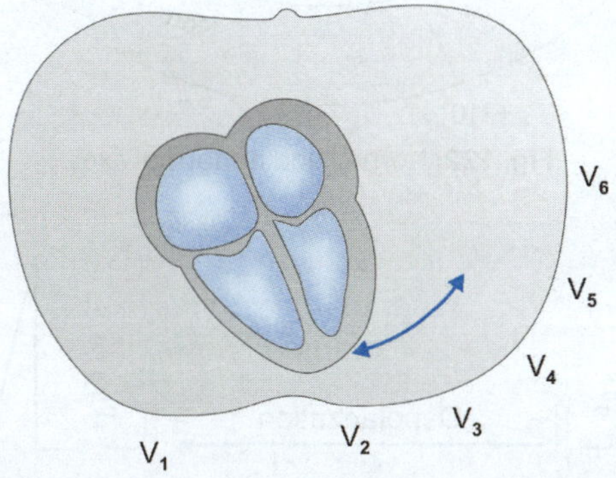

Fig. 120: This figure shows the counterclockwise rotation of heart: A left ventricular epicardial complex is seen in V2 indicating the counterclockwise rotation of heart.

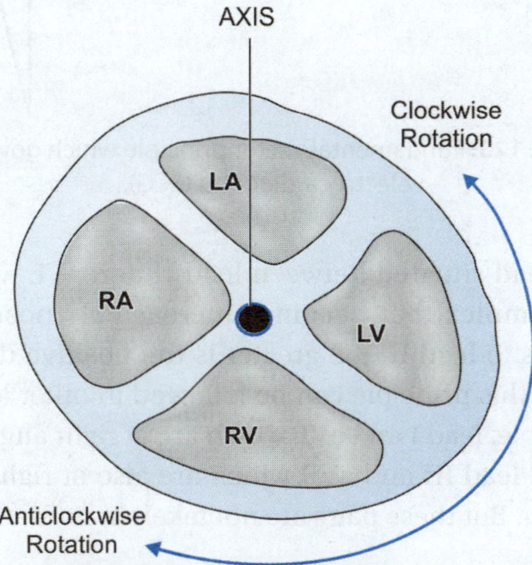

Fig. 121: Rotation of a heart around its long axis. If the electrical activity of a heart has turned more toward the right side of a patient, then it is called the *counterclockwise rotation of heart*. On the other hand, if the electrical activity of a heart has turned more toward left side of a patient, then it is called the *clockwise rotation of heart*. (LA: left atrium; LV: left ventricle; RA: right atrium; RV: right ventricle)

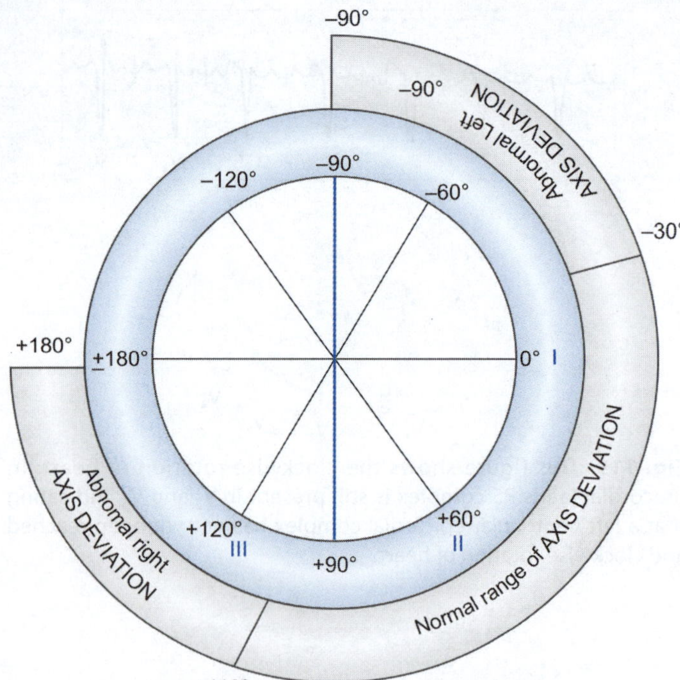

Fig. 122: Normal and abnormal axes.

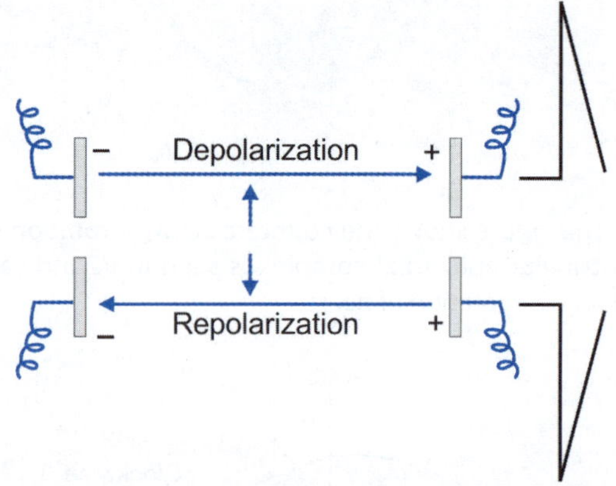

Fig. 123: Fundamental vector principle which govern electrocardiogram (ECG).

Any lead situated between lead II and aVL will record a QRS complex that becomes increasingly positive. The closer it is to lead II, the greater is the positive deflection. Similarly, this principle can be followed in other leads also. For example, lead I and aVF which are at right angle to each other and lead III and aVR which are also at right angle to each other. But these pairs are not taken in normal situation **(Fig. 124)**.

Determination of Cardiac Axis

The two ways of calculating cardiac axis are:
1. A quick but less precise way
2. A slow but more precise way.

A Quick But Less Precise Way to Work Out Cardiac Axis

This technique helps us to decide within a moment, if the cardiac axis is normal or abnormal. For this, we will have to look only at two limb leads and that is lead I and lead II. If the QRS complex in lead I is mainly positive, then it indicates that the axis or the main direction of flow of impulse of ventricular depolarization lies anywhere between −90° and +90°. A cardiac axis situated exactly at −90° or +90° would produce a precisely isoelectric QRS complex in lead I. Hence, a predominantly positive QRS complex found in lead I rules out right axis deviation (beyond +110°), because if the axis goes beyond +90° **(Fig. 125)**, then the deflection in lead I will become negative. But, positive deflection in lead I does not exclude left axis deviation (does not exclude an axis beyond −30°).

On the other hand, if the QRS complex in lead II is mainly positive, then it confirms that the axis lies anywhere between −30° and +150° **(Fig. 126)**. Thus, a positive deflection of QRS complex in lead II rules out the left axis deviation (beyond −30°), because if the axis is beyond −30°, then the deflection in lead II will be negative. But, positive deflection in lead II does not rule out right axis deviation (beyond +110°) because if there is a right axis deviation, i.e., beyond +90°, there will also be positive deflection in lead II.

So, now depending on whether the QRS complex is positive or negative in these two standard limb leads I and II, we are able to say immediately whether the axis is normal or deviated to the left or right (abnormal).

Summary
- A mainly positive QRS complex in both standard limb leads I and II means the axis is normal.
- A mainly positive QRS complex in lead I and mainly negative QRS complex in lead II indicates that there is left axis deviation.
- A mainly negative QRS complex in lead I and mainly positive QRS complex in lead II indicates a right axis deviation **(Table 2)**.

A Slow But More Precise Way to Calculate the Cardiac Axis

For more practical purposes, it is sometimes very necessary to determine accurately the axis of heart, because it is not always sufficient to know simply whether the axis is normal or abnormal. Contrarily, the calculation of cardiac axis precisely is not difficult. But, it does take a little time.

The principle for the precise calculation of axis is that the net amplitude and the direction of QRS complex in any two of frontal plane leads that look at the heart at right angles

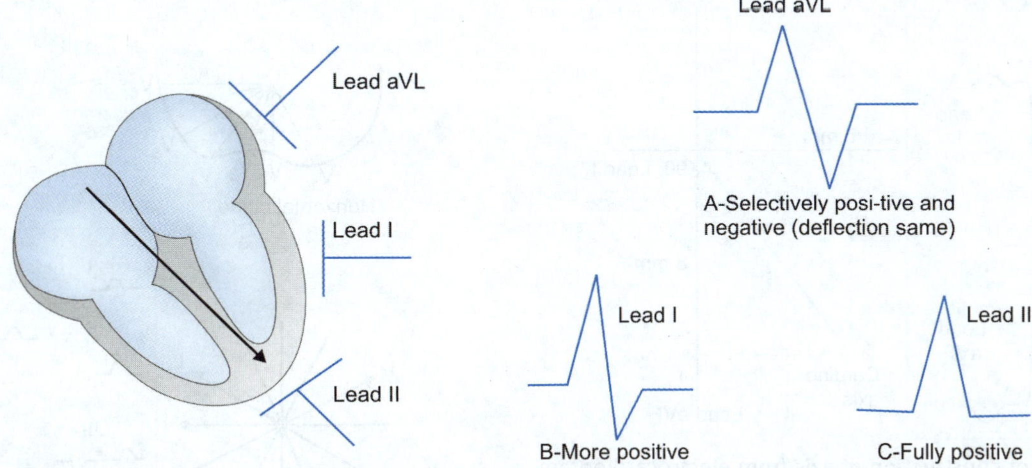

Fig. 124: If a current flows at right angles to the +pole of a lead, then the generated electrocardiogram (ECG) complex will be isoelectric, because the positive and negative deflections will cancel each other. Here, in this figure, it is applicable in the aVL lead. So, it can be explained how the lead II records ventricular depolarization. As the flow of current in ventricle is entirely toward it (lead II), the QRS complex is entirely positive in this lead II. Any lead looking toward the heart, between leads II and aVL will record a complex that will become increasingly positive, the closer it is toward lead II.

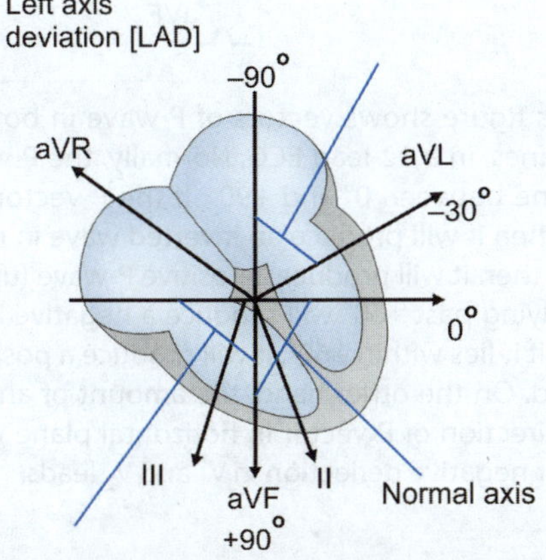

Fig. 125: A predominantly positive QRS in lead I puts the axis between −90° and +90°. So, a predominantly positive QRS complex in lead I excludes right axis deviation. Right axis deviation occurs when the axis goes beyond +110°.

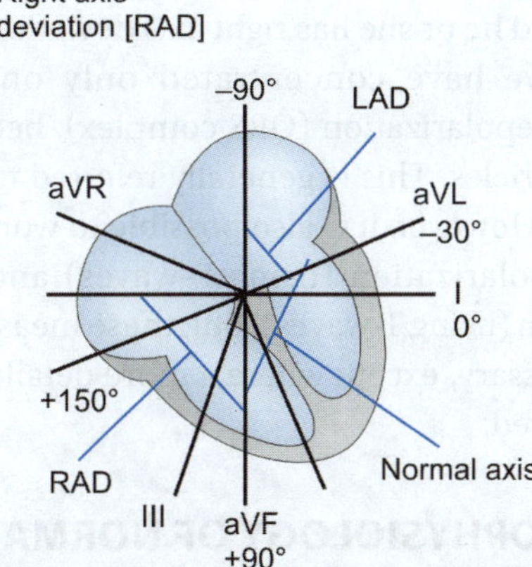

Fig. 126: A predominantly positive QRS complex in lead II and so it puts the axis in-between -30° and +150°. So, a predominantly positive QRS complex in lead II excludes left axis deviation. (LAD: left axis deviation; RAD: right axis deviation)

to each other are plotted along the axis of these two leads. For example, we usually take lead I and lead aVF for the calculation of cardiac axis, as they are at right angles to each other. The overall size and the polarity of QRS complexes in these two leads should be worked out by subtracting the depth of S-wave from the height of R-wave of that lead. This polarity (positive or negative) will tell us whether the impulse is moving toward or away from the +ve pole of that lead. The two QRS vectors should, then, be plotted according to their amplitude and direction (polarity, i.e., +ve or –ve) in the lead axes of these two leads **(Fig. 127)**. Perpendicular lines are next drawn at these two locations (points). A line is then drawn from the center of reference system to the

TABLE 2: Determination of cardiac axis.		
Lead I	**Lead II**	**Cardiac axis**
• Positive QRS deflection	• Positive QRS deflection	• Normal axis
• Positive QRS deflection	• Negative QRS deflection	• Left axis deviation
• Negative QRS deflection	• Positive QRS deflection	• Right axis deviation

intersection of these two perpendiculars and this represents the direction of approximate mean QRS vector (axis). Its angle is the frontal plane axis. We can thus finally derive an angle in degrees that determines the cardiac

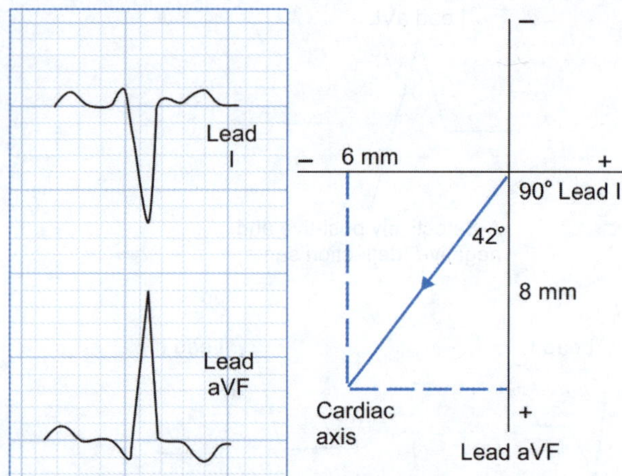

Fig. 127: Method of construction of axis from electrocardiogram (ECG). First, the overall size and polarity of QRS complexes in lead I and aVF is determined. Here, the overall QRS height is -6 mm, with negative polarity in lead I. On the other hand, the overall QRS height is +8 mm, with positive polarity in lead aVF.

(QRS) axis. The axis in this patient is, therefore, +132° (90° + 42°) and he or she has right axis deviation.

So far, we have concentrated only on the axis of ventricular depolarization (QRS complex), because it flows through ventricles. This is generally referred to as the main cardiac axis. However, it is also possible to work out the axis of atrial depolarization (using P-waves) and ventricular repolarization (using T-waves). But, these measurements are seldom necessary, except where a more detailed analysis of ECG is required.

ELECTROPHYSIOLOGY OF NORMAL HEART AND PRODUCTION OF NORMAL ECG

Atrial Complex

The initial impulse in cardiac cycle begins at SA node due to its depolarization. This depolarization of SA node cannot be recorded in clinical ECG. But, it can be recorded by a special electrode placed within the SA node. The impulse arising from SA node, then, traverses through internodal pathways to depolarize whole atria, producing P-wave in ECG and then reaches AV node. Normally, the impulse is delayed in AV node by 0.07 seconds and then passes on to bundle of His **(Fig. 128)**.

So, the P-wave represents the atrial depolarization and *its vector or axis (P vector) is directed leftward and inferiorly in frontal plane and slightly anteriorly in horizontal plane.* The polarity (negative or positive deflection) of P-wave in any given lead will, therefore, depend on the relation between the direction of P vector (axis) and the positive pole of the respective lead.

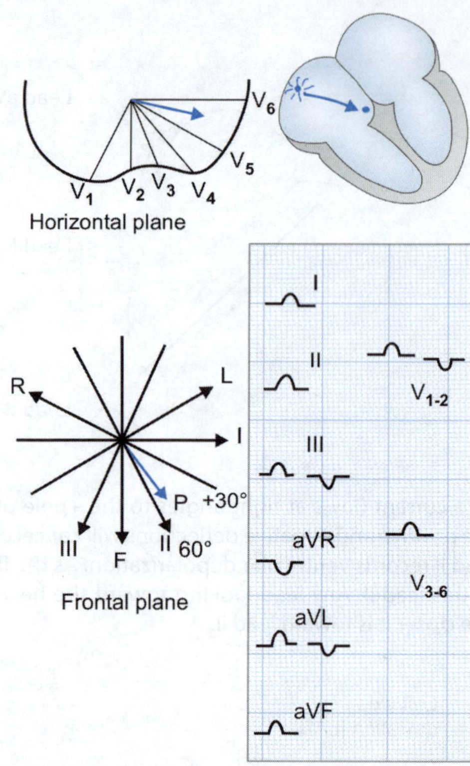

Fig. 128: This figure shows vectors of P-wave in both frontal and horizontal planes, in a 12-lead ECG. Normally, the P vector remains in frontal plane between 0° and +90°. If the P vector lies between 0° and +30°, then it will produce an inverted wave in lead III. If it lies beyond +30°, then it will produce a positive P-wave (upright) in ECG. The P vector lying past +60° will produce a negative P-wave in aVL. Alternatively, if it lies within +60°, it will produce a positive P-wave in same aVL lead. On the other hand, the amount of anterior and the right or left direction of P vector in horizontal plane will determine the positive or negative deflection in V_1 and V_2 leads.

P-wave in Frontal Plane Leads (I, II, III, aVR, aVL, and aVF)

Normally, the P vector is oriented inferiorly and leftward in frontal plane between 0° and +90°. Therefore, the P vectors are upright in leads I, II, aVF, and inverted in aVR. The P vector is upright in lead III, when its axis is greater than +30°. It is inverted in lead III, when its axis is lesser than +30°. In lead aVL, the P vector is upright, if its axis is lesser than +60° and inverted if its axis is greater than +60°.

P-wave in Horizontal Plane Leads (Precordial Leads V_1 to V_6)

In the horizontal plane, the normal P vector is directed leftward and anteriorly. Depending upon the degree of anterior or leftward orientation, the P-wave may be upright, biphasic or inverted in lead V_{1-2}. But it is always upright in leads V_{3-6}. After the impulse reaches AV node from SA node, it is normally delayed for 0.07 seconds, before the impulse passes on to the bundle of His. This delay of impulse at AV node produces an isoelectric PR segment in all the leads.

Ventricular Complex

Ventricular Complex (Initial)

The initial conduction of impulses to ventricle from AV node and bundle of His via the septal fibers of left bundle branch results in the primary depolarization of left side of interventricular septum which next spread to the right side of it (interventricular septum). *This produces a septal depolarization from left to right. This vector is, therefore, oriented rightward in horizontal plane.* Due to the anatomical disposition of septum, the septal depolarization force is oriented anteriorly and superiorly or sometimes even inferiorly in frontal plane. It is of a small magnitude.

Initial ventricular complex in frontal plane leads: This initial left-to-right septal vector records a small negative deflection as "q" in lead I. Its recording and deflection in ECG in the other frontal plane leads will also depend on its relationship with other frontal plane axis. *Lead II will record an upright deflection "r-wave", if it lies inferiorly between 30° and +150° and a negative deflection, if it lies superiorly between –30° and +150°.* Lead aVF will record an upright deflection "r", if the septal vector lies inferiorly between 0° and +180° and a negative deflection, if the septal vector lies superiorly between 0° and –180°. In other leads like aVL, aVR, and lead III, the same principle is applied **(Fig. 129)**.

Initial ventricular complex in horizontal plane leads: The left to right and anterior initial septal vectors will record a small positive deflection as "r-wave" in leads V_{1-2}. Reciprocally, it records a small negative deflection as "q-wave" in leads V_{5-6}.

Ventricular Complex (Major)

After depolarization of interventricular septum, the impulse goes down the right and left bundle branches. Then, it passes through the fibers of Purkinje system and activates the right and left ventricles. After that, the impulses traverse through ventricular myocardium from endocardial to epicardial surfaces.

Vectors of major ventricular QRS complex in frontal plane leads **(Fig. 130)**: *The axis (vector) of major QRS complex is directed leftward between –30° and +90° in frontal plane and results in a large upright deflection (R-wave) in leads I and II.* On the contrary, it produces a large negative deflection (S-wave, in place of R-wave) in lead aVR. The recording in other frontal plane leads will depend on the relation between the axis of frontal plane leads and the axis (vector) of this major ventricular QRS complex. Lead aVF will record

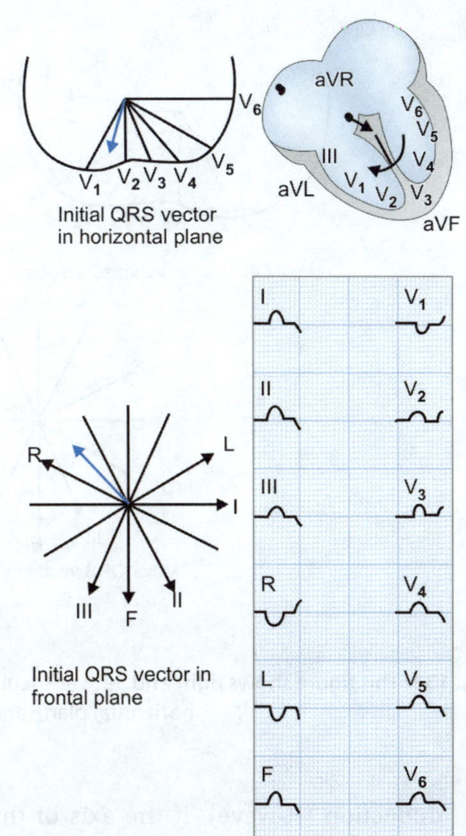

Fig. 129: This figure shows septal activation which is the beginning of ventricular QRS complex. This force is normally oriented toward right and anteriorly in horizontal plane. It may also be directed superiorly (shown in figure) or inferiorly in frontal plane.

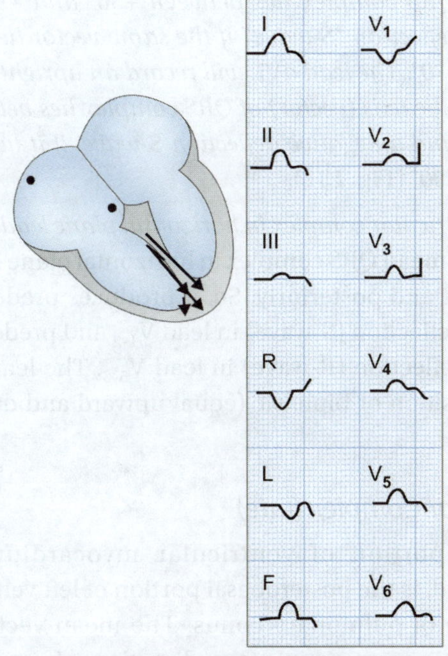

Fig. 130: This figure shows the activation of anteroseptal region of myocardium, after septal activation. Like septal activation, this also produces a mean force, oriented toward right and anterior.

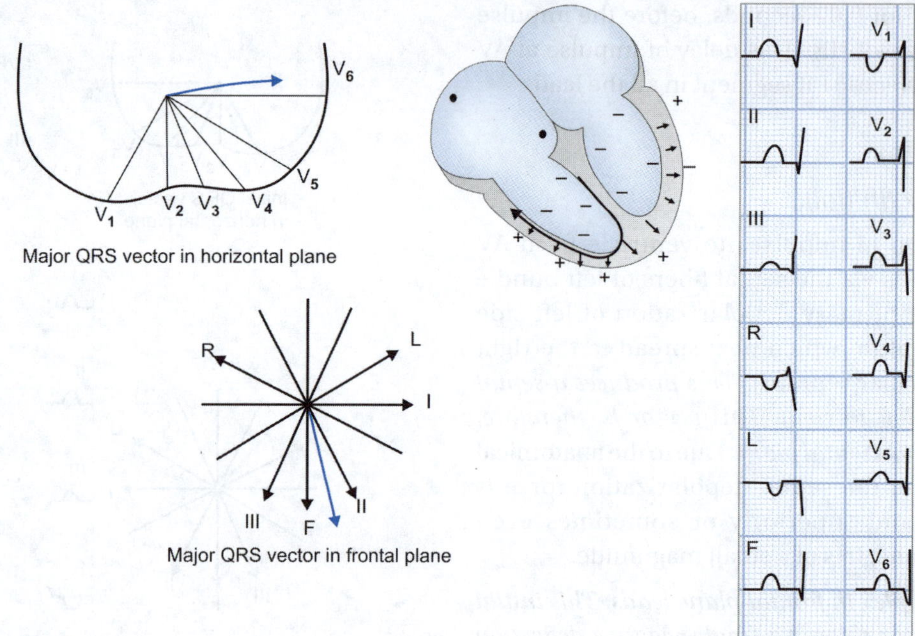

Fig. 131: This figure shows right and left ventricular activation. The mean vector (axis) of this force is directed toward left in horizontal plane and inferiorly and posteriorly in frontal plane.

an upright deflection (R-wave), if the axis of this major ventricular QRS complex lies between 0° and +90°. It will record a RS or "rs" complex wave, if the mean axis is at 0°. It will also record a negative deflection S-wave, if the axis (vector) of QRS complex is directed between 0° and –30°. *Lead III will record an upright deflection "R-wave", if the axis of major QRS complex lies between +30° and +90°, and a negative deflection "S-wave", if the same vector lies between +30° and –30°. The lead aVL will record an upright deflection R-wave, if the axis (vector) of QRS complex lies between –30° and +60° and a negative deflection S-wave, if it lies between +60° and +90°* **(Fig. 131)**.

Major ventricular complex in horizontal plane leads: The axis (vector) of mean QRS complex in horizontal plane is directed toward left and posteriorly. So, it produces predominantly negative deflection (S-wave) in lead V_{1-2} and predominantly positive deflection (R-wave) in lead V_{5-6}. The lead V_{3-4} will show transition or biphasic (equal upward and downward) deflection.

Ventricular Complex (late)

The last portion of ventricular myocardium, to be depolarized, is the posterobasal portion of left ventricle and the region of pulmonary conus. The mean vector of this activation is oriented in many directions. If it is directed rightward, then a small negative deflection's wave' will be recorded in leads I and V_{5-6}. If it is directed superiorly, then

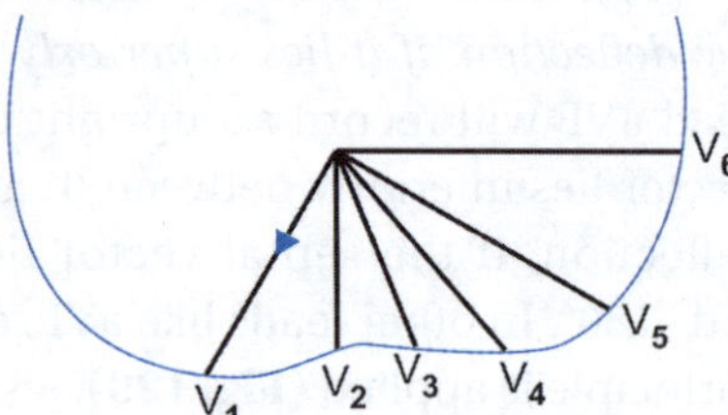

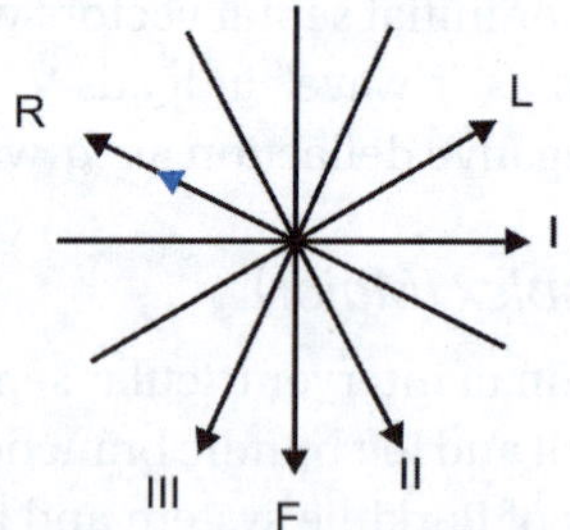

Fig. 132: Late major QRS vector is due to the activation of posterobasal portion of left ventricle, pulmonary conus, and the uppermost portion of interventricular septum. This figure illustrates the mean vector of this force (late major QRS) which is oriented rightward, superiorly, and anteriorly.

a small negative deflection's wave' will be recorded in lead aVF. If it is oriented anteriorly, a small positive deflection "r-wave" will be recorded in leads V_{1-2} **(Fig. 132)**.

Repolarization: The sequence of events of ventricular repolarization is very complex. Simply, it can be said that

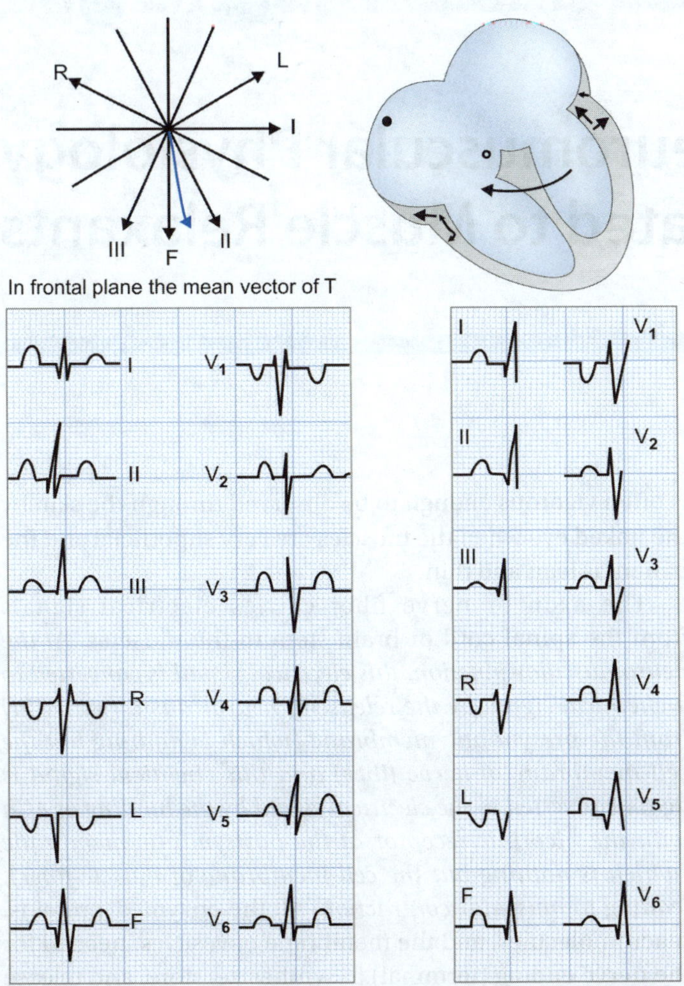

Fig. 133: Repolarization: The mean T vector is oriented toward left (in horizontal plane) and inferiorly and anteriorly (in frontal plane).

both the right and left ventricular cavities are negative during ventricular repolarization. The epicardial surface of left ventricle is positive. That of right ventricle may be positive or negative. The ST segment will be isoelectric in all leads. *The usual normal axis of mean T vector is oriented to the left and inferiorly (between 0° and +90°). So the frontal plane leads will record upright T-waves in leads I and II and inverted T-wave in lead aVR* **(Fig. 133)**.

The polarity of T-wave (upward or downward deflection) in other frontal plane leads (aVL, aVF, and II) will depend on the relation between the axis (vector) of T-wave with the axis of this lead in frontal plane, like the P and QRS axis, described before. In the leads of horizontal plane, the mean T vector is oriented anteriorly. Depending on the degree of anterior orientation, the T-wave may be inverted, biphasic, or upright in lead V₁ and upright in leads V₃₋₆.

Neuromuscular Physiology Related to Muscle Relaxants

MORPHOLOGY OF NEUROMUSCULAR JUNCTION

A single myelinated axon or nerve fiber, after arising from the body of a motor nerve cell, situated at the ventral horn of gray matter of the spinal cord, runs uninterruptedly through the spinal or cranial nerves and supplies the skeletal muscles. There (at the supply point to muscle) it makes multiple branches and ultimately ends into several expanded complicated structures which are known as the *axon terminals or sole feet*. These axon terminals ultimately end on each muscle cell (fiber) as a *neuromuscular junction or motor endplate*. Actually, the motor endplates are small depressions on the muscle cell membrane, where a branch of the nerve terminal ends. *It (the depression on muscle cell membrane) contains many nicotinic cholinergic receptors which are sensitive to Ach*. The diameter of this typically discoid or oval-shaped neuromuscular junction or motor endplate is 20–30 μm **(Fig. 1)**. The number of muscle cells (fibers) supplied by the multiple terminal branches of a single axon or nerve fiber together form *one motor unit*. In a single motor unit, there may be 5–2,000 muscle fibers (cells). Synchronous contraction of all these muscle cells of a motor unit is called as the *fasciculation*. Fasciculation usually cannot be seen by the naked eye, but sometimes it is often vigorous enough to be observed through the skin by the naked eye when the muscles are very superficial and the patient is lean and thin.

The axon or nerve fiber carries electrical signals from the spinal cord or brain stem to the muscles. *At the neuromuscular junction, this electrical signal is converted to a chemical signal by the release of neurotransmitter (ACh) from the presynaptic membrane (which is nothing but the cell membrane of nerve fiber) and this chemical signal is again converted to the electrical signal by the binding of ACh with the nicotinic receptor at the postsynaptic membrane (which is nothing but the cell membrane of muscle fiber), leading to muscular contraction*. All the enzymes, proteins, macromolecules, and the membrane of vesicles, needed for the nerve ending (terminal) to synthesize, store, and release ACh for chemical signals are made into the cell body of nerve fiber and are then transported to the nerve ending by axonal transport. Only the chemical substances such as choline and acetate are obtained locally at the nerve ending to synthesize ACh **(Fig. 2)**. *The nerve ending is itself nonmyelinated because the myelin sheath ends before the nerve terminal touches the endplate on muscle cells. But, it is covered with the cell membrane and the cytoplasm of the Schwann cell with its nucleus.* The axoplasm of axon fiber, at its terminal end, is filled with numerous mitochondria, endoplasmic reticulum, and other materials and cell organelles which are required for chemical synthesis of neurotransmitter and numerous vesicles to store it **(Fig. 3)**. It is claimed that mitochondria, present in the axoplasm of nerve terminal, take part in the synthesis of ACh which is then subsequently stored in a synaptic vesicle (of nerve terminal) and released when the propagated impulse through nerve fiber reaches the nerve terminal **(Fact file I)**.

The gap between the nerve cell membrane (presynaptic membrane) and the muscle cell membrane (postsynaptic membrane) at the neuromuscular junction is called the *junctional cleft or synaptic cleft* which is measured at about 20 nm. This synaptic cleft is filled with an extracellular

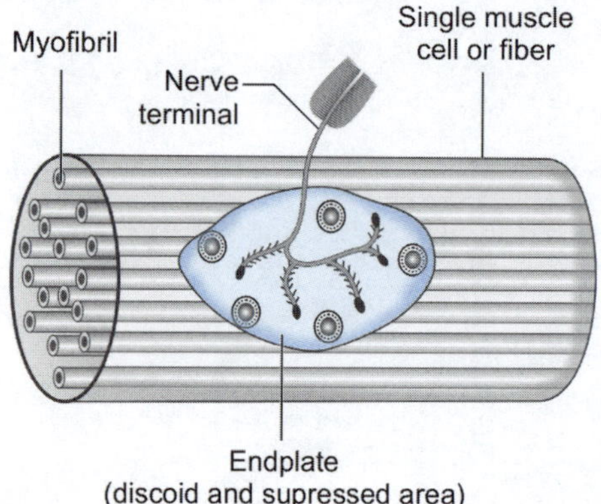

Fig. 1: Motor endplate in relation to a muscle fiber—surface view.

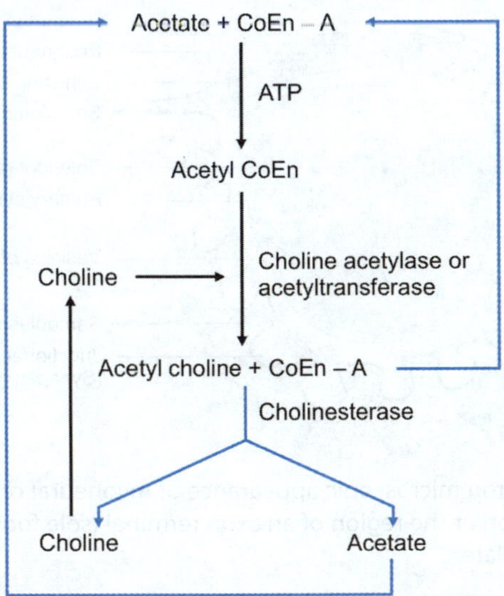

Fig. 2: Acetylcholine (ACh), after its synthesis, is released from the nerve terminal and is broken down locally by true cholinesterase enzyme, present at the synaptic cleft into acetate and choline. Then, this choline is absorbed again into the nerve terminal and takes part in the synthesis of ACh at the nerve endings. For this further synthesis of ACh, acetate comes from the metabolism of glucose by glycolytic pathway. There are two types of cholinesterase enzymes—(1) true cholinesterase and (2) pseudocholinesterase. The difference between them is given in **Table 1**.

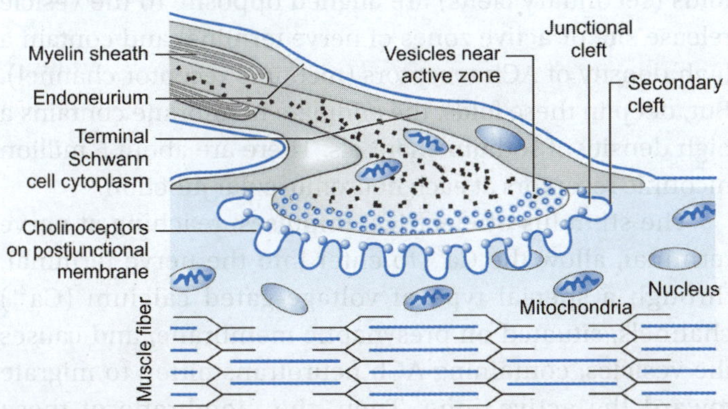

Fig. 3: Neuromuscular junction or motor endplate with an axon terminal containing vesicles of acetylcholine. The neurotransmitter is released on the arrival of an action potential (AP) (electrical impulse) and crosses the junctional cleft to stimulate the postjunctional nicotinic receptors, present on the shoulders of secondary clefts of the postsynaptic membrane.

fluid which is called the *gap substance*. This synaptic cleft, separated by the cell membrane of both the nerve cell (presynaptic membrane) and muscle cell (postsynaptic membrane) also contains: (i) many fibrous strands, linking the nerve and muscle cell membrane and (ii) enzyme, called the acetylcholinesterase (AChE) (it is commonly called as cholinesterase or ChE). It is also called true cholinesterase. There is another cholinesterase, circulating in plasma. It is called the plasma cholinesterase or pseudo cholinesterase

FACT FILE I

The shoulder of secondary cleft is densely populated with acetylcholine (ACh) receptors (nicotinic type). But, the depth of these secondary folds or cleft is populated with Na^+ channel, which transforms the depolarization (electrical signal), produced by the ACh-receptor into the muscle action potential (electrical signal) and triggers the contraction of muscle. Muscle cell membrane surrounding the endplate at the periphery is also rich in Na^+ channel and functions as the same, i.e., endplate depolarization into a muscle action potential.

TABLE 1: Differences between two types of cholinesterase.

	True cholinesterase (acetylcholinesterase)	*Pseudo (butyryl) or plasma cholinesterase*
Distribution	All cholinergic synapses (in synaptic cleft) and RBC	Plasma, liver, and GI (not found in synaptic cleft)
Hydrolysis of ACh	Very fast	Very slow or nil
Hydrolysis by butyrylcholine	Not hydrolyzed	Hydrolyzed
Inhibition	More sensitive to physostigmine	More sensitive to organophosphates
Function	Termination of action of ACh	Hydrolysis of synthetic esters such as succinylcholine

(ACh: acetylcholine; GI: gastrointestinal; RBC: red blood cell)

or butyryl cholinesterase. It is synthesized in liver and it breaks the succinylcholine which is used as depolarizing muscle relaxant during intubation. The differences between the true and plasma cholinesterase is shown in **Table 1**. Multiple secondary clefts also arise from the postsynaptic membrane (of muscle cell membrane), extending from the main junctional cleft and thus the total surface area of the postsynaptic of endplate increases many folds. The branched and expanded nerve terminals, which come in contact with the muscle fiber, lie within this corrugated postsynaptic membrane (muscle cell membrane) of the endplate and this corrugation is due to the formation of this multiple secondary clefts from the main synaptic cleft. Numerous nuclei and mitochondria are also seen in the sarcoplasm (cytoplasm) of muscle cells near the motor endplate.

There is only one neuromuscular junction on each muscle cell or fiber, except some extraocular muscles and internal laryngeal muscles which have several neuromuscular junctions or endplates on each muscle cell, locating at short distance from each other and maintain a steady contraction in response to stimulus. These muscles are important to anesthetists because instead of causing brief contraction (fasciculation), and followed by paralysis, the depolarizing muscle relaxants cause long-lasting contractions in these types of muscles and contribute to a rise in intraocular pressure. Virtually all human skeletal muscles (except the extraocular and possibly some internal laryngeal muscles) contract in the all-or-none principle.

The peripheral surrounding area of the muscle cell membrane, around the neuromuscular junction, is called as the *perijunctional area*. It actually indicates the transitional area between the postsynaptic membrane of endplate and the true cell membrane of muscle fiber. It is a *very critical area* for the function of the neuromuscular junction. Because, it is here where the action potential, developed at the endplate, is converted to an electrical impulse that sweeps along the whole muscle cell membrane and initiates muscular contractions. It contains a mixture of a smaller number of nicotinic types of ACh receptors and a higher number of Na$^+$ channels. The perijunctional area also participates actively in the modulation of neuromuscular transmission and an individual's response to the muscle relaxant. Moreover, some special variants (isomers) of nicotinic receptors and Na$^+$ channels can appear in this area at different stages of life which are responsible for abnormal decreases or increases in nerve-muscle activity. This variability seems to contribute to quantitative and qualitative differences in the response to the muscle relaxants that are seen in patients at different clinical statuses and ages. Congenital abnormalities, regarding the number and morphology of these ACh receptors (nicotinic receptors) and Na$^+$ channels are also known.

The vesicles, containing the ACh neurotransmitter, at the nerve ending, are arranged or congregated toward the presynaptic membrane of the neuromuscular junction. On the other hand, the microtubules, mitochondria, and the other structures of nerve terminal are located on the opposite side of the junctional surface of nerve ending. The vesicles, containing neurotransmitter, are arranged in a pattern of triangular arrays, with their apex directing toward the small, thickened electron-dense patch of the presynaptic membrane which is referred to as the *active zone*. In cross-section, these thickened areas (or active zone) of the presynaptic membrane shows many bands, running across the width of the synaptic surface of nerve ending. The vesicles make an attachment to the active zone before they are ruptured into a junctional cleft. The attachment sites of these vesicles lie on the sides, rather than in the center of the active zone. Many small particles are also seen, along the active zone, between the vesicles. Actually, these particles are the special voltage-gated calcium channels that also allow the Ca^{2+} to enter the nerve ending from the extracellular space and cause the release of ACh neurotransmitter from these vesicles **(Fig. 4)**.

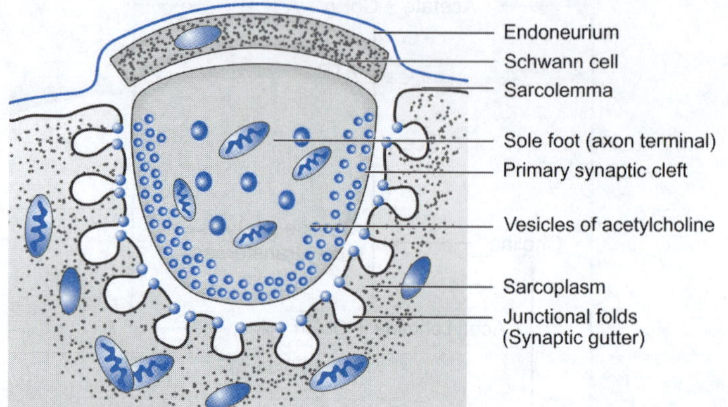

Fig. 4: Electron microscopic appearance of myoneural or neuromuscular junction at the region of an axon terminal (sole foot) ending in motor endplate.

The endplate area of muscle cell membrane, which is a part of neuromuscular junction and forms the postsynaptic membrane, is very convoluted and this convolution is due to the presence of multiple secondary cleft or folds which are already discussed before. Thus, the muscle cell membrane, which is a part of neuromuscular junction, exposes a very large area of it to the nerve terminal for the better transmission of impulses. The crests or the shoulders of these folds (secondary clefts) are aligned opposite to the vesicle release site or active zones of nerve terminal and contain a high density of ACh receptors (nicotinic receptor channel). But, deep in these folds, the endplate membrane contains a high density of sodium channels. There are about 5 million nicotinic receptors at each neuromuscular junction.

The stimulus or electrical impulses, reaching at nerve terminal, allow the Ca^{2+} to enter into the nerve terminal, through a special type of voltage-gated calcium (Ca^{2+}) channels, situated on presynaptic membrane, and causes the vesicles, containing ACh neurotransmitter, to migrate toward the active zone. Then, the membrane of these vesicles fuses with the neural membrane of nerve terminal (presynaptic membrane) and discharges their contents of ACh into the synaptic cleft. Since, the release sites of ACh are located along the sides of active zones and immediately opposite to the nicotinic receptors on postjunctional surface, so normally little transmitter is wasted and the response of muscle is coupled very directly with the electrical signal from nerves **(Fig. 5)**.

Normally, the endplate potential that is produced continuously at rest, by the continuous release of uniformly sized packages or quanta of neurotransmitter, is called as the *miniature endplate potential (MEPP)*. This is 1/100th of the amplitude of *evoked endplate potential* when the motor nerve is stimulated and muscle contraction occurs. For each nerve impulse, to produce the contraction of a single

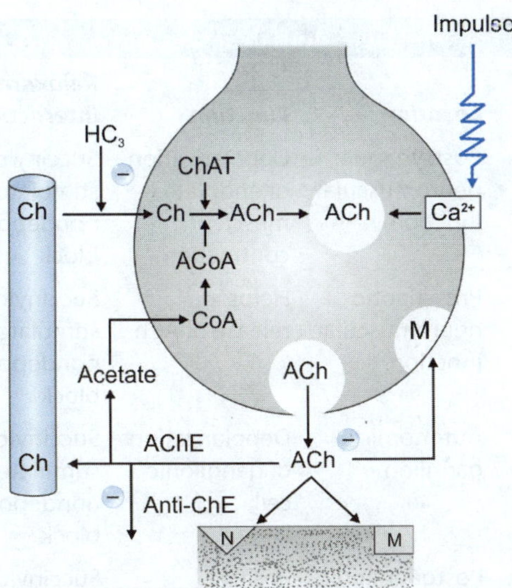

Fig. 5: The process involved in synthesis, release, and deposit of acetylcholine at cholinergic nerve terminals and receptor site during transmission of nerve impulses. (ACh: acetylcholine; AChE: acetylcholinesterase; ACoA: acetyl coenzyme A; anti-ChE: anticholinesterase; ChAT: choline acetyltransferase; BoT: botulinus toxin; HC$_3$: hemicholinium; M: muscarinic receptor; N: nicotinic receptor)

muscle fiber, 200 quanta or vesicles, containing 5,000 ACh molecules in each vesicle, is released. Thus, the number of ACh molecules, released by each impulse, is 1,000,000. Each ACh or nicotinic receptor needs two ACh molecules for its activation. Thus, the number of receptors activated by the neurotransmitter (ACh) released by a single nerve impulse is also large and is about 500,000. But, actually, each impulse activates only 300,000 receptors, requiring only 600,000 molecules of ACh (each vesicle activates 1,500 receptors requiring 3,000 ACh molecule, but they have an extra amount). Thus, the rest of ACh molecule is either destroyed by acetylcholinesterase or binding single, instead of pairs to a receptor. After coupling of neurotransmitter such as ACh, with the postjunctional ACh and nicotinic receptor, the Na$^+$ ions that flow through the channel of activated receptor, cause the maximum depolarization of endplate, which is greater than the threshold for stimulation of muscle fiber and causes a full cycle of endplate action potential.

The entry of Ca^{2+} inside the nerve ending is the most important step for the release of neurotransmitter, ACh. Neither only Na$^+$ in flux, nor only the depolarization of presynaptic nerve membrane will produce the release of neurotransmitter from nerve ending if Ca^{2+} is not entered in nerve endings. The introduction of Ca^{2+} into the nerve ending by micropipette will also release neurotransmitter, even if the nerve terminal is not depolarized by an electrical impulse. The Ca^{2+} enters the nerve terminal from extracellular fluid (ECF) via a special type of protein channels which are called as the *Ca^{2+} channels*. Among the several types of these

calcium channels, only P and L type of Ca^{2+} channels are most important for the release of neurotransmitter from the presynaptic membrane. Again, among the P and L type of Ca^{2+} channels, the P channels are found only in motor nerve endings, adjacent to the active zones of nerve terminals and are responsible (not L type of Ca^{2+} channel) for Ca^{2+} entry and subsequent transmitter release from nerve terminal for neuromuscular transmission.

These Ca^{2+} channels are voltage-dependent which means that they are opened and closed only by the changes in membrane voltage caused by the propagated nerve action potential. On the other hand, many bivalent organic cations such as Mg^{2+}, cadmium, and Mn^{2+} can also block this Ca^{2+} channel and thus profoundly impair neuromuscular transmission. This is the mechanism for muscle weakness in the mother and fetus when magnesium sulfate is administered to treat preeclampsia. The Eaton–Lambert myasthenic syndrome is another acquired autoimmune disease in which antibodies are detected against this voltage-gated calcium protein channel at the nerve ending. Patient with this myasthenic syndrome exhibit an increased sensitivity to depolarizing and nondepolarizing muscle relaxants. Normally, the P-type of Ca^{2+} channel cannot be blocked by organic calcium channel-blocking drugs such as verapamil, diltiazem, and nifedipine. Because these drugs have profound effects only on the slower L type of Ca^{2+} channels, present in the cardiovascular system (CVS). So, the L-type calcium channel blockers, at their therapeutic doses, have no significant effect on the normal release of ACh from the nerve terminal or on the strength of normal neuromuscular transmission.

The exact mechanism by which the Ca^{2+} causes the release of neurotransmitter from nerve terminals is not yet known. But, its entry into the nerve terminal seems to trigger a series of phosphorylation reaction which disrupt the resting state of nerve terminal and causes the release of neurotransmitter. An effect, of the increased level of calcium at nerve terminal, is also seen as clinically important in *post-tetanic potentiation*, which occurs when a nerve of a paralyzed patient, paralyzed with a nondepolarizing muscle relaxant, is stimulated by the current of high tetanic frequencies. During tetanic stimulation, Ca^{2+} enters the nerve ending with every stimulus, but it cannot be excreted out as quickly as the nerve is stimulated and Ca^{2+} enters. Thus, it is gradually accumulated during tetanic period. So, when a strong stimulus is applied post-tetanically, then the nerve ending causes the release of more than the normal amount of ACh, due to the more availability of Ca^{2+} at nerve terminals. This abnormally large amount of released ACh antagonizes the effect of muscle relaxants and causes the characteristic increase in the size of post-tetanic twitch which is known as *post-tetanic potentiation* (**Fig. 6**).

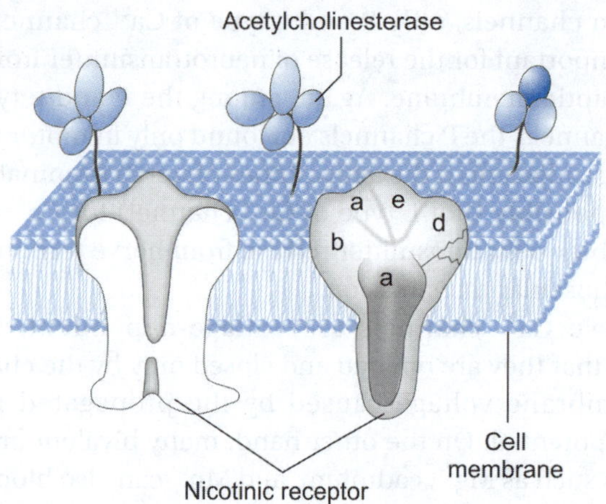

Fig. 6: Postsynaptic membrane. It shows two structures in the center that represent nicotinic acetylcholine receptors. Each is made up of five subunits, arranged as a ring around a channel. The three balloons-like structures represent the true acetylcholinesterase (AChE) enzyme.

Two types of vesicles (containing ACh neurotransmitters are found at nerve endings). One is readily releasable smaller vesicles, called VP2vesicles. They are situated very close to the synaptic cleft at nerve terminal, attaching to the active zones, and are ready to release neurotransmitter, present within them. Another is large reserve or store vesicles, called VP$_1$ vesicles. They are majority in number and are firmly tethered to the cytoskeleton of cells by proteins, called *synapsins.*

After releasing ACh in the synaptic cleft, few of these vesicles have been recycled for further storing of neurotransmitter. But, most of these vesicles are newly synthesized. They are formed in the cell body of a neuron and are transported to the nerve ending. The release of neurotransmitter from the vesicles involves many steps and all of these steps are regulated by the vesicular or *synaptic membrane proteins.* First the vesicle has to unbind from its storage position and then it binds to a *docking protein* which is situated on the inner side of presynaptic membrane. There, then, fusion occurs between the vesicular and synaptic neural membrane. Next, Ca^{2+} enters the nerve ending through the P type of Ca^{2+} channel which is lined up on the sides of the active zone, and activates a protein, called *the synaptophysin,* which is situated on the vesicle wall. These activated vesicle wall protein synaptophysin, then, reacts with nerve membrane to form a pore through which the vesicles discharge its contents. Thus, ACh is poured into synaptic cleft. Hence, there is some delay in the propagation of impulse from nerve fiber to muscle fiber through synaptic cleft. This delay of propagation of impulses between the nerve ending and that of the endplate of muscle cell is called as

TABLE 2: Cholinergic receptors; their sites and action of relaxants.

Receptors	Location	Function	Relaxant interactions
Nicotinic	Postsynaptic neuromuscular junction	Depolarization of endplate—muscle contraction	Succinylcholine—stimulates, nondepolarizer block
Nicotinic	Presynaptic neuromuscular junction	Helps in release of ACh	Succinylcholine—stimulates nondepolarizers block
Nicotinic	Autonomic ganglion	Depolarization of ganglionic cell	Succinylcholine—stimulates nondepolarizer block
Nicotinic	Postganglionic neuron terminal	Positive feedback for transmitter release	Succinylcholine—stimulates nondepolarizer block
Muscarinic	SA node of the heart	↓Heart rate	Succinylcholine stimulate—↓HR nondepolarizer block—↑HR
Muscarinic (M1)	Autonomic ganglionic interneuron cell bodies	Inhibition of depolarization	Nondepolarizer block
Muscarinic (M2)	Autonomic ganglia: Ganglion cell bodies	Depolarization	Atropine blocks, nondepolarizers do not act

(ACh: acetylcholine; HR: heart rate; SA: sinoatrial)

synaptic delay which is about 0.1 milliseconds. When the nerve is called upon to work **(Table 2)** hard due to repeated stimulation at high frequencies, then these reserved VP1 vesicles replace the worn-out VP$_2$ vesicles and participate in the transmission of the impulse. Under such circumstances, Ca^{2+} enters the nerve terminal more deeply, also through the L-type of Ca^{2+} channel, in addition to the P-type of Ca^{2+} channel, and activates the calcium-dependent enzymes. These enzymes, then, phosphorylate and cause the breakage of synapsin links that hold the vesicles to cytoskeleton, and thereby allowing the vesicles to move toward release sites.

After the discharge of neurotransmitter into the synaptic cleft, the vesicular membrane temporarily becomes the part of nerve cell membrane at nerve ending (i.e., presynaptic membrane). Then, a special protein that is present in vesicular membrane detaches it from the nerve cell membrane and makes it return back again into the cytoplasm of nerve terminal as a rudimentary vesicle. These rudimentary vesicles, then, again become filled with ACh neurotransmitter and moves into the previous position for release. Thus, these membranes of vesicles are used again and again until finally worn out and transported back to the nerve's cell body for complete destruction. The complex molecules, such as enzymes, proteins, and new membranes which are used for the synthesis and storage of ACh in vesicles are made in the nerve's cell body and are transported back through the axon to nerve terminal. For the synthesis of ACh the simple molecule, choline is only obtained by the nerve cell body from the extracellular fluid and is transported to the cytoplasm of nerve ending by a special system.

But, the acetate for the synthesis of ACh is available from the acetyl coenzyme A (acetyl CoA) molecule which is present in the mitochondria of nerve ending and is obtained during the metabolism of glucose, fat, and amino acid. Choline and acetate, then, react with the help of an enzyme, named *choline acetyltransferase* to form ACh in the cytoplasm which is then transported and stored into the vesicles. At rest, as the lipid bilayer of the cell membrane is more permeable to K^+ than Na^+, so more K^+ leaks out of the cell than Na^+ gets in. Thus, it creates a slight excess positive charge on the outside and negative charges on the inside of the cell membrane of nerve terminal, leading to a resting membrane potential of about -70 to -90 mV. During the action potential of nerve fiber, Na^+ flows inside the cell, and thus resulting depolarization opens the voltage-gated Ca^{2+} channel. This allows the entry of Ca^{2+} ion into nerve ending and causes a release of ACh from vesicles.

In a resting situation, the concentration of Ca^{2+} ion is many times greater at the outside than the inside of a nerve cell membrane, which facilitate the influx of it (Ca^{2+}) from the extracellular fluid, after the depolarization had reach the nerve ending. This concentration gradient of Ca^{2+} ion between the intracellular and extracellular fluid of nerve ending is maintained by:

- A very efficient system, which transports the Ca^{2+} ion from the inside to the outside of a cell.
- Sequestrating a huge amount of Ca^{2+} inside the intracellular organelles (e.g. sarcoplasmic reticulum).
- Binding Ca^{2+} with intracellular proteins **(Fact file II)**.

After the release of ACh as neurotransmitter, it reacts with the ACh receptor protein (or nicotinic receptor) on the motor endplate to initiate muscular contraction. *Acetylcholinesterase enzyme* remains attached to the motor endplate by a thin stalk of collagen fiber, like bundles of balloons attached to strings. So, most of the ACh molecule, after its release from nerve terminals, passes between these acetylcholine esterase enzymes to reach the postjunctional nicotinic receptor. Hence, they (ACh) are hydrolyzed by enzyme acetylcholinesterase, during their passage

Depolarization or opening of Na^+ channel of nerve cell membrane activates Ca^{2+} channel and causes the transient and localized rise of intracellular Ca^{2+} concentration in nerve terminal. This inward Ca^{2+} current persists until the membrane potential is returned to normal by outward fluxes of K^+ from the nerve cell. Thus, calcium current can be prolonged by potassium channel blockers (e.g., 4-aminopyridine) which slow or prevent K^+ efflux out of the nerve. Thus, the prolongation of action potential by K^+ channel blockers causes the increase in quantal discharge of acetylcholine (Ach) and improved muscular contraction.

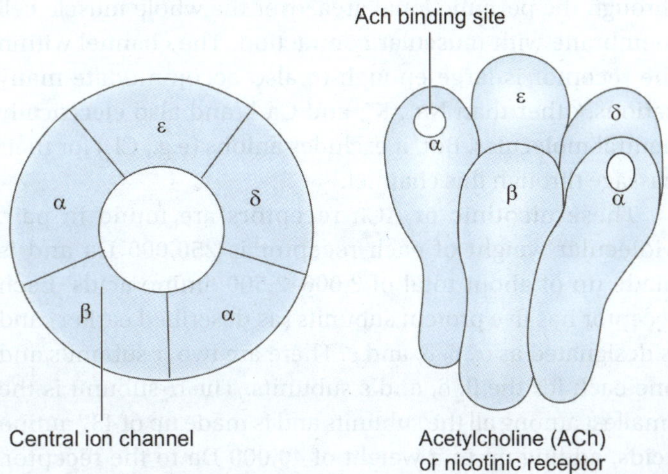

Fig. 7: Cholinergic nicotinic receptor.

through synaptic cleft. Acetylcholine molecules that are not hydrolyzed during their passage through synaptic cleft react with nicotinic type of ACh receptor and are later hydrolyzed by acetylcholinesterase enzyme. So, the action of ACh is very short-lived and is destroyed in <1 millisecond. Two ACh molecules react with one receptor only for the function of later (i.e., ACh) **(Fig. 7)**.

The ACh or nicotinic receptors are synthesized at the motor endplate of muscle cell membrane, under the guidance of messenger ribonucleic acid (mRNA). After synthesis, each receptor is inserted into the muscle cell membrane at motor endplate (postsynaptic membrane) and are held firmly there by 43Kd protein in such a way that each receptor crosses from the one side of cell membrane to the another side. Each ACh receptor is made up of five subunits which are protein in nature and are assembled like a funnel-shaped cylinder with a channel within it. Each of these protein subunits consists of 400–500 amino acids. Normally, the channel within these nicotinic types of ACh receptors remains closed. But, if the neurotransmitter ACh molecules react on their specific sites at the extracellular end of these receptors, then these protein subunits of ACh nicotinic receptor undergo some conformational changes and open the channel, present in the center of the receptor. Thereafter, when the channel is opened, then the Na$^+$ and Ca^{2+} flow from outside into the inside of the endplate membrane and the K$^+$ flow from inside to the outside of the cell, resulting in an *endplate potential* (action potential) that stimulates the muscle to contract. The current that passes through each opened channel is very minimal and this is only of few Picoampere. However, a burst of each vesicle from nerve terminal, liberating ACh neurotransmitter normally opens about 500,000 ACh nicotinic receptor channels. Hence, the produced total current is more than adequate to cause the depolarization of motor endplate and helps its subsequent spread, passing through the perijunctional area, over the whole muscle cell membrane with muscular contraction. The channel within the receptor is large enough to also accommodate many cations, other than Na$^+$, K$^+$, and Ca^{2+}, and also electrically neutral molecules. But, it excludes anions (e.g., Cl$^-$) for their passage through this channel.

These nicotinic or ACh receptors are found in pair. Molecular weight of each receptor is 250,000 Da and is made up of about total of 2,000–2,500 amino acids. Each receptor has five protein subunits (as described earlier) and is designated as α, β, δ, and ε. There are two α subunits and one each for the β, δ, and ε subunits. The α-subunit is the smallest among all the subunits and is made up of 437 amino acids, adding up to a weight of 40,000 Da to the receptor. The molecular weight of other subunits ranges between 50 and 70,000 Da. One of the likely configurations of nicotinic receptor, looking clockwise from the outside of motor endplate is α, ε, α, δ, and β.

All the five subunits of this nicotinic receptor have four membrane-spanning domains. It means their (the subunits of nicotinic receptor) string of amino acids traverse the cell membrane four times and both the end of this string are being on the extracellular side. The ion channel within the receptor is funnel-shaped and is only lined by the second membrane domain of each subunit. At rest, the channel is closed, because the membrane-spanning domains of subunits, lining the channel in the center, touch each other at one point. The length of each receptor is 11 nm and half of this length protrudes in the extracellular space and only 2 nm protrudes into the cytoplasm of cell. The larger end of this funnel-shaped channel of this receptor remains on the outside of the cell. The ACh binding site on the receptor is situated only on both the α-subunit. They are also the site for binding of both the agonist and antagonist. When only both the α-subunit is occupied by ACh (agonist), then all the subunits of this receptor undergo some conformational changes and the ion channel within the receptor opens. On the other hand, if only one of the two α-subunits is occupied by agonist, then channel does not open and also remains closed.

The nondepolarizing muscle relaxants (antagonist of receptor) act by attaching at the binding site of ACh on one or both the two α-subunits of nicotinic receptor and prevent the ACh molecule to attach with the α-subunit of receptor. So, the channel within the receptor remains closed and thus prevents the depolarization of motor endplate and muscular contraction. The interaction between the agonist and antagonist on the receptor site is competitive in nature and the final outcome depends on the relative concentration and the binding characteristic of these agents (agonist and antagonist) involved. There is also ACh receptors on the presynaptic membrane which play the role in mobilizing the vesicles, containing neurotransmitter ACh, from its reserve site to its immediately releasable position. These receptors are also of nicotinic cholinergic type and can also be blocked by the small doses of nondepolarizing agents (antagonists). Presynaptic receptors also can bind with agonists such as succinylcholine. This presynaptic action of succinylcholine accounts for the fasciculation of skeletal muscles and the effectiveness of pretreatment with small doses of nondepolarizing agents.

SUMMARY OF THE MECHANISM OF MUSCULAR CONTRACTION BY NEUROMUSCULAR TRANSMISSION

Structure of Skeletal Muscle

The muscles which are attached to the skeleton (bones) are called as the skeletal muscles. They are supplied by somatic nerves, so they are under voluntary control. Hence, these muscles are also called as voluntary muscles. The skeletal muscles are formed by long and narrow fiber-like muscle cells. So, these *muscle cells are also named as the muscle fibers.* Here, we will have to remember that the muscle fibers are the muscle cells, but the nerve fibers are not the nerve cells. They are only the processes (or extensions) of nerve cells.

The individual muscle fibers (muscle cells) are electrically separated from each other. Because, *on the wall of the muscle fibers, there is no gap* junction. The cell membrane and the cytoplasm of muscle fibers are called as *sarcolemma* and *sarcoplasm*, respectively. Within the sarcoplasm, *each muscle fiber (cell) contains multiple nuclei.* Because, each skeletal muscle fiber develops from the fusion of many myoblasts which are the embryonic precursor of muscle fibers. The skeletal muscle fibers cannot divide after birth. Hence, its damage is replaced by fibrosis.

Each skeletal muscle fiber contains plenty of contractile filaments and these filaments are arranged in bundles. These contractile filaments are called as the *myofibrils.* These myofibrils are divided into two groups—(1) thick filaments which are called as the *myosins* and (2) thin filaments which are called as the *actins.* Each thick myosin filament is made up

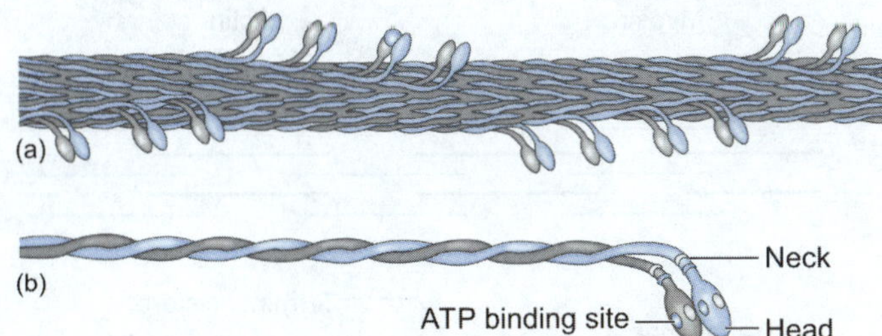

Fig. 8: This figure shows myosin filament (a) and myosin molecule (b).

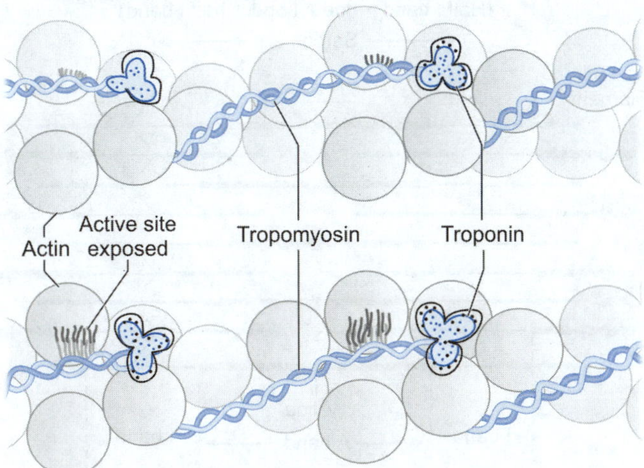

Fig. 9: This figure shows actin filaments with troponin and tropomysin.

of many myosin molecules (myosin-II type of molecules). Each myosin molecule is composed of *two heavy chains* and *four light chains*. The heavy chains are long thick thread-like structures with a long tail at one end and two globular heads at another end. In one myosin molecule, the two heavy chains are twisted over one another and are arranged in a double-helix manner. The each globular head of myosin molecule is attached with two light chains. Therefore, as one myosin molecule has two globular heads, so it has four light chains. *These light chains have adenosine triphosphatase (ATPase) activity.* The globular head and the thick body of myosin molecule are joined by a side chain which is called as the *cross bridge.* These cross-bridges are arranged in six different directions. So, when the thick body of myosin molecules is bundled together, the side chains are directed to six different directions and can attach with six thin actin filaments around it **(Fig. 8)**.

Each thin actin filament is composed of three types of proteins, named: (1) actin, (2) tropomyosin, and (3) troponin. The *actin protein molecules* are globular in shape and are arranged in two chains. In one actin filament, there are two such actin chains and each actin chain is called F-actin. These two F-actin chains are twisted one over another and form a double-helix structure. The *tropomyosin protein molecule* is a thread-like structure and is situated in the groove, formed in the double-helix of the F-actin chain. These tropomyosin threads cover the active sites, present on the chain of actin molecules, where the myosin heads are attached. The *troponin protein molecules* hold the tropomyosin molecules in position so that the latter can cover the active sites of actin filament.

When Ca²⁺ binds to troponin molecules, then the tropo-myosin molecules are released and move away slightly to expose the active sites on actin. Troponin molecule is formed of three parts: (1) *Troponin-C*, (2) *Troponin-T*, and (3) *Troponin-I*, with their distinct individual function. *Troponin-C binds with Ca²⁺. The Troponin-T holds the three parts of troponin together with the tropomyosin. Troponin-I binds with actin in such a way that tropomyosin is kept in position, covering the active sites of actin. Therefore, tropomyosin and troponin are called as the regulatory* proteins, *as they regulate the interactions between the actin and myosin filaments (or muscle contraction). On the other hand, the actin and myosin filaments are called as the contractile proteins* **(Fig. 9)**.

Sarcomere

Each muscle fiber (each muscle cell) is divided into several segments by transverse partitions (lines), which are called as the *Z-lines.* This line is formed by an interconnected protein molecule. Each of these segments, i.e., *the portion of a muscle fiber between the two consecutive Z-lines is called as the sarcomere. It (sarcomere) is the contractile unit of a muscle fiber.* The thin actin filaments are attached with the Z-line, on its either side, in two groups. The thick myosin filaments are present in the center of sarcomere, interdigitating with the thin actin filaments at its free ends (another end of actin filaments are attached with Z line). The part of the sarcomere, through which the myosin filaments extend (are present) is called the *A-band* (the letter "A" stands for the ward anisotropic which means dark. Hence, under the light microscope these A-band are looked at as dark bands). The ends of the sarcomere (the part of sarcomere near the Z-line) contain only thin actin filament and this area is called as the *I-band* (the letter "I" stands for the word isotropic which means light. Under the light microscope, these I-bands are looked as light area or light bands). Within the A-band of the sarcomere, at its central portion, the absence of thin actin filaments in between the myosin filaments produces a lighter area which is called the *H-zone.* In H-zone only the myosin filaments are present, without any actin filaments. In the center of this H-zone, again there is a dark line which is called the *M-line.* It is due to the central thickening of thick myosin filaments. The myosin filaments are remained attached to

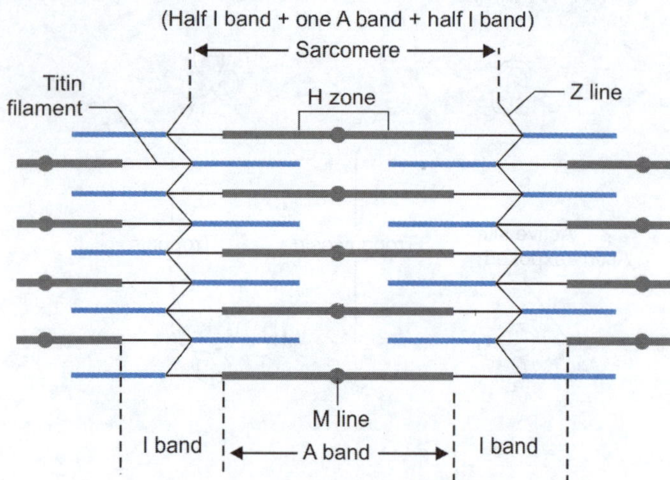

Fig. 10: This figure shows the structure of sarcomere.

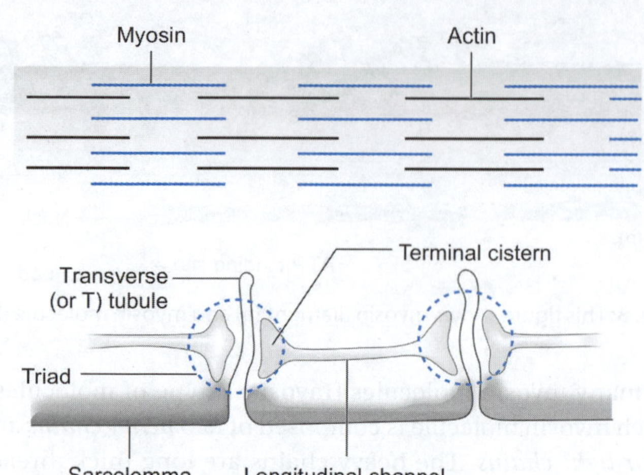

Fig. 11: The longitudinal channel (tubules), transverse tubule, and triad. This triad is the connection between the surface of muscle fiber and the sarcoplasmic (endoplasmic) reticulum.

the Z-line by protein filaments which are called as the *titin*. On the other hand, the actin filaments remain attached to Z-line by another protein filaments which are called as the *actinin*. In summary, we can say that *one sarcomere contains one A-band in the middle and ½ of I-band on the either side of it (A-band). Within the A-band, at its center, there is a lighter H-band (zone). Further, within this H-band, at its center, there is a dark M-line* **(Fig. 10)**.

When the muscle fibers contract, then the thin actin filaments are pulled firmly toward the center of sarcomere. *Therefore, as the thin actin filaments are firmly attached to Z-lines, so the Z-lines are brought closer and the sarcomere shortens.* Obviously, therefore the I-band and H-band become narrower, but the darker *A-band remains constant*. As a result, the shortening of sarcomere leads to the shortening of muscle fiber and this reflects on the whole muscle. However, we have to keep in my mind that the shortening of muscle occurs in isotonic contraction, but not in isometric contraction. *At rest, the length of a sarcomere varies between 2 and 2.6 µm. When its length becomes <2 µm, then there is an overlapping of thin actin filaments. On the other hand, when the length of sarcomere is >3.6 µm, then thin actin filaments are completely pulled out of A-band (myosin filaments).*

Sarcotubular System (Sarcoplasmic Reticulum or SR System)

This system is a complex network of tubules, formed of unit membranes. It is well-developed in skeletal muscle. In this system, there are two components: (i) a set of T tubules, and (ii) a set of sarcoplasmic reticulum. The set of T (means transverse) tubules which is formed due to the invagination of sarcolemma (muscle cell membrane) are present at the junction of A-band and I-band (in cardiac muscle, the T tubules are situated along the Z-lines). The containing space within the T tubules is obviously the extracellular space and

contains the extracellular fluid. Thus, the extracellular space extends into the interior of cells through T tubules. The other component of this sarcoplasmic reticulum system is the sarcoplasmic reticulum (SR) which is formed by a complex network of longitudinal tubules around the myofibrils (contractile elements, i.e., myosins and actins). These are like the endoplasmic reticulum (ER), found in other cells. *These longitudinal tubules have lateral swellings (near the T tubules) on their either side and these are called as the terminal sacs or terminal cistern. One T tubules with two terminal sacs on its (T tubules) on both sides together form a triad* **(Fig. 11)**.

The SR (sarcoreticular system) plays a very important role in muscle contraction. Intracellular Ca^{2+} ions are stored in terminal sacs with the help of a protein, called *calsequestrin*. Action potential, after its formation at motor endplate, spreads along the whole muscle cell membrane (sarcolemma) and then spreads further down in the interior of cell along the T tubules, up to the vicinity of terminal sacs (triad). Then, Ca^{2+} is released from the terminal sacs and causes the muscle to contract by increasing the concentration of intracellular Ca^{2+}. After the contraction of muscle is over, this Ca^{2+} is again pumped back into the longitudinal portion of SR and then finally into the terminal cisterns of triad by the help of the Ca^{2+}-Mg^{2+}-ATPase enzyme.

Mechanism of Muscle Contraction

Muscle contraction occurs due to the interaction between the thick myosin and thin actin filaments and this process is as follows. When an impulse reaches the nerve terminals or sole feet, then the depolarization of motor endplate takes place by the help of the liberation of ACh from the presynaptic vesicle into the synaptic cleft through the presynaptic membrane, with the participation of the entry of Ca^{2+} from the outside extracellular fluid within the nerve terminal. The ACh, thus, liberated diffuses across the synaptic cleft and reacts with the ACh or nicotinic receptor on the postjunctional membrane (PJM), forming the ACh-receptor complex. Due to the enough release of ACh, a large number of nicotinic receptors in PJM are activated and now this activated state of nicotinic receptor facilitates the entry of enough Na$^+$ through the channel within this receptor, producing the depolarization of PJM. If the depolarizing potential of PJM attains a threshold level, then an impulse of action potential is developed and is propagated in both directions, along the sarcolemma (the cell membrane of muscle cell).

After the formation of an action potential at motor endplate, it (action potential) spreads in all the direction along the sarcolemma and also spreads down into the interior of muscle fiber (cell) along the T tubules. When this action potential reaches the terminal sac, then the Ca^{2+} are released from the terminal sac into the sarcoplasm (cytoplasm of muscle cell) and binds with troponin C.

Sarcoplasm normally contains Ca^{2+}. But, it (Ca^{2+}) combines maximally with troponin C, when its concentration increases to 5 mmol/L. The mechanism of release of Ca^{2+} from terminal sac is like that the voltage-gated Ca^{2+} channels (receptors), named *dihydropyridine receptor*, present in T tubules, are activated by AP. These activated Ca^{2+} channels (receptors), then, open the another set of channels, called the *ryanodine receptor*, in the terminal sac through which Ca^{2+} of terminal sac comes out into the sarcoplasm.

Troponin C and Ca^{2+} complex, then, undergoes conformational changes, and the *troponin I* is loosened. This releases tropomyosin from its position and then subsequent lateral movement of tropomyosin molecule *exposes the active site on the actin molecule.* Now, the myosin heads are attached to these active sites of actin filaments and form *cross-bridges.* After that *forceful bending (movement) of myosin heads occurs (it is called as power stroke) and this causes the sliding of thin actin filaments over the thick myosin filaments (Fact file III).* The myosin heads, then, detach and reattach to the next active sites on the actin filaments. *As the myosin heads, at the two ends of myosin bundles are in opposite direction, so the power stroke draws the actin filaments of both sides toward the center of sarcomere. This process of attachment, bending, detachment, and again attachment of myosin head with actin filament is called as the recycling of cross-bridges.*

There are many active sites on thin actin filaments and the myosin head goes on reacting with them one after another, causing the movement of actin filaments toward the center of sarcomere. This action is like a ratchet mechanism (Ratchet is a device with a set of angled teeth in which a cog or tooth fits, allowing movement in one direction).

FACT FILE III

Propagated action potential along the axon → the depolarization of neuron terminals → ACh is released from the synaptic vesicles of nerve terminal with the help of Ca^{2+} entry → released ACh diffuses across the synaptic cleft → ACh forms a (ACh–receptor) complex with the nicotinic receptor on PJM → the opening of channel within the receptor → increased permeability of Na$^+$ and K$^+$ of PJM → depolarization of endplate → depolarization of Na$^+$ channel at the perijunctional zone which is a very critical area where potential, developed at the endplate, is converted to an action potential which sweeps along the muscle sarcolemma (cell membrane) → transmission of such action potential from sarcolemma to the triads (sarcotubular system—T system + sarcoplasmic reticulum) → release of Ca^{2+} from sarcoplasmic reticulum → binding of Ca^{2+} with troponin → troponin with Ca^{2+} activate myosin ATPase → myosin ATPase is activated → cross-bridges are formed → actin filament slides along the myosin filament → contraction of muscle is developed.

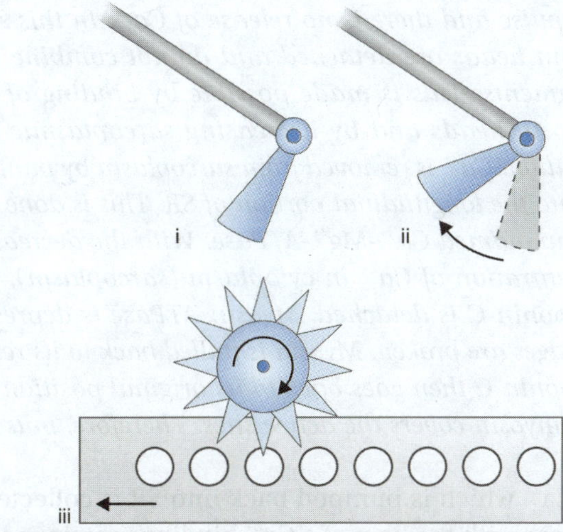

Fig. 12: The figure i, ii, and iii shows the ratchet mechanism of muscular contraction.

Hence, it is called as the *ratchet theory of muscle contraction.* One such cycle leads to a 1% shortening of sarcomere in isotonic contraction. In isometric contraction (where muscles shortening does not occur), there is no recycling of cross-bridges. Here, the cross-bridges remain formed and power stroke leads to force generation or tension development. **(Fig. 12)**

Role of Adenosine Triphosphate in Muscle Contraction

Adenosine triphosphate is required at all the steps of muscle contraction. The energy, released by the hydrolysis of ATP, is essential for the power stroke (bending of myosin head). ATP is also required for the detachment of myosin heads. Furthermore, to cause relaxation, Ca^{2+} is to be pumped back into the SR system which also requires ATP. Presently, it is believed that on binding with one ATP (till it is not hydrolyzed and energy is not released), the myosin head is detached from the actin. Subsequently, the hydrolysis of ATP energizes the myosin head which is then attached to the next active site on actin filament. Then, the release of energy from the myosin head leads to a power stroke. After binding with another ATP the myosin head again begins to detach from the cross bridge to repeat the cycle.

Attachment of ATP → detachment of myosin head → troponin with Ca^{2+} activate myosin ATPase → myosin ATPase is activated → *hydrolysis of ATP → myosin head is energized → attachment of myosin head with actin → release of energy → power stroke → attachment of another ATP with myosin head → cycle goes on.*

Relaxation of Muscle

Relaxation of muscle means returning to the state before its contraction. It occurs when the muscle is not excited by nerve impulse and there is no release of Ca^{2+}. In this state, the myosin heads are detached and do not combine with actin filaments. This is made possible by binding of ATP with myosin heads and by decreasing sarcoplasmic Ca^{2+} concentration. Ca^{2+} is removed from sarcoplasm by pumping it back into the longitudinal portion of SR. This is done by a Ca^{2+} pump, named Ca^{2+}-Mg^{2+}-ATPase. With the decrease in the concentration of Ca^{2+} in cytoplasm (sarcoplasm), Ca^{2+} from troponin-C is detached. Myosin ATPase is depressed. Cross-bridges are broken. Myosin is pulled back to its resting site. Troponin-C then goes back to its original position and the tropomyosin covers the active sites. Therefore, muscle is relaxed.

The Ca^{2+} which is pumped back into SR is collected in terminal sac with the help of a Ca^{2+} binding protein, named *calsequestrin.* Therefore, it is obvious that muscle relaxation also requires ATPs and is an active process. It can be said that the relaxed muscle is like a loaded gun (binding of ATPs with myosin heads). If the trigger is released (AP reaches the terminal sac and the ryanodine receptors are activated), then it fires (action starts) due to the release of Ca^{2+} from the terminal sacs and hydrolysis of ATP. If the Ca^{2+} cannot be removed from cytosol (sarcoplasm) or there is no supply of ATPs for the detachment of myosin heads, then the muscle remains in a state of continued contraction. This condition of continued contraction is called as *contracture* and it occurs even in absence of any stimulus. *Rigor mortis* is a similar condition due to the failure of relaxation of skeletal muscles after death. This is because after death ATPs are not available for binding with myosin heads.

Under normal conditions, the impulses may be excitatory or inhibitory. When there is a preponderance of excitatory impulses over the inhibitory impulses, then there will be depolarization of postsynaptic motor neuron membrane and the discharge of action potential will be of excitatory postsynaptic potential (EPSP) type. But, when there is predominance of inhibitory impulses, over the excitatory impulses, then there will be hyper-polarization of the postsynaptic motor neuron membrane. Thus, inhibitory postsynaptic potential (IPSP) will be developed and this will inhibit the discharge of any impulses.

Energy for Muscle Contraction

The immediate energy source for muscle contraction is ATP. Because, ATP is hydrolyzed to adenosine diphosphate (ADP), and the energy is released. This ADP is, then, converted to ATP again by creatine phosphate (CP) as follows and energy is stored. ADP + CP ↔ ATP + C. *This reaction is known as Lohman's reaction and it is catalyzed by creatine kinase.* These two high-energy phosphate compounds (ATP and ADP) can provide energy for some time and then these are to be resynthesized. ATP is provided partly by the glycolytic pathway, but mainly from the mitochondria. ATP then converts the creatine (C) to CP. Now, the stored energy in CP is carried to ADP, forming ATP. So, both the ATP and CP are replenished by metabolism within the cells. The major fuel for this ATP formation, particularly in red muscles, is the metabolism of free fatty acids and carbohydrates, when the contraction is prolonged and exhaustive. But, in the case of white muscles, carbohydrate is the main source of energy. The pattern of metabolism, during muscular contraction, e.g., exercise, depends not only on the type of muscles but also on the rate of muscle contraction, i.e., type of exercise.

Lactic acid is produced as a result of muscle contraction, due to anaerobic glycolysis. It is normally produced from pyruvic acid after glycolysis in fast (white) muscles and also in slow (red) muscles when O_2 supply cannot keep pace with demand. This lactic acid is mainly disposed of through the *Cori cycle.*

A muscle containing more white fibers is called as *white muscle.* It looks pale (white) because this type of muscle has less or no myoglobin. These muscles are very rapid in their action and are also called as the *fast muscles.* These muscles have very high ATPase activity. This type of muscle derives their ATP requirement from glycolysis (anaerobic), so cannot continue contraction for a longer time. The typical example of this type of white muscle is extrinsic muscles of eyeball. The muscles, moving the fingers of hand, are also of this category.

A muscle, containing more red fibers, is called as the *red muscle.* It looks dark (red), because this type of muscle has more myoglobin. These muscles are slow in their action and so are also called as the *slow muscles.* These muscles have low ATPase activity. This type of muscle derives their ATP requirement from tricarboxylic acid (TCA) cycle (aerobic or oxidative), so can continue contraction for a longer time. The typical examples of this type of red muscle are postural muscles, leg muscles, etc. However, most of the muscles of our body are of mixed types. But, a single motor unit is always composed of the same type of muscle fibers **(Fig. 11)**.

Endplate Potential

It is defined as the changes in electrical potential at motor endplate, induced by the activation of ACh receptors which cause the increase in endplate permeability to Na^+ and K^+. This endplate potential can be recorded by inserting a microelectrode into the motor endplate. When an impulse reaches the neuromuscular junction through an axon, then ACh is liberated from the terminal nerve endings and depolarizes the motor endplate of muscle cell membrane. When this local depolarization exceeds −30 to −40 mV (threshold level), then a spike potential (depolarization) in muscle cell is initiated with an amplitude of +35 mV, and the muscle contracts.

At rest, the neurotransmitter substances are continuously liberated from the vesicles at a very slow rate from nerve terminal which is incapable of producing any depolarization up to threshold level and failed to initiate a full action potential with any propagated impulse and contraction of muscle. This small endplate potential is called as the *miniature endplate potential (MEPP)* and it is not >0.5 mV. However, when the nerve action potential reaches axon terminals, then there is synchronous release of several vesicles, full of transmitter substance, causing a *threshold endplate potential (TEPP)* and muscle contraction.

ACTIONS OF DRUGS ON NEUROMUSCULAR TRANSMISSION

Neuromuscular transmission can be blocked by two ways: (i) by inhibiting the release of neurotransmitter, ACh, from presynaptic neuron through the presynaptic membrane, or (ii) by inhibiting the action of ACh, after its release, on its nicotinic receptor at motor endplate (a) through a competitive inhibition or (b) by a persistent depolarization **(Fig. 13)**.

Botulinum toxin blocks the neuromuscular transmissions by inhibiting the release of ACh from nerve terminals through its action on presynaptic membrane. Whereas, the curare muscle relaxants such as tubocurarine, pancuronium, atracurium, etc., block the neuromuscular transmissions by competitive inhibition of ACh for binding at the level of nicotinic receptor, present at the motor endplate on postsynaptic membrane. It means, the curare competes with ACh for binding with nicotinic receptor, but does not prevent the release of it (ACh) from the presynaptic nerve terminal. *As the curare prevents the onset of depolarization of motor*

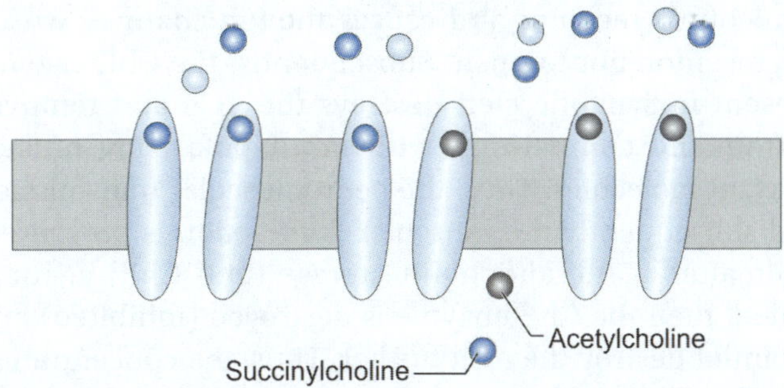

Fig. 13: The classical action of agonists (acetylcholine and succinylcholine) on endplate nicotinic acetylcholine receptors. Any combination of two agonist molecules causes the channel in nicotinic receptor to open. But, different agonists cause action potential of different durations, depending upon the duration of binding of agonists with the receptors. ACh causes a few milliseconds of binding on receptor, with depolarization and paralysis. Succinylcholine causes a long duration of binding on receptors, with prolonged depolarization (better to say prevent repolarization) and paralysis than Ach.

endplate, leading to the relaxation of skeletal muscle, so these curare are called as the nondepolarizing muscle relaxants.

The drugs which block the neuromuscular transmission and produce muscular paralysis by persistent depolarization of postsynaptic membrane of motor endplate are called as the depolarizing muscle relaxants. The examples of such depolarizing muscle relaxants are—decamethonium and succinylcholine. They act on nicotinic receptor at postsynaptic membrane of motor endplate, like ACh. But, their duration of action is many times longer than ACh and so causes prolonged depolarization of motor endplate. Thus, they prevent the further action of neurotransmitter ACh on nicotinic receptor at postsynaptic membrane of motor endplate and produce muscular relaxation (because ACh cannot act on the already depolarized nicotinic receptor). So, they are called as the depolarizing muscle relaxant. The prolonged depolarization, produced by succinylcholine or decamethonium, is because these drugs are metabolized and eliminated very slowly by *pseudocholinesterase* in comparison to ACh. The ACh which is found in normal neuromuscular transmission cannot produce prolonged depolarization and muscular paralysis, because the elimination of it is very rapid (fraction of a second) as the *true cholinesterase*, not pseudocholinesterase, present in the synaptic cleft destroys it within few milliseconds.

Nondepolarizing Muscle Relaxants and Nicotinic Receptor

The nondepolarizing muscle relaxants prevent the depolarization of endplate, because they bind to the ACh recognition site of the α-subunit of nicotinic receptor. Thus, it prevents the ACh, from its binding to the α-subunit of nicotinic receptor and causes the ion channel, within the receptor, not to open. Subsequently, the ChE enzyme present in synaptic cleft destroys the ACh and removes it from the competition with nondepolarizing muscle relaxant molecules. Thus, the neuromuscular transmission and subsequently the muscular contraction is prevented. Thereafter, if the anticholinesterase (anti-ChE) agent is added, then the ChE enzyme is destroyed (inhibited) and it cannot destroy the ACh further. Thus, the concentration of ACh will gradually increase in synaptic cleft and will shift the competition between the ACh and nondepolarizing muscle relaxant molecules in favor of ACh, though the molecules of nondepolarizing muscle relaxants are still present in the extracellular fluid. Therefore, the molecules of nondepolarizing muscle relaxant are replaced from their binding site on nicotinic receptor and the molecules of ACh are attached with the receptor, as the binding site of ACh and nondepolarizing agents on nicotinic receptor is the same. Hence, the neuromuscular transmission will be improved and muscles will contract **(Table 3)**.

Nicotinic receptor channels will not open, unless ACh is attached to two α-subunits of this receptor at a time, i.e., two molecules of ACh per receptor is needed for the activation and the opening of channel within a nicotinic receptor. Whereas, the attachment of a single molecule of nondepolarizing muscle relaxant to the ACh binding site of one α-subunit of nicotinic

receptor is adequate to prevent the opening of receptor channel. So, the competition between the agonist (ACh) and antagonist (nondepolarizing relaxants) is biased in favor of antagonist. Mathematically, this biasness is equivalent to the second power effect of the number of molecules of antagonist (i.e., for two molecules of relaxants four molecules of ACh is needed). All these explanations indicate that the block (muscular paralysis), produced by high concentration of nondepolarizing muscle relaxants, is more difficult to reverse than a low concentration of it and sometimes impossible **(Fig. 14)**.

There are typical features (or characteristics) of nondepolarizing and depolarizing muscular relaxation (or block) by which we can differentiate them. The characteristic features of nondepolarizing and depolarizing block or muscular relaxation are:

- Generally, in normal neuromuscular physiology, at least 10 seconds must be allowed to elapse between the two successive single twitch stimuli (or pulse) for the complete recovery of motor endplate and subsequent transmission of impulse and the contraction of muscle. Therefore, if the interval of two pulses is >10 seconds, i.e., if the frequency of impulses is <0.1 Hz, then there is full recovery of motor endplate and there is no depression (or fade) for transmission of impulses with the contraction of muscle, by successive impulses, will be found.

  On the other hand, if the frequency of impulses is >0.1 Hz, i.e., the interval between two successive impulses is <10 seconds and the endplate does not get adequate time to recover completely from the effect of first impulse, then fades appear after successive impulses. Fade increases with the increase of frequency up to 2 Hz, when a plateau is reached. This plateau is maintained up to 50 Hz. Fade reaches its maximum value by the fourth impulse from where the idea of train-of-four (TOF) has come. In the both nondepolarizing and depolarizing block, when the block is very intense, i.e., one hundred percent (100%) and all the nicotinic receptors at motor endplate are involved; and then there is no twitch response of muscle to any type of stimulus. This is called as the *period of no response*. Thereafter, with the passing of time, when the intensity of block gradually declines and some receptors become free from the molecule of relaxant (nondepolarizing or depolarizing), then the muscular twitch response to stimulus (whatever is the type of stimulus) starts to appear *(responsive phase)*. Then, *if the frequency of stimulus is <0.1 Hz*, then in the muscular response against the stimulus there will be no fade, but only the depression of height of all the responses will be found. But, *if the frequency of stimulus is >0.1 Hz*, then the gradual depression of responses, i.e., the gradual decrease in the height of

TABLE 3: Characteristics of depolarizing and nondepolarizing block (muscular paralysis).

Feature	Depolarizing or (phase I) block	Nondepolarizing and phase II block
Effect on single twitch height	Reduced	Reduced
TOF fade	Height of twitch response of muscle against stimulus is reduced, but not it is gradual. So, fade is not found	Height of twitch response of muscle against stimulus is gradually reduced which is called as fade. So, fade is found
Tetanic fade	Height of twitch response of muscle against stimulus is reduced, but fade is not found	Height of twitch response of muscle against stimulus is gradually reduced. So, fade is found
Post-tetanic facilitation	Not found	Found
Effect of anti-ChE agent	Potentiation	Reverse
Effect of nondepolarizing agent	Reduction of block	Potentiation

(anti-ChE: anticholinesterase; TOF: train-of-four)

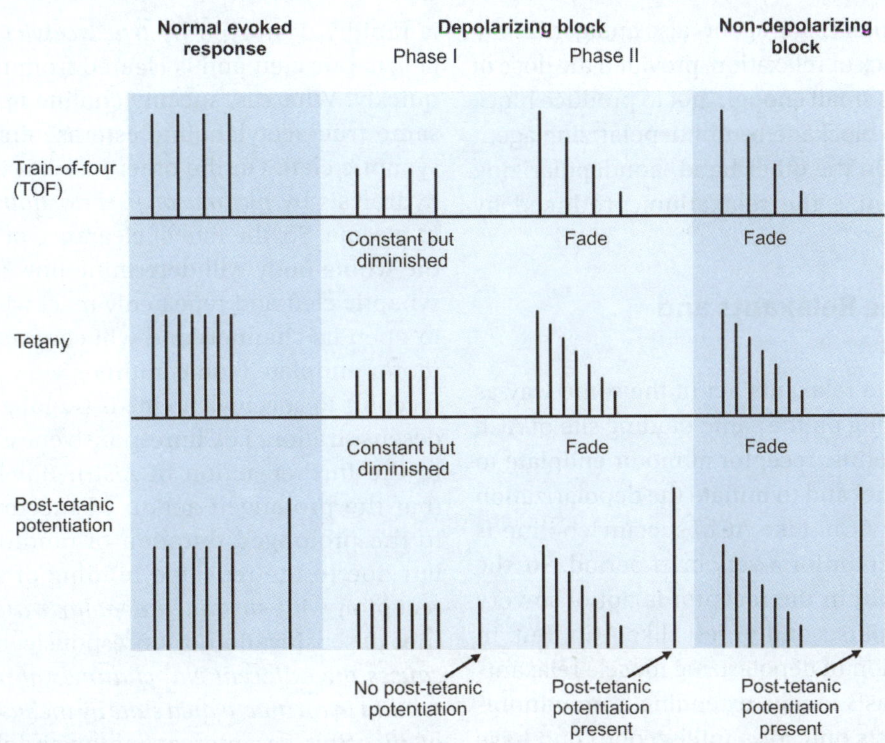

Fig. 14: Evoked responses during depolarizing (phase I and phase II) and nondepolarizing block.

responses or *fade appears in nondepolarizing type of block, but not in the depolarizing type of muscle relaxant.* Clinically, in surgical state of anesthesia, patients usually stay in responsive phase, because the intensity of block is not so high (not 100%, i.e., all the nicotinic receptors are not blocked) that any stimulus will not respond. So, in the therapeutic clinical dose of relaxants, for the surgical stage of anesthesia, any single twitch stimulus will produce a response, but of low amplitude in both depolarizing and nondepolarizing muscle relaxants (block), but will so fade in nondepolarizing relaxant and no fade in depolarizing relaxant, provided the stimulus is >0.1 Hz (NB 1 Hz = 10 impulses in 10 seconds or 1 impulse in 1 second. 0.1 Hz = 1 impulse in 10 seconds. About 2 Hz = 20 impulses in 10 seconds or 1 impulse in 0.5 seconds).

In TOF stimulation, the frequency of impulse is 2 Hz and is consists of subsequent four impulses, separated by 0.5 seconds. With nondepolarizing relaxants, fade, i.e., the gradual depression of the height of response after subsequent four stimuli is seen with TOF stimulus, after the first response has appeared, and this fade is maximum at the fourth response. In contrast, with depolarizing muscle relaxants, there is no fade after TOF stimuli. But, all the responses are of same low in amplitude (equal depression in all the responses, not gradual depression, or fade-like nondepolarizing relaxant) than the previous nonblock response (2 Hz = 20 impulses in every

10 seconds. So, the interval between two impulses is 0.5 seconds).

- *Tetanic stimulation* (here, frequency is 30–100 Hz and the gap between impulses is 0.3–0.1 seconds) is also characterized by fade (gradual depression) in nondepolarization relaxation. However, in depolarizing relaxation, the response to tetanic stimulation is sustained like a normal muscle, but with of low amplitude (only depression, but not gradual).

- *When a single twitch or TOF stimulus is applied after a tetanic stimulation,* then the response by a single twitch or TOF stimulation in nondepolarizing block is exaggerated or facilitated. This is called as the *post-tetanic facilitation* and the probable explanation of this facilitation is the displacement of nondepolarizing muscle relaxant molecules from the motor endplate, by the ACh which is released maximally during the tetanic stimulation. This post-tetanic facilitation is absent in depolarizing blocks, like normal muscle. This post-tetanic facilitation should not be confused with the *post-tetanic potentiation,* applied in post-tetanic count (PTC) which is an augmented stimulus of single twitch or TOF stimulation after a tetanic stimulation.

- *Nondepolarizing block (muscle relaxation) is reversed by anti-ChE agents,* but depolarizing block (muscle relaxation) becomes intense due to the potentiation of depolarization by increased levels of ACh by these anti-ChE agents. Depolarizing agents also antagonize the nondepolarizing block or relaxation, provided the dose of depolarizing agent is small enough, not to produce block in its own right, and blockade by nondepolarizing agent is intense enough. On the other hand, nondepolarizing agents also antagonize the relaxation, produced by depolarizing agents.

Depolarizing Muscle Relaxants and Nicotinic Receptors

The depolarizing muscle relaxants act in the same way as ACh. They act by attaching on the same binding site of ACh on the α-subunit of nicotinic receptor at motor endplate to open the receptor channel and to initiate the depolarization of motor endplate, like ACh. Like ACh, succinylcholine is not attached to the receptor for a very brief period. So, the opening of a channel within the receptor is not of so very short duration, i.e., 1 millisecond or less, like ACh. But, in contrast to ACh, the action of depolarizing muscle relaxants (e.g., succinylcholine) lasts longer, extending from minutes to hours (ACh action lasts only for a millisecond) and have a biphasic action on skeletal muscles, causing it to contract initially and then to relax finally, (the explanation of which is discussed underneath). The difference between the duration of action of ACh and succinylcholine (structurally, which is actually two molecules of ACh) is because ACh

is rapidly destroyed by *true acetylcholinesterase,* present at synaptic cleft and is cleared from the synaptic cleft very quickly. Whereas, succinylcholine is not destroyed by the same true acetylcholine esterase enzyme, present in the synaptic cleft. On the other hand, it is eliminated through hydrolysis by *plasma or pseudocholinesterase,* circulating in plasma. So, the rate of clearance of succinylcholine from the whole body will determine how long it will last in the synaptic cleft and repeatedly react with nicotinic receptors to open its channels and will continuously depolarize the motor endplate (some author's view is that binding of the receptor to succinylcholine is prolonged and this produces desensitization, i.e., unresponsiveness of nicotinic receptor to the further action of ACh). But here, it is explained that the prolonged action of succinylcholine is not due to the prolonged duration of binding with the receptor, but due to the repeated binding of succinylcholine with receptor, with *sustained depolarization of motor endplate* (not desensitization or unresponsiveness of receptor) *that causes the adjacent Na$^+$ channels of perijunctional area to remain in an inactivated state by the sustained depolarization of nicotinic receptor at motor endplate and not getting time for repolarization* which normally help the adjacent Na$^+$ channels at perijunctional area to be activated and to help further transmission of impulses, causing muscular contraction. So, after first muscle contraction (fasciculation) paralysis prevails **(Fig. 15A to C)**.

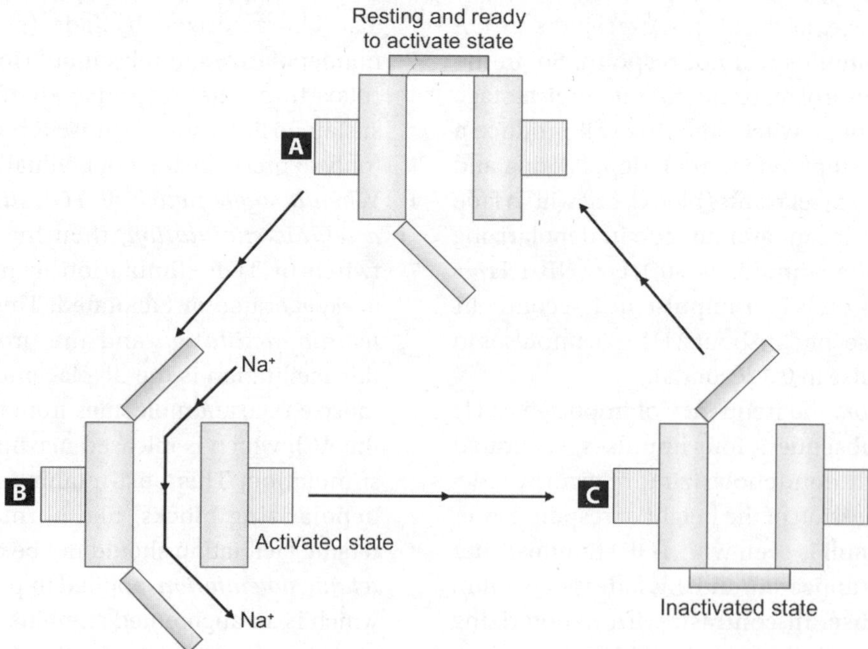

Figs. 15A to C: Sodium (Na$^+$) channel. Each Na channel has two bars. One is upper and another is lower. These two bars represent the gate of the channel. The upper one is voltage-dependent. But the lower one is time-dependent. (A) Represents the resting state of the Na$^+$ channel. With upper gate is closed and lower gate is opened; (B) Represents the activated state with both the gates open; (C) Represents the inactivated state with upper gate open and lower gate closed. Then it again passes to the resting state where upper gate is closed and lower gate is opened. Thus, the cycle repeats and becomes ready for next impulse.

In case of succinylcholine, there is a quick shift from brief muscle contraction, which is seen as fasciculation, to relaxation. This is because at the edge of motor endplate, i.e., at the perijunctional area, two different kinds of membrane, such as the endplate membrane and the true muscle membrane (which is also called perijunctional membrane) with their different types of channels, come in contact. The endplate membrane contains ACh nicotinic receptors whose channels open by ACh or succinylcholine and the perijunctional muscle membrane contains Na^+ channels that do not respond to chemicals such as ACh and succinylcholine, but open when they are exposed to postsynaptic transmembrane voltage change at motor endplate, due to the depolarization of endplate by nicotinic receptor and ACh. Thus, the two types of channels (channel in nicotinic receptor and Na^+ channel) on the two parts of membrane (endplate area and perijunctional area) respond to two different types of stimuli, i.e., chemical and electrical. Endplate area responds to chemical stimuli, such as ACh due to nicotinic receptor and the perijunctional area responds to electrical stimuli due to the Na^+ channel.

Na^+ channel, at perijunctional membrane (area) like ACh receptor, is also a cylindrical protein tube, residing across the cell membrane. It responds only to the sharply changing electrical voltage of perijunctional membrane, due to the opening of adjacent nicotinic receptor of endplate by ACh, but not due to the direct responses to chemical (ACh), like nicotinic receptor. These Na^+ channels are made up of three protein subunits, called as α, β_1 and β_2. The α-subunit of this Na^+ channel is the shape of a doughnut and is thicker than the perijunctional membrane itself. The intracellular portion of Na^+ channel is larger than the extracellular portion of it. The β_1 and β_2 subunit, each lie on the outside of α-subunit. They are smaller than the α-subunit and occupy only the external half of cell membrane. The overall size of a Na^+ channel is approximately 13.5 nm in thickness and 10 nm in its largest diameter. The molecular weight of a Na^+ channel is approximately of 30,000 da.

The Na^+ channel of perijunctional area has two gates that act sequentially. *The upper gate of it is voltage-dependent and responds only to the voltage changes of motor endplate. The lower gate of it is time-dependent and closes or opens for a fixed time period (1–2 milliseconds). In a resting (ready to be active) state, the upper gate of it remains closed and the lower gate remains opened.* So, the sodium (Na^+) ion cannot pass through this incompletely opened resting, but ready to be active, Na^+ channel of perijunctional area. When these Na^+ channels of perijunctional area are subjected to sudden voltage changes, by the depolarization of the adjacent endplate membrane, by the activation of nicotinic receptor channel of endplate area by ACh, then the top gate of these

Na^+ channels opens and they become activated. Therefore, since the lower gate is still open, so Na^+ ion starts to flow through this activated Na^+ channel (its both gates are opened), driven by the favorable high extracellular Na^+ concentration and electrical gradients. This state of Na^+ channel is called as its *activated state*. Thus, this entry of Na^+ into the muscle cells from outside initiates the depolarization of muscle cell membrane and subsequently this depolarization spreads from one Na^+ channel to the next as action potential (AP). *In that way, a wave of depolarization (action potential) moves along the whole muscle cell membrane and triggers the muscle contraction which is seen as fasciculation shortly after the administration of succinylcholine.* Shortly after that, the time-dependent lower gate of Na^+ channel closes, with still the upper gate open, after a fixed time from the onset of Na^+ flow, i.e., after 1–2 milliseconds, and cuts off the flow of Na^+ ions inside the muscle cell. This state of these Na^+ channel at perijunctional membrane is called as the *inactivated state. When the activation of ACh or nicotinic receptor and the depolarization of motor endplate stops and the endplate membrane potential is brought back to its resting value by the quick hydrolysis of neurotransmitter ACh, then the Na^+ channel again comes to the previous resting and ready to be activated state, with the voltage-dependent upper gate closes and lower gate opens from the inactivated lower gate closed and upper gate open state.* But, during continuous depolarization of motor endplate by succinylcholine, the perijunctional Na^+ channels remain in this inactivated state (as the lower time-dependent gate must close after a fixed time under any condition and the upper gate will still remain open as the motor endplate is in still depolarized state) after the first activated state for which muscle contraction (that is seen as fasciculation) occurs and does not come back to the resting and ready to be activated state. This inactivated state of Na^+ channel (lower gate is closed, but the upper gate is open) prevents the further spread of depolarization from the motor endplate which is still now in depolarized state, by succinylcholine, to the other part of the muscle cell membrane causing muscle relaxation.

Since the Na^+ cannot flow through a channel that has a closed lower gate and an opened upper gate (inactivated state) in perijunctional area, so the adjacent Na^+ channels, beyond the perijunctional area in muscle membrane, is not further depolarized and due to that the other downstream Na^+ channels on muscle cell membrane are freed of depolarizing influence. So, the muscle remains paralyzed, as long as the endplate remains depolarized by succinylcholine and Na^+ channel of perijunctional area stays in inactivated state. In fact, in junctional zone the first line of Na^+ channels acts as a buffer which shields the rest of the Na^+ channel of muscle membrane from the events of motor endplate (**Figs. 16A to C**).

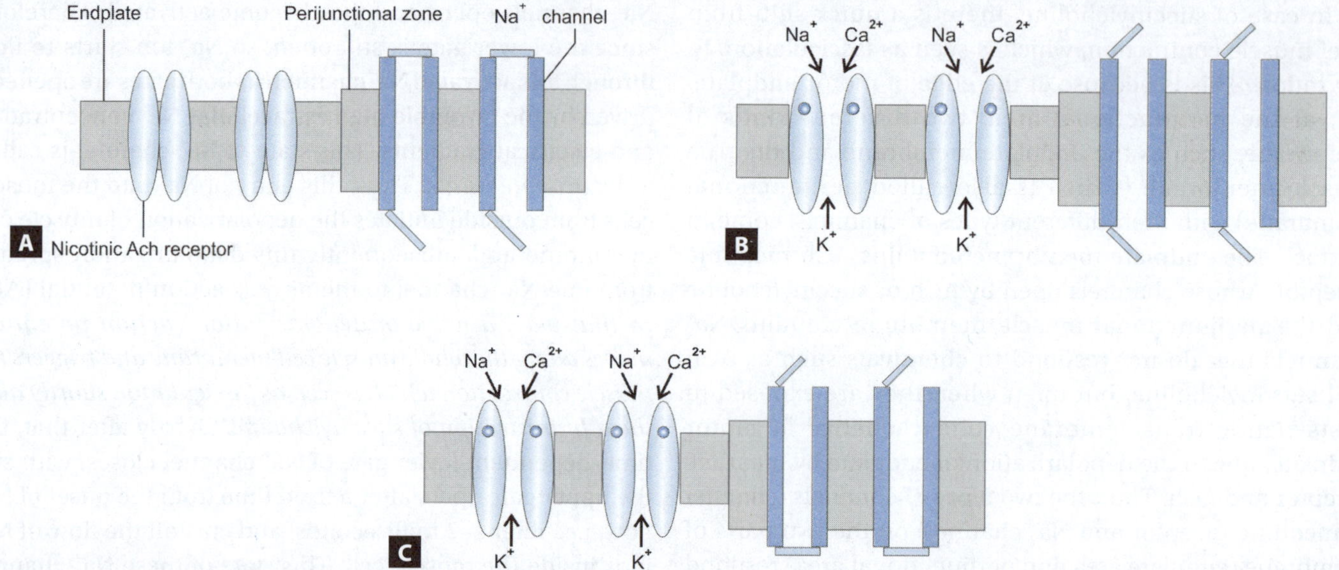

Figs. 16A to C: Nicotinic acetylcholine (ACh) receptors (spindle shaped) in the endplate membrane, and Na$^+$ channels (rectangular shaped) in the muscle membrane at perijunctional area. The spindle shaped ACh receptors are chemically sensitive, but voltage insensitive. On the other hand, the rectangular shaped Na$^+$ channels are chemically insensitive, but voltage sensitive. The upper and lower bars within Na$^+$ channel represent gates. The top gates remain closed. But, it opens when voltage is applied across the membrane. This top gate of Na$^+$ channel is called as the *activation gate*. The lower gate of this Na$^+$ channel is called as the *inactivation gate* and normally it remains open. But, it closes spontaneously after the voltage-dependent upper gate opens and after a fixed time. So, it is called as the time-dependent gate. To flow Na$^+$ through the sodium channel both the gates must be opened. (A) Resting membrane. Here, no current flows through any ACh or Na$^+$ channel, as they remain in resting state; (B) Activation of chemically sensitive ACh-receptor of endplate by ACh or succinylcholine (blue dot) by nerve impulse or applied. Thus, the voltage potential which is developed by the flow of current through the ACh receptor channel causes the upper gate of the adjacent voltage sensitive Na$^+$ channel in the perijunctional zone to open. Therefore, the first Na$^+$ channel is activated and current (Na$^+$ ions) starts to flow through this Na$^+$ channel. This causes the subsequent voltage changes and opens the next Na$^+$ channels. Thus, a wave of depolarization spreads along the surface of muscle cell membrane which starts first at the endplate and then by Na$^+$ channel at the perijunctional zone. This wave of depolarization causes muscle contraction and is shown as fasciculation when succinylcholine is used; (C) The ACh receptors in the endplate are still in depolarized state due to the long duration of action of *succinylcholine*. So, the voltage-dependent upper gate of the Na$^+$ channel in the perijunctional zone next to the endplate remains open. But, the time-dependent inactivation lower gate closes spontaneously after a fixed time interval. So, no ion flows through this Na$^+$ channel, situated in the first row of the perijunctional zone. Therefore, there will be no change of voltage potential in the muscle membrane around the endplate. Thus, the gates of the next second, third, fourth, and the subsequent rows of Na$^+$ channel return to their resting state. So, the *inability* of the Na$^+$ channels which are situated just by the side of the endplate, in the perijunctional zone to pass sodium current due to continuous depolarization of the ACh receptor by succinylcholine, causes the blockade of neuromuscular transmission and muscular paralysis.

During the depolarization of endplate by ACh, the activation of Na$^+$ channel of perijunctional area also causes the activation of adjacent K$^+$ channel and opening of it. These K$^+$ channels are selective only for K$^+$ ions and it exit the muscle cell, driven by high intracellular concentration of it (K$^+$) and electrical gradient (the inside of the cell becomes electrically positive, due to the influx of Na$^+$). Thus, the waves of action potential (AP) spread along the muscle cell membrane. So, the excitability of resting muscle cell can also be modified by K$^+$ channels. For example, the continuous opening of K$^+$ channel produces a hyperpolarization state (inside of the cell is more negative) and the cell becomes less excitable **(Fact file IV)**.

Thus, during the action of depolarizing muscle relaxant, such as succinylcholine, the muscle membrane is divided into three zones: (1) the motor endplate with nicotinic receptor,

FACT FILE IV

Normally, acetylcholine (Ach) is hydrolyzed quickly within the synaptic cleft and so the depolarization of endplate is very short. But, this Ach-induced depolarization of endplate causes the Na$^+$ channel in the adjacent muscle membrane (perijunctional area) to open which subsequently activates the adjacent K$^+$ channel and depolarizes the muscle membrane. This depolarization on muscle membrane spreads from one Na$^+$ channel to another Na$^+$ channel and like waves spreads all over the muscle cell and muscle contracts. Upon the hydrolysis of ACh, endplate repolarizes and the adjacent Na$^+$ channels quickly complete their cycles. Then, it returns to their resting state and becomes ready to send further the next depolarization wave.

which is depolarized by succinylcholine, (2) the junctional zone where Na$^+$ channels are frozen in inactivated state (lower gate is closed and upper gate is opened) after a brief *activated state (both the lower and upper gate is opened and Na⁺ flows), producing a wave of depolarization and muscular contraction (that is seen as fasciculation), and (3) the rest of the muscle membrane where the Na⁺ channels are in resting state (upper gate is closed and the lower gate is opened) after passing an impulse (action potential) and producing fasciculation.*

Since a further burst of ACh from nerve terminal, due to the passing of impulses through nerve, cannot produce further depolarization of motor endplate, due to the still presence of succinylcholine at endplate and cannot overcome the inactivated state of Na⁺ channel in perijunctional area, due to the continuous depolarization of endplate. So, the neuromuscular transmission is blocked and the muscle remains in paralyzed (relaxed) state. *This phenomenon is called as the accommodation.* During accommodation, when the synapse is unexcitable via the nerve, then the direct electrical stimulation of muscle will cause muscle contraction. This is because, since, the sodium channel beyond the perijunctional area are in the resting excitable (ready to be activated) state.

However, the extraocular muscles are tonic muscles that are multiply innervated with numerous motor endplates. So, most of its surface is chemically excitable, like a continuous sheet of motor endplate, with no resting and relaxation zone. Thus, in these muscles accommodation does not occur. So, these muscles undergo sustained contraction in the presence of succinylcholine, and causes increased intraocular pressure. There is also evidence that the extraocular muscles contain a special type of receptor that does not become desensitized in the continued presence of succinylcholine or another depolarizing agent.

Succinylcholine also has presynaptic action. The binding of succinylcholine to the presynaptic nicotine receptors depolarizes the nerve terminals and action potential may be generated which travels backward retrogradely along the nerve terminals to invade its neighboring branches and thus produce the contraction of a whole motor unit. Fasciculation is probably (some school thought) due to this mechanism, rather than the sustained transient depolarization of motor endplate receptors because small doses of nondepolarizing agents are effective in preventing this phenomenon. Another probable explanation of this fasciculation is the special sensitivity of muscle spindles (intrafusal fibers) to succinylcholine which may produce muscular contractions via gamma afferents.

There are many drugs that act on nicotinic receptors, but are not classically as competitive of ACh, like succinylcholine. Because, they cannot be antagonized by increased level of ACh by anti-ChE. They act by: (i) desensitization of nicotinic receptor molecule and (ii) blockade of ion channel.

These drugs react with the ACh receptors directly or via its lipid environment to change their functional integrity and impair transmission, but not acting via the ACh binding site of the nicotinic receptors. This reaction between the drugs and the receptor causes changes in the dynamics of nicotinic receptor, so that the modified receptor channels, instead of opening and closing sharply, become fixed or sluggish. They open more slowly and stay open longer or they close slowly in several steps or both. This effect of drugs on nicotinic receptor causes corresponding changes in the flow of ions and distortion of endplate potential. *Procaine, ketamine, inhaled anesthetic agents, and other drugs which dissolve in the membrane lipid act in that way. If the channel is prevented from the opening, then the transmission is weakened. On the other hand, if the channel is prevented from slow in closing, then transmission may be enhanced. Such drugs can be involved in two clinically important reactions: (1) receptor desensitization and (2) channel blockade.*

Receptor Desensitization

The ACh or nicotinic receptors are macromolecules. They are not rigid, static, and fixed receptors. Actually, they are flexible, dynamic, and set in a fluid lipid content of muscle cell membrane and be in many states. One of these states is a desensitized state. In this state, agonists bind with these receptors with exceptional avidity and it does not undergo any conformational changes that open the channel. *This is known as the desensitization state of nicotinic receptor.* The mechanism by which the desensitization of nicotinic receptor occurs are not known. Some evidence suggests that this desensitization is accompanied by the phosphorylation of tyrosine unit, present in the receptor protein. Indeed, normally, the receptor molecules undergo spontaneously the transformation between its sensitized and desensitized state and at a particular time the sensitized and desensitized receptors remain in a certain proportion at the motor endplate. Therefore, at a certain time, the intensity of neuromuscular transmission depends on the ratio of these sensitized (resting normal) and desensitized (abnormal) receptor concentrations. This is because desensitized receptors are not able to take part in neuromuscular transmission. If only a few receptors are desensitized, then the system will be more susceptible to blockade of neuromuscular transmission by antagonist (nondepolarizing relaxants) and vice versa **(Figs. 17A to E)**.

Agonist such as ACh or succinylcholine binds tightly with the nicotinic receptor and promotes the transition from a sensitized to desensitized state. Antagonist also binds tightly to desensitized receptors and its action is augmented by ACh. Many drugs such as halothane, alcohol, thiopentone, succinylcholine, neostigmine, local anesthetic,

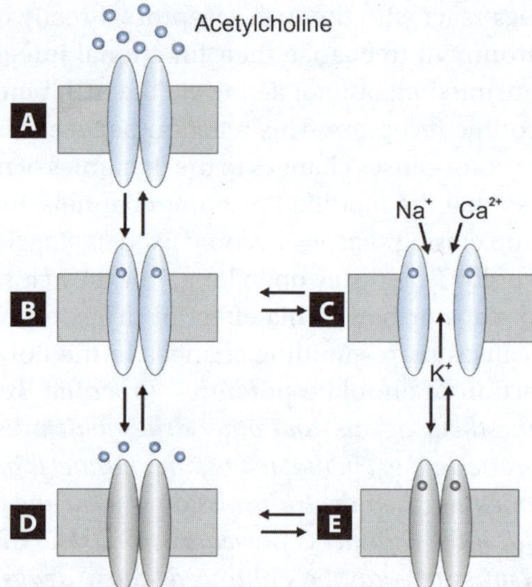

Figs. 17A to E: Different states of endplate nicotinic acetylcholine receptors. (A) Resting receptor; (B) Resting receptor with agonist (acetylcholine) bound to the recognition site. But the channel is not yet opened; (C) Active receptor with an opened channel which allows the flow of ion; (D) Desensitized receptor without agonist bound to the recognition site; (E) Desensitized receptor with agonist bound to the recognition site. Both (D) and (E) are nonconducting. All states of the receptors are in dynamic equilibrium.

> **BOX 1:** Some drugs that can cause desensitization of nicotinic cholinergic receptors.
>
> - *Anticholinesterases (anti-ChEs) inhibitors:* Neostigmine, pyridostigmine, edrophonium, physostigmine, and organophosphorus compounds
> - *Agonists:* Acetylcholine, succinylcholine, decamethonium, and carbachol
> - *Volatile anesthetics:* Halothane, isoflurane, and methoxyflurane
> - *Antibiotics:* Polymyxin B
> - *Alcohols:* Ethanol, butanol, and propranolol.
> - *Barbiturates:* Thiopental and pentobarbital
> - *Local anesthetics:* Lignocaine, dibucaine, prilocaine, and etidocaine
> - *Phenothiazines:* Chlorpromazine and trifluoperazine prochlorperazine
> - *Ca^{2+} channel blocker:* Verapamil

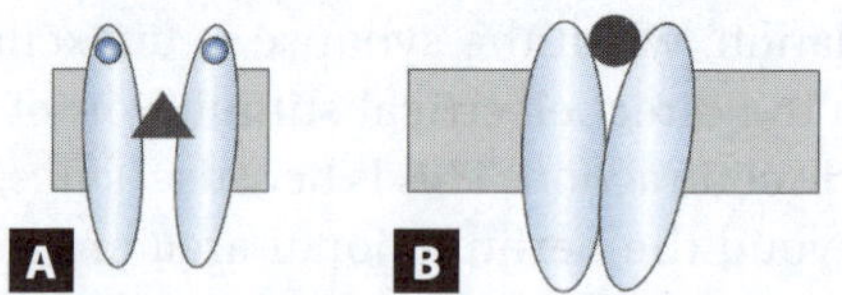

Figs. 18A and B: Nicotinic receptor channel blockade. (A) Open and (B) Closed.

chlorpromazine, etc., promote the shift of the receptor from normal sensitized to abnormal desensitized state and reduce the neuromuscular transmission, augmenting nondepolarizing agent's action. These drugs also can weaken the neuromuscular transmission by reducing the margin of safety that normally exists at the neuromuscular junction or they can cause an apparent increase in the sensitivity of the nondepolarizing agents to block neuromuscular transmission. As these actions are not based on a competition between the drug and ACh and based on the making of more desensitized receptors from a sensitized one, so it cannot be reversed by anti-ChE **(Box 1)**.

Channel Blockade

The molecules of many drugs (such as local anesthetics and Ca^{2+} channel blockers) may enter the channel of nicotinic receptor and block the flow of ions through this channel, preventing depolarization. These are called as the channel blockers. There are two types of channel blockade: (1) *open channel blockade* and (2) *close channel blockade*. In both opened and closed channel blockade, the normal flow of ions through the nicotinic receptor is impaired, resulting in the prevention of depolarization of the motor endplate and a weak or no neuromuscular transmission. However, since the action of these agents is not at the ACh recognition site of receptor, so it is not a competitive antagonist of ACh and

is not relieved by the action of anti-ChE that increases the concentration of ACh **(Figs. 18A and B)**.

Open Channel Blockade

Some drugs like muscle relaxants, also enter up to the middle of the channel of a nicotinic receptor, while it is opened by ACh, and block it. So, it impedes the flow of ions through it (channel). Thus, it prevents the depolarization of motor endplate. The nondepolarizing muscle relaxant is the best example of it. Even though they act at the ACh recognition site, they also block the nicotinic receptor channel directly or physically by this way. A given drug may act preferentially at one or other site. Pancuronium acts preferentially at ACh recognition site. Gallamine acts equally at two sites. Tubocurarine, at a low dose, purely acts at ACh recognition site of nicotinic receptor and at a higher dose at both the sites (recognition site and enter the receptor to block the channel). Increasing the concentration of ACh may cause the channel to open more and it (more opening of the channel) make the receptor more susceptible to open channel blockade. So, neostigmine and other cholinesterase inhibitors (ChEIs) also can act as open-channel blocking drugs. Decamethonium and succinylcholine act as agonist and open the channels by binding at the selective ACh binding site of α-subunit of nicotinic receptor. They also enter the channel and block them (channels) as open channel blockers. But, decamethonium and some other drugs also can penetrate

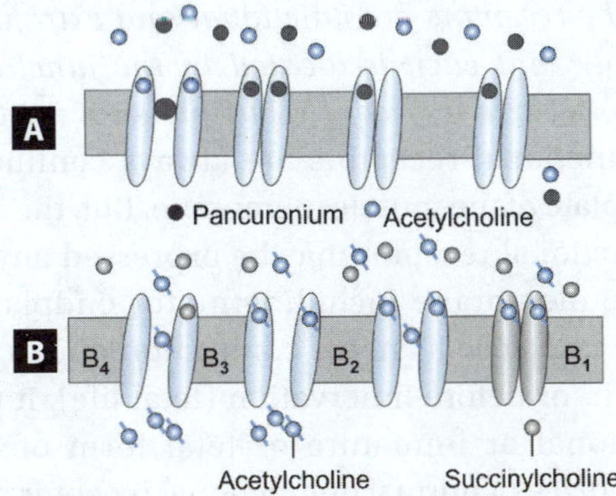

Figs. 19A and B: (A) Some effects due to prolonged exposure of ACh receptor to high concentrations of antagonists (pancuronium). The three receptors at the right side of the picture have recognition site, blockade by pancuronium. The single receptor at the left side of the picture has open channel blockade; (B) Some effects due to prolonged exposure of ACh receptor to high concentrations of agonists (succinylcholine). The right-most single receptor (B₁) is desensitized (blue). While that to the right of center (B₂) has open channel blockade. At left (B₃ and B₄) succinylcholine has penetrated the open channels of two ACh receptors and entered the cytoplasm.

all the way through the open channel of a nicotinic receptor and enter the muscle cytoplasm where they interfere the intracellular process and prevent depolarization. Whether prolonged administration of nondepolarizers, as in the intensive care unit, can result in the entry of relaxant in channel and blockade of it or finally entry of a drug into the cytosol is unknown. This effect may partially explain the muscle weakness associated with prolonged relaxant therapy in the intensive care unit. In such a situation neuromuscular block is complex. At the end, we can conclude that some drug molecules cause depolarization due to action on the recognition site, while others cause—channel blockade, promote desensitization of the receptor, or interfere with the intracellular process **(Figs. 19A and B)**.

Close Channel Blockade

In closed channel blockade, the molecules of a drug block the mouth of a channel, while it is closed. Thus, by their (drug) presence at the mouth of a channel, they prevent the physiological ions from passing through the channel to depolarize the motor endplate. This process of blocked can take place, even when the channel is not open. This type of blocked is the part of action of cocaine, quinidine, tricyclic antidepressants, etc.

Phase-II Blockade

This is a complex phenomenon, which occurs if the neuromuscular junction is continuously exposed to a depolarizing agent. The characteristic features of this

phase II block are similar to that of nondepolarizing block, but cannot be reversed by anti-ChE agents. Normally, the neuromuscular transmission usually remains blocked throughout the period of exposure with a depolarizing agent by the continuous opening of the nicotinic receptor channel. But, the continuous and repeated opening of receptor channels by large or repeated doses of a depolarizing agent allows the continuous efflux of potassium and influx of sodium. This result in the abnormal electrolyte balance of the motor endplate which distorts the function of perijunctional membrane and Na⁺ channel and thus it explains the mechanism of phase II block. The Ca²⁺, entering the muscle fiber (cell) via an open channel, also cause the disruption of the function of receptor and sub-endplate element. This also contributes to the mechanism of phase II block.

On the other hand, the activity of Na⁺- K⁺-ATPase pump on the muscle cell membrane is increased due to the increased intracellular Na⁺ and extracellular K⁺ concentration. Thus, by pumping more Na⁺ out of the cell and more K⁺ into it, it works hard to restore the normal ionic balance and membrane potential as a compensatory mechanism. In such circumstances, the return of the ratio of Na⁺ and K⁺ to normal level restores the membrane potential toward normal level, even though the channel remains open. If the depolarizing muscle relaxant is applied in high concentration and is allowed to remain at neuromuscular junction for a long time, other things also occur which further explain the mechanism of phase II block. These are like that the drug itself enters into the receptor channel to obstruct it or pass through the channel into the cytoplasm of cell, like the open and close channel blockade. Similar actions also occur on the prejunctional structure. Thus, the combination of pre- and postjunctional effects plus the secondary changes on the muscle and nerve homeostasis results in the complicated phenomenon, known as the phase II blockade. The phase II block is a complex and ever-changing phenomenon. Though, the phase II block shows response to tetanic or TOF stimulation, like nondepolarizing agent, still it is best not to take any attempt to reverse this type of block by anti-ChE agents. The development of phase II block depends on—(i) the type of depolarizing drug, (ii) the duration of its exposure, (iii) the concentration of the drug, and (iv) the type of muscle **(Table 4)**.

Atypical Receptors

In contrast to other cells, muscle cells have hundreds of nuclei. Each of these nuclei have genes which direct to make two types of ACh (nicotinic) receptors at the motor endplate—*mature or junctional* and *immature or fetal or extrajunctional.* Other than gene, multiple other factors,

TABLE 4: Difference between phase I and phase II block by succinylcholine.

Features	Phase I	Transition	Phase II
Tetanic stimulation	No fade	Slight fade	Fade
TOF	No fade	Slight fade	Fade
TOF ratio	>0.7	0.4–0.7	<0.4
Post-tetanic facilitation	Nil	Slight	Yes
Anti-ChE	Potentiate	Little effect	Antagonize
Recovery	Rapid	Rapid	Prolonged
Dose requirement (mg/kg)	±2	±4	≥6

(Anti-ChE: anticholinesterase; TOF: train-of-four)

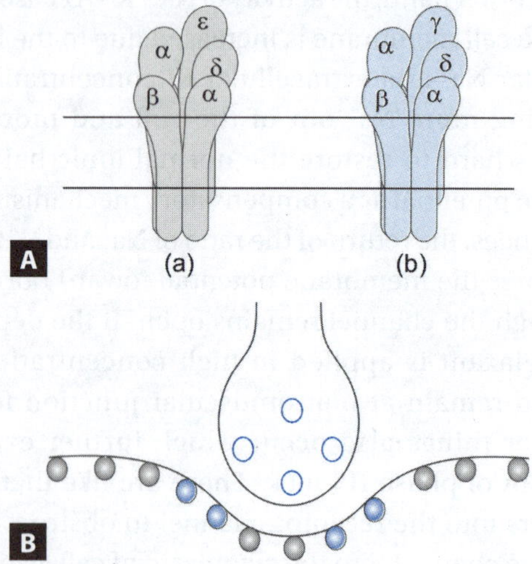

Figs. 20A and B: (A) Junctional (a) and extrajunctional (b) ACh-receptors. Junctional receptors contain ε-subunits and extrajunctional receptors contain γ-subunits; (B) Neuromuscular junction with deficient activity. Muscle membrane contains extrajunctional receptors (ash coloured circle). Endplate contains both junctional (blue circle) and extrajunctional (ash coloured circle) receptors.

such as electrical signal coming to the muscle (innervation), growth factor, etc., also determine which type of receptor will be formed on the endplate of muscle fiber in every individual **(Figs. 20A and B)**.

The difference in the structure of these two types of receptors (junctional and extrajunctional) cause significant qualitative variations in the response, among the individual patient, to muscle relaxants and also seem to be responsible for some of the abnormal results to muscle relaxants. At molecular level, these two types of nicotinic receptor differ at ε-subunit of junctional receptor which is replaced by γ-subunit in extrajunctional receptor. This difference is of great enough to affect the physiology and the pharmacology of nicotinic receptor and ion channel within it. *Although the*

names of the receptors are junctional and extrajunctional, which imply that each is located in the junctional and extrajunctional area respectively, but this is not strictly correct. Because junctional receptors are always confined to the motor endplate of the muscle membrane. But, the immature or extrajunctional receptor may be expressed anywhere in the muscle membrane including motor endplate. When the muscle cells lose its nerve connection due to avulsion, stroke, burn, or before innervation (fetal life), it produces extrajunctional or immature or fetal form of nicotinic receptor in place of normal or junctional receptor.

In fetus, before innervation, muscle cells only synthesize the extrajunctional receptors throughout the whole muscle membrane, including the motor endplate. Then, as the fetus develops, muscle become innervated and begins to manufacture junctional receptor at the motor endplate and over the whole muscle. In this stage, at the endplate, there is a mixture of both the junctional and extrajunctional receptor. In a child of about 2 years old, before nerve muscle units are matured, both the types of receptors are found. Then, as the child grows and nerve muscle unit matures, extrajunctional receptor diminishes in concentration and disappear, both from the periphery of the muscle and the endplate. The process of making and removing the extrajunctional receptor is very fast. They appear within an hour after the diminution of neuromuscular activity and are removed within half-life of 18 hours when the activity returns to normal.

Although ACh does not bind with the γ- or ε-subunit of receptor, still these subunits influence the ways in which these two kinds of receptors respond to the drug. The extrajunctional receptors are activated by the lower concentration of agonist (succinylcholine) than are junctional receptor. So, the extrajunctional receptors are more sensitive to depolarizing agents. In contrast, the extrajunctional receptors are less sensitive than junctional receptor to the nondepolarizing drugs. In some circumstances, the nondepolarizing muscle relaxants act as a partial agonist and muscle contracts.

As extrajunctional receptors develop within few hours of stoppage of muscle activity, so due to denervation or paralysis, patient becomes resistant to nondepolarizing agents and then it is become more difficult to block them than usual. So, the patient with deficient neural activity, demand more than usual dose of nondepolarizing agent. On the other hand, as the extrajunctional receptor is sensitive to depolarizing agent, so less amount of agonist such as succinylcholine is needed. Patient's receptor mixture and sensitivity to relaxants can began to change within a day after a nerve injury or hospitalization. Well-built heavy muscular person who exercises vigorously are resistant to nondepolarizing agent. This is because their nerve secret more ACh than normal and so transmission is more vigorous and hardened to block.

Patient with muscular paralysis, due to denervation, are more prone to succinylcholine induced hyperkalemia. This is because in these patients, the extrajunctional receptors predominate over the muscle cell membrane which are sensitive to depolarizing agent. So, they remain open for long time by the agonist succinylcholine and allow the more K^+ to escape from muscle and enter the blood.

In infant and children, the neuromuscular junctions are not mature. So, there are mixtures of junctional and extrajunctional receptor at the motor endplate. Their ratio varies with chronological age (with increasing age extrajunctional receptors disappear), muscular activity, health, vigor of child, and from the one group of muscle to another. Since, the junctional and extrajunctional receptor differ in their sensitivity to depolarizing and nondepolarizing agent, so, the amount of relaxant needed to produce muscle paralysis differs from one child to another, but in poorly predictable ways. Muscular paralysis produced by succinylcholine is not due to the continuous depolarization of whole muscle. But it is due to the inactivated Na^+ channel ring at perijunctional zone due to the continuous depolarization of endplate which insulate the depolarized motor endplate from the rest of muscle. Therefore, in infant and children, as the insulating Na^+ channel ring is not developed properly, so the effect of depolarizing relaxant may not be the same as that of an adult.

■ ANTAGONISM OF NEUROMUSCULAR BLOCK

The competitive neuromuscular block, caused by the action of (antagonist) nondepolarizing muscle relaxants on the nicotinic receptor is overcome by increasing the concentration of competitor, i.e., ACh (agonist). Increasing the number of molecules of ACh in the synaptic junctional cleft changes the agonist: antagonist ratio and increases the probability of agonist molecules, such as ACh, to bind with the unoccupied recognition (binding) site of it (ACh) on its nicotinic receptor. Normally, only about 500,000 out of 5 million available receptors are activated by a single nerve impulse. So, a large number of receptors remain in reserve and could be occupied by a competitor agonist (ACh). *Actually, ACh cannot displace the already bound molecule of nondepolarizing agent (antagonist) from its nicotinic receptor and has to wait for the antagonist (nondepolarizing muscle relaxant) to dissociate spontaneously from the receptor, before it (ACh) can compete with the antagonist (nondepolarizing agent) for its attachment at the site where the antagonist was attached. So, the length of time, for which the nondepolarizing agents present in the synaptic cleft, is also important.* The nondepolarizing muscle relaxing agents bind to the nicotinic receptor for longer period than the life span of ACh. It indicates that most of the ACh is destroyed before any significant number of antagonist molecules have dissociated. So, prolonging the time for which ACh remain in synaptic junction, allows the time for dissociation of antagonist from receptor and the receptor to be freed and made available for the attachment of ACh.

The neuromuscular block can be antagonized by two classes of drugs such as: *(i) K^+ blocking agents and (ii) acetylcholinesterase inhibitors.* The K^+ blocking agent, such as 4-aminopyridine, acts on the prejunctional area. So, by impeding the efflux of K^+, it also prolongs the action potential of nerve ending. So, the duration of depolarization of nerve endings is prolonged. Thus, the indirectly prolonged action potential of nerve endings, caused by K^+ blocking agents, increases the influx of Ca^{2+} into the nerve ending. Therefore, the nerve releases more ACh and for a longer time than usual, causing antagonism of neuromuscular blockade, produced by nondepolarizing agents. As the K^+ blocking agent acts only on prejunctional area, so it also antagonizes the blockade, produced by some antibiotics that act on prejunctional nerve endings, such as polymyxin B. So, 4-aminopyridine and this class of drugs are used very restrictedly to antagonize some specific neuromuscular block. However, these drugs are not specific and act on all the nerve endings, including the motor nerves, autonomic nerves, central nervous system (CNS), etc., and are so associated with many side effects. So, this group of drugs is not used routinely to antagonize the neuromuscular block produced by nondepolarizing muscle relaxing agents.

Acetylcholine is inhibited or hydrolyzed by an enzyme, called true acetylcholinesterase (which is also commonly called as cholinesterase or ChE). It is only present in synaptic cleft, but not in plasma (pseudocholinesterase is present in plasma). So, the acetylcholinesterase inhibitors (also called as anti-ChE), such as, the neostigmine, pyridostigmine, edrophonium, etc., (all carbamates and organophosphorus compounds), increase the level of ACh in the synaptic cleft and improve the neuromuscular transmissions by inhibiting the true acetylcholinesterase enzyme (by inhibiting the hydrolysis of ACh).

Anticholinesterases or acetylcholinesterase inhibitors (commonly called as cholinesterase inhibitors or ChEIs) are esters of carbamic acid. So, they are also called as the carbamates. Acetylcholine is inactivated after its combination with the enzyme, acetylcholinesterase, at its (ChE) two sites—(i) an anionic site, bearing a negative charge which attracts the quaternary nitrogen atom (N^+) of ACh molecule and (ii) an esteratic site which attracts the carboxyl group (–COOH) of ACh molecule. As a result of the union of ACh molecule with both the sites of ChE enzyme, the esteratic site of ChE enzyme is acetylated by the acetyl radical of ACh molecule and this results in the splitting of this ACh molecule. Then, the acetyl group from the esteratic site of ChE enzyme is immediately removed (in a fraction of a second) as a result of the combination of acetyl group with water, forming acetic acid. Thus, this sets the esteratic site of ChE enzyme free. Now, the anionic site of ChE is also freed of quaternary nitrogen atom (N^+) of ACh molecule spontaneously. *Therefore, the subsequent events of the attachment of one ACh molecule with both the anionic and esteratic sites of ChE molecule are like that—attachment of ACh molecule with ChE enzyme molecule → acetylation of esteratic site of ChE enzyme → formation of acetic acid → free of esteratic site of ChE → free of anionic site of ChE from quaternary N^+ atom → free of whole ChE molecule for further inactivation of another ACh molecule.*

The molecules of anti-ChE or ChEIs such as neostigmine, pyridostigmine, etc., attach with the ChE enzyme molecule in the same way as that of ACh molecule. Hence, the ACh molecule cannot be attached with the ChE enzyme molecule and is not destroyed, sparing the ACh molecule and increasing its concentration into synaptic cleft.

Anticholinesterase or cholinesterase inhibitors (anti-ChEs or ChEIs) are usually of two types—reversible and irreversible. Once irreversible anti-ChE combines with the molecules of ChE enzyme, then this binding is not reversed, until the whole complex of ChE and anti-ChE molecule is metabolized. The examples of these irreversible anti-ChEs are organophosphorus compounds.

Reversible anti-ChE are also capable of combining with the anionic and esteratic sites of ChE enzyme molecule like ACh, but does not form fixed ChE and anti-ChE complex like irreversible anti-ChE. So, they are called as the reversible anti-ChE. The complex which anti-ChE form with the esteratic site of ChE enzyme is hydrolyzed, but much less readily **(Fig. 21)** (after many minutes) than the acetyl-esteratic site complex formed with ACh. Thus, this produces a temporary inhibition of true ChE enzyme and prevents the breakdown of ACh and increases its concentration into synaptic cleft. Like ACh, both the reversible and irreversible anti-ChEs also can directly act on ACh-receptor and may produce muscle relaxation like depolarizing agents, but it needs very higher doses. In contrast to other reversible anti-ChE, edrophonium forms reversible complex only with the anionic site of ChE enzyme and hence has a shorter duration of action.

Organophosphorous compound (irreversible anti-ChE) combines only with the esteratic site of ChE enzyme and consequently the esteratic site is phosphorylated. Then the hydrolysis of this phosphorylated esteratic site of ChE

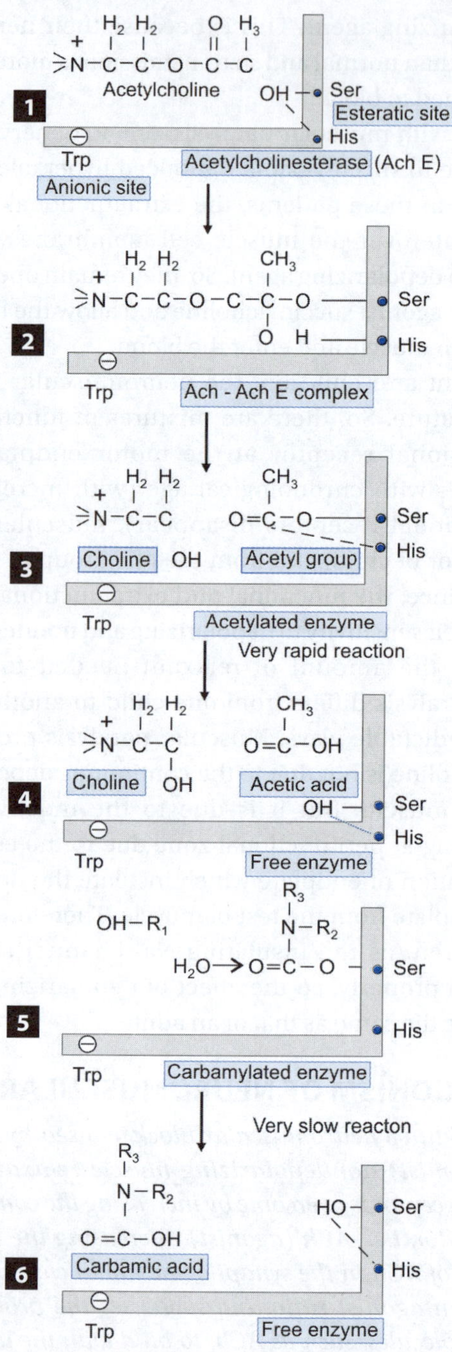

Fig. 21: Breakdown of ACh (1–4) and mechanism of action of carbamate anticholinesterase (3 and 4). (His: histidine; Ser: serine; Trp: tryptophan)

enzyme is extremely slow and in certain cases does not occur at all. This produces an almost irreversible permanent inhibition or destruction of ChE enzyme. So, they are called as the irreversible anti-ChEs or ChEIs. Echothiophate (irreversible anti-ChE) forms complexes with both the anionic and esteratic site of ChE enzyme and hence is much more potent than other organophosphorus compounds. Thus, organophosphorus compounds, permanently inhibiting the ChE enzyme, gradually raises the body ACh level which causes prolonged depolarization of motor endplate → skeletal muscle paralysis → respiratory arrest → cardiac arrest and death.

Edrophonium (a reversible anti-ChE) is neither an ester, nor a carbamate compound. It is attracted and only bound to the anionic site of ChE enzyme molecule by an electrostatic attraction between the positively charged nitrogen atom in the drug (edrophonium) and the negatively charged anionic site of enzyme. Without any hydrolysis of edrophonium molecule, it is removed from the enzyme molecule, as an intact form and excreted through kidney. Other than the inhibition of ChE enzyme, edrophonium also enhances the release of ACh from prejunctional site (membrane) and so helps in the reversal from deep neuromuscular block. The blocking (inhibition) action of ChE enzyme by edrophonium is very short lived and departs the enzyme from edrophonium-enzyme complex in a very short time. So, for decades edrophonium was considered to have the shortest duration of action and to be useful in anesthesia. But, now it is understood that the duration of action of any anti-ChE is not determined by the duration of molecular reaction with the ChE enzyme, but by the existence of drug (ChEI or anti-ChE) in our body which depends on renal clearance. One edrophonium molecule attaches with enzyme (cholinesterase) for short time, but as the one molecule departs from the enzyme molecule, it is immediately replaced by another edrophonium molecule, so that the ChE enzyme remains inhibited for as long as the drug edrophonium is in the body. The elimination of edrophonium from our body is same as that of neostigmine and pyridostigmine. So, the duration of acetylcholinesterase-inhibition and blockade reversal is same for all the three drugs.

However, as the patient has normal true choline esterase enzyme level in synaptic cleft, so the pharmacokinetic properties of anti-ChE agents are the principle determinant factor of the reversal of neuromuscular blockade (paralysis), caused by the nondepolarizing muscle relaxing agents. The activity of serum or plasma ChE or the lack of it plays a minor role in the recovery of nondepolarizing agent by anti-ChE. Of the three commonly used anti-ChE, edrophonium shows by far the greatest selectivity between the true acetylcholinesterase and butyryl or plasma cholinesterase.

Butyrylcholinesterase is the serum esterase that hydrolyzes only the succinylcholine and mivacurium, but not ACh. Edrophonium greatly favors the true ChE enzyme and the most desirable agent to reverse mivacurium. If the patient has atypical pseudocholinesterase that does not destroy mivacurium, the inhibition of true ChE by neostigmine has no result, till mivacurium will be present in our body. Mivacurium, like succinylcholine, is metabolized by pseudocholinesterase. It is only minimally metabolized by true cholinesterase. This introduces the possibility of prolonged action in patients with low pseudocholinesterase levels or variants of the *pseudocholinesterase* gene. In fact, patients who are heterozygous for the atypical gene will experience a block approximately twice the normal duration. Whereas atypical homozygous patients will remain paralyzed for several hours. As atypical homozygotes cannot metabolize mivacurium, the neuromuscular blockade may last for 3–4 hours. In contrast to succinylcholine-induced paralysis, in these patient's pharmacological antagonism with ChEIs will quicken reversal of mivacurium blockade once some response to nerve stimulation becomes apparent. Edrophonium more effectively reverses mivacurium blockade than neostigmine because it inhibits true ChE activity only. Again, there is no reason to choose one anti-ChE over another.

Neostigmine, pyridostigmine, and edrophonium do not cross the blood-brain barrier as they are the quaternary ammonium compound. So, they have less CNS effects. Similarly, quaternary ammonium derivative of atropine such as glycopyrrolate also cannot cross the blood-brain barrier. So, frequently glycopyrrolate is used to limit the cholinergic effects of anti-ChE agents on the periphery. Atropine cross blood-brain barrier and may cause CNS problems.

Anticholinesterases are not only selective for the neuromuscular junction, producing the nicotinic action of ACh which causes removal of neuromuscular blockade. But it also acts on ChE in other sites of the body producing muscarinic action of ACh. So, atropine- or glycopyrrolate-like drug is used to counter the muscarinic effects of ACh that accumulates in the synapses of gut, bronchi, salivary gland, and CVS, etc. Anticholinesterase such as physostigmine and tacrine are not quaternary ammonium compound. So, they cross blood-brain barrier and have profound CNS effect. Anticholinesterase such as physostigmine and tacrine also inhibit phosphodiesterase enzyme in addition to ChE enzyme which plays important role in transmitter release at many synapses in CNS. This action is used in the treatment of Alzheimer's dementia.

Many anti-ChE agents have methyl group on its positively charged nitrogen atom. So, it also acts as agonist like ACh on the nicotinic receptor channel, initiating ion flow and enhancing neuromuscular transmission. Mixing of different anti-ChEs (neostigmine, edrophonium, etc.) is not advisable. Because they do not potentiate each other. Therefore, when additional doses of anti-ChE are needed for treatment of incomplete reversal, then it is better to continue the original drug.

ANTICHOLINESTERASES OR CHOLINESTERASE INHIBITORS

Though the matter under this heading has already been discussed under the previous heading, still it lacks some points which are elaborated here. The anti-ChEs or ChEIs are the agents which inhibit the ChE enzymes from destroying the ACh and thus they protect it and promote neuromuscular transmission. Except for increasing the concentration of ACh at motor endplate level, the anti-ChEs have additional direct and indirect action (by increasing the concentration of ACh) on cholinergic nicotinic and muscarinic receptors situated at other places in our body. So, the actions of anti-ChEs are qualitatively similar to that of ACh and other directly acting choline receptor agonists. Hence, the action of anti-ChEs, which is mediated by the action of increased concentration of ACh, are divided into two groups, like the action of ACh and these are the *muscarinic action and nicotinic actions*. However, the relative intensities of action of anti-ChEs, mediated by ACh, on muscarinic receptors [present on the smooth muscles, gastrointestinal tract (GI) tract, respiratory tract, urinary system, exocrine glands, etc.] and nicotinic receptors (present on autonomic ganglia, skeletal muscles, CNS, etc.) vary among the different agents.

Classification of Anticholinesterases

Anticholinesterases are primarily grouped into two groups such as reversible and irreversible anticholinesterase:

- *Reversible anticholinesterases:*

Carbamates	Acridine
• Neostigmine	• Tacrine
• Pyridostigmine	
• Physostigmine	
• Edrophonium	
• Rivastigmine	
• Donepezil	
• Galantamine	

- *Irreversible anticholinesterases:*

Carbamates	Organophosphates
• Carbaryl (Sevin)	• Parathion
• Propoxur (Baygon)	• Dyflos (DFP)
	• Malathion
	• Diazinon (TIK-20)
	• Echothiophate
	• Tabun
	• Sarin
	• Soman

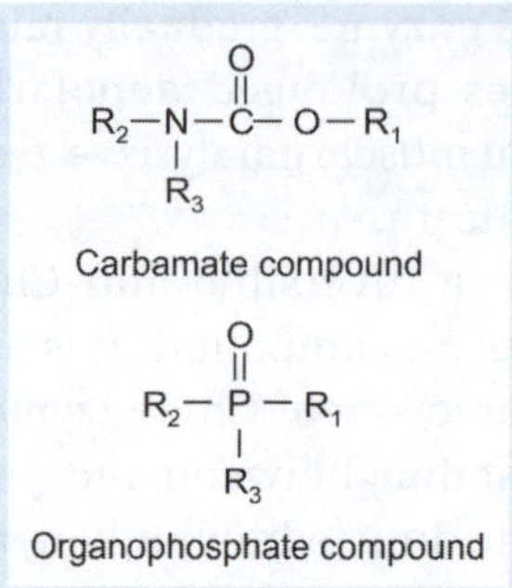

Fig. 22: Basic structure of anticholinesterase.

Chemistry of Anticholinesterases

All anti-ChEs are either esters of carbamic acid (carbamates) or derivatives of phosphoric acid (organophosphates). **(Fig. 22)**.

All organophosphates are highly lipid-soluble, except echothiophate which is water soluble. Among the carbamates, in physostigmine the R_1 may have a nonpolar *tertiary* amino N atom and render the compound lipid-soluble. Whereas, in other carbamates (e.g., neostigmine) the R1 has a *quaternary* N^+ ion and render them lipid-insoluble.

Mechanism of Action of Anticholinesterases

The main mechanism of action of anti-ChEs are the inhibition of ChE enzyme which destroy the ACh by hydrolysis. This results in an increased concentration of ACh at synaptic cleft and thereby increases in the likelihood of ACh, occupying the unblocked nicotinic receptors at motor endplate and improved the neuromuscular transmission. The reaction between the anti-ChE compound and ChE enzyme differs from the reaction between ACh and ChE enzyme in that in previous reaction the complex molecules (formed by the anti-ChE and ChE) have a longer dissociation half-life and is about 7 minutes, as the anti-ChE and ChE complex molecules are hydrolyzed at very slow rate. Whereas the ACh and ChE complex molecule breaks down by hydrolysis within a fraction of second and ChE enzyme is freed immediately for further action (hydrolysis) on other ACh molecules. Thus, it (ChE) quickly breaks all the ACh molecules. In the reversible group of anti-ChE compounds, the ChE enzyme is freed after a long time, during which period the level of ACh is increased sufficiently to produce muscular contraction. Then, the free ChE enzyme again hydrolyzes the ACh molecules like normal circumstances. In the irreversible group of anti-ChE compounds, the complex formed by the anti-ChE and ChE enzyme is permanent and ChE enzyme is not freed by hydrolysis (so they are called as irreversible anti-ChE). So, the ChE enzyme does not become free and gradually excessive ACh accumulates and death occurs due to high concentration of ACh at synapses by the irreversible group of anti-ChE compounds.

For the attachment and destruction of ACh, the active region of ChE enzyme (acetylcholinesterase enzyme) makes a groove that contains an aromatic anionic site near its tryptophan molecule at 86 positions and an ester site near its serine and histidine molecule at 203 and 447 positions, respectively. First the quaternary nitrogen atom (N^+) of ACh is attached with the negatively charged anionic site of ChE enzyme and then the carboxyl group ($-COOCH_3$) of ACh is attached with the ester site of ChE enzyme. As soon as the carboxyl group of ACh molecule is attached with the ChE enzyme molecule at its ester site, then the choline part is splitted out from the ACh molecule, forming an acetylated ChE enzyme complex only. Then, this acetylated ChE enzyme complex reacts with a water molecule extremely rapidly and the ester site of ChE is freed, in a fraction of millisecond, forming acetic acid, and free ChE enzyme (cholinesterase is here known as acetylcholinesterase). Thus, at the end of reaction, we get choline, acetic acid, and a free ChE enzyme molecule for further action on ACh molecule.

Neostigmine and pyridostigmine (carbamate compounds) combine with both the anionic and esteratic sites of ChE enzyme, in almost the same way, as ACh reacts with ChE enzyme, but with a longer dissociation half-life of about 7 minutes. The carbamate and ChE complex (carbamylated ChE enzyme) undergo hydrolysis like ACh + ChE enzyme complex molecule, so it (carbamate) is *reversible,* but this hydrolysis occurs very slowly. Whereas, the organo-phosphate and ChE enzyme complex (phosphorylated ChE enzyme) molecules does not undergo hydrolysis at all, (so, the organophosphates are called as *irreversible anti-ChE*). *It is noteworthy that edrophonium (carbamate) in difference with neostigmine (another carbamate) attaches only to the anionic site of ChE enzyme, while organophosphates attach only to the ester site of ChE enzyme. Dissociation of edrophonium from ChE enzyme (the reactivation of inhibited enzyme) does not involve hydrolysis of edrophonium, but involve only its detachment from the ChE enzyme. The dissociation of edrophonium from the enzyme occurs more readily with much shorter dissociation half-life of about 20 seconds.*

Anticholinesterase agents such as neostigmine, pyridostigmine, and edrophonium, may also have a direct stimulating effect on the nicotinic receptor, facilitating neuromuscular transmission. Another action of these agents is at the presynaptic level, involving the direct enhanced liberation of ACh. This effect is particularly marked with edrophonium which is thought to act mostly by increasing the liberation of ACh, rather than by the inhibition of acetylcholinesterase enzyme.

If anti-ChE agents are administered in large doses or in the absence of muscle relaxants, then they produce fasciculation and even a depolarizing type of block (neuromuscular paralysis), similar to that produced by succinylcholine. However, this is unlikely to occur if a nondepolarizing muscle relaxant is used, even if almost complete recovery appears to have occurred. The likely explanation of it is that a large proportion of nicotinic receptors are still occupied by the muscle relaxant.

After treatment with anti-ChEs, the ACh accumulated and released by a single nerve impulse, is not immediately destroyed, but rebinds to the same receptor, diffuses to act on neighboring receptors and activates the prejunctional fibers causing repetitive firing, twitching, and fasciculation. The force of contraction in particularly curarized and myasthenic muscles is increased. Higher doses of anti-ChE cause persistent depolarization of endplates, due to high level of ACh at that site, result in blockade of neuromuscular transmission with further weakness and paralysis.

Pharmacokinetics of Anticholinesterases

Neostigmine and its congeners (except physostigmine) are poorly absorbed orally, as they are water soluble (lipid-insoluble). So, the oral doses of them is 20–30 times higher than their parenteral dose. They do not penetrate the blood-brain barrier. They are partially hydrolyzed and partially excreted unchanged through urine. Elderly patients show reduced rate of clearance of all these three agents with prolongation of their half-life. The dose-response curves of these three anti-ChE agents show that pyridostigmine is five times and edrophonium is 10 times less potent than neostigmine. It has also been shown that the dose-response curves of neostigmine and edrophonium are not parallel which indicates that edrophonium has a different mode of action. The elderly requires a larger dose of neostigmine to attain the same rate of recovery, while the dose should be reduced in children.

Doses of Anticholinesterases

The commonly recommended dose for neostigmine is 0.3–0.5 mg/kg (30–50 µg/kg), for pyridostigmine is 0.2–0.25 mg/kg, and for edrophonium is 0.5–1 mg/kg. Among these three anti-ChE agents, edrophonium is the most rapid-acting agent, with peak effect between 2 and 4 minutes, after its administration. While the peak effect of neostigmine is 10 minutes and pyridostigmine is 15 minutes, after their administration. Pyridostigmine is, therefore, too slow in the onset of action for routine use. On the other hand, although the edrophonium is faster acting, but it is not always effective in antagonizing a relatively deep neuromuscular block.

It is also true that higher doses of anti-ChE is sometimes required to antagonize the higher depth of the block, more rapidly and more completely, than their smaller doses. But, this is true up to a limit. Beyond which, the increase in the dose of anti-ChE does not produce any greater antagonism. Thus, the maximum dose of neostigmine and pyridostigmine is 60–80 µg/kg and 1–15 mg/kg, respectively.

Other Effects of Anticholinesterases

It is previously stated that the actions of anti-ChEs are qualitatively similar to that of directly acting choline receptor agonists (cholinergic agents), i.e., Ach, and therefore, these actions of anti-ChEs are classified as muscarinic, nicotinic, and CNS effects. The muscarinic actions of anti-ChEs are consisting of the actions on heart, mucous membrane, blood vessels, smooth muscles, exocrine glands, and eyes. On the other hand, the nicotinic actions of anti-ChEs are consisting of the actions on autonomic ganglia and skeletal muscles. The effects of neostigmine (also other anti-ChEs) on the cardiovascular system are variable and depend upon the prevailing autonomic tone. As a general rule, the anti-ChE agents cause bradycardia, leading to a fall in cardiac output. They decrease the effective refractory period of cardiac muscles and decrease the conduction time in conducting tissues of heart. In higher doses, the neostigmine may cause hypotension, secondary to its central effect. Actually, the cardiovascular effects of neostigmine are complex. This is because the muscarinic actions of it would produce bradycardia and hypotension, while the ganglion-stimulating nicotinic effect of neostigmine would tend to increase the heart rate and blood pressure (BP). The action of neostigmine on medullary centers further complicates the picture, as the ganglion-blocking effect of it with high doses. Thus, the overall effects of anti-ChEs are often unpredictable and depend on the agent and its dose.

Neostigmine increases bronchial secretion and may cause bronchoconstriction. This drug also increases salivation, decreases esophageal and gastric tone, increases gastric acid output, and increases gastrointestinal tract motility. So, nausea and vomiting may occur.

In therapeutic doses, the anti-ChE agents have action on skeletal muscles, leading to muscular contraction. But, in higher doses, neostigmine may block the neuro-muscular transmission by the combination of its direct effect on nicotinic receptor and by allowing the excessive accumulation of ACh.

Lipid-soluble anti-ChE agents, such as physostigmine and organophosphates, have more marked muscarinic and CNS effects. They also stimulate ganglia, but their action on skeletal muscles is less prominent. Whereas the lipid-insoluble agents such as neostigmine and other quaternary ammonium compounds have more nicotinic effects, producing more marked action on the skeletal muscles (direct action on muscle endplate choline receptors as well) and autonomic ganglia, with less muscarinic effects. They do not penetrate CNS and have no central effects.

In ganglion, the local hydrolysis of ACh is less important. But, the inactivation of ACh in ganglia occurs partly by diffusion and partly by hydrolysis in plasma. The anti-ChEs stimulate the ganglia primarily through nicotinic receptors, present there. High doses of anti-ChEs cause the persistent depolarization of ganglionic nicotinic receptors and blockade of transmission in ganglion.

The muscarinic actions of anti-ChE agents result in bradycardia, hypotension, increased mucous secretions, and increased smooth muscle contractions. These effects (muscarinic actions of anti-ChEs) can be prevented by the simultaneous or prior administration of antimuscarinic (anticholinergic) agents such as atropine (20–30 µg/kg or 0.02–0.03 mg/kg) or glycopyrrolate (10 µg/kg or 0.01 mg/kg). These anticholinergic agents only have antimuscarinic actions (so-called antimuscarinic agents) without any antinicotinic actions. Nicotinic antagonists are generally referred to as "ganglion blockers" and "neuromuscular blockers."

Atropine and glycopyrrolate are highly selective for muscarinic receptors. But, some of its synthetic substitutes do possess significant nicotinic-blocking properties, in addition to their antimuscarinic property. Atropine and glycopyrrolate only block the Ach-induced muscarinic actions, but not the actions evoked by histamine and 5-hydroxytryptamine (5-HT). The use of glycopyrrolate is associated with greater stability of heart rate when neostigmine is used. But, atropine is the preferred agent with edrophonium, because of their similar speed of onset of action. Edrophonium requires a lower dose of anticholinergic agent, as its muscarinic effects are less. Glycopyrrolate has distinct advantages over atropine, as it does not cross the blood-brain barrier.

Neostigmine and pyridostigmine, but not edrophonium, cause the prolongation of the effect of subsequently administered succinylcholine and mivacurium, by inhibiting plasma ChE activity. Administration of neostigmine also may be associated with increased incidences of postoperative nausea and vomiting (PONV).

Acid–Base Balance

■ INTRODUCTION

In our body, the amount of H^+ cation is very small in comparison to other common physiologically important cations and anions such as Na^+, K^+, HCO^-, Cl^-, etc. In normal plasma, their concentration is respectively near about 140, 4, 24, and 100 mmol/L (mEq/L), whereas the H^+ concentration in normal plasma is only 0.00004 (or 4×10^{-6}) mmol/L or 0.00000004 (or 4×10^{-9}) mol/L. So, this small numerical number of H^+ ion concentration is commonly expressed either as pH (negative logarithm of H^+ ion concentration) or as nmol/L. *The concentration of H^+ ion in normal arterial blood is 40 nmol/L (nEq/L) or pH is 7.4 which is considerably an easier expression to write than 0.00004 mmol/L or 0.00000004 mol/L.*

Life is an acid-producing process because for the continuation of life, during the production of energy by the catabolism of glucose, fatty acids, amino acids, etc., different acids are produced continuously, for example, during the metabolism of glucose, amino acids, and fatty acids through the citric acid cycle, CO_2, and water are produced. This again form carbonic acid ($CO_2 + H_2O \rightleftharpoons H_2CO_3$ $H_2CO_3 = H^+ + HCO_3^-$) giving H^+ ion in plasma. At the pulmonary alveolar level, this H_2CO_3 is then broken down and CO_2 is excreted through lungs. Thus, lung is the main channel for the excretion of *carbonic or nonmetabolic acids*. During the metabolism of amino acids through other cycles, different *noncarbonic or metabolic acids* such as H_2SO_4 and H_3PO_4 are also produced. These also produce H^+ ion and these H^+ ions, produced from metabolic acids, are mainly excreted through kidneys.

Diet also contains large amount of H^+ ion, normally in the form of sulfur containing amino acids in protein. Urine is the main channel for the excretion of these noncarbonic or metabolic acids, whereas lung is the main channel for the excretion of nonmetabolic or carbonic acid, such as CO_2. In a normal **(Table 1)** adult, the average daily oral H^+ intake is 50–80 mmol/day (the normal blood concentration of

H^+ ion is 0.00004 mmol/L. So, the body has to handle a huge burden of H^+ ions which are taken as food and are produced by metabolism).

In a resting subject, the catabolism of carbohydrates and fats produces an acid load (volatile acids $\rightarrow$ H_2CO_3) approximately of 18,000–20,000 mmol/day, which is excreted by the lungs as CO_2. Protein catabolism also leads to additional production of 60–80 mmol/day of nonvolatile acids, mostly in the form of sulfuric and phosphoric acids, which are excreted by the kidney. Again, the oxidation of carbohydrates and fats in a diseased state or in an anaerobic metabolic state leads to the production of more nonvolatile acids such as lactic acid (in anaerobic metabolism) and keto acids (in diabetes mellitus) **(Table 2)**.

During intracellular metabolism, various acids, produced from the catabolism of different substrates, flow into alkaline extracellular fluid and thus maintains a normal intracellular H^+ ion concentration. Then, this H^+ ion is excreted through urine as a titrable acid or through lungs as CO_2. Hence, our body constantly balances this H^+ input by an efficient process of H^+ output, but when this balance of H^+ ion is not maintained, then small changes in this normal H^+ concentration (pH) can produce significant alteration in the body enzymatic activity. This presents clinically, then, as organ dysfunction. As the metabolic processes lead to a change in H^+ concentration, similarly

TABLE 1: Daily normal input and output of acids.

	Input (mmol/day)	Output (mmol/day)
• *Nonvolatile acids*	By metabolism	*By liver and kidney*
– Lactate	1,500	1,500
– Protein	50–80	30
– Phospholipid	30	40
– Other	12	
• *Volatile acids*	By metabolism	By lungs
– Carbon dioxide	13,000	13,000

TABLE 2: The mechanism by which the primary acid–base changes are compensated. If the pH of blood has been fully returned to normal, then the primary change is said to be fully compensated. Otherwise, it is said to be partially compensated.

Type of acidosis or alkalosis	Compensating organ	Mechanism of compensation
Respiratory acidosis	Kidney	Metabolic alkalosis with a further rise in plasma [HCO_3^-] by increasing its absorption through kidney or with further fall in plasma [H^+] by increasing its (H^+) excretion through kidney
Respiratory alkalosis	Kidney	Metabolic acidosis with a further fall in plasma [HCO^-] by increasing its excretion through kidney or with a further rise in plasma [H^+] by decreasing its excretion through kidney
Metabolic acidosis	Lungs	Respiratory alkalosis with a further fall in plasma [H^+] by eliminating more CO_2 through lungs
Metabolic alkalosis	Lungs	Respiratory acidosis with a further rise in plasma [H^+] by decreasing the excretion of CO_2 through lungs

the changes in H^+ concentration (or acid–base balance) lead to alteration of metabolic processes. Also, these changes in H^+ ion concentration are an indicator of current status of metabolic processes, occurring in human body and a real-time predictor of the utility of critical therapy. So, a complete understanding of acid–base balance is very important, but unfortunately, most anesthetists avoid this chapter. This is because pH is defined complicatedly as a negative logarithm (–log) of H^+ ion concentration and there is widespread of use of multiple, complex, overlapping, irrelevant terms such as "standard bicarbonate", "negative base excess (BE)", and "alkali reserve" to describe this acid–base status.

Various buffer systems in cells and in extracellular fluid work against this excessive accumulation of H^+ ion or against any disruption of the balance between the amount of intake and output of H^+ ions. The buffer capacity capable of absorbing this accumulating H^+ ion is up to 10 mmol/kg of body weight, i.e., 500–700 mmol in an adult per day. Tissue hypoxia, starvation, diminished ventilation, diabetes, heart failure, renal failure, etc., which cause increased input of H^+ in body, cause strain to this buffer capacity of our body. Therefore, it is important that all this should be brought under control before any surgery as far as possible, with least possible encroachment on buffer capacity. This is because to deal in future with acute rises of H^+ concentration, due to any cause, during surgery by buffer system.

The normal arterial H^+ concentration is 40 nmol/L, yielding pH of 7.4. This arterial H^+ concentration reflects the present dynamic balance between the input (from ingestion and metabolism of food) and the output (through lungs as CO_2 and through kidney as nonvolatile acids) of it (H^+ ion). Thus, when an imbalance between this normal input and output of H^+ ion occurs, then the H^+ concentration in blood will deviate from the normal to its range of viable variability, roughly 160–20 nmol/L (pH 6.8–7.7) beyond which life is not possible.

Two types of acids are produced during the metabolism of substrates in our body:

1. *Volatile or carbonic or respiratory acids:* This is carbonic acid (H_2CO_3) which is formed by the hydration of CO_2 by the following equation like that $CO_2 + H_2O \leftrightarrow H_2CO_3 \rightleftharpoons H^+ + HCO_3^-$. This CO_2 is produced by the metabolism of glucose, fatty acids, and amino acids through a tricarboxylic acid cycle (TCA) cycle in mitochondria. CO_2 is produced at an average rate of about 200 mL/min or 288 L/day. This gas is eliminated via lungs and, so, is referred to as the "volatile" or "respiratory" acid.

2. *Nonvolatile or noncarbonic or metabolic acids:* These are lactic acid, pyruvic acid, acetoacetic acid, β-hydroxybutyric acid, phosphoric acid, sulfuric acid, hydrochloric acid, keto acids, and a variety of other organic acids. The lactic acid is produced from pyruvic acid during glycolysis in the absence of O_2. So, lactic acid is often used as a clinical marker of anaerobic metabolism from hypoxia, poor perfusion of tissues, or other disturbances of tissue oxygenation. Also, it is important to realize that in our body about 1,400 mmol of lactic acid is normally produced each day, principally by skeletal muscles, red blood cells (RBCs), and skin. This lactic acid is, then, converted into liver to form CO_2 and H_2O. A smaller amount of lactate is also cleared through renal excretion or by conversion through gluconeogenesis in liver.

Keto acids are produced in diabetes mellitus from the metabolism of glucose and fatty acids. Phosphoric, hydrochloric, and sulfuric acids are produced during the metabolism of amino acids. Hydrochloric acid (HCl) is produced during the metabolism of lysine, arginine, and histidine amino acids. Sulfuric acid (H_2SO_4) is the product of cysteine and methionine amino acid metabolism. Phosphoric acid (H_3PO_4) is derived from the normal metabolism of dietary phosphate (**Table 3 and Fig. 1**).

TABLE 3: Sets of pH–PCO₂ acid–base data forming CO₂ titration curve.

SL	PaCO₂ (mm Hg)	pH	Metabolic status	Respiratory status	Overall status
N	40	7.4	Normal	Normal	Normal
M	70	7.1	Acidosis	Acidosis	Acidemia
O	70	7.4	Alkalosis	Acidosis	Normal (compensated)
P	30	7.3	Acidosis	Alkalosis	Acidemia (uncompensated)
Q	30	7.6	Alkalosis	Alkalosis	Alkalemia

(PaCO₂: partial pressure of arterial carbon dioxide; PCO₂: partial pressure of carbon dioxide; CO₂: carbon dioxide)

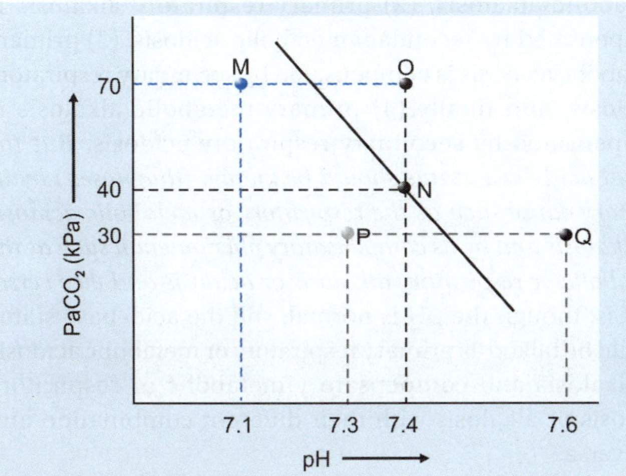

Fig. 1: CO₂ titration curve formed by sets of pH–PaCO₂ acid–base data. (PaCO₂: partial pressure of arterial carbon dioxide; CO₂: carbon dioxide)

A part of these loads of metabolic acids is balanced by the production of bicarbonate (HCO₃⁻) from the metabolism of aspartate, glutamate, and citrate, and a part of these loads of metabolic acids is balanced by the excretion of these acids through kidney. The sum of these additions and loses of these metabolic acids and bases (HCO₃⁻) results in a net positive balance of H⁺ of about 70 mmol/day or approximately 1 mmol/kg/day, i.e., normal pH of blood. Metabolic acids are either further metabolized in liver or excreted primarily through kidney. Pyruvic acid, acetoacetic acid, and β-hydroxybutyric acids, which are also obtained from other sources, are further degraded to CO₂ and H₂O in liver.

The changes (increase or decrease) in carbonic acid component of blood reflect an imbalance between the production of CO₂ and its elimination by alveolar ventilation. *It is represented by the changes in partial pressure of arterial carbon dioxide (PaCO₂) and is termed the respiratory or carbonic acid–base abnormalities (respiratory acidosis or alkalosis)*, whereas the changes (increase and decrease) in the handling of metabolic acid or alkali result in metabolic or noncarbonic acid–base abnormalities which is termed the *metabolic acidosis or alkalosis* and *is represented by the changes of HCO₃⁻ level in blood.*

The goals of the assessment of acid–base balance:
- To define the types of acid–base imbalance, whether respiratory (carbonic) and/or metabolic (noncarbonic).
- To quantify the magnitude of respiratory abnormality in respiratory acidosis or alkalosis by the measurement of PaCO₂.
- To quantify the magnitude of metabolic acid–base abnormality (metabolic acidosis and alkalosis) by the estimation of plasma HCO₃⁻ level or the extracellular fluid base excess.
- To quantify the buffer capacity.

■ TERMINOLOGY

An acid is usually defined as a chemical compound that can act as a proton (H⁺) donor, whereas a base is defined as a chemical compound that can act as a proton acceptor (*Bronsted–Lowry definition*). In physiological solutions, it is probably better to use *Arrhenius's definitions*. According to this definition, an acid is a compound that contains hydrogen ion (H⁺) or reacts with water to form hydrogen ion (H⁺), whereas a base is a compound that contains hydroxide ion (OH⁻) or reacts with water to form hydroxide ion (OH⁻).

Chemically, the *acidity of a substance* is defined by its ability to ionize in solution and to give an amount of H⁺ ion and base (A⁻). Thus, the relationship between the acid and base can be written by the equation as: HA (acid) = H⁺ + A⁻ (base). In this reaction HA is termed "acid" or "H⁺ (proton) donor" and the anion A⁻ is termed "H⁺ (proton) acceptor" or "conjugate base". The acid which dissociates more in an aqueous solution is called strong acid, e.g., HCl. The *stronger is the acid, the weaker is its conjugate base*, that is, the less ability of the base to accept H⁺ ion, e.g., HCl → H⁺ + Cl⁻. The acid which dissociates less in an aqueous solution is called weak acid. The *weaker is the acid, the stronger is its base*, for example, lactic acid: CH₃CHOHCOOH → CH₃CHOHCOO⁻ + H⁺. Other examples of weaker acids are: H₂CO₃ → H⁺ +

HCO_3^-, $H_3PO_4 \rightarrow H^+ + H_2PO_4^-$, etc. In our body, only 1/100 of lactic acid remains in ionized form, while 99/100 of it remains in unionized form.

The equation of acid–base balance follows the *law of mass action* which states that the product of a reaction on one side is proportional to the products of reaction on the other side. The degree to which a certain acid will remain in dissociated condition in a solution is constant for that specific acid and this degree of dissociation (ability of dissociation) is known as *dissociation constant*. This law of mass action can be expressed in the following formula:

$$HA \underset{k_1}{\overset{k}{\rightleftharpoons}} H^+ \times A^-$$

Here, the dissociation constant (k or k_1) determines the point at which equilibrium is reached in a specific equation. If k is larger than k_1, then the reaction will proceed preferentially toward the right (due to more dissociation) and will result in more H^+ and A^- ions than HA. This means HA is more acidic in nature. Reversely, if k_1 is larger than k, then this reaction will proceed preferentially toward the left (due to less dissociation) and there will be more HA than the amount of H^+ and A^- is formed. This means HA is less acidic in nature.

Acidity of a solution is also defined by the concentration of H^+ in that solution which is measured by the pH electrode. The normal value of arterial plasma pH is 7.4 at $PaCO_2$ of 40 mm Hg which usually (normally) varies within the range in between 7.35 and 7.45. The range of pH of venous blood varies in between 7.32 and 7.42. Acidemia occurs when the arterial blood pH is <7.35 or H^+ ion concentration is >44 nmol/L. Alkalemia occurs when the arterial blood pH is >7.45 or H^+ ion concentration is <36 nmol/L.

A clear understanding of acid–base disturbances and their compensatory physiological responses requires some precise terminology. The suffix "-osis" is used to denote any *pathological process* that alters the arterial pH. Thus, any disorder (or process) that tends to reduce blood pH to less than normal is termed *acidosis*, whereas any disorder or process that tends to increase arterial pH is termed *alkalosis*. If the disorder primarily affects (increase or decrease) the HCO^- ion, then it is termed "metabolic". On the other hand, if the disorder primarily affects (increase or decrease) the partial pressure of carbon dioxide (PCO_2), then it is termed "respiratory". The suffix "-emia" is used to denote the net effect on the arterial pH of all the primary processes (acidosis or alkalosis) and their compensatory physiological responses (alkalosis or acidosis), for example, the pH of arterial blood normally runs in between 7.35 and 7.45. When the pH of blood runs below 7.35, then it is called the "acidemia".

On the other hand, when the blood pH runs above 7.45, then it is called the "alkalemia".

Acidosis or alkalosis are abnormal conditions that cause acidemia and alkalemia in blood respectively, provided if no secondary changes occur to compensate for the primary changes. Usually, the acidosis or alkalosis of one system (e.g., respiratory or metabolic system) is compensated by the alkalosis or acidosis of other systems (metabolic or respiratory system respectively), so that the resulting blood pH still lies within its normal ranges (7.35–7.45). It means (1) primary respiratory acidosis is compensated by secondary metabolic alkalosis, (2) primary respiratory alkalosis is compensated by secondary metabolic acidosis, (3) primary metabolic acidosis is compensated by secondary respiratory alkalosis, and finally (4) primary metabolic alkalosis is compensated by secondary respiratory acidosis. *But the actual acid–base status should be known (diagnosed) by its primary cause such as the respiratory or metabolic acidosis or alkalosis and by its compensatory phenomenon such as the metabolic or respiratory alkalosis or acidosis and vice versa.* That is, though the pH is normal, still the acid–base status should be talked as primary respiratory or metabolic acidosis or alkalosis and compensatory metabolic or respiratory acidosis or alkalosis with their different combination and vice versa.

A respiratory acidosis or alkalosis is said to be present, when the $PaCO_2$ is above 45 mm Hg (6 kPa) or below 35 mm Hg (4.7 kPa) respectively (kPa means kilopascal, 1 mm Hg = 0.13 kPa). Also, if the value of a set of pH and $PaCO_2$ values produces a point to the left or right of the normal arterial $PaCO_2$ titration curve **(Fig. 1)**, then a respiratory acidosis or alkalosis, respectively, is present, but one has to keep in mind that there is no specific center for H^+ ion regulation in the central nervous system (CNS).

Though the concentration of H^+ ion in aqueous body solution is very low (40 nmol/L), still the range of concentration of it varies normally, is large enough which extends from 10^{-1} to 10^{-15} mol/L. So, for convenience, these H^+ concentration or $[H^+]$ is expressed by the way of an exponential arithmetic method such as: $[H^+] = 10^{-P} = 1/10^P$. As pH is the negative logarithm (to base10) of H^+ concentration (P means negative log), so the pH $= -\log_{10} [H^+] = -\log_{10} [10^{-P}] = P$ (negative logarithm of $10^{-P} = P$).

The term pH was introduced by Sorensen, in 1909. It is a more convenient way of expression of H^+ ion concentration than molar expression of it in mol/L or mmol/L, or nmol/L. Here, the exponent (power) of H^+ concentration in mol/L, i.e., "p" stands for the initial letter of ward "potenz" or "puissance" or "power".

The hydrogen ion concentration of pure water is 10^{-7} mol/L. Using the pH notation, the pH of pure water is 7, because $pH = -\log_{10}[H^+] = -\log_{10}(10^{-7}) = 7$. The negative log of 10^{-7} is 7. For various reasons, the H^+ concentration of our body is conventionally expressed as pH which is the negative logarithm (base 10) of the concentration of H^+ ion in mol/L. Thus, this pH scale indicates the number of H^+ in mol/L logarithmically.

According to the System of International (SI) nomenclature, the acidity is expressed as H^+ concentration in nmol/L, instead of mol/L or pH unit, but such expression of H^+ concentration in favor of nmol/L is sometimes criticized. This is because:

- The biological activity of a solution is related to the chemical potential of it (solution) which is again exerted by the activity of its H^+ ion and this is logarithmic in nature. It means the relation between the biological activity and H^+ concentration of a solution is logarithmic in nature.
- The measurement of H^+ concentration of a solution is made according to a standard, operational pH scale.
- The blood pH values in the population are probably evenly distributed, but the distribution of H^+ concentration in $nmol^{-1}/L$ in a population is distorted.

Thus, ideally, the H^+ concentration of a solution should be converted to its pH units, before any statistical analysis, for *easy and correct results*. But the pH system has a great source of confusion because unlike the direct concentration of H^+ in *nmol or mmol/L* which is usually expressed as a *linear*, positive numerical scale, the pH scale is logarithmic which is *not linear*. On the other hand, the number used to express the pH becomes *smaller* as the H^+ concentration becomes *greater*. So, this counter molar system makes the clinician awkward, but once understood, the concept of molar system, expressed as *nmol/L* is quite workable in a clinical setting **(Table 4)**.

TABLE 4: Conversion of H^+ concentration in mol/L and nmol/L to pH units.		
1 nanomole (nmol) = 10^{-9} mol or 10^{-6} mmol (1 mol = 1,000 mmol, 1 mmol = 1,000 μ mol, 1 μ mol = 1,000 nmol) 1 mol = 10^9 nanomole or 1 nanomole = 10^{-9} mol		
H^+ (mol/L)	*pH*	*H^+ (nmol/L)*
$0.001 = 10^{-3}$	3	1,000,000
$0.0001 = 10^{-4}$	4	100,000
$0.00001 = 10^{-5}$	5	10,000
$0.000001 = 10^{-6}$	6	1,000
$0.0000001 = 10^{-7}$	7	100
$0.00000001 = 10^{-8}$	8	10
$0.000000001 = 10^{-9}$	9	1
$0.000000000000001 = 10^{-15}$	15	0.000001

Some important points regarding the pH scale are:

- As pH scale is expressed as the negative logarithmic of (base 10) the concentration of H^+ ion in mol/L, so it means *there is a 10-fold change of H^+ ion concentration, expressed in nmol/L or mmol/L or mol/L for every one unit change in pH*, for example, a solution with a pH of 4 has 10 times more H^+ ion concentration in nmol/L or mmol/L or mol/L than a solution with a pH of 5 and 100 times more than a solution with a pH of 6.
- The changes in H^+ concentration in nmol/L differ vastly at different points of the pH scale, depending upon at which point of the scale these changes occur.
- Though the H^+ concentration in nmol/L scale is easier to visualize, still the pH scale is deeply infixed in our mind and is the standard with which we can function.

INTERCONVERSION OF H^+ CONCENTRATION AND PH

This can be shown best by two examples:

1. If the normal pH of whole blood is 7.4, then what will be the H^+ concentration or $[H^+]$.
   [ ] is the symbol of concentration.

$$pH = 7.4$$
$$Or, \quad -\log_{10}H^+ = -\log_{10}10^{-7.4}$$
$$Or, \quad H^+ = 10^{-7.4}$$
$$So, \quad [H^+] = 10^{-7.4}\ mol/L$$
$$= 10^{-7.4} \times 10^9\ nmol/L$$
$$= 10^{1.6}\ nmol/L$$
$$= 40\ nmol/L$$

2. If the hydrogen ion concentration is 100 nmol, what is the pH?

$$100\ nmol/L = 100 \times 10^{-9}\ mol/L\ (1\ nmol = 10^{-9}\ mol)$$
$$\therefore \quad [H^+] = 100 \times 10^{-9}\ mol/L$$
$$\therefore \quad pH = -\log[H^+]$$
$$= -\log(100 \times 10^{-9})$$
$$= -\log[1/100^{-1} \times 1/10^9]$$
$$= -\log[1/10^{-2} \times 1/10^9]$$
$$= -\log[1/10^7]$$
$$= -\log[10^{-7}]$$
$$= 7$$

In other simple way, it can also be calculated by:

$$[H^+] = 100\ nmol/L$$
$$= 100 \times 10^{-9}\ mol/L$$
$$\therefore \quad pH = -\log[H^+]$$
$$= -\log(100 \times 10^{-9})$$
$$= -\log 100 - \log^{-9}$$
$$= -2 + 9$$
$$= 7$$

[The negative log of 100 is –2 and the negative log of 10^{-9} is 9. Thus, taking the advantage of log we can add instead of multiplication **(Table 5)**].

TABLE 5: Relation between H^+ ion concentration and pH. Life exists in pH in between 7.8 and 6.8.

[H⁺] nmol/L	pH	
10	8	Alkalosis
15	7.8	Alkalosis
20	7.7	Alkalosis
25	7.6	Alkalosis
30	7.5	Alkalosis
40	7.4	*Normal*
50	7.3	Acidosis
65	7.2	Acidosis
80	7.1	Acidosis
100	7	Acidosis
160	6.8	Acidosis

Another way of interconversion between pH and $[H^+]$ is:

- If the $[H^+]$ of a solution is 2.86×10^{-4} mol/L, then the pH can be calculated as follows:

$$[H^+] = 2.86 \times 10^{-4} \text{ mol/L}$$
$$pH = -\log_{10} 1/[H^+]$$
$$= -\log_{10} [1/(2.86 \times 10^{-4})]$$
$$= -\log_{10} [1/(10^{0.456} \times 10^{-4})]$$
$$= -\log_{10} (1/10^{3.544})$$
$$= -\log_{10} 1/10^{3.544}$$
$$= -\log_{10} 10^{-3.544}$$
$$= 3.544$$

Or,
$$pH = -\log [H^+]$$
$$= -\log (2.86 \times 10^{-4})$$
$$= -\log (10^{0.456} \times 10^{-4})$$
$$= -\log 10^{-3.544}$$
$$= 3.544$$

- For the calculation of $[H^+]$ from a known pH value, the calculation will be reversed. Suppose, the pH value of a solution is 3.544, then the $[H^+]$ will be:

$$pH\ 3.544 = \log 10^{3.544}$$
$$= \log (1/10^{-3.544})$$
$$= \log (1/10^{0.456} \times 10^{-4})$$
$$= \log (1/2.86 \times 10^{-4})$$

Antilog of 0.456 = 2.86

$\therefore$ H^+ concentration of $[H^+]$
$$= 2.86 \times 10^{-4} \text{ mol/L}$$
$$= 286,000 \text{ nmol/L}$$

An easy formula for the conversion pH to [H⁺].
At a pH of 7.40, the [H⁺] is 40 nEq/L. Below 7.40 pH, for each 0.01 decrease in pH, there is a 1.25 nEq/L increase in [H⁺]. Above 7.40 pH, for each 0.01 increase in pH, there is a 0.8 nEq/L decrease in [H⁺].

Calculation of pH of a Neutral Pure Water

According to the law of mass action the equilibrium, governing the ionization of water is as follows:

$$H_2O \rightleftharpoons [H^+] \times [OH^-]$$

Or,
$$K[H_2O] = [H^+] \times [OH^-]$$

[ ] is the symbol of concentration.

At a particular temperature (23°C) the product of the number of hydrogen ions multiplied by the number of hydroxyl ions is constant for pure neutral water and this is known as the *dissociation constant* (dissociation constant is designated as Ka. The pKa is the negative logarithm to base ten of Ka value. The pKa number shows how weak or strong an acid is, i.e., how completely an acid dissociates in its aqueous solution). The dissociation constant of water can be denoted as K_W ("w" stands for water) and its value in case of pure water is 10^{-14}. Thus, by the law of mass action:

$$[H^+] \times [OH^-] = K_W = 10^{-14}$$

In pure water, the concentration of H^+ ions is equal to the concentration of OH^-.

Hence, $[H^+] = 1 \times 10^{-7}$, $[OH^-] = 1 \times 10^{-7}$

Therefore, pH of the pure neutral water will be:

$$pH = -\log [H^+]$$
$$= \log [1/H^+]$$
$$= \log (1/1 \times 10^{-7})$$
$$= 7$$

So, pure water, having an equal number of $[H^+]$ and $[OH^-]$ ions, is neutral with pH 7.0. Here, one thing is to notice that the reduction of pH of 0.3 units represents a doubling of $[H^+]$ and vice versa.

One basic difficulty, during the measurement of pH *in vivo*, is that it is not possible to measure either the actual H^+ concentration or its activity in a biological system. On the other hand, the pH numbers which are produced by electrometric measurement *in vitro* are defined by an operational scale which is based upon the standard buffer solution and fixed temperature. They do not relate precisely to H^+ concentration and its activity.

◼ ACID–BASE HOMEOSTASIS

The acid–base homeostasis means the addition or elimination of acid to compensate the elimination or addition of base and vice versa. But as life is an acidogenic process, so there is a continuous formation of acids. Hence, in normal situation, acid–base homeostasis means elimination of acid (respiratory carbonic acid as CO_2 and metabolic acids through urine) and addition or recovery of base (as HCO_3^-) to balance that small portion of acid that is normally not eliminated or added. In pathological state, this normal homeostasis may be failed, causing alkalosis (metabolic or respiratory) or moves in opposite direction causing acidosis (metabolic or respiratory). Despite the regulating mechanisms, the H^+ concentration in tissue varies up to 10-fold from 16 to 160 nmol/L (pH 6.8–7.8) which is compatible to life. Beyond that range, life is not compatible. However, usually, the normal range of H^+ ion concentration in blood is 36–44 nmol/L (pH 7.35–7.45) after homeostasis. No other ion in the tissues has such a wide range of variability within which life can exist.

There are three mechanisms that maintain this pH homeostasis. These are (1) *buffering,* (2) *compensation,* and (3) *correction. Buffering* is the process in which a chemical as a buffer agent is used by the body to immediately neutralize or minimize the change in pH or H^+ ion concentration. *Compensation* is a process where the other systems are activated to restore the HCO_3^-/H_2CO_3 ratio to normal, for example, when there is a retention of CO_2 or H_2CO_3 due to any downward adjustment of ventilation, then there is an excessive loss of H^+ or retention of HCO_3^- by the kidney and maintain the normal acid–base (HCO_3^-/H_2CO_3) ratio. *Correction* refers to any exogenous medical management of the primary metabolic derangement responsible for this abnormality in pH.

Buffer System

Buffer system is composed of: (1) a weak acid and its salt as a strong base or (2) a strong acid and its salt as a weak base. It resists the changes of H^+ concentration in a solution after addition of a stronger acid or base (which causes the changes in pH) in this solution. Stronger acids that are added in the solution and cause the changes in pH are buffered by the base part of the buffer system to form weak acids. Similarly, stronger bases which are added in the solution are buffered by the acid part of buffer system to produce weak bases, for example, HCl is a strong acid that is largely dissociated as H^+ and Cl^- ion. This H^+ combines with $NaHCO_3$ (weak base part of the *bicarbonate buffer system*) to produce H_2CO_3, which is a weaker acid than HCl. It is less dissociated, and therefore less H^+ is released by its dissociation than if the HCl was present alone in the solution without a buffer. Similarly, a strong base such as NaOH is buffered by the weak acid part of a *bicarbonate buffer system* to produce a weak base, for example, $NaOH + H_2CO_3 = NaHCO_3 + H_2O$. If NaOH is not buffered, then the large amount of dissociated OH^- ion from the strong base of NaOH would combine with a large amount of H^+ and will decrease the huge concentration of it, thus it will raise the pH much. On the other hand, after buffering as the $NaHCO_3$ is a weaker base than NaOH, it is less dissociated and thereby causes less change in H^+ ion concentration. To be maximally effective, a buffering system

must be adequate enough to be able to buffer a large amount of acid or alkali which is eliminated or added, and have a pK value which is close to the initial pH of the solution to be buffered. It is known that weaker acids and their salts (Na-salts of acids are base) as strong base are more effective buffers than the buffer system which is composed of strong acid and their salts as weak base.

About three-fourths of the chemical buffering power of our body lies within the cells. It is due to the high concentration of intracellular proteins, phosphates, hemoglobin (Hb) (in RBC), and other inorganic compounds. So, proteins, phosphates, and Hb buffer systems are more important intracellularly. On the other hand, the remaining one-fourth of the buffering power of our body lies in extracellular fluid. The acid–base disturbances due to the respiratory causes are buffered mainly by the intracellular buffers, whereas the acid–disturbances due to the metabolic causes are buffered mainly by the extracellular buffers. The preferential utilization of this extracellular buffer occurs in the initial phase of metabolic acidosis, with the contribution of intracellular buffer, which is becoming gradually greater as the metabolic acidosis increases in severity. *The buffer pair of greatest importance in extracellular fluid is carbonic acid (H_2CO_3) and bicarbonate ($NaHCO_3$ or $KHCO_3$), i.e., bicarbonate buffer system.* In both the intracellular and extracellular environment, the power of action of a buffering system depends on (1) the pK value of this buffer system, (2) the pH at which it is working, and (3) on the concentration of buffer elements.

Although, both the carbonic (bicarbonate) and noncarbonic (nonbicarbonate) buffer systems are located throughout the body in both the intracellular and extracellular fluid, but *blood is the only window* through which we can view the acid–base derangements. So, the pH and PCO_2 electrodes only measure the plasma pH and $PaCO_2$, but cannot tell anything about the inside of a cell. On the other hand, plasma is in close equilibrium with interstitial fluid as far as the pH, PCO_2, and $[HCO_3^-]$ are concerned. Thus, the measurement of acid–base status of blood gives a reasonable assessment of the acid–base status of extracellular fluid (interstitial plus blood) but offers only an indirect insight of the intracellular status from which the actual acid–base disorder is originating.

The tendency of an acid to dissociate in water may be described quantitatively by *the law of mass action.* Thus, [HA] (acid) $\propto [H^+] \times [A^-]$, A^- is the conjugate base of the acid HA. Or K [HA] = $[H^+] \times [A^-]$. Here, K is the dissociation constant which describes the tendency of an acid to dissociate. Large K means stronger acid and vice versa. This equation is called the *Henderson equation.* So, $[H^+] = K [HA] (acid)/[A^-]$ (base) **(Fact file I)**.

FACT FILE I

From the Henderson equation, such as $[H^+] = K\,[HA]/A^-$, we can calculate any one factor, if other two factors are known. This is as follows:

- For bicarbonate buffer system, the Henderson equation can be written as: $[H^+] = K\,(PaCO_2\text{ mm Hg})/HCO_3^-$
- If $PaCO_2 = 50$ mm Hg, $HCO_3^- = 24$ mEq/L, and $K = 24$ (dissociation constant of carbonic acid), then:

$$[H^+] = (24 \times 50)/24 = 50$$

- Therefore, the $[H^+]$ concentration is 50 nmol/L. Now, from Table 5 we can read the pH as 7.3 when the $[H^+]$ is 50 nmol/L.
- When the pH is 7.4 and $PaCO_2$ is 50 mm Hg, then the HCO_3^- level can be calculated like this:

$$H^+ = K\,(PaCO_2)/HCO_3^-$$
Or, $$CO_3^- = K\,(PaCO_2)/H^+$$
Or, $$HCO_3^- = (24 \times 50)/40\ (H^+ \text{ concentration at pH 7.4}$$
$$= 40\text{ nmol/L})$$
Or, $$HCO_3^- = 30\text{ mEq/L}.$$

The negative logarithmic expression of this equation is:

$$-\log[H^+] = -\log k\,[HA]\,(acid)/[A^-]\,(base)$$
Or $$pH = p^K + \log[A^-]\,(base)/[HA]\,(acid)\ (p = -\log).$$

From this equation, it is apparent that the pH of a solution is related to the ratio of dissociated anion to undissociated acid.

Here, p^K is the negative logarithm of K and also reflects the strength of an acid.

Therefore, $$pH = p^K + \log base/acid$$

This is called the *Henderson–Hasselbalch equation*. This equation is used for the determination of pH of a buffer solution or for the determination of the relative concentration of salt (base) and acid which is required to achieve the normal pH, for example, the pH of a buffer solution prepared by mixing 35 mL of (N/10) acetic acid with 15 mL of (N/10) NaOH can be determined by the Henderson–Hasselbalch equation: $pH = p^K + \log$ (salt A^-/acid HA) where p^K is log $(1/k)$, k is the dissociation constant of acid.

When these two solutions are mixed up, then 15 mL of (N/10) NaOH will neutralize 15 mL of (N/10) acetic acid to form 15 mL of the salt, Na-acetate. So, 20 mL of acetic acid will remain unneutralized. Thus, in the buffer solution, the salt and unneutralized acid ratio will be (15/20). The dissociation constant (k) of acetic acid is (1.86×10^{-5}) and so the p^K will be log $(1/k)$ and that is 4.73.

So, in the Henderson–Hasselbalch equation:

$$pH = 4.73 + \log(15/20)$$
$$= 4.73 + \log 0.75$$
$$= 4.73$$
$$= 4.6$$

If the ratio of salt and unneutralized acid ratio becomes 1:1, then the pH value of this buffer mixture will be equal to the p^K value of acid, for example, if 30 mL of (N/10) acetic acid and 15 mL of (N/10) NaOH are mixed up, then the 15 mL of Na-acetate salt will be formed and 15 mL of acetic acid will remain as an unneutralized acid, so the salt and acid ratio will be (15/15) = 1. So, interpolating this value in the Henderson–Hasselbalch equation, the result will be:

$$pH = p^K + \log(salt/acid)$$
$$= 4.73 + \log(15/15)$$
$$= 4.73 + \log 1$$
$$= 4.73 + 0$$
$$= 4.73$$

So, the buffering action in this case is at its maximum and can react either as acid or as base.

Each unit change in pH represents a 10-fold change of $[H^+]$ in nmol or mmol or mol per liter. So, when the pH number decreases, the $[H^+]$ increases and vice versa. For any given buffer system, the p^K is constant for this buffer system. So, the pH will depend on the log of the ratio of [base]/[acid]. If acid or alkali is added in this buffer system, then the smallest change in this ratio and therefore the smallest change in pH will result, if the initial [base] is equal to the [acid] or base/acid ratio is 1. Under these circumstances, pH $= p^K$ [since base/acid = 1 and log1 = 0]. So, a buffer system resists the pH changes best, when it is operating at a pH close to its p^K value.

In the plasma, tissue fluids, and within the cells many buffer systems exist. These important buffer systems are *bicarbonate (HCO_3^-/H_2CO_3), phosphate ($HPO_4^{2-}/H_2PO_4^-$), ammonia (NH_3/NH_4^+), protein (Pr^-/PrH), and hemoglobin (Hb^-/HbH)*. The effectiveness of these buffers in various fluid compartments is related to their concentration. Bicarbonate buffer is most important in an extracellular fluid compartment. Hb though is restricted inside the red blood cells (intracellular), also functions as an important buffer in blood (extracellular fluid). Proteins (other than Hb) probably play a major role in buffering the intracellular fluid compartment. *Phosphate and ammonium are important urinary buffers.*

The buffering of H^+ in extracellular compartment can also be accomplished by the exchange of this extracellular H^+ for Na^+ and Ca^{2+} from bone and intracellular K^+. *Thus, acid loads demineralize the bone and release alkaline compounds such as $CaCO_3$ and $CaHPO_4$. Contrary, alkaline loads increase the deposition of carbonate in bone.* Further, acidosis is associated with hyperkalemia ($\uparrow K^+$). The buffering in plasma by bicarbonate is *immediate*, whereas the buffering in interstitial fluid compartment by bicarbonate takes *15–20 minutes* and buffering by intracellular proteins and bone *takes 2–4 hours. Up to 50–60% acid loads may ultimately be buffered by intracellular buffers and bone.*

Bicarbonate Buffer System (HCO$_3^-$/H$_2$CO$_3$)

$$H^+ + HCO_3^- \rightleftharpoons H_2CO_3 \rightleftharpoons CO_2 + H_2O \qquad ...I$$

This is the *main buffer system in blood and interstitial fluid (extracellular compartment)*. This bicarbonate buffer system consists of a mixture of H$_2$CO$_3$ (weak acid) and its salt NaHCO$_3$ (strong base). Usually, NaHCO$_3$ remains in extracellular fluid, and KHCO$_3$ or Mg (HCO$_3$)$_2$ is present in intracellular fluid. The relationship between the concentration of carbonic acid and their salt (bicarbonate buffer system) and the pH can be described by the Henderson–Hasselbalch equation:

$$pH = pK + \log [HCO_3^-]/[H_2CO_3]$$
$$= 6.1 + \log [HCO_3^-]/P_aCO_2 \times 0.03$$

(0.03 is the solubility coefficient of CO$_2$ and 6.1 is the negative log of dissociation constant of H$_2$CO$_3$ or p^K value of bicarbonate buffer system).

So, the pH of blood is determined by the ratio of [HCO$_3^-$]/[H$_2$CO$_3$]. The reaction curve of bicarbonate buffer system, i.e., the relation between the relative concentration of HCO$_3^-$ and H$_2$CO$_3$ with pH is S-shaped. The buffering power of this system is greatest where the slope of this curve is the steepest. This is because the addition of a certain amount of acid or base causes a smallest change of pH to occur in this part. This buffer system is most efficient when the concentration of HCO$_3^-$ and H$_2$CO$_3$ are equal or when pH = p^K or log [HCO$_3^-$]/[H$_2$CO$_3$] = 1.

The p^K value of bicarbonate buffer system is 6.1; therefore it is most effective at pH 6.1. Its chemical buffering capacity at pH 7.4 (which is its usual working pH) is poor, but its efficiency increases when the pH of blood decreases. Normally, when this buffer system functions at a pH of around 7.4, then the ratio of bicarbonate to carbonic acid is 20:1 which is well outside its optimum working range (once the relative concentration of bicarbonate and carbonic acid exceeds 8:1 in either direction, then the buffering power of this system falls rapidly) **(Fig. 2)**.

But on the other hand, at physiological pH of 7.4, the importance of this bicarbonate buffer system lies in the ability of carbonic acid to produce CO$_2$ which is excreted via lungs. The addition of H$^+$ and the elimination of CO$_2$ drive the *Equation-I* to the right and compensate for the acidosis.

The bicarbonate–carbonic acid buffer system, i.e., the bicarbonate buffer system forms the cornerstone of acid–base balance. This is because carbonic acid (H$_2$CO$_3$) can be formed by the addition of nonvolatile acids (metabolic or nonrespiratory load), as seen in equation-II. Then, this H$_2$CO$_3$ ultimately converts to CO$_2$ which is then eliminated by ventilation through lungs. CO$_2$ (or H$_2$CO$_3$) remains in

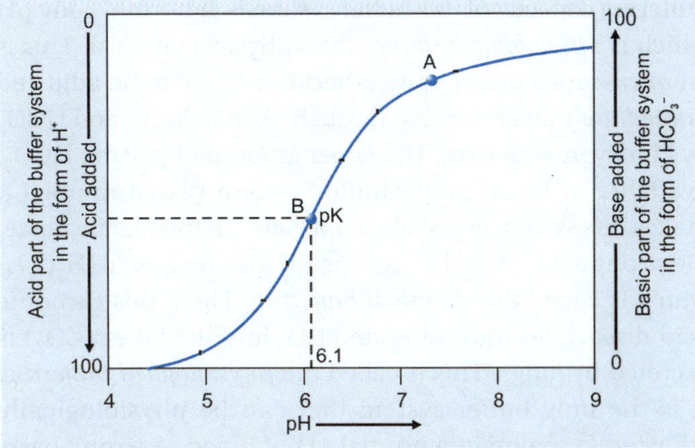

Fig. 2: Reaction curve of bicarbonate buffer system. Point A indicates the normal operating condition where this bicarbonate buffer system works in the body. Point B indicates pK value of this buffer system at which it works maximally.

equilibrium with HCO$_3^-$. More H$^+$ leads to more consumption of HCO$_3^-$ and more excretion of CO$_2$ through stimulated ventilation. It is clinically important to note that the change in HCO$_3^-$ in the body reasonably reflects the amount of H$^+$ added to or removed from the system (in a short time at least until other slower buffer systems have had time to start work and compensate).

Mechanism of action of bicarbonate buffer system: Carbonic acid and its salt, primarily NaHCO$_3$ [other salts are KHCO$_3$, Mg (HCO$_3$)$_3$] which is present in extracellular fluid constitutes the bicarbonate buffer system. It buffers only the metabolic (noncarbonic) acid or alkali. This system does not function to buffer the respiratory acid load or deficit that is CO$_2$ or H$_2$CO$_3$ load or their deficit.

$$\text{Excreted through lungs} \leftarrow CO_2 + H_2O$$
$$\downarrow\uparrow$$
$$HCl + NaHCO_3 \rightleftharpoons H_2CO_3 + NaCl \qquad ...II$$
$$\downarrow\uparrow$$
$$H^+ + HCO_3^-$$

Due to the addition of noncarbonic acid (let HCl), during metabolic process, the resulting carbonic acid (due to reaction of HCl with NaHCO$_3$ of bicarbonate buffer system) is a weaker acid than the hydrochloric acid which is added in this system of our body. The carbonic acid, thus formed, escapes from the blood as CO$_2$, causing a constant PaCO$_2$ of 40 mm Hg. The changes in HCO$_3^-$ level or the amount of consumed HCO$_3^-$ in the form of NaHCO$_3$ to neutralize the acid equals to the amount of acid added. *Thus, for the bicarbonate buffer system, which works in metabolic acidosis or alkalosis, the change in [HCO$^-$] provides a good measure to know the quantity of H$^+$ added or removed from the plasma by metabolic acids (not respiratory acids).* The major buffering capacity of this buffer system is at normal body pH which is *physiological*, rather than physicochemical. This is an *open-ended* buffer system because CO_2 can be adjusted *immediately* by ventilation through normal lungs and HCO_3^- by kidney in *long term*. The larger amount of plasma HCO_3^-, available in bicarbonate buffer system (24.28 mmol/L), makes this system especially important. In the first instance, the strong acid (let HCl) is "swapped" for a weak acid (H_2CO_3) which is called the *chemical buffering*. Then, this carbonic acid dissociates into water and CO_2 and the latter (CO_2) is excreted by lungs. This is called the *physiological buffering*. It is the only buffer system that can be physiologically adjusted to maintain a normal pH of blood. A strong base, such as NaOH may also be buffered by carbonic acid (H_2CO_3) of this bicarbonate buffer system.

$$NaOH + H_2CO_3 \rightleftharpoons NaHCO_3 + H_2O$$

$NaHCO_3$ is a weaker base than NaOH, so it will less dissociate, causing the less change in H^+ and OH^- concentration (explained before).

The bicarbonate buffer system functions to neutralize the metabolic acid and base only which is discussed earlier. It does not buffer the respiratory acids such as H_2CO_3 produced from the accumulation of CO_2 due to lung dysfunction. This is because if carbonic acid is added to a bicarbonate buffer solution, then the H^+ and HCO^- level does not change. They are produced in equal amounts.

$$CO_2 + H_2O + NaHCO_3 = H^+ + HCO_3^- + NaHCO_3$$

Changes in the absolute value of $[HCO_3^-]$ from normal indicate the amount of metabolic (noncarbonic) acid or H^+ is added to or removed from the solution. *But the changes in $PaCO_2$ which is an indicator of respiratory acidosis or alkalosis do not cause any measurable alteration in the bicarbonate $[HCO_3^-]$ level in plasma which is an indicator of metabolic acidosis or alkalosis.*

A working formula of Henderson–Hasselbalch equation for bicarbonate buffer system is: $H^+ = 24 \times (H_2CO_3)$ or $PaCO_2/[HCO_3^-]$. *Another simple theory is that below 7.4 pH, for every 0.01 unit decrease in pH there is 1.25 nmol/L increase of H^+ concentration, and above 7.4 pH for every 0.01 increase in pH there is 0.8 nmol/L decrease of H^+ concentration.* These two theories are very helpful clinically, because the H^+ concentration, pH of blood, $PaCO_2$, and HCO_3^- concentration all can be calculated easily from the above, for example, if pH of arterial blood is 7.26, then the $[H^+] = 40 + [(40 - 26) \times 1.25] = 57.5$ nmol/L. If $PaCO_2$ in the arterial sample is 30 mm Hg, then

$$57.5 = 24 \times 30/[HCO_3^-]$$

or $\quad [HCO_3^-] = (24 \times 30)/57.5 = 12.52$ mEq/L

The two important characteristics of bicarbonate buffers are that (1) the bicarbonate buffer is effective against metabolic, but not against respiratory acid–base disturbances and (2) The bicarbonate buffer is not effective against increases in $PaCO_2$ and changes in the concentration of HCO_3^- do not reflect the severity of respiratory acidosis.

Let 3 mEq/L of a strong nonvolatile acid (let HCl) is added to extracellular fluid. This acid will be neutralized by plasma HCO_3^-. The normal value of plasma HCO_3^- is 24 mEq/L. Now, the reaction will be: 3 mEq/L H^+ + 24 mEq/L of $HCO_3^- = H_2CO_3 = CO_2 + H_2O + 21$ mEq/L HCO_3^-. After neutralization of nonvolatile acid by HCO_3^- the CO_2 will be produced and will be eliminated by lungs, such that $PaCO_2$ will not change. Now, the plasma HCO_3^- level is 21 mEq/L and H^+ ion concentration is $K \times PaCO_2/HCO_3^-$ or $24 \times 40/21 = 45.6$ nEq/L and pH is 7.34, further this decrease in HCO_3^- level reflects the amount of nonvolatile acid (metabolic acidosis).

In contrast, an increase in $PaCO_2$ (volatile acid) has minimal effect on HCO_3^- concentration, for example, if $PaCO_2$ increases from 40 to 80 mm Hg, then the dissolved CO_2 will increase only from 1.2 to 2.2 mEq/L. Further, the equilibrium constant of the reaction between CO_2 and H_2O ($CO_2 + H_2O \leftrightarrow H_2CO_3 \leftrightarrow H^+ + HCO_3^-$) is such that the increase in magnitude of CO_2 does not or minimally drive the reaction toward the left. Now, if we thought that there is no appreciable change of HCO_3^- concentration, then the concentration of H^+ ion is $24 \times 80/24$ (formula is $K \times PaCO_2/HCO_3^-$) = 80 nEq/L and pH = 7.10. Therefore, the concentration of H^+ ion increases from 40 to 80 nEq/L, and HCO_3^- is produced in 1:1 ratio with H ion, i.e., HCO_3^- concentration also increases by 40 nEq/L (not mEq/L). Thus extracellular HCO_3^- concentration increases negligibly from 24 to 24.000040 mEq/L. This also proves that bicarbonate buffer is not effective against increase in $PaCO_2$ and changes in HCO_3^- concentration do not reflect the severity of respiratory acidosis.

Phosphate Buffer System ($HPO_4^{2-}/H_2PO_4^-$)

$$H + HPO_4^{2-} \leftrightarrow H_2PO_4^-$$

This buffer system consists of NaH_2PO_4 (weak acid) and Na_2HPO_4 (strong base). This buffer system works exactly in the same way as that of a bicarbonate buffer system. The pK value of this buffer system is 6.8. It means this buffer system has the highest working capability at the pH near about 6.8. *It is the largest inorganic chemical buffer system in the body. Its concentration in plasma is much lower and, therefore, its capacity as a buffer in blood is also much less. Its importance predominantly lies in an intracellular environment and in urine.* Unlike bicarbonate buffer system, this buffer system neutralizes both the carbonic (respiratory) and noncarbonic (metabolic) acid or alkali. Thus, this phosphate buffer system neutralizes strong acids and alkalis as seen in the following reactions.

$$HCl + Na_2HPO_4 \rightleftharpoons NaH_2PO_4 + NaCl$$
$$NaOH + NaH_2PO_4 \rightleftharpoons Na_2HPO_4 + H_2O$$

Here, NaH_2PO_4 and Na_2HPO_4 are the weak acid and strong base, respectively. The conversions of strong acids and strong bases which are added to our body by this phosphate buffer system to weaker ones result in the liberation of less H^+ and OH^- ion and therefore smaller changes in pH.

This buffer system has a little effect in extracellular environment. This is because the concentration of this system is <10% of bicarbonate buffer system in the extracellular fluid. The concentration of this system is highest within the cell. Furthermore, the pKa value of this phosphate buffer system is same as that of intracellular pH (intracellular pH is 6.9) which increases its buffering power within the cell (explained earlier). For the similar reasons, this buffer system is also very important in renal tubular fluid. In renal tubular fluid, the phosphate buffer is greatly concentrated and the pH of renal tubular fluid is closer to the pKa value of this phosphate buffer system which increases its efficacy.

Formation of urinary titrable acidity (TA): At pH 7.4, the 80% of circulating phosphate is in monohydrogen (Na_2HPO_4) form and 20% is in dihydrogen (NaH_2PO_4) form. The majority of urinary TA is produced by the conversion of monohydrogen to dihydrogen phosphate ($Na_2HPO_4 \rightarrow NaH_2PO_4$). This occurs throughout the nephron. At maximum urinary acidity, i.e., at pH 4.5, all most 99% of filtered phosphate is in dihydrogen form (as the pKa of this system is 6.8). At this highest urinary pH, 70% of filtered creatinine and 90% of uric acid are in unionized form and may account for the 20% of urinary TA.

Normally, 20–40 mmol of H^+ ion is excreted through urine per day as urinary TA. In diabetic ketoacidosis, the rate of excretion of nonionized β-hydroxybutyric is 60%. In this condition, it (β-hydroxybutyric acid instead of NaH_2PO_4) produces a large component of urinary TA. Acetoacetic acid is excreted, but forms a lesser component of urinary TA. Almost all of the urinary ketone excretion is in the form of β-hydroxybutyric acid. Excretion of nonionized lactic acid in lactic acidosis is also low. Normally, the urinary excretion of phosphate is determined by the need to maintain phosphate balance rather than acid–base homeostasis. Thus, TA appears to play a supportive rather than taking an active role in H^+ balance.

Proteins as Buffer (Prot–/H Prot)

$$H^+ + Prot^- \rightleftharpoons H\ Prot$$

Like hemoglobin (globin part of Hb is protein), plasma proteins also act as an effective buffer. This is because of large total concentration of it in our body and the p^K value of some proteins approximates 7.4 at which they are likely to work most efficiently. *Proteins are most important buffers in side of the cells.* They contain both acidic group (–COOH) and basic group (–NH_2) in one molecule to make up the buffer pairs. Acidic group dissociates into –COO^- + H^+ and donate H^+ to buffer excess base: –$COOH + OH^- \rightleftharpoons$ –$COO^- + H_2O$. Basic group, commonly in the form of –NH_2 buffers excess acid by accepting H^+ to form –NH_3^+.

$$-NH_2 + H^+ \leftrightarrow -NH_3^+$$

As the pK value of most of the protein buffer systems are around 7.4, so at normal condition they work best. *They buffer both carbonic (respiratory) and noncarbonic (metabolic) acid or alkali.*

Hemoglobin as Buffer (Hb^-/HbH)

Hemoglobin is responsible for 50% buffering power of blood (extracellular, though in RBC). It is an effective buffer between pH of 5.7 and 7.7 because its pK value of this buffer system is 6.8. *It buffers respiratory and metabolic acids only. It does not buffer any alkali.* It acts as a buffer because it is a protein in nature and more importantly due to the ability of imidazole group of heme (within the histidine molecules which dissociates less in oxygenated than in deoxygenated blood) to accept H^+. This H^+ for neutralization comes from two sources: One, from the dissociation of metabolic acids and another from CO_2 which is available from metabolism of substrates through TCA cycle. At tissue level, the O_2 is liberated from Hb and CO_2 enters in the erythrocyte. Erythrocyte is rich in carbonic anhydrase which helps in the formation of H_2CO_3 from CO_2 by the reaction:

$$CO_2 + H_2O \rightleftharpoons H_2CO_3 \rightleftharpoons H^+ + HCO_3^-$$

When the H^+ of H_2CO_3 is buffered by Hb, it exists within the erythrocyte as a weak acid (HHb) than carbonic acid (because pK value of HHb is 6.8, whereas the pK value of H_2CO_3 is 6.1). After buffering of H^+ ion by Hb, the level of HCO_3^- within RBC is increased proportionally. Then, the corresponding increase in HCO_3^- concentration in erythrocytes causes a diffusion back of HCO_3^- into plasma, along the concentration gradient. This results in exchange **(Fig. 3)** or shifting of Cl^- into erythrocyte from plasma, which is called the *chloride shift.* Therefore, while most of the H^+ ion is buffered within the cell (RBC), but most of the change in the level of HCO_3^- ion is seen in plasma (so, it is an extracellular buffer system). After entering into erythrocyte, CO_2 molecule is also carried directly as carbamino compound, after combining directly with the terminal amino acids of the globin part of the Hb molecule. The acidity of these imidazole group (or deoxygenation) is influenced by the oxygenation and reduction of Hb. Hemoglobin is a weaker acid in reduced form than when it is oxygenated and increases the availability of buffer sites for H^+. When oxygenated Hb gives up O_2 to the tissue, it becomes reduced (weaker acid) and is therefore becomes more able to accept CO_2 in the form of H^+. In the lungs, reverse effects occur. Upon reaching the lung and becoming oxygenated, the Hb becomes a stronger acid, and buffering capacity (to accept H^+) is reduced. So, H^+ ion which was attached with Hb at tissues is released from Hb in lungs to react with $KHCO_3$, and CO_2 is formed. CO_2 is released directly from the carbamino groups.

$$HHb + O_2 + KHCO_3 \rightleftharpoons KHbO_2 + H_2O + CO_2$$

This effect explains that reduction or deoxygenation of Hb makes it a weaker acid and increases its buffering capacity to accept H^+, whereas oxygenation makes Hb a stronger acid and decreases its buffering capacity to accept H^+. This is known as *Haldane effect*. Reduced Hb (H–Hb) is a better buffer than O_2–Hb. Hemoglobin has three times better buffering capacity than plasma proteins in gram-for-gram comparison and is twice the concentration in blood than plasma protein. Therefore, Hb has six times the total buffering capacity than plasma protein **(Figs. 4A and B)**.

The Bohr effect is the decrease of O_2 binding capacity of Hb with the increase of the concentration of CO_2 or decrease in pH, whereas the Haldane effect is the decrease of CO_2 binding capacity of Hb with the rise in the concentration of O_2. These two effects are the two properties of Hb that help the dissociation of respiratory gases from Hb, based on the physiological conditions of their final destination. The Bohr effect helps in the release of O_2 from oxyhemoglobin (O_2Hb) at the level of metabolizing tissues. While the Haldane effect aids in the release of CO_2 from carboxyhemoglobin in lungs.

Thus, the buffers in order of importance are:

- *In blood:* Hb, bicarbonate, plasma protein, and phosphate
- *In interstitial fluid:* Bicarbonate, phosphate, and interstitial protein.
- *In cells:* Proteins, phosphate, ammonia, and other inorganic substances. Phosphates and ammonia are also important *urinary buffers.*

As nonvolatile acids are released from cellular metabolism, so their effect is mainly buffered by the action of bicarbonate buffer system in extracellular fluid (ECF) and by bicarbonate (50%), Hb (35%), plasma protein (6%), and phosphate buffer system in plasma. In summary, buffering is the mechanism by which an influx of H^+ is initially dealt with by the body and limits the change in pH. Thereafter, the respiratory mechanism becomes activated to eliminate CO_2 and later the renal regulation of acid and alkali secretion increases to increase the buffer capacity.

Compensation

The alteration of H^+ ion concentration also stimulates the compensatory part of pH homeostatic mechanism and maintains a normal pH by restoring the $HCO_3^-/PaCO_2$ ratio or HCO_3^-/H_2CO_3 ratio. So, in addition to buffering mechanism, the homeostasis of acid–base disturbance is also maintained

Fig. 3: Reduced (or deoxygenated) Hb is a better buffer than oxygenated Hb.

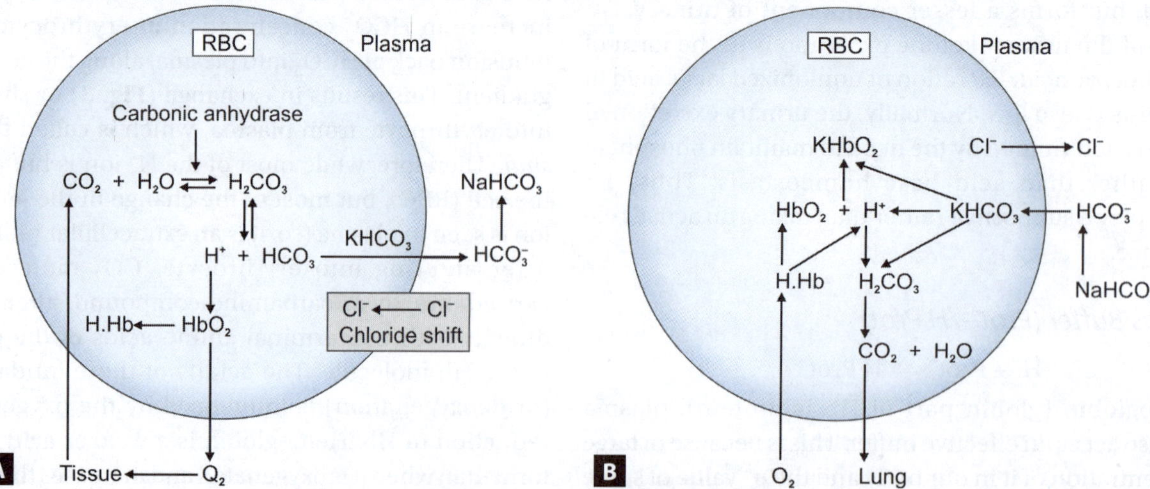

Figs. 4A and B: Chloride shift in (A) tissue and (B) lung.

by compensation, played by the pulmonary and renal excretion or retention of acids or bases.

Pulmonary Compensation

Pulmonary compensation is made by increasing or decreasing the ventilation and is only limited to CO_2 excretion by lungs ($CO_2 \leftarrow H_2O + CO_2 \leftarrow H_2CO_3 \leftarrow H^+ + HCO_3^-$). So, the pulmonary compensation is active only during metabolic acidosis or alkalosis, because respiratory acidosis or alkalosis is caused by the diseases of pulmonary system itself which cannot work now as a compensatory organ. Ventilation is controlled by the chemoreceptor areas of medulla, and by the carotid and aortic bodies. Among them, the medulla plays the primary role and H^+ ion is the predominant mediator, affecting the chemoreceptors of it. The changes in blood PCO_2 cause rapid changes in PCO_2 of cerebrospinal fluid (CSF). This is because the blood–brain barrier is highly permeable to CO_2, but not to H^+ ion. Thus, the rapid increase in CO_2 concentration and subsequently its tension in CSF is associated with rapid increase in H_2CO_3 in CSF which in turn dissociate into a large amount of H^+ ion, but the buffering capacity of CSF to neutralize the H^+ is limited. So, the increase of H^+ in CSF is greater than it would be in tissue and stimulates the medullary chemoreceptor center increasing ventilation and washing out CO_2. Minute ventilation increases 1–4 L/min for every 1 mm Hg increase in $PaCO_2$. Usually, lungs are responsible for eliminating approximately 15 mEq of CO_2, produced everyday as a byproduct of carbohydrate and fat metabolism.

The metabolic acid–base disturbances are only compensated by ventilation. Among these, the metabolic acidosis or alkalosis, caused by the increase or decrease of H^+ from metabolic acid is best compensated by the pulmonary mechanism. The metabolic acidosis or alkalosis caused by the increase or decrease of HCO_3^- concentration is also compensated by pulmonary mechanism. This is described here. Decrease in plasma HCO_3^- level with its concomitant decrease in pH, due to any metabolic causes, will stimulate the ventilation and will excrete more CO_2 and will reduce H_2CO_3 level, despite normal or low PCO_2 in blood. This is only to maintain the ratio of HCO_3^-/H_2CO_3. Conversely, an increase in plasma HCO_3^- concentration with its concomitant increase in pH, due to any metabolic causes will depress the ventilation and retain CO_2. This will increase H_2CO_3 level and maintain the ratio of HCO_3^-/H_2CO_3 and thus pH, though PCO_2 is high. If the decrease of ventilator drive is very strong to cause hypoxia, ventilatory center will be stimulated by the effects of hypoxia on carotid bodies.

Renal compensation: Unlike, the pulmonary compensation which is only limited to metabolic acidosis and alkalosis, the renal compensation extends to both the respiratory and metabolic acidosis and alkalosis; however the renal compensation is three times more active in acidosis than alkalosis. It is performed by four ways: (1) increasing the reabsorption or excretion of filtered HCO_3^-, (2) increasing or decreasing the secretion of H^+ ion from tubular cells in tubular fluid, (3) increasing the excretion of $H_2PO_3^-$ as titrable acids, and (4) increasing the production of ammonia. These four mechanisms of acid–base balance by kidney are probably activated immediately. But their effects are generally not appreciated for 12–24 hours and become maximum at the fifth day.

The amount of HCO_3^- filtered by the kidney is approximately 24 mmol/L and virtually all are reabsorbed. HCO_3^- is not permeable to cell membrane, so it cannot be reabsorbed directly through tubular cell membrane. The *mechanism of reabsorption of filtered HCO_3^- is:* H^+ is passed out into tubular fluid from tubular cells of proximal tubule and reacts with HCO_3^- to form H_2CO_3 which further dissociates into $H_2O + CO_2$. This reaction is catalyzed by carbonic anhydrase, present in large amount in the brush border of tubular cells. Then, this CO_2 is rapidly reabsorbed into tubular cell. Again carbonic anhydrase within the tubular cell converts the CO_2 back into HCO_3^-. The proximal tubules usually reabsorb 80–90% of filtered HCO_3^- along with Na^+ in that process, whereas the remaining 10–20% of HCO_3^- is absorbed in distal tubules. Unlike the secretion of H^+ in proximal tubules, the secretion of H+ in distal tubules is not necessarily linked to absorption of Na^+. The secretion of H^+ in distal tubules is capable of generating a steep gradient of H^+ ion between the tubular fluid and tubular cells. Thus, urinary pH can decrease to as low as 4.4 compared to a pH of 7.4 in plasma **(Fig. 5)**.

Instead of reabsorption of HCO_3^- which is filtered through glomerulus, kidneys also generate new HCO_3^- during the metabolism of glutamine in proximal tubules to compensate acidosis. *The mechanism is:* Metabolism of glutamine produces CO_2 and NH_3. This ammonia constitutes 60% of urinary ammonia, whereas another 40% of NH_3 comes from blood. Acidosis increases markedly the renal production of NH_3 from glutamine. This NH_3 is secreted into tubular fluid. It buffers the H^+ ion of tubular fluid by forming NH_4^+ which is nondiffusible (NH_3 is diffusible) and excreted through urine. Then, CO_2 which is produced by the metabolism of glutamine also diffuses in tubular fluid and combines with H_2O to form HCO_3^- which is then absorbed. If the kidneys are unable to excrete NH_4^+ through urine, the retention of NH_4^+ negates the benefit of the new HCO_3^- generation. Systemic acidosis, hypokalemia, and mineralocorticoids increase ammonia production and thus try to combat (compensate) acidosis.

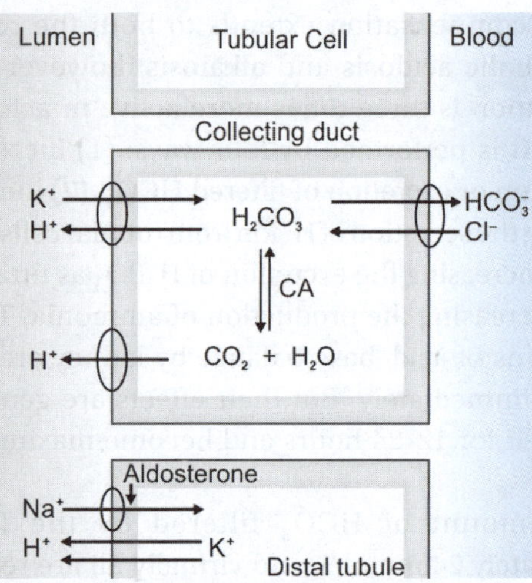

Fig. 5: In the collecting duct, some H⁺ ion secretion occurs in exchange for K⁺, whereas in distal tubule aldosterone helps in the absorption of Na⁺ in exchange of K⁺ and H⁺.

In addition to recovering HCO_3, by reabsorbing it, the kidneys also excrete an amount of acid (H^+) equal to its daily production. It is approximately 70 mmol/day. This may increase to 300 mmol/day in severe acidosis. These acids (H^+) are not excreted directly through urine. Before being excreted directly through urine, these free acids are first buffered by the weaker acids such as ammonia (NH_4^+/ and phosphate ($HPO_4^{2-}/H_2PO_4^-$) in renal tubular fluid. These NH_4^+ and $H_2PO_4^-$ cannot be absorbed due to its charge and are excreted through urine. Therefore, the net result is: H^+ is excreted as $H_2PO_4^-$ and NH_4^+ from body, and the HCO_3^- that is generated in the process of formation of CO_2 from H^+, enter the bloodstream. With a pK value of 6.8, this $HPO_4^{2-}/H_2PO_4^-$ buffer pair is normally present in urine. However, when urinary pH reaches 4.4, then all the phosphates, reaching the distal tubule, is in the form of $H_2PO_4^-$. In such condition, HPO_4^{2-} are no longer available for elimination of more H^+. After complete reabsorption of HCO_3^- and consumption of phosphate buffer, the NH_3/NH_4^+ buffer pair becomes the most important urinary buffer system. However, both the reabsorption of HCO_3^- from tubular fluid and secretion of H^+ in it depends on the active secretion of H^+ which in turn is regulated by the changes in plasma HCO_3^-, plasma pH, and plasma PCO_2.

During metabolic or respiratory acidosis, due to increase in H^+ concentration or decrease in HCO_3^- concentration, there is direct or an indirect increase in concentration of H^+ in tubular cell which in turn stimulates the release of H^+ into the tubular fluids. Increase availability of H^+ in tubular fluid increases the recovery of HCO_3^- ($H^+ + HCO_3^- = H_2CO_3 = CO_2 + H_2O$, $CO_2 \rightarrow$ passed in the tubular cell. Then $CO_2 + H_2O =$

$H_2CO_3 = HCO_3^- + H^+$) and thus try to compensate the acidosis. In acidosis metabolism of glutamine is also stimulated by increasing the availability of H^+ in tubular fluid. But this glutamine mechanism takes up to several days for complete adaptation, because it requires more time for synthesis of new enzymes for more metabolism of glutamine.

Conversely, during metabolic and respiratory alkalosis, there is inhibition of reabsorption of HCO_3^- from the tubular fluid due to reduction of the availability of H^+ in tubular fluid and thus compensates alkalosis.

Since the renal H^+ excretion from tubular cells occurs simultaneously with Na^+ reabsorption for electrical balance, but the process is also affected by aldosterone. Increased aldosterone stimulates reabsorption of Na^+ and simultaneous excretion of H^+ into the tubular fluid, causing increased reabsorption of HCO_3^-, alkalosis, and acidic urine. Thus, Na^+ deficiency and excess of mineralocorticoid is associated with metabolic alkalosis. Na^+ depletion decreases ECF volume and enhances the absorption of Na^+ in the proximal tubule. To maintain neutrality, increased Na^+ absorption causes increased absorption of Cl^-. So, as Cl^- ion decreases in number (<10 mmol/L) reabsorption of HCO_3^- must be increased. Thus, metabolic alkalosis is frequently associated with less urinary Cl^- excretion. The opposite effect occurs with decreased levels of aldosterone.

The excretion of H^+ in proximal tubule is a low gradient, but a high capacity system. The proximal H^+ secretion is increased with hypokalemia, hypercapnia, increased luminal HCO_3^- level, increased tubular Na^+ reabsorption, the presence of nonabsorbable anions (e.g., NO_3^-, SO_4^{2-}, etc.), and increased carbonic anhydrase activity. In the presence of extracellular fluid depletion or metabolic acidosis, the Na^+/ H^+ exchange mechanism is exaggerated, maintaining the extracellular fluid volume at the expense of pH homeostasis Thus, the maximum HCO_3^- reabsorption capacity of the kidney is not a fixed value and varies in response to the above factors.

Contrary to proximal tubules the secretion of H^+ in distal tubule is a high gradient, but a low-capacity system. Unlike proximal tubule, it is influenced by mineralocorticoid activity. In hyperaldosteronism, distal Na^+ reabsorption and in exchange excretion of H^+ and K^+ are increased. In the presence of hypokalemia, H^+ loss is further increased due to maintaining the electroneutrality in tubular fluid. In secondary hyperaldosteronism, the loss of K^+ and H^+ may be less than in primary hyperaldosteronism. This is due to reduction in distal luminal Na^+ flow induced by avid proximal reabsorption of it. Thus, an increase in distal H^+ or K^+ urinary secretion may only become evident when distal Na^+ delivery is increased. An example of it is the use of diuretics.

CARRIAGE OF CARBON DIOXIDE

The discussion regarding the transport of CO_2 in blood is important in this chapter because it is carried in blood as H^+ and HCO_3^- form, which are the important determinants of acid–base balance. Near about, 120 L of CO_2 is contained (stored) in our body at any moment. This CO_2 store can be divided into *three compartments*, depending on the possible rate of exchange of this gas between these compartments. These are: (1) *fast*, (2) *medium*, and (3) *slow compartment*. The fast compartment consists of brain, heart, and kidney with high blood flow, where the tissue PCO_2 levels match with the alveolar PCO_2 very closely. The medium compartment consists mainly of skeletal muscle and the slow compartment consists mainly of fatty tissues. The blood flow in these last two compartments varies from medium (in skeletal muscle) to low (in fatty tissues) **(Table 6)**.

Due to the enormous volume of CO_2 storing capacity in our body, the changes in the arterial PCO_2 will not be sudden due to the sudden changes of ventilation or other causes. It will take much time for a new equilibrium to be attained. But contrary, following a sudden increase in ventilation a new equilibrium is reached after about 20 minutes (the half time is 3–4 minutes). Following a sudden decrease in ventilation the half time for the new equilibrium to reach is 15–20 minutes (i.e., delayed).

After CO_2 is produced into tissues by metabolism, it enters the bloodstream through tissue capillaries and is carried to the lungs where it is liberated. The 100 mL of venous blood carries about 52 mL of CO_2, whereas the 100 mL of arterial blood carries about 48 mL of CO_2. Therefore, the average normal arteriovenous difference of CO_2 content is about 4 mL. In other words, each 100 mL of arterial blood, while passing through tissues, takes up 4 mL of CO_2. Similarly, each 100 mL of venous blood, while passing through lungs, also releases 4 mL of CO_2, so that the blood carries a constant volume (amount) of CO_2 amounting to about 48 mL/100 mL

of blood. This constitutes the "*alkali reserve*", because most of the bicarbonate ion (HCO_3^-) is obtained from it, during equilibrium. Although, much CO_2 is carried in blood, yet blood reaction does not become acid. This proves that, during CO_2 transport, the blood buffers play a very important role.

After CO_2 is produced by metabolism into cell, it comes out through interstitial fluid and enters the plasma. Then, it passes into red cells to reach lungs. The PCO_2 of venous blood, reaching pulmonary capillary, is 46 mm Hg. Whereas the PCO_2 in alveoli is 40 mm Hg. Therefore, a pressure gradient of 6 mm Hg drives CO_2 across the alveolar membrane from venous end of capillary into alveoli.

Carry of CO_2 by Blood from Tissue to Lungs

- *As a physical solution in plasma:* Though, only a small quantity of total CO_2 (5%) is carried in this manner, but it forms a very important portion because this portion is responsible for CO_2 tension (PCO_2) in plasma and acts intermediary between alveolar air and plasma. The solubility coefficient of CO_2 in plasma is 0.03 mmol/L/mm Hg. Therefore, at $PaCO_2$ of 40 mm Hg and at 37°C only $0.03 \times 40 = 1.2$ mmol/L of CO_2 is carried by plasma in this physical form. The CO_2 is also carried in plasma in the form of H_2CO_3, but the concentration of H_2CO_3 in plasma, by which form CO_2 can be carried, is only 1/1,000 of total CO_2 content, due to the lack of carbonic anhydrase (CA) in plasma.

- *As bicarbonate:* The most part of total CO_2 (90%) content in blood is carried in this manner, i.e., in bicarbonate (HCO_3^-) form. Bicarbonates are formed in blood by the following ways **(Fig. 6)**:
  - *In RBC:* Hb remains combined with K and forms potassium bicarbonates in the following way: (1) $CO_2 + H_2O = H_2CO_3$ and (2) $KHb + H_2CO_3 = HHb + KHCO_3$. In RBC carbonic anhydrase helps in this process. In the absence of carbonic anhydrase, the reaction between CO_2 and H_2O to form H_2CO_3 takes 15–30 minutes. But in our body, the RBC in tissue capillaries becomes saturated with CO_2 within 1–2 seconds and the same time is required for the excretion of CO_2 through lungs. This is only possible due to the presence of carbonic anhydrase in RBC. In blood, it is almost exclusively present in red cells. All the other tissues of our body contain it in traces but the pancreas and stomach also contain it in considerable amounts.
  - *In plasma:*
    - *By the phosphate buffers:* Alkaline phosphates combine with carbonic acid and form sodium bicarbonate.

TABLE 6: Differences between venous and arterial blood sample.		
	Venous sample	*Arterial sample*
PO_2	38–42 mm Hg	80–100 mm Hg
PCO_2	44–48 mm Hg	36–44 mm Hg
pH	7.36–7.39	7.38–7.42
SPO_2	75%	95–100%
HCO_3^-	20–24 mEq/L	22–26 mEq/L
Na^+	135–145 mEq/L	Same
K^+	3.5–5.5	Same
Cl^-	95–105 mEq/L	Same

(PCO$_2$: partial pressure of carbon dioxide; PO$_2$: partial pressure of oxygen; SPO$_2$: saturation of peripheral oxygen)

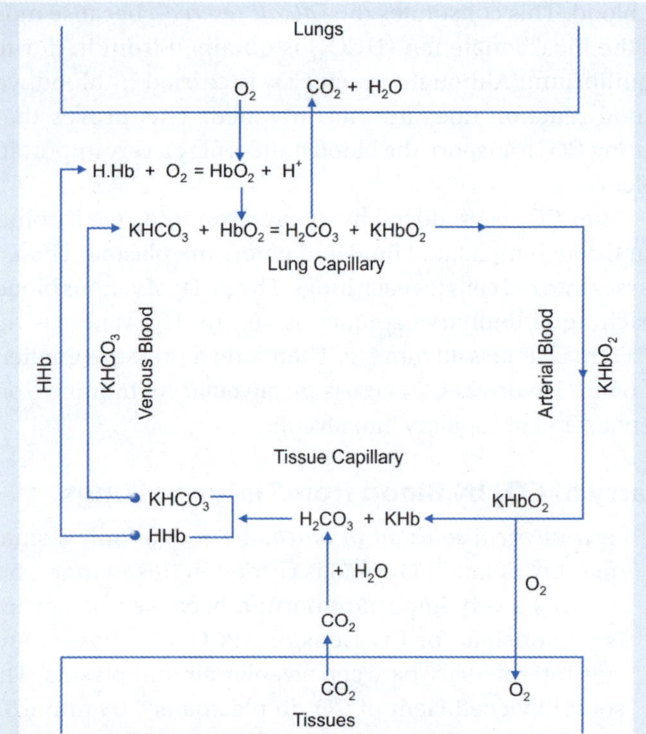

Fig. 6: Schematic representation showing interrelation between the carriage of O_2 and CO_2.

- $Na_2HPO_4 + H_2CO_3 = NaH_2PO_4 + NaHCO_3$
- By plasma proteins: The plasma proteins mostly remain combined with sodium (to be presented as NaPr) and form bicarbonates in the following way: $NaPr + H_2CO_3 = HPr + NaHCO_3$
- Chloride shift or Hamburger phenomenon. This can be described by the following way:

After entering into the plasma from tissue, CO_2 enters the red cell, where with the help of enzyme, carbonic anhydrase (CA), CO_2 reacts with H_2O to form H_2CO_3. This is because RBC is rich in this enzyme. The enzyme carbonic anhydrase is not found in plasma. So, the formation of H_2CO_3 and subsequently bicarbonate cannot take place in plasma or is formed in very little amount. Within the RBC, H_2CO_3 is formed in large amount and dissociates immediately into H^+ and HCO^- ($H_2CO_3 \rightleftharpoons H^+ + HCO_3^-$).

At the tissue level, within red cells, this O_2Hb after giving up the O_2 combine with this H^+ which comes from the dissociation of H_2CO_3 ($Hb + H^+ \rightleftharpoons HHb$) and favors the formation of HCO^- by displacing the equilibrium (of the bicarbonate forming equation) to the right according to the law of mass action ($H_2CO_3 \rightleftharpoons H^+ + HCO^-$). Then, this bicarbonate (HCO^-) diffuses out of the red cell into plasma, and to maintain the ionic equilibrium chloride ions (Cl^-) diffuse back in the opposite direction from plasma into the red cells. This is called the chloride shift or *Hamburger*

effect (phenomenon). Thus, CO_2 is carried to the lungs as bicarbonate (HCO_3^-).

When the blood reaches lung capillaries, then all the reactions occur in reverse direction. Due to pressure gradient of CO_2 of 6 mm Hg (plasma PCO_2 = 46 mm Hg and alveolar PCO_2 = 40 mm Hg), the CO_2 which is dissolved in a physical state in plasma, diffuses out into alveoli across the alveolar membrane from plasma. So, the physically dissolved CO_2 concentration in the plasma falls, then the pressure gradient of dissolved CO_2 between RBC and plasma widens. So, CO_2 leaves the red cells and is dissolved in plasma, and is finally excreted through lungs. To produce more CO_2 in red cells, HCO_3^- again enters the red cells in exchange of Cl^- (Cl^- comes out of red cell → opposite to the chloride shift or Hamburger effect). In the red cell, HCO_3^- combine with H^+ to form CO_2. Here, the equation $CO_2 + H_2O \rightleftharpoons H_2CO_3 \rightleftharpoons H^+ + HCO_3^-$ is shifted to left. H^+ is obtained from Hb, because Hb takes O_2 from alveoli and releases H^+. This explains how CO_2 comes out of the red cells and is excreted through lungs. Plasma bicarbonate (HCO_3^-), therefore, plays a very important role as the principal storehouse of CO_2 and carries it in blood.

- *As a carbamino compound:* 5% of the total body CO_2 is carried within plasma in this manner. Here, CO_2 combines with the amino group of globin (protein) part of Hb to form carbaminohemoglobin. In this process, the NH_2 radicle of the globin part of Hb combines with one molecule of CO_2 as free gas, but not as bicarbonate. It does not require the help of carbonic anhydrase.

$$Hb.NH_2 + CO_2 \rightleftharpoons Hb.NH.COOH$$

Smaller amount of CO_2 also combines with the amino group of plasma protein in similar fashion, like globin (protein) part of Hb to form the carbamino compound. The combination between CO_2 and plasma protein also takes place directly and no enzyme is required.

Thus, it will be seen that the CO_2 is carried out in the blood in three forms and 100 mL of venous blood carries about 52 mL of CO_2 as follows:

- In physical solution (2.7 mL)
- *As bicarbonate (45.7 mL):* Bicarbonates are formed in four ways: (1) with NaPr, (2) with Na_2HPO_4, (3) with Na of NaCl helped by "chloride shift", and (4) with KHb. These are the chief forms in which CO_2 is carried. A large part of this bicarbonate remains permanently in the plasma and constitutes the so called *alkali reserve.*
- *As carbamino compounds (3.7 mL):* These are chiefly formed in red cells (2.6 mL) with the protein of Hb and only in traces in plasma (1.1 mL) with plasma protein. It constitutes about 5–10% of total CO_2 carriage and is responsible for a large part of the normal arteriovenous difference.

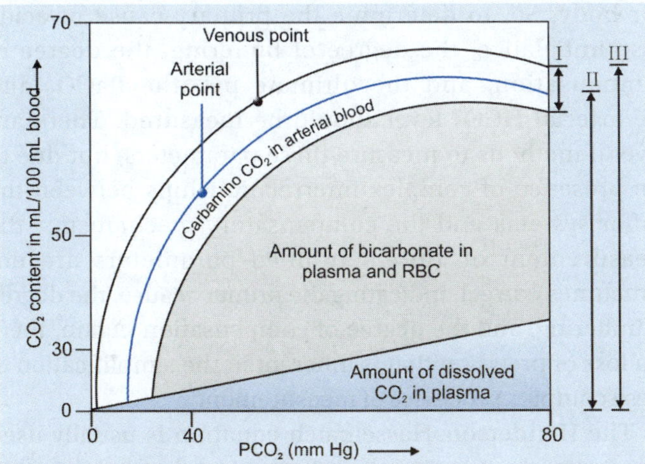

Fig. 7: CO_2 dissociation curve of whole blood. (CO_2: carbon dioxide; PCO_2: partial pressure of carbon dioxide; RBC: red blood cells)

Note:

I. Carbamino CO_2 in venous blood

II. Total CO_2 content in arterial blood

III. Total CO_2 content in venous blood

Carbon Dioxide Dissociation Curve (Fig. 7)

The relationship between the CO_2 concentration and CO_2 tension (PCO_2) in blood is depicted by this curve. Oxygenation of blood is the main determinant of the position of this curve because the more deoxygenated the blood will be, the more CO_2 it will carry at a given PCO_2 and change the curve. This is called the *Haldane effect*. The upper portion of the curve is for the fully deoxygenated blood and the lower portion of the curve is for the fully oxygenated blood. The major part of the Haldane effect is due to the increased carriage of CO_2 by reduced Hb as a carbamino compound. In addition, the carriage of CO_2 as bicarbonate is also increased.

Reduced or deoxygenated Hb buffers the H^+. Thus, by absorbing H^+, the reduced Hb displaces the equilibrium of this equation to the right and increases the concentration of bicarbonate (HCO_3^-), and produces the chloride shift (Hamburger effect). Thus, due to the Haldane effect, at the capillary level CO_2 uptake and due to the Bohr effect, at the lung level CO_2 elimination is facilitated by shifting the equation once to the right (at capillary level) and then to the left (at lung level) respectively.

◼ ELIMINATION OF H^+

Rapid Elimination by Respiration

Carbon dioxide produced by the oxidation of substrates produces H^+ ion load in our body which is excreted again as CO_2 through lungs, leaving H_2O. This equation is like that $CO_2 + H_2O \rightleftharpoons H_2CO_3 \rightleftharpoons H^+ + HCO_3^-$. After production into cell, CO_2 readily diffuses across the cell membrane and produce the changes of pH in both intracellular fluid (ICF) and ECF. The H^+ ion directly cannot diffuse through cell membrane, so it passes through the cell membrane in disguise of CO_2. Thus, increased CO_2 production in a normal situation stimulates respiration and balance H^+ concentration (in turn CO_2 concentration) rapidly. The carbonic acid and bicarbonate chemical buffer or the bicarbonate buffer system is ineffective here. Carbonic acid remains in equilibrium with the dissolved CO_2 content of body fluids and can therefore be eliminated through lungs. Addition of H^+ from the metabolic acids also increases H_2CO_3 at the expense of a reduction in bicarbonate and is eliminated as CO_2. The H^+ (of metabolic origin) + HCO_3^- = $H_2CO_3 = H_2O + CO_2 \rightarrow$ lungs

Slow Elimination by Kidney

Slow and long-term control of H^+ elimination by kidney depends on three mechanisms:

1. *Reabsorption of filtered bicarbonate:* Presence of carbonic anhydrase in renal tubular cells facilitates the production of H^+ from CO_2 load. $CO_2 + H_2O \rightleftharpoons H_2CO_3 \rightleftharpoons H^+ + HCO_3^-$. This H^+ passes in the lumen of proximal tubule. Normally daily 5,000 nmol HCO_3^- is filtered at glomerulus. This HCO_3^- reacts with H^+ and CO_2 is produced which diffuses back in the tubular cells. Thus, there is no net H^+ excretion, resulting from this action, but prevents the loss of filtered base. The smaller amount of H^+ is secreted in the distal and collecting ducts to make the urine acidic with pH of 4.6.

   During acidosis, the excess H^+ passes in the proximal tubular lumen and after preserving all the filtered HCO_3^-, extra H^+ is excreted. This secondary response is slow to develop and takes 5 days for full compensation to occur. In the absence of CA or when acetazolamide is used then nonavailability of H^+ causes HCO^- to be excreted as $NaHCO_3$ and plasma HCO_3^- falls. So, in acidosis acetazolamide should never be used.

2. *Buffers:* 20–30 mmol of H^+ which is excreted daily through urine as titrable acid, is combined to monohydrogen phosphate and excreted as dihydrogen phosphate (titrable acid). $H^+ + HPO_4 \rightleftharpoons H_2PO_4$ ($Na_2HPO_4 \rightarrow NaH_2PO_4$).

3. *Formation of ammonia:* NH_3^+ is formed in renal tubular epithelial cells throughout the nephron. Among this, 60% is formed from glutamine by deamination and 30–35% comes from artery as free NH_3^+. This NH_3^+ then diffuses into the renal tubular lumen and binds to neutralize H^+ by producing a nondiffusible (nonabsorbable) ammonium ion (NH_4^+). This is excreted daily and may rise to 700 mmol/day in severe acidosis. Thus, the maximum renal acid secretion as in diabetic ketoacidosis is approximately 700–750 mmol/day, of which two-thirds is NH_4^+ and one-third is titrable acid (TA) which is discussed earlier.

■ MEASUREMENT OF ACID–BASE BALANCE

The acid–base disturbances in our body occur, when the disease processes cause the disruption of normal pH homeostatic mechanisms or when the acid or alkali burden (more rarely) exceeds the adaptive capacity (or reserve) of compensatory mechanisms.

- The normal arterial pH usually ranges from 7.36 to 7.42 from its mean value of 7.40. It is maintained by intracellular and extracellular buffers. Ultimately, these buffers work through the renal and respiratory regulatory mechanisms.
- The intracellular pH ranges from 6.4 to 7.35.
- The pH is negative logarithm to base 10 ($-\log_{10}$) of the hydrogen ion concentration, expressed in mol/L.
- The pH of 7.4 represents $[H^+]$ of 40 nmol/L.
- The pH rising to 7.5 represents a drop in $[H^+]$ to 32 nmol/L.
- The pH of 7.0 is equal to $[H^+]$ of 100 nmol/L.
- The center of understanding of acid–base disturbance is the understanding of carbonic acid and bicarbonate buffer pairing. This is expressed by Henderson–Hasselbalch equation such as $[H^+] = 181 \times PaCO_2/[HCO_3^-]$, 181 is the dissociation constant or coefficient of carbonic acid in the presence of carbonic anhydrase. This buffer pairing system is ubiquitous. It is also the dominant physiological buffer system in man and most importantly it is in equilibrium with all other buffer systems of our body.
- A combination of both the respiratory and metabolic acidosis, or alkalosis may present at the same time with normal pH value, compensating with each other.
- The dissociation constant (K) is affected by the changes in temperature, for example, the pH of water at 25°C is 7.0, whereas it is changed to 6.8 at 37°C. So, during the measurement of pH, the temperature should be taken into consideration.

The respiratory acidosis or alkalosis is the change or a potential change in pH, resulting from the alteration in $PaCO_2$. The metabolic acidosis or alkalosis is the change or a potential change in pH, resulting from the alterations in nonvolatile acids in blood such as lactic acid, keto acid, β-hydroxy-butyric acid, sulfuric acid, phosphoric acid, pyruvic acid, etc., or when the primary disturbance is in the control of plasma bicarbonate concentration (not primary disturbance is in the control of plasma PCO_2). Though all the types of combination are possible, so the PCO_2 measurement quantifies the respiratory component and the "base excess" or base deficit (BD) (HCO_3^- excess or deficit) measurement quantify the metabolic component of acid–base balance.

Despite the presence of buffer and other compensatory mechanisms, the acid–base disturbances do occur in our body. So, to determine the primary cause of acid–base imbalance, the degree of buffering, the degree of compensation, and the ultimate pH, the $PaCO_2$ and the arterial HCO_3^- level should be measured. There are several methods to measure these parameters, but due to the presence of complex interrelationships between the buffer systems and the compensatory mechanisms, the measurement of aforementioned parameters are not sometimes correct, indicating the primary cause, the degree of buffering, and the degree of compensation. Again, there is a loss of precision that is inherent in the simplification of these complex processes of measurement.

The Henderson–Hasselbalch equation is usually used to measure the bicarbonate buffer system, but several other different methods are also utilized to correct for the presence of other buffer system, by allowing one to evaluate the entire system as a bicarbonate buffer. These include *alkali reserve*, *standard bicarbonate*, *base excess*, and *buffer base*. The alkali reserve and the standard bicarbonate are no longer in use for clinical practice. Base excess and buffer base are still in use and act by compensating the buffering capacity of noncarbonic buffer system. In this compensation, other buffer systems are converted to the equivalent of bicarbonate buffer in which the change in HCO_3^- level directly reflects the change in H^+ ion of the system.

The acid–base disorders also can be evaluated from CO_2 titration curves, derived from the present values of pH, PCO_2, and HCO_3^- concentration. Clinical values are then compared with the normal human values and the deviation is quantified for both the acute and chronic disorders. This *in vivo method (titration curve)* is superior to the *in vitro methods* (measurement of pH, PCO_2, and HCO_3^-), because it recognizes the changes in pH due to specific causes and thus presents a very dynamic scenario.

Partial Pressure of Carbon Dioxide

The PCO_2 of a gas mixture, saturated with water vapor at 37°C is given by the equation: $PCO_2 = FCO_2 \times (P_B - 47)$ mmHg. The FCO_2 is the fractional concentration of CO_2 in this gas mixture, P_B is the barometric pressure (760 mm Hg), and 47 mm Hg is the saturated vapor pressure of water at 37°C. The PCO_2 in plasma is best understood by considering a gas–liquid system which is in equilibrium. The CO_2 tension in a liquid is equal to that in the gas mixture when no net exchange of CO_2 occurs between these two phases. At any given equilibrium, the CO_2 content of plasma is a reflection of PCO_2 of its gas phase. The PCO_2 of blood is thus defined as the PCO_2 in a gas mixture which, when in contact with the blood results in no net exchange of CO_2 between these two phases. The normal value of $PaCO_2$ is 35–42 mm Hg.

Carbon Dioxide Titration Curve

The consideration and the application of the Henderson–Hasselbalch equation is the core to the understanding of the acid–base balance. Both the metabolic and respiratory factors are represented in this unique equation. This equation also links the pH to the molar concentration of bicarbonate and carbonic acid in plasma, but the constants in the equation cannot be predicted accurately **(Fig. 8A)**.

This equation also says us that any alteration of PCO_2 will be associated with a predictable change in pH. If the PCO_2 is either increased or decreased and time is allowed for a steady state or for an equilibrium to be reached, then the CO_2 titration curve (straight line using a pH and PCO_2 plot) is obtained **(Fig. 7)**. When a titration is performed adding deliberately varying amounts of acid, then a family of curves, approximately parallel to and to the left of the normal curve is found. The more acid is added, the further is the curve shifted to the left. Thus, a nonrespiratory (metabolic) acidosis produces curves shifted to the left and a nonrespiratory (metabolic) alkalosis produces curves shifted to the right. With increasing metabolic acidosis, the buffering capabilities will also increase, which causes the left-shifted curves to be more vertical and the right-shifted curves to be more horizontal **(Fig. 8B)**.

During the construction of CO_2 titration curve, arterial blood is tonometered (measured of PCO_2) with CO_2 gases of two known, but of different concentration. If pH is measured after tonometry, then an *in vitro* blood CO_2 titration curve could be constructed **(Fig. 8C)**. Next, the actual PCO_2 of any original blood sample can be determined by interpolation, if its pH is measured. In general, it is realized that the titration curve of blood from acidotic patients lay to the left of this curve, and from alkalosis patients lay to the right. But it was appreciated that the Hb concentration altered the slope of the curve and induces errors. Thus, a number of parameters were used to get rid of these errors. These are base excess, buffer base, and standard bicarbonate **(Fig. 8C)**.

When the normal blood is diluted to different Hb concentration and thereafter is equilibrated with gas mixtures of different PCO_2, then this yields a family of PCO_2/pH curves, intersecting at pH of 7.4 and PCO_2 of 40 mm Hg. After that if a strong acid or alkali is added, then different families of curves are produced **(Fig. 8D)**. Now if the intersections of each family are joined, then a base excess curve is produced. The value of this base excess curve is thus independent of Hb concentration and is a useful index of only patient's metabolic acid–base status (not the patient's respiratory acid–base status). It was found empirically that the correction of metabolic acidosis could often be obtained by the infusion of sodium bicarbonate in mmol/L which can be determined by the formula: 0.3 + base excess × weight in kg **(Fig. 8D)**.

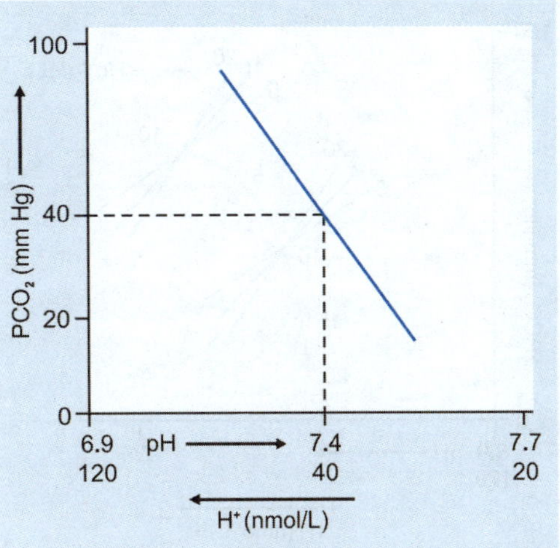

Fig. 8A: In vivo CO_2 titration curve.

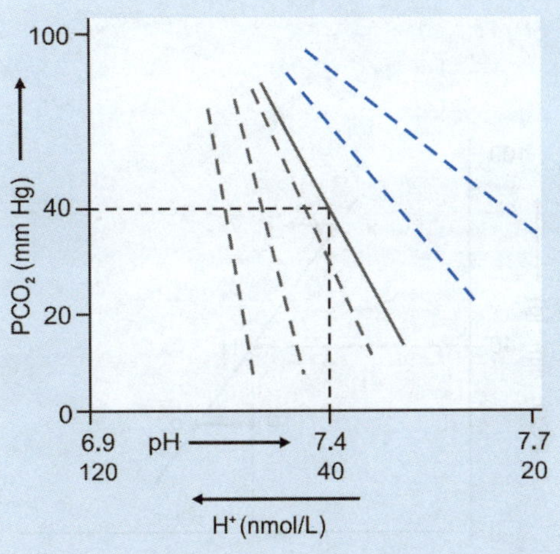

Fig. 8B: Family of *in vivo* CO_2 titration curves in nonrespiratory (metabolic) acidosis (dotted lines on the left side of normal line) and alkalosis (dotted lines on right side of normal line).

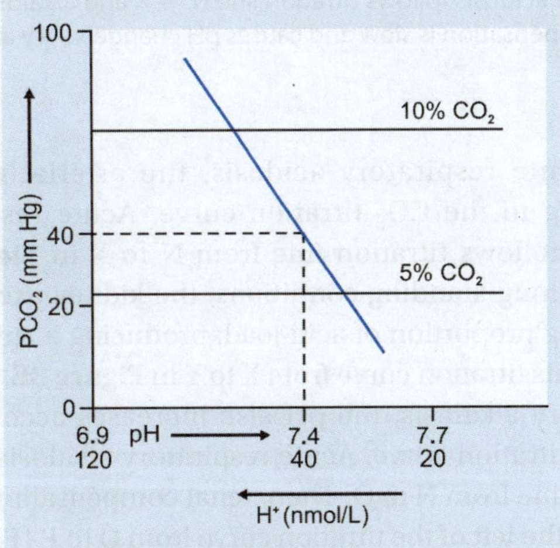

Fig. 8C: Measurement of PCO_2 and construction of in vitro CO_2 titration curve.

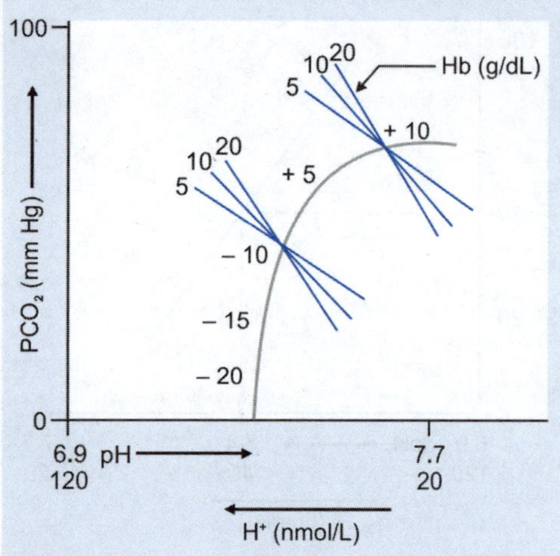

Fig. 8D: Construction of "base excess" curve.

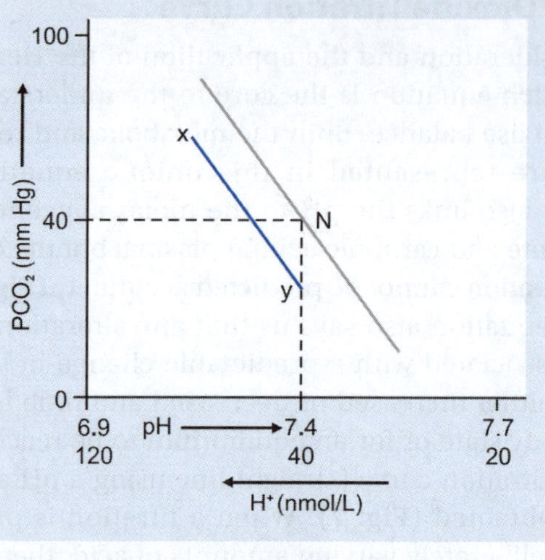

Fig. 8F: Acid–base change during nonrespiratory (or metabolic) acidosis. Respiratory stimulation allows pH to move N → x. In the absence of respiratory compensation, pH would be y.

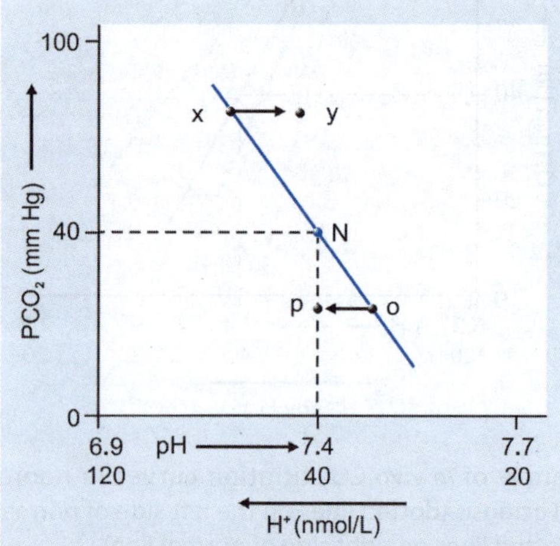

Fig. 8E: pH–PCO₂ changes during respiratory disturbances. Acute respiratory acidosis follows titration line N → X and alkalosis N → O. Renal compensation is slow and causes pH change x → y and o → p.

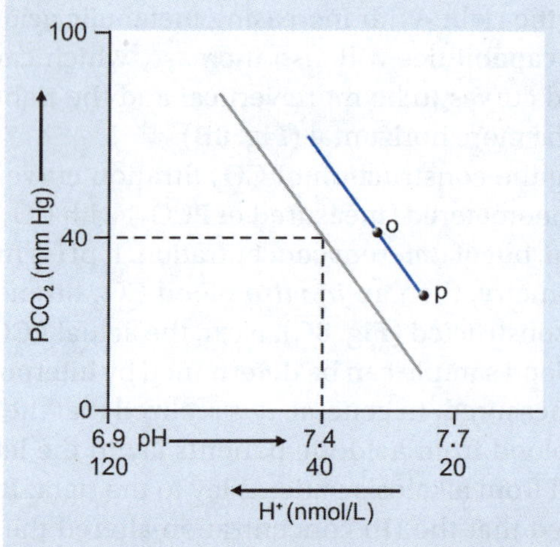

Fig. 8G: Acid–base changes during metabolic alkalosis. Respiratory compensation allows pH to move N → O. In the absence of respiratory compensation pH would be p.

In acute respiratory acidosis, the arterial pH falls according to the CO_2 titration curve. Acute respiratory acidosis follows titration line from N to X in **Figure 8E**. Then, in long-standing conditions, the kidney excretes an increasing proportion of acid load, producing a shift to the right of this titration curve from X to Y in **Figure 8E**. In acute respiratory alkalosis, the pH also increases according to the CO_2 titration curve. Acute respiratory alkalosis follows titration line from N to O. Then, renal compensation causes a shift to the left of the titration curve from O to P **(Fig. 8E)**.

In metabolic acidosis, the CO_2 titration curve is shifted to the left in **Figure 8F**. In metabolic acidosis, the ventilation is stimulated by the peripheral chemoreceptor drive, so that the CSF and arterial PCO_2 and HCO_3^- concentration are lowered until the pH returns almost to normal. If the pH is corrected rapidly by the administration of bicarbonate, then the PCO_2 of CSF will rise and pH will fall stimulating the central chemoreceptors and replacing the arterial metabolic acidosis with a respiratory alkalosis. In metabolic alkalosis, the CO_2 titration curve is shifted to the right in **Figure 8G**.

There is usually the same respiratory compensation, but less than in a metabolic acidosis. So, the PCO_2 is elevated, which reduces the pH of CSF and leads to an increase in CSF the concentration of HCO_3^- **(Fig. 8G)**.

Standard Bicarbonate

It is the bicarbonate concentration (HCO_3^- in mmol/L) in fully oxygenated blood which has been equilibrated at 37°C with a gas mixture having a PCO_2 of 40 mm Hg. The normal range of standard bicarbonate (HCO_3^-) concentration is 22–26 mmol/L (or mEq/L). It is an effective evaluation of only the metabolic status of acid–base balance. A standard bicarbonate level in excess of 26 mEq/L is a sign of the presence of metabolic alkalosis. In case of bicarbonate, the numerical value of mmoL/L and mEq/L is same, as the valency of bicarbonate is one. A standard HCO_3^- level <22 mEq/L is a sign of metabolic acidosis. To determine the metabolic acid–base status, among the parameters such as the base excess, buffer base, and standard bicarbonate, the first one is the most useful and widely used. This can be calculated by extrapolation from the pH and PCO_2 value, using Siggaard-Andersen (SA) nomogram (A nomogram is a graph with several scale lines, laid on the graph, intersects the scale at the related values of variables. The values of any two variables can be used to find the values of others).

Siggaard-Andersen nomogram: pH = pK + log $[HCO_3^-]$/$[H_2CO_3]$. As H_2CO_3 concentration is directly proportional to PCO_2, therefore H_2CO_3 in the above equation, for bicarbonate buffering system, can be replaced by α PCO_2. This α is the solubility coefficient for CO_2 (0.03 mmol/L/mm Hg). The equation then becomes: pH = pK + log $[HCO_3^-]$/α PCO_2. The value of pK for bicarbonate buffer system is 6.1 at 37°C. Again at PCO_2 of 40 mm Hg. the plasma bicarbonate concentration is about 25 mmol/L. So, pH = 6.1 + log 25/(0.03 × 40) = 7.4. Numerous graphic representations of this Henderson–Hasselbalch equation have been suggested. The important graphic representation is a pH–bicarbonate plot and the pH–log PCO_2 plot. Siggaard–Andersen nomogram is the graphic representation of Henderson–Hasselbalch equation in which pH is plotted against log $PaCO_2$.

Lines can be plotted on this nomogram showing the changes in pH which occur when a sample with normal Hb is equilibrated with various concentration of CO_2. An arterial blood sample is taken and equilibrated with two gas mixtures containing different but known concentration of CO_2 and then pH of the sample is measured. Two points are therefore plotted on the nomogram and joined by a straight line. This is called the *buffer line* and it describes the relationship between pH and $PaCO_2$ in that particular blood sample. The pH of the patient's blood is measured anaerobically in the sample. Using this pH value and the buffer line, the CO_2 of the sample can be interpolated from the nomogram. The buffer line will cross the horizontal plasma bicarbonate line at a $PaCO_2$ of 40 mm Hg, where the bicarbonate value can be read. This is the *standard* bicarbonate.

Base Excess

It is not uncommon that there may be a mixed respiratory and metabolic acid–base disturbance. Thus, the base excess measurement is one way of quantifying the metabolic component, when there is presence of mixed acid–base disturbances. The two examples will best illustrate this term, i.e., base excess.

First Example

Let the initial measurements of an arterial blood sample are: pH is 7.6, $PaCO_2$ is 55 mm Hg, and Hb is 15 mg/dL. Then the blood sample is kept at 37°C and equilibrated with a CO_2 gas mixture to make the $PaCO_2$ 40 mm Hg. Therefore, it will remove the respiratory component of acid–base abnormality. The pH is now 7.7. Next, a strong acid is added to titrate the pH back to 7.4. The amount of acid required is found to be 20 mmol/L; therefore the base excess of the original sample is 20 mmol/L

Second Example

Let the initial measurements of an arterial blood sample are: pH is 7.3, and $PaCO_2$ is 20 mm Hg, and Hb is 15 g/dL. Then the blood sample is kept at 37°C and equilibrated with CO_2 gas mixture to make the $PaCO_2$ 40 mm Hg. Now the pH is 7. Then a strong alkali is added to bring the pH to 7.4. The amount of alkali required is 15 mmol/L. Therefore, the base excess is –15 mmol/L. This also can be expressed as *base deficit* which is 15 mmol/L. Both the expressions such as base excess with +ve value or deficit with –ve value are commonly used. Usually, there should normally be neither a base excess, nor deficit. So, the normal valve for base excess or deficit is zero.

Therefore, it is defined as a titrable base that can be titrated to pH 7.4 at PCO_2 of 40 mm Hg and at temperature of 37°C. This is the base concentration of whole blood, measured by titration against a strong acid or base to pH 7.4, at PCO_2 of 40 mm Hg, and at 37°C. For acidosis (base deficit) titration is carried out with a strong base and for alkalosis titration is carried out by strong acid (base excess). Base excess is measured in mmol/L and is an attempt to quantify the excess or deficit of HCO_3^-. The normal range of base excess varies between –2 to +2 mmol/L (or 12 mEq/L). It represents residual buffering capacity.

The BE <–2 signifies the presence of metabolic acidosis, whereas BE more than +2 signifies the presence of metabolic alkalosis. Nowadays, it is not necessary to perform this time-consuming titration to measure the base excess. In practice, the base excess is derived from: (1) Siggaard–Andersen nomogram, (2) acid–base slide rule (Severing Hans), or (3) mathematically as in many automatic blood gas analyzers.

The base excess (unlike buffer base) measurement is independent of Hb concentration. Altering the Hb concentration of a blood sample would result in a change in pH and PCO_2 but no change in base excess.

Buffer Base

It is the sum of concentration of all the buffer anions, present in blood such as HCO_3^-, phosphate, protein, Hb, etc. The normal values of buffer base depend on Hb concentration. So, it is reduced in anemia. Apart from the changes in Hb concentration, it is increased in metabolic alkalosis and decreased in metabolic acidosis. A rise in PCO_2 in respiratory acidosis does not affect it. Because although $[HCO_3^-]$ increases, the extra $[H^+]$ combines with Hb, so that the concentration of this ion is correspondingly reduced **(Table 7)**.

$$CO_2 + H_2O \rightleftharpoons H_2CO_3 \rightleftharpoons H^+ + HCO_3^-$$
$$\downarrow\uparrow$$
$$H^+ + Hb^- \rightleftharpoons H.Hb$$

pH Measurement

H^+ concentration is measured directly by a glass electrode with a membrane that is only permeable to H^+ ions. Then, derived pH is displayed on a meter. Partial pressure of carbon dioxide is measured by the Severinghaus electrode which incorporates a modification of the technique where a CO_2 permeable membrane is used. PO_2 is measured by Clark polarographic electrode **(Table 8)**.

Our concept regarding the acid–base balance is now changing. In the past, we concentrate on the concentration of H^+, pH, PCO_2, standard bicarbonate, base excess/base deficit, etc. But now the world is thinking on strong ion difference (SID), PCO_2, total weak acid concentration (A_{TOT}), etc., to explain in best way the acid–base balance in physiological system. SID is the sum of all strong, completely dissociated cations such as Na^+, K^+, Ca^{2+}, and Mg^{2+} minus the sum of all strong anions such as Cl^-, lactate, HCO_3^-, etc. When we calculate the SID, it indicates some unmeasured ions. PCO_2 is important because it is an independent variable as respiration is going on.

▌ TECHNIQUE FOR ARTERIAL BLOOD–GAS SAMPLING

The acid–base status of most of our body tissues is reflected in that tissue's venous blood. But the brain is an important exception to this rule, as the lactate produced by the anaerobic metabolism of the brain, is confined by the blood-brain barrier, brain cells, and CSF. Thus, the assessment of the whole body acid–base status may be determined by the analysis of mixed venous blood and this can only be achieved by a pulmonary artery or at least, right ventricular sampling which is very difficult. So, most investigators use arterial blood as "oxygenated mixed venous blood" to measure the different parameters of acid–base balance. This has the additional advantage that the arterial PO_2 may be determined from this same sample.

An alternative, which is particularly useful in small children, is to use a sample of capillary blood. If this is taken from a warm, vasodilated part of the periphery, usually the hand or heel, then it has been shown that the PCO_2 is within 0.5 mm Hg and the pH is within 0.005 units of simultaneously obtained arterial samples. But this capillary sampling is unsuitable for the determination of PO_2.

The samples for arterial blood gas analysis are taken into a syringe whose potential dead space is filled with heparin in concentration of 1,000 units/ml. There must not be any air

TABLE 7: Uncompensated changes in acid–base status.

Acid–base state	pH	Plasma bicarbonate	PCO₂
Normal	7.35–7.45	22–28 mmol/L	36–46 mm Hg
• Metabolic acidosis	Low	Low	Normal
• Metabolic alkalosis	High	High	Normal
• Respiratory acidosis	Low	Normal	High
• Respiratory alkalosis	High	Normal	Low

TABLE 8: Acid–base status.

Acid–base state	Standard bicarbonate in mmol/L	Base excess in mmol/L	Total buffer base in mmol/L
Normal	22–26	0 ± 3	44–48
• Metabolic acidosis	Low	Negative	Low
• Metabolic alkalosis	High	Positive	High
• Respiratory acidosis	Normal	Normal	Normal
• Respiratory alkalosis	Normal	Normal	Normal

bubble in this syringe and the blood should be well mixed with heparin. Excess heparin reduces the value of measured pH by virtue of its own acidity. Blood should be taken by direct arterial puncture from a brachial, radial, or femoral artery or withdrawn from an indwelling arterial cannula, taking care to avoid air bubbles.

Measurements should be done immediately, after drawing of blood sample, because the metabolism will continue within the blood cells at room temperature and this will increase PCO_2 and decrease PO_2. Alternatively, the sample should be capped and stored in crushed ice. The temperature of the patient and the inspired O_2 concentration should be noted. The diffusion of CO_2 across the wall of plastic syringes does not produce a change in CO_2 tension within the first three hours of storage.

Capillary samples are often used in babies and are taken into special pre-heparinized glass capillary tubes. The PCO_2 and pH of capillary blood are close to those of arterial blood, taken at the same time. The PO_2 is less reliable.

■ DISTURBANCES OF ACID–BASE BALANCE

During the management of a patient with severe acid–base disturbances, it is very essential to keep in mind the clinical condition of patient, while evaluating the laboratory results. An isolated pH measurement is totally valueless without an arterial PCO_2, and in the case of respiratory disease without an arterial PO_2, as well. Free H^+ are constantly being produced by our body, but changes in H^+ concentration are kept to a minimum by different buffering and compensating mechanisms of the body. Respiratory and renal compensatory mechanism comes into play, when plasma buffering capacity is exceeded, in an attempt to achieve a normal plasma pH.

Classically, the disturbances of acid–base balance are divided into respiratory and metabolic acidosis or alkalosis and should be considered in relation to Henderson–Hasselbalch equation which normally works in the following manner:

$$pH = p^K + log\ [HCO_3^-/H_2CO_3] \qquad I$$
$$= p^K + log\ 24/1.2\ (normal\ plasma\ [HCO_3^-]\ is$$
$$24\ mmol/L\ and\ [H_2CO_3]\ is\ 12\ mmol/L)$$
$$= p^K + log\ 20$$
$$= 6.1 + log\ 20\ (p^K\ of\ bicarbonate\ system\ is\ 6.1)$$
$$= 6.1 + 1.301\ (log\ 20 = 1.301)$$
$$= 7.4\ \textbf{(Fig. 8H)}.$$

Despite the apparent clear-cut disturbances of acid–base balance, in practice, there are often mixed disorders. In such situations, when we are confronted with an estimation of blood gases, then it is important to isolate the most abnormal parameter (primary abnormality), since

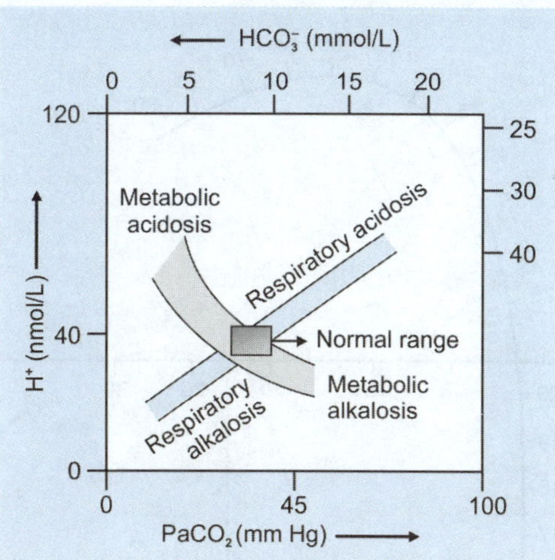

Fig. 8H: This is a Flenley acid–base diagram, which shows the changes in blood H^+ concentration, $PaCO_2$, and HCO_3^- level in stable compensated acid–base disorders. The rectangle, at the center of the diagram, indicates the limits of normal ranges for H^+ concentration and $PaCO_2$. The bands extending from the central rectangle represent 90% confidence limits for a single disturbance of acid–base balance. When the point is obtained by plotting H^+ concentration against $PaCO_2$ and it does not fall within one of the bands, then compensation is incomplete or a mixed disorder is present.

the other abnormalities are possibly secondary to this or of compensatory in nature. So, in these circumstances, an acid–base diagram may be very helpful. The Flenley acid–base diagram is an alternative way of looking at the acid–base disturbances and is in fact a modification of the Siggaard–Andersen nomogram in which bicarbonate buffer system only is considered. In it (Flenley acid–base diagram), the linear relationship between the H^+ ion activity and $PaCO_2$ is plotted on a graph in which the isopleths of equal HCO_3^- concentration radiate out as a fan-shaped manner from the origin or center. The fan-shaped radiation represents 95% of confidence limits which are shown in **Figure 8H**. During acid–base disturbances, the serial values of blood gases are plotted on it to define the nature of disturbances and its progress.

On this acid–base diagram, a point to the left of normal pH (of 7.4) implies an acidosis and a point to the right of the normal pH implies an alkalosis. The plasma bicarbonate can be read directly. **Figure 8H** is of great value during therapy, to monitor the changes in response to the treatment.

Siggaard–Andersen Nomogram

This nomogram is very useful to plot the acid–base characteristics of a sample of arterial blood. This nomogram has a vertical axis which indicates PCO_2 and a horizontal axis which indicates pH. Thus, any point to the right of a vertical line through pH 7.4 indicates alkalosis and any

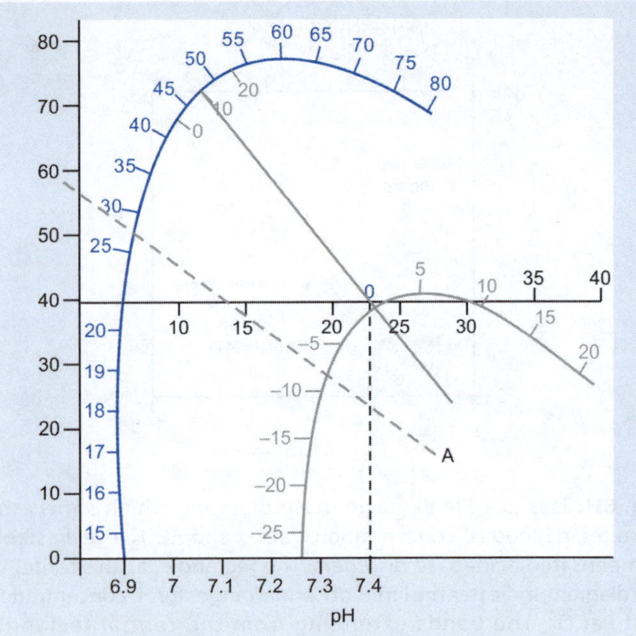

Fig. 9: Siggaard–Andersen nomogram (schematic diagram).

point to the left indicates acidosis. Similarly, the position of a point below or above the horizontal line through PCO_2 of 40 mm Hg indicates the degree of hyper- or hypoventilation, respectively **(Fig. 9)**.

If a solution containing $NaHCO_3$ and no buffer is equilibrated with a blood sample containing a gas mixture of various amounts of CO_2, then at equilibrium the pH and PCO_2 value would fall along the line A or a line parallel to it. If buffers are not present, the steepness of the line will be greater and if buffers are present, the slope of the line will be greater. For normal blood containing 15 g of Hb, the CO_2 titration line will pass through the 15 g/dL mark on the Hb scale (point B) which is situated on the underside of the upper curved scale. This line will also pass through the point where the PCO_2 = 40 mm Hg and pH = 74 lines will interact. When the Hb content of the blood is low, then there is a significant loss of buffering capacity. It will cause the diminished slope of the CO_2 titration line; however blood always contains some buffer in addition to Hb. So, the line drawn from the zero point on the Hb scale and through the normal PCO_2–pH intercept is steeper than the line for a solution containing no buffers.

For clinical use, the arterial blood is drawn anaerobically and its pH is measured. The pH of the same blood is again measured after equilibration with two gas mixtures containing different known amount of CO_2. This pH value at known CO_2 concentration is plotted and connected to provide the CO_2 titration line for the blood sample. The pH of the blood sample before equilibrium is plotted on this line and the PCO_2 of the sample is read from the vertical scale.

The standard bicarbonate content of the sample is indicated by the point at which the CO_2 titration line intersects the bicarbonate scale on the PCO_2 = 40 mm Hg line. The standard bicarbonate is not the actual bicarbonate concentration; rather it indicates the remaining portion of bicarbonate which is present after elimination of any respiratory component. Actually, it is a measure of the alkali reserve of blood and like it; it is also an index of the degree of metabolic acidosis or alkalosis. But the difference is that standard bicarbonate is measured by determining the pH, rather than the total CO_2 content of the sample after equilibration.

The buffer base also can be measured from the additional graduations on the upper curved scale of the nomogram. The point where the CO_2 titration line of the arterial blood sample intersects this scale shows the buffer base in mEq/L. The normal value of it in an individual with 15 g/dL of Hb is 48 mEq/L. The buffer base is equal to the total number of buffer anions such as protein, HCO_3^-, Hb^-, etc., which can accept H^+ in the blood.

Base excess also can be calculated from this nomogram. The point at which the CO_2 titration line intersects the lower curved scale indicates the base excess. It is defined as the amount of acid or base that would restore 1 L of blood to normal acid–base composition at a PCO_2 of 40 mm Hg. It is positive in alkalosis and negative in acidosis.

■ RESPIRATORY ACIDOSIS

The typical blood picture of a pure respiratory acidosis will be like that pH <7.40, $PaCO_2$ >40 mm Hg, and HCO_3^- >24 mEq/L. This (respiratory acidosis) is due to the excess CO_2 in the blood. This excess CO_2 in respiratory acidosis is due to the lack of excretion of it (CO_2) through lungs or due to the excess production of it (CO_2) from hypermetabolism or excess inhalation of CO_2. It may be acute or chronic in nature, but the compensatory response to the *acute elevation of PCO_2* in respiratory acidosis is limited. This is because ventilation cannot be increased to excrete excess CO_2 as the pathology is within the lungs (respiratory system). Buffering is primarily provided by Hb and the exchange of H^+ ion (produced by reaction of CO_2 with H_2O) for Na^+ and K^+ from bone and intracellular fluid. The renal response to retain more HCO_3^- as a compensatory process is also very limited in acute condition, i.e., respiratory acidosis. Latter slowly renal compensation occurs. The normal arterial CO_2 tension in blood is 35–45 mm Hg. The term "respiratory acidosis" means that $PaCO_2$ is higher than this normal value and this CO_2 becomes hydrated to H_2CO_3 so that the value of log $[HCO_3^-]/[H_2CO_3]$ in equation-I falls with a fall in pH. The kidney compensates this respiratory acidosis by retaining more HCO_3^- and excreting more H^+ and thus tries to reduce or compensate the fall in pH. Thus, the renal compensation causes to increase the plasma and CSF bicarbonate (HCO_3^-) level, so as to return pH toward normal. But an acute increase in $PaCO_2$ results in an acute increase in H_2CO_3 which does not get any time for compensation by kidney. For every 10 mm Hg rise of $PaCO_2$, there is a 8 nmol/L rise of H^+ ion but only 0.08 mmol/L rise of HCO_3^- and the relation between PCO_2 and H^+ ion concentration is linear. But the relation between the logarithmic scale of H^+ concentration (pH) and PCO_2 is not linear. The approximate relation between pH and PCO_2 is for every rise of 10 mm Hg of $PaCO_2$, there is a decrease of 0.07 unit of pH within 30–60 mm Hg range of $PaCO_2$. Beyond this range, the decrease of pH is more faster. In *chronic respiratory acidosis* with renal compensation, as the ratio of HCO_3^- to H_2CO_3 (or $PaCO_2$) approaches to normal by the retention of HCO_3^-, so the changes in HCO_3^- is greater and the changes in pH is less than for an acute disturbance **(Box 1)**.

So, in chronic hypercapnia or respiratory acidosis with renal compensation, every 10 mm Hg increase of PCO_2 results in a 4 mmol/L increase of HCO_3^- and a 3.2 nmol/L rise of H^+ with a 0.03 unit decrease of pH. The upper limit of HCO_3^- for compensation in acute respiratory acidosis is 30 mEq/L and in chronic respiratory acidosis is 50 mEq/L. If the measured HCO_3^- is higher than the expected HCO_3^- level, then metabolic alkalosis is also present. On the other hand, if measured HCO_3^- is below than the expected HCO_3^- level, then associated metabolic acidosis is present. The expected HCO_3^- after compensation is acute respiratory acidosis $HCO_3^- = (PCO_2 - 40) \times 0.1 + 24$. In chronic respiratory acidosis this formula is $HCO_3^- = (PCO_2 - 40) \times 0.35 + 24$.

This secondary renal compensatory change, in response to respiratory acidosis, is slow to develop and may take many days for full compensation to occur. The compensatory responses to chronic respiratory acidosis are therefore a metabolic alkalosis (retention of HCO_3^- by kidney) which

tends to return the pH to normal. In the presence of acute hypercapnia which happens during GA, there is no time for any appreciable renal compensation to occur. During apnea, the arterial PCO_2 rises about 3–6 mm Hg/min and H^+ ion accumulates at a rate of 10 nmol/min. This is 20 times faster than the kidney to excrete them.

The high arterial PCO_2 in respiratory acidosis can be produced by:

- If CO_2 production remains constant, but alveolar ventilation (V_A) is reduced, e.g., chronic obstructive pulmonary disease (COPD), parenchymal lung disease, lung injury, acute respiratory depression by narcotics, impaired neuromuscular function such as relaxant drugs, myasthenia gravis, poliomyelitis, and peripheral neuritis.
- If CO_2 production is raised, but V_A does not rise sufficiently to excrete the extra CO_2, e.g., fever.
- If CO_2 tension in inspired air ($FiCO_2$) is raised, e.g., rebreathing of CO_2 from expired air due to malfunctioning of anesthetic apparatus.

Systemic Effects of Respiratory Acidosis (Hypercapnia)

The respiratory acidosis or hypercapnia has multiple systemic effects. The *central nervous system effects* include impairment of mental activity, loss of consciousness, ↑ in the central blood flow due to cerebral vasodilation, ↑ CSF pressure, and stimulation of respiration followed by depression if PCO_2 rises gradually.

The general, *sympathetic overactivity* also occurs due to hypercapnia. If high inspired O_2 concentration is not delivered during hypercapnia, then hypoxemia also follows hypercapnia, and thereafter profound effects of these both (i.e., hypoxia and hypercapnia) are seen on cardiovascular system (CVS). The heart muscles are depressed by high blood CO_2 level. However, this effect is partly offset by increased sympathetic activity, due to hypercapnia. This increased sympathetic activity, accompanied by peripheral vasodilation, causes rise in CO, but causes pulmonary vasoconstriction. As the arterial PCO_2 rises, due to hypoventilation from low to high values, then the cardiac output (CO) increases at first gradually, only due to an increase in stroke volume. But later, the increase in cardiac output is due to an increase in both stroke volume and heart rate. These changes are accompanied by a rise in mean arterial pressure and a fall in peripheral vascular resistance (due to vasodilatation). Thus, the gradual rise of CO_2 tension in blood causes tachycardia. This is followed by bradycardia and depressed conduction in heart, particularly in bundle of His, when plasma PCO_2 rises to very high. So, in severe hypercapnia, the heart block and a slow ventricular rhythm are commonly observed, with an increased myocardial

---

BOX 1: Causes of respiratory acidosis.

- *Parenchymal lung diseases:* Pneumonia, collapse, aspiration, pulmonary emboli, pulmonary edema, interstitial lung disease, etc.
- *Airway obstruction:* Asthma, foreign body, tumor, laryngospasm, COPD, etc.
- *Skeletal abnormalities:* Myopathies, neuropathies, flail chest, kyphoscoliosis, poliomyelitis, myasthenia gravis, tetanus, etc.
- *Pleural abnormalities:* Pleural effusion and pneumothorax
- *CNS depression:* Drug overdose, trauma, tumor, CVA, and obesity hypoventilation (Pickwickian syndrome)
- *Ventilator malfunction and increased CO_2 production:* Thyroid storm, malignant hyperpyrexia, severe shivering, thermal injury, etc.

(CNS: central nervous system; COPD: chronic obstructive pulmonary disease; CVA: cerebrovascular accident)

irritability. A rise in CO_2 tension in blood increases the secretion of catecholamines (mainly epinephrine) from sympathetic nerve ending within myocardium. There is also an increase in plasma epinephrine and norepinephrine level, due to secretion from adrenal glands due to high CO_2 level. At the same time, during anesthesia the sensitivity of target organs to catecholamines by volatile anesthetics is increased by high plasma PCO_2 level. So, many anesthetic agents, primarily halothane cause arrhythmia in presence of high CO_2 level, thus both increased catecholamine level and increased sensitivity of myocardium to catecholamine make halothane responsible for frequent arrhythmia during hypercapnia. In such a situation, improving ventilation and reducing the dose of halothane will help to restore the normal rhythm **(Table 9)**.

During hypercapnia, the blood pressure rises due to sympathetic stimulation. So, increased bleeding is seen through surgical wounds. The patient also presents with warm skin, dilated veins, and a bounding pulse. Bounding pulse is due to increased pulse pressure which is due to increased systolic pressure and decreased diastolic pressure. Increased systolic pressure is due to increased myocardial contractility due to sympathetic stimulation. Decreased diastolic pressure is due to vasodilatation. There is also a rise in plasma potassium level. Oxyhemoglobin dissociation curve is shifted toward right in any acidosis. But it is important to mention that under anesthesia many of the above signs may be masked.

It is important to emphasize that during anesthesia the anesthetists are largely responsible for controlling arterial PCO_2 at about normal level. The main difficulty for anesthetist is to recognize the minor degrees of hypoventilation clinically. The time-honored custom of looking only at reservoir bag and thinking that ventilation is adequate is often grossly erroneous, especially for high-risk patients. Fluctuation of $PaCO_2$ between 40 and 60 mm Hg is probably of little consequence in normal, healthy patients. But when the arterial PCO_2 rises to around 80 mm Hg, it denotes a severe and dangerous hypoventilation. When CO_2 level rises to 110 mm Hg, then CO_2 narcosis occurs. In such a situation, the patient will not regain consciousness, even when the anesthetic drugs are withdrawn. If at this moment, the patient is allowed to breathe room air, simply because the operation is over, then he will be with a disadvantage, because alveoli filled with anesthetic gases (usually N_2O) escaping from circulation will cause diffusion hypoxia. This hypoxia will again increase due to uneven ventilation–perfusion ratio, which normally follows anesthesia and also due to the reduced quantity of available oxygen from lungs due to high CO_2 tension. Thus, hypoxia will occur definitely.

Treatment of Respiratory Acidosis

The treatment of respiratory acidosis is aimed at the underlying causes, for example, (1) improving the ventilation by using intermittent positive pressure ventilation, if respiration is depressed or totally absent, (2) rebreathing of CO_2 should be avoided, and (3) the dead space of anesthetic apparatus should be reduced. Alkali therapy has no place in chronic respiratory acidosis. In COPD, the aim of the

TABLE 9: Characteristic changes in arterial H^+ ion concentration, $PaCO_2$, and HCO_3^- level in different acid–base disturbances.

Disorder	H^+	nmol/L	$PaCO_2$	mm Hg	HCO_3^-	nmol/L
• *Respiratory acidosis:*						
– Acute	+	60	+ +	70	WNR	28
– Compensated	Slight ↑ or WNR	44	+ +	66	+ +	40
(by renal retention of HCO_3^-)						
• *Respiratory alkalosis:*						
– Acute	–	22	– –	20	WNR	22
– Compensated	Slight ↓ or WNR	36	–	30	–	15
(by renal excretion of HCO_3^-)						
• *Metabolic acidosis:*						
– Acute	+	60	WNR	40	– –	12
– Compensated	Slight ↑ or WNR	48	–	30	– –	13
(by ↑ ventilation)						
• *Metabolic alkalosis:*						
– Acute	–	26	WNR	40	+ +	42
– Compensated	Slight ↓ or WNR	35	+	60	+ +	40
(by ↓ ventilation)						

Note: Normal H^+ concentration: 35–45 nmol/L, $PaCO_2$: 35–45 mm Hg, HCO_3^-: 21–28 mmol/L, WNR: within normal range, +: increased, –: decreased treatment of respiratory acidosis should be to lessen H^+ ion activity to just <56 nmol/L (pH >7.25), rather than to normalize it completely. This is because the acidity of blood which is important to maintain ventilation through chemoreceptor-mediated ventilatory drive by CO_2 in COPD patients and this is modified by renal compensatory HCO_3^- retention. It is too difficult to assess the $PaCO_2$, simply by clinical examination, so the repeated blood gas monitoring is of course mandatory. If invasive positive pressure ventilation (IPPV) is used to produce normal $PaCO_2$ then the patient will be left with variant HCO_3^- level and metabolic alkalosis.

The typical blood gases level in *acute situation* of respiratory depression and respiratory acidosis without any compensation are like this: (1) pH → 7.2, (2) $PaCO_2$ → 70 mm Hg, and (3) HCO_3^- → 29 mmol/L.

In the more common COPD, where renal *compensation* has occurred, typical blood gases findings are like this: (1) pH → 7.3, (2) $PaCO_2$ → 60 mm Hg, (3) HCO_3^- → 35 mmol/L, and (4) PaO_2 → 70 mm Hg.

The alveolar gas equation, in case of respiratory acidosis, always predicts that hypoxia is must accompanied with ↑ $PaCO_2$ due to poor ventilation. The resultant fall in PaO_2 (hypoxia) limits hypercapnia to approximately 100–110 mm Hg. Higher level of $PaCO_2$ above 110 mm Hg imposes PaO_2 (hypoxia) so low that it is incompatible to life. Under such circumstances, it is hypoxia, but not hypercapnia, which poses the principal threat to life. So, administration of O_2 along with ventilation (to remove CO_2) is the most critical part of the management of respiratory acidosis.

Naloxone and flumazenil are important to treat hypercapnia, if it is due to an opioid or benzodiazepine overdose. During mechanical ventilation, minute ventilation should be gradually raised in such a fashion that $PaCO_2$ will gradually return to the higher side of the normal base level. Rapid reduction of $PaCO_2$ risks the development of posthypercapnic alkalosis with potential serious consequences. If posthypercapnic alkalosis is developed, then it should be treated with chloride, usually as its K-salt, and administering bicarbonate wasting diuretic such as acetazolamide at the dose of 250–350 mg once or twice daily.

Explanation: In primary respiratory acidosis HCO_3^- is in normal value, as there is no renal compensation. In compensated respiratory acidosis the level of HCO_3^- is elevated. The pH is on the acidotic side of the normal range in compensated respiratory acidosis. The parameters of metabolic alkalosis look-like compensated respiratory acidosis, but the diagnostic point is pH which is on the alkali side. The differences between primary respiratory acidosis and compensated respiratory acidosis and compensated metabolic alkalosis are enumerated in **Table 10**.

TABLE 10: Differentiation between primary respiratory acidosis and compensated respiratory and metabolic alkalosis.

	pH	*PaCO$_2$*	*HCO$_3^-$*
Primary respiratory acidosis	7.30	55	24
Compensated respiratory acidosis	7.38	50	30
Compensated metabolic alkalosis	7.42	50	32

■ RESPIRATORY ALKALOSIS

Respiratory alkalosis is the most frequently found acid–base disorder because it occurs in normal pregnancy and high-altitude dwellers. It is also particularly prevalent among the critically ill patients. In this group of patients, it carries a bad prognosis, because mortality increases in direct proportion to the severity of hypocapnia. The usual blood picture of primary (uncompensated) respiratory alkalosis is like that pH >7.40, $PaCO_2$ <40 mm Hg, HCO_3^- ± 24 mEq/L. In most of the cases pH does not exceed 7.55 and severe manifestation of alkalemia is usually absent. Like respiratory acidosis, the respiratory alkalosis also follows the Henderson–Hasselbalch equation: pH = pK + log $[HCO_3^-]/[H_2CO_3]$. As the value of $[H_2CO_3]$ falls in the respiratory alkalosis, so the value of pH rises, calculated from this equation.

In this situation, CO_2 is washed out due to hyperventilation and this reaction: $CO_2 + H_2O \rightleftharpoons H_2CO_3 \rightleftharpoons H^+ + HCO_3^-$ is shifted to the left leaving HCO_3^- in excess in respect to H^+ ion concentration in plasma. Thus, plasma H_2CO_3 level is reduced in respect to H^+, and the log $[HCO_3^-]/[H_2CO_3]$ value is increased with an increase in pH. Compensatory changes occur, if the disturbance is prolonged. The kidney compensates for this rise in pH by excreting more HCO_3^- ion (**Box 2**) and retaining more H^+ ion and thus restoring pH to normal by reducing the log $[HCO^-]/[H_2CO_3]$ ratio. By reabsorbing less HCO_3^- and secreting less H^+, it produces alkaline urine. The secondary (compensatory) response to a respiratory alkalosis is therefore a metabolic acidosis (retention of H^+). But this secondary compensatory response is reduced in anaesthetized person due to a fall in the renal blood flow. So, it is not uncommon to find mild metabolic acidosis in anesthetized hyperventilated patient with mild respiratory alkalosis.

An *uncompensated* respiratory alkalosis leads to the following changes in blood, such as: (1) low level of $PaCO_2$ (or H_2CO_3), (2) more or less normal level of plasma bicarbonate (HCO_3^-) level, (3) high pH, (4) low level of H^+ ion, (5) but normal buffer base, base excess, and standard bicarbonate level. However, in respiratory alkalosis, the decrease of H^+ in comparison to HCO_3^- is more (reverse of respiratory acidosis). An acute decrease of 10 mm Hg of PCO_2 results in decrease of 2 mmol/L of HCO_3^- and an

---

BOX 2: Causes of respiratory alkalosis.

- *CNS stimulation causing hyperventilation:* Anxiety, pain, fever, infection, drug-induced (salicylates), stroke, tumor, hysteria, etc.
- *Peripheral stimulation causing hyperventilation:* Hypoxemia, anemia, high altitude, shock, pregnancy, pulmonary diseases, etc.
- *Iatrogenic:* IPPV

(CNS: central nervous system; IPPV: invasive positive pressure ventilation)

---

8 nmol/L decrease of H^+. The pH increases by 0.08 unit for every 10 mm Hg decrease of PCO_2.

Renal compensation for chronic respiratory alkalosis causes a decrease in tubular H^+ secretion and diminished HCO_3^- reabsorption. So, after compensation, plasma HCO_3^- level decreases and the ratio of HCO_3^- to H_2CO_3 (pCO_2) approaches to normal. In chronic compensated respiratory alkalosis, each 10 mm Hg decrease in PCO_2 is associated with a 6 nmol/L decrease in H^+ ion and a 0.03 unit increase of pH. *After compensation, if the measured HCO_3^- is higher than the expected level, then metabolic alkalosis is present along with respiratory alkalosis.* On the other hand, if the measured HCO_3^- is lower than the expected level, then associated metabolic acidosis is present along with respiratory alkalosis. The expected HCO_3^- level, after compensation in acute respiratory alkalosis, is $HCO_3^- = 25 - (40 - PaCO_2) \times 0.25$. In chronic respiratory alkalosis, this formula is $HCO_3^- = 25 - (40\ PaCO_2) \times 0.5$.

The main danger of respiratory alkalosis under anesthesia is cerebral vasoconstriction. This is because it is known that arterial PCO_2 largely controls the diameter of cerebral vessels. Thus, severe alkalosis may produce intense cerebral vasoconstriction and decreases intracranial pressure by decreasing cerebral blood flow (CBF). The cerebral effects of hyperventilation or hypocapnia (respiratory alkalosis) such as euphoria and analgesia also have been demonstrated. But whether they are only due to cerebral vasoconstriction or due to direct action of low CO_2 tension on brain cells is not definitely known, however the latter seems to be much more likely. It is also true that long periods of severe respiratory alkalosis, leading to cerebral damage, is still lacking. So, most clinicians believe that mild respiratory alkalosis is more beneficial for the patients, rather than mild respiratory acidosis.

Other features of respiratory alkalosis are: (1) hypokalemia ($\downarrow K^+$), (2) increased neuromuscular excitability producing tetany due to decreased ionic Ca^{2+} concentration, (3) a tendency toward increased ventricular irritability, (4) and a shift to the left of $Hb–O_2$ dissociation curve. This causes increased O_2 affinity to Hb and less unloading of it to tissues which is again prevented by rise in 2,3-disphosphoglycerate (2,3-DPG) level by alkalosis. Decrease in the level of 2,3-DPG, due to acidosis or other causes, tries to shift the $Hb–O_2$ dissociation curve toward right and help in unloading of O_2 to tissues.

Alkalemia reduces the original threshold level and predisposes the patient to refractory supraventricular and ventricular arrhythmias. This cardiac effect is more evident in patients with underlying heart disease. Alkalosis also depresses respiration. This effect is of little consequence in healthy patient, but this effect is very prominent in a patient who is on ventilator. In such patient, even mild alkalemic can frustrate the efforts to wean from ventilator.

Hypokalemia is an almost constant feature of any alkalemic disorder, but it is more prominent in those of metabolic origin. Translocation of K^+ into cells, and renal losses of it are the cause of hypokalemia in alkalosis. This hypokalemia has several adverse effects. These are neuromuscular weakness, polyuria, increased ammonia production (that can increase the risk of hepatic encephalopathy), digitalis-induced arrhythmia, etc. Alkalosis stimulates anaerobic glycolysis and increases the production of lactic acid and keto acids.

Respiratory alkalosis in commonly associated with hyponatremia, hypokalemia, hypocalcemia (ionized Ca^{2+}), and hyperchloremia. During anesthesia with controlled ventilation, the low PCO_2 causes the cardiac output to fall. This is because the main determinant of the cardiac output during anesthesia is the arterial PCO_2 level.

Causes of Respiratory Alkalosis

- Cortical stimulation causing hyperventilation due to pain, fear, anxiety, analeptic drugs, salicylate poisoning, head injury, hepatic failure, pregnancy, labor pain, etc.
- Hyperventilation by hypoxic drive due to high altitude, hemorrhagic shock, or any other shock. A hypoxic drive from peripheral chemoreceptor occurs at a high altitude and probably explains the cause of hyperventilation and respiratory alkalosis.
- Cardiopulmonary diseases, for example, asthma, pulmonary edema, pulmonary embolism, etc. All these factors may also cause respiratory acidosis but will depend on the degree of stimulation of respiration, causing hyperventilation and lung conditions, causing retention of CO_2.
- Excessive IPPV during long-term ventilatory support
- Hysterical over-breathing.

An important and serious clinical hazard of acute hyperventilation or respiratory alkalosis occurs when it is superimposed upon pre-existing metabolic alkalosis because it may result in severe hypokalemia, especially in the presence of digitalis, leading to severe ventricular arrhythmias. In such a situation, severe depletion of the body's CO_2 store occurs. When hyperventilation ceases, then the stores of CO_2 are gradually replaced during the period of hypoventilation. The O_2 consumption is unchanged and the respiratory quotient RQ (CO output/O_2 consumption) is decreased during respiratory alkalosis. The reduction of RQ in respiratory alkalosis causes a decrease in PaO_2 and is thus another reason why patient should receive additional O_2 during weaning from mechanical ventilation if there is hyperventilation.

Treatment of Respiratory Alkalosis

Whenever possible, the management of respiratory alkalosis must be directed toward correcting the underlying cause. In most cases, especially chronic cases pose little risk to health and produce few or no symptoms. So, in such circumstances measures to treat the deranged acid–base status is not required. In anxiety hyperventilation syndrome sedation and psychotherapy is very helpful. Rebreathing into a paper bag on through any closed system provides prompt relief, but it is short-lived.

Explanation: In primary respiratory alkalosis as there is no compensation, so HCO_3^- is in normal range. In its compensated form pH comes down, but on slightly alkali side and HCO_3^- falls. In compensated metabolic acidosis, $PaCO_2$ falls for compensation and pH is slightly on acidic side after compensation.

Differentiation between primary respiratory alkalosis and compensated respiratory alkalosis and compensated metabolic acidosis are enumerated in **Table 11**.

The correction of respiratory alkalosis can be made by preventing the increased central or peripheral respiratory drive, if this is appropriate. Mechanical ventilation should be controlled by monitoring the arterial or end-tidal PCO_2.

■ METABOLIC ACIDOSIS

This occurs when an abnormal amount of metabolic acids (noncarbonic acid) are formed and accumulate or an abnormal loss of base occurs. So, as a compensatory mechanism respiratory alkalosis occurs and the level of PCO_2 (marker of respiratory acid–base status) in blood is

reduced. This is manifested secondarily by hyperventilation which try to mitigate the ratio of HCO_3^-/H_2CO_3 to normal level (compensatory respiratory alkalosis). Here, the sources of H^+ ions are nonvolatile acids or fixed acids and not the H_2CO_3, coming from the reaction of CO_2 with water. Normally, the different types of nonvolatile acids such as lactic acid, acetoacetic acid, hydroxybutyric acid, acetone, and free fatty acids are produced in variable amounts during the metabolism of different substrates (discussed before) and have relatively little renal excretion. They are normally removed by metabolism in liver with regeneration of bicarbonate. However, the fixed acids such as the HCl, H_2SO_4, and H_3PO_4 can only be eliminated by renal excretion. They are not metabolized in liver. If *uncompensated*, then the changes due to metabolic acidosis seen in blood are low pH, low plasma bicarbonate, normal $PaCO_2$, a negative base excess, and a low standard bicarbonate. But typical values *after compensation* are pH <7.36 (H^+ concentration is >44 nmol/L), $PaCO_2$ <35 mm Hg (compensated), and HCO_3^- <18 mmol/L (compensated).

In metabolic acidosis, an increase in an anion gap may occur and an insight of the overall buffering capacity of body during this acid–base disturbance may be available by calculating this *anion gap*. These represent those negative ions that are not normally measured in clinical practice, including phosphate, sulfate, lactate, keto acids, and albumin. *The working formula is anion gap = plasma Na$^+$ – (plasma Cl$^-$ + plasma HCO$_3^-$).* The normal value of anion gap varies between 8 and 14 mmol/L. Where excessive acid is added to the plasma, either by metabolic disorder or by addition of exogenous acid or there is the failure of acid excretion, then this anion gap is increased. In metabolic acidosis, the value of log HCO_3^-/H_2CO_3 will be reduced due to low HCO_3^- or high H_2CO_3 level and hence pH falls. (Metabolic acidosis is due to fall of HCO. Metabolic alkalosis is due to an increase in HCO. Respiratory acidosis is due to an increase in HCO. Respiratory alkalosis is due to fall in.) In metabolic acidosis, though CO_2 does not accumulate excessively to form much H_2CO_3, but it is formed excessively by the reaction of $H^+ + HCO_3^- = H_2CO_3$ where the equation is shifted to the right and further reduces the HCO_3^- level. This H^+ ion comes from metabolic acids, such as lactic acid, keto acids, and pyruvic acid. This H^+ ion stimulates chemoreceptors and increases ventilatory drive to washout CO_2 for compensation (compensatory respiratory alkalosis). Thus, CO_2 is excreted ($H_2CO_3 \rightleftharpoons H_2O + CO_2$) from H_2CO_3 through the lungs as a compensatory process, resulting in a decrease in PCO_2 or H_2CO_3 level and attenuation of the fall in pH. Although the reduction in PCO_2 is rapid, still the respiratory response is only capable of 50–70% compensation for metabolic acidosis. In other word, an uncorrected metabolic acidosis

TABLE 11: Differentiation between primary respiratory alkalosis and compensated respiratory alkalosis and compensated metabolic acidosis.

	pH	PaCO₂	HCO₃⁻
Primary respiratory alkalosis	7.55	30	24
Compensated respiratory alkalosis	7.45	28	15
Compensated metabolic acidosis	7.35	30	17

FACT FILE II

Anion gap (AG): It is a very useful clinical tool for (1) narrowing the differential diagnosis of metabolic acidosis, (2) identifying the variety of acids that originated in metabolic disorder, and (3) recognizing certain mixed acid–base disturbances. The anion gap is generally measured from the concentration of four common electrolytes, such as Na^+, K^+, Cl^-, and HCO_3^-. Sometimes K^+ is excluded from the calculation. Then the calculation will be:

$$Na^+ = Cl^- + HCO_3^- + AG$$

Or,

$$AG = Na^+ - [Cl^- + HCO_3^-]$$

Otherwise, the usual formula is (if K^+ included in the calculation):

$$Na^+ (140) + K^+ (5) = Cl^- (105) + HCO_3^- (25) + AG (15)$$

Or,

$$AG = [Na^+ + K^+] - [Cl^- + HCO_3^-]$$

The normal range of AG is 12 ± 4 mEq.

Some causes of metabolic acidosis release anions in extracellular fluid which are not normally measured, but when this occurs there will be an unexpected discrepancy between the sums of principal cations and anions. When there are some additional unmeasured anions, then they become part of the anion gap which will be larger. An anion gap larger than 30 mEq suggests that there is an increase in the concentration of unmeasured anions. An increased AG is the only clue that metabolic acidosis is present isolatedly or in a mixed acid–base disorder. The AG indicates the quantity of added acids. The fall in HCO_3^- also equals the rise in AG. It is useful in following the response of patient treating for diabetic ketoacidosis or other metabolic disorders.

In metabolic acidosis with anion gap (AG >12 mEq), there is a decrease in HCO_3^- level. This is due to the buffering of an acid whose anions are other than Cl^- (such as H_2SO_4 and lactic acid). Hence, it is called normochloremic acidosis. These acids may be endogenous (lactic acid, keto acid, and uremic acid) or exogenous (salicylates) or the endogenous metabolic products or the exogenous toxins (such as methanol and ethanol). Other unmeasured anions are proteins, phosphates, sulfates, etc.

There is another metabolic acidosis where there is no anion gap (AG = 8–12 mEq), but a decrease in HCO_3^- level. This is due to buffering of an acid whose anion is Cl^- (such as HCl acid), so this is called hyperchloremic acidosis.

that would reduce the pH to 7 is normally compensated to a pH of 7.2–7.3 **(Fact file II)**.

The typical blood picture of a compensated metabolic acidosis is pH <7.40, $PaCO_2$ <40 mm Hg, and HCO_3^- <24 mEq/L. If the measured $PaCO_2$ from a blood sample is higher than the expected $PaCO_2$ (which should be reduced), then it should be thought that additional respiratory acidosis is present. On the other hand, if the measured $PaCO_2$ is less than the expected $PaCO_2$, then an additional respiratory alkalosis is present. There are the mixed disorders. In a compensated metabolic acidosis, the expected $PaCO_2$ is calculated as: $(1.5 \times HCO_3^-) + 8 \pm 2$.

Profound derangements of K^+ level occur in metabolic acidosis. For every decrease in 0.1 pH, there is an equivalent 0.8 increase in K^+ level. Correction of it is usually not required,

unless there is a threat to life, because correction of acidosis will correct it.

Causes of Metabolic Acidosis

The causes of metabolic acidosis are:

- *Accumulation of acid:*
  - Diabetic ketoacidosis is where blood levels of lactic acid, acetoacetic acid, β-hydroxybutyric acid, α-ketoglutaric acid, and acetone are increased.
  - *Following starvation:* Following starvation, there is excessive metabolism of fat, leading to accumulation of different keto acids.
  - *Renal tubular acidosis (RTA):* The RTA is a type of metabolic acidosis where the cause is in the renal tubule. It results either from a defect in reabsorption of bicarbonate in the proximal tubule or from a defect in the failure of secretion of H^+ (failure of acidification of urine) from collecting tubules. Decreased reabsorption of bicarbonate causes large amount of losses of HCO_3^- in urine and a marked reduction in plasma HCO_3^-. In the failure of secretion of H^+, there is also a failure of secretion of Cl^-. So, there is persistent hyperchloremic acidosis. It is also associated with hypercalciuria, hyperphosphaturia, and loss of Na^+ in urine.

- *Salicylate overdose:*
  - *Hypoxia:* It causes metabolic acidosis by metabolizing the pyruvate to lactic acid, but not to acetyl-coenzyme A (acetyl-CoA), which is the gateway of pyruvate to TCA cycle in the presence of O_2.
  - *Low cardiac output (CO)*—producing tissue hypoxia
  - *Following cardiac arrest:* Anaerobic metabolism and acute metabolic acidosis occur in cardiac arrest.
  - *Following transfusion of a large amount of stored blood:* Administration of a large volume of stored blood, where acid–citrate–dextrose (ACD) is used as an anticoagulant. It produces an acute metabolic acidosis, although the hepatic metabolism of citrate in the next 2–3 days will convert this to a nonrespiratory alkalosis.

The substances such as paraldehyde, methyl alcohol, ethylene glycol, fructose, sorbitol, xylitol, and ethanol may also cause metabolic acidosis. There may also be an increase in H^+ concentration from accumulated HCl which is released during the metabolism of arginine and lysine, present in the synthetic amino acid solution and following the therapeutic use of NH_4Cl.

An uncommon (but probably overemphasized) form of metabolic acidosis also occurs when sometimes extracellular bicarbonate is diluted with saline, which is used excessively during over enthusiastic replacement therapy.

Such administration of excessive NaCl only occurs during the resuscitation of a severely hypovolemic patient, in whom the restoration of circulatory volume by an isotonic fluid is an urgent requirement to restore the tissue perfusion and aerobic metabolism. A mild metabolic acidosis occurs in general anesthesia (GA). It is also commonly observed after a period of extracorporeal perfusion, after circulating arrest, after hypothermia, and following temporary occlusion of a major vessel, such as aorta and massive blood transfusion.

- *Loss of bicarbonate:*
  - *From gastrointestinal (GI) tract:*
    - Fistula of small intestine, pancreatic fistula, or biliary fistula
    - Diarrhea
    - Ureteroenterostomy
    - Use of cholestyramine
  - *From kidney:*
    - Renal tubular acidosis
    - Use of carbonic anhydrase inhibitor (CAI), such as acetazolamide (explained before).

In metabolic acidosis, the body will try to compensate for this fall of pH by the stimulation of respiration, leading to fall in $PaCO_2$ which will try to return the pH toward normal, by reducing the level of H_2CO_3 in blood. Although, the fall in pH is modified, but it does not return completely to normal **(Box 3)**.

Effects of Metabolic Acidosis

- Initially, the acidosis stimulates the CVS and increases the CO (cardiac output) and BP. But later the heart muscles are depressed and CO falls. The cardiovascular responses to sympathetic activity or sympathomimetic drugs are initially increased and then reduced. Intense peripheral vasoconstriction occurs initially. These changes further tend to intense the acidosis, so that a vicious cycle is set-up.
- Increase in circulating catecholamines
- Increased intracellular H^+ ion will tend to displace K^+ from the intracellular fluid which will result in hyperkalemia.
- Cardiac arrhythmias and arrest
- Pulmonary hypertension
- Mental changes
- Metabolic acidosis stimulates the peripheral and central chemoreceptors by increased H^+ ion. Thus, ventilation is increased and the PCO_2 and HCO_3^- level of arterial blood and CSF are lowered until the pH returns almost to normal. If the pH is corrected rapidly by $NaHCO_3$, then the PCO_2 of blood and CSF will rise and pH will fall stimulating central chemoreceptor and replacing metabolic acidosis with respiratory alkalosis.
- Hb–O_2 dissociation curve will shift to the right.

Management of Metabolic Acidosis

The treatment of metabolic acidosis is directed toward the underlying causes. It is generally more serious than respiratory acidosis because the etiology of metabolic acidosis is more life threatening. The treatment of metabolic acidosis is also very difficult and more complex than treating respiratory acidosis. Therefore, therapy with $NaHCO_3$ should be reserved for fairly severe disorders, since it is not without hazards.

If the pH is very low (<7.2), then the metabolic acidosis itself becomes life threatening, because of its serious effects on heart or CVS. Therefore, in such circumstances, $NaHCO_3$ should be given through intravenous (IV) without delay. If the acidosis is less severe, then the management depends upon (1) the diagnosis of causes, (2) associated disorder of electrolyte and fluid balance, and (3) whether the acidosis is still developing or not. Thus, for example, a patient with diabetic ketoacidosis and base excess of –12 mmol/L (base deficit 12 mmol/L) will correct his own acidosis, if only saline and insulin is given. It probably does not require any bicarbonate. But a patient with a base excess of –8 mmol/L, during any major surgery, will probably require bicarbonate, because they cannot tolerate the depressing effect of a slight decrease of pH on the myocardium. On the other hand, it is important not to give too much $NaHCO_3$, as this may have several undesirable effects.

■ SODIUM BICARBONATE

Sodium bicarbonate ($NaHCO_3$) solution is available in a variety of concentrations. The concentration of $NaHCO_3$ that is commonly used clinically for resuscitation is 8.4% which contains 1 mmol of Na^+ and HCO_3^-/mL. Therefore, there is a danger of a high Na load, precipitating heart failure. The sodium bicarbonate solution of this concentration is hypertonic and irritating to veins. Thus, it may also result in extensive skin necrosis, if this solution leaks from veins into tissues. Sometimes, a hyperosmolality syndrome may precipitate by 8.4% $NaHCO_3$ solution. Therefore, 8.4% $NaHCO_3$ should be reserved for acute situations such as cardiac arrest and should preferably be given via a central line.

Disadvantages of NaHCO$_3$

The disadvantages of IV administration of $NaHCO_3$ are the following:

- Administration of 8.4% $NaHCO_3$ causes excess of sodium load which is especially dangerous in patients with heart disease. The administration of 50 mL of 8.4% $NaHCO_3$ will increase the serum osmolarity by 3 mmol/L in normal adults **(Fact file III)**.
- During cardiac arrest, there is both respiratory and metabolic acidosis which develops rapidly in tissues. In such a situation of complete absence of circulation and respiration, administration of $NaHCO_3$ evolves large amount of CO_2. This huge amount of CO_2 cannot get its exit through lungs, due to absence of circulation and respiration (if circulation and ventilation is not started). Then, it leads to more severe hypercapnia and acidosis and more and more depression of myocardium. Thus a vicious cycle will set up. $NaHCO_3 + H^+ \rightleftharpoons H_2CO_3 \rightleftharpoons CO_2 + H_2O$.

Ketoacidosis is one of the example of HAGMA. It is found in starvation, alcoholism, and insulin-dependent diabetics. It is characterized by the elevated level of β-butyric acid and acetoacetic acid. The elevation of the level of these two acids are due to:

- An increased hepatic synthesis, caused by an increase in the level of free fatty acid (FFA) which is liberated from adipose tissue due to reduced insulin and increased catecholamine level.
- An altered hepatic metabolism due to reduction in insulin, promoting keto genesis rather than triglyceride synthesis.

Beta-hydroxybutyrate, acetoacetate, and acetone are together called the *ketone bodies*. Among these, the acetoacetate undergoes spontaneous decarboxylation and yields CO_2 and acetone. The acetone is not an acid and is excreted largely through lungs, like CO_2. The acetoacetate and β-hydroxybutyrate remain in equilibrium in plasma and their normal ratio is 3:1 (vary in between 1:1 and 10:1). This level increases during hypoxia. The normal fasting level of β-hydroxybutyrate is <1.2 mEq/L. In prolonged fasting, it may rise up to 2–5 mEq/L. Normally, the FFA concentration in plasma ranges between 0.4 and 0.8 mEq/L and seldom rises >1 mEq/L. But in diabetic ketoacidosis, the FFA level may rise up to 2–4 mEq/L and keto acids may increase up to 10–15 mEq/L.

During cardiac arrest, lactic acidosis results from anaerobic metabolism in tissues and there is no formation of CO_2 due to the stoppage of TCA cycle in the absence of O_2. Therefore, a sudden increase in CO_2 level in blood, after the administration of $NaHCO_3$ reverses the diffusion gradient and CO_2 will easily enter the cell, causing intracellular acidosis. This intracellular hypercapnia (acidosis) will compound the existing intracellular lactic acidosis, which will further reduce the intracellular pH and will further decrease the myocardial contractility. Thus, it will exacerbate an already compromised low cardiac output state. The CO_2, thus, produced in the blood will also easily cross the blood–brain barrier and will cause a disproportionate acidosis of CSF. In fact, 50 mL of 8.4% $NaHCO_3$ will be converted to 200 mL of CO_2 which is equivalent to the production of it by the basal metabolism of a normal adult in 1 minute.

- $NaHCO_3$ administration causes an extracellular alkalosis and movement of oxyhemoglobin dissociation curve toward left. This will impair O_2 delivery to tissues. In uncontrolled diabetes mellitus, the acidosis exists with a high level of 2,3-DPG level. Acidosis itself shifts the O_2 dissociation curve toward right and on the other hand high 2,3-DPG shifts it toward left. Therefore, the net effect of oxygen delivery to the tissue remains normal. If $NaHCO_3$ is administered in these circumstances, then the pH will rise, leaving the unopposed effect of a high 2,3-DPG level and further shifting of O_2 dissociation curve toward left. This will cause the severe impairment of delivery of O_2 to tissues. The 2,3-DPG level takes several days to return to normal and it is important in this respect to ensure a normal plasma phosphate.
- In diabetes acidosis, $NaHCO_3$ may precipitate disequilibrium syndrome.
- Rebound alkalosis may occur if excessive dose of $NaHCO_3$ are used. This alkalosis will also reduce serum ionized Ca^{2+} level by 25% and can further decrease the myocardial contractility.
- Administration of $NaHCO_3$ results in rise of $PaCO_2$. If the patient is able to hyperventilate, then this excess CO_2 will be excreted via lungs. But in a patient with impaired consciousness, mechanical ventilation at high minute volume may be required to washout this excess CO_2 with repeated measurement of blood gas tension.
- In hypokalemic patients $NaHCO_3$ administration will increase pH. This will promote further K^+ uptake by the cell and thus lethal hypokalemia may occur.

In summary, $NaHCO_3$ is a dangerous drug but may be very essential after cardiac arrest for the successful action of inotropic agents, provided if the circulation and ventilation are established.

Doses of Bicarbonate

The doses of bicarbonate for the acute management of metabolic acidosis can be calculated from base excess, assuming that equilibrium will occur throughout extracellular fluid which is about 20% of total body weight or lean body mass (LBM). So, the dose of $NaHCO_3$ (mmol) = [Base excess × Body weight (kg)]/3.

It is often recommended that at initial phase about half of the total calculated dose of $NaHCO_3$ is given. After that blood gases must be checked again. It is much better to undercorrect the acidosis than to overcorrect it. The results, after administering the total dose of bicarbonate as suggested earlier, are not always predictable. This is due to the possible development of further acidosis and because the original blood sample which was taken during altered equilibrium, does not indicate the level of actual base excess. Also, it will have to keep in mind that the measurement of acid–base state of blood may give a very inaccurate index of the actual metabolic state of the whole body, as the measurement of intracellular pH by a clinical procedure is not yet possible. For this reason, it is essential to reassess the acid–base status of arterial blood after half of the recommended dose of bicarbonate has been given and to correct further if it is necessary only. Sodium bicarbonate is a poor buffer in its own right (as explained previously) and acts mainly by combining with H^+ ions to form CO_2 and H_2O. Administration of bicarbonate to correct a metabolic acidosis, therefore, presents a CO_2 load on the lungs. So, the efficient buffering of metabolic acidosis by $NaHCO_3$ depends mainly on adequate pulmonary ventilation.

Tri-hydroxymethyl aminomethane (THAM): It is a nonsodium-containing buffer that has been used in some parts of the world, with a variable degree of success, to treat metabolic acidosis instead of $NaHCO_3$ **(Fig. 10)**.

■ LACTIC ACIDOSIS

Glycolysis is the process of breakdown of glycogen or glucose into pyruvic (in presence of O_2 this pyruvic acid does not accumulate and enters the TCA cycle) or lactic acid (in absence of O_2, this pyruvic acid cannot enter the TCA cycle and is converted into lactic acid and accumulates) through Embden–Meyerhof or glycolytic pathway. Glycogen leaves the liver in form of glucose, but it leaves the muscles in form of pyruvic or lactic acids only and not in the form of glucose. This difference is probably due to the fact that the enzyme systems and chemical reaction, responsible for the metabolism of glycogen and glucose in liver and muscle are not same. The pyruvic or lactic acid that emerges from muscles is carried to the liver through bloodstream where

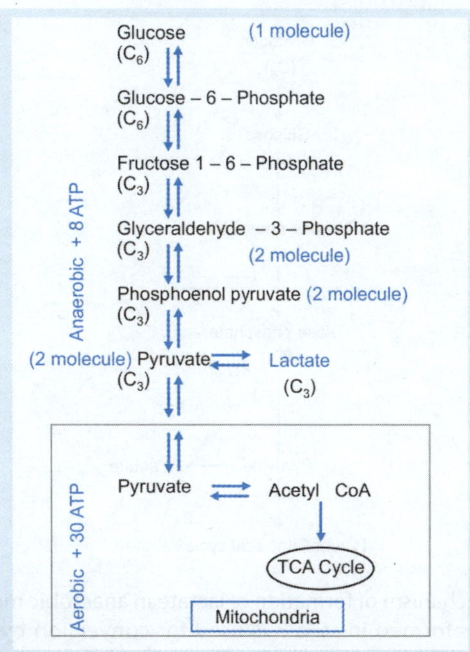

Fig. 10: Pyruvate and lactate metabolism. (ATP: adenosine triphosphate; CoA: acetyl coenzyme A; TCA: tricarboxylic acid cycle)

it is reconverted into glycogen. This glycogen is again remobilized from liver into the bloodstream as glucose. Muscles again take up this glucose from bloodstream and recover its lost glycogen from where again pyruvic or lactic acid is produced due to its metabolism. This cyclic process of circulation of carbohydrate in different forms in different tissues is known as *Cori cycle,* through which muscle lactic acid and liver glycogens become readily interchangeable. In normal condition, one-fifth of the muscle lactate is broken down to CO_2 and H_2O and four-fifths is reconverted into glycogen in the liver **(Fig. 11)**.

In skeletal muscles, pyruvic acid but not lactic acid is the end product of glucose metabolism. In muscle, it (pyruvic acid) is converted into lactic acid only in anaerobic conditions, such as during heavy exercise. This lactic acid, then, from muscles enters the bloodstream, when O_2 supply is inadequate. In muscle, pyruvic acid is also finally oxidized into CO_2 and H_2O through citric acid or TCA cycle in the presence of O_2. Cardiac muscle also utilizes lactic acid directly and completely in preference to glucose. Glucose utilization by the heart of a diabetic person is less than normal, but as regards lactate, the diabetic heart uses it almost as readily as normal heart. On the other hand, there is a very little glycogen store in the brain. It uses sugar in the form of galactose only which is locally synthesized from blood glucose. In the brain, galactose is also metabolized to lactic acid. It is also interesting to note that brain tissue is very rich in fat, but it derives its energy from sugar. The RBC also readily forms lactic acid from sugar.

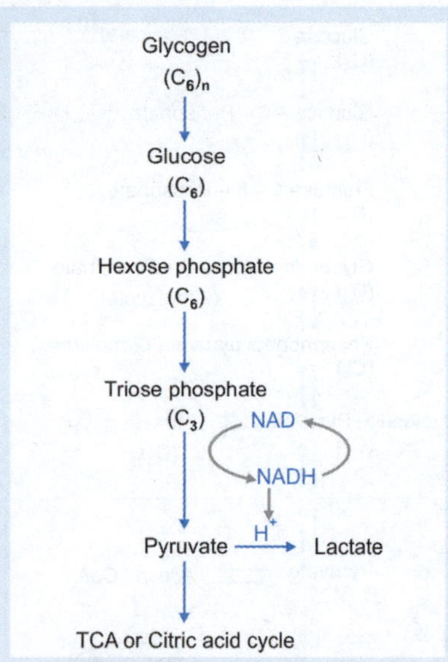

Fig. 11: Mechanism of formation of lactate in anaerobic metabolism. H^+ which is formed in step 3 is used for conversion by pyruvate to lactate. (NADH: reduced nicotinamide adenine dinucleotide; TCA: tricarboxylic acid cycle)

Lactic acidosis is best defined as an acidotic condition when pH is <7.25 and blood lactate concentration is >5 mmol/L. But the care must be taken to exclude other conditions which are responsible for acidosis with increased level of lactic acid such as renal failure, ketoacidosis, and other conditions where the elevation of lactic acid is not alone responsible for acidosis.

Lactic acid is formed from pyruvic acid and is the **(Fact file IV)** final product of glycolytic pathway in the absence of O_2. Thus, glycolytic cycle unlike the citric acid cycle can continue in anaerobic condition also. But normally further metabolism of pyruvate, formed at the end of TCA cycle, requires O_2 for its entry into the oxidative TCA cycle which is present within the mitochondria. In the absence of O_2, the TCA cycle stops and pyruvate accumulates and is converted to lactic acid. In hypoxia, this accumulation of lactic acid and H^+ ion will allow to continue the reaction (Embden–Meyerhof) for some period. Thus, lactate accumulation occurs during anaerobic metabolism by (1) increased production or (2) decreased gluconeogenesis from lactate into the liver and kidney or (3) failure of pyruvate to enter the tricarboxylic acid (TCA) cycle. Hepatic utilization of lactate usually accounts for 1,500 mmol/day with the ability to rise it to 3,400 mmol/day.

Etiology of Lactic Acidosis

Lactic acidosis is classified into two types: (1) *type A* and (2) *type B*. Type A lactic acidosis is due to tissue hypoxia and anaerobic metabolism. Type B lactic acidosis is due to the other causes which will be described further **(Fig. 12)**.

FACT FILE IV

Lactic acidosis may be caused by increased lactate production, due to hypoxia or may be caused by decreased lactate utilization by liver and kidney. Normal arterial lactate level is <2 mmol/L. Lactate level between 2 and 4 mmol/L are abnormal, but of uncertain clinical significance. Plasma lactate level, >5 mmol/L, is used to diagnose lactic acidosis. But in most cases of lactic acidosis, the lactate level runs between 10 and 30 mmol/L. Plasma lactate level is measured in a heparinized arterial blood sample, stored in ice. It should be assayed within 1 hour after the sample is drawn. Lactate level can also be measured from blood, collected in a fluoride oxalate tube which is normally used for glucose estimation. Though lactic acidosis is classified into type A and type B, still some believe that there is a little utility in this division, as both these types often share mechanisms of overproduction or underutilization.

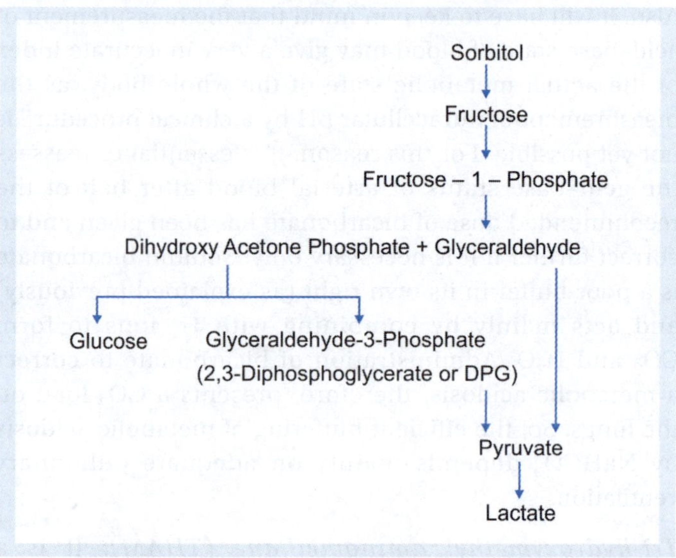

Fig. 12: Metabolism of fructose and sorbitol.

Type A Lactic Acidosis

The association between the metabolic lactic acidosis with the circulatory collapse and hypoxia is well recognized. The impaired tissue perfusion, due to circulatory collapse causing tissue hypoxia, is the result of any form of shock. This tissue hypooxygenation (hypoperfusion) may be further compromised by added severe hypoxemia (low PaO_2) due to respiratory causes and anemia. So, the blood lactate concentration, although seldom measured, closely correlates with the mortality rate. There is a mortality rate of about 75% in patients with blood lactate concentration rising from 4.4 to 8.9 mmol/L, but there is only the 10% mortality rate with lactate concentration rising from 1.3 to 4.4 mmol/L. However, the treatment of type A lactic acidosis entails the removal of causes and the subsequent O_2 and alkali therapy.

Type B Lactic Acidosis

The causes of type B lactic acidosis are:

- *Common disorders:* Diabetes mellitus, renal failure, hepatic failure, severe infection, and leukemia
- *Drugs:* Phenformin, metformin, salicylates, and paracetamol
- *Parenteral nutrition:* Fructose, sorbitol, and xylitol
- *Inherited:* Glycogen storage disease, fructose 1,6-diphosphate deficiency, Leigh's syndrome, methylmalonic acid, and anemia
- *Toxins:* Ethanol and methanol.

The most common cause of acute and serious Type B lactic acidosis is biguanide therapy for diabetes mellitus. Among the biguanides, phenformin is ten times more likely to produce an attack of lactic acidosis than metformin. The mortality of Type B lactic acidosis is 50%. Biguanides produce hypoglycemia by (1) reducing the alimentary absorption of glucose and amino acids, (2) decreasing hepatic gluconeogenesis, and (3) increasing glycolysis. Thus, lactic acidosis by biguanides is inherent and is produced by the hypoglycemic actions of it mentioned in (2) and (3). Usually during biguanide therapy blood lactate is <2 mmol/L, but impaired renal excretion, hepatic dysfunction or cardiovascular disease may easily induce lactic acidosis.

Fructose, sorbitol, xylitol, etc., have been used as energy substrates, instead of glucose, in diabetic patient because they all can be metabolized without insulin. This is of a particular importance in very sick patients who are insulin resistant. In addition, these agents are less irritant to veins than glucose. However, all these agents result in increased production of lactate. About 35% of fructose infusion is converted rapidly into pyruvate and then into lactate by liver.

Ethyl alcohol (ethanol) infusion inhibits hepatic neoglucogenesis. In the presence of hepatic disease or when administered with fructose, sorbitol, or biguanide, then lactic acidosis may result from ethanol.

Treatment of Lactic Acidosis

Like the treatment of type A lactic acidosis, the treatment of type B lactic acidosis should also always be directed at the underlying causes and must always ensure adequate oxygen delivery to tissues. The treatment of type B lactic acidosis is very difficult than type A lactic acidosis. If possible, causes should be removed first then symptomatic treatment is started. Large amounts of alkali are necessary for the treatment of this type B lactic acidosis, due to continuing lactate production. Therefore, alkalinization with $NaHCO_3$ is the mainstay of therapy of this type of lactic acidosis. Isotonic $NaHCO_3$ (1.4%) should be used to bring the pH back to normal, but slowly over about 6 hours. If hyperkalemia coexists, then this therapy will be beneficial for it, as the K^+ will enter the cells with the pH rises. If hyperglycemia exists insulin may be required.

Attempts have also been made to remove the lactate by dialysis or by stimulating the pyruvate dehydrogenase, which will encourage the conversion of lactate to pyruvate and will remove the latter via TCA cycle. Glucose and insulin seldom help in the treatment of type B lactic acidosis, as glycolysis is stimulated and gluconeogenesis is inhibited.

Central venous pressure (CVP) line and urinary catheter should always be inserted to monitor the progress of therapy, as circulatory overload with cardiac failure is a serious complication during the treatment of type B lactic acidosis. Hemodialysis may be required to treat cardiac failure. Repeated estimation of blood-gas is essential in any disturbance of acid–base balance and in these circumstances, it is of great practical value for repeated measurement of lactate levels.

■ METABOLIC ALKALOSIS

Metabolic alkalosis is less common than metabolic acidosis. It occurs due to: (1) excess production of base or (2) excess loss of noncarbonic acid (H^+), preserving HCO_3^-. It is characterized by (1) an increase in plasma bicarbonate, (2) a fall in blood H^+ concentration, (3) rise in plasma pH, and (4) a small compensatory rise in $PaCO_2$. In a healthy normal person when the plasma HCO_3^- rises above normal, then the urinary excretion of HCO_3^- increases rapidly. It is, therefore, very unusual to observe metabolic alkalosis in the presence of normal renal function. Uncompensated severe metabolic alkalosis has a very high mortality rate. The typical findings of uncompensated metabolic alkalosis are pH >7.4, $PaCO_2 \pm 45$ mm Hg, H^+, ion concentration <36 nmol/L, HCO_3^- concentration >32 mmol/L.

In metabolic alkalosis log HCO_3^-/H_2CO_3 component of the Henderson–Hasselbalch equation is increased due to raised HCO_3^- concentration and thus pH rises. Immediately compensation occurs by hypoventilation (respiratory acidosis). This conserves CO_2 and increases $PaCO_2$ so that the concentration of H_2CO_3 rises and thereby modifies the increase in pH by restoring the ratio of HCO_3^-/H_2CO_3 to normal. $H^+ + HCO_3^- \rightleftharpoons H_2CO_3 \rightleftharpoons CO_2 + H_2O$ equation shifts to the left.

This compensation may be limited till hypoxemia results from hypoventilation, particularly if the patient is breathing room air. It appears that respiratory stimulation from hypoxemia is stronger than the compensatory depression due to alkalosis and thus oxygenation is often maintained despite a metabolic alkalosis.

The formula for the expected raised $PaCO_2$ which occurs during respiratory compensation in a metabolic alkalosis is: $0.6 \times$ (measured $HCO_3^- - 24$) + 40. If the measured $PaCO_2$ is higher than expected, then one should think that this present metabolic alkalosis is mixed with respiratory acidosis. On the other hand, if the measured $PaCO_2$ is less than the expected $PaCO_2$, then it can be thought that this metabolic alkalosis is partially compensated or mixed with respiratory alkalosis. The compensation of metabolic alkalosis by elevating $PaCO_2$ is more erratic than that of metabolic acidosis and $PaCO_2$ usually does not rise above the level of 55 mEq/L. This is because the hypoxemia which is caused by hypoventilation will limit the compensatory rise of $PaCO_2$ that is described earlier.

The differential diagnosis of metabolic alkalosis is based on urinary Cl^-, i.e., urinary Cl^- <20 mEq/L and urinary Cl^- >20 mEq/L. This is because due to compulsion of electroneutrality, there are only two methods to add HCO_3^- to a compartment of ECF, i.e., either loss of Cl^- or retention of Na^+. In the ECF, the only anion that is present in sufficient quantity is Cl^-. The Cl^- is lost with H^+ or NH_4^+ ion. So, the loss of H^+ or NH_4^+ ion is equivalent to gain of HCO_3^-. The net effect is loss of Cl^- and gain of HCO_3^- leading to metabolic alkalosis.

Classification of metabolic alkalosis according to urinary Cl^-.
- *Chloride responsive* or urinary Cl^- <20 mEq/L:
  - *Renal loss:* Diuretics and cystic fibrosis
  - *GI loss:* Suction, vomiting, and chloride-wasting diarrhea
- *Chloride-resistant* or urinary Cl^- >20 mEq/L:
  - *Excess mineralocorticoids:* Cushing's and Conn's syndrome
  - Excess steroid administration
  - Bartter's syndrome.

Causes of Metabolic Alkalosis

Loss of H^+ Ions

- *Renal:* Primary and secondary hyperaldosteronism (discussed further).
- *K^+ depletion:* Acid (H^+) may be lost from kidney by hypokalemia with its paradoxical combination of acid urine and alkaline ECF.
- Conn's syndrome and Cushing's syndrome.
- *Drugs:* Diuretics (thiazide and furosemide) and corticosteroids.
- *GI tract:* Vomiting, nasogastric suction, pyloric stenosis, high intestinal obstruction, etc.
- Chloride deficiency **(Fact file V)**.

Gain in Alkali (HCO_3^-)

Metabolic alkalosis is also caused by administration of large amount of alkali by ingestion of oral antacids or infusion of $NaHCO_3$. There is also metabolic conversion of organic acid anions such as lactate and citrate to HCO_3^-, causing alkalosis.

FACT FILE V

Metabolic alkalosis causes hypoventilation and elevates $PaCO_2$ as one compensatory mechanism, but this compensation is more erratic than for metabolic acidosis and generally $PaCO_2$ does not exceed 55 mm Hg. To maintain the electro-neutrality in alkalosis, due to addition of more HCO_3^-, there are two ways: either loss of an anion such as Cl^- or retention of cation such as Na^+. So, the most useful biochemical parameter is to measure the level of urinary chloride which forms the basis of classification of metabolic alkalosis. The only anion that is present in sufficient quantity in ECF to be lost is Cl^-. It is lost with H^+ or NH_4^+. The net effect is loss of HCl or NH_4Cl to gain HCO_3^-. The loss of HCl or NH_4Cl is equivalent to loss of Cl^- for HCO_3^-. The two organs which are capable of inducing a loss of Cl^-, together with gain of HCO_3^- are stomach (vomiting, intestinal obstruction, etc.) and kidney (absorption of Na^+ as bicarbonate to maintain ECF volume).

Hypokalemia is an almost constant feature of alkalemic disorder (alkalosis produces hypokalemia or hypokalemia produces alkalosis), but is more prominent in those of metabolic origin. This is due to renal or extra renal losses of K^+ (diarrhea, suction, vomiting, etc.) in varying degrees. This condition also commonly occurs (1) after several days of IV therapy, where K+ replacement is inadequate; (2) prolonged, and strong diuretic therapy; (3) diarrhea; (4) hyperaldosteronism; and (5) other common causes of hypokalemia.

Normally 98% of total body K^+ remains as intracellular. The K^+ depletion causes metabolic alkalosis by two mechanisms: (1) during K^+ depletion, kidney vigorously attempts to conserve it, causing increased secretion of H^+ and concomitant increase in blood base and (2) K^+ is the major intracellular cation. Hypokalemia induces intracellular K^+ to enter the extracellular space to maintain near-normal serum level. This extracellular migration of K^+ forces the intracellular migration of H^+ and alkalosis. The net result is extracellular increase of HCO_3^-. This explains how mineralocorticoids cause hypokalemia and alkalosis.

This also explains how low serum K^+ level (hypokalemia <3.5 mmol/L) reflects a severe depletion of intracellular K^+. In turn, hypokalemia has several adverse effects. It includes neuromuscular weakness, polyuria, sensitization to digitalis-induced arrhythmia, and increased ammonia production which can heighten the risk of hepatic encephalopathy. Alkalosis stimulates anaerobic glycolysis and increases the production of lactic acid and keto acids. Alkalosis reduces the release of O_2 to the tissues by tightening the bond between O_2 and Hb. But chronic alkalosis negates this effect by increasing the concentration of 2,3-DPG level in RBC.

(2,3-DPG: 2,3 diphosphoglyceric; ECF: extracellular fluid; $PaCO_2$: partial pressure of carbon dioxide; RBC: red blood cell)

This situation is observed after a massive blood transfusion when the citrate is metabolized by liver over the next 48 hours to HCO_3^-, resulting in metabolic alkalosis.

There are important relationships between the handling of Na^+, K^+, and H^+ by kidney. Metabolic alkalosis is perpetuated when there is a reduction in ECF volume. The explanation is that in collecting duct final adjustment of urine composition is made by reabsorption of Na^+ in exchange of secretion of both K^+ and H^+ from tubular cells into the lumen. Thus, if the

BOX 4: Causes of metabolic alkalosis.

- *Chloride responsive (urinary chloride <20 mmol/L):*
  - Renal: Diuretics and hypercapnia
  - GI: Vomiting, diarrhea, nasogastric suction, gastrointestinal (GI) fistula, abuse of antacids, villous adenoma, excessive administration of alkali ($NaHCO_3$), etc.
- *Chloride resistant (urinary chloride >20 mmol/L):*
  - Primary hyperaldosteronism
  - Secondary hyperaldosteronism
  - Severe hypokalemia
  - Cushing's syndrome, Bartter's syndrome, etc.
- *Miscellaneous:* Milk alkali syndrome, alkali therapy, massive blood transfusion, etc.

kidney avidly retains Na^+ (in hypovolemic), it cannot retain K^+ or H^+, leading to metabolic alkalosis **(Box 4)**.

If, in addition to metabolic alkalosis, there is low intracellular K^+ concentration, because of potassium depletion (hypokalemia due to any cause), then there is obligatory more secretion of H^+ in place of K^+ and the resulting alkalosis will be even greater. When aldosterone and other mineralocorticoids (which increase the drive of tubular Na^+ reabsorption) are present in excess such as in primary or secondary hyperaldosteronism, then they have a similar effect.

Chloride is also very important in this context because normally at the various sites in nephron, Na^+ can be reabsorbed along with either chloride or bicarbonate. To maintain neutrality with raised HCO_3^- absorption, the Cl^- is excreted through kidney. So, urinary Cl^- level is increased in hyperaldosteronism, Cushing's syndrome, and in K^+ deficiency. But urinary chloride is low when HCl is lost from stomach or intravenous $NaHCO_3$ and diuretics are administered. In such condition when chloride is deficient, there is a preferential reabsorption of bicarbonate, instead of Cl^- which will make an alkalosis further worse. This will also prevent the additional excretion of bicarbonate by distal renal tubule, which is usually necessary as compensation, to correct an established metabolic alkalosis.

The classic typical example of metabolic alkalosis is sustained vomiting due to any cause. In normal condition, when H^+ are secreted into the gastric lumen, then HCO_3^- (a byproduct of H^+ ion formation) from parietal cells is absorbed into blood. Subsequently, this is neutralized by the reabsorption of secreted H^+ from a small bowel. In sustained vomiting, the initial loss of H^+ from our body initiates alkalosis. But the kidney is unable to restore the homeostasis by retaining H^+ ion because there is also a deficit of Na^+ and water due to constant vomiting, causing enhanced tubular Na^+ reabsorption in exchange of K^+ and H^+ (explained before). As K^+ is also lost in vomiting, there is an intracellular K^+ deficit. So, in the absence of K^+, tubular H^+ ion secretion

or its lost into lumen is magnified and alkalosis is sustained. Chloride is also lost during vomiting, so there is enhanced bicarbonate reabsorption by renal tubule (**Fig. 13**).

Use of diuretics, particularly if it is aggressive leading to ECF volume depletion, may have similar effects. Due to the inhibition of Na^+ absorption at proximal tubule by diuretics, more Na^+ is delivered to the collecting duct for reabsorption which causes more secretion of H^+. The depletion of ECF volume by diuretics also enhances the level of renin, angiotensin, and aldosterone which increases the drive of Na^+ reabsorption at collecting tubule, in exchange of H^+ and K^+ causing sustained alkalosis.

Kidney

In the proximal tubule there is obligatory Na^+ absorption, the extent of which is controlled by ECF volume. In the distal tubule Na^+ is reabsorbed in exchange for K^+ and H^+ under the influence of aldosterone. This is the cause of alkalosis in aldosteronism. Thus, hypokalemia occurs with alkalosis due to the increased excretion of both K^+ and H^+ for increased reabsorption of Na^+. In renal cause of retention of HCO_3^-, causing alkalosis, correction of pH alone without treatment of the underlying disease will result in recurrence and persistence of the metabolic alkalosis.

Clinical Effects of Metabolic Alkalosis

The clinical effects of metabolic alkalosis are tetany, hypocapnic vasoconstriction, left hand shift of O_2 dissociation curve, mental changes, and hypokalemia. It is discussed in more details in the next part of this chapter.

Treatment of Metabolic Alkalosis

Severe metabolic alkalosis may be a life-threatening condition, especially if it is accompanied by hypokalemia but it is uncommon. Treatment of this severe form of alkalosis includes the following:

- *Restoration of ECF volume:* This may involve transfusion of NaCl, plasma, or blood. It is important to say that to give chloride, NaCl is the simplest form, if Na load is not contraindicated.
- *Restoration of plasma K^+ concentration:* It is possible by using KCl or K^+ conserving diuretics such as triamterene and amiloride, if not contraindicated.
- *Inhibition of aldosterone (where appropriate):* This is done by using spironolactone.
- *Inhibition of carbonic anhydrase:* This is performed by acetazolamide which will produce retention of H^+ ions.
- *Direct acidification:* Sometimes HCl, NH_4Cl, lysine, or arginine may be used for the correction of metabolic alkalosis. These may all be given intravenously and will result in the release of free H^+ ions. HCl should only be

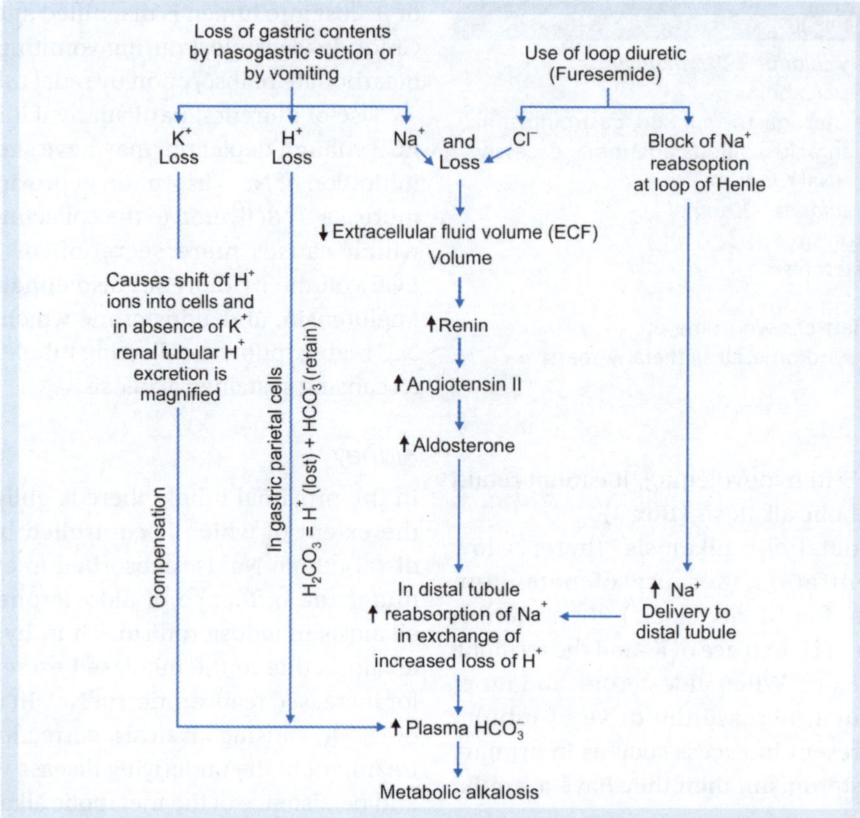

Fig. 13: Pathogenesis of metabolic alkalosis. This is due to the loss of gastric contents or use of loop diuretics.

administered through a central venous line at a rate of 0.2 mmol of H^+/kg/h. The maximum dose of H^+ which is about 300–500 mmol/day should not be exceeded.

One-sixth molar NH_4Cl has also been used as a source of acid because two molecules of NH_4Cl condense to form one molecule of urea and two molecules of HCl, but it is contraindicated in hypokalemic patients, as the further loss of K^+ is induced.

- *Loss of H^+ by vomiting or gastric suction causing alkalosis:* This can be controlled easily by ranitidine which reduces the H^+ concentration of gastric secretion.

■ MORE ABOUT ANION GAP

For electrical neutrality to exist, the number of anions (negatively charged ions such as Cl^-, HCO_3^-, etc.) must be equal to the number of cations (positively charged ions such as Na^+, Mg^+, etc.). When these two numbers are not equal, the difference between them is called the *anion gap*. The anion gap may be calculated in several ways and the normal range will therefore vary between different laboratories. One method of calculation which can be done on a routine electrolyte estimation is $(Na^+ + K^+) - (Cl^- + HCO_3^-)$. This gives a value between 11 and 19 mmol/L. It represents approximately the sum of some anions such as protein, phosphate, lactate, and 3-hydroxybutyrate, etc., which are usually not measured. Some laboratories also exclude K^+ from the calculations of the anion gap which gives a lower normal range.

Causes of High Anion Gap

- Uremic acidosis
- Keto acidosis
- Salicylate poisoning
- Lactic acidosis
- Methanol, ethylene glycol, and paraldehyde toxicity
- All of these afore-mentioned factors cause acidosis with a high anion gap. But there are many other causes of acidosis in which the anion gap is not abnormal because in such cases chloride replaces bicarbonate, for example, diarrhea.
- Dehydration.

Causes of Low Anion Gap

- Dilutional states
- *Hypoalbuminemia:* Albumin, at normal blood pH, has a marked negative charge and therefore accounts for most of the anion gap.
- Hypernatremia, hypermagnesemia, and hypercalcemia

- *Paraproteinemia:* Here, the increased viscosity of blood interferes with blood sampling.
- *Paraprotein:* Immunoglobulin produced by neoplastic plasma cells proliferating abnormally, e.g., myeloma protein.

Minor variations in the anion gap should be interpreted with care since it is calculated from four variables. However, it is of value in detecting an abnormality before a more specific investigation can be undertaken.

EFFECTS OF ACID–BASE DISTURBANCES

Continuously, acid–base disturbances due to metabolic ($\uparrow\downarrow H^+$ and $\uparrow\downarrow HCO_3^-$) or respiratory ($\uparrow\downarrow PaCO_2$) causes are going on in our body. So, homeostatic mechanisms are also acting dynamically to counter these disturbances and to bring back the plasma pH to normal. But the acute or prolonged disturbances can outpace these homeostatic mechanisms and result in a variety of acid–base disorders with their different clinical responses. Among these, the most frequently found acid–base disturbance is acidosis. Alkalosis occurs less frequently but is more harmful than acidosis. Acid–base disturbances cause multiple changes in different organs, with a myriad of interrelations and interactions. So, it is sometimes very difficult to understand (to identify or to differentiate between) the *cause* or *effects of acid–base disturbances* on different systems.

Effects on Cardiovascular System

There are different and separate responses of CVS, due to separate changes for $PaCO_2$ and pH. Again, it is very difficult to separate the responses of CVS due to the changes in CO_2 tension alone from the changes for sympathoadrenal stimulation which occurs during hypercapnia. So, it is very difficult to elucidate the actual effect of acid–base alteration on CVS system. In general, if $PaCO_2$ is maintained constant, then an increase or decrease in pH causes depression of myocardial contractility with fall in stroke volume and cardiac output, associated with a decrease in peripheral vascular resistance. In addition, the responsiveness of heart to catecholamine is also diminished in metabolic acidosis. On the other hand, hypercapnia produces increased stroke volume and cardiac output by increasing sympathetic activity. The effect of hypercapnia on peripheral vascular tissue depends on the degree of sympathetic innervation of it (peripheral vascular tissue). Richly innervated organ (kidney) respond to hypercapnia by vasoconstriction, whereas poorly innervated organs (cerebral cortex) respond by vasodilation. On the other hand, during hypocapnia, there is a generalized vasoconstriction independent of sympathetic innervation **(Table 12)**.

TABLE 12: Clinical effects of acidosis and alkalosis.			
	Direct effect	*Indirect effect*	*Net clinical effect*
Decreased pH (acidosis)			
Heart rate	↓	↑↑	↑↑
Cardiac contractility	↓	↑	0
Arterial resistance	↓↓	↑	↓
Venous resistance	↑	↑	↑↑
Pulmonary resistance	↑	↑	↑↑
Cerebral blood flow	↑	↑	↑↑
Airway resistance	↓	↑↑	↑
Renal circulation	↑	↓↓	↓
Serum K^+	↑	0	↑
Ionized Ca^{2+}	↑	0	↑
Increased pH (alkalosis)			
Heart rate	0	0	0
Cardiac contractility	0	0	0
Arterial resistance	↑	0	↑
Venous resistance	0	0	0
Pulmonary resistance	0	↓	↓
Cerebral blood flow	↓	0	↓
Airway resistance	↑↑	↓	↑
Renal circulation	0	0	0
Serum K^+	↓	0	↓
Ionized Ca^{2+}	↓	0	↓

↓: Decreased; ↑: Increased; 0: No effect

The effects of acid–base disturbances on heart rate (HR) should be discussed in steps: (1) The effect of changes of pH directly on HR and (2) the effect of catecholamine and ACh due to changes in pH (indirectly) on HR. In an isolated heart preparation (denervated or blocked) acidemia causes bradycardia. But in normal heart with intact nerve supply, the effect of acidemia is different. When pH decreases from 7.4 to 7.1, then the HR increases indirectly as a result of the effect of epinephrine which is released from adrenal medulla in response to acidemia. In severe acidosis, when pH further decreases below 7.1 then the effect is bradycardia. This bradycardia is due to increased vagal tone and accumulation of Ach (acetylcholine), as a result of decreased metabolism of it in acidic environment. So, clinically in normal healthy patient, acidosis (respiratory or metabolic) will cause initially tachycardia which is followed later by bradycardia, as the depressant effect of parasympathetic system overworks on the initial stimulating effect of sympathetic system.

Myocardium is also sensitive to the changes in $PaCO_2$ and pH both. So, the atrial and ventricular arrhythmias are common in acid–base disturbances. But it is not clear whether the arrhythmia is directly due to the changes in pH or due to the changes in extracellular K^+, secondary to the changes in pH. Arrhythmia may also be due to pH-related changes in Ca^{2+}, Mg^{2+}, and catecholamine levels. A change in 0.1 unit of pH is related to change in K^+ level of 0.5–1.5 mmol/L in opposite direction. In acidosis, high intracellular H^+ ion concentration causes hyperkalemia, but causes reduction of intracellular K^+ concentration. This alters the resting membrane potential of myocardium and causes arrhythmia. Decreased pH (acidosis) lowers the threshold value for ventricular fibrillation and increased pH (alkalosis) elevates it. Therefore, acid–base disturbances are frequently accompanied by ventricular arrhythmia. Decreased pH also causes an increase in ventricular ectopic by elevating the level of circulating catecholamines. Among all the volatile anesthetic agents halothane sensitizes the myocardium maximally to catecholamines. But in healthy patient, this is of little clinical significance.

Acidosis itself causes depression of myocardial contractility. This direct depression effect of myocardial contractility in acidosis is due to the impairment of Ca^{2+} entry into myocardial cells or decreased release of Ca^{2+} from intracellular storage site such as sarcoplasmic reticulum (SR). On the other hand, acidosis increases the level of circulating catecholamines. This increased level of catecholamines stimulates the myocardial contraction and overcomes the direct depressant effect of acidosis. Therefore, the net result of acidosis is increased myocardial contraction. But this occurs till the fall of pH up to 7, beyond which the direct depressive effect of acidosis predominates over sympathetic stimulating effects. Thus, mild acidosis, i.e., fall of pH up to the level of 7 will increase catecholamine level which will elevate cardiac output as a result of (1) increased in heart rate, (2) increase in myocardial contractility, (3) increase in venous tone (preload), and (4) simultaneous decrease in SVR (afterload). But when the pH goes further down below 7, then the cardiac depressant effects of acidosis are greater than the stimulant effects of catecholamines on myocardium, and cardiac output will fall. This also explains why a patient taking a Ca^{2+} channel blocker will demonstrate a decrease in contractility at a relatively slight change in pH.

Alkalosis does not induce the increased catecholamine secretion, but increases the responsiveness of the myocardium to circulating catecholamines. Thus, it produces an elevation of myocardial contractility and O_2 consumption. On the other hand, alkalosis or hypocapnia constricts coronary vessels and elevates coronary vascular resistance, thereby providing less supply of O_2 to myocardium. On the other hand, hypocapnia or alkalosis shifts O_2 dissociation curve toward the left, providing less extraction of O_2 by myocardium or less tissue unloading.

So, the net effect of alkalosis on myocardium is increased myocardial contractility, less O_2 supply to heart, and small myocardial O_2 reserve. In severe alkalosis, unbound plasma Ca^{2+} level decreases which possibly further reduces myocardial contractility.

The effect of acid–base disturbances on peripheral vasculature is also very complicated. In general, the direct effect of acidosis on systemic arterial bed (not the pulmonary) is vasodilatation, but this is not true in metabolic acidosis which causes vasoconstriction. In respiratory acidosis there is elevation of CO_2 level in blood which crosses the cell membrane of vascular smooth muscle more readily than H^+ ion. Within the cells, this CO_2 is converted to carbonic acid and the resultant decrease in intracellular pH is responsible for the decrease in vascular smooth muscle tone. In metabolic acidosis, the reduction of intracellular pH is not so great as respiratory acidosis, because H^+ ion itself, produced in metabolic acidosis, has the limited intracellular diffusibility, compared with CO_2.

On the other hand, due to release of more catecholamines, vasoconstriction is the result of metabolic acidosis. This vasoconstriction induced by metabolic acidosis continues until the pH falls up to 7.2. Below that level vasodilation will again occur in response to metabolic acidosis. On the other hand, both metabolic and respiratory acidosis causes pulmonary vasoconstriction, but when compared with hypoxic pulmonary vasoconstriction, the vasoconstriction caused by acidosis or alkalosis is less. Acidosis or alkalosis also enhances the normal hypoxic pulmonary vasoconstriction response. Thus, the acidosis increases pulmonary artery pressure and resistance. This is due to the constriction of pulmonary capillary sphincter and also due to the increase in venous return, secondary to acidosis-induced peripheral vasoconstriction. Furthermore, catecholamine-induced increase in cardiac output due to acidosis produces an increase in pulmonary blood flow and causes further increase in pulmonary artery pressure.

The individual vascular bed responds differently to acidosis. This is because of the varying contributions of direct and indirect effect of acidosis, type of acidosis, and the degree of sympathetic innervation. Metabolic acidosis will directly dilate the arterial bed of skin, skeletal muscles, kidney, other different organs, uterus, and coronary vasculature. Indirect effect of acidosis is mediated through the sympathetic system causing constriction. Thus, the net effect of acidosis on vascular bed is (1) richly innervated organ such as kidney responses by vasoconstriction, (2) poorly innervated cerebral cortex responses by vasodilatation, (3) splanchnic beds response by vasoconstriction, and (4) other vascular beds have variable changes.

Normally the coronary vascular constriction or dilatation, its resistance, and its blood flow mainly depend on local myocardial O_2 demand which is controlled by the heart rate, the force of myocardial contraction and afterload, etc. These are again varied by acid–base changes. So, it is very difficult to define the coronary response to acid–base changes. But the general rule is that acidosis causes dilatation and alkalosis causes constriction of the coronary vascular beds, therefore hyperventilation can increase the myocardial ischemia and lactate levels by significantly reducing the coronary blood flow.

The venous side of vascular bed responds by constriction to both the metabolic and respiratory acidosis, acting both by directly and indirectly. Alkalosis also tends to produce vasoconstriction, except pulmonary vasculature which dilates in alkalosis.

Effects on Respiratory System

The alteration of acid–base status also effect the respiration and O_2 delivery to the tissues through the changes on minute ventilation and O_2 dissociation curve. Acidosis increases minute ventilation and causes rightward shifting of O_2 dissociation curve (i.e., better delivery of O_2 to tissues). The increase in minute ventilation is accomplished by a substantial increase in tidal volume and little increase in respiratory rate (Kussmaul breathing, characterized by deep and rapid breathing pattern). The rise of minute volume is about twice as great if the fall in pH is due to rise in $PaCO_2$ (respiratory acidosis) than if the same fall in pH is due to an increase in H^+ ion concentration (metabolic acidosis). This is because CO_2 produced by the respiratory acidosis diffuses more readily across the blood–brain barrier than H^+ ion, produced from metabolic acids.

Hypercapnia increases ventilation by stimulating the central and peripheral chemoreceptor up to a maximum $PaCO_2$ of 80–90 mm Hg (11–12 kPa), but above that level of PCO_2 ventilation decreases. The 80% changes in minute volume are due to the effect of $PaCO_2$ on the medullary chemoreceptors, while the lesser percentage of changes in minute ventilation is due to the stimulus, originating from peripheral chemoreceptors. However, as the peripheral chemoreceptors are stimulated by the changes in both pH (H^+) and PCO_2, but the medullary receptors are stimulated only by the passage of CO_2 across the blood–brain barrier and the subsequent increase in H^+ ion concentration in CSF. CO_2 stimulates centrally-mediated respiration by decreasing the pH of ECF of brain which perfuse central chemoreceptor on the ventrolateral surface of the medulla. This takes place slowly over several minutes, but the increase of PCO_2 and reduction of pH produce a more rapid effect, within seconds, through the peripheral chemoreceptor of the aortic and carotid bodies. The respiratory stimulation by CO_2 among the normal healthy individual varies widely (0.5–5 L/min/ mm Hg), but in the same individual, the CO_2 response curve is similar at different times. The normal CO_2 response curve shows that respiratory acidosis will increase minute ventilation by 2–3 L/min for each 1 mm Hg increase in PCO_2. The CO_2-response curve is shifted toward the left by acidosis and toward the right by alkalosis (opposite to the O_2 dissociation curve). The volatile anesthetic agents decrease the slope of CO_2-response curve in a dose-dependent manner.

The acid–base disturbances also modify the resistance of airway by direct (local) and indirect (through sympathetic and parasympathetic axis) way. Directly, the increased CO_2 level, by easily and directly diffusing inside the cell, increases the intracellular concentration of H^+ ion and causes smooth muscle relaxation and reduction of airway resistance. Indirectly, the effects of hypercapnia cause bronchoconstriction by means of vagal stimulation. In normal healthy patients, the indirect bronchoconstricting vagal effect predominates over direct local bronchodilating effects, causing a net increase in airway resistance and work of breathing. Conversely, reduced PCO_2 level (in hypocapnia or respiratory alkalosis) produces a direct bronchoconstrictive effect, which is partially reduced by a centrally-mediated bronchodilating effect. However, the direct bronchoconstrictive effect of hypocapnia is clinically predominant and useful in matching the ventilation with blood flow in both healthy and pathological lungs such as in pulmonary embolism.

Both the CO_2 level and pH of blood alter the position of O_2 dissociation curve. An increase in PCO_2 or decrease in pH (i.e., acidosis) shifts the O_2 dissociation curve toward the right, causing an increased P_{50} level. The P_{50} is the partial pressure of O_2 in blood when Hb is 50% saturated and the normal value of this P_{50} is 27 mm Hg. An increased P_{50} means high O_2 partial pressure with same 50% saturation of Hb by O_2, which helps in better or more delivery of O_2 to tissues at the same 50% saturation of Hb by O_2. On the other hand, hypocapnia and alkalemia causes a shift to the left of O_2 dissociation curve and decrease in P_{50} level which means low O_2 partial pressure with same 50% saturation of Hb by O_2, i.e., lesser delivery of O_2 to the tissues.

During acidosis, the P_{50} is increased by about 2 mm Hg by a reduction of pH of 0.1 unit (10 nmol/L). Another cause of increased O_2 delivery to the tissues in acidosis is Bohr's effect. The Bohr's effect describes that the affinity of Hb for O_2 decreases as the level of H^+ in Hb increases. Thus, it increases the availability of O_2 to tissues. Contrary, alkalosis or decrease in H^+ concentration in Hb increases the affinity of Hb for O_2. This causes less delivery of O_2 to the tissues and increases its absorption by Hb in the lung. In normal healthy patient, this Bohr's effect has an overall important effect on the absorption of O_2 by Hb at pulmonary level and delivery of O_2 by Hb at tissue level. This is because O_2 affinity of Hb is greater in the normally somewhat alkalotic lung and lesser in the more acidotic tissue.

In acidosis, the rightward shift of the O_2–Hb dissociation curve occurs immediately. But after 20–30 hours, the concentration of 2,3-DPG level falls and restores the O_2 affinity of Hb. Thus, it shifts again the O_2–Hb dissociation curve back toward the left. The 2,3-DPG concentration decreases in acidosis because glycolysis in RBC is impaired in an acid environment and the glycolytic intermediates for the production of 2,3-DPG is depleted. Thus, the right shift of O_2 dissociation curve, produced by a decrease in pH, is partially antagonized by a decrease in 2,3-DPG level, induced by a decrease in intracellular pH.

Tissue oxygen delivery is the product of cardiac output and arterial oxygen content ($CO \times Hb \times SO_2$ and dissolved oxygen). A metabolic acidosis decreases the delivery of O_2 to the tissues by reducing CO which is partially compensated by the right shift of O_2 dissociation curve, whereas a metabolic alkalosis reduces the delivery of O_2 to tissues by both decreasing CO and shifting the O_2 dissociation curve toward the left. So, consequently, the correction of metabolic acidosis should always be undercorrected and not be overcorrected.

Effects on Nervous System

Like other vascular beds, a rise in arterial PCO_2 also results in cerebral vasodilatation and increased cerebral blood flow. At $PaCO_2$ of 80 mm Hg, the cerebral blood flow becomes double. When $PaCO_2$ is reduced to 20 mm Hg, then the cerebral blood flow becomes half of the normal value, due to cerebral vasoconstriction. But below 20 mm Hg of arterial CO_2 tension, the cerebral blood flow does not further reduce. This is due to the accumulation of lactate by hypoxia, which again stimulates vasodilatation and limits the further reduction of the blood flow.

As the H^+ ion cannot cross the blood–brain barrier, so the neurological changes from acid–base imbalance are only due to the changes of PCO_2 which cross the blood–brain barrier. The changes of CO_2 concentration on both the direction also causes the changes in pH of CSF on both the direction which impairs neuronal function and may lead to the changes of mental status and coma. Increasing the pain threshold during hyperventilation is also probably the result of this. These clinical effects are more pronounced in respiratory acidosis or alkalosis than that of metabolic acidosis or alkalosis, because CO_2 originating from respiratory acidosis rather than H^+ ion originating from metabolic acids (H^+) is permeable to blood–brain barrier. Cerebral metabolism

increases with acidosis and is maximum at a pH of 7. But CO_2 has a little direct effect on the cerebral metabolism.

Respiratory acidosis causes hypothermia. It is due to the impairment of function of the central thermoregulation center and also due to the cutaneous vasodilatation, increasing the heat loss.

Acidosis also causes an increase in the level of circulating catecholamines and stimulation of sympathetic nervous system. Epinephrine is released from the adrenal glands and norepinephrine is released from the sympathetic nerve terminals. In mild acidosis, this elevated catecholamine level tends to counteract the direct depressant effects of acidemia on organ function. However, in severe acidosis, the cellular response to catecholamine stimulation decreases and the direct depressant effect of the acidosis on cellular function becomes more apparent, despite increased catecholamine levels.

Effects on Enzyme Activity

Each enzyme has its optimal pH level for its optimum activity. Again, the cellular functional integrity depends upon the balance of the activity of different intracellular enzymes. So, if the pH varies beyond its normal limits, then intracellular enzymatic chaos results, and the cellular functions are deranged. This is because the activity of some intracellular enzymes is enhanced, while that of others is reduced.

Renal Effects

The response of renal vasculature to acidosis is vasoconstriction. As acidosis worsens, the renal vascular resistance also gradually increases and blood flow decreases. This renal vasoconstriction is the ultimate response (effect) after a balance between the direct, indirect, and systemic effects of acidosis on renal vasculature. Metabolic acidosis causes increased renal vascular constriction than the respiratory acidosis for an equal change of pH. This is because increased PCO_2 in respiratory acidosis increases the availability of CO_2 to cross the cell membrane and relaxes the vascular smooth muscle cells, reducing the intracellular pH. Catecholamine-mediated vasoconstriction of renal vasculature predominates over the vasodilatation effect of acidosis **(Fact file VI)**.

Uteroplacental Effects

The acid–base disturbances affect the fetus in two ways: (1) directly and indirectly. Directly the acid–base disturbance acts on the fetus through the changes of PCO_2, as the CO_2 is readily diffusible across the placenta. The passage of H^+ and HCO_3^- ion through placenta is very slow and, therefore, metabolic acidosis or alkalosis will cause little change in fetal

FACT FILE VI

- *Intracellular pH (pHi):* Attempts have been made to measure the pHi by inserting microelectrodes, with their tips smaller than 1 μm in diameter into the cell. Rough estimations of intracellular pH also can be made after the administration of indicator drugs or by examining the rates of pH-dependent intracellular enzymatic reactions. But all these methods, currently available, are open to methodological criticism. In addition, it is unlikely that the cells of all the parts of an organism or indeed all the parts of a single cell are at the same level of pH.

  Nevertheless, many studies have shown that, during normal healthy circumstances, the intracellular pH is roughly related to the extracellular pH (pHe), but is always lower than it, i.e., when pHe is 7.4, the pHi is usually <7.

  During acid–base disturbances the pHi:pHe ratio may alter. CO_2 is freely permeable across the cell membranes, so that respiratory changes are reflected by the similar changes in pHe and pHi ratio. But the highly ionized substances such as HCl and $NaHCO_3$ do not cross the cell membrane. So, the changes in their extracellular concentration have a negligible effect on pHi and pHe ratio.

  Changes in the intra:extracellular ratio of electrolytes such as sodium and potassium also do alter the ratio of pHi:pHe, however as the concentration of H^+ is 1,000–100,000 of the concentration of K^+, so the changes are not the result of a one-to-one exchange (between K^+ and H^+) across the cell membrane. Moreover, the total replacement of intracellular H^+ by extracellular K^+ would produce no measurable change in K^+ concentration. Nevertheless, in potassium deficiency, the intracellular cation deficiency is partly compensated by the movement of H^+ resulting in extracellular alkalosis and intracellular acidosis.
- *CSF pH:* The pH of CSF is controlled within very narrow range than the rest of the ECF of our body. Compared with the arterial blood, the CSF pH is lower by 0.1 units and the PCO_2 is higher by 7–9 mm Hg, but the bicarbonate concentration is similar. As the elevation of PCO_2 increases the cerebral perfusion, thus it eliminates more CO_2. So, the blood–brain PCO_2 difference is decreased in hypercapnia and increased in hypocapnia.

  The CSF acid–base status can be modified only by the changes in PCO_2 of CSF. So, the changes in metabolic acid–base status are not mirrored in the pH of CSF, because the blood–brain barrier is relatively impermeable to H^+ and HCO_3^-, although CO_2 equilibration is rapid. Consequently, respiratory acid–base disturbances cause a plasma equivalent CSF change. So, during longstanding metabolic disturbances, lasting several hours and days, the pH of CSF remains almost unchanged, whilst the change of it in respiratory acidosis or alkalosis is corrected within hours. The compensation for respiratory change is accompanied by a change in HCO_3^- (not H^+) of CSF so that the pH of CSF returns toward normal values. Although occasionally incomplete, such compensation for the respiratory disturbances and the minimal response to nonrespiratory changes result in the relative constant pH of CSF. But till now, the parts played by the active and/or passive mechanism in the adjustment of HCO_3^- of CSF are so far uncertain. Similarly, the role of the brain cells in generating HCO_3^- is not known.

(CSF: cerebrospinal fluid; ECF: extracellular fluid; $PaCO_2$: partial pressure of carbon dioxide; RBC: red blood cell)

pH for several hours. The acid–base disturbances indirectly act on fetus through the changes in placental blood flow. The changes in fetal pH also produce the similar effects on the fetal organ function as seen in adults. The direct effect of acidosis on the uteroplacental blood flow is vasodilatation but in severe acidosis, the overall effect on uterine blood flow is minimum. This is because the vasodilatation effect of acidosis is opposed by the vasoconstricting effects of the sympathetic stimulation, caused by acidosis.

The direct effect of alkalosis on uteroplacental vasculature is vasoconstriction. Alkalosis also causes a leftward change in the maternal O_2–Hb dissociation curve which increases the affinity of maternal Hb for O_2 and less delivery of it to fetus. So, severe maternal alkalosis causes fetal hypoxemia and fetal acidosis, due to the combined effects of uteroplacental vasoconstriction and decreased O_2 delivery to the fetus.

Effects on Ca^{2+} and K^+

There are three forms of Ca^{2+} in plasma (bound to plasma protein and nonbound to plasma protein, this nonbound Ca^{2+} is again in two forms: (1) ionized and (2) nonionized.

Approximately, 50% of plasma Ca^{2+} remains in unionized form and bound to plasma protein which is available for diffusion into the tissues. Another 45% of the plasma calcium remains in ionized form and is chemically active. The remaining 5% of plasma Ca^{2+} is present as nondiffusible form but is bound to other plasma components. In acidosis, H^+ ions compete for the negatively charged binding site of albumin, where Ca^{2+} is attached. Thus, H^+ ion displaces the Ca^{2+} ion from its binding site and increases its ionized serum level. Reversely, alkalosis causes an increase in the available protein binding sites and a reduction of ionized Ca^{2+} concentration with hypocalcemia. This causes tetany or mild disturbances in cardiac contractility.

Serum K^+ and pH levels are usually inversely related. So, when pH falls plasma K^+ level rises and vice versa. In acidemia, H^+ enters the cell along the concentration gradient and displaces the intracellular K^+ to maintain the intracellular electrical neutrality. K^+ comes out of the cell and causes hyperkalemia. It is estimated that for each 0.1 unit change in plasma pH causes a 0.6 mmol/L change in K^+ concentration in plasma. But this relation is not always linear.

DIAGNOSIS OF ACID–BASE DISORDERS AND PRACTICAL APPROACH

Interpretation of acid–base status from the value of parameters of blood gas analysis and subsequent its management requires a step-by-step systemic approach. This step-by-step systemic approach is described here **(Fig. 14)**:

First look at the pH of arterial blood. If this is acidemia (acidosis) or alkalemia (alkalosis). Now, we will have to look at the $PaCO_2$ and if this change in $PaCO_2$ is the cause of change in pH or not. That means, if pH decreases and $PaCO_2$ increases, then this acid–base disorder is respiratory acidosis or if pH increases and $PaCO_2$ decreases, then this acid–base disorder is respiratory alkalosis. On the other hand, if pH decreases, but $PaCO_2$ does not increase, rather decrease, then look at the HCO_3^- level. In such a situation, if HCO_3^- is decreased, then metabolic acidosis is confirmed and $PaCO_2$ is compensatory. Similarly, pH is increased, but $PaCO_2$ does not decrease, rather increases, then we will have to look at the HCO_3^- level. If it is elevated, then metabolic alkalosis is confirmed and elevated $PaCO_2$ is compensatory.

Therefore, the dictum is that if due to change in pH, the change in $PaCO_2$ and HCO_3^- concentration is in the same direction (both decrease or increase), then the acid–base disorder is simple (not mixed) and from the pH, $PaCO_2$ and HCO_3^- level you try to diagnose this type of primary disorder (respiratory acidosis/alkalosis or metabolic acidosis/alkalosis) and its compensatory part. Now, we will have to calculate if compensation is completed or still uncompensated.

If the change in $PaCO_2$ and HCO_3^- concentration is not in same direction, but in opposite direction, then the acid–base disorder is mixed type.

- With the change of pH, if the change of $PaCO_2$ and HCO_3^- concentration is in same direction, i.e., if the acid–base disorder is simple type (not mixed variety), then we will have to calculate if the compensatory response is more or less than expected **(Table 13)**.
- If our diagnosis is metabolic acidosis, then we will have to calculate the plasma anion gap.
- If our diagnosis is metabolic alkalosis, then we will have to calculate urinary Cl^- concentration.
- Now, we will discuss the mixed type of acid–base disorder. The mixed type of acid–base disorder is diagnosed by the following way: (1) With the change in pH, the change in $PaCO_2$ and HCO_3^- concentration is not at the same direction (in opposite direction), for example, pH is decreased and $PaCO_2$ is increased (primary respiratory acidosis), but there is a decreased HCO_3^- level (mixed with metabolic acidosis). Due to decreased level of HCO_3^-, the change in pH will be greater than the change in $PaCO_2$ (if the change in pH is greater or lesser than expected or predicted, a mixed type of acid–base disorder can be suspected); (2) pH is decreased and $PaCO_2$ is increased, but HCO_3^- concentration is increased

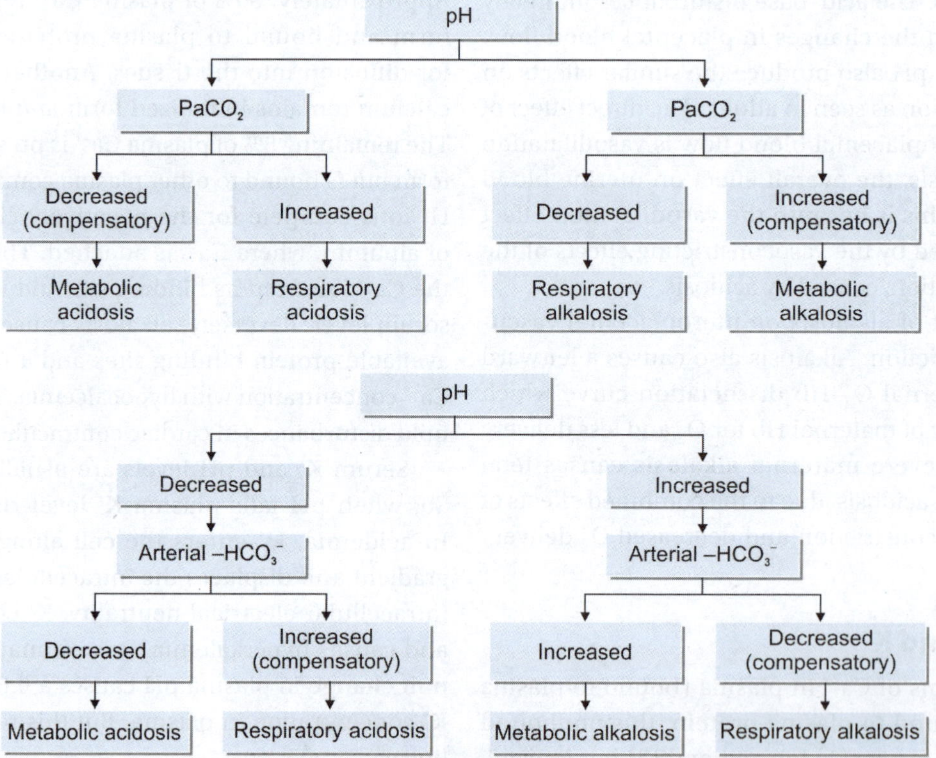

Fig. 14: Easy diagnosis of acid-base imbalance from this algorithm.

TABLE 13: Assessment of primary and compensatory response of different acidosis and alkalosis.

Disturbance	Primary response	Compensatory response	Expected change
Respiratory acidosis			
• Acute	• $\uparrow PaCO_2$	• $\uparrow HCO_3^-$	• 1 mEq/L/10 mm Hg increase in $PaCO_2$
• Chronic	• $\uparrow PaCO_2$	• $\uparrow HCO_3^-$	• 4 mEq/L/10 mm Hg increase in $PaCO_2$
Respiratory alkalosis			
• Acute	• $\downarrow PaCO_2$	• $\downarrow HCO_3^-$	• 2 mEq/L/10 mm Hg decrease in $PaCO_2$
• Chronic	• $\downarrow PaCO_2$	• $\downarrow HCO_3^-$	• 4 mEq/L/10 mm Hg decrease in $PaCO_2$
Metabolic acidosis	$\downarrow HCO_3^-$	$\downarrow PaCO_2$	$1.2 \times$ the decrease in $[HCO_3^-]$
Metabolic alkalosis	$\uparrow HCO_3^-$	$\uparrow PaCO_2$	$0.7 \times$ the increase in $[HCO_3^-]$

(respiratory acidosis mixed with metabolic alkalosis). Due to increase in HCO_3^- concentration, the change (decrease) in pH will be less than expected, according to increase in $PaCO_2$. Here, with the change in pH, the change of $PaCO_2$ and HCO_3^- level in the same direction. So, we thought that the change in HCO_3^- level is due to compensation. But in bicarbonate buffer chapter, we have said that with the increase in $PaCO_2$ the increase in HCO_3^- level will be minimum; and (3) the pH is increased and $PaCO_2$ is decreased and HCO_3^- level is increased. Here, pH is increased means primary disorder is alkalosis (respiratory or metabolic). If we consider this disorder is respiratory alkalosis, due to $\downarrow PaCO_2$, then due to compensation HCO_3^- will also decrease (change in the same direction), but here the change in $PaCO_2$ and HCO_3^- in opposite direction. So, there is a mixed disorder and that is metabolic alkalosis with respiratory alkalosis. Here, we will not discuss which one is primary and which one is secondary (compensatory), here both are primary.

- pH 7.39
  $PaCO_2$ 43 mm Hg
  PaO_2 90 mm Hg
  HCO_3^- 25 mEq/L

This patient has normal acid–base balance or fully compensated any acid–base disorder. History and clinical examination will suggest.

- pH 7.41
  PaO_2 64 mm Hg
  $PaCO_2$ 40 mm Hg
  HCO_3^- 23 mEq/L
  SaO_2 90%
  BE 0

This patient has normal acid–base balance or near fully compensated any acid–base disorder with mild hypoxemia.

- pH 7.20
  $PaCO_2$ 80 mm Hg
  PaO_2 82 mm Hg
  HCO_3^- 26 mEq/L
  BE 0
  SaO_2 92%

This patient is suffering from uncompensated severe respiratory acidosis with no hypoxia. Uncompensated because of HCO_3^- within normal range.

- pH 7.33
  $PaCO_2$ 66 mm Hg
  PaO_2 75 mm Hg
  HCO_3^- 34 mEq/L

This patient has partially compensated respiratory acidosis with mild hypoxia.

- pH 7.39
  $PaCO_2$ 55 mm Hg
  PaO_2 60 mm Hg
  HCO_3^- 38 mEq/L

This patient has completely compensated respiratory acidosis with moderate hypoxia.

- pH 7.50
  $PaCO_2$ 30 mm Hg
  PaO_2 100 mm Hg
  HCO_3^- 25 mEq/L

This patient is suffering from uncompensated respiratory alkalosis; respiratory alkalosis because $PaCO_2$ falls and uncompensated because HCO_3^- does not rise. It is within the normal range.

- pH 7.42
  $PaCO_2$ 32 mm Hg
  PaO_2 98 mm Hg
  HCO_3^- 20 mEq/L

The patient has compensated respiratory alkalosis; respiratory alkalosis because $PaCO_2$ falls to 32 mm Hg and compensated because the HCO_3^- comes down.

- pH 7.44
  $PaCO_2$ 25 mm Hg
  PaO_2 99 mm Hg
  HCO_3^- 20 mEq/L

This patient has partially compensated respiratory alkalosis. If it is fully compensated, then HCO_3^- is expected to fall more.

- pH 7.13
  $PaCO_2$ 42 mm Hg
  PaO_2 140 mm Hg
  HCO_3^- 14 mEq/L

This is a case of uncompensated metabolic acidosis. It is acidosis and uncompensated because the present pH value is far below the normal value, metabolic acidosis because only the HCO_3^- falls far below the normal range, and uncompensated because $PaCO_2$ does not change. In compensated stage it will fall.

- pH 7.26
  $PaCO_2$ 30 mm Hg
  PaO_2 130 mm Hg
  HCO_3^- 10 mEq/L

This is a case of partially compensated metabolic acidosis with hyperoxemia. It is metabolic acidosis because the level of HCO_3^- fall with the fall of pH. In the case of the fully compensated stage the formula for expected $PaCO_2$ is: $(1.5 \times HCO_3^-) + 8 \pm 2$. So, here if it was a fully compensated metabolic acidosis, the expected $PaCO_2$ is: $(1.5 \times 10) + 8 \pm 2 = 23$ mEq/L, but here $PaCO_2$ falls up to 30 mm Hg. So, it is partially compensated.

- pH 7.55
  $PaCO_2$ 38 mm Hg
  PaO_2 120 mm Hg
  HCO_3^- 34 mEq/L

This is a case of uncompensated metabolic alkalosis with hyperoxemia. It is metabolic alkalosis because pH is elevated and HCO_3^- is raised and uncompensated because $PaCO_2$ is not raised. It is within the normal range.

- pH 7.55
  $PaCO_2$ 50 mm Hg
  PaO_2 84 mm Hg
  HCO_3^- 50 mEq/L

This is a case of partially compensated metabolic alkalosis. Why it is metabolic alkalosis is easily understood? In a fully compensated case the formula for expected rise of $PaCO_2$ is: $6 \times (\text{measure } HCO_3 -24) + 40$. So, here if it is a fully compensated metabolic alkalosis, then the expected $PaCO_2$ should be: $6 \times (50 - 24) + 40 = 6 \times 26 + 40 = 55.6$ mEq/L, but here $PaCO_3$ is elevated only up to 50 mm Hg. So, this metabolic alkalosis is partially compensated.

A patient is suffering from congestive heart failure (CHF). He has tachypnea, low urine output, and poor peripheral circulation. He is placed on ventilation and $FiO_2 = 1.0$ (100%). His blood gas analysis report, Hb, and electrolyte measurements are like that: pH = 7.48, $PaCO_2$ = 12 mm Hg, PaO_2 = 210 mm Hg, HCO_3^- = 7.8 mEq/L, base deficit = –11 mEq/L, Hb = 9.4 g/dL, Na^+ = 7.8 mEq/L, K^+ = 5.4 mEq/L, Cl^- = 95 mEq/L, total CO_2 content = 8 mEq/L. Total CO_2 content is measured with electrolytes includes both plasma HCO_3^- concentration and dissolved CO_2 in plasma.

Now the question is what is the acid–base disturbance?
The answer is, using the previous discussion, we can come to a conclusion that clearly the patient has an alkalosis (pH >7.45) and it is respiratory in origin ($PaCO_2$ <40 mm Hg) or respiratory alkalosis. Here, the amount of decrease of $PaCO_2$ is $40 - 12 = 28$ mm Hg. For that the expected decrease of HCO_3^- should be $2 \times 28/10 = 5.6$ mEq/L and HCO_3^- level should be $24 - 5.6 = 18.4$ mEq/L. But here the patient's measured HCO_3^- level is 7.8 mEq/L (much below expected). Therefore, the diagnosis is that the patient has a definite mixed type of acid–base disturbance and it is primary respiratory alkalosis ($\downarrow PaCO_2$) plus primary metabolic acidosis ($\downarrow HCO_3^-$).

The change (decrease) in HCO_3^- level is beyond the expected compensatory change. So, we can conclude that in metabolic acidosis there is not only a compensatory (secondary) part, but also a primary cause (primary metabolic acidosis).

In another way, we also thought, there is a definite alkalosis (pH >7.45). If you look at the HCO_3^- level first (before looking at $PaCO_2$), then we will see that HCO_3^- level is much less than normal. So, it is not metabolic alkalosis. It is compensatory to respiratory alkalosis or associated metabolic acidosis.

Here, another interesting point is that the difference between the patient's HCO_3^- concentration (7.8 mEq/L) and expected HCO_3^- level for pure respiratory alkalosis (18.4 mEq/L) roughly correspond to base excess or negative base deficit, i.e., $18.4 - 7.8 = 10.6$ mEq/L.

Now, the second question is what is the cause of respiratory alkalosis and metabolic acidosis in this patient?
The answer is that the respiratory alkalosis is probably due to tachypnea and hyperventilation by ventilator in CHF and metabolic acidosis is probably due to lactic acidosis which is again due to poor tissue perfusion. The later is suggested by the calculated plasma anion gap. Here, the anion gap is $135 (95 +8) = 32$ mEq/L.

Now, the third question is what treatment is indicated?
The patient was treated with diuretics vasodilator (nitroglycerin) and inotropes. Patient improves slightly. Now, the repeat laboratory measurements are as follows: pH = 7.52, $PaCO_2$ = 23 mm Hg, PaO_2 = 136 mm Hg, HCO_3 = 18 mEq/L, BD = –3.0 mEq/L, Na^+ = 137 mEq/L, K^+ = 3.9 mEq/L, and total CO_2 = 18.5 mEq/L.

These laboratory findings show respiratory alkalosis is still present, but the base deficit has improved. K^+ has decreased due to diuresis. The expected decrease of HCO_3^- should be $17 \times 2/10 = 3.4$ mEq/L and HCO_3^- level should be $24 - 3.4 = 20.6$ mEq/L, but now the patient's HCO_3^- is 18 mEq/L. Hence, patient still has metabolic acidosis (2 mEq/L less). However, this HCO_3^- difference is close to the given BD. The anion gap is still high. Now, the anion gap is $137 - (92 + 18) = 27$ mEq/L. This high anion gap explains why the patient is still not doing well.

Water Balance

■ INTRODUCTION

Water is the most vital and abundant component of our body. It constitutes about 60–70% of our total body weight or lean body mass (LBM). It is better to use the term LBM than the total body weight. In our body, within this water, the major cations like Na^+, K^+, Ca^{2+}, H^+, Mg^{2+}, etc. and the major anions like Cl^-, PO_4^-, HCO_3^- etc. and proteins, carbohydrates, lipoproteins, vitamins, etc. are dissolved. Without water there will be no form of life. It forms the intracellular (IC) medium within which the metabolic reactions of cell, responsible for life, takes place, and it also forms the extracellular (EC) medium through which the transport and exchange of different solutes between the IC and EC spaces take place. Water deprivation brings about death earlier and easily than that of food. If water is given instead of food, then life may continue for several weeks by the loss of body fat and tissue proteins.

Total body water (TBW) in an average human being, weighing about 70 kg, varies between 45 and 50 L. It is 60–70% of 70 kg body weight. In female, it is 10% less than that of male. So, in female, the TBW constitutes about 50–60% of her LBM. Therefore, TBW in female weighting about 70 kg is 40–45 L. But, these above values vary mostly with the relative degree of obesity of an individual, *because body water content is inversely related to the adiposity of any living organism. Hence, as female has more body fat, it contains less TBW in relations to LBM than that of a male and in a lean person the value of TBW is higher than that of an obese person. Therefore, in general, the woman contains more fat and less water than man.*

The total water of a body is considered to be distributed within two main components: (1) the *intracellular (IC)* component and the *extracellular (EC)* component. The water of IC component constitutes about 55% of TBW or 40% of LBM. The remaining 45% of TBW constitutes the extracellular fluid (ECF) component or 20% LBM. Of this 20% EC body water, 15% remains in interstitial compartment and 5% remains in intravascular compartment. The cell membrane actually provides the boundary between these two IC and EC compartments **(Table 1)**.

The IC fluid component represents the sum of fluid contents of all the cells in our body. It is neither in a continuous nor in a homogenous phase with other EC tissue fluid. The cell membrane plays an important role controlling the IC and EC fluid volume and their composition. This is done in the following way. *A membrane-bound ATPase-dependent Na^+-K^+ pump exchanges (pushes) K^+ inside the cell and brings out Na^+ outside of the cell in 2:3 ratio.* This is due to the relative impermeability of cell membrane to Na^+ in relation to K^+. Therefore, *Na^+ is mainly concentrated in the ECF and is the most important determinant factor for EC osmotic pressure and osmolality, whereas K^+ is concentrated mainly in the IC fluid and acts as the most important determinant factor for IC osmotic pressure and osmolality.* This IC and

TABLE 1: Percentage of body fluid compartment of a 70-kg adult male.

Compartment	Fluid as percent (%) of lean body mass (LBM)	Fluid as percent (%) of total body water (TBW)	Fluid volume (L)
Intracellular	40	55	28 L
Extracellular	20	45	14 L
	Total: 60	Total: 100	Total: 42 L
In extracellular: Interstitial including connective tissue, bone, lymph, cartilage, transcellular, etc.	15	37 Connective tissue (7.5), bone and cartilage (7.5), lymph (20), transcellular (2)	10.5 L
In extracellular: Intravascular	5 Total: 20	8 Total: 45	3.5 L Total: 14 L

EC osmotic pressure and osmolality determines the IC and EC fluid volume. Protein (anion) is a nondiffusible solute and impermeable to cell membrane. This results in high IC protein concentration and is *also responsible* for IC osmotic pressure and osmolality. *The unequal exchange of three ion of K^+ going into the cell against the two ions of Na^+ going out of the cell by Na^+-K^+-ATPase pump, situated on the cell membrane, maintains this relative IC hyperosmolar condition and this is critical for the function of cells.* Therefore, the interference of this Na^+-K^+-ATP pump, due to any cause, such as ischemia, hypoxia, poison, etc., leads to a progressive swelling of cells and ultimately its death.

Like IC fluid component, the ECF component is also not a continuous or homogenous phase. Rather, it is a heterogeneous collection of fluids. It is postulated that 55% of TBW is present in IC component and the rest 45% of TBW is in the EC component. The ECF component is again divided into the following subcompartments: interstitial fluid and lymph (20%), intravascular fluid (8%), fluid in dense connective tissue and cartilage (7.5%), inaccessible bone water (7.5%), and transcellular water (2%). The transcellular fluid is the part of ECF component which is separated from other ECF by an epithelial membrane. Thus, the transcellular fluid includes: CSF, joint or synovial fluid, intraocular fluid, fluid in pleural or pericardial or peritoneal cavity, fluid in the duct of digestive gland, intraluminal fluid of gastrointestinal (GI) system, etc. The ECF provides medium for different electrolytes, nutrients, waste products, enzymes, hormones, gases, etc., to move from one place of its origin to another. Therefore, the maintenance of ECF volume is also very critical to maintain the functions of cell. The Na^+ is quantitatively the most important ECF cation and is the major determinant factor for ECF volume and pressure which is parallel to the intravascular fluid volume and pressure. The changes in total body Na^+ content is, therefore, related to EC and intravascular fluid volume and pressure. The total body Na^+ content further depends on its intake through oral or intravenous route and excretion through renal and extrarenal route **(Fig. 1)**.

Normally, very little amount of interstitial fluid remains in free form, because it is usually present in chemical association with EC substances, called *"proteoglycans"* forming a gel. This interstitial or tissue fluid (water) comes from plasma by the process of diffusion or filtration through capillaries. This fluid occupies the intercellular (interstitial) space and forms the connecting link for the transport of nutrition, gases, and metabolic end products between the blood capillaries, tissue cells, and lymph. It constitutes the internal environment of body which surrounds the cells. This interstitial fluid is also derived from cells, due to IC activities.

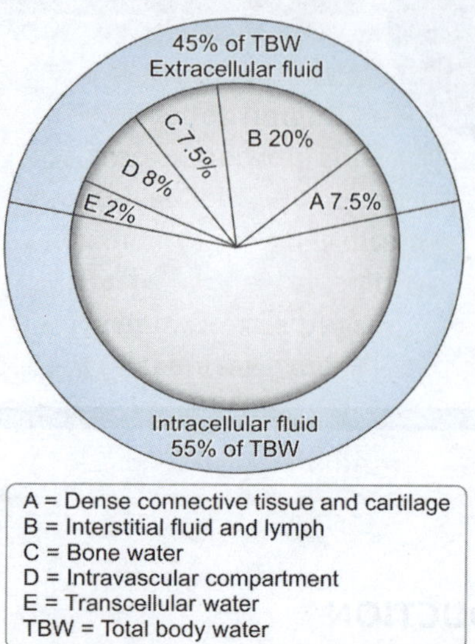

Fig. 1: Schematic representation of distribution of body water in different compartment (in % of TBW or total body water).

The amount of interstitial fluid, coming from plasma, depends upon: (1) the capillary permeability, (2) the differences of hydrostatic pressure between capillary blood and interstitial fluid, (3) the difference of colloidal osmotic pressure of blood and interstitial fluid. It is obvious that anything that increases the capillary permeability will also increase the amount of interstitial fluid that is formed. Regarding the blood pressure and osmotic (colloidal) pressure, it is known that at the arterial end of capillary, the average blood pressure (hydrostatic pressure) is about 32 mm Hg and at the venous end it (capillary) is about 10 mm Hg. On the other hand, the colloidal osmotic pressure of blood at both the ends of capillary is same and is about 25 mm Hg. Therefore, at the arterial end the net filtration pressure is 32–25 = +7 mm Hg which is directed toward the interstitial fluid. On the other hand, at the venous end, due to fall in blood or hydrostatic pressure the net filtration pressure is negative which is 10–25 = –15 mm Hg and in the opposite direction, i.e., from interstitial fluid toward capillary. Thus, at the arterial end of capillary, the water, electrolytes, nutrients, gases, and other solutes pass from the intravascular to interstitial compartment and at the venous end they pass in opposite direction and maintain the homeostasis of water in interstitial compartment.

Moreover, the magnitude of these forces differs at the various tissue beds. The capillary pressure at its arterial end is determined by the precapillary sphincter tone. When the tone of this sphincter increases, then there is less flow of blood through capillaries and the capillary pressure is reduced. Thus, some capillaries which require high pressure (e.g., glomeruli) maintain low precapillary sphincter tone,

TABLE 2: Composition of fluid in different compartment of body.

Intracellular (mEq/L)				↔	Interstitial (mEq/L)				↔	Intravascular (mEq/L)			
Na^+	10	Cl^-	4		Na^+	140	Cl^-	110		Na^+	140	Cl^-	100
K^+	140	HCO_3^-	10		K^+	4	HCO_3^-	30		K^+	4	HCO_3^-	26
Ca^{2+}	1	PO_4^{2-}	100		Ca^{2+}	3	PO_4^{2-}	2		Ca^{2+}	3	PO_4^{2-}	2
Mg^{2+}	40	SO_4^{2-}	2		Mg^{2+}	3	SO_4^{2-}	1		Mg^{2+}	3	SO_4^{2-}	1
		Protein (or 16 g/dL)	50				Protein	6				Protein (or 7 g/dL)	24

while high sphincter tone is maintained for low pressure capillaries of muscles **(Table 2)**.

The amount of interstitial fluid, formed from tissue cells, depends upon the degree of metabolic activity of these cells. It should be noted that the tissue cells produce water as an end product of their carbohydrate, fat, and protein metabolism. This metabolic water is added to the already existing interstitial fluid. More the degree of activity, more will be the metabolic water formed and consequently the amount of interstitial fluid will increase. The two most important exceptions of this usual hemodynamic events of capillary pressure are: (1) the capillaries of lungs where the hydrostatic blood pressure is about 0.6 mm Hg and water does not come out of capillary and (2) the capillaries of kidney where glomerular hydrostatic pressure is about 60–80 mm Hg and large amount of water comes out of capillary. In normal body tissues, if the hydrostatic blood pressure is increased within capillaries, then it will interfere the return of water to the venous end of these capillaries and if it is excess than the amount which is drained by lymphatics, then it will result in excess accumulation of interstitial fluid, causing edema.

It is believed that the composition of interstitial fluid is same as that of lymph, except that its (interstitial fluid) protein content is negligible. So, its colloidal osmotic pressure is very low. The composition and the volume of interstitial fluid are regulated by the constant interchange of it between the blood and lymph. The specific gravity of interstitial fluid varies in-between 1.015 and 1.023. It may contain few or no erythrocytes. But, regarding white cells, the interstitial fluid contains a good number of lymphocytes and a small number of granulocytes. Blood proteins and nutrient contents of it are very low. It does not contain platelets, but may also clot very slowly. It contains higher concentration of waste products, but glucose, salt, and water contents of it are more or less same, as that of plasma **(Fact file I)**.

The interstitial fluid constitutes the internal media or environment in which the tissue cells are bathed. The cells draw O_2 and nutrition from this fluid and excrete their metabolites into it. Hence, the interstitial fluid may be regarded as the medium which supplies all the immediate

FACT FILE I

The capillary endothelium acts as freely permeable membrane to water, anions, cations, and many diffusible substances such as urea, glucose, amino acids, etc., except protein. As a result, the solute concentration between the plasma and interstitial fluid is same. Each contains sodium and chloride as the principal cations and anions, respectively. As protein is a nondiffusible anions, it remains in plasma at a higher concentration. The concentration of Cl^- is slightly higher in interstitial fluid. This is due to maintain electrical neutrality which is called "*Donnan equilibrium*".

requirements of cells. The interstitial fluid also acts as a great reservoir of water, salts, nutrition, etc. This function of interstitial fluid is very important. Because in any condition, when the blood volume is increased or diminished, then the new physical forces are set up by which the blood volume is kept constant with the help of this tissue reserve. For example, during hemorrhage, when the capillary pressure becomes very low and goes below the colloidal osmotic pressure of capillary blood which remains same, then due to this relative higher colloidal osmotic pressure in capillaries, the water is drawn in from interstitial space of tissues, so that blood volume is restored. When water is drawn away from blood, such as due to diuresis, excessive sweating, diarrhea etc., then the blood volume and blood pressure will be lowered. But, the plasma proteins will be more concentrated. This will increase the colloidal osmotic pressure of blood. This increased osmotic (colloidal) pressure of plasma and reduced blood pressure will increase the rate of absorption of water from tissue fluid and thus the blood volume will be kept constant. On the other hand, when blood volume increases, as for instances by intravenous infusion of large quantities of iso-osmotic saline, then the fluid will immediately pass out into tissue spaces, due to two causes: (1) saline will dilute the colloids and reduce the capillary colloidal osmotic pressure and at the same time, (2) by increasing the volume of blood will raise the blood pressure and will cause more filtration. Both these factors will cause more fluid to run out into tissue spaces, until blood volume comes back to its original level.

The intravascular fluid compartment is completely restricted to vascular space, enclosed by endothelium and the fluid, in it, is called "plasma". Most electrolytes, glucose, amino acids, enzymes, hormones, water, etc., can freely pass between this plasma and interstitial space, resulting in nearly identical composition of interstitial fluid and plasma. But, protein cannot pass freely between the plasma and interstitial space. This is due to tight intercellular junction between the adjacent endothelial cells. As a result, plasma protein, mainly albumin, remains in high concentration in intravascular compartment and acts as only osmotically active solute.

DIFFERENT NOMENCLATURES AND DEFINITIONS

To understand the water and electrolyte balance properly, it is mandatory to know the concentration of electrolytes and other solutes in their solution accurately. Usually, the concentration or the quantity of solutes in a solution is expressed as *percentage, gram moles, equivalent, etc., per liter*. Furthermore, to complicate the things, the concentration of solution can be expressed as the quantity of a solute per volume of solution (volume/volume) or per weight of solvent (weight/volume). At present, the concentration of solution is expressed by some systems of international unit (SI). These systems of international units are: *molarity, molality, osmolality, osmolarity, etc.*

According to Avogadro's principle, the number of molecules represented in one mole of substance is 6.023×10^{23}. A mole or gram molecular weight (i.e., molecular weight in gram) is the amount of substance equal to its molecular weight expressed in grams. *When the amount equal to the molecular weight in grams of a solute is dissolved in 1 L of solvent, then it is called the one molar (M) solution.* For example, when 98.016 g of H_2SO_4 (molecular weight of H_2SO_4 is 98.016) is dissolved in 1 L of water, then it produces one molar solutions. *When one molecular weight expressed in gram of a solute is dissolved in 1 kg of solvent, then it is called one molal (m) solution. Therefore, the number of moles of a solute per liter of solution is called "molarity". On the other hand, the number of moles of a solute per kilogram of solution is called "molality".*

Osmosis refers to the movement of solvent (e.g., water) across a semipermeable membrane into the region where there is higher concentration of nondiffusible solute. This nondiffusible solute is known as the osmotically active particles. The term *osmosis* and *osmoles* are only applicable to nondiffusible solutes. The amount of this nondiffusible (or nondissociable or osmotically active particles) solutes present in solution is expressed as osmoles, like moles. *One osmole of nondissociable solute is equal to the one mole or molecular weight in gram of dissociable solute. The number of*

FACT FILE II

Tonicity is a physiological term, whereas osmolality is a chemical term and may be confused with the previous one. But, it should not be done. The critical difference between these two terms is that all solutes contribute to the osmolality, but only solutes which do not cross the cell membrane is responsible for tonicity. Because, the term "tonicity" is used to describe the osmotic pressure created by nondiffusible solid of a solution in relation to that of plasma. The substances such as urea, glucose, ethanol, methanol, etc., can diffuse across the cell membrane freely. Therefore, they do not alter the distribution of water between the IC and EC fluid compartments and cannot contribute to tonicity. But, they contribute to osmolality, whereas the substances such as mannitol and sorbitol cannot cross the cell membrane and is only restricted to the ECF compartment. Therefore, they contribute both to the osmolality and tonicity.

osmoles of nondissociable solute per liter of solution is called "osmolarity". On the other hand, the number of osmoles of nondissociable solute per kilogram of solvent is known as "osmolarity" **(Fact file II)**.

The relation between the *osmole and mole* is that when each mole of dissociable solute ionizes then it results in $n \times$ osmole (Osm), where n represents the number of different types of ions produced by dissociate solutes. *For example, when one mole of highly dissociable solutes such as NaCl is dissolved in water, it produces 1 Osm of Na^+ and 1 Osm of Cl^- or 2 Osm of ions. Therefore, 1 Osm of dissociable solutes (such as NaCl) is equal to the one mole of that substance, divided by the number of freely moving particles or ions that each molecule of that substance liberates in solution. Therefore, 1 mole of NaCl = 2 Osm of NaCl. Hence, 1 Osm of NaCl = 1/2 mole of NaCl. In another example, 1 mole of Na_2SO_4 would dissociate into Na^+, Na^+, and SO_4^{2-}, supplying 3 Osm. So, 1 Osm of Na_2SO_4 is 1/3 mole of it. Therefore, osmolality is the number of particles (different ions) per liter of water and osmolarity is the number of particles per kilogram of water (Fact file II).*

The molecular weight of glucose is 180. Therefore, one mole or one gram molecular weight (gmol) of glucose is 180 g. Hence, if 180 g of glucose is dissolved in 1 L of water, then this solution will represent molar concentration of 1 mol/L and as the glucose is nondissociable and nondiffusible solute (or osmotically active particles), so the solution will also represent osmolar concentration of 1 Osm/L. On the other hand, NaCl is a dissociable solute. It ionizes in solution and each ion represents an osmotically active particle. Molecular weight of NaCl is $23 + 35.5 = 58.5$. Therefore, if 58.5 g of NaCl is dissolved in 1 L of water then the molarity of this solution is 1 mol/L and osmolarity is 2 Osm/L.

In body fluids, the concentration of different solutes is much lower. So, they are expressed as *millimole per liter*

FACT FILE III

A. Molarity, molality, and equivalency:

1. Molarity, molality, and equivalency are applicable to measure the concentration of dissociable substances. Previously (as older method), the term "concentration" was used (still also in common use) to measure (or express) the quantity of solute in a solution and it is expressed as gram per volume (in liter) of solution or per weight (in kg) of solvent. But, now, the system of international (SI) units is used to measure the amount of solute in a solution and these are: molarity, molality, osmolarity, and osmolality.
2. *Molarity* of a substance is defined as the number of moles of a solute per liter of solvent or solution. 1 mole (mol or M) of a substance represent 6.02×10^{23} molecules. Gram molecular weight is the 1 mole of a substance in gram. 1 mole is numerically equivalent to the molecular weight of that substance.
3. *Molality* of a substance is expressed as the number of moles of a solute per kilogram of a solvent or solution.
4. Let, the concentration of a substance in a solution is 5 moles. It means, 5 moles ($5 \times$ molecular weight in gram) of this substance is present in 1 L of solvents or solution. Let, the concentration of a substance is 5 molal. It means, 5 moles of this substance is present in 1 kg of solvent or solution.
5. Equivalency is applicable for the substances which are also ionized (or dissociable) in a solution. Equivalent of a substance (Eq/L) is the number which is obtained by multiplying the number of mole by its charge (valency). For example, 1 mole (M) solution of $MgCl_2$ yields 2 equivalent of Mg per liter and 2 equivalent of Cl per liter. 1 M solution of NaCl yields 1 Eq of Na and 1 Eq of Cl.

B. Osmolarity, osmolality, and tonicity:

1. Osmolarity and osmolality are applicable to measure the amount of substances in their solution which are nondissociable or nonionizable. 1 Osm of nondissociable substance is equivalent to the 1 mole of dissociable substance in its solution. *Osmolarity* of a substance is expressed as the number of osmole (1 Osm of nondissociable substance = 1 mole of dissociable substance) of a nondissociable solute per liter of solvent or solution.
2. *Osmolality* of a nondissociable substance is expressed as the number of osmoles of a solute per kilogram of a solvent or solution.
3. For substances that ionize or dissociate, however, each mole (M) of such substances results in *n Osm* of substance, where *"n"* is the number of ionic species, produced after ionization. For example, 1 mole of NaCl dissolved in solution will produce solution of 2 Osm concentration of NaCl.
4. *Tonicity* is a term that is often used interchangeably with osmolarity and osmolality, refers to the effect a solution has on cell volume. An isotonic solution has no effect on cell volume, whereas hypotonic and hypertonic solutions increase or decrease the cell volume, respectively.
5. *Osmosis* is the net movement of water across a semipermeable membrane as a result of a difference in nondiffusible (only for this membrane), not nondissociable, solute concentrations between the two sides. *Osmotic pressure* is the pressure that is applied on the side of higher solute concentration to prevent the movement of water across the membrane to dilute the solute.

(mmol/L) which is equal to the one-thousandth of one mole per liter. Thus, 1 mole of NaCl is 58.5 g and 1 mmol = 58.5 mg.

In vivo or in the body the dissociation of dissociable solutes remains incomplete. So, a solution of NaCl containing 1 mmol/L of solute contributes osmolarity slightly less than the theoretical 2 mOsm/L.

Equivalent is also commonly used as measuring unit for solutes that ionizes in solution and produces ions. Actually, it is the measuring units of ions in a solution produced from dissociable solutes. *The equivalent number of each ion is the number of moles of these ions divided by its valency or charge.* Thus, 1 mole (M) solution of NaCl yields 1 equivalent of Na^+ and 1 equivalent of Cl^- per liter of solution. Hence, one equivalent of $Na^+ = 23$ and one equivalent of $Cl^- = 35$. Similarly, one molar solution of CaCl2 yields 2 equivalent of Ca^{2+} and 2 equivalent of Cl^-, but 1 equivalent of Ca^{2+} is $40 \div 2 = 20$. *Gram equivalent is the molecular weight in gram divided by the number of valency of ion present or equivalent which is expressed in gram. One milliequivalent (mEq) is one-thousandth of one equivalent.*

The concentration of solution is also measured by *percentage*. This percentage can be expressed as *percent by weight or present by volume*. Weight in grams of a solute per 100 g of solution is known as percent by weight and the same amount of solute in gram dissolved in 100 mL of solution is known as percent by volume **(Fact file III)**.

■ ELECTROLYTES AND COLLOIDS

The *electrolytes* are the compounds which can be dissociated into anions and cations, when they are in molten state or in solution. The examples of electrolytes are: salts, acids, bases, etc. On the other hand, the *nonelectrolytes* are the compounds which cannot be dissociated in its solution of water, after the passage of currents, e.g., glucose.

When sugar, urea, NaCl, etc., are dissolved in water, they result in a clear solution. This is called true or *crystalloids solution*. On the other hand, when the protein, starch, glycogen, etc., are dissolved in water they result in thick, opalescent solution. This is called *"colloidal solution".* But, the *actual difference between a crystalloid and colloid solution depends on the size of the molecules of solute in their solvent. If the size of the molecules of a solute is >200 μm, they remain as suspension. While, if the size of the molecules of a solute is <1 μm they remain as true clear solutions. Therefore, the size* *of the molecules in a colloid solution varies between 1 and 200 μm.* To understand the difference between a crystalloid and a colloid, one should have a *clear idea regarding the forces that help the solute particles to stay in solution* which are roughly as follows:

- The inherent movement of solute particles, i.e., diffusibility of solute.
- The inherent movement of solvent molecules which continuously dash against the solute particles and thus help to keep them in solution.
- The electric charges—positive or negative—carried by the solute particles which by constant attraction or repulsion also help to form uniform solution.
- Hydration or carrying water molecules with the solute molecules.

If the solute particles are very small (below 1 μm), then all these, abovementioned, forces will act to their maximum. Thus, it will result in a permanent true clear solution. Now, if the solute particles be gradually made larger and larger, then their own movement or diffusibility will gradually be reduced and ultimately will be almost nil. Then, the other forces, such as the dashing forces of solvent molecules, electric charges, etc., will further try to keep the large solute particles, somehow in solution and will be able to do so up to a certain extent. This is called the "colloid solution". If then the solute particles be made still larger (over 200 μm), then all the forces will completely fail and the solute particles will not go into solution at all. Then they remain in suspension or as insoluble state. Hence, if the relation between solute and solvent be studied as a series of phenomenon, it will be found that at one extreme end there is complete solubility or true crystalloid solution and at the other extreme end there is complete insolubility. While in the intermediate stages there will be a phenomenon of semisolubility. This is called the "colloidal solution" (**Fact file IV**).

Thus, other factors remaining constant the real difference between a true crystalloid solution and colloid solution lies

FACT FILE IV

The difference between the IC and EC fluid compartment is that in IC fluid the principal cation is K^+ and the principal anion is phosphate (PO_4^{2-}). Further, there is high protein content inside the cell due to impermeability of it to the cell membrane. But the cell membrane is permeable to different ions, glucose, urea, water, etc. Therefore, there is continuous movement of water across the cell membrane and equalizes the osmotic pressure between the IC and EC fluid compartment. However, at equilibrium the osmolality between the IC and EC fluid compartment is not equal. This is also due to the active movement of water and diffusible particles across the cell membrane and produces any induced osmolal gradient. This is the fundamental principle which helps to understand the physiology of fluid and electrolytes.

in the size of the solute particles and not upon their chemical nature. Hence, a colloid may be defined as a substance which by the reason of the size of its molecules is slowly diffusible rather than soluble in water and is incapable of passing through a semipermeable membrane. In this substance, the solute particles are proportionally larger than the solvent molecules.

METHOD OF EXCHANGE OF SUBSTANCES IN BETWEEN DIFFERENT FLUID COMPARTMENTS

The exchange of different substances and water between the different fluid compartments in our body mainly occurs by three processes. These are: *(1) filtration, (2) diffusion, and (3) osmosis.*

Filtration

It is the process by which undissolved particles are separated from a liquid through a membrane, as a result of a mechanical force which is called the "filtering force". It is done through a porous substance. *This filtering force is either gravity or hydrostatic pressure* which may be positive or negative. The important examples of filtration are: (1) the absorption from small intestine, (2) the passage of water, salts, food stuffs, etc. from blood stream into interstitial fluid, and (3) filtration in glomeruli.

Diffusion

The molecules of a substance are continuously in motion. This motion is least in solids, intermediate in liquids, and maximum in gases. When the two such substances are kept in contact or are separated by a membrane, then the molecules of two substances will pass into each other, until a uniform admixture is obtained. *This spontaneous admixture of the molecules of two substances due to their inherent molecular movement is called the "diffusion."* Anything that alters the molecular movement of substances also alters the rate of diffusion, proportionally. *The rate of diffusion of a substance across a membrane depends on:* (1) the concentration of substances on the two sides of membrane, (2) for charged substances the electrical potential (charges) across the membrane, (3) permeability of these substances through membrane, (4) pressure difference between the two sides of the membrane, because the pressure imparts greater kinetic energy. In human, *some clinical examples of diffusion are:* (i) absorption from intestine, (ii) exchange between plasma and red cells, (iii) exchange at the capillary bed such as nutrients, O_2, CO_2, metabolic waste products etc., and (iv) exchange at the lung capillaries of O_2 and CO_2.

The diffusion of substances through cell membrane between the IC and interstitial fluid or space takes place by the following mechanism: (1) through different protein channels in cell membrane, (2) directly by diffusion through cell membrane, (3) by some carrier protein situated on cell membrane such as glucose, amino acids, etc. The water, O_2, CO_2, and many other different lipid-soluble molecules diffuse through cell membrane directly. Different ions such as Na^+, K^+, Cl^-, etc., diffuse through cell membrane poorly. This is because of their unfavorable voltage potential across the cell membrane which is created by Na^+-K^+ pump. Therefore, these ions can diffuse only by the help of specific protein channels.

The capillary endothelial cell wall is only 0.4–0.6 µm thick, consisting of a single endothelial cell layer, situated on a basement membrane. The gap or cleft between the two adjacent endothelial cells is only 5–6 nm. Water, O_2, CO_2, and other many lipid-soluble substances can diffuse directly through the endothelial cell membrane from both sides which is governed by the hydrostatic and colloidal osmotic pressure of tissue and capillary. Only glucose, Na^+, K^+, and other water soluble substances, with low molecular weight, cross the intercellular clefts.

Osmosis

When a solute dissolved in water at two different concentrations is separated by a semipermeable membrane, then the diffusion of water (but not the solute) from lower to higher concentration of solution, through this semipermeable membrane, is called *"osmosis"*, provided the solute itself is not permeable to membrane. The water moves on both direction, but the movement of water from lower solute concentration to higher solute concentration is more. Then, a time will come when the movement of water molecules from both the side is same, so that no further alteration of volume of solution on any side of membrane will take place. At this stage, the *hydrostatic pressure of the solution of previously concentrated side will neutralize the attractive force of this higher concentrated solution for water molecules. This attractive force is called the "osmotic pressure".* This is the force, under which a solvent moves from lower solute concentration to higher solute concentration, when a selectively permeable membrane separates these two solutions of different concentration. The osmotic pressure does not depend on the size of the molecules of solute, but upon the total number of discrete particles of solute per unit volume of solution. If the solute is ionizable, then the osmotic pressure will be proportionately more. If more hydrostatic pressure is applied on the side of the solution of higher concentration, then water will pass from higher concentrated solution to the lower concentrated solution, opposite to osmosis. This is called *"ultrafiltration".*

If the two solutions are separated by a semipermeable membrane and have the same osmotic pressure, then they are called the *"isotonic solutions."* But if one has the less osmotic pressure than another, then it is called the *"hypotonic solution"* and if one has higher osmotic pressure than another, then it is called the *"hypertonic solution".* For example, 0.9% NaCl solution is isotonic with blood or plasma and commonly known as normal saline. A 5% solution of glucose has also similar osmotic pressure like plasma and is isotonic. Therefore, these two solutions such as 0.9% NaCl and 5% dextrose are isotonic, but they are not isosmotic, because they have not similar number of solute particles per unit volume of solutions. Clinical examples of osmosis are: absorption from intestine, exchange in tissue capillary bed, regulation of urine formation in renal tubules, reabsorption of CSF, etc.

■ WATER METABOLISM AND ITS BALANCE

Life first evolved in an aquatic medium. So, there will be nothing to be astonished that water is the most essential component of life. Of the three factors such as water, salt, and food, water is the most important for survival of life. So, deprivation of water will kill a subject much earlier than deprivation of salt and food. It must be remembered that the water content of our body is derived from two sources: (1) from the food and drink, and (2) from the cells as the end product of metabolism. The former is called the *"exogenous water"* and the latter is called the *"endogenous water".* The body water remains in two states: (i) *Free water,* i.e., not combined with anything. Most of the body water remains in this from. Various substances can remain dissolved in this form of water and they can be removed by ultrafiltration. (ii) *Bound water*—this is very small in quantity and remains combined with colloids and other substances.

The endogenous water comes from cells, as an end product of metabolism. Almost the whole amount of H^+, coming from solid food, is converted into water. But, only about 5 g of hydrogen is excreted in the form of ammonia, urea, etc. Different food stuffs yield different amount of water. Its approximate figures are given below:

100 g of fat gives 100 g of water. 100 g of starch gives 50 g of water. 100 g of protein gives 40 g of water. 100 g of alcohol gives 120 g of water. Water is continuously being lost and supplied to our body. But, still the total water content of our body is kept more or less constant, by maintaining a balance between the supply and loss. This indicates that there must be an efficient machinery for maintaining water balance.

Water Requirement and Loss

The total water requirement of an adult under ordinary conditions is about 2,500–3,000 mL/day. This is about 1 mL per calorie of energy intake. Half of this quantity, i.e., 1,500 mL or ½ mL of water per calorie intake should be taken as free drinks.

Supply of water:	
• Drink	1,400 mL
• Solid food	800 mL
(All solid foods contain some water as free form)	
• Metabolism	400 mL
Total	**2,600 mL**
Loss of water:	
• Kidney	1,500 mL
• Skin	600 mL
(Visible and nonvisible perspiration)	
• Lungs	400 mL
• Feces	100 mL
Total	**2,600 mL**

The above figures are average and the approximate gain or loss by any one of these routes may rise or fall under various conditions. The loss of water through skin varies according to the temperature and humidity of atmosphere and also upon the amount of muscular exercise done. In hot climates and with exercise this excretion of water through skin may vary from 3 to 10 L per day. Higher atmospheric humidity reduces the water loss through skin. Water excretion by lungs also increases in hot dry weather. In diarrhea, dysentery, cholera, etc., more water is lost through feces. While in condition of diuresis more water is passed out by kidneys. The water, secreted in digestive juices, is not lost. Because it is completely reabsorbed and about 5–7 L of water circulate in this way per day. The loss of water through saliva and lachrymal secretions is negligible under normal conditions (**Fig. 2**).

Positive and Negative Water Balance

Physiologically water balance is said to be positive in growing infants, children, convalescents, athletes, pregnant women, etc., who are storing water and building their body tissues. During positive water balance, each gram of protein is laid down with about 3 g of water, whereas fat and glycogen are deposited with less amount of water. When diet is changed from higher fat to higher carbohydrate, then more water retention takes place and the balance becomes more positive.

Water balance is negative under following conditions: (1) when the subject is thirsty, (2) when a preexisting edema is clearing up due to diuresis, (3) when diet is changed from high protein to carbohydrate and fat. In any condition of increased water loss, the relative proportion of Na⁺ and K⁺

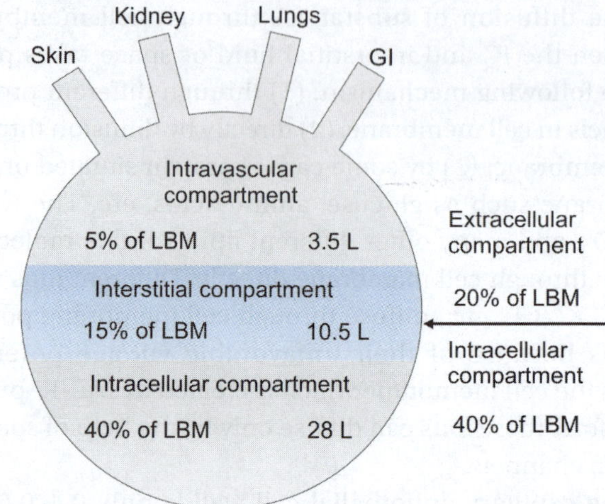

Fig. 2: Distribution of total body water (TBW) in the different compartments of our body. (LBM: lean body mass)

content of this fluid, which is going to be lost, will indicate whether the water is coming chiefly from EC or IC sources. The fluid with high Na⁺ content will indicate EC sources, whereas the fluid with high K⁺ content will indicate IC sources, provided intake of these two electrolytes remains constant.

Regulation of Water Balance

In spite of large amount of water is constantly appearing in and disappearing from our body, a fairly accurate balance is maintained between its gain and loss which indicates that there must be a strong regulating machinery. The mechanism which regulates this water balance in our body is very intricate and is not yet fully known. However, the following factors are closely involved in it. These factors are: *endocrine, renal, respirations,* and *thirst.*

Endocrine

A number of endocrines take part in this water regulation. These are posterior pituitary, hypothalamus, and adrenal cortex.

- *Posterior pituitary and hypothalamus:* From posterior pituitary gland, *antidiuretic hormone (ADH) or vasopressin* is secreted which has got immense influence upon water balance. It increases the reabsorption of water from distal renal tubules and thus reduces urine volume. It is very interesting to note that the secretion of this hormone is controlled by water content of our body. Excess of water input in our body depresses, while the dehydration stimulates the secretion of this ADH hormone. This is constituted through hypothalamus. The *hypothalamus* controls the secretion of ADH from posterior pituitary through supraopticohypophyseal tract. Excess of TBW dilutes blood and reduces the osmolality of ECF, as a result of which the hypothalamus is depressed (the specialized neuron in *supraoptic* and *paraventricular* nuclei of hypothalamus are very sensitive to the osmolality of ECF) leading to less secretion of ADH from posterior pituitary and consequently diuresis is produced with the maintenance of blood volume and the osmolality of tissue fluid. When the body water is reduced, then osmolality of ECF increases and subsequently hypothalamus is stimulated. Thus, more ADH is secreted and consequently urine volume is reduced with maintenance of blood volume and osmolality of tissue fluid. Hypothalamus also controls the formation of urine by regulating renal circulation and general blood pressure through sympathetic nervous system and adrenal cortex through corticotropin-releasing hormone (CRH).

- *Adrenal cortex:* Adrenal cortex secretes aldosterone which plays a very important part in the maintenance of water balance in our body. The secretion of aldosterone is controlled by angiotensin II and also by high serum K^+ and low serum Na^+ level. The aldosterone regulates water balance through the release of ADH from posterior pituitary, mediated through serum K^+ and Na^+ level, causing the retention of water and thus increases blood volume. The function of these two hormones is to tell the kidneys to retain or loss water. The ADH directly increases or decreases the reabsorption of water and aldosterone directly increases or decreases the reabsorption of Na and K through kidney. On the other hand, aldosterone influences the secretion of ADH by influencing the blood volume, by influencing the reabsorption of Na and K. In adrenal cortical insufficiency, there is decreased reabsorption of Na^+ and as a result more Na^+ is lost through urine. This causes increased reabsorption of K^+. Along with the decreased reabsorption of Na^+, the reabsorption of Cl^- is also depressed. Therefore, there is consequential change in the composition of body fluids. The IC crystalloid osmotic pressure exceeds that of EC crystalloid osmotic pressure and water flows from the ECF into IC fluid. Plasma volume decreases and there is hemoconcentration.

Renal

In physiological condition, when the total water content of our body rises, such as by excess intake of water or by the infusion of saline, etc., then the kidneys excrete more water. This effect is due to: (1) Increased blood volume and consequently the rise of blood pressure and thereby increased filtration pressure. (2) Dilution of plasma protein, reducing colloidal osmotic pressure and consequently increasing the available filtration pressure in glomeruli. (3) Increase in the number of active glomeruli which was dormant till now. (4) The depression of reabsorption of water by renal tubules, through the direct inhibition of hypothalamus and pituitary ADH mechanism. (5) Increase of central blood volume enhances the urine output through the inhibition of secretion of ADH. It is also suggested that the inhibition of ADH secretion takes place reflexly, through the stimulation of stretch receptors, present in left atrial wall. (6) Less secretion of renin, angiotensin II, aldosterone, and decreased absorption of water. Among these, the fourth and sixth factors are most important in regulating the excretion of water by the kidneys under physiological conditions.

Lungs and Skin

These channels also take considerable part in regulation of water balance, by excreting the variable amounts of water.

Thirst

When more fluid is lost such as in diarrhea, vomiting, diuresis, sweating, hemorrhage, etc., then the subject feels thirsty and drinks water. So, thirst may be defined specifically as the "hunger for water". In this way, the amount of lost water is replenished. In hibernating animals, the metabolism is so slow that water produced by oxidation of food stuffs within the cells is enough to equalize the water loss. Hence, under such condition no thirst is felt. During thirst, drinking is stimulated by two types of stimuli, acting on hypothalamus. These stimuli are: (1) rise in ECF osmolarity, even with or without any change in blood volume and (2) a fall in blood volume, even with or without any change in ECF osmolarity (**Fig. 3**).

Osmoreceptors, present at the lateral preoptic area of hypothalamus, are very sensitive to the changes in blood volume or ECF osmolarity. Activation of these receptors by decrease in blood volume or increase in ECF osmolarity induces thirst and causes individual to take water. This is the major defense mechanism of body against hypovolemia and hyperosmolarity, because it is the only mechanism that increases water intake voluntarily. On the other hand, ADH and aldosterone are the protective mechanism and act only when the excess water has been accumulated or lost. Contrary, when an appropriate amount of water has been drunk, then the sensation of thirst immediately vanishes, because of the activity of oral and gastric receptors. Unfortunately, the thirst mechanism is only operative in conscious patient who is capable of drinking.

Plasma Osmolality

There is a great confusion regarding the use of apparent interchangeable terms such as the osmolarity (measured

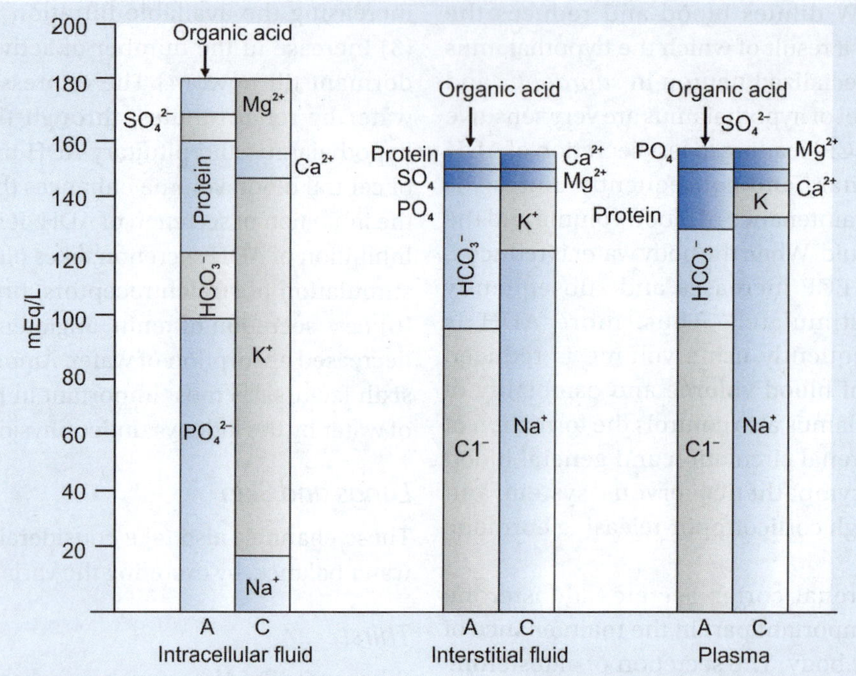

Fig. 3: The distribution of electrolytes in intracellular fluid, interstitial fluid, and plasma. (A = Anion, C = Cation).

in Osm/L) and osmolality (measured in Osm/kg). *The term osmolality is defined as the number of osmoles per unit of total weight of solvent in kilogram, whereas the term osmolarity is defined as the number of osmoles per unit of total volume of solutions in liter. Therefore, unlike osmolarity, osmolality is not affected by the presence of various solutes in solution (as it refers only one solute). In plasma, the osmolality and osmolarity is same and varies between 280–300 mOsm/kg and 280–300 mOsm/L, respectively.* This numerical equivalent is explained by the almost negligible amount of solute, contained in biological fluid and by the fact that most osmotically active particles which are dissolved in water have density of one. Therefore, in plasma mOsm/L is equal to mOsm/kg, but still the more accurate term to use in clinical practice is osmolality.

The osmolality of plasma and ECF is equals (as they remain in equilibrium) and is equivalent to the sum of concentration of all dissolved solutes, but Na⁺ (cation) and its anion such as Cl⁻ and HCO₃⁻ constitutes the major (90%) osmotically active particles in plasma. Plasma glucose and urea make a smaller contribution. *Therefore, the plasma osmolality (pOsm) is estimated from the following formula:*
pOsm = Na⁺ conc. + plasma glucose conc. + plasma urea conc.
= 1.86 (Na⁺) + Glucose/18 + BUN/2.8 (all units in mOsm/kg)
= 290 mOsm/kg.

[NB: NaCl does not dissociate completely in vivo and thus contributes 1.86 mOsm/L. 180 g of glucose contributes 1 mOsm of particles. When glucose concentration is expressed in mg/dL, it is divided by 18 to convert it to mOsm/kg of H₂O. Urea does not dissociate. The molecular weight of urea is not 28 but it contains two atoms of nitrogen per molecule and the concentration of nitrogen is not measured as urea concentration but as blood urea nitrogen (BUN) concentration. Thus, the molecular weight of two nitrogen molecules (14 each) rather than the molecular weight of urea is used in calculation. As urea does not dissociate therefore, 28 mg of urea nitrogen contributes 1 mOsm. BUN concentration is usually expressed as mg/dL. Thus, urea nitrogen concentration is divided by 2–8 to calculate the mOsm/kg].

Osmolal Gap

The difference between the measured and theoretically calculated value of osmolality of plasma is known as the osmolal gap. The normal value of plasma osmolality is 280–300 mOsm/L. This osmolal gap between the measured and calculated (mathematically) values increases, when there is the presence of high concentration of osmotically active abnormal particles in plasma which do not usually come during the measurement of normal osmolality. These abnormal osmotically active particles are: mannitol, ketone bodies, glycine (used during transurethral resection), ethanol, etc. The osmolal gap may also be present and become high during hyperproteinemia and hyperlipidemia. This is because, during both these conditions, there is increase in volume of plasma, without increase in concentration of Na$^+$. This osmolal gap may also increase during renal failure, because of retention of many small solutes which are not measured during the measurement of osmolality.

Calculation of Water Requirement

Assessment

Before calculation of water requirement, it needs the assessment of loss. The loss of water is called "dehydration". It is assessed clinically by history, clinical examinations, and is also assessed by laboratory investigations.

From history we can know how long the patient is suffering from the loss of fluid and its severity, as for example: (1) recent oral intake, (2) the frequency and the volume of vomiting, (3) diarrhea, (4) bleeding, (5) gastric suction, (6) amount of drainage from wound, (7) recent hemodialysis if the patient has renal failure, etc. The specific clinical features of dehydration are: dryness of mouth, thirst, hypotension, loss of skin turgor, tachycardia, ↓jugular venous pressure, ↓urine output, ↓CVP, etc. With normal renal function, the loss of water is associated with less urine output than 0.5 mL/kg/hour. Therefore, by *clinical examination*, the patient can be assessed for the severity of dehydration. Clinically, the severity of dehydration is classified as mild, moderate, and severe. *Mild dehydration* is described as the loss of 3 L of water (4% of total body weight) which is manifested as sunken eyes, dry mucous membrane, and loss of skin turgor. *Moderate dehydration* is described as the loss of 4–6 L of water (5–8% of total body weight) which is manifested as hypotension, oliguria, and tachycardia in addition to the manifestation of mild dehydration. *Severe dehydration* is described as the loss of >7 L of water (8–10% of total body weight) which is manifested as severe oliguria and compromised cardiovascular function **(Table 3)**. Unfortunately, many medications administered during anesthesia, as well as the neuroendocrine stress response to operative procedures, frequently alter these signs, and render them unreliable in the perioperative period. Intraoperatively, in addition to heart rate and BP, (i) the fullness of peripheral pulse, (ii) urinary flow rate, and (iii) indirect signs, such as the blood pressure response to positive pressure ventilation and to vasodilating or negative inotropic effects of anesthetics, are often used for guidance.

The *laboratory investigations* to assess the severity of dehydration include: serial hematocrits, arterial blood pH, urinary specific gravity or osmolality, urinary Na$^+$ and Cl$^-$ concentration, serum Na, and BUN to serum creatinine ratio. The laboratory signs of dehydration may include: rising hematocrit and Hb, progressive metabolic acidosis, urinary specific gravity >1.010, urinary Na$^+$ <10 mEq/L, urinary osmolality >450 mOsm/L, hypernatremia, BUN to creatinine ratio >10:1, etc. In acute blood loss, the hematocrit and Hb level will remain unchanged, because there is insufficient time for extravascular fluid to shift into the intravascular compartment. *Ultrasound* will reveal nearly a collapsed vena cava and incompletely filled cardiac chambers. *Radiographic* indicators of volume overload include increased pulmonary vascular and interstitial markings (*Kerley "B" lines*), diffuse alveolar infiltrates or both.

In very major surgeries, where rapid alterations of volume status are expected, in such situations central venous pressure (CVP) is used to assess the volume status. Pulmonary artery pressure monitoring has been used in settings where CVP readings do not correlate well with the clinical assessment or when the patient has primary or secondary right ventricular dysfunction. Secondary right ventricular dysfunction is due to pulmonary or left ventricular disease. Pulmonary artery occlusion pressure (PAOP) reading of <8–10 mm Hg indicates hypovolemia in patients with normal left ventricular compliance. The value of PAOP >18 mm Hg indicates left ventricular volume overload. The normal relationship between PAOP and left ventricular end-diastolic volume (LVEDV) is altered in the presence of mitral valve disease, severe aortic stenosis, etc., as well as by increased thoracic and pulmonary airway pressure.

All the PAOP measurements should be taken at the end of expiration. However, recently, multiple studies have

TABLE 3: Signs of fluid loss (expressed as the percentage of total body weight).

Signs	5% fluid loss	10% fluid loss	>15% fluid loss
Mucous membrane	Dry	Very dry	Parched
Heart rate	Normal or increased	>100/minute	Markedly increased (130/min)
Blood pressure	Normal	Mildly decreased with respiratory variation	Decreased
Urine output	Mildly decreased	Decreased	Markedly decreased
Sensorium	Normal	Lethargic	Obtunded
Orthostatic changes in heart rate (HR) and blood pressure (BP)	None	Present	Marked

failed to show that pulmonary artery pressure monitoring leads to improved outcome in critically ill patients. In such patients, echocardiography provides more accurate and less invasive estimate of cardiac filling and function. In critically ill patients, another method which accurately guides the fluid therapy is stroke volume variation (SVV). This SVV is calculated by the following formula:

$$SVV = SV_{max} - SV_{min}/SV_{mean}.$$

The maximum, minimum, and mean SV are calculated for a set period of time by the various measuring devices. During spontaneous ventilation, the BP decreases in inspiration. During IPPV, the opposite occurs. The normal value of SVV is <10–15% for patients on controlled ventilation. Patients with greater degrees of SVV are likely to be responsive to fluid therapy.

Calculation

Regardless of the disease process, there is both sensible and insensible loss of water and electrolytes from the body. In normal healthy individual, the sensible water loss occurs through urine, sweat, and feces, but the insensible loss of water occurs through skin and lungs. The insensible water loss per day accounts for about 25–30% of total water loss of a day. The major route of sensible water loss is kidney. Kidney also excretes the solute overload which is taken with food, plus which is produced by metabolism through urine, mixing with water. The final solute concentration in urine varies from 1,200 to 50 mOsmol/Liter or Kg of H_2O.

Protein is catabolized to urea, PO_4^{2-} and SO_4^{2-}. 1 g of protein contains 150 mg of nitrogen and this 150 mg of nitrogen is converted to 5 mmol of blood urea nitrogen (or BUN). Thus, 5 mOsm of solute is yielded from each gram of protein. On the other hand, the normal daily protein requirement is 1–2 g/kg/day. Therefore, the protein used per day produces 5–10 mOsm of solute/kg/day as BUN. The second major solute load comes from electrolyte balance. The daily Na^+ requirement is 1 mmol/kg/day and the daily K^+ requirement is also 1 mmol/kg/day. Hence, the daily total Na^+ and K^+ requirement is 2 mmol/kg/day. This same amount is also excreted per day with the equal amount of added anions to maintain homeostasis. Therefore, the total load of excreted electrolytes is 4 mmol/kg/day (the additional solute of 2 mmol/kg/day is due to other electrolytes such as Cl^-, HCO_3^-, Mg^{2+}, SO_4^{2-}, etc.). In addition, a small amount of osmoles are also produced by the metabolism of lipids which release phosphates and uric acid. Hence, the total solute load which is to be excreted is 10–15 mOsm/kg/day. But, it may be higher in catabolic patients who receive large amount of electrolytes and lower in starving patient. To excrete this normal solute load in

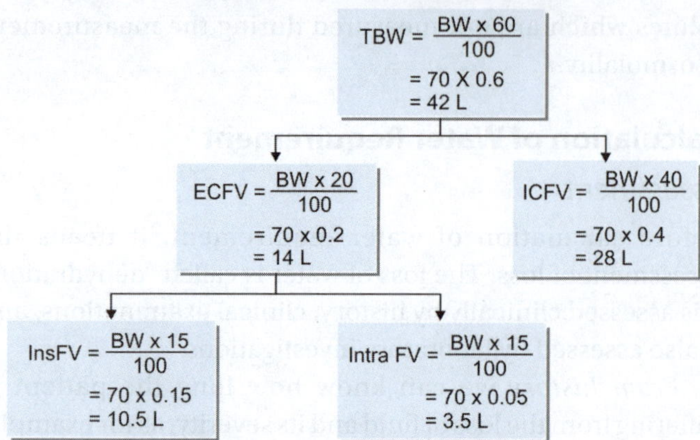

Flowchart 1: Distribution of total body water (TBW) in liter in a 70-kg body weight (BW) adult male.

(ECFV: extracellular fluid volume; ICFV: intracellular fluid volume; Ins FV: interstitial fluid volume; Intra FV: intravascular fluid volume)

a normal individual, the usual urinary output is 0.5 mL/kg/ hour with normal urine osmolality. In extreme cases, it may vary in any direction, such as (1) very low urinary volume (500 mL/day which is called "obligatory urine output") with very high osmolality or (2) very high urinary volume with very low osmolality (**Flowchart 1**).

In the previous part of this chapter, we have already discussed that a 70-kg patient with normal body temperature and normal metabolic rate may loss about 2,600 mL of water per day. So, naturally this patient will need the same amount of water to maintain his water balance. Allowing 400 mL of water to gain from cellular metabolism, now this healthy patient needs 2,600 – 400 = 2,200 mL of water/day from external source. Hence, the thumb rule for daily water requirement of a 70 kg individual is 30–35 mL/kg/day. With this water, the normal Na^+ requirement is 1 mmol/kg/day or 60–80 mmol/day and like Na^+, the K^+ requirement is also 1 mmol/kg/day or 60–80 mmol/day. Thus, a 70 kg healthy individual requires the daily provision of 2,200–2,600 mL of water with approximate 70 mmol of Na^+ and K^+ each. This can be provided by 1,500–2,000 mL of 5% dextrose and 500 mL of 0.9% NaCl with 1 g of KCl (15 mmol) is each 500 mL of fluid.

Perioperative Fluid Therapy

For operative procedures, the patients are kept fasting for prolonged periods before operation, during which time the patient has both sensible and insensible loss of water. Again, during surgical procedures, they also loss blood, loss ECF into third space, and also loss water through kidney as urine. They also loss water from skin, gut, and lungs during the whole perioperative period. So, every patient needs the amount of water which is equal to their normal maintenance plus extra loss. *For the loss of small amount of blood (<20% of total blood volume), the patient does not need any blood transfusion. In such circumstances, only crystalloids electrolyte solution, such as compound sodium lactate is sufficient. But, unfortunately, the crystalloid solutions quickly leave the intravascular compartment and are distributed into EC compartment. Therefore, due to the loss of blood, if the blood volume is maintained only by the infusion of crystalloid, then this crystalloid solution at the rate of at least three times of lost blood volume should be infused. Alternatively, the colloid solution which remains in intravascular compartment for longer period may be infused in a volume equal to that of estimated loss.*

During surgery, at the site of operation, due to tissue injury, there is sequestration of fluid from intravascular compartment into interstitial compartment. But, this fluid does not take part in normal metabolic process and is frequently referred to as *"third space loss"*. The amount of loss of this fluid into third space is proportional to the severity of tissue injury. This (plasma like) third space fluid is not contained in any anatomically separate space and cannot be measured easily. It is reabsorbed 48–72 hours after surgery.

In minor surgery, any IV fluid, in the dose of 1–1.5 mL/ kg/hour is sufficient to meet the requirement for normal maintenance. But, for any major abdominal surgery a volume of 5–6 mL/kg/hour of fluid during operation, in addition to 1.5 mL/kg/hour as normal maintenance is the requirement and transfusion of blood for any excessive blood loss is the rule. For any major surgery, the volume of IV fluid and the volume of blood needed to be transfused should be guided by CVP, urine output, plasma osmolality, cardiac output, preload, intra-arterial blood pressure, serum electrolyte concentration, etc. In the postoperative period, after replacing the total loss, the fluid should be administered only in maintenance dose. Additional fluid in the form of compound sodium lactate or 0.9% NaCl is only needed in the following conditions such as loss of GI fluid through nasogastric tube or fistula, loss of serum or blood through surgical drains, or continued third space loss for first 24–48 hours after very major surgery. *Usually, K^+ is not administered for first 24 hours after surgery. This is because, there is large release of endogenous K^+ from catabolism and tissue trauma which impose restriction of its use.*

During the immediate postoperative period, there is increased release of ADH, cortisol, aldosterone, etc. due to stress. These cause renal retention of Na^+ and water and excretion of K^+. But, still the restriction of water and Na^+ during the immediate postoperative period is inappropriate. This is because, there is increased loss of water and Na^+ by evaporation and into third space during the immediate

postoperative period. Patients with renal failure also require fluid replacement for abnormal losses, but the total volume needed should be determined by urine output and serum electrolyte concentration. Fluid and electrolyte requirement in infants and small children differ from those in adults.

Effect of Different Fluid Load on Extracellular and Intracellular Water Contents

Normal

Normal plasma osmolarity = 280 mOsm/L
Therefore, the total body solute
$$= 280 \times 42 \text{ L (42 L is TBW)}$$
$$= 11,760 \text{ mOsm}$$
Intracellular solute
$$= 280 \times 28 \text{ L (28 L is the IC fluid volume)}$$
$$= 7,840 \text{ mOsm}$$
Extracellular solute
$$= 280 \times 14 \text{ L (14 L is the extracellular fluid volume)}$$
$$= 3,920 \text{ mOsm}$$
Extracellular Na concentration
$$= 280/2 = 140 \text{ mEq/L.}$$

	Intracellular	Extracellular
Osmolarity	280	280
Volume (L)	28	14
Net water gain	0	0

Isotonic Load: 3 L Isotonic NaCl is Infused

New total body water = 42 + 3 = 45 L
Plasma osmolarity = 280 mOsm/L
Total body solute = 280 × 45 = 12,600 mOsm
Intracellular solute = 280 × 28 = 7,840 mOsm
Extracellular solute = 280 × (14 + 3) = 4,760 mOsm

	Intracellular	Extracellular
Osmolarity	280	280
Volume (L)	28	17
Net water gain	0	0
Net effect: Fluid remains in extracellular compartment.		

Free Water (Hypotonic Load): 3 L Distilled Water is Infused

New body water = 42 + 3 = 45 L
New body osmolarity = 11,760 ÷ 45 = 261 mOsm/L
New IC volume = 7,840 ÷ 261 = 30 L
New EC volume = 3,920 ÷ 261 = 15 L

	Intracellular	Extracellular
New osmolarity	261	261
New IC volume (L)	30	15
New water gain (L)	30 – 28 = 2	15 – 14 = 1

Net effect: Fluid is distributed in two compartments, but more in IC than EC. However, the osmolarity is same, so fluid does not move from one to another compartment.

Hypertonic Load: 500 mEq NaCl is Infused (Minimal Water)

Total body solute = 11,760 + 500 = 12,260 mOsm/L
New body osmolarity = 12,260 ÷ 42 = 291 mOsm
New extracellular solute = 3,920 + 500 = 4,420 mOsm
New EC volume = 4,420 ÷ 291 = 15.1 L
New IC volume = 42 – 15.1 = 26.9 L

	Intracellular	Extracellular
Osmolarity	291	291
Volume (L)	26.9	15.1
New water gain	26.9 – 28 = –1.1	15.1 – 14 = +1.1

Net effect: IC to EC movement of water and IC dehydration will result.

■ INTRAVENOUS FLUIDS

Intravenous fluid management may consist of infusions of crystalloids, colloids, or combination of them. The crystalloid solutions are the aqueous solutions of highly dissociable salts (ions), with or without glucose, whereas the colloid solutions are the aqueous solution of nondissociable substances, with high molecular weight such as proteins or large glucose polymers. Crystalloid solutions are rapidly distributed and equilibrate with the entire EC space. But, the colloid solutions remain for long time in the intravascular compartment and help to maintain the plasma oncotic pressure. Slowly, a small part of them is distributed in EC space.

Controversy remains regarding the use of crystalloids versus colloids for surgical patients. The argument in favor of the use of colloids is that in smaller volume they are more efficient in restoring the normal intravascular volume, plasma oncotic pressure, and cardiac output. On the other hand, the argument in favor of crystalloid is that they are equally effective like colloids when given in appropriate amounts and may avoid the disadvantage that colloids may enhance the formation of pulmonary edema fluid in patients with unrecognized increased pulmonary capillary permeability. However, the general opinions are that:

- To replace intravascular volume deficit, the crystalloids generally require 3–4 times of volume than colloids.
- When crystalloids are used in that sufficient amount, then they are as effective as colloids.
- Surgical patients usually have ECF deficit than intravascular fluid deficit. Here, crystalloids help better to maintain the ECF deficit.
- Intravascular fluid deficit is better and more rapidly corrected by colloids.
- Rapid administration of large volume of crystalloids is often associated with tissue edema.

Crystalloid Solutions

Crystalloid are often used as first choice during the initial resuscitation of patients suffering from hemorrhagic shock, septic shock, burn, head injury, and in patients undergoing plasmapheresis, hepatic resection, etc. Colloids are used during the resuscitation of patients, after the administration of crystalloids, depending on the protocols of institution and the preference of anesthesia provider. There are wide varieties of crystalloid solutions available in market **(Table 4)** and their use depends on the type of fluid loss. For example, if the fluid loss primarily involves the loss of water, then it should be replaced by hypotonic crystalloid solutions. But, hypotonic solutions must be administered slowly to avoid inducing hemolysis. On the other hand, when the fluid loss primarily involves the loss of both water and electrolytes, then it should be replaced by isotonic crystalloid electrolyte solutions. Glucose is provided in some solutions to maintain tonicity and to prevent ketosis and hypoglycemia due to fasting or as tradition. Children and diabetic patients are more prone to developing hypoglycemia (<50 mg/dL) following 6–8 hours fasting.

Among the crystalloid solutions available in market the normal saline has high chloride (Cl^-) content and lacks in bicarbonate. So, when it is given in large volume, it produces hyperchloremic metabolic acidosis. Except normal saline, other crystalloid solutions have low Cl^- content and this Cl^- is replaced by lactate, gluconate, or acetate. These low Cl^- content crystalloid solutions are balanced electrolyte solutions (Ringer's lactate, Ringer's acetate, Hartmann's solution, Plasmalyte 148, etc.). Most intraoperative fluid losses are isotonic, so isotonic crystalloid solutions such as normal saline (not preferred) or balanced electrolyte solutions (preferred) are most commonly used for replacement. Normal saline is the preferred solution for hypochloremic metabolic alkalosis and for diluting packed red blood cells, prior to transfusion. The 5% dextrose in water is used for the replacement of pure water deficit and as a maintenance fluid for patients on Na^+ restriction. Hypertonic 3% saline is employed in therapy of severe symptomatic hyponatremia.

TABLE 4: Composition of different crystalloid solutions.

	Plasma	0.9% NaCl	Ringer's lactate	Ringer's acetate	Hartmann's solution	Plasmalyte A	Plasmalyte 148
Osmolarity (mOsm/L)	±270–290	307	275	275	275	290	290
pH	7.35–7.45	±7.0	±7.4	6.0–8.0	5.0–7.0	±7.4	6.5–7.5
Na^+ (mmol/L)	135–145	154	130	130	130	140	140
K^+ (mmol/L)	3.5–5.5	0	5	5	5	5	5
Cl^- (mmol/L)	90–110	154	110	111	109	98	98
Ca^{2+} (mmol/L)	2.2–2.6	0	1.5	1.0	2.0	0	0
HCO_3^- (mmol)	24–32	0	0	0	0	0	0
Lactate (mmol/L)	1–2	0	28	0	28	0	0
Acetate (mmol/L)	1	0	0	28	0	28	28
Gluconate (mmol/L)	0	0	0	0	0	23	23
Mg^{2+} (mmol/L)	1	0	0	1	0	1.5	1.5

Colloid Solutions

Colloid solutions are made of osmotically active substances with high molecular weight. They tend to remain in intravascular compartment. The average intravascular half-life of colloid solutions is 4–6 hours (the average half-life of crystalloid solutions is 20–30 minutes). The indications for the use of colloid solutions are described before. But, relatively greater cost and occasional complications, associated with the infusion of some colloids, limit their use. The generally accepted indications for the use of colloids are: (1) resuscitation in patients with severe intravascular fluid loss such as hemorrhagic shock, prior to the arrival of blood for transfusion and (2) resuscitation in the presence of severe protein loss such as burn. In burn patients, colloids are used after initial resuscitation with crystalloid solutions.

Colloid solutions are generally derived from either plasma proteins or synthetic glucose polymers and are supplied in isotonic normal saline or electrolyte solution. Hence, they may cause hyperchloremic metabolic acidosis. Several colloid solutions are available in market. They are derived from either plasma proteins, collagen protein (gelatin), or synthetic glucose polymers and are supplied in isotonic electrolyte solutions.

The blood derived colloids include albumin (5% and 25% solutions) and plasma protein fraction. The plasma protein fraction include α and β globulins. Plasma is heated in water bath to 60°C for 10 hours to minimize the risk of transmitting hepatitis and other viral diseases. Blood derived colloids sometimes result hypotensive allergic reactions. Gelatin derived colloids (hemaccel) are associated with histamine-mediated allergic reaction and are not available in USA. Synthetic glucose polymers (dextran, hetastarch) are widely used as colloids in practice than albumin and plasma proteins. Dextran is a complex polysaccharide and available as dextran 70 and dextran 40, with their molecular weight of 70,000 and 40,000, respectively. Other than maintaining fluid balance and oncotic pressure, the other advantages of dextran are: it reduces blood viscosity, von Willebrand factor antigen, platelet adhesion, and RBC aggregation. Hence, due to these properties, it improves microcirculation and decreases the risk of microthrombus formation. Anaphylactoid and anaphylactic reactions have been reported after dextran infusion. This can be prevented by using dextran 1 prior to the use of dextran 70/40, because dextran 1 acts as a hapten and binds with any circulating dextran antibodies.

Hetastarch (hydroxyethyl starch) is available as multiple formulations and is designated by its concentration (6–10%), molecular weight (200–670), degree of starch substitution, and the ratio of hydroxylation between the C2 and C6 position. Hetastarch is highly effective as plasma expander, but is less expensive. Smaller starch molecules are eliminated through kidneys, whereas the large molecules remain in circulation. Allergic reactions by it are rare, but anaphylactoid or anaphylactic reactions may occur. It may prolong the prothrombin time and may cause hemorrhagic complications. It is potentially nephrotoxic and should not be administered in patients with kidney disease, elderly, and critically ill.

Electrolyte Balance

■ INTRODUCTION

Although Na$^+$ is abundantly present in drinking water, milk, and all the ordinary diet, *but it is most commonly taken as eating salt.* The normal daily requirement of Na$^+$ in an adult person is 1–1.5 mEq/kg/day (or 5–10 g/day). *But, usually the average daily intake of sodium is much higher than its daily requirement and is about 8–10 g/day. So, naturally Na$^+$ deficiency is very rare.* Daily Na$^+$ excretion is generally same as daily intake. To maintain a normal balance, usually, it is lost through sweat and feces, but the final adjustment is made by kidney through urine. Urinary Na$^+$ excretion may be as little as 2 mEq/day during salt restriction and may go up to 700 mEq/day after salt loading. In case of Na$^+$, the mEq and mmol are numerically same as the valency of Na$^+$ is one and mmol of Na$^+$ is obtained by dividing the mEq of it by its valency **(Fact file I)**. It is discussed in more details in Chapter 9 (Water Balance).

The Na$^+$ in plasma provides the 90% of total base of our body. It works in our body in two forms: (1) sodium ion (dissociable Na$^+$ salt) and (2) sodium compound (nondissociable Na$^+$ salt). All the functions of Na$^+$ ions are usually accomplished by maintaining the normal resting membrane potential (RMP) of cells. *Therefore, the functions of Na$^+$ ions in our body are:*

FACT FILE I

1 g of NaCl gives 17 mEq of Na$^+$ ions, whereas 1 g of sodium itself gives 43 mEq of Na$^+$ ions. In our body, the net Na$^+$ balance is equal to the total Na$^+$ intake which is average 150–200 mEq/day minus both the extra-renal and renal Na$^+$ loss. The kidneys play a very important role in Na$^+$ balance, because it has enormous variable capability to excrete Na$^+$ which varies between 1 mEq/L and >100 mEq/L.

- It initiates and maintains the contraction of heart.
- It is essential for the normal functions of cells.
- It is essential for the contraction of voluntary and involuntary muscles.
- It excites nerves as opposed to Ca^{2+} ions, which reduces the excitation of nerves.

On the other hand, sodium compounds are present in our body as bicarbonate, phosphate, chlorides, proteinates, etc. The functions of sodium compounds in our body are:

- *Maintains blood reaction:* This is done in many ways. For instance (a) sodium bicarbonate is the chief buffer of blood and other body fluids; (b) The acid and alkaline sodium phosphates (NaH$_2$PO$_4$ is acid and Na$_2$HPO$_4$ is alkali) also constitute an important buffer system; (c) Sodium which remains combined with plasma proteins (sodium proteinates) can also act as a buffer; (d) Sodium of NaCl can also fix acids with the help of phenomenon known as chloride shift.
- *Controls reaction of urine:* Kidneys regulate the urine reaction (acid or alkali) by altering the proportion of acid and alkaline sodium phosphate in urine.
- *Reaction of pancreatic juices and bile:* This is due to the presence of sodium carbonate.
- *Maintain osmotic pressure:* NaCl is the chief regulator of osmotic pressure of our body fluids.
- *Helps in the formation of HCl in gastric juices:* NaCl takes part in series of reactions and as a result of which HCl is manufactured by stomach.
- Maintains water balance.

The Na$^+$ balance is intimately related to extracellular fluid (ECF) volume and water balance in our body (discussed in Chapter 9). This is because it is widely distributed primarily in ECF space, including the interstitial and intravascular space (whereas intracellular space is primarily dominated by K^+) and crosses the capillary bed readily. On the other hand, the distribution of Na^+ between the intracellular and ECF space is restricted and determined by Na^+-K^+-ATPase pump, situated on cell membrane. There are two types of disorder of Na^+ balance: *hypernatremia and hyponatremia.*

■ HYPERNATREMIA

It is defined as plasma Na^+ concentration above 150 mmol/L. It is nearly always the result of either (i) loss of water in excess of Na^+, where Na^+ may be lost or not (loss of hypotonic fluid or only loss of water without Na^+) or (ii) retention of large quantities of Na^+ itself with little retention of water or not. In the first condition, the hypernatremia is a *relative* one, because the total Na^+ content in body remains same as only the water is lost and is associated with *reduced ECF volume* (both blood and interstitial fluid are taken as ECF and always they remain in an equilibrium) and its *hyperosmolality.* Contrary, in the second condition, there is true hypernatremia, because the total Na^+ content in the body is increased, even if the water content is increased or not and is associated with increased ECF volume and also hyperosmolality.

Classification of Hypernatremia (Table 1)

So, always the clinical assessment of volume status and osmolality of blood is important in the diagnosis and the management of hypernatremia. Therefore, hypernatremia is classified into three forms: (A) Hypernatremia with increased body Na^+ content (Na^+ is added); (B) Hypernatremia with normal body Na^+ content (only water is lost); (C) Hypernatremia with low body Na^+ content (both Na^+ and water are lost, but loss of water is more than Na^+). Now, though there are different types of hypernatremia, *the common abnormality of all these hypernatremic states is hyperosmolality of ECF* (blood and ECF remain always in an equilibrium) which causes the drawing of excess fluid from intracellular compartment and intracellular dehydration **(Fact file II).**

FACT FILE II

The total body Na^+ content is directly proportional to extracellular fluid (ECF) volume. Therefore, any changes in total body Na^+ content result in variation of ECF volume. A positive Na^+ balance increases ECF volume. Contrary, a negative Na^+ balance reduces ECF volume. On the other hand, Na^+ is the predominant extracellular cation. So, Na^+ in ECF reflects the total body Na^+ content. Na^+ in ECF compartment remains in equilibrium between the interstitial and intravascular fluid compartment. Hence, plasma Na^+ content more or less indicates total body Na^+ content and water balance.

Hypernatremia (Type-I) with Increased Total Body Na^+ Content

Usually, this is an iatrogenic condition in origin and is mainly due to excessive exogenous salt gain. It commonly results from the administration of hypertonic saline or administration of excessive amount of sodium bicarbonate, during cardiopulmonary resuscitation. It is also caused, when the isotonic fluids are given to patients who have only insensible loss of hypotonic fluid, containing less Na^+. Patients suffering from *primary hyperaldosteronism* and *Cushing's syndrome* may also have this condition. Management of this condition is comprised of the induction of diuresis by loop diuretic, which excretes Na^+ through urine, provided the kidney function is normal. Urine or water output is balanced in part by 5% dextrose which does not contain any Na^+. If the patient suffers from renal dysfunction, then dialysis or hemofiltration is the way of management of this type of hypernatremia with high body Na^+ content.

Hypernatremia (Type-II) with Normal Total Body Na^+ Content

This condition occurs when there is only loss of water, containing no or minimal amount of Na^+. Therefore, the total body of Na^+ content remains normal or slightly decreased, but in relation to water its concentration is always higher. *So, there is hypervolemia (drawing of fluid from cells), hyperosmolality, and hypernatremia.* Without loss of Na^+, the excessive loss of pure water via skin and respiratory tract is very rare. But, some examples of this condition are fever, hyperventilation, thyrotoxicosis, etc. However, the most common cause of this condition is diabetes insipidus. In diabetes insipidus, there is either decrease in antidiuretic hormone (ADH) secretion from posterior pituitary gland or the failure of renal tubules to respond to normally circulating ADH. Hence, the first condition is called as the *central diabetes insipidus* and the later is called as the *nephrogenic diabetes insipidus* **(Box 1).**

In *central diabetes insipidus,* the lesion or pathology is usually found in and around the hypothalamus or pituitary

TABLE 1: Classification of hypernatremia.

Hypernatremia	$\uparrow\uparrow Na^+$	$\uparrow$ ECF volume	$\uparrow$ Osmolality with $\uparrow$ body Na^+ content
Hypernatremia	$\downarrow\downarrow H_2O$, $\downarrow Na^+$	$\downarrow$ ECF volume	$\uparrow$ Osmolality with $\downarrow$ body Na^+ content
Hypernatremia	$\downarrow\downarrow H_2O$, no Na^+ loss	$\downarrow$ ECF volume	$\uparrow$ Osmolality with normal Na^+ content

BOX 1: Causes of hypernatremia.

- *Hypernatremia (Type-I) with increased total body Na$^+$ content:*
  - Excessive Na$^+$ salt ingestion
  - Infusion of hypertonic saline
  - Administration of excess NaHCO$_3$
  - Administration of excess of steroid (Cushing)
  - Excess aldosterone (Conn syndrome)
- *Hypernatremia (Type-II) with normal body Na$^+$ content:*
  - *Extrarenal loss of only water without Na$^+$:*
    - Fever
    - Hyperventilation thyrotoxicosis
  - *Renal loss of water without Na$^+$:*
    - Central diabetes insipidus
    - Nephrogenic diabetes insipidus
    - Chronic renal failure
- *Hypernatremia (Type-III) with decreased total body Na$^+$ content:*
  - Renal hypotonic fluid loss
  - Osmotic diuresis (mannitol, urea, and glucose)
  - *Extrarenal hypotonic fluid loss:*
    - Vomiting
    - Diarrhea
    - Excessive sweating

gland. So, it is commonly seen following hypothalamus or pituitary tumor, neurosurgical procedures of brain, head injury, etc. It is also developed following brain death. *The central diabetes insipidus is diagnosed by history of polyuria (volume of urine >8 L/day), polydipsia (even in the absence of hyperglycemia), and low urinary osmolality than plasma. In unconscious patient, the absence of thirst, associated with diabetes insipidus, can easily produce marked water loss and hypovolemia. The diagnosis of central diabetes insipidus can be confirmed by the increase in urinary osmolality by administration of ADH (or vasopressin) from exogenous source.* There are two preparations of vasopressin, such as in aqueous solution and in oil. However, the aqueous preparation of ADH is the treatment of choice. It is used in the dose of 5 U at the interval of every 4 hours through subcutaneous route. Oil preparation of vasopressin is also used in the dose of 0·3 mL/day only through intramuscular route. It is long-acting and therefore frequently causes water intoxication. There is another synthetic analog of vasopressin, called *desmopressin (DDAVP)* with 12–24 hours duration of action. It is available as an intranasal preparation and can be used both for ambulatory or preoperative patient in the dose of 5–10 mg/day or twice daily.

Nephrogenic diabetes insipidus is commonly due to: (i) chronic renal disease, (ii) secondary to side effects of certain drugs, such as lithium, mannitol, amphotericin B, etc., (iii) certain electrolyte disturbances, such as hypercalcemia and hypokalemia, (iv) certain other diseases such as sickle-cell disease, hyperproteinemia, etc., and (v) sometimes congenital. In these conditions, there is normal plasma level of ADH (vasopressin), but the kidneys fail to respond to normally circulating ADH and unable to concentrate the urine, resulting in excretion of huge amount of hypo-osmolal urine. *The diagnosis can be confirmed by the failure of kidney to produce a hyperosmolal urine, still following the administration of exogenous vasopressin.* The *treatment* of this condition is intake of adequate fluid which will try to keep the water balance of our body normal and specific management of underlying etiology. Administration of loop diuretics, in nephrogenic diabetes insipidus, paradoxically reduces the urine output as it reduces the water load to the collecting tubules, where ADH acts. Proteins and sodium restriction can similarly decrease the urine output.

Hypernatremia (Type-III) with Low Total Body Na$^+$ Content

In this condition, the patient has losses of both Na$^+$ and water, but the Na$^+$ loss is less than the loss of water (loss of hypotonic fluid). Therefore, there is low body Na$^+$ content (due to Na$^+$ loss), but still hypernatremia (due to more loss of water than Na$^+$). This loss of hypotonic fluid may be due to renal or extrarenal cause. The example of renal loss of hypotonic urine, causing hypernatremia and low body Na$^+$ content, is osmotic diuresis by mannitol, glucose, etc., where water is lost more than Na$^+$. On the other hand, the example of extrarenal loss of hypotonic fluid causing this condition are vomiting, diarrhea, exercise, excessive sweating, etc., where there is more water loss than Na$^+$ loss.

Clinical Manifestations of Hypernatremia

The clinical manifestation of hypernatremia is mainly due to the hyperosmolality of ECF which causes the shifting of water from intracellular compartment to extracellular compartment and cellular dehydration. The major consequences of hypernatremia and hyperosmolality of ECF involve the central nervous system (CNS) and the severity depends on the rapidity with which this hyperosmolality develops. The cellular dehydration causes the reduction of cell volume and water content of brain which produces restlessness, hyperreflexia, seizures, coma, and ultimately death. The reduction of cell volume and water content of brain causes rapid decrease of brain volume and increased permeability of vascular structure which may produce the rupture of cerebral veins, resulting in focal intra-cerebral and/or subarachnoid hemorrhage. Hence, the patients may present with pyrexia, nausea, vomiting, convulsion, coma, or virtually any type of neurological syndrome. The chronic form of hypernatremia is better tolerated than its acute form. Serious neurological damage and convulsions are more common in children and particularly when the plasma Na^+ concentration exceeds 158 mmol/L.

Treatment of Hypernatremia

The majority of hypernatremic patients are hypovolemic (except in type I iatrogenic condition where there is exogenous salt gain and here water in ECF compartment is increased, though there is intracellular dehydration), and the total water content of body is decreased due to intracellular dehydration. Therefore, the aim of the management of hypernatremia is (i) the restoration of volume of intracellular fluid (ICF) compartment; (ii) the correction of the osmolality of ECF compartment; and (iii) the correction of underlying problem.

If one assumes that hypernatremia is due to the only water loss or due to more water loss than little Na^+ loss (types II and III), then *the total body Na^+ remains more or less normal*. Then, the water deficit can be corrected by the following way: Water deficit = Normal total body water (TBW) – Present TBW. If a 60 kg man, suffering from hypernatremia of type- II and III, is found to have a plasma Na^+ concentration of 160 mmol/L, then the present TBW can be calculated from the following equation, such as: Normal TBW × 140 = Present TBW × 160 (Normal plasma Na^+ concentration = 140 mmol/L)

∴ Present TBW = (Normal TBW × 140) ÷ 160 = (60 × 0.6 × 140) ÷ 160 (0.6 = 60% of body weight is water) = 31.5 L

∴ Water deficit = Normal TBW – Present TBW = (60 × 0.6) – 31.5 L = 36 – 31.5 L = 4.5 L.

This hypernatremia and hypovolemia should be corrected slowly over 48–72 hours. Because rapid correction of hypernatremia and hypovolemia may cause cerebral edema, convulsions, permanent neurological damage, and even death. During this management, serial measurement of Na^+ concentration is performed and plasma Na^+ concentration should not be reduced faster than 0.4–0.6 mmol/h. Regarding the type of fluid, hypernatremic patients with decreased total body Na^+ should be given isotonic saline to restore both the plasma volume and the body Na^+. Because this isotonic saline is taken as relative hypotonic in patients with severe hypernatremia and the Na^+ in normal saline helps to restore the depletion of total body Na^+. Once volume and Na^+ depletion have been corrected, further correction of any water deficit can be accompanied with isotonic 5% dextrose.

Until the etiology of hypernatremia and fluid deficit is corrected properly all elective surgeries should be cancelled in patients suffering from severe hypernatremia (>150 mmol/L).

◼ HYPONATREMIA

It is a very common hospital finding and is defined as plasma Na^+ concentration of <135 mmol/L. It may occur relatively as a result of water retention (dilutional) or as a result of true Na^+ loss (depletion) or both. Therefore, hyponatremia is associated with normal, decreased, or increased ECF volume. *But, in all these forms there is hypo-osmolality of ECF (interstitial plus vascular) compartment*. Due to this reduced osmolality, water moves from ECF compartment to intracellular (IC) fluid compartment and swelling of cells (mainly brain) with water intoxication occurs.

Classification of Hyponatremia (Table 2)

Na^+ ion is present only in the water portion of plasma which constitutes about 93% of whole plasma. But, in the laboratory, it is measured against the whole (100%) plasma and is expressed as mmol/L of whole plasma. In hyperlipidemia and hyperproteinemia, this water portion of plasma is decreased, but the whole plasma volume remains same. Hence, in such condition, the measurement of the concentration of Na^+ against whole plasma is decreased (as water content decreases), but its concentration against only water portion of plasma (which is not constituted by lipids, proteins, etc.) is normal. Therefore, the measurement of Na^+ against the whole plasma in these conditions show false hyponatremia. Hence, this type of hyponatremia is called as the *pseudohyponatremia*. However, the routine measurement of plasma osmolality with Na^+ level in hyponatremic patients rapidly excludes this pseudo form. This pseudo form of hyponatremia will not confuse us, if plasma Na^+ concentration is measured by ion-specific electrodes. Because, this method directly assesses the aqueous phase of Na^+ and produces exact result.

Like hypernatremia, the hyponatremia is also classified according to the presence of relative water retention (dilutional) without loss of Na^+ or true Na^+ loss (depletion) into three forms:

1. Hyponatremia with decreased total body Na^+ content
2. Hyponatremia with normal total body Na^+ content
3. Hyponatremia with increased total body Na^+ content.

TABLE 2: Classification of hyponatremia.

Hyponatremia	↓ Na^+ (Na^+ loss)	↓ ECF volume	↓ Osmolality	↓ total Na^+ content in body
Hyponatremia	↑↑ H_2O gain, ↑ Na^+ gain	↑ ECF volume	↓ Osmolality	↑ Na^+ content in body
Hyponatremia	↑ H_2O gain, no Na^+ gain	↑ ECF volume	↓ Osmolality	Normal Na^+ content in body

Hyponatremia with Decreased Total Body Na⁺ Content

This is caused by progressive loss of both Na^+ and water, but the Na^+ loss exceeds the water loss. Hence, there is hyponatremia and decreased total body Na^+ content (If water loss exceeds the Na^+ loss, then this will cause hypernatremia with decreased total body Na^+ content). The assessment of volume status reveals hypovolemia ($\downarrow$ECF). This Na^+ and water loss may be renal or extrarenal. The examples of renal loss are: the administration of diuretics, Addison's disease, renal tubular acidosis, salt losing nephropathies, etc. In such renal causes of hyponatremia, usually, the urinary Na^+ concentration exceeds 20 mmol/L. The examples of extrarenal Na^+ and water loss are from gastrointestinal (GI) tract, such as diarrhea, vomiting, etc. (these are also the cause of hypernatremia) or in the third space such as during peritonitis, surgery, etc. In such extrarenal cause of hyponatremia, the urinary Na^+ loss is <10 mmol/L, except vomiting. In vomiting, there is metabolic alkalosis which obligates the concomitant excessive excretion of Na^+ and HCO_3^- through kidney to maintain electrical neutrality in urine.

Hyponatremia with Normal Total Body Na⁺ Content

In this condition, there is no Na^+ loss, but hyponatremia is due to only water overload. This situation is caused by: glucocorticoid insufficiency, hypothyroidism, drug therapy by cyclophosphamide and SIADH (syndrome of inappropriate ADH secretion). Hyponatremia, associated with glucocorticoid insufficiency, is due to excessive secretion of ADH along with hypersecretion of corticotrophin releasing factor, in the absence of adequate glucocorticoids. In this condition, there is modest excess of TBW and modest increase of ECF volume with normal total body Na^+ content, showing hyponatremia. It also may be due to iatrogenic origin. This iatrogenic cause is due to excessive administration of intravenous fluids with low Na^+ content in patients with loss of isotonic fluid **(Box 2)**.

Hyponatremia with Increased Total Body Na⁺ Content

In this condition, there is increase in both TBW and total body Na^+ content, but overload of water exceeds that of Na^+. Hence, hyponatremia occurs. The examples of this situation are: congestive heart failure, renal failure, nephrotic syndrome, cirrhosis of liver, etc. In these circumstances, hyponatremia results from the progressive impairment of excretion of both Na^+ and free water by kidney, but the accumulation of water exceeds the accumulation of Na^+. The pathophysiology of this condition parallels the severity of underlying disease process **(Fig. 1)**.

<table>
<tr><td>

BOX 2: Causes of hyponatremia.

- *Hyponatremia with decreased total body Na⁺ content (hypovolemia):*
  - *Renal loss (urine Na⁺ >20 mmol/L) diuretics:*
    - Osmotic diuretics (mannitol and glucose)
    - Mineralocorticoid deficiency
    - Renal tubular acidosis
    - Salt-losing nephropathy
  - *Extrarenal loss (urine Na⁺ <10 mmol/L):*
    - Diarrhea
    - Vomiting
    - Third space loss
- *Hyponatremia with normal total body Na⁺ content (normovolemia or hypervolemia)*
  - *Low plasma osmolality:*
    - Syndrome of inappropriate ADH
    - Glucocorticoid insufficiency
    - Hypothyroidism
    - Drug therapy
  - *Normal plasma osmolality:* Pseudohyponatremia
    - Hyperlipidemia
    - Hyperproteinemia
    - Hyperglycemia
- *Hyponatremia with increased total body Na⁺ content (hypervolemia):*
  - Congestive heart failure
  - Renal failure
  - Nephrotic syndrome
  - Cirrhosis of liver

Group A is a depletion syndrome. So, saline is required. Group B and C (except pseudohyponatremia) is dilutional syndrome. So, fluid restriction is required.

</td></tr>
</table>

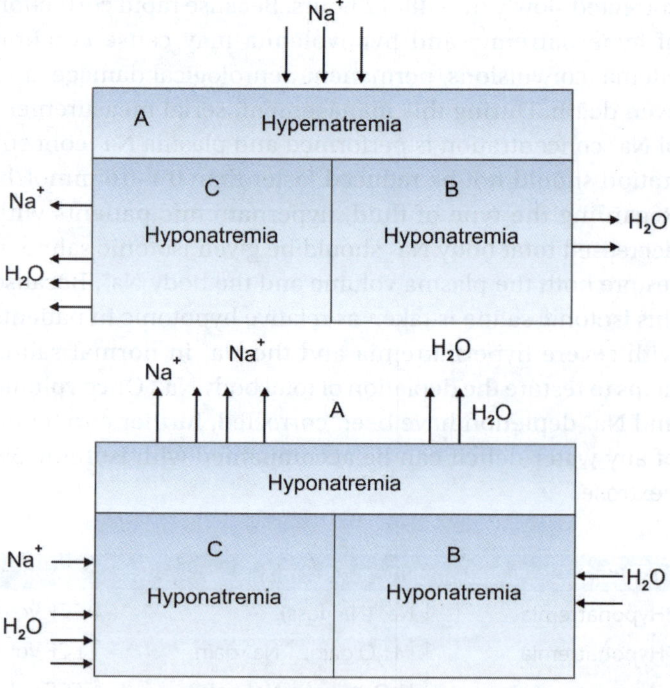

Fig. 1: Pathophysiology of hyponatremia.

Clinical Manifestations of Hyponatremia

The clinical manifestation of hyponatremia is primarily due to increase in ICF volume and affects mainly the brain cells. So, there is subsequent cerebral edema and increase in ICP causing nausea, vomiting, delirium, convulsions, coma, and even death. But, the symptoms vary with the magnitude of the reduction of plasma Na$^+$ level and the rapidity with which plasma Na$^+$ level falls. Patients with *mild hyponatremia (Na$^+$ level between 125 and 135 mmol/L)* are usually asymptomatic or are associated with mild symptoms, such as anorexia, nausea, vomiting, weakness, etc. However, *moderate hyponatremia (Na$^+$ level between 120 and 125 mmol/L)* is associated with symptoms, such as lethargy, confusion, etc. While the *severe hyponatremia (Na$^+$ level <120 mmol/L)* is associated with convulsions, coma, or death. *Chronic hyponatremia is less symptomatic than acute hyponatremia. This is because in previous condition there is enough time for compensation by losing intracellular solutes along with extracellular loss of Na$^+$ which help to restore the cell volume to normal. In chronic hyponatremia, the neurological manifestations are not due to the changes of cell volume, but rather due to the changes in cell membrane potential by low extracellular Na$^+$.*

Treatment of Hyponatremia

Like hypernatremia, the management of hyponatremia also includes the correction of plasma Na$^+$ level and the underlying disease process. Acute symptomatic hyponatremia is a medical emergency condition. So, it needs prompt intervention by using *isotonic saline*, but the rapidity with which hyponatremia is corrected is a matter of controversy. This is because very rapid correction of hyponatremia is associated with serious permanent neurological sequel. But, the general agreement is that correction period should not be <12 hours, and after which the plasma Na$^+$ level should not be <125 mmol/L. The rapidity with which the hyponatremia can be corrected slowly or very slowly depends on the severity of symptoms. *However, the following tailored correction rate is followed: for mild hyponatremia <0.5 mmol/L/h, for moderate hyponatremia <1 mmol/L/h, and for severe hyponatremia <1.5 mmol/L/h.*

In hyponatremia, the amount of Na$^+$, which is needed (Na$^+$ deficit) to make the desired plasma level, can be calculated as follows:

Na$^+$ required or deficit = TBW × (desired or required Na$^+$ concentration − measured Na$^+$ concentration). Here, TBW is total body water and not the total body weight.

If the weight of a patient is 70 kg and the present plasma Na$^+$ concentration is 120 mmol/L.

Then the required total Na$^+$ in mmol/L = 70 × 0.6 × (130 − 120) = 420 mmol/L

(0.6 indicates TBW and is approximately 60% of body weight, 130 mmol/L is the desired level of plasma Na$^+$ level to be raised)

Normal saline contains Na$^+$ = 154 mmol/L.

Hence, the patient should receive 420 ÷ 154 = 2.72 L of normal saline.

Isotonic saline is generally the treatment of choice for hyponatremia with decreased total body Na$^+$ content. On the other hand, hyponatremic patients with normal or increased total body Na$^+$ content should be treated with more water restriction. More specific treatment also can be instituted for hyponatremia. For example, hormone replacement for thyroid or adrenal hypofunction which can be started to correct hyponatremia. For heart failure patient, the aim of management is to increase the cardiac output.

Problems during anesthesia of a patient suffering from altered Na$^+$ balance results from the changed pathophysiology due to hyper- or hyponatremia and as well as from the underlying disorders. Hyper- or hyponatremia present either as hypo- or hypervolemia. Therefore, both these manifestations should be corrected before elective surgery. Hypovolemic patients are sensitive to hypotension. Therefore, vasodilating and negative inotropic agents such as volatile anesthetics, histamine-releasing agents, barbiturates, etc. should be used cautiously. Due to the reduction of the volume of distribution of drugs in hypovolemia the doses of all the therapeutic agents also should be reduced. Regional anesthesia is also very sensitive to develop hypotension due to hypovolemia. If there is hypervolemia, it should also be corrected by diuretics before surgery. Any abnormalities of cardiac, renal, and hepatic function also need proper evaluation and correction before anesthesia and surgery.

POTASSIUM BALANCE

■ INTRODUCTION

K^+ is the major intracellular cation (Na^+ is the major extracellular cation). The intracellular concentration of it is 140–150 mmol/L and this intracellular K^+ constitutes about 98% of total body K^+ content. Only 2% of total body K^+ content remains in extracellular space or fluid. This extracellular K^+ concentration is 4 mmol/L. The regulation of intracellular K^+ concentration is poorly understood. The extracellular K^+ concentration is generally reflected by the plasma concentration of it (or vice versa) and the balance between the K^+ intake and excretion of it. The concentration of K^+ in plasma or ECF does not reflect the concentration of it (K^+) in intracellular compartment. Under physiological condition, the intracellular K^+ concentration more or less remains constant. Under some pathological conditions, the redistribution of K^+ between ECF and ICF compartment can result in marked changes in extracellular K^+ concentration, without any change in total body K^+ content or change in intake and excretion of it. This extracellular concentration of K^+ (not intracellular concentration of K^+) is regulated precisely, because many of the cell functions are very sensitive to this change in ECF potassium concentration. For example, slight changes of plasma K^+ concentration have an important impact on neuromuscular transmission and cell membrane potential, most significantly on myocardial cell. An increase in plasma K^+ concentration (which is in equilibrium with ECF K^+ concentration of only 3–4 mmol/L) from its original value can cause cardiac arrhythmia or even cardiac arrest.

The daily intake of K^+ usually ranges between 50 and 200 mmol/day (average 80 mmol/day). But, in a single meal, this K^+ intake may rise as high as 500 mmol. Therefore, the failure to rapidly rid of ECF from this high ingested K^+ load could cause life-threatening hyperkalemia. Similarly, a small loss of K^+ from ECF may cause severe hypokalemia in the absence of rapid and appropriate compensatory response.

Normally, the daily intake of K^+ is equivalent to the daily excretion of it and vice versa. The renal excretion of K^+ can vary from as little as 5 mmol/L to over 100 mmol/L, according to the intake and output, in the absence of any renal pathology. This maintenance of body K^+ balance depends primarily on its excretion by kidney. *Kidney excretes 90–95% of ingested K^+, whereas the remaining 5–10% K^+ is lost through the feces and sweat. Thus, kidney is the principal organ to control the body K^+ rapidly and precisely in wide variations of intake and abnormal loss.* In the kidney about 90–100% of filtered K^+ is reabsorbed actively by proximal tubules and thick ascending limb of the loop of Henle. Therefore, nil to 10% of filtered K^+ escapes this renal reabsorption and is

excreted through urine. Normally, the K^+ which is excreted through urine is the result of distal tubular secretion. This K^+ secretion in distal tubules is coupled to aldosterone mediated reabsorption of Na^+. Therefore, if GFR is normal, then this amount (secreted by distal tubule) is adequate to maintain K^+ balance by excreting it through urine. For this reason, hyperkalemia is very uncommon in the presence of normal renal function. However, if GFR is reduced then excessive active secretion of K^+ by distal nephron is necessary to avoid the progressive accumulation of K^+ in blood (due to less filtration by glomeruli) and eventual hyperkalemia.

The control of K^+ distribution between the ECF and ICF compartment also plays an important role in K^+ homeostasis. This is because 98% of total body K^+ remains into cells and they can serve as a soaking site for the excess of K^+ from ECF compartment during hyperkalemia or as a source of K^+ during hypokalemia. Thus, the redistribution of K^+ between ICF and ECF compartment provides a first line of defense against the changes in K^+ concentration in ECF compartment. The K^+ of ECF compartment is pumped into cell in exchange of Na^+, pumped out into ECF, by the ubiquitous Na^+-K^+-ATPase pump, situated on cell membrane in a ratio of 3 Na^+ to 2 K^+ ions. This creates a negative intracellular voltage and is responsible for resting membrane potential. The intracellular K^+ concentration remains constant at around 140 mmol/L though this Na^+-K^+-ATPase pump acts continuously. This is because of some passive leakage of K^+ from cells through some separate K^+ selective ion channels, other than Na^+-K^+-ATPase pump. *This Na^+-K^+-ATPase pump is stimulated by insulin and β-adrenergic agonist and this effect is exploited to treat hyperkalemia. It (Na^+-K^+-ATPase pump) is inhibited by acidosis. Therefore, hyperkalemia is commonly associated with acidosis, diabetes, and use of β-blocker. The plasma K^+, therefore, is a very sensitive factors, influencing the shift of K^+ between the ECF and ICF compartment of muscle cells which are the principal storing site of K^+.*

■ URINARY EXCRETION OF POTASSIUM

Generally, the extracellular concentration of K^+ (not intracellular concentration of K^+) parallels with the excretion of it through urine. It is excreted mainly by the secretion of tubular cells of distal nephron and this whole thing of the secretion of K^+ by distal nephron is mediated by aldosterone hormone. On the other hand, the extracellular concentration of K^+ is the major determinant factors of aldosterone secretion from adrenal gland. Hyperkalemia stimulates the secretion of aldosterone, whereas hypokalemia suppresses it. The other major stimulus to aldosterone secretion is angiotensin

II. Thus, any factors that inhibit the renin-angiotensin system will inhibit the secretion of aldosterone and blunt the renal compensatory response to rise in plasma K^+ (hyperkalemia). These include ACE inhibitors, nonsteroidal anti-inflammatory drugs (NSAIDs) (by blocking prostaglandin-mediated renin release) and β-antagonists (by inhibiting the release of renin, mediated by renal nerves). Drugs which block the action of aldosterone such as spironolactone, amiloride, etc. also cause hyperkalemia, particularly if the GFR is low.

INTERCOMPARTMENTAL SHIFTS OF POTASSIUM

It is already discussed that, like urinary excretion, the intercompartmental shifting of K^+ between the ECF and ICF compartment is also very important to maintain the homeostasis of it (K^+) or the concentration of it in ECF which is most important for life. *This intercompartmental shifting of K^+ is mediated by changes in: extracellular pH, levels of circulating catecholamines, level of circulating insulin, hypothermia, and plasma osmolality. Except these, the exercise also transiently increases the plasma K^+ level due to release of it from muscle cells. This increase of plasma K^+ concentration is parallel to the duration and the intensity of muscular activity.*

The changes in extracellular pH directly affect the extracellular K^+ concentration. This is because the ICF buffers up to 50% of an acid load or H^+ and the remaining are excreted through kidney. During acidosis extracellular H^+ enters the cell or is formed within the cells and displaces the intracellular K^+. Thus, K^+ comes out of the cell to maintain the intracellular electrical balance and increases the plasma K^+ level. During alkalosis, the reverse occurs and plasma K^+ concentration decreases. A thumb rule of maintaining the relationship between the plasma K^+ concentration and blood pH is that plasma K^+ concentration changes nearly 0.5–0.7 mmol/L for every 0.1 U change of arterial pH in any direction.

The increased level of catecholamines by sympathetic stimulation also decreases the plasma K^+ level by enhancing the intracellular uptake of it. This is mediated by the Na^+-K^+-ATPase pump which is controlled by β-adrenergic receptors. Catecholamines through β-receptors stimulate this pump which pushes two K^+ ions inside the cell in exchange of drawing three Na^+ ions out of the cell. Therefore, β-adrenergic stimulant decreases the level of plasma K^+ concentration. Contrary, β-blockers increase the concentration of plasma K^+. On the other hand, α-adrenergic activity impairs the intracellular movement of K^+ and increases the concentration of plasma K^+.

Changes in the circulating levels of insulin also alter the plasma K^+ concentration. It also acts the same way through Na^+-K^+-ATPase pump, like catecholamines and increases the uptake of K^+ in the liver and skeletal muscle cells. Thus, administration of insulin decreases the plasma K^+ level and helps to treat hyperkalemia.

Hypothermia decreases the plasma K^+ level by increasing the cellular uptake of it. Contrary, the increased temperature of body reverses this shifting and increases the plasma K^+ level. Changes of plasma osmolality also change the plasma K^+ level. Increased plasma osmolality due to hypernatremia, hyperglycemia, or the administration of mannitol, etc. increases the plasma K^+ concentration. The explanation of it is like that increased plasma osmolality causes the shifting of water from ICF to ECF compartment. This causes cellular dehydration and increased intracellular K^+ concentration which results in movement of K^+ from inside to outside of the cell and increased plasma K^+ level.

There are two types of disturbances of K^+ balance in our body. These are hypokalemia and hyperkalemia.

Hypokalemia

It is defined as plasma concentration of <3.5 mmol/L. It occurs as a result of: (i) inadequate intake or (ii) excessive loss or (iii) both. Excessive loss may be of two types: loss through urine, stool, sweat, or shift from ECF to ICF compartment. In the circumstances of shifting from ECF to ICF compartment, the total K^+ content in our body remains same. While, in the circumstances of inadequate intake and excessive loss of K^+ through urine, stool, vomit, or sweat result in low total body K^+ content.

When the K^+ intake is very low, then its filtration through glomeruli and subsequent reabsorption of it in nephron is enhanced. This causes gradual fall of urinary excretion of K^+ to about 5 mmol/day which is obligatory. But, this continuous minimum loss of K^+ through urine and further daily continuous loss of K^+ which is near about 5–10 mmol/day, through stool and sweat, can result in gradual depletion of total body K^+ content, provided this minimum amount of K^+ loss is not replaced daily by intake. On the other hand, if K^+ reabsorption in renal tubules is impaired, then urinary loss will be greater and there will be quick manifestation of hypokalemia, provided intake of K^+ is still inadequate. As kidneys have enormous ability to reabsorb the filtered K^+ and decrease the urinary K^+ excretion to only 5 mmol/day, therefore marked reduction in K^+ intake is required to produce hypokalemia. In hypokalemia, the low plasma K^+ level correlates very poorly with the total body K^+ deficit. A decrease in plasma K^+ from 4 to 3 mmol/L usually represents 100–200 mmol of deficit. Whereas a plasma K^+ level below 3 mmol/L can represent a deficit between 200 and 400 mmol **(Box 3)**.

BOX 3: Causes of hypokalemia.

- *Reduced intake:*
  - Inadequate dietary intake
  - K⁺-free IV fluid
- *Increased loss through urine:*
  - Conn syndrome (primary hyperaldosteronism)
  - Secondary hyperaldosteronism, such as heart failure, ECF depletion, renal artery stenosis, cirrhosis, nephrotic syndrome, etc.
  - Cushing syndrome
  - Renal tubular acidosis and hypomagnesemia
  - Renin excess
  - Diuretics
  - Batter syndrome
  - Uncontrolled diabetes
  - Amphotericin B, carbenicillin
  - Liddle syndrome
- *Increased loss through GI tract:*
  - Vomiting, diarrhea, and malabsorption syndrome
  - Aspiration of upper GI contents drainage through fistula
  - Villous adenoma of colon
- *Intercompartmental shift:*
  - Metabolic alkalosis
  - Insulin and β-blocker
  - Hypothermia

Hypokalemia also occurs, even though, intake is adequate. This is due to the presence of excessive loss. This excessive loss of K^+ is either through renal route or through gastrointestinal tract. Excretion of K^+ through the urine rises, whenever there is increased delivery of Na^+ to distal tubule. This increased delivery of Na^+ to distal tubule causes increased reabsorption of it, in exchange of increased K^+ secretion, which is lost through urine. This mechanism of excessive renal K^+ loss is found in uncontrolled diabetes, and use of loop diuretics, such as furosemide, thiazides, etc. Excretion of K^+ through urine is also increased, whenever there is high concentration of aldosterone which promotes excessive reabsorption of Na^+ in distal tubule in exchange of excessive secretion and loss of K^+ through urine. The causes of this high concentration of aldosterone are: Conn syndrome, secondary hyperaldosteronism, Cushing syndrome, etc. Most often the secondary hyperaldosteronism results from enhanced secretion of renin in response to inadequate renal perfusion (e.g., heart failure, hypoalbuminemia, renal artery stenosis, cirrhosis, nephrotic syndrome, etc.). Enhanced secretion of renin increases the secretion of aldosterone through angiotensin I and angiotensin II pathway. In patients with ECF depletion, there are high plasma levels of renin, angiotensin I, II, and aldosterone. The GFR is maintained by angiotensin II mediated efferent arteriolar constriction. So, the distal Na^+ delivery is relatively preserved, but the aldosterone drives the urinary losses of K^+.

The other causes of renal loss of K^+ are: renal tubular acidosis, hypomagnesemia, ketoacidosis, some drug therapies such as carbenicillin, amphotericin B, etc., and salt-wasting nephropathies. The causes of increased loss of K^+ through GI route are: vomiting, diarrhea, malabsorption syndrome, abuse of laxative, nasogastric suction, losses of secretin through fistula, villous adenoma, etc. Dialysis, by low K^+ containing fluids, also causes hypokalemia. Continuous increased sweat formation sometimes causes hypokalemia, provided when it is associated with low K^+ intake. Uremic patients have normal or high plasma K^+ concentration, though it has total body K^+ deficit. This is due to acidosis which causes shifting of K^+ from ICF to ECF compartment. Any factor which moves K^+ into cells will cause the increased intracellular K^+ concentration, including that in the cells of distal tubule. This also enhances the secretion of K^+ and hence its urinary losses. This mechanism operates in alkalosis from any cause. Therefore, alkalosis and hypokalemia are commonly associated with each other. Similarly, acidosis and hyperkalemia are commonly associated with each other.

Except alkalosis, the hypokalemia due to intracellular movement of K^+ also occurs during insulin therapy, β-adrenergic agonists, and hypothermia. Hypokalemia also occurs following the transfusion of frozen red cells. Because, these cells lose K^+ during their preservation process and take up K^+ from plasma following reinfusion.

Clinical Manifestations and Diagnosis of Hypokalemia

Hypokalemia can produce widespread dysfunction of organs by increasing the threshold for initiation of action potential. Most patients remain asymptomatic, until plasma K^+ concentration falls below 3 mmol/L. At first the diagnosis of hypokalemia may be suggested by tiredness and muscular weakness. Other neuromuscular effects of hypokalemia include muscle cramping, tetany, and rarely rhabdomyolysis. In extreme cases, the patient may be unable to walk or climb stairs. Reduced intestinal motility or paralytic ileus may occur in hypokalemia. Cardiovascular effects in hypokalemia are most prominent and include ventricular arrhythmia, decreased cardiac contractility, low BP, potentiation of adverse effects of digitalis, etc. Typical ECG changes occur during hypokalemia and these are: (i) sinus rhythm with normal QRS complex, (ii) increased P-wave amplitude, (iii) prolongation of P-R interval, (iv) depression of ST segment, (v) T-wave flattening and inversion, and (vi) increasingly prominent U-wave.

Hypokalemia induced by diuretics is often associated with metabolic alkalosis. This is because kidneys absorb more Na^+ to compensate for intravascular volume depletion due to diuretics in exchange of K^+. In presence of hypokalemia as

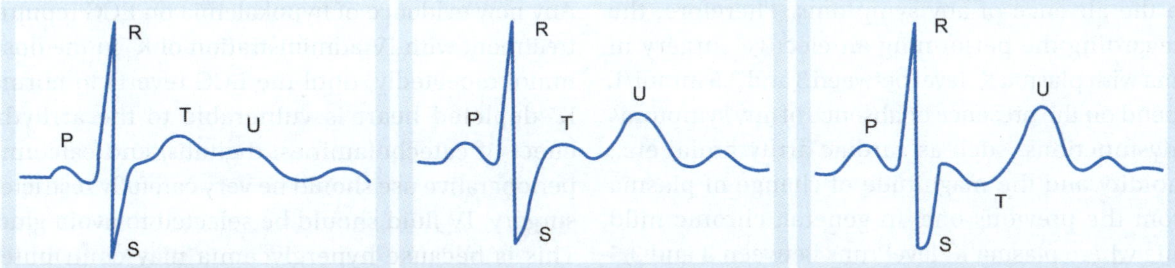

Fig. 2: The effects of hypokalemia on ECG. It is characterized by: gradual increase in amplitude of P-wave, progressive increase of P-R interval, depression of ST segment, progressive flattening of T-wave, and increasingly prominent U-wave.

there is less availability of K^+, so Na^+ will absorb in exchange of H^+ causing alkalosis. Also, bicarbonate is absorbed to compensate the diuretic-induced hypochloremia. Therefore, the end result of diuretics is hypokalemia and hypochloremia, associated with metabolic alkalosis. Long-standing hypokalemia damages renal tubular structure and results in the failure of antidiuretic response to ADH. Therefore, gradually patients with hypokalemia may present with nocturia (nocturnal diuresis) or polyuria and polydipsia **(Fig. 2)**.

In most cases of K^+ depletion, the plasma K^+ concentration is low. But, in some cases the factors that cause to move K^+ out of the cell may help to maintain a normal plasma K^+ level in spite of low body K^+ content as, for example, diabetic ketoacidosis. On the other hand, patients with metabolic alkalosis or who have been taking excessive insulin or β-adreno-receptor agonists may have a low plasma K^+ level despite a normal total body K^+ content. This is because of the movement of K^+ into cells. Therefore, in mentioning the cause of hypokalemia, the measurement of urinary K^+ excretion may be helpful. A value of urinary K^+ concentration <20 mmol/day makes abnormal renal K^+ loss unlikely. While a urinary K^+ excretion >50 mmol/day in the presence of hypokalemia suggests renal cause.

Management of Hypokalemia

Giving K^+ salt orally or through IV route treats hypokalemia. But, the mode of treatment of hypokalemia (either oral or through IV route) depends on the severity of organ dysfunction and the degree of hypokalemia. Intravenous replacement of K^+ should usually be reserved for patients with serious cardiac dysfunction or severe muscle weakness. Otherwise, oral replacement of K^+ is the choice of management. During IV replacement of K^+ continuous ECG monitoring and periodic assessment of muscle strength is mandatory. The goal of intravenous K^+ therapy is to manage the emergency and not necessarily to correct the entire K^+ deficit. For IV K^+ replacement, KCl is usually used. Any other associated salt and water deficit with hypokalemia should be replaced first. This is because any IV administration of K^+ is avoided, until

adequate urine output is established. Dextrose containing solutions should generally be avoided for IV replacement of K^+. Because the resulting hyperglycemia and secondarily increased secretion of insulin may actually lower the plasma K^+ level, even further. During IV replacement, the dose of K^+ should not exceed 10–20 mmol/h or 240 mmol/day.

The oral route for K^+ replacement is most commonly practiced and safer. It is used for nonemergency circumstances. Oral KCl (1 g = 13.4 mmol of K^+) is a satisfactory preparation, unless metabolic acidosis is present. Otherwise, in acidosis $KHCO_3$ is used. This oral KCl preparation may cause GI irritation, esophageal and small bowel erosion, strictures, etc. In alkalosis KCl is preferred, because it also corrects the chloride deficit. The dose of oral preparation of KCl is 80–100 mmol/day. A diet rich in K^+ such as bananas, citrus fruit, milk, chocolate, etc. are also helpful in hypokalemia. If hypokalemia is found to be difficult to correct in patients who have had diuretics, then it should be thought that there may be an associated Mg^{2+} deficiency. Therefore, correction of this Mg^{2+} deficiency is necessary, before hypokalemia is treated to normal. Oral replacement of K^+ deficit usually requires several days.

Anesthetic Considerations of Hypokalemia

Hypokalemia is a very common perioperative finding. It is found that patients with plasma K^+ concentration of <3 mmol/L are at increased risk of cardiac arrhythmia. So, these hypokalemic patients should be taken as serious and all the precautionary measures such as continuous ECG monitoring, IV replacement of K^+, correction of acid-base imbalance, use of nerve stimulator, etc. should be taken. But, the patients who have plasma K^+ concentration between 3 and 3.5 mmol/L produce problem to take the decision, especially in such circumstances, if elective surgery should be done or not. This is because in such circumstances the incidence of intraoperative cardiac arrhythmias does not increase in asymptomatic patient with chronic K^+ level between 3 and 3.5 mmol/L. Further, it is not suggested to infuse K^+ preoperatively, depending solely on plasma

K$^+$ level in the absence of any symptoms. Therefore, the decision regarding the performing an elective surgery in hypokalemia with plasma K$^+$ level between 3 and 3.5 mmol/L should depend on the presence or absence of any symptoms or organ dysfunctions, such as cardiac arrhythmia, etc., and the rapidity and the magnitude of change of plasma K$^+$ level from the previous one. In general, chronic mild hypokalemia where plasma K$^+$ level runs between 3 and 3.5 mmol/L and there is no cardiac arrhythmia or other organ dysfunction does not appear to increase the anesthetic risk appreciably. But, this will not be applicable to patients who are taking digitalis, though their plasma K$^+$ level is near about 4 mmol/L. So, it is reasonable to repeat the measurement of plasma K$^+$ level and to obtain an ECG for detection of cardiac arrhythmia, before any induction of anesthesia in patients who are considered at increased risk from the effects of hypokalemia **(Fig. 3)**.

No specific anesthetic drugs or techniques appear to be superior for use in hypokalemic patient. But, it is important to monitor the ECG continuously, during perioperative period, for any evidence of adverse effect of hypokalemia.

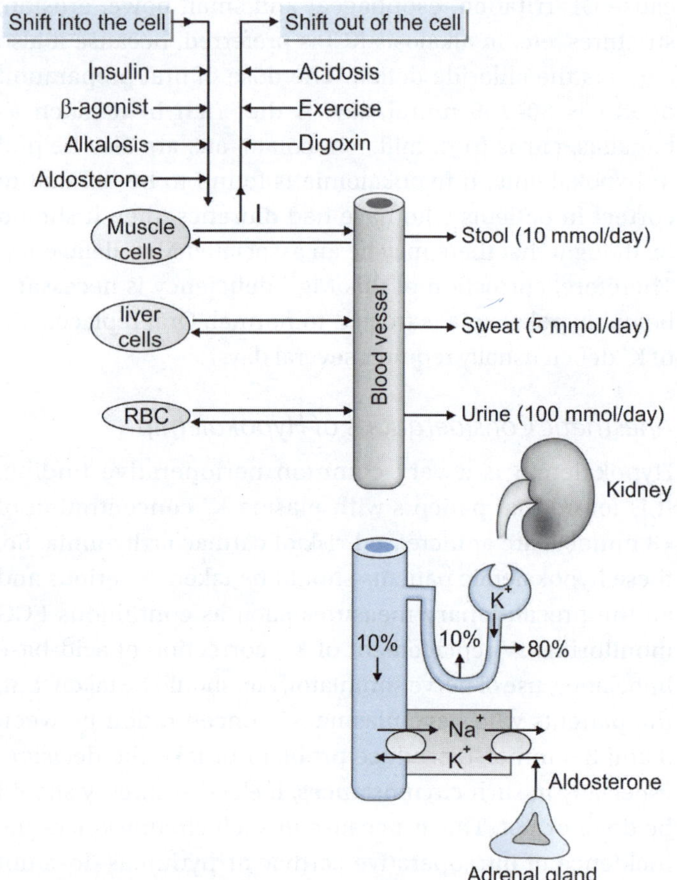

Fig. 3: The total body K$^+$ metabolism by the mechanism of secretion of K$^+$ in distal renal tubule, intercompartmental shifting, and excretion through stool, urine, and sweat.

Any new evidence of hypokalemia on ECG requires prompt treatment with IV administration of K$^+$ in the dose of 0.5–1 mmol repeatedly, until the ECG reverts to normal. As the K$^+$ depleted heart is vulnerable to the arrhythmogenic effect of catecholamines, digitalis, and calcium, so their perioperative use should be very carefully restricted. During surgery, IV fluid should be selected to avoid glucose load. This is because hyperglycemia may contribute to more hypokalemia, the cause of which is explained before. Continuous capnography and measurement of arterial blood gas and pH are helpful for confirming the proper management of ventilation. Because, hyperventilation can produce further alkalosis and hypokalemia. Hypokalemic patients have increased sensitivity to neuromuscular blocking agents. So, a prudent approach is to reduce the dose of muscle relaxant to 30–50% and use of nerve stimulator to follow the degree of muscular paralysis and the adequacy of reversal. Chronic hypokalemia is associated with decreased myocardial contractility and hypotension. Therefore, patient with chronic hypokalemia might be unusually sensitive to cardiac depressant effect of volatile anesthetic agent. There is also evidence that epinephrine, used with local anesthetic agents to perform axillary block in hypokalemic patient, is associated with arrhythmia shown by ECG. So, it is prudent to avoid the use of epinephrine with local anesthetic agent in patient suffering from hypokalemia.

Hyperkalemia

Hyperkalemia is defined as plasma K$^+$ concentration >5.5 mmol/L, where the usual normal plasma value of it varies between 3.5 and 5.5 mmol/L. It is a less common disturbance of K$^+$ balance than hypokalemia, because the kidneys have enormous capacity to excrete K$^+$ which may go up to 400–600 mmol/day (average 500 mmol/day). Usually, the hyperkalemia can result from: (i) decreased renal excretion of K$^+$, (ii) shifting of K$^+$ from intracellular to extracellular compartment, without any change in total body K$^+$ content, (iii) increased intake of K$^+$, and (iv) combination of these factors.

Increased Intake of K$^+$

Increased intake of only K$^+$ is a rare sole cause of hyperkalemia. This is because there are enormous capabilities of adaptation for excretion of K$^+$ by kidneys which ensure rapid elimination of it in response to increased dietary load or consumption. However, iatrogenic hyperkalemia may result from overzealous parenteral K$^+$ replacement or usual amount of replacement of K$^+$ in patients with renal insufficiency or patients taking insulin or β-blockers. Other sources of iatrogenic hyperkalemia are: transfusion of stored blood,

BOX 4: Causes of hyperkalemia.

- *Increased intake:*
  - High K^+ intake through food
  - Chronic ingestion of drugs containing K^+ compound
  - Excessive IV therapy with K^+
  - Na^+ salt substitute by K^+ salt
- *Impaired renal excretion:*
  - *Reduced GFR:*
    - Renal failure and reduced renal blood flow (shock)
    - Urinary tract obstruction
  - *Impaired tubular secretion of K^+ hypoaldosteronism:*
    - Addison disease, 21-hydroxylase deficiency
    - ACE inhibitor, NSAID
    - β-blockers, K^+-sparing agents
    - SLE and sickle-cell disease
- *Intercompartmental shift of K^+:*
  - Acidosis, diabetes, and β-blockers
  - Tissue hypoxia and succinylcholine
  - Strenuous exercise
  - Water depletion (ECF hypertonicity)
  - Rhabdomyolysis
- *Enhanced Cl^- reabsorption:*
  - Cyclosporine
  - Gordon syndrome
- *Pseudohyperkalemia:*
  - Incorrect blood sampling
  - Tissue damage during venipuncture
  - Red cell hemolysis
  - Marked leukocytosis and/or thrombocytosis

(ACE: angiotensin-converting enzyme; ECF: extracellular fluid; GFR: glomerular filtration rate; NSAID: nonsteroidal anti-inflammatory drugs; SLE: systemic lupus erythematosus)

chronic consumption of potassium preparation of any drug (such as potassium penicillin), taking K^+ salt as substitute of Na^+ salt where much Na^+ intake is prohibited, etc. The K^+ concentration in one unit of stored blood can increase from 25 to 35 mmol/L after 24 days of storage. Therefore, where there is risk of hyperkalemia large transfusion of old whole blood should be avoided. On the other hand, this hyperkalemia can be minimized by transfusing only the packed red cells **(Box 4)**.

Decreased Renal Excretion of K^+

Chronic hyperkalemia is also virtually associated with decreased excretion of K^+ by kidney due to: (i) decreased glomerular filtration rate (GFR) and (ii) decreased aldosterone activity or reduced K^+ secretion from distal nephron. The reduced GFR is due to the reduced circulation or hypovolemia which causes acute oliguric renal failure. This acute renal failure causes hyperkalemia due to decreased excretion of K^+. On the other hand, reduced circulation or shock is also associated with acidosis and increased catabolism which again causes hyperkalemia.

Therefore, this hyperkalemia (due to acidosis and increased metabolism) further aggravates the hyperkalemia which is already produced by oliguric renal failure (due to reduced circulation and shock).

Hyperkalemia due to decreased excretion of K^+ from renal tubule may be due to decreased aldosterone activity. At distal nephron, aldosterone causes reabsorption of Na^+ in exchange of K^+ which is excreted through urine. In the absence of aldosterone, Na^+ is not absorbed, so K^+ is not secreted and causes hyperkalemia. Hypoaldosteronism may be due to primary defect in the synthesis of aldosterone hormone or a defect in the renin-angiotensin-aldosterone system. The defect of aldosterone synthesis again may be due to primary adrenal insufficiency (Addison disease) or congenital 21 hydroxylase adrenal enzyme deficiency, which is needed to synthesize the mineralocorticoids. These patients show impaired ability to increase the secretion of aldosterone in response to hyperkalemia as a positive feedback compensatory mechanism. They are usually asymptomatic, but create problem when they are given with K^+ sparing diuretics or their intake of K^+ increases.

Factors which also interfere the action of renin-angiotensin-aldosterone system may cause the hyperkalemia. This is even more apparent when this renin-angiotensin-aldosterone interference is accompanied by impairment of renal function and reduced excretion or secretion of K^+ due to this renal dysfunction. ACE-inhibitors interfere the secretion of angiotensin-II-mediated release of aldosterone and thus also cause hyperkalemia. NSAIDs inhibit the secretion of renin by inhibiting the synthesis of prostaglandin and thus causes hyperkalemia. Heparin, including the low-molecular weight compound, also inhibits the production of aldosterone by the cells of zona glomerulosa and can lead to sever hyperkalemia in a subset of patients with underlying renal disease, diabetes mellitus, and those receiving K^+ sparing diuretics.

Decreased secretion of K^+ by distal and collecting tubules may be the principal cause of hyperkalemia. It results from *either impaired Na^+ reabsorption or increased Cl^- reabsorption*. So, they also often have varying degree of *Na^+ wasting or loss and hyperchloremic metabolic acidosis*. This may be intrinsic or acquired defect. Such defect may even occur in the presence of normal renal function. It is characterized by unresponsiveness or resistance to aldosterone therapy. So, it may be called as *pseudoaldosteronism*. The other acquired causes of decreased secretion of K^+ in distal tubule are SLE, diabetic neuropathy, sickle-cell anemia, etc. The decreased secretion of K^+ is also caused by K^+ sparing diuretics which antagonize the action of aldosterone activity and produce the effect of pseudoaldosteronism.

Shifting of K⁺ from Intracellular Fluid to Extracellular Fluid

The hyperkalemia may also occur due to the movement of K^+ out of cells. *This is commonly due to:* (1) the administration of succinylcholine, intravascular hemolysis, breakdown (lysis) of cells due to any cause, acidosis, excessive exercise, massive tissue trauma, rhabdomyolysis, etc. The average increase of plasma K^+ concentration, after the administration of succinylcholine, is 0.4–0.6 mmol/L. But, it may be exaggerated following severe trauma, massive burn, or following lower motor neuron disease; (2) Insulin deficiency and hypertonicity (e.g., hyperglycemia) promote the shifting of K^+ from intracellular compartment to extracellular compartment; (3) The severity of exercise-induced hyperkalemia is related to the degree of exertion. It is due to increased release of K^+ from muscles and is rapidly reversible which is often associated with rebound hypokalemia; (4) Treatment with β-blockers rarely causes hyperkalemia, but may contribute to elevation in plasma K^+ concentration, seen with other conditions; (5) Hyperkalemia may also occur with severe digitalis toxicity due to the inhibition of Na^+-K^+-ATPase pump; (6) Uremia may also impair the activity of Na^+-K^+-ATPase pump and produce hyperkalemia; (7) Arginine hydrochloride is used to treat metabolic alkalosis. But, it may cause hyperkalemia because the arginine cations enter the cells and potassium anions move out of the cell to maintain electrical neutrality.

Pseudohyperkalemia is a condition where there is artificial or spurious elevation of plasma K^+ concentration during its measurement in laboratory. This is due to the release of K^+ out of red cells, because of hemolysis in a blood specimen immediately following venipuncture. The other contributing factors for pseudohyperkalemia may also include: (i) prolonged use of tourniquet causing hemolysis, (ii) repeated fist clenching, (iii) release of K^+ from lysis of white cells and platelets in marked leukocytosis and thrombocytosis, etc. **(Figs. 4A to C)**.

Clinical Manifestation of Hyperkalemia

The *most important and common effects of hyperkalemia* are found on cardiac and skeletal muscles. Hyperkalemia reduces the threshold for initiation of action potential and thus causes sustained spontaneous depolarization of muscle cells like succinylcholine. This is the mechanism of manifestation of hyperkalemia. Cardiac manifestation of it is likely to occur when the plasma K^+ concentration crosses over 7 mmol/L. In general, the plasma K^+ values over 6 mmol/L should be treated. The *earliest ECG changes* during cardiac manifestations of hyperkalemia include increased T-wave amplitude (peaked T-wave). More severe degree of hyperkalemia may also result in prolonged PR interval, prolonged QRS duration, delay in AV conduction, and loss of P-wave. Then, with gradual increase in plasma K^+ concentration, there is loss of R-wave amplitude with progressive widening of QRS complex which merges with T-wave and produces a *sine wave pattern in ECG*. More severe hyperkalemia produces VF and asystole.

Since the resting membrane potential of a cell is related to the ratio of intracellular and extracellular concentration of K^+, so the hyperkalemia partially depolarizes the cell membrane. This partial, prolonged, and sustained depolarization of cell membrane impairs the membrane excitability which is manifested as muscular weakness. This may progress to flaccid paralysis (like succinylcholine) and hypoventilation, if the respiratory muscles are involved. Hyperkalemia also inhibits the reabsorption of NH_4^+ in thick ascending limb of loop of Henle and renal amino acid synthesis. Therefore, the net renal acid excretion is impaired which results in metabolic acidosis. This may further exacerbate hyperkalemia, due to the movement of K^+ out of cells, in exchange of entry of H^+ into cells.

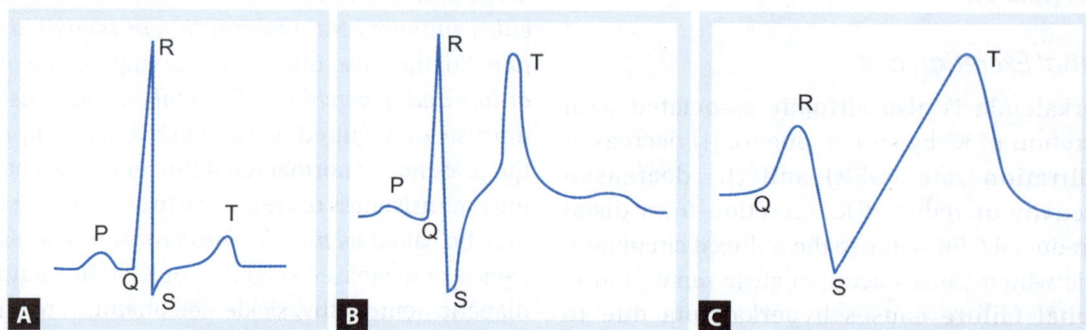

Figs. 4A to C: This figure shows the effects of hyperkalemia on ECG. It is characterized by: (i) loss of P-wave, (ii) decrease in amplitude of R-wave, (iii) ST-segment depression, (iv) widening of QRS complex, (v) shortened QT interval, and (vi) peaked T-waves. Thus, the graph of ECG resembles a "sine wave". (A: normal ECG; B: transition; C: sine wave)

Treatment of Hyperkalemia

Chronic hyperkalemia is *most commonly due to* impaired excretion of K^+ through kidney, except some rare causes. If the etiology of hyperkalemia is not readily apparent and the patient is asymptomatic, then the pseudohyperkalemia should be thought first and excluded. The severe chronic renal insufficiency, due to oliguric acute renal failure, caused by hypovolemia, also should be ruled out. The history will also guide, regarding the excessive intake of K^+ or any drug that impairs the handling of K^+, causing hyperkalemia. The estimation of effective circulating volume, ECF component, or urine output is also the essential part of physical examination which will help to find out the exact etiology of hyperkalemia. The severity of hyperkalemia is determined by the symptoms, plasma K^+ concentration, and ECG abnormalities.

The appropriate renal response to hyperkalemia is to excrete at least 200 mmol/day of K^+. In most cases, the reduced renal K^+ loss is due to impaired K^+ secretion. This impaired K^+ secretion again may be due to either hypoaldosteronism (less synthesis) or resistance to its renal effect. This can be determined by evaluating the K^+ loosing response of aldosterone, after administration of exogenous mineralocorticoids. Primary adrenal insufficiency should be differentiated from secondary hypoaldosteronism (hyporenin hypoaldosteronism) by examining the renin-aldosterone axis. Therefore, the plasma renin and aldosterone levels should be measured.

The approach to therapy for hyperkalemia depends on its degree which is determined by plasma K^+ concentration, associated muscular weakness, and changes on ECG. Potentially the fatal effect of hyperkalemia rarely occurs, unless the plasma K^+ concentration goes above 7 mmol/L which is associated with profound weakness, QRS widening, absence of P-waves, ventricular arrhythmia, and lastly cardiac arrest. Hence, to avoid this lethal outcome, plasma K^+ concentration, exceeding 6 mmol/L, should always be treated immediately. The treatment of hyperkalemia is aimed at; (i) reversing the cardiac manifestation; (ii) removing the muscle weakness; and (iii) restoring the plasma K^+ concentration to normal. The treatment modalities of hyperkalemia should depend on the severity of manifestations and the cause of hyperkalemia.

Severe hyperkalemia requires emergency treatment, directed at: (i) minimizing membrane depolarization; (ii) shifting K^+ into cells; and (iii) promoting K^+ loss. In addition; (iv) the exogenous K^+ intake and anti-kaliuretic drugs (that prevents kaliuresis or K^+ excretion through urine) should be discontinued. In emergency, calcium gluconate is the drug of choice and reduces the membrane excitability.

The usual dose of calcium gluconate is 5–10 mL of 10% solution which is administered over 2–3 minutes. Its effects are very rapid (within minutes) and antagonizes the cardiac effects of hyperkalemia. But, unfortunately, the results are very short lived (30–60 minutes) and the dose should be repeated. If the initial dose of calcium gluconate cannot produce any change in ECG, then the second dose also can be repeated, after 5–10 minutes. Instead of calcium gluconate, calcium chloride also can be used in the dose of 3–5 mL of 10% solution.

Insulin causes K^+ to shift into cells by mechanism, described before, and is so used to treat hyperkalemia. It is used with glucose, because glucose also stimulates the secretion of endogenous insulin and prevents hypoglycemia if occurs. Only glucose also can be used to treat hyperkalemia by stimulating the pancreatic β-cells to release insulin. But, this action is much delayed. The recommended dose of exogenous insulin is 10–20 units of regular variety with 25–50 g of glucose. If effective the plasma K^+ concentration will fall by 1–1.5 mmol/L in 20–30 minutes and the effect will last for several hours. Hyperglycemic patients should not be given glucose. They will only receive insulin. Acidosis causes shifting of K^+ out of the cells and hyperkalemia. Therefore, alkali therapy with intravenous $NaHCO_3$ shifts K^+ into the cells and reduces hyperkalemia. This is administered as an isotonic solution in the dose of 130 mmol/L and will decrease the plasma K^+ concentration within 20 minutes. Ideally, alkali should be reserved for severe hyperkalemia which is associated with metabolic acidosis. The β-adrenergic agonist also promotes the cellular uptake of K^+. Thus, it may be useful in acute hyperkalemia associated with massive transfusions. When it is administered parenterally or in nebulized form, the onset of action is 30 minutes and lowers the plasma K^+ concentration by 0.5–1.5 mmol/L. This effect lasts for 2–4 hours. If the renal function is adequate, then the loop and thiazide diuretics (often in combination) may enhance K^+ excretion. So, they may be used as an adjunct to the management of hyperkalemia. Sodium polystyrene sulfonate is a cation exchange resin. It also promotes the excretion of K^+ in exchange of Na^+ in the gastrointestinal (GI) tract. It is used through oral or rectal route and each gram binds with 1 mmol of K^+ and release 2–3 mmol of Na^+. When given by mouth the usual dose of sodium polystyrene is 25–50 g which is mixed with 100 mL of 20% sorbitol to prevent constipation. This will lower the plasma K^+ concentration by 0.5–1 mmol/L within 1–2 hours of its administration and the action lasts for 4–6 hours. Another way of treating hyperkalemia is dialysis. It is effective in severe and refractory hyperkalemia. Among the dialysis, hemodialysis is more safe and effective than peritoneal dialysis. The rate of decreases of plasma K$^+$ level by hemodialysis is 50 mmol/h, whereas the rate of removal of plasma K$^+$ level by peritoneal dialysis is only 15–20 mmol/h.

Anesthetic Considerations

There is a general agreement that plasma K$^+$ concentration should be kept below 5.5 mmol/L before any elective anesthesia and surgery. If this is not possible, then elective anesthesia and surgery should be postponed in patients with hyperkalemia. In emergency circumstances, anesthetic technique should be adjusted simultaneously at both directions, such as by preventing any further increase and lowering the plasma K$^+$ concentration by previously mentioned different techniques. Ventilation always should be controlled and monitored by capnography to prevent the accumulation of CO_2 causing respiratory acidosis which could result in transfer of K$^+$ from intracellular to extracellular sites. It is found that 10 mm decrease in $PaCO_2$ causes decrease in plasma K$^+$ concentration by about

0.5–1 mmol/L. Metabolic acidosis due to arterial hypoxemia should also be considered which prevents hypokalemia. The use of succinylcholine is contraindicated in the presence of hyperkalemia, because there is no reliable method to prevent succinylcholine induced K$^+$ release.

Care should be given regarding the perioperative intravenous fluid because most of the solutions contain K$^+$, as, for example, the lactated Ringer's solution contains K$^+$ in the concentration of 4 mmol/L. Hyperkalemia accentuates the effect of muscle relaxants and decreases its intraoperative requirements. So, the practical approach, in such circumstances, is to titrate the dose of neuromuscular blocking agent by the use of nerve stimulator. Unlike the plasma Na$^+$ concentration, hyperkalemia is not associated with alterations in the dose requirement of volatile anesthetics.

Intraoperatively, all the patients should be monitored carefully and continuously by ECG. Drugs such as Ca^{2+}, glucose, and insulin should be kept ready for any acute hyperkalemia.

CALCIUM BALANCE

■ INTRODUCTION

Calcium (Ca^{2+}) is the principal component of human skeleton and is the fourth most common inorganic element in our body. The total calcium content of a normal adult human body is about 20–25 g/kg of lean body mass (LBM). *The bone and teeth constitute about 98% of total body calcium.* The remaining 2% of it (Ca^{2+}) is distributed in different tissues of body, such as in muscle, plasma, lymph, liver, etc. In plasma, the Ca^{2+} level (ionized plus nonionized) varies between *9 and 11 mg/100 mL of blood.* This level is maintained fairly constant and is very critical. Calcium (Ca^{2+}) in plasma is remained in the following form: *diffusible* and *nondiffusible.* Diffusible calcium again remains in two forms: (1) *ionized* and (2) *nonionized.* The examples of *ionized* Ca^{2+} in plasma are: CaCl$_2$, Ca-gluconate, etc. and the examples of *nonionized* Ca^{2+} in plasma are Ca-citrate, Ca-bicarbonate, Ca-phosphate, etc. The nondiffusible Ca^{2+} remains in plasma in combination with plasma protein, especially albumin **(Fact file III)**.

Among the total plasma Ca^{2+}, 50% remains as free-ionized form and the remaining 40% stays as protein bound. Then, another 10% remains as complex with anion, such as citrate and amino acids. *Among these, it is the free-ionized Ca^{2+} which constitutes about 50% of total plasma Ca^{2+} and is the most physiologically important. Normally, the concentration of free-ionized Ca^{2+} in plasma is 4.5–5.5 mg/dL or 2.38–2.66 mEq or 1.19–1.33 mmol/L.* (Here, the mEq and mmol are not numerically same, as the valency of Ca^{2+} is two and mmol is obtained by dividing the mEq by valency). Lowering of this free-ionized Ca^{2+} concentration, due to any cause, produces *tetany.* However, the reduction of total calcium content in our body or the reduction of nondiffusible portion of total (Ca^{2+}) in plasma, due to diminished plasma protein, does not cause tetany. *It proves that the changes in plasma protein (mainly albumin) concentration affect the total Ca^{2+} content of our body, but not the ionized Ca^{2+} concentration.* The general rule is that for each increase or decrease of 1 g/dL of albumin, the total plasma Ca^{2+} level increases or decreases approximately 0.8–1 mg/dL, respectively. *The free-ionized plasma Ca^{2+} level also changes directly with the changes of blood pH. This is due to the changes of the degree of protein-binding capacity of Ca^{2+}* **(Fig. 5)**.

Alkalosis decreases the concentration of ionized Ca^{2+} and acidosis increases it. The thumb rule is that the concentration of ionized Ca^{2+} increases approximately 0.16 mg/dL for each decrease in 0.1 unit of plasma pH and vice versa. The

---

FACT FILE III

Molecular weight of calcium is 40. Body content of it is regulated by PTH-related protein, vitamin D and calcitonin. The intracellular Ca^{2+} concentration is very low which is 100 nM/L (100 nano mole per liter). This is due to active pumping out of Ca^{2+} from cell and active pumping it into sarcoplasmic reticulum. The extracellular concentration of Ca^{2+} is 1 mmol/L.

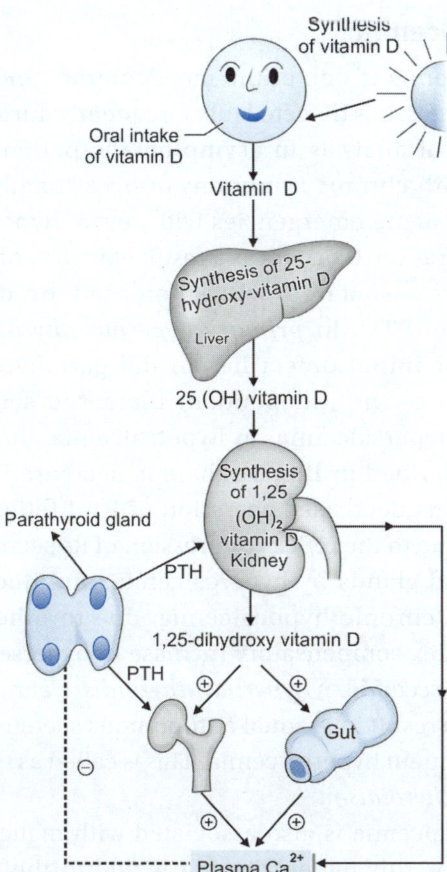

Fig. 5: Homeostasis of Ca^{2+} which is maintained by interaction between parathyroid hormone (PTH) and vitamin D. Only ionized-free Ca^{2+} controls the secretion of PTH. Normally 50% of total plasma Ca^{2+} exists in serum as free-ionized form. Remaining 40% of Ca^{2+} exists as protein bound, mainly with albumin. Next remaining 10% of Ca^{2+} exists as complexed form with organic compound such as citrate, phosphate, etc.

plasma phosphate concentration also varies inversely with plasma Ca^{2+} level. An increase in phosphate ions causes a corresponding decrease in Ca^{2+} ion and vice versa. However, the product of calcium and inorganic phosphate of blood (10 mg Ca^{2+} × 5 mg PO^{2-}) is kept constant and is about 50. This inverse relation of pH and phosphate concentration of plasma with Ca^{2+} in blood may be due to the increased excretion or deposition of Ca^{2+} in bones.

Ca^{2+} has enormous importance for the function of our body. It is involved in nearly all the essential biological functions of cells. These are: (i) contraction of heart muscle, (ii) coagulation of blood, (iii) maintenance of normal neuromuscular excitability (iv) release of different neurotransmitter and hormones, (v) activation of different enzymes, (vi) control of permeability of capillary endothelium, and (vii) formation of bones and teeth, etc. Although, the 2% of total body weight is constituted by calcium and 98% of this total body calcium is in the bone and

teeth, still the maintenance of remaining small extracellular or plasma Ca^{2+} concentration is crucial for its homeostasis. In adult, the Ca^{2+} intake and loss are same. This is called as the calcium balance. When the Ca^{2+} is retained in our body, then the balance is called as positive. It is found during growth, pregnancy, etc. or during recovery after calcium starvation. On the other hand, when the loss of Ca^{2+} is more than the intake, then this balance is called negative. It is found during (i) the hyperactive condition of thyroid and parathyroid, (ii) in calcium deficiency, and (iii) in certain other diseases, such as rickets, osteomalacia, etc.

The average intake of Ca^{2+} in adults is about 700 mg/day. It is absorbed mainly through the upper part of small intestine, under the direct influence of vitamin D and indirect influence of parathyroid hormone (PTH). Its absorption in small intestine varies greatly according to the different types of food. On high protein diet, only 20% of dietary Ca^{2+} is absorbed, while on low protein diet it is only 5%. Up to 80% of daily Ca^{2+} intake is normally lost through feces. Soluble inorganic forms of Ca^{2+} is much better absorbed. It is probable that the organic Ca^{2+} in food is converted to inorganic form, before it can be absorbed. Insoluble Ca^{2+} compounds are never absorbed. Thus, the presence of phytic acid in cereals produces the formation of calcium phytates which is insoluble and does not absorb. Oxalates may have the similar effect. Calcium phosphates are also not absorbed.

Ca^{2+} is also excreted through urine which is about 150–200 mg/day, but it may vary from as low as 50 mg/day to 300 mg/day. About 98% filtered Ca^{2+} is reabsorbed through proximal renal tubules and the ascending limb of the loop of Henle. This is parallel to the reabsorption of Na$^+$. But, the difference is that the distal renal tubular reabsorption of Ca^{2+} is controlled by parathyroid hormone (PTH). This is unlike to that of Na$^+$ whose reabsorption is controlled by aldosterone at the distal site of renal tubule. The PTH is secreted by the chief cells of parathyroid gland. It also increases the absorption of Ca^{2+} from gut indirectly (PTH converts 25-hydroxy D$_3$ to 1,25-dihydroxy D$_3$ and this 1,25-dihydroxy D$_3$ enhances the absorption of Ca^{2+} from small intestine) and mobilizes the Ca^{2+} from bone into plasma. The increased secretion of PTH also enhances the reabsorption of Ca^{2+} in distal nephron and decreases its excretion and vice versa.

■ CONTROL OF CALCIUM METABOLISM

The plasma Ca^{2+} level is normally maintained by equal amount of input and output. In plasma, the input of Ca^{2+} is related to: absorption from GI tract, reabsorption from bone, and reabsorption by kidney. In contrast, from plasma the output of Ca^{2+} is related to: deposition in bone, urinary excretion, secretion into GI tract, and sweat formation.

However, all these input and output and the subsequent constant plasma Ca^{2+} level are closely regulated by three hormones: PTH, vitamin D, and calcitonin which act primarily on bone, distal renal tubules, and small intestine.

Among these factors, PTH is the most important agent for the regulation of plasma Ca^{2+} concentration. Normally, it increases the plasma Ca^{2+} level by: (i) mobilizing the Ca^{2+} from bone, (ii) increasing the renal reabsorption of Ca^{2+} and excretion of PO_4^{2-} at distal tubule, and (iii) increasing indirectly the intestinal absorption of Ca^{2+} via the acceleration of 1,25-dihydroxy-chole-calciferol (DHCC) synthesis in kidney. The secretion of PTH from parathyroid gland is regulated by plasma Ca^{2+} level **(Fact file IV)**. Increase in plasma Ca^{2+} concentration decreases the secretion of PTH and vice versa.

Vitamin D also helps in Ca^{2+} homeostasis in body. It exists in several form, but the most active biological form of it is 1,25-DHCC. It is formed from the cholecalciferol, first in the liver by conversion to 25-cholecalciferol and then in the kidney by conversion to 1,25-DHCC. The last conversion of vitamin D is catalyzed by PTH. Like PTH, the active biological form of vitamin D also helps in intestinal absorption of Ca^{2+}, renal reabsorption of Ca^{2+} and potentiation of the action of PTH on bone.

Calcitonin is another polypeptide hormone whose action is opposite to PTH. It also helps in Ca^{2+} homeostasis in our body. It is secreted from the parafollicular cells of thyroid gland. It inhibits the mobilization of Ca^{2+} from bone and increases the excretion of Ca^{2+} through urine by inhibiting its reabsorption at distal renal tubules. Thus, calcitonin tries to decrease the plasma Ca^{2+} level in oppose to the action of PTH. Hence, hypercalcemia stimulates its secretion and hypocalcemia inhibits its secretion from the parafollicular cells of thyroid glands.

There are two types of disturbances of Ca^{2+} balance: (A) *hypercalcemia,* and (B) *hypocalcemia.*

Hypercalcemia

Hypercalcemia is one of the most common biochemical abnormalities. It is detected most frequently during routine biochemical analysis in asymptomatic patients. It may present with chronic symptoms or occasionally patients present as acute emergencies with severe hypercalcemia and dehydration. It occurs as a result of variety of disorders which are associated with increased or decreased secretion of PTH. In *primary hyperparathyroidism,* the primary or initial defect lies in the parathyroid gland which causes the independent increased secretion of PTH and hypercalcemia. In hypercalcemia, due to other cause (described in **Box 5**), there is decreased secretion of PTH. This decreased secretion of PTH (effect not the cause) is due to the reflex suppression of its secretion from parathyroid glands by hypercalcemia, and due to other causes. In chronic hypocalcemia, due to other causes, there is reflex compensatory increase in hypersecretion of PTH. This *secondary hyperparathyroidism* can, however, sometimes result in gradual autonomous secretion of PTH and subsequent hypercalcemia. This is called as the *tertiary hyperparathyroidism.*

Hypercalcemia is also associated with malignancy. In malignancy, this hypercalcemia is due to the abnormal secretion of some humoral mediators (such as PTH like substances, prostaglandins, cytokines, etc.) from tumor cells which release the Ca^{2+} from bones or due to direct bony metastases of cancer cells. In Paget's disease and chronic immobilization, hypercalcemia is due to increased turnover of Ca^{2+} from bone. Hypercalcemia in the milk alkali syndrome, granulomatous disease (e.g., sarcoidosis), hypervitaminosis of vitamin D, etc. is due to the increased intestinal absorption of Ca^{2+}. Still in many circumstances, the mechanism responsible for hypercalcemia is poorly understood.

FACT FILE IV

Parathyroid hormone (PTH) has direct effect on bone and renal tubules. It promotes reabsorption of Ca^{2+} from bone and renal tubules. It has also indirect effect on small intestine which is mediated by increasing the conversion of 25-hydroxy-chole-calciferal to the most potent hormone 1,25-dihydroxy-chole-calciferol (DHCC). This results in increased Ca^{2+} absorption from food in gut and increased mobilization of Ca^{2+} from bone. In regulating Ca^{2+} homeostasis, PTH plays an important role. This is because, dietary Ca^{2+} and vitamin D are rarely deficient. The 98% of total body calcium is in bone. This remains in dynamic equilibrium between extracellular fluid and store, by the process of deposition and reabsorption.

BOX 5: Causes of hypercalcemia.

- *With elevated parathyroid hormone (PTH) levels:*
  - Primary hyperparathyroidism
  - Tertiary hyperparathyroidism
  - Lithium-induced hyperparathyroidism
- *With low parathyroid hormone (PTH) levels:*
  - Milk-alkali syndrome
  - Malignancy
  - Multiple myeloma
  - Paget disease of bone
  - Vitamin D hypervitaminosis
  - Granulomatous disorder (tuberculosis and sarcoidosis)
  - Thiazide diuretics

Secondary hyperparathyroidism is due to hypocalcemia.

Clinical Manifestations of Hypercalcemia

In most of the patients, hypercalcemia is asymptomatic. About 50% of patients with primary hyperparathyroidism and hypercalcemia may go unrecognized, until the patient presents with some renal calculi. *The 10% of first renal stone formers and 20% of recurrent renal stone formers have primary hyperparathyroidism.* The patients of hypercalcemia, due to malignancy, can have a rapid onset of symptoms or may have clinical features, according to the site of malignancy which will help to localize their pathology. *Hypertension is common in hypercalcemia. Other symptoms and signs of hypercalcemia include polyuria, polydipsia, renal colic, anorexia, nausea, lethargy, dyspepsia, etc.* Other pathologies, like peptic ulcer, pancreatitis, and renal failure may also complicate the hypercalcemia. The *ECG signs of hypercalcemia* include: shortened ST segment, shortened QT interval, and premature ventricular contraction due to depressed cardiac conductions, etc. **(Box 5)**.

Diagnosis and Treatment of Hypercalcemia

The most important step in the management of hypercalcemia is the measurement of PTH level by specific radioimmunoassay. If the PTH and urinary calcium level are elevated, then the *diagnosis about hyperparathyroidism is confirmed.* On the other hand, if the PTH level is low, urinary Ca^{2+} is high and no other apparent cause of hypercalcemia is found, then the malignancy with or without bony metastases is very likely. Low plasma phosphate and increased alkaline phosphatase level support the diagnosis of primary hyperparathyroidism or malignancy. Hypercalcemia may cause nephrocalcinosis and the impairment of renal tubular function, causing hyperuricemia and hyperchloremia. Unless the source of hypercalcemia is obvious, *all the patients should be screened for malignancy* with X-ray, MRI, or isotope bone scan. The patient should also be screened for myeloma by ESR, serum protein electrophoresis, level of immunoglobulin, and urinary Bens–Jones protein.

Symptomatic hypercalcemia is usually associated with dehydration. So, it requires rapid treatment by rehydration which is accomplished by the administration of IV saline (to replace as much as 4–6 L deficit of water or to keep urinary output at 20–30 mL/h). This rehydration should be followed by brisk diuresis to accelerate the excretion of Ca^{2+}. Regarding diuresis, the clinician should be cautious about that premature diuresis or excessive diuresis after rehydration may increase plasma Ca^{2+} level by additional fluid depletion. During rehydration, the patient may need monitoring with CVP in old age or who is suffering from renal impairment. After rehydration and diuresis, the plasma Ca^{2+} level may come down, but still remains above normal level, though the potential risk for cardiovascular and neurological complications of hypercalcemia are removed.

Patients who are not responding to proper rehydration and mild diuresis or have severe hypercalcemia (total Ca^{2+} >15 mg/dL) may require additional therapy by bisphosphonates, glucocorticoids, or calcitonin. Among the bisphosphonates, the pamidronate is used in the dose of 90 mg through IV slowly over 4–6 hours. It is the agent of choice in hypercalcemia, because of its prolonged duration of action. Pamidronate causes a fall in plasma level of Ca^{2+} which is maximum at 2–3 days and lasts for few weeks. Unless the cause of hypercalcemia is removed, such as by the surgical removal of parathyroid gland, the patient should be followed up with an oral bisphosphonate after an emergency IV therapy. Calcitonin for the treatment of hypercalcemia is used in the dose of 2–5 U/kg through subcutaneous route. Hemodialysis for the treatment of hypercalcemia may be necessary in the presence of cardiac or renal failure. Glucocorticoids are helpful in the setting of vitamin D-induced hypercalcemia, such as granulomatous disease states.

Hypercalcemia in patients with primary hyperparathyroidism responds less well to pamidronate and glucocorticoids than the hypercalcemia due to malignancy. Urgent removal of parathyroid gland in primary hyperparathyroidism (such as adenoma and hyperplastic gland) is occasionally required, but strenuous attempts should be made to replace the fluid deficits and lower the plasma Ca^{2+} level, before administering anesthesia in such patient. Postoperative hypocalcemia is not uncommon, after the removal of parathyroid gland, during the first 2 weeks after surgery. But, the residual suppressed parathyroid tissue gradually recovers and the plasma Ca^{2+} level comes to normal.

Anesthetic Considerations of Hypercalcemia

Before and during the operation of a hypercalcemic patient, every attempt should be made to normalize the ionized plasma Ca^{2+} level, if it is already high and to avoid the circumstances which will raise it. So, perioperative acidosis should be checked by any cost. Therefore, ventilation must be controlled and monitored by capnography, during GA. Adequate hydration should be continued pre- and intraoperatively with great care to avoid hypervolemia. So, IV fluid therapy in a hypercalcemic patient should be monitored by CVP or pulmonary artery pressure, especially in patients with decreased cardiac reserve. The periodic measurement of K^+ and Mg^{2+} level in plasma also should be done during rehydration and diuretic therapy for the detection of any iatrogenic hypokalemia and hypomagnesemia in hypercalcemic patients. At last, patient should be monitored periodically by checking the plasma ionized Ca^{2+} level throughout the whole perioperative period.

Hypocalcemia

The incidence of hypocalcemia is less common than that of hypercalcemia. *It should be diagnosed only on the basis of plasma-ionized free Ca^{2+} concentration, but not on the basis of total plasma Ca^{2+} concentration or total body Ca^{2+} content.* Because the most common cause of hypocalcemia is low plasma albumin with *normal free-ionized Ca^{2+} concentration.* Contrary, ionized-free Ca^{2+} level may be low in the face of *normal plasma Ca^{2+} concentration* during alkalosis as a result of hyperventilation. *Therefore, when the direct measurement of plasma free-ionized Ca^{2+} level is not available then the total plasma Ca^{2+} concentration should be corrected for increase or decrease of plasma albumin level.* Hence, as almost all the laboratories routinely report the total serum Ca^{2+} concentration, but it is the ionized concentration which is biologically important and should be measured **(Table 3)**.

Symptomatic *hypocalcemia is most commonly due to* decreased plasma Ca^{2+} concentration, resulting from *hypoparathyroidism.* On the other hand, this hypoparathyroidism may be due to *surgical, idiopathic or pseudo causes.* Surgical hypoparathyroidism commonly occurs during thyroid surgery, but this complication is only permanent in 1% of thyroidectomy. Transient hypocalcemia develops in 10% of patients after 12–36 hours, following subtotal thyroidectomy for Graves' disease. Idiopathic hypoparathyroidism is sometimes occurred with autoimmune disease of adrenal gland, thyroid gland, or ovary at any age. *Pseudohypoparathyroidism* is usually an autosomal dominant syndrome where there is development of tissue resistance to PTH. Hypoparathyroidism may be associated with hypomagnesemia, because deficiency of magnesium is postulated to impair the secretion of PTH and antagonize its effects on bone. *In chronic renal failure, hyperphosphatemia may also be the common cause of hypocalcemia. Hypocalcemia may also occur* as the result of vitamin D deficiency which again may result from malabsorption, reduced intake, or abnormal metabolism of vitamin D.

Acute severe ionized hypocalcemia may also occur when the large amount of Ca^{2+} chelating agents such as citrate are administered during blood and plasma transfusion. The degree of hypocalcemia during transfusion of blood depends on the rate of its administration and the ability of bone to provide additional Ca^{2+} and the liver which metabolizes the citrate. Similarly, *transient hypocalcemia may also result* following rapid infusion of large amount of albumin. Another cause of hypocalcemia is pancreatitis. It is due to precipitation of Ca^{2+} with fats, following the release of lipolytic enzymes and fat necrosis.

Other less common cause of hypocalcemia includes: Hypersecretion of calcitonin (e.g., calcitonin secreting medullary carcinoma of thyroid) and use of large dose of heparin, protamine, glucagon, etc.

CLINICAL MANIFESTATIONS OF HYPOCALCEMIA

The fall of ionized Ca^{2+} concentration increases the relative proportion of neuroexcitatory ions such as Na^+, K^+, PO_4^{2-}, etc., and produces hyperexcitability of peripheral nerves. This is called as tetany. It is the clinical manifestation of hypocalcemia and occurs when *the ionized free Ca^{2+} concentration goes below 0.8 mmol/L (3.2 mg/dL) in the absence of alkalosis or total plasma calcium level is*

TABLE 3: Causes of hypocalcemia.				
	Ionized Ca^{2+} concentration	**Total Ca^{2+} concentration**	**Plasma PTH concentration**	**Plasma phosphate concentration**
Hypoparathyroid	↓	↓	↓	↑
Pseudohypoparathyroid	↓	↓	↑	↑
Alkalosis	↓	N	N	N
Renal failure	↓	↓	↑	↑
Vitamin D deficiency	↓	↓	↑	↑
Hyperphosphatemia	↓	↓	↑	↑
Precipitation of Ca^{2+} • Pancreatitis • Fat embolism	↓	↓	↑	↑
Chelation of Ca^{2+}	↓	↓	↑	↑

↑ = Increased, N = Normal, ↓ = Decreased; PTH: parathyroid hormone

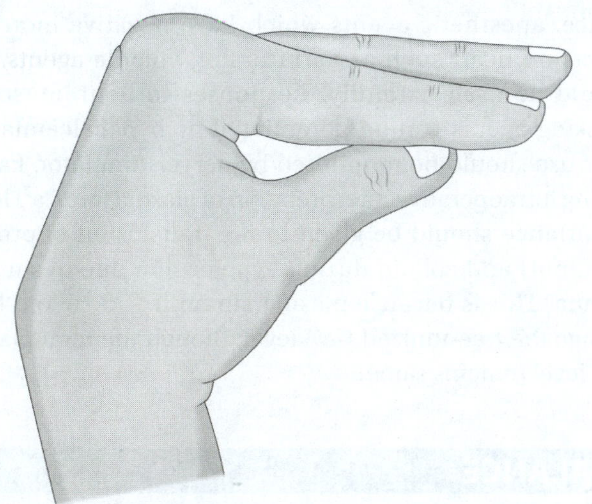

Fig. 6: Carpopedal spasm or Trousseau's sign.

<2 mmol/L (or <4 mEq/L). Alkalosis may be produced by excess intake of alkali, profuse vomiting, or increased breathing. It causes tetany without reducing the total plasma Ca^{2+}. This is because *alkalosis alters the ionic balance and decreases the amount of ionic-free Ca^{2+} without affecting the total Ca^{2+} concentration.* Also, alkalosis increases the proportion of neuro-excitatory ions and makes the peripheral nerve fibers and central nervous system more excitable. Children are more sensitive to tetany than adult. Magnesium depletion should also be considered as a possible contributing factor for hypocalcemia ($\downarrow$ ionized Ca^{2+} concentration) and tetany.

Tetany is commonly manifested in children as a triad of *carpopedal spasm, laryngeal stridor,* and *convulsion,* though one or more of these signs may be found independent of others. In carpopedal spasm, the hand adopts a characteristic figure which include flexed **(Fig. 6)** metacarpophalangeal joint, extended interphalangeal joint of fingers and thumb, and apposition of thumb with fingers. Stridor is caused by the closer of glottis. Furthermore, the adult patients complain of feeling a tingling sensation in their hands and feet, and around their mouth. The latent tetany also may be present when the signs of overt tetany are lacking. It is best recognized by eliciting the carpopedal spasm by inflating the sphygmomanometer cuff on upper arm above their systolic BP. A less specific sign of hypocalcemia is Chvostek's sign where tapping on facial nerve, near the styloid process, causes twitching of facial muscles.

Other clinical manifestations of hypocalcemia include paresthesia, confusion, lethargy, cardiac irritability leading to arrhythmia, decreased cardiac contractility causing hypotension, etc. ECG findings are not characteristic of hypocalcemia.

TREATMENT OF HYPOCALCEMIA

Symptomatic hypocalcemic or tetany is a medical emergency condition. So, it should be treated immediately. Instant IV injection of 10–20 mL of 10% Ca-gluconate will gradually raise the serum free Ca^{2+} concentration and control the situation. Instead of Ca-gluconate, 3–5 mL of 10% $CaCl_2$ also can be used. However, during IV administration of calcium, it should be remembered that 1 g of Ca-gluconate contains 90 mg (or 45 mEq or 225 mmol) of calcium and 1 g of $CaCl_2$ contains 272 mg (136 mEq or 68 mmol) of calcium. Also, it should be kept in mind that 1,000 mg of Ca-gluconate and 400 mg of $CaCl_2$ provides the same 100 mg of elemental calcium and when any commercial preparation of Ca^{2+} is given with equal amount of elemental calcium, then the influence of different preparation on ionized Ca^{2+} is equivalent. During the management of hypocalcemia, serial measurement of ionized free Ca^{2+} level in plasma is mandatory. The Ca^{2+}, Mg^{2+}, PO_4^{2-}, and K^+ are predominantly intracellular ions. So, their abnormalities frequently coexist with hypocalcemia. Therefore, their plasma concentration should be checked periodically, particularly PO_4^{2-} and Mg^{2+}, and should be treated. After the initial bolus dose, repeated bolus doses or continuous infusion of Ca^{2+} in the dose of 0.5–2 mg/kg/h may be necessary to obtain a prolonged effect of calcium therapy.

An intramuscular injection of 10 mL Ca-gluconate may also be given to obtain a more prolonged effect. To control tetany alkalosis should also be reversed acutely. This can be accomplished by encouraging the rebreathing of expired air in a paper bag or administering 5% CO_2 in O_2.

ANESTHETIC CONSIDERATIONS OF HYPOCALCEMIA

During anesthesia of a hypocalcemic patient, in their perioperative period, one should always try to recognize and treat the adverse effects of hypocalcemia. An anesthesiologist will also give his full effort preventing the further decrease of plasma Ca^{2+} level in the face of hypocalcemia, once it is checked. Therefore, alkalosis should be prevented by avoiding hyperventilation and monitoring it by capnometer. During treatment of metabolic acidosis by $NaHCO_3$, hence, one should be careful about the overdrive alkalosis and will repeatedly check the ionized plasma free Ca^{2+} level in patient with the history of hypocalcemia. There is chance of developing life-threatening hypocalcemia during GA, in patient with renal insufficiency, undergoing vascular surgery. In such circumstances, a clinician should be very careful and will take proper measures.

Normally, administration of few units of whole blood, containing citrate as preservative, does not cause any problem. This is because Ca^{2+} is rapidly mobilized from body stores which is kept as reserve and maintain the normal plasma Ca^{2+} level. But, during emergency, when the citrated blood is transfused very rapidly, e.g., 500 mL in every 10 minutes, then there is chance of patient developing hypocalcemia. This chance of hypocalcemia is further aggravated in the presence of cirrhosis of liver, hypothermia, and renal dysfunction where the metabolism of citrate is impaired.

Continuous monitoring by ECG is useful during perioperative period to facilitate the diagnosis of hypo-calcemia. It produces cardiac depression and hypotension.

Hence, anesthetic agents which have negative inotropic effects on heart such as barbiturates, volatile agents, etc. should be used carefully. Responses to neuromuscular blocking agents can be potentiated by hypocalcemia. So, their use should be monitored by nerve stimulator. Lastly, during intraoperative interpretation of plasma free Ca^{2+} level, importance should be given to the transfusion of protein (albumin) and colloid during hypotension due to surgical trauma. This is because plasma albumin and colloid level change the free-ionized Ca^{2+} level, though the total plasma Ca^{2+} level remains same.

PHOSPHORUS BALANCE

■ INTRODUCTION

Like K^+, the phosphorus is also an important intracellular cation (P^{3+}), but it is present mainly in bone, like Ca^{2+}. Out of total phosphorus of our body, only 0.1% remains in ECF. Bone contains 85% of total phosphorus of our body. The remaining 15% phosphorus is present in ICF. Within the cell, its presence is required for the synthesis of: (i) ATP which is used for the storage of energy, (ii) phosphonucleotides which is used for protein synthesis, and (iii) phospholipids and phosphoproteins which are required for the synthesis of cell membrane and intracellular organelle.

The normal P^{3+} concentration in plasma in an adult is 2.5–4.5 mg/dL (0.8–1.45 mmol/L). In children, this normal plasma level may go up to 6 mg/dL. Our daily P^{3+} intake varies between 800 mg and 1,500 mg. It is absorbed maximally from the upper part of small intestine and vitamin D increases its absorption. It is excreted mainly through kidney as urine and this excretion through kidney is responsible for regulating the total body P^{3+} content. PTH controls the P^{3+} content (level) of our body by its excretion through urine by inhibiting its proximal tubular reabsorption. This effect of PTH is again inhibited by the PT-H induced release of phosphate from bones and the excretion of P^{3+} through urine is increased. Unlike PTH, vitamin D increases the reabsorption of P^{3+} through kidney. Serum hypophosphatemia increases the production of vitamin D. Whereas, the hyperphosphatemia decreases the synthesis of vitamin D. In chronic kidney disease, the low active vitamin D (di-hydroxy-cholecalciferol) level in plasma leads to hypocalcemia and secondary hyperparathyroidism.

In plasma, P^{3+} exists in both inorganic and organic form. Of this inorganic form, 20% phosphorus remains as protein-bound nonfilterable form and 80% remains as nonprotein-bound filterable (through kidney) form. The majority of this inorganic phosphorus remains in the form of $H_2PO_4^{1-}$ and HPO_4^{2-} in the ratio of 1:4. On the other hand, organic phosphorus remains in the form of phospholipids. The plasma P^{3+} concentration is usually measured, during fasting condition. Because, recent carbohydrate intake transiently decreases plasma P^{3+} level.

■ HYPERPHOSPHATEMIA

The common causes of hyperphosphatemia are: (i) increased P^{3+} intake through food and drugs, and (ii) decreased P^{3+} excretion through kidney. The examples of excessive phosphorus intake are: excessive use of phosphate containing laxatives and excess administration of potassium phosphate administration. The example of decrease phosphorus excretion is chronic renal disease. Directly, hyperphosphatemia usually does not produce any significant functional disturbances of cell and its manifestations. But, indirectly it (hyperphosphatemia) produces hypocalcemia and its manifestations by chelating plasma Ca^{2+}. It also indirectly produces kidney injury by parenchymal and tubular deposition of Ca^{2+}-phosphate salts.

This hyperphosphatemia is usually managed by: (i) dietary restriction, (ii) use of phosphate binders, such as aluminum hydroxide or aluminum carbonate, (iii) dialysis, and (iv) combination of these methods. During anesthesia, usually the hyperphosphatemia has no direct interaction with it (anesthesia). But, kidney function should be assessed and hypocalcemia should be excluded.

■ HYPOPHOSPHATEMIA

The common causes of hypophosphatemia are: (i) decreased intake, (ii) increased excretion, and (iii) shifting of P^{3+} from extracellular compartment to intracellular compartment. This intercompartmental shifting of P^{3+} usually occurs during alkalosis, following carbohydrate ingestion, and insulin administration. The examples of decreased intake of phosphorus are: use of large doses of aluminum and magnesium containing antacids and insufficient P^{3+} supplementation during total parenteral nutrition. Among the alkalosis, respiratory alkalosis commonly causes hypophosphatemia. Metabolic alkalosis rarely causes it. On the other hand, metabolic acidosis, such as diabetic ketoacidosis commonly causes hypophosphatemia.

The clinical manifestations of hypophosphatemia vary according to the plasma level of P^{3+}. The mild-to-moderate hypophosphatemia (plasma P^{3+} level is 1.5–2.5 mg/dL) usually remains asymptomatic. In contrast, severe hypophosphatemia (plasma P^{3+} level is <1.0 mg/dL) causes metabolic acidosis, hemolysis, platelet dysfunction, arrhythmia, cardiomyopathy, skeletal myopathy, respiratory failure, etc. and is associated with increased morbidity and mortality in critically ill patients.

The mainstay of the treatment of hypophosphatemia is the supplementation of it by oral or parental route.

But, the supplementation of phosphorus through oral route is preferred. Because, the supplementation of phosphorus through parental route causes: (i) precipitation of Ca^{2+}, resulting in hypocalcemia, and (ii) increased risk for hyperphosphatemia, hypomagnesemia, and hypotension. So, the parenteral replacement of phosphorus is only reserved for severe hypophosphatemia (<0.32 mmol/L). When the oral phosphate replacement is utilized, then vitamin D is required for the better absorption of phosphorus through intestine.

During anesthesia of patients, suffering from hypophosphatemia, the following care should be taken and these are: (i) hyperglycemia and respiratory alkalosis should be avoided to prevent the further decrease of plasma phosphorus level, (ii) neuromuscular function should be monitored, when the NMBs are used, (iii) postoperative mechanical ventilation may be required in some patients suffering from severe hypophosphatemia.

Autonomic Nervous System and its Pharmacology

INTRODUCTION

All the functions of our body are controlled by nervous system. It is divided *anatomically* into peripheral nervous system (consisting of peripheral nerves) and central nervous system (CNS) (consisting of brain and spinal cord) and *physiologically (or functionally)* into somatic and autonomic nervous systems (ANS). The somatic nervous system controls the function of our body's voluntary muscles and helps in carrying different somatic sensations from skin, joint, muscles, and the other structures of our body. On the other hand, the ANS is the part of nervous system which controls the different activities of viscera, blood vessels, glands, and other parts of our body which are not under our direct control.

Almost a century ago, in 1898, this ANS was first actually described by Langley. It was called, at that time, as the visceral, vegetative, or involuntary nervous system. Unlike the somatic nervous system, in periphery, the ANS consists of nerves, ganglia, and plexuses which innervate the heart, lungs, blood vessels, glands, viscera, and smooth muscles in various tissues. Therefore, it is widely distributed throughout the body and regulates their function, except the voluntary muscles and somatic sensation, without a person's conscious control. So, its actions are generally independent of a person's will and below the level of consciousness.

Like the somatic nervous system, the ANS also has both the *central* and *peripheral divisions* and *afferent (sensory)* and *efferent (motor) paths*. But, unlike the somatic nervous system, the control of ANS is mostly bilateral. On the other hand, like the somatic nervous system, it has got both the spinal and cranial outflows. The higher centers, such as hypothalamus, thalamus, corpus striatum, and cerebrum control this ANS. Certain other special higher centers, situated in the medulla, pons, and midbrain are also included in this autonomic system and control it **(Flowchart 1)**.

The activities of somatic and ANS always run in parallel. But, at many important levels of CNS, there are free intercommunications between them (these two nervous systems). However, cerebrum controls both these systems. Although involuntary, yet the ANS is not altogether beyond the

Flowchart 1: Classification of the nervous system.

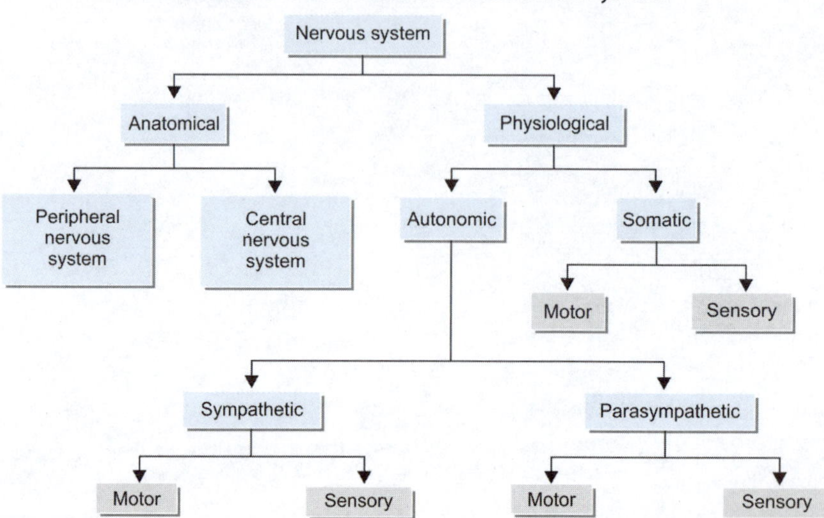

voluntary control. For example, by meditation and yoga, the HR, BP, visceral sensation, etc., which are controlled by the ANS, can be modulated.

All the innervated structures of our body, except some parts of skeletal muscles and cutaneous sensory structures which are innervated by somatic nerves, are supplied by ANS. The single most important difference between the autonomic and somatic nervous system is that the most distal synaptic junction in ANS which occur in ganglia are situated entirely outside the cerebrospinal axis. This is unlike to somatic nervous system, where the most distal synaptic connections lie within the spinal cord, or anywhere within the cerebrospinal axis. These ganglia of ANS, which are situated outside of cerebrospinal axis, are small and complex in structures and contain axon-dendritic synapses between the preganglionic and postganglionic neurons. Whereas the somatic nervous system contains no peripheral ganglia and the most distal synapses between the pre- and postganglionic neurons are located entirely within the cerebrospinal axis.

The autonomic nerves, which are situated outside **(Table 1)** the cerebrospinal axis, form an extensive peripheral plexus on organs, but such network is absent in somatic nervous system. All the nerves of somatic nervous system are myelinated and have no peripheral ganglion. So, there is no question of preganglionic or postganglionic fibers in the somatic nervous system, as it comes directly from the anterior horn cells of spinal cord or from the nuclei of cranial nerves, as postganglionic fibers. On the other hand, the preganglionic fibers of ANS are myelinated, but the postganglionic fibers are nonmyelinated.

TABLE 1: Some differences between autonomic and somatic nervous system.

	Autonomic	Somatic
Organ innervated	All the visceral organs, blood vessels, glands, etc. except skin and skeletal muscles	Skeletal muscles and skin
Nerve fibers	• Preganglionic-myelinated • Postganglionic-nonmyelinated	Myelinated (no pre- or postganglionic fibers)
Distal most synapse	Outside CNS (in ganglia)	Within CNS
Efferent transmitter	Acetylcholine and noradrenaline	Acetylcholine
Peripheral plexus	Present	Absent
Effect of nerve section on organ supplied	Activity maintained and no atrophy of organs	Paralysis and atrophy of skeletal muscle and loss of sensation of skin

A major goal, during the administration of anesthesia on a patient, is to maintain an optimum level of homeostasis or equilibrium between the two divisions of ANS, i.e., sympathetic and parasympathetic, during the maximum surgical stress and strain. This is because the modification and ablation of these stress and strain responses, controlled by ANS, may improve the perioperative outcome.

So, an intelligent administration of anesthetic care to a patient requires a full and comprehensive knowledge of ANS and its pharmacology. In addition, many diseased states, such as diabetes, hypertension, etc., may impair the functions of ANS to a significant extent and may thereby alter the expected responses of a patient to surgery and anesthesia.

Like the somatic nervous system, the ANS is also divided into two parts the centers of ANS in brain and the peripheral autonomic nerves **(Fig. 1)**.

CENTERS OF AUTONOMIC NERVOUS SYSTEMS

Extensive ramifications of ANS normally exist in brain above the level of spinal cord. But, there is no exclusive localized central controlling area for ANS (i.e., center of ANS) in brain. Therefore, considerable intermixing and integration of somatic and ANS occur there (in brain). So, somatic responses are always accompanied by autonomic visceral responses and vice versa. Regarding the highest centers of ANS, the probable theory is that the highest centers in brain, regulating ANS, is situated in hypothalamus. Within it, the posterior and lateral nuclei are primarily *sympathetic*, while the anterior and medial nuclei are primarily *parasympathetic*. Many higher centers of ANS are also located in pons, midbrain, and medulla which are related to the somatic cranial nerves. Therefore, the centers of ANS in the brain and spinal cord consist of the following:

- The area of ANS, controlling the visceral function, is located in cerebral hemisphere. These constitute the limbic system.
- The autonomic centers in brainstem and medulla are located in its reticular formation and is related to its cranial nerves outflow.
- The autonomic centers in spinal cord are located in the intermediolateral column (lateral horns) of gray matter of it. In spinal cord, the intermediolateral group of neurons (lateral horn) are present in the segments of spinal cord, extending from T1 to L2 and S2 to S4 vertebral level, constituting the spinal sympathetic and parasympathetic outflow respectively.

The hypothalamus and nucleus tractus solitarius are generally regarded as the principal loci for the integration of all functions of ANS which include the regulations of

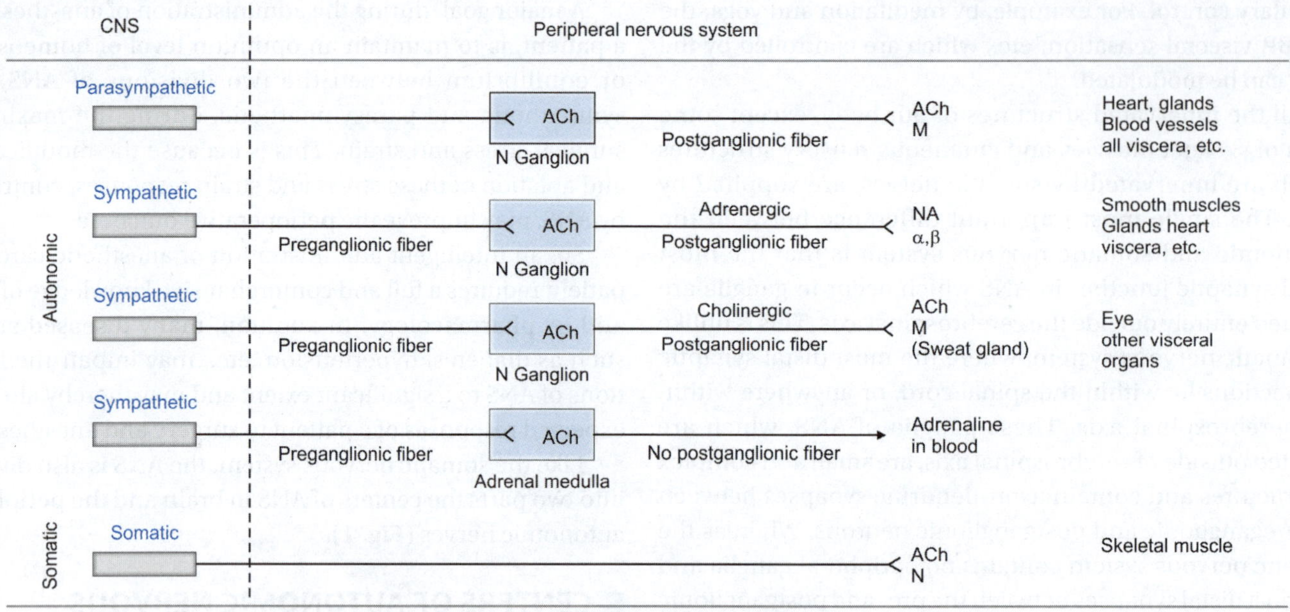

Fig. 1: The general outlay of different part of autonomic and somatic nervous system. (CNS: central nervous system)

body temperature, water balance, metabolism of protein/carbohydrate and fat, regulation of blood pressure, control of emotions, sleep, respiration, control of sexual responses, etc. During the integration of all functions of ANS, signals are received from the different parts of our body through ascending spinobulbar pathways and also from limbic system, neostriatum, cerebral cortex, and other higher brain centers. Then, it reaches to hypothalamus and nucleus tractus solitarius. Subsequently, the stimulation of nucleus tractus solitarius and hypothalamus activates the descending bulbospinal pathways, and stimulates the hormonal output (which are known as the neurotransmitters of sympathetic and parasympathetic system) to mediate autonomic responses.

PERIPHERAL PARTS OF AUTONOMIC NERVOUS SYSTEMS

Like the somatic nerves, the peripheral autonomic nerves also have the afferent (sensory) and efferent (motor) fibers.

Autonomic Afferents (Sensory)

Except some local axonal reflexes, most of the visceral autonomic reflexes are mediated through the afferent autonomic fibers, center of these autonomic nerves in cerebrospinal axis (brain and spinal cord) and efferent autonomic fibers. The afferent autonomic fibers, running from the visceral structures to spinal cord, form the first link of autonomic reflex arc. These autonomic afferent fibers are nonmyelinated and are carried to the cerebrospinal axis by the autonomic visceral nerves, such as vagus, pelvic, splanchnic or other autonomic nerves, through which also the efferent autonomic fibers come out. *For example, most of the fibers (4/5) of vagus nerve are afferent (or sensory) and rest (1/4) of it are efferent (or motor). Many autonomic afferent fibers such as from blood vessels, skeletal muscles, and certain other integumental structures are also carried through their respective somatic spinal nerves, instead of any separate autonomic visceral nerves.*

As most of the autonomic visceral nerves carry the nonmyelinated autonomic afferent (sensory) fibers, the cell bodies of these afferent (sensory) fibers are located in the dorsal or posterior root ganglia of spinal nerves in vertebral canal at the spinal level and the sensory autonomic ganglia of cranial nerves, e.g., nodose ganglion of vagus, trigeminal ganglion, etc. within the skull at cranial level. They transmit different afferent impulses from visceral such as pain, pressure, stretching, etc. and are responsible for the cardiovascular, respiratory, and other visceral reflexes. For sympathetic reflexes the dendrites of the neurons of dorsal root ganglion collect impulses from peripheral receptor and then run through the visceral nerve, sympathetic chain, ganglia (without making any synapse) white ramus and spinal nerve to end in the cell body of dorsal root ganglia. After that the axons of these cells body of dorsal ganglion transmit impulses to the lateral horn cells or the dorsal horn cells of spinal cord.

The neurotransmitter responsible for transmission of these afferent autonomic sensory impulses is not properly known. However, the *substance P* (neuroactive peptide) is present in abundance in the afferent autonomic sensory fibers of dorsal root ganglia and the dorsal horn cells of spinal cord, like the somatic sensory fiber. So, this peptide is considered as the leading candidate among the transmitters that passes the visceral nociceptive stimuli from the periphery to the spinal cord or brain through ANS. Other neuroactive peptides which are also responsible for transmission of autonomic sensory impulses are *somatostatin, vasoactive intestinal polypeptide (VIP),* and *cholecystokinin. Enkephalins,* present in the interneuron of dorsal horn cells of spinal cord (within the area termed "substantia gelatinosa"), also have the visceral antinociceptive effects. It inhibits the release of substance P and diminishes the activity of cells that project from the spinal cord to the highest centers of ANS in CNS. The excitatory amino acids, such as *glutamate* and *aspartate* (which act through the NMDA receptor), also play a major role in the transmission of sensory responses (both autonomic and somatic) in spinal cord.

Autonomic Efferents (Motors)

The efferent or motor pathway of ANS is also functionally divided into the sympathetic and parasympathetic systems. Most of the viscera receives both the sympathetic and parasympathetic innervation and functionally they are antagonistic to each other. However, the level of activity of an innervated internal organ, at a given moment, is the algebraic sum of the sympathetic and parasympathetic activity during that period. Despite the conventional concept of antagonism between these two divisions of ANS, their activities on specific structure may also be either (i) discrete and independent or (ii) integrated and interdependent. For example, the effects of sympathetic and parasympathetic stimulation on heart and iris show a pattern of functional antagonism in controlling the HR and pupillary aperture. But, their actions on the male sexual organs are complementary to each other and are integrated to promote the whole sexual function. On the other hand, most of the blood vessels, spleen, sweat glands, and hair follicles receive only the sympathetic innervation, while the ciliary muscles, gastric and pancreatic glands, receive only the parasympathetic innervation.

The neurotransmitter for (i) all the efferent preganglionic autonomic fibers (both sympathetic and parasympathetic), (ii) all the postganglionic efferent parasympathetic fibers, and (iii) only few postganglionic efferent sympathetic fibers is acetylcholine (ACh). So, they are called the *cholinergic fibers.* Whereas the neurotransmitter for the majority of efferent postganglionic sympathetic fibers is norepinephrine (NE). So, they are called the *adrenergic fibers.*

SYMPATHETIC (ADRENERGIC) NERVOUS SYSTEM

Sympathetic nervous system is also called the *adrenergic nervous system.* Because, the term "adrenergic" is referred to the actions of adrenaline (epinephrine), although noradrenaline (norepinephrine) is the primary neurotransmitter, responsible for most of the adrenergic (epinephrine like) activity of sympathetic nervous system. The activation of sympathetic nervous system elicits reaction what is traditionally called the "fight or flight" response. It includes: (i) the redistribution of blood flow from different nonvital structure such as skin, different splanchnic regions, and skeletal muscles to the vital organs, (ii) increased cardiac function, (iii) sweating, (iv) salivation, (v) pupillary dilatation, etc. Under normal circumstances, the sympathetic system is continuously active and the degree of its activity varies from moment to moment and from organ to organ. The adjustments of our body to a constantly changing environment are usually accomplished by this sympathetic part of ANS. Under the circumstances of stress, the lack of sympathetic function becomes evident by the fall of HR, BP, body temperature, etc. and cannot be regulated. The other examples of lack of these effects of sympathetic nervous system are that the concentration of glucose in blood does not rise when it is needed and compensatory responses to hemorrhage, hypoxia, excitement, exercise, etc. are lacking.

The outflow of the efferent part of sympathetic nervous system takes place only from the lateral horns of the thoracolumbar region of spinal cord. It extends from the first thoracic to the second lumbar segment of spinal cord. The cell bodies of this spinal component of central part of sympathetic nervous system lie in the lateral horns of the gray matter of spinal cord (the intermediolateral columns).

The nerve fibers arising from these cell bodies of lateral horns of spinal cord extend peripherally to three types of ganglia.
1. Paravertebral → ganglia → grouped → as paired sympathetic chain
2. Collateral or prevertebral unpaired ganglia
3. Terminal ganglia near the target organs **(Table 2)**.

The efferent (motor) sympathetic nerve fibers first pass out as axons from the lateral horn cells of spinal cord and then run through the anterior root of spinal nerves. These preganglionic efferent sympathetic fibers are thinly *medulated* and are of β type. So, they are looked white. Then, they leave the spinal nerve in the form of a branch, called the *white ramus communicans,* and enter the ganglion of sympathetic chain. Now, they may end in the corresponding ganglion to create postganglionic fiber or may simply run upward or downward through the sympathetic chain to other ganglia, situated above or below in the same sympathetic chain and

TABLE 2: Some differences between the parasympathetic and sympathetic nervous system.

Origin	Cranio-sacral outflow (III, VII, IX, and X cranial nerves and S2–S4 spinal segment)	Dorso- or thoracolumbar outflow (T1 to L2/L3 spinal segment)
Ganglia	Situated on or close to the organs supplied	Situated away from the organs supplied
Pre : Postganglionic fiber ratio	1:2–1:3 (except in enteric plexus)	1:10–1:100
Postganglionic fiber	Short	Long
Neurotransmitter at target level	Acetylcholine (ACh)	Noradrenaline (most), ACh (sweat gland, pilomotor, and adrenal medulla)
Stability of neurotransmitter	ACh is rapidly destroyed and has very local action	NA is stable, diffuses, and has actions over wider area
Important function	Conservation of energy (anabolic)	In stress and emergency (catabolic)

there they make synapses and produce the postganglionic fibers. The efferent postganglionic sympathetic fibers which arise from the ganglion of sympathetic chain are *nonmedulated.* Hence, they are looked gray. Now, they run back from the ganglion to join again with the spinal nerve in the form of another branch, called the *gray ramus communicans* and then are ultimately distributed along all the spinal nerves, throughout the whole body such as to the pilomotor, sudomotor (sweat gland), blood vessels, skin and to the other organs of extremities which are not controlled by somatic nervous system. It is to be noted that all the spinal nerves, extending from first the cervical to coccygeal nerves, receive gray rami communicantes which carry the postganglionic sympathetic fibers and arise from all the ganglia of sympathetic chain and supply the whole body except viscera. But, only the thoracic and upper two lumbar spinal nerves have the white rami communicantes, which carry the preganglionic fibers to sympathetic chain, arising from the first thoracic to second lumbar spinal segments.

Some preganglionic sympathetic fibers arise directly from the paravertebral ganglia of sympathetic chain, without making any synapses there and run to the *prevertebral or collateral ganglion.* From these collateral ganglia postganglionic sympathetic fibers arise and innervate the visceral structures of thorax, abdomen, and pelvis. The prevertebral or collateral ganglion supplying the thoracic, abdominal, and pelvic viscera contain cell bodies from where the postganglionic fibers arise. They receive preganglionic fibers from the lateral horn cells of T5–T12 thoracic segments of spinal cord, directly through the sympathetic chain, without making synapses there. Many of the upper thoracic sympathetic fibers arising from the paravertebral ganglia of sympathetic chain form terminal plexuses, such as the cardiac, esophageal, and pulmonary plexuses and supply these organs. The sympathetic distribution to head and neck is through the cervical sympathetic chain and its three ganglia. All the postganglionic sympathetic fibers, supplying

head and neck, from this cervical chain arise from the cell bodies located in these three cervical ganglia. But, all the preganglionic sympathetic fibers supplying head and neck arise from the lateral horn cells of the upper thoracic segments of spinal cord, as there are no sympathetic fibers that leave the CNS above the first thoracic level.

Sympathetic Ganglia

There are three types of sympathetic ganglia.
1. Paravertebral ganglia forming the sympathetic chain
2. Unpaired prevertebral or collateral ganglia
3. Terminal ganglia.

Paravertebral Ganglia

They are about 24 pairs in numbers (3 cervical, 12 thoracic, 4 lumbar, 4 sacral, and 1 coccygeal) lying on both the sides of vertebral bodies and are connected with one another by the nerve fibers in the form of a chain which is called the paravertebral sympathetic chain. It extends from the base of the skull to the front of the coccyx. These ganglia are also connected to the spinal nerves by white and gray rami communicantes. The white rami are only restricted to the segments of thoracolumbar outflow (connected to the first thoracic spinal nerve to the second lumbar spinal nerves), because they carry only the preganglionic myelinated sympathetic fibers that exit from spinal cord through the anterior spinal roots, arising from lateral horn cells. The gray rami arise from all the ganglia and carry the postganglionic fibers back to the corresponding spinal nerves for distribution to sweat glands, pilomotor muscles, blood vessels, joints, skeletal muscles of trunk and limbs, and the skin of whole body. Therefore, as a rule, there should be one ganglion for each spinal nerve or vertebral segment of spinal cord. But, they show a tendency to coalesce at cervical, sacral, and coccygeal region. For instance, the eight cervical ganglia in neck are fused to form three ganglia, such as the superior, middle, and inferior cervical ganglia on each side.

In the thoracic region, there are 12 ganglia on each side. The first thoracic ganglion in man sometimes fuses with inferior cervical ganglion, forming the stellate ganglion. In lumbar region, there are usually four and in sacral region there are about four to five ganglia on each side. In coccygeal region, the terminal portions of two sympathetic chains fuse together and form a single ganglion in front of coccyx which is called the coccygeal ganglion.

Unpaired Prevertebral or Collateral Ganglia

They lie in thorax, abdomen, and pelvis in close relation to aorta and its big branches, and supply the postganglionic sympathetic fibers to different viscera. These are *celiac, superior mesenteric, aorticorenal,* and *inferior mesenteric ganglion.* The preganglionic sympathetic fibers to celiac ganglion are supplied by the lateral horn cells of T5–T12 spinal segments. The celiac ganglion innervates the liver, spleen, kidney, pancreas, small bowel, and the proximal colon. The preganglionic sympathetic (**Fig. 2**) fibers after arising from the lateral horn cells of T5–T12 spinal segments bypass the chain of paravertebral sympathetic ganglion, without making synapses there and form the greater splanchnic nerve (containing only the preganglionic fibers). It ends in the celiac ganglion and makes synapses there.

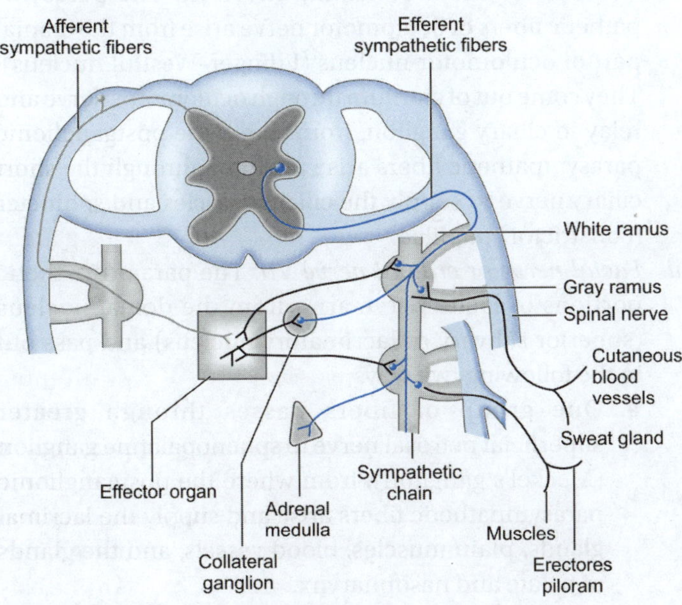

Fig. 2: The principles of peripheral distribution of motor and sensory components of sympathetic nervous system. Blue lines are preganglionic sympathetic fibers, coming out of lateral horn cells, through the anterior root of spinal nerve. Black lines are postganglionic sympathetic fibers, coming out of sympathetic ganglion. Grey lines are sensory sympathetic fibers, running through the posterior root of spinal nerve, with cell body at posterior root ganglion.

Then, the postganglionic fibers from the celiac ganglion innervate all the above-mentioned viscera, forming plexuses over them. Some preganglionic fibers of splanchnic nerves even do not synapse in celiac ganglion and innervate the adrenal medulla directly.

The preganglionic fibers, arising from the lateral horn cells of T10–T11 segment of spinal cord, may bypass the chain of paravertebral sympathetic ganglion and form the lesser splanchnic nerve. It ends in the aorticorenal ganglion which is considered as the lowest detached part of celiac ganglion. The least splanchnic nerve arises from the lateral horn cells of 12th thoracic segment of spinal cord and joins the renal plexus. Then, it ends in a small ganglion from where the postganglionic sympathetic fibers arise and supply the kidney and ureter. The superior mesenteric ganglion innervates the distal colon and the inferior mesenteric ganglia innervate the rectum, urinary bladder, and genitalia.

Terminal Ganglia

They (the terminal ganglia) are situated in close relation to target organs which are supplied by them (these terminal ganglia). They are few in number and include the ganglia, connected with urinary bladder, rectum, and some ganglia in the region of neck. The adrenal medulla and other chromaffin tissues are homologous to sympathetic ganglia. This is because all of them are derived embryologically from neural crest cells, present in spinal cord. But, the adrenal medulla differs from sympathetic ganglia in that the principal catecholamine that is released from adrenal medulla is epinephrine (adrenaline). Whereas, norepinephrine or noradrenaline is the principal catecholamine of other sympathetic ganglia and is also principally released from the postganglionic sympathetic nerve endings.

The characteristics of sympathetic outflow or efferents (motors) are:

- As the sympathetic ganglia are close to CNS, so the preganglionic fibers are short and postganglionic fibers are long.
- The distributions of sympathetic efferent fibers are diffuse in character and their responses are not confined to the organs supplied by spinal segments from which they originate. Thus, this allows a more dramatic and widespread response with diffuse discharge from sympathetic system.
- Sympathetic fibers pass through multiple ganglia, before they finally synapse with postganglionic neurons or fibers.
- Sympathetic system has a system of amplification. This is because a preganglionic terminal fibers synapse with >20 postganglionic cells in one ganglion and thus a large

number of postganglionic neurons arise from a single preganglionic neuron. In addition, synaptic innervation overlaps with each other, so that one ganglion cell may be supplied by several preganglionic fibers. In contrast, the parasympathetic system has its ganglia very near to or within the organs which are innervated by them. Thus, the parasympathetic distribution is much more localized, limited, and circumscribed in its influences. In most organs, the relationship or ratio between the number of preganglionic and postganglionic parasympathetic fibers is 1:2 (i.e., there is localization and least amplification) with exception that the ratio of preganglionic vagal fibers to its postganglionic cells in Auerbach's plexus has been estimated to be about 1:8,000.

The cell bodies of somatic motor neurons lie in the ventral horn cells of gray matter of spinal cord. The axon from this cell body of somatic motor neuron passes through the ventral root of spinal nerve. It, then, passes through the somatic spinal nerves and reaches the muscles where it divides into many terminal branches and each of which innervates a single muscle fiber. Thus, >100 muscle fibers of a muscle may be supplied by one motor neuron (cell body of which is present at anterior horn) to form a motor unit. At each neuromuscular junction, the axonal terminal of each nerve fiber loses its myelin sheath and lies opposite to a specialized surface area on muscle cell membrane, called the "motor endplate". Mitochondria and synaptic vesicles, containing neurotransmitters, are concentrated at this nerve terminal near the endplate. Through the trophic influences of nerve, the nuclei of a skeletal muscle cell, lying in close proximity to synapse, acquire the capacity to activate its specific genes which synthesize the synapse-localized specific proteins or receptor. Thus, nicotinic receptors are synthesized at the motor endplate of muscle cell membrane.

■ PARASYMPATHETIC NERVOUS SYSTEM

The elimination of parasympathetic nervous system is not incompatible with life. This is because it is responsible only for localized and discrete functions which are not essential for life. Like the sympathetic nervous system, this system is not concerned with stress and emergency conditions. It mainly governs those activities of our body which are more associated with digestive and genitourinary functions. The function of parasympathetic nervous system is concerned primarily with the conservation of energy and maintenance of organ functions, during the periods of minimal activity. This system (i) reduces the HR and BP, (ii) stimulates the GI movement and secretion, (iii) helps in the absorption of nutrients, (iv) protects retina from excessive light, and (v) empties the urinary bladder, and rectum, etc. Still, however, many parasympathetic responses are protective in nature.

Parasympathetic outflow or efferent (motor) takes place through the cranial (midbrain and medulla) and sacral nerves only. The cell bodies for the cranial outflow of parasympathetic nervous system lie in the nuclei of cranial nerves, such as III (midbrain), VII, IX, and X (medulla) cranial nerves. Whereas, the cell bodies for the sacral outflow of parasympathetic system lie in the lateral horn cells of sacral segment of spinal cord. Like sympathetic system, the presence of peripheral ganglion is also a characteristic feature of parasympathetic system. But, unlike the sympathetic system, the ganglia of parasympathetic system lie in or near the viscera, except (i) Meckel's ganglion which is situated at a distance from supplying viscera and (ii) Otic ganglion. Hence, the parasympathetic nervous system exerts a more localized action than the sympathetic nervous system.

Parasympathetic Outflow or Efferent (motor)

Cranial Outflow

The cranial outflow of parasympathetic nervous system takes place through four cranial nerves: (i) Oculomotor (III), (ii) facial (VII), (iii) glossopharyngeal (IX), and (iv) vagus (X) nerves.

i. *Oculomotor nerve or cranial nerve III:* The parasympathetic fibers of oculomotor nerve arise from the cranial part of oculomotor nucleus (Edinger–Westful nucleus). They come out of cranium through oculomotor nerve and relay in ciliary ganglion, from where the postganglionic parasympathetic fibers arise and pass through the short ciliary nerve to supply the ciliary muscles and sphincter (constrictor) pupillae.

ii. *Facial nerve or cranial nerve VII:* The parasympathetic portions of facial nerve arise from the dorsal nucleus (superior salivary or lacrimatory nucleus) and pass out in the following two ways:

   a. One group of fibers passes through greater superficial petrosal nerve to sphenopalatine ganglion (Meckel's ganglion), from where the postganglionic parasympathetic fibers arise and supply the lacrimal glands, plain muscles, blood vessels, and the glands of palate and nasopharynx.

   b. Another group of fibers passes out through chorda tympani nerve to join with lingual nerve. Then, at the floor of mouth, these fibers separate from the lingual nerve to end in ganglia, such as sublingual and submaxillary ganglion, close to the sublingual and submaxillary glands. The postganglionic parasympathetic fibers arise from these ganglia and supply the secretory and vasodilator fibers to these glands. Afferent taste fibers from the anterior two-thirds of tongue also end in this dorsal nucleus forming a reflex arc for salivation. Hence, its name is *superior salivary nucleus.*

iii. *Glossopharyngeal nerve or cranial nerve IX:* Preganglionic parasympathetic portion of this nerve arises from the dorsal nucleus (inferior salivary nucleus). Then, it passes along the tympanic and lesser superficial petrosal nerve to otic ganglion. Here, the postganglionic parasympathetic fibers arise which pass along the auriculotemporal nerve and supply the secretory and vasodilator fibers to parotid gland. Taste fibers from the posterior one-third of tongue end in this nucleus and form a reflex arc for salivation. Hence, the name of this nucleus is *inferior salivary nucleus.*

iv. *Vagus nerve or cranial nerve X:* The vagus is the most important parasympathetic nerve in our body. It is widely distributed and carries parasympathetic fibers practically to every corner of our body. The preganglionic fibers of vagus arise from dorsal nucleus, situated in medulla, and run through this nerve. Then, the fibers supplying individual organs pass out of vagus trunk separately to end at ganglia which are situated in or near those viscera, from where the postganglionic parasympathetic fibers arise and supply that viscera, as mentioned below. The vagus nerve, in addition, also carries a far greater number of parasympathetic afferent fibers (but apparently no pain fibers) from viscera to the medulla. The cell bodies of these fibers lie in the nodose ganglion.

- *Heart:* The preganglionic efferent parasympathetic fibers of vagus reach the heart near SA and AV node. Postganglionic parasympathetic fibers arise from the ganglionic cells near SA and AV nodes, and supply inhibitory fibers to the junctional tissues, cardiac muscles, and the dilator fibers of coronary vessels.
- *Lungs:* Vagus supplies the constrictor fibers to bronchial muscles.
- *GI tract:* Vagus supplies the GI tract from the esophagus to cecum. Preganglionic parasympathetic vagal fibers reach the tract at Auerbach and Meissner's plexuses. Postganglionic parasympathetic fibers arise from this Auerbach's plexus and Meissner's plexus. Fibers from the former plexus supply the muscle coats to stimulate intestinal movements and to inhibit sphincters. Fibers from the latter plexus supply the vasodilator and secretomotor fibers to the glands and mucosa.
- *Pancreas:* Parasympathetic vagus fibers supply the secretory fibers to the pancreatic alveoli, as well as to the Islets of Langerhans.

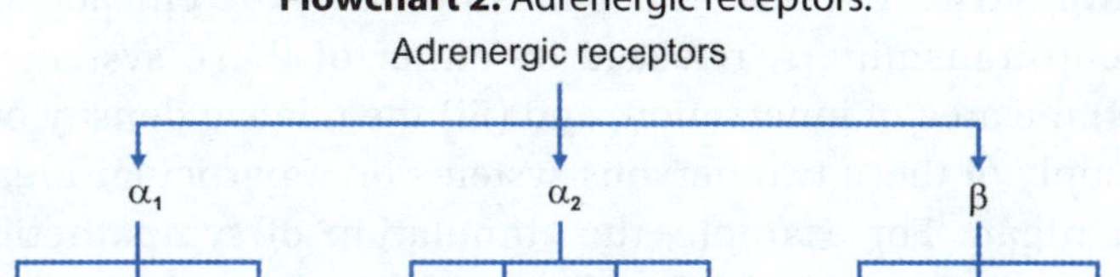
Flowchart 2: Adrenergic receptors.

- *Gallbladder:* Action of vagus on gallbladder is reverse to that of sympathetic fibers.
- *Liver and kidney:* Parasympathetic vagus has no appreciable effect on liver and kidney.

Sacral Outflow

The sacral outflow of the parasympathetic nervous system consists of axons that arise from the lateral horn cells of 2nd, 3rd, and 4th sacral segments of spinal cord. After that, it proceeds as preganglionic fibers through their corresponding anterior roots and the trunk of spinal nerves. Then, they come out of spinal nerves and unite to form a single nerve, on each side, called the *nervi-erigentes (preganglionic).* After that they relay in hypogastric ganglia (parasympathetic terminal ganglia) from where the postganglionic parasympathetic fibers arise to supply the urinary bladder, prostate and whole of large intestine, except cecum, lower part of rectum and anal canal. The actions of the nerves of sacral outflow are:

- Movement of GI tract is stimulated and sphincters are inhibited or relaxed (reverse of sympathetic).
- Supplies dilator fibers to the blood vessels of external genitalia. This vasodilation is an important factor for causing erection of penis (hence the name is "nervi erigentes").

Spinal Parasympathetic

Posterior spinal nerve roots contain certain parasympathetic fibers, which on stimulation produce vasodilatation. These fibers are said to be parasympathetic due to their action. But, unlike that of other vasodilator parasympathetic fibers, their actions are not abolished by atropine. These fibers are known as antidromic vasodilator fibers, as their impulses pass out against the general afferent impulses of posterior nerve roots and extend up to the posterior root ganglion. Local stimulation by irritants, applied to skin, produces vasodilatation through these fibers. This is known as the axon reflex. The vasodilatation is produced due to the liberation of ACh from these nerve endings **(Flowchart 2)**.

■ CONCLUSION

Though the actions of sympathetic and parasympathetic nervous system are antagonistic in nature, but it is not always true. Because, it depends upon: (i) the efficacy of neurotransmitters, released by either of these systems, (ii) the area of innervation, and (iii) the relative density of supply of these two nervous systems on a particular area or organ. For example, the stimulation of sympathetic nervous system markedly enhances the peripheral vascular resistance, but it is not altered appreciably by the activity of parasympathetic system. The explanation is like that generally most of the vessels, involved in the control of blood pressure, are innervated only by sympathetic fibers and these fibers are continuously active. Whereas the parasympathetic fibers which serve the blood vessels are normally restricted to a small area of our body and vasodilatation in these areas does not contribute appreciably to fall of systemic blood pressure. So, to decrease blood pressure, it is more significant to paralyze (block) the continuous sympathetic activity, rather than to stimulate parasympathetic activity **(Box 1)**.

The motor or efferent fibers of ANS is again traditionally classified into *cholinergic* and *adrenergic* nervous systems on the basis of chemical neurotransmitters through which they work. The postganglionic efferent autonomic nerve fibers, accepting ACh as their neurotransmitter at their effective site, is called the *cholinergic nerves* and the postganglionic efferent autonomic nerve fibers, accepting norepinephrine (NE) and epinephrine (EPI) as their neurotransmitter at their effective site, is called the *adrenergic nerves*.

The receptors through which ACh neurotransmitter acts are called *cholinergic receptors*. The cholinergic receptors are protein in nature and are situated on the cell membrane of effector cells. They react with ACh or any other cholinomimetic (like ACh) drugs to cause the cell to respond. Two types of cholinergic receptors are recognized, and these are *muscarinic* and *nicotinic*. The muscarinic receptors are the *G-protein-coupled receptor* in nature (discussed here) and the nicotinic receptors are the *ligand-gated cation channel*

molecules. (Ligand is an organic molecule that donates the necessary electrons to form the coordinate covalent bonds with metallic ions. Also, the ligand is an ion or molecule that reacts with another molecule to form a complex).

The *cholinergic agonists* are agents or drugs that act on cholinergic receptors like ACh. These drugs are also called the cholinomimetic drugs. The *cholinergic antagonists* are the agents or drugs that bind with cholinergic receptors and block the access of ACh or other cholinergic agonist to ACh-receptors and prevent their actions. These drugs are also called the *anticholinergic or cholinergic blocking or cholinolytic drugs.*

The receptors through which NE and EPI neurotransmitter act are called the *adrenergic receptors*. The adrenergic receptors are also protein in nature and situated on the cell membrane of effector cells. They react with NE, EPI, and other adrenergic agonists and cause the cell to respond. Adrenergic receptors have been classified into α- *and* β-*adrenergic receptors* which are further subclassified into α_1, α_2 and β_1, β_2 *and* β_3 *receptors*. Among all these, the α_2-receptors are primarily located on the presynaptic membrane and are inhibitory in nature. On the other hand, the α_1 and β_2-receptors are primarily located on the surface of smooth muscle cells of different organs. The β_1-receptor is primarily located on myocardial (cardiac muscle) tissues. The drugs, mimicking the action of NE, are called the *adrenergic or sympathomimetic drugs* and the drugs inhibiting the effects of NE are called the *antiadrenergic, adrenergic blocking, or sympatholytic drugs.*

Due to the advent of molecular biology, the α_1 receptor is again subclassified into α_1A, α_1B, α_1D, and the α_2 receptor is again subdivided into α_2A, α_2B, and α_2C receptor. But, such subclassification is only for scientific analysis and research. The adrenergic drugs, currently available for clinical use, are still classified as the traditional pattern, such as the α_1, α_2 and β_1, β_2 agonists or antagonists (blockers).

■ RECEPTORS

The autonomic receptors are macromolecules and protein in nature. A large number of these autonomic receptor proteins have been identified, cloned, studied, and their primary sequence of amino acids (AA) have also been worked out. Each of these autonomic receptors has two parts: (1) intramembranous and (2) extramembranous and each receptor is made up of several units which are not identical. Each such unit again has a polar and no-polar portion. The nonpolar portion of each unit [the amino acid (AA) sequence of receptor protein] is buried in the cell membrane and the polar portion of each unit tends to come out in aqueous medium on both sides of the cell membrane. The small

---

BOX 1: Cholinergic and adrenergic nerves.

The cholinergic nerves include:
- All the motor nerves that innervate the skeletal muscles.
- All the postganglionic parasympathetic neurons (fibers). So parasympathetic system is also called the cholinergic system
- All the preganglionic parasympathetic and sympathetic neurons (all the preganglionic autonomic fibers)
- Some postganglionic sympathetic neurons (fibers) supplying the sweat glands and certain blood vessels
- Preganglionic sympathetic neurons that arise from greater splanchnic nerve and directly innervate the adrenal medulla
- Some central cholinergic neurons

The adrenergic nerves include:
- Postganglionic sympathetic neurons
- Some interneurons
- Certain central neurons

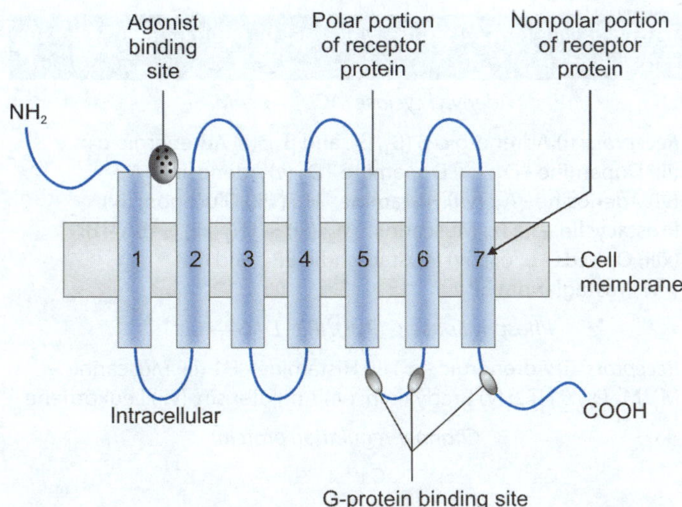

Fig. 3: G-protein-coupled type of receptor which is coupled with G-protein. Each receptor consists of 7 units and each unit represents a membrane spanning chain of amino acids. These units are connected by 3 loops on each side of the membrane. The amino terminus of the receptor lies on the extracellular surface. The carboxy terminus lies on the cytoplasmic side. The approximate location of the agonist or antagonist and the G-protein-binding sites on the receptor are shown in the diagram.

TABLE 3: Several types of G-proteins have been described. They are distinguished by their α-subunits. The important G-proteins and the chemical (second messenger) through which they activate the cells are tabled below. The other G-proteins which are not tabled above are Gn, Gk, G_{13}, Gt, etc.

G-protein	Effector system or second messenger
Gs	Adenylyl cyclase ↑, Ca^{2+} channel ↑
Gi	Adenylyl cyclase ↓, K^+ channel ↑
Go	Ca^{2+} channel ↓
Gq	Phospholipase C ↑

TABLE 4: Some receptors coupled with or act through G-proteins

Receptor	G-protein
β-adrenergic	Gs, Gi, Go, Gn, and Gq
Muscarinic	Gi, Gs, and Gk
α₂-adrenergic	Gi, Gs, Gn, and Go
GABA–B	Gi, Go, and Gk
Dopamine D₂	Gi, Go, and G13
5–HT	Gi, Gq, Gs, Gk, and Gt

(GABA: gamma-aminobutyric acid)

molecules of agonistic or antagonistic agent (ligands) bind to the outer polar site of any unit of these receptor molecules and are capable of tripping the balance of electrical charges of these receptors by altering the distribution of their units **(Fig. 3)**.

Thus, this tripping of balance of electrical charge brings out the conformational changes at the inner polar site of receptor and initiates the binding of G-proteins with these receptors at their inner polar site. This is the mechanism of action of all G-protein-coupled receptors, such as *all the adrenergic receptors* (α- and β-receptors) *and the cholinergic muscarinic (M) receptors*. On the other hand, the binding of agonists and antagonists (ligands) at the outer polar site of some cholinergic receptors bring about changes in their quaternary structure and the relative alignment of their subunits, resulting in the opening of a centrally located cation channel within these receptors. This is the mechanism of action of some receptors with intrinsic cation channel within them, such as the *cholinergic nicotinic (N) receptors*. Thus, the receptors subserve two essential functions. These are:

1. The recognition and the binding of some specific molecules which are called the ligands (or agonistic and antagonistic agents) at outside on the specific binding domain (site) of receptor and the activation of receptor.
2. The transduction of outside signal into the response of cell through a highly complex multistep process **(Table 3)**.

According to the type of receptor activation and its transduction into functional responses within the cell, the responses can be grouped into five major categories. These are *agonistic, partial agonistic, antagonistic, partial inverse agonistic, and inverse agonistic*. The receptors, falling in one category of function, have also been found to possess considerable structural homology among themselves and may be considered to belong to one family. According to the mechanism of action, all the autonomic receptors are broadly classified into two families: (1) the receptors coupled with or acting through the G-protein and (2) the receptors coupled with or acting through the ion (cation) channel.

Receptors Acting Through (Coupled with) G-proteins (Table 4)

These form a large family of receptors which are situated on cell membrane. It includes adrenergic receptors (α₁, α₂, β₁, and β₂), cholinergic muscarinic receptors (M₁, M₂, and M₃), dopamine (DA) receptors (D₁ and D₂), adenosine receptors (A₁ and A₂), gamma-aminobutyric acid (GABA) receptors, opioid—α, κ, δ receptors, and others. They act through one or more *GTP-activated proteins* for the response of cells. So, they are called the G-protein-coupled receptors. All such receptors which act through the G-protein have a common pattern of structural organization. These receptor molecules have two to seven membrane spanning helical structures which are made up of a specific sequence of amino acids and

Flowchart 3: Inside the cell.

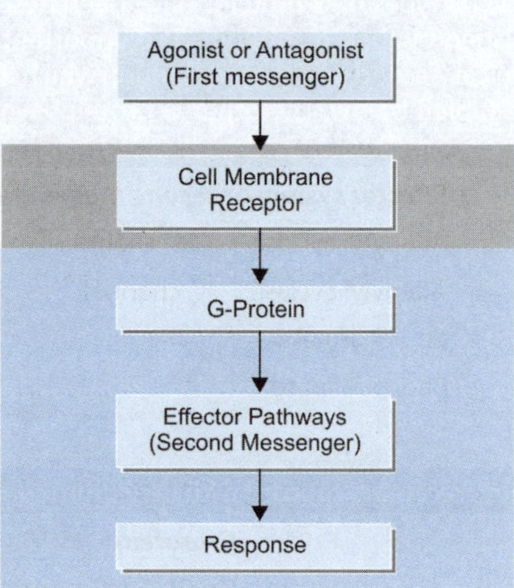

TABLE 5: Different receptors which act through different effector substances.

Adenylyl cyclase (AC) $\uparrow \rightarrow$ *cAMP* $\uparrow$
Receptors: (i) Adrenergic-β (β_1, β_2, and β_3); (ii) Adrenergic-α_2; (iii) Dopamine - D_1; (iv) Dopamine - D_2 (v) Adenosine- A_1; (vi) Adenosine - A_2; (vii) Histamine - H_2; (viii) Glucagon; (ix) Prostacyclin – IP; (x) Muscarinic- M_2; (xi) 5- HT; (xii) GABA – B; (xiii) Opioids - μ, δ; (xiv) Prostaglandin EP_3; and (xv) Prostaglandin EP_2
Phospholipase-C (PLC): IP3 - DAG $\rightarrow$ Ca^{2+} $\uparrow$
Receptors: (i) Adrenergic - α_1; (ii) Histamine - H1 (iii) Muscarinic - M_1, M_3 (iv) 5 HT2; (v) Bradykinin; (vi) Angiotensin; (vii) Leukotriene

Channel-regulation protein			
	$Ca^{2+} \uparrow$	$Ca^{2+} \downarrow$	$K^+ \downarrow$
Receptors	Adrenergic -β_1	Dopamine -D_2 GABA - B Opioid -κ Adenosine - A_1	Adrenergic - α_2 Dopamine - D_2 GABA - B Muscarinic - M_2 Adenosine - A_1

(GABA: gamma-aminobutyric acid)

connected with each other by three extracellular and three intracellular loops. The final amino terminal (–NH2) of the amino acid chain lies on extracellular surface and the final carboxy terminus (–COOH) of the amino acid chain lies on the cytoplasmic site of the receptor. The agonist binding site of the receptor is located somewhere between the helices on its external surface. Whereas, the G-protein binding site of receptor is located at the cytosolic segments of the receptor **(Flowchart 3)**.

The G protein which binds with the intracellular portion of receptor is composed of α, β, and γ subunits. A number of G-proteins, distinguished by their α-subunits, also have been described. These are Gs, Gi, Ge, Gq, etc. Different receptors act through different G-proteins and different G-proteins again next act through different effectors substances (second messenger) or pathways. These effector substances or pathways are called the *second messengers* (first messengers are agonist and antagonists or ligands) and they produce, according to their nature, either stimulatory or inhibitory responses in effector cells. The effector pathways or second messengers through which the G-proteins act are *adenylyl cyclase (AC), phospholipase-C (PLC),* and *channel regulation proteins*. These intracellular channel regulation proteins should not be confused with the nicotinic type of ACh receptors and Na^+ channel protein, which are actually the receptor with their intrinsic ion channel (discussed later) and present at motor endplates or other sites. These channel regulation proteins, through which G-proteins act, have no channel within them, like ACh receptor or Na^+-channel protein. They only regulate different channels, present on the cell membrane.

Effector Substances (Second Messenger)

Adenylyl cyclase: When an agonist binds with a receptor at its extracellular portion, outside of cell membrane, then the receptor makes a coupling with the G-protein at the inside of cell membrane and activates it (G-protein). Subsequently, the activated G-protein causes the activation of AC (effector pathway or second messenger) → it results in the intracellular accumulation of cAMP → causes the phosphorylation or the activation of protein kinase-A (PKA) → causes the alteration of the functions of many enzymes, ion channels, or carrier proteins within the cells. Ultimately, this is manifested as many cellular functions such as the increased contractility, impulse generation, relaxation of smooth muscles, glycogenolysis, lipolysis, hormone synthesis, etc. For example, when the epinephrine acts on β-receptor, situated on the cell membrane of cardiac muscle, then it activates the Gs protein within the cell which in turn stimulates the AC, a type of effector pathway or second messenger. The reverse occurs, when the AC is inhibited by the inhibitory Gi protein (Gi is inhibitory and Gs is stimulatory G-protein), which is activated by the receptor when an antagonist acts on the same β-receptor and stimulates it (β-receptor). As for example, the action of ACh on muscarinic M_2 receptor (located in the myocardial cell membrane) activates an inhibitory G-protein (Gi) inside the cell. Subsequently, the activated inhibitory G-protein (Gi) opposes the activation of AC and inhibits the accumulation of cAMP. Thus, ACh produces inhibitory responses in myocardial cells. The receptors which act through G-protein (Gs or Gi) and AC pathways are adrenergic β ($\uparrow$), adrenergic α_2 ($\downarrow$), muscarinic M_2 ($\downarrow$), dopamine D_1 ($\uparrow$), dopamine D_2 ($\uparrow$), adenosine A_2 ($\uparrow$), adenosine A_1 ($\uparrow$), etc. **(Table 5)**.

Phospholipase-C (PLC): The coupling of receptor with stimulatory G-protein (Gs) at the inner side of cell membrane, after the binding of agonist with the receptor at the outer side of cell membrane, causes the activation of an another-effector pathway (second messenger) which is called the phospholipase-C (PLC). This causes the hydrolysis of phosphatidyl inositol 4, 5-bisphosphate (P1P2, a membrane phospholipid) → causes the generation of inositol triphosphate (IP3) and diacylglycerol (DAG) → results in the mobilization of Ca^{2+} from the intracellular depots by IP3 and DAG → activates protein kinase-C (PKC) → $\uparrow Ca^{2+}$ and activated PKC mediates all the cellular functions, i.e., contraction, secretion, transmitter release, neuronal excitability, etc. Like AC, the PLC can also be inhibited by inhibitory G-protein (Gi) when the opposite responses would be expected. Receptors which act through the G-protein (Gs or Gi) and phospholipase-C pathways are adrenergic α_1 and muscarinic M_1, M_3 receptors **(Fig. 4)**.

Channel regulation proteins: The coupling of receptors with G-proteins on the inner side of cell membrane, due to the binding of agonists (ligands) with receptors on the outside of cell membrane, causes the activation of multiple intracellular channel regulation proteins which subsequently cause the opening or closing of other different ionic channels present on the cell membrane. These ion channels are specific for Ca^{2+}, K^+, Na^+ ions, and are situated on the cell membrane and cause depolarization or hyperpolarization of the cell membrane. The Gs protein opens Na^+ and Ca^{2+} channels on the myocardial and skeletal muscle cell membrane. So, these are stimulatory in nature. On the other hand, Gi and Go open the K^+ channels in the heart and smooth muscles and close the neuronal Ca^{2+} channels. Opening of K^+ channel causes hyperpolarization of cell. So, these are inhibitory in nature. Closing of Ca^{2+} channel is also inhibitory in nature. Physiological responses such as positive or negative inotropic effects, chronotropic effects, transmitter release, smooth muscle relaxation or contraction, etc. also occur through this mechanism (previously mentioned other mechanisms also take part). Examples of these categories of receptors are adrenergic β_1 ($Ca^{2+}\uparrow$), dopamine D_2 ($Ca^{2+}\downarrow$), and adrenergic α_2 ($K^+\uparrow$).

Receptors Acting Through Intrinsic Ion Channels

These receptors, at its intracellular end, do not act through G-protein, and second messenger effector system such as AC, PLC, channel-regulation protein, etc., present within the cell. But, these receptor molecules, present in the cell membrane, are composed of five subunits ($2\alpha + \beta + \gamma + \delta$) and enclose a cylindrical ion channel for the passage of ions such as Na^+, K^+, Ca^{2+}, Cl^-, etc. All the subunits of this type of receptor, with intrinsic ion channel, generally have four membrane spanning amino acid (AA) chains which traverse the full width of cell membrane six times. The subunits of receptor are arranged around the center channel like a rosette and the α-subunit of this receptor usually bears the agonist and antagonist binding sites.

Normally, these receptors, with intrinsic ion channel at its center, remain closed. But, when the agonist molecules bind to the α-subunit of this receptor, then all the other subunits move apart, opening the central channel, and allow the passage of Na^+ ion and other cation through this channel. Anions are prevented from passing through this channel because it is lined with positive charges. Receptors such as nicotinic cholinergic (at motor endplate), GABA-A, glycine, NMDA, 5-HT₃, etc. fall in this category. In these types of receptors, agonists directly operate the ion channels through their binding site, situated within the receptor, without the help of any second messenger or coupling with G-protein. The onset and the offset of responses through this class of receptors are faster than that of the receptors which act through G-proteins.

■ ADRENERGIC RECEPTORS

The chemical structure, classification, subclassification, and the mechanism of action of different types of adrenergic receptors had already been described previously with other receptors. The remaining aspect of individual adrenergic receptors are discussed here.

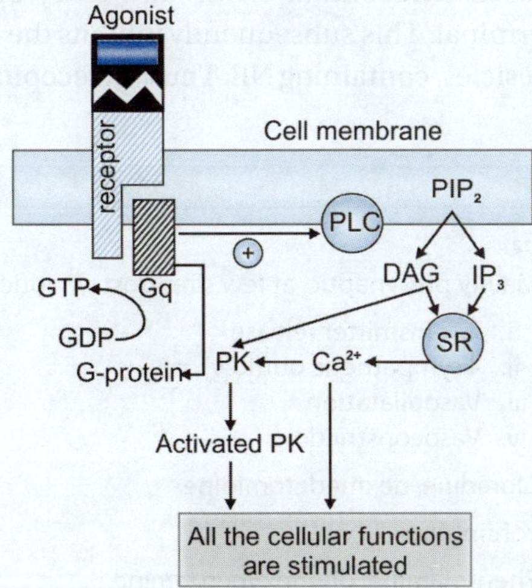

Fig. 4: The phospholipase C effector pathway for cellular response. (DAG: diacylglycerol; GDP: guanosine diphosphate; GTP: guanosine triphosphate; PK: protein kinase; PLC: phospholipase-C; SR: sarcoplasmic reticulum)

α₁ Receptor

These receptors are postsynaptic adrenoreceptors, located on the smooth muscles throughout our body (in blood vessels, eye, lungs, gut, uterus, and genitourinary system). The activation of these adrenergic receptors increases intracellular Ca^{2+} ion concentration (using phospholipase-C →IP-3/DAG as second messenger), leading to the contraction of smooth muscles. Hence, the α_1 agonists are associated with vasoconstriction, mydriasis, bronchoconstriction, gut motility, and the constriction of the sphincters of gut and genitourinary tract. The stimulation of α_1 receptors also inhibits insulin secretion and lipolysis. The location and the responses of α_1 receptors are as follows:

- *Arteriole's smooth muscle:* Coronary arteries → constriction; skin and mucosa → constriction; skeletal muscles → constriction; cerebral vessels → constriction; pulmonary vessels → constriction; abdominal viscera → constriction; renal vessels → constriction.
- *Veins:* Constriction.
- *Heart:* Minimum α_1 receptors → causes positive inotropic effect → may play role in catecholamine-induced arrhythmia.
- *Lung:* Bronchial smooth muscles → no or minimum α_1 receptor → Bronchoconstriction.
- *Bronchial gland* → increased secretion.
- *Eye:* Radial muscle of iris → mydriasis and ↓ aqueous secretion; Lacrimal gland → ↑ secretion.
- *Stomach and intestine:* Motility → Decrease; Sphincter → Contraction.
- *Bladder:* Detrusor muscle → no α receptor, Muscles of trigone → Contraction.
- *Ureter:* Motility → Increase.
- *Uterus:* Pregnant → Contraction.
- *Smooth muscle of prostate and bladder neck:* Contraction and obstruction to urine flow.
- *Male sex organ:* Ejaculation.
- *Spleen capsule:* Contraction.
- *Skin-pilomotor:* Contraction.

- *Sweat gland:* Secretion.
- *Salivary gland:* K^+ and water secretion.
- *Insulin secretion:* Inhibited (α_2 predominant) **(Table 6)**.

Specific agonists of α_1 receptor are methoxamine and phenylephrine and its specific antagonist is prazosin. Prazosin is a selective α_1 antagonist. So, its use in benign prostatic hypertrophy avoids deleterious effects that occur with other less specific α_1-antagonists.

α_2 Receptor

The α_2 receptors are found in CNS, peripheral nervous system, and in variety of other organs which include platelets, liver, pancreas, kidney, and eye, etc. The predominant α_2 receptor which is found at human spinal cord is identified as α_{2A} subtype.

The α_2 receptors can be presynaptic or postsynaptic, but predominantly they present on presynaptic membrane. The presynaptic α_2 receptor may act either as heteroreceptor or autoreceptor (an autoreceptor is a presynaptic receptor that reacts with neurotransmitter which is released from its own presynaptic nerve terminal, providing a feedback regulation. A heteroreceptor is a presynaptic receptor that responds to substances other than the neurotransmitter, released from that specific nerve terminal).

Among many presynaptic receptors that have been identified, the α_2 receptor is of the greatest clinical importance. These presynaptic α_2 receptors regulate the release of NE and ATP through a negative feedback mechanism from its own presynaptic nerve terminal. The stimulation of α_2 receptor on presynaptic membrane, by the released NE from that nerve terminal, inhibits AC activity. This decreases intracellular cAMP and entry of Ca^{2+} into neuronal terminal. This subsequently inhibits the exocytosis of storage vesicles, containing NE. Thus, α_2 receptor creates a

TABLE 6: Differences between α_1 and α_2 receptor.

	α_1		α_2
Location	Mainly postsynaptic, at few sites presynaptic		Mainly presynaptic, at few sites postsynaptic
Function	i. Vascular smooth muscle–contraction ii. Gut smooth muscle–relaxation iii. Gland–secretion iv. Genitourinary–contraction		i. ↓Transmitter release ii. ↓sympathetic outflow iii. Vasodilatation iv. Vasoconstriction
Selective agonists	Methoxamine and phenylephrine		Clonidine, dexmedetomidine
Selective antagonist	Prazosin		Yohimbine
Nonselective antagonist	Phentolamine, phenoxybenzamine		Phentolamine, phenoxybenzamine
Coupling G-protein	G-q		G-i and G-o
Second messenger	↑ IP-3/DAG		↓adenylyl cyclase and ↓cAMP

negative feedback loop and blocks subsequent release of NE from presynaptic neuron. In CNS, stimulation of postsynaptic α_2 receptor causes sedation and reduces sympathetic outflow, leading to peripheral vasodilatation and lowering of BP. Peripherally, stimulation of presynaptic α_2 receptor causes inhibition of release of NE and hypotension. In addition, vascular smooth muscle contains postsynaptic α_2 receptor that produces vasoconstriction. Clonidine is a prototype of α_2 agonist. The action of clonidine in relief of pain and sedation by stimulation of α_2 receptor is discussed in elsewhere. Highly-densed α_2 receptors are found in cortex and medulla. Stimulation of these α_2 receptors at this level is responsible for bradycardia and hypotensive action of α_2 agonist. Presynaptic α_2 receptors and cholinergic receptors inhibit the release of NE, whereas the presynaptic β-receptors stimulate the release of NE.

Location and responses of α_2 receptors at other sites than presynaptic membrane and CNS are:

i. *Coronary artery:*	Constriction
ii. *Artery of skin:*	Constriction
iii. *Renal artery:*	Constriction
iv. *Veins:*	Constriction
v. *Intestine:*	Decreased motility and secretion

β-receptors

Like α-receptors, the β-receptors are also the member of a superfamily G-protein-coupled receptors which act through coupling with G protein. They have seven helices (chains) of amino acids which are passed seven times through cell membrane. These transmembrane domains (helices) are labeled by numbers from M1 to M7. The antagonists have specific binding sites on these receptors, whereas the agonists are more diffusely attached to the hydrophobic site on this receptor. Like other G-protein-coupled receptors, the extracellular portion of these receptors ends as an amino group. A carboxyl group occupies the intracellular terminus of this receptor and it is here where the phosphorylation or activation of receptors occurs. At these cytoplasmic domains, the interaction of receptor with G-proteins occurs. The β-receptors have the structural and functional similarities with the cholinergic muscarinic and adrenergic α-receptors, but not with the cholinergic nicotinic receptors **(Table 7)**.

The β-receptors are subdivided into β_1, β_2, β_3 subreceptors (as already discussed). NE and EPI are equipotent on β_1 receptor. Whereas, EPI is significantly more potent than NE on β_2 receptor. All of them increase the level of intracellular cAMP through the activation of G protein and adenylate cyclase effector pathway (second messenger). Traditionally, the β_1 receptors are thought to be concentrated more on cardiac tissues and initiates a kinase phosphorylation

TABLE 7: Differences among adrenergic β_1, β_2, and β_3 receptor.

	β_1 *receptor*	β_2 *receptor*	β_3 *receptor*
Location	Heart and JG cells of kidney	Blood vessels, bronchi, uterus, liver, intestine, eye, and urinary tract	Adipose tissue, gallbladder, and brain
Selective agonist	Dobutamine	Salbutamol and terbutaline	Mirabegron
Selective antagonist	Metoprolol and atenolol	α-methyl-propranolol	ICI-118551
NE	Strong action	No or very weak action	Strong action
EPI	Strong action	Strong action	Weak action

(EPI: epinephrine; NE: norepinephrine)

cascade. Thus, the β_1 receptors cause positive chronotropic ($\uparrow$HR), positive dromotropic ($\uparrow$conduction) and positive inotropic ($\uparrow$contractility) effects. On the other hand, the β_2 receptors are thought to concentrate on cardiac tissues, vascular smooth muscles, bronchial tissues, glandular tissues, and other smooth muscles of our body, such as the urinary bladder, gut, genital organs, etc. Glycogenolysis, lipolysis, gluconeogenesis, and insulin release are stimulated by β_2 receptor stimulation. But, the interesting finding is that the mechanism of action of both β_1 and β_2 receptor are same (G-protein $\rightarrow$ AC $\rightarrow$ cAMP). The typical model of distribution of β_1 and β_2 receptor is useful for the pharmacological manipulation of them by their specific drugs. But, the role of β_2 receptors is more important during heart failure than normal cardiac function. The β_2 receptor population in ventricles and atria are 15% and 30% of the total β receptors, respectively.

These β_2 receptors play an important role in compensation during cardiac failure and help to maintain the responses to catecholamine stimulation. The β_1 receptors are downregulated during chronic catecholamine stimulation and CHF. But, the β_2-receptor population remains unaffected till the end-stage of congestive cardiac failure. In addition to positive inotropic effects, β_2 receptors in human atria participate in the regulation of heart rate. Thus, β_2 agonism may have a significant effect on cardiac contractility and rate.

Location and Responses of β_1 and β_2 Receptors

- *Heart:* SA node ($\beta_1 > \beta2$) $\rightarrow \uparrow$heart rate; Atria ($\beta_1 > \beta_2$) $\rightarrow \uparrow$contractility, $\uparrow$conduction velocity; AV node ($\beta_1 > \beta_2$) $\rightarrow \uparrow$automaticity, conduction velocity; His-Purkinje system ($\beta_1 > \beta_2$) $\rightarrow \uparrow$automaticity, $\uparrow$conduction velocity;

ventricles ($\beta_1 > \beta_2$) → ↑contractility, ↑conduction velocity, ↑automaticity, ↑ idioventricular pacemaker.

- *Arterioles:* Coronary (β_2) → dilatation; skeletal muscle (β_2) → dilatation; Pulmonary (β_2) → dilatation; abdominal viscera (β_2) → dilatation; Renal (β_1, β_2) → dilatation.
- *Veins* (β_2): Dilatation.
- *Lung, tracheal, and bronchial smooth muscle* (β_2): Relaxation.
- *GI* (β_1, β_2): Decreased motility.
- *Gallbladder* (β_2): Relaxation.
- *Detrusor of bladder* (β_2): Relaxation.
- *Uterus* (β_2): Relaxation.
- *Spleen capsule* (β_2): Relaxation.
- *Skeletal muscle* (β_2): Increased contractility, ↑glycogenolysis, and ↑ lactic acid (lactic acidosis).
- *Liver* (β_2): Glycogenolysis, gluconeogenesis, and ↑ lood glucose.
- *Islets of pancreas* (β_2): ↑ glucagon and ↑ insulin (mild) secretion.
- *Fat cells* (β_2): Inhibition of lipolysis. But, $\beta_1 + \beta_2 + \beta_3 =$ lipolysis and increased FFA.
- *Eye:* No effect on iris, slight relaxation of ciliary muscles, enhanced aqueous secretion.
- *Kidney:* Renin release by β_1.

The β_3 receptors are found on brain, gallbladder, and adipose tissue. Its exact role in gallbladder physiology is not known, but probably it causes relaxation of gallbladder. In adipose tissue, it causes lipolysis and thermogenesis.

Dopamine Receptor

Dopamine is an intermediate product during biosynthesis of norepinephrine (NE) and epinephrine (EPI). It acts through five dopamine receptors. Among them, DA_1 and DA_2 receptors are most prominent. Dopamine also acts on α and β receptors.

DA1 receptors are postsynaptic and are located at renal, mesenteric, and vascular smooth muscles. It mediates vasodilatation response. The DA_2 receptors are presynaptic and inhibits the release of NE. The DA_2 receptors are also located in brain, which mediate nausea and vomiting. The antiemetic action of droperidol and metoclopramide acts through these DA_2 receptors.

■ SUMMARY

After the attachment of adrenergic agonists to adrenergic receptors, the extracellular signal is transformed into an intracellular signal by coupling of a stimulated α_1, α_2, β_1, β_2 adrenergic receptor with intracellular G-proteins. This signal transformation is known as the signal transduction. Each class of adrenergic receptor couples to different type of G protein which in turn is linked to different types of effector pathway or second messengers such as AC, phospholipase-C, etc. Thus, α_1 receptor is linked to Gq protein and in turn is linked to activation of phospholipase-C. In contrast, the α_2 receptor is linked to Gi protein and is responsible for the inhibition of AC. The β-receptor is linked to Gs protein and in turn is linked to stimulation of AC. ACh receptor is linked to Gi protein and in turn is linked to the inhibition of effector system, named adenylyl cyclase.

Mechanism Action of G-Protein

The G protein has three subunits, such as α, β, and γ. The α-subunit of G protein is most variable and determines the type of activity **(Table 8)** of G-proteins. According to

TABLE 8: Responses of effector organs due to adrenergic and cholinergic nerve impulses.			
Organ	**Receptor**	**Adrenergic response**	**Cholinergic response**
		Heart	
SA node	Mainly β_1, β_2 (minimum)	↑Heart rate	↓Heart rate
Atria	Mainly β_1, β_2 (minimum)	↑Contractility, ↑conductivity	↓Contractility/conductivity
AV node	Mainly β_1, β_2 (minimum)	↑Automaticity, ↑conductivity	↓Conduction – AV block
Purkinje system	Mainly β_1, β_2 (minimum)	↑Automaticity, ↑conductivity	Little effect
Ventricle	Mainly β_1, β_2 (minimum)	↑Contractility ↑Conduction velocity ↑Automaticity ↑Idioventricular pacemaker	Little effect Little effect Little effect Little effect
		Arterioles	
Coronary	α_1, α_2 β_2	Constriction + Dilatation + +	Dilatation
Skin and mucosa	α_1, α_2	Constriction + + +	Dilatation

Contd…

Contd...

Organ	Receptor	Adrenergic response	Cholinergic response
Skeletal muscle	α_1, α_2 β_2	Constriction + + Dilatation + +	Dilatation
Cerebral	α_1	Constriction +	Dilatation
Pulmonary	α_1 β_2	Constriction + + Dilatation +	Dilatation
Abdominal viscera	α_1 β_2	Constriction + + + Dilatation +	No effect No effect
Renal	α_1, α_2 β_1, β_2	Constriction + + + Dilatation +	No effect No effect
Vein Systemic	α_1, α_2 β_2	Constriction + + Dilatation + +	No effect No effect
Lung Bronchial muscle Bronchial gland	β_2 α_1 β_2	Relaxation + ↑ Secretion ↓ Secretion	Contraction + + Secretion + + No effect
Intestine Motility/tone Sphincter Gland secretion Gallbladder and bile duct	α_1, α_2, β_2 α_1 α_2 β_2	Decrease + Contraction + Decrease + Relaxation	Increase + + + Relaxation + Increase + + + Contraction +
Eye Iris (radial muscle) Iris (sphincter muscle) Ciliary muscle Lacrimal gland	α_1 – β_2 α	Contraction No effect Relaxation Secretion +	No effect Myosis (contraction) + + + Contraction for near vision + Secretion + + +
Urinary bladder Detrusor Trigone, sphincter	β_2 α_1	Relaxation Contraction + +	Contraction + + + Relaxation + +
Ureter Motility, tone Uterus Sex organs (male)	α_1 α_1 β_2 α_1	Increase Contraction Relaxation Ejaculation	No effect Variable No effect Erection + + +

the variety of α-subunit, G protein may be of stimulatory (Gs), inhibitory (Gi) or inactive (Go). The α-subunit may split off from the mother molecule of G protein and behave independently, whereas β and γ subunit may remain together. In resting state, G protein is attached to a guanosine diphosphate (GDP) molecule. When a G-protein molecule is activated through the receptor [after the (i.e., the attached GDP with G-protein becomes GTP) attachment of receptor with an agonist], then it leads to the displacement of GDP by GTP. Now, the GTP molecule is attached with the α-subunit of activated G-protein molecule. Then, G-protein splits up simultaneously into two parts, consisting of α-GTP and β–γ subunit. The released α-subunit of G-protein with GTP, then binds to the second messenger molecule, such as AC and activates it and then converts its attached GTP to GDP. Therefore, GDP returns to its resting state and is detached from the α-subunit of G protein. Then, the α-subunit rejoins again with the β-γ subunit of G-protein and reconstructs the G-protein, waiting at the inner surface of cell membrane with the receptor for further activation **(Fig. 5)**.

Both the β_1 and β_2 receptor stimulation by an agonist activates the G protein which in turn enhances or activates the AC. Then, this activated AC increases the intracellular concentration of cAMP. Next, this increased intracellular cAMP concentration activates the protein kinase, which then further phosphorylates or activates many other target proteins. Thus, the target phosphorylation elicits a variety of cellular responses and completes the path between the receptor and the responses of cells.

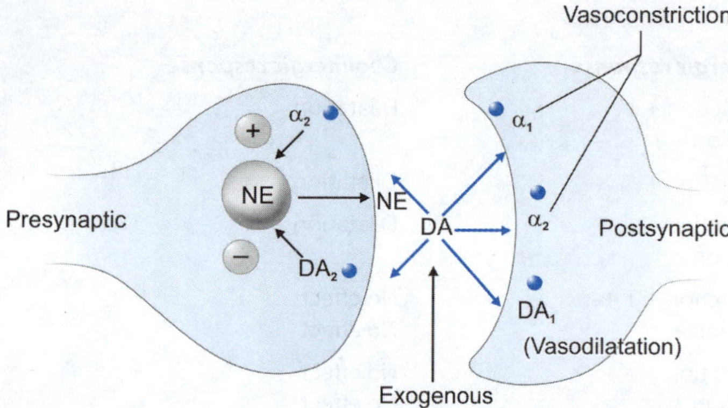

Fig. 5: This is a schematic representation of α_1, α_2, and DA_1 receptors on postsynaptic membrane and α_2, DA_2 receptor on presynaptic membrane. When the dopamine is administered exogenously, then the activation of DA_1 receptor on postsynaptic membrane causes vasodilatation. While the activation of DA_2 receptor on presynaptic membrane causes the inhibition of NE release. The large doses of dopamine also activate the α_1 and α_2 receptor on postsynaptic membrane and cause vasoconstriction. It also activates the α_2 receptor on presynaptic membrane and inhibits the release of NE. Normally, the NE is released from presynaptic sympathetic terminal and acts on α_1 and α_2 receptor on postsynaptic membrane, causing vasoconstriction.

The stimulation of α_1 receptor results in inhibition of the AC and this inhibition is mediated by the Gi protein **(Fig. 6)**.

Actually, the α_1 receptor acts through the G-proteins, but activates phospholipase-C in the inner surface of cell membrane. Activated phospholipase-C, then, increases the hydrolysis of phospho-inositol diphosphate (P1P2) to triphosphate and diacylglycerol (DAG). These two compounds, then, mobilize the intracellular calcium stores from sarcoplasmic reticulum and causes a marked increase in the concentration of intracellular calcium ion. This calcium then binds to calmodulin (calcium sensitive intracellular protein) which subsequently activates the myosin light chain kinase. This myosin light chain kinase, then, phosphorylates the myosin light chain and facilitates the interaction between the actin and myosin filaments, resulting in muscular contraction. In other cells, this calmodulin stimulates other kinases, resulting in other cellular effects.

The myocardial cells respond according to the receptors and their agonist or antagonist (the first messenger), i.e., NE, EPI, dopamine, ACh, etc. which act on their respective receptors **(Table 9)**. The two opposing effects, i.e., inhibition or stimulation depends on the type of agonist/antagonist, their respective receptor, their respective G-proteins, and their respective effectors system or second messenger (i.e., AC, phospholipase-C, etc.).

The negative inotropic action of halothane and other volatile anesthetic agents is mediated through the inhibitory G protein (Gi) and ↓ cAMP concentration. Other possible

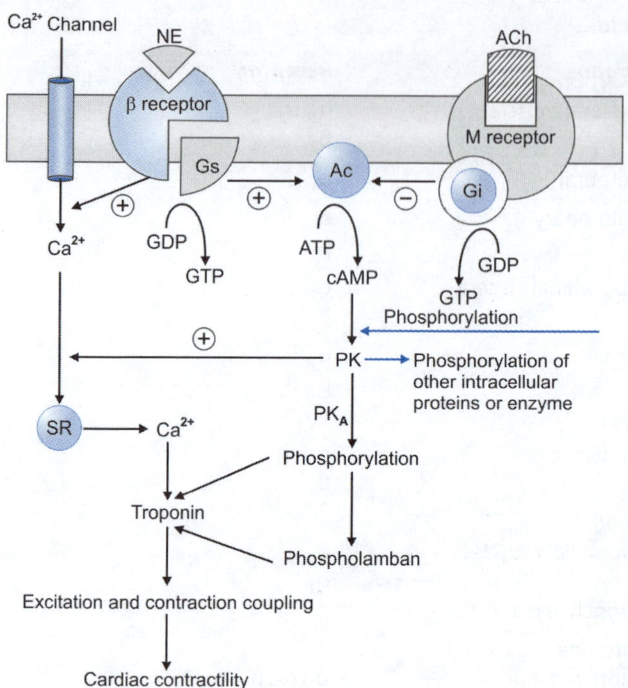

Fig. 6: NE binds to β-adrenergic receptors on the outer surface of cell membrane and induces some conformational changes within the receptor. This permits the attachment of receptor with Gs protein (stimulatory G-protein) and the activation of it. Now, the activated Gs protein binds with GTP and its (G-protein) α active subunit is dissociated. Activated Gs now activates the enzyme AC (adenylyl cyclase), located on the cytoplasmic side of the cell membrane. Then, activated AC hydrolyses ATP to cAMP. Now, cAMP phosphorylates and activates the protein kinase (PK$_A$). The activated PK$_A$ then phosphorylates many intracellular functional proteins, including the troponin and phospholamban. Phospholamban and troponin then interact with intracellular Ca²⁺, resulting in increased force of contraction. This intracellular Ca²⁺ is made available by direct entry from outside as well as from the intracellular stores. The direct entry of Ca²⁺ from outside is through Ca²⁺ channels, situated on the cell membrane, which is again facilitated by Gs protein and the phosphorylation of PK$_A$. The action of ACh on muscarinic receptor (M) activates the inhibitory G-protein (Gi), which opposes the activation of AC by Gs protein.

mechanisms of negative inotropic effects of halothane are the attenuation of release of neurotransmitter from peripheral sympathetic neuron, blockage of calcium channel in heart and thus the alteration of calcium fluxes from sarcoplasmic reticulum and reduction of cardiac contraction. Hence, it proves that the negative inotropic effect of inhalational anesthetics occurs at several sites.

Up- and Downregulation of β-receptors

The number of postsynaptic β-adrenergic receptors is not fixed at their site of action. However, the number of these receptors changes continuously and significantly, matching with the available amount of adrenergic agonists and

TABLE 9: The difference of adrenergic responses mediated through α and β receptors.

α-actions	β-actions
1. Constriction of arterioles and veins→ rise in BP (α_1 and α_2 action, α_1 action predominates)	1. Dilatation of arterioles and veins → fall of BP (β_2 action)
2. Little action on heart	2. Cardiac stimulation (β_1 and β_2, but β_1 action predominates → cause ↑heart rate, ↑force of contraction and ↑conduction velocity)
3. On bronchus—no α action	3. Bronchodilatation (β_2 action)
4. Contraction of radial muscle of iris→ mydriasis (α_1 action)	4. No effect on iris and ciliary muscle
5. Decreased aqueous secretion	5. Enhanced aqueous secretion
6. Intestinal relaxation (α_1, α_2) contraction of sphincter (α_1)	6. Intestinal relaxation (β_2 action)
7. Bladder trigone—contraction (α_1) and sphincter spasm	7. Detrusor—relaxation (β_2)
8. Uterus—contraction (α_1)	8. Uterus—relaxation (β_2)
9. Insulin secretion—inhibited (α_2)	9. i. Insulin secretion—increased (mild) ii. Glucagon secretion—increased (β_2)
10. Liver—no action	10. i. Liver → glycogenolysis (β_2) → hyperglycemia ii. Muscle → glycogenolysis (β_2) → hyperlactacidemia iii. Fat → lipolysis (β_2) → increased FFA
11. Male sex organs—ejaculation	Sex organ → no action
12. Smooth muscle of prostate and bladder neck—contraction with obstruction (α_1)	No effect

antagonists which are released in the synaptic cleft. It is found that 30 minutes after denervation or blockade by an antagonist, there is an increased number of receptors. This is called the *"upregulation of receptor"* and is the explanation for the sudden rebound phenomenon of tachycardia, ischemia, and increased incidence of MI, after sudden discontinuation of β-blocker, e.g., atenolol, propranolol, metoprolol, etc.

Reversely, if the receptors are continuously or tonically exposed to an agonist, then the responses wane rapidly, despite continuous exposure to adrenergic agonists. This is due to the reduction of number of receptors which is called the *"downregulation of receptor"* or the reduction of the sensitivity of receptors to agonists which is called the *"desensitization of receptor"*. There are three underlying mechanisms for the desensitization of receptor: *uncoupling (phosphorylation), sequestration, and downregulation.*

Uncoupling

It is found that when an agonist continuously binds with a receptor, then it promotes the phosphorylation of receptor's serine residues near its intracellular carboxy terminus. This allows it (receptor) to bind with a protein, called β-arrestin, which hinders its (receptor) interaction with Gs protein or coupling, causing desensitization by blocking the signal transduction.

Sequestration

This is a well-described but poorly understood process. It does not appear to be related to phosphorylation. It is reversible if the agonist stimulation ceases with the receptor being returned to cell surface.

Downregulation

It is just opposite to upregulation. Here, the destruction of receptor is increased, or the synthesis of receptor is decreased due to the continuous exposure of receptor to an agonist. It is a slow process than uncoupling and sequestration and refractoriness develops over weeks and months and recedes slowly. CHF is the most important example of downregulation.

Another example of up- and downregulation of β-adrenergic receptors is the disease of thyroid gland. The activity of thyroid gland influences the receptor density with hyperthyroidism decreasing the density and hypothyroidism increasing the density.

■ CHOLINERGIC RECEPTORS

The receptors on which ACh or agents, which actions are like ACh, act are called the cholinergic receptors and these agents are called the cholinergic agonists or agents. There are two types of cholinergic receptors: *muscarinic and nicotinic.*

ACh has no specificity for these two types of cholinergic receptors, but these two types of receptors structurally and functionally are of two completely distinct classes and have significantly different responses to ACh. Lately, specific agonists to these individual cholinergic receptors (muscarinic and nicotinic) have emerged with their definite structure-activity relationship. Chemically, all these cholinergic agonists are of quaternary ammonium compound and have an atom which is capable of forming a hydrogen bond with cholinergic receptor through an unshared pair of electrons. The distance between the two (i.e., the ammonium group and the hydrogen-bond forming atom) determines whether the cholinergic agonism is muscarinic or nicotinic. When the distance is 4.4 Å, then the agonist has muscarinic action and when the distance is 5.9 Å, then the agonist has nicotinic action.

Muscarinic Cholinergic Receptors

These receptors (M-receptors) belong to the superfamily of G-protein-coupled receptors. Therefore, it also consists of 7 helical, membrane spanning, amino acid (chains), where the amino terminus ($-NH_2$) lies outside the cell membrane, and the carboxy terminus ($-COOH$) lies inside the cell membrane. These muscarinic cholinergic receptors (M-receptors) are selectively stimulated by a chemical substance, named muscarine. So, they are called the muscarinic receptors. It can be blocked by atropine. These muscarinic receptors are located in many visceral organs, such as heart, blood vessels, eyes, smooth muscles, glands, CNS, etc.

These muscarinic (M) receptors are also present on presynaptic membrane of postganglionic cholinergic nerve endings. The activation of these presynaptic muscarinic receptor inhibits the further release of ACh. This is also one of the mechanisms of action of α_2-adrenergic agonist which also acts on this prejunctional cholinergic muscarine (M) receptors to decrease ACh release with some clinical relevance. Similar one also has been demonstrated on presynaptic membrane of adrenergic terminals, activation of which inhibits the release of NA. All the blood vessels have muscarinic receptors, located on their endothelial cells, though most of them lack cholinergic innervation. Activation of these endothelial muscarinic receptors releases endothelium-derived relaxing factor (EDRF) which diffuses into the smooth muscles of blood vessels and causes its relaxation with vascular dilatation.

Muscarinic (M) receptors have been divided into five subtypes and named as M-1, M-2, M-3, M-4, and M-5 on the basis of the primary structural variability of these receptors which include a huge cytoplasmic loop, situated between the fifth and sixth membrane spanning domains (amino acid chain). Out of these, the first three receptors (M-1, M-2, and M-3) have been clearly functionally defined, while the responses indicated through M4 and M5 receptor subtypes are not well-defined. Most organs have more than one subtype of muscarinic receptor, but usually one subtype predominates in a given tissue. The M-1 receptors are primarily neuronal receptor, located on ganglionic cells and central neurons; especially in cortex, hippocampus, and corpus striatum (though all the subtypes of muscarinic receptors are present in CNS). It also plays a major role in mediating gastric secretion and relaxation of lower esophageal sphincter on vagal stimulation. Cardiac muscarinic receptors are predominantly of M-2 subtype, while the smooth muscle and glandular ones are of M-3 subtype. Therefore, the M-2 and M-3 subtypes of muscarinic receptors together mediate most of the well-recognized muscarinic actions of ACh (principal neurotransmitter of parasympathetic system).

As described previously, the muscarinic receptors are the G-protein-coupled receptors, so the M-1 and M-3 (and probably M-5) subtypes function through the Gq/11 type of G protein and activate the membrane bound phospholipase-C (as second messenger), generating inositol triphosphate (IP3) and diacylglycerol (DAG). Actually, the stimulation of phospholipase-C causes the immediate hydrolysis of phosphatidyl inositol poly-(tri)-phosphates (PIP3), which are the components of plasma membrane and form inositol triphosphates. This, in turn, releases Ca^{2+} intracellularly from ER and causes the contraction of smooth muscle of GI tract and glandular secretion. The M-2 (and probably M-4) subtype of muscarinic receptor functions through the Gi and Go type of G protein. It inhibits the membrane bound AC which in turn opens the K^+ channels, causing the hyperpolarization and the suppression of the activity of voltage-gated Ca^{2+} channels. Thus, it causes the reduced pacemaker activity of SA node, slowing of conduction through AV node and the decrease of the force of contraction of heart **(Table 10)**.

The responses of muscarinic (M) receptor to its agonists and antagonists are slow. They may be excitatory or inhibitory. However, they are not necessarily linked to the changes in ion permeability through cell membrane, like nicotinic receptor.

Nicotinic Cholinergic Receptors

These receptors belong to the superfamily of ion-gated channel (i.e., there is a channel through the receptor with gates, through which ion passes) and are selectively activated by nicotine. So, they are called the nicotinic (N) receptors. These nicotinic (N) receptors are located only at the motor endplates in neuromuscular junctions and in peripheral autonomic ganglion (e.g., ganglion of sympathetic chain). The nicotinic type of cholinergic receptors which are located

TABLE 10: The sites of cholinergic transmission and type of receptors involved.

Site	Type of receptors	Specific agonist	Specific antagonist
All postganglionic parasympathetic nerve endings	Muscarinic (M)	Muscarine	Atropine
Inside the ganglia (both sympathetic and parasympathetic)	Nicotinic (Nn)	Nicotine DMPP (selective)	Hexamethonium
Few postganglionic sympathetic (sweat gland, some blood vessels, nerve endings)	Muscarinic (M)	Muscarine	Atropine
Adrenal medulla	Nicotinic (Nn)	Nicotine DMPP (selective)	Hexamethonium
Skeletal muscle: motor endplate	Nicotinic (Nn)	Nicotine PTMA (selective)	Curare
CNS (cortex, basal ganglia, spinal cord, and other sites)	Both muscarinic and nicotinic	Muscarine nicotine	Atropine curare

(ACH is agonist to both muscarinic and nicotinic receptors; DMPP: dimethylphenylpiperazinium; PTMA: phenyltrimethylammonium)

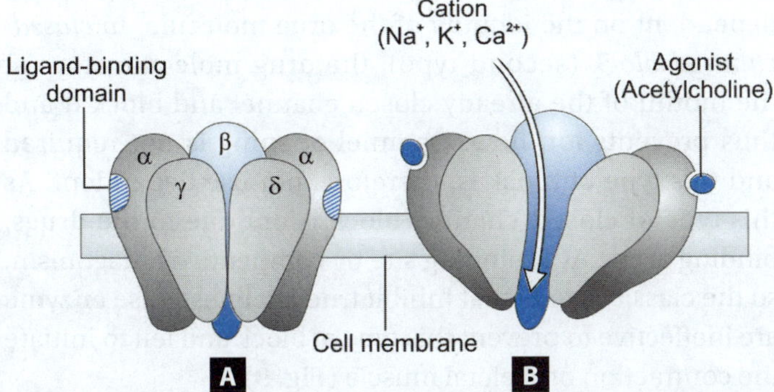

Figs. 7A and B: This is a schematic representation of a nicotinic receptor with an intrinsic ion channel. (A) It shows a closed nicotinic cholinergic receptor. This molecule is composed of five subunits such as: 2α, β, γ, and δ subunits, enclosing a cylindrical ion channel. (B) It shows, when two molecules of ACh bind to the two α-subunits of a nicotinic receptor. When this occurs, then all the subunits of a nicotinic receptor move apart. This opens the central channel of receptor and allows the passage of cation. The anions are blocked from passing through the channel by the positive charges, lining it. In other cases, K^+ and Ca^{2+} ions move through this channel, depending on its ion selectivity.

in the motor endplates, can be blocked selectively by tubocurarine, decamethonium (10 carbon atom structure) or other nondepolarizing muscle relaxants. But, those which are located at the autonomic ganglion can be blocked selectively by hexamethonium (six-carbon atom structure), which has no effect at motor endplates (**Figs. 7A and B**).

The nicotinic receptors or ion-gated channels (channels with upper and lower gate and through these channels ion moves) are a pentameric membrane protein in structure, which form the passage for nonselective cations through this channel and among the cations the most important is Na^+. In each nicotinic receptor, there are two α-subunits and one each of β, ε, and δ subunit. The α-subunit represents the binding site for both agonists (ACh, nicotine, etc.) and antagonists (curarins and decamethonium, etc.). At birth,

γ subunit occupies the position of ε (epsilon) subunit, which is normally present in an adult receptor. But, within the first 2 weeks of life, this γ subunit of nicotinic receptor is replaced by ε subunit. This change in subunit converts the receptor from one with low conductance and a relatively long duration of opening of channel to a high conductance with a brief duration of opening of channel. Therefore, there are important structural and functional differences of nicotinic receptors during their developments in life. But, it is important to mention that the important drug-binding subunit or α-subunit remains constantly present in the receptor throughout the life. Again, there are eight subtypes of this α-subunit which are named as the α_2 to α_9 and there are three subtypes of β-subunit which are named as β_2 to β_4. Although not all the combinations of α and β subunits are functional, but the number of permutations and combinations of these subtypes of α and β subunit, that yield many functional nicotinic receptors, is sufficiently large to produce a pharmacological variation and classifications of all these receptor subtypes.

On the basis of the location and the selective action of agonist and antagonist, two subtypes of nicotinic receptor such as N_M and N_N (previously labeled as N_1 and N_2) are also recognized. The N_M subtype of nicotinic receptors are present at skeletal muscle's endplates and mediate the skeletal muscle contraction. Whereas the N_N subtype of nicotinic receptors are present at autonomic ganglion (sympathetic and parasympathetic), adrenal medulla (embryologically derived from the same site as ganglionic cells), spinal cord, and at the certain areas of brain. The difference between the N_M and N_N subtype of nicotinic receptor is that the pentamer of NN receptor consists only of α- and β-subunits and constitutes the primary pathway for transmission in a ganglion.

These five subunits (2α, β, ε, δ) of a nicotinic receptor surround a channel through which the cations, like Na^+ and Ca^{2+} may enter or K^+ may exit the cell. So, it is called the ion channel. For the channel within this nicotinic to open, both the α-subunit should be occupied by the agonists, such as ACh. The occupation of one α-subunit by ACh will not open the channel. Thus, if one α-subunit is occupied by ACh and the other is empty, then this channel will remain closed with no flow of ions, no change in electrical potential at motor endplate, and no muscular contraction. On the other hand, if one α-subunit is occupied by ACh and another α-subunit is occupied by an antagonist, such as pancuronium, then the channel will also remain close and no contraction of skeletal muscle will occur. Similarly, if both the α-subunits are occupied by pancuronium, the channel also remains closed. From this discussion, it is clear that for the action of agonist (ACh) two molecules are needed which bind with the two α-subunits of nicotinic receptor. But, for the action of antagonist (nondepolarizing muscle relaxant) only one molecule is sufficient which binds with one α-subunit of nicotinic receptor.

The response of nicotinic or ion-channel receptor to ACh is instantaneous, but usually lasts for few milliseconds only. This is because ACh is rapidly destroyed by true acetylcholinesterase, present in synaptic cleft. This ultrashort-acting response of a nicotinic NM receptor to ACh gives the motor endplate a greater flexibility to neural stimulation. This contributes profoundly not only to the viability of an organism or animal, but also to its ability to control its own body movements precisely **(Table 11)**.

In addition to the binding of α-subunit by ACh or its antagonist, there are another two types of channel block: *opened and closed* **(Fig. 8)**.

With open-channel block (first type), a drug enters the channel, after it is opened by ACh. But, the drug molecule cannot travel all the way through the channel. Entering the opened channel, the drug molecule temporarily binds at some point within the wall of the channel. Thus, it blocks the ionic flow through the channel and prevents the depolarization and muscular contraction. So, the intensity of this type of neuromuscular block depends upon the degree of previous opening of channel and the total activity of the system. Thus, this open type of channel block of nicotinic receptor is termed the "use dependent" block. This type of open-channel block is driven by the difference of electrical potential across the membrane and the charge which is inherent to drug, responsible for this type of block. So, the duration of this type of open-channel block is partially dependent on the identity of the drug molecule. In *closed-channel block* (second type), the drug molecule stays at the mouth of the already closed channel and block it and thus prevents ion flow. Channel opening is not required and this type of block is, therefore, not use dependent. As this type of closed-channel block is not due to the drugs, binding at the ACh binding site by competitive antagonism, so the classic agents that inhibit true cholinesterase enzyme are ineffective to prevent this type of block and fell to initiate the contraction of skeletal muscle **(Fig. 9)**.

At motor endplate or on the postsynaptic membrane of ganglia, the nicotinic receptors are present only opposite to the presynaptic area (membrane) and are absent on the rest of the muscle cell membrane. The usual density of this nicotinic receptors at a motor endplate is about 10,000/sq μm and is the center of accomplishing successful neuromuscular transmission. A number of intracellular (utrophin and syntrophin) and extracellular (agrin, laminin, and dystroglycan) proteins have been identified, those direct and help in the formation of nicotinic receptors at motor endplate and on the postsynaptic membrane in ganglia

TABLE 11: Differences of subtypes of nicotinic receptors.		
	N$_M$ nicotinic receptor	**N$_N$ nicotinic receptor**
Location and function	Neuromuscular junction → contraction of skeletal muscle	• Autonomic ganglia → transmission of impulse through ganglia • Adrenal medulla → release of catecholamines • CNS site → action and inhibition
Nature	• Has intrinsic ion channel • Pentamer of 2α, β, δ and ε or γ subunits	• Has intrinsic ion channel • Pentamer of only α and β subunits
Transducer mechanism	Passage of cation (Na$^+$, K$^+$)	Passage of cation (Na$^+$, K$^+$, Ca^{2+})
Agonist	Nicotine	Nicotine
Antagonist	Tubocurarine and other muscle relaxants	Trimethaphan and hexamethonium

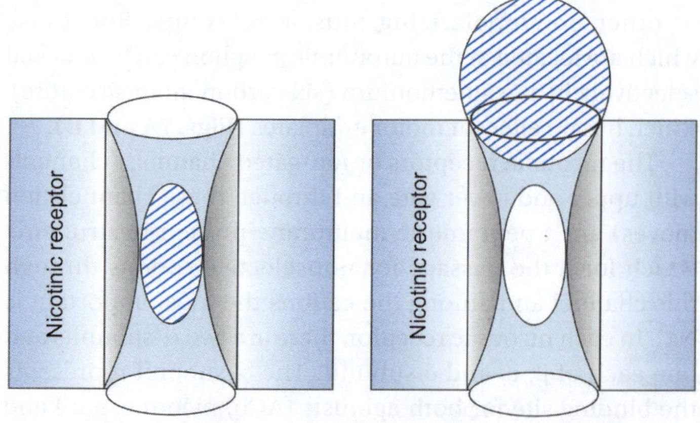

Fig. 8: Opened and closed block of nicotinic receptor.

within the few hours of presynaptic terminals reaching the myocyte (muscle cell) or postsynaptic neurons, during the development of motor endplate or ganglion in intrauterine life. Only the postsynaptic areas of cell membrane are depolarized by ACh and generates an action potential which next spreads along the whole cell membrane of myocyte from that synaptic point, resulting in the contraction of skeletal muscles or the transmission of impulses by postsynaptic neurons through ganglion.

The action of ACh on nicotinic cholinergic receptor can be prolonged by its repeated doses, or by anticholinesterase drugs which destroy the true cholinesterase enzyme or by long-acting cholinomimetic agents, such as succinylcholine. In such circumstances (succinylcholine), the initial depolarization and propagation of impulse along the cell membrane of a skeletal muscle fiber, which is seen as fasciculation, is quickly followed by the blockade of the transmission of impulses and skeletal muscular relaxation. This clinical effect is due to Na^+ channels which are present on the cell membrane of myocyte just around the (at the periphery of) motor endplate area. In normal circumstances, after the first impulse of depolarization, these Na^+ channel at the perisynaptic area (around the endplate area) gets time for rest. During this rest period, they (Na^+ channel) become repolarized and become ready to transmit the

next impulse for next muscular contraction. But, when ACh is used repeatedly or its concentration is increased at the motor endplate by anticholinesterases or when succinylcholine is used, which action is much longer than ACh, then these perisynaptic Na^+ channels remain continuously in depolarized state and do not get time for recovery or repolarization, before the further transmission of impulses. Thus, it blocks the subsequent transmission of impulses which are continuously generated at motor endplate by succinylcholine or anticholinesterase or repeated doses of ACh and produce molecular paralysis. This is discussed more elaborately in Chapter 7.

■ TRANSMISSION OF IMPULSES

New Concept

For many years, the ACh, dopamine, NE, GABA, histamine, etc. were considered as the only neurotransmitters for the transmission of impulses. But, recently many other compounds have also been identified as neurotransmitters. These are purines (ATP, adenosine); peptides (vasoactive intestinal peptide or VIP, neuropeptide-Y or NPY; substance-P or SP; enkephalins; somatostatin; etc.); 5-HT, calcitonin gene-related peptide (CGRP) and many other small molecules, such as NO, etc. Furthermore, a peculiar nonadrenergic and noncholinergic transmission has also been demonstrated in the autonomic innervation of gut, vas deferens, urinary tract, salivary glands, and certain other blood vessels where the nerve stimulation is able to evoke responses, even in the presence of total adrenergic and cholinergic blockade (**Fact file I**).

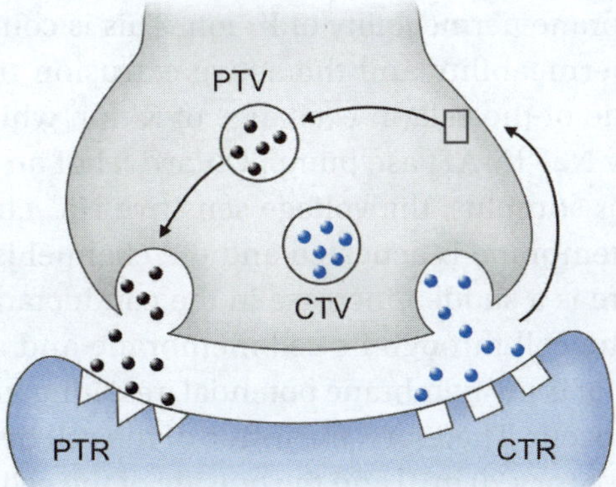

Fig. 9: This is a schematic diagram of transmission by cotransmitter. The cotransmitters are stored in prejunctional nerve terminal like primary transmitter, but in a separate vesicle. Sometimes, the cotransmitter is stored in the same vesicle with primary transmitter. Nerve impulses, coming to nerve terminal, release both the transmitters (primary transmitter and cotransmitter) at the same time, but from the separate vesicles specific for each or from the same vesicle containing both. After release, acting on cotransmitter receptor, the co-transmitters modify the responsiveness or the effects of primary transmitter. Sometimes, they even substitute it. The cotransmitters may also act on prejunctional receptors and modulate the release of primary transmitter. (CTR: contransmitter receptor; CTV: contrasmitter vesicle; PTR: primary transmitter receptor; PTV: primry transmitter vessicle)

FACT FILE I

The diameter of each vesicle or quanta is 300 μm and each vesicle contains 10,000 molecules of ACh (the range of which varies from 1,000 to over 50,000 per vesicles). The difference between the central cholinergic transmission and the cholinergic transmission at neuromuscular junction is that very few vesicles are present in presynaptic terminal at CNS and these vesicles look clear under electron microscope.

The release of the contents of one vesicle causes the opening or stimulation of 2,000 receptors, situated on the postsynaptic membrane, and produces a *miniature endplate potential* of 0.5 mV. Upon the activation of receptor by ACh, its intrinsic Na^+ channel opens for about 1 millisecond. During this brief period, about 50,000 Na^+ ions traverse the channel through thisopened receptor. Thus, each channel that is opened, results in the depolarization of 0.00022 mV. When the impulses arrive at presynaptic nerve terminal, then 100–300 vesicles or quantas release their contents and bring about changes in the normal resting membrane potential of postsynaptic membrane above the threshold level. This is called the *excitatory postsynaptic potential (EPSP)* which is about +50 to +100 mV.

Before the recognition of these newer transmitters, *"one neuron - one transmitter"* model was the accepted theory. But, it has now become apparent that this classical model was an over-simplification. Many peripheral and central neurons have been shown, now, to release more than one active substance when stimulated, i.e., more than one neurotransmitter may be co-localized in same nerve terminal and the synaptic transmission may be mediated by the release of more than one neurotransmitter.

The most common combination of neurotransmitters in nerves are NE, ATP, and NPY in sympathetic nervous system and ACh, VIP in parasympathetic nervous system and SP, CGRP, ATP in sensorimotor nerves. These newer transmitters are called the *cotransmitters* and the transmission caused by them is called the *cotransmission*. The cotransmitter is stored in the same neuron, but in distinct synaptic vesicles and at distinct locations. On being released by the presynaptic nerve impulse, these cotransmitters may serve to regulate the presynaptic release of primary neurotransmitter and/or postsynaptic sensitivity to it (neuromodulator role). The cotransmitter may also serve as an alternative transmitter in its own right.

In case of many, but not all, there is evidence that NE and ATP act as cotransmitters. Being released by the same nerve, they act on α_1-adreno-receptors and P_2-purinoreceptors respectively to produce vasoconstriction. The first component of contraction appears to be mediated by the voltage dependent P2 calcium channels and ATP, while the sustained later part of contraction is mediated by NE through its α1-adreno-receptor.

Neuromodulation also modifies the process of neurotransmission. Such neuromodulators may be the circulating neurohormones, local agents, or neurotransmitter substances, which are released from the same nerve terminal or form other nerves nearby. This neuromodulation can occur either prejunctionally by decreasing or increasing the release of the amount of neurotransmitter from presynaptic membrane or postjunctionally by altering the effect of neurotransmitter on postsynaptic membrane. In all the known examples where both the pre- and postjunctional neuromodulation occur, they act in concert, either to alternate or augment the effective transmission.

Examples

NPY neurotransmitter is localized with NE and ATP transmitters at nerve endings. After release, it acts as a neuromodulator. Prejunctionally, it inhibits the release of NE from nerve terminal and postjunctionally it enhances the action of NE. In spleen, skeletal muscles, cerebral vessels, coronary vasculature, etc., NPY has direct vasoconstrictive actions.

In heart and brain, NPY is used by the local intrinsic neuron as the principal transmitter to cause vasoconstriction. Actually, the release of this type of neurotransmitter depends on the frequency of stimulation or nerve impulse.

ACh and VIP neurotransmitters coexist in parasympathetic nerve endings of many organs. They are stored in separate vesicles and are released separately by stimulation of different frequencies. They both modulate transmission by acting on pre- and postjunctional site.

Steps of Transmission of Impulses

Before discussion of this part of chapter, we will have to define two terms: *conduction of impulse* and *transmission of impulse*. The term *"conduction"* is defined as the passage of an impulse along an axon to the synapse. And the term *"transmission"* is defined as the passage of an impulse across a synaptic junction, i.e., between an axon and a muscle fiber or between two axons. Thus, the term transmission includes the release of transmitter and the action of transmitter on postsynaptic membrane.

Conduction of Impulse to Synapse

At the resting state of a cell, the transmembrane or resting membrane potential (RMP) varies between –70 mV and –90 mV. This is due to the high negativity inside of a cell and the high positivity outside of a cell. It is established and maintained by the high intracellular concentration and the high cell membrane permeability of K^+ ion. This is coupled with the low permeability and the active extrusion of Na^+ ion from inside of the cell, in exchange of K^+ ion which enters the cell by Na^+-K^+-ATPase pump. On arrival of an electrical impulse or stimulus, the voltage sensitive Na^+-channel on the cell membrane is activated and the channel is opened. Thus, there is a sudden increase in the conductance of Na^+ ion into the cell through its cell membrane and a positive overshoot of transmembrane potential, resulting in depolarization to occur. Therefore, the inside of the cell becomes 20 mV positive (or +20 mV) and the outside of the cell becomes negative which are opposite to the resting state of the cell. After this depolarization, rapid inactivation of Na^+ channel and the opening of K^+ channel on cell membrane occurs. This permits the K^+ ions to move out of the cell and repolarization occurs. This means the inside of the cell again becomes –ve, like the resting membrane potential (with the extrusions of K^+), which had become +ve due to the entry of Na^+ during depolarization. Then, after repolarization in refractory period, ionic distribution which is now reversed by Na^+ remaining inside of the cell and K^+ remaining outside of the cell is normalized by the activation of Na^+-K^+-ATPase pump, involving an adenosine triphosphatase (ATPase).

This Na$^+$-K$^+$-ATPase pump is activated by Na$^+$ at the inner surface and by K$^+$ at the outer surface of the cell membrane. Now, Na$^+$ goes out and K$^+$ comes into the cell. Thus, the action potential (AP), which is generated by depolarization and repolarization, sets up a local circuit of current and activates the ionic channels at next excitable part of axonal cell membrane or next node of Ranvier in myelinated nerve fiber and is propagated without any decrement. Although not important in axonal conduction, but Ca^{2+} channels on cell membrane in other tissues (e.g., heart) also contribute to this action potential by prolonging the depolarization by its inward movement. This influx of Ca^{2+} into cell also serves as stimulus to initiate other multiple intracellular events, such as muscular contraction, secretion, etc.

Release of Transmitter

Different neurotransmitters, such as excitatory or inhibitory, are stored at presynaptic nerve endings in different synaptic vesicles. The nonpeptide neurotransmitters (ACh, NE, etc.) are largely synthesized at the terminal regions of axons and are stored there in multiple synaptic vesicles. Peptide neurotransmitters (SP, ATP, NPY, etc.) are found in large dense core vesicles which are transported down the axon from their site of synthesis in the cell body of neurons. After their formation, the vesicles are clustered at nerve terminals in some particular discrete areas, underlying the presynaptic plasma membrane, termed the "active zone". These active zones often are aligned with the tips of postsynaptic fold. After the impulse reaches nerve endings, the vesicles move, and fuse with the presynaptic axonal membrane. Then, all the contents of the vesicles are extruded into the synaptic cleft. This *fusion* and *fluidization* of vesicular cell membrane with the axonal cell membrane is promoted by the impulse itself and by the entry of Ca^{2+} ion into nerve ending from the ECF. A number of proteins like *synaptotagmin, synaptobrevin, neurexin, syntaxin*, etc. are also located on the vesicular and axonal membranes which participate in this fusion and fluidization of vesicular with axonal membrane, resulting in the extrusion of transmitters. This is called *exocytosis*.

This exocytosis or the release of neurotransmitters into synaptic cleft is also modulated by this neurotransmitter itself or some cotransmitter, through the activation of some specific receptors, located on the presynaptic membrane. For example, the release of NE is inhibited by NE itself and by some other cotransmitter such as dopamine, adenosine, etc., acting on the presynaptic α_2 receptors and dopamine receptor, respectively. While isoprenaline, acting on presynaptic β_2 receptor increases the release of NE. Similarly, the α_2 and muscarinic receptor agonists, acting on presynaptic and other α_2 and muscarinic receptors,

inhibit the release of ACh at autonomic neuro-effector site, but not in ganglia and skeletal muscles. The stimulation of presynaptic nicotinic receptors also enhances the release of nerve transmitters in motor neurons. Adenosine, dopamine, glutamate, GABA, PGS (prostaglandins), enkephalins, etc. have also been shown to influence the release of various neurotransmitters.

Action of Transmitters on Postsynaptic Membrane

The released neurotransmitter diffuses across the synaptic cleft and combines with its specific receptors on postsynaptic membrane. Depending on its nature, the neurotransmitters induce an *excitatory postsynaptic potential (EPSP)* or an *inhibitory postsynaptic potential (IPSP)*.

EPSP: In this type of action potential (AP), there is an increase in the permeability of Na$^+$ ions and occasionally Ca^{2+} ions inside the cell, causing depolarization which is followed by the efflux of K$^+$, causing repolarization. This results in an excitatory AP and propagation of impulse.

IPSP: In this type of action potential, there is no increase in the permeability of Na$^+$ ions, but there is only an increase in the permeability of smaller ions such as K$^+$ and Cl$^-$. So, that K$^+$ moves out and Cl$^-$ moves into the cell, resulting in the hyperpolarization of cell. The normal electrical potential difference across the cell membrane is called the polarized state of cell where the inside of the cell is negative and the outside of the cell is positive. Hyperpolarization means inside of the cell becomes more negative, which is normally present during the resting condition of a cell. This is called IPSP. The changes in some special channel permeability that cause this type of potential change, i.e., hyperpolarization, are specifically regulated by some specialized postjunctional receptors and some specific neurotransmitters acting on it. The ligand-gated protein channels which usually belong to a large superfamily and include nicotinic, glutamate, certain serotonin (5-HT3) and purine receptors, etc. conduct primarily the permeability of Na$^+$ from outside into the cells and cause depolarization. So, they are excitatory (of postsynaptic potential) in nature. On the other hand, the GABA and glycine receptors which primarily conduct the permeability of Cl$^-$ from outside into the cells, cause the hyperpolarization of cell and are inhibitory (of postsynaptic potential) in nature.

Without any impulse, in resting state, there is continuous and spontaneous slow release of some isolated quanta of transmitters at synaptic cleft. This produces a minimal electrical response or action potential below the threshold level at postsynaptic membrane. This is called the *miniature endplate potential (MEPP)*. This is associated with the minimum maintenance of the physiological responsiveness of effector organ. Thus, a continuous slow level of electrical activity within a motor unit of skeletal muscle is needed and is very important, since the skeletal muscle lacks its inherent tone.

Postjunctional activity: MEPP cannot generate action potential above the threshold level like EPSP, which is needed to generate a *propagated* postjunctional AP, resulting in nerve impulse (in neuron), contraction (in muscles), secretion (in glands) and other cellular activities. But, multiple MEPP work together to form a clinically effective action potential, resulting in EPSP. An IPSP stabilizes the postjunctional membrane and resists the depolarizing stimuli. Whether a propagated impulse or some other response will occur, it depends on the summation of all the excitatory (EPSP) and inhibitory potential (IPSP).

Termination of Action of Neurotransmitter

Following the attachment with receptor, the transmitter is either locally degraded (e.g., ACh) or is taken back into the prejunctional neurons by active uptake (e.g., NE) or diffuses away into extracellular space and enters the circulation. The rate of termination of transmitter's actions governs the rate at which the responses can be transmitted across the synaptic junction. The termination of the action of only amino acid neurotransmitters results from their active transport into presynaptic neurons and the surrounding glial cells. Peptide neurotransmitters are hydrolyzed by various peptidase enzymes and are also dissipated by diffusion.

■ NEUROTRANSMITTERS

Adrenergic Neurotransmitters

The adrenergic (more precisely called noradrenergic) neurotransmitter is mainly related to postganglionic (postsynaptic) sympathetic nerve endings. There are three structurally closely related *endogenous* adrenergic neurotransmitters. These are *noradrenaline, adrenaline,* and *dopamine.*

Noradrenaline or Norepinephrine

It naturally acts as neurotransmitter in certain areas of brain and at all the postganglionic sympathetic nerve endings, except the sweat glands, hair follicles and some sympathetic vasodilator fibers where the ACh acts as a neurotransmitter.

Adrenaline or Epinephrine

It is mainly secreted from the terminal end of presynaptic neuron in adrenal medulla. Because, it (adrenal medulla) acts as sympathetic ganglia, where only the preganglionic fibers end, but no postganglionic fibers exit from it.

Adrenaline may have some role as neurotransmitter in some places of brain also.

Dopamine

It is normally the major neurotransmitter in basal ganglia, limbic system, CTZ, and the anterior pituitary of CNS and in some places of peripheral nervous system.

Synthesis of adrenergic neurotransmitter or catecholamines (CA): Primarily the adrenergic neurotransmitter such as dopamine, NE, and EPI are synthesized from *tyrosine.* It (tyrosine) is actively transported to preganglionic sympathetic nerve endings, directly from circulation. Tyrosine is first synthesized from *phenylalanine* in liver with the help of an enzyme named *phenylanine hydroxylase.* It is also available directly from diet. In *phenylketoneuric* patients, there is lack of phenylalanine hydroxylase enzyme. So, in these patients, tyrosine is not synthesized in liver. Tyrosine is available for these patients only from diet. The enzymes that participate in the formation of NE from tyrosine at nerve ending are synthesized in the cell bodies of neurons and are then transported along the axons to their nerve terminals. In the nerve endings, as a first step, tyrosine after entering from the circulation, is converted to *dihydroxy phenylalanine (DOPA)* by an enzyme, named *tyrosine hydroxylase (TH)* **(Fig. 10)**.

This is a rate-controlling step for the biosynthesis of NE. Because tyrosine hydroxylase enzyme is activated following the stimulation of adrenergic nerves. This enzyme is activated by cyclic AMP-dependent or Ca^{2+}-calmodulin-dependent protein kinase-C. Thus, this activation or phosphorylation of TH enzyme, catalyzed by protein kinase C, may be associated with increased tyrosine hydroxylase activity. This is an important acute mechanism for increasing the

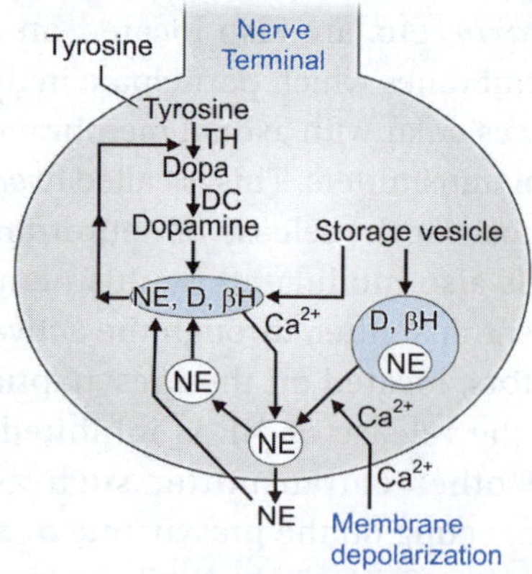

Fig. 10: The synthesis, release, and reuptake of NE at presynaptic sympathetic nerve terminal. (DC: DOPadecarboxylase; DOPA: dihydroxy phenylalanine; DβH: dopamine β-hydroxylase; NE: norepinephrine; TH: tyrosine hydroxylase).

synthesis of catecholamine in response to increased nerve stimulation. On the other hand, high levels of NE inhibit TH enzyme and low levels stimulate this enzyme. During sympathetic stimulation, an increased supply of tyrosine will also increase the synthesis of NE. Chronic stress can also elevate the TH enzyme levels by stimulating the synthesis of new enzyme. When the TH enzyme level is reduced quantitatively, it may reduce NE synthesis significantly and may account for the changes in wakefulness of an individual. The inhibition of TH enzyme by α-methyl-P-tyrosine results in the depletion of catecholamines. Thus, this also can be used in pheochromocytoma before surgery, and also in the inoperable cases **(Fig. 11)**.

In the next step, DOPA is converted to *dopamine* by an enzyme, called *DOPA decarboxylase*. In the course of synthesis of adrenergic neurotransmitter, the hydroxylation of tyrosine to DOPA and the decarboxylation of DOPA to dopamine take place in the cytoplasm of nerve terminal. About half of the dopamine, formed in cytoplasm, is then actively transported into the dopamine-β-hydroxylase (DβH) enzyme containing storage vesicle. In this storage vesicle, the dopamine is converted to *norepinephrine (NE)* by the enzyme, named *dopamine-β-hydroxylase* (DβH). The remaining dopamine in cytoplasm is metabolized to homovanillic acid (HVA).

In Parkinson's disease, the central dopaminergic functions are altered (reduced). So, the administration of DOPA can improve the dopaminergic function in brain. This is because DOPA, but not the dopamine, crosses the blood brain-barrier. Dopamine can act as a neurotransmitter in some cells. But, in most adrenergic neurons, dopamine is catabolized quickly by an enzyme, named *monoamine oxidase (MAO),* which is found in mitochondria.

The enzyme DOPA decarboxylase is nonspecific and can also act on some closely related substances. For example, this enzyme can form 5HT from hydroxytryptophan and α-methyl dopamine from α-methyl DOPA. The latter, i.e., α-methyl dopamine may function as a false neurotransmitter and so the α-methyl DOPA is used in the treatment of hypertension in pregnancy.

In adrenal medulla, in some discrete regions of brain, and in certain ganglia, there is an additional enzyme, named *phenyl-ethanolamine N-methyltransferase (PNMT)*. This enzyme methylates about 85% of NE to EPI. Glucocorticoids from adrenal cortex, passing through adrenal medulla, can activate this system, so that the stress-induced steroid release can cause the increased level of EPI production from adrenal medulla. In adrenal medulla, NE is stored as chromaffin granules into vesicles. These vesicles also contain extremely high concentration of ascorbic acid, ATP, and some other specific proteins, such as chromogranins, enzyme DBH and peptides including enkephalin and neuropeptide Y. In sympathetic nerve terminal under electron microscope two types of storage vesicles are found: (i) large dense core vesicles corresponding to chromaffin granules and (ii) small dense core vesicles containing NE, ATP, and membrane bound dopamine-β-hydroxylase (DBH) enzyme.

Storage of catecholamines:

After synthesis of NE, EPI, or DA it is stored in synaptic vesicles as granules at adrenergic nerve terminal. The vesicular membrane actively takes up the dopamine from cytoplasm. Then, the final step of synthesis and storage of NE takes place inside the vesicles. The vesicles also contain calcium, varieties of peptides or proteins, and ATP which looks under electron microscope as granules. The proteins of synaptic vesicles can be classified functionally into two classes.

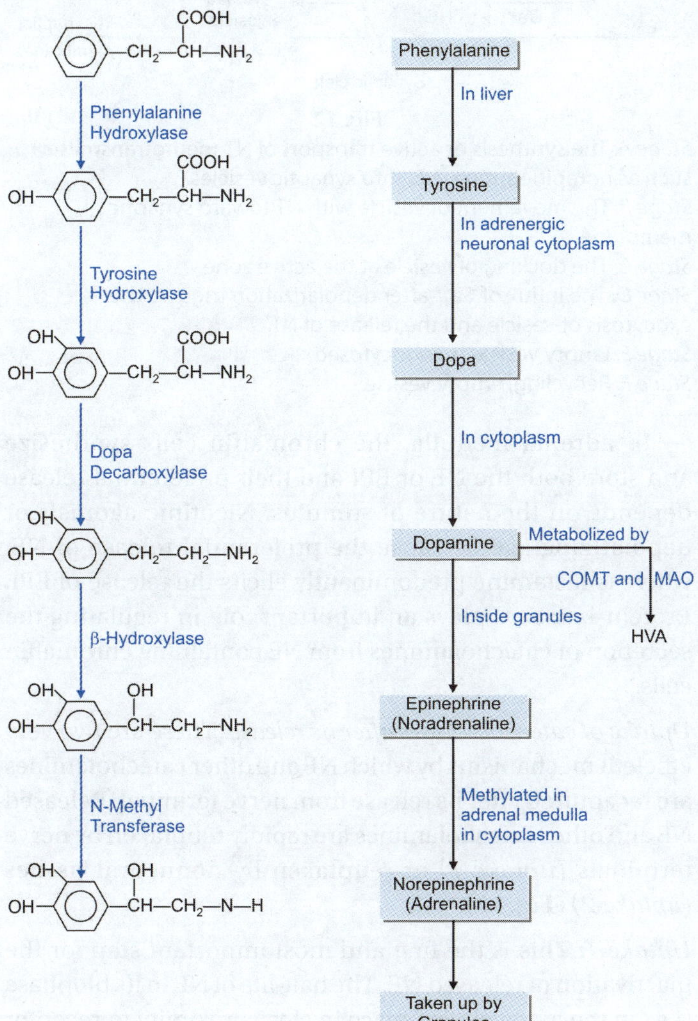

Fig. 11: Biosynthesis of endogenous catecholamines (DA, EPI, and NE). (COMT: catecholamine-o-methyl- transferase; DA: dopamine; EPI: epinephrine; MAO: mono-amino-oxidase; NE: norepinephrine)

One class consists of transport proteins that provide the channels and pumps and are needed for the uptake and the storage of neurotransmitters. Another class consists of proteins that are involved in the direction of movement and the docking reactions of synaptic vesicular membrane with presynaptic membrane.

The NE is stored into vesicle as a complex with ATP (in ratio of 4:1), and is absorbed on the surface of a protein, called chromogranin granules. In adrenal medulla, the NE thus formed within vesicles and absorbed on chromaffin granules, again diffuses out into the cytoplasm of cell, where it is methylated and EPI is formed. Then, the EPI so formed is again taken up by a separate set of vesicles.

Functionally, there are two types of vesicles at nerve terminal: (i) *recycling population* of synaptic vesicles that are used normally and (ii) a *reserve population* of synaptic vesicles that is mobilized only on extensive stimulation during emergency. Transmitters that are newly synthesized or newly taken up from synaptic cleft are preferentially incorporated into the vesicles of recycling population and are released during the normal stimulation of nerve. Sympathomimetic drugs that mimic adrenergic neurotransmitter are also taken up presynaptically and are stored into these recycling vesicles. Among the reserve population of vesicles, only 10% stays in readily releasable condition. But, only 1% out of this 10% readily releasable reserve population is released during each depolarization which implies a significant functional reserve.

Release of catecholamines:

The release of the contents of synaptic vesicles into synaptic cleft is called *exocytosis*. When an AP reaches the nerve terminal, then the presynaptic plasma membrane is depolarized and the voltage-gated calcium channels, situated on it, open at their active zone. As a result, the intracellular Ca^{2+} concentration increases and triggers the *docking, fusion,* and *fluidization* of the vesicular and presynaptic membrane, causing pouring out of all the vesicular contents, such as NE, EPI, ATP, DBH, chromogranin granules, etc. in synaptic cleft. In addition, the vesicles which contain peptides like enkephalin, neuropeptides-Y, etc., as cotransmitters are also simultaneously released. The release of this vesicular content is modulated by many presynaptic receptors, of which α_2-inhibitory control is dominant. Many chemical compounds, such as angiotensin II, prostacyclin, histamine, etc. may also potentiate the release of transmitters. While ACh, prostaglandin E, etc. inhibit this release of transmitter. Tyramine (a sympathomimetic amines) induces the release of NE. But, it is done by displacing the NE from nerve ending binding sites and by exchange diffusion, utilizing *amine carrier of uptake-I.* This process is not called exocytosis and does not require Ca^{2+} **(Fig. 12)**.

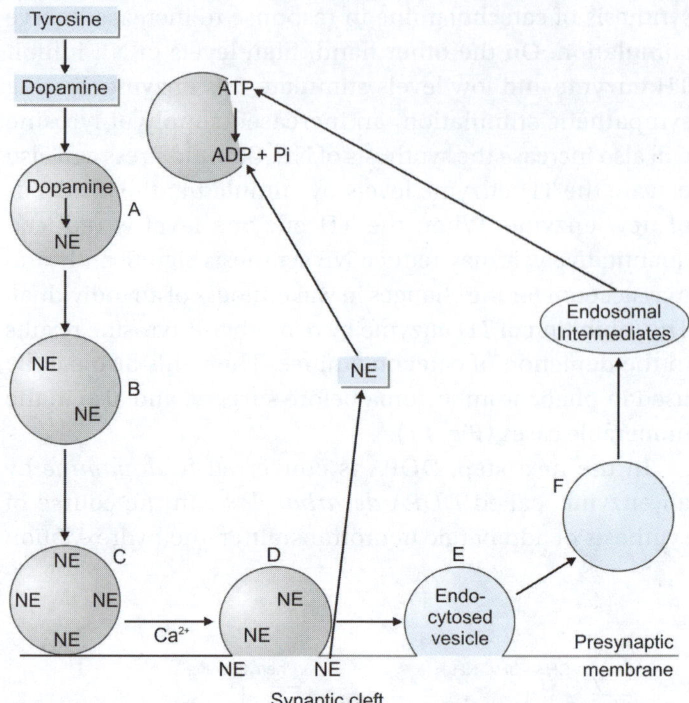

Fig. 12

Stage A: The synthesis or active transport of NT (neurotransmitter) such as norepinephrine (NE) into synaptic vesicles.
Stage B: The movement of vesicle with NT toward synaptic membrane.
Stage C: The docking of vesicle at the active zone.
Stage D: The influx of Ca^{2+} after depolarization triggers the exocytosis of vesicle and the release of NT.
Stage E: Empty vesicle is endocytosed.
Stage F: Recycling, empty vesicle

In adrenal medulla, the chromaffin cells synthesize and store both the NE or EPI and their preferential release depends on the nature of stimulus. Nicotinic agonists or depolarizing agents cause the preferential release of NE, whereas histamine predominantly elicits the release of EPI. Protein-kinase C plays an important role in regulating the secretion of catecholamines from NE containing chromaffin cells.

Uptake of catecholamines after its release: There are two very efficient mechanisms by which NE and other catecholamines are recaptured after its release from nerve terminal. Released NE and other catecholamines are rapidly reuptaken by nerve terminals *(uptake-1)* or reuptaken by nonneural tissues *(uptake-2)* **(Fig. 13)**.

Uptake-1: This is the first and most important step for the inactivation of released NE. The half-life of NE in its biophase (i.e., in the extracellular space in close proximity to receptor after combination with it) is very short. The majority of released NE is transported again back into nerve ending for reuse by an active amine pump (transporter), which is present

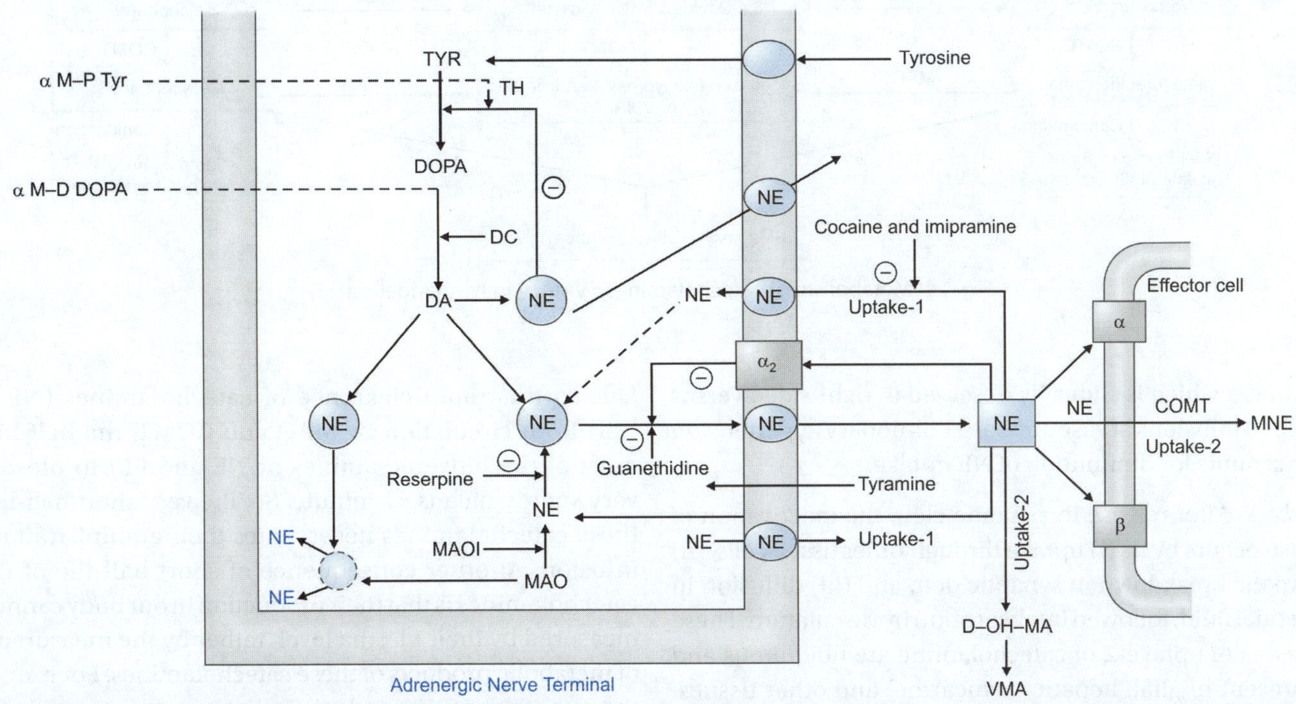

Fig. 13: Schematic representation of adrenergic neurotransmission and its modification by drugs. (1) TYR→ Tyrosine, (2) α M-P-Tyr→ α-methyl-P-tyrosine, (3) α M-DOPA→ α methyl DOPA, (4) D-OH-MA→ Dihydroxy-mandelic acid, (5) MNE→ Metanorepinephrine, (6) VMA→ Vanillyl-mandelic acid, (7) DA→ Dopamine.

at presynaptic neural membrane. This active amine pump is a large hetero-oligomeric molecular complex, containing eight or nine different subunits. This amine transport system, across the axoplasmic membrane, is Na^+ dependent and can be blocked selectively by a number of drugs, including *cocaine* and the *tricyclic antidepressants*, such as imipramine. Thus, they cause an enhanced response to catecholamines, as the most NE is available to receptors on postsynaptic membrane. Cocaine and tricyclic antidepressants also block the reuptake of NE into vesicle from axoplasm.

A number of other highly specific transport system have also been identified for the reuptake of dopamine, norepinephrine, serotonin, and a variety of other amino-acid neurotransmitters. These transport or reuptake system may be viewed as targets for many specific drugs, which are used in clinical practice, such as *cocaine* (block dopamine transport or reuptake), *fluoxetin* (block serotonin transport or reuptake), etc. Then, this NE is driven from axoplasm into vesicle by an electrochemical proton gradient across the membrane of synaptic vesicle. After reuptake into the axoplasm of nerve terminal, a small amount of NE which is not taken up by the vesicle is deaminated by MAO enzyme. There are several organ specific forms of this enzyme. After reuptake or new synthesis, some vesicular NE constantly leaks out into axoplasm and is recaptured or metabolized

by this mechanism. This reuptake of NE into vesicle from axoplasm is inhibited by *reserpine*.

This reuptake of NE into nerve terminal and then into vesicle is not always specific for that neurotransmitter. So, some compounds that are similar to NE in structure may also enter the nerve terminal and vesicle, causing the depletion of actual neurotransmitter. These structurally similar compounds are called the false or pseudotransmitters and have great clinical importance in the management of hypertension.

The integrity of this uptake-1 system varies from tissue to tissue. As for example, the reuptake of NE is lowest or minimum in peripheral blood vessels (where the rate of new NE synthesis is highest). Conversely, the highest rate of reuptake of NE is found in cardiac tissues with less rate of synthesis of NE. Thus, those drugs that inhibit the biosynthesis of NE (e.g., α-methyl dopa) have more effects on blood vessels and blood pressure. While those that affect the reuptake of NE (e.g., cocaine, desipramine, and its congeners, such as guanethidine and many H1 antihistaminics) have more influences on cardiac rate and rhythm.

When NE passes through pulmonary circulation, then 25% of circulating NE is removed by lung tissues, while EPI and dopamine passes unchanged. However, the functional significance of this removal of NE by pulmonary vasculature is not known. This effect may also account for some of the

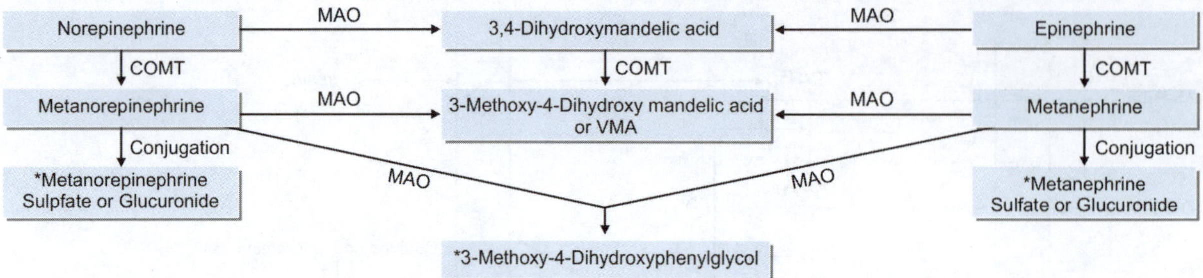

Fig. 14: Metabolism of catecholamines. (VMA: vanilyl-mandelic acid)

differences which is clinically observed in right-sided versus left-sided infusions of vasopressors. Pulmonary hypertension also accounts for diminution of NE uptake.

Uptake-2: After release in synaptic cleft, the inactivation of NE also occurs by its (i) uptake through other tissue cells, (ii) enzymatic breakdown in synaptic deft, and (iii) diffusion in interstitial fluid, followed by absorption by vasculature. These processes of uptake-2 of catecholamine are ubiquitous and are present in glial, hepatic, myocardial and other tissues. This has no physiological or pharmacological importance. It is not inhibited by uptake-1 inhibitors (cocaine, imipramine, fluoxetine, etc.).

Metabolism of catecholamines:

The pathways of metabolism of catecholamines are depicted in **Figure 14**. During storage, release, and reuptake of catecholamines at nerve endings, a small amount always escapes and enters the circulation. In the circulation, NE is metabolized by mono-amino-oxidase (MAO) and catecholamine-o-methyl-transferase (COMT) enzyme very rapidly. So, inhibition of MAO by MAOI greatly increases the sympathetic function. The metabolism of catecholamine also occurs in the intestine and kidney. EPI liberated from adrenal medulla is also metabolized by same pathway. The final product of both NE and EPI metabolism is 3-methoxy-4-hydroxy-mandelic acid or vanilyl-mandelic acid (VMA) which are excreted through urine. The other major metabolites, excreted through the urine, are 3-methoxy-4-hydroxy-phenylglycol, along with some normetanephrine and metanephrine. These metabolites are mostly conjugated with glucuronic acid or sulfate, before excretion through urine. Only 25–50 µg of NE and 2–5 µg of EPI are excreted in free form in 24 hours urine. However, the metabolism of NE and EPI by MAO and COMT in circulation does not play an important role in terminating the action of catecholamines, liberated at nerve terminal. Very quick reuptake of NE and EPI from synaptic cleft and store into vesicles and little metabolism by these two catabolic enzymes account for the efficient clearance of catecholamines, liberated at nerve terminal.

Due to this rapid clearance of catecholamines (NE and EPI) from circulation by MAO and COMT, the half-life of most of the biogenic amines or NE and EPI in plasma is very short which is <1 minute. So, the very short half-life of these catecholamines necessitates their administration by infusion. Another consequence of short half-life of these catecholamines is that their production in our body cannot be measured by their plasma level, rather by the measurement of metabolic products of these catecholamines. For example, the screening of NE producing pheochromocytoma is done by frequently measuring the plasma or urine level of VMA, but not the plasma level of NE **(Fig. 14)**.

Cholinergic Neurotransmitters

Acetylcholine is the cholinergic neurohumoral transmitter and occupies the major portion of autonomic as well as somatic synapses. The sites of synthesis of this cholinergic neurotransmitter and the description of its receptors are discussed before. So, here, we will discuss only the mechanism of synthesis, storage, and the inactivation of ACh.

Synthesis of Acetylcholine

Acetylcholine is synthesized intraneurally from choline (the source of which is described below) and acetyl CoA (formed during the metabolism of glucose, fat, and amino acid) by the enzyme, named *cholineacetyl transferase (ChAT)* situated into mitochondria. The ChAT enzyme, like other protein constituents of neuron, is synthesized within perikaryon (cell body of neuron) and then is transported along the length of axon to its terminal. Axon terminals also contain a large number of mitochondria, where acetyl CoA is synthesized from the metabolism of glucose, fat, and protein.

The sources of choline which is another component of ACh includes:

- Dietary choline – a type of phospholipid.
- Hepatic synthesis of phosphatidylcholine from dietary precursors, such as ethanolamines
- Choline, released by hydrolysis from previously synthesized ACh.

Among these three sources, the hepatic source for choline is the major and most important. After synthesis in liver, the choline is transported as phospholipid to nerve terminal through circulation and is actively taken up by a high affinity transport system, situated on the neuroaxonal membrane. This hepatic synthesis of choline appears to be largely responsible for determining the levels of ACh at nerve terminals. The level of circulating choline in blood also affects the amount of ACh, released from nerve terminals, particularly when the rapid firing (discharge of electrical impulses) takes place at cholinergic motor neurons. There is also some evidence that the availability of precursor for the synthesis of ACh may limit the cholinergic activity.

It is found that despite the presence of high density of choline-acetyl-transferase enzyme (ChAT) in brain tissues, choline itself is not produced there, but is transported from outsources. So, research is going on to develop choline analogs to enhance the neural transmission in brain and to treat Alzheimer's disease.

Choline, after entering into nerve cell, binds with acetyl-coenzyme A, which is present within the cell on the surface of an enzyme, named choline-acetyl-transferase (ChAT). This enzyme facilitates the condensation of choline with the acetyl group of acetyl CoA. Thus, ACh and CoA are produced. After synthesis, ACh is rapidly packed up into vesicles for immediate release during proper stimulation. ChAT enzyme also catalyzes the reaction in a reverse direction between the ACh and CoA producing choline and acetyl CoA, but at a much slower rate than the forward direction **(Fig. 15)**.

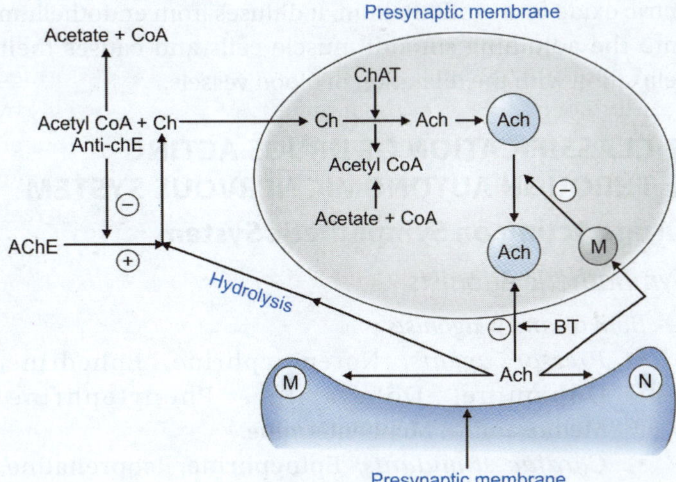

Fig. 15: Cholinergic neuronal transmission. (ACh: acetylcholine; AChE: acetylcholine esterase; Anti-chE: anticholine esterase; BT: botulinus toxin; Ch: choline; ChAT: choline acetyl transferase; H: chemicolinium; M: muscarinic receptor; N: nicotinic receptor)

Storage and Release of Acetylcholine

After synthesis, ACh is rapidly packed in synaptic vesicles at nerve terminals which are called the quanta. It has been calculated that a single motor nerve terminal contains near about 3,00,000 vesicles or quanta. In addition, an uncertain but possibly a significant amount of ACh is also present in extravesicular cytoplasm. When an action potential reaches the nerve ending, then ACh is released from the vesicle into synaptic cleft by the same mechanism as adrenergic neurotransmitters, but at fixed presynaptic release sites (active zone) which are located opposite to the shoulders of the folding of postjunctional membrane. At first, the quantas or vesicles, containing ACh, move toward these specific release sites or active zone of presynaptic membrane which is influenced by the influx of Ca^{2+} like adrenergic transmission and fuse with presynaptic membrane. Then, the fluidization of vesicular and synaptic membranes occurs and throws out their contents into synaptic cleft and on postsynaptic membrane receptors.

Inactivation of Acetylcholine

After release into synaptic cleft, ACh is rapidly broken down by hydrolysis into choline and acetate. But, neither of these metabolites have significant pharmacological actions. This hydrolysis of ACh is catalyzed by an enzyme called *cholinesterase*. There are two most important types of cholinesterases, present in our body. These are tissue cholinesterase or *true cholinesterase* and butyryl or *pseudocholinesterase*.

The tissue or true acetylcholinesterase is a postsynaptic-membrane-bound enzyme which is present at all the cholinergic synapses and destroys the ACh neurotransmitter, after it is released from presynaptic membrane. It is called the "true cholinesterase" or "tissue cholinesterase", because it does not circulate in plasma. It is also found in tissues that are not innervated by nerves, e.g., erythrocytes. But, here its function is not exactly known.

Butyryl or cholinesterase is also called the "plasma cholinesterase" or "pseudocholinesterase" and is found in plasma. It is synthesized in liver and circulates into blood. Its function in plasma in a normal healthy person is not known and the individuals who are genetically incapable of synthesizing these enzymes are normal in all other regards. Only its importance lies in the destruction of some cholinergic drugs, e.g., succinylcholine which is used as muscle relaxant during anesthesia and is not destroyed by tissue cholinesterase or true cholinesterase.

The molecule of true or pseudocholinesterase has two areas: (i) an anionic site which carries a strong *negative charge* and (ii) an esteric site which contains electrophilic amino acids. ACh molecule has a *positive charge* at its quaternary nitrogen atom. During hydrolysis, the positive charge of ACh is attracted by the negative charged site of enzyme (true cholinesterase) and is attached there. Then, an electrophilic attack on the molecule of ACh occurs and the acetate link is transferred from the choline of ACh to the amino acid site of enzyme. After that the choline which is attached, by its positive charge quaternary nitrogen atom, to the negatively charged anionic site of cholinesterase enzyme drifts away, leaving only the acetylated cholinesterase enzyme (because acetate of ACh is already attached with the amino acid site of enzyme). The acetate link on the acetylated cholinesterase enzyme is subsequently attacked and broken down by a hydroxyl group forming water. After that the acetate also drifts away from the cholinesterase enzyme and the regenerated free enzyme becomes again ready to interact with another molecule of ACh.

Inhibition of cholinesterase enzyme prevents the destruction of ACh in cholinergic synapses and subsequently prolongs its action (both muscarinic and nicotinic action) in all the cholinergic systems.

Characteristics of Cholinergic Transmission at Various Sites

The characteristics of cholinergic transmission are not same in different tissues. There are marked differences of cholinergic transmission at various sites. The examples are:

Skeletal muscle: The attachment of ACh molecule with nicotinic (N_M) cholinergic receptor situated at postsynaptic endplate membrane of skeletal muscle causes marked increase in the permeability of Na^+ cations through it, due to the opening of receptor channels. This results in localized depolarization within the endplate (EPP) which triggers the skeletal muscle action potential and contraction.

Cholinergic autonomic nerve endings: Here, the ACh molecule, as first messenger, acts through muscarinic (M) receptor and causes the stimulation or inhibition of autonomic effector cells (smooth muscles and glands) by acting through muscarinic receptor → G protein → effector system or second messenger complex, such as AC and phospholipase-C. In contrast to skeletal muscles, all the cardiac and smooth muscles have their own intrinsic electrical activity. Here, the cholinergic transmission only modulates the intrinsic electrical activity of cardiac and smooth muscles, but does not initiate any new impulse or action potential. In intestinal smooth muscles, the site of pacemaker activity continuously changes. But, in heart this spontaneous depolarization normally arises from the SA node. Under pathological conditions, when SA node activity is depressed, then a new pacemaker activity can arise from any part of conduction system, as all of them have the intrinsic electrical activity. In basal conditions, the individual cell of SA node shows the waves of depolarization. Cholinergic transmission causes the inhibition of this spontaneous depolarization of the cell of SA node by causing hyperpolarization of cell membrane. These effects are, at least in part, due to selective increase in the permeability of K^+ ion.

Autonomic ganglia: The primary pathway of cholinergic transmission in autonomic ganglia is similar to that of neuromuscular junction of skeletal muscles, i.e., through nicotinic (N_N) receptors. Several secondary neurotransmitters or modulators either enhance or diminish the sensitivity of the postsynaptic membrane of ganglionic cells to ACh. But, this sensitivity appears to be related to the membrane potential of postsynaptic nerve's cell body or its dendritic branches.

Action of ACh on presynaptic sites: The action of ACh neurotransmitters on presynaptic cholinergic receptors appear to be present on sympathetic vasoconstrictor or adrenergic nerves. Activation of these presynaptic cholinergic receptors by ACh causes the inhibition of further release of NE and produces vasodilatation. But, practically the cholinergic innervation of blood vessels is limited. So, the clinical dilatation of blood vessels in response to the administration of ACh involves a separate mechanism which includes the presynaptic inhibition of NE release. The vasodilator effect of ACh requires an intact layer of endothelium in blood vessels. The activation of this presynaptic muscarinic ACh receptors results in the liberation of special vasodilator substances, called the endothelium derived relaxing factor (EDRF) or nitric oxide from endothelium. It diffuses from endothelium into the adjoining smooth muscle cells and causes their relaxation with the dilatation of blood vessels.

CLASSIFICATION OF DRUGS ACTING THROUGH AUTONOMIC NERVOUS SYSTEM

Drugs Acting on Sympathetic System

Sympathetic Agonists

a. *Both α- and β-agonists*
   - *Pressor agents:* Norepinephrine, Ephedrine, Dopamine, Dobutamine, Phenylephrine, Methoxamine, Mephentermine.
   - *Cardiac stimulants:* Epinephrine, Isoprenaline, Dobutamine.
   - *Bronchodilators:* Isoprenaline, Salbutamol (Albuterol), Salmeterol, Formeterol, Terbutaline, Bambuterol.

- *Nasal decongestants:* Phenylephrine, Xylometazoline, Oxymetazoline, Naphazoline, Pseudoephedrine, Phenyl propanolamine.
- *CNS stimulant:* Amphetamine, Methylamphetamine, Dexamphetamine, Methylphenidate.
- *Anorectics:* Amphetamine, Fenfluramine, Dexfenfluramine, Sibutramine.
- *Uterine relaxant and vasodilators:* Ritodrine, Isoxspurine, Salbutamol, Terbutaline.

b. *Selective α_1 agonists:* Phenylephrine and Methoxamine.
c. *Selective α_2 agonists:* Clonidine, Dexmedetomidine, Apraclonodine, Guanfacine, Guanabenz, Tizanidine, Brimonidine.

Sympathetic Antagonists (Blockers)

a. *A-receptor antagonists:*
   i. *Noncompetitive type:* Phenoxybenzamine.
   ii. *Competitive type:*
      1. *Nonselective: Ergot alkaloids: Ergitamine,* Ergotoxine.
         Hydrogenated ergot alkaloids: Dihydroergotamine, Dihydroergotoxine.
         Imidazoline: Phentolamine.
         Miscellaneous: Chlorpromazine.
      2. *α_1 selective:* Prazosin, Terazosin, Doxazosin, Alfuzosin, Tamsulosin, Silodosin.
      3. *α_2 selective:* Yohimbine.
b. *B-receptor antagonists:*
   i. *Nonselective (β_1 and β_2):*
      1. Without intrinsic sympathomimetic activity: Propanolol, Sotalol, Timolol.
      2. With intrinsic sympathomimetic activity: Pindolol.
      3. With additional α blocking property: Labetalol, Carvedilol.
   ii. *Cardioselective (β_1):* Atenolol, Metoprolol, Acebutolol, Bisoprolol, Esmolol, Nevibolol. Celiprolol, Betaxolol.

Drugs Acting on Parasympathetic System

Parasympathomimetics

a. *Cholinergic agonist:*
   i. *Choline ester:* Acetylcholine, methacholine, carbachol, and bethanechol.
   ii. *Alkaloids:* Muscarine, pilocarpine, and arecoline
b. *Anticholinesterase:*
   i. *Reversible:*
      1. *Carbamates:* Neostigmine, physostigmine, pyridostigmine, rivastigmine.
      2. *Noncarbamates:* Edrophonium, tacrine, donepezil, and galantamine.

   ii. *Irreversible:*
      1. *Carbamates:* Carbaryl, propoxur.
      2. *Organophosphates:* Malathion, echothiophate, dyflos, diazinon, parathion.

Antiparasympathetics

a. *Muscarinic receptor blockers (Anticholinergics):*
   i. *Natural alkaloids:* Atropine and hyoscine.
   ii. *Semisynthetic:* Homatropine, ipratropium, tiotropium, atropine methonitrate, and hyoscine butylbromide.
   iii. *Synthetic:*
      1. *Mydriatics:* Cyclopentolate and tropicamide.
      2. *Antispasmodics and antisecretory:* Glycopyrrolate, propantheline, aclidinium, pipenzolate, oxyphenonium, isopropamide, dicyclomine, ipratropium, and tiotropium.
      3. *Vasoselective:* Flavoxate, tolterodine, darifenacin, and solifenacin.
      4. *Antiparkinsonian:* Trihexyphenidyl (Benzhexol), procyclidine, and biperiden.
b. *Nicotinic-receptor blockers:*
   i. *Neuromuscular blockers:* Tubocurarine, pancuronium, atracurium, rocurium, and vecuronium.
   ii. *Ganglion blockers:* Hexamethonium, pentolinium, and trimethaphan.

■ CATECHOLAMINES

The parent structure of all the sympathomimetic agents is β-phenyl-ethyl amine which includes a benzene ring and an ethylamine side chain. When the 3rd and 4th position of this benzene ring is substituted by a hydroxyl group (–OH), then this benzene ring is called the *catechol ring* and the β-phenyl-ethyl amine is called the dihydroxy phenylethylamine which is known as catecholamines. The catecholamines which are found naturally in our body are called the *endogenous* catecholamines. They are NE (norepinephrine), EPI (epinephrine), and dopamine. The synthetic sympathomimetic agents, such as isoproterenol, dobutamine, etc. also have similar structure like that of endogenous catecholamines. So, they are called the *non-endogenous* (or *exogenous)* catecholamines. There are other sympathomimetic agents which structures are not like catecholamines. So, they are called the *noncatecholamine sympathomimetic* agents. Some examples of this type of drugs are metaproterenol, albuterol, terbutaline, methoxamine, phenylephrine, mephentermine, metaraminol, etc. **(Fig. 16)**.

Due to hydroxyl group, sympathomimetic agents of catecholamine group are quickly metabolized by COMT. But, the absence of –OH group in noncatecholamine

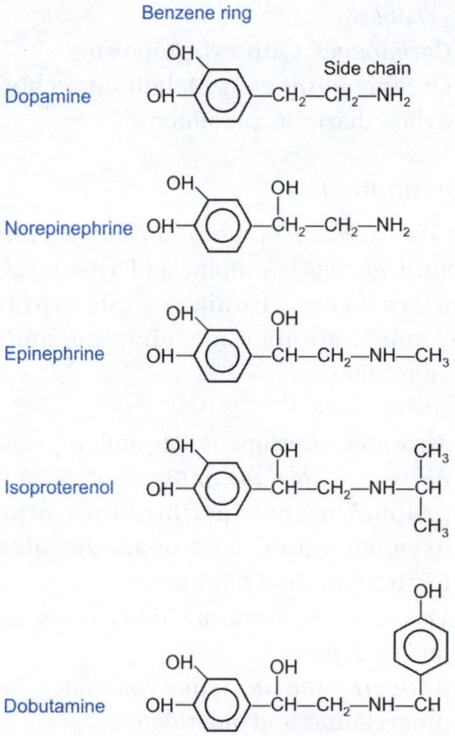

Benzene ring

Side chain

Dopamine

Norepinephrine

Epinephrine

Isoproterenol

Dobutamine

Fig. 16: Structures of some common catecholamines. The catechol nucleus is formed by a benzene ring with two adjacent hydroxyl groups.

sympathetic agents increases their oral effectiveness and duration of action, as they are not metabolized by COMT. They are primarily metabolized by MAO. Noncatecholamine sympathetic agents, that have a substituted α-carbon, have a longer duration of action. This is because they are not metabolized by either COMT or MAO.

Endogenous Catecholamines

Epinephrine (Adrenaline)

The effects of an endogenous catecholamine such as epinephrine (EPI) on its target organs are complex, as it is a potent stimulant of both α_1, α_2 and β_1, β_2 adrenergic receptors. Its particular and prominent actions are found on heart than the vascular and other smooth muscles, although the occurrence of sweating, piloerection, and mydriasis, produced by EPI, depend on the physiological state of a subject. The most potential therapeutic effects of EPI include its positive inotropic effects (β_1), positive chronotropic effects (β_1), enhanced conduction in heart (β_1), smooth muscle relaxation in vascular and bronchial tree (β_2) and peripheral vasoconstriction of resistance vessels (α_1). Various effects of EPI at different sites are:

a. Blood pressure:

EPI is one of the most potent vasopressor agents. On rapid intravenous injection, BP rises rapidly which is proportional to the dose. The increase in systolic pressure is greater than the increase in diastolic pressure.

The mechanisms of rise of BP due to epinephrine and due to its IV administration are:

i. Positive inotropic action—direct myocardial stimulation that increases the force of ventricular contraction.

ii. Positive chronotropic action—increases in heart rate.

iii. Constriction of vascular smooth muscles, particularly precapillary resistance vessels of skin, muscle, mucosa, kidney, and veins.

Initially HR increases, but later it slows down markedly which is proportional to the height of the rise of blood pressure. This is due to compensatory vagal discharge.

On small doses of 0.1 μg/kg through IV, EPI reduces blood pressure and this is due to only β_2 receptor stimulant effect of EPI. But, in higher doses there is a biphasic response of EPI on BP (initially rises of BP, then falls). In higher doses, this biphasic response of EPI on BP is due to greater sensitivity of epinephrine to β_2-receptors in high doses which causes vasodilation than the α_1-receptor effect of it which cause vasoconstriction. The effects of EPI in doses as large as 0.5–1.5 mg through IV (10–30 μg/min) are rise in systolic BP due to increased cardiac contractile force and a rise in the cardiac output. But, the diastolic BP decreases due to the decrease in peripheral resistance, owing to the dominant action on β_2-receptors, causing vasodilatation than α_1-receptors of resistance vessels, causing vasoconstriction. Heart rate, stroke volume, CO, and left ventricular workload are all increased as a result of its direct cardiac stimulant effect and increased venous return to heart. At higher doses, the effects of EPI on peripheral resistance and diastolic pressure depends on the ratio between the amount of presence of α and β responses on the various vascular beds.

b. Vascular effects:

The site of action of EPI on vascular beds is at the smaller resistance arterioles and precapillary sphincters, but various vascular beds react differently. EPI markedly decreases cutaneous blood flow. However, in therapeutic doses, the blood flow to the skeletal muscle increases with EPI. This is due to its powerful and predominant vasodilating β_2-receptor action (β_1 is situated on heart). But, it is particularly counter-balanced by the vasoconstrictory α-receptor action (both α_1 and α_2). In such situations, if an α-adrenergic antagonist is given, then the vasodilatation effect of β_2-receptor predominates and SVR decreases, resulting in acute fall of mean blood pressure. Reversely, EPI increases blood pressure considerably, if the vasodilatation action of β_2-receptor is blocked by some nonselective β-blocker.

c. Cerebral blood flow:

The adrenergic receptors present on cerebral vascular bed is predominantly α_1 (vasoconstrictor). So, the therapeutic doses of EPI cause cerebral vasoconstriction. This is due to the direct effect of EPI on cerebral vessels. But, clinically, the main effect of EPI on cerebral circulation is conducted through the changes in systemic BP and not through these α_1 receptors, present on vascular bed. Again, the cerebral self or local autoregulatory mechanism tends to limit the increase in cerebral blood flow, caused by increase in systemic BP by EPI **(Table 12)**.

d. Renal effects:

Kidney has both the α_1, α_2 and β_1, β_2 adrenergic receptors. Here, the vasoconstrictor effect of α-receptor predominates much more over the vasodilatation action of β-receptor. So, the doses of EPI which cause little effect on mean arterial pressure, cause the tremendous decrease (40%) in renal blood flow due to a consistent increase in renal vascular resistance by the predominant $\alpha1$ action of EPI. In spite of this, GFR is slightly altered and filtration fraction is consistently increased. Its cause is discussed in details in renal chapter. Urine volume may be increased, decreased, or unchanged. Due to the direct effect of EPI on β_1-receptor

of juxta-glomerular apparatus, renin secretion is also increased.

e. Pulmonary effects:

Pulmonary vasculature contains both the α_1 (vasoconstriction) and β_2 (slight vasodilatation) receptors. Due to the predominant α_1 action of EPI on pulmonary vasculature, arterial and venous pulmonary pressure is raised. Still, clinically, the redistribution of blood from pulmonary circulation to systemic circulation does not occur. Rather, redistribution of blood from systemic to pulmonary circulation occurs and this is due to strong vasoconstriction action of more powerful musculature of systemic great veins. Therefore, the total effect is an increase in pulmonary vascular pressure. Thus, by the same mechanism epinephrine in higher concentration may precipitate pulmonary edema by elevating the pulmonary capillary filtration pressure.

f. Coronary circulation:

Coronary vessels contain α_1, α_2 and β_2 receptors (myocardium has β_1 receptors). Here, the vasodilatation action of β_2 receptors predominates over the vasoconstriction action of α receptors. So, coronary blood flow is increased by it or by cardiac sympathetic stimulation. Another mechanism of increased coronary blood flow by EPI is the elevated aortic blood pressure, caused by it. Epinephrine increases the strength of myocardial contraction (β_1 action) and O_2 consumption which also dilates the coronary vessels by their local metabolic effects. This local metabolic dilatation effect of EPI on coronary arteries is mediated by adenosine, released from cardiac myocytes due to hypoxia. Therefore, all these effects tend to overcome the direct coronary vasoconstriction effect of EPI that results from the activation of α receptor in coronary vessels.

g. Cardiac effects:

Heart muscles contain predominantly β_1 receptors. But, β_2 and α receptors are also present in minimum concentration. Therefore, EPI is a powerful myocardiac stimulant and acts mainly through β_1 receptors. It increases heart rate and often the sinus rhythm is altered. All the effects of EPI on cardiac tissue are largely secondary to this increase in heart rate. Because, when the HR is increased, then the duration of action potential is consistently shortened and the refractory period is correspondingly decreased. This increased heart rate by epinephrine is due to the acceleration of slow diastolic depolarization phase or phase 4 of action potential and also due to the increased rate of the rise of transmembrane potential to threshold level, at which point the action potential is triggered. The amplitude of AP and the maximal rate of the rise of depolarization (phase 0) are also increased. Cardiac systole becomes shorter and powerful.

TABLE 12: Comparison of effects of NE and EPI (Intravenous infusion).

Response	NE (norepinephrine)	EPI (epinephrine)
Cardiac responses		
Heart rate	↓ (A)	↑↑
Stroke volume	↓	↑↑
Cardiac output	0, ↓	↑↑↑
Arrhythmias	↑↑↑	↑↑↑
Coronary blood flow	↑↑	↑↑
Blood pressure		
Systolic	↑↑↑	↑↑↑
Diastolic	↑↑	↑0↓
Mean	↑↑	↑
Pulmonary	↑↑	↑↑
Peripheral circulation		
Systemic vascular resistance	↑↑	↑
Muscle blood flow	0, ↓	↑↑↑
Cerebral blood flow	0, ↓	↑
Renal blood flow	↓	↓
Cutaneous blood flow	↓	↓
Splanchnic blood flow	0, ↑	↑↑↑
Metabolic responses		
Blood glucose	0, ↑	↑↑↑
Blood lactic acid	0, ↑	↑↑↑
Oxygen consumption	0, ↑	↑↑↑

0 = No effect, ↓ = Decreased effect, ↑ = Increased effect, A = Increased after atropine.

CO increases. The workload of heart and O_2 consumption is also markedly increased by EPI. But, the cardiac efficiency which is determined by workload relative to O_2 consumption decreases. EPI also increases excitability and automaticity in the specialized tissues of heart. This is also due to the acceleration of slow diastolic depolarization phase of action potential. However, these changes in automaticity usually do not occur in the atrial and ventricular muscle fibers. These occur only in the cells of SA node.

Altered pacemaker activity due to increased automaticity by exogenous EPI is rarely seen with its conventional dose. But, ventricular extrasystole, tachycardia or even ventricular fibrillation may be precipitated by the release of small amount of endogenous epinephrine, when the heart has been sensitized by certain anesthetic agents or in case of MI.

EPI shortens the refractory period of AV nodal tissue and decreases the grade of AV block, which usually occurs by the effect of many diseases, drugs, and vagal stimulation.

Supraventricular arrhythmias may occur from the combination of action of epinephrine and cholinergic stimulation, if these two events occur at the same time due to any reason. Depression of sinus rate and AV conduction by vagal discharge probably plays a part in the EPI-induced ventricular arrhythmias. So, various drugs (e.g., atropine) that block the vagal effect confer some protection against EPI-induced ventricular arrhythmias. The action of EPI in enhancing cardiac automaticity, and causing arrhythmias are effectively antagonized by β-adrenergic receptor antagonist.

h. Bronchial smooth muscle:

Epinephrine has a powerful bronchodilating effect. This is particularly occurred when EPI is administered therapeutically during the acute exacerbation phase of bronchial asthma due to allergic response to various drugs and autacoids. In such situations, EPI has a striking therapeutic effect as a physiological antagonistic agent to the substances that cause bronchoconstriction. The beneficial effect of EPI in asthma also arises from the inhibition of antigen-induced release of inflammatory mediators from mast cells, and to a lesser extent from the diminution of bronchial secretions and congestion within the mucosa. The inhibition of bronchial smooth muscle constriction by EPI which is induced by mast cell secretion (release of inflammatory mediators) is mediated through the stimulation of β_2-adrenergic receptors and the effects EPI on bronchial mucosa (reduction of congestion) are mediated through the stimulation of α_1 adrenergic receptors.

i. Urinary bladder:

The detrusor muscle of urinary bladder is relaxed as a result of the activation of β-receptors by EPI. This causes retention of urine. Again, the α-agonistic activity of epinephrine results in the contraction of trigonal and sphincteric smooth muscles, causing hesitancy and retention of urine. The activation of smooth muscle contraction in prostate by EPI also promotes the urinary retention (α-receptor effect).

j. Effects on uterus:

The response of EPI on uterine muscle varies with species, phases of sexual (menstrual) cycles, state of gestation and the doses of drug given. During last month of pregnancy and parturition, epinephrine inhibits uterine tone and reduces its contraction which is mediated through its β_2-receptor agonistic action. So, β_2-selective agonists (ritodrine and terbutaline) have been commonly used to delay the premature labor by relaxing uterine musculature.

k. Gastrointestinal tract:

The effects of EPI on the smooth muscles of vascular system have more physiological importance than their effect on the smooth muscles of GI tract. In general, GI smooth muscle is relaxed by EPI and this effect is due to the activation of both α and β adrenergic receptors. Tone, frequency, and amplitude of intestinal contraction are all reduced. The stomach is usually relaxed, but the pyloric and ileocecal junction (sphincter) are contracted. However, these effects of EPI on gastrointestinal system depend on the preexisting tone of smooth muscles which is present there from before. If the tone of gastrointestinal tract (GIT) muscular is already high, then EPI causes better relaxation of the smooth muscle of GIT and vice versa.

l. CNS effects:

As the EPI is a polar compound, so it usually does not cross blood-brain barrier and does not enter CNS. Thus, it is not a powerful CNS stimulant. Hence, restlessness, headache, tremor, apprehension, etc. produced by EPI are all due to the secondary effects of it and its metabolites on CVS, skeletal muscle, and other systems. It is not due to the direct effect of epinephrine on CNS. Though EPI does not enter CNS, but some other sympathomimetic drugs can readily cross the blood-brain barrier and may produce these symptoms.

m. Metabolic effects:

The EPI increases the concentration of glucose and lactate in blood. It inhibits the secretion of insulin by its α_2-receptor action and stimulates the secretion of insulin by its β_2-receptor activation on islets of Langerhans. But, both of these actions are contradictory. However, the predominant effect of epinephrine on insulin secretion is inhibition and rise of blood-glucose concentration. Glucagon secretion is enhanced by the action of EPI on β-receptors, present on the α-cells of pancreatic islets. This also causes increased concentration of glucose in blood. The effect of EPI to stimulate glycogenolysis in most of the tissues involves β-receptor stimulation.

EPI raises the concentration of free-fatty acids in blood by stimulating β-receptors in adipocytes. This result is due to the activation of triglyceride lipase (due to the activation of β-receptors in adipocytes) in adipocytes which accelerates the breakdown of triglycerides to form free-fatty acids and glycerol. The plasma-renin activity is also increased by epinephrine (β1 effect). The serum K^+ concentration transiently rises (due to release from liver), following the administration of epinephrine. Later, a more prolonged decrease in K^+ concentration follows. Epinephrine administration increases the basal metabolic rate by 20–30%. So, in combination with cutaneous vasoconstriction (that the drug produces), pyrexia may result due to this increased metabolism by EPI.

n. Effects on secretory glands:

In most of the secretory glands of GI tract, EPI inhibits secretion. This is partly due to reduced blood flow in gland, caused by vasoconstriction and partly due to direct action of EPI on α and β receptors, situated on these glands. On lacrimal glands, it stimulates lacrimation (α-receptor action), but causes scanty mucous secretion from salivary glands. Sweating and pilomotor activity (α1-receptor) is minimal after systemic administration of epinephrine.

o. Effects on eye:

Mydriasis occurs during the systemic administration of EPI. It is due to the contraction of radial muscles of iris (α_1 action). But, it does not occur when the EPI is instilled in conjunctival sac. Because, it (EPI) penetrates the cornea poorly. Epinephrine also lowers the intraocular pressure, especially in wide angle glaucoma. However, the mechanism of this effect is not clear. But, both the reduced production of aqueous humor due to vasoconstriction and enhanced outflow due to mydriasis are the probable causes.

p. Skeletal muscle:

Directly EPI does not excite the contraction of skeletal muscle. But, indirectly it facilitates neuromuscular transmission. In ANS, the stimulation of presynaptic α-receptor by epinephrine causes the inhibition of release of ACh. In contrast, the stimulation of α-receptor by EPI at somatic motor neurons causes a more rapid increase in transmitter release. The greater physiological and clinical importance of EPI on skeletal muscle is its selective β_2 agonistic activity which causes physiological tremor. This is due to the β-receptor-mediated enhancement of discharge of impulses from muscle spindle.

Absorption, fate, and excretion: EPI is not effective by oral administration. This is because it is rapidly metabolized in the mucosa of GIT during its absorption by COMT and is rapidly metabolized in liver by MAO enzymes which are present there when circulates through portal circulation. Because of its local vasoconstriction effect, the absorption of epinephrine from subcutaneous tissues is also very slow. But, after intramuscular injection, the absorption of EPI is more rapid. In emergencies, EPI is always used through IV route. When EPI is used by inhalation or through nebulizer, then its action is largely restricted locally to respiratory tract. However, arrhythmia may also occur, if a large amount of EPI is used through this route.

Epinephrine is metabolized and inactivated by COMT and MAO enzyme which are present in all the body tissues, plasma, and liver. The liver is rich in both the enzymes and is particularly important in this regard.

Administration and preparations: Epinephrine is unstable in alkaline solutions. So, it is always prepared in acidic medium. It should always be protected from air and light. Because, in air and light, the EPI is oxidized to adrenochrome which then turns from pink to brown, due to the formation of its (adrenochrome) polymers.

EPI is used in different clinical conditions and through different routes, such as subcutaneous (most common), intravenous (during emergencies), inhalation and topical (specific). So, a variety of formulation of EPI, with different strength and concentration, are available in market for use through different routes. The epinephrine injection which are available in different strengths are 1:100 (10 mg/mL), 1:1,000 (1 mg/mL), 1:10,000 (0.1 mg/mL), 1:100,000 (10 µg/mL) and 1:200,000 (5 µg/mL). The patients vary tremendously in their response to catecholamines. Therefore, a patient's response should be carefully titrated with the doses of EPI when used through any route. During administration of EPI, appropriate measures should be taken to monitor the renal, cerebral, and myocardial perfusions which are more important than a rigid adherence to a theoretical dosing scheme. An infusion rate of 1–2 µg/min of EPI predominantly activates the β_2 adrenergic receptors, causing vascular and smooth muscle relaxation. On the other hand, a rate of 2–10 µg/min of EPI infusion activates both the β1 and β_2 receptors, causing an increased heart rate, conduction through AV node and contractility of heart. The dose of EPI in excess of 10 µg/min by infusion causes marked α-stimulation with resultant generalized vasoconstriction and ↑BP.

EPI is a potent renal vasoconstrictor, acting directly through stimulation of α-receptor and indirectly by stimulation, causing release of renin. So, to avoid renal ischemia, dopamine in renal dose is frequently combined with IV doses of epinephrine. The usual subcutaneous therapeutic dose of EPI in an adult is 0.3–0.5 mg. However, absorption of subcutaneous EPI is extremely slow. This is due to intense local subcutaneous vasoconstriction.

The effect of very large subcutaneous doses of epinephrine such as 0.5–1.5 mg is roughly equivalent to an intravenous infusion in the dose of 10–30 μg/min which can result in life-threatening ventricular arrhythmias, hypertension, and cerebral hemorrhage.

The normal dose of epinephrine by IV infusion during the management of hypotension or shock is 0.01–0.1 μg/kg/min which is titrated according to the response of patient. In emergency, the IV route for administration of EPI is preferred and the drug is used very slowly and very cautiously by diluting the solution. The IV dose of EPI seldom exceeds 0.25 mg, except in cardiac arrest, when large doses of it can be used (3–5 mg or more) according to the response of patient. In very emergency conditions such as asystole, VF, EMD, and anaphylactic shock the recommended dose of epinephrine is 0.5–1 mg/70 kg through IV. The aim of this higher dose of EPI is to maintain the myocardial and cerebral perfusion by increasing the mean arterial pressure through intense peripheral vasoconstriction. However, higher doses of EPI > 0.1 mg/kg also have been studied during the resuscitation of cardiac arrest, but do not appear to improve the rate of survival in adults. This higher dose of EPI is used only when the usual doses fail to respond. The endotracheal doses of EPI in emergency situations, when IV route is not available, should be at least double of the IV dose and is diluted in 10 mL of normal saline solution in adult patients. This is because epinephrine is well absorbed from tracheal mucosa. The 1% (1:100) formulation of EPI is only used for inhalation and should never be used for parenteral route. This is because inadvertent IV injection of 1:100 solution can be fatal. Inhaled EPI constricts edematous mucosa and may be used in the treatment of severe croup and traumatic airway edema. For inhalation, 1% solution of epinephrine is diluted with water or saline in 1:4 ratio and nebulized. This treatment can be repeated every 2 hours with effects lasting for 30–60 minutes.

Adverse effects and contraindications: EPI causes more or less serious adverse effects. Less serious, but common adverse effects of epinephrine are transient restlessness, palpitation, anxiety, tremors, throbbing headache, etc. On the other hand, more serious, but less frequent adverse effects are cerebral hemorrhage, angina, cardiac arrhythmias, etc. and all these are due to the large doses of EPI. The use of EPI is contraindicated in hypertensive, hyperthyroid, and angina patients. It should be given cautiously during halothane anesthesia and to patients who are receiving nonselective β-blockers. This is because its unopposed actions on vascular α_1-adrenergic receptor may lead to severe hypertension. Halothane is known to sensitize the heart to catecholamines (CAs). So, the dose of epinephrine should be limited to 1 μg/kg/30 min in presence of halothane and to 3 μg/kg/30

min in presence of isoflurane and sevoflurane. CAs decrease refractory period and thus renders the heart more susceptible to arrhythmias. Preexisting use of α_1-blockade can cause the paradoxical phenomenon of EPI reversal, because as the β_2-vasodilating effects are unmasked.

Therapeutic uses of EPI: EPI has limited therapeutic uses. But, its major use is to provide a rapid relief during hypersensitivity reactions including anaphylaxis, arising from drugs and other allergens. Its cardiac effects may be of use in restoring cardiac rhythm in patients with cardiac arrest. Other therapeutic uses of EPI are with local anesthetics or as topical hemostatic agents, or for inhalation in the treatment of postintubation or infectious croup **(Box 2)**.

When used with local anesthetic agents or applied locally on mucosal surfaces to stop bleeding, then α-receptor-mediated vasoconstrictive effect of EPI decreases bleeding in that area and slows vascular uptake of local anesthetic agents. Thus, it decreases the peak serum level of local anesthetic agent and prolongs its duration of action. Several studies have shown that elevation in the plasma levels of EPI after local application is relatively modest, but substantially less than the levels, seen during physiological stress.

Management of patient with suspected anaphylaxis: As soon as an anaphylaxis is suspected in a patient, it should be

---

BOX 2: A general protocol for management of suspected anaphylaxis.

- Suspected drugs, likely to cause anaphylaxis, should be stopped immediately.
- 100% O_2 should be given with maintenance of airway.
- Feet should be elevated with the patient lying flat.
  - Epinephrine should be used immediately. The recommended dose is 50–100 mg (0.05–0.1 mL of 1:1,000 solution) IV over 1 minute, for hypotension with titration for further doses, as required.
  - In patients with severe cardiovascular collapse, 0.5–1 mg (0.5–1 mL of 1:1,000) may be required intravenously, in divided doses by titration. This should be given at a rate of 0·1 mg/min, stopping when a response has been obtained.
  - Alternatively, epinephrine may be given im in a dose of 0.5–1 mg (0.5–1 mL 1:1,000) and may be repeated every 10 minutes according to the arterial pressure and pulse, until improvement occurs.
- Intravascular volume expansion with crystalloid or colloid should be started immediately.
- As a secondary measure, corticosteroids (100–300 mg hydrocortisone IV) and antihistamines (chlorpheniramine 10–20 mg by slow IV) are also given.
- Catecholamine infusion is started:
  - *Epinephrine:* 0.05–0.1 mg/kg/min
  - *Norepinephrine:* 0.05–0.1 mg/kg/min
- Sodium bicarbonate can be considered for acidosis (0.5–1m.mol/kg IV)
- Bronchodilators may be required, if there is bronchospasm.

controlled by the following basic steps, which are given in **Box 2**.

Norepinephrine

Norepinephrine differs structurally from epinephrine by lacking the methyl substitution in amino group and is the major neurotransmitter among all the postganglionic adrenergic nerve endings. Normally, in adrenal medulla NE constitutes about 10–20% of its total catecholamine content. But, in pheochromocytoma, NE constitutes about 97% of its total catecholamine content in adrenal medulla. This is due to the lack of enzyme, named N-methyl transferase.

Like EPI, the NE is also a direct adrenergic agonist, stimulating both the adrenergic α and β receptors on effector cells. But, the action of NE depends mainly on the ratio of its effectiveness on α and β receptors. It is usually used for its potent α-agonism. NE is a potent agonist of α-receptors and has a relatively lesser action on β-receptors (than EPI). So, peripheral or systemic vascular resistance is tremendously raised by NE due to the constriction of resistance vessels (α_1-action > β_2-action) by it. This results in elevation of both systolic (β_1-action on heart, though less potent) and diastolic blood pressure (α_1-action on resistance vessel). Thus, pulse pressure is also increased. Cardiac output is unchanged or decreased (due to increase in systemic vascular resistance). Compensatory vagal reflex activity due to increased mean arterial pressure slows down the heart rate ($\downarrow$HR). The increased systemic vascular resistance causes reduction of blood flow in kidneys, mesenteric vessels, liver, and other splanchnic areas. Coronary blood flow is increased by NE due to local coronary vasodilatation (here β-action predominates over the α-action) and also due to elevated aortic pressure. Patients with Prinzmetal's variant angina may be supersensitive to α-adrenergic vasoconstrictor effects of NE. Unlike EPI, small doses of NE do not cause vasodilatation (in low doses, β-action of EPI predominates over α-action and the vessels dilate and cause reduction in BP) and does not reduce blood pressure. The α-adrenergic blocking agents, therefore, abolish the pressor effects of NE, but do not cause significant hypotension in low doses.

Other effects of NE, such as on bronchial muscles, mast cells, mucosa, eye, uterus, etc. are like EPI, but are not prominent in human beings. This is because these are observed only when much larger doses of NE are given than EPI. So, NE is mainly considered as a pressor agent and is not considered as an effective "hormone"-like epinephrine.

Like epinephrine, NE is also not effective when given orally. It is also poorly absorbed through subcutaneous route. It is rapidly metabolized in our body by COMT and MAO enzymes like EPI. Therefore, due to its short half-life of 25 minutes, a continuous infusion of NE is recommended. With <2 µg/min of infusion dose, the β stimulation effect of NE predominates. While with the usual infusion rate of >3 µg/min, peripheral vasoconstriction is elicited from α stimulation of NE. Small amount of metabolites of NE are normally found in urine. But, in pheochromocytoma the concentration of metabolites of NE in urine is greatly increased.

The complications and contraindications of NE are similar to those of EPI. There is typical greater elevation of blood pressure by NE than EPI. The excessive doses can cause severe hypertension. So, careful monitoring of blood pressure is generally indicated during systemic administration of this agent. Blood pressure must be determined frequently during infusion and particularly during the adjustment of rate of infusion. Reduced blood flow to the organs, such as the kidney and intestine, impose a constant danger to these organs, during the use of NE. So, to ameliorate these renal effects, low dose of dopamine infusion also can be added to NE infusion. Pulmonary vascular resistance may be increased, so NE should be used with caution in patients with pulmonary hypertension. During IV infusion of NE, extravasation of drug can cause necrosis and sloughing of tissues **(Table 13)**

Like EPI, the NE has also limited therapeutic use. Like other sympathomimetic amines, it is mainly used in shock to elevate blood pressure. In the treatment of hypotension, the

TABLE 13: Dose-dependent actions of adrenergic agents.

Drug	*Receptor*	*Dose of infusion*
Norepinephrine	α_1, β_1, >β_2	4–10 µg/kg/min (but much higher doses have been used in clinical practice)
Epinephrine	• β_2 • $\beta_1 + \beta_2$ • α_1 • Cardiac arrest	• 1–3 µg/kg/min • 2–10 µg/kg/min • >10 µg/kg/min • 0.5–1 mg IV (bolus)
Dobutamine	$\beta_1 > \beta_2$, α_1	3–10 µg/kg/min (but much higher doses have been used in clinical practice)
Dopamine	• D_1 • β_1 • α_1	• 1–3 µg/kg/min • 3–10 µg/kg/min • >10 µg/kg/min (or even higher doses)
Isoproterenol	$\beta_1 > \beta_2$	1–10 µg/min
Amrinone	Increase cAMP by PDE inhibition	0.75 mg/kg/loading dose over 2–3 minutes, followed by 5–10 g/kg/min infusion

dose of NE is titrated to the desired pressure response. *Dose:* 2–20 µg/min by IV infusion.

Dopamine

It has been discussed in detail in the chapter of heart failure. It is an endogenous, nonselective, direct, and indirect adrenergic and dopaminergic agonist. The clinical effects of dopamine vary markedly with its dose. It is always used as IV infusion. At low doses (0.5–3 µg/kg/min), DA primarily activates dopaminergic receptors (especially D-1) present on renal vasculature and dilates renal vessels. Thus, it causes diuresis and natriuresis. Although this low dose of DA increases renal blood flow, but actually this "renal dose" of DA does not impart any beneficial effect on kidney function. In moderate dose (3–10 µg/kg/min), DA causes β_1 receptor stimulation and increases myocardial contractility, heart rate, systolic BP, and CO. Myocardial O_2 demand increases more than its supply. In more higher doses (>10 µg/kg/min), DA stimulates α_1 receptor and increases vascular resistance by constricting vessels. This results in increase in BP and fall in renal blood flow. The indirect effect of DA is due to release of NE from presynaptic sympathetic nerve ganglion.

Previously, DA was used as a first-line drug for the treatment of shock to improve CO, BP, and renal blood flow (renal function). But, the chronotropic and proarrhythmic effects of it limit its usefulness. So, it has been replaced by NE for many situations in critical illness.

Fenoldopam

It is a selective D-1 receptor agonist. It has many of the benefits of DA. But, it has little or no α- and β-adrenoreceptors or D-2 receptor agonistic activity. Fenoldopam exerts an antihypertensive effect due to decrease of SVR (systemic vascular resistance), but helps to maintain renal blood flow. Therefore, it causes hypotension along with an increase in renal blood flow, diuresis, and natriuresis. It is mainly used for patients in hypertensive emergencies. It is also principally used for patients undergoing cardiac surgery and aortic aneurysm repair with potential risk of perioperative kidney impairment.

Fenoldopam has a fairly rapid onset of action and is easily titrable because of its short elimination half-life. It is used as continuous infusion and is started in the dose of 0.1 µg/kg/min. Then, this dose is increased by increments of 0.1 µg/kg/min at 15–20 minutes interval, until target BP is achieved.

■ ADRENERGIC AGONISTS

These include (i) endogenous, (ii) exogenous catecholamines, and (iii) noncatecholamine sympathetic amines. Among these the endogenous catecholamines are discussed before. Here, we will discuss only the exogenous catecholamines and noncatecholamine sympathetic amines which are adrenergic agonist.

β-Adrenergic Agonists

The β-adrenergic agonists play a major role in the treatment of heart block and bronchoconstriction such as in patients with asthma or COPD. At first, for many years epinephrine was used as a bronchodilator. Later, ephedrine was introduced, in 1924, as a bronchodilator. It has action on both α- and β-receptors, but the action of ephedrine on β-receptors is more prominent than α-receptors. Then, isoproterenol, a selective β-receptor agonist (both β_1 and β_2), without any α-adrenergic activity was developed, in 1940. The recent development of β_2-selective adrenergic agonist with minimum β_1 cardiovascular effect and lack of α-adrenergic activity has changed the total scenario of management of asthma. But, till now no selective β_1 agonist has been developed to control the cardiac problems. The drugs which are used as specific β_2 agonistic effect, but still in these groups of drugs β_1 effect is greater than β_2 effect.

The specific β_1-adrenergic agonists are used to stimulate the rate and force of cardiac contraction. The chronotropic effect of specific β_1-adrenergic agonist is useful in the emergency treatment of arrhythmias, such as torsades-de-pointes, bradycardia, heart block, etc. Whereas, the inotropic effect of specific β_1-adrenergic agonist is useful when it is desirable to augment the myocardial contractility.

Isoproterenol

It is a potent nonselective β-adrenergic agonist with very low affinity or almost no action on α-receptors. It has powerful effects on both β-receptors (β_1 and β_2), but its β_1-effect is significantly stronger than its β_2 effects. The intravenous infusion of isoproterenol, due to its prominent β_2-stimulating action, relaxes the vascular smooth muscles (β_2-receptor dilates and α_1-receptor constricts the vascular smooth muscles), primarily the blood vessels of skeletal muscles, but also of renal and mesenteric vascular beds and lowers SVR. So, diastolic pressure falls. But, systolic pressure is increased due to positive inotropic and chronotropic effects of it (β_1-stimulating action). CO is increased by isoproterenol, due to the positive chronotropic and inotropic actions, coupled with decreased SVR by it. Large doses of isoproterenol may lead to palpitation, sinus tachycardia, and more often serious arrhythmias. This is due to strong β_1 effect of it. So, due to the development of other safe inotropes, its popularity as inotropes has gradually declined, because of these side effects like tachycardia and serious arrhythmias. Further, myocardial O_2 demand increases, while O_2 supply falls, making isoproterenol or any pure β-agonists a poor inotropic choice in most situations.

Isoproterenol helps in asthma, not only by bronchial smooth muscle relaxation (β₂-action), but also by inhibiting the antigen-induced release of histamine and other inflammatory mediators due to inflammation. But, for many years in the treatment of bronchial asthma, isoproterenol has been replaced by other β₂-selective adrenergic agonists which cause lesser cardiac side effects.

During emergencies, isoproterenol is usually used parenterally by IV route (infusion rates at 0.5–10 µg/min for adults) to increase heart rate in patients, suffering from severe bradycardia on heart block, particularly in anticipation with implantation of cardiac pacemaker or in patients with ventricular arrhythmia like torsades-de-pointes. In the past, it has been used in the treatment of bradycardia or heart block which is resistant to atropine. But, now it is no longer a part of the "Advanced Life Support Protocol". It is readily absorbed when given by other parenteral routes, for example, as an aerosol, subcutaneous injection, etc. It is metabolized primarily in liver and other tissues by COMT. Isoproterenol is a relatively poor substrate for MAO and is not taken up by sympathetic nerve terminals to same extent as NE and EPI. The duration of action of isoproterenol is, therefore, longer than that of EPI, but is still brief.

Dobutamine

Dobutamine is a racemic mixture of its two isomers. It has affinity for both β₁ and β₂ receptors, but possesses higher selectivity for β₁ receptors. Therefore, for higher selectivity for β₁ receptors, its primary cardiovascular effect is rise in CO, as a result of increased myocardial contractility. A decline in peripheral vascular resistance, caused by β₂ activation by dobutamine, usually prevents much of rise in arterial BP, caused by increased cardiac contractility. Left ventricular filling pressure decreases, whereas coronary blood flow increases. Dobutamine is often used as cardiac inotropes. But, it increases myocardial O₂ consumption. So, it should not be used routinely without specific indications. It is often used in pharmacological stress testing. Dobutamine is administered as an infusion at a rate of 2–20 µg/kg/min. It has been discussed in more details in heart failure chapter along with dopamine.

β2-Selective Adrenergic Agonist

As already discussed, nonselective β-adrenergic agonist, used in the treatment of asthma, also causes the stimulation of β₁-adrenergic receptors in heart. So, the drugs with preferential affinity for β₂-receptors than β₁-receptors have been developed. However, this selectivity is not absolute and

at higher doses this preferentiality for β₂ than β₁ receptors becomes blurred. In addition, the β₂-receptor stimulation in SA node causes tachycardia.

The other aim to increase the usefulness of a selective β₂-receptor agonist in the treatment of asthma, by modifying the structure of it, is to lower the rates of metabolism of this drug and thus prolonging the therapeutic benefits and enhancing the oral bioavailability of it. This can be done by placing a hydroxyl group at position 3 and 5 or substituting another moiety for the hydroxyl group at position 3 of phenyl ring of β agonist. Thus, this results in drugs, such as metaproterenol, terbutaline, albuterol (salbutamol), etc. and these are not the substrates for COMT. Thus, the addition of a bulky structure to the amino group of catecholamine increases the β₂ selectivity, decreases the affinity for α-receptor, and protects it against metabolism by COMT.

The other strategy for enhancing the preferential β₂ receptor activity of these drugs is to administer them by inhalation. This activates only the β₂ receptor in airways and causes less systemic drug concentration. Thus, the less systemic drug concentration of β₂ agonist prevents the activation of cardiac β₁ receptors and skeletal muscle β₂ receptor (stimulation of β₂ receptor of skeletal muscle causes tremor and limits the oral therapy). The β₂ adrenergic agonists, given by aerosol, have very rapid therapeutic actions, generally within minutes (except salmeterol which has a delayed onset of action). The response to this aerosol therapy of bronchial asthma by β₂ receptor agonists depends on the technique of delivery of drugs to distal airways which in turn depends on (i) the size of the particles of drug in aerosol, (ii) inspiratory flow rates, (iii) tidal volume, (iv) breath-holding time, and (v) airway diameter. Only about 10% of inhaled dose actually enters the lungs. Much of the remainder of the drug is swallowed and ultimately is absorbed through stomach. The successful therapy of bronchial asthma by inhalation of β₂-adrenergic agonist requires each patient to be master regarding the inhalation technique of drug administration. Whereas, particularly the children and elders fail to use the optimum technique. So, in these patients, spacer devices enhance the efficacy of inhalation therapy.

Other than the activation of pulmonary β₂ receptors and decrease of airway resistance, the selective β₂ adrenergic agonists have other major therapeutic effects in bronchial asthma, such as (i) the suppression of the release of leukotrienes and histamine from mast cells in lung tissues, (ii) the enhancement of mucociliary function, (iii) the decrease in microvascular permeability, and (iv) the inhibition of phospholipase-A₂. It is becoming increasingly clear that airway inflammation is directly involved in airway hyperresponsiveness. So, the use of anti-inflammatory drugs, such as inhaled steroids may also have primary importance.

The adverse effects of selective β_2-adrenergic agonists are due to the additional excessive side activation of β_1-adrenergic receptors. Hence, in patients at risk of underlying cardiovascular diseases, this adverse effect can be reduced by administering the drug by inhalation, rather than orally or through other parenteral routes. Susceptibility to arrhythmia, caused by these selective β_2-agonistic agents, is due to the direct cardiac stimulation by β_1- or by β_2-induced hyperkalemia. Skeletal muscle tremor (β_2 effect) is a relatively common adverse effect of β_2-selective adrenergic agonist. However, tolerance generally develops to this effect, but it is not clear whether this tolerance is due to the desensitization of β_2 receptors on skeletal muscles or adaptation in CNS. Tachycardia is another common adverse effect of β_2-adrenergic agonists and is primarily due to the β_1 receptor stimulation of heart. It is still uncertain, to what extent the increase in heart rate is due to the activation of cardiac β_1 receptor or is due to the reflex effect that stems from the β_2-receptor mediated peripheral vasodilatation. However, during severe asthmatic attack, the HR may actually decrease during the therapy with β_2-adrenergic agonist and it is due to the improvement of pulmonary function with the consequent reduction of endogenous cardiac sympathetic stimulation. In patients with cardiac diseases, β_2-adrenergic agonists rarely cause significant arrhythmias or myocardial ischemia. But, the patients with underlying coronary artery disease or preexisting arrhythmias are at greater risk. The risk of adverse cardiovascular effects also increases in patients who are receiving other sympathomimetic drugs or MAO inhibitors.

The long-term systemic administration of β_2-adrenergic agonists leads to downregulation of this β_2 receptor and decreases its pharmacological responses. Chronic use of these drugs may also increase airway hyperactivity. However, it appears that the tolerance to the pulmonary effect of these drugs is not a major clinical problem for majority of the asthmatic patients who do not exceed the recommended dosage of the β_2-adrenergic agonist and when given by inhalation.

When given parenterally, the selective β_2-adrenergic agonists may increase the concentration of plasma glucose, lactate, and free fatty acid level. Plasma K^+ concentration is increased and it may be especially important in patients with cardiac disease, particularly those taking cardiac glycosides and diuretics. Therefore, hyperglycemia may be worsened by these drugs and higher doses of insulin may be required. All these adverse effects of selective β_2 agonists are far less likely with the inhalation route than with the oral or other parenteral routes.

The examples of some β_2-selective adrenergic agonists are metaproterenol (orciprenaline), albuterol (salbutamol), fenoterol, formoterol, salmeterol, isoetharine, terbutaline, etc.

Metaproterenol

Though metaproterenol is a selective β_2-adrenergic agonist, but less selective than terbutaline and albuterol (salbutamol). It is resistant to methylation by COMT. So, it is absorbed in the active form after oral administration. Effects occur within minute of inhalation of metaproterenol and persists for several hours. However, after oral administration the onset of action is slower and its effects last for 3–4 hours.

Albuterol (Salbutamol)

It is also a selective β_2-adrenergic agonist and all the pharmacological actions of it are similar to that of terbutaline. It may be administered by inhalation or orally. When administered by inhalation, it produces significant bronchodilatation effect within 15 minutes and this action lasts for 3–4 hours. The CVS effects of salbutamol are considerably weaker than those of isoproterenol when the equivalent doses that produce comparable bronchodilatation are administered by inhalation.

Terbutaline

It is also a β_2-selective adrenergic agonist and is not a substrate for methylation by COMT. It can be administered orally or by inhalation or by parenteral (subcutaneous) routes. Effects are very rapid after inhalation or subcutaneous injection. After inhalation, the action of terbutaline persists for 3–6 hours. With oral administration, the onset of action is delayed by 1–2 hours.

α_1-Selective Adrenergic Agonists

The action of α_1-adrenergic receptors is predominant on vascular smooth muscles (though both α_1 and α_2 receptors are present on vascular smooth muscle) and activation of both α_1 and α_2 receptors causes vasoconstriction, causing increased systemic vascular resistance (SVR) and increased BP. So, the α_1-adrenergic agonists are useful in the treatment of hypotension and shock, and where the peripheral vasoconstriction is needed, as in the treatment of hypotension in spinal anesthesia. Phenylephrine and methoxamine are directly acting selective α_1-adrenergic agonists. Whereas, the mephentermine and metaraminol are both the directly and indirectly acting selective α_1-adrenergic agonists. The indirect action means, "a portion of the effect of the drug is mediated through the release of endogenous norepinephrine".

Methoxamine

It is a selective and directly acting α_1-adrenergic agonist and increases the SVR and BP. It has no action on β-adrenergic receptors and does not cause cardiac stimulation. The increase in BP is associated with reflex sinus bradycardia. This is because of the activation of vagal reflexes. So, the atropine can counteract this bradycardia. Methoxamine is administered through IV in the treatment of hypotension and shock.

Phenylephrine

It is also a directly-acting selective α_1-adrenergic agonist. But, at very high concentrations, it may also activate the β receptors. The pharmacological actions of phenylephrine are similar to those of methoxamine and are used by intravenous infusion to raise BP. When given intravenously, the phenylephrine has a rapid onset and relatively short duration of action (5–10 min). It may be given by bolus doses of 40–100 µg or by infusion at a starting rate of 10–20 µg/min. Phenylephrine is also used as a mydriatic, nasal decongestant, and with local anesthetics for local vasoconstriction.

Mephentermine

It acts by both directly and indirectly stimulating the adrenergic α_1 and β_1 receptors. Direct stimulation means, mephentermine produces both cardiac stimulation and vasoconstriction by directly activating α_1 (predominant) and β_1 (lesser extent) adrenergic receptors. Indirect stimulation means, it acts by releasing the endogenous norepinephrine (NE). It enhances the cardiac contraction and increases CO. Both the systolic (due to enhanced cardiac contraction and CO) and diastolic blood pressure (due to peripheral vascular constriction and increase in SVR) are increased. The ultimate increase or decrease in CO depends on the increase in afterload and preload caused by mephentermine. If SVR increases tremendously, then CO may fall. In hemorrhagic shock, naturally as a compensatory mechanism, there is an increase in SVR and in the force of cardiac contraction due to the release of large amount of endogenous CAS. But, still, the CO falls and this is due to the severe reduction of preload reflecting severe hypotension. In spinal anesthesia, there is reduction of SVR (afterload) which may increase the CO. On the other hand, the reduction of venous return (preload) may decrease the CO. But, the ultimate reflection of hypotension in spinal anesthesia is due to ⁻SVR, ⁻preload, and ↓CO. If the reduction of BP is not much below the level of 20% of MAP, then in such situations there is a definite increase in CO, due to ⁻SVR only (after load). But, this small fall of BP is due to the slight reduction of

TABLE 14: Adrenergic agonists and their receptors.	
Epinephrine (EPI)	α_1, α_2, β_1, and β_2 (no β_3 action or weak)
Norepinephrine (EPI)	α_1, α_2, β_1, and β_3 (no β_2 action or weak)
Isoprenaline	β_1, β_2, and β_3 (no α action)
Dopamine	D, β_1, and α_1 (Dopamine receptor-D, predominates)
Dobutamine	α_1, β_1, and β_2 (β_1 predominates)
Salbutamol	β_1 and β_2 (β_2 predominates)
Methoxamine	α_1 and β_1 (α_1 predominates)
Phenylephrine	α_1
Mephentermine	α_1 and β_1 (α_1 predominates)
Metaraminol	α_1 and β_1 (α predominates over β)

preload, which is not up to that extent causing the reduction of CO and severe hypotension. So, mephentermine is used to prevent hypotension which frequently accompanies spinal anesthesia, in titrable doses to keep the BP at preoperative level or within 20–25% of MAP **(Table 14)**.

The direct positive chronotropic effect of mephentermine on heart is generally counterbalanced by the indirect vagal stimulation due to the rise in mean BP. So, the change in HR is variable, depending on the degree of vagal tone which again depends on BP. All the adverse effects of mephentermine are related to the excessive rise of BP causing LVF, pulmonary edema, etc. and arrhythmia (β_1 effect).

Mephentermine is not a substrate for either MAO or COMT. So, it is orally active with longer duration of action (2–6 hours). It can cross the blood-brain barrier partially and so produce excitatory CNS effects at higher doses. During the treatment of hypotension, the dose of mephentermine is usually titrated according to the fall of BP. It is presented as 15 mg in 1 mL amp or 3 mg/mL in 10 mL vial. Mephentermine is now used mainly to prevent and treat hypotension due to spinal anesthesia.

Metaraminol

Metaraminol is a synthetic sympathomimetic amine. Like mephentermine, it is also a direct and indirect-acting adrenergic agent and has agonistic effects on both α- and β-adrenoreceptors, although the α agonistic activity predominates. So, its main action is peripheral vasoconstriction.

Metaraminol causes a sustained increase in systolic and diastolic blood pressure due to the increase in SVR and CO. But, the increase or decrease of CO depends on the elevation of SVR and preload. It also increases the pulmonary vascular resistance. Like mephentermine, a reflex bradycardia also occurs with rise of BP. Like epinephrine the coronary blood flow is increased by metaraminol by an indirect mechanism.

It causes a slight decrease in respiratory rate and an increase in tidal volume. The cerebral blood flow is decreased by the administration of metaraminol. The renal blood flow is also decreased by it due to the renal vasoconstriction. This drug may cause the contraction of pregnant uterus.

Metaraminol increases the glycogenolysis and inhibits the release of insulin, leading to hyperglycemia. Lipolysis is similarly increased by it. The drug may also increase the O_2 consumption and body temperature.

Like mephentermine, metaraminol also causes CNS stimulation and produces headache, dizziness, tremor, nausea, and vomiting. Rapid and large increase in blood pressure, resulting in LVF and cardiac arrest have also been reported after the administration of metaraminol.

Metaraminol is mainly used by intravenous infusion, diluted in saline or dextrose and the dose should be titrated according to the response. Bolus doses of 0.5–5 mg of metaraminol may be administered intravenously, but with extreme caution. Its onset of effect after IV administration occurs within 1–2 minutes with maximum effect at 10 minutes and lasts for 20–60 minutes. The corresponding IM or SC dose of metaraminol for the prevention of hypotension is 2–10 mg.

Metaraminol is used as an adjunct for the treatment of (i) hypotension occurring during general or spinal anesthesia and (ii) for the management of hypotension, occurring during cardiopulmonary bypass.

α_2-Selective Adrenergic Agonists

Many blood vessels contain α_2 receptors that promote vasoconstriction on its stimulation. So, clonidine as a selective α_2-adrenergic agonist was initially developed as a vasoconstricting nasal decongestant. But, later it was found that clonidine reduces the blood pressure by activating the presynaptic α_2-adrenergic receptors, present in the CNS which controls the CVS. Such central presynaptic α_2-adrenergic receptor activation suppresses the outflow of sympathetic nervous system activity from brain. Therefore, there is a contradiction between the peripheral action of clonidine, causing hypertension and its central action, causing hypotension. But, the ultimate or resultant effect of clonidine depends on the predominancy of the site of action of this drug. For example, when the clonidine is given intravenously, then there is acute rise in BP. This is due to the predominant activation of α_2 receptors in peripheral vascular smooth muscles. After IV administration, the transient vasoconstriction and hypertension caused by clonidine is followed by hypotension which results from the decreased central outflow of impulse from central sympathetic nervous system. However, this hypertensive response of clonidine that follows parenteral administration is not seen when the drug is given orally.

Clonidine

When clonidine was first synthesized in 1960, it was used to produce vasoconstriction (as a nasal decongestant) that was mediated through the stimulation of local peripheral α_2-adrenergic receptors on vascular system. But, later when clonidine was used, it was found that clonidine can cause hypotension, sedation, analgesia, and bradycardia. Then, it was postulated that this action of clonidine is mediated through the central presynaptic α_2-adrenergic receptors.

The probable mechanisms of hypotension and analgesic effect of clonidine are:

- The activation of the presynaptic α_2 receptors by clonidine in the lower brainstem region decreases the discharge from sympathetic preganglion fibers in the splanchnic nerve, as well as in the postganglionic fibers of cardiac nerves.
- Clonidine also stimulates the parasympathetic outflow and this may contribute to the slowing of heart rate.
- Some of the antihypertensive effects of clonidine may also be mediated by the activation of presynaptic α_2 receptors that suppress the release of norepinephrine from the preganglionic nerve endings.
- The α_2 receptors are also located on the primary afferent terminals (peripheral and spinal) of the neurons of the superficial laminae of spinal cord, and within several brainstem nuclei which are responsible for analgesia. This explains the analgesic effect of α_2-receptor agonist, clonidine.
- Similar to a local anesthetic agent, α_2-adrenergic agonists have also been found to produce the dose-dependent blockade of conduction in nerve fibers, particularly of C fibers than A-δ fibers. This can explain the local anesthetic property of clonidine.
- Additionally, the clonidine hyperpolarizes some neurons of the dorsal horn and renders them less responsive to afferent impulses. Thus, it can produce analgesia.
- Neuroaxial administration of clonidine directly inhibits the sympathetic preganglionic neurons in the spinal cord. So, local anesthetic agents when is combined with α_2-adrenergic agonists can increase the degree of sympatholysis, resulting in severe hypotension.

- Similar to opioids, clonidine also decreases the afferent noxious inputs through its interaction with the specific receptors in spinal cord which are G-protein-coupled receptors. Like opioids, clonidine also reduces substance P and the excitatory amino acids, which are released by peripheral nerves stimulation at noxious intensities.

Clonidine is well absorbed after oral administration. Bioavailability is 100% through the oral route. The peak effect of clonidine is observed within 1–3 hours after its oral administration and the duration of action is 12 hours.

The major adverse effects of clonidine are dry mouth and sedation. Sexual dysfunction may also occur by clonidine. Marked bradycardia and hypotension are observed in some patients.

The major therapeutic use of clonidine is the treatment of hypertension. Now, clonidine is useful in selected patients receiving anesthesia, because it decreases the requirement of anesthetics agents and increases the hemodynamic stability. Other potential benefits of clonidine in anesthesia include preoperative sedation, anxiolysis, drying of secretions, and analgesia.

Dexmedetomidine

It is the active S-enantiomer of medetomidine and is a selective α_2-adrenergic agonist, like clonidine. But, compared to clonidine, dexmedetomidine is more selective for α_2-adrenergic receptor. The $\alpha_2:\alpha_1$ specificity ratio for clonidine is 200:1, whereas the $\alpha_2:\alpha_1$ specificity ratio of dexmedetomidine is 1,600:1. It has shorter half-life (2–3 h) than clonidine (12–24 h). It has sedative, analgesic, and sympatholytic effects. Hence, it blunts many cardiovascular responses, which are seen during perioperative period. The sedative and analgesic effect of dexmedetomidine is mediated by the activation of presynaptic α_2-adrenergic receptor in brain and spinal cord. When used intraoperatively, it reduces the requirement of intravenous and volatile anesthetic drugs. It is very useful for sedating patients in preparation for awake fiberoptic intubation. It is also very useful for sedating the critically ill and ventilated patients in intensive care unit.

The recommended dosing of dexmedetomidine consists of a loading dose at 1 µg/kg over 10 minutes, followed by an infusion at 0.2–0.7 µg/kg/h. However, the clinicians administer this agent in a great many ways, including intranasally for sedation in children. In this recommended dose, it produces little respiratory depression. The side effect of dexmedetomidine is similar to that of clonidine, i.e., hypotension, bradycardia, and dry mouth. Hence, during ongoing therapy, it may produce hypotension and bradycardia, but rapid administration may cause hypertension. It is metabolized in liver and is excreted through urine and bile. Long-term use of these agents, i.e., clonidine and dexmedetomidine, leads to supersensitization and upregulation of receptors. Hence, abrupt discontinuation of either drug may cause an acute withdrawal syndrome including hypertensive crisis. Because of increased affinity of dexmedetomidine for α_2 receptor, compared to clonidine, hence this withdrawal syndrome will usually manifest 48 hours of discontinuation of dexmedetomidine.

Methyldopa

Methyldopa is also a selective α_2-adrenergic agonist and its antihypertensive action is exerted through its central action like clonidine which is by inhibiting the adrenergic neuronal outflow from the brainstem. Actually, the methyldopa is a prodrug and an analog to DOPA. It is metabolized by decarboxylase in the adrenergic neuron to α-methyl-dopamine which is then converted to α-methyl norepinephrine. After that this α-methyl norepinephrine (which is called false neurotransmitter) is stored in the vesicles at the adrenergic nerve endings and acts as a false adrenergic neurotransmitter, replacing or substituting the true norepinephrine. Thus, when the adrenergic neuron discharges its neurotransmitter, then α-methyl norepinephrine is released instead of NE. As a vasoconstrictor (peripheral α_2-adrenergic agonistic action) α-methyl norepinephrine is as potent as NE (but NE has both α- and β-agonistic action). But, α-methyl norepinephrine acts in the brain to inhibit the adrenergic vasoconstrictive outflow and this central effect, which predominates than the peripheral effect, is principally responsible for its antihypertensive action.

Methyldopa reduces the peripheral vascular resistance (afterload) and preload. Thus, the increase or decrease of cardiac output depends on the intensity of reduction of afterload and preload. If the reduction of afterload is more than preload (younger patients with uncomplicated essential hypertension), then CO increases. Alternatively, if the reduction of afterload is more than afterload (as in older patients), then CO falls with the reduction in stroke volume. Symptomatic orthostatic hypotension is less common with methyldopa than other antihypertensive agents which act on peripheral adrenergic receptors or autonomic ganglia. This is because methyldopa does not block baroreceptor-mediated vasoconstriction. For this reason, it is well tolerated during surgical anesthesia. Any severe hypotension, produced by methyldopa, can only be reversed by volume expansion, but not by a peripheral α-adrenergic agonist. This is because methyldopa does not block the peripheral α-receptors. In hypotension, like spinal anesthesia, where the adrenergic (sympathetic) neurons are blocked, in such condition the peripheral α-adrenergic agonists are antidotes. But, this is not possible in hypotension produced by methyldopa.

Renal blood flow and renal function are maintained during the treatment with methyldopa. Plasma concentration of NE falls in association with the reduction of arterial pressure during the treatment with methyldopa and this reflects the decrease in sympathetic tone, discharged from CNS. In contrast, the reduction of BP by vasodilators is associated with the increased concentration of NE in plasma. Renin secretion is reduced, but this is not the major effect and is not responsible for the hypotensive effect of methyldopa.

In brain, methyldopa acts on α_2-adrenergic receptors and inhibits the centers that are responsible for wakefulness and alertness. Thus, it produces sedation, drowsiness, and depression. The medullary centers, that control salivation, are also inhibited by α_2-adrenergic receptors, and so the methyldopa produces dryness of mouth. Other CNS effects of methyldopa include reduction in libido, parkinsonian signs, hyperprolactinemia, and gynecomastia.

Methyldopa is absorbed actively through GI tract by amino acid transport system, when it is administered orally. Its transport into CNS is also an active process. So, in spite of rapid absorption, the peak action of methyldopa is delayed by about 6–8 hours, even after an IV administration. This is due to the time taken by methyldopa to convert to its active metabolites, α-methyl norepinephrine. The duration of action of a single dose of methyldopa usually lasts for about 24 hours.

Methyldopa is an active antihypertensive agent, but is not usually used as the first line of treatment. This is because of its frequent side effects, such as hepatotoxicity and hemolytic anemia (Coomb's test becomes positive and that is due to the autoantibodies directed agonist the Rh locus on erythrocytes). Therefore, methyldopa is reserved for patients in whom it may have a special value. For example, it is the preferred drug for the treatment of hypertension during pregnancy which is based on its effectiveness and safety for both the mother and fetus.

Receptor Selectivity of Adrenergic Agonists

Refer **Tables 15 and 16**.

TABLE 15: Receptor selectivity of adrenergic agonists.

Drugs	α_1	α_2	β_1	β_2	DA$_1$	DA$_2$
Epinephrine	+ +	+ +	+ + +	+ +	0	0
Norepinephrine	+ +	+ +	+ +	0	0	0
Phenylephrine	+ + +	+	0	0	0	0
Ephedrine	+ +	Not known	+ +	+	0	0
Dopamine	+ +	+ +	+ +	+	+ + +	+ + +
Dobutamine	0	0	+ + +	+	0	0
Clonidine	+	+ +	0	0	0	0
Dexmedetomidine	+	+ + +	0	0	0	0
Fenoldopam	0	0	0	0	+ + +	0
Terbutaline	0	0	+	+ + +	0	0

TABLE 16: The effects of adrenergic agonists.

Drug	Heart rate	MAP	CO	SVR	Renal blood flow	Bronchodilatation
Epinephrine	↑↑	↑	↑↑	↑/–	↓↓	↑↑
Norepinephrine	↓	↑↑↑	↑/↓	↑↑↑	↓↓↓	0
Phenylephrine	↓	↑↑↑	↓	↑↑↑	↓↓↓	0
Ephedrine	↑↑	↑↑	↑↑	↑	↓↓	↑↑
Dopamine	↑/↑↑	↑	↑↑↑	↑	↑↑↑	0
Dobutamine	↑	↑	↑↑↑	↓	↑	0
Isoproterenol	↑↑↑	↓	↑↑↑	↓↓	↑/↓	↑↑↑
Fenoldopam	↑↑	↓↓↓	↓/↑	↓↓	↑↑↑	0

Other Selective α₂-adrenergic Agonists

Apraclonidine

It reduces the formation of aqueous humor and is usually used topically to reduce the intraocular pressure.

Guanfacine

It is a more selective α_2 agonist than clonidine and has less side effects. Its mechanism of action is same as that clonidine and is used in the treatment of hypertension.

Guanabenz

It is also a selective α_2 adrenergic agonist. Its mechanism of action and therapeutic effects are similar to that of clonidine and guanfacine.

Tizanidine

It is also a selective α_2-adrenergic agonist, and is used as a muscle relaxant in the treatment of spasticity, associated with cerebral and spinal disorders.

Brimonidine

Being a α_2 agonist, it is used topically to lower the intraocular pressure in patients with ocular hypertension or open angle glaucoma.

Miscellaneous Adrenergic Agonists

Ephedrine

It is a both α- and β-adrenergic receptor agonist (direct action) and also enhances the release of endogenous NE from sympathetic neurons (indirect action). By its α action it increases the systemic vascular resistance (SVR) and BP, and by its β action it increases the HR and CO. Ephedrine also increases the coronary blood flow. It is a respiratory stimulant and also causes bronchodilatation. It is a potent CNS stimulant. Like amphetamine, it also increases the cerebral blood flow. Mydriasis occurs after its topical use. Ephedrine constricts renal blood vessels and may lead to a decrease in both the renal blood flow and GFR. It is not metabolized by MAO or COMT. So, it is also effective after oral administration and this effect lasts for many hours. Ephedrine is excreted through the urine, largely as an unchanged form.

Previously, ephedrine was used in (i) Stokes Adams attack, (ii) as a CNS stimulant in narcolepsy and depressive states, (iii) as bronchodilator in bronchial asthma, (iv) in urinary incontinence, etc. But, nowadays, ephedrine is replaced by more specific drugs for each disorder. Recently, ephedrine has only been used to treat hypotension, occurring with spinal anesthesia.

The untoward effects of ephedrine include the risk of hypertension, particularly after its parenteral administration or with higher than recommended oral dose. The parenteral dose of ephedrine is 3–30 mg which is titrated according to the response.

Other Miscellaneous Adrenergic Agonists

Other miscellaneous adrenergic agonists are amphetamine, methylamphetamine and methylphenidate.

Several sympathomimetic drugs, used primarily as a vasoconstrictor of nasal mucous membrane, when used topically are propylhexedrine, naphazoline HCl, tetrahydrozoline HCl, oxymetazoline HCl, and xylometazoline HCl.

Phenylephrine, pseudoephedrine, and phenylpropanolamine are the sympathomimetic drugs that have been used as oral preparation for the relief of nasal congestion.

USES OF SYMPATHOMIMETIC AGENTS IN HYPOTENSION AND SHOCK

The drugs, with predominant α adrenergic activity, can be used to raise BP in patients with decreased SVR, due to the failure of sympathetic nervous system, such as spinal anesthesia, overdose of antihypertensive medications, etc. However, slight hypotension is not an indication for treatment by these agents, if there is adequate perfusion of vital organs, such as brain, kidney, heart, and lungs. But, in patients with spinal anesthesia, where there is severe or total failure of sympathetic nervous system, then in such cases, the use of vasopressor drugs to increase SVR and to maintain perfusion in the vital organs is indicated. A number of sympathomimetic agents have been used for this purpose. But, the ideal agents would cause arterial constriction, with relatively little arteriolar constriction (the primary side for systemic vascular resistance), which would not increase the afterload and will not reduce CO, although will maintain the BP. However, no such ideal agent is currently available. Only midodrine shows promise in treating hypotension with this idea.

In other forms of shock, such as hemorrhage, loss of fluid, etc., where the sympathetic nervous system does not fail, but the accompanying fall in BP generally leads to the marked activation of sympathetic nervous system. This, in turn, causes increased peripheral vasoconstriction and SVR and also an increase in the rate and force of cardiac contraction. In the initial stage of shock, this mechanism tries to maintain BP and cerebral blood flow, but blood flow to the kidneys, skin, and other organs may be decreased, leading to impaired production of urine and metabolic acidosis. But, later when the SVR tremendously increases and the preload severely falls, due to more hemorrhage and loss of fluid, then CO drastically reduces, causing more hypotension. Thus, a vicious cycle sets up.

So, the initial therapy of shock involves basic life support and a specific therapy, such as fluid or blood for hypovolemic shock, antibiotics for septic shock, emergency cardiac catheterization, or surgical revascularization or even angioplasty for cardiogenic shock. Mechanical left ventricular assisting devices, such as the intra-aortic balloon pump (IABP) also may be important in maintaining CO and coronary perfusion in critically ill patients. In the setting of severely impaired CO, the failing blood pressure leads to intense discharge of sympathetic outflow (provided the sympathetic system is not blocked) and vasoconstriction. This may further decrease CO, as the damaged heart had to pump against a higher peripheral systemic resistance or afterload. In such situations, medical intervention is designed to optimize the CO by the manipulation of cardiac filling pressure (preload), myocardial contractility (pump), and peripheral vascular systemic resistance (afterload).

Preload may be increased by the administration of IV fluid or reducing the dose of diuretics and nitrates (nitrates reduce the preload by dilating the venous side of the vascular system). If these measures do not lead to an adequate therapeutic response, then it may be necessary to use vasoactive drugs in an effort to improve abnormalities of BP and flow. Many of these pharmacological approaches, while apparently clinically reasonable, are of uncertain efficacy. The adrenergic agonist may be used in an attempt to increase the myocardial contractility or to modify the peripheral vascular resistance. In general terms, (i) the β adrenergic agonist increases the HR and the force of contraction, (ii) the α-adrenergic agonist increases the SVR, and (iii) the dopamine (in renal doses) promotes the dilatation of renal and splanchnic vascular beds, in addition to activating β- and α-adrenergic receptors (in higher doses).

A number of sympathetic amines have been used to increase the force of cardiac contraction. But, some of these drugs have disadvantages. For example, isoproterenol is a powerful chronotropic agent and can greatly increase the myocardial O_2 demand. NE intensifies peripheral vasoconstriction and EPI increases the heart rate and may predispose the heart to dangerous arrhythmias. Dopamine is an inotropic agent that causes less increases in heart rate and promotes renal arterial dilatation. When dopamine is given in higher doses ($>10–20\ \mu g/kg/min$), it activates α-adrenergic receptors, causing peripheral and renal vasoconstriction. Dobutamine has complex pharmacological actions to increase the myocardial contractility with little increase in HR and peripheral resistance.

In the most forms of shock, except few, where there is vasodilatation (e.g., spinal anesthesia, septicemia, and anaphylaxis), there is intense reflex vasoconstriction. In such situations, the use of α-adrenergic agonists may further compromise blood flow to the vital organs, such as kidneys, brain, heart, guts, etc. as well as adversely increase the work of heart. Indeed, in such situations, vasodilating drugs such as nitroprusside are more likely to improve blood flow in vital organs and decrease cardiac work by decreasing the afterload, if a minimally adequate blood pressure is maintained.

■ ADRENERGIC RECEPTOR ANTAGONISTS

α-Adrenergic Receptor Antagonist

Endogenous catecholamines (CAS), exogenous catecholamines, and other noncatecholamine sympathomimetic or adrenergic agents mediate their actions through both α and β or only through α or β receptor.

Among these, the α_1-receptor-mediated actions are confined only to the arterial and venous smooth muscle contraction. Whereas the α_2-receptor-mediated actions are:

- Suppression of central sympathetic outflow
- Increment of vagal tone
- Facilitation of platelet aggregation
- Inhibition of the release of NE and ACh from presynaptic nerve endings
- Regulation of metabolic effects, including the suppression of insulin secretion, inhibition of lipolysis, etc.
- Contraction of smooth muscles of some arteries and veins.

So, the α-adrenergic-receptor antagonists have a wide range of pharmacological actions and every agent has different affinity for both the α_1 and α_2 receptors. For example, prazosin as α-receptor antagonist has greater affinity for α_1 than α_2 receptors. Whereas yohimbine is a selective α_2 antagonist and phentolamine has the same affinity for both the α_1 and α_2 receptors. The α-receptor antagonists are also heterogenous in nature because they vary widely in structure.

α₁-Adrenergic Receptor Antagonist

Clinically, the most important effect of α_1-receptor antagonist is observed in cardiovascular system. The blockade of α_1 receptor causes vasodilatation and decrease in BP with reduction in SVR. This fall of blood pressure is more marked in upright than in supine position and in hypovolemia. This fall in BP by α_1-receptor antagonist is usually counteracted (compensated) by rise in HR and CO by compensatory reflex baroreceptor mechanism. There is also fluid retention during the use of α_1-adrenergic-receptor antagonist.

The interaction between the α_1-receptor antagonist and the sympathomimetic amine (which sometimes occur in clinical practice) depends on the adrenergic agonist that is administered. For example:

(i) The pressor response of phenylephrine can be completely suppressed by α_1-receptor antagonist. (ii) The action of NE can be incompletely blocked by the α_1-receptor antagonist, because of the residual stimulation of cardiac β_1 receptor by NE. (iii) The pressure response of EPI can be transformed to hypotension effects by the concomitant use of a α_1-receptor antagonist. This is because of the residual stimulation of β_2 receptors by EPI on vasculature with resultant vasodilatation and hypotension.

The α_1-receptor antagonist also inhibits the smooth muscle contraction of bladder trigone, bladder sphincter, and prostate, leading to decreased resistance to urinary outflow. Recent evidence suggests that there are two types of α_1 receptors such as α_{1A} and α_{1B}. Among these α_{1A} receptors are important in mediating catecholamines-induced prostatic smooth muscle contraction which can be inhibited by a specific α_{1A} receptor blocker, such as tamsulosin. Although, theoretically, some α_1 receptors promote bronchial smooth muscle contraction, but the importance of α_1-receptor antagonist in asthma is minimal.

α_2-Adrenergic Receptor Antagonist

The α_2 receptors have an important role in the regulation of the activity of sympathetic nervous system, both peripherally and centrally. The activation of presynaptic α_2 receptors inhibits the release of NE from sympathetic nerve endings. Thus, block of presynaptic α_2 receptors withdraw this inhibition and causes increased release of NE from nerve endings, leading to activation of both α and β receptors in heart and contraction of peripheral vascular smooth muscles with consequent rise in BP and SVR. Whereas the activation of presynaptic α_2 receptors in pontomedullary region of CNS inhibits sympathetic outflow and causes fall in BP. The α_2 antagonist thus reverses this action and increases the sympathetic outflow and BP. Thus, on one side, the α_2-receptor antagonist increases the sympathetic outflow by acting peripherally on the receptors at presynaptic membrane and acting centrally at pontomedullary region. Thus, it increases BP and SVR. On the other side, α_2 antagonist directly blocks the peripheral vascular α_2 receptor which causes vasoconstriction and thus produces vasodilatation with decrease in BP.

Some α-Adrenergic Antagonists and their Therapeutic Uses

Phenoxybenzamine

It irreversibly blocks both the α_1 and α_2 receptors (irreversible because further restoration of cellular responsiveness to α-adrenergic agonists probably requires the synthesis of new receptors) and causes the progressive lowering of BP and SVR. It is predominantly an arterial vasodilator. Thus, it increases the HR and CO (up to a certain level of fall of blood pressure) and this is due to the reflex baroreceptor stimulation. During the use of phenoxybenzamine, pressor response of exogenously administered CAs is impaired and the hypotensive response to EPI occurs. This is because of the unopposed β-adrenergic receptor mediated vasodilatation by EPI. In normotensive subjects, BP in supine position is little affected by phenoxybenzamine. But, there is a marked fall in BP in standing position (orthostatic hypotension) and this is because of the antagonism (absence) of α-receptor-mediated compensatory vasoconstriction which is essential for maintaining BP in standing condition. In addition, the normal ability of a patient to respond to hypovolemia and to anesthesia-induced vasodilatation is impaired by phenoxybenzamine, causing severe hypotension. The drug also increases the rate of peripheral turnover of NE. This is because the amount of NE that is released per nerve stimulation is increased by the blockade of presynaptic α_2 receptor. Phenoxy benzamine inhibits CAs induced cardiac arrhythmias. It also causes a shift of fluid from the interstitial to vascular compartment and it is due to the vasodilatation of pre- and postcapillary resistance vessels.

The major clinical use of phenoxybenzamine is the treatment of pheochromocytoma. A vast majority of patients, suffering from pheochromocytoma, are treated surgically. But, this drug is used frequently to treat the patient where surgery is contraindicated or to prepare the pheochromocytoma patient, waiting for operation preoperatively. Initially phenoxybenzamine is started in the dose of 10 mg twice daily for 1–3 weeks before operation. Then, the dose is gradually increased till the desired lower level of BP is achieved. But, the therapy by phenoxybenzamine may be limited by postural hypotension. The usual total daily dose of phenoxybenzamine in patient with pheochromocytoma is 40–120 mg which is given in two or three divided doses. The corresponding dose of phenoxybenzamine by intravenous infusion (diluted in dextrose or saline) over 1 hour is 10–40 mg. After its intravenous administration, the drug acts within 1 hour and has a duration of action for 3–4 days. Some anesthesiologists do not routinely use phenoxybenzamine preoperatively for the preparation of patient before pheochromocytoma surgery. In patients with inoperable and malignant pheochromocytoma, prolonged treatment with phenoxybenzamine may be necessary. Another approach for the management of pheochromocytoma, particularly with a malignant disease, is the administration of metyrosine. It is a competitive inhibitor of tyrosine hydroxylase which is the rate limiting enzyme in the synthesis of catecholamines.

The β-adrenergic receptor antagonists or β-blockers are also used to treat pheochromocytoma, but only after the administration of α-receptor antagonist.

Phenoxybenzamine is the first α-receptor antagonist which was also used previously for the treatment of benign hypertrophy of prostate (BHP). The mechanism of action of phenoxybenzamine in the treatment of BHP is the blockade of α receptors, situated on the smooth muscle of prostate and bladder base. Thus, it decreases the obstructive symptoms and decreases the need to urinate at night (α-receptor activation is responsible for the spasm of muscle of bladder trigone, bladder neck and prostate, causing urinary obstruction). However, terazosin, doxazosin, alfuzosin, tamsulosin, and silodosin are safer and more preferred than phenoxybenzamine, as they are more specific α_1-adrenergic antagonists for this disorder.

The major side effects of phenoxybenzamine is postural hypotension which is accompanied by reflex tachycardia. Hypotension produced by α-antagonist may be severe, if there is hypovolemia and there is history of concomitant use of vasodilator drugs.

Phentolamine and Tolazoline

Like phenoxybenzamine, phentolamine is also a competitive α-adrenergic antagonist and have same affinity for both the α_1 and α_2 receptors. The α_1 agonism and direct smooth muscle relaxation are responsible for peripheral vasodilatation and decline in arterial blood pressure. This drop in BP provokes compensatory reflex tachycardia. This tachycardia is augmented by antagonism of presynaptic α_2 receptor in heart. Because, the α_1 blocked promotes the release of NE by eliminating negative feedback. These cardiovascular effects are usually apparent within 2 minutes and last up to 15 minutes. It also causes the blockade of 5-HT receptors and causes the release of histamine from mast cells. Tolazoline has similar function like phentolamine, but is less potent. Phentolamine and tolazoline both increase the motility of GI which can be antagonized by atropine.

Phentolamine can be used for a short-term basis to control hypertension in pheochromocytoma. It is administered intravenously as intermittent bolus doses (1–5 mg in adults) or as infusion. The infusion of phentolamine is used very cautiously. It is administered by IV infusion (diluted in dextrose or saline) at the rate of 0˙1–0˙2 mg/min. Like other adrenergic antagonists, the extent of the response to receptor blockade by phentolamine depends on the degree of the existing sympathetic tone. Excessive reflex tachycardia and postural hypotension limit the usefulness of phentolamine to the treatment of hypertension, caused by the excessive stimulation of α_1 receptor (pheochromocytoma, clonidine withdrawal, etc.).

To prevent or to minimize tissue necrosis, following the extravasation of IV fluids, containing an α-agonist (e.g., norepinephrine), 5–10 mg of phentolamine in 10 mL normal saline can be infiltrated locally. This is another indication for therapeutic use of phentolamine.

Prazosin and Related Drugs

Prazosin

It is also a potent selective α_1-adrenergic antagonist, with 1,000-fold greater affinity for α_1 than α_2 receptor. But among the subtypes of α_1 receptors (α_{1A}, α_{1B}, and α_{1D}) it has same affinity to all.

The pharmacological effects of prazosin are due to the result of blockade of α_1 receptors in arterioles and veins, leading to ↓ BP, ↓ SVR and ↓ preload. However, like other vasodilating drugs, it does not reflexly increase the HR at clinical level. Again, it does not block the presynaptic α_2 receptor. Hence, it does not promote the release of NE from presynaptic sympathetic nerve endings in heart. As the prazosin decreases preload more than afterload, so it does not increase CO (in contrast to vasodilators, such as hydralazine that have minimal dilatory effect on veins). It also acts in CNS and suppresses the central sympathetic outflow.

Prazosin is well absorbed when given orally with bioavailability of about 50–70%. Peak serum concentration through oral route is generally reached within 1–3 hours after its administration. The plasma half-life of prazosin is 2–3 hours and the duration of action is typically 7–10 hours. For the treatment of hypertension, prazosin is started initially in smaller doses, such as 1 mg at bedtime, so that the patient is recumbent for at least several hours after its administration. Thus, it reduces the risk of syncopal reaction due to hypotension that may follow the first dose of prazosin. Then, the dose is titrated upward, depending on blood pressure. The maximum effect of prazosin is generally observed with the total daily dose of 20 mg in patient with severe hypertension. For the treatment of benign prostatic hypertrophy (BPH), prazosin in the dose of 1–5 mg twice daily is usually used.

Terazosin: It is structurally an analog of prazosin, but less potent than it. Like prazosin it is highly selective to α_1 receptors than α_2, with no discrimination among α_{1A}, α_{1B}, α_{1D} receptors regarding affinity. The oral bioavailability of terazosin is 90% and half-life of elimination is approximately 12 hours with duration of action of 18 hours. The drug is taken as once daily dose to treat hypertension and BPH. An initial first dose of 1 mg of terazosin is recommended. Then, the doses are titrated upward gradually, depending on the therapeutic responses. Terazosin in the dose of 10 mg/day may be required for maximal effect in BPH.

Doxazosin: It is another long-acting (half-life 18 hours) congener of prazosin with pharmacological profile similar to terazosin. It has also apoptosis promoting effect on the cells of prostate. It is used in both hypertension and BHP.

Tamsulosin: It is a relative uroselective α_{1A}/α_{1D} blocker. It is as effective as terazosin in improving BHP symptoms, because α-subtype predominates in the base of bladder and prostate. However, it lacks the apoptosis promoting property of prostate, such as terazosin and doxazosin. It is not used as hypertensive because it does not cause significant change in BP at doses which relieve urinary symptoms. Postural hypotension and retrograde ejaculation are the only significant side effects of tamsulosin. Problem of floppy iris has been encountered during cataract surgery in patients taking tamsulosin.

Silodosin: It is another selective α_{1A} blocker. All the pharmacological actions of it similar to that of tamsulosin. Terazosin and doxazosin, not others, have apoptosis action on prostate. Terazosin, doxazosin, alfuzosin, and tamsulosin are used once daily dose.

β-Adrenergic Receptor Antagonists

It has been discussed in more details in the hypertension chapter. Here, we will discuss only few.

Propranolol: It is a nonselective β blocker. It blocks both β_1 and β_2 receptors. Arterial blood pressure is lowered by propranolol through several mechanisms. These include (i) decreased myocardial contractility, (ii) lowering of HR, and (iii) diminished renin release. Vessels do not dilate and peripheral vascular resistance does not reduce by propranolol. However, the CO and myocardial O_2 demand are reduced by it. Propranolol slows AV conduction and slows the ventricular response to supraventricular tachycardia.

The side effects of propranolol include bronchospasm (β_2 antagonism), acute congestive heart failure, bradycardia, and AV heart block (β_1 antagonism). The concomitant administration of propranolol and verapamil or diltiazem synergistically depress HR, myocardial contractility, and AV conduction. The half-life of propranolol is quite long (100 min). Generally, the IV dosage of propranolol is titrated as 0.5 mg after every 3–5 minutes, according to its effect. But, its total dose rarely exceeds 0.15 mg/kg.

Esmolol: It is a selective β_1-receptor blocker. It mainly reduces HR and BP. It is mainly used to prevent or minimize tachycardia and hypertension, induced during laryngoscopy or perioperative surgical stimuli. It is also used in controlling ventricular rate in atrial fibrillation and atrial flutter. Like all β_2 antagonists, esmolol also should not be used (i) with sinus bradycardia, (ii) greater than first degree heart block, (iii) low ejection fraction heart failure, etc.

It is used as an IV bolus (0.2–0.5 mg/kg) for short-term therapy, e.g., attenuation of cardiovascular response to laryngoscopy and intubation. For long-term therapy, it is started as loading dose of 0.5 mg/kg over 1 minute. This is followed by continuous infusion of 50 µg/kg/min to maintain therapeutic effect.

Mixed α- and β-Adrenergic Antagonists

Labetalol: It blocks α_1, β_1, and β_2 adrenergic receptors. The ratio of α-blockade to β-blockade activity of labetalol is approximately 1:7, following its IV administration. The α_1 blockade by labetalol causes vascular dilatation and reduction of peripheral vascular resistance. The β_1 blockade by labetalol causes reduction in HR and CO. But, CO may increase by the reduction of vascular resistance. The β_2 blockade prevents the dilatation of blood vessels. But, the ultimate result is that heart rate and cardiac output are usually slightly depressed or unchanged. BP is lowered without reflex tachycardia because of combined α and β blocking effect which is beneficial to patients with coronary artery disease.

Labetalol is always administered through intravenous route. The initial recommended dose is 2.5–10 mg over 2 minutes. After the initial dose, depending on response, 5–20 mg may be given at 10 minutes interval, until the desired level of BP is reached. The peak effect of labetalol usually occurs within 5 minutes of its intravenous dose.

Carvedilol: It is also an α_1, β_1, and β_2 adrenergic receptor blocker and produces vasodilatation due to α_1-receptor blocking action as well as Ca^{2+}-channel-blocking action. Its cardiovascular effect is similar to that of labetalol. It is used in the management of chronic heart failure secondary to cardiomyopathy (cardioprotective β-blocking effect), left ventricular dysfunction following acute MI, and hypertension. Carvedilol is started as 3.25 mg BD doses for 2 weeks. Then, its dosage is gradually increased and individualized maximally up to 25 mg twice daily, as required, and tolerated.

CHOLINERGIC RECEPTOR (MUSCARINIC AND NICOTINIC) AGONIST AND ANTAGONIST

The cholinergic-receptor agonists are the drugs or agents that act like ACh on its both muscarinic and nicotinic cholinergic receptors. ACh is the endogenous cholinergic neurotransmitter which acts on its both muscarinic and nicotinic receptors (so, ACh is a nonspecific cholinergic agonist). But, there are other agents which also act selectively only on the muscarinic or nicotinic receptors. So, they are called the selective muscarinic or nicotinic receptor cholinergic agonists, respectively.

Nonspecific Cholinergic Agonist

Acetylcholine

It is an endogenous cholinergic neurotransmitter. It acts at all the cholinergic synapses in central and peripheral nervous system of our body. Its actions are mediated through both the muscarinic and nicotinic receptors. The *muscarinic cholinergic receptors* in peripheral nervous system are primarily found (i) on all the cells that are innervated by preganglionic autonomic (sympathetic and parasympathetic) nerve fiber except the ganglionic cells, (ii) the postganglionic parasympathetic nerve fibers, and (iii) some postganglionic sympathetic fibers that supply the sweat gland, hair follicle, and erector piloris muscle. The muscarinic receptors are also present in CNS and on certain other cells such as endothelial cells of blood vessels that receive little or no cholinergic innervation. Certain centers of our brain, such as hippocampus, cortex, thalamus, etc. also have a high density of muscarinic receptors. The *nicotinic cholinergic receptors* are only found (i) at neuromuscular junctions, causing skeletal muscle contraction, and (ii) at peripheral autonomic ganglia (both sympathetic and parasympathetic) including the adrenal medulla, because adrenal medulla itself is an autonomic ganglion.

As ACh acts on both the muscarinic and nicotinic receptors, so its pharmacological actions can also be divided into muscarinic and nicotinic actions.

Muscarinic actions: It is due to stimulatory action on muscarinic receptors. In general, the muscarinic actions include actions on heart, blood vessels, smooth muscles, glands, eyes, viscera, mucous membrane, etc., where muscarinic receptors are abundantly present. Whereas, nicotinic actions include only actions on skeletal muscles and autonomic ganglia where nicotinic receptors are only present.

a. On CVS:

The main muscarinic effects of ACh on CVS are vasodilatation, $\downarrow$ HR, $\downarrow$ conduction in heart, $\downarrow$ contractility of cardiac muscle, etc. ACh is not given systemically for any therapeutic indication. But, its importance lies within the mechanism of action of many cardiac glycosides, many antiarrhythmic drugs, following afferent stimulus from viscera, during surgical intervention, etc. Intravenous small dose of ACh causes the reduction of BP, due to vasodilatation and reflex tachycardia, due to this reduction of BP. A relatively higher dose of ACh causes bradycardia and $\downarrow$ conduction in cardiac tissues. However, intravenous large dose of ACh causes $\uparrow$ BP,

especially after the administration of atropine, which blocks the muscarinic receptors. This is caused by the stimulation of adrenal medulla and sympathetic ganglia by ACh which releases CAs into circulation from adrenal medulla and postganglionic sympathetic nerve endings (nicotinic actions).

ACh causes the dilatation of both pulmonary and coronary vasculature. This dilatation of coronary blood vessel is caused by the baroreceptor and chemoreceptor mediated reflex or by the release of NO. However, neither the parasympathetic vasodilator nor the sympathetic vasoconstrictor fiber plays any major role in the regulation of coronary blood flow. It is principally affected by local O_2 tension and local autoregulatory metabolic factors, such as adenosine that determines the blood flow through coronary vessels. Though, most of the blood vessels of our body do not receive any cholinergic innervation, still the vasodilatation of it (blood vessels) is mediated in response to ACh by the presence of muscarinic receptors on their endothelial cells, primarily of M_3 subtypes. When these receptors are stimulated by ACh, then the endothelial cells release endothelium-dependent releasing factor (EDRF) or nitric oxide, which diffuses into the adjacent smooth muscles and causes them to relax. The vasodilatation may also arise secondarily from the inhibition of the release of NE from adrenergic nerve ending by ACh.

Cholinergic parasympathetic fibers are extensively distributed in SA node, AV node, atrial muscle, bundle of HIS, right and left bundle branch, and specialized conducting tissue of heart, like Purkinje fibers. The cholinergic innervation to ventricular myocardium is sparse. ACh acts on this cardiac conducting tissues directly by stimulating parasympathetic activity and indirectly by inhibiting the effects of adrenergic activity. The inhibition of adrenergic activity by ACh depends on the present level of sympathetic drive on heart. Inhibition of this adrenergic drive by ACh results partly from the inhibition of cyclic AMP formation and partly from the reduction in L-type Ca^{2+} channel activity. In SA node, the pacemaker activity of SA nodal cells is caused by the presence of spontaneous slow diastolic depolarization phase or phase 4 of action potential. At a critical level (i.e., at the level of threshold potential), this spontaneous slow diastolic depolarization automatically initiates a full action potential and a full cardiac cycle. ACh slows the heart rate by decreasing the rate of this spontaneous slow diastolic depolarization and by increasing the repolarizing current (i.e., resting membrane potential becomes more negative) of SA nodal cells and thus delaying the attainment of threshold potential from RMP and delaying the cardiac cycle.

ACh also reduces the force of contractility of cardiac muscles, slows the conduction in conducting cardiac tissues, and increases the refractory period. The decrement in AV nodal conduction by ACh is usually responsible for complete heart block that may be observed when a large number of quantities of cholinergic agonists are administered systemically. With an increase in vagal tone (which acts through ACh neurotransmitter) such as produced by digitalis glycosides, the increased refractory period of AV node and bundle of HIS can contribute to the reduction in frequency, with which the aberrant atrial impulses are transmitted to the ventricle and thus decreases ventricular rate during atrial flutter and fibrillation.

b. Gastrointestinal, urinary tract, and other smooth muscles:

The smooth muscles of most of the organs are contracted by ACh, as they are rich in muscarinic receptors. Thus, the tone and the peristalsis of GI tract are increased and their sphincters are relaxed, causing abdominal cramps and the evacuation of bowel by ACh. Bronchial smooth muscles also contract by ACh, causing the attack of bronchial asthma. Peristalsis of ureter is also increased by ACh. The detrusor muscles of urinary bladder contract, while the bladder trigone and sphincter relaxes by ACh, causing the voiding of bladder (this is opposite to the stimulation of sympathetic system).

c. Glands:

Secretion from all the cholinergically innervated glands is increased by ACh, causing increased salivation, sweating, lacrymation, etc. Tracheobronchial and gastric secretion are also increased by ACh. The secretion of pancreatic and intestinal glands also increases, but is not so marked. The secretion of milk and bile is not affected by ACh.

d. Eye:

The contraction of the constrictor muscle of iris by ACh causes miosis (constriction of pupil). The contraction of ciliary muscles by ACh also causes loss of accommodation, increased outflow facility, and reduction in intraocular tension.

e. Central nervous system:

The naturally occurring cholinomimetic alkaloids, such as pilocarpine, muscarine and aerocholin, etc. can cross the blood-brain barrier and evoke a characteristic cortical arousal and CNS stimulating response which are similar to that produced by the injection of anticholinesterase agents. The arousal response of all of these three drugs can be reduced or blocked by atropine and related agents. But, cholinesters, e.g., ACh, being a quaternary compound, does not cross the blood-brain barrier and does not produce any CNS symptoms.

Nicotinic actions: This is due to the stimulatory actions of nicotinic receptors. The nicotinic receptors are present in all the autonomic ganglia (both sympathetic and parasympathetic) and at the neuromuscular junctions of skeletal muscle.

- *Autonomic ganglia:* Nicotinic receptors which are situated in both the sympathetic and parasympathetic (autonomic) ganglia can be stimulated by ACh, but only in higher doses. Higher dose of ACh, after IV atropine (to block the muscarinic action of ACh) causes ↑BP and tachycardia. This is called the nicotinic action.
- *Skeletal muscle:* ACh causes the contractions of skeletal muscles through the nicotinic receptor at motor endplate.

Nonspecific Cholinergic Antagonist

There is no such nonspecific single agent which blocks the action of ACh on both muscarinic and nicotinic cholinergic receptor. All they are either muscarinic receptor or nicotinic receptor blocker. The specific muscarinic receptor antagonists and specific nicotinic receptor antagonists are discussed later.

Specific Muscarinic Receptor Agonists

The specific muscarinic receptor agonists can be divided into two groups:

1. Some synthetic cholinesterase → such as methacholine, carbochol, bethanechol, etc.
2. Naturally occurring cholinomimetic alkaloids → such as pilocarpine, muscarine, arecoline, etc.

Therapeutic uses of muscarinic agonist: Among the above-mentioned muscarinic agonists, very few are used therapeutically. These are:

Pilocarpine

Pilocarpine is obtained from the leaves of pilocarpus microphyllus and some other of plants. It has prominent muscarinic actions and also stimulates the ganglia mainly through the ganglionic nicotinic receptors. It causes marked increase in sweating, salivation, and other secretions as well. The cardiovascular effects of pilocarpine are complex. Small doses generally cause a fall in BP. But, higher doses elicit a rise in BP and tachycardia, which is probably due to ganglionic stimulation (through nicotinic receptors). Due to its high systemic toxicity, it is only used in ophthalmic medicine as topical form. Applied to eye, it penetrates the cornea and promptly causes miosis and ciliary muscle contraction. Thus, it reduces intraocular pressure. So, the strength of 0.5–4% solution of pilocarpine is used in the treatment of glaucoma. It is usually better tolerated than anticholinesterase agents which by inhibiting the cholinesterase enzyme increases the level of ACh and produce the muscarinic actions. Pilocarpine is also used in the treatment of xerostomia, following head and neck radiation and in Sjögren's syndrome by increasing the secretion from salivary and lacrimal glands.

Bethanechol

As bethanechol stimulates the smooth muscle contraction of GI tract, so it is used in certain cases of postoperative abdominal distention, gastric atony or gastroparesis, in certain cases of congenital megacolon, adynamic ileus, etc. But, due to its many side effects prokinetic agents like metoclopramide (due to its combined cholinergic agonist and dopamine antagonist activity) and serotonin antagonist like ondansetron, have largely replaced bethanechol in the management of previously mentioned disorders.

Bethanechol is also used in the treatment of urinary retention and inadequate emptying of bladder, when any organic obstruction is absent. These α-adrenergic receptor antagonists are also useful in reducing the outlet resistance at the internal sphincter of urinary bladder.

Specific Muscarinic Receptor Antagonists (Anticholinergic Agents)

Specific muscarinic receptor antagonists (also called anticholinergic agents) only prevent the muscarinic action of ACh or other agonists by blocking their action only on muscarinic receptors which are present at the neuroeffector sites of smooth muscles of different organs, cardiac muscles, glands, eye, and CNS. These specific muscarinic receptor antagonists cannot block the action of ACh on its nicotinic receptor. In CNS, cholinergic transmission occurs both by muscarinic and nicotinic receptors. These CNS muscarinic actions can also be blocked by specific muscarinic antagonists which can pass the blood-brain barrier. Therefore, at high-toxic doses muscarinic receptor antagonist causes CNS stimulation followed by depression. But, the anticholinergic agents that are quaternary compounds cannot penetrate the blood-brain barrier and have no effect on CNS.

Though the specific nicotinic receptor antagonists block the nicotinic actions of ACh (which are mediated through their nicotinic receptors), but they are generally referred to as the ganglion blockers and neuromuscular blocking agents. However, they are usually not called the anticholinergic agents. Anticholinergic agents are those which can block only the muscarinic receptors of ACh. All anticholinergic agents are competitive antagonists to ACh **(Fig. 17)**.

Classification of Anticholinergic Agents

- *Natural alkaloids:* Atropine, hyoscine (scopolamine).
- *Semisynthetic derivatives:* Homatropine, ipratropium, and atropine methonitrate.

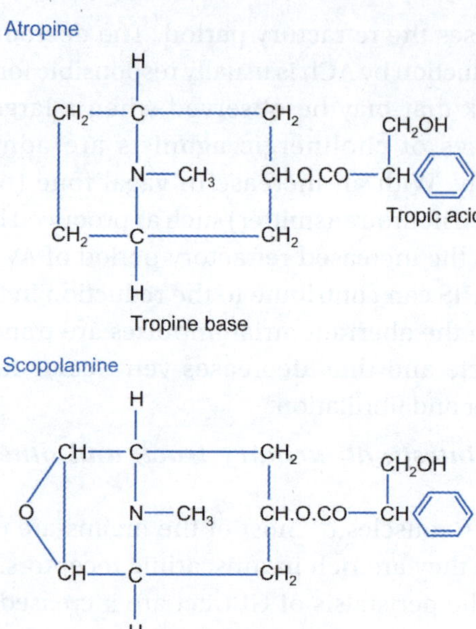

Fig. 17: Structure of anticholinergic agents.

- *Synthetic derivatives:*
  - *Specific antisecretory and antispasmodics:*
    - *Tertiary amines:* Dicyclomine, pirenzepine, atropine (also available naturally).
    - *Quaternary compound:* Glycopyrrolate, propanthelin, oxyphenonium, and clidinium.
  - *Specific mydriatics:* Cyclopentolate and tropicamide.
  - *Specific anti-parkinsonian:* Benzhexol, procyclidine, and benztropine.

In addition, many other drugs, such as tricyclic antidepressants, phenothiazines, antihistaminics, etc. also possess significant antimuscarinic or anticholinergic actions.

Atropine

Naturally, atropine and its related alkaloids are obtained from many plants such as Atropa belladonna (which means deadly nightshade), *Atropa acuminata, Hyoscyamus niger,* and *Datura stramonium* (Datura), etc. The name Atropa belladonna represents a paradox. Because the term "Atropos" comes from the oldest name of "Three Fades", who cut the thread of life (i.e., death) and the term "Belladonna" is derived from a type of practice of beauticians of Venetian court who put the extract of these plants in their eyes to impart them a "luster". For many centuries the belladonna preparations were also known to ancient Hindus. In Roman Empire and in medieval ages, this deadly nightshade shrub (*Atropa Belladonna*) was also frequently used to produce obscure or darkness and prolonged poisoning. During the ancient times, in India, the roots and the leaves of some weeds, named Jimson which also contain atropine alkaloids, were burnt and this smoke was inhaled to treat asthma.

British Colonist observed this and introduced the belladonna alkaloids in western medicine as early as 1780 to treat asthma. From this idea, ipratropium is used now as inhalation to treat chronic asthma. Then, Dr Mein, in 1831, first isolated atropine in pure form and in 1867, Dr Bezold first showed that atropine blocked the cardiac muscarinic effects, caused by vagal stimulation.

Chemically, atropine is the ester of an organic aromatic acid named "tropic" and an aromatic base named "tropin" (so, it is also an organic aromatic compound). The semisynthetic atropine ester, named homatropine, is an ester of "tropine" base and "Mandelic acid". Its quaternary derivatives are obtained by adding a second methyl group to the nitrogen atom of this ester. The tropine base and tropic acid themself are devoid of any antimuscarinic activity. So, the formation of an ester is essential for their antimuscarinic activities. The presence of free OH group at the acyl portion of this ester is also important for the antimuscarinic activity of atropine. When given parenterally, the quaternary derivatives are more potent than their parent ester compounds on both muscarinic and nicotinic receptors (ganglionic blocking activities). But, these quaternary derivatives lack the CNS activity, because they cannot cross the blood-brain barrier. The conversion of nitrogen from its tertiary group to a quaternary group also increases their blocking action at nicotinic receptors.

Mechanism of action of atropine: Atropine blocks the muscarinic effect of ACh by competing with it at the binding site on muscarinic receptors. So, it is called the competitive antagonist. The binding site of atropine (competitive antagonist) and ACh on muscarinic receptor is situated in a cleft which is formed by the seven transmembrane helices (subunits) of muscarinic receptor. An aspartic acid which is present at the N-terminal portion of third transmembrane helix of muscarinic receptor is believed to form an ionic bond with the cationic quaternary nitrogen atom of ACh (agonist) and the tertiary or quaternary nitrogen atom of its antagonist. However, atropine does not interfere with the synthesis or release of ACh at cholinergic nerve endings. It has no intrinsic ACh like activity. So, atropine and its receptor combination does not produce any muscarinic response, like ACh. As the antagonism between ACh and atropine is of competitive type, so the direction of their action depends on the relative concentration of these two compounds at their muscarinic neuroeffector site and the action of agonist (ACh) can be reversed by increasing the concentration of antagonist (atropine) and vice versa.

The dose of atropine, required to produce the antimuscarinic action (also called anticholinergic action) by the blockade of muscarinic receptor, varies from organ to organ. Salivary secretion is extremely sensitive to the blockade by atropine, while the smooth muscle of GI tract, eye, and heart muscles are less affected or blocked by atropine. In CNS, the cholinergic transmission at their subcortical and cortical level is predominantly muscarinic and can be blocked by atropine (atropine can penetrate the blood-brain barrier).

Pharmacological properties of atropine

i. Central nervous system:

Atropine has almost no detectable effect on CNS in doses which are used clinically. In this dose, it produces the peripheral effects only. At therapeutic doses (0.5–1 mg), atropine causes only mild stimulation of medulla (including vagal, respiratory, and vasomotor centers) and some higher cerebral centers. But, with higher toxic doses, atropine can produce severe cortical excitation, restlessness, disorientation, hallucination, and delirium. With still higher doses, this stimulation of CNS is followed by depression, leading to circulatory collapse, respiratory failure, and coma. The belladonna alkaloids and other related muscarinic receptor antagonists are also used to suppress the tremor and rigidity of Parkinsonism (extrapyramidal symptoms) by blocking the relative muscarinic cholinergic overactivity in basal ganglia. Muscarinic receptor antagonists are also used to treat the extrapyramidal symptoms that commonly occur as side effects, after antipsychotic drug therapy. Atropine also depresses the vestibular excitation which works through the muscarinic cholinergic pathway and thus exerts an antimotion sickness property.

ii. Cardiovascular system:

The most prominent effect of atropine on CVS is tachycardia. It is due to the blocking of vagal action, mediated by their muscarinic M2 receptors on SA node. Sometimes, initial transient bradycardia often occurs before this tachycardia. There are no accompanying changes in blood pressure or CO by atropine. This is because the cholinergic impulses are not involved in the maintenance of vascular smooth muscle tone and BP.

The influence of atropine on HR is most noticeable in healthy young adults, in whom the vagal tone is highest. Contrary in infancy and old age, even large doses of atropine may fail to produce tachycardia. This is because in this age group vagus has minimum action on heart. Atropine often produces cardiac arrhythmias, but without any significant cardiovascular symptoms.

Vagus nerve mediated many reflexes, such as the bradycardia or asystole, caused by oculo-cardiac reflex, anal stretching, peritoneal reflexes, etc. can be abolished by atropine. Atropine shortens the functional refractory period of AV node and facilitates AV conduction, provided it is caused by the increased vagal tone. Thus, in some 1st and 2nd degree heart block, caused by increased vagal tone, atropine may lessen the degree of this type of block. In some patients with complete heart block, the idioventricular rate may be increased by atropine. Occasionally, in therapeutic doses atropine causes cutaneous vasodilatation and flushing. This may be a compensatory reaction, permitting the loss of heat to balance the atropine-induced rise in body temperature, due to the inhibition of sweating.

iii. Glands:

Atropine markedly decreases lachrymal, tracheal, bronchial, salivary, and other secretions of our body by blocking the muscarinic M3 receptors which are responsible for these secretions. Atropine also inhibits the activity of sweat glands, innervated by sympathetic cholinergic fibers. Because, it acts as an anticholinergic agent. Thus, the skin, mouth, and eyes become dry; talking and swallowing become difficult. Cephalic and fasting phase of gastric secretion is also markedly reduced, but the intestinal phase is partially inhibited by atropine. As both the HCO^- and H^+ secretion are blocked, so the pH of gastric secretion does not increase, i.e., does not become more alkaline. The secretion of mucin and proteolytic enzymes in stomach are more directly under the control of the vagus nerve than the acid secreting cells. So, atropine inhibits the secretion of mucin and enzyme more than the acid in stomach. Intestinal and pancreatic secretions are not significantly reduced by atropine. Bile secretion is not under cholinergic control, so it is not affected by atropine.

iv. Smooth muscles:

All the visceral smooth muscles that receive parasympathetic or cholinergic motor innervation are relaxed and the sphincteric smooth muscles are contracted by atropine. This is mediated by the muscarinic M3 receptor blockade action caused by atropine, because parasympathetic cholinergic nerves enhance both the smooth muscle tone and motility of GI tract and relax the sphincteric smooth muscle, acting through M3 receptor. However, the peristalsis of GI tract is only incompletely suppressed by atropine. This is because the intestine has a complex system of intramural local nerve plexuses that regulate its motility and is not completely dependent on parasympathetic or cholinergic control. It (intestinal motility) is also regulated by some local reflexes and other neurotransmitters (5-HT, enkephalin, etc.) and hormones. Cholinergic impulses from CNS through vagus which can be blocked by atropine, only modulate these intrinsic reflexes of intestine.

In a normal subject and in a patient with GI disease, atropine produces prolonged inhibitory effect on the motor activity of stomach, duodenum, jejunum, ileum, and colon.

This inhibitory effect of atropine on GI tract is characterized by a reduction in tone, amplitude, and frequency of peristaltic contractions, resulting in relief from spasm and causing constipation. However, relatively large doses of atropine are needed to produce such inhibition.

In regulating bronchomotor tone, the parasympathetic neurons play a major role. Vagal fibers make synapses and activate the nicotinic receptors in parasympathetic ganglia, located in the wall of the airway. Short postganglionic parasympathetic fibers come out from this ganglion and release ACh which finally acts on the M3 muscarinic receptors on airway smooth muscles. The submucosal glands are also innervated by these postganglionic parasympathetic neurons and have predominantly M3 receptors. So, vagal stimulation causes airway smooth muscle contraction and increased tracheobronchial secretion. Thus, atropine causes bronchodilatation and reduces airway resistance, especially in COPD and asthma patients, by inhibiting this vagal cholinergic activity. Inflammatory mediators such as histamine, prostaglandins, kinins, etc. also increase vagal activity in addition to their direct actions on bronchial smooth muscles and glands, causing bronchoconstriction and increased airway resistance. Atropine also partially blocks their action by antagonizing the reflex vagal component (mediated by histamine, prostaglandins, kinins, etc.) and forms the basis of the use of anticholinergic agents, along with β-adrenergic agonists in the treatment of bronchial asthma. Thus, with the introduction of inhaled ipratropium (semisynthetic anticholinergic agent), anticholinergic therapy in COPD and asthma has been revived.

Atropine by its anticholinergic activity also decreases the normal tone and amplitude of the smooth muscle contraction of ureter and bladder. So, urinary retention may occur in older males, especially with prostatic hypertrophy during the use of anticholinergic agent (atropine).

Atropine also exerts mild antispasmodic action on gallbladder and bile ducts. But, this effect is not usually sufficient to prevent its marked spasm and increased biliary duct pressure, induced by opioids. In such circumstances, the nitrates are more effective than atropine.

v. Eye:

The muscarinic receptor antagonists or anticholinergic agents block the responses of cholinergic neurotransmitter such as ACh on the sphincter pupillae muscle of iris and the ciliary muscle of lens, which are responsible for constriction of pupil and accommodation of vision. Thus, atropine dilates the pupil (mydriasis) and paralyzes the accommodation reaction (cycloplegia) of eye. The wide dilatation of pupil causes photophobia. Due to the blockade of ciliary muscles, the lens become fixed for far vision and the near objects become blurred. This is called the paralysis of accommodation or cycloplegia.

Thus, the topical instillation of atropine causes mydriasis, loss of light reflex, cycloplegia, photophobia, and blurring of near vision, lasting for 7–10 days. The IOP (intraocular pressure) tends to rise, especially in narrow angle glaucoma by atropine. However, all these effects are caused by topical application of atropine and the conventional systemic dose of atropine produces minor ocular effects. Muscarinic receptor antagonists such as atropines, used as a mydriatic, differ from the sympathomimetic agents, such as epinephrine which also causes mydriasis. This difference is that the latter causes only pupillary dilatation without any loss of accommodation. Because sympathomimetic agents act only on the dilator muscle of pupillae and have no action on the accommodating ciliary muscle of lens.

Absorption rate and excretion: All the anticholinergic agents, such as the natural belladonna alkaloids, semisynthetic derivatives, and tertiary synthetic derivatives are well absorbed rapidly from the GI tract. But, the quaternary synthetic derivatives are poorly absorbed orally and their effects on CNS are lacking. This is because these quaternary agents do not cross the blood-brain barrier. The half-life of atropine on parenteral administration is approximately 4 hours. Half of the doses of atropine is metabolized in liver and the remainder is excreted unchanged through urine.

Atropine Substitutes

Many semisynthetic and large number of fully synthetic derivatives of belladonna alkaloids have been introduced in clinical practice with the aim of producing more selective antimuscarinic actions. These synthetic derivatives are again classified as *quaternary compounds, tertiary compounds, mydriatics,* and *anti-parkinsonians.*

Quaternary Anticholinergic Agents

The characteristics of quaternary anticholinergic compounds are:

- Poor oral absorption
- Do not produce CNS and ocular effects, after parenteral or oral administration, due to their poor penetration in brain and eye.
- Have higher nicotinic receptor blocking property which may even occur at clinical doses, causing postural hypotension and impotence.
- At higher doses, the neuromuscular blocking effect may also occur due to the blocking of nicotinic receptor at motor endplate.

The following are the quaternary anticholinergic agents:

- *Hyoscine butylbromide:* It is used as antispasmodic.
- *Atropine methonitrate:* It is used for abdominal colic and hyperacidity. As an aerosol, it is also used in the treatment of bronchial asthma.
- *Ipratropium bromide:* It is also used in the treatment of bronchial asthma by inhalation. The ipratropium bromide acts on muscarinic receptors, located mainly on the large central airways (in contrast, sympathomimetic agents such as β_2 agonists which act primarily on the peripheral bronchioles). The increased parasympathetic (cholinergic) tone is the major reversible factor in **(Figs. 18A to C)** chronic obstructive pulmonary disease (COPD). Therefore, it is more effective in COPD than in acute bronchial asthma. The another desirable feature of ipratropium is that in contrast to atropine, it does not depress the mucociliary clearance of bronchial epithelium. It has gradual onset of action and late peak (60–90 minutes) bronchodilating action in comparison to inhaled sympathomimetic agents. So, it is more suitable for regular prophylactic use, rather than for rapid symptomatic relief, during an acute attack.
- *Tiotropium bromide:* It is a congener of ipratropium with high bronchial selectivity in action.
- *Propantheline:* It is used for the treatment of gastric ulcer by reducing gastric secretion.
- *Oxyphenonium:* It is used for the treatment of peptic ulcer by reducing gastric secretion.
- *Clidinium:* It is used with diazepam as antispasmodic in nervous dyspepsia, irritable colon, etc.
- *Pipenzolate:* It is used for infantile colic.

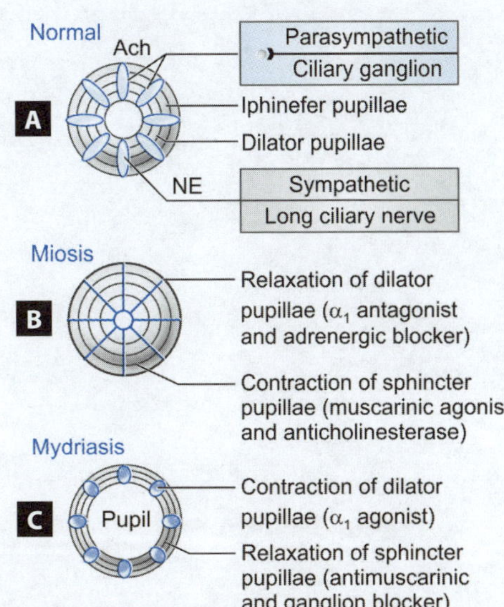

Figs. 18A to C: Autonomic control of pupil. (A) Normal pupil; (B) Miotic pupil; (C) Mydriatic pupil.

- *Isopropamide:* It is used in hyperacidity, nervous dyspepsia, irritable bowel syndrome, etc.
- *Glycopyrrolate:* It is a potent and rapidly acting antimuscarinic agent, lacking the central and ocular effects. Otherwise, all its (glycopyrrolate) clinical actions are like atropine. The dose of glycopyrrolate to control the muscarinic effects of neostigmine is 10–15 µg/kg.

Tertiary Anticholinergic Agents

- *Synthetic atropine:* Already discussed.
- *Dicyclomine:* Due to direct smooth muscle relaxation effect, it is used as an antispasmodic.
- *Pirenzepine:* It selectively blocks the M1 muscarinic receptors and inhibits gastric secretion, without producing typical atropine like side effects which are due to the blockade of M2 and M3 receptor. The exact location of M1 receptors through which pirenzepine exerts its antisecretory action is not definite. The most likely site of action of pirenzepine is the intramural plexuses and the ganglionic cells, rather than the parietal cells of stomach.

Mydriatics

- *Homatropine:* It is 10 times less potent than atropine as mydriatic agent and its peak onset of action is 40–60 minutes. The mydriasis, caused by homatrophine, lasts for 1–3 days, while the accommodation recovers in 1–2 days.
- *Cyclopentolate:* It is also a potent and rapidly acting mydriatic agent. Mydriasis and cycloplegia occur in 30–60 minutes and lasts for a day.
- *Tropicamide:* It has the quickest (20–40 minutes) and briefest (3–6 hours) mydriatic and cycloplegic action.

Nicotinic Receptor Agonists and Antagonists

As described before, the nicotinic receptors are rosette-like pentameric (have five subunits) structures, enclosing a cation (Na^+) channel. The activation of this receptor causes the opening of this channel and the rapid flow of cations such as Na^+ resulting in depolarization and action potential of cell membrane. Specifically, these receptors are activated by nicotine (so it is such named) and blocked by tubocurarine or hexamethonium. These nicotinic receptors are classified into N_N and N_M (previously as N_1 and N_2) subtypes on the basis of their location and their selective agonists and antagonists.

i. N_M nicotinic receptor:

These are located at the endplate of skeletal muscle and are activated by ACh, but they are selectively activated by phenyltrimethylammonium (PTMA). Activation of these receptors mediates skeletal muscle contractions. Activation of these receptors by ACh is antagonized by tubocurarine and other nondepolarizing muscle relaxants.

ii. N_N nicotinic receptor:

They are present on the cell membrane of (i) the sympathetic and parasympathetic ganglionic cells, (ii) the cells of adrenal medulla (as the adrenal medulla is derived embryologically from the same site as ganglionic cells), (iii) the cells of spinal cord and in certain areas of brain. They are also stimulated by ACh, but are selectively stimulated by dimethylphenylpiperazinium (DMPP) and blocked by hexamethonium. They constitute the primary pathway for the transmission in ganglia.

Preoperative Evaluation and Preparation

■ INTRODUCTION

The diversity and versatility of the subject of anesthesia makes proper preoperative evaluation of each patient a major issue. This is because, a single anesthetic procedure cannot meet all the various demands of all the patients. The ultimate need of preoperative assessment, in patients about to undergo anesthesia care, is to reduce morbidity and mortality, to improve the quality of anesthesia, to optimize the patient's health, and to return the patient to normal functioning, as early as possible. So, an anesthesia program should be made, keeping in mind the specific patient's physiological status, psychological built-up, past and present medical conditions, previous surgical history, present complaints, drug allergy and intolerance, anesthetic experiences of the past, and, of course, the planned surgical procedure. We should remember that improper and inadequate preoperative evaluation is one of the major causes of all anesthetic complications. So, every time surgery is planned in a patient, he should be evaluated thoroughly in the preanesthetic clinic by an anesthesiologist preferably, treated for any existing medical pathology and his health should be optimized, that is he should be made fit for anesthesia.

■ PREOPERATIVE ASSESSMENT

Preoperative assessment is traditionally done by arranging a meeting between the patient and the anesthesiologist. This facilitates certain important purposes, and helps to make the patient comfortable, by rendering a healthy patient–doctor relationship.

Goals Achieved by Preoperative Assessment

1. It helps to know the medical history and the psychological make-up of the patient, to assess any known or unknown underlying pathology, to determine the required laboratory tests and specialized consultations, for optimizing the patient's health. This decreases hospital-stay and unnecessary delay in scheduling of surgery.

2. It helps the anesthesiologist to select the proper anesthesia care or program for the operation planned by understanding the patient's mental make-up and the medical history.

3. In this age of information technology, a preoperative meeting between the patient and the anesthesiologist helps to inform and educate the patient about the anesthesia services rendered, perioperative care, and postoperative pain management. Patient education also helps to reduce the patient's anxiety, allay his fears, and makes recovery faster and better.

4. It helps to maintain a more optimal health of the patient by managing preexisting medical pathologies efficiently. Detection and treatment of conditions such as respiratory tract infection, diabetes mellitus, congestive cardiac failure, etc. prior to delivery of anesthesia, by proper and meticulous preoperative assessment, improves the quality of anesthesia and optimizes the health of the patient, thus reducing perioperative morbidity and mortality. The presence and severity of underlying medical problems may require consultation with specialists, for obtaining an optimal medical condition, before anesthesia is actually delivered. The specialist's help can also be extended for better perioperative care.

5. It facilitates better perioperative care management and even helps to make it less costly by proper planning.

6. It helps to obtain an informed consent from the patient, in the true sense, for all medicolegal purposes.

Routine Preoperative Anesthetic Assessment

1. History
   - Name, age, sex, and weight
   - Present complaints
   - Past medical history

- *Treatment history:*
  - Medicines being used currently
  - Medicines that had been used in the past
  - Drug allergy and intolerance
- *Social history:*
  - History of addiction and habits, drugs, alcohol, tobacco, etc.
- *Nonspecific factors:*
  - Obstetric history in females, pain history, etc.
- *Family history:*
  - For malignant hyperpyrexia, porphyria, cholinesterase abnormality, etc.
- History of previous surgery and anesthesia.

2. History to have an Overall Review of All Systems
   - *Respiratory system:* History of smoking, bronchitis, common cold, asthma, chronic cough, etc.
   - *Cardiovascular system:* History of hypertension, palpitation, chest pain, syncope, dyspnea, etc.
   - Gastrointestinal system
   - Genitourinary system
   - Musculoskeletal system
   - Neurology
   - Hematology
   - Endocrinology
   - Orthopedics
   - Dermatology
   - Psychiatry

3. Physical Examination of the Patient
   - *General condition:* Pallor, cyanosis, jaundice, edema, consciousness, aptitude, cooperativeness, activity level, etc.
   - *Vital signs:* Arterial blood pressure in both hands, examination of peripheral pulses, jugular and carotid pulsations, etc.
   - *Airway:* Neck mobility, jawbone size, tongue size, etc. for intubation.
   - *Pulmonary evaluation:* Auscultation for rhonchi, wheeze, crepts, or other sounds of lung pathology.
   - *Cardiovascular evaluation:* Auscultation for murmurs, thrust, gallop, and other adventitious sounds.
   - *Extremities:* Edema, clubbing, varicosity of veins, etc.
   - *Neurological examination:* Peripheral neuropathy, tremor, convulsion, seizure, etc.

4. Laboratory Investigations
5. American society of anesthesiologists classification.

■ HISTORY TAKING

History taking is the most vital part of preoperative evaluation. It helps to establish all known past and present medical problems of the patients, plan the anesthetic program, laboratory tests, and postoperative management efficiently. The medication history often reveals significant drug allergies, (rash and dyspnea), drug interaction, and drug intolerance (GIT or gastrointestinal tract problems). Even herbal medicines cause drug interactions, like garlic, often used to reduce blood pressure and cholesterol level, inhibit platelet aggregation and should be discontinued 7 days prior to surgery. Ginseng, a root, is often used as an antistress factor is known to produce hypoglycemia and inhibition of coagulation cascade, and should be discontinued 7 days prior to surgery. Meticulous history to review the various systems and their pathologies, if present, is one of the best tools for optimal assessment of a patient, along with optimal choice of laboratory investigations required and subsequently the perfect choice of anesthesia care. Preoperative interview helps to bring out important information and gives the anesthesiologist enough time to motivate a patient for a healthy lifestyle, like maintaining blood pressure and blood sugar, reducing or even quitting smoking, if required, etc. This naturally improves the quality of the anesthesia service and helps to reduce morbidity and mortality due to anesthesia **(Box 1)**.

Laboratory Investigation

Preoperative laboratory testing and its results had so far been the primary source of information of a patient's vital characteristics. But now, they are considered ineffective as screening devices. The tests are considered useful only when the anesthesiologist changes the anesthesia plan according to the laboratory test results for the benefit of the patient and helps to optimize the health of the patients. But, it is not always true that the results of the laboratory tests

---

BOX 1: The rule of three for history taking.

1. The three aspects of acute history that affect preoperative evaluation of a patient waiting for anesthesia are:
   - i. History of present health problems
   - ii. Tolerance to exercise
   - iii. How long ago the patient had visited his primary care physician?
2. The three aspects of chronic history that affect preoperative evaluation of a patient waiting for anesthesia are:
   - i. Medicines being used currently and allergy, if any, to any medicine
   - ii. Family history
   - iii. Social history
   - iv. History of past illness
3. The three features of clinical examination are:
   - i. Vital signs of the patient
   - ii. Pulmonary assessment
   - iii. Cardiovascular evaluation

are necessarily adjuvants to the patient's medical history and physical examination for meticulous preoperative assessment.

Preoperative test with borderline or false-positive results can merely distract the anesthesiologist's attention and cause no benefit at all. The anesthesiologist may then pursue and treat this border-line or false-positive cases unnecessarily, causing unwanted delay in scheduling of surgery and also making the procedure expensive. Thus, unindicated routine laboratory testing can decrease the overall quality of anesthesia care, by causing sheer confusion and is often harmful for the patients. So, laboratory tests should only be implemented in patients in whom it may decrease health hazards, mortality, and morbidity due to anesthesia. Extra-testing hardly provides medicolegal protection to the anesthesiologist. When too many tests are ordered, the anesthesiologist often tends to overlook the slightly positive or borderline cases, and that poses greater medicolegal risk to the doctor. Only those patients who actually suffer from a disease may benefit from the test specific for the disease.

American Society of Anesthesiologists Classification

The ASA (American Society of Anesthesiologists or American Association of Anesthetists) had classified the pre-operative patients into seven groups (**Box 2**) and in 2002, had set up a set of guidelines to be followed by anesthesiologists during routine preoperative evaluation (**Box 3**).

This helped the anesthesiologists to do a meticulous and justified preoperative assessment, of a patient waiting for anesthesia and surgery. It was not mandatory to follow these guidelines, but they were there to help the anesthesiologists, whenever they were in a dilemma to take decisions.

The guidelines were:
1. In patients undergoing minimally invasive surgery, the anesthesiologists' opinion, based on the history and physical examination, should be considered more important than the results of the laboratory tests.
2. In patients undergoing surgery other than the minimally invasive ones, or if patient is not presently healthy, preoperative evaluation should always occur one day prior to the day of surgery.
3. Certain laboratory tests to be done as routine procedures in most invasive surgeries.
4. Pregnancy test to be done in all female patients of the reproductive age group.

■ ANESTHETIC PLAN

The choice of the final anesthetic plan should be safe, comfortable for the patient, suit the competence and

---

BOX 2: American Society of Anesthesiologists classification of patients waiting for surgery.

- *Grade 1:* Normal, healthy patients, no preexisting medical pathology, other than the disease for which surgery is planned
- *Grade 2:* Patients with mild systemic disease, without any functional handicap
- *Grade 3:* Patients with severe systemic disease, with functional handicap
- *Grade 4:* Patients with severe life-threatening systemic disease
- *Grade 5:* Moribund patients who would die without the surgery
- *Grade 6:* Brain-dead patients who are being operated for removal of organs, for donor purposes
- *Grade E:* Emergency procedures—here the physical status is followed by E, e.g., -3E

BOX 3: Routine preoperative laboratory investigations.

- *Full blood count:*
  - All male patients above 50 years of age
  - All female patients
  - All major surgical procedures whenever pallor is detected clinically
- *Routine urine examination (for sugar, blood, and protein):*
  - All patients
- *ECG (an ECG tracing is valid for a year, if there is no recent history of cardiac pathology):*
  - All patients above 50 years of age
  - All patients with cardiac diseases, hypertension, and chronic pulmonary diseases
- *Blood glucose (FBS and PPBS):*
  - All patients with diabetes mellitus
  - All patients with glycosuria
- *Urea and creatinine electrolytes:*
  - All patients >60 years of age
  - All major surgical procedures
  - All patients with diabetes mellitus
  - All patients taking diuretic drugs
  - All patients with renal diseases
- *Blood coagulation tests:*
  - All patients with bleeding tendencies
  - All major surgeries
- *Chest X-ray:*
  - All patients of acute cardiac diseases
  - All patients of acute pulmonary diseases
  - Chronic-on-acute cardiac or pulmonary diseases
  - Malignant diseases
  - Suspection of pulmonary tuberculosis
- *Pregnancy test:*
  - All female patients in the reproductive age

(FBS: fasting blood sugar; PPBS: postprandial blood sugar)

---

experience of the anesthesiologist, and, of course, depend on the type of surgery and the convenience of the surgeon. A detailed and meticulous preoperative evaluation enables the anesthesiologist to draw an anesthetic plan (**Box 4**) and discuss it in details with the patient. This helps to assure

BOX 4: A routine anesthetic plan.

- Fasting premedication
- Plans of airway maintenance anesthesia planned:
  - *General anesthesia:* Induction
    - Muscle relaxation maintenance reversal
  - *Regional anesthesia:* Technique
    - Drugs
  - *Monitored anesthesia care:* Oxygen supplementation intraoperative management
  - Monitoring of the patient
  - Positioning of the patient depending on the surgery
  - *Fluid management:* Ventilation
  - Special procedures, if required postoperative management
  - Fluid management pain management
  - Postoperative ventilation, if required, special care, if required
- Complication management

BOX 5: Routine preanesthetic preparation.

- Patient education and psychological support, regarding all procedures planned
- Sedation to be given the previous night, for a restful sleep
- Fasting
- Evacuation of the urinary bladder
- Removal of false teeth and eyes, artificial limbs, contact lenses, jewelleries, nail varnish, etc.
- Loose OT dress to be worn
- Identification tag to be put on the patient
- Signature on the informed consent
- Premedication
- All resuscitative measures to be started, like intravenous line, noninvasive monitoring, etc.
- *Documentation:* Preoperative notes

quality of anesthesia service, reduce the patient's anxiety and fear, and reduce mortality and morbidity.

■ PREANESTHETIC PREPARATION

Routine preanesthetic preparation is a must for every patient ready to undergo anesthesia and surgery **(Box 5)**.

Fasting

It is an important event during the postoperative preparation of a patient for surgery or anesthesia. Aspiration of gastric contents into the lungs is associated with high morbidity and mortality. Some very common causes for regurgitation of gastric contents and subsequent pulmonary aspiration are: pregnancy, obesity, full stomach, difficult airway, emergency surgery without proper preoperative medication, etc. Even 20–30 mL of gastric content aspirated can cause severe irreversible pulmonary damage. So, one of our main aims during preoperative preparation of a patient is to decrease the volume of gastric content, so that regurgitation is prevented.

Gastric emptying time may be delayed due to metabolic disorders (diabetes mellitus or renal failure), head injury, pyloric stenosis, opioids, trauma, etc. Whereas, pregnancy and obesity increase the intra-abdominal pressure and cause passive regurgitation.

Antacids (not the particulate ones), like sodium citrate solution, given shortly before induction of anesthesia, neutralizes the acid in the stomach, but is not at all preferred by most anesthesiologists as it increases the volume of gastric contents, causing further complications. Proton-pump inhibition and H_2 blockers decrease acid secretion in the stomach and are very effective. Gastric motility increasing agents, like metoclopramide, are very effective, especially in trauma patients being put up for emergency operation, more

TABLE 1: American Society of Anesthesiologists guidelines for preoperative fasting in healthy patients presenting for elective surgeries.

Clear liquid	Water, clear tea, fruit juice without pulp	2 hours
Breast milk		4 hours
Infant formula milk		4–6 hours
Animal milk	Cow, goat, and buffalo	6 hours
Light meal	Toast	8 hours
Solid meal	Fish, chicken (high fat or protein content)	8 hours

by the intravenous route than orally. Ranitidine may also be used routinely, especially in pregnant patients **(Table 1)**.

Premedication

A preoperative interview between the doctor and the patient, thorough explanation of all planned and anticipated procedures, and support-cum-compassion of the anesthetic team are not always enough to allay the fears and concern of the patient, and reduce all the unwanted stress factors. Certain drugs are often used to treat anxious patients preoperatively. Preoperative medication helps the anesthesiologist to travel a comfortable road during the course of anesthesia, and decreases morbidity and mortality to a great extent.

Special care should be taken to select the drugs for premedication of each patient individually, depending on the history and clinical examination of the patient, the surgery planned, and the anesthetic program decided.

Metoclopramide

It is essentially a prokinetic drug, i.e., it increases the gastroduodenal motility and hastens gastric emptying.

Though it is structurally similar to procainamide, its pharmacological properties are absolutely different from procainamide. Metoclopramide is now widely used as an antiemetic.

It relaxes the pylorus and the first part of the duodenum, and thus hastens gastric emptying. It increases the lower esophageal sphincter (LES) tone, and prevents gastroesophageal reflux. It also increases intestinal peristalsis but has no action on gastric secretion. It has certain antidopaminergic actions, prolactin-secretion inducing action, and blocking of vomiting induced by narcotics. So, it is considered to be a relatively selective D_2 antagonist and its antiemetic action is due to D_2 antagonism in the chemoreceptor trigger zone (CTZ). Peripherally, it has cholinomimetic actions, i.e., it increases acetylcholine release from the myenteric neurons. This, in turn, promotes gastroduodenal peristalsis, speeds up gastric emptying, and increases the LES tone. Metoclopramide also blocks the $5HT_3$ receptors present in the CTZ and the vagal efferents in the GIT, but only in higher doses.

Metoclopramide is absorbed very rapidly when given orally, crosses the blood-brain barrier and the placental **(Fact file I)** barrier, and is secreted in the breast milk. Its half-life is 4–6 hours. It is partly conjugated in the liver and is excreted through the urine. It speeds up absorption of drugs like aspirin and diazepam, reduces the absorption of digoxin, and decreases the effects of levodopa, by blocking the DA receptors in the basal ganglion.

Metoclopramide is well tolerated but certain extrapyramidal symptoms such as dizziness, sedation, muscle dystonias, and diarrhea are not uncommon. Galactorrhea, gynecomastia, and parkinsonism may occur, when the drug is used continuously for a long time. The dose is 10 mg orally, IM or IV.

It is an effective antiemetic agent for many types of vomiting such as drug-induced, postoperative, radiation sickness, chemotherapy-induced, migraine, etc. It is not very effective in motion sickness and should be used very cautiously in pregnancy, as the safety factor is still not very well-defined. It should also be used cautiously in lactating mothers since it is secreted in the breast milk. It is the most effective gastrokinetic agent used to accelerate gastric emptying, especially when general anesthesia has to be given in a patient posted for emergency surgery, when he has taken solid food <4–5 hours ago.

Ondansetron

This is a $5HT_3$ antagonist, first developed to control intense nausea and vomiting induced by chemotherapy or radiotherapy, in patients undergoing treatment for cancer.

But, later it was found to be equally effective in controlling postoperative nausea and vomiting. Ondansetron blocks both the peripheral origin in the gut and the central pathway in the CTZ, of the emetogenic reflex. But, neither does it reduce motion sickness induced nausea and vomiting nor does it block the dopaminergic receptors. Unlike procainamide, it does not have any prokinetic action in the GIT. It blocks the $5HT_3$ receptors, thus inhibiting the action of 5HT in the GIT as well as in the CTZ. Thus, it is useful in combating the multifactorial origin of postoperative nausea and vomiting **(Table 2)**.

Due to first pass metabolism, bioavailability of ondansetron after oral intake is about 60–70%. CYP1A2, 2D6, and 3A can hydroxylate ondansetron. Drug interactions are rare. It is secreted through the urine and feces as metabolites. The half-life of ondansetron is 2–5 hours and duration of action is 4–10 hours. Side effects are rare. Dose to control postoperative nausea and vomiting is 4–8 mg IV and may be repeated after 4 hours.

(The other drugs have been discussed in the relevant chapters).

Informed Consent

All conscious, educated, and competent patients have the right to either give or withhold consent for their treatment, or even a physical examination. A competent person is an adult, who is intelligent enough to understand his problems, remember the information given to him, and weigh out the risk–benefit ratio rationally, to make a decision regarding his treatment. No other person can interfere with the decisions of such a competent person. To get the consent of the patient, all details of the anesthetic procedures with its alternatives and complications should be discussed, so that the intelligent and competent person can understand and choose the best procedure for his treatment. A thorough discussion of the benefits versus the risks often helps the patient to choose the best option. All theoretical risks need

---

FACT FILE I

A good premedicant should:
- Help to decrease the patient's anxiety and stress.
- Decrease the secretion of the respiratory tract.
- Decrease salivary secretion.
- Decrease undesirable vagal reflexes.
- Reduce intraoperative awareness of the patient.
- Facilitate smooth recovery from anesthesia.
- Reduce postoperative nausea and vomiting.
- Reduce postoperative restlessness of the patient.
- Reduce postoperative pain.
- Be safe for the patient.
- Protect the patient from the toxic effects of anesthetics.
- Keep the patient optimized.

TABLE 2: Some commonly used preoperative drugs.

Drugs			Route	Dose
Drugs increasing gastric	pH	Ranitidine Omeprazole Sodium citrate solution	Oral IM/IV Oral IV Oral	• 150–300 mg previous night and 2 hours before surgery • 50 mg 2 hours before surgery • 40 mg previous night and 2 hours before surgery • 40 mg slow IV over 40 minutes • 30 mL 10 minutes before surgery
Sedatives	BDZ	Temazepam	Oral	10–30 mg
		Lormetazepam	Oral	0.5–1.5 mg
	Non-BDZ	Lorazepam	Oral	1–2.5 mg
		Midazolam	Oral	0.2–0.5 mg
			IM	2–10 mg
		Zopiclone	Oral	3.75–7.5 mg
Antiemetics		Metoclopramide	Oral/IM/IV	10 mg
		Ondansetron	IV	4–8 mg before surgery
Analgesics	Opioids	Morphine	IM/SC	10–15 mg
		Pethidine	IM	50–100 mg
	NSAIDs	Diclofenac	Oral/PR	50–100 mg
	Others	Paracetamol	Oral/PR	1 mg
Anticholinergics		Atropine	IM/IV	0.6–2 mg
		Glycopyrrolate	IM/IV	0.1–0.3 mg
Anxiolytics		Diazepam	Oral	5–10 mg

(BDZ: benzodiazepine; IM: intramuscular; IV: intravenous; NSAIDs: nonsteroidal anti-inflammatory drugs)

not be detailed, instead the common and realistic ones should be explained. Life-threatening complications, if likely, should always be enumerated. This often helps the patient and his guardian to accept the inevitable and prepares them mentally, allay their concern and anxiety to some extent.

Competent young adults over the age of 16 years can give their own consent regarding their treatment. Competent children even below the age of 16 years can give their own consent, especially if they can weigh out the risk–benefit ratio appreciably. If a competent child refuses treatment, the consent of the parents enables the doctor to proceed with all life-saving procedures. The consent of the parents is enough to start treatment in patients below the age of 18 years, who are not competent. Verbal consent may be accepted in life-threatening and emergency conditions, but written ones are always preferred for medicolegal purposes. When the child or even the parent refuses treatment in an emergency and life-threatening condition, a court order may be sought to continue with the necessary treatment legally. Unconscious adults may be given essential treatment without consent, but it is always better to discuss the procedures with his guardian. Patients hospitalized with mental disorders may be treated without consent for his mental problems, but never for his associated physical ailments. But, electroconvulsive therapy (ECT) always requires the consent of the patient or his guardian.

Restricted Consent

Some competent patients may give consent for the treatment in general, but refuse certain aspects of the treatment, e.g., blood transfusion. This is called restricted consent. The risks and the benefits of the procedures should be discussed in details with the patient, always in presence of a witness. All details of the patients' restrictions and refusals should be noted in the consent form, duly signed by the patient and the witness. But, in the end, the desire of a competent patient should be honored.

Any procedure performed without a proper consent can lead to medicolegal assault of the anesthesiologist. Treatment without consent is allowed only in dire emergencies or in life-saving procedures.

Documentation

Maintenance of pre-, intra- and postoperative anesthesia record is of utmost importance in present day scenario. It helps to monitor the patient intraoperatively, deal with postoperative complications if any, and is the best document for all medicolegal purposes. Thus, proper documentation ensures quality service.

Preanesthetic Record

A preanesthetic record maintenance is absolutely mandatory nowadays. It should contain all the information about the preoperative evaluation of the patient by the anesthesiologist and his team, including medical history, treatment history, laboratory test results, ASA classification of the patient, and advice of the specialist, if required, for optimizing the health of the patient. It should have the detailed anesthetic plan with all the alternatives clearly stated. All common and probable complications should be mentioned. It should also contain an informed anesthesia consent, duly signed by the patient or his guardian. This record may be handwritten, narrative, or printed forms may also be filled up with all the details.

Intraoperative Record

This is a useful intraoperative monitor and assures quality anesthesia service. It also helps to guide future anesthesia care. Hence, this document should be accurate and precise.

It should include the following:

- Checking of the anesthesia machine and other instruments, required to provide quality anesthesia delivery and service, often referred to as the "cockpit drill".
- Final evaluation of the patient before the induction of anesthesia.
- Checking for the duly signed anesthesia consent, newer laboratory results, if any, and specialist's advice for optimizing the health of the patient, if required.
- All information about the important and vital anesthesia procedures such as intubation, positioning of the patient, attachment of all invasive and noninvasive monitors, Ryle's tube placement, etc.
- Details of intraoperative fluid management and blood product transfusion.
- Details of all drugs administered with their dosage used and time of administration.
- Details of findings of all intraoperative monitoring and assistance.
- All vital signs recorded every 5 minutes, if possible, graphically.

- Timing of all vital events such as intubation, excision, extubation, etc.
- Complications, if any, and how they were managed.
- The patient's condition during extubation and recovery from anesthesia.

Postoperative Record

The anesthesiologist should always accompany the patient to the postanesthesia care unit (PACU) and look after the patient till all the vital signs become normal and the patient is considered stable. He should give a detailed discharge note before the patient leaves the PACU, including the pain management procedures and the general condition of the patient during discharge from the PACU. Only then, does the responsibility of the anesthesiologist end.

■ CONCLUSION

The primary goal of an anesthesiologist is to deliver quality anesthesia service to the patient, decreasing morbidity and mortality in the process and most important, returning the patient to his normal stable status as soon and as efficiently as possible. This whole procedure is a teamwork. A balanced harmony among the anesthesiologist, surgeon, internist, and specialist ensures the best possible outcome. For the anesthesiologist, the show is the longest, starting from meticulous preoperative evaluation and ending with the discharge of the patient from the PACU, and hence the job is the toughest. Thus, preoperative evaluation and meticulous and thoughtful patient preparation facilitate achieving the most sought-after goals, improve quality care, and reduce the cost of treatment. Perhaps the most productive and enjoyable part of clinical anesthesia practice is interaction with the patient during preoperative evaluation in the preanesthetic clinic (PAC). Inefficient and inadequate preoperative assessment is nowadays the main reason for medicolegal assault against anesthesiologists.

Local Anesthetic Agents

■ HISTORY

The *local anesthetics* (LAs) are drugs or agents which temporarily prevent or cause the reversible loss of generation of impulses from any part of a neuron or temporarily stop the conduction of impulses through a nerve fibers, when they come in contact with it, but without causing any structural damage of it. The term *"local anesthesia"* is restricted to the technique of infiltration of local tissue with a LA agent, where only the nerve endings, supplying that particular tissue, are blocked. Whereas the term *"regional anesthesia"* signifies the temporary block of conduction of impulses through a specific nerve or a group of nerves, supplying a particular region of the body such as hands, legs, face, etc.

Before the days of LA agents, in the 16th and 17th centuries, Ambroise Paré (French surgeon) obtained the effect of local anesthesia, by producing direct mechanical compression on nerve trunks. Then, other European and American surgeons also followed this procedure of Ambroise during this period for local anesthesia. For many centuries, the leaves of an indigenous shrub, called Erythroxylum coca, were chewed by the people of Peru and Bolivia of South America, as a central nervous system (CNS) stimulant and appetizer. During this chewing of these leaves, they were used to feel numbness of their oral mucous membrane. But, at that period this associated numbness (the LA effect) of their oral mucous membrane was not given much importance by them. They also never knew that this effect (numbness) is primarily due to the LA effect, caused by the principal alkaloid, named cocaine, present in the leaves of these shrubs.

However, it was first understood, and this alkaloid (cocaine) was isolated by Niemann in 1860. Then, the physiological or LA effects of *cocaine* were studied in detail by Sigmund Freud, in 1880. But, he did not publish it. In 1884, when S. Freud was visiting his fiancé, then his colleague Carl Koller took the opportunity and in his absence Carl Koller

first declared and introduced the LA properties of cocaine in an Ophthalmological Congress. Thus, he (C. Koller) himself took all the credit of discovery of cocaine immediately.

Then, he performed an impressive series of experiments on himself and his colleagues, using the suspension of cocaine powder in distilled water. After that, this news of Koller's work spread rapidly all over the world and subsequently cocaine solution was injected locally or applied topically by a wide variety of practitioners for local anesthesia in both Europe and America. But, the high systemic toxicity and addictive properties of cocaine had engineered the search for a better substitute of it. Thus, *procaine* came in 1905, which was synthesized first by Einhorn, in 1904. It was less toxic than cocaine, but unfortunately it was quite unreliable and had a very short duration of action.

Then, gradually many other nonpromising LA drugs came and phased out. Such as, in 1930, *dibucaine* and *tetracaine* arrived which despite being much longer acting, still proved to be toxic in large volumes. Furthermore, these compounds, being esters like their predecessors, were unstable at high temperature and thus could not be autoclaved. Another great disadvantage of these ester groups of LA agents was that their metabolites had frequently caused allergic reaction which was sometimes very serious.

The next great milestone in local anesthesia was the introduction of *lignocaine*, in 1943. It was first synthesized by two scientists, named Lofgren and Lundquist in the laboratory of Astra. However, the beauty of lignocaine is that it was not an ester compound like their predecessors. Therefore, this drug was stable at high temperature and less toxic. It did not have such metabolites that could be implicated for allergic reactions. Hence, during that period it became the first prototype of a new class of LA agents, called the "amides". However, it is still now the most widely used LA agent all over the world. Subsequently, the late 1950s saw the appearance of *mepivacaine* and *prilocaine*.

In 1963, the introduction of *bupivacaine* in clinical practice was the beginning of an era of long-acting LA agents in anesthesia which are amides. But, the potential more cardiotoxicity of bupivacaine than lignocaine had provided the impetus for the development of *ropivacaine* which is the newest lesser cardiotoxic, but long-acting amide LA agent. It became available by 1997 in most of the countries.

Other than LA agents, the LA action can also be produced by many other compounds, such as some tertiary amines, certain alcohols, and few other drugs such as propanol, antihistamines, quinidine, chlorpromazine, etc. But, they are not used for this purpose, because of their local irritation and other undesired prominent systemic effects. Local anesthesia can also be produced by deep cooling, as for example by the application of ice, CO_2 snow, ethyl chloride spray, etc. on the surgical site.

■ CHEMISTRY OF LOCAL ANESTHETIC AGENTS

A general molecular structure of a LA agent and their salt with HCl is depicted in **Figures 1 and 2**. All the LA agents bear the suffix "caine". Structurally, they have two groups: (1) a *lipophilic aromatic* group and (2) a *hydrophilic amine* group. This amine group may be a secondary or a tertiary amine. An intermediate chain (alkyl or acyl) links these two groups through an *ester or amide linkage*. On the basis of this ester or amide linkage, the LA agents are classified into two broad groups.

When this linkage chain is an ester (–COO–), then they are called the *ester LA agents* (esters of aromatic acids with amino alcohols). The examples of ester LA agents are *cocaine, procaine, chloroprocaine, amethocaine (tetracaine), etc.* Esters are unstable in solution and cannot be autoclaved, because of their relatively unstable ester-linkage. They are also too short acting, because of their rapid metabolism.

When the linkage chain is an amide (–NHCO–), then they are called the *amide LA agents*. These amide LA agents are again of two types: (1) amides of aromatic acid with aliphatic di-amines (aminoalkyl amides) and (2) amides of aromatic acids with amino amines (aminoacyl amides). The examples of aminoalkyl amides are *cinchocaine (dibucaine or nupercaine) and procainamide*. The examples of aminoacyl amides are *lignocaine, prilocaine, mepivacaine, bupivacaine, etidocaine, ropivacaine, etc.* **(Fig. 3)**. Among all the amide LAs, only the hydrophilic amine group in prilocaine is a secondary amine. Otherwise, all others have tertiary amines.

The amine group in the structure of an amide LA molecule confers it the property of an insoluble weak base (or proton acceptor). Thus, it can combine with an acid to form a water soluble acid salt which is shown in **Figure 2**. This water soluble acid salt remains in more ionized form in

Aromatic lipophilic group	Intermediate linking chain (ester –COO– or amide –NHCO–)	Amine hydrophilic group, secondary or tertiary amine

Fig. 1: Linkage of an anesthetics.

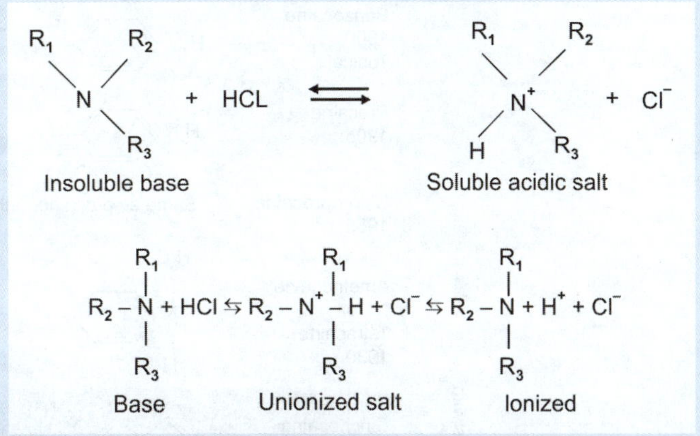

Fig. 2: Chemistry of an anesthetics.

its commercially available aqueous solution than its alkaline salt, which is not soluble in water.

All the LA drugs, except ropivacaine, are of racemic mixtures. However, ropivacaine is unique, in that, only it is available in its pure chiral form. This is important, because all the racemic mixtures have more toxicities and variable potencies, when compared to its chiral form. So, one of the major advantages of ropivacaine, in clinical use, is its less systemic toxicity than any other LA agents, but with similar duration of action.

Features of Amide Local Anesthetics in Comparison to Ester LAs

- The amide groups of LA agents produce more intense and long lasting local anesthesia than the ester group of LA agents.
- The amide groups of LA agents bind to α_1 acid glycoprotein and albumin in plasma.
- The amide groups of LA agents are not hydrolyzed by plasma esterase like ester group of LA agents.
- The amide groups of LA agents very rarely cause hypersensitivity reactions than the ester group of LA and have no cross sensitivity with ester group of LA.

Carbonated Local Anesthetic Agents

From the previous discussion, we already come to know that the original amide groups of LA agents are insoluble weak base. So, the commercial preparations of these drugs are produced as soluble acidic salt (mainly *hydrochloride salt*, by reacting with HCl), with pH values ranging in between

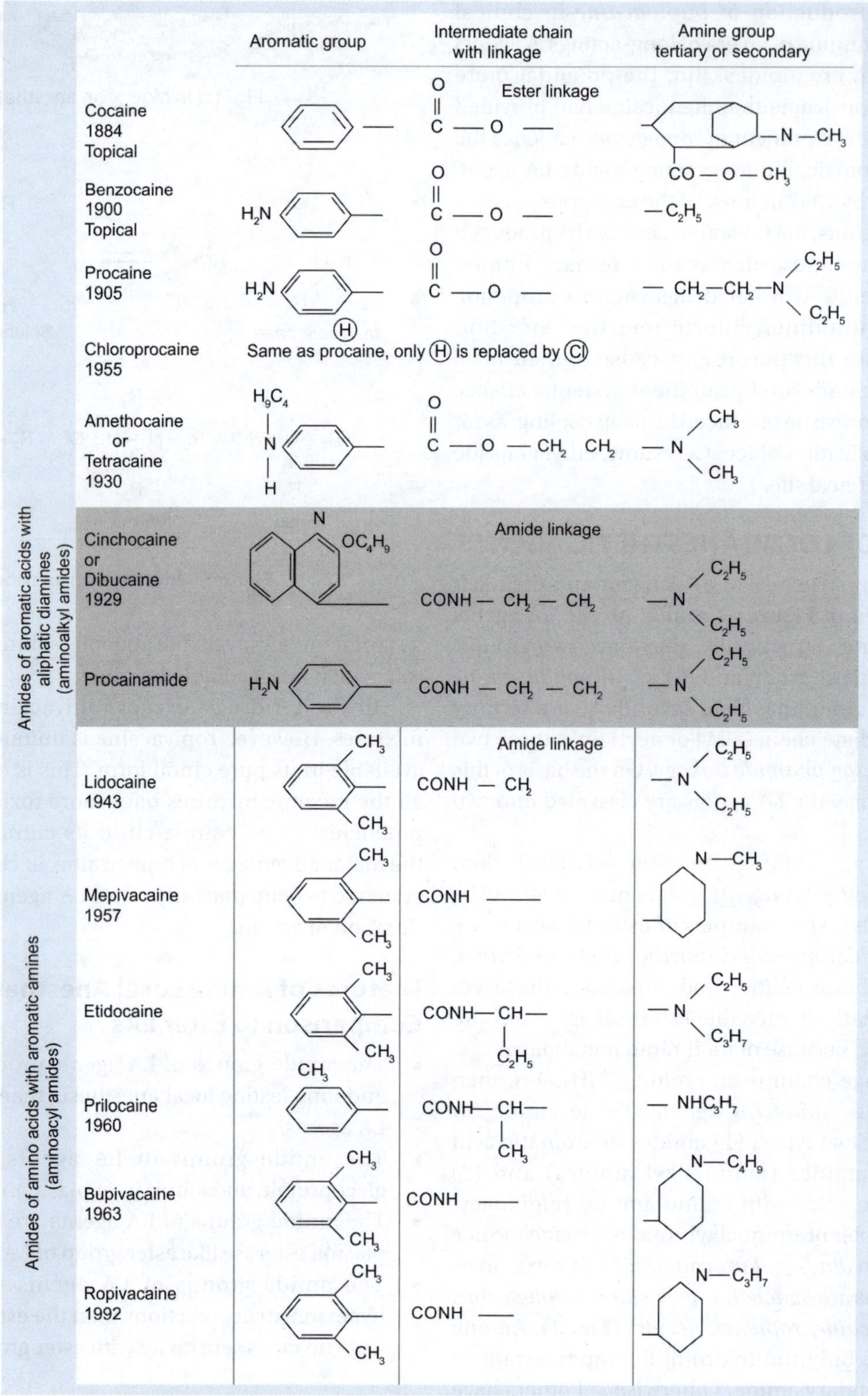

Fig. 3: Structures of various local anesthetic agents.

3 and 7. It is also clear from the previous discussion that in the solution of lower pH (i.e., in acidic situations), these drugs remain mainly in ionized form, and the ion of which cannot penetrate or diffuse the nerve cell membrane easily. On the other hand, we also come to know that only the unionized form of a molecule of LA agent penetrates or diffuse the nerve cell membrane easily and for its action from the inner side of the cell membrane of an axon, it further undergoes

intracellular ionization. Thus, the unionized molecule of a LA agent helps its penetration through the nerve cell membrane, and for its final action, this unionized molecule of LA agent ionizes first within the cell cytoplasm and then this ionized form acts at the inner side of the Na^+ channel which is situated on the cell membrane. The inner side of a Na^+ channel which is situated on the cell membrane is the principal site of action of LA agent. So, one would easily predict that due to more ionization of acid salt in the acidic solutions of LA agents it will have less penetrable form of LA molecule (i.e., unionized LA molecule). So, acidic hydrochloride preparation of LA agent will less penetrate the cell membrane and its intracellular concentration will be less. Hence, the acidic solution of a LA agent would take longer time for its onset of action, produce less intense block, and have an increased incidence of missed block. Therefore, it can be predicted that the alkalinization of a LA solution, with $NaHCO_3$ (which is called carbonated LA) prior to its injection, will result in its better action than its acidic solution, in respect to the onset, duration and density of action. This is because in an alkaline carbonated form LA agent remains more in the cell membrane-penetrable unionized form. But the main problem of this alkalization of LA agent is that the formation of original molecule of LA agent by adding $NaHCO_3$ are weak base and are so insoluble in water solution of it.

A number of factors contribute to the enhanced effect of a carbonated LA agent over its hydrochloride form. These are:

- When the pH of the solution of a LA agent is more alkaline, then there is an increased concentration of uncharged or unionized base form of this LA agent which can easily penetrate the cell membrane.
- CO_2 diffuses rapidly into the interior of the cell through its cell membrane. Within the cell the CO_2 lowers the intracellular pH (make acidic) by forming H_2CO_3 and increases the ionization of the LA agent.

The intracellular ionization of a LA agent helps in two ways:

- The release of more cations after the intracellular ionization of a LA agent enhances the nerve blocking activity of it.
- The reduction of the concentration of the unionized base inside the cell increases the gradient of this form of LA agent and helps for further diffusion of this unionized form of this LA agent into the cell.

Carbonated lignocaine is also superior to its hydrochloride form for epidural block in respect to the speed of onset, reduction in the incidence of missed segment and increased incidence of deep motor block.

Compounds with more lipophilic nature are obtained by increasing the size of the alkyl substitutes. These agents are more potent and produce long-lasting effects than their less lipophilic congeners. For example, etidocaine has three more carbon atoms than lignocaine in the amine end of the molecule and is four times more potent and five times more long lasting.

CLASSIFICATION OF LOCAL ANESTHETIC AGENTS

Local anesthetic agents can be classified under different headings as described here.

Injectable

- *Low potency and short duration of action:* Cocaine, procaine, and chloroprocaine.
- *Intermediate potency and medium duration of action:* Lignocaine, prilocaine, and mepivacaine.
- *High potency and long duration of action:* Tetracaine, bupivacaine, ropivacaine, dibucaine, and etidocaine.

Surface Anesthetic

- *Soluble:* Cocaine, lidocaine, tetracaine (amethocaine), and proparacaine.
- *Insoluble:* Benzocaine, oxethazaine, and butyl aminobenzoate (butamben).

Chemistry

- *Ester:* Cocaine, amethocaine (tetracaine), benzocaine, butamben, chloroprocaine, and procaine.
- *Amide:* Prilocaine, lidocaine, mepivacaine, bupivacaine, etidocaine, and ropivacaine.

As the amide groups of LA agents are structurally base, so it combines with acids to make a water soluble acidic salt which is stable in its aqueous solution and can be autoclaved. Otherwise, the amide group of LA itself, being a base, is not water soluble and is only soluble in relatively lipophilic organic solvents. So, for convenience, most of the LA drugs are marketed as its soluble acidic hydrochloride salts. On the other hand, the ester linked LA agents are unstable in its aqueous solution and cannot be autoclaved. The ester linked LA agents are degraded in plasma by hydrolysis, except cocaine, and their metabolites are more prone to produce anaphylactoid reaction. Cocaine is metabolized predominantly by hepatic carbonyl esterase. The para-aminobenzoic acid (PABA) is one of the important metabolites of all the ester type compounds that can induce anaphylactoid or allergic reactions. But, the amides are degraded by oxidative dealkylation in liver and hence anaphylactoid reactions are extremely rare, produced by them.

The lipophilic or lipid-soluble unionized form of amide LA agent (base or unprotonated) is the active form which can penetrate the nerve cell membrane. This unionized form of amide LA agent after entering the cell membrane is ionized and acts at the intracellular pole of Na^+ channel to exert their LA action. In a marketed acidic solution of amide LA agent, the unionized and ionized form of a LA compound remain in certain ratio. The equilibrium of this ratio, between the unionized and ionized portions of a particular LA agent, depends on the pKa value of that particular drug.

The pKa value of a LA agent is the pH, at which the unionized and ionized forms of this LA agent remain in 50:50 proportion. Most of the LA agents in clinical use are weak bases with pKa values varying between 7.5 and 9.5 (mainly around 8). The higher the pKa value of a drug, the stronger is its action as a base. Therefore, little of it will be available in the unionized (more will be ionized) form at normal body pH. As for example, the pKa value of lignocaine is 7.86. So, at a tissue pH of 7.8, lignocaine will have unionized and ionized forms in the ratio 50:50. But, at a pH of 7.4, only 25% of lignocaine will remain in the active unionized form and the rest 75% will remain in the nonactive ionized form. In an inflamed tissue, the pH is more acidic. So, the percentage of the active unionized form of LA agent will be lesser and the anesthetic effect will be also low in the same concentration or dose for a given drug. The relation between the pKa value, degree of ionization and the pH of a LA agent is shown in **Figure 4**.

The pKa value of procaine is 9. So, at pH 9 the unionized and ionized forms of this drug are at the proportion of 50:50. But, at pH 7.4, only 25% of procaine will remain in unionized active and penetrable to cell form and the rest will be in the ionized form. As, it is the unionized, lipid soluble moiety of a LA agent that can penetrate most rapidly the lipid rich

barriers protecting the axon, so one would easily predict that procaine would penetrate the body tissues slowly at normal body pH. Thus, the clinical utility of procaine is confined primarily to the circumstances in which the large lipid barriers are not encountered, such as during the direct topical anesthesia of cornea or conjunctiva and spinal anesthesia.

After injection in the tissue, the LA drug first moves from the site of injection to the area which is immediately outside the target nerve fiber. This movement of LA agent is probably through the subcutaneous or other tissues. The factors, governing this first stage of journey of a LA agent, from the site of injection to the site of action at nerve fiber are: (i) the concentration gradient, (ii) the total mass or volume of drug, (iii) the degree of ionization, and (iv) the solubility of LA agent.

The concentration gradient at the site of injection and the total mass depend on the volume and concentration of the drug injected. Greater concentration and bigger volume of injected drugs will cause a rapid increase in the therapeutic concentration of the drug at the nerve site. According to the theory of drug diffusion, the drug molecules of larger size will have more difficulty in moving rapidly through the extracellular space. In fact, the speed of drug movement is more closely related to the square root of the size of the drug molecules. The molecular weight of all the LA agents usually varies between 236 and 250 Da. Therefore, this factor (molecular weight) plays a little role in the difference, regarding the speed of onset of action among the LA drugs.

According to the previous discussion, it is found that at physiological pH most of the LA agents exist in a protonated or ionized form, while a much smaller portion exists as unprotonated or unionized form. Consequently, the sodium channel which is responsible for the cellular action potential (AP) is a protein in nature and is embedded in the lipid-rich cell membrane. It is the inner intracellular pole of this Na^+ channel which is the site of action of LA agents. Unprotonated LAs are lipophilic in nature. Therefore, these molecules move easily and rapidly through the cell membrane (but not through the Na^+ channel) to arrive inside the cell. Subsequently, this unprotonated or unionized form of LA agent, then, becomes protonated or ionized inside the cell and traverses through the water and electrolyte-rich cytoplasm of the cell to attach to the inner side of Na^+ channel. This protonated or ionized or cationic form of the LA agent is responsible for most of the nerve blocking or Na^+ channel blocking effect, which acts from the interior of the cell membrane. Whereas, the unprotonated or unionized or the base form of LA agent is responsible for penetration of the nerve fiber for its lipid solubility. Thus, the unionized form is more important and active form than the ionized form.

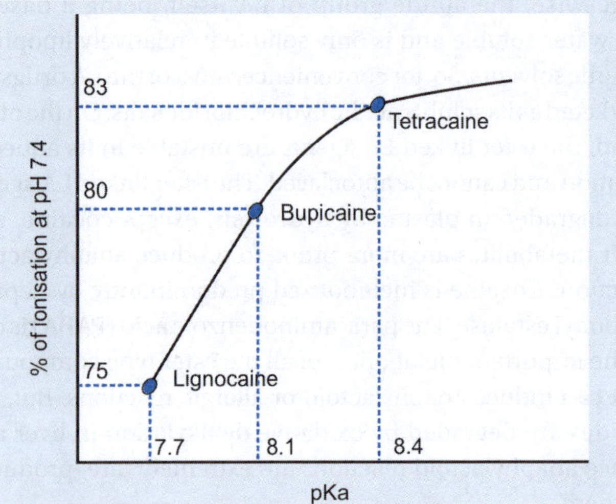

Fig. 4: This schematic diagram shows the percentage of charged ion of different local anesthetic agents with different pKa value at pH 7.4.

Once attached to the intracellular part of the sodium channel, it appears that the LA molecule can act on any one of the functional states of Na^+ channel. However, the LA inhibits only the active sodium channels more strongly than the inactive sodium channels. Actually, the sodium channels pass through a cycle of different stages. This corresponds to the different functional states depending on the different phases of the AP. The ability of a LA molecule to bind with any given form of sodium channel is said to be the function of the position of that sodium channel in its cycle of AP. It is also a dynamic process that channels are rapidly occupied and unoccupied by LA agents during a single AP.

The pH of a tissue into which LA agent is injected also directs the drug activity by altering the relative percentage of uncharged or unionized (unprotonated) and charged or ionized (protonated) molecule of the agent according to its pKa value. The uptake of drug by tissues largely results from the lipophilic absorption. So, as more of the drug will be lipophilic the more of this drug will be absorbed. Alkaline tissues alter the drug activity by matching the tissue pH with the drug pKa values and thereby favoring the unionized base for its absorption. The tissues also alter the effect of the drug by limiting the diffusion of the LA agent from its site of injection. The tendency of the drug to be protonated (ionized) also depends on many other environmental factors such as temperature and the medium surrounding the drug.

When the pH of a LA solution is lowered by the addition of adrenaline, sodium metabisulfite (antioxidant), glucose, etc. then the tissue pH becomes more acidic (this is because the buffering effect of local tissue is low) and the availability of unionized form of LA agent will be less. Thus, the power of penetration and intracellular concentration of LA agent decreases which in turn decreases the intracellular ionized form and hence the blocking action of the Na^+ channel from inside of the cell membrane. The mucous membrane also has minimal buffer reserve and so needs higher concentration of drugs for topical anesthesia. The pH of all marketed plain solutions of LA agents varies from 4.4 (etidocaine) to 6.3 (lignocaine).

■ ANATOMY OF NEURON

The term "neuron" means a nerve cell. It consists of a body and some processes which are coming out from this body. These processes are called the dendrites and axon. The dendrites are usually multiple in numbers, but axon is usually single in number. The neurons vary in their shapes and sizes in the different parts of our body. For example, its diameter varies from 5 μm (in cerebellum) to 120 μm (at the anterior horn cells of spinal cord). The length of axons also varies from a few micromillimeter to about 90 cm.

Within the cell body of a neuron, there is cytoplasm (in axon it is called axoplasm) and nucleus. The cytoplasm in the cell body of a neuron is again differentiated into two parts, such as under the cell membrane a superficial gel layer and a relatively fluid core at the center. The outer gel layer of cytoplasm has a contractile property. This contractile property of the outer gel layer results in a continuous flow of axoplasm from the cell body to the periphery into the axon and dendrites. A large vesicular nucleus with a single prominent nucleolus is seen in the every cell body of a neuron. In the cell body adjacent to the nucleus, there is often seen a large granule, representing sex chromatin. In the cytoplasm of the cell body of a neuron, near the nucleus, there are also found many Nissl's granules, numerous rod-like mitochondria, Golgi apparatus, and some fine long filaments which are called the neurofibrils. The neurofibrils and mitochondria can enter into the axons from cell body, but the Nissl's granules are not found in axon.

Nissl's granules are actually the endoplasmic reticulum and the granules covering them are called the ribonucleoprotein (RNP). The RNPs are one of the most striking morphological features of a neuron and it indicates intense protein production by it with high activity. In dendrite, the Nissl's granules are rod shaped. In motor neurons they are coarse and flocculent, while in sensory neurons they are almost dust like. The fatigue, poisons, and sectioning of the axon cause the Nissl's granules to disintegrate into fine dust and eventually disappear.

Dendrites are the processes that carry impulses toward the nerve cell body from outside (centripetally). They are generally shorter than the axon and contain many branches with Nissl's granules. The number of dendrites of a cell body varies from nil to numerous. But, as a rule they are multiple, relatively short, and follow a specific branching pattern.

According to the number of processes, the neurons can be classified in the following ways **(Fig. 5)**:

- *Apolar neurons:* They have no processes.
- *Unipolar neurons:* All the developing neuroblasts pass through this stage when they have only one process, and this single process is considered as the axon. In the adult humans such true unipolar neurons are not commonly seen. They are only found in the mesencephalic nucleus of 5th cranial nerve.
- *Bipolar neurons:* Typically these neurons are spindle shaped, possessing an axon at one pole and a dendrite at the other. Neurons, developing from neuroblasts, pass through this stage. In adults, they are usually found in the retina, vestibular ganglion, spiral ganglion of cochlea, and olfactory neuroepithelium.
- *Pseudounipolar neurons:* Such typical bipolar neurons are found in all the spinal ganglia and in the ganglia of

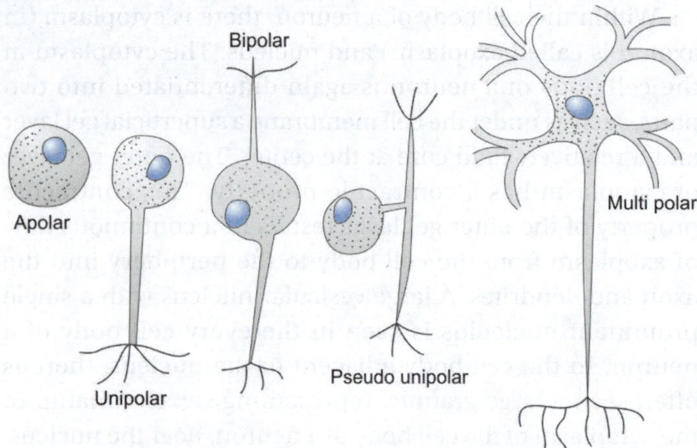

Fig. 5: Basic morphological features of different types of neurons.

cranial nerves, other than the 8th cranial nerves. In this type of neuron, there is a single process with T-shaped divisions. One branch of this T is a dendrite coming from the periphery and the other is the axon, extending centrally.

- *Multipolar neurons:* These neurons have most varied forms. They are the Purkinje cells of cerebellar cortex, the pyramidal cells of motor cortex, the small neurons of the spinal nucleus of trigeminal nerve, the motor neurons of the ventral horn of spinal cord, etc. Usually, the shape of these neurons depends mainly on the number and the position of dendrites.

Axon is the process of a nerve cell body which carries impulses away from it. The term nerve fiber usually refers to the bundle of axons. The axon arises from that part of the nerve cell body, which is called the axon hillock. The axon contains no Nissl's granules. The number of axon arising from the cell body of a neuron is single, but constant. If a neuron has only one process, then it will be the axon. The axis cylinder of an axon contains cytoplasm which is called the axoplasm. It is a semifluid substance and is essential for the nutrition and the growth of nerve fiber. The axon also contains many neurofibrils and mitochondria within its axoplasm and ends in numerous terminal button-like structures, which are called the telodendria.

So long as the nerve fiber or axon remains within the gray matter of CNS, it remains naked, without myelin sheath. Then, as soon as, it enters the white matter of CNS, it gets the first covering, called the myelin sheath (white). After that, when it comes out of the CNS, it receives a second covering called the neurilemma. When the nerve fiber terminates at the periphery on a target cell, then the neurilemma sheath is lost first and next the myelin sheath. Lastly, as axis cylinder, the axon ends on its target cell as a naked process without any coverings.

Each motor nerve fiber at its termination breaks up into about 150 branches and each of these branches ends on a separate muscle cell (fiber). One motor nerve fiber (axon) with all the muscle fibers that it supplies constitutes one motor unit. Each motor unit is controlled by one motor nerve cell of the CNS. In the CNS, the nerve fibers do not contain any neurilemma sheath. The myelination of nerve fiber in CNS does not take place by Schwann cells. It is occurred by oligodendroglia cells which surround the axon in CNS and form the myelin sheath. Schwann cells take part in the formation of myelin sheath in the periphery. Like the peripheral nerves, the nerve fibers of CNS also possess the nodes of Ranvier, but these are not so obvious as in the peripheral nerves.

Medullated (or Myelinated) Nerve Fiber and Myelinogenesis

In a myelinated nerve fiber, the central core is the axon and it is surrounded by myelin sheath. The cell or plasma membrane of this axon, which is called the axolemma, is here the actual impulse conducting membrane. The axon is filled with a viscous intracellular fluid, called the axoplasm. In a myelinated nerve fiber, the axolemma is surrounded by a sheath of lipid material, which is known as the myelin sheath. The myelin sheath is present in all the thick somatic nerve fibers, but not over the postganglionic autonomic nerve fibers. The somatic nerve fibers of 1 μ diameter or less are not medullated. All the preganglionic autonomic fibers are also medullated. The myelin sheath is again lined by a delicate membrane which is known as the neurilemma sheath. However, this is nothing but the last turn of the Schwann cell and is formed during the formation of myelin sheath. In the last turn of the Schwann cell, there is a nucleus which is located near the most outer membrane of the Schwan cell. Thus, the most outer Schwann cell membrane, nucleus, and the irregular cytoplasmic strands inside the Schwann cell membrane constitute the Schwann cell sheath of neurilemma in all the matured nerve fibers.

In a medullated nerve, the myelinogenesis is caused by the deposition of myelin sheath around the axon by the Schwann cells. The axon is first enveloped completely by a Schwann cell. The Schwann cell then gives several turns around the axon by many concentric layers of cytoplasm and its plasma membrane. Then, the cytoplasm disappears from the concentric layers, leaving only the plasma membrane of Schwann cells, wrapping one on another. Thus, the compact myelin sheath consists only of several concentric layers of plasma membrane of Schwann cell. Only the outer turn of the plasma membrane of Schwann cell persists as the sheath of neurilemma with some cytoplasm and nucleus inside the

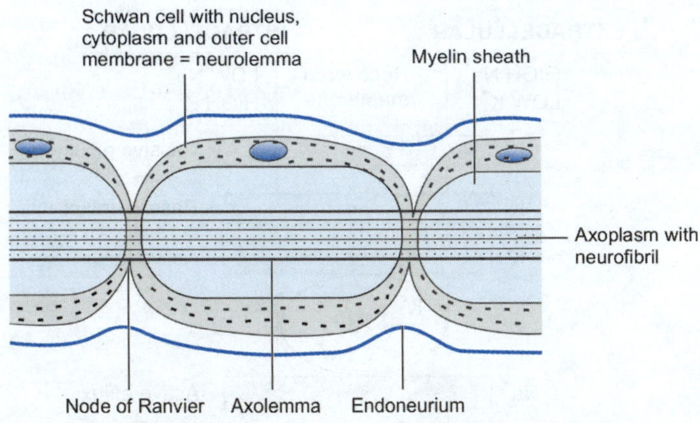

Fig. 6: Longitudinal section of a myelinated peripheral nerve.

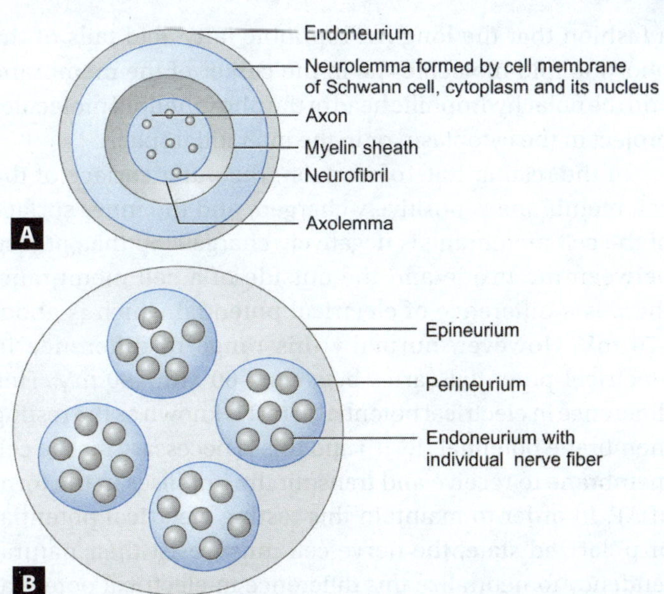

Figs. 7A and B: Organization of a single peripheral nerve fiber and a nerve trunk in cross section: (A) Cross section of a single nerve fiber and (B) Cross section of a nerve trunk.

neurilemma. This myelin sheath acts as an insulator and prevents the flow of almost all the ions across the axolemma. The myelin sheath is not continuous all over the whole axon, but is interrupted regularly at an interval by the nodes of Ranvier. In the nodes of Ranvier, the myelin sheath is absent, and the outer turn of the Schwann cell membrane (neurilemma) is dipped inward over the axon. In comparison with the myelin sheath, the axolemma and neurilemma in this region of the nodes of Ranvier are highly permeable to all ions and takes part in the conduction of impulse along the axon.

In case of unmyelinated nerve fibers, the axons are also buried within the Schwann cells. Here, the axons are enclosed by a Schwann cell, but it does not spin a myelin sheath around them. Nonmyelinated nerves exist in large amount in CNS and in the dorsal nerve root. In small number of myelinated nerve fiber which is present in CNS, myelination occurs by different processes. Here, the cell is oligodendroglia, but not the Schwann cells which take part in the process of myelination (or myelinogenesis).

Thus, a medullated nerve fiber consists of the following structures from within outward (Fig. 6):

- A central core of axon with semifluid axoplasm, which flows from the cell body of a neuron to the periphery. If the axon is sectioned, then the axoplasm pours from its cut ends. The axoplasm contains numerous fibrils like structure called the neurofibril and mitochondria. The axolemma (the cell membrane of the axon) separates the axoplasm from the surroundings structures.
- The axon is surrounded by a myelin sheath, which is interrupted regularly at the nodes of Ranvier.
- The neurilemma represents the outer most plasma membrane of Schwann cell and under it lies a thin layer of Schwann cell cytoplasm with its peripheral nucleus.
- At the most periphery, outside the neurilemma sheath, (which is the outermost single turn of a Schwann cell),

and a single axon is wrapped by a layer of permeable connective tissue, called the *endoneurium*. Several of these units are further bundled together within a sheath of squamous cells, known as the *perineurium*. This layer is more resistant than the endoneurium to the passages of chemical molecules. The perineural bundles can be seen with the naked eye. These multiple perineural bundles are packed by another outermost connective tissue covering and constitute a nerve. This outermost connective tissue covering of a nerve is called the *epineurium*. This layer protects the nerve from the external damage. It is more permeable than the perineurium and contains the nerve's blood vessels **(Figs. 7A and B)**.

ACTION POTENTIAL OF NERVE FIBER AND TRANSMISSION OF IMPULSES

Initiation of Action Potential

Action potential is the sequence of changes of intracellular and extracellular electrical charges which accompanies the passage of an impulse along the cell membrane. This is the mechanism by which the nerve cells transmit the electrical signals. A typical cell membrane is a molecular lipid bilayer which is composed of phospholipids and cholesterol in the ratio of about 5:1. This lipid bilayer of a cell membrane also contains many proteins which are absorbed on the surface or embedded in it. These proteins are known as the receptors or ion channels and are used for the communication between the intracellular and extracellular environment. The lipid bilayer character of a cell membrane is arranged in such a fashion that the long hydrophobic fatty acid tails of the phospholipid molecules lie in the center of the membrane and the polar hydrophilic head of the phospholipid molecules project in the cytoplasm or in the interstitial space.

In the resting state of an axon, the outer surface of the cell membrane is positively charged, and the inner surface of the cell membrane is negatively charged. So that, at rest, between the inside and the outside of a cell membrane, there is a difference of electrical potential which is about –70 mV. However, normally this range of difference in electrical potential varies between –60 and –90 mV. This difference in electrical potential at rest is known as the resting membrane potential (RMP) and this is necessary for the cell membrane to receive and transmit the impulses in the form of AP. In order to maintain this resting electrical potential or polarized state, the nerve cell must resist their natural tendency to neutralize this difference in electrical potential by opposing the diffusion of ions across the cell membrane according to their concentration gradient. So, this diffusion is opposed and the polarized state or the concentration gradient of ions between the inside and the outside of the cell is maintained by an ATP energized Na^+ and K^+ membrane pump (Na^+-K^+-ATPase pump) which actively push the Na^+ ion out of the cell and K^+ ion into the cell. For every three Na^+ ion is pushed out, two K^+ ion is pushed in.

In the resting state, the concentration of Na^+ ion at the outside of a cell membrane is higher than that of the inside of a cell membrane. Again, the concentration of K^+ ion at the inside of a cell membrane is higher than that of the outside of a cell membrane. On the other hand, K^+ can penetrate easily through a cell membrane at the resting state, but not the Na^+ ion. The positivity at the outside of a cell membrane which is due to higher Na^+ ion concentration and other reasons also cause the K^+ ion to be pushed inside the nerve cell, producing higher K^+ concentration inside the cell. The axoplasm (the cytoplasm of an axon) is also rich in proteins and organic acids, which are negatively charged and are too large to pass through the membrane **(Fig. 8)**.

These are also responsible for the negativity of the inside of a cell in the resting state. Not all the ions are equally important for the maintenance of RMP. But, each ion contributes to the aggregate potential difference across the cell membrane which is based on the ratio of their concentration gradient between the inside and the outside of a cell and also based on the permeability of cell membrane to that particular ion. The Na^+-K^+-ATPase pumps which are straddled in the cell membrane and require high energy phosphate (ATP) for their action are only responsible for maintaining Na^+ and K^+ gradient across the cell membrane at resting state. This gradient is again responsible for the influx of Na^+ into the cell and the movement of K^+ out of

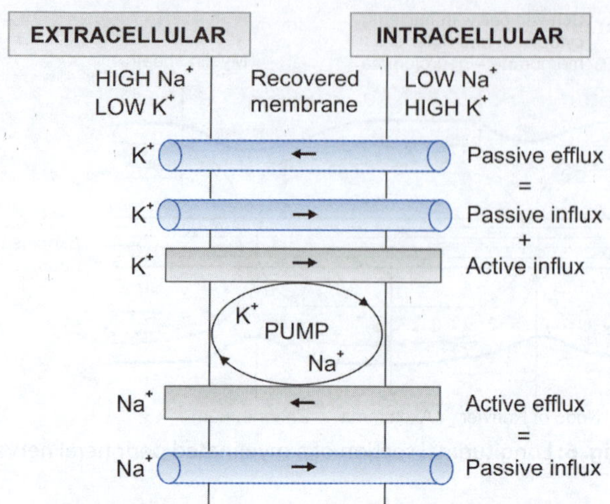

Fig. 8: Sodium pump is required to expel Na^+ from the interior of an axon, so that the internal Na^+ concentration is held to about 7% that of external fluid. At the same time, this pump also drives K^+ uphill from a lower external concentration of it to about 28 times higher its internal concentration.

the cell, during AP. If this gradient is not maintained, then AP is not possible.

In the resting state, the nerve fiber remains in a polarized state and the RMP lies around –70 mV. The inside of the nerve cell is negative and the outside of the nerve cell is positive. The permeability of Na^+ through the cell membrane is increased only when the stimulus reaches the cell membrane. It is the first event of the AP. It has been postulated that in the resting state the calcium ions (Ca^{++}) remain bound to the protein surfaces of the membrane pores. It does not allow the Na^+ ion to permeate these resting pores. During excitation, this Ca^{++} is dislodged from its binding sites, and the permeability of Na^+ inside the cell is increased.

With the entry of Na^+ inside the cell, the membrane potential gradually decreases. However, when the potential difference across the cell membrane comes to a critical or threshold level (approximately –20 to –40 mV for most cells), then there is a sudden and spontaneous increase in Na^+ permeability and Na^+ rushed inside the cell membrane. Thus, the depolarization starts with the onset of the increase in Na^+ permeability of the cell membrane. This tremendous increase in Na^+ conductance during this period is known as the activation of membrane. During depolarization, this change in transmembrane potential is accompanied by a further increase in Na^+ permeability with the creation of a positive feedback loop by which the influx of Na^+ facilitates further Na^+ influx.

Thus, due to the influx of Na^+ during depolarization, the reversal of electrical potential across the cell membrane is occurred with the development of positivity inside of the cell membrane and negativity outside of the cell membrane. With the increase of positivity, inside of the cell, the further entry of Na$^+$ is prevented and the calcium begins to bind with the proteins of membrane pores. So, at the end of depolarization, as soon as the transmembrane potential attains the voltage of approximately +50 mV, then Na$^+$ influx stops. In that situation, the cell attains an unstable condition, because both the Na$^+$ and K$^+$ are inside of the cell with reverse potential (positivity inside of the cell and negativity outside of the cell). But, this unstable condition cannot be allowed to continue indefinitely. So, at this point a less rapid but more sustained change in the permeability of the cell membrane to K$^+$ occurs and this is the beginning of repolarization. With the beginning of repolarization K$^+$ flows, along its concentration gradient, from inside to the outside of the cell, taking positive (+ve) charges with it. Thus, the loss of +ve ions from inside of the cell causes a fall in the electrical potential of the inside of a cell and reach the normal resting negative (–ve) value. But, indeed, the change in this K$^+$ permeability is sustained for a sufficient time and this is for the net potential difference across the cell membrane to reach –75 mV which is somewhat below the RMP (–70 mV). This hyperpolarization combined with the inactive sodium ion channel is responsible for the brief refractory period that each segment of a neuron requires following the generation of an AP.

In this hyperpolarization phase, though the RMP (i.e., negativity inside the cell and positivity outside the cell) is achieved, but the resting ionic status is not established (Na$^+$ inside and K$^+$ outside of the cell). So, the resting ionic status is achieved now by the active Na$^+$-K$^+$-ATPase pump mechanism and Na$^+$ begins to come out of the cell. Increased concentration of Na$^+$ outside the cell now causes the K$^+$ to diffuse back into the interior of the nerve cell.

Thus, the AP cycle is completed with the establishment of a normal electrical potential status and normal ionic status. Now, the Na$^+$-K$^+$-ATPase pumps maintain this concentration gradient of Na$^+$ and K$^+$ across the cell membrane. This whole process of AP is shown in **Figure 9**.

Transmission of Impulses

The *impulses* are actually the *propagated waves of depolarization*, caused by the continuous *coupling* between the excited and the nonexcited regions of the cell membrane of a nerve fiber. It has already been discussed earlier that a resting nerve fiber remains in a polarized state (not in a depolarized state) with positive charges lined up along the outside of the cell membrane and negative charges along the

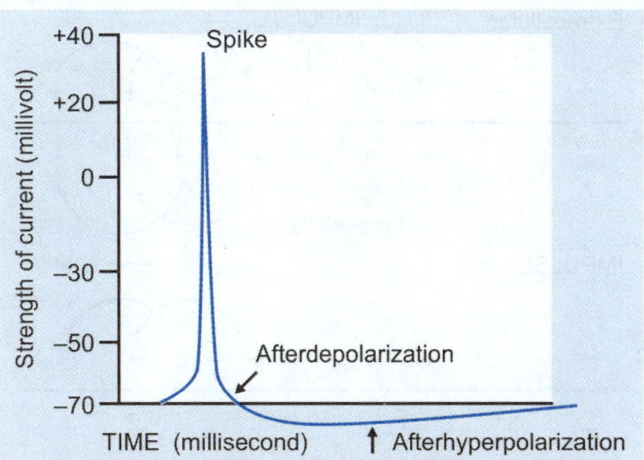

Fig. 9: A complete action potential. The first manifestation of action potential is the depolarization of membrane, i.e., the influx of Na$^+$ ion into the cell. After an initial –20 to –40 mV depolarization, the rate of depolarization increases. The point where this change of rate occurs is called the threshold or firing level. After the threshold level, the depolarization level overshoots and crosses the isopotential (or zero potential), to reach +40 mV. Then, the membrane potential reverses and falls rapidly toward the resting level. This is called the "repolarization". When this repolarization is 70% completed, then the rate of change decreases, and the tracing approaches the resting level more slowly. The sharp rise and the rapid fall of membrane potential are called the "spike". The slower fall at the end of the repolarization is called the "afterdepolarization". After reaching the resting level, the membrane potential slightly moves in the hyperpolarizing direction, to form a small but prolonged "afterhyperpolarization" state.

inside of the cell membrane. Then, as soon as the nerve fiber is excited at any point, then the polarity is changed (reversed) at that point of excitation for a brief period. However, this reversed polarity of cell membrane at that point of stimulation is due to the increased inward permeability of Na$^+$ through the cell membrane. Thus, a small area of depolarization develops at the point of excitation.

Then, a local circuit sets up and current flows between the depolarized area of the membrane which is developed at the point of the excitation and the adjacent resting polarized area of the membrane. Thus, an ionic current entering the axon through the excited depolarized region, flows down the axoplasm and exits through the surrounding resting membrane, causing the depolarization of the adjacent resting regions. Thus, a positive current flows inward through the depolarized membrane and a negative current flows outward through the resting membrane and in this way a small circuit of current or a wave of depolarization is completed whereas an impulse travels in all directions along the entire length of the nerve fiber.

Though, this circuit of local current or the wave of depolarization spreads away from the excited zone in both directions, *but the regions behind the impulse, having just been depolarized, is absolutely refractory*. So, the

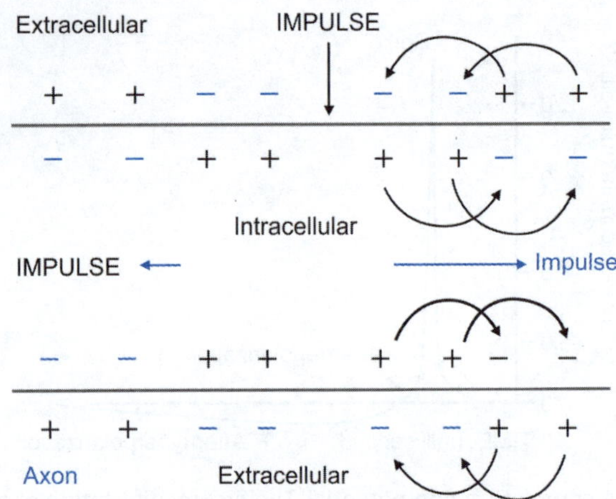

Fig. 10: Current flowing along the cell membrane of an axon (axolemma) in an unmyelinated nerve fiber.

impulse propagation is *unidirectional*. After the wave of depolarization, a repolarization wave first occurs at the point of stimulus, within a fraction of a second later than the depolarization wave and spreads progressively along the membrane, following the similar directions, as the depolarization wave had spread previously. This type of conduction is observed in the nonmedullated nerve fibers. This whole description is depicted in **Figure 10**.

However, in the myelinated nerve fiber, the conduction occurs in a similar pattern as described above. But the myelin sheath is an effective insulator. So, ions cannot pass through the myelin sheath. Therefore, the nodes of Ranvier only allow the ions to penetrate through it more easily. The nodes of Ranvier are 500 times more permeable than unmyelinated fibers. For this reason, the impulse or the wave of depolarization is transmitted from one node of Ranvier to another, rather than continuously along the entire length of the medullated nerve fiber. Thus, the depolarization in a myelinated axon (nerve fiber) jumps from one node of Ranvier to the next. So, this jumping or leaping of depolarization from one node to another is known as the saltatory (saltare means to jump or dance) conduction of impulse.

MECHANISM OF ACTION OF LOCAL ANESTHETIC AGENTS

The LA agents block the generation or conduction of nerve impulses by decreasing or stopping the entry of Na$^+$ ions through its channel inside the cell, during the depolarization phase of AP. As the concentration of LA agent is increased, then the rate of the rise of depolarization potential to the threshold level and subsequently the initiation of AP is inhibited, causing the slowing or total block of generation and conduction of nerve impulses.

The LA agent acts through its binding at a specific site which is situated at the intracellular portion of the voltage sensitive Na$^+$ channel and raises the threshold value of the opening of this channel. This binding site of LA agent at the intracellular portion of Na$^+$ channel is called the LA receptor. This Na$^+$ channel is nothing but a special protein through which Na$^+$ enters the cell, and also called the ion channel. Thus, the Na$^+$ channel fails to open, after binding with the LA agent and the Na$^+$ permeability fails to increase in response to an oncoming impulse or stimulation.

These Na$^+$ channels are situated in the cell membrane with a small portion protruding inside and outside of it. It has an activation gate (A) near its extracellular mouth and an inactivation gate (B) at the intracellular mouth. In the resting state, the activation gate (A) is closed and inactivation gate (B) remains open. During the depolarization of AP when the threshold level of membrane potential has been reached, then the activation gate opens and allows the Na$^+$ ions to flow inside the cell, along the concentration gradient. Because, at the resting state, the concentration of Na$^+$ outside the cell is higher than the inside of the cell. At resting state, the cell membrane is normally permeable to K$^+$ through the K$^+$ channel, but not permeable to Na$^+$ through the Na$^+$ channel. But, during the depolarization phase of AP the nerve membrane transiently switches its permeability from K$^+$ selectivity to Na$^+$ selectivity.

After the opening of the activation gate, within a few milliseconds, the inactivation gate (B) closes and ion flow ceases. But, in this phase, the activation gate is still open. After that, the channel recovers to the resting state in a time-dependent manner with the closed activation gate (A) and opened inactivation gate (B). This whole process is shown in **Figure 11**.

At a physiological pH, the LA molecule is partly ionized and partly unionized. However, the equilibrium between the unionized or unprotonated base form (BH) and the ionized or protonated or cationic form (B) of a LA agent depends on the pKa value of it, the pH of the solution, and also the pH of the local tissue. The LA agent traverses the nerve cell membrane in its lipophilic unionized form (BH).

Then, it (the LA agent) reionizes in the axoplasm and its ionized form approaches the LA receptor situates at the intracellular mouth of Na$^+$ channel. At the receptor site, the LA agent binds with the Na$^+$ channel and prevents its opening. It is the cationic or ionized form (B) of the LA agent which primarily binds to the receptor and is responsible for its action. The activated receptor has higher affinity or is more accessible to the LA agent, compared to the resting state of it. The binding of a LA agent molecule to its receptor site stabilizes the Na$^+$ channel in its inactive state and thus

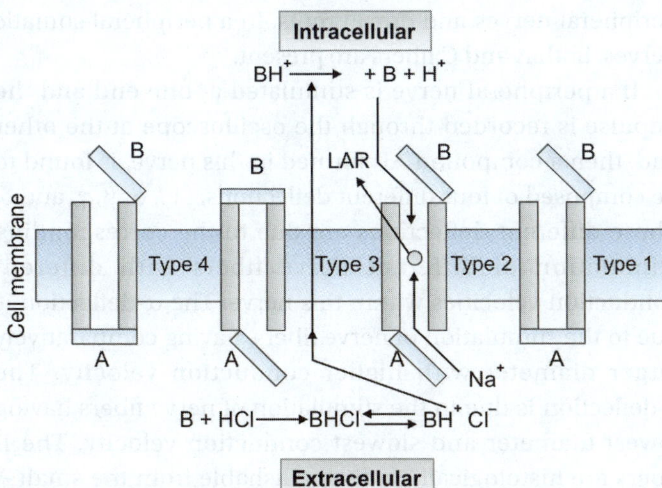

Fig. 11: This is a schematic diagram of axonal Na⁺ channel in different phases of action. The picture also shows the site and the mechanism of action of local anesthetic agents. The Na⁺ channel has an activation gate (A), near its extracellular mouth and an inactivation gate (B), at its intracellular mouth. In the resting state, the activation gate (A) remains closed, while the inactivation gate (B) is open **(Type 1)**. When the resting membrane potential (RMP), reaches the threshold level and depolarization shoots up, then the activation gate opens and allows the Na⁺ to flow into the cell along the concentration gradient **(Type 2)**. Within a few milliseconds the inactivation gate (B) closes and the flow of Na⁺ stops **(Type 3)**. After that the Na⁺ channel recovers to the resting stage **(Type 4)** by the opening of inactivation gate (B) and the closing of activation gate (A). B = Insoluble local anesthetic base, BHCl = Soluble hydrochloride of local anesthetic (LA), but nonionized, BH⁺ = Ionized form of LA, LAR = Local anesthetic receptor.

reduces the probability of the opening this Na⁺ channel and prevents the influx of Na⁺ inside the cell. Thus, it prevents the depolarization part of AP to be initiated and block the conduction of impulses through a nerve fiber. With the gradual increased concentration of LA agent, how the AP of nerve fiber is inhibited, is shown in **Figure 13**.

Moreover, the exposure of LA receptor to higher concentration of Ca²⁺ reduces the inactivation of Na⁺ channels and lessens the degree of block. Here, the generation of blockade of any conduction of impulses by the LA agent is not due to the hyperpolarization of cell membrane. In fact, RMP is also unaltered, because the K⁺ channels are not affected. These are blocked only by higher concentrations of the LA agent **(Fact file I)**.

Thus, a resting nerve is rather resistant to blockade and blockade develops rapidly when the nerve is stimulated repeatedly. The degree of blockade is also frequently dependent on higher frequency of stimulation. The onset of blockade is primarily related to the pKa value of the LA agents. Those with lower pKa values (7.6 to 7.8), such as lidocaine, mepivacaine, etc., are fast acting, because 30–40%

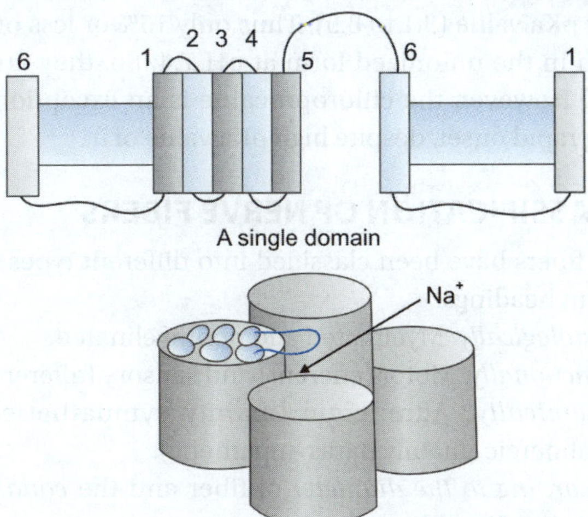

Fig. 12: Four domains forming the Na⁺ channel.

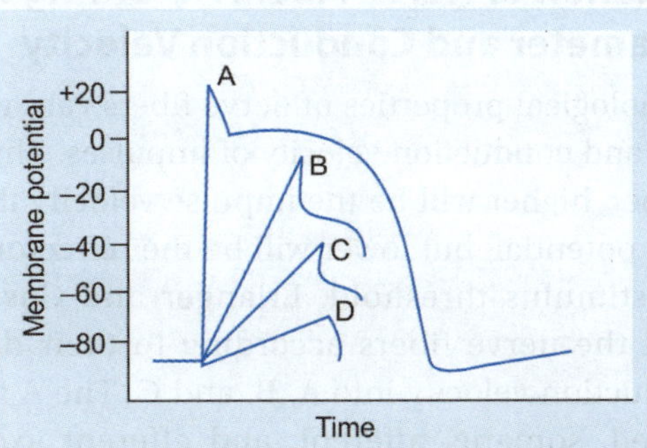

Fig. 13: This is the schematic diagram of action potential of different nerves, untreated or treated by LA agents. A = Action potential of a nerve untreated by a local anesthetic, B, C, D = Show the effects of LA agents on the generation of action potential of a nerve fiber by progressively increasing its (LA agent) concentration.

FACT FILE I

The molecular weight of a neuronal Na⁺ channel has been found to be of 300 KDa. Chemically, it is a glycoprotein and is composed of one large (α) and two small (β₁, β₂) subunits. The α-subunit encloses the Na⁺ selective pore within its four homologous domains (I to IV) where each domain has six membranes spanning helical segments (S₁–S₆) connected alternately by intracellular and extracellular loops. The wall of the pore is formed by the S₅ and S₆ segment of all the four domains, while the short nonhelical loops connecting S₅–S₆ segments on the extracellular surface fold into the pore and serve as the activation gate. The voltage sensor, located in the S₄ segment, move vertically on depolarization, and open the activation gate by allosteric conformational change. A few milliseconds later, the short intracellular loop connecting the domains III and IV folds into the inner mouth of the pore, activating the channel. The LA receptor is located in the S₆ segment of domain IV. This is shown in **Figure 12**.

of these LA agents remain in the unionized base form at pH 7.4 and it is this form of LA agent which only penetrates the axon membrane. Procaine, tetracaine, and bupivacaine have higher pKa value (8.1 to 8.9). Thus only 15% or less of them remain in the unionized form at pH 7.4. So, they are slow acting. However, the chloroprocaine is an exception of it, having rapid onset, despite high pKa value of it.

■ CLASSIFICATION OF NERVE FIBERS

Nerve fibers have been classified into different types under different headings:
- *Histologically:* Myelinated and nonmyelinated.
- *Functionally:* Motor (efferent) and sensory (afferent).
- *Chemically:* Adrenergic (mainly sympathetic) and cholinergic (mainly parasympathetic).
- *According to the diameter* of fiber and the *conduction velocity* of impulses.

Classification of Nerve Fibers According to their Diameter and Conduction Velocity

The physiological properties of nerve fibers vary with their diameter and conduction velocity of impulses. Thicker will be the fiber, higher will be the impulse velocity through it and peak potential, but lower will be the refractory period and the stimulus threshold. Erlanger and Gasser have classified the nerve fibers according to their diameters and conduction velocity into A, B, and C. The A fibers are myelinated, somatic, afferent, and efferent axons. The B fibers are the preganglionic, myelinated, efferent, and sympathetic axons. The C fibers are the sympathetic, somatic, and unmyelinated axons. Again the C fibers are of two types, i.e., the s C group and d r C group. The s C groups of fibers are the efferent, postganglionic sympathetic axons, and the d r C groups of fibers are the small afferent axons, found in the peripheral nerves and dorsal roots. In a peripheral somatic nerves, both A and C fibers are present.

If a peripheral nerve is stimulated at one end and the impulse is recorded through the oscilloscope at the other end, then a compound AP, formed in this nerve, is found to be composed of four different deflections, i.e., α, β, γ, and δ. These different deflections are due to the corresponding stimulation of different nerve fibers with different conduction velocities within this nerve. The α-deflection is due to the stimulation of nerve fibers, having comparatively larger diameter with higher conduction velocity. The δ-deflection is due to the stimulation of nerve fibers having lowest diameter and slowest conduction velocity. The B fibers are histologically indistinguishable from the small A fibers, but distinguishable principally from A fibers by the absence of negative AP. The C fibers in a somatic nerve are stimulated only when the threshold stimulus is higher than the stimulus which is used in case of A fibers. Functionally, the C nerve fibers are distinguishable from the A fibers by slow conduction velocity, long spike duration, and a high threshold value.

The classification of nerve fibers according to their conduction velocity and diameter is given in **Table 1**. For the clinical blockade of a myelinated nerve fiber a segment or a length of at least 6 mm (or preferably 10 mm), representing 2–3 nodes of Ranvier must be exposed to the LA agent. Because, it will deter the impulses from skipping over the blocked segment by a process which is known as the saltatory conduction. The motor nerves have greater internode distances, than the sensory nerves. This may account for the differential blocked, favoring the affection of more sensory

TABLE 1: Classification of nerve fibers according to their diameter and conduction velocity.

Types of fiber	Diameter of fiber in μm	Velocity of conduction in m/sec	Location	Sensory function	Motor function
(Myelinated) A					
A-α	12–20	70–120	Afferent and efferent from joints and muscles	Proprioception	Somatic motor
A-β	5–12	30–70	Afferent and efferent from joints and muscles	Touch, pressure	Somatic motor
A-γ	3–6	15–30	Efferent to muscle spindle	No sensory	Motor to muscle spindle
A-δ	2–5	12–30	Afferent sensory nerves	Pain, temperature, and touch	No motor
(Myelinated) B	<3	3–15	Preganglionic sympathetic and parasympathetic fibers	–	Various autonomic functions
(Nonmyelinated) C-dorsal root (d r C)	0.4–1.2	0.5–2	Afferent sensory fibers	Pain, temperature, and reflex response	No motors
C-sympathetic (s C) (Nonmyelinated)	0.3–1.3	0.7–2.3	Postganglionic sympathetic	–	Various autonomic functions

than the motor fibers in certain circumstances. Where the length of a nerve fiber, available for exposure to LA agent is short, then the decision to use a higher concentration of LA agent may be necessary in order to achieve desired effects. Whereas, if longer sections of a nerve are available for action, then the contact with LA agent with less concentrations of drug would be sufficient. However, a certain minimum concentration of a LA agent is necessary to block a nerve fiber of a given type. Hence, the clinical emphasis should always be on using the least effective concentration in the smallest volume that produces the desired degree of blockade. Motor and proprioceptive nerve fibers require higher minimum concentration of the LA agent for effective block, than the other modalities such as pain and temperature. Hence, if the achievement of motor akinesia is used as the yard stick for block effectiveness, then pain will never be experienced if there is full motor block. In such situation, touch and tissue movement appreciation (proprioceptive mediation) may be occasionally experienced as pain or discomfort in nervous patients.

POTENCY, DURATION OF ACTION, AND SENSITIVITY OF DIFFERENT NERVE FIBERS TO LOCAL ANESTHETIC AGENTS

Certain physicochemical conditions control the important biological properties of LA agents. Among these: (i) the protein binding; (ii) dissociation ratio; and (iii) lipid solubility are the most important ones. The affinity for protein (protein binding) is the predominant property that governs the *duration of action of LA* agents. The agents with high protein affinity occupy the active binding sites of the receptor for a longer period of time and therefore have a prolonged duration of action (e.g., bupivacaine and etidocaine). Drugs with somewhat lesser affinity for protein receptor have an intermediate period of action (e.g., lignocaine and mepivacaine). Whereas, procaine which is poorly protein bound is a short-acting LA agent.

The dissociation ratio between the unionized and the ionized form of a LA agent is largely responsible for the *speed of onset* and the tissue penetration ability of the drugs. Those, being presented in more highly ionized form have inferior properties in this regard.

High potency of a LA agent is associated with high lipid solubility of it. This property also facilitates the solution of a LA agent to enter into the cell through its cell membrane and to reach the nerve fiber (site of action) from the site of injection. So, the lipid solubility or hydrophobicity is the prime determining factor for intrinsic anesthetic potency of LA drugs. After entering the cell, the ionized form of the LA drug is again attached to the hydrophobic LA receptor

site of Na⁺ channel which is also related to the potency of a LA agent. But, clinically the correlation between the lipid solubility and potency of the drug is not precise. There are some differences between the in vitro and in vivo results. *These differences in result, between the in vitro and in vivo studies, are related to a number of factors, such as: (i) the volume of the drug; (ii) the concentration of the drug; (iii) the local vasodilatation or constriction property of the drug; and (iv) the tissue redistribution property of the drug.*

Usually, the injected volume and the concentration of a LA drug are important in the process of the spread of this LA agent and achieving the adequate concentration of it around the nerves. The concentration of the drug around the nerve fiber is also of prime importance in the development of diffusion gradient for nerve penetration. So, though high potency and long duration of action depend primarily on the lipid solubility of the drug, but the action of less lipophilic drugs can be prolonged by increasing the concentration and the volume of it at the injection site or near the nerve fibers. The vasoconstrictive effects of a LA drug also tend to prolong its action by reducing the rate of removal of it from the site of action by vascular absorption. The vasodilatation property of the drug has opposite effects. Lignocaine causes greater degree of vasodilatation than prilocaine, causing more rapid vascular uptake and shorter duration of action. So, fewer molecules are available for nerve blockade and have a reduced potency, though lipid solubility of lignocaine is greater than prilocaine. High-lipid solubility of etidocaine results in greater uptake of this agent by adipose tissue in the epidural space, leaving fewer molecules available for nerve blockade, as compared to bupivacaine.

All the types of nerve fibers are affected by LA agents, but fine and slower conducting nerve fibers are more readily blocked than the thicker and fast conducting fibers. This is because the sensitivity of block is determined by the diameter of the fiber. So, the fine fibers are blocked more easily than the thick fibers. But, these rules do not always hold good. For example, the myelinated preganglionic B fibers are more sensitive than the nonmyelinated preganglionic C fibers, though the former is thicker than the latter. The preganglionic myelinated B fibers are most sensitive to all. So, vasodilatation and consequent hypotension is the first effect of spinal anesthesia than the sensory blockade.

Though the thick A fibers are certainly more resistant to LA agents, but the fibers within them also differ in the critical length that must be exposed to the LA agent for effective block. Fine fibers have shorter critical length and so are more sensitive to LA agents. Frequency-dependent block also makes the fine sensory fibers more vulnerable to LA agents. This is because they generate high frequency, long lasting AP than that of motor fibers. The fibers subserving the pain and temperature (A-δ) are more sensitive than C pain fibers. So, sometimes pathological pain, e.g., impending uterine rupture which is conducted by C fibers may break through an epidural block, which is relieving the physiological pain of labor. This is called the epidural sieve. Sensory A fibers are more sensitive than motor A-fibers.

Thus, the order of sensitivity of nerve fibers to LA agents (starting from most sensitive to less sensitive) are: preganglionic (myelinated B fibers) → Pain (dr-C followed by A-δ) → Temperature (dr-C followed by A-δ) → Touch (A-β fibers) → Proprioception (pressure) → Motor (A-α fibers).

PHARMACOLOGICAL EFFECTS OF LOCAL ANESTHETIC AGENTS

The pharmacological effects of LA agents are described under three headings: (1) local; (2) regional; and (3) systemic.

Local Effects

The block of conduction of impulses through nerve and the relaxation vascular smooth muscle is the two most important local direct effects of LA agents.

Regional Effects

Loss of pain, temperature, touch, and pressure sensation are the regional effects of LA agents. Loss of motor power and vasomotor tone are also the regional effects of LA agents.

Systemic Effects

The LA agent, injected locally is ultimately absorbed by the blood and produces systemic effects. However, this systemic effect depends on the plasma level of this drug. The production of nerve block by systemic administration of a LA agent requires very high doses, rather than local infiltration and is so systemically highly toxic. Hence, it is not used for conduction block of nerves by systemic administration. For example, lethal doses of lignocaine are necessary to block the sensory nerve endings when used systemically. Another example is that the analgesic properties of procaine infusion are due to its action on the CNS, rather than peripheral nerve blocking effect.

The chief systemic toxicities of LA agent are mainly divided into cardiovascular system (CVS) and CNS effects, and this is principally due to its membrane stabilizing property. Therefore, the toxic effects when they occur affect mainly the organs which have excitable membranes such as the brain and myocardium. The incidence of systemic toxicity with LA agent when used locally is also related to the total dose of drug given, vascularity of the site of injection, type of drugs used, speed of injection and whether the adrenergic agents have been used as an additive with the LA agent to delay the systemic absorption or not. However, in clinical practice the systemic toxicity is most likely to be encountered following the unintentional intravascular injection.

Action on Cardiovascular System

Infiltration of the LA agent in conventional doses has no significant effect on the CVS. Infiltration in higher doses or inadvertent IV injection of the LA agent causes all the problems. They depress automaticity of sinoatrial (SA) node and suppress cardiac rhythms. They prolong the AP of myocardium, increase effective refractory period, slow down conduction through atrioventricular (AV) node, bundle of His and Purkinje fibers and depress the myocardial force of contraction. All the LA agents reduce cardiac sensitivity to adrenaline.

The LA agent such as procaine and procainamide has quinidine like effects. However, procaine is not used as an antiarrhythmic agent for its short duration of action, but procainamide is a classical antiarrhythmic drug. The electrophysiological properties of the heart muscles are markedly altered by the high plasma concentration of LA agent, and then can itself induce cardiac arrhythmias. Lignocaine is not so cardiotoxic and used clinically as an antiarrhythmic agent. Bupivacaine is more cardiotoxic and may cause ventricular tachycardia, fibrillation, or even cardiac arrest. Cardiac toxicity of bupivacaine usually does not occur in subconvulsive doses or in the absence of severe electrolyte disturbances or respiratory and metabolic acidosis. Large doses of LA agent may also produce circulatory collapse, as a result of the medullary depression.

Action on Vascular Smooth Muscles

Local anesthetic agent acts on the smooth muscles of blood vessels through different levels: local, regional, and systemic. But the ultimate effect is both complicated and confusing. At the local level procaine is a vasodilator and cocaine is a vasoconstrictor. Mepivacaine is a vasoconstrictor at clinical concentration than prilocaine, lignocaine, bupivacaine in that order. Lignocaine exists in two isomers and the vasoconstrictive effect appears to be vested only on one of the isomers. In case of mepivacaine, both the isomers have vasoconstrictive property.

However, at the regional level all the LA agents cause vasodilatation in the area, supplied by the blocked sympathetic fibers. At the systemic level, the effects of LA agents on vascular smooth muscle are produced by reflex mechanism or through CNS involvement.

Action on Central Nervous System

Cocaine is primarily a CNS stimulant, producing euphoria, excitement, restlessness, tremor, twitching, or convulsions. This is due to the inhibition of the inhibitory neurons of CNS, as the inhibitory neurons are more susceptible than the excitatory neurons. So, after inhibition of the inhibitory neurons, the excitatory neurons of CNS take an upper hand and produce convulsions. In the second phase with increasing dose of cocaine, when the excitatory neurons are also blocked after the inhibitory neurons, then the total depressive effects of the LA agents become prominent. This is manifested by unconsciousness, respiratory depression, cardiac depression, coma, and death. Cardiac depression of LA agents may be the result of medullary depression, other than direct action on myocardium and is compounded by convulsion with associated hypoxia.

Procaine and other LA agents are much less potent. At the safe clinical doses, they produce little or no CNS effect. But, at higher doses or after accidental IV injection it produces CNS stimulation, followed by depression like cocaine.

Lignocaine, on the contrary as CNS effect, causes sedation and higher doses produce excitation, followed by depression. The sedative effect of lignocaine which is observed after epidural administration is well recognized. Hypoxia and acid-base disturbances lower the threshold, both to the CNS and to the cardiac toxicity of the LA agent.

Action on Autonomic Nervous System

Cocaine potentiates the action of autonomic sympathetic nervous system by inhibiting the catecholamine uptake at the synaptic level and then produces excitement, tachycardia, hypertension, etc. However, other LA agents block both the cholinergic and adrenergic receptors (but not found in clinical doses).

Hypersensitivity

The true hypersensitivity reaction against the modern amide group of LA agents is very rare. But, it is reported and is more common in atopic individuals than the normal population. On the other hand, this term is frequently misused to describe the other adverse reactions of LA agents which are due to the accidental intravenous injection or frank over doses of it. The other modalities of reactions of LA agents which may be mistaken as allergic reactions are vasovagal attacks, which are often found during injection (may be due to fear) in a person with strong vagal activity. The hypersensitivity reaction of a LA agent is manifested as local edema, urticaria, angioneurotic edema, etc. However, the anaphylactic reaction against a LA agent is less common than its atopic reaction.

The hypersensitivity reactions to the ester group of LA agents are not rare and are more common than the amide group of LA agents. This is because the PABA, produced by the enzymatic cleavage of it in plasma, is the principal metabolic product of the ester-linked LA agents and this product is thought to trigger off the allergic reactions in certain individuals. Amide-linked LA agents, on the other hand, are broken down into liver, but not into plasma like the ester type of LA agent, producing PABA. However, as the methyl para-aminobenzoic acid (methyl paraben) which is used as a preservative in the multidose vials preparation of certain amide-linked LA drug is related to PABA and may produce hypersensitivity reaction. So, it is better to use preservative-free vials, where the history of the problem of allergic reaction exists. There is also a history of cross-sensitivity between the ester group of LA drugs and PABA used in sunscreen, cosmetics, different food preservatives, etc. This is because all the benzoic acid esters are highly antigenic.

PHARMACOKINETIC EFFECTS OF LOCAL ANESTHETIC AGENTS

Absorption

All the LA agents are totally absorbed in systemic circulation, after their parenteral use through local tissue infiltration. But, the systemic absorption of all the LA agents, after their local infiltration in tissues, depends on several factors.

Solubility of the Agent

It determines the proportion of the aqueous part of a LA agent which is available for rapid removal by blood and the proportion of the lipid soluble part of this LA agent which is taken up by the tissues and thereafter slowly released into systemic circulation.

Vascularity of the Tissue

The vascularity of local tissues where the LA agents are infiltrated also dictates the absorption of LA agents in circulation. The more vascular is tissue, the more is the absorption of LA agent into circulation and its systemic effects. This is also altered by the LA agent itself by its vasodilator or vasoconstrictor property and by the adrenaline, added into the LA solution. The absorption of a LA agent through a trachea and inflamed urethra is also as good as IV injection.

Absorption Through Various Tissues and the Gastrointestinal Tract

It is only good for LA agent like procainamide and so it is useful as oral antiarrhythmic agent. But, for lignocaine, after oral administration, 70% of it is metabolized during its single passage through liver. So, this route is ineffective for lignocaine. A comparison of the blood concentration of LA agents, after their absorption following various routes of administration, reveals that the plasma level of LA drug is highest after the intercostal blocks, followed by caudal epidural, lumbar epidural, brachial plexus, and subcutaneous tissue infiltration in a decreasing order. Thus, the use of a fixed dose of LA agent may be toxic in one area, but not in others. For example, 400 mg of lignocaine in intercostal block may easily cause the peak plasma level of 7 µg/mL, which is sufficiently high for CNS toxicity. Whereas, the same dose in brachial plexus block causes peak plasma level of only 3 µg/mL, which is rarely associated with CNS toxicity. A large volume of diluted solutions of a LA agent cause higher blood level than the same dose in milligram in smaller volume. This is because the large volume of a LA drug causes larger spread with large surface area for its absorption. With same anesthetic profile lignocaine absorb more quickly than prilocaine, and bupivacaine than etidocaine.

Distribution of Local Anesthetic Agents

After infiltration of a LA agent into tissues, it is gradually absorbed into blood. In the blood, LA agent is bound to the plasma protein, such as α1-acid glycoprotein. But, a quantitatively more important contribution is made by the plasma albumin and a small proportion remains free which enters the red cells. Then, the LA is very rapidly removed from the blood by other tissues and it is so rapid that even before proper mixing of the drug in circulation, the removal of LA agents by the other tissues is complete. So, a full equilibrium, after the distribution among different tissues, takes many hours to develop. LA agents readily cross the blood-brain barrier and the placenta. It is distributed throughout all the body tissues, but the relative concentration in different tissues varies. A highly perfused organ shows higher concentration and a less perfused organ shows less concentration. The LA agent is rapidly extracted by the lung tissue, so that the whole blood concentration of a LA agent decreases markedly, as these agents pass through the pulmonary circulation. The lung tissue has a lower pH than the plasma and thus favors the transformation of LA agent into its ionized form.

The highest percentage of an injected dose of a LA agent is found in skeletal muscles. At tissue level, LA agents are also metabolized by tissue enzymes. This is important for the esters than the amide LAs, but this has minimal clinical significance. The kinetics of this total process varies from drug to drug. But, more prominently, this kinetics varies greatly with the anatomical site of the injection. The relative speed of absorption of a LA agent from the site of injection are determined by the vascularity of that site, and by the amount of local fat at the site of injection that bind the LA agent and makes its absorption into the blood stream slow. Nevertheless, different drugs given at the same site will also result in different plasma concentrations. The degree of ionization and the solubility of individual drug play some role in this process. Other important factors that play a role in this process are: the total dose of drug in milligram, the speed of injection, the presence or absence of additives such as bicarbonate or adrenaline, the presence or absence of concomitant end-organ diseases and the effect of surgical lesion on homeostasis. It is very interesting to know that the plasma level of LA agent does not correlate well with age, body habitus, or gender.

Metabolism of Local Anesthetic Agents

The LA agents are metabolized in liver to form more water soluble compounds and so are rapidly excreted through kidney than other agents. The amide LAs are mainly metabolized into liver, whereas the most ester group of LA agents are hydrolyzed in plasma. In liver, the several pathways of metabolism that are mainly involved are: N-dealkylation, hydroxylation, and hydrolysis. Now, most of the LAs agents are tertiary amines. So, the N-dealkylation of a tertiary amine (e.g., lignocaine) produces a more water soluble secondary amine and renders it more susceptible to amide hydrolysis, like secondary amine such as prilocaine.

The hydroxylation of the aromatic nucleus of a tertiary amine is also believed to occur in the case of lignocaine, mepivacaine, bupivacaine, etc. However, hydroxylations of these agents produce a compound which can be conjugated and so become solely water soluble. Thus, as much as, 70% of all the amide LA agents may be broken down during their single passage through liver. This high first-pass clearance of lignocaine in liver yields mainly its N-dealkylated product, such as monoethylglycinexylidine, which is itself moderately toxic and effective antiarrhythmic agent. However, the high clearance rate of lignocaine is markedly reduced in the presence of low cardiac output. There is a strong relation between the class of LA drug and the rate of hepatic metabolism. In addition, a small fraction of the injected dose of a LA agent is excreted unchanged directly through kidney.

Procainamide (aminoalkylamides → diamines) is metabolized more slowly than lignocaine (aminoacylamide → tertiary amines) and a larger proportion of it is excreted unchanged through kidney. Some degradation of amide type of LA agent also occurs in tissues other than the liver. Less than 5% unchanged drug is excreted via kidney through the urine. Procaine and amethocaine are hydrolyzed by pseudocholinesterase in plasma and compete with suxamethonium. Cocaine is not broken down by cholinesterase.

The water soluble metabolites of LA agents are rapidly excreted through the urine. But, the lipid soluble LA base once filtered through glomerulus is reabsorbed by the renal tube. In an acidic urine, it becomes highly ionized, then tubular reabsorption is inhibited and renal clearance increases.

■ TOXICITY OF LOCAL ANESTHETIC AGENTS

The toxicity of LA agent mainly affects the CNS and CVS. The subconvulsive doses do not cause the circulatory depression, but may depress the CNS. However, like other drugs, the toxicity of LA agents is not the mere extension of their therapeutic action, but has a distinct mechanism. It depends on the speed of vascular absorption, and trouble starts when the absorption and elimination of the drug does not balance. The occurrence of toxicity of a LA agent is not related to the concentration of the solution injected, but rather to the total dose of the drug. Similarly, the site of injection and its vascularity also affect the speed of absorption of LA agent, as well as its toxicity. The relative overdose for a given plasma concentration in case of very young or old patients is not due to their raised sensitivity. So, widespread field block and excessive surface application should be avoided in such group of patients. The cause of toxicity of LA agents in correctly administered dose is due to gradual accumulation in body due to the continuous or repeated administration of gradual accumulation in body due to the short-acting drugs. So, the long duration of action of bupivacaine and the rapid elimination of etidocaine has clear advantage for their continuous infusion.

Central Nervous System Toxicity

Subjective Signs

These are: light headedness, dizziness, visual, and auditory disturbances such as difficulty in focusing, tinnitus, disorientation, and drowsiness.

Objective Signs

These are shivering, twitching, tremor, convulsion, respiratory depression, respiratory arrest, coma, and death. There is an inverse relationship between the intrinsic anesthetic potency of a LA agent and the doses required to induce CNS toxicity.

An increase in $PaCO_2$ decreases the convulsive threshold level of a LA agent by approximately 50%. The explanation is like that an elevation of $PaCO_2$ increases the cerebral blood flow and so more anesthetic agent is delivered to the brain rapidly. In addition, the diffusion of CO_2 in the neural cell decreases the intracellular pH and thus facilitates the conversion of the unionized form of a LA drug to ionized form within the cell, which only binds with the hydrophobic receptor site of the intracellular part of Na^+ channel. Thus, the cationic or ionized form does not cross the nerve cell membrane, so that ion trapping occurs and increases CNS toxicity.

On the other hand, hypercapnia or acidosis decreases the plasma protein binding capacity of LA agents, and so increases the proportion of free drug in plasma, available for diffusion into the brain. Seizure and CNS depression again produce hypoventilation and respiratory acidosis, which further exacerbates the CNS toxicity, establishing a vicious cycle. So, during the management of LA, CNS toxicity prompt assisted ventilation, correcting acidosis, is essential.

Cardiovascular Toxicity

The direct cardiac effects of LA agents are:

- The LA agents decrease the rate of depolarization in the fast conducting tissues such as the Purkinje fibers and ventricular muscles. This reduction in the rate of depolarization in the fast conducting tissues of heart is believed to be due to the decrease in the availability of fast Na^+ channel in these cardiac tissues, causing myocardial depression.
- The duration of AP and effective refractory **(Fact file II)** period is decreased, leading to ventricular tachycardia, ventricular fibrillation, ventricular ectopic, etc.
- The ratios of effective refractory period and the duration of AP are increased.
- Bupivacaine depresses the rapid phase of depolarization to a greater extent than lignocaine.
- The rate of recovery from the use dependent block is slower in bupivacaine than lignocaine. This slow rate of

---

FACT FILE II

The cardiac toxicity of the more potent LA agents, such as bupivacaine appears to differ from that of lignocaine in the following ways:
- The CC/CNS ratio, i.e., the ratio of the dose that is required to produce cardiac collapse (or toxicity), and the CNS toxicity is lower for bupivacaine than lignocaine.
- Ventricular fibrillation or any other ventricular arrhythmia usually occurs following the IV administration of bupivacaine, but not lignocaine
- Cardiac resuscitation is more resistant following bupivacaine-induced cardiac collapse than that of lignocaine.
- Pregnant patients are more sensitive to cardiac toxicity of bupivacaine than lignocaine.
- Cardiac toxicity of bupivacaine is markedly potentiated by acidosis and hypoxia.

recovery of blocked Na^+ channel results in incomplete restoration of some Na^+ channel and less availability of it between two subsequent AP. In contrast, recovery from lignocaine is complete. The effect of this differential recovery explains the antiarrhythmic properties of lignocaine and arrhythmogenic property of bupivacaine.

- The LA agents prolong the conduction time and thus increase the PR interval and the duration of QRS complex.
- The extremely high concentration of LA agents depress the spontaneous pacemaker activity in the SA node, causing sinus bradycardia and sinus arrest.
- All the LA agents have dose-dependent negative inotropic action on cardiac muscles. This negative inotropic effect on myocardium is due to the inhibition of release of Ca^{2+} from the sarcoplasmic reticulum and also inhibition of Na^+ currents.

Local Tissue Toxicity

The volume and concentration of LA agent, used clinically, rarely produce localized nerve damage. But, the evidence of local neurotoxicity caused by LA agents is occasionally seen and depends on: (i) the type of agent used (the ester-linked may be more neurotoxic than the amide-linked anesthetics); (ii) its concentration; (iii) the site of injection; (iv) the osmolarity and pH of solution; and (v) the presence of other certain additives with it such as the vasoconstrictors, antioxidants, and preservatives. Electron microscopy studies indicate that the perineurium, Schwann cells, and axons themselves may be damaged, due to the neurotoxicity of LA agents. The advanced age and diseased states of the nervous tissue also enhance the susceptibility of LA agents to the neurotoxicity.

The neurotoxicity in clinical practice is most commonly seen with spinal anesthesia. Adrenaline has also been investigated as a possible contributor to LA neurotoxicity. The suspected mechanism is decreased intraneural blood supply, due to vasoconstriction by adrenaline. The admixture of LA agent with antioxidant, such as sodium bisulfite, in the presence of a low pH has also been shown to be neurotoxic. So, for a safer and more effective alternative to these commercial solutions, the adrenaline may be added to the LA solution freshly before use.

There are many reports of inadvertent needle penetration into the globe of eyeball, during the peribulbar or retrobulbar block, which is followed by the injection of LA agent in clinical concentration within the eyeball. But, the retina which is a specialized nerve tissue does not undergo toxic changes in these circumstances. The concentration of lignocaine, required to produce irreversible conduction blockade and permanent damage of nerve fiber in experimental conditions,

overlap the concentration which is used clinically, such as 2% lignocaine. But, practically this does not happen. This is because the LA agents are not applied clinically directly to the nerve fiber in such concentrations.

So, although the LA is injected clinically at a much higher concentration than their physiological effective range, but they are usually diluted in the tissues during the process of transport (spreading) from the site of injection to the site of action and hence no harm is produced. If this dilution does not occur, then a permanent neural deficit does result. Thus, the application of 5% lignocaine in hyperbaric solution into subarachnoid space, through a narrow intrathecal catheter, is associated with the high incidences of cauda equina syndrome. However, anesthetists should keep in mind that the concentrations of marketed LA solutions are neurotoxic and their dilution in tissue is essential for safe use.

Continuous spinal anesthesia using a microcatheter is associated with the high incidences of neurotoxicity, such as radicular irritation and cauda equina syndrome. Studies suggest that microcatheter facilitates a localized deposition of high concentration of drug which is inadequately dispersed or diluted in the CSF, leading to direct contact of a high concentration of drug around the sacral roots and consequent neurotoxicity.

THE ADJUVANT DRUGS TO AUGMENT THE CLINICAL EFFECTS OF LOCAL ANESTHETICS

The most commonly used adjuvant drugs with LA agents to increase their efficacy and duration of action are adrenaline, noradrenaline, felypressin, hyaluronidase, and sodium bicarbonate.

Adrenaline

By its α-stimulant action, adrenaline constricts the vessels at the site of the injection of LA agents and thus reduces its absorption through blood (circulation). So, the LA action is prolonged, the depth of block is increased and the toxicity of drug is reduced. As a whole, the quality and the reliability of the block are improved. Adrenaline added to the LA solution also provides a marker for inadvertent intravascular injection of it. Because, if the needle is placed unwillingly and unknowingly into the vessels, then the small amount of test dose of LA agent containing adrenaline will produce tachycardia. Other vasoconstrictors, such as norepinephrine and phenylephrine also have been used with LA agents, but they are not superior to adrenaline in this purpose. The α-adrenergic receptors in spinal cord are also known to activate the endogenous analgesic mechanism and thus adrenaline also increases the depth of analgesic action of LA agents in the central neuraxial block. Therefore, where prolonged block is necessary, the addition of adrenaline with LA agents reduces the number of repeated doses of it, and thus delays the onset of chronic toxicity and tachyphylaxis of LA agents. Particularly, it is very valuable in highly vascular areas, e.g., intercostal space, pelvic floor, etc. than the less vascular areas, e.g., the epidural space. So, the aim of use of adrenaline differs from time to time. Sometimes, it is to reduce the toxicity and sometimes it is to prolong the effect of LA agent.

However, the presence of adrenaline in the LA solution makes the injection more painful. It also increases the chances of subsequent local tissue edema and necrosis, as well as delays the wound healing by reducing the oxygen supply and enhancing the O_2 consumption in the injected area. Sometimes, the LA agent with adrenaline may raise BP and promote arrhythmia in susceptible individuals. The effect of adrenaline on long-acting drugs such as bupivacaine and etidocaine is less marked. In dentistry, always some form of vasoconstrictor is essential with most LA agents to diminish bleeding during the extraction of teeth. The inclusion of adrenaline in LA solution necessitates the addition of antioxidants such as sodium metabisulfite or ascorbic acid. This is because adrenaline is stable in acidic solution only and this is provided by Na-metabisulfite or ascorbic acid. But, these agents more reduce the pH of a LA solution even <4 and increase its toxicity. In Britain, bupivacaine with adrenaline contains fewer additives and the pH is around 4.5 **(Fact file III)**.

Dose of Adrenaline in a LA Solution

Adrenaline should not be used in concentration >5 µg/mL (1:200,000) which causes the optimal degree of vasoconstriction. But, in dentistry as the total volume of drug used is small, so a higher concentration of adrenaline such as 12.5 µg/mL (1:80,000) is used. When injected IV accidentally, then adrenaline is more dangerous than the LA itself. If the total volume of LA agent, containing 100–150 µg of adrenaline, is inadvertently injected

<table>
<tr><td>FACT FILE III</td></tr>
</table>

Advantages and disadvantages of addition of vasoconstrictors in local anesthetic agents may be as follows:
- Prolongs the duration of action by decreasing the rate of removal of a LA agent from the site of injection in the circulation
- Reduces the systemic toxicity
- Increases the dose of the drug
- Increases the chances of local tissue edema and tissue necrosis
- Delays wound healing by decreasing the oxygen supply, while increasing its consumption in the affected area
- Makes the injection more painful
- Increases the blood pressure and chances of arrhythmias in susceptible persons

intravenously, then it produces severe systemic effects such as tachycardia, arrhythmia, ventricular fibrillation, and sweating for a brief duration. But, in a correctly placed block, adrenaline is absorbed slowly from the tissue and no systemic effect occurs. Adrenaline is contraindicated in patient: (i) taking certain antihypertensive drugs; (ii) taking tricyclic antidepressants; (iii) with thyrotoxicosis; (iv) for digital block; and (v) for penile block, etc. Its use may be dangerous in epidural analgesia or anesthesia for anterior spinal artery syndrome.

Noradrenaline

It is also an α-adrenergic stimulant and constricts the vessels but less potent than adrenaline. So, in dentistry for the purpose of vasoconstriction and to reduce the bleeding, noradrenaline in high doses, such as 20–40 µg/mL (1:50,000 to 1:25,000) may be necessary. But, this high dose of noradrenaline produces severe hypertension.

Felypressins

It is a synthetic polypeptide, related to vasopressin. As a vasoconstrictor it is also suitable agent like adrenaline, but less toxic. For example, it produces no changes in CVS in conditions where adrenaline in the dose of 12.5 is likely to produce tachycardia. With prilocaine it is more effective in prolonging the action of LA agents with less toxicity than adrenaline.

Hyaluronidase

The enzyme hyaluronidase is frequently added to LA agents for regional ophthalmic anesthesia to promote the spread of drug (LA agents) through the intraorbital tissues. It breaks down the collagen bonds and thus allows the anesthetic solution to spread across the fine septal barriers of connective tissues. This action of hyaluronidase is accomplished by the reversible hydrolysis of hyaluronic acid which is the most common cement substance of intercellular connective tissues. However, to maintain the full activity of this product, the refrigeration of hyaluronidase is important. Prolonged exposure of hyaluronidase to room temperature (>48 hours) results in the deterioration of its enzyme potency. Autoclaving of solutions also results in the destruction of this enzyme strength.

Hyaluronidase is added to the LA solution in a concentration of 7.5–15 turbidity units/mL. The higher concentrations of it have no added advantage. Prior to its introduction, the volume of LA agent, injected into the orbital cavity for ophthalmic regional anesthesia, was limited (cannot be increased). This is due to the raised intraorbital and subsequently the intraocular pressure as the LA solution does not spread quickly into the intraorbital tissues after its administration into the orbit. Then, the greatly improved standards of effective local infiltration anesthesia for ophthalmic surgery (especially cataract extraction), without compromising the intraocular pressure was made possible by adding the hyaluronidase with a large volumes of LA injection.

However, the hyaluronidase reduces the duration of local anesthesia. This is because it increases the spread of LA agent and subsequently increases its absorption through the blood vessels. But, adrenaline reverses that tendency. It has allergic potential and is more myotoxic than enzyme-free solutions. However, the use of hyaluronidase enzyme is not a substitute for less precise anatomical knowledge and poor technique for high quality ophthalmic regional anesthesia, as it only facilitates the spread of LA solution along the path of least resistance of tissue. So, the LA solution should be placed accurately within the appropriate compartment. Hyaluronidase does not enhance brachial plexus block, nor does it influence the plasma levels of LAs agents.

Sodium Bicarbonate

The tissue penetration and the onset of action of a LA agent are enhanced by adjusting the pH of its aqueous solution toward the nonionized base by the addition of small amount of sodium bicarbonate. For each LA agent, there is a pH at which the amount of nonionized molecules (which only penetrate the cell membrane) of a LA agent in solution becomes saturated. Increase in pH beyond that point results in the precipitation of the free base, after which no further clinical benefit is achieved. In fact, a nuisance factor, such as the blockage of needles by free base precipitate creates problems. There are also many literatures which are equivocal about the effectiveness of pH adjustment of LA agents by just mere adding $NaHCO_3$ in LA solution in various clinical circumstances. So, many anesthetists fail to see any benefit in their practice, after pH adjustment of LAs with sodium bicarbonate. However, alkalinized solutions should be used within 6 hours of their preparation. There is definite lesser pain during injection, when bicarbonate is used with LA agents.

GENERAL CONSIDERATION OF LOCAL ANESTHETIC AGENTS

Onset of Action

The speed of onset of block (action) by a LA agent is the specific property of that individual agent. But, it also depends on the concentration of that particular agent. For example: (i) 0.25% bupivacaine has slow onset of action. But, increasing the concentration of it to 0.75% hastens the onset of action. Beyond that concentration limit, the onset of action does not improve further. (ii) The onset of action of chloroprocaine (pKa 9) is slow. This is due to the less

availability of nonionized molecule of chloroprocaine in normal tissue pH. But, its low systemic toxicity allows its use in higher concentration (3%), and thus obviously improves the onset of action. So, in clinical use, 3% chloroprocaine has faster onset of action than 2% lignocaine.

Duration of Action

As we know that the duration of action of a LA agent depends on the peripheral vascular effects of that agent, but most of the LA agents have biphasic effects on the vascular smooth muscles. At a low concentration, these agents tend to cause vasoconstriction and at clinical concentrations they cause vasodilatation. Lignocaine is a potent vasodilator than mepivacaine and prilocaine, and has a shorter duration of action than these two. The vessels of pia mater are dilated by bupivacaine, but constricted by ropivacaine.

Differential Sensory and Motor Block

Differential block means sensory block (loss), without affecting the motor nerves (muscular paralysis). This is ensured only with the lower concentration of LA agents. Bupivacaine and etidocaine profoundly have this property. Bupivacaine in a concentration of 0.125% produces adequate sensory loss by affecting only the sensory fibers and without profound inhibition of motor activity. So, the bupivacaine is widely used in epidural space for obstetric analgesia (not anesthesia) and for postoperative pain management without muscle weakness or paralysis.

There are two probable explanations for this differential block:
- The length of nerve fiber which is exposed to LA drug in epidural space can explain clinically the differential block. Because if the drug-exposed region of a nerve fiber is longer, then it yields a block by lower concentration of LA drug which is found in case of sensory nerve fiber. However, this does not explain the functional differential loss from peripheral nerve block.
- Selective ability to inhibit Na^+ channels over K^+ channels by the lower concentration of LA agent, which itself can produce a differential block. Because, these channels are present in very different proportions in different types of nerves.

Site of Injection

The most rapid onset, but shortest duration of action occurs following the intrathecal or subcutaneous administration of a LA agent. The longest latency of onset and the prolonged duration of action of a LA agent are observed following brachial plexus block. For example, bupivacaine in intrathecal route has the onset of action within 5 minutes and the duration of action is 3–4 hours. But, in brachial plexus block the onset of action of bupivacaine is 20–30 minutes and duration of action is ±10 hours.

Explanation

The lack of connective tissue sheath around the spinal nerve and the deposition of drug in the immediate vicinity of the cord and the nerve are responsible for this rapid onset of action. But, relatively the small amount of drug used for intrathecal block is responsible for this short duration of action. On the other hand, in brachial plexus block the LA agent has to diffuse through the various tissue barriers, before reaching the nerve which causes the delayed onset of action. This also needs a large volume of drug and this larger dose is responsible for prolonged action.

pH Adjustment of Local Anesthetic Solution

The addition of $NaHCO_3$ to a LA solution causes the rapid onset of its action. This is because the increase of pH of a LA solution increases the amount of drug in its unchanged base (nondissociated) form in this aqueous solution and enhances its diffusion across the cell membrane, resulting in a more rapid onset of action. It happens with bupivacaine also. But, still now, there is a controversy about the efficacy of technique of carbonation (just merely adding $NAHCO_3$ in acidic LA solution. I do not believe in this process because if causes precipitation) and pH adjustment of LA agent.

Mixture of Local Anesthetic Agents

The use of a mixture of two or three LA agents has become popular in recent years. The basis (principle) for making of this mixture is to compensate the delayed onset of action of one LA agent by the early onset of action of another LA agent and also to compensate the shorter duration of action of one LA agent by the longer duration of action of another. But recently, confusing results have come to the forefront. For example, a mixture of 3% chloroprocaine and 0.5% bupivacaine was used to produce short latency and prolonged duration in brachial plexus block. But, subsequent studies indicate that the duration of epidural anesthesia produced by this mixture is significantly shorter than bupivacaine alone. However, the clinicians should be cautioned not to use the maximum doses of two LA agents in the mixture, with the mistaken belief that toxicities of these agents are independent.

Pregnancy

Except mechanical factors (dilatation of epidural veins, causing decreased epidural space, and subsequently the greater spread of LA agent through the epidural space in pregnancy), increased sensitivity of LA agent of the nervous tissue during pregnancy, due to the alteration in the maternal hormonal level, causes greater intensity of epidural anesthesia. However, this greater spread of epidural anesthesia (the cause of which is explained above) only occurs during the first trimester of pregnancy.

Pharmacokinetic Alterations of LA Agent by Patient's Age

Patient's age influences the pharmacological characters of LA agents. For example, the half-life of lignocaine, following IV administration, is twice in old age than in young adults. The newborns and infants have immature hepatic enzyme system and so they experience a prolonged elimination half-life of lignocaine and bupivacaine.

On this basis, a maximum infusion rate of 0.4 mg/kg/hour for bupivacaine in adults during epidural anesthesia has been proposed. Whereas during continuous epidural anesthesia by bupivacaine the rates of infusion for neonates and young infants should not exceed 0.2 mg/kg/hour. Similarly, lignocaine infusion in neonates should not exceed 0.8 mg/kg/hour.

Methemoglobinemia

Large doses of prilocaine are associated with methemoglobinemia. In general, 600 mg of prilocaine is required for the development of clinically significant levels of methemoglobinemia. This is because the metabolism of prilocaine in liver results in the formation of *O*-toluidine which is responsible for the oxidation of Hb to methemoglobin. This methemoglobinemia is spontaneously reversible or may be treated by IV methylene blue. The effect of methemoglobin is that the patient appears to be cyanotic, but will have normal oxygen saturation level. The effect of methemoglobin on oxygen carrying capacity is not so important in a healthy adult, but can be significant in infants. So, prilocaine is generally avoided in infants.

Summary

The LA agents act by causing selective reversible restriction of permeability of sodium ions through its Na^+ channel, but without interfering the free movement of potassium through its K^+ channel. Usually, the sodium ions are restricted to the extracellular space, except when the sodium ion channels are open, allowing diffusion through it. Potassium ion is freely diffusible across the membrane. But, it selectively accumulates inside the nerve cell to preserve the electrical neutrality by balancing the cations. In an unexcited state, the electrical potential inside the cell is negative in reference to the outside of the cell. During the conduction of impulses

(AP), these ion gradients are altered along the nerve cell membrane by opening of the sodium channels.

Thus, sodium enters into the cell and increases the intracellular Na^+ concentration. This is called the depolarization of cell. The Na^+ channels are lipoprotein in nature and are embedded in the cell membrane of nerve fiber along the entire width. The gate that opens and closes these channels is present at the intracytoplasmic side of these channels. These Na^+ channels are most susceptible to LA agents in an open active state and remain inactive in this open state, preventing the further depolarization of cell.

The changes in the configuration of Na^+ channel is voltage dependent. But, the LA molecule prevents this voltage shift which activates the Na^+ channel. So, LA molecule stabilizes the Na^+ channel in nonconducting configuration.

The LA molecule also has some minor effects on both K^+ and Ca^{2+} channels, which modulate the action of Na^+ channels. However, the K^+ and Ca^{2+} channels blockade by clinically available LA agents are so low that they do not contribute significantly to the conduction blockade.

The LA molecule in its nonionic (nondissociated) form crosses the lipophilic hydrocarbon part of the nerve cell membrane to reach the cytoplasmic end of Na^+ channel. Within the cell, in cytoplasm the LA molecule becomes active (dissociates) in its ionic state and attach to the hydrophilic LA receptors (binding site) of Na^+ channel. This dual requirement of a LA molecule (undissociated and dissociated form) determines the chemical characteristic of LA agent. One LA molecule blocks only one Na^+ channel.

When the nerve cell membrane is rapidly depolarized from its RMP of –70 mV to +20 mV (i.e., to the threshold level), then there is a rapid increase in the permeability of sodium channels. The greater the magnitude of depolarization, the greater is the permeability of Na^+ channels.

The LA molecules have an aromatic ring (lipophilic), connected to a tertiary amine (hydrophilic) by a short alkyl chain and a hydrophilic bond (amide or ester). So, the LA agents are amines and are called amino-amides or amino esters. All the LA molecules are amphipathic, i.e., possessing both the lipophilic and hydrophilic action at the opposite sides of the molecule. All the LA agents are weak bases and are able to accept proton or H^+ to change (to dissociate) into their cationic form at pH below their pKa value. This can be calculated from the following formula: pKa = pH + Log (cation/free base).

The aromatic (lipophilic) group or side of a LA molecule provides most of the lipophilic properties of a LA molecule. Its size restricts the movement of the amine (hydrophilic) group to an axis, perpendicular to the aromatic ring. This linear relationship between the amine (hydrophilic) and aromatic (lipophilic) group seems necessary to block the hydrophilic binding site of the receptor (LA binding site of Na^+ channel) by the hydrophilic amine group. This also explains the movement of the amine group toward the receptor, while the aromatic lipophilic group of a LA molecule is still embedded in the lipophilic nerve cell membrane.

The intermediate chain of LA molecule allows the reversible action of clinically useful LA agent. Since, without the intermediate chain and an amide or ester bond, the metabolism of LA agent would be very difficult and toxicity would be unacceptable. The potency of a LA agent increases as the lipid coefficient of these lipophilic bonds increase.

The amines (hydrophilic group) are situated at the side of the LA molecule. It accepts proton and in cationic state the LA molecule is mostly involved in the blockade of Na^+ channel. It is probable that the ionic movement of the hydrophilic group away from the lipophilic side of the molecule orients the amine group into a configuration that fits into the sodium channel receptor.

The lipophilic portion of a LA agent is involved in the molecular passage through the lipid cell membrane. So, this facilitates the penetration of perineurium and as well as the nerve cell membrane. The bigger the lipophilic portion greater the potency of a LA agent. The equilibrium of dissociation between the ionic and the nonionic form of LA molecule occurs inside the nerve cell. The hydrophilic group in the ionic form is the part of the molecule which is involved in entering the Na^+ channel to interrupt the Na^+ conduction. A specific distance is required between these two different groups and this is served by the intermediate chain. If the length is too short or too long, then there is minimal or no LA activity.

Between the LA molecule and the receptor at the Na^+ channel, a semispecific binding of reversible nature occurs. The speed of entry and the exit of LA molecules through these Na^+ channels is agent specific. The short and intermediate acting LA agents are short-in and short-out of Na^+ channels in character (e.g., lignocaine, procaine, mepivacaine). So, they are of early onset and shorter duration of action. The long-acting agents (e.g., bupivacaine) are slow-in and slow-out of the Na^+ channels in character. So, they have a delayed onset and a longer duration of action. The bond between the receptor and the molecule of LA agent is weak in case of closed channels, but strongest and most rapid in open sodium channels.

When the lipophilic butyl group is added to the aromatic ring of procaine, then tetracaine is created which is 40 times more potent than procaine. Thus, 40 times increase in potency confirms that the lipophilic property of a LA molecule is the principle determinant of its potency. If the same butyl group is added with a hydrophilic tertiary amine group, then the resultant molecule has a potency lower than procaine. It may be due to that, the hydrophilic region (receptor) near the Na^+ channel orients the hydrophilic amine group of the LA molecule in that channel. So, the addition of lipophilic butyl group with the hydrophilic amine group of LA molecule prevents its orientation in Na^+ channel and reduces the potency.

Protein binding capacity of LA agent determines the duration of action. Agents with greater protein binding capacity have a greater attraction for receptors and remain binding with the Na^+ channel for a longer period of time, causing longer duration of action, e.g., bupivacaine, etidocaine, etc. Agents with poor protein binding capacity such as procaine, chloroprocaine, etc. are readily washed out from the channel causing shorter duration of action.

Regarding the alkalization by adding sodium bicarbonate to the LA solution, wherever it is possible without precipitation (because the addition of sodium bicarbonate to lignocaine hydrochloride causes precipitation of lignocaine bicarbonate), decreases the latency to onset (has been reported in numerous series). For example, in mepivacaine where the pKa value is 7.6 and the pH of its commercial preparation is 5.5, then the alkalization of mepivacaine is possible without precipitation. This alkalization increases the concentration of the unionized portion of LA agent in its aqueous solution which is from <0.1% to about 40%. However, in more lipophilic agents, like bupivacaine, this precipitation limits the amount of alkalization and results are more equivocal.

Regarding the toxicity of LA agents, the main determinants of it include the total concentration versus the free concentration which is again determined by the protein binding capacity of it and the ionization capability of it. The subarachnoid injection of a LA agent for spinal anesthesia is associated with its lowest blood level.

Regarding the relation between the lipid solubility and the toxicity, the CNS toxicity of a LA agent in clinical setting is directly related to its lipid solubility. The penetration of lipid cell membrane is the limiting step for the CNS toxicity of a LA agent. So, more lipid soluble means more CNS toxicity. While the highly lipid soluble LA agents are more potent, but their therapeutic and toxic ratio is narrow and the degree of safety is less. Toxic form of a LA agent is the unionic unbound fraction in the blood which is available for penetration of the blood-brain barrier. The early signs of CNS toxicity are reported in patients, when the unbound fraction begins to cause ionic changes within the CNS. The intra-arterial injection of a small amount of LA agent cause vary rapid onset of massive CNS reaction, because the agent is delivered directly in high concentration to the CNS.

Regarding tissue toxicity, all the LA molecules are directly cytotoxic to nerve cells at some concentration. The balance between the ideal concentration to facilitate conduction block and cause nerve damage determines its therapeutic safety index. In addition to the cytotoxicity of anesthetic agents itself, various buffers and preservatives added to the LA agents have been found in some cases to be cytotoxic.

Regarding allergy, the true allergy to LA agents is rare. The most common allergies are due to the ester agents and their metabolites like PABA. This may be due to the ubiquitous presence of this aromatic PABA molecule in food preservatives, pharmaceuticals, cosmetics, and in sunscreen lotions. Thus, any previous exposure to PABA, through these chemical agents, may prime the immune system in some individuals for an immunologically mediated response to the metabolites of ester group of LA agent.

Regarding the cardiac toxicity, the specific CVS depression with highly lipid soluble agents, such as bupivacaine and etidocaine, is not only associated with their increased lipid solubility, but also the specific binding of these agents to the cardiac conduction system magnifies their cardiac toxicity. Bupivacaine has a quinidine like blocking action on the conduction system of heart. This increases the activity in re-entrant pathways and predisposes the heart to the development of ventricular arrhythmia.

■ INDIVIDUAL LOCAL ANESTHETIC AGENTS

Procaine and Procainamide

Procaine is a LA agent with poor penetrative power and a short duration of action. This is due to its vasodilator activity and high pK value. This high pK value renders the procaine to remain in highly ionized state at a physiological pH of 7.4. So, after injection, it is rapidly absorbed into circulation and has less penetrative power in the tissues and nerve. Hence, it is inactive as a surface anesthetic agent. It is less potent than lignocaine and its duration of action is half than that of lignocaine. But, the potency and the duration of action of procaine can be greatly extended by the addition of adrenaline.

It is hydrolyzed in plasma by pseudocholinesterase and in liver to PABA and diethylaminoethanol.

There are several drug reactions with procaine or procainamide. These are:

- PABA which is one of the metabolites of this group of LA agents is a potent inhibitor of the bacteriostatic action of sulfonamide group of antibiotics.
- PABA itself acts as an allergen and causes allergy.
- PABA prolongs the effect of suxamethonium by competing for the same enzyme, i.e., pseudocholinesterase which is responsible for the termination of action of them by hydrolysis.

- Anticholinesterase agents potentiate the toxicity of procaine and procainamide. So, it should not be used in patients suffering from myasthenia gravis.

Procaine and procainamide has antiarrhythmic effects like quinidine. But, the procaine is replaced by procainamide which too has antiarrhythmic properties and is not broken down by pseudocholinesterase, like procaine. At present, procaine has no indication for use as LA or antiarrhythmic agent. It has been replaced by many newer and better drugs.

Lignocaine HCl

It was first synthesized, in 1943, by Lofgren in Sweden at AB Astra laboratory. But, it was first introduced in clinical practice, in 1948. It is of moderate potency and has intermediate duration of action which varies with: (i) the site of injection; (ii) the concentration and volume of drug; (iii) the presence or absence of adrenaline, etc. It causes local vasodilatation which again causes quick absorption of it through the circulation and reduces the duration of action. Repeated injection of lignocaine causes tachyphylaxis. Now, it is one of the most widely used LA agent in the world. It works rapidly and reliably to give both motor and sensory blockade. It can be used virtually by any route and is a standard antiarrhythmic agent when given IV without any preservative.

Lignocaine is commonly marketed as its hydrochloride salt. But, the carbonate (salt) of lignocaine has remarkable penetration power, rapid onset of action, and high incidence of deep motor and sensory blockade. The absorption of lignocaine through mucosal surface is very rapid and gives rise to high blood level. The absorption of it from the inflamed urethra is also as good as IV injection. An iontophoretic system (a needle-free drug delivery system) for the delivery of lignocaine and epinephrine is also available. But, this system is generally used for superficial dermal procedures and provides anesthesia up to the depth of 10 mm from skin surface.

As lignocaine stabilizes the membrane of damaged and excitable cells, so it is used for the treatment of ventricular ectopic foci. In therapeutic antiarrhythmic doses, it causes no change in heart rate, does not depress the conduction in Purkinje tissue, does not widen the QRS complex, and has no apparent myocardial depression. Instead, improvement in cardiac output and BP is observed when lignocaine is used in the treatment of dysrhythmias. But, it is less useful in supraventricular dysrhythmias. The great value of lignocaine is observed in the acute treatment of ventricular arrhythmias after myocardial infarction (MI) and cardiac surgery and this is due to the lack of myocardial depressant effect of it.

Doses of Lignocaine

Lignocaine in the concentration of 0.5–1% is used for local infiltration anesthesia. The maximum dose of lignocaine for this infiltration anesthesia is 4.5 mg/kg without adrenaline, and when adrenaline is used this amount can be increased by one-third. When extensive block with high volume of drug is required, then 0.25% lignocaine with adrenaline should be used. For intravenous regional anesthesia 40 mL of 0.5% lignocaine without adrenaline is used. 1% lignocaine is sufficient for local nerve block. A concentration of 2% lignocaine with adrenaline (1:80,000 or 12.5 µg/mL) is used in dentistry. 1–2% lignocaine with or without adrenaline (1:200,000 or 5 µg/mL) is used in epidural anesthesia. For surface application, 4% lignocaine is used as a liquid or 10% as a spray or 5% as a gel.

For cardiac arrhythmias, mainly ventricular, lignocaine is used in the dose of 1 mg/kg IV as bolus, then 4 mg/kg for next 20 minutes, which is gradually slowed down to 1 mg/minute as tissues begin to take up lignocaine less rapidly. Such infusion continued for days may give rise to systemic toxicity.

The safe upper limit of the dose of lignocaine for infiltration anesthesia is of much dispute. Most commonly accepted view is 200 mg plain and 500 mg with adrenaline. But, here there is no mention of body weight and the site of injection. Another recommended maximum safe dose of lignocaine is 6 mg/kg, but is possibly lesser for plain solution in vascular areas, while greater with adrenaline in less vascular areas. Toxic symptoms of lignocaine may occur at a plasma level of 3–5 µg/mL. Yet such a level is not uncommonly produced after a single shot epidural block using 20 mL of 2% lignocaine without adrenaline.

Lignocaine is metabolized in liver to monoethylglycinexylidine and glycinexylidine. The later can be metabolized further to monoethylglycine and xylidine. Both the monoethylglycinexylidine and glycinexylidine retain the LA property.

Mepivacaine HCl

Regarding clinical activity and toxicity, mepivacaine is similar to that of lignocaine. But, it has a lesser inherent vasodilator property. So, the duration of action of mepivacaine is 50% longer than lignocaine. The addition of adrenaline also prolongs its action by about 75%. Topically, unlike lignocaine, mepivacaine is not effective.

Bupivacaine HCl

It was first introduced in clinical practice, in 1963. Its structure is similar to that of lignocaine, except that the amine containing group is a butyl piperidine. It is 3–4 times more potent than lignocaine and has longer duration of action. Its long duration **(Table 2)** of action and tendency to provide more sensory than motor blockade, has made it a popular drug for providing prolonged analgesia, during labor or postoperative pain. Analgesia by bupivacaine for postoperative pain usually lasts for 4 hours or more, when it is used through epidural route. While caudal administration of bupivacaine usually produces perineal analgesia for 8 hours or more.

When bupivacaine is given by repeated injections, then tachyphylaxis is much less common than that of lignocaine. Thus, a safe and effective analgesia can usually be provided indefinitely (for several days) by taking the advantage of catheter and continuous infusions through it by epidural route.

Bupivacaine is more cardiotoxic than equieffective doses of lignocaine. It causes severe ventricular arrhythmias and myocardial depression, than lignocaine, if there is sudden inadvertent IV injection of it. Lignocaine and bupivacaine both rapidly block cardiac Na^+ channels during systole. But, bupivacaine dissociates from these Na^+ channels much more slowly than lignocaine, during diastole. So,

significant number of Na^+ channels remains blocked at the end of diastole with bupivacaine. Thus, this block caused by bupivacaine is cumulative and is responsible for more cardiac toxicity than lignocaine. A part of cardiac toxicity produced by bupivacaine is also mediated through centrally, as it is observed that small quantities of bupivacaine injected in the medulla produce malignant ventricular arrhythmias.

Different doses of bupivacaine in spinal and epidural anesthesia is discussed in their specific chapters. Bupivacaine crosses the placenta, but very little in amount. So, it has a unique value in obstetrics. It is used extensively for lumbar epidural blockade in the concentration of 0.125–0.5%. Bupivacaine in a concentration of 0.125%, usually produces only sensory blockade, without affecting the motor function. So, for painless labor or walking epidural, where motor function is preserved, but only analgesia is provided, then 0.125–0.25% of bupivacaine is the choice. When the concentration of bupivacaine is gradually increased from 0.125 to 0.25%, then there is gradually lesser chance of failure of sensory blockade, but more chance of motor blockade and vice versa. For a single dose epidural, the maximum safe dose of bupivacaine is 2 mg/kg. To provide prolonged or continuous analgesia, 30 mg bupivacaine at 2 hours

TABLE 2: Physicochemical properties of local anesthetic agents.

	Procaine	Lignocaine	Mepivacaine	Bupivacaine	Etidocaine
Year of introduction	1905	1943	1957	1963	1972
Site of metabolism	Plasma (ester hydrolysis)	Liver (amide hydrolysis)	Liver	Liver	Liver
Onset of action	Slow	Fast	Fast	Intermediate	Fast
Duration	Short	Intermediate	Intermediate	Long	Prolonged
Equieffective anesthetic concentration	2% (slow potency)	1% (intermediate potency)	1% (intermediate potency)	0.25% (high potency)	0.5% (high potency)
Protein binding	6%	65%	75%	95%	95%
Duration of action	(Short)	(Intermediate)	(Intermediate)	(Long)	(Long)
Dissociation constant (pKa)	8.9	7.7	7.6	8.1	7.7
Time of onset of action	Slow onset	Fast onset	Fast onset	Intermediate onset	Fast onset
Tissue penetration	Poor	Good	Good	Intermediate	Good
% of base at pH of 7.4	2%	35%	35%	20%	35%
Lipid/water coefficient	0.6	2.9	0.8	27.5	14.1
Partition coefficient (anesthesia potency)	Low potency	Intermediate potency	Intermediate potency	High potency	High potency
Maximum single dose (plain solution)	800 mg	250 mg	300 mg	150 mg	300 mg
Maximum single dose (with adrenaline)	1,000 mg	500 mg	500 mg	250 mg	400 mg

interval is sufficient and this dose can be repeated for indefinite period. The maximum safe dose of bupivacaine is 2–3 mg/kg without adrenaline for infiltration. When adrenaline is added with bupivacaine, then this amount can be increased by one-third.

Etidocaine HCl

Etidocaine is an engineered modification of lignocaine molecule with high potency and prolonged duration of action. It is mainly used in the Scandinavian countries and USA. Unlike bupivacaine, it has a rapid onset of action. So, because of its fast onset and prolonged action, compared to bupivacaine, etidocaine is in vogue in ophthalmological practice. It is used clinically in 0.5%, 1%, and 1.5% concentrations for any type of regional and infiltration block. This drug can also be used topically, but is rarely used by this route. It is less potent than bupivacaine in producing sensory block, but is more potent for motor block. So, it is usually recommended where prolonged epidural with high degree of motor blockade is necessary. For this purpose, 20 mL of 1% etidocaine with adrenaline (1: 200,000 or 5 µg/mL) is used and the motor blockade lasts for 3–5 hours, though the sensory blockade is not always adequate. Hence, for obstetric pain relief etidocaine is less reliable than bupivacaine. This is because no concentration of etidocaine can produce effective sensory blockade without affecting motor block.

Prilocaine

It emerged first, in 1960, from the AB Astra laboratory, though it had already been synthesized previously by Lofgren. Chemically, it is an amino-amide compound and its pharmacological profile is similar to that of lignocaine. But, its penetrative power is very good. It can be used for all types of local anesthesia in the same concentration like lignocaine. When used in epidural anesthesia, it produces higher incidences of motor blockade and a longer duration of action than lignocaine. However, it has lesser vasodilatation action than lignocaine and thus it is used without any vasoconstricting agent. For its increased volume of distribution (high therapeutic index), it is less CNS toxic and so also very suitable for IV regional anesthesia. The administration of prilocaine gives rise to much lower plasma concentration than that of lignocaine. This is because of its more rapid metabolism, greater tissue uptake, and lesser protein binding property. It is only about 2/3 as toxic as lignocaine after a single dose. It is considerably less cumulative.

Prilocaine is unique, among all the LA agents, for its greater propensity to cause methemoglobinemia. It is due to the metabolism of its aromatic ring to O-toluidine in liver which induces methemoglobinemia. The chances of development of methemoglobinemia, after the local administration of prilocaine, dependents on its total dose administered which is usually above 8 mg/kg of body weight. In a healthy person, it is not a problem and can be treated by methylene blue in the dose of 1–2 mg/kg of body weight by infusion. However, methemoglobinemia following prilocaine has restricted its use in obstetric anesthesia. The maximum concentration of methemoglobin normally occurs between 4 and 6 hours, after the administration of prilocaine. Then, it decreases gradually to the normal value in 24 hours. Though the occurrence of methemoglobinemia contraindicates the use of prilocaine in many circumstances, but a transient rise to its maximum level, which occurs in most of the people after its use, is harmless.

Ropivacaine

It is a derivative of bupivacaine and consists of a single enantiomer, such as the S-stereoisomer. Whereas, the bupivacaine consists of both isomers and lignocaine has no stereoisomer. Ropivacaine is intrinsically less cardiotoxic. It is cleared more quickly from circulation, if the drug is injected IV erroneously and cardiac resuscitation is easy. An important mechanism for the cardiotoxic action of any LA is the very slow reversal of Na^+ channel from its blocked condition by this LA agent. This is the hallmark of bupivacaine, and such slow Na^+ channel reversal with bupivacaine is associated with the persistent slowing of conduction of the conducting pathways of heart, resulting in re-entry circuits, ventricular tachycardia, and ventricular fibrillation.

The difference between the ropivacaine and bupivacaine is that the negative inotropic potency of ropivacaine is less than that of bupivacaine and the therapeutic index of ropivacaine is greater than that of bupivacaine. Again, ropivacaine is slightly less potent and has a shorter duration of action than bupivacaine and the convulsant dose of ropivacaine is larger than that of bupivacaine. The cardiotoxic effect of ropivacaine in pregnancy is not greater than in the nonpregnant state which is most advantageous for it. All this makes the ropivacaine a significantly safer drug for local and regional anesthesia in obstetric patients. Interestingly, it seems to have even more motor sparing effect than bupivacaine.

Eutectic Mixture of Prilocaine (2.5%) and Lignocaine (2.5%)

The depth of action of a mixture of LA agents, such as prilocaine and lignocaine, in the ratio of 1:1 by weight, is in between the topical and infiltration anesthesia. The efficacy of this combination lies in the fact that the

TABLE 3: Local anesthetics commonly used for topical ophthalmic anesthesia (except cocaine).

Drug	Concentration (%)	Maximum dose	Duration (minute)	Corneal toxicity
Cocaine	1–4	1 mg/kg (20 drops 4%)	30	+++
Lignocaine	2–4	4 mg/kg, (up to 60 drops, 4%)	20	Nil to least
Amethocaine (tetracaine)	0.5	5 mg total (15 drops)	20	++
Proparacaine (proxymetacaine)	0.5	10 mg total (30 drops)	20	+ –
Benoxinate	0.4	4 mg total (up to 15 drops)	20	Least

mixture of prilocaine and lignocaine has a melting point less than that of either compound taken alone, i.e., below the room temperature and can exist at room temperature as an oil rather than as crystal, which can penetrate more the intact skin. The maximum depth of penetration of this mixture in the skin is 5 mm. The onset of action of this mixture of two LA agents is 1 hour. It is effective for surgical procedures involving the skin and superficial structures. The components of this LA mixture are also absorbed into systemic circulation. This eutectic mixture of two LA agents should not be used on the mucous membrane or abraded skin, as rapid absorption of their component may result in systemic toxicity.

LOCAL ANESTHETICS LARGELY RESTRICTED TO OPHTHALMOLOGICAL USE

Topical Anesthetics in Ophthalmology

Topical anesthesia is very essential in ophthalmological practice. It is used for the measurement of intraocular pressure, removal of sutures and foreign bodies, and for other superficial surgeries of the conjunctiva and cornea. Topical anesthesia is also invaluable in preparing the conjunctiva for subsequent painless transconjunctival injections. Also, like the early part of this century, many cataract surgeries by phacoemulsification technique are now done under topical anesthesia. The onset of action of all the commonly used LA agents as topical drop is 15–20 seconds and last for 15–20 minutes. The initial stinging sensation of conjunctiva is the chief side effect of topical anesthesia, especially in pediatric group of patients. A most useful means of avoiding this stinging sensation is to use 5% proparacaine drops, diluted by a sterile balanced salt solution, prior to the instillation of full strength LA agent. Physiological corneal protective mechanism will be in abeyance in topical anesthesia **(Table 3)**.

So, any rubbing of the eye must be prohibited. Prolonged use of any topical anesthetic agent may result in corneal toxicity. Healing is delayed and cell division will be inhibited by topical anesthesia. The alteration of lacrimation and tear film instability may also occur. Certain preservatives, such as benzalkonium and chlorobutanol, which are present in topical anesthetic agents, may be implicated for this effect. Idiosyncratic reactions to any topical anesthetic agent may also occur. The rate of drug absorption in topical anesthesia is intermediate between intravenous and subcutaneous injection and cannot be influenced by the addition of adrenaline. Therefore, topically administered LA agents are also capable of attaining clinically significant serum concentrations. The digital occlusion of lacrimal puncta is a useful method of preventing the drugs from entering the nasolacrimal duct and thus gaining access to further mucosal surfaces from which additional absorption can occur. In topical anesthesia, it is also important not to exceed the safe clinical dose. As serious and even fatal reactions do occur with overdosing.

Local Anesthetics used Primarily on Mucous Membrane and Skin

Some LAs are too irritating or too ineffective to be applied on eye. But, they are useful as topical anesthetic agents on skin and mucous membrane. Their preparations are effective for the symptomatic relief for anal and genital pruritus, many acute and chronic dermatoses, etc. They are sometimes combined with glucocorticoids or antihistamines. LAs used for these purposes are dibucaine, xylocaine hydrochloride, and pramoxine hydrochloride.

Intravenous Anesthetics

■ INTRODUCTION AND HISTORY

At the beginning of the 17th century, some farsighted pioneers conceived the idea of anesthesia through the intravenous (IV) route. But they lacked suitable anesthetic agents and appropriate technology for their IV administration. So, the time delay, between the pioneers thought and the appearance of an appropriate anesthetic agent and appropriate technology for the administration of IV anesthesia was about 200 years. After that, there was a further delay of about five to six decades. This is because suitable drugs were not invented to make IV anesthesia *popular*. Thus, the arrival of hexobarbitone, in 1932, marked the birth of a new age of anesthesia, after which IV induction of anesthesia and its supplementation became the norm. However, during this period, it results in more comfort to the patient, but not necessarily more safety.

If we travel back in the past, we will see that, in 1665, for IV anesthesia Johann Sigismund (a German physician) first injected rude opium intravenously to produce unconsciousness. Then, Francis Rynd of Dublin, in 1845, used trocar and cannula for the IV administration of morphine for the treatment of trigeminal neuralgia. After that, in 1872, Pierre, a professor of Physiology at Bordeaux, used chloral hydrate intravenously in a patient, suffering from tetanus. But the Alexander Wood of Edinburgh was the true founder of IV anesthesia by first using the Ferguson syringe ("syringe" came from a Greek word named "syrinx" which means a tube or pipe).

During that period, IV ether also had been tried on animals by Nikolai Ivanovich of Russia, in 1847, for IV anesthesia. This was a year after Morton's use of ether by inhalation. A 25–5% solution of ether in normal saline or in 5% glucose was used by him. He also used chloroform intravenously on animals in that way.

After that barbituric acid was first synthesized by Adolf Baeyer of Munich, in 1864, but its sedative and hypnotic effects were not realized at that time. Then, in Munich, diethyl barbituric acid was also synthetized by Fischer and Von, in 1903. At that time, this was known as Veronal. Then, phenobarbitone was discovered, in 1912, at elsewhere in the world and only oral preparation of it was used for sedation. But somnifaine was the first barbiturate to be given intravenously. It was a combination of diethyl and diallyl barbituric acids and was used in France by Bardet in 1924.

During this period, Noel and Souttar also tried paraldehyde intravenously for sedation. Intravenous morphine and hyoscine were also employed by them for "twilight sleep" in 1916. In 1923, Bumm introduced Pernocton, while 2 years later Zerfas in the USA used sodium amytal intravenously. This was soon followed by IV preparation of pentobarbitone (Nembutal). Magill was the first person who demonstrated their clinical effects through the IV route in Britain. Then, John Silas Lundy of the Mayo Clinic attempted to popularize Nembutal in the USA, in 1931. In between this time, Martin Kirschner tried bromethol intravenously, in 1929, with moderate success.

Then, the invention of hexobarbiturate was a great breakthrough in the history of IV anesthesia. It was the first drug to make IV anesthesia popular and was first used, in 1932, by Helmut. He was a professor of pharmacology at Dusseldorf (Germany) and was director of pharmacology at Beyer. The historical significance of this event, also, was that it was the first happy partnership between an academic house and a big business house for any invention in medical science. Later, this partnership became a model which had been copied many times for the benefit of mankind. Thus, Helmut was the true father of IV anesthesia, though hexobarbitone was first synthetized, in 1931, by Kropp and Taub in Elberfeld. It was first used in Great Britain, in 1933, by Ronald Jarman.

BARBITURATES

History

Barbituric acid was first synthesized, in 1864, by Baeyer which has no hypnotic property. Then, Fisher and Von first synthesized diethylbarbituric acid in 1903 which had hypnotic property. After that, in between 1903 and 1932, many barbiturates with hypnotic property were synthesized, but their onset of action is slow and had a long duration of action, so they could not be used for IV anesthesia. Thus, up to 1932, no IV drug was getting a strong foothold in IV anesthesia. Finally, in 1932, the synthesis of methylated oxybarbiturate (hexobarbiturate) set the stage. It had a very good hypnotic property, with a very rapid onset of action and short duration of action, but it had many excitatory side effects. Then, in 1934, the actual breakthrough was done by the discovery of thiopentone.

However, during the first report, the proper pharmacokinetic and pharmacodynamic property of this drug (thiopentone) was not known. At that time, it was thought (wrongly) that the short duration of action of thiopentone is due to its rapid metabolism in our body. Thus, at that time, hexobarbitone and thiopentone were used intravenously for the induction and maintenance of anesthesia such as ether and chloroform by inhalation. So, the overdose of these drugs (hexobarbitone and thiopentone) was frequently used due to their short duration of action which was thought at that time due to quick elimination from the body by metabolism) causing many deaths, resulting from hypotension. Hence, during that period, IV anesthesia was described as *"an ideal method of euthanasia".* One such example of many deaths by thiopentone is during the treatment of multiple casualties of war by thiopentone at *Pearl Harbor.* So, at that time it was also thought that though thiopentone has a rapid onset and short duration of action, but it has also a great toxic effect, but later it was proved that the dose and the method of administration of the drug, rather than the drug's inherent toxicity, caused the adverse outcome. *Then, Brodie first demonstrated that the effects of thiopentone were quickly terminated not by its rapid metabolism in our body, but by its redistribution, from their sites of action to other body tissues. However, in 1960, Price explained that during large dose administration of thiopentone, as the peripheral redistribution site of it (thiopentone) approached to saturation and equilibrium, then redistribution from the effector site to other tissues was less effective and blood concentration rose quickly which ultimately causes cardiovascular system (CVS) collapse and death* **(Fig. 1).**

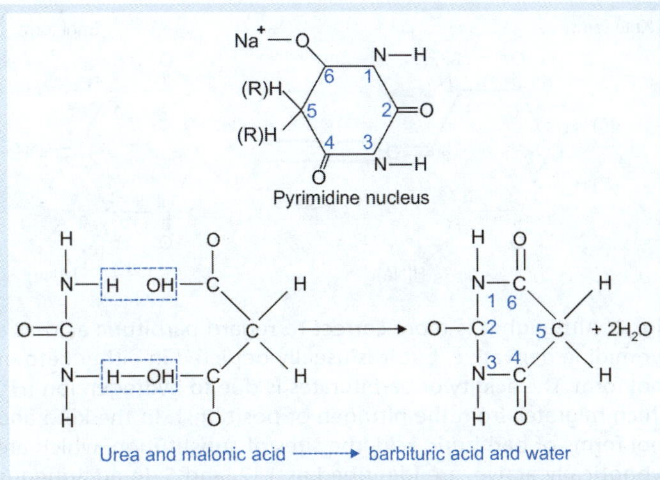

Fig. 1: Synthesis of barbituric acid from urea and malonic acid.

Chemistry of Barbiturates

The barbiturates are the salt (usually Na^+) of barbituric acid. It is synthesized from urea and malonic acid, so it is also called malonylurea. Barbituric acid actually has a pyrimidine nucleus. It (barbiturate) is termed in North America, *by using the ending as "al"* (for example, thiopental) and in Britain *by using the ending as "one"* (for example, thiopentone). It is available either in keto or enol form and it is acidic in nature, due to the presence of H^+ ion at position 1 in the pyrimidine ring. However, the Na^+ salt (at position 3) of barbituric acid is water soluble, yielding a highly alkaline solution. The presence of the carboxyl group, in the structure of barbituric acid, at position 2, is responsible for the acidic character of barbiturates. This is because of the keto–enol tautomerization, which is also favored by its location between two electronegative amido nitrogens. The enol form of barbiturates is favored in alkaline solution and salts result. Barbiturates, in which the oxygen atom at C_2 is replaced by a sulfur atom, are called *thiobarbiturates.* These are more lipid soluble than the corresponding oxybarbiturates.

Depending on the H, O, and S atoms, and the CH_3 group in 1 and 2 positions; the barbiturates are classified into four distinct groups as follows:

1. Oxybarbiturates (1 = H, 2 = O)
2. Methylated oxybarbiturates (1= CH_3, 2 = O)
3. Thiobarbiturates (1 = H, 2 = S)
4. Methylated thiobarbiturates (1= CH_3, 2 = S) **(Fig. 2).**

The sodium salt of thiopentone (thiobarbiturates) is a pale yellow colored hygroscopic powder, with a bitter taste. It is readily soluble in water and alkaline in property. The commercial preparation of thiobarbiturates contains six parts of anhydrous Na^+ carbonate.

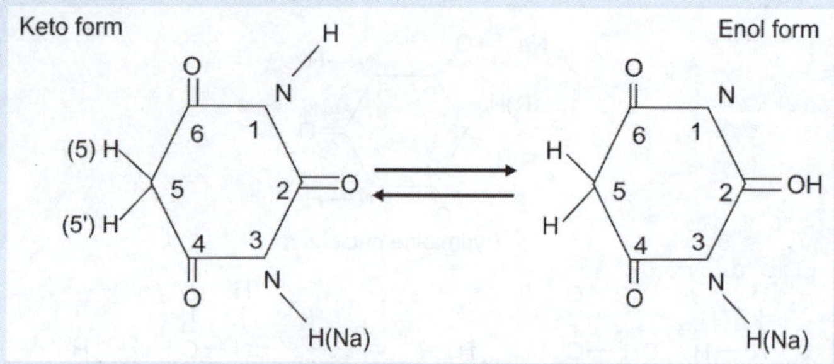

Fig. 2: Although it is more correct to regard barbituric acid as a pyrimidine derivative, but it is usually depicted in either keto or enol form. The acidity of barbiturates is due to hydrogen ion (H⁺) which migrates from the nitrogen of position 1. In the keto and enol forms of barbituric acid, the sites of substitution, which are hypnotically active, are identified as 1, 2, and 5. In an aqueous solution, it dissociates into hydrogen ion and barbiturate ions. The Na-salts (in position 3) of barbituric acid are water soluble and can be administered parenterally.

TABLE 1: Classification of barbiturates.

Ultrashort-acting	Short-acting	Long-acting
• Methohexitone	• Secobarbitone	• Mephobarbitone
• Hexobarbitone	• Butobarbitone	• Phenobarbitone
• Thiopentone	• Pentobarbitone	

This prevents the formation of insoluble free barbituric acid from thiopentone by its reaction with atmospheric CO_2 and subsequent precipitation. The aqueous solution of thiobarbiturates is strongly alkaline and the pH of 2.5% thiopentone is about 10.5. The solution of thiobarbiturate (thiopentone) in water may remain stable at room temperature for up to 2 weeks, after its aqueous preparation, but it should not be used, if they become cloudy **(Table 1)**.

Structure–Activity–Relationship

The barbituric acid itself originally lacks the central depressant activity.

- The barbituric acid itself has no hypnotic property. The hypnotic activity is introduced into barbituric acid, if a side chain, consisting of an alkyl or aryl group (at least if one of them is branched), is added at position 5 or 5′ in its (barbituric acid) structure.
- Sleep cannot be produced very rapidly (in one arm–brain circulation time) after an IV injection of an effective dose of any oxybarbiturate. So, these have very limited use in clinical anesthesia and are mainly employed as oral hypnotics and sedatives.
- Replacing the O atom of oxybarbiturates with the S atom, at position 2, produces thiobarbiturates which are more lipid soluble and have a more rapid onset and shorter duration of action, for example, thiobarbiturates (thiopentone and thiamylal) have a faster onset and shorter duration of action than oxybarbiturates (pentobarbital and secobarbital).

- The increased length of the side chain, in position 5, increases both the potency and the duration of action of barbiturates, for example, secobarbital and thiamylal are more potent than pentobarbital and thiopentone.
- Methylation and sulfuration of barbituric acid increases lipid solubility and the rate of penetration of barbiturates in the central nervous system (CNS).
- The addition of methyl group at position 1 of oxy barbiturates (oxymethyl barbiturate) not only produces the rapid onset and short duration of action but also increases the excitatory side effects.
- Methylated thiobarbiturates combine the rapidity of onset of action and the convulsive activity of such severity as to preclude their use in clinical anesthesia.
- Only thiobarbiturates and methylated oxybarbiturates are used in anesthesia practice.
- The stereoisomerism has an important effect on the structure-activity relationship of barbiturate. The L-isomer of pento, seco, thio, and thiamylal are twice as potent as the D-isomers of it. These barbiturates are marketed as a racemic mixture. Methohexital has four stereoisomers.

Barbiturates are weak acids and in the stomach (where pH is 1 or 2) they remain practically in a unionized state. Hence, in aqueous solution, they cannot be absorbed orally. So, their rate of absorption through gastric mucosa is related to their lipid solubility which helps the barbiturate molecules to pass through the lipid cell membrane of gastric mucosal cells. Thus, methylated and thiobarbiturates are very rapidly absorbed by mouth and cause brief period of intense hypnosis, when used orally, as they are highly lipid soluble. The approximate potency of available barbiturate compounds, relative to thiopentone are (1) thiamylal 1.1, (2) thialbarbitone 0.5, (3) thiobutobarbitone 0.7, (4) metho-hexitone 2.5–3, (5) enibomal 1, and (6) hexobarbitone 0.5.

Mechanism of Action of Barbiturates

The barbiturates act throughout the whole CNS. In nonanesthetic doses, it preferentially suppresses the polysynaptic responses. So the facilitation is diminished and inhibition is enhanced. The site of inhibition of barbiturates in CNS is either the postsynaptic area, for example, the cortical and cerebellar pyramidal cells, cuneate nucleus, substantia nigra, and thalamic relay neurons or the presynaptic area, for example, the spinal cord. The enhancement of the inhibition of conduction of impulses by barbiturates occurs primarily

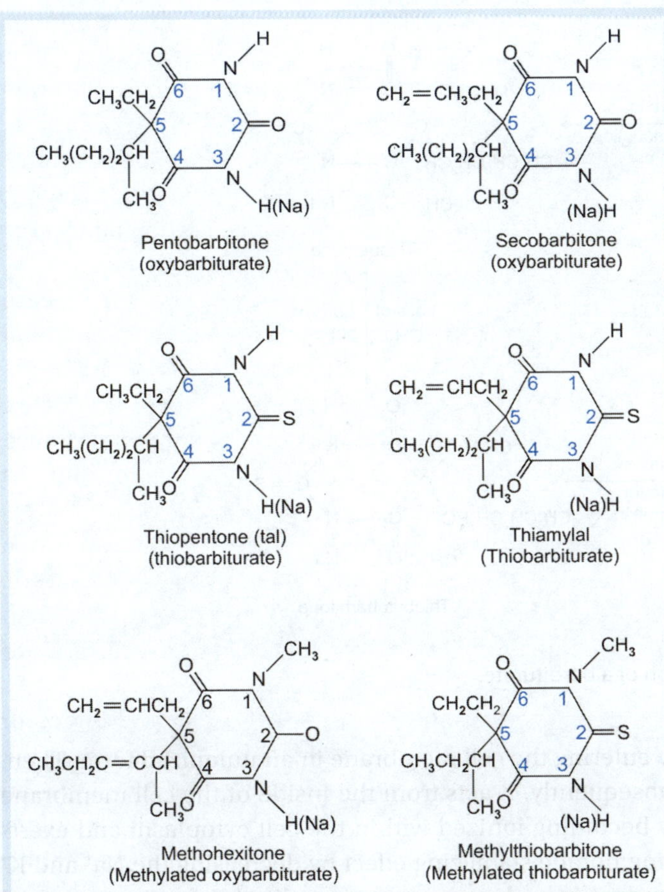

Fig. 3: Structure of various barbituric agents.

at synapses where the neurotransmission is mediated by inhibitory γ-aminobutyric acid (GABA) neurotransmitter, acting through γ-aminobutyric acid type A (GAB$_A$) receptors **(Fig. 3)**.

Barbiturates act mainly through the GABA$_A$ receptor complex at clinical concentration and correlate well with anesthetic potency of this agent. GABA is the principal inhibitory neurotransmitter in CNS which also acts through GABA$_A$ receptor. GABA$_A$ receptor has five glycoprotein subunits which assemble to form an internal chloride ion channel and has one GABA, benzodiazepine (BZD), and barbiturate-binding sites on its subunits. The activation of this GABA$_A$ receptor, by binding with barbiturates, at its own binding site, increases chloride ion conduction through its ion channel within GABA$_A$ receptor and causes the hyperpolarization of the cell membrane of neurons. Thereby, it reduces the excitability of postsynaptic neuron (GABA$_A$ receptors are referred to as the ligand-gated chloride ion channel) **(Fig. 4)**.

The barbiturates enhance or mimic the action of inhibitory neurotransmitter, such as GABA. By attaching to

their binding site on GABA$_A$ receptor, barbiturates decrease the rate of dissociation of GABA from their binding site on the receptor and increase the duration of GABA-activated chloride ion channel opening. Thus, barbiturates enhance the action of an inhibitor neurotransmitter, named GABA (*GABA-enhancing activity of barbiturates*). However, at higher concentration, but still in the clinical range, these barbiturates directly activate the GABA$_A$ receptor (chloride ion channel) after attaching to their barbiturate-binding site on the receptor, even in the absence of GABA. This is known as the *GABA-mimetic effect of barbiturates*. The enhancement of the action of GABA by barbiturates is responsible for its sedative and hypnotic effect. But the GABA-mimetic effect of barbiturates at higher concentration is responsible for the anesthetic activity of barbiturates. The mechanism of underlying actions of barbiturates on the GABA$_A$ receptor appears to be distinct from the action of either GABA or BZD on the same receptor.

These differences include the following:
- Although the barbiturates enhance the binding of GABA neurotransmitter to GABA$_A$ receptor, they also promote (rather than displace) the binding of BZD.
- The barbiturates potentiate the GABA-induced chloride currents by prolonging the suppression of burst periods, rather than increasing the frequency of suppression of bursts as the BZDs do.
- Only the α- and β-subunits of GABA$_A$ receptors are required for the action of barbiturates, but not the γ-subunit.
- Barbiturate's action on GABA$_A$ receptor is not affected by the deletion of tyrosine and threonine residue of the β-subunit of GABA$_A$ receptor that governs the sensitivity of GABA$_A$ receptor to activation by its agonist GABA **(Fig. 5)**.

Except for GABA receptor mechanism, there are other proposed mechanisms through which the barbiturates also act. These are:
- Barbiturates also act on the glutamate receptors and reduce glutamate-induced depolarization. Only the α-amino-3-hydroxy-5-methyl-4-isoxazolepropionic acid (AMPA) subtypes of glutamate receptors are blocked by barbiturates.
- At higher concentration that produce anesthesia, the barbiturates also suppress the high-frequency repetitive firing of a neuron as the result of the direct inhibition of the function of the voltage-dependent Na$^+$ channel.
- Still, at higher concentrations, the barbiturates also suppress the voltage-dependent K$^+$ channel and its conductances.

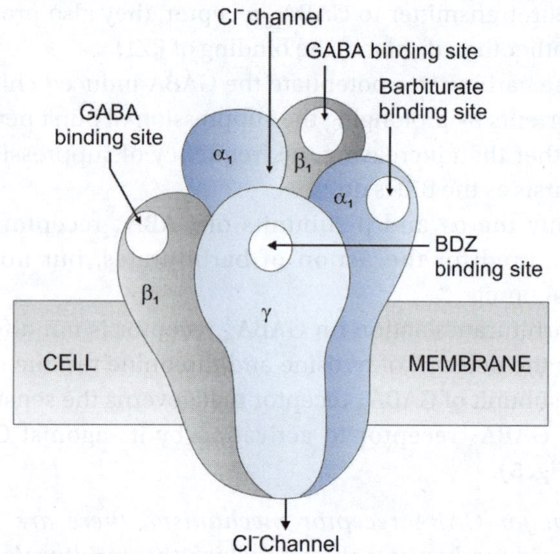

Fig. 4: Mechanism of action of a barbiturate.

Fig. 5: GABA–BZD–barbiturate receptor complex (GABA$_A$ receptor) with a chloride channel inside it. It is a pentameric protein composed of two α, two β, and one γ–subunits. There are total of two sites for GABA binding on the two β–subunits. There is a single-binding site, each for BZD, and barbiturate on the γ– and α–subunit, respectively. There is a similarity between the GABA$_A$ receptor and the nicotinic acetylcholine receptor. (BZD: benzodiazepine; GABA: γ-aminobutyric acid; GABA$_A$: γ-aminobutyric acid type A)

In summary, the barbiturates activate the inhibitory GABA$_A$ receptors, inhibit the excitatory AMPA receptors, and also inhibit the voltage-dependent Na$^+$ and K$^+$ channels, like local anesthetic agents. The barbiturates or thiopentone may act in a manner analogous to that of local anesthetic agents

by entering the cell membrane in an unionized form. Then, subsequently, it acts from the inside of the cell membrane by becoming ionized within the cell cytoplasm and exerts a membrane stabilizing effect by decreasing the Na$^+$ and K$^+$ conductance, decreasing the amplitude of action potential and slowing the rate of conduction of impulse in excitable tissues. In high concentration, the barbiturates also depress the enzyme, involved in glucose oxidation which inhibit the formation of adenosine triphosphate (ATP) and thus depress the Ca^{2+}-dependent action potential.

Pharmacokinetics of Thiopentone

Following an IV injection of thiopentone, the blood concentration of it rises rapidly. The concentration of thiopentone in highly perfused organ, but with less tissue volume such as the brain, heart, and kidney also rises equally rapidly in parallel to its rise in concentration in blood and equilibrate quickly between blood and brain, resulting in the induction of anesthesia.

Thus, the rapid onset of action of thiopentone is due to:
- The high blood flow in the brain.
- The high lipophilicity of the drug.
- Its low degree of ionization in the blood.

The thiopentone remains as 60% nonionized and diffusible form in blood, at pH 7.4. This helps it to diffuse into the brain quickly in increased amount because only this nonionized fraction of thiopentone is able to cross the blood–brain barrier. Hyperventilation increases the pH of blood and hence increases the nonbound or nonionized fraction of thiopentone. Thus, it increases the anesthetic effect of it. So, thiopentone concentration in cerebral spinal fluid (CSF) reaches a level almost as high as that of the unbound portion of the drug in plasma and is responsible for induction of anesthesia very rapidly. After that, the amount of drug, which is present in the blood after its first distribution to brain, is distributed rapidly to the other next highly perfused organ with a large tissue volume such as the liver, muscle, and spleen. Thus, within a few minutes, after IV injection, the blood (central pool) has given up about 90% of the injected dose of thiopentone to the tissues. First, the drug is given up by the blood to the brain and the patient becomes unconscious. Later, the drug is given up by the blood to the other highly perfused tissues. As a result, the concentration of thiopentone in the blood falls rapidly. At that moment, as the concentration of the drug in the brain tissue is still high than that of blood, so it diffuses back again into the blood from the brain tissue and is redistributed to other tissues such as the muscles and fat, thus the decrease in the brain concentration of thiopentone terminates its effect on the brain (induction of anesthesia) and helps in the arousal of a patient from sleep. With thiopentone, this whole event, resulting in awakening of patient, occurs within 5–15 minutes, after a single bolus injection of usual anesthesia induction dose **(Fig. 6)**.

Equilibrium with muscle tissue is not attained, until a quarter of an hour, after an IV injection has passed and thereafter its concentration declines at a higher rate parallel to that of plasma. Despite its higher affinity for thiopentone, adipose tissue which is responsible for the final redistribution of this drug, takes up thiopentone very slowly, because of its poor perfusion. With a fat/blood partition coefficient of 11:1, thiopentone will move from the blood into fat, as long as the concentration of thiopentone in fat is <11 times than that of blood. The maximum deposition of thiopentone into fat occurs, approximately 2.5 hours after its IV administration. The irreversible removal of thiopentone from our body, i.e., elimination clearance by metabolism contributes little to the termination of the anesthetic effect of the induction dose of it. Thus, in summary, it can be concluded that the relatively brief duration of anesthesia, following a bolus induction dose of thiopentone is due to its redistribution from the brain to muscle tissue and later to fat tissue, but not due to elimination from the body by metabolism.

In the compartmental pharmacokinetic model, the central volume of distribution (V_C) of thiopentone exceeds its volume of distribution in intramuscular space. This indicates that the brain, like the intramuscular compartment, is also a part of V_C and also explains the rapid onset of action of thiopentone.

When thiopentone is administered in large doses, i.e., by repeated multiple bolus doses or by continuous infusion, then the capacity of lean tissue (muscle) to reduce the plasma concentration of the drug (thiopentone) by absorption or redistribution in it, decreases progressively, as the concentration of drug in tissue slowly approaches an equilibrium with blood concentration. Then, after the completion of distribution and redistribution and reaching on equilibrium, the termination of the action of drug gradually depends on the slower process of reuptake of thiopentone into adipose tissues from muscles and its metabolism in liver, resulting in prolonged drug effect. When thiopentone was administered continuously by infusion for 3–5 days for cerebral resuscitation, then the redistribution sites (muscle, fat, etc.) reach equilibrium with a blood concentration, and the enzymes, responsible for the metabolism of thiopentone in the liver, also soon approach saturation. Then, the recovery from thiopentone depends entirely on the nonlinear drug metabolism process and its subsequent excretion through the kidney and bile, which took nearly about 5 days. The first-pass pulmonary uptake of thiopentone is only 14%.

In hypovolemic (hemorrhagic) shock patients, the anesthetic dose requirement of thiopentone is very less. This is because the fraction of the administered dose removed from the brain tissue by distribution and redistribution to other tissues is very less. This is due to the decreased blood flow to other tissues which is again due to peripheral vasoconstriction for hypotension. In such a situation, the induction dose of thiopentone should be based on the lean body weight (BW), rather than the total body mass. The usual dose of thiopentone which is based on the total body mass shows an increased response in aged, obese, and female patients. This is because the lean body mass which represents the principal site for distribution and

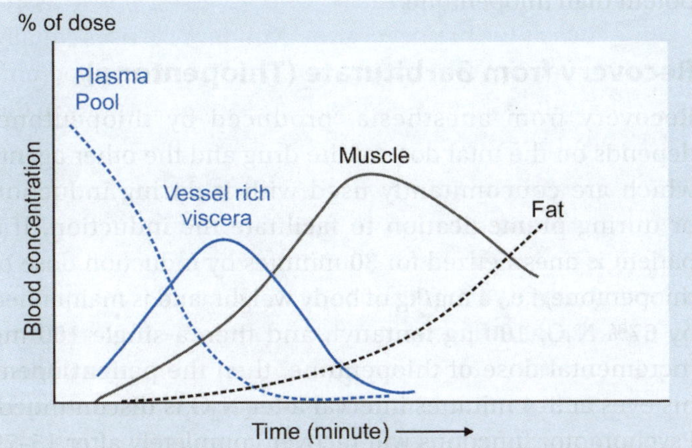

Fig. 6: Distribution of thiopentone in different tissues and organs at various times after its IV injection.

redistribution represents smaller proportion of the total body mass in these patients.

Acute tolerance was seen in thiopentone, i.e., the plasma thiopentone concentration, at which the patient awakes, is proportional to the initial dose used. The higher the induction dose of thiopentone is used, the lesser sensitive a patient will be to the subsequent doses. On the other hand, when a large amount of thiopentone is given, then the subsequent incremental dose, necessary to maintain a sleep, becomes gradually less. This is because tissue equilibrium gradually occurs when small doses are required at long intervals. These not only replace the drug which has been detoxicated by metabolism but compensate for the increasing tolerance to metabolism.

The thiopentone is 60–80% protein bound in plasma, predominantly to albumin. However, 40% of the injected dose is sequestrated in red blood cells (RBCs).

Detoxification and Biotransformation of Thiopentone

The 10–15% of the inducing dose of injected thiopentone is broken down in liver per hour. About 30% of the drug may remain in the body for 24 hours, after the IV administration of an inducing dose of thiopentone. Liver has an important role in metabolism and also in the recovery from the excess doses of thiopentone which is rapidly removed from the brain by redistribution. The metabolism (oxidation and reduction) of thiopentone is occurred by the cytochrome P_{450} system, situated in the endoplasmic reticulum (ER) of liver cells. Liver is the largest reservoir of ER and removes 50% of thiopentone from the hepatic blood. Thus, it also plays a definite role for the short duration of action of thiopentone, after its distribution and redistribution in different tissues.

The pathways involved in the metabolism of barbiturates in liver are threefold:

1. *Side chain oxidation at C_5 position:* The oxidation of radicals at the C_5 position of thiopentone molecule is the most important step of biotransformation of thiopentone and is responsible for the termination of its biological activity. This oxidation of thiopentone results in the formation of alcohols, ketones, phenols, or carboxylic acid which may appear in urine as such, or as conjugates of glucuronic acid.
2. *Oxidative replacement of sulfur at C_2 position:* It forms a small quantity of the drug's oxygen equivalent such as pentobarbitone.
3. *Ring cleavage to form urea and three carbon fragments:* The uptake and reuptake of thiopentone by muscle is mainly responsible for the early fall of its arterial concentration, with a modest (but imprecisely defined)

contribution from metabolism in the liver and the uptake and reuptake by fat. The excretion of thiopentone occurs predominantly through urine as its inactive metabolites. The elimination half-life of thiopentone is 4–22 hours and cannot be removed by dialysis.

Dosage and the Duration of Action of Thiopentone

When thiopentone is injected intravenously, the maximum effect of it is found within about 1 minute. The duration of effect of a single induction dose of thiopentone in 4–5 mg/kg is about 5–8 minutes. The induction dose of thiopentone for a healthy adult is 2.5–4.5 mg/kg, for children, this induction dose of thiopentone is 5–6 mg/kg, and for infant, it is 7–8 mg/kg. The premedicated geriatric patient may require a 30% reduction in dose, as compared with the younger patient. Concomitantly, when midazolam, opiates, inhalational anesthetics, ketamine, etc., are given with thiopentone, then these drugs shift the dose-response curve of thiopentone to the left, in proportion to the dose of midazolam, opiates, inhalational agents, etc., which are administered. In the hypothermia and circulatory failure state, the circulation time is decreased and the induction time is prolonged. Therefore, much lower doses of barbiturate are needed in such conditions. An acutely inebriated patient by alcohol requires less thiopentone to induce anesthesia, while chronic alcoholic patients require a higher dose of thiopentone than normal. This is due to the induction of enzyme, responsible for the metabolism of thiopentone in the liver. Clinically, there are no differences between the thiopentone and thiamylal in relation to their dose, duration of action, potency, incidences of laryngospasm, respiratory depression, and cardiotoxicity during induction. On the contrary, the induction dose of methohexital is 1–2 mg/kg of body weight. This is because methohexital is 2.5 times more potent than thiopentone.

Recovery from Barbiturate (Thiopentone)

Recovery from anesthesia, produced by thiopentone, depends on the total dose of the drug and the other agents which are concomitantly used with it during induction or during premedication to facilitate the induction. If a patient is anesthetized for 30 minutes by induction dose of thiopentone, i.e., 4 mg/kg of body weight, and is maintained by 67% N_2O, 100 μg fentanyl, and then a single 100 mg incremental dose of thiopentone, then the patient opens his eyes at 3–4 minutes interval after N_2O is discontinued. Psychomotor functions will recover completely after 15–75 minutes and the psychophysiological functions will recover completely after 8 hours. However, the abnormal sleep pattern in electroencephalographic (EEG) is found for 12 hours after thiopentone anesthesia. All these data recommend not to drive vehicles for 24 hours after thiopentone-induced general anesthesia (GA).

Complications during the Injection of Thiopentone

- *Pain:* The incidence of pain is 1–2% when thiopentone is injected into small veins on the back of the hand or wrist, but there is no incidence of pain when this thiopentone is injected into large veins. If any extravasation of thiopentone occurs, then reactions ranging from slight pain, edema, erythema, and mild soreness to extensive local tissue necrosis can occur, depending on the concentration and the total amount of drug injected. Venous sequelae such as thrombosis and phlebitis may not be seen, until a few days postoperatively and its incidence is 3–4% in a patient, receiving thiopentone.
- *Intra-arterial injection:* If inadvertently thiopentone, in concentration >2.5%, is injected intra-arterially, then intense arterial spasm results, causing immediate excruciating pain, spreading distally from the site of injection to the hand or fingers. This intense arterial spasm may also cause edema, hyperesthesia, anesthesia, motor weakness, and even gangrene or loss of tissues of hand. But the severity of all these complications depends on the concentration, dose, total volume, and the rate of injection of the thiopentone into artery.

The pathology of these complications, following intra-arterial injection of thiopentone, is (1) the chemical endarteritis, induced by high concentration (>2.5) of it, leading to the damage of endothelial, subendothelial, and even muscle layer of artery and (2) the intra-arterial thrombosis, causing gangrene, or necrosis. Usually, the pulse is not felt, but the presence of a pulse does not rule out the development of thrombosis. The aim of management of this dangerous complication, following intra-arterial injection of thiopentone, is to relieve the arterial spasm and to prevent the formation of thrombus, leading to the resumption of circulation of blood. These can be achieved by (1) intra-arterial injection of papaverine (40–80 mg in normal saline) or 5–10 mL of 1% lignocaine which will dilute the thiopentone and will relieve the spasm, (2) blocking the sympathetic supply to upper extremity by stellate ganglion or brachial plexus block, (3) using heparin intravenously to prevent thrombosis, and (4) using analgesic and α-adrenergic antagonists, but the prevention is better than cure. So, as a prophylactic measure, to avoid this complication, thiopentone should always be used maximally at a concentration of 2.5%.

Pharmacodynamics of Thiopentone

Effect on Central Nervous System

Thiopentone reversibly depresses the activity of all excitable tissues such as the brain and heart, so it produces a smooth and rapid induction of anesthesia. The CNS is highly sensitive to thiopentone, but its direct effects on peripheral excitable tissues are weak. The antianxiety property of barbiturates is not equivalent to those, exerted by BZDs, especially with respect to the degree of sedation that is produced by BZDs with equivalent doses. Thus, thiopentone has a small therapeutic window; therefore due to this small therapeutic window of thiopentone, it is not possible to achieve the desired effect, regarding sedation, like BZD, without the evidence of much general depression of CNS, like GA. Thiopentone produces a dose-related depression of EEG. During the induction of the anesthesia, by the effect of thiopentone, the wake α-pattern of EEG is gradually replaced by higher amplitude, slower frequency delta, and theta waves which then gradually progresses to burst suppression and finally a flat EEG. This flat EEG, produced by thiopentone can be maintained by continuous infusion of it in the dose of 4 mg/kg/h, after a loading dose. As there is a depression of central neuronal electrical activity, so the cerebral O_2 demand which is necessary for and parallel to the cerebral electrical activity, is also reduced, but this does not indicate the reduction of cerebral O_2 demand, necessary for other cellular metabolic activity which only can be reduced by hypothermia. Along with this reduction of cerebral electrical activity and its parallel cerebral O_2 demand, there is also a parallel reduction of cerebral blood flow and reduction of intracranial pressure (ICP) by thiopentone (provided there is no CO_2 retention, following administration of it), but the cerebral perfusion pressure remains uncompromised because ICP decreases more than the mean arterial pressure. So, the thiopentone is considered as a best drug for neurosurgical anesthesia.

As thiopentone or other barbiturates have no analgesic property, so pain perception and reactions against this pain remain relatively unimpaired by thiopentone, until the final and very deep stage of anesthesia is reached. Contrary, in small doses, the barbiturates increase the reactions against painful stimuli. So, thiopentone has a hyperalgesic effect by a subanesthetic dose. This hyperalgesia or antanalgesic effect of a subanesthetic dose of thiopentone may result only from the depression effect of barbiturate on some inhibitory systems (centers) of the brain, (inhibition on inhibition causes excitation), but in full anesthetic concentration, it inhibits both the inhibitory and the excitatory part of the nervous system, both at the spinal and cerebral level and thus produce the total depression of CNS instead of excitation.

Effect on Cardiovascular System

In sedative or hypnotic doses, barbiturates (thiopentone) do not produce significant cardiovascular depression, except for a slight decrease in blood pressure (BP) and heart rate (HR) which occur normally during a natural sleep. But thiopentone itself is a direct myocardial depressing agent and depresses myocardial contractility; however this is less than that of the equivalent concentration of any volatile anesthetic agent. The fall in pH of blood (acidosis) increases this cardiovascular depressing activity of barbiturates, however the mechanism of this myocardial depressant effect of thiopentone is unknown. It is not due to the alteration of Ca^{2+} uptake by the cardiac sarcoplasmic reticulum, like halogenated inhalational anesthetic agents, but the probable explanation is like that in addition to depressing Na^+ channels; they also reduce the function of at least two types of K^+ channels of myocardium. However, the direct depression of cardiac contractility by thiopentone occurs only when large doses of it, which is several times greater than those required to cause GA, are administered.

Thiopentone produces venodilatation and thus reduces preload and cardiac output (CO). Therefore, the HR increases via the baroreflex mechanism, due to this decrease of BP, but cannot compensate for this reduced CO. The systemic vascular resistance (SVR) remains unchanged by thiopentone. But in higher doses, there is also a reduction of SVR and much reduction of BP. This is due to the decreased sympathetic tone and dilatation of peripheral resistance vessels. In a normal person, the slow pulse rates are usually quickened (due to a fall in BP) and the fast pulse rates are slowed (if it is due to sympathetic stimulation due to tension and anxiety, but not due to shock) by thiopentone during the induction of anesthesia. Cardiovascular depression is also obtained by partial inhibition of sympathetic transmission by higher doses of thiopentone. This is most evident in patients with congestive heart failure or hypovolemic shock, whose sympathetic reflexes already are operating maximally and in whom the barbiturates can cause an exaggerated fall in BP.

In higher doses, thiopentone itself decreases sympathetic outflow from CNS, resulting in decreased catecholamines level in the blood, but it does not sensitize the heart to catecholamines. So there is no arrhythmia during the induction of anesthesia by thiopentone, if hypoxia and hypercarbia are avoided.

The thiopentone-induced tachycardia caused by hypotension increases myocardial O_2 demand, but this is meted by the proportional decrease in coronary vascular resistance and increase in myocardial blood flow (if aortic pressure is maintained) by thiopentone. So, thiopentone should be used cautiously in increased HR, low BP, and ↓ preload [e.g., hypovolemia, congestive heart failure (CHF), ischemic heart disease (IHD), heart block, etc.]. The hypotensive effect of thiopentone is also exaggerated in a patient who receives β-blocker. This is due to blunted baroreflex, preventing tachycardia. The IV bolus injection of thiopentone leads to a high plasma concentration of a drug, suddenly coming into contact with the heart, vasomotor center, and respiratory center. So, in hypotensive patients, with decreased CV reserve, thiopentone may lead to a further decrease in venous return (preload), which in turn causes a further fall in CO and decreased coronary blood flow. Thus, a vicious cycle can easily be established and may have disastrous effects. So, IV bolus thiopentone anesthesia is relatively contraindicated in cardiac patients, where rapid hypotensive action is harmful. In contrast, inhalation induction technique has a more gradual depressant effect and can be rapidly reversed.

Effect on Respiratory System

Thiopentone reduces both the rate and the depth of respiration until apnea occurs. This depends on the dose and the speed of the injection of thiopentone. The stimulatory respiratory response to both hypercarbia and hypoxia, by reflex mechanism, mediated by chemoreceptor, are depressed by thiopentone. The neurogenic stimulatory drive for respiration is diminished by hypnotic doses of thiopentone, but usually not more than during natural sleep. This neurogenic respiratory drive can essentially be eliminated completely by a dose that is three times greater than that normally used to induce sleep. However, such doses of thiopentone do not suppress the hypoxia drive, but eliminate the chemoreceptor drive by hypercarbia for respiration. At still higher doses, powerful hypoxic drive also fails.

Coughing, sneezing, hiccough, and laryngospasm may also occur when barbiturates are employed as IV anesthetic agents. Among these, laryngospasm is one of the chief complications of barbiturates anesthesia. This laryngospasm, which sometimes occurs, is due to the direct effect of thiopentone only on the inhibitory system of the brain, leaving behind the excitatory part in low doses of it (inhibition on inhibition which is described earlier). The laryngospasm may also be due to insertion of artificial airways, laryngeal mask airway (LMA), or endotracheal (ET) tube in a lightly anesthetized patient (inadequate doses of thiopentone). Laryngeal reflexes are less depressed after thiopentone than the equivalent dose of propofol. There is also a low incidence of hypersalivation and rarely bronchospasm due to thiopentone, still thiopentone is safe for asthmatic patients, though it does not cause bronchodilation.

Effect on Gastrointestinal Tract, Kidney, and Liver

Hypoproteinemia, in patient with liver and renal disease, leads to the circulation of a greater amount of unbound portion of thiopentone in blood than in normal persons. This causes an exaggerated response of thiopentone, even with same doses. In hepatic failure patient, the duration of action of thiopentone is more prolonged in contrast to renal failure patient, where recovery is more rapid. Thiopentone also causes decreased urine output due to a decrease in renal blood flow and GFR. This is because thiopentone causes renal vasoconstriction due to sympathetic stimulation from hypotension. So, the correction of hypotension by the administration of adequate IV fluid prevents the renal effect of thiopentone from becoming a clinical problem. But controversy exists, whether there is an increase in secretion of antidiuretic hormone (ADH) from pituitary in response to thiopentone which may be responsible for decreased urine output.

There is also a clinically insignificant increase in blood glucose levels and impairment of glucose tolerance testing (GTT) after thiopentone anesthesia. The incidence of nausea and vomiting after thiopentone anesthesia is less than that of inhalational anesthesia, but the incidence of nausea and vomiting is even less, after midazolam and propofol than thiopentone.

Peripheral Nervous Structures

The barbiturates selectively depress transmission of impulses through autonomic ganglia and reduce excitation of nicotinic receptor at the motor end plate which is responsible for muscular action. So, at the skeletal neuromuscular junction, the blocking effects of nondepolarizing muscle relaxants are enhanced during barbiturate anesthesia. These depressing actions of thiopentone, at the neuromuscular junction, probably result from the inhibition of the passage of current through nicotinic cholinergic receptors.

Miscellaneous Actions

Heat loss, due to thiopentone-induced muscular and cutaneous vasodilatation, leads to postoperative shivering. It reduces the plasma cortisol level but does not suppress the adrenocortical stimulation, during the stress and strain of surgery. Thiopentone causes dose-related release of histamine, but it is rarely of any clinical significance. After an injection of thiopentone, there may be an anaphylactoid reaction (urticarial rash, hives, edema, bronchospasm, and shock), but the incidence of it is very infrequent. The

treatment of this thiopentone-induced anaphylactoid reaction includes epinephrine, IV fluid, steroid, and aminophylline.

Sometimes, the thiopentone causes mild muscular excitatory movements, i.e., hypertonicity, tremor, twitching, and respiratory excitatory effect including cough and hiccup. This is probably due to inadequate induction doses of thiopentone which evoke an excitatory response because inhibitory areas of the brain are the first to be depressed. Atropine and opioids, given as premedication prior to thiopentone, may help to reduce this muscular activity, but phenothiazines and scopolamine, used as premedication, may exaggerate it.

Thiopentone does not have curariform action and does not block the motor impulses directly. Muscular relaxation, caused by thiopentone, can be explained only through its CNS depression actin. Thiopentone reduces the degree of hyperkalemia, caused by suxamethonium. This drug also causes some depression of intestinal activity and the constriction of splanchnic vasculature, by sympathetic stimulation, due to hypotension.

Obstetric Effects of Thiopentone

Thiopentone does not depress uterine tone or contraction. During cesarean section (CS), when thiopentone is used in the doses of 6 mg/kg of body weight, then the fetus is not usually depressed during delivery. This is due to the placental factors and due to the redistribution of thiopentone in mother and fetal tissue. The maximum concentration of thiopentone in fetal blood occurs at about 3 minutes after its IV injection, during which there is an equilibrium between the maternal and fetal blood concentration. This also explains why the umbilical cord blood concentration of thiopentone is half than that of maternal blood, during delivery. If delivery is done within 10 minutes of induction by thiopentone or ketamine, then the baby usually remains safe, but the neurobehavioral test of newborn shows better results after induction by ketamine than thiopentone.

Continuous Infusions of Thiopentone

The continuous infusion of thiopentone for the maintenance of hypnosis is not generally used in anesthesia practice. This is because of prolonged recovery, after completion of infusion of thiopentone. However, this can be explained by the context-sensitive half-time graph (time taken by a drug to decrease to 50% of its plasma concentration) of thiopentone, in relation to other IV hypnotic agents, used for GA. This CSHT graph is nothing but the representation of pharmacokinetic property of a particular agent which is discussed before. The successful continuous infusion by thiopentone can be achieved by maintaining its blood concentration at the level of 10–20 µg/mL during induction and 5–10 µg/mL during maintenance which is only obtained by IV administration of 2–3 mg/kg/h of thiopentone.

Action of Thiopentone as Anticonvulsants

Barbiturates (thiopentone) and BZDs (diazepam, midazolam, etc.) can abruptly stop seizures in convulsive patient, but BZDs have largely replaced thiopentone in acute treatment of seizures. This is because, though barbiturates have anticonvulsant property, but it (except phenobarbital) possesses a high degree of selectivity and a low therapeutic index. Thus, it is not possible by barbiturates to achieve the desired anticonvulsion effect without the evidence of general depression of CNS, like GA.

The mechanism of actions of barbiturates as anticonvulsant:

- Both the barbiturates and BZDs, acting on $GABA_A$ receptors, facilitate the action of inhibitory neurotransmitter, named GABA, and prolong the hyperpolarization of postsynaptic membrane. Thus, it inhibits conduction of impulses and stops convulsions.
- Barbiturates alter the postsynaptic membrane conductance of chloride ions and thus antagonize the glutamatergic and cholinergic excitation.
- They presynaptically block the entry of Ca^{2+} into nerve terminals and thus diminish the release of neurotransmitter.
- They increase the threshold for convulsion in the brain, by inhibiting the kindling process, more effectively.

Action of Thiopentone as Brain Protection

Thiopentone protects the brain by the following mechanisms:

- It decreases cerebral metabolism (which is only responsible for electrical activity) till the EEG becomes flat, after which no further suppression of metabolism (responsible for other cellular activities, other than electrical) occurs, even with an increased dose.
- Thiopentone enhances *reversed steal phenomenon* in which vasoconstriction in healthy area of the brain shunts the blood to diseased areas. Thus, the nonhealthy tissue of the brain becomes less ischemic.
- Thiopentone reduces both ICP and BP supplying the brain, but the reduction of ICP is greater than BP. Thus, it maintains the cerebral perfusion pressure. So, arterial hypotension should be avoided, during thiopentone anesthesia, to maintain adequate cerebral perfusion pressure.
- It causes the stabilization of liposomal membrane and free radical scavenging of the cell.

- It attenuates cerebral edema, resulting from cranial surgery, head injury, or cerebral ischemia. They may decrease the size of cerebral infarction and increase the survival rate.

Contraindications of the Use of Thiopentone

There are some occasions, where it is necessary to use thiopentone with particular care (relative contraindications) or sometimes to avoid it completely (absolute contraindications).

These occasions are:

- Thiopentone should not be used on outpatients who have to leave hospital alone. After regaining of consciousness, from thiopentone anesthesia, there is a stage of euphoria, when the patient is not fit to take care of or to perform responsible actions by himself. So, driving a car by the patient himself is forbidden for 24 hours following thiopentone anesthesia.
- Children are unsuitable for thiopentone, as a sole anesthetic agent, because they need relatively larger doses to produce a satisfactory depression of all reflex activities.
- When the adequacy of airway is in doubt, then thiopentone should be used cautiously.
- Thiopentone should not be used in patients with a history of hypersensitivity to barbiturates and bronchial asthma. Allergic reactions to thiopentone occur, especially in persons who tend to have asthma, urticaria, angioedema, or similar conditions. Hypersensitivity reactions in this category generally include localized swellings, particularly of eyelids, cheeks, or lips and erythematous dermatitis.
- During anesthesia on patient, suffering from cardiac and peripheral circulatory failure, the benefit of smooth and pleasant induction by thiopentone should be balanced against the deleterious effect of vasomotor and respiratory depression, caused by it. In cardiac diseases with fixed and low CO, such as in AS (aortic stenosis), the vasodilation and consequent hypotension caused by thiopentone may lead to cardiac arrests. In shock patient where BP is maintained by sympathetically stimulated vasoconstriction, then vasodilation and depression of sympathetic system, by barbiturates, can produce a fatal effect; however such conditions are not necessarily absolute contraindications to the use of thiopentone but should be used very cautiously by an experienced person.
- Severe uremia, where small doses of barbiturates produce prolonged effects, are relative contraindications for the use of thiopentone.

- Porphyria: In the latent stage of this disease, any barbiturate may cause an acute exacerbation of symptoms with porphyrinuria, respiratory paralysis, and frequent death. This is because barbiturates enhance porphyrin synthesis. So, the use of thiopentone, in a patient with a history of porphyria, is absolutely contraindicated.
- Untreated adrenocortical insufficiency: This is due to the inability of such patient to respond to any form of stress by secreting an adequate amount of adrenocortical steroids, though the thiopentone does not depress the release of adrenocortical steroids itself.
- Abnormal severe respiratory depression may follow after the use of thiopentone in dystrophia myotonica.
- Untreated myxedematous patients are very sensitive to any IV anesthetic agents, but the thiopentone is most sensitive among them.

Porphyrias

The porphyrins are chemical compounds that are formed by the binding of four pyrrole rings. Examples of porphyrins are heme and its precursor compounds such as protoporphyrin, protoporphyrinogen, coproporphyrinogen, and uroporphyrinogen. During the biosynthesis of heme, multiple steps are involved which are governed by a particular enzyme in every step. Deficiency of these enzymes results in an increased concentration of that particular precursor of heme (or porphyrins) in blood and urine. This condition is called the *porphyrias*. Porphyria is classified according to the site of defective enzymes such as hepatic porphyrias and erythrocytic porphyria.

The acute attack of porphyria is precipitated by various triggering factors which include general anesthetic agents such as barbiturates and sulfonamides. An acute attack of porphyria is characterized by abdominal (intermittent) pain, neurological symptoms, psychiatric symptoms, etc. The diagnosis can be confirmed by examining urine during an acute attack. The finding of raised aminolevulinic acid (ALA) and porphobilinogen (PBG) in urine establishes the diagnosis, but the urine should be protected from light, during its collection, however, the concentration of ALA and PBG in urine will be normal in between the attacks.

■ BENZODIAZEPINES

History

Since antiquity to the beginning of the 19th century, alcoholic beverages and some potions (containing laudanum and various herbals) had been used to induce sleep. Then, in the middle of the 19th century, the first pharmacological agent to be introduced as a *sedative* and soon, thereafter, as *hypnotic* was bromide. After that, as sedative and hypnotic came chloral hydrate (in 1869) and paraldehyde (in 1882) which are rarely used now. Then, Fischer and Von Mering introduced barbiturates in the form of *barbitone*, in 1903, and *phenobarbitone,* in 1912. After that, barbiturates reigned supreme, till 1960. Then, BZDs had started eroding their (barbiturates) position, after the first discovery of *chlordiazepoxide*, as BZD, in 1957, and have now totally replaced them (barbiturates) as sedatives and hypnotics in anesthesia practice.

Then, the discovery of partial separation of sedative, hypnotic, and anesthetic properties from anticonvulsant properties which was a characteristic of phenobarbital (it has only anticonvulsant properties) had led to the search for agents which have more selective effects on CNS. As a result, *phenytoin* with relatively nonsedative and high anticonvulsant property was developed, in 1930 and then *chlorpromazine*, in 1950, without any anticonvulsant property, but only with the taming properties, was developed.

The introduction of barbiturates in clinical practice starts the era of IV anesthesia, after an initial setback, but the *barbiturates have only hypnotic property*. So, the search for an ideal IV anesthetic drug that should have hypnotic, amnestic, and analgesic property was started. On that searching, many drugs were gradually introduced in clinical anesthetic practice, with varying degree of acceptance. Thus, with the increasing number of better IV drugs and discoveries of superior methods of IV drug delivery system, the use of IV anesthesia continues to grow. But as not a single IV drug has all the ideal properties of general IV anesthesia, so the future of IV anesthetic management involves the *simultaneous use of several drugs*, with their specific properties. In 1988, a survey of mortality among 100,000 GA reveals that the practice of combined anesthetic drugs, in small doses with their specific property, may be safer than the use of only one or two drugs in high doses, to extract the all properties, which are exerted by many drugs in small doses. This is because a single drug in high doses has many side effects and increases mortality.

In 1955, as the first generation of BZD, *chlordiazepoxide* was synthesized and, in1957, its hypnotic and sedative effects were first discovered. Then, in 1960, it was released as the first orally used BZD, but as chlordiazepoxide has no parenteral form, so it was not used for IV anesthesia. After that, as BZD, the *diazepam* was synthesized, in 1959, and was used in anesthesia through the IV route. Then, gradually *oxazepam*, a metabolite of diazepam, was synthesized, in 1961, and *lorazepam*, a substitution of oxazepam, was synthesized in 1971. Next, the major achievement was the synthesis of water-soluble BZD, named *midazolam*, in 1976. Its water solubility is pH dependent and formulated in a buffered acidic medium (pH 3.5), but it is most lipid-soluble

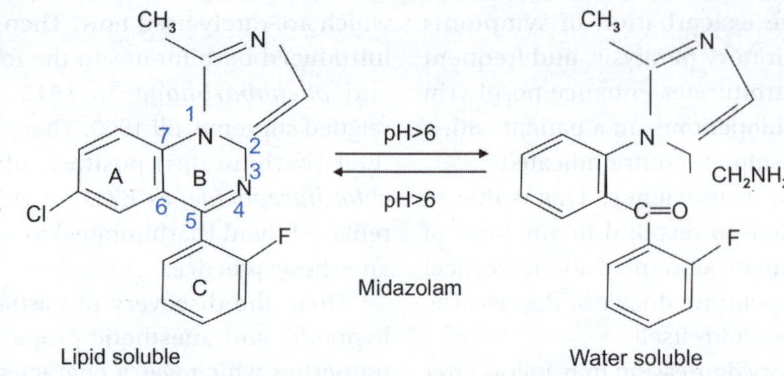

Fig. 7: Change in the solubility of midazolam in lipid and water.

in vivo than diazepam and lorazepam. After that, in 1977, BZD receptor was described. However, this (BZD receptor) is better termed *BZD, GABA, and barbiturate receptor complex* which is discussed later in this chapter.

Chemistry

The term "*benzodiazepine*" is referred to the structure of a molecule that is composed of a benzene ring fused to a seven-membered 1,4-diazepine ring. However, since all the important BZDs compounds contain a 5-aryl substituent ring, so the term "benzodiazepine" has come to mean the 5-aryl-1,4-benzodiazepine. Then, various modifications, in the structure of this ring system, have produced different compounds with similar activities, but the substitutions, at various positions on these rings, affect the potency and the mechanism of biotransformation of these compounds. A special BZD ring, named the "*imidazole ring of midazolam*", contributes to its water solubility at low (acidic) *pH*. The insolubility of diazepam and lorazepam in water requires propylene glycol, for their parenteral preparations, which has been associated with venous irritation and pain during their IV injection **(Fig. 7)**.

BZD–GABA–Barbiturate Receptor Complex or GABA$_A$ Receptor

Benzodiazepines act by occupying the BZD receptors. Barbiturates and another inhibitory neurotransmitter, named GABA, also act by occupying their respective barbiturate and GABA receptors, but actually, they are not any separate receptor structure. They (separate receptor structure) are truly the binding site of BZD, barbiturate, and GABA compound on a single large receptor complex, situated on postsynaptic membrane which is called the BZD–GABA–barbiturate receptor complex or GABA$_A$ receptor. This large GABA$_A$ receptor complex exerts the pharmacological action of barbiturates, BZDs, and GABA, after their binding with this receptor complex at their each specific-binding site and ultimately by promoting and modulating the action of GABA compound. This large receptor complex (GABA$_A$ receptor) is found in higher concentration at cerebral cortex, cerebellum, olfactory bulb, hippocampus, and the substantia nigra of the brain. In lesser density, this large receptor complex is also found at spinal cord, brain stem, and corpus striatum of CNS. The barbiturates and BZDs both act through this receptor, but in contrast to barbiturates, the BZDs selectively inhibit the activity of this receptor in limbic system, particularly at hippocampus.

These GABA receptors are membrane-bound protein structure that can be divided into two major subtypes such as GABA$_A$ and γ-aminobutyric acid type B (GABA$_B$). The GABA$_A$ receptor is composed of five subunits that coassemble to form an integral chloride channel. These receptors are responsible for most of the inhibitory neurotransmission in CNS. The BZD does not act on GABA$_B$ receptor, but acts only on GABA$_A$ receptor. Unlike barbiturates, the BZD do not directly activate the GABA$_A$ receptor, but require inhibitory neurotransmitter GABA to express their own effects, i.e., BZD only modulates or promotes the action of inhibitory neurotransmitter, named GABA. The BZD modulates the GABA-binding site and GABA alters the BZD-binding site in an allosteric fashion **(Fig. 8)**.

Each GABA$_A$ receptor complex is believed to be consisted of five homologous subunits. Mainly, these subunits are α, β, and γ and they are coassembled to form this receptor, but there may be other subunits in this GABA$_A$ receptor such as δ, ε, π, and θ. Again 16 several isoforms of each subunit of this GABA$_A$ receptor have also been cloned. These subunits and their isoform composition of the receptor complex may differ at different sites. The multiplicity of these subunits and their isoform generates an enormous heterogeneity in this large

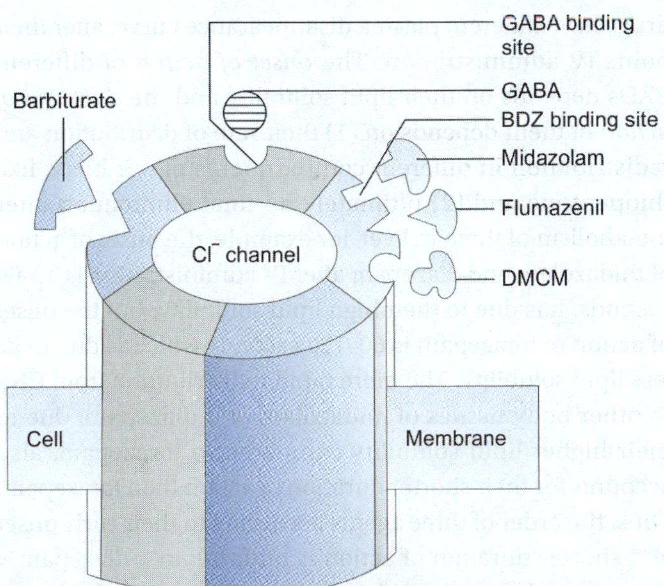

Fig. 8: GABA–BZD–barbiturate receptor complex (GABA$_A$ receptor) with chloride channel within it. A part of it, i.e., the BZD-binding site (or BZD-receptor) modulates the action of GABA$_A$ receptor in either direction. The agonist like midazolam facilitates the opening of GABA-mediated Cl⁻ channel in the GABA$_A$ receptor complex and produces all the actions of BZD, whereas the inverse agonist like methyl 6,7-dimethoxy-4-ethyl-β-carboline-3-carboxylate (DMCM) hinder GABA-mediated Cl⁻ channel opening, producing the opposite action of midazolam, whereas the BZD antagonist flumazenil blocks the action of both midazolam and DMCM. The barbiturate receptor is located in the other part of GABA$_A$ receptor. It also facilitates the action of GABA and is capable of opening the chloride channel directly. (BZD: benzodiazepine; DMCM: methyl-6,7-dimethoxy-4-ethyl-β-carboline-3-carboxylate; GABA: γ-aminobutyric acid)

GABA$_A$ receptor complex and is responsible for their huge pharmacological diversity. The macromolecular complex of this GABA$_A$ receptor and chloride channels within it also may be the site of action of many general anesthetic agents, ethanol, and inhaled anesthetic drugs. The subunits of GABA$_A$ receptor complex contain various ligand-binding sites such as BZD, GABA, and barbiturate. The BZD-binding site is located on the γ-subunit and GABA-binding site is located on the β-subunit of this GABA$_A$ receptor complex. With the activation of this GABA$_A$ receptor (GABA–BZD–barbiturate receptor complex) after binding of BZD or barbiturates or GABA with this receptor at their respective binding site, the opening of chloride channel is triggered and hyperpolarization of postsynaptic membrane is occurred. This leads to the resistance of neuronal excitation which is responsible for inhibition of transmission.

The pharmacological spectrum of intrinsic activity of BZD has been classified into five different classes and these are *agonist, partial agonist, antagonist, partial inverse agonist, and inverse agonist.* The *antagonist* blocks all the action of

TABLE 2: The relationship between the different effects of midazolam and its receptor occupancy.

Effect	*Receptor occupancy (%)*
• Anticonvulsant	20–25
• Anxiolysis	20–30
• Slight sedation, amnesia, and reduced attention	30–50

• Intense sedation:
  – Unconsciousness
  – Muscle relaxation
	60–90

• Anesthesia	>95

agonist, whereas the *inverse agonist* expresses no action from itself, but causes all the opposite action of agonist, for example, an agonist, such as midazolam, has full positive intrinsic action of BZD and produces hypnosis, sedation, amnesia, etc., because it alters the configuration of GABA$_A$ receptor complex, after binding with BZD-binding site of this receptor complex which is called the BZD receptor. Thus, the binding affinity of GABA neurotransmitter to the GABA-binding site of GABA$_A$ receptor complex is increased and the chloride channel within the GABA$_A$ receptor is fully opened, whereas the antagonist (e.g., flumazenil) occupies this BZD receptors, i.e., the BZD-binding site on GABA$_A$ receptor complex and have a very little intrinsic action, expressed by itself, after binding with the receptor. Contrary, it blocks all the action of both agonist and inverse agonist by preventing the binding of them with BZD receptor (BZD-binding site of GABA$_A$ receptor complex). Therefore, there is no action of BZD agonist and inverse agonist. In the absence of agonist and inverse agonist, antagonist does not itself cause any GABA$_A$ receptor function, so they are also called *neutral in function.* On the other hand, the *inverse agonist* has opposite intrinsic activity to agonist, i.e., produces opposite effect of agonist, in the absence of it. It reduces or inhibits the GABA synaptic transmission (agonist enhances GABA synaptic transmission) and since GABA is inhibitory, so the result of this inhibition of inhibitory GABA (inhibition on inhibition) causes CNS stimulation. The potency of these agonist, antagonist, and inverse agonist is dictated by their affinity for BZD receptor and the duration of effect of these compounds is dictated by the rate of clearance of these drugs from receptor **(Table 2)**.

It is still not known how the different effects of BZD (hypnosis, sedation, anxiolytic, amnesia, anticonvulsant, and sleep) are mediated by the same receptor. For this, there are two probable theories and these are (1) the different receptor subtypes mediate different actions and (2) the different actions of a single BZD are due to the different blood levels of a particular drug, as for example, the anxiolytic effect of

BZD occurs at 20% $GABA_A$ receptor occupancy, the sedation effect of BZD is observed with 30–50% receptor occupancy and the unconsciousness effect of BZD is observed with 60% receptor occupancy.

Different compounds of BZDs differ in their potency and efficiency. This is due to the different chemical structure of each drug which again dictates its particular physicochemical, pharmacokinetics, and receptor-binding characteristics, for example, the order of receptor affinity (thus potency) of three BZD agonists from higher to lower is lorazepam > midazolam > diazepam. So, the midazolam is 3–4 times and lorazepam is 5 times more potent than diazepam.

Chronic administration of BZD produces tolerance to their pharmacological effects and causes increased dose requirement of it. This is due to downregulation of GABA–BZD–barbiturate receptor complex ($GABA_A$ receptor). After the cessation of chronic use of BZD, there is again upregulation of these receptor complexes, causing increased susceptibility to BZDs.

Pharmacokinetic of Benzodiazepines

Benzodiazepines compounds, used in anesthesia, are classified as (1) long-acting, with a half-life >24 hours (one example is lorazepam), (2) intermediate-acting, with a half-life 6–24 hours (one example is diazepam), and (3) short-acting, with half-life <6 hours (one example is midazolam) according to their plasma clearance. The clearance rate of lorazepam is 0.2–0.5 mL/kg/min, the clearance rate of diazepam is 0.8–1.8 mL/kg/min, and this same for midazolam is 6–11 mL/kg/min. So, all these drugs have different plasma disappearance curve, after their bolus IV administration. The *onset of action* of different BZDs depends on their lipid solubility and the *duration of action* of them depends on (1) their rate of distribution and redistribution in different compartments of our body, like thiopentone and (2) ultimately on final elimination after metabolism of them in liver, for example, the onset of action of midazolam and diazepam after IV administration is 30–60 seconds. It is due to their high lipid solubility, but the onset of action of lorazepam is 60–120 seconds which is due to its less lipid solubility. The more rapid redistribution from CNS to other body tissues of midazolam and diazepam, due to their higher lipid solubility compared to lorazepam, also accounts for their shorter duration of action than lorazepam. Thus, the order of three agents according to their early onset and shorter duration of action is midazolam < diazepam < lorazepam. Although, midazolam is more water soluble and less lipid soluble at low (acidic) pH, but its imidazole ring closes at physiological (alkaline) pH and causes an increase in its lipid solubility **(Table 3)**.

Again, after prolonged infusion of BZDs, when the redistribution site of them becomes saturated and is in equilibrium with their primary site of action, then the blood levels of midazolam will decrease more rapidly than other BZD. It is due to its greater hepatic metabolic clearance rate than the other BZDs. So, the patients will awake faster, after midazolam infusion, than others. The more lipid-soluble member of BZD enters the brain rapidly and has two phases of plasma concentration decay curve, like thiopentone. The *first decay curve* is due to the redistribution and the *later decay curve* is due

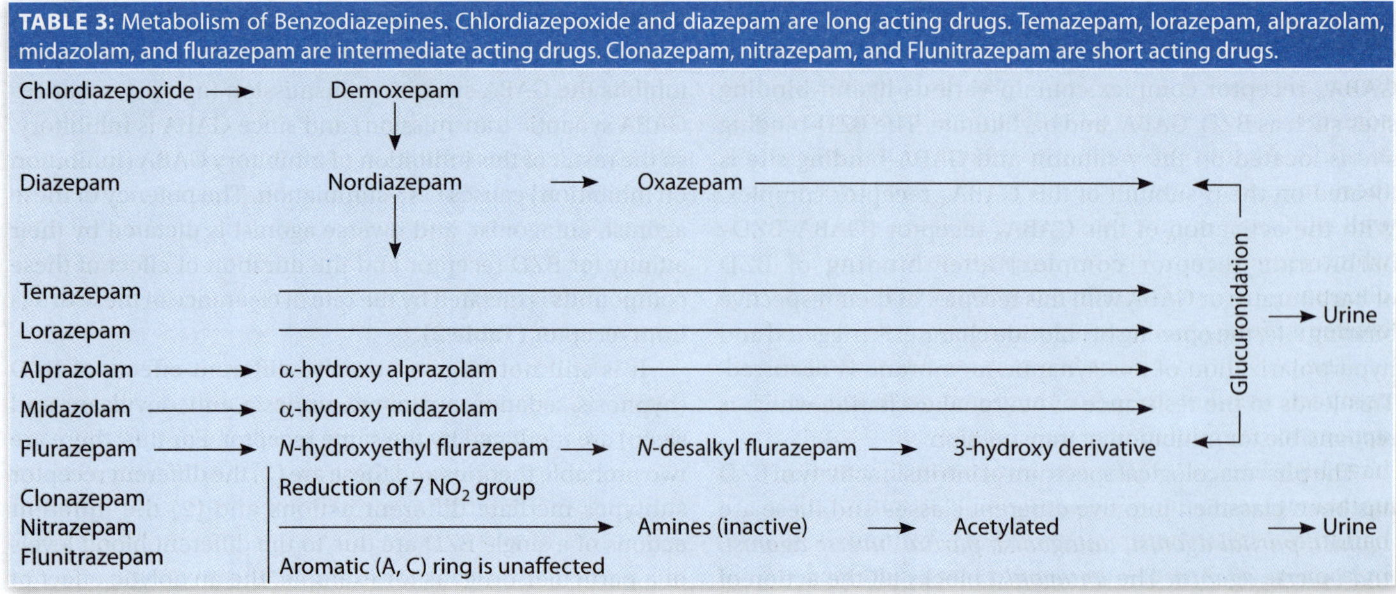

TABLE 3: Metabolism of Benzodiazepines. Chlordiazepoxide and diazepam are long acting drugs. Temazepam, lorazepam, alprazolam, midazolam, and flurazepam are intermediate acting drugs. Clonazepam, nitrazepam, and Flunitrazepam are short acting drugs.

to the elimination of this BZD by metabolism or directly through urine. A relatively shorter duration of action is seen with a single dose of any BZD compound that is rapidly redistributed, even though it may have a long elimination half-life (t½). So, only using the elimination t½ (half-life) alone to predict the duration of action may be misleading, however the plasma t½ determines the duration of action of drugs whose elimination is by far the dominant feature or when the drug is given repeatedly in bolus doses or by continuous infusion.

Benzodiazepines are metabolized in liver by dealkylation and hydroxylation to many metabolites, however some of which are also active. This explains why the effect or biological half-life of some BZDs are much longer than the actual plasma t½ of administered compound. Some BZDs (e.g., diazepam) undergo enterohepatic circulation and is also responsible for their long duration of action. The BZDs are commonly administered orally or intravenously for premedication, sedation, or induction of GA. Midazolam, diazepam, and lorazepam are well absorbed from gastrointestinal tract (GIT) and their peak plasma level is usually achieved within 30 minutes, 1 hour, and 2 hours, respectively. The midazolam also can be used through intranasal (0.2–0.3 mg/kg), buccal (0.07 mg/kg), and sublingual (0.1 mg/kg) route to provide effective preoperative sedation. The intramuscular injection of diazepam is very painful and its action in this route is unreliable, due to very erratic absorption of its oily preparation from the muscle. In contrast, midazolam and lorazepam are well absorbed after intramuscular injection, with peak levels achieved within 30 and 90 minutes, respectively. However, the induction of GA by BZDs requires only IV administration of them.

Metabolism of Benzodiazepines

Benzodiazepines and their metabolites, which are sometimes more potent than their parent compound, bind to some plasma proteins. The extent of this binding of these metabolites with plasma protein correlates strongly well with their lipid solubility and their duration of action which ranges from 70% for alprazolam to nearly 99% for diazepam. The concentration of BZDs in CSF is equal to the concentration of free drugs in plasma.

The plasma concentration of most BZDs exhibits two-compartmental models, but three-compartmental models appear to be more appropriate for the compounds which have high lipid solubility, like midazolam. There is a rapid uptake of BZDs by CNS, after their IV administration, like barbiturates. This rapid uptake of BZDs by brain is followed by a phase of redistribution to less well-perfused tissues,

like muscles. Next, this muscle uptake is followed by again redistribution to fat.

As the metabolites of some BZDs are more active and biotransformed more slowly than their parent compounds, so the duration of action of many BZDs bears little relationship with their actual half-life or elimination of drug that has been administered. All the BZDs cross the placental barrier and are secreted into breast milk.

Benzodiazepines are metabolized extensively into the liver by the enzymes of the cytochrome P_{450} family. Some BZDs such as oxazepam and lorazepam are not metabolized by these enzymes but is conjugated directly into the liver. The midazolam is rapidly metabolized by hydroxylation of its methyl group to α-hydroxymidazolam which has appreciable biological activity (elimination half-life 1 hour), and then is conjugated with glucuronic acid into the liver.

Diazepam, in the first phase, is metabolized by the cytochrome P_{450} system in liver to N-desmethyl diazepam (nordiazepam) which is a long-acting active metabolite. In the second phase, this nordiazepam is again metabolized to oxazepam which is then conjugated with glucuronic acid and excreted through bile. The half-life of diazepam in plasma is between 1 and 2 days, while that of N-desmethyl diazepam (nordiazepam) is about 60 hours. The half-life of lorazepam in plasma is about 14 hours.

Pharmacodynamics of Benzodiazepines

Effects on Central Nervous System

The most prominent effects of BZDs on CNS are sedation, hypnosis, decreased anxiety, anterograde amnesia, and anticonvulsion. The muscle relaxation effect of BZDs is independent to their sedative action and is due to their action on the spinal cord and brain stem. They affect the activity of neural axis at all levels (CNS and spinal cord), but some structures are affected by much greater extent than the others. They are not capable of producing the same degree of neuronal depression at all the centers of CNS, as the barbiturates and volatile anesthetics do.

All the BZDs have very similar pharmacological profiles, but nevertheless, they differ in selectivity to their different effects (actions). So, the clinical usefulness of individual BZD varies considerably. The BZDs alone do not cause true GA, since the awareness usually persists and relaxation which is sufficient to allow surgery cannot be achieved by them. During the induction of anesthesia by BZD, with inducing doses, the patients become clinically asleep, but the EEG changes are not typical to sleep. In a dose-related manner, the BZDs gradually reduce cerebral metabolic rate, with a reduction of O_2 consumption cerebral metabolic rate of oxygen ($CMRO_2$), and cerebral blood flow (CBF).

They increase seizure threshold and thus inhibit seizure. They have also a cerebral protective effect against hypoxia-like barbiturates. In this respect, midazolam is superior to other BZDs but is inferior to thiopentone.

All the BZDs have antiemetic effect and among them the lorazepam has highest result. As the BZDs produce anxiolysis, amnesia, sedation, and hypnosis gradually, so they should be titrated for these effects by increasing their doses gradually and the end point of this titration is sedation or hypnosis. The onset of action is most rapid in case of midazolam, than diazepam and is slowest in case of lorazepam, but recovery with midazolam is faster than diazepam, after its bolus IV administration. With all the three BZDs (midazolam, diazepam, and lorazepam) there is amnesia, but there is a different level of sedation, hence the patient remains conscious and coherent but amnestic for the events and instruction (conscious sedation). With IV preparation, the loss of memory by BZDs can occur independent of loss of consciousness. When taken by mouth, it is not possible to demonstrate the amnestic action of BZDs in the absence of drowsiness and the usual small tranquilizing doses of BZDs (diazepam 5 mg and lorazepam 1 mg) produce no amnesia. There is synergistic action between the midazolam and the regional anesthesia in respect to ventilation. They do not cause hyperalgesia like barbiturates.

Anticonvulsant Property of Benzodiazepines

All the BZDs have anticonvulsant properties. Among them, midazolam, diazepam, and lorazepam have well-defined roles in the management of status epilepticus. This action is due to their (BZDs) strong ability to enhance the GABA-mediated synaptic inhibition through their BZD-binding site (or BZD receptor) which is an integral part of a $GABA_A$ receptor.

Effects on Cardiovascular System

Benzodiazepines display minimal cardiovascular depressant effects, even at their induction doses. The peak hemodynamic effects of BZDs occur within the first 10 minutes, after their IV administration. They all decrease the BP and increase HR. With midazolam, these effects appear to be secondary to the decrease in peripheral SVR, but with diazepam, these effects are secondary to the decrease in left ventricular workload and CO. The diazepam increases the coronary blood flow, possibly by increasing the interstitial concentration of adenosine. The accumulation of cardio-depressant metabolite may also explain the negative inotropic effects of all the BZD groups of drugs. The predominant hemodynamic changes, produced by BZDs, are:

- The reduction of mean arterial pressure (MAP) (in midazolam 12–26%) due to the decrease in SVR. In this respect, midazolam has the highest effect than other BZDs and is similar to thiopentone. The reduction of SVR by diazepam is up to 0–8% and for midazolam, it is up to 0–18%. Still, they are safe and effective for the induction of anesthesia with severe aortic stenosis (AS).
- Pulmonary artery pressure (PAP) and pulmonary vascular resistance (PVR) remain unchanged or slightly reduced by BZDs. In midazolam both are unchanged, but in diazepam, the effect varies between unchanged to minimum reduction.
- The right atrial pressure remains unchanged by BZDs.
- The variable response to cardiac index (CI) remains unchanged in case of diazepam, but there is 0–25% reduction of CI in case of midazolam.
- In patient, with elevated left ventricular filling pressure, diazepam, and midazolam produce nitroglycerin (NTG)-like effect, by lowering the ventricular filling pressure and increasing CO.

The mechanism, by which BZDs maintain a stable hemodynamic condition, is due to preservation of homeostatic reflex by them. Midazolam or any BZD can block the stress response, due to intubation or surgery; however the addition of N_2O with BZDs has a slight synergistic effect to block this stress response, during intubation and surgery. But the addition of opioids with BZD has a supra-additive synergistic effect and causes a greater decrease of BP and stress response than when used alone, during intubation and surgery. However, the mechanism of this synergistic effect is not known but probably is due to reduction of sympathetic tone. Benzodiazepines cause coronary vasodilatation which is seen after the administration of their therapeutic doses.

Effect on Respiratory System

The hypnotic doses of BZDs produce minimal effect on respiration in normal subjects, but special care should be taken for children, aged, and alcoholics. It depresses ventilatory response both to hypoxia and CO_2. This depression is usually insignificant unless the drugs are administered intravenously in large doses or in association with other respiratory depressing agents, although the incidence of apnea may be less common after BZD induction than after barbiturate induction, still sometimes even a small IV dose of diazepam and midazolam have resulted in respiratory arrest. Respiratory arrest or apnea is more likely to occur, during the concomitant presence (use) of opioids. The steep dose-response curve of midazolam shows a slightly prolonged onset (compared with thiopentone) and high potency of it, necessitating careful titration to avoid overdose and apnea. So, ventilation must be monitored in all the patients, receiving IV BZDs and resuscitation equipment must be immediately available.

The hypnotic doses of BZDs may also worsen sleep-related breathing disorders, by adversely affecting the tone of upper airway muscles and by decreasing the ventilatory response to CO_2. The latter effect may be sufficient to cause hypoventilation and hypoxemia in some patients, especially with severe chronic obstructive pulmonary disease (COPD). In some patients, with obstructive sleep apnea (OSA) syndrome, the hypnotic doses of BZDs may decrease upper airway muscular tone and exaggerate the incidence of apneic episodes. Thus, many physicians consider OSA as a contraindication for the use of sedative and hypnotic agents like BZDs. So, during the administration of BZDs caution should be exercised in a patient who snores regularly. This is because partial airway obstruction may be converted to OSA under the influence of these drugs.

The central respiratory depression, produced after administration of BZDs, is greater in midazolam than in diazepam. However, the slope of ventilatory response curve to CO_2 for BZD is flat than normal and is not shifted to the right, like opioids. The peak onset of ventilatory depression effect with midazolam is about 3 minutes and remains for about 60–120 minutes. The faster the drug is given, the quicker is the peak depression. The combination of opioids with BZDs produces a supra-additive respiratory depression effect. Apnea is more common to midazolam than other BZDs and its incidence is similar to thiopentone.

Effects on Gastrointestinal Tract

Benzodiazepines markedly decrease nocturnal gastric secretions in human beings.

Induction and Maintenance Doses of Benzodiazepines

Among all BZDs, midazolam is the choice for the induction of anesthesia, because for its rapid onset, rapid recovery, and lack of venous complications. The induction of anesthesia is complete when there is unresponsiveness to command and loss of eyelash reflexes of patient. On the other hand, the induction of anesthesia with midazolam occurs less rapidly than thiopentone, but amnesia caused by it is more reliable than thiopentone. The dose, the speed of injection, premedication, the age of patient, the ASA (American Society of Anesthesiologists) status of patient, and many other factors influence the induction time of BZDs. For example, midazolam in the dose of 0.2 mg/kg induces anesthesia within 28 seconds, if given through IV, whereas the diazepam in the dose of 0.5 mg/kg takes 39 seconds for induction of

TABLE 4: The uses and the doses of commonly used benzodiazepines (BZDs).

Agent use	Route	Dose (mg/kg)
• Diazepam premedication	Oral	0.2–0.4
– Sedation	IV	0.04–0.3
– Induction	IV	0.3–0.5
• Midazolam premedication	Oral	0.5
	IM	0.07–0.2
– Sedation	IM	0.07–0.1
– Induction	IV	0.1–0.4
• Lorazepam premedication	Oral	0.05
– Sedation	IM	0.025–0.05
	IV	0.025–0.05

(IM: intramuscular; IV: intravenous)

anesthesia if it is given through the same route and in the same speed **(Table 4)**.

Due to increased susceptibility to BZD receptors, the elders need lower doses of BZDs. In premedicated patient, the induction dose of midazolam is reduced to 0.1–0.2 mg/kg. Emergence (defined as oriented to time and pace) in healthy young patient after 10 mg midazolam is 15 minutes. In comparison between midazolam and thiopentone for hypnotic component in balanced anesthesia, midazolam is superior for this purpose. This is because of better amnesia and lesser hemodynamic changes, produced by it. Midazolam reduces opioid requirement than thiopentone. The amnestic period, after an induction dose of midazolam, is 1–2 hours. The bolus loading dose of midazolam is 0.05–0.15 mg/kg which maintains the plasma level of it at 50 μg/mL. This is sufficient to keep the patient asleep and amnestic, but the patient is arousable at the end of infusion.

■ INDIVIDUAL BENZODIAZEPINE (FIG. 9)

Diazepam

Chemically, diazepam is a BZD derivative. The main actions of it are hypnosis, sedation, anxiolysis, anterograde amnesia, anticonvulsion, and muscular relaxation. Like other BZDs, the diazepam is also thought to act via their specific BZD receptors, found at synapses throughout the CNS, but is concentrated especially in cortex and midbrain; however the individual receptor cannot directly act. They are closely linked with a large complex $GABA_A$ receptor and appear to facilitate the activity of inhibitory GABA neurotransmitter. The activated $GABA_A$ receptors by diazepam, then, open its own chloride ion channels within the receptor which then either hyperpolarize or short-circuit the postsynaptic membrane. Thus, the hyperpolarization of postsynaptic membrane reduces the action potential and inhibits the transmission of impulses.

The main action of diazepam on cardiovascular system is the transient decrease of BP and a slight decrease of CO, but only following its IV administration. The coronary arterial blood flow is increased by diazepam, but this is secondary to the coronary arterial vasodilatation, caused by the accumulation of adenosine. A decrease in myocardial O_2 consumption has also been reported by it. The large dose of diazepam causes respiratory depression, causing decreased tidal volume, decreased respiratory rate, and decreased minute volume. It may also cause apnea, necessitating invasive positive pressure ventilation (IPPV). The hypoxic ventilatory drive is depressed by diazepam to a greater extent than the hypercarbic drive. Diazepam is anxiolytic and so it decreases aggression, although sometimes paradoxical excitement may occur. Sedation, hypnosis, and anterograde amnesia also occur after the administration of diazepam. The drug also has anticonvulsion and slight analgesic property and depresses spinal reflexes.

The toxicity or the side effects of diazepam are nothing, but the excessive depression of CNS, including drowsiness, ataxia, and headache. Tolerance and dependence to diazepam may occur with prolonged use of it, like other BZDs. So, acute withdrawal of diazepam in these circumstances may produce insomnia, anxiety, confusion, psychosis, or perceptual disturbances. Rashes, gastrointestinal (GI) upset, and urinary retention also have been reported as the side effects of it. The commercially available lipid preparation of IV diazepam is highly irritant to vein. So, it produces intense pain during IV injection, but its water-soluble preparation is not so irritant to do so. However, this water-soluble preparation of diazepam is not available commercially.

Diazepam is rapidly absorbed after its oral administration. The bioavailability of it (diazepam) by oral route is 90–100%. On the other hand, the absorption of diazepam, after intramuscular (IM) administration of its lipid preparation, is slow and erratic. This drug is 99% protein bound in plasma. Diazepam is metabolized into liver to its active metabolites. The major active metabolite of diazepam

is desmethyldiazepam (nordiazepam) whose half-life is >100 hours. The other active metabolites of it (diazepam) are oxazepam and temazepam which are further metabolized by glucuronidation. Due to these active metabolites, diazepam is a long-acting agent. All these metabolites of diazepam are excreted through urine. Diazepam decreases the value of minimum alveolar concentration (MAC) of volatile anesthetic agents and potentiates the action of nondepolarizing muscle relaxants. It is absorbed on plastic and cannot be removed by dialysis. The diazepam is used in anesthesia (1) for premedication in the dose of 0.2–0.5 mg/kg orally, (2) for sedation in the dose of 0.04–0.2 mg/kg IV, and (3) for induction of anesthesia in the dose of 0.3–0.6 mg/kg IV.

Midazolam

Chemically, it is a water-soluble imidazobenzodiazepine compound. Its main actions and mode of action is same as that of diazepam. The midazolam decreases systolic BP by 5%, diastolic BP by 10%, and SVR by 20–30%. The HR, increased by midazolam, is 20%. Midazolam in combination with fentanyl obtunds the pressure response during intubation to a greater extent than the thiopentone in combination with fentanyl. It decreases tidal volume, but this is offset by the increase in respiratory rate. The minute volume is thus little changed by midazolam; however, this does not occur with an increased dose of midazolam. However, with increased dose of midazolam, there is a leukocyte reduction of both the tidal volume and respiratory rate with the reduction of minute volume. Apnea occurs in 10–70% of patients when midazolam is used as an induction agent with appropriate doses. The drug impairs ventilatory response both to hypercapnia and hypoxia **(Fig. 10)**.

The anticonvulsion properties of midazolam in man are like that of other BZDs. Both the cerebral O_2 consumption and cerebral blood flow are decreased in a dose-related manner by midazolam, but a normal relationship is maintained between the two. When administered intrathecally or epidurally, this drug has good antinociceptive

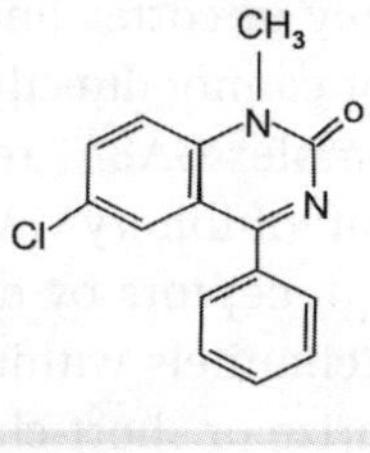

Fig. 9: Diazepam.

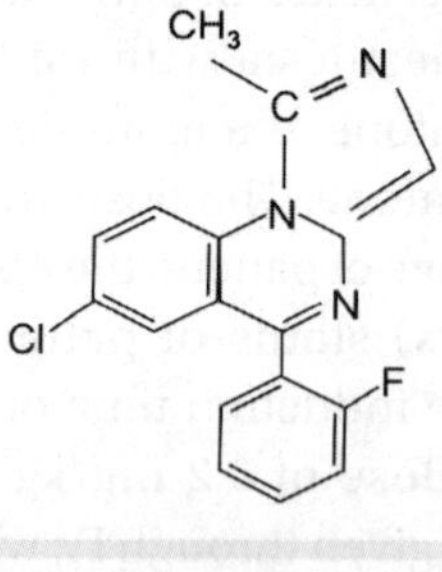

Fig. 10: Midazolam.

effects. A midazolam fentanyl induction sequence is associated with a lower incidence of postoperative vomiting than with the thiopentone–fentanyl sequence. This drug decreases the adrenergic responses, but not the cortisol and renin responses to stress during intubation and surgery. It causes significant inhibition of phagocytosis and bactericidal activity of leukocytes.

The oral dose of midazolam is 0.5 mg/kg. The intramuscular dose of it is 0.07–0.15 mg/kg. The IV dose of midazolam for sedation is 0.07–0.1 mg/kg which is titrated according to the response. During titration, the endpoint of this sedation is drowsiness and slurring of speech, but patient's response to a command, however, is maintained. The dose of midazolam for the induction of anesthesia through the IV route is 0.1–0.4 mg/kg. The drug may also be administered intrathecally in an adult in a dose of 0.3 to 2 mg or epidurally in a dose of 0.1–0.2 mg/kg. The bioavailability of midazolam, when is administered by the oral route is only 45%, and by the intramuscular route is 80–100%. It is 96% protein bound in the plasma.

The midazolam is virtually completely metabolized into liver to its active hydroxylated derivatives which are then conjugated to glucuronide and excreted through bile and urine. These metabolites of midazolam also bind to CNS BZD receptors and are pharmacologically active. The excretion of midazolam occurs through urine, predominantly as hydroxylated derivatives which are formed in the liver. In the absence of renal function, it can be excreted solely through bile. So, renal impairment has little effect on the excretion of midazolam. It produces little discomfort at the site of the injection. Withdrawal phenomenon may also occur in children after prolonged infusion of midazolam.

The short duration of action of midazolam is due to its high lipophilicity, rapid redistribution (but less than thiopentone and propofol), high metabolic clearance, and rapid rate of elimination, however, this may not be true after prolonged infusion in the intensive care unit. The use of midazolam as premedication decreases the value of MAC of volatile anesthetic agents by approximately 15%. The clinical effects of this drug can be reversed by physostigmine, flumazenil, and glycopyrronium.

Lorazepam

Chemically, lorazepam is a lipid-soluble hydroxybenzodiazepine compound. Its mode of action is same as that of diazepam and midazolam, but the only difference is that the prolonged duration of action of lorazepam makes it unsuitable for outpatient (daycare) surgery. It appears to have no direct cardiac effects. Mild respiratory depression occurs following the administration of this drug which is of clinical

Fig. 11: Lorazepam.

significance only for the patients with lung disease, elderly, children, and neonates. Like other BZDs, it also produces sedation, anterograde amnesia, and anticonvulsion effects, but the slow rate of the onset of action of lorazepam would make it unsuitable, even through the IV route, for the control of status epilepticus, though it could be given as an anticonvulsant. However, the clonazepam, which is an another BZD, is recommended as a more specific agent for the control or the prevention of convulsions. This drug has no effect on basal gastric acid secretion. When lorazepam is used as premedication, the circulatory cortisol and glucose levels fall. This is probably secondary to its anxiolytic effect. The prolonged action of lorazepam makes it the most dependable agent for minimizing the emergence sequelae which are found, after the use of ketamine in adults. This can be achieved by IV injection of lorazepam near the end of operation, but not by its premedicant use. So, to be effective lorazepam has to be given in the doses of 2.5 mg through IV, but this may delay the complete recovery from anesthesia **(Fig. 11)**.

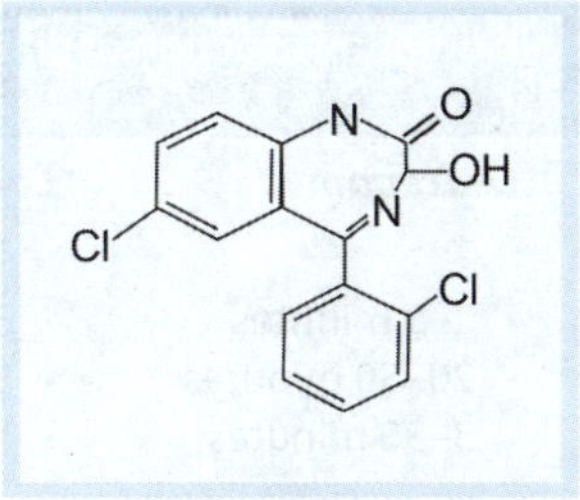

In adults, the oral or sublingual dose of lorazepam is 1–4 mg/day in divided doses. For premedication in anesthesia the lorazepam is used orally in a dose of 0.05 mg/kg. The IV or intramuscular dose of it for sedation is **(Table 5)** 0.025–0.05 mg/kg. Intramuscular injection of lorazepam is painful. The bioavailability of this drug is 90% when administered by the oral or IM route. It is 80–90% protein bound in the plasma. Lorazepam is less extensively distributed in tissues than diazepam. Thus, it has a longer duration of action than diazepam, despite a shorter elimination half-life of it. It is conjugated directly in liver to glucuronide to form an inactive water-soluble metabolite. About 80% of an orally administered dose of lorazepam appears in the urine as the glucuronide. The elimination half-life of it is 8–25 hours. This is unaffected by the renal disease.

The side effects of lorazepam are like that of other BZDs which are drowsiness, sedation, confusion, impaired coordinated movements, etc., in a dose-dependent manner. Paradoxical stimulation of CNS has also been reported after lorazepam and occurs more frequently when hyoscine

TABLE 5: Difference in duration of action of diazepam (10 mg) and lorazepam (2 mg).

	Diazepam	Lorazepam
Intravenous		
• Peak effect	• 2–5 minutes	• 30–40 minute
• Duration of sedation	• 20–50 minutes	• 3–6 hours
• Duration of amnesia	• 3–30 minutes	• ½–4 hours
Oral		
• Onset of action	20–40 minutes	40–50 minutes
Route differences	Oral more rapid than intramuscular	Intramuscular more rapid than oral

is administered concurrently with it. The tolerance and dependence in lorazepam may occur with prolonged use of it and acute withdrawal in these circumstances may produce insomnia, anxiety, confusion, psychosis, and perceptual disturbances.

PHENCYCLIDINE–KETAMINE

Phencyclidine was the first agent among this group of drugs. It was first synthesized by Maddox and was introduced into clinical practice by Johnstone, in1959. During that period, it was a very useful IV anesthetic agent, but it had high adverse psychological effect, so it was withdrawn from market gradually. Then, came *cyclohexylamine* which was a congener of phencyclidine. It had the same anesthetic property like phencyclidine, but it had less analgesic property and had more adverse psychological effects than cyclohexadiene, so it was also abandoned.

Then, *ketamine* as a derivative of phencyclidine was first synthesized, in 1962, by Stevens and was first used in human beings, in 1965. However, it was released for clinical use, in 1970, and is still now the most promising agent among the 200 phencyclidine derivatives.

Chemistry

Chemically, ketamine is an arylcyclohexylamine compound and is a congener of phencyclidine. It is a partially water soluble, white crystalline salt, with a pKa value of 7.5. It is highly lipid soluble which is 5–10 times greater than that of thiopentone. Ketamine is available commercially as its hydrochloride salt (pH 3.5–5.5) in concentration of 10 and 50 mg/mL in NaCl solution, with benzethonium chloride as a preservative. It has two optical isomers and the commercial preparation of ketamine is a racemic mixture of both the isomer [S(+) and R(–)] in equal amounts, despite the S(+) isomer being more potent and having less side effects than that of R(–) isomer **(Fig. 12)**.

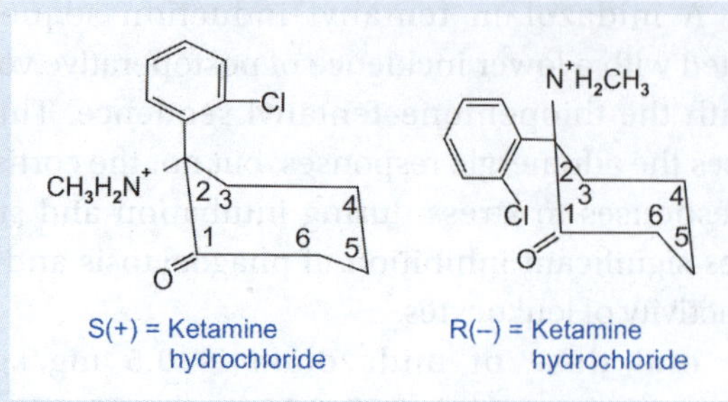

Fig. 12: Two stereoisomers of ketamine.

Pharmacokinetics

The onset and the duration of action of an induction dose of ketamine is also determined by the same distribution and redistribution mechanism which is found in other highly lipid-soluble parenteral anesthetics agents such as thiopentone, propofol, benzodiazepines, etc. Ketamine's pharmacokinetic action has been studied in detail, after bolus administration of an anesthetizing (2–2.5 mg/kg), subanesthetizing (0.25 mg/kg), and a continuous infusion dose of it. However, regardless of dose, ketamine's plasma disappearance can be described by a two-compartmental model. The high lipid solubility of ketamine is reflected by its relatively large volume of distribution. The clearance rate of ketamine is also relatively high which accounts for its relatively short elimination half-life of 2–3 hours. Ketamine's large volume of distribution and rapid clearance make it suitable for continuous infusion, without drastic lengthening of its duration of action, as seen with thiopentone. The protein binding capacity is much lowers with ketamine than that of other parenteral anesthetic agents. Thus, the bolus administration of ketamine results in quick entry of it into CNS and a very fast onset of action.

Metabolism

Ketamine is principally metabolized in liver by hepatic microsomal enzyme and the principal metabolic pathway of it is N-demethylation which forms norketamine (metabolite-I) from ketamine first. Norketamine is then hydroxylated to hydroxyl norketamine (metabolite-II) which is then next conjugated to water-soluble glucuronide derivative and excreted through urine and bile. Norketamine is an active metabolite of ketamine and has 20–30% activity of its parent compound.

Pharmacodynamics

Effects on Central Nervous System

The primary site of action of ketamine is a *thalamo-neocortical projection* in the brain. It depresses the cortex (association area) and thalamus, but simultaneously stimulates the limbic system and hippocampus of the brain. Thus, it creates a functional disorganization between the midbrain, thalamus, and cortex.

For ketamine's anesthetic effect Na$^+$ channel blockade is not the mechanism of action, but its interaction with N-methyl-D-aspartate (NMDA) receptor in the brain mediates general anesthetic and analgesic effect of it. The interaction of ketamine with opioid receptors in the brain and spinal cord also accounts for its analgesic effect. The S(+) enantiomer of ketamine has also been shown to have some opioid μ-receptor activity, accounting for part of its analgesic effect. The inhibition of the wide dynamic range (WDR) of neuronal activity in dorsal horn cells of the spinal cord also account for ketamine's analgesic activity at the spinal level.

The cerebral metabolic rate, cerebral O$_2$ demand, CBF, and ICP are all increased by ketamine during its anesthesia. There is also a generalized increase in sympathetic nervous system activity by ketamine and all the aforementioned CNS effect of ketamine is due to this increased sympathetic activity, but thiopentone and BZDs prevent all these responses of ketamine.

Ketamine produces both the dose-related unconsciousness and strong analgesia. During unconsciousness produced by ketamine, the patient remains in a cataleptic state, i.e., he is in sleep, but his eyes are opened. So, this anesthetic state of ketamine is termed "*dissociative anesthesia*". Although ketamine does not produce a classical anesthetic state, still patients are remained in an amnestic and unresponsiveness state to the painful stimuli. During ketamine anesthesia, the corneal, coughing, and swallowing reflexes are present, but they are not protective. There is amnesia during ketamine anesthesia, but it is less than BZDs. The low molecular weight, pKa value near physiological pH, and high lipid solubility of ketamine, allow it to cross the blood–brain barrier very rapidly. So, the onset of action of ketamine is very rapid, which is about 30 seconds, after its IV administration. Lacrimation, salivation, ↑muscle tone, purposeless movement of body, dilated pupil, nystagmus, etc., are all very common events during ketamine anesthesia.

The duration of action of 2 mg/kg IV bolus dose of ketamine is 15 minutes and then full recovery (orientation to place and time) occurs within 30 minutes. The plasma level of ketamine of 0.6–2 μg/mL is considered as its minimal plasma concentration for GA. The short duration and early termination of action of ketamine is thought to be due to its redistribution from the brain (well perfused) to the other body tissues (less perfused) such as thiopentone and BZDs. Analgesia due to ketamine occurs considerably

at lower blood concentration than GA. This analgesic effect of ketamine also occurs at subanesthetic dose like 0.25–0.5 mg/kg through IV. This analgesia due to ketamine even occurs at plasma level, as low as 0.1 μg/mL.

There are various undesirable psychological reactions during awakening from ketamine anesthesia which are termed the *emergence reaction* or *emergence delirium*. This emergence delirium of ketamine, which are characterized by hallucination, vivid dreams, or illusions, etc., may sometimes result in serious patient dissatisfaction and can complicate the postoperative management. The incidence of this emergence reaction after ketamine anesthesia ranges from 5 to 100% and abates within first postoperative hour. Though, the exact mechanism of this emergence reaction, during awakening from ketamine anesthesia, is not known, but it is postulated that the psychic reactions that occur secondary to ketamine anesthesia during recovery is due to induced depression of auditory and visual relay nuclei, leading to misperception and/or misinterpretation of auditory and visual stimuli. Many factors affect this emergence reaction of ketamine such as age (less incidence in pediatric group), sex (women are more susceptible than man), dose (larger dose and rapid administration predisposes to higher incidence), and psychological susceptibility of person. Benzodiazepines and among them lorazepam is still the best drug to attenuate this ketamine-induced emergence reaction. The S-enantiomer of ketamine enables quicker recovery than the racemic mixture of it. This is because lower doses of S(+) enantiomer of ketamine is necessary to produce the equianesthetic effect of a racemic mixture of it and has a 10% faster hepatic clearance rate.

Effects on Cardiovascular System

Due to increased sympathetic activity, during ketamine anesthesia, there is an increase in BP, HR, CO, myocardial O$_2$ consumption, and demand, but this increased myocardial O$_2$ consumption and demand is fulfilled by ↑CO and ↓ coronary vascular resistance in a normal heart by ketamine so that the coronary blood flow is appropriate for the increased myocardial O$_2$ demand and consumption. This hemodynamic change, caused by ketamine is not related to the dose of it, i.e., a very small dose of ketamine also can produce the same effect like the higher doses of it. On the other hand, the ketamine-induced hemodynamic changes are same in healthy patient and in those with varieties of acquired and congenital heart diseases (CHDs). In patient with CHD, there are no significant changes in direction through shunt after induction with ketamine. Ketamine seems to cause a more pronounced increase in PVR than SVR.

Ketamine enhances sympathetic responses by its centrally-mediated action, but the exact mechanism by which ketamine enhances the sympathetic activity is not known. But the probable explanation is that ketamine attenuates the pressure-controlling baroreceptor function by affecting the NMDA receptor of nucleus tractus solitarius of vagus. Directly ketamine is depressant to heart muscle, but the centrally-mediated enhanced sympathetic response of it overrides this direct response of it on myocardium. So, the ketamine anesthesia experiences all the CVS effects which are described earlier. The sympathetic cardiovascular effects of ketamine are also mediated by the inhibition of both central and peripheral catecholamine reuptake.

The raised sympathetic response during ketamine anesthesia can be attenuated in clinical practice by:

- Use of adrenergic antagonists (both α and β)
- Use of vasodilator
- Prior administration of BZDs or thiopentone
- Very slow and continuous infusion of ketamine
- Use of inhalation anesthetics along with ketamine.

Effect on Respiratory System

The central respiratory drive is minimally affected by ketamine, with an unaltered response to O_2 (hypoxia) and CO_2 (hypercarbia). But there is a transient decrease in minute ventilation, due to respiratory depression, after an IV bolus dose of it. Seldom, very unusual high dose of ketamine produces apnea. Usually, O_2 and CO_2 levels in blood are maintained at a normal level by a conventional dose of ketamine, provided no other sedative is used along with it. By its sympathomimetic action, ketamine produces bronchodilatation. In patient with reactive airway disease and bronchospasm, pulmonary compliance is also improved by ketamine. So it is a useful drug to treat status asthmaticus which is unresponsive to conventional therapy. Increased salivation caused by ketamine may also produce upper airway obstruction and laryngospasm. Although the laryngeal, pharyngeal, and swallow reflexes are preserved in ketamine anesthesia, they are not coordinated and not protective. So, there is evidence that silent aspiration can occur during ketamine anesthesia.

Uses

The poor-risk patients with severe cardiovascular and respiratory disorders (except ischemic heart disease and hypertension) are best suitable for ketamine induction and maintenance of anesthesia. Hemodynamically compromised patients, with hypovolemia and cardiomyopathy, are also better subjects for ketamine anesthesia, but not the patients suffering from coronary artery disease. Profound analgesia; allowing the use of high inspired O_2 concentration without using N_2O and inhalational anesthetics; and bronchodilatation make the ketamine an excellent agent for induction of anesthesia in asthma patient. However, for extensive trauma or severe septic shock patients, we have to keep in our mind that ketamine has an intrinsic myocardial depressant effect and it (myocardial depression) may be manifested if the sympathetic store is completely depleted, due to this extensive trauma and severe septic shock in these groups of patients, before ketamine induction. The cardiac problems which can better be managed by ketamine than thiopentone are cardiac tamponade, restrictive pericarditis, congenital heart disease, and especially those in whom the propensity for right to left intracardiac shunt exists. Ketamine is also a very useful drug for induction and maintenance of anesthesia in patients with the history of potential malignant hyperthermia. It is not arrhythmogenic.

When ketamine is combined with BZDs and fentanyl or sufentanil in continuous infusion, then they attenuate the unwanted tachycardia as well as hypertension, caused by ketamine alone and produce very satisfactory condition in cardiac anesthesia for valvular disease and IHD. This combination is also associated with (1) minimum hemodynamic changes, (2) profound analgesia, (3) dependable amnesia, and (4) uneventful convalescence. Ketamine also can be used for postoperative analgesia in subanesthetic dose ($\leq$1 mg/kg), when one wishes to avoid narcotics, because of their (narcotics) respiratory depression, and when there is also a reason to avoid nonsteroidal agents such as ketorolac.

Ketamine is mainly used for short pediatric outdoor procedures such as cardiac catheterization, radiation therapy, radiological diagnostic procedure, and dressing changes. But caution is advised, during the use of ketamine in patient with elevated PVR. When used as supplementation for regional anesthesia, ketamine (0.5 mg/kg IV) combined with diazepam (0.15 mg/kg IV) is better accepted by the patient and is not associated with greater side effects, as compared with the unsedated patient (**Box 1**).

Doses and Route of Administration

Ketamine can be administered through IV, IM, oral, or rectal route, however the dose of it depends on this route of administration and the desired therapeutic effect. The oral dose of ketamine is 5–10 mg/kg, and the onset of action of this oral dose is 20–40 minutes. However, the corresponding IV dose of it is 1.5–2 mg/kg, which is administered over a period of 60 seconds. The onset of action of ketamine through

BOX 1: Uses and doses of ketamine.

- Induction of GA
  - 0.5–2 mg/kg IV
  - 4–6 mg/kg IM
  - 3–10 mg/kg oral
- Maintenance of GA
  - 0.5–1 mg/kg IV (bolus) with $N_2O + O_2$
  - 10–50 µg/kg/min IV
  - 30–90 µg/kg/min IV without N_2O
- Sedation and analgesia
  - 0.2–0.8 mg/kg IV over 3–4 minutes
  - 2–4 mg/kg IM
  - 10–20 µg/kg/min IV (maintenance)

Note: Lower doses are used if other drugs such as opioids, BZDs, or thiopentone are also given with ketamine
(BZDs: benzodiazepines; IM: intramuscular; IV: intravenous)

the IV route is within 30–60 seconds and the duration of action is 5–10 minutes. Through the IM route the onset of action of ketamine is about 5 minutes and the peak effect is obtained at about 20 minutes after its administration. Ketamine may be infused intravenously at the rate of 50 µg/kg/min. The drug is also effective when it is administered extradurally (in an adult the dose is 10 mg) or intrathecally.

Side Effects and Contraindication

The side effects of ketamine are its contraindication for use. These are:

- Increased intracranial lesion, increased ICP, and cerebral ischemia
- IHD due to increased myocardial O_2 consumption and demand
- Open globe injury
- Vascular aneurysm
- Psychiatric disease such as schizophrenia
- Eclampsia
- Hypertension.

■ PROPOFOL

History

In 1970, the worldwide extensive search for the derivatives of phenol, as a disinfectant substituent of it, suddenly resulted in the development of 2,6-diisopropylphenol (commonly named as propofol) which has a strong hypnotic property. Then, the first clinical trial of 2,6-diisopropylphenol as a hypnotic, in 1977, confirmed the potentiality of it as an anesthetic-inducing agent. Initially, it was prepared in Cremophor EL due to its insolubility in water. But due to the increased incidence of anaphylactoid reaction, because of Cremophor EL, the drug was reformulated as an emulsion in soybean oil and egg white.

Chemistry

Chemically, propofol is a 2,6-diisopropylphenol. Its chemical structure is given in **Figure 13**. As it is an alkylphenol derivative, so it is insoluble in water and remains as liquid oil at room temperature. It is highly lipid soluble. Therefore, the present emulsion formulation of propofol consists of 1% propofol, 10% soybean oil, 2.25% glycerol, and 1.2% purified egg phosphatide, without any preservative. But disodium ethylenediaminetetraacetic acid (EDTA) or sodium metabisulfite is added as a preservative to inhibit bacterial growth in the USA. Without EDTA or metabisulfite, the emulsion preparation of propofol should be used shortly after the removal from its sterile packaging; otherwise significant bacterial contamination can cause serious infection, as there is no preservative. This emulsion preparation of propofol is milky white in appearance and slightly viscous due to soybean oil and egg white. It is stable at the room temperature and is not light-sensitive. This emulsion preparation is compatible with 5% dextrose solution for continuous infusion. The pH of propofol is 7 and it is commercially available as a 1% solution.

Pharmacokinetics

Propofol is only available as IV preparation for induction and/or for the maintenance of GA. It is also used for conscious sedation to deep sedation by continuous IV infusion. The high lipid solubility character of it results in the onset of action that is almost as rapid as that of thiopentone. The duration of action, after a single equivalent bolus dose of propofol, is also similar to or even shorter than that of thiopentone. This is due to the rapid decline of plasma concentration of propofol, after an IV bolus dose, which can be fitted to a typical three-compartment model of thiopentone and explain its rapid distribution, redistribution, and clearance rate (elimination).

The initial volume of distribution of propofol is 20–40 L and the initial distribution half-life of it is 2–8 minutes. Following an IV bolus dose of propofol, the plasma level initially declines rapidly, due to the redistribution from highly perfused but lower capacity tissues such as brain,

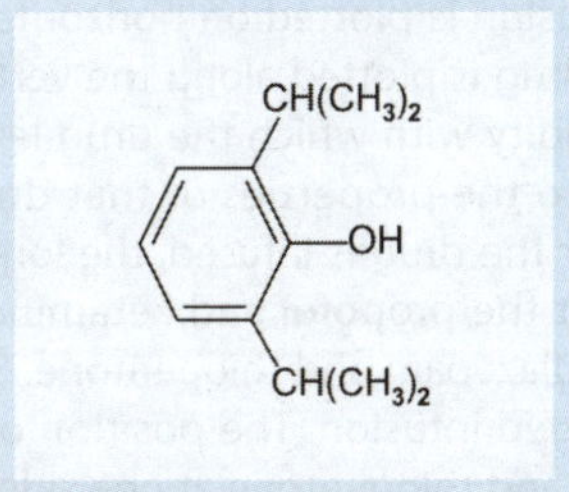

Fig. 13: The structure of propofol. It is an alkyl phenol derivative.

heart, etc., to high capacity but lower perfusion sites such as muscles, liver, and spleen. This initial clearance of propofol from central compartment to peripheral compartment by redistribution is rapid (3–4 L/kg/min) and is responsible for quick awakening and less hangover from a single bolus dose of it. Thus, this makes it a better agent for outpatient anesthesia than thiopentone and methohexitone **(Fig. 14)**.

Propofol's pharmacokinetics may be altered by a variety of factors such as age, gender, weight, other medications, preexisting diseases, etc. A lower induction dose is recommended in elderly patients. This is because of their smaller initial volume of distribution. Women may require higher dose of propofol than men and appear to awaken faster, due to higher volume of distribution. Recovery after multiple doses or infusions of propofol is much faster than thiopentone. This can be explained by its very high metabolic clearance rate in liver which is about 1.5–2.5 L/min and it is 10 times higher than that of thiopentone. This high metabolic clearance rate of propofol exceeds hepatic blood flow. This implies the existence of some extrahepatic metabolic clearance site of propofol which is still unknown. But the lung does not take part as an extrahepatic metabolic site for the metabolic clearance of propofol.

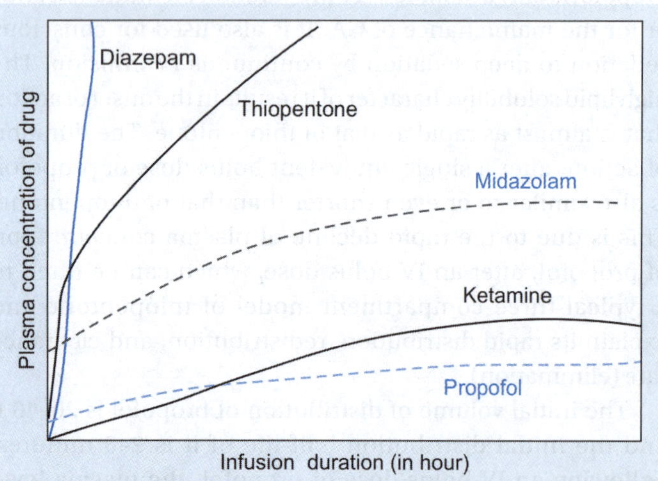

Fig. 14: The context-sensitive half-time (CSHT) is the time for the plasma level of a drug to drop 50%, after the cessation of infusion. This figure shows context sensitive half-time (CSHT) for diazepam, thiopentone, midazolam, ketamine, and propofol. In this figure, the duration of infusion is plotted on horizontal axis and the drop of plasma level of drug is plotted along the vertical axis. This figure shows that the rapidity with which the drug level in plasma drops is directly related to the properties of that drug and the time of infusion. The longer the drug is infused, the longer is the half-time. It is also noted that the propofol and ketamine have significantly shorter CSHT than diazepam and thiopentone. So, this makes them suitable for prolonged infusion. The position of midazolam lies in between diazepam and thiopentone at one side and ketamine with propofol at another side.

In the liver, propofol is metabolized by conjugation to water-soluble glucuronide and sulfates, which are excreted through bile and kidney. The metabolites of propofol are not active one, although the metabolites of propofol are primarily excreted through urine, but chronic renal failure does not affect the clearance of parent drug. The pharmacokinetic of propofol do not appear to be affected by moderate cirrhosis. Use of continuous propofol infusion for long-term sedation in children, who are critically ill, has been associated with the cases of lipedema, metabolic acidosis, and death.

Pharmacodynamics

Effect of Propofol on the Central Nervous System

The primary actions of propofol are *hypnosis* and *sedation*, but the exact mechanism of these actions is not known. Probably, it acts by enhancing the function of GABA-activated chloride channel such as BZDs and thiopentone (barbiturates).

Unlike thiopentone, propofol is *not antianalgesic*. The onset of action (hypnosis), following IV administration of propofol in the doses of 2.5 mg/kg, is 30 seconds (though it depends on the speed of injection), and the duration of action (though dose-dependent) is 10–15 minutes **(Table 6)**. The onset and the duration of action of propofol also depend on the type and the dose of premedication, used along with it. Propofol can also be used in subanesthetic or subhypnotic dose. A subhypnotic or subanesthetic dose of propofol will only produce conscious sedation and amnesia, but not hypnosis or anesthesia. The infusion of propofol in the dose of 2 mg/kg/h is necessary to provide amnesia in unstimulated patients. But during surgery, a higher infusion rate is necessary to prevent awareness, if propofol is used alone.

The effect of propofol on epileptogenic activity is in controversy because the results from multiple studies on anticonvulsion effects of it are mixed, however propofol-induced convulsion is very rare. The amplitude of EEG

TABLE 6: Uses and doses of commonly used drugs for sedation and induction of anesthesia.			
Thiopentone (2.5%)	Sedation	IV	0.5–1.5 mg/kg
	Induction	IV	4–5 mg/kg
Propofol (1%)	Sedation (infusion)	IV	25–100 µg/kg/min
	Induction	IV	1–2 mg/kg
	Maintenance	IV	50–200 µg/kg/min
Ketamine	Induction	IV	1–2 mg/kg
Methohexital (1%)	Sedation	IV	0.2–0.4 mg/kg
	Induction	IV	1–2 mg/kg
		Rectal	25 g

increases, when the propofol blood concentration varies between 3 and 8 µg/mL, but when the propofol concentration in the blood rises above 8 µg/mL, then the amplitude of EEG decreases, rather than increases, and there is a burst suppression. The induction of GA by propofol is occasionally accompanied by excitatory phenomenon such as muscle twitching, spontaneous movement, opisthotonus, and hiccup. This may be due to the subcortical antagonism of inhibitory glycine by propofol, although these reactions (muscle twitching, spontaneous movement, opisthotonus or hiccup, etc.) may occasionally mimic tonic–clonic seizure, but actually, propofol appears to have predominantly anticonvulsion property. So, propofol can be successfully used to terminate status epilepticus and may safely be administered in epileptic patients.

Propofol decreases ICP (30–50%) both in normal and in a patient with already raised ICP, however this decrease in ICP is also associated with a decrease in cerebral perfusion pressure, both in normal and elevated ICP patient, and therefore may not be beneficial, like barbiturates. This is due to the much reduction of systemic BP in comparison to the reduction of ICP. So, steps should be taken to support the mean arterial pressure and to elevate the cerebral perfusion pressure (>50 mm Hg). Propofol also provides cerebral protective effects, following ischemic brain injury like thiopentone. It also acutely reduces intraocular pressure (IOP) by 30–40% and a small second dose is more effective in preventing the rise of IOP secondary to succinylcholine or endotracheal tube (ET) intubation.

The blood concentration of propofol (Cp50) needed for the loss of response to verbal command is 3.5 µg/mL and to skin incision is 16 µg/mL (propofol alone without narcotics, inhalational agents, etc.). This propofol Cp50 value for skin incision comes down to 2.5 µg/mL when it is combined with BZDs (as premedication) and 66% N_2O. This value again comes down to 1.7 µg/mL, if narcotic is used in place of BZDs. Awakening from induction, caused by propofol, usually occurs when the plasma concentration of propofol comes down to or below 1.6 µg/mL, and orientation comes back when the plasma concentration of it comes down to 1.2 µg/mL.

Effects of Propofol on Cardiovascular System

Propofol produces a dose-dependent decrease in BP which is significantly greater than that produced by thiopentone. Propofol has both vasodilation (venous and arterial) and myocardial depression effects. This appears to be due to the reduction in sympathetic tone and also due to the direct negative effect of propofol on intracellular Ca^{2+} mobilization in smooth muscle. Thus, there is a decrease in vascular smooth muscle tone and a reduction in preload and afterload. As a result, there is a decrease in systolic BP, a decrease in diastolic BP, and a decrease in SVR (due to vasodilation). However, the changes in CO, stroke volume, cardiac index, etc., produced by propofol depend on the multitude of changes in preload, afterload, and SVR. The pulmonary artery pressure and pulmonary wedge pressure are also reduced by propofol.

The HR does not change significantly with the reduction of BP, after an induction dose of propofol. This suggests that propofol either resets or inhibits the baroreceptor reflexes and thus reduces tachycardia response to hypotension. Changes in HR and CO, caused by the induction dose of propofol are usually transient and insignificant in healthy patients, but it may be severe enough and lead to asystole, particularly in patients who are at extreme of age, on negative chronotropic medications, undergoing surgical procedures, associated with ocular cardiac reflex, etc.

When the patients are allowed to breathe air or air plus O_2 and hypnosis is maintained only by propofol infusion in the dose of 50–100 µg/kg/min, then SVR, BP, CO, and CI are reduced, but when these same patients are intubated and hypnosis is maintained by N_2O and propofol infusion of the same dose, then SVR and BP do not reduce, but CO and CI falls. This is due to the presence of N_2O or surgical stimulus. So, the intraoperative BP cannot be reduced in intubated hypertensive patients by propofol only. Infusion of propofol results in a significant reduction in both myocardial blood flow and myocardial O_2 consumption, but the global O_2 supply/demand ratio is preserved. Though the reduction of BP (due to vasodilation) and myocardial depression effect of propofol is blood concentration-dependent, but the decrease in BP from propofol during infusion is much less than that seen following an induction bolus dose.

Effects of Propofol on Respiratory System

Propofol's effects on the respiratory system are similar to that of barbiturates. So, like barbiturates, it depresses respiration and may produce apnea. The onset, duration, and the incidences of apnea due to propofol depend on the dose, speed of injection, and the concomitant use of premedication. The incidence of propofol-induced apnea is greater than any other IV-inducing agents and is preceded by a marked reduction in tidal volume (40% decrease) and respiratory rate (20% decrease). So, there is an unpredictable change in minute ventilation (decreased or increased).

During the infusion of propofol, the respiratory rate gradually decreases. Then, when this respiratory rate is fixed at a lower level and still if the concentration of infusion is gradually increased, then there is a gradual decrease in tidal volume, but no change in respiratory rate. This is followed by apnea. Propofol infusion inhibits hypoxic ventilatory drive. Ventilatory response to CO_2 (hypercarbia) is also decreased by propofol. Propofol induces bronchodilatation in patients with COPD, although it can cause histamine release. So, the induction with propofol is sometimes accompanied by few incidences of wheezing in asthmatic and nonasthmatic patients, compared to barbiturates, but is not contraindicated in asthmatic patients. The propofol-induced depression of upper airway reflexes exceeds than that of thiopentone and can prove helpful during intubation or LMA placement in the absence of muscular paralysis by a muscle relaxant.

Miscellaneous Effects

Like thiopentone, propofol does not potentiate the neuromuscular blockade, produced by muscle relaxants. Propofol does not trigger malignant hyperpyrexia and so is the anesthetic of choice in such condition. It does not affect corticosteroid synthesis or does not alter the responses to adrenocorticotropic hormone (ACTH) stimulation. The incidence of anaphylactoid reaction, following the administration of propofol, has been reported at about the same low frequency as that of thiopentone. But a high percentage of the patient who develops an anaphylactoid reaction against propofol has a previous history of allergic response. So, propofol should be used cautiously for the patients who will give a history of multiple drug allergies. It has significant antiemetic property and is a good choice for sedation or anesthesia on the patient who have a high risk for nausea and vomiting. Sometimes, postoperative nausea can be treated successfully by IV bolus doses of 10 mg propofol. Although propofol does cross the placental barrier, still it is considered safe for use in the pregnant patients and transiently depresses the activity of newborns as thiopentone.

Doses of Propofol

The doses and the indications for the use of propofol are enumerated in **Box 2**. The premedication of patients with opiates and/or BZDs markedly reduces the induction and maintenance dose of propofol. Increased age also reduces the dose of propofol with or without premedication. It can also be used successfully for patient-controlled sedation (PCS), like patient-controlled analgesia (PCA), but in this respect, it is better than midazolam and it is due to its rapid onset and offset action. Propofol by its continuous infusion provides a readily titratable level of sedation and rapid recovery, once the infusion is terminated, irrespective of the duration of infusion.

■ DROPERIDOL

History

In 1950, Laborit and Hugnenard thought of a new anesthetic technique (concept) that will produce a state of "artificial hibernation or neurolept". This new anesthetic technique was without the need of muscular paralysis and was devoid of CVS and respiratory depression effects. Their concept, regarding this new anesthetic technique was to block centrally the autonomic, endocrine, and other centers which normally are activated in response to stress during surgery. This central block can be performed *selectively* by drugs which will produce artificial hibernation, in contrast to the entire depression of CNS which causes GA. The first drug which was evolved for this purpose and was used in this concept was *"lytic cocktail".* It was a mixture of meperidine (analgesic), chlorpromazine or promethazine (tranquilizer), and atropine (antisialagogue). It can produce conscious sedation, but not the full GA. Then, Janssen first synthesized haloperidol [which was the first member of the butyrophenones group of drugs and the primary neuroleptic component of neuroleptic anesthesia (NLAN)] and phenoperidine (which is the derivative of meperidine). After that in 1959, De Castro and Mundeleer combined these and used them as a forerunner of NLAN. Then, Janssen synthesized droperidol (a derivative of haloperidol) and fentanyl (phenoperidine congener). So, De Castro and Mundeleer again used these combinations and reported that these (droperidol and fentanyl) combination is superior to the previous combination. Now, droperidol and fentanyl are the currently used combination for NLAN.

The term "neuroleptic" is synonymous with the term "antipsychotic". Initially, the term *"neuroleptic"* was used to denote the effect of chlorpromazine and reserpine which reduce the initiative and the interest of the patient for the external environment as well as decrease the manifestation of emotions. The term "neuroleptic" is still used now as a synonym for antipsychotic effect. But the more general term *"antipsychotic"* is preferred nowadays than neuroleptic. Despite their sedation effects, neuroleptic drugs generally are not used to treat anxiety disorders. This is largely because of their autonomic and neurological side effects, which paradoxically include severe anxiety and restlessness.

Mechanism of Action

Like all antipsychotic drugs, droperidol acts by its potent dopamine (DA) D_2 receptor blocking action. The blockade of the dopaminergic projection to the temporal, prefrontal (constituting the limbic system), and mesocortical areas of the brain are probably responsible for the antipsychotic action of droperidol because the dopamine overactivity at the limbic system is responsible for the psychiatric condition. Dopaminergic blockade in the basal ganglia also appears to cause the extrapyramidal symptoms of droperidol, while that in CTZ is responsible for the antiemetic action of it. Droperidol, like other antipsychiatric drugs, also has the α-adrenergic blocking action, weak H_1-antihistamine action, and anti-5-hydroxytryptamine (anti-5-HT) action.

Pharmacokinetics

The clearance rate of droperidol is 14 mL/kg/min and its elimination half-life is 103–134 minutes, which indicates its short duration of action. The time course of the disappearance of fentanyl and droperidol from plasma is the same.

Pharmacodynamics

Effects of Droperidol on Central Nervous System

The effects of droperidol on CNS differ in normal and psychotic individuals. In normal individuals, it produces indifferences to the surroundings, paucity of thought, psychomotor slowing, emotional quietening, reduction in initiative, and tendency to go to sleep from which the subject is easily arousable. The spontaneous movements are minimized, but the slurring of speech, ataxia, or motor in coordination does not occur. These have been referred to as the "neuroleptic syndrome". Now, there is a tendency to use the term "neuroleptic" to emphasize the more neurological aspects of this syndrome. The neuroleptic agents also have characteristic of neurological effects including bradykinesia, mild rigidity, tremor, and restlessness which resemble Parkinson's disease and are quite different from the sedative action of barbiturates and other similar drugs. These effects are appreciated as unpleasant by most of the normal individuals.

On the other hand, in psychotic individuals, it reduces irrational behavior, agitation, aggressiveness and controls the psychotic symptomatology. The disturbed thought and behavior are gradually normalized and anxiety is relieved. Hyperactivity, hallucinations, and delusions are suppressed.

It potentiates the action of hypnotics, opioids, etc. Performances and intelligence of an individual are relatively unaffected, but vigilance is impaired by droperidol. The medullary respiratory center and other vital centers are not affected. It has profound antiemetic action, exerted through CTZ.

Effects of Droperidol on Cardiovascular System

Droperidol has vasodilating properties and a decrease BP. This is due to the α-adrenergic blocking action of it. Directly, it has no action on myocardial contraction, but it possesses some antiarrhythmic properties like quinidine.

Effects of Droperidol on the Respiratory System

Droperidol has very little effect on RS. So, no significant effect on respiratory rate and tidal volume is found.

Use of Droperidol

Droperidol is used as a component of NLAN. It is also used as antiemetic in the dose of 10–20 µg/kg through IM or IV route. It reduces the incidence of nausea and vomiting in up to 50% of cases. The indications for the use of droperidol and its doses are enumerated in **Box 3**.

Droperidol and Fentanyl Combination

In the clinical practice of NLAN, the droperidol and fentanyl combination is used in a ratio of 50:1 (droperidol 2.5 mg/mL and fentanyl 50 µg/mL). In this combination, the droperidol produces the hypnotic, sedative, and antiemetic effect, while the fentanyl produces the analgesic effect. The action of these two components in their combination is simply additive, but not synergistic. Consciousness returns after NLAN very promptly within 3–5 minutes.

Due to the presence of fentanyl, this combination produces respiratory depression. This respiratory depression can be antagonized by the administration of a narcotic antagonist. This combination also produces ↓BP (droperidol effect) and ↓HR (fentanyl effect–fentanyl-induced increased vagal tone), however there is no reduction in CO if adequate blood volume is maintained. The combination of droperidol and fentanyl, used as NLAN (neurolept anesthesia) is very helpful for short outdoor surgeries, diagnostic procedures, and sedation during local anesthesia or conduction anesthesia. This combination can also be used

BOX 3: Uses and doses of a combination of droperidol and fentanyl in the ratio of 50:1 (droperidol 2.5 mg/mL and fentanyl 50 µg/mL).

- *Induction of general anesthesia:*
  - 0.1–0.15 mL/kg with N_2O and O_2
- *Maintenance of general anesthesia:*
  - Fentanyl 0.02–0.05 µg/kg/min
- *Sedation and analgesia:*
  - 0.5–1 mL IV repeated according to the desired effect
  - 1–2 mL IM

as an inducing agent in GA, performed by N_2O and muscle relaxant in the dose of 0.1–0.15 mL/kg. The components of NLAN can be given separately or as a mixture. When given separately, then droperidol should be given first in the dose of 5–10 mg (5–15 µg/kg). This is followed by incremental doses of fentanyl which varies between 50 and 100 µg. These drugs should be used with caution for the possibility of vasodilatation and hypotension. So, a test dose of 1–2 mL is always recommended before the bolus induction dose. It is also recommended to give 200–300 mL of balanced salt solution and correct hypotension prior to induction. The customary dose of this combination for sedation is about 2–4 mL in divided doses, titrated to the desired level of sedation. It is very helpful for surgeries that are associated with a high incidence of postoperative nausea and vomiting.

Neuroleptic anesthesia has several adverse effects and these are as follows:
- *Muscle rigidity:* This is due to fentanyl which can be treated by muscle relaxants.
- *Respiratory depression:* This is due to fentanyl which can be treated by opioids antagonist. But this may reverse the analgesic effect of opiates and precipitate hypertension.
- *Hypotension:* This is due to droperidol which can be treated by IV fluid and or α-adrenergic agonist.
- *Prolonged somnolence:* This is due to droperidol which is dose-related and is reversed by physostigmine (2 mg). Physostigmine is not the specific antagonist of droperidol. Physostigmine clearance is rapid than droperidol, so resedation can occur.
- *Extrapyramidal symptom:* It is manifested by dyskinesia of the face and neck with speech and swallowing difficulties. It is due to droperidol which can be treated by diphenhydramine or benztropine.
- Psychological reactions sometimes occur, when used as a premedicant and manifested as the patient refuses to have surgery.
- *Hallucination,* e.g., weightlessness and loss of body image
- Rare complication such as malignant neuroleptic syndrome.

■ FLUMAZENIL

The chemical structure of Flumazenil (imidazobenzodiaz-epine) is depicted in **Figure 15**. It was first synthesized, in 1979, as *BZD receptor antagonist* or *blocker*. The benzodiaz-epine *agonists* (BZDs) have both the affinity for binding with the BZD receptor and have the ability to produce maximal intrinsic activity such as hypnosis, sedation, and amnesia. On the other hand, BZD antagonists have the same affinity to a BZD receptor for binding but have no ability to produce

Fig. 15: Flumazenil.

any intrinsic activity. They just only block the physiological effects of BZD agonists, inverse agonists, and other molecules, by preventing them to bind with the BZD receptor. *Inverse agonists* have an also affinity to the BZD receptor and have an intrinsic activity which is opposite to the physiological effect of BZD agonist. *Partial agonists* have an affinity to BZD receptor and produce submaximal intrinsic activity in the same direction of the agonist.

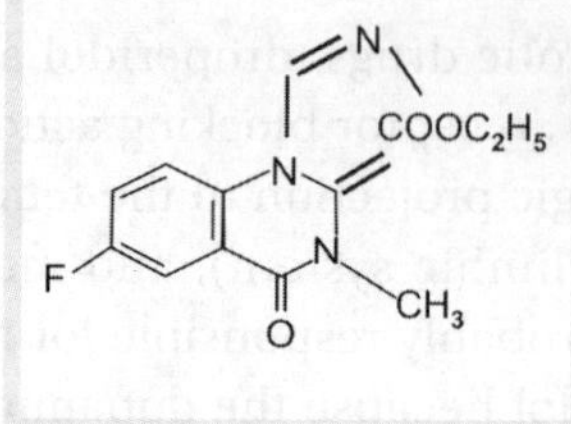

Partial inverse agonists have an affinity to BZD receptor and produce submaximal intrinsic activity in the opposite direction to the agonist. However, as flumazenil is a BZD receptor antagonist, so its structure is similar to that of classical BZD, except for a phenyl group which is replaced by a carbonyl group and blocks all the activities of BZDs and its inverse agonists. It was released for clinical use, in 1991. The mechanism of action of agonist, inverse agonist, antagonist, etc., is explained in **Figure 16**.

Flumazenil is a BZD analog and forms a complex with BZD receptor with high affinity and great specificity and blocks all the effects of BZD agonists and inverse agonists, which also binds with this BZD receptor. So, both the electrophysiological and behavioral effects of BZD (agonist) and DMCM (inverse agonists) are blocked; hence it blocks both the depressant effect of BZDs and the stimulant effect of DMCM. The DMCM has a stimulant effect because it is an inverse agonist of the BZD receptor. So, it (DMCM) produces all the opposite effects of BZDs. Flumazenil replaces BZD agonists at the receptor level in a competitive (competitive antagonist) and concentration-dependent manner. Flumazenil, like other competitive antagonists, does not displace the agonist from the receptor which is already attached with the receptor, but rather it occupies the receptor when an agonist dissociates from it and prevents the agonists from further attachment with the receptor. The half-life of a bond between a BZD receptor and antagonist (flumazenil) is a few seconds and new bonds are then immediately formed. So, it is a dynamic situation, where agonists and antagonists continuously compete with each other to occupy the BZD receptor. The proportion of receptor occupancy by agonists and antagonists obeys the law of mass action and depends on the affinity and concentration of agonists and antagonists.

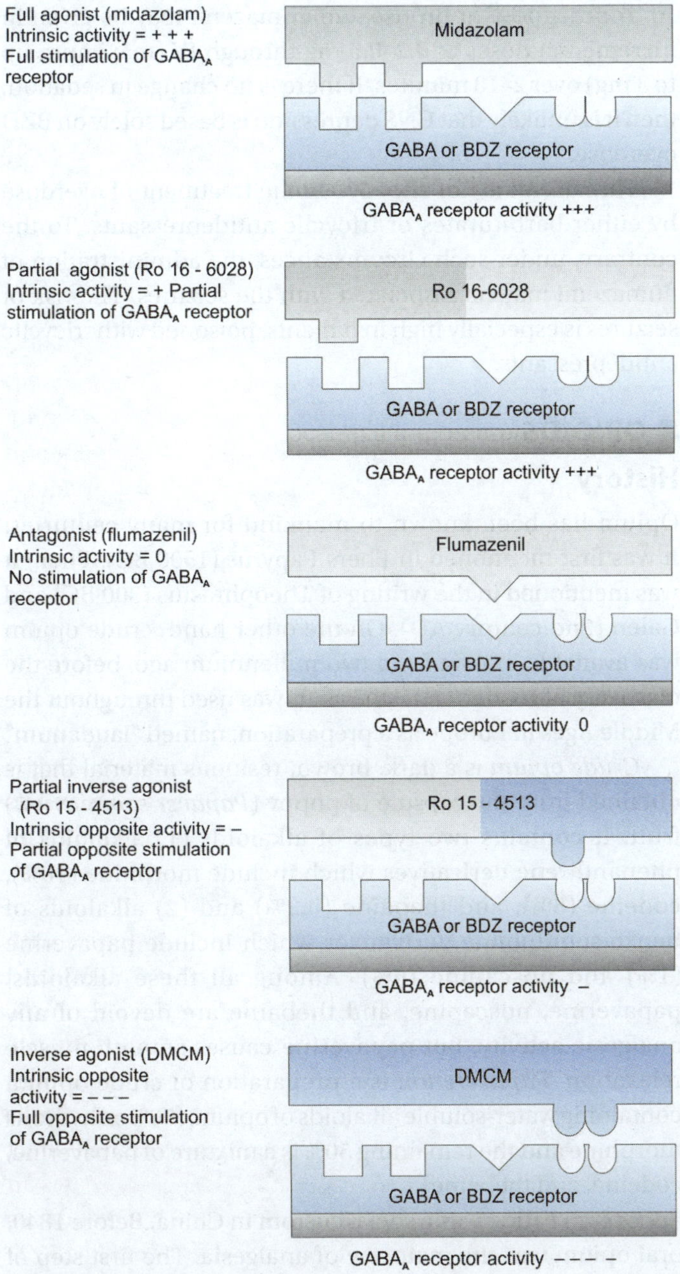

Fig. 16: GABA$_A$ receptor activity.
(DMCM: methyl 6,7-dimethoxy-4-ethyl-β-carboline-3-carboxylate; GABA$_A$: γ-aminobutyric acid type A)

As flumazenil (antagonist) is cleared from plasma relatively rapidly, so, though it has a high affinity to the receptor, but the chances of receptor reoccupied by agonist (BZDs) will increase and the potential for resedation will exist. Low dose of flumazenil in the presence of high doses of agonist will only attenuate the deep CNS depression of agonist (unconsciousness and respiratory depression), but without attenuating other agonistic effects which occur at lesser receptor occupancy (drowsiness and amnesia). On the contrary, only high doses of flumazenil, in the presence of low doses of agonist (BZD), will completely reverse all the effects of BZD and can precipitate withdrawal symptoms in dependent patients.

Pharmacokinetics of Flumazenil

In comparison with BZD receptor agonists, flumazenil (BZD receptor antagonist) has the highest clearance and shortest elimination half-life. The plasma half-life of flumazenil is only 1 hour. This shorter half-life of it (flumazenil) than its agonist counterpart causes the potential risk of resedation, due to the still presence of agonist (BZD) in plasma and binding of it with a receptor. So, to avoid this drawback and to maintain a constant therapeutic blood level of the antagonist (flumazenil), the repeated administration or continuous infusion of flumazenil is required in the rate of 30–60 mg/min or 0.5–1 µg/kg/min. Flumazenil is not used orally, because it is rapidly absorbed after oral administration, but <25% of this drug reaches the systemic circulation, as a result of its extensive first-pass hepatic metabolism or clearance. This is explained in **Figure 17**.

Pharmacology of Flumazenil

When flumazenil is given alone in the absence of any administration of any BZD, then its intrinsic effects on the BZD receptor are difficult to observe or nil because flumazenil only binds with the receptor by replacing the BZD molecules which are attached before, but it does not elicit any action by binding with a receptor. As previously described, the flumazenil acts by replacing the BZDs from its receptor, so its onset and duration of action are governed by the law of mass action. The onset of action of flumazenil is very rapid and the peak effect reaches within 1–3 minutes, after its IV administration. It rapidly reverses unconsciousness, respiratory depression, sedation, amnesia, and psychomotor dysfunction, produced by BZDs according to the dose. It has no effect on EEG and cerebral metabolism. The flumazenil itself has no epileptogenic or anticonvulsant property, but it reverses the anticonvulsant property of BZDs. Higher dose of flumazenil is required to reverse the effects of lorazepam than diazepam and this is because of the greater potency of the former. The duration of action of flumazenil is determined by its dose and the dose and type of agonist (BZD). Usually, the duration of action of flumazenil is 45–90 minutes, after a dose of 3 mg through IV; however, flumazenil will not reverse the opioid-induced respiratory depression. It is completely devoid of cardiovascular side effects.

Metabolism of Flumazenil

Like BZDs, flumazenil is also rapidly taken by the liver from plasma and is metabolized to N-desmethyl flumazenil

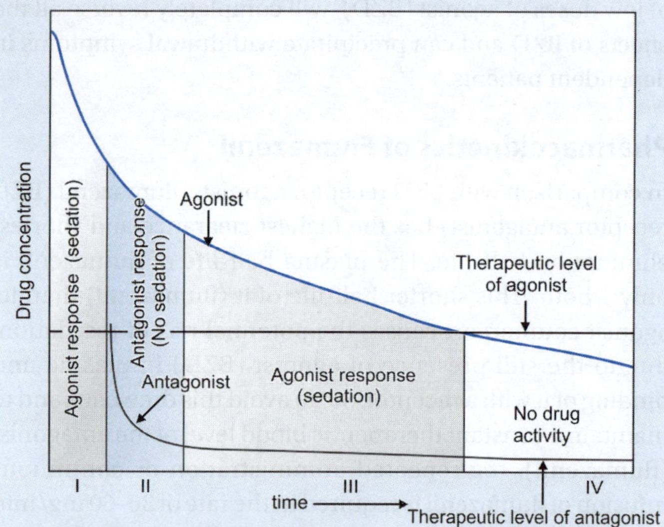

Fig. 17: The interaction between the duration of action of the short-acting antagonist and the long-acting agonist, causing resedation. The above agonist curve shows the gradual disappearance of agonist from blood. The below antagonist curve shows the gradual disappearance of the antagonist from the blood. This agonist–antagonist interaction is represented by four conditions:
I: Full agonistic response or sedation. In this phase, antagonist is not administered.
II: Full antagonistic response or awake from sedation. In this phase, antagonist is administered and the plasma level of both the agonist and antagonist is above their respective therapeutic level. Patient awakes from sedation, because the antagonist completely blocks the action of the agonist.
III: Reagonist response or resedation. This is because the plasma level of antagonist goes below its therapeutic level, but the plasma level of the agonist still remains above its therapeutic level.
IV: No drug effect, with the disappearance of both the action of the agonist and antagonist. This is because the plasma level of both drugs go below their respective therapeutic level.

and N-desmethyl flumazenil which are later conjugated to glucuronic acid and excreted through bile and urine.

Uses and Doses of Flumazenil

Flumazenil is successfully used to reverse the effect of sedation, respiratory depression, and amnesia, produced by BZDs during the practice of anesthesia and BZD poisoning. The dose of flumazenil varies with the particular type of BZD, being reversed. The duration of reversal is dependent on both the kinetics of the agonist (BZD) and antagonist (flumazenil). To prevent resedation, caused by longer-acting BZDs, flumazenil may be administered by continuous infusion. The useful dose of flumazenil is 0.1–0.2 mg which is repeated up to a total 1–3 mg over 1–3 minutes. This dose is usually sufficient to abolish the effects of therapeutic doses of BZDs; however the administration of a series of small doses of flumazenil is preferred to a single bolus injection of it.

For diagnostic purpose, the flumazenil may be given in incremental doses of 0.2–0.5 mg through IV (maximum up to 3 mg) over 2–10 minutes. If there is no change in sedation, then it is unlikely that CNS depression is based solely on BZD overdose.

Flumazenil is not effective in the treatment of overdose by either barbiturates or tricyclic antidepressants. To the contrary, under such circumstances, the administration of flumazenil may be associated with the seizures. The risk of seizures is especially high in patients, poisoned with tricyclic antidepressants.

■ OPIOIDS

History

Opium has been known to mankind for many centuries. It was first mentioned in Ebers Papyrus (1500 BC). Then, it was mentioned in the writing of Theophrastus (300 BC) and Galen (2nd century AD). On the other hand, crude opium was available in Asia from two millennium ago, before the discovery of modern anesthesia. It was used throughout the Middle Ages in Europe as a preparation, named "laudanum".

Crude opium is a dark, brown, resinous material that is obtained from the capsule of poppy (*Papaver somniferum*) fruit. It contains two types of alkaloids (1) alkaloids of phenanthrene derivatives which include morphine (10%), codeine (5%), and thebaine (0.2%) and (2) alkaloids of benzoisoquinoline derivatives which include papaverine (1%) and noscapine (6%). Among all these alkaloids, papaverine, noscapine, and thebaine are devoid of any analgesic activity, but papaverine causes smooth muscle relaxation. *Papaveretum* is a preparation of crude opium, containing water-soluble alkaloids of opium, (50% anhydrous morphine and the remaining 50% is a mixture of papaverine, codeine, and thebaine).

Opium eating was a social custom in China. Before 1840, oral opium was the mainstay of analgesia. The first step of success, for the introduction of opioids in anesthesia, was the isolation of morphine from opium by Serturner, in 1803. It was named "morphine" after the name of a Greek god of dreams named "Morpheus". After isolation, morphine was first given hypodermically, using a vaccination lancet, in 1836. Then, the introduction of syringe and hollow needle in clinical practice by Wood, in 1853, finally permitted opioids to be administered in more precisely measured doses.

Morphine was frequently injected at that time intramuscularly as premedication or as a supplement during ether or chloroform anesthesia or as postoperative analgesia. Then, in late 19th century, a high dose of morphine (3 mg/kg) with scopolamine was used as one complete anesthetic agent. After that, though this technique initially gain popularity, but rapidly again fell into disfavor for its high perioperative morbidity and mortality. So, for the next 30–40 years, anesthesiologists never used opioids. Later, the introduction of thiopentone, as an IV anesthetic agent and the introduction of the concept of balanced anesthesia led to renewed enthusiasm for the intraoperative use of opioids.

Diamorphine (heroin) was the first synthetic opioid that was synthesized in the laboratory, in 1875. This event marked the first chemical manipulation of natural opioids for the production of analgesia. Then, papaveretum was prepared, in 1909, as a pharmaceutically standardized preparation of crude opium. It was one of the first opiates to become available as solutions in ampoules.

The next important step, in the history of opioids, was the development of a completely synthetic opioid, named pethidine, in 1939 (meperidine) in Germany. Later, during World War II methadone was also developed in Germany and was originally named as "Dolophine" in the honor of Adolf Hitler. Then, fentanyl and alfentanil were produced, in 1962. Sufentanil followed soon after this.

Opioid receptors, which are peptides in nature, were also first discovered in 1979. The word "opium" is derived from the term "opos". This is a Greek word that means juice. So, the opium means drugs that are obtained from "opos" or juice of poppy capsule. The term *"opioids"* (which literally means opium-like) is used to describe the drugs (irrespective of their chemical structure and nature) that specifically bind to any of the several subtypes of opioid receptor and share the same pharmacological properties of morphine (opium), whereas the compounds which are derived from opium or are chemically related to morphine are called *"opiates".* They may not have morphine-like action. The term "narcotic" is derived from the Greek word for stupor. At one time the term "narcotic" was referred to as any drug that induced sleep and then it (the term "narcotic") became associated with opioids, but now it is often used in the legal context to refer varieties of substances that have abuse or addictive potential. They may be opioids or not.

Classification

Opioids are usually classified into two groups (1) according to their availability and (2) mode of action.

According to their Availability

- *Naturally occurring:* These include morphine and codeine.
- *Semisynthetic:* These include codeine, heroin (diacetylmorphine), dihydromorphine, thebaine derivatives (etorphine and buprenorphine), pholcodine, ethylmorphine, hydromorphone, oxymorphone, hydrocodone, and oxycodone.

These semisynthetic products are obtained from morphine by the following several changes:

- Esterification of one hydroxyl group of morphine results in *codeine* (methyl morphine).
- Esterification of both the hydroxyl group of morphine results in *heroin,* (it is diacetylmorphine, made from morphine by acetylation at 3 and 6 position).
- Reduction of the double bond in the benzene ring of morphine results in *hydromorphone.*
- Thebaine differs from morphine in that both the hydroxyl groups of it are methylated and the ring has two double bonds. It is an inactive opium derivative. It is the precursor of several clinically used compounds such as *oxymorphone, oxycodone,* and *naloxone.* Etorphine which is a thebaine derivative, is thousand times more potent than morphine and is used for immobilization and anesthesia in wildlife management **(Figs. 18A to D)**.
- *Completely synthetic:*
  - *Morphinan series:* Levorphanol and butorphanol
  - *Diphenylpropylamine series:* Methadone
  - *Benzomorphinan series:* Pentazocine
  - *Phenylpiperidine series:* Meperidine, fentanyl, sufentanil, alfentanil, and remifentanil.

Many of these synthetic opioids are used experimentally for analgesia and anesthesia. But only the morphinan, benzomorphinan, and phenylpiperidine series are used clinically and play an important role in anesthesia.

Classification of opioid compounds is enumerated in **Box 4**.

According to their Mode of Action on Opioid Receptor (Figs. 18A to D)

- *Agonists:* They produce full morphine-like physiological effect in a dose-dependent manner. They act on one or two or all types of opioid receptors and do not block (antagonist) any type of opioid receptor, e.g., morphine, pethidine (meperidine), fentanyl, and its congeners.
- *Mixed agonists and antagonists:* They act as an agonist at one type of opioid receptor and as an antagonist (block) at another type of opioid receptor, e.g., pentazocine and nalbuphine. These are further classified into two:
  1. *μ antagonist + κ agonist:* Nalorphine, pentazocine, butorphanol, nalbuphine, and levallorphan
  2. *μ agonist + κ antagonist:* Buprenorphine
- *Pure antagonists:* They act competitively and displace the agonists from their receptors by attaching with it (receptor), while they (antagonists) attach with their receptor, they elicited no or little effect on their own at clinical doses (intrinsic effect), e.g., naloxone, naltrexone, and nalmefene.

BOX 4: Classification of opioid compounds.

- *Natural occurring:*
  - Codeine (methyl morphine)
  - Morphine
- *Semisynthetic:*
  - Heroin (diacetylmorphine)
  - Codeine* and pholcodine
  - Ethyl morphine
  - Thebaine derivatives (e.g., etorphine and buprenorphine)
  - Hydromorphone, di-hydromorphone, oxymorphone, hydrocodone, and oxycodone
- *Synthetic:*
  - Morphinan series (e.g., levorphanol and butorphanol)
  - Phenylpiperidine series (e.g., meperidine, fentanyl, sufentanil, alfentanil, and remifentanil)
  - Benzomorphan series (e.g., pentazocine)
  - Diphenylpropylamine series (e.g., methadone)
  - Dextromoramide and dipipanone

*codeine is obtained both by naturally and by synthesis

Phenylpiperidine skeletal

Meperidine

Fentanyl

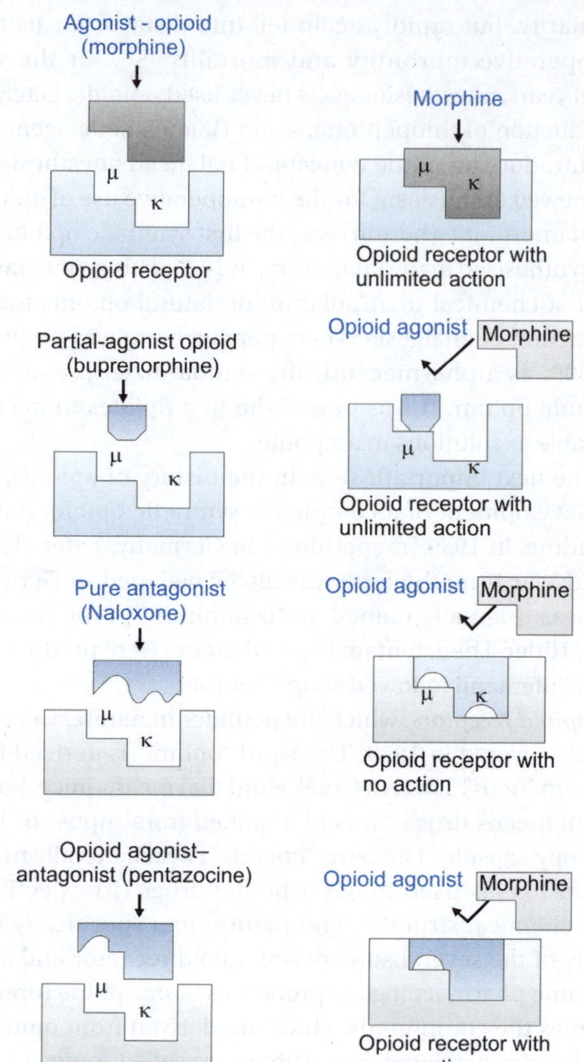

Figs. 18 A to D: Opioid receptor interactions with agonist, partial agonist, mixed agonist and antagonist, and antagonist at two receptor sites (1) mu (μ) and (2) kappa (κ). (A) A pure opioid agonist stimulates both the μ and κ receptor and analgesic action is unlimited; (B) A partial opioid agonist only combines with the μ-receptor with limited analgesic activity. κ-site remains unoccupied. It also prevents morphine to act; (C) An opioid antagonist occupies both the μ and κ receptors and prevents the agonist from to attach with the receptor but it has no intrinsic activity; and (D) The action of agonist and antagonist opioid which has mixed effect on μ- and κ-receptors. Analgesia is κ–receptor related, while blockade occurs at μ-receptors.

Opioid Receptor

In 1973, opioid receptors were first conceptualized from a hypothesis that all opioids act on some macromolecules, present on the cell membrane. These macromolecules are protein in nature and modulate pain, mood, hedonic (pleasure-related) behavior, motor behavior, emesis, pituitary hormone release, GIT motility, etc., however, later this hypothesis was confirmed and these macromolecules were described as opium receptor.

Morphine and all other opioids exert their action by interacting with these opioid receptors. Radioligand binding studies have divided this opioid receptor into three types (1) μ (mu), (2) κ (kappa), and (3) δ (delta) and each has its own specific pharmacological profile. They also have distinct pattern of anatomical distribution in the brain, spinal cord, and peripheral tissues. Three subtypes of each receptor have also been proposed, but have not yet been cloned **(Table 7)**.

- *μ (morphine or mu) receptor:* This receptor is named after the drug morphine which was used in the study of this receptor. This μ-opioid receptor manifests a high affinity for morphine, pethidine, fentanyl, and its congeners. On the other hand, other opioid peptides such as β-endorphin, enkephalins, and dynorphins also bind to this μ-receptor, but with low affinity. These μ-receptors are located both in the brain and spinal cord, with a highest concentration at the periaqueductal gray region, thalamus, nucleus tractus solitarius, nucleus

TABLE 7: Location of μ- and δ–receptors.

μ-receptor	δ-receptor	μ and δ receptor
Cortex (laminae I and IV)	Cortex (laminae II, III, and V)	Cortex (lamina IV)
Thalamus	Amygdala	Nucleus ambiguous
Hypothalamus	Olfactory tubercle	Nucleus tractus solitarius
Corpus striatum	Corpus striatum	Vagal fibers
Periaqueductal gray matter	Nucleus accumbens	Trigeminal nucleus
Hippocampus	Pontine nuclei	Substantia gelatinosa of the spinal cord
Colliculus (superior and inferior)		
Interpeduncular nucleus		
Midbrain		

TABLE 8: Nature of interactions of opioid ligands on the three major types of opioid receptors.

Opioids	μ (mu)	κ (kappa)	δ (delta)
Morphine	Ago (St)	Ago (W)	Ago (W)
Meperidine	Ago (St)	Ago (W)	Ago (W)
Pentazocine	P. ago, Anta (w)	Ago (W)	P. ago
Buprenorphine	P. ago	Ago (M)	P. ago
Butorphanol	P. ago	Anta (M)	Ago
Nalorphine	Anta (St)	Ago (St)	Not known
Nalbuphine	Anta (M)	Ago (M)	Ago
Naloxone	Anta (St)	Ago (M)	Anta (W)
Naltrexone	Anta (St)	Anta (M)	Anta (W)
Enkephalin	Ago (M)	Anta (St)	Ago (St)
β-endorphin	Ago (St)	–	Ago (St)
Levorphanol	Ago (St)	–	–
Fentanyl	Ago (St)	–	–
Sufentanil	Ago (St)	–	Ago (W)

(Ago = agonist; Anta: antagonist; M: moderate action; P. ago: partial agonist; St: strong action; W: weak action)

ambiguus, and substantia gelatinosa region of the brain. The stimulation of these μ-receptors causes analgesia, respiratory depression, euphoria, miosis, reduced GI motility, physical dependence, etc. The two subtypes of μ-receptor have been described. These are $μ_1$ and $μ_2$. Among these, the $μ_1$ has more affinity for morphine. It mediates supraspinal analgesia and can selectively be blocked by naloxonazine, whereas the $μ_2$-receptor has a lower affinity for morphine. It mediates spinal analgesia, respiratory depression, and constipation.

- *(Ketocyclazocine or kappa) receptor:* This receptor is named for its high affinity for ketocyclazocine drug which is used for the study of this κ-*receptor*. The activation of κ-receptor causes mild to moderate analgesia, ceiling respiratory depression, dysphoria, hallucination, miosis, sedation, physical dependence, etc. Two subtypes of κ-receptor such as $κ_1$ and $κ_3$ are functionally important. Analgesia caused by κ-agonists (opioids) is primarily spinal and acts through the $κ_1$ receptor. However, $κ_3$-receptors mediate supraspinal analgesia and are of lower ceiling character **(Table 8)**.

- δ *(delta) receptor:* This receptor has a high affinity for enkephalins and is present both in the spinal cord (dorsal horn) and brain (limbic area). The activation of this receptor causes analgesia, respiratory depression, affective behavior, reduced GI motility, etc. The δ-mediated analgesia is mainly spinal (as δ-receptors are present mainly in the dorsal horn of the spinal cord), but the affective component of supraspinal analgesia appears to involve the δ-receptor present in the limbic areas. They

are also responsible for dependence. The proconvulsant action is more prominent in δ-receptor agonists. The myenteric plexus neurons expresses a high density of δ-receptor which mediates reduced GI motility.

- σ *(sigma) receptor:* Now, it is no longer considered an opioid receptor, because it is neither activated by morphine nor blocked by naloxone. However, certain opioids such as pentazocine and butorphanol bind to σ-receptor. Certain effects such as dysphoria, psychotomimetic action, tachycardia, mydriasis, etc., caused by pentazocine-like drugs, are believed to be mediated by σ-receptor and are not reversed by naloxone **(Table 9)**.

Cellular Mechanism of Action of Opioid Receptor

All three types of opioid receptors (μ, κ, and δ) have been cloned and their functions are studied extensively. All these receptors have belonged to the family of G-protein coupled receptor. However, this group of opioid receptors constitutes about 80% of all the known G-protein coupled receptors family in our body which also includes muscarinic, adrenergic, GABA, and somatostatin receptors. The amino acid sequence of these opioid receptors is very similar to somatostatin receptors than other receptors. The opioid receptors have three parts such as extracellular, transmembrane, and intracellular. The amino acid sequences of these three opioid receptors (μ, κ, and δ) are

TABLE 9: Action of different types of opioid receptors.

μ (mu receptor)	κ (kappa receptor)	δ (delta receptor)
Analgesia: • μ_1-supraspinal • μ_2-spinal	*Analgesia:* • κ_3-supraspinal • κ_1-spinal	*Analgesia:* • No supraspinal • Only spinal
Respiratory depression (μ_2)	Respiratory depression	Respiratory depression
Euphoria	Dysphoria, hallucination	Affective behavior
Miosis	Miosis	Do not cause miosis
Reduced GI motility	Do not reduce GI motility	Reduced GI motility
Sedation	Sedation	Do not cause sedation
Physical dependence	Physical dependence	Do not cause physical dependence

TABLE 10: Receptor subtypes and action of various opioids.

Functions	Receptor subtypes	Actions	
		Agonist	**Antagonist**
Analgesia: • Supraspinal • Spinal	• μ, κ, and δ • μ, κ, and δ	• Analgesic • Analgesic	• No effect • No effect
Respiratory depression	μ	Decrease	No effect
GI tract	μ, κ	Decrease motility	No effect
Psychomimetic	κ	Increase	No effect
Sedation	μ, κ	Increase	No effect
Diuresis	κ	Increase	
Hormone regulation: • Prolactin • Growth hormone	• μ • μ and/or δ	• Increase • Increase	• Decrease • Decrease
Neurotransmitter release: • Acetylcholine • Dopamine	• μ • μ, δ	• Inhibit • Inhibit	

60% identical, and greater similarities among them exist in the transmembrane and intracellular part of them. However, the specific amino acid sequence in the extracellular part of these opioid receptors is the key factor in determining the ligand-specific action.

The opioid molecules exert their actions by modulating synaptic transmission through opioid receptors by both presynaptic (indirect) and postsynaptic (direct) facilitatory and inhibitory actions. Inhibitory action is mediated by Gi/Go protein and excitatory effect is mediated by Gs protein. G-protein coupled receptors are situated mostly on the prejunctional neurons. They generally exercise inhibitory modulation by decreasing the release of the junctional transmitter. Various monoadrenergic [norepinephrine (NA), DA, and 5-HT], GABA, and glutamate (NMDA) pathways are also intricately involved in opioid actions **(Table 10)**.

Opioid receptor-activated G-protein effector system can also be divided into two categories (1) short-term effectors, acting through K^+ and Ca^{2+} channels and (2) long-term effectors, acting through cyclic adenosine monophosphate (cAMP) and adenylyl cyclase system. All opioid receptors inhibit the opening of the Ca^{2+} channel and activate the K^+ channel. Thus, the decrease in intracellular Ca^{2+} influx can inhibit the mobilization of neurotransmitter with the inhibition of release of it and become a component of the mechanism of opioid-induced analgesia. The K^+ channel effect results in the hyperpolarization of the neuronal membrane and decreases synaptic transmission by inhibiting the release of neurotransmitter. The changes in cAMP may underline the opioid-induced modulation of the release of neurotransmitter, such as substance P.

Mechanism of Analgesia

The opioids, when are used systemically, act through many higher CNS centers such as the amygdala, mesencephalic reticular formation, periaqueductal gray matter (PAG), and rostral ventral medulla, but the role of these higher centers of the brain, containing opioid receptor in opioid analgesia, is still in controversy. The action of opioids at PAG results in impulses that modulate the degree of inhibition, coming from different neuronal pools, and contribute in reducing the transmission of nociceptive (perception of pain) information from peripheral nerves to the spinal cord. The rostral ventromedial region of the medulla also modulates the transmission of nociceptive information in the dorsal horn of the spinal cord. Opioid action at PAG controls this region of the medulla by direct neural connection. Thus, the opioids by systemic administration activate the total analgesic system in CNS **(Fig. 19)**.

Spinal opioids, given through the spinal or epidural route, produce analgesia by their direct action on the spinal cord only at their level of administration. Substantia gelatinosa of the spinal cord possess dense collection of opiate receptors (μ, κ, and δ), and the direct application of opioid to these receptors of the spinal cord creates intense analgesia by their action at the presynaptic level, by reducing the release of substance P from the cells of substantia gelatinosa. Opioid in the spinal cord also acts on the opioid receptors

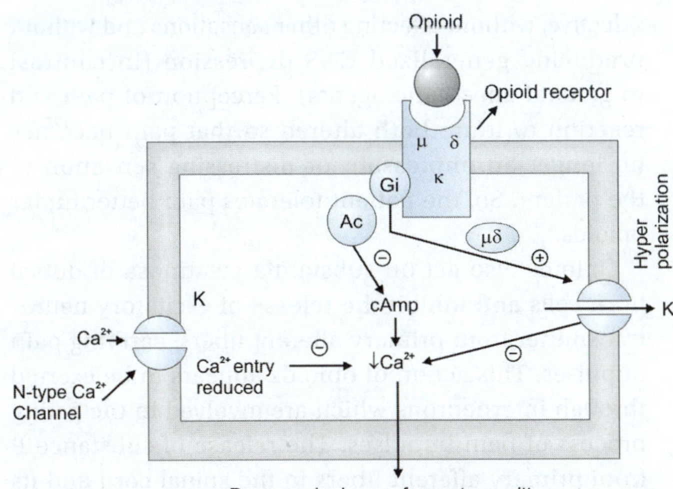

Fig. 19: All these three types of opioid receptors (μ, κ, and δ exercise inhibition and decrease the release of junctional neurotransmitter. Various monoaminergic pathways such as NA, DA, 5-HT, GABA, and glutamate (NMDA) pathways are intrinsically involved in opioid actions. Opioid receptor activation reduces intracellular cAMP formation. It also opens K⁺ channel mainly through μ and δ receptors. It also suppresses the voltage-gated N type of Ca²⁺ channel, mainly through κ receptors. All these actions result in hyperpolarization and reduced availability of intracellular Ca²⁺. Thus, it causes a decrease in the release of neurotransmitter from the CNS and myenteric neurons and blocks the pain pathway. (cAMP: cyclic adenosine monophosphate; CNS: central nervous system; DA: dopamine; GABA: gamma-aminobutyric acid; NA: norepinephrine; NMDA: N-methyl-D-aspartate; 5-HT: 5-hydroxytryptamine)

of dorsal horn cells and inhibits the sharp pain stimulation, conducted by the A-δ fibers. At the dorsal horn cells, opioids also block the excitatory postsynaptic potential summation of pain transmission and thus inhibit the dull persistent pain sensation, transmitted via the C fibers. This summation is much easier to block before the pain occurs than to treat. This concept explains why preemptive analgesia is more effective than analgesia after stimulation. Opioids also modulate the pain sensation by preventing the excitatory threshold reduction at the dorsal horn cells.

By some peripheral mechanisms, acting outside the CNS, opioids also produce analgesia. At the periphery, the opioid receptors are located at the nerve terminals of the presynaptic afferent neurons and the immune cells, infiltrating the inflamed tissues and producing endogenous opioids for peripheral opioid receptors. Opioids act on these receptors at the periphery and produce analgesia. Opioid agonists also produce local anesthetic-like effect on the surface of excitable cell membrane and reduce pain. Serotonergic (5-HT) and monoadrenergic pathways may also take part in opioid-mediated analgesia. Some opioids also act through GABA$_A$ receptors such as BZD and barbiturates.

The concentration of opioid receptors and the proportion of its subtypes can change with age and this explains the variation of pain sensitivity with age. Certain opioids can have a duration of action that extends beyond its plasma half-life and it is because of a high affinity of these drugs to μ-receptor, for example, buprenorphine has a very high affinity for μ-receptor and a very slower dissociation rate from it, which explains the cause for difficulty in reversing its respiratory depression effect by naloxone.

The other parts of CNS which also contain opioid receptors are basal ganglia, limbic area, etc., and they are responsible for the action of endogenous opiates. Cardiovascular system also contains opioid receptors which are responsible for receptor-mediated opioid's actions in myocardial ischemia, shock, and other cardiovascular events.

Endogenous Opioids

In 1970, a number of peptides that also have an affinity for opioid receptors (μ, κ, and δ) and have morphine-like actions were isolated from the brain, spinal cord, plasma, GIT, and placenta. So, it was hypothesized that these peptides constitute an endogenous opiate system that normally modulates the pain perception, mood, hedonic (pleasure-related) behavior, motor behavior, emesis, pituitary hormone release, GIT motility, diuresis, modulation of respiratory responses to stimuli and drugs, reduction of stress, etc. These endogenous opioid peptides are active in very small amounts and their actions can also be blocked by naloxone. These endogenous opioid peptides are classified into three different families and each is derived from a distinct large precursor polypeptide. These three families of endogenous opioid system are (1) *endorphin family*, (2) *encephalin family*, and *dynorphin family*.

Endorphins (Endorphin Family)

There are many endorphins in this family, but β-endorphin (β-END) is the most important, among all these endorphins, in this family. It has 31 amino acids and *proopiomelanocortin* is its precursor. This precursor is cleaved to form ACTH and β-lipotropin (β-LPH). Then, β-LPH is again cleaved to form β-END and other endorphins. The highest concentration of β-END occurs in the pituitary gland, and in medial, basal, and arcuate regions of hypothalamus. However, the presence of β-END in the spinal cord is debatable. Outside CNS, the β-END exists in GIT, placenta, and plasma.

Enkephalins (Enkephalin Family)

The most important enkephalins are methionine–enkephalin (met–ENK) and leucine–enkephalin (leu–ENK). They are penta peptides. *Proenkephalin* is the precursor of met-ENK. The *prodynorphin* is the precursor of leu-ENK and dynorphin. The enkephalins are widely distributed in many areas of CNS such as the amygdala, globus pallidus, striatum, hypothalamus, thalamus, brain stem, and dorsal horns that receive afferent nociceptive information. Enkephalins have also been isolated in the peripheral nervous system such as peripheral ganglia, ANS, adrenal medulla, GIT, and plasma. Enkephalins may also elicit analgesia through the modulation of the release of substance P from dorsal horn cells.

Dynorphins (Dorphin Family)

The prodynorphins are the precursor of dynorphins and are found in hypothalamic–neurohypophyseal axis. Dynorphin functions primarily as neuromodulators in CNS by interacting with μ, δ, and κ-receptors. Dynorphin also appears to be distributed in other areas of CNS which are relevant to nociception, such as the periaqueductal grey region, limbic system, thalamus, dorsal horn of the spinal cord, etc. Dynorphin is thought to play a more important role for nociception at the spinal cord level (by activation of κ-receptor) than in the brain. It may also control centrally the function of CVS.

A functional interaction (correlation) occurs between the nociception and the level of endogenous opioids. The preliminary processing of afferent nociceptive (painful) information (impulses) first occurs at the dorsal horn cells of the spinal cord. Both endogenous opioids such as dynorphins and enkephalins are active in these areas. Then the second processing station for nociception resides in the midbrain, brainstem, and thalamus. High concentration of dynorphins, enkephalins, and β-endorphin can be found in these areas. Higher brain centers such as the limbic system, amygdala, and cortex where final processing of pain occur and are involved in affective dimensions of pain, contain a significant population of neurons where dynorphin, enkephalin, and β-endorphins are found.

■ PHARMACOLOGICAL ACTIONS OF OPIOIDS
Pharmacodynamics of Opioids
Neurophysiological Actions of Opioids

- *Analgesia:* The dull and visceral pain than the somatic pain is better relieved by opioids. The nociceptive impulses (pain impulses) arising from the peripheral receptor is better relieved than neurotic pain, arising from neural structure, due to its damage. The other associated reactions to intense pain such as apprehension, fear, autonomic effects, etc., are also reduced by opioids. Suppression of pain perception by opioids is also selective, without affecting other sensations and without producing generalized CNS depression (in contrast to general anesthetic agents). Perception of pain and reaction to it are both altered so that pain becomes no longer an unpleasant or distressing sensation to the patient. So, the patient tolerates pain better under opioids.

  Opioids also act on substantia gelatinosa of dorsal horn cells and inhibit the release of excitatory neurotransmitter from primary afferent fibers, carrying pain impulses. This action of opioids appears to be exerted through interneurons which are involved in the gating process of pain impulses. The release of substance P from primary afferent fibers in the spinal cord and its postsynaptic action on dorsal horn neurons is also inhibited by opioids. The action of opioids at supraspinal sites such as the medulla, midbrain, limbic system, and cortical areas may also alter the processing and interpretation of pain impulses, as well as send inhibitory impulses through descending pathways to the spinal cord. Several aminergic (NA and DA) and other neuronal (5-HT, GABA, NMDA, etc.) systems also appear to be involved in the action of opioids. Simultaneous, action at spinal and supraspinal sites greatly amplifies the analgesic action of opioids.

- *Sedation:* Sedation or hypnosis, produced by opioids, is different from sedation and hypnosis produced by other sedatives or hypnotics such as BZD and barbiturates. This difference is that the drowsiness and indifference to the surroundings as well as to his own body, produced by opioids, occurs without any motor incoordination, ataxia, or apparent excitement (in contrast to alcohol). Opioids have a weaker amnestic effect compared to propofol, barbiturates, midazolam, or other BZDs.

- *Mood and subjective effects:* Opioids relieve anxiety and produce calmness. It causes a loss of apprehension and a lack of initiative. Limbs feel heavy. It causes transient flushing and hot sensation, due to the release of histamine. There is mental clouding and an inability to concentrate. Patients who are suffering from pain, anxiety, and those who are addicted, perceive it as a great pleasure. It produces euphoria or dysphoria.

- *Cetirizine (CTZ):* Nausea and vomiting can result from opioids. It especially occurs, if the stomach is full and the patient stands or moves. The mechanism of action of nausea and vomiting, produced by opioids, is due to the sensitization of the CTZ center by vestibular and other impulses.

- *Edinger–Westphal (EW) nucleus:* Opioids stimulate the EW nucleus or release cortical inhibition on it and thus produce miosis. However, no miosis is found by the topical application of opioids on the conjunctiva. It proves that the miosis, caused by opioids, is completely due to the central mechanism of action.

- *Other cortical areas and hippocampal cells:* The excitation of CNS by opioids is seen in some individuals. This is due to the stimulation of some cortical areas and hippocampal cells by it (opioids). So, opioids have no anticonvulsant action, rather they may precipitate it. Muscular rigidity is another feature of opioids. The proconvulsion action of opioids also has been ascribed, due to the inhibition of the release of GABA inhibitory neurotransmitter from hippocampal interneurons.
- *EEG changes:* The neurophysiological changes produced by large doses of opioids and inhaled anesthetic agents are different. In contrast to *gradual* burst suppression and ultimately a flat EEG, which is found as the effect of inhalational anesthetic agents; a *ceiling effect* is reached by opioids. Once the ceiling effect has been reached then the subsequent increased dose of opioid does not affect the EEG. Low doses of opioids produce minimal changes in EEG. Higher doses result in high voltage (δ-delta) waves, suggesting a state of consistent with anesthesia. The transient, isolated (not generalized) sharp wave activity is also seen after large doses of opioids.
- *Neuroprotection effect:* The role of opioids in neuroprotection is controversial.
- *Cerebral blood flow:* Opioids decrease (10–25%) cerebral metabolic rate and ICP, by causing cerebral vasoconstriction.
- *Neuroexcitatory phenomenon:* Opioids cause neuroexcitatory phenomenon, ranging from delirium to grand mal seizure-like activity. Opioids also cause other types of neuroexcitation ranging from nystagmus to only flexion or extension of a single extremity to a repetitive clonic–tonic activity. Initially, on IV injection opioids frequently stimulate coughing, which is of brief duration. This is followed by suppression of cough. Meperidine is notorious for its CNS excitability. However, the mechanism of neuroexcitability, caused by meperidine, is unique which is described here. It is related to its N-demethylation metabolite, named *normeperidine,* which is twice as likely to cause CNS excitation and convulsion as meperidine and has half the analgesic potency. The CNS adverse effects associated with meperidine include disorientation, hallucination, tremors, twitching, myoclonus, psychosis, and seizures. The treatment of CNS excitability, produced by meperidine, is supportive and includes cessation of administration of meperidine, substitution with another opioids for analgesia, and administration of BZD for

signs and symptoms of CNS irritability. For the treatment of CNS excitability, caused by opioids, naloxone should be avoided, because it can further precipitate seizure by unmasking the excitatory effects when depressant effects are antagonized (inhibited). Normeperidine has a long elimination half-life (15–40 hours) and is excreted via the kidney after its hydrolysis to normeperidinic acid which is inactive.

The probable mechanisms for the neuroexcitatory phenomenon of opioids are:

- The opioids cause an increase in the excitatory glutamate activated current.
- They change in central catecholamine concentration through dopaminergic pathways.
- The opioids cause an increase in the release of excitatory neurotransmitter such as met-enkephalin and leu-enkephalin, which possess epileptogenic property.
- The opioids cause disinhibition of pyramidal cells of the hippocampus.
- More recent work suggests that certain excitatory actions of opioids may be related to their coupling to mitogen-activated protein kinase cascades **(Box 5)**.

If opioids are anesthetics?

It is a debatable question for many years and still now is not resolved. High incidences of awareness, during large doses of only opioid anesthesia highlighted this potential problem. Unconsciousness, defined by unresponsiveness to verbal command, can be produced with opioids but is very unpredictable and inconsistent. On the other hand, all the opioids cause reduction of MAC value of inhaled anesthetic agents. Thus, the potency ratio of fentanyl/sufentanil/alfentanil/remifentanil, which is based on MAC reduction, is approximately 1:12:1/16:1.2. Opioid's analgesic effects reach a ceiling that is subanesthetic. The exact mechanism of opioids for amnesia and anesthesia is in doubt. The ability of opioids to produce full analgesia

BOX 5: Factors responsible for intraoperative awareness.

- No premedication
- Obstetric anesthesia
- Improper anesthetic plan
- Excessive use of muscle relaxants
- Inadequate use of analgesic
- Morbidly obese patient
- American Society of Anesthesiologists (ASA) grade III and IV, where less-anesthetic drugs are used
- Prolonged time for intubation
- Cardiac surgery
- Laryngoscopy, bronchoscopy, etc.

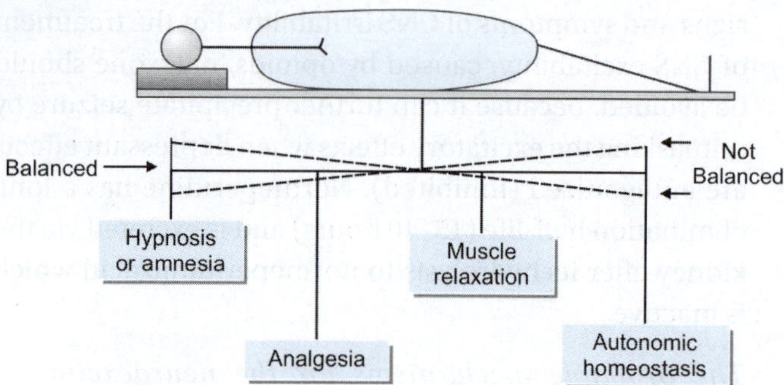

Fig. 20: Four components of a balanced anesthesia.

in subanesthetic concentration and loss of consciousness in higher concentration may be mediated by different mechanisms. A dual mechanism for the anesthetic effect of opioids has been proposed in addition to receptor-mediated effects which are responsible for the analgesic effects of opioids **(Fig. 20)**.

Intraoperative awareness is defined as "spontaneous recall of events occurring during GA and surgery". The conscious recollection of this intraoperative memory is called *explicit memory*. When the patient cannot recollect its intraoperative memory in a conscious state, then this intraoperative awareness is called *implicit memory*. Usually, an auditory function is left largely intact by opioids and is responsible for awareness during anesthesia. The overall incidence of intraoperative awareness is 1%. There are also other factors that are responsible for intraoperative awareness. Clinically, intraoperative awareness is monitored by motor and autonomic function. Motor functions, during anesthesia such as eyelid motion, coughing, movements of limbs, facial grimacing, etc., are the signs of inadequate amnesia, whereas autonomic functions during anesthesia such as hypertension, tachycardia, mydriasis, tearing, sweating, and salivation indicate a light level of anesthesia. The monitoring of muscular activity, as an indicator of awareness is useful because muscle movements usually occur before awareness occurs. Central nervous system activity also can be measured by auditory evoked response and EEG. Raw EEG has limited value for awareness monitoring. Bispectral analysis (it is a mathematical power spectrum analysis of EEG) obtains an index number, after using processed EEG and correlates well with sedation or anesthesia by hypnotic or anesthetic drugs, but not by opioids. Opioids do not alter BIS, except in high doses.

- *Muscle rigidity:* Opioids often increase muscle tone and produce muscular rigidity. Sometimes, this may progress to severe stiffness. The incidence of it may vary from 0 to 100%. In a conscious state, this rigidity is often manifested

as hoarseness of voice. Clinically, the significant opioid-induced muscular rigidity begins usually after the patient loses consciousness. Rigidity of abdominal and/or thoracic muscles (wooden chest syndrome) impairs both spontaneous and controlled ventilation in a nonparalyzed patient. Rigidity of chest muscles causes ↓pulmonary compliance, ↓functional residual capacity (FRC), ↓ventilation, hypercarbia, hypoxemia, etc. It also causes ↑CVP, ↑PAP, and ↑PVR. Rigidity also causes ↑ICP and ↑O_2 consumption. The rigidity and abnormal muscle movement may also occasionally occur during the emergence from opioid anesthesia. This abnormal muscle movement ranges from only flexion or extension of a single extremity to multiple tonic–clonic movements of the whole body.

The precise mechanism for this opioid-induced abnormal muscle movement and muscular rigidity is not known, however the probable hypothesis are (1) alteration of dopamine concentration within the striatum area of the brain by opioids and (2) stimulation of GABAergic interneurons.

- *Pruritus:* The exact mechanism of opioid-induced pruritus is not known, but definitely, it is not due to the release of histamine or allergic manifestation by opioids which was previously thought, because naloxone reverses this pruritus and confirmed the opioid receptor-mediated central mechanism of action of it. Face, particularly the nose is the most common site for the opioid-induced pruritus. Nasal scratching may stimulate ventilation and counter the opioid-induced respiratory depression. This may be the mechanism why the nose is the most common site for pruritus, induced by opioids. Pruritus on nose, by spinal opioid, may also be due to opioid-triggered neural transmission at the distant sites.

- *Thermoregulation and shivering:* Shivering is a common phenomenon in patients, recovering from anesthesia. Its physiological role is to produce heat, but its occurrence in relation to anesthesia is inconsistent and is incompletely understood. Nevertheless, postoperative shivering can cause several undesirable physiological consequences. These are an increase in O_2 consumption, increase in CO_2 production, ↑in minute ventilation, ↑in CO, ↓in mixed venous O_2 saturation, and difficulty to measure O_2 saturation of hemoglobin (Hb) by pulse oximetry. Opioid ligands and their receptors have a great functional role in thermoregulation, for example, μ-receptor stimulation produces hyperthermia, whereas κ-receptor agonists result in hypothermia. Opioids like inhaled anesthetic agents also reduce thermoregulatory threshold and cause shivering.

Meperidine is unique among all opioids in its ability to effectively terminate or at least attenuate shivering in approximately 70–80% of patients. Shivering related to blood transfusion can also be controlled with meperidine. Usually, 25–50 mg slow IV administration of meperidine is effective; however in the presence of an opioid antagonist larger dose of meperidine may be necessary. Intravenous fentanyl, sufentanil, and morphine are not as effective as meperidine to reduce this postoperative shivering. The cause of this underlying difference and the mechanism for the ability of opioids to attenuate shivering is unclear. Meperidine administered spinally or epidurally is also effective in treating shivering that occurs during epidural anesthesia.

Action of Opioids on Respiratory System

All the opioids, stimulating μ-receptors cause dose-dependent depression of respiration. This is because a high concentration of opioid receptors is found in supraspinal respiratory centers, such as nucleus solitarius, nucleus retroambigualis, and nucleus ambiguus. Opioids also depress the respiratory rate through pontine and medullary respiratory center, because endogenous opioid receptors are also present in high concentration in the brain stem nuclei, regulating respiration. Opioid-induced effects on respiratory rate and respiratory pattern include delays in expiration, long respiratory pauses, irregular and/or periodic breathing, apnea, and decreased tidal volume. Prolonged expiratory pause, induced by opioids, causes a greater reduction in the respiratory rate than in the tidal volume **(Fig. 21)**.

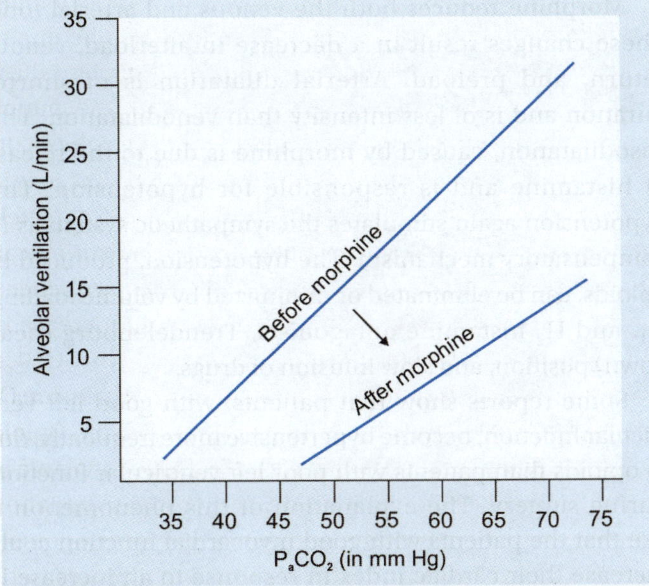

Fig. 21: The displacement or shifting of the CO$_2$ curve downward and to the right after the use of morphine. (CO$_2$: carbon dioxide; PaCO$_2$: partial pressure of arterial carbon dioxide)

The stimulating effect of CO$_2$ on ventilation is significantly reduced by opioids. Resting partial pressure of carbon dioxide (pCO$_2$) in plasma increases and the ventilatory response to CO$_2$ challenge is blunted, resulting in the shift of CO$_2$ response curve downward and to the right. These effects are mediated through respiratory centers in the brain stem. The apneic threshold, i.e., highest partial pressure of arterial carbon dioxide (PaCO$_2$) at which a patient remains still apneic, is elevated. Opioids also decrease the carotid body chemoreceptor and hypoxic ventilatory drive. High doses of opioids can eliminate spontaneous respiration, without producing unconsciousness. So, the patient will still follow the verbal command and often breathe when directed to do so. Gender differences may exist in these effects, with women demonstrating more respiratory depression by opioids.

Opioids decrease pain and anxiety-induced hyperventilation and thus prevent respiratory alkalosis, though large doses of opioids decrease pulmonary compliance and impair ventilation due to thoracic muscular rigidity and respiratory depression effect. On the other hand, opioid analgesic therapy improves breathing, by alleviating pain and decreasing voluntary muscle tone, related to pain which results in improved dynamic of total respiratory compliance.

Opioids, especially dextromethorphan, have centrally-mediated antitussive action, but are not necessarily linked to respiratory depression. Again, cough may be precipitated after IV bolus opioids. It is due to the stimulation of irritant receptors in tracheal smooth muscles; however this cough is not vagally mediated because atropine pretreatment does not affect it. Pretreatment with inhaled β-adrenergic agonists significantly reduces this incidence of cough, associated with IV opioids injection.

Opioids blunt the somatic and autonomic responses, during tracheal intubation, by depressing the upper airway and tracheal reflexes. Thus, it allows the patient to tolerate endotracheal (ET) tube better, without coughing and bucking. Hence, during emergence from GA where the patient was anesthetized only with potent inhalational agents and no opioid, routinely cough and buck, prior to regaining consciousness, whereas when the patients are adequately treated with opioids, then they can awake without such disturbances, even while they are still intubated. Morphine and meperidine can cause histamine-induced bronchospasm in susceptible patients. Although opioids can affect the contractile responses of airway smooth muscles, but the clinical significance and relevance of these opioid-induced effects on airway resistance remain controversial, because opioids can also help by avoiding increases in bronchomotor tone in asthma. Opioids can decrease airway smooth muscle tone and have long been used in the management of asthma. Fentanyl has antimuscarinic, antihistaminergic, and antiserotoninergic actions. So, it may be more effective than morphine in patients with asthma or other bronchospastic diseases.

Certain IV anesthetic agents, including opioids, minimally alter the pulmonary function of gas exchange. The minimal impact of opioids on the hypoxic pulmonary vasoconstriction effect (in contrast to the effect of the potent inhaled anesthetics), associated hemodynamic stability, and the stability of bronchomotor tone, all contribute to minimal interference with pulmonary gas exchange which is observed after the use of opioids and many other IV anesthetic agents.

Factors affecting the opioid-induced respiratory depression:
- *Dose:* Opioids cause dose-dependent respiratory depression and have no ceiling effect.
- *Sleep:* Sleeping patients are more sensitive to opioids and sleep apnea is an additional risk factor.
- *Old age:* Respiration of an aged patient is more sensitive to opioids for depression and its probable causes are decreased clearance, increased elimination half-life, and increased brain sensitivity.
- *Neonates:* Neonates are more sensitive to morphine on the basis of weight than adults. Low lipid solubility of morphine limits its penetration to blood–brain barriers. But in neonates and infants, morphine easily penetrates the brain and this is due to immature blood–brain barriers which make the neonates and infants more sensitive to morphine than adults. On the other hand, children are not more sensitive to more lipid-soluble opioids (meperidine, fentanyl, and sufentanil) because the penetration of these drugs into the brain is not affected by blood–brain barrier maturity, but depends on their lipid solubility.
- *Other CNS depressants:* Potent inhaled anesthetic agents, alcohol, barbiturates, BZDs, etc., potentiate the respiratory depression action of opioids, however exceptions are droperidol and clonidine.
- *Pain:* Pain counters the respiratory depression effects of opioids.
- Hyperventilation with hypocarbia enhances the activity of opioids. On the other hand, hypercarbia has the opposite effect, however the possible explanation of this response is the increased unionized state of opioids with hypocarbia which facilities its brain penetration and vice versa.

Action of Opioids on the Cardiovascular System

The opioids not only provide analgesia but also promote stable hemodynamic conditions both in the presence and absence of noxious stimuli. Large doses of opioids, administered as the sole primary anesthetic agent, result in a stable hemodynamic situation throughout the operative period. The close association between the distribution of opioid receptors, cardiovascular regulatory centers (nucleus solitarius, dorsal vagal nucleus, nucleus ambiguous, and parabrachial nucleus), and autonomic regulatory center in CNS, explain the cause of this stable hemodynamic condition by opioids. Endogenous opioid peptides are also associated with the sympathetic and parasympathetic centers in the brain, and also control cardiovascular function. Different opioid receptors, occupying the ventrolateral portion of the periaqueductal gray region of the brain which is the key central site for analgesia also affect hemodynamic control.

The activation of the μ-opioid receptor suppresses the somatosympathetic reflexes which are transmitted by unmyelinated C-afferent fibers at the level of the spinal cord and modulate them at the brain stem. These actions also contribute to anesthetic capabilities of opioids. Opioids thus modulate the stress responses by their action on the hypothalamic–pituitary–adrenal axis. Most opioids reduce sympathetic tone and enhance vagal tone. The ablation of sympathetic tone can occur by all modern opioids.

The direct actions of opioids on the myocardium are significantly less than other IV and inhalational anesthetic agents. However, the direct effects of different opioids on myocardial contractility are different and controversial. Meperidine has been reported to produce decreased, increased, or mixed effects on myocardial contractility. On the other hand, morphine has a positive inotropic effect. However, most hemodynamic variables including HR, BP, CO, SVR, PVR, etc., usually remain unchanged after fentanyl, sufentanil, and remifentanil.

Morphine reduces both the venous and arterial tone. These changes result in a decrease in afterload, venous return, and preload. Arterial dilatation is of shorter duration and is of less intensity than venodilatation. This vasodilatation, caused by morphine is due to the release of histamine and is responsible for hypotension. This hypotension again stimulates the sympathetic system as its compensatory mechanism. The hypotension, produced by opioids, can be eliminated or minimized by volume loading, H_1, and H_2 histamine antagonists, Trendelenburg (head down) position, and slow infusion of drugs.

Some reports show that patients, with good left ventricular function, become hypertensive more frequently, due to opioids than patients with poor left ventricular function, during surgery. The explanation of this phenomenon is like that the patients with good myocardial function could increase their cardiac index in response to an increase in SVR, induced by surgical stimuli. Thus, the patients with limited myocardial reserve could not always maintain CO in the face of ↑SVR. So, their BP does not increase and at times decreases. This rise of BP after opioids, especially during intubation and surgical stimulation, has been most often due to light GA which is resulted from underestimation of opioid dose and faulty timing of drug administration. So, opioids should be administered in a fashion that will permit the establishment of peak effect before noxious stimuli.

The predominant and usual effect of opioids on HR is to produce bradycardia, resulting from the stimulation of the central vagus nucleus. Hence, opioid-induced bradycardia can be prevented by vagal block with atropine. The blockade of sympathetic chronotropic actions by opioids may also play an important role in opioid-induced bradycardia. Meperidine, in contrast to other opioids, rarely results in bradycardia, but it can cause tachycardia. Tachycardia after meperidine may be due to its structural similarity to atropine or normeperidine or due to its early toxic CNS manifestation.

Opioids depress cardiac conduction. Thus, it slows AV nodal conduction, prolongs PR interval, increases AV nodal refractory period, prolongs the duration of the action potential of Purkinje fibers, and prolongs QT interval. This effect may be related to (1) enhanced Ca^{2+} entry into myocardial cells, during the plateau phase of action potential or (2) depression of outward K^+ current during terminal repolarization of action potential. Clinically, the disturbances of cardiac conduction due to opioids are very rare, but they may be more likely to occur in the presence of a Ca^{2+} channel blocker or β-adrenergic blocker.

Compared with inhalation anesthetic agents, opioids cause better preservation of myocardial function. The hypotension, produced by morphine, is not due to myocardial depression, like inhalational agents. Myocardial opioid receptor stimulation results in the reduction of infarction size. High doses of opioids maintain better myocardial perfusion and O_2 supply/demand ratio than inhalational agents.

Morphine and meperidine cause the release of histamine which causes sympathoadrenal activation. This is documented by a significant increase in plasma epinephrine and norepinephrine level in response to opioids. This hormonal alteration contributes to cardiovascular changes, which are seen after morphine and it includes an increase in cardiac index. A decrease in arterial BP and SVR is also due to this histamine effect. Meperidine causes histamine release more frequently than most other opioids, including morphine, fentanyl, sufentanil, and remifentanil. Unlike morphine and meperidine, fentanyl, sufentanil, and remifentanil do not produce an increase in plasma histamine and hypotension. Although, the μ-opioid agonists modulate the adrenal secretory response to pain, still the adrenal secretory response to hemorrhage is preserved.

Hormonal Response of Opioids

Stress response is totally a physiological process that occurs when a patient encounters a significant insult from injury and/or surgery. The main part of this stress response is the neuroendocrine component which works through some centers, situated in the brain and releases corticotropin-releasing hormone (CRH) from the paraventricular hypothalamic nucleus and locus coeruleus, responsible for nor epinephrine/autonomic nervous system. During stress or surgical insult, the hypothalamus secrets trophic hormones which stimulate pituitary to release ACTH, growth hormone (GH), renin, prolactin, ADH, etc., thus the level of cortisol, catecholamines, glucagon, and thyroxine are increased after stress. However, the plasma level of anabolic hormones such as insulin and testosterone is decreased. This increased level of stress hormones during GA and surgery causes hemodynamic instability and perioperative catabolic metabolism which contribute to operative mortality.

In general, inhalational anesthetic agents cannot suppress this stress response but only mask it. But opioids can do it to a certain degree. Only the combinations of different anesthetic agents and different anesthetic techniques can control this stress response best. Opioids are potent inhibitors of the hypothalamus pituitary adrenal axis. It reduces the stress responses by blocking the nociception at different levels of the neural axis.

Fentanyl and its congeners are more effective than morphine and meperidine in modifying these hormonal responses to surgery. Increased stress response is detrimental to very ill patients, undergoing major surgical procedures. Increased catecholamine increases cardiac risk, increases protein catabolism, and delays recovery. So, the reduction of stress responses by opioids, during surgery, reduces morbidity and mortality.

Renal Effects of Opioids

Morphine and meperidine prevent the release of ADH from the posterior pituitary gland which occurs in response to stress. Thus, the absence of an increase in plasma ADH, renin, and aldosterone level, following the administration of opioids, indicate that opioids most likely preserve or minimally alter the renal function in human subject in response to stress. Opioids reduce the tone of the bladder's smooth muscle, but increase the tone of bladder sphincter, causing the retention of urine. Opioids also cause increased contraction of the ureter smooth muscle.

Gastrointestinal Effects of Opioids

The opioid receptors and endogenous opioids are found throughout the GI tract. So, opioids produce widespread effects on the GIT by supraspinal (vagus nerve-mediated), spinal, and by peripheral nervous mechanism. Opioids increase the tone of smooth muscle and decrease the motility of the GI tract and are more likely to have a full stomach, regardless of their NPM (nothing per mouth) status. Opioids lower the esophageal sphincter activity, causing relaxation, but cause the spasm of the pyloric, ileocecal, and anal sphincter. It causes a decrease in all GI secretion. Epidural and intrathecal opioids also reduce the GI tract motility. Naloxone reverses the opioid-induced delays of gastric emptying.

Opioids induce the spasm of the common bile duct (CBD) and sphincter of Oddi. Thus, opioids reduce the caliber of CBD and increase the pressure of the biliary duct. The opioid-induced reduction of the caliber of CBD is greatest with morphine and is insignificant after fentanyl or sufentanil. This opioid-induced spasm of the biliary tree can completely be countered by naloxone, glucagon, nitrates, theophylline, and partially by atropine. The meperidine has a dual effect. In lower concentration, it produces an antimuscarinic effect, i.e., the relaxation of the biliary tree, and in higher concentration it produces biliary spasm. Neither of these responses of meperidine are affected by naloxone.

The little, but big problem, during the perioperative period, is the postoperative nausea and vomiting which is caused by opioids. Opioids stimulate the center of CTZ, situated at the postrema area of medulla in the brain, and possibly through δ-receptor. This central action of opioid combined with their action on GI tract promotes nausea and vomiting. There is very little evidence to suggest that any one opioid is constantly more emetogenic than other. Nevertheless, in one particular patient, changing from one opioid to another opioid influenced the incidence of associated nausea and vomiting. Factors that increase the incidence of nausea and vomiting are age (the pediatric group is more susceptible), sex (females are more prone), obesity, history of motion sickness, anxiety, certain surgical procedures (laparoscopy), opioid premedication, intensity of pain, gastric distension, and N_2O. Propofol significantly reduces the incidence of nausea and vomiting, caused by opioids.

Nausea and vomiting caused by opioids are of great concern to postoperative patients, so, attempts should always be taken to minimize their occurrence. Some efficient antiemetic therapies, commonly used in anesthesia, are:

- Anticholinergic drug, such as scopolamine, which can be given through IM or IV, or transdermal patch to reduce postoperative nausea and vomiting. Glycopyrrolate is ineffective in this respect, as it cannot penetrate the blood–brain barrier. Atropine is effective to some extent.
- Droperidol (0.005–0.07 mg/kg IV) which is very effective to reduce postoperative nausea and vomiting, caused by opioids. It acts by its antidopaminergic action.
- Dopamine antagonist, such as metoclopramide, which is also effective. It acts centrally by blocking D2 receptor at CTZ and peripherally at the GI tract.
- Serotonin antagonist such as ondansetron may be highly effective, but it is associated with low incidences of headache (3%), liver enzyme elevation, and high-cost benefit ratio.

Obstetric Effects of Opioids

Morphine and meperidine (not fentanyl, sufentanil, alfentanil, etc.) adversely affect IVF (*in vitro fertilization*) due to their teratogenic potentiality, so they are not used for this purpose. The parenteral administration of opioids, prior to delivery in obstetrics practice, remains a commonly used method of analgesia, despite the known adverse maternal, fetal, and neonatal effects of it and it is due to the arguably superior alternatives other than epidural analgesia. Meperidine (50 mg IV) has been suggested to result in less neonatal depression than morphine. This is because of the immaturity of the fetal blood–brain barrier which allows greater than normal brain penetration of relatively less lipophobic morphine, compared with meperidine. Soon after injection, the morphine and meperidine rapidly cross the placenta barrier and cause its significant blood level in a newborn. The elimination half-life of meperidine in newborns can be as long as 23 hours.

Sufentanil is highly bound to plasma protein and thus impedes its placental transfer. Placenta takes up more sufentanil, compared to other opioids, and acts as a drug depot. Thus, the placental transfer is reduced in the case of sufentanil, and transfer to the fetus may be least when delivery occurs within 45 minutes of this drug administration. Meperidine increases uterine contraction and shortens the duration of labor in a dose-dependent fashion which is not reversed by naloxone.

Though, traditionally opioid is not used in GA for cesarean section but recently patient with severe pregnancy-induced hypertension (PIH) and CVS problems are induced with newer congener of opioids to promote CVS stability. Maternal effects are deemed beneficial because naloxone is used for the reversal of neonatal respiratory depression. Opioids excrete through breast milk and depress neonatal neurobehavior. The newborn of an addicted mother exhibits opioid withdrawal symptoms and requires appropriate treatment.

Ocular Effects of Opioids

All the opioids prevent the increase in intraocular pressure, associated with succinylcholine and/or tracheal intubation.

Allergic Reaction

True anaphylactoid reactions to opioids are rare, but most commonly local allergic reactions occur and this may be due to preservatives or histamine release. Naloxone and antihistamines partially attenuate these histamine-induced local opioid allergic reactions.

Pharmacokinetics of Opioids

Opioids are weak base. So, when they are dissolved in solution, then they dissociate into protonated or ionized fraction. The relative proportion of these protonated (on ionized) and free base (on nonionized fraction) part depends on the pH of the solution and the pKa value of this agent. Free base or nonionized form is more lipid soluble than the ionized or protonated form. High lipid solubility increases the entry of opioids at its site of action, i.e., CNS, and facilitates its rapid onset of action. On the other hand, opioid receptors recognize an opioid molecule in protonated form and the intensity of the opioid effect is closely related to the concentration of this ionized portion of the drug in the cell. Thus, the speed of onset and intensity of action is a complex function of lipid solubility and the percentage of ionization which again depends on the tissue pH and pKa value of the drug, like the local anesthetic agent which is discussed in respective Chapter No. 13.

Opioids are bound to plasma proteins (albumin and α_1-acid glycoprotein) to some extent. Opioid molecules that are bound to plasma protein cannot pass from blood into CNS or any other tissues. Only the unionized and unbound fraction (free base) passes from blood into tissues, where it is ionized and makes a concentration gradient of a nonionized form of this drug which promotes further diffusion. Hence, the concentration gradient, lipid solubility, and the plasma tissue partition coefficient determines the rate at which the diffusion of opioid into tissue will take place. Morphine has a low diffusible fraction and is an opioid of slow onset of action. This is because of its low lipid solubility. On the other hand, alfentanil has a high diffusible fraction and is an opioid of rapid onset of action. This is because of its high lipid solubility than morphine.

After IV injection, the plasma concentration (central compartment) of opioids rises to a peak level within one circulation time such as thiopentone and propofol. Thereafter, the plasma concentration of opioids first falls very rapidly due to the distribution and redistribution of it in peripheral tissues and later slowly due to the metabolism and excretion of it through the liver and kidney. This is also like barbiturates, propofol, and BZD.

In general, the opioids are cleared from plasma by biotransformation (conjugation with glucuronic acid) in liver. Kidneys also play a role in the conjugation of opioids. Blood and tissue esterase are also responsible for the metabolism of remifentanil. The subtle difference of pharmacokinetic of different opioids is also due to their uptake by pulmonary tissue. This is because the time taken to reach to peak concentration in plasma by an opioid is influenced by the percentage of pulmonary uptake of it. About 75% of fentanyl is taken up by the lung due to its high lipophilicity and is subsequently released rapidly.

Pharmacokinetic of Individual Opioid

Pharmacokinetic of morphine: The pharmacokinetic of morphine is notably different from its fentanyl congeners. Due to its low lipid solubility, there is a little first-pass uptake of morphine by the lungs. The pKa value of morphine is 8 which is greater than the physiological pH of blood. So, after IV injection only 10–20% of morphine remains as unionized form and 80–90% remains as ionized form. This property and low lipid solubility limit the ability of morphine to penetrate into tissues, particularly CNS, and explain its slow onset of action. But in neonates and infants, where the blood–brain barrier is not properly built up, in such cases morphine has high penetration power in CNS. These pharmacokinetic properties of commonly used opioids are given in **Table 11**.

Morphine is principally metabolized in liver by glucuronide conjugation. Kidney is also an important site for the extrahepatic metabolism (40%) of morphine. The morphine-3-glucuronide (M3G) is a major metabolite of morphine, without its any analgesic property. Another important metabolite of morphine, named morphine-6-glucuronide (M6G) accounts for 10% of the total metabolites of morphine, however, it is more potent analgesic than morphine itself and also acts through μ-receptor.

TABLE 11: Physical characteristics of opioids that determine its tissue distribution.

Agent	Protein binding	Unionized (diffusible) fraction	Lipid solubility
Morphine	+ +	+ +	+
Meperidine	+ + +	+	+ +
Fentanyl	+ + +	+	+ + + +
Alfentanil	+ + + +	+ + +	+ + +
Sufentanil	+ + +	+ + +	+ + +
Remifentanil	+ + +	+ + +	+ +

The bioavailability of orally administered morphine is significantly lower than the pareneral route and is only 20–30%. This is due to the hepatic first-pass effect on morphine. The M6G is the primary active component when morphine is administered orally due to its high hepatic extraction.

Pharmacokinetic of meperidine: Unlike morphine, after IV injection, the first-pass uptake of meperidine by the lungs is approximately 65%. Meperidine's physicochemical properties are not like morphine, but more similar to those of fentanyl. Its pKa value is 8.5. So, it is less unionized (<10%) at the physiological pH of the blood. Meperidine is more lipid soluble than morphine, but it is more highly bound to plasma protein than morphine, i.e., 70% of meperidine is bound to α_1-glycoprotein. In contrast to morphine, meperidine binds to plasma albumin in a minor extent.

The principal metabolites of meperidine are normeperidine, normeperidinic acid, and meperidinic acid. All these are produced by N-demethylation and diesterification of meperidine in liver. Only <5% meperidine is excreted unchanged through the kidney. Normepridine has analgesic and neuroexcitatory property (twice as potent as the parent compound in producing seizures). Hence, the meperidine has some convulsion-producing property and this epileptogenic property of meperidine make its therapeutic index low than that of morphine.

Normeperidine is excreted through the kidney and has a greater elimination half-life than meperidine itself. So, the repeated administration of meperidine causes the accumulation of this toxic metabolite (normeperidine) of it (meperidine) in patients with renal failure and produces seizures.

Pharmacokinetic of fentanyl: A three-compartmental model is typically used to describe the pharmacokinetic property of fentanyl, instead of two-compartmental models which are used to describe the pharmacokinetic property of morphine and meperidine. Like meperidine, after IV injection, the first-pass uptake of fentanyl by the lungs is 75%. Its pKa value is 8.4. So, like meperidine at the physiological pH of blood, the unionized diffusible form of fentanyl is <10% and ionized form is >90%, so the diffusible fraction of fentanyl (unionized base) is less. But fentanyl's high lipid solubility increases its large volume of distribution in tissues than morphine and meperidine. Less unionized forms also explain less availability form of fentanyl for brain tissue and delayed onset of action (than alfentanil). On the other hand, high lipid solubility explains the quick transfer of it into CNS and rapid onset of action. So, the actual onset of action of fentanyl is the resultant effect of these two properties. High lipid solubility of fentanyl also explains more uptake of it by peripheral tissues and prolonged action. About 80% of injected fentanyl is bound to plasma protein and 40% is taken up by RBC.

Fentanyl is metabolized mainly in liver by N-dealkylation and hydroxylation. It has a high hepatic clearance rate. Norfentanyl, the primary metabolite of fentanyl is detectable in urine for up to 48 hours after a single bolus IV administration of fentanyl. It (norfentanyl) is inactive and has no analgesic or toxic property.

Pharmacokinetic of alfentanil: The unique physicochemical property of alfentanil is its pKa value which is only 6.5. So, at the physiological pH of blood, it is mostly (90%) in unionized and diffusible form. But alfentanil is highly protein bound and is of low lipid soluble. Thus, despite intense protein binding and lower lipid solubility diffusible fraction of alfentanil makes its early penetration into CNS. This explains alfentanil's short latency to peak effect (early onset of action) after its IV injection. Alfentanil's lower lipid solubility, compared with fentanyl, causes its less amount of uptake by lipid-rich brain tissue. This mechanism explains alfentanil's rapid offset of action (short duration of action).

The volume of distribution of alfentanil is 0.4–1 L/kg, whereas that of fentanyl is 3–6 L/kg. This is due to the low lipid solubility of alfentanil than fentanyl and causes the less tissue accumulation of this drug. This mechanism is also largely responsible for the short elimination half-life of alfentanil in spite of its lower clearance rate than fentanyl (alfentanil's clearance rate is 4–9 mL/kg and fentanyl's is 10–20 mL/min/kg)

Noralfentanil is the major metabolic product of alfentanil. Other metabolites of alfentanil metabolism are desmethyl alfentanil, desmethyl noralfentanil, etc. Any of the metabolites of alfentanil have little or no analgesic activity.

Pharmacokinetic of sufentanil: It is often reported that sufentanil is 5–10 times more potent than fentanyl. The pKa value of it at the physiological pH of blood is same as that of morphine, i.e., 8, therefore only a small amount (20%) of it exists in unionized form. After IV injection, first-pass pulmonary extraction and retention of sufentanil in lungs are similar to those of fentanyl.

However, this physiochemical property is of little clinical importance to sufentanil. This is because sufentanil is twice as lipid-soluble as fentanyl and is highly protein bound (93%) including α_1-acid glycoprotein. The major *metabolic pathways* of sufentanil include N-dealkylation, oxidative N-dealkylation, oxidative O-demethylation, and aromatic hydroxylation in liver. The major resultant metabolites of sufentanil include N-phenylpropanamide. Sufentanil is tightly bound to receptor. This property, along with the high degree of plasma protein binding capacity and lower volume of distribution, are the probable explanation of sufentanil's shorter elimination half-life and shorter duration of action as compared to fentanyl, despite the fact that it is highly lipophilic. In fact, after intraoperative infusion of sufentanil, for <6–8 hours of duration, the effects of this opioid would dissipate as rapidly as those produced by similar infusions of alfentanil.

Pharmacokinetic of remifentanil (G187084B): Remifentanil is the first ultrashort-acting opioid for clinical use as a supplement to GA. The pharmacokinetic properties of remifentanil are best described by three-compartmental models like fentanyl and its congeners such as alfentanil and sufentanil, *although it is chemically related to fentanyl congeners, but it is structurally unique, because of its ester linkage. Remifentanil's ester structure contributes its susceptibility to hydrolysis by plasma and tissue nonspecific esterases, resulting in rapid metabolism of it.* Like fentanyl, it is not significantly metabolized or sequestrated in the lungs. Its metabolic clearance is several times greater than that of hepatic blood flow. This explains its widespread extrahepatic metabolism, i.e., in plasma.

Remifentanil is a weak base with a pKa value of 7. Its free base is formulated as a solution in glycine. As glycine has been shown to act as an inhibitory neurotransmitter and causes reversible motor weakness when injected intrathecally, *so remifentanil is not approved for spinal or epidural use.* Remifentanil is highly protein bound (70%), mainly with α-acid glycoprotein. In blood, remifentanil is metabolized primarily by enzymes that are present in erythrocytes, *therefore it is not a substrate for pseudocholinesterase and is not influenced by pseudocholinesterase deficiency.* The primary metabolic pathway of remifentanil is de-esterification to form a carboxylic acid, which has a very low analgesic property and is inactive. This metabolite is excreted through urine, though its pharmacokinetic is not appreciably influenced by renal and hepatic failure. The context-sensitive half-time (CSHT) of different opioids is shown in **Figure 22**.

Factors that Alter the Pharmacokinetics and Pharmacodynamics of Opioids

Factors that change the pharmacokinetics and pharmacodynamics of opioids are:

- *Age:* Neonate exhibits a reduced rate of elimination of opioid. This is due to the immature mechanism for metabolism of opioid, resulting in extended elimination half-life of them. At the end of the first year, this initial extended elimination of opioid is quickly normalized and at the end of the first decade of life, maximum opioid metabolic capacity is achieved.

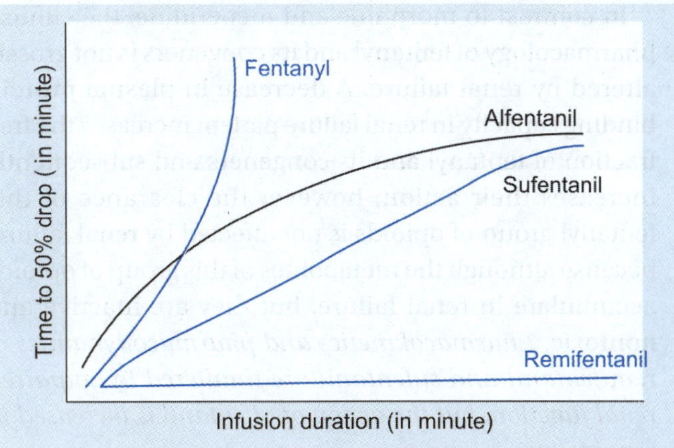

Fig. 22: The context-sensitive half-time (CSHT) of different opioids. Among all the opioids, the time necessary to achieve a 50% decrease in the plasma concentration (CSHT) of remifentanil is very short and is not influenced by the duration of its infusion.

However, at the old age, the pharmacokinetic changes play a little role, rather the pharmacodynamic changes which are primarily responsible for the decreased dose requirement of opioid in old age. The small pharmacokinetic change in old age that results in higher peak concentration, after a bolus dose of opioid, is due to low CO and small central volume of distribution.

- *Weight:* The pharmacokinetic parameters of opioids are more closely related to our lean body mass than our total body weight. This is because >90% of our body's metabolic process is thought to occur in lean body tissues. So, the dose regimens should be based on lean body mass than total body weight. But the estimation of lean body mass is a cumbersome calculation and total body weight closely relates to lean body mass. So, the dose regime based on the total body weight is a clinically acceptable alternative.
- *Renal failure:* Renal failure has a major implication on the duration of action of morphine and meperidine, but renal failure has a less marked implication on the duration of action of fentanyl and its congeners.

Patient with renal failure develops a very high level of M6G after morphine administration. This M6G is μ-agonist with similar or greater potency than morphine. So, there is every chance of life-threatening respiratory depression in renal failure patient, after the administration of morphine. The clinical pharmacology of meperidine is also significantly altered by renal failure. So, the morphine and meperidine is not a good choice for the renal failure patients, however if they are used at all, then their dose should be decreased and patient should be carefully monitored.

In contrast to morphine and meperidine, the clinical pharmacology of fentanyl and its congeners is not grossly altered by renal failure. A decrease in plasma protein binding capacity in renal failure patient increases the free fraction of fentanyl and its congeners and subsequently increases their action; however the clearance of this fentanyl group of opioids is not affected by renal failure, because although the metabolites of this group of opioids accumulate in renal failure, but they are inactive and nontoxic. *Pharmacokinetics and pharmacodynamics of remifentanil and sufentanil are unaltered by impaired renal function, but the action of alfentanil is increased in renal failure.*

- *Hepatic failure:* Even though liver is the primary responsible organ for the metabolism of opioid, but the degree of liver failure that is commonly observed in perioperative patient, does not have a major impact on the pharmacokinetic of most of the opioids, except liver transplantation. The possible explanation of this is the huge metabolic reserve of the liver.

There are numerous ways by which liver disease can influence the pharmacokinetics of opioids and these are:

- Reducing metabolic capacity (cytochrome P450 system and conjugation)
- Reducing hepatic blood flow
- Reducing plasma protein binding capacity
- Edema and increasing the total body water; thus increasing the distribution characteristic of a drug (volume of distribution)
- Increasing metabolic capacity by enzymatic induction in early alcoholism.

Because of these numerous mechanisms, by which liver disease may alter the pharmacokinetics of opioids, it can be difficult to predict exactly how an individual patient with liver disease will respond to opioid administration.

The pharmacokinetic of morphine is relatively unchanged by the liver failure because the substantial amount of metabolism of morphine is done by the kidney. On the other hand, the pharmacokinetic of meperidine is altered by liver failure. Like meperidine, the pharmacokinetics of alfentanil is also altered by hepatic failure. The pharmacokinetic of fentanyl is not altered by hepatic failure. Remifentanil is perhaps the prototype example of an opioid whose pharmacokinetic is completely unchanged by the liver disease.

Anesthetic Technique Using Opioids

The routine anesthetic induction is usually achieved by combining a loading dose of fentanyl (2–6 µg/kg) with any sedative or hypnotic, such as most commonly thiopentone or propofol and a muscle relaxant. The doses of sedative or hypnotic should be significantly reduced for induction of anesthesia if opioids are used. Ketamine (0.5–2 mg/kg) provides more hemodynamic stability, compared with thiopentone or propofol, after fentanyl or other opioids, especially in patients with cardiovascular diseases. Opioids can ameliorate or eliminate the cardiovascular responses to noxious stimuli and thus control the changes in HR, BP, pulmonary capillary wedge pressure, and other aspects of stress responses that occur during laryngoscopy, intubation, and surgery. Fentanyl and sufentanil should be administered 4–6 minutes and alfentanil and remifentanil should be administered 1–2 minutes prior to any stress or stimulation. Once, the stress response is achieved and catecholamines are released, then the opioids are less effective in maintaining the hemodynamic stability. However, it is confirmed that the responses to laryngoscopy is better controlled with opioids than with esmolol, but everyone has its advantages and disadvantages.

After induction, anesthesia is usually maintained by N_2O with O_2 and a low concentration of any potent inhalation anesthetic agent, plus intermittent boluses (25–50 µg after every 15–30 minutes) or continuous infusion (0.5–5 µg/h/kg) of fentanyl or other opioids. For short surgical procedures, lower doses of fentanyl, as bolus or infusion, can be used. Premedication by any BZD may also reduce the dose of this supplementation. Propofol infusion may also be used, during maintenance, as a part of balanced anesthesia.

Fentanyl plasma concentration of 1–2 ng/mL provides analgesia, but fentanyl levels of at least 2–3 ng/mL is usually required, during surgery for adequate analgesia, if N_2O as the only inhaled agent is used. This plasma level can easily be achieved by initial bolus dose of fentanyl as 4–8 µg/kg, followed by a continuous infusion of 2–4 µg/kg/h. This will often result in adequate plasma levels of fentanyl at 3–6 ng/mL.

Excessive doses of fentanyl or other congeners of it may result in postoperative respiratory depression. This is more likely, however, if fentanyl is given empirically without making titration with pain to some clinical endpoint. Somebody gives additional fentanyl in the dose of 1–2 µg/kg, during the closing of peritoneum to attenuate the hemodynamic response during extubation, but it may lead to troublesome respiratory depression postoperatively. Another useful clinical approach to attenuate hemodynamic responses, during extubation, is to wait for spontaneous ventilation to resume. Then, an additional titrated dose of fentanyl at the dose of 25–50 µg is administered to produce a respiratory rate at 10–12/min prior to tracheal extubation. Sufentanil, alfentanil, and remifentanil are also can be used in place of fentanyl.

Continuous Opioid Infusion

Continuous infusions of modern opioids are better alternatives to the intermittent bolus technique. It maintains continuously (1) a desired plasma level, (2) a desired drug concentration at the effected site, and (3) a steady state condition by replacing the drug in plasma that is removed by redistribution and metabolism. The advantages of continuous infusion of newer opioids such as fentanyl and its congener over intermittent bolus doses are (1) better hemodynamic stability, (2) decreased total dose, (3) decreased side effects, (4) more rapid recovery of consciousness, (5) less respiratory depression and less need for opioid antagonist, and (6) decrease in discharge time.

The dose of continuous infusion of opioid is often reduced gradually to obtain a lower effective plasma concentration level and thus it avoids accumulation, when the redistribution of the drug declines and the peripheral compartment comes to an equilibrium with the central compartment, after being fully saturated. The computer-assisted continuous infusion [computer-controlled infusion pump (CCIP)] delivers the drugs, based on the pharmacokinetic data of a particular agent which feeds in the computer. CCIP calculates the necessary infusion rate from the population-based pharmacokinetic data of this particular drug to achieve the targeted concentration and then CCIP gradually decreases the rate of infusion, based on this particular drugs pharmacokinetics. Now, CCIP is becoming increasingly popular.

High-Dose Only Opioid-Based Anesthesia

The popularity of high-dose only opioid-based anesthesia was first established by morphine and it has most commonly been employed in cardiac anesthesia. But this popularity of high-dose only opioid-based anesthesia had been gradually diminished due to several factors.

These include:

- Lack of significant benefit from a very large dose of opioid
- Recent trend toward the "first track" anesthesia
- Opioid as a sole anesthetic agent is not consistently reliable for sedation
- The frequent need to intervene hypotension, caused by high dose opioid-based anesthesia, with vasoactive agents
- Excessive postoperative respiratory depression
- Intraoperative hemodynamic instability (only by a high dose of morphine). So, this morphine is not recommended for high dose opioid anesthesia.

But now newer opioids are administered in higher doses by continuous infusion with other anesthetic agents and are still important and effective anesthetic agents for patient, undergoing cardiac and other extensive operations.

Fentanyl: Many different techniques are used for fentanyl with high doses. Initial bolus injection of fentanyl range from 5 to 75 µg/kg, but there is little benefit of administering loading bolus doses of fentanyl >5–30 µg/kg. These doses will establish plasma fentanyl concentration between 10 and 30 ng/mL, which is sufficient to provide stable hemodynamic condition during induction and intubation. Then continuous infusion in the dose of 0.1–1 µg/kg/min is used for cardiac surgery.

This high-dose fentanyl anesthesia is very effective and safe for pediatric cardiac surgery also. It reduces the incidence of intraoperative ventricular fibrillation in neonates, undergoing cardiac surgery.

Alfentanil: Large doses of alfentanil (150 µg/kg) may be used with or without thiopentone or propofol for the induction of anesthesia, but only large doses of alfentanil are not suitable for induction. For cardiac surgery induction and maintenance of anesthesia with alfentanil (25–75 µg/kg loading dose plus 1–2 µg/kg/min infusion) and propofol (0.25–1 mg/kg bolus plus 80–100 µg/kg/min) is reliable and stable.

Sufentanil: Sufentanil is superior to fentanyl for high-dose opioid anesthesia in cardiac surgery. The advantages are more rapid induction, better attenuation of intubation reflexes, greater reduction of left ventricular stroke work, more stable hemodynamic condition intraoperatively and postoperatively, early recovery and extubation, and more decrease of BP than equivalent doses of fentanyl.

- *Dose:* For induction, sufentanil is used as a bolus dose of 2–20 µg/kg or infused over 2–10 minutes.

For significant cardiovascular disease, etomidate is a better drug combination with sufentanil. Alternative to etomidate, propofol can be used. Interestingly, sufentanil requirements become triple when midazolam is employed instead of propofol for induction. Etomidate (0.1–2 mg/kg) plus sufentanil (0.5–1 µg/kg) provide excellent hemodynamic stability during induction. The maintenance of anesthesia by infusion of sufentanil (1–2 µg/kg/h) in a balanced anesthetic technique, achieves the advantages of an opioid-based anesthesia and avoids prolonged opioid action postoperatively.

Remifentanil: In high-dose opioid anesthesia, the data regarding remifentanil is insufficient and nothing can be commented. Remifentanil has been employed in cardiac anesthesia. The pharmacokinetics of remifentanil were studied in patients undergoing coronary artery bypass grafting (CABG) with cardiopulmonary bypass (CPB).

The volume of distribution of remifentanil increases by 86% with the institution of CPB. The elimination clearance also decreases by 7% for each degree of decrease of temperature below 37°C. So, infusion rate of remifentanil should be changed accordingly to maintain a constant plasma remifentanil level. It was shown that the induction with remifentanil (2 µg/kg) together with propofol and maintenance with remifentanil at the dose of 0.25–0.5 µg/kg/min provides appropriate anesthesia for minimally invasive CABG surgery.

Transdermal and Transmucosal Route for Opioid Delivery

These two routes, for opioid delivery system, have enormous potentialities (1) to improve analgesic therapy by increasing patient's compliance, (2) to reduce pain associated with drug delivery, (3) to increase drug bioavailability, and (4) to increase their analgesic efficacy.

Transdermal Route

The transdermal opioid delivery technique requires both the high water-soluble (for passage through dermis) and high lipid soluble (for passage through corneum) property of that agent. Again, the drug should also be of low molecular weight, highly potent (little amount causes clinical effect), and have no skin irritation effect.

At present, fentanyl (but no other opioids) is only available for transdermal delivery system. The advantages of it are (1) no first-pass metabolism by the liver, (2) improved patient's compliance, (3) consistent analgesia, (4) simple noninvasive type of delivery in nature, and (5) giving no pain during the administration of drug.

After the application of fentanyl transdermal patch, the plasma fentanyl level reaches its plateau level very slowly, extending between 8 and 16 hours and then its plasma level also falls very slowly after the removal of the patch, because the absorption of the drug, which is deposited in the skin, still continues. The half-life for the decline of fentanyl level after the removal of its patch is 17 hours. This transdermal route for the administration of fentanyl is very effective for the pain management in cancer patient. Faster-acting route should be used initially during the acuteness of situation and then to switch over to this transdermal route. This transdermal drug delivery system can also be enhanced by iontophoresis (external electric current). So, the patient, receiving opioid by iontophoresis, requires fewer additional opioid analgesics.

Transmucosal Route

This route for drug delivery through mucosa can be achieved through oral, lingual, oropharyngeal, nasopharyngeal, sublingual, rectal, or tracheobronchial mucosa (by inhalation). Among them, the sublingual route is the most convenient for patients. But increased salivary secretion and subsequent swallowing of this saliva may convert this route to oral and prevent the increased systemic availability of drug, due to hepatic fast pass metabolism, but if this saliva is not allowed to swallow, then this sublingual route increases systemic availability, by eliminating hepatic first-pass metabolism and improves patient's compliance. As mucosa is rich in blood vessels and lymphatics, so absorption of drug will be faster, and onset of action will be rapid if drug is administered through this route. This route of administration of drug is usually used for premedication, postoperative pain management, and treatment of chronic pain. Highly lipid-soluble opioids such as buprenorphine, fentanyl, and their congener such as methadone are more effectively absorbed sublingually.

- *Sublingual buprenorphine:* Buprenorphine is a (1) potent, (2) synthetic, (3) mixed agonist and antagonist opioid with a long half-life, and (4) is readily absorbed by a sublingual route. When the tablet of buprenorphine is swallowed, then it is almost completely metabolized by the liver, after absorption due to its first-pass metabolism. So it is not used orally. But the systemic bioavailability of buprenorphine, after the sublingual route is 50% of that following its IV administration. When sublingual buprenorphine (0.3 mg) is given 1 hour prior to surgery, then it provides a reliable preoperative sedation, intraoperative and postoperative analgesia, which is similar to IM, morphine, but as the onset of action is slow (3 hours), so the sublingual buprenorphine is not effective for immediate postoperative pain relief. The percentage of postoperative pain relief by sublingual buprenorphine is 80%, requiring supplementation for higher success rate (if required).
- *Transmucosal morphine:* Buccal morphine for analgesia is not so promising (initial report was promising, but subsequent report disproved it), like buprenorphine, because low lipid solubility than other opioids makes it (morphine) a bad candidate for this route. In addition, the bitter taste of morphine initiates salivation and subsequently the swallowing of this saliva, containing morphine; make it an easy prey to the first-pass liver metabolism. The bioavailability of sublingual morphine is 6 times lower than the equivalent dose of it by IM route.
- *Transmucosal fentanyl:* The oral transmucosal (not sublingual) preparation of fentanyl is made of fentanyl citrate which is incorporated in a sweet lozenge. This is called oral transmucosal fentanyl citrate (OTFC). When consumed, it partly absorbed through oral mucosa and partly swallowed and absorbed through the GI

tract, but drug bioavailability is greater through oral transmucosal route than GI tract. The recommended dose for this transmucosal fentanyl ranges from 5 to 15 µg/kg, depending on the desired degree of sedation and analgesia. The peak plasma concentration, after OTFC administration, occurs at 15–30 minutes and then declines after 1 hour. The speed of onset of analgesia with OTFC is equal to that of IV morphine and elimination half-life is 7 hours which is similar to that of IV route also.

However, unlike transdermal route, OTFC does not leave any depot in mucosa, after it is removed. As some fraction of OTFC is swallowed and absorbed through GI tract, so the total systemic bioavailability is only 50% as buprenorphine, but much greater than sublingual morphine. Like systemic fentanyl, OTFC also causes nausea, vomiting, and respiratory depression.

Other routes through which opioids can also be administered are intranasal, intratracheal, inhalation, and rectal.

■ INDIVIDUAL µ-RECEPTOR AGONIST

Morphine

The molecular structure of morphine is depicted in **Figure 23**. Still, now, morphine is the gold standard µ-receptor agonist, among all the opioids. So, against this gold standard opioid agonist, i.e., morphine, the potency of other newer opioid analgesic drugs are measured, though individual response may vary dramatically, for example, some patients cannot tolerate morphine, but have no problem with equianalgesic doses of methadone, however the actual underlying mechanism of it is still not known. Chemically, morphine is a phenanthrene alkaloid derivative. It is an agonist on all the opioid receptors such as the µ, κ, and δ receptors, but its affinity for µ-receptors is much higher than that for other two opioid receptors. The effects of morphine, therefore, are primarily due to the result of µ-receptors activation. Like other opioids, morphine also appears to extend their effects by decreasing intracellular Ca^{2+} concentration, which in turn increases K^+ conductance and causes the hyperpolarization of excitable cell membrane. Thus, the decrease in membrane excitability by morphine may decrease both the pre- and postsynaptic responses.

Due to difficulties, morphine is not synthesized, it still now, in the laboratory and is obtained from *opium* (extract of an unripe capsule of the poppy plant, named *Papaver somniferum*). The milky juice, opium, is dried and powdered to make opium powder which contains a number of alkaloids, and these alkaloids are divided into two distinct chemical classes such as *phenanthrenes* and *benzylisoquinolines* **(Table 12)**.

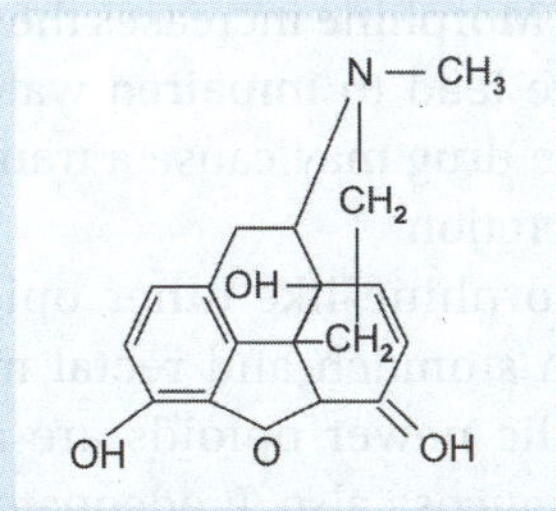

Fig. 23: Molecular structure of morphine.

TABLE 12: Derivatives of phenanthrene and benzoisoquinoline.

Phenanthrene derivatives	Benzoisoquinoline derivatives
Morphine (10%)	Papaverine (1%)
Codeine (0.5%)	Noscapine (6%)
Thebaine (0.2%)	

Note: Thebaine, papaverine, and noscapine are nonanalgesic

BOX 6: Causes of morphine-induced hypotension.

- Release of histamine
- Bradycardia due to vagal stimulation
- Decrease in sympathetic tone (centrally mediated)
- Arterial and venous dilatation (direct and indirect)
- Large doses and rapid administration
- Sequestration of blood in splanchnic area

The morphine has minimal effects on CVS. The predominant effect of morphine on CVS is orthostatic hypotension, secondary to a decrease in SVR, at least part of which is mediated by the histamine release. The drug may also cause bradycardia when it is administered in high doses. The causes of hypotension, produced by morphine are depicted in **Box 6**. The principal effect of morphine on respiration is depression with decreased ventilatory responses to hypoxia ($\downarrow O_2$) and hypercarbia ($\uparrow CO_2$). It also has potent antitussive action. Bronchoconstriction may occur with the use of high doses of it.

Morphine is a potent analgesic agent. So, along with the relief of pain, the morphine also causes drowsiness, relief of anxiety, and euphoria. Miosis, produced by morphine, is the result of the stimulation of Edinger–Westphal nucleus in the brain by it. Seizures and muscular rigidity may occur with the use of high doses of morphine. It decreases GI motility and also decreases gastric, biliary, and pancreatic secretion. It increases common bile duct pressure by causing the spasm of sphincter of Oddi. The drug may also cause nausea, vomiting, and constipation. Morphine increases the tone of ureters, detrusor muscle of bladder, and its sphincter, thus it may precipitate urinary retention. Mild diaphoresis and pruritus may result from morphine and it is due to histamine release. Morphine increases the secretion of ADH and may therefore lead to impaired water excretion and hyponatremia. The drug may cause a transient decrease in adrenal steroid secretion.

In general, morphine-like other opioids are quickly absorbed through stomach and rectal mucosa; however the more lipophilic newer opioids are absorbed by the nasal and buccal mucosa also. It adequately penetrates the tissue of the spinal cord, following its epidural or intrathecal administration, and produces profound analgesia which lasts for about 12–24 hours. As, the nature of morphine is more hydrophilic and its absorption by the nerve tissues of the spinal cord is less than that of other highly lipophilic opioid agents (fentanyl, sufentanil, etc.), so the rostral spread of morphine, after its intrathecal administration in CSF, is more and this increases the incidences of respiratory depression by morphine. In contrast, highly lipophilic opioid agents such as fentanyl and its congeners produce many localized effects on spinal cord, due to their quick absorption in local nerve tissue (due to high lipid solubility) and produce more segmental analgesia than morphine. The bioavailability of morphine by oral route is only 25%, due to its first-pass metabolism in liver. The shape of the time-effect curve of morphine varies with the different routes of its administration. Compared with other more lipid-soluble opioids such as codeine, heroin, methadone, fentanyl congeners, etc., morphine crosses the blood–brain barrier at a considerably lower rate and equilibrates very slowly between the plasma and CSF.

About one-third of absorbed morphine is protein bound, predominantly to albumin. It does not persist in tissues for 24 hours or tissue concentration remains very low after the last dose. The major pathways for morphine metabolism are its conjugation with glucuronic acid into the liver. The major metabolites of morphine metabolism are M6G, M3G, and a small amount of morphine 3,6-diglucuronide. Both the M3G and M6G compounds are polar and cross the blood–brain barrier easily to produce significant clinical effects. The M6G is responsible for most of the morphine's analgesic activity in patient receiving chronic oral morphine. Very little morphine is excreted unchanged through urine. It is eliminated by glomerular filtration primarily as M3G. However, 90% of the total excretion of morphine takes place during the first day of its administration.

Morphine should be used with caution in the presence of hepatic failure, because the drug may precipitate hepatic encephalopathy. Similarly, the use of morphine in patients with hypopituitarism may precipitate coma. Like other opioids, it also decreases the apparent MAC value of coadministered volatile anesthetic agents. Most of the actions of this drug are reversed by naloxone, although the analgesia, afforded by the epidural administration of morphine, is well preserved after the administration of naloxone. Morphine cannot be removed by hemodialysis or by peritoneal dialysis.

Meperidine (Pethidine)

The molecular structure of meperidine is depicted in **Figure 24**. It is a synthetic phenylpiperidine derivative and predominantly μ- and κ-opioid receptor agonist. It was first synthesized as an atropine substitute in 1939 and has same actions like anticholinergics. So, though chemically unrelated to morphine, still it (meperidine) has many similar actions like it (morphine) and has been shown to interact with many opioid receptors. Its actions can also be blocked by naloxone. The mechanism of action of meperidine is same as that of morphine. It decreases intracellular Ca^{2+} concentration which in turn increases K^+ conductance and causes the hyperpolarization of excitable cell membrane, especially of neuron. Thus, the decrease in membrane excitability by meperidine results in the decrease of both pre- and postsynaptic responses (transmission).

Like morphine, meperidine also causes orthostatic hypotension. This is due to the combination of the effect of histamine release and α-adrenergic blockade that it produces. The drug also has a mild quinidine-like effect and anticholinergic properties (dry mouth, tachycardia, blurred vision, urinary retention, etc.). Meperidine is a potent respiratory depressant, having a greater effect on tidal volume than on respiratory rate. It obtunds the ventilatory response to both hypoxia and hypercapnia. It has little antitussive action and chest wall rigidity may occur by it.

Meperidine is one-tenth as potent as an analgesic than morphine. It appears to cause more euphoria, but less nausea and vomiting than the equipotent doses of morphine. Miosis and corneal anesthesia may follow the topical application of it. In common with other opioids, meperidine decreases the rate of gastric emptying. This drug appears to cause a less marked increase in bile duct pressure and less depression of intestinal activity (and therefore it causes constipation) than the equipotent doses of morphine. This drug is less responsible for the increase in ureteric tone. It may increase the amplitude of contractions of the pregnant uterus.

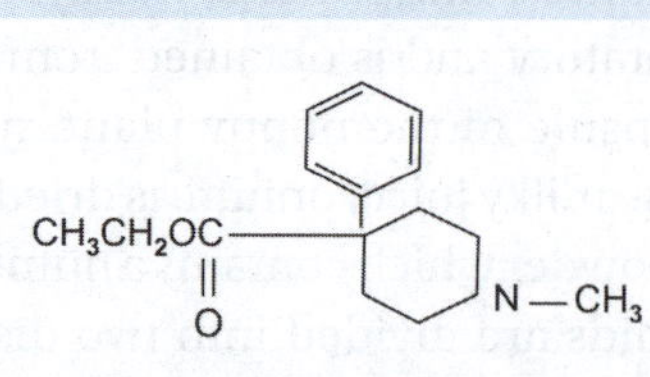

Fig. 24: Meperidine.

The important differences between meperidine and morphine are:

- Meperidine has a dose to dose one-tenth analgesic potency of morphine.
- After an IM injection of meperidine, the onset of action is more rapid, but the duration of action is shorter (2–3 hours) than morphine.
- It does not effectively suppress the cough.
- The spasmodic action on smooth muscles by meperidine is less marked. So, the miosis, constipation, urinary retentions, etc., caused by meperidine, are less prominent than morphine. The liability to induce biliary spasm by meperidine is low.
- As meperidine is equally sedative and euphoriant like morphine, so it has similar abuse potential.
- The degree of respiratory depression, produced by meperidine at equianalgesic doses, is equivalent to morphine.
- It causes less histamine release, so it is safer in asthmatics than morphine.
- It has also local anesthetic actions. Corneal anesthesia may also be seen after its systemic administration.

Meperidine (pethidine) can be absorbed by all routes, but the absorption of it may be erratic after its intramuscular injection. The adult oral dose of meperidine is 50–150 mg at 4 hours intervals. The corresponding dose of meperidine by IM route is 25–150 mg and by IV route is 25–100 mg. Meperidine may also be administered via the epidural route and a dose of 25 mg is usually employed. The drug acts within 15 minutes when it is administered orally and within 10 minutes when it is administered intramuscularly. The duration of action of meperidine is 2–4 hours. The bioavailability of meperidine when administered orally is only 40–70%. It is due to its significant fast pass metabolism in liver. This drug has a bioavailability of 100% when administered intramuscularly.

Meperidine is 50% protein bound in plasma. It crosses the placenta and the mean cord blood concentration at delivery is 70–90% of maternal blood concentration.

Meperidine is mainly metabolized in liver. It is hydrolyzed to meperidinic acid which in turn is conjugated. Meperidine is also N-demethylated to *normeperidine* which may then be hydrolyzed to normeperidinic acid and subsequently conjugated. This conjugated meperidinic and normeperidinic acid is excreted through bile and kidney. This *normeperidine* may accumulate in the presence of renal or hepatic failure. It has 50% analgesic potency of its parent compound and *has marked convulsant property*. Meperidine also appears to be effective in the treatment of postanesthetic shivering.

Severe reactions may follow after the administration of meperidine to a patient, being treated with monoamine oxidase (MAO) inhibitors. The reactions are delirium, hyperthermia, hypo or hypertension, rigidity, convulsion, coma, and death. This reaction is due to the blockade of neuronal reuptake of serotonin by meperidine and the resultant serotonergic overactivity at the synaptic level. So, meperidine and its congener (diphenoxylate and loperamide), dextromethorphan, and tramadol should not be used in patient taking monoamine oxidase inhibitor (MAOI). However, similar interaction with other currently used opioids have not been observed clinically.

Promethazine enhances meperidine-induced sedation. Amphetamine enhances the analgesic property of meperidine while counter acts its sedation effect.

Tramadol

Tramadol is a synthetic codeine analog with a dual mechanism of action. It is a weak opioid μ-receptor agonist and to a lesser extent a δ- and κ-receptor agonist. A part of its analgesic effect is also produced by the inhibition of the reuptake of norepinephrine and serotonin. So, the inhibition of pain perception by tramadol partly involves the activation of the descending serotonergic and noradrenergic pathways. Tramadol as an analgesic is one-fifth to one-tenth as potent as morphine and can be given by various parenteral routes. So, in the treatment of mild to moderate pain, it is effective, but for the treatment of severe chronic or acute pain, tramadol is less effective. Tramadol has no clinically significant cardiovascular effects, after its IV administration. Respiratory rate, minute volume, and $PaCO_2$ remain essentially unchanged following the IV administration of the therapeutic doses of this drug. It has no demonstrable effect on bile duct and its sphincter activity. The tramadol is 20% protein bound in plasma and 80% of its administered dose crosses the placenta. The bioavailability of tramadol following oral administration is 70–100%.

The primary O-demethylated metabolite of tramadol is 2–4 times as potent as its parent drug and may account for part of its analgesic effect. The tramadol is supplied as a racemic mixture. The (+) enantiomer of tramadol binds to the μ-receptor and also inhibits serotonin uptake, while the (–) enantiomer of tramadol only inhibits norepinephrine uptake and stimulates the adrenergic receptor.

The recommended dose of tramadol ranges from 50 to 100 mg after every 4–6 hours interval, with a maximum daily dose of 400 mg through all the routes of administration. The pediatric dose of tramadol is 1–2 mg/kg at 4–6 hours intervals.

This compound undergoes hepatic metabolism and renal excretion with an elimination half-life of 6 hours. It is less respiratory depressant, compared with equianalgesic dose of morphine and the degree of constipation is less than that which is seen after the equivalent dose of codeine.

Its abuse potential is unclear. By reducing seizure threshold, it can cause seizure. Because of its inhibitory effect on serotonin uptake, tramadol should not be used in patient taking MAOI. The use of tramadol is not recommended in patients with end-stage renal failure. The dosage interval of tramadol should be increased to 12 hours in patients with renal or hepatic failure. The drug is not licensed for intraoperative use, as it may enhance intraoperative recall during N_2O anesthesia. Tramadol appears to be effective in the treatment of postoperative shivering. It can be slowly removed by hemodialysis.

Fentanyl and its Congeners (Sufentanil, Alfentanil, and Remifentanil)

Fentanyl

Fentanyl is a synthetic amine opioid and is structurally related to the phenylpiperidine nucleus. It is a pure μ-receptor agonist and 100 times more potent than morphine as an analgesic in an equivalent dose. The molecular structure of fentanyl is shown in **Figure 25**.

The mechanism of action of fentanyl is the same as that of morphine and meperidine. The adult dose of fentanyl for premedication by the intramuscular route is 50–100 µg. For the induction or the supplementation of GA, an IV dose of 1–100 µg/kg fentanyl may be used. Fentanyl may also be administered via the epidural or spinal route and a dose of 25–50 µg is usually employed through these routes. The drug acts within 2–5 minutes when is administered intravenously. A small dose of fentanyl has the duration of action of 30–60 minutes, whereas high doses of fentanyl (>50 µg/kg) may be effective for 4–6 hours. The doses of fentanyl and other opioids are given in **Table 13**.

It has a rapid onset and rapid termination of action, after a small bolus dose and has relative cardiovascular stability. The recovery from the analgesic effect of fentanyl is very fast, however with a large dose or after prolonged infusion, the action of fentanyl is prolonged and recovery is delayed, like the long-acting opioids. All the effects of fentanyl are like pure μ-receptor agonist such as morphine. Muscle rigidity such as chest wall rigidity (wooden chest phenomenon) is also common after IV bolus doses of fentanyl and its congeners. This muscle rigidity is centrally-mediated and may be an effect of the drug on μ-receptors, located on GABAergic interneurons. This rigidity can be mitigated by the slower administration (avoiding bolus) or by the pretreatment with nonopioid anesthetics such as IV-inducing agents, e.g., thiopentone, propofol, etc., or by the muscle relaxants. The higher dose of fentanyl also can cause neuroexcitation.

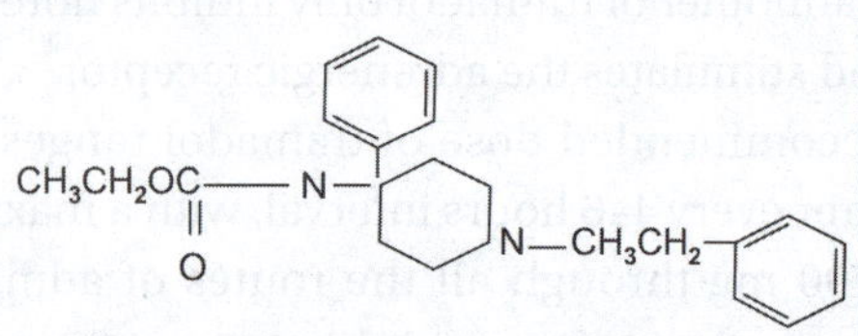

The most significant cardiovascular effect of fentanyl is bradycardia which is of vagal in origin. Cardiac output, mean arterial pressure, systemic and pulmonary vascular resistance, and pulmonary capillary wedge pressure are all unaffected or slightly decreased by the administration of fentanyl. It also obtunds the cardiovascular responses to laryngoscopy and intubation.

Fentanyl is a potent respiratory depressant opioid causing a decrease in both the respiratory rate and tidal volume. It also diminishes the ventilatory response to hypoxia or hypercarbia. The drug is also a potent antitussive agent.

TABLE 13: Doses of commonly used opioids in different routes for different purposes.

Drugs	Use	Route	Doses
Morphine	Premedication	IM	0.04–0.25 mg/kg
	Intraoperative	IV	0.2–1 mg/kg
	Postoperative	IM	0.04–0.25 mg/kg
		IV	0.02–0.1 mg/kg
Meperidine	Premedication	IM	0.5–1.5 mg/kg
	Intraoperative	IV	1–2 mg/kg
	Postoperative	IM	0.5–1.5 mg/kg
		IV	0.2–0.5 mg/kg
Fentanyl	Intraoperative	IV	1–100 µg/kg
	Postoperative	IV	0.5–2 µg/kg
Sufentanil	Intraoperative	IV	0.2–30 µg/kg
Alfentanil	Intraoperative	IV	5–100 µg/kg
	Maintenance	IV	0.5–3 µg/kg/min
Remifentanil	Intraoperative (loading dose)	IV	1 µg/kg
	Maintenance	IV	0.5–10 µg/kg/min

Note: Opioids have large therapeutic window. This is indicated by a wide range of doses of opioids. The doses of opioids also depend on other anesthetics which are administered simultaneously. During IV infusion of it, tolerance develops rapidly, usually within 2–3 hours, and infusion rates should be increased gradually. For obese patients, the doses of opioids should be calculated according to their lean body weight or ideal body weight but not on total body weight.

Fig. 25: The molecular structure of fentanyl.

It causes minimal release of histamine. Bronchospasm is thus rarely precipitated by the drug.

Fentanyl though is 100 times more potent as an analgesic than morphine, but has little hypnotic or sedative activity. Miosis is produced as a result of stimulation of the Edinger–Westphal nucleus. There have been several reports of seizure-like motor activity, occurring in patients who receives fentanyl, however no epileptic-like spike-wave patterns are demonstrable on EEG after the use of fentanyl.

Fentanyl decreases GI motility and decreases the gastric acid secretion. It also doubles the CBD pressure by causing spasms of the sphincter of Oddi. The drug increases the tone of ureters, detrusor muscle of the bladder, and vesicular sphincter. High doses of fentanyl will obtund the metabolic stress response to intubation and surgery. Unlike morphine, fentanyl does not increase the activity of ADH. Like other opioids fentanyl also decreases the apparent MAC value of coadministered volatile anesthetic agents and increases the effect of nondepolarizing muscle relaxants. The drug fentanyl is pharmaceutically incompatible with thiopentone. So they should not be mixed in the same syringe. It is unknown whether fentanyl is removed by hemodialysis or not.

As fentanyl is highly lipid soluble, so it rapidly crosses the blood–brain barrier, and an equilibrium between the plasma and CSF concentration is rapidly approximated within 5 minutes. Then, the concentration of fentanyl in plasma and CSF rapidly declines due to the redistribution of it from a low volume but a highly perfused group of tissues (brain) to other high-volume but a less perfused group of tissues such as muscle and fat. The short duration of action of a single dose of fentanyl is due to this quick distribution and redistribution of it to other tissues from the brain or nervous tissues, rather than the quick metabolism and elimination of it through the liver and kidney. So, this is like thiopentone, propofol, and ketamine. When the saturation and the equilibrium of high volume, but less well-perfused tissues, such as muscles and fats occurs, then the duration of fentanyl's effect prolongs and its elimination half-life reaches about 3–4 hours.

Therefore, after higher doses or prolonged infusions, fentanyl becomes a long-acting opioid. Fentanyl is absorbed orally, but the bioavailability of it by this route is only 33%. The drug is 90% protein bound in plasma. Fentanyl undergoes both the hepatic metabolism and renal excretion. It appears to be metabolized primarily by N-dealkylation to norfentanyl with subsequent hydroxylation of it. The parent compound is metabolized to hydroxypropionyl derivatives. The drug may also undergo hydroxylation and amide hydrolysis in liver. Some enterohepatic circulation of fentanyl may also occur. The 10% of an administered dose of fentanyl is excreted through urine. The elimination half-life of fentanyl is 1.5–6 hours.

Sufentanil

All the pharmacokinetic and pharmacodynamic properties of sufentanil are similar to that of fentanyl, except it is 10 times more potent than fentanyl (i.e., 1,000 times more potent than morphine). The chemical structure of sufentanil is similar to that of fentanyl and is related to the phenylpiperidine nucleus. The pharmacokinetic properties of sufentanil are also adequately described by a three-compartmental model like fentanyl. After IV injection, the first-pass pulmonary extraction, retention, and release of sufentanil are also similar to those of fentanyl **(Fig. 26)**.

The IV dose of sufentanil is 0.5–50 µg/kg. The dose via the epidural route is 10–100 µg. The optimal postoperative dose of sufentanil is 30–50 µg. When administered intravenously, the drug acts within 1–6 minutes, and the duration of effect is 0.5–8 hours. Though the drug is normally administered intravenously, it is 20% absorbed when administered transdermally. Sufentanil is 92% protein bound in the plasma, predominantly to α-1 acid glycoprotein. It is twice as lipid-soluble as fentanyl. The major metabolic pathway of sufentanil includes N-dealkylation, oxidative O-demethylation, and aromatic hydroxylation. Major metabolites of sufentanil include N-phenylpropanamide. About 60% of an administered dose of sufentanil appears in the urine and 10% in the bile. The elimination half-life of sufentanil is 119–175 minutes.

Like other opioids, sufentanil also decreases the MAC value of the coadministered volatile anesthetic agents by 60–70%. The drug should be used with caution in the presence of renal or hepatic failure, although the kinetics appears to be unaltered.

Remifentanil (G187084B) and Alfentanil

They are also synthetic pure µ-opioid receptor agonist, related to phenylpiperidine nucleus. The pharmacological properties of these two opioids are the same as fentanyl, except few differences. These compounds have very rapid onset and predictable termination of effects. The potency of remifentanil is equal to fentanyl, but 20–30 times greater than that of alfentanil. Analgesic effect of both of these compounds

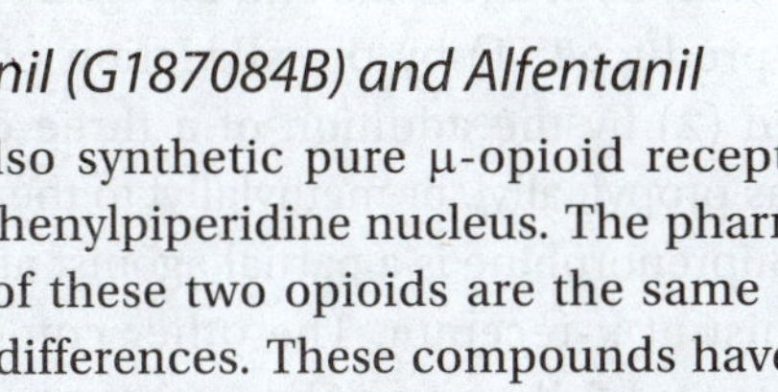

Fig. 26: Sufentanil.

occurs within 1–1.5 minutes after IV administration. Alfentanil is metabolized in liver and its elimination half-life is 1–2 hours. Remifentanil is unique in that it is metabolized by plasma esterase enzyme. So, elimination of remifentanil from our body is independent of hepatic metabolism and renal excretion and the elimination half-life of it is only 8–20 minutes. Therefore, there is no prolongation of effect of remifentanil after repeated doses or prolonged infusion. After 3–5 hours of infusion of remifentanil, recovery of respiratory function can be seen within 3–5 minutes, while full recovery from all the effects of remifentanil occurs within 15 minutes. The major metabolite of remifentanil is remifentanil acid which is 2,000–4,000 times less potent than its parent compound and is excreted through the kidney. Remifentanil is ideally suited for short surgical procedures where rapid recovery is the goal. It is also very useful in longer surgical procedures where rapid emergence from anesthesia is important, such as neurosurgery. However, due to the short duration of action, remifentanil alone is a poor choice for postoperative analgesia. It is generally given by continuous IV infusion because its short duration of action makes bolus administration impractical.

Alfentanil can be used intraspinally, but remifentanil is not being used intraspinally, because glycine used in commercial preparation of it as a preservative can cause temporary motor paralysis.

Individual Opioid with Both Agonistic–Antagonistic Activity and only Antagonistic Activity

The opioids with both agonistic and antagonistic property are usually produced (1) by the alkylation of piperidine nitrogen and (2) by the addition of a three-carbon side chain such as propyl, allyl, or methylallyl to the structure of morphine. Buprenorphine is a partial agonist at μ-receptor, but antagonist at κ-receptor. The other compounds are μ-antagonists and full or partial agonists at κ-receptors. Agonists and antagonistic opioids are less prone to abuse because they cause less euphoria and are associated with less drug-seeking behavior and physical dependence.

Classification of Opioid Agonists and Antagonists

- *μ agonist + κ antagonist:* Buprenorphine
- *μ antagonist + κ agonist:* Nalorphine, pentazocine, butorphanol, levallorphan, and nalbuphine.
- *μ, κ, and δ antagonist (pure antagonists):* Naloxone, naltrexone, and nalmefene.
  Nalorphine, levallorphan, and nalbuphine are not used now, due to their high toxicity.

Pentazocine

It is a benzomorphan derivative of morphine and has both agonistic action on κ-receptor and weak antagonistic action on μ-receptor. So, it is an agonistic and antagonistic opioid. It is also called κ-analgesic as its analgesic action is exerted through κ-opioid receptor.

The CNS effect of pentazocine is like morphine, including analgesia, sedation, and respiratory depression. It is ½–¼ as potent as morphine. The analgesic action of pentazocine is due to its agonistic action on κ-receptor. Higher doses of it (60–90 mg) elicit dysphoric and psychotomimetic effect. The possible mechanism for this side effect, caused by pentazocine, is the activation of supraspinal κ-receptor which can be reversed by naloxone. Ceiling to both the analgesia and respiratory depression effect of pentazocine occurs after the administration of 30–70 mg of it.

Pentazocine depresses myocardial contractility but causes ↑BP, ↑HR, ↑SVR, ↑pulmonary artery pressure, ↑left ventricular end-diastolic pressure, and ↑cardiac workload (left ventricular work index). It also increases the blood catecholamine level, hence all these changes show that pentazocine increases myocardial O_2 demand and may precipitate myocardial ischemia. Hemodynamic effects of opioid agonists and antagonists, compared with morphine are given in **Table 14**. Pentazocine appears to cause less *nausea* and vomiting and a less marked rise in biliary tract pressure than an equivalent dose of morphine. The drug decreases both the gastric and small intestinal motility.

Though pentazocine has weak antagonistic action on μ-receptor, but it does not antagonize the respiratory depression effect, produced by morphine. But when pentazocine is given in patient dependent on morphine or other μ-receptor agonist, then it may precipitate withdrawal or reduce its analgesic effect.

However, the potentiality for the abuse of pentazocine is less than that of morphine, but the prolonged use of it can lead to physical dependence on it. The drug is also well absorbed when administered orally. Orally the bioavailability of pentazocine is only 20%. It is due to significant hepatic first-pass metabolism of it. The adult oral dose of pentazocine is

TABLE 14: Hemodynamic effects of opioid agonist–antagonist compared with morphine.

Drug	Cardiac workload	Blood pressure	Heart rate	Pulmonary artery pressure
Morphine	↓	↓	↓	↓
Pentazocine	↑	↑	↑	↑
Buprenorphine	↓	↓	↓	↓
Butorphanol	↑	↑	=	↑

50–100 mg, given at 3–4 hours intervals. The corresponding parenteral dose of it is 30–60 mg at 3–4 hours intervals. The drug is irritant when is injected intramuscularly or subcutaneously. The pentazocine acts within 2–3 minutes, when is administered intravenously, and within 20 minutes when is administered intramuscularly. The duration of action of this dose of pentazocine is 3–4 hours. The metabolism of pentazocine occurs in liver by the oxidation and glucuronidation; however, 60% of the administered dose of it is excreted through urine within 24 hours. Among this 2–10% remains unchanged. The elimination half-life of pentazocine is 2 hours and can be removed by hemodialysis.

Buprenorphine

It is a semisynthetic, highly lipophilic agonist–antagonist opioid which is derived from thebaine. It is a partial or weak μ-receptor agonist and κ-receptor antagonist. It dissociates very slowly from its opioid receptor, leading to a prolonged duration of action (analgesia). Buprenorphine substitutes for morphine at low level of dependence on later, but precipitates withdrawal in a highly-dependent subject, thus it reflects its partial agonistic action at μ-receptor. Being a partial agonist, buprenorphine like other agonist–antagonistic group of opioids may antagonize the effects of morphine and cause symptoms of abstinence in patient who is receiving pure μ-agonist (morphine-like drug) for several weeks, thus it restricts its usefulness, if other μ-agonists are used. Buprenorphine also appears to have high affinity for κ-receptors which are antagonistic in nature.

The structure of buprenorphine is similar to morphine, but is 33 times more potent than it. Its high lipophilicity and high receptor affinity cause its receptor's association and dissociation action very slow. So, it possesses a much longer half-life which is near about 160 minutes (fentanyl half-life is 6 minutes), hence the plasma level of buprenorphine does not correspond to its CNS effect. Buprenorphine's onset of action is slow. Its peak action may not occur until 3 hours. Its duration of action is also prolonged ($\leq$10 hours). Metabolism of it occurs in liver, with biliary excretion of most of its metabolites such as buprenorphine-3-glucuronide, norbuprenorphine, and buprenorphine which are less potent and have lower affinities for the opioid μ-receptor. Thus, most of the drug is excreted through feces.

Buprenorphine produces analgesia and other CNS effects like morphine. It has minimal cardiovascular effects. The HR may decrease by up to 25% and the systolic BP may fall by 10%, following the administration of it. Buprenorphine produces respiratory depression and has antitussive effects, similar to that produced by morphine. The respiratory depression effects of buprenorphine are not completely reversed by even larger doses of naloxone. This is probably because of more tight binding of buprenorphine with its opioid receptors. Doxapram, however, will do so. Severe respiratory depression has occurred when BZDs have been coadministered with buprenorphine. It may cause the release of tryptase and histamine from the lung parenchymal mast cells and may increase pulmonary vascular resistance. It also produces miosis and decreases cerebral glucose metabolism by up to 30%.

It is well absorbed by most of the routes. The recommended analgesic dose of buprenorphine is 0.3–0.4 mg by oral, IM, IV, or sublingual route (1) for premedication, (2) as an analgesic component in balanced anesthesia, and (3) for postoperative pain control. The drug is also effective when administered by epidural route and a dose of 0.3 mg buprenorphine has been recommended for this. The drug is well absorbed when is administered orally but undergoes a significant first-pass liver metabolism. Therefore, the sublingual route is preferred than oral, when parenteral route is not used. The bioavailability of buprenorphine is 40–90% when administered intramuscularly and 44–94% when administered sublingually. It is not removed by hemodialysis. Opioid withdrawal symptoms develop slowly (5–10 days) after buprenorphine is discontinued following long-term administration.

Butorphanol

Chemically it is morphine congener, with a profile of action similar to that of pentazocine. Like pentazocine, it is an antagonist at μ-opioid receptor and agonist at κ-opioid receptor which is responsible for its analgesic effect, but it is more potent than pentazocine (2 mg butorphanol = 30 mg pentazocine). However, the antagonistic property of butorphanol at μ-receptor are weak and do not usually interfere with the use of other opioid agonist in anesthesia.

In a healthy subject, the butorphanol produces no or minimal CVS changes, but in cardiac-diseased patient, the butorphanol causes changes, similar to that produced by pentazocine. It causes $\uparrow$cardiac index, $\uparrow$left ventricular end-diastolic pressure, and $\uparrow$pulmonary artery pressure. So, butorphanol is not useful in patients with CCF or at increased risk for myocardial ischemia or with a history of previous myocardial infarction (MI). The major side effects of butorphanol are drowsiness, weakness, sweating, nausea, and CNS stimulation, while the incidence of psychotomimetic side effects (quantitatively) of butorphanol is lower than that of equianalgesic doses of pentazocine, but they are qualitatively similar.

Butorphanol is subject to less abuse and has less addictive potential. It is only available in parenteral form.

The recommended dose of butorphanol is 1–4 mg through IM or 0.5–2 mg through the IV route.

Nalorphine

It is *N*-allylnormorphine. It was the first opioid antagonist, introduced in 1951, to reverse the action of morphine (for μ-receptor antagonist), but later it was found that it possesses agonistic action on the κ-opioid receptor as well, producing lower ceiling analgesia. It is not used clinically, because it has strong dysphoric and psychotomimetic effects.

■ OPIOID ANTAGONISTS

The antagonists of opioid receptors (specific or nonspecific) are important armors for the scientific research of opioids and its receptors. In early 1950, nalorphine and levallorphan were evaluated as an opioid antagonist for clinical use, though they have agonistic in action, but later they were discarded due to their high incidences of side effects. Then, in 1960, naloxone was introduced and had established its efficacy as a pure antagonist (without any agonistic action on any opioid receptors) for opioid-induced respiratory depression.

Classification of Agonist–Antagonist Opioids

- *Not used as analgesic:* Nalorphine (μ-antagonist + κ-agonist) and levallorphan (μ-antagonist + κ-agonist)
- *Used as analgesic:* Pentazocine (μ-antagonist + κ-agonist) and nalbuphine (μ-antagonist + κ-agonist)
- *Partial/weak agonists:* Buprenorphine (μ-agonist + κ-antagonist) and butorphanol (μ-antagonist + κ-agonist)
- *Pure antagonists:*
  - *Block μ, κ, and δ receptor:* Naloxone and naltrexone
  - *Block only μ receptor:* Nalmefene

Naloxone

The molecular structure of naloxone is shown in **Figure 27**. Slight minor changes in the structure of an opioid molecule can convert its agonistic action into an antagonistic action on its opioid receptors. The most common example of such a substitution is the N-methyl group which is typical for μ-receptor agonist. So, such substitution transforms morphine to *nalorphine*; levorphanol to *levallorphan*, and oxymorphone to *naloxone* or *naltrexone*. Some of these substituted opioid congeners are completely competitive antagonist at μ-receptor, but agonist at κ-receptor. So, they can be used as agonist–antagonistic opioid. Hence, these nalorphine, levallorphan, and nalbuphine, etc., can also be used as analgesics such as pentazocine, butorphanol, and buprenorphine, because though they are antagonistic at μ-receptor, but are agonistic at κ-receptor, however some

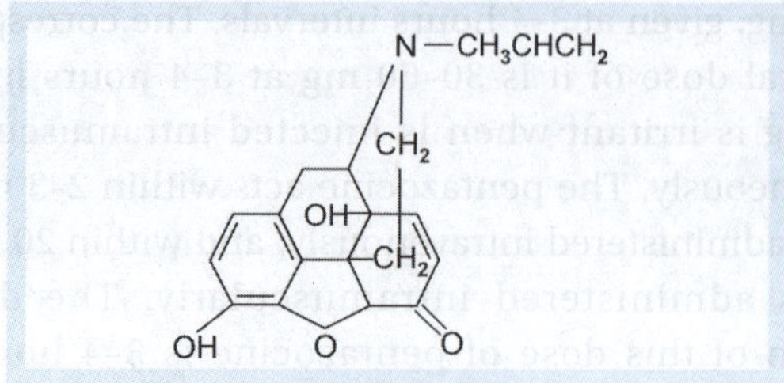

Fig. 27: Naloxone.

of the substituted opioid congeners have antagonistic action on all the opioid receptors (μ, κ, and δ) without any agonistic action on any opioid receptor. These are *naloxone* and *naltrexone*. Later specific opioid receptor antagonists were developed which are not congeners of opioids, for example, *nalmefene* which is a pure μ-receptor antagonist. *Norbinaltorphimine* and *naltrindole* are specific κ- and δ-receptor antagonist, respectively.

Thus, naloxone chemically is a substituted oxymorphone derivative. Its mode of action is competitive antagonist at μ, κ, and δ receptors. Naloxone itself produces no effects on any opioid receptor. It means it has no intrinsic effects like morphine, when it combines with opioid receptors independently or if opioids with μ-receptor agonistic action are not administered previously. If an opioid is used previously, then naloxone, injected intravenously (0.4–0.8 mg) will rescue the respiratory depression effect of opioids. Respiration will not only be normalized but will be stimulated (probably due to sudden sensitization of the respiratory center to retained CO_2). In addition, it can reduce or reverse opioid-induced analgesia, nausea, vomiting, pruritus, urinary retention, rigidity, biliary spasm, etc. Hence, these drugs may precipitate acute withdrawal symptoms in opiate addicts and pupils will dilate, however sedation will be less completely reversed.

The mechanism of action of naloxone is that it binds with all the opioid receptors and prevents the binding of opioid agonists, thus it prevents the manifestation of actions of opioid agonist, which work through these receptors. At 4–10 mg dose, it antagonizes the agonistic action of nalorphine, pentazocine, etc., but the dysphoric and psychotomimetic action of some of them will be incompletely suppressed. The actions of buprenorphine are suppressed, but will not be effectively reversed by naloxone, because it fails to displace buprenorphine that has already been bound to opioid receptors.

In shock and certain forms of stress, when the endogenous opioid system is activated, then the opioid antagonist naloxone also has visible consequences. It attenuates the hypotension associated with shock of diverse origins, including that caused by anaphylaxis, endotoxin, hypovolemia, etc.

Naloxone also apparently acts to antagonize the actions of endogenous opioids that are mobilized by pain, stress, and that are involved in the regulation of BP by CNS.

However, a high dose of naloxone (12 mg) alone has an intrinsic agonistic effect, but this is of little clinical significance. Dose of naloxone in excess of 0.3 mg/kg shows increased systolic BP.

Endogenous opioid peptides usually participate in the regulation of pituitary secretion, by exerting tonic inhibitory effects on the release of certain hypothalamic hormones. Thus, administration of naloxone by removing this inhibition increases the secretion of corticotropin-releasing factor and elevates the plasma concentration of ACTH. Thus, the elevated ACTH increases the plasma concentration of cortisol and catecholamines.

Naloxone can also be administered through IV, IM, or subcutaneous route, but the drug should be administered intravenously in small incremental doses until the desired end point of reversal of respiratory depression without reversal of analgesia is reached. This is because at different blood level naloxone antagonize the different actions of morphine. Small dose (0.4–0.8 mg) of naloxone given IM or IV does not reverse the μ-receptor-mediated analgesic effects of opioids, but it reverses only the respiratory depression effect and so the respiratory rate increases within 1–2 minutes. Higher dose of naloxone is needed to antagonize the respiratory depression effect of buprenorphine. Sedative effect of opioid is also reversed and BP, if depressed, returns to normal. If IV access is not available, then naloxone in a dose similar to that given by IV is effectively absorbed after intratracheal administration. Naloxone also reverses the psychotomimetic and dysphoric effects of agonist–antagonistic agents, such as pentazocine, but for this much higher doses of naloxone are required.

Opioids decrease the sympathetic outflow through their action on CNS (brain and spinal cord). The α-adrenergic agonist (clonidine) and opioids perform this through their action on preganglionic sympathetic neurons. Opioid antagonists block this action of opioids and increase sympathetic outflow. This explains clonidine's effectiveness in blocking hemodynamic stimulation following naloxone.

The side effects such as increased HR, BP, and more serious complication like pulmonary edema may follow the administration of naloxone, due to this sympathetic stimulation. So, opioid reversal by naloxone should be avoided in patients in whom the increased HR and BP could be detrimental. Patient with coronary artery disease could be adversely affected by naloxone, because of this sympathetic stimulation. Opioid reversal by naloxone may be hazardous in patients with pheochromocytoma.

The onset of action of naloxone after IV administration is 1–2 minutes and duration of effect is about 30–60 minutes, although naloxone is rapidly absorbed through GI tract (91%), but it is almost completely metabolized by the liver, before reaching in systemic circulation (only 2%). So it must be administered parenterally. It is mainly metabolized by glucuronidation.

Recurrence of respiratory depression after administration of naloxone is due to its short half-life and reuptake of opioid by μ-receptor from peripheral compartmental tissues. So, renarcotization occurs more frequently, after the use of naloxone, during the reversal of longer acting opioids, such as morphine.

Naloxone acts through μ, δ, and κ-receptor, but has greatest affinity on μ-receptor, through which antirespiratory depression and antianalgesic action of it are mediated. It is unlikely that analgesia is always spared, but careful titration by naloxone often restores adequate spontaneous ventilation without reversal of analgesia.

The other probable conditions where naloxone can be used are:

- Hemorrhagic shock
- Septic shock
- Postanesthetic apnea in infants, where opioid is not used
- Primary apnea and periodic breathing associated with hypoxia
- In the treatment of alcoholism (alcohol interacts with many neurotransmitters and endogenous opioid system in the brain. Mesolimbic dopamine system is mainly affected and the links between alcohol and opioid system play an important role in alcohol addiction).
- To reverse the effects of some nonopioid CNS depressants (BZD and barbiturates → opioid–GABA receptor interactions).
- To ameliorate neurological deficits in the spinal cord and brain trauma
- To reduce obesity and clonidine overdose
- To diagnose the suspected opioid overdose
- Naloxone may also partially antagonize the ketamine- and N_2O-induced analgesia.

Sometimes naloxone enhances the analgesia and morphine requirements are significantly less in patients receiving it. Proposed possible mechanism for this paradoxical effect of naloxone is the enhanced release of endogenous opioids by it and the upregulation of opioid receptors.

Naltrexone

It is a pure μ, δ, and κ-receptor antagonist. It is chemically related to naloxone but differs from naloxone by: (1)

naltrexone is more potent than naloxone and longer acting, (2) its half-life is 8–12 hours, and (3) it can be used by oral route. Naltrexone is not subjected to much first-pass hepatic metabolism as naloxone, so its duration of action approaches 24–48 hours, after its moderate oral dose. Oral naltrexone, in the dose of 5–10 mg, reduces the severity and frequency of respiratory depression, pruritus, nausea, and vomiting associated with morphine, without diminishing analgesia. Like naloxone, naltrexone also stimulates CVS. *It is mainly used for the treatment of opium addiction and alcoholism due to its longer acting and effectiveness by oral route.* Its long duration of action makes it suitable for "opioid blockade" therapy of postaddicts. If 50 mg is given per day orally, then if the subject takes his usual shot of opioids, then no subjective feeling will be produced and the craving for opioids will subside. Common side effects of naltrexone are nausea and headache.

Methyl naltrexone: This derivative of naltrexone does not penetrate the blood–brain barrier, so it only effectively blocks the peripheral μ-opioid receptors. Hence, it is being used to reverse constipation in cancer patients, receiving chronic opioid analgesia, and in those taking methadone maintenance therapy.

Nalmefene

The structure of nalmefene is similar to that of naloxone and naltrexone, but it has a greater affinity to opioid μ-receptor. It has nil or minimal effect on opioid δ- and κ-receptor. It is long-acting both after oral and parenteral administration. The bioavailability of it after oral administration is 50% (highest). It lacks the hepatotoxicity of naltrexone. The plasma half-life of nalmefene varies from 3 to 8 hours. It produces little or nil intrinsic effect by itself when administered without previous administration of opioids.

Interaction in Between Inhaled Anesthetic and Opioid

During N_2O administration, cardiovascular function is usually preserved. But the N_2O–opioid combination cause ↓CO, ↓HR, ↓BP and ↑SVR, ↑PVR, and ↑coronary vascular resistance, resulting in impaired coronary blood flow. Deterioration of cardiac function with N_2O–opioid combination is due to an increase in afterload (↑SVR and ↑PVR). This deterioration is not evident during routine monitoring of BP, due to elevated SVR.

Analgesia produced by N_2O is mediated partly by opioidergic system and cause infra-additive interaction between N_2O and opioid. So, the advent of short-acting IV anesthetics (e.g., propofol) and volatile anesthetics with blood–gas partition coefficient equal to that of N_2O (e.g., sevoflurane) has recently decreased the popularity of N_2O in balanced anesthesia. Except halothane, combination of a low concentration of other volatile anesthetics and opioid is beneficial for compromised ventricular function. New volatile anesthetics such as isoflurane, desflurane, and sevoflurane cause only little myocardial depression.

Low concentration of isoflurane and a high dose of sufentanil is very effective and safe to treat intraoperative hypertension, without producing myocardial depression and without decreasing CO in coronary artery surgery. Halothane plus opioid anesthesia to control hypertension produces ↓BP and ↓CO which exacerbate regional myocardial hypoperfusion and increase lactate production. Some potent newer inhaled anesthetics (isoflurane and desflurane) increase sympathetic nervous system activity, but this can be attenuated by opioid.

Interaction In between Sedative–Hypnotic and Opioid

Benzodiazepines are the ideal agents to combine with opioids. This combination acts as synergistic fashion (supra-additive) and potentiates to reduce the dose of opioid. The BZD and opioid combination preserve ventricular function, but reduces BP, SVR, CI, and HR due to sympathetic depression and venodilatation. So, in patients with poor ventricular function, this drug regime may be hazardous. Fluid loading can attenuate a decrease in BP, ventricular filling, and CO.

Barbiturates, droperidol, ketamine, etomidate and propofol are some of the other sedative–hypnotics which can be combined with opioids. Hypotension after a barbiturate-opioid combination is due to vasodilatation, causing decreased cardiac filling and myocardial depression, due to decreased sympathetic nervous activity.

Propofol and opioid combination has the same effect such as BZD and opioid combination. Together they provide unconsciousness and block the responses to noxious stimuli; whereas neither drug alone reliably does both. Propofol + fentanyl or sufentanil anesthesia provide acceptable conditions for coronary artery bypass surgery. Sometimes, mean arterial pressure can decrease to a level that may jeopardize coronary perfusion. Mean arterial pressure and HR can decrease up to 35 and 16% respectively.

Etomidate and ketamine can be combined with opioid without loss of cardiovascular stability in cardiac surgery. Etomidate and fentanyl combination cause less hypotension than propofol–fentanyl combination.

CHAPTER 15

Inhalational Anesthetic Agents

INTRODUCTION AND HISTORY

In ancient times, the main anchors of analgesia and anesthesia during surgery, especially before 1800, were the *oral opium, laudanum* (an opium derivative), *mandragora* (a juice from "mandrake" plant) and the liberal use of *alcohol*. Then, Anton Mesmer had given much importance to psychological preparation of patient and he had first introduced *mesmerism* in Europe, as a mode of anesthesia in surgery. This was in between 1750 and 1800. At that time, many literatures were also full of references with many wondrous sleeping positions, ranging from Snow White's apple to mandrake plant, used by Shakespeare's Cleopatra. But, modern inhalational anesthesia was dawned by the introduction of inhalational anesthetic agents, such as N_2O *in 1844, ether in 1846, and chloroform in 1847.*

Around 1628, William Harvey had first discovered circulation. He also had first observed difference in color between the pulmonary venous and pulmonary arterial blood. But, he was unable to draw any firm conclusion, regarding the functions of lungs and the cause of difference in color between the pulmonary venous and arterial blood. Then, in-between 1660 and 1670, Robert Boyle and Robert Hooke had thought or imagined that there is some component of air which is absorbed by lungs and is responsible for that difference in color between the blood of pulmonary vein and artery. After that, Harvey had discovered the different components, circulating in blood and had developed an intravenous technique for therapeutic purposes. At that time, the basic scientific work on respiration by *Priestly, Lavoisier,* and *Laplace* had also led to the possibility of the use of different breathing gases and vapors for therapeutic reasons (for the treatment of different pulmonary diseases, e.g., tuberculosis) **(Fig. 1)**.

When Priestley was in Birmingham, he experimented with many gases for therapeutic (treatment) purposes of pulmonary diseases. During this period, his friend, Pearson

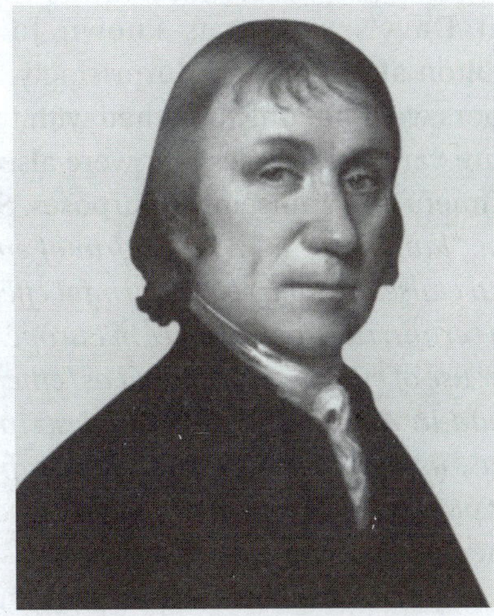

Fig. 1: Joseph Priestley.

had recommended the inhalation of ether for the recovery of different lung diseases. Then, in the period between 1780 and 1800, Thomas Beddoes, a physician and chemist of Oxford and a friend of this group of scientists, founded a Pneumatic Institution in Bristol for the study of this pneumatic therapy for the treatment of different lung diseases of patients. Among these gases that Beddos had used for the therapy of patients were oxygen, CO_2, water gas (mixture of H_2, CO, and CO_2) and hydrogen. But, Chaussier had first used O_2 in medicine in 1780 for neonatal asphyxia. In 1798, Beddos and Humphrey Davy met each other, while they were on a holiday at Cornwall. There, Beddos invited Davy to be the superintendent of this Pneumatic Institution in Bristol.

Davy was then only 19 years old. Here, Davy undertook a series of experiments on the effects of breathing of N_2O. Once he had severe inflammation of his gum with acute pain. During an experiment with this pain, he breathed three large doses of N_2O. The pain was diminished and then Davy had suggested the probable use of N_2O as analgesic, with definite advantages, during surgical operations.

This was the first experiment and suggestion in 1800 by Davy that surgical analgesia might be achieved by inhalation of N_2O. So, inhalational anesthesia can be dated back to that very suggestion, with dawn of modern inhalational anesthesia, where many modern volatile anesthetics were delivered with sophisticated electronic vaporizers. Davy also realized the pulmonary blood flow. He also suggested that cardiac output and pulmonary blood flow could be measured by estimating the rate, at which N_2O is taken up by the lungs. During that period, to assist the work of Davy, Sir James Watt also made a special N_2O container. But, after few years, due to some unknown reason, Davy or his contemporaries did not further pursue the idea of deliberately inhaling N_2O to produce surgical analgesia **(Fig. 2)**.

After that Davy's work was known to many and influenced Colton after 44 years. Surprisingly, at that time gases and vapors were not only breathed with the hope that they might cure various diseases, but were also inhaled for pure entertainment and amusement purposes. *So, Davy also named N_2O as "laughing gas". As this form of entertainment did not seem to cause any long-term harmful effects, so it was widespread in certain rich social circles in Europe. During that period, similar use of ether vapor, named as "ether frolics" was also widespread in America. We get the description of such entertainments, using laughing gas and ether frolics, in the works of great poets, like Samuel Taylor and Robert Southey.*

In 1824, the first deliberate use of inhaled gas, to produce anesthesia, was performed by Hickman on an animal for surgical operation. He used CO_2 for anesthesia. But, his experiment and contribution in medical science was not recognized by medical body at that time. Thus, it was he (Hickman) who introduced the concept of anesthesia using an inhaled substance. The first recorded general anesthesia, administered by the inhalation of gases in humans was, in 1842, by Long and Clarke, using ether. *Then, on 16th October in 1846, Morton first successfully demonstrated publicly ether anesthesia at Massachusetts General Hospital. The operation was the removal of a vascular tumor from just below the mandible and was held at place, what is now called as the "Ether Dome", at Massachusetts General Hospital. The patient, who gave the informed consent for operation, was a young man, named Edward Gilbert Abbott, a printer and journalist and Mr Warren was the surgeon.*

Then, in 1847, Pierre Flourens, a Paris physiologist, suggested that ether gradually affects first the higher cerebral centers, then the cerebellum and spinal cord, and finally the medulla oblongata where the cardiovascular and respiratory centers are situated as anesthesia is gradually deepened. Flourens had also previously demonstrated that the cardiovascular and respiratory centers were located in the medulla.

After that, *John Snow*, an eminent physician of London, also became interested in ether, soon after its introduction. Even before Gudell, he described the five stages of ether anesthesia in his own publication in 1847. According to him, the first three stages were of light anesthesia. The fourth stage is comprised of what we call as surgical anesthesia **(Fig. 3)** and, in fifth, respiration would become progressively shallow and eventually stopped. Snow quickly realized that the method of administration of ether was faulty. So, he developed many apparatuses for delivering ether vapor to patients, with different known concentration, in an attempt to increase safety. *At that time, in 1847, two deaths associated with ether anesthesia were reported. The first was a young woman at Grantham of Lincs and the second was a 52-year-old man at Essex in Colchester Hospital.* Snow's inventory work was stimulated further by these first report of deaths. Then, Snow investigated many other potential volatile agents

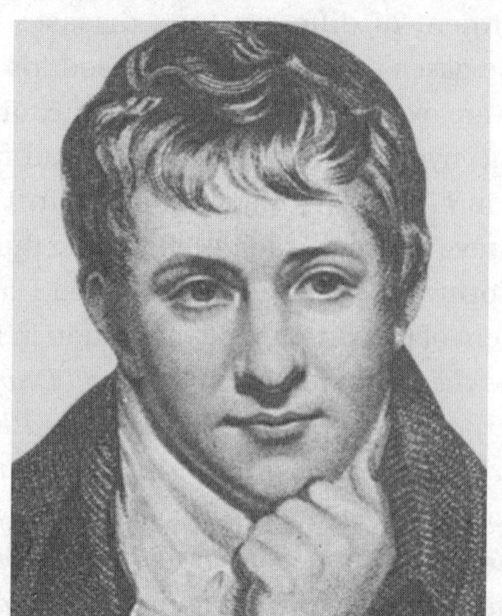

Fig. 2: Humphrey Davy.

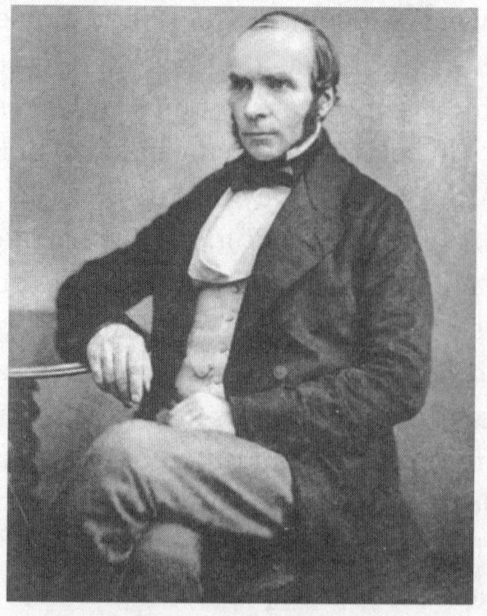

Fig. 3: John Snow.

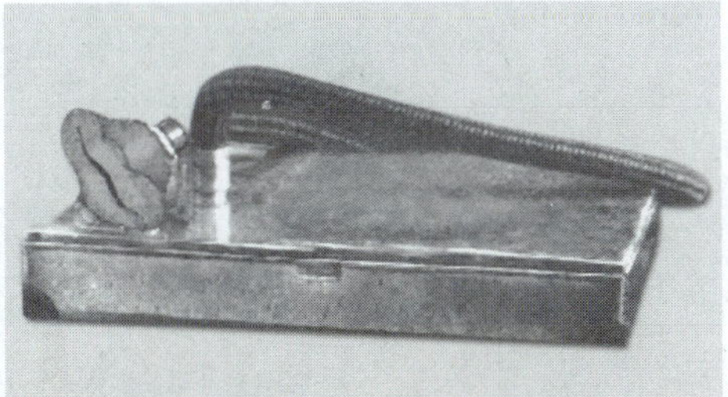

Fig. 4: Snow's inhaler.

for inhalational anesthesia, instead of ether such as benzene, bromoforms, ethyl bromide, ethyl nitrate, and amylene, in last 10 years of his life, from 1848 to 1858. During this time, in 1857, two patients had also died, while he was administering amylene to the patients. *Then, he was the first to suggest that there was an inverse relationship between the lipid solubility and the potency of inhalational anesthetic agents.* During that period, around 1850, many different types of apparatus were also developed to improve the vaporization of ether. It was also tried by preventing the cooling of liquid ether which occurs when it is evaporated. Many scientists also tried to prevent the dilution of ether vapor, which occurred with air, during the administration of it **(Fig. 4)**.

Chloroform was first identified in 1831. But, in 1847, the anesthetic properties of chloroform in animals were first described by Pierre Flourens. *It was first used on humans at St Bartholomew's Hospital of London by Dr Lawrence, under the name of "chloric ether", in one spring of 1847. But, the use of chloroform in clinical practice was first made in vogue by Simpson. Then, it was popularized by his two assistants, who experimented with chloroform, by inhaling it themselves in Simpson's house. Simpson then read a report in Edinburgh Medical Society and described chloroform as a new anesthetic agent which could be used as a substitute for sulfuric ether in surgery and midwifery. Gradually, after 1847, due to the works of Simpson and Snow chloroform became a favored anesthetic agent in Britain than ether. Simpson who had worked more on chloroform also had been impressed by ether, but was trying to overcome the disadvantages of ether associated with its administration. He had also been trying for inhalational anesthesia with other organic volatile agents before chloroform. Then, he finally considered that chloroform had major advantages over ether* **(Fig. 5)**.

Snow, who had worked more on ether, later also abandoned ether and accepted chloroform as better inhalational anesthetic agent. But, he recognized the dangers of chloroform, if its vapor was too strong. To overcome this danger, Snow invented an instrument by which a fixed percentage of chloroform could **(Box 1)** *be delivered. Then, within a few months, chloroform displaced ether and became the most popular inhalational anesthetic agent in Britain.*

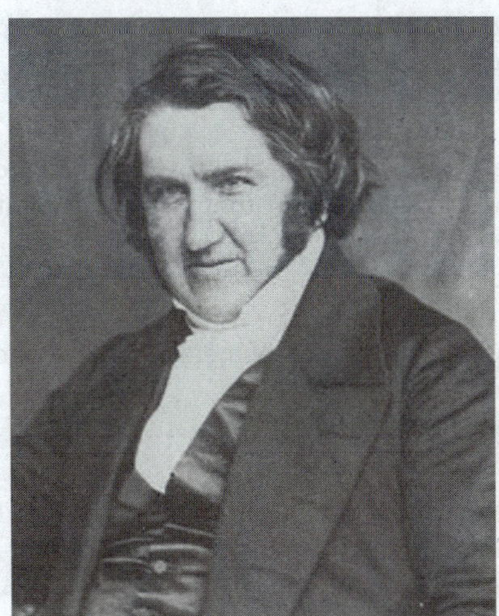

Fig. 5: Young Simpson.

BOX 1: The advantages of chloroform over ether (as thought by Simpson).

- Less volume was needed and it was therefore cheaper
- It was more pleasant than ether for patient and induction was quicker

BOX 2: The toxicities for which chloroform lost it popularity.

- Gradual fall of BP with deepening of anesthesia
- Sudden cardiac arrest during light anesthesia due to ventricular fibrillation or vagal inhibition
- Severe sensitization of myocardium to chloroform

On 28th January of 1848, just little more than 2 months after the introduction of chloroform, first death due to chloroform was reported. The patient was a 15-year-old boy, named Hannah Greener of New Castle. The anesthesia was given for a minor operation by Dr Meggison. Then, Snow gave 5,000 anesthesia by chloroform with only one death. So, he recommended not to use chloroform in concentration of >4% in an air-mixture. Then, due to toxicity, chloroform gradually lost its favor in England **(Box 2)**.

Ether did not regain much popularity in Britain, until *B. Jeffries* came from America and advocated ether as being much safer than chloroform in 1872. Then, 2 years later, in 1874, Clover introduced his gas-ether sequence. After that, ether became accepted as a safe inhalational anesthetic agent than chloroform for all-purpose anesthesia.

The major war, in which inhalational anesthetic agents were used first, was the Crimean War in the period of 1850. Even after the introduction of ether for anesthesia in surgery by Morton, surgeries were still being rampantly performed without any form of anesthesia in European Teaching Hospitals. At that time, different countries had also adopted

BOX 3: The advantages and disadvantages of ether vapor over chloroform.

Advantages
- A relative lack of toxicity, especially in light planes of anesthesia
- Excellent muscle relaxation, without severe respiratory depression
- Lack of cardiac depression, even if overdose produced respiratory depression
- Relatively nontoxic products of metabolism (alcohol, acetaldehyde, and acetic acid)
- Little tendency to cause dysrhythmias

Disadvantages
- The risk of explosion and fire, although explosions have never been described during the administration of ether and air mixture, even when diathermy has been used.
- Stimulation of the secretion of mucus
- Postoperative nausea and vomiting
- A slow induction and recovery due to its high solubility in blood

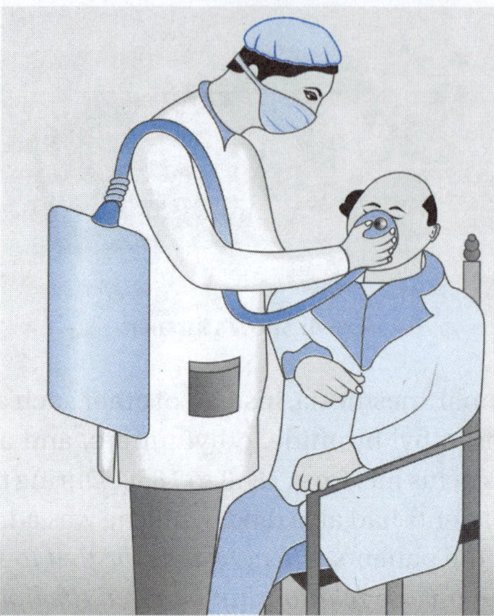

Fig. 6: Joseph Clover monitoring the patients pulse while giving anesthesia by chloroform vapor from a bag.

one of these two anesthetic agents, i.e., ether or chloroform and different methods of their administration. *Thus, chloroform was very popular and was used more frequently in Scotland, greater part of Europe, and South America. While ether was favorite in England and North America. At that time, there was also much controversy, regarding which is more safe among these two* **(Box 3).**

Then, a committee was set up in 1864, which drew attentions to the dangers of chloroform. But, the committee also considered ether to be impractical, because it provided a lengthy induction and a prolonged excitatory phase. *This committee also recommended the use of mixture of ether and chloroform or the only use of chloroform for the induction of anesthesia and then switching over to ether for its maintenance. Then, ACE mixture (alcohol, chloroform, and ether in the ratio of 1:2:3) was introduced in anesthesia practice and also had gained considerable acceptance.* This also opened the door for other important new concepts and the committee suggested that different anesthetic agents may be needed for different types and stages of a surgical operation. Because, till that period, there was no single perfect universal inhalational anesthetic agent.

Clover had worked intensively both on chloroform and ether in 1862. He invented a chloroform inhaler which had enabled the anesthetists for accurate measurement and administration of desired percentage of a mixture of air and chloroform to reduce the risks of chloroform. This took the form of a large bag which was slung over the back of an anesthetist, containing the mixture of 45% chloroform vapor with air. So, Clover was selected in the committee which had investigated chloroform extensively and he realized its danger. So, he abandoned chloroform and set to work to make the administration of ether simpler, easier, and accurate.

He later worked on inducing anesthesia with nitrous oxide, before adding ether. Next, in 1877, Clover had also invented his portable regulating ether inhaler which had made ether more popular at the expense of chloroform. Another Clover's achievements were his teaching that ether could safely be given over long periods with desired and adequate depth of anesthesia. *Thus, by 1870, in this way ether had largely won the game. Then, the two agents N_2O and ether remained the mainstays of inhalational anesthesia for the next 80 years (up to 1950)* **(Fig. 6).**

After the experiment with chloroform and ether, the amylene was also used successfully for inhalational anesthesia by Snow. But, it was quickly abandoned following two deaths. Then, came *ethylchloride* for its rapid action and relative freedom from side effects. But, ethylchloride in its active pure chemical form was difficult to obtain, as it is a highly volatile agent. Again, at that time, there was no such technically improved vaporizer for the use of ethylchloride. So, ethylchloride was introduced as local anesthetic spray, especially for dentistry, rather than general inhalational anesthesia. In 1894, this local use of ethylchloride, by dental surgeons, resulted in accidental general anesthesia. Thus, the apparent ease for the use of ethylchloride had led some surgeons to adopt it for GA. However, the first death, associated with use of ethylchloride, was reported in 1899. Then, gradually, the dangers of ethylchloride soon became apparent, as general anesthetic agent over chloroform and ether. *So, several anesthetists used ethylchloride just for induction of anesthesia and then changed over to ether or chloroform for its maintenance.*

Next, toward the end of 19th century, after a rush of innovation, the development in anesthesia became dramatic. At that time, antiseptic methods were also developed in surgical fields which was parallel to the development of anesthesia. The combination of this development of antisepsis in surgery and the development of anesthesia gradually had allowed to perform prolonged and delicate surgery that could not have been possible before the beginning of 20th century or at the end of 19th century. *But, during that period, still it was very difficult to convince a surgeon that anesthesia required its own specialist. It required someone who was perfectly skilled to select the anesthetic agents and apparatus which are most suitable for that patient, according to his physical conditions and the proposed operation. However, though late, still this realization came first from Britain, followed by America and much later from the other parts of Europe. Then, from 1800s to 1900s there were many significant changes in inhalational anesthesia. But, it was more a period of consolidation.*

At the end of 19th century, two German pharmacologists, named Meyer and Overton suggested that the potency of inhalational anesthetic agents increase with their lipid solubility. This hypothesis was based on the assumption that anesthetic agents act on the brain which is rich in lipids. In 1922, the 5th edition of Hewitt's book was published which helped to uphold the standard of British anesthesia. The influence of this book was widespread. Hewitt emphasized in his book that N_2O anesthesia was possible without hypoxia. He also suggested that chloroform was especially dangerous during induction. *During that time, ether and chloroform were still the main anesthetic agents, but ethylchloride and N_2O were often used for induction. During this period Simpson's open-drop method for ether administration was most popular, though, in 1917, the first Boyle's machine had already appeared. From this time onward, the speed of progress in anesthesia was very fast and was continued to do so. Before 1930s the anesthetists administered the mixture of only volatile anesthetic agents as balanced anesthesia which produced unconsciousness, muscle relaxation, and analgesia. This balanced method of anesthesia by mixture of gases had reduced the amount of a particular toxic drugs and also reduced the hazards of anesthesia.*

However, the actual concept of balanced anesthesia had started in 1911 by George Crile. He taught that "psychic stimuli" must be obliterated by light general anesthesia with volatile anesthetic agents while the noxious stimuli due to surgery must be blocked by local anesthesia. In 1926, Lundy of the Mayo's Clinic had first introduced the term *"balanced anesthesia"* by combination of premedication, regional analgesia, and general anesthesia, using one or more volatile anesthetic agents, so that pain relief was obtained by judicious mixing of agents and techniques. *While anesthesia was first divided into three basic components such as narcosis,*

- The popularization of endotracheal intubation by Magill and Rowbotham
- The appearance of bromethol, divinyl ether, cyclopropane, and trichloroethylene
- The induction of anesthesia by intravenous barbiturates

analgesia, and relaxation by Rees and Gray of Liverpool. Gray named these components of GA as the "triad" of narcosis, reflex suppression, and relaxation **(Box 4)**.

In the early part of 1930s, there were also certain important innovations in anesthesia. During that period, blind nasotracheal intubation only under the volatile anesthetic agents was increasingly used. But, there was difficulty in obtaining good relaxation of the jaw and larynx with ether only. So, controlled respiration with muscle relaxation was used with cyclopropane during that period. Thus, when Griffith at Montreal first used curare in 1942, to deal with hypoventilation and apnea by controlled ventilation, then it was already well established and so intermittent positive pressure ventilation (IPPV) became a routine procedure.

The two World Wars had greatly influenced and changed the scenario of both surgery and anesthesia. The doctors had learnt a lot during their army tenure and had practised those anesthetic procedures, learnt during army tenure, later during their next civilian life. That led to massive development in anesthesia speciality. Then, technical improvement in anesthesia and academic recognition of it was followed gradually. *In 1935, in London, the first examination for Diploma in Anesthesia was held successfully.*

In 1917, *Haldane* had first popularized the modern medical use of oxygen. In 1995, *Helium* was first isolated by a British chemist and Nobel Prize winner, named Sir W Ramsay. The respiratory stimulating effect of CO_2 was first shown by Herman and Escher, in 1870. This was followed by recommended use of 5% CO_2 in anesthesia by Haggard and Henderson, in 1921. However, then many fatal accidents had occurred with accidental overdosage of CO_2. So, *Waters* pointed out that the ill effects of inadequate ventilation were not due to hypoxia, but also due to excess of CO_2 in 1920s. When Waters started to use cyclopropane, he extensively developed a CO_2 absorption system, though this CO_2 absorption system during anesthesia was introduced first by John Snow.

In the first half of 20th century, a number of other volatile anesthetic agents also enjoyed immense popularity. These included: *ethylene, acetylene, premixed O_2 and N_2O (or Entonox), trichloroethylene, cyclopropane, methyl-n-propyl ether, ethyl-vinyl ether, etc.* Ethylene was more potent than N_2O and had shorter induction period. Therefore, more oxygen could be used with it than N_2O which was the main disadvantage of the use of N_2O. But, the main disadvantage of ethylene was that it was highly inflammable. During that period, it was used mainly in the USA and 20 massive explosions were reported with the use of ethylene. So, ethylene was abandoned and paved the way for *acetylene*.

Characteristics of anesthetic properties of acetylene were similar to that of ethylene. There was rapid induction and recovery by acetylene, and also there was possibility of administering O_2 up to 50% with it. It was used mainly in Germany and the USA. It was also highly inflammable and multiple explosions were reported with the use of acetylene.

Then, in 1945, premixed N_2O and O_2 (80:20) in a cylinder at a pressure of 700 lbs/in^2 was used in the USA. Later, it was found that at room temperature and at a pressure of 2,000 lbs/in^2 certain proportions of N_2O in O_2 remain as a gaseous phase due to the solvent action of O_2 at this pressure. *This is called as the Poynting effect. Tunstall had described this phenomenon making the point that up to 75% of N_2O remains in gaseous phase with O_2 under this condition. He also first reported the clinical use of a mixture of 50% N_2O and 50% O_2, contained in one cylinder for the relief of pain during childbirth. Cooling of such a mixture of N_2O and O_2 produces liquid N_2O at the bottom of cylinder. This remains liquid even when the cylinder is rewarmed. In these circumstances, if the cylinder is used, it will first deliver the gas mixture with high O_2 content and later with high N_2O content. So, delivery of constant mixture of N_2O and O_2 from the cylinder can only be assured either by preventing cooling or by inverting the cylinder many times, after rewarming, if cooling occurs. Thus, Entonox (50:50 mixture of N_2O and O_2) was prepared and sold commercially* (**Fig. 7**).

The *trichloroethylene* had long been used in industries, both as fat solvent and for dry cleaning. Its poisonous properties had also long been recognized and this poisonous property of trichloroethylene was used therapeutically, especially to produce numbness and anesthesia, along the distribution of fifth cranial nerve, to relieve trigeminal neuralgia. But, its general anesthetic properties were later described in 1911 and 1933. Then, it was used to anesthetize 300 patients in 1935. If trichloroethylene was used in a closed circuit with soda lime, then toxic substances were formed. Among these, the most important toxic product of trichloroethylene in a closed circuit with soda lime is dichloroacetylene which is a very potent nerve poison and produces the paralysis of cranial nerves or even death. Also, it is decomposed into phosgene at a temperature above 125°C during cautery, and had caused death of many patients. But, cardiovascular stability provided by trichloroethylene was good, although dysrhythmias were often seen. The heart was sensitized to adrenaline by trichloroethylene. It had an

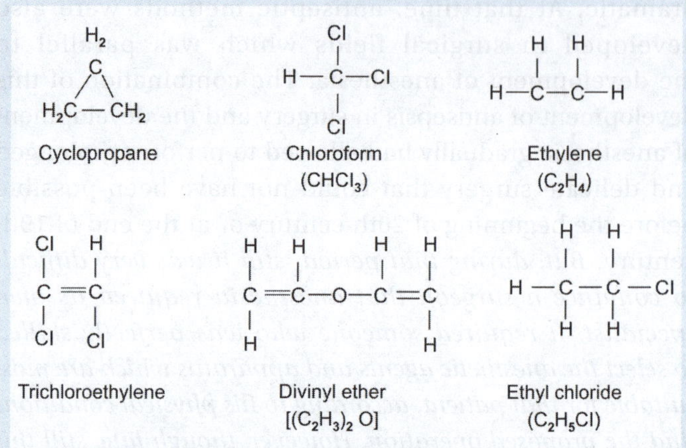

Fig. 7: Commercial anesthetic agents.

BOX 5: Advantages of cyclopropane.
- Very rapid induction
- Cardiac output and arterial pressure are well maintained, even in very ill patients.

excellent analgesic property and was used in both surgery and in obstetrics, but was abandoned after the 1st half of 20th century.

Cyclopropane was first synthesized in 1882, but nobody knew its anesthetic property. Its anesthetic property was first discovered in 1929. It was stored in orange cylinders as liquid, at a pressure of five bars, without requiring any reducing valves during delivery. It was highly explosive and inflammable (**Box 5**).

*Though, it had a powerful respiratory depressant effect, and also produced ventricular dysrhythmias with some deaths from ventricular fibrillation, still it was used for many years in the practice of inhalational anesthesia, since its introduction, due to some advantages which are described in **Box 5**.* The high incidences of postoperative nausea and vomiting (PONV) was common after anesthesia with cyclopropane. Some anesthetists found it immensely useful for very old, ill, and shocked patients, as it provides a strong hemodynamic stability. It was also popular for induction in children, till 1980s (**Figs. 8A and B**).

In 1950, Kety and Eger had first described the pharmacodynamic of inhalational anesthetic agents, and determined the rate at which arterial partial pressure of a volatile anesthetic agent approached that of its inspired concentration. *During that period, the occurrence of diffusion hypoxia during the emergence from N_2O anesthesia was also described by Fink.*

Booth and Bixby, in 1932, observed that the greatest potential of an inhalational anesthetic agent lay within its organic fluoride compound. This is because the substitution

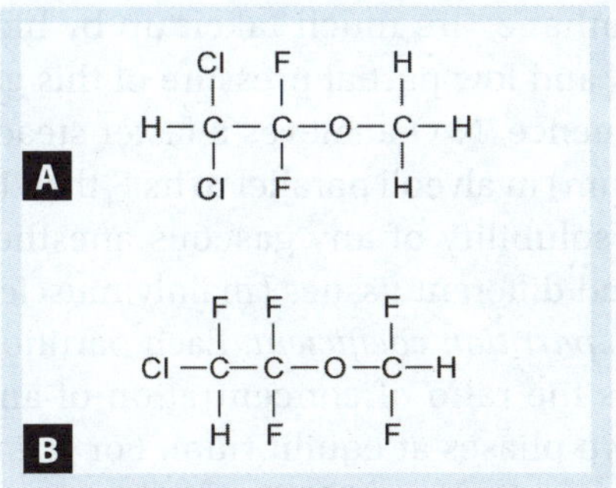

Figs. 8A and B: (A) Methoxyflurane and (B) Enflurane.

of fluoride ion for other halogenions in the compound reduced the boiling point, increased the stability, and generally reduced the toxicity of gases. Then, a large number of fluorinated volatile anesthetic compounds were produced over the next 20 years. At last, it had culminated in 1950 with the development of fluroxene and then, in 1952, with the synthesis of halothane, the first of the truly modern inhalational anesthetic agents.

Then, the first great jump-forward in modern anesthesia was the introduction of halothane into clinical practice with calibrated vaporizers in 1956. Then, gradual progress in the field of anesthesia depended mainly on pharmaceutical companies, developing the various inhalational anesthetic agents. In 1960, *methoxy-flurane* arrived. It had good analgesic properties, but had an unpleasant smell. It was noninflammable and nonexplosive. It had no reaction with soda lime. However, a significant amount of methoxyflurane was metabolized to fluoride which was toxic to the kidneys and caused high output renal failure. So, methoxyflurane was abandoned after its introduction.

Then came *enflurane*, in 1963, in the USA. After that, *isoflurane* entered into the anesthetic arena. It was a fluorinated methyl-ethyl ether which was originally synthesized in 1965, but was first used in clinical anesthesia in 1971. Then, *sevoflurane* was first synthesized in late 1960s at Baxter Travenol laboratory and was first used experimentally on animals in 1971 in North America. The first published record of its use in humans came out in the year of 1981. *Then, the results of phase I trial of this drug on six healthy adults were published. It had two drawbacks. The metabolism of sevoflurane resulted in the production of potentially significant level of fluoride ions. And, it had also been found to be chemically unstable in the presence of soda lime. So, Baxter Company decided not to develop this drug commercially. Then it had contracted with a Japanese pharmaceutical firm. There more extensive experiments were being done. After that, it was approved for clinical use in Japan in 1990 and eventually became the most popular inhalational anesthetic agent there. Its success in Japan was subsequently*

followed by its introduction in Europe. But, the potential toxic degradation products of sevoflurane delayed its release in the USA, until 1994.

Then came *desflurane*. It was first synthesized by Dr Ross Terrell who had also developed isoflurane and enflurane. But, due to its some peculiar physical properties and some technical difficulties the subsequent research of desflurane was delayed. Later, a safer process for the synthesis of desflurane was developed, and the result of phase I trial was published in 1990. Subsequently, it was approved for clinical use in the USA in 1992 **(Fig. 9)**.

PHARMACOKINETICS OF INHALATIONAL ANESTHETIC AGENTS

To attain the ultimate therapeutic effects of any inhalational anesthetic agent, a therapeutic tissue concentration in central nervous system (CNS) of this agent should be reached. For this purpose, the inhalational anesthetic agents are delivered to patients from the cylinders or vaporizers, attached to an anesthetic machine. Then, from this anesthetic machine they (inhalational agents) reach to the alveoli of lungs of a patient through the inspired gas mixture. Next, they enter into the blood at the arterial end of pulmonary capillary and is carried to CNS. In CNS, they enter the brain cells (neurone) and produce therapeutic effects (unconsciousness, amnesia, analgesia, etc.)

Factors Affecting the Inspiratory Concentration (Fi) of Inhalational Agents

Different gases (inhalational agents) are released from different components of an anesthetic machine. For example, N_2O and O_2 are delivered from cylinders. Volatile anesthetic liquids are delivered from vaporizers. After final mixing, all these gases produce a final gas concentration which comes out from the final outlet of machine. Then, the final concentration of each gas in the gas mixture, coming out of the final outlet of machine, depends on the flow rate of these gases through rota meter and dial setting of vaporizer by anesthetist.

Next, the fresh gases, leaving anesthetic machine mixes with the gases, present in breathing circuit, before being inspired by the patient. Therefore, the actual composition of inspired gas mixture or the concentration of each gas in their mixture is changed and reaches to alveoli. Therefore, this concentration of each gas, reaching to alveoli, is known as the inspired concentration (F_i) of this gas. *Now, this inspired concentration (F_i) of each gas, reaching alveoli, depends on: (i) fresh gas flow rate, (ii) volume of breathing circuit, and (iii) any absorption of gas by machine/breathing circuit.* The difference between the concentration of any inhalational anesthetic agent in fresh gas flow, coming out of the final outlet of machine and the actual inspired concentration of this agent in alveoli, can be narrowed by: (i) increasing FGF, (ii) lowering the volume of breathing circuit, and (iii) lowering the circuit absorption rate of this gas.

Factors Affecting the Alveolar Concentration (F_A) of Inhalational Anesthetic Agents

It depends on the following factors: (a) Uptake from alveoli into blood, (b) Ventilation, and (c) the inspired concentration (F_i) of inhalation anesthetic agent.

Uptake from Alveoli into Blood

After reaching alveoli, inhalational gaseous agents are taken up by pulmonary circulation and then the alveolar concentration (F_A) of this gas falls below its inspired concentration (F_i) level. As a result, the equation will be $F_A < F_i$ or $F_A/F_i < 1$. If there are no uptake of inhalational anesthetic agent by blood from alveoli, then the alveolar gas concentration (F_A) will rapidly approach to inspired gas concentration (F_i). Then, the equation will be $F_A = F_i$ or $F_A/F_i = 1$. The greater the uptake of gaseous anesthetic agent by blood from alveoli, the slower will be the rise of alveolar concentration of anesthetic agent. So, the F_A/F_i ratio will be much lower than 1.

The concentration of inhalational anesthetic agents in alveoli (F_A) is directly proportional to the partial pressure of this agent in alveoli. Therefore, with the greatest uptake of inhalational anesthetic agent from alveoli into blood will reduce the partial pressure of this agent in alveoli. On the other hand, the partial pressure of any inhalational anesthetic agent in alveoli is important. Because it determines the partial pressure of inhalational anesthetic agent in blood and ultimately in CNS or brain which determines the clinical effect.

Therefore, the inhalation anesthetic agent which has high blood solubility ($\uparrow$ blood/gas partition coefficient) will be taken up by blood more, leading to $\downarrow F_A$ of this agent and $\uparrow$ in the difference between F_i and F_A of this agent and the slower rate of induction of anesthesia. *Here, three factors affect the uptake of inhalation anesthetic agent from alveoli to blood. These three factors are: (i) solubility of this gaseous agent in blood, (ii) alveolar blood flow, and (iii) the difference in partial pressure between the alveolar gas and venous blood.*

The inhalation anesthetic agents which are relatively insoluble in blood (low blood/gas partition coefficient), such as N_2O, are little taken up by blood and will cause high F_A and high partial pressure of this gas in alveoli. On the other hand, the inhalation anesthetic agents which are relatively soluble in blood (high blood/gas partition coefficient), such as halothane, are much taken up by blood and will cause low F_A and low partial pressure of this gas in alveoli. As a consequence, N_2O achieves a faster steady state level (or equilibrium) in alveoli parallel to its F_i than halothane.

Relative solubility of any gaseous anesthetic agent in air, blood, and different tissues (mainly muscle and fat) are expressed as *partition coefficient*. Each partition coefficient is defined as the ratio of concentration of anesthetic gas in each of two phases at equilibrium. For example, blood/gas partition coefficient of N_2O at 37°C is 0.47. It means, at equilibrium, 1 mL of blood contains 0.47 times N_2O as does 1 mL of alveolar gas. Blood/gas partition coefficient of halothane is 2.4 at 37°C. It means, at equilibrium, 1 mL of blood contains 2.4 times of halothane than that of 1 mL of alveolar gas. Stated in another way, blood has only 47% capacity for N_2O to hold in comparison to full 100% capacity in alveolar gas and blood has 240% capacity for halothane to hold in comparison to 100% capacity of halothane in alveolar gas. It indicates N_2O is the least soluble and halothane is the highest soluble in blood. Therefore, higher the blood/gas partition coefficient, greater is the anesthetic's solubility in blood $\rightarrow$ greater uptake by pulmonary circulation $\rightarrow$ slow rise of partial pressure to a steady state level (equilibrium) in alveoli $\rightarrow$ slow induction. Moreover, more solubility of a gas in blood will cause less increase in partial pressure of this gas in blood and less partial pressure of a gas in blood will cause less transfer of gas into brain and slow induction.

The second factor that affects uptake of gaseous (inhalation) anesthetic agent from alveoli to blood is alveolar blood flow and they are directly proportional (in absence of pulmonary shunting). So, when cardiac output increases $\rightarrow$ anesthetic uptake from alveoli into blood increases $\rightarrow$ slow rise of alveolar partial pressure of that gaseous anesthetic agent $\rightarrow$ induction of anesthesia is delayed. Similarly, when cardiac output decreases (shock) the induction of anesthesia is rapid. Therefore, low cardiac output condition predisposes patients to overdoses with soluble gaseous anesthetic agents, as the rate of rise in alveolar concentration will be markedly increased. The effect of changing cardiac output on the duration of induction of anesthesia is less pronounced for water insoluble gaseous anesthetic agents, as little is taken up by blood from alveoli, regardless of alveolar blood flow.

Ventilation

Increase in alveolar ventilation increases alveolar concentration (partial pressure) of that gaseous anesthetic agent. This is because the lowering of alveolar concentration (partial pressure) of a gaseous anesthetic agent by uptake by blood from alveoli can be countered by increasing alveolar ventilation. Or, in other ward, increased ventilation constantly replaces anesthetic agent in alveoli which is taken up by blood. This effect of ventilation on partial pressure (or F_A/F_i ratio) of a gaseous anesthetic agent in alveoli is most obvious for soluble inhalation anesthetic agent, as they are more subject to uptake by blood. Because, F_A/F_i ratio of an inhalation anesthetic agent very rapidly approaches to 1 for insoluble agents with increasing ventilation of little effect. An anesthetic agent which decreases cardiac output and decreases the uptake by blood from alveoli, with ↑ alveolar concentration, also depresses spontaneous ventilation and decreases the rate of rise of alveolar concentration of this anesthetic agent.

Concentration of Inhalation Anesthetic Agent

Increased inspired concentration of inhaled anesthetic agent counters the slowing of induction, due to uptake of it from alveoli. Also, it is found that increased inspired concentration of gaseous anesthetic agent not only increases the alveolar concentration (partial pressure) of it, but also increases its rate of rise (↑ F_A/F_i ratio). This ↑ F_A/F_i ratio is due to two phenomena that produce a so-called "concentrating effect".

(i) Phenomenon-1: First, if 50% of an inhaled anesthetic is taken up by pulmonary circulation, then 20% inspired concentration of an inhaled anesthetic drug will result in an alveolar concentration of 11%. Similarly, if the inspired concentration of an anesthetic agent is raised to 80%, then the alveolar concentration will be 67%. Thus, even though 50% of anesthetic agent is taken up in both cases, but a higher inspired concentration results in a disproportionately higher alveolar concentration. The principle is increasing inspired concentration fourfold results in sixfold increase in alveolar concentration.

(ii) Phenomenon-2: This second phenomenon, responsible for the concentrating effect of inhaled anesthetic agent, is the augmented inflow effect. Using the example above, the 10 parts of absorbed gas must be replaced by an equal volume of 20% mixture to prevent alveolar collapse. Thus, alveolar concentration becomes 12% (10 + 2 parts of anesthetic in a total 100 parts of gas). Similarly, after absorption of 50% anesthetic agent in 80% gas mixture, 40 parts of 80% gas must be inspired. This further increases the alveolar concentration from 67 to 72% (40 + 32 parts of anesthetic agent in a total 100 parts of gas).

This concentration effect is more significant for N_2O than other inhaled anesthetic agents. Because, the former is used in much higher concentration. Furthermore, a high concentration of N_2O will augment, by the same mechanism, not only its own uptake, but that of concurrently administered volatile anesthetic agent. Thus, this concentration effect of one gas on another gas is called as the *second gas effect.*

Factors Affecting Arterial Concentration (Fa) of Inhaled Anesthetic Agents

Theoretically, the partial pressure of a gaseous anesthetic agent in alveoli and artery is assumed to be equal at a steady state level (at equilibrium). But, practically, the arterial partial pressure (Pa) of a gaseous anesthetic agent is consistently less than that of alveoli. The causes of this are venous admixture, alveolar-dead space, nonuniform alveolar gas distribution, and ventilation/perfusion mismatch. Thus, bronchial intubation, right to left intracardiac shunt, etc. will slow the rate of induction by N_2O more than sevoflurane.

Factors Affecting Elimination of Inhalation Anesthetic Agents

Recovery from anesthesia depends on the lowering of concentration of anesthetic agents in brain tissue. Any anesthetic agent can be eliminated by biotransformation and subsequent excretion through bile and urine, transcutaneous loss or exhalation. The most important route for elimination of inhalation agent is alveolus. The factors that speed induction by inhalation agent also speed its recovery. These factors are: elimination of rebreathing, high fresh gas flow, low anesthetic circuit volume, low absorption by anesthetic circuit, decreased solubility, high cerebral blood flow, increased ventilation, etc. Elimination of N_2O is so rapid that O_2 and CO_2 concentration in alveolus gas are diluted. The resulting diffusion hypoxia is prevented by administering 100% O_2 for 5–10 minutes, after discontinuing N_2O. The rate of recovery is usually faster than induction, because tissues that have not till reached the level of equilibrium, will continue to take up that anesthetic agent, until the alveolar partial pressure falls below the tissue partial pressure level. For instance, fat will continue to take up the inhaled anesthetic agent and will speed up the recovery until the partial pressure of inhaled anesthetic agent in fat is same as that of alveoli. However, this redistribution is not as useful after prolonged anesthesia. Because, after prolonged anesthesia by inhalational anesthetic agent, the partial pressure of this anesthetic agent in fat and arterial blood remains at equilibrium, during recovery. Therefore, the speed of recovery from anesthesia of a gaseous anesthetic agent will also depend on the length of time, the anesthetic agent has been administered.

PHARMACODYNAMICS OF INHALATIONAL ANESTHETICS

Theories of the Action of Inhalational Agents

General anesthesia is defined as an altered physiological state which is characterized by the reversible loss of consciousness, analgesia, amnesia, and some degree of muscular relaxation. The spectrum of chemical structure of agents which produces general anesthesia is very wide and varies from a simple inert element xenon (Xe) to a simple inorganic compound (N_2O) to a halogenated hydrocarbon (halothane) to ethers (isoflurane, sevoflurane, and desflurane) to organic compound with complex structures (propofol and ketamine). Therefore, obviously, various anesthetic agents probably act by various sets of molecular mechanisms, including the voltage-gated ion channels, ligand-gated ion channels, second messenger functioning system, neurotransmitter receptors, etc. But, all of them act on CNS. The Xe and N_2O are believed to act (inhibit) on excitatory *N*-methyl-*D*-aspartate (NMDA) receptors. Ether, halothane, isoflurane, sevoflurane, and desflurane interact with GABA ion (Cl^-) channels, leading to the inhibition of neuronal activity.

Previously, it was thought that all inhalational agents share a common mechanism of action at molecular level. This was previously supported by the observation that the anesthetic potency of inhalational agents correlates directly with their lipid solubility (Meyer–Overton rule). But, this theory was rejected, because all the lipid soluble agents are not anesthetic agents, rather some are convulsants and the correlation between the anesthetic potency and the lipid solubility of anesthetic agents is only slightly approximate. Another point is that neuronal membrane contains numerous hydrophobic (lipophilic) sites in their phospholipid bilayer. General anesthetic agents binding to these sites expand the bilayer beyond a critical volume, altering membrane function (critical volume hypothesis). However, this theory is almost certainly an oversimplification of the mechanism of action of general anesthetic agents.

Regarding the site of action of general anesthetic agents, there is no single macroscopic site in brain or spinal cord where all the inhalational agents act. Various anesthetic agents act on various sites in brain, including reticular activating system, cuneate nucleus, hippocampus, cerebral cortex, etc. and even spinal cord. In spinal cord, the general anesthetic agents depress the excitatory transmitter, particularly at the level of dorsal horn interneurons that are involved in pain transmission. The different components of general anesthesia, exerted by a single agent, may be due to the different sites of action of this single agent. For example, unconsciousness and amnesia are probably mediated by cortical anesthetic action. Analgesic action is probably mediated by the actions on subcortical structures, such as brain stem and spinal cord.

Anesthetic Neurotoxicity, Neuroprotection, and Cardiac Preconditioning

Recently, multiple studies are going on, regarding the effect of anesthetic agents on a developing brain of newborn, infants, and children and it is found that the early exposure to general anesthetic agents can cause cognitive impairment in later life. But, still it is not confirmed. Because, conducting a randomized-controlled trials, for that purpose on newborn, infants, and children are unethical. However, the huge data from one large study had demonstrated that the children who underwent surgery and anesthesia had a greater likelihood of carrying CNS developmental disorder. But, this finding is always not supported by other small studies. The causes for this cognitive impairment, due to the exposure to general anesthetic agents are: anesthetic exposure causes delay in development and elimination of synapses in newborn and infant brain. For example, isoflurane exposure promotes neuronal apoptosis and subsequent learning disability. This apoptosis is probably due to the alteration of cellular Ca^{2+} homeostatic mechanism. Also, it has been suggested that the general anesthetic agents cause Tau protein hyperphosphorylation, leading to the progression of Alzheimer disease (AD). Because, AD is associated with Tau protein hyperphosphorylation.

Although the inhalational general anesthetic agents have been suggested to contribute to neurotoxicity, but they have also been shown to provide both neurological and cardiac protective effects against any ischemic perfusion injury. However, various molecular mechanisms have been suggested for this protection of cells. But, among these, one important mechanism is opening of K_{ATP} channels, resulting in less mitochondrial Ca^{2+} ion concentration and the reduction of reactive oxygen species (ROS) production. ROS contributes to cellular injury. The general anesthetic agents also cause the increased production of antioxidants. In addition, the excitatory NMDA receptors are responsible for the development of neuronal injury. Hence, NMDA antagonists, such as the noble anesthetic gas xenon, have been shown to be neuroprotectors. The xenon also has an antiapoptotic effect that may be secondary to its inhibition of Ca^{2+} ion influx, following cell injury.

Minimum Alveolar Concentration

Minimum alveolar concentration (MAC) of an inhaled anesthetic agent is defined as the lowest concentration of this agent in alveoli by which the response (movement) to a standard stimulus (e.g., surgical incision) is prevented in 50% of patients. The usefulness of MAC is: (i) It mirrors the partial pressure of inhaled anesthetic agent in brain tissue, (ii) It compares the potency among inhaled anesthetic agent, (iii) It provides a standard for experimental evaluation. But, the limitation of the usefulness of MAC is it indicates only a median value. The MAC value of different inhalational anesthetic agents is additive. It means when two gaseous anesthetic agents are used together, then their individual MAC values are reduced.

MAC values are altered by several physiological and pharmacological variables. Among these, the age is the most important variable. For example, there is 6% decrease in MAC for the increase of every decade of age, regardless of the type of volatile anesthetic agent. But, MAC is relatively unaffected by species, sex, or the duration of anesthesia.

■ NITROUS OXIDE (FIG. 9)

History

N_2O was first prepared by Priestley in 1772. But, Humphrey Davy had first demonstrated its anesthetic property in 1800. At that time, Davy was only 21 years old. However, from 1800 to 1844 it was absent from anesthetic practice, though the exact reason behind this is still not known. Then, on 10th December in 1844, Gardner Colton **(Fig. 10)** again demonstrated the anesthetic property of N_2O in front of a big audience at Hartford. He was a lecturer in chemistry. Horace Wells **(Fig. 11)**, a dentist, was among these audience, during the demonstration of anesthetic property

of N_2O by Colton. He (Horace Wells) was very much impressed by seeing the anesthetic property of N_2O. So, this demonstration was again repeated on himself on the next day, privately. During this demonstration, an assistant from a local druggist's shop, named Samuel Cooley banged the shin bone of Mr Wells and made it bleed, while he was under the effect of N_2O.

Then, Wells after recovery, stated that he had experienced no pain. He also commented that N_2O could be used for tooth extraction painlessly. During this time, the wisdom teeth of Mr Wells was producing trouble. So, he requested Mr Colton to extract it and to try N_2O gas on him, during this dental surgery.

So, on 11th December in 1844, this experiment with N_2O was carried out, again where Colton was an anesthesiologist, John M Rigg was dental surgeon and Wells was the patient. It was also a big success, when Mr Wells had recovered from the anesthetic effect of N_2O. Then he declared it as the new era of dental medical science. So, he asked for some N_2O from Colton and on the next day he used it on one of his patients for extraction of tooth. This procedure was also painless. By the middle of January, in 1845, Wells then performed 15 successful cases of painless extraction of tooth at his clinic. Next, Wells had tried to demonstrate this technique, at Massachusetts General Hospital, in front of a big audience. But, the patient complained of pain and Wells was dubbed as a fraud. The low lipid solubility of N_2O was the cause of this failure and it may be the cause of suicide of Wells, at the age of 33 years.

These series of events antedate the first public demonstration of ether, as an anesthetic agent, by only 21 months. So, at that time, the introduction of both ether and N_2O delayed the full appreciation of analgesic effect of latter

Fig. 9: Nitrous oxide.

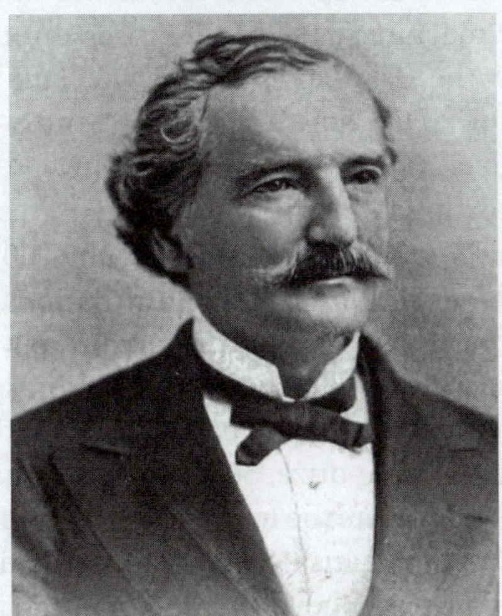

Fig. 10: Gardner Colton.

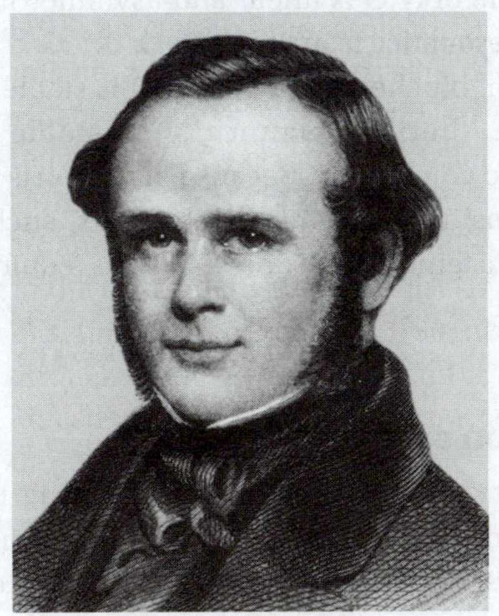

Fig. 11: Horace Wells.

(N$_2$O). Again, 20 years later, Colton reintroduced it in dental practice.

So, after a temporary period of eclipse by ether, N$_2$O was reintroduced in anesthesia practice and then again was widely used from 1867 onward. By 1868, the gas was first available in London, as compressed gas in metal cylinders. 2 years later, it was available as liquid nitrous oxide in metal cylinders. Then, a reducing valve was attached in 1873 to its cylinder. During this period, the main difficulty was in the technique of administration of N$_2$O in its pure form (100%), as asphyxia was inseparable by this use. This difficulty was first overcome by Edmund Andrew, who, in 1868, used 80% N$_2$O with 20% O$_2$ for prolonged anesthesia, avoiding asphyxia. Then, in 1868, Clover first proved that N$_2$O had true anesthetic properties. Subsequently, in 1876, he first introduced N$_2$O-ether sequence in anesthesia.

N$_2$O is the only gas which was used continuously from the era of chloroform, till the present day. In view of other large number of volatile anesthetic compounds that have been used as inhalational anesthetic agents and which use had been discontinued after a shorter or longer period, it is remarkable that the use of N$_2$O is still continuing. More patients have been anesthetized with N$_2$O than with any other inhalational agent and at present it still continues to be the most widely used agent than any other volatile anesthetic.

Chemistry of N$_2$O

Except xenon, nitrous oxide is the only *inorganic compound* which has been used to produce analgesia and general anesthesia. This is not only due to some unusual pharmacological property of N$_2$O, but is also due to the consequence of its degree of solubility in blood and lipid, and due to its chemical stability in our body. The structure of a molecule of N$_2$O is linear and asymmetrical, having a significant resonance feature: N=N=O.

Although, biochemically, the N$_2$O is stable compound, but it is a thermodynamically unstable and is an endothermic compound. Because, it supports combustion by decomposing itself into its elements, such as N$_2$ and oxygen. But, a temperature above 450°C is required to initiate this reaction.

$$2\,N_2O \rightarrow 2\,N_2 + O_2 + 163\ kJ$$

Preparation of N$_2$O

In laboratory, N$_2$O is prepared by allowing the reaction between iron and nitric acid. In this reaction, nitric oxide is produced first which is then reduced to N$_2$O by excess iron.

$$Fe + 2\,NO \rightarrow N_2O + FeO$$

Commercially, it is produced by heating ammonium nitrate between 245°C and 270°C temperature.

$$NH_4NO_3 \rightarrow N_2O + H_2O + 58.4\ kJ$$

The major part of world's supply of N$_2$O gas is usually obtained by this method. In older plants, this was performed by heating solid ammonium nitrate. But, now in more modern plants, an aqueous solution of 83% ammonium nitrate is being used. This is available as by product, during the large-scale manufacturing of ammonia.

Accurate temperature control, during the preparation of N$_2$O, is essential. Because, the reaction for the preparation of N$_2$O is exothermic and above 270°C, the level of impurities with N$_2$O increases. Again above 290°C, this reaction becomes very explosive. So, the accurate control of temperature during the preparation of N$_2$O is very necessary. Serious explosions may also occur in a nitrous oxide manufacturing plant, if the temperature goes out of control. In the older type of plants, where the solid ammonium nitrate was used, the retort in which the exothermic reaction is occurred, had to be externally cooled by ice-water. But, in newer plants, where ammonium nitrate solution is used, the temperature control is done only by the addition of more solution.

During the preparation of N$_2$O by heating NH$_4$NO$_3$, other higher components of nitrogen, such as ammonia, nitric acid, N$_2$, NO, and NO$_2$ are also produced as impurities. But, by different processes, adopted by different companies, N$_2$O is separated, dried, and purified from this mixture. Then, the pure N$_2$O is compressed to its liquid form and filled in cylinders. However, during purification, a great care should be taken, so that the content of higher oxide of nitrogen, mixed with N$_2$O, should not exceed 1 vpm (volume per million). Greater care is also taken to prevent the moisture, from being included with N$_2$O, in gas cylinder. Because, if water vapor is present in cylinder with N$_2$O gas, then this water vapor will tend to freeze within the pipelines of anesthetic machine, as the N$_2$O passes through reducing valves, when the cylinder is turned on, and may lead to the obstruction of gas flow. About nine-tenths of a full N$_2$O cylinder is filled with the liquid form of N$_2$O.

Nitrous oxide is stored and supplied in cylinders for anesthetic purpose under the pressure of 5,000 kPa at 20°C. A full N$_2$O cylinder at room temperature contains liquid N$_2$O. For this reason, cylinder should be kept upright when it is in use. When the cylinder is turned on and the gaseous portion of N$_2$O above its liquid form leaves the cylinder, then the liquid N$_2$O starts to vaporize. So, the pressure gauge on N$_2$O cylinder cannot indicate the total content of liquid N$_2$O, until all the liquids are exhausted and cylinder is filled only by N$_2$O gas. Nevertheless, they do warn about the failure of gas flow when all the liquids are exhausted. For vaporization of

N$_2$O, during its flow from the cylinder, latent heat is obtained from the metal cylinder. So, it rapidly cools, and water vapor of air outside the cylinder freezes on the cylinder forming a layer of ice.

Physical Properties of N$_2$O

N$_2$O is a nonirritating, odorless, and colorless gas. Its molecular weight is 44. It is neither inflammable nor explosive. Specific gravity of N$_2$O is 1.527 (air = 1). At 50 atmospheric pressure and at 28°C, N$_2$O becomes a clear and colorless liquid with boiling point at −89°C. It is stable in soda lime. Its partition coefficient at 37°C is: oil/water 32, water/gas 0435, oil/gas 14, blood/gas 0468. The critical temperature of N$_2$O is 36°C and the critical pressure of it is 72 bar. Its MAC value is 105.

Importance of N$_2$O as Anesthetic Agent

This is remarkable that N$_2$O has stood the test for a long time, since its inception, as an anesthetic agent. The other volatile anesthetic agent which also stood the test of time with contemporary history is only the diethyl ether. But, since the introduction of halothane, in 1950, ether has been of little use in Europe, and recently its production has also been stopped. Therefore, it is expected that N$_2$O would still have the considerable virtues as an inhalational anesthetic agent which are listed in **Box 6**.

The speed of onset and the recovery from anesthesia of any volatile anesthetic agent is regulated by its blood solubility. The lower the blood solubility, the faster will be the onset and recovery. The blood-gas partition coefficient of N$_2$O is only 0.46. This is the lowest for all the inhalational agents that are currently used. So, the speed of onset and recovery from N$_2$O anesthesia is fastest. This lowest blood-gas solubility of N$_2$O has another advantage. This advantage is the lowest blood gas solubility of N$_2$O makes easier to control the depth of N$_2$O anesthesia. Because, any slight change in inspired concentration of N$_2$O rapidly results in the change of its partial pressure in blood and subsequently in the brain, due to this less blood gas solubility of it. Thus, the lightening and deepening of anesthesia by N$_2$O is quickly achieved, which is parallel to the partial pressure

of this agent in blood and brain. So, after a few breaths, the alveolar concentration of N$_2$O becomes equivalent to the inspired concentration of it, and the alveolar concentration or the partial pressure of N$_2$O in alveoli (which is parallel to the partial pressure of the agent in blood and brain) reflects the depth of anesthesia **(Fig. 12)**.

So, from the above discussion, it is now clear that the low blood gas solubility of N$_2$O or any inhalational agent is a great asset for it. But, low blood-gas solubility of N$_2$O is also associated with low fat solubility of it, which indicates that the N$_2$O is of low anesthetic potency. Because, it is known that the anesthetic potency of any volatile agent depends on its fat solubility. This is the disadvantage of N$_2$O or any such agent with low fat solubility and is the reason for high MAC value of N$_2$O which is 104.

Impurities of N$_2$O

During the manufacturing of N$_2$O, the main impurity in it is one higher oxide of nitrogen, i.e., NO$_2$. In addition to nitrogen dioxide (NO$_2$), at least seven other oxides of nitrogen are also known to be present in it during commercial preparation of N$_2$O. But, among these impurities, those of importance as contaminants are: nitric oxide (NO) and nitrogen trioxide (NO$_3$). This is because nitric oxide (NO) combines with air to form an even more toxic, nitrogen dioxide, which remains in equilibrium in the mixture and this point of equilibrium depends on the temperature of mixture. The European and US standards for the maximum permissible limit of NO and NO$_2$ in the medical preparation of N$_2$O is 5 ppm. The higher oxides of nitrogen in N$_2$O can be detected by smell at a concentration above 5 ppm. The consequences of inhaling higher oxides of nitrogen, as impurities with N$_2$O, in concentrations above 50 ppm are: reflex inhibition of

BOX 6: Virtues of N$_2$O as an anesthetic agent.

- Have no irritant properties
- Have good analgesic property
- No metabolism in body
- Minimal adverse effects
- Have advantages when used with other volatile agents
- Low blood solubility
- Accuracy of administration

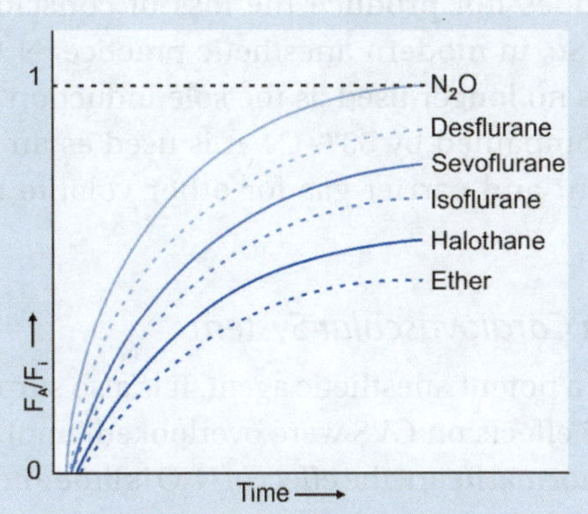

Fig. 12: F$_A$/F$_i$ ratio of different volatile anesthetic agents. In case of N$_2$O the alveolar fractional concentration (F$_A$) rises rapidly and reaches the value of inspired fractional concentration (F$_i$) quickly. Thus, the F$_A$/F$_i$ ratio reaches to the value of 1 most rapidly with least soluble agent such as N$_2$O.

breathing, laryngospasm, cyanosis, methemoglobinemia, and pulmonary edema. An insidious feature of these manifestations is pulmonary damage, which may not become apparent until the pulmonary edema is developed and this usually occurs many hours later. If the patient does not die immediately from pulmonary damage, then chronic chemical pneumonitis may follow with the resultant pulmonary fibrosis. Hypotension may be marked and results from the effect of nitrates on vascular smooth muscles. Other impurities in N_2O, except the higher oxides of nitrogen, are: ammonia, carbon monoxide, and chlorine. So, after production scrubbing of N_2O with permanganate solution, sulfuric acid solution and water are important to remove all these impurities.

Pharmacological Actions

N_2O is very rapidly absorbed from alveoli into blood and only remains in plasma as dissolved state. 100 mL of plasma can carry 45 mL of N_2O. It does not combine with Hb. Also, it does not undergo any chemical combination with any body tissue. It remains in blood just as physical solution. So, elimination of N_2O from body is as speedy as absorption through lungs. It is 15 times more soluble in plasma than N_2, and 100 times more so than O_2. As far as anesthetic action is concerned, N_2O is a weak anesthetic agent. To produce a surgical anesthesia (stage III) only with N_2O, a plasma partial pressure of 760 mm Hg of it is required. However, 80% N_2O in mixture with O_2 at normal atmospheric pressure produces a partial pressure of only 600 mm Hg in blood. So, surgical anesthesia cannot be produced without hypoxia when N_2O is used alone. Only a 50:50 mixture of N_2O and O_2 at two atmospheric pressure can rapidly produce this surgical anesthesia with complete saturation of arterial blood by O_2. Whereas, the same concentration of N_2O at one atmospheric pressure does not produce the loss of consciousness in a patient. So, in modern anesthetic practice, N_2O alone at sea level is no longer used as the sole induction agent. But when accompanied by 33% O_2, it is used as an important supplement and carrier gas for other volatile anesthetic agents.

Effects on Cardiovascular System

N_2O is not a potent anesthetic agent. It is also surprising that its adverse effects on CVS were overlooked, until the recent years. On normal heart, the effect of N_2O is little and is entirely obscured by sympathetic stimulation with concomitant rise in plasma noradrenaline concentration which is an important pharmacological action of N_2O. If there is no sympathetic stimulation or it is prevented, then it reduces cardiac output which is suggestive of its cardiac depression effect. It also causes fall in heart rate and decreases in limb blood flow. So, it is said that N_2O has negative inotropic and chronotropic effect on heart and at the same time produces α-adreno-receptor stimulation on peripheral circulation which neutralizes the depressive action on heart.

In spite of this cardiac depression effect, normal arterial pressure appears to be maintained by N_2O. This is because of the increased peripheral resistance by concomitant sympathetic stimulation by N_2O. It is also suggested that the depressant effect of N_2O on heart is enhanced by the cardiac depressant effect of other anesthetic agent, when they are used concomitantly. This N_2O-induced myocardial depression may be offset by concomitant increase in sympathetic nervous system tone, caused by it. The 70% N_2O decreases myocardial contractility to approximately same extent as that of 1 MAC isoflurane. The negative inotropic action of N_2O may be more pronounced in the presence of preexisting left ventricular (LV) dysfunction. N_2O also produces LV diastolic dysfunction in a patient undergoing coronary artery bypass graft surgery. The N_2O-induced myocardial depression is due to the decrease in Ca^{++} availability to contractile element of myocardial tissue. But, it does not affect myofibril sensitivity to Ca^{++} or in Ca^{++} uptake and its release from sarcoplasmic reticulum (SR).

N_2O increases venous tone and decreases venous capacitance. It modestly increases pulmonary artery pressure and pulmonary vascular resistance (PVR). But, in a normal patient, this pulmonary artery pressure and PVR are not significantly affected by N_2O. When pulmonary hypertension is already present, then N_2O causes marked increase in mean pulmonary artery pressure and PVR. Thus, the combined effects of enhanced venous return; elevated PVR and depressed myocardial contractile function, probably contribute to increase in central venous pressure (CVP) during N_2O anesthesia. Such an increase in PVR may adversely enhance the right (R) to left (L) atrial or ventricular shunt (if they are present) and compromises arterial oxygenation in a patient with congenital heart disease. So, in such circumstances, the use of N_2O is inadvisable.

The addition of N_2O to halothane lowers the threshold value in which halothane-induced arrhythmia occurs. This results from the combination of both sympathetic nervous system stimulation by N_2O and myocardial sensitization by halothane. As the N_2O activates sympathetic nervous system, it also causes capillary dilation, diaphoresis, ↑SVR and increased central blood volume. These findings suggest that N_2O-induced direct myocardial depression is partially offset by sympathetic nervous system stimulation, and may be partially responsible for the relative stability of hemodynamic during N_2O anesthesia.

The sympathomimetic action of N_2O on heart normally exceeds its direct depressant effect. The administration of drugs that tend to block this sympathetic stimulation, such as narcotics, may reveal the underlying cardiac depressant action of N_2O. For this reason, the addition of N_2O to high-dose narcotic anesthesia (to reduce the risk of awareness) has been found to cause depression of cardiac function, which is not seen when either drug is given alone. However, this effect of N_2O is only of importance when the cardiac performance is compromised by some cardiac disease. Thus, it is safe to conclude that in such conditions where there is need of strong sympathetic stimulation, such as hypovolemia, then N_2O is considered as a cardiodepressant. Again, in more complex situations, its cardiac effects are not always predictable. This is because of an uncertain balance between its direct depressant and indirect stimulant (through sympathetic activation) action.

Effects on Respiratory System

Nitrous oxide is pleasant to inhale. Its pharmacokinetic properties make it very useful to act as supplement to other volatile anesthetic agents, particularly during inhalational induction. This is done by increasing the uptake and reducing the MAC value of other volatile or inhalational anesthetic agents. When given alone, N_2O has minimal effect on ventilation. Like other inhalational agents, N_2O also increases respiratory rate and decreases tidal volume. However, this increase in respiratory rate is sufficient enough to compensate for the decrease in tidal volume. So that, despite the unfavorable change in the ratio of dead space to tidal volume, during N_2O anesthesia, alveolar ventilation is well maintained and $PaCO_2$ does not rise. This remains true even up to 2 MAC value of nitrous oxide, when the respiratory rate has been found to be two to three times greater than the normal value. N_2O does not alter compensatory ventilatory responses to the changes in $PaCO_2$, but it significantly reduces the ventilatory responses to hypoxia.

Effects on Central Nervous System

When N_2O is used alone, it produces significant increase in both cerebral blood flow (CBF) and intracranial pressure (ICP) in normal, head injury, and brain tumor patients. If N_2O is added to any volatile anesthetic agent, there is also significant rise in CBF and ICP. However, the interesting finding is that when the intravenous anesthetic agents are administered in conjunction with N_2O, then these effects of N_2O on CNS may be greatly attenuated. N_2O also increases cerebral metabolism. When the N_2O is used during neurosurgery, then it should be kept in mind that it may diffuse into any air pockets, left within the skull, following the closure of wound and may later increase the intracranial pressure. Despite all these potential disadvantages, the use of N_2O in patients undergoing neurosurgery remains an established and accepted practice **(Box 7)**.

Analgesic Properties

From the first observations of Humphrey Davy, it has been demonstrated that even when N_2O is inhaled at sub-anesthetic concentrations, it has a strong analgesic action. The analgesic effect of 30% nitrous oxide has been found to be equivalent to that produced by 10 mg of morphine subcutaneously. So, the 50:50 nitrous oxide and oxygen mixture (Entonox) is widely used, all over the world, to alleviate labor pain and to facilitate minor surgical procedures. But, it has a very weak anesthetic property. Anesthesia is likely to be inadequate, when N_2O is used alone as a sole anesthetic agent.

It is unclear why some inhalational anesthetic agents have an analgesic effect at subanesthetic concentrations and others do not. However, in case of N_2O (but not in case of other agents) there is evidence that the analgesic effect or at least a part of it is brought about by an interaction of N_2O with the opiate receptors. The chief evidence in support of this view is that the partial, but significant, reversal of analgesia, produced by nitrous oxide, is possible by naloxone. Also, depletion of endogenous opiate stores may play a part in the acute tolerance to N_2O **(Box 8)**.

BOX 7: Advantages when N_2O is used in combination with a second volatile anesthetic agent.

- It reduces the MAC of second agent
- It also reduces the amount of second agent required for effect
- It also increases the uptake and elimination of second volatile agent by second gas effect
- It increases the rate of induction and recovery

BOX 8 : Adverse effects of N_2O.

Harmful effects which have been clearly demonstrated:
- Adverse circulating effects
- Diffusion in close (compliant or noncompliant) spaces
- Oxidation of vitamin B_{12} causing:
  - Abnormalities in hemopoietic system
  - Abnormalities in nervous system

Harmful effects which are insignificant:
- Impaired wound healing
- Impaired leukocyte function
- Malignant hyperpyrexia
- Postoperative nausea and vomiting
- Teratogenicity
- Carcinogenicity
- Mutagenicity

However, the naloxone neither reverses the effect of anesthesia nor increases the MAC value of N_2O. In case of N_2O, although analgesia is partially reversed, but the ED_{50} of nitrous oxide as assessed by loss of righting reflex in mice (= MAC) is unaffected by naloxone. It is therefore evident that the effect of anesthesia is separable from analgesia in case of N_2O.

Not only, naloxone does not affect the anesthetic effect, produced by other inhalational agent, but it also does not affect the analgesia produced by such volatile anesthetic agents, other than N_2O. This shows the further evidence of the existence of other nonopiate pain control systems. It also suggests that the opiate receptor and endorphin system is not directly involved in the mechanism of general anesthesia.

Metabolism of N_2O

N_2O is metabolized very minimally in our body. Hence, the metabolites of N_2O in liver has been detected, though in very low concentration. So, it can be concluded that with the probable exception to xenon, nitrous oxide is least metabolized in our body among all the anesthetic agents.

The two small loci, responsible for N_2O metabolism, have been identified in our body. One is the reduction of this gas to nitrogen by bacteria, which is present in gut. This has been estimated to be about 0.004% of the total quantity of N_2O taken by the body. It has also been shown that during this reduction of N_2O into bacteria, free intermediate radicals may also be formed. These compounds are potentially harmful, but there is no evidence of any such toxic effects, resulting from these compounds, due to their very low concentrations. Some bacteria in gut may also synthesize N_2O themselves.

The other identified metabolic process of N_2O is the interaction between N_2O and vitamin B_{12}. The amount of gas taking part in this reaction is also too small to be of any significance. Interestingly, the reduction of nitrous oxide by intestinal bacteria may result, at least in part, from the same chemical reactions in body, since these organisms synthesize vitamin B_{12}.

Toxicity of N_2O

N_2O has no direct toxic activity. However, its long-term use can indirectly produce some hematological, neurological, and gestational defects.

Hematological Toxicity

Use of N_2O for a long period may cause pancytopenia (aplastic anemia) and megaloblastic anemia. Mild depression of bone marrow, seen after the exposure of N_2O for 6 hours, may become severe after 24 hours of exposure. The mechanism of this response is probably due to N_2O-induced inactivation of vitamin B_{12}, which leads to the impaired synthesis of methionine and deoxythymidine, and also an impaired folate metabolism. However, all these are very essential factors for normal hematopoiesis.

Neurological Toxicity

These have been found after long-term unintentional inhalation of N_2O by anesthesiologist, OT assistant, and habitual abuser. Neurological toxicity caused by N_2O appears in the form of motor and/or sensory incoordination and/or reflex defects. These effects are due to the demyelination of posterior column, lateral spino-thalamic tract, and spinocerebellar tract of spinal cord. However, the mechanism of this toxicity is like hematological toxicity, i.e., inactivation of vitamin B_{12}. The failure to synthesis S-adenosyl-methionine from methionine and adenosine triphosphate (ATP) leads to the failure of methylation of basic protein in myelin sheath.

Gestational Toxicity

Increased incidences of gestational defects, abortion, fetal death, etc. are found among OT personnel who continuously inhale N_2O for prolonged period. The mechanism of this gestational toxicity, caused by N_2O, is similar to that of hematological and neurological effects of N_2O, i.e., inactivation of vitamin B_{12} and impaired folate metabolism.

Interaction between N_2O and Vitamin B_{12}

The introduction of long-term IPPV by a ventilator, after 1952, facilitated the use of N_2O for long-term sedation. Then, several workers described granulocytopenia in cases where N_2O had been used continuously for several days. On long-term administration of N_2O, even at low concentration, leukopenia will occur after about 3 days which may develop into agranulocytosis in 5–7 days. However, if the patient does not succumb due to his or her primary illness, then the recovery of bone marrow from its depression effects of N_2O occurs within 4–5 days, after withdrawal of N_2O. In such circumstances, the treatment with vitamin B_{12} was found to have no result.

In 1968, a paper was published describing the interactions between N_2O and vitamin B_{12}. Then, in 1978, it was established that giving N_2O for 24 hours affects DNA synthesis. Shortly after this, it was shown that the selective inhibition of synthesis of vitamin B_{12} by N_2O is due to the inhibition of the action of an enzyme named methionine synthetase which is responsible for DNA synthesis. Thus, it affects DNA synthesis **(Fig. 13)**.

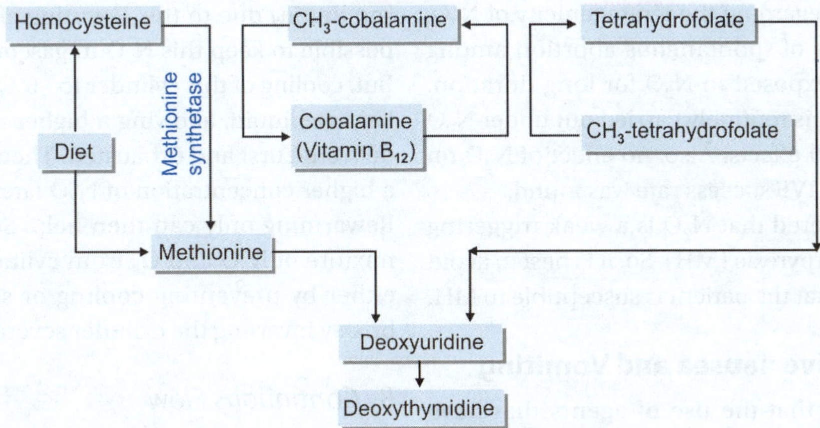

Fig. 13: The mechanism of synthesis of methionine from homocysteine with the help of vitamin B_{12} and folic acid.

Vitamin B_{12} is a cobalamine. The function of cobalt in the structure of vitamin B_{12} can be compared with that of iron in Hb. The oxidation of cobalt in vitamin B_{12} by N_2O is analogs to the oxidation of Fe in Hb, by any chemical oxidizing agents, to form methemoglobin. In the case of cobalt, the N_2O converts the monovalent cobalamine to bivalent cobalamine, in which form it can no longer function as a methyl carrier. Methionine is a sulfur containing essential amino acid. It is available from food and also by the metabolism of homocysteine. Folate, which is also of dietary origin, is necessary for this conversion.

The enzyme methionine synthetase together with vitamin B_{12} transfers the methyl group from methyl-tetra-hydro-folate to homocysteine, and converts the later (homocysteine) to methionine. At the same time, by losing its methyl group, methyl-tetra-hydro-folate becomes simply tetra-hydro-folate. Following this transmethylation, methionine and tetra-hydro-folate take part in several reactions and result in the formation of deoxy-thymidine from deoxy-uridine. Deoxythymidine is an essential component of synthesis of DNA. The 90% of this deoxy-thymidine, incorporated into DNA, comes from the metabolism of deoxy-uridine. Thus, the inhibition of DNA synthesis by N_2O is thought to cause the hematological and the neurological toxicity effects of N_2O. The neurological effects may result from the depletion of methionine.

The duration of exposure of N_2O which is required to produce significant bone marrow depression is very clearly important. In man, this time course is slower. No inactivation of methionine synthetase activity in human placenta was found, following N_2O administration for up to 30 minutes during cesarean section. Presumably, this duration of exposure for N_2O is inadequate. The intermittent exposure to N_2O, such as entonox, during physiotherapy, has been found to produce megaloblastic bone marrow.

It is clearly important to discover the extent up to which the biochemical lesions produced by N_2O can be prevented or reversed by restoring the levels of deficient metabolites by folinic acid (5-formyl tetra-hydro-folate, leukovorin, citrovorum factor, etc.). These compounds are freely available. They are used in chemotherapy as an antidote to folic acid antagonists, such as methotrexate. They are converted to methylene tetra-hydro-folate and thus restores the metabolic pathway which leads to DNA synthesis. It is also seen that the two parenteral doses of 20 mg folinic acid prevent the development of an abnormal deoxyuridine suppression test and megaloblastic changes in the bone marrow in 8 out of 10 patients, ventilated for 36 hours with 50% N_2O. It is also seen that in patients subjected to N_2O anesthesia for up to 12 hours, the abnormal deoxyuridine suppression test is corrected almost to the normal limit within 2 hours of giving of 15 mg folinic acid.

In addition to the impairment of DNA synthesis, a clinical feature of N_2O toxicity is vitamin B_{12} deficiency. This N_2O-induced B_{12} deficiency is characterized by inability to synthesize myelin, causing a neuropathy. This usually develops insidiously in peripheral nerves and gradually progresses to involve the posterior and lateral columns of the spinal cord. But, it may be concluded that neuropathy is unlikely to be developed during clinical use of N_2O within the normal dose range in normal subjects.

The evidences regarding the effects of N_2O on chemotaxis, phagocytosis, and wound healing are not entirely consistent. But, it seems likely that the stress metabolic responses due to surgery and anesthesia on wound healing are more important than the effects of N_2O itself on it. The N_2O does not have any direct negative effect on wound healing.

Multiple reports have failed to show any carcinogenic potential of N_2O. The teratogenicity or other effects of N_2O on the reproductive process is also less clear. The only agreed positive finding, regarding the teratogenicity of N_2O, is an increase in the rate of spontaneous abortion among the personnel who are exposed to N_2O for long duration. However, oocyte retrieval is routinely carried out under N_2O anesthesia without any ill effects. Also, no effect of N_2O on human spermatozoa and IVF success rate was found.

It is generally considered that N_2O is a weak triggering agent for malignant hyperpyrexia (MH). So, it is best to avoid its use, if it is suspected that the patient is susceptible to MH.

N_2O and Postoperative nausea and Vomiting

It is generally accepted that the use of agents that have sympathomimetic effects, such as cyclopropane or trichloro-ethylene results in more postoperative nausea or vomiting than the use of agents that lack such effects. For this reason and also due to the effects on middle ear (that is already described) it has been suspected that nitrous oxide might produce increased incidence of PONV.

Methods of Administration of N_2O

By Intermittent Flow

This method of delivery of N_2O by intermittent flow is important for economy of this gas. For intermittent flow, two techniques are adopted. *In first technique,* a demand valve is commonly used where N_2O and O_2, coming from separate sources, are combined in variable concentration in a mixing chamber and this is situated on the high-pressure side of demand valve. The characteristic of this demand valve is that it will deliver a flow of gas at low pressure, but up to peak inspiratory flow rate, in response to the slight negative pressure, developed by the patient's own inspiratory effort. Since, as this type of valve is capable of delivering gas flows equal to that of peak inspiratory flow rate, so no reservoir bag is needed. Sometimes a low resistance vaporizer, such as Goldman's vaporizer may be placed between the valve and the patient if anesthetist wants to use volatile anesthetic agents to anesthetize his patients. Such an assembly may be classified as an intermittent flow machine and these are commonly used for dental anesthesia.

The second technique depends on premixed cylinder, containing N_2O and O_2 under pressure with a demand valve, which allows the gas mixture to flow to patient, only during inspiration. In room temperature and at a certain pressure (2,000 lbs./sq. in) some N_2O remains in gaseous phase (25% in liquid form and 75% in gaseous) with O_2 due to the solvent action of later. This solvent action of O_2 is called as the Poynting effect. In a premixed N_2O and O_2 cylinder, with 50:50 proportion (Entonox) under the pressure of 15,000 kPa at 20°C, N_2O remains fully in gaseous phase (no liquid) due to this Poynting effect. Without O_2 it is not possible to keep this N_2O in gaseous phase under pressure. But, cooling of this cylinder to –6°C causes the part of N_2O to become liquid, allowing a higher concentration of O_2 to be delivered first and exhausted. Then, the cylinder will deliver a higher concentration of N_2O later and will cause hypoxia. Rewarming only can then help. So, delivery of a constant mixture of N_2O and O_2 from cylinder can only be assured, either by preventing cooling or should cooling occur, by briskly inverting the cylinder several times after rewarming.

By Continuous Flow

The continuous flow of N_2O is supplied from Boyel's anesthetic machine through an open, semi-closed (frequently used), or completely closed system (circuit). The semi-closed technique is frequently used with CO_2 absorber to make the gas flow economical. The completely closed system with CO_2 absorber is not indicated when N_2O is used. Because, it is extremely difficult to ensure adequate oxygenation of that patient, if N_2O is used in a completely closed system. However, the development of an accurate oximeter with a high and low alarm and also a digital display of FiO_2 has brought the completely closed circuit for N_2O delivery into the realms of clinical anesthesia. In the absence of such sophisticated instruments the only safe way of the use of N_2O by continuous flow is to maintain a spontaneous respiration and to stop using N_2O once the system (circuit) is completely closed.

In a completely closed circuit, if low-gas flow (e.g., 1 L flow of 75:25 N_2O/O_2) is used, then it will not render the patient unconscious, even after 10 minutes of breathing of this mixture. This is because, the volume of air in lungs and the apparatus dead space is great enough and leads to the dilution of inspired N_2O to a level which is insufficient for narcosis. So, a high flow (e.g., 8 L) of N_2O and O_2 gas mixture is used first. Then, when the consciousness is lost within few minutes, as the apparatus dead space is rapidly flushed out, it is switched over to a low-flow technique. So, if low flow and a completely closed N_2O technique is to be used, it should always be started with a high flow for few minutes, before reducing to low flow. Once, on a low flow and the circuit is completely closed, then we will have to keep in mind that the inspired O_2 concentration is not at the same level for certain constant flow, like at the beginning. Because, during every inspiration, O_2 will be taken up from alveoli into blood, while the N_2O will not be taken up (when body is completely saturated with N_2O). So, the concentration of O_2 in alveoli will gradually fall and N_2O concentration will gradually increase. This emphasizes the paramount importance of using an O_2 analyzer in a completely closed circle system, when a low flow of N_2O and O_2 mixture is being administered into circuit. Provided that the concentration of O_2 in the inspired mixture does not fall below 25% and the total minute volume is adequate, then this technique can safely be used. It is best not to use an inspired mixture containing <33% of O_2.

Diffusion of N_2O into Closed Space

The diffusion is defined as the physical process of intermingling of molecules, when the different gases and liquids are kept in close contact. This process results from the random movement of the molecules, present in the gases and the liquids. This is called the Brownian movement.

The factors which regulate the rate of diffusion are:
- The concentration gradient or partial pressure of gases
- The molecular size
- The solubility of gases in the liquid when the passage of gas through liquid is involved.

Fick's law dictates that the rate of diffusion is directly proportional to the concentration or the gradient of partial pressure of the gases.

Graham's law dictates that the rate of diffusion of gases of identical partial pressure through some membranes is inversely proportional to the square root of their molecular weight. Therefore, a difference in gas density has only a small effect on the rate of diffusion. Finally, where the transfer of gas across the blood or water film is involved, the rate of diffusion is proportional to the solubility of the gas in that liquid. This is the principal factor for regulating the rate of diffusion of gases into or out of the spaces within the body, which can be seen from the **Table 1**.

The body is normally in equilibrium with the atmospheric nitrogen. So, the N_2 present in the air of any closed cavity within the body will contain approximately the same concentration of N_2 as in the atmosphere. But, if the subject breathes a nitrogen-free gas mixture, containing 60–70% N_2O and 30–40% O_2, then it can be seen from the table that N_2O will diffuse into such spaces 25 times faster than the rate at which N_2 can diffuse out. But if the space is compliant, such as the gut, then there will be an increase in volume without an increase in pressure. But, if the space has rigid walls and is noncompliant, such as the middle ear, then there will be a rise in pressure without an increase in volume.

Some cavities, e.g., the pneumothorax will fall between these two clearly defined cases, where there is both an increase in volume and an increase in pressure. Such an increase in volume and pressure may take place at the expense of other tissues, namely the lungs and mediastinal structures in the case of the pneumothorax.

There are some sites within the body where the air-filled cavities are normally present (such as the middle ear, sinus, etc.) or where air has been accidentally pushed or injected, (such as pneumothorax) or deliberately introduced (such as air encephalogram) and they cause an increase in volume and/or pressure, following the administration of N_2O. If the administration of N_2O is continued for a long time, then all the nitrogen of the body will diffuse out of the space, and the pressure and/or volume after having risen to a peak will return to normal. This is because, all the nitrogen would be replaced by the nitrous oxide and an equilibrium will be reached. Also, when the N_2O is withdrawn and air breathing is started, then the process goes into a reverse order and a subatmospheric pressure is created for a while in any cavity, until all the nitrogen diffuse back into the cavity. This low-pressure phase during recovery is only seen in the case of the noncompliant middle ear **(Box 9)** .

Stomach and Gut

Under normal situations the volume of gas in the gut is not large enough. So, little-to-moderate increase in its volume due to diffusion of N_2O into the gut is not important in the absence of obstruction. But, when the intestinal obstruction is present, then the volume of gas within the lumen of intestine may be much greater and then even a little expansion of it by N_2O could cause problems. Imagining that no nitrogen is absorbed through the gut, so the theoretical increase in the volume of the gut that could result from the breathing of 66% nitrous oxide is almost 200%.

The effects of nitrous oxide on the motility of post-operative bowel have been extensively investigated. It is found that any excess of gas (N_2O) is absorbed long before

TABLE 1: Diffusion of gases.			
Gas	**Density relative to O_2**	**Diffusion capacity relative to O_2**	**Water solubility relative to O_2**
O_2	1	1	1
N_2O	137	14	163
N_2	0.88	0.55	0.5

BOX 9: Types of air-filled cavities in our body.

Noncompliant
- Nasal sinuses
- Middle ear
- Vitreous cavity
- Intercranial—subdural and cisternal

Compliant
- Stomach and gut
- Pneumoperitoneum
- Pneumothorax
- Air embolus
- Surgical emphysema

the peristalsis of gut is re-established. So, the use of N_2O does not delay the return of gastrointestinal function or motility in patients undergoing bowel surgery.

Pneumoperitoneum

The gas which is most commonly introduced in the peritoneal cavity during laparoscopy surgery is CO_2. However, N_2O anesthesia does not produce any problem during this CO_2 pneumoperitoneum, because (i) N_2O and CO_2 have similar diffusing capacity, and (ii) the abdominal cavity is always vented out through some leak.

Pneumothorax

When GA is maintained by continuous flow of N_2O, then the risk of accumulation of N_2O in the cavity of pneumothorax, producing tension pneumothorax has long been investigated. The similar risk is also applied when the subpleural blebs or lung cysts are present. Such cavities are noncommunicating or communicate with airways only through a very narrow orifice, which becomes valvular when there is an increase in the volume of cavity. But during breathing air, the volume of these cavities does not increase and does not cause any problem. However, the volume increases in the pneumothorax or in the subpleural blebs when N_2O is breathed in. It is found experimentally that during breathing of 70% N_2O, the volume of a pneumothorax is doubled in 15 minutes and tripled in 35 minutes.

Surgical Emphysema

During maintenance of GA by N_2O, if surgical emphysema is produced, then air bubbles in the subcutaneous tissue will be expanded by N_2O, diffusing within it. But, problems have not been reported from this phenomenon, perhaps because even extensive surgical emphysema is not life-threatening.

Air Embolism

It is predicted that during N_2O anesthesia N_2O would enter and enlarge the venous air emboli, which may occur during neurosurgery and also open-heart surgery. In such situations, stopping the administration of N_2O should produce a rapid decrease in the size of such air bubbles.

Middle Ear and Nasal Sinuses

The skull cavities such as the middle ear, frontal sinus, maxillary sinus, etc. are normally vented to atmosphere via Eustachian tube or various other ostia. These may be blocked by inflammatory processes or other lesions previously. Then, pressure changes within these closed cavities, following diffusion of N_2O, during the maintenance of GA by continuous inflow of N_2O within these cavities may be

expected. The nasal sinuses remain to be investigated. But, in case of middle ear, the effects have been observed which is attributable to both the raised pressure during nitrous oxide administration and subatmospheric negative pressure, after its removal. These effects include: (i) rupture of drum, (ii) graft displacement, (iii) stapes displacement, (iv) hematotympanum, and (v) temporary or permanent hearing loss. Low pressure in middle ear after N_2O administration is particularly common in children. This is probably because the Eustachian tube is compliant and it collapses when ear pressure is subatmospheric. Thus, fails to maintain equilibrium of pressure on both sides.

Pneumoencephalus

The presence of air pockets or air bubbles anywhere within the brain or within the rigid skull raises the possibility of harmful pressure changes, due to diffusion of N_2O into these cavities if NO_2 is administered during GA. This is called tension pneumoencephalus. It is very common after posterior cranial fossa surgery, particularly in sitting position. This condition is also found, if air is injected into ventricle for radiological investigations, which is followed by general anesthesia with N_2O. Intermittent drainage or aspiration of CSF from ventricle during surgery via a shunt or ventriculostomy is also associated with this type of complication.

The Eye

During surgery for retinal detachment, some ophthalmic surgeons may often inject gas bubbles into vitreous cavity to tamponade the retina in place. So, it is desirable that this gas bubble remains in place for several days. For this purpose, sulfur hexafluoride (SF_6) and perfluoropropane (C_3F_8) gas have been used. They have very low blood-gas solubility. So, they are very slowly absorbed by blood. A bubble of 40% SF_6 and 60% air maintains a constant volume for several days. But, if N_2O is given for maintenance of anesthesia in such cases, then a considerable rise in intraocular pressure may occur due to the diffusion of N_2O into this C_3F_8 or SF_6 gas bubble. So, it is recommended that N_2O should be discontinued 20 minutes before the injection of SF_6 or C_3F_8 gas into vitreous cavity. However, practically the rise in intraocular pressure is not much, if N_2O is withdrawn simultaneously as the gas is injected.

Cuffs and Balloons and N_2O

The cuffs of endotracheal tube, balloons of Swan–Ganz catheters, and other balloons and cuffs which are used in anesthesia are all permeable to N_2O gas. When these balloons and cuffs are in situ and filled with air, then they are subjected to pressure and/or volume changes in the same way, as other gas-filled cavities in our body, during N_2O anesthesia. These changes are clearly a complex one and many variables determine the rate of change of volume and pressure in these cuffs or balloons. These variables include the permeability of the material of balloons or cuffs to N_2O, elasticity, the contents of cuff, its initial volume and pressure, inspired N_2O concentration, temperature, etc.

Although sore throat is common after effect of intubation, but serious problems do not commonly occur as a result of increased endotracheal tube cuff pressure, after routine N_2O anesthesia. However, it is clearly undesirable to expose the tracheal mucosa to unnecessary pressure. Thus, care must be taken to inflate the cuff of endotracheal tube to not more than the sealing pressure. We should also remember that the pressure may go on rising which needs certain adjustments accordingly, after every interval of 3 hours. The suggestions to minimize the pressure changes in cuffs include: inflating the cuff with inspired gas mixture (such as with N_2O and air), or perhaps best of all with water and saline. Recently, several constant pressure inflating devices also have been developed.

Second Gas Effect of N_2O

When a high concentration of N_2O is given with O_2 and other accompanying volatile anesthetic agents, then N_2O quickly replaces the nitrogen of air, which was previously present in alveoli. Then, though N_2O has a low blood-gas solubility, compared to other volatile agents, still it is more soluble in blood than nitrogen. So, the volume of N_2O taken up by blood is greater than the volume of nitrogen entering the alveoli from blood. Therefore, the alveoli become smaller and the fractional concentration of second volatile anesthetic agent (which is given along with N_2O and mixture O_2) in alveoli increases. This phenomenon is called as the "second gas effect". After absorption of N_2O into blood, although the volume of N_2O in alveoli decreases, but its concentration does not diminish to previous level, because the volume of alveoli also decreases.

At the end of anesthesia, the opposite phenomenon occurs. The supply of N_2O is stopped and the patient is allowed to breathe air. At that time, N_2O diffuses back into alveoli from blood more rapidly than the rate at which blood can take up nitrogen from alveoli (as patient is breathing air). So, the concentration of N_2O in alveoli increases with the volume of alveoli. This increase in volume of alveoli will cause relative reduction of the concentration of second volatile anesthetic agent, also in turn will help in recovery.

Diffusion Hypoxia or Fink Effect

While a patient is breathing N_2O mixed with O_2 during anesthesia, then a relatively large amount of this gas will replace the less soluble N_2 which is already present in the body tissues and fluids during breathing of air. Again, at the end of anesthesia when the patient starts breathing air, then the alveoli soon become filled with N_2 and O_2 from air. But, there is still an appreciable quantity of N_2O dissolved in the blood and body tissues. Although N_2O is always referred to as an insoluble anesthetic agent, it is 34 times more soluble than N_2. It means blood can carry much more N_2O than N_2. So, during the first few minutes after the end of anesthesia, when the patient starts breathing in room air, then large quantities of N_2O leave the body tissue and enter into the alveoli and N_2 (now being breathed with air) diffuses from the alveoli back into the tissues. As the solubility of N_2O is much greater than that of N_2, so a relatively small amount of N_2 passes from the alveoli to the blood and tissues, but much larger amount of N_2O passes back from the tissues and blood to the alveoli. This mass movement of N_2O into the alveoli causes dilution of the alveolar O_2 concentration and reduces its tension. This is called the diffusion hypoxia or Fink effect. Normally in an alveolus, when the patient breathes in room air, then O_2 concentration is 14%. But, under these conditions, this O_2 concentration may drop to as low as 10% and result in a severe degree of hypoxia, which may be dangerous for elderly and critically ill patients. Clinically, diffusion hypoxia is only significant for N_2O anesthesia, because N_2O is the only anesthetic agent which is used in high concentrations and this diffusion hypoxia usually persists for about 10 minutes after the stoppage of flow of N_2O. However, it is of little significance in healthy patients and can be prevented by giving 100% O_2 for 5 minutes in the immediate postoperative period.

■ DIETHYL ETHER $(C_2H_5)_2O$ (FIG. 14)

History

It is commonly called as ether and was first prepared by Valerius Cordus in 1540. But, at that time it was not used as an anesthetic agent and during this period, it was called as "Sweet Oil of Vitriol". Then, Sigmund August, a German chemist, botanist, and physician, named it as ether. Previously, instead of being used as an anesthetic agent, the vapor of it was being mostly used as a drug of amusement, together with N_2O, in both America and Europe. However,

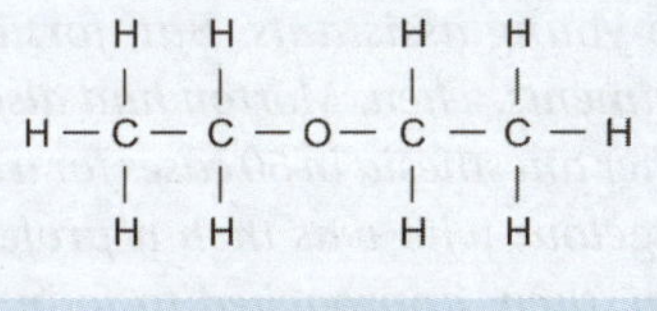

Fig. 14: Diethyl ether.

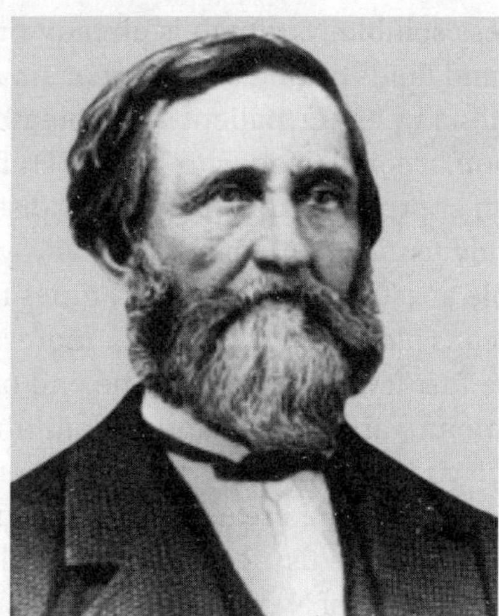

Fig. 15: Crawford Long.

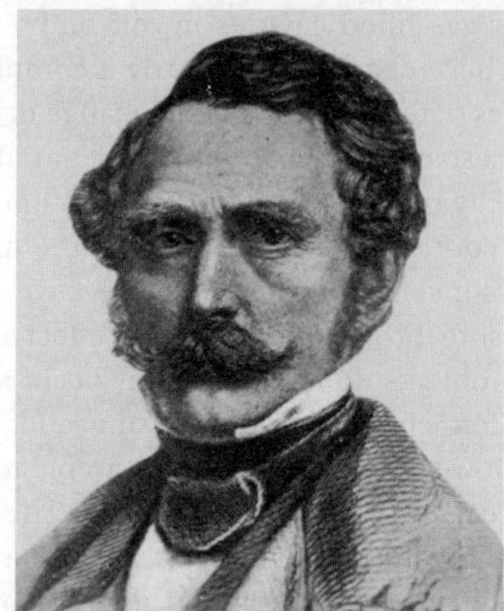

Fig. 16: Green Morton.

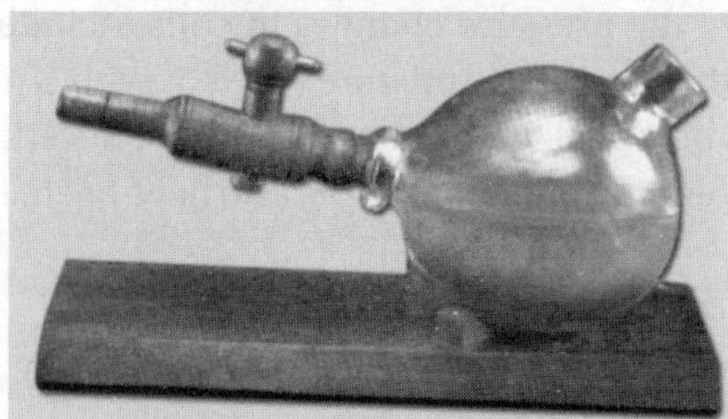

Fig. 17: Morton's inhaler.

analgesic effects of ether were accidentally discovered in 1833 by an unknown chemist. He was wiping freely the face of his wife with ether during her prolonged labor. Then, he observed that her distress passed away. So, he understood that ether had analgesic property. After that, ether was probably first used for clinical anesthesia by Clarke, an anesthetist, in the January of 1842 when a dentist named Elijah Pope extracted a tooth from his patient, named Miss Hobbie. But, this was not published by Clarke and did not attract attention during that period.

Crawford Williamson Long **(Fig. 15)**, a general practitioner of Jefferson in Georgia, was used to inhale ether vapor frequently for amusement. Like Mr Wells, he also noted that he could acquire painless trauma on his body, while he is under the influence of ether, without remembering it (trauma) later on. He applied this experience to remove one or two cysts from the back of his patient's neck, after administering ether from a towel. Thus, he used ether over next few years for minor surgeries. But, even he did not publish the results of his work.

*During the period of 1843, Green Morton **(Fig. 16)**, a specialist in dental prosthetic works, had moved from Hartford to Boston and at Boston he had set up his dental practice. He had observed both Well's demonstration of N_2O and his failure at Massachusetts General Hospital in 1845. He had also observed anesthetic effect of ether on his patients, when they breathed the vapor of ether which was applied as liquid to deaden the painful tooth sockets. Subsequently, Morton had tried ether vapor on himself, on his pet dog, and on his two young assistants. But, fortunately all were successful experiments. Then, Morton had also gained further experience of ether anesthesia in 50 cases for a surgeon, named Henry Jacob Bigelow, who was then a professor of Materia Medica. Morton, then, approached to John Warren who at that time was a senior surgeon of Massachusetts General Hospital, for an opportunity to make a public demonstration of ether anesthesia. However, this was arranged within 2 days and on 16th October, in 1846, Morton successfully demonstrated the anesthetic properties of ether publicly on a patient, named Gilbert Abott, for removal of a congenital vascular malformation from the floor of mouth under tongue. It was operated by surgeon, named JC Warren. The operation took place in what is now known as the "Ether Dome" at Massachusetts General Hospital **(Fig. 17)**.*

Williamson Long had also discovered the anesthetic property of ether, even before Morton. But, he did not demonstrate this in public. So, when Mr Long had reported his work in 1849, then Morton's fame was already well established. In science, ironically the recognition for new discovery goes to the man who demonstrates, publishes, and convinces the world first, but not to the man in whom the idea came first. Hence, as Morton convinced the world regarding the advantages of ether anesthesia, though late, so he bagged the crown.

Preparation of Ether

Ether is prepared by the reaction between ethyl alcohol and sulfuric acid at 140°C. $C_2H_5OH + H_2SO_4 \rightarrow C_2H_5HSO_4 + H_2O$
$C_2H_5HSO_4 + C_2H_5OH \rightarrow (C_2H_5)_2O + H_2SO_4$.

Physical Properties of Ether

Ether is a colorless, volatile liquid, with a very characteristic pungent smell. At room temperature (20°C), its vapor pressure is 425 mm Hg. This vapor pressure helps to calculate the inspired concentration (Fi) of ether, delivered to patient by bubble-through type of vaporizer (copper Kettle or Vernitrol). But, this vapor pressure is not helpful for a blow-over type of vaporizer (Boyel's ether bottle) to calculate the inspired concentration (Fi) of ether. If Boyle's ether bottle is converted to bubble-through type of vaporizer, by dipping the plunger into the liquid of ether, then also the constant change of temperature of liquid ether, due to the latent heat of vaporization, makes the calculation of inspired concentration of ether difficult. On the other hand, in a copper kettle the temperature of ether is kept constant. The cooling of Boyle's ether bottle due to latent heat of vaporization and freezing of moisture outside the glass bottle is prevented in Oxford Vaporizer Mark II, where the ether bottle is surrounded by a chemical crystal with a melting point more than ether, and it helps the ether to vaporize constantly. So, the ether vapor in Oxford vaporizer remains under pressure and emits spontaneously and continuously at a set concentration (Fi).

Ether and its vapor is highly inflammable and ignites at 154°C. Low concentration of ether vapor burns itself with a clear blue flame and at higher concentrations it explodes. Ether vapor is 2.5 times heavier than air and spreads like an invisible blanket over the floor. So, a spark from any electric point near the floor can ignite this ether blanket, causing a cold blue-like flame which is invisible in daylight. The zone of inflammability of ether vapor is usually confined to 25 cm around the expiratory valve. So, if diathermy is kept outside this area and an efficient gas exhaust system is maintained in OT, then there is little risk of explosion **(Table 2)**.

The decomposition of ether is favored by air, light, and heat and it is prevented by copper and hydroquinone. So, ether is always kept in a dark and airtight bottle in cool place.

The main impurities due to decomposition of ether are: acetic aldehyde, ether peroxide, alcohol, sulfuric acid, SO_2, mercaptans, ethyl ester, etc. The systemic effects (toxicity) due to these impurities of ether in man are doubtful. The probable problems, due to these impurities of ether on human body, are gastric irritation (due to peroxide) and tachycardia with hypotension (due to mercaptans). During ether anesthesia, the presence of mercaptans can be suspected, if the patient's expired air has a peculiar fishy odor.

Pharmacological Properties of Ether

Ether's blood/gas solubility coefficient is 12.1. So, it indicates that ether is highly absorbable (soluble) in blood. Therefore, as it is constantly being removed from alveoli, by dissolving in plasma and without increasing its tension in plasma due to its high-blood solubility, it takes a longer time to raise the plasma and alveolar tension. On the other hand, the alveolar and plasma tension of any inhalational anesthetic agent is synonymous with its brain tension. So, the induction of anesthesia by ether will be slow (15–20 minutes) and may take a longer time to achieve deep anesthesia than other volatile anesthetic agents, whose blood/gas solubility coefficient is very less. Similarly, the recovery from ether anesthesia will also be slow. The oil/gas solubility of ether is only 65, indicating that it is less potent than halothane and other volatile agents (halothane's oil/gas solubility 224). This is because, the potency of any volatile anesthetic agent depends on its lipid solubility, i.e., oil/gas solubility coefficient.

The 90% of inspired ether vapor is excreted unchanged through lungs. Rest of it is metabolized or excreted through skin, body secretions, and urine. About 4% of inhaled ether is metabolized in liver to acetaldehyde and ethanol. Like phenobarbitone, ether is also a powerful inducing agent of hepatic microsomal enzymes. So, its prolonged exposure increases the rate of metabolism of other drugs

TABLE 2: Characteristic features of various anesthesia.							
Agent	**Molecular weight**	**Boiling point (°C)**	**Vapor pressure at 20°C (mm Hg)**	**Blood-gas solubility**	**Oil-gas solubility**	**MAC**	**Metabolism**
Nitrous oxide (N_2O)	44	–88	–	0.42	1.4	105	0
Diethylether (C_2H_5–O–C_2H_5)	74	36.5	440	12.1	65	1.92	4
Halothane ($CF_3CHClBr$)	197.4	50.2	243.3	2.5	224	0.75	20
Isoflurane (CHF_2–O–$CHClCF_3$)	184.5	48.5	250	1.4	99	1.15	0.2
Sevoflurane (CF_3–CHO–CH_2F–CF_3)	200.5	58.5	160	1.69	50	2	4
Desflurane (CHF_2–O–CHF–CHF_2)	168	22.8	664	0.42	19	6	0.02
Xenon (Xe)	131.3	–107	–	0.11	–	71	0

in liver. Ether is irritant to mucosa of respiratory tract and so it increases bronchial secretion. It also stimulates the vagal afferent fibers in bronchial tree, leading to increased depth and rate of respiration. Ether itself is a bronchodilator. It does not affect surfactant production. So, it does not reduce the surface tension of alveoli and does not help in the formation of atelectasis. As respiratory rate increases during ether anesthesia, till a very deep level is achieved when the paralytic action supervenes with steady decline of minute volume, leading to apnea. So, $PaCO_2$ level does not rise till a very deep level of anesthesia is reached with ether. Thus, in spontaneous respiration during ether anesthesia, controlled or assisted ventilation is not usually needed till a very deep level of anesthesia is reached.

Ether minimally depresses the ventilation than the other inhalational anesthetic agents. It diminishes the ventilatory response to inhaled CO_2 at an anesthetic depth at which $PaCO_2$ is maintained at normal levels. The action of ether on CVS is explained by increased sympathetic activity, caused by it. Ether anesthesia produces a small alteration in BP and pulse rate. Very rarely, it leads to cardiac irregularities, because it does not sensitize the myocardium to adrenaline. With a very deep anesthesia, CVS is also depressed by ether. This is due to reduced catecholamine secretion from exhausted sympathetic system and at this situation it should be used very cautiously with β-blocking agents.

Ether causes skeletal muscle relaxation by: (i) depressing the CNS, (ii) affecting the motor end plate, and (iii) affecting the muscle itself similar to tubocurarine. Ether is secreted through saliva and passes to stomach. It also stimulates the vomiting center in medulla and is responsible for higher incidences of PONV. Smooth muscle motility of the intestine is depressed during ether anesthesia. As ether stimulates sympathetic activity, so it leads to an increased release of catecholamines. Hence, glycogen is mobilized from both the liver and muscles and a marked rise in blood sugar follows, due to endogenous catecholamine-induced glycolysis. Ether reduces the tone of gravid uterus, even in slight concentration.

Clinical Uses of Ether

Ether is associated with the lowest death rate in a properly conducted anesthesia and is associated with the lowest incidences of liver damage. Still, it is gradually going out of vogue, because (i) it does not attenuate intubation induced sympathetic over activity, (ii) it possesses a strong pungent odor, (iii) it causes increased secretion, (iv) it causes delayed induction and recovery of anesthesia, etc. It alone produces all the three major components of anesthesia such as sedation, analgesia, and depression of reflexes. So, though modern anesthetic techniques go far beyond this maxim, ether still remains as very popular and the most effective means of anesthesia in many underdeveloped countries, mainly at rural area.

Guedel's Classification of Ether Anesthesia

As the depth of ether anesthesia increases, then gradually the respiratory pattern of anesthetized patient changes, more and more reflexes are suppressed and some characteristic changes in the size of pupil occur. So, in 1920, these slow progressions of changes made it possible for Guedel to divide these various alterations in reflex activity, during deepening of anesthesia, into four stages, after an exhaustive study of open-drop ether anesthesia **(Fig. 18)**.

GA by only ether vapor causes an irregular or regular depression of CNS in descending order, i.e., higher functions of brain are involved (lost) first and progressively the lower areas of brain are involved. But, in spinal cord the lower segments are affected somewhat earlier than the higher segments. The vital centers located in the medulla are paralyzed at last, as the depth of anesthesia increases. However, these clear-cut stages of anesthesia, produced by inhalational agents other than ether, are not seen nowadays with the use of muscle relaxants, faster-acting inhalational anesthetic agents, premedications, and employment of many drugs together. These precise sequences of events also differ somewhat with other inhalational anesthetics than ether. However, as still ether continues to be widely used in India and so the descriptions of these stages still serve us to define the level of anesthesia such as the light and deep anesthesia **(Fig. 19)**.

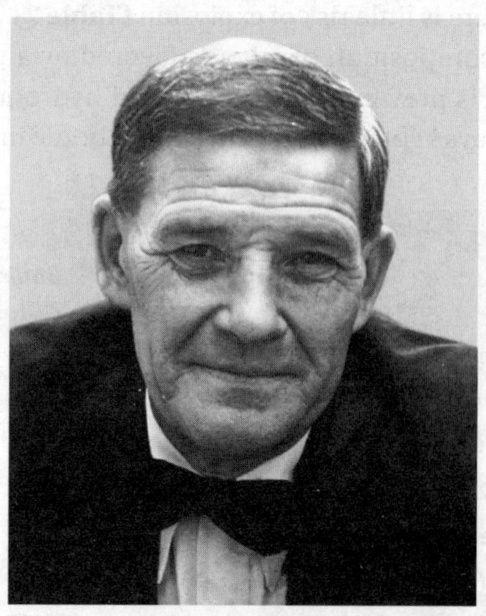

Fig. 18: Guedel.

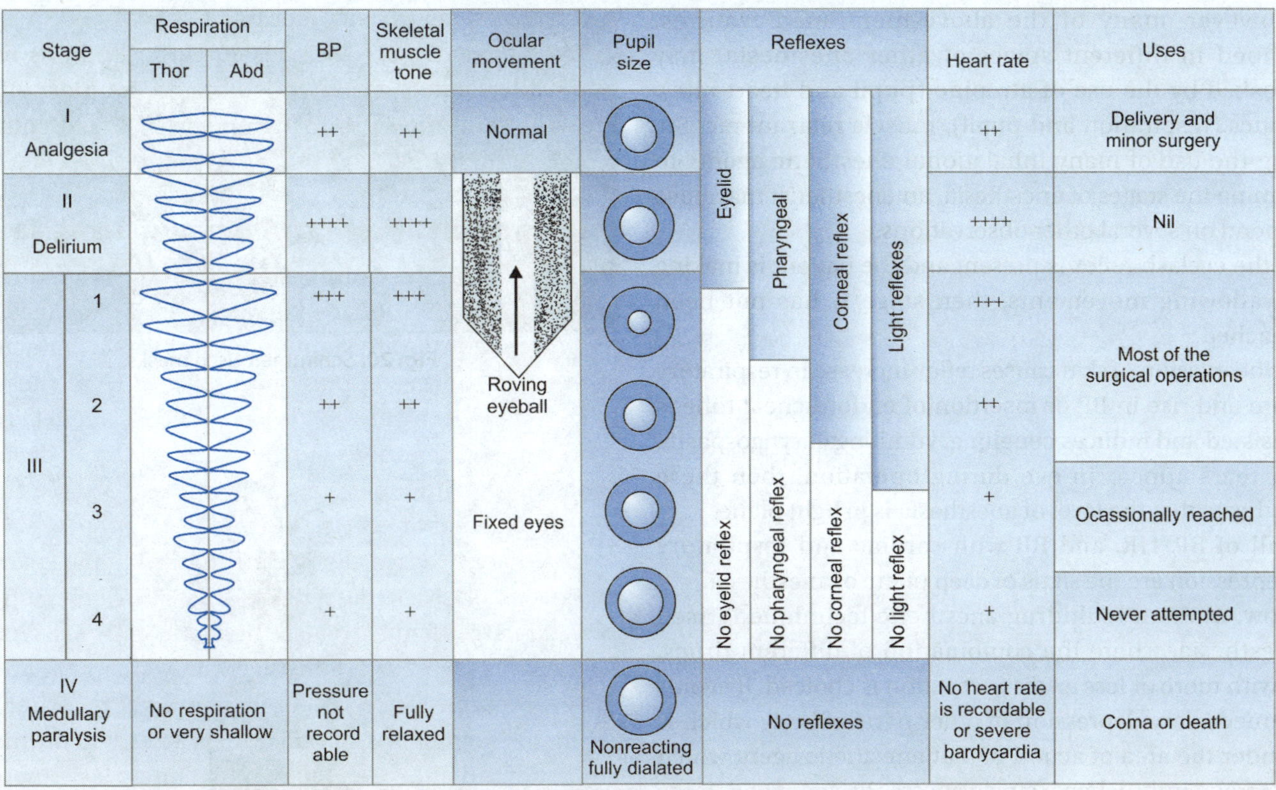

Fig. 19: Stages of general anesthesia.

Stage I or Stage of Analgesia

It starts from the beginning of inhalation of ether vapor to the loss of consciousness. Pain is progressively abolished during this stage. Thus, this stage is named so. But, the patient remains conscious or semiconscious. At the end of this stage, the patient becomes unconscious. He can hear, see, and feel a dreamlike state. The reflexes and respiration remain normal in this stage. Though some minor operations of short duration can be carried out during this stage, but it is rather difficult to maintain this stage. So, its use is limited to very short procedures only.

Stage II or Stage of Delirium

It extends from the loss of consciousness to the beginning of regular respiration. Apparent excitement with irregular respiration is seen in this stage. The patient may shout, struggle, or hold his breath. Muscle tone increases. Jaws are remained tightly closed. Breathing is jerky and vomiting, involuntary micturition, or defecation may occur in this stage. Heart rate and BP may rise and pupils may dilate due to sympathetic stimulation. No stimulus should be applied or no operative procedure should be carried out during this stage. This stage can be cut short by rapid induction and premedication. However, this stage is inconspicuous in modern anesthesia due to the use of IV anesthetic agents, muscle relaxants, very rapidly acting inhalational anesthetic agents, etc.

Stage III or Surgical Anesthesia

This stage extends from the onset of regular respiration to the cessation of spontaneous breathing. This has been again divided into four planes which are well distinguished as:

i. *Plane I:* Moving the eyeballs. This plane ends when the eyeballs become fixed.
ii. *Plane II:* Loss of corneal or laryngeal reflexes.
iii. *Plane III:* Pupil starts dilating and light reflex is lost.
iv. *Plane IV:* Intercostal paralysis, shallow abdominal respiration, and dilated pupils.

In this stage of anesthesia, as the level passes on from superficial to deeper planes progressively, then the muscle tone gradually decreases, BP falls, pulse becomes weak, and heart rate increases. After that respiration gradually decreases in depth and later in frequency.

Stage IV or Stage of Medullary Paralysis

It extends from the cessation of breathing to the failure of circulation and death. In this stage of anesthesia, pupil is widely dilated, muscles are totally paralyzed, pulse is imperceptible and BP is very low to nonrecordable.

However, many of the above-mentioned features, described in different stages of ether anesthesia, may be masked by the use of atropine (pupil and heart rate), narcotics (respiration and pupil), muscle relaxant etc. So, during the use of many inhalational anesthetic agents to determine the stages of anesthesia, an anesthetist may have to depend on several other observations.

i. If the eyelash reflex is present and the patient is making swallowing movements, then stage II has not been reached.

ii. If the incision of skin causes reflex increase in respiratory rate and rise in BP or insertion of endotracheal tube is resisted and induces coughing, vomiting, laryngospasm, or tears appear in eye during operation, then these indicate that the level of anesthesia is in light plane.

iii. Fall of BP, HR, and RR with cardiac and respiratory depression are the signs of deep plane of anesthesia.

Now, modern multidrug anesthetic technique is used in anesthesia, where the combination of different drugs, each with more or less its distinct action is choiced. It avoids the unnecessary depression of other parts of body which is not under the area of action of that anesthetic agent which occurs frequently, when a single anesthetic agent with large doses is used. This type of multidrug anesthesia is called as the *control or balanced anesthesia,* utilizing more than one agent to offset the disadvantage of another. Now, we choose a mixture of drugs that best fits with the anticipated needs of that operation.

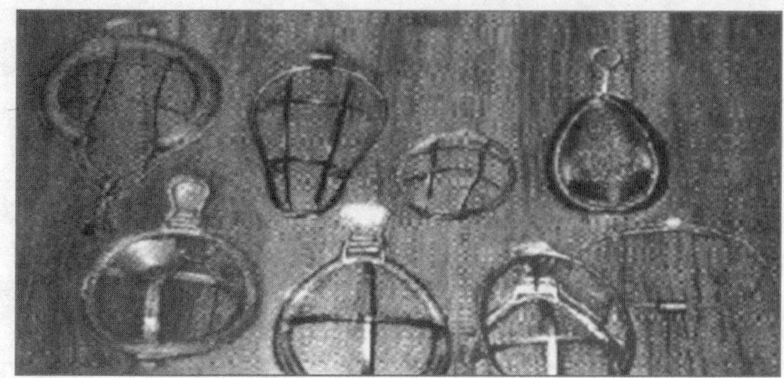

Fig. 20: Schimmelbusch masks.

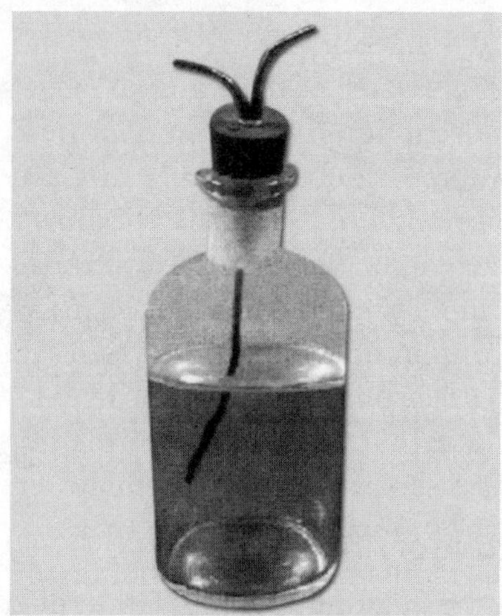

Fig. 21: Bellamy Gardner dropper bottle of ether.

Method of Administration of Ether

Ether can be administered mainly by three methods such as *open, semiclosed,* and *closed with CO_2 absorption.* The open technique is used by a Schimmelbusch mask and ether is dropped from a Bellany Gardner dropper bottle. As the patient inspires only the mixture of air (which contains only 20% O_2) and ether vapor, so in this mixture the exact inspired O_2 concentration (FiO_2) falls below 20%, which cannot be calculated accurately. Hence, extra O_2 supply by a catheter is mandatory to rise the FiO_2 >33%. Patient inhales air and anesthetic ether (ether vapor) mixture which is at low temperature due to vaporization of liquid ether. So, the respiratory tree is called upon to perform heavy duty to raise the temperature of air-ether mixture to 37°C and also to saturate it with water vapor. It has also been estimated that there is heat loss of about 300 calories/minute from the patient, using ether vapor **(Fig. 20)**.

In a semi-closed technique, ether is vaporized by blowing the mixture of N_2O and O_2 gas over it or bubbling through it (ether) that is contained in a marked glass bottle vaporizer. The example of this technique is ether anesthesia by Boyel's machine, using Boyel's ether bottle vaporizer. Safety of this technique lies in the fact that, as the vaporization of ether increases, then the temperature of liquid ether and vaporizing bottle falls which in turn slows the rate of vaporization of ether from bottle. Therefore, the control knob which is set to deliver a certain concentration of ether vapor cannot perform this job. This is because after sometime, with the control knob still in same position, there is reduction in vapor concentration of ether due to the cooling of anesthetic agent and bottle. In a circle system, higher concentration of ether is built-up very quickly (only if vaporizer is within the circuit), because the whole volume of expired gas passes through vaporizing ether bottle and vaporization of ether is assisted by heat, both from the patient and the C_2O absorbing canister **(Fig. 21)**.

EMO Vaporizer

Basically, this is a draw-over or blow-over type of vaporizer, which is used to vaporize the ether. To deliver a required concentration of ether, the ether bottle is kept in a water bath which acts as heat buffer and supply the latent heat for the vaporization of ether and allows the delivery of a fixed concentration of anesthetic ether vapor, set by the dial. This discussion is only for historical interest.

■ HALOTHANE

(2-bromo 2-chloro 1, 1, 1 tri-fluoro-ethane) **(Fig. 22)**.

CW Suckling had first synthesized halothane in the laboratory of Imperial Chemical Industries at Manchester in 1951. Then, Raventos had studied its pharmacological properties in succeeding years. After that, it was first used clinically, in 1956, by Johnstone at Manchester and that was followed by Bryce–Smith and O'Brien at Oxford.

Physical Properties of Halothane

Halothane is a colorless, noninflammable, and potent anesthetic liquid with very sweet smell. Its commercial preparations contain 0.01% thymol for stability. Boiling point of halothane is 50.2°C and it does not react with soda lime. It decomposes to HCl, HBr, free chlorine, free bromine, and phosgene gas, when it is exposed to bright light for several days. So, presence of thymol prevents this decomposition. It is suitable for vaporization in a bubble-through vaporizer (copper kettle) or temperature and flow compensated vaporizer (flutec vaporizer).

If water vapor is present in halothane vapor, then it can attack some metals such as aluminum, brass, and lead. But, copper and chromium are not attacked by halothane vapor. So, the previous metals are not used to build the halothane vaporizers. Halothane is readily soluble in rubber, but less so in polythene. Significant rubber solubility and large amount of rubber, used in anesthetic delivery system, make the uptake of halothane by rubber very significant. The concentration of vapor of halothane in an anesthetic gas mixture can be estimated by gas chromatography or by infrared analyzer or by ultraviolet light analyzer.

Pharmacological Properties of Halothane

The MAC value of halothane is 0.8. Its blood gas solubility co-efficient is 2.3 (N_2O is 0.46, ether is 12.1, isofluorane is 1.4, and sevoflurane is 0.69). So, the solubility of halothane in blood is of medium range. Thus, as it is relatively insoluble in blood (in comparison to ether), so it is not taken up by

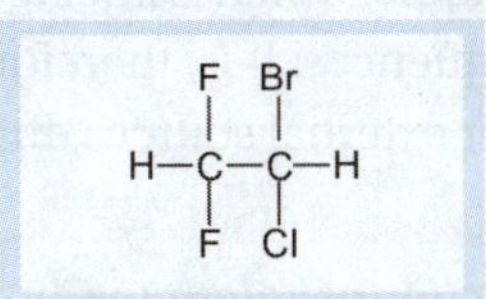

Fig. 22: Halothane.

blood very rapidly from alveoli. This means that alveolar concentration and tension of halothane can soon approach to its inspired concentration (Fi) and tension very rapidly. On the other hand, the alveolar concentration and tension is virtually synonymous with the brain concentration and tension of any volatile anesthetic agent. So, a high concentration and tension of halothane is rapidly achieved in brain. This means the induction of anesthesia by halothane is relatively rapid in comparison to ether. During the first few minutes of halothane anesthesia, most of it goes to heart, brain, liver, kidney, and later comes to an equilibrium with these tissues. After that, muscles tend to remove their quota from the circulation and take a few hours to come to an equilibrium. Then, one of the principal reasons for the prolonged uptake of halothane by our body is the remarkable capacity of human fat to absorb it, due to its high solubility coefficient in fat (60 for halothane and 1 for N_2O). So, the fat is capable of removing almost all the halothane, that is received in circulation. In this manner, the body continues for almost indefinite period to keep removing halothane vapor from lungs. In fact, a complete equilibrium between the inspired and alveolar concentration of halothane is probably never reached, because a small amount of it is continuously lost through skin.

Metabolism of Halothane

The 12% of total inspired halothane is metabolized in our body by liver through the oxidation and dehalogenation mechanism, forming tri-fluoro-acetic acid, bromide radicals, and chloride radicals, etc. which are excreted through urine. Then, the remaining part of inhaled halothane is expired through lungs.

Pharmacological Actions of Halothane

Effects on Cardiovascular System

Halothane is a potent volatile anesthetic agent. It reduces the force of myocardial contraction, stroke volume, cardiac output, and heart rate by its direct negative (–ve) chronotropic action on SA node and by its direct negative (–ve) inotropic action on myocardium. Thus, during halothane anesthesia, BP goes down without any change in SVR. The 2 MAC value of halothane results in 50% decrease in blood pressure and cardiac output. As halothane also attenuates baroreceptor reflexes, so the HR does not change (increase) with the fall in BP that is normally expected in response to hypotension. At 1.1% end-tidal concentration of halothane, the baroreceptor reflex is completely inhibited, but the SVR is very slightly affected. However, atropine can reverse this bradycardia, induced by halothane, but not arterial hypotension or

BOX 10: Mechanism of actions of hypotension due to halothane.

- It gradually blocks the action of noradrenaline at the effector sites in heart, central nervous system (CNS), and peripheral tissues
- It gradually reduces the secretion and activity of noradrenaline at the sympathetic nerve endings in the myocardium
- It sensitizes the parasympathetic nerve endings, leading to bradycardia

cardiac output. Thus, it indicates that the hypotension during halothane anesthesia is due to its direct myocardial depression effect and not due to bradycardia **(Box 10)**.

The major cause of arterial hypotension, during halothane anesthesia, is fall in cardiac output, due to the depression of myocardial contractility. During halothane anesthesia the limbs remain warm and dry with prominent peripheral superficial veins, suggesting vasodilatation of both arteriolar and venous component of vascular tree. But, this does not cause the reduction in SVR and hypotension. The plasma catecholamine level is not raised during halothane anesthesia. The decreased catecholamine level during halothane anesthesia is due to the diminished release of adrenaline and noradrenaline from adrenal medulla and sympathetic nerve endings. Marked reduction of coronary vascular resistance also occurs by halothane. So, although halothane is a potent coronary vasodilator, but the coronary blood flow actually decreases. It is due to the fall of systemic arterial pressure. However, adequate myocardial perfusion is still usually maintained, as its oxygen demand also drops.

Arrhythmia and Halothane: Most of the changes in cardiac rate and rhythm, which occur during halothane anesthesia, may be explained on the basis of altered autonomic balance, i.e., the preponderance of either vagal or sympathetic activity, induced by halothane. The vagal stimulation produced by halothane causes the slowing of sinus rate. If the sinoatrial (SA) node is sufficiently depressed, then the role of pacemaker activity of SA node may be taken over by atrioventricular (AV) node. There may also be some independent activation of atria or ventricles, while intense vagal stimulation may lead to partial or complete SA block, bundle branch block, or even asystole. The relative sympathetic stimulation, induced by halothane, also causes sinus tachycardia or occasional ventricular extrasystole, although the actual plasma catecholamine level does not increase. When this relative sympathetic activation caused by halothane becomes more profound, then the multifocal ventricular extrasystoles, ventricular tachycardia and VF may occur **(Table 3)**.

It has also long been known that the general anesthetic agents, which have a hydrocarbon structure in some form,

sensitize myocardium to the effects of catecholamines. So, like other hydrocarbons, halothane also sensitizes the myocardium to the effects of catecholamines, though the actual level of catecholamines does not increase. However, the manner by which halothane produces this effect (arrhythmia) is not clear, but it would seem that a reduction of HR and increase of ventricular automaticity plays an important role.

The halothane anesthesia is accompanied with the shifting of natural pacemaker site from SA node to AV node. It is probable that these changes are mainly due to increased vagal activity and can often be countered by the action of atropine. It is believed that some form of re-entry mechanism is also likely the cause for the production of halothane-induced arrhythmia. The respiratory depression and the retention of CO_2 during halothane anesthesia also may give rise to bigeminal rhythm, multi-focal ventricular extrasystoles, and VT. The higher degree of hypercarbia is required to provoke ventricular extrasystoles and their incidence is not related to the concentration of inspired halothane. The correction of respiratory acidosis will often abolish these ventricular irregularities, even though the concentration of halothane is unaltered.

It is essential that the changes in heart rate and rhythm during halothane anesthesia should not be treated indiscriminately with atropine. Because, the random abolition of any restraining vagal tone may accentuate the severity of arrhythmia and may even induce VF. It has long been suggested that if ventilation is adequate and the concentration and the total dose of adrenaline is kept within prescribed limits, then the SC injection of adrenaline may safely be given during halothane anesthesia. It has been found that ED_{50} (the dose producing a positive response in 50% of patients) of epinephrine that produces arrhythmia during halothane anesthesia is 2.5 µg/kg. So, it is considered that a maximum dose of 10 mL of 1:100,000 epinephrine for 10 minutes period is safe. In vast majority of patients, the incidence of arrhythmia can also be diminished, if isoflurane is substituted for halothane. The endogenous catecholamines are also an important factor for the causation of arrhythmia, when their concentration is elevated during light anesthesia by surgical stimulation. In such circumstances, the absorption of even a small amount of exogenous adrenaline, which is injected from outside, may have serious consequences. It is, therefore, best to avoid the use of adrenaline for external sources during light halothane anesthesia.

The mechanism of action of halothane on cardiac contraction: Halothane, like other inhaled anesthetic agents, depresses

TABLE 3: Clinical pharmacology of inhalational anesthetics.

	N_2O	Halothane	Isoflurane	Sevoflurane	Desflurane
CVS					
i. Blood pressure	0	↓↓	↓↓	↓	↓↓
ii. Heart rate	0	↓	↑	0	0/↑
iii. SVR	0	0	↓↓	↓	↓↓
iv. Cardiac output	0	↓	0	↓	0/↓
Respiratory					
i. Respiratory rate	↑	↑↑	↑	↑	↑
ii. Tidal volume	↓	↓↓	↓↓	↓	↓
iii. PaCO₂	0	↑	↑	↑	↑↑
Cerebral					
i. Blood flow	↑	↑↑	↑	↑	↑
ii. ICP	↑	↑↑	↑	↑	↑
iii. Cerebral mechanism	↑	↓	↓↓	↓↓	↓↓
iv. Seizures	↓	↓	↓	↓	↓
Renal					
i. Renal blood flow	↓	↓↓	↓↓	↓	↓
ii. GFR	↓	↓↓	↓↓	↓	↓
iii. Urinary output	↓	↓↓	↓↓	↓	↓
Hepatic					
Blood flow	↓	↓↓	↓	↓	↓
Neuromuscular					
Nondepolarizing blockade	↑	↑↑	↑↑	↑↑	↑↑
Metabolism	0.004%	15–20%	0.2%	5%	<0.1%

No change = 0, Elevated = ↑, Reduced = ↓

(CVS: cardiovascular system; GFR: glomerular filtration rate; ICP: intracranial pressure; SVR: systemic vascular resistance)

myocardial contraction by decreasing the free intracellular Ca^{2+} level by:

- Interfering with Ca^{2+} movement through sarcolemma and by decreasing the release and availability of Ca^{2+} from the sarcoplasmic reticulum.
- Altering the sensitivity of regulatory and contractile proteins to the available Ca^{2+}. The order of potency of inhalational anesthetic agents, regarding myocardial depression, is halothane >enflurane >isoflurane >N_2O.

Halothane and pulmonary vascular resistance: In the absence of underlying pathology, halothane has little effect on pulmonary blood flow and pulmonary arterial pressure. However, halothane in general decreases PVR and increases left atrial pressure.

Halothane and hypoxic pulmonary vasoconstrictive response: The mechanism by which halothane interferes the hypoxic pulmonary vasoconstrictive (HPV) response remains still a mystery. The possible theories are:

- Halothane acts by interfering with the action of local vasoactive metabolic substances, responsible for vasoconstriction.
- Direct relaxing effect of halothane on vascular smooth muscles, counteracting the locally or systemically mediated vasoconstrictive response.
- Interfering with Ca^{++} uptake by the cells of vascular smooth muscle.

Halothane and baroreceptors: Due to normal protective baroreceptor reflexes, the changes in blood pressure result in an alteration in peripheral vascular resistance, heart rate, venous tone, and CO. Halothane (like other anesthetics) depresses this baroreceptor reflex. So, hypovolemic or CVS compromised patients are less able to compensate the hypotension, when they are anesthetized by halothane. Another importance of this baroreceptor attenuation is that the clinical signs of hypovolemia or reduced CO, e.g., tachycardia are masked under halothane anesthesia.

So, sophisticated monitoring is required during halothane anesthesia, especially when there is associated hypotension.

Effects on the Respiratory System

Halothane is a nonirritating respiratory depressant and progressively decreases tidal volume, rather than rate of respiration. Actually, halothane increases rate of respiration. But, still the minute volume is reduced and this is due to relative much reduction of tidal volume. Halothane used in clinical practice produces bronchodilatation and this is probably not mediated through β_2-adrenoreceptor stimulation. This is proved by the fact that this bronchodilating action of halothane is not inhibited by propanolol or β-adrenergic blocking agents. Halothane attenuates airway reflexes and relaxes bronchial smooth muscles by inhibiting intracellular mobilization of Ca^{2+} within these bronchial smooth muscle cells.

Halothane is most potent bronchodilator among all the available volatile anesthetic agents. There may even be a decrease in effective alveolar ventilation. It has no effect on the synthesis of surfactant in alveoli of lungs. In normal healthy unstimulated airway, the resting muscle tone is minimal. So, the bronchodilating properties of halothane is also nil (during normal condition). Only during bronchoconstriction, bronchodilating property of halothane is well demonstrated. Systemic administration of halothane via a bypass pump does not cause bronchodilatation which suggests that halothane acts directly on airway musculature and/or through local reflex arc, rather than via centrally controlled reflex pathways.

Halothane does not inhibit the release of histamine from mast cells, causing bronchoconstriction. So, histamine level is not affected. Patients, resistant to other bronchodilators, promptly respond to halothane.

Halothane and mucociliary function of respiratory tract: All the halothane-like inhaled anesthetic agents diminish the rate of mucous clearance by diminishing the ciliary movement and also by altering the quality and quantity of mucous production. Halothane anesthesia decreases the mucous velocity by 7.7 mm/min. So, no mucous movement seen after 90 minutes of halothane anesthesia. Hence, prolonged halothane anesthesia could lead to the pooling of mucus into the airways, resulting in the atelectasis and infection. Patients with greater risk are those who are susceptible to excessive mucous production such as asthma, bronchitis, RT infection, cystic fibrosis, etc. So, the patients of chronic obstructive pulmonary disease (COPD) who are anesthetized by regional block, show the less incidence of respiratory failure, than those who are undergone general anesthesia with volatile anesthetic agent.

Halothane and ventilatory response to CO_2: Measuring of minute ventilation in response to varying levels of $PaCO_2$ is a common method of measuring the effects of anesthetic drugs on ventilatory drive, caused by $PaCO_2$. Compensatory changes in ventilation, secondary to the alteration in $PaCO_2$, are believed to be mediated chiefly via chemoreceptors, located in medulla. In normal subjects, there is increase in ventilation by approximately 3 L/min for every mm Hg increase in $PaCO_2$. All inhaled anesthetic agents, including halothane, generally depress this CO_2 response curve. At sedating concentrations, halothane has little effect on this response curve. But, 1 MAC halothane has a profound depressant effect. At 2.5 MAC halothane level, there is no increase in ventilation in response to any altered blood CO_2 level. The slope of ventilatory response curve, during halothane anesthesia, usually returns toward normal after 6 hours of anesthesia. N_2O is a relatively weak inhaled anesthetic and does not depress the ventilatory drive or response to CO_2, even at its (N_2O) concentration of 50%.

Halothane and ventilatory response to hypoxemia: Increased ventilation in response to progressively lowered PaO_2 is also mediated entirely by peripheral chemoreceptors. Ventilatory response curve to hypoxemia is hyperbolic. This hyperbolic response curve rises most sharply at a PaO_2 of approximately 40 mm Hg. At 1 MAC level of halothane, significant depression of ventilatory responsiveness to hypoxia is observed. Synergistic effect of hypoxia and hypercarbia on ventilation is also profoundly attenuated by halothane. The peripheral chemoreceptors are remarkably sensitive to the depression effect of halothane. Patients with chronic respiratory failure, in whom the level of $PaCO_2$ may represent an important determinant of minute ventilation, may be drastically affected by halothane.

Effects on Cerebral Blood Flow and Intracranial Tension

Halothane decreases cerebral vascular resistance by dilating the cerebral vessels. Thus, it increases the cerebral blood flow, provided the systemic BP is maintained. Hence, the intracranial and CSF pressure increases, especially in a case of space occupying intracranial lesion. So, headache may occur following halothane anesthesia. Cerebral blood flow is further increased by the addition of N_2O, because the autoregulation of cerebral blood flow is completely abolished by halothane. The net effect on ICP and cerebral perfusion pressure depends on the systemic blood pressure and brain compliance. CSF production is decreased by 30% by halothane. This increase in ICP and cerebral blood flow by halothane can be prevented by hypocapnia. But, if there is any intracranial lesion, then this rise of ICP by mixture of halothane, N_2O and O_2 cannot be prevented by hypocapnia or hyperventilation. Halothane also reduces the cerebral O_2 consumption by 25% with greatest reduction at an inhaled concentration of halothane in between 0.5 and 0.8%. There is little further change in cerebral O_2 consumption with a further increase in halothane concentration, until the toxic levels are reached.

Effects on the Gastrointestinal Tract

Halothane inhibits the motility of the stomach, jejunum, small intestine, and colon like other inhalational anesthetic agents.

Effects on the Skeletal Muscle

Halothane has direct neuromuscular blocking action and also potentiates the action of other neuromuscular blocking agents. Thus, halothane produces moderate skeletal muscle relaxation with increasing depth of anesthesia. It is postulated that the postjunctional membrane is the structure which is most sensitive to the neuromuscular blocking effects of halothane **(Box 11)**.

Shivering caused by halothane: Shivering is sometimes observed, during the early postoperative period, after halothane anesthesia. *This is probably due to the vasodilatory action of drug and the cool environment of operation theater.* This shivering and muscle spasticity which occurs during the emergence, particularly from the halothane anesthesia, also occurs with other halogenated volatile agents and is often referred to as the *"halothane shakes"*. Due to this shivering, oxygen consumption and the incidence of hypoxia are markedly increased. Its incidence may be as high as 80%. Patients are commonly hypothermic due to the cutaneous vasodilatation by halothane and the chilled OT environment. Thus, there is significant heat loss during anesthesia, *as the thermoregulatory response is also impaired by halothane.* So, the shivering is a normal physiological response during recovery (when muscle relaxation is gradually withdrawn).

However, this is not the complete explanation. There are also some central and spinal effects of halothane which may cause altered muscular activity during the emergence from halothane anesthesia, producing shivering. A number of agents have been experimented to reduce this shivering, such as opiates, magnesium sulfate, muscle relaxants and clonidine, etc. But among these, *meperidine is most effective in reducing such shivering.*

Effects on the Uterus

Halothane relaxes the uterine muscles. It is due to the stimulation of uterine adrenergic β_2-receptors. But, uterine contraction is recovered twice as quickly as ether when halothane is stopped. So, it is not so liable to produce postpartum hemorrhage (PPH) as has been stated before. It readily crosses the placental barrier.

Effects on the Liver

It is the most controversial issue. Although no consistent abnormal histological pattern of liver parenchyma after the exposure to halothane has emerged in the National Halothane Study, still it appears that some cases exhibited a lesion which simulate the fatal viral and drug-induced forms of hepatitis, after the exposure to halothane. It is more often associated with the administration of halothane than those associated with the administration of other inhalational anesthetic agents. It is written in details later in the chapter of "liver diseases and anesthesia".

Clinical Use of Halothane

Due to a high vapor pressure (243.3 mm Hg at 20°C), low boiling point (50.2°C), high lipid gas solubility (224), and low blood gas solubility, the halothane can be regarded as a potent anesthetic agent. So, a low concentration, such as 0.4% halothane is capable of maintaining unconsciousness. Thus, it is widely used in anesthesia for all types of surgeries, including general, ENT, orthopedic, pediatric, neuro, etc. The reduction of blood pressure by halothane is used as an advantage in major surgeries. Halothane is also used to reduce the blood loss and to control the intubation-induced hypertension. It has a low incidence of PONV. During abdominal surgery, if halothane is combined with muscle relaxant, then a very good skeletal muscle relaxation is achieved, without restoring to high concentration of halothane, which prolongs the recovery.

Method of Vaporization of Halothane

High cost of halothane demands reasonable economy during its use. So, it cannot be used by open-mask method,

---

BOX 11: The mechanism of relaxation of bronchial smooth muscles by halothane in asthma.

- Direct dilatation of the bronchial smooth muscles, involving increased cyclic AMP
- Blocking the effects of various bronchoconstricting mediators by reducing the free Ca^{++} level in the cytoplasm and suppressing the influx of Ca^{++} across the cell membrane. This action is also common to vascular smooth muscles for relaxation and cardiac muscles for depression by halothane
- Bronchodilatation of halothane is not caused by β_2 stimulation
- Attenuation of centrally mediated bronchoconstriction reflexes by increasing the depth of anesthesia (depresses the airway reflexes), which occurs in light anesthesia

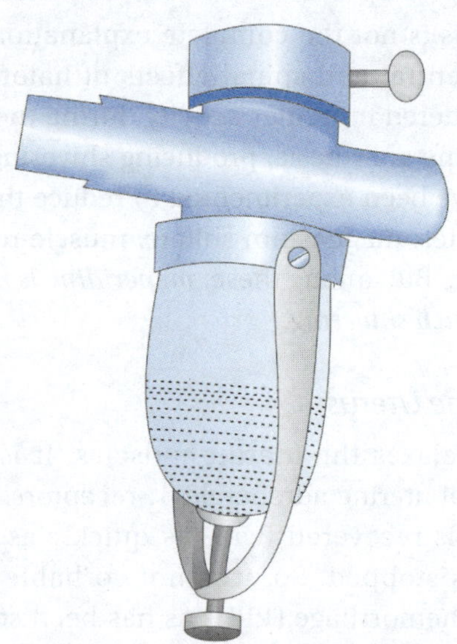

Fig. 23: Goldman's halothane vaporizer.

pouring drop by drop on Schimmelbusch mask, like liquid ether. Previously, halothane was used in copper kettle (bubble through) vaporizer with a flow of 100 mL O_2 through vaporizer at room temperature. When this is added to 5 L of $N_2O:O_2$ gas mixture, we get an inspired concentration of 1% halothane. Similarly, 200 mL of O_2 will give 2% halothane concentration.

But, at present halothane is used by Flutec vaporizer. It is a temperature and flow-compensated vaporizer. It receives a part of inspired gas mixture, enroutes to the patient, and adds a predicted amount of halothane vapor to this gas mixture. It is now the most sophisticated and satisfactory vaporizer for halothane administration.

A small, convenient, inexpensive Goldman vaporizer, which delivers a maximum of 2.3 volume % of halothane, is generally used in developing countries. It is not temperature or flow-compensated vaporizer **(Fig. 23)**.

■ ISOFLURANE

Chemically, isoflurane is a methyl-ethyl-ether **(Fig. 24)** and is an isomer of enflurane.

Physical Properties of Isoflurane

It is a clear, colorless, and noninflammable liquid. Specific gravity of isoflurane is 1.52 at 25°C. Its boiling point is 48.5°C and vapor pressure is 250 mm Hg (like halothane) at room temperature (20°C). It is noncorrosive and does not attack any metal, which are commonly used in the construction of anesthetic apparatus and vaporizers. *It has three fluorine atoms on its terminal ethyl carbon which makes it resistant to chemical and biological degradation.* It is stable in warm soda lime and ultraviolet radiation. It can also be stored

Fig. 24: Di-ethyl-ether.

without any preservative at room temperature. Though, it is stable in soda lime, but like enflurane and desflurane it contains some moiety. So, it may undergo some degradation when exposed to soda lime or baralyme, resulting in the production of carbon monoxide, although not to same degree as enflurane or desflurane.

Isoflurane has very pungent smell like ether. The pungent odor of isoflurane limits its speed of induction due to coughing, breathholding, laryngospasm, etc. But, the low blood-gas solubility coefficient of isoflurane theoretically indicates its rapid induction like halothane. However, premedication, use of intravenous inducing agents, or step-by-step increase in inspired concentration of isoflurane can overcome this problem. The low blood/gas solubility coefficient of isoflurane (isoflurane 1.4 and halothane 2.3) suggests a swift induction and emergence from anesthesia, compared to halothane. It takes only 4 minutes to reach a F_A/F_i (ratio of the alveolar concentration to the inspired concentration) ratio of 0.5, compared to 30 minutes required by halothane.

Greater chemical stability of isoflurane is reflected by its lesser metabolism in our body tissues (0.2%). This may, in turn, reduce the likelihood of its toxicity due to the low level of its metabolites. The rate of metabolism of isoflurane is considerably less (<1/5th of halothane) and near about 95% of inspired volume is excreted unchanged through expired air. The metabolism of isoflurane is occurred in liver by oxidation through hepatic cytochrome P_{450} system with the production of inorganic fluoride and trifluoroacetic acid (TFA).

Pharmacology of Isoflurane

The MAC value for isoflurane is 13. It decreases to 1 in elderly patients and decreases further to 0.6, when N_2O is used with it. For example, the addition of 70% N_2O roughly halves the MAC value of isoflurane, which further can be reduced by opioid analgesics. The premedicant drugs also reduce the requirement of isoflurane and its MAC value. Its oil/gas solubility coefficient is 98, which is much lower than that of halothane (halothane is 224). This suggests isoflurane is a weaker anesthetic agent than halothane. Its vapor pressure is 250 mm Hg at room temperature (halothane's vapor pressure 243 mm Hg) and thus allows the delivery of desired concentration of isoflurane from the same vaporizer which is usually used for halothane. But, for obvious reasons this practice is not encouraged. Isoflurane is absorbed in the plastics and rubber used in the anesthetic circuits, although not to the same extent as halothane.

Action of Isoflurane on Respiratory System

Isoflurane is a potent respiratory depressant and this effect is more than halothane. For this reason, there is lack of increase in respiratory rate, when a high concentration of isoflurane vapor is inhaled. This is in contrast to halothane, sevoflurane, and desflurane anesthesia where respiratory rate increases. However, at a lower concentration of isoflurane, respiratory rate is increased, but the tidal volume is decreased with the net reduction of minute ventilation. Ventilatory responses to hypercarbia, progressively and linearly approaches to zero at about 2 MAC value of isoflurane. Ventilatory response to hypoxia disappears at 1 MAC concentration of isoflurane. So, reduction of ventilatory response to hypercarbia and hypoxia may lead to a grossly impaired ventilation and gas exchange. Isoflurane produces a small drop in total lung compliance and FRC. The bronchodilating effect of isoflurane is as good as halothane. As isoflurane is quite irritating (due to its ether-like pungent odor) to airway, so it is not particularly suitable for the inhalational induction of anesthesia.

Action of Isoflurane on Cardiovascular System

Isoflurane is less myocardial depressant than halothane, even up to the concentration of 2 MAC value. But, the arterial blood pressure and peripheral vascular resistance [systemic vascular resistance (SVR)] are much reduced in a dose-related manner by isoflurane than halothane. It is due to the direct relaxation of vascular smooth muscles, produced by isoflurane. However, cardiac output is maintained close to control value by isoflurane. This well-maintained cardiac output with isoflurane and sevoflurane is accompanied by or due to dose-related decrease in SVR by them, without the depression of myocardium. Whereas we have seen that there is little change in SVR, but a greater decrease in cardiac output, due to greater depression of cardiac contractility with increasing doses of halothane. Thus, in contrast to isoflurane and sevoflurane, halothane lowers BP by reducing the myocardial contractility and cardiac output, but not reducing the SVR. For this reason, deep isoflurane anesthesia has been suggested as an appropriate technique for controlled hypotension (being preferable to halothane, in which hypotension is accompanied by decreased cardiac output and hence decreased perfusion).

Isoflurane depresses baroreceptor function, but very less quantitatively than other inhaled anesthetics. This less depressed responsiveness of baroreceptors probably better maintains cardiac output in the face of hypovolemia. So, there is wide margin of cardiovascular safety with isoflurane than with halothane. Isoflurane increases HR in response to lowered BP and maintains cardiac output. This is because, the baroreceptor reflexes are relatively preserved. The isoflurane-induced tachycardia is more pronounced in pediatric patients or in the presence of vagolytic agent. This CVS stimulation and tachycardia by isoflurane may result from sympathetic stimulation. It is achieved by the activation of tracheopulmonary and systemic adrenoreceptors by isoflurane, and can be attenuated by pretreatment with β_1-adrenoreceptor antagonist, α_1-adrenoreceptor antagonist or opioids.

Isoflurane is also a coronary vasodilator. Ventricular work and myocardial oxygen consumption are reduced by isoflurane. Thereby, it improves myocardial oxygen supply and demand ratio. The coronary vasodilatation, produced by isoflurane, is mediated through ATP-gated potassium channel (K_{ATP}). In the presence of adequate O_2, where intracellular level of ATP is high, these channels open and cause hyperpolarization. In turn, this hyperpolarization reduces cellular activity. Therefore, in vascular smooth muscles, the muscle tone is reduced, and blood flow is increased in coronary vessels (also in other vessels). In myocardial cells, the activation of these channels results in reduced action potential duration, reduced calcium entry, and reduction in myocardial contractility. But, this is very insignificant. Thus, this helps to protect the myocardial cells from the effects of ischemia. Although the isoflurane causes some slowing of myocardial conduction, but it is less than halothane. So, cardiac rhythm is more stable during isoflurane anesthesia.

Isoflurane preserves the regulation of autonomic nervous system on circulation to a greater extent than other volatile anesthetic agents. During halothane anesthesia, there is dose-related increase in right atrial pressure and it is as a result of direct negative inotropic action of halothane on heart. Whereas the pronounced venodilatation properties of isoflurane and sevoflurane cause less increase in right atrial pressure than halothane.

So, there appears to have a wide margin of cardiovascular safety with isoflurane. Cardiac index (ratio of doses producing circulatory arrest versus MAC) of isoflurane is 5.7, which is significantly higher than halothane which is only about 3. Isoflurane does not affect cardiac rhythm and so dysrhythmia, following injection of adrenaline, is less likely with isoflurane than with halothane. This is the major advantage of isoflurane over halothane in plastic surgery, where there is widespread use of adrenaline. The doses of epinephrine, required to produce arrhythmia in patients receiving isoflurane, are three times greater than the dose required in patients receiving halothane.

In normal doses and concentration, as isoflurane does not evoke sympathetic activity, so β_1-adrenoreceptor blocking agents are unlikely necessary. The vast majority of disorders of ventricular rhythm during isoflurane anesthesia usually disappears when the concentration of inspired isoflurane is reduced and ventilation is improved. The use of β_1-adrenoreceptor blocking compounds should be reserved for intractable tachyarrhythmias which is liable to progress to ventricular fibrillation. But, these drugs are contraindicated in the management of disorders of heart, arising from excessive vagal activity.

Isoflurane tries to maintain myocardial contractility near normal and does not sensitize the heart to adrenaline. But, it maintains CVP very well. During isoflurane anesthesia, BP falls due to decrease in SVR, but not due to myocardial depression and HR increases. It maintains peripheral blood flow and tissue perfusion very well. Ventricular work is reduced by isoflurane, due to the reduction of after load. Pulmonary artery and wedge pressure remain normal during isoflurane anesthesia.

Action of Isoflurane on Central Nervous System

Isoflurane produces dose-dependent depression of CNS activity. Concentration of isoflurane above 0.25 MAC produces amnesia. It does not promote convulsive activity. Cerebral metabolism is decreased which may lead to decrease in cerebral blood flow. This property of isoflurane is very helpful in conditions, where there is elevated intracranial pressure. Isoflurane does not increase CBF in normocapnia patients, provided the mean arterial pressure does not increase. If MAP is allowed to fall, then ICP and CBF are both reduced. The increase in ICP, if occurs with isoflurane, is easier to reverse with hypocapnia than with halothane. Isoflurane with hypocapnia does not increase ICP associated with intracranial mass.

Neuromuscular Effects of Isoflurane

Isoflurane produces adequate muscle relaxation. It also enhances the action of suxamethonium. The neuromuscular effect of isoflurane is dose-related, but is more pronounced than that observed with halothane. Shivering also occurs during emergence from isoflurane anesthesia like halothane, due to thermoregulatory response to hypothermia. But, this can be suppressed with meperidine.

Effects of Isoflurane on Uterus

As isoflurane relaxes the muscles of uterus in dose-related manner and increases bleeding, so it is not recommended in obstetrical anesthesia.

Metabolism and Toxicity of Isoflurane

Isoflurane is physico-chemically very stable and this is reflected by its resistance to biodegradation. So, 95% of administered dose of isoflurane is excreted unchanged through expired air. Only <0.2% of administered isoflurane (much less than halothane) is metabolized in liver and is excreted as urinary metabolites. Thus, the near absence of metabolism of isoflurane implies that the possibility of liver and kidney toxicity by the metabolites of isoflurane is remote. The main metabolites of isoflurane metabolism are TFA and inorganic fluoride ions. The peak serum inorganic fluoride level after prolonged isoflurane anesthesia was found to be only 4.4 μmole/L, a concentration which renders the possibility of nephrotoxicity very little or almost nil. At a comparable anesthetic exposure, there is 10 times more production of fluoride ions with methoxyflurane which is known for nephrotoxicity. Production of TFA, responsible for hepatotoxicity, is also 10 times less, during isoflurane anesthesia than during comparable exposure to halothane.

The Ames test which is widely accepted as a test for the mutagenicity and carcinogenicity for both the mother drug and its metabolites is negative for isoflurane, but positive for halothane and its metabolites.

Indications for Use of Isoflurane

The use of isoflurane is clearly of benefit in circumstances where:

- The disturbance of cardiac rhythm is very likely.
- The neurosurgical patients who are known to have raised intracranial pressure.
- The patient presents with preexisting renal and liver diseases.
- The patient who needs frequent exposure to an inhalational anesthetic.

It is less useful, if an increase in heart rate is not desirable, but would be deleterious in the presence of multivessel coronary artery diseases.

■ SEVOFLURANE

Chemically, it is a halogenated (fluorine only) methyl-propyl-ether. Its molecular structure is like that 1, 1, 1, 3, 3, 3-hexafluoro-2-(fluoromethoxy) propane **(Fig. 25A)**. As it does not contain any chlorine or bromine atom, so like halothane, isoflurane, and desflurane it has no effect on the

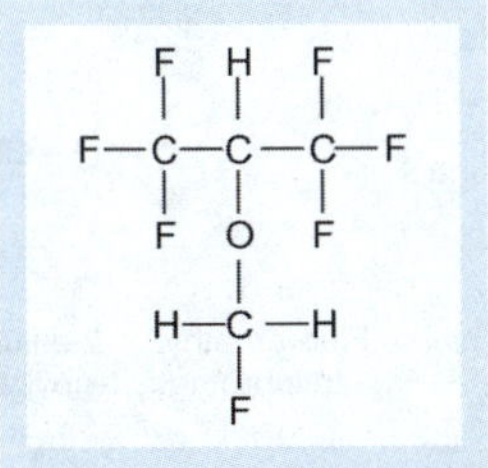

F H F
F—C—C—C—F
F O F
H—C—H
F

Fig. 25A: Structure of sevoflurane.

ozone layer of environment. The first report of this agent appeared in 1970. It has no asymmetrical carbon atom, so it has no optical isomer. In this respect, sevoflurane is unique among all the currently available inhaled anesthetics.

Physical Properties of Sevoflurane

Molecular weight of sevoflurane is 200.1(Da) and boiling point is 58.5°C. Its vapor pressure at 20°C is 160 mm Hg. So, it can be administered by using a conventional temperature and flow compensated vaporizer. Rubber/gas partition coefficient of sevoflurane is 31(halothane 120 and isoflurane 62). So, it is less soluble in rubber and plastic (which are present in anesthetic circuits) than halothane and isoflurane. The MAC value of sevoflurane with O_2 is 2 and with 70% N_2O is 0.8. The MAC value of sevoflurane also decreases with increase in age, like other inhalational agents. So, in neonates the MAC value of sevoflurane is 3.3, while in adults it is only 1.48. The MAC value of sevoflurane is also reduced with narcotics and hypnotics. No preservative is needed for sevoflurane to keep it in bottles (in halothane, thymol is used as preservative). Most of the administered sevoflurane is excreted unchanged by exhaled air through lungs and only 3–5% is recovered as metabolites **(Table 4)**.

The blood/gas partition coefficient of sevoflurane is 0.6, which is substantially lower than the other inhalational anesthetic agents. So, alveolar anesthetic concentration of sevoflurane is very rapidly achieved, resulting in fast induction. Within 5 minutes, after starting of induction of anesthesia, the F_A/F_i (ratio of alveolar concentration to inspired concentration) value for sevoflurane is 0.5, which is reached by halothane only after 30 minutes. This F_A/F_i ratio of sevoflurane is same as isoflurane. So, it also indicates very quick induction of anesthesia by sevoflurane like isoflurane. However, sevoflurane blood-gas solubility, unlike that of halothane and isoflurane, does not alter with age. Sevoflurane has also lower distribution coefficient than other agents. So, elimination of it is very quick. Hence, it may prove ideal for outpatient anesthesia due to fast recovery. Sevoflurane is nonirritant to the upper airway.

TABLE 4: Effect of age on MAC of sevoflurane.

Age (years)	Sevoflurane with O_2	Sevoflurane with N_2O and O_2
<3	2.5–3.5	2
3–5	2.5	NA
5–10	2.5	NA
10–25	2.5	1.4
25–35	2.2	1.2
40	2	1.1
50	1.8	0.95
60	1.6	0.85
80	1.4	0.7

NA: not applicable

So, it is very suitable as an inhalational-inducing agent for children. It is noninflammable.

Sevoflurane breaks down with soda lime. Metabolism of sevoflurane occurs in liver by its cytochrome P_{450} system. It is broken down into inorganic fluoride ions and organic fluoride compounds, such as hexafluoroisopropanol (HFIP). Next, HFIP is conjugated with glucoronic acid to form HFIP glucuronide, which is then excreted through bile and kidneys. There is no evidence of hepatic and renal toxicity, associated with HFIP.

Pharmacological Actions of Sevoflurane

Cardiovascular System Effects

Sevoflurane has effects on CVS which is similar to that of isoflurane, but it may cause less marked changes in heart rate. That is, unlike isoflurane which causes tachycardia, sevoflurane causes minimal tachycardia or none. It causes decrease in pulmonary arterial pressure and systemic arterial pressure, where decrease in diastolic pressure is more than systolic. This is due to the vascular smooth muscle relaxation and the reduction of SVR, but not due to much reduction of cardiac contractility and cardiac output, like halothane. It causes dose-related minimal decrease in myocardial contractility and cardiac output. Renal and hepatic blood flow is also well-maintained. Sevoflurane does not sensitize myocardium to catecholamines.

Respiratory Effects

Sevoflurane has no irritant effect on airway, unlike ether and isoflurane, and is very pleasant to inhale. So, these two qualities (nonirritant and pleasant smell), along with its low blood/gas solubility coefficient, make the sevoflurane a very suitable agent for inhalational induction in children, infant, and neonate. It is least respiratory tract irritant among all the currently available inhalational anesthetic agents. But, for induction, it is less potent than halothane (MAC value of sevoflurane is 2, whereas MAC value of halothane is 0.75). This can be overcome by using initially a higher inspired concentration of sevoflurane which is also very well-tolerated.

Like other halogenated volatile ether anesthetics, sevoflurane is also a respiratory depressant. Tidal volume is reduced and respiratory rate is increased. But, this increased respiratory rate cannot compensate the reduction in tidal volume. Thus, it causes reduction of minute volume. Both, the ventilatory response to CO_2 (more than halothane) and hypoxia (30–40%) is depressed by sevoflurane. Sevoflurane also reduces the protective hypoxic pulmonary vasoconstriction reflexes in dose-dependent manner. But, there is no change in arterial O_2 concentration, when sevoflurane or isoflurane is used in anesthesia during one-lung ventilation. Sevoflurane is also an effective bronchodilator, but is not as effective as halothane.

Central Nervous System Effects

Sevoflurane may cause less cerebral vasodilatation than isoflurane. But, the other effects of it on CNS are similar to that of isoflurane. Sevoflurane causes minimal increase in CBF in normocapnia, like isoflurane. Both the sevoflurane and isoflurane can reduce the cerebral metabolic rate. Cerebral perfusion pressure (CPP) is better maintained by sevoflurane than isoflurane. Sevoflurane, like isoflurane, also causes a slight increase in ICP in normocapnic patients. The cerebrovascular response to CO_2 and cerebral autoregulation are both preserved under sevoflurane anesthesia.

Metabolism and Toxicity of Sevoflurane

Sevoflurane is less significantly metabolized than halothane (but more than isoflurane and desflurane) by defluorination in liver and the plasma fluoride and HFIP concentration reaches a level of 15–25 µmol/L, after 1 MAC exposure of this drug for 1 hour. But, it is much less than the nephrotoxic level. Approximately 3–5% of inhaled dose of sevoflurane undergoes biotransformation in liver. But, this is one-fourth than that of halothane and 20–25 times more than that of isoflurane and desflurane. After prolonged anesthetic exposure (13–14 hours) in five out of 10 patients, the serum fluoride concentration exceeds >50 µmole/L **(Fig. 25B)**.

This is a level (50 µmole/L) which was previously thought to be nephrotoxic. But, still there have been no reports of renal failure. In vitro, sevoflurane undergoes extensive metabolism. But, clinically (in vivo), it is not a problem, because it is very less soluble in blood. When

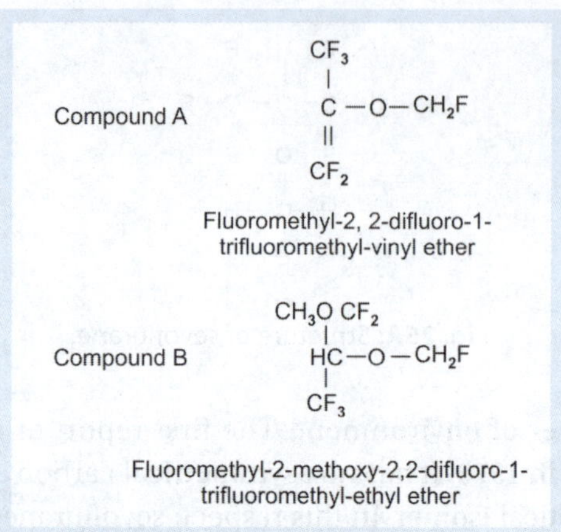

Fig. 25B: Sevoflurane compounds A and B.

sevoflurane is exposed to baralyme or soda lime, it breaks into methanol, formaldehyde, carbon monoxide, compound A and compound B. Both of these compounds (compound A and compound B) are hepatotoxic and nephrotoxic. But, still there is no evidence of long-term serious renal or hepatic injury, after exposure to sevoflurane with baralyme or soda lime. Of the halogenated anesthetic agents, which are currently in widespread use, the sevoflurane is only one which is not metabolized to TFA, implicated in hepatotoxicity. Sevoflurane can also be degraded to hydrogen fluoride. This is due to the metal or environmental impurities which are present in manufacturing equipment. This hydrogen fluoride may produce an acid burn, when it comes in contact with respiratory mucosa.

Potential Indications for Use of Sevoflurane

Sevoflurane has prominent place in pediatric anesthesia for inhalational induction and maintenance of anesthesia. Though, the induction and recovery from sevoflurane is quick, like isoflurane and has no pungent smell, so there is a definite advantage of sevoflurane over isoflurane. Sevoflurane offers good hemodynamic stability (like isoflurane) than halothane. As sevoflurane does not contain any chloride ion, so it is environment friendly. Although sevoflurane has fewer side effects than halothane, but there are some concerns about its hepatotoxicity (like halothane). There is also some concern about renal toxicity of compound A, formed as a result of degradation of sevoflurane by CO_2 absorbers. But, this is not proved to be of any clinical problem.

■ DESFLURANE

After the appearance of sevoflurane in 1971, hundreds and hundreds of halogenated volatile anesthetics agents were synthesized and analyzed. Then, desflurane came in this effort. Initially, several factors had delayed the

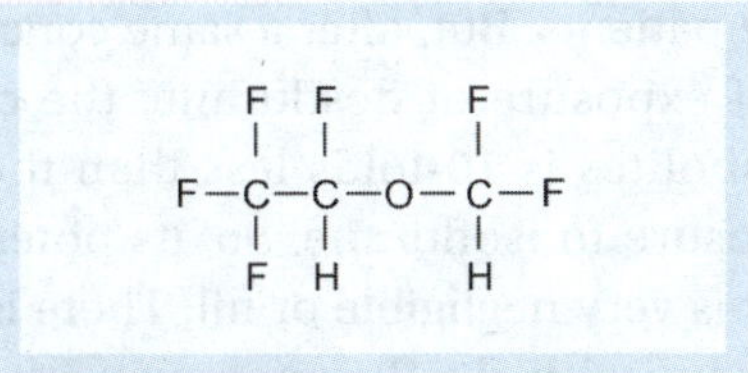

$$F-C-C-O-C-F$$

Fig. 26: Structure of desflurane.

development of desflurane. These were: (i) the potentially hazardous process of handling only fluorine in the synthesis of desflurane (in desflurane there is no chlorine or bromine ion), and (ii) the peculiar vapor pressure of desflurane which is very close to atmospheric pressure at room temperature. This is because the boiling point of desflurane is 22.8°C which is near about to room temperature. So, it starts to boil in normal room condition. This precludes the use of conventional vaporizers for its administration. Later, a safer process of synthesizing desflurane was developed and thereafter Aladdin cassette vaporizer was invented for its administration. Then, desflurane was subsequently approved for clinical use in the USA in 1992. Desflurane is a halogenated (fluorine only) methyl-ethyl-ether **(Fig. 26)**. Structurally, it differs from isoflurane by the substitution of chlorine by fluorine on α-ethyl-carbon. Desflurane exists in different optical isomers. So, the clinically used desflurane is a racemic mixture of its different optical isomers.

Physical Properties of Desflurane

The desflurane has very pungent odor. So, it (pungent odor) makes desflurane very irritating and unpleasant to inhale, like isoflurane. The molecular weight of desflurane is 168, boiling point is 22.8°C and vapor pressure at 20°C is 664 mm Hg. The low boiling point of desflurane which is near about to room temperature indicates that it cannot be administered by using a standard vaporizer. The MAC value of desflurane varies, depending on stimulus and other co-agents used, along with it. It also decreases with age. The MAC value of desflurane with O_2 is 6–9 and with 70% N_2O is 2.5–3.5. The blood/gas partition coefficient of desflurane is 0.42. It needs no preservative for its storing in bottle and is stable in alkali, ultraviolet light, and metal. Only 0.02% of inhaled drug (desflurane) is recovered, as its metabolites. Desflurane has lowest blood and other tissue partition coefficient, compared to other inhaled anesthetics. So, it is unique, as an inhalational anesthetic agent, for very fast induction and recovery from anesthesia than other inhalation anesthetic agents. But, unfortunately, as it is irritant to upper respiratory tract and causes cough, breathholding, laryngospasm, etc., so induction by desflurane is automatically slowed. Hence, it is not the drug of choice for induction of anesthesia.

Desflurane is relatively less potent than other agents. It is extremely stable and is presented as clear liquid in amber bottles without preservatives. Its one unique physical property (i.e., boiling point of desflurane is around room temperature) does not allow its use by a standard vaporizer. So, special Tec-6 vaporizer is needed for its use. Like sevoflurane, as it is entirely fluorinated, so ozone depletion of environment by desflurane is minimal. Thus, it is environment friendly. Both soda lime and baralyme can degrade it with the production of carbon monoxide.

Pharmacological Action of Desflurane

Cardiovascular System Effects

The effect of desflurane on CVS is same as that of isoflurane. It causes the reduction of SVR and mean arterial pressure, but increase of HR. The decrease in MAP by desflurane is due to the decrease in SVR, but not due to the reduction in cardiac contractility, like halothane. Therefore, there is a very small change in cardiac output. The arrhythmogenic potency of desflurane is like that of isoflurane. The decrease of SVR by desflurane is due to peripheral vasodilatation. However, the cardiac index remains unchanged or increased. The hepatic blood flow is maintained by desflurane. When desflurane is used for the maintenance of anesthesia, then there is no change in renal blood flow at its concentrations are up to 2 MAC. The desflurane is direct coronary vasodilator. But, the potential improvement in coronary blood flow, due to coronary vasodilation, is offset by tachycardia, caused by desflurane and also by fall of coronary perfusion pressure, resulting from peripheral vasodilatation, caused by desflurane and hypotension. Like isoflurane, use of desflurane is associated with rapid increase in HR. But, this can be reduced by small doses of opioids, esmolol, clonidine, and N_2O. Desflurane does not sensitize the myocardium to epinephrine. It can slow atrioventricular (AV) conduction or induce junctional bradycardia.

Respiratory Effects

Like other inhaled anesthetic agents, the ventilatory response of desflurane is accompanied by increase in respiratory rate and decrease in tidal volume. But, ultimately there is reduction in minute volume and increase in $PaCO_2$. However, desflurane does not significantly reduce minute ventilation, until a concentration of it >1.6 MAC value has been used. Thus, at higher concentrations of desflurane respiratory rate decreases, but it is less than that of halothane. At higher concentrations, the respiratory depression effect of desflurane is similar to that of isoflurane and sevoflurane. Ventilatory response to CO_2 and hypoxia are also reduced.

Intrapulmonary shunt fraction and physiological dead space are also increased by desflurane. Induction by desflurane is associated with coughing, salivation, and laryngospasm due to its very pungent odor, like ether and isoflurane. This outweighs the benefit of its direct bronchodilating action and rapid induction. And, it is postulated that this causes early sympathetic stimulation. Thus, desflurane is unsuitable for inhalational induction of anesthesia, both for children and adults.

Central Nervous System Effects

Desflurane decreases cerebrovascular resistance. Thus, it increases cerebral blood flow and intracranial pressure. But, it also decreases cerebral O_2 requirement. Desflurane increases CSF pressure to a greater extent than isoflurane. In a comparative study, carried out on patients with intracranial mass, 1 MAC desflurane or isoflurane was given. Then, it was observed that ICP had increased progressively in desflurane group, even with hypocapnia. Whereas, there was no increase in ICP in isoflurane group. Of the commonly employed volatile anesthetic agents, the order of cerebral vasodilating potency is as follows. Halothane >>Enflurane >Isoflurane = Sevoflurane = Desflurane

Desflurane causes increased CSF production, under condition of ↑ICP and even in hypocapnia. To date, no clear advantage has been seen for any given inhalation anesthetic agent over another in neurosurgical anesthesia. But, very rapid recovery characteristic of desflurane may offer a definitive advantage for its use in neurosurgical patients, in whom rapid postoperative neurological assessment is desirable. An EEG change, caused by desflurane, is comparable with that of isoflurane, but no epileptic form of activity is seen.

Effects on Muscle

Like other inhaled anesthetic agents, desflurane depresses neuromuscular function and augments the action of both nondepolarizing and depolarizing muscle relaxants. Thus, it can provide sufficient skeletal muscle relaxation to allow tracheal intubation.

Metabolism and Toxicity of Desflurane

Desflurane has a very low blood-gas and blood-tissue solubility. So, it is very stable and undergoes minimal metabolism in our body. These are the properties of desflurane that favor its low systemic toxicity. However, still a very small amount of desflurane is metabolized in our body, with the production of difluoroacetic acid, which may interact with hepatic proteins and may induce an immune response

in susceptible patients. But, after a same concentration and same hour of exposure of desflurane, the concentration of toxic metabolites is 10-folds less than the levels, seen after the exposure to isoflurane. So, its potential to cause organ toxicity is very negligible or nil. There is no evidence of renal toxicity with desflurane, even after prolonged exposure. Desflurane may trigger malignant hyperthermia. So, it is prudent not to use desflurane in susceptible patients. The magnitude of carbon monoxide production in soda lime or baralyme absorber from greatest to lowest is: Desflurane >>Enflurane >Isoflurane >>Halothane = Sevoflurane.

Indications for Use of Desflurane

The recovery from desflurane anesthesia is more rapid and complete than following recovery from either propofol, isoflurane or sevoflurane anesthesia. This suggests that it is very suitable for day-case anesthesia. Insolubility of desflurane makes it eminently suitable for use in low-flow, closed circuit anesthesia delivery systems. The lack of effect on atmospheric ozone layer also makes desflurane environmental friendly. Though, desflurane is metabolized in fraction to isoflurane, this advantage is theoretical than practical, as the use of isoflurane is not associated with significant incidence of organ toxicity.

■ XENON (XE)

This element was first discovered, in 1898, by W Ramsay and M W Travers. It is present in atmosphere to an extent of about only one part out of 20 million part. Thus, the concentration of xenon in atmosphere is only 0.00000087%. Before 1962, it was generally assumed that xenon and other noble inert gases were unable to form compounds with other elements. But, evidence has been mounting in last few years that xenon and other zero-valency elements can form compounds with other elements. However, xenon is not toxic. But, its compounds are highly toxic, because of their strong oxidizing characteristics.

By 1950, studies had proved that there was some hypnotic effect of this noble gas, xenon. Then, in 1951, xenon was first used as an anesthetic agent by Cullen and Groa and the patient was an 81-year-old man, undergoing orchidectomy. They used xenon of 80% concentration. After that and till now, different attempts have been taken to make feasible to use xenon in clinical practice. But, due to different reasons which are described later, it was not technically possible. At that time, different isotopes of xenon were also isolated and used in different industries, such as in X-ray tubes for high intensity lights and in many biological experiments such as measurement of cerebral blood flow and lung volumes, etc. **(Box 12)**.

BOX 12: Advantages and disadvantages of Xenon (Xe) anesthesia.

Advantages:
- Inert—has no metabolism
- Nontoxic
- Minimal CVS effects
- Very low blood gas solubility coefficient
- Very rapid induction and recovery
- Does not trigger malignant hyperpyrexia
- Nonexplosive
- Environment friendly

Disadvantages:
- Very high cost
- Low potency (MAC = 71)
- At present, no commercially available anesthetic equipment using xenon

Atomic number of xenon is 54 and its molecular weight is 131.3. It is a colorless, odorless, nonirritating gas, and is four times heavier than air. It is more viscous than nitrogen. It freezes at $-111.9°C$ and boils at $-107.1°C$. It is noninflammable and does not support combustion. As it is extremely inert, so it does not react with soda lime. It can diffuse readily through rubber. The MAC value of xenon is 71. It indicates that xenon is a more potent anesthetic agent than N_2O. Therefore, it is possible to use xenon as a sole anesthetic agent, at least in some patients. Its blood/gas partition coefficient is 0.115 and is lowest among all the available inhalational anesthetic agents. So, it provides very rapid induction and very rapid emergence from anesthesia. Its oil/gas partition coefficient is 0.14–0.2, which is lower than that of N_2O (0.47).

Xenon is extracted, as side product, during air liquefaction (Linde process). Then, the gas is stored in cylinders, similar to those, used to store O_2 or N_2O. As xenon only makes up a very small percentage of atmospheric air, so it is extremely expensive to extract Xe from air. It exerts analgesic effects, independent of α_2-adrenergic and opioid receptors. Although the most intravenous general anesthetics agents enhance the inhibitory activity of gamma-aminobutyric acid (GABA) receptors, but the action of xenon on these receptors is also negligible. Xenon potentially inhibits the excitatory N-methyl-D-aspartate (NMDA) receptor channels, like ketamine and this may account for xenon's anesthetic property. Though, xenon has more potent analgesic action than N_2O, but it is not always possible to use xenon as a sole anesthetic agent. However, less supplementation by intravenous or inhalational anesthetic agents is needed than N_2O. Like N_2O, xenon has the same potential for diffusion hypoxia during recovery and has the same implications regarding diffusion into gas-filled cavities within our body.

Xenon, being a chemically inert gas, does not enter into any metabolic process of our body, and therefore leaves behind no metabolic products. It is completely excreted through lungs. Even in high concentrations, xenon is completely non-toxic. Xenon has no or minimal systemic and pulmonary effects. As xenon is odorless, so like N_2O, it is very useful for inhalational induction. Xenon is four times greater in density than that of nitrogen and three times denser than that of N_2O. Also, it has a higher viscosity than that of both nitrogen and N_2O. Thus, both the high density and high viscosity property of xenon have significant effects on pulmonary mechanics, i.e., increasing airway resistance and airway pressure. So, xenon should not be used in patients with respiratory diseases, especially during obstruction of airway. Respiratory rate is slowed by xenon, but there is compensatory increase in tidal volume, with little change in minute ventilation. It preserves myocardial contractility in humans. Xenon attenuates increased plasma epinephrine and cortisol level, associated with surgical stimulus. It has very minimal effect on LV systolic and diastolic functions of both normal and cardiomyopathy heart. In conclusion, we can say that xenon provides good hemodynamic stability with almost little change in myocardial contractility, SVR, PVR, blood pressure and heart rate (slight reduction of heart rate) than other inhalational anesthetic agents.

Xenon causes an increase in the CBF and an increase in the ICP, but a reduction of CPP. So, xenon should be used with caution in patients who are at risk from raised ICP. Xenon does not cause malignant hyperthermia. S-100 is a protein that is found in high concentration in the nervous system of vertebrates. Any structural damage of the glia cells causes leakage of this protein S-100 into the extracellular compartment and finally into the serum, where the β-subunit of the protein S-100 can be measured. But, there is no increase in S-100 values during xenon anesthesia. Thus, it can be concluded that xenon does not impair cerebral integrity.

When exposed to xenon, the patient loses consciousness within a very short period and the patient's state remains stable throughout the anesthetic procedure. Pain is alleviated. Unlike other commonly used anesthetic agents, patient's blood pressure does not drop. Patient becomes fully conscious without any side effects within 2 minutes of completion of the operation and cessation of the supply of xenon. The depth of anesthesia is also sufficient at a xenon gas concentration of about 55%.

Till now, xenon is too expensive to use in routine anesthesia practice. Only when the reuse of this gas within low-flow, closed circle system becomes true, then the clinical application of xenon will become both possible and economical. Now, at the end of the process of anesthesia, xenon gas is recollected in a container, compressed, and filled again into cylinders. Then it is returned again to gas supplier to prepare for reuse. Roughly, 15–20 L of xenon gas is consumed during an operation, lasting for 2–3 hours. Xenon anesthesia is mainly used in pediatric and cardiac anesthesia. It is environmental friendly, as it is an atmospheric gas. Now, it is routinely used for anesthesia in Germany, Netherlands, Sweden, and Russia.

ANESTHETIC DELIVERY SYSTEM OR CIRCUITS

History

The administration of volatile anesthetic agents by open-drop method was first introduced by Sir James Y. Simson, in 1847, for chloroform. He had first used a folded handkerchief as mask on patient's face, on which liquid chloroform was instilled drop by drop. Later, it was modified by different persons to ultimately Schimmelbusch mask, which is still used now. But, the disadvantages of this open-drop method are: (i) an uneven anesthesia due to variations in concentration of vapor of volatile anesthetic agent which is inhaled, (ii) risk of fire, wastefulness, and pollution of atmosphere, (iii) fall in O_2 concentration under the mask (which could be remedied by giving O_2 under the mask via a small catheter), and (iv) risk of damage to eyes and skin of patient from direct contact of anesthetic liquid.

Then, the administration of ether by a simple inhaler was developed by Morton. In 1846, he had used a glass draw-over vaporizer for his public demonstration of general anesthesia by ether. In 1862, Thomas Skinner, who was a general practitioner and obstetrician of Liverpool had first invented a wire frame mask, covered with a cotton domette, which could be carried in the top of a hat. After that, these masks gained a wide acceptance. Then, in 1890, Sir Schimmelbusch, a Berlin surgeon, developed a trough-shaped rim, around this wire frame, to prevent the anesthetic liquid from flowing over directly on patient's skin of face, during this open drop method of administration of volatile liquid anesthetic agent. It was used both for ether and chloroform liquid. During these first 80 years of general anesthesia, many millions of patients were managed satisfactorily using this face mask and dropping liquid ether or chloroform on this face mask (open drop method).

What is now called as anesthetic face mask, was originally called as face-piece and was first invented by Cloquet and Sibson. Sibson's original mask was made of mackintosh (waterproof coat) and was lined internally with silk. Later, it was improved by Mr Snow whose version was made of a thin lead sheet, covered with leather on outside and velveteen inside. It was fitted with valves and was used with his newly invented ether inhaler. During that period, nasal masks were

also developed instead of face masks for dental anesthesia. In 1859, Faure of Paris gave chloroform vapor through a rubber tube and inserted it into one of the patient's nostrils for oral surgery.

The history of anesthetic machine dates back to 1880, when both O_2 and N_2O were available as compressed gases in iron bottles (cylinders) for industrial purposes. From this period, the development of basic anesthetic machine began. In late 19th century, Sir Frederick Hewitt had described a machine, in which both the O_2 and N_2O from their cylinders, was stored in two rubber bags and was delivered in variable concentrations to patient via a stopcock that he designed. Then, in 1912, Cotton and Boothby developed a N_2O, O_2, and ether apparatus with compressed gas cylinders, where in addition, they had incorporated, reducing valves, bubble flow meters, and a bubble-through ether vaporizer. During that period, many machines were also developed by many scientists. But, the First World War had stimulated the major developments in anesthetic machine.

In 1912, James Gwathmey of the USA had developed the first practical anesthetic machine. Then, in 1917, Henry Boyle modified this American Gwathmey Apparatus and from that period his name became synonymous with this anesthetic machine. One of the Boyle's most important modifications of Gwathmey Apparatus was the addition of reducing valves. During that time, another modification of Gwathmey's Apparatus was done by Marshall in London. Thus, a major advantage of this Marshall and Boyle's modification over the Gwathmey's Apparatus was the use of Hewitt stopcock to prevent rebreathing.

The original Boyle's machine of 1917 was rebuilt by an engineering firm, named *Coxeters,* for commercial use, making a company. In its original form, it housed two N_2O and two O_2 cylinders in a wooden box. There also was a water-sight flow meter and an ether vaporizer. It had **(Table 5)** a pressure gauge on O_2 cylinders and had fine adjustment reducing valves. It also had a spirit lamp to warm these cylinders and to prevent the obstruction of gas flow

TABLE 5: Modifications of the Boyle's machine.	
1920	Addition of the first Boyle's vaporizing bottle to flowmetres
1926	Addition of second vaporizing bottle and bypass controls
1927	Addition of third water-sight flowmeter, for CO_2
1930	Addition of a plunger device to the Boyle's vaporizing bottle
1933	Dry bobbin type of flowmeter instead of the water-sight meter
1937	Rotameters displaced dry bobbin flowmeters
1952	Introduction of the pin-index system

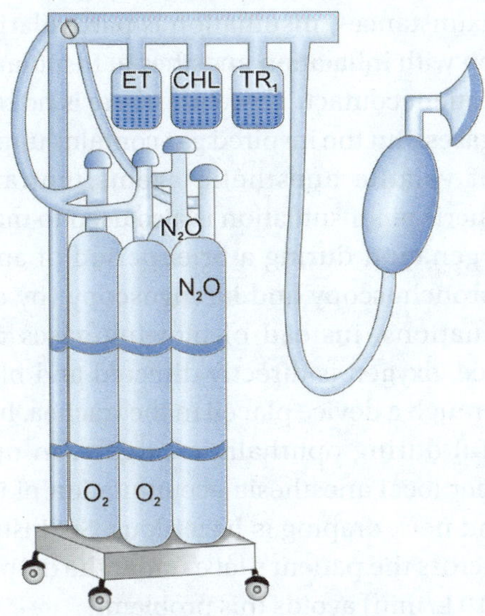

Fig. 27: Early Boyle's machine.

from cylinder due to freezing of water vapor which remained as an impurity in early gas, supplied in cylinder. A reservoir bag, a three-way stopcock and a facemask completed the apparatus. A portable form of this Boyle's apparatus was also designed for the use of British army in France, and was then popularized very rapidly. However, the modern Boyle's apparatus bears little resemblance to this original model and subsequent modifications were included in the original one **(Fig. 27)**.

In the meantime, many developments in anesthesia had continued between the wars. For example, Jackson in the UK introduced a circle system in 1915. Waters in the USA developed CO_2 absorption system, in 1924, using granular sodium and calcium hydrate. At this time, water sight feed-meters and bubble bottles were used in industry to indicate the gas flow. In the early 1930s, Coxeter introduced the dry gas flowmeter. The rotameter which is still used today had been first designed by Kuppers, in 1908, and was first widely used in the industry for gas and fluid. It was not until 1937, when it was introduced into anesthetic machines.

After that, during next 50 years or more, much of the development of Boyle's apparatus was focused on patient's safety and the standardization of its design. However, since early 1990s, the introduction of sophisticated electronic patient monitoring devices in anesthetic arena has placed a new set of demands on machine's design.

So, the design of an anesthetic machine has now changed much for patient's safety and monitoring purposes from its introduction at the end of last century. However, the modern anesthetic machine is a highly sophisticated piece of mechanical, pneumatic, and electronic engineering tools which is built to maintain good safety standards and

incorporate a state-of-the-art monitoring and ventilator system. Now, the anesthetic machine is called as anesthetic work-station and is a part of a larger system incorporating: decision support, central monitoring, and automated anesthetic record keeping. Now, the most dangerous part of an anesthetic machine is the operator. Therefore, it is the obligation of the manufacturer to make the new machines absolutely easy to use and also to help the anesthesiologists to understand how to use them safely. The Inhalational anesthetic system has basically two parts:

 i. Anesthetic machine, itself, and
 ii. Anesthetic delivery system or breathing system.

The breathing system is defined as a conduit which is situated between the pressure-reduced and flow-restricted gas source of anesthetic machine and the patient's airway. The term "breathing system" is nowadays the preferred term, rather than the former term "circuit". Because the flow of gases does not necessarily circulate in a fashion of circle repeatedly. Many breathing systems also incorporate the facility of artificially ventilating the patient, a system of humidification and also a facility of connecting the machine to a scavenging system.

Here, we will discuss only the anesthetic delivery or breathing systems (circuits), but not the whole anesthetic machines. The whole anesthetic machine is discussed in details in Chapter 1. All the anesthetic delivery systems have some standard common features. These are:

- Source of O_2 may be atmospheric or compressed.
- Source of anesthetic gases is compressed cylinders (N_2O) or vaporizers (for volatile anesthetic agents).
- A method of CO_2 elimination—either by venting it to atmosphere or by absorbing with in a chemical.
- A reservoir to meet the demand of high peak gas flow during inspiration.
- A steady inflow of fresh gas both during inspiration and expiration.

The breathing system has three main functions and these are:
 i.   The supply of O_2 to the patient
 ii. The supply of anesthetic gases and vapors to the patient
 iii. The elimination of CO_2.

Classification of Anesthetic Delivery System (Anesthetic Circuit)

It is not possible to classify all the anesthetic delivery systems (anesthetic circuits) in a completely logical or water-tight manner. Also, there is no justification in using the two near most similar terms, i.e., "semi-closed" and "semi-opened" creating confusion, instead of one in a single test book. The term "semi-open" is most commonly used in North America. Any system (circuit) may function in different modes, according to (i) rate of inflow of fresh gas, (ii) pattern of ventilation, (iii) whether patient is in spontaneous or controlled ventilation, and (iv) different interchanging positions of the entry point of fresh gas, reservoir bag, expiratory valve, etc.

The main classifications of anesthetic delivery systems are:

- Open or non-rebreathing system.
- Semi-closed or semi-opened system, where partial rebreathing may occur, as there is no CO_2 absorption, such as Mapleson circuits.
- Closed circuit rebreathing system with CO_2 absorption.

The main difference between the semi-open and semi-closed system is that the *semi-open systems* are valveless and entrainment of room air can occur. But, in modern anesthesia, this should not be happened. On the other hand, a *semi-closed system* cannot entrain room air. Because it uses an APL valve and there is an airtight seal between the breathing system and patient's face, either through a tight-fitting mask or by a connection between breathing system (circuit) and an airway device such as an ET tube or laryngeal mask airways (LMA). In a semi-closed system, the problem of peak inspiratory flow is overcome by the incorporation of a reservoir bag. The bag collapses during inspiration to compensate the differences between the fresh gas flow (FGF) rate and peak inspiratory flow rate. As long as the FGF rate is sufficient to replace the loss from system (circuit) which occurs through APL valve during expiration, the bag will return to its original full state after expiration.

Open or Nonrebreathing System

This system ensures that each breath gets full fresh gas flow and all the expired gas is vented out to atmosphere. This classification includes:

- Open drop mask
- Insufflation
- A nonrebreathing valve with or without an inspiratory reservoir bag.

Open drop mask: This is the simplest form of anesthetic delivery system. If supplementary O_2 is not given under the mask, then some rebreathing does occur from the space under the mask which becomes an extension of the anatomical dead space. Schimmelbusch mask and Gardner ether bottle are the best examples of this system.

Insufflation: Insufflation means the blowing of anesthetic gases across the patient face or any part of the patient's airway. Although it is categorized as a breathing circuit, but actually it is considered as a technique that avoids the direct connection between a breathing circuit and the patient's face or airway. Children often resist the direct placement of facemask or an intravenous line before induction.

In such circumstances, insufflation is particularly valuable for induction with inhalation anesthesia. Insufflation avoids any direct patient contact. Therefore, there is no rebreathing of exhaled gases. But the inspired gas contains unpredictable amounts of volatile anesthetic agents, entrained with the atmospheric air. Insufflation is also used to maintain the arterial oxygenation during a brief period of apnea, such as during bronchoscopy and laryngoscopy (by oxyscope). In such situations, instead of blowing gases across the patient's face, oxygen is directly directed and blowed into the lungs through a device placed in the trachea. Insufflation is also useful during ophthalmic surgery. In ophthalmic surgery under local anesthesia accumulation of CO_2 under the head and neck draping is hazardous. So, insufflation of O_2 and air across the patient's face under the drape at a high flow rate (>10 L/min) avoids this problem.

Nonrebreathing valve: Nonrebreathing valve is a modification of semi-closed system. It prevents rebreathing by allowing the unidirectional flow of all the expired gases to atmosphere. Thus, it enables the patient to inspire a constant proportion of fresh gas flow from the machine or the air, as there is no mixing of inspired and expired gases. Hence, any moment the anesthesiologist can tell the exact proportion of gases that the patient is inspiring. The examples of this type of nonrebreathing valves are: *Frumin valve, Ruben valve, Demand valve, etc.*

Frumin valve: It can be used both for spontaneous and controlled ventilation. It is so designed that any sudden rise of pressure in the bag which is filled with fresh gases, like squeezing it during controlled ventilation, closes the expiratory valve and all the gases pass on to the patient. On release of pressure at the end of inspiration the expiratory gases escape fully to the atmosphere through the expiratory valve which open during expiration only. This valve can be used either with a facemask or with the ET tube. Resistance and dead space of this valve are minimal.

Ruben valve: The mechanism of action of this valve is same as that of Frumin valve, but it differs from the latter only by very little dead space. Like the Frumin valve, during inspiration this valve automatically closes in both controlled and assisted ventilation, but opens during expiration only allowing expiratory gases to escape fully to the atmosphere. The main advantage of this valve is the small dead space which is only 9 mL. Resistance is also very low in this valve. If it is used with a continuous gas supply, then an inspiratory reservoir bag must be incorporated into the system to supply the peak inspiratory flow rate and the gas flow into the system must be equal or should exceed the patient's minute volume **(Fig. 28)**.

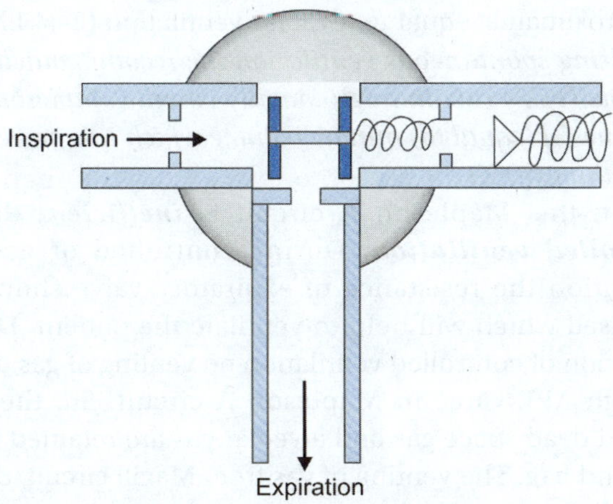

Fig. 28: Nonbreathing Ruben's valve.

When the patient draws air from the atmosphere (i.e., when compressed gas supply is absent), then no reservoir bag is needed. But, the system must have a low resistance circuit to meet the peak inspiratory flow rate. Low resistance vaporizers, such as an EMO vaporizer, may be placed in the circuit to deliver the volatile anesthetic agent and this constitutes a draw-over anesthetic apparatus. This type of equipment is very useful in remote areas where compressed gas supply is absent. Useful addition to such a system is (i) an extra inlet to permit O_2 enrichment of the inspired air and (ii) a bellows with additional valves to permit manual controlled ventilation when needed. The space between the nonrebreathing valve and the patient constitutes the apparatus dead space and for this reason the valve should be mounted as close to the patient as possible. The valve disk and the spring must be made as light as possible to reduce the resistance. The valve should be specially constructed to prevent the formation of water by condensation of its vapor which is present in the expired air. This is because the presence of water may prevent proper functioning of the valve due to sticking (back flow) and may cause serious accidents.

Demand valve: This is a valve which is attached to a cylinder of a compressed gas and will deliver the gases at a low pressure up to the peak inspiratory flow rate in response to the slight negative pressure developed by the patient's inspiratory effort. Demand valve is commonly used in connection with the cylinder containing N_2O and O_2 mixture (Entonox). As the valve is capable of delivering gas flows equal to the peak inspiratory flow rate, so no reservoir bag is needed. Such an assemble is classified as an intermittent-flow machine, because the valve allows the gas to flow intermittently, corresponding only with the patient's inspiratory effort.

Semi-closed System

The best example of this breathing system is the series of Mapleson circuits. In 1954, Mapleson described and analyzed *five different types of semi-closed systems or circuits, depending on five different arrangements* of the following factors, such as: (a) entry point of fresh gas flow, (b) length of tubing, (c) position of face mask, (d) position of reservoir bag, and (e) position of expiratory valve. The aim of five different arrangements of the above-mentioned factors, on which basis the series of Mapleson circuits are developed is to prevent rebreathing maximally during both spontaneous and controlled ventilation. However, in general, the elimination of CO_2 depends also on many other factors, other than these above-mentioned five factors. *These are (i) fresh gas flow rate, (ii) minute volume, (iii) tidal volume, (iv) pattern of breathing (spontaneous or controlled), (v) apparatus dead space, (vi) resistance of circuit, (vii) respiratory rate, (viii) I:E ratio, (ix) duration of expiratory pause, (x) peak inspiratory flow rate, (xi) volume of breathing tube, and (xii) volume of breathing bag.*

The five Mapleson semi-closed circuit is classified as A, B, C, D, and E. Willis added an extra F-system to these original classifications. Recently these six types of Mapleson systems were grouped functionally into three. These include: (i) group A, (ii) group B, C, and (iii) group D, E, and F. The Mapleson A circuit has a spring-loaded pop-off (APL) valve, located near face mask and the fresh gas flow enters into circuit from the opposite end of patient site, distal to reservoir bag. In B and C groups, the spring-loaded pop-off (APL) valve is located near face mask, but the fresh gas inlet is located near the patient site, close to APL valve, but proximal to reservoir bag. The reservoir tubing and the breathing bag serve as a closed blind limb where the fresh gas, dead space gas, and alveolar gas are collected. In Mapleson D, E, and F groups, which is also called as T-piece group, the fresh gas enters the circuit near the patient end, proximal to APL valve or an exhalation port, where there is no valve and the excess gas is popped-off from the opposite end of circuit.

Mapleson-A: It is the most familiar semi-closed breathing circuit to anesthesiologists and is also known as Magill's circuit. In this circuit the entry of fresh gas flow is distal to reservoir bag, opposite to patient's end at a distant from patient. The expiratory (or pressure relief or APL) valve is near patient's end. The type of expiratory value which is used in Mapleson circuit is Heidbrink. Rebreathing *during spontaneous respiration* in this circuit can be prevented by a relatively low fresh gas flow than any other Mapleson circuits. *During anesthesia with spontaneous respiration, the Magill's attachment is still the best in an adult for economy in total gas flow and for virtual elimination of rebreathing. During spontaneous expiration*, the first part of expired gas comes from anatomical dead space (upper airway) and contains no CO_2. It travels down the corrugated tube, toward reservoir bag and fills it, mixing with fresh gas, coming from machine. In next part of expiration, when the volume of expired gas from patient increases, then the pressure in circuit also rises. Thus, the expiratory valve is lifted up (opening pressure of Heidbrink valve should not be >1–2 cmH$_2$O) and expired gas escapes. Gas, escaping at this expiratory part of respiratory cycle, is alveolar gas, containing maximum amount of CO_2. *During spontaneous inspiration*, the fresh gas flushes the dead space gas (which collects in the tubing during first part of expiration) through tubing toward patient for rebreathing. But, rebreathing of this dead space gas by patient poses no problem, as it does not contain any CO_2. If the fresh gas flow is adequate, then the dead space gas during expiration cannot go up to reservoir bag, but meets with the fresh gas flow at the earlier part of tube and escapes with alveolar gas at the end of expiration, pushed by FGF. So, this circuit preferentially eliminates alveolar gas first, and then the dead space gas later. If the fresh gas flow is gradually reduced, still then rebreathing does not occur, until the fresh gas flow falls below 70% of minute volume, a figure **(Figs. 29A to F)** which

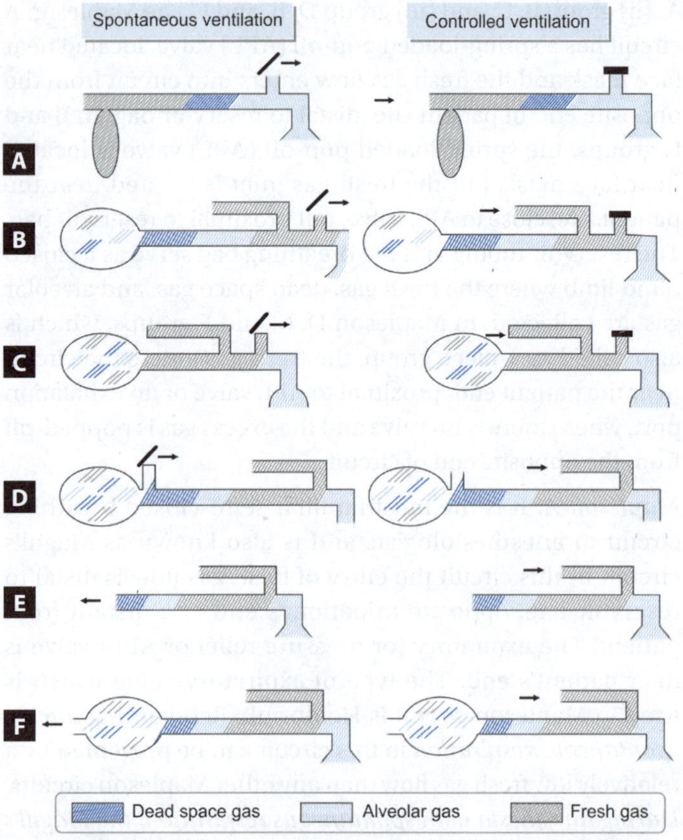

Figs. 29A to F: Gas disposition at the end of expiration, during both spontaneous and controlled ventilation in Mapleson circuits.

is approximately equal to alveolar ventilation (2– 4 L/min). *So, during spontaneous ventilation the recommended fresh gas flow (FGF) rate through Magill's circuit (Mapleson A) is one times of (equal to) minute volume which can prevent the rebreathing of CO_2.*

But, this Mapleson A circuit is ***inefficient during controlled ventilation***. During controlled or assisted ventilation the resistance of expiratory valve should be increased which will help to ventilate the patient. During expiration of controlled ventilation no venting of gas occurs through APL valve in Mapleson A circuit. So, the total expired dead space gas and alveolar gas are retained in the tube and bag. The venting of gas from Magill circuit, during controlled ventilation, occurs only during inspiration by the manual compression of reservoir bag. During squeezing of reservoir bag, the alveolar gas with CO_2 which is retained during expiration in tube is rebreathed first (goes into patient's lung), before the pressure in circuit increases enough to force the expiratory valve open. Then, this opened expiratory valve causes the dead space gas (without CO_2) with fresh gas to vent out in last part of inspiration, through pop-off valve. So, adequate CO_2 elimination or prevention of rebreathing during controlled ventilation with Mapleson A system requires a fresh gas flow >20 L/min or three times of minute volume. *Hence, in practice, Magill (Mapleson A) circuit should not be used for controlled ventilation. But, it is the circuit of choice for spontaneous ventilation.*

Mapleson-B: In this system, the fresh gas inlet is near to patient, but just distal to expiratory valve and proximal to reservoir bag. Unlike Mapleson A, this system functions similarly (equally effectively) both during spontaneous and controlled respiration. During the first part of expiration (both during spontaneous and controlled ventilation), fresh gas with the dead space gas accumulates in circuit tube and bag. Then, the expiratory valve opens, when the pressure in circuit increases and a mixture of alveolar with fresh gas is discharged. Some CO_2-containing alveolar gas, dead space gas, and fresh gas are also collected in reservoir circuit tube and bag. During the next inspiration (in both spontaneous and controlled) patient receives the fresh gas flow from machine and a mixture of retained dead space gas and alveolar gas from the tubing and reservoir bag. The composition of this inhaled mixture depends on the fresh gas flow rate. In this circuit rebreathing of expired gas (acceptable level of inspired CO_2 is 0.2–1%) can be prevented, if the fresh gas flow rate is >2.5 times of minute ventilation during both spontaneous and controlled ventilation. Therefore, as this circuit does not offer any extra advantage than other circuits and so is not used more for both spontaneous and controlled ventilation. The amount of FGF needed for proper functioning of this circuit (i.e., prevention of rebreathing of CO_2) is >D, E, and F group of circuit.

Mapleson-C: This system (circuit) is also known as "Water's circuit". It is also called as "Westminster face piece". Arrangement of this system is similar to that of Mapleson B, except that the expiratory or reservoir tube is of large bore and very short. This change reduces the reservoir volume and allows good mixing of fresh gases with exhaled gases. However, this system is less efficient than Mapleson B system. Because, as there is no tube to maintain the separation of alveolar and dead space portions of expired gas, therefore the whole expired volume is mixed in reservoir bag. So, the inspired mixture contains more expired alveolar gas than that of Mapleson B. *Thus, a fresh gas flow >2.5 times of minute volume is required to prevent rebreathing. This mechanism of action is similar both during spontaneous and controlled ventilation. So, with FGF of 2.5 times of minute volume, this circuit is efficient for both spontaneous and controlled ventilation. Hence, it does not provide any extra advantage than other circuits and is no more used now. It is, however, a very convenient arrangement for ventilating a patient before intubation or to assist chest physiotherapy in intensive care unit.*

Mapleson-D: Actually, this circuit looks like a T-piece. The T-piece has three-way tubular connections and these three connections are: (i) a patient connection port, (ii) a fresh gas connection port, and (iii) a port for connection to corrugated tubing with a reservoir bag and an APL valve for expiration. The Mapleson D system is popular, because the scavenging of expiratory gases is relatively easy in this circuit and it is most efficient of all the Mapleson circuits, during controlled ventilation. For scavenging, a large bore tube can be attached to adjustable pressure limiting (APL) valve. The fresh gas inlet is located near the patient end of circuit and the pop-off expiratory valve is close to reservoir bag, i.e., away from patient end. While in A, B, and C Mapleson circuit the pop-off expiratory valve is situated close to the patient. The length of expiratory tube is determined by the distance which an anesthesiologist wants to maintain from the patient, but this length has minimal effects on ventilation. The sensor or sampling site for respiratory gas monitoring may be placed between the bag and its mount, between the corrugated tubing and T-piece or between the corrugated tubing and APL or pop-off valve. In adults, it may be placed between the T-piece and patient.

During the early part of *expiratory phase of spontaneous ventilation,* first dead-space gas, then alveolar gas, and then fresh gas flow subsequently down the expiratory limb. As the expiration continues and pressure increases, then expiratory valve opens and a portion of this gas mixture containing dead space and alveolar gas is expelled. Patient receives a mixture of fresh gas and expired gas from the expiratory limb

during next *inspiration phase of spontaneous ventilation.* The composition of this inspired gas mixture is determined by the rate of fresh gas flow, patient's tidal volume, and the duration of expiratory pause. *Slow respiratory rate with long expiratory pause allows the fresh gas to drive out all the expired alveolar gas, moving down the expiratory limb. High respiratory rate with short expiratory pause provides inadequate time to flush out all the alveolar gas and allows rebreathing to occur. Rebreathing in this situation can be prevented by high fresh gas flows.*

During the inspiratory phase of *controlled ventilation,* the alveolar gas and the dead space gas are also forced out of expiratory valve instead of fresh gas like spontaneous ventilation. Therefore, this system also causes less rebreathing than Mapleson A, B, and C systems during controlled ventilation. *Recommended fresh gas flow rates during spontaneous ventilation with Mapleson D system is approximately 2.5 times of minute ventilation. So, this circuit is not used for spontaneous ventilation. The recommended fresh gas flow-rate for Mapleson D circuit during controlled ventilation are: (i) 1.6 times of minute ventilation at normal respiratory rate (10–12 breath/minute) or (ii) 70–100 mL/kg/min (which is almost equal to minute ventilation), if respiratory rate is increased to 16 breath/min. Many clinicians prefer to (ii) method.*

Bain's circuit: It is a modification of Mapleson D circuit and is named after the name of scientist, Bain who modified this Mapleson D circuit. It is also called as coaxial circuit because the fresh gas flows through a narrow inner tube which is situated within the outer corrugated wide bore tube used for expiration and delivers fresh gas flow directly at the patient end of circuit. The expired gas enters the corrugated outer wide bore tube and is vented out through expiratory APL valve, near reservoir bag, situated opposite to the patient end of circuit. The expiratory gas does not enter the inner narrow tube, carrying the fresh gas, because the pressure inside the narrow inner tube is high. The Bain's circuit may be used for both spontaneous and controlled ventilation. Like Mapleson D, to maintain normocarbia and to prevent rebreathing in Bain's circuit, the fresh gas flow of 2.5 times of minute volume is needed during spontaneous ventilation. But, only 70 mL/kg/min of fresh gas flow will produce normocarbia in Bain's circuit during controlled ventilation. Functional analysis of Bain's circuit during spontaneous and controlled ventilation is like that of Mapleson D circuit. In spontaneous ventilation during exhalation the expired gas mixes with fresh gas and moves through the corrugated outer tube toward the bag. After the bag is filled with expired gas, the gas exists via the pop-off or APL valve. Then, during expiratory pause the fresh gas also flows down the outer corrugated tubing from narrow inner tubing and pushes the exhaled gas in front of it **(Figs. 30A and B)**.

In spontaneous ventilation then during inspiration, patient inhales the fresh gas from fresh gas inlet, corrugated outer tubing (filled with fresh gas) and reservoir bag (filled with fresh gas). If the FGF is high, then all the gases which are inspired by patient, during inspiration from the corrugated tube and reservoir bag will also be fresh gas. If the FGF is low, then some exhaled gas which is present in outer corrugated tubing and reservoir bag will be inhaled. So, the ventilatory pattern, the FGF rate, and the rate of breathing will also help to determine the amount of rebreathing.

In controlled ventilation during expiration, the expired gas flows down the corrugated outer tubing from patient's end. At the same time, fresh gas flow also enters the corrugated outer tubing. During expiratory pause, the fresh gas flow continues and pushes the exhaled gas down the corrugated outer tubing toward the APL valve and reservoir bag. During inspiration of controlled ventilation, helped by squeezing of reservoir bag, the fresh gas, mixed with expired gas from corrugated outer tubing, enters the patient. If the fresh gas flow is low, then some exhaled gases may be inhaled from corrugated tube with fresh gas from the narrow inner tube. If the FGF is high, then it fills up the whole outer corrugated tube and reservoir bag, driving out all the expired gases and the patient inhales only the fresh gas from inner tube, outer corrugated tube, and reservoir bag. Prolonging inspiratory time, increasing respiratory rate, adding an inspiratory plateau, etc. will increase rebreathing. Rebreathing also can

be decreased by allowing a long expiratory pause, so that the fresh gas can get adequate time to flush out all the exhaled gas from outer corrugated tubing through APL valve. When the fresh gas flow is high, there is little rebreathing. The $ETCO_2$ is determined mainly by minute ventilation. The rate of FGF is the main determining factor, controlling CO_2 elimination. The higher will be FGF, the lower will be $ETCO_2$ level.

Bain's circuit (coaxial modification, i.e., tube within tube modification of Mapleson D system) is also available with a metal head and channels, drilled into it for permanent attachment with anesthetic machine. This provides a fixed position of reservoir bag and APL valve in relation to anesthetic machine. Some metal heads also have a pressure manometer. Mechanically, controlled ventilation can also be achieved by connecting the hose of an anesthetic ventilator in the place of reservoir bag and completely closing the APL valve. Excess gas is vented out through ventilator.

Positive end-expiratory pressure (PEEP) valves or devices can also be applied with Bain's system. A bidirectional PEEP device or valve may also be used between the APL valve and corrugated outer tubing. This allows PEEP to be administered both during mechanical and manual ventilation. However, some PEEP valves close when a negative pressure is applied. So, spontaneous breathing is impossible, when such a valve is present in this system. The PEEP valve may be applied in hose pipe, leading to anesthetic ventilator. In this location, it will only be effective during mechanical ventilation. A unidirectional PEEP valve can also be attached at the attachment site of reservoir bag, using special connectors and unidirectional valves. Such an arrangement allows application of PEEP both during mechanical and spontaneous ventilation, but not during manual ventilation **(Fig. 31)**.

The advantages of Bain's circuit are: lightweight, convenient, less resistance (<0.7 cmH$_2$O) can easily be sterilized, reusable, and easy scavenging of expired gases. The exhaled gases in outer corrugated reservoir tube add warmth to the cold inspired gases passing through narrow inner tube. Another advantage is this circuit is long (1.8 meters), making it useful for head and neck surgeries where an anesthetist is away from patient. In a patient weighing <40 kg, the fresh gas flow should not be reduced below 3 L/min, otherwise higher

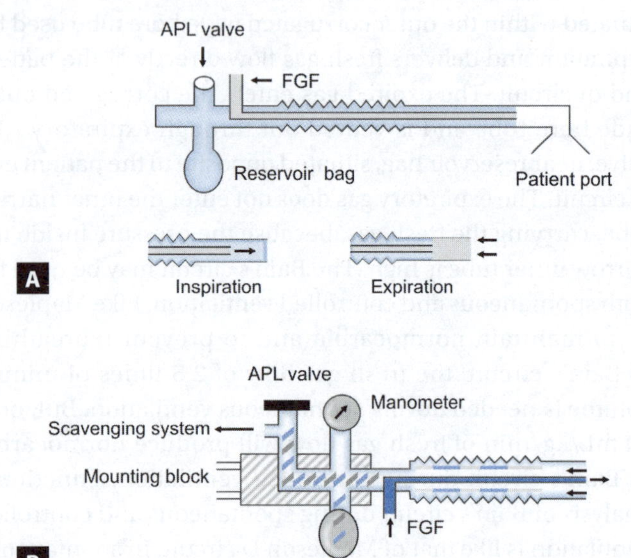

Figs. 30A and B: Bain's modification of the Mapleson D system. The fresh gas supply tube is inside the corrugated tubing (coaxial version). (APL: adjustable pressure limiting valve (A) is the simple Bain's circuit, (B) is the ventilator compatible Bain's circuit permanently mounted on the anesthetic machine; FGF: fresh gas flow)

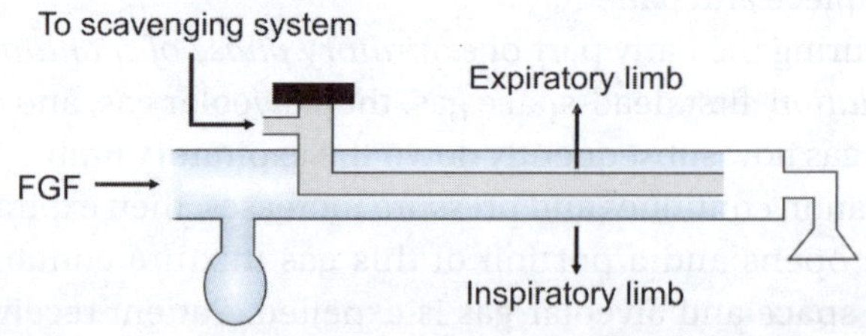

Fig. 31: This shows Lack's modification of the Mapleson A system.

PaCO$_2$ (ETCO$_2$) values will result. This is a reflection of higher metabolic rate in children and infants. *Disadvantage of Bain's* circuit includes unrecognized disconnection or kinking of inner fresh gas tube. So, the outer tube should be transparent for inspection of inner tube.

Another alternative arrangement of coaxial tubing (circuit) is *Lack's circuit*. Here, the fresh gas flows through outer wide corrugated tube and the expired gas flows down the central narrow inner tube. This central narrow tube runs from the connection at patient's end to APL valve at the machine end of circuit. This makes it easier to adjust the valve and facilitates the scavenging of excess gas. However, it slightly increases the work of breathing. Actually, this is a modified configuration of Mapleson A (Magill) circuit, where the central inner tube extends from the patient's end to APL valve. However, the same considerations, like Bain circuit, will govern the fresh gas flow rate, which is required to prevent rebreathing in Lack's circuit. The diameter and length of tube used in this circuit should be of low-flow resistance. The Lack circuit is suitable for spontaneous respiration and requires a lower fresh gas flow, than Magill's circuit. The Lack system is also available in both dual tube (parallel arrangement) or tube within a "tube" (coaxial arrangement) arrangements, in which the narrow expiratory limb runs inside the outer wide inspiratory limb. For spontaneous ventilation, the APL or expiratory valve is kept in fully opened position. Excess gas comes out of it during the later part of expiration. For controlled or manual ventilation, intermittent positive pressure is applied to the bag. Then, the APL valve is tightened accordingly, so that when the bag is pressed, sufficient pressure can be built-up which will be able to inflate the lungs. APL valve opens during inspiration and closes during expiration in controlled ventilation. It is opposite to spontaneous ventilation.

Humphrey ADE system (using Mapleson A, D, and E Principle): This is a recently described system or circuit which is available in both coaxial and noncoaxial form. It is claimed that Humphrey circuit functions with efficiency like Lack's system for spontaneous respiration and like Bain's system for controlled ventilation. But, it is heavier and less convenient to use. As the name implies, this ADE system works on the principle of Mapleson A, D, and E circuits. In A configuration, it acts similar to the Lack's modification of Mapleson A system. In D configuration, its action resembles to that of Bain's modification of Mapleson D system. It also has a system which allows the APL valve to be bypassed in D configuration, so that it resembles to Mapleson E system. It has two levers and their positions determine the functioning of a particular circuit (system). There is also a self-locking mechanism which prevents the accidental displacement of

any lever from their selected position. In the coaxial version, the expiratory limb runs inside the inspiratory limb (Lack system). In noncoaxial or parallel version, the inspiratory and expiratory tubes are held together at machine end by a metal bridge. The expiratory limb consists of: (i) a long tube which extends from the patient's end to machine, (ii) an APL valve, (iii) a reservoir bag, (iv) a valve-bypass outlet, (v) a fresh gas inlet, and (vi) a lever that directs the flow of gases through either APL valve or valve bypass outlet. When the liver is kept at a vertical position, then the gases can flow in and out of the reservoir bag and pass through APL valve. On the other hand, when it is kept in horizontal position, then the APL valve is isolated and reservoir bag is blocked and gases flow through valve-bypass outlet, like Mapleson E system. Both the outlets have 30-mm external diameters for attachment to scavenging devices. The valve-bypass outlet also has a 22-mm internal diameter for the attachment of a hose, leading to a ventilator or a reservoir bag. A pressure limiting device may also be fitted near APL valve **(Figs. 32A and B)**.

Later, a single lever Humphrey ADE system has also been developed. It is again available in both parallel (noncoaxial) and coaxial forms. Here, there is a single lever controlled rotating cylinder which passes through both the inspiratory and expiratory limbs. When the lever is at an upright position, then the reservoir bag and APL valve are in the circuit. Thus, the valve-bypass outlet is excluded from circuit. On the other hand, when the lever is turned down, then the bag and APL valve are excluded from circuit. Thus, the valve-bypass outlet is connected to circuit.

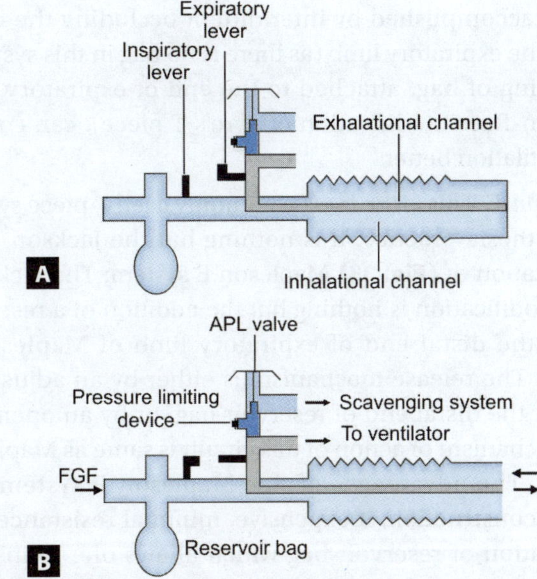

Figs. 32A and B: Humphrey ADE system. The dual lever coaxial version of this system is shown here. (A) A mode ventilation, with vertical levers; (B) D and E mode of ventilation, with horizontal levers.

Mapleson-E: The classical example of Mapleson E breathing system is Ayre's T-piece with one modification of expiratory limb. Phillip Ayre had first developed Ayre's T-piece in 1937 for use in pediatric patients, undergoing cleft palate repair and intracranial surgery. Mapleson E is the *modification of this Ayre's T-piece with the addition of an expiratory limb, but without any reservoir bag.* As it has no reservoir bag, so it cannot be considered as a complete circuit. The picture shows the relationship between the fresh gas inlet, patient's end, expiratory limb, and the gas exit point. It has minimum dead space, no valves, and exerts very little resistance. The expiratory limb constitutes or acts as reservoir, as there is no reservoir bag in this original Mapleson E system. If the volume of expiratory limb exceeds the tidal volume, then the breathing of room air through it does not occur and thereby prevents the dilution of anesthetic gases with room air, which can also occur in original simple T-piece (without expiratory limb) developed by Philip Ayre. On the other hand, if the volume of expiratory limb is less than the tidal volume of patient, then the reverse will occur. If fresh gas inflow equals to two and half (2.5) times of minute volume of patient, then rebreathing will not occur. The actual length of expiratory limb is irrelevant, provided it does not cause appreciable resistance to expiration and rebreathing. During expiration of spontaneous ventilation, the fresh gas and the exhaled gas flow down the expiratory limb. Then, at the end of expiration, fresh gas accumulates at the patient's end of expiratory limb. During next breath, this fresh gas is drawn by patient, both from the fresh gas inlet and expiratory limb. As there is no reservoir bag, it is used only for spontaneous ventilation. But, controlled ventilation can be accomplished by intermittent occluding the distal end of the expiratory limb (as there is no bag in this system). Squeezing of bag, attached to the end of expiratory limb (Jackson-Rees modification of Ayre's T piece), can control the ventilation better.

Mapleson-F: This is the most commonly used T-piece system in anesthesia practice. It is nothing but the Jackson–Rees modification of **(Fig. 33)** Mapleson E system. The Jackson–Rees modification is nothing but the addition of a reservoir bag at the distal end of expiratory limb of Mapleson E system. The release mechanism is either by an adjustable valve at the distal end of reservoir bag, or by an open tail. The mechanism of action of this circuit is same as Mapleson D or E. The advantages of this Mapleson F system are: simple construction, inexpensive, minimal resistance and observation of reservoir bag which allows one to inspect the respiratory excursion and also judge the depth of anesthesia. Controlled ventilation can also be instituted easily by squeezing the bag, if needed. Scavenging system of

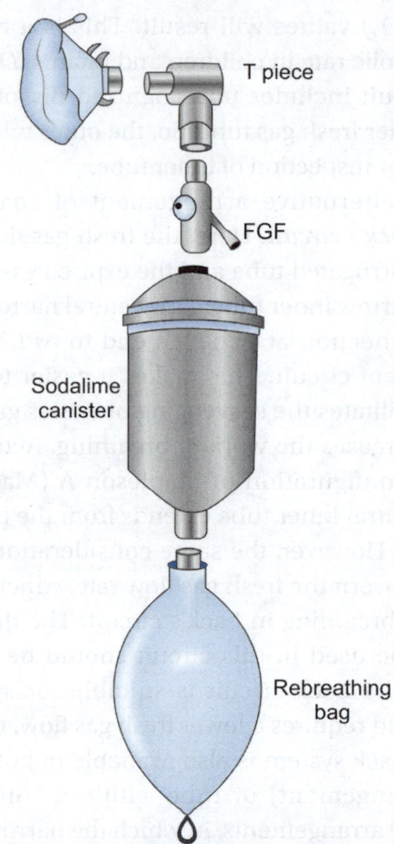

Fig. 33: Water's To and Fro T-piece system with carbon dioxide absorption canister which was first introduced in 1923, in clinical anesthesia practice by Ralph Waters. It is discussed here only for its historical interest. In this system, a canister filled with soda lime was placed between the face mask and the rebreathing bag. Both inspiration and expiration took place through this canister.

this circuit is also easy. It is accomplished by enclosing the reservoir bag in a plastic chamber.

This "To and Fro System" had some definite advantages. It was cheap, simple, easy to operate, and easy to sterilize. It offered very low resistance and a low gas flow. Heat loss was also low as the exhaled gases were kept warm by the heat generated by a reaction during carbon dioxide absorption. It also helped in the conservation of moisture. But, it also had some disadvantages. As the canister lays close to the head of the patient (especially a small baby), alkaline dust easily passed on to the patient. Also, a heavy canister near the head of the patient was inconvenient.

The disadvantage of this Mapleson F system is lack of humidification. This problem can be overcome by allowing the fresh gas to pass through an online-heated humidifier. Another disadvantage of this Mapleson F (Jackson–Rees modification of Mapleson E system) is the need of high fresh gas flow. This system is used mainly in pediatric patients and for transportation of anesthetized patients.

T-piece system: This is defined as a breathing circuit or system where the fresh gas flow acts as the vertical limb of T and enters at a place between the patient's end and the expiratory end of a tube which acts as the horizontal limb of T. So, Mapleson A, B, and C systems do not come under this T-piece system. But, this functional definition is sometimes confusing as there does not necessarily have a separate limb, leading to expiratory port. It thus also includes some circuits or systems which physically do not look like T-piece. As the T-piece breathing system is commonly used in paediatric anesthesia, so resistance is of great importance. Highest resistance in this system occurs at a peak expiratory flow, to which must be added the fresh gas flow.

T-piece system without expiratory limb: Devices of this type of breathing circuit are mainly used with endotracheal tube or tracheostomy tube. If the patient breathes spontaneously, then no rebreathing occurs in this system, as there is no expiratory limb where the expired gas can accumulate. So, the total amount of expired air is breathed out in atmosphere. But, when anesthesia is provided by inhalational agents, then to prevent the breathing of room air due to the absence of expiratory limb, the fresh gas flow must be equal to or exceed the peak inspiratory flow rate. This is widely used for resuscitation purposes. If necessary, for controlled ventilation, the intermittent occlusion of expiratory orifice by operator's finger affords a compact and convenient method of inflating patient's lungs. But, in such conditions a pressure-relief valve with a water manometer is essential, as the pressure of fresh gas supply is applied directly to the patient's lungs.

Most of the T-pieces have a fresh gas entry port of narrow bore which enters the T-piece at right angles to main respiratory channel. If high flow of fresh gas enters at an acute angle, within the T-piece, then it is found that gases can be entrained in main tube by venturi principle. But, this results in an impedance of expiration with dangerously high intrapulmonary pressure. This principle is used in a rigid bronchoscope to permit ventilation under general anesthesia with muscle relaxants. A fine tube, mounted at the eyepiece of a rigid bronchoscope, is used for O_2 delivery intermittently. The jet of O_2 entrains air and generates sufficient pressure to inflate the patient's lungs, which deflates as soon as the gas flow through fine tube is stopped.

Now, at the end of discussion, we can conclude that the relative efficiency of different Mapleson systems with respect to prevention of rebreathing during spontaneous ventilation is like the following: Mapleson A > D, E, F > B, C and during controlled ventilation is like the following: Mapleson D, E, F > B, C > A.

The Mapleson A, B, and C systems are rarely used now, but D, E, and F systems are commonly employed. There is also some confusion regarding the recommendation of FGF in different breathing systems with multiple variable predictions **(Table 6)**. So, monitoring of end-tidal CO_2 is the best method of determining optimal fresh gas flow. But, during monitoring it should be noted that $PaCO_2$ to $ETCO_2$ gradient decreases with rebreathing.

Pressure limiting properties of rubber reservoir bag: The pressure/volume or elastic characteristic of rubber bag, which is commonly used as reservoir in anesthetic circuit, constitutes a useful safeguard against the accidental build-up of dangerously high pressure in patient's lungs. Otherwise, which might occur if an expiratory valve is accidentally occluded. For example, if gas starts to flow at a rate of 8 l/min into a 2-l rubber bag, then the pressure rises quickly within few seconds to a peak value of 25–30 mm Hg and thereafter falls slightly, until it bursts after reaching a volume of >144 l.

Tubing of circuits: Tubing in anesthetic system is usually made up of corrugated walls, so that it can bend at acute angles without kinking. Regarding size, 20 mm is the

TABLE 6: Fresh gas flow in spontaneous and controlled ventilation with Mapleson's A, B, C, D, E, and F systems.

Circuit	Fresh gas flow in spontaneous ventilation	Fresh gas flow in controlled ventilation	Comments
Mapleson A	Equal to minute ventilation	Very high flow (3 × minute volume	Circuit of choice for spontaneous ventilation. Not used for controlled ventilation
Mapleson B	2.5 × minute volume	2.5 × minute volume	No more used
Mapleson C (Water circuit)	2.5 × minute volume	2.5 × minute volume	No more used
Mapleson D (Bain circuit)	2.5 × minute volume	1.5 × minute volume	Circuit of choice for controlled ventilation. Not used for spontaneous ventilation. Most commonly used semi-closed circuit
Mapleson E (Ayre's T piece)	2.5 × minute volume	2.5 × minute volume	Pediatric use, and incomplete circuit
Mapleson F (Jackson–Rees circuit)	2.5 × minute volume	1.5 × minute volume	Most commonly used pediatric circuit

recommended minimum internal diameter of tube, used in anesthetic circuit. It must be sufficiently electrically conductive (conduct or transfer static electric charges from machine to ground) by adding carbon to rubber and will prevent static charges to build up (accumulate) during anesthesia procedure, otherwise which might produce sparking. The compliance of tube may also become an important factor. If the tube has high compliance, then a larger portion of ventilator's stroke volume may be lost in tubing. In patient with very stiff lung, this may be a great problem.

The advantages of Mapleson system (circuits)

i. The Mapleson circuits are most simple and inexpensive. In this system, without APL valve, there is no moving parts. The components of this system are easy to disassemble for disinfection or sterilization.

ii. This system has multiple buffering effects. So, any variation in minute volume affects end-tidal CO_2 tension less than a circle system.

iii. Rebreathing will result in retention of heat and moisture. In coaxial system, the gases in inner inspiratory limb are heated by the warm exhaled gas in large outer coaxial expiratory tube.

iv. The resistance of this system is usually within recommended ranges, at a given fresh gas flow, which is usually used in clinical practice. So, the work of breathing during spontaneous ventilation is significantly less with these systems than with circle system. However, this is not always true. The work of breathing increases, if the APL valve is not oriented properly.

These systems (circuits) are of light-weight and not bulky. So, they are not likely to produce excessive pull-on endotracheal tube or cause accidental extubation.

They are easy to position in relation to patient. A long Mapleson D system with an aluminum APL valve may also be used to ventilate a patient undergoing MRI investigation.

The disadvantages of Mapleson system

i. The Mapleson system requires a high gas flow. So, it results in higher costs, increased atmospheric pollution and difficulties in assessment of spontaneous ventilation.

ii. In this system, it is difficult to determine the optimum fresh gas flow. On the other hand, it is necessary to change the fresh gas flow matching with respiratory rate from time to time during spontaneous ventilation and also while changing from spontaneous to controlled ventilation or vice versa.

iii. Anything that causes accidentally the fresh gas flow to be low then it presents a hazard, because dangerous rebreathing may occur. This has been reported with unnoticed emptying of N_2O cylinder, a leak in humidification device or leak of gas through a loose vaporizer-filler cap.

iv. If extra components, such as respiratory gas monitor, heat exchanger, moisture exchanger, etc. are placed between the fresh gas inlet and the patient, then a tremendous increase of dead space area will occur. Therefore, this will cause dangerous rebreathing.

v. In Mapleson A, B, and C systems, the APL valve is located close to patient, where it is inaccessible to user. In addition, scavenging is also difficult from this inaccessible APL valve. This disadvantage can be overcome by using Lack's modification of Mapleson A circuit.

vi. The Mapleson systems are not suitable for patient with increased CO_2 load, such as malignant hyperthermia. Because it may not be possible to increase enough the fresh gas flow to remove increased CO_2 load.

vii. Mapleson E system is notorious for air dilution, as the expiratory limb is short and there is no reservoir bag. It is also difficult to scavenge the Mapleson E and F systems.

Respiratory Gas Monitoring Site and Mapleson systems: All the Mapleson systems, except "A", have the fresh gas inlet near patient-connection port. This may make it difficult to get a reliable sample of exhaled gases for analysis and monitoring **(Fig. 34)**.

There are four possible sites from where the sampling of gases is done. These are:

i. At the junction of breathing system and elbow connector to ET tube

ii. At the corner of elbow connector

iii. 2 cm distal to elbow connector

iv. In the tracheal tube connector.

It is found that if sampling is carried out at two sites which are close to patient, i.e., at point 3 and point 4 of table above, then the values are more accurate. Significant errors are

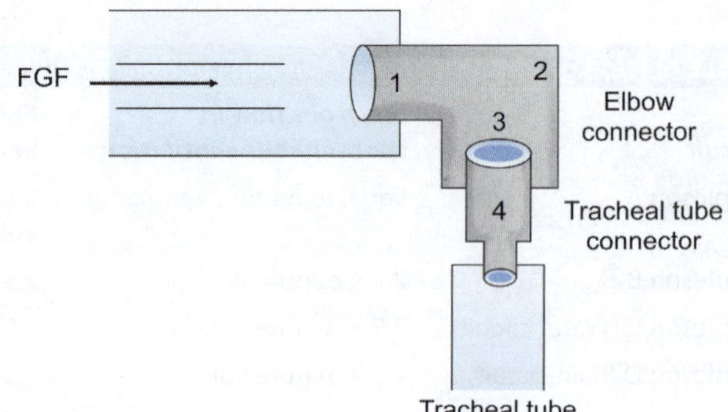

Fig. 34: Respiratory gas sampling site in a Mapleson system. Accurate values for expiratory concentration of gases are obtained by sampling at the sites of 3 and 4. Sampling at the site 2 will yield accurate values, only if the fresh gas flow (FGF) is not high. Sampling at the site 1 will yield inaccurate values, even at low fresh gas flows.

noted when the samples are taken from the corner of elbow connector (site 2). But, this error occurs only if a high fresh gas flow is used and not in low fresh gas flow. Significant errors are also noted when the sampling is performed at the junction of breathing system and elbow connector (site 1), even if a low fresh gas flow is used. On the other hand, a cannula that projects into airway can be used to improve sampling. In another study, involving infants and children, sampling at the junction of tracheal tube and breathing system resulted in a falsely low end-tidal CO_2 values in patients weighing <8 kg. The accuracy of measurement can also be improved by inserting a small heat and moisture exchanger, between the breathing system and tracheal tube connector. But, the use of device at this site will result in an increase in dead space and may result in excessive resistance so that spontaneous respiration cannot be used.

Closed Circuit Rebreathing System

In closed circuit expiratory gases pass through the expiratory limb to reach canister, containing soda lime/barylime/lithium hydroxide. In this canister, CO_2 is absorbed from expired gases and then this expired gas is reused by patient. Since no gases are vented out in atmosphere, these are considered as closed circuit. As the same gases are being reused, only the O_2 consumed by body needs to be replaced, requiring very low flows and that is why the anesthesia given with closed circuit is called as the *"low flow anesthesia"*. The differences between the closed circuit and semi-closed circuit are depicted in **Table 7**.

There are two types of closed circuits: (i) *Circle system* which is commonly used and (ii) *To and fro system of Water's* which is no more used. Closed circuit was first introduced in human anesthesia by Water's in 1923.

Universal-F system (circuit): It is a single limb closed circuit system, intended to decrease the cumbersomeness of circle system.

The circle system is the most popular breathing system in anesthesia practice and is free from most of the drawbacks which are found in to and fro Mapleson arrangements. It is so named because its components are arranged in a circular manner. The circle system may be completely closed or semi-closed. The completely closed circle system prevents rebreathing of CO_2 by CO_2 absorber, but allows rebreathing of other exhaled gases. The extent of rebreathing of CO_2 in this system depends on the CO_2 absorption power of absorbent, component arrangement, and the rate of fresh gas flow **(Fig. 35)**.

In a semi-closed system the APL valve is partially open and there is no rebreathing of expired gases and requires a very high fresh gas flow. Whereas a completely closed system is one in which the fresh gas flow exactly matches the volume being consumed by patient. There is complete rebreathing of all other exhaled gases after absorption of CO_2, as all the valves are completely closed.

The circle system consists of nine components:

  i. Entry site of fresh gas flow
 ii. *Inspiratory and expiratory unidirectional valve:* These valves maintain unidirectional flow of gases and ensure

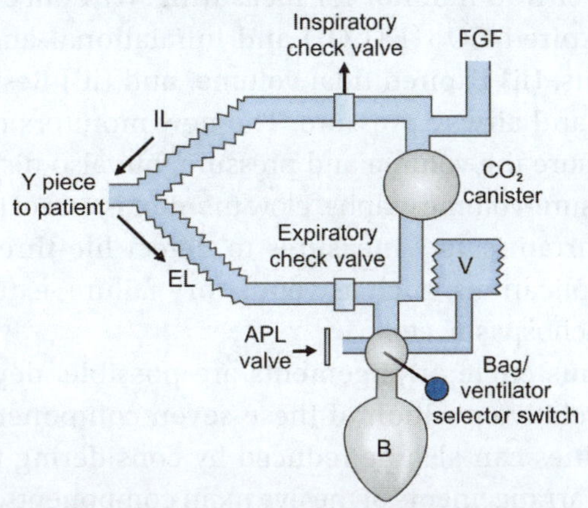

Fig. 35: Components of a simple form of circle system. (APL: adjustable pressure limiting valve; B: bag; EL: expiratory limb; FGF: fresh gas flow; IL: inspiratory limb; V: ventilator)

TABLE 7: Differentiation between closed system (circuit system) and semi-closed system (Mapleson system).	
Closed system (Circle system)	***Semi-closed system (Mapleson system)***
Advantages: (i) Economical as same gas and inhalational anesthetic agents are reused. (ii) Less theater pollution. (iii) Humidity is well preserved. (iv) In conditions in which there is very high production of CO_2, then only closed circuit can eliminate such high CO_2, e.g., malignant hyperthermia	*Disadvantages*: (i) Not economical as high gas flow is required. (ii) High theater pollution. (iii) Humidity is not preserved. (iv) Cannot eliminate all CO_2 if its production is very high in body
Disadvantages: (i) Heavy weight due to tubing, canister, and accessories. (ii) If soda lime is exhausted or expiratory valve gets stuck, there can be dangerous hypercapnia. (iii) Production of toxic compound A with sevoflurane. (iv) Desiccated soda lime can produce CO with desflurane. (v) Cross infection from apparatus may occur. (vi) High-breathing resistance and high dead space. (vii) As low flow is used, so high level of monitoring is needed	*Advantages*: (i) Light weight. (ii) No risk of soda lime exhaustion and no risk of sticking of expiratory valve. (iii) No risk of production of toxic compound. (iv) Chances of cross infection is less. (v) Breathing resistance and dead space is low. (vi) High-level monitoring is not needed

that expiratory gases do not enter the inspiratory limb and vice versa.

iii. Inspiratory and expiratory corrugated tube

iv. Y-piece connector

v. An overflow or pop-off or damp valve, which is also called the APL valve

vi. Reservoir bag

vii. Canister, containing CO_2 absorbent

viii. *Oxygen analyzer:* It is fitted in inspiratory limb. It is one of the most important safety measures as it measures the final delivered concentration of O_2 to patient. The O_2 analyzers, used in most of the modern machines, are electrochemical (galvanic cell or polarographic cell). The O_2 passes through the sensor membrane, gets reduced, and generates current. The amplitude of current generated is proportional to the partial pressure of O_2 which is converted into percentage by software.

ix. *Flow sensor:* The use of flow sensor is considered mandatory by the American Society of Anesthesiology. It is connected at the end of breathing circuit. It collects sample from expiratory gases during expiration and deliver it to monitor for measuring: (i) Concentration of expired CO_2 (ETCO$_2$) and inhalational anesthetic agents, (ii) Expired tidal volume, and (iii) Respiratory rate and airway pressure. The new monitors not only measure the volume and pressure, but also display the pressure-volume graphs. Flow monitor is one of the most important safety measures to detect life-threatening complications, such as ventilatory failure, extubation, bronchospasm, etc.

Various circle arrangements are possible, depending on the relative position of these seven components. The possibilities can also be reduced by considering the best possible arrangements of the five main components, such as unidirectional valve, APL valve, reservoir bag, CO_2 absorber, and the site of fresh gas entry.

To prevent rebreathing of CO2, three rules must be followed. They are:

- *Rule I:* Unidirectional valve must be located both in inspiratory and expiratory limbs, between the patient and reservoir bag.

- *Rule II:* Fresh gas inflow will not enter the circuit between the expiratory valve and patient. Fresh gas inflow is best placed on the downstream side of relief valve and after the canister containing CO_2 absorbent. This arrangement conserves the fresh gas which would otherwise be lost through relief valve. It has been argued that placing the inflow site before canister would allow the fresh gas to become humidified by water, which is evolved with the absorption of CO_2-by-CO_2 absorbent. However, this

water is needed to ensure that the reaction takes place at a maximum rate. If the inlet of fresh gas is placed anywhere on the downstream side of inspiratory valve, then the fresh gas will become mixed with expiratory gas during expiration and part of it will be ejected. If, however, the inlet is placed on the upstream side of inspiratory valve, then during inspiration any changes in the concentration of anesthetic gases are made effective immediately, while during expiration (when inspiratory valve is closed) the fresh gas will fill up the reservoir bag. This is the position of fresh gas inlet for maximum economy and efficiency.

- *Rule III:* The overflow (pop-off) valve cannot be located between the patient and inspiratory valve, but it must be located on the downstream side of expiratory valve. If these rules are followed, then any arrangement of other components does not increase the rebreathing of CO_2. The most efficient arrangement of circle system is shown in the picture, and this arrangement conserves the dead space gas and preferentially eliminates the alveolar gas. But, the most practical arrangements, used in all the contemporary anesthetic machines, are less efficient, because it allows the alveolar and dead space gas to mix before venting. Even, with the fresh gas flow inlet fixed, there are several alternative options for position of the relief valve: (i) in the inspiratory limb, after the reservoir bag, (ii) in the expiratory limb, before the reservoir bag, or (iii) after the expiratory valve **(Fig. 36)**.

There are two factors which determine the choice of the position of relief or APL valve. First, although the expired air will be blown-off in any of these three positions, but the closer the valve is to the patient, the more the gas

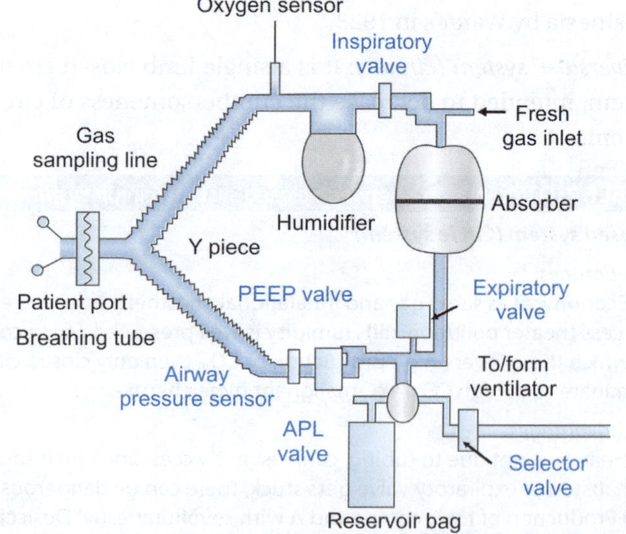

Fig. 36: Option for position of relief valve.
(APL: adjustable pressure limiting valve; PEEP: positive end-expiratory pressure)

will be pure alveolar air and also depends at the point in respiratory cycle when the valve opens. Second, if the relief valve is placed before the expiratory valve, there is possibility of ejecting fresh gas, during the inspiratory phase of controlled and assisted ventilation. Thus, combination of these two conditions such as having the relief valve as close to the patient as possible and also on the upstream side of expiratory valve, can be obtained if the inspiratory valves are a made part of patient's T-piece. The practical disadvantage of this arrangement is that the connection to the patient becomes cumbersome and the operation of the valves may not be reliable, in practice. The alternative arrangement of retaining the relief valve on the T-piece connection to the patient, but moving the inspiratory and expiratory valves back to the anesthetic machine, is economical only when the respiration is spontaneous. If the relief valve is also moved away from the patient, both alveolar and dead space gases are ejected, but the efficiency of the system is maintained only during controlled ventilation.

Circle System with Low Gas Flow

In a circle system where components are arranged with optimum efficacy, then the expired alveolar gas is preferentially expelled from the circuit. Here, the circle system behaves like the Magill's circuit and rebreathing of CO_2 will not take place until the fresh gas flow falls below the alveolar ventilation. It is found that in the Magill's circuit the minimum fresh gas flow needed to prevent rebreathing in a spontaneously breathing patient is 3–4.5 L/min. Magill's circuit loses this efficiency when the above calculation is used for controlled ventilation. But, in an optimum arrangement of circle system the preferential elimination of the alveolar gas continues during controlled ventilation also with the same low gas flow which is sufficient to prevent rebreathing in Magill's circuit during spontaneous breathing. During commonly used conditions such as "closed circuit with leak" and with a fresh gas flow of 4 L/min, it is unnecessary to have any soda lime in the canister at all. Under this condition the fresh gas flow takes over the role of the alveolar ventilation in controlling $PaCO_2$ without soda lime, even in controlled ventilation.

When the fresh gas flow is reduced to a level below the alveolar ventilation (or in some other arrangement of components where the system is not optimum) then soda lime is required in the circle system to prevent the rebreathing of CO_2. Without soda lime, when the fresh gas flow falls below the alveolar ventilation, then discrepancy develops between the inspired and delivered O_2 concentration in controlled ventilation. Calculation of the inspired O_2 concentration during the low fresh gas flow (N_2O:O_2 mixture)

with considerable accuracy is possible only when a steady state has been achieved. For this reason, monitoring of the inspired O_2 concentration in the circuit is necessary.

Totally Closed System

The circle system can also be used in a completely closed manner. After a period of about 10 minutes of breathing with high inflow of fresh gas, which brings about denitrogenation, the expiratory valve can be completely closed and the only fresh gas flow into the system is the patient's basal O_2 requirement together with anesthetic agent. Such a system was widely used when cyclopropane was in extensive use and if the O_2 (not N_2O) is the only gas which is flowing, apart from other liquid anesthetics. In such circumstances no monitoring is required, except for the usual close observation of patient.

Advantages of the Circle System (Totally Closed or Partially Closed)

- *Reduction of atmospheric pollution:* Once the expiratory valve is totally closed, then no anesthetic gas escapes into the air to pollute the environment except a very small percentage which is lost through the different leaks. During totally closed halothane anesthesia, concentration of halothane in the theater does not rise above 0.03 ppm. In a partially closed system, there is some atmospheric pollution, but this can be prevented by a scavenging system.
- *Economical:* In a totally closed system, the consumption of any volatile anesthetic agent and fresh gas flow is very low. For example, the consumption of halothane in an adult patient is about 3.5 mL/h and the fresh gas flow is about 250 mL O_2/min. So, it is very economical.
- *Humidification:* Intubation by passes the normal physiological mechanism for humidification of the inspired gas. But, in the circle system with a CO_2 absorber, the inspired gas will be fully saturated with water vapor nearly at a body temperature.
- *Reduction of heat loss:* Close circuit conserves the loss of heat of body. Because the soda lime gets hot during use and thus the circuit actively assists in maintaining the temperature of inspired gas and thus the patient's body temperature.
- *Ease of monitoring:* If O_2 is the only fresh gas flow into the completely closed circuit, then the patient's O_2 uptake is easily determined. Then, it is just the flow which is required to keep the volume in the circuit constant. Any change in this rate would be quickly noticed by the volume and movement of the bag. This would give an early warning of the onset of malignant hyperpyrexia. Patient's tidal volume can be assessed more accurately

by the observation of the reservoir bag in a totally closed circuit, because there is no high flow of gas to affect the bag's movement.

Disadvantages of the circle system: The major disadvantage of the circle system stems from its complex design. Misconnections, disconnections, obstructions, and leaks are the principal problems of this system. Malfunctioning of the valves can also cause serious problems. If the valves stick in an open position, then rebreathing occurs. On the other hand, if the valves are stuck closed, total occlusion of the circuit with high expiratory resistance occurs. In such circumstances, breath stacking and tension pneumothorax can occur.

N_2O in a totally closed system: The N_2O agent can be used in a totally closed system, but very cautiously and in a sophisticated manner. It is found that uptake of N_2O by body is about 500 mL/min in the first 2 minutes. Then, it falls to about 200 mL/min after 0.5 hour, and 100 mL/min after about an hour. After that, it tends to remain constant at about 50–100 mL/h, due to inevitable losses through the skin and the wound. The complete saturation of body tissues by N_2O takes about 5 hours. At the end of a 3-hour operation, during which an inspired concentration of 70% N_2O has been used, an average adult will absorb 20–26 L of N_2O, dissolved in his tissues. The fall in uptake of N_2O by the body from a closed circle system will be indicated by a gradual decrease in the inspired O_2 concentration, and the gradual increase in the inspired N_2O concentration in the circuit, which necessitates continuous readjustment of the $O_2{:}N_2O$ ratio. So, N_2O should never be used in a totally closed circuit, without O_2 and N_2O analyzer.

CARBON DIOXIDE ABSORPTION

History

The idea of CO_2 absorption techniques in anesthesia by the soda lime or other agents came from submarine and chemical warfare. It was first applied during World War I, necessitating effective gas masks. Then, in 1915, Wilson had patented new soda lime with increased efficiency. But, CO_2 absorption technique in anesthesia was slow to gain popularity, until the cyclopropane, which was then an expensive gas, was introduced in this discipline **(Box 13)**.

Chemistry

Sodalime and *Baralyme* are the two most important agents which are commonly used for CO_2 absorption in anesthesia practice. The recently introduced chemical as CO_2 absorbent is *calcium hydroxide lime* (Amsorb) and *lithium hydroxide.* Of these four agents, the most commonly used agent is soda

lime. Calcium hydroxide lime consists primarily of $Ca(OH)_2$, $Ca(Cl)_2$, and two other setting agents, such as calcium sulfate and polyvinyl pyrolidine. The latter two chemicals enhance the hardness and porosity of granules of calcium hydroxide lime and increase its efficacy. The most significant advantage of calcium hydroxide lime (*Amsorb*) over the other two agents, used for absorption of CO_2, is its lack of sodium and potassium hydroxides as its compositions. The absence of these two chemicals in calcium hydroxide lime eliminates the undesirable production of (i) carbon monoxide and (ii) nephrotoxic substance, such as compound A, by the reaction of halogenated anesthetic agents with it.

Sodalime consists of 94% $Ca(OH)_2$, 5% NaOH, and 1% KOH. But, the precise proportion of these compounds differs for different manufacturers. The composition of "best effective", and "highly moisture" soda lime is 80% $Ca(OH)_2$, 15% H_2O, 4% NaOH, and 1% KOH. Some silica is also added in it to produce calcium and sodium silicate which makes the product hard and reduces dust formation. But, the hardness and CO_2 absorption power of any agent varies inversely. In this CO_2 absorbent (soda lime), the NaOH acts as the most active component for CO_2 absorption and KOH acts as an activator. In the first step, CO_2 reacts with water to form carbonic acid which then reacts with sodium and potassium hydroxide to form sodium and potassium carbonate. This chemical change requires the presence of some moisture which is provided by patient's expired gases and at the same time produces heat. The $Ca(OH)_2$ then reacts with Na_2CO_3 and K_2CO_3 to form calcium carbonate and regenerate NaOH or KOH.

$$CO_2 + H_2O \leftrightharpoons H_2CO_3$$
$$H_2CO_3 + NaOH \text{ (or KOH)} \rightarrow Na_2CO_3 \text{ (or } K_2CO_3) + H_2O + Heat$$
$$Na_2CO_3 \text{ (or } K_2CO_3) + Ca(OH)_2 \rightarrow CaCO_3 + 2\,NaOH \text{ (or KOH)}$$

Some CO_2 directly reacts with $Ca(OH)_2$ to form **(Table 8)** calcium carbonate. But, this reaction is very slow. In early days, it was noted that soda lime could regenerate its efficacy automatically, even after being exhausted. But, the explanation for this regeneration is very complex and is of little clinical importance today. Regeneration is rarely seen nowadays. This is because of the improved quality of soda lime with less silica and addition of more potassium hydroxide.

TABLE 8: Specifications of soda lime.

Contents	$Ca(OH)_2$	94%
	NaOH	5%
	KOH	1%
Moisture		>14%
		<19%
Hardness		>75
Size of granules		4–8 mesh

TABLE 9: Different colors of indicators.

Indicators	*Soda lime*	
	Fresh	Exhausted
Mimosa-Z	Red	White
Phenolphthalein	Colorless	Pink
Clayton yellow	Pink	Yellow
Methyl orange	Orange	Yellow
Ethyl violet	Colorless	Purple (violet)

Water is required in every step of reaction, during CO_2 absorption. But, moisture which is provided to soda lime from patient's expired air does not chemically combine with it. It is probably present as a thin film of NaOH solution on the surface of $Ca(OH)_2$. The sodium and potassium hydroxide are hygroscopic, but calcium hydroxide is not. The moisture threshold of both the soda lime and baralyme for their effective absorption of CO_2 is 10%, and the optimum efficiency for the absorption of CO_2 by soda lime is obtained with hydration of 14–19%. When the soda lime is exposed to room air, then it loses its moisture and subsequently its efficacy falls rapidly. So, it must be stored properly.

Baralyme is composed of 80% $Ca(OH)_2$ and 20% $Ba(OH)_2$. It may also contain some KOH. It is more stable than soda lime and does not need any silica binder. But, it is 15% less efficient than soda lime, based on weight basis. Baralyme contains water as barium hydroxide in octa-hydrate form, i.e., $Ba(OH)_2$ 8 H_2O, on its surface. So, it may perform better in dry climate. Because of this, baralyme is more stable, when it is exposed to dry atmosphere than soda lime. For this reason, baralyme is used to absorb CO_2 in space capsule, despite it is being less efficient than soda lime. The optimum water content for best reaction of baralyme is 11–14%. The reaction of CO_2 with baralyme differs from soda lime in that more water is liberated during direct reaction of barium hydroxide with carbon dioxide. This CO_2 next reacts with water to form H_2CO_3. $Ba(OH)_2 + 8H_2O + CO_2 \rightarrow BaCO_3 + 9H_2O + Heat. H_2O + CO_2 \rightarrow H_2CO_3$

Then, by a direct reaction like with KOH and NaOH, carbonic acid (H_2CO_3) reacts with $Ca(OH)_2$ to form a carbonate. $H_2CO_3 + Ca(OH)_2 \rightarrow CaCO_3 + H_2O + Heat$

Like soda lime, baralyme too has no regeneration capability. The size of the granules of soda lime or baralyme, used in anesthesia practice, varies between 4 and 8 mesh. This is the optimum size, at which resistance to airflow is negligible. This is also the optimum size of granules, balancing between the resistance and its absorptive capability. The smaller the granules, the more is the surface area, available for absorption of CO_2, but the airflow resistance will also increase. The larger the granules, the reverse occurs.

Mesh refers to the number of openings per linear inch in a sieve, through which the granular particles can pass. A 4-mesh screen means that there are four 0.25-inch openings per linear inch. An 8-mesh screen means that there are eight 0.125-inch openings per linear inch. The hardness number of granules is 75.

Theoretically, the amount of CO_2 that should be absorbed is 26 L/100 g of absorbent (soda lime or baralyme). However, this is not true in practice, because direct channeling of gas through the granules of absorbent decreases its efficiency. Thus, it actually allows only 10–20 L of CO_2 to be absorbed with an average of only 15 L. The 100 g of soda lime will absorb about 15 L of CO_2 before the concentration of CO_2 in exit gas exceeds 1%. From this it can be calculated that 1 kg of soda lime is sufficient for 8 hours. On the other hand, the absorptive capacity of calcium hydroxide lime has been reported to be 10 L of CO_2 per 100 g of absorbent **(Table 9)**.

Like Amsorb, *lithium hydroxide* does not produce carbon monoxide and compound A. Moreover, they are believed to have more absorbing capacity than soda lime. However, they are more expensive and can cause burn to skin and respiratory tract.

Indicators

The indicators are the chemical compounds which are used to assess the functional integrity of another chemical compound. The pH indicators act on the principle of changes in pH. The pH indicator which is commonly used for both soda lime and barylime, to assess their functional integrity, is ethyl violet or tri-phenyl methane dye. The critical pH value of this indicator is 10.3. It means that above or below this pH level, the color of this indicator will change. The pH of fresh absorbent is alkaline and remains above this critical value and the ethylviolet indicator in this pH of CO_2 absorbent exists in colorless form. Ethyl-violet changes from colorless to violet when the pH of CO_2 absorbent decreases below 10.3 as a result of CO_2 absorption (acid formation). In such circumstances, the base of indicator reacts with carbonic acid, which is produced in absorbent, after absorption of CO_2 to form a soluble carbonate, which is violet in color. Indicators are not always reliable for functional status of absorbent. Fluorescent light can also deactivate the indicator, so that the absorbent appears white even though it is exhausted.

The final proof of efficacy of a particular soda lime canister's contents can only lie in periodic testing of gases, flowing through it, for the possible presence and percentage of CO_2. Examples of other indicators are: methyl orange, phenolphthalein, clayton yellow, etc.

Canister

It is a container made up of transparent plastic to see the **(Fig. 37)** changes of color of its contents such as soda lime or baralyme with indicators. It is mounted vertically in anesthetic machine. The size of a canister is no longer critical and it can be made considerably larger for a longer period of life. But, the optimum size of a canister, which is commonly used clinically, is 18 cm in height and at least 12 cm in diameter. The capacity of canister of this size is 2 L and there is an annular ring which prevents the channeling of gases between soda lime and canister wall.

The gas flow in canister is from above downward and the upper chamber is exhausted first. Once the upper chamber of canister is exhausted, the lower chamber is placed up and fresh soda lime should be placed in lower compartment, resulting in a highly efficient use of soda lime. To reduce condensation in canister and to prevent the soda lime from becoming caked, air spaces are provided at the top and at the bottom of canister. The heat which is produced inside the canister due to the absorption of CO_2 is known as the "heat of neutralization". The rise in temperature of up to 60°C has been recorded inside the canister.

The production of some heat is a sign that soda lime is functioning efficiently. There is also an overall increase in weight of the contents of canister which amounts to about 33% when they are completely worn out.

Absorbents and Anesthetic Agents

There are always some reactions between CO_2 absorbents and the newer halogenated volatile anesthetic agents. Halothane, isoflurane, sevoflurane and desflurane are all degraded to some extent by CO_2 absorbents. But among them, the most extensive degradation occurs with sevoflurane and this degradation product is called 'compound A.' There are some factors which increase this degradation products. These are:

- Higher concentration of sevoflurane
- Low fresh gas flow
- Higher temperature of absorbent
- Use of baralyme instead of soda lime
- Drying of absorbent.

The significance of these degradation products is still controversial. The CO_2 absorbents also absorb some amount of volatile anesthetic agents. So, they cause slower induction of anesthesia and later subsequent exposure of patient to these volatile anesthetic agents when their use is stopped. Dry absorbents absorb more volatile anesthetic agents, than the wet one. When the volatile anesthetic agents are used with absorbents, there is more production of carbonmonoxide (CO).

The concentration of CO increases in following condition:

- Increased length of time of use
- Dry absorbents
- Use of baralyme, instead of soda lime
- Increased concentration of anesthetic agent
- Higher temperature of absorbents.

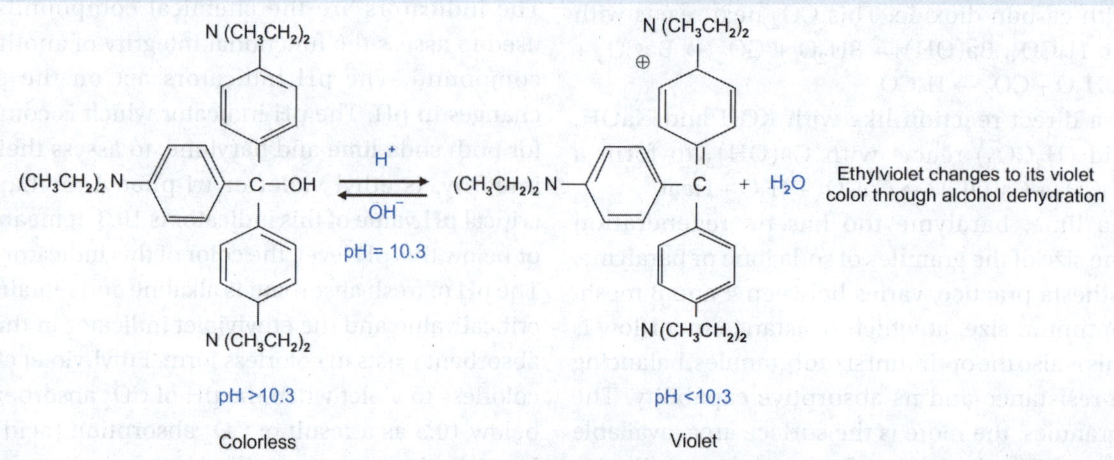

Fig. 37: The mechanism of changes of colored of soda lime.

The carbon-monoxide (CO) formation is maximum with desflurane which is followed by isoflurane. The amount of CO formed by sevoflurane and halothane is same and very little. Sevoflurane mainly produces 'compound A'. Moisture in absorbent reduces this CO formation. However, the respiratory gas monitors which are used currently cannot detect this CO directly.

Factors affecting CO_2 absorption in closed circuit:

- Freshness of soda lime.
- *Tidal volume of patient:* Tidal volume of patient should be equal or less than airspace in canister. Otherwise, large tidal volume will pass through canister without CO_2 being absorbed.
- *High flows:* High flow will allow less time for CO_2 absorption.
- *Dead space:* Increased dead space in canister will decrease CO_2 absorption.
- *Inadequate filling of soda lime:* Too loosely filled soda lime will allow gas to pass through the gap between soda lime granules and canister wall without absorption of CO_2. This is called as channeling. Too tightly filled soda lime will decrease air space and CO_2 absorption will be decreased.
- *Resistance to outflow:* Increasing the resistance to outflow permit gases to remain in contact of soda lime for more time and thus allowing more CO_2 absorption.

Induction and Nitrogen Elimination

The elimination of body N_2 by O_2 during induction is very essential. So, for the first 3–5 minutes a high flow of 100% O_2 is necessary. This will reduce the nitrogen concentration in the lungs and breathing system to <5%. Fresh 100% O_2 flow can then be reduced. Only the N_2 is dissolved in the tissues, then is diffused back into the alveolar gas. The volume of the dissolved N_2 in an average adult is approximately 1 L and it takes about 5 hours for the entire body N_2 to be abstracted. In a low flow and semi-closed system, N_2 escapes through the release valve. In a totally closed system, N_2 will accumulate and may constitute as much as 15% of the circuit gas after an hour. However, this is of no consequence, provided N_2O is not given in a totally closed system.

■ VAPORIZERS

Introduction

Most inhalational anesthetic agents, which are used today, are liquids at normal atmospheric pressure and room temperature. So, they must be converted into gas or vapor, before they are used. Vapor is the gaseous phase of a chemical agent that is liquid at room temperature and normal atmospheric pressure. Thus, a vaporizer is an instrument which is developed to change a liquid (phase of) anesthetic agent into its vapor or gaseous form (phase) and to deliver a controlled amount of this vapor or gas to the fresh gas flow. As many as three types of vaporizers are now commonly used and are attached to a modern anesthetic machine. *These three types of vaporizers are: TEC-7 vaporizer, TEC-6 vaporizer, and Aladdin cassette vaporizer.*

Simultaneously, with the development of different types of volatile anesthetic agents, different types of vaporizers also have been evolved. It has initially started from rudimentary open-mask ether inhalers. Then, it (vaporizer) passes through EMO and copper kettle vaporizer to finally reach **(Table 10)** the temperature-compensated, variable-bypass vaporizers (TEC-3/4/5/7 vaporizers). In 1993, with introduction of desflurane in anesthesia practice, even more sophisticated vaporizers (TEC-6 and Aladdin cassette vaporizer) were also introduced to handle the unique physical properties of this agent (desflurane). But, the operating principles of every vaporizer depend on some basic physical characteristics of volatile anesthetic agents. *These basic physical characteristics of volatile anesthetic agents, on which vaporizers work, are: boiling point, vapor pressure, latent heat, specific heat, and thermal conductivity.*

Physics of Vaporizers

Boiling Point and Vapor Pressure

When a volatile liquid is kept inside a container, closed to atmosphere, then few molecules of this liquid break away from the upper surface of liquid and enter the air space above it. Thus, the vapor of this liquid is formed. If the temperature of this container is kept constant, then a dynamic equilibrium is developed between the liquid phase and the vapor phase

TABLE 10: Properties of common volatile anesthetic agents important for vaporizers.

Agent	Boiling point (°C)	Vapor pressure (mm Hg)	Heat of vaporization (calorie/mL)	Specific heat of liquid (calorie/mL)	MAC in
Halothane	50.2	243	65	0.35	0.75
Isoflurane	48.5	238	63	0.35	1.15
Sevoflurane	58.6	157	–	–	2
Desflurane	22.8	669	–	–	6.4

of this liquid anesthetic agent (above its liquid surface) at that temperature. In that situation, the number of molecules in vapor phase of this volatile agent remains constant and the pressure, created by the bombardment of vapor molecules against the wall of container is also constant. *Now, the pressure of this vapor is called as the "saturated vapor pressure of this liquid anesthetic agent" at that temperature and pressure. After that, if more heat is applied to liquid, then the equilibrium is shifted more toward the vapor phase of liquid, so that the more and more molecules enter the vapor phase from the liquid phase of this liquid anesthetic agent and the vapor pressure rises.*

On the contrary, if the heat is taken away from this anesthetic liquid, then more and more molecules enter from its vapor phase into its liquid phase of this liquid anesthetic agent and vapor pressure falls. This causes the shifting of equilibrium towards liquid phase. During delivery of anesthesia, when a carrier gas (N_2O and O_2) is passed over a volatile anesthetic liquid, then the equilibrium shifts toward its vapor phase. *The saturated vapor pressure of a volatile liquid depends on the temperature and atmospheric pressure and the character of this liquid. So, it is useless to talk about the vapor pressure without mentioning the temperature and pressure. At the boiling point of a liquid, the vapor pressure and the atmospheric pressure are same at that temperature.* It means, at 100°C the number of water molecules, which are coming out of its liquid phase to gaseous phase, are such that they are capable of producing normal atmospheric pressure (760 mm Hg). At 80°C, the number of water molecules, which is coming out of its liquid phase to gaseous phase, is such that they are not capable of producing normal atmospheric pressure. If the boiling point of a liquid is 150°C, then the number of molecules of that liquid, which is coming out of its liquid phase to gaseous phase, is such that they are capable of producing normal atmospheric pressure (760 mm Hg). When pressure over a liquid is increased, the boiling point is increased. It means at that pressure (let two atmospheric pressure) and temperature (boiling point or boiling temperature), the number of molecules, which are coming out of its liquid phase to gaseous phase, are such that they are capable of producing that increased atmospheric pressure (let two atmospheric pressure).

Boiling Point

Boiling point of a liquid is defined as the temperature at which its vapor pressure becomes equal to the atmospheric pressure. Or conversely, during gradual increase in temperature of a liquid when the vapor pressure of the gaseous phase of this liquid and atmospheric pressure becomes same, then this temperature will be called as

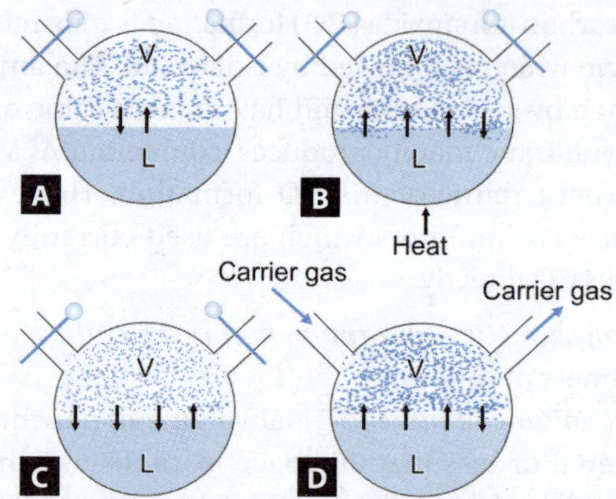

Figs. 38A to D: This figure depicts the changes in vapor pressure, with variations in temperature. (A) shows that the vapor and liquid phases are in equilibrium. (B) shows that the equilibrium shifts toward the vapor phase. Because, heat is applied and more molecules enter from the liquid into the vapor phase. (C) shows that the equilibrium shifts to the liquid phase. Because, cooling of liquid causes more molecules of vapor to enter the liquid and thus reduces the vapor pressure. (D) also shows that the equilibrium shifts to the vapor phase. This is because the carrier gas passes over the liquid. The liquid takes the energy for the molecules to break away and to form vapor. Thus, vaporization gradually removes the molecules from the liquid, which have more energy and the temperature of the liquid falls, as vaporization proceeds. So, a gradient of temperature will be created between the liquid with the surroundings, and heat will flow from the surroundings to the liquid. This heat is called the heat of vaporization. It is defined as the number of calories necessary to convert 1 mL of liquid into vapor.

the boiling point of this liquid. The lower the atmospheric pressure, the lower will be the boiling point and higher the atmospheric pressure, the higher will be the boiling point **(Figs. 38A to D)**.

Concentration of Gases

To express the concentration of a gas or vapor in a mixture of gases, two methods are commonly used. These are: partial pressure in mm Hg or volume in percent (%). A mixture of many gases in a closed container will exert a total constant pressure on the walls of it (container). A part of this total pressure, which is exerted on the wall of the container by an individual gas in the mixture, is called as the partial pressure of that individual gas in this mixture. Hence, the total pressure of the gas mixture is the sum of the partial pressures of each of the constituent gases. Now, the partial pressure of an individual gas depends on the concentration of that gas in this gaseous mixture and these parameters are directly proportional.

Volume in percent, to express the concentration of a gas in a mixture of gases, is defined as the number of units of volume of a particular gas in relation to the total 100 units of volume of total gas mixture. In a mixture of gases, each constituent gas exerts pressure which is directly proportional to its percentage of volume of that gas in the total volume of mixture, i.e., concentration of that gas in total mixture. The volume percent (%) expresses the relative ratio of volume out of total 100% volume of different gases in a gas mixture. Whereas, partial pressure of a gas expresses an absolute value. Partial pressure ÷ Total pressure = volumes percent ÷ 100.

Although, the concentration of an anesthetic gas or a vapor in a mixture is most commonly expressed as volume in percent, but patient uptake or the depth of anesthesia caused by an anesthetic gas are directly related to the partial pressure of that anesthetic gas in inspired gas mixture or in alveoli of lungs.

Latent Heat

Latent heat of vaporization is defined as the number of calories, required to change 1 g of liquid into vapor, but without any change in its temperature. This latent heat for vaporization comes from the liquid itself, or from outside sources. In the absence of outside energy (heat) sources, the surrounding air gives the required heat to anesthetic liquid for its vaporization. So, the water vapor in air condenses outside the Boyle's vaporizing glass ether bottle and Goldman vaporizer which are not used now in modern anesthetic machine. Thus, the temperature of an anesthetic liquid falls and vaporization is reduced.

Specific Heat

The specific heat of a substance is the number of calories (heat), required to increase the temperature of 1 g of that substance by 1°C. The concept of specific heat is important for the design and construction (metal) of vaporizers by the following two ways:

1. It (specific heat) indicates how much heat should be supplied to the anesthetic liquid to maintain a constant temperature when the heat is lost during vaporization.
2. Manufacturers select the metal to build a vaporizers that have a high specific heat. Because, it will supply more heat to minimize the decrease in temperature, associated with vaporization.

Thermal Conductivity

The thermal conductivity of a metal is defined as the speed with which the heat flows through this substance (metal). Vaporizers are made of metals of high thermal conductivity which helps to maintain a uniform temperature.

Types of Vaporizers

The vaporizers are classified according to the table **(Box 14)**.

BOX 14: Classification of different vaporizers.

According to method of vaporization
- Open drop
- Bubble through
- Flow over
- Injection

According to the regulation of output concentration
- Concentration calibrated
- Bypass flow calibrated

According to the compensation of temperature
- Thermocompensation
- Supplied heat

Open Mask

The basic requirement of all the anesthetic vaporizers is that they should convert the volatile liquid anesthetic agents into a continuous flow of vapor of this anesthetic liquid. Then, it is mixed with air or some other carrier gases under controlled conditions (concentration). The simplest form of vaporizer is a gauze pad which is usually fitted on a wire frame. It acts as wick and a partial reservoir of volatile anesthetic liquid. The patient's respiration (inspiration) through this gauze pad, which is soaked with a liquid volatile anesthetic agent, results in a continuous flow of anesthetic vapor which is present at saturated vapor pressure level near the gauze. But, it is subsequently diluted as air is entrained, passing though the gauze. The temperature of anesthetic liquid in gauze pad will drop below the atmospheric level, because the heat required for vaporization will be greater than that available from the immediately surrounding air. Some control of this situation can be obtained by controlling the rate, at which the anesthetic liquid is dropped onto the gauze of mask, and the distance between the gauze pad and patient's face (i.e., the amount of diluting air that is entrained). It is also fortunate that the main agent administered by open-mask is diethyl ether which does not dramatically depress the respiration **(Figs. 39A and B)**.

Uncalibrated Vaporizers

When the use of compressed anesthetic gases in metal cylinders was introduced into anesthesia practice, then it became necessary to contain the liquid anesthetic agents into bottle. Then, it also became necessary to bubble the anesthetic carrier gases through this liquid anesthetic agents, or to blow it (anesthetic carrier gases) over its (liquid anesthetic agents) surface for vaporization. Thus, this bottle or container, containing liquid anesthetic agent, is called as the vaporizer. This simple vaporizer is sometimes also called as *plenum vaporizer*. Because, gas is being forced into a

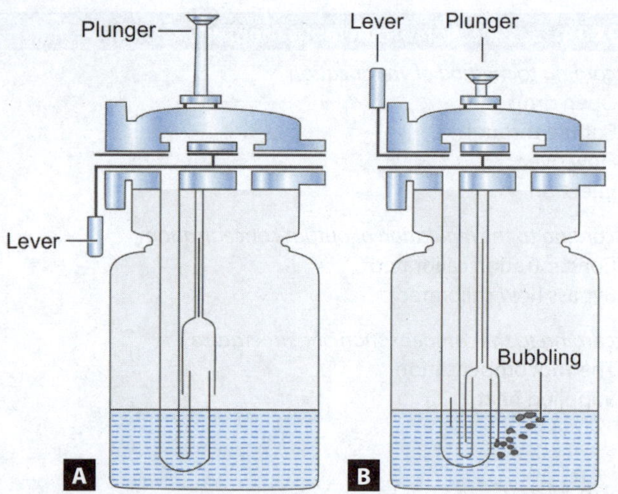

Figs. 39A and B: This figure shows uncalibrated vaporizers. (A) The cowl is not fully impinged in the liquid, so it is a Blow-Over type of vaporizer. (B) The cowl is fully impinged in the liquid, so it is a Bubble-Through type of vaporizer.

chamber or container and plenum is a chamber or container in which pressure is greater than outside.

Simple glass bottle ether vaporizer is the ideal example of uncalibrated plenum vaporizer. In old Boyle's anesthetic machine, such *simple uncalibrated, plenum, glass bottle vaporizer is used for anesthetic liquid ether*. Here, the stream of fresh gas flow which is directed to patient is divided into two, after coming out of rota meter. The main bypass stream of FGF passes straight to machine outlet, without coming into contact with anesthetic liquid, present in glass bottle which is called here as vaporizer. The second bypass stream of FGF is allowed to pass over the surface or is allowed to bubble through the liquid anesthetic agent, kept in vaporizing glass bottle and is reunited with the main bypass stream. The ratio of main bypass stream of FGF, not passing through vaporizing chamber and second bypass stream of FGF, passing through vaporizing chamber is determined by the position of control knob.

Again, the position of plunger and control knob, manipulated by anesthesiologist will determine how closely the stream of carrier gas will pass over the surface of liquid anesthetic (blow-over) agent or whether it actually bubbles through anesthetic liquid. In this kind of simple vaporizers, the control of splitting ratio of carrier gas by the control knob, is not accurate. It is usually very nonlinear and there is wide variation between different instruments. Also, as the latent heat of vaporization (for vaporization of liquid anesthetic agent) is taken from this liquid anesthetic agent, glass bottle and environment, so there is also cooling of liquid anesthetic agent, which will reduce vaporization, resulting in low vapor concentration with passing of time. A number of factors, such

as gas flow rate, volume of liquid in bottle and atmospheric temperature also influence the rate of vaporization.

So, the resulting concentration of anesthetic vapor, received by patient, cannot be predicted with accuracy, as it will not match with the number of position of control knob. Agitation of vaporizing bottle, due to any cause, will produce increase in vapor concentration, even without bubbling. Finally, when the bottle is not used for long time, then the total internal gas space over the volatile anesthetic liquid becomes filled with saturated anesthetic vapor. Then, the initial concentration of anesthetic agent, when the control lever is first turned on, will be unexpectedly dangerously high. This happens particularly when the bottle is surrounded by warm water bath, which is sometimes done, to avoid the reduction in anesthetic vapor concentration, produced by cooling of both liquid and bottle.

Though, there are considerable drawbacks, still the widespread use of these types of uncalibrated vaporizers indicates their relative safety. Their safety feature lies in the fact that the anesthetic vapor concentration falls with time due to cooling of anesthetic liquid. Since, the concentration of vapor, they produce, is not accurately known, so its anesthetic effect can only be estimated by noting the volume of anesthetic liquid being used (vaporized) and close continuous observation of patient.

The *Goldman halothane vaporizer* is another example of this type of very simple uncalibrated plenum vaporizer, which is most commonly used, even today, for halothane in less sophisticated machine and all the physics, which is discussed till now, should also be applied here. Actually, it was designed for use in an intermittent flow machine. It can also be used inside a circle anesthetic system. It has a small volume. It offers a low resistance to gas flow, because it was initially intended for use during spontaneous respiration. It is an inefficient vaporizer without temperature compensation. The maximum halothane output of this vaporizer is about 3%. It has also been used successfully in a totally closed anesthesia circuit.

Oxford vaporizer (Fig. 40)

This vaporizer is discussed, here, only for its historical interest. It was developed by Robert Macintosh, in collaboration with Morris Motors, for use by the Armed Forces, in 1940. To increase the concentration of ether vapor the condensation of moisture outside the ether bottle, during its vaporization at the expense of latent heat, can be prevented by placing a jacket of warm water around the ether glass bottle. Alternatively, the ether can be kept constantly above its boiling point (36.5°C), so that the ether vapor in

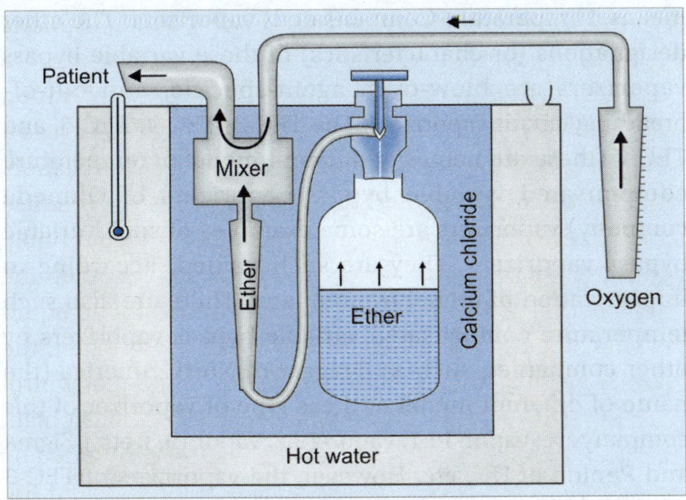

Fig. 40: Oxford vaporizer.

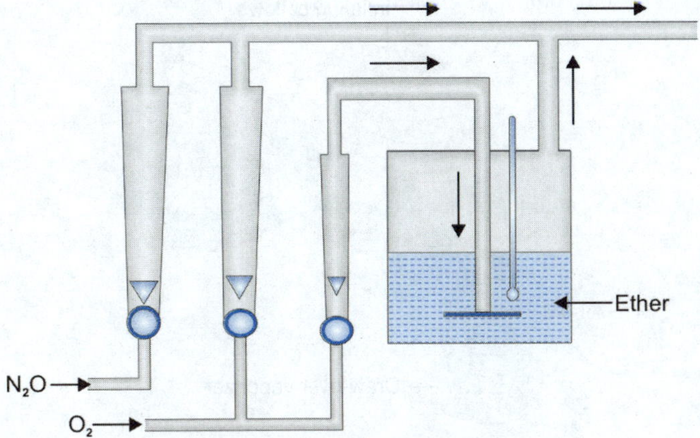

Fig. 41: A copper kettle vaporizer.

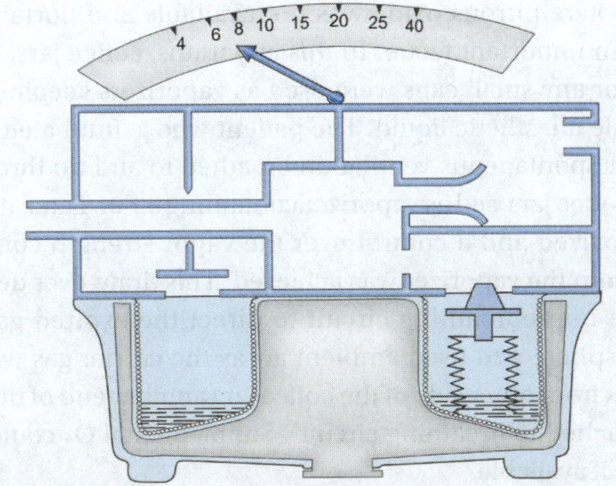

Fig. 42: Epstein Macintosh Oxford (EMO) vaporizer.

container is under pressure and is trying to escape. Then, a fixed amount of ether vapor, controlled by a knob, is allowed to come out and is mixed with carrier gas, to obtain a known percentage of ether vapor which is delivered to patient. This principle was used in the construction of Oxford vaporizers. Here, ether was surrounded by chemical crystals of calcium chloride with a melting point above that of ether, which was again surrounded by warm water. Once these crystals melted due to warm water, ether vapor would come out spontaneously.

Copper Kettle Vaporizer (Fig. 41)

This was commonly used in the past at North America. It is also discussed here for historical interest. In this type of vaporizer an O_2 supply, separate from the main supply, is metered, and is passed through a copper vessel (for rapid heat transfer) containing a liquid anesthetic agent. The gas passes through a fenestrated bronze disk which breaks it up into very fine bubbles. Thus, the gas becomes fully saturated during its passage through the anesthetic liquid. The temperature of the anesthetic liquid is measured by a thermometer. From the graph of saturated vapor pressure against this temperature, the concentration of the anesthetic vapor coming out from the vaporizer can be calculated. Now the volume of gas passing through the vaporizer fully saturated with anesthetic vapor is known. So, the final concentration of anesthetic vapor in the mixture reaching the patient can be simply calculated. It may be adjusted finely as required by changing the gas flow rate through the vaporizer. This type of vaporizer is capable of a high degree of accuracy than the simple Boyle's glass bottle vaporizer. The same apparatus may be used for all the types of volatile anesthetic agents.

Draw-over Vaporizers

Any vaporizer where the inspired gases is drawn over the surface of a volatile anesthetic liquid which is kept in a container and offers sufficiently low resistance (1–2 cmH$_2$O is a satisfactory figure) to gas flow at a normal respiratory flow rate, may be called as a draw-over **(Fig. 42)** vaporizer. The patient inspires air via the vaporizer and expiration is directed to the atmosphere by a nonrebreathing valve. A simple tin can, filled with an anesthetic liquid, through which a patient inspires air, may be used as a draw-over vaporizer. A vaporizer, which has been specially designed for this purpose, is Epstein Macintosh Oxford (EMO) vaporizer. In this vaporizer, ether is used as anesthetic agent. In this system a tank of water is used as a heat reservoir and the temperature compensation is made by a bellows filled with ether. It can be combined with an Oxford inflating bellows for IPPV. When the plunger is not dipped in anesthetic liquid, then the uncalibrated glass bottle ether vaporizer, used in old Boyle's machine, also acts as the draw-over type of vaporizer.

Draw-over apparatus **(Fig. 43):** This equipment was developed during the First World War, especially for field

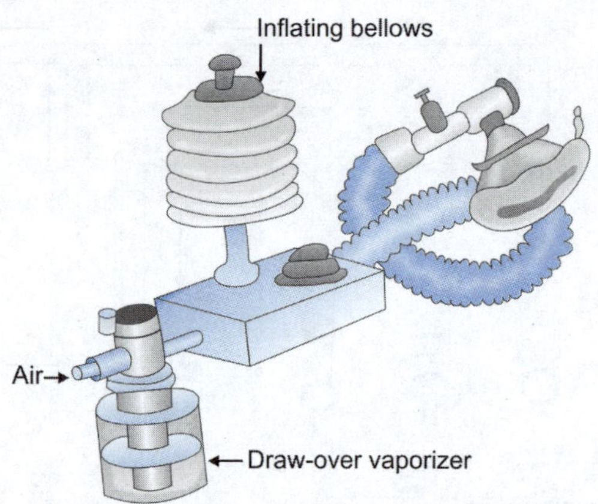

Fig. 43: Draw-over apparatus.

use where nitrous oxide was not available and portability was an important factor. In this apparatus, coffee jars, food tins, or any small cans were used as vaporizers keeping the volatile anesthetic liquid. The patient who is intubated and under spontaneous ventilation breathed to and fro through this coffee jar used as vaporizer containing ether. Later, it was improvized and a control over the vapor strength coming out from the vaporizer was achieved. This draw-over device had a nonrebreathing circuit to direct the expired gas to atmosphere and used ambient air as the carrier gas which enters from other side of the coffee jar (another end of the jar is attached to breathing circuit). Supplemental O_2 could be used, if available.

In its most basic application, air is drawn through a low resistance draw-over vaporizer which may be made of a glass bottle or coffee jar, food tins, or any small can which was used in First World War. For vaporization, a suitable low resistance vaporizer, such as the EMO vaporizer may also be placed in the circuit instead of food tins. The device can be fitted with connections and equipment that allow IPPV as well as CPAP and PEEP with a scavenging system. The N_2O can never be used with draw-over devices. Patients often manifest an oxygen saturation (SpO_2) <90%. This can be treated with supplemental O_2, attached to a T-piece at the upstream side of the vaporizer. Across the clinical range of tidal volume and respiratory rate, an O_2 flow rate of 1 L/min gives FiO_2 of 30– 40% or with 4 L/min FiO_2 of 60–80%. The greatest advantage of the draw-over system is its simplicity and portability. But, the main disadvantage is the absence of a reservoir bag. So, the depth of the tidal volume is not well appreciated during spontaneous ventilation.

Variable Bypass Vaporizers

The variable bypass vaporizer is also called as concentration-calibrated, direct-reading, dial-controlled, automatic-planum, percentage-type, and TEC-type (TEC type means TEmperature Compensated) vaporizers. The other designations (or characteristics) of these variable bypass vaporizers are blow-over, agent-specific, and out-of-breathing circuit vaporizers. The TEC-3, TEC-4, TEC-5, and TEC-7 (these are names of different model of temperature compensated variable bypass vaporizers of Ohmeda company) vaporizers are some examples of such variable bypass vaporizers. They are such named, according to improvization of model by company. There are also such temperature compensated variable bypass vaporizers by other companies, such as Dragger of North America (the name of different model of these type of vaporizer of this company are: Vapor-19.1, Vapor-19.2, Vapor 19.3, etc.), Sigma and Penlon of UK, etc. However, the vaporizers of TEC-3 model of Ohmeda and similar model of other companies, such as: Flutec Mark-3, Fortec-3, Enfluratec-3, Sevotec-III, etc. are no longer manufactured at present.

The term *"variable bypass"* refers to the method of regulating the output of vapor of volatile anesthetic agent in different concentration. When the delivered gas, after rota meter, flows through vaporizer's inlet, then the setting of concentration control dial of vaporizer determines the ratio of flow that goes through bypass channel without entering the channel that goes through vaporizing chamber. The gas, which is channeled through vaporizing chamber, flows over the surface of liquid anesthetic agent, and becomes saturated with the vapor of anesthetic liquid. So, the term "blow-over" is referred to the method of vaporization in these variable bypass type of vaporizers (in contrast to bubble-through type of vaporization in Copper Kettle). The term "temperature-compensated" is applied to this type of vaporizer, because every vaporizer is equipped with an automatic temperature compensating device that helps to maintain a constant vaporizer output concentration of volatile anesthetic agent over a wide range of temperature variation. The mechanism is discussed in Chapter 1 and in this chapter. All these types of vaporizers are agent specific, because all the volatile anesthetic agents have their own different vapor pressure at certain temperature. So, the control dial, controlling the entry of carrier gas into vaporizing chamber and then thus subsequently controlling the concentration of output of anesthetic agent is marked accordingly. Hence, they are designed to accommodate a single agent and any agent cannot be used in any vaporizer. However, desflurane cannot be used by this variable bypass type of vaporizers, the cause of which is explained later. These variable bypass vaporizers are usually calibrated using O_2 as the carrier gas. But, even if air is used instead of O_2 then there is no change in output also. On the other hand, addition of N_2O as a carrier gas results in change of vaporizer output **(Fig. 44)**.

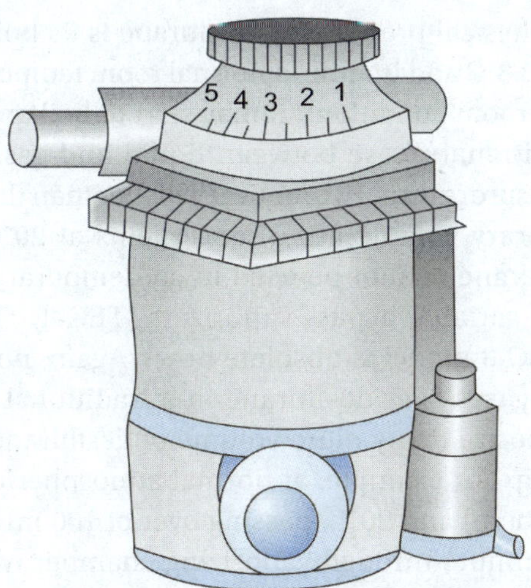

Fig. 44: Tec-3 halothane vaporizer.

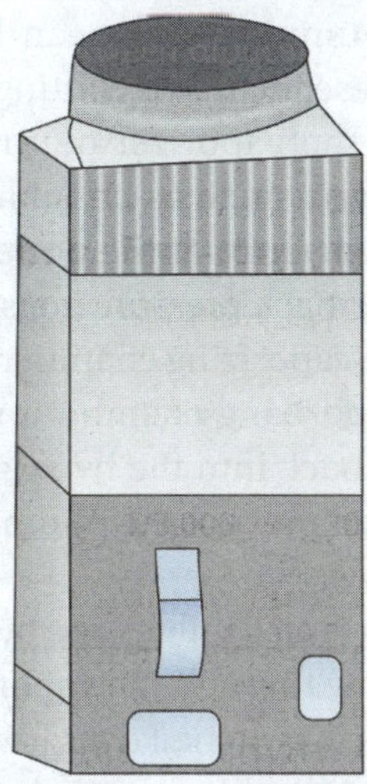

Fig. 45: Tec-5 vaporizer specific for isoflurane, halothane, and sevoflurane.

These vaporizers are also called as level-compensated vaporizers. Because, one of the causes of variability of output from a simple vaporizers, which is not level compensated, is the change in the level of anesthetic liquid in vaporizer, as it is used up. To prevent this variability of output, with the change in the level of anesthetic liquid in vaporizer, these level-compensated vaporizers use wicks. If the vaporizing chamber contains wicks which are constantly wetted by contact with anesthetic agent, then not only the vaporization will be more efficient, but the output will also be constant (apart from temperature effect) until the level of the liquid anesthetic falls so low that the wicks are no longer wetted. The vaporizer using wicks in this way is described as the level-compensated vaporizer **(Fig. 45)**.

The vapor pressure of a particular volatile anesthetic agent depends on the temperature. For example, at 20°C the vapor pressure of isoflurane is 238 mm Hg, whereas at 35°C the vapor pressure of isoflurane is 450 mm Hg (almost double). So, at a fixed dial setting with variation of temperature, the output of the anesthetic gas will also vary. So, all the modern vaporizers should be temperature-compensated to keep the outflow constant by regulating the gas entry into the vaporizer. Actually, the temperature compensating devices are bimetallic strips. At an increased temperature, this bimetallic strip changes its shape and moves in one direction.

This movement allows more flow to pass through the bypass chamber, and less flow to pass through the vaporizing chamber. On the other hand, when the temperature falls due to vaporization of the liquid anesthetic, the opposite occurs. Thus, the net effect is a constant vaporizer output. So, vapor pressure at a certain fixed temperature which is a physical principle of individual anesthetic agents is important for a constant vaporizer output.

At 760 mm Hg pressure (normal atmospheric pressure), the boiling point of desflurane, isoflurane, halothane, and sevoflurane are approximately 22.8°C, 48.5°C, 50.2°C, and 58.5°C, respectively. Desflurane boils at a temperature that may be encountered at normal room conditions. So, this unique physical characteristic alone mandates a special vaporizer (Tec-6) for desflurane to vaporise and control the delivery of that agent. From the above discussion it is clear that the output of an individual volatile agent depends on its vapor pressure and the temperature. Thus, the resetting dial is graduated accordingly depending on vapor pressure of that agent. So, every vaporizer is agent specific.

Though these variable bypass vaporizers have many advantages, but still they have some limitations. These limitations are: noncompensated for flow-rate, noncompensated for intermittent back pressure, and dependent on the carrier gas composition. As these variable bypass vaporizers are not flow-rate compensated so the output variation of the volatile anesthetic agent is particularly noticeable at the extremes of flow rate. The output from these types of vaporizers is less than the dial setting, when the flow rate is <250 mL/min. Similarly, at an extremely high flow rate (15 L/min) the output is also less than the dial setting.

Intermittent back pressure during IPPV or O_2 flushing can cause lower or higher vaporizer output than the dial setting. This phenomenon is called the pumping effect. The pumping effect is more pronounced at low flow rates, low dial setting, low level of liquid anesthetic agent in the vaporizing chamber, high respiratory rate, and high peak inspired pressure. The proposed mechanism for this pumping effect is the retrograde pressure transmission from the patient's circuit to the inside of the vaporizer during the inspiratory phase of positive pressure ventilation, i.e., when the bag is compressed.

However, this pumping effect can be minimized in a number of ways. These include the fitting of a small pressure regulating valve at the vaporizer output and keeping the vaporizing chamber as small as possible. The Tec-3 model has a controlling resistance at the outlet of the vaporizing chamber, so that the back pressure goes around the bypass and not through the vaporizing chamber. In addition, a long inlet pipe to the vaporizing chamber prevents vapor from the chamber to get back into the bypass gas stream by this route. This method to prevent the pumping effect is used in the *Draeger vaporizer.*

Vaporizer output is also influenced by the composition of carrier gases that flow through the vaporizers. For example, when the carrier gas is switched over from 100% O_2 to 100% N_2O, then there is a rapid transient decrease in vaporizer output due to slow vaporization of anesthetic liquid followed by a slow increase to a new steady state value. This is because other than temperature, atmospheric pressure, and character of anesthetic liquid. The vaporization of an anesthetic liquid depends on the composition of gas that blows over it. Most vaporizers are calibrated using O_2 as the carrier gas. Generally, a little change in output occurs if air is substituted for O_2. Addition of N_2O to the carrier gas typically results in both a temporary and a long-lasting effect on vaporizer output. The temporary effect is usually a decrease in vapor concentration. The duration of this effect depends on the gas flow rate and the volume of liquid in the vaporizer. The permanent effect may be an increase or decrease, depending on the construction of the vaporizer **(Fig. 46)**.

TEC-6 Vaporizer

It is a different kind of variable bypass vaporizer and is only used for desflurane for its peculiar physical properties. This peculiar physical property of desflurane is its boiling point which is 22.8°C and is around normal room temperature. So, in normal room conditions, it may start to boil and remains in a transitional phase between liquid and gas. Thus, its vapor pressure is three to four times higher than that of other contemporary volatile anesthetic agents at 20°C. That is why desflurane cannot be used in contemporary different models of variable bypass vaporizers (TEC-4, TEC-5, and TEC-7; TEC-3 model is obsolete now). Again, normal flow of carrier gases over desflurane in a traditional vaporizer would vaporize many more volume of desflurane than the dial setting. For example, at normal atmospheric pressure (1 atmosphere) and 20°C, passing over of 100 mL of carrier gas for 1 minute through vaporizing chamber will entrain 735 mL/min of desflurane vapor in comparison to 46 and 47 mL/min of isoflurane and halothane vapor, respectively. This is due to difference in vapor pressure at 20°C of desflurane, isoflurane, and halothane which is 669, 240, 244 mm Hg, respectively. Under the same condition, the amount of bypass flow to dilute the flow which is coming over anesthetic fluid and necessary to achieve 1% concentration of an anesthetic desflurane output is approximately 73 L/min, compared to 5 L/min for isoflurane, halothane, and sevoflurane.

The MAC value of desflurane is 6–7 which is four to nine times higher than the commonly used volatile anesthetic agents. So, the absolute amount of desflurane, needed over a given period of time, is considerably higher than other volatile anesthetic agents. Thus, the supplying of desflurane in higher concentration causes excessive cooling of vaporizer. So, in the absence of an external heating source, the temperature compensation by using traditional temperature compensated variable bypass vaporizer, where simple bimetallic strip is used is almost impossible. Hence, Tec-6 vaporizer requires an external electrical source for heat.

The TEC-6 vaporizer is also flow-compensated. So, at a specific dial setting with different fresh gas flow rates, vaporizer output is constant (other variable bypass vaporizers are only temperature-compensated but not flow-compensated. Actually, the traditional vaporizers are flow compensated in certain limited range such as 250 mL/min–15 L/min). Thus, to conclude we can say that the TEC-6 vaporizer is an electrically heated, temperature and flow compensated, pressurized, electromechanically coupled, and dual-circuit vaporizer. This is not a blow-over type of vaporizer (other all TECs are blow-over type of vaporizer).

In Tec-6 vaporizer, two circuits for gas flow are used (dual circuit). One circuit carries the main gas flow (carrier gas) without any bypass chamber. In another circuit, there is a container which contains the desflurane in vapor

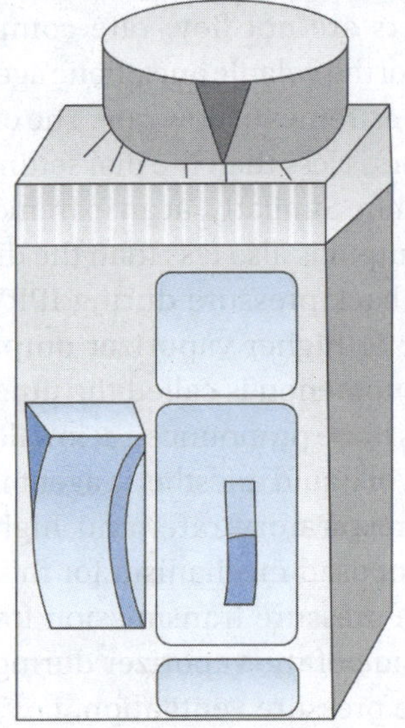

Fig. 46: Tec-6 vaporizer (specific for desflurane).

phase. This is done by heating the desflurane electrically and controlling thermostatically at 39°C (a temperature well above the desflurane boiling point). Then the output flow and concentration of desflurane vapor is controlled electronically and is mixed with the main carrier gas flow at the main vaporizer outlet.

- Cassette pressure censor
- Cassette temperature censor
- Cassette flow censor
- *CPU:* Central processing unit.

Aladdin Cassette Vaporizer (Fig. 47)

It is a very sophisticated and electronically-controlled vaporizer which is designed to deliver five different types of volatile anesthetic agents, including halothane, enflurane, isoflurane, sevoflurane, and desflurane. This type of vaporizer has two main components: (1) a permanent internal control unit or anesthetic delivery unit (ADU) and (2) an interchangeable Aladdin agent specific cassette unit that contains the volatile anesthetic liquids.

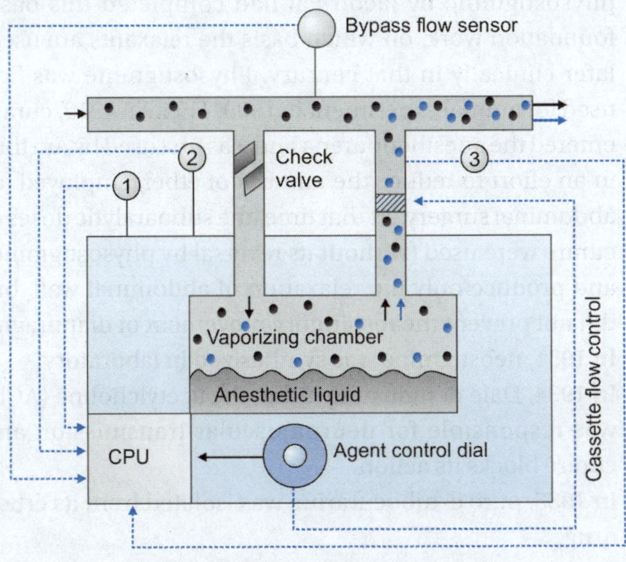

Fig. 47: Aladdin's cassette vaporizer.

Aladdin agent-specific cassettes are color-coded, so that the control unit (ADU component) can identify the specific anesthetic cassette (containing specific anesthetic agent) which is inserted. The heart of control unit has an electronically regulated flow-control valve, located at vaporizing chamber outlet. This electronically regulated flow-control valve is controlled by a computer [central processing unit (CPU)] which receives information from multiple sources, such as (i) agent's concentration control dial, located by the side of CPU and set by an anesthetist, (ii) a pressure sensor, located inside the vaporizing chamber, (iii) a temperature sensor, located inside the vaporizing chamber, (iv) a flow measurement unit, located in bypass chamber, (v) a flow measurement unit, located at the outlet of vaporizing chamber, and (vi) a gas analyzer, analyzing the composition of carrier gas. Using data from all these multiple sources, the CPU of vaporizer is able to precisely regulate the flow control valve to attain the desired output of vapor concentration of anesthetic agent.

Technically, the Aladdin cassette vaporizer is a combination of Tec-4, -5, and -7 variable bypass vaporizers, along with the Tec-6 vaporizer and a computer. When desflurane is not used in Aladdin vaporizer, then the carrier gas passes over the anesthetic liquid in cassette and vaporizer works like blow-over type (like Tec-4, -5, and -7 vaporizers). But, all the parameters are controlled by the computer. On the other hand, when desflurane is used, then Aladdin works like Tec-6 vaporizer, where carrier gas does not pass over anesthetic liquid. The bypass chamber is cut off from the cassette containing desflurane and the whole unit works as dual circuit (like Tec-6). One circuit carries carrier gas and another circuit carries desflurane anesthetic vapor from cassette, where like in Tec-6 the desflurane is always kept in a vapor form by a computer-controlled electronically heating system at 39°C. Now, the flow and output of concentration of desflurane is under computer control and at outlet it mixes with carrier gas.

Muscle Relaxants and their Antagonists

■ HISTORY

- The hint of the presence of these types of drugs, such as curare or nondepolarizing muscle relaxants, first came to the ears of the world, in 1596, when Sir Walter Raleigh mentioned an *"arrow poison"* in his book named *"Discovery of the Large, Rich and Beautiful Empire of Guiana"*.
- Then 200 years later, in 1812, Sir Benjamin first showed that the life of animals could be maintained (continued) by artificial respiration, after they were paralyzed or curarized by arrow poison. His source of curare was the bark, leaves, or vines of a tree named *Chondrodendron tomentosum*, growing near Amazon. Also, before that it had long been used by Amazonian Indians to poison the heads of arrow (arrow poison) for hunting of animals. Later on, they transported this poison to the different parts of the world in bamboo tubes, from where the name *tubocurarine (curare in tube)* was derived.
- Curare was first brought to the Europe by Charles Waterton. He also described a classic experiment, in which he kept alive a curarized she-ass by artificial ventilation with bellows and a tube, introduced through a tracheostomy wound.
- Then, in 1850, the great French physiologist named, Claude Bernard had laid the most important scientific foundation stone, regarding the muscle relaxant. He demonstrated that curare acts by paralyzing the myoneural junction. Later, this led to the discovery of concept of motor endplate.
- During this period, George Harley also showed that curare can be used as an antidote to the convulsion of strychnine poisoning.
- After that, in 1858, a decade after the anesthetic use of ether, Lewis Albert used curare and artificial verification through a tracheostomy wound to treat the muscular rigidity of tetanus in New York.

- Then, in 1862, curare was first used in American Civil War as chemical weapon.
- After that another foundation stone of anesthesia was laid in 1864, when physostigmine was isolated from the calabar bean, by Sir TR Fraser. But, at that time, he was not aware of the anticurare action of physostigmine.
- Then, in 1900, the discovery of anticurare action of physostigmine by Jacob Pal had completed this basic foundation work, on which basis the relaxants are used, later clinically in that century. Physostigmine was first used for animal experiment in 1909. Then, in 1912, curare entered the anesthetic arena and was first used by Aurthur in an effort to reduce the amount of ether, employed for abdominal surgery. At that time, the subparalytic doses of curare were used (without its reversal by physostigmine) and produce only the relaxation of abdominal wall, but did not prevent the respiratory movement of diaphragm.
- In 1931, neostigmine was synthesized in laboratory.
- In 1934, Dale demonstrated that the acetylcholine (ACh) was responsible for neuromuscular transmission and curare blocks its action.
- In 1935, pure d-tubocurarine was isolated from its crude drug.
- On January 23rd of 1942, at Montreal of Canada, appendectomy was done under cyclopropane anesthesia, where d-tubocurarine was first used through IV route, deliberately to give skeletal muscle relaxation during surgery. This was a famous day in the history of anesthesia. During this period, the muscle relaxant was used with the idea to provide a greatly relaxed surgical field, without the need for large doses of hypnotics and opiate drugs. Thus, the cardiovascular side effects of these anesthetic agents could be minimized and allowed the very sick patients to get the benefit of surgery.
- The first reported use of curare, in routine anesthesia practice, was from Britain in 1945.

- Gallamine was first used in 1948.
- In 1948, decamethonium was also described.
- In 1952, succinylcholine or suxamethonium was first used as muscle relaxant and had revolutionized the anesthesia practice.
- In 1958, alcuronium was first described and used in man.
- In 1967, pancuronium had first come into the anesthetic arena.
- In 1980, atracurium and vecuronium had further revolutionized the clinical anesthetic practice.
- The early 1990 had witnessed the introduction of pipecuronium and doxacurium.
- Mivacurium was introduced in 1993 and rocuronium in 1994.

CHEMISTRY OF MUSCLE RELAXANT

According to chemical structure, most of the muscle relaxants have two positive charged N^+ atoms. So, they mimic the quaternary nitrogen (N^+) atom of ACh which acts as neuromuscular transmitter at motor endplate. This is the main reason for the attraction of the molecules of muscle relaxing agents to the cholinergic or ACh (nicotinic) receptors at the motor endplate, like ACh. The cholinergic or ACh receptors are broadly classified as muscarinic and nicotinic type. In peripheral nervous system, the nicotinic receptors are found postsynaptically at neuromuscular junction and at autonomic ganglia. On the other hand, the muscarinic receptors are found at all the postganglionic parasympathetic nerve endings and some postganglionic sympathetic nerve endings, such as sweat gland, erector pile, etc. The muscle relaxants act on the postsynaptic nicotinic receptors at neuromuscular junction and autonomic ganglion. Most modern muscle relaxants are specific for these nicotinic receptors at motor endplate with limited effects on other cholinergic receptors (both nicotinic and muscarinic receptors), found at peripheral nervous system, autonomic ganglia, and parasympathetic effector organs. As all the neuromuscular blocking agents have a quaternary ammonium structure, containing nitrogen (N^+) atom, so these are maximally ionized at the physiological pH and therefore penetrate the blood-brain barrier poorly **(Table 1)**.

The two positive charged N^+ atoms in a molecule of muscle-relaxing agent are separated by a bridging structure which is lipophilic in nature. This bridging structure is different in size for different muscle relaxant molecules and is the major determinant factor for the potency and other the pharmacokinetic properties of these group of drugs. *Most of the muscle relaxing agents are highly water soluble. This is due to the positive charge of their molecules and contain various O_2 bearing group. Because of their water solubility, most of the muscle relaxing agents are easily excreted through urine by glomerular filtration and are generally not reabsorbed through renal tubules. The high-water solubility of muscle relaxants also prevents their passage through the lipoid blood-brain barrier, placental barrier, and lipoid cell membrane of most of the cells, such as renal tubular cells, hepatocytes, nerve cells, muscle cells, etc.*

Except few steroidal muscle relaxants, most are not metabolized by liver, due to two reasons: (i) the water solubility of most of the muscle relaxants inhibits their uptake by the hepatocytes, and (ii) the cytochrome p-450 oxidative enzyme system in liver microsome requires lipophilic substrates for

TABLE 1: The cholinergic receptors and its sites and the action of muscle relaxants on it.

Receptors	Location	Function	Relaxant—interactions
Nicotinic	Postsynaptic neuromuscular junction	Depolarization of endplate–muscle contraction	• Succinylcholine—stimulates • Nondepolarizers—block
Nicotinic	Presynaptic neuromuscular junction	Helps to release of ACh	• Succinylcholine—stimulates • Nondepolarizers—block
Nicotinic	Autonomic ganglion	Depolarization of ganglionic cell	• Succinylcholine—stimulates • Nondepolarizer—block
Nicotinic	Postganglionic neurons terminal	Positive feedback for transmitter release	• Succinylcholine—stimulates • Nondepolarizers—block
Muscarinic	SA node of heart	↓ Heart rate	• Succinylcholine stimulates— ↓ Heart rate (HR) • Nondepolarizers block—↑ HR
Muscarinic (M_1)	• Autonomic ganglionic • Interneuron cell bodies	Inhibition of depolarization	Nondepolarizers—block
Muscarinic (M_2)	Autonomic ganglia: Ganglion cell bodies	Depolarization	• Atropine blocks • Nondepolarizers do not act.

their metabolism. The muscle relaxants, used in anesthesia practice, are broadly classified under two headings according to their mode of action. These are *depolarizing muscle relaxants and nondepolarizing muscle relaxants.* Among the depolarizing group of muscle relaxants, there are many drugs, but succinylcholine is only and mostly used clinically.

SUCCINYLCHOLINE OR SUXAMETHONIUM (DIACETYLCHOLINE)

Succinylcholine is a quaternary ammonium compound. It is entirely a synthetic product. In contrast to the heavy bulky rigid molecules of nondepolarizing muscle relaxants, the structure of this depolarizing molecule is long, thin, and flexible. *It is made up of two ACh molecules, which are linked back-to-back. Like ACh, it also depolarizes the postsynaptic membrane. But, its effect on motor endplate is more persistent than that of ACh. However, though the action of succinylcholine is like that of ACh, such as muscular contraction, but the prolonged action of it on nicotinic receptor at motor endplate produces muscular paralysis,* the mechanism of which is discussed in specific chapter. Now, succinylcholine is the only depolarizing muscle relaxing agent which is still in clinical use. Though, the demise of succinylcholine has been forecasted many times, but it is still widely used in clinical practice, because of some unique properties of it, such as earliest (still now) onset and the shortest duration of action.

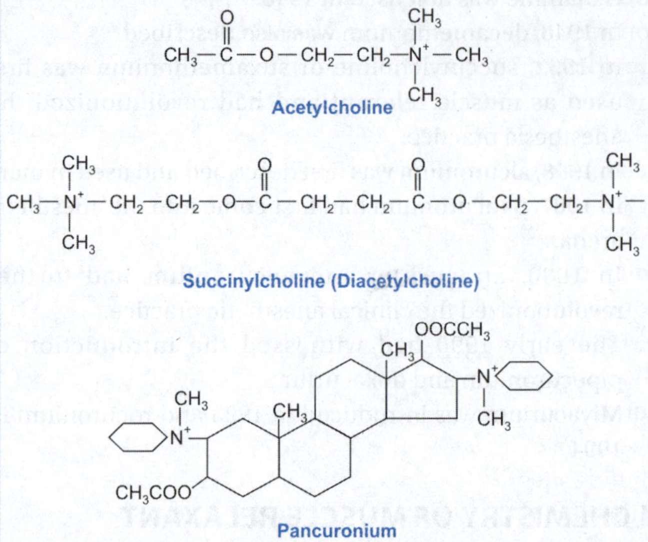

Succinylcholine produces depolarizing block which is characterized by:

- The absence of fade in response to train-of-four (TOF) and tetanic stimulation **(Fig. 1)**.
- The absence of posttetanic facilitation
- The increased intensity of block in the presence of anticholinesterase or cholinesterase inhibitors.

Mechanism of Action of Succinylcholine

Like ACh, succinylcholine is not metabolized at motor endplate by true cholinesterase enzyme which is present there (in synaptic cleft). So, the concentration of succinylcholine does not fall, as rapidly as ACh, in synaptic cleft. Thus, it causes the prolonged depolarization of motor endplate and muscle relaxation, till it swept away from the synaptic cleft. The continuous depolarization of motor endplate by succinylcholine causes muscle relaxation. This is due to the Na^+ channels which are present around the motor endplate (perijunctional area) and which have time-sensitive lower gate which opens only during the depolarization for a fixed-time period. During the passing of first wave of depolarization, from the motor endplate to the whole muscle fiber (casing fasciculation), these perijunctional Na^+ channels are also depolarized, and their time-sensitive lower gate opens that

Acetylcholine

Succinylcholine (Diacetylcholine)

Pancuronium

Fig. 1: The structural relationship between the acetylcholine, succinylcholine, and pancuronium. The succinylcholine is simply two molecules of acetylcholine, linked through the acetate methyl groups. So, it is called as the di-acetylcholine. Like acetylcholine, succinylcholine also stimulates the nicotinic-cholinergic receptors at neuromuscular junction, at the ganglionic sites, and also on the muscarinic receptors at other autonomic sites. The pancuronium is also made up of acetylcholine like fragments, but properly oriented like a steroid nucleus. But, in contrast, the pancuronium and other nondepolarizing agents block the nicotinic receptors or inhibit the actions of acetylcholine at the motor endplate (neuromuscular junction) and autonomic cholinergic sites.

allows the passage of Na^+ which is a process of depolarization. Then, it closes after a fixed time period and enters in inactivated state and cannot further reopen until the endplate repolarizes. The motor endplate, due to prolonged action of succinylcholine on it, does not quickly repolarize, after its depolarization, caused by it. Thus, the perijunctional Na^+ channel which makes a barricade around the motor endplate, remains in inactive state. Hence, this line of Na^+ channel at the perijunctional area prevents the passage of subsequent impulse, which comes through nerve fiber to spread on the surface of muscle fiber, and prevents the contraction of it producing paralysis. On the other hand, the muscle endplate does not repolarize and continue depolarization till the succinylcholine is present there and thus maintain the muscular relaxation. This is called as the "phase I block".

If the depolarization of muscle endplate is prolonged further due to repeated injection and/or large doses of succinylcholine, then the ACh (or nicotinic) receptors at motor endplate undergo an ionic and conformational changes that result in *"phase II block"* like nondepolarizing muscle relaxant, i.e., the ion channel within the ACh (nicotinic) receptor closes permanently with no flow of ions and becomes insensitive to ACh and its effect (muscular contraction), even in the absence of succinylcholine, providing prolonged muscular paralysis. On the contrary, the mechanism of action of nondepolarizing muscle relaxing agents, producing phase II block, is like that of the nondepolarizing muscle relaxants which act on the α-subunit of ACh nicotinic receptors and do not allow them to open their channel for ion movement from the very beginning and thus produce muscle relaxation. When the molecules of nondepolarizing muscle relaxant are moved away from the receptor (nicotine), then the ACh again acts on the receptor and resume muscular contraction. The site of the action of nondepolarizing agents is the same Ach-binding site on the α-subunit of nicotinic ACh receptors. However, there are two binding sites of nondepolarizing muscle relaxant on the ACh (nicotinic) receptor, as there are two α-subunits in one ACh receptor. But, the occupancy of only one α-subunit by one nondepolarizing agent molecule is sufficient for their action.

This explains the difference in action or the effects of depolarizing and nondepolarizing muscle relaxing agents in different disease states. For example, during the denervation of muscles, there is decrease in the release of ACh. Hence, it stimulates the compensatory increase in ACh (nicotinic) receptors at motor endplate on muscle cell membrane. *This upregulation of this receptor causes an increase in the sensitivity of muscle to the depolarizing agents, as more receptors are being depolarized. But, the nondepolarizing agents show a resistance in response, as the most receptors are presented for the same amount of drugs to be blocked. For another example, in myasthenia gravis there are fewer ACh receptors. This downregulation of these ACh receptors demonstrates a resistance to the depolarizing agents and an exaggerated response to the nondepolarizing agents.*

There are also some agents which act on the ACh (or nicotinic) receptors at motor endplate and block these receptors to produce neuromuscular paralysis, but not like agonistic (succinylcholine) or antagonistic (nondepolarizing) agents. They function by not disturbing the ACh-binding sites of ACh nicotinic receptors. The examples of such agents are inhalational anesthetic agents, local anesthetic agents, ketamine, some antibiotics, neostigmine, quinidine, etc. There are of two types of blocks of ACh (or nicotinic) receptor through which the above-mentioned agents act. These are *close-channel blockade and open-channel blockade*. In close-channel blockade, the molecules of the agents plug the mouth of the channel of ACh receptor and prevent the ion movement, whether or not the receptors are activated by ACh. In open-channel blockade, these neuromuscular blocking agents enter the ACh receptor channel after its opening and plug it (channel), preventing ion movement. So, it is use dependent and acts after the ACh activates the receptor and opens the channel. The significance of this channel blockade (closed or opened) is that such neuromuscular block cannot be overcome by increasing the concentration of ACh by cholinesterase inhibitors. All these are discussed in more details in Chapter 7.

Pharmacokinetics and Pharmacodynamics

Succinylcholine is the only available depolarizing muscle relaxing agent which is still used clinically and is still very popular, though the popularity is under eclipse now. The popularity of it is due to: (i) the very rapid onset of action (30–60 seconds), and (ii) the very short duration of action (5–10 minutes for the dose of 1–1.5 mg/kg IV). According to the initial bolus dose, the duration of action of succinylcholine varies. For example, in the dose of 0.5 mg/kg through IV, the duration of action is only 3–5 minutes, though the onset of action remains same.

It is assumed that the rapid onset of action of succinylcholine is due to the relatively large dose that is administered initially. As the succinylcholine is more water soluble and less lipid soluble, so this property of it prevents the drug to pass easily through the lipoid cell membrane and hence it needs higher doses. After an initial IV bolus dose, a large portion of succinylcholine is rapidly hydrolyzed by pseudocholinesterase, presents in plasma, and then a small portion of it is distributed to the motor endplate in tissues. This also explains why a large dose of succinylcholine is needed initially.

The plasma cholinesterase (pseudocholinesterase) enzyme is synthesized in liver and has a half-life of 5–12 days. It hydrolyzes or metabolizes 70% of a 100-mg bolus dose of succinylcholine within 1 minute. Other drugs, metabolized by plasma cholinesterase, include mivacurium, cocaine, and diamorphine. Only a small fraction of the injected dose of succinylcholine (10–15%) reaches neuromuscular junction. *As there is no pseudocholinesterase enzyme at motor endplate, so the neuromuscular blockade, by the action of succinylcholine at neuromuscular junction, is terminated only by its diffusion away from the endplate into the extracellular fluid, where it is hydrolyzed by pseudocholinesterase.* Only the action of ACh is terminated at motor endplate by the action of true cholinesterase which is present there. The rapid hydrolysis of succinylcholine by pseudocholinesterase (synthesized by liver) in plasma is the cause of the brief duration of action of it. Other than plasma-cholinesterase, the succinylcholine is also metabolized in liver. In the liver, succinylcholine is metabolized first to succinylmonocholine. Much of this succinylmonocholine has weak neuromuscular blocking effect and appears in urine.

The neuromuscular blocked produced by succinylcholine can be prolonged by (i) the reduced quantity of normal (typical) pseudocholinesterase enzyme (acquired cause) due to the reduction of synthesis of this enzyme by liver due to disease process of it, or (ii) by the normal quantity of atypical pseudocholinesterase enzyme (inherited cause), replacing the normal enzyme due to congenital error. The *acquired factors* that cause lower typical pseudocholinesterase level in plasma are liver disease, pregnancy, oral contraceptive pill (due to high-estrogen level), echothiophate, neostigmine, edrophonium, cytotoxic drugs, neoplasia, burns, metoclopramide, bambuterol (a prodrug of terbutaline), malnutrition and elderly, etc. The reduced typical plasma cholinesterase activity can also occur when some drugs which share the same metabolic pathway as succinylcholine (therefore compete with succinylcholine for the cholinesterase enzyme) are administered such as esmolol, monoamine oxidase inhibitors (MAOI), methotrexate, etc. **(Table 2)**. However, the prolongation of neuromuscular block, by succinylcholine, in these conditions is not very long. *Very prolonged block by succinylcholine is, however, usually associated with the presence of "silent or atypical genes" in homozygous individuals, producing atypical pseudocholinesterase enzyme "(inherited cause)". The neuromuscular block in these cases (atypical enzyme) lasts for several hours, until the succinylcholine is broken down completely by the presence of little amount of normal enzyme (if present any) and eliminated very slowly through urine.*

Ranitidine has no effect on pseudocholinesterase level. In a study, it is found that when the pseudocholinesterase level was reduced to 20% of its normal value, then the only duration of apnea caused by succinylcholine is increased from 3 minutes to 9 minutes.

TABLE 2: Drugs which cause the decrease of pseudo (or plasma) cholinesterase level.

i.	AChE inhibitors	• Neostigmine • Pyridostigmine
ii.	Organophosphate use in glaucoma	Echothiophate
iii.	Cancer agent	Cyclophosphamide
iv.	MAOI	Phenozine
v.	β-blocker	Esmolol
vi.	Antiemetic agent	Metoclopramide
vii.	Oral contraceptive	• Estrogen • Progesterone
viii.	Nondepolarizing muscle relaxant	• Pancuronium • Vecuronium • Atracurium, etc.

(AChE: acetylcholinesterase; MAOI: monoamine oxidase inhibitors)

Atypical Plasma or Pseudocholinesterase (Table 3)

Though the vast majority of population possess *normal gene*, responsible for the normal level of typical plasma or pseudocholinesterase enzyme, but rarely some patients are encountered who are either heterozygous or homozygous for the *atypical gene,* responsible for synthesis of atypical pseudocholinesterase. There are four principal autosomal dominant genes which are associated with the normal and atypical plasma or pseudocholinesterase enzyme. But, more genes are also described recently. These four principal autosomal genes, responsible for normal and atypical plasma or pseudocholinesterase enzyme synthesis, are designated as: E^u, E^a, E^f, and E^s. Among these the only E^u gene is responsible for the synthesis of typical pseudo- or plasma-cholinesterase enzyme and the normal hydrolysis of succinylcholine. Over the 95% of whole population have these normal genes and are homozygous who are designated as (E^u and E^u). Whereas the E^a, E^f, and E^s genes are responsible for the synthesis of atypical type of pseudocholinesterase enzyme and cannot hydrolyze the succinylcholine at all or cause hydrolysis of it partially. Normally, the succinylcholine is not resistant to inhibition by dibucaine and in homozygous person (E^u and E^u) the dibucaine number is 70–85. This is a method of assessment of the level or activity of typical pseudocholinesterase. The significance of which is discussed in more detail later. The duration of action of succinylcholine will be prolonged, if the varieties of atypical genes are present and typical pseudocholinesterase is not produced in normal quantity. The most common of these variations is the presence of atypical gene E^a in heterozygous form which is present in about 4% of the population. An individual who is heterozygous for this atypical gene (E^u and E^a) may have a slightly prolonged neuromuscular block, following a bolus dose of succinylcholine (up to 30 minutes). But, if the patient is homozygous for this atypical E^a gene (E^a E^a), then he will remain paralyzed for several hours, after administration of succinylcholine whose prevalence is approximately 1 in 2,500 population **(Table 4)**.

The atypical pseudocholinesterase enzyme, produced by atypical gene, is resistant to dibucaine. Other atypical

TABLE 3: Different genotype of plasma- or pseudocholinesterase.

Genotype	Figure	Action
Usual (or typical)	E^u	Normal hydrolysis of succinylcholine
Atypical	E^a	Dibucaine resistant
Atypical	E^f	Fluoride resistant
Atypical	E^s	Complete lack of cholinesterase activity (silent)

TABLE 4: Incidence of genotype.

Genotype	Zygosity	Incidence
$E^u E^u$	Homozygous	95%
$E^u E^a$	Heterozygous	5%
$E^u E^f$	Heterozygous	0.5%
$E^u E^s$	Heterozygous	0.5%
$E^a E^a$	Homozygous	0.05%
$E^a E^f$	Heterozygous	0.005%
$E^f E^f$	Homozygous	0.0003%
$E^f E^s$	Heterozygous	0.0005%
$E^s E^s$	Homozygous	0.002%

TABLE 5: Different genotype and dibucaine number.

Genotype	Dibucaine number
$E^u E^u$ $E^u E^a$	70–80 (70–80% enzyme is inhibited, 30–20% enzyme is resistant to dibucaine)
$E^u E^f$ $E^u E^s$ $E^a E^a$	50–60 (50–60% enzyme is inhibited, 50–40% enzyme is resistant to dibucaine)
$E^a E^f$ $E^f E^f$ $E^f E^s$	15–30 (15–30% enzyme is inhibited, 85–70% enzyme is resistant to dibucaine)
$E^s E^s$	0–5 (Only 5% enzyme is inhibited by dibucaine)

TABLE 6: Relationship between dibucaine number and duration of neuromuscular blockade by succinylcholine.

Type of pseudocho-linesterase	Genotype	Frequency	Dibucaine number	Response to succinyl-choline
Typical homozygous	$E^u E^u$	Normal	70–80	Normal
Typical heterozygous	$E^u E^a$ $E^u E^f$	1/500	50–60	Slightly prolonged
A typical homozygous	$E^a E^a$ $E^s E^f$ $E^s E^s$	1/3,000	20–30	Markedly prolonged

genes are fluoride resistant gene (E^f) and silent gene (E^s). Fluoride-resistant gene produces atypical pseudo- or plasmacholinesterase enzyme which are not resistant to dibucaine, but is resistant to fluoride. Homologous persons with silent gene ($E^s E^s$) completely lack the plasma cholinesterase activity in their plasma. Persons may be homologous or heterologous of these types of genes which are responsible for atypical pseudocholinesterase enzyme with different dibucaine number. These are shown in **Table 5**.

The most variants of atypical pseudocholinesterase are due to the single amino acid substitution or error at or near the active site of the enzyme, e.g., substitution of glycine for aspartic acid at position 70 in atypical dibucaine-resistant pseudocholinesterase.

The activity of plasma cholinesterase enzyme can be measured by using the spectrophotometric technique. Phenotype classification is also possible by adding different inhibitors such as dibucaine, sodium fluoride, etc. which cause different enzyme inhibition depending upon the types of enzyme present. Dibucaine inhibits the normal pseudocholinesterase enzyme to a greater extent than the abnormal enzyme. This observation had led to the development of a test by dibucaine and had made possible to create a number. Dibucaine test examines the amount of inhibition of particular plasma cholinesterase (or pseudocholinesterase) activity by dibucaine. If a specimen has high normal (typical) enzyme content then it will be inhibited to a larger extent by dibucaine. *This percentage of inhibition can then be expressed as the dibucaine number. For example, if dibucaine inhibits normal enzyme about 80%, then the dibucaine number is 80. It means in that person the amount of typical pseudocholinesterase is 80% and the amount of atypical pseudocholinesterase is 20%. On the contrary, if the dibucaine inhibits normal enzyme about 20%, then the dibucaine number is 20. It means in that person the amount of typical pseudocholinesterase is 20% and the amount of atypical pseudocholinesterase is 80%.* Thus, the dibucaine number indicates the genetic makeup of an individual patient with respect to typical pseudocholinesterase level in plasma. It does neither measure the concentration of enzyme in plasma nor does it indicate the efficiency of the enzyme **(Table 6)**.

Fluoride test will also reveal a few instances where the samples may show a normal looking dibucaine number, yet an abnormally low-fluoride number and prolonged duration of action of succinylcholine. The significance of fluoride test and its number is same as dibucaine. This is due to some variants of gene which produce such plasma pseudocholinesterase which is inhibited by dibucaine but not by fluoride. Such a situation would be evident in the presence of $E^f E^f$ genotype. The incidence of genotype will play an important part in the number of cases of prolonged response to succinylcholine. If it is accepted that the enzyme formed from $E^u E^u$ genotype can hydrolyze the clinical dose of succinylcholine in about 4 minutes, then $E^u E^a$ and $E^u E^f$ genotype would take 10–20 minutes. However, in $E^a E^a$, $E^f E^f$, and $E^s E^s$ genotype, more prolonged muscular paresis will persist.

Doses of Succinylcholine

Succinylcholine is usually administered intravenously, but it can also be given through intramuscular (IM) and subcutaneous (SC) route. However, by IM or SC route, the onset of action of succinylcholine is delayed and the duration of action is long lasting. By IV route, the arrival of succinylcholine at any group of muscle is heralded by brief fasciculation which represents this agent's ACh-like agonist activity. This usually happens within 30–40 seconds, with maximum effect of block, occurring in 30–60 seconds, following the administration of succinylcholine in the dose of 1 mg/kg through IV. This dose represents approximately the three times of ED_{95} value of this agent. The fasciculation following IV administration of succinylcholine is first observed in the eyebrow and in the eyelid group of muscles, passing later to the shoulder girdle and abdominal musculature, and finally to the hands and feet. However, this muscle fasciculation is less obvious in deeply anesthetized patient.

The average single bolus dose of succinylcholine in man is 1–1.5 mg/kg by IV with the duration of action for only about 5–10 minutes. For continuous infusion, the dose of succinylcholine is 20–40 µg/kg/min. Repeated small bolus doses such as 10 mg at small intervals (when effects of relaxation of the previous dose wane out) can also be used during short surgical procedures which require brief, but intense skeletal muscle relaxation, such as endoscopies, dilatation and curettage of uterine cavity, EUA, etc. When the succinylcholine infusion is used, then sometimes methylene blue dye is used as an indicator in the drip. Because, it prevents the confusion between the solution of succinylcholine in bottle and other intravenous fluids. But, in modern anesthesia practice, the availability of short-acting nondepolarizing muscle relaxants, such as mivacurium has decreased the popularity of this continuous infusion technique of succinylcholine. However, to avoid the overdose of succinylcholine by infusion, it is essential to monitor the neuromuscular transmission continuously, whenever an infusion of succinylcholine or intermittent repeated bolus doses of it are used.

Adverse Effect of Succinylcholine

Cardiovascular System

As succinylcholine is agonist to ACh, so it stimulates all the cholinergic receptors which are constituted by both the nicotinic and muscarinic types. The action of succinylcholine on the nicotinic receptors of ACh at neuromuscular junction produces fasciculation and subsequent muscular paralysis. The actions of succinylcholine on the muscarinic receptors of ACh on various tissues vary accordingly. The action of succinylcholine on the muscarinic receptors of cardiac tissues produces sinus bradycardia, junctional rhythm, conduction block, and ventricular arrhythmias,

ranging from unifocal premature ventricular contraction to ventricular fibrillation, etc. However, sinus bradycardia is more common, after a second dose of succinylcholine and particularly it is found in children. This can be prevented by blocking the vagus nerve or attenuating the muscarinic effect by atropine or by small dose of nondepolarizing muscle relaxing drug. The higher incidence of bradycardia and other cardiac complications, after a second dose of succinylcholine, suggests that the hydrolyzed product of succinylcholine (succinyl-mono-choline and choline) may sensitize the heart to the subsequent doses of it. However, bradycardia is not observed when succinylcholine (suxamethonium) is infused slowly.

The nodal rhythm, caused by succinylcholine, is due to the greatest activation of muscarinic receptor in SA node and thus suppressing the sinus mechanism and allowing the emergence of AV node as pacemaker. It is also common after second dose and can be prevented by atropine or small doses of nondepolarizing muscle relaxing agent. *Succinylcholine also induces ventricular arrhythmias because:*

- It lowers the arrhythmia threshold of ventricle.
- It increases the level of catecholamine and K^+ (due to fasciculation) which also increases the incidence of arrhythmia.
- Other associated autonomic stimulation due to intubation, hypoxia, hypercarbia, etc. also increases the incidence of arrhythmia, induced by succinylcholine.
- Different anesthetic drug, such as halothane (most common) also lowers the ventricular threshold level for ectopic beat or increases the arrhythmogenic effect of catecholamine. When this effect of halothane combines with the arrhythmogenic property of succinylcholine, then the incidence of arrhythmia increases manyfold. Glycopyrrolate is also effective in preventing the bradycardia and dysrhythmia, produced by succinylcholine.
- Other drugs which interact with succinylcholine and predispose ventricular arrhythmias are digitalis, MAOI, tricyclic antidepressant, exogenous catecholamine, etc.

Hyperkalemia

The administration of succinylcholine is associated with high rise of plasma K^+ level and it is believed to be due to the efflux of K^+ from muscle fibers, during fasciculation. In normal patients, this increase in plasma K^+ level is about 0.5 mmol/L and is of little significance. But, this may be significant for patients with preexisting elevated serum potassium level. Under certain abnormal circumstances, this rise of plasma K^+ level is very high and it is due to the spread of ACh receptors (nicotinic receptor) away from the restricted motor endplate area to the whole outer surface of muscle cell membrane.

BOX 1: Conditions where succinylcholine causes more hyperkalemia.

- Massive trauma
- Massive burn injury
- Tetanus
- Stroke
- Spinal cord injury (hemiplegia or paraplegia)
- Encephalitis
- Severe Parkinson's disease
- Guillain–Barré syndrome
- Polyneuropathy
- Head injury
- Severe infection or septicemia
- Prolonged immobilization of whole body
- Multiple myopathies (Duchenne muscular dystrophy)
- Hemorrhagic shock with metabolic acidosis

So, in these patients, succinylcholine acts vigorously by binding with all the nicotinic receptors, causing excessive fasciculation and tremendous rise of plasma K^+ level. The abnormal circumstances where this type of reaction occurs are massive burn, massive muscle trauma, lower motor neuron lesion, upper motor neuron lesion, any lesion of the spinal cord, skeletal muscle diseases, bed-ridden subjects, intra-abdominal infection, renal failure, etc. **(Box 1)**. But, among these both the burn and massive muscle trauma patients are most susceptible to hyperkalemia following succinylcholine. This susceptibility to hyperkalemia lasts for at least 60 days, following burn or trauma or until the adequate healing of damaged muscle occurs. So, in the above-mentioned conditions, succinylcholine should not be used, or if used in unavoidable condition, then anesthetist should be very cautious. Otherwise, subsequent cardiac arrest can occur which is quite refractory to the routine CPR.

If there is rise of plasma K^+ level due to any renal cause, then the use of succinylcholine is definitely contraindicated. Otherwise, the use of succinylcholine in renal failure is a controversial subject. Because many studies have failed to demonstrate the rise of plasma K^+ level by succinylcholine in renal failure patient. To them, succinylcholine is the muscle relaxants of choice, as it does not depend on the renal excretion. Since, a number of nondepolarizing muscle relaxants are now available that depend little or not at all on the kidney for their elimination (e.g., atracurium, mivacurium, and vecuronium), so they may be an alternative to succinylcholine as muscle relaxants in patient with renal disease.

Intraocular Pressure

Succinylcholine causes *tonic contraction* of extraocular muscles and thus increases intraocular pressure (IOP).

But, it has no clinical significance in most of the patients, where globe is not opened. IOP increases within 1 minute of the administration of succinylcholine, reaches peak value at an interval of 4 minutes and the duration for this action ($\uparrow$IOP) lasts for about 6 minutes. The mechanism for this tonic contraction of extraocular muscles by succinylcholine is discussed in the previous chapter. The use of nondepolarizing drugs before the administration of succinylcholine to prevent the rise of IOP is controversial. But, the use of succinylcholine alone is not contraindicated if the anterior chamber is not opened. Still, there are many studies, where the succinylcholine has successfully been used in penetrating eye injuries, without any loss of global contents. Other than succinylcholine, additional factors such as cough, vomiting, bucking, etc. also raise IOP. So, to prevent a raised IOP, the patient should be anesthetized deeply and should not strain, which can be achieved by an adequate dose of IV anesthetic drug, deeper level of inhalation anesthesia, application of topical anesthesia on trachea, additional muscle relaxants (nondepolarizing), etc.

But, in conclusion, we can comment that in open globe eye surgery or lacerated globe injury, the succinylcholine should be avoided. However, if for any reason the use of succinylcholine is mandatory for rapid sequence intubation due to full stomach or due to any other causes, then the above-mentioned measures should be taken to prevent an increase in IOP.

Intragastric Pressure

The succinylcholine increases IGP maximum up to 30 cmH$_2$O. But, the rise of IGP, up to 12 cmH$_2$O, is often normally found, following the use of succinylcholine in adult. However, this effect is inconsistent, because many patients even show no rise of IGP, after the use of succinylcholine. Again, this effect is insignificant, provided the esophageal sphincter mechanism is properly intact. The increase of IGP by succinylcholine is due to: (i) fasciculation of abdominal muscles, (ii) Ach-like effect of succinylcholine which causes vagal stimulation and subsequently increase IGP (4–7 cmH$_2$O). The increased IGP caused by succinylcholine can be prevented by prior curarization and atropinization. Normally, an increase in IGP is not important, as the opening pressure of lower esophageal sphincter also subsequently increases due to succinylcholine.

Usually, IGP above than 28 cmH$_2$O is necessary to overcome the competence of gastroesophageal junction. But, except in few cases, normally this limit does not exceed by succinylcholine. However, only when the normal oblique entry angle of esophagus into the stomach is altered or distorted due to pregnancy, abdominal distention by ascites or any other causes, intestinal obstruction, obesity, hiatus hernia, etc. then the IGP, required to cause the incompetence of gastroesophageal junction, becomes frequently low and is <15 cmH$_2$O. So, for the above-mentioned causes, precautionary measure should be taken to prevent regurgitation or the use of appropriate nondepolarizing drug, instead of succinylcholine, should be thought. Succinylcholine does not increase IGP in infant and children. This is due to minimum or absent of fasciculation in this group of patients.

Muscle Pain and Fasciculation

The incidence of muscle pain, which is most commonly observed as the side effects, following the administration of succinylcholine, varies from 25 to 89%. It develops mostly in chest wall, upper abdomen, shoulder, and back. Sometimes, this muscle pain becomes very debilitating, necessitating analgesics, and bed rest. However, it is more common after minor surgeries, in women and in ambulatory patients than the bed-ridden patients. It is also more common in young and fit patients and in those who are mobilized early. Extremes of age and pregnancy are seemed to be protective. This muscle pain is due to the fasciculation and it can be substantiated by finding myoglobinemia and increase in serum creatine phosphokinase (CPK), following the administration of succinylcholine, especially in children anesthetized with halothane.

The prior administration of subparalyzing dose of nondepolarizing muscle relaxant, before the administration of succinylcholine, prevents this fasciculation and muscle pain and substantiates this hypothesis. But, this prior treatment with nondepolarizing drug, mainly pancuronium, reduces the effectiveness of succinylcholine by about 30% and also causes the prolongation of the effect of depolarizing drug by virtue of its anticholinesterase properties. However, due to the reduction of effectiveness a larger dose of succinylcholine (1.5 mg/kg) is then required. Muscle pain can also be reduced by premedication with diazepam, lignocaine, thiopentone, and bed rest. Raised CPK level, due to the rupture of muscle cell fiber, associated with muscle pain supports that fasciculation produced by succinylcholine is the cause of muscle pain.

So, it may be a better practice to use a small dose of nondepolarizing muscle relaxants, before the administration of succinylcholine, due to the following reasons: (i) fasciculation, which is the root of many problems can be prevented, (ii) postoperative whole body muscle pain, elevated IOP, and increased IGP—all can be decreased or eliminated, (iii) succinylcholine-induced increase in serum-creatine phosphokinase (CPK) and myoglobinuria may be better attenuated. The relation between the muscle spasm and malignant hyperthermia is variable.

Masseter Spasm

Succinylcholine may cause contraction of certain group of muscles, especially masseters, leading to masseter spasm, while other muscles are relaxed. Probably, this is an exaggerated response of succinylcholine at neuromuscular junction of certain specific group of muscles and mainly found in children. Sometimes, this masseter spasm may be severe enough, making the laryngoscopy and intubation difficult. In such cases, a smaller dose of nondepolarizing agent is not of much benefit. It is not the diagnostic sign of malignant hyperthermia, because it is not invariably associated with this syndrome, though it has been suggested that this is an early warning sign of the development of malignant hyperthermia.

Intracranial Pressure

Succinylcholine transiently increases ICP, though the mechanism and significance of it is unknown.

Malignant Hyperpyrexia

Succinylcholine often triggers the mechanism of malignant hyperpyrexia in susceptible patient who is anesthetized with halothane. Malignant hyperthermia is a hypermetabolic disorder of skeletal muscles. But, the signs and symptoms of it resemble those of neuroleptic malignant syndrome (NMS), though the pathogenesis is completely different. However, there is no need to avoid the use of succinylcholine in patients with NMS.

Allergic Reaction

Of all the drugs used in anesthesia, the frequency of allergic and/or anaphylactic reactions is probably highest with succinylcholine. If there is a history of previous allergic reactions, then the likelihood of further reaction is very high. Succinylcholine may also give rise to cross-sensitivity with other muscle relaxants in this respect.

Phase II Block

It occurs if the ACh (nicotinic) receptors are exposed to succinylcholine, either in excess doses or for prolonged period. The phase II block is nothing but (like) nondepolarizing block with some exception. The transition from a depolarizing or phase I block to phase II block is gradual and usually occurs, after the administration of large dose, such as 7–10 mg/kg of succinylcholine intravenously. The recovery from phase II block is much slower and for it the cholinesterase inhibitor (anticholinesterase) should not be used. If used, it may prolong the effects of succinylcholine and phase II block will be more intense.

Interaction between Succinylcholine, Nondepolarizing Muscle Relaxants and Neostigmine

Interaction between the succinylcholine and the nondepolarizing muscle relaxants are antagonistic and/or additive, i.e., complex. These complex interactions are:

- If succinylcholine is given first to facilitate the intubation, then it enhances the depth of block caused by the subsequent dose of nondepolarizing muscle relaxant and reduces the dose of it. But, there is no effect when the nondepolarizing drug is given after the block from succinylcholine has dissipated.
- If the nondepolarizing agent is given first, then it antagonizes the depolarizing phase I block, produced by the subsequent administration of succinylcholine. This is because the nondepolarizing agents occupy some of the ACh-nicotinic receptor at motor endplate and partially prevent the agonistic action of succinylcholine. An exception to this phenomenon is pancuronium. It augments the blockade of succinylcholine by inhibiting the pseudocholine esterase enzyme and thus by increasing the concentration of succinylcholine.
- When succinylcholine is used after neostigmine, then the duration of succinylcholine action is prolonged. This is due to the inhibition of pseudocholinesterase by neostigmine.
- If neostigmine (AChE–inhibitors) is used to antagonize or to recover the phase I block, produced by succinylcholine, then it markedly prolongs the effect of succinylcholine. This happens by two mechanisms: (a) by inhibiting acetylcholinesterase (AChE) enzyme, they cause higher ACh concentration at motor endplate which intensifies the depolarization and phase I block. (b) They also reduce the hydrolysis of succinylcholine by inhibiting the pseudo-(plasma) cholinesterase enzyme and potentiate the phase I block.

Difference between Phase I and Phase II Block

Train-of-four is the best guide to detect the transition from phase I to phase II block **(Table 7)**. It helps to avoid the succinylcholine overdose by detecting the development of phase II block, observing the rate of recovery and assessing the effect of neostigmine on recovery from phase II block. Attempt to antagonize the phase II block by neostigmine is controversial. If TOF ratio is <0.4, administration of neostigmine causes prompt antagonism of phase II block.

TABLE 7: Difference between phases I and II block by succinylcholine.

	Phase I	*Transition*	*Phase II*
Train-of-four (TOF)	No fade	Moderate	Marked fade
TOF ratio	>0.7	0.4–0.7	<0.4
Tetanic stimulation	No fade	Moderate	Marked fade
Posttetanic facilitation	No	Moderate	Marked present
Recovery	Rapid	Less rapid	Prolonged
AchE inhibitor	Increase (agonist)	Little effect	Decrease (antagonize)
Dose requirement (IV)	1–2 mg	3–4 mg	>5 mg

(AChE: acetylcholinesterase)

■ NONDEPOLARIZING MUSCLE RELAXANTS

Classification

Classification According to Chemical Structure

A. *Steroidal compounds* (Pancuronium, pipecuronium, vecuronium, rocuronium, and ORG 9487, or rapacuronium).

Steroidal compounds have the following characteristics:
- High potency
- Lack of histamine release
- *Exhibits vagolytic property:* It is moderate for pancuronium, slight to moderate for rocuronium, absent in clinical dose for pipecuronium and vecuronium.
- Excreted by kidney
- Duration of action depends on the balance between the lipophilic and hydrophilic activity of the molecule.

B. *Benzyl-iso-quinolinium compound* [d-tubocurarine (dTc), metocurine, doxacurium, atracurium, cisatracurium (51W89), and mivacurium]

Benzyl-iso-quinolinium compound has the following characteristic **(Table 8)**:
- High potency
- Lack of vagolytic effect
- Tendency to release histamine. It is prominent for d-tubocurarine, moderate for metocurine, slight in atracurium and mivacurium, absent in doxacurium and 51W89 (cis-atracurium)
- Excreted by kidney—also have unimportant biliary excretion for dTc and doxacurium
- Degradation by Hoffmann elimination (atracurium and 51W89) or hydrolysis by pseudocholinesterase (mivacurium) in plasma.

TABLE 8: Summary of pharmacology of nondepolarizing muscle relaxants.

Drugs	Chemical structure	Primary excretion	Histamine release	Vagal blockade	Autonomic ganglion block
d-tubocurarine	B	Renal	+++	+	++
Gallamine	B	Renal	++	+++	0
Pancuronium	S	Renal	0	++	0
Pipecuronium	S	Renal	0	0	0
Vecuronium	S	Biliary	0	0	0
Atracurium	B	Insignificant	+	0	0
Cisatracurium	B	Insignificant	0/+	0	0
Doxacurium	B	Renal	0	0	0
Mivacurium	B	Insignificant	+	0	0
Rocuronium	S	Biliary	0	+	0
Rapacuronium	S	Biliary	++	0	0

(B: benzyl-iso-quinolinium compound; S: steroid compound)

However, the choice of a particular drug, during anesthesia practice, depends upon their unique pharmacodynamic and pharmacokinetic characteristics which are related to their molecular structures. This can be explained by the fact that steroidal compounds tend to be more vagolytic, whereas the benzyl-iso-quinolinium compounds release more histamine. Again because of the same chemical structure allergic history to one group of muscle relaxants may precipitate allergic reactions to other group of muscle relaxants.

Classification According to Duration of Action

- *Long-acting nondepolarizing muscle relaxants:* It includes d-tubocurarine (dTC), metocurine, doxacurium, pancuronium, pipecuronium, gallamine, and alcuronium. They have slow onset of action and maximum blockade occurs at 3–6 minutes, following an intubating dose which is two to three times of their ED_{95} dose. The average duration of action of these groups of muscle relaxants is 80–120 minutes (measured as recovery of twitch response to the 95% of baseline) following an intubating dose. In clinical practice, selection of these long-acting nondepolarizing muscle relaxant depends on their effect on CVS and the duration of surgery. Careful antagonism of residual paralysis at the end of operation is very important when these long-acting muscle relaxants are used. All these long-acting muscle relaxing agents are primarily excreted unchanged through urine with little or no-metabolism.
- *Intermediate acting nondepolarizing muscle relaxants:* It invites vecuronium, rocuronium, atracurium, and cisatracurium (51W89). The onset of action of this group of drugs occurs is 2–3 minutes, following administration of an intubating dose which is two to three times of their ED_{95} dose. The duration of action of these group of drugs is average 45–75 minutes (90–95% twitch recovery). The vecuronium and rocuronium have dual excreting pathway (liver and kidney). However, the atracurium and 51W89 undergo Hoffmann elimination.
- *Short-acting nondepolarizing muscle relaxants:* It includes only mivacurium and rapacuronium (ORG9487). Onset of action of these agents is 2–3 minutes, following their tracheal intubating dose and their clinical duration of action is about 12–15 minutes. After intravenous administration of these agents 95% twitch recovery occur between 25 and 35 minutes. Mivacurium is destroyed spontaneously in plasma by pseudocholinesterase like succinylcholine, though it is a nondepolarizing drug. Only 5% of these drugs are excreted unchanged in urine.

Pharmacokinetics and Pharmacodynamics of Nondepolarizing Muscle Relaxants

The nondepolarizing muscle relaxing agents act by competitive antagonism with ACh at nicotinic ACh receptor on the postsynaptic membrane of neuromuscular junction. The dose-response relationship of this group of drugs is sigmoid in shape. From this sigmoid-shaped dose-response curve, like any other agent, the potency of any nondepolarizing neuromuscular blocking agent can also be estimated **(Fig. 2)**.

The potency of any agent is expressed as effective dose (ED) value. The effective dose or ED value that results in 50, 90, or 95% neuromuscular block is termed (expressed) as the ED_{50}, ED_{90}, and ED_{95} of muscle relaxant respectively. In general, a dose that is two to three times of ED_{95} value is administered for the facilitation of tracheal intubation.

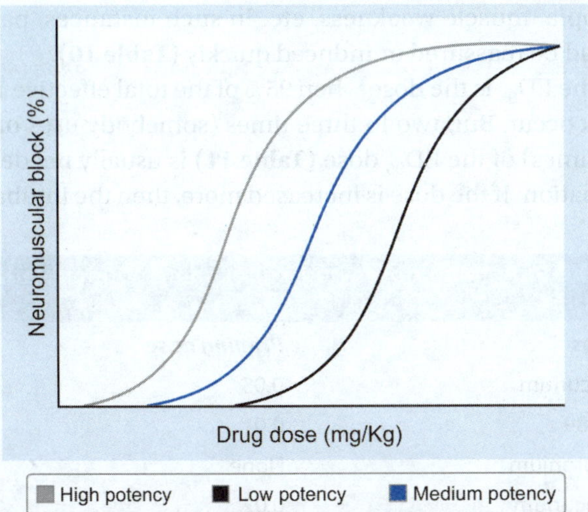

Fig. 2: This is a schematic representation of relationship between the dose of a muscle relaxant and the percentage of neuromuscular block. A drug of high potency would be represented by pipecuronium, medium potency by atracurium, and a low potency by gallamine.

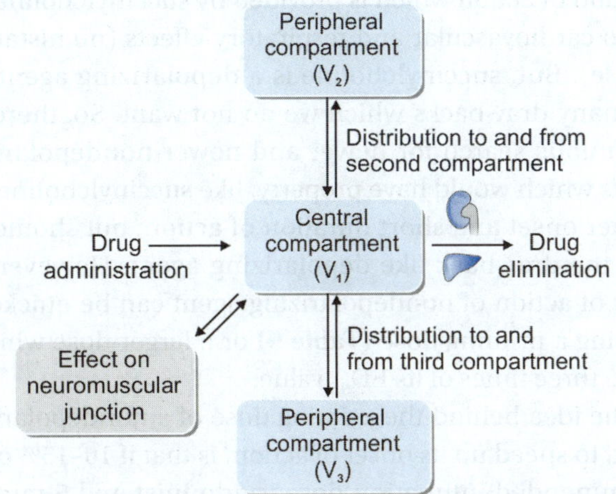

Fig. 3: This is a schematic representation of drug distribution into the different compartments of our body. These compartments are mathematical concepts only. It does not represent the real physiological space. The effect compartment in this case is the neuromuscular junction.

Clinically, the onset of neuromuscular block is the time which is taken for a drug to produce a depression of measurable response which is the contraction of muscles for a muscle-relaxing agent. During the onset of response (muscular paralysis), nearly 70% of the nicotinic receptors must be occupied by the drug. *The speed of onset of action of a muscle-relaxing agent depends upon the* (i) cardiac output, (ii) muscle blood flow, (iii) the potency of this drug, (iv) the dose of this agent, and (v) some kinetic characteristic (e.g., distribution, clearance, etc.) of this muscle relaxant. *It is now established that the drugs with low potency have a more rapid onset of action and the drugs with high potency have a slow onset of action. This is because as potency increases less amount of drugs (fewer molecules) are injected and the concentration gradient of the acting drug at their acting receptor site will be low, causing delayed onset of action.* For example, doxacurium is the most potent muscle-relaxing agent, but has the slowest onset of action. Potent muscle relaxants also have high affinity for the receptors. So, their effects wear off very slowly, resulting in long duration of action.

The distribution profile of the currently used nondepolarizing muscle relaxants can be described *by two or three compartmental models.* First, the relaxants are distributed from their central compartment (blood) to the peripheral compartment (tissue). Then, it is followed by one or two elimination phases, when the drugs are metabolized in liver and excreted through urine. After intravenous injection, the concentration of muscle relaxant in plasma (central compartment) rises rapidly. After that this drug moves into the tissues from plasma and the

concentration of it in the blood fall rapidly. When this fall in plasma level goes beyond the tissue concentration level, then the drug again returns into plasma from tissues. Now, the plasma concentration of this muscle relaxing agents depends on two factors: (i) the rate of re-entry of it into plasma from tissues and (ii) the elimination of it from the plasma by metabolism and/or excretion. Ultimately, an equilibrium between the tissue concentration and the plasma concentration reaches and after that there is slow decrease in the concentration of drug in plasma, constituting terminal elimination phase **(Fig. 3)**.

After an intravenous injection, the plasma concentration of muscle relaxants falls gradually. But, in contrast to the decrease in plasma concentration of a muscle-relaxing agent, the neuromuscular block begins to occur and does not recover, even after many minutes of the gradual decrease of plasma concentration of muscle relaxant. This discrepancy between the plasma concentration and the drug effect (muscular paralysis) is because the action of muscle relaxants is not in the plasma, but at the neuromuscular junction.

The potency of nondepolarizing muscle relaxants is increased by prior administration of succinylcholine. But, this potency is decreased in patients with burn, injury, neonates, and infants than the older children and adults.

Choice of Nondepolarizing Agents for Tracheal Intubation

None of the recently available nondepolarizing muscle-relaxing agent can fulfill all the desired conditions, necessary for tracheal intubation, i.e., (i) rapid onset and short duration of action which is provided by succinylcholine and (ii) no cardiovascular and respiratory effects (no histamine release). But, succinylcholine is a depolarizing agent and has many drawbacks which we do not want. So, there is a continuous search for newer and newer nondepolarizing agents which would have property, like succinylcholine, i.e., quicker onset and short duration of action, but should not have the drawback like depolarizing agent. However, the onset of action of nondepolarizing agent can be quickened by using a priming dose **(Table 9)** or a larger dose which is two to three times of its ED_{95} value.

The idea behind the priming dose of a nondepolarizing agent, to speed up its onset of action, is that if 10–15% of the recommended intubation dose is administered 5 minutes before induction, then it will occupy the enough receptors, so that the paralysis will quickly occur when the balance or remaining 85–90% of the recommended dose is given after induction and before intubation. The use of this technique enables to perform intubation quickly within 60–90 seconds after the administration of the principal dose of muscle relaxant. However, it is applicable mainly for the short- and intermediate-acting nondepolarizing agents. Priming dose occupies usually 20–25% of the nicotinic receptors at neuromuscular junction. So, it does not produce any clinically significant muscular paralysis and its symptoms before induction which requires 75–80% receptor occupancy. However, in some patients priming dose produces clinical paralysis, manifested by dyspnea or heaviness of breath, diplopia, muscle weakness, etc. In such instances, patient should be reassured or induced quickly **(Table 10)**.

The ED_{95} is the dose when 95% of the total effective 100% block occur. But, two to three times (somebody uses one to two times) of the ED_{95} dose **(Table 11)** is usually needed for intubation. If the dose is increased more, then the intubation

TABLE 9: Priming doses (mg/kg) of some nondepolarizing relaxants.

Drugs	Priming dose
Atracurium	0.05
51W89	0.01
Rocuronium	None
Mivacurium	0.02
Vecuronium	0.01

TABLE 10: Doses of some nondepolarizing muscle relaxants for rapid tracheal intubation in mg/kg.

Drugs	Intubating dose (mg/kg)	Clinical duration (minutes)	Full recovery (minutes)
Atracurium	0.7–0.8	45–60	60–90
51W89	0.2–0.25	50–70	70–100
Rocuronium	0.6–1.0	30–60	60–120
Vecuronium	0.15–0.2	60–70	90–120
Mivacurium	0.25	15–20	20–30

TABLE 11: Doses, onset of action, duration of action and potency of different nondepolarizing agents.

Drug	ED_{95} (mg/kg)	Intubation dose (mg/kg)	Onset of action of intubating dose (min)	Duration of action of intubating dose (min)	Supplemental dose (mg/kg)	Potency
Long-acting						
Tubocurarine	0.5	0.5–0.6	1–2	30–60	0.1–0.2	7
Gallamine	3.0	4–6	2–3	90–120	0.5–1	40
Pancuronium	0.07	0.08–0.12	2–3	60–120	0.01–0.02	1
Pipecuronium	0.05	0.08–0.1	2–3	60–120	0.01–0.15	0.8
Doxacurium	0.025	0.05–0.08	4–5	90–150	0.01–0.05	0.4
Intermediate-acting						
Vecuronium	0.05	0.1–0.2	2–3	45–90	0.01–0.02	0.8
Atracurium	0.23	0.5–0.6	2.5–3	30–45	0.1	3.5
Cisatracurium (51W89)	0.05	0.1–0.15	2–3	30–60	0.02	1
Rocuronium	0.3	0.6–1	1–1.5	30–60	0.1–15	6
Short-acting						
Mivacurium	0.08	0.2–0.25	2.5–3	15–20	0.05–0.1	1.6
Rapacuronium (ORG9487)	0.75	1.5–2	1.5	14–20	0.05	–

will be more rapid. But, it exacerbates the side effects and prolongs the duration of action of this muscle-relaxing agent. For example, pancuronium in high doses of 0.15 mg/kg (usual dose 0.08 mg/kg) produces an excellent intubating condition within 90 seconds and its irreversible duration of action lasts for >60 minutes, but at the cost of pronounced tachycardia and hypertension.

It is also important to understand that the different muscle groups of our body vary in their sensitivity to different nondepolarizing muscle relaxants. The relaxation of laryngeal muscles is important for intubation. But, it recovers from blockade more quickly than adductor pollicis muscle which is commonly monitored for neuromuscular paralysis.

Doses of Nondepolarizing Muscle-relaxing Agents—the Principle

- The dose of nondepolarizing muscle relaxants for tracheal intubation is two to three times than that of their ED_{95} dose.
- If the patient has already been intubated, then the dose slightly less than that of ED_{95} dose is needed to produce the surgical relaxation.
- The maintenance doses for nondepolarizers range from 20 to 30% of their initial bolus dose.
- The intermediate and short-acting nondepolarizing muscle relaxants can be used by continuous infusion **(Table 12)** to keep the relaxation smooth. It also helps in rapid adjustment in the depth of relaxation, according to surgical needs and prompt recovery at the end of surgery.
- Somebody thought that if the subparalyzing dose of a nondepolarizing agent is given 2–4 minutes before the final second dose for tracheal intubation after induction, then the onset of action of this second dose will be accelerated and intubation can be performed within 90–120 seconds. *This procedure is called as the "priming".* When rapid tracheal intubation is performed by nondepolarizing relaxants, then "priming" is recommended. But, long-acting nondepolarizing drugs are not advised for this priming and rapid intubation.

TABLE 12: The doses of different nondepolarizing agents when they are used by continuous infusion.

Continuous infusion	µg/kg/minute
Mivacurium	6–8
Atracurium	4–12
Cisatracurium (51W89)	1–2
Rocuronium	10
Vecuronium	0.8–2

Metabolism and Elimination of Nondepolarizing Muscle Relaxants (Table 13)

All the nondepolarizing muscle relaxants contain quaternary nitrogen (N^+) atom. So, they are positively charged cation. This chemical characteristic conforms them a high degree of water solubility and only a slight degree of lipid solubility. So, this hydrophilic character enables the nondepolarizing muscle relaxants to eliminate completely via kidney with no tubular reabsorption. Hence, they depend little or nothing for metabolism in liver for exit from our body. Therefore, the elimination of these drugs depends only on glomerular filtration and makes them long-acting in renal disease.

Effect on Central Nervous System

The nondepolarizing muscle relaxants can hardly enter into cerebrospinal fluid (CSF) and brain tissue and so their clinical significance on central nervous system (CNS) is not clear. When inadvertently neuromuscular blocking agent is administered into CSF (during spinal anesthesia) then myotonia, autonomic changes, convulsion, etc. have been observed. However, prolonged administration of rocuronium, atracurium, and vecuronium in ICU results in the entry of sufficient amount of these drugs into CSF. Laudanosine, a metabolite of atracurium, crosses the blood barrier and causes CNS stimulation. In case of cisatracurium which is an isomer of atracurium and five times more potent than it, the measured quantities of laudanosine in CSF is five times lower than that of atracurium. However, the CNS effect of nondepolarizing muscle relaxant, due to prolonged use, on the morbidity and mortality ICU patients is unclear.

Pediatric Group of Patient and Nondepolarizing Muscle Relaxant

- At birth, the development of neuromuscular unit is immature. It becomes mature at 2 months of age. So, the newborns are more sensitive to nondepolarizing muscle relaxants than adult and a lower plasma concentration of it can achieve the desired neuromuscular block, like adult. But, the dose of nondepolarizing muscle relaxant should not be reduced, due to its large volume of distribution, in neonates and infants. The slower clearance rate by kidney also contributes to the longer elimination half-life of nondepolarizing agents in children. In spite of these, the nondepolarizing muscle relaxants can safely be used in neonates and infants.
- Atracurium, cisatracurium, vecuronium, and rocuronium are the commonly used nondepolarizing muscle relaxants in children due to their faster onset, intermediate duration of action, and minimum residual paralysis.

TABLE 13: Metabolism and elimination of muscle relaxants.

Drug	Duration of action	Metabolism	Elimination by kidney	Elimination by liver
Succinylcholine	Ultra short	Pseudocholinesterase (99%)	<2% metabolites eliminated in urine	None
Mivacurium	Short	Pseudocholinesterase (90%)	<10% metabolites eliminated in urine	None
Atracurium	Intermediate	Hoffmann elimination and esterase hydrolysis (60–90%)	10–40% metabolites eliminated in urine	None
51W89 (cisatracurium)	Intermediate	Hoffmann elimination (90%)	10–40% metabolites eliminated in urine	–
Rocuronium	Intermediate	None	40% relative excretion by liver and kidney	60%
Vecuronium	Intermediate	Liver (20–40%)	40–60%	60–40%
Pancuronium	Long	Liver (10–30%)	85%	15%
Pipecuronium	Long	None	>90%	<10%
Tubocurarine (dTc)	Long	None	80%	20%
Gallamine	Long	None	100%	0

- The mivacurium can safely be used in children and needs larger doses than adult. However, the duration of action of mivacurium is shorter in children than adult. It is best used by infusion in children for its shorter duration of action and infusion rate should be twice than that of adult.
- The status of rocuronium in children is same as that of the adult. Rocuronium in the dose of 0.6 mg/kg has the earliest onset of action (60–90 seconds) among all the nondepolarizing agents and produces an excellent intubating condition for rapid tracheal intubation than vecuronium and atracurium, both for the adult and children. For rapid sequence intubation (within 30–60 seconds) in the presence of full stomach, rocuronium in the high dose (1.2–1.5 mg/kg) are also suggested.
- The succinylcholine should be discontinued in pediatric group of patients because of many side effects of it such as rhabdomyolysis, hyperkalemia, acidosis, and even cardiac arrest, particularly in patient with unsuspected muscular dystrophy of Duchenne type.
- The antagonism of nondepolarizing block in children is similar to adult.

Geriatric Group of Patients and Muscle Relaxant

The duration of action of most of the nondepolarizing muscle relaxants is prolonged in older group of patients. This is due to many geriatric physiological changes which occur in body and neuromuscular junction with increasing age.

The physiological changes in geriatric group of patients which affect the action of muscle relaxants are:
- ↓ Splanchnic and renal blood flow
- ↓ Glomerular filtration rate (GFR)
- ↓ Hepatic function
- ↓ Total body water
- ↓ Cardiac reserve.

With increased age, the physiological and anatomical changes of neuromuscular junction which affects the action of muscle relaxants are:
- ↑ Junctional cleft
- Flattening of folds of motor endplate
- ↓ Concentration of ACh receptors
- ↓ Amount of ACh in vesicle.

In old age, the sensitivity of nicotinic receptor to the muscle-relaxing agents at myoneural junction is not altered. But, the decreased clearance of each drug from plasma explains the prolonged duration of action of it in old age. The decreased clearance of drug in elderly is due to the ↑ volume of distribution. Atracurium and cisatracurium depend on ester hydrolysis and Hoffmann degradation for their clearance. So, the duration of action of atracurium and cisatracurium is not influenced by age. The plasma cholinesterase activity of older patients is reduced by 26% than the younger ones. So, as mivacurium is metabolized by plasma cholinesterase, its activity is prolonged by 20–25% in the aged.

Obesity

The doses of nondepolarizing muscle relaxing agents should be precisely calculated in obese patient. In obese, the doses of a drug depend on their lean body mass rather than the actual body weight of them and will be 20% more. However, the recovery from atracurium does not depend on obesity. The duration of action of rocuronium is prolonged in obese, but the duration of action of pancuronium is unaffected by obesity.

Renal Disease

The renal failure prolongs the duration of action of nondepolarizing muscle-relaxing agents by causing decreased elimination of these drugs or their metabolites via kidney or by decreasing the activity of enzymes which metabolize the drugs. The long-acting nondepolarizing muscle relaxants, such as pancuronium, pipecuronium, doxacurium, gallamine and metocurine, etc. are associated with decreased plasma clearance and increased elimination half-life, with prolonged duration of action in renal failure. So, because of the prolonged duration of action and the availability of intermediate and short-acting muscle relaxants which depend much less on the kidney for their elimination, use of long-acting nondepolarizing muscle-relaxing drugs in renal failure is not recommended now. The duration of action of atracurium is unaffected by renal failure. Vecuronium depends on both liver and kidney for its excretion. So, its clearance is also reduced and action is prolonged in renal failure patient. In renal failure patient, due to decreased activity of plasma cholinesterase, the duration of action of mivacurium is also prolonged by 50% (10–15 minutes).

However, the duration of action of rocuronium is not prolonged and is not cumulative in renal failure. As only 16% of the total excretion of cisatracurium depends on kidney (77% by Hoffmann degradation), so the renal failure has little impact on the duration of action of cisatracurium.

Liver Disease

Hepatobiliary diseases prolong the duration of action of pancuronium, doxacurium, vecuronium, rocuronium, and mivacurium. The relationship between the liver disease and the pharmacokinetics of nondepolarizing muscle relaxants is complex. Liver disease is associated with increased volume of distribution and decreased plasma clearance. As a result, there is apparent resistant to the effect of drug and prolonged action. So, the initial dose is increased to reach the desired level of effect in plasma and thus the subsequent recovery is slower. On the other hand, the decreased synthesis of plasma cholinesterase in liver disease causes prolonged action of mivacurium and almost is tripled. But the clearance of atracurium and cisatracurium is little affected by liver disease, and so also their duration of action.

Inhaled Anesthetics

In a dose-dependent manner all the inhaled anesthetic agents potentiate the action of nondepolarizing muscle relaxants. But, the extent of potentiation is different for different inhaled anesthetic agents.

The proposed several mechanisms for the augmentation of neuromuscular blockade by inhaled anesthetic agents are:

- The increased blood flow, caused by inhaled anesthetic agents, causes the most availability of injected muscle relaxants at neuromuscular junction.
- Due to the depressive action on CNS, the volatile anesthetic agent itself often produces adequate muscle relaxation. Thus, this augments the action of muscle relaxants without producing any direct neuromuscular block by itself.
- The decreased sensitivity of postjunctional membrane to depolarization by inhaled anesthetic agent augments the neuromuscular blockade.
- Some specific effects of inhaled anesthetic on ACh-receptor channel which reduces the average duration of opening of it (channel) during its activation. The effect of inhaled anesthetics on nondepolarizing blockade is a pharmacodynamic one (i.e., blood concentration of muscle relaxants to produce paralysis is decreased) but not a pharmacokinetic one.

Temperature

Hypothermia invariably lengthens the duration of neuromuscular blockade, produced by nondepolarizing muscle relaxants.

Antibiotics

Some antibiotics enhance the neuromuscular blockade, caused by the nondepolarizing muscle relaxants. The mechanism of potentiation of neuromuscular blockade by these antibiotics is prejunctional (depression of the evoked release of ACh) or postjunctional or mixed. Calcium is not used for the reversal of this neuromuscular blockade, caused by antibiotic for two reasons: (i) antagonism produced by calcium is not sustained, and (ii) the calcium antagonizes the antibacterial effect of antibiotics also. The antibiotics that potentiate the neuromuscular blockade are streptomycin, gentamicin, kanamycin, neomycin, tetracycline, polymyxin A and B, lincomycin, clindamycin, etc.

Magnesium

Magnesium sulfate, used in the treatment of preeclampsia and eclampsia, also has the neuromuscular blocking property and enhances the action of both nondepolarizing and depolarizing muscle-relaxing agents. The enhancement of succinylcholine blockade by magnesium also involves the same mechanisms as that of succinylcholine. Magnesium also inhibits the action of plasma cholinesterase enzyme.

The mechanism of actions of magnesium in neuromuscular blockade are:

- It reduces the amount of ACh, released from presynaptic membrane at nerve terminal.
- It reduces the depolarizing action of ACh on postjunctional membrane.
- It reduces the excitability of muscle fiber.
- It reduces the amplitude of motor endplate potential.

Local Anesthetic and Antiarrhythmic Agents

Local anesthetic agents enhance the effect of neuromuscular blocking agents, produced by both nondepolarizing and depolarizing muscle relaxants. So, when the local anesthetic agent is given as antiarrhythmic agent in intraoperative or postoperative period, then the muscular relaxation effect produced by the muscle relaxants is prolonged. It acts by stabilizing the postjunctional membrane and thus by blocking the ACh-induced muscular contraction. In addition, procaine inhibits the plasma cholinesterase action and enhances the effect of succinylcholine.

The antiarrhythmic agents (e.g., quinidine) also augment the neuromuscular blocking effect, caused by muscle relaxants. Any drug that influences the conduction of impulse and electrical properties of heart, e.g., β-blocker, Ca^{2+} channel blocker, etc. also influence the ion transport at neuromuscular junction and enhance the action of muscle relaxants. But, in clinical level these interactions are insignificant.

Antiepileptic Agents

Antiepileptic agents, e.g., phenytoin, carbamazepine, etc. reduce the action of both depolarizing and nondepolarizing muscle relaxants and accelerate the recovery from muscular paralysis. Patients receiving anticonvulsants are somewhat resistant to the blocking effect of muscle relaxants.

Diuretics

The diuretics in their clinical dose augment the effect of nondepolarizing muscle relaxants. They inhibit the production of cyclic AMP $\rightarrow$ leads to $\downarrow$ ATP $\rightarrow$ $\downarrow$ output of neurotransmitter $\rightarrow$ $\uparrow$ blocking effect. Mannitol and other osmotic and tubular diuretics have no effect on the nondepolarizing muscle relaxants. Because the excretion of relaxants depends primarily on GFR. Mannitol, being an osmotic diuretic, exerts its effect in proximal tubules, so that the water is retained within the tubules, but does not $\uparrow$ GFR and does not increase the excretion of nondepolarizing relaxants.

Interactions Between the Nondepolarizing Drugs (Change from Short- to Long-acting Agents and *Vice Versa*)

The effects of some nondepolarizing muscle relaxants may be potentiated by simultaneous or prior administration of other nondepolarizing agents. This usually happens if the combinations of aminosteroidal and benzyl-iso-quinolinium group of muscle relaxants are used together. In modern anesthetic practice, there is no reason to combine the drugs from different group of nondepolarizing relaxants. But, the sequential administration of long- and short-acting drugs can be considered. However, the general rule for the change over from one group of nondepolarizing agent (steroidal or isoquinolinium) to another group (steroidal or isoquinolinium) of agents is that 95% of the drug of first group should be cleared. If anybody wants to change from short- to long-acting muscle-relaxing agent (for example, mivacurium to doxacurium), then the second drug should be given, when the TOF response, from the first group of drugs, has begun to recover, i.e., two to three twitches, out of four twitches, are visible. Similarly, if anybody wants to change from the long- to the short-acting group of drugs for maintenance, then very small dose should be given.

Anaphylactic or Allergic Reaction

Due to quaternary structure and previous natural sensitization to such molecules, the muscle relaxants are the most commonly responsible drug for allergic or anaphylactic reaction during anesthesia. The manifestations of some reactions, such as flushing, urticaria, tachycardia, and hypotension, etc. may sometimes be severe enough and can lead to cardiac arrest. In some patients, this reaction is manifested as severe bronchospasm. Succinylcholine is the most commonly implicated agent for allergic reaction, though any muscle-relaxing agent may be responsible for that. Recently, rocuronium and cisatracurium have also been implicated for allergic reactions. However, the preoperative determination for this probable anaphylactic or allergic reaction, caused by a muscle relaxant, involves the demonstration of specific antibodies against this muscle-relaxing agent or skin testing by this agent.

Effects on Autonomic Ganglia and Release of Histamine

Within the range of therapeutic doses, the different nondepolarizing muscle-relaxing agents differ in their effects on autonomic ganglia. The older muscle-relaxing agent, like tubocurarine, has marked ganglion (which also contains nicotinic receptor) blocking effect. Thus, it compromises

TABLE 14: Interactions of depolarizing and nondepolarizing muscle relaxants with other drugs.

Other drugs	Depolarizing muscle relaxant	Nondepolarizing muscle relaxant
A. *Antibiotics:* Streptomycin, kanamycin, neomycin, polymyxin, colistin, aminoglycosides, tetracycline, clindamycin, lincomycin, etc.	Potentiation	Potentiation
B. *Anticonvulsants:* Carbamazepine, phenytoin, valproate, primidone, etc.	Resistant	Resistant
C. *Antiarrhythmics:* Ca-channel blocker, quinidine, etc.	Potentiation	Potentiation
D. *Cholinesterase inhibitors:* Neostigmine, edrophonium, pyridostigmine, etc.	Potentiation	Resistant
E. *Inhalational anesthetics:* Halothane, isoflurane, sevoflurane, desflurane, etc.	Potentiation	Potentiation
F. *Magnesium sulfate*	Potentiation	Potentiation
G. *Lithium carbonate*	Potentiation	Not known
H. *Ketamine*	Not known	Potentiation
I. *Local anesthetics*	Potentiation	Potentiation

the ability of sympathetic nervous system to increase the heart rate and myocardial contractility in response to hypotension and other perioperative stresses. On the other hand, gallamine and pancuronium have marked vagal blocking or vagolytic (muscarinic-receptor blocking) effect, causing tachycardia. All the newer nondepolarizing muscle relaxants, such as atracurium, cisatracurium, rocuronium, vecuronium, etc. are devoid of significant ganglion blocking effects in their recommended clinical dose range. Many nondepolarizing agents release histamine from mast cells, causing bronchospasm, peripheral vasodilatation, hypotension, skin flushing, urticaria, etc. But, these are insignificant in their recommended clinical dose range, except the atracurium and mivacurium where these incidences are high **(Table 14)**.

Other Factors that may Interfere with the Action of Muscle Relaxants

Acid-base State

Acidosis (respiratory or metabolic) augments the effect of nondepolarizing block. So, antagonism of neuromuscular block is difficult in such situation. Administration of narcotics in recovery room, to relieve pain, may cause hypoventilation and respiratory acidosis → more augmentation of residual block → again more hypoventilation → more acidosis → vicious cycle.

Electrolyte Imbalance

The low extracellular K^+ concentration increases the endplate resting transmembrane potential (due to higher ratio of intracellular to extracellular K^+ concentration). This hyperpolarization increases the resistance to depolarization and neuromuscular transmission. Thus, hypokalemia enhances the block produced by nondepolarizing muscle relaxants. This also diminishes the ability of neostigmine to antagonize the block. Thus, K^+ imbalance due to other diseases also increases the response to muscle relaxants. Severe dehydration also causes increased concentration of muscle-relaxing agents in the plasma, thereby increases their muscle-relaxing activity.

Myasthenia Gravis and Muscle Relaxants

In myasthenia gravis (autoimmune disease), as there is less number of postjunctional nicotinic receptor, so the patients are more sensitive to nondepolarizing muscle relaxants and resistant to succinylcholine. However, not all the muscles are affected in the same way. So, only the short- and intermediate-acting nondepolarizing muscle relaxants should be used in low dose, guided by the monitoring with nerve stimulator. About 1/5 to 1/10th of ED_{95} value should be given initially as test dose to estimate the patient's requirement.

If patients have already received pyridostigmine for the treatment of myasthenia gravis, it should be continued preoperatively. It modifies the response of muscle relaxants as follows: (i) the sensitivity to nondepolarizing muscle relaxants will be diminished, (ii) the response to succinylcholine and mivacurium are lengthened, because pyridostigmine inhibits plasma cholinesterase, (iii) the reversal of block is ineffective as AChE inhibitor already exists in plasma. So, it will probably be safer to allow the spontaneous recovery.

Eaton-Lambert Syndrome (Myasthenic Syndrome)

This syndrome resembles to myasthenia gravis and is associated with carcinoma and motor neuropathy. The patients with this syndrome are usually sensitive to both the nonpolarizing and depolarizing muscle relaxants.

Lower and Upper Motor Neuron Disease

- The lower motor neuron diseases result in increased resistance to nondepolarizing muscle relaxants. It is because of the proliferation of ACh (or nicotinic) receptors on motor endplate and muscle cell membrane.

- In upper motor neuron lesions (hemiplegia and paraplegia) the patients are more susceptible to succinylcholine.

Burns and Muscle Relaxants

The burn patients show abnormal response to depolarizing muscle relaxants. Because, after burn there is proliferation of extra-junctional ACh (or nicotinic) receptor throughout the surface of the muscle cell membrane. It means the nicotinic receptors are now not limited at the motor endplate, it spreads all over the cell membrane of a muscle cell. This occurs 48 hours after burn injury and returns to its normal state after 1–2 years, according to the injury. Thus, massive stimulation of these receptors by normal dose of succinylcholine can cause the massive release of potassium, producing ventricular tachycardia, ventricular fibrillation, or cardiac arrest. So, succinylcholine can safely be administered within first 24 hours following burn injury or 1–2 years after the burn, when the skin has healed completely. Burned patients also show abnormal response to nondepolarizing muscle relaxant. Due to increased hepatic and renal clearance and due to hypermetabolic state, burn injury shortened the duration of action of nondepolarizing agent. Dose requirement of nondepolarizing agent is also increased. This resistant is due to the increased population of extra-junctional ACh (nicotinic) receptors by burn injury.

INDIVIDUAL NONDEPOLARIZING MUSCLE RELAXANT

d-Tubocurarine

The d-tubocurarine (dTc) is the first nondepolarizing neuromuscular blocking agent which is found in the arena of anesthesia. It was clinically first used by Griffith and Johnson in 1942 at Montreal during an appendectomy operation. It was first described by King, in 1935, as bisquaternary compound. But, the correct formula of it is monoquaternary compound, which is described recently. Despite many side effects, it was very popular till 1970. But, after that, pancuronium and other short-acting drug, like gallamine, takes place of this long-acting muscle relaxant. However, now it was only indicated for prolonged operation and where hypotension is desired which is due to the huge release of histamine by it **(Fig. 4)**.

The release of histamine is profound by dTc than any other nondepolarizing neuromuscular blocking agent, when it is given in bolus doses. However, it (release of histamine) can be prevented by the slow administration of dTc, but not by H_1 and H_2 blockers. Histamine release may go up to 10-folds,

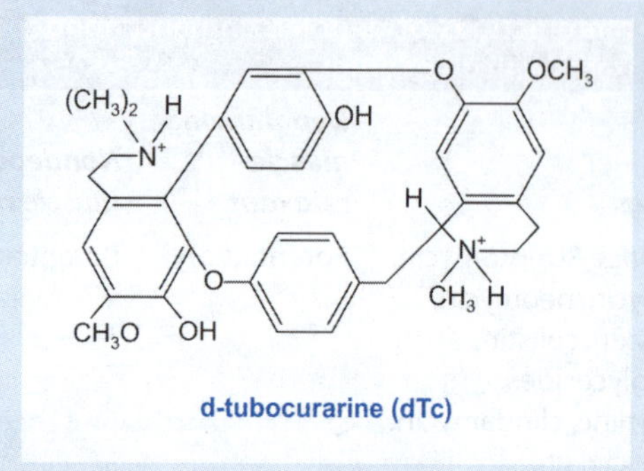

Fig. 4: The chemical structure of d-tubocurarine.

causing severe hypotension (30–50% drop of BP). Though, theoretically it causes anaphylactoid reaction, but clinically it is extremely rare, even in atopic individuals. Although, it was widely used in asthma without any adverse effect, still it may produce bronchospasm and should be avoided in these patients. The dTc has profound ganglion blocking effect, as the ganglion has nicotinic receptors. But, this side effect of dTc is probably beyond the clinical dose range of it. Increase in HR by dTc is uncommon and may be due to hypotension which is again due to the release of histamine.

As the hypotension, caused by dTc, is usually due to the release of histamine, but it also may be due to very slight ganglion blocking and cardiac depressant effect.

There is no active metabolism of dTc. It is mainly excreted unchanged through the urine. So, the kidney is the primary and the liver is the second alternative route for elimination of it. In the presence of renal failure, biliary excretion of dTc is increased to provide a satisfactory alternative means of its excretion. So, this drug is not indicated when both the renal and hepatic failure are present at a time.

Clinical Use of d-tubocurarine

The dTc is not used now due to the discovery of many other safe nondepolarizing muscle relaxants. But, the prolonged experience on this drug, since 1946, has established its safety. However, it should be avoided in atopic and hypovolemic patients. It should be avoided or used with caution in those patients in whom a modest fall of BP may endanger his/her cardiac functions. The effective neuromuscular blocking dose of dTc is 0.3–0.5 mg/kg through IV which provides good skeletal muscle relaxation for about 45–75 minutes.

Gallamine Triethiodide

Chemically, gallamine is a tribenzene triethiodide compound. In 1947, Bovet and his coworkers had first described the muscle-relaxing property of this synthetic product. It is the first synthetic neuromuscular blocking

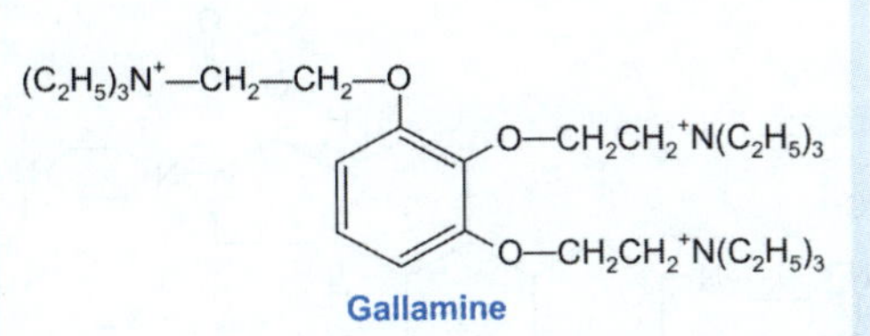

Fig. 5: It is a triquaternary ether of gallic acid. Its strong vagolytic property is probably due to the triquaternary structure of it. Gallamine is the only triquaternary compound, available in clinical anesthesia.

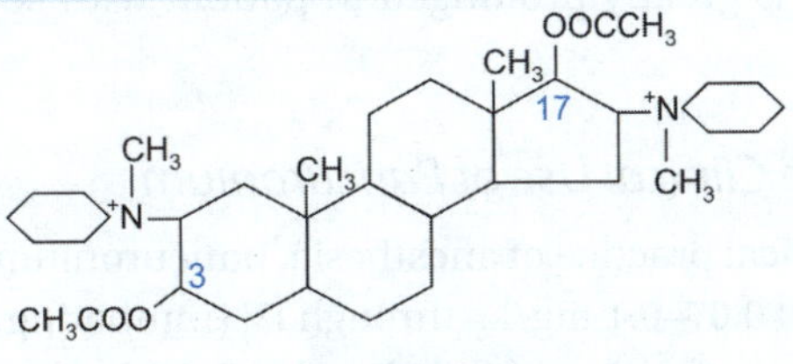

Fig. 6: The chemical structure of pancuronium.

agent, which is used in the practice of anesthesia. But, the effect of this muscle relaxant in man was first described in 1948 **(Fig. 5)**.

Like dTc, it is also a nondepolarizing muscle-relaxing agent. The triquaternary structure of gallamine confers a strong vagolytic property on it and the degree of tachycardia, caused by it, due to its vagolytic action, goes up to 20–60% over the control value. This property of gallamine is useful, when it is used in combination with halothane, as halothane reduces the HR by stimulating the vagus. This tachycardia, caused by gallamine, can be accompanied by ↑BP and ↑CO. This may probably be due to the increased release of catecholamines. The gallamine causes very little (1/2 to 1/5 quantity of histamine as compared to dTc) release of histamine and less block of autonomic ganglia. Therefore, it does not cause the decrease in BP. It crosses the placenta in appreciable concentrations. It is not metabolized in liver. So, it is entirely excreted through urine as unchanged form and has no biliary excretion. Hence, in absence of renal function, there is no alternative way of lowering the blood concentration of this drug. The effective neuromuscular blocking dose of gallamine is 4–6 mg/kg through IV for intubation and 1–1.5 mg/kg of bodyweight through infusion for maintenance of relaxation.

Pancuronium

It was introduced in the practice of clinical anesthesia by Baird and Reid, in 1964, by the addition of 2-ACh-like groups on the rigid nucleus of a steroid molecule, at 2 or 3 and 16 or 17 position. Thus, the pancuronium is a bisquaternary aminosteroidal nondepolarizing muscle-relaxing agent which was ultimately introduced into the market in 1967. It is 10 times more potent than dTc with an ED_{95} value of about 0.06 mg/kg. (i) High potency, (ii) Lack of hypotensive effect, and (iii) Mild-to-moderate vagolytic property, in contrast to then only available drugs, i.e., dTc and gallamine, make the pancuronium an instant success in clinical anesthesia practice. It was the first muscle relaxant, introduced in

clinical practice, which did not have the ganglion blocking or histamine releasing properties, like dTc and gallamine, but has a long duration of action like them. So, its administration was ideally suited for longer operation, lasting for 3–4 hours and in which prompt extubation was not necessary. It is also suited for operation in which increased HR and BP is desirable, as it has no ganglion blocking and histamine-releasing property. Pancuronium also causes transient mild depression of pseudocholinesterase enzyme **(Fig. 6)**.

Cardiovascular System Effects of Pancuronium

Pancuronium stimulates the sympathetic nervous system (i) by inhibiting the reuptake and increasing the release of catecholamines at nerve ending and (ii) by causing the muscarine receptor blockade action. Thus, the level of catecholamines is increased by the use of pancuronium. All these effects result in tachycardia, ↑SVR, ↑CO, ↑after load, etc. So, the pancuronium should not be used in patient with coronary artery diseases and myocardial failure. It may be associated with arrhythmias and cardiac ischemia in susceptible individuals. So, the use of pancuronium is only advantageous in some situations, where increase in HR, BP, and CO is needed. Two such situations are when high dose of opium is used in cardiac surgery or in shock patients. Hence, the use of pancuronium has been decreased remarkably following the introduction of other new short- and intermediate-acting muscle relaxants. But, still it is a popular choice with many anesthetists for use during cardiac surgery. This is because, it tends to counteract the vagal effects which are found in high-dose opiate anesthesia. It causes very little release of histamine.

Metabolism and Excretion of Pancuronium

85% of the injected dose of pancuronium is cleared unchanged by kidney and 15% is metabolized in liver to 3-hydroxy or 17-hydroxy or 3,17-hydroxy compound which are excreted through both the kidney and bile. The first and principal metabolite of pancuronium is 3-hydroxy derivative, which potency is half than that of the mother compound. Due to the limited metabolism and limited biliary excretion, its action is greatly prolonged in patient with severe renal disorder.

Dose and Clinical Use of Pancuronium

In the clinical practice of anesthesia, pancuronium is used in the dose of 0.07–0.1 mg/kg through IV (intubating dose) and the duration of action of this dose is 60–120 minutes. In this clinical dose (which is about 1–1.5 times of its ED_{95} value) intubating condition only reach after 3–4 minutes of its IV administration. However, higher doses of pancuronium have faster onset and much longer duration of action. As pancuronium has the markedly cumulative action, so the top-up maintenance dose, only in the range of 0.01–0.015 mg/kg, should be used with the duration of action of 30–40 minutes. With repeated administration, progressive increase in the duration of action of pancuronium occurs.

Pipecuronium

Chemically, pipecuronium is also an aminosteroidal compound. Though, it is a pancuronium derivative, but still its vagolytic property is 1/10 of that of pancuronium. The another advantage of pipecuronium is that it is 20–30% more potent than pancuronium, but still it is free from cardiovascular side effects of the latter. Pipecuronium is a long-acting muscle relaxing drug with the duration of action depending on the size of the dose. Spontaneous recovery from pipecuronium is very slow. Hence, it is only used when early extubation is unnecessary and cardiovascular stability is required.

In the clinical dose range, pipecuronium does not release histamine. It has nonvagolytic action and does not block autonomic ganglia. The ED_{95} dose of pipecuronium during balanced anesthesia is about 0.04 mg/kg. In comparison with pancuronium, increase in HR and cardiac index was observed only when the two times of ED_{95} dose of pipecuronium is administered. Hemodynamic changes are also minimal following pipecuronium up to the doses of three times of ED_{95} value **(Fig. 7)**.

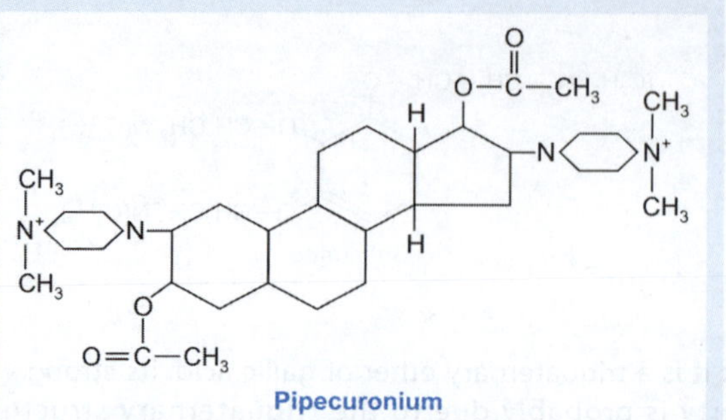

No metabolism of pipecuronium occurs in body. So, it is mainly excreted unchanged through the kidney. Liver is possibly a minor secondary pathway for the elimination of pipecuronium. Intubating dose of pipecuronium is 0.08–0.12 mg/kg with duration of action 60–120 minutes. The onset of action of this intubating dose is 2.5–4.5 minutes and this dose is 1–2 times of ED_{95} value. The time of onset of neuromuscular block also decreases with increasing the dose. Maintenance dose of pipecuronium is 0.005–0.01 mg/kg with the duration of action of 30–45 minutes. Like all other muscle relaxants, renal elimination is also basic to pipecuronium. But, this additional process of clearance

Fig. 7: The positive charge of the quaternary nitrogen atom in the Pipecuronium molecule is separated by two carbon atoms from the carboxyl group in comparison to pancuronium. This chemical change reduces the vagolytic effect of pipecuronium by 10 times than pancuronium.

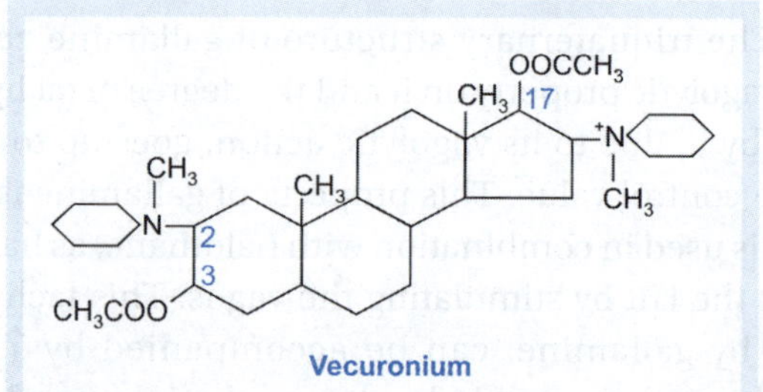

Fig. 8: The chemical structure of vecuronium.

shortens the duration of effect of this nondepolarizing muscle-relaxing agent.

Vecuronium

Chemically, vecuronium is a 2-desmethyl analog (or 16-monoquaternary derivative) of pancuronium, with ED_{95} value of 0.04–0.05 mg/kg. However, the stereoisometric relationship of the 3-acetyl group on the molecule of vecuronium makes it structurally dissimilar from pancuronium. It is more lipid soluble than pancuronium. This is because of the absence of methyl group in the molecule of vecuronium **(Fig. 8)**.

The loss of quaternizing methyl group at position 2 also destabilizes the 3-acetyl group present in the molecule of it. *As a result, the vecuronium compound in the form of solution has very short half-life and should be prepared in alkaline buffer solution, shortly before its use. But, the powder of it does not need refrigeration.* It is the first nondepolarizing muscle relaxing agent with intermediate duration of action and the most popular muscle relaxant in clinical practice at present. *The reasons of the popularity of vecuronium are:* (i) It helps in more facile tracheal intubation, (ii) It causes easy administration by infusion for maintenance, (iii) It possesses intermediate duration of action, (iv) It has faster and more complete recovery, (v) It causes a remarkable lack of cardiovascular side effect, throughout a wide clinical dose range from one to eight times (0.05–0.4 mg/kg). It is more potent than pancuronium, because ED_{90} value of vecuronium is 0.03 mg/kg, compared to 0.05 mg/kg for pancuronium.

It has 20 times less vagolytic action than pancuronium. It possesses no ganglion blocking, histamine releasing, and cumulative effect. The drug is rapidly cleared from plasma. It has a short α-half-life, compared to pancuronium. However, its β-half-life is similar to that of pancuronium **(Fig. 9)**.

Vecuronium has two major routes of elimination. These are liver and kidney, and they are of approximately equal importance. The 30–40% of the injected dose of vecuronium is deacetylated at 3 and 17 position by liver, producing 17-OH vecuronium, 3-OH vecuronium and 3,17-OH vecuronium. But, the major metabolite is 3-OH vecuronium which is as potent as the mother compound and is excreted through both urine and bile. For this reason, the effects of vecuronium are prolonged in patients with hepatic or renal failure. These metabolites may also be responsible for prolonged paralysis, seen after long-term administration of vecuronium in patients at ICU. Because of the lack of cumulative effect, vecuronium can be used as continuous IV infusion and rapid recovery is ensured after infusion has stopped.

Doses of Vecuronium

The intubating dose of vecuronium is 0.1–0.2 mg/kg through IV route with the duration of action ranging between 45 and 90 minutes. It provides acceptable intubating condition within 90–120 seconds, after the administration of above-mentioned dose. However, both the onset and the duration of action are dose related. The onset of action of vecuronium can also be accelerated by inducing anesthesia with a potent volatile anesthetic agent, such as sevoflurane. The maintenance dose of vecuronium is 0.01–0.02 mg/kg through intravenous, as intermittent bolus with duration of action only 15–30 minutes. The infusion dose of vecuronium is 0.8–2 mg/kg/min. Because of the safety factor, the top-up dose of vecuronium can also be given in multiples of ED_{95} value for maintenance.

Of all the neuromuscular blocking drugs available, vecuronium is the most specific for neuromuscular junction and, therefore, has the least side effect. So, even when used in large doses, it is associated with extremely good cardiovascular stability. There is a wide separation between the vagal and neuromuscular blocking dose (68:1) of vecuronium. It has little sympathetic stimulation activity. Larger doses of vecuronium ($1–4 \times ED_{95}$) can also be administered to achieve a faster onset of action and good intubating conditions for rapid sequence intubation.

Atracurium (BW33A)

Like vecuronium, the atracurium also has revolutionized the clinical anesthesia practice due to same reasons. Chemically, it is a synthetic bisquaternary benzyl-iso-quinolinium ester **(Fig. 10)** and is of intermediate duration of action. It is the first nondepolarizing muscle relaxant which is degraded in plasma by spontaneous chemical reaction, called the *Hoffmann elimination,* but not by biological process, i.e., metabolism in liver and excretion through urine or bile.

The cardiovascular effects of atracurium are same as that of vecuronium. But, it has a strong potential for the release of histamine. However, it (release of histamine) is evident only when higher doses (two times of ED_{95} value) of atracurium are injected very rapidly. The release of histamine causes ↓BP and facial erythema. But, the combined H_1 and H_2 receptor blocker effectively blocks the CVS manifestation of histamine, released by atracurium. The atracurium has no vagolytic action. It also does not block autonomic ganglia. The pharmacodynamics of atracurium are unchanged with advancing age.

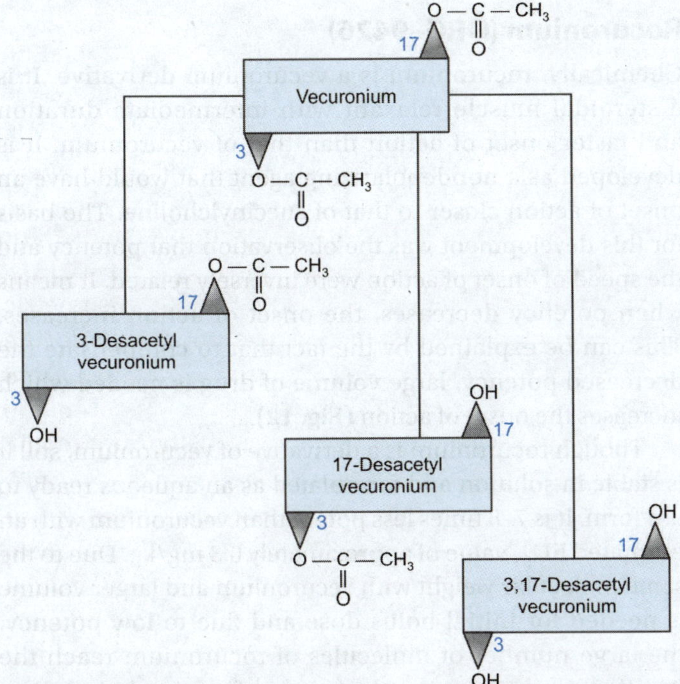

Fig. 9: This is a schematic diagram of the metabolism of vecuronium. The metabolism of vecuronium occurs in liver. About 30–40% of injected vecuronium is deacetylated at its 3 and 17 position. The major metabolite is 3-OH vecuronium. Other metabolites are 17-OH vecuronium and 3,17-OH vecuronium. All these metabolites are excreted through urine and bile.

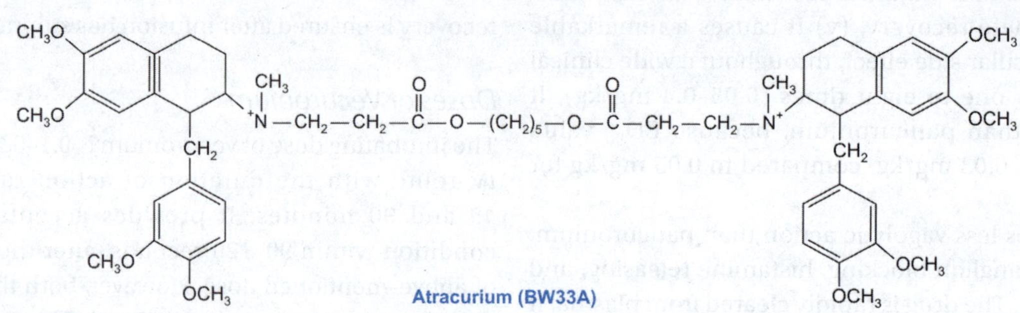

Fig. 10: It is a benzyl-iso-quinolinium diester and undergoes Hoffmann elimination. This reaction is facilitated by the orientation of the ether oxygen of the carboxyl group toward the center of chain.

Atracurium is spontaneously degraded by (i) Hoffmann elimination and (ii) ester hydrolysis. *The Hoffmann elimination is a pure chemical process, where the parent molecule of atracurium is fragmented by itself to laudanosine (a tertiary amine) and a monoquaternary acrylate at physiological pH and temperature of plasma, i.e., at pH of 7.4 and a temperature of 37°C.* However, this spontaneous degradation of atracurium is slowed down with the fall in pH (acidic condition) and temperature (hypothermia) of plasma. Whereas, the degradation of it is accelerated by alkaline pH and rise in temperature of plasma. So, atracurium is stored at 4°C and is buffered to a pH of 3, where it is stable. Atracurium becomes unstable when it is injected in bloodstream and breakdown from itself in blood's normal pH and temperature. The alteration of pH and temperature of blood within its physiological range does not decrease the rate of Hoffmann's elimination of atracurium and does not cause clinically significant increase in the duration of action of it. The duration of action of atracurium is prolonged markedly by hypothermia. The ester hydrolysis which is a second pathway for the degradation of atracurium may be of more importance than was originally thought. The steps of this hydrolysis of atracurium are shown in **Figure 11**. Laudanosine which is formed by Hoffmann's degradation of atracurium is excreted through urine and bile. It can cross the blood-brain barrier and enter into CNS. Very high doses of laudanosine can cause CNS excitation. But, no clear-cut cases have been noted in human.

The duration of action of atracurium is not prolonged by absence of hepatic and renal pathways for excretion. So, it is the relaxants of choice for patient with renal and hepatic failure. 90% atracurium is destroyed in plasma. Only 10% of this drug is excreted unchanged through urine.

Doses of Atracurium

The intubating dose of atracurium is 0.5–0.6 mg/kg through IV with duration of action only 30–45 minutes. Actually, the ED_{95} value of atracurium is approximately 0.2 mg/kg and the onset of action of this ED_{95} value is 3–5 minutes. So, this onset of action can be reduced by increasing the intubating dose from 0.2 mg/kg to 0.5 mg/kg. The maintenance dose of atracurium is 0.1–0.15 mg/kg as intermittent bolus with duration of action only 15–20 minutes. The infusion dose of atracurium is 4–12 µg/kg/min. The repeated administration of atracurium does not lead to any increase in its duration of action. The unique type of metabolism of atracurium makes it suitable for use in the critically ill patient, as it is associated with rapid recovery.

Rocuronium (ORG–9426)

Chemically, rocuronium is a vecuronium derivative. It is a steroidal muscle relaxant with intermediate duration and faster onset of action than that of vecuronium. It is developed as a nondepolarizing agent that would have an onset of action closer to that of succinylcholine. The basis for this development was the observation that potency and the speed of onset of action were inversely related. It means when potency decreases, the onset of action increases. This can be explained by the fact that to compensate the decreased potency, large volume of drug is needed which increases the onset of action **(Fig. 12)**.

Though rocuronium is a derivative of vecuronium, still it is stable in solution and formulated as an aqueous ready to use form. It is 7–8 times less potent than vecuronium with an estimated ED_{95} value of approximately 0.3 mg/kg. Due to the same molecular weight with vecuronium and larger volume is needed for initial bolus dose and due to low potency, the large number of molecules of rocuronium reach the junctional nicotinic receptors within few circulation time, causing faster onset of action. The faster onset of action of rocuronium also can be improved by the addition of opiates, ketamine, or a small dose of ephedrine which maintains a better cardiac output and thus improves the rapid delivery of muscle relaxant to the neuromuscular junction. The weaker

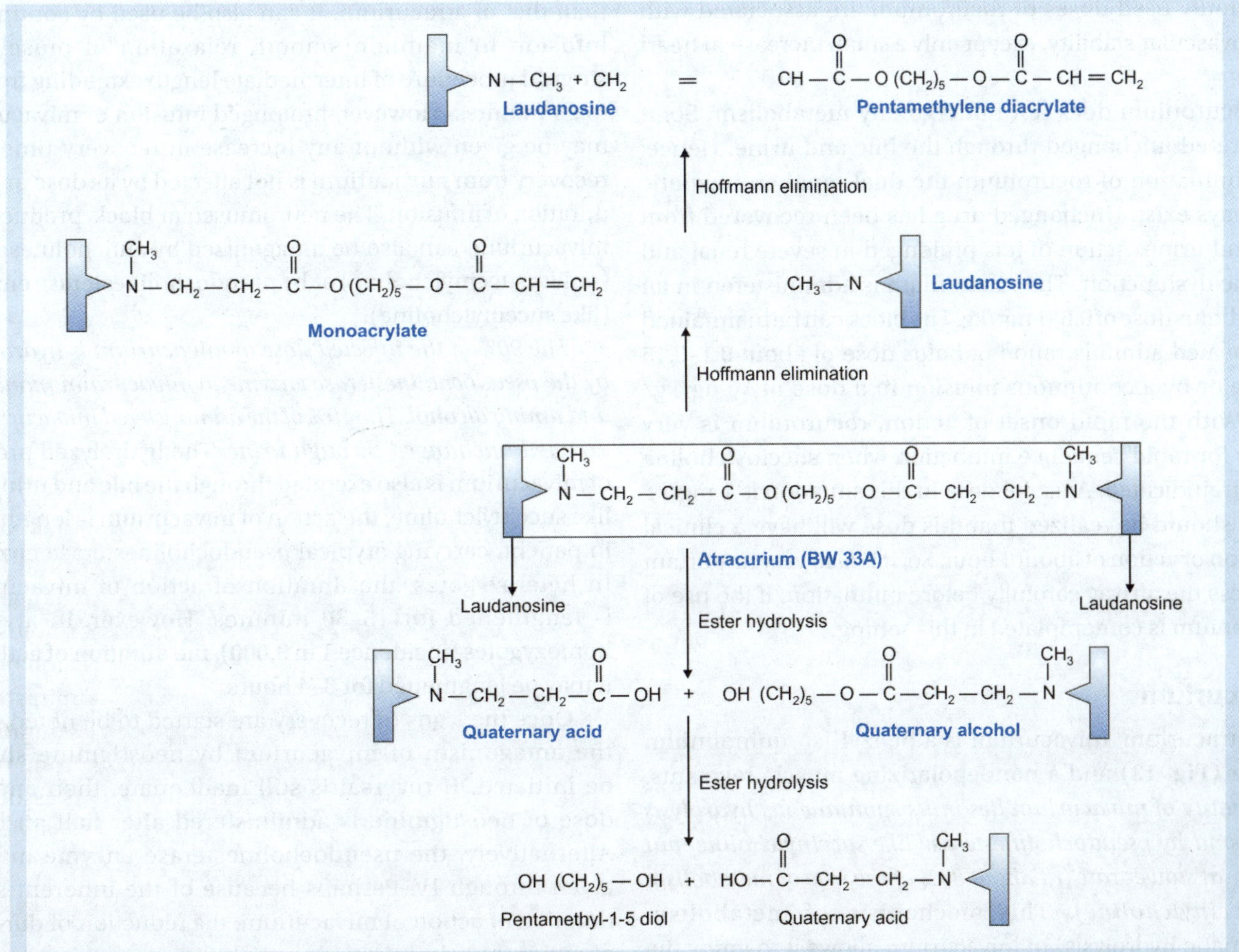

Fig. 11: Schematic diagram of metabolism of atracurium. The major metabolite of atracurium is laudanosine. It is excreted through urine and bile. Laudanosine may enter the CNS as it is a tertiary amine. Less than 10% of the administered atracurium is excreted unchanged as the parent compound.

Fig. 12: A vecuronium derivative of faster onset and intermediate duration of action. The faster onset is conferred by lower potency. The lower potency is largely due to the D-ring substitutions with respect to vecuronium.

binding ability of rocuronium molecule with receptor allows repetitive binding and unbinding and thus easy diffusion of drugs is away from the receptor site which limits the duration of action.

Rocuronium is peculiar for its lower potency with faster onset of action. The onset of maximum block following an intubating dose of 0.6 mg/kg occurs in about 60–90 seconds, which is near similar to that of succinylcholine. More larger doses have a more rapid onset of action. However, a dose of about 1 mg/kg is required to obtain a good intubating condition during a rapid sequence induction. The duration of action of rocuronium is similar to that of vecuronium and atracurium in comparable doses. The clinical duration of action of 0.6 mg/kg of rocuronium is 30 minutes. The repeated administration of it does not usually result in a prolonged effect. With adequate dose, rocuronium may enable tracheal intubation within 60 seconds and make it an ideal substitute for succinylcholine during rapid sequence intubation.

It has no ganglion blocking effect and no histamine releasing property, but has mild vagal blocking effect, resulting sometimes in increase in heart rate. So, the commonly used doses of rocuronium are associated with cardiovascular stability, except only a small increase in heart rate.

Rocuronium does not undergo any metabolism. So, it is excreted unchanged through the bile and urine. Hence, for elimination of rocuronium the dual renal and hepatic pathways exist. Unchanged drug has been recovered from bile and urine. Action of it is prolonged in severe renal and hepatic dysfunction. The rocuronium is administered in an initial bolus dose of 0.6–1 mg/kg. The block can be maintained by repeated administration of bolus dose of about 0.1–0.15 mg/kg or by a continuous infusion in a dose of 10 µg/kg/ min. With the rapid onset of action, rocuronium is very useful for rapid sequence intubation when succinylcholine is contraindicated. A useful dose in this situation is 1 mg/kg and it should be realized that this dose will have a clinical duration of action of about 1 hour. So, it is also very important to assess the airway carefully before intubation, if the use of rocuronium is contemplated in this setting.

Mivacurium

Like atracurium, mivacurium is a benzyl-iso-quinolinium diester **(Fig. 13)** and a nondepolarizing muscle relaxants. *The beauty of mivacurium lies in its spontaneous hydrolysis in plasma by pseudocholinesterase like succinylcholine, but slightly at slower rate (at about 80% of the rate of metabolism of succinylcholine).* This mechanism of metabolism (enzymatic hydrolysis) of mivacurium allows it to enjoy the shorter duration of action than vecuronium and atracurium, but 2–2.5 times than that of succinylcholine.

It has neither autonomic ganglion blocking action nor any vagolytic action. Like atracurium, it has the potential to cause histamine release, resulting facial erythema and ↓BP. The duration of action of mivacurium is 2–2.5 times longer than that of succinylcholine, but 1/2 to 1/3 times longer

than that of atracurium. It can also be used by continuous infusion to maintain smooth relaxation of muscle for surgical procedure of intermediate length extending from 30 to 90 minutes. However, prolonged infusion of mivacurium may be given without any increase in recovery time. The recovery from mivacurium is not affected by its dose or by its duration of infusion. The neuromuscular block, produced by mivacurium, can also be antagonized by anticholinesterase (unlike succinylcholine) or by pseudocholinesterase enzyme (like succinylcholine).

The 90% of the injected dose of mivacurium is hydrolyzed by the pseudocholinesterase enzyme to mivacurium monoester and amino alcohol. The 10% of the administered mivacurium is excreted unchanged through urine. The hydrolyzed product of mivacurium is also excreted through the bile and urine. So, like succinylcholine, the action of mivacurium is lengthened in patient, carrying atypical pseudocholinesterase enzyme. In heterozygotes, the duration of action of mivacurium is lengthened for 15–30 minutes. However, in atypical homozygotes (incidence 1 in 3,000), the duration of action of it may be lengthened for 3–4 hours.

Once the signs of recovery are started to be noted, then the antagonism of mivacurium by neostigmine should be initiated. If reversal is still inadequate, then another dose of neostigmine is administered after half an hour. Alternatively, the pseudocholinesterase enzyme may be given through IV. Perhaps because of the inherent short duration of action of mivacurium, the reduction of duration of action by administering anticholinesterase is relatively small. Theoretically, anticholinesterase (neostigmine) may prolong the action of mivacurium like succinylcholine. But, this has not been found to occur, when the neostigmine has been administered to antagonize the neuromuscular block, produced by mivacurium. However, the previously administered neostigmine may prolong the effects of subsequently administered mivacurium **(Fig. 14)**.

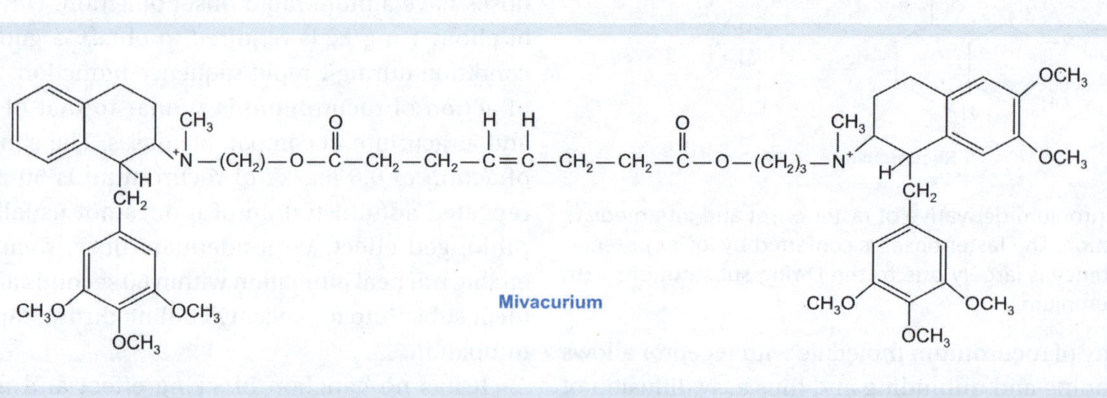

Fig. 13: It is a benzyl-iso-quinolinium diester which is hydrolyzed by pseudocholinesterase at the rate of about 80% of succinylcholine. This hydrolysis of mivacurium is facilitated by the orientation of the ether oxygen of its carboxyl group toward its quaternary nitrogen atom.

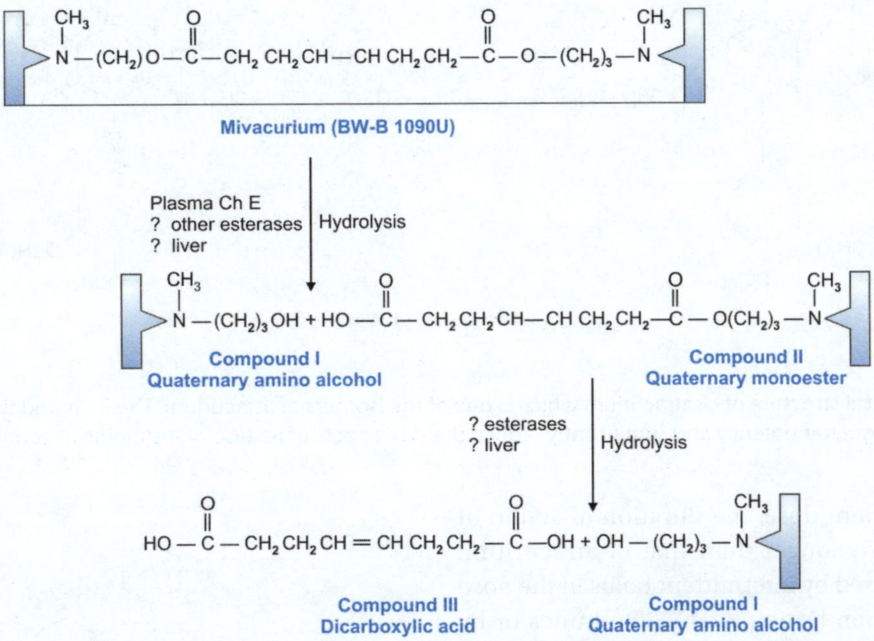

Fig. 14: Schematic diagram of metabolism of mivacurium. It is metabolized by plasma cholinesterase. The reaction occurs at the rate of about 70–80% of succinylcholine. These metabolites are inactive and carry positive charges. So, their CNS entry is minimal.

Doses of Mivacurium

The ED_{95} dose of mivacurium is 80 µg/kg and like other nondepolarizing muscle relaxant, the onset of action is dose dependent. It is the currently available shortest acting nondepolarizing muscle relaxant and this duration of muscle relaxation lasts only for about 15 minutes, following a dose of 0.15 mg/kg ($2 \times ED_{95}$) through IV. The increase in the duration of action of mivacurium, with increasing doses, is not as marked as with other nondepolarizing relaxants. The intubating dose of mivacurium is 0.2–0.25 mg/kg through IV with the duration of action of only 15–20 minutes. The maintenance dose of mivacurium is 0.05–0.1 mg with the duration of action of 5–10 minutes. Mivacurium is the most suitable agent for maintaining relaxation by infusion. Continuous infusion is the preferred method of administration of mivacurium for anything, but for brief surgical procedures. The recovery from mivacurium does not change significantly by the repeated administration of bolus doses of it or infusion of mivacurium in varying doses and duration. It suggests that the mivacurium has minimal or no cumulative property. Infusion dose of mivacurium is 6–8 µg/kg/min.

There exist three isomers of mivacurium. Among these cis-cis isomer is hydrolyzed by pseudocholinesterase very slowly, but fortunately constitutes only 5% of the commercial preparation. However, 95% of the commercial preparation is made up of cis-trans and trans-trans isomer of mivacurium which is hydrolyzed very rapidly (t 1/2 β is 2–3 minutes). Another advantage of cis-cis isomer is that it is of less potent, about one-tenth of the neuromuscular blocking potency of other two isomers. It (cis-cis isomer) undergoes some renal excretion as well as is broken down by plasma cholinesterase. In renal failure, the duration of action of mivacurium is prolonged. In hepatic failure, the action of mivacurium is also prolonged due to the reduction of plasma cholinesterase activity. The same is true for elderly patient also.

Cisatracurium (51W89)

Cisatracurium constitutes about 15% of the commercially available preparation of atracurium. It is one of the 10 stereoisomers of atracurium and is very potent. It liberates only minimum amount of histamine than its parent compound. It is in clinical practice only for about last few years. In comparison to atracurium, the ED_{95} value of cisatracurium is 0.05 mg/kg which indicates that it is four times more potent than atracurium (ED_{95} value of atracurium is 0.2 mg/kg). However, being more potent, the drug has slower onset of action. In the dose of 0.1 mg/kg (intubating dose 0.1–0.15 mg/kg) the onset of maximum neuromuscular block in cisatracurium takes about 3–5 minutes. Although increasing the dose (0.15 mg/kg) accelerates the onset of action, but it is still slower than that of atracurium. The duration of action of cisatracurium is 30–60 minutes at its initial bolus dose of 0.1–0.15 mg/kg and it depends

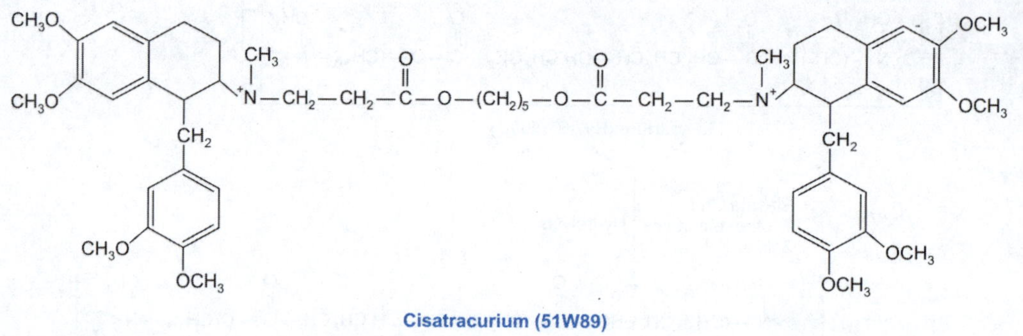

Fig. 15: This is the chemical structure of cisatracurium which is one of the isomers of atracurium. The R-cis and the R'-cis conformation of the structure provide greater potency and significantly reduce the side effects of release of histamine in comparison to atracurium.

on the dose. At equivalent dose, the duration of action of cisatracurium is slightly longer than that of atracurium. Cisatracurium can be used by intermittent bolus in the dose of 0.02 mg/kg with action lasting for 15–20 minutes or by continuous infusion in the dose of 1.5 µg/kg/min for longer procedures **(Fig. 15)**.

As cisatracurium releases the negligible amount of histamine, so it gives us a stable cardiovascular activity. Even, when administered in higher doses (eight times the ED_{95} dose), the cisatracurium does not give rise to any significant changes in arterial pressure and heart rate. It is eliminated predominantly by Hoffmann degradation like atracurium. So, the pharmacokinetics of cisatracurium are independent of its dose, in healthy adult patients. The renal clearance is responsible for 10% of total elimination of this drug from our body. So, the recovery profile is not altered in patients with liver failure, but becomes slightly slower in renal failure patient. Compared with atracurium, the cisatracurium produces much less laudanosine, even when the drug is given by continuous infusion.

Rapacuronium (ORG–9487)

Chemically, rapacuronium is also a steroidal nondepolarizing muscle relaxant. The introduction of rocuronium in clinical practice had stimulated the search for such a nondepolarizing muscle relaxants which have rapid onset, but short duration of action like succinylcholine. This is because rocuronium has rapid onset of action like succinylcholine, but does not have short duration of action. So, it has instigated the advent of rapacuronium which has both the rapid onset and shorter duration of action, like succinylcholine **(Fig. 16)**.

Rapacuronium is analog of vecuronium and is of low potency with an ED_{95} value of about 0.75 mg/kg. In the dose of 1.5 mg/kg, rapacuronium produces complete block

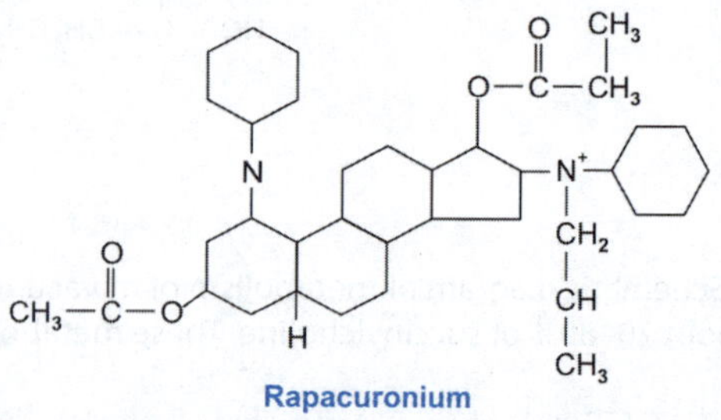

Fig. 16: The chemical structure of rapacuronium.

(neuromuscular paralysis) in 80 seconds, compared with 60 seconds for succinylcholine, in the dose of 1 mg/kg. The rapid onset of rapacuronium is possibly due to its low potency, necessitating higher doses and facilitating a rapid access to the site of action. Though, initially rapacuronium was thought to have short duration of action of only 8–9 minutes in the dose of 1.5 mg/kg, but recent studies have reported that this value will be about 14–20 minutes. This drug also showed cumulative properties, especially after repeated doses or administration by infusion. Rapacuronium causes higher rate of respiratory side effects, especially bronchospasm both in adults and children, though its exact cause has not yet been determined. But, histamine release and muscarinic receptor stimulation in the airways may be the probable explanation of bronchospasm by rapacuronium. So, the drug was withdrawn from clinical use finally, in March 2001, due to its higher risk of bronchospasm.

ANTAGONISM OF NEUROMUSCULAR BLOCKADE

The neuromuscular blockade (paralysis) produced by nondepolarizing muscle relaxant can be antagonized by allowing the neurotransmitter, ACh to accumulate in synaptic cleft by temporarily inhibiting true cholinesterase enzyme which is present in synaptic cleft and inactivates the neurotransmitter, ACh. Thus, anticholinesterase antagonizes this true cholinesterase enzyme and increases the concentration of ACh in synaptic cleft and improves the neuromuscular transmission. The agents which inhibit this true cholinesterase enzyme are called the *anticholinesterase or AChE-enzyme inhibitor (commonly called cholinesterase inhibitor)*. The clinically commonly used cholinesterase enzyme inhibitors are edrophonium, pyridostigmine, and neostigmine. They indirectly antagonize the nondepolarizing block: (i) by increasing the concentration of neurotransmitter, such as ACh at motor nerve terminals, and (ii) by blocking the neuronal potassium channels and thus preventing hyperpolarization.

Reversal of nondepolarizing paralysis by AChE inhibitor depends on five major factors.

Depth of Block at the Time of Administration of Acetylcholinesterase Inhibitor

The deeper will be the neuromuscular block, the longer will be the time interval, required between the administration of nondepolarizing muscle relaxant and the administration of a standard dose of antagonist (AChE-inhibitor) in restoring the twitch or TOF response to a level which is compatible with the clinically normal function of skeletal muscles (respiratory muscles). Usually, the deeper block requires much longer time interval between the administration of muscle relaxant and the administration of anticholinesterase, such as 15–30 minutes for adequate reversal of neuromuscular paralysis. The relationship between the reversal time and the depth of block is hyperbolic. The maximum antagonistic effect of neostigmine is likely to be reached within 10 minutes, after its administration.

Type of Antagonist Administered

Under standard condition and in moderate depth of neuromuscular paralysis, the order of rapidity of action of antagonist is: edrophonium > neostigmine > pyridostigmine. But, edrophonium is not as effective (or potent) as neostigmine in antagonizing profound muscular paralysis which is >90% of twitch depression. As the depth of block becomes more intense, edrophonium becomes less potent than neostigmine. The dose-response curves between edrophonium and neostigmine are not parallel and become increasingly divergent as the depth of block intensifies. It indicates that edrophonium is less effective than neostigmine at very deep level of block.

AchE inhibitor acts indirectly by increasing the level of ACh at synaptic cleft by inhibiting true cholinesterase.

ACh has both nicotine and muscarinic response as it acts on its both the receptors. So, AChE inhibitor also have indirect both nicotinic and muscarinic effects. But, the nicotinic effect that is muscular contraction or reversal of neuromuscular blockade is only desired. So, the muscarinic effect of AChE inhibitor, which is not desired, should be blocked by anticholinergic (antimuscarinic) agents, such as atropine or glycopyrrolate. Atropine acts more rapidly than glycopyrrolate. So, atropine is better suited with rapid acting edrophonium, whereas glycopyrrolate is better suited with slower acting neostigmine.

It was initially thought that edrophonium is not suitable for antagonism of neuromuscular block, because of its too short duration of action. But, when it is used in standard large dose of 0.5–1 mg/kg, then a sustained action of antagonism results. In fact, elimination half-life of edrophonium in this dose is similar to that of neostigmine. So, use of edrophonium in this dose is more justified for faster onset of action, fewer muscarine side effects and standard duration of action like neostigmine.

The highly purified preparation of human pseudocholinesterase enzyme is also available. This enzyme antagonizes the block produced by mivacurium and succinylcholine in patients with abnormal pseudocholinesterase enzyme activity and this antagonism may be 100%.

Dose of Antagonist

It is commonly thought that larger dose of AChE inhibitor can antagonize any level of depth of block more rapidly and more completely than smaller dose and this dose of AChE inhibitor is parallel to the depth of block. But, this is true up to a certain point, i.e., up to a certain maximum dose of AChE inhibitor, beyond which this is not true. For neostigmine, this maximum dose limit is 0.06–0.08 mg/kg (or 60–80 µg/kg) and for edrophonium this limit is 1–1.5 mg/kg. The maximum effect of both these drugs occurs between 5 and 10 minutes, after their IV administration. Further recovery that occurs slowly beyond that period is largely dependent on the rate of clearance of muscle relaxants from the body.

If 30 minutes, after neostigmine administration, adequate reversal of block does not occur, then good rules of practice are that: (a) continue the support of airway and ventilation, (b) wait for another 30–45 minutes which is 50% of the half-life of both muscle relaxants and neostigmine, (c) administer another dose of same antagonist equal to 50% of original dose (30 µg/kg of neostigmine). This repeat dose of AChE inhibitor would help to return the function of muscle power satisfactorily within subsequent 30 minutes. Neostigmine and edrophonium do not potentiate each other and should not be mixed and repeat dose should be of the original drug.

Concentration of Inhaled Anesthetic Agents

The inhaled anesthetic agents retard the antagonism of neuromuscular block, produced by AChE inhibitors.

Rate of Clearance of Muscle Relaxants

The clearance rate (CR) from our body for different muscle relaxants are different. Usually, for long-acting drugs the CR is 1.2–2 mL/kg/min and reversal time interval is 20–40 minutes from deep depth of block which is about 95% of twitch depression. CR of intermediate acting drugs is 3–6 mL/kg/min and reversal time interval is 12–15 minutes from 95% block. For mivacurium CR is 50 mL/kg/min and reversal time interval is 7–8 minutes from 95% block by neostigmine. So, higher the plasma clearance of muscle relaxant, shorter the time interval will be required for antagonism of block. If adequate reversal time interval from 95% block is not elapsed and neostigmine is administered, then after 10 minutes when the maximum antagonistic effect of neostigmine occurs, little amount of long-acting drug is removed from plasma. Therefore, there is chance of re-paralysis. So, in such circumstances, restoration of adequate neuromuscular function depends entirely on the action of neostigmine, and large doses (50–70 µg/kg) is recommended for antagonism of long-acting drug. This larger dose of AChE inhibitor maximally inhibits true AChE, but may cause a transient neuromuscular block by themselves.

INDIVIDUAL NEUROMUSCULAR ANTAGONIST

Neostigmine

Chemically, neostigmine is a quaternary amine compound and is also an ester of an alkylcarbamic acid. It is a reversible (acid transferring) cholinesterase enzyme inhibitor. It acts by binding to the esteratic site of acetylcholinesterase or AChE (true cholinesterase) enzyme, presents at synaptic cleft and thus temporary blocks and subsequently prevents the ACh from hydrolysis by this enzyme. Later, the AChE inhibitor (neostigmine) is hydrolyzed by this true cholinesterase enzyme like ACh and makes free the true cholinesterase (AChE) enzyme, but at a much slower rate than the ACh. So, the AChE enzyme remains engaged by neostigmine, till the neostigmine is hydrolyzed completely by it (enzyme) and cannot attack the ACh which will accumulate gradually into synaptic cleft. Thus, the accumulation of ACh at neuromuscular junction allows it (ACh) to make competitive antagonism with any nondepolarizing muscle relaxant that is present there. Hence, the mode of action of neostigmine is to let the accumulation of ACh at motor endplate and the reversal of neuromuscular blockade (paralysis) by nondepolarizing agent **(Fig. 17)**.

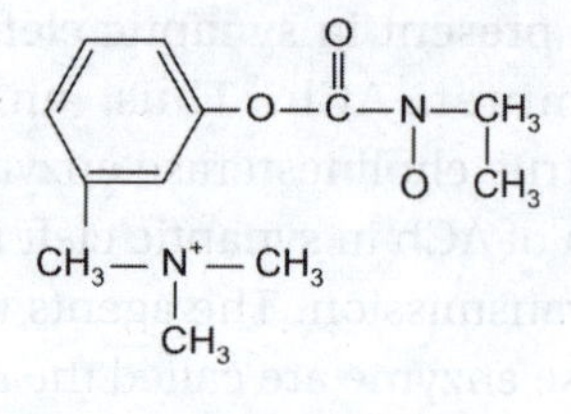

Neostigmine

Fig. 17: The chemical structure of neostigmine.

TABLE 15: Comparison between physostigmine and neostigmine.

		Physostigmine	Neostigmine
1.	Source	Natural alkaloid, obtained from calabar bean	Synthetic
2.	Chemistry	Tertiary amine derivative	Quaternary ammonium compound
3.	Oral absorption	Good	Poor
4.	CNS effect	Present	Absent
5.	Topical action on eye	Good corneal penetration	Poor corneal penetration
6.	Direct action on cholinergic receptor	Absent	Present
7.	Prominent effect on	Autonomic target organ such as eye	Myasthenia gravis
8.	Important use	In glaucoma (miotic)	Myasthenia gravis

The pharmacological effects of neostigmine are indirect and are due to the accumulation of excess ACh which has both the nicotinic and muscarinic action. So, the nicotinic action of neostigmine, caused by the nicotinic action of ACh, is manifested as the removal of neuromuscular blockade or the initiation of muscular contraction. Whereas, the muscarinic action of neostigmine, caused by the muscarinic action of ACh, is manifested on different organs, where there is presence of muscarinic receptors, such as heart, bronchial glands and its smooth muscles, intestinal glands and its smooth muscles, blood vessels, urinary bladder, salivary glands, etc. The effects of neostigmine on cardiovascular system (CVS), due to the accumulation of ACh, are variable and depend upon **(Table 15)** the prevailing autonomic tone. The drug may cause bradycardia, leading to a fall in cardiac output. It increases the duration of effective refractory period of cardiac muscle and decreases the conduction time in conducting tissue. In high doses, neostigmine may cause hypotension, secondary to its central CNS effect also. It increases the bronchial secretion and may cause bronchoconstriction. Miosis and the failure of accommodation may be precipitated by the administration of this drug. Neostigmine increases salivation, elevates esophageal and gastric tone, increases gastric acid output, and increases gastrointestinal tract motility. Nausea and vomiting may occur. It increases ureteric peristalsis and may lead to involuntary micturition. Sweating and lacrimation are increased by neostigmine. All these effects are due to the muscarinic action of accumulated ACh, caused by neostigmine.

The side effects of neostigmine are due to the excess manifestations of its pharmacological actions, as described above. The cardiac arrest also has been reported after the use of large dose of neostigmine. In small doses, the drug has an indirect action on skeletal muscle, leading to muscular contraction by the accumulation of ACh. But, in higher doses, neostigmine like other anticholinesterase may also block the neuromuscular transmission, by allowing the accumulation of excess ACh which acts like succinylcholine.

It is very poorly absorbed when administered orally and the bioavailability of this drug by this route is only 1–2%. This drug is highly ionized in aqueous solution and therefore does not cross the blood-brain barrier to any significant extent. Neostigmine is 6–10% protein bound in the plasma and the volume of distribution is 0.4–1 L/kg. It is predominantly metabolized or broken down by plasma cholinesterase enzyme (described above) to a quaternary alcohol. Some hepatic metabolism of neostigmine with subsequent biliary excretion may also occur. The 50–60% of an administered dose of neostigmine is excreted through urine. The rate of the clearance of neostigmine is 5–10 mL/min/kg and the elimination of half-life is 15–80 minutes. The clearance of neostigmine is decreased and the elimination half-life of it is increased in the presence of renal impairment.

It is available for oral use as 15 mg neostigmine bromide tablet and as a clear, colorless solution for injection in ampule, containing 0.5 mg/mL of neostigmine methylsulfate. A fixed-dose combination, containing 0.5 mg of glycopyrrolate and 2.5 mg of neostigmine methylsulfate per 5 mL of injection, is also available for the reversal of neuromuscular blockade at the end of surgery. The adult oral dose of neostigmine is 15–30 mg at regular interval of 2–4 hours. The intravenous dose of neostigmine for the reversal of nondepolarizing neuromuscular blockade is 50–70 µg/kg. It is administered slowly and in combination with an appropriate dose of an anticholinergic agent such as atropine or glycopyrrolate to counteract its muscarinic effect. The peak effect of the drug, when administered intravenously, started 5–10 minutes after its injection. A single dose of neostigmine has a duration of action for only 50–60 minutes.

Neostigmine prolongs the duration of the action of succinylcholine by also inhibiting the plasma (pseudo) cholinesterase enzyme. There is also some evidence that the use of neostigmine to reverse the neuromuscular blockade is associated with an increased incidence of gastrointestinal anastomotic breakdown due to increased intestinal motility. Pyridostigmine resembles neostigmine in all these respects, but in dose-to-dose comparison it is less potent and longer acting. So, less frequent dosing of pyridostigmine is required in myasthenia gravis. The dose of pyridostigmine in myasthenia gravis is 60–180 mg orally and 1–5 mg IM or SC.

The indications for the use of neostigmine are:
- For the reversal of nondepolarizing neuromuscular block
- For the treatment of myasthenia gravis
- For the treatment of paralytic ileus
- In urinary retention.

Edrophonium

Chemically, the edrophonium is a synthetic ammonium compound. Like neostigmine, it is also a prosthetic reversible inhibitor of true AChE enzyme, present at synaptic cleft. So, it also acts by competing with ACh, like neostigmine, for the anionic esteratic site of enzyme true cholinesterase and reversibly binds to it. Thus, it left ACh unbroken and accumulates to facilitate the neuromuscular transmission. A part of the effect of this drug also appears to be exerted through the prejunctional receptors and increases the liberation of ACh **(Fig. 18)**.

Thus, the mode of action of edrophonium is like neostigmine, i.e., nicotinic and cholinergic (muscarinic). The nicotinic action of edrophonium improves neuromuscular transmission and prevents muscular paralysis. The cholinergic (muscarinic) action is like ACh. So, the drug may cause bradycardia, leading to a fall in cardiac output, increase in effective refractory period of cardiac muscle, and decrease in conduction time. Like muscarinic action of ACh, the edrophonium also increases bronchial secretion and may cause bronchoconstriction. For CNS effect, agitation and dreaming may occur by this drug and has a predictable

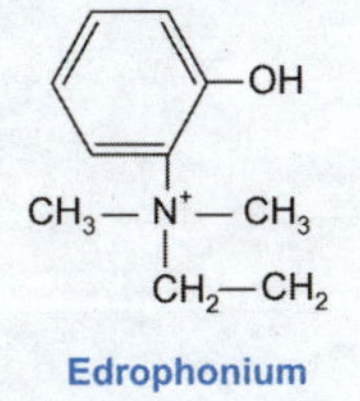

Fig. 18: Chemical structure of edrophonium.

miotic effect. The weakness of muscle due to fasciculation and paralysis may also occur due to the accumulation of excessive ACh when edrophonium is administered to normal subjects. The drug increases the salivation and lower esophageal and gastric tone. It increases the gastric acid output and gastrointestinal tract motility. Nausea and vomiting may occur. Like neostigmine, edrophonium also increases the ureteric peristalsis and may lead to involuntary micturition. Lacrimation and sweating are increased by this drug.

The metabolic fate of edrophonium is uncertain. It is not hydrolyzed by cholinesterase, like ACh or neostigmine. The volume of distribution of edrophonium in tissue is 0.9–1.3 L/kg. The details of excretory pathways of this drug are unknown. The clearance rate of edrophonium is 6–12 mL/kg/min and the elimination of half-life is 110 minutes. The toxic effects of edrophonium are nothing, but only the exaggerated manifestations of its pharmacological actions which are described above. Cardiac arrest has also been reported after the use of edrophonium. Edrophonium is usually administered intravenously. It has a more rapid onset (peak effect occurring at 0.8–2 minutes) and shorter duration of action (10 minutes) than neostigmine. The "Tensilon Test" for the diagnosis of myasthenia gravis consists of slow IV administration of 2 mg edrophonium, followed by further injection of 8 mg, if clinical deterioration does not occur. When it is used in the differentiation between myasthenic crisis and cholinergic crisis, then a dose of 2 mg of edrophonium is used first. If the weakness increases, then the diagnosis is cholinergic crisis and if the weakness improves then the diagnosis is myasthenia gravis. An anticholinergic agent (e.g., atropine) must be immediately available when these tests are performed. In anesthetic practice, the dose of edrophonium for reversal of neuromuscular blockade is 0.5–0.7 mg/kg and is used by slow intravenous injection. This is preceded by an appropriate dose of an anticholinergic agent to counter the peripheral muscarinic side effects of this drug. The potency of edrophonium is 12–16 times less than that of neostigmine. The muscarinic effects of this drug are relatively easier to counteract than those of neostigmine.

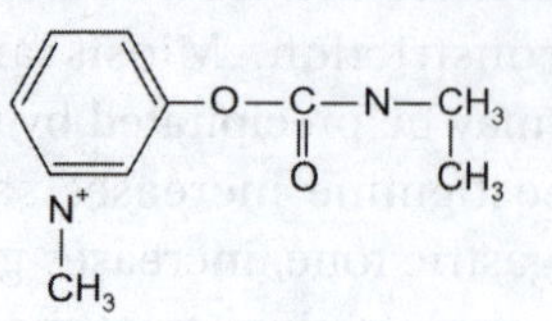

Fig. 19: Chemical structure of pyridostigmine.

Edrophonium is less predictable than neostigmine when used to reverse the profound competitive neuromuscular blockade.

The edrophonium is used for:

- The reversal of nondepolarizing neuromuscular blockade
- The diagnosis of suspected phase II block
- The diagnosis of myasthenia gravis (Tensilon test)
- The differentiation between myasthenia gravis and cholinergic crisis in myasthenic patient.

Pyridostigmine

It is an analog of neostigmine. It was introduced for the treatment of myasthenia gravis. It has one-fourth potency of neostigmine. So, 10 mg of pyridostigmine through IV route is equivalent to 2.5 mg of neostigmine through same route. But, the action of pyridostigmine on intestine and heart is less marked. The muscarinic action of pyridostigmine is less than the equivalent dose of neostigmine. The action of pyridostigmine on neuromuscular junction is less reliable than neostigmine and takes longer time, near about 5 minutes, to start its action. So, it is not used in anesthesia practice **(Fig. 19)**.

Physostigmine

It is also analog of neostigmine and acts as cholinesterase inhibitor. But, clinically it is only used in ophthalmology as eye drops for the management of glaucoma. The difference between physostigmine and neostigmine is given in the **Table 15**.

Pharmacology of Perioperative Arrhythmia

◼ INTRODUCTION

The agents or drugs which are used to prevent the irregularities of cardiac rhythm are called antiarrhythmic agents or drugs. Abnormal automaticity or impaired conduction of impulse or both underlie the cardiac arrhythmias. This may be paroxysmal or present continuously. It may cause sudden death, syncope, heart failure, palpitation, or no symptoms. Arrhythmias are often a manifestation of an underlying structural heart disease. But it may also occur in the context of an otherwise normal heart. The two most common forms of abnormal cardiac rhythm are tachycardia and bradycardia, respectively. When the heart rate is >100/min, it is called tachycardia and when the heart rate is <60/min, it is called bradycardia. Tachycardia is caused by two mechanisms: Increased automaticity due to increased repeated spontaneous depolarization or re-entry due to repeated nonspontaneous depolarization by a closed loop or re-entry circuit. But most tachyarrhythmias are due to this re-entry mechanism. Bradycardia is also caused by two mechanisms: Reduced automaticity or abnormal slow conduction (due to block).

According to the site of origin, the arrhythmias may also be supraventricular (sinus, atrial, junctional, or nodal) or ventricular. Arrhythmias arising from the supraventricular site usually produce narrow QRS complexes. This is because the ventricles are depolarized by impulses which pass normally through the atrioventricular (AV) node, bundle of His, and Purkinje fibers. In contrast, ventricular arrhythmias produce broad bizarre QRS complexes. This is because the ventricles are activated by impulses which arise from any side of the ventricular wall and pass through an abnormal pathway such as the myocardium. However, occasionally, supraventricular arrhythmias can produce broad or wide QRS complexes due to coexisting bundle branch block or the presence of accessory conducting tissue.

The incidence of perioperative arrhythmias varies and depends on the definition (any minor cardiac arrhythmia or any potentially dangerous arrhythmia), the mode of surveillance, patient's characteristics, and the nature of surgery. The factors that determine how a patient tolerates a cardiac arrhythmia usually include the heart rate, duration of arrhythmia, the presence and severity of any underlying cardiac disease, etc. However, more or less, the importance of a specific arrhythmia depends on its effects on the cardiac output and the possible interactions of the antiarrhythmic drugs which the patients are already taking with the drugs that are used in the perioperative period for anesthetic and analgesic purposes.

◼ CLASSIFICATION

Perioperative cardiac arrhythmias are mainly divided according to their etiology under two headings:
1. Disturbances of impulse formation
2. Disturbances of impulse conduction.

Disturbances of Impulse Formation

- *Sinus rhythm:* Sinus bradycardia, sinus tachycardia, sinus arrhythmia, sinus arrest, sick-sinus syndrome
- *Atrial rhythm:* Paroxysmal supraventricular tachycardia (PSVT) (atrial tachycardia), atrial extrasystole, atrial flutter (AFL), atrial fibrillation (AF)
- *AV nodal rhythm:* AV nodal extrasystole, AV nodal tachycardia, AV junctional escape rhythm
- *Ventricular rhythm:* Ventricular extrasystole, ventricular escape rhythm, ventricular tachycardia (VT), idioventricular tachycardia, ventricular flutter, ventricular fibrillation (VF), torsades-de-pointes, ventricular asystole.

Disturbances of Impulse Conduction

Sinoatrial (SA) block, AV block, and Wolff–Parkinson–White (WPW) syndrome cause cardiac arrhythmia. The bundle branch block (right or left) does not cause any cardiac arrhythmia. So, it is not included in this classification.

■ MECHANISM OF ARRHYTHMIA (FACT FILE I)

At rest, in a cell, there is a potential difference of −70 to −90 mV across the cell membrane. This is known as the resting membrane potential (RMP). It is due to the Na^+–K^+-ATPase pump which brings out three Na^+ from the cell and pushes two K^+ inside the cell. So, there is a high concentration of Na^+ outside of the cell and a high concentration of K^+ inside of the cell. In this stage, the fast Na^+ channels remain closed. But the K^+ channels remain open. Therefore, the cell membrane in resting condition is relatively impermeable to Na^+ but permeable to K^+. Thus, K^+ can also move passively into the cell by an electromotive force other than the Na^+–K^+-ATPase pump. When the cell becomes active by an impulse from outside or due to automaticity (explained later), the RMP rises to the threshold level and then the permeability of the cell membrane to Na^+ suddenly increases. This is due to the opening of fast response Na^+ channels and inactivation of the Na^+/K^+-ATPase pump. Thus, Na^+ rapidly moves along the concentration gradient from outside into the cell, producing a rapid and complete depolarization (phase 0). After this rapid and complete depolarization, there is a short period of repolarization or phase 1. Deactivation of inward Na^+ current and activation of outward K^+ current are responsible for this short period of repolarization or phase 1. Then, this phase 1 is followed by plateau phase (phase 2) during which complex ionic movement chiefly involving Ca^{2+} takes place. Ca^{2+} channels open during phase 0. They remain open for 30–300 ms and account for this plateau phase. In this phase, Ca^{2+} enters the cell and balances the outward K^+ current maintaining the plateau.

After that, a more rapid phase of repolarization (phase 3) occurs. During this phase, the slow inward Ca^{2+} current is inactivated and more K^+ channels open causing exit of more K^+ from the cell and restoring the transmembrane potential to its resting state. But the nature of ionic distribution across the cell membrane is opposite to the resting state, i.e., K^+ outside of the cell and Na^+ inside the cell **(Fig. 1)**. At the end of this process or phase 3, the Na^+/K^+-ATPase pump is again reactivated and restores the resting ionic balance which has already become opposite during the whole action potential, i.e., Na^+ is inside and K^+ is outside of the cell. This is called

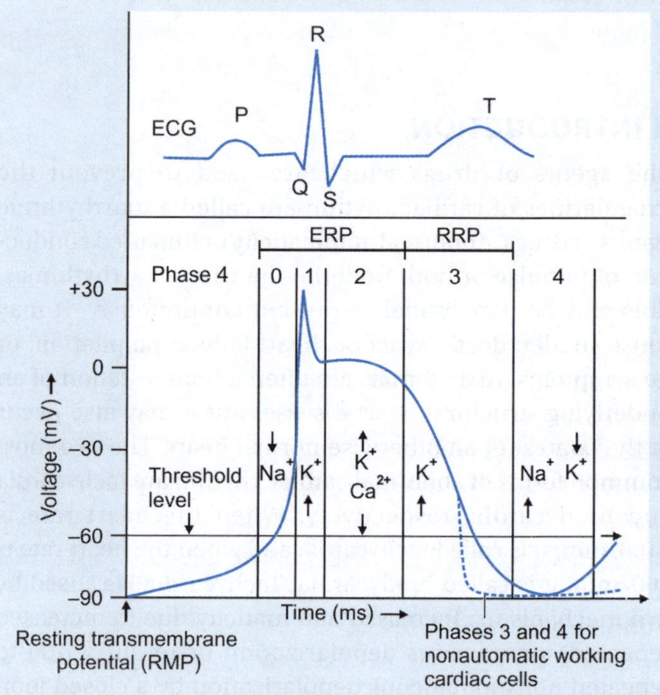

Fig. 1: Sequence of action potential of an automatic sinoatrial (SA) nodal cell (unbroken line) and a nonautomatic ventricular muscle cell (broken line) and its relationship with electrocardiogram (ECG). Phase 4 undergoes spontaneous depolarization from the RMP (−90 mV) until the threshold potential is reached, which is the characteristic of an automatic SA nodal cell or any pacemaker cell. Then, depolarization (phase 0) occurs. Depolarization of the ventricle corresponds to the QRS complex of ECG. Depolarization of the atrium corresponds to the P-wave. Phases 1, 2, and 3 represent repolarization. Among them, phase 3 of the ventricular cell corresponds to the T-wave on the ECG. The repolarization of the atrium is masked by the QRS complex (depolarization of the ventricle) in ECG. The effective refractory period (ERP) is the time during which extracardiac impulses cannot be conducted, whatever may be the intensity of the impulses or stimulus. During the relative refractory period (RRP), a stronger than normal stimulus can initiate an action potential. The action potential of nonautomatic working cardiac cells differs from an automatic cardiac cell such as the SA node, in that, phase 4 of nonautomatic cardiac cell does not undergo spontaneous slow depolarization during the diastolic period which corresponds with phase 4 of action potential. In the figure, the downward arrow indicates that the ion enters the cell and upward arrow indicates that the ion exits the cell.

FACT FILE I

Genesis of RMP

The different distribution of ions across the cell membrane and the different nature of the ion channels on the cell membrane provide the explanation of the RMP. At resting condition, the increased concentration gradient of K^+ inside the cell facilitates its exit out of the cell via K^+ channels passively, without any help of a pump. But its electrical gradient is in the opposite direction (inward). Ultimately, an equilibrium is reached when the tendency of K^+ to move out of the cell is balanced by its tendency to move into the cell. At that equilibrium, there is a slight excess of cations on the outside and anions on the inside which is responsible for RMP varying between −70 and −90 mV. This condition is maintained by the Na^+–K^+-ATPase pump which pumps three Na^+ out of the cell for every two K^+ pumps in. This pump is electrogenic as it works against the electromotive force. It should be emphasized that the number of ions responsible for RMP is a small fraction of the total number of ion present and also the total concentration of negative and positive ions is equal everywhere except along the cell membrane.

phase 4. During this phase, the Na$^+$/K$^+$-ATPase pump reestablishes the normal baseline concentration gradient of the relevant cations, with two K$^+$ ions moving into the cell for every three Na$^+$ ions moving out.

This sequence of events (RMP-depolarization-repolarization-RMP) is the pattern for nearly all the myocardial cells. But certain cells, particularly the specialized conducting tissues of the SA and AV nodes and the His–Purkinje system, have the property of automaticity. In them, the RMP in phase 4 constantly drifts upward until it reaches a threshold level (usually about –40 to –60 mV). So, phase 4 of these cells is called the slow diastolic depolarization phase. When RMP in the slow diastolic depolarization phase drifts to the threshold level, then the Na$^+$/K$^+$-ATPase pump is automatically inhibited and the fast response Na$^+$ channels reopen. This is responsible for the further massive influx of Na$^+$ ions into the cell and increases the transmembrane potential from –70 to –90 mV (RMP) to +20 mV (depolarization or phase 0). Thus, again, active electrical and mechanical events of action potential are triggered off. It is thus important to realize that this threshold level can be raised or lowered by drugs or injury and that automaticity in working cells also may be inhibited or induced by these influences **(Box 1)**.

Thus, for cardiac arrhythmias, five principal mechanisms have been identified. These are enhanced automaticity, after depolarization, re-entry, fractionation of impulse, and conduction block. Among these, the first four factors are clubbed under the heading of disturbances of impulse formation, and the last factor is put under the heading of disturbances of impulse conduction.

Enhanced Automaticity

The heart has many potential pacemaking cells and are situated in the SA node, AV node, bundle of His–Purkinje fibers, and atria (atrial cells). The SA node has the fastest inherent spontaneous discharge rate, which usually ranges around 80 beats/min. The inherent automatic discharge rate of the potential AV nodal and the bundle of His pacemaking cells is about 60 and 50 beats/min, respectively. The inherent automatic discharge rate of the Purkinje cells is about 40 beats/min. Pacing or automaticity of cells is due to phase 4 slow diastolic depolarization **(Figs. 2A to E)**. Decreasing the time to reach the threshold potential or increasing the slope of phase 4 (slow diastolic depolarization phase) or elevating the RMP (i.e., making it less negative) leads to enhanced automaticity and is manifested as an accelerated heart rate. Hypoxia, hypercarbia, hypokalemia, hyperthermia, mechanical stretching of cardiac muscle, catecholamines, sympathomimetic drugs, etc., increase the slope of phase 4

BOX 1: Factors causing arrhythmias during the perioperative period.
• Hypoxemia
• Hypercarbia
• Electrolyte disturbances
• Hypokalemia
• Hypomagnesemia
• Acid–base disturbances
• Imbalance of the autonomic nervous system
• *Increased stretching of myocardial fiber:*
– Systemic hypertension
– Valvular diseases
– Congenital heart diseases
– Cardiomyopathy
• Myocardial ischemia
• *Drugs:*
– Catecholamines
– Volatile anesthetics
• Coexisting cardiac diseases
• Valvular diseases
• *Hypertrophy:*
- Ventricular preexcitation [Wolff–Parkinson–White (WPW) syndrome]
- Prolonged QT interval syndrome
- Hypo- or hyperthermia
• Types of surgery
• Tracheal intubation

or decrease the time to reach the threshold potential. Thus, they induce or accelerate the pacemaking or automaticity, producing tachyarrhythmias whereas acetylcholine, hyperkalemia, hypothermia, etc., cause a decrease in the slope of phase 4 or increase the time to reach the threshold potential. Thus, they reduce automaticity and produce bradyarrhythmia.

Hyperpolarization, i.e., making the RMP more negative, also produces bradyarrhythmia. The automaticity also results from the sites that ordinarily lack spontaneous pacemaking activity, e.g., ventricular cells. This is due to the ventricular myocardial cell damage by ischemia causing depolarization and automaticity. A current thus flows between these depolarized injured fibers and the normally polarized fibers (current of injury) and initiates automaticity. Thus, cardiac arrhythmia results.

After Depolarization

Under some pathophysiological conditions, a normal cardiac action potential may be followed or interrupted by a sudden abnormal premature depolarization. If this abnormal premature depolarization reaches the threshold level, then it may give rise to a secondary upstroke, which then can propagate and create an abnormal rhythm. Two major forms of secondary upstroke or after depolarization

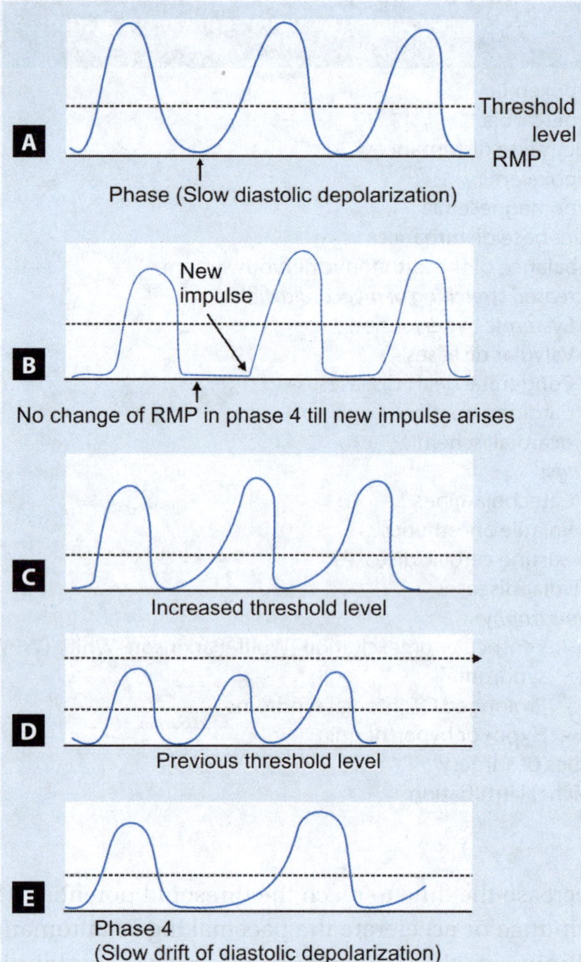

Figs. 2A to E: The action potentials from different cardiac muscle cells with the property of (A) automaticity and (B) without automaticity. (A) Sinoatrial (SA) node cell. In these cells, the resting membrane potential (RMP) is continuously and spontaneously drifting in phase 4 toward the threshold level. This explains the electrical basis of automaticity of the SA nodal cells or any pacemaker cells. (B) Normal working myocardial cell. In these cells, RMP does not spontaneously drift to the threshold level. For the next depolarization, they wait for an impulse coming from outside; (C) Working myocardial cells damaged by injury. Like the SA node, here also the RMP drifts spontaneously due to injury to the threshold level, which represents a tendency to automaticity; (D) Class IA drugs reduce the peak of the rise of action potential. It also raises the threshold level by inactivation of the Na^+ pump. This results in reduced automaticity; (E) Class IB drugs produce the same effect by slowing the rate at which the drift of phase 4 takes place so that it takes longer time to reach the threshold level.

are recognized. These are delayed after depolarization and early after depolarization (EAD).

Delayed After Depolarization

After a full action potential and attaining the RMP, a secondary premature deflection or depolarization may occur

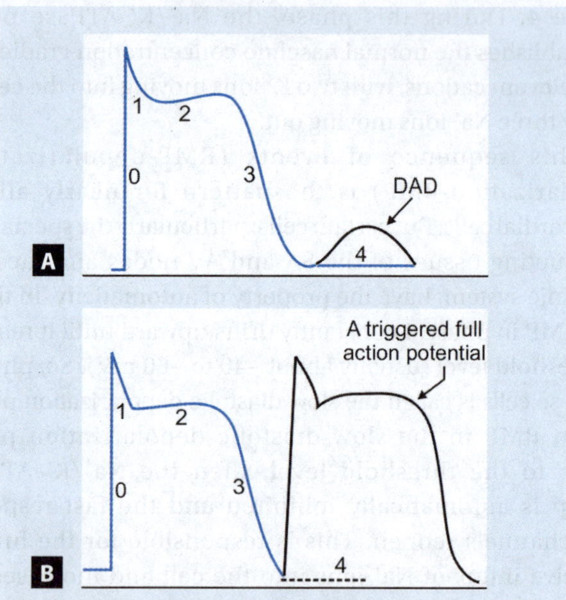

Figs. 3A and B: (A) Delayed after depolarization (DAD), arising after full repolarization; (B) A DAD that reaches the threshold results in a triggered upstroke and causes a full action potential.

at phase 4 which can reach the threshold level and initiate a single premature action potential. As this premature action, potential is needed to trigger the arrhythmias, this type of arrhythmias is called "trigger arrhythmias". Examples of such trigger arrhythmias are some tachycardias, coupled beats, etc. **(Figs. 3A and B)**.

Early After Depolarization

Sometimes, phase 3 or repolarization part of action potential is interrupted by an early premature depolarization and thus the membrane potential oscillates. If the amplitude of oscillation of this membrane potential is sufficient enough, then a series of impulses are propagated and neighboring tissues are activated, causing arrhythmia **(Figs. 4A and B)**. They are frequently associated with abnormally prolonged action potential such as bradycardia, low extracellular K^+, and certain drugs that prolong the duration of action potential (APD). When EAD is present, then subsequent sympathetic stimulation (α and β) can increase the likelihood of triggered beats. Again, if the cardiac repolarization is markedly prolonged, then VT with a long QT interval, known as "torsades-de-pointes" syndrome, may occur **(Fig. 5)**.

Re-entry

Primarily due to some abnormality in the conduction pathway, an impulse which is normally generated may recirculate in the heart muscle and can cause repetitive activation of it without the need for any new impulse to be generated.

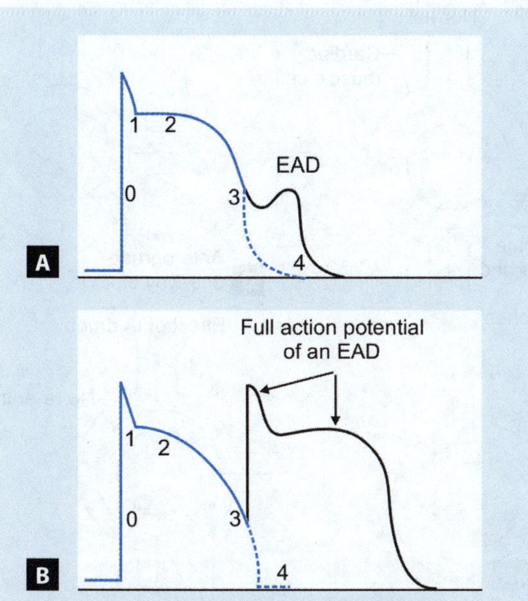

Figs. 4A and B: Early after depolarization (EAD), interrupting the phase 3 part of repolarization of action potential. (A) Under some conditions, EAD cannot reach the threshold level and becomes unable to give a full action potential; (B) But sometimes, EAD reaches the threshold level and initiates a full action potential causing arrhythmia.

These are called re-entry arrhythmias. It also has two mechanisms: Circus movement and micro re-entry.

Circus Movement Mechanism

When an impulse propagates by more than one pathway between two points of the heart, then part of the impulse may recirculate again and again in the heart muscle, causing repetitive activation of it without the need for any new impulse to be generated. These are called the circus variety of reentrant arrhythmias. One of the examples of this re-entry arrhythmia is WPW syndrome. In WPW syndrome, there is an accessory conducting path between the atrium and the ventricle. With each sinus node depolarization, the impulses can excite the ventricle via the normal structure (AV node) or the accessory pathway. But the electrophysiological properties of the AV node and the accessory pathways are different. Accessory pathways consist of fast-response tissue, whereas the AV node is composed of slow-response tissue. Thus, with every atrial beat, conduction may fall in both the accessory pathway and the AV node. Then, the impulse passing through the accessory pathway depolarizes a part of the ventricle first (as it is fast-conducting tissue) and produces delta waves. Then, it meets the ventricular depolarization caused by the impulse passing through the AV node and produces total QRS complex. During this

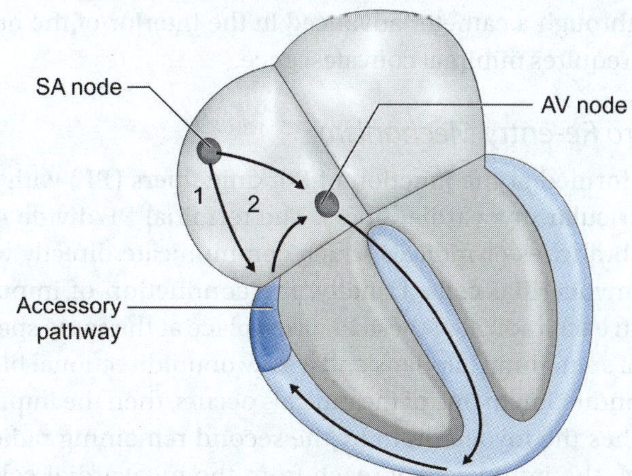

Fig. 5: In this patient, an accessory pathway connecting between the atrium and the ventricle is present and is shown by the black area. This picture explains a retrograde re-entry circuit mechanism of arrhythmia through the accessory pathway. A normal or premature atrial beat (1) cannot pass through the accessory pathway as it is refractory by the previous sinus beat. Thus, the atrial beat propagates slowly through the AV node as usual. Then, it reaches the accessory pathway through the Purkinje fibers and ventricular wall. Upon reaching the accessory pathway through the ventricular wall, which is by now no longer refractory, the impulse reenters the atrium (2). It then again reenters the ventricle via the AV node and thus becomes a self-sustained circuit. AV nodal-blocking drugs readily terminate this tachycardia or arrhythmia. Recurrences can also be prevented by drugs that prevent the atrial premature beats or by drugs that alter the electrophysiological characteristics of tissues in the circuit (i.e., they prolong the AV nodal refractoriness) or by nonpharmacological techniques that cut the accessory pathway. (AV: atrioventricular; SA: sinoatrial)

period, the accessory pathway is no longer refractory. Thus, the impulse which comes through the AV node reenters the atrium via the accessory pathway, and then it can again re-enter the ventricle via the AV node. It then again reenters the atrium via the accessory pathway and such goes on again and again. Re-entry arrhythmia of this type is, therefore, determined by: (1) the presence or absence of an anatomically defined accessory circuit, (2) heterogeneity in refractoriness among the regions of these circuits, and (3) slow conduction in one part of the circuit than the other.

Similarly, an "anatomically defined" re-entry circuit commonly occurs (1) in the region of the AV node causing AV nodal re-entry tachycardia and (2) in the atrium causing AFL. This is discussed in more detail in Chapter 6. The term paroxysmal supraventricular tachycardia includes both AV re-entry and AV nodal re-entry tachycardia as both of them share the many same clinical features. In some of these cases, it is now possible to identify this re-entry circuit and to ablate the critical portions of this reentrant pathways. It thus cures the patient nonpharmacologically and obviates the need for long-term drug therapy. This ablation procedure is carried out through a catheter advanced in the interior of the heart and requires minimal convalescence.

Micro Re-entry Mechanism

It is formed at the junction of Purkinje fibers (PF) with the ventricular myocardial fibers. The terminal PF divide into two branches or radicals which communicate directly with the myocardial cells. Usually, the conduction of impulse down each radical of these PF takes place at the same speed. But if something happens and a slow or unidirectional block of conduction in one of the radicals occurs, then the impulse reaches the myocardium by the second remaining radical. Then, the impulse may reach from the myocardial cell to the blocked radical. Under this circumstance, the retrograde conduction occurs through the blocked segment **(Figure C)** as the block is unidirectional and the impulse crosses the block. Then, the impulse passes again through the undamaged or unblocked radical (which is now nonrefractory) back to reach the myocardial cell and again to the blocked radical. Thus, a self-creating micro re-entry circuit is set up, causing arrhythmia. Examples of this micro re-entry mechanism are ventricular ectopic, VT, VF, etc. **(Figs. 6A to E)**.

There is another re-entry mechanism which is called the functionally defined re-entry mechanism. This can happen in the absence of any anatomically distinct accessory pathway or certain block-like micro re-entry mechanism. An example of this mechanism is VT in myocardial infarction (MI). Here, the ischemic area is divided into two parts: rapid longitudinal and slow transverse segments, which are electrophysiologically different. These two parts also have different refractory periods. Thus, the formation of these two different refractory areas results in alternate cyclical changes of refractoriness which allow the impulse to circulate repeatedly among these two types of tissues with different refractory periods causing arrhythmias.

Fractionation of Impulse

When the ERP of atrial or ventricular muscular fiber is brief and inhomogeneous, then a generated impulse is conducted irregularly over the atrium or ventricle. It means that the impulse moves rapidly through the fibers with short ERP (which have recovered completely) or slowly through the fibers with long ERP (which have recovered partially) or does not move at all through the still refractory fibers. Thus, an asynchronous activation of atrial or ventricular fibers occurs, causing arrhythmia.

Conduction Block

Different types of blocks in the SA node and the AV node, but not the bundle of His and PF, can also cause arrhythmia.

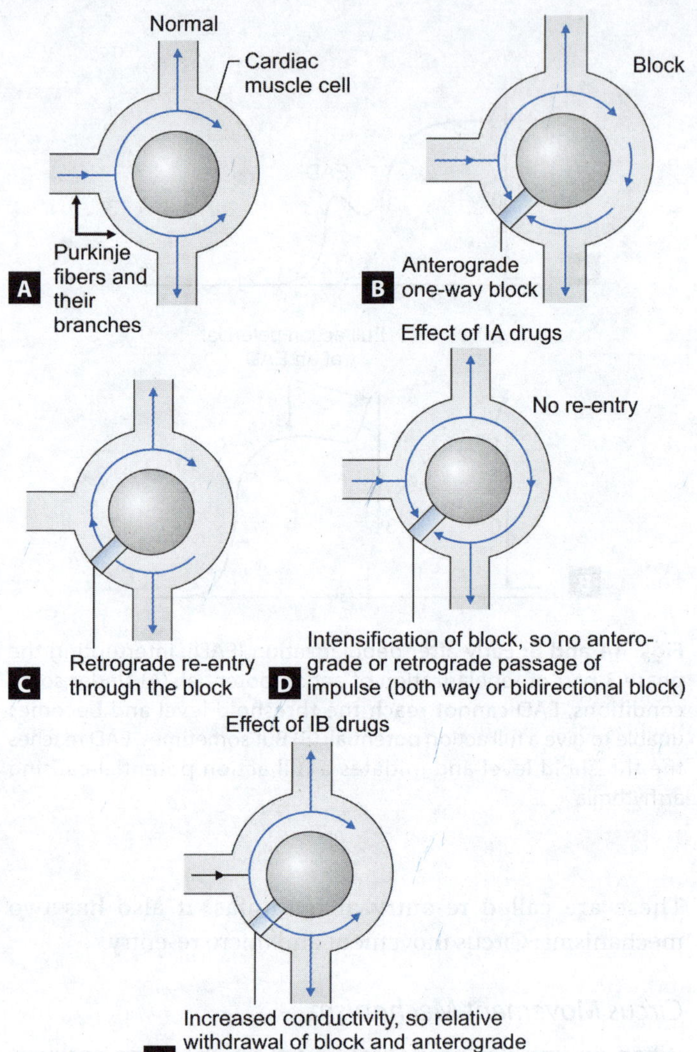

Figs. 6A to E: The micro re-entry mechanism causing cardiac arrhythmia and the effects of antiarrhythmic drugs. (A to C) The mechanism in which a local microentry circuit rhythm is established between the Purkinje fiber and the cardiac muscle cell. (A) The normal conduction of impulse between the Purkinje fibers and cardiac muscle cells; (B) There is a unidirectional block in one of the branches of Purkinje fiber, which prevents the anterograde passage of impulse. But when another impulse which passes through the normal branch of Purkinje fiber comes to the other end of the block such as in (C), within this time this tissue is no more refractory to the impulse and it passes retrogradely. This phenomenon goes on repeatedly, producing a local micro re-entry circuit and arrhythmia; (D) The effect of class IA drugs which induces a bidirectional block and so interrupts re-entry; (E) The effect of class IB drugs which raises conductivity so that antegrade conduction can take place and interrupt micro re-entry.

DRUGS USED IN THE TREATMENT OF CARDIAC ARRHYTHMIAS (FIG. 7)

Drugs used in the treatment of cardiac arrhythmias are mainly grouped under two headings. These are: (1) Drugs

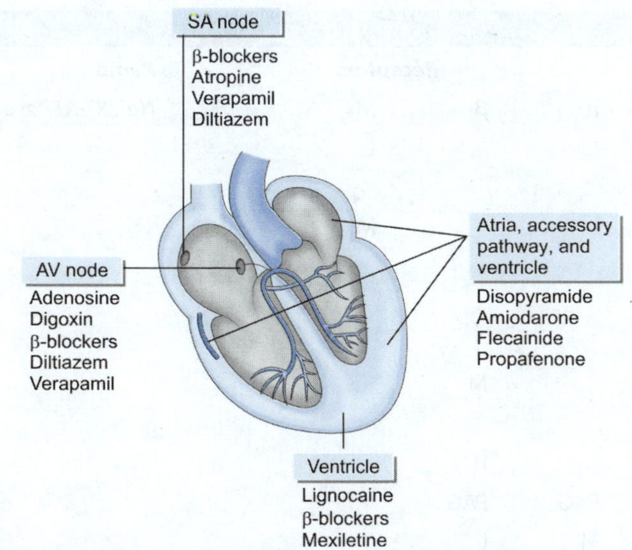

Fig. 7: Classification of antiarrhythmic drugs by their site of action. (AV: atrioventricular; SA: sinoatrial)

TABLE 1: William's classification.	
	Membrane-stabilizing drugs (fast Na⁺ channel blockers)
Class I	
IA	Quinidine, procainamide, and disopyramide. They block Na⁺ channel and prolong action potential
IB	Lignocaine and mexiletine. They block Na⁺ channel and shorten the duration of action potential
IC	Flecainide, encainide, and propafenone. They block Na⁺ channel with no effect on action potential
Class II	β-adrenoreceptor antagonist, i.e., propranolol, metoprolol, esmolol
Class III	Drugs which increase the duration of action potential and the refractory period (antifibrillatory drugs), e.g., amiodarone, bretylium
Class IV	Calcium channel blockers, e.g., verapamil, diltiazem
Others	Cardiac glycosides, adenosine, dofetilide, ibutilide, propafenone, etc.
For atrioventricular (AV) blocks	Anticholinergic—atropine Sympathomimetics—isoprenaline, etc.

NB: Some drugs have properties of more than one class. For example, amiodarone has actions of all four classes.

used to treat disturbances in impulse formation and (2) drugs used to treat disturbances in impulse conduction.

Drugs Used to Treat Disturbances in Impulse Formation

Antiarrhythmic drugs used to treat disturbances in impulse formation act in different ways. These are by blocking (1) different ionic channels (Na⁺, K⁺, Ca²⁺), (2) different receptors, and (3) different pumps. There are many classifications of antiarrhythmic drugs, but none of them is satisfactory. Till now, only the useful classification of antiarrhythmic drugs is William's classification. However, this classification also has several limitations in practice. This is because (1) many drugs have more than one mechanism of action, (2) there are considerable variations in the mechanism of action of drugs in the same class, and (3) there are distinct similarities between the drugs of supposedly different classes.

So, an alternative new classification of antiarrhythmic drugs such as "Sicilian Gambit" was introduced in 1990. Unlike William's classification which is purely based on the electrophysiological characteristic of the mechanism of action of drugs, this new approach is a gambit as in chess, rather than a finalized structure. It is based on the consideration of three factors which influence the antiarrhythmic effects of various drugs **(Table 1)**. These three factors are (1) the molecular targets on which the drug acts, (2) the mechanism of action responsible for the antiarrhythmic property of this agent, and (3) the clinical considerations.

However, this classification is more complex and less easy to memorize than William's classification. But it has the advantage of allowing better visualization of some complex effects of newer drugs, which is unhindered by the constraints, imposed by the purely electrophysiological basis of earlier classification.

Arrhythmogenic Potentiality of Antiarrhythmic Drugs

Most antiarrhythmic agents which are used clinically may themselves precipitate serious arrhythmias. Two multicentric trials have shown that the post-MI patients, randomized to receive encainide, flecainide, moricizine, and other antiarrhythmic agents on a long-term basis, had a higher incidence of sudden death, though initially, the same drugs had suppressed ventricular extrasystole (VES) in these patients. It is possibly due to the marked intraventricular conduction slowing action of these drugs, resulting in VT and VF. It is, therefore, not prudent to try and suppress all the extrasystoles or arrhythmias with the drugs perioperatively **(Table 2)**.

Class I—Membrane stabilizing drugs: Drugs in this class are known as membrane stabilizers. So, they act by blocking the fast Na⁺ channels, across the cell membrane at phase 0 of action potential like local anesthetic agents. Thus, they

TABLE 2: "Sicilian Gambit" table.

Drug	William's classification	Channels			Receptors				Pump
		Na⁺	K⁺	Ca²⁺	α	β	M₂		Na⁺/K⁺-ATPase
Quinidine	IA	A	H		L		L		
Procainamide	IA	A	H						
Disopyramide	IA	A	H				M		
Lignocaine	IB	H							
Mexiletine	IB	H							
Tocainide	IB	H							
Propafenone	IC	A				M			
Flecainide	IC	A	H						
Propranolol	II	M				H			
Bretylium	III		H		PAG	PAG			
Amiodarone	III	I	H	L	M	L			
Verapamil	IV	M		H	L				
Diltiazem	IV								
Adenosine								AG	
Digoxin							AG		H
Atropine							H		

H: high; I: inactivated state blockers; M: medium; A: activated state blocker; L: low; AG: agonist; PAG: partial agonist.

interfere with the onset of depolarization and decrease the responsiveness to excitation. They also reduce the rate of phase 4 slow diastolic depolarization in automatic or pacemaker cells. There are pharmacologically diverse groups of drugs in this class (class I) which have been subclassified into IA, IB, and IC. However, the primary antiarrhythmic effect of all these drugs is related to their effect on decreasing the maximum rate of voltage change during phase 0 of action potential. Several other mechanisms may also be involved in this group of drugs, such as abolishing the re-entry currents.

This is a new classification of antiarrhythmic drugs. It is based on the activities of the membrane channels, receptors, and pumps. This classification also offers a different perspective of the William's classification which only considers the electrophysiological effects.

Subclass IA: They are open-state Na⁺ channel blockers with moderate delay in channel recovery. Hence, they suppress the AV conduction and prolong the PR, QRS, and QT interval and APD. The drugs that fall into this group are given in the following text.

- *Quinidine:* Chemically, it is a dextro-isomer of quinine and an alkaloid which is available from cinchona bark. A Dutch merchant had first noticed the beneficial effect of cinchona bark on irregular pulse, taken during malaria. Then, he demonstrated this to British cardiologist

Wenckebach, in 1912, and subsequently quinidine was synthesized.

It reduces the rate of depolarization or phase 0 of action potential and its overshoot, i.e., it decreases the membrane responsiveness. Thus, it depresses the cardiac excitability by: (1) raising the threshold potential level, (2) prolonging the APD, and (3) prolonging the ERP of His–Purkinje cells. Thus, it slows the intra-atrial, AV, and intraventricular conduction of impulses. It extinguishes the extrasystole and is important in the prophylaxis of reentrant arrhythmias. Quinidine has little effect on "after depolarization". SA nodal automaticity is little affected by quinidine at therapeutic concentration. As ERP is prolonged, the tissue remains refractory even after the full repolarization. The QT interval in the electrocardiogram (ECG) is prolonged by quinidine. Therefore, monitoring by ECG may provide a useful guide to its dosage. Prolongation of the QT interval with quinidine therapy may also have been associated with severe tachyarrhythmias.

Quinidine has anticholinergic effects. The cardiac anticholinergic effects include an increase in the sinus rate. It has a variable effect on AV nodal conduction which may be depressed or enhanced, depending on the balance between direct depression and anticholinergic enhancement (**Box 2**).

BOX 2: Principles of use of antiarrhythmic drugs.

The drugs used to treat different cardiac arrhythmias are potentially toxic. So, they should be used carefully according to the following principles:

- Many arrhythmias are benign and do not produce any hemodynamic instability. So, they do not require specific treatment and only need observation
- Precipitating or causal factors for arrhythmia should always be searched and corrected first, if possible. These may include myocardial ischemia, drug effect, hyperthyroidism, acidosis, hypokalemia, hypomagnesemia, excess alcohol or caffeine consumption, etc.
- If drug therapy is required at all, it is best to use as few drugs as possible
- In difficult cases, electrophysiological study may help to identify the optimum therapy
- Patients on long-term antiarrhythmic drugs should be reviewed regularly. Attempts should always be made to withdraw the therapy if the factors which precipitate the arrhythmias are no longer operative
- Nonpharmacological antiarrhythmic therapy such as pacing or radiofrequency ablation of the accessory path is often preferred to long-term drug therapy

Then, anticholinergic effects of quinidine are also responsible for a variety of noncardiac effects. These are gastrointestinal (GI) irritation, nausea, vomiting, tinnitus, and visual disturbances which are found in mild overdosage whereas severe central nervous system (CNS) symptoms such as confusion and psychosis may occur with major over dosage.

Mechanism of action: Quinidine blocks the myocardial fast Na^+ channel in the open state. Thus, it reduces the automaticity by decreasing the maximal rate of depolarization or phase of action potential. Some prolongations of action potential by quinidine are also due to the K^+ channel-blocking action. Lengthening of ERP by quinidine is due to its effect on the recovery of Na^+ and K^+ channels. As quinidine has some α-adrenergic blocking properties at higher doses, so it also directly dilates the blood vessels and causes a fall in blood pressure (BP).

Uses: Quinidine has been used to treat atrial and ventricular arrhythmias but is not in common use today. It is usually administered orally because of the adverse hemodynamic consequences on parenteral use. Absorption from the GI tract of quinidine is rapid and effective. Presently, quinidine is used only for maintenance and prophylaxis purposes, after AF and AFL which have been terminated by DC shock or by other measures. Recently, it is also used to prevent the recurrence of VT. *Dose:* 200–400 mg TDS orally.

- *Procainamide:* It is the amide derivative of a local anesthetic agent named procaine. Procaine was also found to have antiarrhythmic activity but is not suitable clinically due to the rapid hydrolysis and marked CNS effects of it. So, in 1951, procainamide (analog of procaine) was developed and had circumvented some of the limitations of procaine.

Like quinidine, it also decreases the rate of rise of depolarization during phase 0 and phase 4 of action potential. However, less prolongation of QT interval than quinidine is observed by procainamide. Procainamide also has anticholinergic effect but is less marked than quinidine. It has no α-blocking activity, so there is no fall in BP. It is better tolerated than quinidine when given intravenously.

Uses: Procainamide is orally active and is an alternative drug to quinidine, having the same spectrum of efficacy. Some patients not responding to other antiarrhythmic agents may respond to procainamide. Procainamide is more likely to increase the ventricular rate in a patient with AF than quinidine. Thus, it is not used in the treatment of AF and AFL like quinidine. Therefore, its use is usually confined to the treatment of ventricular extrasystole. In this respect, it is usually used as a second line of drug after lignocaine and may be used for the treatment of multiple ventricular extrasystole, R on T phenomenon, and VT.

Initially, procainamide is used as an intravenous (IV) loading dose and later with maintenance by IV infusions during the acute therapy of many supraventricular (except AF and AFL) and ventricular arrhythmias. But long-term oral treatment by procainamide is often stopped because of the many adverse effects.

Doses: For abolition of arrhythmia, procainamide in the dose of 0.5–1 g orally or intramuscularly (IM) is started fast. This is followed by 0.25–0.5 g orally at every 2-hour interval. It can reduce the antimicrobial effect of sulfonamides, probably by generating para-aminobenzoic acid (PABA). Hypotension and marked slowing of conduction are the major adverse effects of procainamide at high concentration, especially during IV use.

- *Disopyramide:* Like quinidine, it is also the drug of class IA and has prominent cardiac depressant and anticholinergic effects (which account for many of its adverse effects). It has no α-adrenergic blocking property. Disopyramide usually has no effect on sinus rate because of opposing both the direct depressant and antivagal actions on the SA node. It is used to treat both the supraventricular (AFL and AF) and the ventricular arrhythmias (VT and ventricular flutter).

It may also cause atypical VT with prolongations of QT interval. Disopyramide may also be effective in slowing conduction through the accessory pathway in a patient with WPW syndrome. It has marked negative inotropic effect on the heart.

The anticholinergic effects of disopyramide include precipitation of glaucoma, constipation, dry mouth, and urinary retention. The latter is more common in males. Sometimes, the negative inotropic effects of disopyramide may precipitate heart failure. It can also cause torsades-de-pointes.

Disopyramide is orally active and is better tolerated than quinidine. The primary indication of use of disopyramide is the prevention of recurrences of ventricular arrhythmias. It may be better tolerated as the maintenance agent after cardioversion of AFL and AF.

Subclass IB: These groups of drugs block Na^+ channels in both the activated and inactivated states, but do not delay the recovery of the channel. They do not depress the AV conduction. Also, they do not prolong the APD, ERP, and QT interval. Class IB groups of drugs have virtually no autonomic effects. By this group of drugs, the rate of rapid depolarization or phase 0 of action and the slope of slow depolarization in phase 4 are decreased in PF.

- *Lignocaine:* It is the most commonly used local anesthetic agent and is also the most popular antiarrhythmic agent in the intensive care unit (ICU).

  Lignocaine blocks both the open and the inactivated cardiac Na^+ channels, but the recovery from this block is very rapid. So, it exerts greater effects on the depolarized (ischemic) tissues. It is not useful in atrial arrhythmias. This is possibly because the atrial action potentials are so short that the Na^+ channel remains in an inactivated state only for a brief period as compared to the diastolic (recovery) times, which are relatively long.

  The most prominent cardiac action of lignocaine is the suppression of automaticity of ventricular ectopic foci, but the SA nodal automaticity is not depressed. It has, practically, no effect on APD and ERP of atrial fibers. Atrial re-entry is also not affected. So, lignocaine is ineffective in treating supraventricular arrhythmias. However, it can suppress the re-entry mechanism responsible for ventricular arrhythmias either by abolishing the one-way block or by producing the two-way block. It also increases the threshold for VF. So, lignocaine is used in the treatment of all forms of ventricular arrhythmias. The normal ventricular muscle fibers and conducting tissues are minimally affected, while depolarized or damaged fibers are significantly affected. This is due to the higher preferential distribution of lignocaine within the ventricular myocardium which has been shown to be more damaged than the normal healthy ventricular myocardium, and the concentration of lignocaine within the ischemic arrhythmic areas of myocardium is the relevant factor for determining its efficacy. Lignocaine acts preferentially on the ischemic myocardium and is more effective in the presence of high extracellular K^+ concentration. Thus, hypokalemia must be corrected before the use of any class IB drugs, other than phenytoin.

Lignocaine has minimal effect on normal ECG. It has no significant effect on PR interval or QRS duration. It causes little depression of cardiac contractility and no reduction of BP. There are no significant actions of lignocaine on the autonomic nervous system. So, all the cardiac effects of lignocaine are due to its direct actions of it on the myocardial cells.

Lignocaine is well absorbed orally. But because of its high first-pass metabolism in the liver, adequate and constant blood levels of lignocaine are not attained by this route. So, it is not used orally. Actions of lignocaine by IV bolus dose lasts only for 10–20 minutes. This is because of its rapid redistribution in the tissues. On the other hand, therapeutic plasma concentration of lignocaine lies within the range of 1.5–5 µg/mL and plasma concentration >9 µg/mL is likely to produce toxic effects. So, the normally accepted therapeutic scheme to maintain the desired therapeutic plasma level of lignocaine requires a loading IV dose of 1–1.5 mg/kg which is followed by an infusion of 150 µg/kg/min for 20 minutes and finally is maintained by infusion at the rate of 3 µg/kg/min.

When rapidly large doses of lignocaine are administered intravenously, then seizures may occur. But during maintenance therapy, wshen the plasma concentration of the drug rises slowly above the therapeutic level, then tremor, dysarthria, and altered level of consciousness occur. Hence, it proves that the main toxicity of lignocaine is its dose-dependent neurological effects. Other neurological symptoms of lignocaine are drowsiness, nausea, twitching, tinnitus, disorientation, nystagmus, etc. Only excessive dose of lignocaine causes cardiac depression and hypotension.

As lignocaine is ineffective in atrial arrhythmias, it is used only in ventricular arrhythmias. It is also said that because of rapidly developing and titratable action, it is a good drug in the emergency setting such as ventricular arrhythmias following acute MI, cardiac surgery, and other acute conditions. Given prophylactically by infusion in acute MI, it also reduces the occurrence of VF. However, a recent meta-analysis has shown that prophylactic lignocaine fails to improve survival rate and may even increase the short-term mortality. Therefore, it is no longer administered routinely to all MI patients. This increased mortality may be due to the lignocaine-induced exacerbated heart block or congestive heart failure (CHF).

- *Mexiletine:* Chemically, it is a lignocaine analog. So, like lignocaine, mexiletine is a local anesthetic and an active antiarrhythmic agent. But, unlike lignocaine, it is active orally. This is because the structure of mexiletine and tocainide which is also analog to lignocaine is modified to reduce the first-pass hepatic metabolism and to make them effective for oral therapy.

  Pharmacologically, mexiletine is also similar to lignocaine. It increases the threshold voltage, reduces the rate of "phase 0" of action potential or depolarization, and decreases the "phase 4" slope. Thus, it converts the one-way block to two-way block. But it has little effect on the heart rate, BP, and ventricular function.

  Mexiletine is almost completely absorbed orally. The incidence of adverse effects of mexiletine is relatively high than lignocaine. These adverse effects are bradycardia, hypotension, AV block, etc.

  Doses: Mexiletine is used orally as the loadding dose of 400–600 mg stat and which is then followed by 150–200 mg thrice daily. Parenterally, it is used in a dose of 100–200 mg IV over 10 minutes, which is then followed by 1 mg/min through infusion. Parenteral mexiletine is effective in postinfarction ventricular arrhythmias as an alternative to lignocaine in resistant cases. Orally, it is used to keep the VES and VT suppressed over a long duration.

- *Tocainide:* Like mexiletine, tocainide is also a lignocaine analog and is active both orally and parenterally. It may be effective against severe ventricular arrhythmias which is refractory to other class I antiarrhythmic drugs. But tocainide is rarely used now because of the risk of severe agranulocytosis, thrombocytopenia (due to potentially fatal bone marrow depression), and pulmonary fibrosis.

- *Phenytoin and dilantin:* These are mainly antiepileptic drugs and are used very infrequently in cardiac arrhythmias. So, they are not discussed in detail here.

Subclass IC: Class IC antiarrhythmic drugs are highly effective and are the most potent Na^+ channel blockers. They suppress the "phase 0" activity of action potential and causes a marked reduction in conduction velocity. They also prolong the PR interval and broaden the QRS complex. They have a profound effect on the His–Purkinje system and accessory pathways for conduction. They markedly retard the anterograde as well as the retrograde conduction through the accessory pathway in the WPW syndrome.

However, recently it has been discovered that this subclass of antiarrhythmic drugs has the ability to be proarrhythmic. Proarrhythmia is a phenomenon which is identified as the development of new arrhythmias or exacerbation of preexisting arrhythmias in response to treatment with an antiarrhythmic drug. Both flecainide and encainide of the subclass IC drugs have been specifically implicated as proarrhythmic agents, and sudden deaths occur. The precise mechanism for proarrhythmogenesis by this group of drugs is not fully understood, but it may be due to the decreased conduction in abnormal areas of the myocardium which favors a re-entry mechanism.

- *Flecainide:* It blocks the Na^+ current and delays the rectifier K^+ current (IKr). It suppresses the phase 0 activity and increases the APD. Thus, it suppresses the VES, VT, and WPW syndrome and prevents the recurrence of AF and PSVT. In a recent study, it was found to increase the mortality in patients recovering from MI and so has been withdrawn from the market in many countries. But in the UK, it is still licensed for the treatment of AF and ventricular arrhythmias which are unresponsive to other therapies and in whom structural heart disease is absent.

  Encainide, a drug with remarkably similar electrophysiological actions like flecainide, is no longer used and available.

- *Propafenone:* It is mainly a Na^+ channel blocker. But, like flecainide, it also blocks the K^+ channels. It also prolongs the PR and QRS interval, but its major action is to slow the conduction in fast response tissue. Propafenone is mainly used orally to maintain the sinus rhythm in patients with supraventricular tachycardia and AF. In ventricular arrhythmias, it is modestly effective.

  The adverse effects of propafenone therapy include increased ventricular response in patients with AF, increased frequency and/or severity of reentrant VT, and exacerbation of heart failure. It has a β-adrenergic blocking effect and causes sinus bradycardia and bronchospasm.

  Propafenone undergoes extensive first-pass hepatic metabolism. It produces a metabolite named 5-hydroxy propafenone which is equipotent like its mother compound as a Na^+ channel blocker but is much less potent as a β-adrenergic receptor antagonist.

Class II—β-Adrenoreceptor antagonist: The primary action of drugs in this class is to suppress the adrenergic-induced automaticity by their specific membrane stabilizing effect like local anesthetic agents which is mediated through the fast Na^+ channels blocking action.

The electrophysiological effects of β-adrenoreceptor antagonists are:

- Decrease in automaticity
- Increase in APD, especially in ventricular conducting tissues
- Increase in ERP in the AV node.

The latter effect is the most important for the antiarrhythmic effect of β-adrenoreceptor antagonists. Automaticity is decreased in both the SA node and AV junctional tissues. There is potent inhibition of catecholamine-induced tachycardia and arrhythmia by this class of drugs.

In the clinically used dose range, the antiarrhythmic action of this class of drug is exerted primarily through their β-adrenergic blockade. It is only in very high doses that the antiarrhythmic action of this group of drug is exerted by their membrane stabilizing property through fast Na^+ channel blocking action. Automaticity is decreased by this class of drug when it is due to the adrenergic influence; otherwise, there is little or no action.

The most important ECG change by the effect of this group of drug is the prolongation of PR interval. Depression of cardiac contractility and hypotension is less marked.

Individual drugs in this class such as propranolol, metoprolol, and esmolol are discussed elsewhere.

Class III: The characteristic actions of this group of drugs in the class are prolongation of repolarization, widening of action potential, and increase in the ERP. Tissue remains refractory even after full repolarization. So, reentrant arrhythmias would also be terminated. Drugs in this class are bretylium and amiodarone.

- *Bretylium:* Bretylium tosylate is a quaternary ammonium compound. After IV injection, it produces a biphasic response. Initially, it displaces or releases noradrenaline from the adrenergic nerve terminals and produces transient sympathomimetic effects. As a result, initially, bretylium can produce transient hypertension and increased arrhythmias. But this effect is rarely observed. Later, it produces adrenergic blockade and hypotension. The major direct action of bretylium is prolongation of action potential and ERP, and this is probably due to the action of the K^+ channel blockade. It is not a Na^+ channel blocker and does not depress the automaticity. In theory, bretylium should be avoided in patients who are especially prone to increased arrhythmias with norepinephrine release. In contrast, hypotension due to inhibition of noradrenaline reuptake is a common problem during bretylium therapy. Bretylium-induced hypotension should be managed with judicious fluid replacement, but not by catecholamines. Since bretylium effectively causes sympathetic denervation, the administration of normal doses of catecholamine such as dopamine may cause marked hypertension.

Oral absorption of bretylium is very poor. So, it is always used through the IV route. It is excreted unchanged in the urine.

Bretylium is mainly used in the treatment of VT and VF which is refractory to lignocaine and/or defibrillation. The first IV loading dose of bretylium is 5–10 mg/kg which is given over 10 minutes. Then, it is repeated up to a total dose of 30 mg/kg. The onset of action of bretylium is very slow. So, resuscitative measures for VT and VF should be continued for 20–30 minutes after administration of bretylium. An infusion of bretylium in the dose of 2 mg/min is used for maintenance of its action.

The efficacy of bretylium in the treatment of acute ventricular arrhythmia is still controversial because of its slow onset of action. But it is still regarded as a second line of drug after lignocaine for the treatment of VT and VF.

- *Amiodarone:* Chemically, amiodarone hydrochloride is a di-iodinated benzofuran derivative and is a highly lipophilic agent. It is a long-acting antiarrhythmic drug and is a structural analog to thyroid hormone. So, some of the antiarrhythmic actions and toxicity of amiodarone may be due to the interaction of it with thyroid hormone receptors. As amiodarone is highly lipophilic, so it is concentrated mainly in the fat-containing tissues and is eliminated very slowly. Hence, the adverse effects of it may be awfully slow to resolve.

Amiodarone exerts multiple actions. It has been suggested that amiodarone's main effects are mediated by the perturbation of lipid milieu of cell membrane in which all the ion channels are situated. On the other hand, amiodarone is a potent inhibitor of abnormal automaticity and in most tissues, it prolongs APD and ERP. The mechanisms of actions of amiodarone are as follows:

- Block K^+ channels and prolongs APD and ERP
- Blocks Na^+ channels (lignocaine like action) and conduction is slowed and automaticity is depressed
- Blocks Ca^+ channel and β-adrenergic blocking property
- Also acts by partial antagonism of alpha- and beta-agonists by reducing the number of receptors and by inhibiting the coupling of agonists with receptors

The SA node is depressed by amiodarone. So, sinus rhythm is slowed by 15%. It is secondary to the reduction of slow diastolic depolarization in SA nodal cells by amiodarone. AV nodal automaticity is also depressed, and AV nodal conduction is also slowed by 25% in the face of atrial tachycardia by amiodarone. It is due to the decreased speed of depolarization of cells and increase in APD. Amiodarone has no effect on the conduction through bundle of His and PF and the ventricular myocardium. It has little effect on the BP and left ventricular contractility. The systemic vascular resistance (SVR) is decreased and coronary blood flow is increased by it.

The SA node is affected slightly by amiodarone. The effect of the oral dose of amiodarone on cardiac contractility and BP is minimal. But IV injection of it frequently causes myocardial depression and hypotension. There are clear differences in the electrophysiological study when the drug is given IV and in chronic oral therapy. Following IV administration, the ERP is prolonged particularly in conducting and ventricular muscle tissue, but there is no prolongation of the QTc interval. In contrast, during chronic oral therapy, the refractory period is prolonged, chiefly in AV nodal tissue with the prolongation of QTc interval.

Amiodarone is now widely used to treat supraventricular arrhythmias, preexcitation syndrome such as the WPW syndrome, and ventricular arrhythmias including VT, VF, etc. Its long duration of action makes it suitable for long-term prophylactic use, but close monitoring is required.

Amiodarone is incompletely and slowly absorbed from the GI tract. So, by daily oral ingestion, the action develops slowly over several days and weeks. But, on IV injection, the action develops rapidly. Amiodarone has very poor and variable bioavailability (20–80%). It undergoes extensive enterohepatic circulation before entry into the central compartment, from where it undergoes extensive tissue distribution. This is due to the exceptionally high tissue/plasma partition coefficient of amiodarone. Its distribution half-life from the central to the peripheral compartment may be as short as 4 hours. But its terminal half-life is both long and variable (9–77 days). This is due to the result of slow mobilization of this highly lipophilic drug out of the adipose tissue. The main metabolite of amiodarone is mono-N-desethylamiodarone which also exerts antiarrhythmic effects and has a long terminal half-life.

Amiodarone is mainly used orally in the dose of 400–600 mg/day for few weeks, and this is followed by 100–200 mg OD for maintenance therapy. In the IV route, 100–300 mg of amiodarone is given slowly over 30–60 minutes. For clinical action, a therapeutic plasma amiodarone concentration in the range of 0.5–2 µg/mL has been suggested. However, the efficacy appears to depend as much as on the duration of therapy and on the plasma concentration of it. But the elevated plasma concentration is not useful in predicting toxicity. As amiodarone accumulates in tissue, so initially a high oral loading dose is usually administered for several weeks and then a maintenance dose is started. The maintenance dose is adjusted on the basis of adverse

effects and the response of arrhythmias for which it is used. If the presenting arrhythmia is life-threatening, then the higher dose of amiodarone which is >300 mg/day is also used, unless clear toxicity occurs. On the other hand, the maintenance dose of amiodarone which is <200 mg/day is used, if recurrence of arrhythmia is tolerated.

Amiodarone treatment may result in supratherapeutic level of iodine in plasma, which may result in either hyper- or hypothyroidism. This is because amiodarone is a potent inhibitor of T_4 and thus it inhibits the peripheral change of T_4 to T_3, causing a dose- and duration-dependent increase in serum reverse T_3. This may account for many of the actions of amiodarone which are similar to those seen after thyroid ablation.

Amiodarone increases the concentration of serum transaminases, indicating hepatic damage secondary to phospholipidosis. A similar mechanism is also believed to account for alveolitis (pulmonary fibrosis) which occurs in about 5–7% of patients receiving amiodarone. This alveolitis (pulmonary fibrosis) produced by amiodarone may be insidious in onset and may present with cough, dyspnea, and diffuse pulmonary infiltration. It may occur acutely, especially after surgery in patients receiving a high dose of IV amiodarone, and may present as a postoperative adult respiratory distress syndrome.

Almost all patients receiving amiodarone develop corneal microdeposits and one-third develop signs of CNS toxicity. Peripheral neuropathy, photosensitivity, and GI upsets are also well-recognized complications of amiodarone. Hypotension, cardiovascular collapse, and AV block have been reported after IV injection of it. Other dysrhythmias may arise, especially in the presence of hypokalemia due to the use of amiodarone.

Serious and prolonged hypotension has been described in patients who are pretreated with amiodarone alone or in combination with angiotensin-converting enzyme (ACE) inhibitors during anesthesia. It is due to the decrease in SVR (due to vasodilation and myocardial depression) caused by chronic amiodarone therapy and is enhanced by the effects of ACE inhibitors. This exaggerated hypotensive effect produced by the combination of action of amiodarone and ACE inhibitor is mainly unmasked during the blood loss in surgery. Hypotension described in these cases is resistant to α-adrenoreceptor agonists such as metaraminol or phenylephrine and requires high infusion rates of noradrenaline to maintain adequate arterial pressure. Hypotension associated with the IV form of amiodarone is also partially due to the action of solvent which is used in its preparation.

Bradycardia and complete heart block which is resistant to atropine, adrenaline, and noradrenaline have also been reported in patients who are receiving amiodarone and undergoing general anesthesia (GA). So, it has been suggested that such patients may require temporary pacing in the perioperative period. The drug is contraindicated in porphyria.

Class IV—Calcium channel blockers: Calcium antagonists inhibit the inward flow of Ca^{2+} ions into the cell which usually occurs during the mid and late phases (i.e., late phase of phase 0, phase 1, and predominantly phase 2) of action potential. The classification of Ca^{2+} channel antagonists recognizes three subclasses. These are:

1. Papaverine derivatives (verapamil)
2. Dihydropyridines derivatives (nifedipine, nicardipine, isradipine, felodipine, nimodipine)
3. Benzothiazepines derivatives (diltiazem).

All the drugs in each subclass of calcium channel blockers have some specific activity on cardiac conducting tissue, cardiac muscle cells, and vascular smooth muscles. But the dihydropyridine derivatives (nifedipine) and benzothiazepine derivative (diltiazem) have some special activity profiles which render them ineffective as antiarrhythmic agents. So, only verapamil is used clinically as an antiarrhythmic agent. The comparisons of electrophysiological actions of these three subclasses of main calcium channel blockers are shown in **Table 3**.

- *Verapamil:* Of the many Ca^{2+} channel blockers, verapamil has the most prominent antiarrhythmic action. It predominantly acts on the SA and AV nodes as these tissues are mainly calcium-dependent for their actions during both phase 0 and phase 4 of action potential. It causes the competitive blockade of slow calcium ion channels of the cell membrane leading to a decreased influx of Ca^+ into the cell. So, the rate of discharge in

the SA node is reduced and the recovery is prolonged by verapamil. The AV nodal conduction is also strongly inhibited, and the ERP is prolonged by it. Because of the powerful AV-blocking effect, some drugs such as β-adrenoreceptor antagonist and halothane should be used very cautiously in patients receiving verapamil during anesthesia **(Table 3)**.

Verapamil is absolutely contraindicated in patients with digoxin toxicity. It also causes a decrease in the influx of Ca^{2+} into the vascular smooth muscle and myocardial cells. This results in the inhibition of contraction and relaxation of cardiac and vascular smooth muscle fibers, leading to coronary and systemic arterial vasodilatation. So, the drug causes a decrease in the SVR and is a potent coronary artery vasodilator. Therefore, verapamil is used in the management of mild-to-moderate types of hypertension and angina.

Verapamil is mainly used in the treatment of supraventricular arrhythmias such as PSVT, AF, and AFL. By the effects of reduction of AV conduction, it also reduces the ventricular rate in AFL and AF such as digoxin. But the rapid action of verapamil makes it preferable than digoxin in the acute management of AFL and AF or other causes of supraventricular tachycardia to reduce the ventricular rate. It also may be combined with digoxin for the treatment of AF to achieve a synergistic effect of low doses of both drugs, with good control of heart rate and minimum undesirable side effects of both drugs. Verapamil should not be used in the treatment of WPW syndrome associated with PSVT because of the increased risk of ventricular rate. It is only effective in treating supraventricular tachycardia when conduction is anterograde through the AV node and retrograde through the accessory pathways. In reverse condition, verapamil is ineffective. It should never be used in broad complex tachycardia because there is a chance of VF. Adenosine is the best drug to distinguish between broad complex tachycardia and supraventricular arrhythmias. Amiodarone is more effective in treating broad complex tachycardia than narrow complex tachycardia.

Intravenous administration of verapamil may cause a negative inotropic effect, and this may be due to the synergistic effect with the hypotensive property of volatile anesthetic agents such as halothane. Thus, profound hypotension and serious cardiac conduction disorders may occur when verapamil and halothane or other halogenated volatile anesthetic agents are used in combination. Verapamil has poor efficacy in the treatment of ventricular arrhythmias. In contrast to β-blockers, verapamil prophylaxis does not reduce mortality in post-MI patients.

TABLE 3: Electrophysiological effects of three commonly used calcium channel blockers.

	Verapamil	Nifedipine	Diltiazem
SA node automaticity	D	Nil	D
Ventricular automaticity	D	Nil	Nil
ERP:			
• Atrial	Nil	Nil	Nil
• AV nodal	I	D/I	I
• Ventricular	Nil	Nil	Nil
• Bypass tract	I	Nil	Nil
ECG:			
• RR interval	I	D	D/I
• PR interval	I	Nil	I

(AV: atrioventricular; D: decreased; ECG: electrocardiogram; ERP: effective refractory period; I: increased; Nil: no effect; SA: sinoatrial)

Uses and doses:
- Verapamil is the drug of choice for terminating an attack of PSVT. Only 5–10 mg of it through an IV route over 2–3 minutes is effective in 80% of cases. Adverse effects such as bradycardia, AV block, and cardiac arrest should be checked during the use of verapamil. For prevention of recurrence of PSVT, it is used in a dose of 60–120 mg thrice daily orally.
- To control the ventricular rate in AFL and AF (as an alternative to digoxin or an addition to it), verapamil should be used in a dose of 60–120 mg TDS.

Side effects: Verapamil can cause first- or second-degree heart block. IV administration of it may precipitate heart failure in patients with impaired left ventricular function. It also precipitates VT or VF in patients with WPW syndrome. The effects of volatile anesthetic agents and β-adrenergic antagonists on myocardial contractility and conduction system of the heart are synergistic with those of verapamil. This drug increases the serum concentration of coadministered digoxin.

If verapamil and dantrolene are administered concurrently, then they may cause hyperkalemia leading to VF. So, these drugs are not recommended to be used together in patients. The drug decreases the minimum alveolar concentration (MAC) value of halothane. Chronic exposure to this drug may potentiate the actions of both depolarizing and nondepolarizing muscle relaxants. Verapamil attenuates the pressor response to laryngoscopy and intubation.

Other antiarrhythmic agents:
- *Cardiac glycosides (digoxin):* It has been discussed in the heart failure chapter.
- *Adenosine:* Adenosine and its physiological effects were first described in 1929. But it has only recently been used as a therapeutic and diagnostic agent. In the human body, it is a naturally occurring compound (nucleoside) composed of adenine (a purine base) which is bonded to D-ribose. It is formed in the body by two major mechanisms: depolarization of adenosine monophosphate (AMP) and breakdown of S-adenosyl homocysteine (SDH). The effects of adenosine in the cardiovascular system (CVS) are mediated by its high affinity to some adenosine receptors such as A1 and low affinity to other adenosine receptors such as A2.

The activity of the A1 receptor inhibits the adenyl cyclase and subsequently inhibits the production of cyclic adenosine monophosphate (cAMP). Thus, adenosine causes depression of cardiac contractility. On the other hand, activation of the A2 receptor causes vasodilation throughout the body, especially pulmonary, renal, and coronary vessels, producing hypotension. The pharmacological actions of theophylline, caffeine, and methylxanthines are also mediated by their competitive antagonistic actions on A1 and A2 receptors. Part of the vasodilating effects of adenosine may be related to prostacyclin (PGI$_2$) synthesis. Though the main role of adenosine is as a diagnostic and therapeutic tool in the management of supraventricular arrhythmias, it may also have important roles as a coronary and pulmonary vasodilator.

Mechanism of action of adenosine as an antiarrhythmic agent:
- Action of adenosine on the A1 receptor activates the acetylcholine-sensitive potassium conductance in sinus, AV nodal, and atrial cells. Thus, it causes hyperpolarization of the cell membrane and hence slows down or completely blocks the spontaneous activity of these cells.
- Adenosine also blocks the slow inward movement of Ca^{2+} current which is responsible for the upstroke (phase 0) of the action potential in the sinus, AV nodal, and atrial cells. Thus, it increases the refractoriness.
- Adenosine also inhibits the release of noradrenaline from the presynaptic terminals. Thus, it enhances the antiadrenergic effect.
- Adenosine also exerts its antiarrhythmic action by blocking the re-entry pathways, either through the AV node or through an accessory pathway.

Despite the availability of different types of sophisticated ECG machines, still the diagnosis of tachyarrhythmias sometimes becomes exceedingly difficult because broad complex tachycardia may be due to VT or supraventricular tachycardia with bundle branch block. If verapamil is used for the treatment of a patient with VT mistaken for PSVT with broad QRS complex due to bundle branch block, then cardiac arrest may occur. Another therapeutic problem of verapamil is that the 15% of narrow QRS complex tachycardia is other than PSVT, where it may can create problem. In such a situation, if adenosine is injected rapidly in large peripheral veins, then it helps in differentiation between supraventricular tachycardia and VT with 90% accuracy because VT remains unaffected by adenosine.

So, currently, the only indication for the use of adenosine is the conversion of PSVT (including that associated with WPW syndrome) to sinus rhythm. IV bolus administration of adenosine for PSVT may induce the onset of AF and thus should be administered only in an appropriate setting with cardioversion capability. Wide complex tachycardia arising from the ventricle, as opposed to the AV node, will not be affected by adenosine. Similarly, atrial arrhythmias (e.g., AF, AFL, multifocal atrial tachycardia) will demonstrate only a transient slowing of the ventricular rate.

Adenosine has no clinically important effects on BP except transient hypotension when administered in a therapeutic dose by bolus. But a continuous high dose of infusion may result in a decrease of SVR and BP. Thus, it causes a dose-dependent reflex tachycardia and an increase in stroke volume and cardiac output. Adenosine also causes a dose-dependent increase in myocardial blood flow which is secondary to coronary vasodilation and mediated via endothelial A2 receptors. But this is without an increase in O_2 consumption and workload. However, the unfavorable changes in the distribution of regional coronary blood flow (intracoronary steal) by adenosine have led to myocardial ischemia in patients with coronary artery disease, which may greatly limit its usefulness during anesthesia **(Table 4)**.

Adenosine also slows the AV conduction and increases the PR interval. It can interrupt the reentrant arrhythmias that involve the AV node. Large doses of adenosine depress the SA node and ventricular automaticity, leading to brief periods of sinus pause, but it resolves spontaneously. Though adverse reactions of adenosine are rare and of brief duration, still it is best avoided in patients with second- or third-degree heart block or sick sinus syndrome. The bolus administration of adenosine is associated with an increase in both the depth and rate of respiration. This is probably mediated by A2 receptor, situated in the carotid body. It decreases pulmonary vascular resistance (PVR), increases intrapulmonary shunt, and can lead to a drop in arterial O_2 saturation because of the inhibition of pulmonary hypoxic vasoconstriction reflex. It may rarely cause bronchospasm in predisposed individuals.

Hypotensive dose of adenosine stimulates A2 receptors, resulting in renal and hepatic arterial vasodilatation, although low doses have no effect on the glomerular filtration rate and urine output.

Adenosine has a very short half-life which is <10 seconds. It is due to rapid uptake of it by the red blood cells (RBC) and endothelial cells where it is converted to 5-AMP and inosine. Almost complete elimination of adenosine occurs in a single passage through coronary circulation. Dipyridamole potentiates the actions of adenosine, while theophylline and caffeine antagonize the action of it by blocking the receptors. So, higher doses of adenosine are required for a tea or coffee drinker.

The advantages of adenosine over verapamil for termination of PSVT are as follows:

- Efficiency of adenosine is greater than verapamil; there is 100% efficacy for adenosine compared with 73% for verapamil.
- Action of adenosine lasts <5 seconds. So, adverse effects of adenosine, even if cardiac arrest occurs, are transient and are in fact the therapeutic goal.
- Adenosine causes no hemodynamic deterioration. So, it can be given to patients with hypotension or those receiving β-blockers. But verapamil is contraindicated in these situations.
- Adenosine is safe in wide QRS tachycardia, while verapamil is unsafe in such conditions.
- Adenosine is effective in patients who do not respond to verapamil.

TABLE 4: The best choice of drugs for different cardiac arrhythmias, during their acute and chronic course.

Arrhythmia	Acute		Chronic	
	First choice	**Second choice**	**First choice**	**Second choice**
Atrial extrasystole	Not necessary		Quinidine	• Propranolol • Disopyramide
PSVT	• Adenosine • Verapamil	• Digoxin • β-blocker	• Verapamil • Digoxin	• β-blocker • Disopyramide
Atrial flutter and atrial fibrillation	• Cardioversion • Verapamil	Esmolol	• Amiodarone • Digitalis	Any of the previous drugs
Ventricular extrasystole	• Lignocaine	• Mexiletine • Disopyramide • Propranolol	Amiodarone	• Mexiletine • Propranolol
VT	• Cardioversion • Lignocaine	• Mexiletine • Amiodarone	• Mexiletine • Amiodarone	• Disopyramide • Quinidine
VF	Cardioversion	• Lignocaine • Bretylium	• Bretylium • Amiodarone	Same
WPW syndrome	Cardioversion	Amiodarone	Amiodarone	Propranolol

(PSVT: paroxysmal supraventricular tachycardia; VF: ventricular fibrillation; VT: ventricular tachycardia; WPW: Wolff–Parkinson–White)

It may produce transient dyspnea, chest pain, and flushing. VF or ventricular standstill may occur in some patients, but it lasts only for few seconds. Bronchospasm may be precipitated in asthmatics. As adenosine has very short duration of action, it is not suitable for recurrent cases. It is very expensive.

Doses: The therapeutic dose of adenosine is 6–12 mg through IV in bolus. Due to rapid metabolism in few seconds, slow administration of adenosine results in the elimination of the drug from the circulation prior to its arrival at the heart. So, adenosine is administered as a rapid IV bolus, followed by a saline flush. The initial adult dose of adenosine is 3 mg which is followed, if necessary, by 6 mg and then 12 mg bolus at 1- to 2-minute intervals, until the desired effects are observed. The pediatric dose of adenosine is 0.05 mg/kg, which is increased by 0.05 mg/kg to a maximum of 0.3 mg/kg. The drug acts within 10 seconds and has a duration of action of 10–20 seconds. No dose adjustment of adenosine is necessary in the presence of renal or hepatic impairment.

- *Dofetilide:* It is a potent, specific, and delayed IKr blocker. So, it acts only on the heart without any extracardiac pharmacological action. Dofetilide is very effective in maintaining sinus rhythm in AF. The use of dofetilide does not increase mortality in patients with advanced heart failure and acute MI.

  Dofetilide is excreted unchanged by kidneys. So, in renal failure, lower doses of dofetilide should be used cautiously. It is marketed first in 2000 and is currently available only in few centers in the world. The incidence of its adverse effects is still unknown.

- *Ibutilide:* It also prolongs the APD by blocking the IKr and inward Na$^+$ current. For immediate conversion of AFL and AF to sinus rhythm, ibutilide is used as rapid infusion (1 mg in 10 minutes). The major drawback of ibutilide is torsades-de-pointes which required immediate cardioversion.

Drugs for Atrioventricular Block (Disturbances for Impulse Conduction)

- *Atropine:* Atropine sulfate (0.6 mg IV, repeated if necessary, to a maximum of 3 mg) increases the sinus rate and SA and AV conduction. It is the treatment of choice for severe bradycardia and/or hypotension due to vagal overactivity. Atropine may also be of important value during the initial management of symptomatic bradyarrhythmia complicating the early stages of inferior MI and cardiac arrest due to asystole. Repeated doses may be necessary because the drug disappears rapidly from the circulation after parenteral administration. Side effects include dry mouth, thirst, blurred vision, and both atrial and ventricular extrasystole.

- *Sympathomimetics:*
  - *Adrenaline:* It is discussed in the chapter "Autonomic Nervous System".
  - *Isoprenaline:* It is discussed in the chapter "Autonomic Nervous System".

Hypertension: Pharmacology and Anesthesia

■ INTRODUCTION

Any definition of systemic hypertension is *arbitrary*. Because, in contrast to any specific disease, hypertension is often taken as a trait or characteristic and represents a *quantitative* rather than a *qualitative* deviation from a normal value of systemic arterial blood pressure (BP). It is the most common, asymptomatic, readily detectable, and easily treatable disease, which, if untreated, often leads to lethal complications. These complications depend also on other risk factors such as age, gender, weight, physical activity, smoking, family history, blood cholesterol, and diabetes. Therefore, the effective management of hypertension requires a holistic approach, which is based on all the identifiable risk factors and adoption of multifactorial intervention. Some patients with mild hypertension require only single-drug therapy, which may consist of a thiazide diuretic, angiotensin-converting enzyme (ACE) inhibitor, ARB (angiotensin receptor blocker), β-adrenergic blocker, or calcium channel blocker (CCB), while some patients with moderate-to-severe hypertension often require combination of these drugs. The combination of a diuretic plus a β-adrenergic blocker and an ACE inhibitor is often effective, when single drug therapy is not. *All the patients with prior myocardial infarction (MI) should receive a β-adrenergic blocker and an ACE inhibitor or an ARB to improve outcome, irrespective of the presence of hypertension.* ACE inhibitors (or ARBs) prolong survival in patients with congestive heart failure (CHF), left ventricular dysfunction, or a prior MI.

Effective drug therapy reduces the progression of hypertension and the incidences of stroke, CHF, coronary artery disease (CAD), and kidney damage. Effective treatment can also delay and sometimes reverse the concomitant pathophysiological changes of hypertension, such as left ventricular hypertrophy (LVH) and altered cerebral autoregulation. Although the understanding of the pathophysiology of elevated arterial pressure has increased, but, still in 80–95% of cases, the etiology of elevated arterial pressure is largely unknown. So, the treatment of hypertension in most of the cases is nonspecific, resulting in large number of minor side effects and a high compliance rate. Hence, in the light of these observations, *hypertension is now defined as the value of arterial BP at which level the benefit of treatment outweighs the cost and complications. The **Table 1** shows the range of normal blood pressure and the grading of hypertension.*

■ CLASSIFICATION OF HYPERTENSION (BASED ON ETIOLOGY)

- *Systolic and diastolic hypertension:*
  - *Primary (essential):* 80–95%
  - *Secondary (5–20%):* Renal disease, renal artery stenosis, primary hyperaldosteronism, Cushing disease, acromegaly, pheochromocytoma, pregnancy estrogen therapy
- *Only systolic hypertension:*
  - Increased cardiac output (CO)
- Aortic regurgitation
- Patent ductus arteriosus
- Arteriovenous fistula
- Fever
- Thyrotoxicosis
  - Rigidity of aorta

TABLE 1: Range of normal blood pressure and grading of hypertension.

Category	Diastolic (mm Hg)	Systolic (mm Hg)
Normal	<80	<120
High normal or prehypertension	80–89	120–139
Hypertension:		
• Mild	90–99	140–159
• Moderate	100–109	160–179
• Severe	110–119	180–209
• Very severe	>120	>210

- Arteriosclerosis
- Only diastolic hypertension.

CLASSIFICATION OF HYPERTENSION (BASED ON NUMERICAL VALUE)

Blood pressure measurements are affected by many variables, including posture, time of day, emotional state, recent activity, and drug intake, as well as the equipment and technique used. *The diagnosis of hypertension cannot be made with only one preoperative reading, but requires confirmation by a history of consistently elevated measurements.* Although preoperative anxiety or pain may produce some degree of hypertension in normal patients, patients with a history of hypertension generally exhibit greater preoperative elevations in BP.

ESSENTIAL OR PRIMARY OR IDIOPATHIC HYPERTENSION

Arterial hypertension, with no definite cause or explanation for its pathophysiology, is said to be essential hypertension. Usually, it constitutes 80–95% of the total cases of hypertension. *Several abnormalities of varying systems* that are mainly involved in the regulation of BP such as kidneys, peripheral resistance vessels, and sympathetic nervous system *have been described in patients with essential hypertension.* But, it is still uncertain, whether these abnormalities of varying system, which are mentioned above, are responsible for the development of hypertension (secondary) or are due to hypertension (primary) caused by an unknown etiology. Also, we do not know if it (hypertension) is the different expressions or pathophysiology of different organs to a single disease process or it (hypertension) is one common sign of multiple expressions (signs) of multiple disease processes which are not known. However,

the second explanation is gradually getting ground. So, the distinction between the primary hypertension and secondary hypertension is gradually becoming blurred. The **Figure 1** shows the evolution of uncomplicated and complicated primary hypertension, related to age.

Individuals in whom the defect of *any specific structural organ* is responsible for the development of systemic hypertension are defined as having a secondary form of hypertension. In contrast, where the *generalized functional abnormalities* are the cause of hypertension (even if the abnormalities are very discrete), it is defined as the essential hypertension.

Hypertension is associated with an abnormal elevation of baseline CO, systemic vascular resistance (SVR), or both. An evolving pattern is commonly seen over the course of disease, where CO gradually returns to normal, but SVR becomes abnormally high. Therefore, this chronic increase in cardiac afterload (SVR) results into construct LVH and altered ventricular diastolic function. Hypertension also alters the cerebral autoregulation, such that normal cerebral blood flow (CBF) is maintained in the face of high BP. This cerebral autoregulation works in the range of mean blood pressure (MBP) of 110–180 mm Hg (explained in more details below).

The mechanisms, responsible for the *changes,* observed in hypertensive patients, seem to involve—(1) vascular hypertrophy, (2) hyperinsulinemia, (3) abnormal increase in intracellular calcium, and (4) increased intracellular Na^+ concentration in vascular smooth muscle cells and renal tubular cells. (5) Sympathetic nervous system overactivity and (6) enhanced responses to sympathetic agonists are present in some patients. (7) Hypertensive patients sometimes display an exaggerated response to vasopressors and vasodilators.

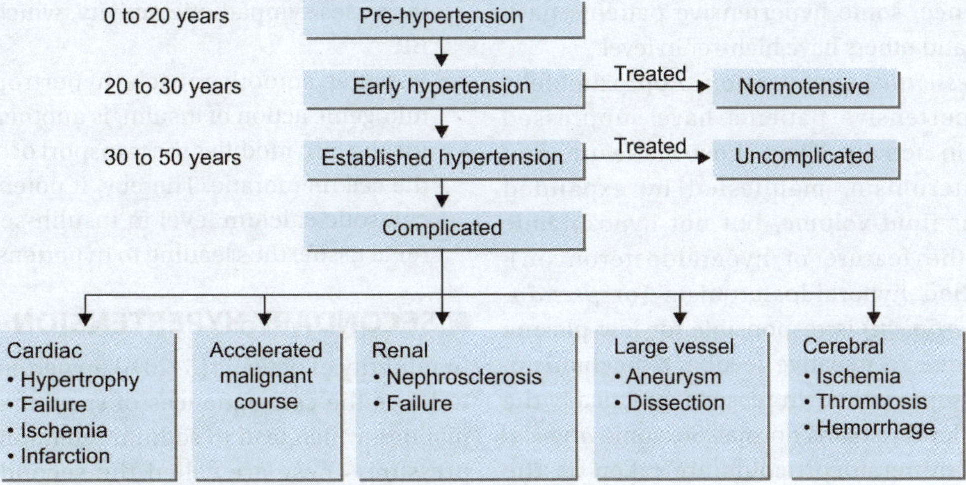

Fig. 1: The evolution of uncomplicated and complicated primary hypertension.

The probable theories of primary or essential hypertension are:

- *Heredity:* It is probably heterogeneous in nature and is multifactorial in origin. Monogenic defects (Liddle's syndrome) and susceptible genes (angiotensinogen gene) are also now reported.
- *Environment:* Environment that is responsible for high BP includes excessive salt intake, obesity, sedentary occupation, smoking, alcohol intake, etc. BP increases with age in more affluent societies and decreases with age in less affluent societies. This explains that environment has great influence on the genesis of hypertension.
- *Sensitivity to salt:* It is gradually receiving much attention, but pathophysiology of it is still uncertain. This hypothesis explains that the sensitivity of an individual to salt varies, which is responsible for hypertension.
- *Renin:* Renin–angiotensin–aldosterone system is an important contributory factor for the genesis of hypertension. Renin is an enzyme, which is secreted by the juxtaglomerular (JG) cell of kidney. It is linked with the secretion of aldosterone through a negative feedback loop. The varieties of factors can modify the rate of secretion of this renin. But, the primary determinant is the circulatory volume status of individual, which is again particularly related to the changes in dietary Na^+ intake. The end product of the action of renin on its substrate (angiotensinogen) is the generation of angiotensin I and angiotensin II, which is responsible for controlling the BP by constricting blood vessels. The intake of Na^+ normally modulates the adrenal and renal vascular response to angiotensin II. With sodium restriction, the adrenal responses are enhanced and the renal vascular responses are reduced; whereas, the sodium loading has the opposite effect. The plasma renin activity is wider in hypertensive subject than in normotensive. As a consequence, some hypertensive patients have low-renin level and others have high-renin level.

    - *Low-renin essential hypertension:* Approximately, 20% of hypertensive patients have suppressed plasma renin activity. They show the features of hyperaldosteronism, manifested by expanded extracellular fluid volume, but not hypokalemic (which is the feature of hyperaldosteronism). This so-called hyperaldosteronism (or *pseudo-hyperaldosteronism*) is responsible for low-plasma renin level due to negative feedback mechanism. But, due to some unknown reasons, practically the aldosterone level remains normal. So, some *atypical* (unknown) mineralocorticoids are taken as the responsible for low-renin hypertension.

    - *Nonmodulating essential hypertension:* This type of hypertension constitutes about 25–30% of population. Here, the plasma renin level is normal to high and adrenal defect is opposite to that observed in low-renin patients. In these patients, Na^+ intake does not modulate either adrenal or renal vascular responses to angiotensin II. So, this type of hypertension is named so.

    - *High-renin essential hypertension:* Here, the plasma renin levels are higher than the normal range, which suggests that plasma renin plays an important role in the pathogenesis of elevated BP. However, some investigators postulate that this elevated renin and increased BP are secondary to the increase in the activity of adrenergic system. It is proposed that angiotensin-dependent high-renin hypertension is nonmodulating defect.

- *Cell membrane defect:* Another postulated explanation for essential hypertension is generalized cell membrane defect, where there is both increase and decrease in the activity of different transport systems. Among these, some abnormalities are primary and some are secondary. The abnormality in sodium transport reflects an undefined alteration in cell membrane. This defect leads to the abnormal accumulation of Na^+ in vascular smooth muscle cells, resulting in higher vascular responsiveness to vasoconstrictor agents.
- *Insulin resistance:* Insulin resistance and/or hyperinsulinemia are/is one of the etiological factors for essential hypertension. Insulin resistance is common both in noninsulin-dependent diabetes mellitus (NIDDM) and obesity. Both obesity and NIDDM are common in hypertensive than normotensive subjects.

Hyperinsulinemia elevates BP by the following mechanism:

- Hyperinsulinemia produces renal sodium retention and increases sympathetic activity, which lead to increased BP.
- Vascular smooth muscle hypertrophy, secondary to mitogenic action of insulin, is another mechanism.
- Insulin also modifies the transport of different ions across the cell membrane. Thereby, it potentially increases the cytosolic calcium level in insulin-sensitive vascular or renal tissue, thus leading to hypertension.

■ SECONDARY HYPERTENSION

In minority of patients (5–20%), hypertension can be shown to be as the consequences of specific diseases or abnormalities, which lead to sodium retention and/or peripheral pressure. These are called the secondary hypertension. These specific causes can be identified and correction of these causes can cure the hypertension. The causes of secondary hypertension are:

1. *Renal:* Acute and chronic glomerulonephritis, chronic pyelonephritis, polycystic renal disease, stenosis of renal artery, diabetic nephropathy, chronic renal failure, renin-producing tumor, etc. are the renal causes for secondary hypertension.
2. *Endocrinal:* Acromegaly, oral contraceptive, pheochromocytoma, Cushing's disease, primary aldosteronism, congenital adrenal hyperplasia, hyperthyroidism, etc. are the endocrinal causes for secondary hypertension.
3. *Neurogenic:* Increased intracranial pressure, psychogenic, polyneuritis, autoimmune vascular diseases, etc. are the neurogenic causes for secondary hypertension.
4. *Miscellaneous:* Coarctation of aorta, pregnancy-induced hypertension, polyarteritis nodosa, increased intravascular volume, polycythemia, excess transfusion, medications by glucocorticoids, etc. are the miscellaneous causes for secondary hypertension.

■ EFFECTS OF HYPERTENSION

Hypertension is one of the common causes of death. Patient dies prematurely due to hypertension. The adverse effects of hypertension mainly involve the cardiovascular system (CVS), kidney, retina, central nervous system (CNS), etc., which often can be detected by simple clinical means.

Effects on CVS

In hypertension, heart has to work against excessive afterload, due to increased SVR. So, the first compensatory change in heart is the concentric LVH to maintain the same CO. Then, gradually myocardial ischemia develops and it damages the myocardium. Thus, the function of left ventricle gradually deteriorates, its cavity dilates, and the signs and symptoms of heart failure appear. During this compensatory phase, angina may appear and this is because of the combination of associated coronary arterial disease, reducing myocardial O_2 supply, and increasing myocardial O_2 demand. Other findings, which are often associated with hypertension, are: (1) the sound of aortic closure is accentuated and a faint murmur of aortic regurgitation is observed, (2) presystolic (4th) heart sound and protodiastolic (3rd) heart sound may be present. Electrocardiography (ECG) and echocardiographic changes show LVH and ischemia. Atrial fibrillation is common. It may be due to diastolic dysfunction, caused by LVH.

Effect on Kidney

The most common renal vascular effects, due to hypertension, are the arteriosclerotic changes in the afferent and efferent arterioles and in the glomerular tuft of capillaries. These changes cause decreased glomerular filtration rate (GFR), proteinuria, and microscopic hematuria. Renal failure contributes 10% of death, caused by hypertension.

Retinal Changes

Retina is the only tissue in which the arteries and arterioles can be examined directly. It also provides the opportunity to observe the progress and the effects of hypertension on vessels. When there is no arteriosclerotic change in retinal vessels, then gradually the increasing severity of hypertension is associated with focal spasm and progressive general narrowing of the arterioles. After that, there is appearance of hemorrhage, exudates (cotton wool), and papilledema. These retinal lesions often produce scotoma, blurred vision, and even blindness, especially when there is papilledema or hemorrhage on macular area. These hypertensive lesions in retina may also develop very acutely. If therapy started immediately and results in significant reduction of BP, then these above-mentioned retinal changes show rapid resolution.

If there are retinal arteriosclerotic changes, which result from the endothelial and muscular proliferation, then it also reflects the similar changes in other organs. These sclerotic changes do not develop as rapidly as hypertensive lesions, nor do they regress easily with therapy. As a consequence, the increased wall thickness and rigidity, caused by the sclerotic arterioles, distort and compress the veins where the two types of vessels cross in their common fibrous sheath. Due to these arteriosclerotic changes, the reflected light streak from the arterioles is changed by the increased opacity of vessel wall.

Hypertensive retinopathy:
- *Grade I:* Arteriolar tortuosity, thickening of arterial wall, and increased reflectiveness (silver wiring).
- *Grade II:* Grade I plus the nipping or constriction at arteriovenous crossing.
- *Grade III:* Grade II plus retinal ischemia, evidenced by flame-shaped hemorrhage and cotton wool exudate.
- *Grade IV:* Grade III plus papilledema.

Effects on CNS

The common symptoms of patients with moderate-to-severe hypertension are headache, dizziness, vertigo, tinnitus, dimness of vision, and syncope. The more serious manifestations of CNS for hypertension are due to vascular occlusion, hemorrhage, or encephalopathy. The pathogenesis of cerebral infarction (vascular occlusion) is secondary to increased cerebral atherosclerosis. The pathogenesis of cerebral hemorrhage or stroke is the result of both elevated cerebral arterial pressure and the development of cerebral vascular microaneurysms. Stroke is the most common complication of hypertension and it may be due to cerebral hemorrhage or cerebral infarction. Hypertensive encephalopathy is a rare condition.

SOME TERMINOLOGIES REGARDING HYPERTENSION

Hypertensive Emergency

It is defined as the elevation of both systolic and diastolic BP with the presence of any acute end organ disease. The organs at particular risk for hypertensive emergency are those that receive greater proportion of CO, that is, heart, brain, and kidneys. *So, the examples of hypertensive emergencies include—hypertensive encephalopathy, dissecting aortic aneurysm, cerebrovascular accidents, severe hypertension with progressive renal insufficiency, and acute left ventricular heart failure.* Hypertensive emergencies may also be caused by pheochromocytoma, preeclampsia, and eclampsia. It may even be drug-related [monoamine oxidase (MAO) inhibitor and tyramine ingestion, withdrawal of α_2 agonist such as clonidine, and use of sympathomimetic agents] or occur postoperatively. Hypertensive emergency is not distinguished by an arbitrarily chosen BP value. It may occur at any level of BP.

Hypertensive Urgency (or Pseudoemergency)

It is described as an elevated BP (diastolic >120 mm Hg) without any acute end organ disease. *The examples of hypertensive urgencies include—perioperative hypertension, intractable nasal bleeding, hypertension associated with increased circulation of catecholamines, and most commonly severe diastolic hypertension without any complications.*

Hypertensive Crisis

Hypertensive emergency and urgency are together encompassed in this term. Hypertensive crisis is rare and treatment must balance the risks of lowering BP too rapidly against the persistent hypertension with continued end organ dysfunction. As for example, in case of left ventricular failure (LVF), blood pressure should be reduced very rapidly, but in cerebral vascular accident (CVA), reduction of BP should be over hours.

Malignant Hypertension

In addition to marked elevation of BP in association with (1) papilledema, (2) retinal hemorrhages, and (3) exudates, the full blown picture of malignant hypertension may include the manifestation of hypertensive encephalopathy, such as (1) severe headache, (2) vomiting, (3) visual disturbances, (4) transient paralyses, (5) convulsions, (6) stupor, and (7) coma.

Accelerated Malignant Hypertension

Until recently, the term "malignant" hypertension was used for the presence of papilledema [grade IV Keith–Wagener (KW) retinopathy], whereas the term "accelerated" was used for the presence of hemorrhages and exudates in retina (grade III KW retinopathy), both with markedly high BP (diastolic BP usually above 140 mm Hg). But, these fundoscopic differences do not establish different clinical features or prognosis, so the term "accelerated malignant" hypertension is recommended and will be used from now on.

Hypertensive Encephalopathy

In addition to the marked elevation of BP associated with papilledema, retinal hemorrhage and exudates, etc., the full-blown picture of malignant hypertension may also include manifestation of hypertensive CNS disturbances, transient paralysis, convulsion, stupor, and coma. This is known as hypertensive encephalopathy. With or without structural defects of accelerated–malignant hypertension, progressively higher BP can lead to hypertensive encephalopathy.

The above-mentioned manifestations have been attributed to spasm and dilatations of cerebral vessels and cerebral edema. In some patients who have died, multiple small thrombi have also been found in cerebral vessels. Cerebrospinal fluid (CSF) is clear but usually under increased pressure. Magnetic resonance imaging (MRI) shows hemorrhage in and around the basal ganglia. However, the neurological deficit is usually reversible if the hypertension is promptly treated.

MECHANISM OF HYPERTENSIVE ENCEPHALOPATHY

With changes in BP, the cerebral vessels constrict or dilate to maintain a relatively constant level of CBF. This is called as the process of cerebral autoregulation and is regulated by sympathetic nervous activity. The cerebral vessels dilate progressively as the pressure decreases and progressively constrict as the pressure increases. During the increase of BP, when mean arterial pressure (MAP) reaches a critical level, say around 180 mm Hg, then the previously constricted vessels are unable to withstand such high pressure and become stretched and dilated. It occurs first in areas, where the vessels are with less muscular tone, thus producing an irregular sausage string pattern and later diffusely producing generalized vasodilatation. This vasodilation allows an

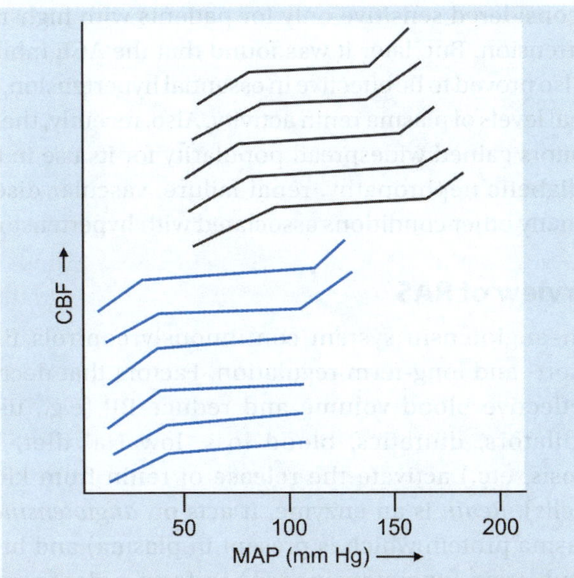

Fig. 2: The relation between cerebral blood flow (CBF) and mean arterial pressure (MAP) in both normotensive and chronic hypertensive patients.

increase of CBF and hyperperfusion of brain under high pressure. This causes the leakage of fluid into perivascular tissue, leading to cerebral edema and the clinical syndrome of hypertensive encephalopathy.

Figure 2 relating the relationship between MAP and CBF demonstrates that CBF is constant between MAP of 60 and 120 mm Hg in normotensive subject, i.e., the lower six curves. Of these lower six curves, the upper two curves show breakthrough hyperperfusion, when the pressure is raised beyond the limit of autoregulation in normotensive subject. These autoregulation curves in chronic hypertensives, whose blood vessels adapt chronically the elevated BP with structural thickening, mediated by sympathetic nerves, are shifted to the right (shown in the upper six curves). Even with this shift, the breakthrough will occur, if the pressure is raised very high to the levels of 170–180 mm Hg.

These findings explain a number of clinical observations. At the upper portion of these autoregulatory curves of the previously normotensive people (lower six curves), who suddenly become hypertensive, may develop encephalopathy at relatively low levels of hypertension. These include the children with acute glomerulonephritis and young women with eclampsia. On the other hand, chronically hypertensive patients less commonly develop encephalopathy and if so only at much higher level of BP.

When BP is lowered by antihypertensive drugs too rapidly, then the chronic hypertensive patients are often unable to tolerate this reduction of BP, without experiencing cerebral hypoperfusion (manifested by weakness, dizziness, etc.). These symptoms appear at the levels of BP that are still

above the upper limit of normal and that are well tolerated by normotensives. The reason is that the entire curve of autoregulation shifts to the right, so that the lower end is also shifted to the right with fall of CBF at the levels of 100–120 mm Hg of MAP **(Fig. 2)**.

If the BP is lowered gradually, then the curve shifts back again toward its normal position, so that the greater reduction in pressure can eventually be tolerated. Unfortunately, chronic hypertensives may lose their ability to autoregulate their CBF and increase the risk of brain damage when BP is lowered acutely. In infarcted brain tissue, autoregulation is lost. Therefore, with high BP, cerebral perfusion would be accentuated through the damaged tissue, leading to edema and compression of normal brain. *Thus, hypertensive encephalopathy is a consequence of progressively rising arterial pressure that breaks through the protection of blood–brain barrier and the autoregulation of CBF.*

DIAGNOSIS OF PRIMARY AND SECONDARY HYPERTENSION

Primary hypertension is diagnosed by the exclusion of secondary causes. But, during the diagnosis of primary hypertension, we will have to keep in mind that the majority of abnormal signs are due to the complications of hypertension, which may be mistaken as the secondary causes. However, certain clues from history, clinical examination, and routine laboratory tests may suggest the secondary form of hypertension which dictates the need for special investigations for the confirmation of it. For example:

- The abrupt onset of severe hypertension, under the age of 25 years or after the age of 50 years, should lead to laboratory tests to exclude renovascular hypertension and pheochromocytoma.
- The history of headache, palpitation, sweating, hyperglycemia, and weight loss suggests pheochromocytoma.
- The presence of abdominal bruit suggests renovascular hypertension.
- The elevated creatinine, ↑BUN, proteinuria, and hematuria suggest renal insufficiency.
- The therapeutic failure with initial drug therapy also suggests secondary hypertension.
- The characteristic faces and habitus suggest Cushing's syndrome. There are also many nonspecific findings which include—LVH, accentuation of the aortic component of 2nd heart sound, 4th heart sound, etc.

Pheochromocytoma

The easiest and best screening procedure for the diagnosis of pheochromocytoma is the measurement of catecholamines or their metabolites in a 24-hour collected urine sample, while patient is hypertensive. Measurement of plasma catecholamine levels is also useful.

Cushing Syndrome

A 24-hour urine test for cortisol: A urine cortisol level of <2,750 number of mole (100 µg) excludes Cushing syndrome. Administration of 1 mg dexamethasone at bedtime, followed by measurement of plasma cortisol at 7–10 AM, is the best screening test for Cushing syndrome. Plasma cortisol level below 140 number of mole/L (5 µg/dL) rules out Cushing syndrome.

INVESTIGATIONS FOR ALL HYPERTENSIVE PATIENTS

- Blood glucose
- Blood urea and creatinine
- Blood electrolytes (hypokalemic alkalosis is usually due to diuretic therapy, but it may indicate primary aldosteronism)
- Serum total and high-density lipoprotein (HDL) and cholesterol
- Urine analysis for glucose, protein, and blood
- 12-lead ECG to diagnose LVH, CAD, etc.
- Microscopic urine analysis
- White blood cell count
- Serum calcium, phosphate, and uric acid.

INVESTIGATIONS FOR SELECTED HYPERTENSIVE PATIENTS

- Ambulatory BP recording to assess "white coat" or borderline hypertension
- Chest X-ray to detect coarctation of aorta, cardiomegaly, heart failure, etc.
- Echocardiography to detect and quantify the left ventricular function
- Urinary catecholamine measurement to detect pheochromocytoma
- Urinary cortisol measurement and dexamethasone suppression test to diagnose Cushing's syndrome
- Renal ultrasonography to detect the possible renal diseases
- Renal angiography to diagnose renal artery stenosis
- Plasma renin activity and measurement of aldosterone to diagnose primary aldosteronism.

RENIN–ANGIOTENSIN SYSTEM

To know the hypertension properly, renin–angiotensin system (RAS) should be known in detail. So, this system is discussed here. Initially, in 1970, the inhibition of RAS

was considered sensitive only for patients with high-renin hypertension. But, later it was found that the ACE inhibitor was also proved to be effective in essential hypertension, with normal levels of plasma renin activity. Also, recently, the ACE inhibitors gained widespread popularity for its use in CHF, MI, diabetic nephropathy, renal failure, vascular disease, and many other conditions associated with hypertension.

Overview of RAS

Renin–angiotensin system continuously controls BP by its short- and long-term regulation. Factors that decrease the effective blood volume and reduce BP (e.g., use of vasodilators, diuretics, blood loss, low Na^+ diet, liver cirrhosis, etc.) activate the release of renin from kidney (JG cells). *Renin* is an enzyme. It acts on *angiotensinogen* (a plasma protein which is present in plasma) and breaks this substrate (angiotensinogen) to form a decapeptide, named *angiotensin-I* (AT-I). This decapeptide is then cleaved by *angiotensin-converting enzyme (ACE)* to yield an octapeptide, named *angiotensin II* (AT-II). This AT-II now acts via diverse and coordinated way to raise or maintain arterial BP. This AT-II causes vasoconstriction and increases peripheral vascular resistance. Thus, it contributes to the short-term regulation of arterial BP. The AT-II also inhibits the excretion of Na^+ and water by kidney. Thus, AT-II causes the changes in renal function, which play an important role in the long-term stabilization of BP.

Renin

It is a glycosylated single chain polypeptide and is secreted from granular JG cells, which lie on the walls of afferent arterioles, as they enter the glomeruli. It is the major determinant factor for angiotensin II (AT-II) production. Its principal substrate is a circulating α_2-globulin, which is called as angiotensinogen and converts it to angiotensin I (AT-I). The first product during the synthesis of renin is *preprorenin*, which is further processed in the ER of JG cells to *prorenin*. This prorenin, then, may be secreted directly from JG cells or is packaged into immature granules where it is further processed to form active mature *renin*.

Control of Renin Secretion

The secretion of renin is controlled predominantly by three pathways. Among these, the two pathways are locally acting within the kidney. The third pathway acting through CNS is the *adrenergic receptor pathway*. The locally acting two pathways within the kidney are—macula densa (MD) pathway and intrarenal baroreceptor pathway **(Fig. 3)**.

1. *Macula densa pathway:* It is composed of some specialized columnar epithelial cells that are called as

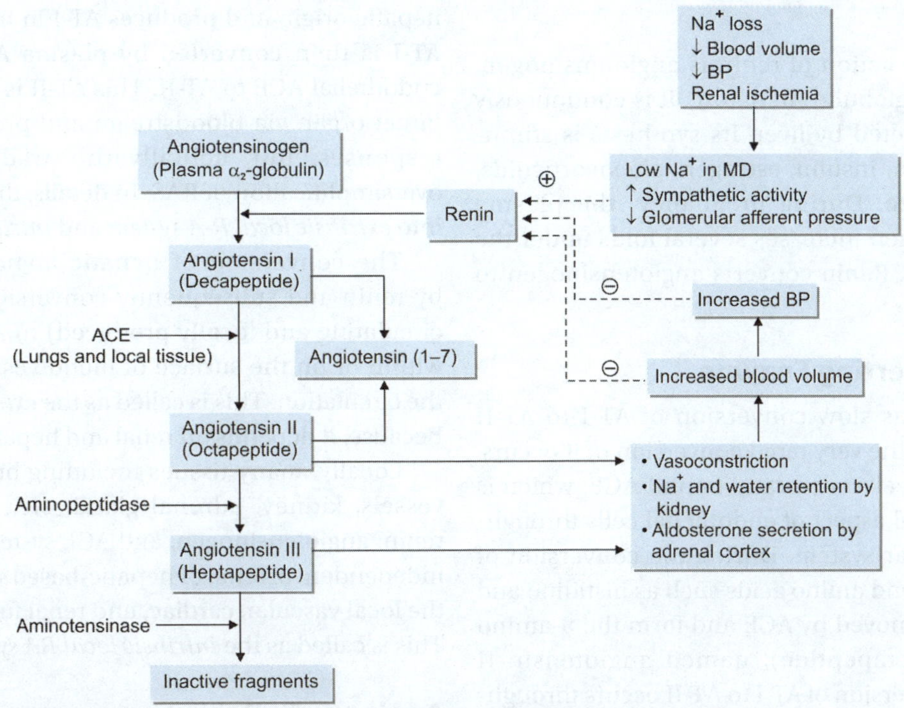

Fig. 3: Control of renin secretion. (ACE: angiotensin-converting enzyme; BP: blood pressure)

the *macula densa* cells. They are located on the wall of the thick ascending limb (TAL) of loop of Henle (LOH) that passes between the afferent and efferent arterioles of glomerulus, adjacent to JG cells. A change in the reabsorption of NaCl by MD cells results in the transmission of chemical signals to the nearby JG cells of afferent arteriole, which modify the release of renin from them. Increase in NaCl influx across the MD cells inhibits the release of renin and decrease in NaCl influx increases the release of renin. This chemical signal pathway involves both the adenosine and prostaglandin chemicals. *Adenosine*, after being released when NaCl transport is increased, inhibits the secretion of renin. Whereas, *prostaglandin* after being released, when NaCl transport is decreased, stimulates the secretion of renin.

2. *Intrarenal baroreceptor pathway:* The increase or decrease of BP in preglomerular vessels inhibits or stimulates the release of renin, respectively. It also acts through PG pathway.

3. *β-adrenergic receptor pathway:* It is mediated by the release of norepinephrine from postganglionic sympathetic nerve terminals. Then, the activation of β1 receptor, situated on JG cells by this released norepinephrine, enhances renin recreation. These three pathways regulating the release of renin are embedded in a physiological network. Increase in renin secretion enhances the formation of angiotensin II (AT-II). Subsequently, this

AT-II (angiotensin-II) stimulates angiotensin subtype I (AT$_1$) receptors on JG cells and inhibits the release of renin. This feedback system has been termed as the *short-loop negative feedback* mechanism. Next, AT-II also increases systemic BP via the stimulation of AT$_1$ receptor, situated on the peripheral vessels of our body. Now, this ↑BP inhibits the release of renin by—(1) activating the baroreceptors, thereby reducing the renal sympathetic tone, (2) increasing the pressure in preglomerular vessels, and (3) reducing the reabsorption of NaCl in proximal tubule (PT) (pressure natriuresis), which increases the tubular delivery of NaCl to MD. This inhibition of release of renin, due to AT-II-induced increase in BP, has been termed as the *long-loop negative feedback* mechanism.

Renin release also can be influenced by a number of pharmacological agents. These are:

- Loop diuretics stimulate the release of renin by blocking the reabsorption of NaCl at MD.
- Nonsteroidal anti-inflammatory drug (NSAID) inhibits the formation of PG and decreases the release of renin.
- ACE inhibitor and AT$_1$ receptor blocker (ARB) interrupt both the short- and long-loop negative feedback mechanism and increase the release of renin.
- Diuretics and vasodilators increase the release of renin by decreasing BP.
- β-adrenergic receptor antagonists decrease the secretion of renin by inhibiting the β$_1$-adrenergic receptor pathway.

Angiotensinogen

The substrate for the action of renin is angiotensinogen. It is glycoprotein (α_2-globulin) in nature. It is continuously synthesized and secreted by liver. Its synthesis is stimulated by inflammation, insulin, estrogen, glucocorticoids, thyroid hormone, etc. During pregnancy, the plasma level of angiotensinogen increases several folds under the influence of estrogen. Renin converts angiotensinogen to angiotensin-I (AT-I).

Angiotensin-converting Enzyme

Although spontaneous slow conversion of AT-I to AT-II occurs in plasma, but the very rapid conversion of it occurs, due to the activity of cell membrane-bound ACE, which is present on the luminal aspect of endothelial cells throughout the whole vascular system. During the conversion of AT-I to AT-II, the two end amino acids such as histidine and leucine of AT-I are removed by ACE and form the 8-amino acid polypeptide (octapeptide), named angiotensin-II (AT-II). Thus, the conversion of AT-I to AT-II occurs throughout the body, but particularly it occurs in the blood vessels of lungs. The angiotensin II is then converted to *angiotensin III (AT-III)* by an enzyme, named aminopeptidase.

Angiotensin Peptides

There are three angiotensin peptides. These are—angiotensin-I (AT-I), angiotensin-II (AT-II), and angiotensin-III (AT-III). The AT-I is <1% as potent as AT-II on vascular smooth muscle, heart, and adrenal cortex. The AT-III is formed by the action of aminopeptidase on AT-II. The AT-II and AT-III have qualitatively similar effects, but quantitatively AT-III is only 25% and 10% as potent as AT-II in elevating BP and stimulating the adrenal medulla, respectively. On the other hand, AT-III is as potent as AT-II (angiotensin-II) in stimulating the secretion of aldosterone.

The AT-I and AT-II are metabolized to *angiotensins (1–7)*. ACE inhibitors increase, rather than decrease, the tissue and plasma levels of angiotensin (1–7). This is because the level of AT-I is increased and is diverted away from AT-II formation to the formation of angiotensin (1–7). Unlike AT-II, the angiotensin (1–7) does not cause vasoconstriction, aldosterone release, or the facilitation of adrenergic neurotransmission, causing the elevation of BP. The angiotensin (1–7) inhibits the proliferation of vascular smooth muscle cells also. The enzymes named aminopeptidases, endopeptidases, and carboxypeptidases also cause the degradation and inactivation of AT-I and AT-II to angiotensin (1–7).

The traditional view of RAS is that the circulating renin of renal origin acts on the circulating angiotensinogen of hepatic origin and produces AT-I in blood. The circulating AT-I is then converted by plasma ACE and pulmonary endothelial ACE to AT-II. This AT-II is then delivered to the target organ via bloodstream and produces physiological responses. But, actually this traditional view is the oversimplification of RAS. In details, the RAS can be divided into *extrinsic local R-A system* and *intrinsic local R-A system*.

The conversion of hepatic angiotensinogen to AT-I by renin and subsequently conversion of this AT-I (both circulating and locally produced) to AT-II occur primarily within or on the surface of blood vessel wall, but not into the circulation. This is called as the *extrinsic local RA system*. Because, it depends on renal and hepatic-based system.

Locally, many tissues including brain, pituitary, blood vessels, kidney, adrenal gland, etc., express mRNAs for renin, angiotensinogen, and ACE system. This system exists independent of renal or hepatic-based system and influences the local vascular, cardiac, and renal function and structure. This is called as the *intrinsic local RA system*.

Angiotensin Receptor

The effects of angiotensin are exerted through some specific receptors, situated on cell surface. It is identified as two types and designated as AT_1 and AT_2. Both the AT_1 and AT_2 receptors are the members of G protein-coupled receptor family. Most of the biological effects of AT-II (angiotensin-II) are mediated by the AT_1 receptor. Whereas, the functional role of AT_2 receptors is still ill defined. AT_2 receptor is widely distributed in fetal tissues, but its distribution in adult is restricted. The AT_1 receptor has high affinity for losartan (AT_1 receptor blocker) than AT_2 receptor. In adult, some tissues contain primarily either AT_1 or AT_2 receptor. Whereas, other tissues contain both these receptors in similar amount.

Preeclampsia is associated with the development of agonistic autoantibodies against AT_1 receptor and thus produces exaggerated response, causing hypertension. The AT_1 receptor activates a large array of intracellular signal transduction system, including the intracellular Ca^{2+} release, influx pathways, phospholipases, mitogen-activated protein kinase pathways, etc. Additional Ca^{2+} also enters the cell from outside, due to the opening of voltage-sensitive Ca^{2+} channels, located on cell membrane. This Ca^{2+} binds now to calmodulin and then the Ca^{2+}/calmodulin complex activates a number of intracellular enzymes that contribute to ultimate cellular responses. This is discussed in more details in autonomic nervous system (Chapter 11).

Function of Renin–Angiotensin System

This RAS plays an important role in regulating BP for both short- and long-term basis. The AT-II is 40 times more potent

TABLE 2: The mechanisms of function of angiotensin II.

Altered renal function	Altered SVR	Altered CV function and its structure
1. Increased reabsorption of Na$^+$ from PT	1. Direct vasoconstriction	1. Increased proliferation, hyperplasia, and hypertrophy of myocardium
2. Increased secretion of aldosterone → increased reabsorption of Na$^+$ and increased excretion of K$^+$ from DT	2. Indirect vasoconstriction through peripheral noradrenergic neurotransmission	2. Increased fibrosis
3. Increased renal vasoconstriction	3. Increased sympathetic discharge from CNS	3. Increased extracellular matrix
4. Increased noradrenergic neurotransmission in kidney	4. Release of catecholamines from adrenal medulla	4. Increased arterial wall thickness, ↑wall tension and ↑after load
5. Increased renal sympathetic tone through CNS		
↓	↓	↓
Slow pressure response	Rapid pressure response	Hypertrophy and remodeling of heart

(CNS: central nervous system; CV: cardiovascular; DT: distal tubule; PT: proximal tubule; SVR: systemic vascular resistance)

than norepinephrine, in respect to increase in BP. This severe pressure response of AT-II is due to severe vasoconstriction and increase in SVR. The AT-II also increases directly cardiac contractility, acting through voltage-gated Ca^{2+} channel and indirectly increases heart rate, acting through the facilitation of sympathetic tone. It also enhances the noradrenergic neurotransmission and increases the release of adrenal catecholamines. But, this increase in BP activates the baroreceptor reflex that decreases sympathetic tone and increases vagus tone. Therefore, in summary, the main functions of RAS are—increase in BP, increase of SVR, alteration of renal function, and alteration of cardiac function with structure **(Table 2)**.

Mechanism by which AT-II (angiotensin-II) Increases the Systemic Vascular Resistance

The AT-II increases SVR via direct effects on blood vessels and via indirect effect through CNS and adrenal medulla by catecholamines.

Direct vasoconstriction: The AT-II contracts the precapillary arterioles (greater extent) and postcapillary venules (lesser extent). This is due to the activation of AT$_1$ receptor, which is located on the smooth muscle cells of blood vessels, by AT-II. But, the intensity of this contraction is different in different vascular beds. Strongest contraction occurs in kidney and somewhat lesser contraction occurs in other splanchnic vascular bed. The AT-II-induced vasoconstriction is much less in the vessels of brain. It is further weaker in those (vessels) of lung and skeletal muscle. But, in these regions, the blood flow actually increases, because the relatively weak vasoconstrictor response in these areas is opposed by

elevated systemic BP and the ultimate blood flow depends on—(1) the intensity of contraction and (2) the rise of BP.

Indirect enhancement of peripheral noradrenergic neurotransmission: The AT-II facilitates the peripheral noradrenergic neurotransmission and increases BP by—(1) augmenting the release of norepinephrine from sympathetic nerve terminals, (2) by inhibiting the reuptake of norepinephrine into presynaptic nerve terminals, and (3) by enhancing the vascular response to norepinephrine.

Through effects on CNS: The AT-II increases arterial BP by its action on CNS. This effect is mediated by increased sympathetic outflow **(Flowchart 1)** from brain due to the effect of AT-II on circumventricular nuclei that are not protected by a blood–brain barrier. The CNS is affected both by blood-borne angiotensin II and by angiotensin II formed locally within the brain. The brain contains all the components of RAS and here the AT-II serves as neurotransmitter or modulator.

Through the release of catecholamines from adrenal medulla: The AT-II stimulates and releases catecholamines from adrenal medulla by depolarizing the chromaffin cells.

Mechanism by which Angiotensin II alters Renal Function

The AT-II reduces the renal excretion of Na$^+$ (increases the renal reabsorption of Na$^+$) and increases the renal excretion of K$^+$. It stimulates the Na$^+$/H$^+$ exchange protein in PT and thus it increases the reabsorption of Na$^+$, Cl$^-$, HCO$^-$ in PT. The AT-II also stimulates the secretion of aldosterone from zona glomerulosa of adrenal cortex, which acts on the

Flowchart 1: The function of renin–angiotensin system (RAS).

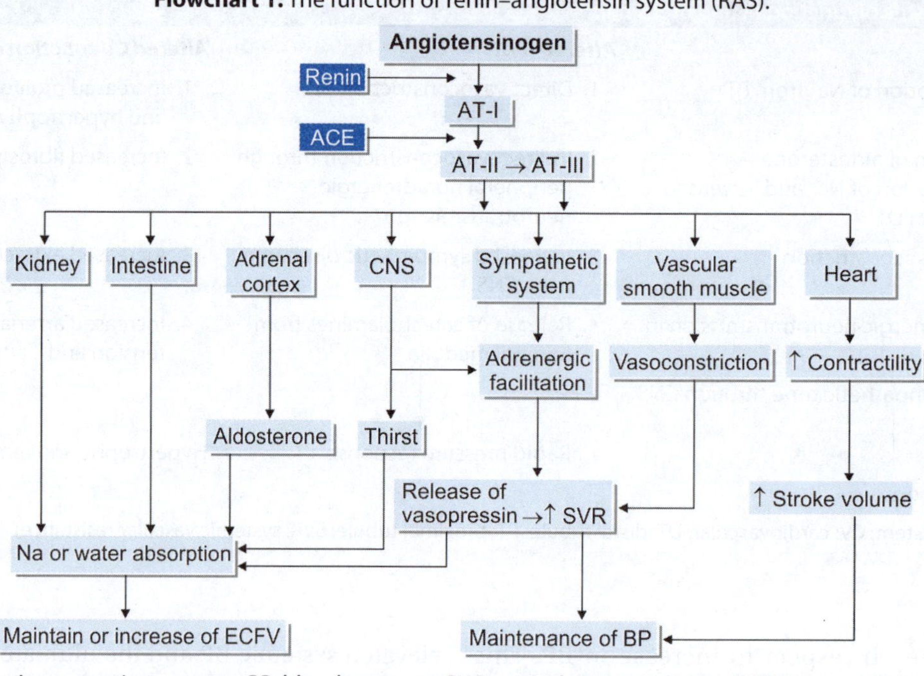

(ACE: angiotensin-converting enzyme; BP: blood pressure; CNS: central nervous system; ECFV: extracellular fluid volume; SVR: systemic vascular resistance)

distal and collecting tubule to cause the retention of Na$^+$ and the excretion of K$^+$ and H$^+$. Aldosterone secretion is usually increased under the condition of hyponatremia and hyperkalemia and is decreased in opposite condition. Such changes are due to the alterations in the number of receptor of AT-II at zona glomerulosa and adrenocortical hyperplasia in Na$^+$-depleted state.

The AT-II reduces the renal blood flow (RBF) by directly constricting the renal vascular smooth muscle or by facilitating the renal noradrenergic neurotransmission. The AT-II influences the GFR in variable way by the following mechanisms: (1) the constriction of afferent arterioles reduces GFR, (2) the contraction of mesangial cells reduces the filtration surface area, and subsequently GFR, (3) the contraction of efferent arterioles causes the increase in intraglomerular pressure and subsequently increases GFR.

The outcome of these opposing effects on GFR depends on the present physiological state. Normally, the AT-II reduces GFR slightly. But in hypotension, the effects of AT-II on efferent arterioles predominate and increase GFR to a greater extent. *So, the blockade of RAS causes renal failure in patient with renal artery stenosis.*

Mechanism by which AT-II (angiotensin-II) alters the Cardiovascular Function and Structure

Several pathological changes occur in cardiovascular structure and its function by AT-II and pose an increased risk of morbidity and mortality. These changes include—(1) increased wall thickness to lumen ratio in blood vessels, (2) cardiac concentric hypertrophy, (3) cardiac eccentric hypertrophy and fibrosis which is associated with congestive failure and infarction, and (4) thickening of the intimal surface of the wall of blood vessel. All these changes are due to increased proliferation, hyperplasia, hypertrophy of smooth muscle cells, and increased extracellular matrix caused by AT-II. The cells which are involved in these changes include vascular smooth muscle cells, cardiac myocytes, and fibroblasts. All these changes in cardiovascular structure cause increase in cardiac contractility, stroke volume, and BP.

Renal pressure–natriuresis curve: The intake of Na$^+$ and its excretion determines the arterial BP. When the relation between Na$^+$ intake, Na$^+$ excretion, and the arterial BP is drawn graphically, then this graph is called as the renal pressure–natriuresis curve. At a stable condition, Na$^+$ intake is equal to Na$^+$ excretion. At some set point, the arterial BP can be obtained from the intersection of a horizontal line (representing Na$^+$ intake) with the renal pressure–natriuresis curve **(Fig. 4)**.

When the dietary Na$^+$ intake is low, then renin release is stimulated and then the subsequent increased angiotensin II acts on the kidney to decrease the excretion of Na$^+$. Thus, this renal "pressure–natriuresis" curve is shifted to the right to maintain the same BP. Conversely, when the dietary Na$^+$

intake is high, then the secretion of renin is inhibited and subsequently the withdrawal of angiotensin II causes the increase in excretion of Na$^+$. Thus, this curve is now shifted to the left and the BP is maintained at normal level. The intersection of salt intake curve with the Na$^+$ excretion line remains near the same set point, despite the large swings in dietary Na$^+$ intake (shown in curve as Na$^+$ excretion). If the curve does not shift, then the arterial BP swings tremendously with different intake of Na$^+$. When pharmacologically the modulation of RAS or the swings of the curve are prevented, then any changes in salt intake markedly affect the long-term levels of arterial BP.

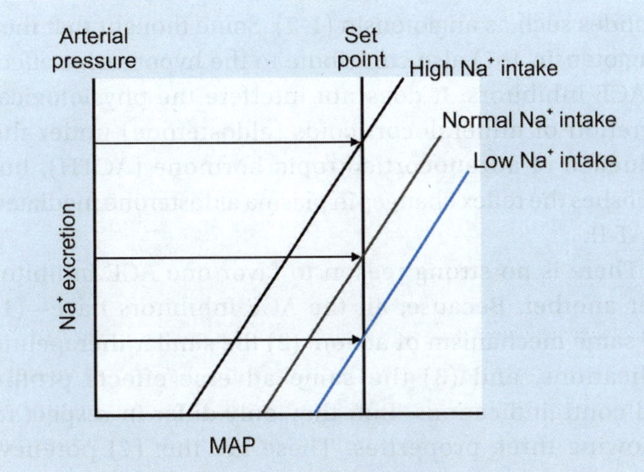

Fig. 4: This figure shows the renal *"pressure–natriuresis"* curve. (MAP: mean arterial pressure)

Inhibition of Renin–Angiotensin System

The inhibition of RAS is the mainstay of the management of hypertension and its complication. It can be achieved by:

- *Decreasing the release of renin:* This can be achieved by sympathetic blockers such as β-blockers and other adrenergic neuron blockers.
- *Blocking the action of renin:* This can be achieved by renin inhibitory peptides or renin-specific antibodies. They interfere the rate-limiting step, producing AT-I from angiotensinogen by renin. But, they are not used clinically **(Flowchart 2)**.
- *Blocking the action of ACE:* These are called as the ACE inhibitor and prevent the generation of active principle AT-II from AT-I. These groups of drugs are used extensively in clinical practice.
- *Blocking the angiotensin receptor (AT$_1$):* They block the action of AT-II on the target cells.
- *Blocking the action of aldosterone:* They block the mineralocorticoid receptors.

ANGIOTENSIN-CONVERTING ENZYME INHIBITORS

In 1960, Ferreria and his colleagues observed that the venom of pit vipers has some factors which increase the responses to bradykinin. These factors are called as the *bradykinin-potentiating factors* and reduce systemic BP. Following the discovery of these factors, the *teprotide* was first synthesized. It was a nonpeptide and inhibits the generation of AT-II from AT-I (angiotensin-I). It was found to lower the BP in many

Flowchart 2: The mechanism of secretion of renin and angiotensin.

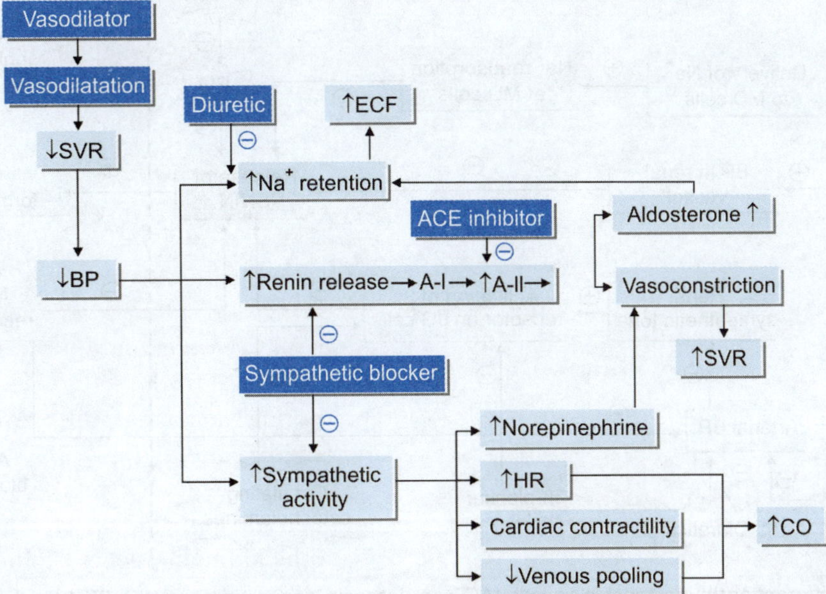

(BP: blood pressure; CO: cardiac output; ECF: extracellular fluid; HR: heart rate; SVR: systemic vascular resistance)

patients with essential hypertension. It also exerts beneficial effect in patients with heart failure. But, it had limitations of parenteral administration and brief duration of action. So, these observations had led to the search for other ACE inhibitors which could be active orally.

Then, in 1977, captopril came which was orally active dipeptide and had quickly gained wide usage. After that, many ACE inhibitors were synthesized and out of that only six are currently available in India. These are *captopril, lisinopril, enalapril, ramipril, benazepril,* and *perindopril.* But, many other ACE inhibitors are also marketed in other countries such as quinapril, fosinopril, cilazapril, zofenopril, etc. However, among all these, the captopril is described as prototype, because most of its effects are common to all the ACE inhibitors **(Fig. 5)**.

Captopril

Chemically, it is a sulfhydryl-containing dipeptide. It blocks the pressure action of AT-I, but not that of AT-II. It does not also block the AT_I receptors. The main pharmacological action of captopril is reduction of BP by inhibiting the conversion of AT-I to AT-II. But, the magnitude of this response in an individual depends on the Na^+ status and the renin–angiotensin activity of that individual. In individual with dietary Na^+ restriction and diuretics, the response of ACE inhibitor is higher. It causes greater fall of BP in renovascular, accelerated, and malignant hypertension.

Captopril decreases SVR. It causes arterioles to dilate. The compliance of large arteries is increased. Both the systolic and diastolic pressures fall and CO increases. Cardiovascular reflexes are not impaired due to any ACE inhibitor and there is little dilatation of capacitance vessels (venules). So, there is no postural hypotension. The RBF is not reduced, even when BP falls substantially. This is due to much dilatation of renal vessels, as AT-II markedly constricts it. The coronary and cerebral blood flows are also not reduced by any ACE inhibitors or captopril.

Since the conversion of AT-I to AT-II is blocked by captopril, so the plasma renin and AT-I levels are increased. AT-I, then, is redirected (metabolized) through another metabolic route, resulting in the increased production of peptides such as angiotensin (1–7). Some thought that they (angiotensin 1–7) also contribute to the hypotensive effect of ACE inhibitors. It does not interfere the physiological secretion of mineralocorticoids (aldosterone) under the influence of adrenocorticotropic hormone (ACTH), but abolishes the reflex changes in plasma aldosterone mediated by AT-II.

There is no strong reason to favor one ACE inhibitor over another. Because, all the ACE inhibitors have—(1) the same mechanism of action, (2) the similar therapeutic indications, and (3) the same adverse effects profile and contraindications. But, they only differ in respect to following three properties. These are the: (1) potency,

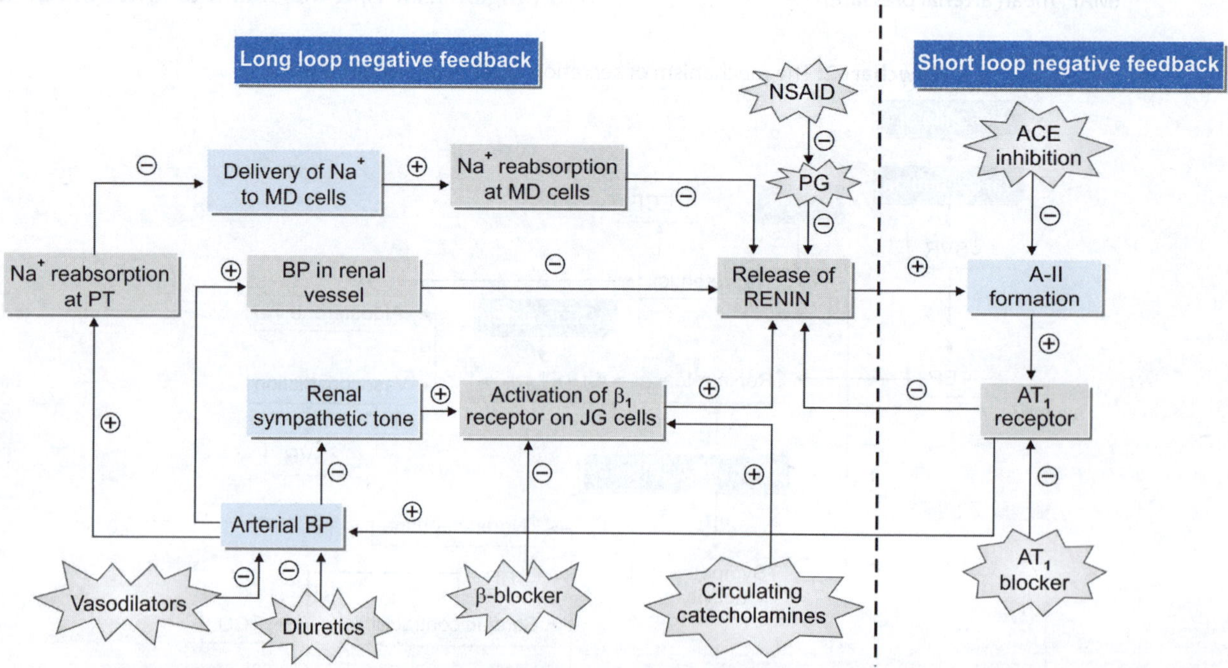

Fig. 5: The site of action of different antihypertensive agents. (ACE: angiotensin-converting enzyme; BP: blood pressure; MD: macula densa; NSAID: nonsteroidal anti-inflammatory drug; PG: prostaglandin; PT: proximal tubule)

BOX 1: ACE inhibitors.

- *Especially suited for:*
  - Young and physically, intellectually, and sexually active person
  - Left ventricular hypertrophy with LV systolic dysfunction
  - Diabetics, gout, and dyslipidemia
  - Nephropathy, high-renin cases
  - Coexisting angina, peripheral vascular diseases
  - Potential MI
  - Chronic heart failure
- *Contraindicated:*
  - Pregnancy
  - Renal artery stenosis
  - Dry cough (relative)
  - Hyperkalemia

(LV: left ventricular; MI: myocardial infarction)

(2) whether ACE inhibition is primarily due to drug itself or due to conversion of a prodrug to its active metabolites, and (3) pharmacokinetics.

Regarding the pharmacokinetics, all the ACE inhibitors differ markedly among themselves, regarding their (1) absorption, (2) tissue distribution, and (3) elimination. This characteristic is exploited clinically to inhibit some local RASs while leaving the other relatively intact. Except the fosinopril and spirapril, which are eliminated by liver and kidney by equal proportion, the other ACE inhibitors are eliminated predominantly by kidney. Therefore, the impaired renal function significantly reduces the plasma elimination of most ACE inhibitors. So, the doses of these ACE inhibitors should be decreased in patients with renal failure. Increased plasma renin activity makes the patient hypersensitive to hypotension, induced by ACE inhibitor. So, the initial dose of it should be reduced in patients who have high plasma renin level, such as salt depletion, heart failure, etc.

Captopril is well absorbed orally (70%), but the presence of food in stomach reduces its bioavailability. It is mainly excreted unchanged through urine. Plasma half-life of captopril is about 2 hours. But, its action usually lasts for 6–12 hours.

The usual dose of captopril is 25 mg twice daily which is increased gradually up to 50 mg thrice daily, according to the response. Sometimes, it is wise to start with small doses such as 6.25 mg twice daily in such patients who are in diuretics and in CHF patients to avoid marked fall in BP initially **(Box 1)**.

Adverse Effects of Captopril

The profile of adverse effects of all ACE inhibitors is same and serious untoward reactions are rare. Captopril is well tolerated by most of the patients, especially if the daily dose of it is kept below 150 mg. The metabolic side effects of captopril are usually not encountered, even during prolonged use. All ACE inhibitors, like captopril, improve insulin sensitivity in patients who are suffering from insulin resistance. They decrease the cholesterol and lipoprotein level in renal disease patients. These drugs do not alter the plasma uric acid and Ca^{2+} level.

- *Hypotension:* Sometimes, sharp fall of BP occurs after the initiations of captopril or any ACE inhibitor therapy. This is particularly true for patients with persistent high-renin activity, such as previous diuretic therapy and CHF.
- *Hyperkalemia:* Captopril or any ACE inhibitors may produce *hyperkalemia*, particularly in patients who is taking K^+-sparing diuretics, K^+ supplement, renal insufficiency, taking β-blocker, or NSAID. But, significant retention of K^+ is rarely encountered in patients with normal renal function and who is not taking any medications.
- *Cough:* In 10–20% patient, captopril or any other ACE inhibitor may produce troublesome cough. It occurs within 1–8 weeks after the starting of treatment of hypertension by ACE inhibitor and is not dose related. Sometimes, the cough is so intense that it requires discontinuation of therapy. However, once the therapy is stopped, the cough disappears. This cough usually is due to accumulation of bradykinin and/or substance P and/or prostaglandin in lungs which are normally degraded by ACE. Thromboxane antagonism reduces this captopril-induced cough.
- *Acute renal failure:* Sometimes, any ACE inhibitor or captopril may induce acute renal failure in patients— (1) with bilateral renal artery stenosis or (2) renal stenosis in single remaining kidney or (3) with heart failure or (4) with dehydration. Normally, AT-II constricts the efferent arteriole and maintains adequate glomerular filtration when renal perfusion pressure is low. So, in the presence of above-mentioned causes, ACE inhibitors precipitate the acute renal failure.
- *Other less serious side effects:* These are rashes, urticaria, angioedema, granulocytopenia, proteinuria, headache, dizziness, nausea, vomiting, etc.
- *Fetal damage:* The ACE inhibitors are not teratogenic in first trimester of pregnancy. But, if these are continued during the second and third trimester of pregnancy, then ACE inhibitors may produce different fetal anomalies such as intrauterine growth restriction (IUGR), pulmonary hypoplasia, oligohydramnios, and IUD. These fetal anomalies are due to fetal hypotension. So, while the ACE inhibitors are not contraindicated during reproductive age, but should be stopped once pregnancy is diagnosed.

Therapeutic Uses of ACE Inhibitors

Hypertension

In hypertension, ACE inhibitors lower the mean, systolic, and diastolic BP and SVR, *except in cases of primary hyperaldosteronism (effective in secondary hyperaldosteronism)*. The change in the level of BP correlates well with the plasma renin–angiotensin level. There is variable vasodilator effect of ACE inhibitors at different vascular beds. But, *kidney is the only exception where there is definite vasodilation and increased RBF.* However, this increased RBF does not increase GFR, because both the afferent and efferent vessels dilate and effective filtration pressure does not increase. Blood flow in cerebral and coronary beds is usually well maintained due to their powerful autoregulatory mechanism. Besides causing systemic arteriolar dilatation, the ACE inhibitors increase the compliance of large arteries, which contributes to the reduction of systolic BP and afterload **(Fact file I)**.

FACT FILE I

The advantages of ACE inhibitor as antihypertensive agent are:
- It is safe for diabetic, asthmatic, and peripheral vascular disease patient
- Renal blood flow is well maintained
- It is not associated with postural hypotension and electrolyte disturbances
- It prevents secondary hyperaldosteronism
- It prevents K^+ loss due to diuretics
- There is no rebound hypertension after withdrawal of ACE inhibitors
- It does not cause hyperuricemia
- It does not produce any deleterious effect on plasma lipid profile
- It reverses left ventricular hypertrophy
- It also reverses the increased wall-to-lumen ratio of blood vessels that occur in hypertensive patients

(ACE: angiotensin-converting enzyme)

Stroke volume and CO increase in uncompromised heart. Baroreceptor and cardiovascular reflexes are usually well maintained. Still with substantial lowering of BP, the heart rate and concentrations of catecholamines in plasma increase only slightly, if at all. This perhaps reflects slight alteration of baroreceptors function with increased arterial compliance and the loss of normal toxic influence of angiotensin II on sympathetic nervous system.

Aldosterone secretion is normally reduced in hypertensive individuals, but is not seriously impaired by ACE inhibitors. Excessive retention of K^+ is encountered by ACE inhibitors only in patients who are—(1) taking supplemental K^+, (2) suffering from renal impairment, or (3) taking other medications that reduce K^+ excretion. It has synergistic action with Ca^{2+} channel blocker, β-adrenergic receptor blocker, or diuretics. Diuretics, in particular, augment the antihypertensive response of ACE inhibitors by rendering the patient's BP renin dependent.

All we have to consider that the goal of antihypertensive therapy **(Table 3)** is not just the lowering of BP, but to diminish the patient's overall risk from cardiovascular complications. ACE inhibitors reduce these incidences of cardiac complications in hypertensive patients more than do other antihypertensive agents such as diuretics, β-blockers, Ca^{2+} channel blockers, etc. This is because other agents have their adverse metabolic effects and due to their inability to reverse the structural changes of heart and/or blood vessels that may be mediated by circulatory catecholamines and/or RAS.

ACE Inhibitors in Left Ventricular Systolic Dysfunction

The left ventricular systolic dysfunction ranges from asymptomatic reduction in left ventricular systolic performance (CO) to symptomatic severe impairment of left ventricular systolic function (Grade IV, LVF). The ACE

TABLE 3: Pharmacokinetics of different ACE inhibitors.

	Captopril	*Enalapril*	*Perindopril*	*Lisinopril*	*Ramipril*
Chemical structure	Sulfhydryl	Carboxyl	Carboxyl	Carboxyl	Carboxyl
Activity	Active	Prodrug	Prodrug	Active	Prodrug
Peak action	½–1 hour	3–6 hours	3–6 hours	8 hours	3–6 hours
Elimination half-life	1–2 hours	12 hours	30–40 hours	12 hours	40–60 hours
Bioavailability	80%	60%	30%	30%	70%
Duration of action	6–12 hours	12–24 hours	>24 hours	>24 hours	>40 hours
Mode of excretion	Renal	Renal	Renal	Renal	Renal
Daily doses (mg)	25–100	5–30	2–8	5–130	2.5–10

(ACE: angiotensin-converting enzyme)

inhibitors should be given to all these patients, whether or not they are experiencing symptoms of overt heart failure. The inhibition of renin–angiotensin–aldosterone system by ACE inhibitors in patients with systolic dysfunction prevents or delays—(1) the progression of heart failure, (2) decreases the incidence of sudden death, and (3) the onset of MI.

The ACE inhibitors commonly reduce the afterload and systolic tension. Both the CO and cardiac index increase, as do the indices of stroke work and stroke volume in heart failure. The heart rate generally is reduced. This is due to the improvement of LV failure and the withdrawal of sympathetic overactivity. The excess volume of body fluids contracts, which reduces the excess venous return to right heart. This reduction of preload results from the venodilatation and increased capacity of venous bed. The ACE inhibitors also reduce pulmonary arterial pressure, pulmonary capillary wedge pressure (PCWP), left atrial pressure, and left ventricular filling volumes and pressure, etc. Consequently, the preload and diastolic wall stress are diminished. The better hemodynamic performance, caused by ACE inhibitors, results in increased exercise tolerance and suppression of sympathetic nervous system. *However, the role of ACE inhibitors on the diastolic dysfunction of left ventricle is still uncertain.*

The ACE inhibitors reduce the overall mortality, when the treatment is best started during the peri-infarction period. Unless contraindicated (e.g., cardiogenic shock and severe hypotension), the ACE inhibitors should be started immediately during the acute phase of MI.

Myocardial Infarction

The ACE inhibitors definitely reduce the early as well as the long-term mortality from MI. However, this is true, if it is administered, while MI is evolving and then continued for another 6 weeks. But, during treatment, it should be noted that hypotension should be avoided. The ACE inhibitor is beneficial for MI, irrespective of the presence or absence of ventricular systolic dysfunction.

Diabetic Nephropathy

The ACE inhibitors also help to prevent or delay the progress of an end-stage renal disease, both in insulin- or noninsulin-dependent diabetes. Albuminuria remains stable during therapy. Those patients who are treated with ACE inhibitors require less dialysis and have higher creatinine clearance. They have longer life expectancy also. So, all the patients suffering from diabetic nephropathy need ACE inhibitors therapy, whether they are hypertensive or not.

MANAGEMENT OF HYPERTENSIVE EMERGENCY

Hypertensive emergency requires immediate reduction of BP to prevent or to minimize the end organ damage. It needs to be distinguished from *severe hypertension or urgency* where there is no possibility of acute end organ damage. Because, aggressive therapy for hypertensive emergency and sudden reduction of BP (to prevent or to minimize the end organ damage) may result in potentially hazardous reduction in myocardial and cerebral perfusion with more end organ damage. Therefore, hypertensive emergency requires immediate lowering of BP, but in a *controlled and predictable manner*. The goal is to lower the mean arterial blood pressure (MAP) by approximately 20–25% of the previous value in first hour, while maintaining adequate perfusion to vital organs. Dropping of BP too quickly or too much can worsen the target end organ damage. With cerebral ischemia, when autoregulation is lost, then CBF is directly proportional to systemic BP. Therefore, if BP is lowered too much, then cerebral perfusion pressure in ischemic areas is also lowered, risking further damage.

The recommendations for the reduction of BP during the management of hypertensive emergency are:
- It should be reduced over 60–90 minutes to a mean BP of 120 mm Hg.
- 20–30% reduction in MAP (MAP = diastolic BP + 2/3rds of pulse pressure).
- Reduction of diastolic pressure by one-third, but not to a level below 95 mm Hg.

This goal should also be modified (i.e., more gradual reduction of BP) in those patients who are more susceptible to loss of CBF, e.g., the elderly, patients with chronic hypertension, and patients with atherosclerotic cerebrovascular diseases.

The ideal drug for treatment of hypertensive emergency should have the following characteristics:
- Rapid onset (controlled not precipitous) and rapid cessation of clinical effects
- Predictable dose–response relationship
- Restoration of cerebral autoregulation
- Lack of side effects
- Convenience to use.

Reasons against the use of oral agents in the management of hypertensive emergency include:
- Unpredictable effect on MAP
- Unpredictable time to peak effect
- Higher failure rate than with parenteral therapy
- Lack of ease in titration.

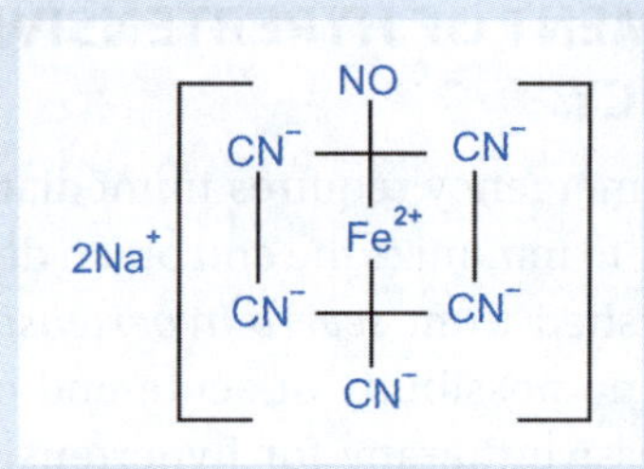

Fig. 6: Sodium nitroprusside.

In addition, there is no less importance for the patient to be monitored vigorously with oral therapy, compared with intravenous therapy. Institution of appropriate oral therapy may be required once hypertension has been controlled by parenteral agents and it is gradually withdrawn. *The drugs used for control of hypertensive emergency are given here.*

Sodium Nitroprusside

The molecular structure of sodium nitroprusside is given in **Figure 6**. It is used primarily to treat hypertensive emergency. But, the drug also can be used in many situations where the short-term reduction of cardiac preload and/or afterload is required. So, the nitroprusside is used to:

- Lower BP during acute aortic dissection
- Increase CO in CHF
- Decrease myocardial O_2 demand, after acute MI
- Induce controlled hypotension during anesthesia.

The β-adrenergic receptor blocker should also be used along with nitroprusside. This is because:

- It counteracts the tachycardia due to hypotension, induced by nitroprusside.
- Reduction of BP by nitroprusside alone can increase the rate of rise of pressure in aorta, as a result of increased myocardial contractility, thereby enhancing the propagation of dissection.

Mechanism of Action of Na-Nitroprusside

The mechanism of the action of Na-nitroprusside is shown in **Figure 7**. Na-nitroprusside is metabolized by the cells of the wall of blood vessels to its active metabolite which is known as nitric oxide (NO). Then, this NO activates the guanylyl cyclase enzyme to form the cyclic guanosine monophosphate (GMP) which in turn causes vasodilatation. Thus, the mechanism of action of nitroprusside is same as that of nitroglycerin. But, the metabolic activation of nitroprusside is catalyzed by *a different NO-generating system*, which is not used for nitroglycerin. Hence, this probably accounts for the difference in the potency of these drugs at different vascular sites. But, the fact is that tolerance develops to nitroglycerin, whereas not to nitroprusside.

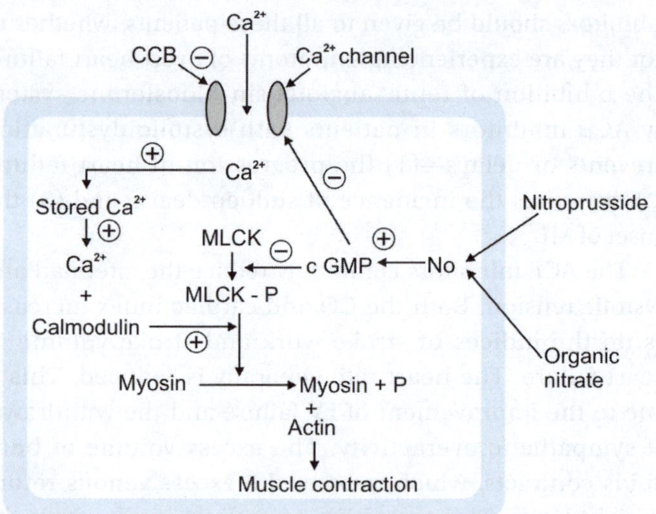

Fig. 7: This figure shows the mechanism of action of calcium channel blocker (CCB), organic nitrates, and nitroprusside. (cGMP: cyclic guanosine monophosphate; MLCK: myosin light-chain kinase)

Pharmacological Effects of Na-Nitroprusside

Nitroprusside dilates both the arterioles and venules. Thus, the total hemodynamic response and CO produced by Na-nitroprusside depend on the combination of the reduction of venous pooling (↓preload) and reduction of arterial impedance (↓afterload). In patient with normal left ventricular function, the effect of reduction of venous pooling which decreases the CO is more than the effect of the reduction of afterload which increases CO. Thus, ultimately, the CO tends to fall. In contrast, for patient with severe impaired left ventricular systolic and diastolic function, the reduction of arterial impedance or afterload is the predominant effect, which leads to the rise in CO. The reduction of preload is also beneficial in this group of patient, suffering from impaired left ventricular systolic and diastolic function.

Nitroprusside is a nonselective vasodilator. So, the regional distribution of blood flow is little affected by this drug. RBF and glomerular filtration are maintained by nitroprusside. Plasma renin activity is increased due to hypotension and subsequent sympathetic stimulation. Unlike hydralazine, diazoxide, minoxidil, and other arteriolar vasodilators, the sodium nitroprusside usually causes only a modest increase in heart rate in respect to the reduction of BP. But, still there is an overall reduction in myocardial O_2 demand.

Absorption, Metabolism, and Excretion

The onset of action of IV nitroprusside is 30 seconds. Peak hypotensive effect of IV nitroprusside occurs within 2 minutes after the starting of its infusion. When infusion is stopped, hypotensive effect disappears within 3 minutes. It is an unstable molecule and decomposes under alkaline conditions and when is exposed to light. The metabolism of nitroprusside occurs within the smooth muscle cells of blood vessel and is initiated by its reduction to cyanide and NO molecule. This cyanide is further metabolized in liver to thiocyanate and almost is eliminated through urine.

Metabolism of Nitroprusside

After injection, nitroprusside (NP) enters the RBC → here, it (NP) receives an electron from iron of oxyhemoglobin ($OHbFe^{2+}$) → as a result, there is formation of methemoglobin ($OHbFe^{3+}$) and unstable nitroprusside radicle (NP^-) → then, this unstable NP^- (nitroprusside radicle) spontaneously breaks into five cyanide ions (CN^-) and active NO (nitric oxide) group → next, the CN^- ions are involved in three reactions: (1) can bind with methemoglobin to form cyanmethemoglobin, (2) can undergo in reaction with thiosulfate, forming thiocyanate in liver and kidney, (3) can bind with tissue cytochrome oxidase system, interfering normal oxygen utilization and producing cyanide toxicity.

$NP + OHbFe^{2+} \rightarrow NP^- + OHbFe^{3+}$; $NP^- \rightarrow 5$ types $CN^- + NO$; (1) $CN^- + HbFe^{3+} \rightarrow CNHbFe^{2+}$; (2) $CN^- + $ Thiosulfate $\rightarrow$ Thiocyanate; $CN^- + $ Cytochrome oxidase $\rightarrow$ Cyanide toxicity

Toxicity of Nitroprusside

The main side effect of nitroprusside is sudden excessive vasodilatation and severe hypotension. Hence, during infusion of NP, continuous close monitoring of BP is mandatory. So, the use of sophisticated variable rate infusion pump will prevent this excessive hemodynamic response of this drug. Toxicity may also result from the excessive conversion of nitroprusside to cyanide and thiocyanate. The excessive accumulation of cyanide, leading to severe lactic acidosis, can also occur, if sodium nitroprusside is infused at the rate of >5 µg/kg/min. But, the concomitant use of sodium thiosulfate can prevent this accumulation of cyanide in a patient who receives more than usual doses of sodium nitroprusside. This is because the limiting factor in the metabolism of cyanide is the less availability of substrate like thiosulfate. The risk of cyanide toxicity also increases when the nitroprusside is infused for >24–48 hours and especially if renal function is impaired. Plasma concentration of cyanide also should be monitored during prolonged infusion of nitroprusside and should not be allowed to exceed >0.1 mg/mL.

Nitroprusside may worsen arterial hypoxemia in patient who is suffering from chronic obstructive pulmonary disease. Because, this drug (nitroprusside) interferes with the compensatory hypoxic pulmonary vasoconstriction reflex and, therefore, promotes the mismatching of ventilation with perfusion. Rebound hypertension may also occur after abrupt the cessation of short-term nitroprusside infusion. This may be due to the persistently elevated concentration of renin in plasma caused by hypotension.

Dose

Nitroprusside should be used in variable, controlled, and continuous infusion according to patient's response. The usual dose of nitroprusside (NP) ranges from 0.25 to 1.50 µg/kg/min.

Organic Nitrates and Nitrites

The organic *nitrates* are the ester of *nitric acid* (–C–O–NO_2). On the other hand, the organic *nitrites* are the ester of *nitrous acid* (–C–O–NO). Their chemical structure is depicted in **Figure 8**. The common organic nitrites and nitrates, which are clinically used, are—*amyl nitrite, nitroglycerin (glyceryl trinitrate), isosorbide dinitrate, isosorbide-5-mononitrate, erythrityl tetranitrate, pentaerythritol tetranitrate*, etc. Glyceryl trinitrate is widely and officially accepted as nitroglycerin which has an explosive property. But, actually it is not nitro compound. Because, nitro compound possesses carbon–nitrogen bonds (C–NO_2) and is highly explosive. So, glyceryl trinitrate is erroneously called as nitroglycerin. For the actions of organic nitrates and nitrites, they are denitrated to release NO by NO synthetase enzyme. These NO synthetase enzymes are found in vascular endothelial and smooth muscle cells, as well as in other types of cells throughout our body including CNS. When the activity of NO synthetase and the production of NO are reduced, then the individual suffers from atherosclerosis. This NO, then, activates cyclic GMP in vascular smooth muscle cells and produces vasodilation like nitroprusside. So, the organic nitrates and nitrites are called as *nitrovasodilators*. Normally, in vascular endothelial and smooth muscle cells, endogenous NO is also formed by NO synthases enzyme, by converting L-arginine to citrulline.

Another organic nitrite, such as *amyl nitrite*, is highly volatile liquid and is administered by inhalation. This is because, usually the low-molecular weight *nitroglycerin* is oily liquid and moderately volatile. *Erythrityl tetranitrate, pentaerythritol tetranitrate, and isosorbide dinitrate* are solids and of high-molecular weight without inert carrier such as lactose. Pure nitroglycerin is highly explosive.

Mechanism of Action of Nitrates and Nitrites

The organic nitrites, nitrates, nitroso compounds, and a variety of other nitrogen oxide containing substances, including nitroprusside, etc. ultimately lead to the formation of a reactive free radical, such as NO. This NO activates cytosolic guanylyl cyclase enzyme → increased cGMP → inhibition of cGMP-dependent protein kinase → dephosphorylation of myosin light chain → relaxation → vasodilation. The phosphorylation of myosin light chain regulates and is responsible for the maintenance of the contractile state of the smooth muscle of vessels. The raised intracellular cGMP may also reduce the entry of Ca^{2+} into cells and contribute the relaxation of the smooth muscles of veins.

Pharmacological Action of Nitrates and Nitrites

Low therapeutic concentrations of nitroglycerin (plus other nitrates and nitrites) produce predominantly venodilatation and reduce preload. Thus, the reduction of venous pooling causes reduction of end-diastolic ventricular volume **(Fig. 8)** and end-diastolic ventricular pressure and reduction of CO. Whereas, the effects of nitroglycerin (and other nitrates and nitrites) on arterioles are minimal, causing little changes in SVR. Hence, systemic arterial pressure may fall slightly. Pulmonary vascular resistance also falls slightly. As preload falls much more than afterload, so CO falls. The doses of nitroglycerin, which do not alter systemic arterial pressure, often produce arterial dilation of face, neck, and meningeal vessels, resulting in flushing and headache. The enzymes, which convert nitrates to NO, are abundant in venous smooth muscles, as compared to arterial smooth muscles cells. This is the cause of predominant venoselective properties of nitrates. On the other hand, the higher doses of organic nitrates cause both the venous and arteriolar dilation which lead to the reduction of both systolic and diastolic BP and increase or decrease of CO, according to the balance between the degree of reduction of preload and afterload. The resultant compensatory tachycardia and peripheral arteriolar vasoconstriction, due to the reduction of CO, tend to restore the SVR. But, this is superimposed by sustained venous pooling. Thus, coronary blood flow may increase transiently as a result of coronary vasodilation. But, it subsequently decreases, if CO and BP fall sufficiently, causing severe reduction of coronary perfusion pressure.

- *Coronary blood flow:* Ischemia is the most powerful stimulus for coronary vasodilation. Regional coronary blood flow is adjusted by the local autoregulatory mechanism. Thus, blood flow is directed from the nonischemic nondilating vessels to the dilated ischemic areas. Organic nitrates do not impair this autoregulation. *The small coronary arterioles, which are responsible for about 90% of overall coronary vascular resistance, are not dilated by nitrates and nitrites. Therefore, the organic nitrates and nitrites do not directly increase myocardial*

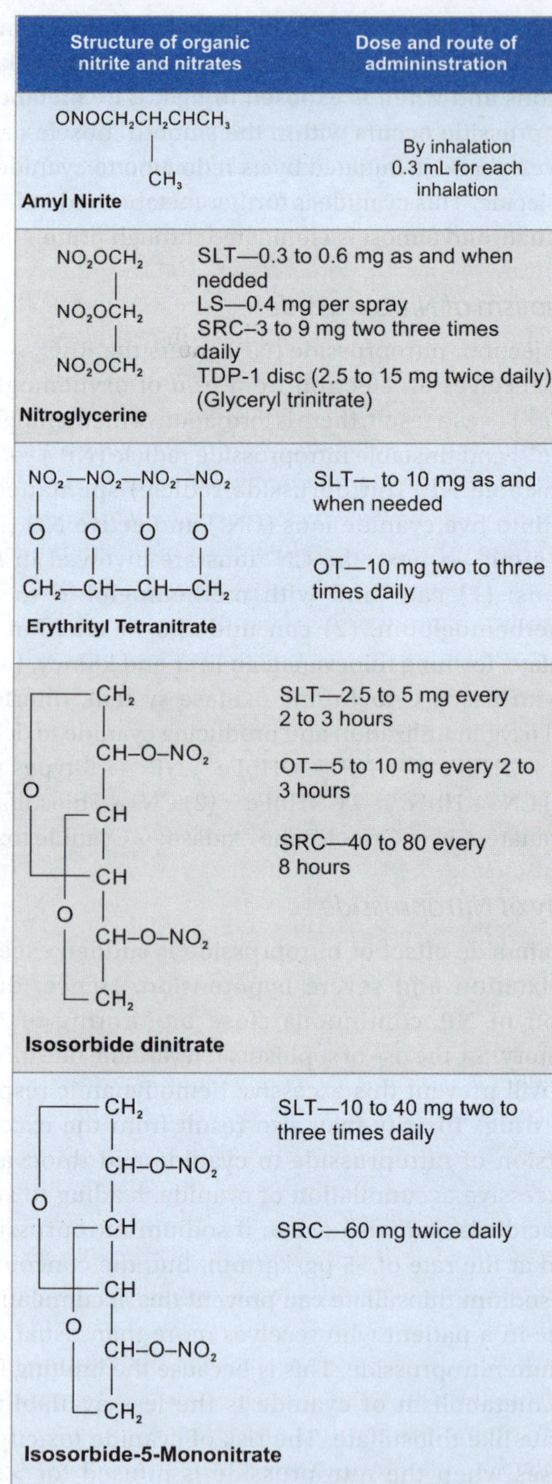

Structure of organic nitrite and nitrates	Dose and route of adminstration
ONOCH₂CH₂CHCH₃ | CH₃ **Amyl Nirite**	By inhalation 0.3 mL for each inhalation
NO₂OCH₂ | NO₂OCH₂ | NO₂OCH₂ **Nitroglycerine**	SLT—0.3 to 0.6 mg as and when nedded LS—0.4 mg per spray SRC–3 to 9 mg two three times daily TDP-1 disc (2.5 to 15 mg twice daily) (Glyceryl trinitrate)
NO₂—NO₂—NO₂—NO₂ | O O O O | CH₂—CH—CH—CH₂ **Erythrityl Tetranitrate**	SLT— to 10 mg as and when needed OT—10 mg two to three times daily
CH₂ | CH–O–NO₂ | CH | CH | CH–O–NO₂ | CH₂ **Isosorbide dinitrate**	SLT—2.5 to 5 mg every 2 to 3 hours OT—5 to 10 mg every 2 to 3 hours SRC—40 to 80 every 8 hours
CH₂ | CH–O–NO₂ | CH | CH | CH–O–NO₂ | CH₂ **Isosorbide-5-Mononitrate**	SLT—10 to 40 mg two to three times daily SRC—60 mg twice daily

Fig. 8: The chemical structure of different organic nitrates and nitrites. (SLT: sublingual tablet; LS: lingual spray; SRC: sustained release capsule; TDP: transdermal patch; OT: oral tablet)

O₂ supply. Vessels >200 µm in diameter, which are responsible for 10% of overall coronary vascular resistance, are highly responsive to organic nitrates. But, the vessels <100 µm are not or minimally responsive.

Thus, organic nitrates and nitrites are only able to cause dilations and prevent constriction of large epicardial vessels. In fact, nitrates do not increase the total coronary blood flow in angina patients. *However, it causes only the redistribution of blood flow when the coronary circulation is partially occluded and area is ischemic.*

Collateral flow to ischemic regions also is increased by nitrates. On the other hand, due to redistribution, there is disproportionate reduction in blood flow to the subendocardial regions of heart, which are subjected to greatest extravascular compression during systole. *Hence, practically, an important indirect mechanism for maintaining subendocardial blood flow is the nitroglycerin-induced reduction in intracavity systolic and diastolic pressure by reducing the preload that opposes the blood flow to subendocardium.* Thus, indirectly the organic nitrates decrease the myocardial oxygen requirement. Increased blood flow in ischemic regions is balanced by decreased flow in nonischemic areas. The explanation for the increased blood flow to ischemic area and decreased blood flow to nonischemic area by nitrates is like that the nitrates dilate the large epicardial vessels. At ischemic area, the resistance vessels are also automatically dilated by their autoregulatory mechanisms and at nonischemic area, the resistance vessels are constricted. Therefore, the blood preferentially flows through dilated epicardial vessels and dilated ischemic area. However, overall total increase in coronary blood flow does not occur. Dilatation of cardiac veins may result in an improvement in perfusion of coronary microcirculation. *In patients, suffering from angina due to coronary spasm, the capability of organic nitrates to dilate the epicardial coronary arteries and particularly at the regions which are affected by spasm may be the primary mechanism by which they are benefited.*

- *Effect on myocardial O_2 demand: Organic nitrates reduce myocardial O_2 demand.* The O_2 demand of heart muscle is directly proportional to the ventricular wall tension, heart rate, and contractility of myocardium. This ventricular wall tension is again directly proportional with preload and afterload. Because, according to Laplace's law: Tension $\propto$ Pressure $\times$ Radius. Preload is determined by the end-diastolic ventricular filling, i.e., end-diastolic left ventricular volume and pressure. Increased venous capacitance with *nitrates decreases venous return to the heart and decreases ventricular end-diastolic volume which in turn decreases the wall tension and O_2 consumption (demand). Reduction of preload also increases the pressure gradient for perfusion across the ventricular wall and favors the subendocardial perfusion.*

Afterload is the impedance against which the left ventricle contracts and ejects its contents. Thus, it is related to the SVR. Decrease of SVR by organic nitrites and nitrates also reduces the afterload and thus reduces the left ventricular wall tension during myocardial contraction. Hence, myocardial O_2 demand is also reduced. An interesting finding is that angina occurs with or without nitroglycerin at the same value of "triple product" (aortic pressure × heart rate × ejection time), which is proportional to myocardial O_2 consumption. *It suggests that beneficial effects of nitroglycerin are the result of reduced cardiac O_2 demand, rather than an increase in the delivery of O_2 to ischemic regions of myocardium.* But, it does not exclude the possibility that direct coronary vasodilation may be the major effect of nitroglycerin where vasospasm is the cause of angina. Organic nitrates have no direct positive inotropic or chronotropic effect on heart, but may affect indirectly. The main therapeutic uses of organic nitrites and nitrates are— angina, CHF, unstable angina, MI, variant (Prinzmetal's) angina, etc.

Absorption, Fate, and Excretion of Nitrates and Nitrites

The lipid-soluble organic nitrates are metabolized to water-soluble inorganic nitrates and denitrated compounds by nitrate reductase enzyme in liver. The denitrated metabolites of nitrates and nitrites are less potent vasodilators than parent compounds. Since the liver has enormous capacity for the metabolism of organic nitrates and nitrites, so the oral bioavailability of them is much less.

The velocity of metabolism of *erythrityl tetranitrate* is three times faster than nitroglycerin (glyceryl trinitrate), while isosorbide dinitrate and pentaerythritol tetranitrate are metabolized at the rate of one-sixth and one-tenth of that of nitroglycerin. After sublingual administration, peak concentration of nitroglycerin in plasma reaches within 3–4 minutes and half-life is 1–3 hours. The onset of action is more rapid, if nitroglycerin is delivered by sublingual spray. Sublingual administration of *isosorbide dinitrate* produces maximal concentration of drug in plasma by 6 minutes and half-life is 45 minutes. Its primary initial metabolites are isosorbide-2-mononitrate and isosorbide-5-mononitrate, which have longer half-life (3–6 hours) and these are presumed to be responsible for the therapeutic efficacy and prolonged action of isosorbide dinitrate. *Isosorbide-5-mononitrate* has excellent bioavailability after oral administration. It does not undergo significant first-pass liver metabolism. So, it has longer half-life and formulated as plain tablet or sustained release capsule, both of which have longer duration of actions.

TABLE 4: Dose, route, and duration of action of different nitrates.

Drugs	Dose and route	Duration of action
GTN (nitroglycerin) Nitrocontin 2.6 mg CR tablet	• 0.5 mg SL (sublingual) • 0.4–0.8 mg SL spray • 5–15 mg SR tablet oral • 5–20 µg/min IV • 5 or 10 mg patch	• 10–30 minutes • 10–30 minutes • 4–8 hours • Till infused • Till applied
Isosorbide dinitrate	• 5 mg SL • 10–20 mg oral • 10–40 mg SR oral	• 20–40 minutes • 2–4 hours • 6–10 hours
Isosorbide-5-mononitrate	• 10–40 mg oral • 10–40 mg SR oral	• 6–10 hours • 12–16 hours
Erythrityl tetranitrate	15–60 mg oral	4–6 hours
Pentaerythritol tetranitrate	• 10–40 mg oral • 80 mg SR oral	• 3–6 hours • 10–12 hours

(CR: controlled-release; SR: sustained-release)

Doses and route of administration of nitrates (Table 4): Nitroglycerin (or glyceryl trinitrate) is the most useful drug among the other organic nitrates that can be given sublingually. It is because of its rapid onset of action, long established efficacy, and low cost. The onset of action of initial 0.3 mg nitroglycerin, administered through sublingual route, is within 1–2 minutes and effects do not last for >1 hour after its administration. So, it can be used as needed. Other nitrates that can be used sublingually are not more effective and do not appear to be longer acting than nitroglycerin. But, they are more expensive.

Oral nitrates are often used to provide prophylaxis against angina episodes. They are given initially in higher doses to provide effective plasma levels due to first-pass hepatic degradation. So, to obtain a continuous plasma therapeutic level of nitroglycerin, the sustained release preparation of it should be used better. The effects of this sustained released form of nitroglycerin reach the peak level at 60–90 minutes and last for 3–6 hours. The dose of isosorbide dinitrate through oral route is 5–10 mg for every 2–3 hours and through sublingual route is 2.5–5 mg for every 2–3 hours.

Application of nitroglycerin ointment also relieves angina. The nitroglycerin disk utilizes nitroglycerin-impregnated polymer for transdermal use that permits gradual absorption and a continuous steady plasma nitrate concentration over 24 hours. But, the onset of action of nitroglycerin through this route is slow with peak effects at 1–2 hours. IV route for nitroglycerin is only used for the management of hypertensive emergency and the dose is 2.5–5 µg/min with increments of 2.5 µg/min.

■ CALCIUM CHANNEL BLOCKERS

Introduction

The Ca^{2+} channel antagonists or blockers are putative coronary vasodilators and possess negative inotropic and chronotropic effects that were not seen with nitroglycerin. The negative inotropic effect of CCBs results from the inhibition of excitation and contraction coupling between the action and myosin filaments, due to the reduction of the movement of Ca^{2+} ion into the cardiac myocytes. They also alter the plateau phase (phase 2) of cardiac action potential that is due to the entry of Ca^{2+} into the myocardial cells.

At present, all the CCBs are divided into three chemical classes, which have distinct pharmacodynamic profiles. This is depicted below:
- *Phenyl alkylamine:* Verapamil
- *Benzothiazepine:* Diltiazem
- *Dihydropyridine:* Nifedipine, amlodipine, cilnidipine, lacidipine, benidipine, felodipine, nimodipine, nicardipine, and nitrendipine.

Among all these three classes of CCBs, only the dihydropyridine class is the most potent Ca^{2+} channel blockers and has proliferated exceptionally.

Practically, there are three types of Ca^{2+} channels present on the cell membrane. These are:
1. *Voltage-sensitive Ca^{2+} channels:* These act (open) due to the changes of action potential in cell membrane. These voltage-sensitive Ca^{2+} channels are again subdivided into three types. These are—*(1) L-type, (2) T-type, and (3) N-type of Ca^{2+} channels.*
2. *Receptor-operated Ca^{2+} channel:* These Ca^{2+} channels are actually receptor. They act independent of the changes in action potential of cell membrane (depolarization). They act like receptors when agonist or antagonist is attached with these types of Ca^{2+} channels.
3. *Leak Ca^{2+} channel:* Small amounts of Ca^{2+} continuously enter into resting cell and again are forced out by Ca^{2+} ATPase pump through some tiny Ca^{2+} channels, which are present on cell membrane. These are called as the leak channels. They are activated (open) by membrane depolarization or act like receptor **(Table 5)**.

Mechanism of Action of CCBs

The increased contraction of the striated cardiac smooth muscle cells and nonstriated vascular smooth muscle cells is caused by the increased concentration of cytosolic Ca^{2+} ion. This increased intracellular or cytosolic concentration of Ca^{2+} is caused by the increased entry of extracellular Ca^{2+} ion into the cells and release of more Ca^{2+} from its intracellular storage site, triggered by this entry of extracellular Ca^{2+} ion into the cells. Hence, the final cytosolic Ca^{2+} concentration

TABLE 5: Difference between three types of voltage-sensitive Ca^{2+} channels.

	L-type	T-type	N-type
1. Activation threshold	High	Low	High
2. Inactivation	Slow	Fast	Medium
3. Location and function	(i) Cardiac and smooth muscle → excitation and contraction (ii) SA and AV node → rate and conduction (iii) Endocrine cells → hormone release (iv) Neurons → release of transmitter	(i) SA node → pacemaker activity (ii) Thalamus and other neurons → T current (iii) Endocrine cells → release of hormone	(i) CNS, sympathetic, and myenteric plexuses → release of transmitter
4. Blocker	Nifedipine, verapamil, and diltiazem	Flunarizine and ethosuximide	Conotoxin

(CNS: central nervous system)

can be increased by initial influx of Ca^{2+} from outside by various stimuli. Many hormones and neurohormones, as stimuli, act through the receptor-operated Ca^{2+} channel and increase the initial Ca^{2+} influx. While some other stimuli, such as high extracellular K^+ concentration and depolarizing electrical stimuli, work through the "voltage-sensitive" or "potential-operated" Ca^{2+} channels and increase the Ca^{2+} influx. Again, small amount of Ca^{2+} continuously leaks into the resting cell through leak channel and is continuously pumped out through "leak channel" by Ca^{2+} ATPase pump.

The Ca^{2+} channels are made up of many subunits such as α1, α2, β, γ, and δ. The *voltage-sensitive Ca^{2+} channels* have been divided at least three subtypes based on their conductance and sensitivity to voltage. These are L, N, and T subtypes of voltage-sensitive Ca^{2+} channels, although P/Q and R types of voltage-sensitive Ca^{2+} channels have also been identified. However, among these, only the L type of Ca^{2+} channels is blocked by the above-mentioned Ca^{2+} channel blockers such as (1) nifedipine and their congeners, (2) verapamil, and (3) diltiazem.

The α1 subunit shares a common topology of four homologous domains (I, II, III, and IV) and each of which is composed of six putative transmembrane segments (S_1-S_6). The phenyl alkylamine group of Ca^{2+} channel blockers (verapamil) binds to the transmembrane segment 6 of domain IV (IVS_6). The benzothiazepine group of Ca^{2+} channel blockers (diltiazem) binds to the cytoplasmic bridge between domain III (IIIS) and domain IV (IVS). However, the dihydropyridine group of Ca^{2+} channel blockers (nifedipine) binds to the transmembrane segments of both domain III ($IIIS_6$) and domain IV (IVS_6).

Pharmacological Properties of CCBs

Action on Vascular Tissue

Although there is some involvement of Na^+ current for the depolarization of vascular smooth muscle, but it primarily

BOX 2: Calcium channel blocker.

- *Especially suited for:*
  - Asthma, COPD patients
  - Pregnancy-induced hypertension
  - Physically and mentally active patient
  - Peripheral vascular disease (e.g., Raynaud's)
  - Isolated systolic hypertension
  - Elderly with low renin
- *To be avoided:*
  - CHF, conduction defects, and sick sinus syndrome
  - Receiving β-blockers
  - Prostate enlargement
  - LVH
  - Gastroesophageal reflux

(CHF: congestive heart failure; COPD: chronic obstructive pulmonary disease; LVH: left ventricular hypertrophy)

depends on the influx of Ca^{2+} current, which occurs through some voltage-sensitive Ca^{2+} channels. Due to depolarization, activation of these Ca^{2+} channels results in the hydrolysis of membrane-bound phosphatidylinositol with the formation of inositol triphosphate (IP_3) which acts as a second messenger to release the intracellular Ca^{2+} ion from sarcoplasmic reticulum. Then this increased intracellular Ca^{2+} ion binds to protein calmodulin → activates myosin light-chain kinase → phosphorylation of light-chain of myosin → promotes interaction between actin and myosin → contraction of smooth muscle. CCBs inhibit these "voltage-sensitive" Ca^{2+} channels → inhibit the influx of Ca^{2+} into the smooth muscle cells → do not trigger the release of Ca^{2+} from intracellular SR → intracellular Ca^{2+} concentration does not rise → myosin light-chain kinase is not activated → actin does not bind with myosin → smooth muscle relaxes. Thus, all the Ca^{2+} channel blockers relax the arterial smooth muscle, but have little effects on venous smooth muscles. So, CCBs do not affect the venous return and cardiac preload does not decrease significantly **(Box 2)**.

TABLE 6: Electrophysiological actions of calcium channel blockers.

	Verapamil	Diltiazem	Nifedipine
SA node automaticity	↓	↓ −	No action
Ventricular automaticity	↓−	No actions	No action
Effective refractory period:			
• Atrial	• No action	• No action	• No action
• AV nodal	• ↑↑	• ↑	• ↑↓
• Ventricular	• No action	• No action	• No action
ECG:			
• PR interval	• ↑	• ↑	• No action
• RR interval	• ↑	• ↑↓	• ↓

(ECG: electrocardiography)

Action on Cardiac Cell

There are some differences in excitation–contraction coupling between the cardiac muscle cells and the vascular smooth muscle cells. The difference is that among the two inward currents, required for the initiation of action potential (depolarization or phase 0 of action potential), one is carried through fast Na^+ channel, and the other is carried through the slow Ca^{2+} channel. In SA and AV node, the depolarization is largely dependent on the movement of Ca^{2+} through this slow Ca^{2+} channel. In the cardiac myocyte, troponin inhibits the actin and myosin interaction which causes muscle contraction. Ca^{2+} binds to this troponin and withdraws this inhibition and initiates contraction. CCB, thus, acts to cause negative inotropic effect, by preventing the binding of Ca^{2+} ion with troponin and by decreasing the entry of Ca^{2+} into the myocardial cells.

The pacemaker activity of SA node and atrioventricular (AV) conduction is dependent mainly on these slow Ca^{2+} channels. Nifedipine does not affect these slow Ca^{2+} channels on myocardial cells. Thus, it has no effect on heart rate and conduction through AV node. It mainly acts on Ca^{2+} channels, present on the smooth muscle of blood vessels in a dose-dependent manner. In contrast, verapamil reduces the slow inward current and the rate of recovery of slow Ca^{2+} channel. Thus, verapamil and diltiazem both reduce the rate of sinus node pacemaker activity and slow the AV conduction **(Table 6)**. This is the basis for their use in the treatment of PSVT. It also causes the prolongation of AV nodal effective refractory period and the prolongation of QT_C interval. In the presence of hypokalemia, this prolongation of QT_C interval may precipitate "torsades de pointes"—a potentially lethal ventricular arrhythmia.

Hemodynamic Effect

Calcium channel blockers decrease the coronary vascular resistance and, therefore, increase the coronary blood flow. Among all the CCBs, the nifedipine is more potent systemic vasodilator than verapamil and diltiazem. The nifedipine dilates resistance arterial vessels, but not the veins. This decrease in arterial BP stimulates sympathetic reflexes and produces tachycardia (positive chronotropic effect) with positive inotropic effect (via sympathetic stimulation). Nifedipine relaxes the vascular smooth muscle at significantly lower concentration than those required for the prominent direct effects (negative inotropic) on heart. Arteriolar resistance and BP are lowered; contractility and segmental ventricular function are improved. So, the heart rate and CO are increased. After oral administration of nifedipine, arterial dilatation increases peripheral blood flow, but venous tone does not change. Because of the lack of myocardial depression and the lack of negative inotropic and chronotropic effect, nifedipine is less effective as monotherapy in a stable angina than verapamil, diltiazem, and β-blocker.

Therapeutic Uses of CCBs

Hypertension

Essential hypertension is the result of increased SVR, caused by the contraction of vascular smooth muscles, mainly arteriole, which is dependent on the free intracellular concentration of Ca^{2+} ion. Therefore, all the CCBs decrease the BP—(1) by reducing SVR and (2) by relaxing the arteriolar smooth muscle. As a consequence of this reduction of BP, the CCBs evoke a baroreceptor-mediated sympathetic discharge. So, in case of nifedipine, tachycardia ensues. Whereas, tachycardia is absent with verapamil and diltiazem, because of their direct negative chronotropic effect on the SA node of the heart. The increased compensatory adrenergic stimulation of heart serves to counter the hypotensive effect of CCB. So, the hypotensive effect of CCB is excessive, when it is used concurrently with β-blocker. As a consequence of peripheral vasodilatation (more arterial dilatation than venodilatation), the CCBs also increase venous return, which will result in increased CO, except in case of verapamil and diltiazem, which exert substantial negative inotropic effect. This increased venous return is beneficial for normal heart, but not for the patient with diastolic dysfunction due to hypertensive cardiomyopathy who is at increased risk of LVF. The CCBs do not improve the diastolic function of ventricle. So, it is not the first choice of treatment in hypertension with LVH. All CCBs are equally effective when used alone in the treatment of mild-to-moderate hypertension, like β-blocker or diuretics.

There is special set of concern, regarding the use of CCB, in presence of ischemic heart disease (IHD) with hypertension. The CCBs do not improve the survival rate in patients, following the MI. Therefore, it is not the first or second drug of choice in the treatment of hypertension in patient who has an MI. The sublingual administration of CCB does not achieve the maximum plasma concentration any more quickly than does oral administration. It is proved that nifedipine is not absorbed by buccal mucosa, when is used by sublingual route. With saliva, it goes to upper gastrointestinal (GI) tract and through stomach, it is absorbed. Hence, oral or sublingual administration of standard formulation of nifedipine (immediate release capsule) as an approach to urgent reduction of BP has been abandoned. Only the short-acting and the parenterally administered CCB agents should be used in the setting of hypertensive urgencies.

In the treatment of emergency of hypertension, there is no place of standard formulation of immediate release capsule of nifedipine with short half-lives through oral route, because it causes great oscillation in BP and concurrent surges in sympathetic reflex activity at the interval of each dosage. Thus, nifedipine is a suboptimal choice for treatment of cardiogenic pulmonary edema. In contrast, nitroprusside causes a greater reduction in left ventricular end-diastolic pressure than equipotent doses of nifedipine and the pharmacological effect of nitroprusside can be regulated more effectively. So, it is a better choice than CCB for treatment of cardiogenic pulmonary edema.

The CCBs are especially effective in low-renin hypertension. The long-acting dihydropyridine group of CCBs reduces the cardiovascular mortality. CCBs should not be used in patient with SA and AV nodal abnormalities and overt CF. It can be used in hypertensive patient with asthma, diabetes, and renal dysfunction. Unlike β-blocker, CCB does not alter the exercise tolerance.

Variant Angina

Variant angina is due to the reduction of blood flow in myocardium, rather than an increase in O_2 demand. So, CCB protects the variant angina by attenuating the coronary spasm and dilating the coronary artery, rather than the alterations in peripheral hemodynamics.

Exertional Angina

The CCBs also are effective in the treatment of exercise or exertional induced angina. The effectivity of these agents may result from—(1) an increase in blood flow due to coronary arterial dilation, (2) from a decrease in myocardial O_2 demand (secondary to a decrease in arterial BP, heart rate, and myocardial contractility), or (3) from both. Numerous double-blind and placebo-controlled studies have shown that these drugs reduce the number of anginal attack and decrease the exercise-induced depression of ST segment.

The "double product", which is calculated from "heart rate multiplied by systolic BP", is an indirect measure of myocardial O_2 demand. Since these agents reduce the level of double product, so the demand of O_2 is also reduced at a given external workload. The beneficial effect of CCB is primarily due to the reduction of O_2 demand, rather than the increase in coronary blood flow. The concurrent therapy of nifedipine with the β-adrenergic receptor antagonist has proven more effective than when the either agent is given alone. Because, the β-blocker suppresses the reflex tachycardia, produced by CCBs, other than verapamil and diltiazem.

■ BETA-BLOCKERS

These drugs inhibit adrenergic responses, which are only mediated through β-receptors and are used in the treatment of *hypertension, ischemic heart disease (angina), CHF,* and *certain arrhythmias.* All the β-blockers are competitive antagonist at the level of their receptors (β-receptors). The β-blocker such as propranolol was first introduced in 1963, and was a great therapeutic breakthrough. Then, it remains the prototype to which the other β-blockers are compared. After that, subsequently more and more new, β-blockers were developed and they are classified by their some properties. These properties are—(1) relative affinity of them for β_1- and β_2-receptors, (2) intrinsic sympathomimetic activity, (3) additional blockade of α-adrenergic receptor, (4) difference in lipid solubility, (5) capacity to induce vasodilatation, and (6) general pharmacokinetic properties. Some of these characteristics have clinical significance. These help to guide the appropriate choice of β-blockers for individual patient.

The *main effectiveness of β-blocker* is found in the treatment of *exertion angina.* This effectiveness is primarily— (1) due to the reduction of myocardial O_2 consumption or demand, during both rest and exercise and (2) due to some tendency for increased coronary flow toward ischemic areas. The decrease in O_2 consumption and demand by β-blocker is again primarily due to—(1) its negative inotropic action, (2) negative chronotropic action, and (3) the reduction of arterial BP during exercise. Not all the actions of β-blockers are beneficial for all patients. Because, the decrease in HR and the decrease in force of myocardial contraction by β-blockers cause an increase in systolic *ejection period*, due to an increase in left ventricular end-diastolic volume with pressure, due to subsequently increase in diastolic period, and due to subsequent decrease in HR. This tends to increase O_2 consumption. But, the net result for the effect of β-blocker is the reduction of O_2 consumption during exercise. On the other hand, some patients with limited cardiac reserve are dependent on adrenergic stimulation. In these patients, the use of β-blocker and the depression of adrenergic stimulation can result in profound decrease of left ventricular function. Despite this, the β-blockers definitely reduce the mortality in patients with CHF.

Classification of Beta-Blocker (Table 7)

- *Nonselective (Acting on both β_1 and β_2-receptors)*
  - *Without intrinsic sympathetic activity:* Propranolol, sotalol, timolol, and nadolol
  - *With intrinsic sympathetic activity (partial agonist):* Pindolol, oxprenolol, and alprenolol
  - *With additional α-blocking property:* Labetalol and carvedilol.

(Some β-blockers intrinsically activate β-receptors in the absence of catecholamines. However, this intrinsic sympathetic activity of these drugs is less than that of full agonist such as isoproterenol. These partial agonistic effects of β-blockers are said to have the intrinsic sympathetic activity.)

- *Cardioselective (acting only on β_1-receptors):*
  - Metoprolol
  - Esmolol
  - Atenolol
  - Acebutolol
  - Celiprolol
  - Bisoprolol
  - Nebivolol
  - Betaxolol
- *Selective β_2-blocker:* Butoxamine. It has no clinical application.

  The partial agonistic β-blockers (β-blockers with intrinsic sympathomimetic action) are those which themselves activate β_1 and/or β_2-receptors submaximally. The probable benefits of these β-blockers are:
- Bradycardia and depression of contractility at rest are not prominent, but exercise-induced tachycardia is

attenuated. Hence, these types of β-blockers are preferred in those who are prone to severe bradycardia.
- Rebound hypertension and angina are less after withdrawal of these β-blockers. This is due to continued agonistic action on β-receptors by the drugs themselves which prevents the development of supersensitivity.
- Plasma lipid profile is less or not worsened by these partial agonistic β-blockers.
- These partial agonistic β-blockers are not suitable for secondary prophylaxis of MI.
- These partial agonistic β-blockers are ineffective for migraine prophylaxis, because they dilate cerebral vessels.

This above classification of β-blockers is not absolute. Because, some selective β_1 antagonists, even though selective for this receptor, have some affinity for β_2-receptors also and block them, e.g., metoprolol, acebutolol, atenolol, etc. *Therefore, this selectivity of β_1-blockers is only relative and is lost at high doses. For this reason, by blocking β_2-receptor, still the selective β_1-blockers have lower propensity to cause bronchoconstriction. Hence, these drugs (β-blockers, even selective β_1-receptor blockers) should be avoided, if possible, in asthmatics.* Third-generation *acebutolol* has some intrinsic sympathomimetic activities. Some β-blockers also have the property of inverse agonism and decrease the basal activation of β-receptor. *Celiprolol* is a β_1-selective blocker that acts on heart and a β_2-selective agonist that promotes vasodilatation. Some β-blockers have membrane-stabilizing or antiarrhythmic action, but this appears to be significant only at higher doses.

In addition to β-receptor blockade, the nebivolol activates the endothelial NO synthase enzyme and enhances the synthesis of NO. Thus, it causes vasodilatation and has the potential to improve endothelial function, which may delay atherosclerosis. The absence of deleterious effect on plasma lipids and on carbohydrate metabolism is another advantage of nebivolol. It also tends to increase insulin sensitivity, instead of decreasing it.

Pharmacological Properties of β-blocker

Cardiovascular System

Heart: The β-blocker has relatively little effect on *normal* heart at rest. But, it has profound effects, when the sympathetic control on heart is dominant, e.g., during exercise and stress. At rest, usually the tonic stimulation of sympathetic β-receptor is low, so the effect of β-blocker is correspondingly low or modest. But, during exercise and stress when the sympathetic system is activated, then the effects of β-blockers are also increased. *Therefore, in the presence of β-blocker, the exercise- or stress-induced*

TABLE 7: Classification of β-blockers.		
First-generation	*Second-generation*	*Third-generation*
β-blockers (nonselective, block both β_1 and β_2)	β-blockers (selective, block β_1 receptor)	β-blockers (with additional property)
Propranolol, timolol, sotalol, pindolol, nadolol, alprenolol, and oxprenolol	Metoprolol, atenolol, acebutolol, bisoprolol, and esmolol	Labetalol, carvedilol, celiprolol, nebivolol, and betaxolol

increase in HR and myocardial contractility is attenuated. However, CO is not affected due to this decrease in HR. This is because of the increase in stroke volume, corresponding with the reduction of heart rate.

In hypertension, propranolol increases SVR and decreases CO. *This increase in SVR by nonselective β-blocker is due to the blockade of peripheral vascular β_2-receptor, which normally dilates the peripheral vessels, especially in skeletal muscles.* The increased SVR is also due to compensatory increase in sympathetic activity due to the lowering of BP and subsequent stimulation of vascular α-adrenergic receptor. *The blockade of β-receptor also causes the α-receptor to take upper hand and increases SVR. However, labetalol and carvedilol, which are both β-receptor and α_1-receptor antagonists, maintain CO with greater fall of SVR. The indications and the contraindications for the use of β-blockers are mentioned in **Box 3**.*

The β-blockers reduce *heart rate*. This is due to the decrease in automaticity of SA node. The β-blockers also cause slow conduction through atria and AV node and increase in the functional refractory period of AV node. Although it has been thought that these effects are exclusively due to the blockade of β_1-receptor, but β_2-adrenergic receptors in small extent are also likely to be involved in regulating the heart rate in human beings.

The *total coronary blood flow* is reduced by β-blockers. This is due to the blockade of coronary dilator β-receptors. But, these are largely restricted to the vessels of subepicardial region. While the vessels of subendocardial area, which is the chief site of origin of ischemia in angina, are not affected. *But the overall effect of β-blockers in angina patient is the improvement of O_2 supply/demand status (supply does not change, but demand is decreased) and the improvement of exercise tolerance, by balancing the reduction of myocardial O_2 demand by decreasing the catecholamine-induced*

increase in heart rate, cardiac contractility, and systolic BP. Ventricular dimensions are decreased in normal subjects, but the dilatation of it can occur in those with reduced reserve. So, CHF may be precipitated or aggravated. As the β-blockers decrease the HR by reducing the rate of slow diastolic depolarization, so they also reduce the risk of ectopic foci, especially if it had been augmented by adrenergic stimuli. They (β-blockers) block the cardiac stimulant action of adrenergic drugs, but not that of digoxin, methylxanthines, or glucagon.

As hypertensive agents, the β-blockers do not generally reduce BP in normotensive patient, but lower it in patient with hypertension. On oral administration, there is little acute change in BP. But, on prolonged oral administration, BP gradually falls. *Initially, the total SVR is increased due to the blockade of β-mediated vasodilatation and CO is reduced with net little change in BP. But with continued treatment, the resistance vessels gradually adapt to chronically reduced CO, so that SVR decreases and both the systolic and diastolic BPs fall.* But, all these are hypothesis and the actual cause of reduction of BP by β-blockers is not known. The probable hypotheses for antihypertensive effects of β-blockers are:

- β-blockers cause decreased renin release from kidney (β_1-mediated). Propranolol causes a more marked fall in BP in hypertensive individual who has high or normal plasma renin levels. Such patients respond at relatively lower doses of β-blocker than those with low-plasma renin. However, pindolol does not decrease plasma renin actively, but is still an effective antihypertensive.
- Inhibition of presynaptic β-adrenergic receptors, which normally cause the release of norepinephrine from sympathetic neurons. Therefore, ultimate result is reduction of NA release from sympathetic terminals.
- By acting centrally and reducing sympathetic outflow from brain. However, the β-blockers which cannot penetrate the blood–brain barrier are also effective antihypertensive.
- The β-blockers cannot decrease the contractility of vascular smooth muscle. But, the long-term use of it can cause reduction of SVR (mechanism is not known), even in the face of persistent reduction of CO and appears to account for much of the antihypertensive effect of these drugs.

Some β-blockers have additional properties that may contribute to their ability to lower BP by peripheral vasodilatation. For example:

- Labetalol and carvedilol directly block α_1-receptor and ↓SVR.
- Celiprolol appears to have partial β_2-receptor agonist and causes vasodilatation.

BOX 3: Relative indications and contraindications of β-blockers.

- *Especially suited for:*
  - Tense young patients
  - Coexisting anxiety and tachycardia
  - Angina
  - Post-MI patients
  - High-renin hypertension
  - Nonobese
  - Low cost
- *To be avoided:*
  - Bradycardia, conduction block, elderly patients
  - Asthma, diabetic
  - Peripheral vascular diseases, abnormal lipid profile
  - LVF
  - Who needs high-physical and mental activities

(LVF: left ventricular failure; MI: myocardial infarction)

- Nonadrenergic receptor-mediated vasodilatation by some β-blockers also contributes to decrease in SVR.

Respiratory System

Stimulation of adrenergic β_2-receptor causes relaxation of bronchial smooth muscles. However, in normal individual, this sympathetic β_2-receptor mediated bronchodilator tone is minimal. So, β-blocker has little effect on normal individual. However, in patient with asthma or chronic obstructive pulmonary disease (COPD), such β_2 blockade can lead to life-threatening bronchoconstriction. *Propranolol*, which is both β_1- and β_2-receptor blockers, is notorious for that. While the β_1-selective antagonist is less likely to increase airway resistance, but should be used very cautiously. *Celiprolol* with β_1-receptor-selective blocker and β_2-receptor partial agonism is of potential promise, but still now is of little clinical experience.

Metabolic Effects

All the β-blockers modify the metabolism of lipids and carbohydrates. Although insulin secretion is enhanced by β-adrenergic agonist, but β-blocker only rarely impairs insulin release. So, there is no effect on normal blood sugar. However, prolonged β-blocker therapy reduces carbohydrate tolerance by decreasing insulin release.

As the catecholamines, through their β-receptor, promote glycogenolysis and mobilize glucose from liver in response to hypoglycemia, so the nonselective β-blocker may adversely affect the recovery from hypoglycemia and should be used cautiously in diabetic patient receiving insulin. On the other hand, all the β-blockers will mask the tachycardia that is typically seen with hypoglycemia.

Beta-blockers block the catecholamine-induced lipolysis and reduce the consequent increase in plasma-free fatty acid levels. Therefore, as there is no lipolysis, so there will be no fat synthesis. Hence, the plasma triglyceride level and low-density lipoprotein (LDL)/high-density lipoprotein (HDL) ratio will be increased during β-blocker therapy.

Local Anesthetic Effect

Propranolol acts as potent local anesthetic agent like lignocaine. But it is not clinically used for this purpose, because of its irritant property.

Uterus

Relaxation of uterus in response to selective β_2 agonist can be blocked by β-blocker. But, the normal uterine activity in presence or absence of β_2 agonist or antagonist (blocker) is not significantly affected by these groups of drugs.

Skeletal Muscles

The β-blockers, especially propranolol, inhibit adrenergically provoked muscle tremor. This peripheral action of β-blockers is exerted directly on muscle fibers, because stimulation of β_2-receptor, present on muscle fibers, produces tremor.

Eye

The adrenergic receptors present in eye are like that (1) α_1-receptors: vasoconstriction of ciliary vessels → reduced aqueous formation → ↓ intraocular pressure (IOP). (2) α_2-receptors: ↓ secretory activity of ciliary epithelium. (3) β_2-receptors: enhanced secretory activity of ciliary epithelium and facilitation of trabecular outflow. (4) β_1-receptors: no effect. (5) α_1-receptors: on radial muscles of iris → contraction → dilatation of pupil. (6) M_3 cholinergic receptors: on constrictor muscle of iris → contraction → constriction of pupil. On ciliary muscle → contraction → ↓ IOP due to increased aqueous outflow due to improved patency of trabeculae.

The β-blockers reduce the secretion of aqueous humor and IOP is lowered. They have no consistent effect on pupil size or accommodation.

Individual Drug

Sotalol

It is a nonselective β-blocker. It has an additional cardiac rectifier K^+ channel blocking and class III antiarrhythmic property. Dose: 40–80 mg OD or BD.

Pindolol

It is a potent nonselective β-blocker with prominent intrinsic sympathomimetic activity. Hence, as antihypertensive agent, it provides advantage for the patients who develop marked bradycardia with propranolol. The chances of rebound hypertension on withdrawal are also less with pindolol. Dose: 10 mg OD or BD.

Timolol

It is also a potent nonselective β-blocker. Orally, it is also used for the management of hypertension, angina, prophylaxis of MI, etc. But, as β-blocker, it is preferred for topical use in eye in glaucoma. Other β-blockers, which are exclusively employed for topical application to eye, are: *betaxolol, levobunolol, carteolol, metipranolol*.

Atenolol

It is one of the most commonly used β-blockers for hypertension and angina. It is a relatively selective

β_1-receptor blocker, without any intrinsic sympathomimetic activity. It is incompletely absorbed orally and has low-lipid solubility. Its duration of action is long, so once daily dose is often sufficient. It has no as such deleterious effects on lipid metabolism (profile). Atenolol in combination with diuretics is very effective for elderly patients with isolated systolic hypertension. The initial dose of it is 50 mg per day, given orally and can be increased to 100 mg per day. But, higher doses are unlikely to provide any greater antihypertensive effect. S(-) atenolol is the pure active enantiomer of atenolol. It is effective at half the dose and is better tolerated. Dose: 12.5–50 mg OD.

Acebutolol

It is a cardioselective β-blocker (only β_1-receptor blocker) with some significant partial agonistic and membrane-stabilizing properties. So, its effect on resting heart rate is less (due to partial adrenergic agonistic activity). Acebutolol is rapidly metabolized in liver to its active metabolite, named diacetolol, which is primarily excreted through kidney and has longer duration of action. So, a single daily dose of acebutolol is sufficient in many patients. Dose: 200–400 mg OD.

Labetalol

It is both α_1 and β ($\beta_1 + \beta_2$) receptor blockers. It has two optical isomers. So, the clinical formulation of labetalol contains four isomers and each of which displays different relative activities. This explains why the pharmacological activities of this drug are so complex. The resultant effect of the mixture of these isomers includes selective blockade of α_1 (as compared to α_2-receptor) and blockade of β_1- and β_2-receptor. There are also some partial agonistic activity on β_2-receptor and inhibition of neuronal uptake of norepinephrine. This is cocaine-like effect. The potency of β-blocking mixture effect of labetalol is fivefold higher than for α_1-blocker effect of it.

The antagonistic action of labetalol on both α_1- and β-adrenergic receptors results in fall of BP in hypertensive patient. The α_1-receptor blockade causes relaxation of arterial smooth muscle and reduction of BP by vasodilation. The β_1-receptor blockade also causes fall in BP. This is caused by blocking of reflex sympathetic stimulation of heart. In addition to these, the intrinsic sympathetic activity of labetalol at β_2-receptor may cause vasodilatation and reduction of BP.

It is available in both oral and intravenous forms (for hypertensive emergency). The oral preparation of labetalol is completely absorbed from gut and goes through extensive first-pass hepatic clearance, with bioavailability of only 20–40%. The elimination half-life of clinical formulation of labetalol is 8 hours.

Carvedilol

It is also a nonselective β ($\beta_1 + \beta_2$) receptor and selective α_1-receptor antagonist and action is like labetalol. Bioavailability of carvedilol is only 20–30% and half-life is 10 hours.

Metoprolol

It is a selective β_1-adrenergic receptor blocker and is devoid of any intrinsic sympathetic activity. After oral administration, it is completely absorbed, but due to first-pass hepatic metabolism, the bioavailability of metoprolol is only 40%. The half-life of metoprolol is 3–4 hours. The use of metoprolol is contraindicated in patient with acute MI with HR <46 beats/min, heart block greater than first degree, systolic BP <100 mm Hg, and moderate-to-severe heart failure. It is less likely to worsen the bronchial asthma but is not entirely safe. It is preferred in diabetics, receiving insulin or oral hypoglycemic agents. Patients who complain of cold hand and feet, while on propranolol, do better on metoprolol. The usual initial dose of metoprolol is 50–100 mg once daily, but frequently it is used in two divided doses. *S(-) metoprolol* is the active enantiomer of metoprolol and is used at half the dose (12.5–50 mg OD or BD) of original metoprolol.

Bisoprolol

It is also a cardioselective β_1-receptor blocker, but without any intrinsic sympathomimetic activity. It is suitable for once daily administration in angina, hypertension, and CHF. Dose: 5–10 mg OD.

Nebivolol

It is also a highly cardioselective β_1-receptor blocker. Additionally, it also acts as NO donor and produces vasodilatation. Due to production of NO, it has also a potential to improve the function of vascular endothelium and delay the formation of atherosclerosis. Absence of deleterious effect on plasma lipids and on carbohydrate metabolism is another advantage. In contrast to other β_1-receptor blockers, nebivolol has rapid onset of action. Dose: 2.5–5 mg OD.

Esmolol

It is an ultra-short acting, selective β_1-receptor antagonist with little (if any) intrinsic sympathomimetic activity and without any membrane-stabilizing property. The beauty of esmolol is that it can be administered intravenously and is of very short duration of action. The half-life of esmolol is 8 minutes. The drug contains an ester linkage and is hydrolyzed rapidly by an enzyme, named esterase present in erythrocyte. The onset of action of esmolol is also very rapid, within 1–2 minutes. The peak hemodynamic effect of esmolol occurs within 6–10 minutes, after IV administration of a loading dose of it and the effect is substantially attenuated within 20 minutes of the stopping of infusion. Strikingly, the esmolol has hypotensive effect on normal individual, but the mechanism of this action is unclear. In urgent setting, where immediate reduction of BP is needed, a partial loading dose is administered which is followed by a continuous infusion of this drug. The half-life of carboxylic metabolites of esmolol is much higher than that of parent compound. So, it can accumulate after prolonged infusion. But, these metabolites have very low potency. Since, in urgent setting where immediate action is desired, esmolol is very helpful. The typical loading dose of esmolol is 0.5 mg/kg and for maintenance, the infusion dose is 0.05–0.2 mg/kg/min. Esmolol is mainly used to terminate supraventricular tachycardia, episodic atrial fibrillation, or flatter, arrhythmia during anesthesia, to prevent excessive adrenergic surge during laryngoscopy and intubation, and to decrease HR and BP during and after cardiac surgery and in early part of the treatment of MI.

Therapeutic Uses of β-blocker

The β-blockers are extensively used in the treatment of *hypertension, angina, acute MI, CHF and cardiac arrhythmias, hypertrophic obstructive cardiomyopathy, and dissecting aortic aneurysm*. The other uses of β-blocker are—*thyrotoxicosis, pheochromocytoma, anxiety, migraine, glaucoma, essential tremor*, etc. The detailed discussion of treatment of these diseases by β-blocker is not possible here.

Myocardial Infarction

The use of β-blocker in the treatment of acute MI and for the prevention of recurrence of MI has been well studied. It is confirmed that when the β-blockers are administered during the early phase of acute MI and are continued for long-term after recovery, then these may decrease the mortality by about 25%. The precise mechanism of it is still not known. But the favorable effects of β-blockers in the management of acute MI and its prophylaxis may arise from the decreased myocardial O_2 demand, redistribution of myocardial blood flow from nonischemic to ischemic area and its antiarrhythmic action. Thus, the β-blockers prevent sudden death from ventricular fibrillation during primary or subsequent attack of MI. However, there is likely much less beneficial effect, if the β-blockers are administered only

for a short period. So, the β-blockers should be used for prolong period in high-risk patients, except those who are not in shock, symptomatic cardiac failure, have heart rate <50 beats/min and with higher than first-degree heart block.

Congestive Heart Failure

It is a very common clinical understanding that β-blockers can worsen or precipitate the CHF in a compensated patient. On the other hand, from the mechanism of action, it is also clear that β-blocker might be effective in the treatment of heart failure. Again, it is clear that some but not all the β-blockers are beneficial in patient with mild-to-moderate heart failure. So, it is interesting to note how a class of a drug (β-blockers) can move from being completely contraindicated to being almost the standard of modern care in many heart failures. The proposed mechanism of beneficial effect of β-blockers in heart failure is that the catecholamines are toxic to heart and inhibitions of their effects through β_1-receptor pathway may help to preserve the myocardial function. Again, the β_1-receptor blocker in heart may attenuate cardiac remodeling, which might have deleterious effects on cardiac function. It also prevents the myocardial cell death caused by continuous activation of β-receptor by sympathetic overactivity in heart failure. Some β-blockers have α_1-antagonist properties and improve cardiac function by reducing the after load. So, the key point of the use of β-blocker in congestive cardiac failure (CCF) is that it should be started with very low doses and should be increased slowly over time, depending on each patient's response.

Arrhythmias

The β_1-blocker is also used in the treatment of arrhythmias. When arrhythmia is associated with hypertension, then α_1-receptor antagonist should be used before β-receptor antagonist. Otherwise, hypertension may be exacerbated, due to upper hand action of α-receptor (vasoconstriction) in the presence of β-receptor block. This exacerbation of hypertension is further because of the loss of β_2-receptor-mediated vasodilation due to their block.

Hypertension and Angina

All the β-blockers are relatively mild antihypertensives and are nearly equally effective. They are one of the drugs of first choice because of their good patient acceptability and cardioprotective potential. All the β-blockers benefit angina of effort (exertion angina). Taken on regular basis for prolonged period, they decrease the frequency of anginal attack and increase exercise tolerance. Higher doses, however, may worsen angina in some patients by increasing ventricular size ($\uparrow O_2$ demand) and reducing coronary flow ($\downarrow O_2$ supply).

Hypertrophic Obstructive Cardiomyopathy

Here, the subaortic left ventricular region of heart is hypertrophied. During systole, more forceful contraction of this region (due to hypertrophy) under sympathetic stimulation, such as during exercise and emotion, increases outflow resistance with severe decrease in CO and other bad hemodynamic consequences. The β-blockers by decreasing force of myocardial contraction reduce left ventricular outflow obstruction and improve CO during sympathetic stimulation. However, they have little effect at rest.

Dissecting Aortic Aneurysm

In such a grave situation, β-blocker (IV esmolol) helps by reducing cardiac contractile force and aortic pulsation. Nitroprusside infusion is often added with β-blocker.

There are many other therapeutic uses of β-blocker. But, there is no scope for discussion of these uses here.

Adverse Effects and Contraindications of β-blockers

- The β-blockers may precipitate or accentuate myocardial insufficiency, leading to CHF by blocking sympathetic support to the heart. When CHF sets on, then sympathetic system comes forward to compensate the failure by increasing CO. During that period, β-blockers may aggravate the failure by cutting down sympathetic compensation. However, when compensation has been restored, then careful addition of certain β_1-blocker is now established therapy to prolong survival.
- Resting heart rate may be reduced to 50 beats/min or less by β-blockers, leading to severe bradycardia. The patients of sick sinus are more prone to develop severe bradycardia.
- Nonselective β-blockers worsen chronic obstructive lung diseases. Even, they can precipitate life-threatening attack of bronchial asthma. The selective β_1-blockers are less likely to produce such situation. But, still all the β-blockers should be avoided in asthmatic and COPD patients.
- Carbohydrate tolerance may be impaired by β-blockers in prediabetic patients. For this purpose, the selective β_1-blockers are less harmful than nonselective β-blockers, because insulin secretion is augmented by β_2-receptor. In liver, the glycogenolysis is mediated by β_2-receptors, leading to the pouring out of glucose from liver during starvation or hypoglycemia, as compensatory mechanism. In diabetic patients who are taking β-blockers, this compensatory mechanism fails and they suffer from severe hypoglycemia. Further, tachycardia in response to hypoglycemia is blocked.
- Blood lipid profile is altered on long-term use of β-blockers (lipolysis is conducted by β_1 + β_2 + β_3 receptors). Total triglyceride and LDL-cholesterol level increases, while HDL-cholesterol level falls. As a result, the risks for coronary diseases increase. The cardioselective β_1-blockers, with their strong intrinsic sympathetic activity, have little or no deleterious effect on blood lipids.
- The β-blockers are completely contraindicated in any degree and any form of heart block, which are greater than first degree. Patients with pacemaker can take β-blockers, if indicated.
- The withdrawal of β-blockers, after their chronic use, should be gradual. Because, rebound hypertension, worsening angina, and even sudden death may occur. This is due to the development of supersensitivity of β-blockers, as a result of the long-term suppression of agonistic stimulation.
- Tiredness and reduced exercise capacity develop frequently after the continuous use of β-blockers. It is due to the blunting (reduction) of β_2-receptor-mediated increase in blood flow to the exercising muscles, as well as the attenuation of glycogenolysis and lipolysis in these muscles. The selective β_1-blockers are less likely to cause it. However, these selective β_1-blockers are ineffective in suppressing the essential tremor, which is mediated by β_2 action on muscle fibers.
- The β-blockers (even cardioselective) may exacerbate vasospastic (variant) angina, due to the unopposed α-mediated vasoconstriction of coronary arteries.
- Cold hands and feet, with the worsening of peripheral vascular diseases, are noticed due to the blockade of vasodilator β_2-receptors by nonselective β-blockers. Selective β_1-blockers are less likely to cause it and there is less chance of precipitating Raynaud's phenomenon.
- Patients often complain of nightmares, forgetfulness, and rarely hallucination after prolonged use of β-blockers. Males often complain of sexual distress.

■ HYDRALAZINE/DIHYDRALAZINE

The molecular structure of hydralazine is given in **Figure 9**. It causes greater decrease of diastolic than systolic BP. Because, it is a directly acting arteriolar vasodilator, but without any effect on capacitance vessels (veins) and coronary arteries. This hydralazine-induced arteriolar dilatation is associated with powerful stimulation of sympathetic nervous system, which causes tachycardia, increased myocardial contractility, increased plasma renin activity → increased aldosterone secretion → increased Na^+ and water retention. Although most of the increased sympathetic activity is due to baroreceptor-mediated reflex, caused by hydralazine-induced hypotension, still hydralazine itself may stimulate the release of norepinephrine from sympathetic nerve terminals and augments myocardial contractility directly. Thus, during the use of hydralazine, a hyperdynamic circulatory state is present, *which may precipitate angina.* There is no decrease in RBF by hydralazine, despite the fall in BP.

The sympathetic stimulation induced by hydralazine increases O_2 demand and precipitates myocardial ischemia. Hydralazine does not dilate the coronary arteries. On the contrary, coronary arteriolar dilation, produced by it, may cause steal effect on myocardial blood flow (drawing away blood from ischemic to nonischemic region). So, hydralazine is contraindicated in hypertensive patient with CAD and age >40 years. As it causes salt retention, hydralazine also may produce high-output CHF. Tolerance to the hypotensive action of hydralazine develops, unless diuretics and β-blockers are given individually or together which block the compensatory sympathetic stimulation mechanism.

Because of the preferential dilation of arterioles over veins, the postural hypotension is not a common problem of hydralazine. Although hydralazine reduces the pulmonary vascular resistance, still the greater increase in CO can cause mild pulmonary hypertension. The exact mechanism of arteriolar smooth muscle relaxation by hydralazine is still not known. The probable mechanism may involve the generation of NO and stimulation of cGMP.

Hydralazine is also well absorbed orally, but its oral bioavailability is low. The peak hypotensive effect of hydralazine occurs within 30–120 minutes after its oral ingestion and half-life is 1 hour. The chief metabolic pathway of hydralazine is acetylation in liver, which is genetically determined. So, half of the population metabolizes hydralazine rapidly (fast acetylators) and half of the population metabolizes it slowly (slow acetylators) in liver. Therefore, oral bioavailability of it is higher in slow acetylators. Though the half-life of hydralazine is 1 hour, still

its hypotensive effect lasts longer (12 hours). This is probably because of its persistent presence in the wall of vessels.

Two types of toxicity against hydralazine may develop. The first one is the extension of pharmacological effect of drug itself, which includes—hypotension, palpitation, angina, flushing, headache, etc. *The second one is the autoimmune. So, lupus erythematosus or rheumatoid arthritis-like syndrome may develop on prolonged use of hydralazine.* Serum sickness, hemolytic anemia, vasculitis, etc. also may develop and all these are immunological reactions. Other less serious adverse effects of hydralazine are—facial flushing, throbbing headache, palpitation, conjunctival injection, etc. and all these are due to vasodilatation. *Dose:* The dose of hydralazine is 25–50 mg orally, once or thrice daily. For hypertensive emergency, 10–20 mg hydralazine is given very slowly through IV route.

■ MINOXIDIL

The molecular structure of minoxidil is given in **Figure 10**. It is very effective in patient who is suffering from severe and some resistant forms of hypertension. Minoxidil itself is inactive *in vivo*. But, it is metabolized in liver to minoxidil-N-O-sulfate which is the active form of it. *Minoxidil sulfate, like hydralazine, is a very powerful arteriolar dilator, but has very little effect on venous capacitance vessels.*

The mechanism of action of minoxidil is like that it first activates the ATP-modulated K-channel → opening of K^+ channel in arteriolar smooth muscle → K^+ efflux → hyperpolarization → relaxation of arteriolar smooth muscles.

Like hydralazine, the marked arteriolar vasodilation by minoxidil elicits strong compensatory elevated adrenergic activity, causing tachycardia and increased myocardial contractility, with increased myocardial O_2 consumption. Thus, myocardial ischemia can be induced by minoxidil in patients with CAD. Like hydralazine, as minoxidil dilates the arteriolar site only, so it increases the venous return to the heart and simultaneously increases CO.

Minoxidil has complex effect on kidney. Though it dilates the renal vessels, but due to hypotension, the RBF is actually reduced. The marked arteriolar vasodilation by minoxidil elicits strong compensatory increased sympathetic reflexes

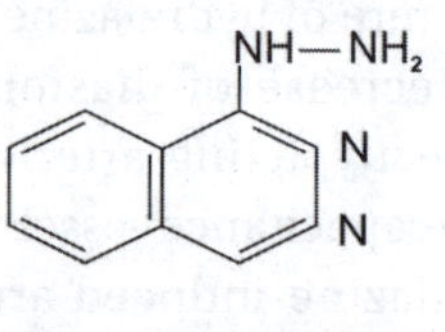

Fig. 9: Hydralazine.

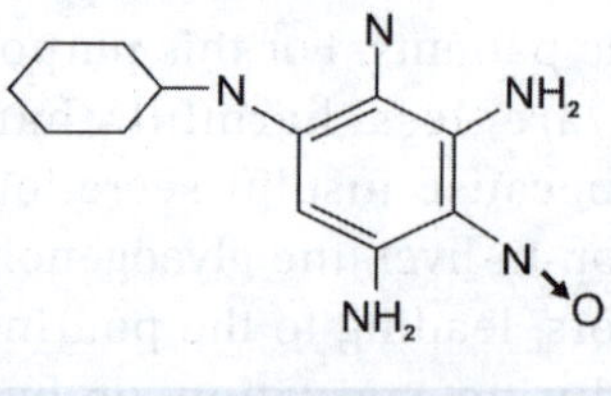

Fig. 10: Minoxidil.

(as said before). *Therefore, there are increased renin release → marked Na⁺ and water retention → edema and CHF may precipitate.* In case of minoxidil, the retention of salt and water is mainly secondary to reduced renal perfusion pressure and reflex stimulation of renal tubular α-adrenergic receptors. All these effects of minoxidil are like hydralazine and diazoxide. So, like hydralazine to offset these effects, it is always practically used along with any loop diuretics and β-blockers. Used in this manner, *it is effective even in severe hypertension, which is resistant to the combination of other drug.* Thus, the adverse effects of minoxidil are divided into three categories: (1) CVS effects, (2) salt and water retention, and (3) hypertrichosis.

Hypertrichosis occurs in all the patients who receive minoxidil for an extended period and is particularly offensive to female patients. It is due to potassium channel activation. The growth of hair occurs in face, back, arms, and legs. Minoxidil is absorbed very well from GI tract and peak concentration of it in blood occurs 1 hour after its oral administration. But, the maximum hypotensive effect of it occurs later, because this time is needed by liver to transform inactive minoxidil to its active form. Its half-life is 3–4 hours, but its action persists for 24 hours or more, as it accumulates in the wall of vessels. *Now, minoxidil is indicated only rarely in severe life-threatening hypertension, where other drugs fail to work.*

■ DIAZOXIDE

The chemical structure of diazoxide is shown in **Figure 11**. Like thiazide diuretics, chemically diazoxide is also a compound, derived from benzothiadiazine. But, it does not contain any diuretic effect, because it lacks the sulfonamide group. Only by IV injection, it promptly decreases the tone of smooth muscles of resistance vessels (arterioles), but without any effect on capacitance vessels (veins). *So, though nitroprusside is the drug of choice, but diazoxide is also used in the treatment of hypertensive emergency and had a definite place in some situations, where the accurate delivery of nitroprusside by infusions pump is not available and/or regulated IV infusion with close monitoring of BP is not possible.*

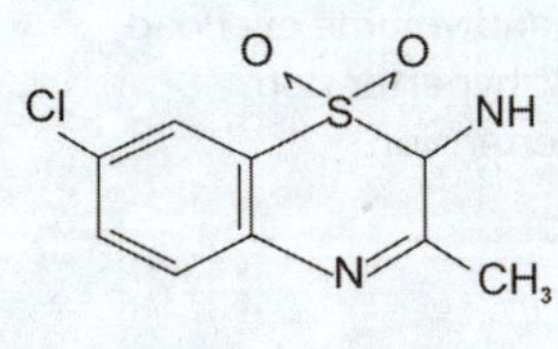

Fig. 11: Diazoxide.

Like minoxidil, it also causes the activation of ATP-sensitive K⁺ channel → increased influx of K⁺ into arterial smooth muscle cells → hyperpolarization of cells → relaxation of the smooth muscles of arterioles. It also produces the reflex activation of sympathetic nervous system and increases heart rate and myocardial contractility. Hence, it also increases CO. Sympathetic stimulation also causes → increase renin release → increased salt and water retention → increased level of angiotensin II. Thus, all these changes ultimately counteract the antihypertensive effect of diazoxide. Diazoxide increases the coronary blood flow. Renal and cerebral blood flow is maintained by autoregulation during diazoxide therapy.

Although well absorbed orally, still diazoxide is used only intravenously in the treatment of hypertensive emergency. The initial recommended dose of diazoxide is 300 mg IV in bolus. But, this bolus dose sometimes causes severe hypotension with resultant cerebral and cardiovascular damage. So, this hypotension can be prevented by the administration of diazoxide in mini bolus doses of 50–150 mg at intervals of 5–15 minutes, until the desired BP level is achieved. After IV bolus dose, the action of diazoxide starts within 30 seconds and maximum effect is achieved within 3–5 minutes. Diazoxide also can be given by slow intravenous infusion at a rate of 15–30 mg per minute.

The *most common side effects of diazoxide* are myocardial ischemia, salt and water retention, and hyperglycemia. This is because diazoxide inhibits insulin secretion from β-cells of pancreas. The myocardial ischemia, due to diazoxide, results from the reflex adrenergic stimulation of heart and the increased coronary flow to nonischemic regions (steal phenomenon). The salt and water retention by diazoxide also causes increased plasma volume and increased cardiac load. But, the routine use of diuretics with diazoxide in the management of hypertensive emergencies is not recommended, because these patients are frequently of volume depleted. The diazoxide solution is highly alkaline. So, pain and necrosis of tissues occur on extravasation.

It is partly metabolized and partly excreted unchanged through urine. Slow IV injection (infusion) of diazoxide is less effective because it binds tightly to plasma proteins, before bindings to the wall of vessels. The plasma half-life of diazoxide is 20–60 hours. The duration of hypotensive action of this drug is variable. It can be as short as 5 hours or as long as 20 hours.

■ DIURETICS

Diuretics are also called as *natriuretics*. They are defined as the drugs which facilitate the loss of Na⁺ and water through urine. However, with continuing their use (diuretic action), the Na⁺ balance in body is soon restored to some extent by compensatory homeostatic mechanisms. But, the ultimate result of their continued diuretic therapy is the small degree of definite Na^+ deficit and the greater degree of the reduction of extracellular fluid volume. Diuretics are mainly used for the management of hypertension, heart failure, and edema. However, the application of diuretics for the management of hypertension has outstripped their use in edema.

Classification of Diuretics

- *Diuretics with high efficacy (Na^+-K^+-$2Cl^-$ cotransporter inhibitors):* Furosemide, bumetanide, and torasemide
- *Diuretics with medium efficacy (Na^+-Cl^- symporter inhibitors):*
  - *Thiazides:* Hydrochlorothiazide, benzthiazide, hydroflumethiazide, and bendroflumethiazide
  - *Thiazide like:* Chlorthalidone, indapamide, clopamide, and xipamide
- *Diuretics with low efficacy:*
  - *K^+-sparing diuretics:*
    - *Aldosterone antagonists:* Spironolactone and eplerenone
    - *Renal epithelial Na^+ channel inhibitor:* Triamterene and amiloride
  - *Osmotic diuretics:* Mannitol and glycerol
  - *Carbonic anhydrase inhibitor:* Acetazolamide.

Furosemide

It is a Na^+-K^+-$2Cl^-$ symporter (cotransporter) inhibitor and acts on TAL of LOH. So, it is also called as the *loop diuretics*. Other diuretics in this group are bumetanide and torasemide. The diuretics acting on Na^+-K^+-$2Cl^-$ symporter at TAL (TAL of LOH) level are highly effective. So, they are often called as the high-ceiling diuretics. This is because: (1) as the 65% of glomerular filtrate is absorbed in PT, so the diuretics acting on PT have limited efficacy. The TAL reabsorbs most of the rejected materials from PT and has a large reserved reabsorptive capacity. So, the diuretics which act on TAL are highly effective. (2) The diuretics acting predominantly on post-TAL site have limited efficacy, because only a small percentage of filtered Na^+ load reaches the post-TAL site and does not possess the reserved reabsorptive capacity.

Mechanism of action furosemide: The Na^+-K^+-$2Cl^-$ cotransporters are a glycoprotein in nature with 12 membrane-spanning domains (units). It is only responsible for the influx (entry) of Na^+, K^+, and $2Cl^-$ ion from the lumen of renal tubule into the epithelial cell of TAL. These cotransporters capture free energy from Na^+ electrochemical gradient, which is established within the epithelial cells by the basolateral Na^+ pump (which extrude Na^+ from cell into the extracellular space) and provides an "uphill" for

the transport of K^+ and Cl^- along with Na^+ into the cell. The presence of K^+ channels on the luminal surface of tubular cell provides a pathway for recycling of K^+ between the cell and the lumen. Also, the presence of basolateral Cl^- channels provides a basolateral exit pathway for Cl^-. The movement of K^+ and Cl^- through their channels maintains an electrical gradient which is approximately 10 mV positive within the lumen, in respect to interstitial space. This positive potential difference repels the intraluminal cations such as Na^+, Ca^{2+}, and Mg^{2+} and thereby provides an important driving force for the paracellular flux of these cations into interstitial space.

Furosemide acts as inhibitors of Na^+-K^+-$2Cl^-$ cotransporter channels. It binds to the Cl^--binding site of these channels located on the transmembrane domain of the cotransporter and blocks the function of these cotransporters. Thus, it brings salt transport in this segment of nephron to standstill and causes diuresis. It prevents the reabsorption of 25% filtered load that is absorbed in TAL. The inhibitors of Na^+-K^+-$2Cl^-$ symporter also inhibit Ca^{2+} and Mg^{2+} reabsorption in TAL by abolishing the transepithelial potential difference, which is a dominant driving force for the reabsorption of these cations. Thus, furosemide also causes marked increases in the excretion of Ca^{2+} and Mg^{2+}. Furosemide has also weak carbonic anhydrase inhibiting activity and increases urinary excretion of HCO_3^-. It also increases the urinary excretion of K^+ due to the increased delivery of Na^+ load to the distal tubule (DT) (increased Na^+ load in the DT enhances the absorption of it and in exchange enhances the excretion of K^+ and H^+). However, K^+ loss by furosemide is less than that with thiazides diuretics. Increased HCO_3^- excretion may cause urinary pH to rise (alkaline). But, the predominant urinary anion is Cl^- whose excretion may increase in response to the action of furosemide. Acidosis does not develop by furosemide or causes minimum distortion of acid–base status. Mild alkalosis develops at high doses **(Box 4)**.

Furosemide tends to raise blood uric acid level by decreasing its renal excretion (increased reabsorption and decreased secretion). Increased uric acid reabsorption in PT is the consequence of volume depletion, caused by

---

BOX 4: Diuretics.

- *Especially suited for:*
  - Renal disease with Na^+ retention
  - Elderly, obese, and volume overload
  - Isolated systolic hypertension
  - Low-renin hypertension
  - Low cost
- *To be avoided:*
  - Gout, diabetic
  - Pregnancy-induced hypertension
  - Abnormal lipid profile

furosemide. However, reduced uric acid secretion is due to competition between the diuretics and uric acid for their secretion through same secretory mechanism in PT, as the furosemide is secreted at PT, passes down the lumen of the LOH, and acts on epithelial cells at TAL (thick ascending limb of LOH) from their luminal side. By blocking the active NaCl reabsorption in TAL, the inhibitors of Na^+-K^+-$2Cl^-$ cotransporter such as furosemide interfere with (impair) the critical step in the mechanism that produces a hypertonic medullary interstitial environment and prevents to concentrate the urine. RBF is transiently increased. There is redistribution of blood flow from outer to midcortical zone of kidney. Here, prostaglandin may be suspected as the cause. NSAID diminishes the diuretic response of loop diuretics, most likely by preventing the prostaglandin-mediated increase in RBF. GFR generally remains unaltered due to compensatory mechanism, despite increased RBF.

Furosemide also acutely increases systemic venous capacitance and, thereby, decreases the left ventricular filling volume and its pressure, even before diuresis ensues. This is responsible for quick relief of symptoms of LVF and pulmonary edema by furosemide. These actions also may be mediated by prostaglandin. Furosemide also causes hyperglycemia, but less marked than thiazides diuretics. It also causes hyperuricemia, which is lower than that of thiazide diuretics. The therapeutic uses of furosemide are— systemic edema, acute LVF, pulmonary edema, cerebral edema, forced diuresis, hypertension, hypercalcemia of malignancy, etc.

Pharmacokinetics of furosemide: Furosemide is rapidly absorbed orally. The bioavailability of furosemide through this route is about 60%. It is mainly excreted unchanged through urine. As it is extensively bound to plasma proteins, so the delivery of these drugs to the tubular cells by glomerular filtration is limited. On the other hand, for the action of furosemide, it should be effectively secreted by the organic acid transporter (OAT) system present on the epithelial cells of PT, and then it flows down through the tubular lumen with tubular fluid to gain the access to their binding sites on Na^+-K^+-$2Cl^-$ cotransporter system, present on the luminal membrane of TAL. It is partly conjugated with glucuronic acid in liver and is excreted through bile. The plasma half-life of furosemide is 1–2 hours.

Dose: Usually, furosemide is used in the dose of 20–80 mg, once daily at the morning orally. In pulmonary edema, 40–80 mg IV bolus may be given or according to the patient's response. In acute renal insufficiency, 200 mg 6 hourly may be given through IV route.

Toxicity, adverse effect, and contraindications: The adverse effects of furosemide are rare and are mostly due to fluid and electrolyte imbalance. So, the overzealous use of loop diuretics causes serious depletions of total body Na^+, resulting in hyponatremia, extracellular fluid depletion, hypotension, circulatory collapse, etc. Increased delivery of Na^+ load to DT from TAL (due to reduction of reabsorption in TAL), particularly when combined with activation of RAS, leads to increased urinary excretion of K^+ and H^+, causing a hypochloremic alkalosis. Increased Mg^{2+} and Ca^{2+} excretion may result in hypomagnesemia and hypocalcemia. Due to reduction of circulation, furosemide may precipitate thromboembolic episode and hepatic encephalopathy in patient with liver disease.

Furosemide can cause ototoxicity, tinnitus, hearing impairment, deafness, etc. It can also cause hyperuricemia (gout) and hyperglycemia. Other Na^+-K^+-$2Cl^-$ symporter inhibitors or loop diuretics are bumetanide and torasemide. But, individual discussion of these agents is not possible here and furosemide should be taken as their prototype.

Thiazide Diuretics

The primary site of action of these diuretics is the early DT. Here, they inhibit the Na^+-Cl^- symporter system at the luminal membrane of the epithelial cells of DT. These groups of drugs also like furosemide gain access to their site of action at DT, after their secretion from PT. After secretion through the organic secretory pathway in PT, they pass along the lumen of the LOH with tubular fluid and finally bind to their specific receptor site, i.e., Na^+-Cl^- symporter system, located on the luminal membrane of the epithelial cells of DT. Like the Na^+-K^+-$2Cl^-$ cotransporter system, the Na^+-Cl^- symporter system is also glycoprotein in nature, with 12 membrane-spanning domains (units). But, it (Na^+-Cl^- symporter) does not bind to furosemide or any other class of diuretics, except thiazides. Due to their action, Na^+ is not absorbed at the proximal part of DT. Hence, an increased amount of Na^+ is presented to the distal nephron, where it is reabsorbed in exchange with K^+ or H^+ (in absence of K^+ or in hypokalemia). So, the urinary excretion of K^+ or H^+ is also increased (alkalosis and hypokalemia) in parallel to the intensity of natriuretic effect of these groups of thiazide diuretics like furosemide. Nevertheless, they are moderately effective, because near about 90% of glomerular filtrate has already been absorbed in PT and LOH, before it reaches their site of action at the proximal of DT. They have a flat dose–response curve. Therefore, little additional diuretics occur, when the dose is increased beyond their maximum dose. They do not cause any significant alteration in acid–base balance of our body. They are not effective in patient with low GFR. They decrease the excretion of urate and Ca^{2+} by the same mechanism as furosemide and elevate blood sugar, due to the decreased release of insulin.

TABLE 8: Thiazide group of diuretics.

Drugs	Dose (daily, in mg)	Duration of action (hour)	Relative efficacy
Hydrochlorothiazide	12.5–100	10–12	2
Polythiazide	1–3	24–48	2.5
Benzthiazide	25–100	12–18	1.5
Hydroflumethiazide	5–100	12	1.5
Bendroflumethiazide	5–10	12	2
Chlorthalidone	50–100	48	2
Xipamide	20–40	24	1.5
Indapamide	2.5–5	24–36	1
Clopamide	10–60	12–18	2

All the thiazides and related drugs are well absorbed orally, and their action starts within 1 hour. The doses of different diuretics, their duration of action, and their relative efficacy are given in **Table 8**. Their duration of action is variable. The more lipid-soluble agents have larger volume of distribution, slower rates of tissue clearance, and therefore, are longer acting. Most of the thiazide agents undergo little hepatic metabolism and are excreted mainly through kidney as such. This is because they are filtered at glomerulus as well as secreted in the PT, like furosemide.

Thiazide diuretics are used mainly in the treatment of edema, hypertension, diabetes insipidus, and hypercalciuria (hypercalciuria means excess Ca^{2+} in urine). In contrast to furosemide, thiazides reduce excretion of Ca^{2+} through urine. Mild-to-moderate edema responses better by thiazides. For the mobilization of edema fluid, the more effective diuretics are employed initially, and thiazides are considered later for maintenance therapy. They are best for cardiac edema and less effective for hepatic or renal edema. They are not responsive in the presence of renal failure.

Most of the *adverse effects of thiazide group of drugs* are due to fluid and electrolyte changes caused by them. Among these, hypokalemia is the most significant problem. But, it is rare in low doses and short period of therapy. The consequence becomes grave, if the thiazide therapy is prolonged and the dietary K^+ intake is low. The hypokalemia associated with thiazide diuretics can be prevented by: (1) high dietary K^+ intake, (2) supplement of KCl (24–72 mEq/day), and (3) concurrent use of K^+-sparing diuretics. The last two measures are not routinely indicated, but only when the hypokalemia is documented or in special risk situations such as cardiac patients, cirrhosis, etc. Other adverse effects of thiazide diuretics are hyponatremia, hyperuricemia, hyperglycemia, hypercalcemia, etc.

There are multiple interactions among thiazides/other high-ceiling diuretics with other drugs. For example: (1) all thiazides, thiazide-related compounds, and high-ceiling diuretics potentiate all other antihypertensives. (2) Hypokalemia induced by these diuretics enhances digitalis toxicity. (3) High-ceiling diuretics and aminoglycoside antibiotics are both ototoxic and nephrotoxic → produce additive effect → should be used together cautiously. (4) Cotrimoxazole, given with diuretics, has caused higher incidence of thrombocytopenia. (5) Antihypertensive action of thiazides and furosemide is also diminished by NSAIDs. (6) Serum lithium level rises due to enhanced reabsorption of Li^+ (and Na^+) in PT.

Spironolactone

It is a K^+-sparing diuretic and is chemically related to aldosterone. Aldosterone acts on DT and CD by combining with a receptor, which promotes the reabsorption of Na^+ and excretion of K^+. Spironolactone acts on this receptor and inhibits the action of aldosterone in a competitive manner. Therefore, it antagonizes the reabsorption of Na^+ and excretion (loss) of K^+ induced by other diuretics. Spironolactone is a weak diuretic, because most of the Na^+ has already been reabsorbed proximal to its (spironolactone) site of action. The K^+-retaining action of spironolactone develops over 3–4 days after its administration. It also increases the excretion of Ca^{2+} by direct action on renal tubules.

The oral bioavailability of spironolactone is 80%. It is highly protein bound and completely metabolized in liver. As it is weak in diuretic action, so is used only in combination with other more strong diuretics. It is more effective in cirrhotic and nephrotic edema, because it breaks the resistance to thiazide diuretics that develop due to secondary hyperaldosteronism. Therefore, it is particularly employed in refractory edema. Given together with K^+ supplements, dangerous hyperkalemia can occur **(Table 9)**.

Eplerenone

It is a more selective and newer spironolactone-like aldosterone antagonist. But, unlike spironolactone, it has lower affinity for other steroid receptors. Therefore, eplerenone is much less likely to produce hormonal disturbances such as menstrual irregularities, gynecomastia, and impotence. Hence, these features of eplerenone make it particularly suitable for long-term use in the therapy of hypertension and chronic CHF. However, the risk of hyperkalemia and gastrointestinal symptoms, produced by eplerenone, are similar to that of spironolactone.

It is well absorbed orally. It is metabolized in liver and excreted through urine. Its half-life is near about

TABLE 9: Urinary excretion of electrolytes by some diuretics and their efficacy.

Diuretic	Na$^+$	K$^+$	Cl$^-$	HCO$_3^-$	Ca^{2+}	pH	Efficacy
Furosemide	+++	+	++	+	++	Alkalosis	High
Thiazide	++	+	+	+	−	Alkalosis	Intermediate
Spironolactone	+	−	+	±	++	Alkalosis	Low
Triamterene	+	−	+	±	−		Low
Mannitol	++	+	+	+	+	Acidosis	High
Acetazolamide	+	++	±	+		Acidosis	Mild

+ = increased, − = decreased

4–6 hours. Eplerenone is especially indicated for moderate-to-severe CHF, postinfarction left ventricular dysfunction, and hypertension.

Triamterene and Amiloride

The most important action of these two diuretics is to decrease the excretion of K$^+$ along with small increase in excretion of Na$^+$. Therefore, their action is similar to spironolactone, but independent of aldosterone. Their site of action is the luminal side of epithelial cells of late DT and CD. At this site of cells, there are some distinct Na$^+$ channels through which Na$^+$ enters the cell down its electrochemical gradient, generated by the Na$^+$-K$^+$-ATPase pump situated at the basolateral side of these epithelial cell membranes. This entry of Na$^+$ into the tubular cells from lumen promotes the secretion of K$^+$ into the lumen. Therefore, if there is more delivery of Na$^+$ to the distal nephron, then there will be more reabsorption of Na$^+$ and more excretion of K$^+$. Thus, all the diuretics acting proximally such as furosemide and thiazides decrease the reabsorption of Na$^+$ proximally and increase the load of Na$^+$ in DT and CD and so they increase the reabsorption of Na$^+$ and excretion of K$^+$ at the level of DT. Triamterene and amiloride act on these Na$^+$ channels on DT and CD, and block the reabsorption of Na$^+$ (diuresis) and reduce the excretion (loss) of K$^+$.

Both these diuretics are used in conjunction with thiazide or other high-ceiling diuretics to prevent hypokalemia. They should not be given with K$^+$ supplements, because dangerous hyperkalemia may develop. Triamterene is partly absorbed orally and largely metabolized in liver. Its duration of action is 6–8 hours. Amiloride is 10 times more potent than triamterene. It decreases the excretion of Ca^{2+} and increases the excretion of urate also. Thus, the hypercalcemic action of thiazides is augmented, but the hyperuricemic action of thiazide is partly annulled. It is partly absorbed orally, not metabolized in liver, and duration of action is 8–10 hours.

Mannitol

- *It is a nonelectrolyte osmotic diuretic with the following properties:*
  - Low-molecular weight (182)
  - Freely filtered at glomerulus
  - Limited reabsorption by renal tubule
  - Pharmacologically inert and minimally metabolize in our body
  - Extremely suitable for osmotic diuresis.
- *Mechanism and site of action of mannitol:* Mannitol acts both at PT and at the TAL of LOH (primary site of action). It mainly acts by—(1) increasing the osmolality of plasma, (2) increasing the osmolality of tubular fluid, and (3) reducing the tonicity of medulla. By the mechanisms of (2) and (3), it limits the tubular water and electrolyte reabsorption, leading to *osmotic diuresis.*

  Mannitol does not enter into the cell. Therefore, it extracts water from intracellular compartment and expands extracellular fluid volume. Thus, it increases the volume and blood, decreases the viscosity of blood, and inhibits renin release. All these effects cause increased RBF (both in cortex and medulla). Therefore, this increased renal medullary blood flow removes NaCl and urea from renal medulla and reduces medullary hypertonicity. Thus, the corticomedullary osmotic gradient is removed. So, there is decreased reabsorption of water from descending thin limb (DTL), causing the dilution of NaCl concentration in tubular fluid entering the ascending thin limb (ATL) and diminishes the reabsorption of NaCl with water in ATL. Thus, an osmotic diuresis sets up and this osmotic diuresis also inhibits the reabsorption of Mg^{2+} and Ca^{2+}. Osmotic diuretics increase urinary excretion of nearly all electrolytes, including Na$^+$, K$^+$, Ca^{2+}, Mg^{2+}, Cl$^-$, HCO$_3^-$, and phosphate.
- *Administration of mannitol:* Mannitol is not absorbed orally and is always given through IV as 10–20% solution. 80% of this drug is excreted as intact form by kidney. Next 20% is excreted after metabolism in liver or is excreted as

intact drug through bile. The plasma half-life of mannitol is 0.25–1.7 hours and in renal failure, it may rise up to 6–36 hours.

- *Adverse effects, indications for use, and contraindications:* As the mannitol does not enter the cell and is only distributed in extracellular (mainly intravascular) compartment, so water is extracted from interstitial compartment to intravascular compartment and then from intracellular compartment to interstitial compartment. Hence, the intravascular fluid volume is expanded. In a patient with incipient heart failure and pulmonary congestion, this *may cause frank pulmonary edema.*

Mannitol should never be used in the treatment of chronic edema or as natriuretic. Because, the loss of water in excess of electrolytes can cause hypernatremia and dehydration. Mannitol is used to maintain GFR and urine flow in impending renal failure, e.g., in shock, severe trauma, hemolytic reaction, cardiac surgery, etc. But, if acute renal failure (anuria) has already set in and kidney becomes incapable of forming urine, even after an initial osmotic load (test dose) by mannitol, then mannitol is *contraindicated* (who are unresponsive to test doses of this drug mannitol). In such circumstances, large plasma volume expansion by mannitol may precipitate pulmonary edema. Sometimes, 45% NaCl is as good as or better than either mannitol or furosemide for forced diuresis in protection against the acute tubular necrosis (ATN) which may lead to acute renal failure. It (mannitol) is not recommended to use repeatedly in case of nonresponders (no urine formation). Nowadays, the loop diuretic such as frusemide is more frequently used to convert oliguria to nonoliguria ATN than mannitol.

By increasing the osmotic pressure of plasma, mannitol extracts water from eye (aqueous humor) and CSF (brain). So, it is frequently used in acute attack of glaucoma and increased ICP (intracranial pressure), during both preoperatively or postoperatively to control IOP and acute rise in intracranial pressure, during head injury, stroke, etc. But, it should not be used in intracranial hemorrhage with an opened blood vessel. Because, in such situation, the mannitol present in the blood clot will draw water from brain tissue and will act as expanding space-occupying lesion.

Mannitol is sometimes used to counter the low osmolality of plasma or extracellular fluid, during rapid hemodialysis or peritoneal dialysis (dialysis disequilibrium). Mannitol, along with large volume of saline, was infused IV to produce "forced diuresis" in acute poisoning with the aim of enhancing excretion of poison. But, this is found ineffective and only causes dehydration and electrolyte imbalance. *Mannitol is contraindicated* in acute LVF (pulmonary edema), CHF, ATN, anuria, cerebral hemorrhage, etc. Hypersensitivity reaction to mannitol is very rare.

Acetazolamide

It is a compound, *derived from sulfonamide*, and is the prototype of a group of agents which have limited diuretic effect, but greatly help to draw a fundamental picture of renal physiology. When sulfonamides are used as chemotherapeutic agents, then they cause *metabolic acidosis* by inhibiting an enzyme named CAase (carbonic anhydrase). This leads to an enormous study and development of *acetazolamide* (sulfonamide derivative) as *carbonic anhydrase inhibitor.*

The main site of action of acetazolamide is the epithelial cells of PT, which are rich in CAase enzyme at their luminal side of cell membrane, basolateral side of cell membrane (type IV carbonic anhydrase), and in cytoplasm (type II carbonic anhydrase). Through the luminal side of cell membrane, Na^+ enters into the cell in exchange of H^+ ion, which is excreted into the tubular lumen by Na^+-H^+ antiporter system (also called Na^+-H^+ exchanger) by free of energy, available from Na^+ gradient, established by the basolateral Na^+-K^+-ATPase pump which extrudes Na^+ from the cell of PT into extracellular fluid and creates low concentration of Na^+ into the cell which further drives the entry of Na^+ from lumen into the cells of PT. Now, the H^+ in the lumen reacts with filtered HCO_3^- to from H_2CO_3, which rapidly breaks into CO_2 and H_2O by the help of CAase and is present at the brush border luminal side of cell membrane of proximal tubular cells. Due to lipophilicity, CO_2 rapidly diffuses into the proximal tubular cells and within the cell, this CO_2 again reacts with H_2O to form H_2CO_3 and subsequently HCO_3^- ion by the help of cytoplasmic carbonic anhydrase.

$$CAase$$
$$CO_2 + H_2O \leftrightarrow H_2CO_3$$

The continuous use of Na^+-H^+ antiporter system causes low H^+ concentration in the cell, which stimulates intracellular H_2CO_3 to ionize spontaneously to H^+ and HCO_3^-. The increased HCO_3^- concentration in the cell (simultaneously increased electrochemical gradient of HCO_3^-) is used by Na^+-HCO_3^- cotransporter system at the basolateral side of cell membrane to transport $NaHCO_3$ into the interstitial space. The net effect of this process is the transport of $NaHCO_3$ from the tubular lumen into the interstitial space, followed by the movement of water (isotonic reabsorption). Thus, the removal of water concentrates Cl^- in the tubular lumen and consequently the Cl^- diffuses into the interstitial space by its concentration gradient via paracellular pathway.

Acetazolamide, thus acting as carbonic anhydrase inhibitors at cell membrane and cytoplasmic level, reduces the availability of H^+ to exchange the luminal Na^+ by the Na^+-H^+ antiporter system and results in nearly complete abolition of $NaHCO_3$ reabsorption (*loss of HCO_3^-*) which ensues *alkaline diuresis.* The secretions of H^+ in DT and CD are also inhibited. Though, H^+ is secreted at these sites (DT and CD) by an H^+-ATPase pump (proton pump), it is generated in the cell by CAase-mediated reaction. Thus, this is a secondary site for the action of CAase inhibitor or acetazolamide. In the DT, the reabsorption of Na^+ takes place in exchange of the excretion of H^+ and K^+. In the absence of H^+, the K^+ is lost in excess to preserve Na^+, producing *hypokalemia.*

Among all the diuretics, acetazolamide causes the *most marked kaliuresis.* Urine produced under acetazolamide action is alkaline and rich in HCO_3^- which is matched by both Na^+ and K^+. The fractional excretion of Na^+ may be as much as 5% and the fractional excretion of K^+ can be as much as 70%. The inhibition of transport mechanism in PT results in increased delivery of Na^+ and Cl^- to the LOH, which has large reabsorptive capacity and captures most of the Cl^- and a portion of the Na^+.

The CAase inhibitors also increase the excretion of phosphate. The effects of acetazolamide on renal excretion are self-limiting. This is probably because, as gradually the metabolic acidosis is developed, then the filtered load of HCO_3^- decreases to the point that the uncatalyzed reaction (reaction without the help of CAase enzyme) between CO_2 and water is sufficient to achieve HCO_3^- reabsorption and then there is no loss of HCO_3^-, no metabolic acidosis, no diuresis.

Extrarenal actions of acetazolamide:
- Other extrarenal tissues such as eye, gastric mucosa, RBC, and CNS are also rich in CAase. Ciliary process of eye is responsible for the formation of aqueous humor by the help of CAase. Acetazolamide, thus inhibiting CAase, reduces the formation of aqueous humor and ↓ intraocular tension.
- CAase inhibitors also decrease gastric HCl and pancreatic $NaHCO_3$ secretion but need very high dose. So, it is not applicable therapeutically for the management of peptic ulcer.
- Due to interference with carbonic anhydrase activity in RBC, acetazolamide increases CO_2 levels in peripheral tissues and decreases CO_2 excretion by lungs.
- Acetazolamide causes increased level of CO and decreased level of pH in brain, leading to sedation and elevation of seizure threshold.

The oral bioavailability of acetazolamide is 100%. The plasma half-life of it is 6–9 hours and is excreted unchanged through urine. The adverse effects of it are very infrequent like other sulfonamides. It may cause bone marrow depression and skin (allergic) reaction in patients who are hypersensitive

to sulfonamides. The adverse effects of acetazolamide are mainly due to the secondary effects of urinary alkalization and metabolic acidosis. So, there is a chance of precipitation of salt of calcium phosphate in alkaline urine and calculus formation. It also causes the worsening of metabolic and respiratory acidosis. Thus, it is contraindicated in COPD patient. Precipitation of hepatic coma by interfering with urinary elimination of NH_3 (due to alkaline urine) may also occur.

The therapeutic uses of acetazolamide are—glaucoma, alkalization of urine for urinary tract infection, acute mountain sickness (only as prophylactic), etc. The probable mechanism of action is by producing metabolic acidosis, or indirectly correcting a metabolic alkalosis, especially caused by decreased excretion of H^+ ion through urine.

■ ANESTHESIA IN HYPERTENSIVE PATIENT

Perioperative management of patients with essential hypertension, scheduled for both the elective and emergency surgeries, is same, i.e., to maintain an appropriately stable range of BP. Patients with border hypertension may be treated as normotensive patients. Those with longstanding or poorly controlled hypertension have an altered autoregulation for CBF, where higher than normal MAP is required to maintain adequate CBF. The MAP should not be reduced >20% of its preoperative value.

During perioperative management of patient suffering from hypertension, it should be kept in mind that the raised intra-arterial pressure is either due to essential hypertension or secondary hypertension, associated with the following conditions, such as renal disease, coarctation of aorta, pheochromocytoma, and Cushing's disease. A severe intraoperative uncontrolled rise in BP is particularly dangerous and may cause cerebrovascular injury, myocardial ischemia, or LVF with pulmonary edema. If the intramural coronary arteries have been affected previously by the atheromatous process, the raised diastolic pressure may jeopardize the myocardial blood flow especially in the subendocardial region and produce ischemic changes in ECG that is performed for monitoring during the whole perioperative period. Decrease of workload on the ventricle by lowering the SVR may relief the failure and restore an adequate myocardial blood flow with reversal of the ECG changes.

Drugs that effectively control the systemic BP in treated individual should be continued throughout the perioperative period. In general, hypertensive patients where BP is not controlled preoperatively should not be scheduled for outpatient or ambulatory (day-case) surgery under general anesthesia because of their tendency to hemodynamic fluctuation.

Preoperative Evaluation of Hypertensive Patient

The aim of preoperative evaluation of patient suffering from hypertension is to determine the adequacy of control of systemic BP. It is very general concept that hypertensive patient should be treated to normotensive before undergoing elective surgery. The point behind this concept is that the incidence of hypertensive emergencies, myocardial ischemia, and other complications is increased in patients who remain hypertensive or not controlled prior to the induction of anesthesia, although the increase in BP during intraoperative period occurs regardless of the degree of preoperative control of BP. On the other hand, it is also evidenced that there is no increased incidence of perioperative complications when hypertensive patients with diastolic pressure as high as 110 mm Hg undergo elective operations, provided there is stringent perioperative control of BP. Therefore, from the above two statements, it is clear that whatever may be the preoperative status of patient regarding the systemic BP, i.e., controlled or uncontrolled, it is the stringent immediate perioperative control of BP which is most important.

Pressure obtained in the hospital setting may not represent patient's usual levels. But, high BP during the admission of a hypertensive patient, who was previously treated and controlled, clearly can predict larger possible fluctuation of it (BP) intraoperatively. It is also very common that BP increases during admission in hospital due to patient's anxiety. This is called "white coat syndrome" and this group of patients also displays exaggerated pressure responses to direct laryngoscopy during tracheal intubation and surgical stimuli during intraoperative period.

The presence of end-organ disease, due to longstanding hypertension, should be evaluated preoperatively by different investigations, e.g., ECG, renal function test, echocardiography, etc. Among them, the most important is the investigation for CAD. ECG for hypertensive patient with LVH, intraventricular conduction blocks, or repolarization abnormality should also be considered. Echocardiogram is more sensitive and informative than 12-lead ECG for the diagnosis of LVH. Previous history of infarction has great significance. Essential hypertension is associated with the shifts of autoregulation curve of CBF to the right. This shift suggests that CBF is more dependent on perfusion pressure in hypertensive patient than in normotensive patient. Urgent revaluation and treatment of hypertension are necessary for patients with presence of fundal hemorrhage, exudates, and particularly papilledema on examination of the optic fundus.

Antihypertensive drugs used in the preoperative management usually do not alter the course and the conduct of anesthesia. But, the abrupt discontinuation of antihypertensive drugs immediately in pre- or postoperative period causes rebound hypertension. This may be another cause for the continuation of antihypertensive drugs during the whole perioperative period. Despite the acceptance of the concept that antihypertensive drug therapy should be continued throughout the perioperative period to reduce the morbidity and mortality, there is still risk that hemodynamic instability and hypertension or hypotension may occur during anesthesia. During the anesthesia of a hypertensive patient, the exaggerated decrease in BP, which is sometimes associated with increase in blood loss, excessive positive airway pressure, or sudden change in body position, could reflect the impaired compensatory peripheral vasoconstriction due to inhibitory effect of antihypertensive drugs on the sympathetic nervous system.

Induction of Anesthesia

There is a general agreement that all the hypertensive patients should receive an oral anxiolytic agent (e.g., benzodiazepine) in addition to their normal morning doses of antihypertensive drugs as a preoperative medication, before the induction of anesthesia. The induction of anesthesia and ET intubation are often associated with hemodynamic instability in hypertensive patients. Regardless of the level of preoperative BP control, many patients with hypertension display an accentuated hypotensive response to induction of anesthesia, followed by an exaggerated hypertensive response to intubation. Many, if not most, antihypertensive agents and general anesthetic agents are vasodilators, cardiac depressants, or both. In addition, many hypertensive patients present for surgery in a volume-depleted state. Sympatholytic agents attenuate the normal protective circulatory reflexes, reducing sympathetic tone, and unmasking vagal activity.

There is also little evidence that any particular inducing agent or technique is better than other during the induction of a hypertensive patient. Still, it should be kept in mind that the *etomidate* has the lowest cardiovascular effects, but thiopental is acceptable, if it is administered carefully. Propofol may produce excessive hypotension in hypertensive patient. The induction of anesthesia with rapidly acting intravenous drug is the standard practice for hypertensive patient, but keeping in mind that exaggerated decrease in BP may occur and this is due to excessive peripheral vasodilatation. This is because all the inducing agents cause widespread venodilatation causing a large decrease in venous return and CO, but a minor decrease in SVR. Ketamine is contraindicated as inducing agent in hypertensive patient.

Direct laryngoscopy and tracheal intubation are associated with exaggerated increase in BP and tachycardia for patients suffering from hypertension. This occurs even if these patients are treated with antihypertensive drugs and rendered normotensive preoperatively. Because, the hypertensive patients usually cause a greater increase in plasma catecholamine concentrations than normotensives, during laryngoscopy and intubation. And, it is also true that the intravenous inducing agents cannot adequately and predictably suppress the responses evoked by tracheal intubation.

This hemodynamic response evoked during laryngoscopy and intubation can be attenuated adequately by:

- Increasing the concentration of inhaled volatile anesthetic agents
- Using adequate bolus dose of IV opioids prior to initiating laryngoscopy and intubation. Intravenous opioid administration should be timed, so that peak effects of the opioids are predictably matched with the stimulus of laryngoscopy and intubation.
- Topical laryngotracheal administration of lignocaine, immediately prior to intubation.
- Administering lignocaine IV in the dose of 1.5 mg/kg about 1 minute before induction and intubation.
- Using nitroprusside 1–2 µg/kg/min through IV just before laryngoscopy.
- Using esmolol 100–200 mg through IV.

As the hemodynamic response is primarily from sympathoadrenal axis against a noxious stimulus, so it is most logical to use either opioids or β-adrenoreceptor antagonists to suppress the hemodynamics response and decrease the incidence of arrhythmias and myocardial ischemia during and after intubation. Excessive autonomic activity may also be avoided when local anesthetic techniques are employed as an adjunct to GA.

Regardless of the drugs that are used to blunt the circulatory effect of laryngoscopy and intubation, it is generally appreciated that excessive depressant effect of drugs producing hypotension during attempts to blunt or reduce the circulatory effect is more undesirable than the transient hypertension effect produced by direct laryngoscopy and tracheal intubation.

Monitoring during Anesthesia of a Hypertensive Patient

Most hypertensive patients do not require any special intraoperative monitors. Direct intra-arterial pressure monitoring should be reserved for patients with wide swings in BP and those undergoing major surgical procedures, associated with rapid or marked change in cardiac preload or afterload. ECG monitoring should focus on detecting the signs of ischemia and arrhythmia. Urinary output should generally be monitored with an indwelling urinary catheter in patients with pre-existing kidney impairment who are undergoing procedures expected to last >2 hours. Ventricular compliance is typically reduced in patients with ventricular hypertrophy. Excessive intravenous fluid administration in patients with decreased ventricular compliance can also result in elevated pulmonary arterial pressure and pulmonary congestion.

Maintenance of Anesthesia of a Hypertensive Patient

Anesthesia may safely be maintained with volatile or intravenous agents. Regardless of primary maintenance technique, the addition of a volatile agent or intravenous vasodilator generally allows a convenient intraoperative BP control. There is no evidence that any anesthetic technique is better than others in hypertensive patient. However, also no limits for the deviation of arterial pressure have been proven to be safe. But, the deviation not >20% from preoperative MAP value is generally accepted. The goal during the maintenance of anesthesia in a hypertensive patient is to adjust the depth of anesthesia and to minimize the wide fluctuations of BP. Indeed, the control of perioperative BP fluctuation with different anesthetic techniques and agents is more important than the preoperative control of hypertension. So, an anesthetist should be trained enough in controlling the perioperative fluctuation of BP than controlling the preoperative BP, before conducting anesthesia on a hypertensive patient.

Chronic hypertension is usually associated with hypovolemia and IHD. Regional anesthesia is an acceptable alternative method for hypertensive patient. But, it should be kept in mind that the sympathetic denervation, proved by RA, may unmask the unsuspected hypovolemia (if present) and cause severe hypotension, which may result in myocardial ischemia. The untreated or poorly controlled hypertensive patient may suffer with greater decrease in BP and abrupt or dangerous bradycardia. The combination of α- and β-adrenoreceptor agonist or a vagolytic drug combined with α-adrenoreceptor agonist is better than α1-adrenoreceptor agonist alone for treating the hypotension after RA.

The intraoperative increase in BP is mainly due to sympathetic stimulation, caused by painful surgical stimuli. The incidence of intraoperative hypertensive episodes is high in patients with history of essential hypertension. This is also evident even in patients who were previously rendered normotensive by drug therapy. Volatile anesthetics are important agents to decrease this sympathetic overactivity, which is responsible for intraoperative pressure response. It acts in dose-depended manner by decreasing SVR and to a lesser extent by decreasing the force of cardiac contraction and CO. There is no evidence that one volatile anesthetic agent is better than another in that respect. The poor blood solubility of desflurane and sevoflurane, compared with that of isoflurane and halothane, may permit more rapid changes in their alveolar concentration and hence the depth of anesthesia with good control of BP. Intraoperative nitroprusside by infusion pump is a very good way of maintaining normotension in a hypertensive patient. There is no evidence that a specific muscle relaxant is better than another for intraoperative management of patient with hypertension. Pancuronium is not absolutely contraindicated in anesthesia of a hypertensive patient, but somebody avoids it in severe hypertension.

Hypotension often occurs during intraoperative control of high BP. This hypotension can be treated by decreasing the concentration of delivered volatile anesthetic agents and decreasing the dose of antihypertensive drugs which are using intraoperatively. Intraoperative hypotension may be caused by a low circulating blood volume (in hypertensive patient blood volume is low). So, a marked fall in arterial pressure may be produced by only a modest blood loss. The assessment of blood and other intravenous fluid requirements should be made from present circulatory status, rather than by relying solely on the eye estimation of volume of blood loss. Measurement of pulmonary wedge pressure is of particular value in assessing intravenous fluid requirements in some patients with diseased left ventricle. Sometimes, sympathomimetic drugs can be used to restore the minimum perfusion pressure in vital organ. The response to sympathomimetic drugs should be both appropriate and predictable and can be titrated with hypotension. But care must be taken when vasopressor drugs are administered because they can interact with some antihypertensive agents.

Intraoperative monitoring of a hypertensive patient depends on the patient's condition and the complexity of surgery. The monitoring can extend from simple manual BP monitoring to intra-arterial BP monitoring to automatic noninvasive blood pressure (NIBP), ECG, pulse oximeter, capnography, PAWP, transesophageal echocardiography, etc. Intraoperative myocardial ischemia is usually evident from the conventional 12-lead ECG. But in some instances, only one lead can be monitored during anesthesia and intensive therapy. In such situation, the CM_5 bipolar lead would appear to be the best to show ischemia changes in ST segment and give a good demonstration of P-wave and QRS complex. In this lead, the reference electrode (right arm lead) is placed over the manubrium of sternum. The exploring electrode (left arm lead) is placed on V_5 position and the earthing wire or electrode (right lower limb lead) may conveniently be placed on left shoulder. The ECG may then be displayed by selecting lead I position.

Management of Intraoperative Hypertension

Intraoperative hypertension, not responding to an increase in anesthetic depth, by increasing the doses of volatile anesthetic agents, opioids, etc., can be treated with a variety of parenteral agents. The common causes of intraoperative hypertension, such as hypoxemia, hypercapnia, and inadequate anesthetic depth, should always be excluded before initiating antihypertensive therapy. The selection of hypotensive agent depends on the severity, acuteness, presence or absence of tachycardia, baseline ventricular function, presence or absence of asthmatic pulmonary disease, and cause of hypertension. The β-adrenergic blockers, such as labetalol, esmolol, and metoprolol, alone or as a supplement to other hypotensive agent are good choice for a patient with good ventricular function and elevated heart rate. But, they are relatively contraindicated for patients with reactive airway diseases. In such cases, the CCBs such as Nicardipine or Clevidipine are preferred. Nitroprusside is the most rapid and effective agent for the intraoperative management of severe hypertension. Nitroglycerin is also useful, but less effective than nitroprusside, in treating severe intraoperative hypertension in the presence of IHD. Fenoldopam, a dopaminergic agonist, is also a useful agent for controlling intraoperative hypertension. Furthermore, it increases the RBF. Hydralazine provides sustained BP control, but its onset of action is not so fast like nitroprusside or nitroglycerin and causes reflex tachycardia. Reflex tachycardia is not seen with labetalol, as it has both α- and β-adrenergic blocking effect.

Postoperative Management

Extubation under light plane of anesthesia or allowing the patient to cough on the tube during extubation can provoke a marked sympathomimetic response with undesirable tachycardia and hypertension. So, extubation should be done under adequate or deep plane of anesthesia.

Hypertensive patient usually responds with elevated BP during early postoperative period. It is usually due to exaggerated sympathetic activity due to postoperative pain. So, postoperative elevation of BP needs prompt assessment and treatment of postoperative pain to decrease the risk of myocardial ischemia, cardiac arrhythmias, LVF, stroke, postoperative bleeding, etc., which may also be seen in postoperative period. When the intraoperative analgesia derived from the N_2O or opiates or others is worn off, the resultant increase in sympathetic activity due to pain can cause a marked rise in systemic BP and thereby heart failure. In addition, sometimes the intraoperative tendency toward pulmonary edema may have been masked by intermittent positive pressure ventilation (IPPV) because of the raised intra-alveolar pressure. So, on return to the spontaneous ventilation, the LVF and pulmonary edema may then become apparent and result in early postoperative collapse.

The postoperative BP control can be done by the agents, which are also used during the intraoperative period such as analgesics, GTN, nitroprusside, labetalol, hydralazine, etc. NSAIDs, though effective as postoperative analgesics, are one of the most common causes of acute renal failure. So, care should be taken in their use in hypertensive patients who are possibly at the risk of renal dysfunction. The use of vasodilator drugs to treat the patient with high systolic BP and normal diastolic pressure is not usually indicated.

If hypertension must be treated and controlled in hypertensive patient before operation:

Till now, it is the most debatable question, because a number of studies have failed to show that hypertension is an independent perioperative risk factor. The questions that center around are:

- Does adequate control of preoperative hypertension could prevent perioperative complications?
- How much preoperative control of BP is needed?
- Should elective surgery be postponed due to preoperative elevated BP, so that treatment can be instituted for hypertension and patient can be optimized?

Now, several schools of thoughts exist and several studies have been carried out. But, unfortunately all the studies have failed to establish a definite answer. Prys–Robert's school believes that the preoperative management of hypertension lowers the incidence of perioperative morbidity and mortality. But others do not. Patients with atherosclerotic disease who present with raised systolic pressure, but normal or low diastolic pressure, should not be considered as true hypertensive and should not have their surgery delayed (Prys–Robert–Brown).

Postponement of surgery due to hypertension is only necessary when there is an indication that the patient will benefit certainly from introducing antihypertensive therapy or modification of existing therapy (Prys–Robert–Brown). Only patients with severe hypertension with clear evidence of end-organ damage need postponement of surgery for

further work-up and treatment for optimization unless minor surgery is planned (Prys–Robert–Brown).

The school represented by Goldman and Caldera views that the perioperative management of patients presenting with untreated hypertension depends upon the level of the diastolic BP and the surgical circumstances. For elective surgery, if the diastolic pressure does not exceed 110 mm Hg, there is no evidence of increased cardiac and CNS complications. Patients with persistent diastolic BP above this level should be referred to a physician for treatment. The occurrence of severe untreated hypertension (a diastolic pressure >130 mm Hg) in the perioperative period is known to be associated with an increased morbidity and mortality.

Bedford, Feinstein, Wolfsthal, and their supporters believe that fluctuation of BP is the condition which is most frequently predicts the rate of perioperative complications. So, according to their opinion by careful titration, the fine control of perioperative BP is more important than only the preoperative treatment of hypertension. Despite the desire to render the patients normotensive before elective surgery, there is no evidence that the incidence of perioperative complication increases if fine control of BP is done when hypertensive patients (diastolic BP as high as 110 mm Hg) undergo elective operations (RK Stoelting and SF Dierdorf).

■ CONCLUSION

Although preoperative BP has been thought to be a significant predictor of the perioperative morbidity and mortality, no data establish definitely whether the preoperative control of hypertension reduces the perioperative risk. Preoperative treatment of patient suffering from hypertension is based on the following concepts that: (1) patient should be educated regarding the importance of hypertension and its management which usually extends postoperatively and life-long; (2) incidence of perioperative hemodynamic fluctuations is less in treated than untreated group; and (3) hemodynamic fluctuation has definitive relationship to morbidity.

The main aim of preoperative management of hypertensive patient is to search for end-organ damage secondary to hypertension, i.e., changes in CNS, coronary arteries, myocardium, aorta, kidneys, peripheral blood vessels, etc., and modulations of anesthetic management accordingly.

Heart Failure and Its Pharmacology

■ INTRODUCTION

The term *"myocardial failure"* is better than the term *"heart failure".* On the other hand, *"heart failure"* is, though an unimpressive term, still most commonly used. *It is a pathophysiological state in which, due to some abnormality of cardiac function, myocardium fails to pump out blood at a rate corresponding to the requirement of metabolizing tissue, and/or can do so (in compensated stage) at the expense of an elevated filling pressure from an abnormally elevated diastolic volume.* This failure of the myocardium to pump out the required amount of blood, which is needed for our body at that moment, may be due to *primary causes*, where the myocardium itself is responsible, or may be due to *secondary causes*, where the myocardium itself is not diseased [e.g., sudden increase of blood pressure (BP), pulmonary diseases, valvular diseases, arrhythmia].

In primary causes, the abnormalities of the heart muscle may be due to (1) cardiomyopathies, (2) viral myocarditis, (3) myocardial ischemia, (4) infarction, or (5) abnormalities of heart valves where the heart muscle has been damaged due to long-standing hemodynamic burden. But, in secondary causes, there is no such detectable abnormality of myocardial function. In such circumstances, the normal heart is suddenly presented with an excessive mechanical load that exceeds its capacity. Secondary heart failure may also occur without any excessive load on myocardial function, but there is chronic impairment of ventricular filling during diastole due to some mechanical abnormalities, such as tricuspid stenosis, constrictive pericarditis, and endocardial fibrosis, which causes the failure to pump out an adequate amount of blood by heart according to the requirement of metabolizing tissue.

However, in most patients, the combination of impaired myocardial function (or primary heart failure) and mechanical abnormality (or secondary heart failure) both coexist because like a vicious cycle, they affect each other. For example, in one form, such as with volume overload, when the myocardium of the ventricle, without any pathology, is called on to deliver an elevated cardiac output for prolonged periods (secondary failure), then it gradually develops myocardial pathology, leading to primary failure. Similarly, systolic and diastolic failure (discussed later) affect each other and run in a vicious cycle.

In the mildest form of heart failure, the cardiac output is adequate at rest but becomes inadequate and is manifested only when the metabolic demand is increased, such as during exercise or some other form of stress. In practice, heart failure or myocardial failure may be diagnosed whenever a patient with significant heart disease develops the signs and symptoms of low cardiac output, pulmonary congestion, or systemic venous congestion.

In summary, the causes of heart failure can be grouped under two headings:

1. *Underlying or primary causes:* Here, the pathology is within the heart muscle itself, e.g., coronary heart disease (CHD), long-standing valvular lesion, ischemia, infarction, myocarditis, arrhythmias.
2. *Precipitating or secondary causes:* Here, the pathology is not within the heart muscle itself but away from it, such as systemic hypertension, fluid overload, anemia, and thyrotoxicosis.

In the presence of different underlying causes of heart failure, initially, the heart usually remains in a *compensated stage* with little additional reserve. So, later, the additional load imposed by precipitating or secondary causes results in further deterioration of cardiac reserve and is manifested as frank or overt failure when this reserve is completely exhausted. In the absence of underlying primary causes, if the secondary factors become acute, then the heart may also undergo failure. Therefore, the identification of such precipitating causes is of very clinical importance because their prompt alleviation may be lifesaving.

In the absence of an underlying primary heart disease, the precipitating or secondary factors by themselves usually do not lead to heart failure, except in an acute stage. Examples of some precipitating factors are anemia, infection, pregnancy, thyrotoxicosis, emotion, physical exertion, fluid excess, pulmonary embolism, hypertension, etc. Precipitating causes of heart failure should also be recognized and treated more effectively than the underlying causes because, the prognosis of heart failure, where a precipitating cause can be identified, treated, and eliminated, is more favorable than it is in the patient in whom the underlying disease process is advanced enough to the point of producing heart failure. The primary and secondary causes of heart failure are given in **Table 1**.

■ TYPES OF HEART FAILURE

The different types of heart failures are classified under different headings. But this different classification of heart failure under different headings is only useful in its early pathophysiological course. Because, late in the course of failure, these differences between them often become blurred. The classifications are given in the following text.

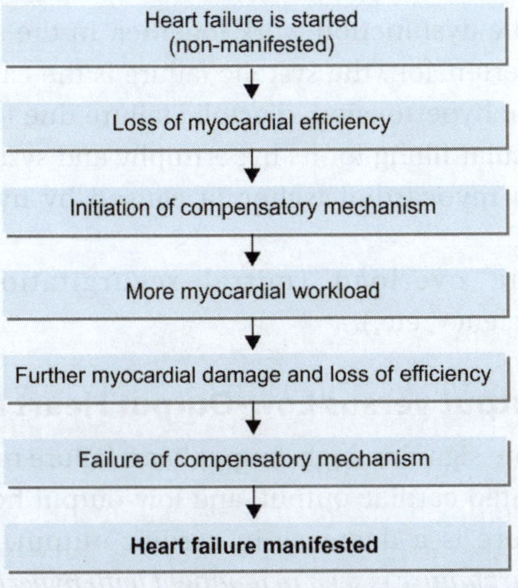

Acute versus Chronic Heart Failure

These two broad classifications of heart failure depend on the suddenness of the onset or the rate of development of it. With this, the causative factors for their development and the effects of these two types of failure are also different. Acute heart failure develops instantaneously within hours to a few days, *without giving any time for any compensatory mechanism to develop*. But chronic heart failure takes weeks or months to develop *with full-blown compensatory pictures*.

The main causative factor of acute heart failure is *acute coronary arterial occlusion* with infarction and/or *arrhythmia*. The other etiologies of acute heart failure are *pulmonary embolism, acute toxic myocarditis, acute rise of BP (malignant hypertension)*, etc. On the other hand, chronic heart failure is the consequence of *chronic hypertension, chronic valvular diseases, chronic lung diseases, chronic anemia, myocardial fibrosis, etc*. In acute conditions, the system does not get enough time for the compensatory mechanism to develop. So, the patient suddenly presents with acute symptoms and signs of heart failure without any hypertrophy of myocardium, dilatation of cardiac chambers, systemic edema, etc., which are found as compensatory mechanisms whereas in chronic heart failure, the compensatory mechanism has got time to develop with full force. So, there is always the presence of myocardial hypertrophy of atriums and/or ventricles, dilatation of cardiac chambers, chronic systemic venous congestion, edema, etc.

Actually, acute and chronic heart failure are two opposite ends of a spectrum of a single disease. But they merge with one another by treatment procedures or natural compensatory processes, which is shown in **Figure 1**.

Systolic versus Diastolic Heart Failure

In systolic heart failure, there is impairment of myocardial contractile function during systole, leading to the reduction in stroke volume, inadequate ventricular emptying, and gradual cardiac dilation. There is no abnormality

TABLE 1: Causes of heart failure.	
Primary	*Secondary*

Diseases primarily affecting the myocardium
Causes:
• Ischemic heart disease: Most common and very serious disease of the heart. It leads to myocardial damage, fibrosis, or infarction
• Inflammation and toxic degeneration of myocardium—myocarditis
• Infiltration of myocardium fatty infiltration, amyloidosis, etc.
• Cardiomyopathies:
  – Primary
  – Secondary due to beriberi, alcoholism, thyroid abnormality, etc.
	Diseases of other cardiac and circulatory components except myocardium leading to secondarily myocardial failure
	Causes:
	• Defects in the control mechanism of the heart, e.g.,
	  – Valvular heart diseases
	  – Cardiac arrhythmias
	• Defects in circulatory components, e.g.,
	  – Systemic hypertension
	  – Chronic lung diseases causing pulmonary hypertension. Both systemic hypertension and chronic lung diseases cause increased cardiac workload

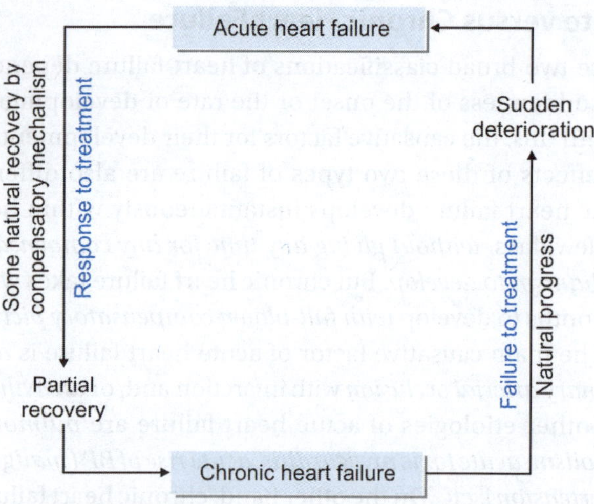

Fig. 1: Acute versus chronic heart failure.

of venous return and ventricular filling during the diastolic period of cardiac cycle (preload). *A decreased ejection fraction with normal preload*, diagnosed by an EDV within normal limit, is the hallmark of ventricular systolic failure. So, measuring the ventricular ejection fraction via echocardiography provides the quantification of the severity of ventricular systolic function. An ejection fraction of <0.45 (45%) is often viewed as evidence of ventricular systolic dysfunction. Examples of systolic heart failure are *ischemic heart disease (IHD), cardiomyopathy, myocarditis, etc.* In IHD, there is gradual loss of the number of myocytes, leading to localized defects in ventricular wall motion and impaired systolic contraction. Myopathies, especially idiopathic dilated cardiomyopathy, result in global ventricular systolic dysfunction. Systemic hypertension, cardiac valvular disease, etc., also may produce systolic failure due to the chronic presence of increased afterload and the gradual damage of cardiac muscle fibers.

But they gradually produce diastolic failure due to their subsequent effects, causing *ventricular hypertrophy* and leading to filling defects. However, actually, in diastolic heart failure, there is impaired relaxation and defect in the filling of the ventricle during its diastole, leading to the elevation of EDP at any given diastolic volume or preload of the ventricle. The failure of the relaxation of the ventricle in diastolic failure can also be caused by stiffened and/ or thickened ventricle, which impaired the filling of it. With diastolic heart failure, the ventricle has decreased compliance and cannot adequately be filled up during the diastolic period. *Examples of diastolic heart failure are restrictive cardiomyopathy, infiltrative conditions of the heart such as amyloidosis and myocardial edema, hypertrophic*

cardiomyopathy, constrictive pericarditis, ventricular hypertrophy due to essential hypertension or aortic stenosis, etc. The symptomatic congestive heart failure with normal ventricular systolic function is most likely due to diastolic dysfunction. In many patients, cardiac hypertrophy and dilatation, i.e., diastolic and systolic failure, can also coexist. Here, the ventricle both fills and empties abnormally.

Though systolic heart failure may result primarily from the abnormality of the heart muscle, such as in cardiomyopathy, it may also result secondarily from chronic excessive cardiac workload, such as in hypertension or valvular heart disease. In IHD, systolic heart failure results from the loss in quantity of normally contracting myocardial cells.

Congestive heart failure is a condition that is coupled with multiple etiologies. These etiologies may be described as:

- Abnormality in cardiac contraction (systolic heart failure, e.g., dilated cardiomyopathies)
- Abnormalities in diastolic filling (diastolic heart failure, e.g., restrictive cardiomyopathy, hypertrophic cardiomyopathy, constrictive pericarditis, cardiac tamponade)
- Pressure overload (afterload abnormalities, e.g., severe hypertension, aortic stenosis). Here, the systolic and diastolic dysfunction work together. In the acute form of hypertension, the systolic failure is the cause. But in chronic hypertension, diastolic failure due to impaired ventricular filling for its hypertrophy and systolic failure due to myocardial ischemia caused by hypertrophy coexist.
- Volume overload (mitral regurgitation, aortic insufficiency, etc.).

High-Output versus Low-Output Heart Failure

As the name signifies, high-output heart failure means there is an elevated cardiac output, and low-output heart failure means there is a decrease in cardiac output. *The high-output heart failure is seen in a patient with hyperthyroidism, anemia, pregnancy, beriberi, arteriovenous fistula, transfusion overload, etc.* In high-output heart failure, though the cardiac output is high, it is still insufficient to maintain the body requirement. So, the heart has to work more and more to meet the tissue requirement, and ultimately it fails like a tired horse.

On the contrary, low-output heart (cardiac) failure due to systolic or diastolic causes is seen in patients with IHD, hypertension, dilated cardiomyopathy, valvular diseases, pericardial diseases, etc. *In low-output failure, the arterio - venous O_2 tension $(A - V)O_2$ tension difference is widened, but in high-output failure, the A-VO_2 difference is normal or low.*

Left-sided versus Right-sided Heart Failure

In the human body, the cardiovascular system consists of two circulations situated in series where the right and left heart act both as a pump in the connecting link for each of the series. The right ventricle (RV) acts as a pump for the pulmonary circulation and the left ventricle (LV) acts as a pump for the systemic circulation. The pulmonary circulation is a low-pressure system. In it, the mean systolic arterial pressure is 15 mm Hg, and the pressure gradient between the pulmonary artery and its (pulmonary) vein is 8 mm Hg. The systemic circulation is a high-pressure system. In it, the mean systolic arterial pressure is 120 mm Hg, and the pressure gradient between the systemic artery and its (systemic) vein is 90 mm Hg. The ratio of the right ventricular mass with its coronary blood supply to the left ventricular mass with its coronary blood supply is 1:4.

The right-sided heart failure is referred to the condition when the RV fails to pump out the blood in the pulmonary circulation and the blood accumulates in and behind it (RV). The causes of this right ventricular failure are as follows:

- Lung diseases causing pulmonary hypertension, such as emphysema, fibrosis, and chronic obstructive pulmonary disease (COPD)
- Some form of cardiac valvular diseases, e.g., pulmonary stenosis, mitral stenosis.
- Some congenital heart diseases with a left-to-right shunt
- As a consequence of left ventricular failure.

The left-sided heart failure is referred to the condition when the LV fails to pump out the blood in systemic circulation and the blood accumulates in and behind it. The causes of this left ventricular failure are as follows:

- Weakness of the muscle of LV due to IHD
- Excessive workload due to systemic hypertension
- Some valvular diseases, such as aortic stenosis and mitral incompetence
- Some congenital heart diseases with a right-to-left shunt.

The causes of right- or left-sided heart failure are given in **Box 1**. The consequences or effects of right- or left-sided heart failure are mainly due to the low output from that ventricle and backward pressure.

In right-sided heart failure, the low output to the lungs from the RV is usually not significant unless the right ventricular failure is a sequel to the left ventricular failure. On the other hand, due to backward pressure in RV failure, the overfilling of right atrium, systemic veins, and capillaries produces systemic edema. Cyanosis in RV failure is the result of excess reduced hemoglobin in systemic capillaries and venules, but not due to defective oxygenation of blood in the lungs. *The measurement of pulmonary artery pressure is very important for the diagnosis of these two types of heart failure.*

BOX 1: Causes of heart failure.

- *Reduced ventricular contractility:* Myocarditis, cardiomyopathy, IHD, myocardial infarction
  Main features: Gradual ventricular dilatation, impaired ventricular wall motion
- *Ventricular inflow obstruction:* Mitral stenosis, tricuspid stenosis, constrictive pericarditis, myocardial fibrosis, and other disorders that cause stiff myocardium (e.g., ventricular hypertrophy)
  Main features: Small vigorous ventricle → dilated hypertrophied atrium
- *Ventricular outflow obstruction:* Hypertension and aortic stenosis (left heart failure), pulmonary stenosis, pulmonary hypertension (right heart failure)
  Main features: Concentric ventricular hypertrophy → try to maintain normal output → secondary changes in myocardium → ventricular dilatation
- *Ventricular volume overload:* Mitral and aortic regurgitation (LV overload), pulmonary and tricuspid regurgitation (RV load), ASD, VSD, increased metabolic demand (high output)
  Main features: Hypertrophy and dilatation of ventricle → maintain normal output → secondary changes in myocardium → impaired contractility → dilatation of ventricle
- *Arrhythmia:* Atrial fibrillation, severe tachycardia, complete heart block

(ASD: atrial septal defect; IHD: ischemic heart disease; LV: left ventricle; RV: right ventricle; VSD: ventricular septal defect)

The increase in pulmonary artery pressure may be the cause of RV failure or may be the effect of LV failure. But, in most cases, the increased pulmonary artery pressure is due to LV failure leading to RV failure (combined failure). In mitral stenosis, RV failure is caused by this mechanism but without LV failure. In chronic pulmonary diseases, pulmonary hypertension and RV failure are the causes of death. In pulmonary stenosis, there is isolated RV failure that later leads to LV failure. Thus, the distinction between right and left ventricular failure is valid and certainly useful from some clinical point of view.

However, when the heart failure exists for a long time, then such classification of failing heart may no longer exist. For example, a patient with long-standing aortic valve disease may have ankle edema and congestive hepatomegaly late in the course of this disease, showing the features of RV failure, even though the abnormal hemodynamic burden initially was placed on the LV. This occurs in part because of secondary pulmonary hypertension and resultant right-sided heart failure arising from left-sided heart failure. But this is also because of the retention of salt and water, characteristic of all forms of heart failure. On the other hand, the muscle bundles comprising both ventricles are continuous, and both ventricles share a common wall, i.e., the intraventricular septum. So, the failure of one of the ventricles precipitates the failure of another. Also, the biochemical changes that occur in heart failure and the factors that are involved in the impairment of myocardial function, such as norepinephrine depletion and alterations in the activity of myosin adenosine triphosphatase (ATPase), occur in the myocardium of both the ventricles, regardless of the specific chamber on which the abnormal hemodynamic burden is placed initially.

Backward versus Forward Heart Failure

The concept of backward heart failure indicates that one or other ventricle fails to discharge its full contents. As a consequence, the pressure on the atrium or venous system behind the failing cardiac chamber rises and by the result of which retention of sodium and water occurs. As a consequence of the elevation of systemic venous and capillary pressure, fluid transudates into the interstitial space. In contrast, the concept of forward heart failure indicates that one or other ventricle discharge inadequate blood into the arterial system. As a consequence, there is also salt and water retention due to diminished renal perfusion, excessive proximal tubular Na^+ reabsorption, and excessive distal tubular water reabsorption through the activation of the renin–angiotensin–aldosterone system.

A rigid distinction between the backward and the forward heart failure is not possible because both the above-explained mechanisms appear to operate to varying extents at a given time in most patients with both types of heart failure. For example, in case of massive left ventricular infarction, stroke volume, cardiac output, and BP are suddenly reduced due to myocardial damage, which is manifested as forward failure, and then the patient may succumb to acute pulmonary edema, which is a manifestation of backward failure.

COMPENSATORY MECHANISMS IN HEART FAILURE

Before the development of signs and symptoms of heart failure, the myocardial reserve comes forward into action to maintain the circulation of blood and to fulfill the normal tissue O_2 demand. This myocardial reserve comes forward by three different mechanisms, which are called the compensatory mechanisms. These are (1) increase in pumping rate or heart rate, (2) dilatation of the ventricular chamber executing the Starling law (dilatation of atrial chamber is ignored here), and (3) hypertrophy of the musculature of the ventricle, executing increased contractility. In the heart, during pathological strain, all these three compensatory mechanisms come into action and try to cope for the considerable derangement. This compensatory mechanism is mediated through the activation of sympathetic and renin–angiotensin–aldosterone systems. The compensatory mechanisms in heart failure are shown in **Flowchart 1**.

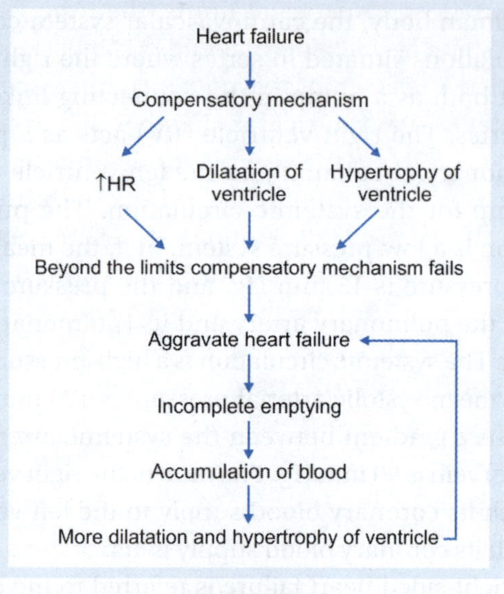

Flowchart 1: Different compensatory mechanisms of heart failure.

(HR: heart rate)

Increase in Heart Rate

Heart rate is an important determining factor of cardiac output because cardiac output = heart rate × stroke volume. When stroke volume is reduced, then with increased heart rate, the cardiac output is maintained. This increase in heart rate is performed by the increase in the activity of the sympathetic system due to reduced cardiac output through baroreceptors, situated in the different parts of our body. Again, this chronic long-standing increased sympathetic activity gradually further deteriorates the ventricular function (which is discussed later) and accelerates the failure. So, what is beneficial and compensatory now will be harmful later.

Dilatation of Ventricle

Under physiological condition and within a limit, the volume of the ventricular chamber at the end of diastole influences the pumping or contractile force of ventricular musculature (Starling law). The larger will be the chamber size of the ventricle due to filling by blood in diastole, the longer will be the length of the ventricular muscle fiber before contraction. Again, the longer will be the length of muscle fiber, the greater will be the contractile force of these muscle fibers. This is called the *Starling law*. In this way, the heart will try to maintain cardiac output to its normal value before it fails. Thus, the conditions where the Starling law mainly comes into action are the early stages of valvular incompetence, valvular stenosis, fluid overload, or other conditions where the venous return or regurgitation starts to increase. In the later stages, when the EDV and subsequent stretching of ventricular muscle fiber increase more and go beyond the physiological limits, then the ventricular chamber starts to dilate permanently. The best example of this ventricular dilatation is valvular incompetence. In aortic incompetence, the ventricular chamber dilates because it has to accommodate the regurgitant blood from the aorta as well as the normal input from the atrium. In valvular stenosis, the ventricular chamber also dilates because it has to accommodate the residual blood from the present contraction as well as from the normal input.

Hypertrophy of Ventricle

Ventricular hypertrophy is another mode of compensatory mechanism of heart failure, where the *increase in the number of muscle fiber* (not the length of the muscle fiber) comes into action and is able to deal with the greater workload. The only pure form of ventricular hypertrophy is best seen during the increased afterload.

Left ventricular hypertrophy is most common in essential hypertension and aortic stenosis. Right ventricular hypertrophy is seen in pulmonary stenosis, in pulmonary hypertension due to chronic lung diseases, and also in mitral valve disease, which secondarily causes pulmonary hypertension. But in the clinical scenario, both hypertrophy and dilatation come into action in different combinations with their different magnitudes to compensate the failure, accompanied by an increased heart rate or not.

Failure of Compensatory Mechanism

The increased cardiac efficiency derived from all three compensatory mechanisms is limited. Beyond this limit, a serious deficiency of the compensatory mechanism ensures cardiac failure with definite signs and symptoms. The heart rate increases mainly at the expense of the duration of diastole. So, when the heart rate increases above 160–180/min, then the period of diastole becomes very much shorter, and ventricular filling is severely jeopardized, and cardiac output does not increase. Similarly, the Starling law also works within a physiological limit (plateau of the curve), beyond which the further dilatation of the ventricle or the stretching of the muscle fiber does not increase the force of contraction. Then, the residual blood gradually accumulates in the chamber, which further helps in the dilatation of the ventricle and failure. Thus, a vicious cycle sets up. Hypertrophy also fails to compensate beyond its maximum limit when the muscle mass has outgrown than its necessary blood supply, causing the impairment of the supply of nutrients, the impairment of chemical and neural stimuli, and inotropic activity. All these lead to further heart failure.

The effects of heart failure are principally seen in the peripheral organs. These are due to hypoxia and/or venous congestion. Hypoxia is well exemplified in the acute form of left ventricular failure, where the cerebral function is seriously disrupted with transient loss of consciousness. In the chronic form of heart failure, weakness and fatigue (which are so common symptoms) are probably the effects mainly of chronic hypoxia. But the damage to the organs due to chronic hypoxia is more difficult to define in chronic heart failure. This is because the effects of venous congestion and water retention in chronic heart failure are added to compensate for the impaired circulation causing hypoxia. Venous congestion is responsible for edema. Breathlessness or dyspnea, which is almost a constant feature of heart failure, is essentially due to venous congestion and fluid retention within the lungs.

DETERMINANTS OF VENTRICULAR FUNCTION

Ventricular function is determined mainly by the three principal cardiac parameters. These are (1) cardiac output, (2) ejection fraction, and (3) ventricular end-diastolic volume or pressure.

Cardiac Output

The main single function of the heart is to eject blood. It is measured in liter per minute and is the product of *stroke volume* and *heart rate*. Stroke volume is again determined by (1) venous return (preload), (2) myocardial contractility (force–velocity curve), (3) afterload, (4) myocardial size (hypertrophy and dilatation), (5) wall motion abnormalities, and (6) valvular dysfunction. In addition, (7) any alterations in the activity of the sympathetic nervous system and (8) humeral-mediated response control the cardiac output. In the presence of mild heart failure, the resting cardiac output may be normal or adequate for the *resting tissues*, without any signs and symptoms of heart failure, *but it becomes unable to meet the demand during stress* whereas in severe heart failure, the *resting cardiac output is even inadequate for resting tissues*. When the cardiac output does not increase in heart failure corresponding with the demand of O_2 by tissues, then the usual O_2 extraction from the blood by the peripheral tissues is increased, and the O_2 content in the venous blood is reduced, producing an increased arteriovenous O_2 tension difference [or $P(a-v)O_2$] in decompensated heart failure.

Venous Return (Preload)

At any fixed level of contractile status of the ventricle (i.e., contractility) and afterload, cardiac performance is profoundly influenced by the ventricular end-diastolic fiber length or the end-diastolic volume (EDV), which is closely related to the end-diastolic pressure (EDP). *This EDP or indirectly the EDV is called the preload. So, terms such as EDV, EDP, venous return, and preload are all interchangeable.* Therefore, cardiac performance is governed by the Frank–Starling law or principle. This Frank–Starling principle dictates the relationship between the initial length of the muscle fiber of the ventricle and the tension or force of contraction developed within it. It means that the stroke volume due to more forceful contraction of the ventricular is increased when the tension developed in the ventricular muscle fiber before contraction is increased, which is again increased when the resting length of that muscle fiber (or volume of the ventricle) due to increased filling is increased. Therefore, the preload is the intraventricular pressure which is closely related to the intraventricular volume at the end of the diastole and governed by the Starling law. On the other hand, the *other major determinants of ventricular preload are* (1) total circulating blood volume, (2) distribution of blood volume in different organs, and (3) atrial contraction.

1. *Total circulating blood volume:* During severe hemorrhage or in hypovolemic shock or in any other conditions where vasodilation occurs, there is absolute or relative reduction in the circulating blood volume. It causes a decrease in venous return → decrease in EDV (preload) → decrease in ventricular EDP → decrease in the length of ventricular muscle fiber → decrease in the tension of ventricular muscle fiber before contraction → decrease in force of contraction → decrease in stroke volume → decrease in cardiac output for a given heart rate.

2. *Distribution of blood volume:* For any given blood volume, the ventricular end-diastolic volume or pressure, which determines the cardiac output, is influenced by the distribution of the total blood volume between the intrathoracic and extrathoracic compartments. This distribution of the total blood volume between the intrathoracic and extrathoracic compartments in turn is influenced by the following factors:

   i. *Body position:* Upright position augments the extrathoracic blood volume and reduces the preload.

   ii. *Intrathoracic pressure:* Increased intrathoracic pressure impedes the venous return and thus reduces the EDV and stroke volume, such as during Valsalva maneuver, intense coughing, and intermittent positive pressure ventilation (IPPV).

   iii. *Intrapericardial pressure:* During increased intrapericardial pressure such as in cardiac tamponed, there is interference for cardiac filling and reduction of stroke volume.

   iv. *Venous tone:* The smooth muscles of the walls of the veins respond to a variety of neural and humoral stimuli and control venous tone, which in turn controls the venous return, preload, and cardiac performance, i.e., cardiac output.

3. *Atrial contraction:* It in ventricular filling and is of particular importance in patients with concentric ventricular hypertrophy. So, the loss of atrial systole, such as in atrial fibrillation, tends to reduce the ventricular filling. Thus, the ventricular end-diastolic volume and pressure (preload) and in turn the stroke volume are reduced.

Thus, now we have come to the conclusion that for all the striated muscle fiber, including the cardiac muscle fiber, the force of contraction depends on the initial length of this muscle fiber. The optimum sarcomere length (the length of a muscle cell) associated with the most powerful contraction of muscle fiber is 2.2 μm. At this length, the actin and myosin are situated in such a fashion that they are able to provide the greatest area of their interaction, and at this length, the myofilaments are maximally sensitive to Ca^{2+} ion. When the sarcomere length (the length of a muscle cell) is increased to 3.65 μm, then the thin actin filaments are entirely withdrawn from the myosin filament and no tension can be developed. Similarly, when the sarcomere is shorter than 2 μm, then the thin actin filaments will pass over one another and are doubly overlapped. So, it reduces both the sensitivity of Ca^{2+} to the contractile sites and the capacity of force to develop. Therefore, the relation between the initial length of cardiac muscle fibers and the subsequent development of the force of contraction is of prime importance for the functional integrity of the myocardium, which is stated by the Frank–Starling law.

Myocardial Contractility or Inotropic State of Ventricle (Force–Velocity Curve)

The state of mechanical contractility of all the striated muscle fibers can be expressed by a relation between the velocity or the rate of shortening and the development of force during contraction within the muscle **(Flowchart 2)**.

The maximum velocity of contraction of a muscle is written as V_{max}, and in the presence of catecholamines when the inotropic state of the heart is increased, then this V_{max} is also increased. This velocity of contraction also depends on the intracellular Ca^{2+} concentration during systole and other neural, humoral, and pharmacological factors. On the other hand, the myocardial contractility is depressed due to anoxia, acidosis, depletion of catecholamine stores, and loss of functioning muscle mass as a result of ischemia

Flowchart 2: Schematic representation of interactions among the various components that regulate cardiac activity. The broken line represents an inhibiting effect.

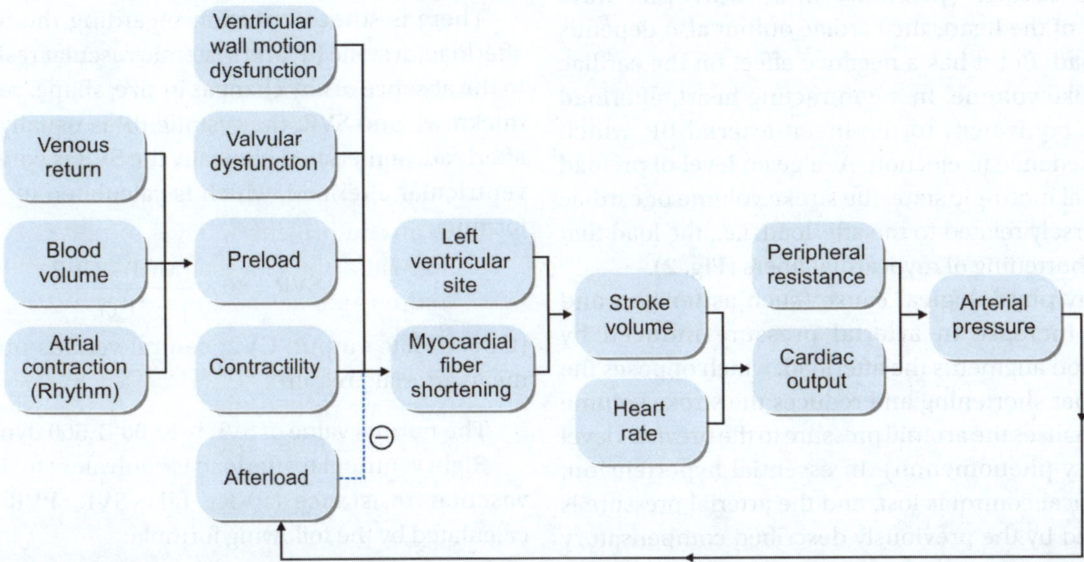

and infarction. Most anesthetic and antiarrhythmic agents decrease myocardial contractility. Alternatively, the V_{max} will decrease when the myocardial contractility is impaired due to some factors which are responsible for heart failure. As for example, volatile anesthetics decrease V_{max}, and this effect is additive to the decreased contractility in the presence of heart failure. In clinical practice, the rate of decrease or increase of intraventricular pressure indicates the decrease or increase of V_{max} and is used as an important guide for the understanding of the inotropic state of the heart.

At any given ventricular end-diastolic volume or pressure (preload), a number of factors described below determine the state of myocardial contractility or V_{max} and the level of ventricular performance, reflecting the change of the ventricular function curve. All these factors act by modifying the myocardial force–velocity relation or curve and by altering the concentration of Ca^{2+} in the vicinity of the myofilaments, which in turn trigger the cross-bridge between the actin and myosin.

These factors are as follows:
- *Adrenergic nerve activity:* Normally, norepinephrine is released from the adrenergic nerve endings in the heart. Its action on the β-adrenergic receptor in the myocardium depends on the adrenergic nerve impulse traffic. This factor is most important for myocardial contractility under physiological conditions.
- *Circulating catecholamines:* After adrenergic nerve stimulation of the adrenal medulla, it releases catecholamines which reach the heart and augment myocardial contractility.

- *Force–frequency relation:* The contractility of the normal (but not the failing) heart is augmented by the increase in the frequency of adrenergic impulse.
- *Exogenously administered inotropic agents:* All inotropes improve the myocardial force–velocity relation and are used to stimulate ventricular performance.
- *Pharmacological depressants:* These include calcium channel blocker, β-blockers, lignocaine, procainamide, etc.
- *Physiological depressants:* Hypoxia, ischemia, acidosis, electrolyte imbalance, etc., acting either singly or in combination, depress the myocardial force–velocity curve or contractility and left ventricular performance at any given EDV.
- *Loss of myocytes:* Ventricular performance or stroke volume is also depressed at a given end-diastolic volume when there is loss of some myocardial cells as in myocardial ischemia (transient loss), infarction (permanent loss), and apoptosis (programmed cell death—can cause scattered loss of myocytes and when sufficiently widespread can impair ventricular function and cause heart failure).
- *Intrinsic myocardial depression:* The fundamental mechanism responsible for depression of myocardial contractility in most cases of chronic heart failure, which is secondary to prolonged ventricular overload or cardiomyopathy, is still unknown. It is now apparent that in this condition, the inotropic state of individual surviving myocytes is depressed, and as a consequence, the ventricular functional curve at any given ventricular preload and afterload is lowered.

Ventricular Afterload

Like venous return (preload) and inotropic state (contractility) of the heart, the cardiac output also depends on the afterload. But it has a negative effect on the cardiac output or stroke volume. In a contracting heart, afterload is commonly equivalent to the mean arterial BP, which produces impedance to ejection. At a given level of preload and myocardial inotropic state, the stroke volume or cardiac output is inversely related to the afterload, i.e., the load that opposes the shortening of myocardial fibers **(Fig. 2)**.

Due to any physiological cause (such as tension and anxiety), an increase in arterial pressure induced by vasoconstriction augments the afterload, which opposes the myocardial fiber shortening and reduces the stroke volume and thus normalizes the arterial pressure to the previous level (compensatory phenomenon). In essential hypertension, this physiological control is lost, and the arterial pressure is not normalized by the previously described compensatory mechanism.

With age, myocardial contractility is impaired, cardiac output falls, and the ventricle dilates. Then, afterload or arterial pressure may rise as a result of the compensatory neural and humoral stimuli that occur in response to a fall in cardiac output. This increased afterload may further reduce cardiac output, while myocardial O_2 consumption is increased. This can set a vicious cycle.

There is some confusion regarding the terms such as afterload, systolic BP, and systemic vascular resistance (SVR). In the absence of any changes in size, shape, ventricular wall thickness, and SVR, the systolic BP is usually taken as the afterload. Sometimes, clinically the SVR is considered as left ventricular afterload, which is calculated by the following formula:

$$SVR = 80 \times \frac{MAP - CVP}{CO}$$

(CO: cardiac output; CVP: central venous pressure; MAP: mean arterial pressure)

The normal value of SVR is 1,000–1,500 dyn s/cm^{-5}.

Right ventricular afterload is equivalent to the pulmonary vascular resistance (PVR). Like SVR, PVR can also be calculated by the following formula:

$$SVR = 80 \times \frac{PAP - PCWP}{CO}$$

(PAP: pulmonary artery pressure; PCWP: pulmonary capillary wedge pressure)

The normal value of PVR is 50–100 dyn s/cm^{-5}.

Myocardial Size (Hypertrophy and Dilatation)

Like the preload, contractility, and afterload, the hypertrophy and dilatation of the ventricular wall also determine the amount of stroke volume. Initially, they represent the compensatory mechanism and help to maintain the cardiac output. But later, they become the causes of further deterioration with a reduction of output and heart failure. Hypertrophy helps to overcome the pressure overload. But it has limitations because hypertrophied muscle functions at a lower inotropic state than the normal cardiac muscle. Dilatations also lead to a compensatory increase in output by the Starling mechanism. But later, both hypertrophy and dilatation are associated with increased O_2 requirement and decreased cardiac efficiency. Ventricular hypertrophy develops in response to chronic pressure overload, such as aortic stenosis, systemic hypertension, mitral stenosis, and pulmonary hypertension whereas the ventricular dilatation develops in response to volume overload, such as aortic incompetence and mitral incompetence.

Wall Motion Abnormalities

For adequate stroke volume, it requires all the ventricular muscle fibers to contract symmetrically at a time. But due to some abnormalities of muscle fiber such as ischemia, hypertrophy, and fibrosis, all portions of the ventricular

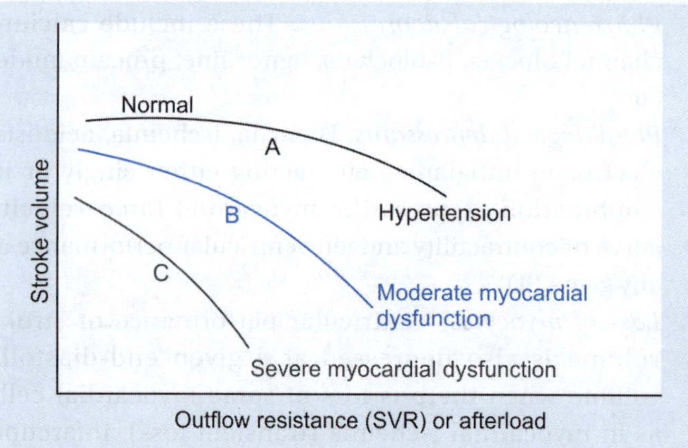

Fig. 2: Relationship between the stroke volume and the ventricular outflow resistance in patients with normal, hypertensive, and systolic ventricular dysfunctional heart. Cardiac outflow resistance is the principal determinant factor of afterload. An increase in systemic vascular resistance (SVR) has little effect on stroke volume in a normal heart (curve A). In contrast, in patients with systolic ventricular dysfunction, an increase in outflow resistance or afterload is often accompanied by a sharp decline in stroke volume (curve B). With severe ventricular dysfunction, the curve becomes steeper (curve C). So, the reduction of SVR, one of the components of outflow resistance, by a vasodilator markedly increases the stroke volume in patients with severe myocardial dysfunction. The decrease in SVR is resulted by an increase in stroke volume and subsequently prevents a fall in BP, which is caused by reduced SVR. Thus, the increase in stroke volume offsets the effect of reduced SVR.

walls do not contract symmetrically and fully. So, ventricular emptying or output becomes impaired. The principal types of ventricular wall motion abnormalities found during echocardiography are akinesia (fully failure to contract), hypokinesia (decreased contraction), and dyskinesia (paradoxical contraction). The severity of impairment of stroke volume depends on the size, number, and type of abnormality of the contracting areas of the ventricular wall.

Valvular Dysfunction

The types of valvular dysfunctions are stenosis, incompetence (regurgitation), or both and can involve any of the four valves. The stenosis of atrioventricular (AV) valves, such as the mitral and tricuspid valve, causes reduction in stroke volume by reducing the preload, but not by altering the afterload. On the other hand, stenosis of the aortic and pulmonary valves reduces the stroke volume by increasing the afterload, which subsequently causes compensatory ventricular hypertrophy, but not by altering the preload. However, the regurgitation of any valve decreases the stroke volume and increases the preload, which subsequently causes compensatory ventricular dilatation.

Ejection Fraction

The ejection fraction of a ventricle is defined as the ratio of the stroke volume to the end-diastolic volume. It signifies the amount of blood filling the ventricle at the end of diastole, the amount of blood is stroked out, and the amount of blood resides in the ventricle at the end of systole. Normally, the ventricle ejects 55–80% of its end-diastolic volume during systole, resulting in an ejection fraction of 0.55–0.8 **(Fig. 3)**.

During rest, even in the presence of heart failure, the value of cardiac output or stroke volume may be within normal limits due to the compensatory mechanism, though it is depressed. Hence, the amount of stroke volume or cardiac output always cannot properly give the idea of cardiac performance. So, a more sensitive index of heart failure or cardiac activity is the ejection fraction than the

total cardiac output or stroke volume. In systolic heart failure, the ejection fraction is depressed even when the stroke volume remains normal. It means with an increase in end-diastolic volume (EDV) due to compensation, the stroke volume may be normal, but the full amount of blood coming into the ventricle cannot be ejected out, and some blood will always remain in the ventricle after ejection. Alternatively, abnormally elevated EDV (normal value 70 ± 20 mL/m^2) in the presence of normal stroke volume signifies impaired left ventricular systolic function.

There are limitations in the isolated measurement of the stroke volume, cardiac output, and ejection fraction for the assessment of the systolic performance of the heart. The limitations are that these parameters are influenced strongly by some factors such as the ventricular filling conditions (preload) and afterload. Thus, a decreased ejection fraction and low cardiac output may be observed in patients with normal ventricular function (contractility) but with reduced preload, such as in hypovolemia, or with increased afterload, as occurs during acutely elevated arterial pressure. So, the measurement of end-systolic ventricular pressure and volume may be a useful index of ventricular performance than ejection fraction, since it is independent of both the preload and afterload. If the ventricular contractility declines, the end-systolic ventricular pressure and volume rises.

The diastolic performance of the ventricle is best assessed by continuously measuring the flow velocity across the mitral valve using Doppler echocardiography. Normally, the flow velocity across the mitral valve is more rapid in early diastole (A) than during atrial systole (E). With impaired relaxation of the ventricle, the rate of early diastolic filling declines, while the rate of presystolic filling, due to atrial contraction, rises. With severe impairment of filling, the pattern is again pseudo-normalized and the early ventricular filling becomes more rapid.

End-Diastolic Pressure

The EDP of a ventricle runs parallel with the end-diastolic volume (EDV) of it. It is also called the preload. It increases in the presence of heart failure. In the absence of failure, this EDP can also increase in the presence of poorly compliant or stiff ventricle. In such circumstances, an increase in EDP does not run in parallel to the EDV of the ventricle, which remains normal or decreases. The normal value of EDP of the LV and RV are 12 and 5 mm Hg, respectively. In the absence of mitral valve disease, the pulmonary artery pressure and the left atrial pressure are equivalent to the left ventricular EDP. In electrocardiogram (ECG), the manifestation of left atrial enlargement correlates

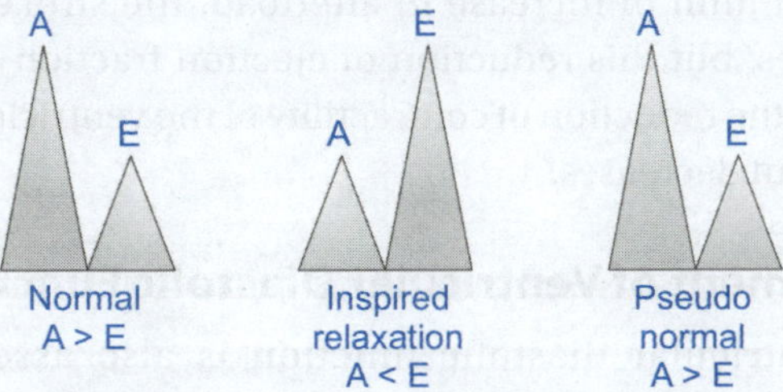

Fig. 3: Patterns of left ventricular filling, as recorded by diastolic Doppler mitral flow velocities. A is the early diastolic filling and E is the late diastolic filling due to atrial contraction.

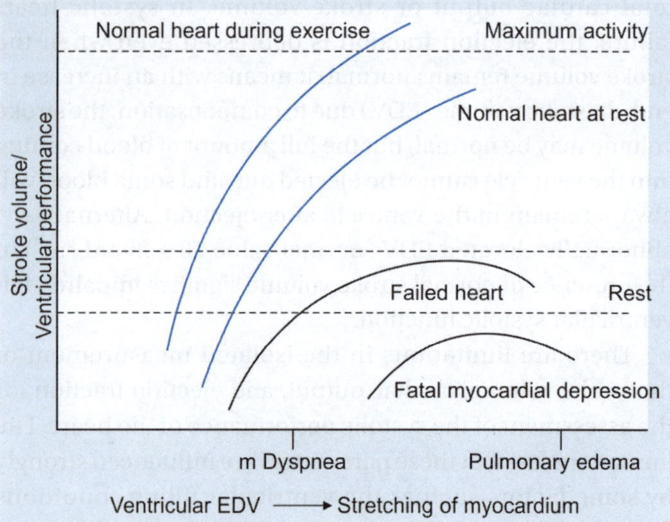

Fig. 4: Normal and abnormal ventricular function curves. It shows the interrelations between the ventricular end-diastolic volume (EDV) by stretching of the myocardium and the contractile state of the heart. Ventricular EDV and resultant filling pressure are plotted on the abscissa and ventricular performance on the ordinate. Blue lines indicate the performance or function of the normal heart during rest and exercise while the black lines indicate the depressed performance of the failing heart.

well with the increased left atrial pressure and subsequently the increased left ventricular EDP **(Fig. 4)**.

The analysis of the heart as a pump is classically centered on the relation of the end-diastolic volume of a ventricle (which is related to the length of the muscle fibers) with its stroke volume (Frank–Starling relation). The EDP of a ventricle is sometimes used as a synonym for its end-diastolic volume. In a normal heart, when the stroke volume remains within its limits, then it correlates directly well with the end-diastolic fiber length or the volume of a ventricle (preload) and inversely with the arterial pressure (afterload). But failed heart delivers a smaller than normal stroke volume from a normal or elevated end-diastolic volume.

So, the relation between the EDP and stroke work (the ventricular function curve) needs a good and useful definition of contractility (i.e., the force of contraction) of the ventricle. An increase in ventricular contractility shifts the ventricular function curve upward and toward the left. It means that with increased contractility, there is a greater stroke volume at any level of EDP (or volume). However, depression of contractility shifts the ventricular function curve downward and to the right. An example of shifting of the ventricular function curve to the left is exercise. During the adrenergic stimulation of the myocardium, accompanying exercise, there is relatively little change in EDV, while cardiac output, aortic flow velocity, stroke volume, and the rate of ventricular

pressure development are all augmented, reflecting an increase in myocardial contractility.

Adrenergic stimulation of the myocardium through an adrenergic neurotransmitter such as norepinephrine has long been recognized. Norepinephrine activates the myocardial β-receptors and thereby increases the concentration of intracellular cyclic adenosine monophosphate (cAMP). The latter in turn causes a more rapid forceful contraction by phosphorylating the Ca^{2+} channel in the myocardial sarcolemma and thereby enhancing the influx of Ca^{2+} into the myocyte, which in turn acts on the contractile apparatus.

■ ASSESSMENT OF VENTRICULAR FUNCTION

The assessment of ventricular function is divided into three parts: (1) Assessment of the systolic function, (2) assessment of diastolic function, and (3) assessment of both ventricular systolic and diastolic function by the ventricular function curve.

Assessment of Ventricular Systolic Function

The ventricular systolic function means the ventricular contractility, and it is best assessed by the changes in intraventricular pressure over time during systole. It is designated as dP/dt. The measurement of this value is difficult and requires a high fidelity ventricular catheter. The usefulness of dP/dt is also limited. It may be influenced by preload and afterload.

The ventricular systolic function or contractility can also be assessed by the ejection fraction (EF), which has been discussed before. In practice, this EF is the most commonly used parameter for the assessment of contractility of the ventricle by the formula:

$$EF = \frac{EDV - ESV}{EDV}$$

(EF: ejection fraction; ESV: end-systolic volume)

The importance of this parameter is that it can be measured noninvasively by echocardiography. The limitation of the importance of ejection fraction is that after a certain limit of increase in afterload, the stroke volume decreases, but this reduction of ejection fraction does not indicate the reduction of contractility of the ventricle, though the output decreases.

Assessment of Ventricular Diastolic Function

The ventricular diastolic function is also assessed by measuring the flow velocity of blood across the mitral or tricuspid value during the ventricular diastole by Doppler echocardiography. The velocity of flow of blood across the mitral or tricuspid valve is measured or assessed by (1) isovolumetric relaxation time (IVRT), (2) the ratio of peak early diastolic flow (PEDF)/peak atrial systolic flow (PASF) (discussed before), and (3) the deceleration time of peak early diastolic flow (DTe) **(Figs. 5A to D)**. The normal value of IVRT is 70–90 ms. It is >100 ms means impaired relaxation and diastolic dysfunction of the ventricle. The normal value of the PEDF/PASF ratio is 0.8–1.2. When this value is <0.8, it also means impaired relaxation and diastolic dysfunction. The normal value of DTe is 150–300 ms, but the value >300 ms means impaired relaxation.

Assessment of Ventricular Systolic and Diastolic Function by Ventricular Function Curve

The graph of Starling law, which plots the stroke volume against the preload (described before), is useful for understanding the pathological states of the heart and the effects of drug therapy on it. But the ventricular pressure–volume curve is more useful than the previous curve because it dissociates the state of contractility from preload and afterload. **Figure 5A** shows the pressure–volume curve of a normal ventricle. **Figure 5B** shows the pressure–volume curve with increasing preload, where contractility and afterload (or intraventricular tension) is like normal. **Figure 5C** shows the pressure–volume curve with increasing afterload (or intraventricular tension) where the preload and contractility are like a normal heart. **Figure 5D** shows the pressure–volume curve with increased or decreased contractility, where the preload and afterload (or intraventricular tension during contraction) are constant.

PROBABLE THEORIES OF HEART FAILURE

There is no single unified theory that can explain all the biochemical basis of all the types of heart failure. Low-output cardiac failure (the most common form) due to coronary ischemia, coronary atherosclerosis, hypertension, cardiomyopathy, valvular lesions, etc., is characterized by reduced external work done by the heart in exchange of elevated O_2 consumption; that is, the ratio of external work performed by the heart to the energy consumed by the heart is depressed.

The probable theories of heart failure are as follows:

- Myocardial energy, which is stored in the form of creatine phosphate (CP), is depleted. Also, the activity of enzyme such as creatine kinase, which is required for the shuttling of high-energy phosphate between the creatine and adenosine diphosphate, is reduced. Hence, it suggests that the reduction of myocardial energy reserves is one of the possible mechanisms of heart failure.

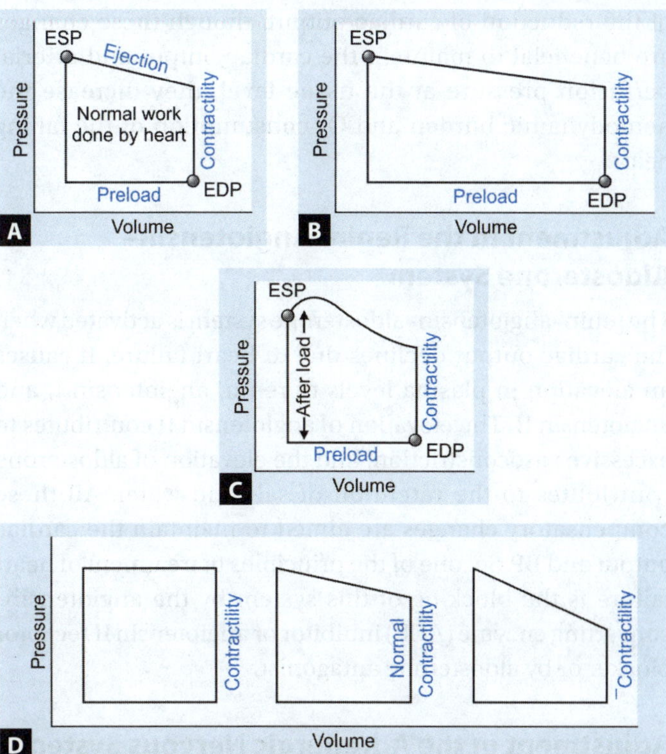

Figs. 5A to D: Volume–pressure curve of single ventricular contraction. (A) Normal heart; (B) Increased preload with constant contractility (intraventricular pressure) and afterload; (C) Increased afterload with constant preload and contractility; (D) Increased and decreased contractility with constant preload and afterload. (EDP: end-diastolic pressure; ESP: end-system pressure)

- Another possible theory of heart failure is the reduction of myosin ATPase activity, which could be caused by an alteration in the expression of troponin-T and/or of myosin light kinase 2 activity. It could also be responsible for lowering the rate of interaction between the myosin and the actin myofilaments.
- The third theory explains that in many forms of heart failure, the delivery of Ca^{2+} to the contractile site is reduced, thereby impairing cardiac performance. The abnormalities actually involved the sarcolemma, T-tubules, or sarcoplasmic reticulum, which is yet to be identified.

NEUROHORMONAL AND BIOCHEMICAL ADJUSTMENT OF HEART FAILURE

The reduction of stroke volume and the reduction of cardiac output in heart failure induce a series of neurohormonal adjustments, which may be considered to be both adaptive (helpful) and maladaptive (not helpful). This neurohormonal adjustment involves (1) the renin–angiotensin–aldosterone system and (2) the adrenergic nervous system. In the face of the reduction of cardiac output, though these changes are beneficial to maintain the cardiac output and arterial perfusion pressure at the tissue level, they increase the hemodynamic burden and O_2 consumption of the failing heart.

Adjustment in the Renin–Angiotensin–Aldosterone System

The renin–angiotensin–aldosterone system is activated when the cardiac output declines due to heart failure. It causes an elevation in plasma levels of renin, angiotensin I, and angiotensin II. The elevation of angiotensin II contributes to excessive vasoconstriction, and the elevation of aldosterone contributes to the retention of salt and water. All these compensatory changes are aimed to maintain the cardiac output and BP. So, one of the principles of treatment of heart failure is the blocking of this system by the angiotensin-converting enzyme (ACE) inhibitor or angiotensin II receptor blocker or by aldosterone antagonist.

Adjustment in the Adrenergic Nervous System

The circulating norepinephrine level is markedly elevated in heart failure patients, which reflects the increased activity of the adrenergic nervous system. This increased adrenergic activity in one way is adaptive (helpful) in supporting ventricular contractility in heart failure. In another way, it is maladaptive as the increased adrenergic activity increases the afterload by raising the vascular resistance and causing further myocardial damage. This latter can be prevented by the cautious use of gradually increasing the doses of β-blocker **(Flowchart 3)**.

Conclusion

The density of the adrenergic receptor and, therefore, the activity of norepinephrine on these cardiac adrenergic receptors (but not the circulating catecholamine or norepinephrine level) are reduced in heart failure. These changes lead to reduction in the activity of adenyl cyclase and lower the intracellular concentration of cAMP. The latter in turn reduces the activation of protein kinase and subsequently the phosphorylation of Ca^{2+} channel, which then reduces the transsarcolemmal Ca^{2+} entry into the cell, as well as the phosphorylation of phospholamban, a protein in the sarcoplasmic reticulum. Thereby, it depresses the reuptake of Ca^{2+} by the latter. The changes in G-protein (or guanine receptor or GR), which couple the β-receptor with the catalytic adenyl cyclase (which is responsible for the production of cAMP), may also occur in heart failure with increased inhibitory activity.

Flowchart 3: Neurohormonal adjustment or compensatory mechanism of heart failure.

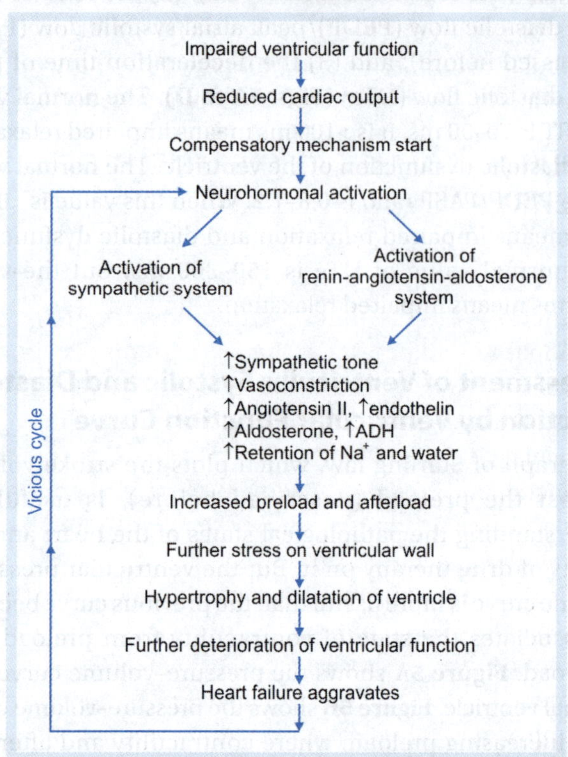

(ADH: antidiuretic hormone)

Finally, we can tell that the basic problem of heart failure is the depression of myocardial contractility (or the force-velocity relationship) and the length–tension curve (or the Starling law), reflecting the reduction of the contractile state of the myocardium. Usually, at rest, the cardiac output and ventricular performance are maintained within their normal limits by an elevated EDV and subsequently increased end-diastolic fiber length through the operation of the Frank–Starling mechanism. This elevation of left ventricular preload is associated with elevation of pulmonary capillary pressure, contributing to dyspnea experienced by patients with heart failure. During exercise, the improvement of contractility of the myocardium due to augmented adrenergic activity is attenuated by norepinephrine depletion and downregulation of myocardial β-receptor, which occur in severe heart failure. The factors that tend to augment ventricular filling during exercise in a normal individual push the failing myocardium along its flattened part of the length–tension curve. Although the LV may perform somewhat better during exercise, but this occurs only as a consequence of an inordinate elevation of the EDV and pressure, and therefore of the pulmonary capillary pressure. The latter intensifies dyspnea and, therefore, plays an important role in limiting the intensity of exercise that the patient can perform. The left ventricular failure becomes fatal when the myocardial length–tension curve is depressed to such a point at which the cardiac performance fails to satisfy the requirements of peripheral tissues, even at rest, and/or the left ventricular end-diastolic and pulmonary capillary pressure are elevated to levels that result in pulmonary edema.

PHARMACOLOGICAL TREATMENT OF HEART FAILURE

The next part of this chapter will discuss the drug therapy of heart failure due to systolic and/or diastolic ventricular dysfunction. The systolic ventricular dysfunction, due to idiopathic, dilated, or ischemic cardiomyopathies, is characterized by a large dilated ventricular chamber. Contrary, the systolic ventricular failure, due to infarction, has the normal ventricular chamber. On the other hand, diastolic ventricular dysfunction, due to long-standing hypertension, or stenotic valvular disease, or primary hypertrophic cardiomyopathy, generally leads to thickened hypertrophied poorly compliant ventricular walls with small ventricular volumes. In practice, many patients have abnormal hemodynamics, comprising different degrees of systolic and diastolic dysfunction. The treatment should, therefore, be according to the underlying pathophysiological process of an individual patient. So, the pharmacological treatment of heart failure can be described under two headings. The *first* heading describes the use of oral drugs in ambulatory patients. The *second* heading will describe the intravenously administered agents for the treatment of acutely hospitalized patients. We will only deal with the second heading here. For the first heading, dealing with only oral drugs in an ambulatory patient suffering from chronic heart failure, we will have to consult any textbook of medicine.

Primarily, the treatment of any heart failure had three aims:
1. Removal of precipitating causes, e.g., the treatment of hypertension, sepsis
2. Correction of underlying causes, e.g., mitral valvotomy, replacement of valve
3. Control of a congestive acute heart failure state.

We will discuss here only the third component of the treatment of acute heart failure. This third component of heart failure treatment again can be divided into three categories: (1) Reduction of cardiac workload, including both preload and afterload, (2) control of excessive retention of salt and water, and (3) the enhancement of cardiac contractility.

Diuretics

A variety of diuretic agents are available in practice, and in patients with mild heart failure, almost all are effective. But in patients with acutely decompensated heart, with failure of sufficient severity, it is generally desirable to initiate an effective diuresis by using the intravenous (IV) doses of a loop diuretic. All the diuretics act by reducing the extracellular fluid volume or by decreasing the ventricular diastolic filling pressure (preload) due to the dilatation of peripheral veins. But, usually, they do not cause a clinically important reduction in cardiac output, except particularly in patients with very advanced heart failure. However, overtreatment must be avoided since the resultant hypovolemia may severely reduce the preload and then cardiac output and may impair the renal function. Examples of common clinically used loop diuretics are frusemide, bumetanide, and torsemide. They are extremely powerful and reversibly inhibit the absorption of Na^+, K^+, and Cl^- through the renal epithelial cells of the thick ascending limbs of loop of Henle by inhibiting the specific protein named the Na^+-K^+-$2Cl^-$ symporter. They depend for their efficacy of action on adequate renal plasma flow and their proximal tubular secretion. Then, they are delivered to their site of action, i.e., the thick ascending limb of the loop of Henle, through the lumen of renal tubule. These loop diuretics also induce renal cortical vasodilation and increase the rates of urine formation that may be as high as one-fourth of the glomerular filtration rate. These drugs also reduce the toxicity of medullary interstitial tissue by preventing the reabsorption of solute in excess of water through the thick ascending limb of the loop of Henle. The excessive use of these loop of diuretics may also cause the development of hyponatremia in a heart failure patient. The increased delivery and subsequently the increased absorption of Na^+ and fluid at the distal segment of nephron, i.e., distal and collecting tubule, due to their less absorption at the thick ascending limb of the loop of Henle, also markedly enhance the excretion of K^+, particularly in the presence of elevated aldosterone levels, which are typically found in the case of heart failure.

When the other diuretics lose their effectiveness when the blood volume is severely constricted due to any cause, then the loop diuretics still remain effective despite the elimination of excessive amount of extracellular fluid volume **(Flowchart 4)**. The major side effects of these loop diuretics are due to their marked diuretic potency, which on rare occasions may result in the contraction of plasma volume, circulatory collapse, reduction of renal blood flow, reduction of the glomerular filtration rate, and the development of prerenal azotemia. The metabolic alkalosis and hypokalemia produced by these loop diuretics are due to the large increase in urinary excretion of Cl^-, H^+, K^+ ions, etc. Hyperuricemia and hyperglycemia are also sometimes observed in loop diuretics. These extremely effective loop diuretics are useful in all the forms of heart failure, particularly in refractory condition and pulmonary edema. They also produce diuresis

Flowchart 4: Pathophysiological mechanism of heart failure and the different sites of action of different drugs used for its treatment. Initially, heart failure is accompanied by compensatory (adaptive) neurohormonal response. It includes the activation of sympathetic and renin–angiotensin–aldosterone systems. These responses initially help to maintain cardiovascular (CV) function by increasing systemic vascular tone and ventricular preload. But with time, decompensation (maladaptive) occurs, and the adaptive mechanism further helps to progress to myocardial failure. Increased ventricular afterload (due to sympathetic vasoconstriction) and gradual cardiac dilatation (due to reduced cardiac output causing gradual elevated ventricular diastolic volume or filling pressure) cause depression in the systolic function. In addition, the direct effect of epinephrine, norepinephrine, and angiotensin on ventricular myocardium causes further dilatation and the loss of myocardial contractile function.

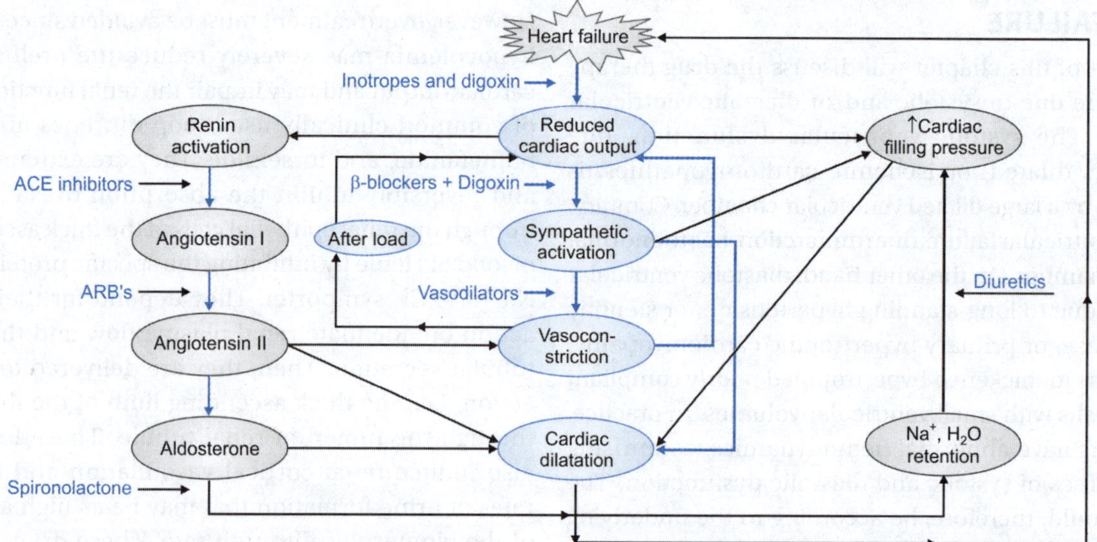

(ACE: angiotensin-converting enzyme; ARB: angiotensin receptor blocker)

in a patient in whom thiazide diuretics and aldosterone antagonist, alone or in combination, are ineffective **(Box 2)**.

The loop diuretics may be administered as repetitive bolus doses or by constant infusion, titrated against the desired response. The advantage of the latter approach is that the same total daily dose of diuretics, when given as continuous infusion, can result in a more sustained and continuous natriuresis due to the continuous maintenance of desired high drug levels within the lumen of renal tubules. A typical continuous furosemide infusion is initiated with 40 mg bolus IV injection, followed by a constant infusion of 10 mg/h, with upward titration as necessary. When there is a poor response to diuretics due to reduced renal perfusion (due to hypotension), then a short-term administration of sympathomimetic drugs or phosphodiesterase (PDE) inhibitors, which act by increasing the cardiac output, may be necessary to achieve the response. Another useful approach for diuresis is the IV administration of dopamine at the so-called low renal doses (<2 µg/kg/min) that causes selective renal dopaminergic receptor stimulation and renal vasodilatation. Therefore, it acts by causing a selective increase in renal blood flow without causing any systemic arterial and venous constriction via α-adrenergic receptor stimulation, which occurs at higher infusion rates of dopamine.

Thiazides and metolazone (a thiazide-related diuretics) diuretics are the agents of choice for the treatment of a chronic ambulatory heart failure patient with a severity

> **BOX 2:** Causes of resistance to diuretics in heart failure.
>
> - Excess dietary Na⁺ intake
> - Noncompliance
> - Decreased renal perfusion and glomerular filtration rate
>   - Hypotension or excessive intravascular fluid depletion
>   - Decline in cardiac output due to severe heart failure
>   - Aggressive diuretics and/or vasodilator therapy
> - Primary renal pathology
> - NSAID agents
>
> (NSAID: nonsteroidal antiinflammatory drugs)

of mild-to-moderate degree and when there are no contraindications of their use, e.g., hyperglycemia, hyperuricemia, hypokalemia, or when the complications are treated. When used alone, other diuretics such as spironolactone, amiloride, and triamterene, act as a weak agent, but they potentiate any thiazide and loop diuretics if they are already used. For heart failure with severe secondary hyperaldosteronism, spironolactone or eplerenone is very effective. In a very severe degree of heart failure, which is refractory to common diuretics, the combination of thiazide diuretics, loop diuretics, and potassium-sparing diuretics is also very effective.

Vasodilators

In heart failure patients, the left ventricular afterload is increased as a consequence of several neural and hormonal influences for low cardiac output, as a compensatory mechanism that tries to increase the BP by constricting the peripheral vascular bed. These neural and hormonal influences include the increased activity of the adrenergic nervous system, the increased circulation of catecholamines, and the increased activity of the renin–angiotensin–aldosterone system. In addition to the vasoconstriction, the EDV and end-systolic volume also rise in systolic heart failure. Vasoconstriction is a compensatory mechanism that tries to maintain adequate flow of blood to the vital organs. But this has no serious effect on cardiac function with normal heart, as for example, hypovolemia due to blood loss with increased sympathetic activities. But, on the other hand, in a low cardiac output state due to impaired cardiac function, this vasoconstriction, which increases the afterload, may further reduce the cardiac output and set a vicious cycle.

We know that afterload is a major determinant factor of cardiac output. With normal cardiac function, moderate elevation of afterload does not reduce the cardiac output or stroke volume. But when the myocardial systolic function is impaired, then such an increase in afterload cannot maintain the stroke volume; instead, it decreases the stroke volume. With the reduction of cardiac output, there is an increase in pulmonary capillary pressure, leading to pulmonary congestion, edema, dyspnea, and all other signs and symptoms of heart failure. In heart failure, the ventricle usually works at the peak flat portion of the Frank–Starling curve. So, any additional increase in afterload (aortic impedance) will reduce the stroke volume. Alternatively, the modest reduction of afterload in a normal individual has no effect on stroke volume, but in a patient with heart failure, it tends to restore the stroke volume toward normal.

So, vasodilation and the reduction of impedance to left ventricular ejection, i.e., the reduction of the afterload, are an important adjustment in the management of heart failure. This vasodilation is very helpful for a patient with *systolic heart failure*. This approach is also helpful for *diastolic failure* by reducing the left EDP, left EDV, and O_2 consumption, while raising the stroke volume and cardiac output, and causing only the modest reduction in systemic BP. A vasodilator should not be used in a patient with severe hypotension because it may impair tissue perfusion and oxygenation, which does not occur after a critical lower value of BP in a hypertensive subject **(Table 2)**. When chronic and acute heart failure patients are treated with vasodilators, then the cardiac output rises, pulmonary wedge pressure falls, and a new steady hemodynamic state is achieved in which the cardiac output increases and the afterload decreases with no or only mild reduction of arterial pressure. Moreover, the reduction of left ventricular end-systolic pressure improves the subendocardial perfusion, which further improves the myocardial contractility.

There are many available vasodilators that are used clinically. But they differ in their hemodynamic effects, site of action, duration of action, and mode of administration. Hydralazine, minoxidil, and α-adrenergic blocking agents

TABLE 2: Vasodilator drugs used to treat heart failure.

Drug class	Examples	Mechanism of action	Afterload reduction	Preload reduction
ACE inhibitor	Captopril, enalapril, lisinopril	Inhibition of formation of angiotensin II	+ +	+ +
Angiotensin receptor blocker	Losartan, candesartan	Blockade of angiotensin II receptor	+ +	+ +
Organic nitrates	Nitroglycerin, isosorbide-dinitrate	Nitric oxide (NO)-mediated vasodilatation	+	+ + +
NO donors	Nitroprusside	NO-mediated vasodilatation	+ + +	+ + +
Direct acting on arterial smooth muscle	Hydralazine, minoxidil	Unknown	+ + +	+
Phosphodiesterase inhibitors	Milrinone, amrinone	Inhibition of cAMP degradation	+ +	+ +
Ca^{2+} channel blocking drugs	Amlodipine, nifedipine	Blocking of L-type Ca^{2+} channel	+ + +	+
Nonselective α-adrenergic receptors antagonist	Phentolamine	α-blocking vasodilatation	+ + +	+ + +
Selective α_1-adrenergic receptor blocker	Prazosin, doxazosin	Selective α_1-blocking vasodilatation	+ +	+ + +
Vasodilating β/α_1-adrenergic receptor antagonist	Carvedilol, labetalol	Selective β_1 and α_1 adrenergic receptor blockade	+ +	+ +

(ACE: angiotensin-converting enzyme; cAMP: cyclic adenosine monophosphate)

(prazosin) act mainly on the arterial system and decrease the afterload and increase the stroke volume. On the other hand, nitroglycerine and isosorbide dinitrate act mainly on the venous site of circulation and reduce preload. ACE inhibitors and nitroprusside are balanced vasodilators. They act on both the arterial and venous beds. Nitroprusside reduces the ventricular filling pressure by directly increasing venous compliance and resulting in the redistribution of blood volume from the central to the peripheral veins. It is also the most effective afterload-reducing agent. It causes a fall in peripheral vascular resistance and an increase in aortic wall compliance. These effects of nitroprusside decrease the left ventricular afterload, resulting in an increase in cardiac output. Nitroprusside also dilates the pulmonary arterioles and reduces the right ventricular afterload. These combinations of reduction of preload and afterload by nitroprusside improve the myocardial function by reducing the wall tension, provided the BP does not fall to the point where the diastolic coronary blood flow is compromised or there is no marked reflex increase in sympathetic nervous system tone causing tachycardia. Nitroprusside is particularly effective in a patient with congestive heart failure due to mitral regurgitation or left-to-right shunt through the ventricular septal defect (VSD). The increase in renal blood flow that accompanies an increase in cardiac output, following initiation of administration of nitroprusside in a patient with severe heart failure, may improve the glomerular filtration rate and increase the effectiveness of diuretics.

Nitroglycerine, like nitroprusside, is also a potent vasodilator. But, in contrast to nitroprusside, nitroglycerine is relatively selective for veins, particularly at low infusion rates. Thus, IV nitroglycerine is most often used in the treatment of acute heart failure when particularly decrease in ventricular filling pressure is desired. At higher infusion rates, nitroglycerine also causes a decrease in systemic and pulmonary arterial resistance, thereby decreasing the ventricular afterload.

Sympathomimetic Amines

The enhancement of cardiac contractility is the cornerstone of the treatment of heart failure. Epinephrine, norepinephrine, isoprenaline, dopamine, and dobutamine are the five sympathomimetic amines that are generally used to improve myocardial contractility in the various forms of heart failure. Among them, dopamine and dobutamine are the most commonly used agents and effective in the management of heart failure, particularly in those patients who have undergone cardiac surgery, in some myocardial infarction (MI), shock, pulmonary edema, etc. Their administration should also be accompanied by careful and

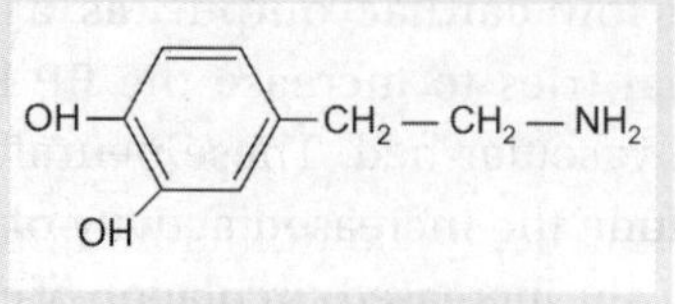

Fig. 6: Dopamine.

continuous monitoring of ECG, arterial pressure, and, if possible, pulmonary artery wedge pressure (PAWP).

Dopamine (3,4-dihydroxyphenyl Ethylamine)

The molecular structure of dopamine is shown in **Figure 6**. It is an endogenous catecholamine, and like dobutamine, it is also a strongly positive inotropic agent that is most often used for the short-term support of circulation in advanced heart failure. Epinephrine, norepinephrine, and isoprenaline, though strongly positive inotropic agent and useful in specific circumstances, have little role in the treatment of most cases of severe heart failure.

Dopamine is an important natural central neurotransmitter and an intermediate metabolic precursor for the synthesis of norepinephrine, epinephrine, and other centrally mediated neurotransmitters. It possesses important intrinsic pharmacological properties. It is ineffective when administered orally because dopamine is a substrate for both the monoamine oxidase (MAO) and catechol-O-methyltransferase (COMT) enzymes, present in the intestinal wall **(Flowchart 5)**.

Dopamine receptor: The action of dopamine is mediated by a family of dopamine receptors. Among them, five subtypes of dopamine receptors are identified. These are designated as D_1, D_2, D_3, D_4, and D_5. Of these, the D_1 and D_5 receptor proteins have a long intracellular carboxy-terminal tail and are the members of pharmacologically defined D_1 class. This D_1 class receptor stimulates the synthesis of intracellular second messenger called cAMP and causes the hydrolysis of phosphatidylinositol. The D_2, D_3, and D_4 receptor proteins share a common large third intracellular loop and are of the D_2 class. The D_2 class receptor inhibits the synthesis of cAMP as well as suppresses the Ca^{2+} currents and activates the receptor-operated K^+ currents.

All the dopamine receptors share the common structural features, including the presence of seven α-helical segments capable of spanning throughout the cell membrane **(Fig. 7)**. This structure identifies the dopamine receptors as the members of a large superfamily, which includes other important receptors such as β-adrenergic receptors, olfactory receptors. All the members of this superfamily act through the guanine nucleotide-binding protein or G-protein and are discussed in more detail in the autonomic nervous system (Chapter 11).

Cardiovascular effects of dopamine: Due to several distinct types of dopamine receptors and different affinity of dopamine to these receptors, the cardiovascular effects of dopamine vary with different doses. At low concentration (<2 µg/kg/min), dopamine acts through its vascular D_1-dopaminergic

Flowchart 5: Synthesis and metabolism of dopamine and levodopa. Levodopa is first synthesized from tyrosine, which is transported into the cell by an active process present on the cell membrane. The conversion of tyrosine to levodopa is a rate-limiting step and is catalyzed by tyrosine hydroxylase (TH). Levodopa is then rapidly converted to dopamine by an enzyme called aromatic amino acid decarboxylase (AAD). After that, this dopamine is taken up into the vesicles of dopaminergic nerve terminals by transporter protein, which can be blocked by reserpine. After its release into the synaptic cleft, the action of dopamine may be terminated by (1) the reuptake, which can be blocked by cocaine, or (2) the degradation by monoamine oxidase (MAO) or catechol-*O*-methyltransferase (COMT) enzyme. The metabolism of dopamine by MAO or COMT produces two metabolic products: DOPAC and homovanillic acid (HVA). But, in human beings, HVA is the primary product of the metabolism of dopamine.

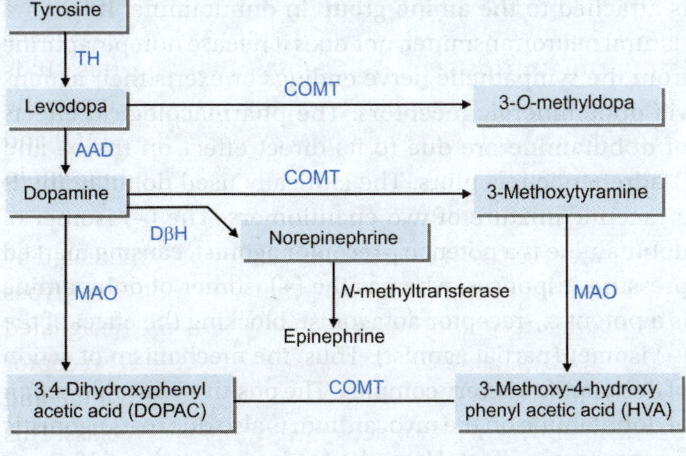

receptors, especially in the renal, mesenteric, and coronary beds. By activating adenyl cyclase and raising intracellular concentration of cAMP, D_1-receptor stimulation leads to vasodilation. So, the infusion of dopamine in low doses increases the renal blood flow, glomerular filtration rate, and Na^+ excretion. Thus, dopamine is often used in these small doses in the management of compromised renal function due to low cardiac output in severe heart failure. At somewhat higher concentration (2–5 µg/kg/min), dopamine acts on β1-adrenergic receptors and produces a positive inotropic effect on the myocardium. In this dose, dopamine also releases norepinephrine from nerve terminals and accounts for its effects on the heart. But the tachycardia induced by dopamine in this dose is less prominent than isoprenaline. At this level, dopamine increases systolic BP but has no effect on diastolic BP, and the total peripheral resistance remains unchanged or is reduced (probably because of the ability of dopamine to reduce regional arterial resistance in some vascular beds). At more higher concentration (5–15 µg/kg/min or higher), dopamine activates the vascular α_1-adrenergic receptor, leading to peripheral arterial and venous constriction, which sometimes may be desirable for the support of critically reduced arterial pressure. But this may further suppress the ventricular systolic function due to the increase in afterload.

As dopamine does not cross the blood–brain barrier readily, it has no central effects, even though there are specific dopamine receptors at the different areas of the central nervous system (CNS).

Precautions, adverse reactions, and contraindications of dopamine: The adverse effects of dopamine are mainly due to its excessive sympathomimetic activity. The tachycardia, anginal pain, arrhythmias, severe hypertension, headache, nausea, vomiting, etc., may be encountered during an infusion of dopamine. Hypovolemia should be corrected by

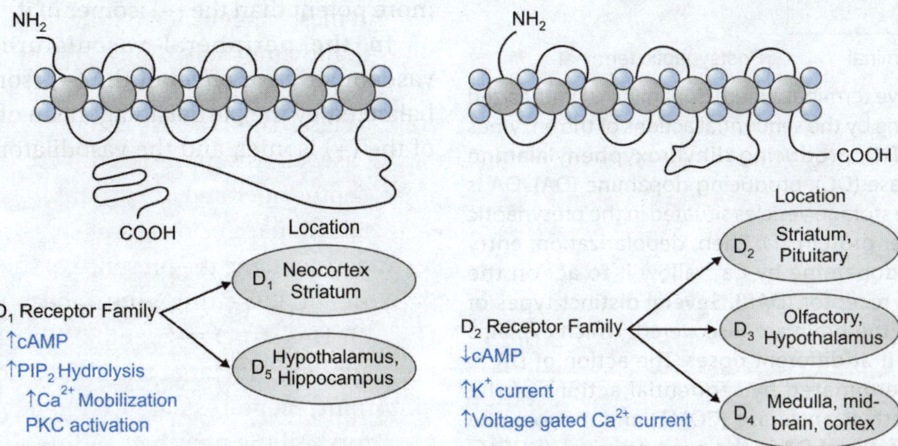

Fig. 7: Distribution and characteristics of different dopamine receptors. (cAMP: cyclic adenosine monophosphate; PKC: protein kinase C)

plasma, whole blood, or appropriate fluids in shock patients before starting the dopamine infusions. Dopamine should be avoided in patients taking MAO inhibitors or tricyclic antidepressant compounds **(Fig. 8)**.

Therapeutic uses and doses of dopamine: The indications where dopamine is mainly used are congestive heart failure with oliguria, low peripheral vascular resistance, cardiogenic shock, septic shock, and during different cardiac surgeries.

Initially, the dopamine infusion is usually started at the rate of <2 µg/kg/min (low dose), and then gradually, it is increased to 2–5 µg/kg/min (intermediate dose). The infusion rate of dopamine may be increased to 20–50 µg/kg/min or more as the clinical situation dictates. During the infusion of dopamine, patients should be continuously monitored for myocardial function, perfusion of vital organs, production of urine, arterial and venous pressure, ECG, etc. The reduction in urine output, tachycardia, or the development of arrhythmias indicates the immediate termination of dopamine infusion. As the duration of action of dopamine is brief, so the rate of administration of it through infusion should be adjusted continuously to control the intensity of its effect.

Usually, an alteration of cardiac responsiveness to catecholamines has been found in the different stages of heart failure. So, the doses of the infusion of sympathomimetic amines should be titrated according to the response of the patient. Increased sympathetic nervous system activity is observed in a patient during the early part of congestive heart failure. At that stage, the infusion of any β or dopa adrenergic agonist has been found to be toxic to the heart. Then, gradually, the overexpression of β or dopa adrenergic receptor lead to dilated cardiomyopathy. After that, a number of changes in β-adrenergic receptor signaling occur in the myocardium in patient with long-standing heart failure. Decreased numbers and functioning of β_1-adrenergic receptor consistently have been found in chronic heart failure, leading to attenuation of β-adrenergic receptor-mediated stimulation or positive inotropic response in the failing heart.

Dobutamine

The molecular structure of dobutamine is shown in **Figure 9**. The structure of dobutamine and dopamine is more or less the same except a bulky aromatic substituent, which is attached to the amino group in dobutamine. It is not a natural neurotransmitter, nor does it release norepinephrine from the sympathetic nerve endings or exerts their actions via dopaminergic receptors. The pharmacological effects of dobutamine are due to its direct effect on the α- and β-adrenergic receptors. The clinically used dobutamine is a racemic mixture of two enantiomers. The (–) isomer of dobutamine is a potent α_1-receptor agonist, causing marked pressure responses, whereas the (+) isomer of dobutamine is a potent α_1-receptor antagonist, blocking the effect of the (–) isomer (partial agonist). Thus, the mechanism of action of dobutamine is very complex. The positive inotropic action of dobutamine on the myocardium is also due to its agonistic β_1-adrenergic effect. Here, the (+) isomer is about 10 times more potent than the (–) isomer of it.

In the peripheral vasculature, the α_1-adrenergic vasoconstrictive effect of the (–) isomer of dobutamine is balanced by the partial antagonism of the α_1-receptor effect of the (+) isomer, and the vasodilatory effect is mainly due

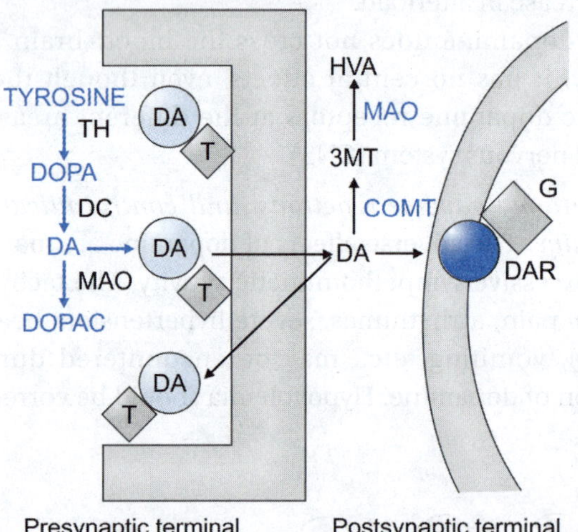

Fig. 8: Dopaminergic nerve terminal, where dopamine is synthesized from the precursor tyrosine by the sequential actions of the enzymes tyrosine hydroxylase (TH), producing dihydroxyphenylalanine (DOPA), and decarboxylase (DC), producing dopamine (DA). DA is then transported into the storage vesicles situated in the presynaptic terminal by a transporter protein (T). Then, depolarization, entry of Ca^{2+}, and release of dopamine by Ca^{2+} allow it to act on the postsynaptic dopamine receptor (DAR). Several distinct types of DA receptors present in the brain are discovered, which explains the different actions of it at different doses. The action of DA at the nerve terminal is terminated by sequential actions of the enzymes catechol-*O*-methyltransferase (COMT) and monoamine oxidase (MAO) or by reuptake of DA in the nerve terminal. (DOPAC: dihydroxyphenyl acetic acid).

Fig. 9: Dobutamine.

to the β_2-receptor stimulation by dobutamine. Thus, the net pharmacological effect of dobutamine is to increase the stroke volume and cardiac output by positive inotropic action on the myocardium (β_1-effect) and to decrease the SVR and venous filling pressure by both α and β effects. Dobutamine has no action on the renal dopaminergic receptor, so it does not dilate the renal vessels. But the increase in renal blood flow and glomerular filtration rate by dobutamine is due to the increase in cardiac output. Dobutamine causes no or little increase in heart rate. It has relatively more prominent inotropic effect than chronotropic effects on the heart. So, at doses that increase cardiac output, there is little increase in heart rate and O_2 consumption of myocardium than dopamine.

Dobutamine is used by infusion and is started with the dose of 2–3 µg/kg/min. Then, it is titrated upward according to the patient's symptoms and hemodynamic goals, which depend on cardiac contractility, cardiac output, and peripheral vascular resistance. Depending on vascular resistance and cardiac output, BP may increase, decrease, or remain the same. In response to improved cardiovascular function by dobutamine, the heart rate often declines due to the withdrawal of reflex sympathetic tone. The measurement of PCWP and cardiac output, using a pulmonary arterial catheter, often allows the more effective use of dobutamine alone or in conjunction with other vasodilators and diuretics. However, the continuous infusion of dobutamine over several days reduces its efficacy due to the development of tolerance. When tolerance develops to dobutamine after prolonged use, then it is necessary to switch over to an IV class III cAMP PDE inhibitory agent, e.g., amrinone or milrinone.

Like other sympathomimetic drugs, the side effects of dobutamine are also severe tachycardia, hypertension, arrhythmia, ventricular ectopic, etc. Patients with a history

of hypertension may be at a greater risk of developing an exaggerated pressure response to dobutamine. As dobutamine facilitates AV conduction (enhancement of AV and intraventricular conduction by isoprenaline and dobutamine is the same), so patients with atrial fibrillation are at an increased risk of marked ventricular response rates. Dobutamine, like other inotropic agents, may also increase the size of myocardial infarct by increasing the myocardial O_2 demand. This risk must be balanced against the patient's overall clinical status. The infusion of dobutamine in a patient receiving β-blocker fails to increase cardiac output as the total peripheral vascular resistance is increased by it. The effect of dobutamine on different cardiovascular parameters is shown in **Figures 10A to C**.

The main therapeutic indication for the use of dobutamine is the short-term treatment of cardiac decompensation with severe hypotension that occurs after cardiac surgery or in a patient with congestive heart failure or in patient suffering from acute MI, because it increases the cardiac output and stroke volume without increasing the heart rate. The half-life of dobutamine is 2 minutes. The onset of action of dobutamine is rapid, so no loading dose is required. Steady-state concentration of dobutamine is generally achieved within 10 minutes of starting an infusion.

Phosphodiesterase Inhibitors (Amrinone and Milrinone)

Adrenaline, in the form of physiological signals, binds with adrenergic receptors on the cell surface and induces the conformational changes of its receptor. These conformational changes of receptor permit interaction of it with stimulatory G-protein (G_S) at its binding site. This G_S-protein is now activated. The activated G_S-protein now activates the enzyme, adenyl cyclase, located on the cytoplasmic site of

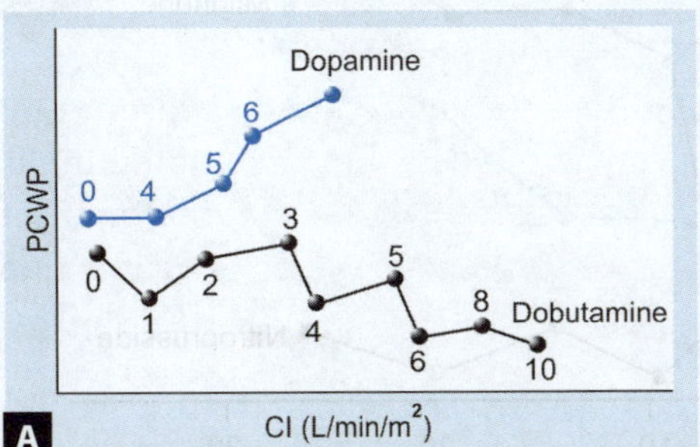

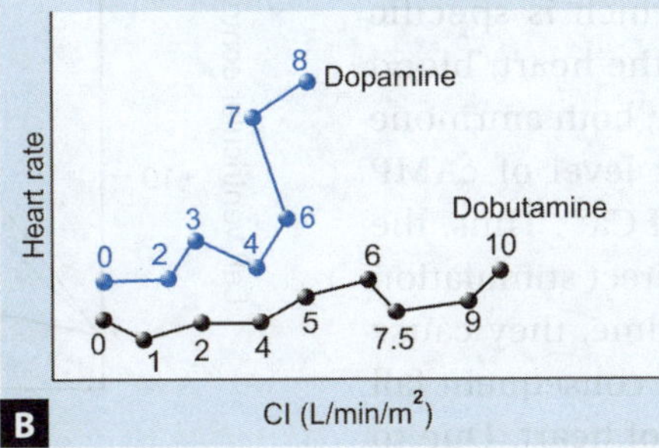

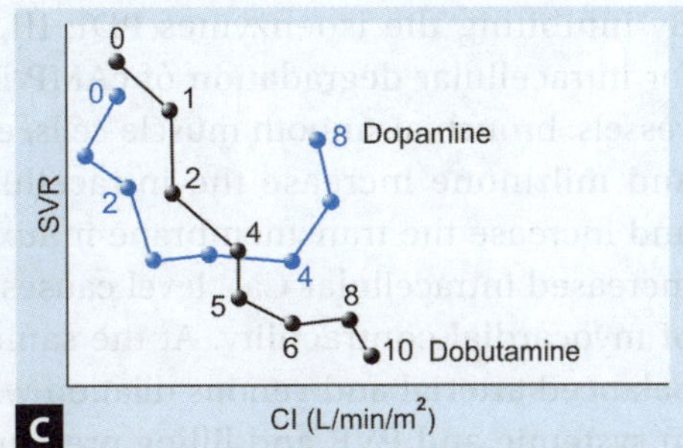

Figs. 10A to C: The effects of dopamine and dobutamine on pulmonary capillary wedge pressure (PCWP), heart rate, and systemic vascular resistance (SVR) were shown in a patient with severe heart failure. Dobutamine increases both cardiac output and cardiac index due to an increase in stroke volume. This effect of dobutamine is associated with a decrease in both PCWP and SVR. It reflects both the direct vasodilation effect of dobutamine due to the stimulation of β_2-adrenergic receptors and the withdrawal of reflex sympathetic tone due to improved cardiovascular function. At infusion rates of dopamine exceeding 2–4 µg/kg/min, it exerts a potent vasoconstrictor effect. It is evidenced by the increase in SVR and PCWP. It also decreases the left ventricular function caused by the increase in afterload. The numbers shown in the figures are infusion rates in µg/kg/min. (CI: cardiac index)

the cell membrane (cytoplasmic signaling protein). Activated adenyl cyclase now hydrolyzes (not dephosphorylation) ATP to cAMP and its intracellular concentration increases. This cAMP, in turn, then, phosphorylates and activates the protein kinase A (PKA), which again phosphorylates many other functional proteins within the cell, including troponin and phospholamban so that they interact with Ca^{2+}, resulting in increased force of contraction. This intracellular Ca^{2+} is also made available for contraction by entry from outside by direct activation of the Ca^{2+} channel, situated on the myocardial cell membrane, by both G_S protein and phosphorylated active PK_A, as well as from intracellular stores in SR.

Now, the physiological signals outside the cell in the form of adrenaline, noradrenaline, acetylcholine, etc., are integrated within the cell as second messenger, such as cAMP, cyclic guanosine monophosphate (cGMP), Ca^{2+}, inositol phosphates, and nitric oxide, and do all the cellular function. Normally, cAMP is eliminated by hydrolysis, which is catalyzed by the cyclic nucleotide PDE. Thus, the PDE inhibitors mimic the effects of adenyl cyclase activation by β-agonists and act through increasing the level of cAMP by inhibiting the hydrolysis of it. Hence, the increased level of intracellular cAMP by PDE inhibitors increases myocardial contractility and causes the vasodilation of both arteries and veins. The first group of PDE inhibitors, e.g., theophylline and aminophylline, has been identified many years ago. But their use at a hemodynamically effective dose for heart failure is plagued by side effects. In 1980, the introduction of amrinone and subsequently later other PDE inhibitors, e.g., milrinone, has become the cornerstone of the treatment of heart failure, alleviating the previous problems.

Amrinone and milrinone: Chemically, both these drugs are bipyridine derivatives and are selective PDE III isoenzyme inhibitors. Pharmacologically, they are distinct from digitalis and catecholamines and form a new class of inotropic drugs. By inhibiting the isoenzymes PDE III, which is specific for intracellular degradation of cAMP in the heart, blood vessels, bronchial smooth muscle cells, etc., both amrinone and milrinone increase the intracellular level of cAMP and increase the transmembrane influx of Ca^{2+}. Thus, the increased intracellular Ca^{2+} level causes direct stimulation of myocardial contractility. At the same time, they cause balanced arterial and venous dilation with consequent fall in systemic and PVR and filling pressure of heart. Due to the stimulation of myocardial contraction and a decrease in afterload, cardiac output increases. As a result of these dual mechanisms of action (vasodilatation and increased cardiac contraction), the increase in cardiac output with milrinone and amrinone is greater than the pure vasodilator agent, such as nitroprusside, when compared for a given

decrease in systemic arterial pressure. Again, the arterial and venous dilatation effects of these two PDE inhibitors are greater than the arterial and venous dilatation caused by dobutamine when compared for a given increase in cardiac output. However, amrinone and milrinone do not inhibit the Na^+-K^+-ATPase pump like digitalis. Their actions are also independent of tissue catecholamine levels and adrenergic receptors (such as β-receptor) concentration (direct action). The effect of milrinone, nitroprusside, and dobutamine on SVR and cardiac contractility is shown in **Figure 11**. The effect of vasodilators, diuretics, and inotropes on a failed heart is shown in **Figure 12**.

Both amrinone and milrinone are commonly used as single agent or in combination with other oral and/or IV drugs for short-term treatment of a patient with severe systolic right or left ventricular failure. Both the drugs are used intravenously, initially by a loading dose which is then followed by a continuous infusion. For amrinone, the initial IV bolus dose is 0.75 mg/kg and is given over 2–3 minutes. Then, it is followed by 2–20 µg/kg/min through continuous infusion. As milrinone is 10 times more potent than amrinone, so the initial loading dose of it is 50 µg/kg IV, which is followed by 0.25–1 µg/kg/min by continuous infusion. The IV action of both these drugs starts within 5 minutes. The half-lives of amrinone and milrinone in healthy subjects are 2–3 hours and 30–60 minutes, respectively. This half-life becomes doubled in a patient with severe heart failure.

Thrombocytopenia is the most common and prominent dose-related side effect of amrinone. But it is mostly transient and asymptomatic. However, thrombocytopenia is rare with milrinone **(Fig. 12)**.

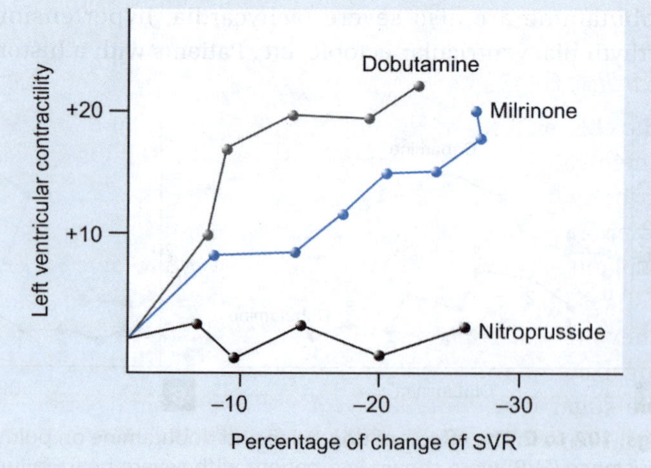

Fig. 11: Comparative study on the effects of nitroprusside, milrinone, and dobutamine on the gradual reduction of systemic vascular resistance (SVR). Among these compounds, dobutamine and milrinone (but not nitroprusside) also increase ventricular contractility with reducing SVR.

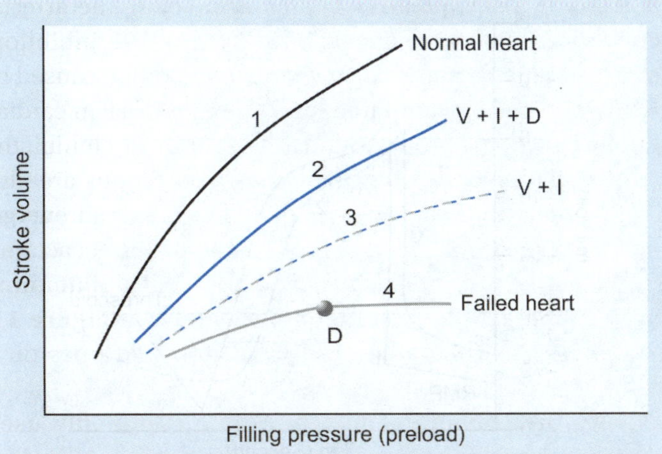

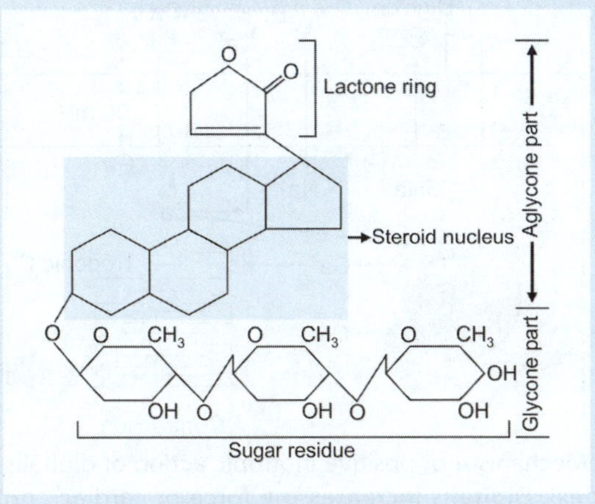

Fig. 13: Structure of digoxin.

Fig. 12: Hemodynamic responses of a failed heart to different pharmacological interventions. Line 1 represents the normal heart, and line 4 represents the failed heart due to systolic dysfunction, with the effects of diuretics (D) alone. The other two curves (line 2 and line 3) show the effect of V + I and V + I + D on the failed heart. The combination of drugs produces the synergistic effect on hemodynamic responses more toward the normal heart. The diuretics alone improve the symptoms of congestive heart failure by reducing only the filling pressure of the heart but not improving the cardiac output with the same ventricular function curve. The use of inotropic agents such as dobutamine and glycosides moves the patients to a higher ventricular function curve (line 1). (I: inotropes; V: vasodilators)

Milrinone is now the agent of choice among the currently available PDE inhibitors for short-term parenteral inotropic support in severe heart failure. This is because of greater selectivity of milrinone for (1) the inhibition of isoenzyme PDE III, (2) shorter half-life, and (3) fewer side effects of it. Hence, in chronic heart failure, these inotropes have no role for long-term use but even increase mortality.

Cardiac Glycosides

The chemical structure of glycoside is shown in **Figure 13**. Chemically, glycosides are compound that contain both a carbohydrate (sugar) and a noncarbohydrate (nonsugar) component. They are particularly found as natural products in plants. They can be converted by hydrolytic cleavage into a sugar (glycone) and a nonsugar (aglycone) component. They are also named specifically according to the type of sugar component, present in it, such as glycoside (when the sugar component is glucose), pentoside (when the sugar component is pentose), or fructoside (when the sugar component is fructose). The glycoside compounds, which have cardiac inotropic effects, are called cardiac glycosides.

All the cardiac glycosides have a common molecular structure, i.e., a steroid (cyclopentanoperhydrophenan-threne) nucleus and an unsaturated lactose nucleus (or ring)

attached to the steroid nucleus at its C_{17} position. This steroid nucleus and the lactose ring together form the aglycone part. One or more sugar residue is attached to the steroid nucleus and constitutes the glycone part of the glycoside molecule. The pharmacological properties of cardiac glycosides reside on the aglycone part of the glycoside molecule. But the sugar or glycone component of the glycoside molecule modifies the water solubility and the cell membrane permeability of it. There are many cardiac glycosides available in practice. But, among them, only digoxin and digitoxin are orally active, and between them only digoxin has widespread clinical use today. Digitoxin differs from digoxin only by the absence of hydroxyl group at C_{12} position, resulting in a less hydrophilic compound with altered pharmacokinetic property (but the same pharmacodynamics) compared to digoxin.

The beneficial effects of cardiac glycosides in heart failure are derived from (1) the positive inotropic effect of it on failing myocardium, (2) the efficacy of it in controlling the ventricular rate in response to atrial fibrillation, and (3) the modulating sympathetic nervous system activity of it, which may be an additional mechanism and contribute significantly to their efficacy in heart failure.

Mechanism of action of glycosides (digitalis): The mechanism of action of cardiac glycoside is shown in **Figure 14**. The cardiac glycosides selectively bind to their specific site of attachment, present on the extra-cytoplasmic part of the α-subunit of Na⁺–K⁺-ATPase pump, situated on the cell membrane and inhibit it. As a result, there is reduction in the rate of active Na⁺ extrusion and rise in intracellular Nas⁺ concentration.

The relationship between the intracellular Na⁺ and Ca^{2+} concentrations is such that a small percentage of increase in intracellular Na⁺ concentration results in a large percentage of increase in intracellular Ca^{2+} concentration. Thus, the resulting increase in intracellular Ca^{2+} interacts

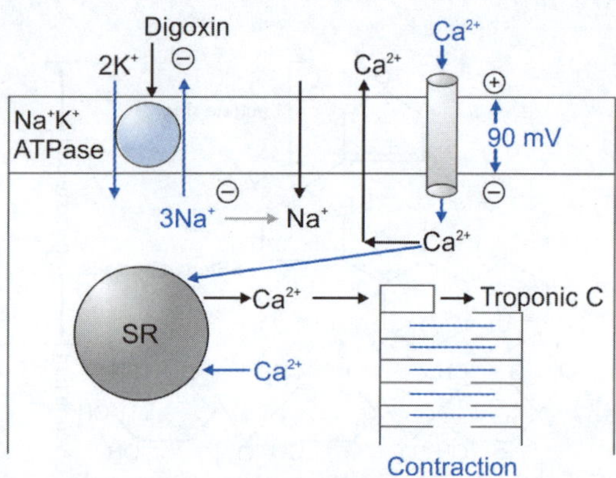

Fig. 14: Mechanism of positive inotropic action of digitalis (cardiac glycosides). Digitalis increases the force of cardiac contraction by not acting through catecholamine's receptor, but by its direct action on the Na⁺–K⁺-ATPase pump. It binds selectively with Na⁺–K⁺-ATP system on the cell membrane and inhibits it. Then, inhibition of this system causes gradual accumulation and increase in the concentration of Na⁺ intracellularly. By the side of the Na⁺–K⁺-ATPase system, there is Na⁺–Ca²⁺ exchange protein which extrudes Ca²⁺ in exchange of influx of Na⁺. Increased intracellular concentration of Na⁺ inhibits the further influx of Na⁺ and extrusion of Ca²⁺ through this Na⁺–Ca²⁺ exchanger, and thus indirectly the digitalis increases the intracellular concentration of Ca²⁺, which gradually store in the SR. During depolarization, Ca²⁺ further enters the cell through the voltage-sensitive Ca²⁺ channel (A). This triggers the more release of excess stored Ca²⁺ from SR and thus helps in more forceful contraction. The more intracellular Ca²⁺ concentration, the more the force of muscular contraction. After contraction is over, Ca²⁺ is further taken back by SR. The portion of Ca²⁺ that enters the cell from outside during depolarization is also extruded by the 3Na⁺–1Ca²⁺ exchanger. This excess Ca²⁺ remains in cytosol and is taken up by SR. Thus, SR is progressively loaded with more and more Ca²⁺, and subsequently, Ca²⁺ store is augmented. (ATP: adenosine triphosphate; SR: sarcoplasmic reticulum)

with troponin-C and activates the cross-bridge interaction between the actin and myosin filaments that results in forceful contraction and sarcomere shortening. Moreover, the raised intracellular Ca²⁺ concentration induces a greater reentry of Ca²⁺ through the voltage sensitive Ca²⁺ channel during the plateau phase of action potential. Hence, this increased intracellular level of Ca²⁺ is taken up by SR, and its storage capacity is increased, which is available for the contractile elements during the subsequent depolarization of myocytes. Thus, the contractility of the myocardium is augmented, and this is the mechanism of action of digitalis.

The binding of glycosides to the Na⁺–K⁺-ATPase pump is slow. So, the Ca²⁺ loading in SR occurs gradually, and the inotropic effects of digitalis take hours to develop, even after its IV administration. As the digitalis inhibits the Na⁺–K⁺-ATPase pump activity, there is gradual depletion of intracellular K⁺ (as K⁺ does not enter), and this is responsible for the mechanism of all toxicities of digitalis. So, the toxicity

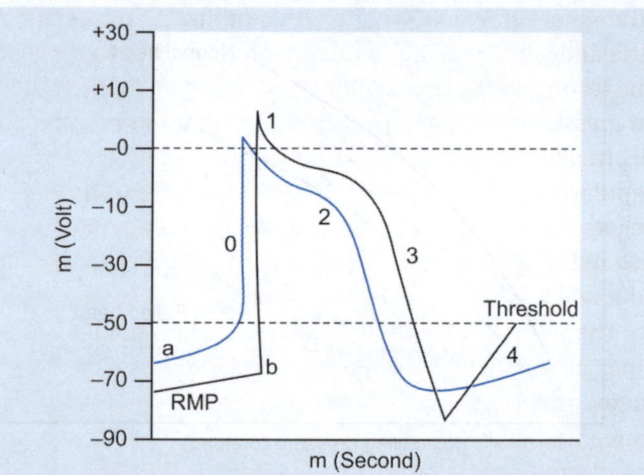

Fig. 15: Effects of digitalis on the action potential (AP) of Purkinje fibers (PF). The effects of digitalis differ qualitatively and quantitatively according to the types of cardiac muscle fibers. PFs, sinoatrial (SA) node, and other conducting tissues are more sensitive to cardiac glycosides. For the action of glycosides, direct action and indirect autonomic influences are both important. Resting membrane potential (RMP) gradually shifts to the isoelectric level (i.e., decreased). So, the excitability or automaticity increases due to the reduction of gap between the RMP and the threshold level. But this occurs in higher doses. At therapeutic concentration, automaticity is reduced [SA and atrioventricular (AV) node] by indirect vagal action, which hyperpolarizes these cells. In therapeutic concentrations, the slope of phase 4 also reduces, i.e., becomes more flat, which explains the reduction of automaticity in SA and AV nodes. In toxic doses RMP also decreases, i.e., becomes less negative. This is due to the depolarization running below the critical potential value, which inactivates the fast Na⁺ channel. In therapeutic concentration, the height of the 0 phase of AP is also reduced by digitalis. This is due to more negative value of RMP at which excitation occurs. This reduction of height of AP is responsible for slow conduction and is most marked in AV node and bundle of His. In high doses, the slope of phase 4 is increased in PFs, which is responsible for enhanced automaticity and ectopic focus. Line-a indicates digitalis treated fiber and line-b indicates digitalis untreated fiber.

of digitalis is partially reversed by K⁺ supplementation. Excessive Ca²⁺ loading in SR during the spontaneous cycles of Ca²⁺ release and reuptake of it produces an oscillation after every contraction or depolarization. So, both the therapeutic and toxic effects of digitalis are due to this myocardial Ca²⁺ overloading. These are inseparable and also explain the low therapeutic index (window) of digitalis.

Electrophysiological effects of glycosides (digitalis): The effects of digitalis on the action potential are shown in **Figure 15**. The electrophysiological effects of digitalis on different types of cardiac tissues, such as atrial muscle, ventricular muscle, pacemaker cells, and conducting fibers, are different due to their different action potential, different sensitivities, and different responses to glycosides. The Purkinje fibers and the other specialized automatic and conducting tissues in the atria and ventricles are more sensitive to cardiac glycosides. The resting membrane potential (RMP) of all these tissues is progressively reversed, i.e., shifted away more from the iso-electrical level. So, the rate and the amplitude of "0" phase depolarization are reduced, primarily as the result of less negative value of RMP. The duration of action potential is also reduced (primarily at phase 2). The amplitude of action potential is also diminished by digitalis.

The action of digitalis on cardiac muscle is mediated by its direct action on cells and also by the indirect action through vagus and sympathetic nervous system. At therapeutic concentration, digoxin reduces the automaticity, increases the diastolic RMP, prolongs the effective refractory period, and decreases the conduction velocity, predominantly in the atrial and AV nodal tissues. All these are due to the increased vagal tone and decreased sympathetic nervous system activity. At higher or toxic serum concentration, digoxin causes sinus bradycardia and/or prolongation of AV conduction, resulting in heart block or arrest. On the other hand, paradoxically, at more higher concentration of digoxin, sympathetic activity increases. This increases the automaticity of cardiac muscle cells that contributes to the generation of atrial and ventricular arrhythmias. Both the increased intracellular Ca^{2+} concentration and increased sympathetic activity by glycoside result in an increase in the spontaneous rate of diastolic depolarization (phase 4) leading to ventricular ectopic, tachycardia, and fibrillation. Nonuniform simultaneous increase in automaticity and depression in conduction through the bundle of His and Purkinje system by glycoside causes arrhythmias, which may lead to ventricular tachycardia and fibrillation.

Pharmacological action of cardiac glycosides: All the cardiac glycosides have similar pharmacodynamic actions. But they differ in only quantitative and pharmacokinetic properties. Digoxin is the prototype of all the cardiac glycosides and is so described here. By convention, the term "digitalis" is applied as a collective name to the whole group of cardiac glycosides.

Digoxin has positive inotropic action and causes the dose-dependent increase in the force of myocardial contraction of failing heart, which is exquisitely sensitive to it. Systole is shortened and diastole is prolonged. When a normal cardiac muscle fiber is subjected to increased impedance to outflow, then by the Starling principle, increased tension is generated in it (cardiac muscle fiber), and its force of contraction is increased, so that the stroke volume is maintained considerably up to certain higher values of impedance while the failing heart, where this limitation is crossed, will not be able to do so and the stroke

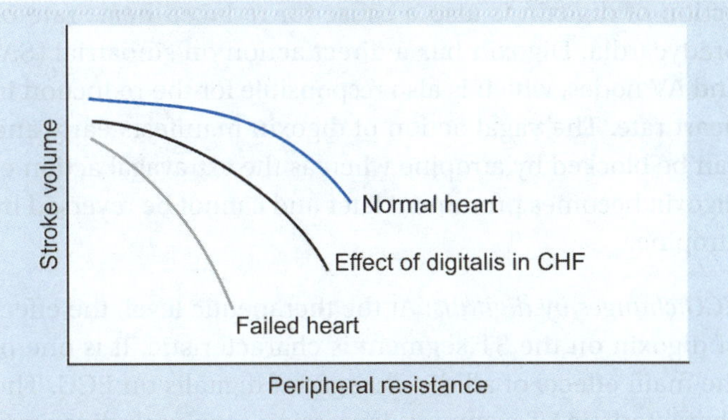

Fig. 16: Relationship between the peripheral resistance (impedance) and the stroke volume in the normal and failing heart. The figure also shows the effect of digitalis on that failed heart. (CHF: congestive heart failure)

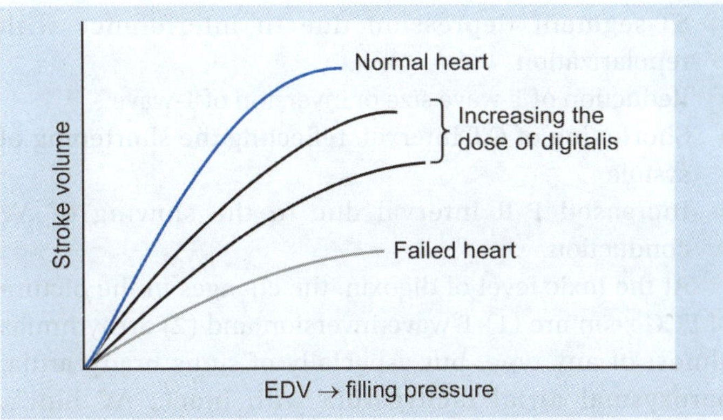

Fig. 17: Relationship between the filling pressure in the ventricle and stroke volume in normal and failed heart. It also depicts the effect of an increased dose of digitalis, which shifts the curve toward normal. (EDV: end-diastolic volume)

volume progressively decreases. This is shown in **Figure 16**. But, under the influence of digoxin, the failing heart regains some of its capacity to contract more forcefully, when it is subjected to increased resistance for ejection (impedance). Therefore, there is more complete emptying of failing and dilated ventricles, and cardiac output is increased. This is shown in **Figure 17**.

Digoxin also increases the force of contraction in the normal heart. But this is not translated into increased output because the normal heart empties almost completely (even otherwise), and therefore further reduction of end-diastolic volume is counterproductive.

Digoxin causes a decrease in heart rate, and it is due to improved circulation. This is more marked in failing heart, where the heart rate is increased as a mechanism of compensation (sympathetic stimulation). The improved circulation reduces the compensated sympathetic activity and thus decreases the heart rate. The direct vagal mimetic action of digoxin is also a cause for reduced heart rate or bradycardia. Digoxin has a direct action on sinoatrial (SA) and AV nodes, which is also responsible for the reduction in heart rate. The vagal action of digoxin manifests early and can be blocked by atropine whereas the extravagal action of digoxin becomes prominent later and cannot be reversed by atropine.

ECG changes by digitalis: At the therapeutic level, the effect of digoxin on the ST segment is characteristic. It is one of the main effects of all the changes of digitalis on ECG. The characteristic ST segment depression seen with digoxin is described as a reverse tick and is most obvious in leads with a tall R-wave.

Therefore, the effects of digoxin on ECG at therapeutic levels are:
- ST-segment depression due to interference with repolarization
- Reduction of T-wave size or inversion of T-wave
- Shortening of QT interval, reflecting the shortening of systole
- Increased P-R interval due to the slowing of AV conduction.

At the toxic level of digoxin, the changes in the picture of ECG seen are (1) T-wave inversion and (2) arrhythmias almost of any type, but especially of sinus bradycardia, paroxysmal atrial tachycardia with block, AV block, ventricular ectopic, ventricular bigeminy, ventricular tachycardia, etc. The abnormal QRS complex of Wolff–Parkinson–White (WPW) syndrome, under the influence of digoxin, is widened because conduction through the normal AV bundle is slowed, but not through the aberrant pathways.

Pharmacokinetics: The most oral preparation of digoxin available in the market has 70–80% oral bioavailability. The presence of food in the stomach delays its absorption. The bioavailability of oral preparation of digoxin differs considerably for different manufacturers. So, it is advisable to stick to one brand. The liquid-filled digoxin capsules have greater bioavailability than its tablets and require dose adjustment if a patient switches over from tablet to liquid-filled capsule. Parenteral digoxin is also available for IV use when only the oral route is impractical. Intramuscular (IM) digoxin administration causes pain and necrosis as all the glycosides are irritant to local tissues. It gets bound to muscle tissues after the IM injection, and so the absorption from the injection site is erratic as well as poor. Hence, the IM route for the administration of digoxin is not recommended.

All the cardiac glycosides have cumulative properties. The elimination half-life ($t\frac{1}{2}$) of digoxin is 36–48 hours in a patient with normal renal function. So, digoxin is given once a day, and the steady-state level with full therapeutic effect is attained after ($4 \times t\frac{1}{2}$) 7 days of initiation of maintenance therapy.

It is primarily excreted unchanged by the kidney, mainly by glomerular filtration. The rate of excretion of digoxin through the kidney is altered in renal disease but is parallel to the creatinine clearance. So, the half-life of digoxin is prolonged in elderly and renal failure patient. Thus, the dose of digoxin has to be reduced, in elderly and renal failure patient.

Doses of digitalis: The dose and the route of digoxin administration depend on the speed of action desired by the clinician. In many patients, the therapeutic response can occur at doses well below the maximum tolerated dose, but in some patients, the reverse is observed. Generally, higher doses of digoxin are needed for a severe heart failure patient. According to the therapeutic need, any digitalis can be used by three methods. These are (1) slow oral digitalization, (2) rapid oral digitalization, and (3) emergency IV digitalization.

Slow Digitalization (oral)
In mild-to-moderate heart failure cases, the digoxin is started orally in the dose of 0.125–0.250 mg/day, depending on the lean body mass, as digoxin concentrates mainly in the heart, skeletal muscle, liver, and kidney, but not in fat. The full therapeutic response of digoxin is developed within 5–7 days after its initiation of therapy. If an adequate response is not seen after 1 week, then the dose is increased to 0.375 mg/day and then to 0.5 mg/day after another 1 week.

The relief of signs and symptoms of heart failure and the reduction of heart rate are the best guide to judge the response of digitalis.

Rapid digitalization (oral)
It is done when the result is expected within few hours. It is started in the dose of 0.5–1 mg, followed by 0.25 mg at every 6-hour interval, with careful monitoring of toxicity, till the response occurs. It generally takes 6–24 hours, and the total dose needed is about 0.75–1.5 g. But this is seldom practiced now.

Emergency IV digitalization
This is also rarely practiced now. It is only taken as a desperate measure in acute heart failure or in atrial fibrillation producing acute symptoms. In such a situation, digoxin is used in the dose of 0.25 mg IV stat, followed by 0.1 mg IV slowly at the interval of every hour, with close ECG, BP, and CVP monitoring, till the response occurs. Usually, IV digitalis takes 2–6 hours for its full action to onset, and the total dose needed is 0.5–1 mg.

CURRENT STATUS OF CLINICAL USE OF DIGITALIS

Before the introduction of (1) high ceiling IV loop diuretics and (2) different specific arterial, venous and mixed vasodilators such as nitroprusside, nitroglycerine, ACE inhibitors, and PDE inhibitors, digitalis was thought as an indispensable agent for the treatment of heart failure. But its importance has been gradually waned away in cardiac failure. All acute, mild, and moderate heart failure are now treated by diuretics, ACE inhibitors, and vasodilators. The emergency IV use of digoxin is practically extinct now. But, as there are no oral inotropes for prolonged use in chronic heart failure, digitalis is still a prominent drug in chronic heart failure patients, those not controlled by diuretics and ACE inhibitors.

Only one question exists, during the prolonged use of digitalis, in chronic heart failure is: after decompensation, how long it should be used? The answer is that with the availability of diuretics, vasodilators, and ACE inhibitors, there has been a trend to discontinue digitalis once compensation has been restored, especially in mild-to-moderate cases. Thus, if a stable clinical state has been maintained for 2–3 months, withdrawal of digitalis may be attempted, and early reinstitution of digitalis is recommended if the cardiac status declines again. There is no coincidence that digitalis prolongs the survival of chronic heart failure patients. The two major limitations for the use of cardiac glycosides are the low margin of safety and the inability to reverse or retard the process that causes the heart to fail. Based on all these discussions, the international recommendation is that digoxin should be reserved for patients with chronic heart failure who have AF or for patients with sinus rhythm who remain symptomatic despite adequate treatment with diuretics, ACE inhibitors, and β-adrenergic receptor antagonists.

ADVERSE EFFECTS OR TOXICITY OF DIGITALIS AND ITS MANAGEMENT

The adverse effects or toxicity of digitalis is very high, and the margin of safety is low. The adverse effects of digitalis are divided into the following:

- *Extra-cardiac effect:* These are anorexia, nausea, vomiting, fatigue, malaise, mental confusion, restlessness, disorientation, psychosis, visual disturbances, etc.

- *Cardiac effect:* Almost all types of arrhythmias can be produced by digitalis. These are pulsus bigeminus, ventricular extrasystole, ventricular fibrillation, ventricular tachycardia, AV junctional ectopic, partial to complete AV block, severe bradycardia, atrial extrasystole, atrial filtration, flutter, etc.

However, the management of all these complications often requires only dose adjustment and appropriate monitoring. Sinus arrest and second- or third-degree AV block are usually treated by IV atropine injection. In extreme cases, temporary ventricular pacing may be needed. Even when the serum K^+ level is in the normal range, still potassium supplementation should be considered for completely digitalized patients with AV junctional and ventricular ectopic beats, unless a higher degree AV block is present. Extracellular K^+ promotes the dephosphorylation of Na^+K^+-ATPase enzyme and decreases the affinity of this enzyme for binding with cardiac glycosides. This provides one explanation for why increased extracellular K^+ reverses some of the toxic effects of digitalis. As extracellular K^+ depletion precipitates digitalis toxicity, this toxicity again causes high plasma K^+ levels.

Lignocaine is used for the treatment of ventricular automaticity of digitalis toxicity that threatens hemodynamic compromise. But it does not accentuate the AV block. Electrical cardioversion carries an increased risk of inducing severe rhythm disturbances in a patient with overt digitalis toxicity, and it should be used with particular caution.

Recently for the treatment of digitalis toxicity, antidigoxin immunotherapy is very promising and is now a great breakthrough. Purified Fab fragment from ovine antidigoxin antisera is an effective antidote for digoxin toxicity. The Fab fragment has been marketed in Europe as "Digibend" (40 mg/vial). It is nonimmunogenic. Given by IV infusion, it markedly improved the survival of digitalis-intoxicated patients. The total neutralizing dose of Fab is calculated from either the estimated total dose of the drug ingested or the total body digoxin burden. This antidigoxin antisera can be administered intravenously with saline solution over 30–60 minutes. After administration, this Fab fragment of antidigoxin antibody binds with the molecule of digoxin and makes a digoxin–Fab complex. Now, this digoxin–Fab complex is rapidly excreted by the kidney. However, it is very expensive.

Management of Airway

■ HISTORY

Tracheal intubation in animals was first described by Mr Vesalius of Padua, in 1543, and by Mr R Hooke of UK, in 1667. But after that, there was a prolonged silence and nobody had tried to intubate trachea. Then, after a long interval, the end of the 18th century had again seen a flurry of researches and publications on tracheal intubation. It was triggered by unhygienic and unethical humanitarian factor, for the resuscitation of drowned persons, by mouth-to-mouth breathing, because during that period mouth-to-mouth resuscitation of a drowned person was condemned due to the unhygienic ground. So, there was a continuous search for an alternative way to resuscitate a drowned person, other than this unhygienic mouth-to-mouth artificial ventilation.

Then, again after a century, in 1776, John Hunter had described tracheal intubation. He had performed it by a metal tracheal tube. After that, in 1788, C Kite had also described an oral and nasal intubation for resuscitation of an apparently drowned person. This was followed by James Curry who had also described several different metal endotracheal tubes (ETTs), in 1792. But in 1827, Leroy had first shown that pneumothorax may result from high intrapulmonary pressures, during this artificial ventilation by tracheal tube. Then, John Snow used a tracheal catheter to resuscitate a newborn baby.

All these works, described earlier, were directed at that time with an aim, either for resuscitation of a drowned person or for the relief of an upper airway obstruction. Then, from 1848, the passage of a metal tube or a catheter into the trachea was routinely practiced to resuscitate only the anesthetic causalities, but not to administer sole anesthesia. Then, gradually, there was significant technical advancement to contemplate for the deliberate administration of anesthetic vapors through this tracheal tube for sole anesthetic purpose. So, John Snow, in 1852, had made a historical leap by intubating animals via a tracheostomy wound and providing inhalational anesthesia through this tube. After that, in 1871, Friedrich Trendelenburg of Rostock used this method in humans while he was a surgical assistant to a surgeon, named Dr Langenbeck, residing in Berlin. He used this method for operation in the mouth. After performing a tracheostomy, he introduced a tube into the trachea and inflates the cuff for administering anesthesia.

At that time, it had been assumed that if a tube was passed through the larynx, then it would not be tolerated, except for tracheostomy. So, they were used to do tracheostomy routinely for intubation. But in 1878, William Macewen of Glasgow had first decided and tried to avoid tracheostomy for intubation, if otherwise inevitable. So, after practicing on a cadaver, he passed a flexible metal tube through the mouth into the trachea, using his fingers as a guide, in a conscious patient. Through this tube, he gave a chloroform and air mixture for the removal of a malignant tumor from the base of the tongue. A sponge was packed by him around the tube at the laryngeal inlet to protect the lungs from contamination. He had also previously used rubber and gum elastic catheters into the trachea for the relief of obstruction in laryngeal diphtheria. Next, in 1901, Franz Kuhn of Kassel had extended and developed this technique by using a flexible metal tube and introducing it through the larynx with the help of a curved guide wire, after palpating the epiglottis with the fingers of his left hand. His preference was for inhalation anesthesia and the patient was breathing to and fro through the tube in the trachea. Then, in 1907, Barthelemy and Dufour of Nancy, in France, blew the mixture of chloroform vapor and air into the lungs from a Vernon Harcourt inhaler through a rubber catheter which was guided into the trachea by hand, as laryngoscope was not invented at that time. It was the first kind of endotracheal (ET) insufflation technique of anesthesia and was subsequently widely used in forth coming World War I, in 1914.

Largely after that, due to their experience as an anesthetist, during World War I, Mr Gillies, Mr Rowbotham, and Mr Magill had first used ether inhalational anesthesia through one narrow gum elastic tube, passed into the trachea via larynx with the help of a laryngoscope. During that period, a laryngoscope had already been invented which is described later. After that, the first blind nasal intubation was performed by Rowbotham. Then, Mr Magill had also published his results of blind nasal intubation, by using a wide-bore rubber catheter, during the years, following 1928. This technique revolutionized the use of ETTs in anesthesia because not only it provides anesthesia, but also gained early control of the airway and protected it. Inflatable cuffs had been used for many years but were again reintroduced by Guedel and Waters in 1928. A pilot balloon had been described first, in 1893, by Eisenmenger. It was also described, in 1906, by Green and was reintroduced by Langton, in 1939.

While the methods of intubation by Magill and Rowbotham had earned the support and approval of surgeons, with whom they worked, but many other surgeons discouraged the use of tracheal intubation through the larynx. This was partly because of the possibility of tissue damage and partly due to conservatism. Thus, it took many years before intubation was accepted by all anesthetists. Those who learned how to perform blind nasal intubation, soon realized its great advantages, especially due to the fact that it (tracheal intubation) would enable a patient to be taken to a necessary level (depth) of anesthesia very quickly by the use of relaxant and intermittent positive pressure ventilation (IPPV) than by the use of only volatile anesthetics which at that time was the rule. In addition, they also realized that tracheal intubation provides a clear airway, prevents laryngeal spasm, and enables the lungs to be protected against aspiration of foreign materials.

During the previous period, tracheal intubation was performed only by deepening anesthesia by volatile anesthetic agents such as ether and chloroform which was only available at that time. After that, when the muscle relaxants became available, then it was possible to perform oral intubation easily and rapidly by direct laryngoscopy because intubation by only an inhalational anesthetic agent was difficult and needed a long time to reach the necessary deep plane of anesthesia for it (intubation). The use of muscle relaxants, to facilitate intubation in UK, was pioneered by Bourne. This turning point in anesthesia was long overdue, so the credit was given to Bourne for convincing the value of muscle relaxants for rapid and easy intubation, to the postwar generation of anesthetists.

The traditional ETTs, for either nasal or oral intubation, were Magill ETTs, made of mineralized red rubber. The red color of this tube is due to the presence of preservatives. The oral tubes had thicker walls than the nasal ones. The angled Oxford tube was thicker in the pharyngeal part and thinner in the tracheal part. Then, polyvinyl chloride (PVC) tubes had started to replace these red rubber tubes, progressively from 1950. The toxicity of the PVC tube was tested by implantation test (IT) in rabbit muscle or by cell culture. The Z79 was the committee in USA that originally approved anesthetic equipment to maintain a standard and was formed first in 1956. Ring–Adair–Elwin (RAE) preformed tubes were first developed in 1980.

During the evolution of direct laryngoscope, indirect laryngoscopy was also evolving. The indirect laryngoscopy, with a mirror, was first introduced by M Garcia who was a teacher of singing in London. Then, it (indirect laryngoscope) was widely used for diagnostic purposes. But direct laryngoscopy was pioneered, in 1895, by Alfred Kirstein. After that Jackson himself designed a laryngoscope which was later modified by Magill, in 1926, and by Miller and Macintosh, in 1932. The light was originally powered from electric mains, but later the light was supplied by a 3 V battery which was incorporated into the handle of the laryngoscope or by a fiber-optic cable. In Macintosh direct laryngoscope, the blade was shorter, curved, and Z-shaped on cross section. Its tip entered into the vallecula, lifted the base of the tongue, and with it lifted the epiglottis so that vocal cords could be visualized. It does not generate so much laryngospasm, as it does not pass over and stimulate the posterior surface of the epiglottis. Then, it was an immediate success and has continued to be so, as it can be used in lighter planes of anesthesia. Macintosh also had developed a laryngeal forceps which bear his name and was used for directing the tip of nasal tubes under direct vision into the larynx.

Without using muscle relaxant, cocaine was first used to suppress laryngeal reflexes during general anesthesia (GA) by Rosenberg, in 1895, and by Magill, in 1928, to aid intubation, then many sprays also have been described such as applying local anesthetic to the larynx to suppress the reflexes for intubation. But lignocaine is now generally preferred, because of its lower toxicity.

To remove the different disadvantages of ET intubation, initially, a small mask had been tried in the pharynx, but it was rejected. Then, the invention of the laryngeal mask airway (LMA) had completed the cycle of the history of airway management in anesthesia. It was first developed by an anesthetist, named Mr A Brain and was later manufactured by an equipment company, named Colgate Medical. After that, improved materials and different designs of LMA, coupled with the timely arrival of propofol which deeply suppresses the pharyngeal and laryngeal reflexes, allowed a successful outcome of it.

■ INTRODUCTION

An airway is defined as a passage through which air passes into and out of the lungs during respiration. Any artificial device, with a lumen inside of it and which serves as a conduit, connecting between the atmosphere and lungs, is also *considered an airway*. These include oropharyngeal airway, nasopharyngeal airway, LMA, other supraglottic airways, ETT, ventilator's breathing circuit, etc. It is estimated that about 600 patients die each year, in a developed country from complications related to airway management. This picture in underdeveloped countries is further grimmer. On the contrary, about 98% of difficult airways in relation to the mask ventilation or ET intubation can be predicted by proper preoperative evaluation or assessment of the airway in a patient. **Box 1** is the list of conditions where the situations such as difficult airway, difficult laryngoscopy, difficult intubation, and difficult musk ventilation may arise.

BOX 1: Preoperative evaluation of the patient.

- *Facial anomalies:*
  - Apert syndrome, Crouzon disease, and maxillary hypoplasia
  - Mandibular hypoplasia and Pierre–Robin syndrome
  - Treacher Collins syndrome and Goldenhar syndrome
  - Mandibular hyperplasia, acromegaly, and cherubism
- *Affection of temporomandibular joint:* Ankylosis, rheumatism, trauma, infection, previous surgery, etc.
- *Problems with teeth:* Loose teeth, false teeth, protruding incisor, and edentulous
- *Problems with tongue:* Macroglossia due to Down syndrome, hypothyroidism, hemangioma, lymphangioma, tumor, scarring, etc.
- *Problems with mouth:* Microstomia due to burns, trauma, scarring, etc.
- *Problems with palate:* Cleft palate, narrow arched palate, palatal swelling, hematoma, etc.
- *Problems with pharynx:* Hypertrophic tonsils, large adenoids, pharyngeal tumors, abscess, retropharyngeal or para pharyngeal abscess, etc.
- *Problems with larynx:*
  - *Supraglottic:* Epiglottitis, tumor, injury, etc.
  - *Glottic:* Laryngomalacia, granuloma, foreign body, and papillomas
  - *Infraglottic:* Congenital stenosis, traumatic stenosis, and edema due to inflammation.
- *Problems with nose:* Choanal atresia, hypertrophic turbinates, deviated nasal septum, polyp, foreign bodies, etc.
- *Problems with trachea:* Tracheal stenosis, tracheal webbing, mass at neck deviating trachea, mediastinal mass deviating trachea, trachea esophageal fistula, tracheomalacia, foreign bodies, etc.
- *Problems of neck and spine:*
  - *Neck:* Large goiters, skin contractures
  - *Spine:* Klippel–Feil syndrome, surgical fusion, fracture of cervical vertebrae, traumatic subluxation, etc.

The difficult airway is defined by the American Society of Anaesthetist (ASA) as the clinical situation in which a conventionally trained anesthesiologist experiences difficulty during mask ventilation or experiences difficulty during tracheal intubation or both. *Difficult mask ventilation* is defined by ASA as the clinical situation in which it is not possible by an unassisted trained anesthesiologist to maintain O_2 saturation >90%, using 100% oxygen and mask for ventilation, provided preventilation O_2 saturation level was within the normal range. *Difficult laryngoscopy* is defined by ASA as the clinical situation in which it is not possible to visualize any portion of the vocal cords with a conventional laryngoscope. ASA also defines *difficult ET intubation* as a situation when insertion of ETT into the larynx requires more than three consecutive attempts or >10 minutes with a conventional laryngoscope and experience. The later definition of ten minutes provides a margin of safety for preoxygenated patients who are undergoing elective intubation in the operating room because such patients in stable circumstances can usually tolerate 10 minutes of attempts without any bad consequences. *"Zero class airway view"* is defined as the inability to see any portion of epiglottis after opening the mouth and tongue protrusion. Approximately 1.8% of patient of the total population belongs to this class of airway view. *Failed intubation* is defined as the clinical condition when the placement of ETT fails after multiple attempts of intubation.

The airway is divided into an upper and lower airway. The *upper airway* is comprised of the oral cavity, nose, and pharynx (nasopharynx, oropharynx, laryngopharynx, and larynx). There are two openings in the upper airway (1) *nose* and (2) *mouth*. The nose leads posteriorly to the nasopharynx and the mouth leads posteriorly to the oropharynx. These two passages are separated anteriorly by the hard palate. The nose is again comprised of an *external nose* and *nasal cavity*. The *lower airway* includes the trachea, bronchi, bronchiole, and its subsequent divisions and subdivisions which terminate into alveoli. The upper airway serves to warm, humidify, and filter the air or gases before it enters the lower airway. Bypassing these structures, by ET intubation or tracheostomy, makes an anesthetist essential to provide warm, humidified, and filtered air to the patient. Among the two airways, the upper airway is more vulnerable to obstruction during anesthesia. This is because, in an anesthetized patient, there is a loss of muscle tone which leads to (1) the tongue to fall back on pharynx, (2) the pharyngeal wall to collapse and occlude the upper airway at the level of laryngopharynx, and (3) then subsequently allows the epiglottis to occlude the airway at the level of larynx.

There are many different acquired and congenital conditions that affect the upper and lower airways and cause the difficult management of it. These are listed in the **Box 1**.

ANATOMY OF THE UPPER AIRWAY

Nose

Nose consists of the external nose and nasal cavity.

External Nose

It is a pyramid-like projection on the face. It presents a free tip or apex and a root at its junction with the forehead. The rounded border between the tip and the root of the nose, along with the adjoining area, is known as the *dorsum of the nose*. The inferior surface of the external nose presents a pair of pyriform apertures which are called *nostrils* or *nares*. Each nostril is bounded medially by the mobile part of nasal the septum and laterally by the ala of nose **(Fig. 1)**.

The framework of the external nose is formed by some bones and cartilages. Among them the upper part is supported by bones and the lower part is supported by cartilages. The upper part of the external nose is supported on each side by the following bones such as nasal bone, frontal process of the maxillary bone, and the nasal part of the frontal bone. The lower part of the external nose is contributed by the following cartilages:

- Anterior border of septal cartilages
- Superior nasal cartilages, which is continuous with septal cartilages
- Inferior nasal cartilage (or alar cartilage) which presents a septal process to form the mobile part of the nasal septum
- A few minor alar cartilages
- Fibrofatty tissue in the lower part of the ala.

The skin overlying the bones at the root of the nose is thin and mobile, but below the root of the nose, it (skin) is thick and adherent to underlying cartilages and fibrofatty tissue. The skin of nose is provided with multiple sebaceous glands. The sensory nerves of external nose are derived from (1) the external nasal and infratrochlear branches of ophthalmic nerve and (2) the infraorbital branch of maxillary nerve.

Nasal Cavity

The nasal cavity is triangular in shape and has an irregular surface. It is divided into the right and left halves (right and left nasal cavity) by the nasal septum. Each half of *nasal cavity extends* anteriorly from the mucocutaneous junction of anterior nares to the nasopharynx posteriorly (posterior nares and choanae). Each nasal cavity has a roof, floor, lateral wall, and medial wall. The *roof of each nasal cavity* slopes downward both in front and behind from its middle horizontal part. The *middle horizontal part of the roof of the nasal cavity* is formed by the cribriform plate of the ethmoid bone. The *anterior slope of the roof of the nasal cavity* is formed by the nasal part of the frontal bone, nasal bone, and nasal cartilages. The *posterior slope of the roof of the nasal cavity* is formed by the inferior surface of the body of the sphenoid bone. The *floor of the nasal cavity* is formed by the palatine process of maxilla and the horizontal plate of the palatine bone. The area of the nasal cavity close to the nostrils or anterior nares is known as *vestibule*. It is lined by skin and provided with coarse hairs, sebaceous glands, and sweat glands. Except vestibule, rest of the nasal cavity is lined by mucous membrane **(Fig. 2)**.

The *lateral wall of each nasal cavity* is irregular and it is due to the presence of three shelf-like or scroll-like bony

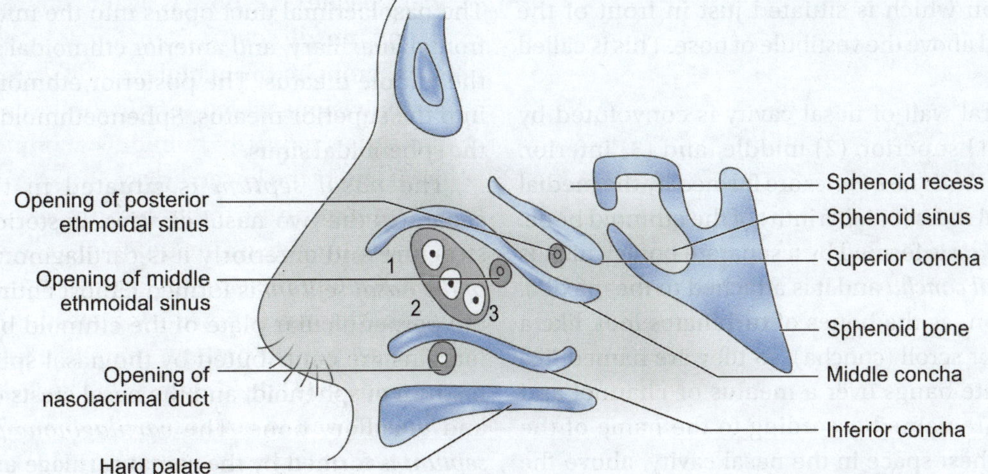

Fig. 1: Structures that open on the lateral wall of the nose. The cut margins of conchae are seen.
(1. Opening of frontal sinus; 2. Opening of anterior ethmoidal sinus; 3. Opening of the maxillary sinus)

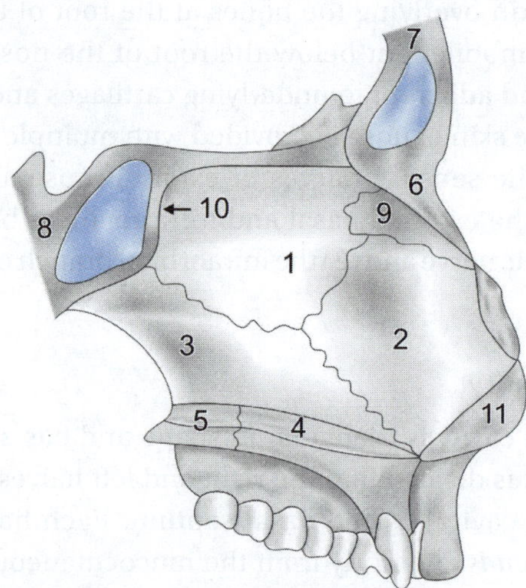

Fig. 2: The formation of nasal septum. (1. Perpendicular plate of ethmoid; 2. Septal cartilage; 3. Vomer; 4. Nasal crest of the maxilla; 5. Nasal crest of the palatine bone; 6. Nasal spine of the frontal bone; 7. Frontal bone; 8. Sphenoid; 9. Nasal crest of nasal bone; 10. Rostrum of the sphenoid; 11. Septal process of the inferior nasal cartilage)

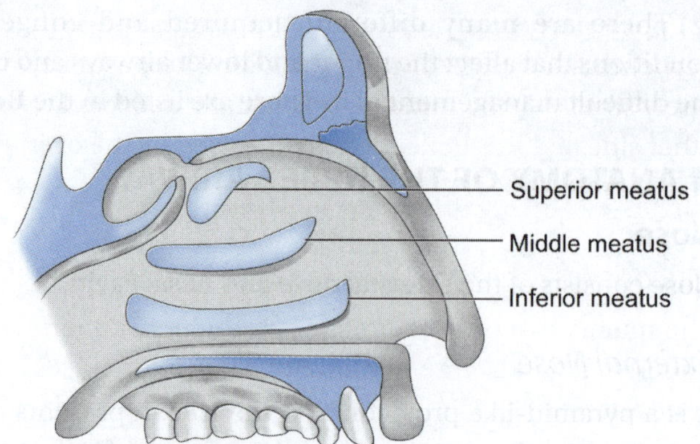

Fig. 3: The lateral wall of the nose.

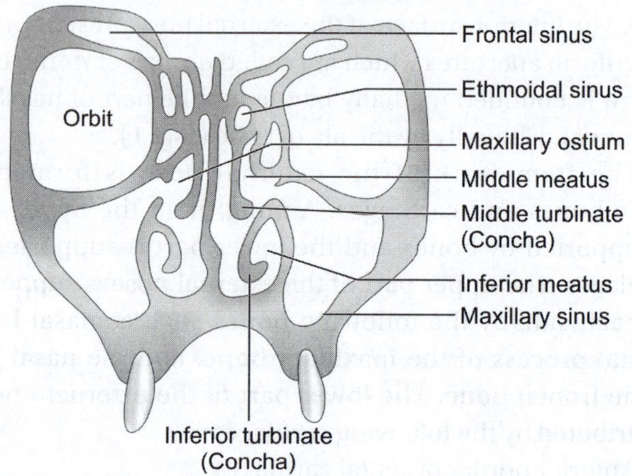

Fig. 4: Coronal section through the nose and sinuses at the plane of the maxillary ostium.

projections. These projections increase the surface area of the nose (nasal cavity) and ensure effective conditioning (warming and humidification) of inspired air. This lateral wall separates the nasal cavity (1) from orbital cavity above, while the ethmoidal air sinuses intervene between them, i.e., between nasal and orbital cavity, (2) from maxillary sinus below, and (3) from lacrimal groove with lacrimal sac and nasolacrimal canal with the nasolacrimal duct in front **(Fig. 3)**.

The *lateral wall of nasal cavity* is formed by some bones. These are nasal, frontal process of the maxilla, lacrimal, labyrinth of ethmoid with superior and middle conchae, inferior nasal concha, perpendicular plate of palatine, and medial pterygoid plate of the sphenoid bone. There is a shallow depression which is situated just in front of the middle meatus and above the vestibule of nose. This is called *atrium* **(Fig. 4)**.

The bony lateral wall of nasal cavity is convoluted by three *turbinates* (1) superior, (2) middle, and (3) inferior. The *superior* and *middle turbinates* are formed by the medial aspect of the lateral mass (or labyrinth) of the ethmoid bone. The *inferior turbinate* is formed by a separate bone which is called *inferior nasal concha* and it is attached to the maxilla. In the cross section, as the bones of turbinates look like a whorl (turbinate) or scroll (concha), so they are named like that. Each turbinate hangs over a meatus or channel and so the meatuses are named according to the name of the turbinate. The highest space in the nasal cavity, above the superior turbinate, is called the sphenoethmoidal recess and sphenoidal sinus opens in this recess.

The *olfactory cleft of nasal cavity* is the area which lies between the superior turbinate, cribriform plate of ethmoid, and the corresponding area of septum. It is lined by specialized olfactory epithelium. Several ducts drain on the lateral wall of the nose at meatuses under the respective turbinate. The nasolacrimal duct opens into the inferior meatus. The frontal, maxillary, and anterior ethmoidal sinuses drain into the middle meatus. The posterior ethmoidal sinuses drain into the superior meatus. Sphenoethmoidal recess receives the sphenoidal sinus.

The *nasal septum* is situated in the midline and separates the two nasal cavities. Posteriorly, it is bony in structure and anteriorly it is cartilaginous. The *bony part of the nasal septum* is formed almost entirely by vomer and the perpendicular plate of the ethmoid bone; however, its margins are contributed by the nasal spine of frontal, the rostrum of sphenoid, and the nasal crests of nasal, palatine, and maxillary bone. The *cartilaginous part of the nasal septum* is formed by the septal cartilage and septal process of inferior nasal cartilage. The attachment of cartilaginous part of nasal septum are (1) inferiorly to maxillary crest,

(2) posteriorly to vomer, and (3) posterosuperiorly to the perpendicular plate of the ethmoid. The nasal septum is rarely strictly in the midline. It is usually deflected to one or other side and this deflection is produced by the overgrowth of one or more constituent parts of it.

Mucous Membrane

The mucus membrane of nose is intimately adherent to its underlying periosteum or perichondrium with the exception at olfactory area. At the olfactory area, it is loosely attached to its underlying bone. The nasal mucous membrane is subdivided into three parts (1) *vestibular part, (2) olfactory part, and (3) respiratory part.*

Vestibular part: This part of mucous membrane lies just inside the aperture of nostril. It is lined by skin with coarse hairs, sweat glands, and sebaceous glands. The hairs (vibrissae) which are curved forward, here, are moistened by the secretion of sebaceous gland and arrest the foreign particles, carried by inspired air.

Olfactory part: This part of mucous membrane contains olfactory cells and its hair. From these olfactory cells, 15–20 olfactory nerves start. Then, these olfactory nerves pass through the cribriform plate of the ethmoid bone and end in the olfactory bulb of the cerebrum.

Respiratory part: The remaining part of the mucous membrane of nose, except the vestibular and olfactory part constitutes the respiratory part. It is lined by thick, vascular, ciliated, and columnar epithelium. This ciliated columnar epithelium is interspersed by goblet cells. It is thickest and most vascular over the lower aspect of septum and over the turbinates. Actually, over the inferior concha, this mucous membrane contains masses of the erectile tissues with numerous arteriovenous shunts. Thus, it permits vascular engorgement to regulate the temperature and humidity of inspired air. The secretion from subepithelial thin-walled vessels, serous glands, and mucous glands contribute to the formation of mucous in nose.

The mucous secreted in nose has two phases, they are (1) the *gel phase* and (2) the *sol phase.* The sol phase is less viscous and is closely applied to the columnar cells of mucous membrane. The gel phase lies over the sol phase and is more viscous. It moves backward by the hooks of beating cilia which are situated at the end of the ciliated columnar cells. The cilia move the mucous of nose back to the nasopharynx. This mucous and nasal vibrissae (hair) helps to trap contaminants or foreign particles from inspired air. The vascularity of nasal mucosa helps in warming and moistening (conditioning) of the inspired air.

Arterial Supply of Nose

The arterial supply of nose consists of (1) the arterial supply of its medial wall (or nasal septum) and (2) the arterial supply of its lateral wall.

- *Arterial supply of medial wall of nose or nasal septum:* The nasal septum is supplied by the following arteries:
  - *The mobile part of nasal septum* is supplied by the septal branches of superior labial artery which is the branch of facial artery **(Fig. 5)**.
  - *The anterosuperior part of the nasal septum* is supplied by the anterior ethmoid artery which is the branch of ophthalmic artery.
  - *The posteroinferior part of the nasal septum* is supplied by the sphenopalatine and greater palatine artery which are the branches of ophthalmic artery.

An area on the anteroinferior part of the septum is highly vascular and known as the *Little's area of epistaxis,* because this is the common site for profuse arterial hemorrhage from nose. Here, the septal branch of facial artery, long sphenopalatine, and terminal branches of greater palatine arteries anastomose.

- *Arterial supply of lateral wall:* Similar to the arterial supply of the nasal septum, the lateral wall of the nose is also supplied by the branches of ophthalmic, maxillary, and facial arteries. These branches are arranged into four quadrants.
  1. *Anterosuperior quadrant:* It is supplied by the anterior ethmoid artery, branch of the ophthalmic artery.
  2. *Posterosuperior quadrants:* It is supplied by the posterior ethmoidal artery, branch of the ophthalmic artery, and sphenopalatine artery, branch of the maxillary artery.
  3. *Anteroinferior quadrant:* It is supplied by the alar branch of facial and terminal branches of greater palatine arteries.
  4. *Posteroinferior quadrant:* It is supplied by the greater palatine artery **(Fig. 6)**.

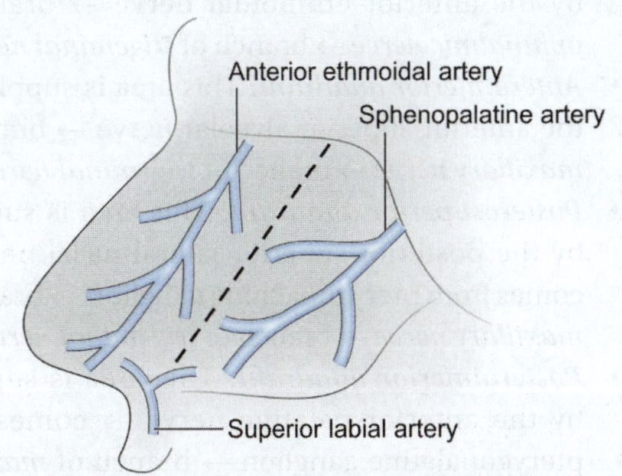

Fig. 5: Arterial supply of nasal septum.

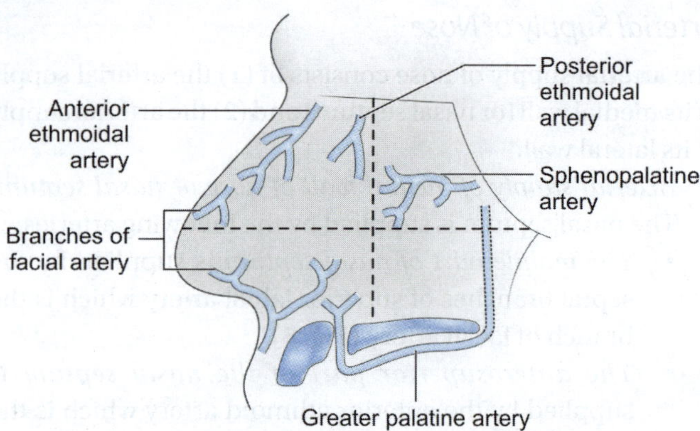

Fig. 6: The arterial supply of the lateral wall of the nose.

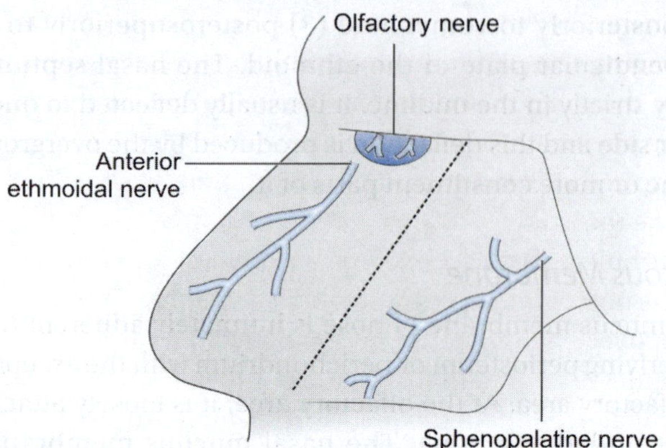

Fig. 7: Nerve supply of the nasal septum.

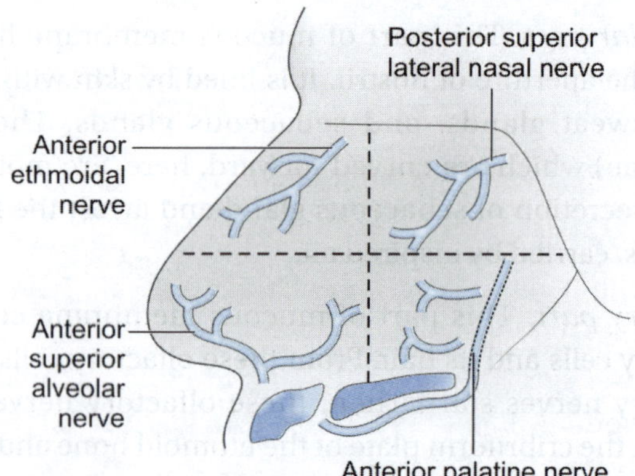

Fig. 8: Nerve supply of the lateral wall of nose.

Nerve Supply of Nose

- *Medial wall of the nose (nasal septum):*
  - *General sensory nerves:* They come from the ophthalmic and maxillary divisions of trigeminal nerve and supply the whole septum.
    - *Anterosuperior part of septum:* This area is supplied by the internal nasal branch of the anterior ethmoidal nerve → branch of ophthalmic nerve → branch of trigeminal nerve.
    - *Posteroinferior part of septum:* This area is supplied by the sphenopalatine branch of pterygopalatine ganglion → branch of maxillary nerve → branch of trigeminal nerve.
    - *Mobile part:* This area of nasal septum is supplied by the external nasal nerve, branch of the ophthalmic division of the trigeminal nerve.
  - *Special sensory olfactory nerves:* They supply the upper olfactory area **(Fig. 7)**.
- *Lateral wall of nose:*
  - *General sensory nerves:* Like nasal septum, the nerve of the lateral wall of nose comes from trigeminal nerve and distribute to the whole portion of it.
    - *Anterosuperior quadrant:* This area is supplied by the anterior ethmoidal nerve → branch of *ophthalmic nerve* → branch of *trigeminal nerve.*
    - *Anteroinferior quadrant:* This area is supplied by the anterior-superior alveolar nerve → branch of *maxillary nerve* → branch of *trigeminal nerve.*
    - *Posterosuperior quadrant:* This area is supplied by the posterior-superior lateral nasal nerve → comes from pterygopalatine ganglion → branch of *maxillary nerve* → branch of *trigeminal nerve.*
    - *Posteroinferior quadrant:* This area is supplied by the anterior palatine nerve → comes from pterygopalatine ganglion → branch of *maxillary nerve* → branch of *trigeminal nerve.*
  - *Special sensory olfactory nerves:* It supplies to the upper part, just below the cribriform plate of ethmoidal bone, up to the superior concha **(Fig. 8)**.

Summary of sensory supply of nose:
- Lateral wall:
  - *Upper olfactory area:* Olfactory nerve.
  - *Rest of lateral wall:*
    - *Anterosuperior:* Ophthalmic division of the trigeminal nerve
    - *Rest of the area:* Maxillary division of the trigeminal nerve
- *Medial wall (nasal septum):*
  - *Upper olfactory area:* Olfactory nerve.
  - *Rest of medial wall:*
    - *Anterosuperior:* Ophthalmic division of trigeminal nerve
    - *Rest of medial wall:* Maxillary division of trigeminal nerve.

Function of Nose

The nose does the following important functions:
- *Respiration:* An adult patient usually takes inspiration through the nose, provided there are no obstructions.

Then, this inspired air passes through a wide curve which begins at nostril and continues through the upper part of the nose to the end at the posterior choanae. This inspired air is laminar in flow by character. However, the expired air does not follow this laminar flow in character, like the inspired air, but it is broken up by turbinates into turbulent and eddies flow and then passes out through the nostrils. It has been postulated that this (the difference between the inspired and expired flow) is because the outlet is smaller than the inlet, as the posterior choana is much larger than the nostril. Inevitably, always there is a certain degree of recirculation of air also.

In a normal adult subject, the resistance for air to flow through the nose is one and half times greater than that of mouth and accounts for nearly two-thirds of the total airway resistance. This explains why a patient takes mouth breathing when high air flow rates are necessary. So, it is always advisable to taste the patency of nasal passage, before nasal intubation is performed. The deflection of nasal septum sometimes becomes severe and diminishes the lumen of respiratory airway, thus it prevents the passage of all, but the smallest of ETT.

- *Defense:* (1) The presence of stiff hairs in the anterior part of nasal fossa (vestibule), (2) the thick and highly vascular (spongy) mucous membrane, the ciliated columnar epithelium, (3) the extensive lymphatic supply, and (4) the bactericidal property of the secreted mucous provide a powerful defensive action of nose against the invasion of any organism, directly from air. The intermittent flushing action of the watery secretion of the nose by sneezing also lies in the reserve of defense action of it.

- *Warming and humidification (conditioning):* The most important work that the nose has to perform is the warming and the humidification of inspired air, which is about 10,000 L in 24 hours in a normal healthy adult. This is only possible due to the high vascularity of nasal mucous membrane, for example, if the temperature of inspired air is 17°C which is equivalent to the normal room temperature, is raised to normal body temperature which is equivalent to 37°C, during its passage through the nose and upper airway. This temperature of inspired air also may vary from 25 to 0°C according to the temperature of environment, but its passage through the nose produces more or less 1°C difference than that of the body temperature when it reaches the laryngeal inlet or alveoli.

When the air passes through the air passages, then with the rising of temperature, also the quantity of water, needed to saturate the air by water vapor increases.

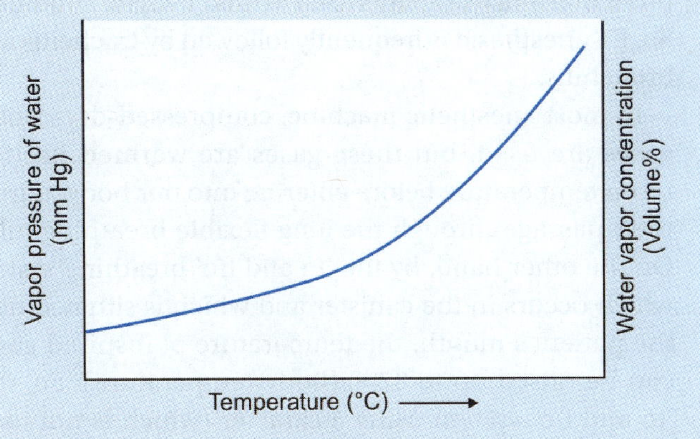

Fig. 9: Relationship between the tension of water vapor and temperature.

This is shown in **Figure 9**, for example, at room temperature of 17°C the air normally contains 2 volume percent of water to become fully saturated. But at a body temperature of 37°C the air should contain 6 volume percent of water vapor to become fully saturated (because the saturation point of air by water vapor rises with the rise of temperature). The nose and the respiratory tract, therefore, have to perform this heavy task of warming and humidification of inspired air by adding large quantities of heat and water vapor in the inspired air to make it warm and saturated with water vapor. Warming and humidification of inspired air is achieved by the dilatation of vessels of large vascular mucosal beds of the turbinates of nose. They normally change their volume after every 4 hours of interval (nasal cycle) and each side alternates.

The humidification of inspired air in air passage is done by the supply of moisture (or water vapor) which comes as transudation of fluid from the mucosal epithelium of the nose, pharynx, and larynx, and to a lesser extent from the secretion of mucous glands and goblet cells, present in the nasal and pharyngeal mucous membrane. The daily volume of nasal secretions is about 1 L. Of which about three-fourths is used to humidify the inspired air. The nose also collects moisture from expired air to prevent the excessive loss of water from our body.

During intubation and tracheostomy, relatively dry and cool anesthetic gases or air reach the trachea directly because the nose and pharynx are bypassed and so proper warming and humidification of inspired air are not done. This compels the mucosa of trachea and bronchus to perform the heavy duties of nasal and pharyngeal mucous membrane, therefore the mucosa of lower airways becomes dry and ciliary activity ceases in such circumstances. Later the tracheal and bronchial mucosa adapts itself to this changed condition. So, ET anesthesia is frequently followed by tracheitis and bronchitis.

In most anesthetic machine, compressed-dry-cooled gases are used, but these gases are warmed itself to room temperature before entering into our body, during their passage through the long flexible breathing tube. On the other hand, by the 'to and fro' breathing system which occurs in the canister and which is situated near the patient's mouth, the temperature of inspired gases can be raised up to 37°C (body temperature). So, this 'to and fro' system using a canister (which is not used now, due to many disadvantages) provides a very efficient method for the warming and humidification of inspired air. But during the passage of expired air through CO_2 absorber in circle system, the expired air gains some heat and water vapor, produced during the absorption of CO_2. In a nonrebreathing valve system, such as if Ruben and Frumin's valve is attached with the circuit, then the inspired air is always at room temperature (17°C) and contains only 2 volume percent of water vapor at full saturation, in this temperature, which is the normal content of air. But as there is no rebreathing, so the expired air at 37°C, containing 6 volume percent of water vapor at full saturation, passes out through the nonrebreathing valve. In the absence of rebreathing, heat with water vapor is also lost from our body to the atmosphere, thus it does not help to warm and humidify the inspired air.

In the circle absorption system, the inspired gas mixture contains fresh dry gases coming from cylinder and pipelines and also some expired gases containing water vapor at room temperature. The expired gas leaves the patient at body temperature containing water vapor. But by the time they have traversed the breathing tube of apparatus; they become cool to the room temperature and so have lost the major part of their water content in the breathing tube of apparatus. Dry, cool, fresh gas is again added to the system for inspiration and is mixed with the expired gas coming from the absorber. So, the circle absorption system does much help in warming and humidifying the inspired gases.

- *Resonance:* Nose, as surrounded by multiple air cavities, so gives some resonance to voice and helps in talk. It also protects the transmission of sound of one's own speech to his own ears. It also equalizes the pressure during respiration between internal (in our body) and external environment.
- *Filter:* Nose also helps in filtering and clearing the suspended particles from inspired air. It also transports mucus posteriorly to lubricate the pharynx.
- *Olfaction:* Nose also acts as an integral part of the olfactory system.

Some Artificial Methods of Humidification of Inspired Air

The inspired air can be humidified by various ways. These are:

- *Direct instillation of water:* Inspired air can be humidified directly by instilling normal saline drop-by-drop into an ET or tracheostomy tube.
- *Water bath:* Here, inspired air is passed over the surface of water, kept in a thermostatically controlled and heated water bath. This type of humidifier should be placed on the inspired limb and the gases will flow from water bath to the patient by the shortest possible route. The tube, in this shortest route, should be insulated to prevent the loss of heat with consequent condensation of water, during the passage of heated and humidified inspired air through this tube. Another method to deliver the inspired gas at body temperature, with full saturation by water vapor, but without condensation in the breathing circuit, is to raise the temperature of water bath few degrees above the body temperature for compensation to loss that occurs during passage through the inspiratory limb. The exact temperature setting of water bath depends on the surface area of water, flow rate of gases, and the amount of cooling and condensation which takes place in the inspiratory limb after the water bath. This type of humidifier should always be kept below the level of patient to prevent the water from blown accidentally into the patient **(Table 1)**.
- *Moisture exchanger:* It is also called an "artificial nose". It mainly consists of a replaceable condenser that can be taken out and cleaned. It is a very light and a moderately efficient method of humidification of inspired air. As this system works at room temperature which is much below the body temperature, so a part of water vapor in expiratory gases is condensed on its inner surface and this condensed water again humidifies the dry-inspired gases. It cannot, of course, achieve full saturation owing

TABLE 1: The percentage of humidity of inspired gases in different anesthetic system.

Anesthetic system	Percentage (%) of humidity
Nose	100
Close circuit	40–60
"To-and-fro" system	60–100
Nonrebreathing valve	0
T-piece	0

to lower temperature. There are two demerits of this system. One is the colonization of bacteria and another is the increase of airway resistance, due to the condensation of moisture. These disadvantages can be overcome by using disposable and sterilized unit.

- *Mechanical nebulizer:* This is operated by pneumatic power and breaks up the drops of water into very small particles. In this system, the water passes up through a capillary tube to its summit, where it is crushed by the jet of air into microparticles. *In this type of nebulizer, 80% of water particles are in the range of 2–4 μm and the remainders are smaller. So, most of these water particles are deposited around the bronchial level and for many patients this is sufficient. Contrary, the 20% water particles, which are <2 μm, reach the small bronchi and alveoli.* Those water particles which are above 4 μm do not float. They coalesce and fall back in the reservoir. This type of nebulizer for humidification of inspired air can be used pre- and postoperatively with a face mask to improve lung function.

- *Ultrasonic nebulizer:* This is the most efficient instrument for humidification of inspired air. Here, the drops of water are passed through a capillary tube and are completely nebulized to aerosol by a vibrating transducer head which is activated by a high-frequency ultrasonic energy. Here, 70% of the water particles get size of 0.8–1 μm. So, usually, most of the particles of <1 μm are deposited in the lower airways and alveoli of the lungs. At the maximum rate of 12 drops of water/min, falling on the transducer head and with a ventilator, delivering of 10 L of gas/min, 72 mL of water as vapor can be provided with each liter of gas. This corresponds to the relative humidity of 160% at 37°C.

Among all the methods of humidification of inspired air, the ultrasonic nebulizer produces the most satisfactory humidification. It can also be used for the administration of water-soluble aerosol drugs. *The two demerits of this instrument are* (1) overhydration, due to extreme efficiency and (2) difficulty to sterilize by a conventional method.

Ciliary Activity of Airway

Throughout the upper and lower respiratory tract, the continuous ciliary activity of the cilia, present on the epithelial cells of the mucous membrane, plays a very important function. This is the prevention of the accumulation of mucus secretion which is needed for the different efficient functions of nose, pharynx, and larynx. By ciliary action in nose, the mucous secretions are swept posteriorly toward the pharynx and in the bronchial tree, the mucous secretions are carried upward toward the larynx.

The microscopic structure of cilia is shown in **Figure 10**. The cilia are fine hair-like structures. They are 7 μm in length and 0.3 μm in width. The tips of cilia are always bent toward the direction of the flow of mucous. *In the shaft of the cilia, which are occupied by cytoplasm, there are multiple longitudinal fibrils or microtubules containing dynein arms. These longitudinal fibrils or microtubules in the shaft of the cilia are arranged in a fashion like that a pair of microtubules is situated in the center and it is surrounded by nine pairs of microtubules at the periphery.* The activity of these cilia which is shown in **Figure 11** depends mainly on a mucous blanket, covering it. This covering mucous blanket on cilia consists of two layers. The *outer gel layer* is thick and viscous. It is designed to entrap the floating particles from inspired gas such as dust, soot, and microorganisms. The *inner sol layer* is thin serous like fluid. It is designed to lubricate the action of ciliary movement of cilia. The tips of cilia come just in contact with the outer gel layer with each beat. *Acting in a union, the cilia set the outer gel layer in motion.* Thus, gathering momentum, the mucous flows toward the pharynx from nose and toward the larynx from bronchus and trachea. They beat forward in an effective stroke, pulling

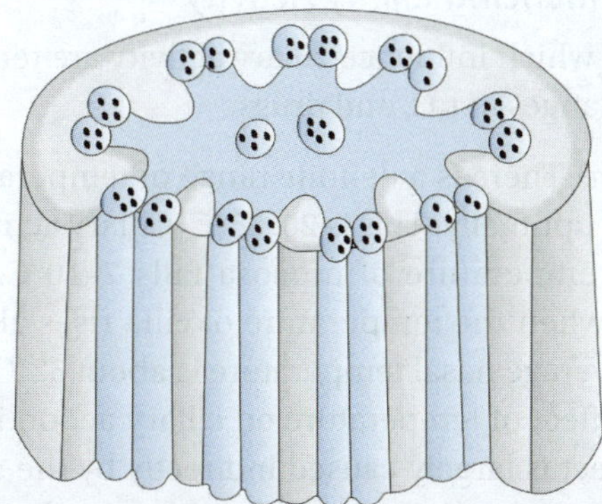

Fig. 10: Transverse and longitudinal section of a nasal cilium (a single cilia) at the middle of the shaft of it.

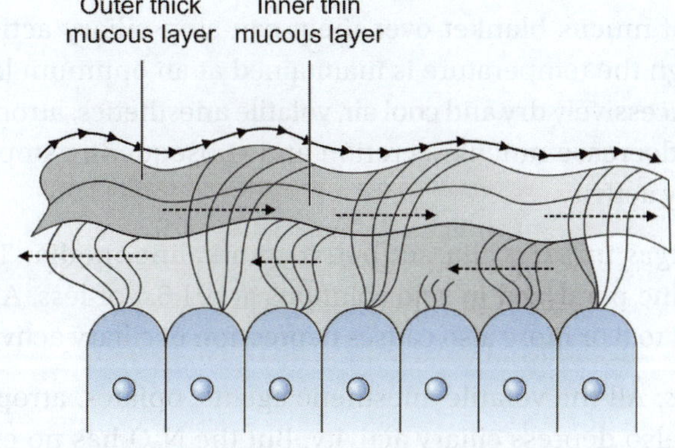

Fig. 11: Ciliary movement (activity).

the gel phase by the action of hooks at the end of the cilia, and then beat backward during the recovery stroke. Their action is reminiscent of a cornfield, being blown by the wind. This movement of cilia is called *metachrony*, as opposed to synchrony where all the cilia beat together. At 37°C, the cilia of nasal mucosa beat about 10–16 times per second. The average estimated speed of movement of a mucous blanket over the mucous membrane is 0.25–1 cm/min, thus the entire mucous content of the nose takes 20–30 minutes to be emptied into the pharynx.

In some conditions, the *ciliary action may be defective, for example, Kartagener's syndrome.* This is a genetic disorder in which there is a defect in the ultrastructure of cilia. This is due to the failure of the synthesis of protein which forms the dynein arm of cilia. The congenital absence of this dynein arm, which normally contains ATP and powers the cilia, makes the cilia immobile. So, these patients have a constantly running nose, secretory otitis media, chronic sinusitis, bronchiectasis, and often situs inversus. The tail of sperms has a similar structure like cilia. So that in this syndrome, there is also male infertility due to reduced sperm motility.

Factors Influencing Ciliary Activity

The factors which influence ciliary activity are temperature, mucous, changes in pH, and drugs.

Temperature: There is a definite range of temperature when the cilia act optimally. This is 28–35°C. Ciliary activity ceases when the temperature of mucosa falls 7–10°C. It is also depressed when the temperature of cilia rises above 35°C, while the average nasal temperature is about 32°C. Actually, the direct effect of temperature on ciliary action is minimal and the effect is largely caused indirectly by the alterations in the amount of mucus, which is secreted at different temperatures.

Mucous: Cilia cannot work without the optimum temperature and the blanket of mucus covering it. Drying out of mucus blanket over them can stop ciliary activity, though the temperature is maintained at an optimum level. So, excessively dry and cool air, volatile anesthetics, atropine, etc., decrease mucus secretion and subsequently stop the ciliary activity.

Changes in pH: Cilia act better in alkaline media. They become paralyzed in acid solutions at pH 6.4 or less. A rise of pH to 8 or more also causes depression of ciliary activity.

Drugs: All the volatile anesthetic agents, opiates, atropine, etc., also depress ciliary activity. But the N_2O has no effect on it.

Pharynx

The pharynx or pharyngeal airway is a U-shaped fibromuscular structure. It extends proximally from the base of the skull at the posterior aspect of nose to distally up to the level of the sixth cervical vertebra or the lower border of the cricoid cartilage, where it becomes continuous with the esophagus (posteriorly) and larynx (anteriorly). Anteriorly the pharynx communicates with nasal cavities, oral cavity, and larynx from above downward. Thus, the pharynx is divided anatomically into the *nasopharynx, oropharynx,* and *laryngopharynx (hypopharynx).* The soft palate separates the nasopharynx from oropharynx and a horizontal plane, drawn at the upper border of epiglottis, separates the oropharynx from laryngopharynx. Except for the nasopharynx which is covered by ciliated columnar epithelium, the oropharynx and laryngopharynx are covered by stratified squamous epithelium. The middle fibrous layer of pharynx consists of pharyngobasilar fascia. The outer muscular layer of pharynx is comprised chiefly of three constrictor muscles such as *superior, middle, and inferior constrictor muscle of pharynx* and they overlap one on another from below upward.

Nasopharynx

Different divisions of the pharynx in the sagittal section are depicted in **Figure 12**. It (nasopharynx) extends from the base of the skull above to the level of hard palate and soft palate below. Anteriorly, the nasopharynx communicates with nasal cavities through the posterior nares and posteriorly it is bounded by the body of C_1 and C_2 vertebrae. *Nasopharyngeal isthmus* is the aperture situated between the nasopharynx and oropharynx and is surrounded by the free margin of soft palate anteriorly and the posterior wall of the pharynx posteriorly. This opening is closed, during the second stage of deglutition, by soft palate. At the junction of the roof and the posterior wall of nasopharynx and at the base of the skull, there lies a small mass of lymphoid tissue, embedding in the mucous membrane of nasopharynx. It is called the *pharyngeal tonsil* or *adenoids*.

On both side of this adenoid, there is an *opening of the Eustachian tube,* which connects the middle ear cavities with nasopharynx. It is also lined by ciliated columnar epithelium and is continuous with the nasopharynx. There is also a collection of lymphoid tissue, around the Eustachian tube opening, which is called the *Eustachian tonsil.* Lying close to the base of adenoids, there is a small recess which is called the *pharyngeal bursa.* It often impedes the passage of a nasal ETT. If force is applied, the tube may, then, penetrate the bursa and can create a false passage. This may lead to the collection of blood and postoperative sepsis. As the pharynx is riched with the lymphatic supply, so the enlargement of

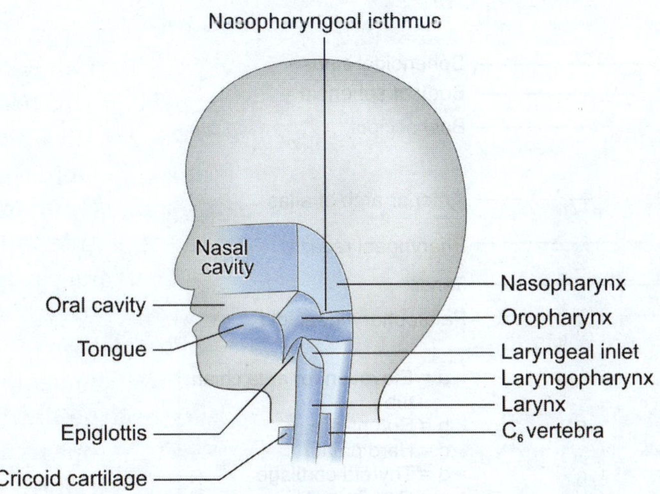

Fig. 12: Sagittal section of the head showing different parts of the pharynx.

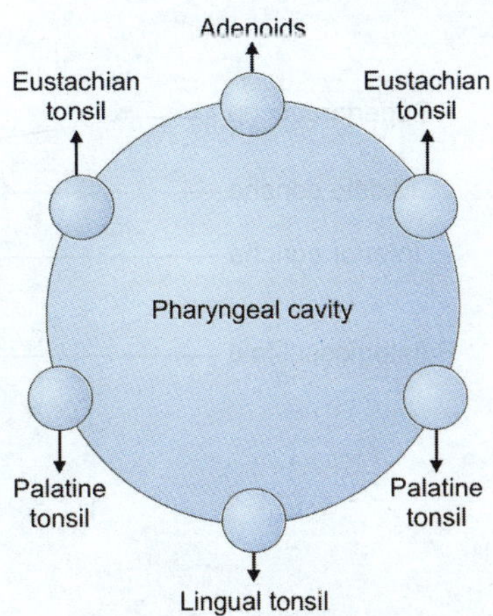

Fig. 13: Ring of Waldeyer.

these lymph glands and the swelling of overlying mucosa may lead to partial obstruction of airway.

All the lymph glands of nasopharynx are arranged in a circular fashion which is called the *Waldeyer ring*. It consists of (1) adenoids (A), (2) Eustachian tonsil (E), (3) palatine tonsil (P) lying between the pillars of fauces, and (4) small lingual tonsil (L) situated at the base of the tongue. The picture of Waldeyer ring is shown in **Figure 13**. The motor nerve, supplying the constrictors muscle of pharynx comes, from vagus. The sensory nerve, supplying the pharynx comes from the maxillary division of trigeminal nerve (nasopharynx) and glossopharyngeal nerve (oropharynx and hypopharynx).

Oropharynx

This part of the pharynx extends from the level of hard palate and soft palate *above* to the level of hyoid bone *below*. At the level of hyoid bone below, by a plane drawn at the upper border of epiglottis, oropharynx is separated from the hypopharynx. It is bounded *above and in front* by the soft and hard palate; *below and in front* by the dorsal surface of the base of the tongue (up to the upper border of epiglottis). It is bounded *posteriorly* by the bodies of C_2 and C_3 vertebrae. The free edge of soft palate forms an arch which is called the *palatine arch*. From the center of this palatine arch, *uvula* hangs downward. From the side of this palatine arch, on either side, two folds of mucous membrane run downward. These two folds of mucous membrane are raised up by the bands of muscle fibers, named the *palatoglossus* and *palatopharyngeus muscle*. They form the pillar of fauces and in this fauces, between these two pillars lies the *palatine tonsil. The glossopharyngeal nerve supplies the sensory of the oropharynx.*

Hypopharynx (Laryngopharynx)

It is a part of the pharynx, lying below oropharynx. It extends from a horizontal plane, drawn at the upper border of epiglottis *above*, to the lower border of cricoid cartilage or C_6 vertebrae *below*. It is continuous with the larynx in front and with esophagus below **(Fig. 14)**. The inlet of larynx, and the posterior surface of cricoid and arytenoid cartilage lie in *front* and the body of fourth, fifth, and sixth cervical vertebrae lies *behind* the hypopharynx. Laterally, the hypopharynx presents the *pyriform fossa* on each side of the inlet of larynx. Pyriform fossa is bounded medially by the *aryepiglottic or quadrate membrane* (the upper border of this membrane is called the *aryepiglottic fold*), extending between epiglottis and arytenoid cartilage, and laterally by the thyroid cartilage and thyrohyoid membrane. Beneath the mucosa of pyriform fossa lies the *internal laryngeal nerve* which is a branch of superior laryngeal nerve.

The motor supply of hypopharynx comes from the *cranial accessory nerve* through the *pharyngeal branches of glossopharyngeal nerve*. The vasomotor of pharynx is supplied by the superior cervical sympathetic ganglion. *The vagus nerve supplies the sensory to the airway below the level of epiglottis. The superior laryngeal nerve*, a branch of vagus, divides into an external (motor) laryngeal nerve and an internal (sensory) laryngeal nerve. The *internal laryngeal nerve* supplies sensory to the hypopharynx and larynx between the epiglottis and vocal cord. Another branch of vagus, named the *recurrent laryngeal nerve*, supplies the sensory to the larynx below its vocal cord and to the trachea.

Summary of sensory supply of pharynx:

- *Nasopharynx:* Maxillary branch of trigeminal nerve. From maxillary nerve, the fibers come through the branches of pterygopalatine ganglion
- *Oropharynx:* Glossopharyngeal nerve

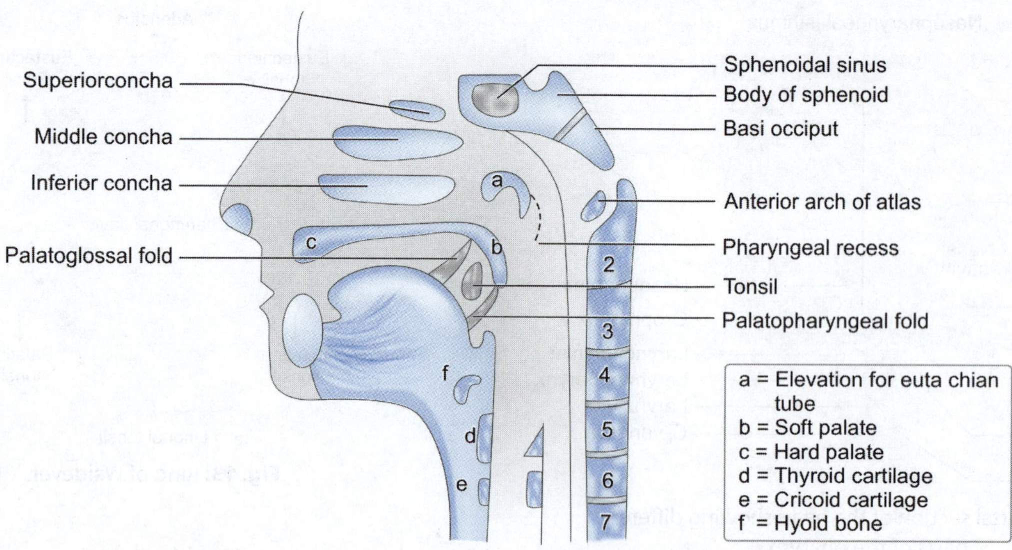

Fig. 14: Sagittal section through the mouth, nose, pharynx, and larynx.

- *Laryngopharynx:* Internal laryngeal nerve → branch of superior laryngeal nerve → branch of vagus
- *Posterior one-third of tongue:* Both taste and general sensation → glossopharyngeal nerve
- *Tonsil:* General sensory → glossopharyngeal
- *Soft palate:*
  - *Oral surface:* Taste and general sensation → glossopharyngeal
  - *Nasal surface:* General sensation → Maxillary branch of trigeminal.

Larynx

Larynx acts as (1) an organ of voice, (2) air passage, and (3) an inlet valve for lower respiratory tract. It extends from laryngeal inlet at the base of the tongue *above* to the trachea *below*. *It lies opposite to the body of C_3–C_6 vertebrae. In children, it lies more anteriorly and at a higher level than adults.* Larynx consists of cartilages, ligaments, muscles, and membranes. These cartilages are total of nine in number. Among them, three are paired (arytenoid, corniculate, and cuneiform) and three are unpaired (epiglottis, thyroid, and cricoid). The epiglottis is a leaf-shaped cartilage with a broad and free upper margin. The lower end of it is pointed and is attached at the angle between the two laminae of thyroid cartilage. Anteriorly the epiglottis is connected to the base of the tongue by three mucosal folds. These three mucosal folds are *a median glossoepiglottic fold* and a *pair of lateral glossoepiglottic folds.* The depression between the median and lateral glossoepiglottic fold is called the *vallecula* and *this is the site where the tip of the blade of Macintosh laryngoscope rests.* The epiglottis projects into the hypopharynx and overhangs on laryngeal inlet.

The epiglottis prevents aspiration by covering the glottis (the opening of larynx) during swallowing. But this sealing of laryngeal inlet by epiglottis, during swallowing and deglutition, is not absolutely necessary. The lateral margins of epiglottis are attached to the *quadrate membrane* (aryepiglottic membrane) which extends from the arytenoid cartilage (situated posteriorly) to the margins of epiglottis (situated anteriorly). The lower free border of this quadrate membrane forms the vestibular fold and the upper free border forms the aryepiglottic fold. Arytenoid is a small pyramidal-shaped cartilage situated at the upper border of the lamina of the cricoid cartilage. The apex of arytenoid cartilage again articulates with corniculate and cuneiform cartilage. Vocal cord is attached to the vocal process of this arytenoid cartilage. Corniculate and cuneiform cartilage lie in the posterior part of aryepiglottic fold **(Figs. 15 and 16)**.

The *thyroid cartilage* is a V-shaped cartilage and is made up of two quadrilateral laminae. They are fused at >90° angle in males and >120° angle in females anteriorly. This line of junction of these two laminae of thyroid cartilage forms in male the *Adam's apple.* The posterior border of thyroid cartilage is free and projects both upward and downward as superior and inferior cornu. The inferior cornu articulates with the cricoid cartilage. On the outer surface of the laminae of thyroid cartilage, there is an *oblique line* that gives attachment to sternothyroid, thyrohyoid, and inferior constrictor muscle of the pharynx. The Upper border of the laminae of thyroid cartilage gives attachment to the *thyrohyoid membrane* which is pierced by the internal laryngeal nerve and superior laryngeal vessels. This thyrohyoid membrane forms the outer boundary of the pyriform fossa.

The *cricoid cartilage* is looked like a signet-shaped ring and encircles the lower part of larynx. The narrow anterior part of this ring-shaped cricoid cartilage is called the *arch* and the broad posterior part is called the *lamina*. *Superiorly this lamina of cricoid cartilage is attached with arytenoid cartilage and at the side with the inferior cornu of thyroid cartilage.* A membrane named the *conus elasticus or cricovocal membrane* extends (but not attached) upward and medially from the upper border of the arch of cricoid cartilage to the lower border of the laminae of thyroid cartilage *in front* and the vocal process of arytenoid cartilage

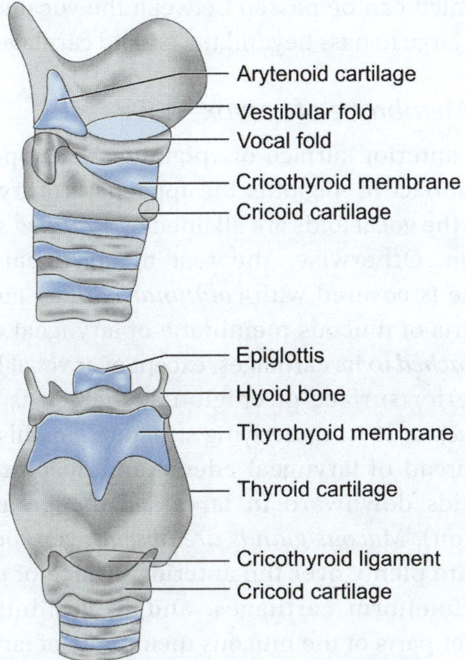

Fig. 15: Cartilages and ligaments of larynx.

behind. The anterior part of this membrane is thick and is known as the cricothyroid ligament. The upper free border of this conus elasticus membrane forms the *vocal cord* (**Fig. 17**).

Cavity of Larynx

The cavity of larynx extends *above* from the inlet of larynx to the lower border of cricoid cartilage *below* where it is continuous with trachea. The *inlet of larynx* opens above in laryngopharynx or hypopharynx. This inlet of larynx is bounded *anteriorly* by epiglottis; *posteriorly* by interarytenoid fold of mucous membrane and *on each side* by an aryepiglottic fold which is the upper border of a quadrate membrane (**Fig. 18**).

Within the cavity of the larynx, on each side, there are two folds of mucous membrane. The upper folds are called the *vestibular folds* and the space between these two vestibular folds is called *rima vestibuli*. The lower folds are called the *vocal cords* and the space between these two vocal cords is called *rima glottidis*.

The vestibular folds and the vocal folds divide the cavity of larynx into three parts. The part of larynx above vestibular fold is called the *vestibule of the larynx*. The space between the vestibular folds and the vocal folds is called the *sinus of larynx*, and the part below the vocal folds is called the *infraglottic part of larynx*. The anterior part of the sinus of larynx is prolonged upward as a diverticulum between the vestibular fold and the lamina of thyroid cartilage. This extension of sinus of larynx is called the *saccule of larynx* and contains mucous glands which help in the lubrication of vocal folds (**Fig. 19**).

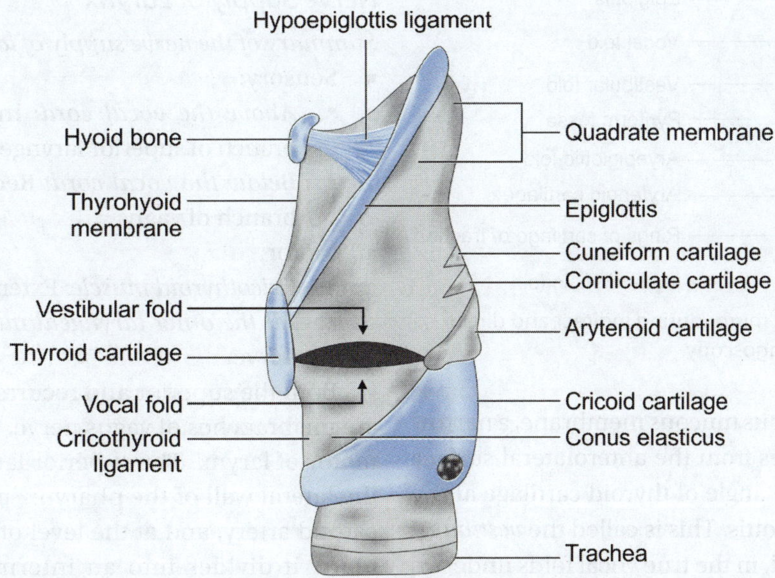

Fig. 16: Ligaments and membranes (mainly quadrate membrane and conus elasticus) of larynx.

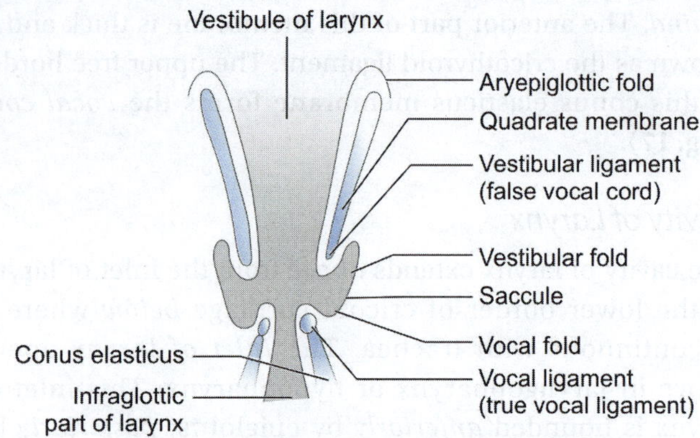

Fig. 17: Coronal section revealing the parts of the cavity of larynx.

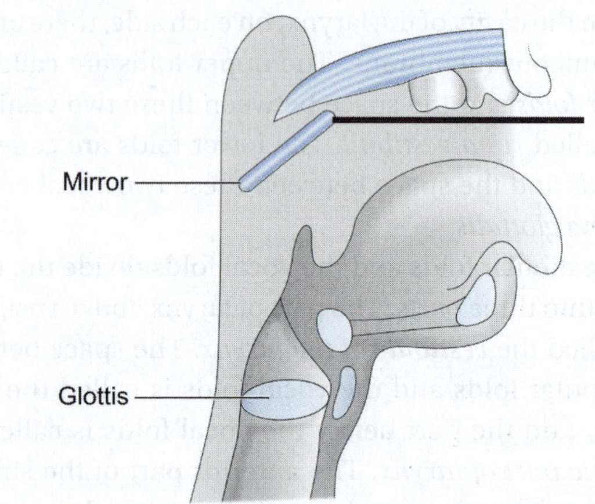

Fig. 18: Indirect laryngoscopy by mirror.

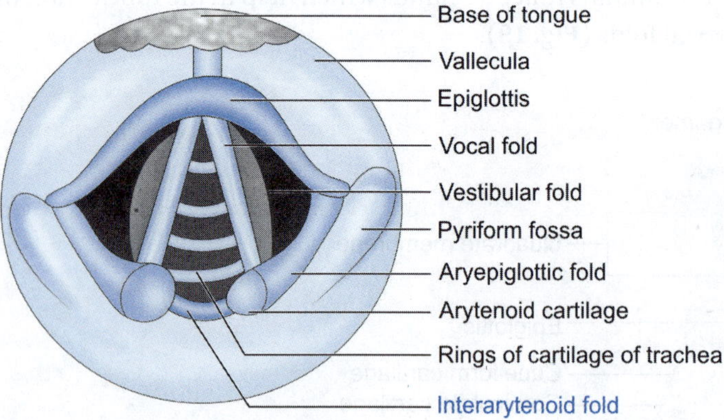

Fig. 19: Laryngeal image on mirror during indirect and direct laryngoscopy.

In vestibular folds, under its mucous membrane, a narrow band of fibrous tissue passes from the anterolateral surface of arytenoid cartilage to the angle of thyroid cartilage at the point of attachment of epiglottis. This is called the *vestibular ligament*. On the other hand, in the true vocal folds under its mucous membrane, a tough fibrous *vocal ligament* extends from the vocal process of arytenoid cartilage to the angle of thyroid cartilage. Since, there is no true submucous layer, with the usual network of blood vessels, within it, the true vocal cords or folds have the characteristic pale appearance.

In an adult, the narrowest part of the laryngeal cavity is the area that is situated between the vocal cords. But in children, under 10 years of age, the narrowest part of larynx is just below the vocal cords at the level of cricoid cartilage. The clinical significance of this anatomical difference in larynx between an adult and a child is found when small children are intubated. The significance is that in children an ETT which can be passed between the vocal cords may yet be too large to pass beyond the cricoid cartilage.

Mucous Membrane of Larynx

The total anterior surface of epiglottis, the upper half of posterior surface of epiglottis, the upper parts of aryepiglottic folds, and the vocal folds are all lined by *stratified squamous epithelium*. Otherwise, the rest of laryngeal mucous membrane is covered with *columnar ciliated epithelium*. All the parts of mucous membrane of laryngeal cavity are *loosely attached* to its cartilages, except over vocal ligaments and posterior surface of epiglottis where it is thin and *firmly adherent* to its underlying structure. So, this prevents further spread of laryngeal edema and accumulation of tissue fluids downward in larynx, causing suffocation (obstruction). *Mucous glands are absent* over vocal cords, but they are plenty over the anterior surface of epiglottis, around cuneiform cartilages, and in vestibular folds. In the other parts of the mucous membrane of larynx these mucous glands are scanty.

Nerve Supply of Larynx

Summary of the nerve supply of larynx.
- Sensory:
  - *Above the vocal cord:* Internal laryngeal nerve → branch of superior laryngeal nerve → branch of vagus.
  - *Below the vocal cord:* Recurrent laryngeal nerve → branch of vagus
- Motor:
  - *Cricothyroid muscle:* External laryngeal nerve
  - *All the other laryngeal muscles:* Recurrent laryngeal nerve.

Both the superior and recurrent laryngeal nerves, which are the branches of vagus nerve, supply the sensory and the motor of larynx. The superior laryngeal nerve descends on the lateral wall of the pharynx, passes posterior to internal carotid artery, and at the level of the greater cornu of hyoid bone; it divides into an internal and external laryngeal branch.

TABLE 2: Laryngeal innervation.		
Nerve	**Sensory**	**Motor**
Internal branch of superior laryngeal nerve (internal laryngeal nerve)	Laryngopharynx and part of the larynx above vocal cord	None
External branch of superior laryngeal nerve (external laryngeal nerve)	None	Cricothyroid (a tensor of vocal cord)
Recurrent laryngeal nerve	Larynx below vocal cord, trachea, and bronchi	• Posterior cricoarytenoid (abductor), • Lateral cricoarytenoid (abductor), • Interarytenoid (abductor), and • Thyroarytenoid (abductor)

The *internal laryngeal* branch of superior laryngeal nerve is entirely sensory and descends on thyrohyoid membrane. It then pierces this thyrohyoid membrane above the superior laryngeal artery and then again divides into two branches: (1) The *upper branch* supplies the mucous membrane of the lower part of the pharynx, epiglottis, vallecula, and the vestibule of larynx and (2) the *lower branch* passes medial to pyriform fossa, beneath its mucous membrane, and supplies the aryepiglottic fold, pyriform fossa and the mucous membrane of the posterior part of the rima glottidis. The *external laryngeal* branch, carrying only the motor fibers, innervates the cricothyroid muscle, therefore the sensory supply of the larynx above the vocal cord is by the superior laryngeal nerve **(Table 2)**.

The *recurrent laryngeal nerve* travels upward deep to the lower border of inferior constrictor muscle of pharynx, accompanying with the laryngeal branch of inferior thyroid artery. Apart from the sensory fibers which supply the mucous membrane of larynx below the level of vocal cords, this nerve innervates all the muscles of larynx, except cricothyroid (adductor of vocal cord) and a small part of arytenoid muscles.

Summary

The upper airway derives its sensory supply from cranial nerves **(Fig. 20)**. This can be summarized as follows. *Anteriorly the nose* gets its sensory supply from the anterior and posterior ethmoidal branch of ophthalmic division of trigeminal nerve (fifth cranial nerve). *Posteriorly the nose* is supplied by the sphenopalatine branch of maxillary division of trigeminal nerve. The *soft and hard palate* gets its sensory

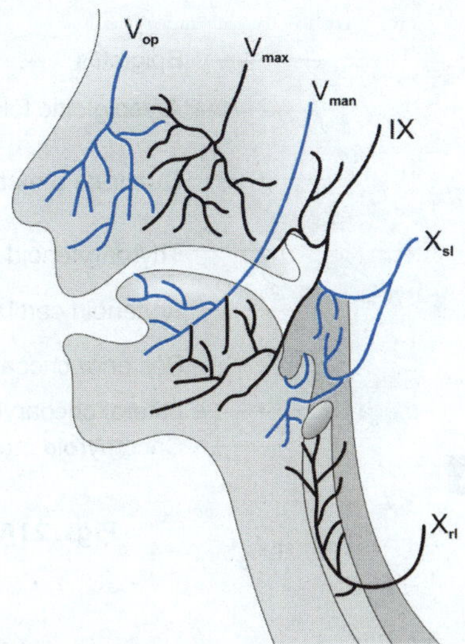

Fig. 20: Sensory supply of airway. (V_{op}: ophthalmic division of trigeminal nerve (anterior ethmoidal nerve); V_{max}: maxillary division of trigeminal nerve (sphenopalatine nerve); V_{man}: mandibular division of trigeminal nerve (lingual nerve); IX: glossopharyngeal nerve; X_{sl}: vagus superior laryngeal nerve; X_{rl}: vagus recurrent laryngeal nerve)

supply from palatine nerve which is the branch of trigeminal nerve. The lingual nerve, a branch of the mandibular division of trigeminal nerve supplies the sensory to the *anterior two-thirds of tongue*. The glossopharyngeal nerve or ninth cranial nerve supplies the sensory to the *posterior one-third of the tongue*. The facial and glossopharyngeal nerve provides the *sensation of taste* to the anterior two-thirds and posterior one-third of the tongue, respectively. The glossopharyngeal nerve also provides sensory supply to the *roof of pharynx, tonsils, and under surface of soft palate*. The vagus nerve or 10th cranial nerve, supplies the sensory of airway *below the epiglottis* through its superior laryngeal (divides into internal and external branch) and recurrent laryngeal branch which is described above.

*The actions of the intrinsic muscles of the larynx (**Figs. 21 and 22**)*

- *The muscles for closing and opening of laryngeal inlet:*
  - Closing—aryepiglottic
  - Opening—thyroepiglottic
- *The muscles for closing and opening of rima glottidis:*
  - Closing—lateral cricoarytenoids, transverse arytenoid, cricothyroid, and thyroarytenoids
  - Opening—posterior cricoarytenoids
- *The muscles which tense and relax the vocal cords:*
  - Tense (adduction)—cricothyroid
  - Relax—thyroarytenoids and vocalis.

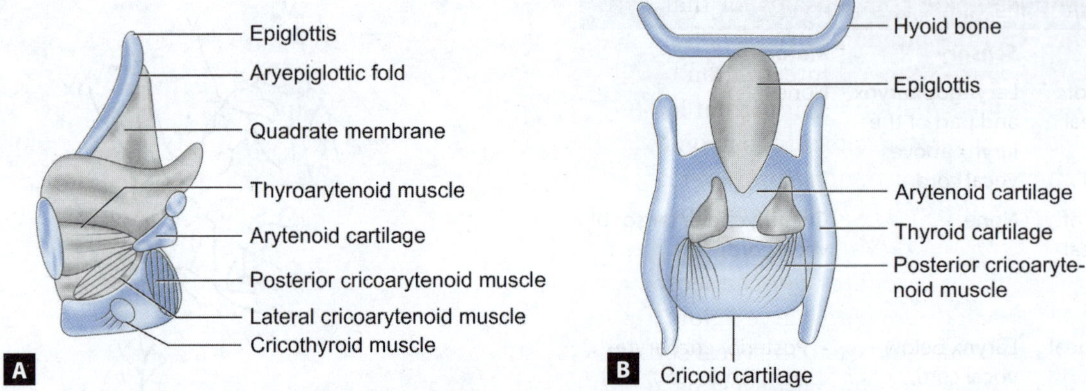

Figs. 21A and B: The intrinsic muscles of the larynx.

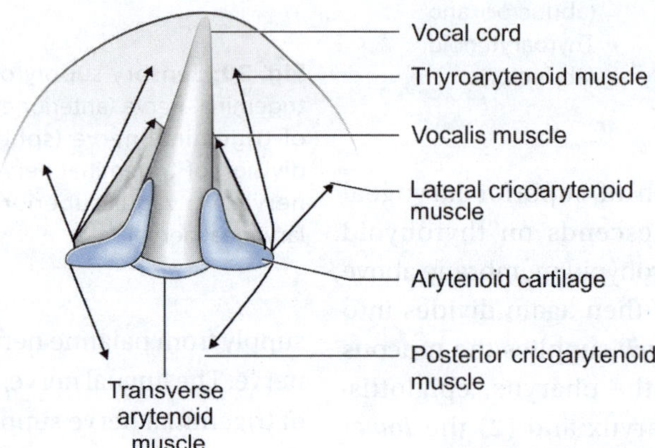

Fig. 22: The different directions of the movement of muscles of the vocal cord.

The movements of vocal cords:

The movements of vocal cords affect the shape and size of rima glottidis and they are as follows:

- During quiet breathing (in resting condition), the intermembranous part of rima glottidis is triangular and the intercartilaginous part of rima glottidis is quadrangular in shape.
- During forced inspiration both the parts of rima glottidis (intermembranous and intercartilaginous) are triangular in shape, so that the entire rima is lozenge-shaped and the vocal cords are fully abducted.
- During phonation (speech), the rima glottidis is reduced to a chink by adduction of vocal cords.
- During whispering, the intermembranous part of the rima glottidis is closed, but the intercartilaginous part is widely open **(Fig. 22)**.

■ APPLIED ANATOMY

- Damage or block of internal laryngeal nerve, which is a branch of superior laryngeal nerve, produces anesthesia of the mucous membrane of supraglottic part of larynx.

So, any foreign body can readily enter into the laryngeal inlet as reflexes do not work. But the function of vocal cord is not jeopardized.

- Damage to the external laryngeal nerve, which is another branch of superior laryngeal nerve, causes some weakness of phonation. It is due to the loss of the tightening effect of vocal cord by the paralysis of cricothyroid muscle which is supplied by it. On the contrary, the bilateral damage of superior laryngeal nerve results in hoarseness and easy tiring of voice. But airway control by vocal cord is not jeopardized, though the reflexes of laryngeal inlet are impaired like the injury of the internal laryngeal nerve.
- When both the recurrent laryngeal nerves are interrupted or blocked, then the vocal cords lie in the position of complete adduction, due to the unopposed action of the cricothyroid muscle. So, the patient will suffer from stridor and respiratory distress. But the airway problem is less frequent in chronic bilateral recurrent nerve interruption. This is because of various compensatory mechanisms which always develop. When only one recurrent laryngeal nerve is paralyzed, then the vocal

cord of the opposite side compensates for that. Then, there is no difficulty in respiration, but only deterioration of voice quality occurs. Bilateral interruption of vagus nerve affects both the superior and recurrent laryngeal nerve. Thus, it produces a flaccid, midpositioned vocal cord as seen after the administration of muscle relaxants.

- Larynx can be seen directly by a laryngoscope (direct laryngoscopy) or by a laryngeal mirror (indirect laryngoscopy). By these procedures, one can see the base of the tongue, valleculae, epiglottis, aryepiglottic folds, pyriform fossae, vestibular folds, and the vocal cords.
- Since the glottis of a larynx is the narrowest part of the respiratory passage in an adult, so if any foreign body enters the respiratory passage, then it will usually lodge at glottis. Once it crosses glottis, then it would easily pass through the trachea to lodge in some peripheral narrow bronchus or bronchiole.
- Laryngeal edema may occur due to a variety of causes which may be traumatic, allergic, infective, etc. This produces inspiratory stridor, dyspnea, and symptoms of hypoxia.
- Laryngismus stridulus is a condition that is characterized by attacks of laryngeal spasms in children, usually during the night. In between the attacks, the child is normal.

PHYSIOLOGY OF AIRWAY PROTECTION

The pharynx, epiglottis, and larynx protect the lower airway from aspiration of foreign bodies. An important defense mechanism, for expelling or preventing the entry of foreign bodies into the lower respiratory passage, below the vocal cord, is *cough*, although the epiglottis covers the laryngeal inlet, but it is not always absolutely essential for airway protection. The closure of vocal cords by reflex mechanism is the most vital mechanism for lower airway protection, which also produces protective laryngeal closure during deglutition. The physiological exaggeration of this reflex closure of vocal cord is called the *laryngospasm;* therefore laryngospasm consists of prolonged intense glottic closure in response to the stimulation by inhaled agents, foreign bodies or stimulation from viscera. Laryngospasm is associated with sound, ranging from high-peached squeaky to total absence of sound, depending on the degree of spasm. Complete laryngospasm is usually silent and should be diagnosed and treated immediately.

The *ideal treatment for complete laryngospasm* is the use of muscle relaxant and mask ventilation or intubation. But before muscle relaxants, the forward displacement of the mandible, and IPPV by mask and bag with 100% O_2 should be tried. In most of the cases, it is effective, because strong pressure applied manually with the help of a bag,

which is full of O_2 can force the gas effectively through the adducted vocal cords. Thus, tracheal intubation can be avoided. In such a situation, the traditional view, regarding limiting the pressure, to avoid barotrauma of lungs are not important and the stomach should be watched closely for if the air is entering the esophagus forcefully or not. Another way of management of laryngospasm is intravenous (IV) administration of propofol or thiopentone, making the patient deeply sedated, provided the airway is clear of any foreign body. A patient who is scheduled for elective surgery, but experiences repeated intermittent laryngospasm and arrhythmia is a poor candidate for continued attempt of intubation.

UPPER AIRWAY OBSTRUCTION

One of the foremost duties of an anesthetist is to maintain an unobstructed airway in an unconscious patient. This obstruction of airway may be total or partial. *Partial obstruction of airway* is associated with (1) diminished tidal volume (but not completely absent), (2) retractive movement of rib cages and neck muscles, (3) tugging movement of diaphragm and snoring sound. If the obstruction is near the laryngeal inlet, then there will be (4) inspiratory stridor. The *total obstruction of airway* is characterized by (1) a complete lack of movement of air in and out of the lungs, or zero tidal volume which is recognized by (2) no movement of breathing bag, and (3) *see-saw paradoxical movement of chest and abdomen*. The entry and exit of air from lungs should be perceived by the feeling with hand, placed over the nose and mouth, looking at the nonparadoxical movement of chest and abdomen, and seeing the movement of breathing bag. An inexperienced person will, usually, wrongly interpret this retractive movement of chest, abdomen (a see-saw paradoxical movement), and neck as a breathing effort. So, the recognition of airway obstruction depends on the close observation of the movement pattern of chest and abdomen and the high index of suspicion **(Figs. 23A and B)**.

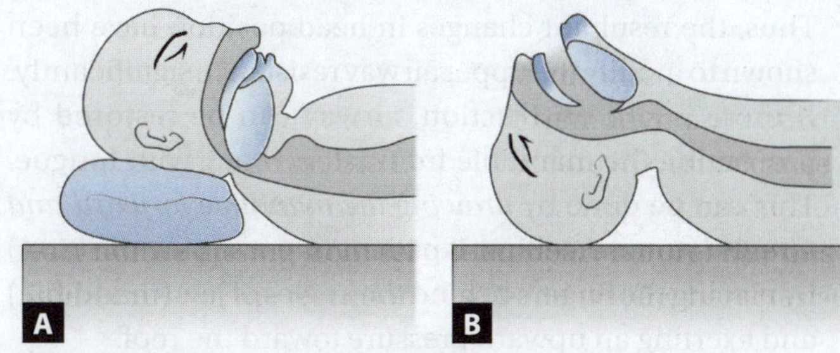

Figs. 23A and B: (A) The fall of a tongue on the posterior pharyngeal wall and the collapse of pharyngeal wall due to the relaxation of the muscles of airway (mainly genioglossus) and (B) The extension of neck and the elevation of the angle of mandible removes the falling base of the tongue from the posterior pharyngeal wall and maintains a clear airway.

Upper airway obstruction is commonly due to soft tissue obstruction, by falling back of tongue, on posterior pharyngeal wall. It may also be due to tumor, foreign bodies or laryngospasm, etc. But here we will only discuss the obstruction of upper airway by the base of falling tongue (obstruction of airway by laryngospasm is discussed earlier). Because it is the most common cause of upper airway obstruction during anesthesia and is due to the relaxation of tongue (mainly genioglossus muscle) and jaw muscles. This occurs as soon as the consciousness is lost and the muscles, supporting the tongue, relax, so the tongue falls back on the posterior wall of oropharynx or hypopharynx or on the inlet of larynx. If the tongue is brought forward by manipulation, then the laryngeal opening once again is cleared and opened. This can be achieved by the following methods.

- *Positioning:* Before any manipulation of airway, correct positioning of patient is very helpful and a must. This correct positioning of patient means the relative alignment of oral, pharyngeal, and laryngeal axes and this is achieved by having the patient in a "sniffing position". When cervical spine pathology is suspected, then the head must be kept in a neutral position, during all airway manipulation. Patient, with morbid obesity, should be positioned on a 30° upward (toward the head) ramp, as the functional residual capacity (FRC) of obese patients deteriorates in a supine position, leading to more rapid deoxygenation if ventilation is impaired.

- The *simple extension of neck* will clear the airway in 75% of cases. It causes the forward movement of mandible and the stretching of anterior tissues of the neck which, in turn, produces the forward traction of tongue. Thus, this simple extension of neck releases the airway obstruction.

- The *extension of neck* also causes the mouth to fall open due to the downward pull of neck tissues. In such condition, the *simple closing of mouth* in an extended position of neck will often improve the airway by straightening the anterior tissues of neck still further. Thus, the resultant changes in head position have been shown to modify the upper airway resistance significantly.

- If there is still obstruction, airway can be restored by preventing the mandible from falling back with tongue. This can be done by *drawing the mandible forward and upward* (toward ceiling, if patient is in a supine position) by placing the fingers behind the angles of jaw (mandible) and exerting an upward pressure toward the roof.

- If the aforementioned procedures also fail, then the removal of obstruction of airway can be accomplished with some *mechanical contrivances*, termed the oropharyngeal or nasopharyngeal airway, though other types of airways are discussed further. The idea behind

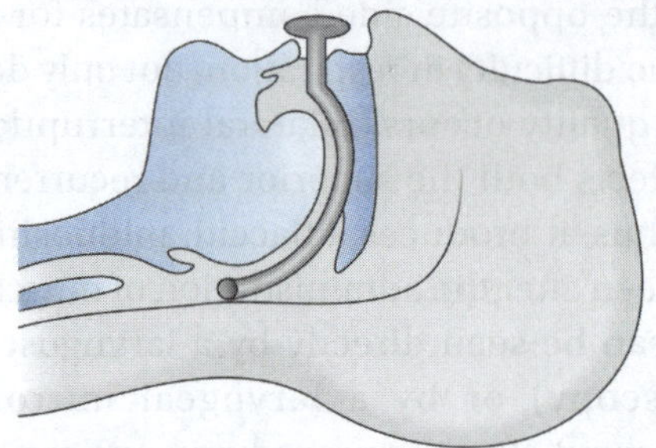

Fig. 24: Oropharyngeal airway elevating the tongue.

both the oropharyngeal and nasopharyngeal airway is to lift the base of the tongue from posterior wall of pharynx and to maintain an air passage and thus to remove obstruction. The nasopharyngeal airway is better tolerated in a light plane of anesthesia than the oropharyngeal airway. But the mere placement of any of the aforementioned airway does not guarantee an unobstructed airflow. This is because these airways do not get any support from relaxed mandible due to the relaxation of jaw muscles and is displaced. So, it is often necessary with oropharyngeal or nasopharyngeal airway to support the mandible further by forward traction or by pressing upward toward ceiling (in a supine position) at the angles of it (mandible). In anesthetized patient, the pharyngeal and laryngeal reflexes are obtunded. If these reflexes are still active, then insertion of any airway to prevent obstruction may precipitate further gagging, emesis, or laryngeal spasm, causing more obstruction **(Fig. 24)**.

The most commonly used oral airway is the *Guedel airway*. The Guedel oral airways are generally made up of plastic and their size (according to length in mm) ranges from Guedel number: 0, 1, and 2 (50, 60, and 70 mm in length, respectively) for children to 3, 4, and 5 (80, 90, and 100 mm in length, respectively) for adults. The appropriate length of this Guedel oral airway for a particular patient is determined by the distance between the tip of a nose and the tragus plus 1 cm or 10 mm. It is inserted first with the upside-down direction while passing through the oral cavity and then it is rotated 180° into the position of function. During the insertion of the oral airway, teeth can be injured and the airway itself can push the base of the tongue into the pharynx, thus it can actually increase the airway obstruction instead of removing it, hence an anesthetist must be careful during the insertion of the oral airway.

To remove the obstruction of the upper airway, by falling tongue, soft nasal airways are useful for patients who are not deeply anesthetized. However, contraindications to the use of nasal airways include coagulopathy, basilar skull fracture, large adenoids, nasal infections, nasal deformities, etc. Because of the risk of epistaxis, the nasal airways are less desirable for anticoagulated and thrombocytopenic patients. The introduction of nasopharyngeal airway can be facilitated by phenylephrine nasal drops (causing vasoconstriction of nasal mucosa) or by lubricating the airway with lignocaine or K–Y gel. During introduction, the tip of a nasal airway should be perpendicular to the face and is advanced slowly along the floor of the nasal passage. Under any circumstances, the tip of the airway should not be directed upward toward the cribriform plate. The length of the nasopharyngeal airways is roughly estimated by the distance from the tip of the nose to the meatus of the ear and it is approximately 2–4 cm longer than oral airways. When such maneuvers and the use of artificial airways provide inadequate relief of upper airway obstruction by soft tissues, then the insertion of an ETT or other methods to bypass the upper airway obstruction should be contemplated.

ROUTINE AIRWAY MANAGEMENT

Routine airway management associated with general anesthesia consists of:

- Preanesthetic airway assessment
- Checking of all anesthetic equipment and accessories
- Proper positioning of the patient
- Preoxygenation
- Mask and bag ventilation
- ET intubation or placement of LMA
- Confirmation of ET intubation
- Extubation.

EVALUATION OF THE AIRWAY (AIRWAY ASSESSMENT)

Introduction

One of the most important thing that an anesthetist has to learn is the *efficient management of airway*. On the other hand, *proper evaluation of an airway* is an essential part for the *efficient management of airway*. So, before every induction for anesthesia, the airway of a patient should be evaluated or assessed properly by an anesthetist. Thus, the discussion regarding the assessment and the evaluation of airway for the efficient management of airway has been widely accepted in anesthesia for a long time, although multiple predictive methods and scoring system for the evaluation of airway has been suggested, but nothing can give a 100% correct prediction. So, we will take only true scientific *predictive protocol* that all anesthesiologists can depend upon it. This is because, still now, sometimes the unanticipated difficult airway in apparently normal patients sends us the signals for our inability to solve this problem.

The questions in these predictions tell us about different terms which are frequently used such as *difficult airway, difficult ventilation, difficult laryngoscopy, or difficult intubation*, because the answers to these questions are different. These three different technical skills are (1) unable to expose the glottis by a conventional laryngoscope (difficult airway), (2) unable to ventilate the patient maintaining SPO_2 >90% (difficult ventilation), (3) and unable to insert an ETT into the trachea through the larynx (difficult intubation). The former is generally termed difficult, if one gets a poor view of the target organ, i.e., glottis (Cormack–Lehane grade 3 or 4). The second is termed difficult if one without any assistance cannot maintain SPO_2 >90% by ventilating an anesthetized patient with a bag and mask and 100% O_2. The third is termed difficult, if after an arbitrary number of attempts (usually three), the ETT cannot be placed into the trachea (difficult intubation). All these three should be evaluated together or separately based on the *history, clinical examination, and radiological diagnostic tests (investigations).* For easy and quick intubation, a good view of the larynx is mandatory. So, difficult laryngoscopy and a bad view of the larynx (difficult airway) is associated with difficult intubation, hence the assessment of difficult airway and difficult intubation should be discussed together. The assessment for difficult ventilation will be discussed under a separate heading.

An airway can be classified on the basis of predictions and ultimate difficulties or outcomes into three categories.

1. A predicted normal airway
2. A predicted abnormal airway
3. An apparently normal and unpredicted difficult airway.

Among them, the patients of group three are the most dangerous. Even, among the patients of group three, those which have failed intubation and mask ventilation are also not adequate (not intubated and not ventilated), actually presents the life-threatening condition.

Evaluation of the airway can be performed under three headings (1) History, (2) Physical examination, and (3) Investigation.

History

One of the most important point during history taking for the evaluation of airway is if there is any difficulty during previous general anesthesia, more specifically during mask ventilation or ET intubation. This history should be properly documented and passed on to the next anesthesia caregiver.

BOX 2: Common congenital syndrome causing difficult airway and intubation.

- *Pierre Robin syndrome:* Micrognathia, macroglossia, and cleft palate
- *Treacher Collins syndrome:* Auricular and ocular defects and mandibular hypoplasia
- *Down's syndrome:* Poorly developed nasal bridge, large tongue, and smallmouth
- *Klippel–Feil syndrome:* Fusion of vertebra and restricted neck movement
- *Goldenhar syndrome:* Mandibular hypoplasia, cervical spine abnormality, occipitalization of the atlas, and auricular and ocular defects
- *Goiter:* Compression and deviation of trachea

Note: There are many other diseases such as rheumatoid arthritis which may progress gradually and may cause airway problems during present anesthesia which might have no airway complications during previous anesthesia.

BOX 3: Conditions associated with difficult airway and intubations.

- *Tumors:* Large goiter, cystic hygroma, lipoma, hemangioma, hematoma, adenoma, papillomatosis, any tumors of pharynx or larynx, etc.
- *Arthritis:* Rheumatoid arthritis, temporomandibular (TM) joints ankylosis, restricted spine. Ankylosing spondylitis, cervical spine ankylosis, and restricted cervical spine mobility
- *Infections:* Abscess (peritonsillar, retropharyngeal, submandibular, etc.), Ludwig's angina, epiglottitis, trismus, laryngeal edema, laryngitis, etc.
- *Trauma:* Maxillary fracture, mandibular fracture, basilar skull fracture, cervical spine fracture, inhalation, burn, laryngeal fracture, edema of airway, etc.
- *Foreign body:* Anywhere in the pharynx and larynx
- *Obesity:* Short neck, sleep apnea, and extra tissue in oropharynx
- *Acromegaly:* Macroglossia and prognathism
- *Other anatomical variations:* Micrognathia, high arched palate, prominent upper incisor, scleroderma, and sarcoidosis
- *Congenital syndrome:* Discussed earlier in **Box 2**.

The history of other previous and present diseases such as infection, trauma, neoplasia, and inflammation which may affect the airway, and subsequently the mode of anesthesia should be taken properly. Some other present conditions that could predispose to a difficult airway are edema of face and neck, burn, active bleeding in oral cavity, tracheal and esophageal stenosis, aspiration of gastric contents, etc. There are many other congenital syndromes that are associated with airway problems and intubation difficulty during anesthesia should also be kept in mind. These common congenital syndromes causing difficult airway and intubation are enumerated in **Box 2**.

Physical Examination

After history taking, every patient should be properly examined physically to predict any difficulty of airway management (difficult laryngoscopy, difficult intubation, and difficult ventilation) during anesthesia **(Box 3)**. Many additional clinical tests to predict difficult laryngoscopy and difficult intubation have also been described, but none of these tests is totally reliable. Their use may complement each other and also the routine physical examination of airway.

The routine physical examination of airway *should start* from the simple inspection of patient for *obesity*. The morbidly obese patients with a BMI of >30 kg/m^2 or more are frequently associated with difficult laryngoscopy and difficult intubation. However, some morbidly obese patients have relatively normal head and neck anatomy and others have much redundant pharyngeal tissue and increased neck circumference. The next routine physical examination of a patient includes the inspection of *his/her head and neck* to identify any obvious problem such as cervical

collars, external injury, burns, contracture, restricted jaw movement, receding mandible, bucked teeth, etc., to *whole body inspection* to some comprehensive *scoring system*, for example, the congenital presence of some ear and hand abnormalities suggest the associated presence of some congenital cardiovascular disorders and abnormal airway. Adequate nasal airway should also be evaluated before any nasal intubations **(Table 3)**.

Regarding the teeth, loose teeth, protuberant upper incisors, false teeth, and other dental works such as crowns, bridges, and braces should be noted. Edentulous patients present seldom difficulty to intubate unless other associated problems are severe. Protuberant upper incisors may make laryngoscopy difficult and can cause damage to the teeth. Severe loose teeth should be removed or fixed by ligature, before laryngoscopy, to avoid aspiration of it. Artificial dentures should be removed.

Next, the *opening of the mouth* should be assessed and it depends on the function of temporomandibular (TM) joint. Any previous and present disease of TM joint makes the mouth opening difficult and visualization of any pharyngeal and laryngeal structure is impossible. Normally, an adult should be able to open their mouth, so that there is a 50 mm distance between the upper and lower incisor teeth **(Fig. 25)**.

After assessment of mouth opening, *oral cavity* should be examined for a large tongue, high-arched palate, long narrow mouth, etc., which may cause difficult laryngoscopy and subsequent difficult intubation. *In 1983, Mallampati has evaluated a scoring system* by observing the structure of oral cavity, through an opened mouth, by which difficulty of laryngoscopy and subsequent difficult intubation can be

TABLE 3: Wilson has identified five risk factors on the basis of which 0, 1, and 2 points are awarded and a scoring system has been developed. A score of 5–10 would predict severe laryngoscopy and intubations difficulty.

	Risk factors	Scoring
Weight	<90 kg	0
	90–110 kg	1
	>110 kg	2
Angle between head and neck	>90°	0
	±90°	1
	<90°	2
Jaw movement (interincisor gap = GP)	>5 cm	0
	±5 cm	1
	<5 cm	2
Receding mandible	Normal	0
	Moderate	1
	Severe	2
Bucked teeth	Normal	0
	Moderate	1
	Severe	2

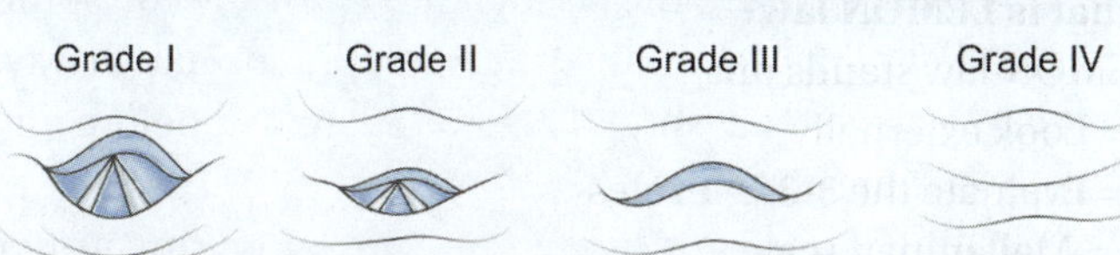

Fig. 25: Grading of laryngeal view (Cormack–Lehane).

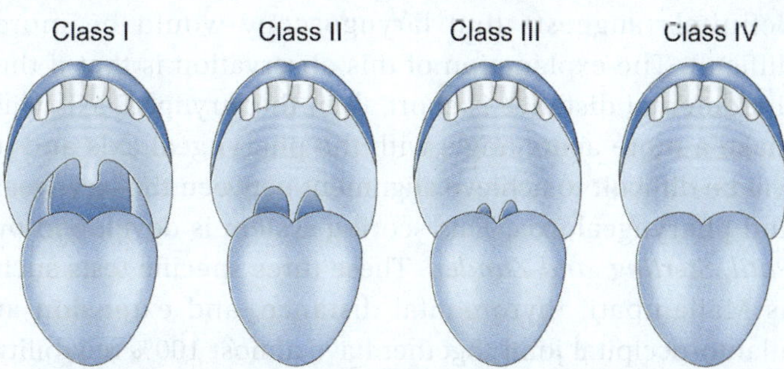

Fig. 26: Mallampati classification or test of oral opening.

BOX 4: Mallampati grading.

- *Grade I:* Anterior and posterior faucial pillar, soft palate, and uvula are visible
- *Grade II:* Only soft palate and uvula are visible
- *Grade III:* Only soft palate is visible
- *Grade IV:* Soft palate is not visible

BOX 5: Mallampati grading for neck extension.

- *Grade I:* >35°
- *Grade II:* 22–34°
- *Grade III:* 12–22°
- *Grade IV:* <12°

assessed or predicted. *This is based on the visualization of soft palate, uvula, and faucial pillar, i.e., to examine the size of the tongue in relation to the size of oral cavity.* The more the tongue obstructs the view of pharyngeal structures; the intubation may be more difficult. This test is performed with the patient sitting upright, head in a neutral position, mouth opened as wide as possible and tongue protruded as far out as possible. Originally, there were three grades (grade-I, grade-II, and grade-III) in the Mallampati scoring system. The scoring system of Mallampati predicts approximately 50% difficult intubation. Then, in 1987, Sampson and Young in their modification of the Mallampati scoring system further added grade IV **(Fig. 26 and Box 4)**. However, the presence of these examination findings may not be very sensitive for detecting difficult laryngoscopy and difficult intubation, but the absence of these findings is predictive for relative ease of intubation.

Another way of assessing the difficulty in laryngoscopy or visualization of glottis and subsequent difficult intubation is to measure the *distance from symphysis of mandible to hyoid bone.* This distance should be at least two large finger breaths in adults. The space between the mandible and hyoid bone is important because during laryngoscopy the tongue is displaced into this place for visualization of glottis. If this space is narrow, then glottis cannot be seen properly.

Then, the neck should be examined for its mobility, particularly for extension. A thick short muscular neck may result in difficult mask ventilation as well as difficult laryngoscopy and intubation. The normal amount of neck extension is 35°. The measurement can be made by simple visual estimation or more accurately with a goniometer. Any reduction in extension of neck is expressed in grades **(Box 5)**.

Cervical spondylosis, ankylosis, rheumatoid arthritis of cervical vertebral joint, etc., may restrict the flexion–extension of intercervical vertebrae or atlanto-occipital joint and may cause difficulty in visualization of glottis by laryngoscope. Thus, difficult intubation may precipitate. *The extension of neck also can be quantified by measuring the distance from symphysis of mandible to thyroid notch (thyromental distance) with the head fully extended.* If the distance is >65 mm (three large finger breaths), then visualization of larynx and intubation will not be difficult. If this thyromental distance varies between 60 and 65 mm (or 6 and 6.5 cm) then visualization of larynx would be slightly difficult. The thyromental distance, below 60 mm, definitely suggests that laryngoscopy would be more difficult. The explanation of this observation is that if the thyromental distance is short, then the laryngeal axis will make a more acute angle with the pharyngeal axis and it will be difficult to achieve alignment between the laryngeal and pharyngeal axis. This scoring system is developed *by Patil, Sterling, and Zanden*. These three specific tests such as Mallampati, thyromental distance, and extension at atlanto-occipital joint together have almost 100% reliability in predicting airway difficulty. Another way of assessment of neck mobility is the *measurement of sternomental distance*. If the sternomental distance is <12.5 cm, then intubation will be difficult. Lesser the distance greater will be the difficulty. This distance should be measured with the head in full extension and the mouth closed **(Fig. 27)**.

It should be noted that the combination of several minor physical anomalies may result in a difficult laryngoscopy and difficult intubation, even when no single factor or test is severely abnormal. Difficult intubation may occur occasionally for reasons that are currently unexplained and none of the available indices predicts it. Even though the airway may look normal on external assessment, one may come across difficulty during laryngoscopy and intubation, due to the variations in internal anatomy of upper airway. *Cormack–Lehane* has defined four grades of laryngoscopic view and predicts subsequent difficult intubation which is given here.

- *Grade I:* Visualization of entire laryngeal aperture, including full length of vocal cord and arytenoid cartilage
- *Grade II:* Visualization of epiglottis, arytenoid cartilage, and posterior part of vocal cord only
- *Grade III:* Visualization of epiglottis only
- *Grade IV:* Epiglottis not visible

Comparison of Mallampati and Cormack–Lehane grading:
- Grade I of Mallampati = Grade I of Cormack–Lehane.
- Grade IV of Mallampati = Grade III and IV of Cormack–Lehane.

- Grade II and III of Mallampati = Relatively uniform distribution in all grades.

The application of external pressure can reduce the incidence of grade III view from 9% to between 5 and 1%.

Investigations

Except clinical, the other ways of assessing the airway are laboratory investigations such as *X-ray, CT scan, and magnetic resonance imaging (MRI) of head and neck*. The lateral X-ray of head and neck, along with distance marking between two bony landmarks have been used to predict the difficult laryngoscopy and difficult intubation. In radiology plate, the measurement of atlanto-occipital distance and interspinous gap between C_1 and C_2 vertebrae may also have a good predictive value. Other radiological examinations for airway assessment include decreased posterior depth of mandible (PDM) and increased anterior depth of mandible (ADM). *A ratio of >3.6 between the mandibular length and posterior depth of mandible (PDM)* has also been shown to indicate the difficult intubation by *White and Kander* **(Fig. 28)**.

Some Rules and Laws

What is LEMON law?

LEMON law stands on:

L = Look externally
E = Evaluate the 3-3-2-1 rules
M = Mallampati scale
O = Obstruction
N = Neck mobility

- *Look externally:* It is the external indicator of either difficult laryngoscopy or difficult ventilation or difficult intubation. It includes presence of a huge beard or large moustache, abnormal facial shape, extreme

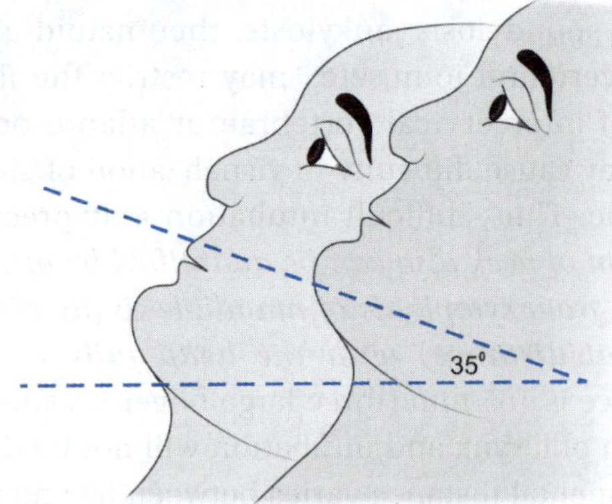

Fig. 27: Assessment of neck mobility by measuring sternomental distance.

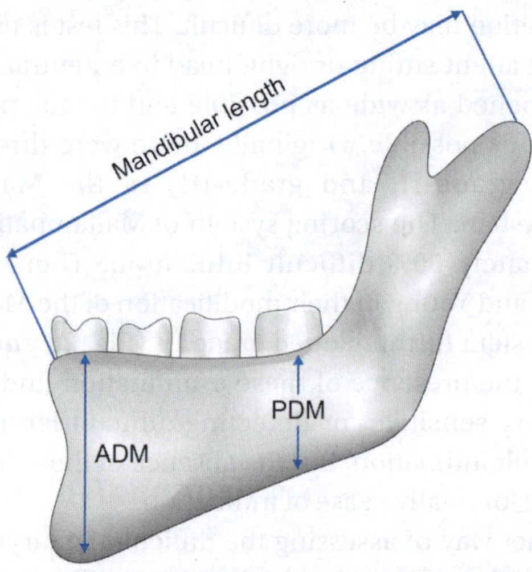

Fig. 28: A ratio between the mandibular length and posterior mandibular depth. (ADM: anterior depth of mandible, PDM: posterior depth of mandible).

malnourishment or overnourishment, a person without teeth, facial trauma, obesity, large front teeth, high-arched palate, receding mandible, short-bull neck, severe contracture, etc.

- *Evaluate the 3-3-2-1 rule:*
  - Three finger mouth opening. The normal interincisor distance is 4.6 cm or more. While <3.8 cm of interincisor distance predicts a difficult airway and <3 cm of interincisor distance indicates TM joint dysfunction. If this distance is <2.5 cm, then it indicates the difficult laryngoscopic view and <2 cm indicates laryngoscopy and intubation is impossible.
  - Three fingers is the normal distance between the tip of the jaw and the beginning of the neck (hypomental distance), while it (neck) is fully extended. The alignment of laryngeal and pharyngeal axis is difficult if this distance is <3 fingers breath (or <6 cm) in adults. If the length varies between 6 and 6.5 cm, then alignment is less difficult and while if the distance is >6.5 cm, it (alignment) is normal.
  - Two fingers breath is the normal distance between the thyroid notch and the floor of the mandible. When this distance is <2 fingers breath, then difficult airway and intubation is predicted **(Fig. 29)**.
  - One finger is the normal subluxation of the lower jaw anteriorly.
- *Mallampati scale:*
  - *Grade I:* About 80–100% easy intubation
  - *Grade II:* Intubation is possible with proper positioning and optimal laryngeal maneuver technique
  - *Grade III:* Intubation is still possible with a special laryngeal blade or with the use of a gun elastic bougie

- *Grade IV:* Intubation is almost impossible. This test should be repeated twice to avoid false positive and false negative results.
- *Obstruction:* For obvious difficulty during laryngoscopy and intubation anesthetist must consider the obstruction of airway with a foreign body, tumor, abscess, epiglottitis, expanding hematoma, etc.
- *Neck mobility* (movement of atlanto-occipital joint and flexion–extension of the neck): Normally the atlanto-occipital (A-O) joint movement ranges around 35°. Limited A-O joint movement is present in cervical spondylosis, rheumatoid arthritis, halo-jacket fixation, etc. The grading of A-O joint movement is done as follows:
  - *Grade I:* >35°
  - *Grade II:* 22–34°
  - *Grade III:* 12–21°
  - *Grade IV:* <12°.

Airway assessment based on LEMON law or method is able to stratify successfully the risk of difficult laryngoscopy and subsequent intubation or ventilation by mask.

What is the LMMAP rule of airway assessment?

It stands for:

L = Look for external deformity of the face and neck
M = Mallampati
M = Measurement 3-3-2-1 or 1-2-3-3 fingers
- 3 fingers mouth opening
- 3 fingers hyomental distance
- 2 fingers distance between the thyroid notch and the floor of the mandible
- 1 finger subluxation of the lower jaw
A = Atlanto-occipital (A-O) extension
P = Pathological airway obstruction.

What are 4Ds?

The following 4Ds also suggest difficult airways:

- *Dentition filtered:* Prominent upper incisors, receding chin, etc.
- *Distortion filtered:* Edema, blood, vomit, tumor, infection, etc.
- *Disproportion filtered:* Short chin to laryngeal distance, bull neck, large tongue, small mouth, etc.
- *Dismobility:* TM joint and cervical spine

What are Magboul 4 Ms?

There is another easier way to memorize the prediction of difficult laryngoscopy and intubation. This is described as Magboul 4 Ms with STOP sign. The 4 Ms are:

- Mallampati
- Measurement
- Movement of neck
- Malformation.

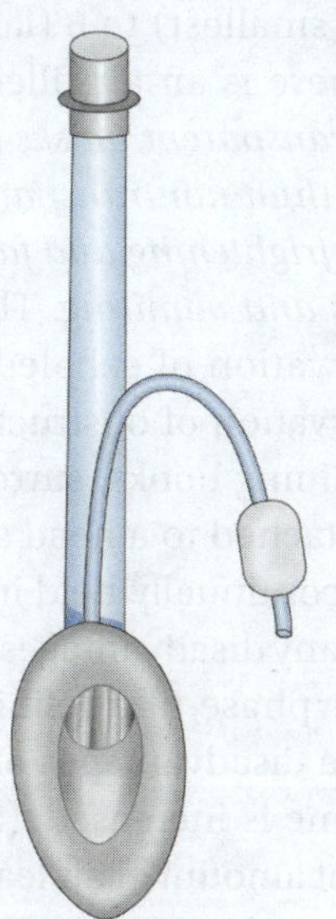

Fig. 29: Laryngeal mask (classic).

The STOP signs are:

S = Skull (hydro and microcephalus)

T = Teeth (buck, protrude, and loose)

O = Obstruction

P = Pathology.

(*Craniofacial abnormality and syndrome:* Treacher Collins, Pierre Robin, Goldenhar's, Waardenburg's syndrome, etc.)

Cass and James risk stratification

In 1965, they summarized six common anatomical causes for difficult intubation and stratification of risk. These are:

- Short muscular neck
- Receding jaw with an obtuse mandibular angle
- Protruding upper incisor teeth
- Long and high-arched palate
- Poor mobility of the mandible
- Decreased distance between alveolar and mental ridge which is required for wide opening of the mandible for the introduction of laryngoscope.

Rapid assessment of airway by "1-2-3 rule"

- *Rule 1:* Ability to insinuate at least one finger in front of tragus when the patient opens his mouth. This establishes the integrity of the movement of TM joint.
- *Rule 2:* Determining the adequacy of the opening of mouth by measuring the interincisor gap. This should be at least of two finger breadths.
- *Rule 3:* Measurement of thyromental distance. It should be at least of three finger breadths.

Type variable score

- *Receding chin or TM distance <7 cm:* 3 points
- *Mallampati Grade IV:* 2 points
- *Restricted head extension:* 2 points
- *Protruding teeth:* 2 points
- *Mouth opening <4 cm:* 2 points
- *Vertical neck length <7.5 cm:* 1 point
- *Neck circumference >33 cm:* 1 point.

The study reveals that a score of 6 or more correctly identifies 22 out of 23 difficult intubations.

Ultrasound Examination of Airway

The ultrasound examination of airway has also been suggested as an assistance of the airway assessment and its management. Ultrasound can be used as an adjunct to confirm ETT placement as well as to assist in the identification of cricothyroid membrane, during emergency cricothyroidotomy.

EQUIPMENT FOR AIRWAY MANAGEMENT

The following equipment should always routinely be available for airway management. These equipment are:

- An oxygen source
- Oral and nasal airways, masks of different types and sizes for bag and mask ventilation
- Laryngoscopes of different types
- ETT of different sizes and shapes
- Stylets and bougies of different sizes
- Supraglottic airway devices
- Suction
- Pulse oximetry and capnometer
- Stethoscope
- Tape.

▌AIRWAY MANAGEMENT BY FACE MASK AND BAG VENTILATION

In emergency situations, where the patient is apneic, after giving muscle relaxant and patient is unintubated or we fail to intubate them, then ventilation by face mask and a bag are lifesaving. Usually, an anesthetic face mask and a bag is employed for ventilation by administering air or O_2 and/or anesthetic gases.

The rim of a face mask is contoured or conformed to a variety of facial features to create an airtight seal with the patient's face. The 22 mm orifice of these face masks is attached to breathing circuit of an anesthetic machine through a right-angle connector. These face masks are made of different materials which may vary from rubber or plastic to silicon. It is also available in different shapes and sizes for newborn to large adult faces. The available sizes of face masks are marked from 0 (smallest) to 6 (largest). At the bottom of the face mask, there is an air-filled cuff that has a soft cushioning effect. *Transparent masks (silicon or plastic) are more advantageous than nontransparent rubber face mask because they are less frightening and facilitate observation of patients for cyanosis and vomiting.* The transparent masks also allow the observation of exhaled humidified gas, i.e., observation of observation of obstructed and unobstructed respiration. The retaining hooks, surrounding the orifice of face mask, can be attached to a head strap so that the mask does not have to be continually held in place. Though mask ventilation carries many disadvantages, still it is used as a life-saving tool in tide over phase, till a definite airway (intubation) is accomplished. The disadvantages of mask ventilation are (1) dead space volume is increased, (2) ventilation mask is tiring, (3) a significant amount of air leaks into the esophagus and can easily increase the intragastric pressure, significant enough (>28 cmH$_2$O) to cause aspiration.

Mask can be held with one hand or both hands (to fit the mask tightly over face, if necessary). If both the hands of an anesthetist are used to fit the mask on patient's face, then an assistant is needed to ventilate the bag or an anesthetic ventilator can be used to supply positive pressure breaths. By the thumb and first (index) finger of anesthetist's left hand, the mask should be held tightly on the patient's face, while the other three fingers of anesthetist's hand will displace the mandible upward by giving an upward thrust on the angle of it (mandible). Of these three fingers, the middle and ring finger will grasp the mandible to facilitate the extension of atlanto-occipital joint, and the little finger is placed under the angle of the jaw and is used to thrust the jaw anteriorly which is the most important maneuver to lift the base of the tongue from the posterior pharyngeal wall (to open the airway). *Care should be taken that fingers should be kept on the ramus of mandible, but not on the soft tissues of neck and the floor of the mouth. Because pressure on the soft tissues of neck by fingers produces discomfort and pushes the base of the tongue toward posterior pharyngeal wall, causing more airway obstruction.* The upward displacement of mandible, along with the upper cervical vertebral extension and lifting of chin upward by fingers, tend to pull the tongue and soft tissues away from the posterior pharyngeal wall. Thus, it relieves upper airway obstruction that occurs in the paralyzed and anesthetized or unconscious patient. During the bag and mask ventilation (BMV), care should also be taken to avoid giving pressure on or contact with the open eye by mask or fingers. So, the eyes should be taped shut as soon as possible to minimize the risk of corneal injury.

But this *mask ventilation is difficult for morbidly obese patients, beards, thick necks, short necks, big faces, edentulous patients, craniofacial deformities, etc.* In edentulous patients, the mask ventilation can be helped by leaving the dentures in place or by using packs or employing the mask strap to pull up the sagging cheeks. Mask ventilation in pediatric patients is easy than in adult patients, provided there is no laryngospasm. Though mask ventilation is very helpful in emergency conditions and easier than ET intubation, but the most serious problems with mask ventilation include failure, distension of the stomach by air, pulmonary aspiration, and pressure damage to the eyes.

If the mask is properly fitted on the face of the patient and the mandible is lifted upward with an extension of atlanto-occipital joint, i.e., the airway is kept patent, then the squeezing of the bag will result in the rise of patient's chest. By this simple maneuver, if the ventilation is found ineffective (no sign of chest rising, no or little end-tidal CO is detected on capnometer, no condensation of clear mask), then oral or nasal airway can be placed to relieve airway obstruction, secondary to lax upper airway muscle tone or redundant pharyngeal tissues.

Artificial Manual Breathing Unit Bag Resuscitation

AMBU stands for *artificial manual breathing unit.* It is usually used to ventilate the patient with a face mask. It also can be attached with ETT for ventilation in the absence of an anesthetic machine. The AMBU unit consists of one self-inflating bag, made up of a rubber or silicon, nonrebreathing valve, and face mask. The nonbreathing valve closes the expiratory port when the bag is manually squeezed, letting the air, which is inside the bag, to pass to face mask. During expiration, the bobbin of valve comes to a normal position and opens the expiratory port, letting the expired air to void to atmosphere. AMBU bags are available in a capacity of 1,200 mL for adults, 500 mL for children, and 250 mL for newborns. About 100% O_2 also can be delivered by AMBU bag by attaching an O_2 source with AMBU bag. By attaching the AMBU bag with an ETT, ventilation also can be done in the absence of a face mask and anesthetic machine.

How do we predict difficult BMV?

Langeron et al., suggested five recognized criteria as independent predictors of difficult BMV and that can be summarized as the word **OBESE**. It is a simple visual way to remember what to look for when evaluating and assessing the airway for difficult mask and bag ventilation.

O = Obese (body mass index >40 kg/m^2)
B = Bearded
E = Elderly (older than 55 years)
S = Snorers
E = Edentulous.

The presence of any two of these criteria is best indicated as a difficult mask and bag ventilation with a sensitivity of 0.72 and specificity of 0.73.

Obesity is associated with decreased posterior airway space behind the base of the tongue. This is due to the accumulation of fat in the pharyngeal soft tissue. Thus, it causes more impairment of airway patency during sleep, due to the fall of a tongue on the posterior pharyngeal wall and is a risk factor for obstructive sleep apnea syndrome. Upper airway obstruction can occur early after induction of anesthesia with the posterior displacement of soft palate, base of tongue and epiglottis in morbidly obese patients (BMI >40 kg/m^2). Age is also closely related with an increased pharyngeal and laryngeal resistance to airflow and is more common in men than women. Lack of teeth and presence of a beard are also associated with difficult mask ventilation. It is due to the decrease in the airtight seal of the facemask and increased air leak around the mask with more difficult positive pressure ventilation.

AIRWAY MANAGEMENT OTHER THAN FACE MASK VENTILATION

If we go to manage the airway other than face mask ventilation, then we have to use different devices for ventilation. These airway devices for ventilation are first divided into two groups (1) *supraglottic airway devices (SADs) and (2) infraglottic airway devices (IADs)*. As the name suggests, the supraglottic devices are placed above the glottis and the infraglottic devices are placed below the glottis. The SADs are used during both spontaneously breathing and ventilated patients during anesthesia. They are also employed as conduits to aid ET intubation when both the BMV and ET intubation have failed. All the SADs consist of a tube that is connected to a breathing circuit with a ventilating bag at their one end and at the another end this tube is attached to a hypopharyngeal device (a device below the pharynx) that seals and directs the airflow to glottis. Additionally, these SADs occlude the esophagus with varying degrees of effectiveness, reducing the distension of stomach by ventilating gas. Some SADs are equipped with a port for the suction of gastric contents; however, no SADs offer 100% protection from aspiration pneumonitis, offered by a properly sited, cuffed ETT. In few years past, anesthesia was routinely delivered solely by mask or ETT administration, but in recent decades a variety of SADs have permitted both airway rescue (when adequate BMV is not possible) and routine anesthetic airway management (when intubation is not necessary). There are >10 kinds of supraglottic airway devices, but among them, only few are used now. Further, among these few supraglottic airway devices, which are used now, the LMA type of supraglottic device is extensively used now. Again, this supraglottic device (LMA) is so extensively used nowadays that the present era is called the *era of supraglottic device*. The airway devices which are included in supraglottic division are LMA, peripharyngeal airway (Cobra-PLMA), Combitube, Pharyngeal Airway Xpress (PAX), Streamlined Linear of the Pharyngeal Airway (SLIPA), etc.

The infraglottic airway devices are further classified as definitive and emergency airway management devices. The definitive infraglottic airway management devices include *ETT* and *tracheostomy tube*. The emergency infraglottic airway device includes a *cricothyroidotomy device.*

Airway Management by Laryngeal Mask Airway

Laryngeal mask airway is a new supraglottic device. It is discovered by Archie Brain, so it is also called *Brain Mask*. Like other SADs, it also consists of a wide-bore tube whose proximal end connects to a breathing circuit through a standard 15 mm connector and whose distal end is attached to an elliptical cuff that can be inflated through a pilot tube. The deflated cuff is lubricated and is inserted blindly into the hypopharynx. Then, the cuff is inflated by air and now this inflated cuff forms a low-pressure seal around the entrance of larynx. An ideally positioned cuff is bordered by the base of the tongue superiorly, pyriform sinuses laterally and the upper esophageal sphincter inferiorly. If the opening of esophagus lies within the rim of the cuff, then gastric distension and regurgitation can occur. The insertion of LMA requires anesthetic depth and muscle relaxation slightly greater than that required for the insertion of an oral airway. For insertion of LMA, a muscle relaxant is not required. If an LMA is not functioning properly, after the attempts to improve the "fit" of the LMA have failed, then we will have to try by another LMA, one size larger or smaller.

The status of LMA, regarding the management of airway, is somewhere between the face mask with oropharyngeal airway at one end and the ETT at another end. This is because it provides a more definite airway than the former, but not more reliable airway protection and maintenance of it than the later. It sometimes acts as an essential airway device to provide a lifesaving emergency airway and intermittent positive pressure manual ventilation, when the conventional mask ventilation and attempts to intubation fails. Although LMA was originally developed for airway management in routine cases with spontaneous ventilation, but it is now listed in the ASA difficult airway algorithm at five different places, as a ventilatory device or as a conduit, for ET intubation.

It is a new device, designed to maintain a seal around the laryngeal inlet for spontaneous ventilation and also permits positive pressure-controlled ventilation at a modest level of pressure (up to 15 cmH$_2$O). But because of the limited ability of LMA to seal off the laryngeal inlet tightly, the elective use of this device is *contraindicated* in any of the condition, where there is an increased risk of gastric aspiration, and where ventilation under high pressure is needed. In patients, without these predisposing factors, the risk for pharyngeal regurgitation appears to be low and the use of LMA is safe. Other *relative contraindications* for LMA include (1) patients with pharyngeal pathology, (2) pharyngeal obstruction, (3) aspiration risk (pregnancy and hiatal hernia), (4) low pulmonary compliance requiring peak inspiratory pressure >30 cmH$_2$O. The LMA may be associated with less frequent bronchospasm than ETT.

Now, LMA is available in seven different sizes for neonates to large adults. In some countries, 8th size (extra-large) is also available **(Table 4)**. The *LMA classic* **(Fig. 29)** is a reusable device. It is made of medical-grade silicone and is free from latex. It is to be discarded after 40 autoclaving.

TABLE 4: Different sizes of LMA for neonates to large adults.

Size of different LMA	Used in patients on the basis of body weight	Cuff volume (air needed)
Size 1	Up to 5 kg	4 mL
Size 1.5	5–10 kg	7 mL
Size 2	10–20 kg	10 mL
Size 2.5	20–30 kg	14 mL
Size 3	30–50 kg	20 mL
Size 4	50–70 kg	30 mL
Size 5	>70 kg (or 70–100 kg)	40 mL
Size 6 (available only in few countries)	>100 kg	50 mL

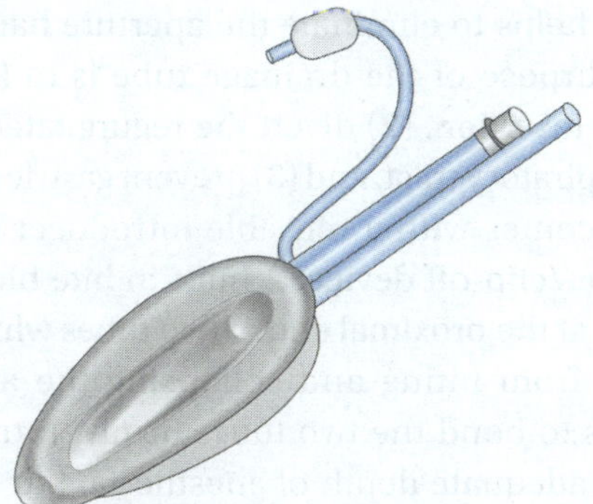

Fig. 30: ProSeal LMA (PLMA).

Now, disposable LMAs are available which are made of polyvinyl or plastic. There are three main components of an LMA classic (1) an airway tube, (2) a laryngeal mask with an inflating cuff, and (3) a cuff inflating pilot catheter with a balloon. The airway tube is of large bore, with a 15 mm standard male adaptor at its distal end, which can be connected with the patient's end of any breathing circuit. It's (large bore airway tube) other end is fitted to a *laryngeal mask* which has an *inflatable cuff*. The cuff can be inflated or deflated via a *valve*, located on the *pilot catheter*. Two aperture bars guard the distal end of a large-bore airway tube. The mask of LMA is specially designed to conform with the contour of hypopharynx (laryngopharynx).

Classification of Laryngeal Mask Airway

Now, several new variants of LMA, except classic LMA, are available. So, the LMAs are classified like that:

- *First-generation LMA:*
  - *LMA classic:* Described earlier
  - *LMA unique:* It is single use disposable LMA
  - *LMA flexible:* Here, the tube of LMA is enforced with a wire, making it flexible, i.e., nonkinkable, and making it useful for head and neck surgeries
- *Second-generation LMA:*
  - *Intubating LMA (also called LMA Fastrach):* In difficult intubation, up to 8 number ETT can be introduced into the trachea through this LMA.
  - *ProSeal LMA:* It has a larger posterior cuff which provides a better seal. Moreover, it has a drain tube which can be used to deflate the stomach. It is described underneath **(Fig. 30)**.
  - *Supreme LMA:* It is like a ProSeal LMA, but with an additional bite block to avoid damage to the LMA tube if the patient bites.
  - *I-gel LMA:* Here, instead of air the cuff is prefilled with gel. Hence, it avoids the complications of air-filled

cuff, such as cuff leakage, damage, and puncture. Like a ProSeal LMA, it also contains a drain tube that can be used to deflate the stomach.

- *LMA C-Trach:* Like a video laryngoscopy, here the patient end of LMA is also attached with a video screen to visualize the laryngeal structure and the process of LMA insertion. Different types of LMA are depicted in **Figure 30**.

All variants of LMA, except the unique variety, are made of silicone or latex-free rubber. The unique variety of LMA is made of medical-grade PVC. Just enough air to seal the laryngeal inlet can raise the intracuff pressure around 60 cmH$_2$O. During cuff inflation, after the introduction of LMA, the tube should not be held by hand, as this prevents the mask from setting into its own correct location from itself in hypopharynx. A small outward movement of the tube is often noted during the inflation of the cuff, as the device seats and adjusts itself in the hypopharynx.

The ProSeal Laryngeal Mask Airway (PLMA) is the latest addition to the various modification of original LMA. Like a classic LMA, the PLMA is also made of latex-free silicone and is reusable. The mask and the inflation assembly of this variety of LMA are identical to the classic variety of it. Here, the original larger ventral cuff is fixed to a second cuff which is attached to the dorsal surface of the first cuff. The dorsal cuff, when inflated, improves the seal by pushing the ventral cuff more firmly on the periglottic tissues. So, a properly placed PLMA can withstand a leak pressure of approximately 35 cmH$_2$O, as against 25 cmH$_2$O, offered by LMA Classic. The PLMA airway tube is flexible, wire-reinforced, and has double-lumen. One lumen is used as an airway tube for ventilation and another lumen is used as a gastric drainage tube for aspiration of gastric contents during regurgitation. The rationale to place the two tubes side by side, except at the level of the mask (bowl) is to give greater stability to the device, while once it is placed into the oral cavity.

The bowl of PLMA is deeper through which traverses the drainage tube and opens most distally. This drainage tube in the bowl helps to eliminate the aperture bars. However, the main purpose of the drainage tube is to (1) facilitate gastric tube insertion, (2) divert the regurgitated fluid away from the respiratory tract, and (3) prevent gastric insufflation. The PLMA comes with a reusable introducer which is an easily clip-on/clip-off device. A built-in bite block has also been added at the proximal end of two tubes which prevents the patient from biting and collapsing the airway tube. It also helps to bond the two tubes firmly. Introduction of LMA needs adequate depth of anesthesia, but not so deep as required for tracheal intubation. So, it is not suitable for conscious emergency room patients **(Fig. 30)**.

Procedure of LMA insertion: LMA insertion requires an anesthetic depth that is slightly greater than that required for the insertion of an oral airway, but lighter than ETT intubation. Under an adequate depth of anesthesia, a LMA of appropriate size is gradually introduced blindly into the mouth and then is gradually pushed into the cavity of the laryngopharynx, with the aperture facing toward the base of the tongue. It is performed by pressing the tip of the cuffed of LMA against the posterior pharyngeal wall and guided by the index finger of dominant hand. The LMA is pushed in hypopharynx till a resistance is felt which indicates that the tip of the cuff has reached the upper esophageal sphincter. Some anesthetists prefer to introduce LMA with deflated cuff and some with a fully inflated one. But it is better to introduce LMA with a partially deflated cuff and when the tip felt the resistance, then the cuff is fully inflated again with the addition of an appropriate volume of air (30–40 mL for adult size) and is secured with tape. Inflated cuff seals the lateral and posterior pharyngeal wall and patient is ventilated through the ventilation ports.

The correct position of the cuff should be checked by the auscultation of lungs and capnography. The other signs for the correct placement of the LMA cuff include one or more of the following (1) the slight outward movement of tube, after the inflation of LMA cuff, (2) the presence of a smooth oval swelling on the neck around the thyroid and cricoid area, (3) no portion of the cuff should be visible in oral cavity **(Fig. 31)**. Before taping (fixing) the LMA in place, a bite block should be inserted. It not only stabilizes the LMA but also prevents the occlusion of a tube from biting. Reinforced flexi LMA are more prone to biting and a bite block should be placed until the LMA is removed.

One of the principal cause for obstruction during the use of LMA is the downward displacement of epiglottis by LMA or curling up of tongue's base on laryngeal inlet. An ideally positioned cuff of LMA is bounded by (1) the base of the tongue superiorly, (2) the pyriform fossa laterally, and (3) the upper esophageal sphincter inferiorly. If the inlet

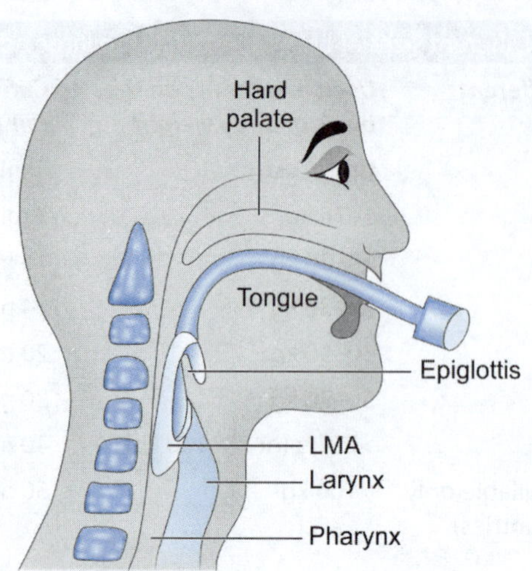

Fig. 31: Laryngeal mask airway (LMA) in position.

of esophagus lies within the rim of the cuff, then gastric distension and regurgitation become a distinct possibility. The anatomic variations of hypopharynx prevent adequate functioning of LMA in some patients. So, if an LMA is not functioning properly after attempts to improve the condition, most anesthetists will try another LMA which is one size larger or smaller. However, the introduction of LMA under direct vision with the help of a laryngoscope or a fiber-optic scope may prove beneficial in difficult cases.

Indications for the use of LMA:

- It provides an *emergency airway* in patients, where either the mask ventilation or tracheal intubation has already been failed. It is also used *as an alternative to intubation* where difficult intubation is anticipated.
- *As an elective method*, in cases where the ET intubation is not mandatory and the operation can simply be performed by spontaneous face mask ventilation, but airway cannot adequately be maintained by simple Guedel's oropharyngeal airway and face mask. *As an elective method* for minor to moderate surgeries with controlled ventilation, but anesthetist electively wants to avoid ET intubation.
- Introduction of LMA eliminates the presence of a relatively large face mask and anesthetist's hand on the patient's face that may interfere with surgical access, especially when the surgical site is situated over the head and neck. On the other hand, the availability of a new flexible LMA provides an easy connection with an anesthetic machine at any angle from the patient's mouth, while resisting kinking and displacement.
- LMA also provides an emergency airway *in awkward positions* such as in lateral and prone position of the patient and in emergency settings when a laryngoscope

TABLE 5: Advantages and disadvantages of LMA over face mask and ETT.

	Advantages	Disadvantages
Advantages and disadvantages of LMA over face mask	• Hands-free area over the face • Better seal in bearded patient • Possible for ophthalmic and ENT surgeries • Easier to maintain airway • Ventilation is better • Protects against airway secretion • Less operating room pollution	• More invasive • Requires new skill • More risk for airway trauma • Some opening of the mouth is required • Requires deeper anesthesia • Many contraindications
Advantages and disadvantages of LMA over ETT	• Less invasive • Less tooth and laryngeal trauma • Useful in difficult intubation • Does not require muscle relaxant • Less bronchospasm and bronchospasm • No chance of esophageal and endobronchial intubation	• Limits PPV, ventilation under high pressure is not possible • Increased risk of gastric aspiration • Airway is less secure • Less safe in a prone position • More gas leaks and OT pollution

(ETT: endotracheal tube; LMA: laryngeal mask airway; PPV: positive pressure ventilation; OT: operation theater)

and other equipment for intubation are not available. Instead of mouth-to-mouth breathing, mouth-to-larynx breathing through LMA in emergency condition is a better alternative.

■ LMA sometimes provides a *conduit to facilitate* fiber-optic-guided or gum bougie-guided or blind oral tracheal intubation during difficult situations of intubation. LMA, specially designed to facilitate such tracheal intubation, is now available and is called *intubating LMA.*

Advantages of LMA: (1) Easy to insert (even a paramedical staff can insert), (2) does not require any laryngoscope and muscle relaxant, (3) does not require any specific position of a cervical spine, therefore can be used in cervical injuries, (4) less sympathetic stimulation as compared to a conventional laryngoscopy and ET intubation, (5) complications of intubation can be avoided, (6) patient's awakening is smooth as compared to intubation, and (7) reusable (40 times).

Disadvantages or complications of LMA: (1) As the air can leak by the side of the cuff into esophagus, so LMA increases the risk of pulmonary aspiration by distending the empty stomach by air during controlled ventilation. Moreover, if gastric distension occurs due to the leakage of air in esophagus, then it is not possible to decompress the stomach by passing a suction tube into the stomach through esophagus, as there is no place to pass a suction catheter or Ryle's tube. This is because of the occupation of oropharynx by the cuff of LMA, (2) as LMA does not provide airtight seal around laryngeal inlet like an ETT, so it increases the risk of pulmonary aspiration during anesthesia with an already full stomach in emergency anesthesia, (3) it can cause laryngospasm, and airway obstruction if is displaced

anteriorly, (4) it may fail to function in the presence of pharyngeal and laryngeal disease, (5) it may fail to provide high inflation pressure during decreased compliance of lungs and thorax and also due to resultant leak around the cuff by high-pressure ventilation, (6) it may cause trauma to the oral cavity and injury to the hypoglossal and lingual nerve if excessive cuff pressure is being used. So, the cuff pressure for LMA should be kept in between 40 and 60 cmH$_2$O, and (7) it may cause sore throat (incidences are 10–20%).

Therefore, the *contraindications for the use of LMA are* full stomach (e.g., in an emergency after taking a full meal, pregnancy, hiatal hernia, intestinal obstruction, etc.) pharyngeal pathology (e.g., tumor, abscess, etc.), and pharyngeal obstruction, low pulmonary compliance [e.g., asthma, chronic obstructive pulmonary disease (COPD), etc.] requiring peak inspiratory pressure >30 cmH$_2$O, etc.

Advantages and disadvantages of LMA over face mask and ETT are enumerated in **Table 5**.

Airway Management by Combitube (Esophageal–Tracheal Combine Tube)

Like an LMA, Combitube is another supraglottic airway device that provides an emergency airway when tracheal intubation is failed and mask ventilation is also not effective or fails. It is a double-lumen tube that combines the features of both a conventional tracheal tube and that of an esophageal obturator airway. Of these double lumen, one lumen is for a conventional tracheal tube and another is for an esophageal obturator airway. Both the lumens of tube are connected at its proximal (outer) end separately with a 15 mm connector that helps it to be attached with main anesthetic machine separately. It is especially useful

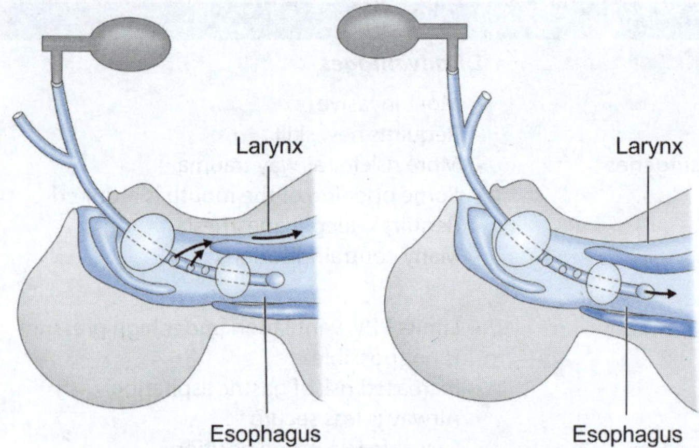

Fig. 32: The mechanism of action of Combitube.

for patients in whom direct visualization of vocal cords is not possible, as in patients with massive airway bleeding or regurgitation, limited access to the airway, and in patients in whom neck movement is contraindicated. As the Combitube is made of natural rubber or latex, so it may cause allergic reactions. It has two latex cuffs or balloons for each tube. One is an esophageal cuff for the esophageal obturator airway tube and another is oropharyngeal cuff for a conventional tracheal tube. The oropharyngeal cuff or balloon is blue in color and larger in volume (100 mL) than the esophageal cuff or balloon (15 mL). The longer lumen is blue in color and ends at the patient's side with multiple apertures between the two cuffs while the shorter lumen ends at the most distal end of this device **(Fig. 32)**.

Combitube can function effectively whether is placed in trachea or much more commonly in esophagus when it is introduced blindly. Ventilation is usually started first through the *blue longer tube*. This is because the placement of the distal end which *proximally begins with a shorter tube* is usually in the esophagus when the Combitube is introduced blindly through the oral cavity. Then, if the auscultation of breath sound is positive and the auscultation of gastric insufflation is negative, ventilation is continued. In this situation, *the multiple apertures which are continuous with the longer blue lumen are situated at the laryngopharynx between the two cuffs and air passes from laryngopharynx through laryngeal inlet into the lungs.* Under this condition, the shorter tube which ends at distal aperture and now is in the esophagus may be used to remove the gastric fluid with a suction catheter.

In such circumstances, if the inflation of lung is absent and the stomach is being insufflated, then *ventilation should be started through the transparent shorter tube* which communicates with the distal single aperture beyond the esophageal balloon. Under this situation, the multiple apertures which are continuous with the longer blue tube

and through which ventilation was done before are situated above the laryngopharynx and the distal end which is connected with the transparent shorter tube is situated in the trachea. So, the air is passing from blue tube through oropharynx and esophagus to the stomach. Then, ventilation should be continued through the transparent shorter tube which can be confirmed by the auscultation of breath sound and the absence of gastric insufflation.

The Combitube has also been successfully used during emergency cardiopulmonary resuscitation and in such circumstances; esophageal balloon provides protection from aspiration which may represent a distinct advantage of it, over the LMA. But care must be taken to avoid excessive deep placement of Combitube in the esophagus, which can further obstruct the glottic opening by the pressure of distal cuff from esophagus. Though, it is listed in the management of difficult airway in the advanced life support algorithm, still Combitube is rarely used by anesthetists now, because they prefer LMA or other devices in such difficult situations.

King Laryngeal Tube

It consists of a single tube (in contrast to Combitube) with a small esophageal balloon for placement in esophagus and a large pharyngeal balloon for placement in hypopharynx. But both the balloons are inflated by one cuff inflation system, consisting of (1) one valve, (2) one pilot balloon, and (3) one inflating tube. Between the two balloons, there are multiple apertures through which gas exits and inflates the lungs. There is a suction port, distal to the esophageal balloon, and permits the decompression of the stomach. The working principle of this tube is that after insertion in >90% of cases the esophageal balloon enters the esophagus and pharyngeal balloon rest in hypopharynx. Now, in this situation, if these balloons are inflated and ventilation is done through this tube, then the lungs will be inflated with gas that exits between these two balloons. If the ventilation is found difficult, after its insertion and cuffs are inflated, then it is likely that the tube is likely inserted too deeply. In such circumstances, slow withdrawal of device improves the ventilation. In rare cases, if the esophageal balloon enters the larynx, then ventilation of the lungs will not be possible. In such circumstances, the king laryngeal tube should be taken out for reintroduction.

Airway Management by Endotracheal Tube–Tracheal Intubation

The introduction of an ETT into the tracheal lumen through the glottic opening is called *tracheal intubation* (commonly called *intubation*). This is the best way of airway management, but not without any disadvantages or complications.

There are many indications for ET intubation, but the principle head lines are:

- Maintenance of unobstructed airway
- Protection of airway from aspiration
- Application of positive pressure ventilation
- Adequate oxygenation and delivery of anesthetic gases.

Equipment for Intubation

The main equipment, needed for intubaton, are *ETT, laryngoscope, and some accessories in difficult situations such as stylate, bougie, light weight, etc.*

Endotracheal tube: In present practice, the commonly used ETTs are, now, made of clear polyvinylchloride (PVC) with *high volume low-pressure cuff,* though red rubber tubes with *low volume and high pressure cuffs* are still manufactured. The differences between the red rubber and PVC tube are given in **Table 6**. The distinct advantage of a clear PVC made ETT is that it helps to observe the condensation of water vapor in expired air which occurs, during expiration and confirm the ET tube is in trachea. They are numbered according to the internal diameter (ID) of their lumen, measured in mm, as for example the internal diameter of the lumen of a 7 number. ETT is 7 mm. The external diameter of ETT varies with the thickness of tube's wall which again varies according to different manufacturers. Less commonly, some ET tubes are numbered in French scale which indicates the external diameter of its lumen in mm, multiplied by 3. The choice of diameter of an ETT for a particular patient always runs through a compromise between maximizing the flow of gases through a large size and minimizing trauma with a small size. The tubes are manufactured in 0.5 mm ID increments from 2.5 to 9 mm. A radiopaque line is impregnated into the wall of the tube which aids its later visualization by X-ray in case of displacement or aid in determination of tube position, after intubation. The radiopaque barium sulfate stripe also significantly lowers the temperature at which the ignition of tube occurs and thus decreases the risk of fire during laser surgery. A diagrammatic picture of an ETT is given in **Figure 33**.

An American Society for Testing and Materials (ASTM) standard, for the manufacturing of tracheal tube, recommends the following things which include (1) the material from which the tube should be constructed, (2) the inside diameter of tube, (3) the length of tube, (4) inflation system, (5) cuff, (6) the radius of the curvature of the tube, (7) markings, (8) Murphy eye, (9) packaging and labeling, etc. A separate standard also covers the testing of the shaft of the tracheal tube for less resistance.

The ASTM standard specifies that the radius of curvature of a conventional ETT should be 140 ± 20 mm. The internal

TABLE 6: Difference between ETT tube of red rubber and PVC.

ETT of Red Rubber	ETT of PVC
• Costlier, reusable (can be autoclaved up to six times without damage), and radiolucent (cannot be visualized in X-ray)	• Cheap, disposable (cannot be autoclaved), and radiolucent but contains a radiopaque line to visualize in X-ray
• Cuff is of low volume and high-pressure type, so there are more chances of tracheal mucosal injury	• Cuff is high volume and low-pressure type, so there are less chances of tracheal mucosal injury
• More rigid (more chances of injury), nontransparent, and has no Murphy eye	• Less rigid (less chances of injury), transparent (secretions and mist can be seen), and has Murphy eye
• Less incidences of sore throat (due to small cuff) and contain lead as preservative	• More incidences of sore throat (due to large cuff) and it does not contain lead as preservative

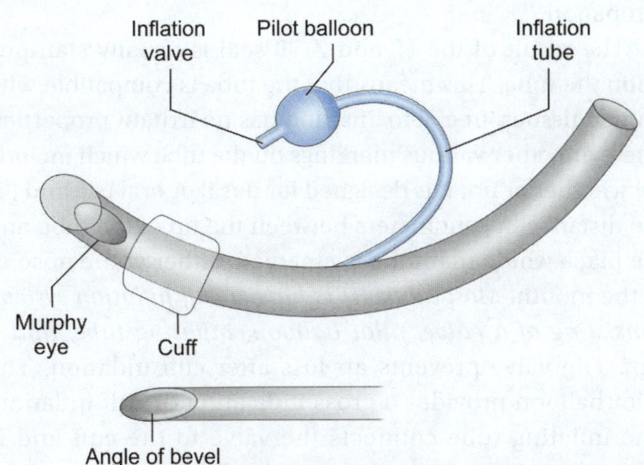

Fig. 33: Cuffed ETT with Murphy eye.

and external walls should be circular. A tube whose lumen is oval or elliptic in shape is more prone to kinking than one that is circular. The machine end of an ETT receives the connector and projects from the patient's mouth or nose. By cutting with scissors, it (the shaft of the tube) should be possible to shorten this machine end of the tube, if necessary. The patient end of an ETT is inserted into the trachea. It usually has a slanted opening which is called the *bevel*. The angle of this bevel is acute which is formed between the axis of the bevel and the longitudinal axis of the tracheal tube. A standard tracheal tube has a bevel with angle of 38 ± 10° (or 45° in oral tubes and 30° in nasal tubes). The opening of the bevel looks left when the tube is viewed from its concave aspect. This is because most often the ETT is introduced into the larynx from the right side of the patient. So, as the bevel faces left, it facilitates better visualization of the larynx (does not obstruct the view) when the tube is being inserted.

Sometimes, there is a hole at the patient end, on the side opposite to the bevel. This is known as the Murphy's eye and an ETT with this feature is called the *Murphy-type tube*. The purpose of this eye is to provide an alternate pathway for the gas flow, if the bevel is occluded, sometimes due to any reason. Some anesthetists think that having such an eye is a disadvantage because secretions may accumulate there and forceps, tube changers, fiberscope, etc., which are sometimes used for different purposes through the ET tube, may inadvertently advance through this Murphy's eye, instead of passing through the main bevel. Some ETTs also have a second eye on their bevel side. This Murphy eye may also provide a measure of safety if the tube accidently advances into the right main stem bronchus. The ETTs, lacking Murphy's eye, are known as the *Magill-type ETTs*. The lack of Murphy's eye allows the cuff to be placed closer to the tip. This may decrease the chance of inadvertent bronchial intubation.

The result of the IT and Z-79 seal is usually stamped upon the tube. This means that the tube is compatible with human tissues, free of toxins, and has no irritant properties. There are other various markings on the tube which include (1) whether or not it is designed for nasal or oral use and (2) the distance in centimeters between the tip of the tube and the place where that tube is emerged, either at the nose or at the mouth. *Most adult ETTs have a cuff inflation system, consisting of a valve, pilot balloon, inflating tube, and a cuff.* The valve prevents air loss after cuff inflation. The pilot balloon provides a gross indication of cuff inflation. The inflating tube connects the valve to the cuff and is incorporated into the wall of the tube. By creating a tracheal seal, the cuff of ETT permits positive pressure ventilation and reduces the likelihood of aspiration. Uncuffed tubes are often used in infants and young children. However, in recent years, the cuffed pediatric ETTs have been increasingly favored.

The ETT may be cuffed or uncuffed. In cuffed ETT, the cuff is present at the patient's end, above Murphy's eye (if present), or few centimeters above the proximal end of the bevel. The aim of inflating the cuff is to prevent aspiration. Usually, 4–8 mL of air is required to fill the cuff. During the inflation of the cuff, it should be ensured that the *cuff pressure would be <30 cmH$_2$O* to prevent the ischemia of tracheal mucosa. The pressure in the cuff of ETT is important. This is because high pressure in the cuff is transmitted to tracheal mucosa and can cause ischemic injury. So, the cuff should be inflated to such a minimum volume and pressure that there is just no leak of air during positive pressure ventilation,

through the gap, between the cuff and tracheal mucosa. This will allow for reasonable airway protection from aspiration without excessive lateral wall pressure on tracheal mucosa that may cause ischemic injury due to pressure and subsequent complication later. The cuff pressure that affords good protection from aspiration is 20–25 mm Hg and it is just below the perfusion pressures of tracheal mucosa which is about 25–35 mm Hg, therefore this 20–25 mm Hg cuff pressure does not cause ischemic injury to tracheal mucosa. The cuff should be filled with saline (instead of air), when the ETT is used for laser surgeries, and when hyper-boric O$_2$ is used. The proximal end of the cuff should be 2–2.5 cm below the vocal cord. The traditional approach, of not using cuffed tubes in children up to 10 years of age, does not always hold true in present-day practice.

The N$_2$O, used during the maintenance of anesthesia, can also diffuse into this cuff of an ETT and can increase cuff pressure which in turn can increase the risk of ischemic tracheal mucosal injury. But if a high volume and low-pressure cuff are used for <24 hours, then it (ischemic injury of tracheal mucosa) is of no clinical significance or importance. On the other hand, tubes with a high volume and low-pressure cuff produces more difficulty during insertion, because the high volume (large) cuff often obscures the view of the tip of ETT and larynx. So, trauma to the airway by this tube is more common. The other way to avoid this problem (ischemic injury of mucosa) is to remove the air from cuff intermittently, guided by the tension of pilot balloon. Alternatively, cuff should be inflated by N$_2$O of clinical concentration or N$_2$O should be totally avoided from the maintenance of anesthesia. The inflation of cuff by 5–10 mL of air would be sufficient to achieve an effective seal if the selection of the ET tube is correct. If the amount of air required is >10 mL, then the ETT should be changed to a size of 0.5–1 mm internal diameter (ID) larger than that had already passed. High volume and low-pressure cuff also increase the incidence of sore throat (due to larger mucosal contact area), aspiration, spontaneous extubation, and difficult insertion due to floppy cuff. But, still because of low incidence of mucosal injury, high volume and low-pressure cuff are more commonly recommended now **(Fig. 34)**.

In younger children, below 8 years of age, uncuffed tubes **(Fig. 34)** have generally been used. This is because the narrowest subglottic area in children, below 8 years of age, is believed to limit the use of a cuffed tube, due to difficulty in its introduction, and in pediatric patient's tracheal mucosa is more sensitive to ischemic injury. In such circumstances, *ETT leak pressure* is a clinically useful guide to confirm the proper selection of an *uncuffed tube size* in children. Leak should occur in a properly selected uncuffed tube at 15–20

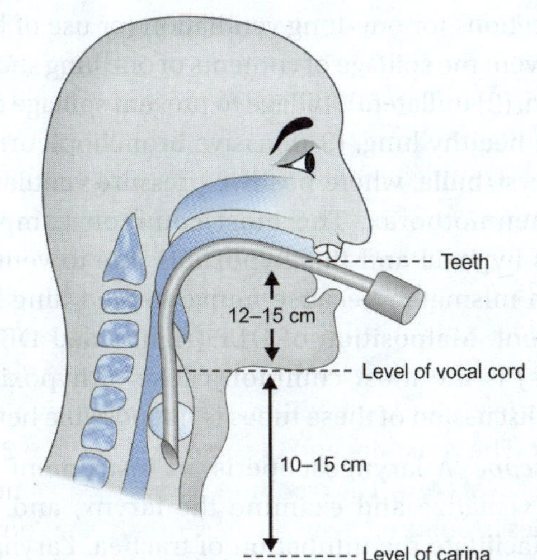

Fig. 34: Distances, relating to endotracheal (ET) tube position.

cmH_2O pressure and above. Below this pressure, there should be no leak, if the uncuffed tube's size is properly selected. In this pressure, there is no ischemic injury of tracheal mucosa and aspiration.

Now, the use of a cuffed ETT in a pediatric group of patients has brought new discussion, keeping in mind the following advantages of it (cuffed tube), i.e., it requires low fresh gas flow, reduces waste gas exposure to operation theater (OT) personnel, and avoid repeat laryngoscopy without any increased incidence of croup.

Deciding the ID of ETT: Generally, larynx is smaller in females than males. So, in an adult male, an ETT of 8 mm ID is appropriate, whereas for an adult female an ETT of 7 mm ID tube is appropriate. In adults, the glottic aperture limits the size of an ETT, but in children, the subglottic area (cricoid cartilage) is the narrowest part of larynx and limits the size of an ETT. The tube size or the ID of an ETT for children up to the age of 14 years is calculated from the formula: [(16 + age in years, not in months) ÷ 4]. But practically, a tube of 0.5–1 mm ID size, smaller or larger than the estimated, must be immediately available.

There are other three popular formulae, for calculating the probable size or ID of ET tube, to be used for pediatric patients and these are:

1. For premature: ETT of 2.5 mm ID. For 0–6 months: ETT of 3–3.5 mm ID. For 6 months to 1 year: ETT of 3.5–4 mm ID
2. For children from 1 to 6 years: Age/3 + 3.5 = ID of tube in mm
3. For children 6 years and above: Age/4 + 4.5 = ID of tube in mm, for example, for a 5-year-old child, the tube size required will be: 5/3 + 3.5 = 1.6 + 3.5 = 5.1 (means 5 number tube). Or (16 + 5) ÷ 4 = 5.2 (means 5 number tube). Smallest size of tube available is 2.5 mm and

largest size of tube available is 10.5 mm. However, a crude clinical guide to calculate the outer diameter of an ET tube, appropriate for a pediatric patient, is that of his little finger.

Deciding the optimal length of ETT: The optimal length of an ETT is the length at which air entry is equal on both sides of the chest (lung). Usually, it is 23 cm in adult males and 21 cm in adult females. In other words, the tip of an ETT should lie 4–5 cm above the carina (the distance between incisors and carina is 26–28 cm). A rough guide is that the optimal length of an ETT is twice the length from the tip of the patient's nose to his or her ear lobule. In children, the length of an oral ETT is calculated by formula: [Age (in years) ÷ 2] + 12 cm. For calculating the optimal length of a nasal ETT in children 3 cm is added to oral length, for example, for a 4-year-old child the optimal oral length will be: [4 ÷ 2] + 12 = 14 cm.

A special type of ETT is used (1) in prone patients, (2) in head and neck surgery, (3) in neurosurgery, or (4) in other surgeries, where there is every possibility of the kinking of it, due to the acute flexion or extension of neck, required for surgery. This type of ETT is called the *armored ETT* **(Fig. 34)**. Here, the wall of the ETT is reinforced with a spiral wire to reduce the chance of kinking and collapse of it. This armored ETT is also useful when it is placed through a tracheostomy or laryngectomy stoma to provide a clear airway. The disadvantage of this armored ETT is that if it becomes kinked from extreme pressure (e.g., an awake patient biting it), then its lumen is permanently occluded due to the deformity of spiral wire, and the tube needs replacement.

Another type of special ET tube, called *RAE tube*, also popularly called the *Oxford tube*, is sometimes used which is available as both oral and nasal versions **(Fig. 34)**. It is best used when it is necessary to keep the tube out of the respective surgical fields. There is a preformed bend in these type of tubes (the curvature of these tubes are predefined to facilitate surgery over the head and neck) that helps the outer portion of it to pass directly over the chin (*oral version or south facing,* used for upper lip, palate, and upper dental surgery) or forehead (*nasal versions or north facing,* used for lower lip, tongue, and lower dental surgery). It may be temporarily straightened during intubation and again the tube takes its preformed shape automatically, after its introduction into the trachea. Like nasal and oral versions, they are also available in *cuffed and uncuffed versions*. As the internal diameter (or size) of this type of tube increases, simultaneously the length (or distance) from the distal tip (patient's end of the tube) to the curve (bend) of the tube also increases. Usually, there is a mark at the bend. In the majority of cases, when this mark is at the teeth or naris, it is assumed that the distal end of the tube is correctly positioned into the trachea, provided the proper size of a tube for that patient is selected; however, this mark is taken only as a general guide, but should not be used as sole criteria for confirming the correct positioning of the tube into the trachea.

The nasal preformed RAE tube has a curvature opposite to the curvature of oral RAE tubes. It is because when this nasal version is in place, then the outer portion of the tube is directed over the patient's forehead. This helps to reduce the pressure on nares. Thus, an RAE tube may be useful for oral intubation of patients who are to be placed in a prone position or are scheduled for otolaryngologic procedures. The oral-preformed RAE tubes are shorter than nasal ones. The external portion of an oral RAE tube is bent at an acute angle, so when it is in place, it rests on the patient's chin.

These RAE tubes are easy to secure. Their use may reduce the risk of unintended extubation. The curvature of the tube allows breathing system to remain away from surgical field during operation, especially around head and neck surgeries, without use of any special connectors. It also helps to protect against kinks. The long length of an RAE tube may also make them useful for insertion through an LMA.

The main disadvantage of preformed RAE tubes is difficulty in passing a suction catheter through them. When necessary, suctioning can be accomplished by cutting the tube at the preformed curvature and reinserting the connector of the anesthetic machine into that cut end. They offer more resistance to airflow than conventional ETTs of comparable size. As the lengths of these tubes are designed to fit the average group of patients, so a tube may be either too short or too long for a given patient.

When selecting the tube size, the reference to the height and weight of a patient may be more useful than the age in years and the user should always be alert to the possibility of bronchial intubation or accidental extubation.

Other varieties of ETTs are (1) microlaryngeal and laryngotracheal surgery tube, (2) double-lumen ETT (to facilitate lung isolation and one lung ventilation), (3) ETTs equipped with bronchial blockers (to facilitate lung isolation and one lung ventilation), (4) Parker Flex-Tip tube, (5) Cole tube, (6) spiral embedded tube, (7) Carden bronchoscopy tube, (8) Carden laryngoscopy tube, (9) Injectoflex tube, (10) different laser resistant metal tubes, etc. As the name suggests, the microlaryngeal and laryngotracheal tubes are used for microlaryngeal surgeries. They are of small size with cuff. *Double-lumen tubes* (DLT) are used when one lung ventilation or lung separation is required for surgery on lungs. The most commonly used DLT is Robertshaw disposable tube. They have two lumens, tracheal, and bronchial. Based on bronchial lumen, they are named right-sided (a bronchial lumen is placed right bronchus) and left-sided (bronchial lumen is placed in left bronchus).

The indications for one-lung ventilation (or use of DLT) are (1) to prevent the spillage of contents of one lung such as pus and blood, (2) unilateral spillage to prevent spillage of lavage fluid to a healthy lung, (3) massive bronchopleural fistula or large cyst/bulla, where positive pressure ventilation can cause pneumothorax. The most common complication of DLT is hypoxia and this hypoxia is due to ventilation–perfusion mismatch because nonventilated lung behaves like a shunt. Malposition of DLT (right-sided DLT in left bronchus) is the most common cause of hypoxia. More detailed discussion of these tubes is not possible here.

Laryngoscope: A laryngoscope is an instrument that (1) helps to visualize and examine the larynx, and (2) also helps to facilitate the intubation of trachea. Laryngoscopy (visualization of larynx) may be direct where glottis is directly visualized or indirect where glottis is visualized indirectly through the optic channel. Based on these methods of laryngoscopy procedures, the laryngoscopes are classified as three types (1) direct rigid laryngoscope, e.g., Macintosh, Miller, Magill, McCoy laryngoscope; (2) indirect (fiber optic) rigid laryngoscope, e.g., Bullard and WuScope laryngoscope, video laryngoscope; and (3) indirect (fiber optic) flexible laryngoscope/bronchoscope. The standard direct rigid laryngoscope consists of two parts (1) a detachable blade with a bulb and (2) a handle containing two batteries. Each direct rigid standard laryngoscope blade has (1) a spatula that compresses the tongue in submandibular space, (2) a flange for displacing the tongue to one side, and (3) an open side for the visualization of larynx by elevating the epiglottis indirectly by pressing on glossoepiglottic fold or directly by pressing on the posterior surface of epiglottis. The batteries in the handle light the bulb at the tip of the blade, alternatively it powers a fiber-optic bundle that terminates at the tip of the blade and acts like a bulb. This light, emitting from the end of this fiber-optic bundle, is less diffused, more intense, and more direct. This rigid laryngoscope with a fiber-optic bundle in the blade also can be made MRI-compatible.

According to the different shapes of the blade, the laryngoscope may be of different types which are not possible to discuss in detail here, however among these few are discussed underneath:

- *Macintosh laryngoscope:* It is the most popular laryngoscope for use in adults. Its blade is curved and Z-shaped on the cross section. Its tip lies beneath the pharyngeal (or anterior) surface of epiglottis. The sizes of the blade of these laryngoscope range from 1 (smallest blade) to 4 (largest blade). Among these, the number 3 blade is most frequently employed for adult use, but the number 4 blade is reserved for unusually large or

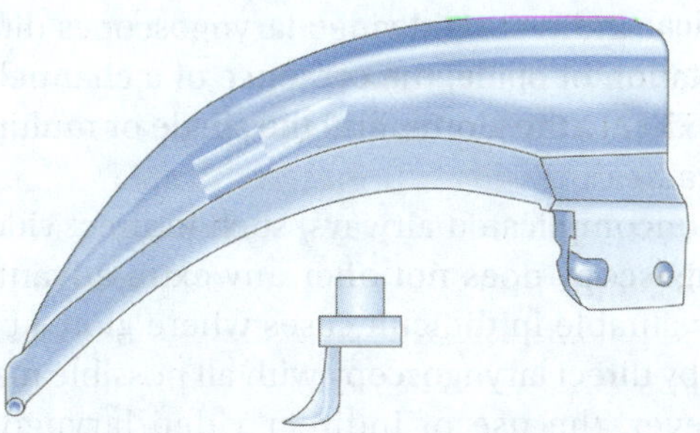

Fig. 35: Macintosh laryngoscope.

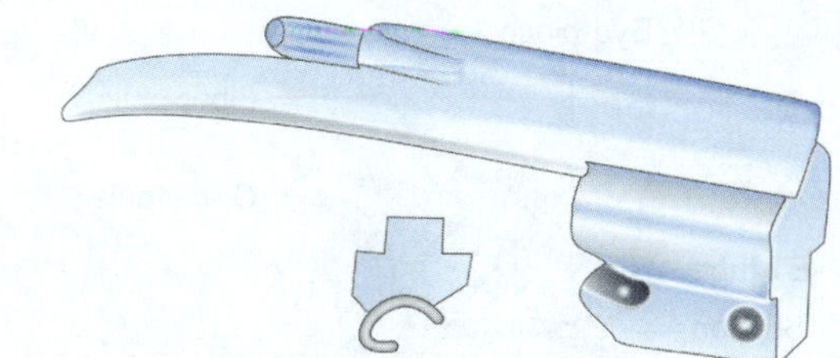

Fig. 36: Miller laryngoscope.

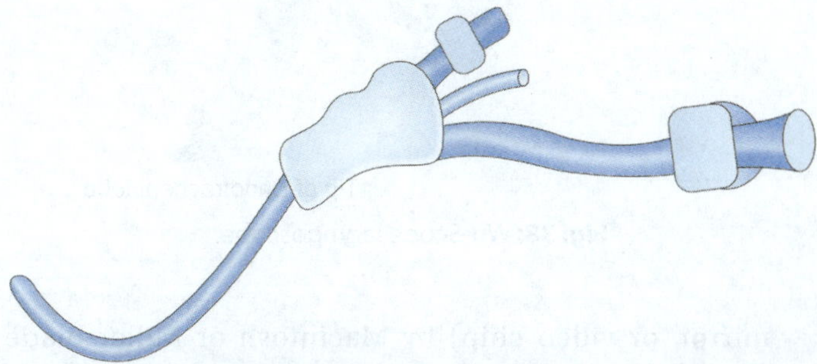

Fig. 37: Bullard laryngoscope.

different patients. The smaller size blades are used for pediatric patients. The tip of Macintosh blade enters the valeculla and lifts the base of the tongue and pharyngeal subtissues from the front of the epiglottis. Thus, it elevates the epiglottis indirectly, so that the vocal cords can be visualized. **Figure 35** depicts a Macintosh laryngoscope.

- *Miller laryngoscope:* Unlike the Macintosh laryngoscope, its (Miller laryngoscope) blade is straight with a slightly curved tip. The size of the blade ranges from 0 (smallest blade) to 4 (largest blade). Neonatal epiglottis is large, leafy, and more anteriorly placed; therefore it needs to be lifted directly by a straight blade to visualize the glottis. Hence, the tip of the blade of this Miller laryngoscope elevates the epiglottis directly from behind (of it) and thus the vocal cords are visualized. Another commonly used straight-blade laryngoscope is the Wisconsin blade which has a straight tip. Although, the straight blades may be advantageous in younger children, but the choice of blade (curved or straight) in older children and adults is really a matter of familiarity and the taste (choice) of an anesthetist. Sometimes, in adults, this straight-blade Miller laryngoscope is also recommended for use in patients with a more anteriorly placed larynx. But an anesthetist should have a habit of using both the curved and straight blades, because when laryngoscopy becomes difficult with one type of blade, then the use of other type of blade may permit adequate visualization of glottis. For neonates and babies, another type of straight blade such as *Oxford infant blade* is also very useful. **Figure 36** depicts a Miller laryngoscope.
- *Magill laryngoscope:* It is similar to a straight-blade Miller laryngoscope, but the tip of its straight blade is not curved. It is also used for neonates and infants.
- *McCoy laryngoscope (Flexi tip laryngoscope):* The peculiarity of this laryngoscope is that it has a hinged tip, assembled by a lever which is positioned alongside the length of the handle on the opposite side of the blade **(Fig. 36)**. After insertion, once the tip of the blade is in vallecula, then pressure on the lever elevates the hinged tip with epiglottis. This becomes especially useful for

grade 3 intubation (of course in combination with cricoid pressure).

- *Bullard laryngoscope:* Bullard intubating laryngoscope is an example of an indirect rigid fiber-optic laryngoscope. By this laryngoscope, glottis is not visualized directly, but indirectly through the fiber-optic channel. It is useful, when the neck is immobile, and mouth opening is very restricted. It has a long curved blade with a fiber-optic illuminating system, suction port, and intubating channels. It is made as both adult and pediatric versions. **Figure 37** shows a Bullard laryngoscope.
- *Wu-Scope laryngoscope:* Like Bullard laryngoscope, it is also an indirect rigid fiber-optic laryngoscope. It has also a curved blade with an elongated tip, fiber-optic light source, suction port, oxygen port, and intubating channels through which an ETT is passed. It is designed to help to see the glottis in a patient with a very large tongue or whose glottis is very anteriorly placed. Anesthetists should gain experience in using this Bullard and Wu-laryngoscope in normal patients, before using it in urgent conditions on patients with difficult airway. Many anesthetists thought that these devices are preferred in patients where a difficult airway is anticipated, but others are not, as they have no experience. **Figure 38** depicts a Wu-Scope laryngoscope.
- *Indirect and video laryngoscope:* In recent years, multiple indirect laryngoscopy devices, utilizing further video technology, have revolutionized the management of the airway. The direct laryngoscopy (directly viewing the larynx by lifting the base of the tongue and epiglottis, without taking the help of fiber-optic cable, lens,

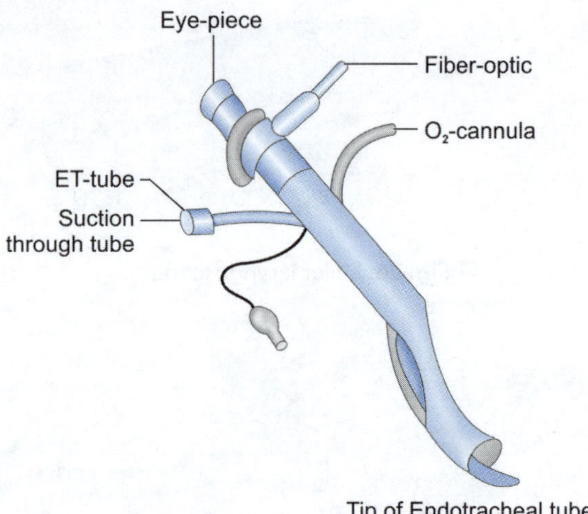

Fig. 38: Wu-Scope laryngoscope.

mirror, or video chip) by Macintosh or Miller blade needs appropriate alignment of oral, pharyngeal, and laryngeal axis to facilitate a direct view of glottis. So, it (direct laryngoscopy) also needs various maneuvers such as "sniffing position" of neck and head, external pressure over cricoid cartilage, etc., to improve the direct view of larynx. But in indirect laryngoscopy, without viewing the larynx directly, by using fiber optic cable (rigid or flexible), lens, mirror, video chips, etc., the larynx is viewed indirectly, without any head and neck maneuver and cricoid pressure. Video laryngoscopy is just one step ahead of indirect laryngoscopy, where the video of a real-time refracted (indirect) image of larynx is obtained on the screen. This indirect laryngoscopy, with or without video, may be rigid or flexible. The flexible indirect laryngoscope is commonly called flexible fiber-optic bronchoscope or laryngoscope which is discussed underneath. Here, we will discuss only the rigid indirect laryngoscope with video technology. Some of these indirect rigid or flexible video laryngoscopes have the option to obtain the image on a laptop or smartphone screen. The most commonly used rigid indirect video laryngoscope and its prototype is C-MAC. The design of it is based on Macintosh blade. The names of other rigid indirect video laryngoscopes are: DCI system, Glide Scope, McGrath, Airway, Air-traq, etc. The multiple studies have reported that the intubation success rate of video laryngoscopy, as a rescue modality, after failed direct laryngoscopy, is 95–99%.

The DCI system, GlideScope, McGrath, and Airway use a video chip system at the tip of their laryngoscope blade to transmit the view of the glottis to the operator. On the other hand, the Airtraq uses a lens/mirror at the tip of its blade to transmit the view of glottis to operator.

All these indirect rigid video laryngoscopes differ in the angulation of blade, the presence of a channel to guide the ETT into the glottis, and the single or multiple use of device.

In uncomplicated airways, such indirect video (rigid) laryngoscopy does not offer any extra advantage. It is only valuable in difficult cases where glottis cannot be seen by direct laryngoscopy with all possible maneuvers. However, the use of indirect video laryngoscopy in uncomplicated airway cases is only valuable as a training guide for learners, when the trainee is performing a laryngoscopy with a device, while the instructor is viewing the glottis on a video screen and is giving the instruction. Additionally, the use of indirect video laryngoscopy in uncomplicated cases improves the familiarity with device for use when direct laryngoscopy is not possible.

Indirect video (rigid) laryngoscopy generally improves visualization of laryngeal structures in difficult airways, but this visualization does not always lead to successful intubation. An ETT stylet is always recommended when video laryngoscopy is to be performed. Some devices come with particular stylets, designed to facilitate intubation with that particular device. Bending the stylet and ETT, in a manner similar to the bend in the curve of the blade, often facilitates the passage of ETT into the trachea. Even when the glottic opening is seen clearly, directing the ETT into the trachea may be difficult. Indirect video (rigid) laryngoscopy causes less displacement of the cervical spine than direct laryngoscopy. But still, all precautions, associated with airway manipulation in a patient with a cervical spine fracture, should be maintained. The different types of indirect video (rigid) laryngoscopes include:

- *C-MAC indirect video (rigid) laryngoscope:* The word C-MAC stands for Current Media Access Control. It is the first Macintosh-type video laryngoscope. Since the advent of its original version, video Macintosh system in 1999, this device has been modified several times. A unique feature of C-MAC is its ability to provide both options of direct and video laryngoscope with the same device. The available evidence shows that in patients with normal airway, C-MAC video laryngoscope compared to direct laryngoscope, can provide better laryngeal view and exerts less force on maxillary incisors, but does not provide conclusive benefits with regard to intubation time, intubation success, number of attempts of intubation, the use of adjuncts and hemodynamic responses to intubation. In patients with predicted or known difficult airway, the C-MAC video laryngoscope achieves a better laryngeal view, higher intubation success rate, and shorter intubation time than a direct laryngoscope.

- *Storz DCI system:* Here, in this system, Macintosh and Miller blades of different adult and pediatric sizes with video capability are incorporated. These blades are similar to conventional intubation blades, permitting direct laryngoscopy, and indirect video laryngoscopy. This system also incorporates an optical intubating stylet. Instructor and assistant are able to see the view obtained by the operator, hence the instructor can guide and the assistant can adjust his maneuvers accordingly to facilitate intubation.
- *McGrath MAC indirect video (rigid) laryngoscope:* It is a portable video laryngoscope and combines both direct and indirect video (rigid) laryngoscopy into a single device, designed to handle the unique challenges of airway management. Its blade length can be adjusted to accommodate the airway of a child of age 5 years up to an adult. The blade can be disconnected from the handle to facilitate its insertion in morbidly obese patients in whom the space between the upper chest and head is reduced. The blade is inserted in the midline and the laryngeal structures are viewed from a distance to enhance intubation success. It is a versatile intubation tool that delivers exceptional first-attempt success.
- *GlideScope indirect video (rigid) laryngoscope:* It comes with disposable pediatric and adult-sized blades. The blade is inserted in midline and is advanced until the glottis structures are found. The GlideScope has a 60° angle and so direct laryngoscopy is not possible by it. For intubation, it always necessitates the use of a stylet that is similar in shape to the blade.
- *Airtraq indirect video (rigid) laryngoscope:* It is a single-use optical laryngoscope, available in pediatric and adult sizes. This device has a channel to guide the ETT into the glottis. It is inserted through the midline and its success rate is high when this device is not too close to glottis.
- *Video intubating stylet:* It is a stylet with a light source and video capability. The stylet is introduced in the midline and the glottis is identified. Then, the ETT is pushed into the trachea. Intubation with this video intubating stylet causes less cervical spine movement than with other techniques.
- *Flexible fiber-optic laryngoscope:* Intubation done under the guidance of a fiber-optic laryngoscope/bronchoscope is called *flexible scope intubation (FSI)*. It is considered as the gold standard technique for the management of difficult or failed intubation. It is (1) less traumatic, (2) does not require any specific position of neck, and (3) can be performed in awake patients. The limitations of flexible fiber-optic laryngoscope are (1) cost, (2) technical expertise, and (3) time-consuming (not used in an emergency). It is discussed in more detail further.

Complications of laryngoscopy: The complications of laryngoscopy are (1) dental injury—most vulnerable are upper incisors, (2) damage to soft tissues and nerves, (3) injury to cervical spinal cord in case of aggressive manipulation of a preexisting injury, (4) hemodynamic alterations; tachycardia, hypertension, cardiac arrhythmias, etc., and (5) breakage and aspiration of the bulb.

Reflex responses to laryngoscopy and intubation:
- During laryngoscopy, there occurs sympathetic stimulation which can cause tachycardia, hypertension, cardiac arrhythmias, etc.
- Intubation can precipitate laryngospasm, particularly if airways are hyperactive or patient is in light anesthesia.
- Methods that can be used to blunt these responses are adequate depth of anesthesia, use of opioids (sufentanil is the choice), IV or topical lignocaine, and β-blockers (esmolol) or calcium channel blockers.

Stylet and bougie:

Stylet: It is made up of flexible metal and is inserted into an ETT in order to maintain a chosen shape of it **(Fig. 38)**. This will facilitate intubation when the visualization of glottis is minimal or absent. It should be remembered that the tip of a stylet should not cross the tip of an ETT; otherwise, it will injure the trachea. The other uses of stylet are rapid sequence intubation and when the hemodynamically stressful time for laryngoscopy should be minimized, e.g., in cardiac patients. During use, the stylet should be lubricated to facilitate its movement within the ETT. The stylet should be removed when the tip of the ETT enters the larynx to avoid undue trauma.

A special type of stylet with a light source at its tip is called the light wand. The advantage of this light wand is that it can be guided with an ETT (light wand is within the tube) into the trachea by observing the movement of light under the skin of neck from outside. Generally, the room should be dark, as the light can be seen adequately from the skin's surface. The ETT is placed over the light wand and is then introduced in the midline, through the hypopharynx, with the patient in a standard sniffing position. The wand is then manipulated until a flare of light down the trachea is seen illuminating the neck. When the ETT with the light wand (within the tube) is correctly positioned above the vocal cord in the midline, a distinct glow is seen in the anterior neck. Then, the tube is gently pushed into the trachea, and the light wand is withdrawn. A special type of light wand is called the "*Trachlight*".

Bougie: It is most commonly known as the gum elastic bougie. But it is neither made of gum, nor elastic, and nor a bougie. It is actually called the *Eschmann introducer* and is such designed that it provides both stiffness and flexibility. The length of this introducer is 60 cm and the external diameter of it is 5 mm. At its tip, it has a 35° bend, 2.5 cm from the patient's end which is inserted into the trachea **(Fig. 38)**.

Like a stylet, it is also a very useful instrument to facilitate intubation when the laryngoscopic view of the glottic is very poor. It is also very useful in limiting the degree of necessary neck movement during intubation with potential cervical spine injuries. It can also be used as a tube exchanger. When the bougie is used, the tip of it is introduced first into the larynx through the glottic inlet, blindly under reduced vision by a laryngoscope. Then, keeping the laryngoscope in place, the ETT is glided over the bougie up to laryngeal inlet. After that 90° anticlockwise turn facilitates the glottic passage of ETT, by presenting the bevel posteriorly. Then, the bougie is withdrawn.

Technique of Intubation

In the technique of intubation the usual sequences are (1) preoxygenation, (2) induction by administering rapid-acting IV or volatile inducing agent, (3) IV administration of rapid-acting neuromuscular blocking agent, (4) cricoid pressure, (5) mask ventilation, and (6) laryngoscopy followed by intubation. Both laryngoscopy and intubation are noxious stimuli and are sometimes more powerful than the surgical stimuli. So, deeper level of anesthesia is required to blunt the stress responses of laryngoscopy and intubation. This stress response has deleterious effects on respiratory, cardiovascular (CV), and neurological systems. Thus, during laryngoscopy and intubation, these stress effects should be blunted to maximum degree if possible, especially when the patient falls into a high-risk category (e.g., hypertension, coronary artery disease (CAD), ↑ICP), cerebral aneurysm, asthma, etc.).

Before giving IV neuromuscular blocking agent, every anesthesiologist must assess his or her own patient, if mask ventilation will be possible or not when the patient will be fully paralyzed and respiration is stopped. Therefore, if there is any doubt, regarding the maintenance of patient's airway and any doubt regarding the ventilation by only mask, after induction and paralysis, then a conscious intubation with mild sedation and/or with local anesthetic agent should be considered, before inducing skeletal muscle paralysis.

The general view, regarding preoxygenation, is that breathing of 100% O_2 for 3 minutes or four vital capacity breaths with 100% O_2 before induction of anesthesia, provides added margin of safety. So, routine preoxygenation is optional, but strongly recommended before induction of anesthesia and intubation of trachea for high risk group of patients. In patients with full stomach, where "rapid sequence" intubation is chosen, there preoxygenation and cricoid pressure (*Sellick maneuver*) is mandatory and mask ventilation is not provided before tracheal intubation, after IV administration of muscle relaxant, unless unsuccessful intubation necessitates it. Preoxygenation also can be omitted in patients (1) who object to accept face mask, (2) who are free of pulmonary diseases, and (3) who do not have any difficult airway.

Once the decision for induction and intubation is taken, then varieties of drugs can be used for setting induction and muscular paralysis and a variety of methods can be chosen to achieve the acceptable intubating conditions. For induction of anesthesia IV, inhalation or oral route can also be used, but usually IV route for adult and inhalation route for pediatric group of patients for induction of anesthesia are chosen. For IV induction, thiopental and propofol are most widely used now. But other rapidly acting barbiturates (methohexital and thiamylal), benzodiazepines, narcotics, ketamine, etomidate, etc., also can be used. However, the choice of inducing agents depends on the status of cardiovascular system (CVS), the status of central nervous system (CNS), effects on bronchomotor tone, presence of allergy, pharmacokinetics, and pharmacodynamics of inducing agent, etc., but among these the most important is the experience of clinicians.

Both the depolarizing and nondepolarizing muscle relaxants can be used for muscular paralysis, needed for tracheal intubation. But due to some disadvantages such as masseter spasm, malignant hyperthermia, hyperkalemia, burns, ↑IOP, and ↑intracranial pressure the choice of succinylcholine for tracheal intubation has recently been questioned. *However, still it is routinely used in many centers, due to some of its advantages* such as (1) excellent intubating condition within a minute (very rapid onset of action), (2) rapid offset of action by ester hydrolysis, if airway cannot be secured, and (3) the patient's own ventilation will return much more quickly than any of the currently available nondepolarizing muscle relaxants. So, still it (succinylcholine) is the relaxant of choice in many potentially difficult intubation cases, unless there are contraindications, however recently rapid onset and excellent intubating condition, produced by a nondepolarizing drug, such as rocuronium, is achieved instead of succinylcholine. Other alternative nondepolarizing drugs such as atracuronium, vecuronium, and cisatracuronium are not quite as rapid in onset of action as rocuronium.

Tracheal intubation may also be accomplished with only IV or inhalation anesthetic agent, without muscle relaxants, when there is any doubt of difficult airway and failed intubation, but this approach posses difficulties, such as the potential for laryngospasm. So, a very deep level of anesthesia should be achieved to avoid untoward laryngospasm, if one wants to intubate the trachea only by IV or inhalational anesthetic agents. In practice, if one wants to intubate only by IV or volatile anesthetic agent, still the majority of clinicians employ lesser degree of muscle relaxation by reducing the dose of muscle relaxants (one-fourth of the usual dose for quick recovery) which will facilitate intubation, but with very quick recovery, if failed intubation occurs.

Oral intubation: For successful oral intubation, the position of head and neck is also very important. Unless there is any contraindication for oral intubation, the head and neck is maintained in classical "sniffing position" to align the oral, pharyngeal, and laryngeal axes in a single straight line. The elevation of head by a small pillow, with the shoulders remaining on table, will first cause the alignment of pharyngeal and laryngeal axes. It will cause the flexion of neck by about 25–35°. Then, the subsequent extension of head at atlanto-occipital joint (85°) causes the alignment of oral axis with pharyngeal and subsequently with laryngeal axis **(Figs. 39A to C)**. Thus, it serves to create the shortest

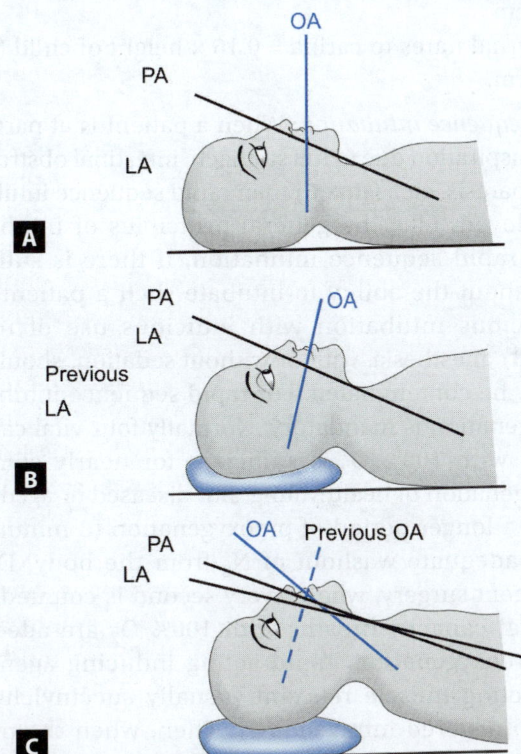

Figs. 39A to C: (A) The OA, PA, and LA in usual position; (B) Elevation of head about 10 cm by a pillow, with the shoulders remaining on table, aligns the LA with PA; and (C) Extension of head at atlanto-occipital joint aligns the OA with PA. So, these three axes such as OA, PA, and LA more or less comes on a single straight line. (LA: laryngeal axis; OA: oral axis; PA: pharyngeal axis)

possible distance and most nearly a straight line from the incisor teeth to the glottic opening. But no such head elevation is required in pediatric age group (<8 years) as their large head circumference keeps their neck in flexion position.

Usually, the laryngoscope is held by the left hand of an anesthesiologist and by the right hand of anesthetist the mouth of the patient is opened. Then, the blade of the laryngoscope is gently inserted into the patient's mouth from the right side of it and the tongue is kept left by the flange of the laryngoscope. During this procedure, any pressure on the teeth, gums, or lips, by the blade of the laryngoscope, should be avoided. After visualization of epiglottis, the tip of the curved blade of laryngoscope (Macintosh) is inserted into the vallecula and the laryngoscope is pulled forward and upward to elevate the epiglottis indirectly which will expose the glottis. During that period, gentle downward pressure on cricothyroid cartilage, from outside by an assistant, may bring a nonvisualized larynx into view.

Then, the ETT is inserted through the right side of the mouth and is then pushed into the trachea between the paralyzed, opened, and abducted vocal cords under direct vision. Instead of curved blade, if the laryngoscope of straight blade is used, then the tip of the blade is usually advanced behind the epiglottis, so that the epiglottis is included within the structures which are lifted up by the laryngoscope blade. Here, the epiglottis is lifted up directly by the blade of laryngoscope. The choice of the blade of laryngoscope depends on clinician's preference and the peculiar anatomy of an individual patient. When one blade does not become successful, then other types of blade become. So, skill should be developed in the use of laryngoscope with different types of blades by an anesthetist.

A failed intubation should not be followed by completely identical repeated attempts. So, some changes of procedure must be made to increase the likelihood of success such as the further repositioning of patient, decreasing the tube size, adding a stylet, selecting different blades, using an indirect laryngoscope, attempting a nasal route, and requesting the assistance of another anesthesia provider.

The cuff of ETT should lie in the upper part of trachea above carina but beyond the larynx or vocal cord. The cuff should be inflated with least amount of air which is just necessary to create an adequate tight seal (not very tight seal) in trachea, during positive pressure ventilation and minimize the injury of tracheal mucosa, caused by pressure transmitted to it (mucosa) from cuff. Feeling of a pilot balloon is not a reliable sign for determining the adequacy of cuff pressure.

After intubation, the chest and epigastrium are immediately auscultated. Capnographic tracing is also monitored to ensure the intratracheal location of the ET tube because the persistent detection of CO_2 by *capnography is the best way for the confirmation of tracheal placement of an ET tube, but it cannot exclude bronchial intubation.* The bronchial intubation is best diagnosed early by an increase in peak inspiratory pressure. The proper placement of an ETT into the trachea also can be confirmed by palpating the cuff on suprasternal notch, while compressing the pilot balloon with the other hand. The cuff of an ET tube also should not be kept above cricoid cartilage because the prolonged intralaryngeal location of cuff between the vocal cords may result in postoperative hoarseness of voice and increase the incidence of accidental intraoperative extubation. The true position of an ETT can also be documented by X-ray, but this is rarely needed except in the intensive care unit (ICU). If there is still any doubt, whether the tube is in esophagus or trachea, then it is prudent to remove the tube and ventilate the patient with a face mask **(Figs. 40A and B)**.

Checking for correct position of ETT (1) the auscultation of chest for air entry, (2) the characteristic feel of bag, (3) the inflation of chest on positive pressure, (4) capnography

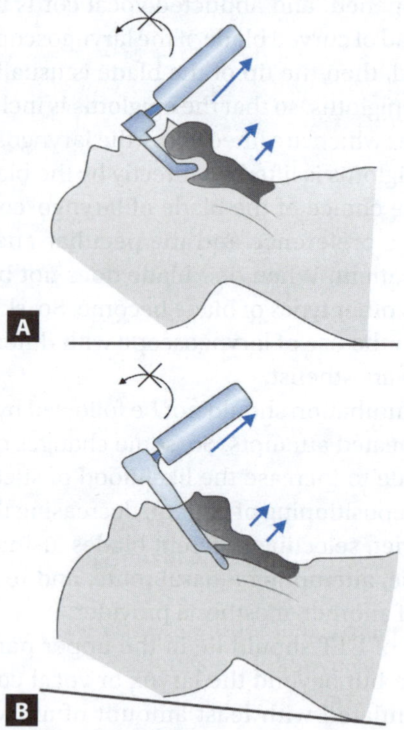

Figs. 40A and B: The proper position of a curved and straight blade of the laryngoscope during the exposure of glottic opening. (A) The tip of curved laryngoscope blade (Macintosh) is placed in the space between the base of the tongue and the pharyngeal surface of epiglottis (vallecula) and (B) The tip of straight laryngoscope blade (Miller or Jackson–Wisconsin) is placed on the laryngeal (posterior) surface of epiglottis. Irrespective of the type of blade, forward and upward force, shown by the arrow, should be applied along the handle of the laryngoscope to elevate the epiglottis and to expose the vocal cord.

(measuring end-tidal CO_2 and tracing), (5) fiber-optic bronchoscopy, (6) X-ray are usually performed, but among these, the capnography is the surest and confirmatory sign.

Under normal conditions, the causes for the non-visualization of vocal cords are mainly due to wrong head position and wrong blade position that is too far advanced, or not enough advanced, or reluctance to apply adequate upward force on the glossoepiglottic fold. The ETT is usually inserted into the trachea by keeping the lip 23 cm away from the tip of an ET tube in an adult male for correct position of cuff in trachea. In that position, the tip of an ETT lies 4 cm above carina. In an adult female, this distance from the lip to the tip of an ET tube is 21 cm. Too far advancement of tube into trachea causes endobronchial intubation (usually right), whereas inadequate advancement of tube causes protrusion of cuff into the glottis (an inlet of larynx) through the vocal cords, leading to the risk of accidental extubation. In children, the distance (in centimeters) between the lips and the tip of a tube can be estimated from the formula: 12 + age/2 **(Table 7)**.

There is also another simple formula to calculate the probable distance of the tip of an ETT from mouth opening or from external nares to carina, which is as follows:

- Mouth opening to carina = 0.16 × height of child (cm) + 2.5 cm
- External nares to carina = 0.16 × height of child (cm) + 4.5 cm.

Rapid sequence intubation: When a patient is at particular risk for aspiration due to full stomach, intestinal obstruction, gastric paresis, etc., **(Box 6)** then rapid sequence intubation is employed. Like the general principles of intubation, during rapid sequence intubation, if there is sufficient doubt about the ability to intubate such a patient, then a conscious intubation with judicious use of topical **(Table 8)** anesthesia, with or without sedation, should also strongly be contemplated. For rapid sequence intubation, preoxygenation is mandatory. Normally four vital capacity breaths with 100% O_2 is sufficient for nearly complete denitrogenation of healthy lung. But diseased or aged lungs require a longer period of preoxygenation (3 minutes) to ensure adequate washout of N_2 from the body. During very urgent surgery, where every second is counted, then four vital capacity breaths with 100% O_2 are adequate. After preoxygenation, rapid-acting inducing agent and rapid-acting muscle relaxant (usually succinylcholine) are administered intravenously. Then, when the patient becomes unconscious, proper cricoid pressure is applied to prevent aspiration, whether muscle relaxant is administered or not. Proper cricoid pressure (or Sellick maneuver) is applied by giving gentle downward pressure with thumb and first finger on the cricoid cartilage. This downward pressure on cricoid cartilage occludes the

TABLE 7: Magboul et al., scoring system.

Score	1	2	3	4
Mallampati	Grade 1	Grade 2	Grade 3	Grade 4
Measurement	3 fingers mouth open	3 fingers hypomental	2 fingers thyromental	1 fingers subluxation
Movement of neck	Left	Right	Flexion	Extension
Malformation	Skull hydrocephalus	Buck teeth, loose teeth, and macro and micro jaw	Obstruction, obesity, and neck swelling	Syndrome and pathology

Note: If the patient scores 8 or higher, he is likely to be a subject of difficult intubation. Magboul et al., reported a 100% correct prediction from this score, but obviously, more multicenter study and data will be needed to support this opinion.

BOX 6: Risks factors for aspiration of gastric contents.

- *Full stomach:*
  - <8 hours fasting in solid food
  - <6 hours fasting in milk
  - <4 hours fasting in breastfeeding
  - <2 hours in clear fluid pregnancy, obesity, and trauma
- Intra-abdominal pathology and intestinal obstruction
- Gastric paresis (peritonitis, infection, diabetes, drugs, and uremia)
- Esophageal diseases and symptomatic reflex motility disorders
- Uncertainty about the intake of food and drink

TABLE 8: Endotracheal tube (ETT) size and length calculated based on patient's age.

Age	ID (mm)	French unit	Distance from teeth to the tip of tube in trachea (cm)
Premature	2.5	10	10
Newborn	3	12	11
1–6 months	3.5	14	11
6–12 years	4	16	12
1–2 years	4.5	18	13
2–4 years	5	20	14
4–6 years	5.5	22	16
6–8 years	6	24	17
8–10 years	6.5	26	18
10–12 years	7	30	20
12–14 years	7 (Female)	30	22
	7.5 (male)	32	
>14 years	7.5 (female)	32	24
	8 (male)	34	

esophageal lumen behind the cartilage because only the cricoid cartilage forms a complete ring or has a posterior cartilaginous bar that can press and occlude the esophagus and thus prevents regurgitation. But this pressure cannot prevent the regurgitation, resulting from forceful vomiting. Only the force of vomiting is blunted by the muscle relaxant.

Laryngoscopy and intubation in a rapid sequence setting are performed without any preceding manual mask bag ventilation, if possible. If intubation is not possible in the first attempt, then only mask ventilation should be started and continued while the cricoid pressure is maintained. It is important to say that the cricoid pressure should be correctly applied, such that it actually does not impede the visualization of glottis or the passage of tube through it by any means. Cricoid pressure also decreases the flow of gas into the stomach and in turn limits the regurgitation.

Nasal intubation (Table 9): In the operating room, oral intubation is the usual method. But in some conditions, when the surgery is performed within oral cavity or on mandible, or at anywhere on the face, when both the surgeon and anesthetist struggle for the same space, then nasal intubation is the choice. Nasal intubation is usually performed under direct vision. But it also can be accomplished in difficult airway conditions blindly or with the help of fiber-optic scope under sedation and topical anesthesia. Blind or fiber-optic nasal intubation is also chosen, where direct laryngoscopy is impossible. The indications, contraindications, advantages, and disadvantages of nasal intubation are discussed in **Table 9**.

In any case when both the oral and nasal intubation has one or more contraindication, then the anesthetist must take any one decision, after discussing the relative risks and benefits of tracheostomy, oral intubation, and nasal intubation with a surgeon, to arrive at an acceptable compromise. Nasal intubation is sometimes chosen, because it may be quicker and more comfortable than oral intubation in topicalized and less-sedated patients.

Technique of nasal intubation: Nasal intubation may be blind or under direct vision by a laryngoscope. It will be helpful, if phenylephrine (0.5% or 0.25%) or tolazoline, as a vasoconstrictor, is applied on nasal mucosa before nasal intubation. After induction of anesthesia and administration of muscle relaxant and mask ventilation (but not always), the nasal ETT, lubricated with water-soluble jelly (K-Y jelly) is introduced into the nose through the nostril, in a plane

TABLE 9: Indications, contraindications, advantages and disadvantages of nasal intubation.

Indications	(1) Oral surgery; (2) oral mass; (3) inadequate mouth opening, due to any cause such as fracture mandible, temporomandibular joint ankylosis, Ludwig angina, quinsy, tetanus, and postburn contracture; (4) for awake intubation, nasal intubation is preferred over oral intubation; and (5) when tube is to be kept for prolonged periods in intensive care units and patient is going to remain awake for most of the time, nasal tube is preferred, because it is better tolerated by patient
Contraindications	(1) Basal skull fracture and CSF rhinorrhea, (2) bleeding disorders (nasal and septal mucosa are highly vascular), (3) nasal polyp, nasal abscess, foreign body in the nose, (4) adenoid hypertrophy, and (5) previous nasal surgery (relative contraindication)
Advantages of nasal over oral intubation	(1) Better fixation of ETT and therefore less chances of accidental extubation, (2) no possibility of tube occlusion by biting, (3) oral hygiene can be better maintained, and (5) better tolerated than oral intubation by patient
Disadvantages	(1) Increased chances of bleeding and trauma to nasal structures. So, to avoid trauma to inferior turbinate, the bevel of the tube should be toward the septum; (2) increased chances of bacteremia such as sinusitis, otitis, meningitis, etc.; and (3) nasal deformities on long-term use
Contraindications for both oral and nasal intubation	As such there is no absolute contraindication for oral or nasal intubation. The very simple rule is *"intubate where you can"*. Therefore, the relative contraindications are (1) *laryngeal edema:* It may get aggravated by intubation, but intubation is lifesaving in such cases and (2) acute epiglottitis and *laryngotracheobronchitis:* As the airway is hyperactive, so intubation can precipitate laryngospasm, but intubation is lifesaving in these cases

(CSF: cerebrospinal fluid; ETT: endotracheal tube)

perpendicular to the face (along the floor of the nose), below the inferior turbinate. The tube's bevel should be directed laterally away from the turbinate. Now, the tube is gradually advanced up to a certain length when the tip of a nasal ET tube reaches the oropharynx. Then, direct laryngoscopy is performed (in case of under direct vision nasal intubation) in the usual fashion and will reveal the vocal cords. After that, the tip of ETT which is seen in the oropharynx is directed into the glottis, by holding and manipulating the machine end of the tube from the outside of the nose.

If this is not possible then a Magill forceps may be used through the mouth and oropharynx to direct the tip of ETT into the glottis, under direct vision laryngoscopy, often with the help of an assistant who will push the machine end of the ET tube. If the glottis cannot be visualized by direct laryngoscopy, then this Magill forceps can still be used to guide the tip of this ETT blindly into the area of glottis.

Blind nasal intubation is usually done in an anesthetized spontaneously ventilated patient, where spontaneous respiration facilitates the intubation blindly. This procedure is described underneath. While the patient is taking spontaneous respiration, under deep sedation or anesthesia (to prevent laryngospasm) or under proper topical anesthesia, the ET tube is gradually advanced through the nasal cavity and then gradually through the nasopharynx, oropharynx, and laryngopharynx, until the maximum breath sounds are heard from the outer end of the ET tube. It implies that the tip of the tube is just above the glottis. The tube is then inserted blindly into the glottis (by manipulating the portion of the tube which is now outside of the nose), during the next inspiration, which tends to be deepest immediately following a cough. During the forward movement of ETT through the laryngopharynx, if breath sounds through the nasal end of the tube disappears, then it should be thought that the tube has passed into the esophagus or in pyriform fossa and must be withdrawn slightly above the level of the glottis. It is then reintroduced blindly into the larynx again and such several attempts can be tried.

If still the tube does not enter the glottis, then the patient's head should be extended, flexed, or turned left or right to guide the tip of the ETT into the glottis. Usually, the tip of the ET tube enters into the esophagus and so the extension of the head is useful. If still, intubation is not possible, then the help of direct laryngoscopy or fiber-optic bronchoscopy should be taken. As in blind procedure, the entry of ETT into the glottis is not seen directly, so it is helpful to have capnographic or bronchoscopic confirmation for the ET placement of tube, because at times, all the indirect signs of intubation may be misleading.

Blind nasal intubation in an anesthetized, apneic, and paralyzed patients may also be attempted, very rarely, but as in this case, there are no spontaneous breath sounds to help the placement of tube into the larynx, so this is only guided by the external observation of tip location into the larynx.

Complications of intubation are enumerated in **Table 10**.

Intubation Failure

Despite the most meticulous preoperative assessment of airway, sometimes few patients present sudden and great difficulty during intubation. No matter, how skilled, every practitioner has to encounter such patients in his practicing life. So, the induction of anesthesia and use of muscle relaxant should be approached with this possibility (failed intubation) in mind, as if a clear plan of action can be persuaded without unnecessarily panicking if intubation failed.

These patients may be of (1) *elective* or (2) *emergency* cases. Failed intubation in *emergency cases* is potentially life-threatening because there is a greater possibility of hypoxia both from regurgitation with aspiration (as these patients are not properly prepared by restricting the intake of food) and failed intubation. *The cardinal rule under such conditions is oxygenation first and everything later*, i.e., regurgitation, aspiration, etc., are secondary. In such cases, the majority of opinion is that it would be wiser to allow the patient to come back to spontaneous respiration or even better to regain consciousness. Then, as the surgery is an emergency and unavoidable, so one can review, rethink, replan, and proceed again. *The objective for these difficult patients should be not to use muscle relaxant-producing apnea until intubation*

has been successfully accomplished at the beginning of any anesthesia or where the intubation has failed and the patient is backed to spontaneous respiration. For such patients, conscious or "awake" intubation by topical/infiltration local anesthesia or intubation under spontaneous respiration under deep sedation or general anesthesia (GA) by a volatile anesthetic agent is ideal.

Indications for Awake Intubations

Indications for awake intubations are (1) previous history of difficult or failed intubation, (2) findings on physical examination that can indicate difficult or failed intubation, and (3) severe risk for aspiration. Actually, the term "awake intubation" is applied to intubation on nonanesthetized conscious emergency patients outside the operating room. But this term is a misnomer in OT, where it is used after appropriate sedation, topical anesthesia, and/or nerve blocks to avoid laryngeal reflexes. If awake intubation has to be performed due to a severe risk of aspiration, then narcotics and other IV sedatives should be used sparingly. **Flowchart 1** shows an algorithm in difficult intubation.

Promoting local anesthesia for awake intubation, the nerves that need to be blocked are trigeminal (area of the nasal cavity and oral cavity), glossopharyngeal (area

TABLE 10: Complications of intubation.	
Perioperative	• *Esophageal intubation:* If not detected in time, can cause severe hypoxia and death • Ischemia, edema, and necrosis at the local mucosal site, especially with red rubber tube • Aspiration, if cuff is not properly inflated • Bronchial intubation and collapse of other lung • Tracheal tube obstruction by secretions, kinking, etc. • Accidental extubation • Trauma to gums, lips, epiglottis, pharynx, larynx, and nasal cavity • Reflex disturbances such as laryngospasm, bronchospasm, tachyarrhythmia, and hypertension
Postoperative	• Sore throat (pharyngitis and laryngitis): This is the most common postoperative complication. It usually subsides in 2–3 days without any treatment • *Laryngeal edema:* It usually presents after 1–2 hours of extubation • Laryngeal nerve palsies • Surgical emphysema and mediastinal emphysema • *Infection:* Pneumonia, lung abscess, mediastinitis, etc. • Lung atelectasis
Delayed	Vocal cord granuloma, laryngotracheal web, subglottic or tracheal stenosis, tracheal collapse. *Delayed complications usually occur after prolonged intubation in intensive care patients. Therefore, the maximum permissible time for which an endotracheal tube (ETT) can be kept is 14 days*

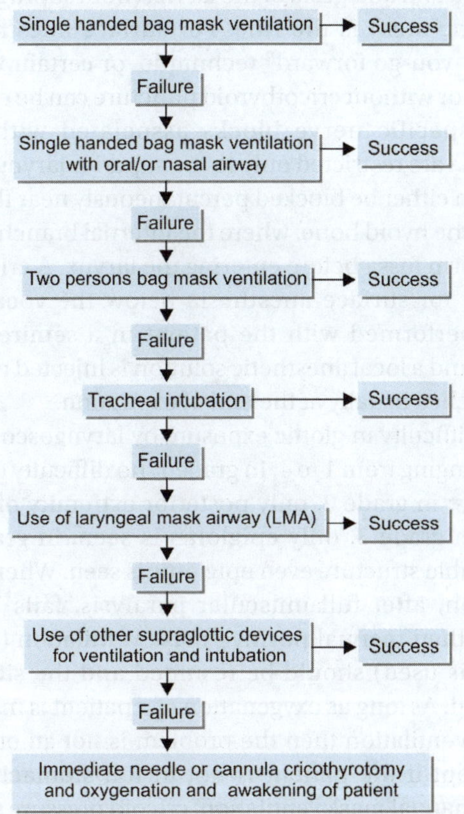

Flowchart 1: Strategy in case of predicted or unpredicted difficult bag-mask ventilation.

of nasopharynx, oropharynx, and laryngopharynx), and vagus (supraglottic and infraglottic region). Woods and Lander describe a technique of glossopharyngeal nerve block that only anesthetizes the sensory supply over the back of the tongue which is innervated by this cranial nerve (glossopharyngeal IX). For this technique, by a 24 G needle, a 2 mL anesthetic drug is injected at the junction, where the base of the tongue opposes with the palatoglossal fold. This causes local anesthesia of the base of the tongue and does not appear to affect airway integrity when performed bilaterally. This block is acceptable with a full stomach also. This type of local anesthesia allows a more comfortable laryngoscopy with lower doses of sedation. It has also been seen that if a larger volume of local anesthetic is given at that site, then the *superior laryngeal nerve (SLN) which is the branch of vagus will also be blocked with glossopharyngeal nerve, because both the nerves lie in the same tissue plane.*

The SLN innervates the epiglottis, aryepiglottic fold, and the laryngeal structure up to the false vocal cords. This nerve can also be blocked isolatedly by giving an injection of 2–3 mL local anesthetic agent *percutaneously* between the greater cornu of hyoid bone and thyroid cartilage. But this block is contraindicated in full stomach patients, *as it impairs the protective mechanism of airway and cannot prevent the regurgitation and aspiration of stomach contents if vomiting occurs.* So, in a full stomach where regurgitation and aspiration have a possibility, then surface anesthesia and analgesia of the larynx (both supraglottic and infraglottic area) is the rule. For surface anesthesia, the "spray-as-you-go forward" technique, or certain variations of it, with or without cricothyroid puncture can be employed.

The specific nerve blocks associated with surface anesthesia are restricted only to the superior laryngeal nerve which can either be blocked percutaneously near the greater cornu of the hyoid bone, where the internal branch traverses the pyriform fossa before entering the larynx. A cricothyroid puncture for surface anesthesia below the vocal cord is usually performed with the patient in a semirecumbent position and a local anesthetic solution is injected or sprayed in the trachea usually at the end of expiration.

The difficulty in glottic exposure by laryngoscopy can be graded ranging from 1 to 4: In grade 1, no difficulty of viewing the glottis; in grade 2, only posterior extremity of glottis is visible; in grade 3, only epiglottis is seen; in grade 4, no recognizable structure even epiglottis is seen. When tracheal intubation, after full muscular paralysis, fails by initial attempt, then manual positive mask ventilation (if muscle relaxant is used) should be resumed and the situation is reassessed. As long as oxygenation of a patient is maintained by mask ventilation then the problem is not an emergency one, except if the patient is not in full stomach. During positive manual mask ventilation, cricoid pressure should be

maintained, if the stomach is full. However, in case of topical anesthesia and/or nerve block, if awake intubation is failed, then the patient's spontaneous respiration is maintained only by giving 100% O_2. After that, slight sedation can be added and fiber-optic intubation can be tried.

During the reassessment of upper airway, after failed intubation in first attempt, the following things that should be brought in mind and corrections should be done are head position, laryngoscopy technique, change in the shape (curved to straight), and size of the blade. If repeated laryngoscopy and failed intubation by an experienced practitioner is unsuccessful, then the first aim should be efficient mask ventilation (obviously in paralyzed patient) to prevent hypoxia and attempts to bring back the patient to spontaneous respiration.

If mask ventilation is efficient, then before bringing back to spontaneous ventilation the anesthesiologist can also again try intubation by the help of stylet, bougie, Flexi tip laryngoscope, light wand (Trachlight), etc. LMA-aided intubation, indirect rigid fiber-optic laryngoscope-assisted intubation, pharyngeal airway Xpress-aided intubation, etc., also can be tried.

If all the previous methods are failed, then patient should be brought back to the spontaneous respiration. After resumption of spontaneous respiration, there are *three options:* One, the patient may be allowed to awaken and the surgical procedure is postponed, if the *case is not emergency*; second, the patient is awakened and intubation is further attempted with topical anesthesia if the case is *emergency*; third, after resumption of spontaneous respiration, not awakening the patient, try again to intubate the patient by previously described methods such as using stylet, bougie, fiber-optic bronchoscope, blind oral or nasal intubation, etc., then the muscle relaxant can be used, if the *operation is emergency.* Actual life-threatening emergency condition arises when after the use of muscle relaxants, the tracheal intubation is failed and mask ventilation is also ineffective. The management of this extremely emergency condition is discussed further.

All anesthetists should develop a skill for conscious (actually under light sedation) oral intubation with a direct laryngoscopy. Blind nasal intubation that avoids the discomfort of laryngoscopy is also equally important to learn.

Intubation failed mask ventilation is effective or patient is breathing spontaneously (no hypoxia–oxygenation is maintained), an operation is urgently needed.

This group of patients can be managed by the following ways:
- If the manual positive bag-mask ventilation is effective enough and the patient is properly prepared from the point of view of an empty stomach and the anesthetist

thinks that he will be able to carry on the operation by only mask ventilation with *muscle relaxation* (if that operation needs relaxation), then he can proceed.

- Operation also can be carried out on an anesthetized patient with spontaneous respiration through the mask, if *muscle relaxant is not so needed* to complete that emergency surgical procedure. So, after muscle relaxation and failed intubation, when spontaneous respiration is reestablished, the anesthesia can be continued with volatile inhalational agents by mask, without muscle relaxant.

- After reestablishment of spontaneous respiration in an anesthetized patient, if the patients fall in the group *where operation is urgent and the full muscle relaxation is required for completion of surgical procedure and mask ventilation is though effective, but cannot be carried out for a prolonged period or the surgical site does not allow the mask ventilation, then the patients should be managed by intubation first after reestablishment of spontaneous respiration and later followed by full muscle relaxation.*

Intubation in this group of patients is tried first with the help of different intubation accessories. In such a situation, another option is the use of LMA. By LMA we can maintain anesthesia by spontaneous ventilation with the inhalational agents or we can ventilate if a muscle relaxant is needed. Mask ventilation or ventilation with LMA (spontaneous or IPPV) is usually satisfactory for short minor procedures such as cystoscopy, exam under anesthesia (EUA), inguinal hernia repair, etc., but not for long complicated procedures or where high pressure for IPPV is needed.

Accessories for Intubation

- *Using stylet:* Difficult orotracheal or nasotracheal intubation can be performed by employing direct laryngoscopy and using stylet which is passed through ETT. With the stylet, the shape and the direction of the tip of the ETT can be modulated according to the wish of an anesthetist. Usually, the tip of the ETT is directed anteriorly with the stylet.

- *Difficult oral intubation using bougie:* Difficult oral intubation may also be attempted by gliding the ETT over a long flexible "bougie", inserted blindly first into the glottis under direct laryngoscopy. Sometimes, the subsequent passage of an ETT by gliding over the bougie is difficult. In such a situation, the laryngoscope should be kept in position and the tracheal tube is rotated 90° anticlockwise, in order to prevent the "fork" created by the beveled end of the tube and the bougie, from impacting on the posterior rim between the arytenoid cartilages.

A white plastic bougie with a soft metal core is said to be easier most to place in the glottis than the older

BOX 7: Recognition of correct placement of ET tube.

- Direct visualization of tube passing through the larynx
- Auscultation of chest
- Auscultation of epigastrium
- Observation of chest movement
- Observation of abdominal movement
- Tension of CO_2 in expired air, confirmed by capnography
- Observation of condensation of water vapor in expired air in PVC ETT
- Movement of reservoir bag in up paralyzed spontaneously breathed patient

(ETT: endotracheal tube; PVC: polyvinylchloride)

gum elastic bougie. Advancement of the distal end of the bougie over the tracheal rings produces a clicking sensation and confirms its placement in the trachea. If the bougie is hollow, then jet ventilation can also be done through this channel or capnography can be attached with it which will show the characteristic pattern of PCO_2 in expired air associated with the breathing. The confirmation of an ETT into the trachea is done by the following signs which are listed in **Box 7**.

- *Using light wands:* Light wand was originally introduced for blind intubation, but it can be used with a direct laryngoscope also (semiblind technique). If the light at the distal end of the tracheal tube is seen to transilluminate brightly through the cricothyroid membrane, then it is confirmed that the ETT is in the larynx. If no transillumination is seen, then the tube is considered to be in the esophagus. The *advantages of the light wand* or trach light are easy technique, relatively inexpensive, useful adjunct in difficult airway, does not require much neck manipulation, useful in cervical spine injury, useful in patient with limited mouth opening, less traumatic than blind nasal intubation, presence of secretion is of no problem, etc. The *disadvantages of the light wand* are it should not be used with laryngeal or tracheal polyps, tumors, inflammation, retropharyngeal abscess, foreign body, etc. In morbidly obese patients, the ability to see the glow of light may be diminished. On the contrary, in thin and frail patients some transilluminations may also occur, even when the tube tip with the light source is in the esophagus, and will confuse the anesthetist.

- *Blind nasal intubation:* For blind nasal intubation, the patient should normally have the head and neck, placed in the classical "sniffing the morning air" position. The anesthetist will have to first decide which of the nasal passage is to be used. Then, as a first step, a well-lubricated nasal tracheal tube is gradually passed along the floor of the nose into the nasopharynx, oropharynx, and hypopharynx (as the patient is breathing spontaneously). After that, it is ultimately introduced blindly into the trachea. But unfortunately this is very uncommon, and commonly these tubes end up either in the pyriform fossae or in the esophagus. In such circumstances, several blind attempts with or without the help of any accessories are tried. Occasionally, they can also cause various degrees of hemorrhage. Chances of successful blind nasal intubation can be increased by the following methods:

- Listening to the proximal end of the nasal tube and feeling the air being breathed out of the tube.
- Using capnography to guide the distal (patient) end of the tube into the larynx.
- Using the light wand which can be manipulated, so that the long shaft of the wand follows the contours of the upper nasal passage and enter the larynx.
- A fiber-optic laryngoscope or bronchoscope can be passed through the nasal tube to guide it into the larynx.

■ *Using LMA:* LMA has also been used on many occasions for difficult intubation because it itself has enabled effective oxygenation by spontaneous ventilation (when muscle relaxants are not used) or manual positive pressure ventilation (when muscle relaxants are used). Laryngeal mask airway has also enabled the passage of bougie and/or fiber-optic scope into the trachea which is again followed by the passage of an ETT in trachea with the help of these bougies or fiber-optic scope. There is also a special type of intubating LMA (ILMA) which is called *"Fastrach LMA"*. It consists of an anatomically curved, short, wide-bore tube, and a laryngeal cuff with a guiding stainless steel handle. It has a single moveable epiglottis elevation bar in place of fixed aperture bars. It is available in three sizes and can accommodate 7, 7.5, and 8 sizes ETT within its wide-bore tube for intubation. The picture of a Fastrach LMA is shown in **Figure 41**.

■ *Combitube:* The most recent method of accomplishing emergency intubation or more correctly ventilation is the use of Combitube or King's tube. Combitube is the modern version of the older esophageal obturator airway. The principle of Combitube is that this tube is inserted blindly and artificial ventilation is started through any one of the distal two ports. Depending on the results of auscultation, any one of the two tubes is selected to ventilate the lungs. The use of King's tube has been described earlier.

■ *Fiber-optic instruments:* Recently fiber-optic laryngoscope or bronchoscope has become an extremely important piece of instrument in the management of difficult airway. Due to their extreme flexibility, they easily can be passed either through the nose or through the mouth into the trachea and assist in intubation. The observer can also see the tip of ETT into the trachea with the help of fiber-optic scope and confirm intubation.

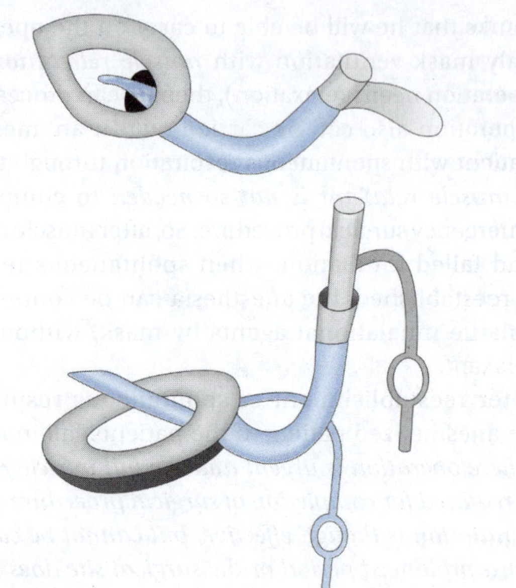

Fig. 41: Intubating laryngeal mask airway (ILMA).

When used for nasal intubation, the fiber-optic laryngoscope or bronchoscope with an ETT can be passed through the nose into the larynx followed by the tracheal tube. Alternatively, the nasotracheal tube or airway can be passed into the pharynx and the fiber-optic scope is passed through it into the larynx, followed by the tracheal tube. The latter technique is used to prevent the tip of the fiberscope from toileting with blood, secretions, or water vapor condensation to get a clear view. By contrast, the usual practice of fiber-optic scope through the oral route is to pass it first using the conventional laryngoscope, followed by an ETT. Once the intubation has been accomplished by either of these two routes or methods, the fiber-optic scope can also confirm the ETT in the trachea by observing the tip of the tube against the tracheal ring or wall.

One of the disadvantages of fiber-optic techniques for intubation is that the instrument is delicate and expensive and can be quite easily damaged. Even in experienced hands, an intubation using these instruments can take duration which is three times longer than that of the conventional method and may be associated with marked cardiovascular responses to intubation. It is reported that blood pressure and heart rate remain higher for a considerably longer period compared with following a normal intubation.

When Intubation is Failed and also Ventilation by Mask Is Ineffective or Not Possible

The patient who is paralyzed by muscle relaxant and who is also a truly impossible candidate for face mask ventilation, after failed intubation, presents really a life-threatening dire emergency condition. Always the best treatment of such a grave condition is its *prevention*, like the other branches of medicine. So, an anesthetist must always carefully evaluate the airway (1) to determine the safest plan for intubation and (2) to evaluate the plan if both the intubation and face mask ventilation failed, before instituting muscular paralysis and general anesthesia. In the patient who has been thoroughly denitrogenated by preoxygenation, then there should be an adequate time to institute one of the following procedures (described underneath), before serious O_2 desaturation and its consequent hemodynamic deterioration happen if such "nonintubated and nonventilated" condition appears. In reality, when such circumstances will arrive, then everybody has to think that he is often dealing with a severely anoxic patient who is near at the brim of cardiac arrest. So, it is critical to start one of the following procedures before irreversible cardiac arrest or brain damage has ensured. The interventions during *"failed to intubate and failed to ventilate by face mask"* are the followings:

- *Establishment of an emergency nonsurgical airway and ventilation:* After the face mask, the LMA or Combitube or King's tube will probably become the next nonsurgical airway intervention for such emergency ventilation.
- *Establishment of an emergency surgical airway and ventilation: To manage the "failed to intubate and failed to ventilate by face mask" condition, the emergency surgical airways can be established by many ways. These are (1) needle cricothyroidotomy, (2) cannula cricothyroidotomy, (3) surgical cricothyroidotomy, (4) percutaneous tracheostomy (PCT), and (5) conventional surgical tracheostomy (ST), etc. Among these, the needle and cannula cricothyroidotomy is done during an emergency condition when an anesthetist "cannot intubate and cannot ventilate by mask" the patient* **(Fig. 41)**.

Through the needle or cannula, used for cricothyroidotomy, *jet ventilation* is performed for the oxygenation of patient, so this procedure may be called the *transtracheal jet ventilation (TTJV)*. Actually, the term "jet ventilation" means introduction of gas (oxygen) into the tracheobronchial tree under high pressure and speed and has been used in different forms, for example, this technique may also be used during anesthesia for bronchoscopy or laser surgery on larynx. During anesthesia for bronchoscopy and laser surgery on larynx, jet ventilation via a needle or cannula, placed within the lumen of an otolaryngological laryngoscope, permita oxygenation of the patient without a tracheal intubation.

Transtracheal Jet Ventilation through Needle Cricothyroidotomy

In such TTJV through needle cricothyroidotomy, a 12–18 G needle (12 G or 14 G for adults and 16 G or 18 G for pediatric patients) is inserted through the cricothyroid membrane

and is attached to a high pressure O_2 source via a low compliance (less distensible) circuit. For high-pressure O_2 source, an anesthetic machine can also be used. For that, an adaptor of an ETT of 5 mm ID, which is attached to the low compliance O_2 supply tubing, is inserted to the fresh gas outlet of anesthetic machine. At the other end (patient's end) of low compliance O_2 tube (i.e., between the O_2 tube and 16 G or 14 G cannula) a three-way stopcock is attached and then this stopcock is connected to the translaryngeal 16 G or 14 G needle or cannula. The three-way stopcock helps, by preventing the excessive pressure to build-up, by releasing the aperture to the air (environment) in between the jet inspiration. Before starting artificial jet ventilation, it is wise to fix the tube. Otherwise, high pressure through a narrow tube will tend to force the tube out of its position. It is essentially a blind technique and incorrect placement or excessive pressure can produce pneumothorax, pneumomediastinum, pneumotrachea, pneumolarynx, etc. In this era of technological advances, flexible fiber-optic endoscope, Bullard laryngoscope, noninvasive light wand, and different intubation guides are also recommended. Anatomy of the cricothyroid membrane is depicted in **Figure 42**.

This *TTJV by needle* provides adequate ventilation, as well as oxygenation, and serves as an alternative emergency procedure for those who are planning to assemble a *standard TTJV system through the cannula cricothyroidotomy by modified Seldinger technique*. This TTJV, either by needle or cannula, only provides emergency oxygenation. So, always the successful TTJV should be followed up by the provision of making a definite airway and ventilation by tracheostomy (percutaneous or classical) or ET intubation or waking up the patient and resumption of a normal airway. In the technique

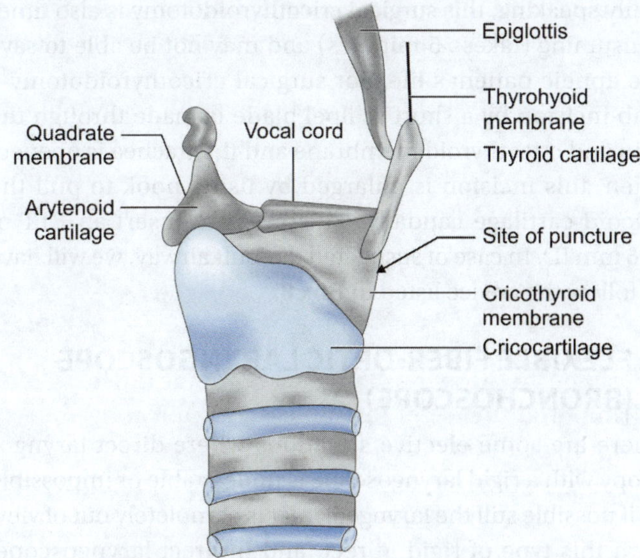

Fig. 42: The anatomy of the cricothyroid membrane.

BOX 8: Difficult airway algorithm.

- *Assessment:*
  - Assessment for difficult mask ventilation
  - Assessment for difficult intubation
  - Assessment for difficulty for patient cooperation and consent
  - Assessment for difficulty for tracheostomy
  - Assessment of opportunities for delivery of supplemental oxygen throughout the process of difficult airway management
- *Consider the relative merits and demerits of the basic choices of management:*
  - Preservation of spontaneous ventilation versus ablation of spontaneous ventilation
  - Awake intubation versus intubation after induction of GA
  - As an initial approach for intubation taking the help noninvasive technique versus the invasive technique
- Difficult airway—recognized or unrecognized
- Develop some other primary and alternative strategies

of cannula cricothyroidotomy, after a needle is introduced into the tracheal lumen, a wire is passed downward through this needle. Then, the needle is withdrawn and a dilator is passed over the wire which is followed by a cannula. The *advantages of this cannula cricothyroidotomy technique* are that it is relatively quick (but not quick than needle cricothyroidotomy) and relatively easy to perform. It is important to comment that neither cricothyroidotomy nor TTJV can relieve obstruction if it occurs below the first few tracheal cartilages.

Surgical cricothyroidotomy: In the "cannot ventilate by mask and cannot intubate" condition, a classical tracheostomy cannot be performed quickly enough to save the life. In such a situation emergency surgical cricothyroidotomy can also be employed to insert a small ET or tracheostomy tube. Truly speaking, this surgical cricothyroidotomy is also time-consuming (takes >5 minutes) and may not be able to save the apneic patient's life. For surgical cricothyroidotomy a stab incision by a short scalpel blade is made through the skin and cricothyroid membrane and the trachea is opened. Then, this incision is enlarged by using hook to pull the cricoid cartilage caudally. This helps to insert an ETT of 5–6 mm ID. In case of suspected difficult airway, we will have to follow the advice listed in **Box 8**.

FLEXIBLE FIBER-OPTIC LARYNGOSCOPE (BRONCHOSCOPE)

There are some elective situations where direct laryngoscopy with a rigid laryngoscope is undesirable or impossible or if possible still the laryngeal inlet is completely out of view with this type of rigid, direct, and indirect laryngoscope. Examples of few such situations are (1) patients with unstable cervical spines due to trauma, (2) there is no movement of the cervical spine, due to severe rheumatoid arthritis, (3) small mouth opening, (4) very poor range of motion of TM joint, (5) severe burn contracture of the neck, (6) certain congenital or acquired upper airway anomalies, (7) upper airway obstruction, such as angioedema or tumor mass, (8) facial deformities and facial trauma, (9) in any situation in which awake intubation is planned, etc.

In such situations, direct visualization of the larynx by flexible fiber-optic scope (laryngoscope or bronchoscope) and intubation, with the help of it, is the only answer. But in contrast to a conventional laryngoscope, its use needs intense practice. Intubation by flexible fiber-optic laryngoscope or bronchoscope requires a longer time. So, it has no role in an emergency situation where the airway has to be established rapidly in the face of severe hypoxia. When the fiber-optic (laryngo) scope-aided intubation is anticipated for the *elective* management of a more difficult airway, then the fiberscope should be employed first, before the visualization of larynx is obscured by edema, secretions, and/or hemorrhage, due to previous repeated attempts and failed intubation.

The flexible fiber-optic laryngoscope or bronchoscope consists of a collection of thin-coated glass fibers whose diameter vary between 5 and 25 µm. These glass fibers transmit light and images by internal reflection, i.e., the light beams are trapped inside the coated glass fibers and exit unchanged through the opposite end. These collections of thin glass fibers are divided into two groups in insertion tube and each group contains 10,000–15,000 glass fibers. Among these two groups, one group transmits image from the target object to our eyes and another transmits light from a powerful source to the object. In addition to all these, a fiber-optic laryngoscope or bronchoscope consists of (1) wires which control the angulation of the tip of insertion tube and (2) ports (aspiration channel) for suction, injection of local anesthetics, and delivery of oxygen. This aspiration channel can be difficult to clean and if not properly cleaned and sterilized after each use, may promote infection.

Flexible fiber-optic intubation (FOI) is usually performed as an elective procedure on awake or asleep via oral or nasal routes in the following scenarios and indications: (1) *Awake FOI*—previously failed intubation or predicted difficult intubation with a predicted inability to ventilate by mask, (2) *asleep FOI*—previously failed intubation patient who refuses awake intubation, (3) *anesthetized paralyzed FOI*—previously failed intubation and anticipated difficult intubation, but when ventilation by mask appears (predicted) easy, (4) *oral FOI*—skull injuries, and (5) *nasal FOI*—poor mouth opening, facial injuries. Other than failed or difficult intubation, an important indication for FOI is cervical cord injury, where the movement of the neck is prohibited. Therefore, different permutations and combinations of FOIs are oral awake, oral asleep, nasal awake, nasal asleep, etc. When FOI is considered, careful planning is necessary. Otherwise, there will be increased complications and increased anesthesia time prior to surgery. Patients should be informed of the need for awake intubation as a part of the informed consent process.

The keys to successful elective intubation by fiber-optic scope (fiber optic intubation) include control of secretions, adequate topical anesthesia, proper sedation, proper defogging of lens, and the aligning of scope at midline. As during any manipulation of airway, a pulse oximeter is also mandatory during this procedure to detect hypoxia. During the use of fiber-optic scope-aided intubation, the use of anticholinergic is strongly recommended, because excessive secretions in the upper airway may obscure the laryngeal view. The tip of the scope should be defogged intermittently and frequently with warm soapy water and its entire length should be lubricated by K-Y jelly to facilitate the passage of scope through an ETT. A patent suction port is important and a 10 mL syringe, filled with 1% lignocaine solution, can be attached for further topical spray through the scope. If O_2 insufflation is desired, then an appropriate O_2 source, adaptable to the fiber-optic scope (bronchoscope) port should be available. This is also useful in keeping the secretions away from the tip of the fiber-optic scope and diminishing fogging, as well as providing a source of 100% O_2, preventing hypoxia during the fiber-optic scope-aided intubation.

The *elective intubation by fiber-optic scope* may be (1) oral or nasal, (2) awake or asleep. But among the oral or nasal route, the nasal route and among the awake or asleep, slightly sedated is preferred. On the other hand, through an *oral route on a completely asleep paralyzed patient, fiber-optic intubation is the most difficult* of the four possible techniques such as oral or nasal fiber-optic intubation in an awake or asleep patient.

During oral intubation by fiber-optic scope on a sedated unparalyzed patient, an endoscopic oral airway or a bite block should be used to protect the scope from biting by teeth. Among the oral airway, the Patil–Syracuse airway or Williams airway or Ovassapian airway have some advantages. It prevents the dorsal displacement of tongue and keeps the instrument in midline and guides the scope past the epiglottis into the larynx. The possible contents in a difficult airway kit are named in **Box 9**.

As a first step, in a conscious or slightly sedated and nonparalyzed patient, the base of the tongue, the oropharynx, and the laryngopharynx is anesthetized topically by 10% lignocaine spray or by the nebulization

- Rigid laryngoscope blades of different sizes and designs
- Endotracheal tube of different sizes and shapes
- Different ET tube guides, such as stylets of different sizes with or without hollow inside for jet ventilation, gum elastic bougies, light wands, and forceps to manipulate the patient's end of the tube in the larynx
- *Various supraglottic airway devices:* LMA of different sizes and types and Combitube
- Fiber-optic intubation device
- Set of a transtracheal jet ventilation
- Set for emergency cricothyrotomy and ventilation
- Set for retrograde intubation
- Capnometer for detection of CO_2 in expired air

(ET: endotracheal; LMA: laryngeal mask airway)

of 4% lignocaine. This is done in a completely conscious patient or with minimum sedation. Patient sedation is provided as tolerated. Dexmedetomidine has the advantage of preserving respiration while providing sedation.

If nasal FOI is planned, then both nostrils are prepared with vasoconstrictive spray. The nostril, through which the patient breathes more easily, is identified. Now, through this nostril, a lubricated ETT, size appropriate to this patient, is introduced as if its tip reaches the hypopharynx. The lubricated shaft of FOB is now introduced through the lumen of this ETT. Oxygen can be insufflated through the suction port and down the aspiration channel of FOB to improve oxygenation and to blow the secretin away from the tip. It is important to keep the shaft of the bronchoscope relatively straight in the midline so that if the head of the bronchoscope is rotated in one direction, the distal end will move to a similar degree and in the same direction. As the tip of the FOB passes through the distal end of ETT, the epiglottis or glottis should be visible. Now, the tip of the bronchoscope is manipulated, as needed, to pass the abducted cords. In difficult cases, forward jaw thrust and/or cricoid pressure may improve the visualization of the vocal cord.

Passing the vocal cord, once into the trachea, the shaft of FOB is advanced to within the sight of the carina. The presence of tracheal rings and carina is the proof of proper positioning of FOB. Now, the ETT is pushed off the FOB into the trachea. The acute angle around the arytenoid cartilage and epiglottis may prevent the easy advancement of ETT. The use of an armored tube usually decreases this problem, due to its greater lateral flexibility and more obtusely angled distal end. The proper position of ETT is confirmed by viewing the tip of the tube at an appropriate distance above the carina (3 cm in adults) before the FOB is withdrawn.

During this whole procedure, oxygenation can be performed in another way. A large nasal airway can be inserted into the contralateral nostril. The breathing circuit can be directly connected to the end of this nasal airway to administer 100% O_2 during fiber-optic laryngoscopy. If the patient is unconscious and not breathing spontaneously, then the mouth can be closed and ventilation is attempted through the single nasal airways. When this technique is used, then the adequacy of ventilation and oxygenation should be confirmed by capnography and pulse oximetry.

If oral FOI is planned, then an intubating airway is inserted through the mouth after topicalization. After that, an ETT is inserted into the mouth, about 8–10 cm, through this airway and then the shaft of the fiber-optic scope is passed through this ETT. Now, the base of the tongue, epiglottis, and finally glottis with vocal cord is visualized in proper sequence. If the tip of the scope is obstructed by the posterior pharyngeal wall (which is diagnosed by pink blur vision), then it should be turned down to visualize the glottis. If the epiglottis obstructs the vision, then the scope should be manipulated, so that the vocal cords (glottis) can be seen. After the visualization of vocal cord, the ETT is introduced into the glottis, by the aforementioned procedure. Passing the vocal cord, once into the trachea, the shaft of FOB is advanced till the carina is seen. Now, the presence of tracheal rings and carina is the proof of proper positioning of FOB. Now, the ETT is pushed off the FOB into the trachea.

Fiber-optic intubation in anesthetized patients may also be done under spontaneous respiration or controlled ventilation in a nonparalyzed and paralyzed patient, respectively. It is obvious that fiber-optic intubation under spontaneous respiration in an anesthetized patient is more technically easier and advantageous than under controlled ventilation in a paralyzed patient. But in spontaneous ventilation, diminished anesthetic level causing cough, vomiting, laryngospasm, bronchospasm, etc., are the definite disadvantages. On the other hand, in fiber-optic intubation under controlled ventilation, apnea is the major headache. Patient should be ventilated with 100% O_2 by mask, in between the intubation attempts by fiber-optic scope, or patient should be ventilated with a special endoscopic mask with a sealing port (through which endoscope is introduced) that allows for the continuous use of mask and ventilation during the attempts of intubation by fiber-optic scope. During endoscopy, additional O_2 from a separate source can be administered through the injection port of the fiber-optic scope.

Nasal intubation by fiber-optic scope has the advantage that the instrument can easily be positioned directly through the nasal route into the hypopharynx to visualize the glottis. If the patient is not anesthetized, the tongue causes less interference, when this route is used. On the contrary, anesthetized intubation by fiber-optic scope through the nasal route is less difficult, due to less upper airway obstruction by soft tissue, caused by anesthesia. In anesthetized patient, a standard nasal airway or a split nasal airway can be used to keep the tongue away from the posterior pharyngeal wall. Usually, the patient is not anesthetized for fiber-optic scope to visualize the glottis, but only anesthesia is employed where the patient is uncooperative and keeping in mind that intubation by fiber-optic scope under anesthesia is usually more difficult. This is because of the development of upper airway obstruction by the falling tongue. If there is any doubt about the ability to maintain ventilation by mask, during fiber-optic laryngoscopy under anesthesia and paralysis, then fiber-optic aided intubation should always be preceded with conscious sedation and/or topical anesthesia, instead of full anesthesia. In topical anesthesia, for nasal fiber-optic intubation the supraglottic, glottis, and tracheal areas may be anesthetized with 1% lignocaine, sprayed through the injection port. After awake sedation, and application of topical anesthesia and vasoconstrictor on nasal mucosa, a nasal ETT or split nasal airway is passed through any nares into the nasopharynx and oropharynx. Then, the fiber-optic scope is passed through it. Thus, in the vast majority of cases glottis can be seen by this scope with minimal tip manipulation. After visualization of glottis, it is very easy to push the tip of an ETT into the larynx with the tip of the fiber-optic scope inside it.

■ OTHER SURGICAL AIRWAY TECHNIQUE

Other surgical airway techniques, except the (1) needle cricothyroidotomy, (2) modified cricothyroidotomy by Seldinger technique (cannula cricothyroidotomy), and (3) surgical cricothyroidotomy are (i) *Percutaneous tracheostomy (PCT),* and (ii) *conventional surgical tracheostomy (ST).* But none is performed under emergency "cannot ventilate and cannot intubate (CVCI)" condition because all these procedures are time-consuming (>5 minutes) and may not be able to save the apneic patient's life. By these aforementioned cricothyroidotomy techniques (including needle, cannula, and surgical cricothyroidotomy) O_2 can be provided on a short-term basis until a definite airway (ET intubation, PCT, and ST) can be placed or the patient resumes spontaneous breathing or wakes up. So, for a *definite airway,* PCT is most commonly performed in ICU on patients who need prolonged ventilatory support for >3 weeks by ETT. The indications, complications, and post surgical care are shown in **Table 11.**

Chevalier Jackson in 1909 first defined the method of surgical tracheostomy. Before that, a patient remains intubated through larynx, till he becomes conscious and cannot maintain his own airway, but prolonged intubation through larynx has many disadvantages. So, if one thinks that a prolonged intubation is needed (>10 days) or if it is

TABLE 11: Indications, complications and post surgical care after surgical tracheostomy.

Indications	• As an elective procedure where prolonged ventilation is required • As a switch-over procedure from intubation • Excessive secretions leading to blockage or frequent change of endotracheal tube • As an alternative when intubation is not possible • To remove upper airway obstruction due to laryngeal edema, impacted foreign body, laryngeal trauma, vocal cord paralysis, Ludwig angina, quinsy, laryngitis, etc.
Tracheostomy tubes	• *Silver tubes:* Not used nowadays • *Cuffed plastic tubes:* Most commonly used nowadays. Cuffs should be of high volume and low pressure • *Montgomery T-tube or Olympic tracheal button:* They have no cuff. So, they produce less tracheal injury and allow air to pass through mouth for speech • *Fenestrated tubes for speaking*
Complications	• *Early:* Malpositioning of tube during insertion, hemorrhage, surgical emphysema, pneumothorax, injury to trachea, larynx, etc. • *Late:* Infection, tracheal ulceration, blockage due to secretion, etc. • *Delayed:* Tracheal stenosis at cuff site or stoma (cuff pressure should be <15 mm Hg), tracheal web, and tracheal dilatation
Care of tracheostomy tube	• Careful aseptic suctioning of secretion at regular interval • Inner cannula should be changed every 4–6 hours • Adjustment of cuff pressure to keep it below 15 mm Hg • Strict asepsis at the time of change. First change should not be done before 5 days, as stoma takes 5 days to establish completely. Change before 5 days creates a false passage

apparent that the patient is unlikely to maintain his airway independently within 3 weeks, then a tracheostomy should be done. Usually, there are two types of *tracheostomy techniques* and these are (1) PCT and (2) ST. The PCT has several advantages over ST (conventional surgical tracheostomy). *These advantages of PCT are* (1) reduced wound complications such as hemorrhage and infection, (2) improved cosmetic results, (3) can easily be done at bedside in ICU, (4) reduced duration of procedure, and (5) it can be performed by a nonsurgical person. The *disadvantage of PCT over ST* is that due to the narrow tract and lack of formal stoma formation in PCT, there is an increased risk of delayed airway loss. Without a formal stoma and with only a narrow

tract between the airway and the skin, tracheostomy tube may be displaced which can lead to death.

First PCT was reported, in 1955, by Sheldon. But because of the high complication rate in this technique, adopted by Sheldon, Ciaglia in 1985 had modified this Sheldon's technique and called it percutaneous dilatational tracheostomy (PDT). This PDT is commonly called PCT. *The PCT differs from conventional ST* in that *in PCT a puncture is made on the trachea in between cartilages* (usually between first and second or between second and third) by needle or scalpel and subsequently the puncture is dilated over a flexible guiding catheter to introduce a small tracheostomy tube or a small ETT, whereas in conventional ST the tracheal cartilages are dissected and cut by the scalpel. On the other hand, in cricothyroidotomy, the site of puncture is a cricothyroid membrane and not on tracheal in between its cartilages. Other different techniques of performing PCT are the Griggs technique, White tusk/Blue Rhino technique, Pere Twist technique, and translaryngeal tracheostomy (TLT) technique.

Percutaneous tracheostomy is performed at an intercartilaginous area in between the first and second tracheal cartilage rings or second and third tracheal cartilage rings. There is an increased incidence of subglottic stenosis when it is performed above the first ring. The area below the third ring is generally avoided to minimize the potential trauma of the isthmus of the thyroid and to prevent the accidental injury of the innominate artery.

In conventional ST, the tracheostomy tube should be placed in such a way that it does not erode the cartilaginous tracheal ring and does not press against the cricoid cartilage. In addition, the opening should not be placed too low, so that the tip of tracheostomy tube or its cuff will be too close to carina. Low placement of tracheostomy tube is also hazardous because the innominate artery crosses anterior to trachea low in the neck. During conventional ST any segment of trachea should not be removed, because this might lead to a greater loss of tracheal wall stability and predispose to stenosis, once healing is accomplished after the removal of tracheostomy tube.

■ SUPRAGLOTTIC AIRWAY DEVICES

These are the devices which, lying above the glottic opening, help in ventilation and avoid the "tube within tube" situation that is produced by intubating trachea by an ETT. It provides a better unobstructed airway during spontaneous respiration than the oropharyngeal or nasopharyngeal airway. It also helps in controlled ventilation, if needed. LMA is such the first supraglottic airway device and has been in practice nearly 30 years, since Dr Archie Brain in UK had first introduced it. The LMA has been used for more than million and million time worldwide, but without a single death attributed to its use. So, now, LMA has a well-established role in the management of patient with both the normal or difficult airways.

Thus, the amazing success trail of LMA has spurred the introduction over a dozen of different supraglottic airway devices, other than LMA, to remove the disadvantages of it, but only some have stood the test of time, while others have dwindled into the oblivion. Some of the supraglottic airway devices which have stood the test of time include (1) Combitube, (2) soft seal and laryngeal airway device, (3) laryngeal tube suction (LTS), (4) Cobra Perilaryngeal Airway (CobraPLA), (5) PAX, (6) streamlined linear of pharyngeal airway (SLIPA), (7) cuffed oropharyngeal airway (COPA), (8) glottic aperture seal airway (GOS airway), and (9) Air-Q laryngeal airway *(Figs. 43A to D)*.

All the supraglottic airway devices (1) produce minimal to nil hemodynamic instability during their placement in larynx, as they avoid the stimulation of infraglottic structures and (2) they offer minimum resistance to patient's airway. Other advantages of supraglottic devices are (1) easy insertion and smooth awakening, (2) no inadvertent bronchial intubation, (3) no vocal cord injury, (4) no translocation of oral or nasal bacterial colony, and (5) no secretions into the lower respiratory tract. Among all the aforementioned supraglottic devices, the LMA and Combitube have been recommended as the rescue of airway in "cannot ventilate, cannot intubate" situations. Again LMA has been recommended at five places in the ASA Task Force Algorithm for the management of difficult airway, either as a ventilating device or as a conduit for ET intubation.

However, today these devices (LMA and Combitube) are not only used during emergency situations, but also during the elective management of the patient's airway. Ambulatory or day case surgery for patients of ASA I and II grade (ASA I patients only according to some anesthetist) are one of the most suitable candidates for the use of these supraglottic devices. These include short procedures, not requiring controlled ventilations with muscle relaxant such as the surgeries of upper and lower limb, ear and nose surgeries, ophthalmic surgeries, short gynecological procedures, etc. These devices are also recommended in patients with ischemic and other heart diseases, coming for short surgical procedures under general anesthesia, as their use is associated with lesser hemodynamic changes, compared to tracheal intubation. At the end of neurosurgery, but prior to termination of anesthesia, ETT can be replaced with LMA as a preventive strategy against hypertension, coughing, bucking, etc., which are associated with extubation and smoother emergence. For these reasons, supraglottic devices also are used during ophthalmic surgery to prevent risk from sudden rise in IOP during intubation and extubation. The supraglottic devices are also extremely popular in patients, undergoing minor therapeutic and diagnostic surgical procedures, outside the OT complex. These include radiotherapy, diagnostic and interventional radiology, endoscopy, ECT, cardioversion, etc. In the ever expanding horizons of supraglottic devices, more and more number of routine general anesthesia, lasting for 2–3 hours are now also being administered, using these devices. Even surgeries associated with increased intra-abdominal pressure (e.g., laparoscopic surgeries) are now being safely done, using ProSeal LMA, LTS, or Combitube.

The factors which prevent the use of supraglottic airway devices include:

Small oral opening and any pharyngeal pathology which prevents the proper fitting of it at the laryngeal inlet, for example, pharyngeal mass and esophageal pathology including caustic injury contradicts the use of supraglottic airway devices such as Combitube and LTS. All the supraglottic airway devices do not offer reliable protection against regurgitation and aspiration of stomach contents, except Combitube and LTS. So, they should not be used in patients with the possibility of reflux of gastric contents and aspiration of it or where retained gastric contents may be present.

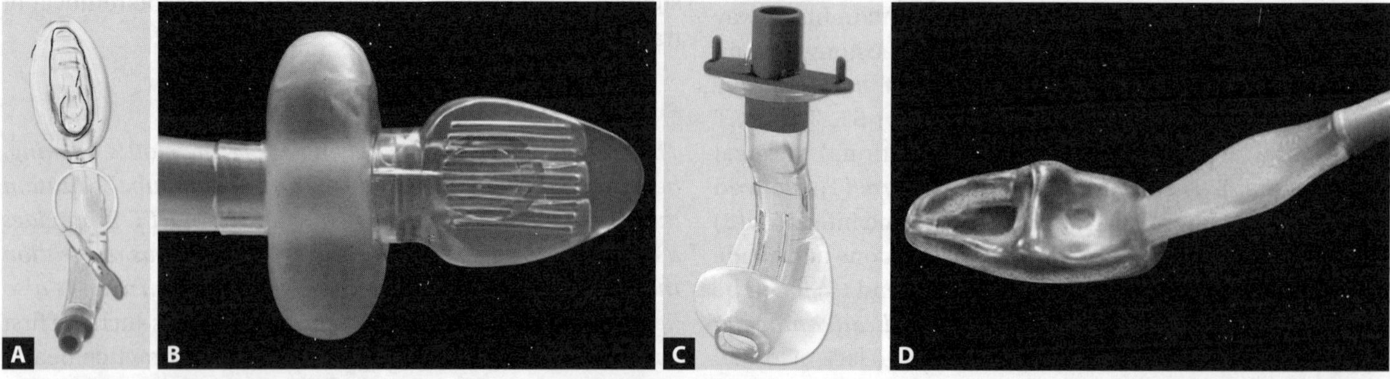

Figs. 43A to D: These figures show some supra-glottic airway devices. (a) Air-Q intubating laryngeal airway; (b) Cobra perilaryngeal airway; (c) COPA (Cuffed oropharyngeal airway); (d) SLIPA (Streamlined linear pharyngeal airway)

These conditions include:

- When fasting is not confirmed
- Morbid obesity
- Pregnancy where there is delayed gastric emptying
- Others conditions associated with delayed gastric emptying such as history of gastroesophageal reflex and hiatus hernia
- Multiple or massive injury
- Acute abdominal or thoracic injury.

But we have to keep in mind that these aforementioned conditions are not the absolute contraindications for the use of supraglottic devices.

Supraglottic airway devices also have the limited value in patients with poor lung compliance as they cannot withstand the high inflation pressure. But it is noted that only the ProSeal LMA can withstand the peak inflation pressure of 35–38 cmH$_2$O without leak from sides.

Individual Supraglottic Device

There are many supraglottic devices, among them which are commonly used are described here.

- *Laryngeal musk airway (LMA):* It has already been discussed earlier.
- *Soft seal and laryngeal airway devices:* Both the soft seal and laryngeal airway device are quite similar to LMA of unique variety, in regards to structure and single use concept. But one major difference between the LMA of unique variety and the soft seal or laryngeal airway device is the removal of the aperture bars from both of these later devices and a softer cuff of soft seal. So, the latter confers a better periglottic seal, which can withstand the higher inflation pressure than the LMA classic.
- *LTS device:* LTS is basically a shorter version of Combitube. It is a newly developed, multiuse, latex free, double lumen, and silicon tube. Like Combitube, it has both oropharyngeal and esophageal low-pressure cuffs, a ventilation outlet in between them and a second tube placed posteriorly. The second tube is situated posterior to the respiratory tube (lumen). The same inflation assembly inflates the two cuffs at a time. When correctly placed, the distal tip along with its opening and the cuff lies in the esophagus. This effectively separates the esophagus from the rest of the airways. Being shorter and blunt, the possibility of the esophageal portion of the tube, entering the trachea, is nonexistent. Laryngeal tube (LT), which is the precursor of LTS has no second tube. So, it has now been replaced by LTS. The method of insertion of LTS is same as that of Combitube. Due to the specially designed inflation line, the proximal cuff is inflated first and stabilizes the tube. Then, once the proximal cuff has

adjusted to the anatomy of the pharynx of the patient, the distal cuff will be inflated automatically. It is usually recommended to use a cuff pressure below 60 cmH$_2$O. Like a Combitube, there is no need to connect both the lumen alternatively for confirmation of ventilation. If ventilation is not adequate, then position of the tube can be changed, by pushing it either distally or pulling it proximally, according to the size of the patient. The fine drained tube allows the insertion of a gastric tube.

- *Cobra PLA:* It is a new device in the field of supraglottic airways. It consists of a tube, a cuff, and a 15 mm standard adaptor for attachment with the anesthetic machine. Distally, the tube ends at an opening, with cobra head design, which holds both the soft tissues and epiglottis out of the way. Thus, it facilitates ventilation through its slotted opening. The cuff, when is inflated gently, seals off the upper airway and allows improved positive pressure ventilation. CobraPLA is usually used as an alternative to face mask and certainly does not protect the airway from the effects of vomiting, regurgitation, and aspiration.
- *PAX:* PAX is a sterile, latex free, single use supraglottic airway device. It is used as an alternative to face mask, LMA, and CobraPLA. The PAX supraglottic device consists of a tube, a cuff and a soft-flexible-gilled tip and is made of medical grade PVC. The tube has a standard 15 mm connector at its proximal end for attachment with anesthetic machine. The soft, flexible, gilled tip is tapered to guide the device and help to rest the device within the cricopharyngeal recess, above the esopharyngeal sphincter. The gilled tip is made of thermoplastic elastomer. A high volume, low-pressure cuff, which volume is 60 mL, stabilizes the PAX within the oropharynx. Approximately, placed cuff lies just below the uvula and pushes the tongue forward for improved ventilation. An open hooded window is situated between the cuff and the gilled tip for aligned to glottic opening. The hood is designed to lift the epiglottis forward. An anatomically curved tube can accept 7.5 mm ETT, if tracheal intubation is indicated.
- *Streamlined Linear Pharyngeal Airway (SLIPA):* The SLIPA is a hollow, preformed, and boot-shaped airway. It is made of soft plastic and blow molded to the shape of pressurized pharynx. As it is fitted tightly in the pharynx, no cuff is provided to seal the device in the pharynx. SLIPA is looked like a boot with "toe bridge and heel" prominences. It is used as an inexpensive single use alternative to LMA and to decrease the risk of aspiration, if limited volume regurgitation should occur. It is available in different sizes to match the patient size **(Flowchart 2)**.

Flowchart 2: Algorithm of airway management.

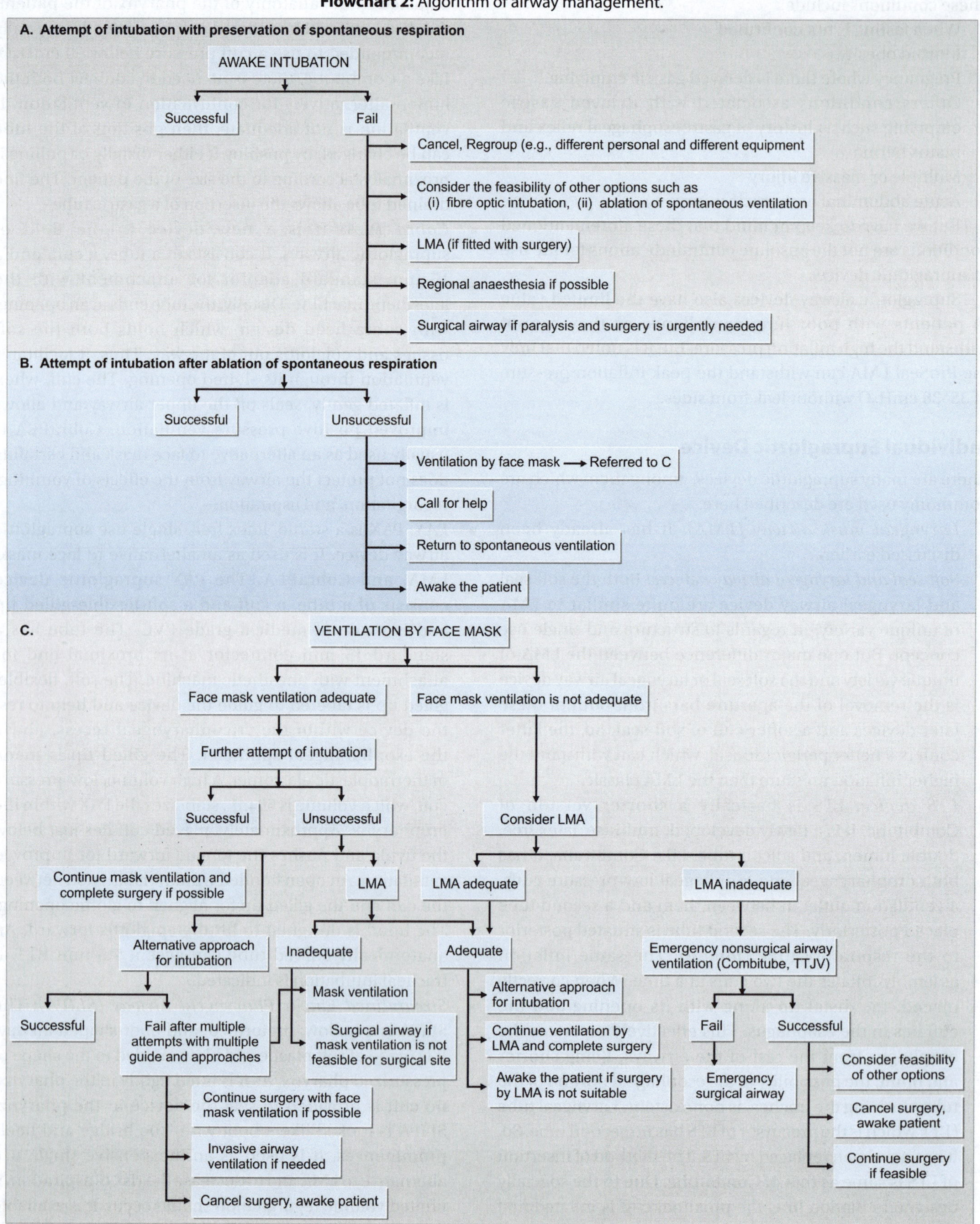

(LMA: laryngeal mask airway; TTJV: transtracheal jet ventilation)